Did you know that you can also...

Get access to www.NaturalDatabase.com

Get everything in this book, plus more - with powerful searches - updated daily - click on references to see actual abstracts

Get Continuing Education credit

Accredited for Physicians, Pharmacists, Nurse Practitioners, and Physician Assistants

For details, see the last pages in this book
or contact the publisher:

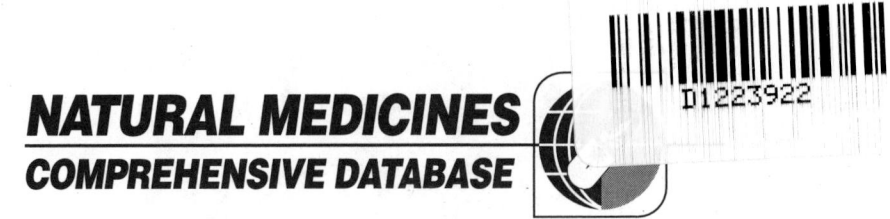

NATURAL MEDICINES
COMPREHENSIVE DATABASE

3120 W. March Lane
PO Box 8190
Stockton CA 95208
Tel: 209-472-2244
Fax: 209-472-2249
Mail@NaturalDatabase.com

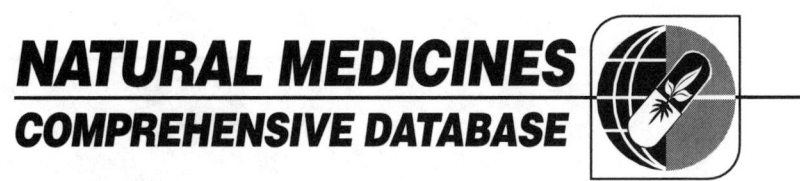

NATURAL MEDICINES
COMPREHENSIVE DATABASE

Consensus of Current Scientific Information of Practical and Clinical Importance to Health Professionals

Covering Herbal Medicines, Dietary Supplements, and other Natural Medicines.

This *Natural Medicines Comprehensive Database* is provided as a Web-based reference. The Web version is being updated every day. This Book contains all the information that was in the Web version on the date the Book was sent to the printer. Of course, new data have been entered into the Web version since then. For the most current data, subscribers are encouraged to go to www.NaturalDatabase.com.

To order a subscription to the Web version, see the order forms at the back of this book.

Continuing education, based on this *Database*, is offered to physicians, pharmacists, nurse practitioners, physician assistants, and registered dietitians. The accredited continuing education is offered through a series of continuing education booklets that are associated with this *Database*. To receive the continuing education booklets and the continuing education credit use the order form at the back of this book.

This *Database* is intended for use by Health Professionals. If a person who is not trained and licensed as a health professional uses the data contained in this *Database*, the publishers strongly encourage seeking appropriate guidance from a Health Professional.

Published by:

Therapeutic Research Faculty
3120 W. March Lane
PO Box 8190
Stockton, CA 95208

Tel: 209-472-2244
Fax: 209-472-2249
E-mail: mail@NaturalDatabase.com
www.NaturalDatabase.com

Compiled by the Editors of:

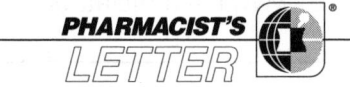 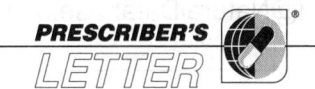

Copyright © 2000 by Therapeutic Research Faculty
3rd Edition

All rights reserved. No part of this book may be reproduced or transmitted in any form or by any means electronic or mechanical, including photocopying, scanning, facsimile, recording, or by any informational storage or retrieval system without written permission from the publisher.

When referencing this *Database*, use the following format for the citation:

Jellin JM, Gregory P, Batz F, Hitchens, K, et al. *Pharmacist's Letter/ Prescriber's Letter Natural Medicines Comprehensive Database*. 3rd ed. Stockton, CA: Therapeutic Research Faculty; 2000:pg xx-xx.

The authors have attempted to compile a comprehensive database of clinically important data on natural medicines. Errors, inaccuracies, or omissions are always possible in a work of this sort. The publisher assumes no responsibility for any patient care based on the application of the data contained in this database. Health professionals who use this database must rely on their own judgment before applying this data to any specific medical situation. People who are not health professionals should seek appropriate professional guidance on the use of any medicinal agent before using it.

For information on obtaining additional copies of this edition, or to receive a subscription to the printed version or the Web version of *Pharmacist's Letter/ Prescriber's Letter Natural Medicines Comprehensive Database*, or the Website, see the last pages of this book, or contact:
Therapeutic Research Faculty, 3120 W. March Lane,
PO Box 8190, Stockton, CA 95208
TEL: 209-472-2244 • FAX: 209-472-2249
E-MAIL: mail@NaturalDatabase.com • WEBSITE: www.NaturalDatabase.com

Printed in the United States of America
ISBN #0-9676136-4-7

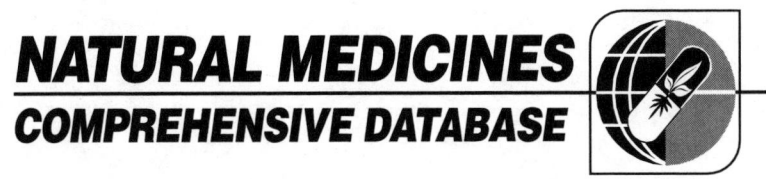

Table of Contents

Research and Writing Team 1

How to get data from this *Database* 3

Data on Natural Medicines 11

References 1153

Brand Names Index 1291

Chart: Drug/Herb Interactions 1427

Chart: Herb/Drug Interactions 1431

Chart: Herbs and Supplements with Therapeutic Efficacy 1437

Chart: Drug Influences on Nutrient Levels and Depletion 1443

General Index 1453

"Tell the Editors" Form 1523

Order Form: *Natural Medicines Comprehensive Database* 1525

Order Form: Continuing Education Credits Based on
    Natural Medicines Comprehensive Database 1527

Order Form: Web Access to *Natural Medicines Comprehensive Database* 1529

The following individuals worked as a team to create this
Natural Medicines Comprehensive Database.

EDITOR

Jeff M. Jellin, Pharm.D.
  Editor, *Pharmacist's Letter*
  Editor, *Prescriber's Letter*

ASSISTANT EDITORS

Philip Gregory, Pharm.D.
  Assistant Editor, *Pharmacist's Letter*
  Assistant Editor, *Prescriber's Letter*

Forrest Batz, Pharm.D.

Kathy Hitchens, Pharm.D., MSBA

Stephen Burson, R.Ph.
  Assistant Editor, *Pharmacist's Letter*
  Assistant Editor, *Prescriber's Letter*

Kay Shaver, Pharm.D.
  Assistant Editor, *Pharmacist's Letter*
  Assistant Editor, *Prescriber's Letter*

Kimberly Palacioz, Pharm.D.
  Assistant Editor, *Pharmacist's Letter*
  Assistant Editor, *Prescriber's Letter*

SPECIAL CONSULTANT

Karen Davidson, Pharm.D.
  Assoc. Editor, *Pharmacist's Letter*
  Assoc. Editor, *Prescriber's Letter*

RESEARCHERS AND WRITERS

Marie Mulligan, M.D.
Jacintha Cauffield, Pharm.D., BCPS
Gayle Nicholas Scott, R.Ph., BCPS
Mary Birchfield, Pharm.D.
Ben Mills, M.D., M.P.H.
James Ables, Pharm.D.
John Cathey, M.S., Pharm.
Gary Holt, R.Ph., Ph.D.
Judith Marshall, R.Ph.
Paul Roberts, R.Ph.
Neeta O'Mara, Pharm.D, BCPS
Lynn Limon, Pharm.D.
John Morozumi, Pharm.D.
Loan Cat, Pharm.D.
Gary Choy, Pharm.D.
Tina Madej, R.Ph.
Sandra Downing, Pharm.D.
Lori Kolczak, R.Ph.
Jennifer Obenrader, Pharm.D.

REVIEWERS

Dan Perri, B.Sc.Phm, M.D.
Barbara Miller, Pharm.D.
Stephen McKernan, B.S. Pharm., N.D., D.O.
Ben Mills, M.D., M.P.H.
Mary Wilson, Ph.D., R.D.
Todd Reynolds, M.D.
Vincent Ferrari, Pharm.
Richard Filice, R.Ph.
John Weeks, M.D.
Joe Pepping, Pharm.D.

DIRECTOR OF CE/CME PROGRAM

Nan Pheatt, M.P.H.

WEBSITE EDITORS

Karen Wilson
  Web Editor
    Pharmacist's Letter and *Prescriber's Letter*
Jessica James
  Web Team Production Manager
Beth MacConnell
  Web Team Production Manager

DATABASE ADMINISTRATORS

Michelle Carlson
  Project Coordinator
Linda Hneitina
  Special Research Coordinator
Timothy Swaim
  Special Research Coordinator
Patrice Verhines
  Editorial Assistant
Pat Harrison
  Editorial Assistant

STAFF

Lisa Shawhan
  Circulation Manager
Connie Johnson
Neng Vang
Tillie Giovannetti
Marilynne Davis
Sandy Harp
Jan Garr
Kathy Webb
Rhonda Bigelow
Russ Johnson
Gloria Rios
Sabrina Coleman
Helen Vann

© Copyright 2000, Natural Medicines Comprehensive Database (209) 472-2244. For updated data, go to www.NaturalDatabase.com • 1

How to Get Data from this
Natural Medicines Comprehensive Database

The idea to create this *Natural Medicines Comprehensive Database* originated from our work in researching and publishing *Pharmacist's Letter* and *Prescriber's Letter*. Over the last 15 years a large number of pharmacists, physicians, and other prescribers have come to rely on the objective drug therapy advice in these publications. In recent years they have been clamoring for reliable and practical scientific data on natural medicines.

Practitioners found that getting good data on herbal medicines and supplements is hard to do. Many studies don't meet rigorous scientific standards. Some studies are corrupted by commercial interests. Some references are biased towards...or against...the use of natural remedies. Some cite anecdotal or unsubstantiated scientific support for certain natural products. This lack of reliable data on natural products results in inappropriate use.

Our goal for the *Natural Medicines Comprehensive Database* is to help patients. We aim to do this by providing health practitioners with the best collection of data and consensus of available scientific information on natural medicines.

We decided that good patient care would be best served by starting with a large database of scientifically reliable and clinically practical data. This *Database* contains a listing for just about every natural medicine sold in the US and Canada, and a listing for every product discussed in any reputable reference. The monograph for each product presents the data that are known, and the editors state when there are insufficient reliable data available.

This *Natural Medicines Comprehensive Database* has been created by a group of over two dozen pharmacists, physicians, researchers, dietitians, and pharmacologists researching and analyzing data. We determined that the data should be divided into categories based on the questions that come up most often. In looking at our *Database*, you'll see that the 15 categories of info for each product address the questions that practitioners face most often.

Name of Product: This *Database* contains all sorts of products that are generally thought of as "natural" medicines. This includes herbal and non-herbal supplements. Some medicines are not harvested or collected from natural sources, but are generally categorized along with natural products, and they are included here. You'll notice that the names of herbs appear in upper case letters, sometimes followed by the part of the plant that is discussed. The plant part makes a big difference. For example, an extract made from horse chestnut seed seems to have a useful role in reducing the symptoms of varicose veins, but horse chestnut flower lacks similar potency.

This Product is Also Known As: Many herbal medicines and non-herbal supplements have a variety of names. Some names are based on the plant species. Some are based on folklore or tradition. Some names are entirely different than the most common name, and some are confusingly similar. All the names appear in the index (at the back of the book) to help you find whatever product you are looking for, no matter what name you use.

Many products have a statement that reads, "CAUTION: See separate listing for xxxxxxx." This is important, and will help make sure you are getting data about the correct product. For example, you might flip to Blue Cohosh thinking that you are getting data on Black Cohosh, but they are different. The "CAUTION" will alert you to the fact that there is a separate entry for each one.

Scientific Names: This field lists the botanical names for herbs, including the family name. For non-herbal supplements the chemical or generic name appears. Common names are separated by commas. Scientific names are separated by semi-colons. If there is also a synonym for a scientific name it will appear with a comma separating the two scientific names. For example, Primula veris, synonym Primula officinalis; Primula elatier.

People Use this Product For: This field does NOT tell you what the product is good for, nor does it tell you what it should, or should not be used for. That information appears in other fields. This field tells you what people use the product for. Often times, products are used for indications even though there is no evidence that they work. For example, goldenseal is used extensively to attempt to mask the results of lab tests for illicit drug use, but it's ineffective. This field is intended to help practitioners understand why a patient might be using, or want to be using a product, and to understand some promotional claims surrounding certain products. In this section you will learn that certain products are used in unexpected ways.

Safety: For each product you will get our assessment of the available data regarding safety. Each product is rated by the following scale: LIKELY SAFE, POSSIBLY SAFE, POSSIBLY UNSAFE, LIKELY UNSAFE, or UNSAFE.

Our team has been very meticulous in analyzing the medical literature to assign the safety ratings. Each rating is assigned according to specific criteria:

> LIKELY SAFE = Reputable references generally agree that the product is safe when used appropriately, or the product is approved for use by a governmental agency such as the FDA or HPB, Health Protection Branch in Canada.

> POSSIBLY SAFE = Reputable references suggest that the product might be safe when used appropriately, or there are human studies reporting no serious adverse effects.

> POSSIBLY UNSAFE = There is some information suggesting the use of this product might be unsafe.

> LIKELY UNSAFE = Reputable references generally agree that the product can be harmful, or there are reliable reports of harm to users.

> UNSAFE = Reputable references generally agree that the product should not be used, or reliable reports show that use of the product often results in clinically significant harm, or a reliable agency has issued a safety warning to avoid using the product.

You will see that different uses of a product often get different safety ratings. For example, camphor is rated "LIKELY SAFE"...when used topically, but it is rated "UNSAFE" ...when used orally.

Questions often come up about using products during pregnancy or lactation, or in children. If there are safety considerations that apply specifically to children, a special mention in the safety field will address the concern. As a matter of editorial policy EVERY listing includes a heading for safety in PREGNANCY and LACTATION. This info is given whenever the data exist.

Effectiveness: This section is handled very similarly to the "Safety" section described above. Our team has been very meticulous in analyzing the medical literature to assign the efficacy ratings. Each product is rated by the following scale:

EFFECTIVE = The product has passed a rigorous scientific review equivalent to a review by the FDA, HPB, or other governmental authority and has been found to be effective for a specific indication as an OTC drug, orphan drug, or prescription drug product.

LIKELY EFFECTIVE = Reputable references generally agree that the product is effective for the given indication, based on two or more randomized, prospective, controlled, adequately large human studies giving positive results for clinically relevant end-points and published in established, refereed journals.

POSSIBLY EFFECTIVE = Reputable references suggest that the product might work for the given indication based on one or more human studies.

POSSIBLY INEFFECTIVE = Reputable references suggest that the product probably doesn't work for the given indication based on one human study giving negative results for clinically relevant end-points.

LIKELY INEFFECTIVE = Reputable references generally agree that the product is not effective for the given indication, based on two or more randomized, prospective, controlled, human studies giving negative results for clinically relevant end-points and published in established, refereed journals. And these studies are not offset by equally convincing positive studies.

INEFFECTIVE = Most reputable references agree that the product is not effective for the given indication, or multiple high-quality studies resulted in negative results. And there are no equally reliable human studies offering convincing contradictory data.

Obviously, the "effectiveness" rating might differ depending on the use, so you will often see more than one rating for a product.

When possible, we have included one very useful bit of information in this effectiveness section...the specific formula or extract that was used in studies that found the product to be effective. This information is not easily found elsewhere, but it is very important. For example, a significant study was published in the *Journal of the American Medical Association* providing evidence that ginkgo has a positive role in delaying the progression of Alzheimer's Disease. Its effects have been likened to *Aricept*. Many published works, and many ginkgo manufacturers have since stated ginkgo's effectiveness in this area. But this information is not useful without knowing what formulation of ginkgo was shown to have a positive effect. This *Natural Medicines Comprehensive Database* states that the formulations of ginkgo that contain Egb 761(Tanakan) or LI 1370 (Lichtwer Pharma), consisting of 24% flavone glycosides and 6% terpene lactones, are the formulations in the prominent studies that were shown to have beneficial effect. It cannot be inferred from this that other formulations of ginkgo will also have the same effect.

Possible Mechanism of Action and Active Ingredients: In the case of herbal medicines, this field will tell you the specific part of the plant that provides active ingredients. It will say if the listing applies to the leaf, bark, root, etc. However, some herbs have a separate listing for different plant parts if these separate parts provide different active ingredients or effects. In these cases, the plant part is not shown in this field, and it is instead listed at the top of the listing along with the product name. For example there is a listing for bilberry leaf, and a separate listing for bilberry dried ripe fruit. Therefore these plant parts do not need to be listed in this field. If the whole plant is used, there will be no mention of plant part.

In this field you will find a very brief description of the known constituents...and actions that might be attributable to these constituents. Keep in mind that most of the natural products are used because people have observed, or think they observed, some benefit to using the product. In many cases there has been relatively little scientific inquiry into the active ingredients and the exact mechanism of action. Also recognize that most herbal medicines are combinations of many constituents. It is quite possible that herbal medicines work by the combined effects of multiple constituents, and the concept of identifying a single specific active ingredient is flawed. Even when a single, specific active ingredient is identified, it is possible that other active ingredients may be discovered later. For example, authorities used to think that St. John's wort exerted its effect due to hypericin content. More recent findings suggest that maybe hyperforin exerts significant activity.

Adverse Reactions Including Known Allergies: This part of the database is more of a collection than a consensus. The editors did not attempt to list only the adverse reactions that are generally agreed to occur when a specific product is used. The editors collected and listed any adverse effects that have been reported, as long as the effects were of practical importance. Known allergies are also listed. For example, people who are allergic to one herb coming from the asteraceae family might also be allergic to other herbs coming from this same family.

Possible Interactions with . . . : You will notice five separate fields listing different categories of possible interactions. For each product, this database lists Possible Interactions with...

Herbs and Other Dietary Supplements
Drugs
Foods
Lab Tests
Diseases and Conditions

Interactions related to "natural medicines" such as herbs are important. There are many potential interactions...many practitioners are not yet on the look-out for them...the usual computerized checking systems do not yet have all this info in their systems...and patients do not recognize the potential problems like they do with drugs. To use the information in these interaction fields, it is important to understand the origin of the data. In some cases it comes from documented reports. In other cases, the data are theoretical, based on animal or in-vitro studies that suggest an interaction might occur. For example, horse chestnut seed contains coumarin derivatives and theoretically increases bleeding time. At this point in time there are very few well-documented interactions. Much of the information regarding potential interactions is theoretical. A synopsis of documented reports and theoretical predictions appears in this field. We have prepared a separate pair of charts in the back of the book to give you a listing of the potential interactions between drugs and commonly used natural medicines.

Drug Influences on Nutrient Levels and Depletion: Some nutrients are known to be depleted from the body by certain drugs. Data about nutrient depletion appears in this field. This is the only field in the *Database* that appears ONLY for those natural medicines that are involved with nutrient depletion interactions. This is because the nutrient depletion interactions are commonly caused by drugs depleting nutrients. The natural medicines listed in this *Database* are typically the ones being depleted, and are not the entities causing the depletion. For this reason, the editors have chosen to only list this field when there are important data to present. In addition, there is an entire chart about nutrient depletion in the back of the book.

Typical Dosages & Routes of Administration that are Commonly Used: The dosages in this field are not necessarily recommended doses, safe doses, or efficacious doses. They are the common and typically used doses. Many products included in this *Database* may not be safe or effective. This needs to be considered even when a typical dose is listed.

Comments: This field presents a potpourri of info. For example, the comments on Siberian ginseng point out that it is a completely different herb than American or Panax ginseng. American or Panax ginseng is considerably more expensive. It is said that the Soviet Union wanted to provide its athletes with any advantage offered by ginseng but wanted a less expensive version. Therefore Siberian ginseng became popular, and this is why most studies on Siberian ginseng are written in Russian.

Scattered throughout the *Database* you will see statements like, "Insufficient reliable information available." This means that data do not exist, or the literature is too contradictory, or the studies are not of high enough quality. This information is valuable because it is important for practitioners to know what is not known. Many references state that certain products are effective, or safe, etc. when data do not exist to support this conclusion. This *Database* states when there is insufficient information to meet the reliability standards of this *Database*.

Tables at the back of the book

References: Statements throughout this *Database* are referenced, and the reference citations are listed at the back of the book. The fact that so many references were used to create this *Database* allows this *Database* to be both a scientific consensus of clinical information and a comprehensive collection of data on natural medicines. This is best explained by describing how the research and writing team used references to get the data that practitioners need.

Brand Names Listing: The brand names of many natural medicine products appear in this listing, and for each one there is a listing of the product's ingredients. This is the one area in which the printed version of this database differs from the web version. There are just plain too many brand name products to list them all with all their ingredients. This book would literally be over 3 inches thick. Therefore many are listed in this printed version, and many more appear in the Web version. Keep in mind that manufacturers can change the ingredients of their brand name products at anytime. This has been creating problems for years. Remember when *Ex-Lax* contained phenolphthalein? Some people did not realize that it was changed to contain sennosides and docusate sodium. The same thing happens frequently with natural medicines. The Web version of the *Database* provides a very powerful tool related to brand names. For every brand name the user can view all the products' ingredients. Then, if the user wants to learn more about an individual ingredient, the user can have the *Database* do a quick search and display detailed information on the ingredient selected. While displaying the detailed information on the ingredient the Web version will invite the user to click a button to view a listing of all the brand name products that contain the ingredient. Within the Brand Name listing, you will sometimes find the term **"Editor's Comments:"** In these instances there will be some commentary from the editors of importance related to this particular brand name product. For example, the listing of all the ingredients in a brand name product may serve to answer some questions about the product, but the use of all these ingredients in COMBINATION form may require additional commentary. Or, there may be some data related to this particular brand that the editors wish for you to know about.

© Copyright 2000, Natural Medicines Comprehensive Database (209) 472-2244. For updated data, go to www.NaturalDatabase.com • 7

Interactions Listing: This chart in the back of the book addresses potential interactions between commonly used natural medicines and drugs. It does not address potential interactions with herbs, foods, lab tests, or diseases or conditions. You'll notice there are actually two charts...one to see if a natural medicine interacts with a drug, and a second one to see if a drug interacts with a natural medicine. For further info on any potential interaction listed, just flip to the listing for the natural medicine in the main body of the *Database*. At this early stage of scientific inquiry on interactions related to natural medicines, it is usually impossible to state the significance of a potential interaction with certainty. Potential interactions are listed if they are known to occur or are theoretical but affect natural medicines that are very commonly used. In the course of preparing these tables we created much longer tables that include potential interactions that do not meet the criteria stated above. We have not included these many potential interactions, because they apply to products that are rarely used, or are less likely to create a problem. As new information is documented, we expect to add more interactions to the published list.

Therapeutically Effective Products List: This listing at the back of the book is a good place to find which products are likely to be useful for certain conditions. To create this listing our editors queried the *Database* to create a list of all products that are listed as "EFFECTIVE" or "LIKELY EFFECTIVE" for any condition. However, any product that is "LIKELY UNSAFE", or "UNSAFE" for this condition is NOT included on this list. Some products that are "LIKELY UNSAFE", or "UNSAFE" for one route of administration may be safer for a different route of administration and may also be "EFFECTIVE" or "LIKELY EFFECTIVE." In these instances a product may be included in the list even if it it unsafe by certain routes of administration. It is interesting to note that the entire listing is relatively short. Some users of this *Database* may feel that more products are truly "EFFECTIVE" or "LIKELY EFFECTIVE," but our editors have followed our scientific criteria and only identified those products where reliable data exist. As more studies are done on these products, it is possible that more "EFFECTIVE" or "LIKELY EFFECTIVE" products will be added to this list.

Nutrient Depletion Chart: A very popular buzz word these days is "Nutrient Depletion." People are interested in the concept that certain drugs will cause the body to lose certain nutrients. There is some documentation of this potential problem in the medical literature related to specific drugs and specific nutrients. Many of the concerns that are popular these days are not based on rigorous science and may not be clinically significant. There are, however, several drugs that do deplete certain nutrients in a manner that is often clinically significant. Data about drugs that influence nutrient levels and depletion are collected into the chart that is located in the Chart Section at the back of the book .

General Index: There are a couple ways you can find data on a particular product in this *Database*. One way is to just flip to the listing. They are in alphabetical order by the most common name. If you don't see a listing for the product you want, use the index in the back of the book. This index is very complete. It includes all the common names and the scientific name(s) of every product. Keep in mind that the general index does NOT include brand names. Brand names are listed separately. Since the brand name index shows the ingredients of each brand name product, it would be confusing to intersperse these listings in the general index.

"Tell The Editors" form: It is unrealistic to believe that all clinicians, researchers, and other experts will always agree with every statement in this *Database*. The editors recognize that new information is surfacing all the time and new interpretations develop all the time. A team of researchers and editors remain employed full-time to constantly update this *Database*. These editors respect intelligent differences of opinion, and in fact, invite and encourage any professional user of this *Database* to share new knowledge, or new interpretations with us. We see this

Database as a central location that is constantly updated and allows all health professionals access to the latest information. If you recommend a change to any statement in this *Database*, please use the form at the back of the book and send it to us. If the form is not available to you, please use the fax, email, or post office address shown in the front of this *Database*. Please include the reference citation. We thank you for helping to make this the best resource possible.

Web Version: Our goal is to provide data that is accurate, timely, clinically practical, and easy to get to. That's why fields are filled in with short concise data. And that's why we offer the data in both printed and Web versions. We want practitioners to have access by whichever format serves them best. The printed version is handy, easy-to-use, and usable anytime anywhere. The Web version allows sophisticated searching and provides you with constantly updated material. Our team monitors all new developments with natural medicines and makes updates to this *Database* constantly. As products and claims for products hit the popular press, our editors make any appropriate updates to the Web version. The Web version also allows licensed health professionals to interact on this subject by posting questions, answers, and relevant citations for colleagues.

Web Version -Reference abstracts: A very ambitious new feature has been added to the Web version at the same time as this third edition of the book is being printed. Both the book and the web version identify thousands of scientific references to support the statements in the *Database*. Users of the Web version will now find thousands of reference citations that can be clicked to bring up the original abstract from the medical literature. This has been a huge effort on the part of our staff to provide the actual abstract readily available for subscribers to view immediately on-line. Our research staff continues to analyze dozens of new scientific articles each week. As reference citations to these articles are posted to the Website, many of them will also be posted with their original abstract.

We anticipate that this *Natural Medicines Comprehensive Database* will be the "go-to" source of reliable data. As such, it deserves a nickname. Our group simply calls it "*Natural Database.*" We hope you find it useful.

The *Natural Database* Team

5-HTP

This Product is Also Known As
5HTP, 5-hydroxytryptophan.
CAUTION: See separate listing for L-tryptophan.

Scientific Names
5-hydroxytryptophan; L-5 hydroxytryptophan.

People Use This For
Orally, 5-HTP is used for sleep disorders (9), depression, anxiety (915), migraine (9), fibromyalgia (913), binge eating associated with obesity (914), attention deficit disorder (ADD) (913), cerebellar ataxia (916), Ramsey-Hunt syndrome (917), Down syndrome (5050), and as adjunctive therapy in seizure disorder and Parkinson's disease (9). In combination with carbidopa, 5-HTP is used for treating intention myoclonus (1403,1404) and as an orphan drug for treating post-anoxia myoclonus (14).

Safety
POSSIBLY UNSAFE ...when used orally. Use of 5-HTP has been associated with eosinophilia myalgia syndrome in one individual and asymptomatic eosinophilia in two others (902,919). 5-HTP used with carbidopa has been associated with an eosinophilia myalgia-like syndrome including scleroderma-like skin changes (1403,1404).
PREGNANCY AND LACTATION: POSSIBLY UNSAFE ...when used orally (919); avoid using.

Effectiveness
LIKELY EFFECTIVE ...when taken orally for treating post-anoxic myoclonus (Land-Adams Syndrome), a rare complication of successful cardiopulmonary resuscitation (903).
POSSIBLY EFFECTIVE ...when taken orally for depression (904,912), fibromyalgia (913), obesity (914), anxiety (915), cerebellar ataxia (916), and Ramsey-Hunt syndrome (917).
LIKELY INEFFECTIVE ...when used orally for Alzheimer's disease (918).
There is insufficient reliable information available about the effectiveness of 5-HTP for its other uses.

Possible Mechanism of Action & Active Ingredients
5-HTP is an intermediate metabolite in the biosynthesis of serotonin from L-tryptophan. 5-HTP readily crosses the blood-brain barrier, increasing CNS synthesis of serotonin, which effects sleep, depression, anxiety, aggression, appetite, temperature, sexual behavior, and pain sensation (901). Some commercial 5-HTP products contain peak x, an impurity that is associated with eosinophilia myalgia in individuals using L-tryptophan (919). Use of 5-HTP has been associated with eosinophilia myalgia syndrome in one individual and asymptomatic eosinophilia in two others (902,919); in these cases the presence of peak x was not confirmed. 5-HTP used with carbidopa has been associated with an eosinophilia myalgia-like syndrome including scleroderma-like skin changes (1403,1404). Researchers believe this might be due to altered 5-HTP metabolism and an increase in either serotonin plasma levels or increased levels of the metabolite kynurenine (1403,1404).

Adverse Reactions Including Known Allergies
Large doses of 5-HTP can cause nausea, vomiting, diarrhea, and anorexia (14). 5-HTP has been associated with eosinophilia myalgia syndrome and asymptomatic eosinophilia (902,919). The combination of 5-HTP and carbidopa has been associated with scleroderma-like skin changes (1403,1404). The scleroderma-like changes partially reversed when 5-HTP and carbidopa are stopped (1403,1404). 5-HTP is reported to cause seizures in patients with Down syndrome (5050).

Possible Interactions with Herbs & Other Dietary Supplements
Insufficient reliable information available.

Possible Interactions with Drugs
CARBIDOPA: Co-administration reduces peripheral 5-HTP metabolism, increasing the amount of 5-HTP available to the brain. Concomitant use can cause hypomania, restlessness, rapid speech, anxiety, insomnia, aggressiveness (14), and an eosinophilia myalgia-like syndrome including scleroderma-like skin changes (1403,1404).
SEROTONIN AGONISTS: Concurrent use of 5-HTP can increase the risk of adverse effects. Serotonin agonist drugs include monoamine oxidase inhibitors (MAOIs), reserpine, SSRIs, tricyclic, and atypical antidepressants (14).
SEROTONIN ANTAGONISTS: Concurrent use of 5-HTP can decrease the effectiveness of these drugs, which include methysergide and cyproheptadine (14).

Possible Interactions with Foods
No interactions are known to occur, and there is no known reason to expect a clinically significant interaction with 5-HTP.

Possible Interactions with Lab Tests
No interactions are known to occur, and there is no known reason to expect a clinically significant interaction with 5-HTP.

© Copyright 2000, Natural Medicines Comprehensive Database (209) 472-2244. For updated data, go to www.NaturalDatabase.com

Possible Interactions with Diseases or Conditions

DOWN SYNDROME: 5-HTP is reported to cause seizures in some patients with Down syndrome. In one case series, 15% of patients receiving long-term 5-HTP treatment experienced seizures (5050).

PEPTIC ULCERS, PLATELET DISORDERS, AND RENAL DISEASE: Some experts caution against using 5-HTP in people with these conditions (14). These cautions appear to be based on indirect reasoning using various in vitro and animal data. Currently, there are no reported animal or human studies to support these cautions.

Typical Dosages & Routes of Administration that are Commonly Used

ORAL: For depression, the typical dose of 5-HTP is 150-300 mg daily (903). For post-anoxic myoclonus, 5-HTP has an orphan drug status. The sponsor of the orphan drug is Circa Pharmaceuticals (516-842-8383).

Comments

5-HTP is promoted for treating insomnia based on the apparent effectiveness of L-tryptophan. Because L-tryptophan converts to 5-HTP, which converts to serotonin, 5-HTP should also be effective for treating insomnia. However, L-tryptophan can produce sleep through a mechanism unrelated to serotonin (946).

7-KETO-DHEA

This Product is Also Known As

7-Keto, 7-keto dehydroepiandrosterone, 7-oxo-DHEA-acetate, 7-oxo-DHEA, 3-acetyl-7-oxo-dehydroepiandrosterone, 7-ketodehydroepiandrostenedione, 5-androsten-3-beta-17-one-DHEA, 3beta-acetoxy-androst-5-ene-7,17-dione, 7-oxo-dehydroepiandrosterone-3-acetate, 7-ODA.
CAUTION: See separate listing for DHEA.

Scientific Names

3-acetyl-7-oxo-dehydroepiandrosterone; 3beta-acetoxy-androst-5-ene-7,17-dione.

People Use This For

Orally, 7-keto-DHEA is used to increase metabolism and thermogenesis and promote weight loss, to improve lean body mass and build muscle, to increase activity of the thyroid gland and immune system, to boost memory, and to reduce aging (5834,5835,5836).

Safety

There is insufficient reliable information available about the safety of 7-keto-DHEA.
Pregnancy and Lactation: Insufficient reliable information available; avoid using.

Effectiveness

There is insufficient reliable information available to rate the effectiveness of 7-keto-DHEA. However, limited clinical evidence from one unpublished study suggest that 7-keto-DHEA might significantly decrease body weight and fat composition compared to placebo. More evidence is needed to rate 7-keto-DHEA for this use.

Possible Mechanism of Action & Active Ingredients

7-keto-DHEA is a metabolite of dehydroepiandrosterone (DHEA) which is formed in the body (5837). Unlike, DHEA, 7-keto-DHEA, is not converted to androgens and estrogens (5837,5840,5842). 7-keto-DHEA is thought to be beneficial in weight loss by increasing metabolism and thermogenesis. Early evidence in animals suggests 7-keto-DHEA can increase thermogenesis, possibly by stimulation of thermogenic enzymes in the liver (5837); however this effect has not yet been reported in humans. Clinical evidence suggests 7-keto-DHEA might increase basal metabolism. One study in obese subjects showed significant increases in thyroid hormone triiodothyronine (T3) when 7-keto-DHEA was used over 4 weeks (5842). Other preliminary studies have shown other effects. In one study in rats, 7-keto-DHEA improved chemically-induced and age-related memory impairment (5839). In another study, 7-keto-DHEA was reported have immunomodulatory effects by stimulating interleukin-2 production by human lymphocytes in vitro (5841).

Adverse Reactions Including Known Allergies

None reported.

Possible Interactions with Herbs & Other Dietary Supplements

Insufficient reliable information available.

Possible Interactions with Drugs

No interactions are known to occur, and there is no known reason to expect a clinically significant interaction with 7-keto-DHEA.

Possible Interactions with Foods

No interactions are known to occur, and there is no known reason to expect a clinically significant interaction with 7-keto-DHEA.

Possible Interactions with Lab Tests

No interactions are known to occur, and there is no known reason to expect a clinically significant interaction with 7-keto-DHEA.

Possible Interactions with Diseases or Conditions

No interactions are known to occur, and there is no known reason to expect a clinically significant interaction with 7-keto-DHEA.

Typical Dosages & Routes of Administration that are Commonly Used

ORAL: For weight loss, 100 mg twice daily were used in one study (5842).

Comments

None.

ABSCESS ROOT

This Product is Also Known As

American Greek Valerian, Blue Bells, False Jacob's Ladder, Sweatroot.
CAUTION: See separate listing for Jacob's Ladder.

Scientific Names

Polemonium reptans.
Family: Polemoniaceae.

People Use This For

Orally, abscess root is used to reduce fevers. It has also been used orally to reduce inflammation, stimulate sweating, as an astringent, and expectorant (18).

Safety

There is insufficient reliable information available about the safety of the oral use of abscess root.
Pregnancy and Lactation: Insufficient reliable information available; avoid using.

Effectiveness

There is insufficient reliable information available about the effectiveness of abscess root.

Possible Mechanism of Action & Active Ingredients

Abscess root contains triterpene saponins. These substances are from colloidal solutions in water that foam when they are shaken. They are often irritating to mucous membranes and could cause symptoms such as sneezing and GI irritation (18,4077).

Adverse Reactions Including Known Allergies

None reported.

Possible Interactions with Herbs & Other Dietary Supplements

Insufficient reliable information available.

Possible Interactions with Drugs

No interactions are known to occur, and there is no known reason to expect a clinically significant interaction with abscess root.

Possible Interactions with Foods

No interactions are known to occur, and there is no known reason to expect a clinically significant interaction with abscess root.

Possible Interactions with Lab Tests

No interactions are known to occur, and there is no known reason to expect a clinically significant interaction with abscess root.

Possible Interactions with Diseases or Conditions

No interactions are known to occur, and there is no known reason to expect a clinically significant interaction with abscess root.

Typical Dosages & Routes of Administration that are Commonly Used

ORAL: A tea is made from the ground root (18).

Comments

Abscess root is also called false Jacob's ladder because it has astringent activity similar to Jacob's ladder (see separate monograph). These two plants are used in similar ways, but differ chemically. Be cautious with use, because one can be confused with the other (18).

ABUTA

This Product is Also Known As
Bejunco de Cerca, Butua, False Pareira, Pareira, Patacon, Velvetleaf.
CAUTION: See separate listing for Pareira.

Scientific Names
Cissampelos pareira; Menispermaceae.

People Use This For
Orally, abuta is used for acne, asthma, dog bites, snake bites, boils, bronchitis, burns, chills, cholera, colds, colic, convulsions, coughs, cystitis, delirium, diabetes, diarrhea, dropsy, dysentery, dyspepsia, erysipelas, fertility in women, fevers, hematuria, hemorrhage, hypertension, itching, jaundice, leukorrhea, malaria, menorrhagia, nephritis, palpitation, parturition, purgative, rabies, rheumatism, sores, stimulating menstrual flow, stomachache, veneral diseases, wounds, a diuretic, expectorant, stimulant, styptic, a tonic (513), for eye infections, nervous children, toothaches, and as an aphrodisiac (3913).

Safety
There is insufficient reliable information available about the safety of abuta.
Pregnancy and Lactation: Insufficient reliable information available; avoid using.

Effectiveness
There is insufficient reliable information available about the effectiveness of abuta.

Possible Mechanism of Action & Active Ingredients
Insufficient reliable information available.

Adverse Reactions Including Known Allergies
None reported.

Possible Interactions with Herbs & Other Dietary Supplements
Insufficient reliable information available.

Possible Interactions with Drugs
No interactions are known to occur, and there is no known reason to expect a clinically significant interaction with abuta.

Possible Interactions with Foods
No interactions are known to occur, and there is no known reason to expect a clinically significant interaction with abuta.

Possible Interactions with Lab Tests
No interactions are known to occur, and there is no known reason to expect a clinically significant interaction with abuta.

Possible Interactions with Diseases or Conditions
No interactions are known to occur, and there is no known reason to expect a clinically significant interaction with abuta.

Typical Dosages & Routes of Administration that are Commonly Used
ORAL: People typically use 1 to 2 grams of powdered abuta bark in tablets or capsules twice daily. Abuta is also taken as a 4:1 tincture in a dose of 2 to 4 mL twice daily (5255).

Comments
Avoid confusion with Abuta grandifolia, which is also referred to as abuta and is a South American medicinal plant used for making arrow poison and other curaré preparations (518).
There is very little scientific information about this product. Our staff is continually analyzing the available information on natural medicines and will add data here as it becomes available.

ACACIA

This Product is Also Known As
Gum Acacia, Gum Arabic, Gum Senegal, Gomme Arabique, Gomme de Senegal, Gummae Mimosae, Kher.
CAUTION: See separate listing for Cassie Absolute.

Scientific Names
Acacia senegal.
Family: Leguminosae/Fabaceae.

People Use This For
Orally, acacia gum is used to reduce cholesterol levels.
In manufacturing, it is used as a pharmaceutical ingredient in making emulsions, troches, demulcent for throat or stomach inflammation, as a masking agent for acrid substances (e.g. capsicum), and as a film forming agent in peel-off skin masks (11).

Safety
LIKELY SAFE ...except in allergic individuals (11).
PREGNANCY AND LACTATION: LIKELY SAFE.

Effectiveness
LIKELY INEFFECTIVE ...when used for reducing cholesterol levels. It may actually elevate serum or tissue cholesterol levels (11).

Possible Mechanism of Action & Active Ingredients
The applicable part of acacia is the gum. Acacia gum consists mostly of arabic acid which becomes arabinose, galactose, and arabinosic acid when hydrolyzed. It is almost completely soluble in twice its weight of water (16).

Adverse Reactions Including Known Allergies
Allergy to acacia dust manifests as skin lesions and severe asthmatic attacks (11).

Possible Interactions with Herbs & Other Dietary Supplements
Insufficient reliable information available.

Possible Interactions with Drugs
ORAL DRUGS: The fiber in acacia can impair absorption of oral drugs (19).
ALKALOIDS: If mixed with certain alkaloids, acacia gum causes partial destruction of them. These alkaloids include atropine, hyoscyamine, scopolamine, homatropine, morphine, apomorphine, cocaine, and physostigmine (11).
IRON: Acacia can be gelatinized by solutions of ferric iron salts (19).
ETHYL ALCOHOL: Mixing acacia with a substance containing greater than 50% concentration of ethyl alcohol can cause acacia to become insoluble (19).

Possible Interactions with Foods
ALCOHOL: Acacia gum used with alcohol or alcoholic solutions can cause precipitation from suspensions (16).

Possible Interactions with Lab Tests
SERUM CHOLESTEROL: Theoretically, acacia might increase serum cholesterol concentrations and test results (11).

Possible Interactions with Diseases or Conditions
No interactions are known to occur, and there is no known reason to expect a clinically significant interaction with acacia.

Typical Dosages & Routes of Administration that are Commonly Used
ORAL: Acacia is usually dissolved in water to make a mucilage. The usual dose is 1 to 4 teaspoons (5263).

Comments
Avoid confusion with sweet acacia (Acacia farnesiana).

ACEROLA

This Product is Also Known As
Barbados Cherry, Puerto Rican Cherry, West Indian Cherry.
CAUTION: See separate listing for Cherokee Rosehip, Rose Hip, and Vitamin C.

Scientific Names
Malpidnia glabra; Malpidnia punicifolia.
Family: Malpighiaceae.

People Use This For
Acerola fruit is used for its high vitamin C content.
Orally, acerola is used to treat or prevent scurvy, colds, heart disease, cancer, pressure sores, retinal hemorrhages, tooth decay, gum infections, atherosclerosis, depression, hay fever, for preventing blood clots, collagen disorders, and to enhance physical endurance (15).

Safety

LIKELY SAFE ...when used orally in individuals with normal kidney function. The vitamin C in acerola is water soluble (6).
POSSIBLY SAFE ...when used orally in patients with diabetes. Large doses may affect blood sugar control (15). ...when used in patients who have kidney stone-forming tendency. Large doses might cause precipitation of urate, cystine, or oxalate stones (15).
PREGNANCY AND LACTATION: POSSIBLY UNSAFE ...because high doses or megadoses of vitamin C from acerola might increase the metabolic rate. Megadoses might also lead to neonatal scurvy (15).

Effectiveness

EFFECTIVE ...when taken orally to prevent scurvy (6).
LIKELY EFFECTIVE ...when taken orally for tyrosinemia of premature infants and idiopathic methemoglobinemia.
POSSIBLY EFFECTIVE ...when taken orally as a urinary acidifier (15). ...in reducing the severity or shortening the duration of the common cold; however, it is unlikely to prevent the common cold. ...when combined with vitamin E for reducing the risk of heart disease.
LIKELY INEFFECTIVE ...when taken orally as a single agent to prevent heart disease.
There is insufficient reliable information available about the effectiveness in cancer prevention (15), and for its other uses.

Possible Mechanism of Action & Active Ingredients

The applicable part of acerola is the fruit. Acerola contains 1000-2330 mg of vitamin C per 100 grams (6). Vitamin C is an essential coenzyme required for normal metabolic function. It is important for collagen formation and tissue repair. Vitamin C is involved in tyrosine metabolism, folic acid conversion, carbohydrate metabolism, synthesis of lipids and proteins, iron metabolism, resistance to infections, and cellular respiration. Vitamin C acts as an antioxidant (6,15). It regenerates and restores oxidized vitamin E (127,128).

Adverse Reactions Including Known Allergies

The vitamin C in acerola can cause nausea, abdominal cramps, fatigue, insomnia, and sleepiness. Doses greater than 1 gram might cause diarrhea (15).

Possible Interactions with Herbs & Other Dietary Supplements

VITAMIN C SUPPLEMENTS: Concomitant use interacts with the vitamin C in acerola and increases total dose of vitamin C which might increase the risk of adverse effects.

Possible Interactions with Drugs

WARFARIN (Coumadin): Concomitant use interacts with the vitamin C in acerola and can reduce anticoagulant activity (506).
IRON: Concomitant use interacts with the vitamin C in acerola and increases GI absorption of iron in foods (ferric) but not from supplements (ferrous) (15).
ESTROGEN: Concomitant use interacts with the vitamin C in acerola and might increase absorption and effects (129,130).
FLUPHENAZINE (Prolixin): Concomitant use interacts with the vitamin C in acerola and decreases blood levels (15).
ACIDIC or BASIC DRUGS: Concomitant use interacts with the vitamin C in acerola and might acidify urine affecting excretion (15).

Possible Interactions with Foods

No interactions are known to occur, and there is no known reason to expect a clinically significant interaction with acerola.

Possible Interactions with Lab Tests

URINE GLUCOSE TESTS: Doses of vitamin C greater than 500 mg can cause false-decreases with glucose oxidase tests (e.g. Clinistix). The vitamin C in acerola might also cause false increases with cupric sulfate tests (e.g. Clinitest) (15).
STOOL OCCULT BLOOD TESTS: The vitamin C in acerola can cause false-negative results if it is ingested 48-72 hours before amine-dependent tests (506).

Possible Interactions with Diseases or Conditions

GOUT: The vitamin C in acerola might increase uric acid levels (15).
KIDNEY STONE FORMING TENDENCY: The vitamin C in acerola in large doses might cause precipitation of urate, cystine, or oxalate stones (15).

Typical Dosages & Routes of Administration that are Commonly Used

The oral RDA for adults is 50-60 mg (the RDA is likely to be raised to 100-200 mg daily) as a dietary supplement. Chronic hemodialysis (adults): 100-200 mg.
Pregnancy: 60 mg. Lactation: 80 mg/day (15). Some experts think the RDA is low. Based on pharmacokinetics, recommend 200 mg daily from fruits and vegetables. Consider daily doses to 1000 mg safe; doses above 400 mg

are of no proven additional benefit (131).

The dry acerola fruit and powder are unlikely to have effectiveness because much of the vitamin C is destroyed during the drying and processing (2,11).

Comments
Acerola fruit also contains vitamin A, thiamine, riboflavin, and niacin (6).

ACETYL-L-CARNITINE

This Product is Also Known As
Acetyl L-Carnitine, Acetyl-Carnitine, Acetyl-Levocarnitine, Acetylcarnitine, ALC, Alcar, ALCAR, Carnitine Acetyl Ester, Gamma-Trimethyl-Beta-Acetylbutyrobetaine, L-acetylcarnitine, Levacecarnine, ST-200, Vitamin B(t) Acetate.
CAUTION: See separate listings for L-Carnitine and Propionyl-L-Carnitine.

Scientific Names
2-(acetyloxy)-3-carboxy-N,N,N-trimethyl-1-propanaminium inner salt; (3-carboxy-2-hydroxy-propyl)trimethylammonium hydroxide inner salt acetate.

People Use This For
Orally, acetyl-L-carnitine is used for Alzheimer's disease (14,1584,1586,3082), age-related memory deficits, senile depression, Down syndrome (1586,1588), alcoholism-related cognitive deficits (1589), cerebrovascular insufficiency after stroke (14), peripheral neuropathies (14), diabetic neuropathy, neuropathy due to anti-viral drugs used in the treatment of AIDS (1585), and facial paralysis (1590).
In combination with L-carnitine, fructose and citric acid (in ProXeed), acetyl-L-carnitine is used to improve sperm quality in male infertility (1587).
Intravenously, acetyl-L-carnitine is used for dementia (14) and cerebral ischemia (1591,1592).
Intramuscularly, acetyl-L-carnitine is used for peripheral neuropathy with pain (1593).

Safety
POSSIBLY SAFE ...when used orally and appropriately. Due to the limited data available, periodic monitoring of blood cell counts and liver and renal function has been recommended during acetyl-L-carnitine therapy (14). ...when used parenterally and appropriately under medical supervision.
PREGNANCY AND LACTATION: Insufficient reliable information available; avoid using.

Effectiveness
POSSIBLY EFFECTIVE ...when used orally for improving memory, slowing the rate of decline in some measures of cognitive function, and improving behavioral performance in people with Alzheimer's disease, especially those less than 66 years of age (1594,1595,1596,1597,1598,1599). Acetyl-L-carnitine may need to be taken between one and six months before any improvement is seen (14). ...when used for improving some measures of cognitive function and memory in elderly people with age-related mental impairment (42,3600,3601). ...when used for decreasing symptoms of depression in elderly people (3602,3603,3604). ...when used for improving some measures of cognitive function in people recovering from strokes, vascular dementia, or other conditions of cerebral insufficiency. (14,43). ...when used intravenously for producing short-term improvements in cerebral blood flow in people with chronic cerebral ischemia after single doses (1591,1592). ...when used orally to improve memory and visuo-spatial capacity in 30 to 60 year-old non-drinking alcoholics with cognitive impairment (1589).
There is insufficient reliable information about the effectiveness of acetyl-L-carnitine for its other uses.

Possible Mechanism of Action & Active Ingredients
Acetyl-L-carnitine occurs naturally in the body, within the inner membrane of mitochondria (14). It is an ester of L-carnitine, and is converted to L-carnitine in the body by carnitine acetyltransferase (14). It is also structurally related to acetylcholine (14). It may act as a cholinergic-enhancing agent by serving as a mitochondrial precursor to acetyl coenzyme A (acetyl CoA), thus contributing acetyl moieties for acetylcholine (14). It is an intracellular carrier of acetyl groups across mitochondrial membranes and promotes acetylcholine release and increases choline acetyltransferase activity (44). These effects have lead to the study of acetyl-L-carnitine in Alzheimer's disease, in which there is substantial cholinergic neuronal loss and acetylcholine depletion (1594). Acetyl-L-carnitine also participates in cellular energy production by acting as a shuttle between the cytoplasm and mitochondria for long-chain fatty acids (1594). Other potentially beneficial actions of acetyl-L-carnitine include neuroprotective actions, enhancement of choline acetyltransferase activity, facilitatory actions on serotonergic pathways, enhancement of synaptic transmission, increased hippocampal binding of nerve growth factor, and reduction of age-dependent losses of hippocampal glucocorticoid receptors (14). An increase in cerebral blood flow has been reported following acetyl-L-carnitine administration to people with cerebrovascular disease (14). In asymptomatic people with AIDS, acetyl-L-carnitine has been reported to slow the loss of CD4 lymphocytes by reducing apoptosis and increasing the serum level of insulin-like growth factor 1 which is protective against apoptosis (3605). Plasma levels of acetyl-L-carnitine have also been reported to be lower in people who developed neuropathy while taking anti-HIV drugs

than in those who did not develop neuropathy (3606). Acetyl-L-carnitine and L-carnitine are present in human sperm and seminal fluid (3607). Their levels increase in sperm during the maturation process in the epididymis and coincide with the acquisition of progressive motility (3608,3609). Levels of acetyl-L-carnitine, and the ratio of acetyl-L-carnitine to L-carnitine, have been reported to be lower in infertile semen and sperm samples with low motility (3610,3611), and an increase in sperm motility is seen in vitro when acetyl-L-carnitine or L-carnitine is added to the sample (3612).

Adverse Reactions Including Known Allergies

When used orally, may cause nausea and vomiting (14,1599), agitation (restlessness and motor overactivity) (14,1596). Side effects reported in people with Alzheimer's disease include psychiatric disturbances, such as depression, mania, confusion and aggression, but it is not clear whether these are due to acetyl-L-carnitine or the disease itself (14).

Possible Interactions with Herbs & Other Dietary Supplements

Insufficient reliable information available.

Possible Interactions with Drugs

No interactions are known to occur, and there is no known reason to expect a clinically significant interaction with acetyl-L-carnitine.

Possible Interactions with Foods

No interactions are known to occur, and there is no known reason to expect a clinically significant interaction with acetyl-L-carnitine.

Possible Interactions with Lab Tests

No interactions are known to occur, and there is no known reason to expect a clinically significant interaction with acetyl-L-carnitine.

Possible Interactions with Diseases or Conditions

HYPERSENSITIVITY: Contraindicated in people with known hypersensitivity to acetyl-L-carnitine or L-carnitine (14).

Typical Dosages & Routes of Administration that are Commonly Used

ORAL: In Alzheimer's disease, 1500 to 4000 mg daily has been used, usually divided into two or three doses during the day (14,1584,1586,1594,1595,1599). In age-related memory impairment, 1500 to 2000 mg daily has been used (1586,3601). In people recovering from stroke, a dose of 1500 mg daily has been used (14). For depression in the elderly, 1500 to 3000 mg daily in divided doses has been used (1586,3602,3603). In Down syndrome 10 mg per pound of body weight has been recommended (1586). In some infertile men, 4000 mg daily has been used to improve sperm function (3607).
INTRAVENOUS: A dose of 20 mg/kg/day has been used in people with dementia (14). Single doses of 1500 mg have been used in people with chronic cerebral ischemia (1591,1592).
INTRAMUSCULAR: In people with peripheral neuropathy, 500 to 1000 mg daily has been used (1593).

Comments

None.

ACKEE

This Product is Also Known As

Akee, Aki, Arbre Fricasse, Seso Vegetal.

Scientific Names

Blighia sapida.
Family: Sapindaceae.

People Use This For

In South America, ackee is used as a treatment for colds, fever, edema, and epilepsy (6).
For food uses, the ripe fruit is eaten (6).

Safety

LIKELY SAFE ...when the ripe fruit is used in traditional Jamaican cooking (6).
UNSAFE ...when the unripe fruit and seeds are ingested. Can cause severe hypoglycemia, convulsions and death (6).
CHILDREN: UNSAFE ...when the unripe fruit and seeds are ingested. Children are more sensitive to the toxic effects of ackee than adults (6). There is insufficient reliable information available about the safety of the ripe fruit for children.

PREGNANCY AND LACTATION: UNSAFE ...when the unripe fruit is ingested (6). There is insufficient reliable information available about the safety of the ripe fruit during pregnancy.

Effectiveness
There is insufficient reliable information available about the effectiveness of ackee.

Possible Mechanism of Action & Active Ingredients
The applicable parts of ackee are the seed and fruit. Unripe fruit and seeds contain liver toxins (hypoglycin A, hypoglycin B). By inactivating flavoprotein acyl-CoA dehydrogenases and inhibiting the oxidation of long-chain fatty acids, the toxins inhibit gluconeogenesis and induce hypoglycemia (5609,5610).

Adverse Reactions Including Known Allergies
There are two forms of toxicity that can occur from after ingestion of the unripe fruit and seeds of ackee. One form is referred to as "vomiting sickness". The symptoms include vomiting, remission for 8-10 hours, renewed vomiting, convulsions, and eventually coma. The second type of toxicity includes convulsions and coma at the onset. Both forms lead to severe hypoglycemia (6) known as toxic hypoglycemic syndrome (THS) (5602). Electrolyte and fluid disturbances may occur due to vomiting (6). Urticaria and anaphylaxis has been reported after ingestion of ackee (5610).

Possible Interactions with Herbs & Other Dietary Supplements
Insufficient reliable information available.

Possible Interactions with Drugs
DIABETES THERAPY: Monitor blood glucose level closely due to claims that ackee has hypoglycemic effects (19).

Possible Interactions with Foods
No interactions are known to occur, and there is no known reason to expect a clinically significant interaction with ackee.

Possible Interactions with Lab Tests
No interactions are known to occur, and there is no known reason to expect a clinically significant interaction with ackee.

Possible Interactions with Diseases or Conditions
DIABETES: Monitor blood glucose level closely due to claims that ackee has hypoglycemic effects (19).

Typical Dosages & Routes of Administration that are Commonly Used
No typical dosage.

Comments
Ackee was brought to Jamaica from West Africa during the end of the 18th century, and the ripe fruit has since become a common ingredient in traditional Jamaican cooking (6). Avoid use of unripe fruit and seeds or water in which unripe ackee has been cooked due to toxicity (5602). Ackee is also found in southern Florida, Central America, and Africa (5602,5609).

ACONITE

This Product is Also Known As
Aconiti Tuber, Blue Monkshood Root, Monkshood, Monkshood Tuber, Wolfsbane.

Scientific Names
Aconitum napellus; Aconitum species.
Family: Ranunculaceae.

People Use This For
Orally, preparations of aconite root have been used for pain, facial paralysis, joint pain, arthritis, gout, rheumatic complaints, inflammation, pleurisy, pericarditis sicca, fever, skin and mucosal diseases, disinfection, and wound treatment (2,11).
Topically, people use aconite root as a counterirritant in liniment (11).
Historically, aconite root has been used orally as a cardiac depressant and an agent to induce mild sweating. Aconite root has been used topically for facial neuralgia, rheumatism, and sciatica (11).

Safety
UNSAFE ...when used orally or topically. Aconite root is a strong, fast-acting poison that affects the heart and CNS (11). All species of this herb are dangerous. Severe poisoning has been reported after ingestion of 0.2 mg of aconitine or 6 g of processed and cured aconite (3490). Aconite can also be absorbed through the skin (11). Even when

used in the therapeutic dose range, aconite can cause toxicity including nausea, vomiting, dizziness, muscle spasms, hypothermia, paralysis of respiratory system, and heart rhythm disorders (2,11).
PREGNANCY AND LACTATION: UNSAFE ...contraindicated for oral or topical use (11,12).

Effectiveness
POSSIBLY EFFECTIVE ...when used topically for severe neuralgia (2).
There is insufficient reliable information available about the effectiveness of aconite for its other uses.

Possible Mechanism of Action & Active Ingredients
The applicable part of aconite is the root. Aconite contains alkaloids (including aconitine, mesoconitine and hypaconitine) which have widespread effects on cardiac, neural and muscle tissue by activating sodium channels (559,3490). Aconitine, the principal alkaloid, is considered to be a fast-acting, lethal poison (2,11).

Adverse Reactions Including Known Allergies
Symptoms of intoxication include nausea, vomiting, weakness, sweating, restlessness, dizziness, numbness, paresthesias beginning in the mouth and then spreading to the limbs, hypotension, palpitations, hypokalemia, metabolic and/or respiratory acidosis, cardiac toxicity (sustained ventricular tachycardia, ventricular fibrillation), reduced consciousness and death (558,559,560,561,562,563,3490). Symptoms of intoxication usually begin 30 minutes after ingestion of aconite (559). Life-threatening symptoms and fatalities have been reported after aconite ingestion (3490,3491). No specific antidote is available. Cardioversion has been reported to be ineffective and the use of antiarrhythmic agents have been successful in some cases (3490).

Possible Interactions with Herbs & Other Dietary Supplements
Insufficient reliable information available.

Possible Interactions with Drugs
No interactions are known to occur, and there is no known reason to expect a clinically significant interaction with aconite.

Possible Interactions with Foods
No interactions are known to occur, and there is no known reason to expect a clinically significant interaction with aconite.

Possible Interactions with Lab Tests
No interactions are known to occur, and there is no known reason to expect a clinically significant interaction with aconite.

Possible Interactions with Diseases or Conditions
No interactions are known to occur, and there is no known reason to expect a clinically significant interaction with aconite.

Typical Dosages & Routes of Administration that are Commonly Used
ORAL: People typically use a homeopathic preparation of aconite of 6c to 30c potency strength (5011). A 6c potency is made by diluting one part of aconite tincture to 99 parts of water or alcohol. One part of the resulting solution is taken and diluted again with 99 parts of water or alcohol. The process is repeated four additional times resulting in a 6c potency (5011).
TOPICAL: No typical dose.

Comments
Aconite is a strong, fast-acting poison that affects the heart and CNS. It should not be used for self-medication because it has an extremely high risk of toxicity (11). Aconite rootstocks can be purchased in Chinese herbstores in western countries and are commonly used as components in Chinese herbal recipes. The rootstocks of aconite are processed and cured in Chinese medicine by soaking in water (with frequent changes to fresh water) and then boiled or steamed for prolonged periods of time. The process hydrolyzes the aconite alkaloids into less toxic derivatives but toxicities and fatalities have been reported after ingestion of cured and processed aconite root (3490).

ACTIVATED CHARCOAL

This Product is Also Known As
Animal Charcoal, Charcoal, Gas Black, Lamp Black, Medicinal Charcoal.
CAUTION: See separate listing for Coffee Charcoal.

Scientific Names
Carbon.

People Use This For
Orally, activated charcoal is used for an antiflatulence, reducing blood lipid levels, acute management of poisonings (6), and cholestasis of pregnancy (126).

Safety

LIKELY SAFE ...when used orally for short term use (6).
PREGNANCY AND LACTATION: POSSIBLY SAFE (126).

Effectiveness

LIKELY EFFECTIVE ...when used as part of a standard treatment for some acute poisonings (15).
POSSIBLY EFFECTIVE ...when used orally for reducing serum cholesterol levels (6). ...for cholestasis of pregnancy (126). ...when used orally as an antiflatulent (15).

Possible Mechanism of Action & Active Ingredients

Activated charcoal has a very large surface area which adsorbs chemicals and therefore prevents their systemic absorption. Activated charcoal may interrupt enterohepatic recirculation of drugs and other compounds that are excreted into the bile (6).

Adverse Reactions Including Known Allergies

Activiated charcoal can cause GI obstruction, pulmonary aspiration, hypernatremic dehydration, and prolonged GI transit time (6). Poisoning cases: Be cautious when using activated charcoal along with an emetic. There is a risk of pulmonary aspiration (6) (see Typical Dosage, Comments).

Possible Interactions with Herbs & Other Dietary Supplements

Activated charcoal may cause reduced absorption of micronutrients (15).

Possible Interactions with Drugs

SYRUP OF IPECAC: Adsorbs/inactivates drug, avoid co-administration (506).
NUMEROUS DRUGS: Avoid co-administration. Activated charcoal may reduce/prevent absorption of drugs including: acetaminophen, barbiturates, carbamazepine, digitoxin, digoxin, furosemide, glutethimide, hydantoins, methotrexate, nizatidine, phenothiazines, phenylbutazones, propoxyphene, salicylates, sulfones, sulfonylureas, tetracyclines, theophyllines, tricyclic antidepressants, and valproic acid (506).

Possible Interactions with Foods

Activated charcoal can reduce absorption of micronutrients (15).
MILK, ICE CREAM OR SHERBET AND OTHER DAIRY PRODUCTS: Co-administration of these foods along with activated charcoal may decrease the adsorptive capacity of activated charcoal (506).

Possible Interactions with Lab Tests

SERUM CHOLESTEROL: Activated charcoal can reduce serum total cholesterol and LDL cholesterol concentrations and test results (6).

Possible Interactions with Diseases or Conditions

GI OBSTRUCTION: Avoid use in conditions of GI obstruction (see Adverse Reactions).

Typical Dosages & Routes of Administration that are Commonly Used

ORAL: Antiflatulent dose; 520-975 mg after meals or at first sign of discomfort. Separate activated charcoal doses from other drugs by at least two hours to avoid interaction.

Comments

In case of POISONING, use caution if an emetic is given, due to the risk of pulmonary aspiration. Laxatives are often co-administered to reduce GI transit time and speed removal of poison from the body (6).

ADAM'S NEEDLE

This Product is Also Known As

Adams Needle.

Scientific Names

Yucca filamentosa.
Family: Liliaceae.

People Use This For

Orally, Adam's needle is used to treat liver and gallbladder disorders (18).

Safety

There is insufficient reliable information available about the safety of the oral use of Adam's needle.
Pregnancy and Lactation: Insufficient reliable information available; avoid using.

Effectiveness

There is insufficient reliable information available about the effectiveness of Adam's needle.

Possible Mechanism of Action & Active Ingredients

The applicable part of Adam's needle is the root of the nonflowering plant. Adam's needle contains saponins, including gitogenin and tigogenin. These substances are from colloidal solutions in water that foam when they are shaken. They are often irritating to mucous membranes and could cause symptoms such as sneezing and GI irritation (18,4077).

Adverse Reactions Including Known Allergies

Oral use of Adam's needle might cause dyspepsia and related abdominal symptoms (18).

Possible Interactions with Herbs & Other Dietary Supplements

Insufficient reliable information available.

Possible Interactions with Drugs

No interactions are known to occur, and there is no known reason to expect a clinically significant interaction with Adam's needle.

Possible Interactions with Foods

No interactions are known to occur, and there is no known reason to expect a clinically significant interaction with Adam's needle.

Possible Interactions with Lab Tests

No interactions are known to occur, and there is no known reason to expect a clinically significant interaction with Adam's needle.

Possible Interactions with Diseases or Conditions

No interactions are known to occur, and there is no known reason to expect a clinically significant interaction with Adam's needle.

Typical Dosages & Routes of Administration that are Commonly Used

The root is ground and taken orally. Sometimes an extract is made from the root and taken orally (18).

Comments

Adam's needle is a native to the southern states in the US, and is used as an ornamental plant in Europe (18). There is very little scientific information about this product. Our staff is continually analyzing the available information on natural medicines and will add data here as it becomes available.

ADRUE

This Product is Also Known As

Guinea Rush.

Scientific Names

Cyperus articulatus.
Family: Cyperaceae.

People Use This For

Orally, adrue is used as an anti-emetic and for digestive disorders, including nausea, colic and flatulence. It is also used orally as a sedative (18).

Safety

There is insufficient reliable information available about the safety of adrue.
Pregnancy and Lactation: Insufficient reliable information available; avoid using.

Effectiveness

There is insufficient reliable information about the effectiveness of adrue.

Possible Mechanism of Action & Active Ingredients

The applicable part of adrue is the root. Adrue produces a volatile oil that contains sesquiterpene alcohols and sesquiterpene hydrocarbons, including cyperenone. At present, we don't know how these components relate to the uses of adrue (18).

Adverse Reactions Including Known Allergies

None reported.

Possible Interactions with Herbs & Other Dietary Supplements

Insufficient reliable information available.

Possible Interactions with Drugs

No interactions are known to occur, and there is no known reason to expect a clinically significant interaction with adrue.

Possible Interactions with Foods

No interactions are known to occur, and there is no known reason to expect a clinically significant interaction with adrue.

Possible Interactions with Lab Tests

No interactions are known to occur, and there is no known reason to expect a clinically significant interaction with adrue.

Possible Interactions with Diseases or Conditions

No interactions are known to occur, and there is no known reason to expect a clinically significant interaction with adrue.

Typical Dosages & Routes of Administration that are Commonly Used

A liquid extract is obtained from the root and taken orally (18).

Comments

Adrue is native to Turkey, Jamaica, and the Nile River region. It has a bitter taste, and an aroma reminiscent of lavender (18).

There is very little scientific information about this product. Our staff is continually analyzing the available information on natural medicines and will add data here as it becomes available.

AFRICAN WILD POTATO

This Product is Also Known As

African Potato, Bantu Tulip, Hypoxis Plant, South African Star Grass, Sterretjie.
CAUTION: See separate listing for potato.

Scientific Names

Hypoxis rooperi.

People Use This For

Orally, the African wild potato is used for bladder and urinary disorders including cystitis, prostate problems including prostatic hyperplasia (7,5943,5944) and prostate cancer (5945), lung disease (5944), and cancer (5943). It is also used in maintaining health in individuals who are HIV positive, for TB, "yuppie flu", arthritis, and psoriasis (5945). Topically, the African wild potato is used for wound healing (5944).

Safety

There is insufficient reliable information available about the safety of the African wild potato. Preliminary human trials indicate the African wild potato glucoside constituent is not toxic (5943).

Pregnancy and Lactation: Insufficient reliable information available; avoid using.

Effectiveness

POSSIBLY EFFECTIVE ...when used orally in increasing volume of urine excreted and improving urine flow in individuals with prostate problems (7).

There is insufficient reliable information available about the effectiveness of African wild potato for its other uses.

Possible Mechanism of Action & Active Ingredients

The African wild potato tuber contains 3.5%-4.5% lignans, particularly norlignan glucoside (5944). It also contains beta-sitosterol and beta-sitosterolin (7). The activity of the African wild potato is attributed to the phytosterols that inhibit the production of prostaglandin synthase (5944). It is also believed to stimulate and regulate the immune system by activating the body's T-cells (5946).

Adverse Reactions Including Known Allergies

The African wild potato constituent beta-sitosterol has been associated with erectile dysfunction and loss of libido (5942).

Possible Interactions with Herbs & Other Dietary Supplements

Insufficient reliable information available.

Possible Interactions with Drugs

No interactions are known to occur, and there is no known reason to expect a clinically significant interaction with African wild potato.

Possible Interactions with Foods

No interactions are known to occur, and there is no known reason to expect a clinically significant interaction with African wild potato.

Possible Interactions with Lab Tests

No interactions are known to occur, and there is no known reason to expect a clinically significant interaction with African wild potato.

Possible Interactions with Diseases or Conditions

No interactions are known to occur, and there is no known reason to expect a clinically significant interaction with African wild potato.

Typical Dosages & Routes of Administration that are Commonly Used

ORAL: To boost the immune system, a typical dose is 15 drops in a glass of water three times daily before meals (5945).

Comments

The African wild potato was originally grown in South Africa (5944).

AGA

This Product is Also Known As

Fly Agaric, Soma.

Scientific Names

Amanita muscaria.
Family: Agariacaceae.

People Use This For

Orally, aga is used as a hallucinogen. It is also used orally in homeopathic dilutions for nerve pain, fever, anxiety, alcohol poisoning, and joint pains (18).

Safety

UNSAFE …when used orally for any reason (see Possible Mechanism of Action) (18).
PREGNANCY AND LACTATION: UNSAFE …contraindicated because of its toxicity (18).

Effectiveness

There is insufficient reliable information available about the effectiveness of aga.

Possible Mechanism of Action & Active Ingredients

The applicable parts of aga are the above ground mushroom parts. Aga is not a true hallucinogen. The illusions which occur with aga ingestion are primarily a misinterpretation of sensory stimuli. These mind altering effects are due to the isoxazoles ibotenic acid, muscimol, muscazone (14) and traces of muscarine (18). Ibotenic acid mimics the neurotransmitter glutamic acid in the brain. It is rapidly converted to muscimol, which imitates the action of the neurotransmitter GABA. Ibotenic acid also acts as a flavor enhancer and may produce an unusual aftertaste in people who take it orally. Toxicity also depends on the isoxazole content. It occurs with about 6 mg of mucsimol and 30-60 mg ibotenic acid. These can occur in a single aga mushroom. Isoxazole content can vary as much as 10 times higher depending on when it is collected. Mind-altering effects have occurred with ingestion of 2-4 mushrooms, and 20 large mushrooms have been ingested with survival. The toxic threshold for humans is approximately 6 mg for muscimol and 30-60 mg for ibotenic acid (14). Death due to aga ingestion is rare (less than 1%). Aga does not contain enough muscarine to produce cholinergic symptoms (14).

Adverse Reactions Including Known Allergies

People develop symptoms within 30-90 minutes of ingesting aga. The effects peak at 2-3 hours. The initial symptom is drowsiness. This is quickly followed by confusion, ataxia, dizziness, euphoria, alcohol-like intoxication, and may proceed to hyperactivity, muscle jerks and spasms, and delirium. In the later stages, deep sleep or coma occurs and usually lasts from 4-8 hours. The whole episode lasts 8-10 hours. Severe vomiting is rare (14).

Possible Interactions with Herbs & Other Dietary Supplements

Insufficient reliable information available.

Possible Interactions with Drugs

No interactions are known to occur, and there is no known reason to expect a clinically significant interaction with aga.

Possible Interactions with Foods
No interactions are known to occur, and there is no known reason to expect a clinically significant interaction with aga.

Possible Interactions with Lab Tests
No interactions are known to occur, and there is no known reason to expect a clinically significant interaction with aga.

Possible Interactions with Diseases or Conditions
No interactions are known to occur, and there is no known reason to expect a clinically significant interaction with aga.

Typical Dosages & Routes of Administration that are Commonly Used
No typical dosage.

Comments
Aga is a mushroom with a red cap spotted with white. It is present in sandy, acid soils in the United States. Aga is also known as "fly agaric" because ibotenic acid and muscimol are toxic to the common housefly (14). Aga is considered unsafe; avoid using.

AGAR

This Product is Also Known As
Agar-Agar, Agarweed, Chinese Gelatin, Colle du Japon, Gelatin, Gelosa, Gelosae, Japanese Isinglas, Layor Carang, Vegetable Gelatin.

Scientific Names
Gelidiella acerosa; Gelidium amanasii; Gelidium cartilagineum; Gelidium crinale; Gelidium divaricatum; Gelidium pacificum; Gelidium vagum; Garacilaria confervoides.
Family: Sphaerococcaceae. Species of the genera Pterocladia; Ahnfeltia; Acanthopeltis; Suhria.

People Use This For
Orally, agar is used as a bulk laxative for chronic constipation.
In dentistry, agar is used to make dental impressions (11).
In manufacturing processes, agar is used as an ingredient in emulsions, suspensions, gels, and hydrophilic suppositories.

Safety
LIKELY SAFE ...when agar is used orally with at least 250 mL of water (12).
PREGNANCY AND LACTATION: Insufficient reliable information available.

Effectiveness
POSSIBLY EFFECTIVE ...when used orally as a bulk laxative (11).

Possible Mechanism of Action & Active Ingredients
Agar consists of two major polysaccharides, neutral agarose and charged agaropectin. Agarose is the gelling fraction (11).

Adverse Reactions Including Known Allergies
Potential to cause esophageal or bowel obstruction if taken with insufficient volume of water (12). Possibly can increase cholesterol levels (11).

Possible Interactions with Herbs & Other Dietary Supplements
Insufficient reliable information available.

Possible Interactions with Drugs
ORAL DRUGS: The fiber in agar can impair absorption of oral drugs (19).

Possible Interactions with Foods
No interactions are known to occur, and there is no known reason to expect a clinically significant interaction with agar.

Possible Interactions with Lab Tests
No interactions are known to occur, and there is no known reason to expect a clinically significant interaction with agar.

Possible Interactions with Diseases or Conditions
BOWEL OBSTRUCTION OR DIFFICULTY SWALLOWING: Contraindicated (12).

Typical Dosages & Routes of Administration that are Commonly Used

ORAL: 4-16 grams, one to two times daily (12). Take each dose with at least 250 mL of water (11) (see Safety).

Comments

OTC products must be labeled: "Warning, taking this product without adequate fluid may cause it to swell and block your throat or esophagus and may cause choking. Do not take this product if you have difficulty swallowing. If you experience chest pain, vomiting, or difficulty swallowing or breathing after this product, seek immediate medical attention" (12).

AGRIMONY

This Product is Also Known As

Agromonia, Agrimoniae herba, Ackerkraut, Cocklebur, Fragrant Agrimony, Funffing, Funffingerkraut, Herba eupatoriae, Herbe d'Aigremoine, Herbe de Saint-Guillaume, Liverwort, Stickwort.
CAUTION: See separate listing for Potentilla.

Scientific Names

Agrimonia eupatoria; Agrimonia procera.
Family: Rosaceae.

People Use This For

Orally, agrimony is used for sore throat, upset stomach, and mild, nonspecific diarrhea.
Topically, agrimony is used as a mild astringent and for mild skin inflammation. The ethanolic extracts of agrimony are used for their antiviral properties (6).
Historically, agrimony has been used for gallbladder disorders, tuberculosis, bleeding, corns, warts, as a gargle, antitumor agent, cardiotonic, diuretic, sedative, and antihistamine.

Safety

LIKELY SAFE ...when the dried above ground parts are used orally and appropriately short-term (2,12). ...when used topically (2).
POSSIBLY UNSAFE ...when used orally or topically in excessive doses due to its high tannin content (12).
PREGNANCY AND LACTATION: POSSIBLY UNSAFE ...when used orally because of the possible effects on the menstrual cycle (4,12).

Effectiveness

POSSIBLY EFFECTIVE ...when taken orally for mild, nonspecific acute diarrhea (2). ...when used topically as a mild antiseptic or astringent (6,8).
There is insufficient reliable information available about the effectiveness of agrimony for its other uses.

Possible Mechanism of Action & Active Ingredients

The applicable parts of agrimony are the dried, above ground parts. The aerial plant parts contain 4-10% condensed tannins which can account for its astringent properties (6).

Adverse Reactions Including Known Allergies

The use of agrimony can cause photodermatitis and can affect blood pressure (6).

Possible Interactions with Herbs & Other Dietary Supplements

Insufficient reliable information available (2).

Possible Interactions with Drugs

ANTICOAGULANTS: Excessive doses of agrimony can potentiate anticoagulant therapy (4).
BLOOD PRESSURE ALTERING DRUGS: Excessive doses of agrimony might cause hypotension, interfering with therapy for hypertension or hypotension (4).
DIABETES THERAPY: Monitor blood glucose level closely due to claims that agrimony has hypoglycemic effects (19).

Possible Interactions with Foods

No interactions are known to occur, and there is no known reason to expect a clinically significant interaction with agrimony.

Possible Interactions with Lab Tests

No interactions are known to occur, and there is no known reason to expect a clinically significant interaction with agrimony.

Possible Interactions with Diseases or Conditions

No interactions are known to occur, and there is no known reason to expect a clinically significant interaction with agrimony.

Typical Dosages & Routes of Administration that are Commonly Used

ORAL: The typical dose of agrimony is 3 grams per day (2).

TOPICAL: A poultice is commonly applied several times daily using approximately 10% water extract, which is prepared by boiling the herb at low heat for 10-20 minutes (8).

Comments

None.

AGROPYRON

This Product is Also Known As

Couch Grass, Cutch, Doggrass, Dog Grass, Dog-grass, Durfa Grass, Graminis rhizoma, Quackgrass, Quack Grass, Quitch Grass, Scotch Quelch, Triticum, Twitchgrass, Witch Grass.

Scientific Names

Agropyron repens, synonyms Elytrigia repens, Triticum repens, Elymus repens.
Family: Gramineae or Poaceae.

People Use This For

Orally, agropyron is used for cystitis, urethritis, prostatitis, benign prostatic hypertrophy, renal calculus, specifically for cystitis with irritation or inflammation of the urinary tract (4), and "irrigation therapy" (use of a mild diuretic and copious fluid intake to increase urine flow) for inflammatory diseases of the urinary tract and prevention of urine stones (2,11). It is also used for common cold, cough and bronchitis, fever and colds, inflammation of mouth and pharynx, and tendency to infection (18).

In folk medicine, agropyron has been used as a diuretic, expectorant, diabetes aid, gout remedy, for liver disorders, for rheumatic pain, and chronic skin problems (11,18).

In foods and beverages, agropyron extracts have been used as a flavoring component (11).

Safety

LIKELY SAFE ...when rhizome or root are used orally in food amounts. Agropyron has Generally Recognized as Safe (GRAS) status in the US. The maximum level used in foods is 0.003% (11).

POSSIBLY SAFE ...when used orally and appropriately for irrigation therapy for short periods of time (2,4).

PREGNANCY AND LACTATION: Insufficient reliable information available; avoid using.

Effectiveness

POSSIBLY EFFECTIVE ...when used orally for irrigation therapy for inflammatory diseases of the urinary tract and prevention of urine stones (2,4,10).

There is insufficient reliable information available about the effectiveness of agropyron for its other uses.

Possible Mechanism of Action & Active Ingredients

Agropyron is a plant that is rich in beta-carotene (19). Agropyrene and its oxidative product seem to have broad antibiotic activity (11). The essential oil has antimicrobial effects (2,6). Agropyron contains flavonoid constituents (4). Agropyron seems to produce diuretic and sedative activity (4,11).

Adverse Reactions Including Known Allergies

Excessive or prolonged use may cause hypokalemia (4).

Possible Interactions with Herbs & Other Dietary Supplements

Insufficient reliable information available.

Possible Interactions with Drugs

POTASSIUM DEPLETING DIURETICS: Theoretically, concomitant use may cause potassium depletion (4).

Possible Interactions with Foods

No interactions are known to occur, and there is no known reason to expect a clinically significant interaction with agropyron.

Possible Interactions with Lab Tests

No interactions are known to occur, and there is no known reason to expect a clinically significant interaction with agropyron.

Possible Interactions with Diseases or Conditions

EDEMA: Irrigation therapy contraindicated in edema due to heart or kidney conditions (2).

Typical Dosages & Routes of Administration that are Commonly Used

ORAL: Dried rhizome: 4-8 grams three times daily, or drink as tea (simmer 1-2 grams herb in 150 mL boiling water 5-10 minutes, strain) three times daily. Liquid extract (1:1 in 25% alcohol) 4-8 mL three times daily. Tincture (1:5 in 40% alcohol) 5-15 mL three times daily (4). Use for "irrigation therapy" requires copious fluid intake (2).

Comments

None.

ALCHEMILLA

This Product is Also Known As

Feuilles d'Alchemille, Frauenmantelkraut, Ladys Mantle, Lady's Mantle, Leontopodium, Lions Foot, Lion's Foot, Marienmantel, Nine Hooks, Silerkraut, Stellaria.
CAUTION: See separate listing for Alpine Lady's Mantle.

Scientific Names

Alchemilla xanthochlora, synonym Alchemilla vulgaris.
Family: Rosaceae.

People Use This For

Orally, alchemilla is used for mild diarrhea (2,8), heavy menstrual flow (8), and diabetes (6).
Topically, alchemilla is used as an astringent for bleeding and to improve wound healing (8).
In folk medicine, alchemilla has been used orally for menopausal complaints, painful menses, gastrointestinal disorders, as a relaxant for muscle spasms, as an anti-inflammatory, as a diuretic (6), and as a gargle for mouth and throat inflammation (18). Alchemilla has been used topically in folk medicine for ulcers, eczema, skin rashes, and as a bath additive for treating lower-abdominal ailments (18).

Safety

POSSIBLY SAFE ...when used orally and appropriately. Alchemilla has been used for many years without reports of significant toxicity (2,6,8,12).
There is insufficient reliable information available about the safety of the topical use of alchemilla.
PREGNANCY AND LACTATION: Insufficient reliable information available; avoid using.

Effectiveness

POSSIBLY EFFECTIVE ...when used for mild diarrhea (2).
There is insufficient reliable information available about the effectiveness of alchemilla for its other uses.

Possible Mechanism of Action & Active Ingredients

The applicable parts of alchemilla are the above ground parts. Alchemilla contains 6-8% tannins (8), which might account for its perceived astringent activity (6). An aqueous extract of Alchemilla xanthochlora demonstrates lipid peroxidation and superoxide anion scavenging activity (6). Flavonoid extracts inhibit proteolytic enzymes, including elastase, trypsin, and alpha-chymotrypsin. This property suggests alchemilla might have a role in protecting conjunctive and elastic tissues (6).

Adverse Reactions Including Known Allergies

Rarely, tannins can cause liver damage (8).

Possible Interactions with Herbs & Other Dietary Supplements

Insufficient reliable information available.

Possible Interactions with Drugs

No interactions are known to occur, and there is no known reason to expect a clinically significant interaction with alchemilla.

Possible Interactions with Foods

No interactions are known to occur, and there is no known reason to expect a clinically significant interaction with alchemilla.

Possible Interactions with Lab Tests

No interactions are known to occur, and there is no known reason to expect a clinically significant interaction with alchemilla.

Possible Interactions with Diseases or Conditions

No interactions are known to occur, and there is no known reason to expect a clinically significant interaction with alchemilla.

Typical Dosages & Routes of Administration that are Commonly Used
ORAL: For diarrhea, one cup tea used up to three times per day between meals. To make tea, steep 1-4 grams above ground parts in boiling water for 10 minutes and strain (8). The average amount used per day is 5-10 grams. Equivalent preparations can also be used (2). Diarrhea persisting for more than 3-4 days should be medically evaluated (8).
TOPICAL: No typical dosage.

Comments
Although the German Standard License warns about possible liver damage, some experts consider the concern to be exaggerated (8).

ALDER BUCKTHORN

This Product is Also Known As
Alder Dogwood, Arrow Wood, Black Dogwood, Buckthorn Bark, Dog Wood, Frangula, Frangula Bark, Frangulae Cortex, Glossy Buckthorn.
CAUTION: See separate listings for European Buckthorn, Sea Buckthorn, and Cascara (California Buckthorn).

Scientific Names
Rhamnus frangula, synonym Frangula alnus.
Family: Rhamnaceae.

People Use This For
Orally, alder buckthorn is used as a laxative (11).
Traditionally, alder buckthorn has been used as a tonic and a component in the Hoxsey cancer cure (11).

Safety
LIKELY SAFE ...when the bark is used orally and appropriately for less than 8-10 days (2,12). Only properly aged bark should be used, and the recommended dose should not be exceeded (12).
POSSIBLY UNSAFE ...when taken orally for more than 8 to 10 days (2,12).
CHILDREN: LIKELY UNSAFE ...contraindicated in children younger than 12 years of age (2,12).
PREGNANCY AND LACTATION: LIKELY UNSAFE ...contraindicated (2,12).

Effectiveness
LIKELY EFFECTIVE ...when taken orally as a laxative (3,4,7,12). Alder buckthorn is comparable to the gentle, laxative effects of cascara (3).
There is insufficient reliable information available about the effectiveness of alder buckthorn for its other uses.

Possible Mechanism of Action & Active Ingredients
The applicable part of alder buckthorn is the bark. The anthraglycosides and particularly the diglycosides are cathartic in the large intestine (1,8,11). They can increase intestinal motility by inhibiting stationary contractions, stimulating propulsive contractions, stimulating active chloride secretion, and increasing water and electrolytes in the intestinal contents (2). The fresh bark contains free anthrone, which can cause severe vomiting and is destroyed by aging the bark naturally for one year or artificially with heat and aeration (2). Anthroid laxative use is not associated with an increased risk of developing colorectal ademoma or carcinoma (6138).

Adverse Reactions Including Known Allergies
Alder buckthorn taken orally can cause cramp-like discomfort (2). Chronic use can cause pseudomelanosis coli (pigment spots in intestinal mucosa) which is harmless, usually reverses with discontinuation (2), and is not associated with an increased risk of developing colorectal ademoma or carcinoma (6138). Chronic use or abuse of the bark can lead to potassium depletion, albuminuria, and hematuria. Potassium depletion can lead to disturbed heart function and muscle weakness (2). The fresh or improperly aged bark can cause severe vomiting due to the presence of the free anthrone, an emetic constituent.

Possible Interactions with Herbs & Other Dietary Supplements
LICORICE: Concomitant use of alder buckthorn can increase the risk of potassium depletion (2).
STIMULANT LAXATIVE HERBS: Theoretically, concomitant use of alder buckthorn with other stimulant laxative herbs can increase the risk of potassium depletion. Stimulant laxative herbs include aloe dried leaf sap, wild cucumber fruit (Ecballium elaterium), blue flag rhizome, butternut bark, cascara bark, castor oil, colocynth fruit pulp, gamboge bark exudate, jalap root, black root, manna bark exudate, podophyllum root, rhubarb root, senna leaves and pods, and yellow dock root (19).
POTASSIUM DEPLETING HERBS: Theoretically, concomitant use of alder buckthorn with horsetail plant or licorice rhizome increases the risk of potassium depletion.

Possible Interactions with Drugs
CARDIAC GLYCOSIDES: Theoretically, overuse or abuse of alder buckthorn increases the risk of adverse effects from cardiac glycoside drugs, like digoxin (Lanoxin).
CORTICOSTEROIDS, POTASSIUM DEPLETING DIURETICS: Concomitant use can increase the risk of potassium depletion (2).
ORAL DRUGS: Theoretically, alder buckthorn can reduce absorption of some drugs due to reduced GI transit time (500).

Possible Interactions with Foods
No interactions are known to occur, and there is no known reason to expect a clinically significant interaction with alder buckthorn.

Possible Interactions with Lab Tests
COLORIMETRIC TESTS: Alder buckthorn can discolor urine (pink, red, purple, orange, rust), interfering with diagnostic tests that depend on a color change, due to its anthraquinone content (1,12,275).
POTASSIUM: Excessive use of alder buckthorn can cause potassium depletion, reducing serum potassium concentrations and test results (1,2,4,12,19).

Possible Interactions with Diseases or Conditions
GI CONDITIONS: Alder blackthorn is contraindicated in individuals with intestinal obstruction, abdominal pain of unknown origin, and intestinal inflammation, including appendicitis, Crohn's disease, irritable bowel syndrome, and ulcerative colitis (12).

Typical Dosages & Routes of Administration that are Commonly Used
ORAL: The typical dose of alder buckthorn is 0.5-2.5 grams of the dried bark (4) or as a tea, which is prepared by steeping 2 grams of the herb in 150 mL boiling water for 5-10 minutes and then straining (12). The average dose per day of the bark is 1 gram (3) or 20-30 mg of the hydoxyanthracene derivatives calculated as glycofrangulin A (2). The common dose of the liquid extract: (1:1 in 25% alcohol) is 2-5 mL three times daily (2). The individual dose of the bark is the minimum amount required to produce a soft stool (2). Limit its use to a maximum of seven to ten days. This preparation should be used only if no effect can be obtained through change of diet or the use of bulk-forming laxative products (2).

Comments
Avoid confusion with European buckthorn. The American Herbal Products Association (AHPA) recommends the following label statement: "Do not use this product if you have abdominal pain or diarrhea. Consult a health care provider prior to use if you are pregnant or nursing. Discontinue use in the event of diarrhea or watery stools. Do not exceed dose. Not for long-term use." (12). Today, alder buckthorn is primarily used as a dye.

ALETRIS

This Product is Also Known As
Ague Grass, Ague Root, Aloerot, Blazing Star, Colic Root, Crow Corn, Devil's-bit, Stargrass, Starwort, Unicorn Root, Whitetube Stargrass.

Scientific Names
Aletris farinosa.
Family: Liliaceae.

People Use This For
Orally, aletris is used for rheumatism (6,11), as a general tonic, as a sedative, to relieve female disorders, as a laxative, as an antiflatulent, as an antispasmodic (6), for colic, as an antidiarrheal, and as a diuretic (11).

Safety
POSSIBLY SAFE ...when used orally and appropriately (6,12).
PREGNANCY AND LACTATION: POSSIBLY UNSAFE ...due to the possibility that aletris contains components that cause estrogenic activity (11) and oxytocin (pitocin) antagonism (12); avoid using.

Effectiveness
POSSIBLY EFFECTIVE ...when used orally to treat menstrual disorders (11).
There is insufficient reliable information available about the effectiveness of aletris for its other uses.

Possible Mechanism of Action & Active Ingredients
Some aletris constituents may have estrogenic activity (6).

Adverse Reactions Including Known Allergies
Small doses may induce colic, stupefaction, and vertigo (6).

Possible Interactions with Herbs & Other Dietary Supplements
Insufficient reliable information available.

Possible Interactions with Drugs
ACID-INHIBITING DRUGS: Theoretically, due to claims that aletris increases stomach acid, it might interfere with antacids, sucralfate (Carafate), H-2 antagonists, or proton pump inhibitors [19].
PITOCIN: Aletris may antagonize activity of Pitocin [12].

Possible Interactions with Foods
No interactions are known to occur, and there is no known reason to expect a clinically significant interaction with aletris.

Possible Interactions with Lab Tests
No interactions are known to occur, and there is no known reason to expect a clinically significant interaction with aletris.

Possible Interactions with Diseases or Conditions
GASTROINTESTINAL DISEASES: Can irritate gastrointestinal tract. Contraindicated in individuals with infectious or inflammatory gastrointestinal conditions [19].

Typical Dosages & Routes of Administration that are Commonly Used
ORAL: Aletris is used as the powdered root, a liquid extract, and an infusion [18]. One common dosage recommendation is 0.3 to 0.6 grams three times daily [18]. The infusion is prepared by adding 1.5 grams of aletris to 100 mL of water, and the fluid extract (1:1) is commonly produced with 45% ethanol water [18].

Comments
None.

ALFALFA

This Product is Also Known As
Feuille De Luzerne, Lucerne, Medicago, Phytoestrogen, Purple Medick.

Scientific Names
Medicago sativa.
Family: Leguminosae or Fabaceae.

People Use This For
Orally, alfalfa is used as a diuretic, for kidney, bladder and prostate conditions, for asthma [6], arthritis, diabetes, indigestion [5,6], and thrombocytopenic purpura. [4]. It is also used as a source of vitamins: A, C, E, and K4, and minerals: calcium, potassium, phosphorous, and iron [4].

Safety
LIKELY SAFE ...when the above ground parts are used orally in moderation [4,5,6,12].
LIKELY UNSAFE ...when large amounts of seeds are consumed. It is associated with pancytopenia [5,6].
PREGNANCY AND LACTATION: POSSIBLY SAFE ...when used in food amounts [4]. Avoid amounts in excess of food because alfalfa contains constituents with possible estrogenic activity [11].

Effectiveness
POSSIBLY EFFECTIVE ...when used orally to lower cholesterol. ...when used for type II hyperlipoproteinemia [4]. There is insufficient reliable information available about the effectiveness of alfalfa for its other uses.

Possible Mechanism of Action & Active Ingredients
The applicable parts are the above ground parts. The alfalfa leaf contains saponins which appear to decrease plasma cholesterol without creating a change in HDL levels [4]. Constituents of alfalfa seem to decrease cholesterol absorption, and increase excretion of neutral steroids and bile acids [4,6]. Alfalfa contains manganese which might be responsible for hypoglycemic effects [4]. Alfalfa contains medicagol which appears to have antifungal properties. Alfalfa also contains coumetrol, genistein, biochanin A, and daidzein which all seem to have estrogenic properties [11].

Adverse Reactions Including Known Allergies
Alfalfa might cause photosensitivity [605]. Ingestion of ground alfalfa seeds is associated with a case of pancytopenia [381].

Possible Interactions with Herbs & Other Dietary Supplements

VITAMIN E: Alfalfa contains saponins which interfere with the absorption or activity of vitamin E (11).
HERBS WITH CLOTTING POTENTIAL: Excessive use of herbs that contain vitamin K, an essential coagulation factor, can increase the risk of clotting in people using anticoagulants. These herbs include: alfalfa, parsley, nettle, plantain, and others.

Possible Interactions with Drugs

ANTICOAGULANTS: Excessive use of alfalfa may interfere with anticoagulant therapy (4).
ORAL CONTRACEPTIVES or HORMONE THERAPY: Excessive doses of alfalfa may interfere with hormone therapy (4).
CHLORPROMAZINE: Excessive doses of alfalfa may potentiate drug-induced photosensitivity (605).

Possible Interactions with Foods

No interactions are known to occur, and there is no known reason to expect a clinically significant interaction with alfalfa.

Possible Interactions with Lab Tests

CHOLESTEROL: Alfalfa seed might lower serum cholesterol concentrations and test results in individuals with type II hyperlipoproteinemia (4).

Possible Interactions with Diseases or Conditions

SYSTEMIC LUPUS ERYTHEMATOSUS (SLE): Consumption of seeds (not stems/leaves) might reactivate latent disease (6,605).
DIABETES: Alfalfa might reduce blood sugar levels; monitor closely (4).
HORMONE-DEPENDENT CONDITIONS: Some constituents of alfalfa have estrogenic properties. Theoretically, these could interact with diseases or conditions that are sensitive to estrogen.

Typical Dosages & Routes of Administration that are Commonly Used

ORAL: 5-10 grams, or as steeped strained tea, three times a day (4). Liquid extract (1:1 in 25% alcohol) 5-10 mL three times a day (4).

Comments

There is some evidence to suggest that saponins from alfalfa stem and leaves might lower cholesterol. Stems and leaves are reportedly free of systemic lupus erythematosus (SLE) triggering substance(s) found in seeds (4). There is one case report of listeriosis traced to the consumption of alfalfa tablets from which Listeria monocytogenes was isolated (5600).

ALGIN

This Product is Also Known As

Alginates, Sodium Alginate.
CAUTION: See separate listings for Laminaria and Bladderwrack.

Scientific Names

Macrocystis pyrifera; Laminaria digitata; Ascophyllum nodosum.
Family: Lessoniaceae.

People Use This For

Orally, algin is used to lower serum cholesterol levels and to reduce absorption of strontium, barium, tin, cadmium, manganese, zinc, and mercury (11).
In folk medicine, algin has been used for the prevention and treatment of hypertension (11).
In pharmacy manufacturing processes, algin is used as a binding and disintegrating agent in tablets, as binding and demulcent in lozenges, and as film in peel-off facial masks (11).

Safety

LIKELY SAFE ...when used orally in amounts typically found in foods. It is approved in the US for use in foods with a maximum use level of 1% in candy, gelatins, puddings, condiments, relishes, processed vegetables, fish products, and imitation dairy products. Algin is believed, but not confirmed, to be indigestible (11).
PREGNANCY AND LACTATION: Insufficient reliable information available.

Effectiveness

POSSIBLY EFFECTIVE ...when used orally to reduce cholesterol and blood pressure. ...when used to reduce absorption of strontium (11).
There is insufficient reliable information available about the effectiveness of algin for its other uses.

Possible Mechanism of Action & Active Ingredients

Algin is comprised of the sodium salt of alginic acid, a linear polymer of L-guluronic and D-mannuronic acid. Although mannuronic acid is the major component, there is variation depending on the algal source (13). Cholesterol lowering effects may be related to viscosity of gel and inhibiting cholesterol absorption (11). Hypotensive effects may be due to laminine dioxalate (11).

Adverse Reactions Including Known Allergies

None reported (11,13).

Possible Interactions with Herbs & Other Dietary Supplements

Insufficient reliable information available.

Possible Interactions with Drugs

ORAL DRUGS: The fiber in algin can impair absorption of oral drugs (19).

Possible Interactions with Foods

No interactions are known to occur, and there is no known reason to expect a clinically significant interaction with algin.

Possible Interactions with Lab Tests

CHOLESTEROL: Theoretically, algin might reduce serum cholesterol concentrations and test results (11). BLOOD PRESSURE: Theoretically, algin might lower blood pressure and blood pressure readings (11).

Possible Interactions with Diseases or Conditions

No interactions are known to occur, and there is no known reason to expect a clinically significant interaction with algin.

Typical Dosages & Routes of Administration that are Commonly Used

No typical dosage.

Comments

Algin is the purified carbohydrate product extracted from brown sea weeds by use of dilute alkali. Algin is isolated from a variety of brown algae (seaweeds, Class: Phaeophyceae), particularly from the genera Ascophyllum, Macrocystis, and Laminaria (11).

ALKANNA

This Product is Also Known As

Alkanet, Alkanna Radix, Anchusa, Dyer's Bugloss, Henna, Orchanet, Radix Anchusae. CAUTION: See separate listing for Henna (Lawsonia inermis).

Scientific Names

Alkanna tinctoria. Family: Boraginaceae.

People Use This For

Historically, alkanna root was used topically by the ancient Greeks to heal skin wounds (18). It was also used as an astringent (6,8), for skin diseases, and diarrhea (6,8).

Safety

POSSIBLY UNSAFE …when the root preparations are used topically on broken or abraded skin (12) because it contains toxic unsaturated pyrrolizidine alkaloids (UPAs) that might be absorbed systemically. LIKELY UNSAFE …when used orally. Repeated exposure to low concentrations of UPAs is linked to serious liver toxicity (4,12). UPAs are also thought to be carcinogenic and mutagenic (12). There is insufficient reliable information available about the safety when used topically on unbroken skin. PREGNANCY: POSSIBLY UNSAFE ...when used topically (12). LIKELY UNSAFE …contraindicated for oral use because it contains UPAs. LACTATION: POSSIBLY UNSAFE ...when used topically. LIKELY UNSAFE …contraindicated for oral use. There is concern that UPAs could be excreted in breast milk (4,12,18).

Effectiveness

POSSIBLY EFFECTIVE …when used topically for enhancing wound healing of leg ulcers (6,18). There is insufficient reliable information available about the effectiveness of alkanna for its other uses.

Possible Mechanism of Action & Active Ingredients

The applicable part of alkanna is the root. Alkanna contains napthazarine esters, pyrrozolidine alkaloids, and tannins (18). Some pyrrolizidine alkaloids have shown carcinogenic and mutagenic properties, and there are reports of renal toxicity. However, the primary concern is veno-occlusive disease (12). Unsaturated pyrrolizidine alkaloids are known to be hepatotoxic (4). The color of alkanna comes from a mixture of 5-6% red pigments which consist mainly of fat-soluble naphthazarin (6).

Adverse Reactions Including Known Allergies

Chronic exposure to plants containing UPA constituents has been associated with veno-occlusive disease (4021). Symptoms of acute veno-occlusive disease are characterized by a dull, dragging ache in the right upper abdomen and marked distention of the abdomen. These symptoms are sometimes accompanied by reduced urine output. Subacute veno-occlusive disease is associated with vague symptoms and persistent liver enlargement (4021).

Possible Interactions with Herbs & Other Dietary Supplements

EUCALYPTUS: Theoretically, concomitant use might increase the risk of unsaturated pyrrolizidine alkaloid toxicity due to enzyme induction by eucalyptus (19).
PYRROLIZIDINE ALKALOID-CONTAINING HERBS: Concomitant use is contraindicated due to the risk of additive toxicity. Herbs containing unsaturated pyrrolizidine alkaloids include: alkanna (12), borage (271), gravel root (4), hemp agrimony (271), hound's tongue (19), petasites (19), comfrey (271), coltsfoot, and the Senecio species plants; dusty miller (19), alpine ragwort (19), groundsel (271), golden ragwort (19), and tansy ragwort (271).

Possible Interactions with Drugs

No interactions are known to occur, and there is no known reason to expect a clinically significant interaction with alkanna.

Possible Interactions with Foods

No interactions are known to occur, and there is no known reason to expect a clinically significant interaction with alkanna.

Possible Interactions with Lab Tests

No interactions are known to occur, and there is no known reason to expect a clinically significant interaction with alkanna.

Possible Interactions with Diseases or Conditions

LIVER DISEASE: Contraindicated due to hepatotoxic potential (19).

Typical Dosages & Routes of Administration that are Commonly Used

No typical dosage.

Comments

Although alkanna is used as a reddish pigment in foods and cosmetics, many countries have banned its use in food (8).

ALLSPICE

This Product is Also Known As

Clove Pepper, Jamaica Pepper, Pimenta, Pimento, West Indian Bay.
CAUTION: See separate listing for Sweet Bay.

Scientific Names

Pimenta dioica, synonyms Pimenta officinalis, Eugenia pimenta.
Family: Myrtaceae.

People Use This For

Topically, allspice is used for muscle pain, toothache, and as an antiseptic.
In dentistry, some dentists use eugenol, an active ingredient in allspice, as a local antiseptic and as an antiseptic for teeth and gums (7200).
In folk medicine, allspice has been used to treat indigestion and flatulence (11), and as a purgative. It is also used for stomachache, menorrhagia, vomiting, diarrhea (6), fever, influenza, and colds.
For food uses, allspice is used as an aromatic spice. It is used in toothpaste as a flavoring.

Safety

LIKELY SAFE ...when used orally and appropriately (12). The maximum levels of sweet bay used in food are 0.1% of the bay leaf and 0.02% of the oil (11).
LIKELY UNSAFE ...if the whole, intact leaf is swallowed because it is indigestible and can become lodged in the esophagus, hypopharynx (132,133,134,137), or perforate the intestinal lining (135,136).
PREGNANCY AND LACTATION: Insufficient reliable information available; avoid using in amounts exceeding those commonly found in foods.

Effectiveness

POSSIBLY EFFECTIVE ...when used orally to improve digestion (11) and as a larvicide (11). ...when used topically as an antiseptic or anesthetic (6).

Possible Mechanism of Action & Active Ingredients

The applicable parts of allspice are the unripe fruit and leaf. The eugenol in allspice may explain this product's effects on the digestive system and its pain relief properties. Eugenol seems to decrease intestinal pain by depressing the CNS and inhibiting prostaglandin activity in the human colon mucosa (11). It also increases the activity of some digestive enzymes, including trypsin (7200). Eugenol may be responsible for allspice's anesthetic effects when the crushed berries are applied topically.

Adverse Reactions Including Known Allergies

Excessive doses may cause nausea, vomiting, CNS depression, convulsions due to eugenol content (6). Topical application may irritate mucous membranes (6).

Possible Interactions with Herbs & Other Dietary Supplements

Insufficient reliable information available.

Possible Interactions with Drugs

ANTICOAGULANT AND ANTIPLATELET DRUGS: Eugenol inhibits platelet activity; individuals on anticoagulant or antiplatelet therapy who choose to use this product should use caution (4).

Possible Interactions with Foods

No interactions are known to occur, and there is no known reason to expect a clinically significant interaction with allspice.

Possible Interactions with Lab Tests

No interactions are known to occur, and there is no known reason to expect a clinically significant interaction with allspice.

Possible Interactions with Diseases or Conditions

No interactions are known to occur, and there is no known reason to expect a clinically significant interaction with allspice.

Typical Dosages & Routes of Administration that are Commonly Used

ORAL: Antiflatulent dose: 0.05-0.2 mL allspice oil (11).
TOPICAL: No typical dose.

Comments

The commercially available spice powder consists of whole ground dried fruit (6). Avoid confusion with sweet bay and California bay.

ALOE dried juice from leaf, latex

This Product is Also Known As

Aloe Juice, Aloe Latex, Burn Plant, Elephant's Gall, Hsiang-Dan, Lily of the Desert, Lu-Hui, Miracle Plant, Plant of Immortality.
CAUTION: See separate listing for Aloe gel.

Scientific Names

Aloe barbadensis, synonym Aloe vera; Aloe perfoliata; Aloe arborescens natalenis; Aloe ferox; Aloe africana; Aloe spicata; Aloe perryi.
Family: Liliaceae.

People Use This For

Orally, aloe juice/latex is used as a laxative or cathartic (5). It is also used for seizures, asthma, colds, ulcers, bleeding, amenorrhea, colitis, depression, diabetes, glaucoma, multiple sclerosis, hemorrhoids, peptic ulcers, varicose veins, bursitis, arthritis, and vision problems.

Safety

POSSIBLY SAFE ...when used orally and appropriately short-term (2,12).
LIKELY UNSAFE ...when used orally long-term (8). Prolonged use can lead to tolerance (2,4). ...when used in high doses. Lethal dose: 1 gram per day for several days (8). ...when used during menstruation (8) or by women who have bleeding between periods, because it might increase blood to the uterus (19).
CHILDREN: LIKELY UNSAFE ...contraindicated in children younger than 12 years (2,4).
PREGNANCY: LIKELY UNSAFE ...contraindicated. It can induce abortions and stimulate menstruation (19).
LACTATION: LIKELY UNSAFE ...contraindicated, genotoxic aloe-emodin might pass into milk (2,4,19).

Effectiveness

LIKELY EFFECTIVE ...when taken orally as a stimulant laxative due to the cathartic effects of the anthraquinones in the aloe (2,4,5,8).

There is insufficient reliable information available about the effectiveness of aloe juice/latex for its other uses.

Possible Mechanism of Action & Active Ingredients

The applicable part of aloe is the dried leaf juice and latex. It is likely that the anthracene derivatives are cleaved into aloe-emodin anthrone in the colon. Anthrones irritate mucous membranes, causing increased mucous secretion and peristalsis. Aloe increases motility of the colon and therefore, increases propulsion and reduces transit time. It also causes fluids and electrolytes to be secreted in the lumen. The effects of aloe cause a feeling of distention. These cathartic effects happen within about ten hours of taking the dose. Water and electrolyte reabsorption are inhibited (8). Aloe juice and latex causes loss of potassium, which paralyzes the intestinal muscles. With continued use, the dose must be increased to maintain a laxative effect (8). Anthroid laxative use is not associated with an increased risk of developing colorectal ademoma or carcinoma (6138).

Adverse Reactions Including Known Allergies

Aloe occasionally leads to abdominal pain and cramps (2,4). Long-term use or abuse of aloe can cause diarrhea, sometimes with blood and sometimes without blood; nephritis; potassium depletion; albuminuria; hematuria; muscle weakness; weight loss; pseudomelanosis coli; and heart disturbances (4). Pseudomelanosis coli (pigment spots in intestinal mucosa) is harmless, usually reverses with discontinuation (2), and is not associated with an increased risk of developing colorectal ademoma or carcinoma (6138).

Tolerance: Aloe juice and latex causes loss of potassium, which paralyzes the intestinal muscles. With continued use, the dose must be increased to maintain the laxative effect (8).

Possible Interactions with Herbs & Other Dietary Supplements

CARDIAC GLYCOSIDE-CONTAINING HERBS: Theoretically, overuse of aloe can increase the risk of cardiac glycoside toxicity. Watch for possible interactions with herbs that contain cardiac glycosides such as black hellebore, Canadian hemp roots, digitalis leaf, hedge mustard, figwort, lily of the valley roots, motherwort, oleander leaf, pheasant's eye plant, pleurisy root, squill bulb leaf scales, and strophanthus seeds (2,18,19,500).

STIMULANT LAXATIVE HERBS: Theoretically, concomitant use of aloe with other stimulant laxative herbs may increase the risk of potassium depletion. Stimulant laxative herbs include: wild cucumber fruit (Ecballium elaterium), blue flag rhizome, alder buckthorn, European buckthorn, butternut bark, cascara bark, castor oil, colocynth fruit pulp, gamboge bark exudate, jalap root, black root, manna bark exudate, podophyllum root, rhubarb root, senna leaves and pods, and yellow dock root (19).

LICORICE/HORSETAIL: Theoretically, concomitant use of aloe with horsetail plant or licorice rhizome increases the risk of potassium depletion (19).

Possible Interactions with Drugs

CARDIAC GLYCOSIDES: Theoretically, overuse of aloe increases the risk of adverse effects from the cardiac glycoside drugs. Overuse of aloe along with drugs that contain cardiac glycosides, such as digoxin (Lanoxin) (19), can increase the risk of toxicity from increased cardiac glycoside effects.

ANTIARRHYTHMIC DRUGS: Overuse of aloe can increase the risk of drug toxicity (664).

DIURETICS: Overuse of aloe can compound potassium loss (2).

CORTICOSTEROIDS: Overuse of aloe can compound potassium loss (2).

OTHER DRUGS: Aloe can reduce drug absorption of some other drugs because aloe causes shorter GI transit time (500).

Possible Interactions with Foods

No interactions are known to occur, and there is no known reason to expect a clinically significant interaction with aloe dried juice from leaf, latex.

Possible Interactions with Lab Tests

BLOOD GLUCOSE: Small amounts of dried aloe juice might reduce blood glucose concentrations and test results (4).

COLORIMETRIC DIAGNOSTIC TESTS: Dried aloe juice discolors alkaline urine (red) and can interfere with diagnostic tests that depend on a color change (2,4).

SERUM POTASSIUM: Excessive use of dried aloe juice can cause potassium depletion, reducing serum potassium concentrations and test results (2,4,5,8,19).

Possible Interactions with Diseases or Conditions

GI CONDITIONS: Contraindicated in individuals with intestinal obstruction, acute intestinal inflammation (Crohn's disease, ulcerative colitis, appendicitis), ulcers, abdominal pain of unknown origin, nausea, or vomiting (2,4) due to the irritating effect of anthranoid aloins (19).

HEMORRHOIDS: Contraindicated due to the possibility of causing stenosis, thrombosis or prolapse (19).

HEART CONDITIONS: Theoretically, overuse of aloe vera dried juice/latex might lead to potassium depletion (8).

KIDNEY DISORDERS: Contraindicated; theoretically, excessive doses can cause nephritis (19).

Typical Dosages & Routes of Administration that are Commonly Used
ORAL: The common laxative dose is 100-200 mg aloe or 50 mg aloe extract taken in the evening (8). People also typically use 50-200 mg daily of the capsules (5011) that contain aloe leaf gel and/or latex, which is the residue resulting after the liquid from cut aloe evaporates (5012). Aloe juice product manufacturers suggest taking 1 to 8 ounces of the juice containing 99.7% of the whole leaf aloe vera juice daily (5015).

Comments
Aloe juice/latex is obtained from the cells beneath the plant's skin and contains cathartic laxative anthraquinones (101). Avoid confusion with aloe, which is obtained from the thin-walled mucilaginous cells of the inner central zone of the leaf. Aloe gel products sold for internal consumption might be contaminated with aloe juice/latex which can cause cathartic laxative effects (5). Aloe of the Bible is an unrelated fragrant wood used as incense (5).

ALOE gel

This Product is Also Known As
Aloe, Aloe Capensis, Aloe Leaf Gel, Aloe Vera, Salvia.
CAUTION: See separate listing for Aloe dried juice from leaf, latex.

Scientific Names
Aloe vera; Aloe barbadensis; Aloe ferox; Aloe africana; Aloe spicata.
Family: Liliaceae.

People Use This For
Orally, aloe gel is used as a general tonic, by which it is utilized as a cleanser, anesthetic, antiseptic, antipyretic, antipruritic, moisturizer, vasodilator, anti-inflammatory agent, and promoter of cell proliferation (5). Aloe gel has also been used orally for gastroduodenal ulcers, diabetes, and asthma.
Topically, aloe gel is used to promote burn or wound healing (5) and to treat cold sores.
In manufacturing of non-laxative drugs and cosmetic products, which include moisturizing preparations, aloe gel is used for its tonic effects (5).

Safety
LIKELY SAFE ...when applied topically, although the maximum duration of treatment is not established (4).
POSSIBLY UNSAFE ...when taken orally due to potential contamination with the anthraquinone constituents (4). Anthraquinones act as stimulant laxative.
PREGNANCY AND LACTATION: LIKELY SAFE ...when used topically (4). POSSIBLY UNSAFE ...when used orally; avoid using because of the potential for anthraquinone contamination (4).

Effectiveness
POSSIBLY EFFECTIVE ...when applied topically for reducing pain and inflammation and enhancing the healing of burns, skin ulcerations, dermabrasion, psoriasis, and frostbite injury (4,5,6,101).
There is insufficient reliable information available about the effectiveness of aloe gel for its other uses.

Possible Mechanism of Action & Active Ingredients
The carboxypeptidase and salicylate components of aloe gel can inhibit bradykinin, which is a pain-producing agent. The magnesium lactate component can inhibit histamine to reduce itching. Other components appear to slow the formation of thromboxane and thereby speed the healing of burns. Some evidence suggests aloe gel has antibacterial and antifungal properties (101).

Adverse Reactions Including Known Allergies
None reported for topical use (4), but the potential exists for adverse reactions with orally ingested aloe gel products that are contaminated with anthraquinones, which act as cathartic laxatives.

Possible Interactions with Herbs & Other Dietary Supplements
Insufficient reliable information available.

Possible Interactions with Drugs
GLYBURIDE: Concomitant use with glyburide (Diabeta, Micronase, Glynase) may increase hypoglycemic effects. Monitor blood glucose (19).
DIABETES THERAPY: Monitor blood glucose levels closely due to claims that aloe vera has hypoglycemic effects (19).
HYDROCORTISONE: Theoretically, concomitant topical use with hydrocortisone might increase anti-inflammatory effects (19).

Possible Interactions with Foods

No interactions are known to occur, and there is no known reason to expect a clinically significant interaction with aloe gel.

Possible Interactions with Lab Tests

No interactions are known to occur, and there is no known reason to expect a clinically significant interaction with aloe gel.

Possible Interactions with Diseases or Conditions

GI OR KIDNEY CONDTIONS: Because aloe gel could be contaminated with aloe latex, it should be used cautiously or avoided by individuals with intestinal obstruction, Crohn's disease, ulcerative colitis, appendicitis, peptic ulcers, abdominal pain of unknown origin, nausea, vomiting, hemorrhoids (2,4). and kidney disease (2,4). DIABETES: Monitor blood glucose level closely due to claims that aloe vera has hypoglycemic effects (19).

Typical Dosages & Routes of Administration that are Commonly Used

ORAL: People typically use 50-200 mg daily of the capsules that contain aloe leaf gel (5011,5012). Some people take 30 mL of aloe gel internally three times daily (5011) or 15-60 drops of an aloe tincture (1:10, 50% alcohol) as needed (5013). Many strengths of capsules are available, such as 75 mg, 100 mg and 200 mg (5008).
TOPICAL: People apply aloe gel liberally as needed three to five times daily (5011). The aloe gel is available in 99.5%, 99.6%, 98% (5008), and 100% purity strengths (5014).

Comments

Aloe gel is the clear, jelly-like substance that is obtained from the thin-walled, sticky cells of the inner portion of the leaf. Avoid confusion with aloe juice or latex which is obtained from the cells beneath the plant's skin and contains the cathartic laxative anthraquinones (101). Aloe gel products sold for internal consumption can be contaminated with aloe juice or latex (5). Stabilized aloe gel is not always topically effective (5).

ALPHA HYDROXY ACIDS

This Product is Also Known As

Dihydroxysuccinic Acid, Gluconolactone, Glycolic Acid, Hydroxyacetic Acid, Hydroxypropionic Acid, Hydroxysuccinic Acid, Lactic acid, Malic Acid, Monohydroxysuccinic Acid, Tartaric Acid.

Scientific Names

Hydroxysuccinic acid; Monohydroxysuccinic acid (Malic acid); 2-hydroxypropionic acid (Lactic acid); Hydroxyacetic acid (Glycolic acid); Dihydroxysuccinic acid (Tartaric acid); Gluconolactone.

People Use This For

Orally, malic acid (an alpha hydroxy acid) is used with magnesium for treating pain and tenderness associated with fibromyalgia (3262).
Topically, alpha hydroxy acids are used for moisturizing and removing dead skin cells (6), for treating acne (947), improving the appearance of photo-aged skin (952,953,954), and for xerosis (pathologic dry skin) (949,955).

Safety

LIKELY SAFE ...when alpha hydroxy acids are used topically and appropriately (947,949,952).
POSSIBLY SAFE ...when malic acid (an alpha hydroxy acid) is used orally with magnesium hydroxide (3262).
PREGNANCY AND LACTATION: LIKELY SAFE ...when alpha hydroxy acids are used topically and appropriately in cosmetic amounts (947,949,952). There is insufficient reliable information available about the safety of the oral use of malic acid; avoid using.

Effectiveness

LIKELY EFFECTIVE ...when alpha hydroxy acids are used in a lotion or cream topically and daily for treating photo-damaged skin (952,953,954). ...when alpha hydroxy acids are used in a lotion or cream topically for treating dry skin (949,955).
POSSIBLY EFFECTIVE ...when alpha hydroxy acids are used topically for treating acne (947). ...when malic acid (an alpha hydroxy acid) is used orally with magnesium hydroxide (Super Malic tablets) for reducing pain and tenderness associated with fibromyalgia (3262).
LIKELY INEFFECTIVE ...when alpha hydroxy acids are used topically in short-contact skin peels for treating photo-damaged skin (953).

Possible Mechanism of Action & Active Ingredients

Hyperkeratinization is thought to contribute to acne, dry skin, and the cosmetic results of photo-aging. Alpha hydroxy acids enhance removal of dead skin cells (948,950). They can enhance skin barrier function (951), and they can decrease cohesiveness of corneocytes by weakening intracellular bonding (6). One study found that malic acid (an alpha hydroxy acid) and magnesium hydroxide can decrease pain and tenderness in patients with fibromyalgia; the mechanism is currently unknown (3262).

Adverse Reactions Including Known Allergies

In nonprescription concentrations, alpha hydroxy acids are generally well tolerated (947,949,952) (see Typical Dosage). Higher concentrations can cause severe skin irritation, burning and sloughing (6).

Possible Interactions with Herbs & Other Dietary Supplements

MAGNESIUM: Malic acid (an alpha hydroxy acid) is used with magnesium hydroxide for reducing pain and tenderness associated with fibromyalgia (3262).

Possible Interactions with Drugs

MAGNESIUM: Malic acid (an alpha hydroxy acid) is used with magnesium for reducing pain and tenderness associated with fibromyalgia (3262).
TOPICAL DRUGS: Theoretically, alpha hydroxy acids can increase irritant effects of other topical agents.

Possible Interactions with Foods

No interactions are known to occur, and there is no known reason to expect a clinically significant interaction with alpha hydroxy acids.

Possible Interactions with Lab Tests

No interactions are known to occur, and there is no known reason to expect a clinically significant interaction with alpha hydroxy acids.

Possible Interactions with Diseases or Conditions

INDIVIDUALS WITH SENSITIVE SKIN: Alpha hydroxy acids can worsen skin conditions by causing skin irritation and sloughing (6).

Typical Dosages & Routes of Administration that are Commonly Used

ORAL: For reducing pain and tenderness associated with fibromyalgia, malic acid (an alpha hydroxy acid) 800-1200 mg per day is taken orally with magnesium hydroxide 200-300 mg twice daily, equivalent to 4-6 Super Malic tablets twice daily (3262).
TOPICAL: For treating photo-aged skin: 8% lactic acid, or 8% tartaric acid, or 8% gluconolactone, or 8% glycolic acid applied to facial or other photo-aged skin twice daily (950,952); 14% gluconolactone solution or 12% lactic acid lotion is also used (955).

Comments

Alpha hydroxy acids are fruit acid compounds, including: malic acid, lactic acid, glycolic acid, tartaric acid, and gluconolactone. Alpha hydroxy acid-containing cosmetic products may lack concentration information on labeling. Try to use products that identify the concentration of active ingredients.

ALPHA-KETOGLUTARATE

This Product is Also Known As

Alpha Ketoglutarate, Alpha-Ketoglutaric Acid, Alpha KG.

Scientific Names

2-Oxopentanedoicic acid, 2-Oxoglutaric acid.

People Use This For

Orally, alpha-ketoglutarate is used for treating chronic kidney and gastrointestinal dysfunction, bacterial overgrowth, intestinal toxemia, liver dysfunction, and chronic candidiasis (5305). It is also used as an adjunct to diet and training for improving peak athletic performance (5307), and improving amino acid metabolism in hemodialysis patients (5311).
Intravenously, alpha-ketoglutarate is used for preventing ischemic injury during heart surgery (5312,5313), improving renal blood flow after heart surgery (5308), and preventing muscle protein depletion after surgery or trauma (5309,5310).

Safety

POSSIBLY SAFE …when used orally and appropriately (5311). …when used intravenously and appropriately (5308,5309,5310,5311,5312,5313).
PREGNANCY AND LACTATION: Insufficient reliable information available; avoid using.

Effectiveness

POSSIBLY EFFECTIVE …when used intravenously for preventing ischemic injury during heart surgery (5312,5313). …when used for preventing muscle protein depletion after surgery or trauma (5309,5310). There is insufficient reliable information available about the effectiveness of alpha-ketoglutarate for its other uses.

Possible Mechanism of Action & Active Ingredients

Alpha-ketoglutarate, the carbon skeleton of glutamate and glutamine, is an intermediate compound in the Krebs cycle (5308). As a precursor of glutamate, alpha-ketoglutarate is taken up by fibroblasts involved in wound healing (5314). The availability of alpha-ketoglutarate determines the recovery of muscle protein synthesis after surgical trauma (5309). Some evidence suggests that rapidly growing cells use alpha-ketoglutarate when cellular glutamine uptake is limited (5314). Hemodialysis patients who take alpha-ketoglutarate with calcium carbonate have improved amino acid metabolism and reduced hyperphosphatemia (5311).

Adverse Reactions Including Known Allergies
No adverse reactions were reported in clinical studies (5308,5309,5310,5311,5312,5313).

Possible Interactions with Herbs & Other Dietary Supplements
Insufficient reliable information available.

Possible Interactions with Drugs
No interactions are known to occur, and there is no known reason to expect a clinically significant interaction with alpha-ketoglutarate.

Possible Interactions with Foods
No interactions are known to occur, and there is no known reason to expect a clinically significant interaction with alpha-ketoglutarate.

Possible Interactions with Lab Tests
No interactions are known to occur, and there is no known reason to expect a clinically significant interaction with alpha-ketoglutarate.

Possible Interactions with Diseases or Conditions
No interactions are known to occur, and there is no known reason to expect a clinically significant interaction with alpha-ketoglutarate.

Typical Dosages & Routes of Administration that are Commonly Used
ORAL: A typical dose of alpha-ketoglutaric acid is 500 mg 10 to 30 minutes before a workout, then again with food 30 minutes after a workout (5307). To improve amino acid metabolism in hemodialysis patients, 1.187 grams are used three times daily (5311).
INTRAVENOUS: For cardiac surgery, a dose of 28 grams of alpha-ketoglutarate has been added to blood cardioplegia (5312,5313). For preventing muscle protein depletion after surgery or trauma, 280 mg/kg of body weight is added to parenteral nutrition (5310).

Comments
Suppliers of athletic nutritional supplements claim alpha-ketoglutaric acid may be an important adjunct to proper diet and training for the athlete desiring peak performance. They base this claim on studies that show excessive ammonia in the body can combine with alpha-ketoglutarate to reduce ammonia toxicity. So far, the only studies that show alpha-ketoglutarate can reduce ammonia toxicity have been performed in hemodialysis patients (5311).

ALPHA-LIPOIC ACID

This Product is Also Known As
Acetate Replacing Factor, a-Lipoic Acid, Alpha Lipoic Acid, Alpha-Lipoic Acid Extract, ALA, Biletan, Lipoic Acid, Lipoicin, Thioctacid, Thioctan, Thioctic Acid.

Scientific Names
Alpha Lipoic Acid; 1,2-dithiolane-3-pentanoic acid; 1,2-dithiolane-3-valeric acid; 6,8-thioctic acid; 5-(1,2-dithiolan-3-yl) valeric acid; 6,8-dithiooctanoic acid.

People Use This For
Orally, alpha-lipoic acid is used as an antioxidant (1547). People with diabetes use alpha-lipoic acid to decrease blood glucose, treat and prevent peripheral neuropathy (1547,3540,3541,3557) and cardiac autonomic neuropathy (3543), and to improve insulin resistance in type 2 diabetes (3544,3545). Alpha-lipoic acid is used for preventing retinopathy (3543), cataracts (3546), and treating glaucoma (1551,1552). Alpha-lipoic acid is also used orally for treating HIV/AIDS, cancer, liver disease, Wilson's disease, cardiovascular disease, and lactic acidosis caused by inborn errors of metabolism (1554,1555,1556,1557,1570).
Intravenously, alpha-lipoic acid is used for improving insulin-resistance and glucose disposal in type 2 diabetes (3557,3874,3875), diabetic neuropathy (3540,3557), and Amanita mushroom poisoning (1547,1548,1549,3871).

Safety
POSSIBLY SAFE ...when used orally and appropriately. Oral alpha-lipoic acid has been used safely in clinical trials lasting from 4 months to 2 years (3540,3541,3542). ...when used intravenously and appropriately. Intravenous alpha-lipoic acid has been used safely in clinical trials lasting up to 3 weeks (3540,3557).
PREGNANCY AND LACTATION: Insufficient reliable information available; avoid using.

Effectiveness

POSSIBLY EFFECTIVE ...when given intravenously for improving symptoms of diabetic peripheral neuropathy (3540,3557). Clinical trials demonstrated significant improvement in Total Symptom Scores when diabetics with peripheral neuropathy were given alpha-lipoic acid 600 mg or 1200 mg intravenously daily. Improvement was seen after 5 days of treatment and continued until treatment was discontinued after 3 weeks (3540,3557). Lower doses have not been shown to be effective (3869). ...when given orally or intravenously for improving insulin sensitivity and glucose disposal in type 2 diabetics (3545,3846,3874,3875,3876). Type 2 diabetics taking alpha-lipoic acid 600 to 1800 mg orally or 500 to 1000 mg intravenously daily had significant improvement in insulin resistance and glucose effectiveness after 4 weeks of oral treatment or after a single dose to 10 days of intravenous administration (3545,3846,3874,3875,3876).

POSSIBLY INEFFECTIVE ...when used orally for improving symptoms of diabetic peripheral neuropathy (3540,3541,3868). Placebo-controlled clinical trials demonstrated significant improvement in neuronal conduction measurements in diabetics with neuropathy who took alpha-lipoic acid orally, but this did not translate into significant symptom reduction (3540,3541,3868). ...when used orally for improving symptoms associated with cardiac autonomic neuropathy in diabetics (3542). A placebo-controlled clinical trial showed that autonomic nerve function indices measured by ECG improved in patients with cardiac autonomic neuropathy who took alpha-lipoic acid orally, but this did not translate into significantly improved symptoms (3541). ...when used orally for lowering glycosylated hemoglobin (HgbA1c) levels in patients with type 2 diabetes (3540). In one human study, alpha-lipoic acid failed to lower HgbA1c after 6 months of oral treatment in patients with type 2 diabetes (3540). ...when used orally for alcoholic liver disease (3880). People with alcohol-related liver disease taking alpha-lipoic acid 300 mg per day for 6 months did not demonstrate significant improvement compared to placebo (3880)...when taken orally for HIV-related dementia (1556). Alpha-lipoic acid had no effect on HIV-associated cognitive impairment in a small trial comparing alpha-lipoic acid alone or in combination with selegiline (Deprenyl) and placebo (1556). There is insufficient reliable information available about the effectiveness of alpha-lipoic acid for other uses.

Possible Mechanism of Action & Active Ingredients

Alpha-lipoic acid was identified as a vitamin when it was isolated 50 years ago, but was reclassified upon the finding that it is synthesized in humans and animals (3871). Endogenous alpha-lipoic acid is a coenzyme that, together with pyrophosphatase, is involved in carbohydrate metabolism and production of adenosine triphosphate (ATP) (6). Exogenous alpha-lipoic acid and the metabolite, dihydrolipoic acid (DHLA), have antioxidant activity and can scavenge free radicals both intra- and extra-cellularly (3871). Alpha-lipoic acid is both water and fat soluble and can regenerate endogenous antioxidants, such as vitamin E, vitamin C and glutathione, and prevent oxidative damage (1547,1550,3546,3871). Alpha-lipoic acid is about 30% absorbed from dietary or supplemental sources, and is reduced to DHLA in many tissues (1561,3871,3872). Preliminary data suggests that these antioxidant effects might provide protection in cerebral ischemia, excitotoxic amino acid brain injury, mitochondrial dysfunction, diabetes, diabetic neuropathy, and other causes of damage to brain or neural tissue (1561,3546,3871). In experimental diabetic models, alpha-lipoic acid increases neuronal blood flow, improves neuronal glucose uptake, increases amounts of reduced glutathione in neurons, and improves neuronal conduction velocity (3873,3878). Preliminary evidence suggests that DHLA in combination with vitamin E might prevent oxidative stress in cardiac ischemia-reperfusion injury (3871,3877). The antioxidant effects of alpha-lipoic acid might be beneficial in liver diseases in which oxidative stress is a factor (3879). Alpha-lipoic acid has been used in combination with other treatments for Amanita mushroom poisoning (105,1548,1549,3871). Evidence of effectiveness in humans is anecdotal, and alpha-lipoic acid has been ineffective in laboratory models of Amanita poisoning, leading some groups to recommend eliminating it from treatment regimens for this condition (3871,3879). Alpha-lipoic acid has shown promise in experimental models to prevent aminoglycoside-induced cochlear damage, and metal (lead, arsenic, cadmium, mercury) and chemical (hexachlorobenzene, n-hexane) poisoning (3871,3879,3881,3882,3883,3884). Children treated with alpha-lipoic acid, alone or in combination with vitamin E, showed normalized organ function and lessened indices of oxidative damage following radiation exposure in the Chernobyl accident (3871). Case reports indicate that it may be helpful in various inborn errors of metabolism which result in lactic acidosis (1554,1555,1557). Preliminary data suggests that alpha-lipoic acid can inhibit replication of the human immunodeficiency virus (HIV) by inhibiting reverse transcriptase (1280,3871). Reactive oxygen species may act as intracellular messengers for HIV gene expression and transcription, and the antioxidant effects of alpha-lipoic acid could inhibit this process (1562,1563). Alpha-lipoic acid supplementation might improve blood antioxidant status and blood peroxidation products, and increase T-helper lymphocytes and T-helper to T-helper suppressor cell ratio, based on a small open trial in HIV positive patients (3885).

Adverse Reactions Including Known Allergies

Skin rash has been reported after oral use of alpha-lipoic acid and local allergic reactions have occurred at the injection site with IV administration (14,1547). Paresthesias have been reported to worsen temporarily at the beginning of therapy. Rarely, platelet disorders and purpura have been observed after IV therapy (14). Intravenously, alpha-lipoic acid can cause gastrointestinal upset, including nausea, vomiting, and headache. Adverse effects are more common in patients receiving higher intravenous doses (3557). Preliminary evidence suggests that high doses of alpha-lipoic acid might cause thiamine deficiency. For people taking high doses of alpha-lipoic acid and who are at risk for thiamine deficiency (e.g., alcoholism), thiamine supplementation may be warranted (3871).

Possible Interactions with Herbs & Other Dietary Supplements

HERBS WITH HYPOGLYCEMIC POTENTIAL: Theoretically, alpha-lipoic acid might have additive effects with herbs that decrease blood glucose levels (devil's claw, fenugreek, garlic, guar gum, horse chestnut seed, Panax ginseng, psyllium, and Siberian ginseng).

HERBS WITH HYPERGLYCEMIC POTENTIAL: Theoretically, herbs that increase blood glucose levels might antagonize the antidiabetic effects of alpha-lipoic acid (ephedra, ginger, gotu kola, and the above ground parts of the stinging nettle).

Possible Interactions with Drugs

ANTI-DIABETES DRUGS: Theoretically, concomitant use might cause additive hypoglycemic effects (6,3545). Dosing adjustments for insulin or oral hypoglycemic agents may be necessary. However, in one study, co-administration of single doses of alpha-lipoic acid and glyburide or acarbose did not cause detectable drug interactions in healthy volunteers (3870).

CHEMOTHERAPEUTIC AGENTS: Theoretically, concomitant use might decrease the effectiveness of chemotherapy. Preliminary evidence from an unpublished study suggests antioxidants may decrease the effectiveness of chemotherapy (14,391).

ETHANOL: Concomitant use decreases the effects of alpha-lipoic acid (14).

Possible Interactions with Foods

FOOD: Administration with food decreases bioavailability (14). Alpha-lipoic acid should be taken on an empty stomach.

Possible Interactions with Lab Tests

BLOOD GLUCOSE: Alpha-lipoic acid might decrease blood glucose levels and test results in patients with type 2 diabetes. Alpha-lipoic acid reduces insulin resistance and improves blood glucose disposal in patients with type 2 diabetes (3545). However, alpha-lipoic acid has no effect on glycosylated hemoglobin (HgbA1c) levels (3540,3557).

T HELPER/SUPPRESSOR LYMPHOCYTE RATIO: Alpha-lipoic acid might increase the T helper/suppressor ratio in patients infected with the human immunodeficiency virus (HIV) (6).

Possible Interactions with Diseases or Conditions

BLOOD DYSCRASIAS: Intravenous alpha-lipoic acid has rarely been associated with platelet disorders and purpura (14). Theoretically, in these cases, alpha-lipoic acid may affect existing blood disorders.

DIABETES: Alpha-lipoic acid can decrease blood glucose levels (6,3545). Dosing adjustments for insulin or oral hypoglycemic agents may be necessary.

Typical Dosages & Routes of Administration that are Commonly Used

ORAL: For treatment of diabetes and peripheral neuropathy, doses of 1200 mg daily or 600 mg three times daily have been used (3540,3541). For cardiac autonomic neuropathy in patients with type 2 diabetes, 800 mg daily has been used (3542). As a general antioxidant, people typically take 20 to 50 mg per day (3894).

INTRAVENOUS: For peripheral neuropathy in patients with type 2 diabetes, doses of 100 mg, 600 mg, or 1200 mg daily have been used (3540,3557). However, doses of 600 mg and 1200 mg daily appear to be more effective than 100 mg daily (3557).

Comments

High doses of alpha-lipoic acid are approved in Germany for the treatment of diabetic neuropathy. Clinical trials using alpha-lipoic acid in higher doses, which might be more effective, and of sufficient duration to show any long-term therapeutic effects are needed (3871). Good dietary sources of alpha-lipoic acid are yeast and liver; other sources include spinach, broccoli, potatoes, and kidney (6).

ALPINE CRANBERRY

This Product is Also Known As

Cowberry, Dry Ground Cranberry, Foxberry, Lingenberry, Lingen, Lingon, Lingonberry, Lowbush Cranberry, Moss Cranberry, Partridgeberry, Red Bilberry, Redberries, Red Whortleberry, Rock Cranberry, Shore Cranberry, Vine of Mount Ida.

CAUTION: See separate listings for Cranberry, Cramp Bark (European Cranberry-Bush), and Uva Ursi (Mountain Cranberry).

Scientific Names

Vaccinium vitis-idaea.
Family: Ericaceae.

People Use This For

Orally, alpine cranberry is used for urinary tract irritation, gout, arthritis and kidney stones. It is also used orally as a urinary tract disinfectant, diuretic, and antiviral (18).

Safety

LIKELY UNSAFE …when the preparations of the leaves are used orally long-term because the arbutin constituent could be toxic (18).

There is insufficient reliable information available about the safety of the short-term oral use of alpine cranberry leaf.

CHILDREN: LIKELY UNSAFE ...contraindicated for oral use in children under 12 years of age because alpine cranberry might be hepatotoxic (18).

PREGNANCY AND LACTATION: LIKELY UNSAFE ...contraindicated for oral use because constituents have mutagenic effects (18).

Effectiveness

There is insufficient reliable information available about the effectiveness of alpine cranberry.

Possible Mechanism of Action & Active Ingredients

The applicable part of alpine cranberry is the leaf or berry. When ingested, alpine cranberry releases hydroquinones. In alkaline urine, the hydroquinones act as a disinfectant. Because hydroquinones can cause liver damage, long-term use is not recommended. There is also concern about long-term use because the constituents, arbutin and hydrochinon, are mutagenic and carcinogenic. (18).

Adverse Reactions Including Known Allergies

Alpine cranberry may cause nausea and vomiting due to its high tannin content (18).

Possible Interactions with Herbs & Other Dietary Supplements

Insufficient reliable information available.

Possible Interactions with Drugs

ANTIGOUT AGENTS: Theoretically, medications that increase uric acid concentrations in the bladder may counteract effects (18).

Possible Interactions with Foods

Theoretically, foods that increase urine uric acid concentrations will counteract any urinary disinfectant effects of alpine cranberry (18).

Possible Interactions with Lab Tests

No interactions are known to occur, and there is no known reason to expect a clinically significant interaction with alpine cranberry.

Possible Interactions with Diseases or Conditions

LIVER DISEASE: Theoretically, the hydroquinones in alpine cranberry may worsen liver disease (18).

Typical Dosages & Routes of Administration that are Commonly Used

ORAL: The daily dose is 2 grams of dried leaf or one cup of tea taken orally. The tea is prepared by steeping 2 grams dried leaf in 150 mL of boiling water for 10-15 minutes and straining (18).

Comments

Alpine cranberry leaves are sometimes used as a substitute for bearberry (uva ursi) leaves (18).

ALPINE LADY'S MANTLE

This Product is Also Known As

Alchemillae alpinae herba, Alpine Ladys Mantle.
CAUTION: See separate listing for Alchemilla (Lady's Mantle).

Scientific Names

Alchemilla alpina.
Family: Rosaceae.

People Use This For

Alpine lady's mantle is used as a diuretic, antispasmodic, and cardioactive agent. It is also used for unspecific female complaints (2).

Safety

There is insufficient reliable information available about the safety of alpine lady's mantle.
Pregnancy and Lactation: Insufficient reliable information available; avoid using.

Effectiveness

There is insufficient reliable information available about the effectiveness of alpine lady's mantle.

Possible Mechanism of Action & Active Ingredients

Insufficient reliable information available.

Adverse Reactions Including Known Allergies

None reported.

Possible Interactions with Herbs & Other Dietary Supplements

Insufficient reliable information available.

Possible Interactions with Drugs

No interactions are known to occur, and there is no known reason to expect a clinically significant interaction with alpine lady's mantle.

Possible Interactions with Foods

No interactions are known to occur, and there is no known reason to expect a clinically significant interaction with alpine lady's mantle.

Possible Interactions with Lab Tests

No interactions are known to occur, and there is no known reason to expect a clinically significant interaction with alpine lady's mantle.

Possible Interactions with Diseases or Conditions

No interactions are known to occur, and there is no known reason to expect a clinically significant interaction with alpine lady's mantle.

Typical Dosages & Routes of Administration that are Commonly Used

No typical dosage.

Comments

Avoid confusion with alchemilla (lady's mantle).

ALPINE RAGWORT

This Product is Also Known As

Life Root, Liferoot, Senecio Herb, Squawweed, Squaw Weed.
CAUTION: See separate listing for Golden Ragwort (Senecio aureus).

Scientific Names

Senecio nemorensis.
Family: Asteraceae or Compositae.

People Use This For

Orally, alpine ragwort is used for diabetes mellitus, hemorrhage, high blood pressure, spasms, and as a uterine stimulant (2,18).
In folk medicine, it has been used to control bleeding after tooth extraction (18).

Safety

LIKELY UNSAFE ...when used orally, due to potential for liver toxicity and possible carcinogenicity and mutagenicity (4,12,18).
PREGNANCY: LIKELY UNSAFE ...contraindicated, due to constituent hepatotoxic pyrrolizidine alkaloids (2).
LACTATION: LIKELY UNSAFE ...contraindicated, due to possibility that pyrrolizidine alkaloids might be excreted in milk (19).

Effectiveness

There is insufficient reliable information available about the effectiveness of alpine ragwort.

Possible Mechanism of Action & Active Ingredients

The applicable parts of alpine ragwort are the above ground parts. Alpine ragwort contains the pyrrolizidines senecionine, fuschsisencionine, 7-angeloylretronecin, bulgarsenine, nemorensin, platyphyllin, and sarracin (18). Hepatotoxicity and carcinogenicity may result from the pyrrolizidine alkaloids and the unsaturated parent compounds (18). Some unsaturated pyrrolizidine alkaloids have shown carcinogenic and mutagenic properties, and there are reports of renal toxicity. However, the primary concern is veno-occlusive liver disease (12). Unsaturated pyrrolizidine alkaloids are known to be hepatotoxic in animals and humans (4).

Adverse Reactions Including Known Allergies

Chronic exposure to plants containing UPA constituents has been associated with veno-occlusive disease (4021). Symptoms of acute veno-occlusive disease are characterized by a dull, dragging ache in the right upper abdomen and marked distention of the abdomen. These symptoms are sometimes accompanied by reduced urine output.

Subacute veno-occlusive disease is associated with vague symptoms and persistent liver enlargement (4021). Alpine ragwort can cause an allergic reaction in individuals sensitive to the Asteraceae/Compositae family. Members of this family include ragweed, chrysanthemums, marigolds, daisies, and many other herbs.

Possible Interactions with Herbs & Other Dietary Supplements

EUCALYPTUS: Theoretically, concomitant use may increase the risk of unsaturated pyrrolizidine alkaloid toxicity due to enzyme induction by eucalyptus (19).

PYRROLIZIDINE ALKALOID-CONTAINING HERBS: Concomitant use is contraindicated due to the risk of additive toxicity. Herbs containing unsaturated pyrrolizidine alkaloids include: alkanna (12), borage (271), gravel root (4), hemp agrimony (271), hound's tongue (19), petasites (19), comfrey (271), coltsfoot, and the Senecio species plants; dusty miller (19), alpine ragwort (19), groundsel (271), golden ragwort (19), and tansy ragwort (271).

Possible Interactions with Drugs

No interactions are known to occur, and there is no known reason to expect a clinically significant interaction with alpine ragwort.

Possible Interactions with Foods

No interactions are known to occur, and there is no known reason to expect a clinically significant interaction with alpine ragwort.

Possible Interactions with Lab Tests

No interactions are known to occur, and there is no known reason to expect a clinically significant interaction with alpine ragwort.

Possible Interactions with Diseases or Conditions

LIVER DISEASE: Contraindicated due to hepatotoxic potential (19).

CROSS-ALLERGENICITY: Can cause an allergic reaction in individuals sensitive to the Asteraceae/Compositae family. Members of this family include ragweed, chrysanthemums, marigolds, daisies, and many other herbs.

Typical Dosages & Routes of Administration that are Commonly Used

No typical dosage.

Comments

Alpine ragwort is considered likely unsafe; avoid using. Avoid confusion with golden ragwort (Senecio aureus) also referred to as squaw weed.

ALPINIA

This Product is Also Known As

Catarrh Root, China Root, Chinese Ginger, Colic Root, East India Catarrh Root, East India Root, Galanga, Galangal, Gargaut, India Root, Rhizome Galangae.

Scientific Names

Alpinia officinarum.
Family: Zingiberaceae.

People Use This For

Orally, alpinia rhizome is used as an aromatic, stimulant, antiflatulent (6), antibacterial, antispasmodic, anti-inflammatory agent, and as a fever reducer (18).

Safety

LIKELY SAFE (6,12). There are no reports of health risks or side effects (18).
PREGNANCY AND LACTATION: Insufficient reliable information available; avoid using.

Effectiveness

POSSIBLY INEFFECTIVE ...when taken for inflammation (6).
There is insufficient reliable information available about the effectiveness of alpinia for its other uses.

Possible Mechanism of Action & Active Ingredients

The applicable part of alpinia is the rhizome. The gingerols and diaryheptanoids constituents are potent inhibitors of PG synthetase (prostaglandin biosynthesizing enzyme). Their structures indicate they can also be active against 5-lipoxygenase, an enzyme involved in leukotriene biosynthesis (6).

Adverse Reactions Including Known Allergies

None reported (18).

Possible Interactions with Herbs & Other Dietary Supplements

Insufficient reliable information available.

Possible Interactions with Drugs

ACID-INHIBITING DRUGS: Theoretically, due to claims that alpinia increases stomach acid, alpinia might interfere with antacids, sucralfate (Carafate), H-2 antagonists (Zantac, Pepcid, Tagamet), or proton pump inhibitors (Prilosec, Prevacid) (19).

Possible Interactions with Foods

No interactions are known to occur, and there is no known reason to expect a clinically significant interaction with alpinia.

Possible Interactions with Lab Tests

No interactions are known to occur, and there is no known reason to expect a clinically significant interaction with alpinia.

Possible Interactions with Diseases or Conditions

No interactions are known to occur, and there is no known reason to expect a clinically significant interaction with alpinia.

Typical Dosages & Routes of Administration that are Commonly Used

ORAL: The typical dose of alpinia is 2-4 grams of the herb per day or one cup of the tea 30 minutes before meals (18). The tea is prepared by steeping 0.5-1 grams in 150 mL hot water for 10 minutes and then straining.

Comments

Alpinia is related to ginger in its botanical and pharmacological properties (6002). The uses of alpinia do not reflect its pharmacological properties. Some constituents possess antifungal activity while others inhibit prostaglandin biosynthesis and can inhibit leukotriene biosynthesis. The other Alpinia genus plants are also pharmacologically active (6).

AMARANTH

This Product is Also Known As

Lady Bleeding, Love-Lies-Bleeding, Lovely Bleeding, Pilewort, Prince's Feather, Red Cockscomb, Velvet Flower. CAUTION: See separate listings for Bulbous Buttercup and Lesser Celandine.

Scientific Names

Amaranthus hypochondriacus.

People Use This For

Orally, amaranth is used for ulcers, diarrhea, and inflammation of the mouth and throat (18).
In foods, amaranth fruit is used similarly to wheat as a cereal grain (6189).

Safety

There is insufficient reliable information available about the safety of amaranth.
Pregnancy and Lactation: Insufficient reliable information available; avoid using.

Effectiveness

POSSIBLY INEFFECTIVE ...when amaranth is used orally for lowering cholesterol in hypercholesterolemic adults (6188). Amaranth muffins added to a National Cholesterol Education Program (NCEP) step one low-fat diet failed to reduce cholesterol levels in a group of hypercholesterolemic adults beyond the reduction achieved by a group who ate only the low-fat diet (6188).
There is insufficient reliable information available about the effectiveness of amaranth for its other uses.

Possible Mechanism of Action & Active Ingredients

The applicable part is the complete amaranth plant. Amaranth is considered an astringent (18). The leaf contains a small amount of vitamin C (3833).

Adverse Reactions Including Known Allergies

None reported.

Possible Interactions with Herbs & Other Dietary Supplements

Insufficient reliable information available.

Possible Interactions with Drugs

No interactions are known to occur, and there is no known reason to expect a clinically significant interaction with amaranth.

Possible Interactions with Foods

No interactions are known to occur, and there is no known reason to expect a clinically significant interaction with amaranth.

Possible Interactions with Lab Tests

No interactions are known to occur, and there is no known reason to expect a clinically significant interaction with amaranth.

Possible Interactions with Diseases or Conditions

No interactions are known to occur, and there is no known reason to expect a clinically significant interaction with amaranth.

Typical Dosages & Routes of Administration that are Commonly Used

ORAL: People typically prepare amaranth as a tea, adding 1 teaspoon of leaves to 1 cup of cold water. The tea is taken cold, 1 to 2 cups a day. As a tincture amaranth is dosed up to 1 teaspoon (5263).

Comments

Avoid confusion with bulbous buttercup (Ranunculus bulbosus) or lesser celandine (Ranunculus ficaria), also known as pilewort.

AMBRETTE

This Product is Also Known As

Abelmosk, Ambretta, Egyptian Alcee, Muskmallow, Musk Seed, Okra, Target-Leaved Hibiscus.

Scientific Names

Abelmoschus moschatus, synonym Hibiscus abelmoschus.
Family: Malvaceae.

People Use This For

Orally, ambrette is used as a stimulant, antispasmodic (11), for snakebites, stomach and intestinal disorders with cramps, loss of appetite, and headaches (18).
In folk medicine, it has been used for stomach cancer, hysteria, gonorrhea, and respiratory disorders (6).
For food uses, ambrette is an ingredient in vermouths, bitters, and other food products (11).
In manufacturing, ambrette is often used in cosmetics such as perfumes, soaps, detergents, creams, and lotions (11).

Safety

POSSIBLY SAFE ...when the seeds or extracts are used orally. The extract has Generally Recognized as Safe (GRAS) status in the US. The maximun level is less than 0.001% (11). ...when the oil or absolute are used topically. The maximum use for the oil is 0.12% in perfumes (11).
There is insufficient reliable information available about the safety of larger amounts of ambrette for oral or topical use.
PREGNANCY: Insufficient reliable information available; avoid using.
LACTATION: POSSIBLY UNSAFE ...when used orally or topically ambrette persists in mother's milk (6), but the effect is unknown.

Effectiveness

There is insufficient reliable information available about the effectiveness of ambrette.

Possible Mechanism of Action & Active Ingredients

The applicable part of ambrette is the seed. The volatile oil is high in fatty acids, including palmitic and myristic acids (6). Ambrettolide and (Z)-5-tetradecen-14-olide are thought to be responsible for its characteristic musk-like odor (11).

Adverse Reactions Including Known Allergies

The topical use of ambrette can cause dermal irritation (6).

Possible Interactions with Herbs & Other Dietary Supplements

Insufficient reliable information available.

Possible Interactions with Drugs

No interactions are known to occur, and there is no known reason to expect a clinically significant interaction with ambrette.

Possible Interactions with Foods

No interactions are known to occur, and there is no known reason to expect a clinically significant interaction with ambrette.

Possible Interactions with Lab Tests

No interactions are known to occur, and there is no known reason to expect a clinically significant interaction with ambrette.

Possible Interactions with Diseases or Conditions
No interactions are known to occur, and there is no known reason to expect a clinically significant interaction with ambrette.

Typical Dosages & Routes of Administration that are Commonly Used
Ambrette is used orally and topically as a tea or tincture (18).

Comments
There is very little scientific information about this product. Our staff is continually analyzing the available information on natural medicines and will add data here as it becomes available.

AMERICAN ADDER'S TONGUE

This Product is Also Known As
American Adders Tongue, Dog's Tooth Violet, Dogs Tooth Voilet, Erythronium, Lambs Tongue, Lamb's Tongue, Rattlesnake Violet, Serpents Tongue, Serpent's Tongue, Snake Leaf, Yellow Snakeleaf, Yellow Snowdrop. CAUTION: See separate listing for English Adder's Tongue.

Scientific Names
Erythronium americanum.
Family: Liliaceae.

People Use This For
Topically, American adder's tongue is used for ulcers (18).

Safety
There is insufficient reliable information available about the safety of American adder's tongue used topically. Pregnancy and Lactation: Insufficient reliable information available; avoid using.

Effectiveness
There is insufficient reliable information available about the effectiveness of American adder's tongue.

Possible Mechanism of Action & Active Ingredients
The applicable parts of American adder's tongue are the leaves and tubers. The leaves can have emollient effects and treat skin ulcers when applied as a poultice. Taken internally, they act as an emetic (18).

Adverse Reactions Including Known Allergies
Cross-sensitivity can occur with the use of American adder's tongue in individuals allergic to tulip, fritallaria, lily, alstroemeria, or Bomarea (18).

Possible Interactions with Herbs & Other Dietary Supplements
Insufficient reliable information available.

Possible Interactions with Drugs
No interactions are known to occur, and there is no known reason to expect a clinically significant interaction with American adder's tongue.

Possible Interactions with Foods
No interactions are known to occur, and there is no known reason to expect a clinically significant interaction with American adder's tongue.

Possible Interactions with Lab Tests
No interactions are known to occur, and there is no known reason to expect a clinically significant interaction with American adder's tongue.

Possible Interactions with Diseases or Conditions
PLANT ALLERGIES: Cross-sensitivity can occur in individuals allergic to tulip, fritallaria, lily, alstroemeria, or Bomarea (18).

Typical Dosages & Routes of Administration that are Commonly Used
TOPICAL: The fresh leaves of American adder's tongue are commonly applied as a poultice (18).

Comments
Avoid confusion with English adder's tongue.

AMERICAN BITTERSWEET

This Product is Also Known As
False Bittersweet, Waxwork.

Scientific Names
Celastrus scandens.
Family: Celastraceae.

People Use This For
American bittersweet is rarely used today.
Historically, American bittersweet was used orally for arthritis, menstrual disorders, and liver disorders. It was also used orally as a diuretic and to stimulate sweating (18).

Safety
There is insufficient reliable information available about the safety of American bittersweet.
Pregnancy and Lactation: Insufficient reliable information available; avoid using.

Effectiveness
There is insufficient reliable information available about the effectiveness of American bittersweet.

Possible Mechanism of Action & Active Ingredients
The applicable parts of American bittersweet are the root and bark. American bittersweet contains tannins and a yellow quinoide nortriterpene called celastrol (18).

Adverse Reactions Including Known Allergies
None reported.

Possible Interactions with Herbs & Other Dietary Supplements
Insufficient reliable information available.

Possible Interactions with Drugs
No interactions are known to occur, and there is no known reason to expect a clinically significant interaction with American bittersweet.

Possible Interactions with Foods
No interactions are known to occur, and there is no known reason to expect a clinically significant interaction with American bittersweet.

Possible Interactions with Lab Tests
No interactions are known to occur, and there is no known reason to expect a clinically significant interaction with American bittersweet.

Possible Interactions with Diseases or Conditions
No interactions are known to occur, and there is no known reason to expect a clinically significant interaction with American bittersweet.

Typical Dosages & Routes of Administration that are Commonly Used
No typical dosage.

Comments
None.

AMERICAN CHESTNUT

This Product is Also Known As
None.
CAUTION: See separate listing for European Chestnut.

Scientific Names
Castanea dentata, synonym Castanea americana.
Family: Fagaceae.

People Use This For
Historically, American chestnut has been used orally for cough, pertussis, and respiratory ailments, and as an antirheumatic, sedative, tonic, and astringent agent (11). It has been used topically for pharyngitis (11).
Commercially, an extract of American chestnut is used in beverages (11).

Safety
LIKELY SAFE ...when taken orally in amounts found in beverages (11). American chestnut is approved for food use in the US (11).
There is insufficient reliable information available about the safety of the oral or topical use of American chestnut for medicinal purposes.
PREGNANCY AND LACTATION: Insufficient reliable information available; avoid using.

Effectiveness
There is insufficient reliable information available about the effectiveness of American chestnut.

Possible Mechanism of Action & Active Ingredients
American chestnut contains 8-9% tannins (11), which could theoretically exert an astringent effect on the mucosal tissue. This effect dehydrates the tissue, reducing internal secretions and forming external cells into a protective layer (12).

Adverse Reactions Including Known Allergies
Though no cases have been reported, adverse effects from oral use of American chestnut are theoretically possible. Plants with at least 10% tannins may cause gastrointestinal disturbances, kidney damage, and necrotic conditions of the liver (12). Some animal experiments show that tannins may cause cancer; others show they may prevent it (12). Regular consumption of herbs with high tannin concentrations correlates with increased incidence of esophageal or nasal cancer (12). No adverse reactions to topical use of American chestnut have been reported.

Possible Interactions with Herbs & Other Dietary Supplements
TANNIN-CONTAINING HERBS: Theoretically, herbs that contain high percentages of tannins (such as American chestnut) may cause precipitation of constituents of other herbs (19).

Possible Interactions with Drugs
ORAL DRUGS: Theoretically, concomitant oral administration may cause precipitation of some drugs due to the high tannin content of American chestnut (19). Separate administration of oral drugs and tannin-containing herbs by the longest period of time practical (19).

Possible Interactions with Foods
No interactions are known to occur, and there is no known reason to expect a clinically significant interaction with American chestnut.

Possible Interactions with Lab Tests
No interactions are known to occur, and there is no known reason to expect a clinically significant interaction with American chestnut.

Possible Interactions with Diseases or Conditions
No interactions are known to occur, and there is no known reason to expect a clinically significant interaction with American chestnut.

Typical Dosages & Routes of Administration that are Commonly Used
ORAL: People typically prepare American chestnut as a tea with 1 teaspoon of leaves and bark boiled in a covered container with 2 cups of water for 30 minutes. The liquid is cooled slowly in the closed container and taken cold, 1 to 2 cups per day (5254).

Comments
Recently, American chestnut (Castanea dentata) has been devastated by fungal disease (11). Chestnut leaves used in commerce usually come from European chestnut (Castanea sativa) or other Castanea species (11).

AMERICAN DOGWOOD

This Product is Also Known As
Bitter Redberry, Box Tree, Boxwood, Budwood, Cornel, Cornelian tree, Dog-Tree, Dogwood, False Box, Green Ozier, Osier, Rose Willow, Silky Cornel, Swamp Dogwood.
CAUTION: See separate listing for Jamaican Dogwood.

Scientific Names
Cornus florida.
Family: Cornaceae.

People Use This For
Orally, American dogwood is used for headaches and fatigue. It has been used to increase strength, for fever, chronic diarrhea and to stimulate appetite. It has also been used orally as a tonic.

Topically, American dogwood has been used as an astringent for boils and wounds (18).
Historically, American dogwood was used orally as a substitute for quinine.

Safety
There is insufficient reliable information available about the safety of American dogwood.
Pregnancy and Lactation: Insufficient reliable information available; avoid using.

Effectiveness
There is insufficient reliable information available about the effectiveness of American dogwood.

Possible Mechanism of Action & Active Ingredients
The applicable part of American dogwood is the bark. American dogwood destroys the snails that carry the tropical human parasite species Schistosoma. A methanol extract has a dose-dependent inhibiting effect on heart activity, and stops the heartbeat at high doses. Animal data suggests the water-insoluble fraction of American dogwood has antimalarial effects comparable to quinine and sulfadiazine (18).

Adverse Reactions Including Known Allergies
None reported.

Possible Interactions with Herbs & Other Dietary Supplements
Insufficient reliable information available.

Possible Interactions with Drugs
No interactions are known to occur, and there is no known reason to expect a clinically significant interaction with American dogwood.

Possible Interactions with Foods
No interactions are known to occur, and there is no known reason to expect a clinically significant interaction with American dogwood.

Possible Interactions with Lab Tests
No interactions are known to occur, and there is no known reason to expect a clinically significant interaction with American dogwood.

Possible Interactions with Diseases or Conditions
No interactions are known to occur, and there is no known reason to expect a clinically significant interaction with American dogwood.

Typical Dosages & Routes of Administration that are Commonly Used
ORAL: American dogwood has been used orally as a tincture as a substitute for quinine.
TOPICAL: American dogwood is used as a liquid extract. It is also prepared as a decoction or infusion, but the use of these products is not specified (18).

Comments
American dogwood is rarely used. Be careful not to confuse it with Jamaican dogwood (18).

AMERICAN ELDER

This Product is Also Known As
American Elderberry, Common Elderberry, Elderberry, Elder Flower, Sambucus, Sweet Elder.
CAUTION: See separate listings for European Elder fruit, European Elder flower, and Dwarf Elder.

Scientific Names
Sambucus canadensis.
Family: Caprifoliaceae.

People Use This For
In folk medicine, the American elder flower and ripe fruit have been used for asthma, bronchitis, bruises, cancer, flatulence, colds, edema associated with weak heart function, epilepsy, fever, gout, headache, neuralgia, psoriasis, rheumatism, to stimulate healing, for sore throat, sores, swelling, syphilis, toothache, as a cathartic laxative, to cause sweating, as a diuretic, emetic, eye wash, mouthwash, poultice, "purifier", and stimulant (4017).
For food uses, the American elder fruit is cooked and eaten and used to make elderberry wine (6). American elder flowers are used as flavor components in foods and beverages (11).
In manufacturing, the extracts of the American elder flower are used in perfumes (11).

Safety
LIKELY SAFE …when the fruit or flower are used in amounts found in foods. The flowers have Generally Recognized as Safe (GRAS) status in the US (11). The maximum use level of the flower is 0.049% (11). Cooked, ripe

fruit has few if any adverse effects (6).

POSSIBLY SAFE …when elder flowers are used orally for medicinal purposes (12).

POSSIBLY UNSAFE …when leaves, stems, or unripe fruit are used. All contain cyanogenic glycosides (12). Limit juice consumption to avoid toxicity (6).

PREGNANCY AND LACTATION: POSSIBLY UNSAFE ...when leaves, stems, or unripe fruit are used. There is insufficient reliable information available about the safety of the flower or cooked fruit; avoid amounts greater than found in foods.

Effectiveness

There is insufficient reliable information available about the effectiveness of American elder.

Possible Mechanism of Action & Active Ingredients

The applicable parts of American elder are the flower and ripe fruit. Elder flowers are believed to have diuretic and laxative effects (6). They are a rich source of vitamin C (19). Elder leaves (6) and unripe berries (12) contain cyanogenic glycosides. If ingested, the leaves or unripe berries can cause cyanide poisoning (6). Sambucus species contain plant lectins with hemagglutinin characteristics that might be useful in blood typing and other blood testing (11).

Adverse Reactions Including Known Allergies

Ingesting several glasses of elderberry juice can cause nausea, vomiting, weakness, dizziness, numbness and stupor (6).

Possible Interactions with Herbs & Other Dietary Supplements

Insufficient reliable information available.

Possible Interactions with Drugs

No interactions are known to occur, and there is no known reason to expect a clinically significant interaction with American elder.

Possible Interactions with Foods

No interactions are known to occur, and there is no known reason to expect a clinically significant interaction with American elder.

Possible Interactions with Lab Tests

No interactions are known to occur, and there is no known reason to expect a clinically significant interaction with American elder.

Possible Interactions with Diseases or Conditions

No interactions are known to occur, and there is no known reason to expect a clinically significant interaction with American elder.

Typical Dosages & Routes of Administration that are Commonly Used

No typical dosage.

Comments

Though making a pea shooter from an American elder stem seems innocuous, it is not a good idea. The stem contains cyanogenic glycosides and has been reported to cause toxicity in children (6).

AMERICAN HELLEBORE

This Product is Also Known As

American Veratrum, American White Hellebore, Bugbane, Devil's Bite, Earth Gall, False Hellebore, Green Hellebore, Green Veratrum, Indian Poke, Itchweed, Tickleweed Veratro Verde.

CAUTION: See separate listings for Black Hellebore, Pheasant's Eye, and White Hellebore.

Scientific Names

Veratrum viride.

Family: Liliaceae.

People Use This For

In folk medicine, American hellebore has been used as an antispasmodic, diuretic, sedative, and antipyretic (18). It has also been used for hypertension.

In manufacturing, American hellebore has been used as an insecticide (13).

Safety

LIKELY UNSAFE ...when used orally (18,1502). ...when used topically. The alkaloids can be absorbed through unbroken skin and should be avoided (18).

UNSAFE ...when large amounts are taken orally; can cause death (18).
PREGNANCY AND LACTATION: LIKELY UNSAFE ...when used orally or topically; contraindicated.

Effectiveness
There is insufficient reliable information available about the effectiveness of American hellebore.

Possible Mechanism of Action & Active Ingredients
The applicable part of American hellebore is the rhizome/root. The principal active constituents are steroid ester alkaloids (13,18), which reduce blood pressure even in small doses (13,18,1502). At therapeutic dosages, they have cardiac depressant, bradycardic, and sedative effects (13,18). The alkaloids inhibit inactivation of sodium-ion channels in excitable cells, especially those regulating cardiac activity (18).

Adverse Reactions Including Known Allergies
The oral use of American hellebore in therapeutic amounts can cause numerous adverse effects, including irritation of mucous membranes and cardiac depression (18). Large doses can cause sneezing, lacrimation, salivation, vomiting, diarrhea, burning sensations in the mouth and pharynx, dysphagia, paresthesias, vertigo, possible blindness, paralysis, mild convulsions, bradycardia, arrhythmias, hypotension, and death due to cardiac arrest or asphyxiation (17,18).

Possible Interactions with Herbs & Other Dietary Supplements
There is insufficient reliable information available.

Possible Interactions with Drugs
No interactions are known to occur, and there is no known reason to expect a clinically significant interaction with American hellebore.

Possible Interactions with Foods
No interactions are known to occur, and there is no known reason to expect a clinically significant interaction with American hellebore.

Possible Interactions with Lab Tests
No interactions are known to occur, and there is no known reason to expect a clinically significant interaction with American hellebore.

Possible Interactions with Diseases or Conditions
CARDIAC DISEASE: Theoretically, American hellebore can worsen cardiac disease by depressing cardiac activity or causing bradycardia. (13,18).
GI IRRITATION: American hellebore can irritate the gastrointestinal tract and is contraindicated in individuals with infectious or inflammatory gastrointestinal conditions (19).

Typical Dosages & Routes of Administration that are Commonly Used
No typical dosage.

Comments
American hellebore is considered likely unsafe; avoid using. Avoid confusion with European hellebore and pheasant's eye.

AMERICAN IVY

This Product is Also Known As
American Woodbine, Creeper, False Grapes, Five Leaves, Ivy, Virginia Creeper, Wild Woodbine, Wild Woodvine, Woody Climber.
CAUTION: See separate listings for Gelsemium, Honeysuckle, and Woodbine.

Scientific Names
Parthenocissus quinquefolia.
Family: Vitaceae.

People Use This For
Orally, American ivy is used for digestive disorders. It is sometimes used to stimulate sweating, as an astringent and as a tonic (18).

Safety
There is insufficient reliable information available about the safety of American ivy.
Pregnancy and Lactation: Insufficient reliable information available; avoid using.

Effectiveness

There is insufficient reliable information available about the effectiveness of American ivy.

Possible Mechanism of Action & Active Ingredients

The applicable part of American ivy is the bark. There is insufficient reliable information available about the possible mechanism of action and active ingredients.

Adverse Reactions Including Known Allergies

The berries contain 2% oxalic acid and are considered poisonous. There is one case of a child's death following ingestion of the berries (18).

Possible Interactions with Herbs & Other Dietary Supplements

Insufficient reliable information available.

Possible Interactions with Drugs

No interactions are known to occur, and there is no known reason to expect a clinically significant interaction with American ivy.

Possible Interactions with Foods

No interactions are known to occur, and there is no known reason to expect a clinically significant interaction with American ivy.

Possible Interactions with Lab Tests

No interactions are known to occur, and there is no known reason to expect a clinically significant interaction with American ivy.

Possible Interactions with Diseases or Conditions

No interactions are known to occur, and there is no known reason to expect a clinically significant interaction with American ivy.

Typical Dosages & Routes of Administration that are Commonly Used

A tea is made from the ground bark and taken orally (18).

Comments

Avoid confusion with woodbine (Clematis virginiana). Also, avoid confusing American ivy with gelsemium or honeysuckle, which are also known as woodbine.

AMERICAN MISTLETOE

This Product is Also Known As

Mistletoe.
CAUTION: See separate listing for European Mistletoe.

Scientific Names

Phoradendron leucarpum, synonyms Phoradendron serontium, Phoradendron flavescens; Phoradendron macrophyllum, synonym Phoradendron tomentosum.
Family: Viscaceae.

People Use This For

Traditionally, American mistletoe has been used as a smooth muscle stimulant for increasing blood pressure, and uterine and intestinal contractions (515). It has also been used as an abortifacient (6).

Safety

LIKELY UNSAFE ...when the flower, fruit, leaf, or stem are taken orally (6,515). All American mistletoe plant parts are considered toxic (6).
PREGNANCY: LIKELY UNSAFE ...contraindicated. American mistletoe is considered an abortifacient (19).
LACTATION: LIKELY UNSAFE ...when used orally; avoid using.

Effectiveness

There is insufficient reliable information available about the effectiveness of American mistletoe.

Possible Mechanism of Action & Active Ingredients

The applicable parts of American mistletoe are the flower, fruit, leaf, and stem. Constituent phoratoxins produce dose-dependent hypertension or hypotension, bradycardia, and increased uterine and intestinal motility (6,14). Experimental exposure to phoratoxins causes depolarization of skeletal muscle, contraction of smooth muscle, vasoconstriction, and cardiac arrest (6,14), similar to the effects reported with cardiotoxins from cobra venom (6,14).

Adverse Reactions Including Known Allergies

Some people who have ingested American mistletoe have reported nausea, bradycardia, hypertension, delirium, hallucinations, vasoconstriction, and cardiac arrest (6). Diarrhea and vomiting from ingestion of this product can lead to serious dehydration, hypovolemic shock, and cardiovascular collapse (6,14). Double vision was noted after ingestion of a large amount of bee pollen containing Phoradendron (14). Mild cases of acute gastroenteritis have been observed with ingestion of a few berries (14). Deaths have been reported after ingestion of teas used as an abortifacient (mistletoe species not identified) (6). However, no fatalities were reported in a review of 1754 accidental American mistletoe exposures extracted from the American Association of Poison Control Centers national data collection system from 1985-1992 (3706). The review concluded that the ingestion of one to three berries or one or two leaves of American Mistletoe is unlikely to result in any significant toxicity (3706).

Possible Interactions with Herbs & Other Dietary Supplements

Insufficient reliable information available.

Possible Interactions with Drugs

No interactions are known to occur, and there is no known reason to expect a clinically significant interaction with American mistletoe.

Possible Interactions with Foods

No interactions are known to occur, and there is no known reason to expect a clinically significant interaction with American mistletoe.

Possible Interactions with Lab Tests

No interactions are known to occur, and there is no known reason to expect a clinically significant interaction with American mistletoe.

Possible Interactions with Diseases or Conditions

HEART DISEASE: Avoid in individuals with heart disease; theoretically, may exacerbate.

Typical Dosages & Routes of Administration that are Commonly Used

No typical dosage.

Comments

American mistletoe is considered likely unsafe; avoid using. Avoid confusion with European mistletoe, as well as mistletoe from Australia, Korea, New Zealand, and other areas. Mistletoe is a parasite. Some Australian mistletoe species are reported to extract toxic constituents from the host plant on which they grow (515), suggesting the importance of identifying the host plant before use of mistletoe is considered.

AMERICAN PAWPAW

This Product is Also Known As

Custard Apple.
CAUTION: See separate listings for Papaya and Papain.

Scientific Names

Asimina triloba.
Family: Annonaceae.

People Use This For

American pawpaw is used in remedies for treating fever, vomiting, and inflammation of the mouth and throat (18).

Safety

There is insufficient reliable information available about the safety of American pawpaw.
Pregnancy and Lactation: Insufficient reliable information available; avoid using.

Effectiveness

There is insufficient reliable information available about the effectiveness of American pawpaw.

Possible Mechanism of Action & Active Ingredients

The applicable parts of American pawpaw are the bark, leaf, and seed. American pawpaw contains multiple acetogenin constituents; of these asimin, asiminacin and asininecin are reported to be highly cytotoxic (258). Based on preliminary animal studies and in vitro studies of human cancer lines, scientists report some acetogenins show activity against certain lung and breast cancers (256). An acetogenin mixture also demonstrates pesticide activity (257).

Adverse Reactions Including Known Allergies

American pawpaw can cause nausea and urticaria (18). American pawpaw extract can cause contact dermatitis (1525).

Possible Interactions with Herbs & Other Dietary Supplements
Insufficient reliable information available.

Possible Interactions with Drugs
No interactions are known to occur, and there is no known reason to expect a clinically significant interaction with American pawpaw.

Possible Interactions with Foods
No interactions are known to occur, and there is no known reason to expect a clinically significant interaction with American pawpaw.

Possible Interactions with Lab Tests
No interactions are known to occur, and there is no known reason to expect a clinically significant interaction with American pawpaw.

Possible Interactions with Diseases or Conditions
No interactions are known to occur, and there is no known reason to expect a clinically significant interaction with American pawpaw.

Typical Dosages & Routes of Administration that are Commonly Used
No typical dosage.

Comments
There is very little scientific information about this product. Our staff is continually analyzing the available information on natural medicines and will add data here as it becomes available.

AMERICAN SPIKENARD

This Product is Also Known As
Indian Root, Life-of-Man, Life of Man, Old Man's Root, Pettymorell, Small Spikenard, Spignet.

Scientific Names
Aralia racemosa.
Family: Araliaceae.

People Use This For
Orally, spikenard is used for colds, chronic coughs, asthma, and arthritis. It is also used as an expectorant, to stimulate tissue renewal, and to promote sweating. Topically, spikenard is also used as an alternative to sarsaparilla for treating skin diseases (18).

Safety
There is insufficient reliable information available about the safety of spikenard.
PREGNANCY: UNSAFE ...contraindicated (12).
LACTATION: Insufficient reliable information available; avoid using.

Effectiveness
There is insufficient reliable information available about the effectiveness of spikenard.

Possible Mechanism of Action & Active Ingredients
Insufficient reliable information available.

Adverse Reactions Including Known Allergies
Spikenard could theoretically cause skin sensitization secondary to its polyyne content (18).

Possible Interactions with Herbs & Other Dietary Supplements
Insufficient reliable information available.

Possible Interactions with Drugs
No interactions are known to occur, and there is no known reason to expect a clinically significant interaction with spikenard.

Possible Interactions with Foods
No interactions are known to occur, and there is no known reason to expect a clinically significant interaction with spikenard.

Possible Interactions with Lab Tests
No interactions are known to occur, and there is no known reason to expect a clinically significant interaction with spikenard.

© Copyright 2000, Natural Medicines Comprehensive Database (209) 472-2244. For updated data, go to www.NaturalDatabase.com

Possible Interactions with Diseases or Conditions

No interactions are known to occur, and there is no known reason to expect a clinically significant interaction with spikenard.

Typical Dosages & Routes of Administration that are Commonly Used

ORAL: Spikenard is taken as one cup of tea at a time throughout the day. The tea is prepared by steeping 15 grams root in 500 mL of boiling water for 10-15 minutes and straining. Alternately, it can be taken orally as a liquid extract (equivalent to 0.8-1.9 grams root) (18).

Comments

There is very little scientific information about this product. Our staff is continually analyzing the available information on natural medicines and will add data here as it becomes available.

AMERICAN WHITE POND LILY

This Product is Also Known As

Cow Cabbage, Water Cabbage, Water Lily, Water Nymph.

Scientific Names

Nymphaea odorata.

People Use This For

Orally, American white pond lily is used to treat chronic diarrhea (18).
Topically, American white pond lily is used for vaginal conditions, diseases of the throat and mouth, and as a poultice for burns and furuncles (18).

Safety

There is insufficient reliable information available about the safety of American white pond lily.
Pregnancy and Lactation: Insufficient reliable information available; avoid using.

Effectiveness

There is insufficient reliable information available about the effectiveness of American white pond lily.

Possible Mechanism of Action & Active Ingredients

The applicable part of American white pond lily is the rhizome/root. American white pond lilly contains tannins which are probably responsible for astringent and antiseptic activity (18).

Adverse Reactions Including Known Allergies

None reported.

Possible Interactions with Herbs & Other Dietary Supplements

Insufficient reliable information available.

Possible Interactions with Drugs

No interactions are known to occur, and there is no known reason to expect a clinically significant interaction with American white pond lily.

Possible Interactions with Foods

No interactions are known to occur, and there is no known reason to expect a clinically significant interaction with American white pond lily.

Possible Interactions with Lab Tests

No interactions are known to occur, and there is no known reason to expect a clinically significant interaction with American white pond lily.

Possible Interactions with Diseases or Conditions

No interactions are known to occur, and there is no known reason to expect a clinically significant interaction with American white pond lily.

Typical Dosages & Routes of Administration that are Commonly Used

ORAL: One cup of tea (steep 1-2 grams dried root in 150 mL boiling water 5-10 minutes, strain) (18). Liquid extract (1:1 in 25% ethanol), 1-4 mL (18).
TOPICAL: As a douche, gargle, or hot poultice (18); no additional information available.

Comments

None.

ANDIROBA

This Product is Also Known As
Andiroba-Saruba, Bastard Mahogany, Brazilian Mahogany, Carapa, Cedro, Crabwood, Iandirova, Requia.

Scientific Names
Carapa guianensis.
Family: Meliaceae.

People Use This For
Orally, andiroba bark and leaf are used to treat fevers, herpes, as an antihelmintic, and as a tonic (517,518). Andiroba fruit oil is taken orally for coughs (517).

Topically, andiroba bark and leaf are used as a wash for dermatoses, sores, ulcers, and skin troubles (517,518). It is used topically for removing ticks from the head and for skin parasites (517). The seed oil is used topically to treat inflammation, arthritis (517), for rashes, muscle and joint aches and injuries, wounds, boils, and herpes ulcers (3918). Other uses of andiroba include use as a solvent for extracting plant colorants, as a lamp oil, and in soaps (as an insect repellent) (3918). Seed oil is also used for mummification of human heads (3918).

Safety
There is insufficient reliable information available about the safety of andiroba.
Pregnancy and Lactation: Insufficient reliable information available; avoid using.

Effectiveness
There is insufficient reliable information available about the effectiveness of andiroba.

Possible Mechanism of Action & Active Ingredients
The applicable parts of andiroba are the bark, leaf, fruit oil, and seed oil. There is insufficient reliable information available about the possible mechanism of action and active ingredients.

Adverse Reactions Including Known Allergies
None reported.

Possible Interactions with Herbs & Other Dietary Supplements
Insufficient reliable information available.

Possible Interactions with Drugs
No interactions are known to occur, and there is no known reason to expect a clinically significant interaction with andiroba.

Possible Interactions with Foods
No interactions are known to occur, and there is no known reason to expect a clinically significant interaction with andiroba.

Possible Interactions with Lab Tests
No interactions are known to occur, and there is no known reason to expect a clinically significant interaction with andiroba.

Possible Interactions with Diseases or Conditions
No interactions are known to occur, and there is no known reason to expect a clinically significant interaction with andiroba.

Typical Dosages & Routes of Administration that are Commonly Used
ORAL: As a tea brewed from the bark and/or leaf (517,518).
TOPICAL: As a tea.

Comments
There is very little scientific information about this product. Our staff is continually analyzing the available information on natural medicines and will add data here as it becomes available.

ANDRACHNE

This Product is Also Known As
None.

Scientific Names
Andrachne cordifolia; Andrachne aspera; Andrachne phyllanthoides
Family: Euphorbiaceae.

People Use This For
In Yemen folklore, andrachne is used to treat eye inflammation (6).

Safety
There is insufficient reliable information available about safety of andrachne.
Pregnancy and Lactation: Insufficient reliable information available.

Effectiveness
There is insufficient reliable information available about the effectiveness of andrachne.

Possible Mechanism of Action & Active Ingredients
Insufficient reliable information available.

Adverse Reactions Including Known Allergies
None reported.

Possible Interactions with Herbs & Other Dietary Supplements
Insufficient reliable information available.

Possible Interactions with Drugs
No interactions are known to occur, and there is no known reason to expect a clinically significant interaction with andrachne.

Possible Interactions with Foods
No interactions are known to occur, and there is no known reason to expect a clinically significant interaction with andrachne.

Possible Interactions with Lab Tests
No interactions are known to occur, and there is no known reason to expect a clinically significant interaction with andrachne.

Possible Interactions with Diseases or Conditions
No interactions are known to occur, and there is no known reason to expect a clinically significant interaction with andrachne.

Typical Dosages & Routes of Administration that are Commonly Used
No typical dosage.

Comments
There is very little scientific information about this product. Our staff is continually analyzing the available information on natural medicines and will add data here as it becomes available.

ANDROGRAPHIS

This Product is Also Known As
Andrographolide, Bidara, Carmantina, Chiretta, Chuan Xin Lian, Creat, Fa Tha Lai Jone, Fa-Tha-Lai-Jone, Indian Echinacea, Kalmegh, Kariyat, King of Bitters, Kirta, Nabin Chanvandi, Sadilata, Sambilata, Takila, Vizra Ufar.

Scientific Names
Andrographis paniculata, synonym Justicia paniculata.
Family: Acanthaceae.

People Use This For
Orally, andrographis is used for preventing and treating the common cold, influenza, pharyngotonsillitis, respiratory allergies, and sinusitis (2744,2747,2748).
In traditional medicine, andrographis is also used for anorexia, atherosclerosis, snake and insect bites, bronchitis, cachexia, prevention of cardiovascular disease, cholera, colic, diabetes, diarrhea, flatulence, gastritis, gonorrhea, hemorrhoids, hepatomegaly, drug-induced hepatotoxicity, and other hepatic disorders, myocardial ischemia, jaundice, leprosy, leptospirosis, malaria, pharyngitis, pneumonia, pruritus, pyelonephritis, rabies, skin wounds, unspecified skin diseases, syphilis, tuberculosis, tonsillitis, and ulcers (2743,2745,2746,2749). Andrographis is used as an astringent, antiseptic, antidote, analgesic, antipyretic, anti-inflammatory, antithrombotic, expectorant, anthelmintic, laxative, and tonic (2743,2746,2758). A flavone extracted from andrographis is used for preventing myocardial infarction (2758).

Safety
POSSIBLY SAFE …when used orally and appropriately, short-term (12). Andrographis extracts have been shown to be safe in one clinical trial using low doses lasting 3 months and in others using higher doses lasting 4-7 days (12,2744,2748,2772,2773,2774).

© Copyright 2000, Natural Medicines Comprehensive Database (209) 472-2244. For updated data, go to www.NaturalDatabase.com

There is insufficient reliable information available about the safety of augmented andrographis preparations which contain elevated concentrations of the constituent andrographolide (See Comments).

PREGNANCY: LIKELY UNSAFE …when used orally due to abortifacient effects; contraindicated (12).

LACTATION: Insufficient reliable information available; avoid using.

Effectiveness

POSSIBLY EFFECTIVE …when used orally for decreasing the severity and duration of symptoms of the common cold when started within 72 hours of the onset of symptoms. Placebo-controlled clinical trials have shown significant overall improvement in symptoms of the common cold after 4-5 days of treatment (2744,2773,2774). Some symptoms improved after 2 days of treatment (2744,2773). Two trials excluded patients who had pre-existing symptoms of the common cold for greater than 2 or 3 days (2744,2773). …when used orally for prevention of the common cold. In one clinical trial, andrographis was compared to placebo for prophylaxis against the common cold over a 3 month period. The rate of developing the common cold was significantly lower in those treated with andrographis only during the third month of treatment; however, the overall relative risk of developing a cold was 2.1 times lower in those receiving andrographis (2772). …when used orally to relieve fever and sore throat associated with pharyngotonsillitis. In one study, high doses of andrographis were comparable to acetaminophen after 3 and 7 days of treatment for fever and sore throat associated with pharyngotonsillitis (2748).

Most clinical trials used Andrographis paniculata dried extract (Kan Jang, Swedish Herbal Institute), standardized to contain the constituent andrographolide 4-5.6 mg per tablet (2744,2772,2773,2774).

There is insufficient reliable information available about the effectiveness of andrographis for its other uses.

Possible Mechanism of Action & Active Ingredients

The applicable parts of andrographis are the leaf and occasionally the rhizome (12,2758,2767). Several active andrographis compounds have been identified, including andrographolide, deoxyandrographolide, and other diterpenes (2750,2760,2768,2771). Although andrographis is used for a wide variety of indications in Ayurvedic and herbal medicine, clinical evidence of effectiveness in humans is limited to the common cold. Preliminary evidence suggests that andrographis might have mast cell-stabilizing, antiallergy activity (2750,2751). Other evidence suggests andrographis might have immunostimulant, anti-HIV, and leukemia cell differentiation-inducing activity (2766,2765,2768). Possible analgesic, antipyretic, and anti-ulcerogenic effects of andrographis have been described (2753,2754). Andrographis has traditionally been used for infectious diseases. Antibacterial activity was not detected by one group of investigators, but preliminary evidence suggests potential use against bacteria in raw water, human roundworm (Ascaris lumbricoides), Toxoplasma gondii, malaria, and E. coli enterotoxin secretion (2752,2753,2764,2767,2777,2779,2780,2781). Andrographis might protect the liver against hepatotoxic drugs (e.g., acetaminophen) and chemicals possibly by increasing bile flow, bile salt, and bile acids (2761,2762,2763,2778). The andrographis constituent, andrographolide, is a more potent hepatoprotectant than silymarin, an active constituent of milk thistle (see separate listing for Milk Thistle) (2762,2778). Andrographis may be beneficial in cardiovascular disease. Early evidence suggests that andrographis might lower blood pressure, prevent arteriosclerosis, inhibit platelet aggregation, and reduce myocardial ischemia and reperfusion injury (2755,2756,2757,2758,2759,2760,2782,2783). Andrographis is reported to have abortifacient activity (12). The mechanism of abortifacient action is unknown (2771). Preliminary evidence suggests that andrographis might also have detrimental effects on male and female fertility. In animals, andrographis decreased fertility of both males and females (2769,2770,2776).

Adverse Reactions Including Known Allergies

Large doses of andrographis are reported to cause gastrointestinal distress, anorexia, and emesis (12,2743). Urticaria has also been reported (2743,2773). Preliminary evidence suggests that andrographis might inhibit male and female fertility (2769,2770,2776).

Possible Interactions with Herbs & Other Dietary Supplements

HERBS WITH ANTICOAGULANT/ANTIPLATELET POTENTIAL: Theoretically, concomitant use with herbs that have anticoagulant or antiplatelet activity might enhance therapeutic effects and increase the risk of bleeding (2758,2759). These include angelica, anise, arnica, asafoetida, bogbean, boldo, capsicum, celery, chamomile, clove, danshen, fenugreek, feverfew, garlic, ginger, ginkgo, Panax ginseng, horse chestnut, horseradish, licorice, meadowsweet, prickly ash, onion, papain, passionflower, poplar, quassia, red clover, turmeric, wild carrot, wild lettuce, willow, and others (4,19).

HERBS/SUPPLEMENTS WITH HYPOTENSIVE ACTIVITY: Theoretically, concurrent use might enhance therapeutic effects and increase the risk of hypotension (2755,2760). These include black cohosh, celery seed, Panax ginseng, and others (4).

Possible Interactions with Drugs

ANTICOAGULANT/ANTIPLATELET DRUGS: Theoretically, concomitant use might enhance therapeutic effects and increase the risk of bleeding (2758,2759).

ANTIHYPERTENSIVE DRUGS: Theoretically, concomitant use might enhance therapeutic effects and increase the risk of hypotension (2755,2760).

IMMUNOSUPPRESSIVE DRUGS: Theoretically, andrographis might interfere with immunosuppressive drugs because of its immunostimulant activity (2766).

Possible Interactions with Foods

No interactions are known to occur, and there is no known reason to predict an interaction.

Possible Interactions with Lab Tests

No interactions are known to occur, and there is no known reason to predict an interaction.

Possible Interactions with Diseases or Conditions

BLEEDING DISORDERS: Theoretically, andrographis might have antiplatelet activity and increase the risk of bleeding in patients with bleeding disorders (2758,2759).
HYPERTENSION: Theoretically, andrographis might lower blood pressure and improve hypertension (2755,2760).
HYPOTENSION: Theoretically, andrographis might lower blood pressure and exacerbate hypotension (2755,2760).
INFERTILITY: Theoretically, andrographis might have detrimental effects on male and female fertility (2769,2770,2776). Avoid in couples with infertility.

Typical Dosages & Routes of Administration that are Commonly Used

ORAL: Most clinical trials used andrographis dried extract (Kan Jang, Swedish Herbal Institute), standardized to contain 4-5.6 mg andrographolide. For decreasing symptoms of the common cold, doses of 400 mg three times daily have been used in clinical trials (2744,2773,2774). For preventing the common cold, a dose of 200 mg daily for 5 days each week has been used in a clinical trial (2772). For relieving fever and sore throat in pharyngotonsillitis, doses of 3 grams and 6 grams daily were used (2748).

Comments

Andrographis is native to Asian countries such as India and Sri Lanka, and is cultivated and naturalized in other areas of the world (2775). Andrographis products have reportedly been used in Scandinavia for more than a decade (2722). One writer credits Andrographis with arresting the 1919 flu epidemic in India, although this has not been verified (2774).
Some Internet vendors offer andrographis augmented to contain up to 30% andrographolide (2746). The safety and effectiveness of andrographis preparations with augmented andrographolide content is unknown.

ANDROSTENEDIOL

This Product is Also Known As

Androdiol, 4-Androstenediol, 4-AD, 5-Androstenediol, 5-AD.

Scientific Names

4-androstene-3beta,17beta-diol; 5-androstene-3beta,17beta-diol.

People Use This For

Orally, androstenediol is used to increase endogenous testosterone production for increased energy, enhanced recovery and growth from exercise, heightened sexual arousal and function, and a greater sense of well being (8304).

Safety

There is insufficient reliable information available about the safety of androstenediol; avoid using.
Pregnancy and Lactation: Insufficient reliable information available; avoid using.

Effectiveness

There is insufficient reliable information available about the effectiveness of androstenediol.

Possible Mechanism of Action & Active Ingredients

There is some evidence that exogenous androstenediol is converted to testosterone in humans; but this is not yet scientifically established.

Adverse Reactions Including Known Allergies

May cause masculinization and increased growth of facial hair in women.

Possible Interactions with Herbs & Other Dietary Supplements

Insufficient reliable information available.

Possible Interactions with Drugs

ANDROGENIC DRUGS: Theoretically, may increase activity and risk of side effects.
ESTROGENIC DRUGS: Theoretically, may reduce or inhibit activity (8304).

Possible Interactions with Foods

No interactions are known to occur, and there is no known reason to expect a clinically significant interaction with androstenediol.

Possible Interactions with Lab Tests

No interactions are known to occur, and there is no known reason to expect a clinically significant interaction with androstenediol.

Possible Interactions with Diseases or Conditions

PROSTATE CONDITIONS: Androstenediol might aggravate prostate conditions due to its androgenic activity.
BREAST CANCER : Androstenediol might aggravate breast cancer due to its estrogenic activity (8304).

Typical Dosages & Routes of Administration that are Commonly Used

No typical dosage.

Comments

There is some concern that the potency and purity of androstenediol products are not always the same as is labeled.

ANDROSTENEDIONE

This Product is Also Known As

Andro, Androstene.

Scientific Names

4-androstene-3,17-dione; Androst-4-ene-3,17-dione.

People Use This For

Orally, androstenedione is used for increased endogenous testosterone production for enhanced athletic performance (674), increased energy, to keep red blood cells healthy, enhance recovery and growth from exercise, and for heightened sexual arousal and function.

Safety

POSSIBLY UNSAFE ...when used orally. New data suggests that androstenedione use can increase the risk of cardiovascular disease by increasing serum estrogen levels and decreasing high-density lipoprotein levels (6000). Androstenedione can also lead to breast enlargement and feminizing effects in men (3861). Androstenedione increases the risk of breast cancer, pancreatic cancer, and prostate cancer (6000). The long-term effects of androstenedione are unknown. Some evidence suggests it might stimulate prostate tumor growth (672).
CHILDREN: LIKELY UNSAFE ...androstenedione could potentially cause premature closure of the bone growth plates (674).
PREGNANCY: LIKELY UNSAFE ...some evidence suggests it might induce labor (673).
LACTATION: POSSIBLY UNSAFE; avoid using.

Effectiveness

POSSIBLY EFFECTIVE ...when used orally in high doses (300 mg/day) in young men with normal testosterone levels to increase testosterone levels (3861).
There is insufficient reliable information available about the effectiveness of androstenedione for its other uses.

Possible Mechanism of Action & Active Ingredients

Androstenedione is a steroid hormone produced by the adrenal glands and testes and ovaries (3861). Androstenedione is a direct precursor of testosterone and estrone in both men and women (674). In young healthy men, androstenedione increases estradiol levels at low doses (100 mg per day), but has no significant effect on testosterone concentrations and no anabolic effect on muscle protein metabolism (3861,3862). Higher doses (300 mg as a single daily dose) increase both testosterone and estradiol in young men (3861). The effect of this dose on muscle strength is unknown. A divided dose of 300 mg per day raises estradiol, but not testosterone levels (6000), and does not enhance skeletal muscle adaptations to resistance training (6000). Hormonal responses to androstenedione are variable, and there might be subsets of the population prone to develop androgenic or estrogenic responses to the drug (3861,3862,6000).

Adverse Reactions Including Known Allergies

Testosterone derivatives similar to androstenedione have been associated with hepatic toxicity (3861).
There is one case report of two episodes of priapism associated with oral androstenedione use in a 30 year old man (5089). In men, androstenedione theoretically might decrease endogenous testosterone production and spermatogenesis; cause acne, testicular atrophy, gynecomastia, and behavioral changes; reduce HDL cholesterol; and increase the risk of pancreatic and prostate cancer (674,6000).
In women, androstenedione theoretically might cause masculinization with the deepening of voice, hirsutism, acne, clitoral hypertrophy, menorrhea, male-pattern baldness, and coarsening of the skin (674).
In children, androstenedione theoretically might cause premature bone growth plate closure and decrease adult height (674). Androstenedione might cause early development of secondary sex characteristics in boys; and acne, oligomenorrhea or amenorrhea, hirsutism, and virilization in girls (217).

Possible Interactions with Herbs & Other Dietary Supplements

Insufficient reliable information available.

Possible Interactions with Drugs

ESTROGENIC DRUGS: Because androstenedione is a precursor of testosterone and estrone, androstenedione theoretically can increase the activity and risk of side effects of androgenic drugs and can affect the activity of estrogenic drugs.

Possible Interactions with Foods

No interactions are known to occur, and there is no known reason to expect a clinically significant interaction with androstenedione.

Possible Interactions with Lab Tests

TESTOSTERONE AND ESTRONE ASSAYS: Supplemental androstenedione use may yield increases in testosterone and estrone assays.

Possible Interactions with Diseases or Conditions

PROSTATE CONDITIONS: Androstenedione can stimulate human prostate tumor cell growth and should be avoided in men concerned about prostate problems (672).
HORMONE IMBALANCES: Androstenedione is a precursor of testosterone and estrone, and should be avoided in conditions sensitive to these compounds.
LIVER DISEASE: Steroids similar to androstenedione have been associated with liver abnormalities and should be avoided by people with hepatic disease (3861).

Typical Dosages & Routes of Administration that are Commonly Used

ORAL: The usual oral dose of androstenedione is 50-100 mg twice daily, taken one hour before exercise or upon awakening (5027,6000). A single daily dose of 300 mg raised serum testosterone levels was used in one study (3861).

Comments

Androstenedione gained popularity as the supplement used by homerun-hitter Mark McGwire. Androstenedione is not prohibited by Major League Baseball, but is banned by the International Olympics Committee (IOC), the National Collegiate Athletic Association (NCAA), the National Basketball Association (NBA), the National Football League (NFL), and the World Natural Body Building Federation (217,5041). There are some concerns that the potency and purity of androstenedione products can differ from the product labeling. The use of androstenedione should be avoided and has the potential of being particularly hazardous in women and children (3861). Consider monitoring liver function tests in people who choose to use androstenedione.

ANGEL'S TRUMPET

This Product is Also Known As

Devil's Trumpet
CAUTION: See separate listing for Jimson Weed (Datura stramonium).

Scientific Names

Datura sauveolens.
Family: Solanaceae.

People Use This For

Orally, Angel's trumpet tea prepared from leaves and flowers has been used to induce hallucinations and euphoria (5624,5625,5626,5627).
Historically, Angel's trumpet has been used to treat asthma (5625).

Safety

UNSAFE ...when used orally (5624,5625,5626,5627). All parts of the plant contain tropane alkaloids and are considered poisonous (5624,5625,5627); the foliage and seeds contain the high concentration of toxic alkaloids (5627).
CHILDREN: UNSAFE ...when used orally (5624,5625,5626,5627). Severe toxicity has occurred in cases of accidental ingestion and in teenagers experimenting with Angel's trumpet for recreational use (5626).
PREGNANCY AND LACTATION: UNSAFE ...when used orally. The entire plant is considered poisonous (5624,5627); contraindicated.

Effectiveness

There is insufficient reliable information available about the effectiveness of Angel's trumpet.

Possible Mechanism of Action & Active Ingredients

The applicable parts of Angel's trumpet are the leaf and flower. Angel's trumpet contains tropane alkaloids, particularly atropine, hyoscyamine and hyoscine (scopolamine), which are responsible for the anticholinergic effects and toxicity (5625,5627).

Adverse Reactions Including Known Allergies

Orally, Angel's trumpet can cause severe toxicity. Ingestion of Angel's trumpet can cause acute anticholinergic poisoning, which often requires medical attention (5624,5625,5626,5627). Oral use has been associated with delirium, dilated pupils, hyperactivity, disorientation, intense thirst, dry skin and mucous membranes, flushing, fever, widened pulse pressure, systolic hypertension, tachycardia (5624,5625), AV disassociation (5627), hyperexcitability, visual hallucinations, anxiety, amnesia, combativeness, ataxia, clonus, muscular weakness, expressive aphasia, muscular paralysis, seizure, urinary retention (5624,5625), decreased GI motility (5627), alternating levels of consciousness, convulsions, and coma (5624,5625). Death may result from respiratory arrest (5624). Each flower contains approximately 0.20 mg of atropine and 0.65 mg of scopolamine. Reports suggest ingestion of tea made from 3-6 flowers can produce hallucinations, and 9 flowers can produce total paralysis (5624).

Possible Interactions with Herbs & Other Dietary Supplements

Insufficient reliable information available.

Possible Interactions with Drugs

ANTICHOLINERGIC DRUGS: Concomitant use may increase anticholinergic effects and adverse effects; drugs include amantadine, atropine, belladonna alkaloids, phenothiazines, scopolamine, and tricyclic antidepressants (506).

Possible Interactions with Foods

No interactions are known to occur, and there is no known reason to expect a clinically significant interaction with Angel's trumpet.

Possible Interactions with Lab Tests

No interactions are known to occur, and there is no known reason to expect a clinically significant interaction with Angel's trumpet.

Possible Interactions with Diseases or Conditions

CONGESTIVE HEART FAILURE (CHF): Contraindicated; Angel's trumpet might cause tachycardia and exacerbate CHF due to its hyoscyamine (atropine) and scopolamine content (15).
CONSTIPATION: Contraindicated; Angel's trumpet might cause constipation due to its hyoscyamine (atropine) and scopolamine content (15).
DOWN SYNDROME: Caution, patients with Down syndrome might be hypersensitive to the antimuscarinic effects (mydriasis, positive chronotropic heart effects, etc.) of hyoscyamine (atropine) and scopolamine contained in Angel's trumpet (15).
ESOPHAGEAL REFLUX: Contraindicated; Angel's trumpet might delay gastric emptying and decrease lower esophageal pressure, promoting gastric retention and exacerbating reflux due to its hyoscyamine (atropine) and scopolamine content (15).
FEVER: Contraindicated; Angel's trumpet might increase the risk of hyperthermia in patients with fever due to its hyoscyamine (atropine) and scopolamine content (15).
GASTRIC ULCER: Contraindicated; Angel's trumpet might delay gastric emptying and exacerbate gastric ulcers due to its hyoscyamine (atropine) and scopolamine content (15).
GI INFECTIONS: Contraindicated; Angel's trumpet might suppress GI motility causing retention of infecting organisms or toxins due to its hyoscyamine (atropine) and scopolamine content (15).
HIATAL HERNIA: Contraindicated; Angel's trumpet might delay gastric emptying and decrease lower esophageal pressure, promoting gastric retention and exacerbating reflux due to its hyoscyamine (atropine) and scopolamine content (15).
TOXIC MEGACOLON: Contraindicated; Angel's trumpet might suppress intestinal motility, which might produce paralytic ileus and exacerbate toxic megacolon, due to its hyoscyamine (atropine) and scopolamine content (2,15).
NARROW-ANGLE GLAUCOMA: Contraindicated; Angel's trumpet might increase ocular tension in patients with narrow-angle (angle-closure) glaucoma due to its hyoscyamine (atropine) and scopolamine content (2,15).
OBSTRUCTIVE GI TRACT DISEASE: Contraindicated; Angel's trumpet might exacerbate obstructive GI tract diseases (including atony, paralytic ileus, and stenosis) due to its hyoscyamine (atropine) and scopolamine content (15).
TACHYARRHYTHMIAS: Contraindicated; Angel's trumpet might cause tachycardia due to its hyoscyamine (atropine) and scopolamine content (2,15).
URINARY RETENTION: Contraindicated; Angel's trumpet might increase urinary retention due to its hyoscyamine (atropine) and scopolamine content (2,15).
ULCERATIVE COLITIS: Contraindicated; Angel's trumpet might suppress intestinal motility, which might produce paralytic ileus and precipitate toxic megacolon, due to its hyoscyamine (atropine) and scopolamine content (15).

Typical Dosages & Routes of Administration that are Commonly Used

No typical dosage.

Comments

Angel's trumpet is considered unsafe to use due to its high potential for toxicity. Angel's trumpet is usually cultivated as an ornamental plant in the southeastern United States (5625,5626) and may be confused with Jimson Weed which grows wild throughout the United States (5621,5622).

ANGELICA herb, seed

This Product is Also Known As
Angelicae Fructus, Angelicae Herba.
CAUTION: See separate listings for Angelica root and Dong Quai.

Scientific Names
Angelica archangelica.
Family: Apiaceae/Umbelliferae.

People Use This For
Historically, people used angelica orally as a diuretic and as a diaphoretic (2).
In food use, angelica is used in candied products to decorate cakes and pastries (5,6).

Safety
LIKELY UNSAFE ...due to the furocoumarins contained in the stem and other plant parts (2,12). Angelica contains a volatile oil. The furocoumarins are angelicin, bergapten, imperatorin, and xanthotoxin. These are photosensitizers and photocarcinogenic (5,8).
PREGNANCY AND LACTATION: UNSAFE ...contraindicated because it seems to be a menstrual and uterine stimulant (12).

Effectiveness
There is insufficient reliable information available about the effectiveness of angelica herb and seed.

Possible Mechanism of Action & Active Ingredients
Angelica contains a volatile oil. It contains furocoumarin which consists of angelicin, bergapten, imperatorin, and xanthotoxin which can make the skin more photosensitive (2).

Adverse Reactions Including Known Allergies
Adverse reactions include photosensitivity (2,6,12). Photodermatitis is possible following contact with plant juice (18).

Possible Interactions with Herbs & Other Dietary Supplements
HERBS WITH ANTICOAGULANT/ANTIPLATELET POTENTIAL: Concomitant use of herbs that have coumarin constituents or affect platelet aggregation could theoretically increase the risk of bleeding in some people. These herbs include: anise, arnica, asafoetida, bogbean, boldo, capsicum, celery, chamomile, clove, danshen, fenugreek, feverfew, garlic, ginger, ginkgo, ginseng Panax, horse chestnut, horseradish, licorice, meadowsweet, prickly ash, onion, papain, passionflower, poplar, quassia, red clover, turmeric, wild carrot, wild lettuce, willow, and others (4,19).

Possible Interactions with Drugs
ACID-INHIBITING DRUGS: Theoretically, due to claims that angelica increases stomach acid, it might interfere with antacids, sucralfate (Carafate), H-2 antagonists, or proton pump inhibitors (19).
ANTICOAGULANTS: Excessive doses can potentiate effects and adverse effects of anticoagulants (4).
HEXOBARBITONE: Theoretically, hepatic metabolism of hexobarbitone might be inhibited by furanocoumarin constituents (4).

Possible Interactions with Foods
No interactions are known to occur, and there is no known reason to expect a clinically significant interaction with angelica herb and seed.

Possible Interactions with Lab Tests
No interactions are known to occur, and there is no known reason to expect a clinically significant interaction with angelica herb and seed.

Possible Interactions with Diseases or Conditions
No interactions are known to occur, and there is no known reason to expect a clinically significant interaction with angelica herb and seed.

Typical Dosages & Routes of Administration that are Commonly Used
ORAL: People typically use 1 teaspoon of the powdered seeds or leaves in 1 cup boiling water and drink as a tea twice daily. As a tincture, angelica is dosed up to 1 teaspoon up to twice a day (5250).

Comments

There has been confusion in the past between angelica and water hemlock. Water hemlock is highly toxic (6).

ANGELICA root

This Product is Also Known As

Garden Angelica, European Angelica, Root of the Holy Ghost, Wild Angelica.
CAUTION: See separate listings for Angelica seed, herb, and Dong Quai.

Scientific Names

Angelica archangelica, synonym Archangelica officinalis; Angelica atropurpurea, Angelica sylvestris; Angelica curtisi; Angelica rosaefolia; Angelica pubescens.
Family: Apiaceae/Umbelliferae.

People Use This For

Orally, angelica root is used for loss of appetite, gastrointestinal spasms, feeling of fullness, and flatulence (2). Topically, it is used to create warmth in neuralgia and rheumatism (6,8), and is used for skin disorders (6). It is also used as part of a multi-ingredient preparation for treating premature ejaculation (2537).
Historically, angelica has been used to promote menstrual flow, as an abortifacient, antiseptic, expectorant, diuretic (5,8,11), and as a cure for the plague (6).

Safety

POSSIBLY SAFE …when the root is used as a medicinal tea or a steam-distilled oil. Although the root contains furanocoumarin constituents that can be phototoxic, photomutagenic, and carcinogenic when exposed to UV light, they are only slightly soluble in water (8), and they are absent in the steam-distilled oil (11). …when used in foods. Angelica has Generally Recognized as Safe (GRAS) status in the US but Canada does not allow archangelica as a nonmedicinal ingredient (12). ...when used topically, short-term as part of a multi-ingredient preparation (SS Cream). This preparation was used safely for premature ejaculation in a clinical trial where the cream was applied and left on the glans penis for 1-hour (2537). Further evaluation is needed to determine its safety after prolonged, repetitive use.
POSSIBLY UNSAFE ...when the root or root extracts are used orally in medicinal amounts (2) because they contain photosensitizing furanocoumarin constituents. ...when applied topically in medicinal amounts. The International Fragrance Association recommends limiting angelica root to a maximum of 0.78% in products to be applied to the skin and exposed to the sun (4,8).
LIKELY UNSAFE …when used orally in large amounts Angelica root preparations can cause poisoning (5). …when used topically in high concentrations.
PREGNANCY: LIKELY UNSAFE ... when used orally. Angelica can have an abortifacient effect (4,12); contraindicated.
POSSIBLY UNSAFE ...when used topically; avoid using.
LACTATION: POSSIBLY UNSAFE ...when used topically; avoid using. There is insufficient reliable information available about the safety of oral use during lactation; avoid using (4).

Effectiveness

POSSIBLY EFFECTIVE ...when taken orally for loss of appetite, gastrointestinal spasms, feeling of fullness, and flatulence. It is approved for these uses (2). ...when used topically for pain and inflammation and treating psoriasis and vitiligo (11). ...when used topically as part of a multi-ingredient preparation for treating premature ejaculation. In one controlled clinical trial, a multi-ingredient cream preparation containing Panax ginseng root, Angelica root, Cistanches deserticola, Zanthoxyl species, Torlidis seed, clove flower, Asiasari root, cinnamon bark, and toad venom (SS Cream) was applied to the glans penis 1-hour prior to intercourse and washed off immediately before intercourse. Men suffering from premature ejaculation who were treated with the cream had significantly improved ejaculatory latency compared to placebo (2537).
There is insufficient reliable information available about the effectiveness of angelica root for its other uses.

Possible Mechanism of Action & Active Ingredients

The constituent, alpha-angelica lactone, can have calcium antagonist effects (11). The coumarins in angelica are responsible for its phototoxicity (12). Volatile emissions from the angelica root can have fungistatic activity (6). The coumarin constituents of related Angelica species can inhibit human platelet aggregation in vitro (736). The related species, Angelica sinensis, can lower prothrombin time in rabbits when coadministered with warfarin (737). The multi-ingredient preparation containing Angelica root is thought to work in premature ejaculation by increasing the penile vibratory threshold and reducing the amplitude of penile somatosensory evoked potentials (2537).

Adverse Reactions Including Known Allergies

Angelica is a photosensitizer, and when used, prolonged exposure to sunlight should be avoided (2,12). Severe poisoning can occur from large doses (5). When the multi-ingredient cream preparation (SS Cream) has been applied topically to the glans penis, sporadic erectile dysfunction, excessively delayed ejaculation, mild pain, and local irritation and burning has occurred (2537).

Possible Interactions with Herbs & Other Dietary Supplements

HERBS WITH ANTICOAGULANT/ANTIPLATELET POTENTIAL: Concomitant use of herbs that have coumarin constituents or affect platelet aggregation could theoretically increase the risk of bleeding in some people. These herbs include: anise, arnica, asafoetida, bogbean, boldo, capsicum, celery, chamomile, clove, danshen, fenugreek, feverfew, garlic, ginger, ginkgo, ginseng (Panax), horse chestnut, horseradish, licorice, meadowsweet, prickly ash, onion, papain, passionflower, poplar, quassia, red clover, turmeric, wild carrot, wild lettuce, willow, and others (4,19).

Possible Interactions with Drugs

ACID-INHIBITING DRUGS: Theoretically, due to claims that angelica increases stomach acid, it might interfere with antacids, sucralfate (Carafate), H-2 antagonists, or proton pump inhibitors (19).
ANTICOAGULANTS: Concomitant use of the angelica root can potentiate the anticoagulant effects of these drugs due to its coumarin constituents (737).
ANTIPLATELET DRUGS: Concomitant use can potentiate the antiplatelet effects (736).
PHOTOSENSITIZING DRUGS: Theoretically, angelica can compound photosensitization and side effects, and concomitant use with these drugs should be avoided.

Possible Interactions with Foods

No interactions are known to occur, and there is no known reason to expect a clinically significant interaction with angelica root.

Possible Interactions with Lab Tests

No interactions are known to occur, and there is no known reason to expect a clinically significant interaction with angelica root.

Possible Interactions with Diseases or Conditions

No interactions are known to occur, and there is no known reason to expect a clinically significant interaction with angelica root.

Typical Dosages & Routes of Administration that are Commonly Used

ORAL: The typical dose of angelica is 4.5 grams per day of the crude root or equivalent preparations for appetite loss and digestive problems, including mild GI tract spasms and flatulence (2). The dose of the fluid extract (1:1) is commonly 1.5-3 grams per day (2). The tincture (1:5) is usually dosed as 1.5 grams per day (2). Do not store angelica root preparations in plastic, because plastic can react with the essential oil (8).

Comments

According to legend, humans began to use the angelica root after an angel explained to them that the plant was a cure for the plague (6). Angelica is often planted in herb gardens as a decorative border and to protect other herbs from the wind (6).

ANGOSTURA

This Product is Also Known As

Angustura, Carony Bark, Cusparia, Cusparia Bark, True Angostura.

Scientific Names

Galipea officinalis.
Family: Rutaceae.

People Use This For

Orally, angostura is used for preventing recurrence of malaria, as an antipyretic, antidiarrheal, and antispasmodic (11). Large doses of angostura can be cathartic and emetic (11).

Safety

LIKELY SAFE ...when used orally, in average food amounts. Average maximum use of extract in alcoholic beverages is 0.3% (11).
There is insufficient reliable information available about the safety of the use of angostura in amounts larger than typical food amounts.
PREGNANCY AND LACTATION: Insufficient reliable information available.

Effectiveness

There is insufficient reliable information available about the effectiveness of angostura.

Possible Mechanism of Action & Active Ingredients

The applicable part of angostura is the bark. Contains angostura bitters 1 and 2, alkaloids, and a volatile oil. Researchers report the alkaloids, cusparine and galipine, have antispasmodic properties (11).

Adverse Reactions Including Known Allergies

Large doses of angostura may cause nausea and vomiting (18).

Possible Interactions with Herbs & Other Dietary Supplements

Insufficient reliable information available.

Possible Interactions with Drugs

No interactions are known to occur, and there is no known reason to expect a clinically significant interaction with angostura.

Possible Interactions with Foods

No interactions are known to occur, and there is no known reason to expect a clinically significant interaction with angostura.

Possible Interactions with Lab Tests

No interactions are known to occur, and there is no known reason to expect a clinically significant interaction with angostura.

Possible Interactions with Diseases or Conditions

No interactions are known to occur, and there is no known reason to expect a clinically significant interaction with angostura.

Typical Dosages & Routes of Administration that are Commonly Used

ORAL: People typically use 300 to 1000 mg of the powdered bark. As a liquid extract, angostura is dosed 0.3 to 2 mL (5264).

Comments

"Angostura bitters" which is sometimes used in mixing alcoholic beverages, no longer contains angostura. It is now made from gentian and other bitters.

There is very little scientific information about this product. Our staff is continually analyzing the available information on natural medicines and we will add data here as it becomes available.

ANISE

This Product is Also Known As

Aniseed, Anisi Fructus, Phytoestrogen, Semen Anisi, Sweet Cumin.

Scientific Names

Pimpinella anisum.
Family: Apiaceae or Umbelliferae.

People Use This For

Orally, anise is used for dyspepsia (2) and as a pediatric antiflatulent and expectorant (6).

Topically, it is used for lice, scabies, and psoriasis treatment (6).

In folk medicine, anise has been used to increase lactation, induce menstruation (8), facilitate birth, increase libido, and alleviate the symptoms of male climacteric, which is the period of life after reproduction functions stop (4).

For food uses, anise is used as a licorice flavor substitute (6). It is often used as a fragrance in food.

In manufacturing, anise is often used as a fragrance in soap, creams, and perfumes.

Safety

LIKELY SAFE ...when anise preparations are used in amounts typically found in food. Anise oil has Generally Recognized as Safe (GRAS) status and is approved for food use (4).

POSSIBLY UNSAFE ...when applied topically, because anise contains coumarin constituents that cause photosensitivity reactions when skin is exposed to UV light. The constituent bergapten is also believed to be carcinogenic (4).

LIKELY UNSAFE ...when the undiluted oil is ingested because 1-5 mL can cause nausea, vomiting, seizures, and pulmonary edema (4).

PREGNANCY: LIKELY SAFE ...when used in food amounts. POSSIBLY UNSAFE ...when used in larger amounts because it might have abortifacient activity (4,12).

LACTATION: LIKELY SAFE ...when used in amounts commonly found in foods (4). Excessive amounts should be avoided because anise contains anethole and estragole, which are structurally similar to safrole, a known hepatotoxin and carcinogen (4).

Effectiveness

LIKELY EFFECTIVE ...when taken orally as an expectorant or mild antispasmodic (2,6,7,11). There is insufficient reliable information available about the effectiveness of anise for its other uses.

Possible Mechanism of Action & Active Ingredients

The applicable parts of anise are the dried fruit, seed, and oil. Anise is rich in calcium and iron (19). The trans-anethole, a major component of the anise oil, is responsible for its characteristic taste, smell, and medicinal properties. Anethole has a structure similar to catecholamines, such as adrenaline, noradrenaline, and dopamine (4), and to the hallucinogenic compound, myristicin (4). Estrogenic activity can be due to anethole and the anethole polymers, dianethole and photoanethole (4,11). The other constituents of anise include the coumarins umbelliferone, umbelliprenine, bergapten, and scopoletin (6).

Adverse Reactions Including Known Allergies

Allergic reactions to anise include reactions of the skin, respiratory, and GI tract, and photosensitivity (4). Excessive doses of anise can cause adverse neurological effects (4). The ingestion of 1-5 mL of the oil can cause nausea, vomiting, seizures, and pulmonary edema (4).

Possible Interactions with Herbs & Other Dietary Supplements

HERBS WITH ANTICOAGULANT/ANTIPLATELET POTENTIAL: Concomitant use of herbs that have coumarin constituents or affect platelet aggregation could theoretically increase the risk of bleeding in some people. These herbs include: angelica, arnica, asafoetida, bogbean, boldo, capsicum, celery, chamomile, clove, danshen, fenugreek, feverfew, garlic, ginger, ginkgo, ginseng (Panax), horse chestnut, horseradish, licorice, meadowsweet, prickly ash, onion, papain, passionflower, poplar, quassia, red clover, turmeric, wild carrot, wild lettuce, willow, and others (4,19).

Possible Interactions with Drugs

EXCESSIVE DOSES of anise can interfere with anticoagulant therapy, monoamine oxidase inhibitors (MAOIs), and hormone therapy (4).

Possible Interactions with Foods

No interactions are known to occur, and there is no known reason to expect a clinically significant interaction with anise.

Possible Interactions with Lab Tests

BLOOD PRESSURE: Theoretically, anise might increase blood pressure and blood pressure readings, due to the catecholamine activity of the constituent anethole (4,11).
HEART RATE: Theoretically, anise might increase heart rate and pulse rate due to the catecholamine activity of the constituent anethole (4,11).
INTERNATIONAL NORMALIZED RATIO (INR), PROTHROMBIN TIME (PT): Theoretically, excessive use of anise might prolong coagulation, increasing PT/INR and test results, due to coumarins contained in anise (4).

Possible Interactions with Diseases or Conditions

SKIN REACTONS: Anise oil potentially can be irritating and photosensitizing. Avoid its use in cases of dermatitis and inflammatory or allergic skin reactions (4).
ANTICOAGULANT-, ESTROGENIC-, and CATECHOLAMINE-SENSITIVE: Anise should be used with caution in these conditions. Anise contains coumarin constituents with anticoagulant, estrogenic, and catecholamine-like properties. Theoretically these could interact with diseases or conditions sensitive to such ingredients.

Typical Dosages & Routes of Administration that are Commonly Used

ORAL: The typical dose of anise is 0.5-1 grams of the dried fruit, 50-200 mL of the essential oil, or as a tea, three times per day (4). The tea is prepared by steeping 1-2 teaspoons of the crushed seed for 10-15 minutes and then straining (4). As an expectorant, a cup of the tea is commonly taken in the morning and/or at night. As an antiflatulent, 1 tablespoon of the tea is usually taken several times a day. For nursing babies and infants, the typical dose is one teaspoon of the tea (8).

Comments

Anise is not considered a primary irritant, but its use can be associated with skin and mouth irritation and sensitization. Bergapten, a constituent, can cause photosensitivity and could be carcinogenic (6). As a flavoring agent, anise has a sweet, aromatic taste similar to licorice. It is commonly used in alcohols and liqueurs, such as Ouzo, Benedictine, Boonekamp, and Danziger Goldwasser. It is also used in dairy products, gelatins, meats, candies, breath fresheners, perfumes, soaps, and sachets (8).

ANNATTO

This Product is Also Known As
Achiote, Achiotillo, Annotta, Arnotta.

Scientific Names
Bixa orellana.
Family: Bixaceae.

People Use This For
In food, annatto is used as a coloring agent (11).

Safety
LIKELY SAFE ...when used in food amounts (12).

Effectiveness
There is insufficient information available about the effectiveness of annatto.

Possible Mechanism of Action & Active Ingredients
The applicable part of annatto is the seed. Researchers think the coloring principles are carotenoids, mostly bixin and norbixin (11), which do not have vitamin A activity (11). No pharmacological information available (11).

Adverse Reactions Including Known Allergies
None reported.

Possible Interactions with Herbs & Other Dietary Supplements
Insufficient reliable information available.

Possible Interactions with Drugs
DIABETES THERAPY: Monitor blood glucose level closely due to claims that annatto has hyperglycemic effects (19).

Possible Interactions with Foods
No interactions are known to occur, and there is no known reason to expect a clinically significant interaction with annatto.

Possible Interactions with Lab Tests
No interactions are known to occur, and there is no known reason to expect a clinically significant interaction with annatto.

Possible Interactions with Diseases or Conditions
No interactions are known to occur, and there is no known reason to expect a clinically significant interaction with annatto.

Typical Dosages & Routes of Administration that are Commonly Used
ORAL: People typically use 1 to 2 grams of powdered leaf in tablets or capsules twice daily. Annatto is also taken as a 4:1 tincture in a dose of 2 to 4 mL twice daily (5255).

Comments
No reliable information available for medicinal uses. This product is used commercially as a food coloring agent (11).

APPLE

This Product is Also Known As
None.

Scientific Names
Malus sylvestris
Family: Rosaceae.

People Use This For
Orally, apples are used to control diarrhea or constipation (6).
Orally, apple juice is used for the softening, passage and collection of gallstones (3472).
In folk medicine, apples are used for treating cancer, diabetes, dysentery, fever, heart ailments, scurvy, warts, and cleaning teeth (6).

Safety
LIKELY SAFE ...when eaten without seeds.
PREGNANCY AND LACTATION: LIKELY SAFE; avoid seeds (6).

Effectiveness
LIKELY EFFECTIVE ...when taken orally for diarrhea and constipation (6).
POSSIBLY EFFECTIVE ...when taken orally to maintain good lung function (3469). Preliminary evidence suggests a positive association may exist between lung function (measured as maximum forced expiration volume in one second) and the frequent consumption of apples (five or more apples per week) (3469). ...when taken orally to lower the risk of lung cancer (3470). Another study suggests an inverse association may exist between lung cancer risk and foods containing quercetin, a flavonoid found in high concentrations in apples (3470). ...when taken orally to soften gallstones. A report suggests apple juice taken orally for seven days, with olive oil taken on the seventh day, may be effective for the softening, passage and collection of gallstones in the stool (3472).

Possible Mechanism of Action & Active Ingredients
The applicable part of apple is the fruit. The pectin in apples probably accounts for their effect on diarrhea and constipation. Pectin absorbs water in the GI tract and swells to a gummy mass. As such, it provides bulk which normalizes hard stools or diarrhea (6). Apples also contain phloretin, which has antibacterial activity (6). The exact mechanism by which apples may affect lung function or lower the risk of lung cancer is unknown. The antioxidant effects of quercetin, a flavonoid found in high concentrations in apples, has been theorized as a possible mechanism (3469,3470). Human studies are needed to determine whether an association between apple consumption and lung function or lung cancer risk does exist. It is unknown how apple juice may soften gallstones.

Adverse Reactions Including Known Allergies
No adverse reactions are generally known or predicted to occur with apple fruit. One death is attributed to ingestion of large amount (a cupful) of seeds, which contain hydrogen cyanide (HCN) (6). Ingestion of large amount of seeds may cause cyanide poisoning, leading to death. To release cyanide, seeds must be hydrolyzed in the stomach, and several hours may elapse before poisoning symptoms occur (6).

Possible Interactions with Herbs & Other Dietary Supplements
Insufficient reliable information available.

Possible Interactions with Drugs
No interactions are known to occur, and there is no known reason to expect a clinically significant interaction with apple.

Possible Interactions with Foods
No interactions are known to occur, and there is no known reason to expect a clinically significant interaction with apple.

Possible Interactions with Lab Tests
No interactions are known to occur, and there is no known reason to expect a clinically significant interaction with apple.

Possible Interactions with Diseases or Conditions
No interactions are known to occur, and there is no known reason to expect a clinically significant interaction with apple.

Typical Dosages & Routes of Administration that are Commonly Used
ORAL: People typically use 500 mg apple pectin capsules daily as a supplement. Some sources recommend "an apple a day". A maximum daily dose has not been established. Dried apple peels are used to make a tea: 1 to 2 teaspoons with 1 cup simmering water. The usual dose is from 1 to 3 cups per day (5250,5263,6006). For the softening of gallstones, one liter of apple juice taken daily for seven days with 1 cup of olive oil taken on the seventh day before going to bed has been used (3472).

Comments
None.

APPLE CIDER VINEGAR

This Product is Also Known As
Cider Vinegar.
CAUTION: See separate listing for Apple.

Scientific Names
None.

People Use This For

Orally, people use apple cider vinegar alone or with honey for weight loss, for leg cramps and pain, queasy stomach, sore throats, sinus problems, high blood pressure, arthritis, for helping rid the body of toxins (5904,5906), to stimulate thinking and slow the aging process (5906), to regulate blood pressure, to fight infection, and to fight osteoporosis (5907).

In combination, apple cider vinegar is used orally with grapefruit and kelp for weight loss (5904). Also in combination, apple cider vinegar is used orally with cayenne, ginger, bromelain, and citrin to maintain healthy cholesterol levels and for weight reduction (5903). In combination, apple cider vinegar is also used orally with gotu kola for curbing appetite; detoxifying the body; weight loss; boosting the immune system; treating arthritis; lowering cholesterol; improving circulation; supplying amino acids, minerals, and vitamins; and aiding in the effective metabolism of food (5905).

Topically, apple cider vinegar is used for acne; as a skin toner; as an ingredient in hair rinse (5904,5910); to soothe sunburn, shingles, and bites; and to prevent dandruff, baldness and itchy scalp (5907). It is also used in the bath for vaginitis (5910).

Safety

LIKELY SAFE ...when apple cider vinegar is used orally as food flavoring. ...when used topically, diluted.
POSSIBLY UNSAFE ...when apple cider vinegar is used in amounts of 250 mL per day long term. There is one report of an individual who developed hypokalemia, elevated renin levels, and osteoporosis after 6 years of ingesting 250 mL apple cider vinegar per day (5911).
There is insufficient reliable information available about apple cider tablets.
PREGNANCY AND LACTATION: LIKELY SAFE ...when apple cider vinegar is used orally as a food flavoring.
POSSIBLY UNSAFE ...when used in larger amounts; avoid using.

Effectiveness

There is insufficient reliable information available about the effectiveness of apple cider vinegar.

Possible Mechanism of Action & Active Ingredients

Cider vinegar is fermented juice from crushed apples. Like apple juice, it probably contains some pectin; vitamin B1, B2, B6; biotin; folic acid; niacin; pantothenic acid; and vitamin C. It also contains small amounts of the minerals sodium, phosphorous, potassium, calcium, iron, and magnesium (5912).

Adverse Reactions Including Known Allergies

There is one published report of an individual who developed hypokalemia, high renin levels, and osteoporosis after ingesting 250 mL apple cider vinegar daily for 6 years.

Possible Interactions with Herbs & Other Dietary Supplements

HERBS WITH CARDIAC ACTIVITY: Theoretically, the overuse of apple cider vinegar can increase the risk of cardiotoxicity due to potassium depletion. Cardioactive herbs include digitalis, lily-of-the-valley, pheasant's eye, and squill.
STIMULANT LAXATIVE HERBS: Theoretically, overuse of apple cider vinegar and stimulant laxative herbs can increase the risk of potassium depletion. Stimulant laxative herbs include aloe vera, alder buckthorn, European buckthorn, cascara sagrada, castor oil, rhubarb, and senna.
HORSETAIL, LICORICE: Theoretically, overuse of apple cider vinegar can increase the risk of potassium depletion from overuse of horsetail or licorice.

Possible Interactions with Drugs

POTASSIUM DEPLETING DIURETICS: Theoretically, overuse of apple cider vinegar concomitantly with potassium-depleting diuretics might increase the risk of hypokalemia (5911)
INSULIN: Theoretically, overuse of apple cider vinegar concomitantly with insulin might cause hypokalemia (5911).
CARDIOVASCULAR DRUGS: Theoretically, overuse of apple cider vinegar could decrease potassium levels, increasing the risk of toxicity of cardiovascular drugs such as digoxin (Lanoxin).

Possible Interactions with Foods

No interactions are known to occur, and there is no known reason to expect a clinically significant interaction with apple cider vinegar.

Possible Interactions with Lab Tests

POTASSIUM LEVEL: Theoretically, long-term use or high doses can reduce serum potassium level and increase urine potassium level (5911).
URINARY ANION GAP: In one case report, long-term use of 250 mL apple cider vinegar per day was associated with high positive urinary anion gap (5911).

Possible Interactions with Diseases or Conditions

DIABETES: Theoretically, long-term use or high doses of apple cider vinegar might increase potassium loss of individuals using insulin.
OSTEOPOROSIS: Theoretically, long-term use or high doses might cause osteoporosis (5911).

Typical Dosages & Routes of Administration that are Commonly Used

ORAL: To aid digestion, a 285 mg tablet taken with each meal, has been used (5909). A typical dose for weight loss is 1 ounce apple cider vinegar, 1 teaspoon of honey in 1-4 ounces of warm water before each meal (5904). A dose for a cold is 2 tablespoons cider vinegar in 1 cup water three times daily (5904). A dose for arthritis is 2 teaspoons of apple cider vinegar and two teaspoon of honey in a glass of water daily (5905). A dose for high blood pressure is 2 teaspoons of apple cider vinegar mixed in water in the morning (5905).

IN BATH: For vaginitis add 3 cups of apple cider vinegar to hot bath and soak, spreading legs to allow water into vagina (5910).

Comments

None.

APRICOT

This Product is Also Known As

Chinese Almond, Laetrile, Vitamin B17.

Scientific Names

Prunus armeniaca.
Family: Rosaceae.

People Use This For

In Chinese medicine very small amounts of toxic kernel constituent, hydrocyanic acid, a source of HCN is used for asthma, cough, and constipation (6).

In folk medicine, uses of apricot include hemorrhage, infertility, eye inflammation, spasm, and vaginal infections (6).

Historically, laetrile, the semi-synthetic derivative of amygdalin constituent, has been fraudulently acclaimed as a cancer treatment (4).

In manufacturing, apricot oil is used in cosmetics or as a vehicle for pharmaceutical preparations (6).

Safety

POSSIBLY SAFE …when apricot oil is used topically (6).

LIKELY UNSAFE …when apricot kernels are taken orally because they are a source of cyanide. Acute poisonings may progress to respiratory failure, coma and death within 15 minutes (4). The lethal dose is 50-60 kernels (12) but amount may vary (4). Chronic poisoning can also occur (4).

CHILDREN: POSSIBLY SAFE …when apricot oil is used topically (6). LIKELY UNSAFE …when apricot kernels are ingested. The lethal dose is 7-10 kernels (12) but amount may vary (4).

PREGNANCY AND LACTATION: POSSIBLY SAFE …when apricot oil is used topically (6). LIKELY UNSAFE …when apricot kernels are ingested (4,12).

Effectiveness

INEFFECTIVE …when used to treat cancer (4,5).

There is insufficient reliable information available about the effectiveness of apricot for its other uses.

Possible Mechanism of Action & Active Ingredients

The applicable parts of apricot are the kernel and oil. Apricot contains fruit acids, a variety of sugars, vitamins C, K, beta-carotene, thiamine, niacin, and iron. The seed contains the glycoside amygdalin which yields laetrile and hydrocyanic acid (6). Several popular theories that have now been disproved claimed preferential uptake and conversion of amygdalin to hydrogen cyanide in tumor cells. Actually, research shows that amygdalin is slowly hydrolyzed to HCN in stomach, rapidly absorbed via GI tract, and then diffused through body (4).

Adverse Reactions Including Known Allergies

Apricot may cause acute poisoning, with symptoms including dizziness, headache, nausea, vomiting, drowsiness, dyspnea, palpitations, marked hypotension, convulsions, paralysis, coma, and death (4). Apricot may also cause chronic poisoning, with symptoms of increased blood thiocyanate, goiter, thyroid cancer, optic nerve lesions, blindness, ataxia, hypertonia, cretinism and mental retardation. Demyelinating lesions and neuromyopathies reportedly occur secondary to chronic exposure, including long-term therapy (4).

Possible Interactions with Herbs & Other Dietary Supplements

Insufficient reliable information available.

Possible Interactions with Drugs

No interactions are known to occur, and there is no known reason to expect a clinically significant interaction with apricot.

Possible Interactions with Foods

No interactions are known to occur, and there is no known reason to expect a clinically significant interaction with apricot.

Possible Interactions with Lab Tests

No interactions are known to occur, and there is no known reason to expect a clinically significant interaction with apricot.

Possible Interactions with Diseases or Conditions

No interactions are known to occur, and there is no known reason to expect a clinically significant interaction with apricot.

Typical Dosages & Routes of Administration that are Commonly Used

ORAL: People typically take from 3 to 9 grams of apricot seed (5268).

Comments

In 1984, amygdalin found in the seed was classified prescription-only to protect the general public (4).

ARECA

This Product is Also Known As

Areca Nut, Betel Nut, Betel Quid, Pinlag, Pinag.

Scientific Names

Areca catechu.
Family: Palmaceae.

People Use This For

Areca nut is widely used as a recreational drug (18) because of its CNS-stimulating properties. But it is rarely used therapeutically.

In veterinary medicine, an extract of areca nut is used for expelling tapeworms in cattle, dogs, and horses (6,18), as a cathartic, and for treating intestinal colic in horses (6).

Historically, areca nut has been used for glaucoma and as a mild stimulant or digestive aid (6).

Safety

LIKELY UNSAFE ...when the nut is used long-term. Two constituents, arecaidine and arecoline, have documented carcinogenic potential (6). Precancerous lesions and squamous cell carcinoma are common in long-time users (6,17). Another constituent, arecaine, is poisonous. Ingesting 8-30 grams of areca nut can cause death (6). ...when used by individuals with asthma because areca nut can trigger or aggravate symptoms (6).

There is insufficient reliable information available about the safety of areca for short-term use.

PREGNANCY AND LACTATION: LIKELY UNSAFE ...when the nut is used long-term. Short-term use should be avoided because constituents have CNS stimulant and cholinergic effects (6,17).

Effectiveness

There is insufficient reliable information available about the effectiveness of areca.

Possible Mechanism of Action & Active Ingredients

The applicable part of areca is the nut. Researchers think alkaloid components have cholinergic action similar to pilocarpine (explains use in glaucoma) but greater CNS action (6). The constituent, arecoline, has antihelmintic activity (6). Experimental evidence suggests constituents, arecaidine and arecoline, have carcinogenic potential (6). Consumption of areca is associated with cardiovascular disease, diabetes, asthma (326), and oral cancer (329).

Adverse Reactions Including Known Allergies

Chewing areca nut results in red-stained mouth, lips, and feces (18). Areca nut may cause pupil dilation, increased salivation, vomiting, diarrhea, gingivitis, and periodontitis (6). High doses can cause convulsions and death (6). Chewing betel quids (see COMMENTS) is likely to produce CNS stimulation similar to caffeine and tobacco (6). Areca and betel quid chewing can cause oral submucous fibrosis in susceptible individuals (327,328,329).

Possible Interactions with Herbs & Other Dietary Supplements

Insufficient reliable information available.

Possible Interactions with Drugs

ANTI-CHOLINERGIC DRUGS: Theoretically, due to cholinergic effects (6) areca nut can interfere with anti-cholinergic drug therapy. Avoid concomitant use.

CHOLINERGIC DRUGS: Theoretically, due to cholinergic effects (6) areca nut can increase the effects and risk of side effects of cholinergic drugs. Avoid concomitant use.

PROCYCLIDINE: Concomitant use can reduce anticholinergic effects of procyclidine (Kemadrin) given to treat the extrapyramidal effects of fluphenazine (19).

Possible Interactions with Foods
No interactions are known to occur, and there is no known reason to expect a clinically significant interaction with areca.

Possible Interactions with Lab Tests
FECAL LAB TESTS: Chewing nuts stains feces red (18). This coloration may interfere with fecal lab tests.

Possible Interactions with Diseases or Conditions
ASTHMA: May aggravate asthma (6).

Typical Dosages & Routes of Administration that are Commonly Used
No typical dosage.

Comments
Areca is considered likely unsafe; avoid using. Areca nut is chewed alone or in the form of betel quids, a mixture of tobacco, powdered or sliced betel nut, and slaked lime wrapped in the leaf of "betel" vine (Piper betel) (6).

ARENARIA RUBRA

This Product is Also Known As
Common Sandspurry, Sabline Rouge, Sandwort.

Scientific Names
Spergularia rubra.
Family: Not available.

People Use This For
Orally, arenaria rubra is used to treat urinary tract disorders, cystitis, dysuria, and urinary calculi (18).

Safety
There is insufficient reliable information available about the safety of arenaria rubra.
Pregnancy and Lactation: Insufficient reliable information available; avoid using.

Effectiveness
There is insufficient reliable information available about the effectiveness of arenaria rubra.

Possible Mechanism of Action & Active Ingredients
Arenaria rubra is stated to have diuretic effects (18).

Adverse Reactions Including Known Allergies
None reported.

Possible Interactions with Herbs & Other Dietary Supplements
Insufficient reliable information available.

Possible Interactions with Drugs
No interactions are known to occur, and there is no known reason to expect a clinically significant interaction with arenaria rubra.

Possible Interactions with Foods
No interactions are known to occur, and there is no known reason to expect a clinically significant interaction with arenaria rubra.

Possible Interactions with Lab Tests
No interactions are known to occur, and there is no known reason to expect a clinically significant interaction with arenaria rubra.

Possible Interactions with Diseases or Conditions
No interactions are known to occur, and there is no known reason to expect a clinically significant interaction with arenaria rubra.

Typical Dosages & Routes of Administration that are Commonly Used
ORAL: People typically prepare the herb as a liquid extract and take 2 to 4 mL (5264).

Comments
There is very little scientific information about this product. Our staff is continually analyzing the available information on natural medicines and will add data here as it becomes available.

ARISTOLOCHIA

This Product is Also Known As
Birthwort, Long Birthwort, Pelican Flower, Sangrel, Serpentaria, Snakeweed, Virginia Serpentary, Virginia Snakeroot.

Scientific Names
Aristolochia serpentaria; Aristolochia clematitis.
Family: Aristolochiaceae.

People Use This For
Orally, aristolochia is used as an aphrodisiac, anticonvulsant, immune stimulant, and to promote menstruation (400). It is sometimes used to treat allergic gastrointestinal colic and gallbladder colic (18).

Safety
UNSAFE ...when used orally. Aristolochia contains aristolochic acid which is nephrotoxic and carcinogenic (18,6118,6119). The FDA considers all products containing aristolochic acid to be unsafe and adulterated (6119).
PREGNANCY AND LACTATION: UNSAFE ...when used orally; contraindicated (6118,6119).

Effectiveness
LIKELY INEFFECTIVE ...for any use (400).

Possible Mechanism of Action & Active Ingredients
The applicable parts of aristolochia are the above ground parts and root. Aristolochia contains aristolochic acid which is nephrotoxic and carcinogenic. Aristolochic acid has been associated with cancers of the kidney, bladder, stomach, lung, and lymphoma in rodents and cancers of the bladder, ureter, and/or renal pelvis in people with aristolochic acid-associated nephropathy (see Adverse Reactions) (6118).

Adverse Reactions Including Known Allergies
Use of aristolochia can cause vomiting, gastroenteritis, spasms, severe kidney damage, and death (18). There have been more than 100 cases of nephropathy, referred to as "Chinese herb nephropathy", characterized by interstitial fibrosis and associated with tea believed adulterated with aristolochia. Of these cases, 43 progressed to end stage renal failure requiring dialysis or transplantation (564,6142) and 18 developed urothelial carcinomas of the bladder, ureter, and/or renal pelvis (6142).

Possible Interactions with Herbs & Other Dietary Supplements
Insufficient reliable information available.

Possible Interactions with Drugs
ACID-INHIBITING DRUGS: Theoretically, due to claims that aristolochia increases stomach acid, it might interfere with antacids, sucralfate (Carafate), H-2 antagonists, or proton pump inhibitors (19).

Possible Interactions with Foods
No interactions are known to occur, and there is no known reason to expect a clinically significant interaction with aristolochia.

Possible Interactions with Lab Tests
KIDNEY FUNCTION TESTS: Aristolochia can cause nephropathy and abnormal kidney function results (564).

Possible Interactions with Diseases or Conditions
GI IRRITATION: Can irritate gastrointestinal tract. Contraindicated in individuals with infectious or inflammatory gastrointestinal conditions (19).

Typical Dosages & Routes of Administration that are Commonly Used
ORAL: When the plant is in flower, the entire plant is used. The root alone is also used. A liquid preparation of aristolochia is prepared by adding 2 teaspoons of the fresh plant or root to 1 cup of water and boiling for 10 minutes. A cold extract is prepared by adding 2 teaspoons of the plant or root to 1 cup cold water, which is allowed to stand for 6 to 8 hours. Sources warn against the toxicity of aristolochia and suggest that a dosage should be obtained from a health care professional (5263).

Comments
The FDA considers all products containing aristolochic acid to be unsafe and adulterated (6119). The FDA intends to automatically detain, without physical examination, any product which contains plants known or suspected to contain aristolochic acid, or which might be adulterated with plants known to contain aristolochic acid. Each detained product will be released only after the responsible party provides direct analytical evidence that it is free

of aristolochic acid (6119). Aristolochia is also banned in Germany, Austria, France, Great Britain, Belgium, and Japan (367).

Health Canada, the Canadian health authority, removed five aristolochia-containing Chinese herbal medicine products from sale. The products include, Touku Natural Herbal Rheumatic Pills, two brands of Tri-Snakegall & Fritillary Powder, Tracheitis Pills and Gastropathy Capsules (367).

ARNICA

This Product is Also Known As
Arnica Flos, Arnica Flower, Arnikablüten, Bergwohlverleih, Fleurs d'Arnica, Kraftwurz, Leopard's Bane, Mountain Tobacco, Wolf's Bane, Wundkraut.

Scientific Names
Arnica montana; Arnica fulgens; Arnica sororia; Arnica latifolia; Arnica cordifolia.
Family: Asteraceae or Compositae.

People Use This For
Topically, arnica is used for the inflammation and immune system stimulation associated with bruises, aches, and sprains (5,11), for mouth and throat inflammation (2), insect bites, and superficial phlebitis (2).
Historically, arnica has been used as an abortifacient (8).
For food uses, arnica is a flavor ingredient in alcoholic beverages, nonalcoholic beverages, frozen dairy desserts, candy, baked goods, gelatins, and puddings (11).
In manufacturing, arnica is used in hair tonics and anti-dandruff preparations. The oil is used in perfumes and other cosmetic preparations (11).

Safety
POSSIBLY SAFE ...when used as a flavoring in alcoholic beverages (12), although Canadian regulations do not allow its use as a nonmedicinal ingredient in oral products (12). Flavoring use is allowed in the US (12), but maximum use level is usually 0.03%. ...when used topically for short-term use on unbroken skin (12).
LIKELY UNSAFE ...when taken orally. Arnica is considered poisonous and has caused severe or fatal poisonings (5). It can be cardiotoxic and cause large increases in blood pressure (5,17). Arnica is irritating to mucous membranes and can cause gastroenteritis, muscle paralysis (voluntary and cardiac), an increase or decrease in pulse rate, heart palpitations, shortness of breath, and death (4,17).
PREGNANCY AND LACTATION: LIKELY UNSAFE; avoid using (12).

Effectiveness
There is insufficient reliable information available about the effectiveness of arnica.

Possible Mechanism of Action & Active Ingredients
The applicable part of arnica is the flowerhead. The sesquiterpenoid lactones of arnica are the active principles and produce anti-inflammatory and analgesic effects. They also can have some antibiotic activity (5). Two components of arnica, helenalin and 11 alpha,13-dihyrohelenalin, inhibit human platelet function (104).

Adverse Reactions Including Known Allergies
Arnica taken orally can cause irritation of mucous membranes, drowsiness, stomach pain, vomiting, diarrhea, tachycardia, shortness of breath, coma, and death (4,6,11). It can cause an allergic reaction in individuals sensitive to the Asteraceae/Compositae family. Members of this family include ragweed, chrysanthemums, marigolds, daisies, and many other herbs. Topically, arnica can cause contact dermatitis and mucous membrane irritation (6,11).

Possible Interactions with Herbs & Other Dietary Supplements
HERBS WITH ANTICOAGULANT/ANTIPLATELET POTENTIAL: Concomitant use of herbs that have coumarin constituents or affect platelet aggregation could theoretically increase the risk of bleeding in some people. These herbs include: angelica, anise, asafoetida, bogbean, boldo, capsicum, celery, chamomile, clove, danshen, fenugreek, feverfew, garlic, ginger, ginkgo, ginseng (Panax), horse chestnut, horseradish, licorice, meadowsweet, prickly ash, onion, papain, passionflower, poplar, quassia, red clover, turmeric, wild carrot, wild lettuce, willow, and others (4,19).

Possible Interactions with Drugs
ANTICOAGULANTS AND ANTIPLATELET DRUGS: Theoretically, arnica can potentiate the effects of anticoagulants and antiplatelet drugs.

Possible Interactions with Foods
No interactions are known to occur, and there is no known reason to expect a clinically significant interaction with arnica.

Possible Interactions with Lab Tests
PLATELET FUNCTION: Theoretically, arnica might inhibit platelet function and test results (104).

Possible Interactions with Diseases or Conditions
BROKEN SKIN: Avoid the use of arnica on broken or damaged skin (2,4).
CROSS-ALLERGENICITY: Arnica can cause reactions in individuals allergic to plants in the Asteraceae or Compositae family, which include ragweed, chrysanthemums, marigolds, daisies, and many other herbs (12,17).
GI IRRITATION: Can irritate gastrointestinal tract. Contraindicated in individuals with infectious or inflammatory gastrointestinal conditions (19).

Typical Dosages & Routes of Administration that are Commonly Used
TOPICAL: The typical strength of arnica is 2 grams of the flowerheads in 100 mL water (8). For a poultice, the tincture of arnica is diluted three to ten times with water (8). For a mouthwash, the tincture is diluted ten times (8). The mouthwash should not be swallowed. Ointments commonly have a maximum of 20-25% of the tincture or 15% of the oil (8). The tincture is usually a 1:10 dilution (2), and the oil is usually made with 1 part herb extract to 5 parts vegetable fixed oil (2,8).

Comments
Avoid internal use of arnica because it can be poisonous and cardiotoxic.

ARRACH

This Product is Also Known As
Dog's Arrach, Goat's Arrach, Goosefoot, Netchweed, Oraches, Stinking Arrach, Stinking Goosefoot, Stinking Motherwort.

Scientific Names
Chenopodium vulvaria.

People Use This For
Orally, arrach is used to relieve cramps and induce menstruation (18).
Topically, arrach is used to relieve cramps (18).

Safety
There is insufficient reliable information available about the safety of arrach.
Pregnancy and Lactation: Insufficient reliable information available; avoid using.

Effectiveness
There is insufficient reliable information available about the effectiveness of arrach.

Possible Mechanism of Action & Active Ingredients
The applicable part of arrach is the whole flowering plant. Chenopodium species are stated to be potentially photosensitizing (19).

Adverse Reactions Including Known Allergies
When taken orally, arrach can be potentially photosensitizing. Excessive periods in the sun should be avoided (19).

Possible Interactions with Herbs & Other Dietary Supplements
Insufficient reliable information available.

Possible Interactions with Drugs
PSORALENS: Theoretically, concomitant use of arrach can increase risk of adverse effects, as unspecified Chenopodium species are associated with photosensitivity (19).

Possible Interactions with Foods
No interactions are known to occur, and there is no known reason to expect a clinically significant interaction with arrach.

Possible Interactions with Lab Tests
No interactions are known to occur, and there is no known reason to expect a clinically significant interaction with arrach.

Possible Interactions with Diseases or Conditions
No interactions are known to occur, and there is no known reason to expect a clinically significant interaction with arrach.

Typical Dosages & Routes of Administration that are Commonly Used
ORAL: People typically use a liquid extract of arrach, 2 to 4 mL taken 3 or 4 times daily (5264).

Comments
There is very little scientific information about this product. Our staff is continually analyzing the available information on natural medicines and will add data here as it becomes available.

ARROWROOT

This Product is Also Known As
Maranta.

Scientific Names
Maranta arundinaceae.
Family: Marantaceae.

People Use This For
Orally, arrowroot is used as a nutritional food for infants and convalescents. Babies cut teeth on arrowroot cookies. It is used as an ingredient in cooking. It is also used as a dietary aid in gastrointestinal disorders and acute diarrhea. Topically, arrowroot is used as a soothing agent for painful, irritated or inflamed mucous membranes (18).

Safety
LIKELY SAFE ...when the starch from the root or rhizome are used orally in amounts found in foods (12).
POSSIBLY SAFE ...when used orally or topically in medicinal amounts (12).
PREGNANCY AND LACTATION: POSSIBLY SAFE ...when used in amounts found in foods. There is insufficient reliable information available about the safety of larger amounts used during pregnancy and lactation; avoid using.

Effectiveness
There is insufficient reliable information available about the effectiveness of arrowroot.

Possible Mechanism of Action & Active Ingredients
The applicable part of arrowroot is the starch from the root/rhizome. Animal data suggests that arrowroot may reduce deposited cholesterol in the aorta and heart muscle. This may be due to an increase in the elimination of cholesterol in the form of bile acids (18).

Adverse Reactions Including Known Allergies
None reported.

Possible Interactions with Herbs & Other Dietary Supplements
Insufficient reliable information available.

Possible Interactions with Drugs
No interactions are known to occur, and there is no known reason to expect a clinically significant interaction with arrowroot.

Possible Interactions with Foods
No interactions are known to occur, and there is no known reason to expect a clinically significant interaction with arrowroot.

Possible Interactions with Lab Tests
No interactions are known to occur, and there is no known reason to expect a clinically significant interaction with arrowroot.

Possible Interactions with Diseases or Conditions
No interactions are known to occur, and there is no known reason to expect a clinically significant interaction with arrowroot.

Typical Dosages & Routes of Administration that are Commonly Used
Arrowroot starch is extracted from the chopped root/rhizome by a specific process using water. The powdered starch is then boiled with water and taken orally (18).

Comments
Arrowroot is often replaced with cheaper starches, including potato, corn, wheat, or rice starch (18).

ARTICHOKE

This Product is Also Known As

Alcachofa, Alcaucil, Artichaut Commun, Artischocke, Cardo, Cardo de Comer, Cardon d'Espagne, Cardoon, Garden Artichoke, Gemuseartischocke, Globe Artichoke, Kardone, Tyosen-Azami.

Scientific Names

Cynara scolymus, synonym Cynara cardunculus.
Family: Asteraceae or Compositae.

People Use This For

Orally, artichoke is used for dyspepsia (2), hyperlipidemia (4), and nausea (2056). It is also used as a diuretic and choleretic (4).

Traditionally, artichoke has been used for treating snakebites, renal insufficiency, anemia, edema, arthritis, cystitis, hepatoprotection (3272) and stimulating liver function (4), preventing gallstones, lowering blood pressure, as a hypoglycemic, diuretic, stimulant, and a tonic (3272).

In foods, artichoke leaves and extracts are used as flavoring agents in beverages. The constituents, cynarin and chlorogenic acid, are sometimes used as sweeteners (11).

Safety

LIKELY SAFE ...when used orally in amounts found in food. Artichoke is approved for food use in the US in alcoholic beverages in concentrations up to 0.00016% (16 ppm) (4,11).
POSSIBLY SAFE ...when used orally and appropriately in therapeutic amounts (2,11,2056).
PREGNANCY AND LACTATION: LIKELY SAFE ...when used orally in amounts found in food (11). There is insufficient reliable information about the safety of therapeutic amounts of artichoke used during pregnancy or lactation; avoid using (4).

Effectiveness

POSSIBLY EFFECTIVE ...when used orally for relieving symptoms of dyspepsia (2,2056). Both artichoke leaf (2) and artichoke leaf extract are used (7,2056). In studies, artichoke leaf extract has significantly reduced symptoms such as nausea, vomiting, flatulence, and abdominal pain in idiopathic dyspepsia and dyspepsia associated with biliary disease. Improvement was seen after 2-6 weeks of treatment (2056).
There is insufficient reliable information available about the effectiveness of artichoke for its other uses.

Possible Mechanism of Action & Active Ingredients

The applicable parts of artichoke are the leaf, stem, and root (4,11). The primary constituents include up to 2% phenolic acids, primarily chlorogenic acid, cynarin, and caffeic acid. Also, up to 4% sesquiterpene lactones and 1% flavonoids, including scolymoside, cynaroside, and luteolin (8006,2056). Artichoke's therapeutic benefit in idiopathic dyspepsia and dyspepsia secondary to biliary disease has centered around its choleretic effects, or ability to stimulate bile flow, which has been demonstrated in several studies (8006,2056). Constituents responsible for this effect are thought to be cynarin, chlorogenic acid, and scolymoside (4,2056). Although not clearly demonstrated in humans (1423,1424), artichoke preparations are reported to have an antihyperlipidemic effect. Cynarin and chlorogenic acid are thought to have a cholesterol-lowering effect. Cynaroside and its derivative, luteolin, might also indirectly inhibit HMG-CoA reductase (1425,1426,2056). Several constituents are reported to have antioxidant activity (1422). Preliminary research suggests that artichoke leaf extract protects liver cells from damage (1421,1422,2056,3269). A mixture of polyphenols and flavonoids, including caffeic acid, chlorogenic acid, cynarin, luteolin-7-O-glycoside (cynaroside), and luteolin might contribute to hepatoprotective activity (3269,2056).

Adverse Reactions Including Known Allergies

Allergic contact dermatitis can occur with the use of artichoke. This has been attributed to the constituent cynaropicrin (11). Artichoke can cause an allergic reaction in individuals sensitive to the Asteraceae/Compositae family. Members of this family include ragweed, chrysanthemums, marigolds, daisies, and many other herbs.

Possible Interactions with Herbs & Other Dietary Supplements

Insufficient reliable information available.

Possible Interactions with Drugs

No interactions are known to occur, and there is no known reason to expect a clinically significant interaction with artichoke.

Possible Interactions with Foods

No interactions are known to occur, and there is no known reason to expect a clinically significant interaction with artichoke.

Possible Interactions with Lab Tests

No interactions are known to occur, and there is no known reason to expect a clinically significant interaction with artichoke.

 © Copyright 2000, Natural Medicines Comprehensive Database (209) 472-2244. For updated data, go to www.NaturalDatabase.com

Possible Interactions with Diseases or Conditions

BILE DUCT OBSTRUCTION: Theoretically, artichoke might worsen bile duct obstruction by increasing bile flow (2,11,2056); avoid using.

GALLSTONES: Theoretically, artichoke might worsen gallstones by increasing bile flow (2,11,2056); use with caution.

CROSS-ALLERGENICITY: Artichoke might cause an allergic reaction in individuals sensitive to Asteraceae/Compositae family plants. Members of this family include ragweed, chrysanthemums, marigolds, daisies, and many other herbs (11,2056).

Typical Dosages & Routes of Administration that are Commonly Used

ORAL: A typical dose using artichoke stem or root is 1-4 grams three times daily (4). The typical dose of the dried leaf is 2 grams three times daily (2). The typical dose of 12:1 dry leaf extract is 500 mg daily (8006). For lowering serum cholesterol, the isolated constituent cyanarin 60-1500 mg per day has been used (1423,1424,2056). For preparations that are prepared as extracts, appropriate dosing will vary depending on the specific extract being used.

Comments

Avoid confusion with Jerusalem artichoke (Helianthus tuberosus) (11).

ARUM

This Product is Also Known As

Adder's Root, Bobbins, Cocky Baby, Cuckoo Pint, Cypress Powder, Dragon Root, Friar's Cowl, Gaglee, Kings And Queens, Ladysmock, Lords and Ladies, Parson and Clerk, Portland Arrowroot, Quaker, Ramp, Starchwort, Wake Robin.

Scientific Names

Arum maculatum.
Family: Araceae.

People Use This For

Orally, arum is used for colds and inflammation of the throat. It has also been used orally to stimulate sweating and as an expectorant (18).

Safety

UNSAFE ...for any oral medicinal use (see Mechanism of Action).
PREGNANCY AND LACTATION: UNSAFE ...contraindicated because of its toxicity (18).

Effectiveness

There is insufficient reliable information available about the effectiveness of arum.

Possible Mechanism of Action & Active Ingredients

The applicable part of arum is the root. Arum can cause severe mucous membrane irritation and bleeding. This is probably due to sharp oxalate crystals present in the root. These injure the mucous membranes, and may also introduce impurities into the wounds. Arum also contains cyanogenic glycosides, but the levels are probably too low to cause poisoning (18).

Adverse Reactions Including Known Allergies

Arum can cause swelling of the tongue, bloody vomiting, and bloody diarrhea in people who take it orally (18).

Possible Interactions with Herbs & Other Dietary Supplements

Insufficient reliable information available.

Possible Interactions with Drugs

No interactions are known to occur, and there is no known reason to expect a clinically significant interaction with arum.

Possible Interactions with Foods

No interactions are known to occur, and there is no known reason to expect a clinically significant interaction with arum.

Possible Interactions with Lab Tests

No interactions are known to occur, and there is no known reason to expect a clinically significant interaction with arum.

Possible Interactions with Diseases or Conditions

No interactions are known to occur, and there is no known reason to expect a clinically significant interaction with arum.

Typical Dosages & Routes of Administration that are Commonly Used
No typical dosage.

Comments
Arum is considered unsafe; avoid using.

ASAFOETIDA

This Product is Also Known As
Asafetida, Asa Foetida, Assant, Devil's Dung, Food of the Gods, Fum, Giant Fennel, Heeng.

Scientific Names
Ferula assa-foetida; Ferula foetida; Ferula rubricaulis.
Family: Apiaceae/Umbelliferae.

People Use This For
Orally, asafoetida is used for chronic bronchitis (4), asthma (11), pertussis (4), hoarseness, hysteria, flatulent colic (4), chronic gastritis, dyspepsia, irritable colon (18), and convulsions (11).
Topically, asafoetida is used for corns and calluses (6).
In Chinese medicine, asafoetida is used as a nerve stimulant in treating neurasthenia (11).
In folk medicine, asafoetida has been used for amenorrhea, croup, insanity, and sarcomas (6).
In manufacturing, asafoetida is used as a fragrance or fixative in cosmetics (11), and it is used as a flavoring ingredient in foods and beverages (11).
Other uses for asafoetida include its use as a cat, dog, and wildlife repellent.

Safety
LIKELY SAFE ...when used in amounts typically found in foods. Asafoetida is approved for use in food in the US. Its maximum safe use level is less than 0.004%.
POSSIBLY SAFE ...when used orally in appropriate amounts. It is contraindicated in people with CNS conditions that could result in convulsions (12).
CHILDREN: UNSAFE ...in infants due to the possible risk of methemoglobinemia (4) (see Adverse Reactions).
PREGNANCY: UNSAFE ...when used in amounts greater than typically found in foods, because it might cause abortion (4).
LACTATION: UNSAFE ...due to possible risk of methemoglobinemia in infants (4).

Effectiveness
There is insufficient reliable information available about the effectiveness of asafoetida.

Possible Mechanism of Action & Active Ingredients
The applicable part of asafoetida is the root resin. Asafoetida may contain sulfur compounds in its volatile oil which may protect against fat-induced hyperlipidemia. Asafoetida may contain coumarin constituents with anticoagulant activity (4). There is some evidence to suggest that its constituents treat irritable bowel syndrome (4).

Adverse Reactions Including Known Allergies
Taking 50-100 mg of asafoetida orally may cause convulsions in people with nervousness (12). There is one report of methemoglobinemia in an infant (4). Large amounts are reported to cause swelling of the lips, belching, flatulence, diarrhea, headache, or convulsions (18). Genital organ swelling was reported after external use of asafoetida on the abdomen (18).

Possible Interactions with Herbs & Other Dietary Supplements
HERBS WITH ANTICOAGULANT/ANTIPLATELET POTENTIAL: Concomitant use of herbs that have coumarin constituents or affect platelet aggregation could theoretically increase the risk of bleeding in some people. These herbs include: angelica, anise, arnica, bogbean, boldo, capsicum, celery, chamomile, clove, danshen, fenugreek, feverfew, garlic, ginger, ginkgo, ginseng (Panax), horse chestnut, horseradish, licorice, meadowsweet, prickly ash, onion, papain, passionflower, poplar, quassia, red clover, turmeric, wild carrot, wild lettuce, willow, and others (4,19).

Possible Interactions with Drugs
ANTICOAGULANT, ANTITHROMBOTIC DRUGS: Theoretically, asafoetida might increase the risk of bleeding (4).
ANTIHYPERTENSIVE, ANTIHYPOTENSIVE DRUGS: Theoretically, excessive doses might interfere with blood pressure control (4).

Possible Interactions with Foods
No interactions are known to occur, and there is no known reason to expect a clinically significant interaction with asafoetida.

Possible Interactions with Lab Tests
No interactions are known to occur, and there is no known reason to expect a clinically significant interaction with asafoetida.

Possible Interactions with Diseases or Conditions
BLEEDING DISORDERS: Theoretically, asafoetida might increase the risk of bleeding (4).
HYPERTENSION, HYPOTENSION: Theoretically, asafoetida might interfere with blood pressure control (4).
GI IRRITATION: Can irritate gastrointestinal tract. Contraindicated in individuals with infectious or inflammatory gastrointestinal conditions (19).

Typical Dosages & Routes of Administration that are Commonly Used
ORAL: 300-1000 mg powdered resin three times daily (4). Tincture of asafetida (concentration unspecified), 2-4 mL (4), or 20 drops as a single dose (18).

Comments
Asafoetida resin is produced by solidifying juice exuded from incisions in living roots of Ferula foetida and other Ferula species. Asafoetida is known to have putrid odor and tastes bitter. The acrid taste is the basis for its name, devil's dung (6). Various species of this plant have somewhat different constituents. The related species Ferula communis, contains toxic coumarin constituents. Other related species are Ferula galbaniflua and Ferula rubricaulis. These seem to cause contact dermatitis (4).

ASARABACCA

This Product is Also Known As
Asaroun, Asarum, Azarum, False Coltsfoot, Hazelwort, Public House Plant, Snakeroot, Wild Ginger, Wild Nard.
CAUTION: See separate listings for Bitter Milkwort and Senega.

Scientific Names
Asarum europaeum.
Family: Aristolochiaceae.

People Use This For
Orally, asarabacca is used for acute and chronic bronchitis, bronchial spasms, and bronchial asthma (18).
In folk medicine, it has been used as an emetic, antitussive, menstrual stimulant, abortifacient, and to treat pneumonia, angina pectoris, migraines, liver disease and jaundice, and dehydration (18).

Safety
POSSIBLY SAFE ...when used orally and appropriately short-term (12).
POSSIBLY UNSAFE ...when used orally in large amounts or long-term (12). Large doses have been associated with significant side effects, including burning tongue, gastroenteritis, diarrhea, skin rashes, and partial paralysis (18). ...when the essential oil is taken orally. The essential oil contains a potential hepatocarcinogenic constituent, beta-asarone (12).
UNSAFE ...when aristolochic acid-contaminated asarabacca is used orally. Asarabacca is commonly contaminated with aristolochic acid, which is nephrotoxic and carcinogenic. The FDA considers all products containing aristolochic acid to be unsafe and adulterated. Only products analytically verified to be aristolochic acid-free should be used (6119).
PREGNANCY: LIKELY UNSAFE ...when used orally. Asarabacca might act as a menstrual or uterine stimulant (12); contraindicated.
LACTATION: Insufficient reliable information available; avoid using.

Effectiveness
POSSIBLY EFFECTIVE ...when used for bronchitis (18).
There is insufficient reliable information available about the effectiveness of asarabacca for its other uses.

Possible Mechanism of Action & Active Ingredients
The applicable part of asarabacca is the rhizome. The constituent phenylpropanol may be responsible for the effects of asarabacca on bronchitis/bronchial asthma. Some products are standardized for content of this constituent (18). Researchers think emetic and spasmolytic effects may be due to the constituent trans-isoasarone (18). Local anesthetic effect demonstrated in humans may be due to constituents, trans-isoasarone and trans-isomethyleugenol (18).

Adverse Reactions Including Known Allergies
Asarabacca may cause nausea and vomiting (12). Severe poisoning has also been reported (553). Symptoms of poisoning include burning of tongue, gastroenteritis, diarrhea, skin rashes, and partial paralysis (18). Asarabacca is commonly contaminated with aristolochic acid, which is nephrotoxic and carcinogenic (6119).

Possible Interactions with Herbs & Other Dietary Supplements
Insufficient reliable information available.

Possible Interactions with Drugs
No interactions are known to occur, and there is no known reason to expect a clinically significant interaction with asarabacca.

Possible Interactions with Foods
No interactions are known to occur, and there is no known reason to expect a clinically significant interaction with asarabacca.

Possible Interactions with Lab Tests
No interactions are known to occur, and there is no known reason to expect a clinically significant interaction with asarabacca.

Possible Interactions with Diseases or Conditions
GI IRRITATION: Asarabacca can irritate the gastrointestinal tract; contraindicated in individuals with infectious or inflammatory gastrointestinal conditions (19).

Typical Dosages & Routes of Administration that are Commonly Used
ORAL: 30 mg dry extract is the average daily dose for adults and children over 13 years old (18).

Comments
Asarabacca has been reported as obsolete for medicinal use (18); safer alternatives are available. Avoid confusion with bitter milkwort (Polygala amara), or senega (Polygala senega) also known as snakeroot.
Asarabacca is frequently contaminated with aristolochic acid, which is nephrotoxic and carcinogenic. The FDA considers all products containing aristolochic acid to be unsafe and adulterated (6119). The FDA intends to automatically detain, without physical examination, any product which contains plants known or suspected to contain aristolochic acid, or which might be adulterated with plants known to contain aristolochic acid. Each detained product will be released only after the responsible party provides direct analytical evidence that it is free of aristolochic acid (6119).

ASH

This Product is Also Known As
Bird's Tongue, Common Ash, European Ash, Weeping Ash, White Ash.
CAUTION: See separate listings for Northern Prickly Ash, and Southern Prickly Ash.

Scientific Names
Fraxinus excelsior; Fraxinus americana.
Family: Oleaceae.

People Use This For
Orally, ash leaf is used for fever, arthritis, gout, bladder complaints, as a laxative, as a diuretic (2), and as a tonic (18).

Safety
There is insufficient reliable information available about the safety of ash.
Pregnancy and Lactation: Insufficient reliable information available; avoid using.

Effectiveness
There is insufficient reliable information available about the effectiveness of ash. (2).

Possible Mechanism of Action & Active Ingredients
The applicable parts of ash are the bark and leaf. There is insufficient reliable information available about the possible mechanism of action and active ingredients.

Adverse Reactions Including Known Allergies
None reported.

Possible Interactions with Herbs & Other Dietary Supplements
Insufficient reliable information available.

Possible Interactions with Drugs
No interactions are known to occur, and there is no known reason to expect a clinically significant interaction with ash.

Possible Interactions with Foods

No interactions are known to occur, and there is no known reason to expect a clinically significant interaction with ash.

Possible Interactions with Lab Tests

No interactions are known to occur, and there is no known reason to expect a clinically significant interaction with ash.

Possible Interactions with Diseases or Conditions

No interactions are known to occur, and there is no known reason to expect a clinically significant interaction with ash.

Typical Dosages & Routes of Administration that are Commonly Used

No typical dosage.

Comments

Avoid use due to lack of safety and effectiveness information. Avoid confusion with northern prickly ash, southern prickly ash. There is very little scientific information about this product. Our staff is continually analyzing the available information on natural medicines and will add data here as it becomes available.

ASPARAGUS

This Product is Also Known As

Asparagi Rhizoma Root, Asperge, Garden Asparagus, Spargelkraut, Spargelwurzelstock, Sparrow Grass.

Scientific Names

Asparagus officinalis.
Family: Liliaceae.

People Use This For

Orally, the rhizome and root of asparagus is used along with copious fluid consumption as "irrigation therapy" to increase urine output. It is also used orally for treating urinary tract infections and other inflammatory conditions of the urinary tract, preventing kidney and bladder stones (2,18), rheumatic joint pain and swelling, female hormone imbalances, dryness in the lungs and throat, AIDS, and to prevent anemia due to folic acid deficiency (3900).
Topically, asparagus is used for cleaning the face, drying sores, and acne (6).
In Chinese medicine, it is used orally as a laxative, for neuritis, and for treating parasitic diseases and cancer (11).
For food uses, the newly-formed shoots, or spears, are eaten as a vegetable (11). The seed and root extracts of asparagus are used in alcoholic beverages (11).

Safety

LIKELY SAFE ...when consumed in amounts typically found in food (11).
POSSIBLY SAFE ...when taken orally and appropriately for medicinal purposes (2,12).
There is insufficient reliable information available for the safety of the topical uses of asparagus.
PREGNANCY: LIKELY SAFE ...when consumed as food. POSSIBLE UNSAFE ...when used for medicinal purposes because the extracts have been used as a contraceptive (6).
LACTATION: LIKELY SAFE ...when consumed as food. Insufficient reliable information available for other uses.

Effectiveness

POSSIBLY EFFECTIVE ...when taken orally along with copious fluid consumption as "irrigation therapy" to increase urine output. ...when taken for inflammatory diseases of the urinary tract and for preventing kidney stones (2,18).
There is insufficient reliable information available about the effectiveness of asparagus for its other uses.

Possible Mechanism of Action & Active Ingredients

The applicable parts of asparagus are the rhizome and root. Asparagus is a vitamin E rich plant source (19). The asparagus root has diuretic effects in animal experiments (2). Asparagus also has hypotensive (11), antibacterial, and antiviral effects in vitro (3900). Fibers from the plant can have mutagen-adsorbing (cancer-preventing) activity (11). The saponin constituents can irritate mucous membranes and can be cytotoxic (6,3901). Asparagus can also cause urinary tract irritation (19).

Adverse Reactions Including Known Allergies

Asparagus used orally can cause mucous membrane irritation (3901). Allergic skin reactions can occur with the topical use of asparagus (2).

Possible Interactions with Herbs & Other Dietary Supplements

Insufficient reliable information available.

Possible Interactions with Drugs

No interactions are known to occur, and there is no known reason to expect a clinically significant interaction with asparagus.

Possible Interactions with Foods

No interactions are known to occur, and there is no known reason to expect a clinically significant interaction with asparagus.

Possible Interactions with Lab Tests

No interactions are known to occur, and there is no known reason to expect a clinically significant interaction with asparagus.

Possible Interactions with Diseases or Conditions

KIDNEY DISEASE: Asparagus is contraindicated in individuals with inflammatory kidney disease because the mucosal irritant effect of asparagus can exacerbate this condition (2,6,12).
EDEMA: Irrigation therapy with asparagus is contraindicated in individuals with edema caused by heart or kidney disorders (2).

Typical Dosages & Routes of Administration that are Commonly Used

ORAL: The typical dose of asparagus is 40-60 grams of the cut rhizome or root per day in the form of tea, which is prepared by steeping 40-60 grams in 150 mL of boiling water for 5-10 minutes and then straining (2). Ensure ample fluid intake when used as "irrigation therapy" (2,18).
TOPICAL: No typical dosage.

Comments

Asparagus seeds are used medicinally in a few cultures. The consumption of asparagus spears produces a pungent odor in the urine of some people.

ASPARTATES

This Product is Also Known As

Aspartate Chelated Minerals, Aspartate Mineral Chelates, Mineral Aspartates.
CAUTION: See separate listing for Chelated Minerals.

Scientific Names

None.

People Use This For

Orally, aspartates is used to increase absorption of mineral supplements (5140), and enhance athletic performance (5133).

Safety

There is insufficient reliable information available about the safety of aspartates.
Pregnancy and Lactation: Insufficient reliable information available; avoid using.

Effectiveness

There is insufficient reliable information available about the effectiveness of aspartates.

Possible Mechanism of Action & Active Ingredients

Aspartate is an amino acid that is metabolized in resting muscle (5141). People theorize that aspartate mineral salts of copper, iron, magnesium, manganese, potassium or zinc have better absorption or improve athletic ability. There is no evidence to suggest that this is true (5133). Except in cases of mineral deficiency, such as iron-deficiency anemia, a well-balanced diet typically provides the RDA of minerals (5133).

Adverse Reactions Including Known Allergies

None reported.

Possible Interactions with Herbs & Other Dietary Supplements

Insufficient reliable information available.

Possible Interactions with Drugs

No interactions are known to occur, and there is no known reason to expect a clinically significant interaction with aspartates.

Possible Interactions with Foods

No interactions are known to occur, and there is no known reason to expect a clinically significant interaction with aspartates.

Possible Interactions with Lab Tests

No interactions are known to occur, and there is no known reason to expect a clinically significant interaction with aspartates.

Possible Interactions with Diseases or Conditions

No interactions are known to occur, and there is no known reason to expect a clinically significant interaction with aspartates.

Typical Dosages & Routes of Administration that are Commonly Used

ORAL: Aspartate mineral supplements typically contain the following, either as individual or combination products: copper aspartate 2 mg, iron aspartate 18 mg, magnesium aspartate 400 mg, manganese aspartate 7 mg, potassium aspartate 99 mg, and zinc aspartate 15 mg. The dose is usually once daily (5265).

Comments

None.

ASPEN

This Product is Also Known As

Populi cortex, Populi folium.

Scientific Names

Populus tremuloides; Populus tremula.
Family: Salicaceae.

People Use This For

Orally, the bark and leaf are used as components of various medicinal herbal combinations for treating rheumatic disorders, prostate discomforts, sciatica, neuralgia, and bladder problems (2).

Safety

There is insufficient reliable information available about the safety of aspen.
Pregnancy and Lactation: Insufficient reliable information available; avoid using.

Effectiveness

There is insufficient reliable information available about the effectiveness of aspen or aspen-containing herb combinations.

Possible Mechanism of Action & Active Ingredients

The applicable parts of aspen are the bark and leaf. Aspen contains salicin, a precursor to salicylate (3700), and therefore aspen may have anti-inflammatory activity (2,7).

Adverse Reactions Including Known Allergies

Topically, salicin is associated with skin rashes (4). Pollen sensitization and allergic contact dermatitis may occur following contact with the bud resin (2,14).

Possible Interactions with Herbs & Other Dietary Supplements

SALICYLATE-CONTAINING HERBS: Theoretically, concomitant use may potentiate effects of other herbs that contain salicylates (19).
HERBS WITH ANTICOAGULANT/ANTIPLATELET POTENTIAL: Concomitant use of herbs that have coumarin constituents or effect platelet aggregation could theoretically increase the risk of bleeding in some people. These herbs include: angelica, anise, arnica, asafoetida, bogbean, boldo, capsicum, celery, chamomile, clove, danshen, fenugreek, feverfew, garlic, ginger, ginkgo, ginseng Panax, horse chestnut, horseradish, licorice, meadowsweet, prickly ash, onion, papain, passionflower, poplar, quassia, red clover, turmeric, wild carrot, wild lettuce, willow, and others (4,19).

Possible Interactions with Drugs

No interactions are known to occur, and there is no known reason to expect a clinically significant interaction with aspen.

Possible Interactions with Foods

ALCOHOL: Theoretically, concomitant use increases the incidence, severity, and risk of salicylate-induced gastrointestinal bleeding (15).

Possible Interactions with Lab Tests

Theoretically, salicylate-containing herbs may interfere with lab tests affected by salicylates, such as serum uric acid, urine glucose, vanillylmandelic acid (VMA), and 5-HIAA tests.

© Copyright 2000, Natural Medicines Comprehensive Database (209) 472-2244. For updated data, go to www.NaturalDatabase.com

Possible Interactions with Diseases or Conditions

SALICYLATE HYPERSENSITIVITY: Theoretically contraindicated, due to salicylate (salicin) content. Avoid or use with caution in people with active peptic ulcer disease, diabetes, gout, hemophilia, hypoprothrombinemia, kidney, or liver disease (15).

Typical Dosages & Routes of Administration that are Commonly Used

ORAL: People typically use 1 to 5 grams of powdered aspen bark. A liquid is prepared using 1 to 2 teaspoons of the bark simmered in a cup of water for 10 to 15 minutes. This is taken three times daily. The liquid extract is dosed 1 to 5 mL (5253,5264).

Comments

Contraindicated in people with salicylate hypersensitivity (15).

ASTRAGALUS

This Product is Also Known As

Beg Kei, Bei Qi, Buck Qi, Huang Qi, Huang qi, Hwanggi, Membranous Milk Vetch, Milk Vetch, Mongolian Milk, Ogi.
CAUTION: See separate listing for Tragacanth.

Scientific Names

Astragalus membranaceus; Astragalus mongholicus.
Family: Leguminosae or Fabaceae.

People Use This For

Orally, astragalus is used for treating the common cold and upper respiratory infections, to strengthen and regulate the immune system and to increase the production of blood cells, particularly in individuals with chronic degenerative disease or in individuals with cancer undergoing chemotherapy or radiation therapy. It is used for chronic nephritis and diabetes. It is used as an antibacterial and antiviral; as a tonic; a liver protectant; an anti-inflammatory; an antioxidant; and as a diuretic, vasodilator, or hypotensive agent (11,303).
Astragalus is used orally in combination with Ligustrum lucidum (glossy privet) for treating breast, cervical, and lung cancers (303).
Topically, astragalus is used as a vasodilator and to speed healing (11).

Safety

LIKELY SAFE ...when used orally (12). Toxicity of astragalus root is reportedly "very low" (11). ...when used topically (12).
PREGNANCY AND LACTATION: Insufficient reliable information available.

Effectiveness

POSSIBLY EFFECTIVE ...when used orally for the common cold and upper respiratory tract infections (303). ...when used orally to relieve angina symptoms (303). ...when used orally or intravenously for chronic hepatitis (303). ...when astragaloside, an active constituent, is given intravenously to individuals with congestive heart failure to relieve symptoms and improve exercise tolerance (303). ...when used orally in combination with Ligustrum lucidum (glossy privet) as adjunct therapy to increase the survival rates in individuals receiving radiation therapy for breast cancer and or chemotherapy for lung cancer (303).
There is insufficient reliable information available about the effectiveness of astragalus for its other uses.

Possible Mechanism of Action & Active Ingredients

The applicable part of astragalus is the root. Astragalus contains varied constituents including greater than 40 saponins, e.g., astragaloside; several flavonoids; polysaccharides; multiple trace minerals; amino acids; and coumarins (11,303). Astragalus is an antioxidant. It inhibits free radical production, increases superoxide dismutase and decreases lipid peroxidation (303). Astragalus is promoted for its effects on the immune system, liver and cardiovascular system. It is believed to improve the immune response by potentiating the effects of interferon. Evidence suggests astragalus also increases antibody levels of IgA and IgG in nasal secretions (303). Lower doses of astragalus appear to stimulate the immune system, but doses in excess of 28 grams seem to suppress immunity (303). When administered intravenously, some evidence suggests astragalus extract might increase proliferation and differentiation of bone marrow stem cells and progenitor cells (303). Astragalus also shows evidence of broad-spectrum antibiotic activity (303). In individuals with chronic hepatitis, astragalus seems to improve liver function as demonstrated by improvement in serum glutamate pyruvate transaminase (SGPT) levels (303). Astragalus is also believed to cause vasodilation and increase cardiac output which might be beneficial in angina, congestive heart failure, and post-myocardial infarction (11,303).

Adverse Reactions Including Known Allergies

Toxicity of astragalus root is reportedly "very low" (11). Although side effects have not been reported, doses greater than 28 grams might cause immunosuppression (303).

Possible Interactions with Herbs & Other Dietary Supplements

GLOSSY PRIVET: Adjunctive use of astragalus and Ligustrum lucidum (glossy privet) increases survival rates in individuals receiving radiation therapy for breast cancer and in patients receiving chemotherapy for lung cancer (303).

Possible Interactions with Drugs

ACYCLOVIR (Zovirax): Theoretically, concurrent use might result in additive antiviral effects (303).
IMMUNOSUPRESSANTS: Theoretically, concurrent use might interfere with immunosuppressive therapy (303); avoid concurrent use.
CYLCLOPHOSPHAMIDE: Some evidence suggests astragalus might reduce immunosuppression caused by cyclophosphamide (Cytoxan, Neosar) immunocompromise (303).

Possible Interactions with Foods

No interactions are known to occur, and there is no known reason to expect a clinically significant interaction with astragalus.

Possible Interactions with Lab Tests

No interactions are known to occur, and there is no known reason to expect a clinically significant interaction with astragalus.

Possible Interactions with Diseases or Conditions

ORGAN TRANSPLANT RECIPIENTS: Astragalus might interfere with immunosuppressive therapy; avoid concurrent use (303).
AUTOIMMUNE DISORDERS: Astragalus might increase immune system activity and may not be appropriate for individuals with autoimmune disorders (303).

Typical Dosages & Routes of Administration that are Commonly Used

ORAL: Astragalus powder 9-30 grams per day (11,303). For serious conditions, astragalus powder 30-60 grams per day has been used (303). However, research suggests that doses greater than 28 grams per day may offer no additional benefit and may even cause immune suppression (303). Some recommend astragalus powder 4-7 grams per day for a 79 kilogram human for optimal immune stimulating activity (303). Astragalus decoction 0.5-1 L per day (maximum of 120 grams of whole root per liter of water) (303). As a soup, mix 30 grams in 3.5 L of soup and simmer with other food ingredients (303).

Comments

Astragalus is most commonly used in combination with other herbs (303).

AUTUMN CROCUS

This Product is Also Known As

Colchicum, Crocus, Fall Crocus, Meadow Saffran, Meadow Saffron, Mysteria, Naked Ladies, Upstart, Vellorita, Wonder Bulb.

Scientific Names

Colchicum autumnale; Colchicum speciosum; Colchicum vernum.
Family: Liliaceae.

People Use This For

Orally, autumn crocus is used for arthritis, gout, and familial Mediterranean fever (2,400).

Safety

UNSAFE ...when taken orally for self-medication because it is a potential poison (6,500). Human intoxication can occur when corms, which are the underground bulb-like stems, are mistaken for onions and ingested (6).
PREGNANCY AND LACTATION: UNSAFE ...because autumn crocus is a potential mutagen and toxin (500); avoid using.

Effectiveness

LIKELY EFFECTIVE ...when taken orally for acute gout attacks and familial Mediterranean fever; however, autumn crocus is unsafe for self-medication (8,400).

Possible Mechanism of Action & Active Ingredients

The applicable parts of autumn crocus are the seed, tuber, and flower. The seeds of this plant contain at least 0.4% colchicine, which is the constituent responsible for its therapeutic benefit (2).

Adverse Reactions Including Known Allergies

Autumn crocus taken orally can cause burning of the mouth and throat, thirst, nausea, vomiting, diarrhea, liver necrosis, hypovolemic shock, kidney impairment, multiorgan failure, and death (6,553). Long-term use of colchicine is associated with agranulocytosis, aplastic anemia, and peripheral neuritis (6). Human intoxication can occur when corms, which are the underground bulb-like stems, are mistaken for onions or when contaminated milk is ingested (6). Topically, the handling of fresh corm slices can cause finger numbness (6).

Possible Interactions with Herbs & Other Dietary Supplements

Insufficient reliable information available.

Possible Interactions with Drugs

COLCHICINE: Avoid concomitant use of autumn crocus with colchicine because it can increase therapeutic and adverse effects (2).

Possible Interactions with Foods

No interactions are known to occur, and there is no known reason to expect a clinically significant interaction with autumn crocus.

Possible Interactions with Lab Tests

URIC ACID: Autumn crocus can lower serum uric acid concentrations and test results due to its colchicine content (8,400).

Possible Interactions with Diseases or Conditions

No interactions are known to occur, and there is no known reason to expect a clinically significant interaction with autumn crocus.

Typical Dosages & Routes of Administration that are Commonly Used

ORAL: Dosing is related to the colchicine content (2). Due to its toxic potential, use the standardized, FDA-approved colchicine. Gout and familial Mediterranean fever require diagnosis, treatment, and monitoring by a medical professional.

Comments

Colchicine is available by prescription and used to treat acute gout attacks and familial Mediterranean fever (506).

AVENS

This Product is Also Known As

Benedict's Herb, Bennet's Root, Colewort, Geum, Herb Bennet.

Scientific Names

Geum urbanum.
Family: Rosaceae.

People Use This For

Orally, avens is used to treat diarrhea (4), catarrhal colitis (4), uterine bleeding (4), intermittent fevers (4), and ulcerative colitis (4).

Safety

LIKELY SAFE ...when used in amounts typically found in foods. The Council of Europe allows avens as a natural source of food flavoring (4).
There is insufficient reliable information available about the safety of the medicinal use of avens above ground parts.
PREGNANCY AND LACTATION: POSSIBLY UNSAFE ...because avens seems to have an affect on the menstrual cycle; avoid using (4).

Effectiveness

There is insufficient reliable information available about the effectiveness of avens (4).

Possible Mechanism of Action & Active Ingredients

The applicable part of avens is the above ground parts. The tannin-type constituents of avens have an astringent action; this supports the traditional use of avens for treating diarrhea (4).

Adverse Reactions Including Known Allergies

None reported (4,18).

Possible Interactions with Herbs & Other Dietary Supplements

Insufficient reliable information available.

Possible Interactions with Drugs

No interactions are known to occur, and there is no known reason to expect a clinically significant interaction with avens.

Possible Interactions with Foods

No interactions are known to occur, and there is no known reason to expect a clinically significant interaction with avens.

Possible Interactions with Lab Tests

No interactions are known to occur, and there is no known reason to expect a clinically significant interaction with avens.

Possible Interactions with Diseases or Conditions

No interactions are known to occur, and there is no known reason to expect a clinically significant interaction with avens.

Typical Dosages & Routes of Administration that are Commonly Used

ORAL: 1-4 grams steeped in boiling water, strained, three times a day (4). Liquid extract (1:1 in 25% alcohol) 1-4 mL three times a day (4).

Comments

Avens is very rarely used medicinally today (18).

AVOCADO

This Product is Also Known As

Ahuacate, Alligator Pear, Avocato.

Scientific Names

Persea americana, synonym Persea gratissima; Laurus persea.
Family: Lauraceae.

People Use This For

Orally, the fruit of the avocado is used to reduce serum cholesterol levels (6).
Topically, the oil is applied to soothe and heal skin, treat sclerosis of the skin, pyorrhea, and arthritis (11). The fruit pulp is used topically to promote hair growth and hasten wound healing (6).
In folk medicine, the fruit has been used as an aphrodisiac and to stimulate menstrual flow (11). The seeds, leaves and bark have been used for dysentery and diarrhea (6), and to relieve toothache (11).
For food uses, the fruit pulp is edible.

Safety

LIKELY SAFE ...when the fruit is consumed in amounts commonly found in foods (11,18). The Mexican avocado, a variant available in the US, is reported to contain estragole and anethole (6) which are hepatotoxic in animals and structurally similar to safrole, a known carcinogen (4).
PREGNANCY AND LACTATION: LIKELY SAFE ...when consumed in food amounts.

Effectiveness

LIKELY EFFECTIVE ...when used orally for reducing total serum cholesterol, LDL cholesterol, apolipoprotein B and increasing HDL cholesterol serum levels (668,669,670,671).
POSSIBLY EFFECTIVE ...when used topically as a skin emollient (6,18).
There is insufficient reliable information available about the effectiveness of avocado for its other uses.

Possible Mechanism of Action & Active Ingredients

The applicable parts of avocado are the fruit, leaves, and seed. The cholesterol lowering and skin soothing/healing effects may be due to the high content of unsaturated fatty acids and other compounds (oleic acid, tocopherols, Vitamin E, sterols, volatile oils) in avocado (6).

Adverse Reactions Including Known Allergies

Allergic cross-sensitivity may be seen in latex-sensitive individuals (676).

Possible Interactions with Herbs & Other Dietary Supplements

Insufficient reliable information available.

Possible Interactions with Drugs

WARFARIN: Avocado may antagonize the anticoagulant effects of warfarin, but there has been only one case report of this interaction (667).

Possible Interactions with Foods

No interactions are known to occur, and there is no known reason to expect a clinically significant interaction with avocado.

Possible Interactions with Lab Tests

CHOLESTEROL: Avocado can lower serum total cholesterol, LDL cholesterol and apolipoprotein B concentrations and test results. Avocado can increase serum HDL cholesterol concentrations and test results (668,669,670,671).

Possible Interactions with Diseases or Conditions

Contains constituents with possible estrogenic and catecholamine-like properties. Theoretically these could interact with diseases or conditions sensitive to such ingredients.

Typical Dosages & Routes of Administration that are Commonly Used

ORAL: Variable dosing used; related to dietary calorie content or fat intake (668,669,670,671,675).

Comments

Avocado oil is derived from the fruit pulp (6). The fruit pulp is a good source of potassium and vitamin D (6,11).

BA JI TIAN

This Product is Also Known As

Morinda, Morinda Root, Morindae radix.
CAUTION: See separate listing for Morinda.

Scientific Names

Morinda officinalis.
Family: Rubiaceae.

People Use This For

Orally, ba ji tien is used for cancer, cholecystitis, debility, enuresis, polyuria, hernia, impotence and premature ejaculation, lumbago (mid- and lower-back pain), dorsalgia (upper back pain) (513), depression (3558), increasing white blood cell count, stimulating the endocrine system (445), improving kidney function, and strengthening the skeletal and nervous systems (446,447).

In traditional Chinese medicine, ba ji tian is used as a kidney tonic to strengthen the yang (449).

In some commercial preparations, Morinda officinalis (ba ji tian) is combined with Morinda citrifolia (see separate listing for Morinda).

Safety

LIKELY SAFE ...when used appropriately (12).
PREGNANCY AND LACTATION: Insufficient reliable information available; avoid using.

Effectiveness

There is insufficient reliable information available about the effectiveness of ba ji tian.

Possible Mechanism of Action & Active Ingredients

The applicable part of ba ji tian is the root. The root contains several potentially active constituents, including an iridoid lactone called morindolide, iridoid glucosides including morofficinaloside, anthraquinones, a monoterpene glycoside, sterols including beta-sitosterol, an ursane-type triterpene, a lactone compound, and 24-ethylcholesterol (448,451,452). However, the role of specific constituents for the purported uses has not been described. Constituents reported to have antidepressant activity have been isolated (succinic acid, nystose, 1F-fructofuranosylnystose, inulin-type hexasaccharide, and heptasaccharide) (449). Ba ji tian is thought to work in depression by increasing serotonergic effects (3558). A study in mice reported that ba ji tian had anti-fatigue properties, reversed radiation-induced leukopenia, and reduced excitability of the parasympathetic nervous system associated with hypothyroidism (453).

Adverse Reactions Including Known Allergies

None reported.

Possible Interactions with Herbs & Other Dietary Supplements

Insufficient reliable information available.

Possible Interactions with Drugs

No interactions are known to occur, and there is no known reason to expect a clinically significant interaction with ba ji tian.

Possible Interactions with Foods

No interactions are known to occur, and there is no known reason to expect a clinically significant interaction with ba ji tian.

Possible Interactions with Lab Tests
No interactions are known to occur, and there is no known reason to expect a clinically significant interaction with ba ji tian.

Possible Interactions with Diseases or Conditions
DYSURIA: Theoretically, ba ji tian may exacerbate urinary difficulties. Ba ji tian is reported to stimulate the kidneys. Use with caution (12).

Typical Dosages & Routes of Administration that are Commonly Used
No typical dosage.

Comments
None.

BAEL

This Product is Also Known As
Bel, Bengal Quince, Indian Bael.

Scientific Names
Aegle marmelos.
Family: Rutaceae.

People Use This For
Orally, bael is used for constipation and diarrhea (18).

Safety
There is insufficient reliable information available about the safety of bael.
Pregnancy and Lactation: Insufficient reliable information available; avoid using.

Effectiveness
There is insufficient reliable information available about the effectiveness of bael.

Possible Mechanism of Action & Active Ingredients
The applicable parts of bael are the unripe fruit, root, leaf, and branch. Bael is stated to have digestive and astringent properties. Constituents include tannins and furocoumarins (18). In vitro, the essential oil isolated from the leaves exhibits variable antifungal activity and inhibits spore germination of fungi isolates (3832).

Adverse Reactions Including Known Allergies
Consuming large amounts of bael may cause GI upset and constipation (18).

Possible Interactions with Herbs & Other Dietary Supplements
Insufficient reliable information available.

Possible Interactions with Drugs
No interactions are known to occur, and there is no known reason to expect a clinically significant interaction with bael.

Possible Interactions with Foods
No interactions are known to occur, and there is no known reason to expect a clinically significant interaction with bael.

Possible Interactions with Lab Tests
No interactions are known to occur, and there is no known reason to expect a clinically significant interaction with bael.

Possible Interactions with Diseases or Conditions
No interactions are known to occur, and there is no known reason to expect a clinically significant interaction with bael.

Typical Dosages & Routes of Administration that are Commonly Used
ORAL: People typically use 4 to 8 mL of the liquid extract (5264).

Comments
There is very little scientific information about this product. Our staff is continually analyzing the available information on natural medicines and will add data here as it becomes available.

BAIKAL SKULLCAP

This Product is Also Known As

Baikal Skullcap Root, Huang Qin, Huangquin, Hwanggum, Ogon, Skullcap, Wogon.
CAUTION: See separate listing for Scullcap.

Scientific Names

Scutellaria baicalensis.
Family: Lamiaceae or Labiatae.

People Use This For

In combination with seven other herbs, Baikal scullcap is used in PC-SPES to treat prostate cancer (5548). In combination with shung hua, the Baikal skullcap constituent baicalin is used to treat upper respiratory tract infections (5541). In combination with other herbs, Baikal skullcap is used to treat minimal brain dysfunction (5551). In Chinese medicine, the Baikal skullcap root is used orally to treat respiratory and gastrointestinal infections (5542), jaundice, viral hepatitis, nephritis, pelvitis, sores or swelling, and fever. It is also used for scarlet fever, headache, irritability, red eyes, flushed face, and a bitter taste in the mouth (5541,5544).

Safety

POSSIBLY SAFE ...when Baikal skullcap is used orally (5548,5549,5550,5551).
PREGNANCY AND LACTATION: Insufficient reliable information available; avoid using.

Effectiveness

There is insufficient reliable information available about the effectiveness of Baikal skullcap.

Possible Mechanism of Action & Active Ingredients

Baikal skullcap appears to have antibacterial and antiviral activity as well as diuretic, sedative, and antihypertensive properties. Baikal skullcap shows evidence it can limit hypersensitivity reactions. The Baikal skullcap constituent baicalein has weak antipyretic properties. Baicalin, a Baikal skullcap glycoside constituent, has potent anti-inflammatory and antitumor properties. Some evidence suggests it can inhibit tumor growth and suppresses carcinoma cell proliferation. The baicalin constituent also shows evidence that it can inhibit HIV-1 infection (5541). The Baikal skullcap constituents baicalein and baicalin are more effective free-radical scavengers than alpha-tocopherol (vitamin E) (5541).

Adverse Reactions Including Known Allergies

Several case reports implicate the Baikal skullcap family of Scutellaria in hepatotoxicity (5542), although the use of Baikal skullcap is considered to relatively nontoxic (5541). Use of Baikal skullcap as an intramuscular injection can cause fever and a sudden drop in the leukocyte count (5541).

Possible Interactions with Herbs & Other Dietary Supplements

Insufficient reliable information available.

Possible Interactions with Drugs

No interactions are known to occur, and there is no known reason to expect a clinically significant interaction with Baikal skullcap.

Possible Interactions with Foods

No interactions are known to occur, and there is no known reason to expect a clinically significant interaction with Baikal skullcap.

Possible Interactions with Lab Tests

No interactions are known to occur, and there is no known reason to expect a clinically significant interaction with Baikal skullcap.

Possible Interactions with Diseases or Conditions

STOMACH DYSFUNCTION: Baikal skullcap should not be used by individuals with stomach or spleen dysfunction (5544).

Typical Dosages & Routes of Administration that are Commonly Used

ORAL: A typical dose is 6-15 grams of Baikal skullcap, toasted to moderate the effect (5544). A typical dose of the Baikal skullcap constituent baicalin to treat viral hepatitis is 500 mg three times daily (5541). A typical dose to treat an upper respiratory tract infection is a tablet containing 50 mg of the Baikal skullcap constituent baicalin in combination with 100 mg of shung hua. Two to three tablets are taken four to six times per day (5541).

Comments

Common substitutions for Scutellaria baicalensis (Baikal scullcap) in Chinese medicine include Scutellaria viscidula, Scutellaria amonea, and Scutellaria ikoninikovii (5541).

BAMBOO

This Product is Also Known As
None.

Scientific Names
Arundinaria japonica.
Family: Poaceae.

People Use This For
In Chinese medicine, people use bamboo orally for asthma, coughs and gallbladder disorders (18).

Safety
There is insufficient reliable information available about the safety of the oral use of bamboo.
Pregnancy and Lactation: Insufficient reliable information available; avoid using.

Effectiveness
There is insufficient reliable information available about the effectiveness of bamboo.

Possible Mechanism of Action & Active Ingredients
The applicable part of bamboo is the young shoot. There is insufficient reliable information available about the possible mechanism of action and active ingredients.

Adverse Reactions Including Known Allergies
None reported.

Possible Interactions with Herbs & Other Dietary Supplements
Insufficient reliable information available.

Possible Interactions with Drugs
No interactions are known to occur, and there is no known reason to expect a clinically significant interaction with bamboo.

Possible Interactions with Foods
No interactions are known to occur, and there is no known reason to expect a clinically significant interaction with bamboo.

Possible Interactions with Lab Tests
No interactions are known to occur, and there is no known reason to expect a clinically significant interaction with bamboo.

Possible Interactions with Diseases or Conditions
No interactions are known to occur, and there is no known reason to expect a clinically significant interaction with bamboo.

Typical Dosages & Routes of Administration that are Commonly Used
Juice from the young shoots is hardened into bamboo sugar and is taken orally (18).

Comments
There is very little scientific information about this product. Our staff is continually analyzing the available information on natural medicines and will add data here as it becomes available.

BARLEY

This Product is Also Known As
Hordeum, Mai Ya, Pearl Barley, Pot Barley, Scotch Barley.

Scientific Names
Hordeum vulgare; Hordeum distychum.
Family: Gramineae or Poaceae.

People Use This For
Orally, barley is used for bronchitis; cancer prevention; diarrhea; gastritis; inflammatory bowel conditions; lowering blood sugar, cholesterol, and lipid levels (6); and weight loss (5078).
Historically, barley has been used for boils, gastrointestinal inflammation, and increasing strength and stamina (6).

For food uses, barley grain has been utilized as a source of folic acid, riboflavin (vitamin B2), niacin (vitamin B3), pantothenic acid (vitamin B5), pyridoxine (vitamin B6), vitamin E, carbohydrates, proteins, and fatty oils (13,18). In manufacturing, barley is used as a food grain, natural sweetener, and as an ingredient for brewing beer and making alcoholic beverages (6).

Safety

LIKELY SAFE ...when used orally (18).
PREGNANCY: LIKELY SAFE ...when used in moderate amounts as a food. POSSIBLY UNSAFE ...when used in the relatively high doses found in medicinal products. Excessive amounts of barley sprouts should not be consumed during pregnancy (12,19).
LACTATION: Insufficient reliable information available.

Effectiveness

POSSIBLY EFFECTIVE ...when used orally for reducing blood cholesterol, lipid and sugar levels, and reducing the risk of colon cancer (6). A group of overweight adults who ate barley muffins rich in beta-glucan lost an average of 1/2 pound per week, reduced total cholesterol 11% and LDL-cholesterol 12%, compared to a group who ate wheat muffins containing no beta-glucan and gained 1/2 pound per week. Each group followed the National Cholesterol Education Program's Step I diet supplemented with muffins for 4 weeks. The results of this unpublished study were presented at the Experimental Biology 2000 meeting (5078).
There is insufficient reliable information available about the effectiveness of barley for its other uses.

Possible Mechanism of Action & Active Ingredients

The applicable part of barley is the grain. The fiber content of barley is responsible for the observed reduction of cholesterol levels in healthy and hypercholesterolemic people, the reduction of blood sugar and insulin levels in healthy people, and the reduction of the colon cancer risk in rats (6). Researchers think that the beta-glucan contained in barley helps control appetite by slowing stomach emptying, prolonging the feeling of fullness and stabilizing blood sugar (5078). Hordenine, a sympathomimetic constituent of barley, stimulates peripheral blood circulation and bronchodilation (6). The enzyme, diastase, is responsible for barley's ability to ferment (216).

Adverse Reactions Including Known Allergies

Occupational exposure to barley flour can cause asthma (1300). Beer made with barley can cause anaphylaxis in sensitive individuals (317).

Possible Interactions with Herbs & Other Dietary Supplements

Insufficient reliable information available.

Possible Interactions with Drugs

DRUGS IN GENERAL: Theoretically, fiber can reduce the absorption of some drugs by reducing the gastrointestinal transit time (6).
SYMPATHOMIMETICS: Theoretically, the use of barley with sympathomimetics can result in duplication of activity due to the hordenine component (6). Concurrent use of barley should be avoided.
DIABETES THERAPY: Monitor blood glucose level closely due to claims that barley has hypoglycemic effects (19).

Possible Interactions with Foods

No interactions are known to occur, and there is no known reason to expect a clinically significant interaction with barley.

Possible Interactions with Lab Tests

CHOLESTEROL: Barley might reduce serum total cholesterol and LDL cholesterol concentrations and test results (6).
GLUCOSE: Barley might reduce blood glucose concentrations and test results (6).
The barley constituent, hordenine, can yield false-positive test results with ELISA, RIA and TLC urine assays for a number of opiate drugs. Positive urine test results should be confirmed with the more sensitive GC/MS or HPLC assay (1302).

Possible Interactions with Diseases or Conditions

CELIAC DISEASE: Because the gluten content in barley can exacerbate this disease, its use should be avoided (6).
SYMPATHOMIMETICS: Because barley can contain the sympathomimetic constituent, hordenine, barley should be avoided or used with CAUTION in conditions sensitive to this activity.

Typical Dosages & Routes of Administration that are Commonly Used

The malt extract is used in medicinal preparations and combination products (18).

Comments

Barley is a common grain that is used world-wide as a food and in the brewing processes of alcoholic beverages. Avoid confusion with malt extract products that do not contain the enzyme diastase and are intended for use as bulk laxatives (13).

BASIL

This Product is Also Known As
Basilici Herba, Common Basil, Garden Basil, Holy Basil, St. Josephwort, Sweet Basil.

Scientific Names
Ocimum basilicum.
Family: Labiatae or Lamiaceae.

People Use This For
In Chinese medicine, basil is used for stomach spasms, kidney conditions, before and after childbirth to promote blood circulation, and to treat snakebites and insect bites (11).
In folk medicine, the above ground parts of basil are used as an antiflatulent, diuretic, lactation stimulant, gargle and mouth astringent, and in maggot-infested nasal disease (8). Basil has traditionally been used to treat head colds and worms (11) and as an appetite stimulant and a cure for warts.
For food uses, basil is used as an oil or oleoresin at levels usually below 0.005%.

Safety
LIKELY SAFE ...when the above ground parts are used as a spice. It has Generally Recognized as Safe (GRAS) status in the US. Generally used at low levels, below 0.005% in foods (11).
POSSIBLY SAFE ...when the above ground parts are used orally and appropriately short-term (2,8,12).
POSSIBLY UNSAFE ...when the above ground parts of basil are used orally long-term. ...when the oil of basil is used orally (12). Both the above ground parts and the oil contain estragole which shows evidence that it might be hepatocarcinogenic (8) and mutagenic (2).
CHILDREN: LIKELY SAFE ...when the above ground parts are used as a spice. POSSIBLY UNSAFE ...when used in larger amounts due to the estragole constituents (2,8).
PREGNANCY AND LACTATION: LIKELY SAFE ...when the above ground parts are used as a spice.
POSSIBLY UNSAFE ...when used in larger amounts due to the estragole constituent of the essential oil. Estragole might have mutagenic effects (2,12).

Effectiveness
There is insufficient reliable information available about the effectiveness of basil (2).

Possible Mechanism of Action & Active Ingredients
The applicable parts of basil are the above ground plant parts. The basil plant is a rich source of vitamin C, calcium, magnesium, potassium, and iron (19). The basil constituents methyl cinnamate, methyl chavicol, ocimene, cineole, and linalool have insecticidal activities (11). The volatile oil of basil can have antagonistic activity on worms (11). The essential oil contains up to 85% estragole (2) (methyl chavicol), which can produce liver tumors in mice (11). The constituent, xanthomicrol, can have cytotoxic and antineoplastic activities (11).

Adverse Reactions Including Known Allergies
Basil is known to cause hypoglycemia (214). Due to the adverse effects of the constituents of basil, CAUTION should be used in long-term treatment, which may be unsafe (12).

Possible Interactions with Herbs & Other Dietary Supplements
Insufficient reliable information available.

Possible Interactions with Drugs
No interactions are known to occur, and there is no known reason to expect a clinically significant interaction with basil.

Possible Interactions with Foods
No interactions are known to occur, and there is no known reason to expect a clinically significant interaction with basil.

Possible Interactions with Lab Tests
No interactions are known to occur, and there is no known reason to expect a clinically significant interaction with basil.

Possible Interactions with Diseases or Conditions
No interactions are known to occur, and there is no known reason to expect a clinically significant interaction with basil.

Typical Dosages & Routes of Administration that are Commonly Used
ORAL: The typical dose of basil leaf for distention or flatulence is 1 cup of the fresh brewed tea 2-3 times a day between meals. The tea is prepared by steeping 2-4 grams in 150 mL boiling water for 10-15 minutes and

straining (8). For chronic flatulence the usual oral dose is 1 cup 2-3 times daily between meals for 8 days, then stopped for 14 days, and resumed for another 8 days (8).

Comments

Due to the carcinogenic potential of basil oil; avoid using (18).

BAYBERRY

This Product is Also Known As

Candleberry, Myrica, Southern Bayberry, Southern Wax Myrtle, Tallow Shrub, Vegetable Tallow, Waxberry, Wax Myrtle.
CAUTION: See separate listing for Sweet Gale (Myrica gale) also known as Bayberry.

Scientific Names

Myrica cerifera; Myrica pensylvanica.
Family: Myricaceae.

People Use This For

Orally, the root bark and berries of bayberry are taken for head colds (5), mucous colitis, diarrhea, as an antipyretic, a circulatory stimulant (4), and an emetic in large doses (5).
Topically, bayberry is used for sore throat as a gargle (4), for leukorrhea (vaginal discharge) as a douche (4), indolent ulcers (5), and wound healing (6).
In folk medicine, bayberry is used to treat diarrhea (5).

Safety

POSSIBLY UNSAFE ...when used orally. The root bark and berries contain high amounts of tannins (6). Large doses may have mineralocorticoid activity (4). Root bark can also contain a carcinogen (5).
There is insufficient reliable information available about the safety of the topical use of bayberry.
PREGNANCY AND LACTATION: POSSIBLY UNSAFE ...because of possible carcinogenic, or mineralocorticoid activities; avoid using (4,5).

Effectiveness

POSSIBLY EFFECTIVE ...when used topically as an astringent (5).
There is insufficient reliable information available about the effectiveness of bayberry used orally.

Possible Mechanism of Action & Active Ingredients

The applicable parts of bayberry are the root bark and berry. The tannin constituents of bayberry are responsible for its astringent action (4).

Adverse Reactions Including Known Allergies

Bayberry can cause gastrointestinal irritation, vomiting, liver damage (possibly due to tannin content), and can act as an irritant and sensitizer (6).

Possible Interactions with Herbs & Other Dietary Supplements

Insufficient reliable information available.

Possible Interactions with Drugs

Large amounts of tannin-containing herbs can interfere with HYPERTENSION, HYPOTENSION, or STEROID therapy (4).

Possible Interactions with Foods

No interactions are known to occur, and there is no known reason to expect a clinically significant interaction with bayberry.

Possible Interactions with Lab Tests

No interactions are known to occur, and there is no known reason to expect a clinically significant interaction with bayberry.

Possible Interactions with Diseases or Conditions

HYPERTENSION: Large amounts of tannin-containing herbs can interfere with this condition.
SODIUM AND WATER RETENTION: Avoid bayberry use due to the potential mineralocorticoid activity, which can influence salt metabolism (4).

Typical Dosages & Routes of Administration that are Commonly Used

ORAL: The typical dose of bayberry is 0.6-2 grams powdered bark, steeped in boiling water and strained, used three times a day (4). The liquid extract of bayberry (1:1 in 45% alcohol) is typically used 0.6-2 mL three times a day (4).

Comments
Bayberry is a shrub that is commonly found in Texas and the eastern US. The wax extract taken from the berries is used in fragrances and candles.

BEAN POD

This Product is Also Known As
Common Bean, Green Bean, Kidney Bean, Navy Bean, Phaseoli fructus, Pinto Bean, Seed-Free Bean Pods, Sine Semine, Snap Bean, String Bean, Wax Bean.

Scientific Names
Phaseolus vulgaris varieties.
Family: Fabaceae.

People Use This For
Orally, bean pod is used for urinary tract infections, kidney or bladder stones, and the promotion of urine flow (2,18).
In herbal tea combinations, bean pod is used for kidney and bladder problems (7,18).
In folk medicine, bean pod is used as a diuretic and for diabetes (18).

Safety
POSSIBLY SAFE ...when the ripe, dried pods are used orally and appropriately in medicinal amounts (18).
POSSIBLY UNSAFE ...when large amounts of fresh bean husks are ingested. Raw bean husks contain lectins that can cause gastrointestinal upset. Cooking destroys lectins (18).
PREGNANCY AND LACTATION: Insufficient reliable information available; avoid using.

Effectiveness
POSSIBLY EFFECTIVE ...when used orally as a supportive treatment for the inability to urinate (2).
There is insufficient reliable information available about the effectiveness of bean pod for its other uses.

Possible Mechanism of Action & Active Ingredients
The applicable part of bean pod is the pod without the seeds. Bean pods demonstrate a weak diuretic effect in animals and humans (18). The chromium salts found in bean pods play a role in its antidiabetic effect (18).

Adverse Reactions Including Known Allergies
The ingestion of large amounts of green bean husks, or raw green beans, can cause vomiting, diarrhea, and gastroenteritis due to the content of the plant protein lectin. Cooking usually destroys lectins (18).

Possible Interactions with Herbs & Other Dietary Supplements
Insufficient reliable information available.

Possible Interactions with Drugs
DIABETES THERAPY: Monitor blood glucose level closely due to claims that bean pod has hypoglycemic effects (19).

Possible Interactions with Foods
No interactions are known to occur, and there is no known reason to expect a clinically significant interaction with bean pod.

Possible Interactions with Lab Tests
No interactions are known to occur, and there is no known reason to expect a clinically significant interaction with bean pod.

Possible Interactions with Diseases or Conditions
DIABETES: Monitor blood glucose level closely due to claims that bean pod has hypoglycemic effects (19).

Typical Dosages & Routes of Administration that are Commonly Used
ORAL: The typical dose of bean pod is one cup tea several times per day, and the tea is prepared by simmering 2.5 grams bean pods in 150 mL boiling water for 10-15 minutes and then straining (2,18). The amount of bean pod usually taken is 5-15 grams of bean pods per day (2,18).

Comments
None.

© Copyright 2000, Natural Medicines Comprehensive Database (209) 472-2244. For updated data, go to www.NaturalDatabase.com

BEAR'S GARLIC

This Product is Also Known As
Bears Garlic, Broad-leaved Garlic, Ramsons, Wild Garlic.

Scientific Names
Allium ursinum.

People Use This For
Orally, bear's garlic is used for GI complaints, indigestion accompanied by the fermentation of stomach contents, flatulence, high blood pressure, and arteriosclerosis (18).
Topically, bear's garlic is used for chronic rashes (18).

Safety
There is insufficient reliable information available about the safety of bear's garlic.
Pregnancy and Lactation: Insufficient reliable information available; avoid using.

Effectiveness
There is insufficient reliable information available about the effectiveness of bear's garlic.

Possible Mechanism of Action & Active Ingredients
The applicable parts of bear's garlic are the herb and bulb. The bear's garlic constituents, glucopyranoside, kaempferol, and flavonoids, inhibit human platelet aggregation (3830). In vitro, bear's garlic exhibits cardioprotective properties. In vitro and in vivo, bear's garlic moderately inhibits the angiotensin converting enzyme (ACE), which could contribute to the suggested cardioprotective and blood pressure lowering action. (3831).

Adverse Reactions Including Known Allergies
None reported.

Possible Interactions with Herbs & Other Dietary Supplements
Insufficient reliable information available.

Possible Interactions with Drugs
No interactions are known to occur, and there is no known reason to expect a clinically significant interaction with bear's garlic.

Possible Interactions with Foods
No interactions are known to occur, and there is no known reason to expect a clinically significant interaction with bear's garlic.

Possible Interactions with Lab Tests
No interactions are known to occur, and there is no known reason to expect a clinically significant interaction with bear's garlic.

Possible Interactions with Diseases or Conditions
No interactions are known to occur, and there is no known reason to expect a clinically significant interaction with bear's garlic.

Typical Dosages & Routes of Administration that are Commonly Used
ORAL: People typically use 3 capsules of dried bear's garlic leaf daily. The quantity of garlic in each capsule, which varies from lot to lot, is determined by the potency of active principals. There are claims that bear's garlic must be used fresh, only the bulb may be dried and suggests using the fresh plant in unspecified quantities as an ingredient in soup, salad, or as a vegetable (5263,5266).

Comments
There is very little scientific information about this product. Our staff is continually analyzing the available information on natural medicines and will add data here as it becomes available.

BEE POLLEN

This Product is Also Known As
Buckwheat Pollen, Maize Pollen, Pine Pollen, Pollen D'Abeille.
CAUTION: See separate listings for Honey Bee venom, Honey, and Royal Jelly.

Scientific Names
None.

People Use This For

Orally, bee pollen is used for nutrition, a tonic, appetite stimulant, improved stamina and athletic ability, premature aging, prevention of hay fever or allergic rhinitis, mouth sores, rheumatism, painful urination, prostate conditions, and radiation sickness. It is also used for bleeding problems including coughing or vomiting blood, bloody diarrhea, nosebleed, cerebral hemorrhage, and menstrual problems. Bee pollen taken orally is used for GI problems including constipation, diarrhea, enteritis, and colitis (5,6,11).

Topically, bee pollen is used for skin care and skin softening products (11).

In Chinese medicine, bee pollen is used orally as a diuretic, and for alcohol intoxication (11), and topically for eczema, pustular eruptions, and diaper rash (11).

Safety

LIKELY SAFE ...when used orally and appropriately (5,6,11).

POSSIBLY UNSAFE ...when used orally by individuals with pollen allergies. Bee pollen can cause allergic reactions including anaphylaxis (5,6,11).

There is insufficient reliable information available about the safety of the topical use of bee pollen.

PREGNANCY: POSSIBLY UNSAFE ...when used orally; avoid using. Might have uterine stimulant effects (5,6,11).

LACTATION: Insufficient reliable information available; avoid using.

Effectiveness

LIKELY INEFFECTIVE...when taken orally for increasing athletic stamina (6).

There is insufficient reliable information available about the effectiveness of bee pollen for its other uses.

Possible Mechanism of Action & Active Ingredients

Up to 50% of bee pollen can be polysaccharides. The other constituents include carotenoids, lipids, protein, simple sugars, and vitamin C. None of the identified constituents have been linked to therapeutic effects (5).

Adverse Reactions Including Known Allergies

Oral use of bee pollen has been associated with two cases of acute hepatitis. One case involved ingestion of two tablespoons of pure bee pollen daily for several months, the other case involved ingestion of 14 tablets per day (for six weeks) of a combination herbal product containing bee pollen, chaparral, and 19 other herbs (1351).

An allergy to bee pollen is manifested by itching, swelling, shortness of breath, light headedness, and anaphylaxis. Chronic allergy symptoms due to bee pollen include GI and neurologic symptoms and eosinophilia (5,6,11).

Possible Interactions with Herbs & Other Dietary Supplements

Insufficient reliable information available.

Possible Interactions with Drugs

No interactions are known to occur, and there is no known reason to expect a clinically significant interaction with bee pollen.

Possible Interactions with Foods

No interactions are known to occur, and there is no known reason to expect a clinically significant interaction with bee pollen.

Possible Interactions with Lab Tests

LIVER FUNCTION TESTS: Bee pollen might increase alkaline phosphatase (Alk Phos), alanine aminotransferase (ALT), aspartate aminotransferase (AST), lactate dehydrogenase (LDH), total bilirubin, prothrombin time (PT), and test results. Bee pollen has been associated with two cases of acute hepatitis and abnormally high results for these tests (1351).

Possible Interactions with Diseases or Conditions

LIVER DISEASE: Caution, bee pollen use has been associated with two cases of acute hepatitis (1351).

POLLEN ALLERGIES: Individuals with pollen allergies can be at increased risk for allergic reactions to bee pollen (6).

Typical Dosages & Routes of Administration that are Commonly Used

ORAL: People typically take 500 mg two to three times daily (6006).

Comments

Bee pollen is composed of plant nectars, bee saliva, and plant pollens collected by worker bees. Sources of the pollens come from various plants, including buckwheat, maize, pine (songhuafen), rape, and typha (puhuang) (11). Avoid confusion with honey bee venom, honey, and royal jelly. Bee pollen composition varies by plant source(s) and geographic region. Products vary in bee pollens used for the manufacturing process (5,6). Although bee pollen contains trace amounts of many nutrients, it is an extremely expensive form of nutrition (5).

BEESWAX

This Product is Also Known As
Bleached Beeswax, White Beeswax, White Wax, Yellow Beeswax, Yellow Wax.

Scientific Names
Apis mellifera; Apis cerana.
Family: Apidae.

People Use This For
Orally, beeswax is used for lowering lipids (4051), as an anti-inflammatory (4052) and as anti-ulcer agent (4053). In Chinese medicine, it has been used orally for diarrhea, hiccups, and pain relief (11).
White beeswax and beeswax absolute are utilized in food and beverages (11), as stiffening agents, and as tablet polishing components in pharmaceutical products (11,16).
In manufacturing, yellow and white beeswax are used as thickeners, emulsifiers, and as stiffening agents in cosmetics (11). Beeswax absolute is used as a fragrance ingredient in soaps and perfumes (11).

Safety
LIKELY SAFE ...when consumed in amounts found in foods (11). Beeswax has Generally Recognized as Safe (GRAS) status in the US (11), and is listed in the United States Pharmacopoeia (10) as an inert ingredient (16). ...when used as an oral medicinal agent (11). ...when used topically (11).
PREGNANCY AND LACTATION: LIKELY SAFE ...when consumed in food amounts.

Effectiveness
There is insufficient reliable information available about the effectiveness of beeswax.

Possible Mechanism of Action & Active Ingredients
A natural mixture of high molecular weight alcohols isolated and purified from beeswax, termed D-002, had mild anti-inflammatory effects in experimental animals (4052). In rats, injected D-002 partially inhibited experimentally-induced gastric damage (4053,4054).

Adverse Reactions Including Known Allergies
Allergic reactions may occur (11).

Possible Interactions with Herbs & Other Dietary Supplements
Insufficient reliable information available.

Possible Interactions with Drugs
NONSTEROIDAL ANTI-INFLAMMATORY DRUGS (NSAIDs): Theoretically, concomitant use may protect against NSAID-induced ulcers (4053,4054).

Possible Interactions with Foods
No interactions are known to occur, and there is no known reason to expect a clinically significant interaction with beeswax.

Possible Interactions with Lab Tests
No interactions are known to occur, and there is no known reason to expect a clinically significant interaction with beeswax.

Possible Interactions with Diseases or Conditions
No interactions are known to occur, and there is no known reason to expect a clinically significant interaction with beeswax.

Typical Dosages & Routes of Administration that are Commonly Used
No typical dosage.

Comments
The three major beeswax products are yellow beeswax, white beeswax, and beeswax absolute. Yellow beeswax is the crude product obtained from the honeycomb. White beeswax is derived from yellow beeswax by bleaching, and beeswax absolute is derived from yellow beeswax by extraction with alcohol. Beeswax is obtained from the honeycomb of the honeybee (Apis mellifera) and other Apis species.

BEET

This Product is Also Known As
Fodder Beet, Garden Beet, Mangel, Mangold, Red Beet, Sugarbeet, Yellow Beet.

Scientific Names
Beta vulgaris.
Family: Chenopodiaceae.

People Use This For
Orally, beets are used as a supportive therapy in the treatment of liver diseases and fatty liver (18).

Safety
LIKELY SAFE ...when eaten as a food or in amounts typically found in foods.
There is insufficient reliable information available about the safety of the oral medicinal use of beets.
PREGNANCY AND LACTATION: Avoid using amounts greater than those typically found in foods (18).

Effectiveness
There is insufficient reliable information available about the effectiveness of beets.

Possible Mechanism of Action & Active Ingredients
The applicable part of beet is the root. Animal data suggests that beets may be effective against fat deposition in the liver. A component called betaine may play a role (18).

Adverse Reactions Including Known Allergies
Ingestion of large quantities of beets could lead to hypocalcemia and kidney damage because of the oxaluric acid content (18).

Possible Interactions with Herbs & Other Dietary Supplements
Insufficient reliable information available.

Possible Interactions with Drugs
No interactions are known to occur, and there is no known reason to expect a clinically significant interaction with beet.

Possible Interactions with Foods
No interactions are known to occur, and there is no known reason to expect a clinically significant interaction with beet.

Possible Interactions with Lab Tests
No interactions are known to occur, and there is no known reason to expect a clinically significant interaction with beet.

Possible Interactions with Diseases or Conditions
KIDNEY DISEASE: Ingestion of large quantities of beets could worsen kidney disease (18).

Typical Dosages & Routes of Administration that are Commonly Used
Beet is taken orally as a standardized granular powder (18).

Comments
None.

BELLADONNA

This Product is Also Known As
Deadly Nightshade, Devil's Cherries, Devil's Herb, Divale, Dwale, Dwayberry, Great Morel, Naughty Man's Cherries, Poison Black Cherries.
CAUTION: See separate listings for Bittersweet Nightshade and Henbane.

Scientific Names
Atropa belladonna; Atropa belladonna acuminata.
Family: Solanaceae.

People Use This For
Orally, belladonna is used as a sedative, antispasmodic in bronchial asthma and whooping cough, cold and hay fever remedy, for Parkinson's disease, intestinal and biliary colic, and motion sickness (11).
Topically, belladonna is used in liniments for rheumatism, sciatica, and neuralgia (11).
Rectally, belladonna is used in hemorrhoid suppositories (11).
In Chinese medicine, the hyoscine-containing plants are used as anesthetics (11).
In folk medicine, belladonna is used in topical medicinal plasters for treating psychiatric disorders, hyperkinesis, hyperhidrosis, and bronchial asthma (18).
Historically, belladonna berry juice has been used by Italian women to dilate their pupils giving them a striking appearance.

Safety

POSSIBLY SAFE ...when the standardized extract is used orally and appropriately under the supervision of a medical professional trained in the use of belladonna (2). Belladonna is available as a prescription drug in the US and has a narrow therapeutic index.
LIKELY UNSAFE ...when the standardized extract is used orally without medical supervision (12). ...when the leaf or root or other preparation is used orally (12).
There is insufficient reliable information available about the safety of topical or rectal use of belladonna.
CHILDREN: POSSIBLY SAFE ...when used orally in children older than 6 years old only under medical supervision. LIKELY UNSAFE ...when the leaf, root, or extract is used orally in children under 6 years old (12).
There is insufficient reliable information available about the safety of topical or rectal use of belladonna in children.
PREGNANCY: LIKELY UNSAFE ...when the leaf or root are used orally without medical supervision. There is insufficient reliable information about the safety of the standardized extract of belladonna used orally, topically or rectally during pregnancy.
LACTATION: LIKELY UNSAFE ...when the leaf, root, standardized extract or other preparation are used orally. Use should be avoided because it can reduce milk production and is secreted into breast milk (15). There is insufficient reliable information available about the safety of topical or rectal use during lactation.

Effectiveness

LIKELY EFFECTIVE ...when used orally for spasms and colic-like pain in the GI tract and the bile ducts (2). There is insufficient reliable information available about the effectiveness of belladonna for its other uses.

Possible Mechanism of Action & Active Ingredients

The applicable parts of belladonna are the leaf and root. Its anticholinergic activity is due to the 0.3%-0.5% tropane alkaloid constituents composed mainly of l-hyoscyamine and traces of l-scopolamine and atropine (dl-hyoscyamine) (11). On extraction, most of the l-hyoscyamine is racemized to atropine (11).

Adverse Reactions Including Known Allergies

Oral use of belladonna can cause dry mouth, decreased perspiration, dilation of pupils, blurred vision, red dry skin, hyperthermia, tachycardia, difficulty urinating, hallucinations, spasms, acute psychosis, convulsions, and coma (2,11,553).

Possible Interactions with Herbs & Other Dietary Supplements

Insufficient reliable information available.

Possible Interactions with Drugs

ANTICHOLINERGIC DRUGS: Belladonna can increase the anticholinergic effects and adverse effects of amantadine, antihistamines, phenothiazines, procainamide, quinidine, tricyclic antidepressants, and others (2).

Possible Interactions with Foods

No interactions are known to occur, and there is no known reason to expect a clinically significant interaction with belladonna.

Possible Interactions with Lab Tests

No interactions are known to occur, and there is no known reason to expect a clinically significant interaction with belladonna.

Possible Interactions with Diseases or Conditions

CONGESTIVE HEART FAILURE (CHF): Contraindicated; belladonna might cause tachycardia and exacerbate CHF due to its hyoscyamine (atropine) and scopolamine content (15).
CONSTIPATION: Contraindicated; belladonna might cause constipation due to its hyoscyamine (atropine) and scopolamine content (15).
DOWN SYNDROME: Caution, patients with Down syndrome might be hypersensitive to the antimuscarinic effects (mydriasis, positive chronotropic heart effects, etc.) of hyoscyamine (atropine) and scopolamine contained in belladonna (15).
ESOPHAGEAL REFLUX: Contraindicated; belladonna might delay gastric emptying and decrease lower esophageal pressure, promoting gastric retention and exacerbating reflux due to its hyoscyamine (atropine) and scopolamine content (15).
FEVER: Contraindicated; belladonna might increase the risk of hyperthermia in patients with fever due to its hyoscyamine (atropine) and scopolamine content (15).
GASTRIC ULCER: Contraindicated; belladonna might delay gastric emptying and exacerbate gastric ulcers due to its hyoscyamine (atropine) and scopolamine content (15).
GI INFECTIONS: Contraindicated; belladonna might suppress GI motility causing retention of infecting organisms or toxins due to its hyoscyamine (atropine) and scopolamine content (15).
HIATAL HERNIA: Contraindicated; belladonna might delay gastric emptying and decrease lower esophageal pressure, promoting gastric retention and exacerbating reflux due to its hyoscyamine (atropine) and scopolamine content (15).

TOXIC MEGACOLON: Contraindicated; belladonna might suppress intestinal motility, which might produce paralytic ileus and exacerbate toxic megacolon, due to its hyoscyamine (atropine) and scopolamine content (2,15).
NARROW-ANGLE GLAUCOMA: Contraindicated; belladonna might increase ocular tension in patients with narrow-angle (angle-closure) glaucoma due to its hyoscyamine (atropine) and scopolamine content (2,15).
OBSTRUCTIVE GI TRACT DISEASE: Contraindicated; belladonna might exacerbate obstructive GI tract diseases (including atony, paralytic ileus, and stenosis) due to its hyoscyamine (atropine) and scopolamine content (15).
TACHYARRHYTHMIAS: Contraindicated; belladonna might cause tachycardia due to its hyoscyamine (atropine) and scopolamine content (2,15).
URINARY RETENTION: Contraindicated; belladonna might increase urinary retention due to its hyoscyamine (atropine) and scopolamine content (2,15).
ULCERATIVE COLITIS: Contraindicated; belladonna might suppress intestinal motility, which might produce paralytic ileus and precipitate toxic megacolon, due to its hyoscyamine (atropine) and scopolamine content (15).

Typical Dosages & Routes of Administration that are Commonly Used

ORAL: The belladonna leaf powder is typically an average single dose of 50-100 mg. The maximum single dose is 200 mg, which is equivalent to 0.6 mg total alkaloids, calculated as hyoscyamine. The maximum daily dose is 600 mg, which is equivalent to 1.8 mg total alkaloids, calculated as hyoscyamine. The root powder is commonly taken in an average single dosage of 50 mg. The maximum single dose is 100 mg, which is equivalent to 0.5 mg total alkaloids, calculated as hyoscyamine. The maximum daily dose of the root powder is 300 mg, equivalent to 1.5 mg total alkaloids calculated as hyoscyamine. The belladonna extract has an average single dose of 10 mg. The maximum single dose is 50 mg, equivalent to 0.73 mg total alkaloids calculated as hyoscyamine, and the maximum daily dosage is 150 mg, equivalent to 2.2 mg total alkaloids calculated as hyoscyamine (2).

Comments

The name, belladonna, means beautiful lady. The belladonna berry juice has been used historically in Italy to dilate the pupils of women giving them a striking appearance (11). Avoid confusion with bittersweet nightshade (Solanum dulcamara) and henbane (nightshade).

BENZOIN

This Product is Also Known As

Benzoe, Gum Benjamin, Gum Benzoin, Sumatra Benzoin.

Scientific Names

Styrax benzoin; Styrax paralleloneurus.
Family: Styraceae.

People Use This For

Orally, benzoin is used for throat and bronchial inflammation.
Topically, benzoin is used as an antiseptic, astringent, skin protectant, and styptic on small cuts. Benzoin is also used topically for skin ulcers, bedsores, cracked nipples, and fissures of the lips and anus (11,13).
The inhalation of benzoin is used to treat laryngitis, croup, and other respiratory conditions.
In combination with other herbs, benzoin tincture (benzoin, aloe, storax and tolu balsam) is used as a skin protectant.
In dentistry, benzoin is used for gum inflammation and oral herpes lesions.
In manufacturing, benzoin is used in making pharmaceutical preparations (11).

Safety

LIKELY SAFE ...when benzoin is used as a food flavoring. Approved for food use; the maximum level is 0.014% in candy and baked goods (11).
POSSIBLY SAFE ...when preparations of the gum resin are used orally for medicinal purposes (12). ...when used topically (11). Tincture of benzoin can cause contact dermatitis.
There is insufficient reliable information available about the safety of inhaled benzoin.
PREGNANCY AND LACTATION: Insufficient reliable information available; avoid using.

Effectiveness

POSSIBLY EFFECTIVE ...when used topically, especially as the compound benzoin tincture for skin. ...when the inhaled benzoin is used as an expectorant (13).
There is insufficient reliable information available about the effectiveness of benzoin for its other uses.

Possible Mechanism of Action & Active Ingredients

The applicable part of benzoin is the gum resin. Benzoin has the following effects: antiseptic, stimulant, expectorant, astringent, diuretic, and skin protectant (11,13).

Adverse Reactions Including Known Allergies

The compound benzoin tincture (benzoin, aloe, storax and tolu balsam) can cause contact dermatitis (11) and should be avoided in sensitive individuals.

Possible Interactions with Herbs & Other Dietary Supplements

Insufficient reliable information available.

Possible Interactions with Drugs

No interactions are known to occur, and there is no known reason to expect a clinically significant interaction with benzoin.

Possible Interactions with Foods

No interactions are known to occur, and there is no known reason to expect a clinically significant interaction with benzoin.

Possible Interactions with Lab Tests

No interactions are known to occur, and there is no known reason to expect a clinically significant interaction with benzoin.

Possible Interactions with Diseases or Conditions

SENSITIVE INDIVIDUALS: Avoid contact with benzoin and the compound benzoin tincture due to contact dermatitis (11).

Typical Dosages & Routes of Administration that are Commonly Used

INHALATION: People typically add 5 mL of a compound benzoin tincture (USP) to 473 mL of hot water or place the tincture directly on a handkerchief (5008).
TOPICAL: People apply no more than a few drops of compound benzoin tincture (USP) every two hours (5008).
Compound benzoin tincture contains 100 grams of benzoin powder, 20 grams of aloe powder, 80 grams of storax, and 40 grams of tolu balsam per 1000 mL of tincture (16).

Comments

Benzoin is the gum resin of Styrax species trees. Avoid confusion with Siam benzoin (Styrax tonikensis), which is used only in manufacturing and has no medicinal uses (11,13).

BERGAMOT OIL

This Product is Also Known As

Bergamot, Bergamot Orange, Bergamota, Bergamotier, Bergamoto, Bergamotte, Bergamotto Bigarade Orange, Oleum Bergamotte.
CAUTION: See separate listings for Bitter Orange flower, Bitter Orange peel, Oswego Tea, and Sweet Orange.

Scientific Names

Citrus bergamia, synonym Citrus aurantium bergamia.
Family: Rutaceae.

People Use This For

Topically, bergamot oil is used to treat psoriasis in conjunction with long-wave ultraviolet light (11). Bergamot oil is also used topically for vitiligo, which is the loss of the melanin pigment on the skin (11), and mycosis fungoides (11). Historically, it has been used as an insecticide to protect the body against lice and other vermin (215).
For food uses, bergamot oil is widely used as a citrus flavoring agent, up to 0.02% in gelatins and puddings (11).
In manufacturing of cosmetics, bergamot oil is used (up to 3% in perfumes and 0.25% in creams and lotions), soaps (11), and suntan oils (9).

Safety

LIKELY SAFE ...when bergamot oil is used orally in food amounts (12).
POSSIBLY UNSAFE ...when applied topically, because it can act as a photosensitizer and can induce malignant changes (6).
CHILDREN: POSSIBLY UNSAFE ...when large amounts are ingested. Can cause intestinal colic, convulsions, and death (12).
PREGNANCY AND LACTATION: POSSIBLY UNSAFE ...when used topically. Insufficient reliable information available; avoid using orally in amounts greater than those found in foods.

Effectiveness

POSSIBLY EFFECTIVE ...when used with long-wave UV light for treating psoriasis, vitiligo, and mycosis fungoides (11).
There is insufficient reliable information available about the effectiveness of bergamot oil for its other uses.

Possible Mechanism of Action & Active Ingredients

The applicable part of bergamot is the peel. Bergamot oil is cold-expressed from the peel (11). Further distillation produces rectified (terpeneless) bergamot oil (11). The photosensitivity of bergamot oil is linked to the furocoumarin constituents, bergapten (5-methoxypsoralen) and xanthotoxin (8-methoxypsoralen) (6).

Adverse Reactions Including Known Allergies

OCCUPATIONAL SENSITIZATION: Frequent contact with the peel or oil can cause erythema, blisters, pustules, dermatoses leading to scab formation, and pigment spots (18). Bergamot oil can cause photosensitivity, skin rash, and hyperpigmentation of the face and other areas. Photosensitivity reaches its peak two hours after topical application (6). Some skin changes can be malignant in nature (6).

Possible Interactions with Herbs & Other Dietary Supplements

Insufficient reliable information available.

Possible Interactions with Drugs

PHOTOSENSITIZING DRUGS: Theoretically, topical use of bergamot oil can compound the photosensitizing effects and increase the risk of side effects. Concomitant use should be avoided.

Possible Interactions with Foods

No interactions are known to occur, and there is no known reason to expect a clinically significant interaction with bergamot oil.

Possible Interactions with Lab Tests

No interactions are known to occur, and there is no known reason to expect a clinically significant interaction with bergamot oil.

Possible Interactions with Diseases or Conditions

SUN SENSITIVE INDIVIDUALS: Avoid the topical use of bergamot oil due to its photosensitivity adverse effects.

Typical Dosages & Routes of Administration that are Commonly Used

No typical dosage.

Comments

Avoid confusion with scarlet bergamot (oswego tea, mondara didyma) (6).

BETA-CAROTENE

This Product is Also Known As

Beta Carotene, Provitamin A.
CAUTION: See separate listing for Vitamin A.

Scientific Names

Beta-carotene.

People Use This For

Orally, beta-carotene is taken as a dietary source of vitamin A (15), for treating vitiligo (6), and reducing photosensitivities, including erythropoietic protoporphyria (EPP) and polymorphous light eruption (15). Beta-carotene is also used orally for decreasing exercise-induced asthma (1474), and reducing the risk of some cancers (6,139,1470,1473), cardiovascular disease, and age-related macular degeneration (138,1470).

Safety

LIKELY SAFE ...when consumed in amounts commonly found in foods (139,140).
POSSIBLY SAFE ...when used in therapeutic amounts by nonsmokers (139).
POSSIBLY UNSAFE ...when used orally in doses greater than 20 mg/day by smokers, former smokers, people exposed to asbestos, and people who drink significant amounts of alcohol (15,139,1471,4257).
PREGNANCY: LIKELY SAFE ...when consumed in amounts found in foods. LIKELY UNSAFE ...when used orally in large doses because large amounts of beta-carotene can be fetotoxic (15).
LACTATION: LIKELY SAFE ...when consumed in amounts found in foods. There is insufficient reliable information available for using larger amounts of beta-carotene during lactation; avoid using.

Effectiveness

LIKELY EFFECTIVE ...when used orally for reducing photosensitivity in erythropoietic protoporphyria (rash, itching, or eczema) due to sunlight exposure (15).
POSSIBLY EFFECTIVE ...when a diet high in beta-carotene is consumed to reduce the risk of breast cancer in premenopausal women with a positive family history of breast cancer (1444). This is based on epidemiological data. ...when a diet high in beta-carotene is consumed to reduce the risk of age-related macular degeneration (1470).

This is based on epidemiological data. ...when beta-carotene supplements are taken orally to reduce the risk of prostate carcinoma in men who have plasma beta-carotene concentrations less than 153.25 ng/mL (1473). ...when beta-carotene supplements are taken orally to induce remission in patients with oral leukoplakia. Study data suggest an increased risk of disease progression over 12 months if beta-carotene is stopped (1470,1472). ...when a mixture of beta-carotene is taken orally to prevent exercise-induced asthma (1474). ...when a mixture of beta-carotene is taken orally as a sunscreen in individuals with sensitivity to sun exposure. In this study, 25 mg of mixed beta-carotene daily for 12 weeks reduced skin redness after exposure to UV light in a group of sun-sensitive individuals compared to skin redness after UV exposure without beta-carotene supplementation in the same group (6134). ...when synthetic beta-carotene is taken orally by malnourished women to reduce pregnancy-related mortality. In one trial, 42 mg all-trans beta-carotene taken weekly before, during and after pregnancy by malnourished women in Nepal reduced pregnancy-related mortality by 49% (6153). ...when synthetic beta-carotene is taken orally by malnourished women to reduce the occurrence of pregnancy-related night blindness. In one trial, 42 mg all-trans beta-cartotene taken weekly before, during and after pregnancy by malnourished women in Nepal reduced, but did not eliminate, the occurrence of pregnancy-related night blindness (6154).

POSSIBLY INEFFECTIVE ...when a diet high in beta-carotene is consumed to reduce the risk of heart disease (15,138,139,1440,1448,1470). ...when synthetic beta-carotene supplements (containing cis- and trans-beta-carotene) are used orally to prevent nonmelanoma skin cancer (NMSC), including basal cell carcinoma (BCC) and squamous cell carcinoma (SCC) (1297). ...when synthetic beta-carotene supplements are used orally to reduce the risk of strokes in male smokers. In one clinical trial, synthetic beta-carotene 20 mg/day for a median of six years had no effect on the overall incidence of strokes in male smokers, but increased the risk of intracerebral hemorrhage by 62% (1371,5028). ...when synthetic beta-carotene is taken orally by malnourished women to reduce fetal and early infant mortality. In one trial, 42 mg all-trans beta-carotene taken weekly before, during and after pregnancy by malnourished women in Nepal failed to reduce fetal and early infant mortality (6152).

LIKELY INEFFECTIVE ...when a diet high in beta-carotene is consumed to prevent prostate cancer in men with plasma beta-carotene concentrations greater than 153.25 ng/mL (148,149,1470,1473). ...when dietary beta-carotene and/or beta-carotene supplements are used to prevent breast, lung, colon, rectal, uterine and ovarian cancers in postmenopausal women (1444,1448). ...when beta-carotene supplements are taken orally to prevent lung cancer in smokers (139,1471). Beta-carotene supplements are associated with an increased risk of lung cancer in smokers, former smokers, people exposed to asbestos and those who ingest significant amounts of alcohol (139,1471). ...when a diet high in beta-carotene is consumed to prevent cervical cancer (140). ...when beta-carotene supplements are used orally as a sunscreen in individuals with normal sun sensitivity (15).

Possible Mechanism of Action & Active Ingredients

Beta-carotene belongs to a class of red, orange, and yellow pigments called carotenoids. Carotenoids are present in many fruits and vegetables. Structurally, beta-carotene is closely related to alpha-carotene. Both alpha- and beta-carotene are precursors for vitamin A, but beta-carotene also has activity independent of its conversion to vitamin A (139,1470). Beta-carotene consists of a number of isomers. Synthetic beta-carotene, the form used in most clinical studies, is composed of the all-trans form. Natural beta-carotene sources also contain 9-cis-, 13-cis- and 15-cis-beta-carotene (1474). Human data indicate that 9-cis-beta-carotene is poorly absorbed, and most is converted to all-trans-beta-carotene. However, tissue levels of 9-cis-beta-carotene may be higher than those of all-trans-beta-carotene. Well designed human trials are needed to determine what, if any, effect the various isomers have on medical conditions. Little is known about the pharmacology of beta-carotene. Preliminary evidence suggests that beta-carotene prevents lipid peroxidation and has antioxidant activity (139), but this is not supported by clinical trials using supplemental all-trans-beta-carotene (1448,1470,1471,1473,2042). Short-term use of all-trans-beta-carotene supplements does not affect T-lymphocyte immune function in lactating women (6105). Supplemental beta-carotene is similarly absorbed when taken with high-fat (36 grams) or low-fat (3 grams fat) meals (6133).

Adverse Reactions Including Known Allergies

Orally, beta-carotene can cause yellow or orange skin pigmentation (15).

Possible Interactions with Herbs & Other Dietary Supplements

Insufficient reliable information available.

Possible Interactions with Drugs

No interactions are known to occur, and there is no reason to expect a clinically significant interaction with beta-carotene (see Drug Influences on Nutrient Levels and Depletion).

Drug Influences on Nutrient Levels and Depletion

SOME DRUGS CAN AFFECT BETA-CAROTENE LEVELS:

CHOLESTYRAMINE (Questran): Cholestyramine can reduce dietary beta-carotene absorption and serum levels (4457).

COLESTIPOL (Colestid): Colestipol can reduce dietary beta-carotene absorption and serum levels (4461).

MINERAL OIL: Concomitant administration can reduce supplemental beta-carotene absorption (4495,4496). Separate administration of mineral oil and beta-carotene by 2 hours to avoid this interaction.

ORLISTAT (Xenical): Concomitant administration can decrease supplemental beta-carotene absorption (6001). Separate administration of orlistat and beta-carotene by 2 hours to avoid this interaction.

PROTON PUMP INHIBITORS: Lansoprazole (Prevacid), Omeprazole (Prilosec, Losec), Rabeprazole (Aciphex), Pantoprazole (Protonix, Pantoloc). Loss of stomach acid interferes with the absorption of beta-carotene. Consider supplementation only if clinical judgment warrants it (31).

Possible Interactions with Foods
OLESTRA can decrease the absorption of beta-carotene.

Possible Interactions with Lab Tests
No interactions are known to occur, and there is no known reason to expect a clinically significant interaction with beta-carotene.

Possible Interactions with Diseases or Conditions
SMOKERS: Beta-carotene supplements taken orally are associated with a higher risk of lung cancer in smokers (139,4257).

Typical Dosages & Routes of Administration that are Commonly Used
ORAL: The typical oral dose of beta-carotene for erythropoietic protoporphyria is 30-300 mg daily for adults and 30-150 mg daily for children. The dose is adjusted to individual requirements and response and can be adjusted to maintain blood carotene levels at 4-6 mcg/mL (15). For decreasing the risk of prostate carcinoma in men with plasma beta-carotene concentrations less than 153.25 ng/mL, 50 mg every other day has been used (1473). For oral leukoplakia, 30 mg orally twice day for a total of 6 months has been used (1472). The Institute of Medicine recently reviewed beta-carotene, but did not make recommendations for daily intake, citing lack of sufficient evidence (6268). Supplemental beta-carotene is similarly absorbed when taken with high-fat (36 grams) or low-fat (3 grams fat) meals (6133).

Comments
The American Heart Association recommends obtaining antioxidants, including beta-carotene, from a diet high in fruits, vegetables and whole grains rather than through supplements until more information is known from randomized clinical trials (1440). Similar statements have been released by the American Cancer Society, the World Cancer Research Institute in association with the American Institute for Cancer Research, and the World Health Organization's International Agency for Research on Cancer (1470).

BETA-SITOSTEROL

This Product is Also Known As
24-ethyl-cholesterol, Angelicin, B-sitosterol 3-B-D-glucoside, B-sitosterolin, Beta sitosterin, Beta-sitosterol glucoside, Beta-sitosterol glycoside, Cinchol, Cupreol, Phytosterols, Plant sterols, Quebrachol, Rhamnol, Sitosterin, Sitosterol, Sitosterolins, Sitosterols, Sterinol, Sterolins.
CAUTION: See separate listing for Sitostanol (beta-sitostanol, stigmastanol, dihydro-beta-sitosterol).

Scientific Names
24-ethyl-cholesterol; 3-beta-stigmast-5-en-3-ol; 22,23-dihydrostigmasterol; 24-beta-ethyl-delta-5-cholesten-3beta-ol.

People Use This For
Orally, beta-sitosterol is used for treating hyperlipidemia (9,14,3658,5330,5331,5332,5333,5334,5336), benign prostatic hyperplasia and prostatitis (9,14,5327,5328,5329), and gallstones (14). It is also used for enhancing sexual activity (5323), and for preventing colon cancer (5322).
In combination with other plant sterols (including campesterol and stigmasterol), it is used to lower blood cholesterol levels (3659). Mixtures of beta-sitosterol and its glycoside (sitosterolin) are used orally to boost the immune system, to prevent immune suppression and inflammation that follows participation in a marathon (5335), to reduce the incidence of colds and influenza, to treat AIDS, rheumatoid arthritis, tuberculosis, psoriasis, allergies, cervical cancer, benign prostatic hyperplasia (BPH) (3654), fibromyalgia, lupus, asthma, alopecia, bronchitis, idiopathic thrombocytopenic purpura (ITP) (3655), colon cancer, coronary disease, migraine, chronic fatigue syndrome, menopausal symptoms, and to lower cholesterol levels (3657).
In foods, beta-sitosterol is added to some margarines designed for use as part of a cholesterol-lowering diet.

Safety
SAFE ...when used in amounts found in a normal diet.
LIKELY SAFE ...when used orally and appropriately. There are no reports of toxicity in clinical trials (9,14,5327,5328,5329,5330,5331,5332,5333,5334,5336,5337,5338,5339).
There is insufficient reliable information available about the safety of beta-sitosterol used in very large doses.
PREGNANCY AND LACTATION: Insufficient reliable information available; avoid using (14).

Effectiveness

LIKELY EFFECTIVE ...when used orally short-term to improve lower urinary tract symptoms in men with benign prostatic hyperplasia (BPH), although there is no significant effect on prostate size (7,14,5327,5328,5329).
POSSIBLY EFFECTIVE ...when used orally for treating hyperlipidemia in adults (14,5330,5331,5332,5333,5334,5336).
LIKELY INEFFECTIVE ...when used orally for treating gallstones (14,5338,5339).
There is insufficient reliable information about the effectiveness of beta-sitosterol for its other uses.

Possible Mechanism of Action & Active Ingredients

Beta-sitosterol is a plant sterol whose chemical structure is that of cholesterol with an ethyl group added at position 24 (14). Beta-sitosterolin is a glycoside of beta-sitosterol (7). Beta-sitosterol is thought to inhibit the intestinal absorption of cholesterol, competing for the limited space for cholesterol in mixed micelles (5814). It also accelerates the esterification rate of the lecithin-cholesterol acyltransferase (LCAT) enzyme, resulting in reduction of cholesterol-rich lipoprotein (14). Beta-sitosterol reduces plasma total and LDL cholesterol in adults by variable amounts, but has little or no effect on HDL cholesterol or triglycerides (14,3665,3666,5327,5328,5329,5331,5333,5334,5336,5337, 5338,5339). In children and adolescents, beta-sitosterol slightly reduces total and LDL lipids; however, it reduces HDL more (14,5330,5332). Margarines containing beta-sitosterol reduce cholesterol absorption from the gut by about half and have been shown to reduce serum cholesterol and hence the risk of heart disease despite compensatory increases in cholesterol synthesis in the liver (5814). Note that plant sterols are potentially atherogenic like cholesterol, but atherogenesis does not occur because so little is absorbed (about 5% for beta-sitosterol) (5814). The mechanism of action of beta-sitosterol in prostatic hypertrophy is unknown, although it binds to prostatic tissue, inhibits prostaglandin synthesis in the prostate and has anti-inflammatory activity (7,14). It improves both symptoms and urine flow (5327,5328,5329).

In-vitro studies indicate that beta-sitosterol can inhibit the growth of human colon cancer cells (3667,3668). Mixtures of beta-sitosterol and sitosterolin have been reported to enhance proliferative responses of T-cells in vitro (3669,5342), and also to reduce the mild immune suppression and inflammation seen in marathon runners after a race (5335). Preliminary studies in people with HIV infection suggest that the mixture may help to stabilize CD4 cell counts, reduce plasma levels of pro-inflammatory interleukin-6, and reduce plasma viral loads (5342). In one study, adjunctive treatment of tuberculosis patients with beta-sitosterol/sitosterolin resulted in greater weight gain and recovery of lymphocyte and eosinophil counts than did treatment with placebo, although there was no difference in time to negative sputum cultures (14,5337).

Some evidence suggests that beta-sitosterol also has anti-neoplastic and anti-pyretic activity (5342). Studies are underway using beta-sitosterol/sitosterolin in people with rheumatoid arthritis, human papilloma virus cervical lesions, chronic rhinitis and sinusitis, and hepatitis C virus infection (5342).

Adverse Reactions Including Known Allergies

Beta-sitosterol can cause nausea, indigestion, gas, diarrhea, and constipation (14,5327,5328).

Possible Interactions with Herbs & Other Dietary Supplements

CAROTENE, VITAMIN E: Beta-sitosterol may reduce absorption and blood levels of alpha and beta-carotene and vitamin E (5814).

Possible Interactions with Drugs

LIPID LOWERING DRUGS: The HMG-CoA reductase inhibitor pravastatin (Pravachol) has been reported to lower plasma levels of beta-sitosterol (3672), but simvastatin (Zocor) had no effect (3673).
CAROTENE, VITAMIN E: Beta-sitosterol may reduce absorption and blood levels of alpha and beta-carotene and vitamin E (5814).

Possible Interactions with Foods

CAROTENE, VITAMIN E: Beta-sitosterol may reduce absorption and blood levels of alpha- and beta-carotene and vitamin E (5814).

Possible Interactions with Lab Tests

CHOLESTEROL: Beta-sitosterol decreases total serum cholesterol and LDL levels (5331,5336).

Possible Interactions with Diseases or Conditions

SITOSTEROLEMIA: Contraindicated in sitosterolemia, a rare inherited lipid storage disease (14,5326). People with the rare autosomal recessive disorder sitosterolemia have increased absorption of cholesterol and beta-sitosterol from the diet, and decreased clearance of beta-sitosterol, leading to increases in total body stores of beta-sitosterol up to 17-fold. These people are prone to premature coronary artery disease and xanthomas (3661,3662), and the elevated hepatic beta-sitosterol levels competitively inhibit cholesterol catabolism, contributing to hypercholesterolemia (3663). Beta-sitosterol and sitosterolin are contraindicated in sitosterolemia (14).

Typical Dosages & Routes of Administration that are Commonly Used

ORAL: For the treatment of benign prostatic hyperplasia (BPH) and prostatitis, a typical dose is 20 to 130 mg of sitosterol two to three times daily (9,14). Clinical studies have used approximately 60 mg per day (5327,5328,5329). After clinical improvement, the dose can be reduced to 10 to 65 mg two to three times daily (9,14). For hyperlipidemia, the usual dose is 2 to 6 grams per day before meals along with dietary modification (14,5327,5328,5329,5330,5331,5332,5333,5334, 5336,5337,5338,5339). In severe disease, doses of 10 to 15 grams per day have been used (14). It is stated that doses should be taken at least 30 minutes, but not more than 90 minutes before meals to have the greatest effect on cholesterol absorption (3658). About 175-200 mg of beta-sitosterol is consumed daily in the average diet (14). In trials of margarines containing beta-sitosterol, typical doses were 0.8 to 3.2 grams daily (5814). The recommended dose of a combination product for lowering cholesterol, containing beta-sitosterol 100 mg, campesterol 50 mg, stigmasterol 40 mg, and other phytosterols 60 mg, is one tablet with each meal (3659). A combination product containing 300 mg sitosterols and sitosterolins has recommended doses of two capsules daily for boosting the immune system, and three to six capsules per day for treatment of immune disorders (3657). A combination of 20 mg beta-sitosterol and 0.2 mg beta-sitosterolin three times daily has been used as adjunctive therapy in people with tuberculosis (14).

Comments

Plant sterols, including beta-sitosterol, stigmasterol and campesterol, and sitosterolins are widely distributed in fruits, vegetables, nuts, and seeds (3654,3655,3657). The average diet provides 175 to 200 mg of beta-sitosterol daily (14). Beta-sitosterol is also present in various herbs including stinging nettle root and echinacea purpurea root (2). Margarines containing beta-sitosterol and other plant sterols have been studied as a component of diets to lower serum cholesterol levels (5336). Avoid confusing beta-sitosterol with sitostanol, the saturated beta-sitosterol derivative. Take Control margarine contains beta-sitosterol and Benecol margarine contains sitostanol (5340,5341). Sitostanol may produce slightly greater reductions in total and LDL cholesterol than beta-sitosterol, and it may also raise HDL "good" cholesterol levels (3665,3666,5814). Fats are needed to solubilize plant sterols; therefore margarines are an ideal vehicle, whereas the contents of capsules may not disperse properly in the gut, limiting their ability to reduce cholesterol absorption (5814). Beta-sitosterol/sitosterolin combination products sold in the US include Moducare, which is reported to contain 20.2 mg "sterinols and sterolins" from soy and pine (3656), and Natur-Leaf, which is reported to contain 300 mg of sitosterols/sitosterolins, plus 50 mg of plant-based enzymes, plant-derived vitamins and minerals (3657).

BETAINE ANHYDROUS

This Product is Also Known As
Betaine, Cystadane.
CAUTION: See separate listing for Betaine Hydrochloride.

Scientific Names
Trimethylglycine (anhydrous).

People Use This For
Orally, betaine anhydrous is taken for homocystinuria caused by cystathionine beta-synthase deficiency, 5,10-methylenetetrahydrofolate reductase deficiency, or cobalamin cofactor metabolism defect (15). It is also used orally for homocystinuria not responsive to pyridoxine (145).

Safety
LIKELY SAFE ...when used orally and appropriately. Betaine is an FDA-approved prescription product for oral use.
PREGNANCY AND LACTATION: Insufficient reliable information available (698); avoid using.

Effectiveness
EFFECTIVE ...when used appropriately. Betaine is an FDA-approved orphan drug.

Possible Mechanism of Action & Active Ingredients
In homocystinuria, betaine acts as a methyl group donor in the remethylation of homocystine to methionine and reduces plasma homocystine levels to 20-30% of the pretreatment levels (15). It is unknown if reducing homocystine levels reduces the risk of coronary atherosclerosis, cerebrovascular disease, peripheral vascular disease, and thrombosis (145,146).

Adverse Reactions Including Known Allergies
Betaine can cause nausea, GI distress, and diarrhea (698).

Possible Interactions with Herbs & Other Dietary Supplements
Insufficient reliable information available.

Possible Interactions with Drugs
No interactions are known to occur, and there is no known reason to expect a clinically significant interaction with betaine anhydrous.

Possible Interactions with Foods

No interactions are known to occur, and there is no known reason to expect a clinically significant interaction with betaine anhydrous.

Possible Interactions with Lab Tests

No interactions are known to occur, and there is no known reason to expect a clinically significant interaction with betaine anhydrous.

Possible Interactions with Diseases or Conditions

No interactions are known to occur, and there is no known reason to expect a clinically significant interaction with betaine anhydrous.

Typical Dosages & Routes of Administration that are Commonly Used

ORAL: For homocystinuria, 3 grams is typically taken twice daily in adults and children. Dose titration is preferable in children. For children younger than three years old, the dose is 100 mg/kg per day, increased in weekly intervals in increments of 100 mg/kg daily. All patients can receive dose increases until plasma homocystine concentrations are undetectable or very low, which can require doses up to 20 grams per day. Dissolve the powder in water immediately before administration (15). The medical conditions betaine is used for require diagnosis and treatment by a physician. Betaine anhydrous is an FDA approved orphan drug (Cystadane). For additional information contact manufacturer, Orphan Medical: 1-800-900-4267.

Comments

This product has Orphan Drug status in the US. Avoid confusion with betaine hydrochloride, a dietary supplement with variable purity and potency that has not been demonstrated safe or effective for treating homocystinuria.

BETAINE HYDROCHLORIDE

This Product is Also Known As

Betaine, Betaine HCl.
CAUTION: See separate listing for Betaine Anhydrous.

Scientific Names

Trimethylglycine hydrochloride.

People Use This For

Orally, betaine hydrochloride is used as a supplemental source of hydrochloric acid, to treat hypokalemia, and as a liver protectant (16,144).

Safety

There is insufficient reliable information available about the safety of betaine hydrochloride.
Pregnancy and Lactation: Insufficient reliable information available; avoid using.

Effectiveness

There is insufficient reliable information available about the effectiveness of betaine hydrochloride.

Possible Mechanism of Action & Active Ingredients

Insufficient reliable information available.

Adverse Reactions Including Known Allergies

Theoretically, betaine hydrochloride can irritate gastric or duodenal ulcers or impede ulcer healing by increasing gastric acid (9).

Possible Interactions with Herbs & Other Dietary Supplements

Insufficient reliable information available.

Possible Interactions with Drugs

No interactions are known to occur, and there is no known reason to expect a clinically significant interaction with betaine hydrochloride.

Possible Interactions with Foods

No interactions are known to occur, and there is no known reason to expect a clinically significant interaction with betaine hydrochloride.

Possible Interactions with Lab Tests

No interactions are known to occur, and there is no known reason to expect a clinically significant interaction with betaine hydrochloride.

Possible Interactions with Diseases or Conditions

GASTRIC and DUODENAL ULCERS: Theoretically, betaine hydrochloride can irritate ulcers or impede healing by increasing gastric acid; avoid using in patients with gastric or duodenal ulcers (9).

Typical Dosages & Routes of Administration that are Commonly Used

ORAL: People typically use 325 to 650 mg daily after a meal that contains protein. Do not take on an empty stomach (6006).

Comments

Avoid confusion with betaine anhydrous. Betaine is manufactured in various salt forms around the world, including betaine hydrochloride. The purity and potency of these dietary supplement products can vary. There are no data to support the effectiveness of betaine hydrochloride in any condition, including homocystinuria. Use only the FDA-approved betaine anhydrous for the treatment of homocystinuria (see separate listing for betaine anhydrous).

BETH ROOT

This Product is Also Known As

Birthroot, Coughroot, Ground Lily, Jew's Harp Plant, Indian Balm, Indian Shamrock, Lamb's Quarters, Milk Ipecac, Pariswort, Rattlesnake Root, Snakebite, Stinking Benjamin, Three–Leafed Nightshade, Wake-Robin.

Scientific Names

Trillium erectum.
Family: Liliaceae.

People Use This For

Orally, beth root is used for long, heavy menstruation and pain relief. Sometimes it is also used orally as an astringent and expectorant.
Topically, beth root is used for varicose veins and ulcers, hematomas, and hemorrhoid bleeding (18).

Safety

POSSIBLY UNSAFE …when used orally. Beth root is a gastrointestinal irritant (12).
There is insufficient reliable information available about the safety of the topical use of beth root.
PREGNANCY AND LACTATION: LIKELY UNSAFE …contraindicated for oral use. Beth root might have menstrual or uterine stimulant activity (12,18).

Effectiveness

There is insufficient reliable information available about the effectiveness of beth root.

Possible Mechanism of Action & Active Ingredients

The applicable parts of beth root are the rhizome, and dried root and leaf. There is insufficient reliable information about the possible mechanism of action or active ingredients.

Adverse Reactions Including Known Allergies

Beth root causes extreme topical irritation (18). Ingestion of large amounts of the plant or volatile oil might produce GI irritation severe enough to cause vomiting (12,18). In pregnant women, the drastic purgative effects can cause reflex uterine contractions.

Possible Interactions with Herbs & Other Dietary Supplements

Insufficient reliable information available.

Possible Interactions with Drugs

No interactions are known to occur, and there is no known reason to expect a clinically significant interaction with beth root.

Possible Interactions with Foods

No interactions are known to occur, and there is no known reason to expect a clinically significant interaction with beth root.

Possible Interactions with Lab Tests

No interactions are known to occur, and there is no known reason to expect a clinically significant interaction with beth root.

Possible Interactions with Diseases or Conditions

CARDIAC CONDITIONS: Due to potential cardiotoxicity from the convallamarin-like glycoside, patients with a cardiac condition should be cautioned against the use of this herb (214).

Typical Dosages & Routes of Administration that are Commonly Used
ORAL: No typical dosage.
TOPICAL: The ground plant parts are used as a poultice (18).

Comments
None.

BETONY

This Product is Also Known As
Bishopswort, Bishop Wort, Hedge Nettles, Wood Betony.

Scientific Names
Stachys officinalis; Betonica officinalis.
Family: Labiatae.

People Use This For
Orally, betony is used to treat diarrhea, irritation of mucous membranes (5), stress and tension, headache, facial pain (6), coughs as an expectorant, bronchitis, and asthma (18).
In combination with other herbs, betony is used for treatment of neuralgia and anxiety (18).
In folk medicine, betony is considered a cure-all and thought effective in 47 different diseases (5), as an antidiarrheal, antiflatulent, and sedative. Betony is also used in folk medicine to treat inflammation of the nose, throat and lung air passages, heartburn, gout, nervousness, bladder and kidney stones, and bladder inflammation (18).

Safety
POSSIBLY SAFE ...when the dried above ground parts are used orally in medicinal amounts (5,6,12).
POSSIBLY UNSAFE ...when used in large amounts because it contains 15% tannins and these can cause gastrointestinal irritation (5,12).
PREGNANCY: POSSIBLY UNSAFE ...when used orally; avoid using (6).
LACTATION: Insufficient reliable information available; avoid using.

Effectiveness
POSSIBLY EFFECTIVE ...when taken orally in small doses for headache, nervous tension, facial pain, congestion, and diarrhea (5,6). ...when taken in large doses as a purgative or emetic (6). ...when used topically as a mouth rinse or gargle for gum, mouth, and throat irritations (5,6).
There is insufficient reliable information available about the effectiveness of betony for its other uses.

Possible Mechanism of Action & Active Ingredients
The applicable parts of betony are the dried above ground parts. The high tannin content (15%) is responsible for its astringent properties (5). The glycoside mixture can have a hypotensive effect, possibly explaining its effectiveness in mild anxiety states and headache (5,6). One constituent, stachydrine, is a systolic depressant that is also active against rheumatism (6).

Adverse Reactions Including Known Allergies
Large doses can cause significant GI irritation due to the tannin component (5,6).

Possible Interactions with Herbs & Other Dietary Supplements
Insufficient reliable information available.

Possible Interactions with Drugs
DRUGS THAT ALTER BLOOD PRESSURE: Theoretically, betony can increase the blood pressure lowering effects of antihypertensive drugs and interfere with the activity of pressor drugs.

Possible Interactions with Foods
No interactions are known to occur, and there is no known reason to expect a clinically significant interaction with betony.

Possible Interactions with Lab Tests
No interactions are known to occur, and there is no known reason to expect a clinically significant interaction with betony.

Possible Interactions with Diseases or Conditions
No interactions are known to occur, and there is no known reason to expect a clinically significant interaction with betony.

Typical Dosages & Routes of Administration that are Commonly Used
ORAL: Betony is typically taken as a tea or an infusion (6002). Use small doses to avoid GI irritation.

Comments
None.

BIFIDOBACTERIUM BIFIDUM

This Product is Also Known As
Bifido, Bifidobacterium, Bifidum, Probiotic.
CAUTION: See separate listing for Brewer's Yeast (Hansen CBS 5926), Lactobacillus Acidophilus, Lactobacillus GG, Saccharomyces Boulardii, and Yogurt.

Scientific Names
Bifidobacterium bifidum.
Family: Actinomycetaceae.

People Use This For
Orally, bifidobacterium is used to prevent acute diarrhea in infants (153), to provide healthful bacteria to human adults (154), and to re-seed intestinal bacteria affected by diarrhea, chemotherapy, advancing age, antibiotics, or other causes (154,155).

Safety
POSSIBLY SAFE ...when used orally by adults (162)
CHILDREN: POSSIBLY SAFE ...when used orally in infants (162). It seems to be well-tolerated even in infants who are malnourished or immunocompromised (153,155).
PREGNANCY AND LACTATION: Insufficient reliable information available; avoid using.

Effectiveness
POSSIBLY EFFECTIVE ...when used orally with S. thermophilus to prevent acute diarrhea in infants (153). ...for preventing traveler's diarrhea when used in combination with Lactobacillus acidophilus, Lactobacillus bulgaricus, or Streptococcus thermophilus (155). Daily consumption of bifidobacterium is usually required to maintain effectiveness, although effects may persist a week after discontinuation (154,1731).
There is insufficient reliable information available about the effectiveness of bifidobacterium bifidum for its other uses.

Possible Mechanism of Action & Active Ingredients
Bifidobacterium bifidum is the predominant intestinal flora of breast-fed infants (161). When taken orally, it travels through the colon without multiplication or death, preventing colonization by other organisms (162). Ingestion of yogurt fermented with Bifidobacterium bifidum increases the numbers of stool bifidobacteria and suppresses coliform bacteria (1731).

Adverse Reactions Including Known Allergies
None reported.

Possible Interactions with Herbs & Other Dietary Supplements
Insufficient reliable information available.

Possible Interactions with Drugs
No interactions are known to occur, and there is no known reason to expect a clinically significant interaction with bifidobacterium bifidum.

Possible Interactions with Foods
No interactions are known to occur, and there is no known reason to expect a clinically significant interaction with bifidobacterium bifidum.

Possible Interactions with Lab Tests
No interactions are known to occur, and there is no known reason to expect a clinically significant interaction with bifidobacterium bifidum.

Possible Interactions with Diseases or Conditions
No interactions are known to occur, and there is no known reason to expect a clinically significant interaction with bifidobacterium bifidum.

Typical Dosages & Routes of Administration that are Commonly Used
ORAL: People typically take one to ten billion viable cells daily (5009). Daily consumption is required for effectiveness (154).

© Copyright 2000, Natural Medicines Comprehensive Database (209) 472-2244. For updated data, go to www.NaturalDatabase.com • 115

Comments
Also referred to as a "probiotic" agent.

BILBERRY dried ripe fruit

This Product is Also Known As
Airelle, Black Whortles, Bleaberry, Blueberry, Burren Myrtle, Dwarf Bilberry, Dyeberry, Huckleberry, Hurtleberry, Myrtilli Fructus, Trackleberry, Whortleberry, Wineberry.
CAUTION: See separate listings for Bilberry leaf and Bog Bilberry.

Scientific Names
Vaccinium myrtillus.
Family: Ericaceae.

People Use This For
Orally, the dried, ripe fruit of bilberry is taken to treat non-specific, acute diarrhea, and to improve visual acuity (2,11), including night vision (6). The dried, ripe fruit extracts are used orally for angina, venous insufficiency of the lower limbs, varicose veins, atherosclerosis, and degenerative retinal conditions (11).
Topically, the dried, ripe fruit of bilberry is used for mild inflammation of the mouth and throat mucous membranes (2,11).

Safety
LIKELY SAFE ...when the dried, ripe bilberry fruit is consumed in amounts typically found in foods (11). There is insufficient reliable information available about the safety of the use of bilberry dried ripe fruit for medicinal purposes (2).
PREGNANCY AND LACTATION: LIKELY SAFE ...when the dried, ripe fruit is consumed as food. Insufficient reliable information is available for larger amounts.

Effectiveness
POSSIBLY EFFECTIVE ...when taken orally for non-specific, acute diarrhea (2). ...when used to treat circulatory problems (6). ...when used for mild inflammation of the mouth and throat mucous membranes (2). ...when taken orally to improve retinal lesions from diabetic or hypertensive retinopathy (39,40). Clinical studies of bilberry's effectiveness have used formulations containing 25% of the bioflavonoid complex anthocyanoside.
There is insufficient reliable information available about the effectiveness of bilberry dried ripe fruit for its other uses.

Possible Mechanism of Action & Active Ingredients
The applicable part of bilberry is the fruit. Astringent tannin components of the dried, ripe fruit of bilberry are responsible for the observed benefits in diarrhea and irritation of the mouth and throat mucosa (6). Anthocyanoside (anthocyandin) constituents increase the synthesis of glycosaminoglycans, decrease vascular permeability, reduce basement membrane thickness, and aid in the redistribution of microvascular blood flow and the formation of interstitial fluid (6,41). An anthocyanadin pigment found in bilberry might have anti-ulcer and gastroprotective effects (6).

Adverse Reactions Including Known Allergies
None reported.

Possible Interactions with Herbs & Other Dietary Supplements
Insufficient reliable information available.

Possible Interactions with Drugs
No interactions are known to occur, and there is no known reason to expect a clinically significant interaction with bilberry dried ripe fruit.

Possible Interactions with Foods
No interactions are known to occur, and there is no known reason to expect a clinically significant interaction with bilberry dried ripe fruit.

Possible Interactions with Lab Tests
No interactions are known to occur, and there is no known reason to expect a clinically significant interaction with bilberry dried ripe fruit.

Possible Interactions with Diseases or Conditions
No interactions are known to occur, and there is no known reason to expect a clinically significant interaction with bilberry dried ripe fruit.

Typical Dosages & Routes of Administration that are Commonly Used

ORAL: The typical oral dose of the dried, ripe berries is 20-60 grams daily. People also drink a decoction of the berries, which is prepared by placing 5-10 grams (1-2 teaspoons) of mashed berries in cold water, bringing the water to a simmer for 10 minutes, and then straining the water. A dose of 160 mg of bilberry extract taken twice daily has been used in patients with retinopathy. (39) Clinical studies of bilberry's effectiveness have used formulations containing 25% of the bioflavonoid complex anthocyanoside.
TOPICAL: The berries are usually applied as a 10% decoction, made by boiling the dried berries in water for 10 minutes and straining (2).

Comments

Avoid confusion with bilberry leaf and bog bilberry.

BILBERRY leaf

This Product is Also Known As

Airelle, Black Whortles, Bleaberry, Blueberry, Burren Myrtle, Dwarf Bilberry, Dyeberry, Huckleberry, Hurtleberry, Myrtilli Fructus, Trackleberry, Whortleberry, Wineberry.
CAUTION: See separate listings for Bilberry dried ripe fruit and Bog Bilberry.

Scientific Names

Vaccinium myrtillus.
Family: Ericaceae.

People Use This For

Orally, bilberry leaf is used for diabetes, arthritis, gout, dermatitis, hemorrhoids, poor circulation, functional heart problems, "stimulating metabolism," "purifying the blood," and prevention and treatment of gastrointestinal, kidney and urinary tract symptoms and diseases (2,8).

Safety

POSSIBLY UNSAFE ...when taken orally in high doses or with prolonged use. Death can occur with chronic dose of 1.5 g/kg/day (2).
PREGNANCY AND LACTATION: UNSAFE ...contraindicated, due to potential toxicity.

Effectiveness

There is insufficient reliable information available about the effectiveness of bilberry leaf.

Possible Mechanism of Action & Active Ingredients

Bilberry leaves contain polyphenols, tannins, flavonoids (1265) and a relatively high concentration of chromium (9.0 ppm) (8). Preliminary evidence suggests that a bilberry leaf extract might have blood glucose and triglyceride lowering effects (1264). The chromium in bilberry leaf is theorized to play a role in potential blood glucose lowering activity (8). Some researchers think that flavonoids in bilberry leaf might also be useful for diabetic circulatory disorders (8).

Adverse Reactions Including Known Allergies

Chronic intoxication has been reported in animals. Symptoms include: wasting, anemia, jaundice, acute excitatory states, disturbances of muscle contraction, and death (2).

Possible Interactions with Herbs & Other Dietary Supplements

Insufficient reliable information is available.

Possible Interactions with Drugs

ANTI-DIABETES DRUGS: Theoretically, concomitant use might require dosing adjustment of antidiabetes drugs. Preliminary evidence suggests that a bilberry leaf extract might have blood glucose lowering activity (1264); monitor closely.
DISULFRAM: A disulfram reaction might occur with herbal products containing alcohol. Avoid concurrent use (214).

Possible Interactions with Foods

No interactions are known to occur, and there is no known reason to expect a clinically significant interaction with bilberry leaf.

Possible Interactions with Lab Tests

BLOOD GLUCOSE: Theoretically, bilberry leaf might lower blood glucose and test results. Preliminary evidence suggests that a bilberry leaf extract might have blood glucose lowering activity (1264).
TRIGLYCERIDES: Theoretically, bilberry leaf might lower serum triglycerides and test results. Preliminary evidence suggests that a bilberry leaf extract might have triglyceride lowering activity (1264).

Possible Interactions with Diseases or Conditions

DIABETES: Theoretically, bilberry leaf might lower blood glucose. Preliminary evidence suggests that a bilberry leaf extract might have blood glucose lowering activity (1264); monitor closely.

Typical Dosages & Routes of Administration that are Commonly Used

ORAL: Drink as tea [steep 1 gram (1-2 teaspoons) finely chopped dried leaf in 150 mL boiling water for 5-10 minutes, strain]; avoid prolonged use (8).

Comments

For short-term use only. Avoid confusion with bilberry dried ripe fruit, and bog bilberry.

BIOTIN

This Product is Also Known As

Coenzyme R, D-Biotin, Vitamin H, W Factor.

Scientific Names

Cis-hexahydro-2-oxo-1H-thieno[3,4-d]-imidazole-4-valeric acid.

People Use This For

Orally, biotin is used for dietary supplementation, biotin deficiency associated with pregnancy, long-term parenteral nutrition, malnutrition, rapid weight loss, individuals with multiple carboxylase deficiency (9,1900,1901), hair loss (174), brittle nails (171), seborrheic dermatitis of infancy (173), and lowering blood sugar in diabetes (177).

Safety

LIKELY SAFE ...when used orally and appropriately as a supplement for diagnosed biotin deficiency (9,1900).
CHILDREN: POSSIBLY SAFE ...when used orally and appropriately (173).
PREGNANCY AND LACTATION: POSSIBLY SAFE ...when used orally and appropriately (1901).

Effectiveness

LIKELY EFFECTIVE ...when used orally as a supplement to prevent or treat biotin deficiency (1901).
POSSIBLY EFFECTIVE ...when used for increasing the thickness of finger and toenails in individuals with brittle nails (171). ...for treating seborrheic dermatitis of infancy (173).
There is insufficient reliable information available about the effectiveness of biotin for its other uses.

Possible Mechanism of Action & Active Ingredients

Biotin-containing enzymes are involved in gluconeogenesis, fatty acid synthesis, propionate metabolism, and the catabolism of leucine in mammals. Biotin is recycled endogenously, and this can be the reason why deficiency symptoms take a long time to develop and are rarely seen in humans. Avidin, a constituent of raw egg whites, consumed in large amounts can induce biotin deficiency (173).

Adverse Reactions Including Known Allergies

None reported.

Possible Interactions with Herbs & Other Dietary Supplements

Insufficient reliable information available.

Possible Interactions with Drugs

CARBAMAZEPINE AND PRIMIDONE can reduce biotin absorption in vitro (172,176).
PHENYTOIN AND PHENOBARBITAL can reduce biotin levels (175,176).

Possible Interactions with Foods

No interactions are known to occur, and there is no known reason to expect a clinically significant interaction with biotin.

Possible Interactions with Lab Tests

THYROID STIMULATING HORMONE (TSH): There is one report of a false-low TSH on the assay by the Boehringer Mannheim ES 700 analyzer due to high serum biotin levels in a neonate (170).
FREE THYROXINE (FT4): There is one report of a false-high FT4 on the assay by the Boehringer Mannheim ES 700 analyzer due to high serum biotin levels in a neonate (170).

Possible Interactions with Diseases or Conditions

CONDITIONS ASSOCIATED WITH LOW BIOTIN LEVELS: Biotin can interfere with conditions of children with seborrheic dermatitis, Leiner's disease, burns and scalds, achlorhydria, alcoholism, and epilepsy and in pregnant and lactating women, athletes, and the elderly (173).

Typical Dosages & Routes of Administration that are Commonly Used

ORAL: There is no recommended dietary allowance (RDA) established for biotin. The adequate intakes (AI) for biotin are 5 mcg for infants 0-6 months, 6 mcg for infants 7-12 months, 8 mcg for children 1-3 years, 12 mcg for children 4-8 years, 20 mcg for children 9-13 years, 25 mcg for adults 14-18 years, 30 mcg for adults over 18 years and pregnant women, and 35 mcg for lactating women (3094) . For neonates, 35 mcg per day is recommended (173), and is increased to 30-200 mcg per day for adults (9,1900). Biotin is available as an oral monovitamin, in vitamin B complex products (1902,1903), and in intravenous multivitamin products (1903).

Comments

Severe biotin deficiency is rare and is characterized by skin eruptions, total hair loss, the development of severe metabolic acidosis, and progressive ataxia (174).

BIRCH

This Product is Also Known As

Betulae folium, Downy Birch, Silver Birch, White Birch.

Scientific Names

Betula pendula, synonym Betula verrucosa; Betula pubescens.
Family: Betulaceae.

People Use This For

Orally, birch leaf is used as a diuretic, for rheumatic ailments, and for "irrigation therapy" (use of a mild diuretic along with copious fluid intake to increase urine flow) to treat pyelonephritis, ureteritis, cystitis, and urethritis (8). In folk medicine, the birch leaf is used for arthritis, rheumatism, loss of hair, skin rashes, and in "spring cures" for "purifying the blood" (8).

Safety

LIKELY SAFE ...when used orally and appropriately as irrigation therapy (2,12).
LIKELY UNSAFE ...when irrigation therapy is used by individuals with edema caused by impaired kidney or heart function (2).
PREGNANCY AND LACTATION: Insufficient reliable information available; avoid using.

Effectiveness

POSSIBLY EFFECTIVE ...when used orally as a diuretic for irrigation therapy to treat bacterial and inflammatory diseases of the urinary tract, for small kidney stones, and as supportive therapy for rheumatic ailments (2).
There is insufficient reliable information available about the effectiveness of birch for its other uses.

Possible Mechanism of Action & Active Ingredients

The applicable part of birch is the leaf. The aquaretic and possibly saluretic effects are due to the flavonoid constituents of the birch leaf. Aquaretics increase urine volume (water loss) but not sodium excretion (512). The high vitamin C content of the leaf can enhance the effect (8).

Adverse Reactions Including Known Allergies

None reported.

Possible Interactions with Herbs & Other Dietary Supplements

Insufficient reliable information available.

Possible Interactions with Drugs

DIURETICS: Theoretically, birch leaf might increase sodium retention and interfere with diuretic therapy (512).

Possible Interactions with Foods

No interactions are known to occur, and there is no known reason to expect a clinically significant interaction with birch.

Possible Interactions with Lab Tests

No interactions are known to occur, and there is no known reason to expect a clinically significant interaction with birch.

Possible Interactions with Diseases or Conditions

EDEMA DUE TO HEART OR KIDNEY CONDITIONS: Irrigation therapy is contraindicated (2).
HYPERTENSION: Theoretically, birch leaf might increase sodium retention and worsen hypertension (512).
URINARY TRACT INFECTIONS: Herbal "irrigation therapy" can be insufficient and requires the addition of an antibacterial agent and close monitoring (8).

Typical Dosages & Routes of Administration that are Commonly Used

ORAL: The typical dose of birch leaf is several times daily as a tea, which is prepared by steeping 2-3 grams of finely cut dried leaf in 150 mL boiling water for 10-15 minutes and straining (2,8). The tea should be taken with plenty of water (8).

Comments

None.

BISHOP'S WEED

This Product is Also Known As

Ammi, Bischofskrautfruchte, Bishops Weed, Bishop's Weed Fruit, Fructus Ammi Visnagae, Fruits De Khella, Khella, Khella Fruit, Visnagafruchte, Visnaga Fruit.
CAUTION: See separate listing for Goutweed.

Scientific Names

Ammi visnagae, synonyms Ammi daucoides, Ammi majus.
Family: Apiaceae/Umbelliferae.

People Use This For

Orally, the dried berry of bishop's weed is used as an antispasmodic, for its effects on coronary vessels (8), bronchi (8), GI tract (8), genital system (8), and biliary tract (8).
Topically, bishop's weed extracts have been used to treat psoriasis (214) and vitiligo (6).
Traditionally, bishop's weed is used orally for treating angina, respiratory diseases, diabetes, kidney and bladder stones, and as a diuretic (6).

Safety

POSSIBLY UNSAFE ...when used orally (2). Increases in liver enzymes that occur with high doses cause concern about possible liver damage (2).
PREGNANCY AND LACTATION: POSSIBLY UNSAFE ...when used orally; avoid using (8).

Effectiveness

There is insufficient reliable information available about the effectiveness of bishop's weed.

Possible Mechanism of Action & Active Ingredients

The applicable parts of bishop's weed are the dried, ripe fruits (6). Bishop's weed contains coumarins and psoralens. These include visnadin, khellin, visnagin, all of which can have calcium channel blocking actions (6,2525). Visnadin is the most active of the three, and can inhibit vascular smooth muscle contraction. Visnadin can dilate peripheral and coronary vessels and increase coronary circulation (6,8,2523,2524). Khellin is commercially available in Europe for oral and parenteral use as a vasodilator in the management of bronchial asthma and angina pectoris (6). Khellin can increase HDL without affecting cholesterol or triglyceride concentrations (6,2522). Bishop's weed contains 8-methoxsalen (8-MOP), the first agent used with UVA radiation to treat psoriasis. It can also contribute to phototoxicity (15,2528). Bishop's weed extract can have antimicrobial activity against gram-positive bacteria and Candida species (6). Bishop's weed extract may not have activity against kidney stones (2526).

Adverse Reactions Including Known Allergies

Elevated liver transaminases and gamma-glutamyltransferase (GGT) have been observed when using bishop's weed (2). The bishop's weed constituent khellin is also associated with elevated transaminases, as well as nausea and vomiting (6,2522).
Prolonged use or overdose of bishop's weed can cause nausea, dizziness, constipation, lack of appetite, headache, itching, and insomnia. The psoralens in bishop's weed are associated with photosensitivity and contact dermatitis (6,2520,2521). Bishop's weed rarely can cause reversible jaundice (2). It may also cause severe ophthalmic changes, in particular pigmentary retinopathy (2527). Topically, bishop's weed may cause skin malignancies in patients predisposed to cancer (214).

Possible Interactions with Herbs & Other Dietary Supplements

Theoretically, bishop's weed can have an additive effect with products that increase liver enzymes (6).

Possible Interactions with Drugs

HEPATOTOXIC DRUGS: Bishop's weed can increase liver enzymes (2,6,2522). Theoretically, it can have additive effects with drugs that increase liver enzymes.
DIGITOXIN (Crystodigin): Theoretically, concomitant use of the constituent visnadin might decrease digitoxin toxicity due to the coronary vasodilation and anti-arrhythmic activity (19).

Possible Interactions with Foods

No interactions are known to occur, and there is no known reason to expect a clinically significant interaction with bishop's weed.

Possible Interactions with Lab Tests

HDL: Theoretically, the bishop's weed constituent khellin may cause a true increase in HDL (6,2522).

LIVER FUNCTION TESTS: Theoretically, the bishop's weed constituent khellin may cause a true increase in AST and ALT when used to treat hyperlipidemia (6,2522).

Possible Interactions with Diseases or Conditions

LIVER DISEASE: Theoretically, bishop's weed can interact with liver diseases or conditions due to its potential to increase liver enzymes (6,2522).

Typical Dosages & Routes of Administration that are Commonly Used

ORAL: For increasing HDL, a khellin dose of 50 mg four times daily has been used (2522). For other uses, the average daily dose of bishop's weed is 20 mg gamma-pyrones (calculated as khellin) (8). Prepared remedies and extracts containing khellin or visnadin are the preferred dose form. Bishop's weed is rarely used as a tea (8). The tea is prepared by pouring boiling water over powdered fruit, steeping 10-15 minutes, and straining (8).

Comments

With the addition of an oxygen atom, khella becomes cromolyn sodium, a prescription drug used for the treatment of asthma and other respiratory conditions (214).

BISTORT

This Product is Also Known As

Adderwort, Dragonwort, Easter Giant, Easter Mangiant, Oderwort, Osterick, Patience Dock, Red Legs, Snakeweed, Sweet Dock.

Scientific Names

Polygonum bistorta.
Family: Polygonaceae.

People Use This For

Orally, bistort is used for digestive disorders, particularly diarrhea.
Topically, bistort is used for mouth and throat infections, and for wounds (18).

Safety

There is insufficient reliable information available about the safety of bistort.
Pregnancy and Lactation: Insufficient reliable information available; avoid using.

Effectiveness

There is insufficient reliable information available about the effectiveness of bistort.

Possible Mechanism of Action & Active Ingredients

The applicable parts of bistort are the rhizome and root. Bistort contains 15-21% tannins, which have astringent effects. Tannins work internally by dehydrating mucosal tissue, which reduces secretions. Externally, tannin astringent effects result in a protective layer of constricted, harder cells. Plants with at least 10% tannins can cause gastrointestinal upset, kidney damage, and liver damage. Animal data conflicts with respect to the carcinogenicity of tannins. They may be carcinogenic…or may even have anti-carcinogenic effects. An increased risk of esophageal or nasal cancer may be linked with people who regularly ingest herbs with high tannin concentrations (12).

Adverse Reactions Including Known Allergies

None reported.

Possible Interactions with Herbs & Other Dietary Supplements

TANNIN-CONTAINING HERBS: Theoretically, herbs that contain high percentages of tannins (such as bistort) may cause precipitation of constituents of other herbs (19).

Possible Interactions with Drugs

ORAL DRUGS: Theoretically, concomitant oral administration may cause precipitation of some drugs due to the high tannin content of bistort (19). Separate administration of oral drugs and tannin-containing herbs by the longest period of time practical (19).

Possible Interactions with Foods

No interactions are known to occur, and there is no known reason to expect a clinically significant interaction with bistort.

Possible Interactions with Lab Tests

No interactions are known to occur, and there is no known reason to expect a clinically significant interaction with bistort.

Possible Interactions with Diseases or Conditions

No interactions are known to occur, and there is no known reason to expect a clinically significant interaction with bistort.

Typical Dosages & Routes of Administration that are Commonly Used

ORAL: The rhizome and root are powdered and use to make an infusion (18).
TOPICAL: The powdered root is used as an extract or in ointment (18).

Comments

None.

BITTER ALMOND

This Product is Also Known As

Amygdala Amara, Bitter Almond Oil, Volatile Almond Oil.
CAUTION: See separate listing for Sweet Almond Oil.

Scientific Names

Prunus amygdalus amara, synonym Prunus dulcis amara.
Family: Rosaceae.

People Use This For

Orally, bitter almond oil is used as an antispasmodic, local anesthetic, and for its narcotic properties (11).
Historically, bitter almond has been used as a cough suppressant and antipruritic (11).

Safety

POSSIBLY SAFE ...when small amounts of HCN-free volatile oil are used. HCN (hydrocyanic acid) is also known as FFPA (free form prussic acid). When the oil is HCN-free, it is nearly pure benzaldehyde, which has Generally Recognized as Safe (GRAS) status in the US (11).
LIKELY UNSAFE ...when the volatile oil containing HCN is used orally (11,12). ...when large amounts of HCN-free volatile oil are used orally. Ingesting 50-60 mL benzaldehyde can cause fatal CNS depression and respiratory failure (11).
PREGNANCY AND LACTATION: LIKELY UNSAFE ...when the volatile oil containing HCN is used orally (11). Insufficient reliable information is available about the safety of HCN-free oil used orally; avoid using.

Effectiveness

There is insufficient reliable information available about the effectiveness of bitter almond.

Possible Mechanism of Action & Active Ingredients

The applicable part of bitter almond is the volatile oil. The bitter almond kernel contains 3-4% amygdalin, which is hydrolyzed to poisonous hydrocyanic acid (HCN, prussic acid). The volatile oil contains 95% benzaldehyde and 2-4% HCN. For food and flavor use, HCN is removed. High doses of benzaldehyde can have narcotic properties and the potential for adverse reactions (11).

Adverse Reactions Including Known Allergies

There is a report of one death of an adult after ingestion of 7.5 mL of the volatile oil (11). Ingestion of 50-60 mL of benzaldehyde (sole constituent of HCN-free oil) can have high toxicity and be fatal due to CNS depression with respiratory failure (11).

Possible Interactions with Herbs & Other Dietary Supplements

Insufficient reliable information available.

Possible Interactions with Drugs

CNS DEPRESSANTS: Theoretically, bitter almond oil use with other CNS depressants increases the existing risk of severe or fatal CNS and respiratory depression.

Possible Interactions with Foods

No interactions are known to occur, and there is no known reason to expect a clinically significant interaction with bitter almond.

Possible Interactions with Lab Tests

No interactions are known to occur, and there is no known reason to expect a clinically significant interaction with bitter almond.

© Copyright 2000, Natural Medicines Comprehensive Database (209) 472-2244. For updated data, go to www.NaturalDatabase.com

Possible Interactions with Diseases or Conditions

No interactions are known to occur, and there is no known reason to expect a clinically significant interaction with bitter almond.

Typical Dosages & Routes of Administration that are Commonly Used

No typical dosage.

Comments

The volatile oil is likely unsafe. It is no longer used in the US as a commercial medicinal ingredient (11). The volatile oil of bitter almond contains 95% benzaldehyde and 2-4% poisonous HCN. It is made by water maceration and steam distillation of partially defatted bitter almond (Prunus amygdalus amara), apricot (Prunus armeniaca), peach (Prunus persica), and plum (Prunus domestica) kernels. The fixed almond oil (sweet almond oil) is prepared by pressing the kernels of both sweet almond and bitter almond and contains no benzaldehyde or hydrocyanic acid (HCN). Sweet almond does not yield a volatile oil (11). Bitter almond volatile oil consists of distilled, partially defatted oil of the kernels of bitter almond (Prunus amygdalus amara) and kernels of other Prunus species.

BITTER MELON

This Product is Also Known As

African Cucumber, Balsam-Apple, Balsambirne, Balsam Pear, Balsamo, Bitter Apple, Bitter Cucumber, Bitter Gourd, Bittergurke, Carilla Gourd, Chinli-Chih, Cundeamor, Karela, Kuguazi, K'u-Kua, Lai Margose, Momordique, Pepino Montero, P'u-T'ao, Sorosi, Wild Cucumber.

Scientific Names

Momordica charantia, synonym Momordica murcata.
Family: Cucurbitaceae.

People Use This For

Orally, the fruit and seeds of bitter melon are used to treat diabetes and psoriasis, and as supportive therapy for individuals with HIV (1900).

Safety

There is insufficient reliable information available about the safety of bitter melon.
PREGNANCY: LIKELY UNSAFE ...when used orally; contraindicated. The juice can stimulate menstruation and cause abortion (19).
LACTATION: Insufficient reliable information available; avoid using.

Effectiveness

POSSIBLY EFFECTIVE ...when taken orally to improve glucose tolerance, and reduce blood sugar and glycosylated hemoglobin in type 2 diabetics (34,35,36).
There is insufficient reliable information available about the effectiveness of bitter melon for its other uses.

Possible Mechanism of Action & Active Ingredients

The applicable parts of bitter melon are the fruit and seeds. The bitter melon fruit and fruit extracts exhibit hypoglycemic activity in normal and diabetic animal models (3762,3763,3764,3765). Bitter melon contains an insulin-like polypeptide called polypeptide P, plant insulin, or p-insulin. P-insulin has pharmacologic effects similar to bovine insulin with an onset of action between 30 and 60 minutes and a peak effect at about 4 hours. (6,37,38). The constituents alpha- and beta-momorcharin have immunosuppressive activity in vitro and in mice (3724). A protein constituent designated as MAP-30 exhibits antiviral and antitumor activity in human cells in vitro (3720,3721). Bitter melon extracts show antitumor and antileukemia activity in mice (3722,3723).

Adverse Reactions Including Known Allergies

None reported.

Possible Interactions with Herbs & Other Dietary Supplements

STIMULANT LAXATIVE HERBS: Theoretically, concomitant use of bitter melon with other stimulant laxative herbs can increase the risk of potassium depletion. Stimulant laxative herbs include aloe dried leaf sap, wild cucumber fruit (Ecballium alterium), blue flag rhizome, alder buckthorn, European buckthorn, butternut bark, cascara bark, castor oil, colocynth fruit pulp, gamboge bark exudate, jalap root, black root, manna bark exudate, podophyllum root, rhubarb root, senna leaves and pods, and yellow dock root (19).
POTASSIUM DEPLETING HERBS: Theoretically, concomitant use with horsetail plant or licorice rhizome increases the risk of potassium depletion.
HYPOGLYCEMIC HERBS: Theoretically, concomitant use with other hypoglycemic herbs can have additive effects (19).

Possible Interactions with Drugs

DIABETES THERAPY: Theoretically, concomitant use of bitter melon can enhance hypoglycemic drug effects and alter blood glucose control (19). Monitor blood glucose levels if bitter melon is used.

INSULIN: Insulin dosage adjustments might be necessary due to the hypoglycemic effects of bitter melon (19).

CHLORPROPAMIDE (Diabinese): Concomitant use of bitter melon can cause additive hypoglycemic effects (19).

Possible Interactions with Foods

No interactions are known to occur, and there is no known reason to expect a clinically significant interaction with bitter melon.

Possible Interactions with Lab Tests

BLOOD GLUCOSE: Theoretically, bitter melon can lower blood glucose and test results (19).

Possible Interactions with Diseases or Conditions

DIABETES: Theoretically, bitter melon can alter blood glucose control (19), and blood glucose levels should be monitored with its use.

Typical Dosages & Routes of Administration that are Commonly Used

ORAL: People typically use 1 to 2 grams of powdered leaf in tablets or capsules daily. Bitter melon is also taken as a 4:1 tincture in a dose of 1 to 3 mL twice daily (5255).

Comments

None.

BITTER MILKWORT

This Product is Also Known As

European Bitter Polygala, European Senega, Evergreen Snakeroot, Flowering Wintergreen, Little Pollom, Snakeroot.

CAUTION: See separate listing for Asarabacca and Senega.

Scientific Names

Polygala amara.

People Use This For

Orally, bitter milkwort is used for upper and lower respiratory disorders, cough, and bronchitis (18).

Safety

There is insufficient reliable information available about the safety of bitter milkwort.

Pregnancy and Lactation: Insufficient reliable information available; avoid using.

Effectiveness

There is insufficient reliable information available about the effectiveness of bitter milkwort.

Possible Mechanism of Action & Active Ingredients

The applicable parts of bitter milkwort are the flowering plant and root. Bitter milkwort can have mild expectorant properties (18). The active constituents are saponin (senegin), bitter substances, and methylestersalizylic acid (18).

Adverse Reactions Including Known Allergies

None reported.

Possible Interactions with Herbs & Other Dietary Supplements

Insufficient reliable information available.

Possible Interactions with Drugs

No interactions are known to occur, and there is no known reason to expect a clinically significant interaction with bitter milkwort.

Possible Interactions with Foods

No interactions are known to occur, and there is no known reason to expect a clinically significant interaction with bitter milkwort.

Possible Interactions with Lab Tests

No interactions are known to occur, and there is no known reason to expect a clinically significant interaction with bitter milkwort.

Possible Interactions with Diseases or Conditions

No interactions are known to occur, and there is no known reason to expect a clinically significant interaction with bitter milkwort.

Typical Dosages & Routes of Administration that are Commonly Used

ORAL: People typically prepare a tea, adding 1 teaspoon of the plant to 1 cup of boiling water. This is taken once daily. Four tablespoons of the leaves are also combined with water and boiled for an extended time. This liquid is taken at a dose of 1 tablespoon every 3 hours (5263).

Comments

Avoid confusion with asarabacca (Asarum europaeum) or senega (Polygala senega), also known as snakeroot. There is very little scientific information about this product. Our staff is continually analyzing the available information on natural medicines and will add data here as it becomes available.

BITTER ORANGE flower, flower oil

This Product is Also Known As

None.
CAUTION: See separate listings for Bergamot Oil, Bitter Orange peel, Oswego Tea, and Sweet Orange.

Scientific Names

Citrus aurantium, synonyms Citrus aurantium amara, Citrus bergamia, Citrus bigaradia, Citrus vulgaris. Family: Rutaceae.

People Use This For

Orally, the bitter orange flower and its oil are used for GI disturbances, duodenal ulcers, constipation, regulating blood lipid levels, lowering blood sugar in diabetes, blood purification, functional disorders of liver and gallbladder, stimulation of the heart and circulation, frost bite, as a sedative for sleep disorders, kidney and bladder diseases, general feebleness, anemia, imbalances of mineral metabolism, impurities of the skin, and hair loss (2,11). Topically, bitter orange use includes inflammation of the eye lid, conjunctiva, and retina, retinal hemorrhage, exhaustion accompanying colds, headaches, neuralgia, muscular pain, rheumatic discomfort, bruises, phlebitis, and bed sores (2).
For food use, the oil is used as a flavoring agent (11).
In manufacturing, the oil is used in pharmaceuticals, cosmetics, and soaps (11).

Safety

LIKELY SAFE ...when taken in the amounts found in foods (11). Bitter orange is Generally Recognized as Safe (GRAS) in the US (11).
There is insufficient reliable information available about the safety of the medicinal use of bitter orange.
PREGNANCY AND LACTATION: Insufficient reliable information available; avoid using.

Effectiveness

There is insufficient reliable information available about the effectiveness of bitter orange (2).

Possible Mechanism of Action & Active Ingredients

The oil exhibits antifungal and antibacterial activities in vitro, due to its flavanoid and pectin constituents (11).

Adverse Reactions Including Known Allergies

No adverse reactions have been reported (2). The flower oil is generally non-irritating and non-sensitizing in humans; however, the potential for contact dermatitis exists (11).

Possible Interactions with Herbs & Other Dietary Supplements

Insufficient reliable information available.

Possible Interactions with Drugs

No interactions are known to occur, and there is no known reason to expect a clinically significant interaction with bitter orange flower and flower oil.

Possible Interactions with Foods

No interactions are known to occur, and there is no known reason to expect a clinically significant interaction with bitter orange flower and flower oil.

Possible Interactions with Lab Tests

No interactions are known to occur, and there is no known reason to expect a clinically significant interaction with bitter orange flower and flower oil.

Possible Interactions with Diseases or Conditions

No interactions are known to occur, and there is no known reason to expect a clinically significant interaction with bitter orange flower and flower oil.

Typical Dosages & Routes of Administration that are Commonly Used
No typical dosage.

Comments
Because of the lack of demonstrated effectiveness and safety data (2), the use of bitter orange flower or its oil should be avoided. Avoid confusion with bergamot oil, bitter orange peel, and sweet orange.

BITTER ORANGE peel

This Product is Also Known As
Aurantii Pericarpium.
CAUTION: See separate listings for Bergamot Oil, Bitter Orange flower, Oswego Tea, and Sweet Orange.

Scientific Names
Citrus aurantium, synonyms Citrus aurantium amara, Citrus bergamia, Citrus bigaradia, Citrus vulgaris.
Family: Rutaceae.

People Use This For
Orally, bitter orange peel is taken as an appetite stimulant and for dyspepsia (2).
In Chinese medicine, bitter orange is used for prolapsed uterus, prolapsed anus or rectum, diarrhea, and blood in the stools (11).
Traditionally, bitter orange has been used as a tonic, antiflatulent, and for cancer (11).

Safety
LIKELY SAFE ...when used orally and appropriately (2).
POSSIBLY UNSAFE ...when used by fair-skinned individuals who are exposed to the sun. Bitter orange peel can cause photosensitivity (2).
CHILDREN: POSSIBLY UNSAFE ...when used orally. Large amounts can cause intestinal colic, convulsions, and death (11).
PREGNANCY AND LACTATION: Insufficient reliable information available; avoid using.

Effectiveness
POSSIBLY EFFECTIVE ...when taken orally as an appetite stimulant and for dyspepsia (2).
There is insufficient reliable information available about the effectiveness of bitter orange peel for its other uses.

Possible Mechanism of Action & Active Ingredients
The peel contains essential oils and bitter principles (11). Bitter orange peel exhibits anti-inflammatory activity, which might be due to its naringin and nobiletin components (11,1281). The flavonoid and pectin constituents of bitter orange peel can have antibacterial and antifungal activity. The pectin content can have a lowering effect on cholesterol in humans and animals (11). The furocoumarins found in bitter orange peel can be responsible for photosensitivity (2,11,18).

Adverse Reactions Including Known Allergies
OCCUPATIONAL SENSITIZATION: Frequent contact with the peel or oil can cause erythema, blisters, pustules, dermatoses leading to scab formation, and pigment spots (18). Photosensitivity can occur, especially in fair-skinned people (2). The ingestion of large amounts of bitter orange peel in children can have TOXICITY and cause intestinal colic, convulsions, and death (11).

Possible Interactions with Herbs & Other Dietary Supplements
Insufficient reliable information available.

Possible Interactions with Drugs
ACID-INHIBITING DRUGS: Theoretically, due to claims that bitter orange peel increases stomach acid, it might interfere with antacids, sucralfate (Carafate), H-2 antagonists, or proton pump inhibitors (19).

Possible Interactions with Foods
No interactions are known to occur, and there is no known reason to expect a clinically significant interaction with bitter orange peel.

Possible Interactions with Lab Tests
No interactions are known to occur, and there is no known reason to expect a clinically significant interaction with bitter orange peel.

Possible Interactions with Diseases or Conditions
No interactions are known to occur, and there is no known reason to expect a clinically significant interaction with bitter orange peel.

Typical Dosages & Routes of Administration that are Commonly Used

ORAL: The typical dose of bitter orange is 4-6 grams per day of the dry peel, which is free of the white pulp layer (2). Bitter orange can be used as a tea, which is prepared by steeping the peel in 150 mL boiling water for 10-15 minutes and straining. Typical doses of the peel tincture is 2-3 grams per day and of the peel extract is 1-2 grams per day (2).

Comments

Avoid confusion with bergamot oil, bitter orange flower or oil, and sweet orange peel.

BITTERSWEET NIGHTSHADE

This Product is Also Known As

Bitter Nightshade, Bittersweet, Blue Nightshade, Common Nightshade, Deadly Nightshade, Dulcarara, Fellen, Fellonwood, Felonwort, Fever Twig, Mortal, Scarlet Berry, Snake Berry, Staff Vine, Violet Bloom, Woody, Woody Nightshade.
CAUTION: See separate listings for Belladonna and Henbane.

Scientific Names

Solanum dulcamara.
Family: Solanaceae.

People Use This For

Orally, the stem of bittersweet nightshade is used for chronic eczema, itchy skin conditions, acne, furuncles, skin abrasions, and warts.
Topically, the stem of bittersweet nightshade is used for chronic eczema.
Historically, bittersweet nightshade is used as an antirheumatic, diuretic, narcotic, and sedative, and has been used for nail bed inflammations (2,6,7,18).

Safety

POSSIBLY SAFE …when the stem of bittersweet nightshade is used orally and appropriately (2,18). …when the stem is used topically and appropriately (2).
LIKELY UNSAFE …when the leaves or berries are used orally. The plant contains the toxic compounds solanine, solanidine, and dulcamarin (6).
CHILDREN: LIKELY UNSAFE …unripe berries have caused poisonings. A lethal dose is estimated to be 200 berries (18). There is insufficient reliable information available about the safety of the stem used topically in children.
PREGNANCY: LIKELY UNSAFE …when used orally, the stem, leaf, or berries are contraindicated. The alkaloids of the plant, solasodine, soladulcine, and related compounds have been linked to malformations in animals (6). Some of these constituents might be present in the stem (296). There is insufficient reliable information available about the safety of the stem used topically during pregnancy.
LACTATION: LIKELY UNSAFE …when the leaves or berries used orally; avoid using. There is insufficient reliable information available about the safety of the oral or topical use of the stem during lactation; avoid using.

Effectiveness

POSSIBLY EFFECTIVE …when used topically as supportive therapy for chronic eczema (2). …when used orally for treating itchy skin conditions (2,7).
There is insufficient reliable information available about the effectiveness of bittersweet nightshade for its other uses.

Possible Mechanism of Action & Active Ingredients

The applicable part of bittersweet nightshade is the stem. It has astringent, antimicrobial, and mucous membrane-irritating actions (2). The steroidal alkaloid constituents of the stem can have anticholinergic effects (2). The component, solasodin, can prevent inflammation (2).

Adverse Reactions Including Known Allergies

In adults, toxicity associated with the stem (2,6,7,18) is uncommon due to the low alkaloid content. There are no reports of adverse effects relating to the topical use of the stem (2,6,7,18). Taken orally, the bittersweet nightshade plant can cause the symptoms of solanine poisoning, commonly associated with old potatoes. Symptoms include scratchy throat, headache, vertigo, dilated pupils, speech difficulties, subnormal temperature, vomiting, diarrhea, GI bleeding, cyanosis, convulsions, circulatory and respiratory depression, and even death (6). The ingestion of unripe berries can cause poisoning in children (18).

Possible Interactions with Herbs & Other Dietary Supplements

Insufficient reliable information available.

Possible Interactions with Drugs

No interactions are known to occur, and there is no known reason to expect a clinically significant interaction with bittersweet nightshade.

Possible Interactions with Foods

No interactions are known to occur, and there is no known reason to expect a clinically significant interaction with bittersweet nightshade.

Possible Interactions with Lab Tests

No interactions are known to occur, and there is no known reason to expect a clinically significant interaction with bittersweet nightshade.

Possible Interactions with Diseases or Conditions

GI IRRITATION: Bittersweet nightshade can irritate the gastrointestinal tract. It is contraindicated in individuals with infectious or inflammatory gastrointestinal conditions (19).

Typical Dosages & Routes of Administration that are Commonly Used

ORAL: The typical dose of the bittersweet nightshade stem is 1-3 grams of the dried herb per day, and can be taken as a tea, which is prepared by steeping the herb in 150 mL boiling water for 5-10 minutes and straining (2).
TOPICAL: The stem is used topically as a compress prepared by steeping 1-2 grams of the dried herb in 250 mL boiling water for 5-10 minutes and straining (2).

Comments

Bittersweet nightshade is a perennial vine-like plant that is found throughout the United States, Canada, and Eurasia and is a member of the same family that includes tomatoes and potatoes. Avoid confusion with belladonna (deadly nightshade) and henbane (nightshade).

BLACK ALDER

This Product is Also Known As

Common Alder, Owler, Tag Alder.

Scientific Names

Alnus glutinosa.
Family: Betulaceae.

People Use This For

Black alder is used for streptococcal sore throat, pharyngitis, and intestinal bleeding (18).

Safety

There is insufficient reliable information available about the safety of black alder.
Pregnancy and Lactation: Insufficient reliable information available; avoid using.

Effectiveness

There is insufficient reliable information about the effectiveness of black alder.

Possible Mechanism of Action & Active Ingredients

The applicable part of black alder is the bark. There is insufficient reliable information available about the possible mechanism of action and active ingredients.

Adverse Reactions Including Known Allergies

None reported.

Possible Interactions with Herbs & Other Dietary Supplements

Insufficient reliable information available.

Possible Interactions with Drugs

No interactions are known to occur, and there is no known reason to expect a clinically significant interaction with black alder.

Possible Interactions with Foods

No interactions are known to occur, and there is no known reason to expect a clinically significant interaction with black alder.

Possible Interactions with Lab Tests

No interactions are known to occur, and there is no known reason to expect a clinically significant interaction with black alder.

Possible Interactions with Diseases or Conditions

No interactions are known to occur, and there is no known reason to expect a clinically significant interaction with black alder.

Typical Dosages & Routes of Administration that are Commonly Used

TOPICAL: The bark is prepared as a decoction and used as a gargle (18).

Comments

There is very little scientific information about this product. Our staff is continually analyzing the available information on natural medicines and will add data here as it becomes available.

BLACK BRYONY

This Product is Also Known As

Blackeye Root.

Scientific Names

Tamus communis.

People Use This For

Orally, black bryony root is used for intestinal mucous membrane irritation and as an emetic (18).
Topically, black bryony root is used for agitation and redness of the skin, bruises, strains, torn muscles, gout, rheumatic disorders, hair loss, and improving blood circulation to the scalp (18).

Safety

POSSIBLY UNSAFE ...when the fresh root is used topically. Skin contact can cause severe skin irritation (18).
UNSAFE ...when used orally. Can cause seizures, respiratory and kidney failure (18).
PREGNANCY AND LACTATION: UNSAFE ...when used orally. POSSIBLY UNSAFE ...when used topically; avoid using (18).

Effectiveness

There is insufficient reliable information available about the effectiveness of black bryony.

Possible Mechanism of Action & Active Ingredients

The applicable part of black bryony is the root. It can stimulate external nerve endings. Applied topically, it acts as mechanical irritant, penetrating the skin with tiny, needle-like crystals of calcium oxalate (3829). The rhizome contains histamine (3829), which can have a role in producing skin irritation (3829). In rats, an ethanolic extract of the root exhibited local anti-inflammatory activity (3828).

Adverse Reactions Including Known Allergies

The black bryony root taken orally can cause severe mouth, pharyngeal and GI irritation, as well as vomiting, diarrhea, spasms, colic, decreased kidney function, and respiratory depression (18). The fresh root applied topically can cause reddening of skin (18). The fresh plant used topically can cause skin irritation, rash, swelling, pustules, wheals, and mucous membrane irritation (18).

Possible Interactions with Herbs & Other Dietary Supplements

Insufficient reliable information available.

Possible Interactions with Drugs

No interactions are known to occur, and there is no known reason to expect a clinically significant interaction with black bryony.

Possible Interactions with Foods

No interactions are known to occur, and there is no known reason to expect a clinically significant interaction with black bryony.

Possible Interactions with Lab Tests

No interactions are known to occur, and there is no known reason to expect a clinically significant interaction with black bryony.

Possible Interactions with Diseases or Conditions

No interactions are known to occur, and there is no known reason to expect a clinically significant interaction with black bryony.

Typical Dosages & Routes of Administration that are Commonly Used

ORAL: People typically use 1 to 5 drops of the tincture.
TOPICAL: The fresh root is scraped and the pulp rubbed into affected areas (5264,5267).

Comments

None.

BLACK COHOSH

This Product is Also Known As

Baneberry, Black Snakeroot, Bugbane, Bugwort, Cimicifuga, Phytoestrogen, Rattle Root, Rattle Snakeroot, Rattlesnake Root, Rattleweed, Squawroot.
CAUTION: See separate listings for Blue Cohosh and White Cohosh.

Scientific Names

Cimicifuga racemosa, Actaea racemosa, Actaea macrotys.
Family: Ranunculaceae.

People Use This For

Orally, black cohosh is used as an alternative to hormone replacement therapy for management of menopausal symptoms (6,4614).
Traditionally, black cohosh has been used for dysmenorrhea, dyspepsia, rheumatism, fever sore throat, cough, and as an insect repellent (4,6,4611). The fresh root was applied topically to rattlesnake bites (4621).

Safety

LIKELY SAFE ...when used orally and appropriately for up to 6 months (12).
There is insufficient reliable information available about the safety of the oral use of black cohosh for more than 6 months (2).
PREGNANCY: UNSAFE ...contraindicated because it has menstrual and uterine stimulant effects (4,6).
LACTATION: UNSAFE ...when used orally in large doses (19).

Effectiveness

LIKELY EFFECTIVE ...when taken orally for managing the symptoms of menopause (2,141,4614,4620). The majority of clinical trials published to date are in the German medical literature. Although many trials were open-label, controlled comparisons with estrogens showed similar efficacy (4611). No study lasted longer than 6 months.
POSSIBLY EFFECTIVE ...when used orally for managing premenstrual discomfort and dysmenorrhea (2). To date, no studies have been published using black cohosh for premenstrual discomfort and dysmenorrhea. Case reports suggest efficacy, and the German Commission E has designated black cohosh as effective for this indication (2,4611,6521).
LIKELY INEFFECTIVE ...when used orally for stimulating menstruation (5).
There is insufficient reliable information available about the effectiveness of black cohosh for its other uses. Clinical studies on the effectiveness of black cohosh have used the Remifemin products made by Schaper and Brummer, a German pharmaceutical company.

Possible Mechanism of Action & Active Ingredients

The applicable parts of black cohosh are the rhizome and root. Black cohosh is a member of the buttercup family and is native to eastern North America. Black cohosh contains phytosterin, isoferulic acid, salicylic acid, sugars, tannins, long-chain fatty acids, and triterpene glycosides, including acetin, cimicifugoside, and 27-deoxyacetin (4611). The presence of an isoflavone, formononetin, is questionable (4611,4616). Earlier reports of isoflavone content may have been a result of contamination with other similar plant species (4615). No pharmacokinetic information is available. Laboratory evidence of estrogenic activity has been conflicting (4618,4619). A black cohosh extract competitively inhibits estradiol binding to estrogen receptors (6180). It also increases uterine weight and increases serum ceruloplasmin oxidase activity (a measure of estrogenic activity in the liver) in female rats with their ovaries removed (6180). The mechanism of action of black cohosh remains unknown. Some clinical evidence suggests that black cohosh suppresses LH secretion, while a more recent study showed no change in LH, FSH, sex hormone-binding globulin (SHBG) prolactin, and estradiol in postmenopausal women (4611,4614,4617). Unidentified compounds acting synergistically may be responsible for the pharmacological effect of black cohosh (4617). Whether black cohosh has an estrogen-like beneficial effect on osteoporosis and cardiovascular disease is unknown. Concomitant use with hormone replacement therapy has not been studied. Some authors have suggested that black cohosh can be safely used in women with a history of breast cancer, citing laboratory evidence that black cohosh does not stimulate the proliferation of estrogen receptor-positive breast cancer cells (4611,4616,4621). Large-scale epidemiological studies looking retrospectively at the association of black cohosh with breast cancer have not been performed.

Adverse Reactions Including Known Allergies

The most common complaint in clinical studies has been occasional GI disturbances (4615,4616). Other adverse effects include headache, feeling of heaviness in the legs, and weight gain (4621). An overdose of black cohosh can cause nausea, vomiting, dizziness, nervous system and visual disturbances, reduced heart rate, and perspiration (4). There is one case report of nocturnal seizures in a woman who used black cohosh, evening primrose oil, and chasteberry (588). Studies on mutagenicity, teratogenicity, and carcinogenicity have been negative (4611,4615).

Possible Interactions with Herbs & Other Dietary Supplements

Insufficient reliable information.

Possible Interactions with Drugs

TAMOXIFEN: May have additive antiproliferative effect with tamoxifen.

Possible Interactions with Foods

No interactions are known to occur, and there is no known reason to expect a clinically significant interaction with black cohosh.

Possible Interactions with Lab Tests

LUTEINIZING HORMONE (LH): Black cohosh might reduce serum LH concentrations and test results (1331).

Possible Interactions with Diseases or Conditions

ESTROGENIC CONDITIONS: Black cohosh contains constituents that might have estrogenic properties, although estrogenic activity is controversial. Theoretically, these constituents could interact with diseases or conditions sensitive to such activity.

Typical Dosages & Routes of Administration that are Commonly Used

ORAL: The usual oral dose of black cohosh is 0.3-2 grams of the dried rhizome or root three times daily. A decoction can also be taken three times daily and is prepared by bringing the dried rhizome or root to a boil in water, simmering for 5-10 minutes, and straining (4). The typical dose of the liquid extract (1:1 in 90% alcohol) is 0.3-2.0 mL (4). Tincture of cimicifuga (1:10 in 60% alcohol) is usually taken in a dose of 2-4 mL (4). The German product used in all clinical studies is called Remifemin. Remifemin is distributed by Enzymatic Therapy and Phytopharmica, both of whom claim to be exclusive US sources (4612,4613). The Enzymatic Therapy tablet contains approximately 20 mg black cohosh and rhizome extract, standardized to contain an unspecified quantity oftriterpene glycosides calculated as 27-deoxyactein (4612). The suggested dose is 1 tablet twice daily (4612). The Phytopharmica tablet contains approximately 40 mg of Black cohosh (Cimicifuga racemosa) and rhizome extract standardized to contain 1 mg of Triterpene glycosides calculated as 27-deoxyactein (4613). The suggested dose is 2 tablets twice daily (4613). Most clinical studies used higher doses of the German product Remifemin; however, a more recent study found equal efficacy with 40 mg and 127 mg daily (4614). The German Commission E limits use to no for longer than 6 months (2). Although no clinical study has lasted beyond 6 months, one author suggests that longer use may be safe (4621). Maximum effect is usually achieved within 4 to 8 weeks (4615,4617).

Comments

Black cohosh was first used medicinally by native Americans who introduced it to European colonists (4611). It was introduced into Germany in the late 19th century and is approved by the German Commission E for premenstrual discomfort, dysmenorrhea or menopausal symptoms (2). Remifemin, a branded black cohosh product, has been used in Germany since the mid-1950s to manage menopause (141). Black cohosh was also used as an ingredient in Lydia Pinkham's Vegetable Compound (6).

The genus name of black cohosh, cimicifuga, comes from the Latin words for "bedbug" and "repel". Although less fragrant than other species of the genus, black cohosh was used as an insect repellent, hence the common name "bugbane". Do not confuse black cohosh with 2 unrelated plants, blue cohosh and white cohosh.

BLACK CURRANT berry

This Product is Also Known As

Cassis.
CAUTION: See separate listing for Black Currant Seed Oil, and Black Currant leaf.

Scientific Names

Ribes nigrum.
Family: Grossulariaceae.

People Use This For

Orally, black currant berry is used for coughs.
For food uses, it is utilized as a flavor component in liqueurs and as a food (513).

© Copyright 2000, Natural Medicines Comprehensive Database (209) 472-2244. For updated data, go to www.NaturalDatabase.com

Safety

LIKELY SAFE …when consumed as food or flavoring (513). …when black current berry is used orally in medicinal amounts (12).
PREGNANCY AND LACTATION: LIKELY SAFE …when used orally as food or as medicinal (12).

Effectiveness

There is insufficient reliable information available about the effectiveness of black currant berry.

Possible Mechanism of Action & Active Ingredients

Insufficient reliable information available.

Adverse Reactions Including Known Allergies

None reported.

Possible Interactions with Herbs & Other Dietary Supplements

Insufficient reliable information available.

Possible Interactions with Drugs

No interactions are known to occur, and there is no known reason to expect a clinically significant interaction with black currant berry.

Possible Interactions with Foods

No interactions are known to occur, and there is no known reason to expect a clinically significant interaction with black currant berry.

Possible Interactions with Lab Tests

No interactions are known to occur, and there is no known reason to expect a clinically significant interaction with black currant berry.

Possible Interactions with Diseases or Conditions

No interactions are known to occur, and there is no known reason to expect a clinically significant interaction with black currant berry.

Typical Dosages & Routes of Administration that are Commonly Used

No typical dosage.

Comments

There is very little scientific information about this product. Our staff is continually analyzing the available information on natural medicines and will add data here as it becomes available.

BLACK CURRANT dried leaf

This Product is Also Known As

Ribes nigri folium.
CAUTION: See separate listing for Black Currant Seed Oil and Black Currant berry.

Scientific Names

Ribes nigrum.
Family: Grossulariaceae.

People Use This For

Orally, black currant dried leaf is taken for arthritis, gout, rheumatism, diarrhea, colic, hepatitis, liver ailments, convulsions, and inflammatory disorders of the mouth and throat (18). It is also used for coughs and colds, whooping cough (18), disinfecting the urine (7), promoting diuresis, treating bladder stones (7,18), and as a cleansing tea (18).
Topically, black currant dried leaf is used for the treatment of wounds and insect bites (18).

Safety

There is insufficient reliable information available about the safety of oral or topical use of black currant.
Pregnancy and Lactation: Insufficient reliable information available; avoid using.

Effectiveness

There is insufficient reliable information available about the effectiveness of black currant dried leaf.

Possible Mechanism of Action & Active Ingredients

Black currant leaves can have diuretic, hypotensive, and cooling effects (18). The leaves of black currant contain flavonoids, including astragalin, isoquercitrin, and rutin. The volatile oil contains trace amounts of ascorbic acid (18).

Adverse Reactions Including Known Allergies
None reported.

Possible Interactions with Herbs & Other Dietary Supplements
Insufficient reliable information available.

Possible Interactions with Drugs
No interactions are known to occur, and there is no known reason to expect a clinically significant interaction with black currant dried leaf.

Possible Interactions with Foods
No interactions are known to occur, and there is no known reason to expect a clinically significant interaction with black currant dried leaf.

Possible Interactions with Lab Tests
No interactions are known to occur, and there is no known reason to expect a clinically significant interaction with black currant dried leaf.

Possible Interactions with Diseases or Conditions
CARDIAC DISORDERS: Avoid the use of black currant in individuals with edema associated with reduced cardiac function (18).
KIDNEY DISORDERS: Avoid its use in individuals with edema associated with reduced kidney function (18).

Typical Dosages & Routes of Administration that are Commonly Used
ORAL: The typical does of black currant is 3-4 cups of the tea daily, and the tea is prepared by adding 1-2 teaspoons or 2-4 grams of the black currant leaves into 150 mL of boiling water for ten minutes and then straining (18).
TOPICAL: Black currant is commonly applied to wounds as a compress, which is made using the freshly grated leaves or leaves soaked in warm water and dried (18). The freshly grated leaves are also rubbed onto insect bites (18).

Comments
None.

BLACK CURRANT SEED OIL

This Product is Also Known As
European Black Currant, European Blackcurrant, Casis, Cassis, Ribes Nero.
CAUTION: See separate listings for Borage Seed Oil, Black Currant berry, Black Currant dried leaf, Evening Primrose Oil, Gamma Linolenic Acid, and Omega-6 Oils.

Scientific Names
Ribes nigrum.
Family: Grossulariaceae.

People Use This For
Orally, black currant seed oil is used for menopause symptoms, premenstrual syndrome, dysmenorrhea, mastodynia (512,515), and for boosting immunity (4016).

Safety
POSSIBLY SAFE ...when used orally to boost immunity in the elderly (4016).
There is insufficient reliable information available about the safety of the other uses of black currant seed oil.
PREGNANCY AND LACTATION: Insufficient reliable information available; avoid using.

Effectiveness
POSSIBLY EFFECTIVE ...when used orally for increasing immunity in the elderly (4016).
There is insufficient reliable information available about the effectiveness of black currant seed oil for its other uses.

Possible Mechanism of Action & Active Ingredients
Black currant seed oil contains 6-19% gamma-linolenic acid (GLA) (512,515). Researchers think it may be beneficial in people unable to metabolize cis-linolenic acid to GLA and produce adequate prostaglandin E1 (PGE1). People with this condition have an imbalance in the ratio of inflammatory to noninflammatory prostaglandins. GLA is thought to improve this ratio (512,4016) and researchers think this is why black currant seed oil increases immune response in elderly people (4016).

Adverse Reactions Including Known Allergies
None reported.

Possible Interactions with Herbs & Other Dietary Supplements
Insufficient reliable information available.

Possible Interactions with Drugs
No interactions are known to occur, and there is no known reason to expect a clinically significant interaction with black currant seed oil.

Possible Interactions with Foods
No interactions are known to occur, and there is no known reason to expect a clinically significant interaction with black currant seed oil.

Possible Interactions with Lab Tests
No interactions are known to occur, and there is no known reason to expect a clinically significant interaction with black currant seed oil.

Possible Interactions with Diseases or Conditions
No interactions are known to occur, and there is no known reason to expect a clinically significant interaction with black currant seed oil.

Typical Dosages & Routes of Administration that are Commonly Used
ORAL: People typically use 500-1000 mg black currant oil daily. A 500 mg capsule is typically labeled to contain about 230 mg cis-linoleic acid, 85 mg cis-gamma-linoleic acid, 65 mg alpha-linoleic acid, and 15 mg stearidonic acid (6006). A dose of 4500 mg per day was used to boost immunity in the elderly in a clinical study (4016).

Comments
Black currant seed oil is the fixed oil obtained from seeds of the black currant (Ribes nigrum). Avoid confusion with black currant berry.

BLACK HAW

This Product is Also Known As
Southern Black Haw, Stag Bush, Viburnum.

Scientific Names
Viburnum prunifolium; Viburnum prunifolium ferrugineum, synonym Viburnum rufidulum.
Family: Caprifoliaceae.

People Use This For
Orally, the root bark and extracts of black haw are used as a tonic, uterine sedative, antidiarrheal, diuretic, and antispasmodic (11).
Traditionally, black haw has been used for painful menses, preventing miscarriage, asthma, and as a postpartum antispasmodic (11).

Safety
LIKELY SAFE …when black haw stem bark is used orally in food amounts. It is approved for food use in the US. The maximum level used is 0.001% (11).
POSSIBLY SAFE …when the root bark is used orally and appropriately in medicinal amounts (12).
PREGNANCY: POSSIBLY UNSAFE …some evidence suggests black haw has uterine relaxant effects (11); avoid using.
LACTATION: Insufficient reliable information available.

Effectiveness
POSSIBLY EFFECTIVE …when used orally as an uterine antispasmodic (11,142).
There is insufficient reliable information available about the effectiveness of black haw bark for its other uses.

Possible Mechanism of Action & Active Ingredients
The applicable parts of black haw are the root bark and stem bark. The root bark contains several active constituents, including scopoletin, tannins, oxalic acid, salicin and salicylic acid (11,296). Scopoletin is thought to be a uterine relaxant (11).

Adverse Reactions Including Known Allergies
None reported.

Possible Interactions with Herbs & Other Dietary Supplements
No interactions are known to occur, and there is no known reason to expect a clinically significant interaction with black haw.

Possible Interactions with Drugs
No interactions are known to occur, and there is no known reason to expect a clinically significant interaction with black haw.

Possible Interactions with Foods
No interactions are known to occur, and there is no known reason to expect a clinically significant interaction with black haw.

Possible Interactions with Lab Tests
No interactions are known to occur, and there is no known reason to expect a clinically significant interaction with black haw.

Possible Interactions with Diseases or Conditions
HISTORY OF KIDNEY STONES: Avoid the use of black haw because it contains oxalic acid and might increase stone formation in individuals with a history of kidney stones (11,12).
ASPIRIN ALLERGY: Theoretically, the salicylate constituents in black haw could trigger allergic reaction in individuals with aspirin allergy or asthma.

Typical Dosages & Routes of Administration that are Commonly Used
ORAL: People typically use 2 teaspoons of the dried bark in 1 cup of water, boiled and simmered for 10 minutes. This is taken three times daily. In tincture form, black haw is taken 5 to 10 mL three times daily (5253).

Comments
Black haw is a shrub that has serrated oval leaves, clusters of white flowers, and blue-black berries. It is native to the woodlands of central and southern North America (4201).

BLACK HELLEBORE

This Product is Also Known As
Christe Herbe, Christmas Rose, Christmas Rose Plant, Melampode.
CAUTION: See separate listings for American Hellebore, Pheasant's Eye, and White Hellebore.

Scientific Names
Helleborus niger.
Family: Ranunculaceae.

People Use This For
In folk medicine, black hellebore is used for nausea, worm infestations, regulating menstruation, acute nephritis, head colds, as a laxative, and as an abortifacient (18).

Safety
LIKELY UNSAFE ...when used orally. Black hellebore contains cardiac glycosides with structure, activity, and adverse effects similar to digitalis (3).
PREGNANCY: LIKELY UNSAFE ...when used orally. Black hellebore is contraindicated in pregnancy because it can have menstrual stimulant (19) or abortifacient effects (18).
LACTATION: LIKELY UNSAFE ...when used orally; avoid using.

Effectiveness
There is insufficient reliable information available about the effectiveness of black hellebore.

Possible Mechanism of Action & Active Ingredients
Black hellebore root contains cardioactive glycosides with digitalis-like effects (18). It also contains saponins that irritate mucous membranes and can cause toxicity (18). Black hellebore is a GI irritant (19), and the fresh plant has local irritant properties (19).

Adverse Reactions Including Known Allergies
Oral use of black hellebore can cause GI irritation (19). The symptoms of poisoning from black hellebore include scratchy throat or mouth, salivation, nausea, vomiting, diarrhea, dizziness, shortness of breath, spasm, and asphyxiation (18). Topically, the fresh plant may cause irritation or inflammation when handled (19).

Possible Interactions with Herbs & Other Dietary Supplements
CARDIAC GLYCOSIDE-CONTAINING HERBS: Contraindicated; concomitant use can increase the risk of cardiac glycoside toxicity. Cardiac glycoside-containing herbs, including black hellebore, Canadian hemp roots, digitalis leaf, hedge mustard, figwort, lily of the valley roots, motherwort, oleander leaf, pheasant's eye plant, pleurisy root, squill bulb leaf scales, and strophanthus seeds (2,18,19,500).
OTHER CARDIOACTIVE HERBS: Avoid concomitant use with other cardioactive herbs due to unpredictability of effects and adverse effects. Other cardioactive herbs include: calamus, cereus, cola, coltsfoot, devil's claw,

European mistletoe, fenugreek, fumitory, ginger, Panax ginseng, hawthorn, white horehound, mate, parsley, quassia, scotch broom flower, shepherd's purse, and wild carrot (4).
STIMULANT LAXATIVE HERBS: Theoretically, overuse or misuse of stimulant laxatives with cardiac glycoside-containing herbs increases the risk of cardiac toxicity due to potassium depletion. Stimulant laxative herbs include: aloe dried leaf sap, blue flag rhizome, alder buckthorn, European buckthorn, butternut bark, cascara bark, castor oil, colocynth fruit pulp, gamboge bark exudate, jalap root, black root, manna bark exudate, podophyllum root, rhubarb root, senna leaves and pods, wild cucumber fruit (Ecballium elaterium), and yellow dock root (19).
LICORICE/HORSETAIL: Theoretically, overuse/misuse of licorice rhizome or horsetail plant with cardiac glycoside-containing herbs increases the risk of toxicity due to potassium depletion (19).

Possible Interactions with Drugs
DIGOXIN: Contraindicated; therapeutic duplication increases risk of cardiac glycoside toxicity (2).
CARDIAC DRUGS: Theoretically, concomitant use can increase the risk of cardiac toxicity (152).
STIMULANT LAXATIVES: Theoretically, overuse/misuse can increase risk of cardiac glycoside toxicity due to potassium depletion (2,506).
POTASSIUM DEPLETING DIURETICS, QUININE can increase the risk of digitalis toxicity (2,506).
QUININE: Theoretically, concomitant use can increase risk of cardiac toxicity (2,506).
TETRACYCLINES and MACROLIDE ANTIBIOTICS (erythromycin-like drugs): Theoretically, concomitant use might increase risk of cardiac glycoside toxicity (152,17).

Possible Interactions with Foods
No interactions are known to occur, and there is no known reason to expect a clinically significant interaction with black hellebore.

Possible Interactions with Lab Tests
No interactions are known to occur, and there is no known reason to expect a clinically significant interaction with black hellebore.

Possible Interactions with Diseases or Conditions
GI INFLAMMATION: Because black hellebore can aggravate GI inflammation, its use is contraindicated (19).
HEART DISEASE: Self-use contraindicated; requires diagnosis, treatment, and monitoring (515).

Typical Dosages & Routes of Administration that are Commonly Used
No typical dosage.

Comments
Black hellebore is likely unsafe for self-use (3). Black hellebore is an obsolete and dangerous natural product (18). Avoid confusion with white hellebore (Veratrum album). Black hellebore is an obsolete and dangerous natural product (18).

BLACK HOREHOUND

This Product is Also Known As
Ballota, Black Stinking Horehound.
CAUTION: See separate listing for White Horehound.

Scientific Names
Ballota nigra.
Family: Labiatae or Lamiaceae.

People Use This For
Orally, black horehound is used for nausea, vomiting, sedation in hysteria and hypochondria (4,18), increasing bile flow, whooping cough, and as an antispasmodic (18). It is used in France for symptomatic relief of nervous disorders in adults and children, especially mild sleep disorders, and for cough (18).
Topically, black horehound is used as a mild astringent (4) and for gout (18).
Traditionally, black horehound has been used for nervous dyspepsia (4,18).
Other uses include rectal enemas against ascaridae, or intestinal worms (18).

Safety
POSSIBLY SAFE ...when the above ground parts are used orally and appropriately in medicinal amounts (12).
There is insufficient reliable information available about the safety of the topical use of black horehound.
PREGNANCY: LIKELY UNSAFE ...when used orally because it is believed to affect the menstrual cycle (4).
There is insufficient reliable information available about the safety of black horehound used topically during pregnancy.
LACTATION: Insufficient reliable information available; avoid using.

Effectiveness

There is insufficient reliable information available about the effectiveness of black horehound.

Possible Mechanism of Action & Active Ingredients

The applicable parts of black horehound are the above ground parts. Black horehound has antiemetic (4,18), sedative, mild astringent (4), antispasmodic, and stimulant effects (18). When administered intravenously in dogs, the aqueous extracts of black horehound can reduce arterial blood pressure and heart rate and increase gallbladder secretions (18).

Adverse Reactions Including Known Allergies

None reported.

Possible Interactions with Herbs & Other Dietary Supplements

There is insufficient reliable information available.

Possible Interactions with Drugs

No interactions are known to occur, and there is no known reason to expect a clinically significant interaction with black horehound.

Possible Interactions with Foods

No interactions are known to occur, and there is no known reason to expect a clinically significant interaction with black horehound.

Possible Interactions with Lab Tests

No interactions are known to occur, and there is no known reason to expect a clinically significant interaction with black horehound.

Possible Interactions with Diseases or Conditions

No interactions are known to occur, and there is no known reason to expect a clinically significant interaction with black horehound.

Typical Dosages & Routes of Administration that are Commonly Used

ORAL: The typical dose of black horehound is 2-4 grams of its above ground parts or one cup of the tea three times daily (4). The tea is prepared by steeping 2-4 grams of the above ground parts in 150 mL boiling water for 10-15 minutes and then straining. The usual dose of the liquid extract (1:1 in 25% alcohol) is 1-3 mL three times daily (4). The common dose of the tincture (1:10 in 45% alcohol) is 1-2 mL three times daily (4). TOPICAL: No typical dosage.

Comments

Avoid confusion with white horehound.

BLACK MULBERRY

This Product is Also Known As

Purple Mulberry, White Mulberry.

Scientific Names

Morus nigra.

People Use This For

Orally, black mulberry is taken as a laxative and for chronic rhinitis (18).

Safety

There is insufficient reliable information available about the safety of black mulberry.
Pregnancy and Lactation: Insufficient reliable information available; avoid using.

Effectiveness

There is insufficient reliable information available about the effectiveness of black mulberry.

Possible Mechanism of Action & Active Ingredients

The applicable parts of black mulberry are the ripe berry and root bark. The fruit contains small amounts of vitamin C (0.17%), rutin, and pectin (18). The pectin may have laxative activity (7).

Adverse Reactions Including Known Allergies

None reported.

Possible Interactions with Herbs & Other Dietary Supplements

Insufficient reliable information available.

Possible Interactions with Drugs

DIABETES THERAPY: Monitor blood glucose level closely due to claims that some species of mulberry leaves have hypoglycemic effects (19).

Possible Interactions with Foods

No interactions are known to occur, and there is no known reason to expect a clinically significant interaction with black mulberry.

Possible Interactions with Lab Tests

No interactions are known to occur, and there is no known reason to expect a clinically significant interaction with black mulberry.

Possible Interactions with Diseases or Conditions

No interactions are known to occur, and there is no known reason to expect a clinically significant interaction with black mulberry.

Typical Dosages & Routes of Administration that are Commonly Used

ORAL: The average amount used daily is 2-4 mL of syrup (18).

Comments

None.

BLACK MUSTARD oil

This Product is Also Known As

Mustard Oil.
CAUTION: See separate listings for Black Mustard seed, Hedge Mustard, and White Mustard.

Scientific Names

Brassica nigra.
Family: Brassicaceae.

People Use This For

Topically, black mustard oil is used for symptoms of the common cold including pulmonary congestion (11), rheumatism and arthritis, as a counterirritant (3,272), and in footbaths for aching feet (6).
In manufacturing, black mustard oil is used as a flavoring agent in foods and beverages (11). In soap making, it is utilized as a lubricant and illuminant.
Other uses include black mustard oil as an ingredient in cat and dog repellents (11).

Safety

LIKELY SAFE ...when black mustard oil is used in the amounts commonly found in foods (11,12). The average maximum level should not exceed 0.02% (11).
POSSIBLY SAFE ...when black mustard oil is used topically in concentrations of 0.5-5% applied 3-4 times daily (3,272).
LIKELY UNSAFE ...when black mustard oil is ingested undiluted. Black mustard oil is an extremely powerful topical irritant and ingesting large amounts can cause irritant poisoning (12). ...when black mustard oil is inhaled (11).
CHILDREN: LIKELY UNSAFE ...when used orally, contraindicated in children under 6 years of age (12,19). There is insufficient reliable information available about the safety of the topical use in children.
PREGNANCY: LIKELY UNSAFE ...when used orally. Black mustard oil is contraindicated because it might have abortifacient and menstrual stimulant effects (19). There is insufficient reliable information available about the safety of topical use during pregnancy; avoid using.
LACTATION: Insufficient reliable information available; avoid using.

Effectiveness

LIKELY EFFECTIVE ...when used topically as a counterirritant if applied in concentrations ranging from 0.5-5% (3,272).
There is insufficient reliable information available about the effectiveness of black mustard oil for its other uses.

Possible Mechanism of Action & Active Ingredients

Black mustard oil consists mainly of allyl isothiocyanate, which is produced after the glucosinolate sinigrin is hydrolyzed and distilled (3,6,11). The allyl isothiocyanate of black mustard oil has strong antimicrobial (bacterial and fungi) properties (11), lacrimatory effects, and can act as a counterirritant when diluted (1:50) (6,11). Black mustard oil has powerful irritant properties that can cause pain and increased inflammation of the skin (6,11).

Adverse Reactions Including Known Allergies

The ingestion of large amounts of black mustard oil can lead to vomiting, stomach pain, diarrhea, somnolence, cardiac failure, breathing difficulties, coma, and possibly death (18). Black mustard oil exacerbates stomach and intestinal ulcers (18,19) and causes kidney irritation, although rarely (19). The isothiocyanate constituents can cause endemic goiters (6,11). Topically, the oil can cause skin blistering and necroses (6,11), and can rarely cause contact allergies (18).

Possible Interactions with Herbs & Other Dietary Supplements
Insufficient reliable information available.

Possible Interactions with Drugs
ACID-INHIBITING DRUGS: Theoretically, due to claims that black mustard oil increases stomach acid, it might interfere with antacids, sucralfate (Carafate), H-2 antagonists, or proton pump inhibitors (19).

Possible Interactions with Foods
No interactions are known to occur, and there is no known reason to expect a clinically significant interaction with black mustard oil.

Possible Interactions with Lab Tests
No interactions are known to occur, and there is no known reason to expect a clinically significant interaction with black mustard oil.

Possible Interactions with Diseases or Conditions
GASTROINTESTINAL ULCERS: Black mustard oil can exacerbate stomach and intestinal ulcers by irritating the mucus membranes (19).

Typical Dosages & Routes of Administration that are Commonly Used
TOPICAL: As a counterirritant, black mustard oil is typically used in concentrations from 0.5-5% and as frequently as 3-4 times daily (3,272).

Comments
Avoid confusion with black mustard, hedge mustard, white mustard (Brassica alba or Sinapis alba), brown mustard (Brassica juncea), Indian mustard (Brassica juncea), and Chinese mustard (Sinapis juncea). Derivatives of mustard oil (allyl isothiocyanate) have formed the basis for toxic agents such as the "mustard gases" and antineoplastic agents (11). The volatile oil of mustard is prepared by steam distillation from brown or black mustard after expressing the fixed oil and macerating in water to allow hydrolysis of sinigrin by enzyme myrosin. The volatile oil mainly consists of allyl isothiocyanate.

BLACK MUSTARD seed

This Product is Also Known As
Mustard.
CAUTION: See separate listings for Black Mustard oil, Hedge Mustard, and White Mustard.

Scientific Names
Brassica nigra.
Family: Brassicaceae.

People Use This For
Topically, black mustard seed is used as a poultice for bronchial pneumonia, pleurisy (18), arthritis, lumbago, and aching feet (11). It is also used topically for rheumatism (11,18), and as a counterirritant (3).
Traditionally, black mustard seed has been used as an emetic, diuretic, and appetite stimulant (6,11).
For food uses, black mustard seed is a flavoring agent in condiments, foods, and beverages (6,11) and is a culinary spice (6).

Safety
LIKELY SAFE ...when black mustard seed is used in the amounts commonly found in foods (11,12). Black mustard has Generally Recognized as Safe (GRAS) status in the US (3,11).
POSSIBLY SAFE ...when used topically and appropriately for less than 2 weeks (18).
LIKELY UNSAFE ...when used orally as an emetic. Black mustard seed is an irritant and when used as an emetic, it re-exposes the esophageal tissue to its corrosive effects (19). Ingesting a large amount can cause irritant poisoning (12). ...when pure mustard powder is applied topically for more than 15-30 minutes, it can cause severe burns (12). ...when it is used topically for more than 2 weeks (18).
CHILDREN: LIKELY UNSAFE ...contraindicated for oral use in children under 6 years of age (12,19). There is insufficient reliable information available about the safety of the topical use of black mustard seed in children.
PREGNANCY: LIKELY UNSAFE ...when used orally because it might have abortifacient and menstrual stimulant effects (19). There is insufficient reliable information available for topical use during pregnancy; avoid using.
LACTATION: Insufficient reliable information available; avoid using.

Effectiveness

There is insufficient reliable information available about the effectiveness of black mustard seed.

Possible Mechanism of Action & Active Ingredients

Black mustard powder contains the glucosinolate sinigrin, which produces allyl isothiocyanate when mixed with warm water (3,6,11,18). Allyl isothiocyanate has strong antimicrobial (bacterial and fungi) properties (11), lacrimatory effects, and can act as a counterirritant when diluted (1:50) (6,11). Mustard oil (produced from powder by hydrolysis) is absorbed through the skin and eliminated through the lungs. This could explain its inclusion in liniment preparations to treat lung congestion (11). Black mustard has powerful irritant properties that can cause pain and increased inflammation of the skin (6,11,18). Sinigrin can be toxic to certain insect larvae (11). The glucosinolate products can have protective effects against carcinogens (11).

Adverse Reactions Including Known Allergies

The ingestion of large amounts of black mustard seed can lead to vomiting, stomach pain, diarrhea, somnolence, cardiac failure, breathing difficulties, coma, and possibly death (18). The isothiocyanate constituents can cause endemic goiters (6,11). Topically, the allyl isothiocyanate found in mustard can cause skin blistering and necroses (6,11,18) but rarely cause contact allergies (18).

Possible Interactions with Herbs & Other Dietary Supplements

Insufficient reliable information available.

Possible Interactions with Drugs

ACID-INHIBITING DRUGS: Theoretically, due to claims that black mustard seed increases stomach acid, it might interfere with antacids, sucralfate (Carafate), H-2 antagonists, or proton pump inhibitors (19).

Possible Interactions with Foods

No interactions are known to occur, and there is no known reason to expect a clinically significant interaction with black mustard seed.

Possible Interactions with Lab Tests

No interactions are known to occur, and there is no known reason to expect a clinically significant interaction with black mustard seed.

Possible Interactions with Diseases or Conditions

ASTHMA: Coughing, sneezing, and possible asthma attacks can result from handling mustard flour (18).
GI IRRITATION: Can irritate gastrointestinal tract. Contraindicated in individuals with infectious or inflammatory gastrointestinal conditions (19).

Typical Dosages & Routes of Administration that are Commonly Used

TOPICAL: To prepare a mustard plaster, typically 100 grams of mustard flour (ground mustard) is mixed with warm water to make a paste. The paste is packed in linen and applied to the affected area for 10 minutes (3-5 minutes for children over 6 years old) (18). Mustard plaster applied for longer than 15-30 minutes is associated with severe burns and skin necroses (12). Treatment should not exceed two weeks (19).

Comments

Avoid confusion with black mustard oil, hedge mustard, white mustard (Brassica alba or Sinapis alba), brown mustard (Brassica juncea), Indian mustard (Brassica juncea), and Chinese mustard (Sinapis juncea).

BLACK NIGHTSHADE

This Product is Also Known As

Garden Nightshade, Houndsberry, Petty Morel, Poisonberry.

Scientific Names

Solanum nigrum.
Family: Solanaceae.

People Use This For

Orally, black nightshade is used for gastric irritation and cramps.
Topically, black nightshade is used for psoriasis, hemorrhoids, and abscesses. The bruised, fresh leaves are used topically to treat inflammation, burns and ulcers.
In folk medicine, people used black nightshade orally as an antispasmodic, pain reliever, sedative, and narcotic (18).

Safety

LIKELY UNSAFE ...when used orally (4009).
There is insufficient reliable information available about the safety of the topical use of black nightshade.

PREGNANCY AND LACTATION: LIKELY UNSAFE ...contraindicated for oral use because of concerns it could be teratogenic (4009).

Effectiveness

There is insufficient reliable information available about the effectiveness of black nightshade.

Possible Mechanism of Action & Active Ingredients

Most of the toxic effects of black nightshade can be attributed to the solanine constituent. Solanine concentrations are high in the green fruits and low in the mature fruits, roots, and shoots. This means the green fruits are more toxic than the other plant parts. However, among plant strains, toxicity varies widely (4009).

Adverse Reactions Including Known Allergies

Overdoses can result in people who ingest large quantities of the green berries or fresh foliage with high alkaloid content. Symptoms include nausea, vomiting, headache, and in rare cases, dilation of the pupils (18). At doses of 200-400 mg, solanine can cause gastroenteritis, tachycardia, dyspnea, vertigo, drowsiness, lethargy, twitches of the arms and legs, and cramping. Other symptoms of poisoning include diarrhea, panic, excitation, coma, hyperthermia. This is followed later by a dazed state, paralysis, and rarely, death due to respiratory arrest and hypothermia (4009).

Possible Interactions with Herbs & Other Dietary Supplements

Insufficient reliable information available.

Possible Interactions with Drugs

No interactions are known to occur, and there is no known reason to expect a clinically significant interaction with black nightshade.

Possible Interactions with Foods

No interactions are known to occur, and there is no known reason to expect a clinically significant interaction with black nightshade.

Possible Interactions with Lab Tests

No interactions are known to occur, and there is no known reason to expect a clinically significant interaction with black nightshade.

Possible Interactions with Diseases or Conditions

No interactions are known to occur, and there is no known reason to expect a clinically significant interaction with black nightshade.

Typical Dosages & Routes of Administration that are Commonly Used

ORAL: No typical dosage.
TOPICAL: A handful of herb is placed in boiling water for 10 minutes, and used as a compress or a rinse (18).

Comments

Black nightshade is sometimes referred to as petty morel. This name is a corruption of the original, petit morel. Originally, black night shade was called petit morel to differentiate it from the more poisonous species, deadly nightshade that is known as great morel. Black nightshade has a musk-like fragrance when wilting. (18).

BLACK PEPPER AND WHITE PEPPER

This Product is Also Known As

Black Pepper, Blanc Poivre, Kosho, Pepe, Pepper, Pepper Extract, Peppercorn, Pepper Plant, Pfeffer, Pimenta, Pimienta, Piper, Poivre, Poivre Noir, White Pepper.

Scientific Names

Piper nigrum.
Family: Piperaceae.

People Use This For

Orally, black pepper is used for stomach disorders, digestive problems, and bronchitis. White pepper is used orally for treating stomachache, malaria, and cholera (11).
Topically, black pepper is used for treating neuralgia and scabies (18). Peppers are also used in topical counterirritant preparations (11).
Traditionally, black pepper and white pepper are used orally for treating cancer (11).
In foods and beverages, black pepper, white pepper, and pepper oil are used as flavoring agents (11).

Safety

LIKELY SAFE …when used orally in amounts found in foods (11). Both white and black pepper have Generally Recognized as Safe (GRAS) status in the US (11). Maximum level of white pepper used is 0.42% (11).

POSSIBLY SAFE …when used orally and appropriately in medicinal amounts (12). …when black pepper oil is used topically. It is nonirritating and non-sensitizing. White pepper contains little volatile oil (11).

CHILDREN: POSSIBLY UNSAFE …when large amounts of black pepper are accidentally ingested. Fatal cases of pepper aspiration have been reported (5619,5620).

PREGNANCY: LIKELY SAFE …when black or white pepper are used orally in amounts found in foods. LIKELY UNSAFE …when a large amount of black pepper is ingested because it might have abortifacient effects (11,19). There is insufficient reliable information available about the safety of the oral use of white pepper or the topical use of black pepper oil during pregnancy.

LACTATION: LIKELY SAFE …when black or white pepper are used as a spice. There is insufficient reliable information available about the safety of using larger amounts of black or white pepper during lactation.

Effectiveness

There is insufficient reliable information available about the effectiveness of black pepper and white pepper.

Possible Mechanism of Action & Active Ingredients

The applicable part of black pepper and white pepper is the fruit. Piper nigrum is said to have antiflatulent and diuretic properties (11), antimicrobial and insecticidal effects (18). It is thought to influence liver and metabolic functions (11), stimulate thermal receptors, induce sweating, stimulate taste buds causing a reflex increase in gastric secretions (18). It might also have lipolytic activity related to the outer layer of the fruit (11). Piper nigrum contains piperine which increases oral absorption of drugs and other substances, possibly by modulating intestinal membrane dynamics (3757). Some evidence suggests piper nigrum might protect against colon cancer (3761). However, other evidence suggests black pepper might induce hepatic enzymes (3760) or cause liver tumors (3759).

Adverse Reactions Including Known Allergies

Taken by mouth, pepper can cause a burning aftertaste. Eye contact with ground pepper can cause redness of eyes and swelling of eyelids (5619). Deaths due to aspiration of large amounts of pepper have been reported (5619,5620).

Possible Interactions with Herbs & Other Dietary Supplements

SPARTEINE: Piperine increases the bioavailability of sparteine, a constituent of scotch broom (19).

Possible Interactions with Drugs

PHENYTOIN: Concomitant administration speeds absorption and slows elimination of phenytoin (Dilantin) (537).

PROPRANOLOL: Concomitant administration speeds and increases absorption, and increases serum concentrations of propranolol (Inderal) (538).

THEOPHYLLINE: Concomitant administration increases absorption and serum concentrations of theophylline (Theo-dur) (538).

Possible Interactions with Foods

No interactions are known to occur, and there is no known reason to expect a clinically significant interaction with black pepper and white pepper.

Possible Interactions with Lab Tests

SERUM DRUG ASSAYS: Can increase phenytoin, propranolol, and theophylline serum concentrations and test results (537,538).

Possible Interactions with Diseases or Conditions

No interactions are known to occur, and there is no known reason to expect a clinically significant interaction with black pepper and white pepper.

Typical Dosages & Routes of Administration that are Commonly Used

ORAL: Single dose ranges from 300-600 mg (18) up to 1.5 grams per day (18).

Comments

Black pepper is the dried, full grown but unripe fruit of Piper nigrum (11). White pepper is the dried ripe fruit of Piper nigrum with the outer covering that is known as a pericarp removed (11). Pepper oil is distilled from black pepper (11). Indian long pepper also contains piperine. Red pepper and cayenne contain no piperine.

BLACK PSYLLIUM

This Product is Also Known As

Brown Psyllium, Fleaseed, Fleawort, French Psyllium, Plantain, Psyllion, Psyllios, Psyllium Seed, Spanish Psyllium.

CAUTION: See separate listings for Blond Psyllium, Buckhorn Plantain, Great Plantain, and Water Plantain.

Scientific Names
Plantago psyllium, synonym Psyllium afra; Psyllium indica, synonym Psyllium arenaria.
Family: Plantaginaceae.

People Use This For
Orally, black psyllium seed is used for chronic constipation and for softening stools in conditions such as hemorrhoids, anal fissures, anorectal surgery, and pregnancy. It is also used for diarrhea, irritable bowel syndrome (2,6,11,18), reducing elevated cholesterol (6,11,18), dysentery (6), and treating cancer (11).

Safety
LIKELY SAFE ...when the seed is used orally with appropriate fluid intake (4,12,272).
LIKELY UNSAFE ...when used orally without adequate fluid intake because it can cause esophageal obstruction (2,4,18). ...when the seeds of non-commercial preparations of black psyllium are chewed, crushed, or ground because they release a pigment that deposits in renal tubules (11) and can be nephrotoxic (6). This pigment has been removed from most commercial products (6).
PREGNANCY AND LACTATION: LIKELY SAFE ...when taken orally with appropriate fluid intake (272).

Effectiveness
EFFECTIVE ...when taken orally as a supplemental source of dietary fiber (272). ...when used as a bulk laxative (272).
POSSIBLY EFFECTIVE ...when take orally as a secondary treatment for diarrhea, for treating irritable bowel syndrome (2), for reducing serum total and LDL cholesterol, and reducing the LDL:HDL ratio (6,11).
There is insufficient reliable information available about the effectiveness of black psyllium for its other uses.

Possible Mechanism of Action & Active Ingredients
The applicable part of black psyllium is the seed. Its constituents are not absorbed and have no systemic effects (1). Psyllium seed forms a mucilaginous mass when mixed with water and has a bulk laxative effect (1,4,6). In people with diarrhea, the mucilage absorbs water, provides mass, and prolongs gastrointestinal transit (1,6). In individuals with constipation, the mucilage absorbs water, swells, and stimulates peristalsis, reducing gastrointestinal transit time (1,4,6). Black psyllium can decrease abdominal pain in people with irritable bowel syndrome by reducing rectosigmoidal pressure (405). Psyllium reduces peak blood glucose levels by slowing carbohydrate absorption (1,6) and can decrease cholesterol by absorbing dietary fats in the gastrointestinal tract, thereby preventing systemic absorption. It can also increase cholesterol elimination in the fecal bile acids (1,6,11,12). Chewing or crushing the seeds can release a pigment that deposits in renal tubules (11) and can be nephrotoxic (6). This pigment is removed from most commercial products (6).

Adverse Reactions Including Known Allergies
Black psyllium taken orally can cause transient flatulence and abdominal distention (4). When consumed without water, it can cause esophageal (4) and bowel obstruction (4,604). Chewing or crushing the seeds can release a pigment that deposits in the renal tubules (11) and can be nephrotoxic (6). This pigment is removed from most commercial products (6). Allergic reactions to black psyllium include allergic rhinitis, conjunctivitis, urticaria, and asthma (18). Occupational exposure to black psyllium can cause sensitization, of which symptoms include sneezing, watery eyes, chest congestion, and anaphylactoid reaction (6).

Possible Interactions with Herbs & Other Dietary Supplements
VITAMIN/MINERAL SUPPLEMENTS: The long-term use of psyllium with vitamin or mineral supplements can reduce the absorption of calcium, iron, zinc, and vitamin B12 (1,12). Supplements should be taken one hour before or four hours after psyllium to avoid this interaction (4,12).

Possible Interactions with Drugs
CARBAMAZEPINE (Tegretol): Psyllium can reduce carbamazepine absorption (539).
WARFARIN (Coumadin): Concomitant use might reduce warfarin absorption (1), requiring dose adjustment (12).
DIGOXIN (Lanoxin): Concomitant use might reduce digoxin absorption (1), requiring dose adjustment (12).
LITHIUM: Psyllium use can reduce serum lithium levels (540).
INSULIN: Psyllium can reduce peak blood glucose levels decreasing insulin requirements in individuals with diabetes (1,18).
DIABETES THERAPY: Monitor blood glucose level closely due to claims that psyllium seeds have hypoglycemic effects (19).
ORAL DRUGS: Oral drugs should be administered one hour before or four hours after psyllium to avoid decreased or delayed absorption (4,12).

Possible Interactions with Foods
NUTRIENT ABSORPTION: The long-term use of psyllium with meals can reduce nutrient absorption (12) requiring vitamin or mineral supplementation.

Possible Interactions with Lab Tests
BLOOD GLUCOSE: Theoretically, black psyllium might lower postprandial blood glucose levels and test results (1,6,1405).

SERUM CHOLESTEROL: Black psyllium can lower total cholesterol and LDL cholesterol levels, LDL:HDL ratio, and test results (1,6,1405).

Possible Interactions with Diseases or Conditions

GI CONDITIONS: Black psyllium is contraindicated in people with fecal impaction, GI atony (1), GI tract narrowing, and obstruction or conditions that can lead to obstruction, such as spastic bowel (1,2,4,12,18).
DIABETES: Use with caution and monitor closely in patients with diabetes. Black psyllium might alter blood glucose levels by reducing carbohydrate absorption (1,2). In addition, commercially available psyllium products can contain sugar and other absorbable carbohydrates (272).
KIDNEY DYSFUNCTION: Avoid chewing, crushing, or grinding the seeds, which releases a potentially nephrotoxic pigment (6). This pigment is removed from most commercial products (6).
SWALLOWING DIFFICULTIES: Contraindicated (12).
PSYLLIUM HYPERSENSITIVITY: Contraindicated.
PHENYLKETONURIA: Avoid products containing aspartame (Nutrasweet) (272).

Typical Dosages & Routes of Administration that are Commonly Used

The amount of black psyllium seed required for an individual can vary. For best results, start with small amounts and increase to the desired response. Follow the package labeling when available.
ORAL: As a laxative, the typical dose of black psyllium seed is 10-30 grams per day (2,18), in divided amounts. Mix 10 grams seed in 100 mL water, to be followed by at least 200 mL water (18). Avoid chewing or crushing the seeds which can release a pigment that deposits in renal tubules (11). Adequate fluid intake is necessary and should be at least 150 mL water for each 5 grams of drug. The FDA labeling recommends at least 8 ounces (a full glass) of water or other fluid with each dose. Taking this product without enough liquid can cause choking (12). Black psyllium should be taken 30-60 minutes after a meal or the administration of other drugs (272).

Comments

Black psyllium is an aggressive-growing, perennial weed found throughout the world. The plant was spread with the colonization of the New World and was nicknamed "Englishman's foot" by the North American Indians.
The FDA requires that psyllium be labeled: "WARNING: Taking this product without adequate fluid may cause it to swell and block your throat or esophagus and may cause choking. Do not take this product if you have difficulty in swallowing. If you experience chest pain, vomiting, or difficulty in swallowing or breathing after taking this product, seek immediate medical attention" (12).

BLACK ROOT

This Product is Also Known As

Beaumont Root, Bowman's Root, Culveris Root, Culver's Physic, Culver's Root, Hini, Oxadoddy, Physic Root, Purple Leptandra, Tall Speedwell, Tall Veronica, Veronicastrum Virginicum, Veronica Virginica Root, Whorlywort.
CAUTION: See separate listings for Brooklime (Veronica beccabungo) and Veronica (Veronica officinalis), which are also known as speedwell; Indian Physic which is also known as Bowman's root, and Comfrey which is also known as black root.

Scientific Names

Leptandra virginica.
Family: Scrophulariaceae.

People Use This For

Orally, black root is used for chronic constipation and disorders of the liver and gallbladder (18). It has also been used as an emetic (214).
Historically, early American doctors used black root to treat bilious fever (6002).

Safety

POSSIBLY SAFE ...when the dried root is used orally (12). The dried root has a milder action than the fresh root (18).
POSSIBLY UNSAFE ...when the fresh root is used orally (12).
PREGNANCY: LIKELY UNSAFE ...when the fresh root is used orally because it has abortifacient and teratogenic effects (19). There is insufficient reliable information available about the safety of the dried root, avoid using.
LACTATION: Insufficient reliable information available; avoid using.

Effectiveness

There is insufficient reliable information available about the effectiveness of black root.

Possible Mechanism of Action & Active Ingredients

The applicable parts of black root are the rhizome and root. Black root is stated to have antiflatulent, laxative, and bowel evacuant properties (18). It can stimulate bile flow into the duodenum and induce sweating. It contains tannic acid, which has astringent properties that act on the GI mucosa. Tannic acid can also form insoluble complexes with alkaloids, glycosides, and certain heavy metals (214).

Adverse Reactions Including Known Allergies
Black root can cause abdominal pain or cramps, changes in stool color or odor, drowsiness, headache, nausea, and vomiting. Hepatotoxicity has been reported after ingestion of large amounts (214).

Possible Interactions with Herbs & Other Dietary Supplements
STIMULANT LAXATIVE HERBS: Theoretically, concomitant use with other stimulant laxative herbs can increase the risk of potassium depletion. Stimulant laxative herbs include aloe dried leaf sap, wild cucumber fruit (Ecballium elaterium), blue flag rhizome, alder buckthorn, European buckthorn, butternut bark, cascara bark, castor oil, colocynth fruit pulp, gamboge bark exudate, jalap root, manna bark exudate, podophyllum root, rhubarb root, senna leaves and pods, and yellow dock root (19).
POTASSIUM DEPLETING HERBS: Theoretically, concomitant use with horsetail plant or the licorice rhizome can increase the risk of potassium depletion (19).

Possible Interactions with Drugs
CARDIAC GLYCOSIDES: Theoretically, the overuse or abuse of black root can increase the risk of adverse effects of cardiac glycoside drugs, e.g., digoxin (Lanoxin). It may also reduce their effectiveness if taken concomitantly, due to its chemically binding with the glycosides while in the GI tract (214).

Possible Interactions with Foods
No interactions are known to occur, and there is no known reason to expect a clinically significant interaction with black root.

Possible Interactions with Lab Tests
No interactions are known to occur, and there is no known reason to expect a clinically significant interaction with black root.

Possible Interactions with Diseases or Conditions
GALLSTONES/BILE DUCT OBSTRUCTION: Black root is contraindicated, because it theoretically has bile stimulatory effects and could aggravate these conditions (19).
HEMORRHOIDS/ MENSTRUATION: Theoretically, black root is contraindicated due to its cathartic properties (19).
GI INFLAMMATION: Black root is contraindicated in individuals with inflammation of the GI tract due to the irritant, emetic, and stimulant laxative effects (19).

Typical Dosages & Routes of Administration that are Commonly Used
ORAL: People typically use 1 teaspoon of dried black root in 1 cup boiling water, which is allowed to steep for 30 minutes, to make a tea. The suggested dose is 1/3 cup before each meal. A black root tincture is taken as 2 to 4 drops in water. The powdered root bark is taken in a dose of 1 to 4 grams. (5263,5264).

Comments
Black root grows in the United States and Canada and has a bitter and nauseous taste.

BLACK SEED

This Product is Also Known As
Ajenuz, Arañuel, Baraka, Black Cumin, Black Caraway, Charnuska, Cominho Negro, Cominho-Negro, Fennel Flower, Fennel-Flower, Fitch, Love in a Mist, Nigelle de Crète, Nutmeg Flower, Nutmeg-Flower, Roman-Coriander, Schwarzkümmel, Toute Épice.
CAUTION: See separate listings for Caraway, Coriander, Cumin, Fennel, and Nutmeg.

Scientific Names
Nigella sativa.
Family: Ranunculaceae.

People Use This For
Orally, black seed is used for treating gastrointestinal conditions including gas, colic, diarrhea, dysentery, constipation and hemorrhoids. It is also used orally for respiratory conditions, including asthma, allergies, cough, bronchitis, emphysema, flu and congestion. Additionally, it is used orally as an antihypertensive, immunoprotectant, anticancer agent, and vermifuge. It is used orally for women's health, including as a contraceptive, and for stimulation of menstruation and increasing milk flow (6).
Topically, black seed is used for inflammatory conditions including rheumatism, headache and skin conditions (6).

Traditionally, black seed has been used for headache, toothache, nasal congestion, and intestinal worms. It has also been used for conjunctivitis, abscesses, and parasites (6).

Black seed has been used in combination with cysteine, vitamin E and saffron to decrease cisplatin-induced side effects (6).

Black seed is also used as a flavoring or spice (6).

Safety

LIKELY SAFE ...when used orally in amounts found in foods (6).

There is insufficient reliable information available about the safety of black seed when used for medicinal purposes.

PREGNANCY: LIKELY UNSAFE ...when used orally in amounts exceeding those found in food. Black seed may decrease or inhibit uterine contractions (241) and may have contraceptive activity (242).

LACTATION: Insufficient reliable information available; avoid using.

Effectiveness

There is insufficient reliable information available about the effectiveness of black seed.

Possible Mechanism of Action & Active Ingredients

The applicable part of black seed is the seed itself. In allergic conditions, black seed might have antihistamine effects. Although not yet demonstrated in humans, low concentration of the constituent nigellone has been shown to inhibit the release of histamine from mast cells in animals (233). Black seed is thought to have immunoprotectant effects. Preliminary evidence suggests it may help minimize chemotherapy-induced decreases in hemoglobin and leukocyte counts. It may also enhance the production of certain human interleukins and alter macrophages (234). Black seed is also used as an anticancer agent. According to preliminary studies, black seed may inhibit stomach tumors, carcinoma, and Ehrlich ascites carcinoma (236,239). The black seed constituents thymoquinone and dithymoquinone are actually cytotoxic toward human cells (238). Although some evidence suggests thymoquinone may offer protection against chemically induced hepatotoxicity (237,240), a study in rats indicates that black seed may actually be hepatotoxic. A fixed oil from black seed is reported to have anti-eicosanoid and antioxidant effects, which may support anti-inflammatory activity (235), but this effect has not been studied in humans. The essential oil may have antimicrobial and anthelmintic activity, particularly against staphylococcus as well as other gram-positive and gram-negative bacteria (243,244). Black seed may have anti-oxytocic potential, and may inhibit spontaneous contractions (241). It may also have contraceptive activity (242).

Adverse Reactions Including Known Allergies

Topical use of black seed oil can cause allergic contact dermatitis (6). Black seed may be associated with hepatotoxicity based on preliminary animal research (245).

Possible Interactions with Herbs & Other Dietary Supplements

Insufficient reliable information available.

Possible Interactions with Drugs

No interactions are known to occur, and there is no known reason to expect a clinically significant interaction with black seed.

Possible Interactions with Foods

No interactions are known to occur, and there is no known reason to expect a clinically significant interaction with black seed.

Possible Interactions with Lab Tests

No interactions are known to occur, and there is no known reason to expect a clinically significant interaction with black seed.

Possible Interactions with Diseases or Conditions

No interactions are known to occur, and there is no known reason to expect a clinically significant interaction with black seed.

Typical Dosages & Routes of Administration that are Commonly Used

No typical dosage.

Comments

Black seed is reported to have been used for over 2000 years. Recordings mention it as far back as 1400 years. Black seed was found in the tomb of King Tutankhamen (6).

An issued patent covers the use of black seed to stimulate immune-competent cells in humans. However, this should not be taken as evidence for the safety and efficacy of black seed as an immunostimulant (246).

BLACK TEA

This Product is Also Known As
Chinese Tea, Tea.
CAUTION: See separate listings for Caffeine and Green Tea.

Scientific Names
Camellia sinensis, synonyms Camellia thea, Camellia theifera, Thea bohea, Thea sinensis, Thea viridis.
Family: Theaceae.

People Use This For
Orally, black tea is used for improving cognitive performance (4221,4224), headache (6,18), reducing the risk of cancer (4223), atherosclerosis (3450), and myocardial infarction (4222). It is also used for stomach disorders, vomiting, and diarrhea (6,18), preventing dental caries (4214); preventing kidney stones (4216), and as a diuretic (6,18). In combination with various other products, black tea is used for weight loss (18).
For food use, black tea is consumed as a hot or cold beverage.

Safety
LIKELY SAFE ...when used orally in moderate amounts (12).
POSSIBLY UNSAFE ...when used orally in large amounts. Black tea contains a significant amount of caffeine. Consumption of more than 300 mg caffeine, which is equivalent to approximately 5 cups of black tea per day, has been associated with significant adverse effects (see Adverse Reactions) (18). These effects would not be expected to occur with the consumption of decaffeinated black tea.
CHILDREN: LIKELY UNSAFE ...when taken orally by infants because it has been associated with impaired iron metabolism and microcytic anemia (6). This might be caused by tannins in black tea which bind and prevent iron absorption in the gastrointestinal tract (19). Children are also more susceptible to the adverse effects of caffeine present in black tea (15).
PREGNANCY: POSSIBLY SAFE ...when used in moderate amounts. Due to the caffeine content of black tea, mothers should closely monitor their intake to ensure moderate consumption. Fetal blood concentrations of caffeine approximate maternal concentrations (4260). Caffeine use in pregnancy is controversial; however, moderate consumption has not been associated with adverse fetal effects (6). Some sources suggest keeping caffeine consumption below 200 mg per day (2078). Black tea provides approximately 10-80 mg caffeine per cup (18,4218).
POSSIBLY UNSAFE ...when used orally in large amounts. Caffeine in black tea crosses the placenta, producing fetal blood concentrations similar to maternal levels (4260). Although controversial, some evidence suggests that high doses of caffeine might be associated with premature delivery, low birth weight, and loss of the fetus (6). Some sources suggest keeping caffeine consumption below 200 mg per day (2078). Black tea provides approximately 10-80 mg caffeine per cup (18,4218). Excessive use of black tea in pregnancy should be avoided.
LACTATION: POSSIBLY SAFE ...when used in moderate amounts. Due to the caffeine content of black tea, mothers should closely monitor their intake to ensure moderate consumption. Breast milk concentrations of caffeine are thought to be approximately 50% of maternal serum concentrations. Moderate consumption of black tea would likely result in very small amounts of caffeine exposure to a nursing infant (6). POSSIBLY UNSAFE ...when used orally in large amounts. Consumption of black tea might cause irritability and increased bowel activity in nursing infants (6026). Large doses or excessive intake of black tea should be avoided during lactation.

Effectiveness
POSSIBLY EFFECTIVE ...when used orally to enhance cognitive performance (4221,4224). One study showed that consumption of black tea and other caffeinated beverages prevented a decline in alertness and cognitive capacity when consumed throughout the day (4224). ...when used orally for reducing the risk of severe aortic atherosclerosis, especially in women (3450). A retrospective study found an association between black tea consumption and reduced risk of severe aortic atherosclerosis (3450). ...when used orally for reducing the risk of myocardial infarction. One case-control study found that tea consumption was inversely associated with the risk of myocardial infarction (4222). ...when taken orally for diarrhea and as a diuretic (7,18). ...when used orally for reducing the risk of kidney stones. In a large-scale cohort study, women consuming black tea had a 8% decreased risk of developing kidney stones (4216).
There is insufficient reliable information available about the effectiveness of black tea for its other uses. However, weak epidemiological evidence suggests that black tea might be beneficial for preventing osteoporosis by improving some measures of bone mineral density (6404). Further evidence is needed to rate black tea for this use.

Possible Mechanism of Action & Active Ingredients
The applicable parts of black tea are the leaf and stem. Flavonoids such as catechins, thearubigins, and theaflavins are abundant in black tea, and are thought to be responsible for many of its proposed benefits by acting as antioxidants (6032,6033). Black tea might be beneficial in atherosclerosis due to flavonoid constituents which might reduce lipoprotein oxidation (6032,6033). For osteoporosis, the mechanism is not known, but it is thought that isoflavanoids in black tea have weak estrogenic effects that might become beneficial in postmenopausal women with low endogenous estrogen levels (6404). Black tea also contains 2-4% caffeine (519). The caffeine in black tea

acts as a central nervous system stimulant (12,15,18) and is thought to be responsible for improving cognitive performance (4221,4224). Caffeine also increases blood pressure (1452), heart rate and contractility (7,18), inhibits platelet aggregation (6,18), stimulates gastric acid secretion, causes diuresis (15,18), relaxes extracerebral vascular and bronchial smooth muscle, stimulates the release of catecholamines (18), and might indirectly inhibit histamine release (6130). The tannin constituents in black tea have antidiarrheal effects (7,18). In infants, the tannin constituents can bind and reduce iron absorption, causing microcytic anemia (631).

Adverse Reactions Including Known Allergies

Orally, black tea can cause gastrointestinal upset (12) and constipation (7). High doses of black tea, due to the caffeine constituent, can cause headache, diuresis, anxiety, nervousness, insomnia, restlessness, agitation, tremor, irritability, tachyarrhythmias, palpitations, premature heartbeat, quickened respiration, tremor, heartburn, loss of appetite, nausea, vomiting, diarrhea, dizziness, ringing in the ears, elevated blood sugar, elevated cholesterol, hepatotoxicity, delirium, and convulsions (6,7,15,18,505). Although acute administration of black tea can cause increased blood pressure, regular consumption does not seem to increase either blood pressure or pulse when consumed on a regular basis, even in mildly hypertensive patients (1451,1452). Chronic use of black tea that contains caffeine, especially in large amounts, can sometimes produce tolerance, habituation, and psychological dependence (15). The abrupt discontinuance of black tea that contains caffeine can sometimes result in physical withdrawal symptoms, including headaches, irritation, nervousness, anxiety, and dizziness (15). Some evidence shows caffeine is associated with fibrocystic breast disease in women; however, this is controversial and has been disputed (14,15). The adverse effects of caffeine found in black tea can be more severe in children than adults (15). In infants, black tea can cause microcytic anemia (631).

Possible Interactions with Herbs & Other Dietary Supplements

CAFFEINE CONTAINING HERBS/SUPPLEMENTS: Concomitant use can increase therapeutic and adverse effects. Natural products that contain caffeine include coffee, tea (black or green), guarana, mate, and cola.
EPHEDRA (ma huang): Concomitant use interacts with the caffeine in black tea and can potentiate the stimulant effects and the risk of adverse effects (6).

Possible Interactions with Drugs

ADENOSINE (ADENOCARD): The caffeine in black tea might interact with adenosine and inhibit the hemodynamic and anti-arrhythmic effects of adenosine (19).
ANTIPSYCHOTICS: Theoretically, the caffeine in black tea might decrease absorption of fluphenazine (Permitil, Prolixin) or haloperidol (Haldol) (626,627).
ASPIRIN, ACETAMINOPHEN: The caffeine in black tea might increase the action of these drugs by as much as 40% (3).
BARBITURATES: These drugs might decrease the effects of the caffeine in black tea (151).
BENZODIAZEPINES: The caffeine in black tea might decrease sedative effects of benzodiazepines (19).
BETA-ADRENERGIC AGONISTS: The caffeine in black tea can increase cardiac inotropic effects of these drugs (15). Beta-adrenergic agonists include albuterol (Proventil, Ventolin, Volmax), metaproterenol (Alupent), terbutaline (Bricanyl, Brethine), and isoproterenol (Isuprel).
BETA-BLOCKERS: Concomitant use of propranolol (Inderal) or metoprolol (Lopressor) can increase blood pressure by interacting with the caffeine in black tea (19).
CHLORPROMAZINE: Theoretically, the caffeine in black tea might inhibit the cataleptic effects of chlorpromazine (Thorazine) (19).
CIMETIDINE: Cimetidine (Tagamet) interacts with the caffeine in black tea and decreases caffeine clearance by 30-50% (14).
CLOZAPINE: The caffeine in black tea might interact with clozapine (Clozaril) and cause acute exacerbation of psychotic symptoms. Caffeine can increase effects and toxicity of clozapine (151). Caffeine doses of 400-1000 mg per day inhibit clozapine metabolism (5051).
CNS STIMULANTS: Concomitant use can increase the toxic effects of the caffeine in black tea (151).
DISULFIRAM (ANTABUSE): Concomitant use can decrease clearance and increase the half-life of caffeine, increasing effects and risk of adverse effects (15).
ERGOTAMINE: The caffeine in black tea can increase GI absorption of ergotamine (15).
LITHIUM: Abrupt withdrawal of the caffeine in black tea can increase serum lithium levels (609), worsening lithium tremor (610).
MAO INHIBITORS: The intake of large amounts of the caffeine in black tea can precipitate a hypertensive crisis (500).
ORAL CONTRACEPTIVES: Concomitant use of oral contraceptives interacts with the caffeine in black tea and can decrease caffeine clearance by 40-65%, increasing effects and risk of adverse effects (14).
PHENYLPROPANOLAMINE (PROPAGEST, RHINDECON): Concomitant use can increase blood pressure and/or cause mania through interaction with the caffeine in black tea (19).
PHENYTOIN (DILANTIN): Concomitant use can enhance metabolism and excretion of caffeine (19).
QUINOLONES: Concomitant use can decrease caffeine clearance and increase effects and risk of adverse effects (606,607,608). Quinolones include ciprofloxacin (Cipro), enoxacin (Penetrex), norfloxacin (Chibroxin, Noroxin), sparfloxacin (Zagam), trovafloxacin (Trovan), and grepafloxacin (Raxar).
THEOPHYLLINE: The caffeine in black tea can increase theophylline (Theo-Dur) levels (151).

© Copyright 2000, Natural Medicines Comprehensive Database (209) 472-2244. For updated data, go to www.NaturalDatabase.com

TRICYCLICS: Theoretically, concomitant use might decrease absorption of amitriptyline (Elavil) or imipramine (Tofranil, Janimine) through interaction with the caffeine in black tea (626,627).

VERAPAMIL (Calan, Covera, Isoptin, Verelan): Concomitant use can increase plasma caffeine levels by 25%, increasing effects and risk of adverse effects (14).

Possible Interactions with Foods

GRAPEFRUIT JUICE: Concomitant use can increase caffeine levels and the risk of adverse effects (504).

MILK: When taken together, milk might bind the antioxidants in black tea and reduce their beneficial effects (220); however, in one study this interaction did not occur (6032).

Possible Interactions with Lab Tests

BLEEDING TIME: The caffeine in black tea can prolong bleeding time and increase the results of a bleeding time test (1701).

SERUM URATE (Bittner method): The caffeine in black tea can cause false-positive test results (15).

CREATINE: The caffeine in black tea can increase urine creatine levels (1701).

URINE CATECHOLAMINES, 5-HYDROXYINDOLEACETIC ACID, VANILLYLMANDELIC ACID (VMA): The caffeine in black tea can cause slight increases in these levels (15).

TESTS FOR PHEOCHROMOCYTOMA, NEUROBLASTOMA: High urine catecholamines or VMA can result in false-positive results. The caffeine in black tea should be avoided while testing for these diseases (15).

Possible Interactions with Diseases or Conditions

GASTRIC, DUODENAL ULCERS: The caffeine in black tea can aggravate these conditions and should be avoided (14,16).

HEART CONDITIONS: The caffeine in black tea can induce cardiac arrhythmias in sensitive individuals (14,16).

DEPRESSION, ANXIETY DISORDERS: The caffeine in black tea can aggravate these conditions (14).

KIDNEY DISEASE: The diuretic effect of caffeine in tea might aggravate certain kidney disorders (19).

Typical Dosages & Routes of Administration that are Commonly Used

ORAL: A typical dose as a stimulant is several cups per day. A typical dose as an antidiarrheal is one cup 2-3 times daily. For reducing the risk of heart attack, kidney stones, and improving cognitive functioning, a dose of at least one cup per day has been used (4216,4222,4224). A current trial in women at high risk for breast cancer is using 4 cups of tea per day (4273). For preventing atherosclerosis, consumption of 125-500 mL (1-4 cups) of brewed black tea daily has been used (3450). To make tea pour boiling water over a teaspoon of tea, cover and allow to steep for 2 minutes, strain (8).

Comments

Green tea and black tea are derived from leaves of the same plant. Leaves used for green tea are prepared immediately after harvest, which limits enzymatic changes. Leaves used for black tea are fermented before preparation, promoting enzymatic changes. Consequently, green tea can have higher concentrations of the natural constituents than black teas (6,7).

BLACK WALNUT

This Product is Also Known As

Nogal Americano, Nogueira-preta, Noyer Noir, Schwarze Walnuss.

CAUTION: See separate listing for English Walnut hull and English Walnut leaf.

Scientific Names

Juglans nigra.
Family: Juglandaceae.

People Use This For

Orally, black walnut hulls are used for diphtheria, leukemia, syphilis, and as an anthelmintic (513).

Topically, black walnut hulls are used as a gargle, hair dye, insecticide, and for wounds (513).

Safety

POSSIBLY SAFE ...when used orally and appropriately, short term (12).

POSSIBLY UNSAFE ...when used topically because it contains the constituent juglone (2). Daily use of the juglone-containing bark of a related species (English walnut) is associated with increased risk of tongue cancer and lip leukoplakia (2,12).

PREGNANCY AND LACTATION: POSSIBLY UNSAFE ...when used topically; avoid using (12). There is insufficient reliable information about the safety of the oral use of black walnut hull during pregnancy or lactation; avoid using.

Effectiveness

There is insufficient reliable information available about the effectiveness of black walnut hull.

Possible Mechanism of Action & Active Ingredients

The applicable part of black walnut is the hull. Black walnut hulls contain approximately 45% tannins (19) which exert an astringent effect on the mucosal tissue. Tannins work internally by dehydrating mucosal tissue, which reduces secretions. Externally, tannin astringent effects result in a protective layer of constricted, harder cells. Plants with at least 10% tannins can cause gastrointestinal upset, kidney damage, and liver damage. Animal data conflicts with respect to the carcinogenicity of tannins. They may be carcinogenic or may even have anti-carcinogenic effects. An increased risk of esophageal or nasal cancer may be linked with people who regularly ingest herbs with high tannin concentrations (12).

Adverse Reactions Including Known Allergies

None reported.

Possible Interactions with Herbs & Other Dietary Supplements

TANNIN-CONTAINING HERBS: Theoretically, herbs such as black walnut contain high percentages of tannins, which might cause precipitation of constituents of other herbs (19).

Possible Interactions with Drugs

ORAL DRUGS: Theoretically, concomitant oral administration might cause precipitation of some drugs due to the high tannin content of black walnut hulls (19). Separate administration of oral drugs and tannin-containing herbs by the longest period of time practical (19).

Possible Interactions with Foods

No interactions are known to occur, and there is no known reason to expect a clinically significant interaction with black walnut.

Possible Interactions with Lab Tests

No interactions are known to occur, and there is no known reason to expect a clinically significant interaction with black walnut.

Possible Interactions with Diseases or Conditions

No interactions are known to occur, and there is no known reason to expect a clinically significant interaction with black walnut.

Typical Dosages & Routes of Administration that are Commonly Used

ORAL: A typical oral dose of black walnut hull is 1000 mg three times daily with water (351), not to exceed 6 weeks (352).

Comments

None.

BLACKBERRY leaf

This Product is Also Known As

Bramble, Dewberry, Goutberry, Rubi Fruticosi Folium, Thimbleberry.
CAUTION: See separate listings for Blackberry root and Raspberry.

Scientific Names

Rubus fruticosus.
Family: Rosaceae.

People Use This For

Orally, blackberry leaf is used for non-specific, acute diarrhea.
Topically, blackberry leaf is used as a mouth rinse for mild inflammation of the mucosa of the oral cavity and throat (2,12).

Safety

LIKELY SAFE ...when used orally for short-term use (2,12).
There is insufficient reliable information available about the safety of long-term use of blackberry leaf.
PREGNANCY AND LACTATION: Insufficient reliable information available; avoid using.

Effectiveness

POSSIBLY EFFECTIVE ...when taken orally for non-specific, acute diarrhea (2). ...when used topically as a mouth rinse for mild inflammation of the mucosa of the oral cavity and throat (2).

Possible Mechanism of Action & Active Ingredients

The astringent property of the tannin constituents can relieve mucosal inflammation and diarrhea (2,12).

Adverse Reactions Including Known Allergies
None reported (2).

Possible Interactions with Herbs & Other Dietary Supplements
Insufficient reliable information available.

Possible Interactions with Drugs
No interactions are known to occur, and there is no known reason to expect a clinically significant interaction with blackberry leaf.

Possible Interactions with Foods
No interactions are known to occur, and there is no known reason to expect a clinically significant interaction with blackberry leaf.

Possible Interactions with Lab Tests
No interactions are known to occur, and there is no known reason to expect a clinically significant interaction with blackberry leaf.

Possible Interactions with Diseases or Conditions
No interactions are known to occur, and there is no known reason to expect a clinically significant interaction with blackberry leaf.

Typical Dosages & Routes of Administration that are Commonly Used
ORAL: The usual dose of the blackberry leaf is 2-5 grams per day taken as a tea, which is prepared by steeping 1-2 teaspoons (1.5 grams) dried herb in 150 mL boiling water for 5-10 minutes and then straining. For equivalent preparations, 2-5 grams per day of the leaf is also used (2,18).
TOPICAL: The blackberry leaf tea can be used as a mouth rinse.

Comments
Avoid confusion with blackberry root. The leaf extract of the related species, Rubus ellipticus, has shown uterotropic activity at 300 mg/kg and can potentiate estrogenic activity (11). The related species, Rubus odoratus, has shown antitumor activity against Walker 256 carcinosarcoma (11).

BLACKBERRY root

This Product is Also Known As
Bramble, Dewberry, Goutberry, Rubi Fruticosi Radix, Thimbleberry.
CAUTION: See separate listing for Blackberry leaf.

Scientific Names
Rubus fruticosus.
Family: Rosaceae.

People Use This For
The blackberry root is used to prevent edema (2).

Safety
There is insufficient reliable information available about the safety of blackberry root.
Pregnancy and Lactation: Insufficient reliable information available; avoid using.

Effectiveness
There is insufficient reliable information available about the effectiveness of blackberry root (2).

Possible Mechanism of Action & Active Ingredients
Insufficient reliable information available.

Adverse Reactions Including Known Allergies
None reported.

Possible Interactions with Herbs & Other Dietary Supplements
Insufficient reliable information available.

Possible Interactions with Drugs
No interactions are known to occur, and there is no known reason to expect a clinically significant interaction with blackberry root.

Possible Interactions with Foods
No interactions are known to occur, and there is no known reason to expect a clinically significant interaction with blackberry root.

Possible Interactions with Lab Tests
No interactions are known to occur, and there is no known reason to expect a clinically significant interaction with blackberry root.

Possible Interactions with Diseases or Conditions
No interactions are known to occur, and there is no known reason to expect a clinically significant interaction with blackberry root.

Typical Dosages & Routes of Administration that are Commonly Used
ORAL: People typically use 1 teaspoon of the root added to 1 cup water. The liquid is taken cold, 1 to 2 cups per day. The root in tincture form is taken 15 to 40 drops in water as needed (5263).

Comments
Avoid confusion with blackberry leaf. The related species, Rubus odoratus, has shown antitumor activity against Walker 256 carcinosarcoma (11). The leaf extract of the related species, Rubus ellipticus, has shown uterotropic activity at 300 mg/kg and can potentiate estrogenic activity (11).

BLACKTHORN berry

This Product is Also Known As
Blackthorn Fruit, Pruni Spinosae Fructus, Sloe, Sloe Berry.
CAUTION: See separate listing for Blackthorn flower.

Scientific Names
Prunus spinosa.
Family: Rosaceae.

People Use This For
Blackthorn berry is used as a mouth rinse (gargle) for mild inflammation of the oral and pharyngeal mucosa (2). In folk medicine, the berry juice is utilized as the gargle for mouth, throat, and gum inflammation (18). The syrup and wine of the blackthorn berry is used for purging the bowels and as a diuretic (18). The berry marmalade is used for dyspepsia (18).

Safety
LIKELY SAFE ...when used orally and appropriately as a mouthrinse, short-term (2,12).
POSSIBLY UNSAFE ...not recommended for long-term use (12).
PREGNANCY AND LACTATION: Insufficient reliable information available; avoid using.

Effectiveness
POSSIBLY EFFECTIVE ...when used as an oral mouth rinse for mild inflammation of the oral and pharyngeal mucosa (2).
There is insufficient reliable information available about the effectiveness of blackthorn berry for its other uses.

Possible Mechanism of Action & Active Ingredients
The astringent properties of the tannin constituents can contribute to the reduction of mucous membrane inflammation (2,7).

Adverse Reactions Including Known Allergies
None reported.

Possible Interactions with Herbs & Other Dietary Supplements
Insufficient reliable information available.

Possible Interactions with Drugs
No interactions are known to occur, and there is no known reason to expect a clinically significant interaction with blackthorn berry.

Possible Interactions with Foods
No interactions are known to occur, and there is no known reason to expect a clinically significant interaction with blackthorn berry.

Possible Interactions with Lab Tests
No interactions are known to occur, and there is no known reason to expect a clinically significant interaction with blackthorn berry.

Possible Interactions with Diseases or Conditions

No interactions are known to occur, and there is no known reason to expect a clinically significant interaction with blackthorn berry.

Typical Dosages & Routes of Administration that are Commonly Used

ORAL: The blackthorn berry is typically used as a mouth rinse up to two times per day. The rinse is obtained from the tea, which is prepared by steeping 1-2 grams in 150 mL boiling water for 10-15 minutes and the straining (2,12). No typical dosage for the other uses of blackthorn berry.

Comments

None.

BLACKTHORN flower

This Product is Also Known As

Pruni Spinosae Llos, Sloe Flower, Wild Plum Flower.
CAUTION: See separate listing for Blackthorn berry.

Scientific Names

Prunus spinosa.
Family: Rosaceae.

People Use This For

Orally, blackthorn flower is used for common colds, ailments of the respiratory tract, bloating, general exhaustion, dyspepsia, kidney and bladder ailments, and to treat and prevent gastric spasms. The blackthorn flower is also used orally as a laxative, diuretic, diaphoretic, expectorant, and as a component in "blood cleansing" teas (2,18).
Topically, blackthorn flower is used for rashes, skin impurities, and "blood purification" (2).
In food use, blackthorn flower is utilized in herbal teas as a coloring agent (2).

Safety

POSSIBLY SAFE ...when blackthorn flower is used as a coloring agent for oral herbal tea mixtures (2).
POSSIBLY UNSAFE ...when blackthorn flower is used orally in medicinal amounts. Contains cyanogenic glycosides that could be toxic (12).
LIKELY UNSAFE ...when used orally long-term or in excessive amounts (12).
There is insufficient reliable information available about the safety of blackthorn flower for its other uses.
PREGNANCY AND LACTATION: LIKELY UNSAFE ...when used orally; avoid using. HCN can be teratogenic (12).

Effectiveness

There is insufficient reliable information available about the effectiveness of blackthorn flower (2).

Possible Mechanism of Action & Active Ingredients

Insufficient reliable information available (2).

Adverse Reactions Including Known Allergies

None reported.

Possible Interactions with Herbs & Other Dietary Supplements

Insufficient reliable information available.

Possible Interactions with Drugs

No interactions are known to occur, and there is no known reason to expect a clinically significant interaction with blackthorn flower.

Possible Interactions with Foods

No interactions are known to occur, and there is no known reason to expect a clinically significant interaction with blackthorn flower.

Possible Interactions with Lab Tests

No interactions are known to occur, and there is no known reason to expect a clinically significant interaction with blackthorn flower.

Possible Interactions with Diseases or Conditions

No interactions are known to occur, and there is no known reason to expect a clinically significant interaction with blackthorn flower.

Typical Dosages & Routes of Administration that are Commonly Used

ORAL: Blackthorn flower is usually taken as a tea, 1-2 cups during the day or 2 cups in the evening. The tea is prepared by steeping 1-2 heaping teaspoons (1-2 grams) in 150 mL boiling water for 5-10 minutes and then straining (18). Blackthorn is for short-term use only (12).

Comments

Blackthorn can be stored for up to one year away from light and moisture (18).

BLADDERWORT

This Product is Also Known As

None.
CAUTION: See separate listing for Bladderwrack.

Scientific Names

Utricularia vulgaris.
Family: Lentibulariaceae.

People Use This For

Orally, bladderwort is used for urinary tract disorders. It is also used orally as a diuretic, antispasmodic, anti-inflammatory, and to stimulate gall bladder secretions.
Topically, bladderwort is used for burns, skin and mucous membrane inflammation.

Safety

There is insufficient reliable information available about the safety of the use of bladderwort.
Pregnancy and Lactation: Insufficient reliable information available; avoid using.

Effectiveness

There is insufficient reliable information available about the effectiveness of bladderwort.

Possible Mechanism of Action & Active Ingredients

Insufficient reliable information available.

Adverse Reactions Including Known Allergies

None reported.

Possible Interactions with Herbs & Other Dietary Supplements

Insufficient reliable information available.

Possible Interactions with Drugs

No interactions are known to occur, and there is no known reason to expect a clinically significant interaction with bladderwort.

Possible Interactions with Foods

No interactions are known to occur, and there is no known reason to expect a clinically significant interaction with bladderwort.

Possible Interactions with Lab Tests

No interactions are known to occur, and there is no known reason to expect a clinically significant interaction with bladderwort.

Possible Interactions with Diseases or Conditions

No interactions are known to occur, and there is no known reason to expect a clinically significant interaction with bladderwort.

Typical Dosages & Routes of Administration that are Commonly Used

ORAL: As a diuretic, two cups are taken daily. The tea is prepared by steeping 2 grams dried leaf in 100 mL of boiling water for 10-15 minutes and straining.
TOPICAL: As an anti-inflammatory, a tea is used in mouthwashes, cleansers, cosmetic, and medical packs. The tea is prepared by steeping 6 grams dried leaf in 100 mL of boiling water for 10-15 minutes and straining (18).

Comments

Bladderwort use is nearly obsolete in Germany. It continues to be used in other countries (18).

BLADDERWRACK

This Product is Also Known As
Black Tang, Bladder Fucus, Blasentang, Cutweed, Fucus, Kelp, Kelpware, Kelp-Ware, Knotted Wrack, Meereiche, Quercus Marina, Rockweed, Rockwrack, Schweintang, Seawrack, Tang, Varech.
CAUTION: See separate listings for Bladderwort, Algin, and Laminaria.

Scientific Names
Fucus vesiculosis; other Fucus species and other brown seaweed species; Ascophyllum nodosum.
Family: Fucaceae.

People Use This For
Traditionally, bladderwrack has been used for thyroid disorders [2], iodine deficiency [9], lymphadenoid goiter [4], myxedema [4], obesity, arthritis, and rheumatism [4]. Bladderwrack is used in folk medicine for arteriosclerosis, digestive disorders, "blood cleansing" [2], constipation [9], bronchitis, emphysema, genitourinary disorders, decreased resistance to disease, anxiety, skin diseases, burns, and insect bites [5].

Safety
POSSIBLY UNSAFE ...when taken orally because 1 gram of bladderwrack might contain as much as 600 mcg iodine [12]. Ingesting more than 150 mcg iodine per day can cause hyperthyroidism or exacerbate existing hyperthyroidism [2]. Heavy metal poisoning has also been reported [645].
CHILDREN: POSSIBLY UNSAFE ...when taken orally; avoid using [14].
PREGNANCY AND LACTATION: LIKELY UNSAFE ...when taken orally; contraindicated [4,12].

Effectiveness
There is insufficient reliable information about the effectiveness of bladderwrack.

Possible Mechanism of Action & Active Ingredients
Iodine, which is the essential substrate for the thyroid hormone, can have a concentration that varies from 0.03-1.0% [18]. The constituent algin (sodium alginate) has bulk laxative and demulcent (soothing) effects [4,5]. The isolated fraction, fucoidin, has 40-50% of the blood anticoagulant activity of heparin [4]. Fucus can concentrate heavy metals [4]. There is limited information available for Fucus vesiculosis, but the pharmacological activities are recognized for the individual constituents and other brown seaweed species.

Adverse Reactions Including Known Allergies
Bladderwrack can induce or exacerbate hyperthyroidism [2,12] and acne [4]. Prolonged ingestion can reduce iron absorption [4]. High sodium content can adversely affect individuals with restricted sodium intake [5]. Iodine can cause idiosyncratic or allergic reactions [2,18]. There is one case report of heavy metal poisoning where arsenic poisoning occurred with ingestions of a contaminated kelp product [645].

Possible Interactions with Herbs & Other Dietary Supplements
IRON: Prolonged ingestion of bladderwrack can reduce iron absorption [4].

Possible Interactions with Drugs
DIURETICS: Bladderwrack can decrease the effectiveness of diuretics due to high sodium content [5].
ANTICOAGULANTS: Theoretically, concomitant use might increase bleeding risk [4].
LITHIUM (ESKALITH, LITHOBID): Theoretically, concomitant use might enhance hypothyroid activity due to high iodine content in bladderwrack [19].
THYROID HORMONES: The high iodine content of bladderwrack might interfere with thyroid hormone replacement therapy [4].

Possible Interactions with Foods
IRON: Prolonged ingestion of bladderwrack can reduce iron absorption [4].

Possible Interactions with Lab Tests
ACTIVATED PARTIAL THROMBOPLASTIN TIME (aPPT): Theoretically, bladderwrack might increase aPTT test results due to the heparin-like activity of one of its constituents [4].
THYROID STIMULATING HORMONE (TSH): Theoretically, bladderwrack might increase serum TSH levels and test results [1701].
THYROXINE (T4): Theoretically, bladderwrack might increase serum T4 levels and test results [1701].
RADIOACTIVE IODINE UPTAKE: Theoretically, bladderwrack might interfere with the results of thyroid function tests using radioactive iodine uptake [15].

Possible Interactions with Diseases or Conditions
HYPERTHYROIDISM, ACNE: Bladderwrack can exacerbate these conditions [2,4,12].
CONDITIONS REQUIRING SODIUM RESTRICTION: The high sodium content can exacerbate these conditions [5].

IRON DEFICIENCY: Bladderwrack can exacerbate this deficiency by reducing iron absorption (4).
IODINE ALLERGY: Avoid bladderwrack use in those sensitive to iodine (2,18).

Typical Dosages & Routes of Administration that are Commonly Used

ORAL: The usual dose is 5-10 grams of the plant or as a tea three times a day. The tea is prepared by steeping the herb in 150 mL boiling water for 5-10 minutes and the straining (4). The typical dose of the liquid extract (1:1) is 4-8 mL three times a day. Bladderwrack can contain over 600 mcg iodine per gram seaweed (12).

Comments

Avoid confusion with bladderwort.

BLESSED THISTLE

This Product is Also Known As

Carbenia benedicta, Cardo Santo, Carduus benedictus, Cnici Benedicti Herba, Cnicus, Holy Thistle, St. Benedict Thistle, Spotted Thistle.
CAUTION: See separate listing for Milk Thistle above ground parts and Milk Thistle fruit, seed.

Scientific Names

Cnicus benedictus.
Family: Asteraceae or Compositae.

People Use This For

Orally, blessed thistle is used for loss of appetite and indigestion (2) as an antidiarrheal, expectorant, antibiotic (4), and for promoting lactation (314).
Topically, blessed thistle is used as a poultice for boils, wounds, and ulcers (4,11).
Traditionally, blessed thistle has been used as a diuretic (11), and for treating colds and fever (11).
In manufacturing, it is used as a flavoring in alcoholic beverages (12).

Safety

LIKELY SAFE …when used as flavoring, regulated in the US as an allowable flavoring for alcoholic beverages (12).
POSSIBLY SAFE …when preparations of the above ground parts are used orally and appropriately (12).
PREGNANCY: LIKELY UNSAFE …contraindicated for oral use (4,12).
LACTATION: Insufficient reliable information available; avoid using (4).

Effectiveness

POSSIBLY EFFECTIVE …when taken orally for loss of appetite and indigestion (2).
There is insufficient reliable information available about the effectiveness of blessed thistle for its other uses.

Possible Mechanism of Action & Active Ingredients

The applicable parts of blessed thistle are the flowering top, leaf, and upper stem. The bacteriostatic properties are due to the volatile oil of blessed thistle. The sesquiterpene lactone constituent, cnicin3, can have antibacterial and antitumor activity (11). Metabolism of the constituents, arctiin and tracheoloside, following oral ingestion results in compounds that inhibit cyclic-AMP phosphodiesterase and histamine release from mast cells (11). Blessed thistle contains 8% tannins (4).

Adverse Reactions Including Known Allergies

Blessed thistle taken in high doses, greater than five grams per cup of tea, can cause stomach irritation and vomiting (12). It can cause an allergic reaction in individuals sensitive to the Asteraceae/Compositae family. Members of this family include ragweed, chrysanthemums, marigolds, daisies, and many other herbs.

Possible Interactions with Herbs & Other Dietary Supplements

Insufficient reliable information available.

Possible Interactions with Drugs

ACID-INHIBITING DRUGS: Theoretically, due to claims that blessed thistle increases stomach acid, it might interfere with antacids, sucralfate (Carafate), H-2 antagonists, or proton pump inhibitors (19).

Possible Interactions with Foods

No interactions are known to occur, and there is no known reason to expect a clinically significant interaction with blessed thistle.

Possible Interactions with Lab Tests

No interactions are known to occur, and there is no known reason to expect a clinically significant interaction with blessed thistle.

156 • © Copyright 2000, Natural Medicines Comprehensive Database (209) 472-2244. For updated data, go to www.NaturalDatabase.com

Possible Interactions with Diseases or Conditions

GI IRRITATION: Can irritate the gastrointestinal tract. Contraindicated in individuals with infectious or inflammatory gastrointestinal conditions (19).

CROSS-ALLERGENICITY: Can cause an allergic reaction in individuals sensitive to the Asteraceae/Compositae family. Members of this family include ragweed, chrysanthemums, marigolds, daisies, and many other herbs.

Typical Dosages & Routes of Administration that are Commonly Used

ORAL: The typical dose of the dried, flowering tops is 1.5-3 grams themselves or as a tea three times daily. The tea is prepared by steeping the dried, flowering tops in boiling water and then straining. The liquid extract (1:1 in 25% alcohol) is commonly taken as 1.5-3 mL three times daily (4).

Comments

Blessed thistle was commonly used during the Middle Ages to treat the bubonic plague and as a tonic for monks. Avoid confusion with milk thistle (Silybum marianum).

BLOND PSYLLIUM

This Product is Also Known As

Blond Plantago, Blonde Psyllium, Englishman's Foot, Indian Plantago, Ispaghula, Ispagol, Pale Psyllium, Plantaginis ovatae semen, Plantaginis ovatae testa, Psyllium, Sand Plantain, Spogel.
CAUTION: See separate listing for Black Psyllium seed, Buckhorn Plantain, Great Plantain, and Water Plantain.

Scientific Names

Plantago ovata, synonyms Plantago decumbens, Plantago isphagula.
Family: Plantaginaceae.

People Use This For

Orally, blond psyllium is used for chronic constipation, for softening stools when desirable (including cases of hemorrhoids, anal fissures, anorectal surgery, and during pregnancy), for diarrhea, irritable bowel syndrome (2,6,11,18), reducing elevated cholesterol (6,11,18,1405), reducing blood sugar in people with type 2 diabetes (1405), dysentery (6), and treating cancer (11).

Topically, blond psyllium seed is used as a poultice for furunculosis (boils) (4).

In food manufacturing, blond psyllium seed husk mucilage is used as a thickener or stabilizer in some frozen dairy desserts (11).

Safety

LIKELY SAFE ...when used orally with adequate fluid intake (240 mL fluid per 3.5-5.1 grams of husk or 7 grams of seed) (4,12,272,1376). A meta-analysis of 19 studies involving 966 psyllium-exposed people found that 5.1-20.4 grams/day of blond psyllium husk for 6 weeks to 6 months did not cause serious adverse effects (1376).

LIKELY UNSAFE ...when it is used with inadequate fluid intake because it can cause esophageal obstruction (2,4,18). ...when the seeds of non-commercial preparations of blond psyllium are chewed, crushed, or ground because they release a pigment that deposits in renal tubules (11) and can be nephrotoxic (6). The pigment has been removed from most commercial products (6).

PREGNANCY AND LACTATION: LIKELY SAFE ...when used orally with adequate amounts of fluid (1,4,272).

Effectiveness

EFFECTIVE ...when the seed husk or seed is used orally as a supplemental source of dietary fiber (272). ...when the husk or seed is used orally as a bulk laxative (272). ...when the husk is used orally for reducing serum total cholesterol, LDL cholesterol, and LDL:HDL ratio in patients with high cholesterol, beyond reductions achieved with diet alone (6,11,1376,6262,6263). Psyllium seed husk 10.2 grams daily added to food reduced LDL cholesterol by 5.3% compared with food without psyllium in a well-designed, 24 week study of 286 people with mild to moderate hypercholesterolemia (6262). Another recent study compared a psyllium power (Metamucil) 5.1 grams mixed with liquid and an identical cellulose placebo taken twice daily for 24 weeks by hypercholesterolemic people who also followed the AHA Step I diet (6261). Total cholesterol was 4.7% lower and LDL cholesterol was 6.7% lower in the group using psyllium (6261). A meta-analysis of eight clinical studies found that blond psyllium husk reduces serum total cholesterol 3-6% and LDL cholesterol 5-9% in patients with hypercholesterolemia already eating a low-fat diet (1376). Another meta-analysis of twelve trials that studied psyllium-enriched cereal consumption by adults with mild to moderate hypercholesterolemia described similar results (6263). The FDA has recently allowed psyllium-containing foods, such as certain breakfast cereals, to be labeled with a claim that these foods, as part of a diet low in saturated fat and cholesterol, may reduce the risk of coronary heart disease (CHD), similar to health labeling for oats (6264).

POSSIBLY EFFECTIVE ...when the seed husk or seed is used orally as a secondary treatment for diarrhea (2). ...when the husk or seed is used orally for treating irritable bowel syndrome (2). ...when the seed is used orally for reducing serum total cholesterol, LDL cholesterol, and LDL:HDL ratio in people with high cholesterol (6,11). ...when the husk is used orally for reducing postprandial glucose and serum total and LDL

cholesterol levels in people with type 2 diabetes and hypercholesterolemia (1405).
LIKELY INEFFECTIVE ...when the husk is taken orally for increasing HDL cholesterol concentrations in patents with hypercholesterolemia already eating a low-fat diet (1376).
There is insufficient reliable information available about the effectiveness of blond psyllium for its other uses.

Possible Mechanism of Action & Active Ingredients

The applicable parts of blond psyllium are the seed and seed husk. The blond psyllium husk and intact seed constituents are not absorbed and have no systemic effects (1). Chewing, crushing, or grinding the seeds can release a pigment that deposits in renal tubules (11) and can be nephrotoxic (6). This pigment is removed from most commercial products (6). The husks of the psyllium seed form a mucilaginous mass when mixed with water and have a bulk laxative effect (1,4,6). In people with diarrhea, the mucilage absorbs water, provides mass, and prolongs gastrointestinal transit (1,6). In people with constipation, the mucilage absorbs water, swells, and stimulates peristalsis, reducing gastrointestinal transit time (1,4,6). Psyllium can decrease abdominal pain in people with irritable bowel syndrome by reducing rectosigmoidal pressure (405). Psyllium might decrease serum cholesterol levels by absorbing dietary fats in the gastrointestinal tract, preventing systemic absorption, and increasing cholesterol elimination in fecal bile acids (1,6,11,12,1376). Psyllium reduces postprandial blood glucose levels by slowing carbohydrate absorption (1,6,1405).

Adverse Reactions Including Known Allergies

Blond psyllium taken orally can cause transient flatulence, abdominal pain, diarrhea, constipation, dyspepsia, nausea (4,1376), and esophageal or bowel obstruction when consumed without water (4,604). Headache, backache, rhinitis, increased cough, sinusitis have been reported (1376). Whole body, respiratory, urogenital, musculoskeletal, nervous, skin, cardiovascular, metabolic, and endocrine adverse effects have been reported in clinical trials of blond psyllium (1376). Chewing, crushing, or grinding the seeds can release a pigment which deposits in renal tubules (11) and can be nephrotoxic (6). This pigment is removed from most commercial products (6). Allergy symptoms from blond psyllium include allergic rhinitis, conjunctivitis, urticaria, and asthma (18). Occupational exposure to psyllium can cause sensitization, of which symptoms include sneezing, watery eyes, chest congestion, and anaphylactoid reactions (6).

Possible Interactions with Herbs & Other Dietary Supplements

VITAMIN/MINERAL SUPPLEMENTS: Long-term use of psyllium with vitamin or mineral supplements can reduce nutrient absorption, including calcium, iron, zinc, and vitamin B12 (1,12). Take supplements one hour before or four hours after psyllium to avoid this interaction (4,12).

Possible Interactions with Drugs

CARBAMAZEPINE (Tegretol): Psyllium can reduce carbamazepine absorption (539).
DIABETES THERAPY: Monitor blood glucose level closely due to claims that blond psyllium has hypoglycemic effects (19).
DIGOXIN (Lanoxin), WARFARIN (Coumadin): Concomitant use with psyllium can require warfarin or digoxin dosing adjustment (12) due to retarded drug absorption (1).
LITHIUM: There is one case report of reduced serum lithium levels associated with psyllium use and was reversed when psyllium stopped (540).
INSULIN: Psyllium can decrease insulin requirements in diabetes by reducing peak blood glucose levels (1,18).
ORAL DRUGS: Take oral drugs one hour before or four hours after psyllium to avoid decreased or delayed absorption (4,12).

Possible Interactions with Foods

NUTRIENT ABSORPTION: Long-term use of psyllium with meals can reduce nutrient absorption (12) requiring vitamin or mineral supplementation. However, use of blond psyllium husk for up to six months did not clinically alter vitamin or mineral status in a review of eight human trials (1376).

Possible Interactions with Lab Tests

GLUCOSE: Blond psyllium can reduce postprandial blood glucose levels and test results (1,6,1405).
CHOLESTEROL: Blond psyllium reduces serum total cholesterol and LDL cholesterol levels, LDL:HDL ratio, and test results (1,6,1405,1376).

Possible Interactions with Diseases or Conditions

GI CONDITIONS: Blond psyllium is contraindicated in people with fecal impaction, GI atony (1), and GI tract narrowing, obstruction, or conditions that can lead to obstruction, such as spastic bowel (1,2,4,12,18).
KIDNEY DYSFUNCTION: Avoid chewing, crushing, or grinding blond psyllium seeds, which releases a potentially nephrotoxic pigment (6). This pigment is removed from most commercial products (6).
DIABETES: Blond psyllium can lower blood glucose levels in people with type 2 diabetes by retarding carbohydrate absorption (1,2,1405). Its use should be monitored closely. In addition, commercially available psyllium products can contain sugar and other absorbable carbohydrates (272).
SWALLOWING DIFFICULTIES: Contraindicated (12).
PSYLLIUM HYPERSENSITIVITY: Contraindicated (1).
PHENYLKETONURIA: Avoid products containing aspartame (Nutrasweet) (272).

Typical Dosages & Routes of Administration that are Commonly Used

ORAL (Husk): The typical adult dose is 3.5 grams blond psyllium seed husk one to three times daily (1). The typical dose of the husk for children 6-12 years is half the adult dose (1). For children under 6 years, psyllium should only be used after medical evaluation (1). For irritable bowel syndrome, the usual dose is 7 grams of husk taken one to three times daily (1). For lowering serum cholesterol, the FDA evaluated studies that used 10.2 grams of psyllium see husk (about 7 grams of soluble fiber) daily (6264). Dosage regimens were typically 3.4 grams of husk three times daily, or 5.1 grams of husk twice daily (6261,6262). Some people have used up to 20.4 grams per day (1,1376). Adequate fluid intake is necessary; a minimum of 240 mL per 5.1 grams or less of blond psyllium husk is recommended (1,12,272). Psyllium should be consumed immediately after mixing and followed with additional fluid (1). If abdominal pain occurs, or there is no response after 48 hours, medical evaluation is needed (1). (Seed): The amount of psyllium seed typically taken as a laxative in adults is 7-40 grams per day, in two to three divided doses (1,2,18). For children 6-12 years, half the adult amount is used (1), and for children under 6 years of age, psyllium should be used only after medical evaluation (1). If a non-commercial product is used, avoid chewing, crushing, or grinding the seeds, which releases a pigment that deposits in renal tubules (11) and can be nephrotoxic (6). This pigment is removed from most commercial products (6). Adequate fluid intake is necessary; a minimum of 240 mL water per 7 grams of blond psyllium seed is recommended (1,12,272). Taking psyllium without enough liquid can cause choking. The amount of blond psyllium seed husk or seed required for an individual can vary. For best results, start with small amounts and increase to the desired response.

Comments

Due to the risk of esophageal and small bowel obstruction with bulk-forming products, the FDA requires the following labeling: "WARNING: Taking this product without adequate fluid may cause it to swell and block your throat or esophagus and may cause choking. Do not take this product if you have difficulty in swallowing. If you experience chest pain, vomiting, or difficulty in swallowing or breathing after taking this product, seek immediate medical attention" (12). Great plantain (Plantago major) seed is sometimes used as a substitute for blond psyllium (4).

BLOODROOT

This Product is Also Known As

Blood Root, Coon Root, Indian Plant, Indian Red Paint, Pauson, Red Indian Paint, Red Puccoon, Red Root, Sanguinaria, Snakebite, Sweet Slumber, Tetterwort.

Scientific Names

Sanguinaria canadensis.
Family: Papaveraceae.

People Use This For

Orally, bloodroot is used as an emetic, cathartic, antispasmodic, and expectorant (4).
Topically, bloodroot is used as an irritant and debriding agent (4).
In dentistry, bloodroot is used topically to reduce plaque (4,6).
Traditionally, bloodroot has been used for bronchitis, asthma, croup, laryngitis, pharyngitis, deficient capillary circulation, nasal polyps (4), rheumatism, warts, cancer (Fell technique), dental analgesic (6), fever, and as a general tonic (11).

Safety

POSSIBLY SAFE ...when the rhizome preparations are used orally and appropriately short-term (4).
POSSIBLY UNSAFE ...when excessive doses are used because sanguinarine, although thought to be poorly absorbed, is a toxic alkaloid (6,12).
PREGNANCY: LIKELY UNSAFE ...contraindicated for oral use (12).
LACTATION: POSSIBLY UNSAFE ...when used orally; avoid using (4).

Effectiveness

POSSIBLY EFFECTIVE ...when used topically in dental products for reducing dental plaque (4,6). ...when used topically for treating carcinomas of the nose and ear (6).
There is insufficient reliable information available about the effectiveness of bloodroot for its other uses.

Possible Mechanism of Action & Active Ingredients

The applicable part of bloodroot is the rhizome. The isoquinolone alkaloid constituents, primarily sanguinarine, have antimicrobial, anti-inflammatory, antihistamine, cardiotonic (exerts a favorable effect on the heart), and antiplaque activity (4). The negative ion of sanguinarine can bind to dental plaque (6).

Adverse Reactions Including Known Allergies

Bloodroot can cause nausea, vomiting (12), slight CNS depression, and narcosis (6). High doses can cause hypotension, shock, coma, and glaucoma (6). Skin contact with the fresh bloodroot can cause irritation or contact dermatitis (19).

Possible Interactions with Herbs & Other Dietary Supplements

There is insufficient reliable information available.

Possible Interactions with Drugs

No interactions are known to occur, and there is no known reason to expect a clinically significant interaction with bloodroot.

Possible Interactions with Foods

No interactions are known to occur, and there is no known reason to expect a clinically significant interaction with bloodroot.

Possible Interactions with Lab Tests

No interactions are known to occur, and there is no known reason to expect a clinically significant interaction with bloodroot.

Possible Interactions with Diseases or Conditions

GI IRRITATION: Bloodroot can irritate the gastrointestinal tract and is contraindicated in individuals with infectious or inflammatory gastrointestinal conditions (19).
GLAUCOMA: Bloodroot might affect glaucoma treatment. Do not exceed the recommended dose (12).

Typical Dosages & Routes of Administration that are Commonly Used

ORAL: The dose of the bloodroot rhizome is typically 60-500 mg three times a day (4). The usual dose of the liquid extract (1:1 in 60% alcohol) is 0.06-0.3 mL three times a day (4). The common dose of the tincture (1:5 in 60% alcohol) is 0.3-2 mL three times a day (4). Avoid contact with the eyes and mucous membranes because of its irritant properties.
EMETIC DOSE: As an emetic, 1-2 of the rhizome, 1-2 mL of the liquid extract (1:1 in 60% alcohol), or 2-8 mL of the tincture (1:5 in 60% alcohol) are commonly used (4).

Comments

During the mid-1800s, topical preparations of the bloodroot extracts were used in the Fell Technique for treatment of breast tumors (6).

BLUE COHOSH

This Product is Also Known As

Blue Ginseng, Caulophyllum, Papoose Root, Squaw Root, Yellow Ginseng.
CAUTION: See separate listings for Black Cohosh, White Cohosh, Ginseng American, Canaigre, Codonopsis, Ginseng Siberian, Ginseng Panax, and Withania.

Scientific Names

Caulophyllum thalictroides.
Family: Berberidaceae.

People Use This For

Orally, blue cohosh is used for stimulating the uterus (5), inducing menstruation (5), as an antispasmodic (5), for antirheumatic effects (4), and as a laxative (11).
Historically, blue cohosh has been used for colic, sore throat, cramps, hiccups, epilepsy, hysterics, and inflammation of the uterus (5).
In food use, the roasted seeds of blue cohosh are often used as a coffee substitute (6).

Safety

POSSIBLY SAFE ...when the roasted seeds are used as a coffee substitute because strong heat is reported to denature the seed toxins (6).
LIKELY UNSAFE ...when the root or rhizome are used orally for self-medication (12). Poisonings have also occurred from the leaf and seeds (4). Canadian products do not allow blue cohosh as a nonmedicinal ingredient in oral products (12).
CHILDREN: LIKELY UNSAFE ...when the root or rhizome are used orally (4).
PREGNANCY AND LACTATION: LIKELY UNSAFE ...when the root or rhizome are used orally. Blue cohosh can act as an abortifacient (12). It has been used by practitioners to stimulate childbirth in pregnant women near term (4,12). One report attributes the profound congestive heart failure of a newborn to the mother ingesting blue cohosh during labor (102).

Effectiveness
POSSIBLY EFFECTIVE ...when taken orally as a uterine contraction stimulant (4,5,11).
LIKELY INEFFECTIVE ...when used orally for inflammation (4,5).
There is insufficient reliable information available about the effectiveness of blue cohosh for its other uses.

Possible Mechanism of Action & Active Ingredients
The applicable parts of blue cohosh are the rhizome and root. A crystalline glycoside, caulosaponin, can cause oxytocic effects (4) and can also have anti-fertility actions (4). Methylcytosine, an alkaloid constituent, acts similarly to nicotine, increasing blood pressure, stimulating the small intestine, and producing hyperglycemia (4,11). A blue cohosh extract enhances estradiol binding to estrogen receptors and enhances estradiol-induced transcription activity in estrogen-responsive cells (6180). It also decreases LH (luteinizing hormone) levels and increases serum ceruloplasmin oxidase activity (a measure of estrogenic activity in the liver) in female rats with their ovaries removed (6180).

Adverse Reactions Including Known Allergies
The rhizome or root taken orally can cause mucous membrane irritation (4). There is one report of neonatal acute MI with profound congestive heart failure and shock associated with the maternal use of a blue cohosh-containing product one month before delivery (566). The ingestion of the leaves and seeds can cause severe stomach pain and poisoning (4,6).

Possible Interactions with Herbs & Other Dietary Supplements
There is insufficient reliable information available.

Possible Interactions with Drugs
ANTIANGINAL, ANTIHYPERTENSIVE DRUGS: Blue cohosh can interfere with drug therapy (4).
NICOTINE: Blue cohosh can increase the effects of nicotine (6002).

Possible Interactions with Foods
No interactions are known to occur, and there is no known reason to expect a clinically significant interaction with blue cohosh.

Possible Interactions with Lab Tests
No interactions are known to occur, and there is no known reason to expect a clinically significant interaction with blue cohosh.

Possible Interactions with Diseases or Conditions
GI CONDITIONS: Blue cohosh can irritate these conditions (4).

Typical Dosages & Routes of Administration that are Commonly Used
ORAL: The typical dose of the dried rhizome or root is 0.3-1 grams or as a tea three times daily. The tea is prepared by steeping the herb in 150 mL boiling water and then straining. The usual dose of the liquid extract (1:1 in 70% alcohol) is 0.5-1.0 mL three times daily (4).

Comments
The indications for this herb require medical evaluation and monitoring. Self-medication can be unsafe (4,5).

BLUE FLAG

This Product is Also Known As
Iris, Sweet Flag.
CAUTION: See separate listing for Orris.

Scientific Names
Iris versicolor; Iris caroliniana; Iris virginica.
Family: Iridaceae.

People Use This For
Orally, blue flag is used as a laxative and diuretic and for dermatological, anti-inflammatory, and antiemetic uses. It is also used as a bile stimulant, for liver dysfunction, and specifically for skin eruptions (4).

Safety
LIKELY UNSAFE ...contraindicated in all but small doses (4). The fresh root can cause nausea, vomiting, and mucosal irritation (4,12). The blue flag oil is a mucous membrane irritant (4).
PREGNANCY: LIKELY UNSAFE ...contraindicated (4,12).
LACTATION: LIKELY UNSAFE ...contraindicated (4).

Effectiveness

There is insufficient reliable information available about the effectiveness of blue flag.

Possible Mechanism of Action & Active Ingredients

The applicable part of blue flag is the rhizome. Little is known about blue flag's phytochemical, pharmacological, and toxicological properties, or those of its constituents. Some related species can be toxic (4).

Adverse Reactions Including Known Allergies

Blue flag can cause nausea and vomiting, and the fresh root can irritate mucosa or skin (4,19). The volatile oil constituent irritates mucous membranes and causes lacrimation, eye inflammation, irritation of the throat, or headache (4).

Possible Interactions with Herbs & Other Dietary Supplements

STIMULANT LAXATIVE HERBS: Theoretically, concomitant use of blue flag with other stimulant laxative herbs can increase the risk of potassium depletion. Stimulant laxative herbs include aloe dried leaf sap, wild cucumber fruit (Ecballium elaterium), alder buckthorn, European buckthorn, butternut bark, cascara bark, castor oil, colocynth fruit pulp, gamboge bark exudate, jalap root, black root, manna bark exudate, podophyllum root, rhubarb root, senna leaves and pods, and yellow dock root (19).

POTASSIUM DEPLETING HERBS: Theoretically, concomitant use with horsetail plant or the licorice rhizome increases the risk of potassium depletion.

Possible Interactions with Drugs

CARDIAC GLYCOSIDES: Theoretically, overuse or abuse of this product increases the risk of adverse effects from cardiac glycoside drugs, e.g. digoxin (Lanoxin).

Possible Interactions with Foods

No interactions are known to occur, and there is no known reason to expect a clinically significant interaction with blue flag.

Possible Interactions with Lab Tests

No interactions are known to occur, and there is no known reason to expect a clinically significant interaction with blue flag.

Possible Interactions with Diseases or Conditions

GI IRRITATION: Blue flag can irritate the gastrointestinal tract and is contraindicated in individuals with infectious or inflammatory gastrointestinal conditions (19).

Typical Dosages & Routes of Administration that are Commonly Used

No typical dosage.

Comments

Blue flag is likely unsafe and ineffective; avoid using. Little is known about its phytochemical, pharmacological, or toxicological properties, or those of its constituents. Some related species can be toxic (4). Though orris root is sometimes used as a common name for blue flag, it is also used to describe the Iris species.

BLUE-GREEN ALGAE

This Product is Also Known As

Blue Green Algae, Cyanobacteria, Dihe, Klamath Blue/Green Algae, Spirulina, Tecuitlatl.

Scientific Names

Microcystis aeruginosa, Microcystis wesenbergii, and other Microcystis species; Spirulina maxima, Spirulina platensis, and other Spirulina species; Anabaena species; Lyngbya wollei; Aphanizomenon flos-aquae.

People Use This For

Orally, blue-green algae products are used as a source of dietary protein, B-vitamins, and iron (14). They are also used orally for weight loss, oral leukoplakia (6), obstetric and gynecological disorders (14), attention deficit-hyperactivity disorder, premenstrual syndrome, diabetes, stimulating the immune system, stress, fatigue, anxiety, depression, improving memory, increasing energy and metabolism, lowering cholesterol, decreasing cardiovascular disease, wound healing, and for promoting digestion and bowel health (3532,3533).

Safety

POSSIBLY SAFE ...when non-contaminated, non-microcystin containing Spirulina species of blue-green algae are consumed orally (6). Some manufacturers grow Spirulina species in controlled environments, perform analytical safety testing, and claim their products are uncontaminated and safe (3534).
POSSIBLY UNSAFE ...when contaminated Spirulina species of blue-green algae are used orally. Spirulina species can be contaminated with microbes, heavy metals (including mercury, cadmium, lead, or arsenic), and radioactive

divalent and trivalent metal ions (6). Spirulina species grown in uncontrolled environments, including lakes and ponds, are more likely to be contaminated (3534). ...when Anabaena, Aphanizomenon, or Microcysitis species of blue-green algae are used orally. These types of blue-green algae often contain hepatotoxic microcystins (3534,3535,3536).

LIKELY UNSAFE ...when any microcystin-containing blue-green algae products are used orally; avoid using all untested blue-green algae products.

CHILDREN: LIKELY UNSAFE ...when any microcystin-containing blue-green algae products are used orally. Children are more sensitive to poisoning by microcystins produced by blue-green algae (3536).

PREGNANCY AND LACTATION: Insufficient reliable information available; avoid using.

Effectiveness

LIKELY EFFECTIVE ...when spirulina blue-green algae are used orally as a source of dietary protein and iron (6).

POSSIBLY EFFECTIVE ...when spirulina blue-green algae are taken orally for treating oral leukoplakia (6).

POSSIBLY INEFFECTIVE ...when spirulina blue-green algae are taken orally as a vitamin B12 supplement (6). ...when spirulina blue-green algae are taken orally for weight loss (6).

There is insufficient reliable information available about the effectiveness of non-spirulina blue-green algae.

Possible Mechanism of Action & Active Ingredients

Spirulina blue-green algae consists of approximately 65% crude protein, high concentrations of B vitamins, phenylalanine, and iron and other minerals (6). The B vitamins are thought to be analogs of vitamin B12 and nutritionally insignificant (6). The phenylalanine content is promoted as being responsible for reducing appetite and causing weight loss (6). The FDA reviewed this claim and found no evidence to support using blue-green algae for weight loss (6). The iron in spirulina blue-green algae has been found to be highly bioavailable in humans (6). As much as 1.5–2 mg of iron can be absorbed from a dose of 10 grams of blue-green algae (6). Evidence suggests that spirulina blue-green algae might enhance antibody production, reduce serum lipids, liver triglycerides, and gastric secretions (6). It might also protect against the effects of gamma radiation, enhance the regression of oral carcinoma, and have antiviral effects (6). The blue-green algae Aphanizomenon flos-aquae (AFA) may stimulate the immune system by increasing T lymphocytes, and B lymphocytes (2534). AFA contains 1.9-2.9 times less of the polyunsaturated fatty acid (PUFA) alpha-linolenic acid (LNA), and 32-44 times less linoleic acid than soybean oil. However, an animal study indicates that AFA-supplementation in animals with a PUFA-deficient diet may increase linoleic acid plasma levels to 67-71% of those found in animals consuming a soybean oil-supplemented diet. Furthermore, preliminary evidence suggests that an AFA-supplemented diet may be more effective than the soybean oil-supplemented diet at lowering triglycerides and total cholesterol (2535).

Researchers at the National Cancer Institute have isolated an antiviral protein, cyanovirin-N (CV-N), which might prove useful in treating human immunodeficiency virus (HIV) infection. Isolated from the blue green algae Nostoc ellipsosporum, CV-N binds irreversibly to sites on the viral envelope, inactivating HIV and inhibiting its entry into cells. CV-N has unique temperature (heat and cold) stability which might allow for its use in applications not typical for proteins. The researchers hypothesize that, attached to a solid matrix, CV-N might be used to adsorb and remove HIV from infected blood products. This unpublished research was presented at the Microbicides 2000 International Conference (1375).

Adverse Reactions Including Known Allergies

Adverse effects have not been reported for non-contaminated, non-microcystin-containing Spirulina species blue-green algae products. Microcystin-containing blue-green algae products can cause hepatotoxicity, jaundice, abdominal pain and distention, nausea, vomiting, weakness, excessive thirst, rapid and weak pulse, shock, and death (3535). Symptoms of poisoning usually occur 30 minutes to 24 hours after ingestion (3535). Children are more sensitive to micorcystin poisoning than adults (3536).

Possible Interactions with Herbs & Other Dietary Supplements

Insufficient reliable information available.

Possible Interactions with Drugs

No interactions are known to occur, and there is no known reason to expect a clinically significant interaction with blue-green algae.

Possible Interactions with Foods

No interactions are known to occur, and there is no known reason to expect a clinically significant interaction with blue-green algae.

Possible Interactions with Lab Tests

No interactions are known to occur, and there is no known reason to expect a clinically significant interaction with blue-green algae.

Possible Interactions with Diseases or Conditions

PHENYLKETONURIA: Theoretically, the phenylalanine content of Spirulina species blue-green algae products might exacerbate phenylketonuria (6); avoid Spirulina species blue-green algae products (6).

© Copyright 2000, Natural Medicines Comprehensive Database (209) 472-2244. For updated data, go to www.NaturalDatabase.com • 163

Typical Dosages & Routes of Administration that are Commonly Used

ORAL: The typical dose of spirulina blue-green algae is 3-5 grams daily before meals (6002). Some people mix one or two teaspoons of 100% spirulina blue-green algae powder in fruit juice or smoothies (5022). There is insufficient information available for dosing non-spirulina blue-green algae.

Comments

Blue-green algae are commonly found in tropical or subtropical alkaline waters that have a high-salt content (6002). The natural color of these algae can give bodies of water a dark-green appearance (6). Blue-green algae (cyanophyta) comprises thousands of species, including Spirulina species blue-green algae and non-Spirulina species blue-green algae (3532,3534,3536). Most commercial products contain Aphanizomenon flos-aquae, Spirulina maxima, or Spirulina platensis. Commercial Spirulina species blue-green algae are usually grown under controlled conditions while some non-Spirulina blue-green algae (Klamath blue-green algae and others) are grown in natural setting (lakes, etc.) where contamination and microcystin production is more likely (3536). Select blue-green algae products that have been tested to avoid products contaminated with heavy metals, microbes, or microcystins (3532,3534,3536). A study by Canadian health authorities found all non-Spirulina species blue-green algae products tested were contaminated with hepatotoxic microcystins, while none of the Spirulina species blue-green algae products tested were contaminated (3536). While blue-green algae products are promoted as an excellent source of dietary protein, they are no better than meat or milk and are estimated to cost more than 30 times as much as beef on a per gram basis (6).

BOG BILBERRY

This Product is Also Known As

None.
CAUTION: See separate listings for Bilberry fruit and Bilberry leaf.

Scientific Names

Vaccinium uliginosum.
Family: Ericaceae.

People Use This For

The dried, ripe fruit of bog bilberry is used for mucous membrane inflammation of the gastric and intestinal tract, for diarrhea, and for bladder complaints (18).

Safety

POSSIBLY UNSAFE ...when used orally in large amounts. Poisoning has been reported when individuals ingest fruit from fungus-infested plants (18).
There is insufficient reliable information available about the safety of dried bog bilberry fruit used in medicinal amounts.
PREGNANCY AND LACTATION: Insufficient reliable information available; avoid using.

Effectiveness

There is insufficient reliable information available about the effectiveness of bog bilberry.

Possible Mechanism of Action & Active Ingredients

The applicable part of bog bilberry is the dried, ripe fruit. The active constituents of bog bilberry are tannins, anthocyanoside, and flavonoids (18).

Adverse Reactions Including Known Allergies

Poisonings from the ingestion of large quantities of the bog bilberry fruit are rare and could have been due to contamination with a fungus, Sclerroyina megalospora (18). The symptoms of poisoning include queasiness, vomiting, states of intoxication, feelings of weakness, and visual disorders (18).

Possible Interactions with Herbs & Other Dietary Supplements

There is insufficient reliable information available.

Possible Interactions with Drugs

No interactions are known to occur, and there is no known reason to expect a clinically significant interaction with bog bilberry.

Possible Interactions with Foods

No interactions are known to occur, and there is no known reason to expect a clinically significant interaction with bog bilberry.

Possible Interactions with Lab Tests

No interactions are known to occur, and there is no known reason to expect a clinically significant interaction with bog bilberry.

Possible Interactions with Diseases or Conditions

No interactions are known to occur, and there is no known reason to expect a clinically significant interaction with bog bilberry.

Typical Dosages & Routes of Administration that are Commonly Used

ORAL: The usual dose of bog bilberry is one cup of the unsweetened tea once or twice daily [18]. The tea is prepared by steeping 2 heaping teaspoons of the dried, ripe fruit in 250 mL cold water for 10-12 hours and then straining.

Comments

Avoid confusion with bilberry fruit or bilberry leaf.

BOGBEAN

This Product is Also Known As

Buckbean, Marsh Trefoil, Menyanthes, Water Shamrock.

Scientific Names

Menyanthes trifoliata.
Family: Menyanthaceae.

People Use This For

Orally, bogbean is used for rheumatism, rheumatoid arthritis [4], loss of appetite, and dyspepsia [2].
In food manufacturing, bogbean is used as a flavoring agent [4].

Safety

LIKELY SAFE ...when used orally in amounts commonly found in foods. The Council of Europe lists bogbean as a natural food flavoring [4].
POSSIBLY SAFE ...when the leaf is used orally in medicinal amounts [12].
POSSIBLY UNSAFE ...when used orally in excessive amounts. Bogbean leaf preparations can irritate the GI tract [4].
PREGNANCY AND LACTATION: POSSIBLY UNSAFE ...due to the lack of toxicity information and its possible purgative action [4]; avoid using.

Effectiveness

POSSIBLY EFFECTIVE ...when taken orally as an appetite stimulant [2].
There is insufficient reliable information available about the effectiveness of bogbean for its other uses.

Possible Mechanism of Action & Active Ingredients

The applicable part of bogbean is the leaf. The bitter principles, or iridoids, can stimulate saliva and gastric juices [2,4]. Bogbean can have purgative actions [4]. An unidentified constituent has hemolytic activity [4].

Adverse Reactions Including Known Allergies

Excessive doses of bogbean can irritate the GI tract, and cause diarrhea, pain, nausea, and vomiting. Theoretically, it can cause bleeding [4].

Possible Interactions with Herbs & Other Dietary Supplements

HERBS WITH ANTICOAGULANT/ANTIPLATELET POTENTIAL: Concomitant use of herbs that have coumarin constituents or affect platelet aggregation could theoretically increase the risk of bleeding in some people. These herbs include: angelica, anise, arnica, asafoetida, boldo, capsicum, celery, chamomile, clove, danshen, fenugreek, feverfew, garlic, ginger, ginkgo, ginseng (Panax), horse chestnut, horseradish, licorice, meadowsweet, prickly ash, onion, papain, passionflower, poplar, quassia, red clover, turmeric, wild carrot, wild lettuce, willow, and others [4,19].

Possible Interactions with Drugs

ANTICOAGULANT, ANTIPLATELET DRUGS: Theoretically, bogbean can increase the risk of bleeding.

Possible Interactions with Foods

No interactions are known to occur, and there is no known reason to expect a clinically significant interaction with bogbean.

Possible Interactions with Lab Tests

No interactions are known to occur, and there is no known reason to expect a clinically significant interaction with bogbean.

Possible Interactions with Diseases or Conditions
DIARRHEA, DYSENTERY, COLITIS: Contraindicated (12).
PEOPLE AT RISK FOR BLEEDING: Theoretically, bogbean can increase bleeding risk.

Typical Dosages & Routes of Administration that are Commonly Used
ORAL: The typical dose of bogbean is 1-3 grams of the dried leaf three times daily or as a tea three times daily. The tea is prepared by steeping 1-3 grams of the dried leaf in 150 mL boiling water for 5-10 minutes and then straining (2,4). The common dose of the liquid extract (1:1 in 25% alcohol) is 1-2 mL three times daily (4). The tincture (1:5 in 45% alcohol) is usually given as 1-3 mL three times daily (4).

Comments
The bogbean fruit resembles a small bean and is commonly found in swamps or bogs, which is the reason for its name (6002).

BOIS DE ROSE OIL

This Product is Also Known As
Cayenne Rosewood Oil, Distilled Oil from Aniba Rosaeodora Wood, Rosewood Oil.

Scientific Names
Aniba rosaeodora.
Family: Lauraceae.

People Use This For
No medicinal uses are reported (11).
For food use, bois de rose oil is a flavoring.
In manufacturing, bois de rose oil is used in cosmetics (maximum use level 1.2% in perfumes).

Safety
LIKELY SAFE ...when taken orally in amounts contained in foods; Generally Recognized as Safe (GRAS) status in US (11). ...when used topically, reported to be nontoxic (11).
PREGNANCY AND LACTATION: Insufficient reliable information available.

Effectiveness
There is insufficient reliable information about the effectiveness of bois de rose oil.

Possible Mechanism of Action & Active Ingredients
The major constituent, linalool, is reported to have anticonvulsant activity in mice and rats, spasmolytic activity on isolated guinea pig ileum, antimicrobial properties, and weak tumor promoting properties in mice (11).

Adverse Reactions Including Known Allergies
None reported (11).

Possible Interactions with Herbs & Other Dietary Supplements
Insufficient reliable information available.

Possible Interactions with Drugs
No interactions are known to occur, and there is no known reason to expect a clinically significant interaction with bois de rose oil.

Possible Interactions with Foods
No interactions are known to occur, and there is no known reason to expect a clinically significant interaction with bois de rose oil.

Possible Interactions with Lab Tests
No interactions are known to occur, and there is no known reason to expect a clinically significant interaction with bois de rose oil.

Possible Interactions with Diseases or Conditions
No interactions are known to occur, and there is no known reason to expect a clinically significant interaction with bois de rose oil.

Typical Dosages & Routes of Administration that are Commonly Used
No typical dosage.

Comments
There is very little scientific information about this product. Our staff is continually analyzing the available information on natural medicines and will add data here as it becomes available.

BOLDO

This Product is Also Known As
Boldine, Boldoak Boldea, Boldo Folium, Boldus, Boldus Boldus.

Scientific Names
Peumus boldus.
Family: Monimiaceae.

People Use This For
Orally, boldo leaf is used for mild GI spasms, gallstones [11], rheumatism, cystitis, hepatic disease, and gonorrhea. It is also used as a diuretic, sedative, bile stimulant [4], and antiseptic [4].

Safety
LIKELY SAFE ...when consumed in the small amounts commonly found in food. Boldo is approved for use in alcoholic beverages with a maximum use level of 0.0002% [11].
LIKELY UNSAFE ...when taken excessively for oral medicinal purposes, because of the presence of the volatile oil (2.5% in leaf), which contains ascaridole [4]. If taken by mouth, ascaridole-free preparations should be used [2].
PREGNANCY AND LACTATION: UNSAFE ...when the volatile oil is used, due to ascaridole.

Effectiveness
POSSIBLY EFFECTIVE ...when taken orally as a cathartic or diuretic [4] and used for mild GI spasms and dyspepsia [2].
There is insufficient reliable information available about the effectiveness of boldo for its other uses.

Possible Mechanism of Action & Active Ingredients
The applicable part of boldo is the leaf. The alkaloidal constituents can be responsible for actions that include stimulating bile and bile flow, stimulating stomach function, and diuresis [4]. The diuretic and mild urinary antiseptic properties probably result from the irritant volatile oil [4].

Adverse Reactions Including Known Allergies
Boldo can cause convulsions when taken orally and can irritate the skin when applied externally [4].

Possible Interactions with Herbs & Other Dietary Supplements
HERBS WITH ANTICOAGULANT/ANTIPLATELET POTENTIAL: Concomitant use of herbs that have coumarin constituents or affect platelet aggregation could theoretically increase the risk of bleeding in some people. These herbs include: angelica, anise, arnica, asafoetida, bogbean, capsicum, celery, chamomile, clove, danshen, fenugreek, feverfew, garlic, ginger, ginkgo, ginseng (Panax), horse chestnut, horseradish, licorice, meadowsweet, prickly ash, onion, papain, passionflower, poplar, quassia, red clover, turmeric, wild carrot, wild lettuce, willow, and others [4,19].

Possible Interactions with Drugs
No interactions are known to occur, and there is no known reason to expect a clinically significant interaction with boldo.

Possible Interactions with Foods
No interactions are known to occur, and there is no known reason to expect a clinically significant interaction with boldo.

Possible Interactions with Lab Tests
No interactions are known to occur, and there is no known reason to expect a clinically significant interaction with boldo.

Possible Interactions with Diseases or Conditions
KIDNEY DISORDERS: Avoid boldo products which are not certified as ascaridole-free [4].
LIVER DISEASE: Contraindicated [8,12].
BILE DUCT OBSTRUCTION: Contraindicated [12].
GALLSTONES: Boldo should not be used for self-medication of gallstones, which requires monitoring [12].

Typical Dosages & Routes of Administration that are Commonly Used
ORAL: The typical dose of boldo is 60-200 mg of the dried leaf three times daily or as a tea three times a day. The tea is prepared by steeping 1 gram of the dried leaf in 150 mL boiling water for 5-10 minutes and then straining [2,4]. The common dose of the liquid extract (1:1 in 45% alcohol) is 0.1-0.3 mL three times daily [4]. The tincture (1:10 in 60% alcohol) is usually given as 0.5-2 mL three times daily [4]. The average daily dose of the boldo leaf by infusion is 3 grams [2].

Comments
Fossilized boldo leaves that are over thirteen thousand years old have been found in Chile with the imprints of human teeth on them [6002].

BONESET

This Product is Also Known As
Agueweed, Crosswort, Feverwort, Indian Sage, Sweating Plant, Teasel, Thoroughwort, Vegetable Antimony.
CAUTION: See separate listings for Gravel Root and Sage.

Scientific Names
Eupatorium perfoliatum.
Family: Asteraceae or Compositae.

People Use This For
Orally, boneset is used as an antipyretic (5,6), diuretic, laxative, emesis, and cathartic (6). Traditionally, boneset has been used to treat influenza (especially with aching muscles) (4), acute bronchitis (4), nasal inflammation (4), rheumatism (6), edema (6), dengue fever (6), pneumonia (6), as a stimulant (11), and a diaphoretic (4,5,11).

Safety
POSSIBLY UNSAFE ...when used orally. Large doses are both cathartic and emetic. Though the alkaloids have not been characterized, hepatotoxic unsaturated pyrrolizidine alkaloids are common in this genus (12).
PREGNANCY AND LACTATION: POSSIBLY UNSAFE; avoid using.

Effectiveness
POSSIBLY EFFECTIVE ...when taken orally as an immunostimulant and anti-inflammatory agent (4).
There is insufficient reliable information available about the effectiveness of boneset for its other uses.

Possible Mechanism of Action & Active Ingredients
The applicable parts of boneset are the dried leaf and flowering parts. Researchers think the sesquiterpene lactones may have immunostimulant activity (4).

Adverse Reactions Including Known Allergies
Boneset can cause an allergic reaction in individuals sensitive to the Asteraceae/Compositae family. Members of this family include ragweed, chrysanthemums, marigolds, daisies, and many other herbs.

Possible Interactions with Herbs & Other Dietary Supplements
Insufficient reliable information available.

Possible Interactions with Drugs
No interactions are known to occur, and there is no known reason to expect a clinically significant interaction with boneset.

Possible Interactions with Foods
No interactions are known to occur, and there is no known reason to expect a clinically significant interaction with boneset.

Possible Interactions with Lab Tests
No interactions are known to occur, and there is no known reason to expect a clinically significant interaction with boneset.

Possible Interactions with Diseases or Conditions
CROSS-ALLERGENICITY: Can cause an allergic reaction in individuals sensitive to the Asteraceae/Compositae family. Members of this family include ragweed, chrysanthemums, marigolds, daisies, and many other herbs.

Typical Dosages & Routes of Administration that are Commonly Used
ORAL: Drink 1 cup tea (steep 1-2 grams herb in 150 mL boiling water 5-10 minutes, strain) three times daily (4). Liquid extract (1:1 in 25% alcohol) 1-2 mL three times daily (4). Tincture: (1:5 in 45% alcohol) 1-4 mL three times daily (4).

Comments
Avoid confusion with gravel root (Eupatorium purpureum) also known as boneset. Snakeroot is a common name used for poisonous Eupatorium species (4).

BORAGE flower, dried above ground parts

This Product is Also Known As
Beebread, Bee Plant, Borago, Burrage, Common Borage, Common Bugloss, Cool Tankard, Ox's Tongue.
CAUTION: See separate listing for Borage Seed Oil.

Scientific Names
Borago officinalis.
Family: Boraginaceae.

People Use This For
Orally, borage is used for fever, cough, depression, arthritis, pain relief, phlebitis, and menopausal disorders. It is also used as an agent to restore the adrenal cortex (4), for "blood purification" and diuresis, as a preventative for inflammation of lungs and peritoneum, as an anti-inflammatory agent, a cardiac tonic, a sedative, to induce sweating, and to increase circulatory capacity (2).

Topically, borage is used as a poultice and as an emollient (11).

Historically, borage was used to promote "happiness and courage" (5), increase breast milk production (6), and to treat rheumatism, bronchitis, colds, and breast or facial cancers (11).

For food uses, borage is found in various products including preserved leaves (6), salads, and soups (4).

In manufacturing, borage is used in skin care products (11).

Safety
POSSIBLY SAFE ...when the above ground parts are used orally in food amounts, short-term (6).

LIKELY UNSAFE ...when used orally long-term in food amounts, as an herbal tea, or as a medicinal because they contain hepatotoxic pyrrolizidine alkaloids (4,12). Excessive doses or long-term use increases risk of adverse effects (2,4,12).

PREGNANCY AND LACTATION: LIKELY UNSAFE; avoid using (4,12).

Effectiveness
LIKELY INEFFECTIVE ...when used orally (2,6).

There is insufficient reliable information available about the effectiveness of the topical use of borage.

Possible Mechanism of Action & Active Ingredients
People think high tannin content gives borage astringent properties. The mucilage may contribute to reported expectorant effect. Malic acid and potassium nitrate may have diuretic effect (6). Gamma linolenic acid acts as a precursor to prostaglandin, particularly PGE1 (11). Borage contains variable amounts of toxic pyrrolizidine alkaloids which are organotoxic, hepatotoxic, and carcinogenic in animal experiments (2).

Adverse Reactions Including Known Allergies
Oral use of borage can cause constipation (5,6). The potential for hepatotoxicity (due to presence of pyrrolizidine alkaloids) increases with larger doses and longer periods of use (4,12).

Possible Interactions with Herbs & Other Dietary Supplements
EUCALYPTUS: Theoretically, concomitant use might increase the risk of unsaturated pyrrolizidine alkaloid toxicity due to enzyme induction by eucalyptus (19).

PYRROLIZIDINE ALKALOID-CONTAINING HERBS: Concomitant use is contraindicated due to the risk of additive toxicity. Herbs containing unsaturated pyrrolizidine alkaloids include: alkanna (12), borage (271), gravel root (4), hemp agrimony (271), hound's tongue (19), petasites (19), comfrey (271), coltsfoot, and the Senecio species plants; dusty miller (19), alpine ragwort (19), groundsel (271), golden ragwort (19), and tansy ragwort (271).

Possible Interactions with Drugs
PHENOTHIAZINES: Theoretically, based on reports from evening primrose oil (source of gamma linolenic acid), people treated with phenothiazines for schizophrenia may have increased risk of seizures (597,614).

Possible Interactions with Foods
No interactions are known to occur, and there is no known reason to expect a clinically significant interaction with borage flower and dried above ground parts.

Possible Interactions with Lab Tests
No interactions are known to occur, and there is no known reason to expect a clinically significant interaction with borage flower and dried above ground parts.

Possible Interactions with Diseases or Conditions
SCHIZOPHRENIA: May increase risk of seizures in people with schizophrenia treated with phenothiazines (597,614).

Typical Dosages & Routes of Administration that are Commonly Used
No typical dosage.

Comments
Borage is likely unsafe when used as a medicine; avoid using. Avoid confusion with borage seed oil.

BORAGE SEED OIL

This Product is Also Known As

Bugloss, Burage, Burrage, Huile De Bourrache, Starflower.
CAUTION: See separate listings for Borage flower, Black Currant Seed Oil, Evening Primrose Oil, Gamma Linolenic Acid, and Omega-6 Oils.

Scientific Names

Borago officinalis.
Family: Boraginaceae.

People Use This For

Orally, borage seed oil is used as a dietary source of the essential fatty acid gamma-linolenic acid (GLA) (4), for rheumatoid arthritis (1985), neurodermatitis (18), stress (4), atopic eczema, premenstrual syndrome, diabetes, alcoholism, inflammation, and for preventing heart disease and stroke (11).

Safety

POSSIBLY SAFE ...when used orally and appropriately. Only products that are labeled as unsaturated pyrrolizidine alkaloid (UPA) free should be used (3,214).
LIKELY UNSAFE ...when products containing UPAs are used orally, although borage seed oil is reported to contain only small amounts of UPAs (502). ...when therapeutic doses are used because UPA amounts may reach toxic levels (214). UPAs are associated with serious hepatic and possibly renal toxicity (3). The German Federal Health Agency limits consumption of toxic UPAs to not more than 1 mcg per day (3). Borage seed oil containing UPAs dosed at 1-2 grams per day might provide as much as 10 mcg of UPAs, which exceeds the German recommendation by 10 times (214).
PREGNANCY AND LACTATION: Insufficient reliable information available; avoid using.

Effectiveness

LIKELY EFFECTIVE ...when used orally as a supplemental dietary source of gamma-linolenic acid (GLA) (4,5). Borage seed oil provides 20-26% GLA (3). Borage seed oil was awarded a Canadian Drug Identification Number (DIN) as a GLA dietary supplement for essential fatty acid deficiency (11).
POSSIBLY EFFECTIVE ...when used orally in combination with analgesics or anti-inflammatory agents for improving symptoms of rheumatoid arthritis (1985). Two small-scale studies have suggested that borage seed oil might decrease symptoms of rheumatoid arthritis after 12-24 weeks of treatment in combination with conventional analgesics or anti-inflammatory agents (214). ...when used prophylactically for attenuating a cardiovascular reaction to stress (4,1985). In one small study, men taking borage seed oil for 28 days had a lower heart rate, lower blood pressure, and performed better when subjected to a stressful psychological test (4). ...when used orally for reducing symptoms of atopic dermatitis (3900).
There is insufficient reliable information available about the effectiveness of borage seed oil for its other uses.

Possible Mechanism of Action & Active Ingredients

Borage seed oil is the fatty oil of the seeds of Borago officinalis. Borage oil contains 20-26% of the essential fatty acid gamma-linolenic acid (GLA) (3), making it useful as a supplemental source of fatty acid. For inflammatory conditions such as rheumatoid arthritis and atopic dermatitis, the GLA constituent is thought to act as an anti-inflammatory. In humans, GLA is rapidly metabolized to dihomogammalinolenic acid, which is a precursor to prostaglandin E1 (PGE1). PGE1 has potent anti-inflammatory properties (214). The mechanism of borage seed oil for reducing the cardiac response to stress is not known (4). The GLA constituent of borage seed oil also lowers plasma triglycerides, increases high-density lipoprotein (HDL) levels, and prolongs bleeding time (1979). It has been theorized that low arachidonic acid levels in breast milk of atopic mothers might increase the risk for development of atopy in infants and that maternal supplementation with borage seed oil might increase arachidonic acid levels in breast milk. However, oral borage seed oil supplements failed to increase breast milk arachidonic acid concentrations in lactating, atopic women (6106). Some borage seed oil preparations contain toxic constituents known as unsaturated pyrrolizidine alkaloids (UPAs). The UPA constituents, including amabiline, are hepatotoxic even in minute amounts (3) and there are some reports of renal toxicity (12). Some UPAs have shown carcinogenic and mutagenic properties; however, the primary concern is veno-occlusive disease (12). Borage seed oil preparations are available that are UPA-free (3).

Adverse Reactions Including Known Allergies

Gamma linolenic acid can prolong bleeding time (1979).

Possible Interactions with Herbs & Other Dietary Supplements

HERBS WITH ANTICOAGULANT/ANTIPLATELET POTENTIAL: Concomitant use of herbs that have coumarin constituents or affect platelet aggregation could theoretically increase the risk of bleeding in some people. These herbs include: angelica, anise, arnica, asafoetida, bogbean, boldo, capsicum, celery, chamomile, clove, danshen, fenugreek, feverfew, garlic, ginger, ginkgo, ginseng (Panax), horse chestnut, horseradish, licorice, meadowsweet, prickly ash, onion, papain, passionflower, poplar, quassia, red clover, turmeric, wild carrot, wild lettuce, willow, and others (4,19).

EUCALYPTUS: Theoretically, unless the oil is certified pyrrolizidine-free, concomitant use with eucalyptus can increase the risk of unsaturated pyrrolizidine alkaloid toxicity due to enzyme induction by eucalyptus (19).
PYRROLIZIDINE ALKALOID-CONTAINING HERBS: Concomitant use is contraindicated due to the risk of additive toxicity. Herbs containing unsaturated pyrrolizidine alkaloids include: alkanna (12), borage (271), gravel root (4), hemp agrimony (271), hound's tongue (19), petasites (19), comfrey (271), coltsfoot, and the Senecio species plants; dusty miller (19), alpine ragwort (19), groundsel (271), golden ragwort (19), and tansy ragwort (271).

Possible Interactions with Drugs
PHENOTHIAZINES: Theoretically, concomitant use of the oil can increase the risk of seizures in people with schizophrenia treated with phenothiazines (4). This is based on reports involving evening primrose oil.
ANESTHESIA: Theoretically, concomitant use can increase the risk of seizures based on one case report of evening primrose oil (source of gamma linolenic acid) and possibly other drugs (613).
ANTICOAGULANTS, ANTIPLATELET DRUGS: Theoretically, concomitant use of the oil can increase the risk of bleeding (1979).

Possible Interactions with Foods
No interactions are known to occur, and there is no known reason to expect a clinically significant interaction with borage seed oil.

Possible Interactions with Lab Tests
HEART RATE: Borage seed oil might lower heart rate in individuals with stress-induced increases in heart rate (4).
BLOOD PRESSURE: Borage seed oil might lower systolic blood pressure and blood pressure readings in individuals with stress-induced increases in blood pressure (4).

Possible Interactions with Diseases or Conditions
SCHIZOPHRENIA: Theoretically, concomitant use of phenothiazines and borage seed oil can increase the risk of seizures in people with schizophrenia (4). This is based on reports of evening primrose oil, another source of gamma linolenic acid.
LIVER DISEASE: Unless certified pyrrolizidine alkaloid-free, the oil is contraindicated in liver disease due to its hepatotoxic potential (19).

Typical Dosages & Routes of Administration that are Commonly Used
ORAL: People typically use 1 gram of borage seed oil once or twice daily with meals (6006). For rheumatoid arthritis, studies have used either 1.1 or 1.4 grams borage seed oil daily (214,3900).

Comments
Some sources have suggested that borage seed oil could be used as an alternative to evening primrose oil because both are good sources of gamma-linolenic acid (GLA) (214).

BORON

This Product is Also Known As
None.

Scientific Names
Boron;B; atomic number 5.

People Use This For
Orally, boron is used for promoting bone health (941), treating osteoarthritis (941), as an aid for building muscle and increasing testosterone levels (944), and for enhancing cognitive function and fine motor skills (6,943).

Safety
LIKELY SAFE ...when used orally in trace amounts similar to amounts found in foods. The Recommended Daily Allowance (RDA) for boron is not established. Poisoning has occurred after ingestion of equivalent of 2.12 grams boron per day for 3-4 weeks (17).
PREGNANCY AND LACTATION: Insufficient reliable information available for supplemental use; avoid using.

Effectiveness
POSSIBLY EFFECTIVE ...for promoting bone health (941,945) and treating osteoarthritis (941). ...when used for improving cognitive function and fine motor skills in older people (943).
LIKELY INEFFECTIVE ...when used orally as a supplement for the purpose of building muscle or increasing testosterone levels (944).

Possible Mechanism of Action & Active Ingredients
Boron seems to be important in mineral metabolism and membrane function (943). Diets higher in boron seem to increase serum 17-beta-estradiol levels in postmenopausal women using estrogen replacement therapy (945).

Supplemental boron may increase serum estradiol levels in postmenopausal women (945) and healthy men (937). Boron together with exercise seems to result in lower serum magnesium levels (942) and modestly lower serum phosphorus concentrations. The lower serum phosphorus concentrations are diminished by exercise (940).

Adverse Reactions Including Known Allergies

Adverse reactions in doses below 10 mg per day (937) are unlikely. Large doses can result in acute poisoning. Children who have ingested large quantities have persistent nausea, vomiting, and diarrhea leading to acute dehydration, shock, and coma. Adults who have ingested very large quantities exhibit nausea, vomiting, diarrhea, epigastric pain, hematemesis and blue-green discoloration of feces and vomit (17). Symptoms in adults and children may also include skin erythema, desquamation, exfoliation, hyperexcitability, irritability, tremors, convulsions, weakness, lethargy, headaches, and depression (17).

Possible Interactions with Herbs & Other Dietary Supplements

Insufficient reliable information available.

Possible Interactions with Drugs

ESTROGENIC DRUGS: Concomitant administration may increase serum estrogen levels (945) (see Mechanism of Action).

Possible Interactions with Foods

No interactions are known to occur, and there is no known reason to expect a clinically significant interaction with boron.

Possible Interactions with Lab Tests

BONE MINERAL DENSITY (BMD): Supplemental boron might increase BMD and BMD measurements in young athletic females (942).
PHOSPHORUS: Supplemental boron might reduce serum phosphorus concentrations and test results in some individuals (942).

Possible Interactions with Diseases or Conditions

KIDNEY DISEASE, IMPAIRED KIDNEY FUNCTION: Theoretically, avoid supplements; boron appears largely excreted by kidneys (939).

Typical Dosages & Routes of Administration that are Commonly Used

ORAL: 3.25 mg boron per 2000 kcal/day is a diet high in boron. A diet low in boron would have 0.25 mg boron per 2000kcal/day (943). These dosages are dietary amounts. Supplements would have larger doses of boron.

Comments

There is evidence that boron is an essential nutrient for humans (945), although no RDA has been established. Dietary requirement estimated at approximately 1 mg per day and up to a safe dietary limit approximately 10 mg per day (945). Boron was used as a food preservative between 1870 and 1920, and during World Wars I and II (945). Some references include information about boric acid/borate when discussing boron; an oral dose of 0.3 gram/kg boric acid can be fatal (6).

BOVINE CARTILAGE

This Product is Also Known As

Antitumor Angiogenesis Factor (anti-TAF), Bovine Tracheal Cartilage (BTC), Catrix, Catrix-S, Processed Bovine Cartilage, Psoriacin, Psoriacin-T, Rumalon.

Scientific Names

None.

People Use This For

Orally, bovine cartilage is used for rheumatoid arthritis (2016), osteoarthritis (2016,2017), ulcerative colitis (2009,2017), scleroderma (2017), psoriasis, allergic reactions caused by chemical toxins (2017), herpes infection (2017), glioblastoma multiforme, and cancer (2010).
Topically, bovine cartilage is used for non-healing ulcerated wounds (2009), moist lesions including pruritus ani, external hemorrhoids, acne, poison oak or poison ivy dermatitis (2009), mandibular alveolitis (dry socket) (2009), and psoriasis (2009).
Rectally, bovine cartilage is used for internal hemorrhoids and fissure-in-ano (2009).
Subcutaneously, bovine cartilage is used for osteoarthritis, rheumatoid arthritis, psoriasis, ulcerative colitis, regional enteritis, progressive systemic sclerosis (2009), glioblastoma multiforme (2010), inoperable squamous cancer of the nose (2010), and cancers of the pancreas, lung, ovary, rectum, prostate, cervix, and thyroid (2010).

Safety

POSSIBLY SAFE ...when used orally. Up to 20 kg total have been used without evidence of toxicity (2010). Up to 40 grams per week and 300 grams total have been injected subcutaneously without evidence of toxicity.
PREGNANCY AND LACTATION: Insufficient reliable information available; avoid using.

Effectiveness

POSSIBLY EFFECTIVE ...when used topically for pruritus ani, poison oak and poison ivy dermatitis, acne, mandibular alveolitis, and psoriasis (2009). ...when used rectally for hemorrhoids and fissure-in-ano (2009). ...when used subcutaneously for osteoarthritis, rheumatoid arthritis, and psoriasis (2009).
There is insufficient reliable information available about the effectiveness of bovine cartilage for its other uses.

Possible Mechanism of Action & Active Ingredients

Researchers theorize that bovine cartilage provides the needed biochemical components to support resynthesis of cartilage in individuals with osteoarthritis (2009). Bovine cartilage is also thought to have anti-inflammatory, immunoregulatory, hygroscopic-drying, and wound-healing activity (2009). Churning symptoms (appearance of new papules as the original lesions fade) may occur for 3-6 weeks during psoriasis treatment. These are thought to result from release of "psoriagens" from present lesions. Eventually, "psoriagens" are excreted or metabolized, resulting in symptomatic improvement (2009).

Adverse Reactions Including Known Allergies

Taken orally, bovine cartilage can cause osmotic diarrhea (2009), nausea, and scrotal edema (2019). When used subcutaneously, bovine cartilage might initially cause local redness, swelling, and itching (2010); the appearance of new psoriatic papules (2009); or nephrotic syndrome (2011). Bovine cartilage can cause local allergic reaction (2010).

Possible Interactions with Herbs & Other Dietary Supplements

Insufficient reliable information available.

Possible Interactions with Drugs

No interactions are known to occur, and there is no known reason to expect a clinically significant interaction with bovine cartilage.

Possible Interactions with Foods

No interactions are known to occur, and there is no known reason to expect a clinically significant interaction with bovine cartilage.

Possible Interactions with Lab Tests

No interactions are known to occur, and there is no known reason to expect a clinically significant interaction with bovine cartilage.

Possible Interactions with Diseases or Conditions

No interactions are known to occur, and there is no known reason to expect a clinically significant interaction with bovine cartilage.

Typical Dosages & Routes of Administration that are Commonly Used

ORAL: Ulcerative colitis, 3 grams four times daily (2009). Cancer- typical amount for maintenance following parenteral loading phase, 3 grams every 8 hours (or 9 grams per day in at least two divided amounts), up to 20 kg during a complete course of treatment (2010).
TOPICAL: Pruritus ani, 5% cream applied two or more times daily, with resolution expected in 3 days (2009). Poison ivy/oak dermatitis, 5% cream applied every two hours initially and less frequently as the itching is controlled, with resolution in 1-2 weeks (2009). Acne, 5% cream applied at least twice daily after washing (2009). Mandibular alveolitis, powdered bovine cartilage mixed with saline to form a paste, packed into the dry socket following tooth extraction (2009). Psoriasis, parenteral therapy followed by 5% ointment applied two to three times daily after bathing (2009); bovine cartilage ointment with 0.1% coal tar for elevated, dry, horny lesions or without coal tar for smooth and red skin after initial sloughing has been achieved (2009).
RECTAL: 2.2 grams in the form of a 2% suppository administered at least three times daily with dioctyl sodium sulfosuccinate (DSS) 100 mg twice daily orally as a stool softener (2009).
SUBCUTANEOUS (SC): Bovine cartilage solution (diluted 1:10 with 1% lidocaine to alleviate discomfort) is reportedly used in a concentration 50 mg/mL in humans (2009,2010). In general, 1.25-2.5 grams (25-50 mL) slowly injected per site with an 18-gauge needle for total of 5 grams per treatment, given weekly or biweekly, to a total of 25 grams for most uses; exceptions are osteoarthritis up to 40 grams, psoriasis up to 75 grams, and cancer 100-300 grams (2009,2010). Boosters of 2.5 grams (50 mL) are administered every 3-4 weeks as needed (2009,2010). Potential sites of administration include the flanks, anterior thorax, abdomen, or anterior thighs, where subcutaneous space is readily distensible (2009,2010). Initial local allergic reaction may be prevented by limiting the first treatment to 2.5 grams, and giving diphenhydramine 25 mg orally for the first four treatments (2010).

Comments

Catrix is a name which refers to activated acid-pepsin-digested bovine tracheal cartilage of calf origin (2009).

BOVINE COLOSTRUM

This Product is Also Known As
Bovine Immunoglobulin, Colostrum, Cow Milk Colostrum, Hyperimmune Bovine Colostrum.

Scientific Names
None.

People Use This For
Orally, bovine colostrum is used for stimulating the immune system, healing injuries, repairing nervous system damage, burning fat, building lean muscle, increasing stamina and vitality, elevating mood and sense of well being, slowing and reversing aging, and as an antibacterial and antifungal agent (4902). Oral hyperimmune bovine colostrum is also used in treating AIDS-related diarrhea (FDA Orphan Drug Status) (14), diarrhea associated with graft versus host disease following bone marrow transplant (4907), and rotavirus diarrhea in children (4903,4904,4909).

Safety
LIKELY SAFE ...when used orally and appropriately. There are no reports of significant toxicity in multiple human trials (4901,4903,4904,4905,4906,4907,4908,4909).
PREGNANCY AND LACTATION: Insufficient reliable information available; avoid using.

Effectiveness
POSSIBLY EFFECTIVE ...when used orally for treating infectious diarrhea in people with HIV/AIDS (4905,4906,4907,4908). Hyperimmune bovine colostrum has FDA orphan status for AIDS-related diarrhea (14). ...when used orally for infectious diarrhea associated with graft versus host disease following bone marrow transplant (4907). ...when used orally for diarrhea associated with rotavirus in children (4903,4904,4909). ...when used orally for treating diarrhea due to enterotoxigenic Escherichia coli (2067,2068,2069) or Shigella flexneri (2070). Most clinical trials have used colostrum from pregnant cows which have been immunized against specific pathogens. The hyperimmune colostrum provides high antibody titers against organisms for which the cow has been immunized (4905).
There is insufficient reliable information available about the effectiveness of bovine colostrum for its other uses.

Possible Mechanism of Action & Active Ingredients
Colostrum is the milky fluid produced by mammals within the first few days after giving birth. Most nutritional colostrum preparations come from cows (3567). Bovine colostrum contains proteins, carbohydrates, fat, vitamins, minerals, and immunoglobulin A (IgA) and immunoglobulin G (IgG) in concentrations approximately 100 times higher than dairy milk (4901). Because of the antibody content, bovine colostrum was thought to offer passive immunotherapy to people with enteric infections. However, bovine colostrum contains only low concentrations of antibodies against enteric pathogens and does not provide high enough titers to prevent disease. Hyperimmune bovine colostrum can be produced by immunizing pregnant cows against specific pathogens (e.g. cryptosporidium or rotavirus) resulting in increased specific colostrum antibody titers (4903). Hyperimmune bovine colostrum has been primarily used in clinical trials. However, the small amounts of antibodies that have been recovered from people who ingested hyperimmune colostrum were nonreactive (2072). Bovine colostrum also contains insulin-like growth factors (IGF), and increases serum insulin-like growth factor I (IGF-I) and insulin in athletes (4901). Bovine colostrum reduces indomethacin-induced gastrointestinal injury in rats and addition of colostrum to drinking water prevents experimental small intestinal injury in mice (4911). Bovine colostrum promotes small intestinal growth in newborn piglets (4901). The phosphatidylethanolamine in hyperimmune bovine colostrum may prevent Helicobacter pylori from binding to the gastric mucosa (2065). The effectiveness of hyperimmune bovine colostrum may decrease when it is taken with a meal (2070), possibly due to stomach acid and digestive enzymes (2071).

Adverse Reactions Including Known Allergies
Orally, bovine colostrum has caused nausea and vomiting in an individual with HIV-related cryptosporidiosis. Elevated liver function tests and decreased serum hematocrit have also been reported in HIV patients treated for infectious diarrhea (4905). It may cause allergic reaction in individuals allergic to bovine milk products.

Possible Interactions with Herbs & Other Dietary Supplements
Insufficient reliable information available.

Possible Interactions with Drugs
No interactions are known to occur, and there is no known reason to expect a clinically significant interaction with bovine colostrum.

Possible Interactions with Foods
MEALS: Taking hyperimmune bovine colostrum with food may decrease antibody activity due to the increase in stomach acid and digestive enzyme secretion (2070,2071,2072).

Possible Interactions with Lab Tests
No interactions are known to occur, and there is no known reason to expect a clinically significant interaction with bovine colostrum.

Possible Interactions with Diseases or Conditions
BOVINE MILK ALLERGY: Avoid using.

Typical Dosages & Routes of Administration that are Commonly Used
ORAL: For enhanced athletic training, 125 mL colostrum whey product twice daily has been used. However, this product is not available in the U.S. (4901). For AIDS-related Cryptosporidium parvum diarrhea, 10 grams powder four times daily for 21-days has been used (4905). For AIDS-related cryptosporidial and other infectious diarrhea, 10-20 grams daily for 10 days has been used (4906). For graft versus host disease following bone marrow transplant, 10 grams per day for 10 days has been used (4907). For rotavirus diarrhea in children10 grams, equivalent to 3.6 grams antirotavirus antibodies, per day for 4 days has been used (4903).100 ml four times per day for 4-days has also been used (4904).

Comments
Bovine colostrum is the milk secreted by cows during the first few days after calving (4901). Hyperimmune bovine colostrum is produced by cows immunized against specific pathogens. Bovine colostrum is not on the banned drug list of the International Olympic Committee (4901). Unpublished information indicates that micro-organisms, such as Lyme disease spirochete and human immunodeficiency virus (HIV), can pass from mother to nursing baby via colostrum (4910). Whether micro-organisms can be passed to humans via pasteurized animal colostrum is unknown.

BOXWOOD

This Product is Also Known As
Bush Tree, Dudgeon.

Scientific Names
Buxus sempervirens.
Family: Buxaceae.

People Use This For
Historically, boxwood was used orally for arthritis and as a blood detoxifying agent (18).

Safety
POSSIBLY UNSAFE ...when the leaf is used topically, boxwood can cause contact dermatitis, particularly when the fresh plant is used (18).
LIKELY UNSAFE ...when used orally (12,18). Can cause seizures, signs of paralysis and death by asphyxiation (18). PREGNANCY AND LACTATION: POSSIBLY UNSAFE ...when used topically; avoid using. LIKELY UNSAFE ...contraindicated for oral use; avoid using.

Effectiveness
There is insufficient reliable information about the effectiveness of boxwood.

Possible Mechanism of Action & Active Ingredients
The applicable part of boxwood is the leaf. There is insufficient reliable information available about the possible mechanism of action and active constituents of boxwood. However, boxwood leaf is toxic. Toxicity can include vomiting and diarrhea as well as death by asphyxiation (18).

Adverse Reactions Including Known Allergies
Boxwood can cause contact dermatitis. Ingestion of toxic doses leads to vomiting, diarrhea, severe clonic spasms. This is followed by paralysis and death secondary to asphyxiation (18).

Possible Interactions with Herbs & Other Dietary Supplements
Insufficient reliable information available.

Possible Interactions with Drugs
PHENOTHIAZINES AND ANALEPTICS: Contraindicated during overdoses with boxwood (18).

Possible Interactions with Foods
No interactions are known to occur, and there is no known reason to expect a clinically significant interaction with boxwood.

Possible Interactions with Lab Tests
No interactions are known to occur, and there is no known reason to expect a clinically significant interaction with boxwood.

Possible Interactions with Diseases or Conditions
No interactions are known to occur, and there is no known reason to expect a clinically significant interaction with boxwood.

Typical Dosages & Routes of Administration that are Commonly Used
No typical dosage.

Comments
The medicinal use of boxwood is obsolete (18). Rarely, boxwood is a contaminant of uva ursi (12).

BRAHMI

This Product is Also Known As
Jalanimba, Jalnaveri, Sambrani Chettu, Thyme-Leave Gratiola.

Scientific Names
Bacopa monnieri, synonym Bacopa monniera; Herpestis monniera; Moniera cuneifolia.
Family: Scrophulariaceae.

People Use This For
Orally, brahmi is used to aid learning (6).
Traditionally, brahmi has been used orally for treating asthma, backache, hoarseness, insanity, epilepsy, rheumatism, sexual dysfunction in both men and women, as a nerve tonic, cardiotonic, and a diuretic (6,2085).

Safety
There is insufficient reliable information available about the safety of brahmi.
Pregnancy and Lactation: Insufficient reliable information available; avoid using.

Effectiveness
There is insufficient reliable information available about the effectiveness of brahmi.

Possible Mechanism of Action & Active Ingredients
Pharmacological activity is attributed to the saponin bacoside and bacopasaponin constituents (6). Some evidence suggests that an extract containing saponins has tranquilizing effects without interfering with coordination (6). Other evidence suggests that purified bacosides A and B may facilitate learning ability and cognitive performance in controlled settings (6). Bacosine may have analgesic effects by acting on the opioid pathway (6). Further evidence suggests that an ethanolic extract can relax smooth muscle in arteries, the trachea and the small intestine (6).

Adverse Reactions Including Known Allergies
None reported.

Possible Interactions with Herbs & Other Dietary Supplements
Insufficient reliable information available.

Possible Interactions with Drugs
PHENOTHIAZINES: Theoretically, concomitant use of brahmi may potentiate chlorpromazine's effects (6).

Possible Interactions with Foods
No interactions are known to occur, and there is no known reason to expect a clinically significant interaction with brahmi.

Possible Interactions with Lab Tests
No interactions are known to occur, and there is no known reason to expect a clinically significant interaction with brahmi.

Possible Interactions with Diseases or Conditions
No interactions are known to occur, and there is no known reason to expect a clinically significant interaction with brahmi.

Typical Dosages & Routes of Administration that are Commonly Used
No typical dosage.

Comments
Brahmi is a well-known herb in India and is frequently used in Ayurvedic herbal preparations. Centella asiatica (gotu kola) and Merremia gangetica have also been referred to by the name "bramhi", but most authorities associate brahmi with Bacopa monnieri (6).

BRANCHED-CHAIN AMINO ACIDS

This Product is Also Known As
BCAAs, Branched Chain Amino Acids, Isoleucine, Leucine, L-Isoleucine, L-Leucine, L-Valine, Valine.

Scientific Names
2-amino-3-methylvaleric acid; 2-amino-4-methylvaleric acid; 2-amino-3-methylbutanoic acid.

People Use This For
Orally, people use branched-chain amino acids to enhance exercise performance, reduce protein and muscle breakdown during intense exercise (692,694), for amyotrophic lateral sclerosis (ALS, Lou Gehrig's disease) (678), latent portosystemic encephalopathy (684,685), and chronic hepatic encephalopathy (690).
Intravenously, people use branched-chain amino acids are used for acute hepatic encephalopathy (686), in conditions of high metabolic stress due to severe trauma or sepsis (266).

Safety
LIKELY SAFE …when used appropriately as an FDA-approved injectable product (15).
There is insufficient reliable information available about the safety of oral use in healthy individuals.
PREGNANCY AND LACTATION: Insufficient reliable information available; avoid using.

Effectiveness
LIKELY EFFECTIVE …when used orally for long-term treatment of latent portosystemic encephalopathy (684,685).
POSSIBLY EFFECTIVE …when used for chronic hepatic encephalopathy (690). …when used for reducing muscle breakdown during exercise (694), but not for enhancing exercise performance (692).
LIKELY INEFFECTIVE …when used for amyotrophic lateral sclerosis (ALS). It is commonly believed that branched-chain amino acids are effective for ALS because early research reported this benefit. More recent studies show that there is no benefit, and occasionally there can be a possible detriment caused by using branched-chain amino acids (679,680,681).
There is insufficient reliable information available for the effectiveness of branched chain amino acids used for acute hepatic encephalopathy; use is still controversial (686,687,688,689,4274).

Possible Mechanism of Action & Active Ingredients
The oral administration of branched-chain amino acids before exercises increases serum ammonia levels during exercise (693,694) and decreases muscle breakdown (694).

Adverse Reactions Including Known Allergies
Taken orally there has been one case report of hepatic encephalopathy in a chronic alcoholic, resolved when dietary BCAAs discontinued, and occurred again with rechallenge (691). Increased mortality reported in one study using branched chain amino acids in the treatment of amyotrophic lateral sclerosis (ALS) (679).

Possible Interactions with Herbs & Other Dietary Supplements
Insufficient reliable information available.

Possible Interactions with Drugs
No interactions are known to occur, and there is no known reason to expect a clinically significant interaction with branched-chain amino acids.

Possible Interactions with Foods
No interactions are known to occur, and there is no known reason to expect a clinically significant interaction with branched-chain amino acids.

Possible Interactions with Lab Tests
No interactions are known to occur, and there is no known reason to expect a clinically significant interaction with branched-chain amino acids.

Possible Interactions with Diseases or Conditions
AMYOTROPHIC LATERAL SCLEROSIS (ALS): The use of branched-chain amino acids is associated with increased mortality (679).
CHRONIC ALCOHOLISM: Dietary use may cause hepatic encephalopathy (691).

Typical Dosages & Routes of Administration that are Commonly Used
ORAL: One study of chronic hepatic encephalopathy used 240 mg/kg/day (690). One study of latent portosystemic encephalopathy used 250 mg/kg/day (685).
INTRAVENOUS (IV): A typical dose is 80-120 grams per day (266).

Comments
None.

BREWER'S YEAST

This Product is Also Known As
Brewers Yeast, Faex Medicinalis, Levure De Biere, Medicinal Yeast.
CAUTION: See separate listing for Brewer's Yeast (Hansen CBS 5926).

Scientific Names
Saccharomyces cerevisiae.
Family: Saccharomycetaceae, Candida utilis, or Cryptococcaceae.

People Use This For
Orally, brewer's yeast is used for diarrhea, loss of appetite, chronic acne, furunculosis [2], and high chromium type diabetes [6003]. It has also been used as a source of B vitamins and protein [215].

Safety
POSSIBLY SAFE ...when used orally and appropriately, short-term.
There is insufficient reliable information available about the safety of the long-term use of brewer's yeast [2].
CHILDREN: POSSIBLY SAFE ...when used orally and appropriately. However, diarrhea should be evaluated by a medical professional before using brewer's yeast [2].
PREGNANCY AND LACTATION: Insufficient reliable information available; avoid using.

Effectiveness
There is insufficient reliable information available about the effectiveness of brewer's yeast.

Possible Mechanism of Action & Active Ingredients
Brewer's yeast can have some action against C. difficile and enterotoxic E. coli. It reduces water and electrolyte influx into the intestines stimulated by the C. vibrio toxin. Brewer's yeast can increase the activity of intestinal disaccharidases, saccharidases, maltase, and lactase to alleviate diarrhea symptoms [2]. It can also increase insulin releases [6004].

Adverse Reactions Including Known Allergies
Brewer's yeast can cause migraine-like headaches in sensitive individuals, intestinal discomfort, and flatulence [2]. Allergic reactions to brewer's yeast can occur in hypersensitive individuals and include itching, urticaria, local or general exanthemas, and Quincke's edema [2].

Possible Interactions with Herbs & Other Dietary Supplements
Insufficient reliable information available.

Possible Interactions with Drugs
MONOAMINE OXIDASE INHIBITORS (MAOIs): Brewer's yeast is contraindicated, because concomitant use can increase blood pressure [2].
ANTIMYCOTIC DRUGS can reduce yeast activity [2].

Possible Interactions with Foods
No interactions are known to occur, and there is no known reason to expect a clinically significant interaction with brewer's yeast.

Possible Interactions with Lab Tests
ANTIMICROBIAL TESTS: Brewer's yeast can confound results. Report the use of brewer's yeast to the lab [2].

Possible Interactions with Diseases or Conditions
No interactions are known to occur, and there is no known reason to expect a clinically significant interaction with brewer's yeast.

Typical Dosages & Routes of Administration that are Commonly Used
ORAL: The typical dose is 6 grams of brewer's yeast per day [2].

Comments
Brewer's yeast is obtained as a by-product from the brewing of beer made from an extract of grains and hops. Avoid confusion with brewer's yeast (Hansen CBS 5926).

BREWER'S YEAST (HANSEN CBS 5926)

This Product is Also Known As
Brewers Yeast Hansen CBS 5926, Probiotic, Saccharomyces cerevisiae Hansen CBS 5926.
CAUTION: See separate listings for Bifidobacterium Bifidum, Lactobacillus Acidophilus, Lactobacillus GG, Saccharomyces Boulardii, and Yogurt.

Scientific Names
Saccharomyces cerevisiae Hansen CBS 5926.
Family: Saccharomycetaceae.

People Use This For
Orally, brewer's yeast (Hansen CBS 5926) is used for prevention and treatment of acute diarrhea, traveler's diarrhea, diarrhea associated with tube feedings, and as an adjuvant treatment for chronic acne (2).

Safety
POSSIBLY SAFE ...when used orally and appropriately, short-term.
There is insufficient reliable information available about the safety of the long-term use of brewer's yeast (Hansen CBS 5926) (2).
CHILDREN: POSSIBLY SAFE ...when used orally and appropriately. However, diarrhea should be evaluated by a medical professional before using brewer's yeast (2).
PREGNANCY AND LACTATION: Insufficient reliable information available; avoid using.

Effectiveness
POSSIBLY EFFECTIVE ...when taken orally for symptomatic relief of acute diarrhea, prophylactic and symptomatic treatment of diarrhea during travel, diarrhea during tube feeding, and as an adjuvant treatment for chronic forms of acne (2).

Possible Mechanism of Action & Active Ingredients
Brewer's yeast can have some action against Clostridium difficile and enterotoxic E. coli. It can reduce water and electrolyte influx into the intestines stimulated by the Vibrio cholera toxin. Brewer's yeast can increase the activity of intestinal disaccharidases, saccharidases, maltase, and lactase to alleviate diarrhea symptoms (2).

Adverse Reactions Including Known Allergies
Brewer's yeast can cause flatulence. Symptoms of intolerance to brewer's yeast include itching, urticaria, local or general exanthemas (skin eruptions), and Quincke's edema (2).

Possible Interactions with Herbs & Other Dietary Supplements
Insufficient reliable information available.

Possible Interactions with Drugs
MONOAMINE OXIDASE INHIBITORS (MAOIs): Brewer's yeast is contraindicated, because concomitant use can cause increased blood pressure (2).
ANTIFUNGAL DRUGS reduce the activity of brewer's yeast (2).

Possible Interactions with Foods
No interactions are known to occur, and there is no known reason to expect a clinically significant interaction with brewer's yeast (Hansen CBS 5926).

Possible Interactions with Lab Tests
STOOL TESTS FOR MICROBES: Report the use of brewer's yeast to the lab, because it can confound antimicrobial tests on stool samples, resulting in false positive results (2).

Possible Interactions with Diseases or Conditions
YEAST ALLERGY: Contraindicated (2).

Typical Dosages & Routes of Administration that are Commonly Used
ORAL: For prevention of traveler's diarrhea in adults and children older than two years, the typical dose of brewer's yeast is 250-500 mg daily starting five days before the trip (2). For the treatment of diarrhea, the usual dose is 250-500 mg daily, continued for several days after the diarrhea has stopped (2). For diarrhea associated with tube feedings, add 500 mg of brewer's yeast to each liter of nutrient preparation (2). For acne, the typical dose is 750 mg per day (2).

Comments
Avoid confusion with brewer's yeast. Hansen CBS 5926 is a specifically standardized product.

BROMELAIN

This Product is Also Known As
Bromelains, Bromelainum, Bromelin, Plant Protease Concentrate.
CAUTION: See separate listing for Papain.

Scientific Names
Pineapple: Ananas comosus, synonym Ananas sativus.
Family: Bromeliaceae.

People Use This For

Orally, bromelain is used for acute postoperative and post-traumatic conditions of swelling (960), especially of the nasal and paranasal sinuses (2). It is also used orally for burn debridement, anti-inflammatory action, prevention of epinephrine-induced pulmonary edema, smooth muscle relaxation, stimulation of muscle contractions, inhibition of blood platelet aggregation, enhanced antibiotic absorption, cancer prevention, shortening of labor, and enhanced excretion of fat (11). Bromelain is also used for mild ulcerative colitis (6253).

In combination with trypsin and rutin, bromelain is used orally for osteoarthritis (6252).

Safety

LIKELY SAFE ...when taken orally in appropriate amounts unless allergic to pineapple or bromelain (2).
PREGNANCY AND LACTATION: Insufficient reliable information available (2); avoid using.

Effectiveness

POSSIBLY EFFECTIVE ...when taken orally for treating acute postoperative and post-traumatic conditions of swelling (960), especially of the nasal and paranasal sinuses (2). ...when taken orally in combination with trypsin and rutin for treating osteoarthritis (6252). In a double-blind trial, 73 patients with painful osteoarthritis of the knee were randomly assigned the combination enzyme product (Phlogenzym) or diclofenac (Voltaren) 50 mg three times daily during the first week and then twice daily in weeks 2 and 3. The enzyme product was similar to diclofenac in relieving pain and improving knee function (6252).

POSSIBLY INEFFECTIVE ...when taken orally for reducing swelling after oral surgery (957).

There is insufficient reliable information available about the effectiveness of bromelain for its other uses. However, two case reports indicate improvement of ulcerative colitis symptoms in people with persistent disease despite standard therapy (6253).

Possible Mechanism of Action & Active Ingredients

The observed effects of bromelain are due to an enzyme constituent that causes the release of a kinin, which stimulates the production of prostaglandin E1-like compounds (11). A polyenzyme preparation containing bromelain can increase the release of reactive oxygen species by polymorphonuclear neutrophils in healthy people (962).

Adverse Reactions Including Known Allergies

Taken orally, bromelain can cause GI disturbances or diarrhea. Allergic reactions to bromelain can occur (2) and include a cross-allergenicity between wheat flour and bromelain (959).

Possible Interactions with Herbs & Other Dietary Supplements

ZINC, an oxidizing agent, inhibits bromelain activity (11).
MAGNESIUM is a reducing agent and activates bromelain (11).
HERBS THAT AFFECT BLEEDING: Theoretically, bromelain can increase the risk of bleeding when used concomitantly with herbs that have anticoagulant or antiplatelet potential (2), including alfalfa, angelica, aniseed, arnica, asafoetida, celery, chamomile, clove, fenugreek, feverfew, fucus, garlic, ginger, horse chestnut, licorice, meadowsweet, poplar, northern and southern prickly ash, quassia, red clover, and willow (4).

Possible Interactions with Drugs

ANTIBIOTICS: Concomitant use might improve antibiotic response (19).
ANTICOAGULANT/ANTIPLATELET DRUGS: Theoretically, concomitant administration can increase effects and adverse effects (2).
5-FLUOROURACIL AND VINCRISTINE: Concomitant use can improve efficacy of the chemotherapy agents due to antitumor and fibrinolytic activity of bromelain (19).
TETRACYCLINES: Concomitant therapy increases plasma and urine tetracycline levels (2).

Possible Interactions with Foods

POTATO PROTEIN AND SOYBEAN can inhibit bromelain activity (958,961).

Possible Interactions with Lab Tests

No interactions are known to occur, and there is no known reason to expect a clinically significant interaction with bromelain.

Possible Interactions with Diseases or Conditions

No interactions are known to occur, and there is no known reason to expect a clinically significant interaction with bromelain.

Typical Dosages & Routes of Administration that are Commonly Used

ORAL: The typical dose of bromelain is 80-320 mg (200-800 FIP units) in two or three doses per day for eight to ten days (2). The administration of bromelain can be prolonged longer than ten days if needed (2). For osteoarthritis, a combination enzyme product (Phlogenzym), which contains rutin 100 mg, trypsin 48 mg, and bromelain 90 mg, was given 2 tablets 3 times daily (6252).

Comments

Proteolytic enzyme isolated from the juice of pineapples (Ananas comosus).

BROOKLIME

This Product is Also Known As
Beccabunga, Mouth-Smart, Neckweed, Speedwell, Water Pimpernel, Water Purslane.
CAUTION: See separate listings for Black Root (Leptandra virginica), and Veronica (Veronica officinalis), which are both known as Speedwell.

Scientific Names
Veronica beccabunga.

People Use This For
Orally, brooklime is used for lessening the elimination of urine (2), constipation, liver complaints, dysentery, lung infection, and bleeding gums (18).

Safety
There is insufficient reliable information available about the safety of brooklime.
Pregnancy and Lactation: Insufficient reliable information available; avoid using.

Effectiveness
There is insufficient reliable information available about the effectiveness of brooklime.

Possible Mechanism of Action & Active Ingredients
Brooklime appears to have a diuretic effect (18).

Adverse Reactions Including Known Allergies
None reported.

Possible Interactions with Herbs & Other Dietary Supplements
Insufficient reliable information available.

Possible Interactions with Drugs
No interactions are known to occur, and there is no known reason to expect a clinically significant interaction with brooklime.

Possible Interactions with Foods
No interactions are known to occur, and there is no known reason to expect a clinically significant interaction with brooklime.

Possible Interactions with Lab Tests
No interactions are known to occur, and there is no known reason to expect a clinically significant interaction with brooklime.

Possible Interactions with Diseases or Conditions
No interactions are known to occur, and there is no known reason to expect a clinically significant interaction with brooklime.

Typical Dosages & Routes of Administration that are Commonly Used
ORAL: People typically use from 1 teaspoon to 3 tablespoons of brooklime plant juice 3 times daily. The juice is sometimes mixed in milk (5263).

Comments
Avoid confusion with black root (Leptandra virginica) and veronica (Veronica officinalis), which are both known as speedwell.
There is very little scientific information about this product. Our staff is continually analyzing the available information on natural medicines and will add data here as it becomes available.

BROOM CORN

This Product is Also Known As
Darri, Durri, Guinea Corn, Sorghum.

Scientific Names
Sorghum vulgare.

People Use This For
Orally, broom corn seed is used for digestive disorders.
For food, broom corn is used as a cereal grain (18).

Safety

LIKELY SAFE …when used in food amounts (18). Although the fruit contains cyanogenic glycosides, the concentrations are very low (18).

There is insufficient reliable information available about the safety of broom corn used in amounts larger than found in foods.

PREGNANCY AND LACTATION: Insufficient reliable information available.

Effectiveness

There is insufficient reliable information available about the effectiveness of broom corn.

Possible Mechanism of Action & Active Ingredients

The applicable part of broom corn is the seed. Broom corn contains a high percentage of starch and a small amount of protein and fatty oil. It also contains thiamine and riboflavin. Dhurrin, a cyanogenic glycoside, is present in a very low amount in the fruit, 0.005-5 mg per 100 grams. In contrast, the foliage contains a much higher level, 250-700 mg per 100 grams. Broom corn is thought to have a soothing effect on the alimentary tract (18).

Adverse Reactions Including Known Allergies

None reported.

Possible Interactions with Herbs & Other Dietary Supplements

Insufficient reliable information available.

Possible Interactions with Drugs

No interactions are known to occur, and there is no known reason to expect a clinically significant interaction with broom corn.

Possible Interactions with Foods

No interactions are known to occur, and there is no known reason to expect a clinically significant interaction with broom corn.

Possible Interactions with Lab Tests

No interactions are known to occur, and there is no known reason to expect a clinically significant interaction with broom corn.

Possible Interactions with Diseases or Conditions

No interactions are known to occur, and there is no known reason to expect a clinically significant interaction with broom corn.

Typical Dosages & Routes of Administration that are Commonly Used

No typical dosage.

Comments

None.

BRYONIA

This Product is Also Known As

Bryoniae Radix, Devil's Turnip, English Mandrake, Ladies' Seal, Tamus, Tetterberry, White Bryony, Wild Hops, Wild Nep, Wild Vine, Wood Vine.

CAUTION: See separate listings for European Mandrake and Podophyllum (American mandrake).

Scientific Names

Bryonia cretica; Bryonia alba.
Family: Cucurbitaceae.

People Use This For

Orally, bryonia root is used as a laxative, emetic, diuretic, for gastrointestinal diseases, respiratory tract diseases, arthritis, liver disease, metabolic disorders, and for prophylaxis against infections (2).

Safety

LIKELY UNSAFE …when bryonia root is used orally (2). …when bryonia berries are ingested, 40 berries might be fatal (18).

CHILDREN: LIKELY UNSAFE …when berries are ingested. 15 berries can be fatal (18). …when the root is used orally (2).

PREGNANCY: UNSAFE …when the root is used orally. Contraindicated because it can cause abortion (2). …when berries are ingested (2).

LACTATION: LIKELY UNSAFE …when the root is used orally (2). …when berries are ingested (2).

Effectiveness

POSSIBLY EFFECTIVE ...when used as an emetic and laxative (2).
There is insufficient reliable information available about the effectiveness of bryonia for its other uses.

Possible Mechanism of Action & Active Ingredients

The applicable part of bryonia is the root. The resin from bryonia has strong purgative effects (18). Some evidence suggests the aqueous extract might be effective against tumors (18). Other evidence suggests the methanol extract could have hypoglycemic effects (18).

Adverse Reactions Including Known Allergies

Bryonia can cause dizziness, vomiting, convulsions, colic, bloody diarrhea, abortion, nervous excitement, kidney damage (2). Large doses can cause anuria, collapse, spasms, paralysis, or death (2). Skin contact with fresh bryonia may cause irritation (19). Ingestion of 15 berries is likely to be fatal to a child. Ingestion of 40 berries is likely to be fatal for adult (18).

Possible Interactions with Herbs & Other Dietary Supplements

Insufficient reliable information available.

Possible Interactions with Drugs

No interactions are known to occur, and there is no known reason to expect a clinically significant interaction with bryonia.

Possible Interactions with Foods

No interactions are known to occur, and there is no known reason to expect a clinically significant interaction with bryonia.

Possible Interactions with Lab Tests

No interactions are known to occur, and there is no known reason to expect a clinically significant interaction with bryonia.

Possible Interactions with Diseases or Conditions

GI IRRITATION: May irritate the gastrointestinal tract. Contraindicated in individuals with infectious or inflammatory gastrointestinal conditions (19).

Typical Dosages & Routes of Administration that are Commonly Used

No typical dosage.

Comments

Bryonia is no longer used as an emetic or laxative due to safety concerns (2).

BUCHU

This Product is Also Known As

Barosmae Folium, Bookoo, Bucco, Bucku, Diosma, Round Buchu, Short Buchu.

Scientific Names

Agathosma betulina, synonym Barosma betulina; Barosma crenulata; B. serratifolia.
Family: Rutaceae.

People Use This For

Historically, buchu has been used as a urinary tract disinfectant in cystitis, urethritis, prostatitis, acute cystitis (4), kidney infections (2), and venereal disease (5).
In manufacturing, the oil from buchu is used to give a fruit flavor (often black current) to foods.

Safety

LIKELY SAFE ...when the leaf is used in amounts found in foods; approved for food use in the US. The maximum level used is 0.002% (4,11).
POSSIBLY SAFE ...when the leaf is used orally and appropriately in medicinal amounts (2,12).
POSSIBLY UNSAFE ...when large amounts of buchu leaf are taken orally or when the oil is ingested. Buchu contains pulegone, a known hepatotoxin (4). Pulegone is a major component of the oil.
PREGNANCY: POSSIBLY SAFE ...when used in food amounts. LIKELY UNSAFE ...when used in larger amounts because buchu is reported to be an abortifacient (4).
LACTATION: POSSIBLY SAFE ...when used in food amounts. There is insufficient reliable information available about the safety of using larger amounts; avoid using.

Effectiveness

There is insufficient reliable information available about the effectiveness of buchu (2,4).

Possible Mechanism of Action & Active Ingredients
Buchu camphor (also known as diosphenol) is the principal constituent of the oil. Researchers believe this constituent may be responsible for buchu's reported diuretic and antiseptic effects (5).

Adverse Reactions Including Known Allergies
Buchu leaf can cause GI and kidney irritation (4,6), and increase menstrual flow (6). Buchu is also a reported abortifacient (4).

Possible Interactions with Herbs & Other Dietary Supplements
Insufficient reliable information available.

Possible Interactions with Drugs
ANTICOAGULANTS: May possibly enhance the effects of anticoagulants (7200).

Possible Interactions with Foods
No interactions are known to occur, and there is no known reason to expect a clinically significant interaction with buchu.

Possible Interactions with Lab Tests
No interactions are known to occur, and there is no known reason to expect a clinically significant interaction with buchu.

Possible Interactions with Diseases or Conditions
KIDNEY INFECTION: Contraindicated (4,12).
URINARY TRACT INFLAMMATION: Contraindicated (4,12).

Typical Dosages & Routes of Administration that are Commonly Used
ORAL: 1 cup of tea (steep 1 gram dry leaf in 150 mL boiling water 5-10 minutes, strain) several times per day (8).

Comments
Liver function should be monitored in people who use buchu because of its potential hepatotoxicity.

BUCKHORN PLANTAIN

This Product is Also Known As
Buckhorn, Chimney-Sweeps, English Plantain, Headsman, Hoary Plantain, Plantaginis lanceolatae herba, Plantain, Ribgrass, Ribwort Plantain, Ripplegrass, Soldier's Herb, Spitzwegerichkraut.
CAUTION: See separate listings for Great Plantain, Blond Psyllium, Black Psyllium, and Water Plantain.

Scientific Names
Plantago lanceolata.
Family: Plantaginaceae.

People Use This For
Orally, buckhorn plantain is used to treat inflammation of mucous membranes in the respiratory tract (2,3,7), for the common cold, cough, bronchitis, and fevers (18).
Topically, buckhorn plantain is used for pharyngeal mucous membrane inflammation, inflammation of the skin, and for wound healing (2,3).
In folk medicine, juice pressed from the plant is used to treat wounds, inflammation, and to arrest hemorrhages (18).

Safety
POSSIBLY SAFE ...when used orally in recommended doses. ...when used topically (2).
PREGNANCY AND LACTATION: LIKELY UNSAFE ...some evidence suggests buckhorn plantain affects muscle tone of the uterus (4275).

Effectiveness
POSSIBLY EFFECTIVE ...when used orally for relieving respiratory tract mucous membrane inflammation (2). ...when used topically for relieving oral and pharyngeal mucous membrane inflammation and inflammation of the skin (2).
There is insufficient reliable information available about the effectiveness of buckhorn plantain for its other uses.

Possible Mechanism of Action & Active Ingredients
The applicable parts of buckhorn plantain are the above ground parts. The tannin constituents have an astringent and antibacterial effect (18). Mucilage constituents are believed responsible for reducing local irritation and protecting mucous membranes from irritants (7).

Adverse Reactions Including Known Allergies
Buckhorn plantain is an allergen and a common problem in the early spring (3901).

Possible Interactions with Herbs & Other Dietary Supplements
Insufficient reliable information available.

Possible Interactions with Drugs
No interactions are known to occur, and there is no known reason to expect a clinically significant interaction with buckhorn plantain.

Possible Interactions with Foods
No interactions are known to occur, and there is no known reason to expect a clinically significant interaction with buckhorn plantain.

Possible Interactions with Lab Tests
No interactions are known to occur, and there is no known reason to expect a clinically significant interaction with buckhorn plantain.

Possible Interactions with Diseases or Conditions
No interactions are known to occur, and there is no known reason to expect a clinically significant interaction with buckhorn plantain.

Typical Dosages & Routes of Administration that are Commonly Used
ORAL: One cup tea (steep 2-3 grams chopped plant parts in 150 mL boiling water for 10 minutes, strain) several times daily (8,18); average amount is 3-6 grams per day (2).
TOPICAL: No typical dosage.

Comments
Avoid confusion with common plantain (Plantago major). CAUTION: Digitalis leaves resemble plantain leaves; adulteration of plantain with digitalis has been reported (3905). Be careful not to confuse buckhorn plantain with digitalis which is an unsafe product (2,12).

BUCKWHEAT

This Product is Also Known As
None.

Scientific Names
Fagopyrum esculentum.
Family: Polygonaceae.

People Use This For
Orally, buckwheat is used to improve venous and capillary tone, and prevent hardening of the arteries. It is also used orally to alleviate venous stasis and varicose veins (18).

Safety
There is insufficient reliable information available about the oral safety of buckwheat when it is used medicinally.
Pregnancy and Lactation: Insufficient reliable information available; avoid using.

Effectiveness
There is insufficient reliable information available about the effectiveness of buckwheat.

Possible Mechanism of Action & Active Ingredients
The applicable part of buckwheat are the leaves and flowers. Buckwheat contains naphthadianthrones, which have photosensitizing effects. Phototoxicity has occurred in animals that ingest large quantities of buckwheat (18).

Adverse Reactions Including Known Allergies
None reported.

Possible Interactions with Herbs & Other Dietary Supplements
Insufficient reliable information available.

Possible Interactions with Drugs
No interactions are known to occur, and there is no known reason to expect a clinically significant interaction with buckwheat.

Possible Interactions with Foods
No interactions are known to occur, and there is no known reason to expect a clinically significant interaction with buckwheat.

Possible Interactions with Lab Tests

No interactions are known to occur, and there is no known reason to expect a clinically significant interaction with buckwheat.

Possible Interactions with Diseases or Conditions

No interactions are known to occur, and there is no known reason to expect a clinically significant interaction with buckwheat.

Typical Dosages & Routes of Administration that are Commonly Used

ORAL: Buckwheat is used as a tea, extract or tablet (18).

Comments

There is very little scientific information about this product. Our staff is continually analyzing the available information on natural medicines and will add data here as it becomes available.

BUGLE

This Product is Also Known As

Bugula, Carpenter's Herb, Middle Comfrey, Middle Confound, Sicklewort.

Scientific Names

Ajuga reptans.
Family: Labiatae.

People Use This For

Orally, bugle is used for gallbladder and stomach disorders.
Topically, bugle is used as an astringent for the inflammation of the mouth and pharynx. It is also used topically for wound treatment (18).

Safety

There is insufficient reliable information available about the safety of bugle.
Pregnancy and Lactation: Insufficient reliable information available; avoid using.

Effectiveness

There is insufficient reliable information available about the effectiveness of bugle.

Possible Mechanism of Action & Active Ingredients

The applicable parts of bugle are the above ground parts. There is insufficient reliable information available about the possible mechanism of action and active ingredients.

Adverse Reactions Including Known Allergies

None reported.

Possible Interactions with Herbs & Other Dietary Supplements

Insufficient reliable information available.

Possible Interactions with Drugs

No interactions are known to occur, and there is no known reason to expect a clinically significant interaction with bugle.

Possible Interactions with Foods

No interactions are known to occur, and there is no known reason to expect a clinically significant interaction with bugle.

Possible Interactions with Lab Tests

No interactions are known to occur, and there is no known reason to expect a clinically significant interaction with bugle.

Possible Interactions with Diseases or Conditions

No interactions are known to occur, and there is no known reason to expect a clinically significant interaction with bugle.

Typical Dosages & Routes of Administration that are Commonly Used

No typical dosage.

Comments

Some people use bugle in alcoholic extracts, in teas, and as a water infusion (18). There is very little scientific information about this product. Our staff is continually analyzing the available information on natural medicines and will add data here as it becomes available.

BUGLEWEED

This Product is Also Known As
Archangle, Ashangee, Green Wolf's Foot, Gypsy Weed, Gypsywort, Hoarhound, Lycopi Herba, Paul's Betony, Sweet Bugle, Water Bugle, Water Hoarhound, Water Horehound, Virginia Water Horehound, Wolfstrapp.

Scientific Names
Lycopus virginicus; Lycopus americanus; Lycopus europaeus.
Family: Lamiaceae.

People Use This For
Orally, bugleweed is taken for mild hyperthyroidism, premenstrual syndrome, breast pain, nervousness, and insomnia (2,18).
Traditionally, it has been used for bleeding, especially nosebleeds and heavy bleeding during menses (7).

Safety
POSSIBLY SAFE ...when the above ground parts are used orally and appropriately (12).
PREGNANCY: LIKELY UNSAFE ...when used orally; contraindicated (12,19) because it has anti-gonadotropic and anti-thyrotropic activity (7,19).
LACTATION: LIKELY UNSAFE ...contraindicated for oral use (12,19) because it might have anti-prolactin activity (7,19).

Effectiveness
POSSIBLY EFFECTIVE ...when taken orally for mild hyperthyroidism and breast pain (2).
There is insufficient reliable information available about the effectiveness of bugleweed for its other uses.

Possible Mechanism of Action & Active Ingredients
The applicable parts of bugleweed are the above ground parts. Bugleweed demonstrates anti-gonadotropic and anti-thyrotropic activity. It lowers serum prolactin levels (2,7) and inhibits peripheral deiodination of T4 (2). Bugleweed can also have hypoglycemic activity (19).

Adverse Reactions Including Known Allergies
Taken orally, bugleweed rarely can cause thyroid enlargement during extended therapy or with large amounts (2,7). The sudden discontinuation of bugleweed can result in a sudden increase in thyroid function (2) and prolactin secretion (7).

Possible Interactions with Herbs & Other Dietary Supplements
THYROID-SUPPRESSING HERBS: Theoretically, concomitant use of bugleweed with other thyroid suppressing herbs can have additive therapeutic and adverse effects (19). Herbs with thyroid-suppressing effects include balm leaf and the wild thyme plant (19).

Possible Interactions with Drugs
DIABETES THERAPY: Theoretically, concomitant use of bugleweed can increase the risk of hypoglycemia (19), and blood glucose levels should be monitored closely.
THYROID HORMONES: Concomitant use of bugleweed is contraindicated, because bugleweed reduces the effects of thyroid hormones by blocking peripheral conversion of thyroxin to T3 (19).

Possible Interactions with Foods
No interactions are known to occur, and there is no known reason to expect a clinically significant interaction with bugleweed.

Possible Interactions with Lab Tests
RADIOACTIVE ISOTOPES: Bugleweed can interfere with diagnostic procedures using radioactive isotopes (2).
THYROID FUNCTION TESTS: Bugleweed might improve thyroid function and test results in mildly hyperthyroid patients (2).

Possible Interactions with Diseases or Conditions
THYROID DISEASE: Bugleweed is contraindicated in thyroid enlargement, thyroid hypofunction (2,12,19), and during administration of other thyroid treatments (12).
DIABETES: Theoretically, bugleweed can interfere with blood glucose control and increase the risk of hypoglycemia (19). Blood glucose levels should be monitored closely while using bugleweed in diabetic patients.

Typical Dosages & Routes of Administration that are Commonly Used
ORAL: The typical dose of bugleweed is 0.2-2 grams per day of the above ground parts or equivalent preparations (2,7). The dose must be carefully individualized, taking age and weight into consideration (2).

Comments
None.

BULBOUS BUTTERCUP

This Product is Also Known As
Crowfoot, Cuckoo Buds, Frogsfoot, Frogwort, Goldcup, King's Cup, Meadowbloom, Pilewort, St. Anthony's Turnip.
CAUTION: See separate listings for Buttercup and Poisonous Buttercup.

Scientific Names
Ranunculus bulbosus.
Family: Ranunculaceae.

People Use This For
Orally, bulbous buttercup is used in dilutions for skin diseases, arthritis, gout, neuralgia, influenza, and meningitis (18).

Safety
LIKELY UNSAFE …when the latex or any part of the fresh plant is used for oral or topical use because it can cause severe local irritation (18).
PREGNANCY AND LACTATION: LIKELY UNSAFE …contraindicated for oral or topical use (18).

Effectiveness
There is insufficient reliable information available about the effectiveness of bulbous buttercup.

Possible Mechanism of Action & Active Ingredients
The applicable parts of bulbous buttercup are the latex and the whole fresh flowering plant. When the fresh plant is crushed or cut into small pieces, the glycoside ranunculin is enzymatically changed into a severely irritating protoanemonin, which, in turn, rapidly degrades into the less toxic anemonin (18). Both protoanemonin and ranunculin are destroyed to an unknown extent during the drying process (2). The constituents ranunculin, protoanemonin, anemonin and labenzym can cause drowsiness, fatigue and depressive moods. Protoanemonin present in the fresh-harvested, bruised plant is severely irritating to skin and mucous membranes (18).

Adverse Reactions Including Known Allergies
Ingestion of bulbous buttercup can cause severe irritation of the gastrointestinal tract, with colic and diarrhea. Irritation of the urinary tract can also occur. Skin contact can cause blisters and burns which are difficult to heal (18).

Possible Interactions with Herbs & Other Dietary Supplements
Insufficient reliable information available.

Possible Interactions with Drugs
No interactions are known to occur, and there is no known reason to expect a clinically significant interaction with bulbous buttercup.

Possible Interactions with Foods
No interactions are known to occur, and there is no known reason to expect a clinically significant interaction with bulbous buttercup.

Possible Interactions with Lab Tests
No interactions are known to occur, and there is no known reason to expect a clinically significant interaction with bulbous buttercup.

Possible Interactions with Diseases or Conditions
No interactions are known to occur, and there is no known reason to expect a clinically significant interaction with bulbous buttercup.

Typical Dosages & Routes of Administration that are Commonly Used
No typical dosage.

Comments
This product is rarely used. Avoid confusing bulbous buttercup with lesser celandine and amaranth; these plants are also referred to as pilewort (18).

BUPLEURUM

This Product is Also Known As
Bei Chai Hu, Chi Hu, Chinese Thoroughwax, Hare's Ear Root, Sho-saiko-to, Shrubby Hare's-ear, Sickle-leaf Hare's-ear, Thoroughwax.

Scientific Names

Bupleurum chinense; Bupleurum falcatum; Bupleurum exaltatum; Bupleurum fruticosum; Bupleurum longifolium; Bupleurum multinerve; Bupleurum octoradiatum; Bupleurum rotundifolium; Bupleurum scorzonerifolium. Family: Apiaceae.

People Use This For

Orally, bupleurum is used for fevers, flu, the common cold, cough, fatigue, headache, tinnitus, liver disorders, premenstrual syndrome, dysmenorrhea, depression, anorexia, cancer, inflammation, lung congestion, malaria, angina, epilepsy, pain, muscle cramps, rheumatism, asthma, bronchitis, indigestion, ulcers, hemorrhoids, diarrhea, constipation, as a sedative, antioxidant, antiseptic, antifungal, antiviral, as an immune stimulant, and for reducing cholesterol and triglyceride levels (6,513,3145,3148,3149). It is also used for increasing sweating, to alleviate female problems, as a protectant against kidney problems, as a liver tonic, and as a spleen and stomach toner (6). Bupleurum is used in many combination herbal formulas. It is included in a Chinese herbal formula used for treating thrombocytopenic purpura (3146) and in a Japanese herbal formula (Sho-saiko-to, TJ-9, Xino-chai-hu-tang) used for various chronic liver diseases (3147). Bupleurum is used orally in combination with Panax ginseng and licorice to help stimulate adrenal gland function, particularly in patients with a history of long-term corticosteroid use (3234).

Safety

There is insufficient reliable information available about the safety of bupleurum.

Pregnancy and Lactation: Insufficient reliable information available; avoid using.

Effectiveness

There is insufficient reliable information available about the effectiveness of bupleurum.

Possible Mechanism of Action & Active Ingredients

The applicable part of bupleurum is the root (12). Compounds isolated from Bupleurum species used in traditional Chinese medicine include saikosaponins, polysaccharides and polyacetylenes. Saikosaponins are triterpenoid saponins, known as saikosides (6). While the saikosaponin content of some species is very similar (3151), that of other species varies considerably, as well as pharmacologic activity (3152). The saikosaponin content is highest in Bupleurum falcatum (2-8%) and Bupleurum chinense (1.7%). For infections, including the flu and the common cold, bupleurum is theorized to work by improving immune function. Bupleurum falcatum is reported to cause proliferation of B-lymphocytes and stimulate them to produce immunoglobulins in vitro. It is also reported to stimulate in vitro macrophage activity, possibly by increasing the number of antibody-binding sites on the cell surface (2598). The constituent saikosaponin-d has immunoregulatory actions on T-lymphocytes, including promotion of interleukin-2 (IL-2) production and IL-2 receptor expression (3160). It also increases macrophage activity, IL-1 production and antibody response (3161). Bupleurum also is reported to have antitussive properties (6). For peptic ulcers, bupleurum is thought to decrease gastric acid and pepsin secretion and have mucosal protecting effects (3154,3155). Bupleurum is also reported to have antitumor (3157), antibacterial (3170), antiinflammatory (2597,3166,3167,3168), antispasmodic (3167), antioxidant (3154,3155,3156), antiplatelet (3159), and hepatoprotectant effects (3163,3164,3165). These effects have not been demonstrated in humans.

Adverse Reactions Including Known Allergies

Bupleurum, when taken orally, can cause increased bowel movements, flatulence, and sedation (3148). The Japanese herbal formula, Sho-saiko-to, which contains bupleurum, has been associated with eosinophilic pneumonia (354), pulmonary edema (361), and multiple cases of pneumonitis (355,356,357). Sho-saiko-to, used in combination with interferon-alpha in people with chronic active hepatitis, has been associated with multiple cases of pneumonitis (358,359,360).

Possible Interactions with Herbs & Other Dietary Supplements

Insufficient reliable information available.

Possible Interactions with Drugs

No interactions are known to occur, and there is no known reason to expect a clinically significant interaction with bupleurum.

Possible Interactions with Foods

No interactions are known to occur, and there is no known reason to expect a clinically significant interaction with bupleurum.

Possible Interactions with Lab Tests

No interactions are known to occur, and there is no known reason to expect a clinically significant interaction with bupleurum.

Possible Interactions with Diseases or Conditions

No interactions are known to occur, and there is no known reason to expect a clinically significant interaction with bupleurum.

Typical Dosages & Routes of Administration that are Commonly Used

ORAL: A dose of 1.5 to 6 grams per day of bupleurum root has been used (3148). Fluid extract (1:2), 1.5-3 mL daily, up to 25-60 mL per week (3148).

Comments

The Japanese herbal formula, Sho-saiko-to, which contains bupleurum, enhances the anti-HIV-1 activity of lamivudine (Epivir, 3TC) in vitro (362).

BURDOCK

This Product is Also Known As

Bardana, Bardanae Radix, Bardane, Beggar's Buttons, Burr Seed, Clotbur, Cocklebur, Cockle Buttons, Edible Burdock, Fox's Clote, Great Bur, Great Burdocks, Happy Major, Hardock, Harebur, Lappa, Love Leaves, Personata, Philanthropium, Thorny Burr.

Scientific Names

Arctium lappa; Arctium minus; Arctium tomentosum.
Family: Asteraceae or Compositae.

People Use This For

Orally, burdock is used as a diuretic, "blood purifier" (5), antimicrobial, antipyretic (11), and to treat anorexia nervosa (4), GI complaints (2), rheumatism, gout, cystitis (2,4), and chronic skin conditions including acne and psoriasis (5).
Topically, burdock is used for dry skin (ichthyosis) and eczema (4,18).
In folk medicine, burdock has been used for treating colds, catarrh, cancers, and as an aphrodisiac (6). Burdock has been used in the past in the treatment of gout and syphilitic disorders.
Burdock is consumed as food in Asia (11).

Safety

LIKELY SAFE ...when burdock root preparations are consumed in amounts commonly found in foods. Burdock is listed as a food flavoring by the Council of Europe (4).
POSSIBLY SAFE ...when used orally and appropriately in medicinal amounts (12).
PREGNANCY: LIKELY UNSAFE ...contraindicated for oral use because it could cause uterine stimulation (4,19).
LACTATION: Insufficient reliable information available; avoid using (4).

Effectiveness

There is insufficient reliable information available about the effectiveness of burdock.

Possible Mechanism of Action & Active Ingredients

The applicable part of burdock is the root. The leaf and flower have Gram-positive and Gram-negative antibacterial activity; the root is active against Gram-negative bacteria (4). Arctiopiricin (constituent) is active against Gram-positive bacteria (4). In vivo, burdock has uterine stimulant activity in animals (4). The plant may have some antimutagenic and antitumor activity (4).

Adverse Reactions Including Known Allergies

Burdock can cause an allergic reaction in individuals sensitive to the Asteraceae/Compositae family. Members of this family include ragweed, chrysanthemums, marigolds, daisies, and many other herbs. Topically, sensitization may occur via skin contact (18).

Possible Interactions with Herbs & Other Dietary Supplements

Insufficient reliable information available.

Possible Interactions with Drugs

HYPOGLYCEMIC DRUGS: Theoretically, large amounts of burdock might cause hypoglycemia (4).
INSULIN: Concomitant use might require insulin dosage adjustment due to hypoglycemic effect (19).

Possible Interactions with Foods

No interactions are known to occur, and there is no known reason to expect a clinically significant interaction with burdock.

Possible Interactions with Lab Tests

No interactions are known to occur, and there is no known reason to expect a clinically significant interaction with burdock.

Possible Interactions with Diseases or Conditions
DIABETES: Theoretically, large amounts may affect blood sugar control (4).
CROSS-ALLERGENICITY: Can cause an allergic reaction in individuals sensitive to the Asteraceae/Compositae family. Members of this family include ragweed, chrysanthemums, marigolds, daisies, and many other herbs.

Typical Dosages & Routes of Administration that are Commonly Used
ORAL: 2-6 grams dried root three times daily, or drink 1 cup tea (steep 1-2 grams dried root in 150 mL boiling water 5-10 minutes, strain) three times daily (4). Liquid extract: (1:1 in 25% alcohol) 2-8 mL three times daily (4). Tincture (1:10 in 45% alcohol) 8-12 mL three times daily (4).

Comments
Burdock has been associated with atropine poisoning as a result of being adulterated with root of belladonna or deadly nightshade (4,5).

BURNING BUSH leaf

This Product is Also Known As
Adiptam, Dittany, Fraxinella, Gas Plant, Herba dictamni herba.
CAUTION: See separate listing for Burning Bush root.

Scientific Names
Dictamnus albus.
Family: Rutaceae.

People Use This For
Historically, burning bush was used orally for cramps, stomach disorders, and worm infestations. In the Middle Ages, people used burning bush leaf orally for epilepsy, as an aid for urination, to promote menstruation and aid in the expulsion of the afterbirth. It was also used topically for curing or treating wounds. Burning bush was also used topically for rheumatism (18).
In other uses, people in Greece utilize burning bush orally as a stimulant and tonic.

Safety
POSSIBLY UNSAFE …when used topically. Can cause photosensitivity (18).
There is insufficient reliable information available about the safety of the oral use of burning bush leaf.
PREGNANCY AND LACTATION: POSSIBLY UNSAFE …when used topically. There is insufficient reliable information available about the safety of the oral use of burning bush leaf; avoid using.

Effectiveness
There is insufficient reliable information available about the effectiveness of burning bush.

Possible Mechanism of Action & Active Ingredients
There is evidence to support the use of burning bush in treating worm infestations. It decreases the ability of a tropical liver fluke called Clonorchis sinesis to lay eggs. This same liver fluke can occur in sushi if the fish has been imported from Asia. Burning bush contains psoralen, xanthotoxin, auraptene, and bergapten. These furocoumarins can cause phototoxic reactions when they are applied topically (18).

Adverse Reactions Including Known Allergies
Skin contact can cause phototoxicity (18).

Possible Interactions with Herbs & Other Dietary Supplements
Insufficient reliable information available.

Possible Interactions with Drugs
No interactions are known to occur, and there is no known reason to expect a clinically significant interaction with burning bush leaf.

Possible Interactions with Foods
No interactions are known to occur, and there is no known reason to expect a clinically significant interaction with burning bush leaf.

Possible Interactions with Lab Tests
No interactions are known to occur, and there is no known reason to expect a clinically significant interaction with burning bush leaf.

Possible Interactions with Diseases or Conditions
No interactions are known to occur, and there is no known reason to expect a clinically significant interaction with burning bush leaf.

Typical Dosages & Routes of Administration that are Commonly Used

ORAL: The daily dose is 1 cup of tea taken orally 3 times daily. One cup of tea is also taken after main meals twice daily. The tea is prepared by steeping 20 grams of dried leaf in 1 L of boiling water for 10-15 minutes and straining. Alternately, 1 gram of fresh or 2 grams of dried herb is added to 1 cup of water (18).

Comments

The alternate burning bush name, herba dictamni herba, sounds similar to herba dictamni cretici (dittany of crete, Origanum dictamnus). Use caution to ensure the two are not confused. Avoid confusion with Euonymus, which has also been referred to as burning bush. Euonymus is the dried bark of the root of Euonymus atropurpureus (Fam. Celastracaea). It was used in the past as a diuretic and cathartic. Burning bush has a distinctive lemon or cinnamon scent. Its oil is easily flammable (18).

BURNING BUSH root

This Product is Also Known As

Adiptam, Dittany, Fraxinella, Gas Plant, Herba Dictamni Herba.
CAUTION: See separate listing for Burning Bush leaf.

Scientific Names

Dictamnus albus.
Family: Rutaceae.

People Use This For

Orally, burning bush root is used for digestive and urogenital disorders, and to promote hair growth.
Topically, burning bush root is used for eczema, impetigo, and scabies.
In Chinese medicine (China and Korea), the root is applied topically for arthritis, fever, hepatitis, skin inflammation, thread fungus, uterine hemorrhages, to calm children crying as a result of a nervous state and as a sedative and tonic (18).
In folk medicine, burning bush root has been used as a diuretic and spasmolytic. In the Middle Ages, it was used for desiccation, epilepsy, hysteria, worm infestations, and to promote menstruation.
Other uses include its utilization in India for amenorrhea and birth control.

Safety

POSSIBLY UNSAFE …when used topically (18).
There is insufficient reliable information available about the safety of the oral use of burning bush root.
PREGNANCY AND LACTATION: POSSIBLY UNSAFE …when used topically. There is insufficient reliable information available about the safety of the oral use of burning bush root; avoid using.

Effectiveness

There is insufficient reliable information available about the effectiveness of burning bush.

Possible Mechanism of Action & Active Ingredients

Insufficient reliable information available.

Adverse Reactions Including Known Allergies

Skin contact can cause phototoxicity (18).

Possible Interactions with Herbs & Other Dietary Supplements

Insufficient reliable information available.

Possible Interactions with Drugs

No interactions are known to occur, and there is no known reason to expect a clinically significant interaction with burning bush root.

Possible Interactions with Foods

No interactions are known to occur, and there is no known reason to expect a clinically significant interaction with burning bush root.

Possible Interactions with Lab Tests

No interactions are known to occur, and there is no known reason to expect a clinically significant interaction with burning bush root.

Possible Interactions with Diseases or Conditions

No interactions are known to occur, and there is no known reason to expect a clinically significant interaction with burning bush root.

Typical Dosages & Routes of Administration that are Commonly Used

ORAL: Tea is taken over the course of one day. The tea is prepared by steeping 1 teaspoon dried root in 2 glasses

of hot water for 10-15 minutes and straining . It is also occasionally used in tea mixtures and in Swedish herb mixtures (18).
TOPICAL: No typical dosage.

Comments
Burning bush root is considered possibly unsafe; avoid using (18). The alternate burning bush name, herba dictamni radix, sounds similar to herba dictamni cretici (dittany of crete, Origanum dictamnus). Use caution to ensure the two are not confused. In addition, previous sources report confusion with Carophyllaceen roots. Avoid confusion with Euonymus, which has also been referred to as burning bush. Euonymus is the dried bark of the root of Euonymus atropurpureus (Fam. Celastracaea). It was used in the past as a diuretic and cathartic. Burning bush has a distinctive lemon or cinnamon scent. Its oil is easily flammable. Its use is mostly obsolete (18).

BURR MARIGOLD

This Product is Also Known As
Water Agrimony.

Scientific Names
Bidens tripartitia.
Family: Compositae.

People Use This For
Orally, burr marigold is used for hair loss, colitis, and gout. It is also used orally as an astringent, diuretic, and to promote sweating (18).

Safety
There is insufficient reliable information available about the safety of the oral use of burr marigold.
Pregnancy and Lactation: Insufficient reliable information available; avoid using.

Effectiveness
There is insufficient reliable information available about the effectiveness of burr marigold.

Possible Mechanism of Action & Active Ingredients
The applicable parts of burr marigold are the above ground parts. There is insufficient reliable information available about the possible mechanism of action and active ingredients.

Adverse Reactions Including Known Allergies
Burr marigold can cause an allergic reaction in individuals sensitive to the Asteraceae/Compositae family. Members of this family include ragweed, chrysanthemums, marigolds, daisies, and many other herbs.

Possible Interactions with Herbs & Other Dietary Supplements
No interactions are known to occur, and there is no known reason to expect a clinically significant interaction with burr marigold.

Possible Interactions with Drugs
No interactions are known to occur, and there is no known reason to expect a clinically significant interaction with burr marigold.

Possible Interactions with Foods
No interactions are known to occur, and there is no known reason to expect a clinically significant interaction with burr marigold.

Possible Interactions with Lab Tests
No interactions are known to occur, and there is no known reason to expect a clinically significant interaction with burr marigold.

Possible Interactions with Diseases or Conditions
CROSS-ALLERGENICITY: Can cause an allergic reaction in individuals sensitive to the Asteraceae/Compositae family. Members of this family include ragweed, chrysanthemums, marigolds, daisies, and many other herbs.

Typical Dosages & Routes of Administration that are Commonly Used
No typical dosage.

Comments
There is very little scientific information about this product. Our staff is continually analyzing the available information on natural medicines and will add data here as it becomes available.

BUTANEDIOL (BD)

This Product is Also Known As
1,4-BD, 1,4-butylene glycol, 1,4-dihydroxybutane, 1,4-tetramethylene glycol, 2(3H)-Furanone di-dihydro, BD, BDO, pine needle oil, Butane-1,4-diol, Butylene glycol, Tetramethylene glycol, Tetramethylene-1,4-diol. CAUTION: see separate listings for Gamma Hydroxybutyrate (GHB) and Gamma Butyrolactone (GBL).

Scientific Names
1,4-butanediol.

People Use This For
Orally butanediol has been used to stimulate growth hormone production and muscle growth, for bodybuilding and weight loss, and for insomnia (3677,3678).

Safety
UNSAFE ...when used orally. Butanediol, and the closely related products gamma hydroxybutyrate (GHB) and gamma butyrolactone (GBL) have been linked to at least 122 serious illnesses, including 3 deaths, reported to the FDA (3678).
PREGNANCY AND LACTATION: UNSAFE ...contraindicated.

Effectiveness
There is insufficient reliable information about the effectiveness of butanediol.

Possible Mechanism of Action & Active Ingredients
Butanediol is converted to gamma hydroxybutyrate (GHB, see separate listing) in the body (14,3678,5813). It is a powerful hypnotic, producing potentially dangerous sedative effects (3679). GHB can be converted in the brain to the neurotransmitter gamma aminobutyric acid (GABA) (14,3699), and specific GHB uptake systems, transport systems, and receptors have also been identified (14,713,3699,5800,5801). Stimulation of GHB receptors reduces dopamine release in the brain (14,713,3699,5801), and GHB has also been reported to affect the endogenous opioid system, raising dynorphin levels (3682,5803). GHB produces general anesthesia (14), induces REM and non-REM sleep, hypothermia, abnormalities on the EEG similar to those seen in petit mal epilepsy (5800,5803), and it stimulates growth hormone secretion (5804).

Adverse Reactions Including Known Allergies
Butanediol, like GBL, is metabolized to GHB, and therefore causes similar toxic effects, including breathing problems, respiratory depression requiring intubation, coma, amnesia, combativeness, confusion, agitation, vomiting, seizures, bradycardia, and death (14,3678,3679). Butanediol, GHB, and GBL have been linked to at least 122 serious illnesses, including 3 deaths (3678).
Withdrawal symptoms, including insomnia, tremor and anxiety, can occur in chronic users of gamma hydroxybutyrate (GHB) (1430), and are therefore likely with chronic butanediol use.

Possible Interactions with Herbs & Other Dietary Supplements
PRODUCTS WITH SEDATIVE EFFECTS: Likely to cause additive sedation with butanediol, increasing the risk of serious adverse effects.

Possible Interactions with Drugs
ALCOHOL: Concomitant use with butanediol and its metabolite GHB may increase the risk of serious CNS and respiratory depression (1430,3678).
CNS DEPRESSANTS: Additive sedative effects with butanediol may be dangerous (3679).
NARCOTIC ANALGESICS: Concomitant use with GHB (a metabolite of butanediol) can potentiate the therapeutic and adverse effects of narcotic analgesics (14).
BENZODIAZEPINES, NEUROLEPTICS: Concomitant use with GHB (a metabolite of butanediol) can potentiate the effects of GHB (14,3682).
D-AMPHETAMINE, NALOXONE, HALOPERIDOL, DRUGS USED FOR ABSENCE SEIZURES: Concomitant use with GHB (a metabolite of butanediol) may antagonize the effects of GHB, but these agents have not been assessed as possible treatments for GHB or butanediol overdose (3682).
SKELETAL MUSCLE RELAXANTS: Concomitant use with GHB (a metabolite of GBL) can potentiate the therapeutic and adverse effects of skeletal muscle relaxants (14,3682).

Possible Interactions with Foods
ALCOHOL: Concomitant use with butanediol and its metabolite GHB may increase the risk of serious CNS and respiratory depression (1430,3678).

Possible Interactions with Lab Tests
GAMMA BUTYROLACTONE (GBL) / GAMMA HYDROXYBUTYRIC ACID (GHB): The mass spectrometry assay for GHB (a metabolite of butanediol) used in either urine or serum studies is unable to differentiate between GHB and GBL (14).

Possible Interactions with Diseases or Conditions

HYPERTENSION OR BRADYCARDIA: GHB, a metabolite of butanediol, should be avoided since it may exacerbate these conditions (14).
CARDIAC CONDUCTION DEFECTS: GHB, a metabolite of butanediol, should be avoided due to the risk of bradycardia (14).
EPILEPSY: GHB, a metabolite of butanediol, should be avoided due to its possible capacity to induce seizures (14).
RENAL IMPAIRMENT: GHB, a metabolite of butanediol, should be avoided due to possible accumulation (14).

Typical Dosages & Routes of Administration that are Commonly Used

ORAL: Doses of butanediol of 0.25 to 1 ounce have been used for stimulating growth hormone release and muscle growth and treating insomnia (3677), but are not considered safe (3678).

Comments

Butanediol is used industrially to make floor stripper, paint thinner, and other solvent products (3678). It is illegal to sell any product for human consumption containing butanediol (3678). Some manufacturers have substituted butanediol in products previously containing GHB or GBL, but the effects of butanediol are just as dangerous (3679). GBL, GHB and BD are associated with at least 122 reports of serious adverse effects including dangerously low respiratory rates (intubation might be required), unconsciousness/coma, vomiting, seizures, slowed heart rate, and death (4259).

BUTCHER'S BROOM

This Product is Also Known As

Box Holly, Jew's Myrtle, Kneeholm, Knee Holly, Pettigree, Sweet Broom, Rusci Aculeati Rhizoma.
CAUTION: See separate listings for Scotch Broom flower, Scotch Broom herb, and Spanish Broom.

Scientific Names

Ruscus aculeatus.
Family: Liliaceae.

People Use This For

Orally, butcher's broom is used to relieve the burning and itching of hemorrhoids (18) and for symptoms of chronic venous insufficiency, including pain, heaviness, leg cramps, leg edema, varicose veins, peripheral vascular disease, itching, and swelling (2).
Traditionally, butcher's broom has been used as a laxative (5,6), diuretic (5), an anti-inflammatory (6), for atherosclerosis (6), and to facilitate the healing of fractures (5).
Historically, the rhizome shoots were eaten as food in some cultures in a manner similar to asparagus (6).

Safety

LIKELY SAFE ...when used orally and appropriately (12). The use of butcher's broom is not associated with any significant toxicity (6).
PREGNANCY AND LACTATION: Insufficient reliable information available; avoid using.

Effectiveness

POSSIBLY EFFECTIVE ...when taken orally to relieve the burning and itching of hemorrhoids and for symptoms of chronic venous insufficiency, including pain, heaviness, leg cramps, itching, and swelling (2,5,6).
There is insufficient reliable information available about the effectiveness of butcher's broom for its other uses.

Possible Mechanism of Action & Active Ingredients

The applicable parts of butcher's broom are the rhizome and root. The steroidal saponin constituents, ruscogenin and neuroscogenin, produce vasoconstrictive effects by direct activation of alpha-adrenergic receptors (5).

Adverse Reactions Including Known Allergies

Butcher's broom taken orally can cause GI disorders and rarely nausea (2).

Possible Interactions with Herbs & Other Dietary Supplements

Insufficient reliable information available.

Possible Interactions with Drugs

No interactions are known to occur, and there is no known reason to expect a clinically significant interaction with butcher's broom.

Possible Interactions with Foods

No interactions are known to occur, and there is no known reason to expect a clinically significant interaction with butcher's broom.

Possible Interactions with Lab Tests

No interactions are known to occur, and there is no known reason to expect a clinically significant interaction with butcher's broom.

Possible Interactions with Diseases or Conditions

No interactions are known to occur, and there is no known reason to expect a clinically significant interaction with butcher's broom.

Typical Dosages & Routes of Administration that are Commonly Used

ORAL: The typical dose of the raw extract is equivalent to 7-11 mg of total ruscogenin, which is determined as the sum of neoruscogenin and ruscogenin obtained after fermentation or acid hydrolysis (2). Butcher's broom is available in capsules, ointments, and suppositories (5).

Comments

European butchers historically have used the leaves and twigs of this plant to clean and scrub their chopping blocks, which had led to its name, butcher's broom (6002). Avoid confusion with scotch broom flower, scotch broom herb, and Spanish broom.

BUTTERCUP

This Product is Also Known As

Acrid Crowfoot, Batchelor's Buttons, Blisterweed, Burrwort, Globe Amaranth, Gold Cup, Meadowbloom, Yellows, Yellowweed.
CAUTION: See separate listings for Poisonous Buttercup and Bulbous Buttercup.

Scientific Names

Ranunculus acris.
Family: Ranunculaceae.

People Use This For

Orally, buttercup is used for arthritis, blisters, bronchitis, chronic skin complaints, and nerve pain (18).

Safety

LIKELY UNSAFE …when the fresh above ground parts are used for any oral or topical use because they can cause severe local irritation (18).
There is insufficient reliable information about the safety of the medicinal use of the dried, cut above ground parts of buttercup.
PREGNANCY AND LACTATION: LIKELY UNSAFE …when the fresh above ground parts are used orally or topically. Buttercup might also stimulate uterine contractions (19). There is insufficient reliable information about the safety of the oral or topical use of the dried, cut above ground parts of buttercup during pregnancy and lactation.

Effectiveness

There is insufficient reliable information available about the effectiveness of buttercup.

Possible Mechanism of Action & Active Ingredients

The applicable part is the fresh above ground parts. When the fresh plant is crushed or cut into small pieces, the glycoside ranunculin is enzymatically changed into a severely irritating protoanemonin, which, in turn, rapidly degrades into the less toxic anemonin (18). Both protoanemonin and ranunculin are destroyed to an unknown extent during the drying process (2).

Adverse Reactions Including Known Allergies

Ingestion of buttercup can cause severe irritation of the gastrointestinal tract, with colic and diarrhea. Irritation of the urinary tract can also occur. Skin contact can cause blisters and burns which are difficult to heal (18). Buttercup can also cause phototoxic skin reactions (19).

Possible Interactions with Herbs & Other Dietary Supplements

Insufficient reliable information available.

Possible Interactions with Drugs

No interactions are known to occur, and there is no known reason to expect a clinically significant interaction with buttercup.

Possible Interactions with Foods

No interactions are known to occur, and there is no known reason to expect a clinically significant interaction with buttercup.

Possible Interactions with Lab Tests

No interactions are known to occur, and there is no known reason to expect a clinically significant interaction with buttercup.

Possible Interactions with Diseases or Conditions

No interactions are known to occur, and there is no known reason to expect a clinically significant interaction with buttercup.

Typical Dosages & Routes of Administration that are Commonly Used

No typical dosage.

Comments

Buttercup is considered unsafe for any use (18).

BUTTERNUT

This Product is Also Known As

Lemon Walnut, Oil Nut, White Walnut, Butternussbaum, Nogal Ceniciento, Noyer Cerdré.

Scientific Names

Juglans cinerea.
Family: Juglandaceae.

People Use This For

Orally, butternut bark is used for gallbladder disorders, hemorrhoids and skin diseases. It is also used orally as a stimulant laxative, antimicrobial, antineoplastic, antiparasitic, and tonic. Some people use butternut bark orally as a tonic to invigorate, refresh, or restore body function (18).

Safety

POSSIBLY SAFE …when preparations of the bark are used orally (12).
PREGNANCY AND LACTATION: LIKELY UNSAFE …when used in large amounts, it can be cathartic (12).

Effectiveness

There is insufficient reliable information available about the effectiveness of butternut.

Possible Mechanism of Action & Active Ingredients

The applicable part of butternut is the bark which is reported to have cathartic properties (12,19).

Adverse Reactions Including Known Allergies

Butternut bark can cause diarrhea and gastrointestinal irritation (19).

Possible Interactions with Herbs & Other Dietary Supplements

CARDIAC GLYCOSIDE-CONTAINING HERBS: Stimulant laxative herbs such as butternut bark can cause potassium depletion increasing the risk of cardiac toxicity. Cardiac glycoside-containing herbs include: black hellebore, Canadian hemp roots, digitalis leaf, hedge mustard, figwort, lily of the valley roots, motherwort, oleander leaf, pheasant's eye plant, pleurisy root, squill bulb leaf scales, and strophanthus seeds (2,18,19).
STIMULANT LAXATIVE HERBS: Theoretically, concomitant use with other stimulant laxative herbs may increase the risk of potassium depletion. Stimulant laxative herbs include: aloe dried leaf sap, blue flag rhizome, alder buckthorn, European buckthorn, cascara bark, castor oil, colocynth fruit pulp, gamboge bark exudate, jalap root, black root, manna bark exudate, podophyllum root, rhubarb root, senna leaves and pods, wild cucumber fruit (Ecballium elaterium), and yellow dock root (19).
LICORICE/HORSETAIL: Theoretically, concomitant use with horsetail plant or licorice rhizome increases the risk of potassium depletion (19).

Possible Interactions with Drugs

ANTIARRHYTHMIC DRUGS: Overuse of butternut bark might cause potassium depletion increasing risk of anti-arrhythmic drug toxicity (664).
CORTICOSTEROIDS: Overuse of butternut bark might compound corticosteroid-induced potassium loss (2).
CARDIAC GLYCOSIDES: Theoretically, overuse of butternut bark increases the risk of adverse effects of cardiac glycoside drugs, including digoxin (Lanoxin) and digitoxin (Crystodigin).
LAXATIVE DRUGS: Concomitant use might compound fluid and electrolyte loss.
POTASSIUM-DEPLETING DIURETICS: Overuse of butternut bark might compound diuretic-induced potassium loss (2).
ORAL DRUGS: Concomitant use might reduce absorption of drugs due to reduced GI transit time (19).

Possible Interactions with Foods
No interactions are known to occur, and there is no known reason to expect a clinically significant interaction with butternut.

Possible Interactions with Lab Tests
No interactions are known to occur, and there is no known reason to expect a clinically significant interaction with butternut.

Possible Interactions with Diseases or Conditions
No interactions are known to occur, and there is no known reason to expect a clinically significant interaction with butternut.

Typical Dosages & Routes of Administration that are Commonly Used
ORAL: Butternut extract 1.25 - 6 mL is taken orally three times daily with a meal and plenty of water or juice (3537,3538). Dried bark 2 - 6 grams is taken orally three times daily (3538).

Comments
None.

CABBAGE

This Product is Also Known As
Colewort.

Scientific Names
Brassica oleracea; va. Capitata.
Family: Cruciferae.

People Use This For
Orally, cabbage is used for gastritis, gastric and duodenal ulcers, gastric pain, gastric hyperacidity and Roemheld (gastro-cardiac) syndrome. It is also used orally to protect the stomach lining from gastric hydrochloric acid. Cabbage is eaten as a vegetable (18).

Safety
LIKELY SAFE ...when eaten in food amounts.
There is insufficient reliable information available about the safety of the oral use of cabbage when used medicinally.
PREGNANCY AND LACTATION: Avoid using in amounts greater than those typically found in foods.

Effectiveness
There is insufficient reliable information available about the effectiveness of cabbage.

Possible Mechanism of Action & Active Ingredients
In vitro data suggest that the R-goitrin and various indoles contained in cabbage induce hepatic metabolism and may decrease effectiveness of other medications metabolized by the liver. In vitro animal data also suggest that thiocyanates, isothiocyanates and oxazolidinethione released when cabbage is chopped or crushed decrease iodine uptake by the thyroid gland. Cabbage is considered a rich source of calcium (19).

Adverse Reactions Including Known Allergies
None reported.

Possible Interactions with Herbs & Other Dietary Supplements
Insufficient reliable information available.

Possible Interactions with Drugs
WARFARIN: Cabbage may counteract the anticoagulant effects of warfarin due to its high vitamin K content (19). OTHER: Cabbage may decrease the effectiveness of certain medications by inducing their hepatic metabolism. These medications include hexobarbital, 7-ethoxycoumarin, warfarin, antipyrine, oxazepam, phenacetin and acetaminophen (19).

Possible Interactions with Foods
No interactions are known to occur, and there is no known reason to expect a clinically significant interaction with cabbage.

Possible Interactions with Lab Tests
TSH TEST: Ingesting large quantities of cabbage juice may elevate TSH test results (19).

Possible Interactions with Diseases or Conditions
THYROID DISEASE: Cabbage may worsen goiters and hypothyroidism (19).

Typical Dosages & Routes of Administration that are Commonly Used
ORAL: Cabbage is chopped and pressed for its juice. One liter of juice is taken orally. For gastric pain and hyperacidity, one teaspoon of the juice is taken orally three times daily before meals (18).

Comments
None.

CADE OIL

This Product is Also Known As
Alquitran de Enebro, Goudron de Cade, Juniper Tar, Juniper Tar Oil, Kadeol, Oil of Cade, Oil of Juniper Tar, Oleum Cadinum, Oleum Juniperi Empyreumaticum, Pix Cadi, Pix Juniper, Pix Oxycedri, Pyroleum Juniperi, Pyroleum Oxycedri, Wacholderteer.
CAUTION: See separate listing for Juniper.

Scientific Names
Juniperus oxycedrus.
Family: Cupressaceae or Pinaceae.

People Use This For
Topically, cade oil is used for itching, psoriasis, eczema and seborrhea (14), parasitic skin conditions, as an antiseptic in wound dressings, and in analgesic and antipruritic preparations (11).
Historically, cade oil has been used for treating various skin disorders, scalp conditions, hair loss and cancers (11). In manufacturing, cade oil is an ingredient in dermatologic creams and ointments, and in anti-dandruff shampoos (11).

Safety
POSSIBLY UNSAFE ...when used topically (14). Cade oil might lead to potentially carcinogenic DNA changes (14).
PREGNANCY AND LACTATION: POSSIBLY UNSAFE ...when used topically (14); avoid using.

Effectiveness
There is insufficient reliable information available about the effectiveness of cade oil.

Possible Mechanism of Action & Active Ingredients
Cade oil contains a constituent called creosol. Creosol is a mild to moderate irritant (14). It has antipruritic and keratolytic activity, and antimicrobial activity in vitro (11).

Adverse Reactions Including Known Allergies
Eye irritation (14).

Possible Interactions with Herbs & Other Dietary Supplements
Insufficient reliable information available.

Possible Interactions with Drugs
No interactions are known to occur, and there is no known reason to expect a clinically significant interaction with cade oil.

Possible Interactions with Foods
No interactions are known to occur, and there is no known reason to expect a clinically significant interaction with cade oil.

Possible Interactions with Lab Tests
No interactions are known to occur, and there is no known reason to expect a clinically significant interaction with cade oil.

Possible Interactions with Diseases or Conditions
No interactions are known to occur, and there is no known reason to expect a clinically significant interaction with cade oil.

Typical Dosages & Routes of Administration that are Commonly Used
TOPICAL: Cade oil found in OTC ointments, shampoos, and scalp preparations in concentrations of 1-20%, and in Compound Resorcinol Ointment USP (14).

Comments

Avoid confusion with juniper berry (Juniperus communis). Cade oil is obtained by distilling the wood of the juniper tree (Juniperus oxycedrus).

CAFFEINE

This Product is Also Known As

Anhydrous Caffeine, Caffeine and Sodium Benzoate, Caffeine Citrate, Citrated Caffeine.
CAUTION: See separate listings for Black Tea, Green Tea, Coffee, Cola, Guarana, and Maté.

Scientific Names

1,3,7-trimethylxanthine.

People Use This For

Orally, caffeine is used in combination with analgesics and ergotamine for treating migraine headaches (3). It is also used orally with analgesics for simple headaches and preventing and treating postoperative and postdural puncture headaches (15,2725,2726,2727,2728). Caffeine is used orally for asthma, increasing blood pressure in hypotension (7), increasing mental alertness (15), and enhancing athletic performance (7). It is used in combination with ephedrine or other stimulants and diuretics for weight loss (695,696,1704). Very high doses are used as euphoriants, often in combination with ephedrine as an alternative to illicit stimulants (7,2707).

Rectally, caffeine is used in combination with ergotamine for migraine headaches (15).

Topically, caffeine cream preparations have been used for reducing erythema and itching in dermatitis (14).

Parenterally, caffeine is also used for postoperative and postdural puncture headache, neonatal apnea (15,6023), for acute respiratory depression, and as a diuretic (13). It is also used for extending the length of seizure with electroconvulsive therapy (14).

Caffeine is also used in foods as an ingredient in soft drinks and other beverages.

Safety

LIKELY SAFE ...when used orally, parenterally, or rectally and appropriately. Caffeine is a FDA-approved product and component of several over-the-counter and prescription products (14,15)

POSSIBLY UNSAFE ...when used orally long-term or in high doses. Chronic use, especially in large amounts, can produce tolerance, habituation, psychological dependence, and other significant adverse effects (15). Doses greater than 250-300 mg per day have been associated with significant adverse effects such as tachyarrhythmias and sleep disturbances (see Adverse Reactions) (14,18).

LIKELY UNSAFE ...when used orally in very high doses. Single doses of 3-10 grams have been associated with serious toxicity, including death (7).

CHILDREN: POSSIBLY UNSAFE ...when taken orally in amounts significantly greater than typical food amounts. Children are more susceptible to the adverse effects of caffeine (15).

PREGNANCY: POSSIBLY SAFE ...when used orally in small amounts or amounts found in food. Mothers should closely monitor their intake of caffeine. Use of caffeine in pregnancy is controversial (2708,2709,2710,2711); however, moderate consumption has not been associated with adverse fetal effects (6). Caffeine crosses the human placenta, but is not considered a teratogen. Fetal blood and tissue levels are similar to maternal concentrations (4260). Mothers should keep caffeine consumption below 200 mg per day. This is similar to the amount of caffeine found in 1-2 cups of coffee or tea (2708). POSSIBLY UNSAFE ...when used orally in large amounts. Caffeine crosses the placenta, producing fetal blood concentrations similar to maternal levels (4260). Mothers should avoid consuming more than 200 mg of caffeine daily or more than 1-2 cups of tea or coffee per day (2708). Maternal doses of greater than 200 mg per day throughout pregnancy has resulted in symptoms of caffeine withdrawal in newborn infants (14). High doses of caffeine have been associated with spontaneous abortion, premature delivery, and low birth weight (2709,2711,6).

LACTATION: POSSIBLY SAFE ...when used orally in small amounts or amounts found in food. Nursing mothers should closely monitor caffeine intake. Breast milk concentrations of caffeine are thought to be approximately 50% of maternal serum concentrations. Minimal consumption would likely result in limited exposure to a nursing infant (6). POSSIBLY UNSAFE ...when used orally in large amounts. Caffeine is excreted slowly in infants and may accumulate. Caffeine can cause sleep disturbances, irritability, and increased bowel activity in breast-fed infants exposed to caffeine (18,2708,6026).

Effectiveness

LIKELY EFFECTIVE ...when taken orally for increasing mental alertness (14,15). Caffeine is FDA-approved as a stimulant for improving psychomotor performance (14). ...when used orally in combination with analgesics for simple headache and analgesia (14,15,2718). Caffeine is a FDA-approved product for use with analgesics for improving pain relief (14). ...when used orally in combination with acetaminophen and aspirin to treat migraine headache (2715,2716,2717). Caffeine is a FDA-approved product for use with analgesics for the treatment of migraine (14). ...when used orally or intravenously to prevent postoperative headache (2725,2726). Caffeine is an FDA-approved product for preventing headache in postoperative patients who regularly consume caffeinated products.

POSSIBLY EFFECTIVE ...when used orally for preventing or delaying onset of Parkinson's disease. Epidemiological evidence suggests increasing caffeine consumption from coffee or other sources is associated with decreased risk of developing Parkinson's disease in Japanese-American men (6022). ...when used orally or intravenously to prevent postdural puncture headache (2727,2728). ...when used orally for asthma (14). ...when used orally for increasing blood pressure in hypotension (15). ...when used orally in combination with ephedrine for weight loss (695,696,1704). ...when used intravenously for respiratory depression secondary to CNS depressant overdose (14). ...when used intravenously for neonatal apnea (14,6023).
POSSIBLY INEFFECTIVE ...when taken orally for sustained, submaximal exercise endurance (14).
LIKELY INEFFECTIVE ...when used orally for improving short-term, high-intensity performance and anaerobic capacity or power (14).
There is insufficient reliable information available about the effectiveness of caffeine for its other uses.

Possible Mechanism of Action & Active Ingredients

Caffeine stimulates the central nervous system (CNS), heart, muscles (15), and possibly the pressor centers that control blood pressure (7,15,2722). Possible mechanisms include adenosine receptor blockade and phosphodiesterase inhibition (2722). Caffeine constricts cerebral vasculature (3) and stimulates gastric acid secretion (15). Caffeine can have positive inotropic and chronotropic effects on the heart with a duration of action from one to three hours (7). Caffeine exerts a diuretic effect, with water losses estimated at 1.17 mL per milligram of caffeine (15,2712). Tachyphylaxis to the diuretic effect develops rapidly, diminishing fluid losses associated with caffeine intake (3). Caffeine-containing beverages consumed during moderate endurance exercise do not appear to compromise bodily hydration status (2713). Caffeine's CNS stimulant effects are thought to improve vigilance and psychomotor performance (2720). Caffeine has been reported to cause increases and decreases in blood glucose (14). However, one study found that type 1 diabetics taking 200 mg of caffeine twice daily had increased frequency and intensity of warning signs of hypoglycemia (6024). This may be due to a reduction in blood flow to the brain and increase in glucose utilization by the brain (6024). For prevention of Parkinson's disease, caffeine may prevent adenosine's inhibition of dopaminergic transmission. This may result in a reduction in the clinical expression of Parkinsonism (6022).

Adverse Reactions Including Known Allergies

Caffeine can cause insomnia, nervousness, restlessness (7,15), gastric irritation (7), nausea and vomiting (15), tachycardia, quickened respiration, tremors, delirium, convulsions, and diuresis (15,505). Large doses can produce headache, anxiety, agitation, ringing in the ears, premature heartbeat, and arrhythmias (15). The adverse effects can be more severe in children than adults (15). Caffeine may cause feeding intolerance and gastrointestinal irritation in infants (6023). Some evidence shows caffeine is associated with fibrocystic breast disease in women; however, this is controversial and has been disputed (14,15). Past epidemiological studies on the relationship between caffeine use and the risk for osteoporosis have been conflicting. A recent study of 92 Caucasian, postmenopausal women does not support idea that caffeine use causes an increased risk for osteoporosis (6025). Chronic use of caffeine, especially in large amounts, can sometimes produce tolerance, habituation, and psychological dependence (15). The abrupt discontinuation of caffeine can sometimes result in physical withdrawal symptoms, including headaches, irritation, nervousness, anxiety, and dizziness (15), although some evidence suggests that clinically significant symptoms may be uncommon (2723).

Possible Interactions with Herbs & Other Dietary Supplements

CAFFEINE CONTAINING HERBS/SUPPLEMENTS: Concomitant use can increase the therapeutic and adverse effects. Natural products that contain caffeine include coffee, black or green tea, guarana, mate, and cola.
CREATINE: There is one report of ischemic stroke in an athlete who consumed caffeine 400-600 mg, ephedra 40-60 mg, creatine monohydrate 6 grams, and a variety of other supplements daily for six weeks (1275). Caffeine can interfere with the ergogenic effects of creatine supplementation (2117).
EPHEDRA (Ma Huang): Concomitant use can increase the risk of adverse effects (7). One unpublished report associated jitteriness, hypertension, seizures, temporary loss of consciousness, and hospitalization requiring life support with the use of a combination ephedra and guarana (caffeine) product (1380). There is one report of ischemic stroke in an athlete who consumed caffeine 400-600 mg, ephedra 40-60 mg, creatine monohydrate 6 grams, and a variety of other supplements daily for six weeks (1275).

Possible Interactions with Drugs

ACETAMINOPHEN (Tylenol): Concomitant use can increase the analgesic effect of acetaminophen by up to 40% (512).
ASPIRIN: Concomitant use can increase the analgesic effect of aspirin by up to 40% (512).
BENZODIAZEPINES: Concomitant use reduces the sedative and anxiolytic effects of benzodiazepines (14).
BETA-ADRENERGIC AGONISTS: Concomitant use can increase the positive inotropic effects of beta-agonists on the heart (15). Beta-adrenergic agonists include albuterol (Proventil, Ventolin), metaproterenol (Alupent), terbutaline (Brethine), and isoproterenol (Isuprel).
CIMETIDINE (Tagamet): Concomitant use can increase serum caffeine concentrations and the risk of caffeine adverse effects. Cimetidine decreases the rate of caffeine clearance by 30-50% (14).
CLOZAPINE (Clozaril): Co-administration can acutely exacerbate psychotic symptoms. Caffeine can also increase the effects and toxicity of clozapine (151). Caffeine doses of 400-1000 mg per day inhibit clozapine

metabolism (5051).

CNS STIMULANTS: Concomitant use can increase the risk of adverse CNS effects (151,2719). Some CNS stimulants include nicotine, cocaine, sympathomimetic amines, and amphetamines.

DIABETES THERAPY: Theoretically, concomitant use of caffeine and diabetes drugs might interfere with blood glucose control. Some reports claim that caffeine might have hyperglycemic effects (19).

DISULFIRAM (Antabuse): Concomitant use can increase caffeine serum concentrations and the risk of adverse effects. Disulfiram decreases the rate of caffeine clearance (15).

EPHEDRINE: Concomitant use can increase the risk of stimulatory adverse effects of ephedrine and caffeine (7,19). An unpublished report associated jitteriness, hypertension, seizures, temporary loss of consciousness, and hospitalization requiring life support with the use of a combination ephedra (ephedrine) and caffeine-containing guarana product (1380).

ESTROGEN (Estrace): Concomitant use can increase serum caffeine concentrations and the risk of caffeine adverse effects. Estrogen inhibits caffeine metabolism (2714).

ERGOTAMINE: Concomitant use increases the gastrointestinal absorption of ergotamine (15).

LITHIUM (Eskalith, Lithobid): Abrupt caffeine withdrawal might increase serum lithium levels (609). There are two case reports of lithium tremor that worsened upon abrupt coffee withdrawal (610).

MEXILETINE (Mexitil): Concomitant use can increase serum caffeine concentrations and the risk of caffeine adverse effects. Mexiletine reduces caffeine metabolism (14).

MONOAMINE OXIDASE INHIBITORS (MAOIs): Concomitant intake of large amounts of caffeine with MAOIs might precipitate a hypertensive crisis (19).

ORAL CONTRACEPTIVES (OCs): Concomitant use can increase serum caffeine concentrations and adverse effects. OCs decrease the rate of caffeine clearance by 40-65% (14).

PHENYLPROPANOLAMINE (Dexatrim, Propagest): Concomitant use can cause an additive increase in blood pressure. Phenylpropanolamine can also increase serum caffeine concentrations (14).

QUINOLONES: Concomitant use can increase serum caffeine concentrations and the risk of caffeine adverse effects. Quinolones decrease caffeine clearance (606,607,608). Quinolones (fluoroquinolones) include ciprofloxacin (Cipro), enoxacin (Penetrex), gatifloxacin (Tequin), levofloxacin (Levaquin), lomefloxacin (Maxaquin), moxifloxacin (Avelox), norfloxacin (Noroxin), ofloxacin (Floxin), sparfloxacin (Zagam), and trovafloxacin (Trovan).

RILUZOLE (Rilutek): Concomitant use might increase serum concentrations and the risk of adverse effects of both caffeine and riluzole. Caffeine and riluzole are both metabolized by cytochrome P450 1A2, and concomitant use might reduce metabolism of one or both agents (14).

TERBINAFINE (Lamisil): Concomitant use can increase serum caffeine concentrations and the risk of caffeine adverse effects. Terbinafine decreases the clearance of intravenous caffeine by 19% (14).

THEOPHYLLINE (Theo-Dur): Large amounts of caffeine might inhibit theophylline metabolism, increase serum theophylline concentrations and the risk of adverse effects (14).

VERAPAMIL (Calan, Isoptin, Verelan): Concomitant use can increase plasma caffeine concentrations and the risk of caffeine adverse effects. Verapamil increases plasma caffeine concentrations by 25% (14).

Possible Interactions with Foods

GRAPEFRUIT JUICE: Concomitant use can increase caffeine levels and increase the risk of adverse effects (504).

Possible Interactions with Lab Tests

BLEEDING TIME: Caffeine can prolong bleeding time and increase the results of a bleeding time test (1701).

SERUM URATE (Bittner method): Caffeine can cause false-positive test results (15).

CREATINE: Caffeine can increase urine creatine levels (1701).

URINE CATECHOLAMINES, 5-HYDROXYINDOLEACETIC ACID, VANILLYLMANDELIC ACID (VMA): Caffeine can cause slight increases in these levels and test results (15).

TESTS FOR PHEOCHROMOCYTOMA, NEUROBLASTOMA: High urine catecholamines or VMA can result in false-positive results. Avoid caffeine while testing for these diseases (15).

DIPYRIDAMOLE THALLIUM IMAGING: Caffeine attenuates the characteristic cardiovascular responses to dipyridamole and can alter test results (14).

Possible Interactions with Diseases or Conditions

PEPTIC ULCER DISEASE (PUD): Caffeine can aggravate PUD by increase gastric acid secretion (14,16); avoid using.

CARDIAC CONDITIONS: Caffeine can induce cardiac arrhythmias in sensitive individuals (14,16); use with caution.

DEPRESSION, ANXIETY DISORDERS: Caffeine might aggravate these conditions (14); use with caution.

DIABETES: Caffeine may enhance the frequency and intensity of hypoglycemic warning symptoms in type 1 diabetics. This may increase the ability of diabetics to detect and treat hypoglycemia early. However, it might also increase the frequency of hypoglycemic events (6024); use with caution.

KIDNEY DISEASE: The diuretic effect of caffeine might aggravate some kidney disorders (19).

HYPERTENSION: The pressor effect of caffeine might increase blood pressure in these patients (2722); use with caution.

Typical Dosages & Routes of Administration that are Commonly Used

ORAL: The typical dose of caffeine for headache or restoring mental alertness is up to 250 mg per day (14,15). For fatigue, the common dose is 100-325 mg up to three times a day (13). For increasing exercise performance, 2-10 mg/kg or more has been used (14). However, doses in excess of 10 mg/kg can result in urine levels greater than the 12 mcg/mL allowed by the International Olympic Committee (14). For weight loss, the ephedrine and caffeine combination products are commonly dosed 20 mg/200 mg three times per day (695,696,1704). For postdural puncture headache, 300 mg orally has been used (14).

TOPICAL: For dermatitis, a 30% caffeine cream has been used (14).

INTRAVENOUS: For apnea in infants one study used an initial intravenous dose of caffeine benzoate of 10 mg/kg. Some infants required a second dose of 5 mg/kg 18-24 hours later (6023). Other studies have used a 20 mg/kg loading dose followed by 5 mg/kg daily for maintenance (14). For extended seizure in electroconvulsive therapy (ECT), 500 mg IV 5 minutes before the procedure has been used (14). For postdural puncture headache, 500 mg caffeine sodium benzoate in 1000 mL normal saline infused over 90 minutes following anesthesia has been used. The same dose has also been administered as a bolus dose and repeated in 8 hours as necessary (14).

Comments

People with voice disorders, singers, and other voice professionals are often advised against the use of caffeine; however, this recommendation has been based on anecdotal evidence. Now preliminary research seems to indicate that caffeine ingestion may actually adversely affect subjective voice quality. Further study is necessary to confirm these preliminary findings (2724).

CAJEPUT OIL

This Product is Also Known As

Cajeputi Aetheroleum, Cajuput, Paperbark Tree Oil, Punk Tree.
CAUTION: see separate listings for Niauli Oil and Tea Tree Oil.

Scientific Names

Melaleuca leucodendra, synonym Melaleuca leucodendron; Melaleuca quinquenervia.
Family: Myrtaceae.

People Use This For

Orally, cajeput oil is used as an expectorant (2) or tonic (11).
Topically, cajeput oil is used either alone or in combination with other ingredients in commercially available antiseptic liniments to treat rheumatic and neuralgic discomforts (2).
As an inhalant, it is used as an expectorant (2) and tonic (11).
In dentistry, cajeput oil is used to relieve dry socket discomfort (11).
Historically, cajeput oil has been used to treat colds, headaches, toothache, and indolent tumors (11). It has also been used topically for its anti-parasitic effect in scabies and tinea versicolor (215).
In food and beverages, it is used as a flavoring in very small amounts .

Safety

LIKELY SAFE ...when cajeput oil is used orally in food amounts. The maximum use is less than 0.001% (11).
POSSIBLY SAFE ...when used topically on unbroken skin (2,7).
POSSIBLY UNSAFE ...when inhaled. Inhalation can cause bronchospasm (7). ...when undiluted cajeput oil is taken orally or topically (3527).
There is insufficient reliable information available about the safety of the oral use of cajeput oil in amounts exceeding those found in food.
CHILDREN: LIKELY UNSAFE ...when used topically on facial areas, especially the nose (2,7) because it might cause bronchospasm.
PREGNANCY AND LACTATION: Insufficient reliable information available; avoid using.

Effectiveness

POSSIBLY EFFECTIVE ...when used orally as an expectorant (7). ...when used topically as counterirritant for arthritis and rheumatism (2). A counterirritant is an agent that causes mild inflammation of the skin for the purpose of relieving a deep-seated inflammatory process. (2).
There is insufficient reliable information available about the effectiveness of cajeput oil for its other uses.

Possible Mechanism of Action & Active Ingredients

Cajeput oil contains 14-65% cineole (7,11), which is reported to have antispasmodic, antimicrobial and fungicidal properties (2,7). Cineole may act as a counterirritant (7). Cineole is identical to eucalyptol (215).

Adverse Reactions Including Known Allergies

Taking cajeput oil orally can lead to dyspepsia (7). Topical use can produce hypersensitivity, allergic reactions and irritation of mucous membranes (7). Inhaling it can cause bronchospasm (7).

Possible Interactions with Herbs & Other Dietary Supplements
Insufficient reliable information available.

Possible Interactions with Drugs
No interactions are known to occur, and there is no known reason to expect a clinically significant interaction with cajeput oil.

Possible Interactions with Foods
No interactions are known to occur, and there is no known reason to expect a clinically significant interaction with cajeput oil.

Possible Interactions with Lab Tests
No interactions are known to occur, and there is no known reason to expect a clinically significant interaction with cajeput oil.

Possible Interactions with Diseases or Conditions
ASTHMA: Inhalation may provoke bronchospasm [7].

Typical Dosages & Routes of Administration that are Commonly Used
No typical dosage.

Comments
Avoid confusion with tea tree oil (Maleleuca alternifolia) and niauli oil (Malaleuca viridiflora). Cajeput oil is produced by steam distillation of fresh leaves and twigs of Melaleuca leucodendra and Melaleuca quinquenervia.

CALABAR BEAN

This Product is Also Known As
Chop Nut, Esere Nut, Faba Calabarica, Ordeal Bean, Physotigma.

Scientific Names
Physostigma venenosum.
Family: Leguminosae/Fabaceae.

People Use This For
Calabar bean is a source of the prescription drug physostigmine.
Historically, African tribes used calabar bean, the "ordeal bean," to identify witches and people possessed by evil spirits [6]. They believed that people who regurgitated the bean and lived were innocent.

Safety
UNSAFE ...when taken orally. The calabar bean is extremely toxic. Its active constituent, physostigmine, can cause death by impairing heart contractility and causing respiratory paralysis [6].
PREGNANCY AND LACTATION: UNSAFE ...contraindicated; avoid using [6].

Effectiveness
EFFECTIVE ...when used as a poison. ...when used as prescription drug physostigmine for prolonging the activity of neurotransmitter acetylcholine [6].

Possible Mechanism of Action & Active Ingredients
The applicable part of calabar bean is the dried, ripe seed. The major constituent, physostigmine, prolongs activity of neurotransmitter acetylcholine [6]. It increases parasympathetic nervous system and striated muscle tone, stimulates glandular secretions, increases GI peristalsis, reduces heart rate, and causes pupil contraction leading to a reduction in intraocular pressure [18].

Adverse Reactions Including Known Allergies
Physostigmine overdose causes cholinergic crisis characterized by excessive salivation and sweating, constricted pupils of eye, nausea, vomiting, diarrhea, bradycardia or tachycardia, hypotension or hypertension, confusion, seizures, coma, severe muscle weakness, paralysis and death [15].

Possible Interactions with Herbs & Other Dietary Supplements
Insufficient reliable information available.

Possible Interactions with Drugs
ANTICHOLINERGIC DRUGS: Physostigmine reverses the effect of belladonna and other drugs with anticholinergic action. These drugs include antihistamines, some emetics, some anti-Parkinson agents and phenothiazines [15].

Possible Interactions with Foods

No interactions are known to occur, and there is no known reason to expect a clinically significant interaction with calabar bean.

Possible Interactions with Lab Tests

No interactions are known to occur, and there is no known reason to expect a clinically significant interaction with calabar bean.

Possible Interactions with Diseases or Conditions

Avoid in patients with Parkinson's disease, bradycardia, asthma, gangrene, diabetes, cardiovascular disease, and mechanical obstruction of intestinal or urogenital tract.

Typical Dosages & Routes of Administration that are Commonly Used

No typical dosage.

Comments

Calabar bean is considered unsafe for medicinal use (6); safer alternatives available. Ritual uses continue in Africa despite being outlawed (6). Subjects of the "ordeal" can increase their chance of survival by not chewing the bean and swallowing it whole. Chewing releases the toxic constituents.

CALAMINT

This Product is Also Known As

Basil Thyme, Mill Mint, Mountain Balm, Mountain Mint.

Scientific Names

Calamintha ascendens.
Family: Labiatae or Lamiaceae.

People Use This For

Orally, calamint is used for respiratory illnesses and colds with fever. It is also used orally to promote sweating and as an expectorant (18).

Safety

There is insufficient reliable information available about the safety of the oral use of calamint.
Pregnancy and Lactation: Insufficient reliable information available; avoid using.

Effectiveness

There is insufficient reliable information available about the effectiveness of calamint.

Possible Mechanism of Action & Active Ingredients

The applicable parts of calamint are the above ground parts. There is insufficient reliable information available about the possible mechanisms of action or active ingredients.

Adverse Reactions Including Known Allergies

None reported.

Possible Interactions with Herbs & Other Dietary Supplements

Insufficient reliable information available.

Possible Interactions with Drugs

No interactions are known to occur, and there is no known reason to expect a clinically significant interaction with calamint.

Possible Interactions with Foods

No interactions are known to occur, and there is no known reason to expect a clinically significant interaction with calamint.

Possible Interactions with Lab Tests

No interactions are known to occur, and there is no known reason to expect a clinically significant interaction with calamint.

Possible Interactions with Diseases or Conditions

No interactions are known to occur, and there is no known reason to expect a clinically significant interaction with calamint.

Typical Dosages & Routes of Administration that are Commonly Used

No typical dosage.

Comments

There is very little scientific information about this product. Our staff is continually analyzing the available information on natural medicines and will add data here as it becomes available.

CALAMUS

This Product is Also Known As

Cinnamon Sedge, Gladdon, Grass Myrtle, Myrtle Flag, Myrtle Sedge, Sweet Cane, Sweet Cinnamon, Sweet Flag, Sweet Grass, Sweet Myrtle, Sweet Root, Sweet Rush, Sweet Sedge.

Scientific Names

Acorus calamus.
Family: Araceae.

People Use This For

Orally, calamus is used for digestive disorders including ulcers, gastritis (18), and flatulence (9), and to stimulate appetite and digestion. Some people use calamus to induce sweating (4). Others chew it to remove the smell of tobacco (6).

Historically, calamus has been used orally as a sedative and for acute and chronic dyspepsia, gastritis, gastric ulcer, anorexia (4), rheumatoid arthritis, and strokes and topically for skin diseases (11). Native Americans of the Cree tribe chewed the root for its stimulant, euphoric, and hallucinogenic effects (214).

In food use, calamus is utilized in cooking as a spice (5).

Safety

LIKELY UNSAFE ...when used orally. FDA prohibits calamus use in food products (12) due to the presence of the carcinogenic constituent, beta-isoasarone (5) in three of the four distinct strains. However, the beta-isoasarone content varies widely among strains (from 0% to 96%) (6), so some products may be safer than others.
PREGNANCY AND LACTATION: LIKELY UNSAFE; avoid using (4,500).

Effectiveness

There is insufficient reliable information about the effectiveness of calamus.

Possible Mechanism of Action & Active Ingredients

The applicable part of calamus is the rhizome. The constituent asarone, which is chemically related to reserpine, may explain calamus' sedative effects (6). It is not known exactly which constituent is responsible for calamus' ability to relieve smooth muscle spasms, though it is probably not isoasarone, because preparations without isoasarone have a measurable spasmolytic effect (6).

Adverse Reactions Including Known Allergies

Calamus oil may contain beta-isoasarone, a known carcinogen associated with kidney damage, tremors, and convulsions.

Possible Interactions with Herbs & Other Dietary Supplements

HERBS WITH SEDATIVE PROPERTIES: Theoretically, concomitant use with herbs that have sedative properties might enhance therapeutic and adverse effects. These include calendula, California poppy, catnip, capsicum, celery, couch grass, elecampane, ginseng Siberian, German chamomile, goldenseal, gotu kola, hops, Jamaican dogwood, kava, lemon balm, sage, St. John's wort, sassafras, scullcap, shepherd's purse, stinging nettle, valerian, wild carrot, wild lettuce, withania root, and yerba mansa (4,19).

Possible Interactions with Drugs

ACID-INHIBITING DRUGS: Theoretically, due to claims that calamus increases stomach acid, it might interfere with antacids, sucralfate (Carafate), H-2 antagonists, or proton pump inhibitors (19).
MAO INHIBITORS: Theoretically, calamus might potentiate the effects and adverse effects of monoamine oxidase inhibitor drugs (4).
CNS DEPRESSANTS: Theoretically, concomitant use with drugs with sedative properties can cause additive effects and side effects (4).

Possible Interactions with Foods

No interactions are known to occur, and there is no known reason to expect a clinically significant interaction with calamus.

Possible Interactions with Lab Tests

No interactions are known to occur, and there is no known reason to expect a clinically significant interaction with calamus.

Possible Interactions with Diseases or Conditions

No interactions are known to occur, and there is no known reason to expect a clinically significant interaction with calamus.

Typical Dosages & Routes of Administration that are Commonly Used

ORAL: 1-3 grams rhizome three times daily, or one cup tea (steep 1-3 grams rhizome in 150 mL boiling water 5-10 minutes, strain) three times daily (4). Liquid extract (1:1 in 60% alcohol) 1-3 mL three times daily (4). Tincture (1:5 in 60% alcohol) 2-4 mL three times daily (4).

Comments

Four different types of herbs/volatile oil exist, each in a different geographic region of the world. The North American variety is isoasarone free and the European form contains less than 10% isoasarone in the volatile oil. Others contain up to 96% carcinogenic beta-isoasarone in the volatile oil (5).

CALCIUM

This Product is Also Known As

Bone Meal, Calcium Acetate, Calcium Aspartate, Calcium Carbonate, Calcium Chelate, Calcium Chloride, Calcium Citrate, Calcium Citrate Malate, Calcium Gluconate, Calcium Lactate, Calcium Lactogluconate, Calcium Orotate, Calcium Phosphate, Dicalcium Phosphate, Heated Oyster Shell-Seaweed Calcium, Hydroxyapatite, Oyster Shell Calcium, Tricalcium Phosphate.
CAUTION: See separate listing for Dolomite.

Scientific Names

Calcium; Ca; atomic number 20.

People Use This For

Orally, calcium is used for reducing the risk of colorectal cancer (970,994,1047), for treating diarrhea and rectal epithelial hyperproliferation following intestinal bypass (1826,1827), for reducing excess fluoride levels in children (990), treating hypertension (976), replacement therapy in hypocalcemia, chronic hypoparathyroidism, osteomalacia (15), preventing and treating osteoporosis (9), treating premenstrual syndrome (1822,1823,1824), rickets, and latent tetany (15). Calcium carbonate is used as an antacid (9). Calcium carbonate and calcium acetate are also used as phosphate binders in renal failure (9).
Intravenously, calcium gluconate is used for severe hypocalcemia (15).

Safety

LIKELY SAFE ...when used orally and appropriately. Routine dietary intake and supplementation in recommended doses are not associated with significant adverse effects (15). ...when used intravenously and appropriately (15).
POSSIBLY UNSAFE ...when used orally in excessive doses. Amounts exceeding 2.4 grams per day can cause kidney stones, which might result in renal damage (945,1816). ...when calcium chloride is used orally. Ingestion of calcium chloride has been reported to cause gastrointestinal hemorrhage (15).
PREGNANCY AND LACTATION: LIKELY SAFE ...when used orally and appropriately (945,3263,3264).

Effectiveness

EFFECTIVE ...when used orally for replacement therapy in hypocalcemia (15). ...when calcium carbonate is used as an antacid (9). ...when calcium carbonate or calcium acetate are used as phosphate binders in renal failure (9). ...when calcium gluconate is used intravenously for severe hypocalcemia (15).
LIKELY EFFECTIVE ...when used orally to prevent bone loss and reduce fractures in postmenopausal women and elderly men and women (977,978,981,1835,1836). ...when used orally for primary prevention of osteoporosis (9,15). ...when used in mothers during pregnancy to improve fetal bone mineralization and density (3263,3264). Calcium supplements in pregnant women who have low dietary calcium intake (less than 562 mg elemental calcium/day), increase fetal bone mineralization, but do not appear to have any effect on women who have an adequate dietary calcium intake (3263,3264). ...when used to reduce the risk of colorectal cancer (970,994,1047). ...when used orally for reducing the symptoms of premenstrual syndrome (1822,1823,1824). ...when calcium carbonate is used orally for reducing secondary hyperparathyroidism in people with chronic renal failure (1827,1828,1829).
POSSIBLY EFFECTIVE ...when used in combination with vitamin D as adjunctive therapy for reducing bone mineral density loss in people with conditions requiring long-term corticosteroid use (982,1046,1830,1831,1832,4462,4463, 4464,4465,4466,4467). ...when used for reducing bone turnover during weight reduction in postmenopausal women (987). ...when used orally for hypertension. In studies, calcium supplementation produced a modest reduction in blood pressure; possibly more effective in subpopulations of hypertensive patients, such as salt-sensitive people and African American adolescents with low dietary calcium intake (945,972,974,976,984,1818,1819, 1820,1821). ...when used orally for reducing blood pressure in individuals with end-stage renal disease (975). ...when used orally for preventing pregnancy-related hypertension and pre-eclampsia. Benefits for pregnancy-related hypertension may be limited to women with insufficient calcium intake (971,973,1833,1834). ...when used orally for treating diarrhea and rectal epithelial hyperproliferation due to intestinal bypass (1826,1827). ...when used for treating

excessive fluoride levels in children (990). …when used orally to prevent ischemic stroke (4822). A large epidemiological study associated low calcium intake with increased risk of ischemic stroke in women (4822). POSSIBLY INEFFECTIVE …when used for preventing bone mineral density loss in lactating women (988). …when used orally for preventing bone loss after bone marrow transplantation (1817). …when used orally for preventing bone loss associated with long-term renal transplantation (4823). Calcium carbonate 500 mg per day in combination with calcitriol 0.25 mcg per day did not significantly improve bone loss in renal transplant patients; however, the treatment group had less osteoclast suppression and there was a trend to maintenance of trabecular bone volume and wall thickness, and some improvement in axial bone mineral density (4823).

Possible Mechanism of Action & Active Ingredients

The bones and teeth contain greater than 99% of calcium in the human body. Calcium in bone also serves as a reserve source of calcium that can be mobilized to maintain extracellular calcium concentrations. About half of serum calcium is bound to plasma proteins. The free or ionized calcium is tightly regulated and a useful clinical indicator of calcium status (1834). Calcium is involved in intracellular regulation and has a pivotal role in muscle cell function (945). In heart muscle and nerve terminals, calcium channels open when membranes are depolarized and stored calcium is released (945). The subsequent rise in cytosolic calcium concentration triggers contraction (945). Calcium balance is generally positive during growth, neutral in the mature adult, and negative in older adults (1834). Calcium is lost in varying amounts through the feces, urine, sweat, and sloughed skin cells (1834). Calcium absorption varies with age, environmental and dietary conditions, and race (1837). Asians and Africans absorb calcium more efficiently than Caucasians (1837). Calcium exhibits threshold absorption. Below the threshold, an increase in calcium intake results in improved response; above the threshold, increased calcium intake has no effect. The many variables of calcium absorption complicates interpretation of calcium absorption studies (1834). Some evidence suggests that calcium citrate and heated oyster shell-seaweed calcium are absorbed better than calcium carbonate, while other research indicates similar bioavailability (1838,1839,1840,1841,1842,1847). Contrary to laboratory evidence, lactose does not enhance calcium bioavailability in lactose tolerant people (4824). Researchers report that a high-calcium, low-calorie diet leads to twice as much weight loss as a low-calcium, low-calorie diet in obese mice. Clinical trials are underway to confirm whether high calcium intake has comparable effects in humans. The results of this unpublished study were presented at the Experimental Biology 2000 conference (5056).

Adverse Reactions Including Known Allergies

Calcium given orally can cause gastrointestinal irritation, belching, and flatulence (9,1843). Although constipation is frequently cited as an adverse effect of calcium, there is no scientific substantiation of this purported side effect (1843,1844,1845). Calcium chloride has been reported to cause gastrointestinal hemorrhage when taken orally (15). Calcium carbonate can cause acid rebound (9). Prolonged ingestion of large amounts (greater than 20 grams per day) of calcium carbonate can cause hypercalcemia, milk-alkali syndrome (9,1843,6123), nephrocalcinosis, and renal insufficiency (6122). In patients with impaired renal function, doses as low as 4 grams per day might cause hypercalcemia (1843). Although there are reports of oyster shell calcium contamination with lead or aluminum and bone meal calcium and dolomite contamination with lead (997), there have never been any reports of significant toxicity from lead contamination (996). Epidemiological evidence suggests that a high intake of dietary calcium might increase the risk for prostate cancer (4825,4827).

Possible Interactions with Herbs & Other Dietary Supplements

VITAMIN D: Concomitant administration with vitamin D increases active absorption of oral calcium (945).
IRON, ZINC, MAGNESIUM: Concomitant administration decreases gastrointestinal absorption of iron, zinc, and magnesium, but does not appear to have any clinically significant effect on the status of these minerals in the body (998,1848,1849,1850). Administration of calcium and other mineral supplements should be done at different times.

Possible Interactions with Drugs

BISPHOSPHONATES (alendronate, etidronate, risedronate, etc.): Absorption is decreased by concomitant administration with calcium. Administer alendronate at least 30 minutes before calcium (14).
ESTROGEN: Concomitant use of estrogen increases supplemental calcium absorption in postmenopausal women (995).
FLUOROQUINOLONES (ciprofloxacin, levofloxacin, ofloxacin, etc.): Concomitant administration decreases the absorption of these drugs and calcium (9). Administer these drugs at least two hours before or after calcium supplements.
LEVOTHYROXINE (Synthroid, Levothroid, Levoxyl): Concomitant administration reduces levothyroxine absorption (14). Three cases have been reported of reduced levothyroxine effectiveness with concomitant calcium carbonate administration (5081,5082). Separate the administration of levothyroxine and calcium by at least 4 hours (14). In some studies, long-term levothyroxine therapy has been associated with decreased bone density in the hip and spine in pre- and post-menopausal women. This is thought to be due to increased urinary loss of calcium. There is currently no evidence that calcium supplementation is either helpful or necessary (27,28,29).
TETRACYCLINES (demeclocycline, doxycycline, minocycline, etc.): Concomitant administration decreases the absorption of these drugs and calcium (9). Administer these drugs at least two hours before or after calcium supplements.
THIAZIDE AND THIAZIDE-LIKE DIURETICS (hydrochlorothiazide, indapamide, metolazone, etc.):

Concomitant use of thiazide diuretics along with moderately large amounts of calcium carbonate increases the risk of milk-alkali syndrome (hypercalcemia, metabolic alkalosis, renal failure) (9,14). Reduce the calcium dose and monitor serum calcium level and/or parathyroid function (14).

VERAPAMIL (Calan, Isoptin, Verelan): Pretreatment with intravenous calcium gluconate can prevent or reduce hypotensive effects of intravenous verapamil without affecting the antiarrhythmic effects of verapamil (6124).

Drug Influences on Nutrient Levels and Depletion

SOME DRUGS CAN AFFECT CALCIUM LEVELS:

TETRACYCLINES: Tetracyclines can form complexes with dietary or supplemental calcium in the GI tract and reduce absorption of both tetracyclines and calcium. Tetracyclines should be dosed 2 hours before or after calcium-containing foods/products to avoid calcium malabsorption (4412).

LOOP DIURETICS and THIAZIDE DIURETICS: Use of loop diuretics and thiazide diuretics can increase urinary calcium excretion and possibly reduce serum levels. This is more likely with higher doses or when used in combination with diuretics of another class (4412).

ALUMINUM SALTS: Use of aluminum salts can indirectly lead to increased urinary calcium excretion. Avoid prolonged administration of large doses of aluminum-containing products which might lead to hypocalcemia (4400).

MAGNESIUM SALTS: Use of magnesium salts can indirectly lead to increased urinary calcium excretion. Avoid prolonged administration of large doses of magnesium-containing products which might lead to hypocalcemia (4400).

MINERAL OIL: Mineral oil can reduce dietary calcium absorption. Avoid long-term use of mineral oil (4495).

STIMULANT LAXATIVES: Stimulant laxatives can reduce dietary calcium absorption. Limit stimulant laxatives to short-term use (4425).

CORTICOSTEROIDS: Use of corticosteroids can cause calcium depletion and osteoporosis with long-term administration. Calcium depletion creates a greater need for both supplemental calcium and vitamin D, which is necessary for calcium absorption. It may be prudent to supplement calcium and vitamin D (Calcitriol) before, during, and after long term and/or high dose corticosteroids (4462,4463,4464,4465,4466,4467).

THYROID HORMONES: In some studies, long-term levothyroxine therapy has been associated with decreased bone density in the hip and spine in pre- and post-menopausal women. This is thought to be due to increased urinary loss of calcium. There is not yet any proof that calcium supplementation is either helpful or necessary (27,28,29).

Possible Interactions with Foods

DAIRY FOODS: Foods that are high in phosphorus, mainly dairy products, may reduce calcium absorption by forming insoluble complexes with calcium ions. Separate calcium supplements from dairy products and other high-phosphorus foods by two hours (14).

DIETARY FIBER: Certain constituents of dietary fiber inhibit calcium absorption. These include phytic acid (found in wheat bran), oxalic acid (found in spinach and rhubarb) and uronic acid (a common plant fiber constituent) (14,945). Separate administration of calcium supplements from these foods by two hours (14).

FOOD HIGH IN VITAMIN D: Ingestion of food, especially food high in vitamin D, increases absorption of supplemental calcium (945).

FOOD HIGH IN SODIUM: High sodium intake increases urinary calcium excretion (1834).

Possible Interactions with Lab Tests

GASTRIN: Calcium carbonate can increase serum gastrin concentrations and test results within 30-75 minutes after calcium carbonate ingestion (275).

GLUCOSE: Calcium gluconate can decrease serum glucose concentrations and test results. This interaction was reported in newborns (275).

11-HYDROXYCORTICOSTEROIDS: Calcium gluconate given intravenously can increase plasma 11-hydroxycorticosteroid concentrations and test results (275).

17-HYDROXYCORTICOSTEROIDS: Calcium gluconate can reduce urinary 17-hydroxycorticosteroid concentrations and test results. One case of this interaction is reported (275).

INSULIN: Calcium gluconate can increase plasma insulin concentrations and test results. This interaction was reported in newborns (275).

I-131 UPTAKE: Calcium gluconate can decrease serum uptake of I-131 (275).

LIPASE: Calcium ions can falsely decrease test results when measuring serum lipase concentrations greater than 5 mmol/L using the method of Teitz (275). Calcium ions do not affect test results when measuring serum lipase concentrations up to 5 mmol/L using the method of Teitz (275).

MAGNESIUM: Calcium gluconate can falsely decrease test results for serum magnesium measured by titan-yellow, but will not affect test results measured by the dihydroxyazobenzene method (275). Calcium gluconate can falsely decrease test results for urine magnesium measured by titan-yellow (275).

BONE MINERAL DENSITY (BMD): Supplemental calcium taken orally can prevent or reduce the rate of bone mineral loss as reflected in BMD measures (977,978,981).

Possible Interactions with Diseases or Conditions

HYPERPARATHYROIDISM: Hyperparathyroid activity predisposes individuals to increased calcium absorption (945).

HYPOTHYROIDISM: People taking levothyroxine (L-thyroxine, Levothroid, Synthroid) replacement therapy are cautioned to separate administration of levothyroxine and calcium carbonate by four hours for maximum levothyroxine effectiveness (14). One case of hypothyroidism is reported involving concomitant administration of levothyroxine and calcium carbonate in a hypothyroid patient. Thyroid function normalized when administration of the two agents was separated (5081).

RENAL INSUFFICIENCY: Calcium carbonate supplementation increases the risk of hypercalcemia and alkalosis (9). Renal insufficiency predisposes individuals to reduced calcium absorption (945).

SARCOIDOSIS: This condition results in increased risk of excessive calcium absorption and hypercalcemia (945).

SMOKING: Cigarette smoking decreases intestinal calcium absorption (1846).

Typical Dosages & Routes of Administration that are Commonly Used

ORAL: Patients in clinical studies have taken between 500 mg and 1600 mg elemental calcium per day for prevention of bone loss (979,980). Supplements are usually divided into three to four doses daily (9); absorption of calcium from supplements is greatest when taken with food in doses of 500 mg or less (15,6122). For pregnant women with low dietary calcium intake, the dose for increasing fetal bone density ranges from 300-1300 mg/day beginning at gestation week 20-22 (3263,3264). The daily Dietary Reference Intakes (DRI) for elemental calcium are: Age 1-3 years, 500 mg; 4-8 years, 800 mg; 9-18 years, 1300 mg; 19-50 years, 1000 mg; 51+ years, 1200 mg; Pregnant or Lactating (under 19 years), 1300 mg; Pregnant or Lactating (19-50 years), 1000 mg (998). The daily upper intake level (UL) for calcium is 2.5 grams for everyone over one year of age (3094). Calcium replacement requirements can be estimated by clinical condition or serum calcium determinations (15). Calcium carbonate and calcium citrate are the two most commonly used forms of calcium (945). Calcium carbonate contains 400 mg calcium/gram and calcium citrate contains 211 mg calcium/gram (15) (1000 mg elemental calcium = 2500 mg calcium carbonate = 4700 mg calcium citrate). Calcium carbonate and calcium phosphate should be taken with food (1816,1842). Other calcium salts may be taken without regard to meals and may be preferable in people with achlorhydria or on drugs that reduce gastric acidity (e.g., H2 antagonists, proton pump inhibitors) (1816).

Comments

To assure calcium needs are met, nutrition experts recommend consuming calcium throughout the day as a calcium-rich food or up to 500 mg supplemental calcium at each meal (307). Calcium-rich foods include milk and dairy products, kale and broccoli, as well as the calcium-enriched citrus juices, canned fish with bones, and tofu processed with calcium.

CALCIUM D-GLUCARATE

This Product is Also Known As

Calcium Glucarate, D-Glucarate (GA).

Scientific Names

D-glucaro-1,4-lactone (1,4 GL).

People Use This For

Orally, calcium D-glucarate is taken for preventing breast (773), prostate, and colon cancer (774), and for detoxifying the body of carcinogens, toxins and steroid hormones (771,772).

Safety

There is insufficient reliable information available about the safety of calcium D-glucarate.

Pregnancy and Lactation: Insufficient reliable information available; avoid using.

Effectiveness

There is insufficient reliable information available about the effectiveness of calcium D-glucarate.

Possible Mechanism of Action & Active Ingredients

Dietary glucarate is reported to inhibit beta-glucuronidase activity and chemically-induced mammary tumor development in rats (775). In vitro, D-glucarate decreases tumor cell proliferation; this activity is synergistic with retinoids (776). In dehydrated rats, sodium D-glucaro-1,4-lactone prevented kanamycin-induced renal impairment, possibly by increasing the rate of kanamycin elimination (777). Urinary excretion of D-glucaric acid may be an indicator of drug metabolizing enzyme activity in people with impaired renal function (778). In alcoholics, while drinking alcohol, urinary excretion of D-glucaric acid was increased (779).

Adverse Reactions Including Known Allergies

None reported.

Possible Interactions with Herbs & Other Dietary Supplements
Insufficient reliable information available.

Possible Interactions with Drugs
ALCOHOL: Theoretically, concomitant use with alcohol may reduce D-glucarate activity.
KANAMYCIN: Theoretically, D-glucarate may increase the rate of kanamycin elimination and reduce the risk of drug-induced renal impairment.

Possible Interactions with Foods
ALCOHOL: Theoretically, concomitant administration may reduce D-glucarate activity.

Possible Interactions with Lab Tests
No interactions are known to occur, and there is no known reason to expect a clinically significant interaction with calcium D-glucarate.

Possible Interactions with Diseases or Conditions
No interactions are known to occur, and there is no known reason to expect a clinically significant interaction with calcium D-glucarate.

Typical Dosages & Routes of Administration that are Commonly Used
No typical dosage.

Comments
Glucaric acid is found in human tissues and body fluids. Dietary sources containing glucaric acid range from a low of 1.12-1.73 mg/100 grams (broccoli and potatoes) to a high of 4.53 mg/100 grams (oranges) (772).

CALENDULA

This Product is Also Known As
Garden Marigold, Gold-Bloom, Holligold, Marigold, Marybud, Pot Marigold.

Scientific Names
Calendula officinalis.
Family: Asteraceae/Compositae.

People Use This For
Orally, calendula flower is used as an antispasmodic (3,4), to initiate menstrual periods (4), reduce fever, for treating cancer (6), and inflammation of oral and pharyngeal mucosa (2).
Topically, calendula is used as an anti-inflammatory and for poorly healing wounds and leg ulcers (2).
Traditionally, calendula has been taken orally for gastric and duodenal ulcers and dysmenorrhea. It has been used topically for nosebleeds, varicose veins, hemorrhoids, proctitis, and conjunctivitis (4).

Safety
LIKELY SAFE ...when the flower preparations are used orally and appropriately (4). ...when the flower preparations are used topically and appropriately (4).
PREGNANCY: LIKELY UNSAFE ...contraindicated for oral use because it has spermatocide, antiblastocyst, and abortifacient effects. There is insufficient reliable information available about the safety of the topical use of calendula during pregnancy (4).
LACTATION: Insufficient reliable information available; avoid using.

Effectiveness
POSSIBLY EFFECTIVE ...when taken orally for inflammation of the oral and pharyngeal mucosa (2). ...when used topically for poorly healing wounds and leg ulcers (2).
There is insufficient reliable information available about the effectiveness of calendula for its other uses.

Possible Mechanism of Action & Active Ingredients
The applicable part of calendula is the flower. Some evidence suggests calendula is useful in wound healing. It has an anti-inflammatory effect and it also stimulates tissue granulation (2). The faradiol monoester is believed to play an important role in anti-inflammatory activity. Some evidence suggests the water-soluble flavonoids might be responsible for the wound-healing effects (515). Calendula also shows some evidence of antibacterial, antiviral, and antitumor activity (4).

Adverse Reactions Including Known Allergies
Calendula can cause an allergic reaction in individuals sensitive to the Asteraceae/Compositae family. Members of this family include ragweed, chrysanthemums, marigolds, daisies, and many other herbs. Despite the widespread use of calendula and the occurrence of allergies to other family members, there has been only one report of anaphylaxis (6).

© Copyright 2000, Natural Medicines Comprehensive Database (209) 472-2244. For updated data, go to www.NaturalDatabase.com • 211

Possible Interactions with Herbs & Other Dietary Supplements

HERBS WITH SEDATIVE PROPERTIES: Theoretically, concomitant use with herbs that have sedative properties might enhance therapeutic and adverse effects. These include calamus, California poppy, catnip, capsicum, celery, couch grass, elecampane, ginseng Siberian, German chamomile, goldenseal, gotu kola, hops, Jamaican dogwood, kava, lemon balm, sage, St. John's wort, sassafras, scullcap, shepherd's purse, stinging nettle, valerian, wild carrot, wild lettuce, withania root, and yerba mansa [4,19].

Possible Interactions with Drugs

BARBITURATES: Theoretically, concomitant use of calendula with barbiturates can cause additive therapeutic and adverse effects [19].
OTHER DRUGS WITH SEDATIVE PROPERTIES: Theoretically, concomitant use of calendula with drugs having sedative properties can cause additive therapeutic and adverse effects [19].

Possible Interactions with Foods

No interactions are known to occur, and there is no known reason to expect a clinically significant interaction with calendula.

Possible Interactions with Lab Tests

No interactions are known to occur, and there is no known reason to expect a clinically significant interaction with calendula.

Possible Interactions with Diseases or Conditions

CROSS-ALLERGENICITY: Can cause an allergic reaction in individuals sensitive to the Asteraceae/Compositae family. Members of this family include ragweed, chrysanthemums, marigolds, daisies, and many other herbs.

Typical Dosages & Routes of Administration that are Commonly Used

ORAL: One cup of the tea is commonly taken three times daily, and the tea is prepared by steeping 1-2 grams of the dried flowers in 150 mL boiling water for 5-10 minutes and then straining [2,4]. The typical dose of the liquid extract (1:1 in 40% alcohol) is 0.5-1 mL three times daily [4]. The tincture (1:5 in 90% alcohol) is usually given as 0.3-1.2 mL three times daily [4].
TOPICAL: The tea is commonly used as a gargle, mouthwash, or poured over an absorbent cloth and applied as a poultice to skin ailments [3]. For topical use, 2-4 mL of the tincture is usually diluted into 0.25-0.5 L water. Ointments typically contain 2-5 grams of the herb in 100 grams ointment [2].

Comments

Avoid confusion with ornamental marigolds of the Tagets species, which are commonly grown in vegetable gardens [11].

CALIFORNIA POPPY

This Product is Also Known As

California Poppies, Poppy California.
CAUTION: See separate listing for Corn Poppy.

Scientific Names

Eschscholzia californica.
Family: Papaveraceae.

People Use This For

California poppy is taken for insomnia, sedation, aches, nervous agitation, enuresis in children, and diseases of the bladder and liver [18].
In combination with other herbs, California poppy is used for depression, neurasthenia, neuropathy, various psychiatric conditions, foehn illness (sleep and mood disturbance associated with strong, warm wind in the Alps), vasomotor dysfunction, sensitivity to weather changes, and sedation [2].

Safety

POSSIBLY UNSAFE ...when used orally and appropriately. Although only the dried aerial parts are used medicinally, the freshly harvested plant contains cyanogenic glycosides that could potentially cause cyanide poisoning [18].
PREGNANCY AND LACTATION: POSSIBLY UNSAFE; avoid using [2].

Effectiveness

There is insufficient reliable information available about the effectiveness of California poppy.

Possible Mechanism of Action & Active Ingredients

The applicable parts of California poppy here the dried, above ground parts. The active constituents are thought to be isoquinoline alkaloids [2,18]. One alkaloid, cryptonine, may have uterine stimulating activity in guinea pigs [2].

The tincture is reported to prolong pentobarbital-induced sleep in mice and to prevent chemically-induced spasms in rat jejunum (2).

Adverse Reactions Including Known Allergies
None reported (18).

Possible Interactions with Herbs & Other Dietary Supplements
HERBS WITH SEDATIVE PROPERTIES: Theoretically, concomitant use with herbs that have sedative properties might enhance therapeutic and adverse effects. These include calamus, calendula, catnip, capsicum, celery, couch grass, elecampane, Siberian ginseng, German chamomile, goldenseal, gotu kola, hops, Jamaican dogwood, kava, lemon balm, sage, St. John's wort, sassafras, scullcap, shepherd's purse, stinging nettle, valerian, wild carrot, wild lettuce, withania root, and yerba mansa (4,19).

Possible Interactions with Drugs
MONOAMINE OXIDASE INHIBITORS: May potentiate MAOI activity (12).
BARBITURATES: Theoretically, concomitant use with barbiturates may cause additive effects and side effects (19).
OTHER DRUGS WITH SEDATIVE PROPERTIES: Theoretically, concomitant use with drugs with sedative properties may cause additive effects and side effects (19).

Possible Interactions with Foods
ALCOHOL: Theoretically, may increase the risk of drowsiness and impair motor skills; avoid concomitant use.

Possible Interactions with Lab Tests
No interactions are known to occur, and there is no known reason to expect a clinically significant interaction with California poppy.

Possible Interactions with Diseases or Conditions
No interactions are known to occur, and there is no known reason to expect a clinically significant interaction with California poppy.

Typical Dosages & Routes of Administration that are Commonly Used
ORAL: People drink 1 cup tea (made by steeping 2 grams herb in 150 mL boiling water 10-15 minutes, strain) up to four times daily (12). Liquid extract, 1-2 mL per day (18).

Comments
Avoid use of the freshly harvested plant due to presence of cyanogenic glycosides. Avoid confusion with corn poppy (Papacer Rhoeas). The California poppy (Eschscholzia californica) is sometimes confused with the opium poppy (Paper somniferum). Both are members of the Papaveraceae family, but they are members of a different genera. They are distant relatives and the California poppy does not provide opium like the opium poppy.

CALOTROPIS

This Product is Also Known As
Mudar Bark, Muder Yercum.

Scientific Names
Calotropis procera.
Family: Asclepiadaceae.

People Use This For
Orally, calotropis is used for toothache, syphilis, digestive disorders, dysentery and diarrhea (18).
In inhalation therapy, smoke from the bark is inhaled for coughs, asthma, and to induce sweating (18).
In folk medicine, calotropis is used orally for boils, ulcers, swellings, rheumatism epilepsy, hysteria, cramps, cancer, warts, leprosy, elephantiasis, worms, fever, gout, and snake bites (18). Historically, it has been used for fever, joint pain, muscular spasm, and constipation (3822).

Safety
LIKELY UNSAFE ...when used orally, especially if used in high doses. Calotropis contains cardiac glycosides. High doses can cause vomiting, diarrhea, bradycardia, convulsions, and death (18).
There is insufficient reliable information available about the safety of the topical or inhaled use of calotropis.
PREGNANCY AND LACTATION: LIKELY UNSAFE ...when used orally; avoid using (18).

Effectiveness
There is insufficient reliable information available about the effectiveness of calotropis (18).

Possible Mechanism of Action & Active Ingredients

Calotropis contains cardioactive glycosides (cardenolides) (13,18) that show some antitumor effects on human cells in vitro (18). Calotropis also has expectorant and diuretic properties (18). In animal studies of calotropis extract have shown anti-inflammatory (3823), antibacterial (3824), antipyretic, analgesic, and neuromuscular blocking activity (3822). In one animal study, the extract produced contractions that were blocked by atropine; this supports a use in constipation (3822). In another animal study, an extract of the root showed significant anti-ulcer activity against aspirin, indomethacin, ethanol, indomethacin + ethanol, or stress-induced ulcerations. This anti-ulcer activity may be attributable to the inhibition of 5-lipoxygenase (3825).

Adverse Reactions Including Known Allergies

High oral doses can cause vomiting, diarrhea, bradycardia, convulsions, and death (18).

Possible Interactions with Herbs & Other Dietary Supplements

CARDIAC GLYCOSIDE-CONTAINING HERBS: Contraindicated. Concomitant use can increase the risk of cardiac glycoside toxicity. Cardiac glycoside-containing herbs include black hellebore, Canadian hemp roots, digitalis leaf, hedge mustard, figwort, lily of the valley roots, motherwort, oleander leaf, pleurisy root, squill bulb leaf scales, strophanthus seeds, and uzara (2,18,19,500).

CARDIOACTIVE HERBS: Avoid concomitant use with cardioactive herbs due to unpredictability of effects and adverse effects. These include: calamus, cereus, cola, coltsfoot, devil's claw, European mistletoe, fenugreek, fumitory, ginger, ginseng Panax, hawthorn, white horehound, maté, parsley, quassia, scotch broom flower, shepherd's purse, and wild carrot (4).

LICORICE/HORSETAIL: The overuse or misuse of licorice rhizome or horsetail plant increases the risk of cardiac toxicity due to potassium depletion (19).

STIMULANT LAXATIVE HERBS: The overuse or misuse of stimulant laxatives increases the risk of cardiac toxicity due to potassium depletion. Stimulant laxative herbs include: aloe dried leaf sap, blue flag rhizome, alder buckthorn, European buckthorn, butternut bark, cascara bark, castor oil, colocynth fruit pulp, gamboge bark exudate, jalap root, black root, manna bark exudate, podophyllum root, rhubarb root, senna leaves and pods, wild cucumber fruit (Ecballium elaterium), and yellow dock root (19).

Possible Interactions with Drugs

DIGOXIN: Theoretically, concomitant use increases risk of cardiac glycoside toxicity.
POTASSIUM DEPLETING DIURETICS, STIMULANT LAXATIVES: Theoretically, concomitant use may increase risk of cardiac glycoside toxicity due to potassium loss.

Possible Interactions with Foods

No interactions are known to occur, and there is no known reason to expect a clinically significant interaction with calotropis.

Possible Interactions with Lab Tests

No interactions are known to occur, and there is no known reason to expect a clinically significant interaction with calotropis.

Possible Interactions with Diseases or Conditions

No interactions are known to occur, and there is no known reason to expect a clinically significant interaction with calotropis.

Typical Dosages & Routes of Administration that are Commonly Used

ORAL: As an expectorant or diuretic, 200 to 600 mg daily; as an emetic, 2-4 grams daily (18). It is also smoked and used topically as a powder (18).

Comments

In India, calotropis has been used as a suicidal and infanticidal poison (215).

CAMPHOR

This Product is Also Known As

Camphora, Camphor Tree, Cemphire, Gum Camphor, Laurel Camphor.

Scientific Names

Cinnamomum camphora.
Family: Lauraceae.

People Use This For

Topically, camphor is used to relieve pain. It has been used specifically on warts, cold sores, and hemorrhoids. It has also been applied topically as an analgesic and an antipruritic. It has been used as a counterirritant, and to increase local blood flow (18). Camphor has frequently been used topically to treat respiratory tract diseases involving mucous membrane inflammation. It has sometimes been used topically to treat cardiac symptoms (2). Camphor is also used topically as an eardrop, and for treating minor burns.

In inhalation therapy, camphor is used as an antitussive (272).

Traditionally, camphor has been used orally as an expectorant (272), antiflatulent (16), and for treating respiratory tract diseases.

Safety

LIKELY SAFE ...when used topically short-term in concentrations ranging from 0.1%-11%. ...when used for hemorrhoids in 0.1%-3% concentration (272). ...when used appropriately for inhalation (272).

LIKELY UNSAFE ...when used on broken or injured skin because it can be absorbed and lead to toxicity (272).

UNSAFE ...when used orally. Internal preparations of camphor are no longer available in the US because of numerous poisonings (17,159).

CHILDREN: UNSAFE ...when used orally. One child died after ingesting 1 gram of camphor (17,159). ...when used topically on the faces of infants (12).

PREGNANCY: UNSAFE ...when used orally (2,12). There is insufficient reliable information available about the safety of the topical use of camphor during pregnancy.

LACTATION: UNSAFE ...when used orally (12). There is insufficient reliable information available about the safety of the topical use of camphor during lactation; avoid using.

Effectiveness

LIKELY EFFECTIVE ...when used topically for itching and irritation, cold sores (0.1%-3%), as a counterirritant (3%-11%), for treating minor burns (0.1%-3% or 3%-11% combined with light mineral oil), for hemorrhoids (0.1%-3%), as an antitussive (camphor ointment 4.7%-5.3%) (2,272). ...when used as an antitussive inhalent (272).

POSSIBLY EFFECTIVE ...when used for respiratory tract diseases involving mucous membrane inflammation (2) (see Safety).

LIKELY INEFFECTIVE ...when used topically for treating warts (272).

There is insufficient reliable information available about the effectiveness of camphor for its other uses (16,272).

Possible Mechanism of Action & Active Ingredients

The applicable part of camphor is the wood distillate. Camphor seems to exert its effect as a nasal decongestant because it induces local vasoconstriction (16). Camphor's vasoconstriction effects cause a counterirritant action which often improves local circulation, and therefore provides analgesic and antipruritic effects (16). Camphor also has weak expectorant effects.

Adverse Reactions Including Known Allergies

Adverse reactions caused by camphor occur because a considerable amount of camphor can be absorbed through intact skin (17). A considerable amount of camphor can also be absorbed due to inhalation (17). If too much camphor gets into systemic circulation, symptoms of toxicity can develop. These symptoms begin with nausea and vomiting, a feeling of warmth and headache. Then they can progress into confusion, vertigo, excitement, restlessness, delirium, hallucinations, increased muscular excitability, tremors, jerky movements, tremors progressing to epileptiform convulsions, followed by depression, coma, CNS depression, death from respiratory failure or from status epilepticus. The convalescence following camphor toxicity is slow (17). Camphor products sometimes contain safrole which can be a carcinogen (12,400). When camphor is applied topically, it can cause a topical contact eczema (2,12).

Possible Interactions with Herbs & Other Dietary Supplements

Insufficient reliable information available.

Possible Interactions with Drugs

No interactions are known to occur, and there is no known reason to expect a clinically significant interaction with camphor.

Possible Interactions with Foods

No interactions are known to occur, and there is no known reason to expect a clinically significant interaction with camphor.

Possible Interactions with Lab Tests

No interactions are known to occur, and there is no known reason to expect a clinically significant interaction with camphor.

Possible Interactions with Diseases or Conditions

GI IRRITATION: Might irritate gastrointestinal tract. Contraindicated in individuals with infectious or inflammatory gastrointestinal conditions (19).

Typical Dosages & Routes of Administration that are Commonly Used

TOPICAL: Itching: 0.1%-3% three to four times daily (272). Cold sores: 0.1%-3% topically three to four times daily (272). Counterirritant: 3%-11% three to four times daily (272). Antitussive: (4.7%-5.3% camphor ointment) to

throat and chest as a thick layer. Area may be covered with a warm, dry cloth or left uncovered (272).
Hemorrhoids: 0.1%-3%. Any of these topical uses should be limited to 3-4 times daily (272).
INHALATION: 1 tablespoon of solution per quart of water is placed directly into a hot steam vaporizer, bowl, or washbasin. Sometimes 1.5 teaspoons of solution are added to a pint of water and boiled. The medicated vapors are breathed. This inhalation may be repeated up to three times a day (272).
ORAL: 30-300 mg per day (2,12).

Comments
Camphor is a well-established folk remedy and is commonly used. This presents problems because camphor can cause toxicity. The American Academy of Pediatrics says non-prescription camphor products should not exceed 11% strength. They also recommend that camphor not be used in treating children (272). Camphorated oil (20% camphor in cottonseed oil) has been removed from the US market due to toxicity (272).

CANADA BALSAM

This Product is Also Known As
Balm of Gilead, Balsam Canada, Balsam Fir, Balsam Fir Canada, Balsam of Fir, Canada Turpentine, Canadian Balsam, Eastern Fir.
CAUTION: See separate listing for Oregon Fir Balsam.

Scientific Names
Abies balsamea.
Family: Pinaceae.

People Use This For
Topically, Canada balsam is used for hemorrhoids and as an antiseptic (11).
In dentistry, Canada balsam is used in root canal sealers and dentifrices (11).
Historically, Canada balsam has been used for burns, sores, cuts, tumors, heart and chest pains (11), cancer, mucous membrane inflammation, colds, coughs, warts, wounds, urogenital complaints, and as a pain-reliever (4017).
Canada balsam is an ingredient in foods and beverages (11).
In manufacturing, Canada balsam is used in cosmetics as a fixative and fragrance (11) in ointments and creams. It is also used as a cement for lenses and prepared microscope slides (11).

Safety
LIKELY SAFE ...when the appropriate parts of the plant are used in food; only needles, twigs (and their derivatives) of Canada balsam are approved for food use in the US (11).
POSSIBLY SAFE ...when used topically (11).
There is insufficient reliable information available about the safety of Canada balsam used orally in amounts greater than those found in foods.
PREGNANCY AND LACTATION: Insufficient reliable information available; avoid using.

Effectiveness
There is insufficient reliable information available about the effectiveness of Canada balsam.

Possible Mechanism of Action & Active Ingredients
Insufficient reliable information available.

Adverse Reactions Including Known Allergies
None reported.

Possible Interactions with Herbs & Other Dietary Supplements
Insufficient reliable information available.

Possible Interactions with Drugs
No interactions are known to occur, and there is no known reason to expect a clinically significant interaction with Canada balsam.

Possible Interactions with Foods
No interactions are known to occur, and there is no known reason to expect a clinically significant interaction with Canada balsam.

Possible Interactions with Lab Tests
No interactions are known to occur, and there is no known reason to expect a clinically significant interaction with Canada balsam.

Possible Interactions with Diseases or Conditions
No interactions are known to occur, and there is no known reason to expect a clinically significant interaction with Canada balsam.

Typical Dosages & Routes of Administration that are Commonly Used

ORAL: People typically take 2 to 6 tablespoons of weak tea of Canada balsam. As a tincture (1:5 with 50% ethanol), Canada balsam is dosed 5 to 20 drops.
TOPICAL: A weak liquid is applied to affected areas (5276).

Comments

Avoid confusion with poplar (Populus tacamahacca, P. balsamifera, P. candicans) or spruce (Picea excelsa) also known as balm of Gilead. Oregon fir balsam (Pseudotsuga menziesii) has been detected as an adulterant in Canada balsam (Abies balsamea) (11). Canada balsam is an oleoresin (rather than a true balsam) collected from punctures in the bark of the Canadian balsam tree (Abies balsamea).

CANADIAN FLEABANE

This Product is Also Known As

Canadian Trailing Arbutus, Coltstail, Flea Wort, Horsewood, Prideweed.

Scientific Names

Erigeron canadensis.
Family: Compositae.

People Use This For

Orally, Canadian fleabane is used for bronchitis, diarrhea, dysentery, edema, uterine bleeding, and tumors. It is also used orally as an antihelmintic, mild hemostyptic, and to counteract or prevent inflammation and fever.
In African folk medicine, Canadian fleabane is used for the treatment of granuloma annulare, sore throats, and urinary tract infections (18).

Safety

There is insufficient reliable information available about the safety of the oral use of Canadian fleabane.
Pregnancy and Lactation: Insufficient reliable information available; avoid using.

Effectiveness

There is insufficient reliable information available about the effectiveness of Canadian fleabane.

Possible Mechanism of Action & Active Ingredients

The applicable parts of Canadian fleabane are the above ground parts. There is insufficient reliable information available about the possible mechanism of action and active ingredients.

Adverse Reactions Including Known Allergies

Canadian fleabane can cause an allergic reaction in individuals sensitive to the Asteraceae/Compositae family. Members of this family include ragweed, chrysanthemums, marigolds, daisies, and many other herbs.

Possible Interactions with Herbs & Other Dietary Supplements

Insufficient reliable information available.

Possible Interactions with Drugs

No interactions are known to occur, and there is no known reason to expect a clinically significant interaction with Canadian fleabane.

Possible Interactions with Foods

No interactions are known to occur, and there is no known reason to expect a clinically significant interaction with Canadian fleabane.

Possible Interactions with Lab Tests

No interactions are known to occur, and there is no known reason to expect a clinically significant interaction with Canadian fleabane.

Possible Interactions with Diseases or Conditions

CROSS-ALLERGENICITY: Can cause an allergic reaction in individuals sensitive to the Asteraceae/Compositae family. Members of this family include ragweed, chrysanthemums, marigolds, daisies, and many other herbs.

Typical Dosages & Routes of Administration that are Commonly Used

No typical dosage.

Comments

There is very little scientific information about this product. Our staff is continually analyzing the available information on natural medicines and will add data here as it becomes available.

CANADIAN HEMP

This Product is Also Known As
Bitterroot, Catchfly, Dogbane, Fly-Trap, Honeybloom, Indian-Hemp, Indian Physic, Milk Ipecac, Milkweed, Wallflower, Wild Cotton.
CAUTION: See separate listings for Indian Physic.

Scientific Names
Apocynum cannabinum.
Family: Apocynaceae.

People Use This For
Topically, the fresh juice of Canadian hemp is used for warts.
Historically, Native Americans used the roots orally for arthritis, asthma, coughs, edema, and syphilis.
In folk medicine, the root is used orally for valvular insufficiency, senile heart, and to strengthen weak heart muscles following pneumonia. It is also used orally as a diuretic (18).

Safety
LIKELY UNSAFE …when the root or juice are used orally. Contains digitalis-like cardiac glycosides that can cause toxicity (18).
There is insufficient reliable information available about the safety of the topical use of Canadian hemp.
PREGNANCY AND LACTATION: LIKELY UNSAFE …when used orally; contraindicated due to toxic potential of digitalis-like cardiac glycosides (18).

Effectiveness
There is insufficient reliable information available about the effectiveness of Canadian hemp.

Possible Mechanism of Action & Active Ingredients
The applicable part of Canadian hemp is the root. Canadian hemp contains cardenolide or digitalis-type glycosides, including cymine. These may cause bradycardia with low blood pressure, increased heart contractions, and reflex hypertension. It also may increase diuresis. It is more irritating to the intestinal mucosa than digitalis and strophanthus preparations. It has a lower therapeutic effect on atrial fibrillation than digitalis (18).

Adverse Reactions Including Known Allergies
Canadian hemp causes topical irritation of the gastrointestinal mucous membranes. This can cause nausea and vomiting more commonly than in other cardenolide glycoside containing plants (such as digitalis). It can also cause bradycardia with low blood pressure, increased heart contractions, and reflex hypertension (18).

Possible Interactions with Herbs & Other Dietary Supplements
CARDIAC GLYCOSIDE-CONTAINING HERBS: Canadian hemp is contraindicated with these herbs, and concomitant use can increase the risk of cardiac glycoside toxicity. Cardiac glycoside containing herbs include black hellebore, digitalis leaf, hedge mustard, figwort, lily of the valley roots, motherwort, oleander leaf, pheasant's eye plant, pleurisy root, squill bulb leaf scales, strophanthus seeds, and uzara (2,18,19,500).

Possible Interactions with Drugs
CARDIAC GLYCOSIDES: Concomitant use of Canadian hemp with digoxin (Lanoxin) or digitoxin (Crystodigin) might increase effects and adverse effects.

Possible Interactions with Foods
No interactions are known to occur, and there is no known reason to expect a clinically significant interaction with Canadian hemp.

Possible Interactions with Lab Tests
No interactions are known to occur, and there is no known reason to expect a clinically significant interaction with Canadian hemp.

Possible Interactions with Diseases or Conditions
No interactions are known to occur, and there is no known reason to expect a clinically significant interaction with Canadian hemp.

Typical Dosages & Routes of Administration that are Commonly Used
ORAL: Some people take 10 to 30 drops of the liquid extract three times daily or 0.3 to 0.6 mL of the tincture (1:10) (18).
TOPICAL: No typical dosage.

Comments
The tough, fibrous barks of both Canadian hemp and Indian hemp have been used as a substitute for hemp; hence, both are known as hemp (18).

CANAIGRE

This Product is Also Known As

Red American Ginseng, Wild Red American Ginseng, Wild Red Desert Ginseng.
CAUTION: See separate listings for Ginseng American, Blue Cohosh, Codonopsis, Ginseng Siberian, Ginseng Panax, and Withania.

Scientific Names

Rumex hymenosepalus.
Family: Polygonaceae.

People Use This For

Orally, canaigre is used as an inexpensive alternative to ginseng (6). These uses include improving physical and athletic stamina, cognitive function and concentration, work efficiency or athletic stamina, and as a general tonic to improve well-being. It is also used for soothing irritated or inflamed tissues, as a diuretic, and as an antidepressant. Historically, canaigre has been used as an astringent (5) and for conditions ranging from lack of vitality to leprosy (515).
In manufacturing, it is used for tanning leather and dying wool (5).

Safety

LIKELY SAFE ...when used orally (12). The petioles, or stems, are edible like rhubarb (6). Avoid excessive amounts. There is some speculation that high tannin contents (such as in canaigre) could be carcinogenic (5,6).
PREGNANCY AND LACTATION: Insufficient reliable information available; avoid using.

Effectiveness

There is insufficient reliable information available about the effectiveness of canaigre.

Possible Mechanism of Action & Active Ingredients

The applicable part of canaigre is the root. High tannin content (25%) has astringent effect when applied topically. Leucoanthocyanin fraction may have antitumor activity (6).

Adverse Reactions Including Known Allergies

None reported.

Possible Interactions with Herbs & Other Dietary Supplements

Insufficient reliable information available.

Possible Interactions with Drugs

No interactions are known to occur, and there is no known reason to expect a clinically significant interaction with canaigre.

Possible Interactions with Foods

No interactions are known to occur, and there is no known reason to expect a clinically significant interaction with canaigre.

Possible Interactions with Lab Tests

No interactions are known to occur, and there is no known reason to expect a clinically significant interaction with canaigre.

Possible Interactions with Diseases or Conditions

No interactions are known to occur, and there is no known reason to expect a clinically significant interaction with canaigre.

Typical Dosages & Routes of Administration that are Commonly Used

No typical dosage.

Comments

Avoid confusion with Panax ginseng, Siberian ginseng, and red ginseng. Canaigre root is unrelated to ginseng.
A 1976 Herb Trade Association policy states that "any herb products consisting of whole or part of Rumex hymenosepalus should not be labeled as containing 'ginseng' " (5).

CANANGA OIL

This Product is Also Known As

None.
CAUTION: See separate listing for Ylang Ylang Oil.

Scientific Names

Cangana odorata macrophylla, synonym Canagnium odoratum macrophylla.
Family: Annonaceae.

People Use This For

Cananga oil is used as a flavoring agent in foods such as gelatins, puddings, and also in beverages [11].
In manufacturing, cananga oil is used to make fragrances in cosmetics and soaps [11].

Safety

LIKELY SAFE ...when consumed in amounts typically found in foods. It has Generally Recognized as
Safe (GRAS) status in the US [11]. When used as a flavoring, the maximum level used does not exceed 0.003% [11].
POSSIBLY SAFE ...when used topically. The maximum level allowed is 0.8% in perfumes [11].
PREGNANCY AND LACTATION: Insufficient reliable information available; avoid using.

Effectiveness

EFFECTIVE ...when used as a fragrance or as a flavoring agent in foods.

Possible Mechanism of Action & Active Ingredients

Insufficient reliable information available.

Adverse Reactions Including Known Allergies

None reported [11].

Possible Interactions with Herbs & Other Dietary Supplements

Insufficient reliable information available.

Possible Interactions with Drugs

No interactions are known to occur, and there is no known reason to expect a clinically significant interaction with
cananga oil.

Possible Interactions with Foods

No interactions are known to occur, and there is no known reason to expect a clinically significant interaction with
cananga oil.

Possible Interactions with Lab Tests

No interactions are known to occur, and there is no known reason to expect a clinically significant interaction with
cananga oil.

Possible Interactions with Diseases or Conditions

No interactions are known to occur, and there is no known reason to expect a clinically significant interaction with
cananga oil.

Typical Dosages & Routes of Administration that are Commonly Used

No typical dosage.

Comments

Distilled oil from Cananga odorata macrophylla flower is used. Avoid confusion with ylang ylang oil (oil from
Canangium odorata genuina).

CANELLA

This Product is Also Known As

White Cinnamon, White Wood, Wild Cinnamon.

Scientific Names

Canella alba.

People Use This For

There are no known medicinal uses.
For food uses, canella is utilized as a cooking spice [18].

Safety

There is insufficient reliable information available about the safety of canella.
Pregnancy and Lactation: Insufficient reliable information available; avoid using.

Effectiveness

There is insufficient reliable information available about the effectiveness of canella.

Possible Mechanism of Action & Active Ingredients

The applicable part of canella is the bark. Canella bark is stated to have stimulant, tonic, and antimicrobial properties (18).

Adverse Reactions Including Known Allergies

None reported.

Possible Interactions with Herbs & Other Dietary Supplements

Insufficient reliable information available.

Possible Interactions with Drugs

No interactions are known to occur, and there is no known reason to expect a clinically significant interaction with canella.

Possible Interactions with Foods

No interactions are known to occur, and there is no known reason to expect a clinically significant interaction with canella.

Possible Interactions with Lab Tests

No interactions are known to occur, and there is no known reason to expect a clinically significant interaction with canella.

Possible Interactions with Diseases or Conditions

No interactions are known to occur, and there is no known reason to expect a clinically significant interaction with canella.

Typical Dosages & Routes of Administration that are Commonly Used

ORAL: People typically use 10 to 40 grains which is 650 to 2600 mg (5267).

Comments

There is very little scientific information about this product. Our staff is continually analyzing the available information on natural medicines and will add data here as it becomes available.

CANTHAXANTHIN

This Product is Also Known As

Canthaxanthine, Carophyll Red, CI Food Orange 8, Colour Index No. 40850, E161, Roxanthin Red 10.
CAUTION: See separate listing for Beta-carotene.

Scientific Names

Canthaxanthin; 4,4-diketo-beta-carotene; Beta,beta-carotene-4,4-dione.

People Use This For

Orally, canthaxanthin is used to reduce photosensitivity associated with erythropoietic protoporphyria (EPP) (14,5644,5645), and light-sensitive skin diseases including polymorphous light eruptions, drug-induced photosensitivity and solar urticaria (14). It is also used orally to color the skin and produce an artificial suntan (9,14). In foods, canthaxanthin is used as a food coloring additive (9,14,5630) and added to animal feed to enhance the color of chicken skins, egg yolks (14), salmon and trout (9).
In manufacturing, canthaxanthin has been used in cosmetics (9), and as a tablet excipient (14).

Safety

LIKELY SAFE ...when consumed in amounts commonly found in foods (14). Canthaxanthin is approved for use in human food, has Generally Recognized as Safe (GRAS) status in the US (5637), and is not to exceed 30 mg per pint of liquid food or per pound of solid or semisolid food (5630).
POSSIBLY UNSAFE ...when used orally in doses to treat and reduce photosensitivities. Development of retinal changes has been reported in patients with EPP being treated with canthaxanthin to prevent photosensitization, including deposition of crystals around the macula of the retina (5644), slowing of dark-adaptation curves, and decreased amplitudes in electroretinograms (5632,5638,5645). Deposition of retinal crystals appears dose related (5638). Evidence suggests individuals taking a cumulative dose of 37 grams will have retinal changes 50% of the time, while those taking a total cumulative dose of 60 grams of canthaxanthin will demonstrate definite retinal changes upon examination (5636,5641).
LIKELY UNSAFE ...when used orally in large amounts to color and produce an artificial tan (5628,5629). Retinal changes have been reported in individuals ingesting large amounts of canthaxanthin chronically for tanning purposes (9,14,5636,5639,5641). Altered eye function, decreased visual acuity (5639), and aplastic anemia (5635) have also been reported.

PREGNANCY AND LACTATION: LIKELY SAFE ...when consumed in amounts found in foods (5630). POSSIBLY UNSAFE ...when consumed in doses to treat and reduce photosensitivities due to reported retinal changes with use (9,5632); avoid using. LIKELY UNSAFE ...when used orally in large amounts for artificial tanning purposes due to reported retinal changes with use (9,14); avoid using.

Effectiveness

LIKELY EFFECTIVE ...when used orally for reducing photosensitivity in erythropoietic protoporphyria (rash, itching, or eczema) due to sunlight exposure (5644,5645).
There is insufficient reliable information available about the effectiveness of canthaxanthin for its other uses.

Possible Mechanism of Action & Active Ingredients

Canthaxanthin is a carotenoid that is found naturally and produced synthetically (5637). It is not a precursor of vitamin A, has no vitamin A activity (9), is highly lipid soluble (5635), and accumulates in fatty tissue (5632). Oral canthaxanthin is thought to color the skin by accumulating in the epidermis and subcutaneous fat tissue (5635). Evidence suggests canthaxanthin and other carotenoids protect against photosensitization due to their antioxidant activity against reactive oxygen species by deactivating electronically excited molecules or acting as chain-breaking agents (5645,5649). In-vitro and in-vivo animal studies suggest canthaxanthin may inhibit the growth and transformation of tumor cells (5642,5647,5648) by inducing the gap junctional communication between cells (5649). Animal studies have not shown any toxic, carcinogenic or mutagenic effects with canthaxanthin (14). Human studies are needed to determine whether canthaxanthin has a role in cancer prevention.

Adverse Reactions Including Known Allergies

Orally, large amounts of canthaxanthin can cause orange-brown coloration of the skin (5632), brick-red coloration of stools (5631), orange discoloration of plasma (5632), discolored body secretions (5634), diarrhea, nausea, stomach cramps (14), dry and itchy skin (5634), urticaria (5637), welts (9), gold and yellow crystalline deposits around the macula of the retina (5632,5635,5636,5638,5639,5640,5641), and hepatitis (14,5635). Decreased visual acuity (5639), diminished retinal sensitivity (5641), and aplastic anemia (5635) have been associated with large doses of canthaxanthin ingestion. A fatal case of aplastic anemia (5635) associated with the ingestion of canthaxanthin for tanning purposes has been reported. The patient refused treatment with human blood products due to religious beliefs and died (5635).

Possible Interactions with Herbs & Other Dietary Supplements

Insufficient reliable information available.

Possible Interactions with Drugs

No interactions are known to occur, and there is no known reason to expect a clinically significant interaction with canthaxanthin.

Possible Interactions with Foods

No interactions are known to occur, and there is no known reason to expect a clinically significant interaction with canthaxanthin.

Possible Interactions with Lab Tests

Canthaxanthin can interfere with carotene and vitamin A laboratory assays (14,5634).

Possible Interactions with Diseases or Conditions

HYPERSENSITIVITY TO VITAMIN A AND CAROTENOIDS: Individuals with known hypersensitivities to vitamin A and carotenoids might also be hypersensitive to canthaxanthin (14).

Typical Dosages & Routes of Administration that are Commonly Used

ORAL: The typical dose for reducing and treating photosensitivities associated with erythropoietic protoporphyria is 60 to 90 mg daily on average for three to five months per year (5640). The typical dose for artificial tanning is 120 mg per day for several days (14,5633).

Comments

Orobronze (canthaxanthin) is sold in Canada as a nonprescription drug for artificial tanning purposes as 30 mg oral capsules (5631,5633). Oral tanning preparations containing canthaxanthin have been found to be readily available to consumers in the United States through mail order and tanning salons despite the FDA warning (5635,5638). A combination product containing beta-carotene and canthaxanthin (Phenoro: 10 mg beta-carotene and 15 mg canthaxanthin) is used in Europe for treatment of photosensitivities associated with EPP (5637). Other combination products containing beta-carotene and canthaxanthin are manufactured (Carotinoid-N, Apotrin), but are not available in the United States (5628,5645).

CAPERS

This Product is Also Known As
Cappero.

Scientific Names
Capparis spinosa.
Family: Capparidaceae.

People Use This For
Topically, capers are used for skin disorders, for improving the function of enlarged capillaries, and for dry skin (6). Capers are consumed as food, and used as a flavoring (6).

Safety
LIKELY SAFE ...when taken orally. The pickled flower buds are commonly used without reports of adverse effects.

There is insufficient reliable information available about the safety of the topical use of capers. Compresses soaked in fluid containing capers can cause contact dermatitis (6).

PREGNANCY AND LACTATION: LIKELY SAFE ...when used orally in amounts typically found in foods; avoid large amounts. There is insufficient reliable information available about the safety of the topical use of capers during pregnancy and lactation.

Effectiveness
There is insufficient reliable information available about the effectiveness of capers.

Possible Mechanism of Action & Active Ingredients
The applicable part of capers is the unopened flower bud. Some evidence suggests that unknown constituents of caper extract may improve dry skin and functioning of enlarged capillaries (6).

Adverse Reactions Including Known Allergies
Capers can cause contact dermatitis (6).

Possible Interactions with Herbs & Other Dietary Supplements
Insufficient reliable information available.

Possible Interactions with Drugs
No interactions are known to occur, and there is no known reason to expect a clinically significant interaction with capers.

Possible Interactions with Foods
No interactions are known to occur, and there is no known reason to expect a clinically significant interaction with capers.

Possible Interactions with Lab Tests
No interactions are known to occur, and there is no known reason to expect a clinically significant interaction with capers.

Possible Interactions with Diseases or Conditions
PEOPLE WITH SENSITIVE SKIN: May cause skin irritation (6); avoid topical use.

Typical Dosages & Routes of Administration that are Commonly Used
No typical dosage.

Comments
CAUTION: Leaves of related species (Capparis fasicularis, Capparis tumentosa) are reported to be poisonous (6).

CAPSICUM

This Product is Also Known As
African Chillies, African Pepper, Bird Pepper, Capsaicin, Capsicum Fruit, Cayenne, Chili Pepper, Garden Pepper, Goat's Pod, Grains Of Paradise, Green Bell Pepper, Green Chili Pepper, Hot Pepper, Hungarian Pepper, Ici Fructus, Louisiana Long Pepper, Louisiana Sport Pepper, Mexican Chilies, Paprika, Pimento, Red Pepper, Sweet Pepper, Tabasco Pepper, Zanzibar Pepper.
CAUTION: See separate listing for Grains of Paradise.

Scientific Names

Capsicum frutescens; Capsicum annuum; Capsicum chinense; Capsicum baccatum; Capsicum pubscens; and other Capsicum species.
Family: Solanaceae.

People Use This For

Orally, capsicum is used to stimulate the stomach to digest food (5), as an antiflatulent, GI stimulant, for colic (4), diarrhea, cramps (11), toothache (11), insufficient peripheral circulation (4), reducing blood cholesterol and clotting tendencies (5), seasickness (18), alcoholism (18), malarial fever, yellow fever and other fevers (18), and for preventing arteriosclerosis and heart disease (18).

Topically, capsicum is used for the pain of shingles, and for post-herpetic, trigeminal, diabetic, post-mastectomy, post-surgical neuralgias and HIV-associated peripheral neuropathy (6,3891). It is also used as a counterirritant to desensitize nerves and to create a feeling of warmth (7,11). Capsicum is used to relieve muscle spasms (2), as a gargle for laryngitis (4), and as a deterrent to thumb-sucking or nail biting (11).

For food uses, capsicum is a condiment (3).

In manufacturing, capsicum is the main ingredient used in many self-defense sprays, also referred to as pepper spray (6,1394).

Safety

LIKELY SAFE ...when the fruit is consumed in amounts typically found in food. Capsicum has Generally Recognized as Safe (GRAS) status in the US. ...when the FDA-approved nonprescription product is used topically and appropriately (272).

POSSIBLY SAFE ...when the fruit is used orally and appropriately in medicinal amounts (4,12).

POSSIBLY UNSAFE ...when the fruit is used orally on a regular basis or in large amounts because it can cause hepatic or renal damage (4,12).

There is insufficient reliable information available about the safety of topical products other than the approved nonprescription product.

CHILDREN: POSSIBLY UNSAFE ...when used topically in children under 2 years old (506). The nonprescription topical product is approved for use in children over 2 years old (272). There is insufficient reliable information available about the safety of oral use in children.

PREGNANCY: LIKELY SAFE ...when used orally in the amounts commonly found in foods (4). ...when used as the FDA-approved nonprescription topical product (272). There is insufficient reliable information available about the safety of capsicum used orally in amounts larger those typically found in food.

LACTATION: LIKELY SAFE ...when used topically and appropriately as the FDA-approved nonprescription product. POSSIBLY UNSAFE ...when ingested orally. There are some reports of dermatitis occurring in breast-fed infants whose mothers' food was heavily spiced with red pepper (739).

Effectiveness

EFFECTIVE ...when applied topically for temporary relief of pain from rheumatoid arthritis, osteoarthritis, and relief of neuralgias due to shingles or diabetic neuropathy. Capsicum is approved by the FDA as an OTC drug (506). Capsaicin (a compound purified from Capsicum annuum L.) is the active ingredient in Zostrix - approved as an OTC drug in the US and Canada.

POSSIBLY EFFECTIVE ...when taken orally as a digestive stimulant (4).

POSSIBLY INEFFECTIVE ...when capsaicin is used topically for HIV-associated peripheral neuropathy (distal symmetrical peripheral neuropathy) (3891).

There is insufficient reliable information available about the effectiveness of capsicum for its other uses.

Possible Mechanism of Action & Active Ingredients

The applicable part of capsicum is the fruit (4). Capsicum contains capsaicinoid constituents which stimulate digestion and therefore are said to aid in digestion (4). When used topically, the capsaicin constituent causes the release of substance P in the nerves. This initially causes pain, but after repeated applications, substance P is depleted. This reduces the ability of the nerves to transmit sensations and reduces pain. Some evidence shows the crude juice of fresh capsicum has antibacterial properties (11).

Adverse Reactions Including Known Allergies

ORAL: When capsicum is taken orally, there can sometimes be GI irritation (4). Sweating and flushing of the head and neck, lacrimation, and rhinorrhea have also been reported (7005). Excessive amounts of capsicum can lead to gastroenteritis, and hepatic or renal damage (4). There are also reports of dermatitis in breast-fed infants whose mothers' food is heavily spiced with red pepper (739). Capsicum may cause hypocoagulability (7006).

TOPICAL: When capsicum is applied topically, there can be burning (6), and urticaria (2). Skin contact with fresh cayenne fruit may cause irritation or contact dermatitis (19).

Inhalation of capsicum can cause allergic alveolitis (4). Capsicum can be extremely irritating to the eyes and mucous membranes.

Possible Interactions with Herbs & Other Dietary Supplements

COCA: Theoretically, concomitant use of capsicum (including exposure to the capsicum in pepper spray) and coca might increase the effects and risk of adverse effects of the cocaine in coca (1394).

HERBS WITH SEDATIVE PROPERTIES: Theoretically, concomitant use with herbs that have sedative properties might enhance therapeutic and adverse effects. These include calamus, calendula, California poppy, catnip, celery, couch grass, elecampane, Siberian ginseng, German chamomile, goldenseal, gotu kola, hops, Jamaican dogwood, kava, lemon balm, sage, St. John's wort, sassafras, scullcap, shepherd's purse, stinging nettle, valerian, wild carrot, wild lettuce, withania root, and yerba mansa (4,19).

HERBS WITH ANTICOAGULANT/ANTIPLATELET POTENTIAL: Concomitant use of herbs that have coumarin constituents or affect platelet aggregation could theoretically increase the risk of bleeding in some people. These herbs include: angelica, anise, arnica, asafoetida, bogbean, boldo, celery, chamomile, clove, danshen, fenugreek, feverfew, garlic, ginger, ginkgo, Panax ginseng, horse chestnut, horseradish, licorice, meadowsweet, prickly ash, onion, papain, passionflower, poplar, quassia, red clover, turmeric, wild carrot, wild lettuce, willow, and others (4,19).

Possible Interactions with Drugs

ACE INHIBITORS (ACEIs): Topically applied capsicum might contribute to the cough reflex in patients using ace inhibitors (7002).

ACID-INHIBITING DRUGS: Theoretically, capsicum might interfere with antacids, sucralfate (Carafate, Sulcrate in Canada), H-2 antagonists, or proton-pump inhibitors, due to claims that capsicum increases stomach acid (19).

ANTIHYPERTENSIVE DRUGS: Theoretically, capsicum might interfere with the activity of antihypertensive drugs by increasing catecholamine secretion (4).

ANTIPLATELET DRUGS: Theoretically, capsicum might increase the effects and adverse effects of antiplatelet drugs (19).

ASPIRIN: Chili powder, taken thirty minutes before aspirin, might reduce gastric mucosal damage (19).

BARBITURATES: Theoretically, concomitant use of capsicum with barbiturates might enhance sedative effects and the risk of adverse effects (19).

COCAINE: Theoretically, concomitant use of capsicum (including exposure to the capsicum in pepper spray) and cocaine might increase cocaine effects and the risk of adverse effects, including death (1394).

DRUGS WITH SEDATIVE PROPERTIES: Theoretically, concomitant use of capsicum and drugs with sedative activity might enhance sedative effects and the risk of adverse effects (19).

HEPATICALLY METABOLIZED DRUGS: Theoretically, capsicum might increase hepatic metabolism of drugs by increasing glucose-6-phosphate dehydrogenase and adipose lipase activity (4).

MONOAMINE OXIDASE INHIBITORS (MAOIs): Theoretically, capsicum might interfere with the activity of MAOIs by increasing catecholamine secretion (4).

THEOPHYLLINE (Theo-Dur): Theoretically, oral administration of capsicum before or at the same time as theophylline might enhance theophylline absorption (19).

Possible Interactions with Foods

No interactions are known to occur, and there is no known reason to expect a clinically significant interaction with capsicum.

Possible Interactions with Lab Tests

Capsicum has led to increased fibrinolytic activity and may lead to prolonged times in coagulation studies (7006).

Possible Interactions with Diseases or Conditions

GI IRRITATION: Oral capsicum causes GI irritation but does not interfere with ulcer healing (4). Contraindicated in individuals with infectious or inflammatory gastrointestinal conditions (19).

DAMAGED SKIN: Capsicum is contraindicated in situations involving injured skin. Do not apply capsicum if the skin is open.

PEPPER ALLERGY: Avoid the use of capsicum (2). Contraindicated in individuals with infectious or inflammatory gastrointestinal conditions (19).

Typical Dosages & Routes of Administration that are Commonly Used

ORAL: Fruit: 30-120 mg 3 times daily (4). Capsicum Tincture: 0.3-1 mL (4). Stronger Tincture of Capsicum: 0.06-2 mL (4). Oleoresin: 0.6-2 mg (4).

TOPICAL: Capsaicin cream (the nonprescription product): Apply to affected areas a maximum of 3-4 times daily. If it is applied with fingers, hands should be washed after applying (506). It might take as long as 3 days to deplete substance P and achieve full effect (4). A diluted vinegar solution is used to remove capsicum; it is not water washable (5). Capsicum should not be used near the eyes or on sensitive skin (5). Capsaicin (a compound purified from Capsicum annuum L.) is the active ingredient in Zostrix. It is approved as a nonprescription drug in the US and Canada. It comes in 0.025% and 0.075% capsaicin concentrations. The high potency preparation is usually used for diabetic neuropathy.

Comments

In nature, capsicum occurs only as a trans stereoisomer. However, civamide, the cis isomer also has activity. Products labeled capsaicin sometimes include nonivamide which is an adulterant or pelargonic acid vanillylamide, which is referred to as "synthetic capsaicin" (7007). Capsaicin is being studied for use in treating urinary urgency as an intravesical injection (214).

CARAMEL COLOR

This Product is Also Known As
None.

Scientific Names
None.

People Use This For
Caramel color is used as a food color in medications, cosmetics and foods. It does not have any known medicinal uses (11).

Safety
LIKELY SAFE ...when used in amounts found in foods and medications. It has Generally Recognized as Safe (GRAS) status in the US, and is official in both the FCC and the National Formulary (10,11). The highest average maximum level is 5.4% (11).
PREGNANCY AND LACTATION: POSSIBLY SAFE ...when used orally in food amounts. There is insufficient reliable information available for the safety of caramel color used in larger amounts during pregnancy and lactation.

Effectiveness
There is insufficient reliable information available about the effectiveness of caramel color.

Possible Mechanism of Action & Active Ingredients
Caramel color is burnt sugar coloring and caramel. This is the color obtained by heating sugar with ammonia or ammonium salts under controlled temperature and pressure until the taste is eliminated and the desired color is achieved (11).

Adverse Reactions Including Known Allergies
Some evidence from short-term and long-term studies suggest that large amounts of caramel might suppress immunity (11).

Possible Interactions with Herbs & Other Dietary Supplements
Insufficient reliable information available.

Possible Interactions with Drugs
No interactions are known to occur, and there is no known reason to expect a clinically significant interaction with caramel color.

Possible Interactions with Foods
No interactions are known to occur, and there is no known reason to expect a clinically significant interaction with caramel color.

Possible Interactions with Lab Tests
No interactions are known to occur, and there is no known reason to expect a clinically significant interaction with caramel color.

Possible Interactions with Diseases or Conditions
No interactions are known to occur, and there is no known reason to expect a clinically significant interaction with caramel color.

Typical Dosages & Routes of Administration that are Commonly Used
No typical dosage.

Comments
None.

CARAWAY dried fruit, seed

This Product is Also Known As
Anis des Vosges, Carvi Fructus, Cumin des Pres, Kummel, Kummich, Semences de Carvi, Semen Cumini Pratensis, Wiesen-Feldkummel.
CAUTION: See separate listing for Caraway Oil.

Scientific Names
Carum carvi, synonym Apium carvi.
Family: Apiaceae/Umbelliferae.

People Use This For

Orally, the dried fruit and seed of caraway is used for dyspepsia, distention, flatulence (2,8), and mild spastic conditions of the gastrointestinal tract (2). It is also used orally as an antibacterial (8), laxative, and digestive aid (11). Traditionally, caraway has been used as an expectorant, to promote lactation, to relieve menstrual discomforts, for incontinence, and as a mouthwash (8,11).

For food uses, caraway is a cooking spice (11).

Safety

LIKELY SAFE ...when consumed in amounts commonly found in foods. Caraway is Generally Recognized as Safe (GRAS) and approved for food use in the US with a maximum use level of 0.02% (11). ...when taken orally for medicinal purposes in appropriate amounts (12).

There is insufficient reliable information available about the safety of caraway in large amounts.

PREGNANCY AND LACTATION: LIKELY SAFE ...in the amounts commonly found in food.

Effectiveness

POSSIBLY EFFECTIVE ...when taken orally as an antiflatulent and for dyspeptic problems, such as mild, spastic conditions of the gastrointestinal tract, bloating, and fullness (2). ...when taken for increasing gastric secretion and stimulating appetite (8).

There is insufficient reliable information available about the effectiveness of caraway for its other uses.

Possible Mechanism of Action & Active Ingredients

Caraway produces a warm sensation and promotes postprandial gas elimination (7). The caraway fruits contain 2-7% volatile oil, consisting mainly of carvone and limonene (7). Carvone induces glutathione S-transferase (GST) in mouse tissues, which can inhibit carcinogenesis (11). There is some evidence that caraway oil has antispasmodic effects, but they are probably weak. There may also be some antihistaminic activity. It is possible that the antispasmodic effects are slightly more pronounced with the alcoholic extract, and less pronounced with the essential oil (7,11).

Adverse Reactions Including Known Allergies

Caraway can cause contact dermatitis (19).

Possible Interactions with Herbs & Other Dietary Supplements

Insufficient reliable information available.

Possible Interactions with Drugs

No interactions are known to occur, and there is no known reason to expect a clinically significant interaction with caraway dried fruit and seed.

Possible Interactions with Foods

No interactions are known to occur, and there is no known reason to expect a clinically significant interaction with caraway dried fruit and seed.

Possible Interactions with Lab Tests

No interactions are known to occur, and there is no known reason to expect a clinically significant interaction with caraway dried fruit and seed.

Possible Interactions with Diseases or Conditions

No interactions are known to occur, and there is no known reason to expect a clinically significant interaction with caraway dried fruit and seed.

Typical Dosages & Routes of Administration that are Commonly Used

ORAL: The typical dose of caraway is 1.5-6 grams of the dried fruit per day or one cup of the freshly prepared tea two to four times daily between meals (8). The tea is prepared by steeping 1-2 teaspoons of the freshly crushed fruit in 150 mL boiling water for 5-10 minutes and then straining. The dose for infants and small children is usually one teaspoonful of the tea, and if necessary, given in a bottle (8).

Comments

Superstitions held that caraway had the power to prevent the theft of any object that contained the seed and to keep lovers from losing interest with one another (6002). Avoid confusion with caraway oil (distilled oil of caraway fruit/seed).

CARAWAY OIL

This Product is Also Known As

None.

CAUTION: See separate listing for Caraway dried fruit, seed.

© Copyright 2000, Natural Medicines Comprehensive Database (209) 472-2244. For updated data, go to www.NaturalDatabase.com

Scientific Names
Carum carvi, synonym Apium carvi.
Family: Apiaceae or Umbelliferae.

People Use This For
Orally, caraway oil is used for digestive problems including mild GI spasms, flatulence, and fullness (2). Traditionally, caraway oil has been used in mouthwashes (6) and topically in skin frictions to improve local blood flow (6).

In manufacturing, caraway oil is used as a flavoring agent in pharmaceutical compounding (11). It is a fragrance commonly utilized in the manufacturing of toothpaste, soap, and cosmetics (11).

Safety
LIKELY SAFE ...when used orally and appropriately (2).
PREGNANCY AND LACTATION: Insufficient reliable information available; avoid using.

Effectiveness
POSSIBLY EFFECTIVE ...when taken orally for digestive problems, including mild GI spasms, flatulence, and fullness (2).
There is insufficient reliable information available about the effectiveness of caraway oil for its other uses.

Possible Mechanism of Action & Active Ingredients
Caraway oil can exhibit antibacterial, antifungal, and larvicidal activity in vitro (6,11). The constituent carvone induces glutathione S-transferase (GST) in mouse tissues, which can inhibit carcinogenesis (11). There is disagreement about whether caraway oil has antispasmodic effects. Some say the oil was demonstrated to have antispasmodic and antihistaminic activity in isolated animal organs (11); however, others say the alcoholic extract, but not the essential oil, has antispasmodic effects (7).

Adverse Reactions Including Known Allergies
Caraway oil can cause contact dermatitis (19).

Possible Interactions with Herbs & Other Dietary Supplements
Insufficient reliable information available.

Possible Interactions with Drugs
No interactions are known to occur, and there is no known reason to expect a clinically significant interaction with caraway oil.

Possible Interactions with Foods
No interactions are known to occur, and there is no known reason to expect a clinically significant interaction with caraway oil.

Possible Interactions with Lab Tests
No interactions are known to occur, and there is no known reason to expect a clinically significant interaction with caraway oil.

Possible Interactions with Diseases or Conditions
No interactions are known to occur, and there is no known reason to expect a clinically significant interaction with caraway oil.

Typical Dosages & Routes of Administration that are Commonly Used
ORAL: The typical dose of the oil is 3-6 drops per day (2).

Comments
Distilled oil of caraway fruit/seed (Carum carvi) is used. Caraway has been used as a love potion, because people superstitiously believed that it had a power of retention and could prevent lovers from losing interest in one another (6002). Avoid confusion with the caraway fruit or seed.

CARDAMOM

This Product is Also Known As
Bai Dou Kou, Cardamon, Cardomomi Fructus.

Scientific Names
Elettaria cardamomum, synonym Amomum cardamomum.
Family: Zingiberaceae.

 © Copyright 2000, Natural Medicines Comprehensive Database (209) 472-2244. For updated data, go to www.NaturalDatabase.com

People Use This For

Orally, cardamom seed is used for dyspepsia (2), intestinal spasm, irritable bowel syndrome (1504), common cold, cough, bronchitis, inflammation of the mouth and pharynx, liver and gallbladder complaints, loss of appetite, and tendency toward infection (18). It is also used as an antiflatulent and laxative (11).

In Chinese medicine, cardamom is used as a stimulant and for urinary problems (11).

For food uses, cardamom is consumed as a spice in many parts of the world (11).

Safety

LIKELY SAFE ...when used orally and appropriately (2).

PREGNANCY AND LACTATION: Insufficient reliable information available; avoid amounts in excess of those used in food.

Effectiveness

POSSIBLY EFFECTIVE ...when taken orally for dyspepsia (2,11).

There is insufficient reliable information available for the effectiveness of cardamom seed for its other uses.

Possible Mechanism of Action & Active Ingredients

The applicable part of cardamom is the seed. The active principals of cardamom are thought to be volatile oils, including cineole (2,11). Volatile oils are believed to have antispasmodic (11), antiflatulent, virustatic (2,18), and motility-enhancing effects (18).

Adverse Reactions Including Known Allergies

None reported (2).

Possible Interactions with Herbs & Other Dietary Supplements

Insufficient reliable information available.

Possible Interactions with Drugs

No interactions are known to occur, and there is no known reason to expect a clinically significant interaction with cardamom.

Possible Interactions with Foods

No interactions are known to occur, and there is no known reason to expect a clinically significant interaction with cardamom.

Possible Interactions with Lab Tests

No interactions are known to occur, and there is no known reason to expect a clinically significant interaction with cardamom.

Possible Interactions with Diseases or Conditions

GALLSTONES: The cardamom seed can trigger gallstone colic (spasmodic pain) (18) and is not recommended for self-medication in patients with gallstones (2).

Typical Dosages & Routes of Administration that are Commonly Used

ORAL: The typical dose of cardamom is 1.5 grams of the ground seeds per day. The usual dose of the tincture is 1-2 grams per day (2).

Comments

None.

CARLINA

This Product is Also Known As

Carlinae Radix, Dwarf Carline, Eberwurz, Ground Thistle, Racine de Carline Acaule, Radix Cardopatiae, Radix Chamaeleontis Albae, Silberdistelwurz, Stemless Carlina Root, Southernwood Root.

Scientific Names

Carlina acaulis.
Family: Asteraceae or Compositae.

People Use This For

Orally, carlina is used for gallbladder disease, poor digestion, and alimentary tract spasms (18).

Topically, carlina is used for dermatosis, rinsing wounds and ulcers, and to alleviate cancer of the tongue (18).

Acetic extracts are used for herpes eruptions, skin pustules, and toothaches (8).

In combination herbal products, carlina is used for gallbladder disorders and gastrointestinal spasms (8).

In folk medicine, carlina is used as a diuretic, tonic, gargle, catarrh, and to induce sweat (8).

Safety

There is insufficient reliable information available about the safety of carlina.
Pregnancy and Lactation: Insufficient reliable information available; avoid using.

Effectiveness

There is insufficient reliable information available about the effectiveness of carlina.

Possible Mechanism of Action & Active Ingredients

The applicable part of carlina is the root. Acetone extract and essential oil have antibacterial activity but aqueous extract does not (8).

Adverse Reactions Including Known Allergies

It can cause an allergic reaction in individuals sensitive to the Asteraceae/Compositae family. Members of this family include ragweed, chrysanthemums, marigolds, daisies, and many other herbs.

Possible Interactions with Herbs & Other Dietary Supplements

Insufficient reliable information available.

Possible Interactions with Drugs

No interactions are known to occur, and there is no known reason to expect a clinically significant interaction with carlina.

Possible Interactions with Foods

No interactions are known to occur, and there is no known reason to expect a clinically significant interaction with carlina.

Possible Interactions with Lab Tests

No interactions are known to occur, and there is no known reason to expect a clinically significant interaction with carlina.

Possible Interactions with Diseases or Conditions

CROSS-ALLERGENICITY: Can cause an allergic reaction in individuals sensitive to the Asteraceae/Compositae family. Members of this family include ragweed, chrysanthemums, marigolds, daisies, and many other herbs.

Typical Dosages & Routes of Administration that are Commonly Used

ORAL: One cup tea (steep 1.5-3 grams finely cut dried root in 150 mL boiling water 5-10 minutes, strain) three times daily between meals (8,18). Tincture (steep 20 grams chopped root in 80 grams of 60% ethanol) 40-50 drops, four to five times daily (18). Wine, (steep 50 grams root in 1 L white wine minimum 12 days, strain) one small glass before mealtime (18).
TOPICAL: Tea (simmer 30 grams root in 1 L boiling water 5-10 minutes, strain) applied externally (18).

Comments

Carlina is rarely used today (8).

CAROB

This Product is Also Known As

Locust Bean, Locust Pods, St. John's Bread, Sugar Pods.

Scientific Names

Ceratonia siliqua.
Family: Leguminosae or Fabaceae.

People Use This For

Orally, carob is used for acute nutritional disorders, celiac disease, obesity, diarrhea, dyspepsia, entero-colitis, vomiting during pregnancy, and sprue. In infants, it is used for vomiting, retching cough (18) and diarrhea (11). Carob flour and extracts are used as ingredients in food. Carob is used as a flavoring agent in foods and beverages. It is used in health food products, including weight-loss formulations, "energy" bars, tea formulations, and as a chocolate substitute (11).

Safety

LIKELY SAFE …when used orally in amounts found in foods. It has Generally Recognized as Safe (GRAS) status in the US (6). …when used orally in medicinal amounts (12).
PREGNANCY AND LACTATION: Insufficient reliable information available; avoid using.

Effectiveness

There is insufficient reliable information available about the effectiveness of carob.

Possible Mechanism of Action & Active Ingredients

The applicable part of carob is the fruit. Tannins contained in carob strongly inhibit digestive enzymes. Animal data suggest that a 15% carob gum diet fed for 2-6 weeks may result in weight loss. Decreases in blood glucose levels, cholesterol plasma levels and insulin levels, and an increased glucose tolerance are also suggested (11).

Adverse Reactions Including Known Allergies

None reported.

Possible Interactions with Herbs & Other Dietary Supplements

Insufficient reliable information available.

Possible Interactions with Drugs

No interactions are known to occur, and there is no known reason to expect a clinically significant interaction with carob.

Possible Interactions with Foods

No interactions are known to occur, and there is no known reason to expect a clinically significant interaction with carob.

Possible Interactions with Lab Tests

No interactions are known to occur, and there is no known reason to expect a clinically significant interaction with carob.

Possible Interactions with Diseases or Conditions

No interactions are known to occur, and there is no known reason to expect a clinically significant interaction with carob.

Typical Dosages & Routes of Administration that are Commonly Used

ORAL: 20-30 grams carob is added to water, tea, or milk and taken orally over one day.

Comments

Avoid confusing carob with carob tree, Jacaranda procera and Jacaranda caroba. The term "carat" evolved from the use of carob seeds as weight units for measuring gold (6).

CARRAGEENAN

This Product is Also Known As

Carrageenin, Carragheenan, Chondrus Extract, Irish Moss Extract, Mousse D'Irlande.

Scientific Names

Chondrus crispus; Gigartina mamillosa and other Gigartina species; Euchema species; related red algae. Family: Gigartinaceae.

People Use This For

Orally, carrageenan is used to soothe mucous membranes irritated by coughs, bronchitis, tuberculosis, and intestinal problems. The French use a form that has been degraded by low pH and high temperatures to treat peptic ulcers (11), and as a bulk laxative (13); this degraded form has lost the gelling properties of the original product. Topically, carrageenan is used for anorectal symptoms (14).

Carrageenan is also an ingredient in weight loss products.

In manufacturing, carrageenan is used as a binder, emulsifier, thickening agent, and as a stabilizer in pharmaceuticals, foods, and toothpaste.

Safety

LIKELY SAFE ...when used orally and appropriately for medicinal use (11). ...when used in food amounts; it is approved for food use in the US (11).

LIKELY UNSAFE ...when used in degraded form. The degraded form was associated with lesions in animals (14).

CHILDREN: POSSIBLY UNSAFE ...when used orally in infants. UK Food Advisory Committee recommended against use in infant formulas because some evidence suggests carrageenan could have adverse effects on the immune system (14).

PREGNANCY AND LACTATION: LIKELY SAFE ...when used in food amounts. There is insufficient reliable information available about the safety of using larger amounts; avoid using.

Effectiveness

POSSIBLY EFFECTIVE ...when used orally for peptic ulcers (11).

There is insufficient reliable information available about the effectiveness of carrageenan for its other uses.

Possible Mechanism of Action & Active Ingredients

In animals, carrageenan has been reported to lower blood cholesterol, reducing GI secretions and food absorption, increasing water content of the gut when large amounts are given. Parenterally it has shown anticoagulant, hypotensive, and immunosuppressive activities; it may also have anti-inflammatory properties (11).

Adverse Reactions Including Known Allergies

Carrageenan can cause bleeding, cramping, diarrhea, hypotension, and can lead to infection. Theoretically, carrageenan may be a problem for infants. It can be absorbed by their immature gut and may affect their immune system adversely (14).

Possible Interactions with Herbs & Other Dietary Supplements

Insufficient reliable information available.

Possible Interactions with Drugs

Carrageenan may increase the risk of bleeding in patients taking anticoagulants, and may enhance hypotensive effects of antihypertensive agents. Additionally, it can impair GI absorption of other drugs (214).

Possible Interactions with Foods

No interactions are known to occur, and there is no known reason to expect a clinically significant interaction with carrageenan.

Possible Interactions with Lab Tests

No interactions are known to occur, and there is no known reason to expect a clinically significant interaction with carrageenan.

Possible Interactions with Diseases or Conditions

No interactions are known to occur, and there is no known reason to expect a clinically significant interaction with carrageenan.

Typical Dosages & Routes of Administration that are Commonly Used

ORAL: A one cup decoction of Irish moss is sometimes taken two to three times daily. The decoction is prepared by adding 1 ounce of the dried plant in 1-1.5 pints boiling water, simmering, and then straining. The decoction can be sweetened with lemon, honey, or cinnamon (6002).

Comments

Carrageenan consists of hydrocolloids from various red algae or seaweeds.

CASCARA

This Product is Also Known As

Bitter Bark, California Buckthorn, Cascara Sagrada, Chittem Bark, Dogwood Bark, Purshiana Bark, Rhamni Purshianae Cortex, Sacred Bark, Sagrada Bark, Yellow Bark.

Scientific Names

Rhamnus purshiana, synonym Frangula purshiana.
Family: Rhamnaceae.

People Use This For

Orally, cascara is used most commonly as a laxative (7,11). Cascara is also used for gallstones, liver ailments, cancer, and as a bitter tonic (11).
In foods and beverages, a bitterless extract of cascara is sometimes used as a flavoring agent (11).
In manufacturing, cascara is used in processing of some sunscreens (11).

Safety

LIKELY SAFE ...when the bark preparations are used orally and appropriately for short periods of time (2). Cascara has FDA approval for use as a nonprescription medication.
POSSIBLY UNSAFE ...when cascara is used orally for more than 1-2 weeks. Chronic use can lead to dependence and electrolyte loss, specifically low levels of potassium (6).
CHILDREN: POSSIBLY SAFE ...when used orally and appropriately in children more than 2 years old. Should be used cautiously, if at all, in children less than 2 years old (272).
PREGNANCY: Insufficient reliable information available; avoid using (4258).
LACTATION: POSSIBLY UNSAFE ...when used orally because it is excreted into breast milk and might cause diarrhea (272).

Effectiveness

EFFECTIVE ...when used as a laxative (2,4,272), and has been approved by the FDA.
There is insufficient reliable information available about the effectiveness of cascara for its other uses.

Possible Mechanism of Action & Active Ingredients

The applicable part of cascara is the dried bark. The anthraglycoside constituents in cascara are cascarosides A and B. These stimulate peristalsis and evacuation leading to its stimulant laxative effect (6). Cascara exerts its effect on the large intestine and does not have much effect on the small intestine. Bacteria in the intestine are required to transform the anthraglycosides into stimulant laxatives. The fresh bark contains free anthrone which is an emetic compound that can cause severe vomiting. But the free anthrone is destroyed by aging the bark for at least one year, or by artificial aging with heat and aeration (2). Anthroid laxative use is not associated with an increased risk of developing colorectal ademoma or carcinoma (6138).

Adverse Reactions Including Known Allergies

Orally, cascara can cause mild abdominal discomfort, colic, and cramps (4). Using cascara for long periods of time can lead to potassium depletion, albuminuria, hematuria, and disturbed heart function. Long-term use can also lead to muscle weakness (2), finger clubbing, and cachexia (4). Chronic use can cause pseudomelanosis coli (pigment spots in intestinal mucosa) which is harmless, and usually reverses with discontinuation (2), and is not associated with an increased risk of developing colorectal ademoma or carcinoma (6138). The fresh or improperly aged bark can cause severe vomiting due to the presence of free anthrones.

Possible Interactions with Herbs & Other Dietary Supplements

LICORICE: Using cascara concomitantly with licorice can increase the risk of potassium depletion (2).
DIGITALIS, LILY OF THE VALLEY, SQUILL: Overuse of cascara can increase the risk of cardiac toxicity, because these herbs are also cardiac glycoside-containing herbs (2,500) and because of potassium loss (4).
STIMULANT LAXATIVE HERBS: Theoretically, cascara used concomitantly with other herbs that are stimulant laxatives can increase the risk of potassium depletion. Stimulant laxative herbs include: aloe, wild cucumber fruit (Ecballium elaterium), blue flag rhizome, alder buckthorn, European buckthorn, butternut bark, castor oil, colocynth fruit pulp, gamboge bark exudate, jalap root, black root, manna bark exudate, podophyllum root, rhubarb root, senna leaves and pods, and yellow dock root (19).
POTASSIUM DEPLETING HERBS: Theoretically, concomitant use of cascara along with horsetail plant or licorice rhizome can increase the risk of potassium depletion.

Possible Interactions with Drugs

CARDIAC GLYCOSIDES: Theoretically, overuse of cascara increases the risk of adverse effects of cardiac glycoside drugs, such as digoxin (Lanoxin).
CORTICOSTEROIDS, POTASSIUM DEPLETING DIURETICS: Concomitant use of these drugs along with cascara can increase the risk of potassium depletion (2).
LAXATIVES: Concomitant use of cascara along with many laxatives can cause electrolyte and fluid depletion.
ORAL DRUGS: Theoretically, cascara can reduce the absorption of some drugs due to the reduced transit time through the GI tract (500).

Possible Interactions with Foods

No interactions are known to occur, and there is no known reason to expect a clinically significant interaction with cascara.

Possible Interactions with Lab Tests

COLORIMETRIC TESTS: Cascara can discolor urine (pink, red, purple, orange, rust), interfering with diagnostic tests that depend on a color change, due to its anthraquinone content (1,12,275).
POTASSIUM: Excessive use of cascara can cause potassium depletion, reducing serum potassium concentrations and test results (1,2,4,12,19).

Possible Interactions with Diseases or Conditions

GI CONDITIONS: Cascara is contraindicated in people with intestinal obstruction, or acute intestinal inflammation. This includes people with Crohn's disease, ulcerative colitis, and appendicitis. It is also contraindicated for people who have ulcers, and abdominal pain of unknown origin (2,4,8).

Typical Dosages & Routes of Administration that are Commonly Used

ORAL: 20-30 mg per day of the active ingredient, hyroxyanthracene derivatives. This is calculated as cascaroside A, from the cut bark, powder, or extracts (2). A typical dose includes 1 cup of tea which is made by steeping 2 grams of finely chopped bark in 150 mL of boiling water for 5-10 minutes, and then straining (18). The cascara liquid extract is given in a dose of 2-5 mL three times daily (4). The appropriate amount of cascara is the smallest dose that is necessary to maintain soft stools (2).

Comments

American Herbal Products Association (AHPA) recommends the following label statement: "Do not use this product if you have abdominal pain or diarrhea. Consult a health care provider prior to use if you are pregnant or nursing. Discontinue use in the event of diarrhea or watery stools. Do not exceed recommended dose. Not for long-term use." (12). Non-standardized anthraquinone-containing preparations should be avoided, as their effects are not predictable (4).

CASCARILLA

This Product is Also Known As
Bahama Cascarilla, Sweet Bark, Sweet Wood Bark.

Scientific Names
Croton eleuteria.
Family: Euphorbiaceae.

People Use This For
Orally, cascarilla is used for digestive disorders, diarrhea, and vomiting (18).

Safety
There is insufficient reliable information available about the safety of cascarilla.
Pregnancy and Lactation: Insufficient reliable information available; avoid using.

Effectiveness
There is insufficient reliable information available about the effectiveness of cascarilla.

Possible Mechanism of Action & Active Ingredients
The applicable part of cascarilla is the bark. Constituents reported to have stimulant and tonic properties (18).

Adverse Reactions Including Known Allergies
None reported (18).

Possible Interactions with Herbs & Other Dietary Supplements
Insufficient reliable information available.

Possible Interactions with Drugs
No interactions are known to occur, and there is no known reason to expect a clinically significant interaction with cascarilla.

Possible Interactions with Foods
No interactions are known to occur, and there is no known reason to expect a clinically significant interaction with cascarilla.

Possible Interactions with Lab Tests
No interactions are known to occur, and there is no known reason to expect a clinically significant interaction with cascarilla.

Possible Interactions with Diseases or Conditions
No interactions are known to occur, and there is no known reason to expect a clinically significant interaction with cascarilla.

Typical Dosages & Routes of Administration that are Commonly Used
No typical dosage.

Comments
In the past, cascarilla was added to tobacco before smoking, due to its pleasant odor when burned. It also produced vertigo and intoxication during this process (215).

CASHEW

This Product is Also Known As
East Indian Almond.

Scientific Names
Anacardium occidentale.
Family: Anarcardiaceae.

People Use This For
Orally, cashew is used for gastrointestinal ailments.
Topically, cashew is used as a skin stimulant and cauterizing agent for ulcers, warts and corns (18).

Safety
LIKELY SAFE ...when consumed as a food (18).
There is insufficient reliable information available about the safety of the oral and topical uses of cashew when it is used medicinally in amounts exceeding those found in foods.

PREGNANCY AND LACTATION: LIKELY SAFE ...when consumed as food; avoid using amounts greater than typically found in foods.

Effectiveness
There is insufficient reliable information available about the effectiveness of cashew.

Possible Mechanism of Action & Active Ingredients
The applicable part of cashew is the nut. A dried ethanolic extract is effective in vitro against gram-positive bacteria Bacillus subtilis and Staphylococcus aureus. Alkyl phenols contained in the cashew nut shell are strong skin irritants. Cashew contains alkyl phenols that are chemically related to constituents in poison ivy, poison oak, mango, and ginkgo. The adverse reactions resulting from cashew are related to the adverse reactions that sometimes occur with these other irritants. Contact can lead to redness, nodule and blister formation. Roasted cashew nuts are free of the alkyl phenols [18].

Adverse Reactions Including Known Allergies
None reported.

Possible Interactions with Herbs & Other Dietary Supplements
Insufficient reliable information available.

Possible Interactions with Drugs
No interactions are known to occur, and there is no known reason to expect a clinically significant interaction with cashew.

Possible Interactions with Foods
No interactions are known to occur, and there is no known reason to expect a clinically significant interaction with cashew.

Possible Interactions with Lab Tests
No interactions are known to occur, and there is no known reason to expect a clinically significant interaction with cashew.

Possible Interactions with Diseases or Conditions
No interactions are known to occur, and there is no known reason to expect a clinically significant interaction with cashew.

Typical Dosages & Routes of Administration that are Commonly Used
No typical dosage.

Comments
Acajou oil, oleum anacardiae and fatty oil, are extracted from cashew nuts [18].

CASSIA

This Product is Also Known As
Bastard Cinnamon, Canton Cassia, Cassia Aromaticum, Cassia Bark, Cassia Cinnamon, Cassia Lignea, Chinese Cinnamon, Cinnamomi cassiae cortex, False Cinnamon, Nees, Rou Gui.
CAUTION: See separate listing for Cinnamon flower and Cinnamon bark.

Scientific Names
Cinnamomum aromaticum, synonym Cinnamomum cassia.
Family: Lauraceae.

People Use This For
Orally, cassia bark is used as an antiflatulent, antispasmodic, antiemetic, antidiarrheal, antimicrobial, and for treating the common cold [4] and loss of appetite [2].
Topically, cassia is used in suntan lotions, nasal sprays, mouthwashes, gargles, toothpaste, and as a counterirritant in liniments [11].
In Chinese medicine, cassia bark is used for impotence, diarrhea, enuresis, rheumatic conditions, testicle hernia, menopause syndrome, amenorrhea, immune stabilizer, and as an abortifacient [18].
In folk medicine, cassia has been used for heart pains, kidney troubles, hypertension, cramps, and cancer [11].
In food and beverages, cassia is used as a flavoring [11].

Safety
LIKELY SAFE ...when used orally in amounts found in foods (maximum use level 0.047%) [11]; Generally Recognized as Safe (GRAS) status in the US.
POSSIBLY SAFE ...when used orally in appropriate doses as a medicinal [12].

LIKELY UNSAFE ...when used topically in concentrations greater than 0.2% (4).
PREGNANCY AND LACTATION: Insufficient reliable information available (12); avoid using in amounts higher than those found in food (4).

Effectiveness

POSSIBLY EFFECTIVE ...when used orally for loss of appetite, mild gastrointestinal spasms, bloating, and flatulence (2).
There is insufficient reliable information available about the effectiveness of cassia for its other uses.

Possible Mechanism of Action & Active Ingredients

The applicable part of cassia is the bark. Cinnamaldehyde, found in the volatile oil fraction of Cassia, causes CNS stimulation at a low dose, but sedation at a high dose. Cinnamaldehyde also has antibacterial and antifungal activity. It accelerates catecholamine release from adrenal glands, increases blood flow, reduces blood pressure and heart rate, and causes hyperglycemia (4).

Adverse Reactions Including Known Allergies

Allergic skin reactions and dermal and membrane irritation have been reported (4).

Possible Interactions with Herbs & Other Dietary Supplements

Insufficient reliable information available.

Possible Interactions with Drugs

No interactions are known to occur, and there is no known reason to expect a clinically significant interaction with cassia.

Possible Interactions with Foods

No interactions are known to occur, and there is no known reason to expect a clinically significant interaction with cassia.

Possible Interactions with Lab Tests

No interactions are known to occur, and there is no known reason to expect a clinically significant interaction with cassia.

Possible Interactions with Diseases or Conditions

ALLERGY TO CINNAMON, PERU BALSAM: Contraindicated (2).
SENSITIVE INDIVIDUALS: Avoid contact, may cause contact dermatitis (12).

Typical Dosages & Routes of Administration that are Commonly Used

ORAL: Dried bark: 0.5-1 grams three times daily, or drink 1 cup tea (steep 0.5-1 grams of dry bark in 150 mL boiling water 5-10 minutes, strain) three times daily (2,4). Essential oil: 0.05-0.2 mL three times daily (2,4).

Comments

Reported to be inferior to true cinnamon in flavor (4,11).

CASSIE ABSOLUTE

This Product is Also Known As

Huisache, Popinac Absolute, Sweet Acacia.

Scientific Names

Acacia farnesiana; Mimosa farnesiana.
Family: Leguminosae or Fabaceae.

People Use This For

Orally, cassie absolute used as an antispasmodic, antidiarrheal, stimulant, aphrodisiac, and to treat fever (11).
Topically, cassie absolute is used for dry skin as a bath additive, insecticide, and a fragrance in perfume (11).
In Chinese medicine, cassie absolute is used for rheumatoid arthritis and pulmonary tuberculosis (11).
In other countries, various plant parts are used for medicinal purposes. Tea made from cassie absolute leaves is used for gonorrhea in India (11), and the root is chewed for sore throat in India (11), and used for stomach cancer in Venezuela (11).
For food uses, cassie absolute is a flavor ingredient in foods and beverages (11).
In manufacturing, cassie absolute is used as a fragrance in perfumes (11).

Safety

LIKELY SAFE ...in amounts found in foods (maximum use level 0.002%); approved for use in foods in the US (11).
There is insufficient reliable information available about the safety of the use of cassie absolute in amounts greater than those found in foods.
PREGNANCY AND LACTATION: Insufficient reliable information available; avoid using.

Effectiveness

There is insufficient reliable information available about the effectiveness of cassie absolute.

Possible Mechanism of Action & Active Ingredients

Reported to have antispasmodic, aphrodisiac, astringent, demulcent, antidiarrheal, antipyretic, antirheumatic and stimulant properties (11). Contains glycosides which reportedly have anti-inflammatory and bronchodilator effects (1505).

Adverse Reactions Including Known Allergies

None reported.

Possible Interactions with Herbs & Other Dietary Supplements

Insufficient reliable information available.

Possible Interactions with Drugs

No interactions are known to occur, and there is no known reason to expect a clinically significant interaction with cassie absolute.

Possible Interactions with Foods

No interactions are known to occur, and there is no known reason to expect a clinically significant interaction with cassie absolute.

Possible Interactions with Lab Tests

No interactions are known to occur, and there is no known reason to expect a clinically significant interaction with cassie absolute.

Possible Interactions with Diseases or Conditions

No interactions are known to occur, and there is no known reason to expect a clinically significant interaction with cassie absolute.

Typical Dosages & Routes of Administration that are Commonly Used

No typical dosage.

Comments

Cassie absolute is an extract of Acacia farnesiana flowers. Limited pharmacologic and toxicologic information is available (11).

CASTOR OIL

This Product is Also Known As

African Coffee Tree, Bofareira, Castor, Castor Oil Plant, Mexico Weed, Palma Christi, Tangantangan Oil Plant, Wonder Tree.
CAUTION: See separate listing for Castor seed.

Scientific Names

Ricinus communis; Ricinus sanguines.
Family: Euphorbiaceae.

People Use This For

Orally, castor oil is used as a stimulant laxative (6).
Topically, castor oil is used as an emollient (11). It has also been used topically to dissolve cysts, growths, or warts, and to soften bunions and corns. Castor oil has been used in the eyes to soothe the irritated conjuctiva after the presence of foreign bodies there (214).
Historically, castor oil has been used alone or with quinine sulfate to induce labor at term, and applied topically as a cervical abortifacient and vaginal contraceptive (6).

Safety

LIKELY SAFE ...when castor oil is used orally and appropriately, short-term.
POSSIBLY UNSAFE ...when more than 60 mL per day are used by adults. ...when castor oil is used for more than 8-10 days (272).
There is insufficient reliable information available about the safety of the topical use of castor oil.
PREGNANCY AND LACTATION: LIKELY UNSAFE ...contraindicated for oral use because it might cause abortion (12,18).

Effectiveness

EFFECTIVE ...as a stimulant laxative (6,272).
There is insufficient reliable information available about the effectiveness of castor oil for its other uses.

Possible Mechanism of Action & Active Ingredients

The oil is hydrolyzed in the duodenum to release cathartic ricinoleic acid (6). Ricin (constituent) is a poison and can be fatal when ingested, inhaled, or given IV.

Adverse Reactions Including Known Allergies

Castor oil can cause burning in the mouth and throat, severe stomach pain, dulled vision, renal failure, uremia, and death. Ricinine (constituent) causes nausea, vomiting, hemorrhagic gastroenteritis, hepatic and renal damage, convulsions, and death (6).

Possible Interactions with Herbs & Other Dietary Supplements

CARDIAC GLYCOSIDE-CONTAINING HERBS: Theoretically, castor oil can increase the risk of cardiac glycoside toxicity (2,18,19,500).

LICORICE/HORSETAIL: Theoretically, concomitant use with horsetail plant or licorice rhizome increases the risk of potassium depletion (18).

MALE FERN: Concomitant use with oil-soluble antihelmintic herbs, such as the male fern, should be avoided due to enhanced absorption of castor oil (19).

STIMULANT LAXATIVE HERBS: Theoretically, concomitant use with other stimulant laxative herbs might increase the risk of potassium depletion (19).

WORMSEED: Concomitant use with wormseed oil might reduce both toxicity and efficacy of wormseed oil (19).

Possible Interactions with Drugs

CARDIAC GLYCOSIDES: Theoretically, can increase the risk of adverse effects of cardiac glycoside drugs, e.g. digoxin (Lanoxin).

CORTICOSTEROIDS, POTASSIUM DEPLETING DIURETICS: Concomitant use may increase risk of potassium depletion (18).

LAXATIVES: Concomitant use may lead to electrolyte and fluid depletion.

ORAL DRUGS: Theoretically, may reduce absorption of drugs due to reduced transit time.

Possible Interactions with Foods

No interactions are known to occur, and there is no known reason to expect a clinically significant interaction with castor oil.

Possible Interactions with Lab Tests

No interactions are known to occur, and there is no known reason to expect a clinically significant interaction with castor oil.

Possible Interactions with Diseases or Conditions

INTESTINAL DISORDERS: Contraindicated in intestinal obstruction (appendicitis, Crohn's disease, irritable bowel syndrome, ulcerative colitis), abdominal pain of unknown origin (18), biliary tract obstruction and other biliary disorders (7).

Typical Dosages & Routes of Administration that are Commonly Used

ORAL: Adult dose, 5-10 grams (1-2 teaspoons); takes effect in 8 hours (7). Maximum dose at one time, 30 grams (6 teaspoons) (7). Castor oil is most effective when taken on an empty stomach (7).

Comments

Castor oil is produced by cold pressing ripe seeds of Ricinus communis.

CASTOR seed

This Product is Also Known As

African Coffee Tree, Bofareira, Castor Bean, Mexico Weed, Palma Christi, Tangantangan Oil Plant, Wonder Tree. CAUTION: See separate listing for Castor Oil.

Scientific Names

Ricinus communis; Ricinus sanguines.
Family: Euphorbiaceae.

People Use This For

Orally, raw or roasted castor seeds have been used as a cathartic, an emetic, to treat leprosy, or cure syphilis (5611). Topically, castor seed powder is used as a poultice for inflammatory skin disorders, boils, carbuncles, abscesses, inflammation of the middle ear, and migraines (18).

Safety

UNSAFE ...when used orally if the seed is chewed or the seed coat has been ruptured (6,5611). Ingestion of 3-6 seeds in an adult has been reported to be lethal (5611). However, if the seed is swallowed intact, poisoning is unlikely (6,5611) but prompt medical attention is recommended after ingestion (5611). Survival of individuals requiring

medical attention and support after ingestion of chewed seeds has been reported (5611,5613).
CHILDREN: UNSAFE ...when used orally the chewed or uncoated seeds can cause severe symptoms of intoxication (5611,5612) and death (5611).
There is insufficient reliable information available about the safety of the topical use of castor seed.
PREGNANCY AND LACTATION: UNSAFE ...when used orally if the seed coat is ruptured; avoid using. There is insufficient reliable information available about the safety of the topical use of castor seed during pregnancy and lactation.

Effectiveness
There is insufficient reliable information available about the effectiveness of castor seed.

Possible Mechanism of Action & Active Ingredients
Castor seed contains the glycoprotein ricin which is considered to be fatal when ingested, inhaled or given IV. It interferes with protein synthesis causing cell death (6,5611). Cytotoxic effects may not occur for two to five days after ingestion (5611). Castor seed also contains glycoproteins which are considered to be extremely allergenic such as the allergen called CBA. Some evidence suggests ricin might have analgesic effects and activity against leukemia (6).

Adverse Reactions Including Known Allergies
Taken orally, castor bean can cause nausea, vomiting, diarrhea, abdominal pain, dehydration, shock, red cell hemolysis, severe fluid and electrolyte disturbances, peripheral vascular collapse, renal failure secondary to hypovolemia, and death. Cellular damage to liver, kidneys, and pancreas may occur two to five days later after ingestion (5611,5612). Topically, exposure to the castor plant, crushed seeds, or seed dust can cause dermatitis (5611).
POISONING: Chewed or uncoated seeds may be lethal to humans; poisoning is considered unlikely if the seed is swallowed intact (6.5611). Prompt medical attention is recommended after ingestion of seeds. Serum chemistries should be monitored for at least five days after ingestion in symptomatic patients (5611).
OCCUPATIONAL ALLERGY: Reported to be an inhalant allergen in coffee industry (repeated inhalation of fumes from shipments of coffee beans contaminated with castor beans) (6). Anaphylaxis can occur after exposure to castor beans, plants, or dust (5611).

Possible Interactions with Herbs & Other Dietary Supplements
Insufficient reliable information available.

Possible Interactions with Drugs
No interactions are known to occur, and there is no known reason to expect a clinically significant interaction with castor seed.

Possible Interactions with Foods
No interactions are known to occur, and there is no known reason to expect a clinically significant interaction with castor seed.

Possible Interactions with Lab Tests
No interactions are known to occur, and there is no known reason to expect a clinically significant interaction with castor seed.

Possible Interactions with Diseases or Conditions
No interactions are known to occur, and there is no known reason to expect a clinically significant interaction with castor seed.

Typical Dosages & Routes of Administration that are Commonly Used
TOPICAL: Apply paste made with ground seeds to affected skin twice daily; treatment takes up to 15 days (18). For use on intact skin; avoid use on broken or damaged skin.

Comments
The plant is used mainly for ornamental purposes (6). Ricin has been evaluated as a possible chemical warfare agent. (6).

CASTOREUM

This Product is Also Known As
Canadian Beaver, European Beaver, Siberian Beaver.

Scientific Names
Castor canadensis; Castor fiber.
Family: Castoridae.

People Use This For

In traditional medicine, castoreum is used for absence of menstrual periods, painful menses, hysteria, restless sleep, and as a calming and restorative agent (11).

In foods and beverages, castoreum extract is used as a flavoring agent.

In manufacturing, castoreum tincture is used as a fragrance or fixative in cosmetics and soaps (11).

Safety

LIKELY SAFE ...when used in amounts found in foods; the maximum use level is 0.009% (11). It has Generally Recognized as Safe (GRAS) status in the US (11). ...when used topically. Castoreum tincture is reported to be nontoxic in dermatological tests (11); the maximum use level is 0.4% in perfumes (11).

There is insufficient reliable information available about the safety of castoreum for its other uses.

PREGNANCY AND LACTATION: Insufficient reliable information available; avoid using.

Effectiveness

There is insufficient reliable information available about the effectiveness of castoreum.

Possible Mechanism of Action & Active Ingredients

Reported to have calming and sedating effects (11).

Adverse Reactions Including Known Allergies

None reported.

Possible Interactions with Herbs & Other Dietary Supplements

Insufficient reliable information available.

Possible Interactions with Drugs

No interactions are known to occur, and there is no known reason to expect a clinically significant interaction with castoreum.

Possible Interactions with Foods

No interactions are known to occur, and there is no known reason to expect a clinically significant interaction with castoreum.

Possible Interactions with Lab Tests

No interactions are known to occur, and there is no known reason to expect a clinically significant interaction with castoreum.

Possible Interactions with Diseases or Conditions

No interactions are known to occur, and there is no known reason to expect a clinically significant interaction with castoreum.

Typical Dosages & Routes of Administration that are Commonly Used

No typical dosage.

Comments

Castoreum is a secretion collected from scent glands of Canadian, European, and Siberian beavers. Castoreum from the Canadian beaver is considered superior in quality to that of the Siberian beaver (11).

CAT'S CLAW

This Product is Also Known As

Cats Claw, Griffe Du Chat, Life-giving Vine of Peru, Samento, Uña De Gato.
CAUTION: See separate listing for Cat's Foot.

Scientific Names

Uncaria tomentosa; Uncaria guianensis.
Family: Rubiaceae.

People Use This For

Orally, people use cat's claw for diverticulitis, peptic ulcers, colitis, gastritis, hemorrhoids, parasites, and leaky bowel syndrome.

In combination therapy with zidovudine (AZT), cat's claw is used for individuals who are HIV positive (6). Researchers have been evaluating the use of cat's claw to fight viral infections such as herpes zoster, herpes simplex, and HIV.

Historically, cat's claw was used for wound healing, treating intestinal ailments, gastric ulcers and tumors, gonorrhea, dysentery, cancers of the urinary tract, as an anti-inflammatory, contraceptive, tonic to ward off disease, treat bone pains, and cleanse the kidneys (6).

Safety

There is insufficient reliable information available about the safety of cat's claw root and bark (12).
CHILDREN: POSSIBLY UNSAFE ...when used orally in children under 3 years old (12).
PREGNANCY: POSSIBLY UNSAFE ...when used orally. Cat's claw is sometimes used as a contraceptive and women should be advised to stop using if they become pregnant (12).
LACTATION: Insufficient reliable information available; avoid using.

Effectiveness

POSSIBLY EFFECTIVE ...when taken orally as an immune system stimulant (6).
Clinical studies on the effectiveness of cat's claw have used extracts of the stem and root standardized to 4% alkaloids.
There is insufficient reliable information available about the effectiveness of cat's claw for its other uses.

Possible Mechanism of Action & Active Ingredients

The applicable part of cat's claw is the root and bark. Cat's claw has an immune stimulating effect due to alkaloid constituents, including pteropodine and isopteropodine (6). Some of cat's claw's constituents have specific effects: Rhynchophylline seems to relax endothelial blood vessels, dilate peripheral blood vessels, inhibit sympathetic nervous system activity, and lower heart rate and blood cholesterol (6). Mytraphylline seems to have diuretic activity (6). Hirsutine seems to inhibit bladder contractions, cause local anesthesia at low doses, and provide curare-like actions at high dose (6). Several quinovic acid glycoside constituents seem to have antiviral activity in vitro, and anti-inflammatory activity in rats (6).

Adverse Reactions Including Known Allergies

Occasionally diarrhea results when the dose of cat's claw gets too large. It is possible that cat's claw can lead to hypotension. Tell people to get up slowly to avoid dizziness. There is the possibility that cat's claw can contribute to unusual bruising, or bleeding gums.

Possible Interactions with Herbs & Other Dietary Supplements

Insufficient reliable information available.

Possible Interactions with Drugs

ANTI-HYPERTENSIVES: Since cat's claw may lower blood pressure, exercise caution if it is being used along with an antihypertensive.

Possible Interactions with Foods

No interactions are known to occur, and there is no known reason to expect a clinically significant interaction with cat's claw.

Possible Interactions with Lab Tests

No interactions are known to occur, and there is no known reason to expect a clinically significant interaction with cat's claw.

Possible Interactions with Diseases or Conditions

HYPOTENSION: Cat's claw may further reduce blood pressure and cause problems.

Typical Dosages & Routes of Administration that are Commonly Used

ORAL: People often use 500-1000 mg once to three times a day (5016). Tablets and capsules containing the raw herb are available in many strengths, such as 400 mg, 500 mg, 800 mg, 1 gram, and 5 grams (5008). Some people prepare and consume cat's claw tea by simmering 1 gram of the root bark in 150 mL of boiling water for five to ten minutes and then straining (5011). The tea is consumed three times daily (5011). Clinical studies on the effectiveness of cat's claw have used extracts of the stem and root standardized to 4% alkaloids.

Comments

In commerce, cat's claw represents an interesting situation. It is ranked as the seventh most popular herb in US sales in 1997 (2), but there is very little scientific evidence of its safety or efficacy. In addition, the active constituents vary greatly in concentration, depending on the time of year the cat's claw is harvested (6). And, up to twenty different plants are identified as "cat's claw", so some people who think they are using cat's claw are using something else. Avoid confusing cat's claw with devil's claw.

CAT'S FOOT

This Product is Also Known As

Antennariase Dioicae Flos, Cats Ear Flower, Cat's Ear Flower, Cats Foot, Cudweed, Katsenpfotchenbluten, Life Everlasting, Mountain Everlasting.
CAUTION: See separate listings for Cudweed and Cat's Claw.

Scientific Names
Antennaria dioica.
Family: Asteraceae or Compositae.

People Use This For
Orally, cat's foot is used to treat intestinal disease (2).
In folk medicine, cat's foot is used as a diuretic (18).

Safety
There is insufficient reliable information available about the safety of cat's foot.
Pregnancy and Lactation: Insufficient reliable information available; avoid using.

Effectiveness
There is insufficient reliable information available about the effectiveness of cat's foot (2).

Possible Mechanism of Action & Active Ingredients
The applicable part of cat's foot is the fresh or dried flowers. Mild spasmolytic and choleric effects reported in animals (18).

Adverse Reactions Including Known Allergies
Cat's foot can cause an allergic reaction in individuals sensitive to the Asteraceae/Compositae family. Members of this family include ragweed, chrysanthemums, marigolds, daisies, and many other herbs.

Possible Interactions with Herbs & Other Dietary Supplements
Insufficient reliable information available.

Possible Interactions with Drugs
No interactions are known to occur, and there is no known reason to expect a clinically significant interaction with cat's foot.

Possible Interactions with Foods
No interactions are known to occur, and there is no known reason to expect a clinically significant interaction with cat's foot.

Possible Interactions with Lab Tests
No interactions are known to occur, and there is no known reason to expect a clinically significant interaction with cat's foot.

Possible Interactions with Diseases or Conditions
CROSS-ALLERGENICITY: Can cause an allergic reaction in individuals sensitive to the Asteraceae/Compositae family. Members of this family include ragweed, chrysanthemums, marigolds, daisies, and many other herbs.

Typical Dosages & Routes of Administration that are Commonly Used
ORAL: The fluid extract of cat's foot is sometimes taken as 14-28 grains three times daily (6002).

Comments
Avoid confusion with ground ivy, which is also sometimes referred to as cat's foot (214).

CATECHU

This Product is Also Known As
Black Catechu: Acacia Catechu Heartwood Extract, Black Cutch, Cachou, Cashou, Catechu nigrum, Cutch, Dark Catechu, Pegu Catechu.
Pale Catechu: Cube Gambir, Gambier, Gambir, Gambir Catechu, Terra Japonica, Uncaria Gambier Leaf/Twig Extract.

Scientific Names
Black catechu: Acacia catechu.
Family: Leguminosae or Fabaceae.
Pale catechu: Uncaria gambier.
Family: Rubiaceae.

People Use This For
Orally, catechu is used for diarrhea (6,9,11), chronic mucous membrane inflammation, dysentery, colitis, bleeding (18), and cancer (11).
Topically, catechu is used for skin diseases, hemorrhoids, traumatic injuries, to stop bleeding, and for dressing wounds. Catechu is included in mouthwashes and gargles for gingivitis, stomatitis, pharyngitis, and oral ulcers (11,18).

In Chinese medicine, black catechu is used to treat indigestion in children (11).
In foods and beverages, catechu is used as a flavoring agent (11).
Catechu is used in some parts of the world as an anti-fertility drug (214).

Safety
LIKELY SAFE ...when used orally in amounts found in foods (maximum use level 0.016%); approved for use in foods in US (11).
POSSIBLY UNSAFE ...when used as a medicinal. Catechu contains tannins with possible carcinogenic and hepatotoxic properties (11). Another constituent, (+)-catechin (cianidanol), is associated with fatal hemolytic anemia (9).
PREGNANCY AND LACTATION: POSSIBLY UNSAFE; avoid using.

Effectiveness
There is insufficient reliable information available about the effectiveness of catechu.

Possible Mechanism of Action & Active Ingredients
Both black and pale catechu are applicable. Researchers think the astringent and antibacterial properties of catechu result from its high tannin content (11). Gambrine (in pale catechu) has hypotensive effects (11). D-catechin (in black and pale catechu) causes blood vessel constriction (11). Fisetin (in black catechu) and (+)-catechin (in black and pale catechu) and may protect against liver damage; (+)-catechin (cianidanol) is also thought to protect against experimentally-induced ulcers in animals (11); (+)-catechin (cianidanol) is associated with fatal hemolytic anemia (9).

Adverse Reactions Including Known Allergies
None reported (18).

Possible Interactions with Herbs & Other Dietary Supplements
Insufficient reliable information available.

Possible Interactions with Drugs
No interactions are known to occur, and there is no known reason to expect a clinically significant interaction with catechu.

Possible Interactions with Foods
No interactions are known to occur, and there is no known reason to expect a clinically significant interaction with catechu.

Possible Interactions with Lab Tests
No interactions are known to occur, and there is no known reason to expect a clinically significant interaction with catechu.

Possible Interactions with Diseases or Conditions
No interactions are known to occur, and there is no known reason to expect a clinically significant interaction with catechu.

Typical Dosages & Routes of Administration that are Commonly Used
ORAL: Dose range 0.3-2 grams three times daily, or single 500 mg dose (18).
TOPICAL: Catechu tincture, 20 drops in a glass of lukewarm water (mouth rinse) or applied undiluted with a toothbrush (18).

Comments
Though black catechu and pale catechu differ somewhat chemically, they are used for the same purposes at the same dose (11). Unstandardized products may contain high amounts of aflatoxin, a metabolite of Aspergillus, which is toxic and may lead to certain cancers.

CATNIP

This Product is Also Known As
Catmint, Catnep, Catswort, Field Balm.

Scientific Names
Nepeta cataria.
Family: Labiatae/Lamiaceae.

People Use This For
Orally, catnip is used for insomnia; migraine headaches; cold; flu; fever; hives; and gastrointestinal upset, including indigestion, colic, cramping, and flatulence (5,6). It has also been used orally for conditions associated with anxiety, diuresis, as a tonic (6), for upper respiratory tract infections, and headaches (6121).

Topically, catnip has been used for arthritis, hemorrhoids, and as a poultice to relieve swelling (6).
In folk medicine, catnip has also been used for lung and uterine congestion, eradicating worms, and for initiating menses in girls with delayed onset of menstruation (6). Catnip is smoked for respiratory conditions and recreationally for inducing a euphoric high (6).
Catnip has been used as a pesticide and insecticide (6).

Safety

POSSIBLY SAFE …when used orally and appropriately (6,12). Significant adverse effects have not been reported when catnip tea is used in cupful amounts (6).
POSSIBLY UNSAFE …when used orally in excessive doses. Higher doses may be associated with significant adverse effects (6). …when inhaled by smoking dried leaves. Smoking the dried leaves of catnip has been associated with a euphoric high (6), which might impair judgment; however, whether catnip can truly produce this effect in humans remains controversial (6).
There is insufficient reliable information available about the safety of topically applied catnip.
CHILDREN: POSSIBLY UNSAFE …when used orally. One child developed stomach pain and irritability followed by lethargy and hypnotic state after ingesting catnip leaves and tea (5,2596).
PREGNANCY: LIKELY UNSAFE …when used orally. Catnip tea has been reported to have uterine stimulant properties (12); contraindicated.
LACTATION: Insufficient reliable information available; avoid using.

Effectiveness

There is insufficient reliable information available about the effectiveness of catnip.

Possible Mechanism of Action & Active Ingredients

The applicable part of catnip is the flowering tops. The pharmacological effect that catnip is famous for is the euphoric state it induces in cats. It is thought that the constituent cis-trans-nepetalcatone produces the characteristic stimulation in cats only when they smell it (5). Although humans have used catnip to induce a euphoric high, whether or not this effect actually occurs in humans is controversial. In humans, the constituent nepetalactone is thought to be responsible for catnip's calming effects in insomnia, anxiety, gastrointestinal conditions, and migraine headache. Nepetalactone is the major component (80-95%) of the volatile oil of catnip and is structurally related to the valepotriates found in valerian. Catnip provides approximately 0.2-1% volatile oil. Catnip reportedly also has antipyretic and diaphoretic effects, which have been attributed to its use for colds, flu, and fever. Other reported pharmacological effects, include diuretic and stimulation of gallbladder activity (6).

Adverse Reactions Including Known Allergies

Catnip abuse may result in headache and malaise. Large amounts of tea may cause vomiting (6). One case report exists of a nineteen-month-old child who developed a stomachache and irritability, followed by lethargy and a hypnotic state after ingesting raisins soaked in catnip tea and chewing on the tea bag (5,2596).

Possible Interactions with Herbs & Other Dietary Supplements

HERBS WITH SEDATIVE PROPERTIES: Theoretically, concomitant use with herbs that have sedative properties might enhance therapeutic and adverse effects. These include calamus, calendula, California poppy, capsicum, celery, couch grass, elecampane, ginseng Siberian, German chamomile, goldenseal, gotu kola, hops, Jamaican dogwood, kava, lemon balm, sage, St. John's wort, sassafras, scullcap, shepherd's purse, stinging nettle, valerian, wild carrot, wild lettuce, withania root, and yerba mansa (4,19).

Possible Interactions with Drugs

BARBITURATES: Theoretically, concomitant use with barbiturates may cause additive effects and side effects (19).
OTHER DRUGS WITH SEDATIVE PROPERTIES: Theoretically, concomitant use with drugs with sedative properties may cause additive effects and side effects (19).

Possible Interactions with Foods

No interactions are known to occur, and there is no known reason to expect a clinically significant interaction with catnip.

Possible Interactions with Lab Tests

No interactions are known to occur, and there is no known reason to expect a clinically significant interaction with catnip.

Possible Interactions with Diseases or Conditions

PELVIC INFLAMMATORY DISEASE (PID) AND EXCESSIVE MENSTRUAL BLEEDING: Because catnip is also used to stimulate menstruation, theoretically it is contraindicated in pelvic inflammatory disease (PID) and excessive menstrual bleeding (12).

Typical Dosages & Routes of Administration that are Commonly Used

ORAL: People typically use two 380 mg capsules three times daily at meals or prepared as a tea using 1 to 2 teaspoons in 6 ounces of boiling water (6006).

Comments
Today, in the US, catnip tea is still commonly used in Appalachia for many of the traditional uses (6).

CATUABA

This Product is Also Known As
Caramuru, Catuaba Casca, Chuchuhuasha, Golden Trumpet, Pau De Reposta, Piratancara, Tatuaba.

Scientific Names
Erythroxylum catuaba.
Family: Erythroxylaceae.

People Use This For
Orally, catuaba is used as an aphrodisiac, for male sexual impotency, agitation, exhaustion and fatigue, insomnia related to hypertension, nervousness, neurasthenia, poor memory or forgetfulness, as a tonic (3918) and for skin cancer (513).

Safety
There is insufficient reliable information available about the safety of catuaba.
Pregnancy and Lactation: Insufficient reliable information available; avoid using.

Effectiveness
There is insufficient reliable information available about the effectiveness of catuaba.

Possible Mechanism of Action & Active Ingredients
The applicable part of catuaba is the bark. An alkaline catuaba extract shows antibacterial effects in mice. It also inhibits the human immunodeficiency virus (HIV) in vitro (3916).

Adverse Reactions Including Known Allergies
None reported.

Possible Interactions with Herbs & Other Dietary Supplements
Insufficient reliable information available.

Possible Interactions with Drugs
No interactions are known to occur, and there is no known reason to expect a clinically significant interaction with catuaba.

Possible Interactions with Foods
No interactions are known to occur, and there is no known reason to expect a clinically significant interaction with catuaba.

Possible Interactions with Lab Tests
No interactions are known to occur, and there is no known reason to expect a clinically significant interaction with catuaba.

Possible Interactions with Diseases or Conditions
No interactions are known to occur, and there is no known reason to expect a clinically significant interaction with catuaba.

Typical Dosages & Routes of Administration that are Commonly Used
ORAL: People typically use 450 mg daily (5262).

Comments
Some think that Juniperus brasiliensis is a synonym for Erythroxylum catuaba (Family: Erythroxylaceae) (3918); however, Juniperus genus plants are classified as members of the Cupressaceae plant family (513,815).
There is very little scientific information about this product. Our staff is continually analyzing the available information on natural medicines and will add data here as it becomes available.

CEDAR leaf

This Product is Also Known As
American Arborvitae, Arborvitae, Eastern Arborvitae, Eastern White Cedar, Hackmatack, Northern White Cedar, Swamp Cedar, Thuga, Thuja, Tree of Life, White Cedar.
CAUTION: See separate listings for Cedar Leaf Oil, Cedarwood Oil, and Cedarwood bark, berry, leaf, seed, twig.

Scientific Names
Thuja occidentalis.
Family: Cupressaceae.

People Use This For
Orally, cedar leaf is used to treat respiratory tract infections, in conjunction with antibiotics for bacterial skin infections and herpes simplex, for bronchitis, rheumatism, trigeminal neuralgia, and strep throat. It is also used as an abortifacient (18).
Topically, cedar is used to manage joint pain, arthritis, and muscle rheumatism (18).

Safety
LIKELY SAFE ...when used orally in amounts found in foods; approved for use in foods in the US, if thujone-free (12).
POSSIBLY SAFE ...when taken orally as a medicinal for occasional use in recommended amounts (12); not for long-term use.
There is insufficient reliable information available about the safety of the topical use of cedar leaf.
PREGNANCY: UNSAFE ...contraindicated due to abortifacient activity (12).
LACTATION: Insufficient reliable information available; avoid using.

Effectiveness
There is insufficient reliable information available about the effectiveness of cedar leaf.

Possible Mechanism of Action & Active Ingredients
Cedar leaf is reported to be a urinary irritant (19), a uterine stimulant, and affect menstrual cycle (12). Thujone, a constituent, is a neurotoxin that can cause convulsions (1304). The glycoprotein and polysaccharide fractions have been used therapeutically (18). Some evidence suggests the polysaccharides might have antiviral and immunostimulating (1305) properties, and might inhibit HIV-1-specific antigens and reverse transcriptase activity (1306).

Adverse Reactions Including Known Allergies
Symptoms of oral overdose include queasiness, vomiting, painful diarrhea, and mucous membrane hemorrhage. Deaths have been reported (18). Other side effects include asthma, CNS stimulation, and seizures (214).

Possible Interactions with Herbs & Other Dietary Supplements
THUJONE CONTAINING HERBS: Avoid; concomitant use may increase the risk of thujone toxicity. Thujone-containing herbs include: oak moss (12), oriental arborvitae (12), sage (2,4,12), tansy (2,4,12), tree moss (12), and wormwood (2,12).

Possible Interactions with Drugs
ANTI-CONVULSANTS: Cedar leaf may lower the seizure threshold in those individuals taking anti-convulsants (214).

Possible Interactions with Foods
No interactions are known to occur, and there is no known reason to expect a clinically significant interaction with cedar leaf.

Possible Interactions with Lab Tests
No interactions are known to occur, and there is no known reason to expect a clinically significant interaction with cedar leaf.

Possible Interactions with Diseases or Conditions
GI CONDITIONS: Can irritate gastrointestinal tract. Contraindicated in individuals with infectious or inflammatory gastrointestinal conditions (19).

Typical Dosages & Routes of Administration that are Commonly Used
ORAL: Liquid extract (unspecified concentration) 2-4 mL only for occasional use (12).
TOPICAL: No typical dosage.

Comments
CAUTION: Do not confuse with other Thuja species.

CEDAR LEAF OIL

This Product is Also Known As
American Arborvitae, Arborvitae, Eastern Arborvitae, Eastern White Cedar, Hackmatack, Northern White Cedar, Swamp Cedar, Thuja, Thuja Oil, Tree of Life, White Cedar.
CAUTION: See separate listings for Cedar Leaf, Cedarwood Oil, and Cedarwood.

Scientific Names
Thuja occidentalis.
Family: Cupressaceae.
CAUTION: Do not confuse with other Thuja species.

People Use This For
Orally, cedar leaf oil is used as an immune stimulant, expectorant, and diuretic (11).
Topically, cedar leaf oil is used to treat skin diseases, condyloma, cancers, as an insect repellent, and as a counterirritant to treat warts (11).
In foods and beverages, cedar leaf oil is used as a flavoring (11).
In manufacturing, cedar leaf oil is used as a fragrance in cosmetics and soaps (11).

Safety
LIKELY SAFE ...when used orally in amounts found in foods (maximum use level 0.002% in condiments and relishes); approved for food use in the US if thujone-free (11).
POSSIBLY SAFE ...when used topically. It is used in perfumes at concentrations of less than 0.4% (11).
UNSAFE ...when used orally for medicinal use (11). A constituent, thujone, is a neurotoxin (1304).
PREGNANCY: UNSAFE ...contraindicated due to toxicity and uterine stimulant activity (11).
LACTATION: UNSAFE ...contraindicated due to toxicity (11).

Effectiveness
There is insufficient reliable information available about the effectiveness of cedar leaf oil.

Possible Mechanism of Action & Active Ingredients
Constituent, thujone, is a neurotoxin that can cause convulsions (1304). Polysaccharides have demonstrated in vitro antiviral, immunostimulating (1305), inhibition of HIV-1-specific antigens and reverse transcriptase activity (1306).

Adverse Reactions Including Known Allergies
Oral use of cedar leaf oil can result in poisoning. Symptoms of thujone poisoning include hypotension, convulsion, and death (11). Other side effects include asthma, CNS stimulation, and seizures (214).

Possible Interactions with Herbs & Other Dietary Supplements
THUJONE CONTAINING HERBS: Avoid; concomitant use may increase the risk of thujone toxicity. Thujone-containing herbs include: oak moss (12), oriental arborvitae (12), sage (2,4,12), tansy (2,4,12), tree moss (12), and wormwood (2,12).

Possible Interactions with Drugs
ANTI-CONVULSANTS: Cedar leaf oil may lower the threshold in those individuals taking anti-convulsants (214).

Possible Interactions with Foods
No interactions are known to occur, and there is no known reason to expect a clinically significant interaction with cedar leaf oil.

Possible Interactions with Lab Tests
No interactions are known to occur, and there is no known reason to expect a clinically significant interaction with cedar leaf oil.

Possible Interactions with Diseases or Conditions
No interactions are known to occur, and there is no known reason to expect a clinically significant interaction with cedar leaf oil.

Typical Dosages & Routes of Administration that are Commonly Used
ORAL: People typically use 2 to 4 mL of the liquid extract (5263).

Comments
Avoid confusion with cedar leaf, cedarwood oil, cedarwood bark/berry/seed/stem, and other Thuja species. Cedar leaf oil is produced by steam distillation of Thuja occidentalis leaves and twigs (11).

CEDARWOOD bark, berry, leaf, seed, twig

This Product is Also Known As
Ashe Juniper, Cedar, Eastern Red Cedar, Red Cedarwood, Red Juniper, Texas Cedarwood, Virginia Cedarwood.
CAUTION: See separate listings for Cedar Leaf Oil, Cedar leaf, and Cedarwood Oil.

Scientific Names
Juniperus virginiana.
Family: Cupressaceae.

People Use This For

In traditional folk medicine, cedarwood has been used for cough, bronchitis, rheumatism, venereal warts, and skin rash (11).

Safety

POSSIBLY SAFE ...when the berry or leaf is used orally (12).

There is insufficient reliable information available about the safety of the oral or topical use of the bark, seed or twig.

PREGNANCY AND LACTATION: LIKELY UNSAFE. Virginia cedarwood berry or leaf is contraindicated in pregnancy (12). There is insufficient reliable information available about the safety of the oral or topical use of cedarwood bark, seed, or twig.

Effectiveness

There is insufficient reliable information available about the effectiveness of cedarwood.

Possible Mechanism of Action & Active Ingredients

Steam distillation of Virginia cedarwood produces an oil that contains alpha- and beta-cedrene, cedrol, and cedreol. It also contains the toxic constituent thujone (11).

Adverse Reactions Including Known Allergies

None reported.

Possible Interactions with Herbs & Other Dietary Supplements

THUJONE CONTAINING HERBS: Avoid; concomitant use may increase the risk of thujone toxicity. Thujone-containing herbs include: oak moss (12), oriental arborvitae (12), sage (2,4,12), tansy (2,4,12), tree moss (12), and wormwood (2,12).

Possible Interactions with Drugs

BARBITURATES: Theoretically, inhaling red cedar chip fragrance might reduce efficacy of hexobarbital or pentobarbital (19).

DICOUMAROL: Theoretically, inhaling red cedar chip fragrance might reduce efficacy of dicoumarol (19).

Possible Interactions with Foods

No interactions are known to occur, and there is no known reason to expect a clinically significant interaction with cedarwood bark, berry, leaf, seed, and twig.

Possible Interactions with Lab Tests

No interactions are known to occur, and there is no known reason to expect a clinically significant interaction with cedarwood bark, berry, leaf, seed, and twig.

Possible Interactions with Diseases or Conditions

No interactions are known to occur, and there is no known reason to expect a clinically significant interaction with cedarwood bark, berry, leaf, seed, and twig.

Typical Dosages & Routes of Administration that are Commonly Used

No typical dosage.

Comments

Avoid confusion with cedarwood oil.

CEDARWOOD OIL

This Product is Also Known As

None.

CAUTION: See separate listings for Cedar Leaf, Cedar Leaf Oil, and Cedarwood.

Scientific Names

Juniperus virginiana (Cedarwood Oil Virginia); Juniperus mexicana (Cedarwood Oil Texas).
Family: Cupressaceae.
Cedrus atlantica (Cedarwood Oil Atlas).
Family: Pinaceae.

People Use This For

In manufacturing, all of the cedarwood oils are used as fragrance or fixatives in cosmetics and soaps (11).
In other uses, cedarwood oil is used as an insect repellent (11).

Safety

POSSIBLY SAFE ...when used topically; the maximum use level is 0.8% in perfumes.
PREGNANCY AND LACTATION: Insufficient reliable information available; avoid using.

Effectiveness

There is insufficient reliable information available about the effectiveness of cedarwood oil.

Possible Mechanism of Action & Active Ingredients

Steam distillation of Virginia cedarwood produces an oil that contains alpha- and beta-cedrene, cedrol, and cedreol. It also contains the constituent thujone (11). Dermatological studies have shown that all three cedarwood oils (Virginia, Texas, Atlas) are generally non-toxic (11). However, there is other evidence that cedarwood oil (probably Virginia) can produce tumors on mouse skin (11).

Adverse Reactions Including Known Allergies

There is some evidence that cedarwood oil (Virginia and/or Texas) is allergenic and is a local irritant (11).

Possible Interactions with Herbs & Other Dietary Supplements

THUJONE CONTAINING HERBS: Avoid; concomitant use may increase the risk of thujone toxicity. Thujone-containing herbs include: oak moss (12), oriental arborvitae (12), sage (2,4,12), tansy (2,4,12), tree moss (12), and wormwood (2,12).

Possible Interactions with Drugs

No interactions are known to occur, and there is no known reason to expect a clinically significant interaction with cedarwood oil.

Possible Interactions with Foods

No interactions are known to occur, and there is no known reason to expect a clinically significant interaction with cedarwood oil.

Possible Interactions with Lab Tests

No interactions are known to occur, and there is no known reason to expect a clinically significant interaction with cedarwood oil.

Possible Interactions with Diseases or Conditions

No interactions are known to occur, and there is no known reason to expect a clinically significant interaction with cedarwood oil.

Typical Dosages & Routes of Administration that are Commonly Used

No typical dosage.

Comments

There are several cedarwood oils with different physical and chemical properties, each produced by steam distillation of wood from various trees. The most common are: cedarwood oil Virginia (synonym cedar oil, red cedarwood oil), cedarwood oil Atlas (synonym cedarwood oil Moroccan), cedarwood oil Texas. Avoid confusion with cedar leaf, cedar leaf oil, cedarwood bark/berry/leaf/seed/twig.

CELERY

This Product is Also Known As

Ache des Marais, Apii Fructus, Celery Fruit, Celery Seed, Fruit de Celeri, Smallage, Selleriefruchte, Selleriesamen.

Scientific Names

Apium graveolens.
Family: Umbelliferae/Apiaceae.

People Use This For

Orally, celery is used to treat rheumatism, gout, hysteria, nervousness, headache, weight loss due to malnutrition, loss of appetite, and exhaustion (2). Celery is also used as a sedative (4), mild diuretic, urinary antiseptic (4,6), digestive aid, menstrual stimulant, antiflatulent, aphrodisiac, to reduce lactation (6), for regulating bowel movements, stimulating glands, and for blood purification.
In Oriental medicine, celery is used to treat headaches (6).

Safety

LIKELY SAFE ...when the oil or seeds are consumed in amounts found in foods. Celery seed has Generally Recognized as Safe (GRAS) status in the US. The maximum use of celery seed oil in food is 0.005% in condiments and relishes (11).
POSSIBLY SAFE ...when used orally and appropriately in medicinal amounts (12).
PREGNANCY: LIKELY SAFE ...when consumed in food amounts. LIKELY UNSAFE ...when the oil or seeds are

used orally in larger amounts, because they might have uterine stimulant or abortifacient effects (4,19).
LACTATION: LIKELY SAFE ...when consumed in food amounts. There is insufficient reliable information available about the safety of larger amounts of celery during lactation.

Effectiveness

There is insufficient reliable information available about the effectiveness of celery.

Possible Mechanism of Action & Active Ingredients

The applicable parts of celery are the fruit and seed. Sedative, diuretic, and antispasmodic effects of celery seed could be due to phthalide constituents (d-limonene, selinene, and related phthalides) (4,6). Plant extracts have hypotensive and hypoglycemic effects (4). In preliminary research, five of 23 celery-based preparations show antiarthritis effects, but no anti-inflammatory or antipyretic effects. The celery seed activity is thought to be dependent on processing at low temperatures (6131). Another constituent, apiogenin, shows evidence of antiplatelet activity. The essential oil can increase kidney inflammation by irritating epithelial tissue (8). Celery juice has been reported to show bile stimulating activity (4). Celery seed oil has shown bacteriostatic effects (4). Celery also contains the furocoumarins bergapten and celereodise, a dihydrofurocoumarin glycoside (isoquercitrin), and the coumarin glycoside apiumoside (6). Celery is a rich plant source of calcium, magnesium, and iron (19).

Adverse Reactions Including Known Allergies

Celery can cause contact dermatitis (19). Allergic and anaphylactic reactions have also been documented (4,6). Cross-allergenicity is possible between celery and pollen, carrots, dandelion, or wild carrot (4,6). Consuming large amounts of celery seed oil can induce CNS depression (6). Contact with celery stems could lead to photosensitivity (4).

Possible Interactions with Herbs & Other Dietary Supplements

HERBS WITH SEDATIVE PROPERTIES: Theoretically, concomitant use with herbs that have sedative properties might enhance therapeutic and adverse effects. These include calamus, calendula, California poppy, catnip, capsicum, couch grass, elecampane, ginseng Siberian, German chamomile, goldenseal, gotu kola, hops, Jamaican dogwood, kava, lemon balm, sage, St. John's wort, sassafras, scullcap, shepherd's purse, stinging nettle, valerian, wild carrot, wild lettuce, withania root, and yerba mansa (4,19).
HERBS WITH ANTICOAGULANT/ANTIPLATELET POTENTIAL: Concomitant use of herbs that have coumarin constituents or affect platelet aggregation could theoretically increase the risk of bleeding in some people. These herbs include: angelica, anise, arnica, asafoetida, bogbean, boldo, capsicum, chamomile, clove, danshen, fenugreek, feverfew, garlic, ginger, ginkgo, ginseng Panax, horse chestnut, horseradish, licorice, meadowsweet, prickly ash, onion, papain, passionflower, poplar, quassia, red clover, turmeric, wild carrot, wild lettuce, willow, and others (4,19).

Possible Interactions with Drugs

ANTICOAGULANTS AND ANTIPLATELET DRUGS: Theoretically, celery can potentiate the effects of these drugs.
DRUGS WITH SEDATIVE PROPERTIES: Theoretically, concomitant use with these drugs may cause additive effects (4).
PUVA: Theoretically, celery might increase the phototoxic response to PUVA therapy due to its psoralen content (6178). Drugs used in PUVA therapy include, methoxsalen (8-methoxypsoralen, 8-MOP, Oxsoralen) and Trioxsalen (Trisoralen).

Possible Interactions with Foods

No interactions are known to occur, and there is no known reason to expect a clinically significant interaction with celery.

Possible Interactions with Lab Tests

No interactions are known to occur, and there is no known reason to expect a clinically significant interaction with celery.

Possible Interactions with Diseases or Conditions

KIDNEY CONDITIONS: Contraindicated in kidney disorders; celery might increase inflammation (8).

Typical Dosages & Routes of Administration that are Commonly Used

ORAL: 0.5-2 grams of dried fruit three times daily, or one cup prepared tea (simmer 1 gram of fresh crushed dried fruit in 150 mL boiling water 5-10 minutes, strain) three times daily (4,8). Liquid extract (1:1 in 60% alcohol) 0.3-1.2 mL three times daily (4).

Comments

Furocoumarin (a potential carcinogen) content increases 100-fold in injured or diseased celery (6). Celery is available in capsule form, containing 450 or 505 mg of the oil. The ancient Greeks used celery to make wine, which was served as an award at athletic games (214).

CENTAURY

This Product is Also Known As
Bitter Herb, Common Centaury, Drug Centaurium, Lesser Centauru, Minor Centaury.

Scientific Names
Centaurium erythraea, synonyms Erythraea centaurium; Centaurium umbellatum; Centaurium minus.
Family: Gentianaceae.

People Use This For
Traditionally, centaury has been used as an oral treatment for anorexia and dyspepsia (4).

Safety
LIKELY SAFE ...when consumed in the very small amounts commonly found in food. Centaury is listed by the Council of Europe as a food flavoring. In the US, it is used in alcoholic and nonalcoholic beverages at maximum-permitted doses between 0.0002% and 0.0008% (4).
POSSIBLY SAFE ...when taken orally for medicinal purposes in amounts greater than those found in food (12). There is no documented toxicity (4).
PREGNANCY AND LACTATION: Insufficient reliable information available; avoid the use of centaury in amounts greater than those commonly found in foods.

Effectiveness
POSSIBLY EFFECTIVE ...when taken orally for loss of appetite and peptic discomfort (2).
There is insufficient reliable information available about the effectiveness of centaury for its other uses.

Possible Mechanism of Action & Active Ingredients
The applicable parts of centaury are the dried, above ground parts. The bitter constituents amarogentin, gentiopicroside, swertiamarin, and the related bitters (3,7) can act as an appetite stimulant, although with less activity than comparable bitter herbs (4). Its antipyretic activity can result from the phenolic acid constituents. The constituent, gentiopicrin, can have antimalarial properties. Animal evidence suggests that centaury has anti-inflammatory activity (4).

Adverse Reactions Including Known Allergies
None reported (4).

Possible Interactions with Herbs & Other Dietary Supplements
Insufficient reliable information available.

Possible Interactions with Drugs
No interactions are known to occur, and there is no known reason to expect a clinically significant interaction with centaury.

Possible Interactions with Foods
No interactions are known to occur, and there is no known reason to expect a clinically significant interaction with centaury.

Possible Interactions with Lab Tests
No interactions are known to occur, and there is no known reason to expect a clinically significant interaction with centaury.

Possible Interactions with Diseases or Conditions
No interactions are known to occur, and there is no known reason to expect a clinically significant interaction with centaury.

Typical Dosages & Routes of Administration that are Commonly Used
ORAL: The typical dose of centaury is 2-4 grams or as a tea three times daily. The tea is prepared by steeping 2-4 grams in 150 mL boiling water (4). The average daily dose of centaury is 6 grams (2). The usual dose of the liquid extract (1:1 in 25% alcohol) is 2-4 mL three times daily (4).

Comments
None.

CEREUS

This Product is Also Known As
Night Blooming Cereus, Sweet Scented Cactus.

Scientific Names

Selenicereus grandiflorus, synonyms Cereus grandiflorus, Cactus grandiflorus.
Family: Cactaceae.

People Use This For

Orally, cereus is used for angina pectoris (18), edema associated with weak heart function (4), and as a cardiac stimulant (sometimes instead of digitalis). Cereus is also used orally for urinary ailments (18).

In folk medicine, cereus is used orally for hemoptysis, menorrhagia, dysmenorrhea, hemorrhage, cystitis and shortness of breath (18); and topically as a skin stimulant for rheumatism (18).

Safety

POSSIBLY SAFE ...when the flower or stem are used orally for non-cardiac conditions (12). Although it contains cactine, which may have a digitalis-like effect, there are not reports of human toxicity (12).

POSSIBLY UNSAFE ...when used orally to self-medicate cardiac conditions.

There is insufficient reliable information available about the safety of the topical use of cereus.

PREGNANCY AND LACTATION: Insufficient reliable information available; avoid using.

Effectiveness

There is insufficient reliable information available about the effectiveness of cereus.

Possible Mechanism of Action & Active Ingredients

The applicable parts of cereus are the flower, stem, and young shoots. There is some evidence that cereus can stimulate the heart and dilate peripheral vessels (18), as well as stimulate spinal cord motor neurons (18). Researchers think tyramine, a cardiotonic amine, can strengthen heart muscle action (4). The reputed digitalis effect of cereus is claimed to be non-cumulative (12).

Adverse Reactions Including Known Allergies

Fresh juice used orally may cause burning of the mouth, queasiness, nausea, vomiting, and diarrhea (4,18). Used topically, it may cause itching and skin pustules (18).

Possible Interactions with Herbs & Other Dietary Supplements

Insufficient reliable information available.

Possible Interactions with Drugs

MONOAMINE OXIDASE INHIBITORS (MAOIs): Theoretically, excessive doses may interact with MAOIs, because of the tyramine content (4).

CARDIAC GLYCOSIDES: Cereus may potentiate the actions of cardiac glycosides such as digoxin, and may enhance the effect of other cardiac drugs (214).

Possible Interactions with Foods

No interactions are known to occur, and there is no known reason to expect a clinically significant interaction with cereus.

Possible Interactions with Lab Tests

No interactions are known to occur, and there is no known reason to expect a clinically significant interaction with cereus.

Possible Interactions with Diseases or Conditions

HEART CONDITIONS: Theoretically, may affect individuals with existing heart conditions or interfere with therapy (4).

Typical Dosages & Routes of Administration that are Commonly Used

ORAL: Fluid extract (1:1) 0.6 mL one to ten times daily (4,18). Tincture of cereus (1:10) 0.12-2 mL two to three times daily (4,18). Tincture in sweetened water (1:10) 10 drops three to five times daily (18). Should not be used as self-medication for cardiac conditions.

Comments

None.

CETYL MYRISTOLEATE

This Product is Also Known As

Cerasomal-cis-9-cetylmyristoleate, CM, CMO.

Scientific Names

Cis-9-cetylmyristoleate.

© Copyright 2000, Natural Medicines Comprehensive Database (209) 472-2244. For updated data, go to www.NaturalDatabase.com

People Use This For

Orally, cetyl myristoleate is used for rheumatoid arthritis, osteoarthritis, systemic lupus erythematosus, multiple sclerosis, ankylosing spondylitis, Reiter's syndrome, Behcet's syndrome, Sjogren's syndrome, psoriasis, fibromyalgia, emphysema, benign prostate hyperplasia (BPH), silicone breast disease, leukemia and other cancers, and relief of various types of back pain.

Safety

There is insufficient reliable information available about the safety of cetyl myristoleate.
Pregnancy and Lactation: Insufficient reliable information available; avoid using.

Effectiveness

There is insufficient reliable information available about the effectiveness of cetyl myristoleate.

Possible Mechanism of Action & Active Ingredients

Cetyl myristoleate is a substance isolated from mice that are immune to chemically-induced arthritis (677). Researchers hypothesize that cetyl myristoleate has surfactant effects. They think cetyl myristoleate might cause lubrication of joints and muscles, softening of tissues, and increased pliability. They theorize that cetyl myristoleate might also be a modulator of the immune system and a mediator of inflammatory process. Thus far, the evidence to back these theories is sketchy.

Adverse Reactions Including Known Allergies

None reported.

Possible Interactions with Herbs & Other Dietary Supplements

Insufficient reliable information available.

Possible Interactions with Drugs

METHOTREXATE: May interfere with absorption. Avoid concomitant use.
STEROIDS: May interfere with therapy; avoid concomitant use.
ALCOHOL: May interact with cetyl myristoleate; avoid concomitant use.

Possible Interactions with Foods

No interactions are known to occur, and there is no known reason to expect a clinically significant interaction with cetyl myristoleate.

Possible Interactions with Lab Tests

No interactions are known to occur, and there is no known reason to expect a clinically significant interaction with cetyl myristoleate.

Possible Interactions with Diseases or Conditions

No interactions are known to occur, and there is no known reason to expect a clinically significant interaction with cetyl myristoleate.

Typical Dosages & Routes of Administration that are Commonly Used

No typical dosage.

Comments

There is very little scientific information about this product. Our staff is continually analyzing the available information on natural medicines and will add data here as it becomes available.

CHANCA PIEDRA

This Product is Also Known As

Chancapiedra, Chanca-Piedra Blanca, Child Pick-a-Back, Derriere Dos, Derrière-Dos, Des Dos, Dukong Anak, Feuilles la Fievre, Memeniran, Meniran, Niruri, Pitirishi, Quebra Pedra, Quebrapedra, Quinina Criolla, Quinine Créole, Rami Buah, Sacha Foster, Sasha Foster, Seed on the Leaf, Shatter Stone, Stone Breaker, Stonebreaker, Tamalaka, Turi Hutan.

Scientific Names

Phyllanthus niruri.
Family: Euphorbiaceae.

People Use This For

Orally, chanca piedra is used for urinary tract infections and inflammation (518,3918), kidney stones (517), urethral or vaginal mucous discharge (517,3919), as a diuretic (3913), antiflatulent (517,3919), as an aperitif, appetite stimulant (517,3919), liver tonic, and blood purifier. It is also taken orally for diabetes (3913), gallstones (517), colic (517,3919), stomach ache (3913), dyspepsia (517,3919), intestinal infections (3923), constipation, dysentery, flu (3913), tenesmus (517,3918), jaundice (3913), hepatitis B (3923), abdominal tumors (3913), fever, pain, venereal problems (3913), syphilis, gonorrhea (517,3919), malaria, tumors (3913), caterpillar stings, cough, edema, itching, miscarriage, rectitis, tremors, typhoid, vaginitis, anemia, asthma, bronchitis, thirst, tuberculosis, and vertigo (3918).

Safety

There is insufficient reliable information available about the safety of chanca piedra.
Pregnancy and Lactation: Insufficient reliable information available; avoid using.

Effectiveness

POSSIBLY INEFFECTIVE ...when taken orally for treating hepatitis B (3924,3925).
There is insufficient reliable information available about the effectiveness of chanca piedra for its other uses.

Possible Mechanism of Action & Active Ingredients

Chanca piedra is thought to have multiple properties; that it is antispasmodic, antiviral, bactericidal, antipyretic, and a diuretic. It is also thought that chanca piedra reduces blood sugar and protects the liver (517). However, not all of these properties are supported by scientific evidence. In vitro, the constituent niuriside, inhibits specific HIV-protein binding activity, but does not protect cells from acute HIV infection (3927). In isolated animal tissue, an extract from the related plant, Phyllanthus sellowianus, has antispasmodic activity (3921). Preliminary studies in humans show the related species, Phyllanthus amarus, has diuretic, hypotensive and hypoglycemic effects (3928).

Adverse Reactions Including Known Allergies

None reported.

Possible Interactions with Herbs & Other Dietary Supplements

Insufficient reliable information available.

Possible Interactions with Drugs

DIABETES THERAPY: Monitor blood glucose level closely due to claims that chanca piedra has hypoglycemic effects (19).

Possible Interactions with Foods

No interactions are known to occur, and there is no known reason to expect a clinically significant interaction with chanca piedra.

Possible Interactions with Lab Tests

No interactions are known to occur, and there is no known reason to expect a clinically significant interaction with chanca piedra.

Possible Interactions with Diseases or Conditions

No interactions are known to occur, and there is no known reason to expect a clinically significant interaction with chanca piedra.

Typical Dosages & Routes of Administration that are Commonly Used

ORAL: People typically use 1 to 2 grams of powdered herb in tablets or capsules twice daily. Chanca piedra is also taken as a 4:1 tincture in a dose of 1 to 3 mL twice daily (5255).

Comments

Older studies published in India were reportedly conducted with Phyllanthus niruri, which is thought to be indigenous to the West Indies (514). A report from India mentions Phyllanthus niruri is a synonym for Phyllanthus amarus (3928); however, these appear to be different species (513,816).

CHAPARRAL

This Product is Also Known As

Creosote Bush, Greasewood, Hediondilla.

Scientific Names

Larrea tridentata; Larrea divaricata.
Family: Zygophyllaceae.

People Use This For

Orally, chaparral is used for arthritis, cancer, venereal disease, tuberculosis, bowel cramps, colds (4), and chronic cutaneous disorders (3497), because of its alleged analgesic, expectorant, emetic, diuretic, and anti-inflammatory properties (5). It is also used orally for weight loss (3497).
Historically, chaparral has been used as a tonic, antiparasitic, antiflatulent, a "blood purifier" for genitourinary and respiratory tract infections, and a treatment for musculoskeletal inflammation, skin diseases, GI conditions, CNS conditions (11), chickenpox and snakebite pain (3497).

Safety

LIKELY UNSAFE ...when taken orally; avoid using. There are reports of serious poisoning, acute hepatitis, kidney and liver damage, and irreversible renohepatic failure (4).

PREGNANCY AND LACTATION: LIKELY UNSAFE ...contraindicated due to demonstrated in vitro uteroactivity in addition to reported toxicity (4).

Effectiveness

There is insufficient reliable information available about the effectiveness of chaparral (4,6,11).

Possible Mechanism of Action & Active Ingredients

Nordihydroguaiaretic acid (NDGA), a constituent of chaparral, may have antioxidant properties (4). Reports of antimutagenic and anticarcinogenic activity are largely based on an observation in one patient (11). Theorized anticancer effects are thought to result from blocking of cellular respiration by NDGA (6).

Adverse Reactions Including Known Allergies

Jaundice, fatigue, abdominal pain (right upper quadrant), dark urine, light stools, nausea, diarrhea, weight loss, fever, anorexia, increases in serum liver enzyme levels (alkaline phosphatase, alanine aminotransferase, aspartate aminotransferase, total bilirubin, gamma-glutamyltransferase, lactate dehydrogenase), cirrhosis, cholestasis, cholangitis (3497), acute hepatitis, kidney and liver failure (4,3497) and mesenteric lymph node lesions have been reported after ingestion of chaparral (6). There are multiple reports of hepatotoxicity, including at least two requiring liver transplant (568,569,570,571,3497). Topical use can result in contact dermatitis (4).

Possible Interactions with Herbs & Other Dietary Supplements

Insufficient reliable information available.

Possible Interactions with Drugs

MAO INHIBITORS: Theoretically, excessive amounts may interfere with MAO inhibitor therapy, due to documented amino acid constituents (4).

Possible Interactions with Foods

No interactions are known to occur, and there is no known reason to expect a clinically significant interaction with chaparral.

Possible Interactions with Lab Tests

No interactions are known to occur, and there is no known reason to expect a clinically significant interaction with chaparral.

Possible Interactions with Diseases or Conditions

Theoretically, individuals with impaired liver function or renal function would have increased risk of adverse effects.

Typical Dosages & Routes of Administration that are Commonly Used

No typical dosage.

Comments

Chaparral is considered likely unsafe; avoid using. Anecdotal reports of anticancer effects may justify further testing; however, use may stimulate growth of certain tumors (6). Herp-Eeze is a dietary supplement promoted for preventing and treating herpes infections. The manufacturer states that a patented manufacturing process renders the product nontoxic. However, toxicity information about this product is limited to the manufacturer's claims (267).

CHASTEBERRY

This Product is Also Known As

Agnus Castus, Agnus-Castus, Chaste Tree, Gattilier, Hemp Tree, Monk's Pepper.

Scientific Names

Vitex agnus-castus.
Family: Verbenaceae.

People Use This For

Orally, chasteberry is used for control of menstrual irregularities (2), to reduce painful menstruation (3), to reduce premenstrual complaints (2,3), to reduce breast pain (2), to reduce the symptoms of menopause (3), to reduce sexual desire (6), for the control of postpartum bleeding, to aid in expulsion of the placenta, and to reduce acne (4). Historically, chasteberry has been used orally against impotence, nervousness, mild dementia, rheumatic conditions, colds, digestive discomfort, and as an antiflatulent (11).

© Copyright 2000, Natural Medicines Comprehensive Database (209) 472-2244. For updated data, go to www.NaturalDatabase.com

Safety

POSSIBLY SAFE ...when used orally and appropriately (4,12).
PREGNANCY: UNSAFE ...contraindicated because chasteberry can have uterine stimulant properties (12). It has occasionally been used in the first trimester to prevent miscarriage in cases of progesterone insufficiency (12).
LACTATION: POSSIBLY UNSAFE ...because it appears to increase milk production without affecting the quality of milk (6). However, there is insufficient reliable information available concerning chasteberry when used during lactation, and until this safety issue can be clearly determined, recommend avoiding chasteberry during lactation (4).

Effectiveness

POSSIBLY EFFECTIVE ...when used orally for breast pain, menstrual irregularity, and for symptoms of PMS (2,3,4,6,7). ...when used for menstrual disorders, when used for greater than four months. ...when used for acne, but the evidence is very sketchy (7011).
POSSIBLY INEFFECTIVE ...when used to increase the quantity of breast milk. The quality of the breast milk is variable (7012,7013).
Despite the fact that chasteberry has been used quite a lot, there are very few reliable studies on this herb. There is insufficient reliable information available about the effectiveness of chasteberry for its other uses.

Possible Mechanism of Action & Active Ingredients

Chasteberries are anti-androgenic (6). The extract contains an active principle which binds to dopamine (D1 and D2) receptors, and seems to inhibit prolactin release (4,6,7,7014). A chasteberry extract enhances estradiol binding to estrogen receptors in vitro, and increases uterine weight, decreases LH (luteinizing hormone) levels, and increases serum ceruloplasmin oxidase activity (a measure of estrogenic activity in the liver) in female rats with their ovaries removed (6180). Other research suggests that chasteberry might act centrally to diminish FSH (follicle stimulating hormone) release from the anterior pituitary, but at the same time increase release of LH and prolactin for an overall effect that favors progesterone over estrogen (4), resulting in normalization of the luteal phase by preventing progesterone insufficiency (7015,7016). In Germany, a proprietary chasteberry preparation available since the 1950s is used for breast pain, ovarian insufficiency, and dysfunctional uterine bleeding (4).

Adverse Reactions Including Known Allergies

The oral ingestion of chasteberry rarely can cause GI reactions, itching, rash, alopecia, headaches, tiredness, agitation, tachycardia, dry mouth, and increased menstrual flow (4,6). Allergic reactions can also occur, but they resolve themselves when the chasteberry is stopped (4).

Possible Interactions with Herbs & Other Dietary Supplements

Insufficient reliable information available.

Possible Interactions with Drugs

DOPAMINE ANTAGONISTS [Antipsychotics, Metoclopramide (Reglan)]: Theoretically, chasteberry might interfere with the action of dopamine antagonists due to dopaminergic effects of chasteberry (2,7).
ORAL CONTRACEPTIVES and HORMONE REPLACEMENT THERAPY: Theoretically, chasteberry can interfere with the efficacy of oral contraceptives and hormone replacement therapy because chasteberry seems to have hormone regulating activity (19).

Possible Interactions with Foods

No interactions are known to occur, and there is no known reason to expect a clinically significant interaction with chasteberry.

Possible Interactions with Lab Tests

No interactions are known to occur, and there is no known reason to expect a clinically significant interaction with chasteberry.

Possible Interactions with Diseases or Conditions

No interactions are known to occur, and there is no known reason to expect a clinically significant interaction with chasteberry.

Typical Dosages & Routes of Administration that are Commonly Used

ORAL: Typical dosages are 0.5-1 gram dried fruit three time daily (4); 20-40 mg per day of dry aqueous-alcoholic extract (6115,6116); 40 drops of fluid extract taken on an empty stomach in the morning; however, it may be necessary to take in divided doses after meals due to the alcohol content (4,6115).

Comments

Chasteberry does not have an immediate effect. It would take five to seven months for anovulatory cycles, and up to 18 months for amenorrhea that has lasted for greater than two years (7013). Historians say that monks chewed chaste tree parts to make it easier for them to maintain their celibacy. Progesterone, 17-alpha-hydroxyprogesterone, testosterone, and epitestosterone have been detected in chaste tree flower extract (11). Androstenedione has been detected in chaste tree leaf extract (11).

CHAULMOOGRA

This Product is Also Known As
Hydnocarp, Hydnocarpus, Gynocardia Oil, Oleum Chaulmoograe.

Scientific Names
Hydnocarpus species.

People Use This For
Topically, chaulmoogra is used for skin disorders, psoriasis, and eczema (18).
Parenterally, chaulmoogra is used for leprosy (18).

Safety
LIKELY SAFE ...for parenteral administration.
LIKELY UNSAFE ...when used orally. The seeds are considered very toxic due to their cyanogenic glycoside content (18).
There is insufficient reliable information available about the safety of the topical use of chaulmoogra.
PREGNANCY AND LACTATION: Insufficient reliable information available; avoid using.

Effectiveness
There is insufficient reliable information available about the effectiveness of chaulmoogra. However, chaulmoogra oil has demonstrated efficacy against Mycobacterium leprae in laboratory experiments and in case reports.

Possible Mechanism of Action & Active Ingredients
The applicable part of chaulmoogra is the seed. Chaulmoogra is thought to have sedative, antipyretic, and skin effects (18). In mice, intraperitoneal and subcutaneous administration of chaulmoogra fatty acids demonstrated antimicrobial activity against Mycobacterium leprae (3826). The cyanogenic glycoside content of the seeds renders them extremely poisonous (18).

Adverse Reactions Including Known Allergies
Ingestion of the seed can cause cough, dyspnea, laryngospasms, nephrotoxicity, visual disorders, head and muscle pain, and central paralysis (18). Topical use can cause skin irritation (18). No adverse effects are reported for parenteral use.

Possible Interactions with Herbs & Other Dietary Supplements
Insufficient reliable information available.

Possible Interactions with Drugs
No interactions are known to occur, and there is no known reason to expect a clinically significant interaction with chaulmoogra.

Possible Interactions with Foods
No interactions are known to occur, and there is no known reason to expect a clinically significant interaction with chaulmoogra.

Possible Interactions with Lab Tests
No interactions are known to occur, and there is no known reason to expect a clinically significant interaction with chaulmoogra.

Possible Interactions with Diseases or Conditions
No interactions are known to occur, and there is no known reason to expect a clinically significant interaction with chaulmoogra.

Typical Dosages & Routes of Administration that are Commonly Used
ORAL: No typical dosage.
TOPICAL: When applied topically, chaulmoogra is used as a powder, oil, emulsion, or in ointments.

Comments
Chaulmoogra seeds provided the elemental materials for synthesizing the first antileprostatic agents (214).

CHEKEN

This Product is Also Known As
Arryan, Chekan, Myrtus.

Scientific Names
Eugenia chequen (dried leaf).

People Use This For

Orally, leaf preparations of cheken are used as a tonic, diuretic, and expectorant (18). Preparations of the leaf oil are used orally for hyperlipoproteinemia (18).

In folk medicine, cheken has been used for diarrhea, fever, gout, and as a tonic, diuretic, antihypertensive, and digestive aid (18).

Safety

There is insufficient reliable information available about the safety of cheken.

Pregnancy and Lactation: Insufficient reliable information available; avoid using.

Effectiveness

There is insufficient reliable information available about the effectiveness of cheken.

Possible Mechanism of Action & Active Ingredients

The applicable parts of cheken are the leaf and leaf oil. The essential oil of the leaf affects fat metabolism; it is used to counter hyperlipoproteinemia. It also has antibacterial and antimycotic properties (18).

Adverse Reactions Including Known Allergies

None reported.

Possible Interactions with Herbs & Other Dietary Supplements

Insufficient reliable information available.

Possible Interactions with Drugs

No interactions are known to occur, and there is no known reason to expect a clinically significant interaction with cheken.

Possible Interactions with Foods

No interactions are known to occur, and there is no known reason to expect a clinically significant interaction with cheken.

Possible Interactions with Lab Tests

No interactions are known to occur, and there is no known reason to expect a clinically significant interaction with cheken.

Possible Interactions with Diseases or Conditions

No interactions are known to occur, and there is no known reason to expect a clinically significant interaction with cheken.

Typical Dosages & Routes of Administration that are Commonly Used

Reportedly used as a liquid extract or as tea by boiling the leaves in water for 10-15 minutes and strained (18).

Comments

There is very little scientific information about this product. Our staff is continually analyzing the available information on natural medicines and will add data here as it becomes available.

CHELATED MINERALS

This Product is Also Known As

Chelated Boron, Chelated Calcium, Chelated Chromium, Chelated Cobalt, Chelated Copper, Chelated Iron, Chelated Magnesium, Chelated Manganese, Chelated Molybdenum, Chelated Potassium, Chelated Selenium, Chelated Trace Minerals, Chelated Vanadium, Chelated Zinc.

CAUTION: See separate listings for Aspartates and individual minerals.

Scientific Names

Mineral-amino acid complex.

People Use This For

Orally, chelated minerals are used as dietary mineral supplements (marketed to be more bioavailable than non-chelated minerals)(1163,1164,1165,1166), for supporting normal growth, building strong muscles and bones, improving immune protection, healthy blood, and glowing skin (1163).

Safety

There is insufficient reliable information available about the safety of chelated minerals.

Pregnancy and Lactation: Insufficient reliable information available; avoid using.

Effectiveness

There is insufficient reliable information available about the effectiveness of chelated minerals.

Possible Mechanism of Action & Active Ingredients

Chelated minerals are marketed to be better absorbed and utilized by the body than non-chelated minerals (1163,1164,1165,1166). However, no evidence supports these claims. Fatty liver-hemorrhagic syndrome is reported in commercial chickens which are fed diets containing chelated minerals (1162).

Adverse Reactions Including Known Allergies

None reported.

Possible Interactions with Herbs & Other Dietary Supplements

Insufficient reliable information available.

Possible Interactions with Drugs

No interactions are known to occur, and there is no known reason to expect a clinically significant interaction with chelated minerals.

Possible Interactions with Foods

No interactions are known to occur, and there is no known reason to expect a clinically significant interaction with chelated minerals.

Possible Interactions with Lab Tests

No interactions are known to occur, and there is no known reason to expect a clinically significant interaction with chelated minerals.

Possible Interactions with Diseases or Conditions

No interactions are known to occur, and there is no known reason to expect a clinically significant interaction with chelated minerals.

Typical Dosages & Routes of Administration that are Commonly Used

See separate listings for specific minerals.

Comments

The term, chelated mineral, refers to formation of a complex of a mineral and an amino acid.

CHENOPODIUM OIL

This Product is Also Known As

Epazote, Jesuit Tea, Mexican Tea.
CAUTION: See separate listings for Wormseed, Wormwood Oil, and Wormwood.

Scientific Names

Chenopodium ambrosioides; Chenopodium ambrosioides anthelminticum.
Family: Chenopodiaceae.

People Use This For

Historically, chenopodium oil has been used as an oral antiparasitic against roundworms and hookworms (11).

Safety

UNSAFE ...when used orally; contraindicated, due to toxicity (11).
PREGNANCY AND LACTATION: UNSAFE ...contraindicated, due to toxicity (11).

Effectiveness

POSSIBLY EFFECTIVE ...when used orally as an antihelmintic (11,400) but toxicity precludes use.

Possible Mechanism of Action & Active Ingredients

The constituent ascaridole is thought to paralyze roundworms, hookworms, and dwarf tapeworms (but not large tapeworms) within the intestines (11,400). Chenopodium oil may explode when heated or treated with acids due to high ascaridole content (11). Handle with caution!

Adverse Reactions Including Known Allergies

Ingestion of chenopodium oil can cause skin and mucous membrane irritation, vomiting, headache, vertigo/dizziness, kidney and liver damage, temporary deafness, convulsions, circulatory collapse, paralysis, and death (11,400).

Possible Interactions with Herbs & Other Dietary Supplements

Insufficient reliable information available.

Possible Interactions with Drugs

No interactions are known to occur, and there is no known reason to expect a clinically significant interaction with chenopodium oil.

Possible Interactions with Foods
No interactions are known to occur, and there is no known reason to expect a clinically significant interaction with chenopodium oil.

Possible Interactions with Lab Tests
No interactions are known to occur, and there is no known reason to expect a clinically significant interaction with chenopodium oil.

Possible Interactions with Diseases or Conditions
No interactions are known to occur, and there is no known reason to expect a clinically significant interaction with chenopodium oil.

Typical Dosages & Routes of Administration that are Commonly Used
No typical dosage.

Comments
Chenopodium oil is considered unsafe; avoid using (11,400). Authorities disagree on whether chenopodium oil is the distilled oil of fresh above ground flowering and fruiting parts (11) or seed oil (18) of Chenopodium ambrosioides. Chenopodium oil may explode when heated or treated with acids (11). Handle with caution!

CHEROKEE ROSEHIP

This Product is Also Known As
Chinese Rosehip, Fructus Rosae Laevigatae, Jinyingzi.
CAUTION: See separate listings for Acerola, Vitamin C, and Rose Hip.

Scientific Names
Rosa laevigata, synonyms Rosa sinica, Rosa cherokensis, Rosa ternata, Rosa nivea, Rosa camellia.
Family: Rosaceae.

People Use This For
In Chinese medicine, Cherokee rosehip is used for male sexual dysfunction (nocturnal emission, spermatorrhea, neurasthenia), gynecologic problems (leukorrhea, uterine bleeding), night sweats, polyuria, enuresis, chronic diarrhea, chronic cough, hypertension, and enteritis (11,1506).

Safety
POSSIBLY SAFE ...when used orally and appropriately. Contains vitamin C as major constituent (11).
POSSIBLY UNSAFE ...when used in large amounts. Hyperoxaluria, hyperuricosuria, hematuria, and crystalluria can occur in some people taking 1 gram of vitamin C (67 grams of Cherokee rosehip) or more per day (14,3042). Prolonged use of large amounts of vitamin C can increase its metabolism, and scurvy might occur when intake is reduced (15).
PREGNANCY: POSSIBLY UNSAFE ...when used orally in large doses because it is associated with newborn scurvy (14,15). There is insufficient reliable information available for use in smaller amounts.
LACTATION: Insufficient reliable information available.

Effectiveness
POSSIBLY EFFECTIVE ...when used for diarrhea and enteritis (1506).
There is insufficient reliable information available about the effectiveness of Cherokee rosehip for its other uses.

Possible Mechanism of Action & Active Ingredients
Cherokee rosehip contains vitamin C (approximately 1.5%) (11). An antidiarrheal effect occurs in humans (11).

Adverse Reactions Including Known Allergies
The vitamin C in Cherokee rosehip may cause nausea, abdominal cramps, fatigue, insomnia, sleepiness; doses greater than 1 gram may cause diarrhea (15).

Possible Interactions with Herbs & Other Dietary Supplements
Due to the vitamin C content, concomitant use of Cherokee rosehip with other products containing vitamin C increases total dose of vitamin C and may increase risk of adverse effects.

Possible Interactions with Drugs
ASPIRIN: Theoretically, the vitamin C in large amounts of Cherokee rosehip might decrease excretion of aspirin (15).
ESTROGEN: Theoretically, the vitamin C in large amounts of Cherokee rosehip might increase absorption and effects of estrogen (129,130).
FLUPHENAZINE: Theoretically, the vitamin C in large amounts of Cherokee rosehip might decrease blood levels of fluphenazine (15).

IRON: Theoretically, the vitamin C in large amounts of Cherokee rosehip might increase GI absorption of food iron (ferric) but not supplement iron (ferrous) due to vitamin C content (15).
WARFARIN: Theoretically, the vitamin C in large amounts of Cherokee rosehip might reduce anticoagulant activity (506).
OTHER DRUGS: Theoretically, the vitamin C in large amounts of Cherokee rosehip might acidify urine, affecting excretion of other drugs (15).

Possible Interactions with Foods
No interactions are known to occur, and there is no known reason to expect a clinically significant interaction with Cherokee rosehip.

Possible Interactions with Lab Tests
URINE GLUCOSE TESTS: Theoretically, large amounts of Cherokee rosehip (containing greater than 500 mg vitamin C) may cause false decreases with glucose oxidase tests (e.g. Clinistix) and may cause false increases with cupric sulfate tests (e.g. Clinitest) (15).
STOOL OCCULT BLOOD TESTS: Theoretically, large amounts of Cherokee rosehip may cause a false-negative result if ingested 48-72 hours before amine-dependent tests due to vitamin C content (506).

Possible Interactions with Diseases or Conditions
GOUT: Theoretically, the vitamin C in large amounts of Cherokee rosehip might increase uric acid levels (15).
KIDNEY STONE FORMING TENDENCY: Theoretically, the vitamin C in large amounts of Cherokee rosehip might cause precipitation of urate, cystine, or oxalate stones (15).
DIABETES: Large amounts may affect blood sugar control because of the vitamin C content (15).

Typical Dosages & Routes of Administration that are Commonly Used
ORAL: People typically use 6 to 18 grams (5269).

Comments
Cherokee rosehip contains vitamin C (approximately 1.5%) (11).

CHERRY LAUREL WATER

This Product is Also Known As
Common Cherry Laurel, Laurocerasus Leaves.
CAUTION: See separate listing for Wild Cherry.

Scientific Names
Prunus laurocerasus, synonym Laurocerasus officinalis.
Family: Rosaceae.

People Use This For
Orally, cherry laurel water is used as a sedative, pain reliever, and antispasmodic (11,18).
Topically, cherry laurel water is used in eye lotions (11).
As an inhalant, cherry laurel water is used as an aromatic, and breathing stimulant (18).
In traditional medicine, the leaves of cherry laurel are used for treating cough, colds, insomnia, stomach and intestinal spasms, vomiting, and cancer (11).

Safety
POSSIBLY SAFE ...when used orally and appropriately. Overdose can be fatal (18). Cherry laurel water contains 0.1% hydrocyanic acid (11).
PREGNANCY AND LACTATION: Insufficient reliable information available; avoid using.

Effectiveness
There is insufficient reliable information available about the effectiveness of cherry laurel water.

Possible Mechanism of Action & Active Ingredients
Contains prunasin, a cyanogenic glycoside (11,18).

Adverse Reactions Including Known Allergies
None reported.

Possible Interactions with Herbs & Other Dietary Supplements
Insufficient reliable information available.

Possible Interactions with Drugs
No interactions are known to occur, and there is no known reason to expect a clinically significant interaction with cherry laurel water.

Possible Interactions with Foods

No interactions are known to occur, and there is no known reason to expect a clinically significant interaction with cherry laurel water.

Possible Interactions with Lab Tests

No interactions are known to occur, and there is no known reason to expect a clinically significant interaction with cherry laurel water.

Possible Interactions with Diseases or Conditions

No interactions are known to occur, and there is no known reason to expect a clinically significant interaction with cherry laurel water.

Typical Dosages & Routes of Administration that are Commonly Used

ORAL: People typically use a dose of 2 to 8 mL cherry laurel water (5264,5267).

Comments

Cherry laurel water is produced by water distillation of cherry laurel (Prunus laurocerasus) leaves. Avoid confusion with wild cherry bark, sweet bay leaf (laurel).

CHERVIL

This Product is Also Known As

Garden Chervil, Salad Chervil.

Scientific Names

Anthriscus cerefolium, synonym Anthriscus longirostris.
Family: Apiaceae or Umbelliferae.

People Use This For

In folk medicine, chervil is used as a diuretic, expectorant, digestive aid, and an antihypertensive (11). Juice from fresh chervil is used for eczema, gout, and abscesses (11).
In foods and beverages, chervil is used as a flavoring agent (11).

Safety

LIKELY SAFE ...when the above ground parts are used orally in amounts found in foods. Chervil has Generally Recognized as Safe (GRAS) status in the US. The maximum level used is 0.114% in meat products (11).
There is insufficient reliable information available about the safety of the oral use of chervil in medicinal amounts.
PREGNANCY AND LACTATION: LIKELY SAFE ...when used in food amounts. LIKELY UNSAFE ...when used in larger amounts because it contains estragole which might be mutagenic (12).

Effectiveness

There is insufficient reliable information available about the effectiveness of chervil.

Possible Mechanism of Action & Active Ingredients

The applicable parts of chervil are the dried flowering parts and leaf. Chervil is a plant source rich in calcium and potassium (19). Estragole, the major constituent of the volatile oil, reported to produce tumors in mice (11).

Adverse Reactions Including Known Allergies

None reported.

Possible Interactions with Herbs & Other Dietary Supplements

Insufficient reliable information available.

Possible Interactions with Drugs

No interactions are known to occur, and there is no known reason to expect a clinically significant interaction with chervil.

Possible Interactions with Foods

No interactions are known to occur, and there is no known reason to expect a clinically significant interaction with chervil.

Possible Interactions with Lab Tests

No interactions are known to occur, and there is no known reason to expect a clinically significant interaction with chervil.

Possible Interactions with Diseases or Conditions

No interactions are known to occur, and there is no known reason to expect a clinically significant interaction with chervil.

Typical Dosages & Routes of Administration that are Commonly Used

ORAL: Chervil is typically prepared by adding 1 teaspoon of fresh or dried herb to water. The dose is up to 1 cup a day, unsweetened, consumed a mouthful at a time (5263).

Comments

None.

CHICKEN COLLAGEN

This Product is Also Known As

Chicken Collagen Type II.

Scientific Names

Chicken collagen type II.

People Use This For

Orally, chicken collagen is used to treat pain syndromes associated with rheumatoid arthritis, osteoarthritis, gouty arthritis, juvenile rheumatoid arthritis, post-surgical joint pain, post-traumatic pain, fibrositis, back pain and neck pain (3110,3112).

Safety

There is insufficient reliable information available about the safety of chicken collagen.
Pregnancy and Lactation: Insufficient reliable information available; avoid using.

Effectiveness

There is insufficient reliable information available about the effectiveness of chicken collagen.

Possible Mechanism of Action & Active Ingredients

The rationale of using chicken collagen for pain syndromes is based on the theory of oral tolerance. This theory hypothesizes that oral administration of small quantities of antigens causes biological processes that suppress inflammation at the cellular level, suppress response to delayed-hypersensitivity antigens, and eliminate the cells that respond to antigens. Although evidence suggests this theory might be true in animals, it is unproven in humans (3126). Based on the theory of oral tolerance, when individuals with rheumatoid arthritis take oral collagen, the collagen should cause certain areas of the gut to generate T cells that are absorbed by the body. Then, in the body, these T-cells are activated by joint collagen and they secrete cytokines that suppress inflammation. Cytokines thought to be involved include interleukin 4, 10, and transforming growth factor beta (3111,3112,3125). Oral administration of collagen is also believed to decrease the expression of pro-inflammatory cytokines including interleukins 1, 2, 6, and 8; tumor necrosis factor alpha; and interferon gamma (3111). So far, the studies determining the efficacy of chicken collagen demonstrate conflicting results (3125,3112,3128), but these studies have used microgram doses. Not everyone agrees with the theory of oral tolerance. One supplement manufacturer recommends a dose of 2 grams of chicken collagen per day, attributing effectiveness to the 15% glucosamine sulfate and 15% chondroitin sulfate contained in collagen type II (3110).

Adverse Reactions Including Known Allergies

Although no significant adverse effects have been reported in the small trials of chicken collagen (3111,3112), allergic reactions to other collagen products have occurred, e.g. bovine collagen used in corneal shields, catgut suture for eye surgery, and dietary collagen in the form of gelatin (3127). If large doses are used, side effects associated with glucosamine sulfate or chondroitin might occur. These include nausea, heartburn, diarrhea and constipation, drowsiness, skin reactions, and headache (14,2608).

Possible Interactions with Herbs & Other Dietary Supplements

Insufficient reliable information available.

Possible Interactions with Drugs

No interactions are known to occur, and there is no known reason to expect a clinically significant interaction with chicken collagen.

Possible Interactions with Foods

No interactions are known to occur, and there is no known reason to expect a clinically significant interaction with chicken collagen.

Possible Interactions with Lab Tests

No interactions are known to occur, and there is no known reason to expect a clinically significant interaction with chicken collagen.

Possible Interactions with Diseases or Conditions

ALLERIGES: Theoretically, individuals who are allergic to chicken or eggs should not use chicken collagen. Collagen products have been associated with allergic reactions (e.g. bovine collagen used in corneal shields, catgut suture for eye surgery, and dietary collagen in the form of gelatin) (3127).

Typical Dosages & Routes of Administration that are Commonly Used

ORAL: For rheumatoid arthritis, doses of 20 to 2500 mcg per day of chicken collagen have been used. For juvenile arthritis, doses of 100 mcg per day for the first month then 500 mcg per day thereafter have been used (3111,3112). However, some supplement manufacturers recommend doses of 2 grams per day (3110).

Comments

The manufacturer of Colloral, an oral chicken collagen product, stopped product development because it failed to demonstrate efficacy in humans (3128). Bovine collagen products have also been used in the treatment of rheumatoid arthritis.

CHICKWEED

This Product is Also Known As

Star Chickweed, Starweed.

Scientific Names

Stellaria media.
Family: Caryophyllaceae.

People Use This For

Orally, chickweed is used for constipation, bronchial asthma, stomach and bowel problems, blood disorders, lung disease, obesity, scurvy (5), psoriasis (6), rabies (5), itching, and muscle and joint pain (11).
Topically, chickweed is used for skin problems including boils, abscesses, and ulcers (5).
For food uses, chickweed is eaten in salads or served as cooked greens (5).

Safety

LIKELY SAFE ...when used orally (12).
There is insufficient reliable information available about the safety of the topical use of chickweed.
PREGNANCY AND LACTATION: Insufficient reliable information available; avoid using in amounts larger than those found in food.

Effectiveness

LIKELY INEFFECTIVE ...for all uses (5,6).

Possible Mechanism of Action & Active Ingredients

The applicable part of chickweed is the leaf. There is no indication that any of the constituents have therapeutic value (5,6). While chickweed does contain some vitamin C, the concentrations are too small to be effective (6).

Adverse Reactions Including Known Allergies

Chickweed is generally well-tolerated (6). There are, however, some poorly documented human cases of paralysis from consumptions of large amounts of chickweed tea (6). There is one case of alleged nitrate toxicity leading to paralysis, but the chickweed implicated in this case may have been contaminated (12).

Possible Interactions with Herbs & Other Dietary Supplements

Insufficient reliable information available.

Possible Interactions with Drugs

No interactions are known to occur, and there is no known reason to expect a clinically significant interaction with chickweed.

Possible Interactions with Foods

No interactions are known to occur, and there is no known reason to expect a clinically significant interaction with chickweed.

Possible Interactions with Lab Tests

No interactions are known to occur, and there is no known reason to expect a clinically significant interaction with chickweed.

Possible Interactions with Diseases or Conditions

No interactions are known to occur, and there is no known reason to expect a clinically significant interaction with chickweed.

Typical Dosages & Routes of Administration that are Commonly Used

ORAL: People typically use 1155 to 3450 mg per day in two to three divided doses. One chickweed supplier suggests three daily doses based on body weight: under 100 pounds, 385 mg per dose; 100 to 175 pounds, 770 mg; and over 175 pounds, 1155 mg. Chickweed is also prepared as a tea with 1 to 2 teaspoons in 6 ounces of boiling water. Chickweed is available as a tincture of unspecified concentration with a typical dose of 1 to 5 mL per day (6006).
TOPICAL: No typical dosage.

Comments

None.

CHICLE

This Product is Also Known As

Breiapfelbaum, Chicle, Chico Sapote, Kaugummibaum, Naseberry, Níspero, Sabojira, Sapodilla, Sapodillbaum, Sapote, Sapotier, Sapotillier, Zapote, Zapotillo.

Scientific Names

Manilkara zapota, synonyms Manilkara zapotilla, Manilkara achras, Sapota achras, Achras sapota, Achras zapotilla.
Family: Zapotaceae.

People Use This For

In manufacturing, chicle is an ingredient in hair preparations (11), and a gum base in chewing gum (11).

Safety

LIKELY SAFE ...in amounts found in gum (20%) (11); approved for use in foods as a chewing gum base in the US (11).
PREGNANCY AND LACTATION: LIKELY SAFE ...in amounts found in chewing gum (11).

Effectiveness

There is insufficient reliable information available about the effectiveness of chicle.

Possible Mechanism of Action & Active Ingredients

Insufficient reliable information available.

Adverse Reactions Including Known Allergies

None reported.

Possible Interactions with Herbs & Other Dietary Supplements

Insufficient reliable information available.

Possible Interactions with Drugs

No interactions are known to occur, and there is no known reason to expect a clinically significant interaction with chicle.

Possible Interactions with Foods

No interactions are known to occur, and there is no known reason to expect a clinically significant interaction with chicle.

Possible Interactions with Lab Tests

No interactions are known to occur, and there is no known reason to expect a clinically significant interaction with chicle.

Possible Interactions with Diseases or Conditions

No interactions are known to occur, and there is no known reason to expect a clinically significant interaction with chicle.

Typical Dosages & Routes of Administration that are Commonly Used

No typical dosage.

Comments

Chicle is derived from the latex collected from the trunk of the chicle tree (Manilkara zapota). Refined chicle is not a true gum (11). It has characteristics similar to natural resins and rubber, it is soft and plastic when chewed and insoluble in saliva (11). Chewing gum consists of approximately 20% chicle, plus sugar, corn syrup, and flavorings (11).

© Copyright 2000, Natural Medicines Comprehensive Database (209) 472-2244. For updated data, go to www.NaturalDatabase.com • 265

CHICORY

This Product is Also Known As
Blue Sailors, Cichorii Herba, Cichorii Radix, Common Chicory Root, Hendibeh, Succory, Wild Chicory.

Scientific Names
Cichorium intybus.
Family: Asteraceae or Compositae.

People Use This For
Orally, chicory root is used as a tonic, diuretic, laxative (5), liver protectant, to balance the stimulant effect of coffee (5), for loss of appetite, dyspepsia (2), liver and gallbladder disorders (11), and cancer.
Topically, chicory leaves are used as a poultice for swelling and inflammation (5).
In folk medicine, chicory has been used for tachycardia (5) and as a laxative in children (18).
For food uses, chicory leaves are often eaten like celery, and the roots are boiled and eaten. Chicory is used as a culinary spice (6), and the leaf buds and roots are eaten as vegetables (6,11).
In food manufacturing, chicory is used as a flavoring component in foods and beverages (11). The roasted root is also ground and used in coffee mixes to enhance richness (11) and is used as a coffee substitute (6).

Safety
LIKELY SAFE ...when leaf or root products are consumed in amounts commonly found in food (5). Chicory has Generally Recognized as Safe (GRAS) status for food use in the US (6).
POSSIBLY SAFE ...when the root is used orally in medicinal amounts (2,12).
There is insufficient reliable information available about the safety of chicory for its other uses.
PREGNANCY: LIKELY UNSAFE ...contraindicated for oral use due to concerns that chicory can induce menstruation or miscarriage (19).
LACTATION: Insufficient reliable information available; avoid using.

Effectiveness
POSSIBLY EFFECTIVE ...when taken orally as an appetite stimulant and for dyspepsia (2).
There is insufficient reliable information available about the effectiveness of chicory for its other uses.

Possible Mechanism of Action & Active Ingredients
The applicable parts of chicory are the root and dried, above ground parts. Chicory root has a mild laxative effect and stimulates bile production. It is also believed to slow heart rate (2,11), perhaps due to the presence of a digitalis-like compound (5). Chicory has a sedative effect that has been attributed to the constituent lactucopicrin (5) and other water-soluble components (6). The sedative effect antagonizes the stimulant effects of coffee and tea (6). The sesquiterpene alkaloid constituents show evidence of bacteriostatic properties (11). The extracts seem to have anti-inflammatory activity (11). Chicory is a rich source of beta-carotene (19).

Adverse Reactions Including Known Allergies
Handling the plant can cause contact dermatitis (6,11). It can cause an allergic reaction in individuals sensitive to the Asteraceae/Compositae family. Members of this family include ragweed, chrysanthemums, marigolds, daisies, and many other herbs.

Possible Interactions with Herbs & Other Dietary Supplements
Insufficient reliable information available.

Possible Interactions with Drugs
No interactions are known to occur, and there is no known reason to expect a clinically significant interaction with chicory.

Possible Interactions with Foods
No interactions are known to occur, and there is no known reason to expect a clinically significant interaction with chicory.

Possible Interactions with Lab Tests
No interactions are known to occur, and there is no known reason to expect a clinically significant interaction with chicory.

Possible Interactions with Diseases or Conditions
CHICORY ALLERGY: Contraindicated (11).
GALLSTONES: Chicory should only be used with monitoring due to its bile stimulating effect (2,6,11).
CROSS-ALLERGENICITY: Can cause an allergic reaction in individuals sensitive to the Asteraceae/Compositae family. Members of this family include ragweed, chrysanthemums, marigolds, daisies, and many other herbs.

Typical Dosages & Routes of Administration that are Commonly Used

ORAL: The typical dose of chicory is one cup of the tea, which is prepared by steeping 2-4 grams of the root in 150 mL boiling water for 10 minutes and then straining (18). The average amount of chicory is 3-5 grams of the root per day (18).

Comments

Chicory can be contaminated with bacteria (6,3807) or foreign substances, including fungicides (6).

CHINESE CLUB MOSS

This Product is Also Known As

Huperazon, Qian Ceng Ta.
CAUTION: See separate listing for Huperzine A.

Scientific Names

Huperzia serrata.
Family: Lycopodiaceae.

People Use This For

Orally, Chinese club moss is used for Alzheimer's disease and other memory disorders (3150).
In Chinese medicine, Chinese club moss is used for fever, inflammation, blood loss, irregular menstruation, and as a diuretic (3130,3131).

Safety

There is insufficient reliable information available about the safety of Chinese club moss.
Pregnancy And Lactation: Insufficient reliable information available; avoid using.

Effectiveness

There is insufficient reliable information available about the effectiveness of Chinese club moss.

Possible Mechanism of Action & Active Ingredients

Chinese club moss contains the alkaloid huperzine A, a reversible acetylcholinesterase (AChE) inhibitor which crosses the blood-brain barrier (3082).

Adverse Reactions Including Known Allergies

None reported with Chinese club moss. Orally, huperzine A which is found in Chinese club moss can cause dizziness, nausea and sweating (3140,3143).

Possible Interactions with Herbs & Other Dietary Supplements

Insufficient reliable information available.

Possible Interactions with Drugs

ANTICHOLINERGIC DRUGS: Theoretically, concurrent use of anticholinergic drugs and Chinese club moss might decrease the effectiveness of Chinese club moss or the anticholinergic agent. In an animal model, huperzine A, an active constituent of Chinese club moss, reversed cognitive deficits induced by scopolamine (5537). Other anticholinergic drugs include atropine, benztropine (Cogentin), biperiden (Akineton), procyclidine (Kemadrin), and trihexyphenidyl (Artane) (15).
CHOLINERGIC DRUGS, ACETYLCHOLINESTERASE (AChE) INHIBITORS: Theoretically, concurrent use might have additive effects with drugs that promote acetylcholine activity because huperzine A has AChE inhibitor properties (14). AChE inhibitors and cholinergic drugs include bethanechol (Urecholine), donepezil (Aricept), echothiophate (Phospholine Iodide), edrophonium (Enoln, Reversol, Tensilon), neostigmine (Prostigmin), physostigmine (Antilirium), pyridostigmine (Mestinon, Regonol), succinylcholine (Anectine, Quelicin), and tacrine (Cognex) (14).

Possible Interactions with Foods

No interactions are generally known or predicted to occur, and there is no known reason to expect a clinically significant interaction with Chinese club moss.

Possible Interactions with Lab Tests

No interactions are generally known or predicted to occur, and there is no known reason to expect a clinically significant interaction with Chinese club moss.

Possible Interactions with Diseases or Conditions

VARIOUS DISEASES: Acetylcholinesterase (AchE) inhibitors are used with caution or are contraindicated in people with asthma, chronic obstructive pulmonary disease, cardiovascular disease, obstruction of the intestinal or urogenital tracts, gastrointestinal ulcer disease, or seizures (14). Avoid using Chinese club moss in people with these conditions until more is known about its effects in humans.

Typical Dosages & Routes of Administration that are Commonly Used

ORAL: Currently available products contain isolated huperzine A extracted from Chinese club moss (see separate listing for Huperzine A).

Comments

Don't let your patients confuse club moss and Chinese club moss. Only Chinese club moss contains huperzine A.

CHINESE CUCUMBER fruit

This Product is Also Known As

Chinese Snake Gourd, Compound Q, Gua Lou, Gua-Lou, Trichosanthes.
CAUTION: See separate entries for Chinese Cucumber root and Chinese Cucumber seed.

Scientific Names

Trichosanthes kirilowii.
Family: Curcurbitaceae.

People Use This For

Orally, Chinese cucumber fruit is used for coughing, reducing fever, swelling, tumors, and diabetes.
Intravaginally, Chinese cucumber fruit is used as an abortifacient (6).

Safety

POSSIBLY SAFE ...when the fruit is used orally and appropriately (12).
There is insufficient reliable information available about the safety of intravaginal use of Chinese cucumber fruit.
PREGNANCY: LIKELY UNSAFE ...contraindicated for oral use because it might induce abortion (6).
LACTATION: Insufficient reliable information available; avoid using.

Effectiveness

There is insufficient reliable information available about the effectiveness of Chinese cucumber fruit.

Possible Mechanism of Action & Active Ingredients

Some evidence suggests a 50% ethanolic extract might have protective effects against ulcers (4044). A sponge containing Chinese cucumber juice might induce abortions when inserted intravaginally (6).

Adverse Reactions Including Known Allergies

When taken orally, Chinese cucumber fruit may cause mild diarrhea and gastric discomfort (12).

Possible Interactions with Herbs & Other Dietary Supplements

Insufficient reliable information available.

Possible Interactions with Drugs

No interactions are known to occur, and there is no known reason to expect a clinically significant interaction with Chinese cucumber fruit.

Possible Interactions with Foods

No interactions are known to occur, and there is no known reason to expect a clinically significant interaction with Chinese cucumber fruit.

Possible Interactions with Lab Tests

No interactions are known to occur, and there is no known reason to expect a clinically significant interaction with Chinese cucumber fruit.

Possible Interactions with Diseases or Conditions

GASTRIC ULCERS: Theoretically, Chinese cucumber fruit might protect against ulcer development or enhance ulcer healing (4044).

Typical Dosages & Routes of Administration that are Commonly Used

ORAL: People typically use 10 to 20 grams of the dried fruit (5269).

Comments

None.

CHINESE CUCUMBER root

This Product is Also Known As
Chinese Snake Gourd, Compound Q, Tian Hua Fen, Tian-Hua-Fen, Trichosanthes.
CAUTION: See separate entries for Chinese Cucumber fruit and Chinese Cucumber seed.

Scientific Names
Trichosanthes kirilowii.
Family: Curcurbitaceae.

People Use This For
Orally, Chinese cucumber root is used to treat HIV infection (6).
Intramuscularly, Chinese cucumber root is used to induce abortions (by intramuscular injection) (6).
In Chinese medicine, cucumber root is taken orally to treat coughs, fever, swelling, tumors and diabetes (6). A starch extract is used for treating abscesses, amenorrhea, jaundice, frequent urination, and tumors (6).

Safety
LIKELY UNSAFE ...when used orally or by injection for self-medication; requires monitoring (6). Extracts of Chinese cucumber can be very toxic (6).
PREGNANCY: LIKELY UNSAFE ...contraindicated, due to abortifacient effects and possible teratogenicity (6,12).
LACTATION: LIKELY UNSAFE; avoid using (6).

Effectiveness
POSSIBLY EFFECTIVE ...as an abortifacient when administered parenterally (6).
There is insufficient reliable information available about the effectiveness of Chinese cucumber root for its other uses.

Possible Mechanism of Action & Active Ingredients
Chinese cucumber root contains several constituents that demonstrate anti-HIV activity. Trichosanthin and protein "TAP 29" can block HIV replication and some evidence suggests they might selectively kill HIV infected cells in the immune system. Other constituents of the root, trichosanthin and momorcharin, can have abortifacient effects. Trichosanthin injected intramuscularly or extra-amniotically can induce first-trimester abortions. It has also been used to terminate ectopic pregnancies (6). Some evidence suggests trichosanthin and momorcharin might cause birth defects (12). Trichosanthin also shows antitumor activity. It has been used to treat invasive moles and certain types of liver tumors. Some evidence suggests that a water extract of the root might have hypoglycemic activity in individuals with normal blood glucose. Subsequent fractionation of the extract yielded five compounds. The activity of one of these suggests it might be useful in reducing blood sugars in individuals with diabetes (4045).

Adverse Reactions Including Known Allergies
Chinese cucumber root extracts are extremely toxic, particularly when they are injected. Trichosanthin injections can be fatal. They can also cause severe reactions including seizures, fever, lung and cerebral edema, cerebral hemorrhage, and heart damage. People receiving trichosanthin injections to cause abortion can develop a severe allergy. After a single exposure, the risk of anaphylaxis from a second exposure can persist for more than a decade (6).

Possible Interactions with Herbs & Other Dietary Supplements
ANTIDIABETES HERBS: Theoretically, concomitant use may potentiate effects of other herbs with hypoglycemic effects (6,4045).

Possible Interactions with Drugs
ANTIDIABETES DRUGS: Theoretically, concomitant use may have additive effects and adverse effects (6,4045). Monitor blood glucose closely, dose adjustment may be needed.

Possible Interactions with Foods
No interactions are known to occur, and there is no known reason to expect a clinically significant interaction with Chinese cucumber root.

Possible Interactions with Lab Tests
BLOOD GLUCOSE: Theoretically, may decrease blood glucose levels and test results (6,4045).

Possible Interactions with Diseases or Conditions
DIABETES: Theoretically, use of Chinese cucumber root may alter blood glucose control (6,4045).

Typical Dosages & Routes of Administration that are Commonly Used
ORAL: People typically use 9 to 15 grams of the root (5268).

Comments
Avoid confusion with Chinese cucumber fruit and Chinese cucumber seed.

CHINESE CUCUMBER seed

This Product is Also Known As
Chinese Snake Gourd, Compound Q, Gua Luo Ren, Gua-Luo-Ren, Trichosanthes.
CAUTION: See separate entries for Chinese Cucumber root and Chinese Cucumber fruit.

Scientific Names
Trichosanthes kirilowii.
Family: Curcurbitaceae.

People Use This For
Orally, Chinese cucumber seed is used for coughs, reducing fever, swelling, tumors and diabetes [6].

Safety
POSSIBLY SAFE ...when taken orally [12].
PREGNANCY AND LACTATION: Insufficient reliable information available; avoid using.

Effectiveness
There is insufficient reliable information available about the effectiveness of Chinese cucumber seed.

Possible Mechanism of Action & Active Ingredients
Some evidence suggests three triterpene compounds isolated from the seed might have anti-inflammatory effects [4042]. Other information suggests that a 50% ethanolic seed extract might have anti-inflammatory and analgesic effects [4043].

Adverse Reactions Including Known Allergies
None reported.

Possible Interactions with Herbs & Other Dietary Supplements
Insufficient reliable information available.

Possible Interactions with Drugs
No interactions are known to occur, and there is no known reason to expect a clinically significant interaction with Chinese cucumber seed.

Possible Interactions with Foods
No interactions are known to occur, and there is no known reason to expect a clinically significant interaction with Chinese cucumber seed.

Possible Interactions with Lab Tests
No interactions are known to occur, and there is no known reason to expect a clinically significant interaction with Chinese cucumber seed.

Possible Interactions with Diseases or Conditions
No interactions are known to occur, and there is no known reason to expect a clinically significant interaction with Chinese cucumber seed.

Typical Dosages & Routes of Administration that are Commonly Used
ORAL: People typically use 9 to 15 grams of the seeds [5268].

Comments
None.

CHIRATA

This Product is Also Known As
Bitter Stick, Bitterstick, Chirayta, Chiretta, East Indian Balmony, Indian Bolonong, Indian Gentian.

Scientific Names
Swertia chirata.
Family: Gentianaceae.

People Use This For
In folk medicine, chirata is used as a bitter tonic, antipyretic, laxative, antihelminthic [11], for dyspepsia, loss of appetite, skin diseases, and cancer [11,18].
In manufacturing, chirata is used for alcoholic and non-alcoholic beverages [11].
In India, it has been used as an anti-malarial, combined with the seeds of Guilandina Bonducella [215].

Safety

LIKELY SAFE ...when taken in amounts found in beverages, alcoholic (maximum use level 0.0016%) and non-alcoholic drinks (maximum use level 0.0008%) (11).

At higher levels, there is insufficient reliable information available about the safety of chirata for other uses; however, no adverse reactions reported (18).

PREGNANCY AND LACTATION: Insufficient reliable information available; avoid using.

Effectiveness

There is insufficient reliable information available about the effectiveness of chirata.

Possible Mechanism of Action & Active Ingredients

The applicable parts of chirata are the above ground parts. The extract is reported to have anti-inflammatory activity in animals (11). Constituents and their reported activity include: chirata stimulates gastric juice secretion (18); swerchirin has antimalarial activity (in vivo) (11); amarogentin has hepatoprotective activity (in vitro) (11); xanthones claimed to have antituberculous activity (11).

Adverse Reactions Including Known Allergies

None reported (18).

Possible Interactions with Herbs & Other Dietary Supplements

Insufficient reliable information available.

Possible Interactions with Drugs

No interactions are known to occur, and there is no known reason to expect a clinically significant interaction with chirata.

Possible Interactions with Foods

No interactions are known to occur, and there is no known reason to expect a clinically significant interaction with chirata.

Possible Interactions with Lab Tests

No interactions are known to occur, and there is no known reason to expect a clinically significant interaction with chirata.

Possible Interactions with Diseases or Conditions

DUODENAL ULCERS: May exacerbate (18); avoid using.

Typical Dosages & Routes of Administration that are Commonly Used

ORAL: People typically use 0.5 to 2 grams of the powdered herb or 2 to 4 mL of the liquid extract (5264).

Comments

Adulteration reported with Andrographis paniculata, roots of Rubia cordifolia, and Swertia species, including Swertia angustifolia (11).

CHITOSAN

This Product is Also Known As

Chitosan Ascorbate, N-Carboxybutyl Chitosan, N,O-Sulfated Chitosan, O-Sulfated N-Acetylchitosan, Sulfated N-Carboxymethylchitosan, Sulfated O-Carboxymethylchitosan.

Scientific Names

Chitosan.

People Use This For

Orally, chitosan is used for weight loss (3243). It is also used orally by some people with renal failure on chronic hemodialysis for reducing high cholesterol, improving anemia, enhancing physical strength, appetite, and sleep (1942).

Topically, chitosan is used for treating periodontitis (1945) and promoting donor site tissue regeneration in plastic surgery (1944).

In pharmaceutical manufacturing, chitosan is used as an excipient in tablets, as a disintegrant to improve drug dissolution, as a vehicle for parenteral drug delivery devices, and as a carrier in controlled release drug systems (1940,1941).

Safety

POSSIBLY SAFE ...when used orally (1942). ...when used topically (1944,1945,4269,4270).

PREGNANCY AND LACTATION: Insufficient reliable information available; avoid using.

Effectiveness

POSSIBLY EFFECTIVE ...when taken orally by patients with renal failure on chronic hemodialysis for reducing high cholesterol, improving anemia, enhancing physical strength, appetite, and sleep (1942). ...when used topically for treating periodontitis (1945) and promoting donor site tissue regeneration in plastic surgery (1944).
LIKELY INEFFECTIVE ...when taken orally for weight loss (3243,3244).
There is insufficient reliable information available about the effectiveness of chitosan for its other uses.

Possible Mechanism of Action & Active Ingredients

Reported hemostatic activity is believed to be due to an interaction between erythrocyte cell membranes and chitosan; this appears to be independent of the classical coagulation cascade (1943). Chitosan ascorbate acts as a surgical cement in treatment of periodontitis, protecting periodontal pockets from oxygen and allowing for proliferation of periodontal tissues (1945). While it is theorized that chitosan might aid in weight reduction, clinical trials with chitosan show no effect on weight loss (3243,3244). The effect of chitosan on serum lipids is unclear. In one study, chitosan had no effects (3243), in a second study it was associated with a slight reduction in LDL and a slight increase in triglycerides (3244), and in a third study significantly reduced total serum cholesterol in patients with renal failure on chronic hemodialysis (1942).

Adverse Reactions Including Known Allergies

People with shellfish allergies should use caution (6).

Possible Interactions with Herbs & Other Dietary Supplements

Insufficient reliable information available.

Possible Interactions with Drugs

No interactions are known to occur, and there is no known reason to expect a clinically significant interaction with chitosan.

Possible Interactions with Foods

No interactions are known to occur, and there is no known reason to expect a clinically significant interaction with chitosan.

Possible Interactions with Lab Tests

CHOLESTEROL: May reduce serum cholesterol levels, and test results, in patients with renal failure on chronic hemodialysis (1942).
HEMOGLOBIN: May increase serum hemoglobin levels, and test results, in patients with renal failure on chronic hemodialysis (1942).
UREA/CREATININE: May reduce blood urea and creatinine levels, and test results, in patients with renal failure on chronic hemodialysis (1942).

Possible Interactions with Diseases or Conditions

RENAL FAILURE: May reduce serum cholesterol, urea and creatinine levels, and increase hemoglobin levels in patients on chronic hemodialysis (1942).

Typical Dosages & Routes of Administration that are Commonly Used

ORAL: Renal failure with chronic hemodialysis: 1.35 grams (30 x 45 mg tablets) three times daily (1942).
No typical dosage for other uses and routes of administration.

Comments

Chitosan is a mucopolysaccharide component of crab, lobster, shrimp and other marine organism exoskeletons.

CHIVE

This Product is Also Known As

Chives, Cives.

Scientific Names

Allium schoenoprasum.
Family: Liliaceae.

People Use This For

Orally, chive is used to expel parasitic worms (18).
For food uses, chives are used commonly as a food flavoring agent.

Safety

LIKELY SAFE ...when used in food amounts.
POSSIBLY SAFE ...when used orally in larger amounts (12).
PREGNANCY AND LACTATION: LIKELY SAFE ...when used in food amounts; avoid larger amounts.

Effectiveness

There is insufficient reliable information available about the effectiveness of chive.

Possible Mechanism of Action & Active Ingredients

The applicable parts of chive are the above ground parts. There is insufficient reliable information available about the possible mechanism of action and active ingredients.

Adverse Reactions Including Known Allergies

Intake of large quantities can lead to dyspepsia (18).

Possible Interactions with Herbs & Other Dietary Supplements

Insufficient reliable information available.

Possible Interactions with Drugs

No interactions are known to occur, and there is no known reason to expect a clinically significant interaction with chive.

Possible Interactions with Foods

No interactions are known to occur, and there is no known reason to expect a clinically significant interaction with chive.

Possible Interactions with Lab Tests

No interactions are known to occur, and there is no known reason to expect a clinically significant interaction with chive.

Possible Interactions with Diseases or Conditions

No interactions are known to occur, and there is no known reason to expect a clinically significant interaction with chive.

Typical Dosages & Routes of Administration that are Commonly Used

ORAL: Chive is used fresh, dried, or powdered.

Comments

None.

CHLORELLA

This Product is Also Known As

None.

Scientific Names

Chlorella Vulgaris; Chlorella pyrenoidosa; other Chlorella species.

People Use This For

Orally, chlorella is used as a food supplement and source of nutrients, including protein, nucleic acids, fiber, vitamins, and minerals (5843,5846). Chlorella is also used orally for cancer prevention, stimulating the immune system (5843,5844), increasing white blood cell counts (e.g. in people with HIV infection or cancer) (5843), preventing colds (5843), to protect the body from the effects of radiation (e.g. during cancer therapy) (5843,5844), to protect the body from toxic metals such as lead and mercury (5844), and to slow aging (5843). It is also used to increase beneficial flora in the gastrointestinal tract in order to improve digestion (5843,5844), and help treat ulcers, colitis, Crohn's disease, and diverticulosis (5843). It is also promoted for the prevention of stress-induced ulcers (5844); treatment of constipation, bad breath, and hypertension (5844); as an antioxidant (5844); to reduce serum cholesterol; to increase energy; to detoxify the body (5843); and as a source of magnesium to promote mental health, relieve premenstrual syndrome (PMS), and reduce asthma attacks (5843).

Topically, chlorella has been used for treating ulcers, postirradiation dermatitis, vulval leukoplakias, and trichomoniasis (5851).

Safety

POSSIBLY SAFE ...when used as a food to supplement a normal diet (5846).

There is insufficient reliable information about the safety of chlorella for its other uses.

PREGNANCY AND LACTATION: Insufficient reliable information available; avoid using.

Effectiveness

POSSIBLY EFFECTIVE ...when used as a source of nutrients to supplement a normal diet (5846).

There is insufficient reliable information about the effectiveness of chlorella for its other uses.

Possible Mechanism of Action & Active Ingredients

Chlorella is a single-celled, freshwater green alga, also referred to as a seaweed (5846,5850). The whole plant is processed for medicinal use and is a rich source of chlorophyll (5846). (See separate monograph for Chlorophyll). Chlorella contains significant amounts of protein, lipid, vitamins and minerals (5846). Serum vitamin B12 levels were significantly higher in a group of vegans who consumed large amounts of chlorella, compared with those who did not (5848). However, it has been suggested that the vitamin B12 found in chlorella might be in an inactive form which can raise serum levels without contributing biological activity (5849).

In-vitro and preliminary animal studies have indicated that substances in chlorella may have antitumor, immune system enhancing, and anti-viral activities (5846,5850). The photosensitizing components in chlorella have been identified as pheophorbides (5846,5847).

Adverse Reactions Including Known Allergies

Allergic reactions, including asthma and anaphylaxis, have been reported in people taking chlorella, and in those preparing chlorella tablets (5846,5847). Photosensitivity reactions have also occurred following ingestion of chlorella (5846,5852). There is a case report of human infection with chlorella, and several reports in animals (5853).

Possible Interactions with Herbs & Other Dietary Supplements

Insufficient reliable information available.

Possible Interactions with Drugs

ANTICOAGULANTS: Chlorella contains significant amounts of vitamin K, which may inhibit the anticoagulant activity of warfarin (Coumadin) and related drugs (5846).

Possible Interactions with Foods

No interactions are known to occur, and there is no known reason to expect a clinically significant interaction with chlorella.

Possible Interactions with Lab Tests

No interactions are known to occur, and there is no known reason to expect a clinically significant interaction with chlorella.

Possible Interactions with Diseases or Conditions

ALLERGIES, INCLUDING IODINE SENSITIVITY: Chlorella has been associated with significant allergic reactions (5846,5847), and is also reported to contain iodine (5845).

Typical Dosages & Routes of Administration that are Commonly Used

No typical dosage.

Comments

Commercial producers of chlorella report that it is a source of protein, including the amino acids: lysine, leucine, isoleucine, threonine, valine, methionine, phenylalanine, tryptophan, histidine, arginine, serine, proline, glycine, alanine, glutamic acid, and aspartic acid (5845). It is also reported to contain chlorophyll, saturated and unsaturated fatty acids, RNA, magnesium, potassium, calcium, iron, zinc, phosphorus, iodine, niacin, beta carotene, thiamine, riboflavin, pyridoxine, pantothenic acid, biotin, inositol, folic acid, vitamin B12, vitamin E, and vitamin C (5843,5844,5845). Since chlorella is a naturally occurring organism, its content can vary with growing, harvesting and processing conditions. By varying the cultivation conditions, it has been reported that a dried preparation of chlorella can contain from 7 to 88% protein, 6 to 38% carbohydrate, and 7 to 75% fat (5851). Most chlorella sold in the United States is cultivated in Japan or Taiwan (5846). Processing of the chlorella cultures includes destroying the cell walls, dehydration and sterilization (5851).

CHLOROPHYLL

This Product is Also Known As

None.
CAUTION: See separate listing for Chlorophyllin.

Scientific Names

Chlorophyll a, Chlorophyll b, Chlorophyll c, Chlorophyll d.

People Use This For

Orally, chlorophyll is used for reducing colostomy odor (1322), bad breath, constipation, detoxification, and wound healing (1900).
Intravenously, chlorophyll is used for treating chronic relapsing pancreatitis (1324).

Safety

LIKELY SAFE ...when used orally (1324).
POSSIBLY SAFE ...when used intravenously (1324).

PREGNANCY AND LACTATION: POSSIBLY SAFE ...when used orally.
There is insufficient reliable information available about the safety of the intravenous use of chlorophyll during pregnancy and lactation.

Effectiveness
POSSIBLY EFFECTIVE ...when used intravenously for chronic relapsing pancreatitis (1324).
POSSIBLY INEFFECTIVE ...when used for reducing colostomy odor (1322).

Possible Mechanism of Action & Active Ingredients
Chlorophyll contains components that are activated by light. It appears that chlorophyll can cause a photosensitization when it is taken internally (1326). Derivatives of chlorophyll which have been extracted from silkworm droppings seem to have a cytotoxic effect on certain cancer cells (1314,1315). Certain carotenoids such as beta-carotene and canthaxanthin seem to prevent or lessen the photosensitivity that results from taking chlorophyll (1326).

Adverse Reactions Including Known Allergies
None reported (1324).

Possible Interactions with Herbs & Other Dietary Supplements
CAROTENOIDS (beta-carotene, canthaxanthin): Theoretically, may prevent or lessen chlorophyll-induced photosensitivity (1326).

Possible Interactions with Drugs
PHOTOSENSITIZING DRUGS: Theoretically, may exacerbate effects (1326).

Possible Interactions with Foods
No interactions are known to occur, and there is no known reason to expect a clinically significant interaction with chlorophyll.

Possible Interactions with Lab Tests
No interactions are known to occur, and there is no known reason to expect a clinically significant interaction with chlorophyll.

Possible Interactions with Diseases or Conditions
No interactions are known to occur, and there is no known reason to expect a clinically significant interaction with chlorophyll.

Typical Dosages & Routes of Administration that are Commonly Used
ORAL: No typical dosage.
INTRAVENOUS: Pancreatitis: Infusion of 5-20 mg water soluble chlorophyll-a per day for 1-2 weeks, followed by intermittent administration (1324).

Comments
Avoid confusion with chlorophyllin, a semisynthetic derivative of chlorophyll. Commercial sources of chlorophyll include alfalfa (Medicago sativa) and silk worm droppings (11). Chlorophyll is a group of related green pigments found in photosynthetic organisms including: Chlorophyll a (found in higher plants, red and green algae), Chlorophyll b (found in higher plants), Chlorophyll c (found in brown algae, diatoms, flagellates), Chlorophyll d (found in red algae).

CHLOROPHYLLIN

This Product is Also Known As
None.
CAUTION: see separate listing for Chlorophyll.

Scientific Names
Chlorophyllin.

People Use This For
Orally, chlorophyllin is used for controlling body, fecal, and urine odors, and for treating constipation and flatulence (1321,1323).

Safety
POSSIBLY SAFE ...when used orally (1321,1323).
PREGNANCY AND LACTATION: Insufficient reliable information available; avoid using.

Effectiveness

POSSIBLY EFFECTIVE ...when used orally for controlling body and fecal odors, treating constipation and flatulence in geriatric patients (1321).

POSSIBLY INEFFECTIVE ...when used orally for controlling urinary odor in incontinent geriatric patients with indwelling catheters (1323).

Possible Mechanism of Action & Active Ingredients

Chlorophyllin has antimutagenic activity in human lymphocytes (in vitro) (1312). Mechanisms may include reduced carcinogen DNA-binding (in fish) (1309), reduced chromosome damage (in vitro) (1311), and reduced carcinogen-induced cell transformation (in vitro) (1307). Bacteriologic studies failed to confirm reports of antibacterial properties for chlorophyllin (1321).

Adverse Reactions Including Known Allergies

None reported (1321).

Possible Interactions with Herbs & Other Dietary Supplements

Insufficient reliable information available.

Possible Interactions with Drugs

No interactions are known to occur, and there is no known reason to expect a clinically significant interaction with chlorophyllin.

Possible Interactions with Foods

No interactions are known to occur, and there is no known reason to expect a clinically significant interaction with chlorophyllin.

Possible Interactions with Lab Tests

No interactions are known to occur, and there is no known reason to expect a clinically significant interaction with chlorophyllin.

Possible Interactions with Diseases or Conditions

No interactions are known to occur, and there is no known reason to expect a clinically significant interaction with chlorophyllin.

Typical Dosages & Routes of Administration that are Commonly Used

ORAL: 100 mg per day used in study for controlling urinary odor in incontinent geriatric patients with indwelling catheters (1323).

Comments

Avoid confusion with Chlorophyll.

CHOLINE

This Product is Also Known As

Choline Bitartrate, Choline Chloride, Intrachol, Lipotropic Factor.
CAUTION: See separate listings for Lecithin and Phosphatidylcholine.

Scientific Names

Trimethylethanolamine; (beta-hydroxyethyl) trimethylammonium hydroxide (16,5157).

People Use This For

Orally, choline is used as a supplement in infant formulas (16,4921), as a dietary supplement (9,5158,5159), for treating liver disease including chronic hepatitis and cirrhosis, for treating high cholesterol, for depression (5158), for treating memory loss, Alzheimer's disease and dementia (5159,5168,5169,5170), schizophrenia (5171,5172), for reducing body fat (5160), for delaying fatigue in endurance sports (5164), for treating Huntington's chorea (5167), Tourette's disease (14), cerebellar ataxia (5161,5173), complex partial seizures (5162), and asthma (5165,5166).
For intravenous use, choline has orphan drug status for TPN-associated hepatic steatosis (5163,5173,5174).

Safety

LIKELY SAFE ...when used in food amounts. Generally Recognized as Safe (GRAS) status in the US (4921). ...when used orally for medicinal purposes in amounts less than 30 grams per day (4921). ...when used intravenously for TPN-associated hepatic steatosis (5173,5174).
PREGNANCY AND LACTATION: Insufficient reliable information available; avoid in amounts greater than found in foods or in prescribed doses of prenatal vitamins.

Effectiveness

LIKELY EFFECTIVE ...when used orally as a supplement in infant formulas (16,4921). ...when used intravenously to treat parenteral nutrition-associated hepatic dysfunction (5163,5173,5174).

POSSIBLY EFFECTIVE ...when used orally for asthma (5165,5166), although choline theophyllinate (oxtriphylline) is no more effective than theophylline alone (15).
POSSIBLY INEFFECTIVE ...when used orally for treating cerebellar ataxia, although one case report suggests effectiveness (5161,5173). ...for delaying fatigue in endurance sports (5164).
LIKELY INEFFECTIVE ...when used orally for treating memory loss, Alzheimer's disease, and dementia (9,5170), treating schizophrenia (5171,5172).
There is insufficient reliable information available about the effectiveness of choline for its other uses.

Possible Mechanism of Action & Active Ingredients

Choline is a precursor to acetylcholine and a methyl donor for synthesis of other compounds. It is an essential structural component of many biological membranes and plasma lipoproteins (9,5157,4921). Choline is also a lipotropic agent that mobilizes lipids and removes excess fat from the liver (9,5157,4921). Experimental evidence suggests oral choline does not affect concentrations of choline metabolites in the brain. Researchers hypothesize that this might be the reason oral choline is not effective for neurodegenerative disorders of cholinergic transmission (5175). Although choline has traditionally been considered to be a B vitamin, it can be synthesized by the human body (9,5157,4921). Choline is readily available in the diet (9,5157,4921). Foods that supply large amounts of choline are liver, kidney, brain, muscle meats, fish, nuts, beans, peas, and eggs (16). Deficiency of choline is uncommon except in people receiving long-term parenteral nutrition. This indicates that dietary choline is required in addition to the choline synthesized by the body. (9,5157,4921,5174). Choline is added to infant formulas to approximate human milk content (90 mg/L) (16,4921). Some studies suggest that choline might have a role in cancer prevention (5178,5179,5180).

Adverse Reactions Including Known Allergies

Adverse reactions include sweating, gastrointestinal distress, vomiting, and with large doses diarrhea (4921). Choline can cause "fishy" body odor (5160,5133). Most adults can tolerate up to 20 g per day. Some can tolerate as much as 30 g per day without adverse effects (4921). No adverse reactions are reported from intravenous administration (5174).

Possible Interactions with Herbs & Other Dietary Supplements

Insufficient reliable information available.

Possible Interactions with Drugs

No interactions are known to occur, and there is no known reason to expect a clinically significant interaction with choline.

Possible Interactions with Foods

No interactions are known to occur, and there is no known reason to expect a clinically significant interaction with choline.

Possible Interactions with Lab Tests

No interactions are known to occur, and there is no known reason to expect a clinically significant interaction with choline.

Possible Interactions with Diseases or Conditions

No interactions are known to occur, and there is no known reason to expect a clinically significant interaction with choline.

Typical Dosages & Routes of Administration that are Commonly Used

ORAL: An average diet will supply 200-600 mg of choline daily (4921). The Dietary Reference Intake (DRI), as established by the Food and Nutrition Board of the National Institute of Medicine, for adults is 550 mg per day for males and lactating women; females, 425 mg per day; pregnant females, 450 mg per day (5181). For children 1-3 years the DRI is 200 mg per day; 4-8 years, 250 mg per day; 9- 3 years, 375 mg per day (5181); for infants less than 6 months, 125 mg per day; infants 7–12 months, 150 mg per day (5181). Upper Intake Levels (UL) for choline are 1 gram for children 1-8 years, 2 grams for children 9-13 years, 3 grams for adults 14-18 years, and 3.5 grams for adults over 18 years of age (3094).

Comments

Choline is a component of phosphatidylcholine, which is a component of lecithin (16). Although closely related, these terms are not synonymous. See separate listing for lecithin.

CHONDROITIN SULFATE

This Product is Also Known As

CDS, Chondroitin Sulfate A, Chondroitin Sulfate C, Chondroitin Sulphate A Sodium, Condroitin, CSA, CSC, GAG, Galactosaminoglucuronoglycan Sulfate.

Scientific Names

Chondroitin 4-sulfate; chondroitin 4- and 6-sulfate.

People Use This For

Orally, chondroitin sulfate is used for osteoarthritis (14,1970,1971,1972). It is frequently used in combination with other products, including manganese ascorbate, glucosamine sulfate, glucosamine hydrochloride, or N-acetyl glucosamine for osteoarthritis (760,4237). Chondroitin sulfate is also used orally for ischemic heart disease, osteoporosis, and hyperlipidemia (9). Chondroitin is also used in a complex with iron for treating iron-deficiency anemia (9).

Intramuscularly, chondroitin sulfate is used for osteoarthritis (14,1970,1971,1972).

Topically, chondroitin sulfate is used for keratoconjunctivitis sicca (dry eyes) (14,1974), as a viscoelastic agent in cataract surgery (14), and as a medium for preservation of corneas used for transplantation (9). Chondroitin sulfate is also used topically in combination with other products for osteoarthritis (384).

Safety

LIKELY SAFE ...when used orally and appropriately. Multiple clinical trials have used chondroitin sulfate safely in studies lasting from two months to three years (14,1342,1970,1971,1972,2533). ...when used topically and appropriately as an ophthalmic product, which is an FDA-approved and prescription-only product that also contains sodium hyaluronate (Viscoat).

POSSIBLY SAFE ...when used intramuscularly (14).

PREGNANCY AND LACTATION: Insufficient reliable information available; avoid using.

Effectiveness

LIKELY EFFECTIVE ...when used orally in combination with analgesics or non-steroidal anti-inflammatory drugs (NSAIDs) for reducing the symptoms of osteoarthritis. Several studies have shown that chondroitin sulfate added to conventional analgesics or NSAIDs is significantly better than analgesics or NSAIDs alone for reducing pain and improving functionality indices in patients with osteoarthritis of the hip and knee (14,322,323,324,1342,1970,1971, 1972,2533,4237). Several studies found that patients taking chondroitin sulfate could decrease their use or dose of analgesics and NSAIDs, but could not completely discontinue them. Treatment with chondroitin sulfate for 2-4 months may be required before significant improvement is experienced (1342). One clinical trial has evaluated the combination of chondroitin sulfate, glucosamine HCl, and manganese ascorbate (Cosamin-DS). The combination was superior to placebo, but was not compared to the individual components alone. It is unclear if the combination adds any benefit compared to chondroitin sulfate alone (4237). Although there have been several trials that have shown positive results, many of them have enrolled small numbers of patients and have been methodologically flawed. Two meta-analytical reviews of the literature have pooled and evaluated the data from these studies and found that chondroitin sulfate likely provides significant benefit in patients with hip and knee osteoarthritis (1342,2533). Additional large-scale, high quality studies are needed to clarify the potential role of chondroitin in treatment of osteoarthritis. ...when used in combination with sodium hyaluronate and applied topically to the eye as a surgical aid in cataract extraction or lens implantation. A combination product containing chondroitin sulfate and sodium hyaluronate (Viscoat) is an FDA-approved, prescription ophthalmic product (266).

POSSIBLY EFFECTIVE ...when used intramuscularly for reducing the symptoms of osteoarthritis (14). ...when used as an ophthalmic preparation for dry eyes (1974).

There is insufficient reliable information available about the effectiveness of chondroitin sulfate for its other uses.

Possible Mechanism of Action & Active Ingredients

Chondroitin sulfate belongs to a class of very large molecules called glucosaminoglycans (GAGs) and is a minor component (~4%) of the low molecular weight heparinoid mixture, danaparoid (Orgaran). Concern has been expressed about possible anticoagulant activity of chondroitin sulfate, but no significant hematological changes were noted in a group of patients during six months of oral chondroitin therapy (760). Chondroitin is manufactured from natural sources, such as shark and bovine cartilage, or produced synthetically (6). Chondroitin sulfate is found in cartilaginous tissues of most mammals and serves as a substrate for the formation of the joint matrix structure (1972,1973). Early evidence that chondroitin is not absorbed orally (4202) has been refuted by more recent studies. Studies show that people absorb 8-18% of orally administered chondroitin (760,3242,4203,4205,4237). Lower molecular weight derivatives of chondroitin formed in the gastrointestinal tract are more readily absorbed (3242) and may contribute to the pharmacological activity of orally administered chondroitin.

Adverse Reactions Including Known Allergies

Taken orally, chondroitin sulfate can cause epigastric pain and nausea (14). Diarrhea, constipation, eyelid edema, lower limb edema, alopecia, and extrasystoles have also been reported in clinical trials (1342). There is the potential for allergic reactions from the biological products (14). When used as an ophthalmic product, it can cause intraocular hypertension, discomfort, and corneal edema after cataract surgery (14). Concern has been expressed about possible anticoagulant activity of chondroitin sulfate, but no significant hematological changes were noted in a group of patients during six months of oral chondroitin therapy (760).

278 • © Copyright 2000, Natural Medicines Comprehensive Database (209) 472-2244. For updated data, go to www.NaturalDatabase.com

Possible Interactions with Herbs & Other Dietary Supplements

GLUCOSAMINE SULFATE: Although chondroitin sulfate and glucosamine sulfate are often administered together, no human studies have compared this combination to either product alone; there is no evidence that the combination has greater benefit than either product alone.

Possible Interactions with Drugs

ANTIPLATELET/ANTICOAGULANT AGENTS: Theoretically, concurrent use of parenteral chondroitin sulfate with ardeparin (Normiflo), aspirin, NSAIDs, dalteparin (Fragmin), dextran, dipyridamole (Persantine), enoxaparin (Lovenox), or heparin, warfarin (Coumadin) (15) might increase the risk of bleeding.
HYALURONIC ACID: Concomitant use of chondroitin sulfate provides a beneficial synergistic effect in cataract surgery (14).

Possible Interactions with Foods

No interactions are known to occur, and there is no known reason to expect a clinically significant interaction with chondroitin sulfate.

Possible Interactions with Lab Tests

ANTI-FACTOR Xa: Theoretically, because it is a component of danaparoid, chondroitin sulfate administered by injection might increase the anti-factor Xa level and test results. No significant hematological changes were noted in a group of patients during six months of oral chondroitin therapy (760).

Possible Interactions with Diseases or Conditions

COAGULATION DISORDERS: Theoretically, parenterally administered chondroitin sulfate might affect coagulation and increase the risk of bleeding when used in patients with clotting disorders; avoid use.

Typical Dosages & Routes of Administration that are Commonly Used

ORAL: For osteoarthritis, the typical dose of chondroitin sulfate is 200-400 mg two to three times daily (14,1970,1971, 1972,3278,4237) or 1200 mg as a single daily dose (1971).
INTRAMUSCULAR: For osteoarthritis, the common dose is 50-100 mg/day in a single daily injection or divided into two daily injections (14). Parenteral chondroitin sulfate products are not available in the US.

Comments

Although chondroitin sulfate and glucosamine sulfate are frequently marketed together in combination products (760), there is no evidence that the combination has greater benefit than either product alone. The National Institutes of Health (NIH) is sponsoring a clinical trial of glucosamine sulfate and chondroitin sulfate. The 16-week, parallel group, double-blind RCT includes four separate treatment arms, in which patients will ingest: 1) placebo, 2) 500 mg of glucosamine sulfate 3 times per day, 3) 400 mg of chondroitin sulfate 3 times per day, or 4) a combination of glucosamine sulfate and chondroitin (3573).

CHROMIUM

This Product is Also Known As

Chromic Chloride, Chromium Chloride, Chromium Nicotinate, Chromium Picolinate.

Scientific Names

Chromium; Cr; atomic number 24.

People Use This For

Orally, chromium is used for weight loss (9,14,1900), glycemic control in diabetes (14,1900), for treating corticosteroid-induced hyperglycemia (5039), lowering lipids in hypercholesterolemia (1900), increasing HDL cholesterol in men taking beta-blockers (5040), and enhancing athletic performance (1900).
Intravenously, chromium is used as a supplement in total parenteral nutrition (TPN) (9).

Safety

LIKELY SAFE ...when used orally in amounts of 50-200 mcg per day (14).
POSSIBLY UNSAFE …when added to short-term TPN. Sufficient amounts of chromium (as contaminants) are contained in amino acid products used for TPN (9,14).
PREGNANCY: LIKELY SAFE ...when used as a supplement to improve glycemic control in gestational diabetes (1953).
LACTATION: LIKELY SAFE ...when used orally in a supplement. Chromium supplements do not seem to increase normal chromium concentration in human breast milk (1937).

Effectiveness

POSSIBLY EFFECTIVE ...when used orally for reducing serum cholesterol and triglycerides (9,14). ...when used orally for modestly increasing serum HDL cholesterol in men taking beta-blockers. In one human trial, chromium increased HDL levels by 10% compared to placebo (5040). ...when used for blood glucose control in type 2 diabetes (9,14).

LIKELY INEFFECTIVE ...when used orally for weight reduction (14).

There is insufficient reliable information about the effectiveness of chromium for its other uses.

Possible Mechanism of Action & Active Ingredients

Glucose tolerance factor (GTF) contains a chromium atom in complex with single molecules of glycine, cysteine, and glutamic acid and two molecules of nicotinic acid (14). The chromium atom is considered key to the complex (14), which researchers believe increases insulin receptor sensitivity and enhances glucose transport into cells to maintain normal blood sugar levels (14). Chromium picolinate is more easily absorbed than other forms (14). Researchers theorize (but have not substantiated) that chromium picolinate may sensitize insulin-sensitive glucoreceptors in the brain, resulting in appetite suppression, activation of the sympathetic nervous system to stimulate thermogenesis, and down-regulation of insulin secretion (14). Chromium picolinate lowers fasting insulin levels in insulin resistant, corpulent rats (6170). This finding leads researchers to wonder whether chromium picolinate might be useful for treating Syndrome X (Metabolic Syndrome) which is associated with obesity, insulin resistance and hyperinsulinemia (6170). Preliminary human data suggest that chromium supplements might reverse corticosteroid-induced hyperglycemia in patients with or without pre-existing diabetes (5039). Currently, the American Diabetes Association does not recommend chromium supplementation unless chromium deficiency is present (3890). Reliable tests for chromium deficiency have not been developed (3859). Chromium and zinc administered together orally cause decreased absorption of both minerals in zinc-deficient rats (1950). Chromium picolinate can cause weight gain in young, obese women if it is given to women who do not exercise (1938). Preliminary evidence suggests that chromium picolinate easily enters cells, where it can produce hydroxyl radicals via two mechanisms, causing DNA damage (1299).

Adverse Reactions Including Known Allergies

When chromium is given orally it can lead to cognitive, perceptual, and motor dysfunction at 200-400 mcg/day (14). It can also cause anemia, thrombocytopenia, hemolysis, hepatic dysfunction, and renal failure when given in dosages of 1.2-2.4 mg/day (554). When chromium is given intravenously (IV) there appears to be a decreased glomerular filtration rate (GFR) in children who receive chromium in long-term total parenteral nutrition solutions (9). Occupational inhalation of hexavalent chromium fumes can cause ulceration of the nasal mucosa (chrome ulcers) and perforation of the nasal septum (chrome holes) and has been associated with pneumoconiosis, allergic asthma, and increased susceptibility to respiratory tract carcinomas (14). Chromium picolinate may have an effect on dopamine, serotonin, and norepinephrine metabolism in the brain, due to the picolinic acid component (217).

Possible Interactions with Herbs & Other Dietary Supplements

VITAMIN B3 (niacin): Concomitant chromium use might improve glucose tolerance (1936).

VITAMIN C: Concomitant vitamin C use might increase chromium absorption (1900).

ZINC: Theoretically, co-administration might decrease absorption of both chromium and zinc (animal data) (1950).

Possible Interactions with Drugs

BETA-BLOCKERS: Concomitant use of chromium supplements and beta-blockers, including atenolol (Tenormin) or propranolol (Inderal), modestly increases serum HDL cholesterol concentrations (5040).

CORTICOSTEROIDS: Chromium might reverse corticosteroid-induced increases in blood sugar in patients with or without pre-existing diabetes. In two patients with type 2 diabetes, oral chromium supplements reversed increases in blood glucose associated with dexamethasone (Decadron) or prednisone (Deltasone). In a third case, chromium reduced the insulin dose required by a patient who experienced prednisone-induced diabetes after a kidney transplant (5039).

INSULIN: Theoretically, concomitant use might increase the risk of hypoglycemia (1952).

NICOTINIC ACID: Concomitant use produces a synergistic effect with chromium in improving glucose tolerance (1936).

Drug Influences on Nutrient Levels and Depletion

SOME DRUGS CAN AFFECT CHROMIUM LEVELS:

CORTICOSTEROIDS: use of corticosteroids can increase urinary chromium excretion, which might lead to chromium deficiency and/or corticosteroid-induced hyperglycemia. Three cases are reported of oral chromium supplements reversing dexamethasone (Decadron) or prednisone (Deltasone) induced hyperglycemia in patients with or without pre-existing diabetes. Consider chromium supplements based on clinical judgment (5039).

Possible Interactions with Foods

No interactions are known to occur, and there is no known reason to expect a clinically significant interaction with chromium.

Possible Interactions with Lab Tests

GLUCOSE: Chromium might reduce blood glucose concentrations and test results in some patients' corticosteroid-induced hyperglycemia. Three cases are reported of oral chromium supplements reversing dexamethasone (Decadron) or prednisone (Deltasone) induced hyperglycemia in patients with or without pre-existing diabetes (5039).

CHOLESTEROL: Chromium can reduce fasting serum cholesterol concentrations and test results in patients with type 2 diabetes (14). Chromium can modestly increase serum HDL cholesterol concentrations and test results in men taking beta-blockers, including atenolol (Tenormin) and propranolol (Inderal) (5040).

GLYCOSYLATED HEMOGLOBIN (HbA1c): Chromium can improve blood glucose control and decrease HbA1c values in patients with type 1, type 2, and gestational diabetes (14,1934).

TRIGLYCERIDES: Chromium can reduce serum triglyceride concentrations and test results in patients with type 2 diabetes (14).

Possible Interactions with Diseases or Conditions

BEHAVIORAL DISORDERS: Picolinic acid (contained in chromium picolinate) can alter serotonin, dopamine, and norepinephrine metabolism in the central nervous system (1935).

DIABETES: Chromium can result in lower blood glucose levels (1939); monitor closely.

RENAL INSUFFICIENCY: Chromium supplements can exacerbate renal insufficiency (1951).

Typical Dosages & Routes of Administration that are Commonly Used

ORAL: The recommended daily allowance (RDA) is 50-200 mcg (9,14). Chromium picolinate is better absorbed than the chloride or nicotinate forms (14). For reducing serum triglycerides in type 2 diabetes, 200 mcg three times daily has been used (1934). For increasing serum HDL cholesterol in men taking beta-blockers, 200 mcg three times daily has been used (5040). For reversing corticosteroid-induced hyperglycemia or exacerbation of pre-existing diabetes, 400 mcg per day or 200 mcg three times daily have been used (5039).

Comments

Chromium is an essential trace element that exists naturally in trivalent and hexavalent states. Hexavalent chromium (as chromic oxide, chromate, or dichromate) is extremely irritating and corrosive to skin (14). Trivalent chromium (typically found in food or nutritional supplements) is not reported to cause cutaneous or mucosal injury (14).

Chromium supplementation in short-term TPN is not recommended. Sufficient amounts of chromium (as contaminants) contained in amino acid products are used for TPN (9,14).

CHRYSANTHEMUM

This Product is Also Known As

Florist's Chrysanthemum, Ju Hua, Mum.

Scientific Names

Dendranthema morifolium; Anthemis grandiflorum; Anthemis stipulacea; Chrysanthemum sinense; Chrysanthemum stipulaceum; Chrysanthemum morifolium; Matricaria morifolia.
Family: Asteraceae or Compositae.

People Use This For

In Chinese medicine, the dried chrysanthemum flower is commonly used orally to treat angina and hypertension (5545).

The chrysanthemum product, jiangtangkang, is used to treat non-insulin dependent diabetes (5546).

In folk medicine, the dried chrysanthemum flower was widely used as an antipyretic, to clear the eye and the mind, and as an antitoxin. It has also been used for colds, headache, dizziness, and swelling (5545).

Chrysanthemum is frequently used in herbal combinations. In one specific combination with seven other herbs (PC-SPES), the dried chrysanthemum flower is used to treat prostate cancer (5548). In combination with licorice (Glycyrrhiza uralensis) and Panax notoginseng, the dried chrysanthemum flower is used to treat precancerous lesions (5555).

In southern China, chrysanthemum is very popular as a summertime tea (5545).

Safety

POSSIBLY SAFE ...when used orally in a specific herbal combination (PC-SPES) (5548).
There is insufficient reliable information available about the safety of chrysanthemum for its other uses.
PREGNANCY AND LACTATION: Insufficient reliable information available; avoid using.

Effectiveness

POSSIBLY EFFECTIVE ...when used orally in a specific herbal combination for prostate cancer. Studies using chrysanthemum in combination with seven other herbs (PC-SPES) in prostate cancer patients, found that it significantly decreases prostate-specific antigen (PSA) levels (5548,5122,5913), causes tumor cell death (5913), and causes clinically significant reductions in testosterone (5548). In two reports, PSA levels fell significantly within 1 month of treatment (5548,5122).
There is insufficient reliable information about the effectiveness of chrysanthemum for its other uses.

Possible Mechanism of Action & Active Ingredients

The dried chrysanthemum flower contains the essential oil bornol, chrysantheonon, camphor, the alkaloid stachydrine and several glycosides. It also contains adenine, choline, B vitamins and substances similar to vitamin A. Some evidence suggests the chrysanthemum might increase coronary vasodilatation and blood flow without increasing coronary contractility or oxygen consumption. Chrysanthemum has antibacterial and antipyretic effects. It can also reduce the capillary permeability induced by histamine (5545). Preliminary information suggests the chrysanthemum product jiangtangkang used by individuals with non-insulin dependent diabetes might improve insulin sensitivity and decrease blood viscosity (5546). A preliminary trial suggests Hua-sheng-ping, a combination of chrysanthemum, licorice, and Panax notoginseng can reverse precancerous gastrointestinal lesions (5555). The chrysanthemum constituents chrysin and acetin-7-O-beta-D-galactopyranoside inhibit HIV replication (5545,5547).

Adverse Reactions Including Known Allergies

Chrysanthemum flowers can cause photosensitivity and contact dermatitis (5552,5553,5554,5556,5557). Chrysanthemum flowers can cause an allergic reaction in individuals sensitive to the Asteraceae/Compositae family. Members of this family include ragweed, chrysanthemums, marigolds, daisies and many other herbs.

Possible Interactions with Herbs & Other Dietary Supplements

CARDIOACTIVE HERBS: Avoid concomitant use with other cardioactive herbs due to unpredictability of effects and adverse effects. Cardioactive herbs include: calamus, cereus, cola, coltsfoot, devil's claw, European mistletoe, fenugreek, fumitory, ginger, Panax ginseng, hawthorn, white horehound, mate, parsley, quassia, Scotch broom flower, shepherd's purse, and wild carrot (4). Cardiac glycoside containing herbs include black hellebore, Canadian hemp root, digitalis leaf, hedge mustard, figwort, lily of the valley root, motherwort, oleander leaf, pheasant's eye plant, pleurisy root, squill bulb leaf scales, and strophanthus seeds (2,18,19,500).

Possible Interactions with Drugs

CARDIOACTIVE DRUGS: Theoretically, chrysanthemum could interfere with cardiovascular therapy; avoid using.

Possible Interactions with Foods

No interactions are known to occur, and there is no known reason to expect a clinically significant interaction with chrysanthemum.

Possible Interactions with Lab Tests

No interactions are known to occur, and there is no known reason to expect a clinically significant interaction with chrysanthemum.

Possible Interactions with Diseases or Conditions

No interactions are known to occur, and there is no known reason to expect a clinically significant interaction with chrysanthemum.

Typical Dosages & Routes of Administration that are Commonly Used

ORAL: To make the water extract, 300 mg of the dried chrysanthemum flower are condensed into 500 mL water. A typical dose is 25 mL three times daily or taken as tea (5545).

Comments

None.

CHYMOTRYPSIN

This Product is Also Known As

Alpha-Chymotrypsin, Chymotrypsin A, Chymotrypsin B, Chymotrypsinum, Quimotripsina.

Scientific Names

Alpha-chymotrypsin; chymotrypsinum.

People Use This For

Orally, chymotrypsin is used for reducing inflammation and edema associated with abscesses, ulcers, surgery or traumatic injuries, as an expectorant in asthma, bronchitis, pulmonary diseases, and sinusitis (9). It is used in minimizing initial rise in serum liver enzymes in burn patients, reducing liver stress and associated degradative changes during wound repair (716).

Topically, chymotrypsin is used for inflammatory and infectious disorders (509).

As an inhalant, chymotrypsin is used for inflammatory and infectious disorders (509).

Intramuscularly, chymotrypsin is used to reduce inflammation and edema associated with abscesses, ulcers, surgery or traumatic injuries (9), and as an expectorant in asthma, bronchitis, pulmonary diseases, and sinusitis (9), and for inflammatory and infectious disorders (509).

Ophthalmically, chymotrypsin is used as an adjunct in cataract surgery to reduce trauma to the eye (9,509).

Safety

LIKELY SAFE ...when used ophthalmically, as approved by FDA.
POSSIBLY SAFE ...when used orally for inflammation due to surgery or trauma injuries (9,717,718). ...when used topically for treating burns (716).
There is insufficient reliable information available about the safety of the inhalant or intramuscular use of chymotrypsin.
PREGNANCY AND LACTATION: Insufficient reliable information available.

Effectiveness

EFFECTIVE ...when used as an adjunct in cataract surgery according to FDA approved Rx product labeling (9,509).
POSSIBLY EFFECTIVE ...when used orally for reducing inflammation and edema associated with surgery or trauma injuries (9,717,718). ...when used for treating burns (716).
There is insufficient reliable information available about the effectiveness of chymotrypsin for its other uses.

Possible Mechanism of Action & Active Ingredients

Chymotrypsin has ingredients that have proteolytic (9,509), anti-inflammatory (9,509,715), and antioxidant activities that reduce tissue destruction (715).

Adverse Reactions Including Known Allergies

Chymotrypsin leads to increased intraocular pressure (9,509), corneal edema, striation, moderate uveitis (9), iridoplegia, and filamentary keratitis (509). Anaphylactic reaction (rare) is characterized by dyspnea, urticaria, edema of the glottis or lip, shock and vascular collapse, loss of consciousness, and death (9,509). If hypersensitivity is suspected, a sensitivity test should be made before administration (9).

Possible Interactions with Herbs & Other Dietary Supplements

Insufficient reliable information available.

Possible Interactions with Drugs

No interactions are known to occur, and there is no known reason to expect a clinically significant interaction with chymotrypsin.

Possible Interactions with Foods

No interactions are known to occur, and there is no known reason to expect a clinically significant interaction with chymotrypsin.

Possible Interactions with Lab Tests

No interactions are known to occur, and there is no known reason to expect a clinically significant interaction with chymotrypsin.

Possible Interactions with Diseases or Conditions

Contraindicated in ocular surgery cases involving congenital cataracts, high vitreous pressure and a gaping incisional wound, or if individual is 20 years of age or younger (9).

Typical Dosages & Routes of Administration that are Commonly Used

ORAL: For inflammation, edema and respiratory secretions: As 6:1 ratio (trypsin: chymotrypsin) in a combined amount of 100,000 units USP four times daily (9,717,718). For burns: As 6:1 ratio (trypsin:chymotrypsin) in a combined amount of 200,000 units USP four times daily for 10 days (716).
INTRAMUSCULAR: For inflammation, edema and respiratory secretions: 5000 USP units one to three times daily (9).
OPHTHALMIC: As an adjunct in cataract surgery: 1:5000 or 1:10,000 solution of chymotrypsin in sterile sodium chloride injection (0.9%) injected to irrigate the posterior chamber (9).

Comments

None.

CIGUATERA

This Product is Also Known As

Ciguatera, Ciguatera Poisoning.

Scientific Names

Gambierdiscus toxicus (6).

People Use This For

There are no medicinal uses for this product, but it may be encountered inadvertently by eating tainted fish (6).

Safety

UNSAFE ...when ingested. Up to 20% mortality has been reported (6). A single bite of fish contaminated with this toxin will produce symptoms (6).

PREGNANCY: UNSAFE ...there has been one report of a fetus being aborted during acute phase of maternal poisoning. However, no lasting adverse effects have been reported in liveborn infants (6).

LACTATION: UNSAFE ...ciguatera is excreted in breast milk; GI symptoms and itching reported in infants breast-fed by symptomatic mothers; infant symptoms resolved with discontinuation of breast feeding (6).

Effectiveness

There is insufficient reliable information available about the effectiveness of ciguatera.

Possible Mechanism of Action & Active Ingredients

The applicable part of ciguatera is the toxin. Ciguatoxin increases cell permeability to sodium, causing sustained depolarization (6). Action in humans is dependent on anti-cholinesterase activity and also to a transmitter-like cholinomimetic activity (6).

Adverse Reactions Including Known Allergies

Poisoning has many different manifestations. But in general, poisoning is characterized by abdominal cramps, nausea, vomiting, diarrhea within 1-6 hours of ingestion; itching, numbness of lips, tongue, throat, paresthesias, blurred vision, hypotension, bradycardia; reversal of hot and cold sensations, and coma (rarely). In severe cases, shock, muscular paralysis, and death are possible (6). GI symptoms usually resolve within 24 hours. Muscle weakness/numbness may last weeks to months (6). Tumultuous fetal movements and intermittent fetal shivering have been reported with maternal poisoning. There has been one case of a fetus aborted during the acute phase of maternal poisoning (6).

Possible Interactions with Herbs & Other Dietary Supplements

Insufficient reliable information available.

Possible Interactions with Drugs

No interactions are known to occur, and there is no known reason to expect a clinically significant interaction with ciguatera.

Possible Interactions with Foods

No interactions are known to occur, and there is no known reason to expect a clinically significant interaction with ciguatera.

Possible Interactions with Lab Tests

No interactions are known to occur, and there is no known reason to expect a clinically significant interaction with ciguatera.

Possible Interactions with Diseases or Conditions

No interactions are known to occur, and there is no known reason to expect a clinically significant interaction with ciguatera.

Typical Dosages & Routes of Administration that are Commonly Used

No typical dose.

Comments

Ciguatera poisoning is caused by eating normally safe, bottom-feeding, coral-reef fish that have accumulated ciguatoxin via the marine food chain (6). The red snapper and barracuda and grouper are most often involved. Florida and Hawaii have the greatest incidence of ciguatera poisoning. Avoid consumption of fish in areas of recently disturbed coral reefs (includes waterfront construction). Ciguatoxic fish appear normal, including smell and taste. Local "rules of thumb" for detection are unsubstantiated. Testing for ciguatoxin is available in some areas (6). Over 400 (normally safe) fish species may contain toxin, including red snapper, barracuda, parrotfish, jacks and grouper (6).

CINCHONA

This Product is Also Known As

Chinarinde, Ecorce de Quina, Fieberrinde, Jesuit's Bark, Peruvian Bark, Quinine, Red Cinchona Bark.

Scientific Names

Cinchona pubescens, synonym Cinchona succirubra; Cinchona calisaya; Cinchona ledgeriana.
Family: Rubiaceae.

People Use This For

Orally, cinchona bark is used for stimulating appetite, promoting GI secretions (8), bloating and fullness (2), hemorrhoids, varicose veins, colds, and leg cramps (11).

Topically, cinchona is used in eye lotions for astringent, bactericidal, and anesthetic effects (11).

In folk medicine, the bark has been used for mild attacks of influenza (8), malaria, fever, cancer, mouth and throat diseases (6), enlarged spleen, muscle cramps, and gastric disorders (18). The cinchona extract has been used for hemorrhoids, stimulating hair growth, and managing varicose veins (8).

Safety

POSSIBLY SAFE ...when bark preparations are used orally and appropriately (12).

LIKELY UNSAFE ...when excessive amounts are used orally. 2 to 8 grams of the quinine constituent (505) or 2.5-8 grams quinidine constituent (17) can cause serious toxicity including death (505); however, the amount of these constituents varies according to the cinchona species (13).

PREGNANCY: LIKELY UNSAFE ...contraindicated for oral use (12).

LACTATION: Insufficient reliable information available; avoid using.

Effectiveness

POSSIBLY EFFECTIVE ...when taken orally for loss of appetite and peptic discomforts, such as bloating and fullness (2).

There is insufficient reliable information available about the effectiveness of cinchona bark for its other uses.

Possible Mechanism of Action & Active Ingredients

The applicable part of cinchona is the bark. The cinchona bark can stimulate saliva and gastric juice secretion (2). The antimalarial effects can be attributed to quinine, an alkaloid constituent. The constituents, quinidine and quinine, have cardiac depressant properties (11).

Adverse Reactions Including Known Allergies

Cinchona taken orally can cause thrombocytopenia, bleeding, and hypersensitivity reactions, including hives and fever (2). Overdose or hypersensitivity to cinchona can cause cinchonism; symptoms include headache (505), nausea, diarrhea, vomiting, ringing in the ears (6), and vision disturbance (8,505). Topically, the cinchona bark can cause contact dermatitis (11).

Possible Interactions with Herbs & Other Dietary Supplements

ANTICOAGULANT HERBS: Theoretically, the cinchona bark can potentiate the activity of herbs with anticoagulant or antiplatelet properties, including alfalfa, angelica, aniseed, arnica, asafoetida, celery, chamomile, clove, fenugreek, feverfew, fucus, garlic, ginger, Panax ginseng, horse chestnut, licorice, northern and southern prickly ash, quassia, and red clover (4).

Possible Interactions with Drugs

ACID-INHIBITING DRUGS: Theoretically, due to claims that cinchona increases stomach acid, it might interfere with antacids, sucralfate (Carafate), H-2 antagonists, or proton pump inhibitors (19).

ANTICOAGULANTS: Cinchona can increase the drug effects and risk of bleeding due to its quinine content (2).

CARBAMAZEPINE, PHENOBARBITAL: Cinchona can increase serum drug levels of carbamazepine and phenobarbital due to its quinine content (540).

QUINIDINE, QUININE: Concomitant use of cinchona can increase the therapeutic and adverse effects of these drugs (505).

Possible Interactions with Foods

No interactions are known to occur, and there is no known reason to expect a clinically significant interaction with cinchona.

Possible Interactions with Lab Tests

No interactions are known to occur, and there is no known reason to expect a clinically significant interaction with cinchona.

Possible Interactions with Diseases or Conditions

GASTRIC OR INTESTINAL ULCERS: Cinchona is contraindicated (8,12) in conditions with an increased risk of bleeding.

Typical Dosages & Routes of Administration that are Commonly Used

ORAL: The typical dose of cinchona is one cup of the tea up to three times daily (18). The tea is prepared by steeping 500 mg of the dried bark in 150 mL boiling water for 5-10 minutes and then straining. The maximum amount of cinchona is 1-3 grams of the bark per day (18) or 0.05-0.2 grams of the essential oil per day (12). The usual dose of the cinchona liquid extract (4-5% total alkaloids) is 0.6-3 grams per day (18). The cinchona extract (15-20% total alkaloids) is commonly given as 0.15-0.6 grams per day (18).

Comments

Cinchona bark contains quinine and related alkaloids, including quinidine (a cardiac depressant) and cinchotannic acid (can cause constipation). While quinine is effective for preventing or suppressing malaria caused by susceptible organisms (15), people treated with cinchona bark are exposed to the risks of quinidine, cinchotannic acid, and other alkaloid constituents. It is recommended that only purified quinine, or other appropriate antimalarial agents, be used to prevent or suppress malaria (15). US drug regulations require products containing cinchona derivatives to contain the labeling, "Discontinue use if ringing in the ears, deafness, skin rash or visual disturbances occur" (12).

CINNAMON bark

This Product is Also Known As

Batavia Cassia, Batavia Cinnamon, Ceylon Cinnamon, Padang-Cassia, Panang Cinnamon, Saigon Cassia, Saigon Cinnamon.
CAUTION: See separate listings for Cassia and Cinnamon flower.

Scientific Names

Cinnamomum verum, synonym Cinnamomum zeylanicum.
Family: Lauraceae.

People Use This For

Orally, cinnamon bark is used as an antispasmodic, antiflatulent, appetite stimulant (2,4), antidiarrheal, antimicrobial, antihelmintic, and for treating the common cold and influenza (4).
Topically, cinnamon bark is used as part of a multi-ingredient preparation for treating premature ejaculation (2537). Historically, cinnamon bark has been used for GI upset and dysmenorrhea (6).
For food uses, cinnamon is commonly consumed as a spice in food and a flavoring agent in beverages (11).
In manufacturing, the volatile oil is commonly used in small amounts in toothpaste, mouthwashes, gargles, lotions, liniments, soaps, detergents, and other pharmaceutical products and cosmetics.

Safety

LIKELY SAFE ...when consumed in amounts commonly found in foods (11). Cinnamon bark has Generally Recognized as Safe (GRAS) status in the US (11).
POSSIBLY SAFE ...when used orally and appropriately in amounts slightly greater than those found in foods (4,12). ...when used topically, short-term as part of a multi-ingredient preparation (SS Cream). This preparation was used safely in a clinical trial where the cream was applied and left on the glans penis for 1-hour (2537). Further evaluation is needed to determine its safety after prolonged, repetitive use.
POSSIBLY UNSAFE ...when used orally in large amounts or long-term (4,12). Consumption of up to 700 mcg per kilogram of the constituent, cinnamaldehyde, is considered the highest acceptable level (4).
PREGNANCY: LIKELY UNSAFE ...contraindicated for oral use in amounts greater than those found in foods (4,12).
LACTATION: Insufficient reliable information available; avoid using amounts greater than found in foods.

Effectiveness

POSSIBLY EFFECTIVE ...when taken orally as an antiflatulent, antispasmodic, and appetite stimulant (2,4). ...when used topically as part of a multi-ingredient preparation for treating premature ejaculation. In one controlled clinical trial, a multi-ingredient cream preparation containing Panax ginseng root, Angelica root, Cistanches deserticola, Zanthoxyl species, Torlidis seed, clove flower, Asiasari root, cinnamon bark, and toad venom (SS Cream) was applied to the glans penis 1-hour prior to intercourse and washed off immediately before intercourse. Men suffering from premature ejaculation who were treated with the cream had significantly improved ejaculatory latency compared to placebo (2537).
There is insufficient reliable information available about the effectiveness of cinnamon bark for its other uses.

Possible Mechanism of Action & Active Ingredients

The volatile oil of cinnamon is responsible for the antispasmodic, antiflatulent, and appetite stimulant effects (4). The constituent cinnamaldehyde is a CNS stimulant at low doses and a sedative at high doses. It also has hypothermic, antipyretic, antibacterial, and antifungal activity. It also increases peripheral blood flow, slows the heart rate, reduces blood pressure, and increases the blood sugar level (4). The astringent properties of the tannin constituents are responsible for the antidiarrheal effect (4). Cinnamon bark is also a urinary irritant (19). The multi-ingredient preparation containing cinnamon bark is thought to work in premature ejaculation by increasing the penile vibratory threshold and reducing the amplitude of penile somatosensory evoked potentials (2537).

Adverse Reactions Including Known Allergies

Orally, no adverse reactions tend to occur with the use of the cinnamon bark; however, the oil can irritate mucous membranes and is a skin irritant and sensitizer. Topical preparations in concentrations greater than 0.01% may cause allergic dermatitis in sensitive individuals (4). When the multi-ingredient cream preparation (SS Cream) has been applied topically to the glans penis, sporadic erectile dysfunction, excessively delayed ejaculation, mild pain, and local irritation and burning has occurred (2537).

Possible Interactions with Herbs & Other Dietary Supplements
Insufficient reliable information available.

Possible Interactions with Drugs
ACID-INHIBITING DRUGS: Theoretically, due to claims that cinnamon increases stomach acid, it might interfere with antacids, sucralfate (Carafate), H-2 antagonists, or proton pump inhibitors (19).

Possible Interactions with Foods
No interactions are known to occur, and there is no known reason to expect a clinically significant interaction with cinnamon bark.

Possible Interactions with Lab Tests
No interactions are known to occur, and there is no known reason to expect a clinically significant interaction with cinnamon bark.

Possible Interactions with Diseases or Conditions
GI CONDITIONS: Cinnamon bark can irritate the gastrointestinal tract. Contraindicated in individuals with infectious or inflammatory gastrointestinal conditions (19).
CINNAMON OR PERU BALSAM ALLERGY: Contraindicated due to potential cross-allergenicity (2).

Typical Dosages & Routes of Administration that are Commonly Used
ORAL: The typical dose of cinnamon is one cup of the tea three times daily (4). The tea is prepared by steeping 0.5-1 grams of the bark in 150 mL boiling water for 5-10 minutes and then straining. The maximum dose of cinnamon is 2-4 grams of the bark or 0.05-0.2 grams of the essential oil per day (12). The usual dose of the liquid extract (1:1 in 70% alcohol) is 0.51 mL three times daily (4).

Comments
Avoid confusion with Chinese cinnamon (cassia). Cinnamon has been used as a recreational drug by youth (214).

CINNAMON flower

This Product is Also Known As
Cinnamon Flos, Zimblúten.
CAUTION: See separate listings for Cinnamon bark and Cassia.

Scientific Names
Cinnamomum aromaticum, synonym Cinnamomum cassia.
Family: Lauraceae.

People Use This For
Orally, cinnamon flower is used as a blood purifier.
Historically, cinnamon flower has been used to remove undesirable agents from the blood.
Cinnamon flower is also a flavoring agent (2).

Safety
LIKELY SAFE ...when consumed in amounts commonly found in food (2).
There is insufficient reliable information available about the safety of medicinal uses of cinnamon flower.
PREGNANCY AND LACTATION: Insufficient reliable information available; avoid amounts greater than those used in foods.

Effectiveness
There is insufficient reliable information available about the effectiveness of cinnamon flower.

Possible Mechanism of Action & Active Ingredients
Insufficient reliable information available.

Adverse Reactions Including Known Allergies
Cinnamon flower can cause allergic reactions with skin and mucous membrane contact in people who are sensitive to cinnamon (2).

Possible Interactions with Herbs & Other Dietary Supplements
Insufficient reliable information available.

Possible Interactions with Drugs
No interactions are known to occur, and there is no known reason to expect a clinically significant interaction with cinnamon flower.

Possible Interactions with Foods

No interactions are known to occur, and there is no known reason to expect a clinically significant interaction with cinnamon flower.

Possible Interactions with Lab Tests

No interactions are known to occur, and there is no known reason to expect a clinically significant interaction with cinnamon flower.

Possible Interactions with Diseases or Conditions

No interactions are known to occur, and there is no known reason to expect a clinically significant interaction with cinnamon flower.

Typical Dosages & Routes of Administration that are Commonly Used

No typical dosage.

Comments

None.

CITRONELLA OIL

This Product is Also Known As

None.
CAUTION: See separate listings for Lemongrass and Stone Root.

Scientific Names

Cymbopogon nardus, synonym Andropogon nardus; Cymbopogon winterianus.
Family: Graminaea or Poaceae.

People Use This For

Topically, citronella oil is used as an insect repellent for people and pets (11).
Historically, citronella oil has been used orally as a vermifuge, diuretic, antispasmodic (6), and digestive stimulant (11).
In foods and beverages, citronella oil is used as a flavoring (11).
In manufacturing, citronella oil is used as a fragrance in cosmetics and soaps (110).

Safety

LIKELY SAFE ...when used orally in amounts found in foods. It has Generally Recognized as Safe (GRAS) status in the US (11). The maximum use level is 0.005% (11).
LIKELY UNSAFE ...when taken orally in large amounts (6,11). ...when inhaled. There have been reports of toxic alveolitis (2).
CHILDREN: LIKELY UNSAFE ...when used orally. There are reports of poisoning in children and one toddler died after ingesting insect repellent that contained citronella oil (2,6,17).
PREGNANCY AND LACTATION: Insufficient reliable information available; avoid using.

Effectiveness

There is insufficient reliable information available about the effectiveness of citronella oil (2).

Possible Mechanism of Action & Active Ingredients

Insufficient reliable information available.

Adverse Reactions Including Known Allergies

There has been at least one report of death following ingestion of insect repellent containing citronella oil (2).
Topical use has caused contact dermatitis (6,11). Inhalation has caused toxic alveolitis (2).

Possible Interactions with Herbs & Other Dietary Supplements

Insufficient reliable information available.

Possible Interactions with Drugs

No interactions are known to occur, and there is no known reason to expect a clinically significant interaction with citronella oil.

Possible Interactions with Foods

No interactions are known to occur, and there is no known reason to expect a clinically significant interaction with citronella oil.

Possible Interactions with Lab Tests

No interactions are known to occur, and there is no known reason to expect a clinically significant interaction with citronella oil.

Possible Interactions with Diseases or Conditions

No interactions are known to occur, and there is no known reason to expect a clinically significant interaction with citronella oil.

Typical Dosages & Routes of Administration that are Commonly Used

No typical dosage.

Comments

Avoid confusion with lemongrass (Cymbopogon citratus). Citronella oil is the essential oil produced by steam distillation of lemongrass (Cymbopogon species), Ceylon or Lenabatu citronella oil (Cymbopogon nardus), Java or Maha Pengiri citronella oil (Cymbopogon winterianus).

CIVET

This Product is Also Known As

African Civet, Large Indian Civet, Zibeth.

Scientific Names

African Civet; Viverra civetta, synonym Civettictis civetta; Indian Civet; Viverra zibetha.
Family: Viverridae.

People Use This For

In Chinese medicine, civet is used for pain relief, and as a sedative [11].
In foods and beverages, civet is used as a flavoring agent [11].
In cosmetics, it is used as a fixative and fragrance component of perfumes, cosmetics, and soaps [11].

Safety

LIKELY SAFE ...when used in amounts found in foods (maximum use level less than 0.0014%) [11]; Generally Recognized as Safe (GRAS) status in the US [11].
There is insufficient reliable information available about the safety of the use of civet in amounts larger than those found in foods.
PREGNANCY AND LACTATION: Insufficient reliable information available; avoid using.

Effectiveness

There is insufficient reliable information available about the effectiveness of civet.

Possible Mechanism of Action & Active Ingredients

The applicable part of civet is the secretion. There is insufficient reliable information available about the possible mechanism of action and active ingredients.

Adverse Reactions Including Known Allergies

Reportedly nontoxic [11].

Possible Interactions with Herbs & Other Dietary Supplements

Insufficient reliable information available.

Possible Interactions with Drugs

No interactions are known to occur, and there is no known reason to expect a clinically significant interaction with civet.

Possible Interactions with Foods

No interactions are known to occur, and there is no known reason to expect a clinically significant interaction with civet.

Possible Interactions with Lab Tests

No interactions are known to occur, and there is no known reason to expect a clinically significant interaction with civet.

Possible Interactions with Diseases or Conditions

No interactions are known to occur, and there is no known reason to expect a clinically significant interaction with civet.

Typical Dosages & Routes of Administration that are Commonly Used

No typical dosage.

Comments
Reportedly, crude civet is frequently adulterated (11).
There is very little scientific information about this product. Our staff is continually analyzing the available information on natural medicines and will add data here as it becomes available.

CLARY SAGE

This Product is Also Known As
Clary, Clary Wort, Clear Eye, Eyebright, Muscatel Sage, See Bright.
CAUTION: See separate listings for Sage and Eyebright.

Scientific Names
Salvia sclarea.
Family: Lamiaceae/Labiatae.

People Use This For
Orally, clary sage is used for upset stomach, digestive disorders, and kidney diseases (11,400).
Topically, clary sage mucilage is used to remove foreign objects from the eye, to remove thorns and splinters from the skin, and for treating tumors (11,400).
In foods and beverages, the oil from clary sage is used as a flavoring agent (11).
In manufacturing, the oil from clary sage is used as a fragrance in soaps and cosmetics (11).

Safety
LIKELY SAFE ...when used orally in amounts found in beverages and food products; maximal use level is 0.016% of oil in alcoholic beverages.
There is insufficient reliable information available about the safety of medicinal uses of clary sage.
PREGNANCY AND LACTATION: Insufficient reliable information available; avoid using.

Effectiveness
There is insufficient reliable information available about the effectiveness of clary sage.

Possible Mechanism of Action & Active Ingredients
The applicable parts of clary sage are the flowering top and leaf. The oil has some anticonvulsant activity in animals (11), and it seems to potentiate the effects of hexobarbitone and chloral hydrate (11). The mucilaginous and sticky solution is thought to be able to pull objects from under the eyelid and from the skin (400).

Adverse Reactions Including Known Allergies
None reported.

Possible Interactions with Herbs & Other Dietary Supplements
Insufficient reliable information available.

Possible Interactions with Drugs
CHLORAL HYDRATE, HEXOBARBITONE: Reportedly potentiates narcotic effects (9,11).

Possible Interactions with Foods
No interactions are known to occur, and there is no known reason to expect a clinically significant interaction with clary sage.

Possible Interactions with Lab Tests
No interactions are known to occur, and there is no known reason to expect a clinically significant interaction with clary sage.

Possible Interactions with Diseases or Conditions
No interactions are known to occur, and there is no known reason to expect a clinically significant interaction with clary sage.

Typical Dosages & Routes of Administration that are Commonly Used
No typical dosage.

Comments
Avoid confusion with sage leaf (Salvia officinalis).

CLEMATIS

This Product is Also Known As
Upright Virgin's Bower.
CAUTION: See separate listings for Traveler's Joy and Woodbine.

Scientific Names
Clematis recta.
Family: Ranunculaceae.

People Use This For
Orally, clematis is taken for treatment of rheumatic pains, headaches, and varicose veins (18).
Traditionally, clematis was used to treat syphilis, gout, rheumatism, bone disorders, chronic skin conditions, and used as a diuretic (18). As part of folk medicine, it was used topically for blisters and as a poultice to treat purulent wounds and ulcers (18).

Safety
POSSIBLY UNSAFE ...when the fresh plant is used topically (18).
LIKELY UNSAFE ...when the fresh plant is taken orally because it is severely irritating to mucous membranes and the gastrointestinal tract (18).
There is insufficient reliable information available about the safety of the oral or topical use of dried clematis (4226).
PREGNANCY AND LACTATION: LIKELY UNSAFE ...when the fresh plant is taken orally. There is insufficient reliable information available for the safety of the dried plant; avoid using.

Effectiveness
There is insufficient reliable information available about the effectiveness of clematis.

Possible Mechanism of Action & Active Ingredients
When the fresh plant is crushed or cut into small pieces, the glycoside ranunculin is enzymatically changed into a severely irritating protoanemonin, which, in turn, rapidly degrades into the non-toxic anemonin (18). Both protoanemonin and ranunculin are destroyed to an unknown extent during the drying process (2), and both have fungicidal activity (4). Since Clematis recta contains low levels of protoanemonin-forming agents, the adverse effects and toxicity may not be as severe as compared to other species of Ranunculaceae. Clematis also contains saponins (18).

Adverse Reactions Including Known Allergies
Orally, freshly harvested clematis can cause colic, diarrhea, and severe irritation to the gastrointestinal and urinary tracts (18). After prolonged skin contact, clematis can cause slow-healing blisters and burns(18).

Possible Interactions with Herbs & Other Dietary Supplements
Insufficient reliable information available.

Possible Interactions with Drugs
No interactions are known to occur, and there is no known reason to expect a clinically significant interaction with clematis.

Possible Interactions with Foods
No interactions are known to occur, and there is no known reason to expect a clinically significant interaction with clematis.

Possible Interactions with Lab Tests
No interactions are known to occur, and there is no known reason to expect a clinically significant interaction with clematis.

Possible Interactions with Diseases or Conditions
No interactions are known to occur, and there is no known reason to expect a clinically significant interaction with clematis.

Typical Dosages & Routes of Administration that are Commonly Used
Clematis recta is available orally as drops, extracts, and tea (18). The tea is used for poultices (18).

Comments
Avoid confusion with other Clematis species (6). Clematis recta is considered a poisonous plant and is rarely used today (18). Plants that are grown in the sun have a higher ranunculin content than those grown in the shade, and therefore have stronger effects (18).

CLIVERS

This Product is Also Known As
Barweed, Bedstraw, Catchweed, Cleavers, Cleaverwort, Coachweed, Eriffe, Everlasting Friendship, Gallium, Goosebill, Goose Grass, Goosegrass, Gosling Weed, Grip Grass, Hayriffe, Hayruff, Hedge-Burs, Hedgeheriff, Love-Man, Mutton Chops, Robin-Run-in-the-Grass, Scratchweed, Stick-a-Back, Sweethearts.

Scientific Names
Galium aparine.
Family: Rubiaceae.

People Use This For
Orally, clivers is used as a diuretic, a mild astringent, for dysuria, lymphadenitis, psoriasis, and specifically for enlarged lymph nodes (4).
Topically, clivers is used for ulcers, festering glands, breast lumps, and skin rashes (18).

Safety
POSSIBLY SAFE ...when used orally and appropriately (12). There is no documented toxicity (4).
There is insufficient reliable information available about the safety of the topical use of clivers.
PREGNANCY AND LACTATION: Insufficient reliable information available; avoid using.

Effectiveness
There is insufficient reliable information available about the effectiveness of clivers.

Possible Mechanism of Action & Active Ingredients
The applicable parts of clivers are the dried or fresh above ground parts. Contains tannins, which are reported to have astringent properties (4).

Adverse Reactions Including Known Allergies
None reported (4).

Possible Interactions with Herbs & Other Dietary Supplements
Insufficient reliable information available.

Possible Interactions with Drugs
No interactions are known to occur, and there is no known reason to expect a clinically significant interaction with clivers.

Possible Interactions with Foods
No interactions are known to occur, and there is no known reason to expect a clinically significant interaction with clivers.

Possible Interactions with Lab Tests
No interactions are known to occur, and there is no known reason to expect a clinically significant interaction with clivers.

Possible Interactions with Diseases or Conditions
DIABETES: Use expressed juice with caution (4).

Typical Dosages & Routes of Administration that are Commonly Used
ORAL: 2-4 grams dried above ground parts three times daily, or one cup tea (steep 2-4 grams herb in 150 mL boiling water 5-10 minutes, strain) three times daily (4). Liquid extract (1:1 in 25% alcohol) 2-4 mL three times daily (4). Expressed juice, 3-15 mL three times daily (4).
TOPICAL: No typical dosage.

Comments
None.

CLOVE dried flowerbud, leaf, stem

This Product is Also Known As
Caryophylli, Caryophyllus, Clous de Girolfe, Cloves, Flores Caryophyllum, Gewurznelken Nagelein.
CAUTION: See separate listing for Clove Oil.

Scientific Names
Syzygium aromaticum, synonyms Caryophyllus aromaticus, Eugenia aromatica, Eugenia caryophyllata, Eugenia caryophyllus.
Family: Myrtaceae.

People Use This For

Topically, clove is used for toothache, as a counterirritant (4), and for mouth and throat inflammation (2,8). It is also used topically as part of a multi-ingredient preparation for treating premature ejaculation (2537).

Traditionally, clove has been used for flatulence, nausea, vomiting (4,11), and as an expectorant (6). It is also smoked as a component of clove cigarettes (6,17).

In manufacturing, clove is used as a flavoring in foods, beverages, and cigarettes (6,11).

Safety

LIKELY SAFE ...when consumed in amounts commonly found in foods (11). Clove has Generally Recognized as Safe (GRAS) status for food use in the US (11).

POSSIBLY SAFE ...when taken orally and appropriately for medicinal purposes (12). ...when used topically, short-term as part of a multi-ingredient preparation (SS Cream). This preparation was used safely for premature ejaculation in a clinical trial where the cream was applied and left on the glans penis for 1-hour (2537). Further evaluation is needed to determine its safety after prolonged, repetitive use.

LIKELY UNSAFE ...when inhaled due to its harmful effects. Smoking the clove cigarettes can cause respiratory injury (17). Clove cigarettes contain more tar, nicotine, and carbon monoxide than tobacco cigarettes (6,17).

There is insufficient reliable information available about the safety of cloves for its other uses.

PREGNANCY AND LACTATION: POSSIBLY SAFE ...when taken orally in the amounts found in foods. Avoid amounts that greatly exceed those in foods (4).

Effectiveness

POSSIBLY EFFECTIVE ...when used topically as part of a multi-ingredient preparation for treating premature ejaculation. In one controlled clinical trial, a multi-ingredient cream preparation containing Panax ginseng root, Angelica root, Cistanches deserticola, Zanthoxyl species, Torlidis seed, clove flower, Asiasari root, cinnamon bark, and toad venom (SS Cream) was applied to the glans penis 1-hour prior to intercourse and washed off immediately before intercourse. Men suffering from premature ejaculation who were treated with the cream had significantly improved ejaculatory latency compared to placebo (2537).

There is insufficient reliable information available about the effectiveness of cloves for its other uses.

Possible Mechanism of Action & Active Ingredients

Cloves contain a volatile oil that can be up to 90% eugenol (11). The mild anesthetic and analgesic properties of clove are attributed to eugenol (4,512). Applied topically, eugenol depresses sensory receptors involved in pain perception by inhibiting prostaglandin biosynthesis (512). Eugenol inhibits platelet activity (4). Some evidence suggests the sesquiterpene constituents might have anticancer activity (838). Other evidence suggests whole cloves might have chemoprotective activity against liver and bone marrow toxicity (6). The multi-ingredient preparation containing clove flower is thought to work in premature ejaculation by increasing the penile vibratory threshold and reducing the amplitude of penile somatosensory evoked potentials (2537).

Adverse Reactions Including Known Allergies

The inhalation of cloves can cause respiratory injury including hemoptysis, bronchospasm, hemorrhagic and nonhemorrhagic pulmonary edema, pleural effusion, respiratory insufficiency, respiratory infection, and aspiration of foreign material. There have been two deaths associated with the smoking of the clove cigarettes (17). Used topically on the oral mucosa, it can cause oral tissue sensitivity, local tissue irritation, and damage to dental pulp or the supporting periodontium (214). When the multi-ingredient cream preparation containing clove flower (SS Cream) has been applied topically to the glans penis, sporadic erectile dysfunction, excessively delayed ejaculation, mild pain, and local irritation and burning has occurred (2537).

Possible Interactions with Herbs & Other Dietary Supplements

HERBS WITH ANTICOAGULANT/ANTIPLATELET POTENTIAL: Concomitant use of herbs that have coumarin constituents or affect platelet aggregation could theoretically increase the risk of bleeding in some people. These herbs include: angelica, anise, arnica, asafoetida, bogbean, boldo, capsicum, celery, chamomile, danshen, fenugreek, feverfew, garlic, ginger, ginkgo, ginseng (Panax), horse chestnut, horseradish, licorice, meadowsweet, prickly ash, onion, papain, passionflower, poplar, quassia, red clover, turmeric, wild carrot, wild lettuce, willow, and others (4,19).

Possible Interactions with Drugs

ANTICOAGULANTS AND ANTIPLATELET DRUGS: Theoretically, clove can potentiate the effects of these drugs.

Possible Interactions with Foods

No interactions are known to occur, and there is no known reason to expect a clinically significant interaction with clove dried flowerbud, leaf, and stem.

Possible Interactions with Lab Tests

No interactions are known to occur, and there is no known reason to expect a clinically significant interaction with clove dried flowerbud, leaf, and stem.

Possible Interactions with Diseases or Conditions

No interactions are known to occur, and there is no known reason to expect a clinically significant interaction with clove dried flowerbud, leaf, and stem.

Typical Dosages & Routes of Administration that are Commonly Used

ORAL: A typical dose of cloves is 120-300 mg (4). Limit clove ingestion to the equivalent of 3.6 mg/kg clove oil per day (4). The buds yield 15-18% volatile oil, The stems yield 4-6% (11).
TOPICAL: Clove is commonly used as a mouthwash, and products usually contain 1-5% clove essential oil (8). A 15% clove tincture can be effective in treating athletes foot (4).

Comments

Clove cigarettes, also called kreteks, generally contain 60% tobacco and 40% ground clove (6). Eugenol in clove cigarettes acts as a topical anesthetic to the posterior oropharynx. It reduces the noxious elements of smoking and can facilitate learning of smoking techniques (17).

CLOVE OIL

This Product is Also Known As

Caryophyllum, Caryophyllus, Clous de Girolfe, Flores Caryophylli, Gewurznelken Nagelein, Oil of Clove.
CAUTION: See separate listing for Clove.

Scientific Names

Syzygium aromaticum, synonyms Caryophyllus aromaticus, Eugenia aromatica, Eugenia caryophyllata, Eugenia caryophyllus.
Family: Myrtaceae.

People Use This For

Orally, clove oil is used as an antiemetic (11) and antiflatulent (4).
In Chinese medicine, clove oil is used to manage diarrhea, hernia, and halitosis (11).
In dentistry, clove oil is used topically for toothache (11), as a dental anesthetic (2), for treating postextraction alveolitis (dry socket) (11), and for mouth and throat inflammation (2,8). It is sometimes used as a counterirritant (272). It is also used a component in dental cements and fillings (11).
In foods and beverages, clove oil is used as a flavoring (11).
In manufacturing, clove oil is used for fragrance in toothpaste, soaps, cosmetics, and perfumes (11).

Safety

LIKELY SAFE ...when taken orally in amounts found in foods (11). It has Generally Recognized as Safe (GRAS) status in the US (11).
POSSIBLY SAFE ...when applied topically (272,512). Should not be used for self-medication, especially when undiluted. Repeated application can cause gingival damage, skin and mucous membrane irritation (4,272).
LIKELY UNSAFE ...when taken orally undiluted. 5-15 mL may induce high anion gap acidosis, seizures, coagulopathy, acute liver damage, behavioral changes, and coma (17).
PREGNANCY AND LACTATION: LIKELY UNSAFE ...when used orally and undiluted; avoid in amounts greater than those found in foods (4).

Effectiveness

POSSIBLY EFFECTIVE ...when applied topically as a dental analgesic (2,512), for mouth and throat mucosal inflammation, and for post-extraction alveolitis (dry socket) (6).
There is insufficient reliable information available about the effectiveness of clove oil for its other uses (272).

Possible Mechanism of Action & Active Ingredients

Researchers attribute mild anesthetic and analgesic properties of clove to eugenol (3,4). On contact, eugenol acts to depress sensory receptors involved in pain perception by a profound inhibition of prostaglandin biosynthesis (3). It is also a powerful inhibitor of platelet activity (6). Clove bud oil contains 60-90% eugenol, clove leaf oil contains 82-88% eugenol, clove stem oil contains 90-95% eugenol (11). Clove oil has antihistaminic and antispasmodic properties, most likely due to eugenyl acetate (6). Clove oil inhibits gram-positive and gram-negative bacteria. It also has fungistatic action, antihelmintic and larvicidal properties. One report suggests it suppresses aflatoxin production (6). Another suggests eugenol from clove oil may counter some effects of environmental mutagens found in foods (6).

Adverse Reactions Including Known Allergies

Oral use of clove oil can cause nervous system depression, seizures, lactic acidosis, disseminated intravascular coagulation, hepatic dysfunction (17), and irritation to mucosal tissues (2,4,6,512). This is one report of disseminated intravascular coagulation and liver failure following clove ingestion by a two-year-old (6). There is one report of depression and electrolyte imbalance following accidental ingestion by a seven-month-old (6). Topical use of clove oil can be irritating to mucosal tissues and skin (2,4,6,512). There is one report of permanent local facial anesthesia and absence of sweating after clove spilled on an individual's face (6). Used topically to the oral mucosa, it can cause oral tissue sensitivity, local tissue irritation, and damage to dental pulp or the supporting periodontium (214).

Possible Interactions with Herbs & Other Dietary Supplements
HERBS WITH ANTICOAGULANT/ANTIPLATELET POTENTIAL: Concomitant use of herbs that have coumarin constituents or affect platelet aggregation could theoretically increase the risk of bleeding in some people. These herbs include: angelica, anise, arnica, asafoetida, bogbean, boldo, capsicum, celery, chamomile, clove, danshen, fenugreek, feverfew, garlic, ginger, ginkgo, ginseng (Panax), horse chestnut, horseradish, licorice, meadowsweet, prickly ash, onion, papain, passionflower, poplar, quassia, red clover, turmeric, wild carrot, wild lettuce, willow, and others (4,19).

Possible Interactions with Drugs
ANTICOAGULANT/ANTIPLATELET DRUGS: Theoretically, concomitant use may enhance antiplatelet or anticoagulant effects and adverse effects, due to eugenol content of clove oil (6).

Possible Interactions with Foods
No interactions are known to occur, and there is no known reason to expect a clinically significant interaction with clove oil.

Possible Interactions with Lab Tests
No interactions are known to occur, and there is no known reason to expect a clinically significant interaction with clove oil.

Possible Interactions with Diseases or Conditions
PLATELET ABNORMALITIES: Theoretically, clove oil is contraindicated in people with reduced platelet counts or platelet function abnormalities (6).

Typical Dosages & Routes of Administration that are Commonly Used
ORAL: Dosages for products containing clove oil vary. These dosages can be 5-30 drops of the fluid extract, 1-5 drops of the oil extract, and 1/2-1 ounce of a mouth rinse containing clove oil (6002).
TOPICAL: As mouthwash, products equivalent to 1-5% clove essential oil (8).

Comments
Undiluted clove oil is unsafe for self-use, requires application by a trained professional (512). Clove bud oil is considered more valuable than clove leaf and clove stem oils (11). Clove oil is obtained by distillation of the bud, leaf, or stem of the Clove Tree (Syzygium aromaticum).

CLUB MOSS

This Product is Also Known As
Stags Horn, Vegetable Sulfur, Witch Meal, Wolfs Claw.

Scientific Names
Lycopodium clavatum.
Family: Lycopodiaceae.

People Use This For
In folk medicine, club moss is used orally for bladder and kidney disorders, and as a diuretic (18).

Safety
POSSIBLY UNSAFE …when the spores or fresh plant are used orally. Club moss contains toxic alkaloids but no poisonings are reported (18).
PREGNANCY AND LACTATION: POSSIBLY UNSAFE …when used orally; avoid using.

Effectiveness
There is insufficient reliable information available about the effectiveness of club moss.

Possible Mechanism of Action & Active Ingredients
The applicable parts of club moss are the plant and spores. Club moss contains potentially toxic alkaloids, including lycopodine, dihydrolycopodine and traces of nicotine (18).

Adverse Reactions Including Known Allergies
None reported.

Possible Interactions with Herbs & Other Dietary Supplements
Insufficient reliable information available.

© Copyright 2000, Natural Medicines Comprehensive Database (209) 472-2244. For updated data, go to www.NaturalDatabase.com

Possible Interactions with Drugs

No interactions are known to occur, and there is no known reason to expect a clinically significant interaction with club moss.

Possible Interactions with Foods

No interactions are known to occur, and there is no known reason to expect a clinically significant interaction with club moss.

Possible Interactions with Lab Tests

No interactions are known to occur, and there is no known reason to expect a clinically significant interaction with club moss.

Possible Interactions with Diseases or Conditions

No interactions are known to occur, and there is no known reason to expect a clinically significant interaction with club moss.

Typical Dosages & Routes of Administration that are Commonly Used

No typical dosage.

Comments

Don't let your patients confuse club moss and Chinese club moss. Only Chinese club moss contains huperzine A.

COCA

This Product is Also Known As

Bolivian Coca, Cocaine Plant, Huanuco Coca, Java Coca, Peruvian Coca, Spadic, Truxillo Coca.
CAUTION: See separate listing for Cocoa.

Scientific Names

Erythroxylum coca, synonym Erythroxylon coca; Erythroxylum novogranatense.
Family: Erythroxylaceae.

People Use This For

Coca leaf is used as the source of cocaine. Cocaine is smoked and snorted for mind-altering effects [17].
Topically, people use the prescription drug cocaine for corneal, nasal, throat mucosa anesthesia, severe ophthalmologic pain, and local vasoconstriction [11,15].
Historically, the coca leaf has been chewed for relief of hunger and fatigue [11]. Leaf extracts have been used to stimulate stomach function, as a sedative, and for treating asthma, colds, and other ailments [11].
In manufacturing, decocainized coca leaf extract is used to flavor cola drinks and food products [11].

Safety

LIKELY SAFE ...when decocainized coca extract is used in amounts found in foods (maximum use level 0.055%). It has Generally Recognized as Safe (GRAS) status in the US. ...when the constituent, cocaine, is used as a FDA-approved product for topical use.
LIKELY UNSAFE ...when the constituent, cocaine, is used as an oral medicinal [17].
UNSAFE ...when the constituent, cocaine, is ingested or inhaled as a recreational drug [17]; 1.2 grams of cocaine can be fatal; 20 mg cocaine can cause severe side effects. Cocaine is a Schedule II controlled substance in the US due to extremely high potential for addiction [17].
PREGNANCY: UNSAFE ...when inhaled or used orally. Coca, and the constituent cocaine, are contraindicated because they can have abortifacient and teratogenic effects [17,6187]. ...when used during pregnancy because it is also associated with a high incidence of Sudden Infant Death Syndrome (SIDS) [17].
LACTATION: UNSAFE ...when used orally, coca and the constituent, cocaine, are contraindicated. Cocaine is excreted into breast milk; cocaine intoxication can occur in infants breast-fed by mothers recently exposed to cocaine [17,18].

Effectiveness

EFFECTIVE ...when the constituent, cocaine, is applied topically for ophthalmologic anesthesia, ophthalmologic pain, topical anesthesia and local vasoconstriction [15]. It is an FDA-approved Schedule C-II drug.
LIKELY EFFECTIVE ...when the constituent, cocaine, is used orally as a stimulant [17]. ...when the constituent, cocaine, is inhaled to cause altered consciousness. The risk of toxicity and potential for addiction are extremely high [17].

Possible Mechanism of Action & Active Ingredients

The applicable part of coca is the leaf. Cocaine, the major alkaloid constituent, has local anesthetic, beta-1, beta-2 and alpha adrenergic stimulating properties [17].

Adverse Reactions Including Known Allergies

Adverse effects initially include euphoria, hyperactivity, and restlessness. Later tremors, hyperreflexia, and seizures develop. Finally, coma, hyporeflexia, respiratory depression, cardiovascular depression and death may occur. In the CNS, cocaine can also cause migraine headaches, stroke, and intracranial and intracerebral hemorrhage (17,5092). Cardiovascular adverse effects include extreme elevations of heart rate and blood pressure, vasoconstriction, myocardial ischemia, myocardial infarction, cardiac arrhythmias, cardiomyopathies, myocarditis, endocarditis, aortic rupture, and diffuse micro-aneurysms (17). Gastrointestinal adverse effects include mesenteric ischemia and malnutrition. Cocaine can cause rhabdomyolysis-induced renal failure (17). Liver adverse effects include hepatic necrosis, and elevation of serum transaminase and serum creatinine phosphokinase liver function tests (17). Metabolic adverse effects include lactic acidosis, hyperthermia, hypoglycemia, and hypoxia (17). Obstetric adverse effects include spontaneous abortion, abruptio placentae, and teratogenicity (17). Fetal exposure to cocaine, a constituent of coca, is associated with impaired auditory information processing in newborns (6187). Psychiatric adverse effects include paranoia, depression, and violence (17). Respiratory adverse effects include exacerbation of asthma, thermal airway injury, adult respiratory distress syndrome, pneumothorax, pneumomediastinum, pulmonary thrombosis, bronchiolitis obliterans, pulmonary edema, pulmonary infiltrates, pulmonary vascular disease, and pulmonary hemorrhage (17). Chronic intranasal cocaine abuse is associated with orbital wall (bone) destruction, acquired nasolacrimal duct obstruction, and orbital cellulitis (1258).

Researchers report that cocaine use is associated with an increased risk of hemorrhagic stroke and increased risk of death caused by stroke. These unpublished research results were presented at the 68th annual scientific meeting of the American Association of Neurological Surgeons (5048).

Researchers report a 30% coronary aneurism rate in patients with a history of cocaine abuse and angina, myocardial infarction, or other coronary events (378). The highest incidence of aneurism previously reported was 5% in a study of patients undergoing coronary bypass surgery (378).

Possible Interactions with Herbs & Other Dietary Supplements

CAPSICUM: Theoretically, concomitant use of coca and capsicum (including exposure to pepper spray which contains capsicum) might increase the effects and risk of adverse effects of the cocaine in coca (1394).
MARIJUANA: Concomitant use can have additive effects, including increased heart rate (17).

Possible Interactions with Drugs

NIFEDIPINE: Nifedipine (Adalat, Procardia) use before cocaine use increases the likelihood of seizures and death (17).
PSEUDOCHOLINESTERASE INHIBITORS: Ingesting organophosphate or carbamate insecticides, echothiophate eye drops (Phospholine Iodine), neostigmine (Prostigmin) or pyridostigmine (Mestinon, Regonol) increases risk of cardiovascular side effects, seizures, death (17).

Possible Interactions with Foods

No interactions are known to occur, and there is no known reason to expect a clinically significant interaction with coca.

Possible Interactions with Lab Tests

No interactions are known to occur, and there is no known reason to expect a clinically significant interaction with coca.

Possible Interactions with Diseases or Conditions

ASTHMA: Cocaine use is associated with more severe exacerbations in people with asthma. One study found exacerbations were more severe among cocaine users, compared to non-users, who presented to an emergency room during an asthma attack (6186).
CARDIOVASCULAR DISORDERS: People with cardiovascular disorders might be at increased risk for cocaine-induced cardiovascular side effects (17).
INTRACEREBRAL HEMORRHAGE: Cocaine use is associated with increased morbidity and mortality in patients who sustain intracerebral hemorrhage (5092).
PLASMA PSEUDOCHOLINESTERASE DEFICIENCY (PPD): People with PPD are at increased risk for cocaine-induced cardiovascular side effects, including seizures and death (17).

Typical Dosages & Routes of Administration that are Commonly Used

No typical dosage.

Comments

Coca is considered unsafe and illegal for self-use. Avoid confusion with Cocoa Seed (Theobroma cacao).

COCILLANA

This Product is Also Known As

Grape Bark, Guapi, Trompillo, Upas.

Scientific Names
Guarea rusbyi, synonym Sycocarpus rusbyi; related Guarea species.
Family: Meliaceae.

People Use This For
Orally, cocillana is used as an ingredient in cough syrups (11).
Traditionally, cocillana was used orally as an expectorant (11). The root bark of Guarea spiciflora was used topically for skin indurations, and the leaf of Guarea trichiloides was used for skin tumors (11).

Safety
There is insufficient reliable information available about the safety of cocillana.
Pregnancy and Lactation: Insufficient reliable information available; avoid using.

Effectiveness
There is insufficient reliable information available about the effectiveness of cocillana.

Possible Mechanism of Action & Active Ingredients
The applicable part of cocillana is the bark. Reported (in the late 1800s) to have expectorant and emetic properties; no recent pharmacological or toxicological data available (11).

Adverse Reactions Including Known Allergies
None reported.

Possible Interactions with Herbs & Other Dietary Supplements
Insufficient reliable information available.

Possible Interactions with Drugs
No interactions are known to occur, and there is no known reason to expect a clinically significant interaction with clocillana.

Possible Interactions with Foods
No interactions are known to occur, and there is no known reason to expect a clinically significant interaction with clocillana.

Possible Interactions with Lab Tests
No interactions are known to occur, and there is no known reason to expect a clinically significant interaction with clocillana.

Possible Interactions with Diseases or Conditions
No interactions are known to occur, and there is no known reason to expect a clinically significant interaction with clocillana.

Typical Dosages & Routes of Administration that are Commonly Used
ORAL: People typically use 0.5 to 1 gram of the powdered bark. In liquid extract form, the dose is 0.5 to 1 mL (5264).

Comments
None.

COCOA

This Product is Also Known As
Cacao, Chocola, Cocoa Bean, Cocoa Oleum, Cocoa Seed, Cocoa Semen, Cocoa Testae, Theobroma.
CAUTION: See separate listing for Coca.

Scientific Names
Theobroma cacao.
Family: Sterculiaceae or Byttneriaceae.

People Use This For
Orally, cocoa seed is used for infectious intestinal diseases and diarrhea (18), asthma, bronchitis, and as an expectorant for lung congestion (11). The seed coat is used for liver, bladder and kidney ailments, diabetes, as a tonic, and as a general remedy (18). Cocoa powder, enriched with flavonoid constituents, is used for prevention of cardiovascular disease (1329).
Topically, cocoa butter has been used to treat wrinkles on the skin and to prevent stretch marks during pregnancy (214).
In foods, cocoa seed is used as a flavoring (6). Chocolate is produced from cocoa powder (214).
In manufacturing, cocoa butter is used as a compounding base for various pharmaceutical preparations (6).

Safety

LIKELY SAFE ...when used orally in amounts found in foods (2,6,3900). ...when used orally in moderate amounts for medicinal purposes (2,6). ...when used topically. Cocoa butter is used extensively as a base for ointments and suppositories and is generally considered safe (11,3900).

POSSIBLY UNSAFE ...when used in large amounts. Due to the caffeine content, when used in excessive doses, significant adverse effects may occur, including tachyarrhythmias and sleep disturbances (18).

PREGNANCY: POSSIBLY SAFE ...when used in moderate amounts or in amounts found in foods. Due to the caffeine content of cocoa preparations, mothers should closely monitor their intake to ensure moderate consumption. Fetal blood concentrations of caffeine approximate maternal concentrations (4260). Caffeine use in pregnancy is controversial; however, moderate consumption has not been associated with adverse fetal effects (6). Some sources suggest keeping caffeine consumption below 200 mg per day (2078). Chocolate products provide 2-35 mg caffeine per serving (2078) and a cup of hot chocolate provides approximately 10 mg (3900).

POSSIBLY UNSAFE ...when used orally in large amounts. Caffeine found in cocoa crosses the placenta producing fetal blood concentrations similar to maternal levels (4260). Although controversial, some evidence suggests that high doses of caffeine might be associated with premature delivery, low birth weight, and loss of the fetus (6). Some sources suggest keeping caffeine consumption below 200 mg per day (2078). Excessive use of cocoa in pregnancy should be avoided.

LACTATION: POSSIBLY SAFE ...when used in moderate amounts or amounts found in foods. Due to the caffeine content of cocoa preparations, mothers should closely monitor their intake to ensure moderate consumption. Breast milk concentrations of caffeine are thought to be approximately 50% of maternal serum concentrations. Moderate consumption of cocoa would likely result in very small amounts of caffeine exposure to a nursing infant (6). POSSIBLY UNSAFE ...when used orally in large amounts. Consumption of excess chocolate (16 oz per day) may can cause irritability and increased bowel activity in the infant (6026). Large doses or excessive intake of cocoa should be avoided during lactation.

Effectiveness

There is insufficient reliable information available about the effectiveness of cocoa.

Possible Mechanism of Action & Active Ingredients

The applicable parts of cocoa are the seed, seed coat, cocoa powder, and butter. Cocoa seed contains oils, tannins, and alkaloids, including theobromine 1-4%, caffeine 0.07-0.36%, trigonelline, and others. Cocoa butter, also referred to as theobroma oil, is the fat obtained from roasted cocoa seeds. It contains oleic acid 37%, stearic acid 34%, palmitic acid 26%, and linoleic acid 2% (13). Cocoa also contains flavonoids, tyramine, phenylethylamine (PEA), magnesium, and possibly N-acylethanolamines (6018,6019). Cocoa has CNS stimulant, cardiac stimulant, coronary dilatory, and diuretic actions (6). Theobromine is the major methylxanthine found in cocoa and has only one-tenth of the cardiac activity of caffeine. In one study, consumption of 1.5 g/kg body weight of chocolate had no acute hemodynamic or physiologic effects on the hearts of healthy, young adults (1373). There has been recent analyses of the health effects of stearic acid, which is found in substantial amounts in cocoa. Unlike other saturated fatty acids, stearic acid does not increase total and low-density lipoprotein (LDL) cholesterol. However, it has been shown that stearic acid can lower high-density lipoprotein (HDL) levels and increases lipoprotein(a). Because of this, the stearic acid content in cocoa products is not thought to provide a reduction in the risk for coronary heart disease as was once proposed (6017,6027). However, preliminary research indicates that flavonoid constituents found in cocoa might be beneficial in cardiovascular disease, much like aspirin. In vitro data has shown that cocoa can stimulate the formation of nitric oxide and inhibit cyclo-oxygenase formation. In a human trial, patients receiving cocoa powder enriched with flavonoids had decreased epinephrine- or ADP-stimulated expression of fibrinogen-binding glycoprotein IIb-IIIa, indicating that it might inhibit platelet aggregation (1329). Dark chocolate contains higher amounts of flavonoids than milk chocolate (6018). Preliminary evidence suggests a defatted-cocoa extract might also prevent arteries from constricting in the presence of cholesterol. This effect might be due to the flavonoids contained in cocoa which are eliminated in the chocolate manufacturing process (see Comments) (5057). It has been suggested that stearic acid might activate coagulation factor VII and impair fibrinolysis (6027). In contrast, one study concluded that diets high in stearic acid do not increase the tendency toward thrombosis (6020). PEA found in cocoa is structurally and pharmacologically similar to catecholamines and amphetamine. PEA may be a modulator of mood. N- acylethanolamines are pharmacologically related to anandamide, which activates cannabinoid receptors in the brain (6019).

Adverse Reactions Including Known Allergies

Orally, cocoa can cause allergic skin reactions (18), shakiness, increased urination, rapid pulse (2,6), constipation (2), and might trigger migraine headaches (18). The cocoa in chocolate can cause nausea, gastrointestinal discomfort, borborygmi, and flatus (1373). Topically, cocoa butter has occassionally caused a rash. In animals, it has been shown to be comedogenic; however, this has not been found in humans (11).

© Copyright 2000, Natural Medicines Comprehensive Database (209) 472-2244. For updated data, go to www.NaturalDatabase.com

Possible Interactions with Herbs & Other Dietary Supplements

CAFFEINE CONTAINING HERBS/SUPPLEMENTS: Concomitant use interacts with the caffeine in cocoa and may increase effects and risk of adverse effects. Natural products that contain caffeine include coffee, tea (black or green), guarana, mate, and cola.

EPHEDRA (ma huang): Concomitant use interacts with the caffeine in cocoa and may potentiate stimulant effects and risk of adverse effects (6).

Possible Interactions with Drugs

ACETAMINOPHEN: Theoretically, concomitant use of large amounts of cocoa might increase acetaminophen effectiveness by up to 40%, due to cocoa's caffeine content (3).

ASPIRIN: Theoretically, concomitant use of large amounts of cocoa might increase aspirin effectiveness by up to 40%, due to cocoa's caffeine content (3).

BARBITURATES: Theoretically, concomitant use might decrease the effects of caffeine found in cocoa. Barbiturates can decrease the effects of caffeine (151).

BETA-ADRENERGIC AGONISTS: Theoretically, concomitant use of large amounts of cocoa might increase cardiac inotropic effects of beta-agonists, due to cocoa's caffeine content (15). Beta-adrenergic agonists include albuterol (Ventolin, Proventil), metaproterenol (Alupent), terbutaline (Brethine, Bricanyl), and isoproterenol (Isuprel).

CIMETIDINE (TAGAMET): Theoretically, concomitant use might increase the effects of caffeine found in cocoa. Cimetidine decreases caffeine clearance by 30-50% (14).

CLOZAPINE (CLOZARIL): Theoretically, co-administration of clozapine and large amounts of cocoa might acutely exacerbate psychotic symptoms, due to cocoa's caffeine content. Caffeine increases the effects and toxicity of clozapine (151). Caffeine doses of 400-1000 mg per day inhibit clozapine metabolism (5051).

DIABETES DRUGS: Concomitant use might interfere with blood glucose control. Cocoa is reported to have hyperglycemic effects (19).

DISULFIRAM (ANTABUSE): Theoretically, concomitant use of disulfiram and large amounts of cocoa might increase the effects of caffeine found in cocoa. Disulfiram reduces caffeine clearance (15).

ERGOTAMINE: Theoretically, concomitant use of ergotamine and large amounts of cocoa might increase the GI absorption of ergotamine, due to cocoa's caffeine content. Caffeine increases the GI absorption of ergotamine (15).

FLUCONAZOLE (Diflucan): Theoretically, concomitant use might increase the effects of caffeine found in cocoa. Fluconazole decreases caffeine metabolism (19).

LITHIUM: Theoretically, abrupt withdrawal of large amounts of cocoa might cause lithium toxicity, due to cocoa's caffeine content. Abrupt caffeine withdrawal reportedly increases serum lithium levels (609).

MONOAMINE OXIDASE INHIBITORS (MAOIs): Theoretically, concomitant use of MAOIs with large amounts of cocoa might precipitate a hypertensive crisis due to cocoa's tyramine content (19).

MEXILETINE (Mexitil): Theoretically, concomitant use might increase the effects of caffeine found in cocoa. Mexiletine reduces caffeine elimination by 30-50% (506).

ORAL CONTRACEPTIVES: Theoretically, concomitant use might increase the effects of caffeine found in cocoa. Oral contraceptives reduce caffeine clearance by 40-65% (14).

PHENYLPROPANOLAMINE (Propagest, Rhindecon): Theoretically, concomitant use might increase the effects of caffeine found in cocoa. Phenylpropanolamine might increase serum caffeine concentrations (506).

QUINOLONES: Theoretically, concomitant use might increase the effects of caffeine found in cocoa. Quinolones decrease caffeine clearance (606,607,608). Quinolones (fluoroquinolones) include ciprofloxacin (Cipro), enoxacin (Penetrex), norfloxacin (Chibroxin, Noroxin), sparfloxacin (Zagam), trovafloxacin (Trovan), and grepafloxacin (Raxar).

THEOPHYLLINE: Theoretically, concomitant use of theophylline and large amounts of cocoa might increase the risk of theophylline toxicity, due to cocoa's caffeine content. Caffeine decreases theophylline clearance 23-29% (506).

VERAPAMIL (Calan, Covera-HS, Isoptin, Verelan): Theoretically, concomitant use might increase the effects of caffeine found of cocoa. Verapamil can increase plasma caffeine levels by 25% (14).

Possible Interactions with Foods

GRAPEFRUIT JUICE: Theoretically, concomitant use might increase the caffeine effects of cocoa. Grapefruit might decrease caffeine clearance (4300).

Possible Interactions with Lab Tests

BLEEDING TIME: Theoretically, large amounts of cocoa might prolong bleeding time and increase test results, due to its caffeine content (1701).

BLOOD PRESSURE: Theoretically, large amounts of cocoa might increase blood pressure and blood pressure readings, due to its caffeine content (4).

URATE: Theoretically, large amounts of cocoa might falsely increase serum urate test results determined by the Bittner method, due to its caffeine content. Caffeine causes false elevations in serum urate test results determined by the Bittner method (15).

CATECHOLAMINES: Theoretically, large amounts of cocoa might increase urine catecholamine concentrations and test results, due to its caffeine content. Caffeine can increase urine catecholamine concentrations (15).

CREATINE: Theoretically, large amounts of cocoa might increase urine creatine concentrations and test results, due to its caffeine content (1701).

5-HYDROXYINDOLEACETIC ACID: Theoretically, large amounts of cocoa might increase urine 5-hydroxyindoleacetic acid concentrations and test results, due to its caffeine content. Caffeine can increase urine catecholamine concentrations (15).

VANILLYLMANDELIC ACID (VMA): Theoretically, large amounts of cocoa might increase urine VMA concentrations and test results, due to its caffeine content. Caffeine can increase urine VMA concentrations (15).

Possible Interactions with Diseases or Conditions

ANXIETY: Theoretically, large amounts of cocoa might aggravate anxiety disorders, due to its caffeine content (506).

DEPRESSION: Theoretically, large amounts of cocoa might aggravate depression disorders, due to its caffeine content (506).

GASTRIC ULCERS, DUODENAL ULCERS: Theoretically, large amounts of cocoa might aggravate ulcers, due to its caffeine content (506).

GASTROESOPHAGEAL REFLUX DISEASE (GERD): Avoid cocoa which reduces lower esophageal sphincter pressure (1374).

HEART CONDITIONS: Theoretically, large amounts of cocoa might induce cardiac arrhythmias in sensitive individuals, due to its caffeine content (506). Limit amount ingested; avoid excessive amounts (2).

IRRITABLE BOWEL SYNDROME: Avoid cocoa-containing products including chocolate which might aggravate irritable bowel syndrome (6).

MIGRAINE HEADACHES: Theoretically, cocoa might trigger migraines in sensitive individuals (2).

Typical Dosages & Routes of Administration that are Commonly Used
No typical dosage.

Comments
Avoid confusion with coca leaf (Erythroxylon coca). Bitter chocolate is produced by pressing roasted cocoa kernels between hot rollers. Cocoa powder is produced by expressing the cocoa butter from bitter chocolate and powdering the remaining residue. Sweet chocolate is produced by adding sugar and vanilla to bitter chocolate (13).

The candy company, Mars, Inc., plans to seek a health claim for chocolate from the Food and Drug Administration in the next few years based on preliminary research they sponsored regarding the potential role of cocoa flavonoids in cardiovascular health (1329).

CODONOPSIS

This Product is Also Known As
Bastard Ginseng, Bellflower, Bonnet Bellflower, Dangshen, Radix Codonopsis.
CAUTION: See separate listings for Ginseng American, Blue Cohosh, Canaigre, Ginseng Siberian, Ginseng Panax, and Withania.

Scientific Names
Codonopsis pilosula; Codonopsis pilosula modesta; Codonopsis tangsheng; Codonopsis tubulosa; other Codonopsis species.
Family: Campanulaceae.

People Use This For
Codonopsis is used to treat HIV infection (1510) and as a protective adjuvant to radiotherapy in cancer treatment (1509).
Codonopsis has been studied as a component of an herbal mixture for minimal brain dysfunction (1508).
In Chinese medicine, codonopsis is used as a substitute for ginseng; in tonic formulas; to stimulate the immune system and replenish qi (Chi, vital energy); and for weakness, anorexia, chronic diarrhea, dyspnea, palpitations, asthma, cough, thirst, diabetes, and spleen and blood deficiencies (11).

Safety
POSSIBLY SAFE ...when used orally and appropriately (12).
PREGNANCY AND LACTATION: Insufficient reliable information available; avoid using.

Effectiveness
There is insufficient reliable information available about the effectiveness of codonopsis.

Possible Mechanism of Action & Active Ingredients
Codonopsis seems to be able to stimulate the central nervous system. It seems to promote weight gain, increase endurance, increase tolerance to anoxia, elevate temperature, increase macrophage activity, increase red and white blood cell counts, promote peripheral vasodilation (11). Codonopsis also has hypotensive, adrenergic blocking, radioprotective and ulcer-protective effects (11).

Adverse Reactions Including Known Allergies
None reported.

Possible Interactions with Herbs & Other Dietary Supplements
Insufficient reliable information available.

Possible Interactions with Drugs
No interactions are known to occur, and there is no known reason to expect a clinically significant interaction with codonopsis.

Possible Interactions with Foods
No interactions are known to occur, and there is no known reason to expect a clinically significant interaction with codonopsis.

Possible Interactions with Lab Tests
No interactions are known to occur, and there is no known reason to expect a clinically significant interaction with codonopsis.

Possible Interactions with Diseases or Conditions
No interactions are known to occur, and there is no known reason to expect a clinically significant interaction with codonopsis.

Typical Dosages & Routes of Administration that are Commonly Used
ORAL: People typically use 12 to 15 grams codonopsis added to 3 to 4 cups water and boiled until the volume is reduced by one-half. The cooled liquid is taken in 2 doses on an empty stomach (5251).

Comments
No ginseng saponins have been found in codonopsis (11).

COENZYME Q-10

This Product is Also Known As
Co-Enzyme Q10, Coenzyme Q10, CoQ10, Co-Q10, CoQ-10, CO Q10.

Scientific Names
Ubiquinone; Ubidecarenone; Mitoquinone.

People Use This For
Orally, CoQ-10 is used for congestive heart failure, angina, diabetes, hypertension (1900), preventing cardiotoxicity associated with doxorubicin (Adriamycin) chemotherapy, treating breast cancer (14), Huntington's disease (1357), for muscular dystrophy (2127), increasing exercise tolerance (2109,2110), reducing symptoms of chronic fatigue (2134), stimulating the immune system of people with AIDS (2123,2124,2137), life extension (2137), and male infertility (2135). Topically, people use CoQ-10 for treating periodontal disease (2107,2108).

Safety
POSSIBLY SAFE ...when taken orally in typical doses (6,14). There have been reports of significant toxicity associated with CoQ-10 in studies lasting up to a year (14,6407). ...when used topically for periodontitis (2107). PREGNANCY AND LACTATION: Insufficient reliable information available; avoid using (6,14).

Effectiveness
LIKELY EFFECTIVE ...when taken orally as adjunctive treatment for congestive heart failure (6,14,6407,6408, 6409,7000). Clinical trials have shown that coenzyme Q-10 can significantly improve quality of life (6408) and decrease hospitalization rates, pulmonary edema, cardiac asthma (6407), and other signs and symptoms of CHF such as dyspnea, peripheral edema, enlarged liver, insomnia, and others (6409) in patients with mild to severe (New York Heart Association Class II-IV) congestive heart failure (CHF). However, coenzyme Q-10 does not appear to improve ejection fraction or exercise tolerance (5090,6408).
POSSIBLY EFFECTIVE ...when used orally for improving symptoms of angina (2121). ...when used orally for hypertension (14,2122). ...when used orally for reducing cardiotoxicity associated with doxorubicin (Adriamycin) chemotherapy (14). ...when used orally for improving immune function in people with AIDS (2123,2124). ...when used orally for improving blood sugar control in individuals with diabetes (2125,2126). ...when used orally for treating muscular dystrophy (2127). ...when applied topically for treating periodontal disease (2107).
POSSIBLY INEFFECTIVE ...when used orally for treating Huntington's disease (1357). In a small, open label trial six months of oral coenzyme Q-10 treatment had no clinically significant effect (1357).
LIKELY INEFFECTIVE ...when used orally for improving exercise performance (2109,2110).
There is insufficient reliable information available about the effectiveness of CoQ-10 for its other uses.

Possible Mechanism of Action & Active Ingredients

Coenzyme Q-10 is found in virtually all aerobic organisms, hence, its alternate name, ubiquinone. It is produced in humans and is an essential cofactor in many metabolic pathways, particularly in the production of adenosine triphosphate (ATP) in oxidative respiration (6,14,6410). The therapeutic benefits of coenzyme Q-10 are primarily attributed to its role in the generation of ATP and its antioxidant effects (6,214). CoQ-10 has been shown to help preserve myocardial sodium-potassium ATP-ase activity and stabilize myocardial calcium-dependent ion channels. Coenzyme Q-10 acts as a free radical scavenger and membrane stabilizer. Coenzyme Q-10 is metabolized to ubiquinol, which prolongs the anti-oxidant effect of vitamin E (6,14). In some cases, people with cardiovascular disease, periodontal disease, and AIDS have been found to be coenzyme Q-10 deficient (6410).

Adverse Reactions Including Known Allergies

CoQ-10 used orally can cause to gastritis, loss of appetite, nausea, and diarrhea (6,14). When taken in amounts exceeding 300 mg per day, CoQ-10 can elevate serum aminotransferases (14).

Possible Interactions with Herbs & Other Dietary Supplements

Insufficient reliable information available.

Possible Interactions with Drugs

ORAL HYPOGLYCEMIC AGENTS: Concomitant use of some, but not all, oral hypoglycemic agents might reduce the effects of CoQ-10 supplementation (14) (see Comments).
HMG-CoA REDUCTASE INHIBITORS ("statin"): Concomitant use might reduce the effects of supplemental CoQ-10 (14,2004). "Statin" drugs include cerivastatin (Baycol), lovastatin (Mevacor), simvastatin (Zocor), pravastatin (Pravachol), and fluvastatin (Lescol).
WARFARIN (Coumadin): CoQ-10 can reduce the anticoagulation effects of warfarin. Monitor patients taking warfarin and CoQ-10 (2128).

Drug Influences on Nutrient Levels and Depletion

SOME DRUGS CAN AFFECT COENZYME Q-10 LEVELS:
HMG CoA REDUCTASE INHIBITORS (Statins): HMG CoA reductase inhibitors can reduce serum CoQ-10 levels. The clinical significance is yet to be determined, and the need for supplementation has not been adequately studied (4404,4405,4406,4407,4408,4409,4410). "Statin" drugs include cerivastatin (Baycol), lovastatin (Mevacor), simvastatin (Zocor), pravastatin (Pravachol), and fluvastatin (Lescol).
ORAL HYPOGLYCEMIC AGENTS: Use of oral hypoglycemic agents can reduce serum CoQ-10 levels. These agents include glyburide (Micronase), acetohexamide (Dymelor), and tolazamide (Tolinase). The clinical significance is yet to be determined, and the need for supplementation has not been adequately studied. Consider CoQ-10 supplements based on clinical judgment (4479). NOTE: Chlorpropamide (Diabinese), glipizide (Glucotrol), and tolbutamide (Orinase) have been found not to reduce CoQ-10 serum levels; there is no data concerning glimepiride (Amaryl).

Possible Interactions with Foods

No interactions are known to occur, and there is no known reason to expect a clinically significant interaction with CoQ-10.

Possible Interactions with Lab Tests

LIVER ENZYMES: CoQ-10 doses in excess of 300 mg per day can elevate serum aminotransferase concentrations and test results (14).
T4/T8 RATIO: CoQ-10 can increase the T4/T8 ratio in normal patients and some HIV+ patients (2123).
BLOOD PRESSURE: CoQ-10 can lower blood pressure and reduce blood pressure readings in patients with essential hypertension (2122).

Possible Interactions with Diseases or Conditions

DIABETES: CoQ-10 can decrease insulin requirements in people with diabetes (14).
BILIARY OBSTRUCTION, HEPATIC INSUFFICIENCY: CoQ-10 levels can increase when patients have either biliary obstruction or hepatic insufficiency (14).

Typical Dosages & Routes of Administration that are Commonly Used

ORAL: Heart failure, 50 mg two times per day (14). Angina, 50 mg three times per day (2121). Hypertension, 225 mg per day (2122). Cardiotoxicity associated with doxorubicin (Adriamycin) chemotherapy, 50 mg per day (14). AIDS, 200 mg per day (2123,2124). Diabetes, 150 mg per day (2125). Muscular dystrophy, 100 mg per day (2127). Note that all of these conditions require medical diagnosis and appropriate monitoring.

Comments

CoQ-10 was first identified in 1957. It is widely used in Japan. Millions of Japanese patients receive CoQ-10 as part of their treatment for cardiovascular disease. The Japanese government approved CoQ-10 for the treatment of congestive heart failure in 1974. CoQ-10 is also used extensively in Europe and Russia. Most of the CoQ-10 used in the US and Canada is supplied by Japanese companies. CoQ-10 is manufactured by beets fermenting and sugar cane with special strains of yeast (507).

COFFEE

This Product is Also Known As
Cafe, Caffea, Espresso, Java, Mocha.
CAUTION: See separate listings for Caffeine and Coffee Charcoal.

Scientific Names
Coffea arabica; Coffea canephora, synonym Coffea robusta; Coffea liberica; other Coffea species.
Family: Rubiaceae.

People Use This For
Orally, coffee is used as a common beverage for short-term relief of mental and physical fatigue (7) and to increase performance capabilities (18).

Safety
LIKELY SAFE ...when coffee containing caffeine is used orally in low to moderate amounts. ...when up to 5 cups of coffee (500 mg caffeine) are consumed daily by regular users who have developed caffeine tolerance (18). ...when decaffeinated coffee is consumed.
POSSIBLY UNSAFE ...when caffeine-containing coffee is used in amounts greater than 5 cups/day short-term or long-term. This dose can cause caffeinism with symptoms of anxiety progressing to delirium and agitation (14). Chronic use of caffeine, especially in large amounts, can sometimes produce tolerance, habituation, and psychological dependence (15). The abrupt discontinuance of caffeine can sometimes result in physical withdrawal symptoms.
CHILDREN: POSSIBLY UNSAFE ...when coffee containing caffeine is taken orally in amounts significantly greater than typical beverage amounts. The adverse effects are usually more severe in children than adults (15).
PREGNANCY: POSSIBLY SAFE ...when less than 300 mg caffeine/3 cups of coffee are consumed spread throughout the day (15). Caffeine crosses the human placenta but is not considered a teratogen. Fetal blood and tissue levels are similar to maternal concentrations (4260). POSSIBLY UNSAFE ...when more than 300 mg caffeine consumed daily (15,18,4260).
LACTATION: POSSIBLY UNSAFE; avoid using. Caffeine can cause sleep disturbances in breast-fed infants (18).

Effectiveness
EFFECTIVE ...for increasing mental alertness (14,15).
LIKELY INEFFECTIVE ...for improving short-term, high-intensity performance, anaerobic capacity or power (14).
INEFFECTIVE ...for sustained, sub-maximal endurance exercise (14).
There is insufficient reliable information available about the effectiveness of coffee for its other uses.

Possible Mechanism of Action & Active Ingredients
Coffee contains 1-2.6% caffeine (7,12,13) which acts as a central nervous system stimulant (12,15,18), increases heart rate and contractility (7,18), inhibits platelet aggregation (6,18), stimulates gastric acid secretion, causes diuresis (15,18), relaxes extracerebral vascular and bronchial smooth muscle, stimulates the release of catecholamines (18), and might indirectly inhibit histamine release (6130). The chlorogenic acid constituent is believed to increase gastric acid secretion (13,18); caffeol is believed to have pharmacologic activity (13). The diterpene constituents, cafestol and kahweol, increase serum cholesterol (1353). Drinking one liter of strong, unfiltered coffee daily for two weeks can raise serum cholesterol by 10% and plasma homocysteine levels by 10% (1353).

Adverse Reactions Including Known Allergies
Coffee can increase excretion of calcium and magnesium (12). It can increase cholesterol levels, LDLs and triglycerides, due to the presence of diterpenes (7,12,18); however, the use of coffee filters might decrease this risk as much as 80% (18). Evidence suggests that coffee might increase the risk of pancreatic cancer (12). In women, coffee seems to be associated with increased risk of heart attack (12), breast cancer (in obese women), and ovarian cancer (12). Coffee that contains caffeine can cause headache, increased blood pressure, increased intraocular pressure, diuresis (12), gastric distress, nervousness, vomiting, insomnia (7,18), anxiety, agitation, ringing in ears, diuresis, and heart arrhythmias (15). Adverse effects of caffeine are usually more severe in children (15). Some evidence shows caffeine is associated with fibrocystic breast disease in women; other evidence disputes this (14,15). Chronic use of caffeine, especially in large amounts, can sometimes produce tolerance, habituation, and psychological dependence (15). Abrupt discontinuance of caffeine can sometimes cause physical withdrawal symptoms, including headaches, irritability, nervousness, anxiety, and dizziness (15).
Combining ephedra with coffee increases the risk of adverse effects, due to the caffeine contained in coffee (2729). One unpublished report associated jitteriness, hypertension, seizures, temporary loss of consciousness, and hospitalization requiring life support with the use of a combination ephedra and guarana (caffeine) product (1380). There is one report of ischemic stroke in an athlete who consumed ephedra 40-60 mg, creatine monohydrate 6 grams, caffeine 400-600 mg, and a variety of other supplements daily for six weeks (1275).

Possible Interactions with Herbs & Other Dietary Supplements
CAFFEINE CONTAINING HERBS/SUPPLEMENTS: Concomitant use of coffee and caffeine-containing herbs/supplements constitutes therapeutic duplication (due to the caffeine contained in coffee) which increases the

risk of caffeine-related adverse effects. Other natural products which contain caffeine include black tea, cocoa, cola nut, green tea, guarana, and maté.

EPHEDRA (Ma Huang): Concomitant use can increase the risk of stimulatory adverse effects, due to the caffeine contained in coffee (7). One unpublished report associated jitteriness, hypertension, seizures, temporary loss of consciousness, and hospitalization requiring life support with the use of a combination ephedra and guarana (caffeine) product (1380).

ZINC: Separate coffee consumption and zinc administration by two hours. Concomitant administration reduces zinc absorption by up to 50% (14).

Possible Interactions with Drugs

ACETAMINOPHEN (Tylenol): Theoretically, concomitant use might increase the pain-relieving activity of acetaminophen, due to the caffeine contained in coffee. Caffeine increases the pain-relieving activity of acetaminophen by up to 40% (512).

ACID-INHIBITING DRUGS: Theoretically, concomitant use might interfere with antacids, sucralfate (Carafate), H-2 antagonists, or proton pump inhibitors. This is based on the claim that coffee increases stomach acid (19).

ALENDRONATE (Fosamax): Separate coffee ingestion and alendronate administration by two hours. Coffee reduces alendronate bioavailability by 60% (14).

ASPIRIN: Theoretically, concomitant use might increase the pain-relieving activity of aspirin, due to the caffeine contained in coffee. Caffeine increases the pain-relieving activity of aspirin by up to 40% (512).

BENZODIAZEPINES: Theoretically, concomitant use might reduce the sedative and anxiolytic effects of benzodiazepines, due to the caffeine contained in coffee (14).

BETA-ADRENERGIC AGONISTS: Theoretically, concomitant use might increase the cardiac inotropic effects of beta agonists, due to the caffeine contained in coffee (15). Beta-adrenergic agonists include albuterol (Proventil, Ventolin), metaproterenol (Alupent), terbutaline (Brethine), and isoproterenol (Isuprel).

CIMETIDINE (Tagamet) Theoretically, concomitant use might increase serum caffeine concentrations and the risk of adverse effects, due to the caffeine contained in coffee. Cimetidine decreases the rate of caffeine clearance by 30-50% (14).

CLOZAPINE (Clozaril): Theoretically, co-administration might acutely exacerbate psychotic symptoms, due to the caffeine contained in coffee. Caffeine can increase the effects and toxicity of clozapine (151). Caffeine doses of 400-1000 mg per day inhibit clozapine metabolism (5051).

CNS STIMULANTS: Concomitant use might increase the risk of stimulant adverse effects, due to the caffeine contained in coffee (151,2719). CNS stimulants include nicotine, cocaine, sympathomimetic amines, and amphetamines.

DIABETES THERAPY: Theoretically, concomitant use of coffee and diabetes drugs might interfere with blood glucose control, due to the caffeine contained in coffee. This is based in the claim that caffeine might have hyperglycemic effects (19).

DISULFIRAM (Antabuse): Theoretically, concomitant use might increase serum caffeine concentrations and the risk of adverse effects, due to the caffeine contained in coffee. Disulfiram decreases the rate of caffeine clearance (15).

EPHEDRINE: Concomitant use might increase the risk of stimulatory adverse effects, due to the caffeine contained in coffee (7,19). An unpublished report associated jitteriness, hypertension, seizures, temporary loss of consciousness, and hospitalization requiring life support with the use of a combination ephedra (ephedrine) and guarana (caffeine) product (1380).

ESTROGEN (Estrace): Theoretically, concomitant use might increase serum caffeine concentrations and the risk of adverse effects, due to the caffeine contained in coffee. Estrogen inhibits caffeine metabolism (2714).

ERGOTAMINE: Theoretically, concomitant use might increase the GI absorption of ergotamine, due to the caffeine contained in coffee. Caffeine increases the GI absorption of ergotamine (15).

LITHIUM (Eskalith, Lithobid): Theoretically, abrupt coffee withdrawal might increase serum lithium levels, due to the caffeine contained in coffee. There are two case reports of lithium tremor that worsened upon abrupt coffee withdrawal (609,610).

MEXILETINE (Mexitil): Theoretically, concomitant use might increase serum caffeine concentrations and the risk of adverse effects, due to the caffeine contained in coffee. Mexiletine reduces caffeine metabolism (14).

MONOAMINE OXIDASE INHIBITORS (MAOIs): Theoretically, concomitant intake of large amounts of coffee with MAOIs might precipitate a hypertensive crisis, due to the caffeine contained in coffee. This is based on the claim that intake of large amounts of caffeine with MAOIs might precipitate a hypertensive crisis (19).

ORAL CONTRACEPTIVES (OCs): Theoretically, concomitant use might increase serum caffeine concentrations and the risk adverse effects, due to the caffeine contained in coffee. OCs decrease the rate of caffeine clearance by 40-65% (14).

PHENYLPROPANOLAMINE (Dexatrim, Propagest): Theoretically, concomitant use might cause an additive increase in blood pressure and serum caffeine concentrations, due to the caffeine contained in coffee (14). Concomitant use of caffeine and phenylpropanolamine can cause an additive increase in blood pressure, and increase serum caffeine concentrations (14).

QUINOLONES: Theoretically, concomitant use might increase serum caffeine concentrations and the risk of adverse effects, due to the caffeine contained in coffee. Quinolones decrease caffeine clearance (606,607,608). Quinolones (also referred to as fluoroquinolones) include ciprofloxacin (Cipro), enoxacin (Penetrex), gatifloxacin (Tequin), levofloxacin (Levaquin), lomefloxacin (Maxaquin), moxifloxacin (Avelox), norfloxacin (Noroxin), ofloxacin (Floxin), sparfloxacin (Zagam), and trovafloxacin (Trovan).

RILUZOLE (Rilutek): Theoretically, concomitant use might increase serum caffeine and riluzole concentrations and the risk of adverse effects of both caffeine and riluzole, due to the caffeine contained in coffee. Caffeine and riluzole are both metabolized by cytochrome P450 1A2 and concomitant use might reduce metabolism of one or both agents (14).

TERBINAFINE (Lamisil): Theoretically, concomitant use might increase serum caffeine concentrations and the risk of adverse effects, due to the caffeine contained in coffee. Terbinafine decreases the rate of caffeine clearance (14).

THEOPHYLLINE (Theo-Dur): Theoretically, concomitant use might increase serum theophylline concentrations and the risk of adverse effects, due to the caffeine contained in coffee. Large amounts of caffeine might inhibit theophylline metabolism (14).

VERAPAMIL (Calan, Isoptin, Verelan): Theoretically, concomitant use might increase plasma caffeine concentrations and the risk of adverse effects, due to the caffeine contained in coffee. Verapamil increases plasma caffeine concentrations by 25% (14).

Possible Interactions with Foods

GRAPEFRUIT JUICE: Interacts with the caffeine in coffee and plasma caffeine concentrations can be elevated, increasing effects and risk of adverse effects (504).

Possible Interactions with Lab Tests

BLEEDING TIME: Coffee might prolong bleeding time and increase test results, due to its caffeine content (1701).

BLOOD PRESSURE: Coffee might increase blood pressure and blood pressure readings, due to its caffeine content (4).

URATE: Coffee might falsely increase serum urate test results determined by the Bittner method, due to its caffeine content. Caffeine causes false elevations in serum urate test results determined by the Bittner method (15).

CATECHOLAMINES: Coffee might increase urine catecholamine concentrations and test results, due to its caffeine content. Caffeine can increase urine catecholamine concentrations (15).

CREATINE: Coffee might increase urine creatine concentrations and test results, due to its caffeine content (1701).

DIPYRIDAMOLE THALLIUM IMAGING: Coffee might interfere with dipyridamole thallium imaging studies, due to its caffeine content. Caffeine attenuates the characteristic cardiovascular responses to dipyridamole and has altered test results (14).

5-HYDROXYINDOLEACETIC ACID: Coffee might increase urine 5-hydroxyindoleacetic acid concentrations and test results, due to its caffeine content. Caffeine can increase urine catecholamine concentrations (15).

VANILLYLMANDELIC ACID (VMA): Coffee might increase urine VMA concentrations and test results, due to its caffeine content. Caffeine can increase urine VMA concentrations (15).

TESTS FOR NEUROBLASTOMA: Coffee (due to its caffeine content) might cause false-positive diagnosis of neuroblastoma, when diagnosis is based on tests of urine vanillylmandelic acid (VMA) or catecholamine concentrations. Caffeine can increase urine catecholamine and VMA concentrations (15).

TESTS FOR PHEOCHROMOCYTOMA: Coffee (due to its caffeine content) might cause false-positive diagnosis of pheochromocytoma, when diagnosis is based on tests of urine vanillylmandelic acid (VMA) or catecholamine concentrations. Caffeine can increase urine catecholamine and VMA concentrations (15).

Possible Interactions with Diseases or Conditions

ANXIETY DISORDERS: The caffeine in coffee can aggravate anxiety disorders (14).

CARDIOVASCULAR DISEASE: Consumption of unfiltered coffee increases plasma homocysteine levels, which are associate with an increased risk of cardiovascular disease (1353).

CANCER: Coffee might increase risk of pancreatic cancer, breast cancer (in obese women), and ovarian cancer (12).

DEPRESSION: The caffeine in coffee can aggravate depression (14).

GASTRIC, DUODENAL ULCERS: The caffeine in coffee can aggravate ulcers; avoid using (14,16).

HEART CONDITIONS: The caffeine in coffee can induce cardiac arrhythmias and tachycardia in sensitive individuals (14,16). Theoretically, large amounts of caffeinated coffee might increase the risk of heart attacks (12).

HYPERCHOLESTEROLEMIA: Avoid unfiltered, fresh-brewed coffee which can increase serum cholesterol levels (7,12,18,1353,4200). However, drinking filtered coffee does not increase serum cholesterol levels (18,4200).

HYPERTHYROID: Avoid use of coffee (18).

KIDNEY DISEASE: The diuretic effect of the caffeine in coffee might aggravate some kidney disorders (19).

OSTEOPOROSIS: Coffee can increase excretion of calcium and magnesium, and thus increase the risk of osteoporosis (12).

SEIZURE PREDISPOSITION: Avoid use of coffee (18).

© Copyright 2000, Natural Medicines Comprehensive Database (209) 472-2244. For updated data, go to www.NaturalDatabase.com

Typical Dosages & Routes of Administration that are Commonly Used
Avoid unfiltered coffee. Choice of coffee, grind, ratio of coffee to water, and other factors determine flavor and strength of beverage. Caffeine content of coffee (per average cup): percolated, 100-150 mg caffeine; instant, 85-100 mg caffeine; and decaffeinated, approximately 8 mg caffeine (13). Darker roasts contain less caffeine due to sublimation during roasting (13).

Comments
None.

COFFEE CHARCOAL

This Product is Also Known As
None.
CAUTION: See separate listings for Activated Charcoal and Coffee.

Scientific Names
Coffea arabica; Coffea canephora, Coffea liberica.
Family: Rubiaceae.

People Use This For
Orally, coffee charcoal is used for nonspecific, acute diarrhea (2).
Topically, coffee charcoal is used for inflammation of the oral and pharyngeal mucosa (2).
In folk medicine, coffee charcoal has been used as a topical treatment for festering wounds (18).

Safety
POSSIBLY SAFE ...when used orally or topically (2).
PREGNANCY AND LACTATION: Insufficient reliable information available; avoid using.

Effectiveness
POSSIBLY EFFECTIVE ...when taken orally for nonspecific, acute diarrhea (2). ...when used topically for mild inflammation of the oral and pharyngeal mucosa (2).

Possible Mechanism of Action & Active Ingredients
Coffee charcoal can have adsorbent and astringent properties (2).

Adverse Reactions Including Known Allergies
None reported (2).

Possible Interactions with Herbs & Other Dietary Supplements
Insufficient reliable information available.

Possible Interactions with Drugs
ORAL DRUGS: Coffee charcoal can reduce the absorption of orally administered drugs (2) and should be separated from oral drug administration by at least two hours.

Possible Interactions with Foods
No interactions are known to occur, and there is no known reason to expect a clinically significant interaction with coffee charcoal.

Possible Interactions with Lab Tests
No interactions are known to occur, and there is no known reason to expect a clinically significant interaction with coffee charcoal.

Possible Interactions with Diseases or Conditions
No interactions are known to occur, and there is no known reason to expect a clinically significant interaction with coffee charcoal.

Typical Dosages & Routes of Administration that are Commonly Used
ORAL: The average single dose of coffee charcoal is 3 grams (18), and the total daily dose is 9 grams per day (2). Store coffee charcoal in a well-sealed container (18). Diarrhea persisting beyond 3 to 4 days should be evaluated by a health care professional (2).
TOPICAL: No typical dosage.

Comments
Coffee charcoal is produced by roasting the outer portion of the coffee beans until blackened or charred. Avoid confusion with coffee seed or activated charcoal.

COLA NUT

This Product is Also Known As
Bissy Nut, Cola Seed, Guru Nut, Kola Nut.
CAUTION: See separate listings for Caffeine and Gotu Kola.

Scientific Names
Cola acuminata, synonym Sterculia acuminata; Cola nitida; and related species.
Family: Sterculiaceae.

People Use This For
Orally, cola nut is used for short-term relief of mental and physical fatigue (2) and depressive states, especially those associated with general muscle weakness. It is also used orally for melancholy, atony, exhaustion, dysentery, atonic diarrhea, anorexia, and migraines (4).
In foods and beverages, cola nut is used as a flavoring ingredient (11).

Safety
LIKELY SAFE ...when consumed in amounts commonly found in foods and beverages. The cola nut has Generally Recognized as Safe (GRAS) status in the US (11).
POSSIBLY SAFE ...when used orally and appropriately (12,18).
POSSIBLY UNSAFE ...when used in excessive amounts or long-term due to its caffeine content (12). Chronic use of caffeine, especially in large amounts, can sometimes produce tolerance, habituation, and psychological dependence (15). The abrupt discontinuance can result in physical withdrawal symptoms (15).
CHILDREN: POSSIBLY UNSAFE ...when used orally in amounts significantly greater than typical food amounts. The adverse effects of caffeine can be more severe in children than adults (15).
PREGNANCY: There is insufficient reliable information available about the safety of cola nut during pregnancy. Although the caffeine content of a typical dose should not cause concern, other constituents could be unsafe.
LACTATION: POSSIBLY UNSAFE; avoid using. It can cause sleep disturbances in breast-fed infants (18).

Effectiveness
POSSIBLY EFFECTIVE ...when used orally for mental and physical fatigue (2).
There is insufficient reliable information available about the effectiveness of cola nut for its other uses.

Possible Mechanism of Action & Active Ingredients
Cola nut has CNS stimulant, antidepressant, diuretic, and antidiarrheal effects (4). Cola nut contains 1-3.5% caffeine (13) which acts as a central nervous system stimulant (12,15,18), increases heart rate and contractility (7,18), inhibits platelet aggregation (6,18), stimulates gastric acid secretion, causes diuresis (15,18), relaxes extracerebral vascular and bronchial smooth muscle, stimulates the release of catecholamines (18), and might indirectly inhibit histamine release (6130).

Adverse Reactions Including Known Allergies
Cola nut can cause sleeplessness, anxiety, tremor, palpitations (4), over-excitability, nervous restlessness, and gastric irritation (2). The caffeine constituent can cause a fast heartbeat, quickened respiration, tremors, delirium, vomiting, convulsions, diuresis (15,505), agitation, ringing in the ears, premature heartbeat, and arrhythmias (15). The adverse effects of caffeine are usually more severe in children (15). Some evidence shows caffeine is associated with fibrocystic breast disease in women; other evidence disputes this (14,15). Chronic use of caffeine, especially in large amounts, can sometimes produce tolerance, habituation, and psychological dependence (15). The abrupt discontinuance can sometimes result in physical withdrawal symptoms, including headaches, irritation, nervousness, anxiety, and dizziness (15). The chewing of cola nuts can cause staining of the oral mucosa to a bright yellow. The chewing of these nuts can also increase the risk of oral carcinoma in smokers (214).
Combining ephedra with cola nut increases the risk of adverse effects, due to the caffeine contained in cola nut (2729). One unpublished report associated jitteriness, hypertension, seizures, temporary loss of consciousness, and hospitalization requiring life support with the use of a combination ephedra and guarana (caffeine) product (1380). There is one report of ischemic stroke in an athlete who consumed ephedra 40-60 mg, creatine monohydrate 6 grams, caffeine 400-600 mg, and a variety of other supplements daily for six weeks (1275).

Possible Interactions with Herbs & Other Dietary Supplements
CAFFEINE CONTAINING HERBS/SUPPLEMENTS: Concomitant use of cola nut and caffeine-containing herbs/supplements constitutes therapeutic duplication (due to the caffeine contained in cola nut) which increases the risk of caffeine-related adverse effects. Other natural products which contain caffeine include black tea, cocoa, coffee, green tea, guarana, and maté.
EPHEDRA (Ma Huang): Concomitant use can increase the risk of stimulatory adverse effects, due to the caffeine contained in cola nut (7). One unpublished report associated jitteriness, hypertension, seizures, temporary loss of consciousness, and hospitalization requiring life support with the use of a combination ephedra and guarana (caffeine) product (1380).

Possible Interactions with Drugs

ACETAMINOPHEN (Tylenol): Theoretically, concomitant use might increase the pain-relieving activity of acetaminophen, due to the caffeine contained in cola nut. Caffeine increases the pain-relieving activity of acetaminophen by up to 40% (512).

ASPIRIN: Theoretically, concomitant use might increase the pain-relieving activity of aspirin, due to the caffeine contained in cola nut. Caffeine increases the pain-relieving activity of aspirin by up to 40% (512).

BENZODIAZEPINES: Theoretically, concomitant use might reduce the sedative and anxiolytic effects of benzodiazepines, due to the caffeine contained in cola nut (14).

BETA-ADRENERGIC AGONISTS: Theoretically, concomitant use might increase the cardiac inotropic effects of beta agonists, due to the caffeine contained in cola nut (15). Beta-adrenergic agonists include albuterol (Proventil, Ventolin), metaproterenol (Alupent), terbutaline (Brethine), and isoproterenol (Isuprel).

CIMETIDINE (Tagamet) Theoretically, concomitant use might increase serum caffeine concentrations and the risk of adverse effects, due to the caffeine contained in cola nut. Cimetidine decreases the rate of caffeine clearance by 30-50% (14).

CLOZAPINE (Clozaril): Theoretically, co-administration might acutely exacerbate psychotic symptoms, due to the caffeine contained in cola nut. Caffeine can increase the effects and toxicity of clozapine (151). Caffeine doses of 400-1000 mg per day inhibit clozapine metabolism (5051).

CNS STIMULANTS: Concomitant use might increase the risk of stimulant adverse effects, due to the caffeine contained in cola nut (151,2719). CNS stimulants include nicotine, cocaine, sympathomimetic amines, and amphetamines.

DIABETES THERAPY: Theoretically, concomitant use of coffee and diabetes drugs might interfere with blood glucose control, due to the caffeine contained in cola nut. This is based in the claim that caffeine might have hyperglycemic effects (19).

DISULFIRAM (Antabuse): Theoretically, concomitant use might increase serum caffeine concentrations and the risk of adverse effects, due to the caffeine contained in cola nut. Disulfiram decreases the rate of caffeine clearance (15).

EPHEDRINE: Concomitant use might increase the risk of stimulatory adverse effects, due to the caffeine contained in cola nut (7,19). An unpublished report associated jitteriness, hypertension, seizures, temporary loss of consciousness, and hospitalization requiring life support with the use of a combination ephedra (ephedrine) and guarana (caffeine) product (1380).

ESTROGEN (Estrace): Theoretically, concomitant use might increase serum caffeine concentrations and the risk of adverse effects, due to the caffeine contained in cola nut. Estrogen inhibits caffeine metabolism (2714).

ERGOTAMINE: Theoretically, concomitant use might increase the GI absorption of ergotamine, due to the caffeine contained in cola nut. Caffeine increases the GI absorption of ergotamine (15).

LITHIUM (Eskalith, Lithobid): Theoretically, abrupt cola nut withdrawal might increase serum lithium levels, due to the caffeine contained in cola nut. There are two case reports of lithium tremor that worsened upon abrupt coffee withdrawal (609,610).

MONOAMINE OXIDASE INHIBITORS (MAOIs): Theoretically, concomitant intake of large amounts of cola nut with MAOIs might precipitate a hypertensive crisis, due to the caffeine contained in cola nut. This is based on the claim that intake of large amounts of caffeine with MAOIs might precipitate a hypertensive crisis (19).

MEXILETINE (Mexitil): Theoretically, concomitant use might increase serum caffeine concentrations and the risk of adverse effects, due to the caffeine contained in cola nut. Mexiletine reduces caffeine metabolism (14).

ORAL CONTRACEPTIVES (OCs): Theoretically, concomitant use might increase serum caffeine concentrations and the risk of adverse effects, due to the caffeine contained in cola nut. OCs decrease the rate of caffeine clearance by 40-65% (14).

PHENYLPROPANOLAMINE (Dexatrim, Propagest): Theoretically, concomitant use might cause an additive increase in blood pressure and serum caffeine concentrations, due to the caffeine contained in cola nut (14). Concomitant use of caffeine and phenylpropanolamine can cause an additive increase in blood pressure, and increase serum caffeine concentrations (14).

QUINOLONES: Theoretically, concomitant use might increase serum caffeine concentrations and the risk of adverse effects, due to the caffeine contained in cola nut. Quinolones decrease caffeine clearance (606,607,608). Quinolones (also referred to as fluoroquinolones) include ciprofloxacin (Cipro), enoxacin (Penetrex), gatifloxacin (Tequin), levofloxacin (Levaquin), lomefloxacin (Maxaquin), moxifloxacin (Avelox), norfloxacin (Noroxin), ofloxacin (Floxin), sparfloxacin (Zagam), and trovafloxacin (Trovan).

RILUZOLE (Rilutek): Theoretically, concomitant use might increase serum caffeine and riluzole concentrations and the risk of adverse effects of both caffeine and riluzole, due to the caffeine contained in cola nut. Caffeine and riluzole are both metabolized by cytochrome P450 1A2 and concomitant use might reduce metabolism of one or both agents (14).

TERBINAFINE (Lamisil): Theoretically, concomitant use might increase serum caffeine concentrations and the risk of adverse effects, due to the caffeine contained in cola nut. Terbinafine decreases the rate of caffeine clearance (14).

THEOPHYLLINE (Theo-Dur): Theoretically, concomitant use might increase serum theophylline concentrations and the risk of adverse effects, due to the caffeine contained in cola nut. Large amounts of caffeine might inhibit theophylline metabolism (14).

VERAPAMIL (Calan, Isoptin, Verelan): Theoretically, concomitant use might increase plasma caffeine concentrations and the risk of adverse effects, due to the caffeine contained in cola nut. Verapamil increases plasma caffeine concentrations by 25% (14).

Possible Interactions with Foods

CAFFEINE-CONTAINING BEVERAGES: Concomitant use can have additive therapeutic and adverse effects due to the caffeine content.

GRAPEFRUIT JUICE interacts with the caffeine in cola nut and can increase caffeine levels, its activity, and the risk of adverse effects (504).

Possible Interactions with Lab Tests

BLEEDING TIME: Cola nut might prolong bleeding time and increase test results, due to its caffeine content (1701).

BLOOD PRESSURE: Cola nut might increase blood pressure and blood pressure readings, due to its caffeine content (4).

URATE: Cola nut might falsely increase serum urate test results determined by the Bittner method, due to its caffeine content. Caffeine causes false elevations in serum urate test results determined by the Bittner method (15).

CATECHOLAMINES: Cola nut might increase urine catecholamine concentrations and test results, due to its caffeine content. Caffeine can increase urine catecholamine concentrations (15).

CREATINE: Cola nut might increase urine creatine concentrations and test results, due to its caffeine content (1701).

DIPYRIDAMOLE THALLIUM IMAGING: Cola nut might interfere with dipyridamole thallium imaging studies, due to its caffeine content. Caffeine attenuates the characteristic cardiovascular responses to dipyridamole and has altered test results (14).

5-HYDROXYINDOLEACETIC ACID: Cola nut might increase urine 5-hydroxyindoleacetic acid concentrations and test results, due to its caffeine content. Caffeine can increase urine catecholamine concentrations (15).

VANILLYLMANDELIC ACID (VMA): Cola nut might increase urine VMA concentrations and test results, due to its caffeine content. Caffeine can increase urine VMA concentrations (15).

TESTS FOR NEUROBLASTOMA: Cola nut (due to its caffeine content) might cause false-positive diagnosis of neuroblastoma, when diagnosis is based on tests of urine vanillylmandelic acid (VMA) or catecholamine concentrations. Caffeine can increase urine catecholamine and VMA concentrations (15).

TESTS FOR PHEOCHROMOCYTOMA: Cola nut (due to its caffeine content) might cause false-positive diagnosis of pheochromocytoma, when diagnosis is based on tests of urine vanillylmandelic acid (VMA) or catecholamine concentrations. Caffeine can increase urine catecholamine and VMA concentrations (15).

Possible Interactions with Diseases or Conditions

GASTRIC, DUODENAL ULCERS: The caffeine in cola nut can aggravate these conditions and should be avoided (14,16).

HEART CONDITIONS: The caffeine in cola nut can induce cardiac arrhythmias in sensitive individuals (14,16).

DEPRESSION, ANXIETY DISORDERS: The caffeine in cola nut can aggravate these conditions (14).

KIDNEY DISEASE: The diuretic effect of caffeine in cola nut might aggravate some kidney disorders (19).

Typical Dosages & Routes of Administration that are Commonly Used

ORAL: The typical dose of cola nut is 1-2 grams of the powdered nut or one cup of the tea three times daily (2,4). The tea is prepared by simmering 1-2 grams of the powdered nut in 150 mL boiling water for 5-10 minutes and then straining. The usual dose of the liquid extract of cola nut (1:1 in 60% alcohol) is 0.6-1.2 mL (4). The common dose of the tincture of cola nut(1:5 in 60% alcohol) is 1-4 mL (4).

Comments

Avoid confusion with gotu kola.

COLLOIDAL MINERALS

This Product is Also Known As

Bioelectrical Minerals, Clay Suspension Products, Colloidal Trace Minerals, Humic Shale, Plant-Derived Liquid Minerals.

Scientific Names

Anhydrous aluminum silicates.

People Use This For

Orally, colloidal minerals are used as a supplemental source of trace minerals, a dietary supplement to increase energy, for improving blood sugar levels in diabetes, arthritis symptoms, reducing blood cell clumping, reversing early cataracts, turning gray hair dark again, flushing poisonous heavy metals from the body, improving general well being, reducing aches and pains (1157).

© Copyright 2000, Natural Medicines Comprehensive Database (209) 472-2244. For updated data, go to www.NaturalDatabase.com

Safety

POSSIBLY UNSAFE ...when used orally. These products contain varying amounts of aluminum, arsenic, lead, barium, nickel and titanium (1157). Some products contain as much as 1800-4400 ppm aluminum and 20 ppm arsenic (1159); generally, foods do not contain more than 10 ppm of aluminum (1159). While no cases of toxicity have been reported, there are concerns about colloidal mineral supplements containing unsafe levels of radioactive metals (1161).

PREGNANCY AND LACTATION: POSSIBLY UNSAFE...avoid using.

Effectiveness

There is insufficient reliable information about the effectiveness of colloidal minerals.

Possible Mechanism of Action & Active Ingredients

Commercial colloidal mineral products are derived from clay or humic shale deposits (1159). Clay minerals are layer type aluminosilicates that figure in terrestrial biogeochemical cycles, in the buffering capacity of the oceans, and in the containment of toxic waste materials (1160). Humic shale is a common source of plant-derived colloidal minerals (1157). When mixed with water, the surfaces of clay particles become negatively charged. This allows the particles to bind with ionic minerals, such as magnesium, sodium, calcium, and potassium (1159). The content of trace minerals in individual products depends upon the rock source used (1159). Proponents claim that, due to mineral depletion of soil, many people do not take in the dietary trace minerals once plentiful in the human diet (1158). However, there is no evidence that there is increased bioavailability of ingested minerals in this form (1159).

Adverse Reactions Including Known Allergies

None reported.

Possible Interactions with Herbs & Other Dietary Supplements

Insufficient reliable information available.

Possible Interactions with Drugs

No interactions are known to occur, and there is no known reason to expect a clinically significant interaction with colloidal minerals.

Possible Interactions with Foods

No interactions are known to occur, and there is no known reason to expect a clinically significant interaction with colloidal minerals.

Possible Interactions with Lab Tests

No interactions are known to occur, and there is no known reason to expect a clinically significant interaction with colloidal minerals.

Possible Interactions with Diseases or Conditions

HEMOCHROMATOSIS, WILSON'S DISEASE: Theoretically, colloidal minerals could exacerbate conditions in which metal accumulation is a problem.

Typical Dosages & Routes of Administration that are Commonly Used

No typical dosage.

Comments

Avoid; these products are possibly unsafe and there is no evidence of effectiveness. The medicinal use of clay-based products in modern days was first encouraged by a southern Utah rancher. Historically, some Native American tribes used clay medicinally (1157). There is a tremendous amount of promotional claims for colloidal mineral products. There is no reliable medical evidence to support using these products. Commercial colloidal mineral products are derived from clay or humic shale deposits (1159).

COLLOIDAL SILVER

This Product is Also Known As

Colloidal Silver Protein, Silver Protein.

Scientific Names

Silver in suspending agent.

People Use This For

Orally, colloidal silver is used to treat ear infections, emphysema (5519), bronchitis (5523), fungal infections, Lyme disease, Rosacea, sinus infections, stomach ulcers, yeast infections (5519), chronic fatigue syndrome (5521), AIDS (5522), and tuberculosis (5523). It is used orally for antibacterial properties (5519), for food poisoning (5523), to promote rapid healing and subdue inflammation (5519), and to treat gum disease (5521). It is used to improve digestion, and to prevent flu and colds (5519,5521). Colloidal silver is used during pregnancy to aid the baby's growth and health as well as the mother's delivery and recovery. (5522).

Topically, colloidal silver is used for acne, burns, eye infections, fungal infections, throat infections, skin infections, and Staphylococcus infections (5519).

Traditionally, colloidal silver has been used for allergies; appendicitis; arthritis; blood parasites; bubonic plague; cancer; cholera; colitis; cystitis; conjunctivitis; atopic dermatitis (cradle cap); diabetes; dysentery; eczema; gastritis; gonorrhea; impetigo; hay fever; herpes; leprosy; leukemia; lupus; lymphangitis; malaria; meningitis; parasitic infections; pneumonia; pneumococci; psoriasis; prostatitis; rhinitis; ringworm; scarlet fever; septic conditions of the eyes, ears, mouth, and throat; Salmonella; septicemia; shingles; skin cancer; syphilis; tonsillitis; toxemia; trench foot; viruses; warts; and yeast infections (5520).

Safety

POSSIBLY SAFE ...when colloidal silver is used orally in amounts that do not exceed a total intake (including food and water) of 14 mcg/kg/day of silver (350 microgram/day/70kg person). 2L of water meeting EPA standards could contain up to 200 mcg, plus a regular diet could contain 90 mcg (5525) for a total of 290 mcg without any additional oral or topical silver use.

POSSIBLY UNSAFE ...when colloidal silver is used orally or topically for medicinal use. According to the FDA final rule, no over the counter products containing colloidal silver are generally recognized as safe (5524).

LIKELY UNSAFE ...when colloidal silver is used orally or topically in large amounts or long-term. Silver accumulates in the body causing an irreversible bluish skin discoloration known as argyria. Neurological deficits, diffuse silver deposition in visceral organs, renal damage, and metal flume fever can occur (5526).

PREGNANCY AND LACTATION: POSSIBLY UNSAFE ...when used orally. Epidemiological evidence links increased silver levels to babies born with developmental anomalies of the ear, face, and neck (5525).

Effectiveness

There is insufficient reliable information available about the effectiveness of colloidal silver.

Possible Mechanism of Action & Active Ingredients

Compounds that contain inorganic silver are germicidal. Silver binds to the reactive groups of proteins, causing denaturation and precipitation. Silver can also inactivate enzymes by binding to sulfhydryl, amino, carboxyl, phosphate, and imidazole groups. When absorbed, silver is most concentrated in the skin, liver, spleen, and adrenals with lesser amounts in the muscle and brain. The half-life depends on the silver salt used. Half-life can range from days to months. Silver deposited in the skin has a much longer half-life. Silver primarily leaves the body via fecal elimination with active biliary excretion (5525).

Adverse Reactions Including Known Allergies

Oral or topical use of colloidal silver can lead to argyria, an irreversible bluish skin discoloration. Argyria first appears in the gingiva with a slate-blue silver line. Colloidal silver can also stimulate melanin production in skin. Areas exposed to the sun will become increasingly discolored. Colloidal silver can also cause neurological deficits, diffuse silver deposition in visceral organs, renal damage, and metal flume fever (5525).

Possible Interactions with Herbs & Other Dietary Supplements

Insufficient reliable information available.

Possible Interactions with Drugs

DRUGS THAT COMPLEX WITH IRON: Theoretically, drugs such as tetracycline, ciprofloxacin (Cipro), methyldopa (Aldomet), norfloxacin (Noroxin), ofloxacin (Floxin), penicillamine (Cupramine), and thyroxine replacement therapy might have reduced absorption if given with colloidal silver.

Possible Interactions with Foods

No interactions are known to occur, and there is no known reason to expect a clinically significant interaction with colloidal silver.

Possible Interactions with Lab Tests

No interactions are known to occur, and there is no known reason to expect a clinically significant interaction with colloidal silver.

Possible Interactions with Diseases or Conditions

No interactions are known to occur, and there is no known reason to expect a clinically significant interaction with colloidal silver.

Typical Dosages & Routes of Administration that are Commonly Used

ORAL: A typical dose is 1 teaspoon of a 5 ppm colloid (25 mcg silver) (5520). A typical antibiotic dose is 1-3 teaspoons of 5 ppm colloid up to three times daily (5527). (75-225 mcg silver) which could exceed the total amount/day considered possibly safe for a 70 kg adult.

Comments

Interestingly, there are many internet ads for the components of a generator to produce colloidal silver at home. Those who produce colloidal silver at home will likely have no means to assay the product to assure any standard potency. There are many products that are far safer and more effective than colloidal silver.

COLOCYNTH

This Product is Also Known As

Bitter Apple, Bitter Cucumber, Colocynth Pulp, Colocynthidis Fructus, Koloquinthen.

Scientific Names

Citrullus colocynthis.
Family: Cucurbitaceae.

People Use This For

Orally, colocynth is used in combination products for acute and chronic constipation (including during pregnancy), and for liver and gallbladder ailments (2).

Safety

UNSAFE ...when taken orally. Colocynth was banned by FDA in 1991, due to toxicity (17).
PREGNANCY AND LACTATION: UNSAFE ...contraindicated; avoid using.

Effectiveness

LIKELY EFFECTIVE ...when taken orally for constipation, but risks preclude use.
There is insufficient reliable information available about the effectiveness of colocynth for its other uses.

Possible Mechanism of Action & Active Ingredients

The applicable part of colocynth is the ripe fruit. Contains up to 3% cucurbitacin, a poisonous constituent that irritates mucous membranes, including GI mucosa (2) .

Adverse Reactions Including Known Allergies

Ingestion of 0.6-1 grams of colocynth can cause severe irritation of the gastric mucosa, bloody diarrhea, kidney damage, hemorrhagic cystitis, and diuresis leading to anuria (2,18). Doses of 2 grams or more can cause convulsions, paralysis, and if untreated, death from circulatory collapse (18).

Possible Interactions with Herbs & Other Dietary Supplements

STIMULANT LAXATIVE HERBS: Theoretically, concomitant use with other stimulant laxative herbs may increase the risk of potassium depletion. Stimulant laxative herbs include: aloe dried leaf sap, wild cucumber fruit (Ecballium elaterium), blue flag rhizome, alder buckthorn, European buckthorn, butternut bark, cascara bark, castor oil, gamboge bark exudate, jalap root, black root, manna bark exudate, podophyllum root, rhubarb root, senna leaves and pods, and yellow dock root (19).
POTASSIUM DEPLETING HERBS: Theoretically, concomitant use with horsetail plant or licorice rhizome increases the risk of potassium depletion.

Possible Interactions with Drugs

CARDIAC GLYCOSIDES: Theoretically, overuse/abuse of this product increases the risk of adverse effects of cardiac glycoside drugs, such as digoxin (Lanoxin).

Possible Interactions with Foods

No interactions are known to occur, and there is no known reason to expect a clinically significant interaction with colocynth.

Possible Interactions with Lab Tests

POTASSIUM: Excessive use of colocynth might cause potassium depletion, reducing serum potassium concentrations and test results (19).
URINE OUTPUT: Excessive use of colocynth might lead to cessation of urine output (anuria) (18).

Possible Interactions with Diseases or Conditions

GI CONDITIONS: Can irritate gastrointestinal tract. Contraindicated in individuals with infectious or inflammatory gastrointestinal conditions (19).

Typical Dosages & Routes of Administration that are Commonly Used

No typical dosage.

Comments

Colocynth is considered unsafe; avoid using. The use of colocynth is not justified due to significant risks (2). Death has resulted from the consumption of as little as 1 1/2 teaspoons of the powder. In the management of poisoning, a dilute tannic acid solution should be taken, followed by large quantities of albuminous drinks (215).

COLOMBO

This Product is Also Known As
Calomba Root, Calumba, Calumbo Root.

Scientific Names
Jateorhiza palmata, synonym Wateorhiza palmata.
Family: Menispermaceae.

People Use This For
Orally, colombo is used to treat gastritis, dyspepsia, chronic enterocolitis [18], and diarrhea [18,7].

Safety
There is insufficient reliable information available about the safety of colombo.
Pregnancy and Lactation: Insufficient reliable information; avoid using.

Effectiveness
There is insufficient reliable information available about the effectiveness of colombo.

Possible Mechanism of Action & Active Ingredients
The applicable part of colombo is the root. Colombo contains alkaloids that have narcotic properties [18,7] and side effects [7] similar to morphine. Both increase the resting tone of smooth muscle in the intestinal tract [18,7]. In frogs, the alkaloids appear to act as a CNS paralyzing agent [18]. Palmatine, the main alkaloid component, has a similar effect in mammals [18]. Colombo's use as a digestive aid is empirically based upon the bitter principle content, which is believed to increase stomach acid secretion via vagal nerve stimulation [19].

Adverse Reactions Including Known Allergies
Large doses of Colombo may cause vomiting and epigastric pain [18]. Overdose can lead to paralysis and unconsciousness [18].

Possible Interactions with Herbs & Other Dietary Supplements
Insufficient reliable information available.

Possible Interactions with Drugs
ANTACIDS, H-2 ANTAGONISTS: Antacids and H-2 antagonists decrease stomach acid secretion, which is contradictory to Colombo's theoretical action [19]. H-2 antagonists include cimetidine, famotidine, nizatidine, and ranitidine.

Possible Interactions with Foods
No interactions are known to occur, and there is no known reason to expect a clinically significant interaction with colombo.

Possible Interactions with Lab Tests
No interactions are known to occur, and there is no known reason to expect a clinically significant interaction with colombo.

Possible Interactions with Diseases or Conditions
No interactions are known to occur, and there is no known reason to expect a clinically significant interaction with colombo.

Typical Dosages & Routes of Administration that are Commonly Used
ORAL: 2 teaspoons of the boiled root as tea is taken every hour [18]. For single use, 20 drops of the extract or 2.5 grams of the tincture can be used [18]. The root should be stored in dry area [18].

Comments
Colombo is no longer used as a digestive aid and is rarely used as an antidiarrheal agent because of its morphine-like effects [18].

COLTSFOOT

This Product is Also Known As
Ass's Foot, Brandlattich, British Tobacco, Bullsfoot, Coughwort, Farfarae Folium leaf, Fieldhove, Filuis Ante Patrem, Flower Velure, Foal's Foot, Foalswort, Guflatich, Hallfoot, Horsefoot, Horsehoof, Kuandong Hua, Pas Diane, Pas d'Ane, Pferdefut, Tussilage.

Scientific Names
Tussilago farfara.
Family: Asteraceae or Compositae.

 © Copyright 2000, Natural Medicines Comprehensive Database (209) 472-2244. For updated data, go to www.NaturalDatabase.com

People Use This For

Historically, coltsfoot leaf has been used orally for bronchitis, asthma, laryngitis, pertussis (4), acute respiratory tract mucous membrane inflammation with cough and hoarseness, acute or mild inflammation of the oral and pharyngeal mucosa (2), and sore throat (6). Coltsfoot has also been used as an inhalant for coughs and wheezing (6).

Safety

UNSAFE ...when used orally (2,7,12,515). All parts of coltsfoot contain unsaturated pyrrolizidine alkaloids (UPAs) in varying amounts (2,7). The unsaturated pyrrolizidine alkaloids are considered to be hepatotoxic and hepatocarcinogenic (7,515) UPAs are released into teas when prepared from coltsfoot leaves (7). Repeated exposure to low concentrations of UPAs is linked to veno-occlusive disease (4,12,515). UPAs are considered to be also possibly mutagenic (12). Dietary supplement products sold in the United States are not required to include the amount of UPAs they may contain; therefore, all preparations used orally containing coltsfoot should be considered potentially unsafe (3484).

PREGNANCY AND LACTATION: UNSAFE ...contraindicated due to its potential to be abortifacient (4,19) and hepatotoxic (4,12,575). ...hepatotoxic pyrrolizidine alkaloids may be excreted in breast milk (4,12,18).

Effectiveness

There is insufficient reliable information available about the effectiveness of coltsfoot.

Possible Mechanism of Action & Active Ingredients

The applicable part of coltsfoot is the leaf. Coltsfoot has been documented to have expectorant, antitussive, demulcent, and anti-inflammatory effects on mucous membranes (4). The mucilage content of coltsfoot has a soothing effect on the throat (6,515). Coltsfoot contains the unsaturated pyrrolizidine alkaloids senkirkirine and senecionine (4,7,515). Unsaturated pyrrolizidine alkaloids are known to be hepatotoxic in animals and humans (4,7,515). UPAs destroy and damage centrilobular hepatocytes of the liver and also destroy small branches of the hepatic vein (7). Animals fed various amounts of coltsfoot have been reported to develop cancerous tumors in the liver (515,3484). In animals, coltsfoot has anti-inflammatory and antibacterial activity against gram negative bacteria (4). It also contains an inhibitor of the platelet activating factor (PAF). PAF is known to play a key role in the inflammatory cascade. The presence of a PAF inhibitor in coltsfoot can account for the effect of coltsfoot in asthma (4). The constituent tusilagone has respiratory stimulant and cardiovascular (including pressor) activities (4). Cardiovascular effects are thought to be mediated by peripheral mechanisms and the respiratory effects by central mechanisms (4). An isolated coltsfoot constituent interacts with the cardiac calcium channel blocker receptor complex (dihydropyridine receptor), but it also has calcium channel blocking activity (4). In animals, coltsfoot is reported to have a pressor effect similar to dopamine but without tachyphylaxis and to be phototoxic (4).

Adverse Reactions Including Known Allergies

Nonspecific symptoms such as anorexia, lethargy and abdominal pain can result after chronic use of coltsfoot (7). Further use can lead to hepatotoxicity (4,7). There is one case report of fatal hepatic veno-occlusive disease in a neonate associated with regular maternal consumption during pregnancy of an herb tea containing several pyrrolizidine alkaloid herbs, including coltsfoot (575). It can cause an allergic reaction in individuals sensitive to the Asteraceae/Compositae family. Members of this family include ragweed, chrysanthemums, marigolds, daisies, and many other herbs.

Possible Interactions with Herbs & Other Dietary Supplements

EUCALYPTUS: Theoretically, concomitant use can increase the toxicity of coltsfoot due to enzyme induction by eucalyptus (19).

PYRROLIZIDINE ALKALOID-CONTAINING HERBS: Concomitant use is contraindicated due to the risk of additive toxicity. Herbs containing unsaturated pyrrolizidine alkaloids include: alkanna (12), borage (271), gravel root (4), hemp agrimony (271), hound's tongue (19), petasites (19), comfrey (271), coltsfoot, and the Senecio species plants; dusty miller (19), alpine ragwort (19), groundsel (271), golden ragwort (19), and tansy ragwort (271).

Possible Interactions with Drugs

ANTIHYPERTENSIVE and CARDIOVASCULAR DRUGS: Theoretically, excessive doses of coltsfoot can interfere with antihypertensive or cardiovascular therapy (4).

Possible Interactions with Foods

No interactions are known to occur, and there is no known reason to expect a clinically significant interaction with coltsfoot.

Possible Interactions with Lab Tests

No interactions are known to occur, and there is no known reason to expect a clinically significant interaction with coltsfoot.

Possible Interactions with Diseases or Conditions

HYPERTENSION, CARDIOVASCULAR DISEASE: Excessive amounts of coltsfoot can interfere with therapy for hypertension or cardiovascular disease (4).

LIVER DISEASE: Coltsfoot is contraindicated due to its hepatotoxic potential (19).

CROSS-ALLERGENICITY: Can cause an allergic reaction in individuals sensitive to the Asteraceae/Compositae family. Members of this family include ragweed, chrysanthemums, marigolds, daisies, and many other herbs.

Typical Dosages & Routes of Administration that are Commonly Used
No typical dosage.

Comments
None.

COLUMBINE

This Product is Also Known As
Culverwort

Scientific Names
Aquilegia vulgaris.
Family: Ranunculaceae.

People Use This For
Orally, columbine is used for general gastrointestinal disorders, to stimulate bile flow, and to regulate gallbladder contraction. It is also used for scurvy, jaundice and as a tranquilizer in patients with agitation [18].

Safety
There is insufficient reliable information available about the safety of the oral use of columbine.
Pregnancy and Lactation: Insufficient reliable information available; avoid using.

Effectiveness
There is insufficient reliable information available about the effectiveness of columbine.

Possible Mechanism of Action & Active Ingredients
The applicable parts of columbine are the above ground parts. There is insufficient reliable information available about the possible mechanism of action and active ingredients.

Adverse Reactions Including Known Allergies
None reported.

Possible Interactions with Herbs & Other Dietary Supplements
Insufficient reliable information available.

Possible Interactions with Drugs
No interactions are known to occur, and there is no known reason to expect a clinically significant interaction with columbine.

Possible Interactions with Foods
No interactions are known to occur, and there is no known reason to expect a clinically significant interaction with columbine.

Possible Interactions with Lab Tests
No interactions are known to occur, and there is no known reason to expect a clinically significant interaction with columbine.

Possible Interactions with Diseases or Conditions
No interactions are known to occur, and there is no known reason to expect a clinically significant interaction with columbine.

Typical Dosages & Routes of Administration that are Commonly Used
No typical dosage.

Comments
There is very little scientific information about this product. Our staff is continually analyzing the available information on natural medicines and will add data here as it becomes available.

COMFREY

This Product is Also Known As
Ass Ear, Black Root, Blackwort, Bruisewort, Common Comfrey, Consolidae Radix, Consound, Gum Plant, Healing Herb, Knitback, Knitbone, Salsify, Slippery Root, Symphytum Radix, Wallwort.

Scientific Names

Symphytum officinale.
Family: Boraginaceae.

People Use This For

Topically, comfrey is used for ulcers, wounds, and fractures (4,5). The above ground parts of comfrey are used for bruises and sprains (2).
Traditionally, comfrey has been used as a tea for ulcers, excessive menstrual flow, diarrhea, bloody urine, persistent cough, rheumatism, pleuritis, bronchitis, cancer, angina, as a gargle for gum disease, and pharyngitis (11,18,214).

Safety

POSSIBLY SAFE ...when the above ground parts are used topically on unbroken skin for less than 10 days (4). ...when the above ground parts are used topically for a maximum of 4-6 weeks per year in amounts at or below a daily dosage of 100 mcg of the hepatotoxic unsaturated pyrrolizidine alkaloids (UPAs) (2).
UNSAFE ...when the root or above ground parts are used orally because of its potential for acute or chronic liver toxicity (2,4,5) . Teas made from comfrey leaf contain lesser levels of alkaloids (4), but regular consumption can lead to toxicity (17,515). Dietary supplement products sold in the United States are not required to include the amount of UPAs they may contain; therefore, all preparations used orally containing comfrey should be considered potentially unsafe (3484).
PREGNANCY AND LACTATION: UNSAFE ...when the above ground parts or root are used orally (4,12). There is insufficient reliable information available about the safety of the topical use of comfrey during pregnancy or lactation; avoid using.

Effectiveness

POSSIBLY EFFECTIVE ...when used topically as an anti-inflammatory agent and for treating bruises and sprains (2,9). Comfrey should be used only on unbroken skin (2).
There is insufficient reliable information available about the effectiveness of comfrey for its other uses.

Possible Mechanism of Action & Active Ingredients

The applicable parts of comfrey are the leaf, rhizome, and root. Comfrey contains unsaturated pyrrolizidine alkaloids (UPAs) which are considered to be hepatotoxic and hepatocarcinogenic (4,7,515). UPAs destroy and damage centrilobular hepatocytes of the liver and also destroy small branches of the hepatic vein (7). The pyrrolizidine alkaloid content of the roots is ten times that of the leaves (5). Sarracind and platyphylline, non-hepatotoxic pyrrolizidine alkaloid constituents, have been used for treating gastrointestinal hypermotility and peptic ulcers (4). The healing activity of comfrey is due to its constituent, allantoin (9). The constituent, rosmarinic acid, shows evidence of anti-inflammatory activity (4) and that it can inhibit microvascular pulmonary injury (3).

Adverse Reactions Including Known Allergies

Chronic exposure to plants containing UPA constituents has been associated with veno-occlusive disease (4021). Symptoms of acute veno-occlusive disease are characterized by anorexia, lethargy (7) and a dull, dragging ache in the right upper abdomen with marked distention of the abdomen. These symptoms are sometimes accompanied by reduced urine output. Subacute veno-occlusive disease is associated with vague symptoms and persistent liver enlargement (4021).

Possible Interactions with Herbs & Other Dietary Supplements

EUCALYPTUS: Theoretically, concomitant use might increase the risk of unsaturated pyrrolizidine alkaloid toxicity due to enzyme induction by eucalyptus (19).
PYRROLIZIDINE ALKALOID-CONTAINING HERBS: Concomitant use is contraindicated due to the risk of additive toxicity. Herbs containing unsaturated pyrrolizidine alkaloids include: alkanna (12), borage (271), gravel root (4), hemp agrimony (271), hound's tongue (19), petasites (19), comfrey (271), coltsfoot, and the Senecio species plants: dusty miller (19), alpine ragwort (19), groundsel (271), golden ragwort (19), and tansy ragwort (271).

Possible Interactions with Drugs

No interactions are known to occur, and there is no known reason to expect a clinically significant interaction with comfrey.

Possible Interactions with Foods

No interactions are known to occur, and there is no known reason to expect a clinically significant interaction with comfrey.

Possible Interactions with Lab Tests

No interactions are known to occur, and there is no known reason to expect a clinically significant interaction with comfrey.

Possible Interactions with Diseases or Conditions

BROKEN, DAMAGED SKIN: Contraindicated. Apply only to unbroken skin (2,4).

Typical Dosages & Routes of Administration that are Commonly Used

TOPICAL: Ointments and other external preparations are commonly made with 5-20% of comfrey. The daily use of comfrey should not exceed 100 mcg of the pyrrolizidine alkaloids. Comfrey should not be used for more than ten days (4,5), and the maximum use is four to six weeks per year (2). It only should be applied externally on unbroken skin (4,12).

Comments

Prickly comfrey is more toxic than common comfrey, but either might be labeled comfrey. Some products labeled common comfrey or Symphytum officinale instead contain the more toxic prickly comfrey (3,515). The American Herbal Products Association recommends all products with toxic pyrrolizidine alkaloids be labeled with the statement, "For external use only. Do not apply to broken or abraded skin. Do not use while nursing" (12).

COMMON STONECROP

This Product is Also Known As

Bird Bread, Creeping Tom, Gold Chain, Golden Moss, Jack-of-the-Buttery, Mousetail, Prick Madam, Wall Ginger, Wallpepper.

Scientific Names

Sedum acre.

People Use This For

Orally, common stonecrop is used for coughs and hypertension.
Topically, common stonecrop is used for wounds, burns, hemorrhoids, warts, eczema, and mouth ulcers (18).

Safety

There is insufficient reliable information available about the safety of common stonecrop.
Pregnancy and Lactation: Insufficient reliable information available; avoid using.

Effectiveness

There is insufficient reliable information available about the effectiveness of common stonecrop.

Possible Mechanism of Action & Active Ingredients

None reported.

Adverse Reactions Including Known Allergies

Common stonecrop can cause vomiting and diarrhea if consumed in greater than medicinal amounts(18).

Possible Interactions with Herbs & Other Dietary Supplements

Insufficient reliable information available.

Possible Interactions with Drugs

No interactions are known to occur, and there is no known reason to expect a clinically significant interaction with common stonecrop.

Possible Interactions with Foods

No interactions are known to occur, and there is no known reason to expect a clinically significant interaction with common stonecrop.

Possible Interactions with Lab Tests

No interactions are known to occur, and there is no known reason to expect a clinically significant interaction with common stonecrop.

Possible Interactions with Diseases or Conditions

GI AND LOWER URINARY TRACT INFLAMMATION: Contraindicated (18).

Typical Dosages & Routes of Administration that are Commonly Used

ORAL: Daily, one cup tea (simmer 1 teaspoon or 1.5 grams in 150 mL boiling water for 10-15 minutes, strain) twice daily (18).
TOPICAL: Crush fresh plant and place on eczematous skin or warts.

Comments

None.

CONDURANGO

This Product is Also Known As
Condurango Cortex, Eagle-Vine Bark.

Scientific Names
Marsdenia condurango; Gonolobus condurango.
Family: Asclepiadaceae.

People Use This For
Orally, condurango bark is used as an appetite stimulant and for dyspeptic complaints (2,18).
In folk medicine, condurango has been used for stomach cancer (8,18).

Safety
LIKELY SAFE ...when used orally and appropriately (2).
PREGNANCY AND LACTATION: Insufficient reliable information available; avoid using.

Effectiveness
POSSIBLY EFFECTIVE ...when used orally as an appetite stimulant (2).
There is insufficient reliable information available about the effectiveness of condurango for its other uses.

Possible Mechanism of Action & Active Ingredients
The applicable part of condurango is the bark. The condurango alkaloid constituents, which as a group are referred to as condurangin, stimulate salivation and the secretion of gastric juices (8).

Adverse Reactions Including Known Allergies
Anaphylaxis can occur with the use of the condurango bark (1501).

Possible Interactions with Herbs & Other Dietary Supplements
Insufficient reliable information available.

Possible Interactions with Drugs
No interactions are known to occur, and there is no known reason to expect a clinically significant interaction with condurango.

Possible Interactions with Foods
No interactions are known to occur, and there is no known reason to expect a clinically significant interaction with condurango.

Possible Interactions with Lab Tests
No interactions are known to occur, and there is no known reason to expect a clinically significant interaction with condurango.

Possible Interactions with Diseases or Conditions
LATEX ALLERGY: Cross-sensitivity to condurango can occur in individuals allergic to natural rubber latex (1500), including anaphylaxis (1501). Avoid the use of condurango in these individuals.

Typical Dosages & Routes of Administration that are Commonly Used
ORAL: The typical dose of the bark is 2-4 grams per day (2). The usual dose of the water extract is 200-500 mg per day (2). The common dose of the liquid extract is 2-4 grams per day (2), and the tincture is usually given as 2-5 grams per day (2).

Comments
None.

CONJUGATED LINOLEIC ACID

This Product is Also Known As
CLA.

Scientific Names
cis-9,trans-11 conjugated linoleic acid; trans-10,cis-12 conjugated linoleic acid.

People Use This For
Orally, conjugated linoleic acid (CLA) is used to prevent and treat cancer (5924,5926,5927,5930), to treat obesity (5924,5928,5929), cachexia (5925), for bodybuilding (5937), for limiting food allergy reactions (5940), and for atherosclerosis (5925).

Safety

LIKELY SAFE ...when consumed in food. Conjugated linoleic acid occurs naturally in milk fat, beef, and meat of other ruminant animals.

POSSIBLY SAFE ...when used orally as a supplement short-term (5935). However, there are no long-term safety studies.

PREGNANCY AND LACTATION: LIKELY SAFE ...when consumed in food. There is insufficient reliable information available about the safety of CLA supplements during pregnancy or lactation; avoid using.

Effectiveness

There is insufficient reliable information available about the effectiveness of conjugated linoleic acid.

Possible Mechanism of Action & Active Ingredients

Conjugated linoleic acid (CLA) is a class of positional and geometric conjugated dienoic isomers of linoleic acid. Dairy products and beef are the major dietary sources. Some evidence suggests CLA might reduce atherosclerosis, regulate energy metabolism and nutrient partitioning (5924). Preliminary data suggests CLA could play a role in preventing malignant melanoma; colorectal, breast (5925), and prostate cancer (5926); or diabetes (5936). CLA might be beneficial in reducing body fat (5926), reducing cachexia associated with advanced cancer (5924), enhancing immune function, and inhibiting cyclo-oxygenase and lipoxygenase pathways in tumor cells (5926). It might also have a beneficial effect upon diabetes (5934,5936), platelet aggregation and the immune system (5934). CLA is believed to have two actions: to inhibit lipoprotein lipase, an enzyme that breaks fat down so it can be absorbed, and to increase the activity of enzymes that break down stored fats (5937). Animal studies show CLA supplementation can increase the vitamin A status (retinol in the breast and liver, retinyl esters in the liver) (5931). Although supplementing the diet of cows with linoleic oil (safflower oil) increases the concentration of CLA in cow's milk (5932), supplementing the diet of humans with linoleic oil does not increase plasma CLA level (5933).

Adverse Reactions Including Known Allergies

Oral use of conjugated linoleic acid might cause gastrointestinal upset (5940).

Possible Interactions with Herbs & Other Dietary Supplements

VITAMIN A: Some evidence suggests conjugated linoleic acid might increase vitamin A (retinol) storage in the liver and breast (5931).

Possible Interactions with Drugs

No interactions are known to occur, and there is no known reason to expect a clinically significant interaction with conjugated linoleic acid.

Possible Interactions with Foods

No interactions are known to occur, and there is no known reason to expect a clinically significant interaction with conjugated linoleic acid.

Possible Interactions with Lab Tests

No interactions are known to occur, and there is no known reason to expect a clinically significant interaction with conjugated linoleic acid.

Possible Interactions with Diseases or Conditions

CANCER: The Life Extension Foundation recommends that cancer patients using CLA should take high doses of soy genistein extract. The rationale is CLA could increase tyrosine kinase C activity which cancer cells use for energy metabolism. Genistein (in soy) inhibits tyrosine kinase C (5937).

Typical Dosages & Routes of Administration that are Commonly Used

ORAL: For weight loss, a typical dose is 3-3.6 grams per day taken with meals (5937). For cancer 3-6 grams per day are taken with meals. The Life Extension Foundation also recommends high doses of genistein extract when CLA is used to treat cancer (5937).

Comments

Some information suggests CLA in milk fat is not affected by processing. However, one study showed grilling ground beef could increase CLA content five-fold (5939).

CONTRAYERVA

This Product is Also Known As

None.

Scientific Names

Dorstenia contrayerva.

People Use This For

Orally, contrayerva is used to increase stamina, and as a snakebite antidote (18).

Safety

POSSIBLY UNSAFE ...when root preparations are used orally. Contains cardenolides that are cardioactive steroids and could affect the heart (18).
PREGNANCY AND LACTATION: POSSIBLY UNSAFE ...when used orally; avoid using.

Effectiveness

There is insufficient reliable information available about the effectiveness of contrayerva.

Possible Mechanism of Action & Active Ingredients

The applicable part of contrayerva is the root. Contrayerva is believed to act as a stimulant and induce sweating (18).

Adverse Reactions Including Known Allergies

Contrayerva contains cardioactive steroids (cardenolides). When used topically, skin contact with plant can increase sensitivity to ultraviolet light (18).

Possible Interactions with Herbs & Other Dietary Supplements

Insufficient reliable information available.

Possible Interactions with Drugs

No interactions are known to occur, and there is no known reason to expect a clinically significant interaction with contrayerva.

Possible Interactions with Foods

No interactions are known to occur, and there is no known reason to expect a clinically significant interaction with contrayerva.

Possible Interactions with Lab Tests

No interactions are known to occur, and there is no known reason to expect a clinically significant interaction with contrayerva.

Possible Interactions with Diseases or Conditions

No interactions are known to occur, and there is no known reason to expect a clinically significant interaction with contrayerva.

Typical Dosages & Routes of Administration that are Commonly Used

ORAL: People typically use 1/2 teaspoon of the powdered root. Contrayerva is also prepared as a tea with 1 ounce added to 2 cups boiling water (5267).

Comments

There is very little scientific information about this product. Our staff is continually analyzing the available information on natural medicines and will add data here as it becomes available.

COOLWORT

This Product is Also Known As

Foam Flower, Mitrewort.

Scientific Names

Tiarella cordifolia.

People Use This For

Orally, coolwort is used for urinary tract and digestive disorders (18), as a tonic, diuretic, for bladder diseases and stones, indigestion, and dyspepsia (3821).

Safety

There is insufficient reliable information available about the safety of coolwort.
Pregnancy and Lactation: Insufficient reliable information available; avoid using.

Effectiveness

There is insufficient reliable information available about the effectiveness of coolwort.

Possible Mechanism of Action & Active Ingredients

Coolwort is thought to have diuretic and tonic properties (18).

Adverse Reactions Including Known Allergies

None reported (18).

Possible Interactions with Herbs & Other Dietary Supplements
Insufficient reliable information available.

Possible Interactions with Drugs
No interactions are known to occur, and there is no known reason to expect a clinically significant interaction with coolwort.

Possible Interactions with Foods
No interactions are known to occur, and there is no known reason to expect a clinically significant interaction with coolwort.

Possible Interactions with Lab Tests
No interactions are known to occur, and there is no known reason to expect a clinically significant interaction with coolwort.

Possible Interactions with Diseases or Conditions
No interactions are known to occur, and there is no known reason to expect a clinically significant interaction with coolwort.

Typical Dosages & Routes of Administration that are Commonly Used
Coolwort is used as a tea (18).

Comments
There is very little scientific information about this product. Our staff is continually analyzing the available information on natural medicines and will add data here as it becomes available.

COPAIBA BALSAM

This Product is Also Known As
Copaiba, Copaiba Oleoresin, Copaiva, Jesuit's Balsam.

Scientific Names
Copaifera officinalis; Copaifera langsdorfii; Copaifera reticulata; and other Copaifera species.
Family: Leguminoseae or Fabaceae.

People Use This For
Traditionally, copaiba balsam has been used for chronic bronchitis, hemorrhoids, chronic diarrhea, chronic cystitis (11), urinary tract infections, as a stimulant, and as a laxative (18).
In foods and beverages, copaiba balsam oleoresin is used as an ingredient (11).
In manufacturing, copaiba balsam oleoresin and oil are used in soaps, cosmetics, and perfumes (11).
In pharmaceutical preparations, both the oleoresin and oil are used in cough medicines and diuretics (11).

Safety
POSSIBLY SAFE ...when used orally in food amounts. Maximum use level is usually less than 0.002%. Both the oleoresin and oil have been approved for food use. ...when used topically in cosmetics. Maximum use level in perfumes is 0.8%.
POSSIBLY UNSAFE ...when used orally for medicinal purposes. Copaiba balsam can irritate mucous membranes. Ingesting 5 grams can cause stomach pains (18).
PREGNANCY AND LACTATION: POSSIBLY UNSAFE ...when used orally for medicinal purposes; avoid using.

Effectiveness
There is insufficient reliable information available about the effectiveness of copaiba balsam.

Possible Mechanism of Action & Active Ingredients
Copaiba balsam contains a volatile oil consisting of alpha and beta-caryophyllene, L-cadinenes, and copene. It also has resins, including diterpenoid oleoresins. Some evidence suggests copaiba balsam might have bacteriostatic (18), diuretic, expectorant, disinfectant, and stimulant activity (11). In addition to these properties, the oil exhibits antibacterial activity (11). Some evidence suggests the oleoresin of the Brazilian Copaifera species might have anti-inflammatory effects (11).

Adverse Reactions Including Known Allergies
Ingesting 5 grams of copaiba balsam orally can cause stomach pains (18); repeated doses can cause shivers, tremor, groin pain, and insomnia (18). Large amounts may cause vomiting, diarrhea, and measles-like rash (11). Used topically, copaiba balsam can cause contact dermatitis with erythema, papular or vesicular rash, urticaria, petechiae, and the rash may leave brown spots after healing (18).

Possible Interactions with Herbs & Other Dietary Supplements
Insufficient reliable information available.

Possible Interactions with Drugs
No interactions are known to occur, and there is no known reason to expect a clinically significant interaction with copaiba balsam.

Possible Interactions with Foods
No interactions are known to occur, and there is no known reason to expect a clinically significant interaction with copaiba balsam.

Possible Interactions with Lab Tests
No interactions are known to occur, and there is no known reason to expect a clinically significant interaction with copaiba balsam.

Possible Interactions with Diseases or Conditions
No interactions are known to occur, and there is no known reason to expect a clinically significant interaction with copaiba balsam.

Typical Dosages & Routes of Administration that are Commonly Used
No typical dosage.

Comments
Copaiba balsam is an oleoresin rather than a true balsam collected from the trunk of Copaifera species trees (11). Copaiba oil is distilled from the oleoresin (11). Copaiba balsam is considered obsolete for medicinal purposes (18).

COPPER

This Product is Also Known As
Cuivre, Elemental Copper.

Scientific Names
Copper; Cu; atomic number 29.

People Use This For
Orally, copper is used to treat copper deficiency, anemia due to copper deficiency (505), wound healing, arthritis, inflammation, and osteoporosis (508).

Safety
LIKELY SAFE ...when taken orally as a supplement to treat copper deficiency (505). The current safe dietary intake for adults ranges from 2-3 mg/day (17).
LIKELY UNSAFE ...when used orally in larger amounts. Renal failure and death can occur with ingestion of as little as 1 gram of copper sulfate (17).
PREGNANCY AND LACTATION: Insufficient reliable information available; avoid using.

Effectiveness
LIKELY EFFECTIVE ...when taken orally for treating copper deficiency and anemia due to copper deficiency (505).
There is insufficient reliable information available about the effectiveness of copper for its other uses.

Possible Mechanism of Action & Active Ingredients
Copper is essential for hemoglobin synthesis and is a key constituent of several enzymes, including ceruloplasmin.

Adverse Reactions Including Known Allergies
TOXICITY: Acute exposure symptoms include: nausea, vomiting, bloody diarrhea, hypotension, hemolytic anemia, uremia, cardiovascular collapse. Chronic exposure symptoms include: sporadic fever, vomiting, epigastric pain, diarrhea, and jaundice (159). Renal failure and death can occur with ingestion of as little as 1 gram of copper sulfate (17).

Possible Interactions with Herbs & Other Dietary Supplements
VITAMIN C (ascorbic acid): 1500 mg of Vitamin C taken daily may decrease copper-dependent enzyme (ceruloplasmin) activity significantly (710).
ZINC: Large amounts of zinc can inhibit copper absorption (707,708) and cause copper deficiency (706).

Possible Interactions with Drugs
PENICILLAMINE: Copper inhibits penicillamine (Cuprimine, Depen) activity; avoid concomitant use (15).

Drug Influences on Nutrient Levels and Depletion
SOME DRUGS CAN AFFECT COPPER LEVELS:
PENICILLAMINE (Cuprimine, Depen): Penicillamine chelates copper in the gastrointestinal tract and decreases absorption. Separate administration by at least 2 hours. The need for supplementation has not been adequately studied (4453,4531,4534,4535).

Possible Interactions with Foods
No interactions are known to occur, and there is no known reason to expect a clinically significant interaction with copper.

Possible Interactions with Lab Tests
No interactions are known to occur, and there is no known reason to expect a clinically significant interaction with copper.

Possible Interactions with Diseases or Conditions
WILSON'S DISEASE: Copper supplementation can worsen this condition or interfere with penicillamine therapy (15,505).

Typical Dosages & Routes of Administration that are Commonly Used
ORAL: For copper deficiency, 0.1 mg/kg cupric sulfate per day (505). The copper requirement for young adults can be as low as 0.8 mg per day (17). The current safe and adequate dietary intake for adults ranges from 2-3 mg per day (17).

Comments
There is no evidence that copper supplementation is needed or beneficial for people eating a normal diet, including athletes (505,703,704,705,709). Copper deficiency is seldom observed in humans and has been associated with excessive zinc intake (505,706,707,708), intestinal bypass surgery, parenteral nutrition, and malnourished infants (505).

CORAL

This Product is Also Known As
Calcium Carbonate Matrix, Sea Coral.
CAUTION: See separate listing for Coral Root.

Scientific Names
Goniopora species; Porites species.

People Use This For
In orthopedics, coral is used as a substrate for growing new bone in areas damaged by trauma, maxillofacial reconstruction, cosmetic facial surgery, and damaged weight-bearing bones (6).

Safety
LIKELY SAFE ...when used in orthopedic surgery. Coral may reduce adverse effects inherent in bone graft surgery (6).
PREGNANCY AND LACTATION: Insufficient reliable information available; avoid using.

Effectiveness
LIKELY EFFECTIVE ...when used in orthopedic surgery as substrate for growing new bone in maxillofacial reconstruction (6).
There is insufficient reliable information available about the effectiveness of coral for its other uses.

Possible Mechanism of Action & Active Ingredients
Coral (calcium carbonate matrix) is harvested and treated with heat, pressure, and chemicals to convert it to hydroxyapatite (6). Researchers think it provides a long-lasting matrix that is very similar to natural bone (6).

Adverse Reactions Including Known Allergies
None reported (6).

Possible Interactions with Herbs & Other Dietary Supplements
Insufficient reliable information available.

Possible Interactions with Drugs
No interactions are known to occur, and there is no known reason to expect a clinically significant interaction with coral.

Possible Interactions with Foods
No interactions are known to occur, and there is no known reason to expect a clinically significant interaction with coral.

Possible Interactions with Lab Tests
No interactions are known to occur, and there is no known reason to expect a clinically significant interaction with coral.

Possible Interactions with Diseases or Conditions
No interactions are known to occur, and there is no known reason to expect a clinically significant interaction with coral.

Typical Dosages & Routes of Administration that are Commonly Used
No typical dosage.

Comments
Avoid confusion with coral root (Corallorhiza odontorhiza).

CORAL ROOT

This Product is Also Known As
Chicken Toe, Crawley, Crawley Root, Fever Root, Scaley Dragon's Claw, Turkey Claw.
CAUTION: See separate listing for Coral.

Scientific Names
Corallorhiza odontorihiza.
Family: Orchidaceae.

People Use This For
Coral root is used for colds, and inducing perspiration [18].

Safety
There is insufficient reliable information available about the safety of coral root.
Pregnancy and Lactation: Insufficient reliable information available; avoid using.

Effectiveness
There is insufficient reliable information available about the effectiveness of coral root.

Possible Mechanism of Action & Active Ingredients
The applicable part of coral root is the rhizome/root. Reported to have diaphoretic, antipyretic, and sedative effects [18].

Adverse Reactions Including Known Allergies
None reported [18].

Possible Interactions with Herbs & Other Dietary Supplements
Insufficient reliable information available.

Possible Interactions with Drugs
No interactions are known to occur, and there is no known reason to expect a clinically significant interaction with coral root.

Possible Interactions with Foods
No interactions are known to occur, and there is no known reason to expect a clinically significant interaction with coral root.

Possible Interactions with Lab Tests
No interactions are known to occur, and there is no known reason to expect a clinically significant interaction with coral root.

Possible Interactions with Diseases or Conditions
No interactions are known to occur, and there is no known reason to expect a clinically significant interaction with coral root.

Typical Dosages & Routes of Administration that are Commonly Used
ORAL: People typically prepare coral root as a tea, adding 1 teaspoon of root to 1 cup of water. The tea is taken hot or cold, 1 to 2 cups per day. In tincture form, the coral root dose is 10 to 20 drops [5263].

Comments
Avoid confusion with coral. Scarcity of this plant limits use [18].

© Copyright 2000, Natural Medicines Comprehensive Database (209) 472-2244. For updated data, go to www.NaturalDatabase.com

CORDYCEPS

This Product is Also Known As
Caterpillar Fungus, Cs-4, Dong Chong Xia Cao, Dong Chong Zia Cao, Hsia Ts'Ao Tung Ch'Ung, Vegetable Caterpillar.

Scientific Names
Cordyceps sinensis.
Family: Ascomycetes or Clavicipitaceae.

People Use This For
Orally, cordyceps is used for strengthening the immune system, for reducing the effects of aging (321), promoting longevity, treating lethargy (512), and improving liver function in people with hepatitis B. It is also used to treat coughs, chronic bronchitis, respiratory disorders, kidney disorders (512), frequent nocturia (3408), male sexual dysfunction (512), anemia, heart arrhythmias, high cholesterol, liver disorders (321), dizziness, weakness, tinnitus (3408), wasting, and opium addiction (4017). It is also used as a stimulant, a tonic (4017), and an adaptogen which is used to increase energy, enhance stamina, and reduce fatigue (512,4017).

Safety
POSSIBLY SAFE ...when used orally and appropriately (12). There are no reports of cordyceps toxicity in humans.
PREGNANCY AND LACTATION: Insufficient reliable information available; avoid using.

Effectiveness
POSSIBLY EFFECTIVE ...when taken orally following cancer chemotherapy for improving quality of life and cellular immunity (3417). ...when taken orally by patients with hepatitis B for improving liver function (3435). There is insufficient reliable information available about the effectiveness of cordyceps for its other uses.

Possible Mechanism of Action & Active Ingredients
Cordyceps sinensis has beneficial effects on the immune, endocrine, cardiovascular, respiratory, renal, sexual, hepatic, immunologic, and nervous systems (3403,3404). Preliminary studies suggest cordyceps might stimulate immune function by increasing the number of T helper cells (3431); increasing the natural killer cell activity (3425,3427); stimulating the blood mononuclear cells (3414); increasing the levels of interferon-gamma, tumor necrosis factor-alpha, and interleukin-1 (3414); and prolonging the survival of lymphocytes (3432). Studies in animals with cancer suggest cordyceps improves immune response, reduces tumor size (3409,3431,3434), and lengthens survival time (3434,3437). Some evidence suggests cordyceps might be cytotoxic to cancer cells (3410,3416,3420), particularly lung carcinoma (3407) and melanoma (3427). Other evidence suggests that cordyceps might reduce the risk of renal toxicity from cyclosporin or aminoglycoside drugs (3411,3418,3419), and prove beneficial in chronic renal failure (3428). Cordyceps shows evidence that it can inhibit platelet aggregation and thrombus formation (3429). Other information suggests it might counteract or prevent arrhythmias, while decreasing heart rate and contractility (3436). Cordyceps polysaccharides show evidence that they might increase corticosterone production (3412). Other studies suggest they might reduce blood glucose (3415) without reducing plasma insulin levels (3415,3421), as well as reduce plasma triglycerides and cholesterol (3415). Preliminary animal studies suggest cordyceps could possibly be beneficial in treating systemic lupus erythematosus (3424). Limited human evidence suggests Cordyceps can improve liver function in patients with chronic hepatitis B (3435).

Adverse Reactions Including Known Allergies
None reported.

Possible Interactions with Herbs & Other Dietary Supplements
Insufficient reliable information available.

Possible Interactions with Drugs
CYCLOSPORINE: Concomitant administration can reduce nephrotoxicity in kidney-transplant recipients (3418).
AMINOGLYCOSIDES: Concomitant administration can reduce amikacin-induced nephrotoxicity in older people (3419).
CYCLOPHOSPHAMIDE: Theoretically, concomitant use might protect helper T-cells and natural killer cells from immunosuppressive drug effects (3427,3431).
PREDNISOLONE: Theoretically, concomitant use might protect helper T cells from immunosuppressive drug effects (3431,3437).

Possible Interactions with Foods
No interactions are known to occur, and there is no known reason to expect a clinically significant interaction with cordyceps.

Possible Interactions with Lab Tests
LIVER FUNCTION TESTS: Cordyceps might improve liver function and test results in people with chronic hepatitis B (3435).

Possible Interactions with Diseases or Conditions
HEPATITIS B: Based on limited human evidence, cordyceps might improve liver function and provide other benefits for people with chronic hepatitis B (3435).

Typical Dosages & Routes of Administration that are Commonly Used
ORAL: A typical dosage of fermented Cordyceps sinensis is 3 grams per day (3403,3404).

Comments
Cordyceps sinensis is a fungus parasite that lives on caterpillars in high mountain regions of China (512). For commercial purposes, the cordyceps cells (Cs-4 strain) can be artificially propagated in the laboratory (512). Jinshuibao capsules are the commercially available form of fermented Cordyceps sinensis Cs-4 (3403).

CORIANDER

This Product is Also Known As
Chinese Parsley, Cilantro, Coriandri Fructus, Koriander.

Scientific Names
Coriandrum sativum.
Family: Apiaceae or Umbelliferae.

People Use This For
Orally, coriander is used for dyspepsia, loss of appetite (2), as a stomach function stimulant, spasmolytic, antiflatulent, bactericide, fungicide, and for diarrhea (8).
In Chinese medicine, coriander has been used to treat measles, dysentery, hemorrhoids, and toothaches (11). The whole plant is used for stomachache, nausea, measles, and painful hernia (11).
In folk medicine, coriander is used for worms, rheumatism, and joint pain (8).
For food uses, coriander is used as a culinary spice (11).
In manufacturing, coriander is used as a flavoring agent in pharmaceutical preparations, as a fragrance component in cosmetics and soaps, and for flavoring tobacco (11).

Safety
LIKELY SAFE ...when consumed in amounts commonly found in foods. Coriander is Generally Recognized as Safe (GRAS) for food use in the US and has a maximum use level of 0.52% (11).
POSSIBLY SAFE ...when used orally and appropriately for medicinal purposes (12).
PREGNANCY AND LACTATION: Insufficient reliable information available; avoid amounts in excess of those found in foods.

Effectiveness
POSSIBLY EFFECTIVE ...when taken orally for loss of appetite and dyspepsia (2,11).
There is insufficient reliable information available about the effectiveness of coriander for its other uses.

Possible Mechanism of Action & Active Ingredients
The applicable part of coriander is the seed/fruit. Coriander is a rich source of vitamin C, calcium, magnesium, potassium, and iron (19). The odor and taste of coriander are due to the volatile oil, which consists mainly of linalool (60-70%) (7). In animals, coriander has shown hypoglycemic activity (11). Coriander oil can possess larvicidal properties (11).

Adverse Reactions Including Known Allergies
Powdered coriander and especially the oil can cause allergic reactions and photosensitivity (8). Like other members of the carrot family, coriander can cause contact dermatitis (19).

Possible Interactions with Herbs & Other Dietary Supplements
Insufficient reliable information available.

Possible Interactions with Drugs
No interactions are known to occur, and there is no known reason to expect a clinically significant interaction with coriander.

Possible Interactions with Foods
No interactions are known to occur, and there is no known reason to expect a clinically significant interaction with coriander.

Possible Interactions with Lab Tests
No interactions are known to occur, and there is no known reason to expect a clinically significant interaction with coriander.

Possible Interactions with Diseases or Conditions
No interactions are known to occur, and there is no known reason to expect a clinically significant interaction with coriander.

Typical Dosages & Routes of Administration that are Commonly Used
ORAL: The typical dose of coriander is 3 grams per day of the dried fruit/seed or one cup of the tea between meals, up to three times daily (2,8,18). The tea is prepared by steeping 1 gram of the crushed seed or fruit in 150 mL boiling water for 5-10 minutes. The usual dose of the tincture is 10-20 drops after meals (18).

Comments
None.

CORIOLUS MUSHROOM

This Product is Also Known As
Boletus Versicolor, Coriolus, Kawaratake, Krestin, Polyporus Versicolor, Polysaccharide Peptide, Polysaccharide-K, Polystictus Versicolor, PSK, PSP, Turkey Tail, Yun-Zhi (cloud mushroom).

Scientific Names
Coriolus versicolor, synonym Trametes versicolor.
Family: Polyporaceae.

People Use This For
Orally, coriolus mushroom or its derivatives are used for stimulating the immune system; treating herpes, chronic fatigue syndrome, hepatitis (5495,5496), treating pulmonary disorders; reducing phlegm; improving body building; increasing energy; curing ringworm and impetigo; treating upper respiratory, urinary, and digestive tract infections; curing liver disorders including hepatitis (5497), ameliorating the toxic effects and pain of chemotherapy and radiation therapy; promoting curative effect of chemotherapy; prolonging life and raising the quality of life; increasing appetite (5498), and improving the effectiveness of cancer chemotherapy (1640,1641,1648,1649,1650,1651,1652, 1653,1654,1655,1656,1657,1658,1659,1660,1661,1662).

Safety
POSSIBLY SAFE ...when coriolus mushroom is used orally and appropriately (5477). ...when isolated PSK and PSP are used orally and appropriately (1635,1636,1640,1641,1648,1649,1650,1651,1652,1653,1654,1655,1656,1657,1658,1659,1660,1661,1662).
PREGNANCY AND LACTATION: Insufficient reliable information available; avoid using.

Effectiveness
POSSIBLY EFFECTIVE ...when isolated PSP and PSK which are found in coriolus are used orally as adjuncts in cancer chemotherapy regimens (1640,1641,1648,1649,1650,1651,1652,1653,1654,1655,1656,1657,1658,1659,1660,1661,1662).
There is insufficient reliable information available about the effectiveness of coriolus for its other uses.

Possible Mechanism of Action & Active Ingredients
The applicable parts of coriolus mushroom are the fruiting body and mycelium (5494,5496). Coriolus mushrooms have a long history in folk medicine, but researchers are just beginning to isolate and identify substances in coriolus that have pharmacological activity (5477,1635). Coriolus contains several polysaccharides, including polysaccharide peptide (PSP) and polysaccharide-K (PSK, krestin), shown to have antitumor and immunomodulating effects (5484,5494,5499,1600,1635,1636,1637,1638,1639,1640,1641,1642,1648,1649,1650). PSK has been used in Japan as a biological response modifier in cancer chemotherapy regimens with varying results (1640,1641,1651,1652,1653,1654,1655,1656,1657, 1658,1659) (1660,1661,1662). Coriolus might have activity against the human immunodeficiency virus (HIV) (1643,1644). Preliminary evidence suggests that coriolus might have analgesic activity and protect against acetaminophen-induced hepatotoxicity (1645,1646,1647).

Adverse Reactions Including Known Allergies
None reported with coriolus (1635,1636). Patients receiving PSK as an adjunct to chemotherapy experienced nausea, leukopenia, and liver function impairment (1651); however, this may have been due to the chemotherapy.

Possible Interactions with Herbs & Other Dietary Supplements
Insufficient reliable information available.

Possible Interactions with Drugs
ACETAMINOPHEN: Theoretically, coriolus might protect against acetaminophen-induced hepatotoxicity.

Possible Interactions with Foods
No interactions are known to occur, and there is no known reason to expect a clinically significant interaction with coriolus mushroom.

Possible Interactions with Lab Tests

No interactions are known to occur, and there is no known reason to expect a clinically significant interaction with coriolus mushroom.

Possible Interactions with Diseases or Conditions

No interactions are known to occur, and there is no known reason to expect a clinically significant interaction with coriolus mushroom.

Typical Dosages & Routes of Administration that are Commonly Used

ORAL: People drink a tea prepared with 20 grams of dried coriolus fruiting bodies three times daily, or take capsules containing up to 5 grams per day of the dried fruiting bodies. As an adjuvant to cancer chemotherapy, 3 grams of PSK is taken daily (1650,1654,1656,1658). A typical dose of PSP is 1 gram 3 times daily (5497,5498).

Comments

None.

CORKWOOD TREE

This Product is Also Known As

Pituri.

Scientific Names

Duboisia myoporoides.
Family: Solanaceae.

People Use This For

Orally, corkwood quids (cured and rolled leaves) are chewed to ward off hunger, pain, and tiredness (6). Alkaloids derived from the plant are used as a therapeutic substitute for atropine (6).

Safety

LIKELY UNSAFE ...when used orally. Corkwood tree leaves contain tropane alkaloids that are potent anticholinergics (6). Large doses of scopolamine and related alkaloids can be fatal (6).
PREGNANCY AND LACTATION: LIKELY UNSAFE ...when used orally; avoid using.

Effectiveness

POSSIBLY EFFECTIVE ...when chewed for conditions which would be treated with hyoscyamine and hyoscine, scopolamine, and atropine (6).
There is insufficient reliable information available about the effectiveness of corkwood tree for its other uses.

Possible Mechanism of Action & Active Ingredients

The applicable part of corkwood tree is the leaf. Researchers document tropane alkaloids (atropine, scopolamine, etc.) as constituents (6). Stimulant and hallucinogenic properties are due to anticholinergic effects (6).

Adverse Reactions Including Known Allergies

Central nervous system disturbances (6).

Possible Interactions with Herbs & Other Dietary Supplements

Insufficient reliable information available.

Possible Interactions with Drugs

No interactions are known to occur, and there is no known reason to expect a clinically significant interaction with corkwood tree.

Possible Interactions with Foods

No interactions are known to occur, and there is no known reason to expect a clinically significant interaction with corkwood tree.

Possible Interactions with Lab Tests

No interactions are known to occur, and there is no known reason to expect a clinically significant interaction with corkwood tree.

Possible Interactions with Diseases or Conditions

No interactions are known to occur, and there is no known reason to expect a clinically significant interaction with corkwood tree.

Typical Dosages & Routes of Administration that are Commonly Used
Leaves are cured and rolled into a quid which Australian natives chew (6).

Comments
Although at one time used as a source of scopolamine, other sources are more commercially viable (6).

CORN COCKLE

This Product is Also Known As
Cockle, Corn Campion, Corn Rose, Crown-of-the-Field, Purple Cockle.

Scientific Names
Agrostemma githago.
Family: Caryophyllaceae.

People Use This For
Historically, corn cockle seeds were for treating cancers, hard tumors, warts, and hard swelling of the uterus. They were placed in the conjunctival sac to induce inflammation of the conjunctiva and cornea (6). The root of the corn cockle has been used for exanthemata (acute skin eruptions signifying a viral or coccal infection) and hemorrhoids (6). Various plant parts have also been used as a diuretic, expectorant, menstrual stimulant, poison, vermifuge, and for jaundice (6).

Safety
LIKELY UNSAFE ...when used orally, due to toxicity (6).
There is insufficient reliable information available about the safety of the topical use of corn cockle.
PREGNANCY AND LACTATION: LIKELY UNSAFE ...contraindicated; avoid using (6).

Effectiveness
There is insufficient reliable information available about the effectiveness of corn cockle.

Possible Mechanism of Action & Active Ingredients
The applicable parts of corn cockle are the root and seed. Poisonous constituents, githagin and agrostemmic acid, are reportedly absorbed from the GI tract causing GI irritation, severe muscle pain and twitching, depression, and coma (6).

Adverse Reactions Including Known Allergies
Oral use can cause GI irritation, severe muscle pain and twitching, depression, and coma (6). Acute poisoning symptoms include: diarrhea, salivation, vertigo, vomiting, paralysis, and respiratory depression (6). Repeated poisoning by small doses is referred to as "githagism" (6).

Possible Interactions with Herbs & Other Dietary Supplements
Insufficient reliable information available.

Possible Interactions with Drugs
No interactions are known to occur, and there is no known reason to expect a clinically significant interaction with corn cockle.

Possible Interactions with Foods
No interactions are known to occur, and there is no known reason to expect a clinically significant interaction with corn cockle.

Possible Interactions with Lab Tests
No interactions are known to occur, and there is no known reason to expect a clinically significant interaction with corn cockle.

Possible Interactions with Diseases or Conditions
No interactions are known to occur, and there is no known reason to expect a clinically significant interaction with corn cockle.

Typical Dosages & Routes of Administration that are Commonly Used
No typical dose.

Comments
Corn cockle is considered toxic; avoid use (6).

CORN POPPY

This Product is Also Known As
Copperose, Corn Rose, Cup-Puppy, Headache, Headwark, Red Poppy, Rhoeados Flos.
CAUTION: See separate listing for California Poppy.

Scientific Names
Papaver rhoeas.
Family: Papaveraceae.

People Use This For
Orally, corn poppy is used for respiratory tract diseases and discomforts, disturbed sleep, and pain relief (2).
Historically, corn poppy has been used in children's cough syrup (18).
For food uses, corn poppy is an ingredient in some "metabolic" teas (18). In other teas, it is used as a brightening agent.

Safety
POSSIBLY SAFE ...when the dried corn poppy flower petals are used orally and appropriately in medicinal amounts (2,18).
CHILDREN: POSSIBLY UNSAFE ...when the fresh leaves or blossoms are eaten because this can cause poisoning (18). There is insufficient reliable information available for the safety of dried corn poppy flower petals used in children.
PREGNANCY AND LACTATION: Insufficient reliable information available; avoid using.

Effectiveness
There is insufficient reliable information available about the effectiveness of corn poppy.

Possible Mechanism of Action & Active Ingredients
The applicable part of corn poppy is the flower. There is insufficient reliable information available about the possible mechanism of action and active ingredients.

Adverse Reactions Including Known Allergies
No adverse effects in adults have been reported (2). However, poisonings have been reported in children who consumed the fresh leaves and blossoms. Symptoms include vomiting and stomach pain (18).

Possible Interactions with Herbs & Other Dietary Supplements
Insufficient reliable information available.

Possible Interactions with Drugs
No interactions are known to occur, and there is no known reason to expect a clinically significant interaction with corn poppy.

Possible Interactions with Foods
No interactions are known to occur, and there is no known reason to expect a clinically significant interaction with corn cockle.

Possible Interactions with Lab Tests
No interactions are known to occur, and there is no known reason to expect a clinically significant interaction with corn cockle.

Possible Interactions with Diseases or Conditions
No interactions are known to occur, and there is no known reason to expect a clinically significant interaction with corn cockle.

Typical Dosages & Routes of Administration that are Commonly Used
ORAL: For bronchial irritation drink one cup tea (steep 2 teaspoons dried petals in boiling water 5-10 minutes, strain) 2 to 3 times daily (may be sweetened with honey) (18).

Comments
None.

CORN SILK

This Product is Also Known As
Cornsilk, Indian Corn, Maidis Stigma, Maize Silk, Stigma Maydis, Zea.

Scientific Names

Zea mays.
Family: Gramineae.

People Use This For

Orally, corn silk is used for cystitis, urethritis, nocturnal enuresis, prostatitis, and acute chronic inflammation of the urinary system (4).

In Chinese medicine, corn silk is used as a diuretic for congestive heart failure, to treat diabetes, and hypertension when decocted with watermelon peel and bananas (11).

Safety

LIKELY SAFE ...when consumed in amounts found in foods (maximum use level 0.002%) (11); Corn silk has Generally Recognized as Safe (GRAS) status in the US (11).

POSSIBLY SAFE ...when used orally and appropriately in medicinal amounts (12).

PREGNANCY: POSSIBLY SAFE ...when consumed in food. LIKELY UNSAFE ...contraindicated in larger amounts greater because it might have uterine stimulant effects (4).

LACTATION: Insufficient reliable information available.

Effectiveness

There is insufficient reliable information available about the effectiveness of corn silk.

Possible Mechanism of Action & Active Ingredients

Corn silk contains tannins, which are astringents, and Cryptoxanthin, which has vitamin A activity (4).

Adverse Reactions Including Known Allergies

Prolonged oral use may cause hypokalemia (4). Allergy to cornsilk, corn pollen, or cornstarch may result in contact dermatitis or urticaria (4).

Possible Interactions with Herbs & Other Dietary Supplements

Insufficient reliable information available.

Possible Interactions with Drugs

ANTICOAGULANTS: Corn silk contains vitamin K. Individuals using anticoagulant drug therapy should consume a consistent daily amount to maintain anticoagulation levels (19).

DIABETES THERAPY: Theoretically, because some evidence suggests corn silk can reduce blood glucose level, excessive amounts might interfere with diabetes therapy (4).

BLOOD PRESSURE TREATMENT: Theoretically, excessive doses might cause hypotension and interfere with drugs used to treat hypertension or hypotension (4).

POTASSIUM-DEPLETING DRUGS: Theoretically, prolonged use might have additive effects with drugs that deplete potassium, including diuretics (4).

Possible Interactions with Foods

No interactions are known to occur, and there is no known reason to expect a clinically significant interaction with corn silk.

Possible Interactions with Lab Tests

No interactions are known to occur, and there is no known reason to expect a clinically significant interaction with corn silk.

Possible Interactions with Diseases or Conditions

DIABETES: Theoretically, excessive doses might reduce blood glucose level (4), interfering with control.

HYPERTENSION, HYPOTENSION: Theoretically, excessive doses might interfere with control of these conditions (4).

POTASSIUM DEPLETION: Theoretically, excessive doses might exacerbate this condition (4).

Typical Dosages & Routes of Administration that are Commonly Used

ORAL: 4-8 grams dried style/stigma three times daily, or one cup tea (steep 0.5 grams dried corn silk in 150 mL boiling water 5-10 minutes, strain) several times daily (4,8). Liquid extract of maize stigmas, 4-8 mL (4). Tincture (1:5 in 25% alcohol), 5-15 mL three times daily (4). Syrup of maize stigmas, 8-15 mL (4).

Comments

Corn silk is the so-called "silk" of an ear of ordinary Indian corn or maize.

CORNFLOWER

This Product is Also Known As
Batchelor's Buttons, Bluebonnet, Bluebottle, Bluebow, Blue Cap, Blue Centaury, Cyani Flos, Cyani Flower, Hurtsickle.

Scientific Names
Centaurea cyanus.
Family: Asteraceae or Compositae.

People Use This For
Orally, cornflower is used for fever, menstrual disorders, vaginal candidiasis, as a laxative, diuretic, expectorant, tonic, bitter, and liver and gallbladder stimulant (2).
Topically, cornflower is used for eye irritation or discomfort (1502).
For food uses, cornflower is utilized in herbal teas as a coloring agent (2).

Safety
LIKELY SAFE ...when used in amounts in coloring agent in herbal teas (2).
There is insufficient reliable information available about the safety of the other oral or topical uses of cornflower.
PREGNANCY AND LACTATION: Insufficient reliable information available; avoid using.

Effectiveness
There is insufficient reliable information available about the effectiveness of cornflower (2).

Possible Mechanism of Action & Active Ingredients
The applicable part of cornflower is the dried flower. The color is due to anthocyanin constituents (1502).

Adverse Reactions Including Known Allergies
Cornflower can cause an allergic reaction in individuals sensitive to the Asteraceae/Compositae family. Members of this family include ragweed, chrysanthemums, marigolds, daisies, and many other herbs.

Possible Interactions with Herbs & Other Dietary Supplements
Insufficient reliable information available.

Possible Interactions with Drugs
No interactions are known to occur, and there is no known reason to expect a clinically significant interaction with cornflower.

Possible Interactions with Foods
No interactions are known to occur, and there is no known reason to expect a clinically significant interaction with cornflower.

Possible Interactions with Lab Tests
No interactions are known to occur, and there is no known reason to expect a clinically significant interaction with cornflower.

Possible Interactions with Diseases or Conditions
CROSS-ALLERGENICITY: Can cause an allergic reaction in individuals sensitive to the Asteraceae/Compositae family. Members of this family include ragweed, chrysanthemums, marigolds, daisies, and many other herbs.

Typical Dosages & Routes of Administration that are Commonly Used
ORAL: People typically use the crushed dried flowers to make a tea, adding 1 gram of cornflower per cup of water (5252).

Comments
None.

CORYDALIS

This Product is Also Known As
Early Fumitory, Squirrel Corn, Turkey Corn.
CAUTION: See separate listing for Turkey Corn.

Scientific Names
Corydalis cava.
Family: Fumariaceae.

People Use This For

Orally, corydalis is used for mild depression, neuroses and emotional disturbances, severe nerve damage, and limb tremors. People sometimes use it orally as a mild sedative and tranquilizer, hallucinogen, to lower blood pressure, and to relax small intestine peristalsis (18).

Safety

There is insufficient reliable information available about the safety of corydalis.
PREGNANCY: LIKELY UNSAFE …contraindicated for oral use because corydalis might promote menstrual flow and stimulate uterine contractions (12).
LACTATION: Insufficient reliable information available; avoid using.

Effectiveness

There is insufficient reliable information available about the effectiveness of corydalis.

Possible Mechanism of Action & Active Ingredients

The applicable part of corydalis is the tuber/root. There is insufficient reliable information available about the possible mechanism of action and active ingredients.

Adverse Reactions Including Known Allergies

Clonic spasms and muscle tremors may occur with overdoses (18).

Possible Interactions with Herbs & Other Dietary Supplements

Insufficient reliable information available.

Possible Interactions with Drugs

No interactions are known to occur, and there is no known reason to expect a clinically significant interaction with corydalis.

Possible Interactions with Foods

No interactions are known to occur, and there is no known reason to expect a clinically significant interaction with corydalis.

Possible Interactions with Lab Tests

No interactions are known to occur, and there is no known reason to expect a clinically significant interaction with corydalis.

Possible Interactions with Diseases or Conditions

No interactions are known to occur, and there is no known reason to expect a clinically significant interaction with corydalis.

Typical Dosages & Routes of Administration that are Commonly Used

ORAL: Corydalis is taken as an extract (18).

Comments

There is very little scientific information about this product. Our staff is continually analyzing the available information on natural medicines and will add data here as it becomes available.

COSTUS OIL

This Product is Also Known As

Auckland Costus, Mokko, Mu Xiang.
CAUTION: See separate listing for Costus root.

Scientific Names

Saussurea lappa, synonym Aucklandia costus.
Family: Asteraceae or Compositae.

People Use This For

In Chinese and Indian medicine, costus oil is used as a tonic, gastric stimulant, antiflatulent, for treating asthma, cough, dysentery, and cholera.
In foods and beverages, costus oil is used as a flavoring component (11).
In other manufacturing processes, costus oil is used as a fixative and fragrance in cosmetics (11).

Safety

LIKELY SAFE …when used in amounts found in foods. Costus oil is approved for food use in the US (11).
UNSAFE …when aristolochic acid-contaminated costus oil is used orally. Costus oil is commonly contaminated with aristolochic acid, which is nephrotoxic and carcinogenic. The FDA considers all products containing aristolochic acid to be unsafe and adulterated. Only products analytically verified to be aristolochic acid-free

should be used (6118,6119).

There is insufficient reliable information available about the safety of costus oil when used for medicinal purposes.
PREGNANCY AND LACTATION: Insufficient reliable information available; avoid using.

Effectiveness
There is insufficient reliable information available about the effectiveness of costus oil.

Possible Mechanism of Action & Active Ingredients
Costus oil is reported to inhibit bronchospasm and lower blood pressure in animals (11).

Adverse Reactions Including Known Allergies
Costus oil might cause allergic reactions, including contact dermatitis (11). Costus oil can cause an allergic reaction in individuals sensitive to the Asteraceae/Compositae family. Members of this family include ragweed, chrysanthemums, marigolds, daisies, and many other herbs. Costus oil is commonly contaminated with aristolochic acid, which is nephrotoxic and carcinogenic (6119).

Possible Interactions with Herbs & Other Dietary Supplements
Insufficient reliable information available.

Possible Interactions with Drugs
No interactions are known to occur, and there is no known reason to expect a clinically significant interaction with costus oil.

Possible Interactions with Foods
No interactions are known to occur, and there is no known reason to expect a clinically significant interaction with costus oil.

Possible Interactions with Lab Tests
No interactions are known to occur, and there is no known reason to expect a clinically significant interaction with costus oil.

Possible Interactions with Diseases or Conditions
CROSS-ALLERGENICITY: Costus oil can cause an allergic reaction in individuals sensitive to the Asteraceae/Compositae family. Members of this family include ragweed, chrysanthemums, marigolds, daisies, and many other herbs.

Typical Dosages & Routes of Administration that are Commonly Used
No typical dosage.

Comments
Costus oil is distilled, extracted oil from the root of Saussurea lappa. Avoid confusion with costus root.
Costus oil is frequently contaminated with aristolochic acid, which is nephrotoxic and carcinogenic. The FDA considers all products containing aristolochic acid to be unsafe and adulterated (6119). The FDA intends to automatically detain, without physical examination, any product which contains plants known or suspected to contain aristolochic acid, or which might be adulterated with plants known to contain aristolochic acid. Each detained product will be released only after the responsible party provides direct analytical evidence that it is free of aristolochic acid (6118,6119).

COSTUS root

This Product is Also Known As
Auckland Costus, Mokko, Mokkou, Mu Xiang.
CAUTION: See separate listing for Costus Oil.

Scientific Names
Saussurea lappa, synonym Aucklandia costus.
Family: Asteraceae or Compositae.

People Use This For
Orally, costus root is used as an antinematode therapy (1516).

Safety
POSSIBLY SAFE ...when used orally and appropriately (12).
UNSAFE ...when aristolochic acid-contaminated costus root is used orally. Costus root is commonly contaminated with aristolochic acid, which is nephrotoxic and carcinogenic. The FDA considers all products containing aristolochic acid to be unsafe and adulterated. Only products analytically verified to be aristolochic acid-free should be used (6118,6119).
PREGNANCY AND LACTATION: Insufficient reliable information available; avoid using.

Effectiveness

POSSIBLY EFFECTIVE ...against nematodes when the root or methanol extract of root is taken orally (1516).

Possible Mechanism of Action & Active Ingredients

In children, costus reduces the number of fecal eggs per gram similarly to treatment with pyrantel pamoate (1516).

Adverse Reactions Including Known Allergies

Costus can cause an allergic reaction in individuals sensitive to the Asteraceae/Compositae family. Members of this family include ragweed, chrysanthemums, marigolds, daisies, and many other herbs. Costus root is commonly contaminated with aristolochic acid which is nephrotoxic and carcinogenic (6119).

Possible Interactions with Herbs & Other Dietary Supplements

Insufficient reliable information available.

Possible Interactions with Drugs

No interactions are known to occur, and there is no known reason to expect a clinically significant interaction with costus root.

Possible Interactions with Foods

No interactions are known to occur, and there is no known reason to expect a clinically significant interaction with costus root.

Possible Interactions with Lab Tests

No interactions are known to occur, and there is no known reason to expect a clinically significant interaction with costus root.

Possible Interactions with Diseases or Conditions

CROSS-ALLERGENICITY: Can cause an allergic reaction in individuals sensitive to the Asteraceae/Compositae family. Members of this family include ragweed, chrysanthemums, marigolds, daisies, and many other herbs.

Typical Dosages & Routes of Administration that are Commonly Used

ORAL: Antinematodal, 50 mg/kg root (or equivalent amount of methanol extract of root) as a single dose (1516).

Comments

Avoid confusion with costus oil.

Costus root is frequently contaminated with aristolochic acid, which is nephrotoxic and carcinogenic. The FDA considers all products containing aristolochic acid to be unsafe and adulterated (6119). The FDA intends to automatically detain, without physical examination, any product which contains plants known or suspected to contain aristolochic acid, or which might be adulterated with plants known to contain aristolochic acid. Each detained product will be released only after the responsible party provides direct analytical evidence that it is free of aristolochic acid (6118,6119).

COTTON

This Product is Also Known As

Cotton Root.
CAUTION: See separate listing for Gossypol.

Scientific Names

Gossypium herbaceum; Gossypium hirsutum; other Gossypium species.
Family: Malvaceae.

People Use This For

Orally, cotton is used for amenorrhea; dysmenorrhea; irregular, painful, or profuse menstrual bleeding; climacteric complaints; poor lactation; nausea; fever; headache; diarrhea; dysentery; urethritis; nerve inflammation; hemorrhage; as an oxytocic; and to expel afterbirth (18).
Cotton has been used as an anti-fertility drug in males, as well as in topical, vaginal contraceptive preparations (214).

Safety

POSSIBLY SAFE ...when used orally in medicinal amounts (12). ...when preparations of the root bark are used in amounts found in foods. Canadian regulations limit use to less than 450 ppm of free gossypol (including cotton seed meal and oil) (12).
PREGNANCY: LIKELY UNSAFE ...when used orally; contraindicated because it is a possible abortifacient and uterine stimulant (12).
LACTATION: Insufficient reliable information available; avoid using.

Effectiveness

There is insufficient reliable information available about the effectiveness of cotton.

Possible Mechanism of Action & Active Ingredients

The applicable part of cotton is the root bark. It is believed to stimulate menstrual flow, act as an oxytocic, and male contraceptive (18). Some evidence suggests cotton root can cause histamine release (18). The constituent, gossypol that is extracted from cotton seed is used as a male contraceptive (6).

Adverse Reactions Including Known Allergies

There is insufficient reliable information available for oral uses; no adverse reactions reported (18). However, in animals, long-term feeding with cotton seed cakes has been linked to poisonings and deaths (18).

Possible Interactions with Herbs & Other Dietary Supplements

Insufficient reliable information available.

Possible Interactions with Drugs

No interactions are known to occur, and there is no known reason to expect a clinically significant interaction with cotton.

Possible Interactions with Foods

No interactions are known to occur, and there is no known reason to expect a clinically significant interaction with cotton.

Possible Interactions with Lab Tests

No interactions are known to occur, and there is no known reason to expect a clinically significant interaction with cotton.

Possible Interactions with Diseases or Conditions

UROGENITAL IRRITATION OR SENSITIVITY: Contraindicated (12).

Typical Dosages & Routes of Administration that are Commonly Used

ORAL: People typically prepare cotton root bark using one teaspoon boiled in a covered container with 3 cups of water for 30 minutes. The liquid is cooled slowly in the closed container and taken cold, 1 to 2 cups per day (5254).

Comments

Avoid confusion with gossypol (cotton seed extract).
Cotton's use as a male contraceptive agent is in question because it may potentially cause irreversible sterility (214).

COUCH GRASS

This Product is Also Known As

Couchgrass, Cutch, Dog Grass, Dog-Grass, Doggrass, Durfa Grass, Quack Grass, Quackgrass, Scotch Quelch. CAUTION: See separate listings for German Sarsaparilla, Sarsaparilla, and Tormentil.

Scientific Names

Agropyron repens, synonyms Elytrigia repens, Triticum repens; Elymus repens.
Family: Gramineae or Poaceae.

People Use This For

Orally, couch grass is used for cystitis, specifically with irritation or inflammation of the urinary tract (4). It is also used orally for urethritis, prostatitis, benign prostatic hypertrophy (BPH), renal calculus, and "irrigation therapy," to increase urine flow for inflammatory diseases of the urinary tract and the prevention of urine stones (2,11). Couch grass is used to treat the common cold, cough and bronchitis, fever and colds, inflammation of the mouth and pharynx, and a tendency toward infection (18).
In folk medicine, couch grass has been used as a diuretic and expectorant and for diabetes, gout, liver disorders, rheumatic pain, and chronic skin problems (11,18).
In foods and beverages, couch grass extracts are used as flavor components (11).

Safety

LIKELY SAFE ...when used orally and appropriately for medicinal purposes for short periods of time (2,4). ...when consumed in amounts commonly found in foods. Couch grass is Generally Recognized as Safe (GRAS) in the US for food use (11).
PREGNANCY AND LACTATION: Insufficient reliable information available; avoid amounts greater than those used in foods.

Effectiveness

POSSIBLY EFFECTIVE ...when taken orally for "irrigation therapy," where it is used as a mild diuretic along with copious fluid intake to increase urine flow to treat inflammatory diseases of the urinary tract and for prevention of urine stones (2,4,10).
There is insufficient reliable information available about the effectiveness of couch grass for its other uses.

Possible Mechanism of Action & Active Ingredients

The applicable parts of couch grass are the root and rhizome. Couch grass is a rich source of beta-carotene (19). Couch grass can have diuretic and sedative activities in animals (4,11). The constituent agropyrene and its oxidative product can have broad antibiotic activity (11). The essential oil of couch grass has antimicrobial effects (2,6).

Adverse Reactions Including Known Allergies

Excessive or prolonged use of couch grass can cause hypokalemia (4).

Possible Interactions with Herbs & Other Dietary Supplements

HERBS WITH SEDATIVE PROPERTIES: Theoretically, concomitant use with herbs that have sedative properties might enhance therapeutic and adverse effects. These include calamus, calendula, California poppy, catnip, capsicum, celery, elecampane, ginseng Siberian, German chamomile, goldenseal, gotu kola, hops, Jamaican dogwood, kava, lemon balm, sage, St. John's wort, sassafras, scullcap, shepherd's purse, stinging nettle, valerian, wild carrot, wild lettuce, withania root, and yerba mansa (4,19).

Possible Interactions with Drugs

POTASSIUM-DEPLETING DIURETICS: Theoretically, concomitant use of couch grass with these diuretics can enhance potassium loss (4).
DRUGS WITH SEDATIVE PROPERTIES: Theoretically, concomitant use with drugs having sedative properties can cause additive therapeutic and adverse effects (4).

Possible Interactions with Foods

No interactions are known to occur, and there is no known reason to expect a clinically significant interaction with couch grass.

Possible Interactions with Lab Tests

No interactions are known to occur, and there is no known reason to expect a clinically significant interaction with couch grass.

Possible Interactions with Diseases or Conditions

EDEMA: "Irrigation therapy," or the use of a mild diuretic and copious fluid intake to increase urine flow, is contraindicated in edema due to heart or kidney disease (2).

Typical Dosages & Routes of Administration that are Commonly Used

ORAL: The typical dose of couch grass is 4-8 grams of the dried rhizome or one cup of the tea three times daily (4). The tea is prepared by simmering 1-2 grams of the herb in 150 mL boiling water for 5-10 minutes and then straining. The usual dose of the liquid extract (1:1 in 25% alcohol) is 4-8 mL three times daily (4). The tincture (1:5 in 40% alcohol) is commonly given as 5-15 mL three times daily (4). When used for "irrigation therapy," couch grass requires copious fluid intake (2).

Comments

Avoid confusion with German sarsaparilla, also known as red couch grass.

COUNTRY MALLOW

This Product is Also Known As

Bala, Bariar, Heartleaf, Khareti.
CAUTION: See separate listings for Mallow flower, Mallow leaf, and Marshmallow.

Scientific Names

Sida cordifolia.
Family: Malvaceae.

People Use This For

In herbal combinations country mallow is used orally for weight loss (4307,4309,4316,4318,4320,4323,4324), to burn fat (4319), to increase energy (4308), for impotence (4312,4315), sinus (4305), allergy (4306), throat diseases (4312), asthma and bronchitis (4313), and to promote a strong skeletal system (4317). In combination with ginger, country mallow root is used orally for intermittent fever. In combination with milk and sugar, country mallow root is used for urinary urgency and leukorrhea (4310).
Traditionally, the country mallow root, leaves, and seeds have been used orally to treat bronchial asthma, cold, flu, chills, lack of perspiration, headache, nasal congestion, cough and wheezing, and edema (4304).
Traditionally, the country mallow root is used orally for heart disease, facial paralysis, healing chronic tissue inflammation, sciatica, insanity, neuralgia, nerve inflammation, chronic rheumatism, and emaciation (4311). It is also used orally as a stimulant, an analgesic, a diuretic, a tonic, and before and after cancer chemotherapy to aid recovery (4311).
Traditionally, the country mallow seeds are used orally to treat urinary infections and as an aphrodisiac (4310).

Traditionally, country mallow root is used topically for numbness, nerve pain, muscle cramps, skin disorders, tumors, joint diseases, wounds, and ulcers (4311). It is also used in a massage oil (4325).

Safety

LIKELY UNSAFE ...when the seeds are used orally for self-medication. Country mallow contains ephedrine and it is most concentrated in the seeds. ...when the country mallow constituent ephedrine is used orally in combination with caffeine. The FDA has proposed banning caffeine in combination with ephedrine alkaloids (2729).
There is insufficient reliable information available about the safety of country mallow aerial parts or root.
PREGNANCY: LIKELY UNSAFE ...contraindicated. The country mallow ephedrine constituent can stimulate uterine contractions (12).
LACTATION: Insufficient reliable information available; avoid using.

Effectiveness

There is insufficient reliable information available about the effectiveness of country mallow.

Possible Mechanism of Action & Active Ingredients

Country mallow plant contains 0.8%-1.2% ephedrine (4304,4310), but ephedrine is most concentrated in the seeds (4314). Some evidence suggests country mallow has anticonvulsant, antipyretic, antibacterial, antifungal, and antiviral activity (4310). Other information suggests the extracts of the aerial and root parts have analgesic, anti-inflammatory, and hypoglycemic properties (4299). An aqueous extract shows evidence that it limits the virulence of dental bacteria, reducing the rate of plaque formation (4303).

Adverse Reactions Including Known Allergies

Taken orally, the country mallow ephedrine constituent can cause dizziness, motor restlessness, irritability, insomnia, headache, anorexia, nausea, vomiting, flushing, tingling, difficulty urinating, tachycardia, and heart palpitations (2,6,7,13). Use of botanical sources of ephedrine such as country mallow have been associated with muscle conditions including myalgia, cardiomyopathy, rhabdomyolysis, eosinophilia myalgia syndrome (1270), and hypersensitivity myocarditis (1271). Botanical sources of ephedrine such as country mallow have also been associated with kidney stones (1272), acute hepatitis, (1273), psychosis (1276), and sudden death (1274). The country mallow constituent ephedrine can also cause a drastic increase in blood pressure, cardiac arrhythmias (2), heart failure, asphyxia, and hyperthermia (18).

Possible Interactions with Herbs & Other Dietary Supplements

CAFFEINE: Concomitant use with the country mallow constituent ephedrine can cause increased stimulatory adverse effects (7).
COFFEE, GUARANA, TEA: Theoretically, concomitant use with the country mallow constituent ephedrine can cause additive stimulatory adverse effects (7).
DIGITALIS: Theoretically, using digitalis with the country mallow constituent ephedrine can cause cardiac arrhythmias (2).
SECALE ALKALOID DERIVATIVES (Ergot): Concomitant use with the country mallow constituent ephedrine can cause hypertension (2).

Possible Interactions with Drugs

METHYLXANTHINES (Caffeine/Theophylline): Concomitant use with the country mallow constituent ephedrine can cause increased stimulatory adverse effects (7,19), and can enhance thermogenesis and weight loss (19).
DIGITALIS: Theoretically, concomitant use with the country mallow constituent ephedrine might cause cardiac arrhythmias (2).
SECALE ALKALOID DERIVATIVES (Ergot): Concomitant use with the country mallow constituent ephedrine might cause hypertension (2).
OXYTOCIN: Concomitant use with the country mallow constituent ephedrine can cause hypertension (2).
DIABETES THERAPY: The country mallow constituent ephedrine can raise blood glucose levels, but country mallow extract shows evidence it might reduce blood glucose. Monitor closely (19).
DEXAMETHASONE: The country mallow constituent ephedrine can increase the clearance and reduce the effectiveness of dexamethasone (19).
URINARY ACIDIFIERS: Concomitant use can increase the excretion of the country mallow ephedrine constituent due to reabsorption effects on kidney tubules (19).
URINARY ALKALINIZERS: Concomitant use can slow the excretion of the country mallow ephedrine constituent due to reabsorption effects on kidney tubules (19).
AMITRIPTYLINE (Elavil): Concomitant use can block the hypertensive effects caused by the country mallow ephedrine constituent (19).
RESERPINE: Concomitant use with the country mallow constituent ephedrine can antagonize the sympathomimetic effects of the reserpine (19).
MONOAMINE OXIDASE INHIBITORS (MAOIs): Contraindicated; concomitant use of the country mallow ephedrine constituent with MAOIs might increase the risk of hypertension (15).

© Copyright 2000, Natural Medicines Comprehensive Database (209) 472-2244. For updated data, go to www.NaturalDatabase.com • 339

Possible Interactions with Foods
COFFEE, TEA: Theoretically, concomitant use of the country mallow constituent ephedrine and large amounts of caffeinated coffee or tea might increase the stimulatory effects and adverse effects of caffeine and ephedrine.

Possible Interactions with Lab Tests
URINE: The country mallow ephedrine constituent can cause positive urine tests for ephedrine, a substance banned by many athletic organizations.

BLOOD GLUCOSE: The country mallow ephedrine constituent might increase blood glucose levels [19], or other constituents of country mallow might reduce blood glucose levels [4299].

Possible Interactions with Diseases or Conditions
ANGINA: Contraindicated; the country mallow ephedrine constituent might induce or exacerbate angina due its cardiac stimulant effects [15,512].

ANOREXIA: Contraindicated; the country mallow ephedrine constituent might suppress the appetite [12,19].

ANXIETY: Large doses of the country mallow ephedrine constituent might cause or exacerbate anxiety due to its CNS stimulant effects [2,12,15,512].

BULIMIA: Contraindicated; bulimic patients might be at increased risk for the adverse effects of the country mallow ephedrine constituent due to inadequate nutritional status [12,19].

BENIGN PROSTATIC HYPERTROPHY (BPH): The country mallow ephedrine constituent might exacerbate urinary retention in patients with BPH due its effects on the detrusor muscle [15,512].

CEREBRAL INSUFFICIENCY: Contraindicated; the country mallow ephedrine constituent might further decrease cerebral blood flow because it has vasoconstrictive effects [2,12,512].

DIABETES: The country mallow ephedrine constituent might interfere with blood sugar control, and exacerbate high blood pressure and circulatory problems in people with diabetes [15,19,512]. However, extract of country mallow shows evidence of hypoglycemic effect [4299]. Monitor closely.

ESSENTIAL TREMOR: The country mallow ephedrine constituent could exacerbate tremor [1715].

NARROW-ANGLE GLAUCOMA: The country mallow ephedrine constituent might exacerbate narrow-angle (angle-closure) glaucoma by causing mydriasis [2,12,15,512].

HEART DISEASE: Contraindicated; the country mallow ephedrine constituent might cause tachycardia, arrhythmias, or induce angina in patients with heart disease due to its cardiac stimulant effects [15,512].

HYPERTHYROID, THYROTOXICOSIS: Contraindicated; the country mallow ephedrine constituent might stimulate the thyroid and exacerbate hyperthyroid symptoms [2,12,15,512].

HYPERTENSION: The country mallow ephedrine constituent might exacerbate hypertension [2,12,15,512]; contraindicated in uncontrolled hypertension.

KIDNEY STONES: The country mallow ephedrine constituent can cause kidney stones [1272].

MYASTHENIA GRAVIS: Large doses of the country mallow ephedrine constituent might increase muscle strength in patients with myasthenia gravis [15].

PHEOCHROMOCYTOMA: Contraindicated; the country mallow ephedrine constituent might exacerbate the symptoms of pheochromocytoma [2].

URINARY RETENTION: Large doses of the country mallow ephedrine constituent might exacerbate urinary retention due its effects on the detrusor muscle [2,12,15,512].

Typical Dosages & Routes of Administration that are Commonly Used
ORAL: A typical dose of powder (root, leaves, seeds) is 0.5 -1 gram twice daily. A typical dose of the fresh juice is 15-30 mL twice daily [4310].
TOPICAL: No typical dosage.

Comments
Country mallow is used extensively in Ayurvedic medicine because it is reported to simultaneously balance the three laws of physiology (Vata, Pitta, Kapha) [4321].

COWHAGE

This Product is Also Known As
Couhage, Cowitch, Kiwach.

Scientific Names
Mucuna pruriens.
Family: Fabaceae.

People Use This For
Orally, cowhage is used as an antihelmintic [18].
Topically, cowhage as a cream or ointment has been used as a rubefacient to treat rheumatic conditions, myalgias [18]; and to stimulate cutaneous blood flow [18] in paralytic conditions [3827].

Safety

POSSIBLY SAFE ...when extracts of cowhage are used orally because irritating constituents are not bioavailable (18).
POSSIBLY UNSAFE ...when the hair of the pods is ingested orally (18). ...when the hair of the pods is used topically. The hairs cause aggressive itching and burning followed by long lasting inflammation (18).
PREGNANCY AND LACTATION: POSSIBLY UNSAFE ...when used orally or topically; avoid using.

Effectiveness

There is insufficient reliable information available about the effectiveness of cowhage.

Possible Mechanism of Action & Active Ingredients

The applicable part of cowhage is the hair on pods and seeds. Cowhage reportedly has antihelmintic, antiflatulent, hypotensive, and hypoglycemic and cholesterol lowering properties (18). Some evidence suggests the constituent, prurieninin, might slow heart rate, lower blood pressure, and stimulated intestinal peristalsis (18). Histamine release is believed to be responsible for blood pressure decline; the indole bases appear to resolve smooth muscle spasms (18). Applied topically to skin, cowhage possesses counterirritant and rubefacient properties (18). The stinging hairs of the pod or seed inject serotonin and proteins into the skin, producing blood vessel dilation with subsequent redness and inflammation (18).

Adverse Reactions Including Known Allergies

Applied to skin, cowhage may cause itching, burning, and long lasting inflammation (18).

Possible Interactions with Herbs & Other Dietary Supplements

Insufficient reliable information available.

Possible Interactions with Drugs

No interactions are known to occur, and there is no known reason to expect a clinically significant interaction with cowhage.

Possible Interactions with Foods

No interactions are known to occur, and there is no known reason to expect a clinically significant interaction with cowhage.

Possible Interactions with Lab Tests

No interactions are known to occur, and there is no known reason to expect a clinically significant interaction with cowhage.

Possible Interactions with Diseases or Conditions

No interactions are known to occur, and there is no known reason to expect a clinically significant interaction with cowhage.

Typical Dosages & Routes of Administration that are Commonly Used

ORAL: People typically use 0.5 to 4 grams of the powder (5264).

Comments

There is very little scientific information about this product. Our staff is continually analyzing the available information on natural medicines and will add data here as it becomes available.

COWSLIP

This Product is Also Known As

Arthritica, Buckels, Butter Rose, Crewel, English Cowslip, Fairy Caps, Herb Perter, Key Flower, Key of Heaven, Mayflower, Our Lady's Keys, Paigle, Paigle Peggle, Palsywort, Password, Peagle, Peagles, Petty Mulleins, Plumrocks, Primrose, Primula.

Scientific Names

Primula veris, synonym Primula officinalis; Primula elatier.
Family: Primulaceae.

People Use This For

Orally, cowslip flower is used for respiratory tract mucous membrane inflammation (2), cough, bronchitis, insomnia, nervous excitability, headache, hysteria, neuralgia, tremors, hydroticum, as a diuretic, antispasmodic, and as a heart tonic for sensations of dizziness and cardiac insufficiency (4,18).
Orally, cowslip root is used for respiratory tract mucous membrane inflammation (2), cough, bronchitis, whooping cough, asthma, gout, and neurologic complaints (18).
In combination with gentian root, European elder flower, verbena, and sorrel it is used orally for maintaining healthy sinuses (373) and treating sinusitis (7,374,379).

© Copyright 2000, Natural Medicines Comprehensive Database (209) 472-2244. For updated data, go to www.NaturalDatabase.com

Safety
POSSIBLY SAFE ...when used orally in appropriate amounts (2,12). ...when cowslip flower is used orally with gentian root, European elder flower, verbena, and sorrel (Quanterra Sinus Defense, Sinupret) (7,374,379).
PREGNANCY AND LACTATION: Insufficient reliable information available (4); avoid using.

Effectiveness
POSSIBLY EFFECTIVE ...when the flower is used orally for treating respiratory tract mucous membrane inflammation (2). ...when cowslip flower is taken orally with gentian root, European elder flower, verbena, and sorrel (Quanterra Sinus Defense, Sinupret) for treating acute or chronic sinusitis (7,374,379). ...when the root is used orally for treating respiratory tract mucous membrane inflammation (2).
There is insufficient reliable information available about the effectiveness of cowslip for its other uses.

Possible Mechanism of Action & Active Ingredients
The applicable parts of cowslip are the flower and root. Cowslip is a rich source of beta-carotene and vitamin C (19). Cowslip is reported to have antispasmodic, diuretic, expectorant, hypnotic, laxative, secretion-reducing, and sedative activities (2,4). Evidence suggests the saponin fraction might initially cause hypotension followed by long-lasting hypertension (4). Flavonoid constituents might have anti-inflammatory and antispasmodic effects. The tannin constituents have astringent effects (4).

Adverse Reactions Including Known Allergies
Cowslip can cause gastric discomfort and nausea (2,4,12). It may cause an allergic reaction in sensitive individuals (4). Toxicity, when it occurs, seems to be associated with saponin constituents of the underground parts of the plant (4).

Possible Interactions with Herbs & Other Dietary Supplements
Insufficient reliable information available.

Possible Interactions with Drugs
HYPERTENSIVE, HYPOTENSIVE DRUGS: Theoretically, excessive amounts of cowslip flower might interfere with the actions of these drugs (4).
DOXYCYCLINE (Vibramycin): Concurrent use of cowslip flower, gentian root, European elder flower, verbena, and sorrel (Quanterra Sinus Defense, Sinupret) with doxycycline and a topical decongestant might improve the outcome of conventional (antibiotic/decongestant) therapy for acute bacterial sinusitis (374).
DIURETICS: May potentiate effects (214).
SEDATIVES: May potentiate effects (214).

Possible Interactions with Foods
No interactions are known to occur, and there is no known reason to expect a clinically significant interaction with cowslip.

Possible Interactions with Lab Tests
No interactions are known to occur, and there is no known reason to expect a clinically significant interaction with cowslip.

Possible Interactions with Diseases or Conditions
HYPERTENSION, HYPOTENSION: Theoretically, excessive doses may interfere with control of these conditions (4).

Typical Dosages & Routes of Administration that are Commonly Used
ORAL (flower): One cup tea (1-2 grams dried flowers steeped in 150 mL of boiling water 5-10 minutes, strain) three times daily (4). Liquid extract (1:1 in 25% alcohol), 1-2 mL three times daily (4). Tincture, 2.5-7.5 grams per day (2). For acute or chronic sinusitis, two Sinupret tablets three times daily for up to two weeks has been used in clinical trials (7,374,379), equivalent to gentian root 12 mg, European elder flower 36 mg, verbena 36 mg, cowslip flower 36 mg, and sorrel 36 mg three times daily. For maintaining healthy sinuses, a typical dose is one tablet of Quanterra Sinus Defense three times daily with water, equivalent to gentian root 9 mg, European elder flower 29 mg, verbena 29 mg, cowslip flower 29 mg, and sorrel 29 mg three times daily (373). Each tablet of Quanterra Sinus Defense contains 125 mg of the herbal combination found in Sinupret (373).
ORAL (root): 0.5-1.5 grams dried root per day, or as prepared tea. Tincture, 1.5-3 grams per day (2).

Comments
None.

CRAMP BARK

This Product is Also Known As
Common Guelder-Rose, Crampbark, European Cranberry-Bush, Guelder Rose, Guelder-Rose, high-bush Cranberry, Snowball Bush.
CAUTION: See separate listings for Alpine Cranberry, Black Haw, Cranberry, and Uva Ursi.

Scientific Names
Viburnum opulus.
Family: Caprifoliaceae.

People Use This For
In folk medicine, cramp bark or root bark has been used for relieving cramps, muscle spasms, menstrual cramps, cramps during pregnancy, as a kidney stimulant in painful or spasmodic urinary conditions (862), cancer, hysteria, infection, nervous disorders, scurvy, and uteritis. It has also been used as a diuretic, emetic, purgative, and sedative (4017).

Safety
POSSIBLY SAFE …when used orally (12).
PREGNANCY AND LACTATION: Insufficient reliable information available; avoid using.

Effectiveness
There is insufficient reliable information available about the effectiveness of cramp bark.

Possible Mechanism of Action & Active Ingredients
The applicable parts of cramp bark are the bark and root bark. There is insufficient reliable information available about the possible mechanism of action and active ingredients.

Adverse Reactions Including Known Allergies
None reported.

Possible Interactions with Herbs & Other Dietary Supplements
Insufficient reliable information available.

Possible Interactions with Drugs
No interactions are known to occur, and there is no known reason to expect a clinically significant interaction with cramp bark.

Possible Interactions with Foods
No interactions are known to occur, and there is no known reason to expect a clinically significant interaction with cramp bark.

Possible Interactions with Lab Tests
No interactions are known to occur, and there is no known reason to expect a clinically significant interaction with cramp bark.

Possible Interactions with Diseases or Conditions
No interactions are known to occur, and there is no known reason to expect a clinically significant interaction with cramp bark.

Typical Dosages & Routes of Administration that are Commonly Used
ORAL: A common dose is 2-4 grams of the dried bark, 2-4 ml of a liquid extract (1:1 in 25% alcohol), or 5-10 ml of a tincture (1:5 in 45% alcohol), three times daily (2822).

Comments
Canadian regulations prohibit cramp bark as a non-medicinal ingredient for oral use products (12). Avoid confusion with black haw (Vibernum prunifolium), which is sometimes referred to as cramp bark (214).

CRANBERRY

This Product is Also Known As
American Cranberry, Arandano Americano, Arandano Trepador, European Cranberry, Grosse Moosbeere, Kranbeere, Large Cranberry, Moosebeere, Mossberry, Ronce d'Amerique, Small Cranberry, Trailing Swamp Cranberry, Tsuru-kokemomo.
CAUTION: See separate listings for Alpine Cranberry, Cramp Bark (European Cranberry-Bush), and Uva Ursi (Mountain Cranberry).

Scientific Names

Vaccinium macrocarpon, synonym Oxycoccus macrocarpos; Vaccinium oxycoccos, synonyms Oxycoccus hagerupii, Oxycoccus microcarpus, Oxycoccus palustris, Oxycoccus quadripetalus, Vaccinium hagerupii, Vaccinium microcarpum, Vaccinium palustre.
Family: Ericaceae.

People Use This For

Orally, cranberry fruit is used for prevention and treatment of urinary tract infections (3,5,6) and as a urinary deodorizer for people with incontinence (6).

In traditional medicine, the American cranberry fruit is used for scurvy and cancer treatment (2810) and European cranberry is used as a diuretic, antiseptic, antipyretic, and for cancer treatment in Eastern Europe (11).
Cranberry fruit is used in foods, including fruit juice, jelly, and sauce (11).

Safety

LIKELY SAFE ...when used orally and appropriately (515).
CHILDREN: LIKELY SAFE ...when used orally and appropriately (2811).
PREGNANCY AND LACTATION: LIKELY SAFE ...when used orally in food amounts (5). There is insufficient reliable information about the safety of therapeutic amounts of cranberry in pregnancy or lactation. Avoid using amounts greater than consumed in foods.

Effectiveness

POSSIBLY EFFECTIVE ...when used orally for preventing and treating urinary tract infections and as a urinary deodorizer for incontinent individuals (5,6,11,7008). There is very little evidence that ingestion of cranberry juice can cure an acute urinary tract infection (7008).
POSSIBLY INEFFECTIVE. ...when used orally for reducing the frequency of bacteriuria in children with neurogenic bladder and intermittent catheterization (2811).
There is insufficient reliable information available about the effectiveness of cranberry for its other uses.

Possible Mechanism of Action & Active Ingredients

The applicable part of the cranberry plant is the fruit. The cranberry is acidic, but does not acidify the urine, and has no antibiotic or antiseptic properties, as was previously thought (3). Cranberries contain proanthocyandin and a high-molecular weight compound (as yet unidentified) which interferes with bacterial adherence to the urinary tract (3,2812,2813,2814). Fructose might also contribute to the anti-infective activity (3,2813). Cranberry reduces the adhesion of Escherichia coli and Enterococcus faecalis to silicone rubber (2815). Preliminary data suggest that a high molecular weight cranberry constituent might prevent adhesion of plaque bacteria that cause periodontal disease (2816). Preliminary evidence suggests that the proanthocyanidin fraction of cranberry might have anticarcinogenic activity (7009).

Researchers report that cranberry juice and cranberry products reduced the number of breast cancer tumors, delayed tumor development, and reduced the spread of tumors to the lungs and lymph nodes in mice. Additionally, cranberry juice demonstrated antioxidant activity by inhibiting LDL-cholesterol oxidation in vitro. These unpublished study results were presented at the Experimental Biology 2000 conference (5058).

Adverse Reactions Including Known Allergies

The cranberry fruit taken orally has no significant adverse effects (6). Ingesting more than 3-4 L per day of cranberry juice can result in diarrhea and other GI symptoms (6).

Possible Interactions with Herbs & Other Dietary Supplements

Insufficient reliable information available.

Possible Interactions with Drugs

PROTON PUMP INHIBITORS: Cranberry juice might increase absorption of dietary vitamin B-12 in people taking proton pump inhibitors, due to its acidity (2817). Proton pump inhibitors include lansoprazole (Prevacid), omperazole (Prilosec), and Rabeprazole (Aciphex).

Possible Interactions with Foods

No interactions are known to occur, and there is no known reason to expect a clinically significant interaction with cranberry.

Possible Interactions with Lab Tests

No interactions are known to occur, and there is no known reason to expect a clinically significant interaction with cranberry.

Possible Interactions with Diseases or Conditions

ATROPHIC GASTRITIS: Cranberry juice might increase absorption of dietary vitamin B-12 in people with atrophic gastritis due to its acidity (2817).
DIABETES: Caution patients with diabetes to avoid cranberry juice cocktail products sweetened with sugar and instead to use cranberry juice cocktail products sweetened with artificial sweeteners.

HYPOCHLORHYDRIA: Cranberry juice might increase absorption of dietary vitamin B-12 in people with hypochlorhydria due to its acidity (2817).

Typical Dosages & Routes of Administration that are Commonly Used

ORAL: For urinary tract infections, a typical dose is 3 oz cranberry juice cocktail (33% pure cranberry juice) daily for preventing infections and 12-32 oz per day for treating infections (515). Six capsules of dried cranberry powder are equivalent to 3 oz cranberry juice cocktail (515). Some sources recommend 300-400 mg of concentrated cranberry juice capsules twice daily (7010). Fresh or frozen cranberries may also be used, 1.5 oz is equivalent to 3 oz cranberry juice cocktail (3). Approximately 1500 grams of fresh fruit produce 1 L of juice. Cranberry juice cocktail is approximately 33% pure cranberry juice, sweetened with fructose or artificial sweetener (11,515).

Comments

Avoid confusing cranberry fruit with high-brush cranberry (Viburnum opulus), which is also known as cramp bark (6,11).

The American cranberry (Vaccinium macrocarpon) is native to the northeastern and north central US and eastern Canada, and the fruit is cultivated commercially for food use and as a beverage base (2818). Cranberries, along with blueberries and Concord grapes, are the only fruits native to North America (2821). The Pilgrims called the cranberry "crane berry" because the stem and flower resembled the neck, head, and beak of the crane, and the name was shortened to the word used today (2821).

The European cranberry (Vaccinium oxycoccos) is native to the same areas of North America as its American cousin, as well as central and northern Europe and temperate areas of Asia (2819). The fruit of European cranberry is commercially important in Russia (2820). Approximately 1500 grams of fresh cranberries produce 1 L of pure cranberry juice.

CREATINE

This Product is Also Known As

Creatine Monohydrate.
CAUTION: Do not confuse creatine with its metabolite, creatinine.

Scientific Names

N-amidinosarcosine; N-(aminoiminomethyl)-N methyl glycine.

People Use This For

Orally, creatine is used to increase exercise performance and muscle mass in athletes (2101,2103) and older adults (4570,4571,4572). Creatine has also been used to treat heart failure (4562,4563), neuromuscular disease (4564), and mitochondrial cytopathy (4565), gyrate atrophy of the choroid and retina (4577,4578), and to lower cholesterol (4573). It is also used to slow the progression of amyotrophic lateral sclerosis (ALS, Lou Gehrig's disease) (207,208) and for various muscular dystrophies (6182).

Intravenously, creatine has been used in cardiac surgery (4586,4587).

Safety

POSSIBLY SAFE ...when used orally and appropriately (2100,2101,2103,3996). A one year study of 5-8 grams of creatine per day for 12 months found no adverse effects on blood and urine markers of health in a group of 17 college football players compared to a control group. This unpublished study was presented at the American College of Sports Medicine 2000 meeting (6117).

There is insufficient reliable information available about the safety of the long-term use of creatine or the use of creatine in children. Concerns about prolonged suppression of endogenous creatine have been raised, but not studied (3997).

PREGNANCY AND LACTATION: Insufficient reliable information available; avoid using.

Effectiveness

POSSIBLY EFFECTIVE ...when used orally for enhancing muscle performance during repeated bouts of brief, high-intensity exercise. Numerous studies have shown creatine to be beneficial for certain types of high-intensity exercises (2100,2101,2102,4591,4592,4593,4594,4601,4602,4604,46056015); however, some studies have shown no effect for other exercises (4582,4595,4596,4597,4606,6183). A meta-analysis of 32 creatine studies showed no effect of creatine supplementation on various measures of anaerobic performance, including fatigue, power, speed, strength, and work values. This unpublished study was presented at the American College of Sports Medicine 2000 meeting (6117). Creatine appears to be more effective for repeated maximal energy bursts than for single event performance (4593,4598,4599,4600). Many variables seem to determine the effect of creatine on performance, including whether the subject is well-trained or sedentary, the type of sport being tested, diet, and the dose regimen of creatine. Benefits have been shown in such sports as weight lifting, cycling sprints, and short-term kayaking bouts. Sports that may not benefit from creatine supplementation include sprints in running and swimming. It is possible that the benefit in certain sports is offset by weight gain from creatine supplementation (4576,4601,4604,4605,6015). Acute creatine loading may be more effective than chronic use (4603). Most studies have used 20 grams daily for 5 days for

© Copyright 2000, Natural Medicines Comprehensive Database (209) 472-2244. For updated data, go to www.NaturalDatabase.com • 345

creatine loading; however, various other regimens have been studied. One study used 9 grams daily for 5 days and was beneficial in weight lifters, while another study used 20 grams daily for 3 days and did not show a benefit in single sprints in cyclists (4576,4599,6015). Due to the variety of study methodologies and conflicting findings, it has yet to be determined exactly who can benefit from creatine supplementation and what dosing schedule might be most effective. So far, the data have been inconclusive. All studies have been limited by small sample size; all have involved less than 40 subjects and most less than 25. ...when used orally to increase strength and endurance in patients with congestive heart failure (4562,4563). In two open-label short-term studies, supplemental creatine improved exercise tolerance, but had no effect on ejection fraction (4562,4563). ...when used orally to treat gyrate atrophy of the choroid and retina (4577,4578). Two small studies have shown that creatine supplementation slows visual deterioration (4577,4578). ...when used orally short-term to improve muscle strength and daily-life activity in adults and children with various muscular dystrophies (6182). In a small double-blind, placebo controlled, crossover trial, creatine monohydrate daily for eight weeks mildly improved muscle strength and daily-life activity in a group of children and adults with facioscapulohumeral dystrophy, Becker dystrophy, Duchenne dystrophy, or sarcoglycan-deficient limb girdle muscular dystrophy (6182).

LIKELY INEFFECTIVE ...when used for increasing endurance or for improving performance in highly trained athletes (2103,2105,2106,4607). ...when used to improve isometric strength and body composition in adults over age 60 (4570,4571,4572). In three well-designed studies, creatine dosed at 20 grams per day for 5 days followed by lower maintenance doses had no beneficial effect on exercise except reducing muscle fatigue (4570,4571,4572). In one study it had no effect on quadriceps fatigue after repeated sets of explosive work (6183).

There is insufficient reliable information available about the effectiveness of creatine for its other uses.

Possible Mechanism of Action & Active Ingredients

Creatine is found primarily in skeletal muscle (95%), but also in heart, brain, testes, retina, and other tissues (3997,3998). The body synthesizes 1 to 2 grams of creatine a day primarily in the liver, kidneys, and pancreas (3997). Dietary sources, such as fish and meats, supply an additional 1 to 2 grams (3977). One pound of fresh uncooked steak contains about 2 grams of creatine (4575). Creatine is irreversibly converted to creatinine and excreted by the kidneys (3997). Creatine in skeletal muscles exists in dynamic equilibrium with phosphocreatine (3997). Body stores of phosphocreatine in skeletal muscle serve as a precursor to the energy molecule, adenosine triphosphate (ATP). Higher levels of creatine can enhance the ability to renew ATP for short energy bursts (10 to 20 seconds) and improve resynthesis of phosphocreatine during recovery from intense exercise, although faster resynthesis has been questioned (2103,3997,4576,4580). Supplementation variably increases total creatine (4574,4583). People such as vegetarians, who have lower initial total creatine, are more likely to respond to supplemental creatine, while people with higher initial levels may not respond (4574). Creatine levels return to baseline within 28 days of discontinuing supplementation (2101,4582). Skeletal muscle has a saturation point at which additional supplemental creatine will not increase intracellular creatine levels (3999). Excess supplementation increases urinary creatine and creatinine (4576). In patients with gyrate atrophy, an inherited metabolic disease in which phosphocreatine is depleted, supplemental creatine increased myofibrillar protein synthesis resulting in muscle accretion (4576,4587). Although some laboratory evidence identifies creatine as a muscle builder, most clinical evidence supports increased water retention as the primary cause of creatine-induced weight gain (4575,4576,4579,4588). Five days of creatine loading (20 grams per day) in healthy adults resulted in increases in body weight and fat-free mass, but did not affect blood pressure, renal function, or plasma CK activity (4569). Body mass changes were greater in men than women (4569). One small study suggests that creatine may reduce lactate production, as evidenced by lower increases in blood lactate levels in well trained males who received the supplement (4604). However, another small study did not show a reduction in blood lactate accumulation with creatine (4592). Creatine might have a beneficial effect on lipid levels in some people (4573). Creatine has been used in preliminary clinical studies to increase high-intensity strength in people with neuromuscular disease (4564) and increase the strength of high-intensity anaerobic and aerobic type activities in people with mitochondrial cytopathies (4565). Early laboratory evidence suggests that creatine might be useful in diseases such as amyotrophic lateral sclerosis, Huntington's disease, and Parkinson's disease (4566,4567,4568).

Adverse Reactions Including Known Allergies

Creatine use can cause gastrointestinal pain, nausea, and diarrhea (2103,4576). Although not reported in clinical studies, 25% of male collegiate athletes taking creatine reported muscle cramping (4584). A one year study of 5-8 grams of creatine per day for 12 months in a group of 17 college football players found no adverse effects on blood and urine markers of health. When researchers compared blood and urine samples they found no differences in serum creatinine, urea nitrogen, uric acid, muscle and liver enzymes, blood lipids, electrolytes, and percentage of whole blood red and white cells in the creatine group compared a control group. Also, there was no increase in the incidence of injury or cramping in the creatine group. This unpublished study was presented at the American College of Sports Medicine 2000 meeting (6117). A theoretical increase in the risk of dehydration subsequent to intracellular fluid shifts has led most creatine manufacturers to caution about adequate hydration with creatine supplementation (217,4576). Creatine typically causes a weight gain of 0.5 to 1.6 kg (see Mechanism of Action) that increases with prolonged supplementation (3997). Creatine can also cause renal dysfunction (184,2118), although renal toxicity among people with healthy kidneys appears to be rare (2120,3996). There is one report of acute interstitial nephritis and focal tubular injury after four weeks of creatine at 5 grams four times daily (184). Supplemental creatine, loaded at 15 grams per day for one week, then 2 grams per day, caused a significant decline in creatinine clearance in a man receiving cyclosporine for steroid-resistant focal segmental glomerulosclerosis (2118). A small study of athletes taking an average of 10 grams of creatine daily for 1 to 5 years maintained renal function comparable to control athletes not taking supplements (3996). The effects of chronic creatine administration have not been adequately studied. There is one report of ischemic stroke in an athlete who consumed creatine monohydrate 6 grams, caffeine 400-600 mg, ephedra 40-60 mg, and a variety of other supplements daily for six weeks (1275). The FDA has received a total of 32 complaints of adverse effects linked to creatine, including seizures, cardiomyopathy, arrhythmias, rhabdomyolysis, and cardiac arrest, although causality has not been proven (4585). Theoretically, the lax manufacturing standards for nutritional supplements could put people using high doses of creatine at risk for significant exposure to toxic contaminants.

Possible Interactions with Herbs & Other Dietary Supplements

EPHEDRA: There is one report of ischemic stroke in an athlete who consumed creatine monohydrate 6 grams, caffeine 400-600 mg, ephedra 40-60 mg, and a variety of other supplements daily for six weeks (1275).
CAFFEINE: There is one report of ischemic stroke in an athlete who consumed creatine monohydrate 6 grams, caffeine 400-600 mg, ephedra 40-60 mg, and a variety of other supplements daily for six weeks (1275). Caffeine can interfere with the ergogenic effects of creatine supplementation (2117).

Possible Interactions with Drugs

NEPHROTOXIC DRUGS: Theoretically, creatine should be avoided by people taking drugs with nephrotoxic potential, such as Cyclosporin, Angiotensin-Converting-Enzyme Inhibitors, and Nonsteroidal Anti-inflammatory drugs on a prolonged basis.

Possible Interactions with Foods

CAFFEINE can interfere with the ergogenic effects of creatine supplementation (2117).

Possible Interactions with Lab Tests

SERUM CREATININE: Creatine is metabolized to creatinine. High serum creatinine levels can result despite normal renal function (2100,2103).

Possible Interactions with Diseases or Conditions

KIDNEY DYSFUNCTION: Creatine should be avoided by people with pre-existing renal disease or by people with diseases such as diabetes that increase the risk for renal dysfunction. (4576).

Typical Dosages & Routes of Administration that are Commonly Used

ORAL: For improving physical performance, several dosing regimens have been tried. Creatine is typically acutely loaded with 20 grams per day (or 0.3 grams per kg) for 5 days followed by a maintenance dose of 2 or more grams (0.03 grams per kg) daily (4576). Although 5 day loading is typical, 2 days of loading has also been used (4576). A loading dose of 9 grams per day for 6 days has also been used (6015). Some sources suggest that, instead of acutely loading, similar results can be obtained with 3 grams per day for 28 days (2104). During creatine supplementation, the water intake should be 64 ounces per day (2103,2104). For heart failure, 20 grams per day for 5-10 days was used in clinical trials (4562,4563). For gyrate atrophy, 1.5 grams per day has been used (4577,4578). For muscular dystrophies, 10 grams per day has been used by adults and 5 grams per day has been used by children (6182).

Comments

Creatine is allowed by the International Olympic Committee, National Collegiate Athletic Association (NCAA), and professional sports (3998,4575,4576). However, the NCAA no longer allows colleges and universities to supply creatine to their students with school funds. Students are permitted to buy creatine on their own and the NCAA has no plans to ban creatine unless sufficient medical evidence indicates that it is harmful (6140). With current testing methods, detection of supplemental creatine use would not be possible (4575). Creatine use is widespread among professional and amateur athletes and has been acknowledged by well-known athletes such as Mark McGuire, Sammy Sosa, and John Elway (3998). Following the finding that carbohydrate solution further increased muscle creatine levels more than creatine alone, creatine sports drinks have become popular (4576,4589). Annual consumption of creatine in the US is estimated to exceed 4 million kg (3998).

CROTON SEEDS

This Product is Also Known As
Tiglium, Tiglium Seeds.

Scientific Names
Croton tiglium.
Family: Euphorbiaceae.

People Use This For
Orally, croton seed oil is used as a purgative (3800).

In Chinese medicine, croton seed oil is used orally to treat gallbladder colic, bowel obstruction, and malaria (18); and topically for rheumatism, gout, neuralgia, and bronchitis (3819).

Safety

LIKELY UNSAFE ...when used orally. One drop of the oil can be toxic, and one mL (20 drops) of oil is considered lethal (18). Also, the phorbol esters in the oil are co-carcinogens (18). ...when used topically; avoid using (18).
PREGNANCY: UNSAFE ...contraindicated, due to abortifacient properties (19).
LACTATION: UNSAFE; avoid using.

Effectiveness

POSSIBLY EFFECTIVE ...when used orally as a purgative (3800,3819), but risk precludes use.
There is insufficient reliable information available about the effectiveness of croton seed oil for its other uses.

Possible Mechanism of Action & Active Ingredients

The applicable part of croton seeds is the oil from the seed. Croton seeds possess powerful irritant, cathartic properties due to phorbol esters (3800). The diterpene, TPA, is carcinogenic, affecting prostaglandin metabolism (18).

Adverse Reactions Including Known Allergies

Oral use of croton seeds can cause burning of mouth, vomiting, dizziness, stupor, painful bowel movements, and collapse (18). Topical use can cause itching, burning and blistering of skin (18).

Possible Interactions with Herbs & Other Dietary Supplements

Insufficient reliable information available.

Possible Interactions with Drugs

No interactions are known to occur, and there is no known reason to expect a clinically significant interaction with croton seeds.

Possible Interactions with Foods

No interactions are known to occur, and there is no known reason to expect a clinically significant interaction with croton seeds.

Possible Interactions with Lab Tests

No interactions are known to occur, and there is no known reason to expect a clinically significant interaction with croton seeds.

Possible Interactions with Diseases or Conditions

No interactions are known to occur, and there is no known reason to expect a clinically significant interaction with croton seeds.

Typical Dosages & Routes of Administration that are Commonly Used

No typical dosage.

Comments

Croton seeds are considered likely unsafe; avoid using (18).

CUBEBS

This Product is Also Known As

Cubeba, Cubeb Berries, Java Pepper, Tailed Chubebs, Tailed Pepper.

Scientific Names

Piper cubeba, Cubeba officinaliz.
Family: Piperaceae.

People Use This For

Orally, cubebs is used as a diuretic, urinary antiseptic, and for amoebic dysentery (11).
Traditionally, cubebs was used as an antiflatulent, stimulating expectorant, for gonorrhea, and cancer (11).
For food uses, cubebs oil is used as a flavoring ingredient (11).

Safety

LIKELY SAFE ...when used in amounts found in foods (maximum use level for oil is 0.004%); approved for use in foods in the US (11).
POSSIBLY SAFE ...when used for orally and appropriately for medicinal purposes (12).
PREGNANCY AND LACTATION: Insufficient reliable information available; avoid using.

Effectiveness

There is insufficient reliable information available about the effectiveness of cubebs.

Possible Mechanism of Action & Active Ingredients

The applicable part of cubebs is the dried, fully grown but unripe fruit. Researchers think that the constituent cubebic acid is responsible for stimulant effect on urinary and respiratory tract (11).

Adverse Reactions Including Known Allergies

None reported (18).

Possible Interactions with Herbs & Other Dietary Supplements

Insufficient reliable information available.

Possible Interactions with Drugs

ACID-INHIBITING DRUGS: Theoretically, due to claims that cubebs increases stomach acid, it might interfere with antacids, sucralfate (Carafate), H-2 antagonists, or proton pump inhibitors (19).

Possible Interactions with Foods

No interactions are known to occur, and there is no known reason to expect a clinically significant interaction with cubebs.

Possible Interactions with Lab Tests

No interactions are known to occur, and there is no known reason to expect a clinically significant interaction with cubebs.

Possible Interactions with Diseases or Conditions

GI CONDITIONS: Can irritate gastrointestinal tract. Contraindicated in individuals with infectious or inflammatory gastrointestinal conditions (19).
NEPHRITIS: Contraindicated in individuals with nephritis (12).

Typical Dosages & Routes of Administration that are Commonly Used

ORAL: People typically use 2 to 4 grams of the powdered fruit or 2 to 4 mL of the liquid extract (5264).

Comments

None.

CUDWEED

This Product is Also Known As

Cotton Dawes, Cotton Weed, Dysentery Weed, Everlasting, Mouse Ear, Wartwort.
CAUTION: See separate listing for Cat's Foot and Mouse Ear.

Scientific Names

Gnaphalium uliginosum.
Family: Asteraceae or Compositae.

People Use This For

Topically, cudweed is used as a gargle or rinse for diseases of the mouth or throat (18).

Safety

There is insufficient reliable information available about the safety of cudweed.
Pregnancy and Lactation: Insufficient reliable information available; avoid using.

Effectiveness

There is insufficient reliable information available about the effectiveness of cudweed.

Possible Mechanism of Action & Active Ingredients

The applicable parts of cudweed are the above ground parts. Cudweed has astringent effects, and promotes and improves appetite (18). Unsubstantiated sources report it has antidepressant, aphrodisiac, and hypotensive effects (18).

Adverse Reactions Including Known Allergies

Cudweed can cause an allergic reaction in individuals sensitive to the Asteraceae/Compositae family. Members of this family include ragweed, chrysanthemums, marigolds, daisies, and many other herbs.

Possible Interactions with Herbs & Other Dietary Supplements

Insufficient reliable information available.

Possible Interactions with Drugs

No interactions are known to occur, and there is no known reason to expect a clinically significant interaction with cudweed.

Possible Interactions with Foods

No interactions are known to occur, and there is no known reason to expect a clinically significant interaction with cudweed.

Possible Interactions with Lab Tests

No interactions are known to occur, and there is no known reason to expect a clinically significant interaction with cudweed.

Possible Interactions with Diseases or Conditions

CROSS-ALLERGENICITY: Can cause an allergic reaction in individuals sensitive to the Asteraceae/Compositae family. Members of this family include ragweed, chrysanthemums, marigolds, daisies, and many other herbs.

Typical Dosages & Routes of Administration that are Commonly Used

ORAL: People typically use 2 to 4 mL of the liquid extract (5264).

Comments

Avoid confusion with cat's foot (Antennaria dioica), which is also referred to as cudweed. Avoid confusion with Pilosella officinarum, also known as mouse ear.

CUMIN

This Product is Also Known As

Cummin.

Scientific Names

Cuminum cyminum; Cuminum odorum.
Family: Apiaceae/Umbelliferae.

People Use This For

Orally, cumin is used as an antiflatulent (11).
Traditionally, cumin was used as a stimulant, antispasmodic, diuretic, aphrodisiac, for stimulating menstrual flow (11), treating diarrhea, colic, and flatulence (18).
In spices, foods, and beverages,
cumin is used as a flavoring component (11).
In other manufacturing processes, cumin oil is used as a fragrance component in cosmetics (maximum use level 0.4% in perfumes).

Safety

LIKELY SAFE ...when used in amounts used as spice (cumin maximum use level 0.4%). ...when used in amounts found in foods (cumin oil maximum use level 0.025%); Generally Recognized as Safe (GRAS) status in the US.
POSSIBLY SAFE ...when used orally and appropriately for medicinal purposes (12).
PREGNANCY AND LACTATION: Insufficient reliable information available; avoid in excess of food amounts.

Effectiveness

There is insufficient reliable information available about the effectiveness of cumin.

Possible Mechanism of Action & Active Ingredients

The applicable part of cumin is the fruit/seed. Cumin is a rich source of iron (19). Cumin oil and constituent, cuminaldehyde, have been reported to exhibit strong larvicidal and antibacterial activity (6). Demonstrated phototoxic effects are reportedly not due to cuminaldehyde (11). Some evidence suggests the dried extract might inhibit platelet aggregation (18) and prolong phenobarbiturate hypnosis in mice; however, a higher dose shortened phenobarbiturate hypnosis (18).

Adverse Reactions Including Known Allergies

Undiluted oil has phototoxic effects (6).

Possible Interactions with Herbs & Other Dietary Supplements

Insufficient reliable information available.

Possible Interactions with Drugs

DIABETES THERAPY: Monitor blood glucose levels closely due to claims that cumin has hypoglycemic effects (19).
BARBITURATES: Theoretically, might increase or decrease activity of barbiturates (18).

Possible Interactions with Foods

No interactions are known to occur, and there is no known reason to expect a clinically significant interaction with cumin.

Possible Interactions with Lab Tests

No interactions are known to occur, and there is no known reason to expect a clinically significant interaction with cumin.

Possible Interactions with Diseases or Conditions

No interactions are known to occur, and there is no known reason to expect a clinically significant interaction with cumin.

Typical Dosages & Routes of Administration that are Commonly Used

ORAL: Average single amount used, 5-10 fruits [18].

Comments

Fine grinding of seed can cause loss of 50% of volatile oil, most within 1 hour [6].

CUP PLANT

This Product is Also Known As

Indian Gum, Pilot Plant, Polar Plant, Prairie Dock, Ragged Cup, Rosinweed, Turpentine Weed.
CAUTION: See separate listing for Rosinweed.

Scientific Names

Silphium perfoliatum.

People Use This For

Orally, cup plant is used for digestive disorders [18].

Safety

There is insufficient reliable information available about the safety of cup plant.
Pregnancy and Lactation: Insufficient reliable information available; avoid using.

Effectiveness

There is insufficient reliable information available about the effectiveness of cup plant.

Possible Mechanism of Action & Active Ingredients

The applicable part of cup plant is the root. Cup plant is stated to have tonic and diaphoretic effects [18].

Adverse Reactions Including Known Allergies

None reported.

Possible Interactions with Herbs & Other Dietary Supplements

Insufficient reliable information available.

Possible Interactions with Drugs

No interactions are known to occur, and there is no known reason to expect a clinically significant interaction with cup plant.

Possible Interactions with Foods

No interactions are known to occur, and there is no known reason to expect a clinically significant interaction with cup plant.

Possible Interactions with Lab Tests

No interactions are known to occur, and there is no known reason to expect a clinically significant interaction with cup plant.

Possible Interactions with Diseases or Conditions

No interactions are known to occur, and there is no known reason to expect a clinically significant interaction with cup plant.

Typical Dosages & Routes of Administration that are Commonly Used

ORAL: Cup plant is used to make a tea; typically 1 teaspoon of cup plant root is added to 1 cup of water. The usual dose is 1 cup daily. The powdered root dose is 20 grains which is 1300 mg, and tincture 5 to 20 drops [5263].

Comments

Avoid confusion with Silphium laciniatum, also known as rosinweed.
There is very little scientific information about this product. Our staff is continually analyzing the available information on natural medicines and will add data here as it becomes available.

CUPMOSS

This Product is Also Known As
Chin Cups.

Scientific Names
Cladonia pyxidata.

People Use This For
Orally, cupmoss is used for coughs, bronchitis, and whooping cough (18).

Safety
There is insufficient reliable information available about the safety of cupmoss.
Pregnancy and Lactation: Insufficient reliable information available; avoid using.

Effectiveness
There is insufficient reliable information available about the effectiveness of cupmoss.

Possible Mechanism of Action & Active Ingredients
Cupmoss is stated to have expectorant and antitussive effects (18).

Adverse Reactions Including Known Allergies
None reported.

Possible Interactions with Herbs & Other Dietary Supplements
Insufficient reliable information available.

Possible Interactions with Drugs
No interactions are known to occur, and there is no known reason to expect a clinically significant interaction with cupmoss.

Possible Interactions with Foods
No interactions are known to occur, and there is no known reason to expect a clinically significant interaction with cupmoss.

Possible Interactions with Lab Tests
No interactions are known to occur, and there is no known reason to expect a clinically significant interaction with cupmoss.

Possible Interactions with Diseases or Conditions
No interactions are known to occur, and there is no known reason to expect a clinically significant interaction with cupmoss.

Typical Dosages & Routes of Administration that are Commonly Used
ORAL: A suggested dose is 2 ounces of liquid, prepared by adding cupmoss to water, mixed with honey as needed for cough (5267,5264).

Comments
There is very little scientific information about this product. Our staff is continually analyzing the available information on natural medicines and will add data here as it becomes available.

CYCLAMEN

This Product is Also Known As
Groundbread, Ivy-Leafed Cyclamen, Sowbread, Swinebread.

Scientific Names
Cyclamen europaeum.
Family: Primulaceae (18).

People Use This For
Orally, cyclamen is used for menstrual complaints, "nervous emotional states," and digestive problems (18).

Safety
LIKELY UNSAFE ...when rhizome or root are used orally. Doses as low as 300 mg can cause poisoning (18).
PREGNANCY AND LACTATION: LIKELY UNSAFE ...when used orally; avoid using.

Effectiveness
There is insufficient reliable information available about the effectiveness of cyclamen.

Possible Mechanism of Action & Active Ingredients

The applicable parts of cyclamen are the rhizome and root. There is insufficient reliable information available about the possible mechanism of action and active ingredients.

Adverse Reactions Including Known Allergies

Poisoning has been reported with doses as low as 300 mg; symptoms include stomach pain, nausea, vomiting, and diarrhea (18). High doses can cause severe poisoning; symptoms include spasm and asphyxiation (18,553).

Possible Interactions with Herbs & Other Dietary Supplements

Insufficient reliable information available.

Possible Interactions with Drugs

No interactions are known to occur, and there is no known reason to expect a clinically significant interaction with cyclamen.

Possible Interactions with Foods

No interactions are known to occur, and there is no known reason to expect a clinically significant interaction with cyclamen.

Possible Interactions with Lab Tests

No interactions are known to occur, and there is no known reason to expect a clinically significant interaction with cyclamen.

Possible Interactions with Diseases or Conditions

No interactions are known to occur, and there is no known reason to expect a clinically significant interaction with cyclamen.

Typical Dosages & Routes of Administration that are Commonly Used

ORAL: People typically use 20 to 40 grains (1300 to 2600 mg) of powdered cyclamen root (5267). One source specifies that cyclamen should not be used without medical supervision (5263).

Comments

None.

CYPRESS

This Product is Also Known As

None.

Scientific Names

Cupressus sempervirens.
Family: Coniferae.

People Use This For

Topically, cypress is used for head colds, cough, bronchitis, and as an expectorant (18).

Safety

There is insufficient reliable information available about the safety of the topical use of cypress.
Pregnancy and Lactation: Insufficient reliable information available; avoid using.

Effectiveness

There is insufficient reliable information available about the effectiveness of cypress.

Possible Mechanism of Action & Active Ingredients

The applicable parts of cypress are the branch, cone, and oil. There is insufficient reliable information available about the possible mechanism of action and active ingredients.

Adverse Reactions Including Known Allergies

Cypress may cause kidney irritation if it is taken orally (18).

Possible Interactions with Herbs & Other Dietary Supplements

Insufficient reliable information available.

Possible Interactions with Drugs

No interactions are known to occur, and there is no known reason to expect a clinically significant interaction with cypress.

Possible Interactions with Foods

No interactions are known to occur, and there is no known reason to expect a clinically significant interaction with cypress.

Possible Interactions with Lab Tests

No interactions are known to occur, and there is no known reason to expect a clinically significant interaction with cypress.

Possible Interactions with Diseases or Conditions

No interactions are known to occur, and there is no known reason to expect a clinically significant interaction with cypress.

Typical Dosages & Routes of Administration that are Commonly Used

TOPICAL: Cypress is used as an ointment (18).

Comments

There is very little scientific information about this product. Our staff is continually analyzing the available information on natural medicines and will add data here as it becomes available.

CYPRESS SPURGE

This Product is Also Known As

None.

Scientific Names

Euphorbia cyparissias.

People Use This For

Cypress spurge is used for diseases of the respiratory organs, diarrhea, and skin diseases (18).

Safety

UNSAFE ...when taken orally. The plant contains poisonous white latex (milky liquid) and cocarcinogenic agents (18). Both the fresh and dried latex are toxic (18).
PREGNANCY AND LACTATION: UNSAFE ...contraindicated due to toxicity (18).

Effectiveness

There is insufficient reliable information available about the effectiveness of cypress spurge.

Possible Mechanism of Action & Active Ingredients

The applicable parts of cypress spurge are the flowering plant and root. Cypress spurge contains varied diterpenes and triterpenes. The ingenan esters are potent inflammatory and cocarcinogenic agents (18). Euphorbia species have topical irritant, GI irritant, emetic, and purgative effects (19).

Adverse Reactions Including Known Allergies

Taken orally, cypress spurge which is part of the Euphorbia species may cause GI irritation, nausea, vomiting, and diarrhea (19). Ingestion of the latex can cause burning of the mouth, vomiting, mydriasis, dizziness, painful bowel movements, stupor, cardiac arrhythmias, and collapse (18). When used topically, Euphorbia species may cause contact dermatitis (19). Skin contact with the latex causes reddening, itching, burning, and blisters (18). Eye contact can cause eyelid swelling, conjunctival inflammation, and corneal defects (18).

Possible Interactions with Herbs & Other Dietary Supplements

Insufficient reliable information available.

Possible Interactions with Drugs

No interactions are known to occur, and there is no known reason to expect a clinically significant interaction with cypress spurge.

Possible Interactions with Foods

No interactions are known to occur, and there is no known reason to expect a clinically significant interaction with cypress spurge.

Possible Interactions with Lab Tests

No interactions are known to occur, and there is no known reason to expect a clinically significant interaction with cypress spurge.

Possible Interactions with Diseases or Conditions

DIARRHEA: Avoid; Euphorbia species have purgative effects (19).
GI IRRITATION, INFLAMMATION: Avoid; Euphorbia species have GI irritant effects (19).
NAUSEA, VOMITING: Avoid; Euphorbia species have emetic effects (19).

Typical Dosages & Routes of Administration that are Commonly Used
No typical dosage.

Comments
Cypress spurge is considered unsafe.

DA QING YE

This Product is Also Known As
Quing Dai.

Scientific Names
Isatis indigota.
Family: Brassicaceae.

People Use This For
In Chinese medicine, da qing ye dried leaf is used to treat acute parotitis, upper respiratory infection, encephalitis, hepatitis, lung abscess, dysentery, acute gastroenteritis, and HIV (5541).
In combination with seven other herbs (PC-SPES), da qing ye is used to treat prostate cancer (5548).

Safety
POSSIBLY SAFE ...when used orally in a specific herbal combination (PC-SPES) (5548).
There is insufficient reliable information available about the safety of da qing ye when used in other preparations.
PREGNANCY AND LACTATION: LIKELY UNSAFE ...when used orally. It is reported to cause uterine contractions (5541); contraindicated.

Effectiveness
POSSIBLY EFFECTIVE ...when used orally in a specific herbal combination for prostate cancer. Studies using da qing ye in combination with seven other herbs (PC-SPES) in prostate cancer patients, found that it significantly decreases prostate-specific antigen (PSA) levels (5548,5122,5913), causes tumor cell death (5913), and causes clinically significant reductions in testosterone (5548). In two reports, PSA levels fell significantly within 1 month of treatment (5548,5122).
There is insufficient reliable information available about the effectiveness of da qing ye for its other uses.

Possible Mechanism of Action & Active Ingredients
The applicable part of da qing ye is the dried leaf. The dried leaf appears to have antibacterial and antiviral activity; it can increase the phagocytic activity of leukocytes. It also shows evidence of antipyretic, antiinflammatory and biliary stimulant properties. Da qing ye seems to relax smooth muscles but contracts the uterine muscle. The dried leaf of da qing ye contains the glycosides indican and isatin B. Of the ingested dose of da qing ye, 90% is excreted in the urine (5541).

Adverse Reactions Including Known Allergies
Oral use of da qing ye can cause nausea and vomiting (5541). If given intramuscularly, it could cause blood in the urine (5541).

Possible Interactions with Herbs & Other Dietary Supplements
Insufficient reliable information available.

Possible Interactions with Drugs
No interactions are known to occur, and there is no known reason to expect a clinically significant interaction with da qing ye.

Possible Interactions with Foods
No interactions are known to occur, and there is no known reason to expect a clinically significant interaction with da qing ye.

Possible Interactions with Lab Tests
No interactions are known to occur, and there is no known reason to expect a clinically significant interaction with da qing ye.

Possible Interactions with Diseases or Conditions
No interactions are known to occur, and there is no known reason to expect a clinically significant interaction with da qing ye.

Typical Dosages & Routes of Administration that are Commonly Used
No typical dosage.

Comments

Other herbs considered to be da qing ye include Isatis tinctoria, Baphicacanthus cusia, Clerodendron cyrtophyllum, and Polyconum tinctorium (5541).

DAFFODIL

This Product is Also Known As

Lent Lily.

Scientific Names

Narcissus pseudonarcissus.
Family: Amaryllidaceae.

People Use This For

Orally, daffodil is used to soothe mucous membrane irritation resulting from whooping cough, colds, asthma, and bronchial catarrh (18), and as an emetic (7200).
Historically, a plaster made from daffodil bulbs was used topically for wounds, burns, strains, and joint pain (7200).

Safety

POSSIBLY UNSAFE ...when used topically. Severe cases of dermatitis have been reported (5004).
LIKELY UNSAFE ...when used orally (19). Merely chewing on the stem may be enough to cause a chill, shivering, and fainting. The constituent lycorine can cause salivation, vomiting, diarrhea at low doses, and paralysis and collapse at higher doses (514).
PREGNANCY AND LACTATION: LIKELY UNSAFE; avoid using.

Effectiveness

There is insufficient reliable information available about the effectiveness of daffodil.

Possible Mechanism of Action & Active Ingredients

The applicable parts of daffodil are the bulb, leaf, and flower. Daffodil contains numerous active constituents including alkaloids (lycorine and galanthamine) and chelidonic acid (18). In small amounts, lycorine causes salivation, vomiting, and diarrhea; at higher doses, it causes paralysis and collapse. Galanthamine is a cholinesterase inhibitor and analgesic (514), and it is being investigated for use in the treatment of Alzheimer's disease (5007). Lycorine, narciclasine, and other constituents are cytotoxic (514). The mucus and sap of daffodil plants and bulbs contain calcium oxalate crystals, which are most likely responsible for the skin irritation (5004). "Micro trauma" to the skin from the oxylate crystals allows penetration of other irritants and worsens dermatitis (5004).

Adverse Reactions Including Known Allergies

Oral use of daffodil can cause irritation and swelling of the mouth, tongue and throat (19), as well as vomiting, salivation, diarrhea and central nervous disorders, and respiratory or CV collapse and subsequent death (18). This is due to the lycorine component (214). Topical use can cause dermatitis (5004,5005) . People who simply handle daffodil plants or bulbs can get "Lily rash" or "daffodil itch" (18,5004).

Possible Interactions with Herbs & Other Dietary Supplements

Insufficient reliable information available.

Possible Interactions with Drugs

No interactions are known to occur, and there is no known reason to expect a clinically significant interaction with daffodil.

Possible Interactions with Foods

No interactions are known to occur, and there is no known reason to expect a clinically significant interaction with daffodil.

Possible Interactions with Lab Tests

No interactions are known to occur, and there is no known reason to expect a clinically significant interaction with daffodil.

Possible Interactions with Diseases or Conditions

No interactions are known to occur, and there is no known reason to expect a clinically significant interaction with daffodil.

Typical Dosages & Routes of Administration that are Commonly Used

ORAL: Used as a powder and an extract (amount unspecified) (18).

Comments

None.

DAMIANA

This Product is Also Known As
Damiana Herb, Damiana Leaf, Herba de la Pastora, Mexican Damiana, Mizibcoc, Old Woman's Broom, Rosemary, Turnerae diffusae folium, Turnerae diffusae herba.

Scientific Names
Turnera diffusa, synonyms Damiana aphrodisiaca, Turnera aphrodisiaca, Turnera microphylla.
Family: Bignoniaceae/Turneraceae.

People Use This For
Orally, damiana is used to treat headache, bedwetting (6), depression, nervous dyspepsia, atonic constipation (4), for prophylaxis and treatment of sexual disturbances, strengthening and stimulation during exertion (overwork), boosting and maintaining mental and physical capacity, and as an aphrodisiac (2).
It is also taken as tea or smoked for a subtle "high" (5).

Safety
LIKELY SAFE ...when used orally in amounts found in foods (maximum use level 0.125%.); Damiana is approved for food use in the US (11).
POSSIBLY SAFE ...when used orally and appropriately for medicinal purposes (12).
PREGNANCY AND LACTATION: Insufficient reliable information available; avoid using (4).

Effectiveness
There is insufficient reliable information available about the effectiveness of damiana.

Possible Mechanism of Action & Active Ingredients
The applicable parts of damiana are the leaf and stem. Ethanolic extracts are reported to exhibit CNS depressant activity (4). The quinone arbutin may be responsible for antibacterial properties (4).

Adverse Reactions Including Known Allergies
Tetanus-like convulsions and paroxysms resulting in symptoms similar to rabies or strychnine poisoning occurred following ingestion of 200 grams damiana extract (4).

Possible Interactions with Herbs & Other Dietary Supplements
Insufficient reliable information available.

Possible Interactions with Drugs
HYPOGLYCEMIC DRUGS: Theoretically, may interfere with hypoglycemic therapy (4).

Possible Interactions with Foods
No interactions are known to occur, and there is no known reason to expect a clinically significant interaction with damiana.

Possible Interactions with Lab Tests
No interactions are known to occur, and there is no known reason to expect a clinically significant interaction with damiana.

Possible Interactions with Diseases or Conditions
DIABETES: Theoretically, may interfere with blood glucose control (4).

Typical Dosages & Routes of Administration that are Commonly Used
ORAL: 2-4 grams dried leaf three times daily, or one cup tea (steep 2-4 grams dried leaf in 150 mL boiling water 5-10 minutes, strain) three times a day (4). Liquid extract of damiana, 2-4 mL (4).

Comments
None.

DANDELION above ground parts

This Product is Also Known As
Blowball, Cankerwort, Common Dandelion, Dandelion Herb, Lion's Tooth, Pissenlit, Priest's Crown, Swine Snout, Taraxaci herba, Taraxacum, Wild Endive.
CAUTION: See separate listing for Dandelion entire plant.

Scientific Names
Taraxacum officinale, synonyms, Taraxacum vulgare, Leontodon taracum.
Family: Asteraceae/Compositae.

© Copyright 2000, Natural Medicines Comprehensive Database (209) 472-2244. For updated data, go to www.NaturalDatabase.com

People Use This For
Orally, the above ground parts of the dandelion are used for loss of appetite and dyspepsia, flatulence and feelings of fullness (2). It is also used as a laxative, promoter of healthy circulation, skin toner, blood vessel cleanser and strengthener (5), for rheumatism, arthritic joints, and as a tonic (5).
For food uses, dandelion is used in salad greens, soups, and wine (6).

Safety
LIKELY SAFE ...when taken orally and appropriately for medicinal purposes (12). ...when used in amounts found in foods (12).
PREGNANCY AND LACTATION: Insufficient reliable information available; avoid amounts greater than those in foods.

Effectiveness
There is insufficient reliable information available about the effectiveness of dandelion above ground parts (2,3).

Possible Mechanism of Action & Active Ingredients
The sesquiterpene lactones are responsible for the diuretic effects and can contribute to dandelion's mild anti-inflammatory activity. Dandelion also contains an appetite-stimulating bitter identified as eudesmanolides, which was previously called taraxacin (6). Dandelion can have a slight laxative effect (5).

Adverse Reactions Including Known Allergies
The use of dandelion can cause contact dermatitis in sensitive individuals (6). Dandelion can cause an allergic reaction in individuals sensitive to the Asteraceae/Compositae family. Members of this family include ragweed, chrysanthemums, marigolds, daisies, and many other herbs.

Possible Interactions with Herbs & Other Dietary Supplements
Insufficient reliable information available.

Possible Interactions with Drugs
No interactions are known to occur, and there is no known reason to expect a clinically significant interaction with dandelion above ground parts.

Possible Interactions with Foods
No interactions are known to occur, and there is no known reason to expect a clinically significant interaction with dandelion above ground parts.

Possible Interactions with Lab Tests
No interactions are known to occur, and there is no known reason to expect a clinically significant interaction with dandelion above ground parts.

Possible Interactions with Diseases or Conditions
OBSTRUCTION: The use of dandelion is contraindicated in patients with obstruction of bile ducts or the gallbladder. If gallstones are present, physician consultation is necessary before the use of dandelion (2).
OTHER: Dandelion is contraindicated in patients with puss in the pleural cavity or obstruction of the bowels (2).
CROSS-ALLERGENICITY: Can cause an allergic reaction in individuals sensitive to the Asteraceae/Compositae family. Members of this family include ragweed, chrysanthemums, marigolds, daisies, and many other herbs.

Typical Dosages & Routes of Administration that are Commonly Used
ORAL: The typical dose of dandelion is 4-10 grams of the dried above ground parts three times daily. The common dose of the liquid extract (1:1 in 25% alcohol) is 4-10 mL three times daily (2).

Comments
Dandelions contain more vitamin A than carrots (6002). Avoid confusion with dandelion as a whole plant.

DANDELION entire plant

This Product is Also Known As
Blowball, Cankerwort, Common Dandelion, Lion's Tooth, Pissenlit, Priest's Crown, Swine Snout, Taraxacum, Wild Endive.
CAUTION: See separate listing for Dandelion above ground parts.

Scientific Names
Taraxacum officinale, synonyms Leontodon taraxacum, Taraxacum vulgare.
Family: Asteraceae or Compositae.

People Use This For
Orally, dandelion plant is used for gallstones, bile stimulation, muscle aches, low urine output, indigestion (4), constipation (4,9,11), flatulence, as a tonic (11), and in anti-smoking preparations (11).

In Chinese medicine, dandelion is used for treating breast cancer (6,11).
Traditionally, dandelion has been used for diabetes, rheumatic conditions, heartburn, bruises, gout, stiff joints, eczema, and cancer (11).
For food uses, dandelion leaves are added to salads. The roasted root and extract are used as coffee substitutes (11).
In food manufacturing, dandelion is a flavoring component for foods as well as beverages (11).

Safety

LIKELY SAFE ...when consumed in amounts commonly found in foods. Dandelion is Generally Recognized as Safe (GRAS) in the US for food use with a maximum level of 0.014% for the fluid extract and 0.003% for the solid extract (11).
POSSIBLY SAFE ...when used orally and appropriately for medicinal purposes (12).
PREGNANCY: POSSIBLY SAFE ...when used in food amounts; avoid amounts greater than those found in foods (4).
LACTATION: Insufficient reliable information available; avoid using.

Effectiveness

POSSIBLY EFFECTIVE ...when taken orally for disturbances in bile flow, dyspepsia, loss of appetite, and stimulating diuresis (2).
There is insufficient reliable information available about the effectiveness of dandelion for its other uses.

Possible Mechanism of Action & Active Ingredients

The dandelion constituent taraxacin favorably effects digestion. The bitter constituents in dandelion root are responsible for increasing bile flow (7). The extracts demonstrate diuretic effects in animals and antitumor activity in vitro (4). The root extract has anti-inflammatory activity in animals (4). Hypoglycemic activity can also occur with the use of dandelion in animals (4). The sesquiterpene lactone constituents can be responsible for allergic reactions (4).

Adverse Reactions Including Known Allergies

The dandelion plant taken orally can cause gastric hyperacidity (2). Topically, the plant can cause contact dermatitis (4). It can cause an allergic reaction in individuals sensitive to the Asteraceae/Compositae family. Members of this family include ragweed, chrysanthemums, marigolds, daisies, and many other herbs.

Possible Interactions with Herbs & Other Dietary Supplements

DIURETIC HERBS: Theoretically, dandelion can have additive effects with herbs having diuretic properties. Herbs thought to have diuretic properties include agrimony, artichoke, broom, buchu, burdock, celery, cornsilk, couch grass, elder, guaiacum, juniper, pokeroot, shepherd's purse, squill, uva ursi, and yarrow.
HYPOGLYCEMIC HERBS: Theoretically, dandelion can have additive effects with herbs having hypoglycemic effects.

Possible Interactions with Drugs

DIURETICS, HYPOGLYCEMIC DRUGS: Theoretically, concomitant use of the dandelion plant can interfere with drug therapy (4).
LITHIUM (Eskalith, Lithobid): Theoretically, concomitant use can cause lithium toxicity due to sodium loss brought about by dandelion (19).
ACID-INHIBITING DRUGS: Theoretically, due to claims that dandelion increases stomach acid, it may interfere with antacids, sucralfate (Carafate), H-2 antagonists (Zantac, Pepcid, etc.), or proton-pump inhibitors (Prilosec, Prevacid) (19).
DIABETES THERAPY: Monitor blood glucose levels closely because dandelion can exhibit hypoglycemic effects (19).

Possible Interactions with Foods

No interactions are known to occur, and there is no known reason to expect a clinically significant interaction with dandelion entire plant.

Possible Interactions with Lab Tests

No interactions are known to occur, and there is no known reason to expect a clinically significant interaction with dandelion entire plant.

Possible Interactions with Diseases or Conditions

Contraindicated in cases of acute gallbladder inflammation, bile duct obstruction, and intestinal blockage (2).
DIABETES: Monitor blood glucose levels closely because dandelion can exhibit hypoglycemic effects (19).
GALLSTONES: Professional evaluation is needed before the use of the dandelion plant in individuals with gallstones (2).
CROSS-ALLERGENICITY: Can cause an allergic reaction in individuals sensitive to the Asteraceae/Compositae family. Members of this family include ragweed, chrysanthemums, marigolds, daisies, and many other herbs.

Typical Dosages & Routes of Administration that are Commonly Used

ORAL: The typical dose of the dandelion leaf is 4-10 grams of the dried leaf or one cup of the tea three times daily (4). The tea is prepared by steeping 4-10 grams of the dried leaf in 150 mL boiling water for 5-10 minutes and then straining. The usual dose of the liquid leaf extract (1:1 in 25% alcohol) is 4-10 mL three times a day (4). The typical dose of the dandelion root is 2-8 grams of the dried root or one cup of the tea three times daily (4). The tea is prepared by steeping 3-8 grams of the dried root in 150 mL boiling water for 5-10 minutes and then straining (4). The usual dose of the root tincture (1:5 in 45% alcohol) is 5-10 mL three times daily (4). The common dose of the whole plant is as a tea, which is prepared by steeping 3-4 grams of the powdered whole plant in 150 mL boiling water for 5-10 minutes and then straining (2). The dose of the liquid extract of taraxacum is typically 2-8 mL (4). The juice of taraxacum is given as 4-8 mL (4).

Comments

The dandelion plant contains more vitamin A than carrots (6002). Avoid confusion with the above ground parts of dandelion.

DANSHEN

This Product is Also Known As

Ch'ih Shen, Dan-Shen, Huang Ken, Pin-Ma Ts'ao, Red Rooted Sage, Red Sage, Salvia Root, Shu-Wei Ts'ao, Tan-Shen, Tzu Tan-Ken.
CAUTION: See separate listing for Sage.

Scientific Names

Salvia miltiorrhiza (red sage); Salvia przewalskii (gansu danshen); Salvia przewalskii mandarinorum; Salvia bowelyana (Southern danshen); Salvia yunnanensis.
Family: Labiatae/Lamiaceae.

People Use This For

Danshen is used for circulation problems, ischemic stroke, angina pectoris, and other cardiovascular diseases. Danshen is used for menstrual problems, chronic hepatitis (6), abdominal masses, insomnia due to palpitations and tight chest, acne, psoriasis, eczema, and other skin conditions (11). Danshen is also used to relieve bruising and to aid in wound healing (11).

Safety

LIKELY SAFE ...when used orally and appropriately (12).
PREGNANCY AND LACTATION: Insufficient reliable information available; avoid using.

Effectiveness

POSSIBLY EFFECTIVE ...for chronic hepatitis when taken orally (6).
There is insufficient reliable information available about the effectiveness of danshen for its other uses.

Possible Mechanism of Action & Active Ingredients

The applicable part of danshen is the root. Researchers think the constituents protocatechualdehyde and 3,4-dihydroxyphenyl-lactic acid may play a role in vasoactivity. There is some evidence that danshen weakens muscular action, but it can also cause an increase in coronary flow rate. Antithrombotic effects and blood vessel dilation have been reported in animals (6).

Adverse Reactions Including Known Allergies

Danshen tinctures of herb can cause pruritus, stomachache, and reduced appetite (12).

Possible Interactions with Herbs & Other Dietary Supplements

HERBS WITH ANTICOAGULANT/ANTIPLATELET POTENTIAL: Concomitant use of herbs that have coumarin constituents or affect platelet aggregation could theoretically increase the risk of bleeding in some people. These herbs include: angelica, anise, arnica, asafoetida, bogbean, boldo, capsicum, celery, chamomile, clove, fenugreek, feverfew, garlic, ginger, ginkgo, ginseng Panax, horse chestnut, horseradish, licorice, meadowsweet, prickly ash, onion, papain, passionflower, poplar, quassia, red clover, turmeric, wild carrot, wild lettuce, willow, and others (4,19).
METHYL SALICYLATE OIL: There is one case report of increased international normalized ratio (INR) with concomitant use of topical methyl salicylate oil, oral danshen, and warfarin (612).

Possible Interactions with Drugs

ANTICOAGULANT, ANTIPLATELET DRUGS: Theoretically, concomitant use of danshen with anticoagulant or antiplatelet drugs might increase the risk of bleeding (6); avoid concomitant use of danshen and anticoagulant or antiplatelet drugs.
WARFARIN (Coumadin): Concomitant use increases warfarin anticoagulant effects and risk of bleeding (611,612); avoid concomitant use of danshen and warfarin.

Possible Interactions with Foods

No interactions are known to occur, and there is no known reason to expect a clinically significant interaction with danshen.

Possible Interactions with Lab Tests

LIVER FUNCTION TESTS: Danshen might improve liver function and liver function test results in patients with chronic hepatitis (6).

Possible Interactions with Diseases or Conditions

BLEEDING DISORDERS: Avoid; theoretically, danshen may increase the risk of bleeding.

Typical Dosages & Routes of Administration that are Commonly Used

ORAL: People typically use 5 to 15 grams of danshen (5269).

Comments

None.

DATE PALM

This Product is Also Known As

None.

Scientific Names

Phoenix dactylifera.
Family: Palmae.

People Use This For

In folk medicine, date palm is used for coughs and other respiratory chest symptoms (18).

Safety

There is insufficient reliable information available about the safety of the oral use of date palm fruit in amounts exceeding those found in foods.
Pregnancy and Lactation: Avoid using in amounts greater than those typically found in foods.

Effectiveness

There is insufficient reliable information available about the effectiveness of date palm.

Possible Mechanism of Action & Active Ingredients

The applicable part of date palm is the fruit. There is insufficient reliable information available about the possible mechanism of action and active ingredients.

Adverse Reactions Including Known Allergies

None reported.

Possible Interactions with Herbs & Other Dietary Supplements

Insufficient reliable information available.

Possible Interactions with Drugs

No interactions are known to occur, and there is no known reason to expect a clinically significant interaction with date palm.

Possible Interactions with Foods

No interactions are known to occur, and there is no known reason to expect a clinically significant interaction with date palm.

Possible Interactions with Lab Tests

No interactions are known to occur, and there is no known reason to expect a clinically significant interaction with date palm.

Possible Interactions with Diseases or Conditions

No interactions are known to occur, and there is no known reason to expect a clinically significant interaction with date palm.

Typical Dosages & Routes of Administration that are Commonly Used

ORAL: Juice from the fruits is sun-dried to a "honey" and taken orally (18).

Comments

There is very little scientific information about this product. Our staff is continually analyzing the available information on natural medicines and will add data here as it becomes available.

DEANOL

This Product is Also Known As

Deanol aceglumate, Deanol acetamidobenzoate, Deanol benzilate, Deanol bisorcate, Deanol cyclohexylpropionate, Deanol hemisuccinate, Deanol pidolate, Deanol tartrate, Dimethylaminoethanol, Dimethylethanolamine, DMAE.

Scientific Names

2-Dimethylaminoethanol.

People Use This For

Orally, people use deanol for treating attention disorder (1664,1669,1677,1678,1679), enhancing memory and mood, boosting cognitive function (1664), treating Alzheimer's disease (1665,1680,1681), increasing intelligence and physical energy, improving athletic performance (1666), preventing aging or liver spots, improving red blood cell function, improving muscle reflexes and increasing oxygen efficiency, extending life span (1667,1671), treating autism (1670), and treating tardive dyskinesia (1665,1672,1673,1674,1675,1676,1803).

Safety

POSSIBLY SAFE ...when used orally and appropriately (1668,1669,1671,1672,1673,1674,1675,1676,1677,1678,1679,1680,1681,2706).
PREGNANCY AND LACTATION: Insufficient reliable information available; avoid using.

Effectiveness

POSSIBLY EFFECTIVE ...when deanol is used orally in combination with ginseng, vitamins, and minerals for improving exercise performance (1671). The combination increases total work load and maximal oxygen consumption during exercise (1671).
LIKELY INEFFECTIVE ...when used orally for treating Alzheimer's disease (1680,1681). ...when used orally for treating tardive dyskinesia (1665,1672,1673,1674,1675,1676,1803,1804).
Clinical studies using deanol for treating attention-deficit disorder have produced inconclusive results (1669,1677,1679). There is insufficient reliable information available about deanol for its other uses.

Possible Mechanism of Action & Active Ingredients

Deanol is a precursor to choline and might enhance central acetylcholine formation (9,1669). Deanol has been formulated in a variety of salts and esters, including deanol aceglumate, deanol acetamidobenzoate, deanol bisorcate, deanol cyclohexylpropionate (cyprodenate, cyprodemanol), deanol hemisuccinate, deanol pidolate, and deanol tartrate (9). The hydrochloride salt of deanol benzilate (deanol diphenylglycoate, benzacine) has been included in antispasmodic preparations (9). Preliminary research with deanol has demonstrated no effect on life span (1682,1683).

Adverse Reactions Including Known Allergies

Orally, deanol can cause constipation, urticaria, headache, drowsiness, insomnia, overstimulation, vivid dreams, confusion, depression, blood pressure elevation, hypomania, an increase in schizophrenia symptoms, and orofacial and respiratory tardive dyskinesia (1674,1680,1684,1685,1686,2706).

Possible Interactions with Herbs & Other Dietary Supplements

Insufficient reliable information available.

Possible Interactions with Drugs

ANTICHOLINERGIC DRUGS: Theoretically, concomitant use might decrease the effect of drugs with anticholinergic activity, due to the potential cholinergic activity of deanol.

Possible Interactions with Foods

No interactions are known to occur, and there is no known reason to expect a clinically significant interaction with deanol.

Possible Interactions with Lab Tests

No interactions are known to occur, and there is no known reason to expect a clinically significant interaction with deanol.

Possible Interactions with Diseases or Conditions

SCHIZOPHRENIA: Deanol can worsen schizophrenia symptoms (1674); avoid using in patients with schizophrenia.
DEPRESSION: Deanol might worsen depression. It is reported to cause depression as an adverse effect (1685).
CLONIC-TONIC SEIZURES: Deanol is relatively contraindicated in people with clonic-tonic seizure disorders (2706).

Typical Dosages & Routes of Administration that are Commonly Used

ORAL: People typically begin with 100 mg per day and gradually increase to 500 mg per day (1664). Doses have ranged from 300 to 2000 mg per day in clinical studies (1669,1672,1673).

Comments

Deanol was previously marketed as the prescription drug, Deaner, by Riker Laboratories for the management of children with behavior problems and learning difficulties (1669,2706). According to 3M (Riker), Deaner was removed from the US market in 1983 because of insufficient evidence of efficacy (1895). Deanol is not an approved food additive in the US, nor is it an orphan drug, as some supplement advertising suggests (1805).

DEER VELVET

This Product is Also Known As
Cornu Cervi Parvum, Deer Antler, Deer Antler Velvet, Horns of Gold, Lu Rong, Nokyong, Rokujo, Velvet Antler, Velvet of Young Deer Horn.

Scientific Names
Cervus nippon; Cervus elaphus.

People Use This For
Orally, deer velvet is used to boost strength and endurance, for muscle aches and pains, to promote youthfulness, increase mental clarity, as an aphrodisiac, to treat sexual dysfunction (5507,5509), to boost estrogen and testosterone levels (5516), to counter the effects of stress, to improve immune system functioning, and to promote rapid recovery from illness (5508). It is used to improve fertility, for menstrual and menopause problems, to reduce hormone replacement therapy dose, to reduce cholesterol and high blood pressure, for liver and kidney disorders, to protect the liver from toxins, for migraines, asthma, indigestion, osteoporosis, and acne (5510,5511,5516). It is also used for its anticancer and anti-inflammatory properties, as a source of growth factors IGR-1 & IGF-2 (5508), to stimulate production and circulation of blood (5513), to increase blood count, and lower the level of free radicals (5516).

In herbal combinations, deer velvet is used to improve athletic performance, for an anti-aging effect, for arthritis and osteoporosis, anemia, gonadotropic disorders, gynecological disorders, skin conditions, tissue and bone rejuvenation (5506). It is also used to increase mental capacity and performance, increase blood circulation to the brain, reduce early stages of muscular degeneration, to improve eyesight and hearing, to help PMS, impotence, and reduce stress (5506,5515).

In Chinese medicine, deer velvet is used to treat symptoms of impotence; cold extremities; soreness and weakness in the lower back and knees; leukorrhea; uterine bleeding; chronic skin ulcers; and frequent, copious, clear urination. It has also been used as a tonic for children with failure to thrive, mental retardation, learning disabilities, insufficient growth, or skeletal deformities including rickets (5501).

In Korean medicine, deer velvet is used at the onset of winter to ward off infections (5512).

Safety
There is insufficient reliable information available about the safety of deer velvet.
Pregnancy and Lactation: Insufficient reliable information available; avoid using.

Effectiveness
There is insufficient reliable information available about the effectiveness of deer velvet.

Possible Mechanism of Action & Active Ingredients
By weight, deer velvet is approximately 50% amino acids (5502). Chondroitin sulfate is a major glycosaminoglycan (5517). Deer velvet also contains vitamin A, estrone and estradiol, sphingomyelin, ganglioside, some prostaglandins (5502), and epidermal growth factor (5518). The sex hormones estrone and estradiol can stimulate sexual function in females (5502). Gangliosides and sphingomyelins are thought to be involved with cell metabolism and growth (5514). Deer velvet is believed to stimulate the growth of body tissues, particularly the reticuloendothelial cells and leukocytes. It also appears to stimulate wound healing. Deer velvet seems to reduce fatigue by improving sleep and stimulating appetite. It is believed to improve health, especially in children and the elderly (5502). Preliminary evidence suggests that athletes taking deer velvet experience increased muscular strength and endurance in training. They also seem to recover faster from muscle tissue damage that results from exercise (5505). Other evidence suggests deer velvet extract might counteract certain effects of repeated doses of morphine, such as the development of tolerance (5503).

Adverse Reactions Including Known Allergies
None reported.

Possible Interactions with Herbs & Other Dietary Supplements
Insufficient reliable information available.

Possible Interactions with Drugs
MORPHINE: Some evidence suggests use of deer antler velvet might inhibit the development of tolerance to repeated doses of morphine (5503).

© Copyright 2000, Natural Medicines Comprehensive Database (209) 472-2244. For updated data, go to www.NaturalDatabase.com

Possible Interactions with Foods

No interactions are known to occur, and there is no known reason to expect a clinically significant interaction with deer velvet.

Possible Interactions with Lab Tests

No interactions are known to occur, and there is no known reason to expect a clinically significant interaction with deer velvet.

Possible Interactions with Diseases or Conditions

ESTROGEN-SENSITIVE CONDITIONS: Theoretically, women with conditions sensitive to estrogen, i.e. history of breast or cervical cancer, should avoid using deer velvet.

Typical Dosages & Routes of Administration that are Commonly Used

ORAL: A typical dose of deer velvet powder for a protective effect is 400-600 mg (5512). A typical dose for treatment is 0.9-2.4 grams. Double-boiled, 3-4.5 grams are used. Alternately, it can be soaked in wine (5501) or prepared as a 20% tincture in wine (5502).

Comments

Deer velvet is the epidermis that covers the inner structure of the growing bone and cartilage that will become deer antlers (5504). The velvet is removed either by a veterinarian or a producer who has been accredited by a veterinarian. Tourniquets of rubber or plastic are placed around the pedicles to prevent bleeding (5514).

DEERTONGUE

This Product is Also Known As

Carolina Vanilla, Deer's Tongue, Hound's Tongue, Liatris, Vanilla Leaf, Vanilla Plant, Vanilla Trilisa, Wild Vanilla.
CAUTION: See separate listing for Hound's Tongue (Cyonglossum officinale).

Scientific Names

Trilisa odoratissima, synonyms Carphephorus odoratissimus, Liatris odoratis.
Family: Asteraceae or Compositae.

People Use This For

Orally, deertongue is used for malaria (11).
In manufacturing, deertongue extracts are used to flavor tobacco, as a fragrance in cosmetics and soaps, and as a fixative in some products (11).

Safety

LIKELY UNSAFE ...when used orally for medicinal purposes. ...when used in amounts found in foods. The use of deertongue is not permitted in foods in the US (11).
PREGNANCY AND LACTATION: LIKEY UNSAFE ...contraindicated, due to potential effects of coumarin constituents.

Effectiveness

There is insufficient reliable information available about the effectiveness of deertongue.

Possible Mechanism of Action & Active Ingredients

The applicable part of deertongue is the dried leaf. Coumarin constituents are reported to cause liver injury and hemorrhage (11).

Adverse Reactions Including Known Allergies

Liver injury and hemorrhage are possible due to coumarin content (11). It can cause an allergic reaction in individuals sensitive to the Asteraceae/Compositae family. Members of this family include ragweed, chrysanthemums, marigolds, daisies, and many other herbs.

Possible Interactions with Herbs & Other Dietary Supplements

HERBS THAT AFFECT BLOOD CLOTTING: Theoretically, may enhance effects of other herbs which affect blood clotting, including alfalfa, angelica, aniseed, arnica, asafoetida, celery, chamomile, clove, fenugreek, feverfew, fucus, garlic, ginger, Panax ginseng, horse chestnut, licorice, northern and southern prickly ash, quassia, and red clover (4).

Possible Interactions with Drugs

ANTICOAGULANTS, ANTITHROMBOTICS: Theoretically, concomitant use may increase risk of bleeding.

Possible Interactions with Foods

No interactions are known to occur, and there is no known reason to expect a clinically significant interaction with deertongue.

Possible Interactions with Lab Tests

No interactions are known to occur, and there is no known reason to expect a clinically significant interaction with deertongue.

Possible Interactions with Diseases or Conditions

BLOOD CLOTTING DISORDERS: Theoretically, may increase the risk of bleeding in these condition.
CROSS-ALLERGENICITY: Can cause an allergic reaction in individuals sensitive to the Asteraceae/Compositae family. Members of this family include ragweed, chrysanthemums, marigolds, daisies, and many other herbs.

Typical Dosages & Routes of Administration that are Commonly Used

No typical dosage.

Comments

None.

DELPHINIUM

This Product is Also Known As

Delphinii Flos, Knight's Spur, Lark Heel, Lark's Claw, Larkspur, Lark's Toe, Ritterspornblüten, Staggerweed.

Scientific Names

Delphinium consolida.
Family: Ranunculaceae.

People Use This For

Orally, delphinium is used as an antihelmintic, diuretic, sedative, and appetite stimulant (2).
In herbal teas, delphinium is used as a brightening agent (2).

Safety

POSSIBLY SAFE ...when the flower is used in tea mixtures (less than 1%) (2).
LIKELY UNSAFE ...except in very low doses because it is toxic to the heart and respiratory systems (2,17).
PREGNANCY AND LACTATION: LIKELY UNSAFE ...contraindicated for oral use (2,17).

Effectiveness

There is insufficient reliable information available about the effectiveness of delphinium (2).

Possible Mechanism of Action & Active Ingredients

The applicable part of delphinium is the flower. The alkaloid constituents are cardiotoxic and seem to be responsible for the curare-like, central paralysis of the respiratory system (2).

Adverse Reactions Including Known Allergies

The use of delphinium can cause bradycardia, hypotension, cardiac arrest, and respiratory failure (2); animal deaths from poisoning are common (18).

Possible Interactions with Herbs & Other Dietary Supplements

Insufficient reliable information available.

Possible Interactions with Drugs

No interactions are known to occur, and there is no known reason to expect a clinically significant interaction with delphinium.

Possible Interactions with Foods

No interactions are known to occur, and there is no known reason to expect a clinically significant interaction with delphinium.

Possible Interactions with Lab Tests

No interactions are known to occur, and there is no known reason to expect a clinically significant interaction with delphinium.

Possible Interactions with Diseases or Conditions

No interactions are known to occur, and there is no known reason to expect a clinically significant interaction with delphinium.

Typical Dosages & Routes of Administration that are Commonly Used

No typical dosage.

Comments

None.

DEVIL'S CLAW

This Product is Also Known As
Devils Claw, Devil's Claw Root, Grapple Plant, Griffe Du Diable, Harpagophyti Radix, Harpagophytum, Wood Spider.

Scientific Names
Harpagophytum procumbens.
Family: Pedaliaceae.

People Use This For
Orally, devil's claw root is used for arteriosclerosis (5), arthritis (4,5), gout, myalgia, fibrositis, lumbago, pleuritic pain in the chest, rheumatic disease (4), GI upset (2,5), loss of appetite (2,11), and degenerative disorders of the locomotor system (2).
Traditionally, devil's claw has been used orally for kidney, bladder disease and menstrual difficulties (5), and topically as an ointment for injuries and disorders (18).

Safety
POSSIBLY SAFE ...when preparations of the tuber are used orally and appropriately (4,5,8,12).
There is insufficient reliable information available about the safety of the topical use of devil's claw.
PREGNANCY: LIKELY UNSAFE ...contraindicated because of possible oxytocic properties (4).
LACTATION: Insufficient reliable information available; avoid using.

Effectiveness
POSSIBLY EFFECTIVE ...when taken orally for loss of appetite or indigestion. ...when used as supportive therapy for degenerative joint disorders (2).
There is insufficient reliable information available about the effectiveness of devil's claw for its other uses.

Possible Mechanism of Action & Active Ingredients
The applicable part of devil's claw is the tuber. Devil's claw contains iridoids, including harpagoside, that some researchers believe responsible for an anti-inflammatory effect. However, trials in humans and animals do not consistently demonstrate this effect (4) Some evidence suggests crude methanolic extracts might be cardioactive due to the presence of the harpagide constituent. Low doses slightly slow the heart rate, increasing the strength of contraction. High doses markedly weaken the heart contraction and the coronary blood flow. (4). Devil's claw extracts show evidence of weak antifungal activity (4).

Adverse Reactions Including Known Allergies
There is one case report of throbbing frontal headache, tinnitus, anorexia, and loss of taste with the oral use of devil's claw (4).

Possible Interactions with Herbs & Other Dietary Supplements
Insufficient reliable information available.

Possible Interactions with Drugs
ACID-INHIBITING DRUGS: Theoretically, due to claims that devil's claw increases stomach acid, it might interfere with antacids, sucralfate (Carafate), H-2 antagonists, or proton pump inhibitors (19).
DIABETES THERAPY: Monitor blood glucose levels closely due to claims that devil's claw has hypoglycemic effects (4).
WARFARIN: There is one case report of purpurea associated with the concomitant use of devil's claw and warfarin (613).
CARDIAC DRUGS: Theoretically, due to reports of chronotropic or inotropic effects, devil's claw might interfere with cardiac drug therapy (4).
BLOOD PRESSURE THERAPY: Theoretically, due to claims of hypotensive effects, concomitant use might interfere with therapy for hypertension or hypotension (4).

Possible Interactions with Foods
No interactions are known to occur, and there is no known reason to expect a clinically significant interaction with devil's claw.

Possible Interactions with Lab Tests
No interactions are known to occur, and there is no known reason to expect a clinically significant interaction with devil's claw.

Possible Interactions with Diseases or Conditions
DUODENAL OR GASTRIC ULCERS: Contraindicated (2).
GALLSTONES: Caution should be used when using devil's claw root in individuals with gallstones (2,8).
DIABETES: Avoid the use of devil's claw in diabetics (4).

CARDIAC DISORDERS, HYPERTENSION, HYPOTENSION: Theoretically, devil's claw can interfere with the treatment of these conditions (4).

Typical Dosages & Routes of Administration that are Commonly Used
ORAL: The typical dose of devil's claw for loss of appetite is 1.5 grams of the root per day (2). For other uses, the usual dose is 4.5 grams of the root per day (2) or as a tea consumed in three portions. The tea is prepared by steeping 4.5 grams of the root in 300 mL boiled water for 8 hours at room temperature and then straining.

Comments
The name for this plant is derived from the appearance of its fruit, which is covered with hooks meant to attach onto animals in order to spread the seeds (6002). Devil's claw is an expensive herb with unclear effectiveness in arthritis. There are many less expensive alternatives that can be more effective for arthritis (5).

DEVIL'S CLUB

This Product is Also Known As
Cukilanarpak, Devils Club, Fatsia.

Scientific Names
Oplopanax horridus; Panax horridum; Echiopanax horridum.
Family: Araliaceae.

People Use This For
Traditionally, devil's club was used orally for arthritis, as a purgative, as an emetic, for wound healing, fever, tuberculosis, stomach trouble, coughs, colds, and pneumonia (6). The inner bark has been used topically as a treatment for swollen glands, boils, sores, and skin infections. The ashes have been used to treat burns (4215).

Safety
POSSIBLY SAFE ...when taken orally (12).
There is insufficient reliable information available about the safety of the topical use of devil's club.
PREGNANCY AND LACTATION: Insufficient reliable information available; avoid using.

Effectiveness
There is insufficient reliable information available about the effectiveness of devil's club.

Possible Mechanism of Action & Active Ingredients
The applicable part of devil's club is the root bark. Several animal studies found no evidence of activity (6).

Adverse Reactions Including Known Allergies
Devil's club possibly has a hypoglycemic effect (6).

Possible Interactions with Herbs & Other Dietary Supplements
Insufficient reliable information available.

Possible Interactions with Drugs
DIABETES THERAPY: Monitor blood glucose levels closely due to claims that devil's club has hypoglycemic effects (19).

Possible Interactions with Foods
No interactions are known to occur, and there is no known reason to expect a clinically significant interaction with devil's club.

Possible Interactions with Lab Tests
No interactions are known to occur, and there is no known reason to expect a clinically significant interaction with devil's club.

Possible Interactions with Diseases or Conditions
DIABETES: Might reduce blood sugar levels. There are repeated anecdotal reports of hypoglycemic activity in individuals with diabetes (6).

Typical Dosages & Routes of Administration that are Commonly Used
ORAL: People typically use 15 to 30 drops of the extract mixed in warm water three times daily between meals. The alcohol content is 55 to 65% (6006).
TOPICAL: The inner bark is baked slowly until it is very dry, then rubbed between the hands until broken and soft. The pulp is placed on the affected area to draw out infection (4215).

© Copyright 2000, Natural Medicines Comprehensive Database (209) 472-2244. For updated data, go to www.NaturalDatabase.com

Comments

Devil's club is a common plant in southeastern Alaska. It is considered the most important medicinal and magical plant of the Yakutat Tlingit. Both the shaman and the layman chew the stem bark (with the thorns removed) for its effects as an emetic, a purgative, and a general cure all (4215).

DHA (DOCOSAHEXAENOIC ACID)

This Product is Also Known As

Fish Oil Fatty Acid, N-3 Fatty Acid, Omega Fatty Acid, Omega 3 Fatty Acid, Omega-3 Fatty Acid, W-3 Fatty Acid.
CAUTION: See separate listings for EPA (eicosapentaenoic acid) and Fish Oils.

Scientific Names

Docosahexaenoic acid.

People Use This For

Orally, docosahexanoic acid (DHA) is used as a supplement for preterm infants (1045), as an ingredient in infant formula (5941), during the first four months of life to enhance mental development of infants (5941), for reducing aggressive behavior in stressed individuals (1043), for preventing depression, reducing symptoms of dementia, and enhancing vision (1048).

In combination with eicosapentaenoic acid (EPA), DHA is used for a variety of conditions, including the prevention and reversal of heart disease, decreasing ectopic ventricular beats, asthma, cancer, painful menses, hay fever, lung diseases, lupus erythematosus, lupus nephritis, and IgA nephropathy (507). EPA and DHA are also used in combination for migraine headache prophylaxis in adolescents (5097), atopic dermatitis, Behcet's syndrome, hyperlipidemia, hypertension, psoriasis, Raynaud's syndrome, rheumatoid arthritis, bipolar disorder, and ulcerative colitis (9). DHA is used in combination with arachidonic acid during the first four to six months of life to enhance mental development of infants (424,5941).

Safety

POSSIBLY SAFE ...when used orally and appropriately (9,945,1016).
CHILDREN: POSSIBLY SAFE ...when used orally and appropriately as a supplement to infant formula (5941). ...when used orally and appropriately in combination with arachidonic acid as supplements to infant formula (424,5941).
PREGNANCY AND LACTATION: Insufficient reliable information available; avoid using.

Effectiveness

POSSIBLY EFFECTIVE ...when used orally for reducing aggressive behavior in stressed individuals (1043). ...when given orally to preterm infants for improving visual attention later in childhood (1045). ...when used orally to improve night vision in children with dyslexia. Dyslexic children who received fish oils rich in DHA developed significantly better dark adaptation when compared with controls (5708). ...when used orally in combination with evening primrose oil, thyme oil, and vitamin E (Efalex) to improve movement disorders in children with dyspraxia. One small clinical trial has shown that this combination significantly decreases movement disorders as determined by objective measures (5708).
POSSIBLY INEFFECTIVE ...when used as a supplement in infant formula for improving cognitive and mental development or growth up to 18 months of age (424).
There is insufficient reliable information available about the effectiveness of DHA for its other uses.

Possible Mechanism of Action & Active Ingredients

DHA is a long chain n-3 polyunsaturated fatty acid that competes with arachidonic acid for inclusion in cyclo-oxygenase and lipoxygenase pathways (9). Long-chain polyunsaturated fatty acids make up a third of all lipids in the brain's grey matter (425). DHA decreases blood viscosity and increases red blood cell deformability (9). DHA can be converted into EPA (eicosapentaenoic acid) in humans (1044). Pure DHA reduces serum triglycerides in adults (1014,6143), and increases serum HDL2-cholesterol, LDL-cholesterol, LDL particle size and fasting insulin, but has no effect on total cholesterol or fasting glucose in mildly hypercholesterolemic men (6143). DHA plays a key role in the structural development of retinal, neural and synaptic membranes, and is thought to be important for normal neural function (424,425). DHA is present in human breast milk but not in standard infant formulas. Formula-fed infants have lower plasma and cerebral cortex DHA levels than breast milk-fed infants; the clinical significance of this, if any, is unknown. Animals who are deficient in n-3 fatty acids (such as DHA) develop learning and vision disturbances. These disturbances do not occur when the parent fatty acid, linolenic acid, is adequately supplied (424).

Adverse Reactions Including Known Allergies

There are not usually adverse reactions for DHA alone. Adverse reactions reported for fish oils containing DHA and EPA include fishy taste, belching (507), nosebleeds (9), nausea and loose stools (9). Three people, each with pre-existing familial adenomatous polyposis, were diagnosed with malignant lesions during the course of long-term fish oil use (999). Fish oils containing vitamins A and D could cause toxicity with long-term use (9).

Possible Interactions with Herbs & Other Dietary Supplements

HERBS WITH ANTICOAGULANT/ANTIPLATELET POTENTIAL: Concomitant use of herbs that have coumarin constituents or affect platelet aggregation could theoretically increase the risk of bleeding in some people. These herbs include: angelica, anise, arnica, asafoetida, bogbean, boldo, capsicum, celery, chamomile, clove, danshen, fenugreek, feverfew, garlic, ginger, ginkgo, Panax ginseng, horse chestnut, horseradish, licorice, meadowsweet, prickly ash, onion, papain, passionflower, poplar, quassia, red clover, turmeric, wild carrot, wild lettuce, willow, and others (4,19).

Possible Interactions with Drugs

ANTICOAGULANTS/ANTIPLATELET DRUGS: Theoretically, concomitant use of DHA with anticoagulant or antiplatelet drugs, including aspirin, can increase risk of bleeding (9,507). Drug interactions can occur with fish oils containing EPA and DHA, and fish oils can attenuate cyclosporin-induced hypertension in people with kidney or heart transplants (507,1012,1021).

Possible Interactions with Foods

No interactions are known to occur, and there is no known reason to expect a clinically significant interaction with DHA.

Possible Interactions with Lab Tests

CHOLESTEROL: DHA increases serum HDL2-cholesterol concentrations, LDL-cholesterol concentrations and LDL particle size and test results in mildly hypercholesterolemic men (6143).
INSULIN: DHA increases fasting insulin concentrations and test results in mildly hypercholesterolemic men (6143).
PULMONARY FUNCTION TESTS: Omega-3 fatty acids can cause a decline in pulmonary function tests in aspirin-sensitive individuals (507).
TRIGLYCERIDES: DHA reduces serum triglyceride concentrations and test results in healthy adults and mildly hypercholesterolemic men (1014,6143).

Possible Interactions with Diseases or Conditions

None reported for DHA alone. Interactions with disease conditions have been reported for fish oils containing DHA and EPA, including interfering with blood glucose control in individuals with diabetes (9) and lowering blood pressure in individuals with hypertension (1001,1020,1030,1033). Omega-3 fatty acids can cause a decline in pulmonary function tests in aspirin-sensitive individuals (507).

Typical Dosages & Routes of Administration that are Commonly Used

ORAL: DHA is usually administered with EPA (eicosapentaenoic acid) in fish oil. A wide range of doses have been used. The typical amount is 5 grams of fish oil containing 169-563 mg of EPA and 72-312 grams of DHA per day (9,507). As a supplement in infant formula, 0.32% DHA has been used (424). For improving dark adaptation of vision in dyslexic individuals, a daily oral fish oil dose containing 480 mg DHA has been used (5708). For improving movement disorders in children with dyspraxia, a daily oral tuna fish oil dose containing 480 mg DHA, combined with 35 mg arachidonic acid, 96 mg gamma-alpha linoleic acid from evening primrose oil, 24 mg thyme oil, and 80 mg vitamin E (Efalex) has been used (5708).

Comments

Preliminary evidence suggests that DHA might prevent or reverse some of the effects of cystic fibrosis. In mice with cystic fibrosis, the lungs, pancreas and intestine show high levels of arachidonic acid. This means the organs are at risk for inflammation and mucus secretion. DHA, which regulates the arachidonic acid and the cellular fluid balance, is significantly reduced. When researchers restored a more normal balance of DHA and arachidonic acid, they were able to prevent lung and intestine abnormalities. It's too soon to know if this might work in humans, but it looks promising and trials are planned (309). Avoid confusing DHA with EPA (eicosapentaenoic acid).

DHEA

This Product is Also Known As

Dehydroepiandrosterone, GL701, Prasterone.
CAUTION: See separate listing for 7-Keto-DHEA.

Scientific Names

Dehydroepiandrosterone; Prasterone.

People Use This For

Orally, DHEA is used for slowing or reversing aging; promoting weight loss; increasing strength, energy, and muscle mass; stimulating immunity; treating systemic lupus erythematosus (SLE) and multiple sclerosis; improving cognitive function; preventing heart disease, breast cancer, and diabetes; slowing the progression of Parkinson's disease and Alzheimer's disease; and treating erectile dysfunction and depression (793,2111,2112,2133, 3270,4233). For people with HIV disease, DHEA is used to improve depressed mood and fatigue (3864). It is also used orally by women who have adrenal insufficiency to improve well-being and sexuality (3231).

Vaginally, DHEA is used in postmenopausal women for vaginal atrophy and increasing bone mineral density (4242). Intravenous DHEA is being investigated as an agent to improve skin graft-site healing (1399).

Safety

POSSIBLY SAFE ...when used orally and short-term by individuals with low DHEA levels (3231,2133,4253). ...when used by men aged 50 or older and postmenopausal women for up to a year (4249,4251,4252,4254,4255). ...when used as an adjunct for systemic lupus erythematosus (SLE) treatment (2113,2114). ...when used vaginally by postmenopausal women (4242).

POSSIBLY UNSAFE ...when used long-term or in amounts that cause higher than normal DHEA levels because of concerns it might increase the risk of prostate cancer (2111,2116), breast cancer or other hormone-sensitive cancers (4256).

PREGNANCY AND LACTATION: POSSIBLY UNSAFE ...when used orally because it can cause higher than normal androgen levels (2133,4249,4251,4253) which might affect pregnancy or a nursing infant.

Effectiveness

POSSIBLY EFFECTIVE ...when taken orally for depression and dysthymia (3270,3892,4233). ...when taken orally for erectile dysfunction (793). ...when taken orally as replacement therapy by women with adrenal insufficiency to improve well-being and sexuality (3231). ...when taken orally as an adjunctive treatment for systemic lupus erythematosus (SLE) (2113,2114,2136). In an unpublished phase III study, 66% of patients treated with DHEA for one year achieved a clinical response compared to 49% with placebo with a trend toward significance. Patients reported less fatigue, reduced symptoms of arthritis, and improved quality of life. There was a significant decrease in flare-up frequency and triglyceride levels. However, there was also a significant decline in high-density lipoprotein (HDL) levels. Some patients had a 2% increase in spinal bone density and were able to use lower prednisone doses. The DHEA preparation used in this study was a special pharmaceutical grade product known as GL701 or prasterone (1295). ...when used vaginally to treat vaginal atrophy and increase bone density (4242).

POSSIBLY INEFFECTIVE ...when taken orally to improve cognitive function (3892,3893).

There is insufficient reliable information available about the effectiveness of DHEA for its other uses. However, researchers report that DHEA might be beneficial for autologous skin grafting. In one study, intravenously administered DHEA improved the rate of re-epithelialization in a group of patients undergoing autologous skin grafting for burn wound closure. The results of this unpublished, Phase II study were presented at the 32nd annual meeting of the American Burn Association. More research is needed to rate DHEA's effectiveness for this use.

Possible Mechanism of Action & Active Ingredients

DHEA and its active component, dehydroepiandrosterone sulfate (DHEA-S) are secreted by the human adrenal glands (3232). DHEA is metabolized to androstenedione, the major human precursor of androgens and estrogens. DHEA and DHEA-S levels are higher in men than in women, and naturally decline with age (4248,6013,6014). DHEA supplementation seems to change the circulating androgen/estrogen ratio in a gender-specific manner. That is, there appears to be significant increases in the levels of estrogens, but not the amount of androgens, in the blood of men given DHEA. Conversely, women given DHEA develop significant increases in the levels of androgens, but not estrogens (6010,6011). The androgen-like or estrogen-like effects might be responsible for some of the benefits of DHEA (2115). Although DHEA and DHEA-S declines with age, there does not appear to be an association between prematurely low DHEA-S levels and increased risk for diseases commonly seen with old age (6013,6014). Exercise at maximal and submaximal levels and consuming food naturally increases the endogenous DHEA level. Endogenous DHEA is decreased in anorexia nervosa, depression, end-stage renal disease, non-insulin dependent diabetes mellitus, schizophrenia, and individuals with SLE taking prednisolone. Endogenous DHEA is increased in some individuals taking diltiazem and a single dose of alprazolam. It is decreased by danazol, dexamethasone, insulin, and morphine (4248). Although clinical studies are few, the use of DHEA for HIV disease has been stimulated by reports of modest antiviral effect of DHEA, possible immunomodulating effects, and the finding that DHEA decreases with declining CD4 lymphocyte counts (3865,3866,3867). DHEA does not affect the CD4 counts, even at high doses (2.25 grams per day) (3865). Preliminary research of the effect of DHEA on depressed mood, fatigue, and androgenic and anabolic effects in people with HIV disease has been inconclusive (3864). Male sex hormones appear to have a harmful effect on organ function after trauma hemorrhage. DHEA attenuates depressed cardiac and hepatic function secondary to trauma hemorrhage in male rats, possibly due to estrogenic activity (6101).

Adverse Reactions Including Known Allergies

DHEA use can cause acne, hair loss, hirsutism, voice deepening, insulin resistance, decreased HDL cholesterol, hepatic dysfunction (2111,2116). When used in very high doses it can cause mild insomnia (4248). In individuals with HIV, it is associated with nasal congestion, fatigue, and headache (4248). Doses up to 2.25 grams taken for four months were well tolerated with no serious adverse effects in people with mild HIV (3865).

Possible Interactions with Herbs & Other Dietary Supplements

Insufficient reliable information available.

Possible Interactions with Drugs

TRIAZOLAM: DHEA can increase plasma triazolam concentrations. Administration of DHEA 200 mg/d for two weeks was shown to inhibit cytochrome P450 3A (CYP 3A) metabolism of triazolam and is due to DHEA-S, rather than DHEA (1389).

OTHER DRUGS: DHEA may potentially increase levels of drugs metabolized through cytochrome P450 3A (CYP 3A) due to enzyme inhibition (1389). Drugs that are substrates of CYP 3A include alprazolam (Xanax), amitriptyline (Elavil), amiodarone (Cordarone), buspirone (Buspar), cerivastatin (Baycol), citalopram (Celexa), felodipine (Plendil), fexofenadine (Allegra), itraconazole (Sporanox), ketoconazole (Nizoral), lansoprazole (Prevacid), losartan (Cozaar), lovastatin (Mevacor), ondansetron (Zofran), prednisone (Deltasone, Orasone), sertraline (Zoloft), sibutramine (Meridia), sildenafil (Viagra), verapamil (Calan, Covera-HS, Isoptin), and many others.

Possible Interactions with Foods
No interactions are known to occur, and there is no known reason to expect a clinically significant interaction with DHEA.

Possible Interactions with Lab Tests
TRIAZOLAM: DHEA can increase plasma triazolam concentrations and test results. DHEA-S, the activated form of DHEA, inhibits triazolam metabolism (1389).

Possible Interactions with Diseases or Conditions
DIABETES: DHEA can increase insulin resistance or sensitivity. Monitor blood glucose level closely (2112,4249,4250).
MENTAL ILLNESS: DHEA might increase hypomania, irritability, sexual inappropriateness or psychosis in some individuals with mental illness (4233).
LIVER DYSFUNCTION: DHEA can exacerbate liver dysfunction (2111,2116).

Typical Dosages & Routes of Administration that are Commonly Used
ORAL: In postmenopausal women and in men, doses of 25-50 mg daily have commonly been used (4249,4251,4252, 4254,4255). For depression, clinical trials have used doses of 30-90 mg daily either alone or in combination with conventional antidepressant therapy (3270,4233). For replacement therapy in individuals with adrenal suppression, clinical trials have used 50 mg, either given daily or as a single dose (2133,3231,4253,6012). For systemic lupus erythematosus (SLE), the typical dose is 200 mg per day as an adjunct to conventional medical treatment (2113,2114). For erectile dysfunction, 50 mg per day has been used (793).
VAGINAL: A 10% cream applied daily has been used (4242).

Comments
The wild yam extract is not converted to DHEA in the human body (2112). For most uses, the risks associated with DHEA outweigh the benefits (2111,2112).
Researchers at the University of Washington report that pharmaceutical grade DHEA (GL701) might improve arthritis and fatigue symptoms in patients with systemic lupus erythematosus (SLE). A trend towards clinical significance was noted in the DHEA-treated patients (66%) compared to placebo-treated patients (49%). In this unpublished, one-year, phase III study, DHEA-treated patients had an improved quality of life, fewer flare-ups, decreased HDL cholesterol and triglyceride levels, a 2% increase in bone density, and used lower prednisone doses (1295).
DHEA is banned by the National Basketball Association (NBA) (5041).

DIBENCOZIDE

This Product is Also Known As
Adenosylcobalamin, Cobalamin Enzyme, Cobamamide, Coenzyme B-12.
CAUTION: See separate listing for Vitamin B12.

Scientific Names
None.

People Use This For
Dibencozide is used as an oral or sublingual preparation to stimulate protein metabolism (5132), increase muscle mass and strength (5133), increase mental concentration (5135), treat depression, anxiety, and panic attacks (5134).

Safety
LIKELY SAFE …when used orally. There are no reports of toxicity from excessive amounts of cobalamins (4921,5133). When tissue binding sites are saturated, excessive dibencozide is excreted in urine and bile (5133).
PREGNANCY AND LACTATION: Insufficient reliable information available; avoid using.

Effectiveness
LIKELY INEFFECTIVE …when used orally or sublingually for uses in individuals without vitamin B12 deficiency (5133,5137).
There is insufficient reliable information available about the effectiveness of dibencozide for its other uses.

Possible Mechanism of Action & Active Ingredients

The term vitamin B12 refers to all cobalamins that are active as coenzymes in humans, including dibencozide (adenosylcobalamin), methylcobalamin, and hydroxocobalamin (5133,4921). Cyanocobalamin, the most stable of the cobalamins, is metabolized in the body to an active coenzyme (4921,5133). Vitamin B12 is involved in fat, protein, and carbohydrate metabolism. It is active in all cells, particularly in the bone marrow, CNS, and GI tract (4921). Produced almost exclusively by microorganisms, vitamin B12 is found in animal protein and in some legumes in small amounts (4921). Adults who eat meat in their diet usually ingest more than the RDA of 2.4 mcg (5138). Vitamin B12 is conserved by enterohepatic circulation; deficiency takes about three years to develop in people with normal absorption (4921). No benefit has been shown from taking large quantities of cobalamins unless an individual is deficient (4921).

Adverse Reactions Including Known Allergies

None reported.

Possible Interactions with Herbs & Other Dietary Supplements

ALCOHOL: Excessive alcohol intake lasting longer than two weeks can decrease vitamin B12 absorption from the gastrointestinal tract (14,15).

Possible Interactions with Drugs

AMINOGLYCOSIDES: Aminoglycoside antibiotics can decrease vitamin B12 absorption from the gastrointestinal tract (14,15).
CHLORAMPHENICOL: May impair hematopoietic response to vitamin B12 (15).
COLCHICINE: Colchicine can decrease vitamin B12 absorption from the gastrointestinal tract (14,15).
ACID INHIBITING DRUGS : Cimetidine (Tagamet), ranitidine (Zantac), omeprazole (Prilosec) can decrease vitamin B12 absorption from the gastrointestinal tract (14,15).
POTASSIUM: Extended-release potassium preparations can decrease vitamin B12 absorption from the gastrointestinal tract (14,15).
AMINOSALICYLIC ACID: Aminosalicylic acid and its salts can decrease vitamin B12 absorption from the gastrointestinal tract (14,15).
ANTICONVULSANTS: Phenytoin (Dilantin), phenobarbital, and primidone (Mysoline) can decrease vitamin B12 absorption from the gastrointestinal tract (14,15).
VITAMIN C: Large amounts of vitamin C can destroy vitamin B12 and should not be taken within an hour of oral vitamin B12 (15).

Possible Interactions with Foods

No interactions are known to occur, and there is no known reason to expect a clinically significant interaction with dibencozide.

Possible Interactions with Lab Tests

No interactions are known to occur, and there is no known reason to expect a clinically significant interaction with dibencozide.

Possible Interactions with Diseases or Conditions

GI CONDITIONS: Ileal disease or resection, intrinsic factor deficiency can cause vitamin B12 malabsorption (4921).

Typical Dosages & Routes of Administration that are Commonly Used

No typical dosage.

Comments

Cyanocobalamin and hydroxocobalamin are the only forms of vitamin B12 stable for storage (5139).

DIGITALIS

This Product is Also Known As

Dead Man's Bells, Fairy Cap, Fairy Finger, Foxglove, Lady's Thimble, Lion's Mouth, Purple Foxglove, Scotch Mercury, Throatwort, Witch's Bells, Wolly Foxglove.

Scientific Names

Digitalis purpurea; Digitalis lanata.
Family: Scrophulariaceae.

People Use This For

Orally, digitalis is used for congestive heart failure and atrial fibrillation/flutter.
Historically, digitalis has been used for diureses in edema, asthma, as an emetic, for epilepsy, tuberculosis, constipation, headache, spasm, and wound and burn healing (6,7,400).

Safety

UNSAFE ...when the leaf is used orally for self-medication. Use requires monitoring by a medical professional (12). Can cause heart arrhythmias and death (17). All parts of the plant are toxic (501). US regulations require labeling to inform consumers that digitalis is inappropriate for use as an anti-obesity agent (12); Canadian regulations prohibit digitalis in foods (12). Deaths have occurred when digitalis was mistaken for comfrey (501).

CHILDREN: LIKELY UNSAFE ...sucking on the flowers, ingesting seeds, or parts of the leaves has caused children to become ill (6).

PREGNANCY AND LACTATION: UNSAFE ...when the leaf is used for self-medication; contraindicated (12).

Effectiveness

LIKELY EFFECTIVE ...when taken orally for atrial fibrillation or flutter, congestive heart failure, and removal of edema associated with heart failure (6).

There is insufficient reliable information available about the effectiveness of digitalis for its other uses.

Possible Mechanism of Action & Active Ingredients

Digitalis contains varied glycosides, primarily glycoside A and glycoside B, which are precursors to digitoxin and gitoxin, respectively. Digitalis lanata contains lanatosides A,B,C,D, and E that yield digitoxin, gitoxin, digoxin, digitalin, and gitaloxin, respectively (6). Cardiac glycosides increase cardiac contractility, decrease heart rate and reduce AV node conduction, stabilize the heart rate, increase cardiac output, and relieve pulmonary congestion and peripheral edema (6).

Adverse Reactions Including Known Allergies

Chronic use of digitalis can lead to intoxication symptoms including visual halos, yellow-green vision, and GI upset (6). Acute poisoning of digitalis includes GI upset, contracted pupils, blurred vision, strong slow pulse, nausea, vomiting, dizziness, excessive urination, fatigue, muscle weakness and tremors, stupor, confusion, convulsions, atrial arrhythmias, AV block, and death (6,159,501).

Possible Interactions with Herbs & Other Dietary Supplements

CARDIAC GLYCOSIDE-CONTAINING HERBS: Contraindicated; concomitant use can increase the risk of cardiac glycoside toxicity. Cardiac glycoside containing herbs, including black hellebore, Canadian hemp roots, digitalis leaf, hedge mustard, figwort, lily of the valley roots, motherwort, oleander leaf, pheasant's eye plant, pleurisy root, squill bulb leaf scales, and strophanthus seeds (2,18,19,500).

OTHER CARDIOACTIVE HERBS: Avoid concomitant use with other cardioactive herbs due to unpredictability of effects and adverse effects. Other cardioactive herbs include: calamus, cereus, cola, coltsfoot, devil's claw, European mistletoe, fenugreek, fumitory, ginger, Panax ginseng, hawthorn, white horehound, mate, parsley, quassia, scotch broom flower, shepherd's purse, and wild carrot (4).

STIMULANT LAXATIVE HERBS: Theoretically, overuse or misuse of stimulant laxatives with cardiac glycoside-containing herbs increases the risk of cardiac toxicity due to potassium depletion. Stimulant laxative herbs include: aloe dried leaf sap, blue flag rhizome, alder buckthorn, European buckthorn, butternut bark, cascara bark, castor oil, colocynth fruit pulp, gamboge bark exudate, jalap root, black root, manna bark exudate, podophyllum root, rhubarb root, senna leaves and pods, wild cucumber fruit (Ecballium elaterium), and yellow dock root (19).

LICORICE/HORSETAIL: Theoretically, overuse/misuse of licorice rhizome or horsetail plant with cardiac glycoside-containing herbs increases the risk of toxicity due to potassium depletion (19).

Possible Interactions with Drugs

DIGOXIN (Lanoxin): Contraindicated; therapeutic duplication increases risk of cardiac glycoside toxicity (2).

CARDIOACTIVE DRUGS: Theoretically, concomitant use can increase the risk of cardiac toxicity (152).

STIMULANT LAXATIVES: Theoretically, overuse/misuse can increase risk of cardiac glycoside toxicity due to potassium depletion (2,506).

POTASSIUM DEPLETING DIURETICS, QUININE can increase the risk of digitalis toxicity (2,506).

TETRACYCLINES and MACROLIDE ANTIBIOTICS (erythromycin-like drugs): Theoretically, concomitant use might increase risk of cardiac glycoside toxicity (152,17).

Possible Interactions with Foods

No interactions are known to occur, and there is no known reason to expect a clinically significant interaction with digitalis.

Possible Interactions with Lab Tests

ELECTROCARDIOGRAM (ECG): Digitalis can normalize arrhythmias, and ECG readings, associated with atrial fibrillation or flutter in patients with congestive heart failure (15).

Possible Interactions with Diseases or Conditions

HEART DISEASE: Self-use contraindicated; requires diagnosis, treatment, and monitoring (515,150).

RENAL DISEASE: May reduce excretion of digitalis, increasing the potential for toxicity (150).

Typical Dosages & Routes of Administration that are Commonly Used

No typical dosage.

Comments

Digitalis is unsafe for self-medication. Digitalis lanata is the major source of digoxin in the US (6).

DILL seed

This Product is Also Known As

American Dill, Anethi fructus, Dilly, European Dill.
CAUTION: See separate listing for Dill above ground parts.

Scientific Names

Anetheum graveolens.
Family: Umbelliferae/Apiaceae.

People Use This For

Orally, dill seed is used for loss of appetite, fever and colds, cough, bronchitis, tendency towards infection, liver and gallbladder complaints (18), and as a digestive aid (11).
Topically, dill seed is used for mouth and throat inflammation (18).
Historically, dill seed has been used for flatulence, hemorrhoids, bronchial asthma, neuralgias, renal colic, dysuria, genital ulcers, and dysmenorrhea (11).
In foods, dill seed is used as a culinary spice (11).

Safety

LIKELY SAFE ...when dill seed is used orally in amounts found in foods. It has Generally Recognized as Safe (GRAS) status in the US (11).
POSSIBLY SAFE ...when used orally and appropriately for medicinal purposes (12).
PREGNANCY: LIKELY SAFE ...when used in food amounts. LIKELY UNSAFE ...when used in amounts greater than those found in foods because dill seed might stimulate menstrual flow (19).
LACTATION: Insufficient reliable information available; avoid amounts greater than those found in foods.

Effectiveness

POSSIBLY EFFECTIVE ...when dill seed or dill seed oil is used for dyspepsia (2,18).
There is insufficient reliable information available about the effectiveness of dill seed for its other uses.

Possible Mechanism of Action & Active Ingredients

Dill seed contains an essential oil rich in carvone (2). Dill seed has antibacterial, antispasmodic, sedative, and diuretic effects. They also think it stimulates lactation (2,11) and is a urinary irritant (19). Dill seed oil has spasmolytic effects on smooth muscle (11). Some evidence suggests an intravenous emulsion might increase respiratory volume and lower blood pressure (2,11).

Adverse Reactions Including Known Allergies

Photodermatosis is possible after topical contact with juice from freshly harvested plants (18,19).

Possible Interactions with Herbs & Other Dietary Supplements

Insufficient reliable information available.

Possible Interactions with Drugs

No interactions are known to occur, and there is no known reason to expect a clinically significant interaction with dill seed.

Possible Interactions with Foods

No interactions are known to occur, and there is no known reason to expect a clinically significant interaction with dill seed.

Possible Interactions with Lab Tests

No interactions are known to occur, and there is no known reason to expect a clinically significant interaction with dill seed.

Possible Interactions with Diseases or Conditions

URINARY TRACT INFLAMMATION: Avoid due to claims that dill seed is a urinary irritant (19).

Typical Dosages & Routes of Administration that are Commonly Used

ORAL: People typically use 3 grams of dill seed daily. People also add 2 teaspoons bruised seeds to a cup of boiling water and drink up to 3 cups per day. As a tincture, dill is taken up to 1 teaspoon up to 3 times daily. As a breath freshener, up to 1 teaspoon is chewed. Oil of dill is taken 100 to 300 mg (2 to 6 drops) daily (5250,5252).

Comments

Avoid confusion with dill above ground parts. Dill seed oil is distilled from the crushed, dried fruit (seed) of the dill plant (Anetheum graveolens).

DILL above ground parts

This Product is Also Known As

American Dill, Anethi herba, Dill Herb, Dill Weed, Dillweed, Dilly, European Dill.
CAUTION: See separate listing for Dill seed.

Scientific Names

Anetheum graveolens.
Family: Apiaceae or Umbelliferae.

People Use This For

Orally, dill above ground parts are used for diseases and disorders of the gastrointestinal tract, kidney, and urinary tract. Dill is also used for spasms (2), flatulence, and sleep disorders (11).
In foods, dill and dill oil are used as flavoring agents (11).
In manufacturing, dill oil is used as a fragrance component in cosmetics, soaps, and perfumes (11).

Safety

LIKELY SAFE ...when consumed in amounts commonly found in foods, and is Generally Recognized as Safe (GRAS) for food use in the US (11).
POSSIBLY SAFE ...when used orally and appropriately for medicinal purposes (12).
PREGNANCY AND LACTATION: Insufficient reliable information available; avoid amounts greater than those found in foods.

Effectiveness

There is insufficient reliable information available about the effectiveness of dill.

Possible Mechanism of Action & Active Ingredients

An aqueous dill extract administered intravenously lowers blood pressure, dilates blood vessels, stimulates respiration, and slows heart rate in animals (11). The dill leaf is reported to be a rich source of beta carotene, iron, and potassium (19).

Adverse Reactions Including Known Allergies

When dill is used topically, photodermatosis is possible after contact with juice from the freshly harvested plants (18,19). Dill can also cause contact dermatitis (19).

Possible Interactions with Herbs & Other Dietary Supplements

Insufficient reliable information available.

Possible Interactions with Drugs

No interactions are known to occur, and there is no known reason to expect a clinically significant interaction with dill above ground parts.

Possible Interactions with Foods

No interactions are known to occur, and there is no known reason to expect a clinically significant interaction with dill above ground parts.

Possible Interactions with Lab Tests

No interactions are known to occur, and there is no known reason to expect a clinically significant interaction with dill above ground parts.

Possible Interactions with Diseases or Conditions

CROSS REACTIVITY: The use of dill can cause allergic reactions in people with allergies to the carrot family plants, which include asafoetida, caraway, celery, coriander, and fennel (19).

Typical Dosages & Routes of Administration that are Commonly Used

ORAL: The common dose of the dried fruits is 1 to 4 grams three times daily (6002). The usual dose of the dill oil is 0.05-2 mL three times daily (6002).

Comments

Dill oil (dillweed oil, dill herb oil) is distilled from freshly harvested dill (Anetheum graveolens). During the Middle Ages, people sometimes used dill as a charm against witchcraft and enchantments (6002). Avoid confusion with dill seed.

DIMETHYLGLYCINE

This Product is Also Known As
Dimethyl Glycine, (Dimethylamino)acetic Acid, DMG, N,N-dimethylaminoacetic Acid, N-methylsarcosine.
CAUTION: Dimethylglycine is one of the compounds found in pangamic acid formulations. See separate listing for Pangamic Acid.

Scientific Names
N,N-dimethylglycine.

People Use This For
Orally, dimethylglycine is taken to improve speech and behavior in autism (5817); for attention deficit disorder (ADD) (5818); to treat epilepsy; to reduce physical and environmental stress; to improve oxygen utilization; to enhance liver function; to optimize athletic performance; to improve neurological function; for anti-inflammatory and anti-aging effects; to improve immune response and enhance anti-viral, anti-bacterial and anti-tumor defenses; and to treat tumors, chronic fatigue syndrome, allergies, respiratory disorders, alcoholism, and drug addiction (5816). It is also taken orally to lower blood cholesterol and triglycerides, and to help normalize blood pressure and blood glucose (5815).

Safety
POSSIBLY UNSAFE ...when taken orally. Dimethylglycine may react with nitrites in the gastrointestinal tract to form the potent carcinogen, dimethylnitrosamine (5,5827), although this has been questioned (5830).
PREGNANCY AND LACTATION: POSSIBLY UNSAFE; avoid using.

Effectiveness
POSSIBLY EFFECTIVE ...when used for enhancing humoral and cell mediated immune responses (14).
LIKELY INEFFECTIVE ...when used for improving athletic performance (14).
POSSIBLY INEFFECTIVE ...when used for treatment of epilepsy (14,5823) and autism (5819).
There is insufficient reliable information about the effectiveness of dimethylglycine for its other uses.

Possible Mechanism of Action & Active Ingredients
Dimethylglycine is the dimethylated form of the amino acid glycine, but it only exists in the body for seconds at a time, and in very small quantities (14,5827). It is formed from betaine during methylation of homocysteine (5828). The effects of supplemental doses in excess of naturally occurring amounts are unknown (14).
Preliminary evidence suggests that dimethylglycine enhances humoral and cell-mediated immune responses in humans and some, but not all, animals (5820,5822,5825). Dimethylglycine has been reported to have anticonvulsant effects in animals (5828), including antagonizing strychnine- and penicillin-induced seizures (5824,5829). A single case report described a dramatic improvement in a person with mixed complex partial and grand mal seizures (5826), but a small study in people with generalized or akinetic/myoclonic seizures found no benefit with dimethylglycine 300 to 600 mg per day (5823). Several small studies in athletes have not found any benefit of dimethylglycine on athletic performance (5821), including maximal treadmill performance, as measured by maximal and recovery heart rates, treadmill time, and pre-test and post-test blood glucose and lactate levels (2645). A small study using low-dose dimethylglycine did not find any benefit in children with autism (5819).

Adverse Reactions Including Known Allergies
Dimethylglycine may react with nitrites in the gastrointestinal tract to form carcinogenic substances (5,5827).

Possible Interactions with Herbs & Other Dietary Supplements
Insufficient reliable information available.

Possible Interactions with Drugs
No interactions are known to occur, and there is no known reason to expect a clinically significant interaction with dimethylglycine.

Possible Interactions with Foods
No interactions are known to occur, and there is no known reason to expect a clinically significant interaction with dimethylglycine.

Possible Interactions with Lab Tests
No interactions are known to occur, and there is no known reason to expect a clinically significant interaction with dimethylglycine.

Possible Interactions with Diseases or Conditions
No interactions are known to occur, and there is no known reason to expect a clinically significant interaction with dimethylglycine.

Typical Dosages & Routes of Administration that are Commonly Used
ORAL: As a dietary supplement, divided doses of 125 to 1000 mg per day sublingual dimethylglycine have been recommended (5816).

Comments
Dimethylglycine is found in low levels in such foods as cereal grains, beans, and liver (5816). In the 1980s, a federal court in Chicago forbade interstate sale of a brand of dimethylglycine stating that it was an unsafe food additive (5827).

DIVI-DIVI

This Product is Also Known As
Divi Divi, Nichol Seeds, Nikkar Nuts.

Scientific Names
Caesalpinia bonducella.
Family: Leguminosae.

People Use This For
Orally, divi-divi is used for fever and diabetes (18).

Safety
There is insufficient reliable information available about the safety of divi-divi.
Pregnancy and Lactation: Insufficient reliable information available; avoid using.

Effectiveness
There is insufficient reliable information available about the effectiveness of divi-divi.

Possible Mechanism of Action & Active Ingredients
The applicable part of divi-divi is the seed. Divi-divi is stated to have antipyretic effects (18). In normal rats, ethanolic and aqueous seed extracts exhibited hypoglycemic effects, with the aqueous extract showing a longer duration of action (3834). In rats with experimentally-induced diabetes, both extracts produced antihyperglycemic effects. However, only the aqueous extract demonstrated an effect in reducing cholesterol and triglyceride levels (3834).

Adverse Reactions Including Known Allergies
None reported.

Possible Interactions with Herbs & Other Dietary Supplements
Insufficient reliable information available.

Possible Interactions with Drugs
No interactions are known to occur, and there is no known reason to expect a clinically significant interaction with divi-divi.

Possible Interactions with Foods
No interactions are known to occur, and there is no known reason to expect a clinically significant interaction with divi-divi.

Possible Interactions with Lab Tests
No interactions are known to occur, and there is no known reason to expect a clinically significant interaction with divi-divi.

Possible Interactions with Diseases or Conditions
No interactions are known to occur, and there is no known reason to expect a clinically significant interaction with divi-divi.

Typical Dosages & Routes of Administration that are Commonly Used
No typical dosage.

Comments
The seed is ground or roasted (18). There is very little scientific information about this product. Our staff is continually analyzing the available information on natural medicines and will add data here as it becomes available.

DODDER

This Product is Also Known As
Beggarweed, Devil's Guts, Dodder Of Thyme, Hellweed, Lesser Dodder, Scaldweed, Strangle Tare.

Scientific Names
Cuscuta epithymum.
Family: Convolvulaceae.

People Use This For
Orally, dodder is used for urinary tract, spleen, and hepatic disorders (18).

Safety
There is insufficient reliable information available about the safety of dodder.
Pregnancy and Lactation: Insufficient reliable information available; avoid using.

Effectiveness
There is insufficient reliable information available about the effectiveness of dodder.

Possible Mechanism of Action & Active Ingredients
The applicable parts of dodder are the above ground parts. Dodder is reported to have hepatic and laxative effects (18).

Adverse Reactions Including Known Allergies
Theoretically, oral administration can cause intestinal colic (18).

Possible Interactions with Herbs & Other Dietary Supplements
Insufficient reliable information available.

Possible Interactions with Drugs
No interactions are known to occur, and there is no known reason to expect a clinically significant interaction with dodder.

Possible Interactions with Foods
No interactions are known to occur, and there is no known reason to expect a clinically significant interaction with dodder.

Possible Interactions with Lab Tests
No interactions are known to occur, and there is no known reason to expect a clinically significant interaction with dodder.

Possible Interactions with Diseases or Conditions
No interactions are known to occur, and there is no known reason to expect a clinically significant interaction with dodder.

Typical Dosages & Routes of Administration that are Commonly Used
ORAL: People typically use 7 to 12 grams of dodder added to 3 to 4 cups of water and boiled until the volume is reduced by one-half. The cooled liquid is taken in 2 doses on an empty stomach (5251).

Comments
There is very little scientific information about this product. Our staff is continually analyzing the available information on natural medicines and will add data here as it becomes available.

DOLOMITE

This Product is Also Known As
Dolomitic Limestone.
CAUTION: See separate listings for Calcium and Magnesium.

Scientific Names
None.

People Use This For
Orally, dolomite is used as a mineral supplement of calcium and magnesium (6).

Safety
LIKELY SAFE ...when used orally and appropriately.
CHILDREN: POSSIBLY UNSAFE ...when used orally long-term due to the presence of lead in some products.

Children are more sensitive to lead than adults (152).
PREGNANCY AND LACTATION: Insufficient reliable information available; avoid using unless certain of purity (6).

Effectiveness
LIKELY EFFECTIVE ...when used as a source of calcium and magnesium supplementation (6).

Possible Mechanism of Action & Active Ingredients
Dolomite is a type of limestone. It is rich in magnesium and calcium carbonate, with smaller amounts of several other minerals. Some evidence suggests that the minerals in dolomite are well-absorbed (6).

Adverse Reactions Including Known Allergies
Some dolomite products are contaminated with heavy metals including aluminum, arsenic, lead, mercury, nickel, and others that may cause heavy metal poisoning (6). Contaminated products have induced seizure activity in otherwise well-controlled patients who have seizure disorders (6). Calcium taken orally can cause gastrointestinal irritation and constipation (9). Calcium carbonate can cause acid rebound (9). Large amounts of calcium carbonate can cause hypercalcemia and alkalosis (9). Magnesium can cause gastrointestinal irritation, nausea, vomiting, and diarrhea (9,14,15). Larger amounts may cause hypermagnesemia (9) with symptoms including thirst, hypotension, drowsiness, confusion, loss of tendon reflexes, muscle weakness, respiratory depression, cardiac arrhythmias, coma, cardiac arrest, and death (9).

Possible Interactions with Herbs & Other Dietary Supplements
BORON: Can increase serum magnesium levels (940).
MAGNESIUM: Theoretically, concomitant use with other magnesium containing supplements can cause diarrhea.
CALCIUM: Theoretically, concomitant use with other calcium containing supplements can cause constipation.

Possible Interactions with Drugs
EXCRETION-ENHANCING DRUGS: Magnesium levels can be reduced by concomitant use of drugs that increase renal excretion. These drugs include amphotericin B, cisplatin, aminoglycoside antibiotics, cyclosporine, thiazide and loop diuretics, mannitol, and intravenous glucose (945).
EXCRETION-REDUCING DRUGS: Magnesium levels can be increased by concomitant use of drugs that decrease renal excretion. These drugs include calcitonin, glucagon, and potassium-sparing diuretics (945).
ESTROGEN: Concomitant use of estrogen increases calcium absorption in postmenopausal women (995).
GLUCOCORTICOIDS: Concomitant use can decrease calcium absorption (15).
REDUCED-ABSORPTION DRUGS: Concomitant use of calcium decreases absorption of fluoride, fluoroquinolones, and tetracyclines (9). Separate administration by at least 2 hours.
THIAZIDE DIURETICS: Concomitant use with moderately large amounts of calcium carbonate increases the risk of milk-alkali syndrome (9).

Possible Interactions with Foods
FOOD: Concomitant ingestion with food, and food high in vitamin D, increases absorption of supplemental calcium (945).
DIETARY FIBER: Certain constituents of dietary fiber inhibit calcium absorption, including phytic acid that is found in wheat bran and uronic acid, a common plant fiber constituent (945).
IRON: Calcium carbonate taken with iron supplements and food might decrease supplemental iron absorption. Calcium carbonate taken with iron supplements on an empty stomach appears to have little effect on supplemental iron absorption (945).
VITAMIN D: Concomitant use increases active absorption of oral calcium (945).

Possible Interactions with Lab Tests
ALKALINE PHOSPHATASE: The magnesium component might cause a false increase in serum alkaline phosphatase test results due to enzyme activation (275).
ANGIOTENSIN-CONVERTING ENZYME: The magnesium component might decrease serum ACE levels and test results (275).
CALCIUM: The magnesium component might cause a false increase in serum calcium test results in some procedures using edetate disodium (EDTA) (275).
DIAGNEX BLUE: The magnesium component might increase urine diagnex blue excretion due to heavy metal displacement of diagnex blue (275).
GASTRIN: The calcium component might cause a physiological increase in serum levels 30-75 minutes after using (275).
LIPASE: The calcium component might cause an analytical decrease in serum concentrations above 5 mmol/L on method of Tietz (275).

Possible Interactions with Diseases or Conditions
HEART BLOCK: Magnesium is contraindicated in people with heart block (9).
HYPERPARATHYROIDISM: Primary hyperparathyroidism predisposes individuals to increased calcium absorption (945).
HYPOPARATHYROIDISM: Predisposes individuals to reduced calcium absorption (945).

RENAL INSUFFICIENCY: Magnesium is contraindicated in people with severe renal disease. Use cautiously in individuals with reduced kidney function due to increased risk of hypermagnesemia (9). Calcium supplementation increases the risk of hypercalcemia and alkalosis in people with renal disease (9). Renal insufficiency predisposes individuals to reduced calcium absorption (945).

SARCOIDOSIS: Increases the risk of excessive calcium absorption and hypercalcemia (945).

Typical Dosages & Routes of Administration that are Commonly Used

ORAL: The recommended amount of elemental magnesium as a dietary supplement for adults is 54-483 mg daily in divided doses (14). The daily Dietary Reference Intakes of elemental calcium for adults is 1000 mg to age 50, 1200 mg thereafter (998).

Comments

None.

DONG QUAI

This Product is Also Known As

Chinese Angelica, Dang Gui, Danggui, Dong Qua, Phytoestrogen, Tang Kuei, Tan Kue Bai Zhi.
CAUTION: See separate listings for Angelica root and Angelica seed.

Scientific Names

Angelica sinensis, synonym Angelica polymorpha sinensis.
Family: Apiaceae or Umbelliferae.

People Use This For

Orally, dong quai root is used for gynecological ailments including menstrual cramps, irregularity, retarded flow, weakness during the menstrual period, and menopause symptoms (515). It is also used orally as a "blood purifier", to manage hypertension, rheumatism, ulcers, anemia, constipation, and in the prevention and treatment of allergic attacks (6,515). Dong quai taken orally is used for the treatment of skin depigmentation and psoriasis (6). In Chinese medicine, dong quai is generally used in combination with other ingredients (515).

Safety

POSSIBLY SAFE ...when taken orally and appropriately (12).
POSSIBLY UNSAFE ...when taken orally in large amounts. Large amounts can cause severe photodermatitis (6,515). Dong quai constituents can be carcinogenic, mutagenic, and photocarcinogenic even without light exposure (6). However, the phototoxic constituents are not found in the steam-distilled oils of the root and seed (12).
PREGNANCY: UNSAFE ...contraindicated, due to uterine stimulant and relaxant effects (12,19,515).
LACTATION: Insufficient reliable information available; avoid using.

Effectiveness

POSSIBLY INEFFECTIVE ...when used for treating menopausal symptoms (738). One well designed study found dong quai (as a single agent) had no effect on endometrial wall thickness or menopausal symptoms (738). Human studies are needed to determine the effect(s) of dong quai in combination with other herbs for treating menopausal symptoms.
There is insufficient reliable information available about the effectiveness of dong quai for its other uses.

Possible Mechanism of Action & Active Ingredients

The applicable part of dong quai is the root. Dong quai has several coumarin constituents including osthol, psoralen, and bergapten. Some coumarins can act as vasodilators and antispasmodics. Osthol has central nervous system stimulant effects (5). Psoralen and bergapten are photosensitizing and can cause severe photodermatitis (6). Psoralens are photocarcinogenic and mutagenic (6). Safrole, a constituent of the dong quai essential oil, is carcinogenic (6). A dong quai extract competitively inhibits estradiol binding to estrogen receptors and induces transcription activity in estrogen-responsive cells (6180). It also increases uterine weight, decreases LH (luteinizing hormone) levels, and increases serum ceruloplasmin oxidase activity (a measure of liver estrogenic activity) in female rats with their ovaries removed (6180). Dong quai can improve abnormal protein metabolism in people with chronic hepatitis or hepatic cirrhosis (4). An injected aqueous extract can show efficacy in treating acute ischemic cerebrovascular disease (11). In animals, dong quai speeds neurocyte growth and prevents the decline of process branches in vitro, which suggests it can have some activity in humans for promoting nerve growth and delaying atrophy (6). The related species, Angelica dahurica, can have anti-inflammatory, analgesic, and antipyretic activity (6). Another related Angelica species inhibits human platelet aggregation (736).

Adverse Reactions Including Known Allergies

The use of dong quai can cause photosensitivity and photodermatitis and is potentially carcinogenic and mutagenic (6).

Possible Interactions with Herbs & Other Dietary Supplements

HERBS WITH ANTICOAGULANT/ANTIPLATELET POTENTIAL: Concomitant use of herbs that have coumarin constituents or affect platelet aggregation could theoretically increase the risk of bleeding in some people. These herbs include: angelica, anise, arnica, asafoetida, bogbean, boldo, capsicum, celery, chamomile, clove, danshen, fenugreek, feverfew, garlic, ginger, ginkgo, ginseng (Panax), horse chestnut, horseradish, licorice, meadowsweet, prickly ash, onion, papain, passionflower, poplar, quassia, red clover, turmeric, wild carrot, wild lettuce, willow, and others (4,19).

Possible Interactions with Drugs

ANTIPLATELET DRUGS: Theoretically, dong quai might potentiate the therapeutic and adverse effects of these drugs.
WARFARIN: Dong quai can potentiate warfarin's effects and the risk of bleeding as measured by INR (3526).

Possible Interactions with Foods

No interactions are known to occur, and there is no known reason to expect a clinically significant interaction with dong quai.

Possible Interactions with Lab Tests

PROTHROMBIN TIME (PT), INTERNATIONAL NORMALIZATION RATIO (INR): Dong quai can enhance the effects of warfarin, resulting in increased PT and INR test results (3526).

Possible Interactions with Diseases or Conditions

No interactions are known to occur, and there is no known reason to expect a clinically significant interaction with dong quai.

Typical Dosages & Routes of Administration that are Commonly Used

ORAL: Women typically use 3 to 4 grams per day in divided doses with meals. One dong quai supplier suggests three daily doses based on body weight: under 100 pounds, 520 mg per dose; 100 to 175 pounds, 1040 mg; over 175 pounds, 1560 mg. Dong quai is sometimes prepared as a tea. An extract of dong quai is used in a dose of 1 mL (20 to 40 drops) three times daily. The extract contains alcohol and glycerin, but the concentration is not specified (6006).

Comments

Dong quai is an aromatic herb that is commonly used throughout the Orient (6). Some references classify Angelica atropurpurea and Angelica dahurica as dong quai (Chinese angelica) (6), while others do not (5,11,12).

DOWN SYNDROME NUTRITIONAL SUPPLEMENTS

This Product is Also Known As

Down's Syndrome Nutritional Supplements, Hap Caps, MSB Plus, NuTriVene-D.

Scientific Names

None.

People Use This For

Orally, Down syndrome nutritional supplements are used by people with Down syndrome for improving immune function, decreasing infections, promoting growth, improving health status, enhancing cognitive development, preventing or ameliorating long-term degeneration and disability (5402), for reversing metabolic disturbances, such as low antioxidant enzymes and high superoxide dimutase, replenishing digestive enzymes, and supplementing deficient amino acids (5403).

Safety

There is insufficient reliable information available about the safety of the oral use of Down syndrome nutritional supplements. The quantities of many of the ingredients, which vary among products, exceed the usual recommended dosages for healthy people.
Pregnancy and Lactation: Insufficient reliable information available; avoid using.

Effectiveness

There is insufficient reliable information available about the effectiveness of the oral use of Down syndrome nutritional supplements in the formulations currently marketed, including Hap Caps, MSB Plus, and NuTriVene-D.
LIKELY INEFFECTIVE ...when previously available formulations containing higher amounts of vitamins and minerals were used orally (5410,5412,5413,5414,5415,5416).

Possible Mechanism of Action & Active Ingredients

Nutritional supplementation for Down syndrome has been advocated by various practitioners for the past 50 years without independent proof of benefit (5410,5412,5413,5414,5415,5416,5427,5428). The supplement formulas are based on five main groups of ingredients: vitamins, minerals, amino acids, antioxidants, and digestive enzymes (5399,5400,5401).

Although an occasional report of vitamin deficiency in Down syndrome has been reported, most studies reveal no vitamin deficiency and no benefit from RDA doses or megadoses of vitamins and minerals (5406,5407,5408,5409,5410, 5411,5412,5413,5414,5415,5416). Preliminary studies have shown that zinc and selenium levels are lower in children with Down syndrome. Zinc supplementation might improve thyroid function in zinc-deficient children (5417,5418,5419, 5420,5421,5422). However, long-term treatment with zinc does not improve immune function or reduce infections (5423). No other mineral has been shown to be deficient or helpful in Down syndrome. Amino acid abnormalities have been described in one study and subsequently refuted by another (5424,5425). In vitro data suggest oxidative damage in Down syndrome, but this has not been shown in vivo (5426). Digestive enzyme deficiency has not been demonstrated in people with Down syndrome.

Adverse Reactions Including Known Allergies

Down syndrome nutritional supplements may cause poor taste and stomach upset (5399,5400,5401,5402,5403). One study reports adverse effects on developmental progress (5416). There are anecdotal reports of diarrhea, hyperactivity, insomnia, and loss of appetite (5427).

Possible Interactions with Herbs & Other Dietary Supplements

The ingredients (including amino acids, minerals, and vitamins) in Down syndrome nutritional supplement formulas varies. There might be specific interactions with specific ingredients.

Possible Interactions with Drugs

The ingredients (including amino acids, minerals, and vitamins) in Down syndrome nutritional supplement formulas varies. There might be specific interactions with specific ingredients.

Possible Interactions with Foods

The ingredients (including amino acids, minerals, and vitamins) in Down syndrome nutritional supplement formulas varies. There might be specific interactions with specific ingredients.

Possible Interactions with Lab Tests

The ingredients (including amino acids, minerals, and vitamins) in Down syndrome nutritional supplement formulas varies. There might be specific interactions with specific ingredients.

Possible Interactions with Diseases or Conditions

The ingredients (including amino acids, minerals, and vitamins) in Down syndrome nutritional supplement formulas varies. There might be specific interactions with specific ingredients.

Typical Dosages & Routes of Administration that are Commonly Used

ORAL: Down syndrome nutritional supplement formulas vary from product to product, and are changed periodically (5399,5400,5401). The nutritional programs are based on 5 main groups of ingredients: vitamins, minerals, amino acids, antioxidants, and digestive enzymes (5399,5400.5401); two sources offer customized formulas based on blood analysis (5399,5400). Down syndrome nutritional supplements containing from 37 to 59 ingredients, are available in powder or capsule form, and may be mixed with beverages or foods to mask the unpleasant taste (5399,5400,5401). Doses are based on weight or age and usually administered 2 to 3 times daily (5399,5400,5401). A separate bedtime supplement contains tryptophan and pyridoxine (5399,5400).

Comments

The National Down Syndrome Congress Position Statement on nutritional intervention states there is "no credible scientific evidence for effectiveness" for Down syndrome nutritional supplements (5404). The National Down Syndrome Society has issued a similar statement (5405). Commercial websites promoting Down syndrome nutritional supplement products cite a recent, unpublished study claiming positive evidence for efficacy (5400,5401,5402).

DRAGON'S BLOOD

This Product is Also Known As

Draconis Resina, Dracorubin, Dragons Blood, Sanguis Draconis, Xue Jie.
CAUTION: See separate listing for Herb Robert and Sangre de Grado.

Scientific Names

Daemonorops draco.
Family: Palmae.

People Use This For

Orally, dragon's blood is used for diarrhea, digestive disorders and as a coloring agent. Dragon's blood is sometimes used as an astringent (18).

Safety
POSSIBLY SAFE ...when used orally (12).
PREGNANCY AND LACTATION: Insufficient reliable information available; avoid using.

Effectiveness
There is insufficient reliable information available about the effectiveness of dragon's blood.

Possible Mechanism of Action & Active Ingredients
The applicable part of dragon's blood is the fruit. There is insufficient reliable information available about the possible mechanism of action and active ingredients.

Adverse Reactions Including Known Allergies
None reported.

Possible Interactions with Herbs & Other Dietary Supplements
Insufficient reliable information available.

Possible Interactions with Drugs
No interactions are known to occur, and there is no known reason to expect a clinically significant interaction with dragon's blood.

Possible Interactions with Foods
No interactions are known to occur, and there is no known reason to expect a clinically significant interaction with dragon's blood.

Possible Interactions with Lab Tests
No interactions are known to occur, and there is no known reason to expect a clinically significant interaction with dragon's blood.

Possible Interactions with Diseases or Conditions
No interactions are known to occur, and there is no known reason to expect a clinically significant interaction with dragon's blood.

Typical Dosages & Routes of Administration that are Commonly Used
ORAL: Dragon's blood is used as a powder (18).

Comments
Dragon's blood is the red resin extracted from the fruit of Daemonorops draco (18).

DUCKWEED

This Product is Also Known As
None.

Scientific Names
Lemna minor.
Family: Lemnaceae.

People Use This For
Orally, duckweed is used for inflammation of the upper respiratory tract, jaundice and arthritis (18).

Safety
There is insufficient reliable information available about the safety of duckweed.
Pregnancy and Lactation: Insufficient reliable information available; avoid using.

Effectiveness
There is insufficient reliable information available about the effectiveness of duckweed.

Possible Mechanism of Action & Active Ingredients
Insufficient reliable information available.

Adverse Reactions Including Known Allergies
None reported.

Possible Interactions with Herbs & Other Dietary Supplements
Insufficient reliable information available.

Possible Interactions with Drugs
No interactions are known to occur, and there is no known reason to expect a clinically significant interaction with duckweed.

Possible Interactions with Foods
No interactions are known to occur, and there is no known reason to expect a clinically significant interaction with duckweed.

Possible Interactions with Lab Tests
No interactions are known to occur, and there is no known reason to expect a clinically significant interaction with duckweed.

Possible Interactions with Diseases or Conditions
No interactions are known to occur, and there is no known reason to expect a clinically significant interaction with duckweed.

Typical Dosages & Routes of Administration that are Commonly Used
ORAL: Duckweed is used as a powder or an extract (18).

Comments
There is very little scientific information about this product. Our staff is continually analyzing the available information on natural medicines and will add data here as it becomes available.

DUSTY MILLER

This Product is Also Known As
None.

Scientific Names
Senecio cineraria, synonym Cineraria maritima.
Family: Compositae.

People Use This For
Orally, dusty miller is used in preparations for eyesight problems (spots before the eyes), migraine, and to promote menstrual flow (18).

Safety
LIKELY UNSAFE ...when any parts of the plant are used orally. Dusty miller contains hepatotoxic unsaturated pyrrolizidine alkaloids (UPAs) (18,19). Repeated exposure to low concentrations of UPAs are linked to veno-occlusive disease (4,12). UPAs may also be carcinogenic and mutagenic (12). ...when used topically on abraded or broken skin because it might be absorbed systemically (12,19).
PREGNANCY AND LACTATION: LIKELY UNSAFE ...contraindicated for oral use because it contains UPA constituents (12). There is insufficient reliable information available about the safety of the topical use of dusty miller during pregnancy and lactation; avoid using.

Effectiveness
There is insufficient reliable information available about the effectiveness of dusty miller.

Possible Mechanism of Action & Active Ingredients
Some pyrrolizidine alkaloids have shown carcinogenic and mutagenic properties, and there are reports of renal toxicity. However, the primary concern is veno-occlusive disease (12). Unsaturated pyrrolizidine alkaloids are known to be hepatotoxic in animals and humans (4).

Adverse Reactions Including Known Allergies
When used orally, acute toxicity may result in hepatic necrosis; chronic toxicity may cause veno-occlusive liver disease. The potential for hepatotoxicity (due to presence of pyrrolizidine alkaloids) increases with larger doses and longer periods of use (4,12). It can cause an allergic reaction in individuals sensitive to the Asteraceae/Compositae family. Members of this family include ragweed, chrysanthemums, marigolds, daisies, and many other herbs.

Possible Interactions with Herbs & Other Dietary Supplements
EUCALYPTUS: Theoretically, concomitant use might increase the risk of unsaturated pyrrolizidine alkaloid toxicity due to enzyme induction by eucalyptus (19).
PYRROLIZIDINE ALKALOID-CONTAINING HERBS: Concomitant use is contraindicated due to the risk of additive toxicity. Herbs containing unsaturated pyrrolizidine alkaloids include: alkanna (12), borage (271), gravel root (4), hemp agrimony (271), hound's tongue (19), petasites (19), comfrey (271), coltsfoot, and the Senecio species plants; dusty miller (19), alpine ragwort (19), groundsel (271), golden ragwort (19), and tansy ragwort (271).

Possible Interactions with Drugs

No interactions are known to occur, and there is no known reason to expect a clinically significant interaction with dusty miller.

Possible Interactions with Foods

No interactions are known to occur, and there is no known reason to expect a clinically significant interaction with dusty miller.

Possible Interactions with Lab Tests

No interactions are known to occur, and there is no known reason to expect a clinically significant interaction with dusty miller.

Possible Interactions with Diseases or Conditions

LIVER DISEASE: Contraindicated.
CROSS-ALLERGENICITY: Can cause an allergic reaction in individuals sensitive to the Asteraceae/Compositae family. Members of this family include ragweed, chrysanthemums, marigolds, daisies, and many other herbs.

Typical Dosages & Routes of Administration that are Commonly Used

No typical dosage.

Comments

American Herbal Products Association recommends labeling all botanical products that contain toxic pyrrolizidine alkaloids "For external use only. Do not apply to broken or abraded skin; do not use when nursing" (12).

DWARF ELDER

This Product is Also Known As

Blood Elder, Blood Hilder, Danewort, Walewort.
CAUTION: See separate listings for European Elder flower, European Elder fruit, and American Elder.

Scientific Names

Sambucus ebulus.
Family: Caprifoliaceae.

People Use This For

Orally, dwarf elder is used for arthritis, weight reduction and as a diuretic (18).

Safety

LIKELY UNSAFE …when large quantities of any part of the plant are used orally. Can cause loss of consciousness and death (18).
There is insufficient reliable information available about the safety of the oral use of dwarf elder in small amounts.
PREGNANCY AND LACTATION: LIKELY UNSAFE …when used orally in large quantities (18).

Effectiveness

There is insufficient reliable information available about the effectiveness of dwarf elder.

Possible Mechanism of Action & Active Ingredients

Dwarf elder contains iridoide monoterpene glycosides. The constituents that cause nausea or purgative effects have not been identified (18).

Adverse Reactions Including Known Allergies

People who ingest large quantities of any plant part of dwarf elder may experience vomiting, bloody diarrhea, cyanosis, dizziness, headache and unconsciousness. Death has been reported (18). Cyanide poisoning can be caused by any plant part of dwarf elder. Sambunigrine, a cyanogenic glycoside, is present in the plant.

Possible Interactions with Herbs & Other Dietary Supplements

Insufficient reliable information available.

Possible Interactions with Drugs

No interactions are known to occur, and there is no known reason to expect a clinically significant interaction with dwarf elder.

Possible Interactions with Foods

No interactions are known to occur, and there is no known reason to expect a clinically significant interaction with dwarf elder.

Possible Interactions with Lab Tests
No interactions are known to occur, and there is no known reason to expect a clinically significant interaction with dwarf elder.

Possible Interactions with Diseases or Conditions
No interactions are known to occur, and there is no known reason to expect a clinically significant interaction with dwarf elder.

Typical Dosages & Routes of Administration that are Commonly Used
No typical dosage.

Comments
Dwarf elder is considered unsafe; avoid using. Dwarf elder is considered obsolete as a medicinal herb in many countries (18). Avoid confusion with elderberry (European or Black Elder), which are the berries of other members of the Sambucus genus (214).

DWARF PINE NEEDLE

This Product is Also Known As
None.
CAUTION: See separate listing for Fir Needle Oil, Scotch Pine Needle Oil, Poplar, Fir, and Pine.

Scientific Names
Pinus mugo, synonym Pinus montana; Pinus pumilio, synonym Pinus mugo pumilio.
Family: Pinaceae.

People Use This For
There are no medicinal uses of dwarf pine needle reported (11).
In foods and beverages, dwarf pine needle is used as a flavoring agent (11).
In other manufacturing processes, dwarf pine needle is used as a flavoring and fragrance component in pharmaceutical preparations (cough and cold medicines, vaporizer fluids, nasal decongestants, analgesic ointments), and as a fragrance ingredient in soaps and cosmetics (maximum use level 1.2% in perfumes) (11).

Safety
LIKELY SAFE ...when used in amounts found in foods (maximum use level 0.001%) (11); approved for food use in the US (11).
POSSIBLY SAFE ...when used topically. There is possible human skin irritation and demonstrated sensitizing in some individuals (11).
PREGNANCY AND LACTATION: Insufficient reliable information available; avoid using.

Effectiveness
There is insufficient reliable information available about the effectiveness of dwarf pine needle (11).

Possible Mechanism of Action & Active Ingredients
The applicable part of dwarf pine needle is the oil. Constituents bornyl acetate, dipentene, and limonene are believed to have antibacterial and antiviral properties (11).

Adverse Reactions Including Known Allergies
Used topically, dwarf pine needle can cause skin irritation (11). It also may be sensitizing in some individuals (11).

Possible Interactions with Herbs & Other Dietary Supplements
Insufficient reliable information available.

Possible Interactions with Drugs
No interactions are known to occur, and there is no known reason to expect a clinically significant interaction with dwarf pine needle.

Possible Interactions with Foods
No interactions are known to occur, and there is no known reason to expect a clinically significant interaction with dwarf pine needle.

Possible Interactions with Lab Tests
No interactions are known to occur, and there is no known reason to expect a clinically significant interaction with dwarf pine needle.

Possible Interactions with Diseases or Conditions
ALLERGY: Avoid if allergic or sensitive to pine oil.

Typical Dosages & Routes of Administration that are Commonly Used
No typical dosage.

Comments
Dwarf pine needle oil is produced by distillation of dwarf pine (Pinus mugo) needles and twigs. Avoid confusion with fir needle oil and scotch pine needle oil.

DYER'S BROOM

This Product is Also Known As
Broom Flower, Dyers Broom, Dyer's Greenwood, Dyer's Weed, Dyer's Whin, Furze, Green Broom, Greenweed, Wood Waxen.

Scientific Names
Genista tinctoria.
Family: Leguminosae.

People Use This For
Orally, dyer's broom is used for digestive disorders, gout, as an emetic or purgative, and to remove bladder stones. It is also used to "detoxify" blood, to increase heart rate, strengthen blood vessels, stimulate blood flow to the kidneys and to alter metabolism. It has been used to deepen breathing and alleviate pain in the lower back and pelvis (18).

Safety
POSSIBLY UNSAFE …when above ground parts are used orally (12).
PREGNANCY: LIKELY UNSAFE …contraindicated for oral use because it could have uterine-stimulant activity (12).
LACTATION: POSSIBLY UNSAFE …when used orally; avoid using.

Effectiveness
There is insufficient reliable information available about the effectiveness of dyer's broom.

Possible Mechanism of Action & Active Ingredients
Dyer's broom contains quinolizidine alkaloids, including methylcytisine, anagyrine, isopsparteine, lupanine, tinctorin, and cysisine. It also contains flavonoids (including luteolin glycosides), isoflavonoids (including genistein and genistin), and lectins (18).

Adverse Reactions Including Known Allergies
Dyer's broom may cause nausea and vomiting. Overuse of dyer's broom can lead to diarrhea (18).

Possible Interactions with Herbs & Other Dietary Supplements
Insufficient reliable information available.

Possible Interactions with Drugs
No interactions are known to occur, and there is no known reason to expect a clinically significant interaction with dyer's broom.

Possible Interactions with Foods
No interactions are known to occur, and there is no known reason to expect a clinically significant interaction with dyer's broom.

Possible Interactions with Lab Tests
No interactions are known to occur, and there is no known reason to expect a clinically significant interaction with dyer's broom.

Possible Interactions with Diseases or Conditions
No interactions are known to occur, and there is no known reason to expect a clinically significant interaction with dyer's broom.

Typical Dosages & Routes of Administration that are Commonly Used
No typical dosage.

Comments
None.

ECHINACEA

This Product is Also Known As

American Cone Flower, Black Sampson, Black Susans, Brauneria Angustifolia, Brauneria Pallida, Comb Flower, Coneflower, Hedgehog, Igelkopfwurzel, Indian Head, Kansas Snakeroot, Narrow-leaved Purple Cone Flower, Purple Cone Flower, Racine d'echininacea, Red Sunflower, Rock-Up-Hat, Scurvy Root, Snakeroot, Sonnenhutwurzel.

Scientific Names

Echinacea angustifolia; Echinacea pallida; Echinacea purpurea.
Family: Asteraceae or Compositae.

People Use This For

Orally, echinacea is commonly used for treating or preventing colds and other upper respiratory infections (4,1412,3279,3280,3281,3282). People also use echinacea orally as an antiseptic, antiviral, immune stimulant, peripheral vasodilator (4), for urinary tract infections, yeast infections, and other infections (6121).

Topically, echinacea has been used for skin wounds, chronic skin ulcers (2), psoriasis (11), and herpes simplex (6121).

Historically, it has been used orally for septicemia, nasopharyngeal catarrh, pyorrhea, tonsillitis, boils, abscesses (4), rheumatism, migraines, streptococcus infections, dyspepsia, pain, wounds, eczema, dizziness, rattlesnake bites, syphilis, typhoid, malaria, diptheria, bee stings, and hemorrhoids (5).

In herbal combination products, echinacea is used orally for treating or preventing colds and other upper respiratory problems (1415,1416,1417,3281).

Safety

LIKELY SAFE ...when taken orally and appropriately (12,1412,3279,3280,3281,3282). Limit daily use to eight consecutive weeks (2,12) due to concern that long-term daily use might depress immunity (4). There is no safety data regarding alternating the use of echinacea for several weeks with a holiday from echinacea use for several weeks. ...when used topically and appropriately (12).

PREGNANCY AND LACTATION: Insufficient reliable information available; avoid using.

Effectiveness

POSSIBLY EFFECTIVE ...when Echinacea pallida root extract is used orally as supportive therapy for influenza-like infections (2). ...when Echinacea purpurea above ground parts (herb) extract (Echinagard/Echinacin) or 95% herb/5% root juice (Echinaforce) is used orally for shortening the duration of the common cold (7,1412,3281). Human studies of echinacea and the common cold vary with regard to the species (angustifolia, pallida, or purpurea), plant part (root, above ground parts), and form (fresh pressed juice, alcohol extract) used. Despite the inconsistencies, recent data generally indicate that some echinacea preparations might reduce the severity and duration of colds if taken when symptoms first develop (1412,3280,3281,6206). However, one recent study of 92 healthy volunteers found that echinacea (species unknown) was no more effective than placebo in lessening the severity or duration of cold symptoms, or in preventing infection with rhinovirus type 23 (6207). ...when Echinacea purpurea above ground parts (herb) juice is used orally as supportive treatment for upper and lower respiratory infections (2,1412,3279,3280,3281). ...when Echinacea purpurea above ground parts (herb) juice is used orally as supportive treatment for urinary tract infections (2,1412). ...when an Echinacea purpurea above ground parts (herb) semisolid preparation (containing at least 15% pressed herb juice) is used topically for poorly healing skin wounds and ulcers (2).

POSSIBLY INEFFECTIVE ...when Echinacea (angustifolia or pallida) above ground parts (herb) extract or root extract is used orally for preventing the common cold or respiratory infections (3280,3281). ...when Echinacea purpurea above ground parts (herb) extract or root extract is used orally for preventing the common cold or respiratory infections (3280,3281,3282).

There is insufficient reliable information available about the effectiveness of echinacea for its other uses. There is also insufficient reliable information available about the effectiveness of combination herbal products containing echinacea.

Possible Mechanism of Action & Active Ingredients

The applicable parts of echinacea are the roots and the above ground parts. Researchers report Echinacea angustifolia extracts and the fresh expressed juice from Echinacea purpurea have multiple effects on wound healing. They inhibit tissue and bacterial hyaluronidase, have anti-inflammatory activity, and stimulate the anterior pituitary-adrenal cortex (11,3279). Echinacea purpurea extracts promote the formation of mesenchymal mucopolysaccharides, stimulate histiogenic and hematogenic phagocytes, promote differentiation of fibrocytes from fibroblasts, and exhibit antiviral activity (11,3279). Echinacea angustifolia, Echinacea pallida, and Echinacea purpurea extracts all increase phagocytosis and promote lymphocyte activity resulting in increased release of tumor necrosis factor (TNF); actions that tend to increase the body's resistance to bacterial activity (3). In preliminary clinical research, Echinacea purpurea has increased phagocytosis and slightly increased the percentage of T-lymphocytes able to stimulate cytokine production in healthy subjects serving as their own controls (6206). Preliminary research suggests that high concentrations of Echinacea purpurea might reduce sperm and ova fertility (4239,4240). Researchers have not yet determined the genotoxic, carcinogenic, or toxic potential of Echinacea purpurea even after experiments involving large amounts (1413).

Adverse Reactions Including Known Allergies

Echinacea taken orally can cause allergic reactions, fever, nausea, and vomiting (2). Few adverse effects have been reported in human studies (1412,3279,3280,3282). Allergic reactions to echinacea have included anaphylaxis (638,1358), acute asthma, and urticaria and angioedema (1358). Individuals sensitive to the Asteraceae/Compositae plant family may be more likely to experience an allergic reaction. Members of this family include ragweed, chrysanthemums, marigolds, daisies, and many other herbs. Individuals with atopy (a genetic tendency toward allergic conditions) may also be more likely to experience an allergic reaction. Unpublished case reports, presented at the American Academy of Allergy, Asthma and Immunology (AAAAI) 2000 annual meeting, describe 23 cases of allergic reactions to echinacea consistent with IgE mediated hypersensitivity. Thirty-four percent of the reactions were in patients with atopy. In a related study, 20% of 100 atopic patients tested who had never taken echinacea had positive skin test reactions to echinacea, indicating hypersensitivity without previous exposure (1358). Some evidence suggests that high doses of echinacea might reduce male and female fertility (4239,4240), but this effect has not been demonstrated in humans.

Possible Interactions with Herbs & Other Dietary Supplements

Insufficient reliable information available.

Possible Interactions with Drugs

IMMUNOSUPPRESSIVE DRUGS: Theoretically, echinacea may interfere with immunosuppressant therapy (4) because of its immunostimulating activity. Echinacea stimulates phagocytosis and increases respiratory cellular activity and the mobility of leukocytes.
ECONAZOLE NITRATE (Spectazole): Concomitant use of echinacea and topical econazole can decrease the recurrence rate of vaginal candida infections (19).

Possible Interactions with Foods

No interactions are known to occur, and there is no known reason to expect a clinically significant interaction with echinacea.

Possible Interactions with Lab Tests

No interactions are known to occur, and there is no known reason to expect a clinically significant interaction with echinacea.

Possible Interactions with Diseases or Conditions

ATOPY: Individuals with atopy (a genetic tendency toward allergic conditions) may be more likely to experience an allergic reaction when taking echinacea. Unpublished case reports, presented at the American Academy of Allergy, Asthma and Immunology (AAAAI) 2000 annual meeting, describe 23 cases of allergic reactions to echinacea consistent with IgE mediated hypersensitivity. Thirty-four percent of the reactions were in patients with atopy. In a related study, 20% of 100 atopic patients tested who had never taken echinacea had positive skin test reactions to echinacea, indicating hypersensitivity without previous exposure (1358).
PROGRESSIVE SYSTEMIC DISEASES: Echinacea is contraindicated in individuals with tuberculosis, leukosis, collagenosis, multiple sclerosis, collagen disorders or other progressive systemic diseases, due to potential for stimulating the autoimmune process (2,7,8).
IMMUNE DISORDERS: Echinacea is contraindicated in individuals with AIDS, HIV infection, autoimmune disorders (2,8).
DIABETES: Parenteral administration might worsen metabolic control (8).
CROSS-ALLERGENICITY: Individuals sensitive to the Asteraceae/Compositae plant family may be more likely to experience an allergic reaction to echinacea. Members of this family include ragweed, chrysanthemums, marigolds, daisies, and many other herbs.
INFERTILITY: Preliminary evidence suggests that echinacea might inhibit oocyte fertilization and alter sperm DNA (4239,4240). This effect has not yet been demonstrated in humans; however, until more is known, use with caution in couples attempting to conceive and avoid use in couples having difficulty conceiving.

Typical Dosages & Routes of Administration that are Commonly Used

ORAL: For symptomatic treatment of colds, upper respiratory infections, and urinary tract infections, a daily dose of 6-9 mL Echinacea purpurea fresh above ground parts (herb) juice is used for a maximum of 8 weeks (2). For reducing cold symptoms, a dose of Echinaforce (Bioforce AG) three tablets twice daily (equivalent to 6.78 mg Echinacea purpurea herb extract per tablet) for up to seven days has been used (1412). For reducing cold symptoms, a dose of Echinacin (Madaus AG) or Echinagard (Nature's Way) (equivalent to Echinacea purpurea 95% herb/5%) 20 drops every 2 hours for the first day, then 20 drops three times daily until symptoms resolve (3281) or 4 mL twice daily (3282). A daily dose of Echinacea pallida root tincture, equivalent to 900 mg above ground parts (herb) (2,3281).
TOPICAL: A semi-solid preparation containing at least 15% pressed juice of Echinacea purpurea above ground parts (herb) is used (2).

Comments

There are three Echinacea species of medicinal interest: Echinacea angustifolia, Echinacea pallida, and Echinacea purpurea. Echinacea species are native to North America, were used as traditional herbal remedies by the Great

Plains Indian tribes, and were adopted for medicinal use by settlers (3279). Echinacea angustifolia and Echinacea pallida were official in the National Formulary from 1916 to 1950 (11). They fell out of favor with the discovery of antibiotics and a lack of scientific data supporting their use (3279). The recent advent of antibiotic resistance has contributed to renewed interest in echinacea. While reputable references cite an 8-week limitation on the continual use of echinacea (2,4,12), some authorities state this limitation is unfounded and unsupported by scientific literature (1267).

ECHINACEA PRODUCT QUALITY: Echinacea products have been commonly adulterated. Studies performed prior to 1991 might be unreliable unless the plant material used was positively confirmed (11,3279,1414). The presence of Echinacea purpurea is now confirmable with HPLC analysis (11,1414). Although some echinacea extract products are standardized for their echinacoside content, echinacoside is not a specific marker for Echinacea purpurea, Echinacea angustifolia or Echinacea pallida (11).

ELECAMPANE

This Product is Also Known As
Alant, Elfdock, Elfwort, Horse-Elder, Horseheal, Inula, Scabwort, Velvet Dock, Wild Sunflower, Yellow Starwort.

Scientific Names
Inula helenium, synonyms Helenium grandiflorum, Aster officinalis, Aster helenium.
Family: Asteraceae or Compositae.

People Use This For
Orally, elecampane is used as an expectorant, antitussive, and diaphoretic (4), for diseases of the respiratory tract (2), as an antihelmintic, for improving stomach function, and as a diuretic (11).

In folk medicine, elecampane has been used for asthma, bronchitis, whooping cough (11), cough associated with tuberculosis (4), nausea, and diarrhea (11).

In foods and beverages, elecampane is used as a flavoring ingredient (11).

In other manufacturing processes, elecampane is used as a fragrance component in cosmetics and soaps (11).

Safety
LIKELY SAFE ...when consumed in amounts found in alcoholic beverages (11).
POSSIBLY SAFE ...when the root and rhizome preparations are used appropriately as an oral medicinal agent (12).
POSSIBLY UNSAFE ...when used orally in large amounts. Elecampane can cause gastrointestinal upset and symptoms of paralysis (12).
PREGNANCY AND LACTATION: LIKELY UNSAFE ...contraindicated for oral use (12).

Effectiveness
POSSIBLY EFFECTIVE ...when used orally for treating hookworm, roundworm, threadworm and whipworm infections (4,11); alantolactone is used as an anthelmintic in Europe and the UK (11).
There is insufficient reliable information available about the effectiveness of elecampane for its other uses.

Possible Mechanism of Action & Active Ingredients
The applicable parts of elecampane are the rhizome/root. Alantolactone and isoalantolactone, sesquiterpene alkaloids found in elecampane, show antibacterial and antifungal (11) activity in vitro and antihelmintic activity in humans (11).

Adverse Reactions Including Known Allergies
Large doses taken orally may cause vomiting, diarrhea, spasms, and symptoms of paralysis (12). Topically, elecampane may cause allergic contact dermatitis (4). It can cause an allergic reaction in individuals sensitive to the Asteraceae/Compositae family. Members of this family include ragweed, chrysanthemums, marigolds, daisies, and many other herbs.

Possible Interactions with Herbs & Other Dietary Supplements
HERBS WITH SEDATIVE PROPERTIES: Theoretically, concomitant use with herbs that have sedative properties might enhance therapeutic and adverse effects. These include calamus, calendula, California poppy, catnip, capsicum, celery, couch grass, Siberian ginseng, German chamomile, goldenseal, gotu kola, hops, Jamaican dogwood, kava, lemon balm, sage, St. John's wort, sassafras, scullcap, shepherd's purse, stinging nettle, valerian, wild carrot, wild lettuce, withania root, and yerba mansa (4,19).

Possible Interactions with Drugs
HYPOGLYCEMIC DRUGS: Theoretically, concomitant use may interfere with drug activity and blood glucose control (4).
ANTIHYPERTENSIVE, ANTIHYPOTENSIVE DRUGS: Theoretically, concomitant use may interfere with drug therapy and blood pressure control (4).
DRUGS WITH SEDATIVE PROPERTIES: Theoretically, concomitant use with drugs with sedative properties may cause additive effects (4).

Possible Interactions with Foods

No interactions are known to occur, and there is no known reason to expect a clinically significant interaction with elecampane.

Possible Interactions with Lab Tests

No interactions are known to occur, and there is no known reason to expect a clinically significant interaction with elecampane.

Possible Interactions with Diseases or Conditions

DIABETES: Theoretically, elecampane may interfere with blood glucose control (4).
HYPERTENSION, HYPOTENSION: Theoretically, elecampane may interfere with blood pressure control (4).
CROSS-ALLERGENICITY: Can cause an allergic reaction in individuals sensitive to the Asteraceae/Compositae family. Members of this family include ragweed, chrysanthemums, marigolds, daisies, and many other herbs.

Typical Dosages & Routes of Administration that are Commonly Used

ORAL: 1.5-4 grams of rhizome/root three times daily, or one cup tea (simmer 1.5-4 grams of rhizome/root in 150 mL boiling water 5-10 minutes, strain) three times daily (4). Liquid extract (1:1 in 25% alcohol) 1.5-4 mL three times daily (4).
ANTHELMINTIC: Adults, alantolactone 300 mg daily for 2 courses of 5 days, with an interval of 10 days. Children, alantolactone 50-200 mg daily (4).

Comments

None.

ELEMI

This Product is Also Known As

Elemi Oleoresin, Elemi Resin, Manila Elemi.

Scientific Names

Canarium commune; Canarium luzonicum.
Family: Burseraceae.

People Use This For

In folk medicine, elemi gum is used for improving stomach function, and as an expectorant and local stimulant.
In foods and beverages, elemi gum is used as a flavoring agent (11).
In other manufacturing processes, elemi gum and oil are used as a fixative and fragrance in cosmetics and soaps (11).

Safety

LIKELY SAFE ...when used in amounts found in foods; approved for food use in the US (11).
There is insufficient reliable information available about the safety of oral uses of elemi exceeding the amount found in foods.
PREGNANCY AND LACTATION: Insufficient reliable information available; avoid using.

Effectiveness

There is insufficient reliable information available about the effectiveness of elemi.

Possible Mechanism of Action & Active Ingredients

The applicable parts of elemi are the gum and oil. There is insufficient reliable information available about the possible mechanism of action and active ingredients.

Adverse Reactions Including Known Allergies

None reported.

Possible Interactions with Herbs & Other Dietary Supplements

Insufficient reliable information available.

Possible Interactions with Drugs

No interactions are known to occur, and there is no known reason to expect a clinically significant interaction with elemi.

Possible Interactions with Foods

No interactions are known to occur, and there is no known reason to expect a clinically significant interaction with elemi.

Possible Interactions with Lab Tests
No interactions are known to occur, and there is no known reason to expect a clinically significant interaction with elemi.

Possible Interactions with Diseases or Conditions
No interactions are known to occur, and there is no known reason to expect a clinically significant interaction with elemi.

Typical Dosages & Routes of Administration that are Commonly Used
No typical dosage.

Comments
Elemi gum is resin exuded by the elemi tree (Canarium commune). Elemi oil is produced by distillation of elemi gum resin.

ELM BARK

This Product is Also Known As
Smooth-Leaved Elm.

Scientific Names
Ulmus minor.
Family: Ulmaceae.

People Use This For
Orally, elm bark is used for digestive disorders and severe diarrhea. Sometimes it is used as a diuretic and astringent.
Topically, elm bark is used for cleaning open and/or festering wounds (18).

Safety
There is insufficient reliable information available about the safety of elm bark.
Pregnancy and Lactation: Insufficient reliable information available; avoid using.

Effectiveness
There is insufficient reliable information available about the effectiveness of elm bark.

Possible Mechanism of Action & Active Ingredients
Insufficient reliable information available.

Adverse Reactions Including Known Allergies
None reported.

Possible Interactions with Herbs & Other Dietary Supplements
Insufficient reliable information available.

Possible Interactions with Drugs
No interactions are known to occur, and there is no known reason to expect a clinically significant interaction with elm bark.

Possible Interactions with Foods
No interactions are known to occur, and there is no known reason to expect a clinically significant interaction with elm bark.

Possible Interactions with Lab Tests
No interactions are known to occur, and there is no known reason to expect a clinically significant interaction with elm bark.

Possible Interactions with Diseases or Conditions
No interactions are known to occur, and there is no known reason to expect a clinically significant interaction with elm bark.

Typical Dosages & Routes of Administration that are Commonly Used
ORAL: One cup of tea taken orally 2-3 times daily. The tea is prepared by simmering 2 teaspoons of bark in 150 mL of boiling water for 10-15 minutes and straining. Alternately, 2-5 grams of powdered root is taken orally per day (18).
TOPICAL: A 20% tea is diluted 1:1 with water for topical use (18).

Comments

There is very little scientific information about this product. Our staff is continually analyzing the available information on natural medicines and will add data here as it becomes available.

EMU OIL

This Product is Also Known As

Emu.

Scientific Names

Dromiceius nova-hollandiae.

People Use This For

Orally, emu oil is used for improving cholesterol levels, as a source of polyunsaturated and monounsaturated fatty acids (5914), for weight loss (5920), and as a cough syrup for colds and flu (5914).

Orally, crushed emu shell is used as an aphrodisiac (5916).

Topically, emu oil is used for relief from sore muscles; aching joints, pain or inflammation (5914); carpal tunnel syndrome; sciatica, shin splints (5918); and gout (5921). It is used to improve healing of wounds and incisions, burns from radiation therapy, to reduce bruises and stretch marks (5914), to reduce scarring and keloids, to heal the donor site of skin grafting (5916), to diminish acne inflammation, soften dry cuticles and promote healthy nails (5914), for skin cancers (5916), athlete's foot, diaper rash, canker sores, chapped lips, circulation (5918), dry skin, eczema, psoriasis, wrinkles or age spots, dry or damaged hair (5914), dandruff (5918), in massage therapy (5914), for its anti-aging properties (5915), to protect skin from sun damage (5917), and to promote skin rejuvenation (5916). It is also used to reduce pain and irritation from shingles, bed sores, hemorrhoids, diabetic neuropathy (5914), insect bites (5917), earaches, eye irritation (5918), "growing pains" (5916), and frostbite (5918). It is used for rashes, razor burn and nicks, rosacea, and roseola (5918).

Intranasally, emu oil is used to treat colds and flu (5914).

In combination, emu oil (7%) is used with glycolic acid (10%) for lowering cholesterol, triglycerides and low density lipoprotein; preventing and treating allergies; preventing scarring; treating headaches, especially migraines; preventing nosebleeds; treating and preventing cold and flu symptoms; and relieving discomfort associated with menstruation (5916).

In veterinary practice emu oil is used to reduce swelling in joints, prevent cracked or peeling paws, calm "hot spots", and reduce irritation of flea bites (5914).

In manufacturing, emu oil is used to sharpen and oil industrial machinery, for polishing timber and leather, and for conditioning and waterproofing (5916).

Safety

POSSIBLY SAFE ...when used orally and appropriately. ...when used topically. There are no reports of adverse affects and the Australian government classifies emu meat as fit for human consumption (5916).

PREGNANCY AND LACTATION: Insufficient reliable information available; avoid using.

Effectiveness

There is insufficient reliable information available about the effectiveness of emu oil.

Possible Mechanism of Action & Active Ingredients

Though not standardized, emu oil typically contains myristic, palmitic, palmitoleic, stearic, oleic, linoleic, and linolenic fatty acids (5919). Linoleic acid is believed to ease muscle ache and joint pain; oleic acid is considered to have a local anti-inflammatory effect (5922). Emu oil appears to have the ability to penetrate the skin, perhaps in part because it does not contain phospholipids (5922). Some animal evidence suggests emu oil is more effective in acute inflammation than in chronic inflammation (5923). A combination of 7% emu oil and 10% glycolic acid is patented for therapeutic use in methods for lowering cholesterol, triglycerides and low density lipoprotein; preventing and treating allergies; preventing scarring; treating headaches; preventing nosebleeds; treating and preventing cold and flu symptoms; relieving discomfort associated with menstruation (5916). However, no studies have been published in refereed journals.

Adverse Reactions Including Known Allergies

None reported.

Possible Interactions with Herbs & Other Dietary Supplements

HERBS WITH ANTICOAGULANT/ANTIPLATELET POTENTIAL: Concomitant use of herbs that have coumarin constituents or affect platelet aggregation could theoretically increase the risk of bleeding in some people. These herbs include: angelica, anise, arnica, asafoetida, bogbean, boldo, capsicum, celery, chamomile, clove, danshen, fenugreek, feverfew, garlic, ginger, ginkgo, ginseng Panax, horse chestnut, horseradish, licorice, meadowsweet, prickly ash, onion, papain, passionflower, poplar, quassia, red clover, turmeric, wild carrot, wild lettuce, willow, and others (4,19).

Possible Interactions with Drugs

ASPIRIN AND ANTICOAGULANTS: Some information suggests the concomitant use of the emu oil constituent linolenic acid might increase risk of bleeding (5914).

Possible Interactions with Foods

No interactions are known to occur, and there is no known reason to expect a clinically significant interaction with emu oil.

Possible Interactions with Lab Tests

LIPID LEVELS: Some evidence suggests that emu oil might reduce lipid levels (5916).

Possible Interactions with Diseases or Conditions

No interactions are known to occur, and there is no known reason to expect a clinically significant interaction with emu oil.

Typical Dosages & Routes of Administration that are Commonly Used

ORAL: Emu oil 7% in combination with 10% glycolic acid, the preferable adult dose is 1 teaspoon daily (5916).
TOPICAL: For sore muscles, aching joints, pain or inflammation, apply emu oil to affected area three times daily for at least three days (5914).

Comments

The emu has been a sacred bird to the Australian Aborigines for thousands of years. The emu provided the Aborigines with clothing, food, and oil believed to have special healing properties (5914). The therapeutic uses of emu oil were patented in 1995 by Elf Resources, Inc., New Rochelle, NY (5916).

ENGLISH ADDER'S TONGUE

This Product is Also Known As

Christs Spear, Christ's Spear, English Adders Tongue, Green Oil of Charity, Serpents Tongue, Serpent's Tongue. CAUTION: See separate listing for American Adder's Tongue.

Scientific Names

Ophioglossum vulgatum.

People Use This For

Topically, English adder's tongue is used to treat ulcers (18).

Safety

There is insufficient reliable information available about the safety of English adder's tongue.
Pregnancy and Lactation: Insufficient reliable information available; avoid using.

Effectiveness

There is insufficient reliable information available about the effectiveness of English adder's tongue.

Possible Mechanism of Action & Active Ingredients

The applicable parts of English adder's tongue are the root and leaf. English adder's tongue is stated to have emollient properties when applied. When taken orally, it is has emetic properties (18).

Adverse Reactions Including Known Allergies

None reported.

Possible Interactions with Herbs & Other Dietary Supplements

Insufficient reliable information available.

Possible Interactions with Drugs

No interactions are known to occur, and there is no known reason to expect a clinically significant interaction with English adder's tongue.

Possible Interactions with Foods

No interactions are known to occur, and there is no known reason to expect a clinically significant interaction with English adder's tongue.

Possible Interactions with Lab Tests

No interactions are known to occur, and there is no known reason to expect a clinically significant interaction with English adder's tongue.

Possible Interactions with Diseases or Conditions

No interactions are known to occur, and there is no known reason to expect a clinically significant interaction with English adder's tongue.

Typical Dosages & Routes of Administration that are Commonly Used
TOPICAL: Fresh leaves are applied as a poultice.

Comments
Avoid confusion with American adder's tongue (Erythronium americanum).

ENGLISH HORSEMINT

This Product is Also Known As
None.

Scientific Names
Mentha longifolia.
Family: Labitae or Lamiceae.

People Use This For
Orally, English horsemint is used for digestive disorders, particularly flatulence.
Historically, English horsemint was used for pain in general, and specifically for headaches [18].

Safety
There is insufficient reliable information available about the safety of English horsemint.
Pregnancy and Lactation: Insufficient reliable information available; avoid using.

Effectiveness
There is insufficient reliable information available about the effectiveness of English horsemint.

Possible Mechanism of Action & Active Ingredients
The applicable parts of English horsemint are the above ground parts. There is insufficient reliable information available about the possible mechanism of action and active ingredients.

Adverse Reactions Including Known Allergies
None reported.

Possible Interactions with Herbs & Other Dietary Supplements
Insufficient reliable information available.

Possible Interactions with Drugs
No interactions are known to occur, and there is no known reason to expect a clinically significant interaction with English horsemint.

Possible Interactions with Foods
No interactions are known to occur, and there is no known reason to expect a clinically significant interaction with English horsemint.

Possible Interactions with Lab Tests
No interactions are known to occur, and there is no known reason to expect a clinically significant interaction with English horsemint.

Possible Interactions with Diseases or Conditions
No interactions are known to occur, and there is no known reason to expect a clinically significant interaction with English horsemint.

Typical Dosages & Routes of Administration that are Commonly Used
ORAL: English horsemint is used as a tea [18].
TOPICAL: It is used as a bath additive [18].

Comments
There is very little scientific information about this product. Our staff is continually analyzing the available information on natural medicines and will add data here as it becomes available.

ENGLISH IVY

This Product is Also Known As
Gum Ivy, Hederae helicis folium, Ivy, True Ivy, Woodbind.

© Copyright 2000, Natural Medicines Comprehensive Database (209) 472-2244. For updated data, go to www.NaturalDatabase.com

Scientific Names
Hedera helix.
Family: Araliaceae.

People Use This For
Orally, English ivy leaf is used for inflammation of mucous membranes in respiratory passages, symptomatic treatment of chronic inflammatory bronchial conditions (2), as an expectorant (3), as an antispasmodic (18), and improvement of lung function in children with chronic obstructive bronchitis (3471).

Topically, English ivy is used for burn wounds, calluses, cellulitis, inflammations, neuralgia, parasitic disorders, ulcers, rheumatic complaints, and for phlebitis (18).

In folk medicine, English ivy is used orally for liver, spleen, and gallbladder disorders as well as for gout, rheumatism, and scrofulosis (18).

Safety
POSSIBLY SAFE ...when used orally and appropriately (2).
There is insufficient reliable information available about the safety of the topical use of English ivy.
PREGNANCY AND LACTATION: Insufficient reliable information available; avoid using.

Effectiveness
POSSIBLY EFFECTIVE ...when used orally for inflammation of respiratory passage mucous membranes; symptomatic treatment of chronic inflammatory bronchial conditions (2) and improvement of lung function in children with chronic obstructive bronchitis (3471).
There is insufficient reliable information available about the effectiveness of English ivy for its other uses.

Possible Mechanism of Action & Active Ingredients
The applicable part of English ivy is the leaf. English ivy has expectorant and antispasmodic actions. It irritates skin and mucosa (2). Researchers think the ivy leaf acts on the gastric mucosa to cause stimulation of mucous glands in the bronchi via parasympathetic sensory pathways (7). Fresh leaves contain the contact allergen falcarinol (7). Preliminary evidence suggests ivy leaf dried extract may improve lung function (measured as forced expiratory volume in one second) in children with chronic obstructive bronchitis due to its secretolytic and spasmolytic effects (3471). Human studies are needed to determine whether ivy leaf dried extract is as effective or beneficial as conventional agents used prophylactically to improve and maintain lung function such as bronchodilators and corticosteroids.

Adverse Reactions Including Known Allergies
Fresh leaves can cause skin irritation (7). Saponin constituents, hederacosides, and hederin monodesmosides have acrid and/or bitter taste (7).

Possible Interactions with Herbs & Other Dietary Supplements
Insufficient reliable information available.

Possible Interactions with Drugs
No interactions are known to occur, and there is no known reason to expect a clinically significant interaction with English ivy.

Possible Interactions with Foods
No interactions are known to occur, and there is no known reason to expect a clinically significant interaction with English ivy.

Possible Interactions with Lab Tests
No interactions are known to occur, and there is no known reason to expect a clinically significant interaction with English ivy.

Possible Interactions with Diseases or Conditions
No interactions are known to occur, and there is no known reason to expect a clinically significant interaction with English ivy.

Typical Dosages & Routes of Administration that are Commonly Used
ORAL: 300-800 mg dried leaf per day (2,18), or one cup tea, steep 1 heaping teaspoon of dried leaf in 1/4 cup boiling water 10 minutes, strain, up to three times daily (18). For chronic obstructive bronchitis in children, 35 mg dried leaf extract three times a day or 14 mg dried leaf alcohol-based extract three times a day (3471).
TOPICAL: Fresh leaves placed on festering wounds and burns (18). For rheumatism, prepare tea, simmer 200 grams of fresh leaves in 1 L boiling water 5-10 minutes, strain; for topical application (18).

Comments
English ivy is most often used in the form of an extract and seldom used as a prepared tea (7).

ENGLISH WALNUT hull

This Product is Also Known As
Fructus Cortex, Juglandis Walnussfrüchtschalen, Walnut Hull.
CAUTION: See separate listing for English Walnut leaf.

Scientific Names
Juglans regia.
Family: Juglandaceae.

People Use This For
Orally, English walnut hull is used to treat gastrointestinal mucous membrane inflammation (2,805).
Topically, English walnut hull is used for skin diseases, abscesses, and eye lid inflammation (2,805).
In combination with other herbs, English walnut hull is used to treat diabetes mellitus, gastritis, and anemia (2).
Historically, English walnut hull was used to treat "blood poisoning" and as a "blood purifier" to remove undesirable agents from the blood (2).

Safety
POSSIBLY UNSAFE ...when the fresh hull is used topically because it contains the constituent juglone (2); daily topical use of juglone-containing English walnut bark preparations is associated with increased risk of tongue cancer and lip leukoplakia (2,12).
There is insufficient reliable information available about the safety of the oral use of English walnut hull.
PREGNANCY AND LACTATION: POSSIBLY UNSAFE ...when used topically (2); avoid using. There is insufficient reliable information available about the safety of the oral use of English walnut hull.

Effectiveness
There is insufficient reliable information available about the effectiveness of English walnut hull.

Possible Mechanism of Action & Active Ingredients
English walnut contains tannins (galloylglucose, ellagitannins), naphthalene derivatives including juglone, and flavonoids including hyperoside and quercitrin. Astringent properties can be attributed to tannins. The constituent, juglone, has antifungal effects (8,18).

Adverse Reactions Including Known Allergies
Topical application of juglone-containing walnut preparations to skin and mucous membranes leads to yellow or brown discoloration (2). Daily use of juglone-containing preparations is associated with tongue cancer and lip leukoplakia (2). Juglone is reported to have mutagenic effects in animals (12).

Possible Interactions with Herbs & Other Dietary Supplements
Insufficient reliable information available.

Possible Interactions with Drugs
No interactions are known to occur, and there is no known reason to expect a clinically significant interaction with English walnut hull.

Possible Interactions with Foods
No interactions are known to occur, and there is no known reason to expect a clinically significant interaction with English walnut hull.

Possible Interactions with Lab Tests
No interactions are known to occur, and there is no known reason to expect a clinically significant interaction with English walnut hull.

Possible Interactions with Diseases or Conditions
No interactions are known to occur, and there is no known reason to expect a clinically significant interaction with English walnut hull.

Typical Dosages & Routes of Administration that are Commonly Used
No typical dosage.

Comments
The amount of juglone in dried English walnut hull is currently unknown (2).

ENGLISH WALNUT leaf

This Product is Also Known As
Juglandis Folium, Walnussblätter, Walnut Leaf.
CAUTION: See separate listing for English Walnut hull.

Scientific Names
Juglans regia.
Family: Juglandaceae.

People Use This For
Orally, English walnut leaf is used for treating diarrhea, and as an adjuvant to topical treatment of skin conditions such as acne, eczema, scrophula, pyodermia, and ulcers (8).
Topically, English walnut leaf is used for superficial inflammation of the skin, excessive hand and/or foot perspiration (2), and for skin conditions such as acne, eczema, scrophula, pyodermia, and ulcers (8).
In folk medicine, English walnut leaf was used for gastrointestinal mucous membrane inflammation, as an antihelmintic, and "blood-purifying" agent (8).

Safety
POSSIBLY SAFE ...when the dried leaf is used topically and appropriately, short-term (2,18).
POSSIBLY UNSAFE ...when used topically long-term; contains tannins (2).
PREGNANCY AND LACTATION: Insufficient reliable information available; avoid using (12).

Effectiveness
POSSIBLY EFFECTIVE ...when used topically for mild, superficial inflammation of the skin, excessive perspiration of the hands and feet (2).
There is insufficient reliable information available about the effectiveness of English walnut leaf for its other uses.

Possible Mechanism of Action & Active Ingredients
Walnut leaf contains tannins with astringent effects (2). Juglone and the essential oil have antifungal effects (8,18). Juglone may quickly break down when leaves are handled or dried (18).

Adverse Reactions Including Known Allergies
None reported.

Possible Interactions with Herbs & Other Dietary Supplements
Insufficient reliable information available.

Possible Interactions with Drugs
No interactions are known to occur, and there is no known reason to expect a clinically significant interaction with English walnut leaf.

Possible Interactions with Foods
No interactions are known to occur, and there is no known reason to expect a clinically significant interaction with English walnut leaf.

Possible Interactions with Lab Tests
No interactions are known to occur, and there is no known reason to expect a clinically significant interaction with English walnut leaf.

Possible Interactions with Diseases or Conditions
No interactions are known to occur, and there is no known reason to expect a clinically significant interaction with English walnut leaf.

Typical Dosages & Routes of Administration that are Commonly Used
ORAL: As an adjuvant for skin conditions, one cup tea (simmer 1.5 grams of finely chopped dried leaf in 150 mL boiling water 3-5 minutes, steep) one to three times daily (8).
TOPICAL: For dressing, lotion, poultice or hip bath, simmer 2-3 grams of finely chopped dried leaf per 100 mL boiling water (2,8). Average daily amount is 3-6 grams of dried leaf (18).

Comments
None.

EPA (EICOSAPENTAENOIC ACID)

This Product is Also Known As
Fish Oil Fatty Acid, N-3 Fatty Acid, Omega Fatty Acid, Omega 3 Fatty Acid, Omega-3 Fatty Acid, W-3 Fatty Acid.
CAUTION: See separate listings for DHA (docosahexaenoic acid) and Fish Oils.

Scientific Names
Eicosapentaenoic acid.

People Use This For
Orally, eicosapentaenoic acid (EPA) is used for treating the symptoms of cystic fibrosis, reducing the risk of intrauterine growth retardation, and treating pregnancy induced hypertension in high-risk pregnancies (1027).
In combination, EPA is used with docosahexanoic acid (DHA) in fish oil preparations for a variety of conditions, including preventing and reversing heart disease, decreasing ectopic ventricular beats, asthma, cancer, dysmenorrhea, hay fever, lung diseases, lupus erythematosus, lupus nephritis, and IgA nephropathy (507). They are also used in combination for migraine headache prophylaxis in adolescents (5097), atopic dermatitis, Behcet's syndrome, hyperlipidemia, hypertension, psoriasis, Raynaud's syndrome, rheumatoid arthritis, Crohn's disease, and ulcerative colitis (9).

Safety
LIKELY SAFE ...when used orally and appropriately (9,945,1016).
PREGNANCY AND LACTATION: Insufficient reliable information available for EPA as a single agent; avoid using.

Effectiveness
POSSIBLY EFFECTIVE ...when used orally as an adjunct to standard therapy for schizophrenia. One clinical study has shown EPA to be superior to both docosahexanoic acid (DHA) and linoleic acid (5073).
POSSIBLY INEFFECTIVE ...when taken orally as a single agent for treating symptoms of cystic fibrosis (1006,1027). ...when used orally for reducing the risk of intrauterine growth retardation (1027). ...when used orally for pregnancy-induced hypertension in women with high-risk pregnancies (1027). ...when taken orally to treat asthma. A clinical trial has shown that EPA has no effects on asthma symptoms when given for 4 weeks (1023). ...when taken orally to treat hay fever. A clinical trial has shown that EPA is no more effective than placebo for relieving hayfever symptoms, including wheezing, cough and nasal symptoms (1036).
There is insufficient reliable information available about the effectiveness of EPA for its other uses.

Possible Mechanism of Action & Active Ingredients
EPA is a long chain n-3 polyunsaturated fatty acid that competes with arachidonic acid for inclusion in cyclo-oxygenase and lipoxygenase pathways (9). EPA decreases blood viscosity and increases red blood cell deformability (9). Pure EPA reduces serum triglyceride concentrations, increases fasting insulin concentrations, and has no effect on total, LDL, or HDL-cholesterol or fasting glucose concentrations in mildly hypercholesterolemic men (6143).

Adverse Reactions Including Known Allergies
None reported for EPA alone. Adverse reactions reported for fish oils containing EPA and DHA, include fishy taste, belching (507), nosebleeds (9), nausea, and loose stools (9). Three people with pre-existing familial adenomatous polyposis were diagnosed with malignant lesions during the course of long-term fish oil use (999).

Possible Interactions with Herbs & Other Dietary Supplements
HERBS WITH ANTICOAGULANT/ANTIPLATELET POTENTIAL: Concomitant use of herbs that have coumarin constituents or affect platelet aggregation could theoretically increase the risk of bleeding in some people. These herbs include: angelica, anise, arnica, asafoetida, bogbean, boldo, capsicum, celery, chamomile, clove, danshen, fenugreek, feverfew, garlic, ginger, ginkgo, ginseng (Panax), horse chestnut, horseradish, licorice, meadowsweet, prickly ash, onion, papain, passionflower, poplar, quassia, red clover, turmeric, wild carrot, wild lettuce, willow, and others (4,19).

Possible Interactions with Drugs
ANTICOAGULANTS/ANTIPLATELET DRUGS: Theoretically, concomitant use of EPA with anticoagulant or antiplatelet drugs, including aspirin can increase the risk of bleeding (9,507).
ETRETINATE: Concomitant use can have additive effects for treating psoriasis (1000). Fish oils containing EPA and DHA can attenuate cyclosporine-induced hypertension in people with kidney or heart transplants (507,1012,1021).

Possible Interactions with Foods
No interactions are known to occur, and there is no known reason to expect a clinically significant interaction with EPA.

Possible Interactions with Lab Tests

INSULIN: EPA increases fasting insulin concentrations and test results in mildly hypercholesterolemic men (6143).
TRIGLYCERIDES: EPA reduces serum triglyceride concentrations and test results in mildly hypercholesterolemic men (6143).
PULMONARY FUNCTION TESTS: Omega-3 fatty acids can cause a decline in pulmonary function tests in aspirin-sensitive individuals (507).

Possible Interactions with Diseases or Conditions

None reported for EPA alone. Interactions with disease conditions have been reported for fish oils containing DHA and EPA, including interfering with blood glucose control in individuals with diabetes (9) and lowering blood pressure in individuals with hypertension (1001,1020,1030,1033). Omega-3 fatty acids can cause a decline in pulmonary function tests in aspirin-sensitive individuals (507).

Typical Dosages & Routes of Administration that are Commonly Used

ORAL: EPA is usually administered with DHA (docosahexaenoic acid) as fish oil. A wide range of doses have been used. The usual amount is 5 grams of fish oil containing 169-563 mg of EPA and 72-312 grams of DHA (9,507). As an adjunct to standard therapy for schizophrenia, an oral EPA daily dose of 2 grams has been used (5703). Many fish oil preparations also contain small amounts of vitamin E as an antioxidant (9).

Comments

Avoid confusion with DHA (docosahexaenoic acid) and fish oils, which contain EPA and DHA. Most available data involving EPA are from research and clinical experience with fish oil products containing variable combinations of EPA and DHA. For more information, see the separate listing for Fish Oils. Researchers are investigating oils containing stearidonic acid (SDA) from genetically modified plants as an alternative source of omega-3 fatty acids. SDA is metabolized to EPA and DHA in animals. However, further research is needed on the effects of SDA in humans (6129).

EPHEDRA

This Product is Also Known As

Cao Mahuang, Desert Herb, Ephedrae herba, Ephedra sinensis, Joint Fir, Ma Huang, Ma-Huang, Mahuang, Mahuanggen (ma huang root), Muzei Mahuang, Popotillo, Sea Grape, Teamster's Tea, Yellow Astringent, Yellow Horse, Zhong Mahuang.
CAUTION: See separate listing for Mormon Tea.

Scientific Names

Ephedra sinica; Ephedra intermedia; Ephedra equisetina; Ephedra distachya; Ephedra gerardiana; Ephedra shennungiana; and other Ephedra species.
Family: Ephedraceae.

People Use This For

Orally, ephedra is used for diseases of the respiratory tract with bronchospasm (2), asthma (3,6), bronchitis (18), allergic disorders (4), nasal congestion, as a central nervous system stimulant (3,12,18), cardiovascular stimulant (18), and appetite suppressant (3,11).
In combination with other herbal products, ephedra is used orally for weight loss.
In Chinese medicine, ephedra is used for colds, flu, fever, chills, headache, edema, anhydrosis, joint and bone pain, and as a diuretic (3,6,11).

Safety

POSSIBLY SAFE ...when used orally and appropriately short-term (2,12). The FDA recommends using ephedra-containing products for a maximum of seven days and in amounts not exceeding 8 mg of ephedrine every six hours or 24 mg per day (2729); however, this recommendation has been controversial.
LIKELY UNSAFE ...when used orally in high doses or long-term. Use for greater than seven days, or in doses exceeding 8 mg of ephedrine every six hours or 24 mg per day, has been associated with life threatening adverse effects (2729). Chronic use can also cause the rapid development of tolerance and dependence (2,12).
CHILDREN: LIKELY UNSAFE ...when used orally in children under the age of six (2,12).
PREGNANCY: LIKELY UNSAFE ...when used orally; contraindicated. Ephedra can stimulate uterine contraction (12).
LACTATION: Insufficient reliable information available; avoid using.

Effectiveness

POSSIBLY EFFECTIVE ...when taken orally for the short-term treatment of diseases of the respiratory tract, including asthma, bronchitis, and bronchospasm (2,3,6,7). Doses recommended for these indications often exceed the safe limit (2729).
LIKELY INEFFECTIVE ...when taken orally as a single agent for weight loss (3).

There is insufficient reliable information available about the effectiveness of ephedra for its other uses. Although ephedra is frequently marketed in combination with caffeine products for weight loss, studies to date have actually used ephedrine and caffeine. Studies have not yet described the herb ephedra plus caffeine for weight loss.

Possible Mechanism of Action & Active Ingredients

The applicable part of ephedra is primarily the dried, young branch. Less commonly, the root or whole plant is used (11,13,18). Ephedra found in dietary supplements is usually either a formulation of powdered stems and aerial portions or a dried extract. Dried extracts contain more ephedra alkaloids per unit weight of material, due to the extraction process. The principle alkaloid constituents are ephedrine and pseudoephedrine. Ephedrine is absorbed faster if it is consumed as the powdered extract. However, onset of action and extent of absorption does not differ greatly between the powdered extract and the powdered herb (6008,6009). Ephedrine and pseudoephedrine can directly and indirectly stimulate the sympathetic nervous system (2,3,6,7,9), increasing systolic and diastolic blood pressure (3,11,18), increasing heart rate (3,6,11), causing peripheral vasoconstriction, bronchodilation (3,6,7,11), and central nervous system stimulation (2,3,7,11). Ephedrine shows antitussive (2,7), bacteriostatic (2), and anti-inflammatory (6,11) activity in animals. Ephedrine can have diuretic, hypoglycemic, and hyperglycemic effects. It can stimulate uterine contraction, and theoretically can be catabolized to mutagenic nitrosamines (6,11). Ephedrine causes relaxation of the smooth muscle in the gastrointestinal tract, urinary retention by relaxing the detrusor muscle, and diminishes contraction of the bladder sphincter (11,15). The above ground parts of ephedra can cause sweating, but the root inhibits perspiration (11).

Adverse Reactions Including Known Allergies

Ephedra taken orally can cause dizziness, motor restlessness, anxiety, irritability, insomnia, headache, anorexia, nausea, vomiting, flushing, tingling, difficulty urinating, tachycardia, heart palpitations, hyperthermia, drastic increase in blood pressure, heart failure, asphyxia, and death (2,6,7,13,18,1276,6008). Reports associate the use of botanical sources of ephedrine, including ephedra, with myopathies, including myalgia, cardiomyopathy, rhabdomyolysis, eosinophilia-myalgia syndrome (1270), and hypersensitivity myocarditis (1271). Botanical sources of ephedrine has also be associated with nephrolithiasis (1272), acute hepatitis (1273), psychosis (1276), and sudden death (1274). Between 1993 and late 1998, 685 voluntary reports were filed with the FDA involving adverse effects associated with the use of ephedra-containing products, including jitteriness, insomnia, addiction, chest tightness, hypertension, cardiac arrest, brain hemorrhage, seizures, stroke, and 39 fatalities (1381). The FDA reports that ephedra doses which exceed 8 mg of ephedrine every six hours or 24 mg per day, or use of ephedra longer than seven days, has been associated with myocardial infarction, seizures, stroke, and death (2729); however, this is controversial.

Combining ephedra with caffeine or caffeine-containing herbs increases the risk of adverse effects (2729). One unpublished report associated jitteriness, hypertension, seizures, temporary loss of consciousness, and hospitalization requiring life support with the use of a combination ephedra and the caffeine-containing guarana product (1380). There is one report of ischemic stroke in an athlete who consumed ephedra 40-60 mg, creatine monohydrate 6 grams, caffeine 400-600 mg, and a variety of other supplements daily for six weeks (1275).

Possible Interactions with Herbs & Other Dietary Supplements

CAFFEINE: Concomitant use can increase the risk of stimulatory adverse effects (7). One unpublished report associated jitteriness, hypertension, seizures, temporary loss of consciousness, and hospitalization requiring life support with the use of a combination ephedra and guarana (caffeine) product (1380).

COFFEE: Concomitant use might increase the risk of stimulatory adverse effects, due to the caffeine content of coffee (7). One unpublished report associated jitteriness, hypertension, seizures, temporary loss of consciousness, and hospitalization requiring life support with the use of a combination ephedra and guarana (caffeine) product (1380).

COLA NUT: Concomitant use might increase the risk of stimulatory adverse effects, due to the caffeine content of guarana (7). One unpublished report associated jitteriness, hypertension, seizures, temporary loss of consciousness, and hospitalization requiring life support with the use of a combination ephedra and guarana (caffeine) product (1380).

GUARANA: Concomitant use can increase the risk of stimulatory adverse effects (7). One unpublished report associated jitteriness, hypertension, seizures, temporary loss of consciousness, and hospitalization requiring life support with the use of a combination ephedra and guarana (caffeine) product (1380).

MATE: Concomitant use might increase the risk of stimulatory adverse effects, due to the caffeine content of maté (7). One unpublished report associated jitteriness, hypertension, seizures, temporary loss of consciousness, and hospitalization requiring life support with the use of a combination ephedra and guarana (caffeine) product (1380).

DIGITALIS: Theoretically, co-administration of ephedra with digitalis might cause cardiac arrhythmias (2).

SECALE ALKALOID DERIVATIVES (Ergot): Theoretically, concomitant use might cause hypertension (2).

Possible Interactions with Drugs

AMITRIPTYLINE (Elavil): Theoretically, concomitant use might reduce the hypertensive effects of the ephedrine contained in ephedra. Amitriptyline blocks the hypertensive effects of ephedrine (19).

CAFFEINE: Concomitant use can increase the risk of stimulatory adverse effects of ephedra and caffeine (7,19), enhance thermogenesis and weight loss (19). An unpublished report associated jitteriness, hypertension, seizures, temporary loss of consciousness, and hospitalization requiring life support with the use of an ephedra/caffeine product (1380).

DEXAMETHASONE (Decadron): Theoretically, concomitant use might reduce the effectiveness of dexamethasone, due to the ephedrine contained in ephedra. Ephedrine increases the clearance rate of dexamethasone (19).

DIABETES DRUGS: Ephedra can raise blood glucose levels and interfere with diabetes drug therapy. Monitor blood glucose concentrations closely (19).

DIGOXIN (Lanoxin): Theoretically, concomitant use might cause cardiac arrhythmias (2).

ERGOTAMINE (Migranol, D.H.E. 45, Ergomar): Theoretically, concomitant use of ephedra and ergot alkaloids might cause hypertension, due to the ephedrine contained in ephedra (2).

MONOAMINE OXIDASE INHIBITORS (MAOIs): Contraindicated; concomitant use of ephedra with MAOIs might increase the risk of hypertension (15). A hypertensive crisis and subarachnoid hemorrhage were reported after a patient took a 50 mg dose of ephedrine and an MAOI drug (15).

OXYTOCIN: Theoretically, concomitant use might cause hypertension (2).

RESERPINE: Theoretically, concomitant use might antagonize the indirect sympathomimetic effects of the ephedrine contained in ephedra (19).

THEOPHYLLINE: Theoretically, concomitant use might increase the risk of stimulatory adverse effects of theophylline and ephedrine (contained in ephedra) (7,19).

URINARY ACIDIFIERS: Theoretically, concomitant use of ephedra and urinary acidifying drugs might reduce the ephedrine-related effects of ephedra. Urinary acidifying drugs increase ephedrine excretion (19).

URINARY ALKALINIZERS: Theoretically, concomitant use of ephedra and urinary alkalinizing drugs might increase the ephedrine-related effects of ephedra. Urinary alkalinizing drugs reduce ephedrine excretion (19).

Possible Interactions with Foods

COFFEE, TEA: Theoretically, concomitant use of large amounts of caffeinated coffee or tea might increase the stimulatory effects and adverse effects of caffeine and the ephedrine contained in ephedra.

Possible Interactions with Lab Tests

EPHEDRINE: Ephedra can cause a positive urine ephedrine test due to its ephedrine content. A case of an athlete whose urine tested positive for norpseudoephedrine was attributed to the use of an herbal supplement labeled to contain ephedra. However, the product might also have contained added norpseudoephedrine as an unlabeled ingredient (1259).

GLUCOSE: Ephedra might increase blood glucose levels and test results (19).

AMPHETAMINE, METHAMPHETAMINE: Ephedra might cause false-positive urine amphetamine or methamphetamine test results. One unpublished case involved a false-positive urine methamphetamine assay in a woman who experienced life-threatening adverse effects associated with the use of an ephedra/guarana product (1381).

Possible Interactions with Diseases or Conditions

ANGINA: Contraindicated; ephedra might induce or exacerbate angina due its cardiac stimulant effects (15,512).

ANOREXIA: Contraindicated due to the purported appetite suppressant effects of ephedra. Anorexic patients might be at increased risk for the adverse effects of ephedra due to inadequate nutritional status (12,19).

ANXIETY: Large doses of ephedra might cause or exacerbate anxiety due to its CNS stimulant effects (2,12,15,512).

BULIMIA: Contraindicated; bulimic patients might be at increased risk for the adverse effects of ephedra due to inadequate nutritional status (12,19).

BENIGN PROSTATIC HYPERTROPHY (BPH): Ephedra might exacerbate urinary retention in patients with BPH due its effects on the detrusor muscle (15,512).

CEREBRAL INSUFFICIENCY: Contraindicated; ephedra might further decrease cerebral blood flow due to its vasoconstrictive effects (2,12,512).

DIABETES: Ephedra might interfere with blood sugar control, and exacerbate high blood pressure and circulatory problems in people with diabetes (15,19,512).

ESSENTIAL TREMOR: Ephedra might exacerbate tremor (1715).

NARROW-ANGLE GLAUCOMA: Ephedra might exacerbate narrow-angle (angle-closure) glaucoma by causing mydriasis (2,12,15,512).

HEART DISEASE: Contraindicated; ephedra might cause tachycardia, arrhythmias, or induce angina in patients with heart disease due to its cardiac stimulant effects (15,512).

HYPERTHYROID, THYROTOXICOSIS: Contraindicated; ephedra might stimulate the thyroid and exacerbate hyperthyroid symptoms (2,12,15,512).

HYPERTENSION: Ephedra might exacerbate hypertension (2,12,15,512); contraindicated in uncontrolled hypertension.

KIDNEY STONES: Ephedra and ephedrine can cause kidney stones (1272).

MYASTHENIA GRAVIS: Large doses of ephedra might increase muscle strength in patients with myasthenia gravis (15).

PHEOCHROMOCYTOMA: Contraindicated; ephedra might exacerbate the symptoms of pheochromocytoma (2).

URINARY RETENTION: Large doses of ephedra might exacerbate urinary retention due its effects on the detrusor muscle (2,12,15,512).

Typical Dosages & Routes of Administration that are Commonly Used

ORAL: For adults, the typical dose of ephedra is 15-30 mg of the total alkaloids calculated as ephedrine, and the maximum dose recommended by some sources is 300 mg per day (2,7,12). The FDA recommends that ephedra products not be used for longer than seven days and that doses of ephedra should not provide quantities of the constituent ephedrine exceeding 8 mg every six hours or 24 mg per day. Use for longer periods of time and in doses providing greater amounts of ephedrine has been associated with severe, life threatening adverse reactions. One cup of the tea is commonly taken three times per day. The tea is prepared by steeping 1-4 grams in 150 mL boiling water for 5-10 minutes and then straining (18). The tincture (1:1) is usually given as 5 grams per dose (18). Another tincture (1:4) is given 6-8 mL three times per day (18). The typical dose of the extract is 1-3 mL three times per day (18). For children over the age of six, the usual dose is 0.5 mg/kg up to a maximum of 2 mg/kg per day (2,7,12).

Comments

Avoid confusion with Mormon tea (American ephedra, Ephedra nevadensis). Mormon tea is alkaloid-free and lacks both the therapeutic effects and the toxicity of ephedrine (3,12).

In one study of ephedra preparations there were considerable variances in the alkaloid content of marketed products. The inconsistencies occurred among different brands and within different lots of the same brand. There were also discrepancies with the actual alkaloid content and what is stated on the product label (6008). Several organizations are working on guidelines for good manufacturing practices in the supplement industry to help minimize this kind of variation (6008).

In June of 1997, the FDA proposed restrictions on the ephedrine content of dietary supplements, new warning labels for ephedrine alkaloid-containing products, and a prohibition on combination products containing ephedra and other natural stimulants, such as guarana and cola nut, which both contain caffeine (2729). These proposals were dropped after the link between ephedra use and serious adverse effects was challenged by Congress and the supplements industry (1381). The FDA is currently reviewing 273 adverse event reports involving ephedrine alkaloid-containing products, including 134 cases of serious illness or death, with 140 of the reports receiving in-depth clinical review by FDA and outside experts (1381,5047).

The FDA has announced that street drug alternatives marketed as dietary supplements, including those containing ephedrine alkaloids, are unapproved and misbranded drugs subject to seizure and injunction. The FDA does not consider street drug alternatives to be dietary supplements because they are intended for recreational purposes and are not intended to supplement the diet (5047).

EPIMEDIUM

This Product is Also Known As

Barrenwort, Herba Epimedii, Horny Goat Weed, Japanese Epimedium, Xian Ling Pi, Yin Yang Huo.

Scientific Names

Epimedium acuminatum; Epimedium brevicornum; Epimedium grandiflorum; Epimedium koreanum; Epimedium pubescens; Epimedium sagittatum; Epimedium wushanese; and other Epimedium species.
Family: Berberidaceae.

People Use This For

Orally, epimedium is used for impotence, involuntary ejaculation, weak back and knees, arthralgia, mental and physical fatigue, memory loss, hypertension, coronary heart disease, bronchitis, chronic hepatitis, polio, chronic leukopenia (11) and viral myocarditis (1513), and as a tonic and aphrodisiac (11).
Epimedium is included in some personal care products for its antimicrobial effects (11).

Safety

POSSIBLY SAFE ...when preparations of the leaf are taken orally, short-term (12).
POSSIBLY UNSAFE ...when used orally, long-term (12).
LIKELY UNSAFE ...when large amounts are used. Some species can cause respiratory arrest (12).
PREGNANCY AND LACTATION: Insufficient reliable information available; avoid using.

Effectiveness

There is insufficient reliable information available about the effectiveness of epimedium.

Possible Mechanism of Action & Active Ingredients

The applicable part of epimedium is the leaf. Researchers think flavonoids, icariin, and polysaccharides are the active constituents. Some evidence suggests epimedium might cause peripheral vasodilation, increase coronary blood flow, increase platelet aggregation, and improve male sexual function (11). Epimedium also seems to inhibit catecholamine effects. It seems to have some hypotensive, immunomodulating, antimicrobial, anti-inflammatory, antitussive and expectorant effects (11). Evidence suggests epimedium might have activity against HIV (1512).

Adverse Reactions Including Known Allergies

Extended use of Japanese epimedium may result in dizziness, vomiting, dry mouth, thirst, and nosebleed (12). Large doses of Japanese epimedium may cause respiratory arrest and exaggeration of tendon reflexes to the point of spasm (12). There is insufficient reliable information available for other Epimedium species.

Possible Interactions with Herbs & Other Dietary Supplements

Insufficient reliable information available.

Possible Interactions with Drugs

No interactions are known to occur, and there is no known reason to expect a clinically significant interaction with epimedium.

Possible Interactions with Foods

No interactions are known to occur, and there is no known reason to expect a clinically significant interaction with epimedium.

Possible Interactions with Lab Tests

No interactions are known to occur, and there is no known reason to expect a clinically significant interaction with epimedium.

Possible Interactions with Diseases or Conditions

No interactions are known to occur, and there is no known reason to expect a clinically significant interaction with epimedium.

Typical Dosages & Routes of Administration that are Commonly Used

No typical dosage.

Comments

The leaf of Japanese epimedium (Epimedium grandiflora) is generally used (12). Leaf, petiole, and stem of other Epimedium species are also sometimes used (11). As many as 15 Epimedium species are interchangeable as "yin yang huo" (11).

ERGOT

This Product is Also Known As

Cockspur Rye, Hornseed, Mother of Rye, Secale cornutum, Smut Rye, Spurred Rye.

Scientific Names

Plant host: Claviceps purpurea.
Family: Claviciptaceae.

People Use This For

Orally, ergot is used for obstetric and gynecologic conditions, including hemorrhage, climacteric hemorrhage, menorrhagia, metrorrhagia (before and after miscarriage), expulsion of placenta, shortening of afterbirth period, and atonia of the uterus (2,18).

Safety

UNSAFE ...when used orally; contraindicated, due to poisoning risk and interactions with many disease states (2). PREGNANCY AND LACTATION: UNSAFE ...contraindicated, due to high level of risk (2,400).

Effectiveness

POSSIBLY EFFECTIVE ...when taken orally for hemorrhage, climacteric hemorrhage, menorrhagia, metrorrhagia (before and after miscarriage), expulsion of placenta, shortening of afterbirth period, and atonia of the uterus (2,17). However, high level of risk and availability of safer alternatives preclude use (2).

Possible Mechanism of Action & Active Ingredients

Ergot alkaloids produce vasoconstriction, myometrial stimulation and alpha-adrenergic blockade (17).

Adverse Reactions Including Known Allergies

Oral use of ergot can cause nausea, vomiting, leg weakness, myalgia, numbness of fingers, angina, tachycardia, bradycardia, localized edema, and itching (18). Overdose or long-term use can cause thrombosis, damage to blood vessels in the retina, optic atrophy, gangrene of extremities, convulsions, and hemiplegia (18). The symptoms of acute poisoning are queasiness, vomiting, diarrhea, thirst, skin coolness, itching of skin, rapid weak pulse, paresthesia, extremity numbness, confusion, and unconsciousness (18). The symptoms of chronic poisoning are ergotismus gangrenosus (painful blood flow disorders of the extremities with dry gangrene, angina, aphasia, visual field loss) (18) and ergotismus convulsivus (muscle twitching, followed by clonic spasms, tonic spasms, hemiplegia, loss of consciousness, death) (18).

Possible Interactions with Herbs & Other Dietary Supplements
Insufficient reliable information available.

Possible Interactions with Drugs
ERGOT ALKALOIDS: Co-administration increases risk of adverse effects, avoid.
SYMPATHOMIMETICS: Co-administration may increase risk of adverse effects (17).

Possible Interactions with Foods
No interactions are known to occur, and there is no known reason to expect a clinically significant interaction with ergot.

Possible Interactions with Lab Tests
No interactions are known to occur, and there is no known reason to expect a clinically significant interaction with ergot.

Possible Interactions with Diseases or Conditions
CONTRAINDICATIONS: Raynaud's disease, thromboangitis obliterans, severe arteriosclerotic vascular changes, liver function disorders, coronary insufficiency, kidney disease, infectious disease, sepsis, hypotonia, and hypertonia (18).

Typical Dosages & Routes of Administration that are Commonly Used
No typical dosage.

Comments
Ergot is considered unsafe; avoid using. Ergot is dried fungal growth that occurs on rye (Claviceps purpurea). Alternatives include FDA-approved ergot alkaloid drug products (standardized potency and purity). These prescription drugs show far less toxicity and the same or higher specific effectiveness (2).

ERYNGO above ground parts

This Product is Also Known As
Eringo, Eryngii Herba, Sea Holly, Sea Holme, Sea Hulver.
CAUTION: See separate listing for Eryngo root.

Scientific Names
Eryngium campestre (18), synonyms Eryngium maritinum, Eyrnigium planum, Eryngium yuccifolium.
Family: Apiaceae (12).

People Use This For
Orally, people use eryngo for urinary tract infections, inflammation of the urinary tract, prostatitis, and mucous membrane inflammation of the bronchi (18).

Safety
There is insufficient reliable information available about the safety of eryngo.
Pregnancy and Lactation: Insufficient reliable information available; avoid using.

Effectiveness
There is insufficient reliable information about the effectiveness of eryngo.

Possible Mechanism of Action & Active Ingredients
Eryngo is stated to have a diuretic effect (18).

Adverse Reactions Including Known Allergies
None reported.

Possible Interactions with Herbs & Other Dietary Supplements
Insufficient reliable information available.

Possible Interactions with Drugs
No interactions are known to occur, and there is no known reason to expect a clinically significant interaction with eryngo above ground parts.

Possible Interactions with Foods
No interactions are known to occur, and there is no known reason to expect a clinically significant interaction with eryngo above ground parts.

Possible Interactions with Lab Tests
No interactions are known to occur, and there is no known reason to expect a clinically significant interaction with eryngo above ground parts.

Possible Interactions with Diseases or Conditions

No interactions are known to occur, and there is no known reason to expect a clinically significant interaction with eryngo above ground parts.

Typical Dosages & Routes of Administration that are Commonly Used

ORAL: Administered as an extract (amount used unspecified) (18).

Comments

None.

ERYNGO root

This Product is Also Known As

Eringo, Eryngii Radix, Sea Holly, Sea Holme, Sea Hulver.
CAUTION: See separate listing for Eryngo above ground parts.

Scientific Names

Eryngium campestre, synonyms Eryngium maritinum, Eyrnigium planum, Eryngium yuccifolium.
Family: Apiaceae.

People Use This For

Orally, eryngo is used for kidney and bladder stones, renal colic, kidney and urinary tract inflammation, urinary retention, edema, coughs, bronchitis, and skin and respiratory disorders (18).

Safety

POSSIBLY SAFE ...when used orally and appropriately (12).
PREGNANCY AND LACTATION: Insufficient reliable information available; avoid using.

Effectiveness

There is insufficient reliable information about the effectiveness of eryngo.

Possible Mechanism of Action & Active Ingredients

Eryngo root is reported to have mild expectorant and antispasmodic properties (18).

Adverse Reactions Including Known Allergies

None reported.

Possible Interactions with Herbs & Other Dietary Supplements

Insufficient reliable information available.

Possible Interactions with Drugs

No interactions are known to occur, and there is no known reason to expect a clinically significant interaction with eryngo root.

Possible Interactions with Foods

No interactions are known to occur, and there is no known reason to expect a clinically significant interaction with eryngo root.

Possible Interactions with Lab Tests

No interactions are known to occur, and there is no known reason to expect a clinically significant interaction with eryngo root.

Possible Interactions with Diseases or Conditions

No interactions are known to occur, and there is no known reason to expect a clinically significant interaction with eryngo root.

Typical Dosages & Routes of Administration that are Commonly Used

ORAL: Three to four cups tea (steep until cold 1 teaspoon ground root in 150 mL of boiling water; strain) daily (18). Alternatively, 2-3 cups decoction (boil 4 teaspoons of ground root in 1 L water for 10 minutes, steep for 15 minutes, strain) daily (18); or 50-60 drops tincture (soak 20 grams powdered root in 80 grams of 60% alcohol for 10 days) divided into 3 or 4 doses daily.

Comments

None.

EUCALYPTUS dried leaf

This Product is Also Known As
Blue Gum, Eucalypti Folium, Eucalyptusblatter, Fever Tree, Fevertree, Fieberbaumblatter, Gum Tree, Red Gum, Stringy Bark Tree, Tasmanian Blue Gum.
CAUTION: See separate listing for Eucalyptus Oil.

Scientific Names
Eucalyptus globulus; Eucalyptus smithii; Eucalyptus fructicetorum, synonym Eucalyptus polybractea.
Family: Myrtaceae.

People Use This For
Orally, dried eucalyptus leaf is taken as an antiseptic, antipyretic, expectorant [4], stimulant in respiratory ailments [11], and for treating respiratory tract mucous membrane inflammation [2].
In Chinese medicine the leaf has been used for aching joints, bacterial dysentery, ringworms, and pulmonary tuberculosis [11].
In folk medicine, eucalyptus has been used for asthma, acne, bleeding gums, bladder diseases, diabetes, fever, flu, gonorrhea, liver and gallbladder complaints, loss of appetite, neuralgia, poorly healing ulcers, rheumatism, stomatitis, whooping cough, wounds, as a gastrointestinal remedy [18], for burns, and cancer [11].
In foods, eucalyptus is used as a flavoring agent [4,11].

Safety
POSSIBLY SAFE ...when the dried leaf is used orally and appropriately [12]. ...when preparations of the dried leaf are used topically.
LIKELY UNSAFE ...when used orally by individuals with inflammatory diseases of the bile ducts, GI tract, or severe liver disease [12].
CHILDREN: LIKELY UNSAFE ...when applied topically to the face or in the nose of infants and young children [2,12]. Can cause bronchospasm. There is insufficient reliable information available about the safety of oral use; avoid using in young children.
PREGNANCY AND LACTATION: Insufficient reliable information available; avoid using [4].

Effectiveness
POSSIBLY EFFECTIVE ...when taken orally for respiratory tract mucous membrane inflammation [2]. ...when used as an expectorant, and depending on the species, the product must contain 70-85% eucalyptol or cineole [3]. There is insufficient reliable information available about the effectiveness of dried eucalyptus leaf for its other uses.

Possible Mechanism of Action & Active Ingredients
The leaf can have secretion-stimulating, expectorant, antiseptic, and weakly antispasmodic properties [2,4]. The antiseptic and expectorant properties of the leaf are due to its volatile oils, particularly eucalyptol [4]. Other evidence suggests eucalyptus can be a urinary irritant [19].

Adverse Reactions Including Known Allergies
Taken orally, the eucalyptus leaf rarely can cause nausea, vomiting, and diarrhea [2]. Signs of eucalyptus poisoning include epigastric burning, nausea, vomiting, diarrhea, dizziness, muscular weakness, miosis, feeling of suffocation, cyanosis, delirium, convulsions, and death [4]. The ingestion of 3.5 mL of the eucalyptus oil can be fatal [11].

Possible Interactions with Herbs & Other Dietary Supplements
Insufficient reliable information available.

Possible Interactions with Drugs
HYPOGLYCEMIC DRUGS: Eucalyptus can interfere with blood sugar control [4].
HEPATICALLY METABOLIZED DRUGS: Eucalyptus oil induces liver enzymes which can reduce the activity of drugs metabolized by the liver [2].

Possible Interactions with Foods
No interactions are known to occur, and there is no known reason to expect a clinically significant interaction with eucalyptus dried leaf.

Possible Interactions with Lab Tests
No interactions are known to occur, and there is no known reason to expect a clinically significant interaction with eucalyptus dried leaf.

Possible Interactions with Diseases or Conditions
Contraindicated in cases of GI tract and bile duct inflammation, liver disease [2], hypotension, and kidney inflammation [500].
DIABETES: Theoretically, eucalyptus can interfere with blood glucose control [4].

Typical Dosages & Routes of Administration that are Commonly Used

ORAL: The typical dose of the eucalyptus leaf is one cup of the freshly prepared tea three times daily (3). The tea is made by steeping 2 grams of the dried leaf in 150 mL boiling water and then straining. Limit the daily intake to 4-6 grams per day of the dried leaf or equivalent preparations (2). The usual dose of the tincture is 3-9 grams per day (2), and the fluid extract is dosed 2-4 grams per day (4).

Comments

None.

EUCALYPTUS OIL

This Product is Also Known As

None.
CAUTION: See separate listing for Eucalyptus dried leaf.

Scientific Names

Eucalyptus globulus; Eucalyptus fructicetorum, synonym Eucalyptus polybractea; Eucalyptus smithii.
Family: Myrtaceae.

People Use This For

Orally, eucalyptus oil is taken for inflammation of respiratory tract mucous membranes (2), for suppressing coughs (3), as an expectorant (11), as cough drops, and as gum lozenges (7).
Topically, eucalyptus oil is used for inflammation of respiratory tract mucous membranes, rheumatic complaints (2), nasal stuffiness (7), as a mouthwash (11), antiseptic liniments, ointments, and in toothpaste (11). Traditionally, eucalyptus oil has been used as an antiseptic and antipyretic, for wounds, burns, ulcers, cancer, and in vaporizer fluids (11).
In dentistry, eucalyptus oil is a component of sealers and solvents for root canal fillings (11).
In manufacturing, eucalyptus oil is utilized as a flavoring and a fragrance component in perfumes (11).

Safety

LIKELY SAFE ...when the oil is consumed in amounts commonly found in foods. Eucalyptus oil is approved for food use in the US (11). Eucalyptol is listed as a synthetic flavoring agent. The maximum level used in food is 0.002% (11).
POSSIBLY SAFE ...when used orally and appropriately for medicinal purposes (2,12). It must be used in very small amounts or diluted (2,12).
POSSIBLY UNSAFE ...when the undiluted oil is used topically (4).
LIKELY UNSAFE ...when undiluted oil is ingested orally. Ingesting 3.5 mL of undiluted oil can be fatal (4).
CHILDREN: LIKELY UNSAFE ...when the oil is used topically on the face, especially the nose, of infants and young children (2) because it can cause bronchospasm. ...when the oil is used orally(4).
PREGNANCY: LIKELY SAFE ...when used orally, but only in food amounts. LIKELY UNSAFE ...when used in larger amounts; contraindicated (4).
LACTATION: Insufficient reliable information available; avoid using in amounts greater than found in foods (4).

Effectiveness

POSSIBLY EFFECTIVE ...when taken orally for inflammation of respiratory tract mucous membranes (2). ...when applied topically for inflammation of respiratory tract mucous membranes (2) and rheumatic complaints (2).
There is insufficient reliable information available about the effectiveness of eucalyptus oil for its other uses.

Possible Mechanism of Action & Active Ingredients

Eucalyptus oil contains 70-85% eucalyptol (1,8-cineole) that stimulates production and secretion of saliva (11). This, in turn, activates the swallowing reflex. Voluntary swallowing can suppress an impending cough (7). Taken by mouth, eucalyptus oil aids in expectorating secretions (2,4), has mild antibacterial action (4), and is mildly antispasmodic (2). In vitro, it has antibacterial and fungicidal effects. Topically, it acts as mild counterirritant (2) and inhibits prostaglandin biosynthesis (18). The crude eucalyptus leaf extract has demonstrated hypoglycemic activity in rabbits (4). Eucalyptus can be a urinary irritant (19).

Adverse Reactions Including Known Allergies

Taken orally, eucalyptus oil can cause nausea, vomiting, and diarrhea (2). Signs of eucalyptus poisoning include epigastric burning, nausea, vomiting, dizziness, muscular weakness, constricted pupils of eyes, feeling of suffocation, cyanosis, delirium, and convulsions. The ingestion of 3.5 mL of the oil can be fatal (4).

Possible Interactions with Herbs & Other Dietary Supplements

PYRROLIZIDINE ALKALOID CONTAINING PLANTS: Eucalyptus can potentiate the toxicity of borage, coltsfoot, comfrey, hound's tooth, and Senecio species (500).

Possible Interactions with Drugs
DIABETES DRUGS: Theoretically, concomitant use of eucalyptus oil can interfere with blood sugar control (4).
HEPATICALLY METABOLIZED DRUGS: Eucalyptus oil induces liver enzymes and, theoretically, can alter the effects of drugs metabolized by the liver (2).

Possible Interactions with Foods
No interactions are known to occur, and there is no known reason to expect a clinically significant interaction with eucalyptus oil.

Possible Interactions with Lab Tests
No interactions are known to occur, and there is no known reason to expect a clinically significant interaction with eucalyptus oil.

Possible Interactions with Diseases or Conditions
DIABETES: Theoretically, eucalyptus oil can interfere with blood sugar control (4).
OTHER CONDITIONS: It is contraindicated in cases of GI tract and bile duct inflammation, severe liver disease (2), hypotension, kidney inflammation, or low blood pressure (500).

Typical Dosages & Routes of Administration that are Commonly Used
ORAL: The typical dose is 300-600 mg of the eucalyptus oil per day (2), and about 0.05-0.2 mL per dose (4).
TOPICAL: Semi-solid or vegetable oil preparations usually contain 5%-20% eucalyptus oil (2,4), and aqueous-alcoholic preparations contain 5%-10% eucalyptus oil (2). The oil is also typically used for local application by diluting 30 mL oil to 500 mL lukewarm water (4). Avoid the use of the undiluted essential oil. The essential oil diluted in vegetable oil is preferred for applications on the skin (4). Avoid use on areas of the face, especially the nose, of infants and young children (2).

Comments
Eucalyptus oil is the steam distilled volatile oil from fresh leaves and branch tops of various species of Eucalyptus.

EUPHORBIA

This Product is Also Known As
Pillbearing Spurge, Snakeweed.

Scientific Names
Euphorbia hirta, synonym Euphorbia capitata; Euphorbia pilulifera.
Family: Euphorbiaceae.

People Use This For
Orally, euphorbia is used for respiratory disorders including asthma, bronchitis, catarrh, laryngeal spasm (4), hay fever, and tumors (11), as an expectorant and an emetic (12). It is also used orally for treating worms, dysentery, gonorrhea, and digestive problems in India (11).

Safety
There is insufficient reliable information available about the safety of euphorbia. In Australia this label has been recommended "Warning: Do not exceed the stated dose" (12).
PREGNANCY AND LACTATION: POSSIBLY UNSAFE; avoid using. Euphorbia is reported to cause smooth muscle contraction and relaxation (4).

Effectiveness
There is insufficient reliable information available about the effectiveness of euphorbia.

Possible Mechanism of Action & Active Ingredients
The applicable parts of euphorbia are the above ground parts. Reported to have antispasmodic, histamine potentiator, antitumor, and antibacterial activity against gram positive and gram negative organisms in animals(4). Constituent, choline, is reported to produce contraction of isolated pig ileum; constituent, shikimic acid, to produce relaxation (11).

Adverse Reactions Including Known Allergies
Euphorbia taken orally may cause nausea and vomiting (12). Skin contact with fresh euphorbia can cause irritation or contact dermatitis (19).

Possible Interactions with Herbs & Other Dietary Supplements
Insufficient reliable information available.

Possible Interactions with Drugs
No interactions are known to occur, and there is no known reason to expect a clinically significant interaction with euphorbia.

Possible Interactions with Foods

No interactions are known to occur, and there is no known reason to expect a clinically significant interaction with euphorbia.

Possible Interactions with Lab Tests

No interactions are known to occur, and there is no known reason to expect a clinically significant interaction with euphorbia.

Possible Interactions with Diseases or Conditions

GI CONDITIONS: Can irritate the gastrointestinal tract. Contraindicated in individuals with infectious or inflammatory gastrointestinal conditions (19).

Typical Dosages & Routes of Administration that are Commonly Used

ORAL: 120-300 mg above ground parts (4), or one cup tea (steep 120-300 mg above ground parts in 150 mL boiling water 5-10 minutes, strain) (4). Liquid extract (concentration unspecified), 0.12-0.3 mL (4). Tincture (concentration unspecified), 0.6-2 mL. (4). For use as an expectorant, 2 grams above ground parts; emetic dose may be similar (12).

Comments

None.

EUROPEAN BARBERRY

This Product is Also Known As

Agracejo, Berberidis cortex, Berberidis fructus, Berberidis radicis cortex, Berberidis radix, Berberitze, Berberry, Berbis, Common Barberry, Épine-Vinette, Espino Cambrón, Jaundice Berry, Mountain Grape, Oregon Grape, Pipperidge, Piprage, Sauerdorn, Sow Berry, Vinettier.
CAUTION: See separate listing for Oregon Grape.

Scientific Names

Berberis vulgaris.
Family: Berberidaceae.

People Use This For

Orally, the fruit of European barberry is used for kidney, urinary tract and gastrointestinal tract discomforts such as heartburn, stomach cramps, constipation and lack of appetite, liver and spleen disease, for bronchial and lung discomforts, spasms, as a stimulant for circulation, for people susceptible to infection, and as a supplemental source of vitamin C (2,18). The bark, root, and root bark of European barberry are used orally for ailments and complaints of the GI tract, liver, gallbladder, kidney and urinary tract, respiratory tract, heart/circulatory system, as an antipyretic, "blood purifier" (2), and for narcotic withdrawal (18).
In folk medicine, European barberry root bark has been used for liver dysfunction, gallbladder disease, jaundice, splenopathy, diarrhea, indigestion, hemorrhoids, renal and urinary tract diseases, gout, rheumatism, arthritis, mid and low back pain, malaria, and leishmaniasis (18).
European barberry fruit is used in making jam, jellies, and wine (18).
In manufacturing, the fruit syrup is used for masking tastes in pharmaceutical preparations (18).

Safety

LIKELY SAFE ...when the fruit is consumed in food amounts. The fruit is considered to contain only trace amounts of berberine (2,12,18).
POSSIBLY SAFE ...when the fruit, the root, bark, or root bark are used orally and appropriately for medicinal uses. Amounts of less than 500 mg of berberine are usually considered safe (2,12,18).
LIKELY UNSAFE ...when more than 500 mg of berberine consumed. Berberine is considered moderately toxic (12). The LD50 in humans is reported to be 27.5 mg/kg (12).
PREGNANCY: LIKELY UNSAFE ...European barberry is contraindicated because it can have uterine stimulant properties (11,12).
LACTATION: Insufficient reliable information is available; avoid using.

Effectiveness

There is insufficient reliable information available about the effectiveness of European barberry.

Possible Mechanism of Action & Active Ingredients

The applicable parts of European barberry are the bark, fruit, root, and root bark. European barberry fruit contains vitamin C (18). Researchers think it has mild diuretic activity due to the acid content (18). The bark, root, and root bark of European barberry contain isoquinolone alkaloid constituents, including berberine, berbamine, columbamine, jatorrhizine, palmatine, and oxyacanthine (11,19). The constituents berberine, columbamine, and oxyacanthine show evidence of antibacterial activity (11). Berberine has anticonvulsant, sedative, hypotensive, antifibrillatory, and bile-stimulating effects. In low doses, it is a cardiac and respiratory stimulant. In high doses it is a depressant (11,12,515). Some evidence suggests berberine sulfate might be amebicidal and trypanocidal (11). Other information suggests the constituent berbamine might have antiarrhythmic, hypotensive, spasmolytic, and immunostimulating activity (11,515).

Adverse Reactions Including Known Allergies
Ingestion of greater than 500 mg berberine, which is found in European barberry, can cause lethargy, nose bleed, skin and eye irritation, nephritis and kidney irritation (2). It might also cause dyspnea, hypotension, cardiac damage (12), nausea, vomiting, diarrhea, hemorrhagic nephritis, respiratory spasms and arrest, and death (2).

Possible Interactions with Herbs & Other Dietary Supplements
BERBERINE-CONTAINING HERBS: Concomitant use can increase the risk of berberine toxicity. Berberine-containing herbs include: bloodroot, goldenseal, celandine, Chinese goldthread, goldthread, Oregon grape (Mahonia species), amur cork tree, and Chinese corktree (12).

Possible Interactions with Drugs
No interactions are known to occur, and there is no known reason to expect a clinically significant interaction with European barberry.

Possible Interactions with Foods
No interactions are known to occur, and there is no known reason to expect a clinically significant interaction with European barberry.

Possible Interactions with Lab Tests
No interactions are known to occur, and there is no known reason to expect a clinically significant interaction with European barberry.

Possible Interactions with Diseases or Conditions
KIDNEY DISEASE: Berberine, which is found in European barberry, can cause kidney irritation and nephritis (2). GI IRRITATION: Can irritate gastrointestinal tract. Contraindicated in individuals with infectious or inflammatory gastrointestinal conditions (19).

Typical Dosages & Routes of Administration that are Commonly Used
ORAL : A typical dose of fruit is one cup tea. To make tea, steep 1-2 teaspoons of whole or squashed berries in 150 mL boiling water 10-15 minutes and strain (18). A typical dose of root bark is one cup of tea, sipped. To make tea, steep 2 grams of root bark in 250 mL boiling water 5-10 minutes and strain (18). Root bark is typically used as a tincture (1:10), 20-40 drops per day (18). Root tea is not recommended (2,18).

Comments
None.

EUROPEAN BUCKTHORN

This Product is Also Known As
Buckthorn berry, Hartshorn, Highwaythorn, Kreuzdornbeeren, Ramsthorn, Rhamni cathartica fructus, Waythorn. CAUTION: See separate listings for Alder Buckthorn, Sea Buckthorn, and Cascara (California Buckthorn).

Scientific Names
Rhamnus catharticus.
Family: Rhamnaceae.

People Use This For
Orally, European buckthorn is used for constipation (2,18).

Safety
POSSIBLY SAFE ...when the standardized preparations of the berry are used orally and appropriately for less than eight to ten days (12). It is important not to exceed recommended amounts (12).
POSSIBLY UNSAFE ...when standardized preparations are used more than ten days (12).
LIKELY UNSAFE ...when nonstandardized preparations are used orally (2,12).
CHILDREN: LIKELY UNSAFE ...contraindicated in children younger than 12 years of age (2,12).
PREGNANCY AND LACTATION: LIKELY UNSAFE ...contraindicated (2,12).

Effectiveness
LIKELY EFFECTIVE ...when taken orally as a stimulant laxative for constipation (2,3,4,7,12) and is comparable to the gentle, laxative effects of cascara (3).

Possible Mechanism of Action & Active Ingredients

The applicable part of European buckthorn is the berry. The anthraquinones in the European buckthorn berry can increase intestinal GI motility by inhibiting stationary contractions and stimulating propulsive contractions (2). Stimulation of active chloride secretion increases the water and electrolytes in intestinal contents, increasing the risk of electrolyte loss with overuse or misuse of the berry (2). Anthroid laxative use is not associated with an increased risk of developing colorectal ademoma or carcinoma (6138).

Adverse Reactions Including Known Allergies

European buckthorn used orally can cause abdominal pain, cramps, or watery diarrhea (12). Chronic use or abuse of the berry can lead to potassium depletion, albuminuria, and hematuria. Potassium depletion can lead to disturbed heart function and muscle weakness (2). Chronic use can cause pseudomelanosis coli (pigment spots in intestinal mucosa) which is harmless, usually reverses with discontinuation (2), and is not associated with an increased risk of developing colorectal ademoma or carcinoma (6138).

Possible Interactions with Herbs & Other Dietary Supplements

STIMULANT LAXATIVE HERBS: Theoretically, concomitant use of European buckthorn with other stimulant laxative herbs can increase the risk of potassium depletion. Stimulant laxative herbs include aloe dried leaf sap, wild cucumber fruit (Ecballium elaterium), blue flag rhizome, alder buckthorn, butternut bark, cascara bark, castor oil, colocynth fruit pulp, gamboge bark exudate, jalap root, black root, manna bark exudate, podophyllum root, rhubarb root, senna leaves and pods, and yellow dock root (19).
HORSETAIL/LICORICE: Theoretically, concomitant use of the berry with horsetail plant or licorice rhizome increases the risk of potassium depletion (19).
CARDIAC GLYCOSIDE-CONTAINING HERBS: Theoretically, overuse or abuse of European buckthorn can increase the risk of cardiac glycoside toxicity. Cardiac glycoside containing herbs include black hellebore, Canadian hemp roots, digitalis leaf, hedge mustard, figwort, lily of the valley root, motherwort, oleander leaf, pheasant's eye plant, pleurisy root, squill bulb leaf scales, and strophanthus seeds (2,18,19,500).

Possible Interactions with Drugs

ORAL DRUGS: European buckthorn can decrease bowel transit time, reducing absorption of oral drugs (19).
CARDIAC GLYCOSIDE DRUGS: Theoretically, the overuse or abuse of European buckthorn increases the risk of adverse effects from cardiac glycoside drugs, like digoxin (Lanoxin).
DIURETICS: Concomitant use with potassium-depleting diuretics might result in hypokalemia (19).

Possible Interactions with Foods

No interactions are known to occur, and there is no known reason to expect a clinically significant interaction with European buckthorn.

Possible Interactions with Lab Tests

COLORIMETRIC TESTS: European buckthorn can discolor urine (pink, red, purple, orange, rust), interfering with diagnostic tests that depend on a color change, due to its anthraquinone content (12,275).
POTASSIUM: Excessive use of European buckthorn can cause potassium depletion, reducing serum potassium concentrations and test results (2,12,19).

Possible Interactions with Diseases or Conditions

GI CONDITIONS: European buckthorn is contraindicated in individuals with intestinal obstruction, abdominal pain of unknown origin, and intestinal inflammation, including appendicitis, Crohn's disease, irritable bowel syndrome, and ulcerative colitis (2,12).

Typical Dosages & Routes of Administration that are Commonly Used

ORAL: The typical dose of the European buckthorn berry is 20-30 mg of the hydroxyanthracene derivative per day calculated as glucofrangulin A (2). One cup of the tea is commonly taken in the evening, and if needed, in the morning and afternoon (8,12). The tea is prepared by steeping 2-4 grams of the fruit in 150 mL boiling water for 10-15 minutes and then straining (8,12). Use the smallest amount necessary to achieve a soft stool (2) and discontinue in the event of diarrhea or watery stools (12). Limit the use of European buckthorn to a maximum of eight to ten days (12). This preparation should be used only if no effect can be obtained through a change of diet or use of bulk-forming laxative products (2).

Comments

Avoid confusion with alder buckthorn (Rhamus frangula). The American Herbal Products Association (AHPA) recommends the following label statement: "Do not use this product if you have abdominal pain or diarrhea. Consult a health care provider prior to use if you are pregnant or nursing. Discontinue use in the event of diarrhea or watery stools. Do not exceed dose. Not for long-term use." (12). Today, European buckthorn is primarily used as a dye.

EUROPEAN CHESTNUT

This Product is Also Known As
Castaneae Folium, Husked Nut, Jupiter's Nut, Kastanienblaetter, Sardian Nut, Spanish Chestnut, Sweet Chestnut.
CAUTION: See separate listing for American Chestnut leaf.

Scientific Names
Castanea sativa, synonyms Castanea vesca, Castanea vulgaris.
Family: Fagaceae.

People Use This For
Orally, European chestnut is used for respiratory tract complaints including bronchitis and whooping cough, disorders affecting the legs and circulation (2), diarrhea (18), fever, the passage of bloody stools, hydrocele, infection, inflammation, kidney disorders, myalgias, nausea, paroxysm, sclerosis, inflammation of the lymph nodes due to tuberculosis infection, and stomach disorders (4017).
Topically, European chestnut is used as a gargle for sore throat (18) and for wounds (4017).

Safety
POSSIBLY SAFE ...when used orally and appropriately (12).
There is insufficient reliable information available about the safety of the topical use of European chestnut.
PREGNANCY AND LACTATION: Insufficient reliable information available; avoid using.

Effectiveness
There is insufficient reliable information available about the effectiveness of European chestnut.

Possible Mechanism of Action & Active Ingredients
The applicable part of European chestnut is the leaf. European chestnut contains 9% tannins, which exert an astringent effect on the mucosal tissue. This effect causes localized dehydration that turns the external cells into a protective layer (12). Plants with 10% tannins or more may cause gastrointestinal disturbances, kidney damage, and necrotic conditions of the liver (12). Some animal experiments show that tannins may cause cancer; others show that they may prevent it (12). Regular consumption of herbs with high tannin concentrations correlates with increased incidence of esophageal or nasal cancer (12).

Adverse Reactions Including Known Allergies
None reported.

Possible Interactions with Herbs & Other Dietary Supplements
TANNIN-CONTAINING HERBS: Theoretically, herbs that contain high percentages of tannins (such as American chestnut) may cause precipitation of constituents of other herbs.

Possible Interactions with Drugs
ORAL DRUGS: Theoretically, concomitant oral administration may cause precipitation of some drugs due to the high tannin content of European chestnut (19). Separate administration of oral drugs and tannin-containing herbs by the longest period of time practical (19).

Possible Interactions with Foods
No interactions are known to occur, and there is no known reason to expect a clinically significant interaction with European chestnut.

Possible Interactions with Lab Tests
No interactions are known to occur, and there is no known reason to expect a clinically significant interaction with European chestnut.

Possible Interactions with Diseases or Conditions
No interactions are known to occur, and there is no known reason to expect a clinically significant interaction with European chestnut.

Typical Dosages & Routes of Administration that are Commonly Used
ORAL: People typically prepare European chestnut as a tea with 1 teaspoon of leaves and bark boiled in a covered container with 2 cups of water for 30 minutes. The liquid is cooled slowly in the closed container and taken cold, 1 to 2 cups per day (5254).

Comments
None.

EUROPEAN ELDER flower

This Product is Also Known As

Black-Berried Alder, Black Elder, Boor Tree, Bountry, Common Elder, Elderberry, Ellanwood, Ellhorn, European Alder, Sambucus, Sweet Elder.
CAUTION: See separate listings for American Elder, European Elder fruit, and Dwarf Elder.

Scientific Names

Sambucus nigra.
Family: Caprifoliaceae.

People Use This For

Orally, European elder flower is used as a diuretic, laxative, and to induce sweating (2,11,18). It is also used to treat colds (2,11,18), flu (11), cough, and bronchitis (18).

Topically, European elder flower preparations are used as a gargle/mouthwash for coughs, headcolds, laryngitis, flu, and shortness of breath (18). It is used on the skin as an astringent for rheumatism (11), swelling, and inflammation (4,18).

In combination with gentian root, verbena, cowslip flower, and sorrel, European elder flower is used orally for maintaining healthy sinuses (373) and treating sinusitis (7,374,379).

In foods and beverages, European elder flowers are used as a flavoring component (11).

In manufacturing, European elder flower extracts are used in perfumes (11). European elder flower water is used as a vehicle in eye and skin lotions.

Safety

LIKELY SAFE ...when European elder flower is consumed in amounts used in foods. It has Generally Recognized as Safe (GRAS) status in the US (11). ...when European elder flower is used orally and appropriately (2,4,12) in therapeutic amounts; no adverse effects have been reported (2,4,6,12).
POSSIBLY SAFE ...when European elder flower is taken orally with gentian root, verbena, cowslip flower, and sorrel (Quanterra Sinus Defense, Sinupret) (7,374,379).
PREGNANCY AND LACTATION: Insufficient reliable information available; avoid using (4).

Effectiveness

POSSIBLY EFFECTIVE ...when used orally for treating colds (2). ...when European elder flower is taken orally with gentian root, verbena, cowslip flower, and sorrel (Quanterra Sinus Defense, Sinupret) for treating acute or chronic sinusitis (7,374,379).
There is insufficient reliable information available about the effectiveness of European elder flower for its other uses.

Possible Mechanism of Action & Active Ingredients

European elder may have sweat-inducing, diuretic, and laxative effects. It also soothes mucous membranes and stimulates bronchial secretions (2,4,11). Compounds responsible for diuretic and laxative properties have not yet been isolated. European elder has demonstrated anti-inflammatory, antiviral, and diuretic effects in animals (4). Constituents of a related species, Sambucus formosana, appear to have a hepatoprotective activity against liver damage (6).

Adverse Reactions Including Known Allergies

The bark, leaf, unripe fruit contain toxic cyanogenic glycosides (4,12). Berry juice ingestion reported to cause nausea, vomiting, weakness, dizziness, numbness, and stupor (6). None reported for elder flowers.

Possible Interactions with Herbs & Other Dietary Supplements

Insufficient reliable information available.

Possible Interactions with Drugs

DOXYCYCLINE (Vibramycin): Concurrent use of European elder flower, gentian root, verbena, cowslip flower, and sorrel (Quanterra Sinus Defense, Sinupret) with doxycycline and a topical decongestant might improve the outcome of conventional (antibiotic/decongestant) therapy for acute bacterial sinusitis (374).

Possible Interactions with Foods

No interactions are known to occur, and there is no known reason to expect a clinically significant interaction with European elder flower.

Possible Interactions with Lab Tests

No interactions are known to occur, and there is no known reason to expect a clinically significant interaction with European elder flower.

Possible Interactions with Diseases or Conditions

No interactions are known to occur, and there is no known reason to expect a clinically significant interaction with European elder flower.

Typical Dosages & Routes of Administration that are Commonly Used

ORAL: One cup tea (steep 2-4 grams dried flowers in 250 mL boiling water 10-15 minutes, strain) three times daily (4); average daily dose 10-15 grams dried flowers (2). Liquid extract (1:1 in 25% alcohol), 2-4 mL three times daily (4). For acute or chronic sinusitis, two Sinupret tablets three times daily for up to two weeks has been used in clinical trials (7,374,379), equivalent to gentian root 12 mg, European elder flower 36 mg, verbena 36 mg, cowslip flower 36 mg, and sorrel 36 mg three times daily. For maintaining healthy sinuses, a typical dose is one tablet of Quanterra Sinus Defense three times daily with water, equivalent to gentian root 9 mg, European elder flower 29 mg, verbena 29 mg, cowslip flower 29 mg, and sorrel 29 mg three times daily (373). Each tablet of Quanterra Sinus Defense contains 125 mg of the herbal combination found in Sinupret (373).

Comments

Avoid confusion with American elder (Sambucus canadensis). American elder (sambucus candadensis) and European elder (sambucus nigra), are discussed together despite the fact most of the information available pertains to European elder (11).

EUROPEAN ELDER fruit

This Product is Also Known As

Baccae, Baises De Sureau, Black-Berried Alder, Black Elder, Black Elderberry, Boor Tree, Bountry, Elder, Elderberry, Ellanwood, Ellhorn, European Alder, European Elder, European Elderberry, Holunderbeeren, Sambuci Sambucus.
CAUTION: See separate listings for European Elder flower, Dwarf Elder, and American Elder.

Scientific Names

Sambucus nigra.
Family: Caprifoliaceae.

People Use This For

Orally, European elderberry juice-containing syrup is used for treating the flu (5260).
Historically, European elderberry has been used as a laxative, diuretic, to induce sweating, for catarrhal complaints, sciatica, neuralgia (8), and cancer (11).
In manufacturing, European elderberry is used for making wine (6) and as a food flavoring (4).

Safety

POSSIBLY SAFE ...when the cooked fruit is used orally (4,6,12).
POSSIBLY UNSAFE ...when the fruit is not cooked sufficiently because it can cause nausea and vomiting (8,12).
PREGNANCY AND LACTATION: Insufficient reliable information available; avoid using.

Effectiveness

POSSIBLY EFFECTIVE ...when an European elderberry juice-containing syrup (Sambocul, See Dosage) is used orally for treating symptoms and shortening the duration of the influenza (5260).
There is insufficient reliable information available about the effectiveness of European elderberry for its other uses.

Possible Mechanism of Action & Active Ingredients

European elderberries contain the flavonoids rutin, isoquertin, and hyperoside (4,8). They also contain 3% tannins, as well as anthocyan glycosides, an essential oil, cyanogenic glycosides including sambunigrin (4,8,12), and a lectin (4151). European elderberry extract inhibits hemagglutinin activity and replication of several strains of influenza viruses a and B (5260). In one clinical trial, European elderberry juice-containing syrup (Sambucol, See Dosage) reduced the symptoms and duration of influenza in adults and children (5260).

Adverse Reactions Including Known Allergies

Raw and unripe fruit might cause nausea, vomiting, or severe diarrhea (4,12). Weakness, dizziness, numbness and stupor are reported following ingestion of elderberry juice (6). No adverse effects were reported in a clinical trial of European elderberry syrup in children and adults (5260).

Possible Interactions with Herbs & Other Dietary Supplements

Insufficient reliable information available.

Possible Interactions with Drugs

No interactions are known to occur, and there is no known reason to expect a clinically significant interaction with European elder fruit.

Possible Interactions with Foods

No interactions are known to occur, and there is no known reason to expect a clinically significant interaction with European elder fruit.

Possible Interactions with Lab Tests

No interactions are known to occur, and there is no known reason to expect a clinically significant interaction with European elder fruit.

Possible Interactions with Diseases or Conditions

No interactions are known to occur, and there is no known reason to expect a clinically significant interaction with European elder fruit.

Typical Dosages & Routes of Administration that are Commonly Used

ORAL: Influenza, an adult dose of four tablespoons of European elderberry juice-containing syrup (Sambucol) daily for three days has been used (5260); a dose of two tablespoons of Sambucol daily for three days has been used in children (5260).

Comments

Avoid confusion with American elder (Sambucus canadensis).

EUROPEAN FIVE-FINGER GRASS

This Product is Also Known As

Cinquefoil, European five finger grass, Five-Finger Blossom, Five Fingers, Sunkfield, Synkfoyle.

Scientific Names

Potentilla reptans.
Family: Rosaceae.

People Use This For

Orally, European five-finger grass is used for diarrhea and fever.
Topically, European five-finger grass is used for inflammation of the mucous membranes of the mouth and gums, toothache, and heartburn. It is also used for an astringent and to treat open wounds (18).

Safety

There is insufficient reliable information available about the safety of European five-finger grass.
Pregnancy and Lactation: Insufficient reliable information available; avoid using.

Effectiveness

There is insufficient reliable information available about the effectiveness of European five-finger grass.

Possible Mechanism of Action & Active Ingredients

Astringent effects are most likely secondary to tannin content (18).

Adverse Reactions Including Known Allergies

None reported.

Possible Interactions with Herbs & Other Dietary Supplements

Insufficient reliable information available.

Possible Interactions with Drugs

No interactions are known to occur, and there is no known reason to expect a clinically significant interaction with European five-finger grass.

Possible Interactions with Foods

No interactions are known to occur, and there is no known reason to expect a clinically significant interaction with European five-finger grass.

Possible Interactions with Lab Tests

No interactions are known to occur, and there is no known reason to expect a clinically significant interaction with European five-finger grass.

Possible Interactions with Diseases or Conditions

No interactions are known to occur, and there is no known reason to expect a clinically significant interaction with European five-finger grass.

Typical Dosages & Routes of Administration that are Commonly Used

ORAL: One cup of tea taken 2-3 times daily. The tea is prepared by simmering 3 grams of dried plant in 100 mL of boiling water for 10-15 minutes and straining.

TOPICAL: A tea is made by simmering 6 grams of dried plant in 100 mL of boiling water for 10-15 minutes and strained before use. It is also used in baths as one handful of dried plant to a bathful of water (18).

Comments

European five-finger grass is easily confused with Potentilla canadensis (18).

EUROPEAN MANDRAKE

This Product is Also Known As

Alraunwurzel, Mandrake, Mandragora, Mandragore, Satan's Apple.
CAUTION: See separate listings for Bryonia (English Mandrake) and Podophyllum (American Mandrake).

Scientific Names

Mandragora officinarum, synonym Mandragora vernalis.
Family: Solanaceae.

People Use This For

In folk medicine, European mandrake root has been used orally as an emetic, purgative, sedative, anesthetic, pain killer and aphrodisiac; and for treating stomach ulcers, colic, asthma, hay fever, convulsions, rheumatism, and whooping cough (14,18,3144).

In folk medicine, European mandrake fresh leaves and leaf extracts have been used topically for treating ulcers (3144).

Safety

POSSIBLY UNSAFE …when the root is used orally in small doses due to the presence of atropine, scopolamine and related anticholinergic alkaloids (14).

UNSAFE …when the root is used orally in large doses (14). European mandrake contains atropine, scopolamine and related anticholinergic alkaloids (14) which can cause respiratory and cardiac arrest and death (15,17).

There is insufficient information available for the topical use of European mandrake leaves; avoid using due to the presence of anticholinergic alkaloids.

CHILDREN: LIKELY UNSAFE ….children can be more susceptible to the adverse effects of anticholinergics (15); avoid using European mandrake root.

PREGNANCY AND LACTATION: POSSIBLY UNSAFE …when the root is used orally due to the presence of atropine, scopolamine and related anticholinergic alkaloids (14); avoid using.

Effectiveness

There is insufficient reliable information available about the effectiveness of European mandrake.

Possible Mechanism of Action & Active Ingredients

The applicable parts of European mandrake are the root and leaf. European mandrake contains atropine, belladonnine, hyoscyamine, mandragorine, scopolamine, and scopoletin (513,816). The root contains 0.4% tropane alkaloids, principally hyoscyamine (18). All plant parts contain tropane alkaloids, principally hyoscyamine and scopolamine (17). The tropane alkaloids have anticholinergic effects, inhibiting the actions of acetylcholine principally at muscarinic receptors (15). They reduce saliva and gastric acid production, inhibit gastrointestinal motility, decrease the tone and amplitude of contractions of the ureters and bladder, reduce bronchial secretions, produce bronchodilation, inhibit sweat gland secretions reducing the volume of perspiration, reduce the movement disorders associated with Parkinsonism, prevent motion-induced nausea and vomiting, and block the responses of the sphincter muscle of the iris and the ciliary muscle of the lens, producing mydriasis and cycloplegia (15). In large doses tropane alkaloids cause tachycardia (15).

Adverse Reactions Including Known Allergies

No adverse reactions reported with European mandrake root or leaf. Consumption of 10 European mandrake fruits by an adult caused confusion, tachycardia, mydriasis, blurred vision and facial flushing (17).

Anticholinergic alkaloids contained in European mandrake (atropine, scopolamine, etc.) can cause drowsiness and blurred vision which could interfere with driving or the operation of machinery (15).

Anticholinergic alkaloids contained in European mandrake (atropine, scopolamine, etc.) may cause dose-related flushing, dryness of the mouth, tachycardia, mydriasis, blurred vision, photophobia, decreased sweat production and overheating, micturition disorders and constipation (15,18). Large doses can cause somnolence, central excitation (restlessness, hallucinations, delirium, manic episodes), exhaustion, respiratory and cardiac arrest, and death (17,18). Elderly patients can be more susceptible to the adverse effects of anticholinergics (15); avoid using European mandrake root.

© Copyright 2000, Natural Medicines Comprehensive Database (209) 472-2244. For updated data, go to www.NaturalDatabase.com

Possible Interactions with Herbs & Other Dietary Supplements

HERBS WITH ANTICHOLINERGIC EFFECTS: Theoretically, concurrent use might have additive effects and adverse effects. Anticholinergic herbs include belladonna, henbane, scopolia, and bittersweet nightshade (2).

Possible Interactions with Drugs

ORAL DRUGS: Theoretically, concurrent use might increase absorption of some drugs because of inhibited GI motility caused by European mandrake (15).

ANTICHOLINERGIC DRUGS: Concurrent use can cause additive anticholinergic effects and adverse effects. Anticholinergic drugs include conventional medications containing tropane alkaloids such as atropine, as well as phenothiazines, amantadine, some antiparkinson drugs, glutethimide, meperidine, tricyclic antidepressants, antiarrhythmic agents, and antihistamines (15).

Possible Interactions with Foods

No interactions are known to occur, and there is no known reason to expect a clinically significant interaction with European mandrake.

Possible Interactions with Lab Tests

No interactions are known to occur, and there is no known reason to expect a clinically significant interaction with European mandrake.

Possible Interactions with Diseases or Conditions

NARROW/CLOSED-ANGLE GLAUCOMA: Contraindicated due to the anticholinergic effects of European mandrake (14).

REFLUX ESOPHAGITIS: Contraindicated due to the anticholinergic effects of European mandrake (14).

OBSTRUCTIVE GASTROINTESTINAL DISEASE: Contraindicated due to the anticholinergic effects of European mandrake (14).

ULCERATIVE COLITIS OR TOXIC MEGACOLON: Contraindicated due to the anticholinergic effects of European mandrake (14).

OBSTRUCTIVE UROPATHY: Contraindicated due to the anticholinergic effects of European mandrake (14).

UNSTABLE CARDIOVASCULAR STATUS IN ACUTE HEMORRHAGE OR THYROTOXICOSIS: Contraindicated due to the anticholinergic effects of European mandrake (14).

PARALYTIC ILEUS or INTESTINAL ATONY: Contraindicated due to the anticholinergic effects of European mandrake (14).

MYASTHENIA GRAVIS: Contraindicated due to the anticholinergic effects of European mandrake (14).

HEPATIC OR RENAL DYSFUNCTION: Avoid using European mandrake due to anticholinergic effects (14,15).

HYPERTHYROIDISM: Avoid using European mandrake due to anticholinergic effects (14,15).

CONGESTIVE HEART FAILURE: Avoid using European mandrake due to anticholinergic effects (14,15).

CORONARY ARTERY DISEASE: Avoid using European mandrake due to anticholinergic effects (14,15).

TACHYARRHYTHMIAS: Avoid using European mandrake due to anticholinergic effects (14,15).

PROSTATIC HYPERTROPHY: Avoid using European mandrake due to anticholinergic effects (14,15).

HYPERTENSION: Avoid using European mandrake due to anticholinergic effects (14,15).

GASTRIC ULCER: Avoid using European mandrake due to anticholinergic effects (14,15).

HIATAL HERNIA: Avoid using European mandrake due to anticholinergic effects (14,15).

GI INFECTIONS: Avoid using European mandrake due to anticholinergic effects (14,15).

DOWN SYNDROME: Avoid using European mandrake in people with Down syndrome. They may be hypersensitive to antimuscarinic effects of anticholinergics (15).

SPASTIC PARALYSIS/BRAIN DAMAGE: Avoid using European mandrake in children with spatic paralysis or brain damage. They may be hypersensitive to antimuscarinic effects of anticholinergics (15).

Typical Dosages & Routes of Administration that are Commonly Used

No typical dosage.

Comments

European mandrake has had many superstitions associated with it and has been claimed to have magical properties (3144). It is now considered obsolete as a therapeutic agent (18). The FDA has issued a ban on the sale of mandrake-containing products as aphrodisiacs, due to lack of evidence of their safety or efficacy (14).

EUROPEAN MISTLETOE

This Product is Also Known As

All-Heal, Birdlime Mistletoe, Devil's Fuge, Drudenfuss, Hexenbesen, Leimmistel, Mistlekraut, Mistletein, Mystyldene, Visci, Visci albi folia, Visci albi fructus, Visci albi herba, Visci albi stipites, Vogelmistel.
CAUTION: See separate listing for American Mistletoe.

Scientific Names
Viscum album.
Family: Viscaceae.

People Use This For
Orally, European mistletoe fruit is used for regulating blood pressure, internal bleeding, epilepsy, arteriosclerosis, infantile convulsions, gout, hysteria, "blood purifying", and major blood loss (18). The stem is sued orally for its calming effect, for treating mental and physical exhaustion, and as a tranquilizer. The young branches, along with the flower and fruit, are used for hypertension, epilepsy, whooping cough, asthma, vertigo, amenorrhea, diarrhea, chorea, nervous tachycardia, hysteria, and nervousness (18).

Subcutaneously, injections are used for palliative therapy of malignant tumors, and for degenerative inflammation of the joints (2,18).

In combination with other herbs, the berry of European mistletoe is used for regulating blood pressure, circulatory problems, seizure disorders, nervous conditions, cardiac conditions, bleeding disorders, gastrointestinal disorders, sleep disorders, menopause symptoms, hemorrhoids, depression, and headaches (2). The stem of European mistletoe is used in combination with other herbs for treating nervous conditions, menopause symptoms, cardiac conditions, gastrointestinal disorders, circulatory problems, and liver and gallbladder conditions (2).

Safety
UNSAFE ...when used orally or by subcutaneous injection for self-medication (4,11). Use requires monitoring and regular blood pressure checks (4,12). European mistletoe berries are considered highly poisonous (4).
CHILDREN: UNSAFE ...when used orally. The berries are considered poisonous (2).
PREGNANCY: UNSAFE ...for self-medication and it may also have uterine stimulant activity (4,19).
LACTATION: UNSAFE ...when used for self-medication (4,11).

Effectiveness
POSSIBLY INEFFECTIVE ...when used subcutaneously for treating pancreatic cancer (3707) and bronchial carcinoma (7).
There is insufficient reliable information available about the effectiveness of European mistletoe for its other uses.

Possible Mechanism of Action & Active Ingredients
European mistletoe has hypotensive, cardiac depressant, and sedative effects (4). It might also have anti-inflammatory and immuno-stimulatory activity (11). Crude plant juices exhibit cytotoxic activity (4); the glycoprotein fractions (lectin, viscotoxins) and alkaloid fractions might be responsible for antitumor activity (4). Some evidence suggests that lectins can stimulate T-lymphocytes, induce macrophage cytotoxicity, stimulate phagocytosis and the release of immune mediators (7). Studies show a lectin fraction can have agglutinating activity that is preferential for tumor cells over erythrocytes (4). Other evidence suggests polypeptides isolated from European mistletoe might have cytotoxic activity against tumor cells. These peptides can also be associated with cardiotoxicity (11). Studies suggest the constituent viscotoxins can cause reflex bradycardia, hypotension, and weaken muscular action, as well as depolarize smooth, skeletal, and cardiac muscle (4).

Adverse Reactions Including Known Allergies
When taken orally, European mistletoe can cause vomiting, diarrhea, intestinal cramps, hepatitis (14), hypotension, contraction of the pupil, uncontrollable movement of the eyeball, seizures, coma, and death (4). Berries are highly toxic (2,4,6,18); poisonings have been reported after ingestion by children (2). When injected subcutaneously, European mistletoe can cause chills, high fever, headaches, angina, orthostatic circulatory disturbances, and allergic reaction (2). Necrosis can result from local inflammatory reaction at the site of injection (2,8).

Possible Interactions with Herbs & Other Dietary Supplements
Insufficient reliable information available.

Possible Interactions with Drugs
HYPERTENSION/HYPOTENSION DRUGS: European mistletoe can cause hypotension, interfering with drug therapy for hypertension and hypotension (4).
CARDIAC THERAPY: European mistletoe can have cardiotoxic and negative inotropic (muscle weakening) effects. It can cause reflex bradycardia and hypotension, and can also depolarize cardiac muscle. Theoretically, these effects might interfere with drug therapy (4).
ANTICOAGULANTS/COAGULANTS: Theoretically, European mistletoe might interfere with anticoagulants or coagulants. (4).
IMMUNOSUPPRESSANTS: Theoretically, immunostimulant effects might interfere with immunosuppressant therapy (4).
ANTIDEPRESSANT THERAPY: Theoretically, European mistletoe might interfere with antidepressant therapy (4).

Possible Interactions with Foods
No interactions are known to occur, and there is no known reason to expect a clinically significant interaction with European mistletoe.

Possible Interactions with Lab Tests

No interactions are known to occur, and there is no known reason to expect a clinically significant interaction with European mistletoe.

Possible Interactions with Diseases or Conditions

CARDIOVASCULAR DISEASE: Contraindicated. European mistletoe can have cardiotoxic and negative inotropic (muscle weakening) effects. It can cause reflex bradycardia and hypotension, and can also depolarize cardiac muscle. (4).

COAGULOPATHIES: Avoid. Theoretically, European mistletoe could interfere with anticoagulant therapy (4).

CHRONIC INFECTION: Contraindicated in people with chronic, progressive infections such as tuberculosis and AIDS (4,12,14).

Typical Dosages & Routes of Administration that are Commonly Used

No typical dosage.

Comments

European mistletoe is considered unsafe for self-use (see Safety). European mistletoe toxicity reports include one case of hepatitis in a woman who consumed a combination product containing mistletoe, kelp, motherworth, and scullcap (3932). Originally, hepatitis was attributed to mistletoe but no other reports of hepatitis have been associated with mistletoe (4). In Germany, mistletoe products are available in aqueous whole plant extract (Plenosol, Helixor), and as Iscador (7). Mistletoe is a parasite; some Australian mistletoe species are reported to extract toxic constituents from the host plant on which they grow (515), suggesting the importance of identifying the host plant before use of mistletoe is considered.

EUROPEAN WATER HEMLOCK

This Product is Also Known As

Cowbane.

Scientific Names

Cicuta virosa.
Family: Umbelliferae.

People Use This For

Orally, European water hemlock is used for migraine headaches, painful menstruation, worm infestations, and inflammation of the skin (18).

Safety

UNSAFE ...when taken orally (18).
PREGNANCY AND LACTATION: UNSAFE ...contraindicated due to toxic potential; avoid using (18).

Effectiveness

There is insufficient reliable information available about the effectiveness of European water hemlock.

Possible Mechanism of Action & Active Ingredients

The applicable parts of European water hemlock are the root/rhizome. The freshly harvested root contains the toxin cicutoxin. The rest of the plant is weakly toxic, and toxicity declines after the root has been dehydrated and stored (18).

Adverse Reactions Including Known Allergies

European water hemlock is fatal at a dose of 2-3 grams of root stock. The first symptoms of poisoning are somnolence and nausea, followed by severe tonic-clonic spasms, unconsciousness, and mydriasis. Death occurs through respiratory arrest during convulsions, or by heart failure (18).

Possible Interactions with Herbs & Other Dietary Supplements

Insufficient reliable information available.

Possible Interactions with Drugs

No interactions are known to occur, and there is no known reason to expect a clinically significant interaction with European water hemlock.

Possible Interactions with Foods

No interactions are known to occur, and there is no known reason to expect a clinically significant interaction with European water hemlock.

Possible Interactions with Lab Tests

No interactions are known to occur, and there is no known reason to expect a clinically significant interaction with European water hemlock.

Possible Interactions with Diseases or Conditions

No interactions are known to occur, and there is no known reason to expect a clinically significant interaction with European water hemlock.

Typical Dosages & Routes of Administration that are Commonly Used

No typical dosage.

Comments

European water hemlock is considered unsafe when used orally. The rhizome has an extremely unpleasant smell and is extremely toxic (18).

EVENING PRIMROSE OIL

This Product is Also Known As

EPO, Fever Plant, Huile D'Onagre, King's Cureall, Night Willow-Herb, Scabish, Sun Drop.
CAUTION: See separate listings for Black Currant Seed Oil, Borage Seed Oil, Gamma Linolenic Acid, and Omega-6 Oils.

Scientific Names

Oenothera biennis and other Oenothera species.
Family: Onagraceae.

People Use This For

Orally, evening primrose oil is used for premenstrual syndrome (PMS), cyclical and noncyclical mastalgia, endometriosis (4), and symptoms of menopause such as hot flashes (274,276). It is also used for atopic eczema, psoriasis (4), acne (6121), rheumatoid arthritis, Raynaud's phenomenon, multiple sclerosis, and Sjogren's syndrome (4). Evening primrose oil is used for cancer, hypercholesterolemia and coronary heart disease (4), intermittent claudication (6121), alcoholism, Alzheimer's disease, and schizophrenia (4). Evening primrose oil is used orally for post-viral fatigue syndrome; asthma; diabetic neuropathy (4); neurodermatitis; hyperactivity in children (18); weight loss (5,6); whooping cough; and gastrointestinal disorders, including ulcerative colitis, irritable bowel syndrome, and peptic ulcer disease (4,6121). It has been used orally in pregnancy for preventing pre-eclampsia, shortening the duration of labor, and preventing postdate deliveries (1407,1408,1409,1411).
In foods, evening primrose oil is used as a dietary source of essential fatty acids (11).
In manufacturing, evening primrose oil is used in soaps and cosmetics (11).

Safety

LIKELY SAFE ...when used orally and appropriately. Evening primrose oil is generally considered safe and has been used in several studies without reports of significant side effects (4,5,6,11,1106,6034,6035,6036).
PREGNANCY: POSSIBLY UNSAFE ...when used orally. Evening primrose oil might increase the risk for pregnancy complications, including prolonged rupture of membranes, oxytocin augmentation, arrest of descent, and vacuum extraction (1411); avoid using.
LACTATION: POSSIBLY SAFE ...when used orally. Nursing mothers who supplement their diets with evening primrose oil secrete high levels of gamma linolenic acid into breast milk (1982); however, this essential fatty acid constituent of evening primrose oil is normally present in significant proportions in breast milk (4).

Effectiveness

POSSIBLY EFFECTIVE ...when taken orally for mastalgia (4,6034,6406). In one study, evening primrose oil was found to relieve cyclic mastalgia in 45% of patients and non-cyclic mastalgia in 27% of patients. Evening primrose was compared to conventional therapy and was less effective than danazol, but had similar efficacy as bromocriptine (6406). ...when taken orally for improving symptoms of rheumatoid arthritis (4,6036). In one study, patients experienced a significant reduction in symptoms of arthritis after 6 months of treatment (6036). ...when taken orally for irritable bowel syndrome exacerbated by premenstrual syndrome (PMS) (4,6034). Some clinical studies on the effectiveness of evening primrose have used evening primrose formulations standardized to 9% gamma linolenic acid. This formulation is similar to Efamol's Pure Evening Primrose Oil.
POSSIBLY INEFFECTIVE ...when taken orally for relief of symptoms associated with premenstrual syndrome (PMS) (1105,1106,6034,6035). Multiple small-scale studies have not demonstrated significant benefit when compared to placebo (1105,1106).
LIKELY INEFFECTIVE ...when taken orally for preventing pre-eclampsia (1409). ...when taken orally for shortening duration of labor (1409,1411). ...when taken orally for preventing post-date deliveries in pregnant women (1411). ...when taken orally for treating menopausal flushing (274).
There is insufficient reliable information available about the effectiveness of evening primrose oil for its other uses.

Possible Mechanism of Action & Active Ingredients

Evening primrose oil is obtained from the plant seed. It contains 2-16% gamma-linolenic acid (GLA) and 65-80% linoleic acid. GLA is metabolized to dihomo-gamma-linolenic acid (DGLA). Both GLA and DGLA are precursors of the prostaglandin E2 (PGE2) and the prostaglandin E1 (PGE1). The administration of supplemental GLA increases the resulting concentration of DGLA, which is converted to 15-hydroxy-DGLA, which may competitively inhibit the production of the certain prostaglandins and leukotrienes from arachadonic acid that are responsible for inflammation (4,6036). Supplementation with evening primrose oil also allows bypassing of the rate-limiting conversion of linoleic acid in food to gamma linolenic acid. Avoiding this step improves the inflammatory and noninflammatory ratio of prostaglandin compounds (4). It is through these mechanisms that evening primrose oil may exert beneficial effects in conditions of an inflammatory nature, such as rheumatoid arthritis (6036). Evening primrose oil is thought to improve conditions that result from certain metabolic deficiencies. These conditions can include mastalgia, atopic eczema, and premenstrual syndrome (PMS) (3). Patients with PMS reportedly have lower levels of GLA, possibly due to a defect in the conversion of linoleic acid to GLA (6034).

Evening primrose can reduce elevated plasma lipids and reduce platelet aggregation (6).

Adverse Reactions Including Known Allergies

Evening primrose oil can sometimes lead to indigestion, nausea, soft stools, and headache (4). Large doses of evening primrose oil can lead to loose stools and abdominal pain (4). There is one case report of nocturnal seizures associated with the use of evening primrose oil, black cohosh, and chasteberry (588). Evening primrose oil might increase the risk for pregnancy complications, including prolonged rupture of membranes, oxytocin augmentation, arrest of descent, and vacuum extraction (1411).

Possible Interactions with Herbs & Other Dietary Supplements

Insufficient reliable information available.

Possible Interactions with Drugs

ANESTHESIA: There is a case report of seizures associated with concomitant use of evening primrose oil and anesthesia; however, other drugs were also involved (613).

PHENOTHIAZINES: Seizures have been reported in people with schizophrenia treated concomitantly with phenothiazine drugs and evening primrose oil (614); use with caution.

Possible Interactions with Foods

No interactions are known to occur, and there is no known reason to expect a clinically significant interaction with evening primrose oil.

Possible Interactions with Lab Tests

No interactions are known to occur, and there is no known reason to expect a clinically significant interaction with evening primrose oil.

Possible Interactions with Diseases or Conditions

EPILEPSY/SEIZURE DISORDER: There is concern that evening primrose oil might lower the seizure threshold or unmask undiagnosed temporal lobe epilepsy. However, current reports have only identified seizure in association with phenothiazine (4,614).

SCHIZOPHRENIA: Seizures have been reported in people with schizophrenia treated concomitantly with phenothiazine drugs and evening primrose oil (614); use with caution.

Typical Dosages & Routes of Administration that are Commonly Used

ORAL: For mastalgia 3-4 grams daily has been used (4). For premenstrual syndrome (PMS), 2-4 grams daily has been used (6034). For rheumatoid arthritis, doses ranging from 540 mg daily to 2.8 grams daily have been used (6036). For atopic eczema, 6-8 grams daily has been used (4). Children take about 2-4 grams daily (4). Some clinical studies on the effectiveness of evening primrose have used evening primrose formulations standardized to 9% gamma linolenic acid. This formulation is similar to Efamol's Pure Evening Primrose Oil. Appropriate dosing may vary depending on the specific formulation.

Comments

Evening primrose oil is approved in the United Kingdom as a "Prescription Only Medicine" for treating atopic eczema and is approved in Canada as a dietary supplement for increasing essential fatty acid intake (11).

EYEBRIGHT

This Product is Also Known As

Augentrostkraut, Euphraisiae herba, Euphrasia, Herbed' Euphraise.
CAUTION: See separate listing for Clary Sage.

Scientific Names

Eurphrasia rostkoviana; Euphrasia officinalis.
Family: Scrophulariaceae.

People Use This For

Orally, eyebright is used to treat nasal mucous membrane inflammation and sinusitis (4).

Topically, eyebright is used as an ophthalmic in the form of a lotion, poultice or eyebath. The eye conditions eyebright is used for include: conjunctivitis (4,6), blepharitis (6), eye fatigue (6), inflammation of the blood vessels, eyelids and conjunctiva, and for "glued" and inflamed eyes. Eyebright is also used to prevent mucus and mucous membrane inflammation of the eyes (2).

Historically, eyebright has been used in British Herbal Tobacco, which was smoked for chronic bronchial conditions and colds (6). It was also used for allergies, cancers, coughs, conjunctivitis, earaches, epilepsy, headaches, hoarseness, inflammation, jaundice, ophthalmia, rhinitis, skin ailments, sore throats (6), and as poultice for styes (8,11).

In foods, eyebright is used as a flavoring ingredient (4).

Safety

POSSIBLY SAFE ...when used orally and appropriately (12). ...when used orally in amounts found in foods. Eyebright is listed by the Council of Europe as a natural source of food flavoring (4).
POSSIBLY UNSAFE ...when used as an ophthalmic; avoid, due to hygienic concerns. Eye products may be subject to contamination (8,11).
PREGNANCY AND LACTATION: Insufficient reliable information available; avoid using (4).

Effectiveness

There is insufficient reliable information available about the effectiveness of eyebright (4,6).

Possible Mechanism of Action & Active Ingredients

Tannin constituents may be responsible for astringent properties (4). The constituent caffeic acid has bacteriostatic activity (4). Constituents, aucubin and iridoid glycosides, have purgative activity (4).

Adverse Reactions Including Known Allergies

10-60 drops eyebright tincture (unspecified route of administration) may induce mental confusion, headache, increased eye pressure with lacrimation, itching, redness, swelling of eyelid margins, dim vision, photophobia, weakness, sneezing, nausea, toothache, constipation, cough, dyspnea, insomnia, polyuria, and sweating (4).

Possible Interactions with Herbs & Other Dietary Supplements

Insufficient reliable information available.

Possible Interactions with Drugs

No interactions are known to occur, and there is no known reason to expect a clinically significant interaction with eyebright.

Possible Interactions with Foods

No interactions are known to occur, and there is no known reason to expect a clinically significant interaction with eyebright.

Possible Interactions with Lab Tests

No interactions are known to occur, and there is no known reason to expect a clinically significant interaction with eyebright.

Possible Interactions with Diseases or Conditions

No interactions are known to occur, and there is no known reason to expect a clinically significant interaction with eyebright.

Typical Dosages & Routes of Administration that are Commonly Used

ORAL: 2-4 grams dried above ground parts three times daily (4), or one cup tea (steep 2-4 grams dried above ground parts in 150 mL boiling water 5-10 minutes, strain) three times daily (4). Liquid extract (1:1 in 25% alcohol), 2-4 mL three times daily (4). Tincture (1:5 in 45% alcohol), 2-6 mL three times daily (4).
OPHTHALMIC: No typical dosage.

Comments

Avoid use of nonsterile solutions (including homemade products) in the eye(s), due to high risk of infection. Ophthalmic application of eyebright is not recommended (5).

FALSE UNICORN

This Product is Also Known As

Blazing Star, Fairywand, Helonias, Starwort.

Scientific Names

Chamaelirium luteum, synonyms Chamaelirium carolianum, Helonias dioica, Helonias lutea, Veratrum luteum. Family: Liliaceae.

People Use This For

Orally, false unicorn is used for ovarian cysts, menstrual problems, menopause (4201), threatened miscarriage (4), vomiting from pregnancy (4), digestive problems (4201), and to normalize hormones after oral contraceptive use (4208). It is also used as a diuretic and to rid the intestines of worms (4208).

Safety

POSSIBLY SAFE ...when the root preparations are used orally and appropriately (12).
PREGNANCY: LIKELY UNSAFE ...contraindicated for oral use because it is a potential uterine stimulant (12,18).
LACTATION: Insufficient reliable information available; avoid using.

Effectiveness

There is insufficient reliable information available about the effectiveness of false unicorn.

Possible Mechanism of Action & Active Ingredients

The applicable parts of false unicorn are the rhizome and root. False unicorn reportedly has anthelmintic, diuretic (18), uterine stimulant, and menstruation stimulant activity (12).

Adverse Reactions Including Known Allergies

Large doses of false unicorn taken orally may cause nausea and vomiting (4).

Possible Interactions with Herbs & Other Dietary Supplements

Insufficient reliable information available.

Possible Interactions with Drugs

No interactions are known to occur, and there is no known reason to expect a clinically significant interaction with false unicorn.

Possible Interactions with Foods

No interactions are known to occur, and there is no known reason to expect a clinically significant interaction with false unicorn.

Possible Interactions with Lab Tests

No interactions are known to occur, and there is no known reason to expect a clinically significant interaction with false unicorn.

Possible Interactions with Diseases or Conditions

GI CONDITIONS: Can irritate the gastrointestinal tract. Contraindicated in individuals with infectious or inflammatory gastrointestinal conditions (19).

Typical Dosages & Routes of Administration that are Commonly Used

ORAL: 1-2 grams dried root three times per day, or, one cup tea (steep 1-2 grams dried root in 150 mL boiling water 5-10 minutes, strain) three times daily (4). Liquid extract (1:1 in 45% alcohol), 1-2 mL three times daily (4). Tincture (1:5 in 45% alcohol), 2-5 mL three times daily (4).

Comments

None.

FENNEL fruit, seed

This Product is Also Known As

Bitter Fennel, Carosella, Common Fennel, Finnochio, Florence Fennel, Garden Fennel, Large Fennel, Phytoestrogen, Sweet Fennel, Wild Fennel.
CAUTION: See separate listing for Fennel Oil.

Scientific Names

Foeniculum vulgare, synonyms Foeniculum officinale, Foeniculum capillaceum, Anethum foeniculum.
Family: Apiaceae or Umbilliferae.

People Use This For

Orally, fennel is used to enhance lactation, promote menstruation, facilitate birth, increase libido (6), treat indigestion, upper respiratory tract mucous membrane inflammation (2), cough, bronchitis (18), stimulate appetite, treat visual problems, and colic in infants (6135).
In Chinese medicine, fennel has been used orally in combination formulas for cholera, backache, and bedwetting (11). Fennel powder has been used topically in Chinese medicine as a poultice for hard-to-heal snake bites (11).

Safety

LIKELY SAFE ...when the seed is used orally in food amounts (11,12).
POSSIBLY SAFE ...when used orally and appropriately for short periods of time (2,12).
POSSIBLY UNSAFE ...when used orally in medicinal amounts for prolonged periods of time. The constituent, estragole, is a procarcinogen (12).
PREGNANCY: LIKELY UNSAFE ...contraindicated for oral use (2).
LACTATION: Insufficient reliable information available; avoid using.

Effectiveness

POSSIBLY EFFECTIVE ...when taken orally for treating mild spastic GI symptoms, fullness, flatulence, and upper respiratory tract mucous membrane inflammation (2).
There is insufficient reliable information available about the effectiveness of fennel fruit or seed for their other uses.

Possible Mechanism of Action & Active Ingredients

Fennel is a rich source of beta-carotene and vitamin C (19). The seed contains a volatile oil composed largely of trans-anethole, with lesser amounts of fenchone, estragole, and other constituents. It also contains significant amounts of calcium, magnesium, and iron, and lesser amounts of other metal cations (6135). Fennel seed can promote GI motility, and in higher concentrations, it can act as an antispasmodic (2). The constituents, anethole and fenchone, reduce upper respiratory tract secretions (11). Some evidence suggests the aqueous fennel extract might also increase mucociliary activity (11). The constituent anethole appears to be allergenic, insecticidal, and toxic. Polymers of anethole have estrogenic activity (11). The constituent estragole is a procarcinogen but the carcinogenic risk is minimal. It is not directly hepatotoxic or hepatocarcinogenic but requires activation by liver enzymes to reach full toxicity. In the liver, other enzymes inactivate the carcinogenic metabolites, limiting possible damage to the liver (12).

Adverse Reactions Including Known Allergies

Fennel can cause allergic reactions affecting the skin and respiratory system (2). It can also cause photodermatitis. Avoid excessive sunlight or ultraviolet light exposure while using this product (19). Allergic cross-sensitivity is possible in people with allergies to carrot, celery, mugwort, or other Apiaceae family plants (6,18).

Possible Interactions with Herbs & Other Dietary Supplements

No interactions are known to occur, and there is no known reason to expect a clinically significant interaction with fennel fruit and seed.

Possible Interactions with Drugs

CIPROFLOXACIN (Cipro): Concomitant administration might reduce the effectiveness of ciprofloxacin therapy. Preliminary evidence suggests that fennel reduces ciprofloxacin bioavailability by nearly 50%, possibly due to interaction with the metal cations contained in fennel. Evidence also suggests that fennel increases tissue distribution and slows elimination of ciprofloxacin (6135).

Possible Interactions with Foods

No interactions are known to occur, and there is no known reason to expect a clinically significant interaction with fennel fruit and seed.

Possible Interactions with Lab Tests

No interactions are known to occur, and there is no known reason to expect a clinically significant interaction with fennel fruit and seed.

Possible Interactions with Diseases or Conditions

CELERY, CARROT, MUGWORT ALLERGY: Allergic cross-sensitivity to fennel possible (6,18).

Typical Dosages & Routes of Administration that are Commonly Used

ORAL: The typical dose of fennel is 5-7 grams of the dried fruit or seed per day or one cup of the tea three times daily (2,18). The tea is prepared by steeping 1-2 grams of the crushed or ground fruit or seed in 150 mL boiling water for 5-10 minutes and then straining. The common dose of the tincture compound is 5-7.5 grams per day (2). Fennel should be used on a short-term basis (2).

Comments

None.

FENNEL OIL

This Product is Also Known As

Foeniculi antheroleum, Phytoestrogen.
CAUTION: See separate listing for Fennel fruit, seed.

Scientific Names

Foeniculum vulgare, synonyms Foeniculum officinale, Foeniculum capillaceum, Anethum foeniculum.
Family: Apiaceae or Umbilliferae.

People Use This For

Orally, fennel oil is used for mild spastic disorders of the GI tract, feeling of fullness, flatulence, upper respiratory tract mucous membrane inflammation (2), cough, and bronchitis (18). Fennel honey syrup is used for upper respiratory tract mucous membrane inflammation in children (2).
Traditionally, fennel oil has been used for improving appetite, digestion, and other stomach complaints (11).
In foods and beverages, fennel oil is used as a flavoring agent (11).
In other manufacturing processes, fennel oil is used as a flavoring agent in some laxatives (11), and as a fragrance component in soaps and cosmetics (11).

Safety

LIKELY SAFE ...when consumed in amounts commonly found in foods. Fennel oil has Generally Recognized as Safe (GRAS) status for food use in the US. A maximum level of 0.119% is used in meat products (11).
POSSIBLY SAFE ...when used orally in medicinal amounts for less than 2 weeks (2,18).
POSSIBLY UNSAFE ...when used long-term.
CHILDREN: LIKELY UNSAFE ...contraindicated for oral use in infants and toddlers (2).
PREGNANCY: LIKELY SAFE ...when used in food amounts. LIKELY UNSAFE ...contraindicated in larger amounts (2).
LACTATION: Insufficient reliable information available; avoid using amounts larger than those found in foods.

Effectiveness

POSSIBLY EFFECTIVE ...when taken orally for mild spastic disorders of the GI tract, feeling of fullness, flatulence, and upper respiratory tract mucous membrane inflammation (including the use of the honey syrup in children) (2).
There is insufficient reliable information available about the effectiveness of fennel oil for its other uses.

Possible Mechanism of Action & Active Ingredients

Fennel oil is composed largely of trans-anethole, with lesser amounts of fenchone, estragole, and other constituents. The oil can promote GI motility, and in higher concentrations, it can act as an antispasmodic (2). The constituents, anethole and fenchone, reduce upper respiratory tract secretions (11). The constituent anethole appears to be allergenic, insecticidal, and toxic. Polymers of anethole have estrogenic activity (11). The constituent estragole is a procarcinogen but the carcinogenic risk is minimal. It is not directly hepatotoxic or hepatocarcinogenic but requires activation by liver enzymes to reach full toxicity. In the liver other enzymes inactivate the carcinogenic metabolites, limiting possible damage to the liver (12).

Adverse Reactions Including Known Allergies

Allergic cross-sensitivity is possible in people with allergies to carrot, celery, mugwort, or other Apiaceae family plants (6,18). Allergic reactions that affect the skin and respiratory system are rare (2).

Possible Interactions with Herbs & Other Dietary Supplements

Insufficient reliable information available.

Possible Interactions with Drugs

No interactions are known to occur, and there is no known reason to expect a clinically significant interaction with fennel oil.

Possible Interactions with Foods

No interactions are known to occur, and there is no known reason to expect a clinically significant interaction with fennel oil.

Possible Interactions with Lab Tests

No interactions are known to occur, and there is no known reason to expect a clinically significant interaction with fennel oil.

Possible Interactions with Diseases or Conditions

CELERY, CARROT, MUGWORT ALLERGY: Allergic cross sensitivity to fennel is possible (6,18).
DIABETES: Use caution with the fennel honey syrup in diabetics due to its carbohydrate content (2).

Typical Dosages & Routes of Administration that are Commonly Used

ORAL: The typical daily dose of fennel oil is 0.1-0.6 mL, which is equivalent to 100-600 mg of the dried fruit or seed. It should only be used up to two weeks without professional evaluation (2). The fennel honey syrup, which contains 500 mg fennel oil/kg, is usually dosed 10-20 grams per day (2).

Comments

Fennel oil is the distilled essential oil of the fennel (Foeniculum vulgare) fruit or seed.

FENUGREEK

This Product is Also Known As
Bird's Foot, Bockshornsame, Foenugraeci Semen, Foenugreek, Greek Hay, Greek Hay Seed, Hu Lu Ba, Methi, Trigonella.

Scientific Names
Trigonella foenum-graecum.
Family: Leguminosae.

People Use This For
Orally, fenugreek seed is used for loss of appetite (2,4), for treating dyspepsia, gastritis (4), for lowering blood glucose in people with diabetes (220,622), constipation, atherosclerosis, high serum cholesterol and triglycerides (1900), and for promoting lactation (314).

Topically, fenugreek is used as a poultice for local inflammation (2), myalgia, lymphadenitis, gout, wounds, leg ulcers (6), and eczema (18).

In Chinese medicine, fenugreek is used for nutrition, kidney ailments, beriberi, hernia, impotence, and other male problems (11).

Traditionally, fenugreek has been taken to reduce fever, promote lactation, and treat mouth ulcers, boils, bronchitis, cellulitis, tuberculosis, chronic coughs, chapped lips, and cancer. It is also used as a cure for baldness (6,11).

For food use, fenugreek is included as an ingredient in spice blends. It is also used as a flavoring agent in imitation maple syrup, foods, beverages, and tobacco (11).

In other manufacturing processes, fenugreek extracts are used in soaps and cosmetics (11).

Safety
LIKELY SAFE ...when seed preparations are used in the amounts commonly found in foods, (maximum use level is 0.05% in meat). It has Generally Recognized as Safe (GRAS) status in the US (11).
POSSIBLY SAFE ...when used orally in medicinal amounts (2,4).
POSSIBLY UNSAFE ...when used topically, the repeated use of fenugreek can result in skin sensitization (2,18).
PREGNANCY: LIKELY UNSAFE ...contraindicated for oral use in amounts greater than those found in foods because of its potential oxytocic and uterine stimulant activity (4).
LACTATION: Insufficient reliable information available; avoid using.

Effectiveness
POSSIBLY EFFECTIVE ...when used orally for lowering blood sugar in people with diabetes (4,6) and for the loss of appetite (2). ...when used topically as a poultice for local inflammation (2).
There is insufficient reliable information available about the effectiveness of fenugreek for its other uses.

Possible Mechanism of Action & Active Ingredients
The applicable part of fenugreek is the seed. Fenugreek affects gastrointestinal transit, slowing glucose absorption (163). The constituent, 4-isoleucine, appears to directly stimulate insulin (164). In healthy individuals, whole seed extracts, gum isolate, extracted seeds, cooked seeds, and the constituent, trigonelline, show evidence of a hypoglycemic effect (4). In people with noninsulin-dependent diabetes, the ingestion of the extracted seeds can improve plasma glucose and insulin response (4). In people with insulin-dependent diabetes, the ingestion of the seed powder can reduce plasma glucose, glycosuria, and the daily insulin requirement (4). Some studies suggest the seed powder can reduce serum cholesterol in people with diabetes (4). Other evidence suggests the seed consumption might decrease calcium oxalate deposition in the kidneys (720). The fenugreekine constituent shows evidence of cardiotonic, hypoglycemic, diuretic, anti-inflammatory, antihypertensive and antiviral properties (4).

Adverse Reactions Including Known Allergies
The oral use of fenugreek can cause diarrhea and flatulence (622). With large doses, hypoglycemia is possible (6,164). Occupational exposure to fenugreek can cause asthma (6), and after inhalation of the seed powder, it can cause allergic symptoms, such as runny nose, wheezing, and fainting. The paste of fenugreek applied to the scalp can cause allergic symptoms, including head numbness, facial swelling, and wheezing (719).

Possible Interactions with Herbs & Other Dietary Supplements
HERBS WITH ANTICOAGULANT/ANTIPLATELET POTENTIAL: Concomitant use of herbs that have coumarin constituents or affect platelet aggregation could theoretically increase the risk of bleeding in some people. These herbs include: angelica, anise, arnica, asafoetida, bogbean, boldo, capsicum, celery, chamomile, clove, danshen, feverfew, garlic, ginger, ginkgo, ginseng (Panax), horse chestnut, horseradish, licorice, meadowsweet, prickly ash, onion, papain, passionflower, poplar, quassia, red clover, turmeric, wild carrot, wild lettuce, willow, and others (4,19).

Possible Interactions with Drugs
ANTICOAGULANT: Theoretically, fenugreek can enhance anticoagulant drug activity and increase the risk of bleeding (4).
CORTICOSTEROID: Theoretically, fenugreek can inhibit corticosteroid drug activity (4).

HORMONE THERAPY: Fenugreek theoretically can interfere with hormone therapy (4).
HYPOGLYCEMIC DRUGS: Fenugreek can alter blood glucose control (4), and when used, blood glucose levels should be monitored closely.
INSULIN: Insulin dosage might need to be adjusted due to the hypoglycemic effect of fenugreek (19).
MONOAMINE OXIDASE INHIBITORS (MAOIs): Theoretically, fenugreek can potentiate their drug activity (4).
ALL DRUGS: Theoretically, the high mucilage content of fenugreek can decrease or delay the absorption of oral drugs (4,19).

Possible Interactions with Foods
No interactions are known to occur, and there is no known reason to expect a clinically significant interaction with fenugreek.

Possible Interactions with Lab Tests
URINE ODOR: Fenugreek can cause a maple syrup odor in urine (6). Avoid confusion with "maple syrup urine" disease (6).
BLOOD GLUCOSE: Fenugreek can lower blood glucose and test results (4,6).

Possible Interactions with Diseases or Conditions
FENUGREEK ALLERGY: Contraindicated.
KIDNEY STONES: Theoretically, it can decrease calcium oxalate deposition and stone formation (720).
DIABETES: Fenugreek can alter blood sugar control in people with diabetes (4,6), and blood glucose levels should be monitored closely.

Typical Dosages & Routes of Administration that are Commonly Used
ORAL: The typical dose is 1-2 grams of the seed or equivalent three times daily (2,4) or one cup of the tea several times a day. The tea is prepared by steeping 500 mg seed in 150 mL cold water for three hours and the straining. The maximum amount of fenugreek is 6 grams of the seed per day (2).
TOPICAL: It is typically used as a poultice, which is prepared by mixing 50 grams of the powdered seed in 0.25-1 L of hot water to form a paste (2,18).

Comments
The taste and odor of fenugreek resembles maple syrup, and it has been used to mask the taste of medicines (6).

FEVER BARK

This Product is Also Known As
Alstonia Bark, Australian Febrifuge, Australian Fever Bush, Australian Quinine, Devil's Bit, Devil Tree, Dita Bark, Pale Mara, Pali-Mara.

Scientific Names
Alstonia constricta.
Family: Apocynaceae.

People Use This For
Orally, fever bark is used for treating fever, hypertension, diarrhea, and malaria. It is also used as a stimulant and a uterine stimulant (18).
Historically, fever bark was used to treat rheumatism (18).

Safety
POSSIBLY UNSAFE ...when used orally and appropriately. Fever bark contains reserpine and yohimbine constituents (18) that can cause severe adverse effects including depression, psychosis, and acute renal failure (2,5,6,11,17,18,19).
PREGNANCY AND LACTATION: Insufficient reliable information available; avoid using.

Effectiveness
There is insufficient reliable information available about the effectiveness of fever bark.

Possible Mechanism of Action & Active Ingredients
The applicable part of fever bark is the bark. Fever bark contains various alkaloids including yohimbe. The constituents reserpine and deserpidine are likely responsible for its antihypertensive effects. Fever bark might also have antipyretic and antispasmodic properties (18).

Adverse Reactions Including Known Allergies
The reserpine constituent of fever bark can cause lethargy, nasal congestion, or depression (17). The yohimbine constituent of fever bark can cause salivation, irritability, fluid retention, skin eruptions, eye dilation, allergy, acute

renal failure, and lupus-like syndrome (2,5,6,11,18,19). Yohimbine is reported to trigger psychosis in people predisposed to it (2,5,6,11,18). Symptoms of yohimbine toxicity include paralysis, severe hypotension, cardiac conduction disorders, cardiac failure, and death (6,18).

Possible Interactions with Herbs & Other Dietary Supplements

ST. JOHN'S WORT: Theoretically, concomitant use of extract of St. John's wort might antagonize effects of reserpine, a constituent of fever bark (19).
TURMERIC: Theoretically, concomitant use might reduce the frequency of gastric and duodenal ulcers associated with reserpine, a constituent of fever bark (19).
YOHIMBE: Theoretically, concomitant use of fever bark with yohimbe can cause additive effects or adverse effects.
INDIAN SNAKEROOT: Theoretically, concomitant use can cause additive effects and side effects due to reserpine and deserpidine content of both herbs.

Possible Interactions with Drugs

GENERAL ANESTHETICS: Reserpine can increase the risk of cardiovascular instability in individuals receiving general anesthetics (151).
SYMPATHOMIMETICS: Reserpine might increase or decrease effects of sympathomimetics (151).
PHENOTHIAZINES: Theoretically, phenothiazines might increase the toxicity of yohimbine due to alpha-two adrenoreceptor antagonism (19).
NALOXONE: Concomitant use of yohimbine and naloxone can cause synergistic effects and adverse reactions (19).

Possible Interactions with Foods

No interactions are known to occur, and there is no known reason to expect a clinically significant interaction with fever bark.

Possible Interactions with Lab Tests

FFA: Reserpine can increase serum free fatty acids (275).
GUAIACOLA SPOT TEST: Reserpine can cause a false reading with urine screening test of Rogers (275).
HOMOVANILLIC ACID: Reserpine can increase urine levels of homovanillic acid; maximum on second day (275).
HYDROCHLORIC ACID: Reserpine can increase gastric hydrochloric acid levels (275).
17-HYDROXYCORTICOSTEROIDS: Reserpine can decrease urine levels (275).
5-HYDROXYINDOLEACETIC ACID (5-HIAA): Reserpine can increase test results (275).
NOREPINEPHRINE: Reserpine can decrease urine levels of norepinephrine (275). Yohimbine can increase plasma and cerebrospinal fluid norepinephrine levels and test results (275).
PEPSIN: Reserpine can increase gastric pepsin levels and test results (275).
PLATELETS: Reserpine can decrease blood platelet levels and test results (275).
PROLACTIN: Reserpine can increase plasma prolactin levels and test results (275).
PROTHROMBIN TIME: Reserpine can decrease plasma prothrombin time (275).
SEROTONIN: Reserpine can decrease plasma 5-HT and test results (275).
T-4: Reserpine can decrease thyroxine (T-4) serum levels and test results (275).
TYRAMINE: Reserpine can cause a false positive response to tyramine test (275).
VANILLYMANDELIC ACID: Reserpine can decrease urine levels and test results (275).

Possible Interactions with Diseases or Conditions

MENTAL DEPRESSION: Theoretically, contraindicated in individuals with a history of mental depression due to reserpine constituent (17,18).
PEPTIC ULCER: Theoretically, contraindicated in individuals with active peptic ulcer due to reserpine constituent (17).
SCHIZOPHRENIA: Theoretically, contraindicated in individuals with schizophrenia because yohimbine constituent might induce psychotic episodes (19).

Typical Dosages & Routes of Administration that are Commonly Used

ORAL: A typical dose is 15 to 20 mL of tea daily. Tea can be made by steeping one part ground bark to 20 parts boiling water for 10-15 minutes, strain. Alternatively 2-4 mL tincture (1:8 or 1:10) daily; or 4-8 mL of liquid extract (1:1) daily (18).

Comments

Most of the information available for fever bark concerns its constituents.

© Copyright 2000, Natural Medicines Comprehensive Database (209) 472-2244. For updated data, go to www.NaturalDatabase.com • 429

FEVERFEW

This Product is Also Known As
Altamisa, Bachelor's Button, Featerfoiul, Featherfew, Midsummer Daisy, Santa Maria, Tanaceti parthenii.

Scientific Names
Tanacetum parthenium, synonyms Chrysanthemum parthenium, Leucanthemum parthenium, Pyrethrum parthenium.
Family: Asteraceae or Compositae.

People Use This For
Orally, feverfew is used for fever, headache, menstrual irregularities, migraines, stomachache (5,11,18), nausea and vomiting (6121).
Topically, feverfew is used as an antiseptic, insecticide, and for toothache (4,18). It is also used as a general stimulant and tonic and for intestinal parasites (4,11,18).
Traditionally, feverfew has been used orally for allergies, arthritis, asthma, colic, digestion, earache, flatulence, kidney pain, tinnitus, morning sickness, and difficulty during labor.

Safety
POSSIBLY SAFE ...when the leaf is used orally and appropriately (12). Although it can cause mouth ulcers and GI disturbances, using the encapsulated, dried leaf dosage form decreases the likelihood of oral irritation. There are no known adverse effects with long-term use (12).
CHILDREN: POSSIBLY UNSAFE ...should not be used in children younger than two years old (6).
PREGNANCY: LIKELY UNSAFE ...contraindicated because some evidence suggests it can stimulate uterine contractions and cause abortion (4).
LACTATION: Insufficient reliable information available; avoid using.

Effectiveness
POSSIBLY EFFECTIVE ...when the dried leaf is used orally for preventing and reducing the severity of migraine headaches. Three studies showed feverfew whole leaf products were effective for reducing the frequency or severity of migraines (724,725); however, one study did not find feverfew to be effective (727). The US Headache Consortium 2000 guidelines for preventing migraine headaches discusses the use of feverfew, but rates the evidence of feverfew efficacy lower than the evidence of efficacy for standard first-line agents (5080).
POSSIBLY INEFFECTIVE ...when the dried leaf is used orally for treating rheumatoid arthritis (11). ...when the standardized ethanol extract is used for prophylaxis and treatment of migraines (726).
There is insufficient reliable information available about the effectiveness of feverfew for its other uses.

Possible Mechanism of Action & Active Ingredients
The applicable part of feverfew is the leaf. Feverfew might work in migraine by preventing prostaglandin production. Feverfew is reported to inhibit 86-88% of prostaglandin synthesis. One active constituent is thought to be parthenolide. Products that do not contain at least 0.2% of parthenolide might not have adequate activity (21). Feverfew leaf can cause uterine contractions in full-term, pregnant women and abortions in cattle (4). Some evidence demonstrates the crude extracts might inhibit blood platelet aggregation and the neutrophil and platelet secretory activity (11).

Adverse Reactions Including Known Allergies
Taken orally, feverfew can cause mouth ulceration, tongue irritation and inflammation (with chewed leaves), abdominal pain, indigestion, diarrhea, flatulence, nausea, and vomiting (1). It can also cause "post-feverfew syndrome," and the symptoms include nervousness, tension headaches, insomnia, joint pain or stiffness, and tiredness (4). Allergic contact dermatitis can occur with topical use of feverfew (1). It can cause an allergic reaction in individuals sensitive to the Asteraceae/Compositae family. Members of this family include ragweed, chrysanthemums, marigolds, daisies, and many other herbs.

Possible Interactions with Herbs & Other Dietary Supplements
HERBS WITH ANTICOAGULANT/ANTIPLATELET POTENTIAL: Concomitant use of herbs that have coumarin constituents or affect platelet aggregation could theoretically increase the risk of bleeding in some people. These herbs include: angelica, anise, arnica, asafoetida, bogbean, boldo, capsicum, celery, chamomile, clove, danshen, fenugreek, garlic, ginger, ginkgo, ginseng (Panax), horse chestnut, horseradish, licorice, meadowsweet, prickly ash, onion, papain, passionflower, poplar, quassia, red clover, turmeric, wild carrot, wild lettuce, willow, and others (4,19).

Possible Interactions with Drugs
ANTICOAGULANT, ANTIPLATELET DRUGS: Theoretically, feverfew can enhance the effects of these drugs and increase the risk of bleeding by inhibiting platelet aggregation.
NONSTEROIDAL ANTI-INFLAMMATORY DRUGS (NSAIDs): Theoretically, NSAIDs might decrease the effectiveness of feverfew (6). This potential interaction might be mediated through NSAIDs' effects on prostaglandins (21).

Possible Interactions with Foods
No interactions are known to occur, and there is no known reason to expect a clinically significant interaction with feverfew.

Possible Interactions with Lab Tests
No interactions are known to occur, and there is no known reason to expect a clinically significant interaction with feverfew.

Possible Interactions with Diseases or Conditions
CROSS-ALLERGENICITY: Feverfew can cause an allergic reaction in individuals sensitive to the Asteraceae/Compositae family. Members of this family include ragweed, chrysanthemums, marigolds, daisies, and many other herbs.

Typical Dosages & Routes of Administration that are Commonly Used
ORAL: For migraine prophylaxis, the typical dose of the fresh leaf is 2.5 leaves daily with or after food (4). The freeze-dried leaf is taken at 50-125 mg per day with or after food (4,6,724,725). The encapsulated, dried leaf dosage form decreases the likelihood of oral irritation. Clinical studies on the effectiveness of feverfew have used whole leaf feverfew standardized to 0.6-0.7% parthenolide.
TOPICAL: No typical dosage.

Comments
Some feverfew tablet products can contain little or no feverfew (5). The Health and Welfare Government of Canada issued a Drug Identification Number (DIN) to a feverfew leaf (capsules) product standardized to 0.2% parthenolide, with the labeling claim "used as a prophylactic against migraines" (724).

FICIN

This Product is Also Known As
Doctor Oje, Leche de Higueron, Leche de Oje, Oje.

Scientific Names
Ficus insipida, synonyms Ficin anthelmintica, Ficin glabrata, and Ficin laurfolia.
Family: Moraceae.

People Use This For
Orally, ficin is used as a digestive aid (11).
In medical procedures, ficin is used to clean and prepare intestinal submucosa for the production of sutures, to clean and prepare animal arteries for human implantation, and in serologic testing (e.g. for Rh factor determination) (11).
Historically, ficin has been used as an anthelmintic in South America (11,3766).
In manufacturing, ficin is used in European anti-inflammatory preparations (11), cheese manufacturing, chillproofing beer (11), preparation of protein hydrolysates, edible collagen films, and sausage casings (11). Ficin is sometimes included in meat tenderizers, usually in combination with papain and/or bromelain (11).

Safety
LIKELY UNSAFE ...when used topically. Crude ficin is corrosive to skin and prolonged contact can cause bleeding (11).
There is insufficient reliable information available about the safety of the oral use of ficin.
PREGNANCY and LACTATION: LIKELY UNSAFE ...when used topically (11). There is insufficient reliable information available about the safety of ficin for oral use; avoid using.

Effectiveness
There is insufficient reliable information available about the effectiveness of ficin.

Possible Mechanism of Action & Active Ingredients
Ficin is a sulfhydryl proteinase and can hydrolyze proteins, amides, esters, and small peptides (11). Some evidence suggests ficin might be useful in treating helminthiasis (11,3766). Other evidence suggests ficin has anti-inflammatory activity (11).

Adverse Reactions Including Known Allergies
Large amounts taken orally can cause catharsis (11). When used topically, crude ficin is corrosive to skin and can cause bleeding with prolonged contact (11). Ficin can also cause contact allergies (11).

Possible Interactions with Herbs & Other Dietary Supplements
Insufficient reliable information available.

Possible Interactions with Drugs

No interactions are known to occur, and there is no known reason to expect a clinically significant interaction with ficin.

Possible Interactions with Foods

No interactions are known to occur, and there is no known reason to expect a clinically significant interaction with ficin.

Possible Interactions with Lab Tests

No interactions are known to occur, and there is no known reason to expect a clinically significant interaction with ficin.

Possible Interactions with Diseases or Conditions

No interactions are known to occur, and there is no known reason to expect a clinically significant interaction with ficin.

Typical Dosages & Routes of Administration that are Commonly Used

ORAL: Anthelmintic, 1.0 cc of prepared latex/kg per day for 3 days to be repeated every 3 months (3766).

Comments

Ficin is the latex harvested from the trunk of felled Ficus insipida trees. Crude ficin consists of the latex combined with acetic acid to prevent coagulation and sodium benzoate as a preservative (11). Purified ficin is not pure ficin. Rather, it is a mixture of several proteases and small amounts of other enzymes and other constituents (11).

FIELD SCABIOUS

This Product is Also Known As

None.

Scientific Names

Knautia arvensis.

People Use This For

Orally, field scabious is used for cough and throat complaints (18).
Topically, field scabious is used for chronic skin conditions, eczema, anal fissures, anal itching, urticaria, scabies, favus (roundworm), and cleansing and healing ulcers, bruises and inflammation (18).

Safety

There is insufficient reliable information available about the safety of field scabious.
Pregnancy and Lactation: Insufficient reliable information available; avoid using.

Effectiveness

There is insufficient reliable information available about the effectiveness of field scabious.

Possible Mechanism of Action & Active Ingredients

The applicable parts of field scabious are the above ground parts. Field scabious contains triterpene saponins including knatioside, knautioside A and B, iridoide monoterpenes including dipsacan, flavonoids, and tannins. It is reported to have astringent, antiseptic, expectorant, and purgative properties (18).

Adverse Reactions Including Known Allergies

None reported.

Possible Interactions with Herbs & Other Dietary Supplements

Insufficient reliable information available.

Possible Interactions with Drugs

No interactions are known to occur, and there is no known reason to expect a clinically significant interaction with field scabious.

Possible Interactions with Foods

No interactions are known to occur, and there is no known reason to expect a clinically significant interaction with field scabious.

Possible Interactions with Lab Tests

No interactions are known to occur, and there is no known reason to expect a clinically significant interaction with field scabious.

Possible Interactions with Diseases or Conditions
No interactions are known to occur, and there is no known reason to expect a clinically significant interaction with field scabious.

Typical Dosages & Routes of Administration that are Commonly Used
ORAL: For chronic eczema, drink 2 glasses tea (add 4 teaspoons to 240 mL boiling water, steep for 10 minutes and strain) throughout day (18). Product is used both orally and topically as an alcoholic extract and tea.

Comments
None.

FIG

This Product is Also Known As
Caricae Fructus, Feigen.

Scientific Names
Ficus carica.
Family: Moraceae.

People Use This For
Orally, fig is used as a laxative (2).

Safety
LIKELY SAFE ...when used orally in food amounts as fresh or dried fruit.
PREGNANCY AND LACTATION: LIKELY SAFE ...when used orally in food amounts as fresh or dried fruit.

Effectiveness
There is insufficient reliable information available about the effectiveness of fig (2).

Possible Mechanism of Action & Active Ingredients
The applicable part of fig is the fruit. There is insufficient reliable information available about the possible mechanism of action and active ingredients.

Adverse Reactions Including Known Allergies
Fig use can cause photodermatitis. Avoid excessive sunlight or ultraviolet light exposure while using this product (19).

Possible Interactions with Herbs & Other Dietary Supplements
Insufficient reliable information available.

Possible Interactions with Drugs
No interactions are known to occur, and there is no known reason to expect a clinically significant interaction with fig.

Possible Interactions with Foods
No interactions are known to occur, and there is no known reason to expect a clinically significant interaction with fig.

Possible Interactions with Lab Tests
No interactions are known to occur, and there is no known reason to expect a clinically significant interaction with fig.

Possible Interactions with Diseases or Conditions
No interactions are known to occur, and there is no known reason to expect a clinically significant interaction with fig.

Typical Dosages & Routes of Administration that are Commonly Used
No typical dosage.

Comments
None.

FIGWORT

This Product is Also Known As
Carpenter's Square, Common Figwort, Heal-all, Rosenoble, Scrophularia, Scrophula Plant, Throatwort.

Scientific Names
Scrophularia mailandica; Scrophularia nodosa (Scrophylariaceae).

People Use This For
Orally, figwort is used as a diuretic (4).
Topically, figwort is used for chronic skin diseases (eczema, itching, psoriasis) (4), hemorrhoids, swelling, and eruptions (201).

Safety
There is insufficient reliable information available about the safety of figwort.
Pregnancy and Lactation: Insufficient reliable information available; avoid using.

Effectiveness
There is insufficient reliable information available about the effectiveness of figwort.

Possible Mechanism of Action & Active Ingredients
The applicable parts of figwort are the above ground parts and root. It is reported to have diuretic and laxative effects (18). Constituents, aucubin and catalpol, exert purgative action in mice; harpagide may have cardioactive and anti-inflammatory activity (4).

Adverse Reactions Including Known Allergies
None reported (18).

Possible Interactions with Herbs & Other Dietary Supplements
CARDIAC GLYCOSIDE-CONTAINING HERBS: Contraindicated, and concomitant use can increase the risk of cardiac glycoside toxicity. Cardiac glycoside-containing herbs include black hellebore, Canadian hemp roots, digitalis leaf, hedge mustard, lily of the valley roots, motherwort, oleander leaf, pheasant's eye plant, pleurisy root, squill bulb leaf scales, strophanthus seeds, and uzara (2,18,19,500).

Possible Interactions with Drugs
No interactions are known to occur, and there is no known reason to expect a clinically significant interaction with figwort.

Possible Interactions with Foods
No interactions are known to occur, and there is no known reason to expect a clinically significant interaction with figwort.

Possible Interactions with Lab Tests
No interactions are known to occur, and there is no known reason to expect a clinically significant interaction with figwort.

Possible Interactions with Diseases or Conditions
DIABETES: Theoretically, may alter blood glucose control (4); monitor closely.
VENTRICULAR TACHYCARDIA: Contraindicated (4,12).

Typical Dosages & Routes of Administration that are Commonly Used
ORAL: Prepared tea (steep 2-8 grams dried above ground parts in 150 mL boiling water 5-10 minutes, steep); no additional dosing information available (4). Liquid extract (1:1 in 25% alcohol), 2-8 mL (4). Tincture (1:10 in 45% alcohol), 2-4 mL (4).

Comments
Figwort is stated to be a suitable substitute for devil's claw (due to similar chemical composition) (4).

FIR

This Product is Also Known As
Fir Tree, Norway Spruce, Piceae turiones recentes, Spruce, Spruce Fir.
CAUTION: See separate listings for Dwarf Pine Needle, Fir Needle Oil, Pine Needle Oil, Pine, Poplar, and Scotch Pine Needle.

Scientific Names
Abies alba, synonym Abies pectinata; Picea abies, synonym Picea excelsa.
Family: Pinaceae.

People Use This For

Orally, fir shoot is used for respiratory tract inflammation (2), colds, cough, bronchitis, fever, inflammation of the mouth and pharynx, muscle and nerve pain, and tendency toward infection (18).

Topically, fir is used for mild myalgia, neuralgia, and rheumatic pain (2,18).

In folk medicine, fir shoot has been used orally for tuberculosis (18) and applied externally as a bath additive for mental illness (18).

Safety

POSSIBLY SAFE ...when used orally and topically in appropriate amounts (2).

PREGNANCY AND LACTATION: Insufficient reliable information available; avoid using.

Effectiveness

POSSIBLY EFFECTIVE ...when taken orally for inflammation of the respiratory tract (2). ...when used topically for mild rheumatic pain or neuralgia (2).

There is insufficient reliable information available about the effectiveness of fir shoot for its other uses.

Possible Mechanism of Action & Active Ingredients

The applicable part of fir is the shoot. Fir shoot can reduce secretions, enhance local circulation, and act as a mild antiseptic (2). The essential oil can have secretory and antibacterial effects on bronchial mucous membranes (18). The essential oil also acts as a rubefacient (counterirritant) and improves circulation when applied externally (18).

Adverse Reactions Including Known Allergies

None reported (18).

Possible Interactions with Herbs & Other Dietary Supplements

Insufficient reliable information available.

Possible Interactions with Drugs

No interactions are known to occur, and there is no known reason to expect a clinically significant interaction with fir.

Possible Interactions with Foods

No interactions are known to occur, and there is no known reason to expect a clinically significant interaction with fir.

Possible Interactions with Lab Tests

No interactions are known to occur, and there is no known reason to expect a clinically significant interaction with fir.

Possible Interactions with Diseases or Conditions

ASTHMA, PERTUSSIS (whooping cough): The fir shoot can exacerbate these conditions (18).

Contraindicated for use as a bath additive for individuals with extensive skin injuries, acute skin diseases, feverish or infectious diseases, cardiac insufficiency, or hypertonia (18).

Typical Dosages & Routes of Administration that are Commonly Used

ORAL: The typical dose is 5-6 grams of the fresh fir shoots per day (2,18). The essential oil is usually given as 4 drops in water or on a sugar lump three times daily (18).

TOPICAL: Boil 200-300 grams of the shoots in 1 L water, steep for 5 minutes, strain, and add to a full bath (2,18).

INHALATION: Inhale the vapor of 2 grams of the essential oil in hot water several times per day (18).

Comments

Avoid confusion with fir needle oil.

FIR NEEDLE OIL

This Product is Also Known As

Fichtennadelöl, Piceae aetheroleum, White Spruce Oil.

CAUTION: See separate listing for Dwarf Pine Needle, Scotch Pine Needle Oil, Poplar, Fir, and Pine.

Scientific Names

Picea abies, synonym Picea excelsa; Piceae aetheroleum; Abies alba; Abies sachalinensis; Abies sibirica. Family: Pinaceae.

People Use This For

Orally, fir needle oil is used for upper and lower respiratory tract infections and conditions (2).

Topically, fir needle oil is used for upper and lower respiratory tract infections and conditions (2). It is also used

topically for rheumatic, neuralgic, and muscle pains (2). Fir needle oil is commonly used as a liniment in alcoholic solutions, ointments, gels, emulsions, and oils. It is used as a bath additive (2).
Fir needle oil is also used as an inhalant (2).

Safety
POSSIBLY SAFE ...when taken orally or applied topically (2).
PREGNANCY AND LACTATION: Insufficient reliable information available; avoid using.

Effectiveness
POSSIBLY EFFECTIVE ...when taken orally or applied topically for treating infections and conditions of the upper and lower respiratory tracts (2). ...when applied topically for rheumatic, neuralgic, and muscle pains (2).

Possible Mechanism of Action & Active Ingredients
Fir needle oil is made from the tips of branches or twigs. Fir needle oil has mild antiseptic and counterirritant properties. It also breaks up respiratory secretions (2).

Adverse Reactions Including Known Allergies
Taken orally, the oil can increase bronchospasms (2). Topically, the fir needle oil increases skin and mucous membrane irritation (2).

Possible Interactions with Herbs & Other Dietary Supplements
Insufficient reliable information available.

Possible Interactions with Drugs
No interactions are known to occur, and there is no known reason to expect a clinically significant interaction with fir needle oil.

Possible Interactions with Foods
No interactions are known to occur, and there is no known reason to expect a clinically significant interaction with fir needle oil.

Possible Interactions with Lab Tests
No interactions are known to occur, and there is no known reason to expect a clinically significant interaction with fir needle oil.

Possible Interactions with Diseases or Conditions
ASTHMA, PERTUSSIS (whooping cough): The fir needle oil is contraindicated in individuals with these conditions because it can increase bronchospasms (2).

Typical Dosages & Routes of Administration that are Commonly Used
Dosage is individualized according to the type and intensity of the illness, the special areas of use, and the mode of administration (2).

Comments
None.

FIREWEED

This Product is Also Known As
French-Willow, Great Willowherb, Rosebay, Willow Herb, Willowherb.

Scientific Names
Epilobium angustifolium.
Family: Onagraceae.

People Use This For
In folk medicine, fireweed has been used for inflammation, fevers, tumors, wounds, as an astringent, and as a tonic (4017).

Safety
POSSIBLY SAFE ...when used orally (12).
PREGNANCY AND LACTATION: Insufficient reliable information available; avoid using.

Effectiveness
There is insufficient reliable information available about the effectiveness of fireweed.

Possible Mechanism of Action & Active Ingredients

The applicable parts of fireweed are the above ground parts. Some evidence suggests that aqueous extracts of fireweed might affect reproduction (858). Other evidence suggests that extracts could have anti-inflammatory effects (859,860).

Adverse Reactions Including Known Allergies

None reported.

Possible Interactions with Herbs & Other Dietary Supplements

Insufficient reliable information available.

Possible Interactions with Drugs

No interactions are known to occur, and there is no known reason to expect a clinically significant interaction with fireweed.

Possible Interactions with Foods

No interactions are known to occur, and there is no known reason to expect a clinically significant interaction with fireweed.

Possible Interactions with Lab Tests

No interactions are known to occur, and there is no known reason to expect a clinically significant interaction with fireweed.

Possible Interactions with Diseases or Conditions

No interactions are known to occur, and there is no known reason to expect a clinically significant interaction with fireweed.

Typical Dosages & Routes of Administration that are Commonly Used

No typical dosage.

Comments

Other Epilobium species are also referred to as willow herb (18).

FISH OILS

This Product is Also Known As

Fish Oil Fatty Acids, Marine Oils, N-3 Fatty Acids, N3-polyunsaturated Fatty Acids, Omega Fatty Acids, Omega 3 Fatty Acids, Omega-3 Fatty Acids, PUFA, W-3 Fatty Acids.
CAUTION: See separate listings for DHA and EPA.

Scientific Names

None.

People Use This For

Orally, fish oils are used for hypertension, hyperlipidemia and coronary heart disease, bipolar disorder, rheumatoid arthritis, psoriasis, atopic dermatitis, ulcerative colitis, Behcet's syndrome, and Raynaud's syndrome (9,507,1002, 5709,6005). Fish oils are also taken orally for weight loss (2049), asthma, cancer, painful menses, lung diseases, hay fever, Crohn's disease (507), chronic fatigue syndrome (1019), albuminuria associated with diabetic neuropathy (1025), restenosis after angioplasty (1028), miscarriage (1032), preeclampsia, preterm labor, and intrauterine growth retardation (1026,1027,1042). Fish oils are used for systemic lupus erythematosus (507), cystic fibrosis (1006), gingivitis (1005), renal impairment associated with cirrhosis (1013), and claudication (1002). Fish oil is also used to treat attention deficit hyperactivity disorder (ADHD) and dyspraxia (5708).
In combination with linoleic and gamma-linoleic acid, fish oils are used orally for treating post-viral fatigue syndrome (1019).
Intravenously, fish oils are used to treat psoriasis (1004,1034).

Safety

LIKELY SAFE ...when used orally and appropriately. Fish oils have Generally Regarded as Safe (GRAS) status in the US (4,9,5703).
CHILDREN: POSSIBLY SAFE ...when used orally and appropriately (5708,5711).
PREGNANCY AND LACTATION: Insufficient reliable information available; avoid using.

Effectiveness

LIKELY EFFECTIVE...when used orally for hypertriglyceridemia. Several clinical trials have shown that fish oil significantly reduces triglyceride levels by 20% to 50% (1024,5702,5705,5706). This effect appears to be dose-dependent (5706).
POSSIBLY EFFECTIVE ...when used orally to reduce mortality after acute myocardial infarction. One study has

shown fish oil started within 18 hours after acute myocardial infarction and continued for 1 year to be superior to placebo for reducing total cardiac events, non-fatal myocardial infarction, and total cardiac mortality (1007). ...when used orally for mild hypertension. Clinical trials have shown that fish oils can produce modest but significant reductions in systolic and diastolic blood pressure in individuals with mild hypertension (1001,1020). ...when taken orally with conventional therapy for bipolar disorder. Patients receiving fish oils in combination with conventional treatment had improved symptoms of depression and increased length of remission (7202). ...when used orally to decrease ventricular ectopic beats and risk of sudden cardiac death (507). ...when used orally to prevent cyclosporine-induced hypertension following cardiac transplant. One clinical trial has shown fish oils can maintain pre-cyclosporine blood pressures in patients after initiating cyclosporine (507,1012). ...when used for preventing cyclosporine-induced nephrotoxicity. One study has shown fish oil can significantly improve glomerular filtration rate and renal blood flow in individuals taking cyclosporine (1021). ...when used orally for rheumatoid arthritis. Several small clinical trials have shown fish oils, with or without naproxen (Naprosyn), to be superior to placebo for decreasing the duration of morning stiffness (1017,1039,1041). Use of fish oils may also allow reduction of non-steroidal anti-inflammatory drug (NSAID) requirements when used concomitantly (1031). ...when used orally to prevent recurrent miscarriage associated with antiphospholipid antibodies. When fish oils were given to 22 women with antiphospholipid syndrome (PAPS) and recurrent miscarriage, 19 of 23 pregnancies resulted in live births (1032). ...when used orally with linoleic and gamma-linoleic acid to treat symptoms of postviral fatigue syndrome. One study has shown the fish oil combination to be superior to placebo for improving overall condition, including degree of fatigue, myalgias, dizziness, and concentration (1019). ...when used orally to reduce albuminuria in individuals with diabetic nephropathy (1025). ...when used orally to improve appetite and increase lean body mass in patients with advanced pancreatic cancer (5701). ...when used orally to improve night vision in children with dyslexia. Dyslexic children who received fish oils developed significantly better dark adaptation when compared with controls (5708). ...when used orally in combination with evening primrose oil, thyme oil, and vitamin E to improve movement disorders in children with dyspraxia. One small study has shown that this combination significantly decreases movement disorders (5708). ...when used intravenously to treat specific types of acute and chronic psoriasis. Clinical trials have shown fish oils to be superior to n-6 fatty acids for decreasing symptom severity and inflammatory substances in chronic plaque psoriasis (1004) and acute, extended guttate psoriasis (1034). ...when used orally with simvastatin to decrease postprandial hemostatic risk factors in hyperlipidemia (5704). ...when used orally for migraine headache prophylaxis in adolescents. In an unpublished small-scale, crossover study announced at the Advancing Children's Health 2000 meeting, adolescent migraineurs receiving fish oil preparations containing eicosapentaenoic acid (EPA) 756 mg and docosahexanoic acid (DHA) 498 mg daily for 2 months had reduced frequency, duration, and severity of migraine headaches (5097). ...when used orally from dietary fish consumption in conjunction with a modified diet for weight loss. In one clinical trial, overweight, hypertensive subjects had significantly decreases in blood glucose and insulin concentrations, and lost more weight on a weight loss diet that included fish than controls, or those on either a weight-loss diet or fish alone (2049). ...when used orally from dietary fish to reduce the risk of age-related maculopathy. Epidemiological evidence indicates that fish consumption more than once per week is associated with reduced risk of age-related maculopathy (6260).

POSSIBLY INEFFECTIVE ...when taken orally to reverse progression of atherosclerosis. When taken for 2 years by people with coronary atherosclerosis, fish oils were no more effective than placebo at decreasing atherosclerotic plaque size (1022). ...when taken orally for systemic lupus erythematosus and lupus nephritis (507). ...when taken orally for atopic dermatitis (507). ...when taken orally for psoriasis. In one clinical trial, fish oil was no more effective placebo for decreasing the severity of psoriasis symptoms (1035). ...when taken orally for gingivitis. One small clinical trial has shown fish oils to be no more effective than placebo for reduced gingival inflammation (1005). ...when taken orally for renal impairment associated with advanced cirrhosis. In one clinical study, fish oils were ineffective for improving renal function in cirrhotic individuals with decreased renal function (1013). ...when taken orally for stable claudication. Fish oils were no more effective than placebo for improving walking distance or pressure indices in one clinical study (1002).

LIKELY INEFFECTIVE ...when taken orally with evening primrose oil for preventing pre-eclampsia, preterm labor, and intrauterine growth retardation (1026,1027,1042). ...when taken orally to prevent restenosis after angioplasty (1028,1038).

Many clinical studies of the effectiveness of fish oils have used products similar to ProOmega (Nordic Naturals), which contains 35% EPA and 25 % DHA.

There is insufficient reliable information available about the effectiveness of fish oils for other uses. Although several studies have evaluated fish oil preparations for inflammatory bowel disease, results have been conflicting (1037,1040,5709,6257,6258,6259). Further evidence is needed to rate fish oil for this use.

Possible Mechanism of Action & Active Ingredients

Fish oils contain the long-chain, omega-3 fatty acids, eicosapentaenoic acid (EPA) and docosahexaenoic acid (DHA). In humans DHA can be converted to EPA (1044). These fatty acids compete with arachidonic acid in the cyclooxygenase and lipoxygenase pathways (9). They have anti-inflammatory effects, likely due to inhibition of leukotriene synthesis (9). Fish oils are thought to beneficial in rheumatoid arthritis due to anti-inflammatory effects and epidemiological data that suggests that EPA is decreased in total plasma fatty acids and synovial fluid, and DHA are decreased in the synovial fluid of people with rheumatoid arthritis (5710). Fish oils have been proposed as a treatment for attention-deficit hyperactivity disorder (ADHD) due to epidemiological data suggest that symptoms of ADHD may be inversely related to the n3-fatty acid phospholipid content (5711). In individuals with bipolar disorder, the fatty acids in fish oils are though to have an effect similar to lithium or valproate, slowing nerve signaling (6005). In hypertriglyceridemia, fish oils are thought to lower triglycerides by decreasing secretion of VLDLs, increasing VLDL apolipoprotein B secretion, possibly by increasing VLDL clearance, and reducing triglyceride transport and decreasing VLDL size (5707). Fish oils also increase fatty acid oxidation by peroxisomal and mitochondrial routes, reduces fatty acid synthesis, diverts fatty acids into phospholipid synthesis, increasing hepatic uptake of triglycerides and down regulation of fatty acid esterifying enzymes (5707). Fish oils also decrease cholesterol absorption and cholesterol synthesis (5707). Fish oils also might also increase high-density lipoproteins (HDL) (5707) and improve flow-mediated arterial dilation (5702). Research shows that fish oils increase lipid peroxidation (1011) and might be cytotoxic to cancer cells (1008). Fish oils decrease blood viscosity and increase red blood cell deformability (9). The antithrombotic activity of fish oils results from prostacyclin synthesis effects, vasodilation, platelet adhesiveness reduction, platelet count reduction, and prolonged bleeding time (9). In individuals with non-insulin dependent diabetes, fish oils appear to improve arterial compliance (1029,5707).

Adverse Reactions Including Known Allergies
Fish oils sometimes have a fishy taste. They can cause belching (507), halitosis, heartburn (6258), and nosebleeds (9). High doses can cause nausea and loose stools (9).

Possible Interactions with Herbs & Other Dietary Supplements
VITAMIN E: Theoretically, the risk of vitamin E deficiency increases with long-term use of fish oils (9).
HERBS WITH ANTICOAGULANT/ANTIPLATELET POTENTIAL: Concomitant use of herbs that have coumarin constituents or affect platelet aggregation could theoretically increase the risk of bleeding in some people. These herbs include: angelica, anise, arnica, asafoetida, bogbean, boldo, capsicum, celery, chamomile, clove, danshen, fenugreek, feverfew, garlic, ginger, ginkgo, ginseng (Panax), horse chestnut, horseradish, licorice, meadowsweet, prickly ash, onion, papain, passionflower, poplar, quassia, red clover, turmeric, wild carrot, wild lettuce, willow, and others (4,19).

Possible Interactions with Drugs
ANTICOAGULANTS/ANTIPLATELET DRUGS: Concomitant use with anticoagulant or antiplatelet drugs can increase the risk of bleeding (9,507). Some of these drugs include, aspirin, clopidogrel (Plavix), dalteparin (Fragmin), dipyridamole (Persantine), enoxaparin (Lovenox), heparin, ticlopidine (Ticlid), warfarin (Coumadin), and others.
ANTIDIABETES DRUGS: Theoretically, concomitant use might interfere with blood glucose control (9).
ANTIHYPERTENSIVE DRUGS: Fish oils can lower blood pressure and might have additive effects in patients treated antihypertensives (1001,1020,1030,1033); use with caution.
CYCLOSPORIN: Fish oils can reduce cyclosporin-induced hypertension in individuals after heart transplants, and may help protect against cyclosporine-induced nephrotoxicity (507,1012,1021).
ETRETINATE: Concomitant use of etretinate with eicosapentaenoic (EPA) can enhance the effects in psoriasis treatment (1000).

Possible Interactions with Foods
No interactions are known to occur, and there is no known reason to expect a clinically significant interaction with fish oils.

Possible Interactions with Lab Tests
ELECTROCARDIOGRAM (ECG): Fish oils might normalize ECG readings in some patients with ventricular ectopic beats. Fish oils might decrease ventricular ectopic beats (507).
BLOOD PRESSURE: Fish oils can moderately lower blood pressure and reduce blood pressure readings in patients with hypertension (1001,1020,1030,1033).
TRIGLYCERIDES: Fish oils can reduce serum triglyceride concentrations and test results by 20% to 50% in patients with elevated triglycerides (1003,1009,1014,1024).

Possible Interactions with Diseases or Conditions
ASPIRIN-SENSITIVE INDIVIDUALS: Fish oils should be used with caution because omega-3 fatty acids can decrease pulmonary function in aspirin-sensitive individuals (507).
CIRRHOSIS: Theoretically, use of fish oil may lower mean arterial pressure (MAP) to hypotensive levels, and may increase risk of bleeding (1013); use with caution.
DIABETES: Use fish oils with caution and monitor blood glucose levels because fish oils can interfere with blood glucose control (9).
FAMILIAL ADENOMATOUS POLYPOSIS: Three people, who had pre-existing familial adenomatous polyposis, were diagnosed with malignant lesions during the course of long-term use of fish oils (999).
HYPERTENSION: Fish oils can lower blood pressure and might have additive effects in patients treated antihypertensives (1001,1020,1030,1033).

Typical Dosages & Routes of Administration that are Commonly Used
ORAL: For lowering triglycerides, studies have used 1-2 grams per day (5707). For lowering blood pressure, studies have used either 4 grams of fish oils or fish oils providing EPA 2.04 grams and DHA 1.4 grams daily (1001,1020). For hypertension secondary to cyclosporine in heart transplant patients, 4 grams per day have been used (1012). For

cyclosporine nephrotoxicity, 12 grams per day containing 2.2 grams EPA and 1.4 grams DHA, has been used (1021). For reducing mortality after a myocardial infarction, a daily oral dose of fish oil providing EPA 1.08 grams has been used (1007). For improving endothelial function in individuals with hypercholesterolemia, 4 grams per day has been used (5702). For decreasing duration of morning stiffness secondary to rheumatoid arthritis, fish oils providing EPA 3.8 grams and DHA 2 grams per day has been used (1039). For preventing miscarriage in women with antiphospholipid antibody syndrome and a history of recurrent miscarriage, 5.1 grams fish oils with a 1.5 EPA:DHA ratio has been used (1032). As an adjunct to standard therapy for bipolar disorder, fish oil providing EPA 6.2 grams and DHA 3.4 grams daily has been used (7202). For weight loss, a daily serving of 2-7 ounces of fish containing approximately 3.65 grams omega-3 fatty acids (0.66 gm from EPA and 0.60 gram from DHA) has been used (2049). For improving appetite in individuals with pancreatic cancer fish oil providing EPA 2.2 grams and DHA 1.4 grams daily has been used (5701). For improving dark vision adaptation in dyslexic individuals, fish oil providing DHA 480 mg daily has been used (5708). For improving movement disorders in children with dyspraxia, fish oil providing DHA 480 mg combined with 35 mg arachidonic acid and 96 mg gamma-alpha linoleic acid from evening primrose oil, 24 mg thyme oil, and 80 mg vitamin E (Efalex) has been used (5708).
Fish oil supplements often contain small amounts of vitamin E as an antioxidant (9). They might also be combined with calcium, iron, or vitamins A, B1, B2, B3, C, or D (507).
INTRAVENOUS: For chronic plaque psoriasis, a daily 200 mL intravenous dose of a parenteral a fish oil-based lipid emulsion (Omegavenous), containing 4.2 grams EPA and 4.2 grams DHA, has been used for 14 days (1004). For acute, extended guttate psoriasis, a daily intravenous dose of a parenteral fish oil product, containing 2.1 grams EPA and 21 grams DHA, has been used for 10 days (1034).

Comments

Fish oils come from a variety of marine life including mackerel, herring, tuna, halibut, salmon (945), cod liver, whale blubber, and seal blubber (1048). Products that are commercially available contain varying amounts and ratios of docosahexaenoic acid (DHA) and eicosapentaenoic acid (EPA) (507). Some experts express concern about the high caloric value and cholesterol content of fish oils (9). Daily fish consumption may offer similar benefits for hyperlipidemia (2049). Researchers are investigating oils containing stearidonic acid (SDA) from genetically modified plants as an alternative to fish oil as a source of omega-3 fatty acids. SDA is metabolized to DHA and EPA in animals. However, further research is needed on the effects of SDA in humans (6129).

FLAXSEED

This Product is Also Known As
Flax Seed, Graine De Lin, Leinsamen, Lini Semen, Linseed, Lint Bells, Linum, Phytoestrogen, Winterlien.
CAUTION: See separate listing for Flaxseed Oil.

Scientific Names
Linum usitatissimum.
Family: Linaceae.

People Use This For
Orally, flaxseed is used for chronic constipation, colon damage due to laxative abuse, diverticulitis, irritable colon, gastritis, enteritis (2), reducing serum cholesterol (6), and bladder inflammation (18).
Topically, flaxseed is used as a poultice for skin inflammation (2).
Ophthalmically, flaxseed is used as an agent for the removal of foreign bodies from the eye (18).

Safety
LIKELY SAFE ...when taken orally in appropriate amounts with sufficient fluid intake, which is in a ratio of 1:10 (seed:liquid) (2,12). ...when applied topically (2), although the regular handling of flaxseed can cause sensitization (6).
PREGNANCY AND LACTATION: POSSIBLY SAFE ...but should be used with caution (2,12).

Effectiveness
LIKELY EFFECTIVE ...when taken orally for reducing high serum cholesterol (6).
POSSIBLY EFFECTIVE ...when taken orally as a bulk forming laxative (2). ...when used topically as a poultice for skin inflammation (2).
There is insufficient reliable information available about the effectiveness of flaxseed for its other uses.

Possible Mechanism of Action & Active Ingredients
The bulk-forming product stimulates intestinal peristalsis, producing a laxative effect (18). Flaxseed can reduce platelet aggregation and serum cholesterol in humans, thereby lowering atherogenic risks (6). It contains constituents that can have weak estrogenic and antiestrogenic properties (6) and cyanogenic glycosides, which can cause toxicity in grazing animals (6). Flaxseed can have lupus activity in mice (6).

Adverse Reactions Including Known Allergies

The oral consumption of flaxseed with inadequate liquid can cause intestinal blockage (18). Sensitization to flaxseed can occur with occupational exposure (6).

Possible Interactions with Herbs & Other Dietary Supplements

Insufficient reliable information available.

Possible Interactions with Drugs

ORAL DRUGS: The fiber in flaxseed can impair absorption of oral drugs (19).

Possible Interactions with Foods

No interactions are known to occur, and there is no known reason to expect a clinically significant interaction with flaxseed.

Possible Interactions with Lab Tests

CHOLESTEROL: Flaxseed can lower serum total cholesterol and LDL cholesterol concentrations, and test results (6).

Possible Interactions with Diseases or Conditions

CONTRAINDICATIONS: Bowel obstruction, esophageal stricture, and acute intestinal inflammation (2,12).

Typical Dosages & Routes of Administration that are Commonly Used

ORAL: The typical dose of flaxseed is 1 tablespoon of the whole or bruised seed (not ground) with 6 oz (150 ml) of liquid 2-3 times daily (2,12). Sufficient liquid with each dose is important to prevent possible intestinal blockage.
TOPICAL: 30-50 grams of flaxseed flour is commonly used for a moist and hot poultice or compress (2).
OPHTHALMIC: A single flaxseed is moistened and placed under the eyelid until the foreign body sticks to the mucus secretion (18).

Comments

Flaxseed has been used for more than ten thousand years as a fiber for weaving and clothing (6). Avoid confusion with flaxseed oil (linseed oil).

FLAXSEED OIL

This Product is Also Known As

Flax Seed Oil, Graine De Lin, Linseed Oil.
CAUTION: See separate listing for Flaxseed.

Scientific Names

Linum usitatissimum.
Family: Linaceae.

People Use This For

Orally, flaxseed oil is used as a food oil, as a supplemental source of dietary alpha-linolenic acid, for arthritis, to prevent heart attacks, for cancer (843), anxiety (294), benign prostatic hyperplasia, constipation, vaginitis (844), and for weight loss (293).
In veterinary medicine, flaxseed oil is given orally for constipation and used topically for demulcent and emollient properties (6).
In manufacturing, flaxseed oil is used as a component in paints and varnishes, and as a waterproofing agent (6).

Safety

LIKELY SAFE ...when flaxseed oil is used in food amounts.
There is insufficient reliable information available about the safety of flaxseed oil used in larger amounts than those found in food.
PREGNANCY: LIKELY UNSAFE ...contraindicated for oral use during pregnancy. Theoretically, flaxseed oil might enable onset of menstruation (19).
LACTATION: Insufficient reliable information available; avoid using amounts greater than found in foods (2,12).

Effectiveness

There is insufficient reliable information available about the effectiveness of flaxseed oil.

Possible Mechanism of Action & Active Ingredients

Flaxseed oil contains linolenic, linoleic, and oleic acids (6), and is among the best natural sources of alpha-linolenic acid (6). Linoleic acid and alpha-linolenic acid are required for the structural integrity of all cell membranes. Preliminary evidence suggests that flaxseed oil might reduce serum triglyceride levels in some patients with

© Copyright 2000, Natural Medicines Comprehensive Database (209) 472-2244. For updated data, go to www.NaturalDatabase.com

hyperlipoproteinemia (3911). One study found flaxseed oil to increase platelet eicosapentaenoic acid (EPA) levels and decrease platelet aggregation in healthy young men (845), while another study found flaxseed oil to have no effect on platelet aggregation in patients with hyperlipoproteinemia (3912).

Adverse Reactions Including Known Allergies
None reported.

Possible Interactions with Herbs & Other Dietary Supplements
Insufficient reliable information available.

Possible Interactions with Drugs
No interactions are known to occur, and there is no known reason to expect a clinically significant interaction with flaxseed oil.

Possible Interactions with Foods
No interactions are known to occur, and there is no known reason to expect a clinically significant interaction with flaxseed oil.

Possible Interactions with Lab Tests
TRIGLYCERIDES: Flaxseed oil might decrease serum triglyceride concentrations and test results in some patients with hyperlipoproteinemia (3911).

Possible Interactions with Diseases or Conditions
No interactions are known to occur, and there is no known reason to expect a clinically significant interaction with flaxseed oil.

Typical Dosages & Routes of Administration that are Commonly Used
Flaxseed (linseed) oil is available in commercial preparations for oral and topical use.

Comments
Specific deficiencies from inadequate intakes of essential fatty acids are rare except in individuals with severe, untreated fat malabsorption or those suffering from famine. Symptoms include dry, cracked, scaly and bleeding skin, excessive water loss from the skin, and impaired liver function resulting from the accumulation of lipid in the liver (i.e. fatty liver) (298).

FO-TI cured root

This Product is Also Known As
Fo Ti, Multiflora Preparata, Radix Polygoni Shen Min, Zhihe Shou Wu, Zhihe-Sho-Wu, Zhiheshouwu, Zi Shou Wu, Zi-Shou-Wu, Zishouwu.
CAUTION: See separate listing for Fo-Ti raw root.

Scientific Names
Source: Polygonum multiflorum.
Family: Polygonaceae.

People Use This For
In Chinese medicine, fo-ti is used as a liver and kidney tonic, blood and vital essence toner, and to fortify muscles, tendons, and bones. It is also used for hyperlipidemia, insomnia, limb numbness, lower back and knee soreness or weakness, premature graying, and dizziness with tinnitus (11).
In manufacturing, fo-ti extract is used as ingredient in hair and skin care products (11).

Safety
There is insufficient reliable information available about the safety of cured fo-ti root.
PREGNANCY: LIKELY UNSAFE …contraindicated for oral use because it could contain anthraquinone constituents (4,11).
LACTATION: LIKELY UNSAFE …contraindicated for oral use because if anthraquinone constituents are present, they could be excreted in breast milk, causing adverse effects (4,11).

Effectiveness
There is insufficient reliable information available about the effectiveness of fo-ti.

Possible Mechanism of Action & Active Ingredients
Raw fo-ti anthraquinone constituents (chrysophanol, emodin, rhein) are cathartic (11). Curing fo-ti reduces these constituents by 42-96%. Cured fo-ti shows evidence it might increase the levels of superoxide dismutase (SOD), serotonin, norepinephrine, dopamine, and decrease levels of monoamine oxidase-B (MAO-B), lipid peroxide, malonyl dialdehyde (MDA) (11); these are believed to be markers for anti-aging effects. Some evidence suggests fo-ti might also increase serum ceruloplasmin levels, reduce thymus gland atrophy, and inhibit atrophy of adrenal

glands; enhancing nonspecific and cellular immunity, and antagonizing the immunosuppressive effects of prednisolone or hydrocortisone (11). Other evidence suggests the alcoholic extract might increase high-density lipoprotein (HDL) cholesterol, reduce total cholesterol, free cholesterol, triglycerides, and retard atherosclerosis (11). The aqueous extract appears to inhibit the replication of hepatitis B (11).

Adverse Reactions Including Known Allergies
Taken orally, fo-ti may cause gastric distress (12).

Possible Interactions with Herbs & Other Dietary Supplements
Insufficient reliable information available.

Possible Interactions with Drugs
CORTICOSTEROIDS: Theoretically, concomitant use may antagonize drug effects (4).

Possible Interactions with Foods
No interactions are known to occur, and there is no known reason to expect a clinically significant interaction with fo-ti cured root.

Possible Interactions with Lab Tests
CHOLESTEROL: Theoretically, cured fo-ti might reduce serum total cholesterol concentrations and test results (11).
COLORIMETRIC TESTS: Cured fo-ti might discolor urine (pink, red, purple, orange, rust), interfering with diagnostic tests that depend on a color change, due to its anthraquinone content (11,275). Cured fo-ti contains 42-96% less anthraquinones than raw fo-ti (11).
GLUCOSE: Theoretically, cured fo-ti might increase or decrease blood glucose concentrations and test results (6,19).
POTASSIUM: Excessive use of cured fo-ti might cause potassium depletion, reducing serum potassium concentrations and test results due to its anthraquinone content (11). Cured fo-ti contains 42-96% less anthraquinones than raw fo-ti (11).
TRIGLYCERIDES: Theoretically, cured fo-ti might reduce serum triglyceride concentrations and test results (11).

Possible Interactions with Diseases or Conditions
No interactions are known to occur, and there is no known reason to expect a clinically significant interaction with fo-ti cured root.

Typical Dosages & Routes of Administration that are Commonly Used
ORAL: People typically use 2.5 grams three times daily. A tea is also prepared by adding 3 to 5 grams (1/2 to 1 teaspoon) to water and boiled. Typically, 3 or more cups are consumed daily (5260).

Comments
Avoid confusion with fo-ti raw root. Many references do not distinguish between fo-ti raw root and fo-ti cured root; these are related products with different chemical composition, actions, and uses (11). Avoid confusion with commercial product Fo-ti-Teng, contains no fo-ti (6).

FO-TI raw root

This Product is Also Known As
Chinese Cornbind, Chinese Knotweed, Climbing Knotweed, Flowery Knotweed, Fo Ti, Foti, He Shou Wu, He-Shou-Wu, Heshouwu, Ho Shou Wu, Ho-Shou-Wu, Hoshouwu, Polygonum, Radix Polygoni Multiflori, Shen Min, Shou Wu, Shou-Wu, Shouwu.
CAUTION: See separate listing for Fo-Ti cured root.

Scientific Names
Polygonum multiflorum.
Family: Polygonaceae.

People Use This For
In Chinese medicine, fo-ti is used for treating lymph node tuberculosis, sores, carbuncles, skin eruptions, itching, and constipation (11).

Safety
There is insufficient reliable information available about the safety of the raw root of fo-ti.
PREGNANCY: LIKELY UNSAFE …contraindicated for oral use because it contains anthraquinone constituents (4).
LACTATION: LIKELY UNSAFE …contraindicated, anthraquinone constituents could be excreted in breast milk and cause adverse effects (4).

Effectiveness

POSSIBLY EFFECTIVE ...when used orally as a cathartic laxative (12).
There is insufficient reliable information available about the effectiveness of the raw root of fo-ti for its other uses.

Possible Mechanism of Action & Active Ingredients

Fo-ti contains chrysophanol and emodin along with a small amount of rhein (5). These anthraquinone derivatives are cathartics, which probably accounts for fo-ti's effectiveness in constipation. Some evidence suggests that isolated stilbene glycoside constituents might have liver protectant effects, including inhibition of GOT and GPT (11).

Adverse Reactions Including Known Allergies

Fo-ti taken orally may cause catharsis (12), diarrhea, abdominal pain, nausea, and vomiting. Reported extremity numbness and skin rashes may have been due to other ingredients present in combination formulas (11).

Possible Interactions with Herbs & Other Dietary Supplements

LAXATIVE HERBS: Theoretically, concomitant use may increase risk of fluid and electrolyte depletion. Laxative herbs include aloe, alder buckthorn, European buckthorn, cascara sagrada, frangula bark, senna, and others.
DIGITALIS: Theoretically, concomitant use may increase risk of potassium loss and digitalis cardiotoxicity.

Possible Interactions with Drugs

DIABETES THERAPY: Monitor blood glucose levels closely due to claims that fo-ti has hypoglycemic effects (19).
DIGOXIN: Theoretically, overuse of anthraquinone laxatives, (e.g. fo-ti) can increase the risk of potassium loss and digoxin cardiotoxicity (151,272).
LAXATIVES: Concomitant use can increase the risk of fluid and electrolyte depletion.
POTASSIUM-DEPLETING DIURETICS: Theoretically, concomitant use of anthraquinone laxatives (e.g. fo-ti) and potassium-depleting diuretics can increase risk of potassium depletion (151,272).

Possible Interactions with Foods

No interactions are known to occur, and there is no known reason to expect a clinically significant interaction with fo-ti raw root.

Possible Interactions with Lab Tests

COLORIMETRIC TESTS: Raw fo-ti might discolor urine (pink, red, purple, orange, rust), interfering with diagnostic tests that depend on a color change, due to its anthraquinone content (11,275).
GLUCOSE: Theoretically, raw fo-ti might increase or decrease blood glucose concentrations and test results (6,19).
POTASSIUM: Excessive use of raw fo-ti can cause potassium depletion, reducing serum potassium concentrations and test results (11).

Possible Interactions with Diseases or Conditions

HEART CONDITIONS: Theoretically, overuse/misuse may cause potassium depletion and exacerbate condition.
CONTRAINDICATED in diarrhea, intestinal obstruction, acute intestinal inflammation (Crohn's disease, ulcerative colitis, appendicitis), ulcer, abdominal pain of unknown origin, nausea, and vomiting.

Typical Dosages & Routes of Administration that are Commonly Used

ORAL: People typically use 1.22 grams to 2.44 grams three times daily at meals. The capsule contents may also be used to prepare a tea (5260).

Comments

Avoid confusion with fo-ti cured root. Many references do not distinguish between fo-ti cured root and fo-ti raw root; these are related products with different chemical composition, actions, and uses (11). Avoid confusion with commercial product Fo-ti-Teng, contains no fo-ti (6).

FOLIC ACID

This Product is Also Known As

B Complex Vitamin, B-Complex Vitamin, Folacin, Folate, Vitamin B9.

Scientific Names

Pteroylglutamic acid; Pteroylmonoglutamic acid; Pteroylpolyglutamate.

People Use This For

Orally, folic acid is used for preventing and treating folate deficiency. It is used for megaloblastic anemia resulting from folate or vitamin B12 deficiency and megaloblastic anemia in sickle cell disease, and for folate deficiency in intestinal malabsorption or sprue (14). Folic acid is also used orally in conditions commonly associated with folate deficiency, including ulcerative colitis, liver disease, alcoholism, renal dialysis, and drug-induced deficiency related to phenytoin, primidone, barbiturates, oral contraceptives, and nitrofurantoin. Folic acid is also used orally for preventing neural tube defects, reducing the risk of colon cancer, preventing pregnancy loss, hyperhomocystinemia, fragile-X syndrome, gingival hyperplasia, memory deficit, vitiligo, osteoporosis, restless leg syndrome, insomnia, depression, peripheral neuropathy, myelopathy, and AIDS. It is also used for reducing lometrexol and methotrexate toxicity, and for preventing signs of aging (14,15,16,412,2165,2251).

Topically, folic acid is used for treating gingival hyperplasia (14) and gingivitis (2152).

Parenterally, folic acid is used intramuscularly, subcutaneously, or intravenously for treating folate deficiency, particularly in patients with malabsorption or those who cannot take oral treatment (15).

Safety

LIKELY SAFE ...when used orally or parenterally and appropriately. Folic acid is generally considered safe when used in appropriate doses (14,15). It is recommended that doses should not exceed the tolerable upper limit of 1000 mcg per day. However, in certain malabsorption disorders, such as sprue, larger doses can be safely used (6241).

POSSIBLY UNSAFE ...when used orally in large doses. Doses above the tolerable upper limit of 1000 mcg per day should be avoided. This limit is recommended primarily due to the association between high-dose folic acid and precipitation or exacerbation of neuropathy related to vitamin B12 deficiency (6421,6242,6245). Very high doses of 15 mg per day have been associated with significant central nervous system (CNS) and gastrointestinal side effects (14,15,16,505).

PREGNANCY AND LACTATION: LIKELY SAFE ...when used orally and appropriately. Folic acid is commonly used during pregnancy for prevention of neural tube defects (14,3094).

Effectiveness

EFFECTIVE ...when used orally or parenterally for treating folic acid deficiency (14,15,16,505).

LIKELY EFFECTIVE ...when used orally for reducing the risk of neural tube birth defects (14,15). ...when used orally for treating hyperhomocystinemia (412,2146,2147,2148,2149,3886). The ability of folic acid to lower homocysteine levels has been shown in several clinical trials (2146,2147,2148,2149); however, studies have not shown that folic acid supplementation can prevent morbidity or mortality associated with cardiovascular disease. ...when used orally for reducing methotrexate toxicity in the treatment of rheumatoid arthritis (14,2162,2163,2164).

POSSIBLY EFFECTIVE ...when used orally for reducing methotrexate-related gastrointestinal side effects in the treatment of psoriasis (768). ...when used orally for reducing the risk of colon cancer (505,2140,2141,2142,2143,2144,2145,2250). ...when used orally for treating vitiligo (14,2153,2154). ...when used topically for treating gingival hyperplasia secondary to phenytoin therapy (2151). ...when used topically for treating gingivitis in pregnancy (2152).

POSSIBLY INEFFECTIVE ...when used orally for treating gingival hyperplasia secondary to phenytoin therapy (14,2150,2151,2152). ...when used orally for reducing lometrexol toxicity (14,2161).

LIKELY INEFFECTIVE ...when used orally for treating fragile-X syndrome (14,2155,2156,2157,2158,2159,2160).

There is insufficient reliable information available about the effectiveness of folic acid for its other uses. However, early evidence suggest folic acid might prevent the progression of subclinical atherosclerosis to symptomatic disease in at risk patients (3886,3887). Further evidence is needed to rate folic acid for this use.

Possible Mechanism of Action & Active Ingredients

Folate is the general term that refers to the various chemical forms of the vitamin (6241). Folic acid, or pteroylmonoglutamic acid, is the form used in vitamin supplements and fortified foods (6241). Folate in food is pteroylpolyglutamate, which has a polyglutamate side chain with peptide linkages (6241). Folate in food is about 40% less bioavailable than synthetic folic acid, which is almost 100% bioavailable (6241). Before folate from food can be absorbed, the polyglutamate side chain must be cleaved to form the absorbable monoglutamate form (6241). After folic acid is absorbed, it is converted to tetrahydrofolate. In humans, tetrahydrofolate-based coenzymes play a major role in intracellular metabolism. Tetrahydrofolate plays an indirect role in the rate-limiting step in DNA synthesis. Abnormalities in this process that occur with folic acid deficiency cause megaloblastic anemia. Folic acid supplementation can correct this problem (14). Folic acid can also reduce damage to DNA and prevent replication errors (2139,2144). Tetrahydrofolate-based coenzymes are also involved in the conversion of homocysteine to methionine (14). Supplementation with folic acid increases conversion of homocysteine to methionine, lowering homocysteine levels and making it useful for hyperhomocystinemia (412,2146,2147,2148,2149,3886). Hyperhomocystinemia has been linked to cardiovascular disease, and low folic acid levels have been associated with elevated homocysteine levels and increased risk of myocardial infarction (1899). It is thought that folic acid supplementation might then decrease the risk of cardiovascular disease, but this has not been demonstrated in studies. However, early evidence suggests that folic acid alone or in combination with other B vitamins can reduce arterial endothelial dysfunction in people with elevated homocysteine levels (412,6235,6236). Folic acid also seems to play an important part in pregnancy. Low folate levels have been associated with recurrent spontaneous pregnancy loss (6237). Whether folate supplementation might be beneficial in women with histories of early pregnancy loss has not been studied. Folic acid also supplementation also prevents neural tube defects in the fetus. However, the role of folic in this process is not understood (15). Folic acid might play a role in Alzheimer's disease. Preliminary clinical evidence indicates that low folate concentrations might be related to atrophy of the cerebral cortex, particularly in people with neocortical lesions related to Alzheimer's disease (6234). A study of nuns, who were highly comparable for environmental and lifestyle factors, strongly associated low serum folate levels to cerebral atrophy on autopsy (6234). Functional and mental deterioration have been associated with low folate levels in elderly people (6238). Folate deficiency has also been attributed to melancholic depression and poor response to antidepressants (6239). Crohn's disease has been associated with decreased folate levels (6269). Low red blood cell folate levels have been associated with the development of dysplasia and cancer in ulcerative colitis (6270). Preliminary clinical evidence suggests folate supplementation might protect against cancer in people with ulcerative colitis (6271).

Adverse Reactions Including Known Allergies

Orally, high doses of folic acid can cause altered sleep patterns, vivid dreaming, irritability, excitability, overactivity, confusion, impaired judgment, exacerbation of seizure frequency and psychotic behavior, nausea, abdominal distention, flatulence, bitter taste in the mouth, allergic skin reactions, and zinc depletion (14,15). In one study, these effects were observed after administration of 15 mg per day for 30 days. Large doses of folic acid can also precipitate or exacerbate neuropathy in people deficient in vitamin B12 (6243). Allergic reactions have occurred rarely. Symptoms have included rash, erythema, itching, malaise, and bronchospasm. An anaphylactic reaction has been reported in one patient receiving intravenous folic acid. Use of folic acid for undiagnosed anemia has masked the symptoms of pernicious anemia, resulting in lack of treatment and eventual neurological damage (15). Patients should be warned to not self-treat suspected anemia.

Possible Interactions with Herbs & Other Dietary Supplements

ZINC: Chronic administration of folic acid can decrease zinc levels (14,15).
VITAMIN B12: Long-term use of folic acid can deplete levels of vitamin B12 (15).

Possible Interactions with Drugs

CHLORAMPHENICOL: Concomitant use can reduce the effectiveness of folic acid in the treatment of anemias (15).
CHOLESTYRAMINE (Questran): Concomitant use can decrease bioavailability of supplemental folic acid (4455).
COLESTIPOL (Colestid): Concomitant administration can decrease bioavailability of supplemental folic acid (14,4461).
PANCREATIC ENZYMES (Pancreatin): Concomitant use can interfere with folic acid absorption (14).
METHOTREXATE (MTX, Rheumatrex): Theoretically, concomitant use might interfere with the effectiveness of methotrexate cancer therapy (15). However, when methotrexate is used in rheumatoid arthritis and psoriasis therapy, large amounts of folic acid can reduce methotrexate side effects without interfering with effectiveness (767,768,2162,4492,4493,4494,4546).
PHENYTOIN (Dilantin), FOSPHENYTOIN (Cerebyx), PRIMIDONE (Mysoline), PHENOBARBITAL: Folic acid can increase metabolism and reduce the serum levels of these drugs (14,15,505). These drugs can also affect folic acid (see Drug Influences on Nutrient Levels and Depletion).
PYRIMETHAMINE (Daraprim): Concomitant use can decrease the effectiveness of pyrimethamine (14).
SULFASALAZINE (Azulfidine): Concomitant use can decrease folic acid absorption (14).

Drug Influences on Nutrient Levels and Depletion

SOME DRUGS CAN AFFECT FOLIC ACID LEVELS:
ANTIBIOTICS: Destruction of normal gastrointestinal flora by antibiotics can cause decreased production of B vitamins. The clinical significance of this decreased production is not known. Consider supplementation only if clinical judgment warrants it (4434,4435,4436,4437,4438,4439,4440,4441,4442,4443).
CARBAMAZEPINE (Tegretol): Treatment with carbamazepine is associated with decreased folic acid levels. However, the necessity for folic acid supplementation to prevent peripheral neuropathies or red cell dyscrasias has not been adequately studied (4426,4427,4428,4429).
CYCLOSERINE (Seromycin): Use of cycloserine can impair dietary folic acid absorption and reduce serum folic acid levels. The need for supplementation has not been adequately studied (4531).
FUROSEMIDE (Lasix): Use of furosemide might increase the excretion of folic acid (1898). Long-term furosemide therapy (1894) in people with hypertension has been associated with decreased folic acid levels and increased homocysteine levels (1898). Elevated homocysteine levels are associated with atherosclerotic vascular disease, arterial and venous thromboembolism, coronary, cerebral, and peripheral arterial occlusive diseases, and increased risk of myocardial infarction in smokers (1891,1892,1893,1899). However, the need for folic acid supplementation during furosemide therapy has not been adequately studied.
METFORMIN (Glucophage): Metformin may reduce serum folic acid and vitamin B12 levels (32,4490). A multivitamin preparation may be valuable in some patients.
METHOTREXATE: Methotrexate binds to dihydrofolate reductase and prevents the conversion of folate to folic acid (1716,1717,1718,1719). Consider folic acid supplements for prolonged methotrexate therapy.
ORAL CONTRACEPTIVES: Use of oral contraceptives can impair dietary folic acid absorption and reduce serum folic acid levels. The need for folic acid supplementation has not been adequately studied (4498,4499).
p-AMINOSALICYLIC ACID (PAS, Aminosalicylic acid): Concomitant use can decrease folic acid absorption in the gastrointestinal tract. The need for supplementation has not been adequately studied. Consider supplementation only if clinical judgment warrants it (4557,4558,4559,4560).
PENTAMIDINE (NebuPent): Treatment with pentamidine can impair dietary folic acid absorption and reduce serum folic acid levels. The need for folic acid supplementation during pentamidine therapy has not been adequately studied (4351).
PHENOBARBITAL (Luminal), PRIMIDONE (Mysoline): These drugs can impair dietary folic acid absorption

and reduce serum folic acid levels. The need for folic acid supplementation has not been adequately studied (4453,4530,4531).

PHENYTOIN (Dilantin), FOSPHENYTOIN (Cerebyx): These drugs can reduce serum folic acid levels. Clinical evidence suggests that giving supplemental folic acid with the initial dose of phenytoin might prevent folic acid deficiency (4471,4472,4473,4474,4477,4531).

PYRIMETHAMINE (Daraprim): Treatment with pyrimethamine can reduce serum folic acid levels. At lower pyrimethamine doses, the need for folic acid supplementation has not been adequately studied. However, with larger pyrimethamine doses (those required to treat toxoplasmosis), if signs of folic acid deficiency develop, administer folinic acid (Leucovorin) 5-15 mg/day (orally, IV, or IM) until normal hematopoiesis is restored (4425,4532).

SULFASALAZINE (Azulfidine): Sulfasalazine-induced blood dyscrasias might involve folic acid depletion. Foods high in folic acid rather than folic acid supplements have been recommended (4515,4516,4517).

THIAZIDE DIURETICS: These drugs might increase the excretion of folic acid. Long-term thiazide diuretic therapy (1894) in people with hypertension has been associated with decreased folic acid levels and increased homocysteine levels (1898). Elevated homocysteine levels are associated with atherosclerotic vascular disease, arterial and venous thromboembolism, coronary, cerebral, and peripheral arterial occlusive diseases, and increased risk of myocardial infarction in smokers (1891,1892,1893,1899). The need for folic acid supplementation during thiazide diuretic therapy has not been adequately studied.

TRIMETHOPRIM (Trimpex): Trimethoprim, including trimethoprim contained in the combination antibiotic trimethoprim/sulfamethoxazole (TMP/SMX, Septra) can interfere with folic acid metabolism, reduce serum folic acid levels, and cause mild folic acid deficiency in patients on long-term or high-dose therapy (4468,4531).

TRIAMTERENE (Dyrenium): Use of triamterene can decrease the utilization of dietary folic acid and reduce serum folic acid levels. The need for folic acid supplementation has not been adequately studied (14,4425,4536,4537).

Possible Interactions with Foods

FOODS: Taking folic acid with food slightly decreases the absorption of folic acid (6241). With food, the bioavailability is estimated at 85% compared to nearly 100% when taken without food (6241).

Possible Interactions with Lab Tests

MEAN CORPUSCULAR VOLUME (MCV): Folic acid supplementation can normalize megaloblastic anemia in cases of folic acid and vitamin B12 deficiencies. In cases of vitamin B12 deficiency or pernicious anemia, treatment with folic acid will normalize hematological findings, but will not prevent neurological damage (14).

Possible Interactions with Diseases or Conditions

PERNICIOUS ANEMIA: Folic acid can mask pernicious anemia by decreasing megaloblastic anemia. This can prevent appropriate treatment with vitamin B12 and result in neurological damage (14,15,16,505). Patients should be warned to avoid treating undiagnosed anemia with folic acid.

SEIZURE DISORDERS: Supplemental folic acid can exacerbate seizures in people with seizure disorders. This was reported in a study using 800 mcg folic acid per day in pregnant women with seizure disorders (14).

SCHIZOPHRENIA: Folic acid supplementation might exacerbate psychotic behavior in schizophrenic patients, despite have normal folic acid blood levels initially (14).

Typical Dosages & Routes of Administration that are Commonly Used

ORAL: For folate deficiency, the typical dose is 250-1000 mcg per day (14,15). For preventing neural tube defects, 400 mcg folic acid per day from supplements or fortified food should be taken by women capable of becoming pregnant and continued through the first month of pregnancy (6241,6243). Women with a history of previous pregnancy complicated by such neural tube defect usually take 4 mg per day beginning one month before and continuing for three months after conception (14,15). For reducing colon cancer risk, 400 mcg per day has been used (2250). For hyperhomocystinemia and reducing atherogenesis, 400-1000 mcg per day has been used (412,2146,2147,2148,2149). For vitiligo, 5 mg is typically taken twice daily (14,2153). For the reduction of methotrexate toxicity, 5 mg a week or 1 mg daily is used (14,2162,2163,2164). The adequate intakes (AI) for infants are 65 mcg for infants 0-6 months and 80 mcg for infants 7-12 months of age (3094). The recommended dietary allowances (RDAs) for folate in DFE, including both food folate and folic acid from fortified foods and supplements are: Children 1-3 years, 150 mcg; Children 4-8 years, 200 mcg; Children 9-13 years, 300 mcg; Adults over 13 years, 400 mcg; Pregnant women 600 mcg; and Lactating women, 500 mcg (3094,6243). The maximum daily levels of folate not likely to pose a risk for adverse effects are 300 mcg for children 1-3 years of age, 400 mcg for children 4-8 years, 600 mcg for children 9-13 years, 800 mcg for adolescents 14-18 years, and 1000 mcg for everyone over 18 years of age (3094).

TOPICAL: For gingival hyperplasia secondary to phenytoin therapy, a 0.1% folate mouthwash is used twice daily (2166). For gingivitis in pregnancy, a folate mouthwash is used twice daily (2152).

Dietary folate equivalents (DFE) are used to account for the differences in absorption of folate from food and synthetic folic acid, either from supplements or fortified food (6241,6243). The Institute of Medicine established these equivalencies: 1 mcg DFE equals 1 mcg food folate equals 0.6 mcg folic-acid-fortified food equals 0.5 mcg supplemental folic acid taken on an empty stomach (6243). Thus 1 mcg supplemental folic acid taken on an empty stomach equals 2 mcg DFE (6241).

© Copyright 2000, Natural Medicines Comprehensive Database (209) 472-2244. For updated data, go to www.NaturalDatabase.com

Comments

Beginning in 1998, the US government required folic acid fortification of all cold cereals and baking flour, which extends to breads, pastas, bakery items, cookies, crackers, etc. (6241). Foods that are naturally high in folate content include spinach, okra, asparagus, legumes, beef liver, and orange and tomato juice (6241).

Folic acid is frequently used in combination with other B vitamins in vitamin B complex formulations. Vitamin B complex generally includes vitamin B1 (thiamine), vitamin B2 (riboflavin), vitamin B3 (niacin/niacinamide), vitamin B5 (pantothenic acid), vitamin B6 (pyridoxine), vitamin B12 (cyanocobalamin), and folic acid. However, some products do not contain all of these ingredients and some may include others, such as biotin, para-aminobenzoic acid (PABA), choline bitartrate, and inositol (3022,3060,3061).

FOOL'S PARSLEY

This Product is Also Known As

Dog Parsley, Dog Poison, Fool's-Cicely, Fools Parsley, Lesser Hemlock, Small Hemlock.
CAUTION: See separate listings for Parsley leaf, root, Parsley seed, and Parsley Piert.

Scientific Names

Aethusa cynapium.
Family: Apiaceae or Umbelliferae.

People Use This For

Orally, fool's parsley is used for gastrointestinal complaints in children, infantile cholera, summer diarrhea, and convulsions (18).

Safety

LIKELY UNSAFE ...when used orally; avoid using. Plant parts are considered poisonous and are associated with serious, potentially life-threatening poisonings (18).
PREGNANCY AND LACTATION: UNSAFE ...contraindicated, due to potential for poisoning (18).

Effectiveness

There is insufficient reliable information available about the effectiveness of fool's parsley.

Possible Mechanism of Action & Active Ingredients

Fool's parsley contains varied flavone glycosides (rutoside, narcissine, camphor oil-3-glucorhamnoside). Freshly harvested leaves (only) contain polyenes aethusin, aethusanol A, asthusanol B (18).

Adverse Reactions Including Known Allergies

There are reports that ingestion caused deaths when fool's parsley was mistaken for garden parsley; however, there is some evidence that the botanical to blame was actually spotted hemlock (18). Nevertheless, caution is warranted.

Possible Interactions with Herbs & Other Dietary Supplements

Insufficient reliable information available.

Possible Interactions with Drugs

No interactions are known to occur, and there is no known reason to expect a clinically significant interaction with fool's parsley.

Possible Interactions with Foods

No interactions are known to occur, and there is no known reason to expect a clinically significant interaction with fool's parsley.

Possible Interactions with Lab Tests

No interactions are known to occur, and there is no known reason to expect a clinically significant interaction with fool's parsley.

Possible Interactions with Diseases or Conditions

No interactions are known to occur, and there is no known reason to expect a clinically significant interaction with fool's parsley.

Typical Dosages & Routes of Administration that are Commonly Used

No typical dosage.

Comments

Fool's parsley is considered unsafe; avoid using. Fool's parsley looks a lot like young garden parsley; hence its name. Be careful not to confuse the two, since fool's parsley is poisonous (18).

FORGET-ME-NOT

This Product is Also Known As
Forget Me Not.

Scientific Names
Myosotis arvensis.
Family: Borraginaceae.

People Use This For
Orally, forget-me-not is used for respiratory disorders and nose bleeds (18).

Safety
LIKELY UNSAFE …when the flowering plant preparations are used orally because they contain hepatotoxic unsaturated pyrrolizidine alkaloids (UPAs) (18). Repeated exposure to low concentrations of UPAs is linked to serious liver toxicity. UPAs are also thought to be carcinogenic and mutagenic (12).
PREGNANCY AND LACTATION: LIKELY UNSAFE …contraindicated for oral use because it contains UPAs (12,19).

Effectiveness
There is insufficient reliable information available about the effectiveness of forget-me-not.

Possible Mechanism of Action & Active Ingredients
The applicable part of forget-me-not is the whole flowering plant. Forget-me-not contains unsaturated pyrrolizidine alkaloids that can cause toxicity (18).

Adverse Reactions Including Known Allergies
When used orally, acute toxicity may result in hepatic necrosis; chronic toxicity may cause veno-occlusive liver disease. The potential for hepatotoxicity increases with larger doses and longer periods of use (4,12).

Possible Interactions with Herbs & Other Dietary Supplements
Insufficient reliable information available.

Possible Interactions with Drugs
No interactions are known to occur, and there is no known reason to expect a clinically significant interaction with forget-me-not.

Possible Interactions with Foods
No interactions are known to occur, and there is no known reason to expect a clinically significant interaction with forget-me-not.

Possible Interactions with Lab Tests
No interactions are known to occur, and there is no known reason to expect a clinically significant interaction with forget-me-not.

Possible Interactions with Diseases or Conditions
No interactions are known to occur, and there is no known reason to expect a clinically significant interaction with forget-me-not.

Typical Dosages & Routes of Administration that are Commonly Used
No typical dosage.

Comments
Forget-me-not is considered unsafe; avoid using (18).

FRANKINCENSE

This Product is Also Known As
Bible Frankincense, Olibanum.
CAUTION: See separate listing for Indian Frankincense.

Scientific Names
Boswellia carteri.
Family: Burseraceae.

People Use This For
Orally, frankincense is used for colic and flatulence.
Topically, frankincense is used in hand cream (18).

Safety

POSSIBLY SAFE ...when used orally (12).

There is insufficient reliable information available about the safety of the topical use of frankincense.

PREGNANCY AND LACTATION: Insufficient reliable information available; avoid using.

Effectiveness

There is insufficient reliable information available about the effectiveness of frankincense.

Possible Mechanism of Action & Active Ingredients

The applicable part of frankincense is the resin. There is insufficient reliable information available about the possible mechanism of action and active ingredients.

Adverse Reactions Including Known Allergies

Frankincense can cause mild irritation when used topically (18).

Possible Interactions with Herbs & Other Dietary Supplements

Insufficient reliable information available.

Possible Interactions with Drugs

No interactions are known to occur, and there is no known reason to expect a clinically significant interaction with frankincense.

Possible Interactions with Foods

No interactions are known to occur, and there is no known reason to expect a clinically significant interaction with frankincense.

Possible Interactions with Lab Tests

No interactions are known to occur, and there is no known reason to expect a clinically significant interaction with frankincense.

Possible Interactions with Diseases or Conditions

No interactions are known to occur, and there is no known reason to expect a clinically significant interaction with frankincense.

Typical Dosages & Routes of Administration that are Commonly Used

No typical dosage.

Comments

Frankincense is the hardened gum resin extruded from incisions made in the trunk of Boswellia carteri. Olibanum is a term which refers to the oleogum resin exuded from incisions in the bark of several Boswellia species, including Boswellia serrata (Indian frankincense), Boswellia carterii (Bible frankincense), Boswellia frereana (African elemi), and Boswellia bhau-dajiana (11). The black kohl used by Egyptian women to paint their eyelids is an ingredient from charred frankincense. Frankincense is considered obsolete as a medicinal herb (18).

FRINGETREE

This Product is Also Known As

Chionanthus, Gray Beard Tree, Old Man's Beard, Poison Ash, Snowdrop Tree, Snowflower, White Fringe.

Scientific Names

Chionanthus virginicus.

Family: Oleaceae.

People Use This For

Orally, fringetree is used for the treatment of liver and gallbladder disorders, including gallstones. It is used to stimulate bile flow, as a diuretic, and as a tonic (18).

Safety

There is insufficient reliable information available about the safety of fringetree.

Pregnancy and Lactation: Insufficient reliable information available; avoid using.

Effectiveness

There is insufficient reliable information available about the effectiveness of fringetree.

Possible Mechanism of Action & Active Ingredients

Insufficient reliable information available.

Adverse Reactions Including Known Allergies

None reported.

Possible Interactions with Herbs & Other Dietary Supplements
Insufficient reliable information available.

Possible Interactions with Drugs
No interactions are known to occur, and there is no known reason to expect a clinically significant interaction with fringetree.

Possible Interactions with Foods
No interactions are known to occur, and there is no known reason to expect a clinically significant interaction with fringetree.

Possible Interactions with Lab Tests
No interactions are known to occur, and there is no known reason to expect a clinically significant interaction with fringetree.

Possible Interactions with Diseases or Conditions
No interactions are known to occur, and there is no known reason to expect a clinically significant interaction with fringetree.

Typical Dosages & Routes of Administration that are Commonly Used
ORAL: Fringetree is used as a liquid extract (18).

Comments
Fringetree is almost odorless and very bitter to taste (18).
There is very little scientific information about this product. Our staff is continually analyzing the available information on natural medicines and will add data here as it becomes available.

FROSTWORT

This Product is Also Known As
Frost Plant, Frostweed, Rock-Rose, Sun Rose.

Scientific Names
Helianthemum canadense.

People Use This For
Orally, frostwort is used for digestive disorders (18).
Topically, frostwort is used for ulcers (18).

Safety
There is insufficient reliable information available about the safety of frostwort.
Pregnancy and Lactation: Insufficient reliable information available; avoid using.

Effectiveness
There is insufficient reliable information available about the effectiveness of frostwort.

Possible Mechanism of Action & Active Ingredients
The applicable parts of frostwort are the above ground parts. Frostwort contains tannins and the glycoside helianthinin. It appears to have astringent and tonic effects(18).

Adverse Reactions Including Known Allergies
None reported.

Possible Interactions with Herbs & Other Dietary Supplements
Insufficient reliable information available.

Possible Interactions with Drugs
No interactions are known to occur, and there is no known reason to expect a clinically significant interaction with frostwort.

Possible Interactions with Foods
No interactions are known to occur, and there is no known reason to expect a clinically significant interaction with frostwort.

Possible Interactions with Lab Tests
No interactions are known to occur, and there is no known reason to expect a clinically significant interaction with frostwort.

Possible Interactions with Diseases or Conditions

No interactions are known to occur, and there is no known reason to expect a clinically significant interaction with frostwort.

Typical Dosages & Routes of Administration that are Commonly Used

Used as an extract (18).

Comments

There is very little scientific information about this product. Our staff is continually analyzing the available information on natural medicines and will add data here as it becomes available.

FRUCTO-OLIGOSACCHARIDES

This Product is Also Known As

FOS, Fructooligosaccharides Oligofructose.

Scientific Names

Beta-D-fructofuranosidase.

People Use This For

Orally, fructo-oligosaccharides are used for prebiotic activity, specifically for bifidobacteria in the GI tract (742). Prebiotic refers to the use of a substance to promote the growth of GI flora. Fructo-oligosaccharides are also used orally for reducing serum cholesterol (743) and increasing fecal mass (744).
In foods, fructo-oligosaccharides are used as a sweetener (740,741).

Safety

POSSIBLY SAFE ...when consumed in amounts less than 30 grams per day (741,745).
PREGNANCY AND LACTATION: Insufficient reliable information available; avoid using.

Effectiveness

There is insufficient reliable information available about the effectiveness of fructo-oligosaccharides.

Possible Mechanism of Action & Active Ingredients

Fructo-oligosaccharides (FOS) pass undigested through the small intestine and are fermented in the colon. In the colon, they specifically promote the growth of some species of the indigenous microflora, especially bifidobacteria. FOS are not hydrolyzed by human digestive enzymes (746), yet they are not recoverable in the feces suggesting complete colonic metabolism (747). Colonic fermentation leads to increased fecal biomass, decreased ceco-colonic pH, and production of short chain fatty acids. The short chain fatty acids exert systemic effects on lipid metabolism similarly to dietary fiber (744). FOS can counteract advanced stages of colon carcinogenesis in mice (748).

Adverse Reactions Including Known Allergies

The use of FOS can cause flatulence in amounts exceeding 10 grams (740), excessive flatus at 30 grams per day, GI sounds and bloating at 40 grams per day, and abdominal cramps and diarrhea at 50 grams per day (745).

Possible Interactions with Herbs & Other Dietary Supplements

BIFIDOBACTERIUM BIFIDUM: Concomitant use of FOS can promote the growth of supplemental bifidobacteria.

Possible Interactions with Drugs

No interactions are known to occur, and there is no known reason to expect a clinically significant interaction with fructo-oligosaccharides.

Possible Interactions with Foods

No interactions are known to occur, and there is no known reason to expect a clinically significant interaction with fructo-oligosaccharides.

Possible Interactions with Lab Tests

No interactions are known to occur, and there is no known reason to expect a clinically significant interaction with fructo-oligosaccharides.

Possible Interactions with Diseases or Conditions

No interactions are known to occur, and there is no known reason to expect a clinically significant interaction with fructo-oligosaccharides.

Typical Dosages & Routes of Administration that are Commonly Used

ORAL: For prebiotic effect (to increase fecal bifidobacteria), the typical dose is 4 to 10 grams per day (749,750).

Comments

Fructo-oligosaccharides are non-digestible plant sugars derived from asparagus, Jerusalem artichokes, and soybeans.

FUMITORY

This Product is Also Known As

Beggary, Earth Smoke, Fumiterry, Fumus, Hedge Fumitory, Herba fumariae, Vapor, Wax Dolls.

Scientific Names

Fumaria officinalis.
Family: Fumariaceae.

People Use This For

Orally, fumitory is used for GI spasms (2) and as a bile flow stimulant (4).
Historically, fumitory has been used for skin eruptions (4), eczema (6), conjunctivitis (4), and cardiovascular disorders (6), and as a diuretic and laxative (4,6).

Safety

POSSIBLY SAFE ...when above ground parts are used orally and appropriately. No significant toxicity usually occurs in standard doses (4,6).
POSSIBLY UNSAFE ...when used orally in large amounts because it contains the alkaloid protopine. Other Fumariaceae species that contain alkaloids including protopine can cause convulsions and death when large amounts are ingested (6). ...when homemade, non-sterile products are used for ophthalmic use (4).
PREGNANCY AND LACTATION: Insufficient reliable information available; avoid using (4).

Effectiveness

POSSIBLY EFFECTIVE ...when taken orally for biliary disorders (4,6,280).
There is insufficient reliable information available about the effectiveness of fumitory for its other uses.

Possible Mechanism of Action & Active Ingredients

The applicable parts of fumitory are the above ground parts. Fumitory can have weak antispasmodic effects on the smooth muscle of the bile duct and upper GI tract (2,4,18). The major alkaloid constituent, protopine, has antihistamine, hypotensive, bradycardic, and sedative activity in small doses, and it causes excitation and convulsions in large doses (4). Fumitory can exhibit bactericidal activity against gram-positive organisms, including Bacillus anthracis and Staphylococcus (4).

Adverse Reactions Including Known Allergies

Adverse reactions to fumitory are not common; however, large quantities of alkaloids in other members of this family (Fumariaceae) have caused trembling, convulsions, and death (2).

Possible Interactions with Herbs & Other Dietary Supplements

Insufficient reliable information available.

Possible Interactions with Drugs

No interactions are known to occur, and there is no known reason to expect a clinically significant interaction with fumitory.

Possible Interactions with Foods

No interactions are known to occur, and there is no known reason to expect a clinically significant interaction with fumitory.

Possible Interactions with Lab Tests

No interactions are known to occur, and there is no known reason to expect a clinically significant interaction with fumitory.

Possible Interactions with Diseases or Conditions

EYE INFECTIONS: Avoid non-sterile and homemade products.

Typical Dosages & Routes of Administration that are Commonly Used

ORAL: The typical dose of fumitory is 2-4 grams of the above ground parts per day or as a tea three times daily (4). The tea is prepared by steeping the herb in 150 mL boiling water for 5-10 minutes and then straining. The usual dose of the liquid extract (1:1 in 25% alcohol) is 2-4 mL three times daily, and the tincture (1:5 in 45% alcohol) is commonly dosed 1-4 mL three times daily (4).
NEBULIZERS have been used to administer the extract; no typical dosage. (6).

© Copyright 2000, Natural Medicines Comprehensive Database (209) 472-2244. For updated data, go to www.NaturalDatabase.com • 453

Comments

The fumitory plant is a low shrub with gray pointed leaves, and from a distance the plant can have the wispy appearance of smoke, because of this it received the name "earth smoke" (6).

GABA (GAMMA-AMINOBUTYRIC ACID)

This Product is Also Known As

Gamma Amino Butyric Acid, Gamma Amino-Butyric Acid, Gamma Aminobutyric Acid.

Scientific Names

Gamma-aminobutyric acid.

People Use This For

Orally, GABA is used for relieving anxiety, elevating mood, relieving premenstrual syndrome (PMS), promoting lean muscle growth, burning fat, stabilizing blood pressure, and relieving pain (5111,5112).
Sublingually, GABA is used for increasing feeling of well being, relieving injuries, improving exercise tolerance, decreasing body fat, and increasing lean body weight (5471).

Safety

There is insufficient reliable information available about the safety of GABA.
Pregnancy and Lactation: Insufficient reliable information available; avoid using.

Effectiveness

There is insufficient reliable information available about the effectiveness of GABA.

Possible Mechanism of Action & Active Ingredients

In the central nervous system, GABA is the primary inhibitory neurotransmitter. It is synthesized in the brain by decarboxylation of glutamate (5109,5110). GABA exerts anticonvulsant, sedative, and anxiolytic effects at the cellular level (5109,5110). Single, oral doses of GABA given to people with photo-convulsant epilepsy had no effect (5113). Single, oral doses of 5 or 10 grams of GABA caused a rise in C-peptide, insulin, and glucagon but not serum glucose in healthy people (5114). GABA given intravenously can cause dysphoria and dose-related increases in blood pressure and pulse (5116). In healthy volunteers, a single 5 gram dose of GABA increased growth hormone, but chronic four-day administration of 18 grams of GABA decreased growth hormone and increased serum prolactin (5115).

Adverse Reactions Including Known Allergies

None reported.

Possible Interactions with Herbs & Other Dietary Supplements

Insufficient reliable information available.

Possible Interactions with Drugs

No interactions are known to occur, and there is no known reason to expect a clinically significant interaction with GABA.

Possible Interactions with Foods

No interactions are known to occur, and there is no known reason to expect a clinically significant interaction with GABA.

Possible Interactions with Lab Tests

No interactions are known to occur, and there is no known reason to expect a clinically significant interaction with GABA.

Possible Interactions with Diseases or Conditions

No interactions are known to occur, and there is no known reason to expect a clinically significant interaction with GABA.

Typical Dosages & Routes of Administration that are Commonly Used

ORAL: People typically use 500 to 2250 mg daily, although some products suggest doses ranging from 250 mg to 5000 mg daily (5117,5118,6006). Some products recommend bedtime dosing (6006).
SUBLINGUAL: People typically use 3 to 5 grams 1 to 2 times daily (5471).

Comments

Although GABA is promoted as an alternative to the benzodiazepines (5111,5112), no clinical trials support these uses.

GALBANUM

This Product is Also Known As
Galbanum Gum, Galbanum Gum Resin, Galbanum Oleogum Resin, Galbanum Oleoresin, Galbanum Resin.

Scientific Names
Ferula gummosa.
Family: Umbelliferae.

People Use This For
Orally, galbanum is used for digestive disorders and flatulence. It is used orally as an appetite stimulant, expectorant (18), and antispasmodic (11).
Topically, galbanum is used for wound treatment (18).
In food and beverages, galbanum oil and resin are used as flavor components .
In manufacturing, galbanum oil and resin are used as fragrance components in cosmetics. Galbanum is rarely used in pharmaceuticals (11).

Safety
LIKELY SAFE ...in amounts found in foods (11). Approved for food use in the US.
POSSIBLY SAFE ...when used topically (11).
There is insufficient reliable information available about the safety of the oral use of galbanum in amounts greater than those amounts typically found in foods.
PREGNANCY AND LACTATION: Avoid using in amounts greater than those typically found in foods.

Effectiveness
There is insufficient reliable information available about the effectiveness of galbanum.

Possible Mechanism of Action & Active Ingredients
The applicable part of galbanum is the gum resin from the roots and trunk. In vitro data suggest antimicrobial activity, particularly against Staphylococcus aureus. Galbanum may also be effective as an emulsion preservative. Emulsions containing galbanum were stable for up to 6 months (11).

Adverse Reactions Including Known Allergies
None reported.

Possible Interactions with Herbs & Other Dietary Supplements
Insufficient reliable information available.

Possible Interactions with Drugs
No interactions are known to occur, and there is no known reason to expect a clinically significant interaction with galbanum.

Possible Interactions with Foods
No interactions are known to occur, and there is no known reason to expect a clinically significant interaction with galbanum.

Possible Interactions with Lab Tests
No interactions are known to occur, and there is no known reason to expect a clinically significant interaction with galbanum.

Possible Interactions with Diseases or Conditions
No interactions are known to occur, and there is no known reason to expect a clinically significant interaction with galbanum.

Typical Dosages & Routes of Administration that are Commonly Used
No typical dosage.

Comments
None.

GAMBOGE

This Product is Also Known As
Camboge, Gambodia, Gummigutta, Gutta Cambodia, Gutta Gamba, Tom Rong.
CAUTION: See separate listing for Garcinia.

Scientific Names

Garcinia hanburyi.
Family: Clusiaceae.

People Use This For

Orally, gamboge is used for constipation, generally in combination with other laxatives (18).
Historically, gamboge has been used for the evacuation of intestinal worms (215).

Safety

POSSIBLY UNSAFE ...when used orally. Deaths have been reported with ingestion of 4 grams (18).
PREGNANCY AND LACTATION: POSSIBLY UNSAFE; avoid using.

Effectiveness

There is insufficient reliable information available about the effectiveness of gamboge.

Possible Mechanism of Action & Active Ingredients

The applicable part of gamboge is the resin. It contains resins (benzophenones and xanthones) and mucilages.
Gamboge reportedly has strong laxative effect (18).

Adverse Reactions Including Known Allergies

Abdominal pain and vomiting has been reported with as little as 200 mg; deaths were reported with ingestion of 4 grams (18).

Possible Interactions with Herbs & Other Dietary Supplements

DIGITALIS: Theoretically, overuse/misuse may cause potassium depletion and increase risk of cardiotoxicity.
STIMULANT LAXATIVE HERBS: Theoretically, concomitant use with other stimulant laxative herbs may increase the risk of potassium depletion. Stimulant laxative herbs include: aloe dried leaf sap, wild cucumber fruit (Ecballium elaterium), blue flag rhizome, alder buckthorn, European buckthorn, butternut bark, cascara bark, castor oil, colocynth fruit pulp, jalap root, black root, manna bark exudate, podophyllum root, rhubarb root, senna leaves and pods, and yellow dock root (19).
POTASSIUM DEPLETING HERBS: Theoretically, concomitant use with horsetail plant or licorice rhizome increases the risk of potassium depletion.

Possible Interactions with Drugs

DIGOXIN: Theoretically, overuse/misuse may cause potassium depletion and increase risk of cardiotoxicity.
LAXATIVES: Theoretically, concomitant use may increase risk of fluid and electrolyte loss.
POTASSIUM DEPLETING DRUGS: Theoretically, concomitant use may increase risk of potassium depletion.
CARDIAC GLYCOSIDES: Theoretically, overuse/abuse of this product increases the risk of adverse effects of cardiac glycoside drugs, e.g. digoxin (Lanoxin).

Possible Interactions with Foods

No interactions are known to occur, and there is no known reason to expect a clinically significant interaction with gamboge.

Possible Interactions with Lab Tests

No interactions are known to occur, and there is no known reason to expect a clinically significant interaction with gamboge.

Possible Interactions with Diseases or Conditions

HEART CONDITIONS: Theoretically, overuse/misuse may cause potassium depletion and exacerbate condition.
Contraindicated in intestinal obstruction, acute intestinal inflammation (Crohn's disease, ulcerative colitis, appendicitis), ulcer, abdominal pain of unknown origin, nausea, and vomiting.

Typical Dosages & Routes of Administration that are Commonly Used

ORAL: People typically use 2 to 5 grains (130 to 325 mg) (5269). Some use a maximum dose of 10 mg (5264).

Comments

The resin is extracted from Garcinia hanburyi. Avoid confusion with garcinia (Garcinia cambogia).
Gamboge may be adulterated with rice and wheat starches, sand, and vegetable fragments. These adulterated products are usually coarser and hard (215).

GAMMA BUTYROLACTONE (GBL)

This Product is Also Known As
1,2-Butanolide, 2(3H)-Furanone Dihydro, 3-Hydroxybutyric Acid Lactone, 4-Butanolide, 4-Butyrolactone, 4-Hydroxybutanoic Acid Lactone, Butyrolactone Gamma, Butyrolactone, Dihydro-2(3H)-Furanone, Gamma Butyrolactone, Gamma Hydroxybutyric Acid Lactone, Tetrahydro-2-Furanone.
CAUTION: See seprate listings for Gamma Hydroxybutyrate (GHB) and Butanediol (BD).

Scientific Names
2,3 dihydro furanone; synonyms 2(3H) furanone dihydro, butyrolactone gamma, 2(3H)-furanone dihydro, butyrolactone, 4-butyrolactone, dihydro-2(3H)-furanone, 4-butanolide, tetrahydro-2-furanone.

People Use This For
Orally, gamma butyrolactone is taken for relaxation, calming, increased mental clarity, fat loss, as a body or muscle "builder", recreational drug, for releasing growth hormone, improving athletic performance, inducing and improving sleep, relieving depression and stress, prolonging life, and improving sexual performance and pleasure (682,1430,1432).

Safety
UNSAFE ...when used orally. The use of GBL or the closely related substances gamma hydroxybutyrate (GHB) and butanediol (BD) has been linked to at least 3 deaths and 122 serious adverse effects (3678,3679). GBL can cause dangerously low respiratory rates and heart rates, seizures, and coma (4259).
PREGNANCY AND LACTATION: UNSAFE ...contraindicated.

Effectiveness
There is insufficient reliable information available about the effectiveness of gamma butyrolactone (GBL).

Possible Mechanism of Action & Active Ingredients
Gamma butyrolactone (GBL) is metabolized in the body to gamma hydroxybutyrate (GHB) (see separate monograph) (1430). However, it is more rapidly absorbed than GHB, has greater lipid solubility, and may avoid first-pass metabolism due to its lactone structure (5813). This can lead to higher serum concentrations and more marked hypnotic activity than with similar doses of GHB (5813). GHB can be converted in the brain to the neurotransmitter gamma aminobutyric acid (GABA) (14,3699), and specific GHB uptake systems, transport systems and receptors have also been identified (14,713,3699,5800,5801). Stimulation of GHB receptors reduces dopamine release in the brain (14,713,3699,5801), which may be the mechanism for GBL-induced reductions in dopamine neuronal impulse flow (5811). GBL has been reported to inhibit stereotyped behavior induced by dopamine agonists (5810,5811). The indirect dopamine agonist amphetamine has been reported to partially reverse effects of GBL (5810). GBL may also have some direct GABA agonist activity (5802), although the GABA antagonist bicuculline only partially reverses GBL-induced inhibition of apomorphine activity (5810). GBL, possibly through conversion to GHB, also affects the endogenous opioid system, and the opiate antagonists naloxone and naltrexone attenuate or abolish the electrical seizure activity, behavioral abnormalities, and increased striatal dopamine content produced by GBL (5812). GHB produces general anesthesia (14), induces REM and non-REM sleep, hypothermia, abnormalities on the EEG similar to those seen in petit mal epilepsy (5800,5803), and it stimulates growth hormone secretion (5804).

Adverse Reactions Including Known Allergies
GBL is converted to gamma hydroxybutyrate (GHB, see separate listing) in the body and can therefore be associated with the same life-threatening adverse effects (14). Oral ingestion of GBL has been associated with at least 55 cases of adverse effects (at least five cases involving children), including involuntary muscle movements, fainting and seizures, bowel incontinence, vomiting, slow breathing, respiratory depression, apnea, slow heart rate, mental changes, severe central nervous system depression, agitation, combativeness and amnesia. One death, two cases of respiratory arrest, and one case of cardiac arrest have been reported. Nineteen of the 55 cases involved unconsciousness or coma, and in some cases intubation was required for assisted breathing (665,666,682,1430). Withdrawal symptoms, including insomnia, tremor and anxiety, can occur in chronic users of gamma hydroxybutyrate (GHB), and these withdrawal symptoms are predicted to occur in chronic GBL uses (1430).

Possible Interactions with Herbs & Other Dietary Supplements
PRODUCTS WITH SEDATIVE EFFECTS: Concomitant use is likely to cause additive sedation with GBL, increasing the risk of serious adverse effects.

Possible Interactions with Drugs
ALCOHOL: GHB, formed from metabolism of GBL, acts synergistically with alcohol to produce CNS and respiratory depression (1430).
NARCOTIC ANALGESICS: Concomitant use with GHB (a metabolite of GBL) can potentiate the therapeutic and adverse effects of narcotic analgesics (14).
D-AMPHETAMINE: Theoretically, concomitant use might antagonize the effects of amphetamine (14), and amphetamine has been reported to partially reverse the effects of GBL (5810).

BENZODIAZEPINES, NEUROLEPTICS: Concomitant use with GHB (a metabolite of GBL) can potentiate the effects of GHB (14,3682).

DRUGS WITH SEDATIVE EFFECTS: Any sedative drug could theoretically increase the risk of serious adverse effects with GBL.

D-AMPHETAMINE, NALOXONE, HALOPERIDOL, DRUGS USED FOR ABSENCE SEIZURES: Concomitant use with GHB (a metabolite of GBL) may antagonize the effects of GHB, but these agents have not been assessed as possible treatments for GHB or GBL overdose (3682).

SKELETAL MUSCLE RELAXANTS: Concomitant use with GHB (a metabolite of GBL) can potentiate the therapeutic and adverse effects of skeletal muscle relaxants (14,3682).

Possible Interactions with Foods

ALCOHOL: GHB, formed from metabolism of GBL, acts synergistically with alcohol to produce CNS and respiratory depression (1430).

Possible Interactions with Lab Tests

GAMMA HYDROXYBUTYRATE (GHB): The mass spectrometry assay for GHB used in either urine or serum studies is unable to differentiate between GHB and GBL (14).

Possible Interactions with Diseases or Conditions

HYPERTENSION OR BRADYCARDIA: GHB and GBL should be avoided since they may exacerbate these conditions (14).

CARDIAC CONDUCTION DEFECTS: GHB and GBL should be avoided due to the risk of bradycardia (14).

EPILEPSY: GHB and GBL should be avoided due to their possible capacity to induce seizures (14).

RENAL IMPAIRMENT: GHB and GBL should be avoided due to possible accumulation (14).

Typical Dosages & Routes of Administration that are Commonly Used

No typical dosage.

Comments

FDA WARNING: Avoid all gamma butyrolactone containing products due to safety concerns (682). GBL has been marketed as an alternative to gamma hydroxybutyrate (GHB), but it is illegal to manufacture or market GBL or the related products GHB and butanediol (BD) (3678). Publication of a Federal Register notice on 3/13/00 brought into effect the Hillory J. Farias and Samantha Reid Date-Rape Drug Prohibition Act of 2000, which effected changes to the Controlled Substances Act, making GHB a schedule 1 controlled substance (like heroin), and GBL a list 1 chemical (3681). GBL, GHB and BD are associated with at least 122 reports of serious adverse effects including dangerously low respiratory rates (intubation might be required), unconsciousness/coma, vomiting, seizures, slowed heart rate, and death (4259).

GAMMA HYDROXYBUTYRATE (GHB)

This Product is Also Known As

Gamma Hydrate, 4-Hydroxy Butyrate, Gamma Hydroxybutyrate Sodium, Gamma Hydroxybutyric Acid, Gamma-OH, Sodium gamma-hydroxybutyrate, Sodium Oxybate, Sodium Oxybutyrate.

CAUTION: See separate listings for Gamma Butyrolactone (GBL) and Butanediol (BD).

Scientific Names

Gamma hydroxybutyrate; 4-hydroxybutyric acid; Sodium 4-hydroxybutyrate.

People Use This For

Orally, gamma hydroxybutyrate (GHB) is used for reducing weight, enhancing muscle growth, as an aphrodisiac (712,714), as an hypnotic (3693), for management of opiate withdrawal and alcohol dependence and withdrawal (3684,3686,3694,3695,3696), and for posthypoxic cerebral edema (3682). It is also used for improving pain, fatigue, and the alpha sleep anomaly in patients with fibromyalgia (711).

Traditionally, it has been used as a sedative alternative to the dietary supplement L-tryptophan (3682,3687).

As an investigational orphan drug, it has been designated by the FDA for treatment of narcolepsy (improving nighttime sleep, and the auxiliary symptoms of cataplexy, sleep paralysis, hypnagogic hallucinations, and automatic behavior) (14).

Intravenously, GHB has been used as part of an anesthetic regimen (14), and to reduce intracranial pressure associated with trauma (3685).

Safety

POSSIBLY SAFE ...when used orally under close medical supervision. GHB has FDA investigational orphan drug status (4261).

UNSAFE ...when used orally as a dietary supplement for any use (5,14,712,714). GHB and the chemically-related products gamma butyrolactone (GBL) and butanediol (BD) are associated with at least 122 reports of serious adverse reactions including dangerously low respiratory rates, tonic-clonic seizure, coma and numerous deaths (see

Adverse Reactions) (3678,3679,3680,3688,4259).

There is insufficient reliable information available about the safety of intravenous GHB as a component of general anesthesia.

PREGNANCY AND LACTATION: UNSAFE ...when used orally. GHB has been associated with life-threatening toxicities (3678,3679,3680,3688,4259); avoid using.

Effectiveness

POSSIBLY EFFECTIVE ...when used orally for improving overnight sleep quality and reducing cataplexy in people with narcolepsy (3683,3689,3690,3691,3692). GHB has FDA investigational orphan drug status for treatment of narcolepsy and associated symptoms (4261). ...when used orally as a hypnotic (3693). ...when used orally for fibromyalgia-associated pain, fatigue and alpha sleep anomaly (711). ...when used orally for management of opiate withdrawal and alcohol dependence and withdrawal (3684,3686,3694,3695,3696).

There is insufficient reliable information available about the effectiveness of GHB for its other uses. However, limited evidence suggests that low doses of GHB given intravenously might be effective as a part of an anesthetic regimen (3697,3698). Further evidence is needed to rate the effectiveness of GHB for this use.

Possible Mechanism of Action & Active Ingredients

GHB occurs naturally in several areas of the brain, with the highest concentrations found in the basal ganglia (14), and is also found in peripheral tissues including kidneys, heart, skeletal muscle and brown fat (3682). In the brain, it is formed as a metabolite of the neurotransmitter gamma aminobutyric acid (GABA), and can also be converted back to GABA during metabolism (14,3699). Specific uptake and transport systems have been identified for GHB in the brain (3699,5800), and specific GHB receptors have been identified (14,713,5801). Stimulation of GHB receptors results in a reduction in dopamine release in the basal ganglia (14,713,5801), and it also influences dopamine release in the substantia nigra (3699). Some authors suggest that GHB interacts with GABA(B) receptors (14,713), but others report that GABA formed from GHB is likely involved and that GHB itself is not a GABA agonist (5801,5802). Another GHB metabolite, gamma butyrolactone (GBL) may have some GABA agonist activity (5802). GHB has also been reported to affect the endogenous opioid system, raising dynorphin levels (3682,5803).

GHB produces general anesthesia, possibly by a general suppressant action on the entire cerebrospinal axis, and muscle relaxation by an action on the spinal cord (14). It also induces REM and non-REM sleep, hypothermia, and abnormalities on the EEG similar to those seen in petit mal epilepsy (5800,5803). It stimulates growth hormone secretion which occurs during slow wave sleep (5804), and this has led to claims of anabolic effects (3688). It is also involved in preventing the production of, and scavenging oxygen-derived free radicals in the brain (3682,5805). It decreases brain glucose utilization (3683), lowers cerebral energy requirements and it may play a neuroprotective role, protecting against the effects of anoxia or excessive metabolic demand (3682,5800,5803). It has been suggested that the natural function of GHB may be to induce and maintain physiological states such as sleep and hibernation in which energy utilization is depressed (5803). Some of the effects of GHB are antagonized by the opiate antagonist, naloxone and anticonvulsant drugs (5800), but the stimulation of growth hormone release is antagonized by flumazenil (a benzodiazepine antagonist) and metergoline (a serotonin receptor antagonist) (5806).

The effects of GHB on sleep have been used to improve nighttime sleep quality, sleep continuity, stage 3 and 4 sleep, and cataplexy in people with narcolepsy, with some studies also reporting a reduction in the number of daytime sleep attacks (3689,3690,3691,3692).

Studies in rats indicate that a cross-tolerance can develop between GHB and ethanol with chronic exposure, leading to investigations of GHB for management of ethanol dependence and withdrawal (14,3686). Efficacy has also been reported in the management of opiate withdrawal (3694,3695), although a fatality occurred when GHB and heroin were taken concurrently (5807).

Adverse Reactions Including Known Allergies

Orally, GHB can cause headaches, hallucinations, dizziness, confusion, nausea, vomiting, drowsiness, agitation, and diarrhea. It can also cause sexual arousal, numbing of legs, loss of peripheral vision, tightness of chest, slowed heart rate, depressed respiration, nystagmus, ataxia, eosinophilia-myalgia syndrome, and seizure-like activity (14,6016). The symptoms usually occur within 15 to 60 minutes and subside within 2 to 96 hours, although dizziness can continue for up to 14-days. Doses of GHB greater than 10 mg/kg can cause amnesia and reduced muscle tone (14,6016). Doses between 20-30 mg/kg can cause somnolence (14), and doses greater than 50 mg/kg can cause abrupt unconsciousness and coma (14). GHB and the chemically-related products, gamma butyrolactone (GBL) and 1,4 butanediol, have associated with at least 122 reports of serious adverse reactions including dangerously low respiratory rates, some requiring intubation, unconsciousness and coma, vomiting, seizures, bradycardia, and multiple deaths (3680,4259). At least two deaths involved the use of GHB and alcohol. Death occurred in less than 24 hours after ingestion and was due to circulatory and respiratory collapse. The amount of GHB consumed in these two cases is not known, however the GHB levels in blood and urine were significantly elevated (6016).

Possible Interactions with Herbs & Other Dietary Supplements

HERBS/SUPPLEMENTS WITH SEDATIVE PROPERTIES: Theoretically, concomitant use with herbs that have sedative properties might enhance therapeutic and adverse effects. These include calamus, calendula, California poppy, catnip, capsicum, celery, couch grass, elecampane, ginseng Siberian, German chamomile, goldenseal, gotu kola, hops, Jamaican dogwood, kava, lemon balm, Melatonin, sage, sassafras, scullcap, shepherd's purse, St. John's wort, stinging nettle, valerian, wild carrot, wild lettuce, withania root, and yerba mansa (4,19).

Possible Interactions with Drugs
ALCOHOL: Concomitant use with GHB can potentiate the CNS and respiratory depression effects of alcohol and GHB (3682).
NARCOTIC ANALGESICS: Concomitant use with GHB can potentiate the therapeutic and adverse effects of narcotic analgesics (14); a fatality has been reported with concurrent use of GHB and heroin (5807).
BENZODIAZEPINES, NEUROLEPTICS: Concomitant use with GHB can potentiate the effects of GHB (14,3682).
DRUGS WITH SEDATIVE EFFECTS: Any sedative drug could theoretically increase the risk of serious adverse effects with GHB.
D-AMPHETAMINE, NALOXONE, HALOPERIDOL, DRUGS USED FOR ABSENCE SEIZURES: Concomitant use with GHB may antagonize the effects of GHB, but these agents have not been assessed as possible treatments for GHB overdose (3682).
SKELETAL MUSCLE RELAXANTS: Concomitant use with GHB can potentiate the therapeutic and adverse effects of skeletal muscle relaxants (14,3682).
RITONAVIR (Norvir), SAQUINAVIR (Fortovase, Invirase): Concomitant use of the protease inhibitor-type antiretroviral drugs ritonavir and saquinavir with GHB reportedly caused a near-fatal reaction, probably due to inhibition of GHB metabolism (1431).

Possible Interactions with Foods
ALCOHOL: Concomitant use with GHB can potentiate the CNS and respiratory depression effects of alcohol and GHB (3682).

Possible Interactions with Lab Tests
GAMMA BUTYROLACTONE (GBL): The mass spectrometry assay for GHB used in either urine or serum studies is unable to differentiate between GHB and GBL (14).

Possible Interactions with Diseases or Conditions
HYPERTENSION OR BRADYCARDIA: GHB should be avoided since it may exacerbate these conditions (14).
CARDIAC CONDUCTION DEFECTS: GHB should be avoided due to the risk of bradycardia (14).
EPILEPSY: GHB should be avoided due to its possible capacity to induce seizures (14).
RENAL IMPAIRMENT: GHB should be avoided due to possible accumulation (14).

Typical Dosages & Routes of Administration that are Commonly Used
ORAL: For narcolepsy and associate symptoms, a dose of 25 mg/kg at bedtime, repeated 3-hours later has been used (3689,3690). For treating alcohol dependence, 50 to 150 mg/kg divided into 3 to 6 doses per day has been used (3684,3696). As a hypnotic, 75-100 mg/kg has been used (3693).

Comments
Gamma butyrolactone (GBL) and butanediol (BD) (see separate monographs) are closely related to GHB and produce similar adverse effects (3678,3679). Due to reports of serious adverse effects, the FDA removed GHB from the market in 1990, but clandestine manufacture continued, with the drug being widely available on the Internet, and being implicated as a date rape agent (3687). Publication of a Federal Register notice on 3/13/00 brought into effect the Hillory J. Farias and Samantha Reid Date-Rape Drug Prohibition Act of 2000, which effected changes to the Controlled Substances Act, making GHB a schedule 1 controlled substance (like heroin), which it is illegal to produce, sell or possess (3680,3681). Orphan Medical is expected to submit a new drug application to the FDA during 2001 for GHB under the generic name sodium oxybate and trade name Xyrem, for the treatment of cataplexy associated with narcolepsy (3680). If approved, the drug would be in Schedule 3 of the Controlled Substances Act for this indication (3680,3681). To access information on sodium oxybate (Xyrem) for narcolepsy contact: Orphan Medical (1-888-867-7426).

GAMMA LINOLENIC ACID

This Product is Also Known As
Gamolenic Acid, GLA.
CAUTION: See separate listings for Black Currant Seed Oil, Borage Seed Oil, Evening Primrose Oil, and Omega-6 Oils.

Scientific Names
(Z,Z,Z)-Octadeca-6,9,12-trienoic acid.

People Use This For
Orally, gamma linolenic acid (GLA) is used for rheumatoid arthritis (14,1985), oral mucoceles (mucous polyps) (1978), hyperlipidemia (1979), systemic sclerosis (1977), diabetic neuropathy (1980,1981,1984), and to hasten the response to tamoxifen in individuals with breast cancer (5902).

Safety
LIKELY SAFE ...when used orally (1983).
PREGNANCY AND LACTATION: Insufficient reliable information available; avoid using.

Effectiveness
POSSIBLY EFFECTIVE ...when taken orally for rheumatoid arthritis (14), diabetic neuropathy (1980,1981,1984), and to hasten the response to tamoxifen in individuals with breast cancer (5902).
POSSIBLY INEFFECTIVE ...when taken orally for systemic sclerosis (1977).
There is insufficient reliable information available about the effectiveness of GLA for its other uses.

Possible Mechanism of Action & Active Ingredients
Gamma linolenic acid can be converted to compounds that have anti-inflammatory and antiproliferative properties (1975), including prostaglandins with vasoactive properties. Preliminary evidence suggests GLA can hasten the response to tamoxifen in individuals with primary breast cancer that is estrogen-sensitive (5902). GLA is believed to benefit individuals who have ischemic lesions associated with systemic sclerosis (1977) and individuals with diabetic neuropathy (1980,1981). Some evidence suggests that gamma linolenic acid might lower plasma triglycerides, increase HDL cholesterol, and prolong bleeding time (1979).

Adverse Reactions Including Known Allergies
GLA might prolong bleeding time (1979).

Possible Interactions with Herbs & Other Dietary Supplements
Insufficient reliable information available.

Possible Interactions with Drugs
ANTICOAGULANTS, ANTIPLATELET DRUGS: Theoretically, concomitant use of GLA can increase the risk of bleeding because it has the potential to prolong bleeding time.
TAMOXIFEN: Preliminary evidence suggests GLA hastens the response to tamoxifen in individuals with primary breast cancer that is estrogen-sensitive. However, it is not known whether GLA reduces the recurrence rate or ultimate outcome of breast cancer (5902).

Possible Interactions with Foods
No interactions are known to occur, and there is no known reason to expect a clinically significant interaction with GLA.

Possible Interactions with Lab Tests
LIPID PROFILE: GLA can lower plasma triglycerides and increase HDL cholesterol, altering serum assay results (1979).
BLEEDING TIME: GLA can increase bleeding time and lab assay results (1979).

Possible Interactions with Diseases or Conditions
HYPERLIPIDEMIA: GLA can lower triglycerides and increase HDL cholesterol (1979).
CONDITIONS WITH BLEEDING RISK: Theoretically, GLA can increase the risk of bleeding due to its potential to prolong bleeding time.

Typical Dosages & Routes of Administration that are Commonly Used
ORAL: For rheumatoid arthritis, the usual dose of GLA is 1.1 grams per day (1985). For diabetic neuropathy, the common dose is 360 mg per day (1984); and for hyperlipidemia, the typical dose is 1.5-6 grams per day (1976,1979).

Comments
Borage oil and evening primrose oil are often used as a source of gamma linolenic acid.

GAMMA ORYZANOL

This Product is Also Known As
None.

Scientific Names
Gamma oryzanol.

People Use This For

Orally, gamma oryzanol is used for hypercholesterolemia, dyslipidemia (752,754), stimulating the production and release of testosterone, stimulation and release of human growth hormone (755), increasing strength during resistance exercise training (751), and for climacteric symptoms associated with menopause and aging (757).

Safety

POSSIBLY SAFE ...when used orally and appropriately (751,752,753,754,755). Gamma oryzanol potentially can decrease human testosterone production (see Mechanism of Action).
PREGNANCY AND LACTATION: Insufficient reliable information available; avoid using.

Effectiveness

POSSIBLY EFFECTIVE ...when taken orally for reducing serum cholesterol (752,757).
There is insufficient reliable information available about the effectiveness of gamma oryzanol for its other uses.

Possible Mechanism of Action & Active Ingredients

Gamma oryzanol shows anticholesterolemic activity in animals by decreasing cholesterol absorption from the gut (756). Single, oral doses of 300 mg gamma oryzanol can reduce elevated serum TSH levels in hypothyroid patients, and chronic use can also result in decreased serum TSH levels (753). Research suggests gamma-oryzanol inhibits serum TSH levels in patients with primary hypothyroidism, possibly by a direct action at the hypothalamus rather than the pituitary (753). Gamma oryzanol has no effect on performance or related physiological parameters, such as testosterone, growth hormone, or beta-endorphin during weight training in humans (751). It can be poorly absorbed from the gut (755). Animal studies using parenteral administration indicate gamma oryzanol can be anti-anabolic by suppressing the release of luteinizing hormone and increasing the release of catecholamines, dopamine, and norepinephrine in the brain (755). If this occurs in humans, gamma oryzanol possibly can reduce testosterone production (755).

Adverse Reactions Including Known Allergies

None reported.

Possible Interactions with Herbs & Other Dietary Supplements

Insufficient reliable information available.

Possible Interactions with Drugs

No interactions are known to occur, and there is no known reason to expect a clinically significant interaction with gamma oryzanol.

Possible Interactions with Foods

No interactions are known to occur, and there is no known reason to expect a clinically significant interaction with gamma oryzanol.

Possible Interactions with Lab Tests

THYROID STIMULATING HORMONE (TSH): Gamma oryzanol can reduce serum TSH concentrations and test results (753).
CHOLESTEROL: Gamma oryzanol can reduce serum total cholesterol (752,757) and LDL cholesterol (752) concentrations and test results. Gamma oryzanol can increase serum HDL cholesterol concentrations and test results (757).
TRIGLYCERIDES: Gamma oryzanol can reduce serum triglyceride concentrations and test results (757).

Possible Interactions with Diseases or Conditions

PRIMARY HYPOTHYROIDISM: Gamma oryzanol can decrease TSH serum levels (753).

Typical Dosages & Routes of Administration that are Commonly Used

ORAL: For reducing serum cholesterol, the usual dose of gamma oryzanol is 300 mg daily (752,757), and in one study, 100 mg three times daily was used (752).

Comments

Gamma oryzanol is an extraction product from rice bran oil.

GARCINIA

This Product is Also Known As

Brindal Berry, Brindall Berry, Brindle Berry, Garcinia Cambogi, Garcinia Cambogia, Gorikapuli, Hydroxycitrate, Hydroxycitric Acid, HCA, Malabar Tamarind.
CAUTION: See separate listings for Gamboge, Malabar Nut, and Tamarind.

Scientific Names
Garcinia cambogia.
Family: Clusiaceae.

People Use This For
Orally, garcinia is used for weight loss (728).
In folk medicine, garcinia is used for dysentery, as a purgative, and for treating worms and parasites (729).
For food uses, garcinia is used as a condiment in Thai and Indian cuisine (730).

Safety
POSSIBLY SAFE ...when used orally and appropriately for 12 weeks or less (728).
There is insufficient reliable information available about the safety of the long-term use of garcinia.
PREGNANCY AND LACTATION: Insufficient reliable information available; avoid using.

Effectiveness
POSSIBLY INEFFECTIVE ...when fruit rind extract is taken orally for weight loss (728).
There is insufficient reliable information available about the effectiveness of garcinia for its other uses.

Possible Mechanism of Action & Active Ingredients
The applicable parts of garcinia are the fruit and rind. Garcinia fruit rind extract reported to contain 50% hydroxycitric acid; theorized to interfere with lipogenesis (728).

Adverse Reactions Including Known Allergies
None reported.

Possible Interactions with Herbs & Other Dietary Supplements
Insufficient reliable information available.

Possible Interactions with Drugs
No interactions are known to occur, and there is no known reason to expect a clinically significant interaction with garcinia.

Possible Interactions with Foods
No interactions are known to occur, and there is no known reason to expect a clinically significant interaction with garcinia.

Possible Interactions with Lab Tests
No interactions are known to occur, and there is no known reason to expect a clinically significant interaction with garcinia.

Possible Interactions with Diseases or Conditions
No interactions are known to occur, and there is no known reason to expect a clinically significant interaction with garcinia.

Typical Dosages & Routes of Administration that are Commonly Used
ORAL: Extract containing 50% hydroxycitric acid; 1,000 mg three times daily used in study that found garcinia ineffective for weight loss (728).

Comments
Avoid confusion with gamboge resin (Garcinia hanburyi).

GARDEN CRESS

This Product is Also Known As
None.

Scientific Names
Lepidium sativum.
Family: Cruciferae.

People Use This For
Orally, garden cress is used for coughs and vitamin C deficiency.
In folk medicine, garden cress is used orally for constipation, poor immunity, and as a diuretic (18).

Safety
There is insufficient reliable information available about the safety of garden cress.
Pregnancy and Lactation: Insufficient reliable information available; avoid using.

Effectiveness

There is insufficient reliable information available about the effectiveness of garden cress.

Possible Mechanism of Action & Active Ingredients

The applicable parts of garden cress are the above ground parts. Garden cress may have in vitro antibacterial activity, but the activity appears to be dependent on the age of the plant at harvest. It also appears to have antiviral activity against the encephalitis virus Columbia SH (animal data) (18).

Adverse Reactions Including Known Allergies

People who ingest large amounts of garden cress may experience gastrointestinal irritation (18).

Possible Interactions with Herbs & Other Dietary Supplements

Insufficient reliable information available.

Possible Interactions with Drugs

No interactions are known to occur, and there is no known reason to expect a clinically significant interaction with garden cress.

Possible Interactions with Foods

No interactions are known to occur, and there is no known reason to expect a clinically significant interaction with garden cress.

Possible Interactions with Lab Tests

No interactions are known to occur, and there is no known reason to expect a clinically significant interaction with garden cress.

Possible Interactions with Diseases or Conditions

No interactions are known to occur, and there is no known reason to expect a clinically significant interaction with garden cress.

Typical Dosages & Routes of Administration that are Commonly Used

ORAL: Garden cress is used as a fresh use herb in oral preparations (18).

Comments

Garden cress is rarely adulterated because it is usually cultivated rather than harvested (18).

GARDEN VIOLET

This Product is Also Known As

None.
CAUTION: See separate listing for Sweet Violet.

Scientific Names

Viola odorata.
Family: Violaceae.

People Use This For

Orally, garden violet is used for acute and chronic bronchitis, bronchial asthma, acute and chronic inflammation of the respiratory tract, and cold symptoms.
Topically, garden violet is used in skin lavages for treating various skin diseases (18).
In folk medicine, garden violet is used orally for coughs, hoarseness, tuberculosis, as an expectorant for throat inflammation and bronchitis accompanied by fixed mucous, nervous strain, insomnia, and hysteria.

Safety

There is insufficient reliable information available about the safety of garden violet.
Pregnancy and Lactation: Insufficient reliable information available; avoid using.

Effectiveness

There is insufficient reliable information available about the effectiveness of garden violet.

Possible Mechanism of Action & Active Ingredients

The whole plant and the essential oil form the leaves are used medicinally. There is insufficient reliable information available about the possible mechanism of action and active ingredients.

Adverse Reactions Including Known Allergies

None reported.

Possible Interactions with Herbs & Other Dietary Supplements

Insufficient reliable information available.

Possible Interactions with Drugs

No interactions are known to occur, and there is no known reason to expect a clinically significant interaction with garden violet.

Possible Interactions with Foods

No interactions are known to occur, and there is no known reason to expect a clinically significant interaction with garden violet.

Possible Interactions with Lab Tests

No interactions are known to occur, and there is no known reason to expect a clinically significant interaction with garden violet.

Possible Interactions with Diseases or Conditions

No interactions are known to occur, and there is no known reason to expect a clinically significant interaction with garden violet.

Typical Dosages & Routes of Administration that are Commonly Used

ORAL: One cup tea is taken 2-3 times daily. The tea is prepared by steeping 2 teaspoons of dried herb in 250 mL of boiling water for 10-15 minutes and straining [18].

Comments

There is very little scientific information about this product. Our staff is continually analyzing the available information on natural medicines and will add data here as it becomes available.

GARLIC

This Product is Also Known As

Aged Garlic Extract, Ail, Ajo, Allii Sativi Bulbus, Allium, Camphor of the Poor, Clove Garlic, Garlic Clove, Nectar of the Gods, Poor Man's Treacle, Rust Treacle, Stinking Rose.

Scientific Names

Allium sativum.
Family: Amaryllidaceae or Liliaceae.

People Use This For

Orally, garlic is used for reducing high blood pressure [2,4], prevention of coronary heart disease by improving lipid profiles [4], preventing age-related vascular changes and atherosclerosis [2,4], reducing reinfarction and mortality rate post-myocardial infarction [4], for treating earaches, and menstrual disorders [6121]. Garlic is also used orally for treatment of Helicobacter pylori infection and cancer prevention [14]. Other uses include immune system stimulation, treatment of diabetes, arthritis, allergies, traveler's diarrhea, colds, flu, and prevention and treatment of bacterial and fungal infections [4760]. An aged garlic extract has been used orally for enhancing circulation, fighting stress and fatigue, and maintaining healthy liver function [1872].
Topically, garlic oil is used for tinea pedis [14,5121], tinea corporis, tinea cruris [4766,4767,5121], and onychomycosis [5121].
Intravaginally, garlic is used alone or in combination with yogurt for vaginitis [5121].
In traditional Chinese medicine, garlic is used for diarrhea, amoebic and bacterial dysentery, tuberculosis, bloody urine, diphtheria, whooping cough, scalp ringworm, hypersensitive teeth, and vaginal trichomoniasis [11]. Garlic has also been traditionally used to treat colds, flu symptoms, fever, coughs, headache, stomach ache, sinus congestion, athlete's foot, gout, rheumatism, hemorrhoids, asthma, bronchitis, shortness of breath, arteriosclerosis, low blood pressure, hypoglycemia, hyperglycemia, cancer, old ulcers, snakebites, and as an aphrodisiac [5,11].
In foods and beverages, fresh garlic, garlic powder, and garlic oil are used as flavor components [11].

Safety

LIKELY SAFE ...when ingested in amounts commonly found in foods. Garlic oil, extract, and oleoresin have Generally Recognized as Safe (GRAS) status in the US [11].
POSSIBLY SAFE ...when used orally and appropriately for medicinal purposes [2,4,12]. Garlic has been used in clinical studies lasting up to 4 years without reports of significant toxicity [4797,4798].
POSSIBLY UNSAFE ...when used orally in large amounts [4]. ...when used topically in large amounts [585].
CHILDREN: POSSIBLY SAFE ...when used orally and appropriately, short-term. In one study, garlic extract 300 mg three times daily had side effects comparable to placebo when used in children ages 8-18 years for 8 weeks [4796]. POSSIBLY UNSAFE ...when used orally in large amounts. Some sources suggest that high doses of garlic could be dangerous or even fatal to children [12]; however, the reason for this warning is not known. There are no case reports available of significant adverse events or mortality in children associated with ingestion of garlic.
There is insufficient reliable information available about the safety of topical garlic use in children.
PREGNANCY: LIKELY SAFE ...when used orally in amounts typically found in foods [12]. POSSIBLY

UNSAFE ...when used orally in large amounts (4). Theoretically, large amounts of garlic might act as an abortifacient, enable onset of menstruation, and cause uterine contractions (4,19). One study also suggests that garlic constituents are distributed to the amniotic fluid after a single dose of garlic (4828). However, there are no published reports of garlic adversely affecting pregnancy. There is insufficient reliable information available about the safety of topical garlic use during pregnancy.

LACTATION: LIKELY SAFE ...when used orally in amounts typically found in foods (12). POSSIBLY UNSAFE ...when used orally in amounts greater than those found in foods (2,12). Some authors suggest that use of garlic should be avoided during lactation (4,12); however, the reason for this warning is not known. There are no published reports of adverse effects in nursing infants whose mothers ingested garlic. Two small studies suggest that garlic constituents are secreted in breast milk and that nursing infants of mothers consuming garlic are prone to extended nursing (4829,4830). There is insufficient reliable information available about the safety of topical garlic use during lactation.

Effectiveness

POSSIBLY EFFECTIVE ...when taken orally for hyperlipidemia. Multiple studies published in the early 1990s consistently indicated that garlic was likely effective for significantly reducing total cholesterol, low-density lipoprotein (LDL) levels, and triglyceride levels and increasing high-density lipoprotein (HDL) levels (279,4782, 4783,4784,4785,4787,4789,4790,4791). Two meta-analyses also reported that garlic can lower total serum cholesterol by 12% and 9% respectively (4786,4788). However, more recent studies have reported conflicting findings. Several studies have now reported that garlic appears to be no better than placebo for hyperlipidemia (731,732,4792,4793,4794,4795). In a recent meta-analysis, garlic was also found to be no better than placebo (4795). The reason for the conflicting findings is unclear. Most studies used similar garlic preparations (garlic powder standardized based on alliin content), doses, and treatment duration. However, variations in manufacturing of garlic preparations, lack of consistent control of dietary changes (14,4792,4800), and relatively small study sample sizes may have contributed to the inconsistent findings. The extent of benefit of garlic for hyperlipidemia remains controversial. Although most studies have used garlic powder preparations standardized based on alliin, limited evidence suggests an aged garlic extract might also improve lipid profiles (1873,1875,1876). Two trials have compared garlic to prescription antihyperlipidemic agents. In one trial, a standardized garlic extract 900 mg daily was comparable to bezafibrate (Bezalip - not available in the US) 600 mg daily for reducing total serum cholesterol, LDL levels, triglycerides, and increasing HDL levels after 12 weeks of treatment (4782). In another trial, garlic was found to be inferior to clofibrate (Atromid-S) (4807). ...when taken orally for lowering blood pressure (277,278,279,1873). A meta-analysis of 8 published and unpublished randomized controlled trials of at least 4 weeks duration found a modest reduction in systolic and diastolic blood pressure. Only 3 studies were specifically conducted in hypertensive patients and many studies were methodologically flawed (277). ...when taken orally for preventing age-related vascular changes and atherosclerosis (4797,4798). Garlic powder 300 mg daily lessened age-related decreases in aortic elasticity, and 900 mg daily slowed the development of atherosclerosis in aortic and femoral arteries over 4 years in 152 patients aged 50 to 80 years (4797,4798). ...when taken orally for reducing cancer risk (4770,4771,4772,4775,4776,4777). Several prospective and retrospective epidemiological studies indicate that garlic might reduce colorectal cancer risk (4770,4771,4772); however, one prospective cohort study found no association between consumption of garlic supplements and decreased risk of colorectal cancer (4773). Epidemiological studies also support decreased risk of stomach and prostate cancer, but no protection from lung or breast cancer (4775,4776,4777,4778,4779). ...when the garlic constituent, ajoene, is used topically for tinea infections (4766,4767). In two studies, ajoene 0.4% cream was effective for tinea pedis, and the 0.6% gel was as effective as terbinafine 1% cream for tinea cruris and tinea corporis (4766,4767). In one study, tinea pedis was cured in 79% of patients treated for 7 days (4766).

POSSIBLY INEFFECTIVE ...when taken orally to treat Helicobacter pylori infection (4761,4762,4763). Despite laboratory and epidemiological evidence of activity against H. pylori, several small open studies with garlic cloves, garlic powder, or garlic oil showed no effect on patients infected with H. pylori; however, the testing methodology used has been criticized (4761,4762,4763,4764,4765,4774). ...when taken orally for peripheral arterial occlusive disease (4801,4809). In a 12 week double-blind, placebo-controlled study of 80 patients with stage II peripheral arterial occlusive disease, garlic powder was not significantly better than placebo for increased walking distance; however garlic did decreased spontaneous thrombocyte aggregation beginning in the fifth week of therapy (4801,4809). ...when taken orally for hypercholesterolemia in children. In one study, garlic powder extract standardized based on alliin content did not significantly affect total serum cholesterol, LDL or HDL levels, triglycerides, lipoprotein (a), apolipoprotein B-100, homocysteine, fibrinogen, or blood pressure (4796).

Most clinical studies have used the brand name product Kwai (Lichtwer Pharma), a dried garlic powder preparation standardized to contain 1.3% alliin. Clinical studies on aged garlic extract have used the brand name product Kyolic (Wakunaga of America).

There is insufficient reliable information available about the effectiveness of garlic for its other uses.

Possible Mechanism of Action & Active Ingredients

The applicable parts of garlic are the bulb and clove. Garlic is most commonly used for its antihyperlipidemic, antihypertensive, and antifungal effects. However, it is also reported to have antibacterial, antihelmintic, antiviral, antispasmodic, diaphoretic, expectorant, immunostimulant, and antithrombotic effects (2,4). For hyperlipidemia, garlic might act as a HMG-CoA reductase inhibitor (statin) to reduce serum cholesterol (4810,4811). For hypertension, garlic is thought produce smooth muscle relaxation and vasodilation by activating production of endothelium-derived relaxation factor (EDRF, Nitric oxide) (4812). For age-related vascular changes and atherosclerosis, garlic is thought to be beneficial by reducing oxidative stress and low-density lipoprotein oxidation and through antithrombotic effects (1880,4813). Garlic appears to prevent endothelial cell depletion of glutathione, which may be responsible for its antioxidant effects (1880). Garlic has been found to have antithrombotic properties and can increase fibrinolytic activity, decrease platelet aggregation, and increase prothrombin time (2). Garlic powder and aged garlic preparations have been shown to have antiplatelet properties in both patients with cardiovascular disease and in healthy volunteers (1874,4802,4803). Garlic oil does not appear to effect platelet aggregation (4805). Raw garlic seems to have more potent antiplatelet properties than cooked garlic (4804). Both fried and raw garlic preparations increase fibrinolytic activity in patients with acute myocardial infarction, old myocardial infarction, or healthy volunteers (14,4799). Many of the pharmacological effects of garlic have been attributed to the constituents allicin and ajoene. However, when doses of fresh garlic clove 4 grams per day are used, only allicin appears to have clinically significant activity (4800). Intact garlic cells contain the odorless amino acid, alliin. When intact cells are broken, alliin comes into contact with the enzyme allinase, producing allicin, an unstable, odiferous compound (5,4768). Fresh garlic contains approximately 1% alliin. One milligram of alliin is converted to 0.458 mg allicin (4800). Further conversion yields active principles including E-ajoene and Z-ajoene (13). Garlic is aged to reduce the content of sulfur compounds and the odor commonly associated with garlic. This process significantly decreases alliin content. Odorless aged garlic extract reduces the alliin content to only 3% of what is typically contained in fresh garlic (4800). Several other constituents of garlic and derivatives of alliin have pharmacological activity. The constituent, allylpropyl disulfide, can reduce blood sugar and increase insulin in normal volunteers (4). Fresh garlic, but not aged garlic, has shown activity against Escherichia coli, methicillin-resistant Staph aureus, salmonella enteritidis, and Candida albicans in the laboratory, and has been suggested as a food additive to prevent food poisoning (4808). Preliminary evidence suggests that garlic compounds might have activity against viruses such as herpes simplex virus type 1, herpes simplex virus type 2, parainfluenza virus type 3, vaccinia virus, vesicular stomatitis virus, and human rhinovirus type 2 (4769). S-allyl cysteine and S-allyl mercaptocysteine, garlic derivatives, might protect the liver against acetaminophen and carbon tetrachloride, according to laboratory studies (14). Other preliminary evidence suggests S-allyl cysteine might ameliorate doxorubicin-induced cardiac and hepatic toxicity (4780). An active component of aged garlic, s-allylcysteine, shows effectiveness in preventing experimental physiological aging, age-related immunodeficiency, and atherosclerosis. Another constituent, S-allylmercaptocysteine, has shown activity against erythroleukemic, breast, and prostate cancer cells (1881,1871,1877, 1878,1879,1880,1882). Additionally, garlic might enhance selenium absorption with possible protection against tumorigenesis (4815). Preliminary reports regarding a possible hepatoprotective effect of aged garlic extract have been conflicting (1883,1884). Early evidence suggests a possible protective effect of aged garlic on methotrexate-induced intestinal toxicity (1885).

Adverse Reactions Including Known Allergies

Garlic taken orally can have dose-related effects including breath odor, mouth and gastrointestinal burning or irritation, heartburn, flatulence, nausea, vomiting, and diarrhea. These effects can be more pronounced with consumption of raw garlic or in individuals unaccustomed to eating garlic (4,5,12,4783,4800). The oral use of garlic can also cause changes to the intestinal flora (4800). There is one report of spinal epidural hematoma and platelet dysfunction associated with the ingestion of fresh garlic (586) and one report of postoperative bleeding and prolonged bleeding time associated with high dietary garlic consumption (587). Asthma in people working with garlic has been reported (4816). True IgE-mediated garlic allergy is relatively rare, but seems to affect young subjects with pollen allergy (4816). Topically, application of fresh garlic has caused dermatitis (4833). Eczema has been reported following occupational exposure to garlic (4832). One child developed blisters and subsequently scars on both wrists after several hours of contact with crushed garlic cloves (585).

Possible Interactions with Herbs & Other Dietary Supplements

EICOSAPENTAENOIC ACID (EPA, fish oils): Concomitant use of garlic can enhance antithrombotic effects (4). HERBS WITH ANTICOAGULANT/ANTIPLATELET POTENTIAL: Concomitant use of herbs that have coumarin constituents or affect platelet aggregation could theoretically increase the risk of bleeding in some people. These herbs include: angelica, anise, arnica, asafoetida, bogbean, boldo, capsicum, celery, chamomile, clove, danshen, fenugreek, feverfew, garlic, ginger, ginkgo, ginseng (Panax), horse chestnut, horseradish, licorice, meadowsweet, prickly ash, onion, papain, passionflower, poplar, quassia, red clover, turmeric, vitamin E, wild carrot, wild lettuce, willow, and others (4,19).

Possible Interactions with Drugs

ANTICOAGULANT/ANTIPLATELET AGENTS: Garlic can enhance the effects of warfarin (Coumadin) as measured by the INR (616). Theoretically, it might also enhance the effects and adverse effects of other anticoagulant and antiplatelet drugs, including aspirin, clopidogrel (Plavix), enoxaparin (Lovenox), and others (4). HYPOGLYCEMIC DRUGS/INSULIN: Theoretically, concomitant use might increase effects and adverse effects of hypoglycemic drugs and insulin (4,19). Dose adjustments may be necessary when used concomitantly (19).

Possible Interactions with Foods

No interactions are known to occur, and there is no known reason to expect a clinically significant interaction with garlic.

Possible Interactions with Lab Tests

GLUCOSE: Garlic can lower blood glucose concentrations and test results (4).

INSULIN: Garlic can increase blood insulin concentrations and test results (4).

INTERNATIONAL NORMALIZED RATIO (INR), PROTHROMBIN TIME (PT): Garlic can increase INR in patients anticoagulated with warfarin (Coumadin). There are two case reports of increased INR associated with concomitant use of garlic products and warfarin (616).

CHOLESTEROL: Garlic can lower serum cholesterol concentrations and test results (2,4,277,278,279).

BLOOD PRESSURE: Garlic can lower blood pressure and blood pressure readings (2,4,277,278,279).

Possible Interactions with Diseases or Conditions

BLEEDING DISORDERS: Theoretically, garlic might increase the risk of bleeding (4); contraindicated.

DIABETES: Theoretically, garlic might reduce blood sugar levels and interfere with control (4); use with caution.

GASTROINTESTINAL IRRITATION: Garlic can irritate the gastrointestinal tract; use with caution in individuals with infectious or inflammatory gastrointestinal conditions (19).

SURGERY: Garlic can prolong bleeding time and should be discontinued one to two weeks prior to scheduled surgery (587,4800).

Typical Dosages & Routes of Administration that are Commonly Used

ORAL: For hyperlipidemia and hypertension, doses of 600-900 mg daily have been used in clinical trials. These doses are commonly divided and given three times daily. Most clinical studies have used a standardized garlic powder extract containing 1.3% alliin content. Aged garlic extract 600 mg to 7.2 grams per day has also been used (18,1874,1875). Fresh garlic 4 grams (approximately one clove) taken once daily has also been used. Fresh garlic typically contains approximately 1% alliin (4800). Appropriate doses may vary depending on the preparation.

TOPICAL: For tinea infections, clinical studies have used the garlic constituent ajoene as a 0.4% cream and 0.6% gel (4766,4767). For onychomycosis and other fungal infections, including tinea infections, some sources suggest applying liquified raw garlic or garlic extract to the affected area three times daily (5121).

Comments

The effectiveness of garlic products is determined by their ability to yield allicin which in turn triggers production of other active principles. To be effective, dried preparations of garlic should have enteric coating to protect the active constituents from degeneration by stomach acid (13). One study from Germany reported that only about 25% of the garlic products commercially available generated an amount of allicin equivalent to one clove of fresh garlic (13). Some odorless garlic preparations do not contain active compounds at all, although this is controversial (4,1877).

GELSEMIUM

This Product is Also Known As

Caroline Jasmine, Evening Trumpet Flower, False Jasmin, Gelsemii Rhizoma, Gelsemin, Gelsemiumwurzelstock Jessamine, Woodbine, Yellow Jasmine, Yellow Jessamine Root.

CAUTION: See separate listings for Jasmine, American Ivy, Honeysuckle, and Woodbine.

Scientific Names

Gelsemium sempervirens, synonyms Gelsemium nitidum, Bignonia sempervirens.
Family: Loganiaceae or Spigeliaceae.

People Use This For

Orally, gelsemium is used as an analgesic for trigeminal neuralgia and migraine headaches (9).

Historically, gelsemium has been used for asthma and in respiratory remedies (6).

Safety

UNSAFE ...when the rhizome or root are used orally. All parts of the plant contain toxic alkaloids (14). The adult lethal dose is 2-3 grams or 4 mL of the fluid extract (18).

CHILDREN: UNSAFE ...the lethal dose is 500 mg (18).

PREGNANCY AND LACTATION: UNSAFE ...contraindicated, due to toxicity (6).

Effectiveness

There is insufficient reliable information available about the effectiveness of gelsemium.

Possible Mechanism of Action & Active Ingredients

The applicable parts of gelsemium are the rhizome and root. Researchers think the active components in gelsemium are gelsamine alkaloids and related compounds (gelsemine, gelsemicine, gelsedine) (6). Gelsemium and the principal alkaloid, gelsemine, are reported to have CNS stimulant (6), CNS depressant (9) and analgesic effects (6).

Adverse Reactions Including Known Allergies

Oral use can be deadly. Toxicity symptoms include: headache, dilated pupils, drooping of the eyelid, double vision, difficulty in swallowing, dizziness, muscle weakness/rigidity, seizures (rare), shortness of breath and bradycardia. Death due to failure of respiratory muscles can occur (14). Whole plant can cause contact dermatitis when used topically (14).

Possible Interactions with Herbs & Other Dietary Supplements

Insufficient reliable information available.

Possible Interactions with Drugs

ASPIRIN, PHENACETIN: May potentiate drug effects (6).

Possible Interactions with Foods

No interactions are known to occur, and there is no known reason to expect a clinically significant interaction with gelsemium.

Possible Interactions with Lab Tests

No interactions are known to occur, and there is no known reason to expect a clinically significant interaction with gelsemium.

Possible Interactions with Diseases or Conditions

HEART DISEASE/WEAKNESS: Contraindicated (18).

Typical Dosages & Routes of Administration that are Commonly Used

ORAL: People typically use 0.3 to 1 mL gelsemium tincture (5264).

Comments

There is a very narrow safety margin and medicinal preparations are considered obsolete (18). Avoid confusion with jasmine or woodbine (Clematis virginiana). Also, avoid confusing gelsemium with American ivy or honeysuckle, which are also known as woodbine.

GENTIAN

This Product is Also Known As

Bitter Root, Bitterwort, Gall Weed, Gentiana, Gentianae radix, Pale Gentian, Stemless Gentian, Yellow Gentian, Wild Gentian.

Scientific Names

Gentiana lutea; Gentiana acaulis.
Family: Gentianaceae.

People Use This For

Orally, gentian root is used for digestive disorders, such as loss of appetite, fullness, and flatulence. (2). It is used orally for fever, for hysteria, to stimulate menstrual flow, as an anthelmintic and antiseptic (5).
Topically, gentian root is used for treating wounds and cancer (11).
In combination with European elder flower, verbena, cowslip flower, and sorrel, gentian is used orally for maintaining healthy sinuses (373) and treating sinusitis (7,374,379). It is used in combination with other products for malaria (5).
In traditional medicine, gentian has been used orally for diarrhea, gastritis, heartburn, and vomiting (11).
Gentian is used as an ingredient in foods and beverages (11).
In manufacturing, gentian is used in cosmetics (11).

Safety

LIKELY SAFE ...when the root preparations are consumed in amounts commonly found in foods. Gentian root is approved for food use in the US. The maximum level of gentian extract used is 0.02%; for stemless gentian, 0.001% (11).
POSSIBLY SAFE ...when taken orally in therapeutic amounts (2). ...when gentian root is used orally with European elder flower, verbena, cowslip flower, and sorrel (Quanterra Sinus Defense, Sinupret) (7,374,379).
There is insufficient reliable information available about the safety of the topical use of gentian.
PREGNANCY: LIKELY UNSAFE ...contraindicated for oral use because gentian is a potential mutagen with effects on the menstrual cycle (4).
LACTATION: Insufficient reliable information available; avoid using.

Effectiveness

POSSIBLY EFFECTIVE ...when taken orally for loss of appetite, fullness, and flatulence (2). ...when gentian root is taken orally with European elder flower, verbena, cowslip flower, and sorrel (Quanterra Sinus Defense, Sinupret) for treating acute or chronic sinusitis (7,374,379).

There is insufficient reliable information available about the effectiveness of gentian for its other uses.

Possible Mechanism of Action & Active Ingredients

The applicable part of gentian is the root. The bitter constituents, gentiamarin, gentiopicrin, amarogentin, and swertiamarin, show evidence that they can increase saliva and digestive juice secretion (2,4). Some evidence suggests the constituent gentianine has anti-inflammatory activity (11). The constituents, gentisin and isogentisin, are both mutagenic (4). The constituent gentiopicrin is lethal to mosquito larvae (11).

Adverse Reactions Including Known Allergies

The oral use of the gentian root can cause GI irritation, nausea, and vomiting (6). It can also cause headaches in individuals sensitive to bitter substances (12).

Possible Interactions with Herbs & Other Dietary Supplements

Insufficient reliable information available.

Possible Interactions with Drugs

ACID-INHIBITING DRUGS: Theoretically, due to claims that gentian increases stomach acid, it might interfere with antacids, sucralfate (Carafate), H-2 antagonists, or proton pump inhibitors (19).

DOXYCYCLINE (Vibramycin): Concurrent use of gentian root, European elder flower, verbena, cowslip flower, and sorrel (Quanterra Sinus Defense, Sinupret) with doxycycline and a topical decongestant might improve the outcome of conventional (antibiotic/decongestant) therapy for acute bacterial sinusitis (374).

Possible Interactions with Foods

No interactions are known to occur, and there is no known reason to expect a clinically significant interaction with gentian.

Possible Interactions with Lab Tests

No interactions are known to occur, and there is no known reason to expect a clinically significant interaction with gentian.

Possible Interactions with Diseases or Conditions

DUODENAL AND GASTRIC ULCERS: Contraindicated (2).

GASTRIC IRRITATION OR INFLAMMATION: Contraindicated (12).

HYPERTENSION: The gentian root may not be well-tolerated in hypertensive individuals (5).

Typical Dosages & Routes of Administration that are Commonly Used

ORAL: The typical dose of gentian is 0.6-2 grams of the dried root three times daily with a maximum of 4 grams per day. One cup of the tea is also taken three times daily (2,4,18). The tea is prepared by steeping 0.6-2 grams of the dried root in 150 mL boiling water for 5-10 minutes and then straining (2,4,18). The tea can be sweetened with honey. The common dose of the tincture (1:5 in 45% alcohol) is 1-3 grams daily (2) or 1-4 mL three times daily (4). The usual dose of the fluid extract is 2-4 grams daily (2). The irritating qualities of the gentian root are minimized in the tea and maximized in the tincture form (12).

For acute or chronic sinusitis, two Sinupret tablets three times daily for up to two weeks has been used in clinical trials (7,374,379), equivalent to gentian root 12 mg, European elder flower 36 mg, verbena 36 mg cowslip flower 36 mg and sorrel 36 mg three times daily. For maintaining healthy sinuses, a typical dose is one tablet of Quanterra Sinus Defense three times daily with water, equivalent to gentian root 9 mg, European elder flower 29 mg, verbena 29 mg, cowslip flower 29 mg, and sorrel 29 mg three times daily (373). Each tablet of Quanterra Sinus Defense contains 125 mg of the herbal combination found in Sinupret (373).

Comments

CAUTION: The highly toxic white hellebore (Veratrum album) can grow in proximity to gentian and has caused accidental poisoning when used in home-made preparations (11). A related Gentiana species is used in Chinese medicine for treating jaundice, headache, sores, inflammation, and rheumatoid arthritis (11). The gentian root is unrelated to the gentian violet dye.

GERMAN CHAMOMILE

This Product is Also Known As

Camomilla, Camomille Allemande, Chamomile, Echte Kamille, Feldkamille, Fleur de Camomile, Hungarian Chamomile, Kamillen, Kleine Kamille, Manzanilla, Matricaire, Matricariae Flos, Pin Heads, Sweet False Chamomile, True Chamomile, Wild Chamomile.

Scientific Names

Matricaria recutita, synonyms Chamomilla recutita, Matricaria chamomilla.
Family: Asteraceae or Compositae.

People Use This For

Orally, chamomile is used for flatulence, travel sickness, nasal mucous membrane inflammation, nervous diarrhea, restlessness (4), GI spasms, inflammatory diseases of the GI tract (2,4), and as an antispasmodic primarily for menstrual cramps (5).
Topically, chamomile is used for hemorrhoids, mastitis, leg ulcers (4), skin, anogenital and mucous membrane inflammation, and bacterial skin diseases, including those of the mouth and gums (2).
As an inhalant, chamomile is used to treat inflammation and irritation of the respiratory tract (2).
In foods and beverages, the essential oil and extracts are used as flavor components (11).
In manufacturing, chamomile is used in cosmetics, soaps, and mouthwashes (11).

Safety

LIKELY SAFE ...when used in amounts commonly found in foods. It has Generally Recognized as Safe (GRAS) status for food use in the US (11).
POSSIBLY SAFE ...when preparations of the flower are used orally in medicinal amounts short-term (2,12). ...when used topically; avoid applying it near the eyes (8).
POSSIBLY UNSAFE ...when used as highly concentrated tea German chamomile can cause vomiting (12).
PREGNANCY: LIKELY UNSAFE ...contraindicated for oral use because it is believed to be a teratogen, affect the menstrual cycle and have uterine stimulant effects (4).
LACTATION: Insufficient reliable information available; avoid using.

Effectiveness

POSSIBLY EFFECTIVE ...when used orally for GI spasms, GI tract inflammation (2,3,4,6,7), and inducing sleep (4). ...when used topically for treating skin and mucous membrane inflammation, bacterial skin diseases, as a mouthwash for oral cavity mucosal infections (2,4), and as a bath or irrigation for treating anogenital inflammation (2). ...when used as an inhalant for inflammation and irritation of the respiratory tract (2).
Clinical studies on the effectiveness of chamomile have used extracts and flowers standardized to 1.2% apigenin. There is insufficient reliable information available about the effectiveness of German chamomile for its other uses.

Possible Mechanism of Action & Active Ingredients

The applicable part of German chamomile is the flowerhead. German chamomile possesses multiple actions, including anti-allergic, antiflatulent, antispasmodic, mild sedative, anti-inflammatory, and antiseptic actions. It also soothes mucous membranes (4). Chamomile's anti-allergic and anti-inflammatory actions result from the azulene constituents which inhibit histamine release (4). The sesquiterpene bisabolol constituents are also pharmacologically active and they possess anti-inflammatory and anti-ulcer properties (3,4). The coumarin constituents can have antibacterial properties (4). German chamomile can affect the menstrual cycle and is known to cause animal teratogenicity (4).

Adverse Reactions Including Known Allergies

The highly concentrated tea can cause vomiting (12). Chamomile can cause allergic reactions including contact dermatitis, severe hypersensitivity reactions, and anaphylaxis (6,567). If used near the eyes, it can be irritating (19). It can cause an allergic reaction in individuals sensitive to the Asteraceae/Compositae family. Members of this family include ragweed, chrysanthemums, marigolds, daisies, and many other herbs.

Possible Interactions with Herbs & Other Dietary Supplements

HERBS WITH SEDATIVE PROPERTIES: Theoretically, concomitant use with herbs that have sedative properties might enhance therapeutic and adverse effects. These include calamus, calendula, California poppy, catnip, capsicum, celery, couch grass, elecampane, ginseng Siberian, goldenseal, gotu kola, hops, Jamaican dogwood, kava, lemon balm, sage, St. John's wort, sassafras, scullcap, shepherd's purse, stinging nettle, valerian, wild carrot, wild lettuce, withania root, and yerba mansa (4,19).
HERBS WITH ANTICOAGULANT/ANTIPLATELET POTENTIAL: Concomitant use of herbs that have coumarin constituents or affect platelet aggregation could theoretically increase the risk of bleeding in some people. These herbs include: angelica, anise, arnica, asafoetida, bogbean, boldo, capsicum, celery, clove, danshen, fenugreek, feverfew, garlic, ginger, ginkgo, ginseng (Panax), horse chestnut, horseradish, licorice, meadowsweet, prickly ash, onion, papain, passionflower, poplar, quassia, red clover, turmeric, wild carrot, wild lettuce, willow, and others (4,19).

Possible Interactions with Drugs

ANTICOAGULANTS: Theoretically, concomitant use of large amounts of chamomile might interfere with anticoagulant therapy (4).
BENZODIAZEPINES: Theoretically, concomitant use with benzodiazepines might cause additive effects and side effects (19).
ETHYL ALCOHOL: Theoretically, liquid extract German chamomile might help prevent ulcer formation caused by ethyl alcohol (19).

INDOMETHACIN (Indocin): Theoretically, bisabolol, a constituent of the volatile oil, might prevent ulcer formation caused by indomethacin (19).

DRUGS WITH SEDATIVE PROPERTIES: Theoretically, concomitant use with drugs with sedative properties can cause additive effects and side effects (19).

Possible Interactions with Foods

No interactions are known to occur, and there is no known reason to expect a clinically significant interaction with German chamomile.

Possible Interactions with Lab Tests

No interactions are known to occur, and there is no known reason to expect a clinically significant interaction with German chamomile.

Possible Interactions with Diseases or Conditions

ASTHMA: Chamomile can exacerbate this condition (4).

CROSS-ALLERGENICITY: Can cause an allergic reaction in individuals sensitive to the Asteraceae/Compositae family. Members of this family include ragweed, chrysanthemums, marigolds, daisies, and many other herbs.

Typical Dosages & Routes of Administration that are Commonly Used

ORAL: The typical dose of chamomile is 2-8 grams of the dried flower heads three times daily (4) or one cup of the tea three to four times daily. The tea is prepared by steeping 3 grams of the dried flower heads in 150 mL boiling water for 5-10 minutes and then straining (2). The liquid extract (1:1 in 45% alcohol) is commonly dosed as 1-4 mL three times daily (4). Clinical studies on the effectiveness of chamomile have used extracts and flowers standardized to 1.2% apigenin.

TOPICAL: Chamomile is used as poultices and rinses. The prepared tea is commonly used (steep 4 teaspoons of the dried flower heads in 1.5 cups boiling water for 15 minutes and then strain) (18). The 3-10% ointments and gels are for external use only (18). Avoid topical use near the eyes (12). For inflammation of mucous membranes of the mouth and throat, the freshly prepared tea is commonly used as a mouthwash or gargle (2).

INHALATION: No typical dosage.

Comments

Avoid confusion with Roman chamomile. Although ointments, creams, and lotions containing the volatile oil of chamomile are intended for the treatment of various skin conditions and are used in Europe, they have not been approved in the US (3).

GERMAN IPECAC

This Product is Also Known As
None.

Scientific Names
Cynanchum vincetoxicum.
Family: Asclepiadaceae.

People Use This For
Orally, German ipecac is used for digestive and kidney disorders, and dysmenorrhea.

Topically, German ipecac is used in poultices for healing swelling and bruising.

In folk medicine, German ipecac is used orally for edema. It was also used for kidney disorders, the plague, snake bite, and dysmenorrhea, as a diuretic, emetic, and to promote sweating (18).

Safety
POSSIBLY UNSAFE ...when used orally (18).

There is insufficient reliable information available about the safety of the topical use of German ipecac

PREGNANCY AND LACTATION: POSSIBLY UNSAFE ...when used orally (18); avoid using.

Effectiveness
There is insufficient reliable information available about the effectiveness of German ipecac.

Possible Mechanism of Action & Active Ingredients
The applicable parts of German ipecac are the leaf and root/rhizome. There is insufficient reliable information available about the possible mechanism of action and active ingredients.

Adverse Reactions Including Known Allergies
High doses of German ipecac may cause vomiting, apnea, and cardiac arrest. Seed extracts may cause advancing paralysis of the central nervous system (18).

Possible Interactions with Herbs & Other Dietary Supplements
Insufficient reliable information available.

Possible Interactions with Drugs

No interactions are known to occur, and there is no known reason to expect a clinically significant interaction with German ipecac.

Possible Interactions with Foods

No interactions are known to occur, and there is no known reason to expect a clinically significant interaction with German ipecac.

Possible Interactions with Lab Tests

No interactions are known to occur, and there is no known reason to expect a clinically significant interaction with German ipecac.

Possible Interactions with Diseases or Conditions

No interactions are known to occur, and there is no known reason to expect a clinically significant interaction with German ipecac.

Typical Dosages & Routes of Administration that are Commonly Used

No typical dosage.

Comments

German ipecac is considered unsafe for oral use; avoid using (18).

GERMAN SARSAPARILLA

This Product is Also Known As

Caricis rhizoma, Red Couchgrass, Red Sage, Sandriedgraswurzelstock, Sand Sedge, Sea Sedge.
CAUTION: See separate listings for Couch Grass, Sarsaparilla, Sage, and Tormentil.

Scientific Names

Carex arenaria.
Family: Cyperaceae.

People Use This For

Orally, German sarsaparilla is used for prevention of gout, inducing sweating, arthritis, skin ailments, and as a diuretic (2). It is also used for venereal disease, flatulence, colic, liver disorders, diabetes, edema, pulmonary tuberculosis, and amenorrhea (18).

Safety

There is insufficient reliable information available about the safety of German sarsaparilla.
Pregnancy and Lactation: Insufficient reliable information available; avoid using.

Effectiveness

There is insufficient reliable information available about the effectiveness of German sarsaparilla.

Possible Mechanism of Action & Active Ingredients

The applicable part of German sarsaparilla is the underground stem. German sarsaparilla contains saponins, a volatile oil containing methyl salicylate and cineole, flavonoids, and tannins (18).

Adverse Reactions Including Known Allergies

The saponins contained in the product may cause local irritation (2).

Possible Interactions with Herbs & Other Dietary Supplements

Insufficient reliable information available.

Possible Interactions with Drugs

No interactions are known to occur, and there is no known reason to expect a clinically significant interaction with German sarsaparilla.

Possible Interactions with Foods

No interactions are known to occur, and there is no known reason to expect a clinically significant interaction with German sarsaparilla.

Possible Interactions with Lab Tests

There are no reports of lab interactions with German sarsaparilla. However, because it contains salicylate(s), use caution in interpreting test results known to be affected by salicylates.

Possible Interactions with Diseases or Conditions

ASPIRIN ALLERGY/ASTHMA: Avoid or use cautiously in individuals who are allergic to aspirin or have asthma; contains salicylates.

Typical Dosages & Routes of Administration that are Commonly Used

ORAL: German sarsaparilla is typically prepared as a liquid. For a tea, 3 grams is added to 1 cup boiling water; 1 cup is taken daily. A cold solution is prepared with 2 teaspoons sarsaparilla added to a cup of water; a cup is taken 2 to 3 times daily (5252).

Comments

There is very little scientific information about this product. Our staff is continually analyzing the available information on natural medicines and will add data here as it becomes available.

GERMANDER

This Product is Also Known As

Wall Germander, Wild Germander.

Scientific Names

Teucrium chamaedrys.
Family: Lamiaceae.

People Use This For

Traditionally, germander has been used orally for treating gallbladder conditions, for fever, as a digestive aid (18), for stomachaches (14), for mild diarrhea, as an adjunct for weight loss (18), as an antiseptic (14), and as "a rinse for gout" (18).
Topically, it has been used as a mouthwash for oral hygiene (514).
In manufacturing, germander is used as a flavoring agent in alcoholic beverages (14).

Safety

LIKELY UNSAFE …when used orally. Germander is associated with multiple cases of hepatitis and death (17,18,514,3741,3742,3743,3744). France has banned its sale (17). Canada does not allow germander to be included in oral products as a non-medicinal ingredient (12,14). However, the US still allows germander to be used in small amounts as a flavoring agent in alcoholic beverages (12,14).
PREGNANCY AND LACTATION: LIKELY UNSAFE (17,18,514,3741,3742,3743,3744).

Effectiveness

There is insufficient reliable information available about the effectiveness of germander.

Possible Mechanism of Action & Active Ingredients

The applicable parts of germander are the above ground parts. Germander contains teucrin A, a diterpene, which causes hepatic necrosis in mice (3740).

Adverse Reactions Including Known Allergies

Taken orally, germander has been associated with hepatitis, liver cell necrosis, and death (18,514,3741,3742,3743,3744).

Possible Interactions with Herbs & Other Dietary Supplements

Insufficient reliable information available.

Possible Interactions with Drugs

No interactions are known to occur, and there is no known reason to expect a clinically significant interaction with germander.

Possible Interactions with Foods

No interactions are known to occur, and there is no known reason to expect a clinically significant interaction with germander.

Possible Interactions with Lab Tests

No interactions are known to occur, and there is no known reason to expect a clinically significant interaction with germander.

Possible Interactions with Diseases or Conditions

No interactions are known to occur, and there is no known reason to expect a clinically significant interaction with germander.

Typical Dosages & Routes of Administration that are Commonly Used

No typical dosage.

Comments

Germander is likely to be unsafe; avoid using.

GERMANIUM

This Product is Also Known As
Bis-Carboxyethyl Germanium Sesquioxide, Carboxyethylgermanium Sesquioxide, Ge-132, GE-132, Ge-Oxy 132, Germanium Lactate Citrate, Inorganic Germanium, Organic Germanium.

Scientific Names
Germanium; Ge; atomic number 32; Bis-carboxyethyl germanium sesquioxide; Germanium lactate citrate.

People Use This For
Orally, germanium is used for arthritis, pain relief, osteoporosis, low energy, AIDS, cancer, high blood pressure, high cholesterol, heart disease, glaucoma, and cataracts. It is used orally for rheumatoid arthritis, depression, hepatitis, cirrhosis, food allergies, candidiasis, chronic viral infections, and heavy metal poisoning (including mercury, cadmium). Germanium is used orally for increasing circulation of blood to the brain, supporting the immune system, and as an antioxidant (2356,2357,2358,2359).

Safety
LIKELY UNSAFE ...when used orally; avoid using. There have been 31 reports of renal failure or death caused by ingestion of 15-300 grams over 2 to 36 months (2360).
PREGNANCY AND LACTATION: LIKELY UNSAFE ...contraindicated, due to reported toxicity (2360).

Effectiveness
There is insufficient reliable information available about the effectiveness of germanium.

Possible Mechanism of Action & Active Ingredients
Insufficient reliable information available.

Adverse Reactions Including Known Allergies
Ingestion of germanium can cause renal tubular degeneration, anemia, muscle weakness, peripheral neuropathy, renal failure, and death (2360).

Possible Interactions with Herbs & Other Dietary Supplements
Insufficient reliable information available.

Possible Interactions with Drugs
FUROSEMIDE: One case report of furosemide resistance associated with a ginseng product containing germanium (770).

Possible Interactions with Foods
No interactions are known to occur, and there is no known reason to expect a clinically significant interaction with germanium.

Possible Interactions with Lab Tests
No interactions are known to occur, and there is no known reason to expect a clinically significant interaction with germanium.

Possible Interactions with Diseases or Conditions
No interactions are known to occur, and there is no known reason to expect a clinically significant interaction with germanium.

Typical Dosages & Routes of Administration that are Commonly Used
ORAL: People typically use 150 mg one to five times daily between meals or with meals (directions vary). Available in capsule and tablet form. The tablet form may also be dissolved under the tongue (6006).

Comments
Germanium is likely unsafe and without proven efficacy; avoid using.

GINGER

This Product is Also Known As
African Ginger, Black Ginger, Cochin Ginger, Gingembre, Jamaica Ginger, Race Ginger.

Scientific Names
Zingiber officinale.
Family: Zingiberaceae.

People Use This For

Orally, ginger is used for motion sickness, colic, dyspepsia, flatulence (2,4), rheumatoid arthritis (721), loss of appetite (4), post-surgical nausea and vomiting (722,723), and discontinuing serotonin reuptake inhibitor (SSRI) drug therapy (3451). It is also used for anorexia, upper respiratory tract infections, cough, and bronchitis.

Topically, the fresh juice of ginger is used for treating thermal burns (11).

In Chinese medicine, ginger is used as a diaphoretic, diuretic, and stimulant (5,11). Ginger is also used in Chinese medicine for treating stomachache, diarrhea, nausea, cholera, and bleeding (11). Fresh ginger is taken orally for treating acute bacterial dysentery, baldness, malaria, orchitis, poisonous snake bites, rheumatism, and toothaches (11).

Pharmaceutically, the oleoresin of ginger is used as an ingredient in digestive, laxative, antitussive, antiflatulent, and antacid preparations (11).

In foods and beverages, ginger is used as a flavoring (11).

In manufacturing, ginger is used as a fragrance component in soaps and cosmetics (11).

Safety

LIKELY SAFE ...when the fresh or dried root are used in the amounts commonly found in foods. It has Generally Recognized as Safe (GRAS) status in the US (11). The maximum use level of ginger in food is 0.023%. ...when used topically, the oil of ginger is well tolerated and is not likely to cause phototoxicity (4,11).

POSSIBLY SAFE ...when the dried or fresh root are used orally and appropriately for medicinal use (2).

POSSIBLY UNSAFE ...when used orally in large amounts. Ginger can cause central nervous system depression and cardiac arrhythmias (5).

PREGNANCY: LIKELY SAFE ...when used orally in amounts found in foods. POSSIBLY UNSAFE ...when used orally in amounts greater than those found in foods; avoid using. One case of spontaneous abortion was reported in the 12th week of pregnancy in a woman who used ginger for morning sickness (721). The effect of ginger on the developing fetus is unknown. A related plant (Zingiber cassumunar) can have utero-activity (4).

LACTATION: Insufficient reliable information available: avoid using amounts greater than those found in foods.

Effectiveness

POSSIBLY EFFECTIVE ...when ginger root is used orally for preventing motion sickness, seasickness, or morning sickness (4,721,6111). ...when used orally for dyspepsia (2). ...when taken orally for relieving joint pain and improving joint movement in people with rheumatoid arthritis (4). ...when used orally for preventing postoperative nausea and vomiting in the absence of narcotic anesthesia or analgesia (722,723).

LIKELY INEFFECTIVE ...when used orally for preventing postoperative nausea and vomiting in the presence of narcotic anesthesia or analgesia (3452,3453).

There is insufficient reliable information available about the effectiveness of ginger for its other uses.

Possible Mechanism of Action & Active Ingredients

The applicable parts of ginger are the rhizome and root. Ginger is thought to contain mutagenic and antimutagenic compounds (4). Constituents called gingerols demonstrate antipyretic, analgesic, antitussive, cardiotonic, and sedative properties (5). However, in preliminary research ginger-containing products fail to demonstrate anti-inflammatory, antipyretic, or antiarthritis effects (6131). Ginger shows hypoglycemic, hypotensive or hypertensive, and positive cardiac inotropic activities. It also inhibits platelets and prostaglandins, and improves appetite and digestion (2,4). Research demonstrates that ginger extracts can stimulate vasomotor and respiratory centers, directly stimulate the heart, lower serum cholesterol, kill vaginal trichomonads (11), inhibit gastric lesions (4,11), reduce gastric secretions, and increase bile secretion (4). A related plant (Zingiber cassumunar) demonstrates utero-activity (4). Ginger might be useful for treating disequilibrium and nausea associated with discontinuation or tapering of selective serotonin reuptake inhibitors (SSRIs) (3451).

Adverse Reactions Including Known Allergies

Ginger can cause dermatitis in sensitive individuals (4). Large overdoses can cause central nervous system depression and cardiac arrhythmias (5).

Possible Interactions with Herbs & Other Dietary Supplements

HERBS WITH ANTICOAGULANT/ANTIPLATELET POTENTIAL: Concomitant use of herbs that have coumarin constituents or affect platelet aggregation could theoretically increase the risk of bleeding in some people. These herbs include: angelica, anise, arnica, asafoetida, bogbean, boldo, capsicum, celery, chamomile, clove, danshen, fenugreek, feverfew, garlic, ginkgo, ginseng (Panax), horse chestnut, horseradish, licorice, meadowsweet, prickly ash, onion, papain, passionflower, poplar, quassia, red clover, turmeric, wild carrot, wild lettuce, willow, and others (4,19).

Possible Interactions with Drugs

ACID-INHIBITING DRUGS: Theoretically, due to claims that ginger rhizome increases stomach acid, it might interfere with antacids, sucralfate (Carafate), H-2 antagonists, or proton pump inhibitors (19).

ANTICOAGULANT, ANTIPLATELET DRUGS: Theoretically, excessive amounts might increase the effect or the risk of bleeding (4).

BARBITURATES: Theoretically, ginger might enhance barbiturate effects (6).

 © Copyright 2000, Natural Medicines Comprehensive Database (209) 472-2244. For updated data, go to www.NaturalDatabase.com

BLOOD PRESSURE THERAPY: Theoretically, due to hypertensive or hypotensive effects, ginger might interfere with blood pressure drug therapy (4).
CYCLOPHOSPHAMIDE (Cytoxan): Theoretically, cyclophosphamide-induced vomiting might be prevented by prior administration of the ginger constituent 6-gingerol or an acetone ginger extract (19).
CARDIAC DRUGS: Theoretically, ginger might interfere with cardiac drug therapy due to inotropic effects (2,4).
DIABETES DRUGS: Theoretically, ginger might interfere with diabetes therapy due to hypoglycemic effects (2,4).
SELECTIVE SEROTONIN REUPTAKE INHIBITORS (SSRIs): Case reports suggest that ginger might be effective for treating disequilibrium and nausea resulting from discontinuation or tapering of sertraline (Zoloft) and other selective serotonin reuptake inhibitors (3451).

Possible Interactions with Foods
No interactions are known to occur, and there is no known reason to expect a clinically significant interaction with ginger.

Possible Interactions with Lab Tests
No interactions are known to occur, and there is no known reason to expect a clinically significant interaction with ginger.

Possible Interactions with Diseases or Conditions
GALLSTONES: Individuals with gallstones should not use ginger except after medical evaluation determines ginger will not worsen gallstone symptoms (12).
BLEEDING CONDITIONS: Theoretically, excessive doses of ginger can interfere with increase risk of bleeding (4).
DIABETES: Theoretically, excessive doses of ginger can cause hypoglycemia, necessitating change in dose of diabetes medication (4).
HEART CONDITIONS: Theoretically, excessive doses of ginger might have cardiotonic activity that can interfere with the therapy for heart conditions (4).
HIGH BLOOD PRESSURE, LOW BLOOD PRESSURE: Theoretically, excessive doses of ginger might increase or reduce blood pressure, interfering with blood pressure control (4).

Typical Dosages & Routes of Administration that are Commonly Used
ORAL: 0.25-1 g dried root three times daily (4) or one cup tea three times daily (4,18). The tea is prepared by steeping 0.5-1 grams dried root in 150 mL boiling water for 5-10 minutes and then straining (4,18). The maximum dose of ginger is 4 grams of the root per day (2). A weak ginger tincture is dosed at 1.5-3 mL (4). A strong ginger tincture is dosed at 0.25-0.5 mL (4). For morning sickness, 250 mg ginger four times daily is used (6). As an anti-emetic, 2 g freshly powdered root is taken with some water (18). For nausea and disequilibrium resulting from serotonin reuptake inhibitor discontinuation or tapering, 550-1100 mg ginger has been used three times daily (3451). For preventing postoperative nausea and vomiting (in the absence of narcotic anesthesia or analgesia), 1 g powdered ginger root one hour before induction of anaesthesia has been used (722,723).

Comments
Ginger is commonly found in the warmer climates, including India, Jamaica, and China, and its flowers are similar to orchids. The rhizome is used as the source for the dried, powder spice. In vitro the volatile oil of the related species, Zingiber purpureum, has antihelmintic activity (4). The constituent of the related species, Zingiber cassumunar, has uteroactivity in pregnant rats (4).

GINKGO leaf

This Product is Also Known As
Bai Guo Ye, Fossil Tree, Gingko, Ginkgo Folium, Ginkyo, Japanese Silver Apricot, Kew Tree, Maidenhair Tree, Salisburia Adiantifolia, Yinhsing.
CAUTION: See separate listings for Ginkgo leaf extract and Ginkgo seed. Ginkgo leaf extract (Ginkgo biloba) is the most commonly used form of Ginkgo.

Scientific Names
Ginkgo biloba.
Family: Ginkgoaceae.

People Use This For
In Chinese medicine, ginkgo leaf is used orally for asthma (4,5,6,7,17), bronchitis, poor circulation (4,11,17), arteriosclerosis, angina pectoris, high serum cholesterol, dysentery, and filariasis (11). It is used topically in Chinese medicine as a prepared tea to wash chilblains, which are lesions on the fingers, toes, heels, ears, and nose caused by exposure to extreme cold (11).
In folk medicine, ginkgo leaf has been used as a psychotropic and neurotropic agent, to improve sexual

Performance, prevent premature aging, regulate gastric acidity, improve liver and gallbladder function, regulate bacterial flora, regulate blood pressure, and treat heart disease (2). Ginkgo leaf has also been used for PMS, thrombosis, heart disease, hypercholesterolemia, cardiac reperfusion injury, dysentery, and filariasis (6,11).

Safety

POSSIBLY UNSAFE ...when used orally. The ingestion of plant parts is associated with severe allergic reactions (17).

LIKELY UNSAFE ...when ginkgo leaf is used by individuals who are hypersensitive to Ginkgo biloba preparations (2).

There is insufficient reliable information available about the safety of the topical use of ginkgo leaf.

PREGNANCY AND LACTATION: POSSIBLY UNSAFE ...when used orally; avoid using.

Effectiveness

There is insufficient reliable information available about the effectiveness of ginkgo leaf.

Possible Mechanism of Action & Active Ingredients

The leaf constituents, ginkgolides A, B, C and M, interfere with platelet aggregation, bronchoconstriction, phagocyte chemotaxis, and the release of inflammatory compounds by competitive inhibition of the platelet activating factor (PAF) (2,4,11,13). Ginkgolides antagonize PAF-induced decreases in myocardial contractility and coronary blood flow, prevent cyclosporin-induced nephrotoxicity, and can interfere with eosinophil infiltration in hypersensitivity reactions (4).

Adverse Reactions Including Known Allergies

The ingestion of the whole plant is associated with severe allergic reactions (17). Ginkgo fruit/pulp is a potent contact allergen. It can cause severe allergic skin reactions, irritation of mucous membranes and the gastrointestinal tract (4,12,17). Ingestion of even small amounts of pulp can cause redness around the mouth, rectal burning, and painful anal sphincter spasms (6). Cross-reactivity is possible with ginkgo fruit in individuals allergic to poison ivy, poison oak, poison sumac, mango rind, and cashew shell oil (6,380). The ginkgo pollen is also strongly allergenic (6). Skin contact with fresh ginkgo leaves can cause contact dermatitis (19). Some evidence suggests that high concentrations of ginkgo biloba might reduce male and female fertility (4239,4240); however, this has not been demonstrated in humans.

Possible Interactions with Herbs & Other Dietary Supplements

HERBS WITH ANTICOAGULANT/ANTIPLATELET POTENTIAL: Concomitant use of herbs that have coumarin constituents or affect platelet aggregation could theoretically increase the risk of bleeding in some people. These herbs include: angelica, anise, arnica, asafoetida, bogbean, boldo, capsicum, celery, chamomile, clove, danshen, fenugreek, feverfew, garlic, ginger, ginseng (Panax), horse chestnut, horseradish, licorice, meadowsweet, prickly ash, onion, papain, passionflower, poplar, quassia, red clover, turmeric, wild carrot, wild lettuce, willow, and others (4,19).

Possible Interactions with Drugs

ANTIPLATELET DRUGS: Theoretically, ginkgo leaves might increase the effects and adverse effects of antiplatelet drugs (19).

MAOIs: Theoretically, ginkgo leaf can potentiate the activity of monoamine oxidase inhibitors (MAOIs) (6,12).

Possible Interactions with Foods

No interactions are known to occur, and there is no known reason to expect a clinically significant interaction with ginkgo leaf.

Possible Interactions with Lab Tests

No interactions are known to occur, and there is no known reason to expect a clinically significant interaction with ginkgo leaf.

Possible Interactions with Diseases or Conditions

INFERTILITY: Some evidence suggests that ginkgo biloba might inhibit oocyte fertilization and should be avoided in couples attempting to conceive (4239,4240). This effect has not yet been demonstrated in humans; however, until more is known, use with caution in couples attempting to conceive and avoid use in couples having difficulty conceiving.

Typical Dosages & Routes of Administration that are Commonly Used

ORAL: People typically use 120 mg to 240 mg ginkgo tablets or capsules daily in two or three divided doses (5008). Some people take 0.5 mL of a standard 1:5 tincture of the crude ginkgo leaf three times daily (5011).

 © Copyright 2000, Natural Medicines Comprehensive Database (209) 472-2244. For updated data, go to www.NaturalDatabase.com

Comments

When people talk about ginkgo, they usually mean ginkgo leaf extract. Fossils of the ginkgo tree have been found to be over two hundred million years old, making the tree the oldest living species in the world, and the tree itself can live as long as one thousand years (6). The ginkgo fruit or pulp is a potent contact allergen, causing severe allergic skin reactions, irritation of mucous membranes and gastrointestinal tract (4,12,17). The ingestion of even small amounts of the pulp can cause perioral erythema, rectal burning, and painful anal sphincter spasms (6).

GINKGO leaf extract

This Product is Also Known As

Adiantifolia, Bai Guo Ye, Fossil Tree, Gingko, Ginkgo Biloba, Ginkgo Folium, Ginko Biloba, Ginkyo, Japanese Silver Apricot, Kew Tree, Maidenhair Tree, Salisburia, Yinhsing.
CAUTION: See separate listings for Ginkgo leaf and Ginkgo seed. Ginkgo leaf extract (Ginkgo biloba) is the most commonly used form of Ginkgo.

Scientific Names

Ginkgo biloba.
Family: Ginkgoaceae.

People Use This For

Orally, ginkgo is used for dementia, including Alzheimer's, vascular, and mixed dementia (2,6,7,11,18). People also use ginkgo for conditions associated with cerebral vascular insufficiency, especially in the elderly, including memory loss, headache, tinnitus, vertigo, dizziness, difficulty concentrating, mood disturbances, and hearing disorders (2,5,6,11,13,18). Ginkgo is used for relief of walking pain associated with intermittent claudication, particularly in patients with Fontaine's stage IIa or IIb peripheral arterial occlusive disease (2,6,7,13,3461). Ginkgo is used to reverse sexual dysfunction caused by SSRI depressants (599). It is also used for cognitive disorders secondary to depression; eye problems, including macular degeneration (6,11); attention deficit-hyperactivity disorder (ADHD) (6121); premenstrual syndrome; thrombosis; heart disease; hypercholesterolemia; cardiac reperfusion injury; dysentery; and filariasis (6,11). Ginkgo is also used to improve cognitive behavior and sleep patterns in patients with depression (348). Ginkgo has also been used to prevent acute mountain sickness (6230). Topically, ginkgo is used on wound dressings (7).
Intravenously, ginkgo is used to increase cerebral blood flow, improve cognition, and for psychiatric conditions in the elderly (6).
In Chinese medicine, ginkgo is used to treat asthma (4,5,6,7,17), bronchitis, poor circulation, various disorders of the central nervous system (17), and chilblains (4,11,17).
In folk medicine, ginkgo has been used as a psychotropic and neurotropic agent. It has been used to improve sexual performance, prevent premature aging, regulate gastric acidity, improve liver and gallbladder function, regulate bacterial flora, regulate blood pressure, and treat heart disease (2).
In manufacturing, ginkgo leaf extract has been used in cosmetics (11).

Safety

LIKELY SAFE ...when used orally and appropriately (2,4,5,7,1515). Standardized ginkgo leaf extracts have been used safely in trials lasting from several weeks to a year (1514,1515).
LIKELY UNSAFE ...when used intravenously (6). The German product has been withdrawn from the market due to severe adverse reactions (6).
PREGNANCY AND LACTATION: Insufficient reliable information available; avoid using.

Effectiveness

LIKELY EFFECTIVE ...when used orally for stabilization or improvement in cognitive function in Alzheimer's, multi-infarct, or mixed dementias. Multiple clinical trials and meta-analyses have demonstrated significant improvement or delay in the progression of disease when standardized ginkgo leaf extracts were used over several weeks to a year (1514,1515,6222,6223,6224,6225). Improvement appears to be similar to the effect documented with the prescription drug donepezil (Aricept) (1515,6224). However, ginkgo has not been directly compared to donepezil or other drugs approved for treating Alzheimer's.
POSSIBLY EFFECTIVE ...when taken orally for increasing pain-free walking distance in patients with intermittent claudication (7,3461,6211,6212,6213). In one study, patients with Fontaine's IIb peripheral arterial occlusive disease who were treated with a standardized ginkgo extract experienced significant improvement in pain-free walking distance. Doses of 120 mg per day and 240 mg per day were compared to placebo. Only the higher dose provided significant improvement after 24 weeks of treatment (3461,6212). However, a meta-analysis of controlled trials found improvement even with lower doses of 120 to 160 mg daily (6211). ...when used orally for vertigo and equilibrium disorders (2,6208,6220,6221). Two clinical studies indicate that ginkgo is significantly more effective than placebo (6220) and possibly as effective as betahistine for improving vertigo and dizziness caused by vascular vestibular disorders and vestibular disorders of unknown origin (6220,6221). ...when used orally for premenstrual symptoms (6229). In a double-blind, placebo-controlled study, ginkgo was more effective than placebo in relieving

© Copyright 2000, Natural Medicines Comprehensive Database (209) 472-2244. For updated data, go to www.NaturalDatabase.com

breast tenderness and neuropsychological symptoms associated with premenstrual syndrome (PMS) (6229). ...when used orally to improve cognitive performance and memory in normal subjects and in elderly people with mild to moderate memory loss. Ginkgo improved cognitive and memory test scores in people with or without memory impairment in doses from 120 mg to 600 mg (1263,6214,6215,6216,6244). In one assessment, the 120 mg dose was more effective than higher doses (6214). ...when used orally to prevent acute altitude sickness and vascular reactivity to cold exposure (6230). During a Himalayan expedition, 44 healthy mountain climbers who had previously experienced altitude sickness were randomized to treatment with 160 milligrams ginkgo twice daily or placebo (6230). In the placebo group, 41% of the climbers experienced mountain sickness (headache, fatigue, dyspnea, nausea, vomiting) compared to none in the ginkgo group (6230). Cold tolerance improved by 22.8% in the ginkgo group and deteriorated by 104% in the placebo group (6230). ...when used orally for age-related macular degeneration (6227,6228). In one controlled trial, ginkgo significantly improved distance vision in 10 patients with macular degeneration (6227). ...when used orally to reverse sexual dysfunction caused by selective serotonin-reuptake inhibitors (SSRIs) in both men and women. Preliminary clinical evidence suggests that ginkgo biloba might be helpful for antidepressant-induced sexual dysfunction (212,599,3965,3966,3967,3968,3969). ...when taken orally for improving color vision in diabetic retinopathy. In a small trial, treatment with Ginkgo leaf extract for 6 months significantly improved measures of color vision in patients with early diabetic retinopathy (6175).

Most clinical studies on the effectiveness of Ginkgo biloba have used the standardized extracts Egb 761 (Tanakan) and LI 1370 (Lichtwer Pharma). These two extracts are similar and prepared to contain approximately 24-25% flavone glycosides and 6% terpene lactones. Products with similar ingredients include Ginkai (Lichtwer Pharma), Ginkgo 5 (Pharmline), Ginkgold and Ginkgo (Nature's Way), and Quanterra Mental Sharpness (Warner-Lambert). There is insufficient reliable information available about the effectiveness of ginkgo leaf extract for its other uses. However, in an unpublished study, Swiss researchers report that ginkgo might improve sleep patterns and cognitive behavior in patients with depression. Results of this study were presented at the American Psychiatric Association 152nd annual meeting (348). Ginkgo might also be beneficial for tinnitus; however, current evidence is conflicting (2,6208,6218,6219). Further evidence is needed to rate ginkgo for these uses.

Possible Mechanism of Action & Active Ingredients

Ginkgo biloba leaf extract contains a variety of constituents. It is thought that its pharmacological effects are partly drawn from individual constituents, primarily from synergistic effects of the constituents working together. The whole extract is thought to be more active than any one isolated constituent. Ginkgo is primarily used for cognitive disorders. Ginkgo extract seems to affect cognitive deficiency in two ways: it stimulates populations of nerve cells that are still functional, and it protects nerve cells from pathologic influences (7). Ginkgo flavonoid constituents, which are mainly rutin, are efficient free-radical scavengers. Rutin is known to improve capillary fragility and permeability (7). Ginkgo contains ginkgolide constituents that competitively inhibit platelet-activating factor (PAF) he European Society of Cardiology, found that high-risk men taking vitamin E 200 mg and vitamin C 500 mg daily for hypersensitivity reactions, and circulatory diseases (6). Ginkgolides antagonize PAF-induced decreases in myocardial contractility and coronary blood flow, and prevent cyclosporin-induced nephrotoxicity (4). Ginkgo contains ginkgolides A and B. These exert an anti-stress and neuroprotective effect by decreasing corticosteroid synthesis (6). Ginkgo leaf extract increases cerebral blood flow. There is some evidence that ginkgo might improve cerebral metabolism and protect against ischemia (6). Ginkgo leaf extract decreases blood viscosity (2,6,7), improves microcirculatory blood flow (2,5,6,11), protects neural and retinal tissue from hypoxic or oxidative injury (2,4,7,11), stimulates choline uptake, and prevents age-related decline in muscarinic receptors in the hippocampus (2,18). Ginkgo can improve vascular blood flow in the corpus cavernosum by relaxing vascular smooth muscle, which helps erectile function (213). It has been suggested that ginkgo leaf extract might exert a monoamine oxidase (MAO) inhibiting effect (6). However, studies have found conflicting results (6231,6232,6233). There is also some suggestion that it shows some activity against Pneumocystis carinii (6), arrests fibrosis in damaged hepatocytes (6), and inhibits nitric oxide production in inflammation (6). Pretreatment with a ginkgo product reduced the extent of brain damage caused by induced strokes in mice. They caution that it is too early to recommend the use of ginkgo in humans at risk for stroke. Results of this unpublished study were presented at the American Academy of Neurology 52nd annual meeting (5077).

Adverse Reactions Including Known Allergies

The use of ginkgo leaf extract in therapeutic doses might cause mild gastrointestinal complaints (2,4,12,17), headache (2,4,9,12,17), dizziness (6,9), palpitations (6,9), and allergic skin reactions (2,6,17). Large doses might cause restlessness, diarrhea, nausea, vomiting (5), lack of muscle tone, and weakness (2). Bleeding is often mentioned as a side effect of ginkgo, but there are very few cases reported. There are two case reports of subdural hematoma associated with ginkgo use (577,578); one report of a subarachnoid hemorrhage (4207), and one case report of a bleeding iris associated with ginkgo use (579). Anecdotal evidence suggests that ginkgo might also be associated with seizures. The FDAs Special Nutritionals Adverse Event Monitoring System lists ginkgo preparations in association with seizure in 7 cases. Four cases involve multi-ingredient products and 3 cases involve ginkgo alone. However, because few details are available, it is not possible to determine if ginkgo caused the seizure in these cases (3575). Intravenous use of ginkgo leaf extract can cause skin allergy, circulatory disturbances, and phlebitis (6). The German intravenous product has been withdrawn from the market (6). Ginkgo fruit/pulp is a potent contact allergen. It can cause severe allergic skin reactions, and irritation of mucous membranes and the gastrointestinal tract (4,12,17). Ingestion of even small amounts of pulp can cause redness around the mouth, rectal burning, and painful anal sphincter spasms (6). Some evidence suggests that high concentrations of ginkgo might reduce male and female fertility (4239,4240).

Possible Interactions with Herbs & Other Dietary Supplements

HERBS WITH ANTICOAGULANT/ANTIPLATELET POTENTIAL: Concomitant use of herbs that have coumarin constituents or affect platelet aggregation could theoretically increase the risk of bleeding in some people. These herbs include: angelica, anise, arnica, asafoetida, bogbean, boldo, capsicum, celery, chamomile, clove, danshen, fenugreek, feverfew, garlic, ginger, ginseng (Panax), horse chestnut, horseradish, licorice, meadowsweet, prickly ash, onion, papain, passionflower, poplar, quassia, red clover, turmeric, wild carrot, wild lettuce, willow, and others (4,19).

Possible Interactions with Drugs

ANTICOAGULANT, ANTIPLATELET DRUGS: Ginkgo can increase risk of bleeding with anticoagulant, antiplatelet drugs (5,18).
CYCLOSPORIN: Theoretically, ginkgo might prevent cyclosporin-induced nephrotoxicity (4).
MAOIs: Theoretically, ginkgo might potentiate the activity of monamine oxidase inhibitors (6,12). However, this effect has not been demonstrated in humans.
SELECTIVE SEROTONIN REUPTAKE INHIBITORS (SSRIs): Ginkgo extract might reverse fluoxetine or sertraline-induced sexual dysfunction (599).
THIAZIDE DIURETICS: Ginkgo can increase blood pressure when used concomitantly with thiazide diuretics (613).
WARFARIN: Ginkgo can increase the anticoagulant effects of warfarin (Coumadin) and risk of bleeding (576).

Possible Interactions with Foods

No interactions are known to occur, and there is no known reason to expect a clinically significant interaction with ginkgo leaf extract.

Possible Interactions with Lab Tests

No interactions are known to occur, and there is no known reason to expect a clinically significant interaction with ginkgo leaf extract.

Possible Interactions with Diseases or Conditions

BLEEDING DISORDERS: Ginkgo can decrease platelet aggregation by inhibiting platelet-activating factor (PAF) and may exacerbate bleeding disorders (6); use with caution.
EPILEPSY: Anecdotal evidence suggests ginkgo might be associated with seizure. The FDAs Special Nutritionals Adverse Event Monitoring System lists ginkgo preparations in association with seizure in 7 cases. Four cases involve multi-ingredient products and 3 cases involve ginkgo alone. However, because few details are available, it is not possible to determine if ginkgo caused the seizure in these cases (3575). Theoretically, ginkgo might induce seizure in epileptic patients; use with caution.
INFERTILITY: Some evidence suggests that ginkgo biloba might inhibit oocyte fertilization and should be avoided in couples attempting to conceive (4239,4240). This effect has not yet been demonstrated in humans; however, until more is known, use with caution in couples attempting to conceive and avoid use in couples having difficulty conceiving.

Typical Dosages & Routes of Administration that are Commonly Used

ORAL: For dementia syndromes a dosage of 120-240 mg per day, divided in two or three doses has been used (2,1514,1515). To relieve walking pain in patients with intermittent claudication, a dosage of 120-240 mg per day, divided into two or three doses has been used; however, the higher dose may be more effective (2,3461). For reversing sexual dysfunction due to SSRIs, the typical starting dose is 60 mg twice daily. This dose can be titrated up to 240 mg twice daily, but should be done slowly to decrease gastrointestinal side effects (212). For vertigo or tinnitus dosages of 120-160 mg per day, divided into two or three doses have been used (2). For prevention of altitude sickness, 160 mg twice daily was used (6230). Most trials used specific standardized Ginkgo biloba leaf extracts. Dosing may vary depending on the specific formulation used.

Comments

When people talk about ginkgo, they usually mean ginkgo leaf extract. Ginkgo biloba comes from the Chinese Yin-Kuo, meaning "silver apricot" and biloba, describing its two-lobed, fan shaped leaves (6208). Ginkgo biloba is the oldest living tree species in the world. Ginkgo trees can live as long as one thousand years (6). Ginkgo use for asthma and bronchitis was described in the first pharmacopoeia, Chen Noung Pen T'sao, dating to 2600 BC (6208). Ginkgo is the most frequently prescribed herbal medicine in Germany (6208). The National Center for Complementary and Alternative Medicine (NCCAM) is beginning a 5-year study of 3000 people aged 75 and older (the largest study ever of dementia) to determine if ginkgo 240 mg daily prevents dementia or Alzheimer's disease (6226).

GINKGO seed

This Product is Also Known As
Baiguo, Fossil Tree, Gingko, Ginkyo, Japanese Silver Apricot, Kew Tree, Maidenhair Tree, Yinhsing.
CAUTION: See separate listings for Ginkgo leaf and Ginkgo leaf extract. Ginkgo leaf extract (Ginkgo biloba) is the most commonly used form of Ginkgo.

Scientific Names
Ginkgo biloba.
Family: Ginkgoaceae.

People Use This For
Orally, ginkgo seed is used as an antitussive and expectorant (4,11), for asthma, bronchitis, genitourinary complaints (11), to aid digestion, and prevent drunkenness (6).
Topically, ginkgo seed is used for scabies and skin sores (11).
For food uses, roasted ginkgo seed, which has the pulp removed, is an edible delicacy in Japan and China (11).

Safety
POSSIBLY SAFE ...when the roasted seed is consumed as food. Limit consumption to a maximum of 8-10 per day (11).
POSSIBLY UNSAFE ...when taken orally for medicinal purposes, especially with long-term use (6,12).
LIKELY UNSAFE… contraindicated for use by people with a known hypersensitivity to ginkgo biloba (2).
UNSAFE ...when consumed as the fresh seeds. Fresh seeds are toxic and potentially deadly (11). The ginkgo seed has a regulatory status that is undetermined in the US (11).
There is insufficient reliable information available about the safety of the topical use of the ginkgo seed.
PREGNANCY AND LACTATION: POSSIBLY SAFE ...when the roasted seed is eaten as food. POSSIBLY UNSAFE ...when used orally for medicinal purposes; avoid using (4).

Effectiveness
There is insufficient reliable information available about the effectiveness of the ginkgo seed.

Possible Mechanism of Action & Active Ingredients
The seeds contain cyanogenic glycosides (4), which are reported to have antibacterial and antifungal effects (6). The seeds also contain ginkgotoxin, a compound believed responsible for causing seizures, loss of consciousness, and death (4,11).

Adverse Reactions Including Known Allergies
The ingestion of the fresh seeds can cause stomachache, nausea, diarrhea, restlessness, difficulty breathing, weak pulse, seizures, loss of consciousness, and shock (4,11). The fresh seeds have caused death in children (11). Ginkgo fruit/pulp is a potent contact allergen. It can cause severe allergic skin reactions, irritation of mucous membranes and the gastrointestinal tract (4,12,17). Ingestion of even small amounts of pulp can cause redness around the mouth, rectal burning, and painful anal sphincter spasms (6). Cross-reactivity is possible with ginkgo fruit in individuals allergic to poison ivy, poison oak, poison sumac, mango rind, and cashew shell oil (6,380).

Possible Interactions with Herbs & Other Dietary Supplements
Insufficient reliable information available.

Possible Interactions with Drugs
ANTICONVULSANTS: Theoretically, the use of ginkgo seed might interfere with the effectiveness of anticonvulsant drugs. Consumption of raw ginkgo seeds reportedly causes seizures, due to the presence of ginkgotoxin (4,11).

Possible Interactions with Foods
No interactions are known to occur, and there is no known reason to expect a clinically significant interaction with ginkgo seed.

Possible Interactions with Lab Tests
No interactions are known to occur, and there is no known reason to expect a clinically significant interaction with ginkgo seed.

Possible Interactions with Diseases or Conditions
GINKGO ALLERGY: Contraindicated (2).
SEIZURE DISORDERS: Contraindicated, consumption of raw ginkgo seeds reportedly causes seizures, due to the presence of ginkgotoxin (4,11).

Typical Dosages & Routes of Administration that are Commonly Used
ORAL: People typically use 120-240 mg ginkgo tablets or capsules daily in two or three divided doses (5008).

Comments

When people talk about ginkgo, they usually mean ginkgo leaf extract. Fossils of the ginkgo tree have been found to be over two hundred million years old, making the tree the oldest living species in the world, and the tree itself can live as long as one thousand years [6].

GINSENG, AMERICAN

This Product is Also Known As

American Ginseng, Anchi Ginseng, Canadian Ginseng, North American Ginseng, Ontario Ginseng, Red Berry, Ren Shen, Sang, Tienchi Ginseng, Wisconsin Ginseng.
CAUTION: See separate listings for Blue Cohosh, Canaigre, Codonopsis, Ginseng Siberian, Ginseng Panax, and Withania.

Scientific Names

Panax quinquefolius.
Family: Araliaceae.

People Use This For

In Chinese medicine, American ginseng is used as a tonic, stimulant, diuretic, and digestive aid and for anemia, diabetes, insomnia, neurasthenia, gastritis, impotence, fever, and hangover symptoms [4,11,13].
In folk medicine, American ginseng has been used for improving stress resistance, preventing the effects of aging, improving stamina [4,6,13], blood and bleeding disorders, atherosclerosis, loss of appetite, vomiting, colitis, dysentery, cancer, insomnia, neuralgia, rheumatism, memory loss, dizziness, headaches, convulsions, and disorders of pregnancy and childbirth [4,6,11,13].
In food manufacturing, American ginseng is used in soft drinks [11].
In other manufacturing processes, American ginseng oil and extracts are used in soaps and cosmetics [11].

Safety

POSSIBLY SAFE ...when used orally and appropriately [12]. Young and healthy people have used it in courses of 15-20 days with a two week ginseng-free period between courses [4]. Older and debilitated people have used American ginseng continuously [4].
There is insufficient reliable information available about the use of American ginseng as a food, and it has an undetermined regulatory status for food use in the US [11].
PREGNANCY AND LACTATION: Insufficient reliable information available; avoid using.

Effectiveness

There is insufficient reliable information available about the effectiveness of American ginseng.

Possible Mechanism of Action & Active Ingredients

The principle constituents of Panax quinquefolius are known as ginsenosides (an Asian research term, of which 18 subtypes are identified) or as panaxosides (a Russian research term of which six subtypes are identified) [8,11]. Panax quinquefolius contains primarily ginsenoside Rb-1, which reportedly lowers blood pressure [8,11], has antihemolytic, antipyretic, antipsychotic [11], CNS depressant [8,11], and ulcer protective activity, increases GI motility [11], and decreases islet insulin concentrations [4]. Most research has focused on the related species, Panax ginseng, which contains ginsenosides Rb-1, Rc, and Rg-1 [4] (See separate listing for Panax ginseng). An American ginseng extract decreases LH (luteinizing hormone) levels and increases serum ceruloplasmin oxidase activity (a measure of estrogenic activity in the liver) in female rats with their ovaries removed [6180]. Preliminary research suggests that Panax quinquefolius extract might reduce breast cancer cell growth and that the extract combined with anti-breast cancer drugs might have a synergistic effect [389].

Adverse Reactions Including Known Allergies

No adverse reactions have been reported specifically with the oral use of Panax quinquefolius. Adverse reactions reported for the related species Panax ginseng include insomnia [589], mastalgia [590], vaginal bleeding [591,592], tachycardia [7], mania [594], cerebral arteritis [595], Stevens Johnson syndrome [596], cholestatic hepatitis (associated with a Panax-containing, multi-ingredient product, Prostata) [598], amenorrhea, decreased appetite, edema, hyperpyrexia, pruritus, rose spots, hypotension, palpitations, headache, vertigo, euphoria, and neonatal death [4,12]. Diarrhea or allergic skin reactions can occur, especially with large amounts or prolonged use [4,9,515]. Allergic reactions to ginseng include palpitations, insomnia, and itching [4]. There are reports of ginseng abuse syndrome, hypertension, nervousness, insomnia, and increased libido [7]. The estrogenic effects have been discredited [512].

Possible Interactions with Herbs & Other Dietary Supplements

CAFFEINE, COFFEE, GUARANA, MATE, TEA: Concomitant use of American ginseng can potentiate the stimulant effects of these drugs [4,12].

Possible Interactions with Drugs

ANTIPSYCHOTIC DRUGS: Theoretically, American ginseng can interfere with antipsychotic drugs (4).

DIABETES THERAPY: Some evidence suggests that American ginseng can lower blood glucose. Theoretically, concomitant use with antidiabetes drugs might enhance blood glucose lowering effects (5800). Monitor blood glucose levels closely.

HORMONES: Theoretically, it can interfere with hormone therapy (4).

MONOAMINE OXIDASE INHIBITORS (MAOIs): Theoretically, it can interfere with monoamine oxidase inhibitor therapy. There is one case report of insomnia, headache, and tremors with concomitant phenylzine (Nardil) and unspecified ginseng use (617). There is also one case report of hypomania with concomitant phenelzine (Nardil) and unspecified ginseng use (618).

STIMULANT DRUGS: Theoretically, concomitant use of ginseng can potentiate the activity of stimulant drugs (4,12).

WARFARIN (Coumadin): Theoretically, concomitant use of ginseng can interfere with warfarin therapy. There is one case report of a decreased international normalization ratio (INR) associated with the addition of a Panax ginseng product to warfarin therapy (619).

Possible Interactions with Foods

COFFEE, TEA: Theoretically, concomitant use of ginseng can potentiate the stimulant effects of coffee or tea (4,12).

Possible Interactions with Lab Tests

COAGULATION TESTS: Theoretically, American ginseng can prolong thrombin time (TT) and activated partial thromboplastin time (aPTT), which is based on in vitro studies with the related species, Panax ginseng (1522).

BLOOD GLUCOSE: Theoretically, American ginseng could cause a decrease in blood glucose levels and test results (5800).

Possible Interactions with Diseases or Conditions

BLEEDING CONDITIONS: Ginseng has been reported to decrease blood coagulation (4); contraindicated in cases of hemorrhage or thrombosis.

CARDIAC CONDITIONS: Ginseng is reported to have negative inotropic and chronotropic activity and hypotensive effects. Ginseng might adversely effect patients with cardiac disorders (4); use with caution.

DIABETES: Ginseng is reported to have hypoglycemic activity (4). Use in diabetics might increase the risk of hypoglycemic episodes; use with caution.

INSOMNIA: High doses of ginseng have been associated with insomnia (597). Theoretically, use in patients with insomnia might worsen the condition; use with caution.

SCHIZOPHRENIA: High doses of ginseng have been associated with insomnia and agitation in schizophrenic patients (597); use with caution.

Typical Dosages & Routes of Administration that are Commonly Used

ORAL: For young and healthy people, the typical dose of American ginseng is 0.25-0.5 grams of the root two times daily (4). Some sources suggest that American ginseng should be taken in the morning two hours before a meal and in the evening not less than two hours after a meal (4). However, because American ginseng might lower blood glucose levels, it might be best to take it with a meal to avoid hypoglycemia (5800). Some sources recommend taking American ginseng for a course of 15-20 days with a ginseng-free period of two weeks between consecutive courses (4). For the elderly and debilitated people, 0.4-0.8 grams of the root is usually taken daily and can be used on a continuous basis (4).

Comments

Avoid confusion with eleutherococcus senticosus, also referred to as Siberian ginseng, and Panax ginseng, also referred to as Asian ginseng. Wild American ginseng is so extensively sought that it has been declared an endangered species in the US (515).

GINSENG, PANAX

This Product is Also Known As

Asian Ginseng, Asiatic Ginseng, Chinese Ginseng, Ginseng Asiatique, Ginseng Radix, Ginseng Root, Japanese Ginseng, Jintsam, Korean Ginseng, Korean Red, Korean Red Ginseng, Ninjin, Oriental Ginseng, Panax Ginseng, Red Ginseng, Ren Shen, Sang, Seng.

CAUTION: See separate listings for Ginseng American, Blue Cohosh, Canaigre, Codonopsis, Ginseng Siberian, and Withania.

Scientific Names

Panax ginseng, synonym Panax schinseng.
Family: Araliaceae.

People Use This For

Orally, Panax ginseng is used as a general tonic for improving well-being and stimulating immune function, for improving physical stamina, athletic stamina, cognitive function, concentration, and work efficiency. It is also used orally for soothing irritated or inflamed tissues, as a diuretic, and an antidepressant (2,4,7,11,13,1427). Panax ginseng is also used orally to improve psychological function in postmenopausal women (3863).

In combination with other herbs, Panax ginseng is used orally with licorice and Bupleurum falcatum for stimulating adrenal gland function, particularly in patients with a history of long-term corticosteroid use (3234).

Topically, Panax ginseng is used as part of a multi-ingredient preparation for treating premature ejaculation (2537).

In Chinese medicine, Panax ginseng is used for anemia, diabetes, gastritis, neurasthenia, impotence, improving male fertility, fever, and hangover (4,11,13,4234).

In folk medicine, Panax ginseng has been used for improving stress-resistance, bleeding disorders, loss of appetite, vomiting, colitis, dysentery, cancer, insomnia, neuralgia, rheumatism, memory loss, dizziness, headache, convulsions, disorders of pregnancy and childbirth, hot flashes due to menopause, and to slow the aging process (4,6,11,13,4228,4235).

In manufacturing, Panax ginseng is used to make soaps, cosmetics, and as a flavoring in beverages (11).

Safety

POSSIBLY SAFE ...when used orally and appropriately in medicinal amounts for less than 3 months (12). ...when used topically, short-term as part of a multi-ingredient preparation (SS Cream). This preparation was used safely for premature ejaculation in a clinical trial where the cream was applied and left on the glans penis for 1-hour (2537). Further evaluation is needed to determine its safety after prolonged, repetitive use.

There is insufficient reliable information available about the safety of the continuous use of Panax ginseng for more than 3 months.

CHILDREN: LIKELY UNSAFE ...when given to infants. There are reports of intoxication leading to death in newborns (12). There is insufficient reliable information about use in children; avoid using.

PREGNANCY: Insufficient reliable information available (12); avoid using.

LACTATION: POSSIBLY UNSAFE ...when used orally. Although there is no proof that Panax ginseng is concentrated in breast milk, the reports of newborn intoxication leading to death (12) suggest Panax ginseng should be avoided.

Effectiveness

POSSIBLY EFFECTIVE ...when used orally for improving abstract thinking, selective memory and mental arithmetic skills (1427,2064). ...when used orally for controlling blood glucose levels in people with non-insulin dependent diabetes (4225). ..when used orally for improving resistance to stress (2,8,13,18,6254). A randomized, double-blind, 12-week study of 625 men and women found ginseng in combination with multivitamins and minerals more effective than multivitamins and minerals alone for improving quality of life (6254). ...when used orally for improving immune response (589,1427). ...when red ginseng, which is produced by steam-curing Panax ginseng prior to drying, is used orally for improving hemodynamics in patients with congestive heart failure (4243). ...when used to decrease risk of cancer. ...when used orally for prevention of cancer. Epidemiological data suggests that ginseng consumption, particularly fresh ginseng extract, might decrease the risk for cancer in general, and for stomach cancer particularly (2063). ...when used topically as part of a multi-ingredient preparation for treating premature ejaculation. In one controlled clinical trial, a multi-ingredient cream preparation containing Panax ginseng root, angelica root, Cistanches deserticola, Zanthoxyl species, torlidis seed, clove flower, asiasari root, cinnamon bark, and toad venom (SS Cream) was applied to the glans penis 1-hour prior to intercourse and washed off immediately before intercourse. Men suffering from premature ejaculation who were treated with the cream had significantly improved ejaculatory latency compared to placebo (2537).

POSSIBLY INEFFECTIVE ...when used orally for enhancing athletic performance in healthy, young adults (1427,4230,4231,4236,4244).

There is insufficient reliable information available about the effectiveness of Panax ginseng for its other uses.

Possible Mechanism of Action & Active Ingredients

The applicable part of Panax ginseng is the root. Red ginseng is produced by steam-curing Panax ginseng prior to drying. White ginseng results when the roots are bleached and dried quickly (4245). Panax ginseng contains several active constituents. In some cases these constituents counteract each other's activity. The principle constituents of Panax ginseng are ginsenosides (Asian research term; 18 subtypes identified) or as Panaxosides (Russian research term; six subtypes identified) (8,11). One constituent, ginsenoside Rg1, raises blood pressure and acts as a central nervous system stimulant; ginsenoside Rb1 lowers blood pressure and acts as a CNS depressant (8,11). The active constituents also alter carbohydrate, lipid, nucleic acid, and albumin metabolism (6,7,8,11); and stimulate natural-killer cell activity and possibly other immune-system activity, including antitumor activity (4,6,7,8). Ginsenosides interfere with platelet aggregation and coagulation (4,1522), exhibit papaverine-like effects on smooth muscle (6), as well as analgesic and anti-inflammatory activity (4,6). They potentiate nerve growth factor (11), promote growth of normal intestinal flora while inhibiting Clostridial species (7), lower serum cholesterol and triglycerides (6), and might potentiate adrenal activity (6,13). Panax ginseng reduces the activity of the thymus gland (4). Panax ginseng reduces fasting blood glucose levels and hemoglobin A1C in people with non-insulin dependent diabetes (4225). Red ginseng improves antioxidant plasma levels and antioxidant activity in smokers (4227). Red ginseng might improve

© Copyright 2000, Natural Medicines Comprehensive Database (209) 472-2244. For updated data, go to www.NaturalDatabase.com • 485

hemodynamics in patients with congestive heart failure and might work synergistically with digoxin (4243). Panax ginseng saponins stimulate corticosteroid production (3256). While Panax ginseng appears to enhance the ability of licorice to increase serum cortisol concentrations (3257), there are no clinical reports to support the combination of licorice, Panax ginseng and Bupleurum falcatum for stimulating adrenal function in corticosteroid-dependent patients. A Panax ginseng extract increases serum ceruloplasmin oxidase activity (a measure of estrogenic activity in the liver) in female rats with their ovaries removed (6180). Preliminary evidence suggests that Panax ginseng might improve psychological symptoms in postmenopausal women by increasing dehydroepiandrosterone (DHEA) sulfate levels (3863). The multi-ingredient preparation containing Panax ginseng is thought to work in premature ejaculation by increasing the penile vibratory threshold and reducing the amplitude of penile somatosensory evoked potentials (2537).

Researchers report that Panax ginseng was beneficial in treating Pseudomonas aeruginosa lung infections in mice. A ginseng preparation injected into the lungs of infected mice cleared bacteria from the lungs faster, improved lung conditions, and increased survival compared to saline. The results of this unpublished study were presented at the 2000 annual meeting of the American Society for Microbiology (6108).

Adverse Reactions Including Known Allergies

Panax ginseng can cause insomnia (589), mastalgia (590), vaginal bleeding (591,592), tachycardia (7), mania (594), cerebral arteritis (595), Stevens-Johnson syndrome (596) cholestatic hepatitis (associated with a Panax-containing, multi-ingredient product, Prostata) (598), amenorrhea, decreased appetite, edema, hyperpyrexia, pruritus, rose spots, hypotension, palpitations, headache, vertigo, euphoria, and neonatal death (4,12). Diarrhea or allergic skin reactions may occur, especially with large amounts or prolonged use (4,5,9). When the multi-ingredient cream preparation (SS Cream) has been applied topically to the glans penis, sporadic erectile dysfunction, excessively delayed ejaculation, mild pain, and local irritation and burning has occurred (2537).

In the past, there has been considerable concern regarding "ginseng abuse syndrome". This syndrome has previously been associated with hypertension, nervousness, insomnia, increased libido (7), and estrogenic effects (5,6). In recent years, the actual existence of this syndrome has come into serious question. These symptoms may be symptoms of Panax ginseng use, but there probably is not a ginseng abuse syndrome (7).

Possible Interactions with Herbs & Other Dietary Supplements

COFFEE, GUARANA, TEA: Concomitant use may potentiate effects due to caffeine content of coffee, guarana or tea (4,12).

HERBS WITH ANTICOAGULANT/ANTIPLATELET POTENTIAL: Theoretically, concomitant use of ginseng with herbs that affect platelet aggregation may increase the risk of bleeding. Ginsenosides in ginseng are reported to inhibit platelet aggregation in vitro (4). This effect has not been demonstrated in humans. In two case reports, ginseng has actually been reported to decrease the effectiveness of the prescription drug warfarin (19,619,1288). Herbs with anticoagulant or antiplatelet properties include: angelica, anise, arnica, asafoetida, bogbean, boldo, capsicum, celery, chamomile, clove, danshen, fenugreek, feverfew, garlic, ginger, ginkgo, horse chestnut, horseradish, licorice, meadowsweet, prickly ash, onion, papain, passionflower, poplar, quassia, red clover, turmeric, wild carrot, wild lettuce, willow, and others (4,19).

Possible Interactions with Drugs

ANTICOAGULANT/ANTIPLATELET AGENTS: In two case reports, ginseng has been reported to decrease the effectiveness of warfarin (19,619,1288). However, some studies have shown that ginsenoside constituents in ginseng can actually decrease platelet aggregation in vitro (4). Theoretically, concomitant use of ginseng and antiplatelet agents might increase the risk of bleeding. However, this effect has not been reported in humans. Use with caution in patients concurrently taking anticoagulant or antiplatelet agents.

ANTIPSYCHOTIC DRUGS: Theoretically, Panax ginseng might interfere with antipsychotic drugs, by interfering with neurotransmitters (4).

CAFFEINE: Long-term use of 3 grams of Panax ginseng daily in combination with caffeine can lead to hypertension (19).

DIGOXIN (Lanoxin): Concomitant use might have synergistic effects in people with congestive heart failure (4243).

ANTIDIABETES DRUGS: Theoretically, concomitant use might enhance blood glucose lowering effects (4,4225). Monitor blood glucose levels closely.

FUROSEMIDE: One case has been reported of a germanium-containing ginseng product associated with resistance to furosemide diuresis (770).

HORMONE THERAPY: Theoretically, Panax ginseng can interfere with steroid or hormone drugs, because of ginseng's effect on the thymus gland (4).

INSULIN: Theoretically, dosage adjustments might be necessary due to the hypoglycemic effects of Panax ginseng (19).

MAO INHIBITORS: Theoretically, Panax ginseng can interfere with monoamine oxidase inhibitor therapy. Concomitant use with phenelzine (Nardil) is associated with insomnia, headache, tremors (617) and hypomania (618).

STIMULANT DRUGS: Panax ginseng can potentiate stimulant drug effects (12).

WARFARIN (Coumadin): In two case reports, ginseng has been reported to decrease the effectiveness of warfarin (19,619,1288); however, animal data suggest that ginseng has no effect on the pharmacokinetics or pharmacodynamic effects of warfarin (2531).

Possible Interactions with Foods

COFFEE, TEA: Concomitant use may potentiate effects due to caffeine content of coffee or tea (4,12).

Possible Interactions with Lab Tests

ACTIVATED PARTIAL THROMBOPLASTIN TIME (aPTT), THROMBIN TIME (TT): Theoretically, Panax ginseng might prolong aPTT, TT, and increase test results (1522).
INTERNATIONAL NORMALIZED RATIO (INR), PROTHROMBIN TIME (PT): Panax ginseng can reduce PT/INR and test results in patients treated with warfarin (Coumadin) (619,1288).
GLUCOSE: Panax ginseng might reduce fasting blood glucose concentrations and test results (4225).
GLYCOSYLATED HEMOGLOBIN (HbA1c): Panax ginseng might improve glucose control and reduce HbA1c values in patients with type 2 diabetes (4225).

Possible Interactions with Diseases or Conditions

BLEEDING CONDITIONS: Ginseng has been reported to decrease blood coagulation (4); contraindicated in cases of hemorrhage or thrombosis.
CARDIAC CONDITIONS: Ginseng is reported to have negative inotropic and chronotropic activity and hypotensive effects. Ginseng might adverse effect patients with cardiac disorders (4); use with caution.
DIABETES: Ginseng is reported to have hypoglycemic activity (4). Use in diabetics might increase the risk of hypoglycemic episodes; use with caution.
INSOMNIA: High doses of ginseng have been associated with insomnia (597). Theoretically, use in patients with insomnia might worsen the condition; use with caution.
SCHIZOPHRENIA: High doses of ginseng have been associated with insomnia and agitation in schizophrenic patients (597); use with caution.

Typical Dosages & Routes of Administration that are Commonly Used

ORAL: Root powder is available in 1 ounce and 4 ounce containers. The root itself is also available in bulk by the pound. Cut or powdered root is taken orally 0.6-3 grams one to three times per day (8,12), or one cup tea (Panax ginseng tea bags usually have 1500 mg of ginseng root. The tea is made by steeping 3 grams of root in 150 mL of boiling water for 10-15 minutes, and then straining). People consume this tea one to three times per day for three to four weeks (8). An extract is made using 2 ounces of root extract in an alcohol base. Capsules come in 100 mg, 250 mg, and 500 mg. People typically take from 200-600 mg per day (7). Panax ginseng can also be taken in an extract form or as an oil. People usually take Panax ginseng from three weeks to three months (2,4,12). Sometimes it is taken continuously. A Panax-free period of two weeks is recommended between consecutive courses (2,4).

Comments

Ginseng has been used for medicinal purposes for over two thousand years. Approximately six million Americans use it regularly. Some consider the age of the ginseng roots important. In 1976, a four hundred year old root of Manchurian ginseng from the mountains of China reportedly sold for an incredible $10,000 per ounce (4208). The contents of preparations labeled as containing Panax ginseng can vary greatly; many contain little or no Panax ginseng (5,6,13). Some authorities categorize Panax pseudoginseng, Himalayan ginseng, as a type of ginseng (5,6,9).

GINSENG, SIBERIAN

This Product is Also Known As

Ci Wu Jia, Ciwujia, Devil's Bush, Devil's Shrub, Eleuthera, Eleuthero, Eleuthero Ginseng, Eleutherococ, Eleutherococcus, Eleutherococci radix, Phytoestrogen, Shigoka, Touch-Me-Not, Wild Pepper, Wu-jia, Wu Jia Pi, Ussuri, Ussurian Thorny Pepperbrush, Siberian Ginseng.
CAUTION: See separate listings for Ginseng American, Blue Cohosh, Canaigre, Codonopsis, Ginseng Panax, and Withania.

Scientific Names

Eleutherococcus senticosus, synonym Acanthopanax senticosus.
Family: Araliaceae.

People Use This For

Orally, people use Siberian ginseng as an adaptogen, for increasing resistance to environmental stress. It is also used orally for normalizing high or low blood pressure, atherosclerosis, pyelonephritis, craniocerebral trauma, rheumatic heart disease, neuroses, increasing work capacity (6,11), Alzheimer's disease, attention deficit disorder, chronic fatigue syndrome, diabetes, fibromyalgia, influenza, chronic bronchitis, tuberculosis, improving athletic performance, reducing toxicity of chemotherapy, symptomatic treatment of herpes simplex type II infections, and as an immune system stimulant (1427,1900).
In traditional Chinese medicine, Siberian ginseng is used as a stimulant, tonic, and diuretic; for insomnia, lower

back or kidney pain, lack of appetite, rheumatoid arthritis; enhancing overall resistance to disease; and for stress (11).

In manufacturing, Siberian ginseng is added to skin care products (11).

Safety

LIKELY SAFE ...when used orally and appropriately, short-term. Studies have safely used Siberian ginseng in multiple course treatment regimens. Patients received daily treatment for 35-60 consecutive days followed by a 2-3 week ginseng-free period. Up to 8 treatment courses have been used, each separated by a ginseng-free period (4,12). PREGNANCY AND LACTATION: Insufficient reliable information available; avoid using (4).

Effectiveness

POSSIBLY EFFECTIVE ...when used orally by healthy individuals for increasing speed, quality, and capacity for physical work (2,4) . ...when used orally as an adaptogen in people exposed to high temperatures, hypoxemia, and conditions that cause motion sickness (4). ...when used orally for preventing atherosclerosis (4). ...when used orally for normalizing blood pressure in people with hypertension or hypotension (4). ...when used orally for treating acute pyelonephritis (4). ...when used orally for treating diabetes (4). ...when used orally for treating acute craniocerebral trauma (4). ...when used orally for treating people with various types of neuroses (4). ...when used orally for treating rheumatic heart disease by reducing blood coagulation (4). ...when used orally for treating chronic bronchitis (4). ...when used orally for treating children with abating forms of pulmonary tuberculosis (4). ...when used orally as a tonic for invigoration during times of fatigue and debility and for building strength during convalescence (2). ...when used orally for reducing frequency, severity and duration of herpes simplex type II infections. Studies for management of herpes simplex have used Siberian ginseng extract standardized to contain eleutheroside 0.3%. This extract is found in the product Elagen (1427).

Possible Mechanism of Action & Active Ingredients

The applicable part of Siberian ginseng is the root. It contains active compounds referred to as eleutherosides A through M (515). The eleutherosides include a diverse variety of compounds including saponins, beta-sitosterol glycoside, coumarin derivatives, and others (515). Siberian ginseng seems to exert most of its effects through the pituitary-adrenocortical system (3,4,6). One constituent, dihydroxybenzoic acid, has platelet anti-aggregation activity (4). Siberian ginseng has been shown to have immunostimulatory effects (3,4,6,7,11). In a study in humans, there was a significant increase in lymphocyte count compared to placebo when a daily ginseng extract was given (4). Healthy subjects receiving 25 drops three times daily of a 35% Siberian ginseng preparation (Taiga Wurzel) had increases in lymphocyte and count and phagocytic activity of neutrocytes (6206). The Siberian ginseng preparation also lowered cholesterol indices and improved oxygen consumption on exercise (6206). Immunostimulant effects seem to be due to polysaccharide constituents (11). Some Siberian ginseng constituents act as antioxidants. These constituents are also believed to have anti edema, anti-inflammatory, diuretic, gonadotropic, and estrogenic activity (11). Siberian ginseng also has protein-anabolic activity (11).

Adverse Reactions Including Known Allergies

It is very rare that Siberian ginseng causes adverse reactions. When they happen, the adverse reactions most commonly are insomnia, slight drowsiness, changes in heart rhythm (tachycardia, extrasystole, and hypertonia in some atherosclerotic patients), melancholy, anxiety, mastalgia, and elevated blood pressure at high doses in individuals with rheumatic heart disease (4,6). Long term use of Siberian ginseng is associated with inflamed nerves, often the sciatic nerve (4). Siberian ginseng can also cause muscle spasms. There is a case report of neonatal androgenization with maternal use of Siberian ginseng product (593). Later it was learned that the product contained silk vine (Periploca sepium) bark which does not seem to have androgenic properties (850).

Possible Interactions with Herbs & Other Dietary Supplements

HERBS WITH SEDATIVE PROPERTIES: Theoretically, concomitant use with herbs that have sedative properties might enhance therapeutic and adverse effects. These include calamus, calendula, California poppy, catnip, capsicum, celery, couch grass, elecampane, German chamomile, goldenseal, gotu kola, hops, Jamaican dogwood, kava, lemon balm, sage, St. John's wort, sassafras, scullcap, shepherd's purse, stinging nettle, valerian, wild carrot, wild lettuce, withania root, and yerba mansa (4,19).
COFFEE: Avoid concomitant use (4).
VITAMINS: Concomitant use with vitamins B1, B2 and C may increase the excretion of these vitamins (4).

Possible Interactions with Drugs

ALCOHOL: Avoid concomitant use of Eleutherococcus (4).
ANTICOAGULANT/ANTIPLATELET DRUGS: Theoretically, concomitant use might increase effects or adverse of anticoagulant or antiplatelet drugs (4).
ANTIPSYCHOTIC DRUGS, HORMONES: Avoid concomitant use (4).
BARBITURATES: Theoretically, concomitant use with barbiturates may cause additive effects and side effects (19).
OTHER DRUGS WITH SEDATIVE PROPERTIES: Theoretically, concomitant use with drugs with sedative properties may cause additive effects and side effects (19).
DIABETES THERAPY: Monitor blood glucose levels closely due to claims that Eleutherococcus has hypoglycemic effects (19).

DIGOXIN: One case report of a product stated to contain Siberian ginseng associated with elevated serum digoxin levels, without symptoms of toxicity (543). However, it is not clear if this is due to an interaction or whether the product ingested in this case actually contained cardiac glycoside-like constituents. The product was found to be free of digoxin and digitoxin (543), but was not tested for the presence of eleutherosides (797). It is unclear whether the product actually contained Eleutherococcus. It has been postulated that it may have contained silk vine (Periploca sepium) which is reported to contain cardiac glycosides and silk vine is a common substitute for Eleutherococcus senticosus (797).

KANAMYCIN (Kantrex): Concomitant use might increase antibiotic efficacy, possibly due to increased T-lymphocyte activity (19).

HORMONES: Avoid concomitant use. Reason not specified (4).

INSULIN: Theoretically, the hypoglycemic effects of Siberian ginseng might cause a need for insulin dose adjustment (19).

Possible Interactions with Foods

ALCOHOL, SPICY FOODS, BITTER SUBSTANCES: Avoid concomitant use (4).

Possible Interactions with Lab Tests

No interactions are known to occur, and there is no known reason to expect a clinically significant interaction with Siberian ginseng.

Possible Interactions with Diseases or Conditions

HYPERTENSION: Siberian ginseng is contraindicated in individuals with blood pressures exceeding 180/90. Siberian ginseng can potentially exacerbate hypertension (4,12).

MYOCARDIAL INFARCTION: Theoretically, Siberian ginseng may exacerbate myocardial infarction (4); use with caution.

PSYCHIATRIC CONDITIONS: Theoretically, Siberian ginseng may exacerbate some psychiatric conditions, including hysteria, mania, and schizophrenia (4); use with caution.

OTHER CONDITIONS: Theoretically, Siberian ginseng might exacerbate numerous other conditions; however, documentation for these effects is lacking. Some authors suggest Siberian ginseng should be avoided in patients with hypertonic crises, conditions with fever (6), and in individuals who are highly energetic, nervous, or tense (4).

Typical Dosages & Routes of Administration that are Commonly Used

ORAL: The dry root, 0.6-3 grams daily for up to one month has been used (4). In healthy people, 2-16 mL of an ethanolic extract is taken one to three times daily up to 60 consecutive days. In unhealthy patients, 0.5-6 mL of an ethanolic extract is taken one to three times daily for up to 35 consecutive days. Studies have used a 2-3 week ginseng-free period after every 30-60 days of treatment with Siberian ginseng (4). For herpes type II infections, studies have used Siberian ginseng extract standardized to contain eleutheroside E 0.3%. Doses used were 400 mg per day (1427).

Comments

Adaptogen is a non-medical term used to suggest that a substance can act to strengthen the body and increase general resistance (18). Typically these substances lack toxicity, and have a non-specific action (4). The chemical content and potency of various Siberian ginseng products varies. This variance depends, in part, on time of year the product is harvested. The herb seems to have the highest content of the active ingredients if it is harvested in October, and lesser concentration if harvested in July (6). Siberian ginseng is often misidentified or adulterated (3), Siberian ginseng is a completely different herb than American or Panax ginseng. American or Panax ginseng is considerably more expensive. It is said that the Soviet Union wanted to provide its athletes with the advantage offered by ginseng but wanted a less expensive version. Therefore Siberian ginseng became popular, and this is why most studies on Siberian ginseng have been done in Russia. Exercise caution in differentiating ginseng products. Silk vine is a common substitute for Siberian ginseng (797).

GLOBE FLOWER

This Product is Also Known As

Globe Crowfoot, Globe Ranunculus, Globe Trollius.

Scientific Names

Trollius europaeus.
Family: Ranunculaceae.

People Use This For

Orally, fresh globe flower is used for scurvy (18).

Safety

LIKELY UNSAFE …when any part of the fresh plant is used orally or topically because it can cause severe local irritation (18).

There is insufficient reliable information available about the safety of the dried, cut plant.

PREGNANCY AND LACTATION: LIKELY UNSAFE ...when any part of the fresh plant is used orally or topically (18). There is insufficient reliable information available about the safety of the dried, cut plant during pregnancy and lactation.

Effectiveness

There is insufficient reliable information available about the effectiveness of globe flower.

Possible Mechanism of Action & Active Ingredients

The applicable part is the whole fresh plant. When the fresh plant is crushed or cut into small pieces, the glycoside ranunculin is enzymatically changed into a severely irritating protoanemonin, which, in turn, rapidly degrades into the less toxic anemonin (18). Both protoanemonin and ranunculin are destroyed to an unknown extent during the drying process (2).

Adverse Reactions Including Known Allergies

Ingestion of globe flower can cause severe irritation of the gastrointestinal tract, with colic and diarrhea. Irritation of the urinary tract can also occur. Skin contact can cause blisters and burns that are difficult to heal (18).

Possible Interactions with Herbs & Other Dietary Supplements

Insufficient reliable information available.

Possible Interactions with Drugs

No interactions are known to occur, and there is no known reason to expect a clinically significant interaction with globe flower.

Possible Interactions with Foods

No interactions are known to occur, and there is no known reason to expect a clinically significant interaction with globe flower.

Possible Interactions with Lab Tests

No interactions are known to occur, and there is no known reason to expect a clinically significant interaction with globe flower.

Possible Interactions with Diseases or Conditions

No interactions are known to occur, and there is no known reason to expect a clinically significant interaction with globe flower.

Typical Dosages & Routes of Administration that are Commonly Used

No typical dosage.

Comments

Globe flower is considered unsafe for oral use; avoid using (18).

GLOSSY PRIVET

This Product is Also Known As

Chinese Privet, Dongqingzi, Ligustro, Ligustrum, Ligustrum Fruit, Nu Zhen, Nu Zhen Zi, Nuzhenzi, To-Nezumimochi, Troène De Chine, Trueno, White Waxtree.

Scientific Names

Ligustrum lucidum.
Family: Oleaceae.

People Use This For

Orally, glossy privet fruit is used for promoting growth and darkening of hair, reducing facial dark spots (11), palpitations, rheumatism, swelling, tumors, vertigo, common cold, congestion, constipation, deafness, debility, fever, headache, hepatitis, insomnia, rejuvenation and longevity. It is also used as a diaphoretic and tonic (513), for improving immune function, and reducing the side effects of chemotherapy (415).

In traditional Chinese medicine, glossy privet is used for blurred vision, invigorating the liver and kidney, for dizziness, tinnitus, and for sore back and knees (11).

Safety

POSSIBLY SAFE ...when glossy privet fruit is used orally and appropriately (12).

CHILDREN: UNSAFE ...glossy privet berries and leaves are considered toxic to children (414).

PREGNANCY AND LACTATION: Insufficient reliable information available; avoid using.

Effectiveness

There is insufficient reliable information available about the effectiveness of glossy privet.

Possible Mechanism of Action & Active Ingredients

The applicable part of glossy privet is the ripe fruit (11). It contains triterpenoids, including oleanolic acid (ligustrin), acetyloleanolic acid, and ursolic acid; glycosides (including ligustroside, oleuropein, 4-hydroxy-beta-phenylethyl-beta-D-glucoside); mannitol; fatty oil, consisting mainly of linoleic, linolenic, oleic and palmitic acids; and a volatile oil consisting primarily of esters, alcohols, thioketones and hydrocarbons (11). Ligustrum is used clinically in China for treating leukopenia (11), although data involving experimentally-induced leukopenia did not show any effect (418). Ligustrum might also have immunomodulatory and antitumor effects (11). Preliminary evidence suggests that glossy privet fruit might inhibit growth of renal cell carcinoma, possibly via augmentation of phagocyte and lymphokine-activated killer cell activity (419). Glossy privet extracts inhibit mutagenicity in bacteria (420), stimulate T-cell function in cancer tissue (423), and reverse tumor-induced macrophage suppression (421). Preliminary evidence suggests that glossy privet fruit, and the ingredient ligustrin, might have anti-inflammatory, anti-allergic, mild cardiotonic, diuretic, sedative, lipid-lowering, blood flow enhancing, blood glucose lowering, and liver protectant effects (11).

Adverse Reactions Including Known Allergies

None reported. However, respiratory allergies (allergic rhinitis, asthma) and cross-allergenicity have been reported with the pollen of other Oleaceae species including common privet (Ligustrum vulgare), olive, ash and lilac (416,417).

Possible Interactions with Herbs & Other Dietary Supplements

Insufficient reliable information available.

Possible Interactions with Drugs

No interactions are known to occur, and there is no known reason to expect a clinically significant interaction with glossy privet.

Possible Interactions with Foods

No interactions are known to occur, and there is no known reason to expect a clinically significant interaction with glossy privet.

Possible Interactions with Lab Tests

No interactions are known to occur, and there is no known reason to expect a clinically significant interaction with glossy privet.

Possible Interactions with Diseases or Conditions

No interactions are known to occur, and there is no known reason to expect a clinically significant interaction with glossy privet.

Typical Dosages & Routes of Administration that are Commonly Used

ORAL: A common dose is 5-15 grams of powdered, encapsulated berries per day. Some people drink a tea prepared by steeping 2-5 grams of powdered berries in 250 mL (1 cup) of boiling water for ten to fifteen minutes, up to three times per day. As a tincture, 3-5 mL is taken three times per day (415).

Comments

Avoid confusion with other species of privet such as Japanese privet (Ligustrum japonicum), border Privet (Ligustrum obtusifolium), Chinese privet (Ligustrum sinense), privet (Ligustrum tschonoskii), common privet (Ligustrum vulgare), and golden privet (Ligustrum x vicaryi) (413). The fruits of glossy privet (Ligustrum lucidum) and Ilex chinensis are both referred to by the Chinese name dongqingzi (11).

GLUCOMANNAN

This Product is Also Known As

Konjac, Konjac Mannan.

Scientific Names

Amorphophallus konjac.
Family: Araceae.

People Use This For

Orally, glucomannan is used for moderate constipation (6,9), weight loss in adults and children (6,180,181,182,183), blood glucose control, and reducing serum cholesterol (6).
For food uses, glucomannan is edible (6).

© Copyright 2000, Natural Medicines Comprehensive Database (209) 472-2244. For updated data, go to www.NaturalDatabase.com • 491

Safety

POSSIBLY SAFE ...when the powder or encapsulated form is used (6,180,182).
LIKELY UNSAFE ...when used in oral tablet form. There have been numerous reports of esophageal and gastrointestinal obstruction (6,9). Oral tablets have been banned in Australia since 1985 (6,9).
PREGNANCY AND LACTATION: Insufficient reliable information available; avoid using.

Effectiveness

POSSIBLY EFFECTIVE ...when used for weight loss in obese adults (6,181,182,183), reducing serum cholesterol in obese adults and adults with diabetes (6,181,182,183), reducing blood glucose and triglycerides in obese adults (181,182), reducing insulin or hypoglycemic drug requirements for people with diabetes (6).
There is insufficient reliable information available about the effectiveness of glucomannan for its other uses.

Possible Mechanism of Action & Active Ingredients

Glucomannan relieves moderate constipation in 1-2 days. The effect is believed due to water absorption, increasing intestinal bulk (6). Glucomannan delays glucose absorption and reduces insulin or hypoglycemic agent requirements in people with diabetes (6). It aids in weight loss, improves lipid profile and glucose tolerance in obese adults (6,181,182,183). In obese children, there has been one report of weight loss, reduced triglycerides and cholesterol (180), but there is another report of no weight loss and increased triglycerides (179). Glucomannan reduces total serum cholesterol in healthy men (178), overweight adults and adults with diabetes; activity reportedly due to inhibited active transport of cholesterol in the jejunum and absorption of bile acids in the ileum (animal data) (6). In mice, glucomannan protects against chemically induced lung cancer (6).

Adverse Reactions Including Known Allergies

Esophageal or gastrointestinal obstruction reported with tablet form (6,9).

Possible Interactions with Herbs & Other Dietary Supplements

Insufficient reliable information available.

Possible Interactions with Drugs

HYPOGLYCEMIC DRUGS, INSULIN: Might reduce fasting blood glucose and postprandial blood glucose levels, interfering with blood sugar control in people with diabetes (6), monitor closely.
ORAL DRUGS: The fiber in glucomannan can impair absorption of oral drugs (19).

Possible Interactions with Foods

No interactions are known to occur, and there is no known reason to expect a clinically significant interaction with glucomannan.

Possible Interactions with Lab Tests

CHOLESTEROL: Glucomannan might reduce serum total cholesterol, LDL cholesterol, and test results in obese adults (6,181,182,183).
GLUCOSE: Glucomannan might reduce fasting and postprandial blood glucose concentrations and test results in patients with type 2 diabetes (6).
TRIGLYCERIDES: Glucomannan might reduce serum triglycerides and test results in obese adults (181,182).

Possible Interactions with Diseases or Conditions

DIABETES: May interfere with blood sugar control (6), monitor closely.

Typical Dosages & Routes of Administration that are Commonly Used

ORAL: Adult weight loss, 1 gram three times daily (1 hour before each meal) (182), or 1.5 grams twice daily (6). Child weight loss, 2-3 grams per day (180). Diabetes, 3.6-7.2 grams per day (6), monitor blood glucose carefully. Reducing high cholesterol 3.9 grams per day (6). If glucomannan is used for treatment of diabetes or hyperlipidemia, therapy should be in conjunction with physician evaluation and effectiveness should be monitored.

Comments

Tablet form is unsafe; avoid using. Glucomannan is a polysaccharide derived from underground stems (tubers) of konjac (Amorphophallus konjac).

GLUCOSAMINE HYDROCHLORIDE

This Product is Also Known As

Glucosamine.
CAUTION: See separate listings for Glucosamine Sulfate and N-Acetyl Glucosamine.

Scientific Names

2-amino-2-deoxyglucose hydrochloride.

People Use This For

Orally, glucosamine hydrochloride is used for osteoarthritis (2608).

In combination with other products, glucosamine hydrochloride, chondroitin sulfate, and manganese ascorbate are used orally for osteoarthritis (4237).

Safety

POSSIBLY SAFE ...when used orally and appropriately in combination with chondroitin sulfate and manganese ascorbate (4237).

There is insufficient reliable information available about the safety of the oral use of glucosamine hydrochloride when used alone.

PREGNANCY AND LACTATION: Insufficient reliable information available; avoid using.

Effectiveness

POSSIBLY EFFECTIVE ...when the combination of glucosamine hydrochloride, chondroitin sulfate, and manganese ascorbate (Cosamin-DS) is used orally for treating knee osteoarthritis pain (4237).

There is insufficient reliable information available about the effectiveness of the oral use of glucosamine hydrochloride when used alone for osteoarthritis.

Possible Mechanism of Action & Active Ingredients

Glucosamine is a glycoprotein derived from marine exoskeletons or produced synthetically (6). It is required for the synthesis of glycoproteins, glycolipids, and glycosaminoglycans, also known as mucopolysaccharides, which comprise the body's tendons, ligaments, cartilage, synovial fluid, mucus membranes, and structures in the eye, blood vessels, and heart valves. Glucosamine stimulates metabolism of chondrocytes in the articular cartilage and of synoviocytes in the synovial tissues. Preliminary evidence suggests glucosamine decreases glucose-induced insulin secretion by inhibiting pancreatic glucokinase in the beta cells of the islet of Langerhans (371,372,3406). No human studies have evaluated glucosamine hydrochloride alone for treating osteoarthritis. All reported clinical trials of glucosamine as a viable agent for osteoarthritis have used glucosamine sulfate. One human trial found the combination of glucosamine hydrochloride, chondroitin sulfate, and manganese ascorbate (Cosamin-DS) decreased knee osteoarthritis pain (4237). Because the study compared the combination to placebo, it is not known if the combination has greater benefit than chondroitin sulfate alone, which has shown benefit for treating osteoarthritis (see separate listing for chondroitin sulfate). Evidence suggests glucosamine impairs insulin-mediated glucose uptake and metabolism in skeletal muscle. It is hypothesized that glucosamine desensitizes cell membranes to the effects of insulin (372,3406). Evidence also suggests that type 2 diabetes and glucosamine induce insulin resistance by acting on a common pathway (3405) and glucosamine-induced insulin resistance might be dose-dependent (3406).

Adverse Reactions Including Known Allergies

None reported. There is concern that glucosamine hydrochloride products derived from marine exoskeletons might cause reactions in people allergic to shellfish, although no reactions have been reported. Until more is known, and because the source of glucosamine hydrochloride products is not listed on product labels, use glucosamine hydrochloride with caution in people with shellfish allergy.

Possible Interactions with Herbs & Other Dietary Supplements

GLUCOSAMINE SULFATE, N-ACETYL GLUCOSAMINE: Although glucosamine sulfate and/or N-acetyl glucosamine are marketed together in combination products with glucosamine hydrochloride, no human studies have evaluated these combinations for treating osteoarthritis. Only glucosamine sulfate as a single agent has shown benefit in humans for treating osteoarthritis (see separate listing for glucosamine sulfate).

Possible Interactions with Drugs

ANTIDIABETES DRUGS: Theoretically, glucosamine hydrochloride might decrease the hypoglycemic effects of insulin and oral antidiabetes agents by increasing insulin resistance and/or decreasing insulin production.

Possible Interactions with Foods

No interactions are known to occur, and there is no known reason to expect a clinically significant interaction with glucosamine hydrochloride.

Possible Interactions with Lab Tests

BLOOD GLUCOSE: Theoretically, glucosamine hydrochloride might increase blood glucose levels and test results, by increasing insulin resistance and/or decreasing insulin production. There are also anecdotal reports of poorer control in people with diabetes who take glucosamine (22,1203,1204,3405,3406).

Possible Interactions with Diseases or Conditions

DIABETES: Theoretically, glucosamine hydrochloride might exacerbate diabetes by increasing insulin resistance and/or decreasing insulin production.

SHELLFISH ALLERGY: There is concern that glucosamine hydrochloride products derived from marine exoskeletons might cause reactions in people allergic to shellfish, although no reactions have been reported. Until more is known, and because the source of glucosamine hydrochloride products is not listed on product labels, use glucosamine hydrochloride with caution in people with shellfish allergy.

Typical Dosages & Routes of Administration that are Commonly Used

ORAL: People typically use 1 to 2 grams of glucosamine hydrochloride daily as a single dose or in divided doses (5261,6006). For osteoarthritis, a combination of glucosamine hydrochloride (1500 mg/day), chondroitin sulfate (1200 mg/day), and manganese ascorbate (228 mg/day) has been used (4237); the equivalent to one Cosamin-DS tablet three times daily (3278,4237). The manufacturer, Nutramax Laboratories, recommends one tablet three times daily in people under 200 lbs., and two tablets twice daily in people over 200 lbs. (3278).

Comments

Read glucosamine product labels carefully for content. Avoid confusion with glucosamine sulfate and N-acetyl glucosamine. Glucosamine sulfate shows benefit in people with osteoarthritis (See separate listing for glucosamine sulfate). There is no human evidence to support the use of N-acetyl glucosamine (See separate listing for N-acetyl glucosamine).

GLUCOSAMINE SULFATE

This Product is Also Known As

Glucosamine, Glucosamine Sulphate.
CAUTION: See separate listings for Glucosamine Hydrochloride and N-Acetyl Glucosamine.

Scientific Names

2-amino-2-deoxyglucose sulfate.

People Use This For

Orally, glucosamine sulfate is used for osteoarthrosis (2600) and osteoarthritis (2601). Glucosamine sulfate is frequently used in combination with other products, including chondroitin sulfate, glucosamine hydrochloride or N-acetyl glucosamine (760).
Topically, glucosamine sulfate is used in combination with other products for osteoarthritis (384).

Safety

LIKELY SAFE ...when used orally and appropriately, short-term. Glucosamine has been used safely in multiple clinical trials lasting from four weeks to three months (2533,2600,2602,2603,2604,2606).
POSSIBLY SAFE ...when used orally and appropriately, long-term. Glucosamine has been used safely in one clinical trial lasting three years (350). ...when used intramuscularly and appropriately, short-term. In one clinical trial, intramuscular glucosamine was given twice weekly for six weeks without significant adverse effects (2605).
PREGNANCY AND LACTATION: Insufficient reliable information available; avoid using.

Effectiveness

LIKELY EFFECTIVE ...when used orally, short-term for reducing the symptoms of osteoarthritis. Several clinical trials have found glucosamine sulfate to significantly improve symptoms of pain and functionality indices in patients with osteoarthritis of the knee compared to placebo in trials lasting from four weeks to three years (350,2533, 2600,2602,2603,2604,2606). Some trials have found glucosamine sulfate to be comparable to the non-steroidal anti-inflammatory drugs (NSAIDs) ibuprofen (2602,2604) and piroxicam (Feldene) (2606); however, NSAIDs appear to relieve symptoms within two weeks compared to four weeks with glucosamine sulfate (2602,2604,2606). In one study, ibuprofen provided superior symptom relief compared to glucosamine sulfate after two weeks of treatment, but after eight weeks, glucosamine sulfate was significantly better than ibuprofen (2602). In a meta-analytical review of the literature, most trials were found to have methodological flaws; however, pooled data from the higher quality, larger-scale studies, indicate that glucosamine likely provides significant benefit (2533).
Some clinical trials used a specific patented oral formulation of glucosamine sulfate (Viartril-S, Rottapharm, Italy), which is not available in the US (2604).
POSSIBLY EFFECTIVE ...when used intramuscularly, short-term for reducing the symptoms of osteoarthritis. In one placebo-controlled clinical trial, intramuscular glucosamine sulfate given twice per week for six weeks significantly reduced the severity of symptoms of knee osteoarthritis in patients with mild to moderately severe disease (radiological stage I-III) compared to placebo. Improvement was significant after five weeks of treatment and symptom relief continued for two weeks after discontinuation of treatment (2605).
POSSIBLY INEFFECTIVE ...when used orally for reducing pain in severe, long-standing osteoarthritis. In one study, glucosamine sulfate added to an existing analgesic regimen failed to improve symptoms of osteoarthritis compared to placebo after two months of treatment. Patients in this study were generally older, heavier, and had more severe and a longer-duration of osteoarthritis than patients in previous studies with positive findings (1330). There is insufficient reliable information available about the effectiveness of topically applied glucosamine sulfate.

Possible Mechanism of Action & Active Ingredients

Glucosamine is a glycoprotein derived from marine exoskeletons or produced synthetically (6). It is required for the synthesis of glycoproteins, glycolipids, and glycosaminoglycans, also known as mucopolysaccharides, which comprise the body's tendons, ligaments, cartilage, synovial fluid, mucus membranes, and structures in the eye, blood vessels, and heart valves. Glucosamine stimulates metabolism of chondrocytes in articular cartilage and synoviocytes in synovial tissue. Glucosamine may stop and possibly reverses degenerative joint disease (DJD) (6). Glucosamine sulfate is 90% absorbed after oral administration. The bioavailability is approximately 26% after first pass metabolism (2608). Glucosamine is incorporated into plasma proteins during first-pass metabolism, and unbound glucosamine is concentrated in the articular cartilage (2608). Free glucosamine is undetectable in the plasma (2607). Some glucosamine preparations are provided as topical creams. It is not known if glucosamine is absorbed transdermally. Oral glucosamine might be better tolerated than the non-steroidal anti-inflammatory drugs (NSAIDs) because its mode of action targets the pathogenic mechanisms of DJD rather than affecting cyclooxygenase, which is responsible for anti-inflammatory, analgesic, and adverse gastrointestinal effects of NSAIDs (2604). Preliminary evidence suggests glucosamine decreases glucose-induced insulin secretion by inhibiting pancreatic glucokinase in the beta cells of the islet of Langerhans (371,372,3406). Evidence also suggests glucosamine impairs insulin-mediated glucose uptake and metabolism in skeletal muscle. It is hypothesized that glucosamine desensitizes cell membranes to the effects of insulin (372,3406). Evidence suggests that type 2 diabetes and glucosamine induce insulin resistance through a common pathway (3405) and glucosamine-induced insulin resistance might be dose-dependent (3406). In a recent unpublished study, announced at the Experimental Biology 2000 conference, non-diabetic subjects taking glucosamine sulfate 1500 mg per day for 12 weeks had significantly increased insulin levels compared to placebo (5059). Additional research is needed to determine the effects of glucosamine in people with diabetes.

Adverse Reactions Including Known Allergies

Short-term use can cause mild gastrointestinal problems, including nausea, heartburn, diarrhea, and constipation. Drowsiness, skin reactions, headache (2608) and elevated blood glucose levels in diabetics have also been reported (22). In a recent unpublished study, announced at the Experimental Biology 2000 conference, non-diabetic subjects taking glucosamine sulfate 1500 mg per day for 12 weeks had significantly increased insulin levels compared to placebo (5059). Additional research is needed to determine the effects of glucosamine in people with diabetes. In two clinical trials, glucosamine sulfate 1500 mg per day appeared to be better tolerated than non-steroidal antiinflammatory drugs (NSAIDs) ibuprofen 1200 mg per day and piroxicam (Feldene) 20 mg per day (2604,2606). However, in one study there was no significant difference in adverse effects between glucosamine sulfate 1500 mg per day and ibuprofen 1200 mg per day (2602). There is concern that glucosamine sulfate products derived from marine exoskeletons might cause reactions in people allergic to shellfish, although no reactions have been reported. Until more is known, and because the source of glucosamine sulfate products is not listed on product labels, use glucosamine sulfate with caution in people with shellfish allergy.

Possible Interactions with Herbs & Other Dietary Supplements

Insufficient reliable information available.

Possible Interactions with Drugs

ANTIDIABETES DRUGS: Theoretically, glucosamine sulfate might decrease the hypoglycemic effects of insulin and oral antidiabetes agents by increasing insulin resistance and/or decreasing insulin production.

Possible Interactions with Foods

No interactions are known to occur, and there is no known reason to expect a clinically significant interaction with glucosamine sulfate.

Possible Interactions with Lab Tests

BLOOD GLUCOSE: Theoretically, glucosamine sulfate might increase blood glucose levels by increasing insulin resistance and/or decreasing glucose-induced insulin production. There are also anecdotal reports of poorer blood glucose control in people with diabetes who take glucosamine (22,1203,1204,3405,3406).
INSULIN: Glucosamine might increase blood insulin levels. An unpublished study found that glucosamine sulfate 1500 mg per day for 12 weeks increased blood insulin levels in a group of non-diabetic patients (5059). Additional research is needed to determine the effects of glucosamine in people with diabetes.

Possible Interactions with Diseases or Conditions

DIABETES: Theoretically, glucosamine sulfate might exacerbate diabetes by increasing insulin resistance and/or decreasing insulin production, resulting in elevated blood glucose levels. There have been anecdotal reports of poorer blood glucose control in people with diabetes who take glucosamine (22,1203,1204,3405,3406). In a recent unpublished study, announced at the Experimental Biology 2000 conference, non-diabetic subjects taking glucosamine sulfate 1500 mg per day for 12 weeks had significantly increased insulin levels compared to placebo (5059). Additional research is needed to determine the effects of glucosamine in people with diabetes.
SHELLFISH ALLERGY: There is concern that glucosamine sulfate products derived from marine exoskeletons might cause reactions in people allergic to shellfish, although no reactions have been reported. Until more is known, and because the source of glucosamine sulfate products is not listed on product labels, use glucosamine sulfate with caution in people with shellfish allergy.

Typical Dosages & Routes of Administration that are Commonly Used

ORAL: For osteoarthrosis and osteoarthritis, the typical dose is 500 mg three times daily (2600,2602,2603,2606).
PARENTERAL: In other countries, intravenous, intramuscular, and intra-articular products are used (2601); however, these products are not available in the US. In one trial, glucosamine sulfate 400 mg intramuscularly twice per week was used (2605).

Comments

Although chondroitin sulfate and glucosamine sulfate are frequently marketed together in combination products (760), there is no evidence that the combination has greater benefit than either product alone. The National Institutes of Health (NIH) is sponsoring its first clinical trial of glucosamine sulfate in combination with chondroitin sulfate. The 16 week, parallel group, double-blind RCT includes four separate treatment arms, in which patients will ingest: 1) placebo, 2) glucosamine sulfate 500 mg three times per day, 3) chondroitin 400 mg three times per day, or 4) a combination of glucosamine sulfate and chondroitin (3573).

GLUTAMINE

This Product is Also Known As

Levoglutamide, Levoglutamine, L-Glutamic Acid 5-Amide, l-Glutamine, L-Glutamine.

Scientific Names

L-(+)-2-Aminoglutaramic acid.

People Use This For

Orally, glutamine is used for depression, moodiness, irritability, anxiety, insomnia, short bowel syndrome, Crohn's disease, and enhanced exercise performance. Glutamine is also used for HIV wasting, abnormal intestinal permeability in people with HIV, chemotherapy-induced mucositis, protection of immune and gut barrier function in people with esophageal cancer undergoing radiochemotherapy, cystinuria, peptic ulcer, ulcerative colitis, sickle cell anemia, improving recovery after bone marrow transplant, and for alcohol withdrawal support (2132,2133,2134, 2135,2136,2331,2702,2705,5451,5455,5456,5457,5460,5461,5462,5464,5465,5466). Glutamine is also used orally as enteral nutrition, for preventing morbidity in trauma patients (5449), and preventing infectious complications in critically ill patients (5450). Intravenously, glutamine is administered for improving recovery after surgery (2363,5448) and after bone marrow transplant (2366,2367,5451,5452,5453,5454), and preventing chemotherapy-induced mucositis (5458).

Safety

POSSIBLY SAFE ...when taken orally and appropriately. In studies, glutamine has been well tolerated and without side effects in doses up to 40 grams per day (2337,2338).
PREGNANCY AND LACTATION: Insufficient reliable information available; avoid using.

Effectiveness

POSSIBLY EFFECTIVE ...when taken orally for treating short bowel syndrome (2334,2361,2362,2363,2701,2703). ...when taken orally for chemotherapy-induced stomatitis (2336,2364,2368,2704,5029). In one study, oral glutamine swished and swallowed every four hours around the clock beginning seven days before transplant reduced the severity and duration of oral mucositis, and use of post-transplant parenteral narcotics, associated with high-dose paclitaxel and melphalan preparation for bone marrow transplant (5029). ...when taken orally for preventing morbidity in trauma patients (5449) and infectious complications in critically ill patients (5450). ...when taken orally for treating weight loss and abnormal intestinal permeability in people with HIV disease (2335,2337,2702,5461). ...when taken orally to prevent decreasing lymphocyte counts and attenuate gut permeability in people with esophageal cancer during radiochemotherapy (2705). ...when given intravenously for improving recovery after surgery (2363,5448). ...when given intravenously for improving recovery after bone marrow transplant (2366,2367,5451,5452,5453,5454). ...when given intravenously for preventing chemotherapy-induced mucositis (5458).
POSSIBLY INEFFECTIVE ...when taken orally for 5-fluorouracil (5-FU)-induced oral mucositis (2365,5462). ...when taken orally for treating cystinuria (2339). ...when taken orally for Crohn's disease (2338,6256). Neither supplemental glutamine 7 grams three times daily or a glutamine-enriched diet had any benefit in patients with Crohn's disease in 2 small, well-designed studies (2338,6256). ...when taken orally for enhancing exercise performance (2341,2342,5455,5456,5464,5465,5466).
There is insufficient reliable information available about the effectiveness of glutamine for its other uses.

Possible Mechanism of Action & Active Ingredients

Glutamine is an amino acid produced primarily in skeletal muscle. It acts as an inter-organ nitrogen and carbon transporter (5467). Although traditionally classified as a non-essential amino acid, glutamine is essential for maintaining intestinal function, immune response, and amino acid homeostasis during times of severe stress (5468). Glutamine is an important metabolic fuel for lymphocytes, macrophages, fibroblasts, and small intestine enterocytes (5468,5469). Glutamine also functions as a precursor of other amino acids, glucose, purines and pyrimidines, and glutathione (5468,5469,5470). Glutamine promotes carbohydrate storage after exhaustive exercise (5457).

Adverse Reactions Including Known Allergies

None reported.

Possible Interactions with Herbs & Other Dietary Supplements

Insufficient reliable information available.

Possible Interactions with Drugs

CHEMOTHERAPY: Oral glutamine can reduce oral mucositis associated with chemotherapeutic agents, including carboplatin (Paraplatin), doxorubicin (Adriamycin, Rubex), etoposide (Etopophos, Toposar, VePesid), ifosfamide (Ifex), melphalan (Alkeran), methotrexate (Rheumatrex), and paclitaxel (Taxol) (2364,2368,2704,5029).
METHOTREXATE (Rheumatrex): Methotrexate might reduce the effectiveness of glutamine in decreasing chemotherapy-induced oral mucositis (2368).

Possible Interactions with Foods

No interactions are known to occur, and there is no known reason to expect a clinically significant interaction with glutamine.

Possible Interactions with Lab Tests

No interactions are known to occur, and there is no known reason to expect a clinically significant interaction with glutamine.

Possible Interactions with Diseases or Conditions

No interactions are known to occur, and there is no known reason to expect a clinically significant interaction with glutamine.

Typical Dosages & Routes of Administration that are Commonly Used

ORAL: For short bowel syndrome, 630 mg/kg per day has been used (2334). For HIV wasting, 8-40 g per day has been used (2335,2702,5461). For Crohn's disease, 7 g three times daily has been used (2338). For reducing chemotherapy-induced stomatitis, glutamine suspension 4 g swish and swallow every four hours around the clock (5029), 2 g/meter twice daily (2336,2367), or 500 mg/kg per day (2704) have been used. For preventing drops in lymphocyte counts and attenuating gut permeability in people with esophageal cancer during radiochemotherapy, 30 g per day has been used (2705).

Comments

Glutamine has orphan drug status for use in combination with human growth hormone in the treatment of short bowel syndrome (2701).

GLUTATHIONE

This Product is Also Known As

gamma-Glutamylcysteinylglycine, gamma-L-Glutamyl-L-cysteinylglycine, GSH.

Scientific Names

N-(N-L-gamma-Glutamyl-L-cysteinyl)glycine.

People Use This For

Orally, glutathione is used for treating cataracts (5355,5356), glaucoma (5356), preventing aging (5356), treating or preventing alcoholism, asthma, cancer, heart disease (atherosclerosis and hypercholesterolemia), hepatitis (5356), liver disease (5355), immunosuppression (including AIDS and chronic fatigue syndrome) (5356), maintaining immune function (5365,5366), memory loss, Alzheimer's disease, osteoarthritis, Parkinson's disease, and detoxifying metal and drugs (5356).
Inhaled, glutathione is used for treating lung diseases (9), including idiopathic pulmonary fibrosis (5369), cystic fibrosis (5367), and lung disease in individuals with HIV disease (5368).
Intramuscularly, glutathione is used for preventing toxicity of chemotherapy (5374,5375) and for treating male infertility (5384).
Intravenously, glutathione is used for preventing anemia in patients undergoing hemodialysis (5359), for preventing renal dysfunction after coronary bypass surgery (5360), for treating Parkinson's disease (5344,5354), improving blood flow and decreasing clotting in individuals with atherosclerosis (5385), for treating diabetes (5357,5358), and preventing toxicity of chemotherapy (5373,5374,5375,5376,5377,5378,5379,5380,5381,5382,5383).

Safety

POSSIBLY SAFE ...when used orally (5361,5362), by inhalation (9,5367,5368,5369), by intramuscular (5374,5375,5384), or intravenous injection (5344,5354,5357,5358,5359,5360,5373,5374,5375,5376,5377,5378,5379,5380,5381,5382,5383).
PREGNANCY AND LACTATION: Insufficient reliable information available; avoid using.

Effectiveness

POSSIBLY EFFECTIVE …when used by intravenous injection for preventing chemotherapy toxicity (5373,5374, 5375,5376,5377,5378,5379,5380,5381,5382,5383).

LIKELY INEFFECTIVE …when used orally because it is not absorbed (5362).

There is insufficient reliable information available about the effectiveness of glutathione for its other uses.

Possible Mechanism of Action & Active Ingredients

Glutathione is primarily synthesized in the liver (5387,5388). It is involved in DNA synthesis and repair, protein and prostaglandin synthesis, amino acid transport, metabolism of toxins and carcinogens, immune system function, prevention of oxidative cell damage, and enzyme activation (5344,5386). Cellular glutathione levels increase during exercise (5398,5386). Glutathione deficiency is associated with aging, age-related macular degeneration, diabetes, lung and gastrointestinal disease, pre-eclampsia, Parkinson's disease, and other neurodegenerative disorders, and a poor prognosis in AIDS (5344,5346,5347,5348,5349,5350,5351,5352,5353,5354,5393,5394,5395,5396,5397). Although glutathione is present in fruits, vegetables, and meats, the levels in the body do not seem to correlate to dietary intake. This suggests that oral glutathione might be inactivated by peptidases in the gut (5344,5890,5891). Despite evidence that suggests that glutathione is bioavailable in rodents (5363,5364), oral doses of 3 grams cause negligible increases in human plasma levels (5362). Preliminary evidence suggests glutathione intake from fruits and vegetables might be associated with a reduced risk of pharyngeal cancer (5345). In individuals with cirrhosis, oral glutathione has no effect on liver function tests (5361).

Researchers report that glutathione inhibits the activity of enzymes that help the flu virus colonize cells lining the mouth and throat. They also report that flu-infected mice fed glutathione-enriched drinking water had lower tissue virus levels than untreated mice. The researchers caution that human studies are needed to determine the effects of glutathione on humans with the flu. The results of these unpublished studies were presented at the Experimental Biology 2000 conference (5061).

Adverse Reactions Including Known Allergies

None reported.

Possible Interactions with Herbs & Other Dietary Supplements

Insufficient reliable information available.

Possible Interactions with Drugs

CISPLATIN: Concurrent use can prevent or reduce the severity of cisplatin-induced nephrotoxicity and neurotoxicity without altering the effectiveness of cisplatin (5373,5374,5378,5379,5380,5381).

GLUTATHIONE-DEPLETING DRUGS: Drugs that deplete glutathione (acetaminophen, alcohol, and others) might decrease the therapeutic effects of glutathione (5394).

Possible Interactions with Foods

No interactions are known to occur, and there is no known reason to expect a clinically significant interaction with glutathione.

Possible Interactions with Lab Tests

No interactions are known to occur, and there is no known reason to expect a clinically significant interaction with glutathione.

Possible Interactions with Diseases or Conditions

ASTHMA: Inhaled (nebulized) glutathione can cause bronchospasm in individuals with asthma (5372).

Typical Dosages & Routes of Administration that are Commonly Used

ORAL: Supplemental doses range from 50–600 mg per day, with a typical dose of 250 mg daily (5355,5356,5365,5366); however, orally administered glutathione is probably not bioavailable (5362).

INHALATION: 600 mg, aerosolized twice daily (5367,5368,5369).

INTRAMUSCULAR: Infertility, 600 mg every other day for 2 months (5384); chemotherapy adjunct, 600 mg on days 2 through 5 of chemotherapy (5374,5375).

INTRAVENOUS: Chemotherapy adjunct, 2.5 grams or 1.5 grams/meter squared immediately prior to chemotherapy (5373,5374,5375,5376,5377,5378,5379,5380,5381,5382,5383).

Comments

The role of glutathione is being studied in the wasting of AIDS, heavy metal poisoning, sepsis, myocardial ischemia, renal dysfunction and nephrotoxicity, liver disorders, corneal disorders, and eczema (9,14,5355,5344,5345). Currently, researchers are investigating whether administering glutathione precursors, such as glutamine and n-acetylcysteine might increase glutathione levels (5344,5389,5392).

GLYCEROL

This Product is Also Known As
Glicerol, Glucerite, Glycerin, Glycerolum, Glyceryl Alcohol.

Scientific Names
Glycerol, 1,2,3-propanetriol.

People Use This For
Orally, glycerol is used for weight loss, enhancing exercise performance, improving rehydration during acute gastrointestinal disease, and reducing intraocular pressure (15,2479,2485). Glycerol is also used by athletes as an aid to hydration (217).

Intravenously, glycerol is used for reducing intra-cranial pressure in various conditions including stroke, meningitis, encephalitis, Reye's syndrome, pseudotumor cerebri, CNS trauma, CNS tumors or space-occupying lesions, for reducing brain volume for neurosurgical procedures, and for postural syncope (15,2477).

Ophthalmically, glycerol is an ingredient for reducing corneal edema to facilitate ophthalmic exams (15).

Rectally, glycerol is used as a laxative (15).

Safety
LIKELY SAFE ...when used rectally and appropriately (15). ...when used orally for reducing intraocular pressure; glycerol is an FDA-approved prescription product for this purpose.

POSSIBLY UNSAFE ...when used intravenously. In one study, hemolysis was reported in 98% of people treated for acute ischemic stroke (2482).

There is insufficient reliable information available about the safety of the oral use of glycerol.

PREGNANCY AND LACTATION: Insufficient reliable information available for oral use; avoid using.

Effectiveness
LIKELY EFFECTIVE ...when used rectally for constipation (15).

POSSIBLY INEFFECTIVE ...when taken orally for weight loss (2485).

LIKELY INEFFECTIVE ...when taken orally for enhancing exercise performance (2474,2475). ...when used intravenously for treating acute stroke (2480,2481,2482,2484,2486).

There is insufficient reliable information available about the effectiveness of glycerol for its other uses.

Possible Mechanism of Action & Active Ingredients
Supplemental glycerol increases serum osmolality (2477). It also has hyperosmotic laxative activity (15). Glycerol consumption failed to enhance human exercise performance (2476,2492) or reduce water loss in underwater divers (2478). However, one study reported that following glycerol ingestion, participants had improved exercise tolerance and reduced heart rate during stationary cycling (2479). Intravenous glycerol failed to improve acute ischemic stroke survival in several clinical trials (2480,2481,2482,2484,2486); however, one study of elderly people with acute ischemic stroke found glycerol improved initial survival (2483).

Adverse Reactions Including Known Allergies
The oral use of glycerol can cause mild headache, dizziness, bloating, nausea, vomiting, thirst, and diarrhea (15,2475). The intravenous use of glycerol has caused hemolysis in people treated for acute ischemic stroke (2480,2482).

Possible Interactions with Herbs & Other Dietary Supplements
Insufficient reliable information available.

Possible Interactions with Drugs
No interactions are known to occur, and there is no known reason to expect a clinically significant interaction with glycerol.

Possible Interactions with Foods
No interactions are known to occur, and there is no known reason to expect a clinically significant interaction with glycerol.

Possible Interactions with Lab Tests
No interactions are known to occur, and there is no known reason to expect a clinically significant interaction with glycerol.

Possible Interactions with Diseases or Conditions
No interactions are known to occur, and there is no known reason to expect a clinically significant interaction with glycerol.

Typical Dosages & Routes of Administration that are Commonly Used
ORAL: For enhancing exercise performance, the usual dose of glycerol is 1 gram/kg with 1.5 L fluid 60-120 minutes before competition (2475). For weight loss, 7.5 grams in a 25% solution is typically taken before meals (2485). For reducing intraocular pressure, glycerol is a FDA-approved prescription product.

© Copyright 2000, Natural Medicines Comprehensive Database (209) 472-2244. For updated data, go to www.NaturalDatabase.com

RECTAL: As an adult laxative, the common dose is a 2-3 grams suppository or a 5-15 mL enema (15). For children younger than six years old, the dose is a 1-1.7 grams suppository or a 2-5 mL enema (15).
OPHTHALMIC: FDA-approved prescription product.
INTRAVENOUS: No typical dosage.

Comments
None.

GOA POWDER

This Product is Also Known As
Araoba, Bahia Powder, Brazil Powder, Chrysatobine, Crude Chrysarobin, Ringworm Powder.

Scientific Names
Andira araroba.

People Use This For
Topically, goa powder is used for psoriasis and fungal infections of the skin (18).

Safety
POSSIBLY UNSAFE ...when used topically. Goa powder is severely irritating to skin and mucous membranes. It can also be absorbed through the skin with adverse effects. As little as 10 mg absorbed is associated with vomiting, diarrhea, and kidney inflammation (18).
PREGNANCY AND LACTATION: Insufficient reliable information available; avoid using.

Effectiveness
There is insufficient reliable information available about the effectiveness of goa powder.

Possible Mechanism of Action & Active Ingredients
The applicable part of goa powder is the latex. Goa powder contains anthrone derivatives including chrysophanolanthrone. The powder is a strong reducing agent and inhibits glucose-6-phosphated-dehydrogenization in psoriatic skin conditions. It is considered a potent irritant to skin and mucous membranes and is easily absorbed through the skin (18).

Adverse Reactions Including Known Allergies
Topical application can cause redness, swelling, pustules, and conjunctivitis. If ingested, vomiting, diarrhea, and kidney inflammation can follow (18).

Possible Interactions with Herbs & Other Dietary Supplements
Insufficient reliable information available.

Possible Interactions with Drugs
No interactions are known to occur, and there is no known reason to expect a clinically significant interaction with goa powder.

Possible Interactions with Foods
No interactions are known to occur, and there is no known reason to expect a clinically significant interaction with goa powder.

Possible Interactions with Lab Tests
No interactions are known to occur, and there is no known reason to expect a clinically significant interaction with goa powder.

Possible Interactions with Diseases or Conditions
No interactions are known to occur, and there is no known reason to expect a clinically significant interaction with goa powder.

Typical Dosages & Routes of Administration that are Commonly Used
TOPICAL: People typically use a 2% goa powder ointment.
ORAL: Goa should not be used internally (5264,5269).

Comments
Likely unsafe when used topically and without demonstrated effectiveness; avoid using (18). Goa powder has been replaced by synthetic anthranol (18).

GOAT'S RUE

This Product is Also Known As
Goats Rue, French Honeysuckle, French Lilac, Galegae officinalis herba, Geissrautenkraut, Goat's Rue Herb, Italian Fitch.
CAUTION: See separate listing for Rue.

Scientific Names
Galega officinalis.
Family: Fabaceae.

People Use This For
Orally, goat's rue is used as supportive therapy for diabetes, and as a diuretic (18).
In combinations with other herbs, goat's rue is used for adrenal gland and pancreas stimulation, for glandular disturbances, blood purification, purifying the mesenchyma, digestive fluid secretion disturbances, fermentative dyspepsia, Roemheld syndrome, diarrhea, abnormal colonic bacterial flora, status lymphaticus and exudative diathesis, for stimulating lactation, as a tonic, and as a liver-protectant (2).

Safety
There is insufficient reliable information available about the safety of goat's rue.
Pregnancy and Lactation: Insufficient reliable information available; avoid using.

Effectiveness
There is insufficient reliable information available about the effectiveness of goat's rue.

Possible Mechanism of Action & Active Ingredients
The applicable parts of goat's rue are the above ground parts. In vitro, the constituent galegine has hypoglycemic effects (2,4006,18), but these effects have not been demonstrated with goat's rue (2,18). In experimental rats, an intravenously administered aqueous extract suppresses platelet aggregation (4007). Fatal poisonings have been reported in grazing animals. Toxicity may involve galegine (4008).

Adverse Reactions Including Known Allergies
None reported in humans. However, fatal poisonings have been reported in grazing animals following ingestion of large amounts of goat's rue (2,18); poisoning symptoms in sheep, include salivation, spasms, paralysis, and asphyxiation (2,18).

Possible Interactions with Herbs & Other Dietary Supplements
HYPOGLYCEMIC HERBS: Theoretically, concomitant use could potentiate effects of other herbs that cause hypoglycemia (2,4006).

Possible Interactions with Drugs
ANTIDIABETES DRUGS: Theoretically, concomitant use could potentiate hypoglycemic drug effects. Monitor closely (2,4006).

Possible Interactions with Foods
No interactions are known to occur, and there is no known reason to expect a clinically significant interaction with goat's rue.

Possible Interactions with Lab Tests
BLOOD GLUCOSE: Theoretically, could cause a true decrease in blood glucose levels and test results (2,4006).

Possible Interactions with Diseases or Conditions
DIABETES: Goat's rue may interfere with effective diabetes treatment; avoid using.

Typical Dosages & Routes of Administration that are Commonly Used
ORAL: As prepared tea (steep 2 grams finely cut above ground parts in 150 mL boiling water 5-10 minutes, strain); frequency of use not specified (18).

Comments
Avoid confusion with rue (Ruta graveolens). Goat's rue is not recommended for diabetes mellitus therapy because effectiveness is uncertain.

GOLDEN RAGWORT

This Product is Also Known As

Cocash Weed, Coughweed, False Valerian, Female Regulator, Golden Groundsel, Golden Senecio, Grundy Swallow, Life Root, Liferoot, Ragwort, Squaw Weed, Squawweed.
CAUTION: See separate listings for Alpine Ragwort and Tansy Ragwort.

Scientific Names

Senecio aureus.
Family: Asteraceae/Compositae.

People Use This For

Orally, golden ragwort is used for diabetes mellitus, high blood pressure, spasms, as a uterine stimulant, and to minimize bleeding. It is also used orally as a diuretic and mild expectorant (4).
In folk medicine, golden ragwort has been used orally for treating conditions involving the female reproductive tract, including functional amenorrhea, menopausal neurosis, dysmenorrhea, pain associated with childbirth, and for inducing uterine contractions (6,18). It has also been used topically for the treatment of bleeding after tooth extraction and as a douche for leukorrhea (18).

Safety

LIKELY UNSAFE ...when used orally. Golden ragwort contains hepatotoxic unsaturated pyrrolizidine alkaloids (UPAs) (12,19). Repeated exposure to low concentrations of UPAs linked to veno-occlusive disease, a serious condition (4,12). UPAs may also be carcinogenic and mutagenic (12). ...when used topically on abraded or broken skin, it might be unsafe due to the potential for systemic absorption (12,19).
PREGNANCY: UNSAFE ...contraindicated due to the possibility it might stimulate menstruation, oxytocic activity, or cause teratogenic effects (19).
LACTATION: UNSAFE ...contraindicated due to pyrrolizidine alkaloid content (19).

Effectiveness

There is insufficient reliable information available about the effectiveness of golden ragwort.

Possible Mechanism of Action & Active Ingredients

Some pyrrolizidine alkaloids have shown carcinogenic and mutagenic properties, and there are reports of renal toxicity. However, the primary concern is veno-occlusive disease (12). Unsaturated pyrrolizidine alkaloids are known to be hepatotoxic in animals and humans (4).

Adverse Reactions Including Known Allergies

When used orally, acute toxicity may result in hepatic necrosis; chronic toxicity may cause veno-occlusive liver disease. The potential for hepatotoxicity (due to presence of pyrrolizidine alkaloids) increases with larger doses and longer periods of use (4,12). It can cause an allergic reaction in individuals sensitive to the Asteraceae/Compositae family. Members of this family include ragweed, chrysanthemums, marigolds, daisies, and many other herbs.

Possible Interactions with Herbs & Other Dietary Supplements

EUCALYPTUS: Theoretically, concomitant use might increase the risk of unsaturated pyrrolizidine alkaloid toxicity due to enzyme induction by eucalyptus (19).
PYRROLIZIDINE ALKALOID-CONTAINING HERBS: Concomitant use is contraindicated due to the risk of additive toxicity. Herbs containing unsaturated pyrrolizidine alkaloids include: alkanna (12), borage (271), gravel root (4), hemp agrimony (271), hound's tongue (19), petasites (19), comfrey (271), coltsfoot, and the Senecio species plants; dusty miller (19), alpine ragwort (19), groundsel (271), golden ragwort (19), and tansy ragwort (271).

Possible Interactions with Drugs

No interactions are known to occur, and there is no known reason to expect a clinically significant interaction with golden ragwort.

Possible Interactions with Foods

No interactions are known to occur, and there is no known reason to expect a clinically significant interaction with golden ragwort.

Possible Interactions with Lab Tests

No interactions are known to occur, and there is no known reason to expect a clinically significant interaction with golden ragwort.

Possible Interactions with Diseases or Conditions

LIVER DISEASE: Golden ragwort is hepatotoxic and may exacerbate liver conditions; contraindicated (6).
CROSS-ALLERGENICITY: Can cause an allergic reaction in individuals sensitive to the Asteraceae/Compositae family. Members of this family include ragweed, chrysanthemums, marigolds, daisies, and many other herbs.

Typical Dosages & Routes of Administration that are Commonly Used
No typical dosage.

Comments
Even though golden ragwort is considered unsafe for oral use (12,18), it is still included in some herbal preparations designed to treat irregular menses and other gynecological disorders. Golden ragwort is sometimes confused with other plants credited with broad healing powers, such as mandrake and ginseng (6).

GOLDENROD

This Product is Also Known As
Aaron's Rod, European Goldenrod, Woundwort.
CAUTION: See separate listing for Mullein.

Scientific Names
Solidago virgaurea (European goldenrod); Solidago canadensis (Canadian goldenrod); Solidago serotina, synonyms Solidago gigantea (Early goldenrod).
Family: Asteraceae or Compositae.

People Use This For
Orally, goldenrod is used as a diuretic, anti-inflammatory, and antispasmodic (3). It is also used as "irrigation therapy" where it is taken with copious fluids to increase urine flow to treat inflammatory diseases of the lower urinary tract, urinary calculi, and kidney gravel. As "irrigation therapy," it is also used as prophylaxis for urinary calculi and kidney gravel (2).
Topically, goldenrod is used as a mouth rinse for inflammation of the mouth and throat and externally for poorly healing wounds (8,18).
In folk medicine, goldenrod has been taken orally as a "blood purifying" agent in gout, rheumatism, arthritis, eczema, and other skin conditions (8). It has been used for acute exacerbations of pulmonary tuberculosis, diabetes, enlargement of the liver, hemorrhoids, internal bleeding, nervous bronchial asthma, and prostatic hypertrophy (18).

Safety
LIKELY SAFE ...when above ground parts are used orally and appropriately for "irrigation therapy" (as a mild diuretic along with copious fluid intake) (2).
There is insufficient reliable information available about the safety of the topical use of goldenrod.
PREGNANCY AND LACTATION: Insufficient reliable information available; avoid using.

Effectiveness
POSSIBLY EFFECTIVE ...when taken orally for "irrigation therapy" where goldenrod is used with copious fluid intake to increase urine flow for inflammatory diseases of the lower urinary tract and kidney gravel, and as prophylaxis for urinary calculi and kidney gravel (2).
There is insufficient reliable information available about the effectiveness of goldenrod for its other uses.

Possible Mechanism of Action & Active Ingredients
The applicable parts of goldenrod are the above ground parts. Goldenrod is classified as an aquaretic, a compound that increases urine volume (water loss) but not sodium excretion (512). The anti-inflammatory and aquaretic effects of goldenrod are due to the saponin and flavonoid constituents (8,512). Goldenrod also has bacteriostatic activity (512).

Adverse Reactions Including Known Allergies
Goldenrod can cause an allergic reaction in individuals sensitive to the Asteraceae/Compositae family. Members of this family include ragweed, chrysanthemums, marigolds, daisies, and many other herbs.

Possible Interactions with Herbs & Other Dietary Supplements
Insufficient reliable information available.

Possible Interactions with Drugs
DIURETICS: Theoretically, goldenrod might increase sodium retention and interfere with diuretic therapy (512).

Possible Interactions with Foods
No interactions are known to occur, and there is no known reason to expect a clinically significant interaction with goldenrod.

Possible Interactions with Lab Tests
No interactions are known to occur, and there is no known reason to expect a clinically significant interaction with goldenrod.

Possible Interactions with Diseases or Conditions

EDEMA DUE TO HEART OR KIDNEY CONDITIONS: "Irrigation therapy," where goldenrod is taken with copious fluid intake to increase urine flow, is contraindicated in these conditions with edema (2).
HYPERTENSION: Theoretically, goldenrod might increase sodium retention and worsen hypertension (512).
URINARY TRACT INFECTIONS: Herbal "irrigation therapy" can be insufficient and require the addition of antibacterial agent. "Irrigation therapy" should be monitored closely (8).
CROSS-ALLERGENICITY: Can cause an allergic reaction in individuals sensitive to the Asteraceae/Compositae family. Members of this family include ragweed, chrysanthemums, marigolds, daisies, and many other herbs.

Typical Dosages & Routes of Administration that are Commonly Used

ORAL: The typical dose of goldenrod is one cup of the tea two to four times daily between meals (18). The tea is prepared by steeping 1-2 teaspoons (3-5 grams) of the dried herb in 150 mL boiling water for 5-10 minutes and then straining. The usual dose ranges from 6-12 grams of the herb per day (2). The common dose of the liquid extract (1:1 in 25% ethanol) is 0.5-2 mL two to three times daily (18). The usual dose of the tincture (1:5 in 45% ethanol) is 0.5-1 mL two to three times daily (18). Drink plenty of water, at least 2 liters per day, with the use of goldenrod (18).
CAUTION: In cases of chronic kidney disorders, professional evaluation is needed (12).

Comments

Avoid confusion with mullein (Verbascum densiflorum; also referred to as goldenrod). Early goldenrod, European goldenrod, and Canadian goldenrod are used interchangeably.

GOLDENSEAL

This Product is Also Known As

Eye Balm, Eye Root, Goldenroot, Golden Seal, Goldsiegel, Ground Raspberry, Indian Dye, Indian Plant, Indian Tumeric, Jaundice Root, Orange Root, Sceau D'Or, Turmeric Root, Warnera, Wild Curcuma, Yellow Indian Paint, Yellow Paint, Yellow Puccoon, Yellow Root.
CAUTION: See separate listings for Barberry, Goldthread, Javanese Turmeric, Oregon Grape, Ox-eye Daisy, and Turmeric.

Scientific Names

Hydrastis canadensis.
Family: Ranunculaceae.

People Use This For

Orally, goldenseal is used for urinary tract infections (3), inflammation of vaginal and uretal mucous membranes, hemorrhoids (11), gastritis, anorexia, peptic ulcers, colitis, menorrhagia and dysmenorrhea, post-partum hemorrhage (4), and internal hemorrhage (3). It is also used to treat conjunctivitis, tinnitus, catarrhal deafness (4), malaria (11), nasal congestion (11), upper respiratory tract inflammation (4), and sore gums (11). Goldenseal has been used to mask urine tests for illicit drugs (11), for atonic dyspepsia with hepatic symptoms (4), jaundice (4,6), gonorrhea (6), and cancer (11).
Topically, goldenseal is used for eczema, itching (4), acne, dandruff, ringworm (11), herpes labialis, and wounds (18).
Historically, American Indians have used goldenseal for whooping cough, diarrhea, fever, flatulence, pneumonia and with whiskey for heart disease (11). They also used it to treat arrow wounds, ulcers, as an insect repellent, diuretic, a stimulant, as a wash for sore eyes, and to produce a yellow dye (6).

Safety

POSSIBLY SAFE ...when used orally and appropriately, short-term (12,1740).
LIKELY UNSAFE ...when used orally in high doses or long-term (12,18). Doses providing more than 500 mg of the constituent, berberine, can lead to significant toxicity. This may correspond to 8-100 grams of dry root, depending on the concentration of berberine (12). Overdoses of goldenseal can cause cardiac damage, spasms, and death (4). The LD50 of the berberine constituent in humans is reported to be 27.5 mg/kg (12). Prolonged use has also been associated with significant side effects, including digestive disorders and hallucinations (see Adverse Reactions) (18).
CHILDREN: LIKELY UNSAFE ...when used orally in newborns. The berberine constituent can cause kernicterus in newborns, particularly preterm neonates with hyperbilirubinemia. A berberine-containing Chinese herbal medicine huanglian was banned in Singapore for this reason (2589).
PREGNANCY: UNSAFE ...when used orally. Goldenseal is reported to affect menstruation and have oxytocic effects (4,6,12,18). Berberine and other constituents are also thought to cross the placenta and may cause harm to the fetus. Kernicteris has developed in newborn infants exposed to goldenseal (2589).
LACTATION: UNSAFE ...when used orally. Berberine and other harmful constituents can be transferred to the infant through breast milk (2589).

Effectiveness

POSSIBLY INEFFECTIVE ...when used orally to cause a false negative immunoassay (EMIT and TDx) for marijuana and cocaine urine tests (260). ...when used orally to cause false negative results for Microgenics CEDIA DAU assay for amphetamines, barbiturates, benzodiazepines, cocaine, opiates, phencyclidine, and tetrahydrocannabinol. Drinking one gallon of water with goldenseal did not increase the number of false negatives over water alone (261).

Possible Mechanism of Action & Active Ingredients

The applicable parts of goldenseal are the dried rhizome and root. The alkaloids hydrastine and berberine are the principle active constituents in goldenseal (4). These alkaloids are poorly absorbed when given orally (6,2591). The isolated berberine constituent has been shown to have significant pharmacological effects, primarily antimicrobial. However, these effects have generally not been demonstrated specifically for goldenseal. Berberine constituent has antibacterial and amoebicidal properties (3,4,6). Evidence suggests it has activity against Corneybacterium diphtheriae, Chlamydia aureus, Salmonella typhi, Diplococcus, pneumoniae, Pseudomonas aeruginosa, Shigella dysenteriae, Trichomonas vaginalis, Neisseria gonorrhea, Neisseria meningitidis, Treponema pallidum, Leishmania donovani, and fungi (4,6,2530). However, due to poor absorption, goldenseal preparations are not expected to achieve berberine serum concentrations high enough to be effective in humans. Berberine from goldenseal is thought to concentrate in the bladder, so theoretically, it might have some activity against urinary pathogens (6411); however, this has not been demonstrated in humans. Berberine might also prevent urinary tract pathogens, such as Escherichia coli, from binding to bladder walls (2583). Berberine sulfate may also have activity against the protozoa Entamoeba histolytica and Giardia lamblia, but not Trichomonas vaginalis (2587,2588). Berberine also shows some evidence of antitumor properties (4,6). Berberine increases coronary blood flow and stimulates the heart, although higher doses or long-term use are thought to inhibit cardiac activity (4,12). Berberine has antimuscarinic and antihistaminic activity (4). In low doses, another constituent, hydrastine, is hypotensive (4); however, at higher doses, hydrastine constricts peripheral blood vessels, potentially leading to hypertensive effects and increased cardiac output (4,6). Goldenseal can stimulate IgM antibody production (2530). While goldenseal is ineffective for causing false negatives on urine screens, it also does not cause false positives for the fluorescent polarization immunoassay (FPIA) or thin-layer chromatography (TLC) assays for amphetamines, opiates, cocaine metabolites, methadone, or their metabolites (2590).

Adverse Reactions Including Known Allergies

Orally, prolonged use of goldenseal can cause digestive disorders, constipation, excitatory states, hallucinations, and occasionally delirium (18). Overdoses can cause stomach upset, nausea, vomiting, nervousness, depression, dyspnea, bradycardia, cardiac damage, hypotension, seizures, paralysis, spasms, and death (4,6). High doses of the constituent hydrastine can cause exaggerated reflexes, convulsions, paralysis, and death from respiratory failure (4). The fresh plant can cause mucosal irritation (12). Using goldenseal vaginally as a douche can cause ulceration (4). Use of goldenseal during pregnancy, lactation or in newborn infants can cause kernicteris, and several resulting fatalities have been reported (2589). The LD50 of the berberine constituent in humans is reported to be 27.5 mg/kg (12).

Possible Interactions with Herbs & Other Dietary Supplements

B VITAMINS: Theoretically, prolonged use of goldenseal can decrease B vitamin absorption (4).
HERBS WITH SEDATIVE PROPERTIES: Theoretically, concomitant use with herbs that have sedative properties might enhance therapeutic and adverse effects. These include calamus, calendula, California poppy, catnip, capsicum, celery, couch grass, elecampane, Siberian ginseng, German chamomile, gotu kola, hops, Jamaican dogwood, kava, lemon balm, sage, St. John's wort, sassafras, scullcap, shepherd's purse, stinging nettle, valerian, wild carrot, wild lettuce, withania root, and yerba mansa (4,19).

Possible Interactions with Drugs

ACID-INHIBITING DRUGS: Theoretically, due to claims that goldenseal increases stomach acid, it might interfere with antacids, sucralfate (Carafate), H-2 antagonists, and proton pump inhibitors (19).
ANTIHYPERTENSIVE AGENTS: Theoretically, large amounts of goldenseal might interfere with blood pressure control due to vasoconstrictive action of constituent hydrastine (4).
BARBITURATES: Theoretically, goldenseal might potentiate barbiturate-induced sleep time (4).
HEPARIN: Theoretically, goldenseal can inhibit anticoagulant effects due to the constituent, berberine (4).
HIGHLY PROTEIN BOUND DRUGS: Theoretically, the berberine in goldenseal can displace highly protein bound drugs, such as phenylbutazone and papaverine (2589).
SEDATIVE DRUGS: Theoretically, concomitant use with drugs with sedative properties might cause additive effects and side effects (4).

Possible Interactions with Foods

No interactions are known to occur, and there is no known reason to expect a clinically significant interaction with goldenseal.

© Copyright 2000, Natural Medicines Comprehensive Database (209) 472-2244. For updated data, go to www.NaturalDatabase.com

Possible Interactions with Lab Tests

BILIRUBIN: Theoretically, goldenseal might increase bilirubin levels. This has been demonstrated with isolated berberine constituent, but not specifically with goldenseal. Berberine can cause a true increase in total and unbound bilirubin concentrations because it displaces bilirubin from albumin (2589).

Possible Interactions with Diseases or Conditions

CARDIOVASCULAR DISEASE: Theoretically, low doses can increase coronary blood flow and stimulate the heart, while large doses can inhibit cardiac function (4).
GASTROINTESTINAL IRRITATION: Might irritate gastrointestinal tract. Contraindicated in individuals with infectious or inflammatory gastrointestinal conditions (19).
HYPERBILIRUBINEMIA: The berberine in goldenseal can cause kernicterus in newborns, particularly preterm neonates with hyperbilirubinemia (2589); contraindicated in newborns.
HYPERTENSION: Vasoconstrictive action of the constituent hydrastine might interfere with blood pressure control (4); use with caution.

Typical Dosages & Routes of Administration that are Commonly Used

ORAL: Doses of 0.5 -1 gram three times daily of the dried root or rhizome or as a tea have been used. The tea is prepared by simmering 0.5-1 gram dried root or rhizome in 150 mL of boiling water for 5-10 minutes and then straining (4,12). The liquid extract (1:1, 60% ethanol) is usually taken as 0.3-1.0 mL three times daily (12). The tincture (1:10, 60% ethanol) is dosed 2-4 mL three times daily (12).
TOPICAL: Used as a mouthwash 3-4 times daily. The mouthwash is prepared by steeping 2 teaspoons (6 grams) of dried herb in 150 mL boiling water for 5-10 minutes, straining, and allowing to cool (3).

Comments

Goldenseal is commonly found in the deep woods from Vermont to Arkansas and received its name from the golden-yellow scars on the base of the stem. When the stem is broken, the scar resembles a gold wax letter seal. In the 1900s, goldenseal was immensely popular and has become endangered due to over-harvesting (13). In 1997, goldenseal became listed under Appendix II of the Convention on International Trade in Endangered Species of Wild Flora and Fauna (CITIES), which controls export of the root to other countries. Goldenseal is now being cultivated in Washington state, and is considered a cash crop (6). Because it is so expensive, it is often adulterated. Common adulterants include Coptis and Xanthorrhiza (6). The concept of using goldenseal as an adulterant in drug screens came from the novel Stringtown on the Pike by the pharmacist John Uri Lloyd, but goldenseal caused a false positive for strychnine poisoning in this fictional situation (6).

GOLDTHREAD

This Product is Also Known As

Cankerroot, Coptide, Coptis, Gold Thread, Mouth Root, Yellowroot.

Scientific Names

Coptis trifolia, synonym Coptis groenlandica.
Family: Ranunculaceae.

People Use This For

Orally, goldthread is used for digestive disorders (18).

Safety

POSSIBLY UNSAFE ...when used orally in low doses. The constituent berberine is considered moderately toxic. Its LD50 in humans is 27.5 mg/kg (12).
PREGNANCY: LIKELY UNSAFE ...contraindicated. Goldthread may induce menstruation and uterine contractions (12,19).
LACTATION: Insufficient reliable information available; avoid using.

Effectiveness

There is insufficient reliable information available about the effectiveness of goldthread.

Possible Mechanism of Action & Active Ingredients

The applicable part of goldthread is the rhizome. Goldthread contains the bitter berberine, which stimulates bile secretion (12). Berberine also has antimicrobial, diuretic, smooth muscle relaxant, and cardiac depressant activities (12). Small doses stimulate the cardiac and respiratory systems and decrease intestinal peristalsis (12). High doses stimulate smooth muscle in the intestines and uterus, and depress respiration and cardiac function (12). In animal studies, berberine depresses cardiac function by dilating blood vessels and stimulating the vagal nerve (12).

Adverse Reactions Including Known Allergies

When taken orally purified berberine can cause lethargy, nosebleed, dyspnea, skin and eye irritation, kidney irritation, nephritis, nausea, vomiting, and diarrhea (2).

Possible Interactions with Herbs & Other Dietary Supplements
Insufficient reliable information available.

Possible Interactions with Drugs
ACID-INHIBITING DRUGS: Theoretically, due to claims that goldthread increases stomach acid, it might interfere with antacids, sucralfate (Carafate), H-2 antagonists, or proton pump inhibitors (19).

Possible Interactions with Foods
No interactions are known to occur, and there is no known reason to expect a clinically significant interaction with goldthread.

Possible Interactions with Lab Tests
No interactions are known to occur, and there is no known reason to expect a clinically significant interaction with goldthread.

Possible Interactions with Diseases or Conditions
ANTACIDS, H2 ANTAGONISTS: Contraindicated; theoretically, these oppose stimulation of gastric acid secretion (19).

Typical Dosages & Routes of Administration that are Commonly Used
ORAL: People typically use 0.5 to 1.2 grams of the powdered rhizome (5264). As a liquid, 1 teaspoon is boiled with 1 cup water, and dosed 1 tablespoon 3 to 6 times daily. The liquid is sometimes used as a mouthwash or gargle. The tincture is taken 5 to 10 drops at a time (5263).

Comments
None.

GOSSYPOL

This Product is Also Known As
None.
CAUTION: See separate listing for Cotton.

Scientific Names
Gossypium hirsutum; Gossypium herbaceum; other Gossypium species.
Family: Malvaceae.

People Use This For
Orally, gossypol is used as a male contraceptive (6,9,17).
Topically, gossypol is used as a spermicidal cream or gel (6).
Gossypol is being investigated for possible uses in treating uterine myoma, endometriosis, dysfunctional uterine bleeding, metastatic carcinoma of the endometrium or ovary, and HIV disease (6).

Safety
POSSIBLY UNSAFE ...when the cotton seed extract of gossypol is used orally (6,10). Inhibitory effects on spermatogenesis are not predictably reversible, although sperm counts usually return to normal within 3 months to 2 years after discontinuation (6). Chronic use might cause sterility (12). Gossypol might also be cytotoxic to endometrial cells (6).
There is insufficient reliable information available about the safety of the topical use of gossypol.
PREGNANCY: LIKELY UNSAFE ...contraindicated because it possibly has abortifacient and uterine stimulant effects (6,12).
LACTATION: POSSIBLY UNSAFE; avoid using.

Effectiveness
EFFECTIVE ...for male contraception (6); but adverse effects limit use.
POSSIBLY EFFECTIVE ...when applied topically as a spermicide (6).

Possible Mechanism of Action & Active Ingredients
The applicable part of gossypol is the cotton seed extract. The contraceptive action of gossypol results from inhibition of an enzyme, lactate dehydrogenase X, that is crucial to energy metabolism in sperm and spermatogenic cells (6). Gossypol does not have estrogenic or androgenic activity, but it potentiates the androgenicity of methyltestosterone (6). Gossypol may act as an antifertility agent by inhibiting prostaglandin synthesis (17); it inhibits platelet activating factor and leukotrienes (6). Gossypol has shown activity against HIV and herpes simplex type 2 viruses (6); early evidence suggests possible inhibition of ovarian function and possible endometrial cell cytotoxicity (6).

Adverse Reactions Including Known Allergies

Taken orally, gossypol can cause fatigue (6,9,17), changes in appetite (6,9), loss of libido, persistent oligospermia (9), and hyperkalemia (17). Gossypol can cause hypokalemia resistant to potassium supplementation and potassium-sparing diuretics (9). GI effects associated with gossypol include mucosal sloughing, mucosal necrosis, ileus, and intestinal hemorrhage (21). The inhibitory effects on spermatogenesis are not predictably reversible, although sperm counts usually return to normal within 3 months to 2 years after discontinuation (6). Chronic use may cause sterility (12). High doses (100 to 700 times the contraceptive dose) may cause diarrhea, hair discoloration, malnutrition, circulatory problems, and heart failure (6). Gossypol might inhibit ovarian function (6). Topically, it might cause a burning sensation on the face and hands (9,17).

Possible Interactions with Herbs & Other Dietary Supplements

CARDIAC GLYCOSIDE-CONTAINING HERBS: Theoretically, concomitant use might increase the risk of cardiac glycoside toxicity due to the potassium depleting effects of gossypol. Cardiac glycoside containing herbs, including black hellebore, Canadian hemp roots, digitalis leaf, hedge mustard, figwort, lily of the valley roots, motherwort, oleander leaf, pheasant's eye plant, pleurisy root, squill bulb leaf scales, and strophanthus seeds (2,18,19,500).

STIMULANT LAXATIVE HERBS: Theoretically, overuse or misuse of stimulant laxatives with gossypol might increase the risk of potassium depletion. Stimulant laxative herbs include: aloe dried leaf sap, blue flag rhizome, alder buckthorn, European buckthorn, butternut bark, cascara bark, castor oil, colocynth fruit pulp, gamboge bark exudate, jalap root, black root, manna bark exudate, podophyllum root, rhubarb root, senna leaves and pods, wild cucumber fruit (Ecballium elaterium), and yellow dock root (19).

LICORICE/HORSETAIL: Theoretically, overuse/misuse of licorice rhizome or horsetail plant with gossypol might increase the risk of potassium depletion (19).

Possible Interactions with Drugs

DIGOXIN: Theoretically, concomitant use might increase the risk of digoxin toxicity due to the potassium-depleting effects of gossypol (9).

NONSTEROIDAL ANTI-INFLAMMATORY DRUGS (NSAIDs): Concomitant use might increase the risk of gastrointestinal side effects (21).

POTASSIUM DEPLETING DIURETICS: Concomitant use increases the risk of potassium depletion and hypokalemia (9).

STIMULANT LAXATIVES: Theoretically, overuse or misuse of stimulant laxatives with gossypol might increase the risk of potassium depletion.

Possible Interactions with Foods

No interactions are known to occur, and there is no known reason to expect a clinically significant interaction with gossypol.

Possible Interactions with Lab Tests

No interactions are known to occur, and there is no known reason to expect a clinically significant interaction with gossypol.

Possible Interactions with Diseases or Conditions

UROGENITAL IRRITATION OR SENSITIVITY: Contraindicated (12).
HYPOKALEMIA: Contraindicated; may induce or exacerbate hypokalemia (6) .

Typical Dosages & Routes of Administration that are Commonly Used

ORAL: Male contraception, 20 mg daily for 2.5 to 4 months followed by weekly maintenance dose of 50-60 mg (9,17); one reference mentions maintenance dose of 75-100 mg taken two times per month (6).
TOPICAL: No typical dosage.

Comments

Gossypol is considered unsafe for self-medication due to toxic potential; requires monitoring. Gossypol is found in cotton root, root bark, seed and stem, but is commercially extracted from cotton seed (6).

GOTU KOLA

This Product is Also Known As

Centella, Gota Kola, Hydrocotyle, Indian Pennywort, Indian Water Navelwort, Marsh Penny, Talepetrako, Thick-Leaved Pennywort, White Rot.
CAUTION: See separate listing for Cola Nut.

Scientific Names

Centella asiatica, synonym Hydrocotyle asiatica; Centella coriacea.
Family: Apiaceae or Umbelliferae.

People Use This For

Orally, gotu kola is used for venous insufficiency (6,18), wound healing, to reduce fatigue, promote longevity, and to improve memory and intelligence (4,11,3901).

Topically, gotu kola is used for skin inflammation and skin diseases, including ulcers, psoriasis, and fungal infections (4,6,11,18).

By injection, gotu kola is used to treat the bladder lesions of schistosomiasis (6), post-phlebitis ulcers, and scleroderma (11).

In Chinese medicine, gotu kola is used to treat colds, sunstroke, tonsillitis, pleurisy, urinary tract infection, hepatitis, jaundice, and dysentery, as an antidote for poisoning, and in poultices for snakebite, scabies, trauma, and shingles (11).

Historically, gotu kola has been used for skin diseases (5,6,11), leprosy (4,5,6,11), abscesses (5,6), syphilis (11), fever (5,6,11), jaundice (5,6), ulcers (5,6), rheumatism (4,5,6,11), mental illness (5,6), hypertension (5,6), epilepsy, fatigue, dehydration, urinary retention, diarrhea, eye diseases, inflammation, and asthma (18). It has also been used for amenorrhea, elephantiasis, lupus, tuberculosis, memory loss (11), and as an aphrodisiac (5,6).

In manufacturing, gotu kola leaf extracts are used as an ingredient in cosmetics (11).

Safety

POSSIBLY SAFE ...when above ground preparations are used orally and appropriately (6,12). However, Canadian regulations prohibit gotu kola as a non-medicinal ingredient for oral use products (12). ...when applied topically (4,6,12).

There is insufficient reliable information available about the safety of gotu kola use by injection.

PREGNANCY: LIKELY UNSAFE ...contraindicated for oral use because it might be an abortifacient (4).

LACTATION: Insufficient reliable information available; avoid using.

Effectiveness

POSSIBLY EFFECTIVE ...when the oral extract is taken for chronic venous insufficiency and to improve memory and intelligence (4,5,6,11,18). ...when applied topically for improved wound healing and treating various skin disorders, including psoriasis (4,6). ...when given by injection to treat the bladder lesions of schistosomiasis (bilharzial infections) (6).

There is insufficient reliable information available about the effectiveness of gotu kola for its other uses.

Possible Mechanism of Action & Active Ingredients

The applicable parts of gotu kola are the above ground parts. Tripterpenoid saponins (e.g., asiaticoside, madecassoside) might promote wound healing and decrease venous pressure in venous insufficiency (4,5,6,11,18); asiaticoside and madecassoside have anti-inflammatory activity (4,5,6,11). Preliminary evidence suggests that asiaticosides might promote wound healing by stimulating collagen and glycosaminoglycan synthesis (1890,2700). Asiaticosides elevate blood glucose, triglycerides and cholesterol levels, decrease urea nitrogen and acid phosphatase levels, and increase vital capacity. The asiaticoside derivatives, asiatic acid, asiaticoside 6, and SM2, protect neurons from beta-amyloid toxicity and might have a role in treating Alzheimer's disease (1889).

Adverse Reactions Including Known Allergies

Taken orally, gotu kola can cause whole body pruritus, photosensitivity, and may cause abortion (4). Large amounts may elevate blood pressure (4). Topical application can result in allergic contact dermatitis (6) and burning sensation (4). Pain and discoloration at injection site may occur with subcutaneous administration (6) and may be diminished with intramuscular administration (6).

Possible Interactions with Herbs & Other Dietary Supplements

HERBS WITH SEDATIVE PROPERTIES: Theoretically, concomitant use with herbs that have sedative properties might enhance therapeutic and adverse effects. These include calamus, calendula, California poppy, catnip, capsicum, celery, couch grass, elecampane, ginseng Siberian, German chamomile, goldenseal, hops, Jamaican dogwood, kava, lemon balm, sage, St. John's wort, sassafras, scullcap, shepherd's purse, stinging nettle, valerian, wild carrot, wild lettuce, withania root, and yerba mansa (4,19).

Possible Interactions with Drugs

CHOLESTEROL-REDUCING DRUGS: Theoretically, large doses can increase serum cholesterol, interfering with cholesterol-lowering drug therapy (4).

DIABETES DRUGS: Theoretically, large doses might increase blood glucose levels interfering with hypoglycemic drug therapy (4).

DRUGS WITH SEDATIVE PROPERTIES: Theoretically, concomitant use with drugs with sedative properties might cause additive effects and side effects (4).

Possible Interactions with Foods

No interactions are known to occur, and there is no known reason to expect a clinically significant interaction with gotu kola.

Possible Interactions with Lab Tests

No interactions are known to occur, and there is no known reason to expect a clinically significant interaction with gotu kola.

Possible Interactions with Diseases or Conditions

DIABETES: Can elevate blood glucose levels (4).
HYPERLIPIDEMIAS: Can elevate triglyceride and cholesterol levels (4).

Typical Dosages & Routes of Administration that are Commonly Used

ORAL: 600 mg dried leaves three times per day (18), or, one cup tea (steep 600 mg dried leaves in 150 mL boiling water 5-10 minutes, strain) three times per day (18). Clinical trials for venous insufficiency used 60-120 mg titrated extract per day for two months (780).
TOPICAL: No typical dosage.
INJECTION: No typical dosage.

Comments

Avoid confusion with cola nut.

GOUTWEED

This Product is Also Known As

Achweed, Ashweed, Bishop's Elder, Bishopsweed, Bishopswort, Eltroot, English Goatweed, Gout Herb, Goutwort, Ground Elder, Herb Gerard, Jack-Jump-About, Masterwort, Pigweed, Weyl Ash, White Ash.
CAUTION: See separate listings for Bishop's Weed and Masterwort.

Scientific Names

Aegopodium podagraria.

People Use This For

Orally, goutweed is used for gout and rheumatic disease. It is also used for hemorrhoids, kidney, bladder, and intestinal disorders (18).

Safety

There is insufficient reliable information available about the safety of goutweed.
Pregnancy and Lactation: Insufficient reliable information available.

Effectiveness

There is insufficient reliable information available about the effectiveness of goutweed.

Possible Mechanism of Action & Active Ingredients

The applicable parts of goutweed are the above ground parts. Goutweed contains a volatile oil, flavonol glycosides (hyperoside, isoquercitrin), and caffeic acid derivatives including chlorogenic acid (18).

Adverse Reactions Including Known Allergies

None reported.

Possible Interactions with Herbs & Other Dietary Supplements

Insufficient reliable information available.

Possible Interactions with Drugs

No interactions are known to occur, and there is no known reason to expect a clinically significant interaction with goutweed.

Possible Interactions with Foods

No interactions are known to occur, and there is no known reason to expect a clinically significant interaction with goutweed.

Possible Interactions with Lab Tests

No interactions are known to occur, and there is no known reason to expect a clinically significant interaction with goutweed.

Possible Interactions with Diseases or Conditions

No interactions are known to occur, and there is no known reason to expect a clinically significant interaction with goutweed.

Typical Dosages & Routes of Administration that are Commonly Used

ORAL: People typically use 2 to 4 mL of liquid goutweed extract (5264).
TOPICAL: The fresh herb is squeezed or softened by soaking in water for poultices (18).

Comments
Avoid confusion with bishop's weed (Ammi visnagae) and masterwort (Heracleum sphondylium and Heracleum lanatum).

GRAINS OF PARADISE

This Product is Also Known As
Guinea Grains, Mallaguetta Pepper, Melegueta Pepper.
CAUTION: See separate listing for Capsicum.

Scientific Names
Aframomum melegueta, synonym Amomum melegueta.
Family: Zingiberaceae.

People Use This For
Orally, grains of paradise fruit and seeds are used as a stimulant (18).

Safety
POSSIBLY SAFE ...when used orally and appropriately (12).
PREGNANCY AND LACTATION: Insufficient reliable information available; avoid using.

Effectiveness
There is insufficient reliable information available about the effectiveness of grains of paradise.

Possible Mechanism of Action & Active Ingredients
The applicable parts of grains of paradise are the fruit and seed. Grains of paradise contains a volatile oil and the constituents hydroxyphenylalkanones and hydroxyphenylalkanoles. The seed is said to be a stimulant (18).

Adverse Reactions Including Known Allergies
Theoretically, may cause GI and lower urinary tract irritation when taken orally (18).

Possible Interactions with Herbs & Other Dietary Supplements
Insufficient reliable information available.

Possible Interactions with Drugs
No interactions are known to occur, and there is no known reason to expect a clinically significant interaction with grains of paradise.

Possible Interactions with Foods
No interactions are known to occur, and there is no known reason to expect a clinically significant interaction with grains of paradise.

Possible Interactions with Lab Tests
No interactions are known to occur, and there is no known reason to expect a clinically significant interaction with grains of paradise.

Possible Interactions with Diseases or Conditions
No interactions are known to occur, and there is no known reason to expect a clinically significant interaction with grains of paradise.

Typical Dosages & Routes of Administration that are Commonly Used
ORAL: People typically use 4 to 6 grams added to 3 to 4 cups of water and boiled until the volume is reduced by one-half. The cooled liquid is taken in 3 doses on an empty stomach (5251).

Comments
Avoid confusion with capsicum (Capsicum annuum), also known as grains of paradise.

GRAPE fruit, skin

This Product is Also Known As
Black Grape Raisins, Cabernet Franc, Cabernet Sauvignon, Calzin, Chardonnay, Emperor, Enocianina, Flame Seedless, Grape, Grapes, Grape Fruit, Grape Fruit Skin, Grape Juice, Grape Skin, Grape Skin Extract, Merlot, Petite Sirah, Raisins, Red Globe, Red Malaga, Sauvignon Blanc, Sultanas, Table Grapes, Thompson Seedless, Wine Grapes.
CAUTION: See separate listings for Grape leaf, Grape seed, Grapefruit, Resveratrol, and Wine.

Scientific Names
Vitis vinifera.
Family: Vitaceae.

People Use This For
Orally, grapes and grape preparations, including grape skin and grape juice are used to prevent coronary heart disease (3579). They are also used as a dietary source of antioxidants (3579). Grapes have also been used for varicose veins, hemorrhoids, capillary fragility, and as a mild laxative for constipation. Grape fasts have been used for "detoxification." Dried grapes, raisins or sultanas, have been used as an expectorant for cough (4201). In beverages and drink mixes, including wine, grape skin extract is used as a coloring agent (11).

Safety
LIKELY SAFE ...when used orally in amounts found in foods (11,18). Grape skin extracts have been approved for beverage use only (11).
There is insufficient reliable information available about the safety of grape fruit or skin for its other uses.
PREGNANCY AND LACTATION: LIKELY SAFE ...when used orally in amounts found in foods (11,18). There is insufficient reliable information available about the safety of grape fruit or skin for its other uses.

Effectiveness
There is insufficient reliable information available about the effectiveness of grape fruit or skin.

Possible Mechanism of Action & Active Ingredients
Grapes and grape preparations provide a variety of constituents that are thought to be pharmacologically active. Various types of phenolic compounds, including anthocyanins, cinnamates, and flavan-3-ols, are thought to provide benefit in the prevention of heart disease. These phenolic compounds are thought to have antioxidant properties and play a role in prevention of low-density lipoprotein (LDL) oxidation. In an in vitro study, a variety of grapes were tested for phenol content and ability to prevent LDL oxidation. Inhibition of oxidation ranged from 22% to 91% at higher concentrations. Red grape varieties tended to produce more oxidation protection than white or blush grape varieties. A similar trend has been seen with red versus white wines. There was a significant correlation between total phenol content and anthocyanin content and antioxidant activity. Phenol content in red grapes is primarily from anthocyanins, which are responsible producing the color in red grapes (3579). Grapes are also reported to have laxative and expectorant properties (4201). Black grape raisins are thought to have similar antioxidant potential as red wine (2540). Grape skin extract also contains anthocyanin pigments (11). Some evidence suggests that anthocyanins might strengthen capillaries and have antifungal and antibacterial activity (11). The anthocyanidins delphinidin and delphinidin/cyanidin dimer show some evidence that they might induce chromosomal damage (4074).

Adverse Reactions Including Known Allergies
Excessive consumption of grapes or dried grapes, raisins or sultanas, might cause diarrhea due to laxative effects (4201). There is one report of an anaphylactic reaction to grape skin extract, which included urticaria and angioedema (4073).

Possible Interactions with Herbs & Other Dietary Supplements
LACTOBACILLUS ACIDOPHILUS: Grape anthocyanins can inhibit the growth of Lactobacillus acidophilus. Concurrent administration might prevent Lactobacillus acidophilus colonization of the gastrointestinal tract (11); avoid concurrent use.

Possible Interactions with Drugs
PHENACETIN: Grape juice decreases phenactin, but not acetaminophen plasma levels. It may decrease levels by inducing cytochrome P450 1A2 (CYP 1A2) metabolism (2539).
OTHERS: Grape juice is thought to induce cytochrome P450 1A2 (CYP 1A2) metabolism and may decrease plasma levels of substrates of CYP 1A2. Drugs metabolized by CYP 1A2 include amitriptyline (Elavil), caffeine, chlordiazepoxide (Librium), clomipramine (Anafranil), clopidogrel (Plavix), clozapine (Clozaril), cyclobenzaprine (Flexaril), desipramine (Norpramin), diazepam (Valium), estradiol (Estrace, others), flutamide (Eulexin), fluvoxamine (Luvox), grepafloxacin (Raxar), haloperidol (Haldol), imipramine (Tofranil), mexiletine (Mexitil), mirtazapine (Remeron), naproxen (Naprosyn), nortriptyline (Pamelor), olanzapine (Zyprexa), ondansetron (Zofran), propafenone (Rythmol), propranolol (Inderal), riluzole (Rilutek), ropinirole (Requip), ropivacaine (Naropin), tacrine (Cognex), theophylline (TheoDur, others), verapamil (Calan, Covera-HS, others), warfarin (Coumadin), and zileuton (Zyflo).

Possible Interactions with Foods
No interactions are known to occur, and there is no known reason to expect a clinically significant interaction with grape fruit or skin.

Possible Interactions with Lab Tests
No interactions are known to occur, and there is no known reason to expect a clinically significant interaction with grape fruit or skin.

 © Copyright 2000, Natural Medicines Comprehensive Database (209) 472-2244. For updated data, go to www.NaturalDatabase.com

Possible Interactions with Diseases or Conditions

No interactions are known to occur, and there is no known reason to expect a clinically significant interaction with grape fruit or skin.

Typical Dosages & Routes of Administration that are Commonly Used

No typical dosage.

Comments

None.

GRAPE leaf

This Product is Also Known As

Folia Vitis Viniferae, Grape Leaf Extract, Red Vine Leaf Extract, Red Vine Leaf AS 195.
CAUTION: See separate listings for Grape Seed; Grape Fruit; Skin; Resveratrol; and Grapefruit.

Scientific Names

Vitis vinifera.
Family: Vitaceae.

People Use This For

Orally, grape leaf is used for vascular or circulatory disorders, especially venous diseases (18) such as chronic venous insufficiency (2538), varicose veins, and edema (4201). It is also used for attention deficit-hyperactivity disorder (ADHD) (3578), diarrhea, heavy menstrual bleeding, uterine hemorrhage, hemorrhoids, and canker sores (4201).
Intravaginally, grape leaf infusions are used as a douche (4201).
Grape leaf is used as a food, particularly in Greek cooking.

Safety

LIKELY SAFE ...when used orally in amounts found in foods (18).
POSSIBLY SAFE ...when used orally and appropriately for medicinal purposes. Significant adverse effects have not been reported (18). In one study using a grape leaf extract, no significant adverse events were reported during 12 weeks of treatment (2538).
PREGNANCY AND LACTATION: Insufficient reliable information available; avoid using.

Effectiveness

POSSIBLY EFFECTIVE ...when used orally for mild to moderate chronic renal insufficiency. In one clinical trial, a specific grape leaf extract, known as red vine leaf extract AS 195 (Antistax, Boehringer Ingelheim), was given to 260 patients with stage I and stage II chronic venous insufficiency for 12 weeks. Leg edema significantly decreased after 6 weeks of treatment compared to placebo. Doses of 360 mg and 720 mg daily were both effective, but the higher dose produced a slightly greater effect. Patients also reported significant decreases in subjective complaints such as tired or heavy legs, tension, and tingling and pain after 12 weeks of treatment (2538).
There is insufficient reliable information available about the effectiveness of grape leaf for its other uses.

Possible Mechanism of Action & Active Ingredients

Grape leaf preparations contain flavonoids that are thought to be responsible for its pharmacological effects (18).
The red vine grape extract AS 195 (Antistax, Boehringer Ingelheim) used in one clinical trial primarily contains the flavonoids quercetin-3-O-beta-glucuronide and isoquercitrin (2538). However, its mechanism of action in chronic venous insufficiency is not clearly understood. Grape leaf is reported to have antiinflammatory and astringent properties (18,4201). These properties are reported to be greatest in the red leaves (4201).

Adverse Reactions Including Known Allergies

In one study, the most common adverse effects were gastrointestinal and included abdominal discomfort, diarrhea, dyspepsia, dry mouth, and retching. Other adverse effects included infections, headache and musculoskeletal disorders. One case of leg hematoma following a minor trauma was also reported in a person using grape leaf extract (2538).

Possible Interactions with Herbs & Other Dietary Supplements

Insufficient reliable information available.

Possible Interactions with Drugs

No interactions are known to occur, and there is no known reason to expect a clinically significant interaction with grape leaf.

Possible Interactions with Foods

No interactions are known to occur, and there is no known reason to expect a clinically significant interaction with grape leaf.

Possible Interactions with Lab Tests

No interactions are known to occur, and there is no known reason to expect a clinically significant interaction with grape leaf.

Possible Interactions with Diseases or Conditions

No interactions are known to occur, and there is no known reason to expect a clinically significant interaction with grape leaf.

Typical Dosages & Routes of Administration that are Commonly Used

ORAL: For chronic venous insufficiency, one clinical trial used a standardized red vine grape extract AS 195 (Antistax, Boehringer Ingelheim). The dose used was 360 mg or 720 mg once daily (2538).

Comments

None.

GRAPE seed

This Product is Also Known As

Extrait De Pepins De Raisin, Grape Seed Extract, Grape Seed Oil, Muskat, OPC, OPCs, Oligomeric Proanthocyanidins, Oligomeric Procyanidins, PCO, PCOs, Procyanidolic Oligomers.
CAUTION: See separate listings for Grape leaf; Grape Fruit, Skin; Pycnogenol; and Resveratrol.

Scientific Names

Vitis vinifera; Vitis coignetiae.
Family: Vitaceae.

People Use This For

Orally, grape seed extract is used for treating and preventing vascular or circulatory disorders including venous insufficiency, varicose veins, atherosclerosis, peripheral vascular disease, edema associated with injury or surgery, and myocardial or cerebral infarction (402,3900,3580). Grape seed extract is also used for hemorrhoids (3580), strengthening blood vessels, inflammation, diabetic complications such as neuropathy or retinopathy (3580,3900), improving wound healing, preventing dental caries (6,3900), cancer prevention, macular degeneration, poor night vision, liver cirrhosis, allergies, and prevention of collagen breakdown associated with collagen diseases and aging (3580,3900). Grape seed oil is used as a supplemental dietary source of essential fatty acids and tocopherols (6).

Safety

LIKELY SAFE ...in the amounts commonly found in foods (6,402).
POSSIBLY SAFE ...when used orally and appropriately for medicinal purposes (6,402).
PREGNANCY AND LACTATION: Insufficient reliable information available; avoid amounts greater than those found in foods.

Effectiveness

POSSIBLY EFFECTIVE ...when grape seed oil is used orally as a supplemental dietary source of essential fatty acids and tocopherols. Ground grape seeds produce an oil that is rich in essential fatty acids and tocopherols (6). ...when grape seed extract is used for treating chronic venous insufficiency. Multiple small European clinical trials have shown grape seed extract or its procyanidin constituents to be superior to placebo for reducing subjective symptoms and improving venous tone (2541). ...when grape seed extract is used for decreasing ocular stress from glare (2541). Multiple small European clinical trials have shown grape seed extract containing procyanidin constituents to be superior to placebo (2541).
There is insufficient reliable information available to rate the effectiveness of grape seed for its other uses. However, preliminary research suggests it might also be beneficial for improving night vision. In one 6-week unblinded study, healthy volunteers had improved night vision after using grape seed extract containing procyanidins (3580). Further research is needed to rate the effectiveness of grape seed for this use.

Possible Mechanism of Action & Active Ingredients

Grape seeds are typically obtained as a by-product of the manufacturing of wine (6). Constituents called oligomeric proanthocyanidins (OPCs) or procyanidins are thought to be responsible for grape seed's pharmacological effects. OPCs from grape seed are theorized to be beneficial to prevent and treat cardiovascular and circulatory conditions due to antioxidant and potential antilipoperoxidant activity (6,3900). OPCs are also thought to inhibit the proteolytic enzymes collagenase, elastase, hyaluronidase, and beta glucuronidase, which are involved in the breakdown of structural components of the vasculature and skin (6,3900). For prevention of dental caries, grape seed is thought to work by inhibiting the growth of Streptococcus mutans and preventing glucan formation from sucrose (6). These pharmacological effects have not yet been clearly demonstrated in humans. Ground grape seeds produce an oil that is rich in essential fatty acids and tocopherol (6).

Adverse Reactions Including Known Allergies
None reported (6,402).

Possible Interactions with Herbs & Other Dietary Supplements
Insufficient reliable information available.

Possible Interactions with Drugs
WARFARIN: Theoretically, due to the tocopherol content of grape seed oil, concomitant use with warfarin might increase warfarin's effects and the risk of bleeding (402); use with caution.

Possible Interactions with Foods
No interactions are known to occur, and there is no known reason to expect a clinically significant interaction with grape seed.

Possible Interactions with Lab Tests
No interactions are known to occur, and there is no known reason to expect a clinically significant interaction with grape seed.

Possible Interactions with Diseases or Conditions
No interactions are known to occur, and there is no known reason to expect a clinically significant interaction with grape seed.

Typical Dosages & Routes of Administration that are Commonly Used
ORAL: Grape seed extract as tablets or capsules dosed at 75-300 mg daily for three weeks followed by a maintenance dose of 40-80 mg daily has been suggested by some sources (402,3900). For chronic venous insufficiency, grape seed extract procyanidin doses of 150-300 mg per day have been used (2541). For reducing ocular stress due to glare, grape seed extract procyanidin doses of 200-300 mg per day have been used (2541).

Comments
Pycnogenol (pinebark extract) is similar to the grape seed extract in active ingredients and medicinal uses (7,402). Both pycnogenol and grape seed contain oligomeric proanthocyanidins (OPCs). Several other natural medicines contain constituents that are similar to the OPCs, including wine, cranberries, bilberries, green and black teas, black currant, onions, legumes, parsley, and hawthorn (3580).

GRAPEFRUIT

This Product is Also Known As
Paradisapfel, Pomelo, Toronja.
CAUTION: See separate listing for grapefruit seed extract, grapefruit oil.

Scientific Names
Citrus paradisi.
Family: Rutaceae.

People Use This For
Orally, grapefruit is used for reducing cholesterol and reversing atherosclerosis, as a supplemental source of potassium, vitamin C, and fiber; for reducing hematocrit, as an anti-cancer agent, and as an aid in weight reduction (6).
In combination with cyclosporine, grapefruit is used for treating psoriasis (6).
For food uses, grapefruit is consumed as fruit and juice (6).

Safety
LIKELY SAFE ...when used orally in food amounts.
There is insufficient reliable information available about the safety of very large amounts of grapefruit.
PREGNANCY AND LACTATION: LIKELY SAFE ...when used in food amounts; avoid excessive amounts.

Effectiveness
There is insufficient reliable information available about effectiveness of grapefruit.

Possible Mechanism of Action & Active Ingredients
The applicable parts of grapefruit are the fruit and juice. Whole grapefruit is high in water and fiber. It is a good dietary source of potassium, vitamin C, pectin, and other nutrients (6). Grapefruit juice contains furanocoumarins, including bergamottin and dihydroxybergamottin, which inhibit cytochrome P450 3A4 (CYP3A4) (3769,5070,5071). In addition, bergamottin inhibits CYPs 1A2, 2A6, 2C9, 2C19, 2D6, and 2E1 (5072). Grapefruit juice also contains naringin, naringenin, limonin, and obacunone which are known to inhibit human hepatic microsomes (6). Grapefruit pectin, which is found in whole fruit but not juice, can reduce cholesterol and promote regression of

© Copyright 2000, Natural Medicines Comprehensive Database (209) 472-2244. For updated data, go to www.NaturalDatabase.com

atherosclerosis (6). Studies suggest grapefruit can affect blood components. Some evidence suggests the constituent, naringin, might induce red cell aggregation. Consuming one half to one grapefruit per day can reduce an individual's hematocrit level (6). An analysis of grapefruit's anti-cancer effects suggests that consumption might reduce the risk of pancreatic cancer (6). Grapefruit juice inhibits hepatic and gut wall CYP3A4. Grapefruit juice increases bioavailability and plasma concentrations of numerous drugs (see Interactions with Drugs) (1386). Human research indicates that blended grapefruit segments, and an extract of grapefruit core and peel, also inhibit CYP3A4 activity (1388). Evidence suggests that grapefruit juice inhibits p-glycoprotein counter-transport activity. P-glycoprotein is thought to reduce the absorption of some drugs by pumping them back into the gut (1390). Grapefruit juice might enhance absorption of some drugs affected by p-glycoprotein activity. However, the clinical effect of grapefruit juice on drugs affected by p-glycoprotein activity requires further investigation. It may be necessary to withhold grapefruit juice for 3 days to avoid interactions with felodipine and nisoldipine (5068,5069).

Adverse Reactions Including Known Allergies

Grapefruit has few reported adverse reactions. One study shows it can reduce hematocrit (531). One case report associates grapefruit juice with hypotension (6).

Possible Interactions with Herbs & Other Dietary Supplements

RED YEAST (Cholestin): Concomitant use of grapefruit with red yeast increases the serum levels of lovastatin, a constituent of red yeast (527).

Possible Interactions with Drugs

ARTEMETHER (Artenam, Paluther): Grapefruit juice increases the oral bioavailability of artemether in healthy men by 90-250% (5065,5066).

BENZODIAZEPINES: Some studies suggest that grapefruit juice increases the maximum blood levels and duration of effect of midazolam (Versed) and triazolam (Halcion); other studies suggest there is no effect (4300). Grapefruit juice increases the maximum blood levels and duration of effect of diazepam (Valium), but the clinical significance of this is not known (3228).

BUSPIRONE (Buspar): Grapefruit juice increases absorption and plasma concentrations of buspirone (3771).

CAFFEINE: Some studies suggest grapefruit juice decreases caffeine clearance, possibly increasing the effects or adverse effects; others disagree (4300).

CALCIUM CHANNEL BLOCKERS: Grapefruit juice increases absorption and plasma concentrations of amlodipine (Norvasc) (523), nifedipine (Procardia, Adalat) (528), nisoldipine (Sular) (529), felodipine (Plendil), nimodipine (Nimotop), nicardipine (Cardura), diltiazem (Cardizem) (524,528,1388,4300) and verapamil (Calan, Isoptin, Verelan) (3229). Some references dispute the clinical relevance of the interactions with amlodipine, diltiazem, and verapamil (3230,4300). In healthy older adults, the hemodynamic response to felodipine (Plendil) plus grapefruit juice might be influenced by altered autonomic regulation. In older healthy adults, a single dose of grapefruit juice and felodipine enhanced the blood pressure lowering effects of felodipine. However, after a week of grapefruit juice and felodipine (steady state), the hypotensive activity was reduced, possibly due to compensatory tachycardia (1392). Research suggests it is necessary to withholding grapefruit juice for 3 days to avoid interactions with felodipine and nisoldipine (5068,5069).

CARBAMAZEPINE (Tegretol): Grapefruit juice increases absorption and plasma concentrations of carbamazepine (524).

CARVEDILOL (Coreg): Grapefruit juice is reported to increase the bioavailability of a single dose of carvediolol by 16% (5071).

CISAPRIDE (Propulsid): Grapefruit juice increases absorption and plasma concentrations of cisapride (1383,3226).

CLOMIPRAMINE (Anafranil): Grapefruit juice increases blood levels of clomipramine. Two cases are reported in which trough clomipramine blood levels increased significantly after adding grapefruit juice to the therapeutic regimen (5064).

CYCLOSPORINE (Neoral, Sandimmune): Grapefruit juice increases absorption and plasma concentrations of cyclosporine (522).

ESTROGENS: Grapefruit juice increases absorption and plasma concentrations of 17-beta-estradiol (526) and ethinyl-estradiol (525).

HMG-CO A REDUCTASE INHIBITORS: Grapefruit juice increases absorption and plasma concentrations of lovastatin (Mevacor) (527), simvastatin (Zocor) (3774), and atorvastatin (Lipitor) (3227). It does not affect pravastatin (3227).

ITRACONAZOLE (Sporanox): Grapefruit juice impairs itraconazole absorption (310,3772).

LOSARTAN (Cozaar): Concomitant use of grapefruit juice and losartan might reduce losartan effectiveness, but this requires further study. Losartan is an inactive prodrug which must be metabolized to its active form, E-3174, to be effective. In one human study, grapefruit juice reduced losartan metabolism, increased losartan AUC, and reduced the AUC of the major active losartan metabolite, E-3174 (1391).

QUINIDINE: Grapefruit juice decreases quinidine clearance and prolongs the half-life by about 20% (5067). The clinical effect of this interaction is unknown.

SAQUINAVIR (Fortovase, Invirase): Grapefruit juice increases absorption and plasma concentrations of the protease inhibitor (PI)-type antiretroviral drug saquinavir (3773).

TERFENADINE (Seldane): Grapefruit juice increases absorption and plasma concentrations of terfenadine (530).

WARFARIN (Coumadin): Grapefruit juice might increase warfarin effects. One case is reported of significantly increased international normalized ratio (INR) associated with consumption of 50 ounces of grapefruit juice daily; no evidence of bleeding was reported. In a small clinical trial, consumption of 24 ounces of grapefruit juice daily for one week had no effect on INR in a group of men anticoagulated with warfarin.

Possible Interactions with Foods
No interactions are known to occur, and there is no known reason to expect a clinically significant interaction with grapefruit.

Possible Interactions with Lab Tests
DRUG ASSAYS: Grapefruit juice decreases metabolism, increasing plasma concentrations and test results of amlodipine (Norvasc) (523), nifedipine (Procardia, Adalat) (528), nisoldipine (Sular) (529), felodipine (Plendil), nimodipine (Nimotop), nicardipine (Cardene), diltiazem (Cardizem, Dilacor XR, Tiazac) (524,528,1388,4300), verapamil (Calan, Isoptin, Verelan) (3229), buspirone (BuSpar) (3771), midazolam (Versed) and triazolam (Halcion) (4300), diazepam (Valium) (3228), carbamazepine (Tegretol) (524), cisapride (Propulsid) (3226), cyclosporine (Sandimmune, Neoral) (522), 17-beta-estradiol (526), ethinyl-estradiol (525), lovastatin (Mevacor) (527), saquinavir (Fortovase, Invirase) (3773), simvastatin (Zocor) (3774), atorvastatin (Lipitor) (3227), and terfenadine (530).
LOSARTAN (Cozaaar): Grapefruit juice might increase plasma losartan concentrations, reduce plasma E-3174 concentrations, and test results. Losartan is an inactive prodrug which must be metabolized to its active form, E-3174, to be effective. In one human study, grapefruit juice reduced losartan metabolism, increased losartan AUC, and reduced the AUC of the major active losartan metabolite, E-3174 (1391).

Possible Interactions with Diseases or Conditions
No interactions are known to occur, and there is no known reason to expect a clinically significant interaction with grapefruit.

Typical Dosages & Routes of Administration that are Commonly Used
ORAL: The pharmacologic effects of grapefruit juice seem to be most pronounced when people consume over four glasses of the juice per day. When using grapefruit juice to increase effect and decrease dose of cyclosporine, it is important to avoid fluctuations in grapefruit juice intake, brand used if a commercial product used, variety of grapefruit if juice is freshly made, and the means of processing used to extract juice (6). However, grapefruit juice should not be used to lower the dose of cyclosporine because it is too unpredictable.

Comments
Drug interactions with grapefruit juice are well documented. The chemistry of the grapefruit varies by the species, the growing conditions, and the process used to extract the juice. Because grapefruit juice is not standardized, use as an adjunct to drug therapy is not recommended (3775).

GRAPEFRUIT OIL

This Product is Also Known As
Cold-Pressed Grapefruit Oil, Expressed Grapefruit Oil, Shaddock Oil.
CAUTION: See separate listing for grapefruit, grapefruit seed extract.

Scientific Names
Citrus X paradisi, synonyms Citrus racemosa, Citrus decumana, Citrus maxima.
Family: Rutaceae.

People Use This For
Topically, grapefruit oil is used to relieve muscle fatigue, to promote hair growth, for toning the skin, and for reducing acne and oily skin. It is also used to aid with the common cold and flu.
Inhaled, the vapors are used to help the body retain water and to relieve headache and stress. The aroma is used to relieve depression.
In food and beverages, grapefruit oil is used as a flavoring component (11).
In manufacturing, grapefruit oil is used as a fragrance component in soaps and cosmetics.

Safety
LIKELY SAFE ...when used in amounts found in foods. Grapefruit oil has Generally Recognized as Safe (GRAS) status in the US. The highest concentrations of grapefruit oil in foods is 0.108% (11). ...when used in amounts found in perfumes and cosmetics. The highest concentrations of grapefruit oil in these products is 1.0% (11).
There is insufficient reliable information available about the safety of topical or inhaled grapefruit oil used medicinally.
PREGNANCY AND LACTATION: LIKELY SAFE ...when used in food amounts. There is insufficient reliable information available about the safety of larger amounts used during pregnancy and lactation; avoid using.

Effectiveness
There is insufficient reliable information available about the effectiveness of grapefruit oil.

Possible Mechanism of Action & Active Ingredients

Grapefruit oil is obtained by cold expression from the fruit peel of the Citrus X paradisi tree (11). Antibacterial activity has been suggested. Grapefruit oil contains furocoumarins, including bergaptens, which are photosensitizing, phototoxic, and mutagenic (2). They are responsible for adverse dermatological reactions in other plants that contain them (see separate listings for angelica and rue) (11,515). Animal data suggests that 9,10-dimethyl-1,2-benzanthracene, the primary carcinogen, promoted tumor formation when grapefruit oil was applied directly to the skin. Dermatological studies have suggested that grapefruit oil is nonirritating, nonsensitizing, and nonphototoxic to human skin (11).

Adverse Reactions Including Known Allergies

Contact dermatitis and phototoxic reactions, including skin blisters, have occurred with other furocoumarin-containing herbs following topical exposure and exposure to sunlight (11).

Possible Interactions with Herbs & Other Dietary Supplements

Insufficient reliable information available.

Possible Interactions with Drugs

No interactions are known to occur, and there is no known reason to expect a clinically significant interaction with grapefruit oil.

Possible Interactions with Foods

No interactions are known to occur, and there is no known reason to expect a clinically significant interaction with grapefruit oil.

Possible Interactions with Lab Tests

No interactions are known to occur, and there is no known reason to expect a clinically significant interaction with grapefruit oil.

Possible Interactions with Diseases or Conditions

No interactions are known to occur, and there is no known reason to expect a clinically significant interaction with grapefruit oil.

Typical Dosages & Routes of Administration that are Commonly Used

No typical dosage.

Comments

None.

GRAVEL ROOT

This Product is Also Known As

Joe Pye, Joe-Pye Weed, Kidney Root, Kydney Root, Purple Boneset, Queen of the Meadow, Roter Wasserhanf, Trumpet Weed.
CAUTION: See separate listings for Boneset.

Scientific Names

Eupatorium purpureum.
Family: Asteraceae or Compositae.

People Use This For

Orally, gravel root is used for urinary calculus, renal or vesicular calculi, cystitis, painful urination, urethritis, prostatitis, rheumatism, and gout (4). It is also used orally for fever from malaria, dengue virus, fever, typhus, as an antacid, aperitif, diuretic, emetic, stimulant, tonic, and for inducing sweating (4017).

Safety

UNSAFE ...when used orally. Gravel root contains hepatotoxic unsaturated pyrrolizidine alkaloids (UPAs) (12,19). Repeated exposure to low concentrations of UPAs is linked to veno-occlusive disease, a serious condition (4,12). UPAs may also be carcinogenic and mutagenic (12). Topical use on abraded or broken skin might be unsafe due to potential for systemic absorption (12,19).
PREGNANCY: UNSAFE ...contraindicated (12,19). Animal data suggests gravel root might be an abortifacient (19).
LACTATION: UNSAFE ...contraindicated due to concern that UPAs might be excreted into breast milk (4,12,18,19).

Effectiveness

There is insufficient reliable information available about the effectiveness of gravel root.

Possible Mechanism of Action & Active Ingredients

The applicable parts of gravel root are the above ground parts and rhizome/root. Although people think gravel root has antilithic, diuretic, and antirheumatic properties (4), this has not been studied. Some evidence suggests an ethanolic extract might have anti-inflammatory activity (4020). The above ground parts of gravel root contain echinatine, an unsaturated pyrrolizidine alkaloid (UPA) (4). Pyrrolizidine alkaloids with an unsaturated pyrrolizidine nucleus can be hepatotoxic in animals and humans (4). Herbs containing UPAs have shown carcinogenic, mutagenic, and renal toxic effects. However, the primary concern is veno-occlusive disease (12).

Adverse Reactions Including Known Allergies
Although no adverse effects are reported for gravel root/rhizome, chronic exposure to other plants containing UPA constituents has been associated with veno-occlusive disease (4021). Symptoms of acute veno-occlusive disease are characterized by a dull, dragging ache in the right upper abdomen and marked distention of the abdomen. These symptoms are sometimes accompanied by reduced urine output. Subacute veno-occlusive disease is associated with vague symptoms and persistent liver enlargement (4021). Gravel root can cause an allergic reaction in individuals sensitive to the Asteraceae/Compositae family. Members of this family include ragweed, chrysanthemums, marigolds, daisies, and many other herbs.

Possible Interactions with Herbs & Other Dietary Supplements
EUCALYPTUS: Theoretically, concomitant use might increase the risk of unsaturated pyrrolizidine alkaloid toxicity due to enzyme induction by eucalyptus (19).
PYRROLIZIDINE ALKALOID-CONTAINING HERBS: Concomitant use is contraindicated due to the risk of additive toxicity. Herbs containing unsaturated pyrrolizidine alkaloids include: alkanna (12), borage (271), gravel root (4), hemp agrimony (271), hound's tongue (19), petasites (19), comfrey (271), coltsfoot, and the Senecio species plants; dusty miller (19), alpine ragwort (19), groundsel (271), golden ragwort (19), and tansy ragwort (271).

Possible Interactions with Drugs
No interactions are known to occur, and there is no known reason to expect a clinically significant interaction with gravel root.

Possible Interactions with Foods
No interactions are known to occur, and there is no known reason to expect a clinically significant interaction with gravel root.

Possible Interactions with Lab Tests
No interactions are known to occur, and there is no known reason to expect a clinically significant interaction with gravel root.

Possible Interactions with Diseases or Conditions
LIVER DISEASE: Contraindicated due to hepatotoxic potential (19).
CROSS-ALLERGENICITY: Can cause an allergic reaction in individuals sensitive to the Asteraceae/Compositae family. Members of this family include ragweed, chrysanthemums, marigolds, daisies, and many other herbs.

Typical Dosages & Routes of Administration that are Commonly Used
No typical dosage.

Comments
Gravel root is considered unsafe for oral use; avoid due to hepatotoxic pyrrolizidine alkaloid content.

GREAT PLANTAIN

This Product is Also Known As
Common Plantain, General Plantain, Greater Plantain.
CAUTION: See separate listings for Buckhorn Plantain, Blond Psyllium, Black Psyllium, and Water Plantain.

Scientific Names
Plantago major.
Family: Plantaginaceae.

People Use This For
Historically, great plantain has been used for cystitis with hematuria, bronchitis, colds, irritated or bleeding hemorrhoids (4), dermatological conditions, and eye irritation or discomfort (514).

Safety
POSSIBLY SAFE …when the leaf is used orally and appropriately (12).
POSSIBLY UNSAFE …when used topically. Great plantain can cause allergic contact dermatitis (4).
PREGNANCY: LIKELY UNSAFE …contraindicated because it can increase uterine tone (4).
LACTATION: Insufficient reliable information available; avoid using.

Effectiveness

POSSIBLY EFFECTIVE ...when used orally for treating spastic and nonspastic chronic bronchitis, and for treating symptoms of the common cold (4).
There is insufficient reliable information available about the effectiveness of great plantain for its other uses.

Possible Mechanism of Action & Active Ingredients

The applicable part of great plantain is the leaf. Great plantain contains low levels of tannins (4), and relatively high concentrations of vitamin K, beta-carotene, and calcium (19). It also contains a variety of acids, amino acids, carbohydrates, and iridoids (4). The anti-inflammatory and wound-healing effects demonstrated in animal studies are attributed to the constituents chlorogenic acid and neochlorogenic acid (4). Studies in humans show great plantain is beneficial in treating chronic bronchitis and the common cold (4). In guinea pigs, an aqueous extract had bronchodilator effects; however, effects were less and had shorter duration than salbutamol or atropine (4). In animals, great plantain extract also lowers blood pressure, and decreases total plasma lipids, cholesterol, and triglycerides (4). In vitro, an aqueous extract increases animal uterine tissue tone (4), and fresh juice has antibacterial activity (4). Great plantain inhibits carcinogenesis and mammary tumor formation in experimental animals (6).

Adverse Reactions Including Known Allergies

Excessive amounts taken orally may have laxative and hypotensive effects (4). Topical application can cause allergic contact dermatitis (4).

Possible Interactions with Herbs & Other Dietary Supplements

HERBS WITH CLOTTING POTENTIAL: Excessive use of herbs that contain vitamin K, an essential coagulation factor, can increase the risk of clotting in people using anticoagulants. These herbs include: alfalfa, parsley, nettle, plantain, and others.

Possible Interactions with Drugs

WARFARIN (Coumadin): Theoretically, consumption of large amounts of great plantain may antagonize drug effects due to vitamin K content. Individuals using anticoagulants should consume a consistent daily amount to maintain effect of anticoagulation therapy (19).

Possible Interactions with Foods

No interactions are known to occur, and there is no known reason to expect a clinically significant interaction with great plantain.

Possible Interactions with Lab Tests

BLOOD CLOTTING TESTS: Theoretically, consumption of large amounts of great plantain may reduce clotting time and test results due to vitamin K content (19).

Possible Interactions with Diseases or Conditions

PLANTAIN HYPERSENSITIVITY: Contraindicated.
MELON ALLERGY: Plantago species pollen may cause cross-reactivity in people allergic to melon (4075).

Typical Dosages & Routes of Administration that are Commonly Used

ORAL: 2-4 grams dried leaf three times daily, or one cup tea (steep 2-4 grams dried leaf in 150 mL boiling water 5-10 minutes, strain) three times daily (4). Liquid extract (1:1 in 25% in ethanol) 2-4 mL three times daily. Tincture (1:5 in 45% in ethanol) 2-4 mL three times daily (4).

Comments

Avoid confusion with Buckhorn plantain (Plantago lanceolata), Blond psyllium (Plantago ovata), and Black psyllium (Plantago psyllium).

GREATER BINDWEED

This Product is Also Known As

Bearbind, Bear's-Bind, Devil's Vine, Hedge Bindweed, Hedge Convolvulus, Hedge Lily, Lady's Nightcap, Old Man's Night Cap, Rutland Beauty.

Scientific Names

Calystegia sepium.
Family: Convolvulaceae.

People Use This For

Orally, greater bindweed is used for fever, urinary tract diseases, as a purgative for constipation, and for increasing bile production (18).

Safety

POSSIBLY UNSAFE ...when the whole plant is used orally because it has strong contact cathartic effects (514).
PREGNANCY AND LACTATION: POSSIBLY UNSAFE; avoid using.

Effectiveness

There is insufficient reliable information available about the effectiveness of greater bindweed.

Possible Mechanism of Action & Active Ingredients

Greater bindweed is said to be a potent smooth muscle stimulant and to increase bile production (18). Constituent gluco-resins (glycoretins) are contact cathartics which cause an increase in water elimination and peristalsis (514).

Adverse Reactions Including Known Allergies

Theoretically, large amounts may cause intestinal and stomach pain (18).

Possible Interactions with Herbs & Other Dietary Supplements

STIMULANT LAXATIVE HERBS: Theoretically, concomitant use with other stimulant laxative herbs may increase the risk of potassium depletion. Stimulant laxative herbs include: aloe dried leaf sap, blue flag rhizome, alder buckthorn, European buckthorn, butternut bark, cascara bark, castor oil, colocynth fruit pulp, gamboge bark exudate, jalap root, black root, manna bark exudate, podophyllum root, rhubarb root, senna leaves and pods, wild cucumber fruit (Ecballium elaterium), and yellow dock root (19).
CARDIAC GLYCOSIDE-CONTAINING HERBS: Concomitant use may increase the risk of cardiac glycoside toxicity. Cardiac glycoside-containing herbs include: black hellebore, Canadian hemp roots, digitalis leaf, hedge mustard, figwort, lily-of-the-valley roots, motherwort, oleander leaf, pheasant's eye plant, pleurisy root, squill bulb leaf scales, and strophanthus seeds (2,18,19,500).
LICORICE/HORSETAIL: Theoretically, overuse/misuse of licorice rhizome or horsetail plant with cardiac glycoside-containing herbs increases the risk of cardiac toxicity due to potassium depletion. (19).

Possible Interactions with Drugs

CARDIAC GLYCOSIDE DRUGS: Theoretically, overuse/abuse of this product increases the risk of adverse effects of cardiac glycoside drugs, e.g., digoxin (Lanoxin).

Possible Interactions with Foods

No interactions are known to occur, and there is no known reason to expect a clinically significant interaction with greater bindweed.

Possible Interactions with Lab Tests

No interactions are known to occur, and there is no known reason to expect a clinically significant interaction with greater bindweed.

Possible Interactions with Diseases or Conditions

GI CONDITIONS: Contraindicated in individuals with intestinal obstruction, abdominal pain of unknown origin, or any inflammatory condition of intestines (appendicitis, colitis, Crohn's disease, irritable bowel syndrome) (12).

Typical Dosages & Routes of Administration that are Commonly Used

ORAL: People typically use one level teaspoon of the powdered root once or twice daily. A liquid is prepared by boiling 1 teaspoon of the flowering plant in 1 cup of water. This is taken 1 tablespoon at a time, as needed.

Comments

None.

GREATER BURNET

This Product is Also Known As

Garden Burnet, Sanguisorba.

Scientific Names

Sanguisorba officinalis.
Family: Rosaceae.

People Use This For

Orally, greater burnet is used for heavy menstrual flow during menopause, hot flashes, irregular menstrual flow, ulcerative colitis, diarrhea, dysentery, enteritis, bladder restraint, hemorrhoids, phlebitis, and varicose veins (4,18). Topically, greater burnet is used in a plaster for wounds and boils (18).

Safety

There is insufficient reliable information available about the safety of greater burnet.
Pregnancy and Lactation: Insufficient reliable information available; avoid using.

Effectiveness
There is insufficient reliable information available about the effectiveness of greater burnet.

Possible Mechanism of Action & Active Ingredients
The applicable parts of greater burnet are the flowering above ground parts. Greater burnet appears to have antihemorrhagic, antihemorrhoidal, astringent, and styptic properties (4).

Adverse Reactions Including Known Allergies
None reported.

Possible Interactions with Herbs & Other Dietary Supplements
Insufficient reliable information available.

Possible Interactions with Drugs
No interactions are known to occur, and there is no known reason to expect a clinically significant interaction with greater burnet.

Possible Interactions with Foods
No interactions are known to occur, and there is no known reason to expect a clinically significant interaction with greater burnet.

Possible Interactions with Lab Tests
No interactions are known to occur, and there is no known reason to expect a clinically significant interaction with greater burnet.

Possible Interactions with Diseases or Conditions
No interactions are known to occur, and there is no known reason to expect a clinically significant interaction with greater burnet.

Typical Dosages & Routes of Administration that are Commonly Used
ORAL: 2-6 grams dried above ground parts three times daily (4), or one cup tea (steep 2-6 grams herb in 150 mL boiling water 5-10 minutes, strain) three times daily (4). Liquid extract (1:1 in 25% alcohol) 2-6 mL three times daily (4). Tincture (1:5 in 45% alcohol) 2-8 mL three times daily (4).
TOPICAL: Used as plasters, no additional dosing or administration available (18).

Comments
None.

GREATER CELANDINE dried above ground parts

This Product is Also Known As
Bai Qu Cai, Celandine, Celandine Herb, Chelidonii, Chelidonii Herba, Schollkraut, Tetterwort.
CAUTION: See separate listings for Greater Celandine root, Lesser Celandine, and Jewelweed.

Scientific Names
Chelidonium majus.
Family: Papaveraceae.

People Use This For
Orally, greater celandine is used for spastic discomfort of bile ducts and the gastrointestinal tract (2).
Topically, greater celandine is used for warts, blister rashes, scabies, tooth pain, and to ease tooth extraction (8,18).
In Chinese medicine, greater celandine is used as an analgesic, antitussive, anti-inflammatory, and detoxicant (8).
In folk medicine, greater celandine is used orally for liver and gallbladder complaints, loss of appetite, gastroenteritis, stomach cancer, cramps, intestinal polyps, breast lumps, angina, edema, arteriosclerosis, hypertension, asthma, gout, and arthritis (8).

Safety
POSSIBLY UNSAFE ...when used orally. The above ground parts of greater celandine have been considered safe when used orally and appropriately (2,7,12). However, greater celandine has been strongly implicated in at least ten cases of hepatitis involving five different brand products manufactured in Germany (363). Until more is known, avoid using greater celandine-containing products.
There is insufficient reliable information available about the safety of the topical use of greater celandine above ground parts.
CHILDREN: UNSAFE ...when used orally. Contraindicated (12).
PREGNANCY: UNSAFE ...contraindicated for oral use because the berberine content might stimulate uterine contractions (12).
LACTATION: Insufficient reliable information available; avoid using.

Effectiveness

POSSIBLY EFFECTIVE ...when given orally for spastic discomfort of the bile ducts and gastrointestinal tract (2). There is insufficient reliable information available about the effectiveness of greater celandine for its other uses.

Possible Mechanism of Action & Active Ingredients

Greater celandine contains 0.1-1% isoquinoline alkaloids (7,12), including chelidonine, which reportedly acts as an antispasmodic and weak central analgesic (7,8). This product is thought to have a papaverine-like effect on the upper gastrointestinal tract (2). In animal studies, an alcoholic extract increased bile flow (7), caused non-specific immune stimulation (2), and acted as a hepatoprotectant (8). The above ground parts of greater celandine also contain small amounts of berberine, which is a uterine stimulant and in large amounts can depress cardiac function (12).

Adverse Reactions Including Known Allergies

Greater celandine taken orally has been strongly implicated in at least ten cases of hepatitis (363). Large amounts can cause stomach pain, intestinal colic, urinary urgency, and hematuria accompanied by dizziness and stupor (7).

Possible Interactions with Herbs & Other Dietary Supplements

Insufficient reliable information available.

Possible Interactions with Drugs

DRUGS FOR GLAUCOMA: May affect treatment (12).

Possible Interactions with Foods

No interactions are known to occur, and there is no known reason to expect a clinically significant interaction with greater celandine dried above ground parts.

Possible Interactions with Lab Tests

LIVER FUNCTION TESTS: Greater celandine-induced hepatitis can increase liver enzyme serum levels and results of liver function tests (363).

Possible Interactions with Diseases or Conditions

BILE TRACT OBSTRUCTION: May exacerbate condition (2).
GLAUCOMA: May affect treatment (12).
HEPATITIS/LIVER DISEASE: Greater celandine taken orally has been strongly implicated in causing hepatitis (363); avoid using in people with liver disease.

Typical Dosages & Routes of Administration that are Commonly Used

ORAL: Dried herb or herb powder 2-5 grams per day (equivalent to 12-30 mg total alkaloids calculated as chelidonine) (2). Fluid extract: 1-2 mL three times daily (18). Do not use in children. Greater celandine tea preparations are difficult to dose properly and are not recommended (7).

Comments

Greater celandine has recently been strongly implicated in at least ten cases of hepatitis involving five different brand products manufactured in Germany (363). Until more is known, avoid using greater celandine-containing products. Avoid confusion with greater celandine rhizome, root and lesser celandine (Family: Ranunculus ficaria).

GREATER CELANDINE rhizome, root

This Product is Also Known As

Celandine Root.
CAUTION: See separate listings for Greater Celandine dried above ground parts, Lesser Celandine, and Jewelweed.

Scientific Names

Chelidonium majus.
Family: Papaveraceae.

People Use This For

In Chinese medicine, greater celandine is used orally for irregular menses (18). The powdered root has been applied topically to ease tooth extraction, and the fresh root chewed to relieve toothache (18).

Safety

There is insufficient reliable information available about the safety of greater celandine rhizome/root.
Pregnancy and Lactation: Insufficient reliable information available; avoid using.

Effectiveness

There is insufficient reliable information available about the effectiveness of greater celandine rhizome/root.

Possible Mechanism of Action & Active Ingredients

Insufficient reliable information available.

Adverse Reactions Including Known Allergies

Greater celandine rhizome/root can cause burning in mouth, nausea, vomiting, bloody diarrhea, hematuria, and stupor following oral use (18).

Possible Interactions with Herbs & Other Dietary Supplements

Insufficient reliable information available.

Possible Interactions with Drugs

No interactions are known to occur, and there is no known reason to expect a clinically significant interaction with greater celandine rhizome, root.

Possible Interactions with Foods

No interactions are known to occur, and there is no known reason to expect a clinically significant interaction with greater celandine rhizome, root.

Possible Interactions with Lab Tests

No interactions are known to occur, and there is no known reason to expect a clinically significant interaction with greater celandine rhizome, root.

Possible Interactions with Diseases or Conditions

No interactions are known to occur, and there is no known reason to expect a clinically significant interaction with greater celandine rhizome, root.

Typical Dosages & Routes of Administration that are Commonly Used

ORAL: Standard dose is 500 mg (18). Store carefully (18).

Comments

There is very little scientific information about this product. Our staff is continually analyzing the available information on natural medicines and will add data here as it becomes available.

GREEK SAGE

This Product is Also Known As

None.

Scientific Names

Salvia triloba.
Family: Labiatae or Lamiaceae.

People Use This For

Greek sage is used for inflammation of the mouth and throat (8).

Safety

There is insufficient reliable information available about the safety of Greek sage.
Pregnancy and Lactation: Insufficient reliable information available; avoid using.

Effectiveness

There is insufficient reliable information available about the effectiveness of Greek sage.

Possible Mechanism of Action & Active Ingredients

Greek sage contains 2-3% volatile oil. Of the volatile oil, 60% is cineole, 5% is thujone (8). Greek sage can inhibit smooth-muscle contractions induced by acetylcholine, histamine, serotonin and $BaCl_2$ (4152). Constituents of the leaf can prolong hexobarbital sleep (4152). Some evidence suggests an aqueous extract of Greek sage might have a blood pressure-lowering effect (4152).

Adverse Reactions Including Known Allergies

None reported.

Possible Interactions with Herbs & Other Dietary Supplements

Insufficient reliable information available.

Possible Interactions with Drugs

HEXOBARBITAL: Greek sage can prolong the effects of hexobarbital (4152).

Possible Interactions with Foods
No interactions are known to occur, and there is no known reason to expect a clinically significant interaction with Greek sage.

Possible Interactions with Lab Tests
No interactions are known to occur, and there is no known reason to expect a clinically significant interaction with Greek sage.

Possible Interactions with Diseases or Conditions
No interactions are known to occur, and there is no known reason to expect a clinically significant interaction with Greek sage.

Typical Dosages & Routes of Administration that are Commonly Used
ORAL: Greek sage is used as a tea. The tea is prepared by pouring boiling water over 3 grams of finely chopped leaf. After 10 minutes, strain (8).

Comments
Greek sage is very rare but sometimes it is found as an adulterant of Salvia officinalis (4,5).

GREEN TEA

This Product is Also Known As
Chinese Tea, Tea.
CAUTION: See separate listings for Black Tea and Caffeine.

Scientific Names
Camellia sinensis, synonyms Camellia thea, Camellia theifera, Thea sinensis, Thea bohea, Thea viridis.
Family: Theaceae.

People Use This For
Orally, green tea is used to improve cognitive performance (4221), treat stomach disorders, vomiting, diarrhea, and headaches. It is used as a diuretic and in combination products for weight loss (6,18). Green tea has been used in Crohn's disease to maintain remission (4209), to reduce the risk of prostate cancer (4210), colon cancer (4211), to protect against heart disease (4219), to protect against dental caries (4214), and to prevent kidney stones (4216).
Topically, green tea bags are used as a wash to soothe sunburn, as a poultice for bags under the eyes, as a compress for headache or tired eyes, and to stop the bleeding of tooth sockets (11).
For food uses, green tea is consumed as a beverage (11).

Safety
LIKELY SAFE ...when used orally in moderate amounts (18,733,6031). Green tea is often consumed daily in Asian cultures and has not been associated with significant adverse effects (6031).
POSSIBLY UNSAFE ...when used orally in large amounts. Green tea contains a significant amount of caffeine. Consumption of more than 300 mg caffeine, which is equivalent to approximately 5 cups of green tea, per day has been associated with significant adverse effects (see Adverse Reactions) (18). These effects would not be expected to occur with the consumption of decaffeinated green tea.
CHILDREN: LIKELY UNSAFE ...when taken orally by infants because it has been associated with impaired iron metabolism and microcytic anemia (6). This might be caused by tannins in green tea which bind and prevent iron absorption in the gastrointestinal tract (19). Children are also more susceptible to the adverse effects of caffeine present in green tea (15).
PREGNANCY: POSSIBLY SAFE ...when used in moderate amounts. Due to the caffeine content of green tea, mothers should closely monitor their intake to ensure moderate consumption. Fetal blood concentrations of caffeine approximate maternal concentrations (4260). Caffeine use in pregnancy is controversial; however, moderate consumption has not been associated with adverse fetal effects (6). Some sources suggest keeping caffeine consumption below 200 mg per day (2078). Green tea provides approximately 10-80 mg caffeine per cup (18,4218).
POSSIBLY UNSAFE ...when used orally in large amounts. Caffeine found in green tea crosses the placenta, producing fetal blood concentrations similar to maternal levels (4260). Although controversial, some evidence suggests that high doses of caffeine might be associated with premature delivery, low birth weight, and loss of the fetus (6). Some sources suggest keeping caffeine consumption below 200 mg per day (2078). Green tea provides approximately 10-80 mg caffeine per cup (18,4218). Excessive use of green tea in pregnancy should be avoided.
LACTATION: POSSIBLY SAFE ...when used in moderate amounts. Due to the caffeine content of green tea, mothers should closely monitor their intake to ensure moderate consumption. Breast milk concentrations of caffeine are thought to be approximately 50% of maternal serum concentrations. Moderate consumption of green tea would likely result in very small amounts of caffeine exposure to a nursing infant (6). POSSIBLY

UNSAFE ...when used orally in large amounts. Consumption of green tea might cause irritability and increased bowel activity in nursing infants (6026). Large doses or excessive intake of green tea should be avoided during lactation.

Effectiveness

POSSIBLY EFFECTIVE ...when used orally for improving cognitive performance (4221). ...when used orally to lower cholesterol and triglycerides. In an epidemiological study, higher consumption of green tea was associated with significantly lower serum total cholesterol, triglycerides, low-density lipoprotein (LDL), and increased high-density lipoprotein (HDL) levels (6403). ...when used orally for treatment of oral leukoplakia (4213). ...when used orally for prevention of certain cancers. Evidence from epidemiological studies suggests that green tea might reduce the risk of some cancers (4218), including bladder (1457,1458,1459), esophageal and pancreatic (733,6031). ...when used orally as a diuretic (7,18). ...when used orally for treating diarrhea (7,18).

Possible Mechanism of Action & Active Ingredients

The applicable parts of green tea are the leaf bud, leaf, and stem. Polyphenols such as gallic acid an catechins are abundant in green tea, and are thought to be responsible for many of its proposed benefits (6031). Green tea also contains 2-4% caffeine (519). Brewed green tea usually contains from 10-80 mg caffeine per cup (512,4218). The caffeine in green tea acts as a central nervous system stimulant (12,15,18,6031); increases blood pressure (1452), heart rate, and contractility (7,18); inhibits platelet aggregation (6,733); stimulates gastric acid secretion; causes diuresis (15,18); relaxes extracerebral vascular and bronchial smooth muscle; stimulates the release of catecholamines (18); and might indirectly inhibit histamine release (6130). Caffeine content is thought to be responsible for green tea's use for improving cognitive performance (4221). Antioxidant catechins in green tea are thought to possibly have a protective effect against atherosclerosis and heart disease (1453,1463). Some preliminary studies have shown that flavonoids found in green tea might reduce lipoprotein oxidation (6032,6033). However, benefits have not yet been described in humans. It is unclear exactly how green tea might reduce the risk of some cancers, but preliminary research suggests that the catechins in green tea, particularly epigallocatechin-3-gallate (ECG), might prevent new blood vessel growth in tumors (1454,1455,1456). Another catechin, epigallocatechin (ECC), might prevent radiation-induced increases of liver lipid peroxide (6). Green tea may also reduce oxidative DNA damage, lipid peroxidation, and free radical generation (4212); and might reduce mutagenic activity in smokers (4217). Green tea has also been used for weight loss. Early evidence indicates that a green tea extract rich in ECG can increase calorie and fat metabolism. Caffeine might also contribute to these effects (1453). The impact of ECG and green tea on weight loss remains to be determined. For diarrhea, tannins in green tea can produce antidiarrheal effects (7,18).

Adverse Reactions Including Known Allergies

Orally, green tea can cause gastrointestinal upset and constipation (7,12). There is one report of liver dysfunction with the excessive use of green tea (65 grams of tea leaves daily for five years) (7). High doses of the caffeine constituent of green tea can cause headache, diuresis, anxiety, nervousness, insomnia, restlessness, agitation, tremor, irritability, tachyarrhythmias, palpitations, premature heartbeat, quickened respiration, heartburn, loss of appetite, nausea, vomiting, diarrhea, dizziness, ringing in the ears, elevated blood sugar, elevated cholesterol, hepatotoxicity, delirium, and convulsions (6,7,15,18,505). Although acute administration of green tea can cause increased blood pressure, regular consumption does not seem to increase either blood pressure or pulse when consumed on a regular basis, even in mildly hypertensive patients (1451,1452). The chronic use of caffeine, especially in large amounts, can sometimes produce tolerance, habituation, and psychological dependence (15). The abrupt discontinuation of caffeine can result in physical withdrawal symptoms, including headaches, irritation, nervousness, anxiety, and dizziness (15). Some evidence shows caffeine is associated with fibrocystic breast disease in women; however, this is controversial and has been disputed (14,15). The adverse effects of caffeine from green tea can be more severe in children than adults (15). In infants, green tea ingestion has been associated with impaired iron metabolism and microcytic anemia (6).

Possible Interactions with Herbs & Other Dietary Supplements

CAFFEINE-CONTAINING HERBS/SUPPLEMENTS: Concomitant use interacts with the caffeine in green tea and can increase the effects and risk of adverse effects. Natural products that contain caffeine include coffee, black tea, guarana, mate, and cola.

EPHEDRA (ma huang): Concomitant use interacts with the caffeine in green tea and can potentiate the stimulant effects and risk of adverse effects (6).

IRON: The concomitant use of iron and green tea can impair iron metabolism in infants and children, resulting in a high incidence of microcytic anemia (6). However, a study in the elderly suggests concomitant use does not affect iron absorption (185).

Possible Interactions with Drugs

ADENOSINE (Adenocard): Theoretically, concomitant use might inhibit the hemodynamic effects of adenosine (19).

ANTIPLATELET AGENTS: Theoretically, green tea might increase the risk of bleeding when used concomitantly with these agents. Green tea is reported to have antiplatelet activity (733); however, this interaction has not been reported in humans. Antiplatelet agents include aspirin, clopidogrel (Plavix), dipyridamole (Persantine), ticlopidine (Ticlid), and others.

ASPIRIN, ACETAMINOPHEN (Tylenol): Concomitant administration can increase the effectiveness of these drugs by as much as 40%, due to the caffeine in green tea (3).

ANTIPSYCHOTIC DRUGS: Theoretically, green tea might cause precipitation of fluphenazine (Permitil, Prolixin), chlorpromazine (Thorazine), haloperidol (Haldol), prochlorperazine (Compazine), thioridazine (Mellaril), and trifluoperazine (Stelazine) (626,627).

BARBITURATES: Concomitant administration can decrease the effects of the caffeine in green tea (151).

BETA-ADRENERGIC AGONISTS: Concomitant use can increase the cardiac inotropic effect of beta-adrenergic agonist drugs due to the caffeine in green tea (15). Beta-adrenergic agonists include albuterol (Proventil, Ventolin), metaproterenol (Alupent), terbutaline (Brethine), and isoproterenol (Isuprel).

BENZODIAZEPINES: Concomitant use might reduce the sedative effects of benzodiazepines due to the caffeine in green tea (19).

CHLORPROMAZINE (Thorazine): Theoretically, concomitant use might inhibit the cataleptic effects of chlorpromazine due to precipitation with compounds in green tea (19).

CIMETIDINE (Tagamet): Concomitant use might increase the effects and adverse effects of caffeine in green tea. Cimetidine can reduce caffeine clearance by 30-50% (14).

CLOZAPINE (Clozaril): Theoretically, concomitant administration might cause acute exacerbation of psychotic symptoms due to the caffeine in green tea. Caffeine can increase the effects and toxicity of clozapine (19,151). Caffeine doses of 400-1000 mg per day inhibit clozapine metabolism (5051).

DISULFIRAM (Antabuse): Concomitant use might increase the risk of adverse effects of caffeine in green tea. Disulfiram decreases the clearance and increases the half-life of caffeine (15).

EPHEDRINE: Concomitant use might increase the risk of agitation, tremors, and insomnia due to the caffeine in green tea (19).

ERGOTAMINE (Ergomar): Concomitant administration might increase the GI absorption of ergotamine due to the caffeine in green tea (15).

LITHIUM (Eskalith, Lithobid): Abrupt caffeine withdrawal can increase serum lithium levels (609). Two case of lithium tremor which worsened with abrupt coffee withdrawal have been reported (610).

MAO INHIBITORS: Concomitant intake with large amounts of green tea might precipitate a hypertensive crisis due to the caffeine in green tea (19).

MEXILETINE (Mexitil): Concomitant use might increase the effects and adverse effects of caffeine in green tea. Mexiletine can decrease caffeine elimination by 50% (1260).

ORAL CONTRACEPTIVES: Concomitant use might increase the effects and adverse effects of caffeine in green tea. Oral contraceptives can decrease caffeine clearance by 40-65% (14).

PHENYTOIN (Dilantin): Concomitant use might reduce the effects of caffeine in green tea. Phenytoin enhances metabolism and excretion of caffeine (19).

PHENYLPROPANOLAMINE (Propagest, Rhindecon): Concomitant use might increase blood pressure and/or cause mania, due to the caffeine in green tea (19).

QUINOLONES: Concomitant use might increase the effects and risk of adverse effects of caffeine in green tea. Quinolones decrease caffeine clearance (606,607,608). Quinolones include ciprofloxacin (Cipro), enoxacin (Penetrex), norfloxacin (Chibroxin, Noroxin), sparfloxacin (Zagam), trovafloxacin (Trovan), and grepafloxacin (Raxar).

THEOPHYLLINE (Theodur): Concomitant use might increase the effects and adverse effects of theopylline due to the caffeine in green tea. Caffeine can reduce theophylline clearance, increase elimination half-life, and increase serum levels (151).

VERAPAMIL (Calan, Isoptin): Concomitant use might increase the effects and adverse effects of caffeine in green tea. Verapamil can increase plasma caffeine levels by 25% (14).

WARFARIN: Consumption of large amounts of green tea is reported to antagonize the effects of warfarin. This has been attributed to the vitamin K1 in green tea (4211). However, there is so little vitamin K1 in green tea (0.03 +/- 0.1 mcg/mL) that the interaction is more likely due to other constituents (1460,1461,1462,1463).

Possible Interactions with Foods

GRAPEFRUIT JUICE: Concomitant use can increase caffeine levels and the risk of adverse effects (504).

MILK: When taken together, milk might bind the antioxidants in tea and reduce their beneficial effects (220); however, in one study this interaction did not occur (6032).

Possible Interactions with Lab Tests

BLEEDING TIME: The caffeine in green tea can prolong bleeding time and increase the results of a bleeding time test (1701).

SERUM URATE (Bittner method): The caffeine in green tea can cause false-positive test results (15).

CREATINE: The caffeine in green tea can increase urine creatine levels (1701).

URINE CATECHOLAMINES, 5-HYDROXYINDOLEACETIC ACID, VANILLYLMANDELIC ACID (VMA): The caffeine in green tea can cause a slight increase in these levels and test results (15).

TESTS FOR PHEOCHROMOCYTOMA, NEUROBLASTOMA: High urine catecholamines or VMA can result in false-positive results. Avoid caffeine while testing for these diseases (15).

Possible Interactions with Diseases or Conditions

DIABETES: Theoretically, the caffeine in green tea might have hyperglycemic effects (19); monitor blood sugar.

GASTRIC, DUODENAL ULCERS: Theoretically, the caffeine in green tea might aggravate these conditions by increasing acid secretion (14,16,19).

HEART CONDITIONS: Theoretically, the caffeine in green tea might induce cardiac arrhythmias in sensitive individuals (14,16).

DEPRESSION, ANXIETY DISORDERS: Theoretically, the caffeine in green tea might aggravate depression or anxiety disorders (14).

KIDNEY DISEASE: Theoretically, the diuretic effect of caffeine in green tea might aggravate some kidney disorders (19).

Typical Dosages & Routes of Administration that are Commonly Used

ORAL: Doses of green tea vary significantly, but usually range between 1-10 cups daily (6002). The commonly used dose of green tea is based on the amount typically consumed in Asian countries, which is about 3 cups per day providing 240-320 mg of polyphenols. For improving cognitive performance, tea providing 60 mg of caffeine, or approximately 1 cup, has been used (4221). For reducing cholesterol, only 10 or greater cups per day has been associated with decreased cholesterol levels (6403). To make teas, people typically use 1 teaspoon of tea leaves in 8 ounces boiling water. Tablets and capsules containing standardized extracts of green tea polyphenols, particularly epigallocatechin, are available. Some provide up to 97% polyphenols, equivalent to drinking four cups of brewed green tea (6006). However, no studies have used evaluated tablet formulations and they cannot be considered equivalent to tea preparations.

TOPICAL: No typical dosage.

Comments

Camellia sinensis leaves and stems are used to manufacture green tea (non-fermented), oolong tea (partially fermented), and black tea (fermented) (4218). Leaves used for green tea are prepared immediately after harvest with limited enzymatic changes. Consequently, green teas can have a higher concentration of the natural constituents than oolong teas or black teas (6,7,4218).

GROUND IVY

This Product is Also Known As

Alehoof, Catsfoot, Cat's-Paw, Creeping Charlie, Gill-Go-By-The-Hedge, Gill-Go-Over-The-Ground, Haymaids, Hedgemaids, Lizzy-Run-Up-The-Hedge, Robin-Run-In-The-Hedge, Tun-Hoof, Turnhoof.

Scientific Names

Nepeta hederacea, synonym Glechoma hederacea.
Family: Labiatae.

People Use This For

Orally, ground ivy is used for mild upper respiratory complaints, coughs, arthritis, rheumatism, and as a diuretic in individuals with bladder and kidney stones (4,18).

Topically ground ivy is used for poorly healing wounds, ulcers, and other skin conditions (18).

In Chinese medicine, ground ivy is used for menstrual irregularities (18).

In the past, ground ivy has been used for bronchitis, chronic bronchial inflammation, tinnitus, diarrhea, intestinal inflammation, hemorrhoids, cystitis, and gastritis (4,18).

In food manufacturing, ground ivy is used as a flavoring agent (4).

Safety

POSSIBLY SAFE ...when preparations of the above ground parts are consumed in amounts found in foods; listed by the Council of Europe as natural source of food flavoring (4). ...when used orally in medicinal amounts (4,18).

PREGNANCY: LIKELY UNSAFE ...contraindicated for oral use because of abortifacient activity (4).

LACTATION: Insufficient reliable information available; avoid using (4).

Effectiveness

There is insufficient reliable information available about the effectiveness of ground ivy.

Possible Mechanism of Action & Active Ingredients

Contains rosmarinic acid, which may be an astringent (4). Contains the volatile oil pulegone, which has hepatotoxic, abortifacient, and irritant properties. The concentration of pulegone in ground ivy is low (4). Fatal poisonings have occurred in animals (18).

Adverse Reactions Including Known Allergies

Taken orally, ground ivy in excessive doses may irritate the GI mucosa and kidneys (4).

Possible Interactions with Herbs & Other Dietary Supplements

PENNYROYAL: Avoid concomitant use, both herbs contain potentially hepatotoxic constituent, pulegone (4).

Possible Interactions with Drugs
No interactions are known to occur, and there is no known reason to expect a clinically significant interaction with ground ivy.

Possible Interactions with Foods
No interactions are known to occur, and there is no known reason to expect a clinically significant interaction with ground ivy.

Possible Interactions with Lab Tests
No interactions are known to occur, and there is no known reason to expect a clinically significant interaction with ground ivy.

Possible Interactions with Diseases or Conditions
KIDNEY DISEASE: The volatile oil is contraindicated due to potential for kidney irritation (4).
LIVER DISEASE: Contraindicated, due to presence of hepatotoxic pulegone (4).
SEIZURE DISORDERS: Contraindicated (4).

Typical Dosages & Routes of Administration that are Commonly Used
ORAL: 2-4 grams dried plant three times daily (4), or, one cup tea (steep 2-4 grams dried plant in 150 mL boiling water 5-10 minutes, strain) three times daily (4). Liquid extract (1:1 in 25% alcohol), 2-4 mL three times daily (4). TOPICAL: Apply crushed leaves to affected area(s) (18).

Comments
Ground ivy is a rich plant source of potassium and iron (19).

GROUND PINE

This Product is Also Known As
Bugle, Yellow Bugle.

Scientific Names
Ajuga chamaepitys.
Family: Lamiaceae.

People Use This For
Orally, the above ground parts of ground pine are used for stimulating menstrual flow, for gout, rheumatism, gynecological complaints (18), for edema, malaria, and sclerosis (4017). They are used as a stimulant and diuretic (18), for inducing sweating, and as a tonic (4017).
Topically, ground pine is used for wound healing (4017).

Safety
There is insufficient reliable information available about the safety of the oral or topical use of ground pine.
Pregnancy and Lactation: Insufficient reliable information is available; avoid using.

Effectiveness
There is insufficient reliable information available about the effectiveness of ground pine.

Possible Mechanism of Action & Active Ingredients
The applicable parts of ground pine are the above ground parts. There is insufficient reliable information available about the possible mechanism of action and active ingredients.

Adverse Reactions Including Known Allergies
None reported.

Possible Interactions with Herbs & Other Dietary Supplements
Insufficient reliable information available.

Possible Interactions with Drugs
No interactions are known to occur, and there is no known reason to expect a clinically significant interaction with ground pine.

Possible Interactions with Foods
No interactions are known to occur, and there is no known reason to expect a clinically significant interaction with ground pine.

Possible Interactions with Lab Tests
No interactions are known to occur, and there is no known reason to expect a clinically significant interaction with ground pine.

Possible Interactions with Diseases or Conditions

No interactions are known to occur, and there is no known reason to expect a clinically significant interaction with ground pine.

Typical Dosages & Routes of Administration that are Commonly Used

No typical dosage.

Comments

There is very little scientific information about this product. Our staff is continually analyzing the available information on natural medicines and will add data here as it becomes available.

GROUNDSEL

This Product is Also Known As

Common Groundsel, Ground Glutton, Grundy Swallow, Simson.

Scientific Names

Senecio vulgaris.
Family: Compositae.

People Use This For

Orally, groundsel is used for worm infestations and colic. The pressed juice is used orally in the treatment of dysmenorrhea and epilepsy (18).
Topically, groundsel pressed juice is used as a dental styptic (18).

Safety

UNSAFE ...when taken orally (2,18). Excessive doses or long-term use increases risk of adverse effects due to unsaturated pyrrolizidine alkaloids (UPAs) (4,12). UPAs are linked to veno-occlusive disease (4,12) and are considered to be hepatotoxic and hepatocarcinogenic (7,515). They might also be mutagenic (12). Groundsel is contraindicated in individuals with liver disease (19). Dietary supplements sold in the United States are not required to include the amount of UPAs they contain (3484); therefore, all preparations used orally containing groundsel should be considered potentially unsafe.
PREGNANCY AND LACTATION: UNSAFE ...contraindicated due to pyrrolizidine alkaloid content (12).

Effectiveness

There is insufficient reliable information available about the effectiveness of groundsel.

Possible Mechanism of Action & Active Ingredients

The applicable part of groundsel is the whole flowering plant. Some pyrrolizidine alkaloids have shown carcinogenic and mutagenic properties, and there are reports of renal toxicity. However, the primary concern is veno-occlusive disease (12). Unsaturated pyrrolizidine alkaloids are known to be hepatotoxic and hepatocarcinogenic in animals and humans (4,7). UPAs destroy and damage centrilobular hepatocytes of the liver and also destroy small branches of the hepatic vein (7).

Adverse Reactions Including Known Allergies

Chronic exposure to other plants containing UPA constituents has been associated with veno-occlusive disease (4021). Symptoms of acute veno-occlusive disease are characterized by nausea, vomiting (5606), anorexia, lethargy (7), a dull, dragging ache in the right upper abdomen and marked distention of the abdomen (4021). These symptoms are sometimes accompanied by reduced urine output. Subacute veno-occlusive disease is associated with vague symptoms and persistent liver enlargement (4021). There is one case report of fatal hepatic veno-occlusive disease in an infant resulting from groundsel tea consumption (5606). It can cause an allergic reaction in individuals sensitive to the Asteraceae/Compositae family. Members of this family include ragweed, chrysanthemums, marigolds, daisies, and many other herbs.

Possible Interactions with Herbs & Other Dietary Supplements

EUCALYPTUS: Theoretically, concomitant use might increase the risk of unsaturated pyrrolizidine alkaloid toxicity due to enzyme induction by eucalyptus (19).
PYRROLIZIDINE ALKALOID-CONTAINING HERBS: Concomitant use is contraindicated due to the risk of additive toxicity. Herbs containing unsaturated pyrrolizidine alkaloids include: alkanna (12), borage (271), gravel root (4), hemp agrimony (271), hound's tongue (19), petasites (19), comfrey (271), coltsfoot, and the Senecio species plants; dusty miller (19), alpine ragwort (19), groundsel (271), golden ragwort (19), and tansy ragwort (271).

Possible Interactions with Drugs

No interactions are known to occur, and there is no known reason to expect a clinically significant interaction with groundsel.

Possible Interactions with Foods

No interactions are known to occur, and there is no known reason to expect a clinically significant interaction with groundsel.

Possible Interactions with Lab Tests

No interactions are known to occur, and there is no known reason to expect a clinically significant interaction with groundsel.

Possible Interactions with Diseases or Conditions

LIVER DISEASE: Contraindicated.
CROSS-ALLERGENICITY: Can cause an allergic reaction in individuals sensitive to the Asteraceae/Compositae family. Members of this family include ragweed, chrysanthemums, marigolds, daisies, and many other herbs.

Typical Dosages & Routes of Administration that are Commonly Used

No typical dosage.

Comments

Groundsel is considered unsafe for oral use; avoid using (18).

GUAIAC WOOD OIL

This Product is Also Known As

Champaca Wood Oil.
CAUTION: See separate listing for Guaiac Wood resin, wood.

Scientific Names

Bulnesia sarmienti.
Family: Zygophyllaceae.

People Use This For

There are no known medicinal uses for guaiac wood oil (11).
In foods and beverages, guaiac wood oil is used as a flavoring agent (11).
In other manufacturing processes, guaiac wood oil is used as a fixative, modifier, or fragrance in soaps and cosmetics (11).

Safety

POSSIBLY SAFE ...when consumed in amounts found in foods (maximum use level 0.002% in meat products); approved for food use in the US (11).
PREGNANCY AND LACTATION: Insufficient reliable information available.

Effectiveness

There is insufficient reliable information available about the effectiveness of guaiac wood oil.

Possible Mechanism of Action & Active Ingredients

Insufficient reliable information available.

Adverse Reactions Including Known Allergies

None reported.

Possible Interactions with Herbs & Other Dietary Supplements

Insufficient reliable information available.

Possible Interactions with Drugs

No interactions are known to occur, and there is no known reason to expect a clinically significant interaction with guaiac wood oil.

Possible Interactions with Foods

No interactions are known to occur, and there is no known reason to expect a clinically significant interaction with guaiac wood oil.

Possible Interactions with Lab Tests

No interactions are known to occur, and there is no known reason to expect a clinically significant interaction with guaiac wood oil.

Possible Interactions with Diseases or Conditions

No interactions are known to occur, and there is no known reason to expect a clinically significant interaction with guaiac wood oil.

Typical Dosages & Routes of Administration that are Commonly Used
No typical dosage.

Comments
The distilled oil is obtained from the wood of Bulnesia sarmienti.

GUAIAC WOOD resin, wood

This Product is Also Known As
Guaiac, Guaiac Heartwood, Guaiacum, Guajaci Lignum, Lingum Vitae, Pockwood.
CAUTION: See separate listing for Guaiac Wood Oil.

Scientific Names
Guaiacum officinale; Guaiacum sanctum.
Family: Zygophyllaceae.

People Use This For
Orally, guaiac wood is used for subacute and chronic rheumatism, chronic rheumatoid arthritis, and preventing gout (2,4,11).
Topically, guaiac wood is used as a bacteriostatic agent in mouthwashes (18).
In lab tests, guaiac resin is used as a diagnostic reagent in tests for occult blood (11).
In folk medicine, guaiac wood has been used for respiratory complaints, skin disorders, and syphilis (18).
As a flavoring agent, guaiac wood is used in foods and in edible oils and fats (4,11).

Safety
POSSIBLY SAFE ...when consumed in amounts commonly found in foods. Guaiac wood is Generally Recognized as Safe (GRAS) for food use in the US (11). ...when taken orally for medicinal purposes in appropriate amounts. The resin can have low toxicity (4).
There is insufficient reliable information available about the safety of the topical use of guaiac wood.
PREGNANCY AND LACTATION: Insufficient reliable information available; avoid using.

Effectiveness
POSSIBLY EFFECTIVE ...when taken orally as supportive therapy for rheumatic complaints (2).
There is insufficient reliable information available about the effectiveness of guaiac wood for its other uses.

Possible Mechanism of Action & Active Ingredients
Guaiac wood can have antirheumatic, anti-inflammatory, diuretic, mild laxative, diaphoretic, and fungistatic activity (4,18).

Adverse Reactions Including Known Allergies
Taken orally, guaiac wood can cause skin rashes (18). High doses can cause diarrhea, gastroenteritis, or intestinal colic (18).

Possible Interactions with Herbs & Other Dietary Supplements
Insufficient reliable information available.

Possible Interactions with Drugs
No interactions are known to occur, and there is no known reason to expect a clinically significant interaction with guaiac wood.

Possible Interactions with Foods
No interactions are known to occur, and there is no known reason to expect a clinically significant interaction with guaiac wood.

Possible Interactions with Lab Tests
No interactions are known to occur, and there is no known reason to expect a clinically significant interaction with guaiac wood.

Possible Interactions with Diseases or Conditions
ACUTE INFLAMMATORY CONDITONS: Contraindicated in acute inflammatory conditions and individuals allergic or hypersensitive to the product (4).

Typical Dosages & Routes of Administration that are Commonly Used
ORAL: The typical dose of guaiac wood is one cup of the tea three times daily (2,4,18). The tea is prepared by simmering 1.5 grams of the wood or resin in 150 mL boiling water for 5-10 minutes and then straining. The usual dose of the liquid extract (1:1 in 80% alcohol) is 1-2 mL per dose. The common dose of the tincture of is 1-4 mL, which is about 20-40 drops (4,18).

Comments
Avoid confusion with guaiac wood oil.

GUAR GUM

This Product is Also Known As
Guar Flour, Jaguar Gum.
CAUTION: See separate listing for Guarana.

Scientific Names
Cyamposis tetragonolobus, synonym Cyamposis psoralioides.
Family: Fabaceae or Leguminosae.

People Use This For
Orally, guar gum is used as a laxative, for reducing serum cholesterol, preventing atherosclerosis, for diabetes, and weight loss (6,7,12,403).
In foods and beverages, guar gum is used as a thickening, stabilizing, suspending and binding agent (11).
In manufacturing, guar gum is used as a binding and disintegrating agent in tablets, as a thickening agent in lotions and creams (11).

Safety
LIKELY SAFE ...when consumed in amounts found in foods (maximum use level 1%); it has Generally Recognized as Safe (GRAS) status in the US (11). ...when taken as an oral medicinal with at least 8 oz (250 mL) of liquid (12). Guar gum is the principle component in certain nonprescription laxative products.
PREGNANCY: POSSIBLY SAFE ...non-teratogenic (6).
LACTATION: Insufficient reliable information available.

Effectiveness
EFFECTIVE ...when taken orally as a laxative.
LIKELY EFFECTIVE ...when taken orally for reducing total cholesterol (6,7) and LDL cholesterol (6), and as fiber source (6,7,12).
POSSIBLY EFFECTIVE ...when taken orally for reducing triglycerides (7) and lowering post-prandial glucose levels when taken in large quantities with meals (6).
There is insufficient reliable information available about the effectiveness of guar gum for its other uses.

Possible Mechanism of Action & Active Ingredients
Guar gum is a dietary fiber that swells 10-20 fold in the presence of water, increases gastrointestinal transit time and contributes to decreased glucose and cholesterol absorption. The bulk forming properties may also cause a sense of fullness, leading to decreased appetite (6).

Adverse Reactions Including Known Allergies
Taken orally, guar gum can cause flatulence, diarrhea, nausea, GI discomfort (6,12), and severe esophageal and small bowel obstruction (602); gastrointestinal side-effects generally subside after several days of use (6). Topically, asthma may result from occupational exposure (600,601).

Possible Interactions with Herbs & Other Dietary Supplements
VITAMIN/MINERAL SUPPLEMENTS: Long term use with vitamin and/or mineral supplements may reduce nutrient absorption (12); take supplements one hour before or several hours after guar gum.

Possible Interactions with Drugs
DIABETES THERAPY: Monitor blood glucose levels closely due to claims that guar gum has hypoglycemic effects (19).
ORAL DRUGS: Might decrease absorption of orally administered drugs (6,12), including aspirin, anticoagulants, digoxin, metformin, and penicillin (12,532,533). Take medications one hour before, or several hours after guar gum.
INSULIN: Concomitant use might reduce insulin requirement due to delayed glucose absorption (19).

Possible Interactions with Foods
NUTRIENT ABSORPTION: Long term use with meals may reduce nutrient absorption (12) requiring vitamin/mineral supplementation.

Possible Interactions with Lab Tests
CHOLESTEROL: Guar gum can reduce serum total cholesterol and LDL cholesterol concentrations, and test results (6,7).
TRIGLYCERIDES: Guar gum might reduce triglyceride concentrations and test results (6,7).
GLUCOSE: Guar gum might reduce postprandial serum glucose concentrations and test results (6).

Possible Interactions with Diseases or Conditions

GI OBSTRUCTION: contraindicated in cases of gastrointestinal obstruction or narrowing, anatomical predisposition to luminal obstruction (6,12).

DIABETES: May alter blood glucose control (6).

Typical Dosages & Routes of Administration that are Commonly Used

ORAL: 5 grams three times per day, just before or with meals taken with at least 8 oz. (250 mL) fluid (7,12); up to 15 grams per day (7,12). Begin with small amount (3 grams per day) and slowly increase to reduce GI side effects.

Comments

Guar gum is derived from the seed of Cyamposis tetragonolobus. CAUTION: Due to the risk of esophageal and small bowel obstruction with bulk-forming products, the FDA requires the following labeling: "WARNING: Taking this product without adequate fluid may cause it to swell and block your throat or esophagus and may cause choking. Do not take this product if you have difficulty in swallowing. If you experience chest pain, vomiting, or difficulty in swallowing or breathing after taking this product, seek immediate medical attention" (12). Additional language is required under the directions for use: "DIRECTIONS: Take (or mix) this product (child or adult dose) with at least 8 ounces (a full glass) of water or other fluid. Taking this product without enough liquid may cause choking. See WARNING." (12).

GUARANA

This Product is Also Known As

Brazilian Cocoa, Guarana Bread, Guarana Gum, Guarana Seed Paste, Paullinia, Zoom.
CAUTION: See separate listings for Caffeine and Guar Gum.

Scientific Names

Paullinia cupana, synonym Paullinia sorbilis.
Family: Sapindaceae.

People Use This For

Orally, guarana is used for weight loss (6,11), to enhance athletic performance, and to reduce fatigue (1900).
In folk medicine, guarana has been used as a stimulant (11,18), tonic (11,18), aphrodisiac (6), diuretic, and astringent (11). It has also been used to prevent malaria and dysentery (6), and for chronic diarrhea, fever, heart problems, headache, rheumatism, lumbago, and heat stress (11).
In food manufacturing, guarana has been used as a flavoring ingredient in beverages and candy (11).

Safety

LIKELY SAFE ...when used in the amounts that are typically found in foods. Guarana's usage in foods is approved in the US (11).
POSSIBLY SAFE ...when used orally and appropriately short-term (12).
POSSIBLY UNSAFE ...when large amounts are used. Chronic use of caffeine, contained in guarana, can sometimes produce tolerance, habituation, and psychological dependence (15). The abrupt discontinuation of caffeine can sometimes cause physical withdrawal symptoms (15).
CHILDREN: POSSIBLY UNSAFE ...when taken orally in amounts significantly greater than typical food amounts. The adverse effects due to the caffeine content are usually more severe in children than adults (15).
PREGNANCY: There is insufficient reliable information available about the safety of guarana during pregnancy. Although the caffeine content of a typical dose should not cause concern, other constituents could be unsafe.
LACTATION: POSSIBLY UNSAFE; avoid using. Caffeine can cause sleep disturbances in breast-fed infants (18).

Effectiveness

LIKELY EFFECTIVE ...when taken orally as a central nervous system stimulant (12,15,18).
POSSIBLY EFFECTIVE ...when taken orally as a diuretic (15,18), for headache, increasing blood pressure in hypotension (15), and weight loss (695,696,1704).
POSSIBLY INEFFECTIVE ...when taken orally for sustained, sub-maximal exercise endurance (14).
LIKELY INEFFECTIVE ...when taken orally for improving short-term, high-intensity performance, anaerobic capacity or power (14).
There is insufficient reliable information available about the effectiveness of guarana for its other uses.

Possible Mechanism of Action & Active Ingredients

The applicable part of guarana is the seed. Guarana contains 2.5-7% caffeine (compared to 1-2% in coffee) (5,6,11,12,18) which acts as a central nervous system stimulant (12,15,18), increases heart rate and contractility (7,18), inhibits platelet aggregation (6,18), stimulates gastric acid secretion, causes diuresis (15,18), relaxes extracerebral vascular and bronchial smooth muscle, stimulates the release of catecholamines (18), and might indirectly inhibit histamine release (6130). Guarana also contains theophylline and theobromine, which have actions similar to caffeine (6,18). Guarana contains tannins with possible carcinogenic and hepatotoxic properties (6,11,12,18). It also contains trace amounts of timbonine, which is used as a fish poison (6).

Adverse Reactions Including Known Allergies

Overdose of guarana can cause painful urination, abdominal spasms, and vomiting (18). Caffeine constituents can cause insomnia, nervousness, restlessness, agitation (7,15), gastric irritation (7), nausea, vomiting, diuresis (15), fast heartbeat, arrhythmias, increased respiratory rate, muscle spasms, tinnitus, headache, delirium, and convulsions (15,505). The adverse effects of caffeine can be more severe in children (15). Some evidence shows caffeine is associated with fibrocystic breast disease in women; other evidence disputes this (14,15). The chronic use of caffeine, especially in large amounts, can sometimes produce tolerance, habituation, and psychological dependence (15). The abrupt discontinuation can sometimes result in physical withdrawal symptoms, including irritability, anxiety, headaches, and dizziness (15).

Combining ephedra with guarana increases the risk of adverse effects, due the caffeine contained in guarana (2729). One unpublished report associated jitteriness, hypertension, seizures, temporary loss of consciousness, and hospitalization requiring life support with the use of a combination ephedra and guarana (caffeine) product (1380). There is one report of ischemic stroke in an athlete who consumed ephedra 40-60 mg, creatine monohydrate 6 grams, caffeine 400-600 mg, and a variety of other supplements daily for six weeks (1275).

Possible Interactions with Herbs & Other Dietary Supplements

CAFFEINE CONTAINING HERBS/SUPPLEMENTS: Concomitant use of guarana and caffeine-containing herbs/supplements constitutes therapeutic duplication (due to the caffeine contained in guarana) which increases the risk of caffeine-related adverse effects. Other natural products which contain caffeine include black tea, cocoa, coffee, cola nut, green tea, and maté.

EPHEDRA (Ma Huang): Concomitant use can increase the risk of stimulatory adverse effects, due to the caffeine contained in guarana (7). One unpublished report associated jitteriness, hypertension, seizures, temporary loss of consciousness, and hospitalization requiring life support with the use of a combination ephedra and guarana (caffeine) product (1380).

Possible Interactions with Drugs

ACETAMINOPHEN (Tylenol): Theoretically, concomitant use might increase the pain-relieving activity of acetaminophen, due to the caffeine contained in guarana. Caffeine increases the pain-relieving activity of acetaminophen by up to 40% (512).

ASPIRIN: Theoretically, concomitant use might increase the pain-relieving activity of aspirin, due to the caffeine contained in guarana. Caffeine increases the pain-relieving activity of aspirin by up to 40% (512).

BENZODIAZEPINES: Theoretically, concomitant use might reduce the sedative and anxiolytic effects of benzodiazepines, due to the caffeine contained in guarana (14).

BETA-ADRENERGIC AGONISTS: Theoretically, concomitant use might increase the cardiac inotropic effects of beta agonists, due to the caffeine contained in guarana (15). Beta-adrenergic agonists include albuterol (Proventil, Ventolin), metaproterenol (Alupent), terbutaline (Brethine), and isoproterenol (Isuprel).

CIMETIDINE (Tagamet) Theoretically, concomitant use might increase serum caffeine concentrations and the risk of adverse effects, due to the caffeine contained in guarana. Cimetidine decreases the rate of caffeine clearance by 30-50% (14).

CLOZAPINE (Clozaril): Theoretically, co-administration might acutely exacerbate psychotic symptoms, due to the caffeine contained in guarana. Caffeine can increase the effects and toxicity of clozapine (151). Caffeine doses of 400-1000 mg per day inhibit clozapine metabolism (5051).

CNS STIMULANTS: Concomitant use might increase the risk of stimulant adverse effects, due to the caffeine contained in guarana (151,2719). CNS stimulants include nicotine, cocaine, sympathomimetic amines, and amphetamines.

DIABETES THERAPY: Theoretically, concomitant use of coffee and diabetes drugs might interfere with blood glucose control, due to the caffeine contained in guarana. This is based in the claim that caffeine might have hyperglycemic effects (19).

DISULFIRAM (Antabuse): Theoretically, concomitant use might increase serum caffeine concentrations and the risk of adverse effects, due to the caffeine contained in guarana. Disulfiram decreases the rate of caffeine clearance (15).

EPHEDRINE: Concomitant use might increase the risk of stimulatory adverse effects, due to the caffeine contained in guarana (7,19). An unpublished report associated jitteriness, hypertension, seizures, temporary loss of consciousness, and hospitalization requiring life support with the use of a combination ephedra (ephedrine) and guarana (caffeine) product (1380).

ESTROGEN (Estrace): Theoretically, concomitant use might increase serum caffeine concentrations and the risk of adverse effects, due to the caffeine contained in guarana. Estrogen inhibits caffeine metabolism (2714).

ERGOTAMINE: Theoretically, concomitant use might increase the GI absorption of ergotamine, due to the caffeine contained in guarana. Caffeine increases the GI absorption of ergotamine (15).

LITHIUM (Eskalith, Lithobid): Theoretically, abrupt guarana withdrawal might increase serum lithium levels, due to the caffeine contained in guarana. There are two case reports of lithium tremor that worsened upon abrupt coffee withdrawal (609,610).

MEXILETINE (Mexitil): Theoretically, concomitant use might increase serum caffeine concentrations and the risk of adverse effects, due to the caffeine contained in guarana. Mexiletine reduces caffeine metabolism (14).

MONOAMINE OXIDASE INHIBITORS (MAOIs): Theoretically, concomitant intake of large amounts of guarana with MAOIs might precipitate a hypertensive crisis, due to the caffeine contained in guarana. This is based on the claim that intake of large amounts of caffeine with MAOIs might precipitate a hypertensive crisis (19).

ORAL CONTRACEPTIVES (OCs): Theoretically, concomitant use might increase serum caffeine concentrations and the risk adverse effects, due to the caffeine contained in guarana. OCs decrease the rate of caffeine clearance by 40-65% (14).

PHENYLPROPANOLAMINE (Dexatrim, Propagest): Theoretically, concomitant use might cause an additive increase in blood pressure and serum caffeine concentrations, due to the caffeine contained in guarana (14). Concomitant use of caffeine and phenylpropanolamine can cause an additive increase in blood pressure, and increase serum caffeine concentrations (14).

QUINOLONES: Theoretically, concomitant use might increase serum caffeine concentrations and the risk of adverse effects, due to the caffeine contained in guarana. Quinolones decrease caffeine clearance (606,607,608). Quinolones (also referred to as fluoroquinolones) include ciprofloxacin (Cipro), enoxacin (Penetrex), gatifloxacin (Tequin), levofloxacin (Levaquin), lomefloxacin (Maxaquin), moxifloxacin (Avelox), norfloxacin (Noroxin), ofloxacin (Floxin), sparfloxacin (Zagam), and trovafloxacin (Trovan).

RILUZOLE (Rilutek): Theoretically, concomitant use might increase serum caffeine and riluzole concentrations and the risk of adverse effects of both caffeine and riluzole, due to the caffeine contained in guarana. Caffeine and riluzole are both metabolized by cytochrome P450 1A2 and concomitant use might reduce metabolism of one or both agents (14).

TERBINAFINE (Lamisil): Theoretically, concomitant use might increase serum caffeine concentrations and the risk of adverse effects, due to the caffeine contained in guarana. Terbinafine decreases the rate of caffeine clearance (14).

THEOPHYLLINE (Theo-Dur): Theoretically, concomitant use might increase serum theophylline concentrations and the risk of adverse effects, due to the caffeine contained in guarana. Large amounts of caffeine might inhibit theophylline metabolism (14).

VERAPAMIL (Calan, Isoptin, Verelan): Theoretically, concomitant use might increase plasma caffeine concentrations and the risk of adverse effects, due to the caffeine contained in guarana. Verapamil increases plasma caffeine concentrations by 25% (14).

Possible Interactions with Foods

GRAPEFRUIT JUICE: Interacts with the caffeine in guarana and can increase caffeine levels, and the effects and the risk of adverse effects (504).

Possible Interactions with Lab Tests

BLEEDING TIME: Guarana might prolong bleeding time and increase test results, due to its caffeine content (1701).

BLOOD PRESSURE: Guarana might increase blood pressure and blood pressure readings, due to its caffeine content (4).

URATE: Guarana might falsely increase serum urate test results determined by the Bittner method, due to its caffeine content. Caffeine causes false elevations in serum urate test results determined by the Bittner method (15).

CATECHOLAMINES: Guarana might increase urine catecholamine concentrations and test results, due to its caffeine content. Caffeine can increase urine catecholamine concentrations (15).

CREATINE: Guarana might increase urine creatine concentrations and test results, due to its caffeine content (1701).

DIPYRIDAMOLE THALLIUM IMAGING: Guarana might interfere with dipyridamole thallium imaging studies, due to its caffeine content. Caffeine attenuates the characteristic cardiovascular responses to dipyridamole and has altered test results (14).

5-HYDROXYINDOLEACETIC ACID: Guarana might increase urine 5-hydroxyindoleacetic acid concentrations and test results, due to its caffeine content. Caffeine can increase urine catecholamine concentrations (15).

VANILLYLMANDELIC ACID (VMA): Guarana might increase urine VMA concentrations and test results, due to its caffeine content. Caffeine can increase urine VMA concentrations (15).

TESTS FOR NEUROBLASTOMA: Guarana (due to its caffeine content) might cause false-positive diagnosis of neuroblastoma, when diagnosis is based on tests of urine vanillylmandelic acid (VMA) or catecholamine concentrations. Caffeine can increase urine catecholamine and VMA concentrations (15).

TESTS FOR PHEOCHROMOCYTOMA: Guarana (due to its caffeine content) might cause false-positive diagnosis of pheochromocytoma, when diagnosis is based on tests of urine vanillylmandelic acid (VMA) or catecholamine concentrations. Caffeine can increase urine catecholamine and VMA concentrations (15).

Possible Interactions with Diseases or Conditions

GASTRIC, DUODENAL ULCERS: The caffeine in guarana can aggravate these conditions; avoid using (14,16).

HEART CONDITIONS: The caffeine in guarana can induce cardiac arrhythmias in sensitive individuals (14,16).

DEPRESSION, ANXIETY DISORDERS: The caffeine in guarana can aggravate these conditions (14).

KIDNEY DISEASE: The diuretic effect of caffeine in guarana might aggravate some kidney disorders (19).

Typical Dosages & Routes of Administration that are Commonly Used
ORAL: Guarana is often used along with other ingredients in weight loss products. People use 1-2 capsules or tablets containing 200-800 mg guarana extract (1:4) before breakfast or lunch (5018), not to exceed 3 grams daily (5008).

Comments
None.

GUAYULE

This Product is Also Known As
None.

Scientific Names
Parthenium argentatum.
Family: Asteraceae or Compositae.

People Use This For
Guayule is a source of natural rubber (6). There are no reported medicinal uses.

Safety
LIKELY UNSAFE ...when used orally or topically. Guayule is a potent contact allergen (6).
PREGNANCY AND LACTATION: LIKELY UNSAFE ...when used orally or topically. Guayule is a potent contact allergen (6).

Effectiveness
There is insufficient reliable information available about the effectiveness of guayule.

Possible Mechanism of Action & Active Ingredients
Contact allergenicity may be caused by guayulin A, which is reported equal in potency to poison ivy (6).

Adverse Reactions Including Known Allergies
Guayule is a potent contact allergen (equivalent to poison ivy) and induces strong erythema at very low concentrations (0.003%); avoid contact (6). Guayule can cause an allergic reaction in individuals sensitive to the Asteraceae/Compositae family. Members of this family include ragweed, chrysandthemums, marigolds, daisies, and many other herbs.

Possible Interactions with Herbs & Other Dietary Supplements
Insufficient reliable information available.

Possible Interactions with Drugs
No interactions are known to occur, and there is no known reason to expect a clinically significant interaction with guayule.

Possible Interactions with Foods
No interactions are known to occur, and there is no known reason to expect a clinically significant interaction with guayule.

Possible Interactions with Lab Tests
No interactions are known to occur, and there is no known reason to expect a clinically significant interaction with guayule.

Possible Interactions with Diseases or Conditions
CROSS-ALLERGENICITY: Can cause an allergic reaction in individuals sensitive to the Asteraceae/Compositae family. Members of this family include ragweed, chrysanthemums, marigolds, daisies, and many other herbs.

Typical Dosages & Routes of Administration that are Commonly Used
No typical dosage.

Comments
Avoid physical contact; guayule is a potent contact allergen.

GUGGUL

This Product is Also Known As
Guggal, Guggulu, Gum Guggal, Gum Guggulu, Indian Bdellium-Tree.
CAUTION: See separate listing for Indian Frankincense.

Scientific Names
Commiphora mukul.
Family: Burseracaea.

People Use This For
Orally, guggul gum resin is used for arthritis, lowering high cholesterol (6,3267), nodulocystic acne (3268), and weight loss (6).

Safety
POSSIBLY SAFE ...when the prepared gum resin is used orally and appropriately (12). No significant adverse effects reported in clinical trials (6).
PREGNANCY: LIKELY UNSAFE ...contraindicated for oral use. Guggul gum resin appears to stimulate menstrual flow and the uterus (12).
LACTATION: Insufficient reliable information available; avoid using.

Effectiveness
POSSIBLY EFFECTIVE ...when gugulipid preparations are used orally for lowering serum cholesterol and triglycerides in people with hyperlipidemia (366,3267). ...when used orally for treating nodulocystic acne (3268). There is insufficient reliable information available about the effectiveness of guggul for its other uses.

Possible Mechanism of Action & Active Ingredients
The applicable part of guggul is the gum resin. Guggul extracts contain guggulsterone and gugulipid. Studies indicate that extracts containing these constituents can lower serum total cholesterol, LDL cholesterol, and triglycerides (366,3267). However, the effects on HDL cholesterol are unclear. In one study, guggul increased HDL cholesterol concentrations (366) while in another study it had no effect on HDL levels (3267). The constituent, guggulsterone has thyroid-stimulating activity (6). It also shows protective effects against drug-induced myocardial necrosis (6). Some evidence suggests guggul extracts might have anti-inflammatory activity (6). Guggul was comparable to oral tetracycline in the treatment of nodulocystic acne (3268). Both treatments decreased inflammation and the number of relapses (3268). Co-administration of gugulipid reduces bioavailability of single doses of propranolol and diltiazem in healthy people (383).

Adverse Reactions Including Known Allergies
Guggul can cause gastrointestinal upset (366), headache, mild nausea, belching, and hiccups (3267).

Possible Interactions with Herbs & Other Dietary Supplements
Insufficient reliable information available.

Possible Interactions with Drugs
PROPRANOLOL (Inderal): Concomitant oral administration can reduce propranolol bioavailability and might reduce therapeutic effects (383).
DILTIAZEM (Cardizem): Concomitant oral administration can reduce diltiazem bioavailability and might reduce therapeutic effects (383).
THYROID DRUGS: Theoretically, concomitant use might interfere with therapy to normalize thyroid function; monitor.

Possible Interactions with Foods
No interactions are known to occur, and there is no known reason to expect a clinically significant interaction with guggul.

Possible Interactions with Lab Tests
SERUM CHOLESTROL: Guggul can reduce serum total cholesterol and LDL cholesterol concentrations and test results (366,3267). It is unclear what effect, if any, guggul has on serum HDL cholesterol concentrations or test results (366,3267).
SERUM TRIGLYCERIDES: Guggul can reduce serum triglycerides and test results (366,3267).

Possible Interactions with Diseases or Conditions
THYROID DISORDERS: Theoretically, concomitant use might interfere with therapy for hyperthyroid or hypothyroid conditions; monitor.

Typical Dosages & Routes of Administration that are Commonly Used
ORAL: For hypercholesterolemia, doses of 100-500 mg gugulipid per day have been used (366,3267). For nodulocystic acne, a dose of gugulipid equivalent to 25 mg guggulsterone per day has been used (3268).

Comments
Guggul is of the same genus as Commiphora myrrha, the myrrh of the bible. The plant has been used in Ayurvedic medicine for centuries to treat a variety of disorders, particularly arthritis, and to aid weight loss [6].

GUMWEED

This Product is Also Known As
August Flower, Grindelia, Grindeliae herba, Gumweed Herb, Rosin Weed, Tar Weed.

Scientific Names
Grindelia robusta; Grindelia squarrosa.
Family: Asteraceae or Compositae.

People Use This For
Orally, gumweed is used for cough, bronchitis, and inflammation of the upper respiratory tract mucous membrane [2,18].

Safety
POSSIBLY SAFE ...when used orally and appropriately [2,12].
PREGNANCY AND LACTATION: Insufficient reliable information; avoid using.

Effectiveness
POSSIBLY EFFECTIVE ...when taken orally for treating upper respiratory tract mucous membrane inflammation [2].
There is insufficient reliable information available about the effectiveness of gumweed for its other uses.

Possible Mechanism of Action & Active Ingredients
The applicable parts of gumweed are the dried top and leaf. Gumweed can have antibacterial effects in vitro [2].

Adverse Reactions Including Known Allergies
When used orally, gumweed can cause gastric mucosa irritation [2,12], diarrhea [18], and kidney irritation [12]. Gumweed can cause an allergic reaction in individuals sensitive to the Asteraceae/Compositae family. Members of this family include ragweed, chrysanthemums, marigolds, daisies, and many other herbs.

Possible Interactions with Herbs & Other Dietary Supplements
Insufficient reliable information available.

Possible Interactions with Drugs
No interactions are known to occur, and there is no known reason to expect a clinically significant interaction with gumweed.

Possible Interactions with Foods
No interactions are known to occur, and there is no known reason to expect a clinically significant interaction with gumweed.

Possible Interactions with Lab Tests
No interactions are known to occur, and there is no known reason to expect a clinically significant interaction with gumweed.

Possible Interactions with Diseases or Conditions
CROSS-ALLERGENICITY: Can cause an allergic reaction in individuals sensitive to the Asteraceae/Compositae family. Members of this family include ragweed, chrysanthemums, marigolds, daisies, and many other herbs.

Typical Dosages & Routes of Administration that are Commonly Used
ORAL: The typical dose of gumweed is 4-6 grams of the dried top or leaf per day [2]. The usual dose of the fluid extract is 3-6 grams per day [2]. The common dose of the 1:10 tincture (60-80% ethanol) is 1.5-3 mL per day, and the usual dose of the 1:5 tincture (60-80% ethanol) is 1.5-3 mL per day [2].

Comments
None.

GYMNEMA

This Product is Also Known As
Gur-Mar, Gurmar, Gurmarbooti, Merasingi, Meshashringi.

Scientific Names
Gymnema sylvestre; Asclepias geminate; Gemnema melicida; Periploca sylvestris.
Family: Asclepiadaceae.

People Use This For
Orally, gymnema leaf is used to treat diabetes (6).
In combination with other products, gymnema is used for metabolic control (6).
In Ayurvedic medicine, gymnema is a component in the Tribang shila compound, which contains tin, lead, zinc, gymnema leaves, neem leaves, jambul seeds, and Enicostemma littorale (6).
Traditionally, gymnema has been used as an antimalarial, digestive stimulant, laxative, and diuretic. It has also been used traditionally for coughs and as a snake bite antidote (14).

Safety
There is insufficient reliable information available about the safety of gymnema.
Pregnancy and Lactation : Insufficient reliable information available; avoid using.

Effectiveness
POSSIBLY EFFECTIVE …when taken orally by patients with type 1 or 2 diabetes on insulin or oral hypoglycemics for further reductions in blood glucose and glycosylated hemoglobin (45,46). …when taken orally for reducing total cholesterol and triglycerides in type 1 diabetics (45). Studies have used the GS4 extract.
There is insufficient reliable information available about the effectiveness of gymnema for its other uses.

Possible Mechanism of Action & Active Ingredients
The applicable part of gymnema is the leaf. Gymnema lowers blood sugar (6), serum triglycerides, total cholesterol, and VLDL and LDL cholesterol in animals (14). The constituent, gymnemic acid, inhibits the ability to taste bitter (quinine) or sweet (sugar) without affecting the ability to taste sour, astringent, or pungent flavors (6). Gymnemic acids can reduce intestinal absorption of glucose and may stimulate pancreatic beta cell growth (47,48). Gymnema can increase serum C-peptide levels, suggesting an increase in endogenous insulin secretion (45).

Adverse Reactions Including Known Allergies
None reported.

Possible Interactions with Herbs & Other Dietary Supplements
Insufficient reliable information available.

Possible Interactions with Drugs
DIABETES DRUGS/INSULIN: Gymnema can enhance the blood glucose lowering effects of insulin and hypoglycemic drugs (45,46); blood glucose levels should be monitored closely.
IRON: Some gymnema preparations can decrease absorption of iron. However, the GS4 extract, which has been used in clinical studies, is thought to be free of constituents that can reduce iron absorption (6420).

Possible Interactions with Foods
No interactions are known to occur, and there is no known reason to expect a clinically significant interaction with gymnema.

Possible Interactions with Lab Tests
BLOOD GLUCOSE: Gymnema can lower blood sugar resulting in lower blood glucose test results.

Possible Interactions with Diseases or Conditions
DIABETES: Gymnema can affect blood sugar control, and blood glucose levels should be monitored closely.

Typical Dosages & Routes of Administration that are Commonly Used
ORAL: For lowering blood sugar, the typical dose of the extract GS4 is 400 mg daily.

Comments
The gymnema leaf is commonly found in Africa and India but is readily distributed worldwide (6).

HARONGA

This Product is Also Known As
Harongablädder leaf, Harongarinde bark, Harunganae madagascariensis cortex bark, Harunganae madagascariensis folium leaf.

Scientific Names
Haronga madagascariensis.
Family: Hypericaceae.

People Use This For
Orally, haronga is used for dyspepsia, mild exocrine pancreatic insufficiency, liver and gallbladder complaints, and loss of appetite (2,18).

Safety
POSSIBLY SAFE ...when used orally and appropriately (2). The recommended maximum safe duration of use is two months (2).
PREGNANCY AND LACTATION: Insufficient reliable information available; avoid using.

Effectiveness
POSSIBLY EFFECTIVE ...when taken orally for dyspepsia and mild exocrine pancreatic insufficiency (2).
There is insufficient reliable information available about the effectiveness of haronga for its other uses.

Possible Mechanism of Action & Active Ingredients
The applicable parts of haronga are the bark and leaf. Haronga can have gallbladder stimulating (2), liver protectant, pancreas stimulating, gastric juice secretion stimulating, and antimicrobial effects (18). It can also have possible anti-amoebic activity (1519).

Adverse Reactions Including Known Allergies
Photosensitivity is possible with the use of haronga, especially in fair-skinned people (2). Phototoxicity is theoretically possible with large doses (18).

Possible Interactions with Herbs & Other Dietary Supplements
Insufficient reliable information available.

Possible Interactions with Drugs
No interactions are known to occur, and there is no known reason to expect a clinically significant interaction with haronga.

Possible Interactions with Foods
No interactions are known to occur, and there is no known reason to expect a clinically significant interaction with haronga.

Possible Interactions with Lab Tests
No interactions are known to occur, and there is no known reason to expect a clinically significant interaction with haronga.

Possible Interactions with Diseases or Conditions
CONTRAINDICATIONS: The use of haronga is contraindicated in acute pancreatitis and exacerbations of chronic pancreatitis, severe liver dysfunction, gallstones, biliary obstruction, gallbladder empyema, or obstruction of the bowels (2,18).
FAIR-SKINNED INDIVIDUALS: Haronga can cause photosensitivity in fair-skinned individuals (2).

Typical Dosages & Routes of Administration that are Commonly Used
ORAL: The typical dose of the haronga dry extract is 7.5-15 mg per day, which corresponds to 25-50 mg of the herb (2,18). The recommended maximum safe duration of use is two months (2).

Comments
None.

HARTSTONGUE

This Product is Also Known As
Buttonhole, God's-Hair, Hind's Tongue, Horse Tongue.

Scientific Names
Scolopendrium vulgare.

People Use This For
Orally, hartstongue is used to treat digestive disorders and urinary tract diseases (18).

Safety
There is insufficient reliable information available about the safety of hartstongue.
Pregnancy and Lactation: Insufficient reliable information available; avoid using.

Effectiveness
There is insufficient reliable information available about the effectiveness of hartstongue.

Possible Mechanism of Action & Active Ingredients

The applicable parts of hartstongue are the above ground parts. Hartstongue contains tannins, mucilage, flavonoids (kaempferol-7-rhamnoside-3 coffeoyl-7-diglucoside), thiaminase, and sugars (sucrose and invert sugar) (18). These constituents seem to produce diuretic and mild laxative and purgative actions.

Adverse Reactions Including Known Allergies

None reported.

Possible Interactions with Herbs & Other Dietary Supplements

Insufficient reliable information available.

Possible Interactions with Drugs

No interactions are known to occur, and there is no known reason to expect a clinically significant interaction with hartstongue.

Possible Interactions with Foods

No interactions are known to occur, and there is no known reason to expect a clinically significant interaction with hartstongue.

Possible Interactions with Lab Tests

No interactions are known to occur, and there is no known reason to expect a clinically significant interaction with hartstongue.

Possible Interactions with Diseases or Conditions

No interactions are known to occur, and there is no known reason to expect a clinically significant interaction with hartstongue.

Typical Dosages & Routes of Administration that are Commonly Used

ORAL: People typically use 2 to 4 grams of the dried hartstongue leaves 3 times daily. This is also made into a tea. A liquid extract in a 1:1 concentration with 25% ethanol is dosed 2 to 4 ml three times daily. A liquid extract in a 1:5 concentration with 55% ethanol is dosed 2 to 6 mL three times daily (5269).

Comments

There is very little scientific information about this product. Our staff is continually analyzing the available information on natural medicines and will add data here as it becomes available.

HAWAIIAN BABY WOODROSE

This Product is Also Known As

Baby Hawaiian Woodrose, Baby Wood-rose, Elephant-Climber, Elephant Creeper, Silver-Morning-Glory, Wood-Rose, Woolly Morning Glory, Woolly-Morning-Glory.

Scientific Names

Argyreia nervosa, synonyms: Argyreia speciosa, Convolvulus nervosus, Convolvulus speciosus, Lettsomia nervosa.
Family: Convolvulaceae.

People Use This For

Orally, Hawaiian baby woodrose seeds are used for pain relief, promoting sweating (5299), for sacramental rituals (5300), and as a hallucinogen (5301,5304).

Safety

LIKELY UNSAFE ...when used orally (17,5301). The seeds of Hawaiian baby woodrose have effects similar to the hallucinogen lysergic acid diethylamide (LSD), including flashbacks (5301).
PREGNACY AND LACTATION: LIKELY UNSAFE ...contraindicated (17,5301).

Effectiveness

There is insufficient reliable information about the effectiveness of Hawaiian baby woodrose.

Possible Mechanism of Action & Active Ingredients

The applicable part of Hawaiian baby woodrose is the seeds. Hawaiian baby woodrose, an ornamental plant, has seeds that contain hallucinogens including ergonovine, isoergine (isolysergic acid amide), and ergine (lysergic acid amide) (17,5300,5301,5304). Four to eight seeds are equivalent to 10 to 100 mcg of lysergic acid diethylamide (LSD) (5301), a potent 5-HT1A agonist (17). The hallucinatory effects of Hawaiian baby woodrose are similar to alcohol intoxication with psychedelic visual effects such as enhanced colors. The effects last 6-8 hours (5301,5304).

Adverse Reactions Including Known Allergies

Oral ingestion can cause nausea and vomiting, dizziness, auditory hallucinations, blurred vision, dilated pupils, involuntary, rapid, rhythmic movement of eyeballs, sweating, fast heart rate, and hypertension (5301).

Possible Interactions with Herbs & Other Dietary Supplements

ST. JOHN'S WORT: Theoretically, Hawaiian baby woodrose might increase the effects and adverse effects of products that increase serotonin levels, including St. John's wort (14,17).

Possible Interactions with Drugs

SSRIs: Theoretically, because Hawaiian baby woodrose contains chemicals related to LSD, it might interact with drugs that increase serotonin including sertraline (Zoloft), paroxetine (Paxil), fluoxetine (Prozac) and other antidepressants. Seizures have occurred in people taking the related compound, LSD, with fluoxetine (Prozac) (14,17). Individuals who have previously used LSD have developed flashbacks and hallucinations when treated with selective serotonin reuptake inhibitors (17).

5-HT2 ANTAGONISTS: Theoretically, because selective 5-HT2 receptor antagonists antagonize the effect of LSD, they might also decrease the effect of Hawaiian baby woodrose. 5-HT2 antagonists include cyproheptadine (Periactin), clozapine (Clozaril), and risperidone (Risperidone) (17).

Possible Interactions with Foods

No interactions are known to occur, and there is no known reason to expect a clinically significant interaction with Hawaiian baby woodrose.

Possible Interactions with Lab Tests

No interactions are known to occur, and there is no known reason to expect a clinically significant interaction with Hawaiian baby woodrose.

Possible Interactions with Diseases or Conditions

PYSCHOSIS: Theoretically, because Hawaiian baby woodrose has effects similar to LSD, individuals with psychotic tendencies might experience prolonged psychotic reactions (17).

Typical Dosages & Routes of Administration that are Commonly Used

No typical dosage.

Comments

Hawaiian baby woodrose is likely unsafe for oral use; avoid using. Hawaiian baby woodrose, a relative of the morning glory, grows in Florida, California, and Hawaii (17). Touted as a "natural LSD" in Internet advertising (5302), the seeds are legal (5301) and easily purchased from Internet sources.

HAWTHORN fruit

This Product is Also Known As

Aubépine, Bianco spino, Crataegi Fructus, English Hawthorn, Épine Blanche, Épine de Mai, Haagdorn, Hagedorn, Harthorne, Haw, Hawthorne, Hedgethorn, May, Maybush, Maythorn, Mehlbeebaum, Meidorn, Nan Shanzha, Oneseed Hawthorn, Shanzha, Weissdorn, Whitehorn.
CAUTION: See separate listing for Hawthorn leaf with flower extract and Hawthorn leaf, flower.

Scientific Names

Crataegus laevigata, synonym Crataegus oxyacantha; Crataegus monogyna; Crataegus pinnatifida; Crataegus cuneata.
Family: Rosaceae.

People Use This For

Orally, hawthorn fruit preparations are used for cardiovascular conditions such as heart failure (4,302), decreased cardiac output (2,4), coronary heart disease (2,11,302), circulatory disturbances (2), paroxysmal tachycardia (4,302), bradycardic arrhythmias (302), hypotension (2), hypertension (4,11), hyperlipidemia (11), arteriosclerosis (2,4), Buerger's disease (4,302), and to decrease the dosage requirement and toxicity of digoxin-like cardiac glycosides (302). Fruit preparations are also used orally in gastrointestinal conditions such as indigestion (11,302), enteritis (11), epigastric distention (11), diarrhea, and abdominal pain (11,302). Fruit preparations are also used orally to treat tapeworm infections (11), acute bacillus dysentery (11,302), and amenorrhea (11).
Topically, hawthorn fruit preparations are used as a wash for sores, itching, and frost bite (11).
In manufacturing, hawthorn fruit is used for making candied fruit slices, jam, jelly, and wine (11,302).

Safety

POSSIBLY SAFE ...when taken orally and appropriately short-term (2,12,302). Specific toxicities with hawthorn fruit have not been reported; however it is expected to have effects similar to other hawthorn preparations (302).
There is insufficient reliable information available about the safety of the long-term oral use of hawthorn fruit.

PREGNANCY: UNSAFE ...contraindicated due to potential uterine activity (4).
LACTATION: Insufficient reliable information available; avoid using.

Effectiveness

There is insufficient reliable information available about the effectiveness of hawthorn fruit.

Possible Mechanism of Action & Active Ingredients

The constituents responsible for the pharmacological effects of hawthorn preparations include flavonoids and procyanidins. Other active compounds are vitexin, rutin, and hyperoside (302,406). Fruit preparations contain higher procyanidin concentrations than other preparations (302). Hawthorn preparations act on the myocardium by increasing force of contraction (4,6,7,11,302,406), lengthening the refractory period (7,406), reducing peripheral vascular resistance (18,406), reducing oxygen consumption (406), and increasing nerve conductivity (406). Researchers think the constituent flavonoids and oligomeric procyanidins increase coronary blood flow due to vasodilation (18). They attribute hawthorn's cardiotrophic properties to increased membrane permeability for calcium and phosphodiesterase inhibition that increases intracellular cAMP. Increased cAMP leads to increased coronary blood flow, vasodilation, and positive inotropic effects (259). Hawthorn has also been reported to decrease uterine tone and motility (11), reduce lipid levels (11,302). It also has antibacterial, spasmolytic, and analgesic effects (11).

Adverse Reactions Including Known Allergies

None reported.

Possible Interactions with Herbs & Other Dietary Supplements

CARDIAC GLYCOSIDE-CONTAINING HERBS: Theoretically, concurrent use might potentiate cardiac glycoside activity and potential for toxicity. Cardiac glycoside-containing herbs include black hellebore, Canadian hemp roots, digitalis leaf, hedge mustard, figwort, lily of the valley roots, motherwort, oleander leaf, pheasant's eye plant, pleurisy root, squill bulb leaf scales, and strophanthus seeds (2,18,19).
OTHER CARDIOACTIVE HERBS: Avoid concurrent use with other cardioactive herbs due to unpredictability of effects and adverse effects. Other cardioactive herbs include: calamus, cereus, cola, coltsfoot, devil's claw, European mistletoe, fenugreek, fumitory, ginger, Panax ginseng, white horehound, mate, parsley, quassia, scotch broom flower, shepherd's purse, and wild carrot (4).

Possible Interactions with Drugs

CORONARY VASODILATORS: Using hawthorn with theophylline, caffeine, papaverine, sodium nitrate, adenosine, epinephrine and other coronary vasodilators might cause additive vasodilatory effects (302,406).
CARDIOVASCULAR DRUGS: Hawthorn might potentiate or interfere with conventional drug therapy for heart failure, hypertension, angina, and arrhythmias (4,12,302).
CNS DEPRESSANTS: Concomitant use of hawthorn and CNS depressants might have additive CNS depressant effects (4,406).
DIGOXIN: Concomitant use of hawthorn and digoxin might potentiate digoxin effects requiring digoxin dose reduction (12,302,406).

Possible Interactions with Foods

No interactions are known to occur, and there is no known reason to expect a clinically significant interaction with hawthorn fruit.

Possible Interactions with Lab Tests

No interactions are known to occur, and there is no known reason to expect a clinically significant interaction with hawthorn fruit.

Possible Interactions with Diseases or Conditions

CARDIOVASCULAR CONDITIONS: Concomitant use of hawthorn with conventional cardiovascular drug therapy might potentiate or interfere with the treatment of these conditions (4,12,302).

Typical Dosages & Routes of Administration that are Commonly Used

ORAL: Dried hawthorn fruit powder 300-1000 mg is taken orally three times daily or as a prepared tea after meals (4,302). Hawthorn fruit liquid extract (1:1 in 25% alcohol) 0.5-1 mL is taken three times daily (4,302). Hawthorn fruit tincture (1:5 in 45% alcohol) 1-2 mL is taken three times daily (4,302). Hawthorn fruit syrup is taken as 1 teaspoon two to three times daily (302). A hawthorn fruit solid extract is used in doses of 1/4 to 1/2 teaspoon (1.7-3.3 mL) daily (302).

Comments

Significant clinical evidence exists for the use of hawthorn leaf with flower extract preparations in individuals with NYHA class II heart failure. New York Heart Association (NYHA) stage I and II refers to individuals with heart disease who do not have resulting limitations of physical activity. They are comfortable at rest but ordinary physical activity results in fatigue, palpitations, trouble breathing, or anginal pain. Although similar clinical evidence does not exist for preparations containing individual plant parts, these preparations may have some benefit. Hawthorn fruit, leaves, and flowers are thought to contain the same active constituents, but in differing quantities. See Hawthorn leaf with flower extract.

HAWTHORN leaf with flower extract

This Product is Also Known As
Aubepine, Crataegi Folium Cum Flore, English Hawthorn, Haw, Hawthorne, May, Maybush, Oneseed Hawthorn, Whitehorn.
CAUTION: See separate listing for Hawthorn leaf, flower and Hawthorn fruit.

Scientific Names
Crataegus laevigata, synonym Crataegus oxyacantha; Crataegus monogyna.
Family: Rosaceae.

People Use This For
Orally, hawthorn leaf with flower extract is used for cardiovascular conditions, including heart failure or decreased cardiac output (2,6,7,11,18,406), chronic cor pulmonale (18), circulatory disorders of the coronary arteries (e.g. angina and ischemic heart disease) (5,6,11,406), cardiomyopathy (406), arrhythmias (6,11,18,406), mild hypertension (6,406), hypotension (6), or regulation of blood pressure (18), atherosclerosis (6), cerebral insufficiency (406), and Buerger's disease. It is also used as a spasmolytic (6), for sedation (5,6,11,18), and to enhance the effects of cardiac glycosides, allowing for dose reduction (406).
In traditional medicine, hawthorn has been used as an astringent, antispasmodic, hypotensive, for diuresis, and as an antisclerotic (11).

Safety
LIKELY SAFE …when standardized extract LI132 Faros or WS 1442 Crataegutt are taken orally and appropriately short-term (2,12,406). Although hawthorn extract might be safe for long-term use, current studies have not extended past 56 days.
POSSIBLY SAFE …when other preparations of leaf and flower extract are used appropriately (12). The toxic dose of hawthorn is thought to be between 100-1000 times the therapeutic dose (406).
PREGNANCY: LIKELY UNSAFE …contraindicated for oral use because it could have uterine activity (4).
LACTATION: Insufficient reliable information available; avoid using.

Effectiveness
LIKELY EFFECTIVE …when standardized extract LI132 or WS 1442 are used orally for improving ejection fraction, exercise tolerance, and reducing subjective symptoms associated with New York Heart Association stage II heart failure (2,4,7,406). People with NYHA stage II heart failure have slight limitations in physical activity. Ordinary physical activity can cause fatigue, palpitation, trouble breathing or angina (150).
There is insufficient reliable information available about the effectiveness of hawthorn leaf with extract for its other uses.

Possible Mechanism of Action & Active Ingredients
The constituents responsible for the pharmacological effects of hawthorn preparations include flavonoids and procyanidins. Other active compounds are vitexin, rutin, and hyperoside (406). Hawthorn preparations act on the myocardium by increasing force of contraction (4,6,7,11,406), lengthening the refractory period (7,406), reducing peripheral vascular resistance (18,406), reducing oxygen consumption (406), and increasing nerve conductivity (406). Researchers think the constituent flavonoids and oligomeric procyanidins increase coronary blood flow due to vasodilation (18). They attribute hawthorn's cardiotrophic properties to increased membrane permeability for calcium and phosphodiesterase inhibition that increases intracellular cAMP. Increased cAMP leads to increased coronary blood flow, vasodilation, and positive inotropic effects (259). Human studies using hydroalcoholic extracts demonstrated therapeutic effectiveness by objective standard bicycle ergometry, anaerobic thresholds, ejection fraction, and patients subjective complaints (7). In most trials, the greatest benefit was seen after 6-8 weeks of therapy (7,406). Hawthorn has also been reported to decrease uterine tone and motility, reduce lipid levels. It also has antibacterial, spasmolytic, and analgesic effects (11).

Adverse Reactions Including Known Allergies
Hawthorn preparations may cause nausea and gastrointestinal complaints, palpitations, headache, dizziness, sleeplessness, agitation, and circulatory disturbances when used in therapeutic doses (406).

Possible Interactions with Herbs & Other Dietary Supplements
CARDIAC GLYCOSIDE-CONTAINING HERBS: Contraindicated; concomitant use may increase the risk of cardiac glycoside toxicity. Cardiac glycoside-containing herbs, include black hellebore, Canadian hemp roots, digitalis leaf, hedge mustard, figwort, lily of the valley roots, motherwort, oleander leaf, pheasant's eye plant, pleurisy root, squill bulb leaf scales, and strophanthus seeds (2,18,19,500).
OTHER CARDIOACTIVE HERBS: Avoid concomitant use with other cardioactive herbs due to unpredictability of effects and adverse effects. Other cardioactive herbs include: calamus, cereus, cola, coltsfoot, devil's claw, European mistletoe, fenugreek, fumitory, ginger, Panax ginseng, white horehound, mate, parsley, quassia, scotch broom flower, shepherd's purse, and wild carrot (4).

Possible Interactions with Drugs

CORONARY VASODILATORS: Using hawthorn with theophylline, caffeine, papaverine, sodium nitrate, adenosine, epinephrine, and other coronary vasodilators might cause additive vasodilatory effects (406).
CARDIOVASCULAR DRUGS: Hawthorn might potentiate or interfere with conventional drug therapy for heart failure, hypertension, angina, and arrhythmias (4,12).
CNS DEPRESSANTS: Concomitant use of hawthorn and CNS depressants might have additive CNS depressant effects (4,406).
DIGOXIN: Concomitant use of hawthorn and digoxin might potentiate digoxin effects requiring digoxin dose reduction (12,406).

Possible Interactions with Foods

No interactions are known to occur, and there is no known reason to expect a clinically significant interaction with hawthorn leaf with flower extract.

Possible Interactions with Lab Tests

No interactions are known to occur, and there is no known reason to expect a clinically significant interaction with hawthorn leaf with flower extract.

Possible Interactions with Diseases or Conditions

CARDIOVASCULAR CONDITIONS: Concomitant use of hawthorn with conventional cardiovascular drug therapy might potentiate or interfere with the treatment of these conditions (4,12).

Typical Dosages & Routes of Administration that are Commonly Used

ORAL: Hawthorn powder 200-500 mg is taken three times daily (406). Hawthorn, as a tea is taken three times daily initially, but can be decreased to twice daily (406). To make tea, pour hot water over a teaspoon of hawthorn leaves and flowers, steep for 20 minutes and strain (8). Twenty drops of the tincture is given 2-3 times daily. A dry extract of hawthorn 160-900 mg (3.5-19.8 mg of total flavonoids calculated as hyperoside or 30-160 mg of procyanidins) is divided and taken 2-3 times daily (2,406). Ergonomic parameters suggest that a minimum daily dose of 300 mg extract is needed for efficacy (7).

Comments

Hawthorn might offer some advantages over digoxin in mild heart failure. Compared to digitalis, hawthorn has a wider therapeutic range, lower risk in cases of dosage errors, less arrhythmogenic potential, may be safer for use in renal impairment, and can be safely used with diuretics and laxatives. However, hawthorn leaf with flower appears to be beneficial only for NYHA stage II heart failure and is inappropriate for more advanced stages (7). New York Heart Association (NYHA) stage I and II refers to individuals with heart disease who do not have resulting limitations of physical activity. They are comfortable at rest but ordinary physical activity results in fatigue, palpitation, trouble breathing, or anginal pain (2).

HAWTHORN leaf, flower

This Product is Also Known As

Aubepine, Crataegi Flos, Crataegi Folium, English Hawthorn, Haw, Hawthorne, May, Maybush, Nan Shanzha, Oneseed Hawthorn, Shanzha, Whitehorn.
CAUTION: See separate listings for Hawthorn leaf with flower extract and Hawthorn fruit.

Scientific Names

Crataegus laevigata, synonym Crataegus oxyacantha; Crataegus monogyna.
Family: Rosaceae.

People Use This For

Orally, hawthorn leaf preparations are used to prevent and treat coronary circulation problems; to improve perfusion of the myocardium; to increase cardiac output reduced by hypertension or pulmonary disease; and to treat chronic arrhythmias, hypotension, and other heart conditions (2).
Orally, hawthorn flower preparations are used to improve heart function, for autonomic heart and circulatory disturbances, coronary insufficiency, angina, cardiac neurasthenia, arrhythmias, cardiac asthma (2), and sedation (11).
Topically, hawthorn leaf has been used as a poultice for boils, sores, and ulcers (11).
Various combinations of hawthorn leaf and flower are also used orally for the same purposes as the individual preparations (406).

Safety

POSSIBLY SAFE ...when taken orally and appropriately short-term (2,12,406). The toxic dose of hawthorn is thought to be from 100-1000 times the therapeutic dose (406). Although hawthorn might be safe for long-term use,

controlled studies with standardized extract of leaf and flower do not exceed 56 days.
PREGNANCY: UNSAFE ...contraindicated due to potential uterine activity (4).
LACTATION: Insufficient reliable information available; avoid using.

Effectiveness

LIKELY EFFECTIVE ...when standardized extract LI132 or WS 1442 are used orally for improving ejection fraction, exercise tolerance, and reducing subjective symptoms associated with New York Heart Association stage II heart failure (2,4,7,406).
There is insufficient reliable information available about the effectiveness of its other uses.

Possible Mechanism of Action & Active Ingredients

The constituents responsible for the pharmacological effects of hawthorn preparations include flavonoids and procyanidins. Other active compounds are vitexin, rutin, and hyperoside (406). Hawthorn preparations act on the myocardium by increasing force of contraction (4,6,7,11,406), lengthening the refractory period (7,406), reducing peripheral vascular resistance (18,406), reducing oxygen consumption (406), and increasing nerve conductivity (406). Researchers think the constituent flavonoids and oligomeric procyanidins increase coronary blood flow due to vasodilation (18). They attribute hawthorn's cardiotrophic properties to increased membrane permeability for calcium and phosphodiesterase inhibition that increases intracellular cAMP. Increased cAMP leads to increased coronary blood flow, vasodilation, and positive inotropic effects (259). Human studies using hydroalcoholic extracts demonstrated therapeutic effectiveness by objective standard bicycle ergometry, anaerobic thresholds, ejection fraction, and patient's subjective complaints (7). In most trials, standardized hawthorn extracts were used and the greatest benefit was seen after 6-8 weeks of therapy (7,406). Hawthorn has also been reported to decrease uterine tone and motility and reduce lipid levels. It also has antibacterial, spasmolytic, and analgesic effects (11).

Adverse Reactions Including Known Allergies

Hawthorn preparations may cause nausea, gastrointestinal complaints (4,406), fatigue, sweating, rash on hands (4), palpitations, headache, dizziness, sleeplessness, agitation, and circulatory disturbances (406) when used in therapeutic doses.

Possible Interactions with Herbs & Other Dietary Supplements

CARDIAC GLYCOSIDE-CONTAINING HERBS: Contraindicated; concomitant use may increase the risk of cardiac glycoside toxicity. Cardiac glycoside-containing herbs, include black hellebore, Canadian hemp roots, digitalis leaf, hedge mustard, figwort, lily of the valley roots, motherwort, oleander leaf, pheasant's eye plant, pleurisy root, squill bulb leaf scales, and strophanthus seeds (2,18,19,500).
OTHER CARDIOACTIVE HERBS: Avoid concomitant use with other cardioactive herbs due to unpredictability of effects and adverse effects. Other cardioactive herbs include: calamus, cereus, cola, coltsfoot, devil's claw, European mistletoe, fenugreek, fumitory, ginger, Panax ginseng, white horehound, mate, parsley, quassia, scotch broom flower, shepherd's purse, and wild carrot (4). See individual product listings.

Possible Interactions with Drugs

CORONARY VASODILATORS: Using hawthorn with theophylline, caffeine, papaverine, sodium nitrate, adenosine, epinephrine and other coronary vasodilators might cause additive vasodilatory effects (406).
CARDIOVASCULAR DRUGS: Hawthorn might potentiate or interfere with conventional drug therapy for heart failure, hypertension, angina, and arrhythmias (4,12).
CNS DEPRESSANTS: Concomitant use of hawthorn and CNS depressants might have additive CNS depressant effects (4,406).
DIGOXIN: Concomitant use of hawthorn and digoxin might potentiate digoxin effects requiring digoxin dose reduction (12,406).

Possible Interactions with Foods

No interactions are known to occur, and there is no known reason to expect a clinically significant interaction with hawthorn leaf and flower.

Possible Interactions with Lab Tests

No interactions are known to occur, and there is no known reason to expect a clinically significant interaction with hawthorn leaf and flower.

Possible Interactions with Diseases or Conditions

CARDIOVASCULAR CONDITIONS: Concomitant use of hawthorn with conventional cardiovascular drug therapy might potentiate or interfere with the treatment of these conditions (4,12).

Typical Dosages & Routes of Administration that are Commonly Used

ORAL: Hawthorn leaf is used as a water extract, a water-alcohol extract, wine tea, and fresh juice (2).
CAUTION: People with self-diagnosed heart disease should not self-medicate with hawthorn or any other product. Heart disease should be diagnosed and monitored by a health care expert.

Comments

Significant clinical evidence exists for the use of hawthorn leaf with flower extract preparations in individuals with NYHA stage II heart failure. New York Heart Association (NYHA) stage I and II refers to individuals with heart disease who do not have resulting limitations of physical activity. They are comfortable at rest but ordinary physical activity results in fatigue, palpitation, trouble breathing, or anginal pain (2) (see separate listing for Hawthorn leaf with flower extract). Although similar clinical evidence does not exist for preparations containing individual plant parts, these preparations may have some benefit. Individual hawthorn leaf and flower preparations are thought to contain the same active constituents, but in differing quantities.

HAY FLOWER

This Product is Also Known As

Cat's Tails, Common Couch, Foxtails, Graminis Flos, Grass Flower, Hay Sack, Kniepp Hay Sack, Lop Grass, Meadow Fescue, Perennial Rye-Grass, Rock's-Foot, Sweet Vernal Grass, Timothy.
CAUTION: See separate listing for Sweet Clover.

Scientific Names

Elymus repens; Anthoxantum odoratum; Lolium perenne; Bromus hordeaceus; Festuca pratensis; Phleum species; Alopecurus species; Dactylis species.
Family: Poaceae.

People Use This For

Topically, hay flower is used as heat therapy for degenerative disorders, including arthritis (2). It is used as a bath additive for musculoskeletal and joint disorders (9).
In folk medicine, hay flower has been used as a bath additive for rheumatic conditions, lumbago, chilblains, and neurasthenia. It has also been used as an inhalant for inflammatory conditions of the respiratory tract (8).

Safety

POSSIBLY SAFE ...when used topically (2).
PREGNANCY AND LACTATION: Insufficient reliable information available; avoid using.

Effectiveness

POSSIBLY EFFECTIVE ...when used topically as heat therapy for degenerative diseases such as arthritis (2). There is insufficient reliable information available about the effectiveness of hay flower for its other uses.

Possible Mechanism of Action & Active Ingredients

The applicable parts of hay flower are the fruit, flower, and above ground parts. Applied topically as a heat pack, hay flower produces moist heat (1517) and promotes local blood flow (2). It can also influence internal organs through cuti-visceral reflexes (2). Hay flower contains coumarins and furanocoumarins, which are thought to have a mild sedative effect when inhaled (8,1518).

Adverse Reactions Including Known Allergies

Rare skin reactions (2) and hay fever have occurred with the use of hay flower (8).
CAUTION: Avoid overheating the topical preparations in order to prevent burns.

Possible Interactions with Herbs & Other Dietary Supplements

Insufficient reliable information available.

Possible Interactions with Drugs

No interactions are known to occur, and there is no known reason to expect a clinically significant interaction with hay flower.

Possible Interactions with Foods

No interactions are known to occur, and there is no known reason to expect a clinically significant interaction with hay flower.

Possible Interactions with Lab Tests

No interactions are known to occur, and there is no known reason to expect a clinically significant interaction with hay flower.

Possible Interactions with Diseases or Conditions

No interactions are known to occur, and there is no known reason to expect a clinically significant interaction with hay flower.

Typical Dosages & Routes of Administration that are Commonly Used

TOPICAL: For use as a flower bag, one hay flower bag is commonly heated to 42 degrees C (108 degrees F) and applied directly to the affected area once or twice per day for 40-50 minutes (2). Avoid overheating the flower bag

in order to prevent burns. As a bath additive, 500 grams of hay flower is typically boiled in 3-4 L, or about one gallon, of water for 1 minute, steeped for 30 minutes, strained, and then added to one normal bath. The individual usually bathes in the water for a maximum of 15 minutes followed by one hour bed rest (8).
INHALATION: The vapors from 5-10 grams of hay flower (1 teaspoon is approximately 2.3 grams) in one liter of boiling water is commonly inhaled (8). Remove from heat before inhaling and handle with care to prevent burns.

Comments
Hay flower includes parts of various plants sieved from cut hay grasses, and its composition varies widely (8).

HAZELNUT

This Product is Also Known As
Aveleira, Avelinier, Avellano, Cobnut, Coudrier, European filbert, European Hazel, Haselnuss, Haselstrauch, Hazel, Hazel Nut, Noisetier.

Scientific Names
Corylus avellana; Corylus heterophylla
FAMILY: Betulaceae; Corylaceae.

People Use This For
Orally, hazelnut oil is used to reduce cholesterol and as an antioxidant (5992).
Hazelnuts are commonly consumed as food.

Safety
LIKELY SAFE ...when ingested in food amounts.
PREGNANCY AND LACTATION: Likely Safe ...when used in amounts commonly found in foods. There is insufficient reliable information available about the safety of the use of hazelnut in larger amounts; avoid using.

Effectiveness
There is insufficient reliable information available about the effectiveness of hazelnut.

Possible Mechanism of Action & Active Ingredients
Hazelnuts contain 54.6-63.2% oil, 14.3-18.2% protein, and 9.8%-13.2% fiber (5995). Preliminary information suggests hazelnut oil and beta-carotene together might increase aminopyrine-N-dimethylase activity in the cytochrome P-450 system (5599).

Adverse Reactions Including Known Allergies
Hazelnut can cause an allergic reaction in sensitive individuals (5991). When ingested orally, hazelnut has been associated with exercise-induced anaphylactic reaction (5998) and one outbreak of botulism from contaminated yogurt (5999).

Possible Interactions with Herbs & Other Dietary Supplements
Insufficient reliable information available.

Possible Interactions with Drugs
No interactions are known to occur, and there is no known reason to expect a clinically significant interaction with hazelnut.

Possible Interactions with Foods
No interactions are known to occur, and there is no known reason to expect a clinically significant interaction with hazelnut.

Possible Interactions with Lab Tests
No interactions are known to occur, and there is no known reason to expect a clinically significant interaction with hazelnut.

Possible Interactions with Diseases or Conditions
Hazelnut is believed to be cross reactive with peanuts (5591), mugwort pollen (5993), brazil nut (5994), birch pollen (5996), and macadamia nut (5997).

Typical Dosages & Routes of Administration that are Commonly Used
No typical dosage.

Comments
None.

HEART'S EASE

This Product is Also Known As
European Wild Pansy, Field Pansy, Hearts Ease, Heartsease, Johnny-Jump-Up, Ladies' Delight, Pansy, Pensee Sauvage, Violae Tricoloris Herba, Wild Pansy.

Scientific Names
Viola tricolor.
Family: Violaceae.

People Use This For
Orally, heart's ease is used for promoting metabolism, as a demulcent for respiratory disorders such as throat inflammation and whooping cough, and as a laxative (18,400).
Topically, heart's ease is used for mild seborrheic skin disorders, milk scall (seborrhea of the scalp) in children, warts, mild skin inflammation, acne, exanthema (skin eruption), eczema, impetigo, and itching of the female external genitalia (2,400).

Safety
POSSIBLY SAFE ...when appropriately used for oral or topical medicinal purposes (2,12).
PREGNANCY AND LACTATION: Insufficient reliable information; avoid using.

Effectiveness
POSSIBLY EFFECTIVE ...when used topically for mild seborrheic skin disorders and seborrhea of the scalp in children (2).
There is insufficient reliable information available about the effectiveness of heart's ease for its other uses.

Possible Mechanism of Action & Active Ingredients
The applicable parts of heart's ease are the above ground parts. Heart's ease can have anti-inflammatory and antioxidant properties (18).

Adverse Reactions Including Known Allergies
None known.

Possible Interactions with Herbs & Other Dietary Supplements
Insufficient reliable information available.

Possible Interactions with Drugs
No interactions are known to occur, and there is no known reason to expect a clinically significant interaction with heart's ease.

Possible Interactions with Foods
No interactions are known to occur, and there is no known reason to expect a clinically significant interaction with heart's ease.

Possible Interactions with Lab Tests
No interactions are known to occur, and there is no known reason to expect a clinically significant interaction with heart's ease.

Possible Interactions with Diseases or Conditions
No interactions are known to occur, and there is no known reason to expect a clinically significant interaction with heart's ease.

Typical Dosages & Routes of Administration that are Commonly Used
ORAL: The typical dose of heart's ease is one cup of the tea three times per day (18). The tea is prepared by steeping 1.5 grams of the above ground parts in 150 mL boiling water for 5-10 minutes and then straining.
TOPICAL: Heart's ease is commonly applied externally three times per day as a poultice or the prepared tea (18).

Comments
Store heart's ease in a well-sealed container and away from light (18).

HEATHER

This Product is Also Known As
Callunae vulgaris herba, Calluna vulgaris flos, Ling, Scotch Heather.

Scientific Names
Calluna vulgaris.
Family: Ericaceae.

People Use This For
Orally, heather is taken for ailments of the kidney and lower urinary tract, prostate enlargement, diuresis, gastrointestinal ailments and diseases, diarrhea, gastrointestinal spasm, colic, disease of the liver and gallbladder, gout, arthritis, sleep disorders, respiratory disorders, cough, colds, and diaphoresis (2,18).
Topically, heather is used for wounds and inflamed eyes (2).
In combination with other herbs, heather is used for diabetes, menstrual discomfort, menopause, stimulation of digestion, nervous exhaustion, and regulation of the circulatory system (2).

Safety
POSSIBLY SAFE ...when used orally or topically and appropriately (12).
PREGNANCY AND LACTATION: Insufficient reliable information available; avoid using.

Effectiveness
There is insufficient reliable information available about the effectiveness of heather (2,400).

Possible Mechanism of Action & Active Ingredients
The applicable parts of heather are the flower, leaf, and plant top. There is insufficient reliable information available about the possible mechanism of action and active ingredients of heather.

Adverse Reactions Including Known Allergies
None reported.

Possible Interactions with Herbs & Other Dietary Supplements
Insufficient reliable information available.

Possible Interactions with Drugs
No interactions are known to occur, and there is no known reason to expect a clinically significant interaction with heather.

Possible Interactions with Foods
No interactions are known to occur, and there is no known reason to expect a clinically significant interaction with heather.

Possible Interactions with Lab Tests
No interactions are known to occur, and there is no known reason to expect a clinically significant interaction with heather.

Possible Interactions with Diseases or Conditions
No interactions are known to occur, and there is no known reason to expect a clinically significant interaction with heather.

Typical Dosages & Routes of Administration that are Commonly Used
ORAL: One cup of tea (simmer 1.5 grams of flower/leaf/plant top in 250 mL boiling water 3 minutes, strain) three times daily between meals (18).
TOPICAL: As a bath, 500 grams of flower/leaf/plant top in a few liters of water, strain and add to full bath (18).

Comments
None.

HEDGE MUSTARD

This Product is Also Known As
English Watercress, Erysimum, St. Barbara's Hedge Mustard, Singer's Plant, Thalictroc.
CAUTION: See separate listings for White Mustard, Black Mustard seed, and Black Mustard Oil.

Scientific Names
Sisymbrium officinale, synonym Erysimum officinale.
Family: Brassicaceae.

People Use This For
Orally, hedge mustard is taken to treat urinary tract diseases, coughs, chronic bronchitis, and inflammation of the gallbladder (18).
Topically, it is used as a gargle or mouthwash (18).

Safety
LIKELY UNSAFE ...when the flowering above ground parts are taken orally since they contain cardioactive glycosides (18).

There is insufficient reliable information available about the safety of the topical use of hedge mustard.
PREGNANCY AND LACTATION: LIKELY UNSAFE ...when used orally; avoid using.

Effectiveness
There is insufficient reliable information available about the effectiveness of hedge mustard.

Possible Mechanism of Action & Active Ingredients
The applicable parts of hedge mustard are the above ground parts. The foliage contains vitamin C and 0.05% cardenolides (cardioactive glycosides) including sinigrin and gluconapin. Hedge mustard also contains the volatile mustard oil allyl isothiocyanate and 3-butenylisothiocyanate (18).

Adverse Reactions Including Known Allergies
Theoretically, digitalis-like effects possible (vomiting, diarrhea, headache, and cardiac rhythm disorders) (18).

Possible Interactions with Herbs & Other Dietary Supplements
CARDIAC GLYCOSIDE-CONTAINING HERBS: Contraindicated, and concomitant use can increase the risk of cardiac glycoside toxicity. Cardiac glycoside-containing herbs include black hellebore, Canadian hemp roots, digitalis leaf, figwort, lily of the valley roots, motherwort, oleander leaf, pheasant's eye plant, pleurisy root, squill bulb leaf scales, strophanthus seeds, and uzara (2,18,19,500).
OTHER CARDIOACTIVE HERBS: Avoid concomitant use with other cardioactive herbs due to unpredictability of effects (4).
STIMULANT LAXATIVE HERBS: Theoretically, overuse or misuse of stimulant laxatives with cardiac glycoside-containing herbs increases the risk of cardiac toxicity due to potassium depletion (19).
LICORICE/HORSETAIL: Theoretically, overuse/misuse of licorice rhizome or horsetail plant with cardiac glycoside-containing herbs increases the risk of cardiac toxicity due to potassium depletion (19).

Possible Interactions with Drugs
DIGOXIN: Contraindicated; concomitant use increases risk of cardiac glycoside toxicity (2).
CARDIAC DRUGS: Theoretically, concomitant may increase risk of cardiac toxicity (152).
STIMULANT LAXATIVES: Theoretically, overuse/misuse may increase risk of cardiac glycoside toxicity due to potassium depletion (2).
POTASSIUM-DEPLETING DIURETICS: Theoretically, concomitant use may increase risk of cardiac glycoside toxicity due to potassium depletion (2,506).
QUININE: Theoretically, concomitant use may increase risk of cardiac toxicity (2,506).
TETRACYCLINES AND MACROLIDE ANTIBIOTICS: Theoretically, concomitant use may increase risk of cardiac glycoside toxicity (152,17).

Possible Interactions with Foods
No interactions are known to occur, and there is no known reason to expect a clinically significant interaction with hedge mustard.

Possible Interactions with Lab Tests
No interactions are known to occur, and there is no known reason to expect a clinically significant interaction with hedge mustard.

Possible Interactions with Diseases or Conditions
HEART DISEASE: Contraindicated; theoretically, cardiac glycosides contained in hedge mustard may exacerbate condition or interfere with existing drug therapy.

Typical Dosages & Routes of Administration that are Commonly Used
ORAL: One cup tea (preparation unspecified) 3-4 times daily (18); average amount is 0.5-1 grams above ground parts per day (18).
TOPICAL: Tea is used as a mouthwash or gargle, several times daily (18).

Comments
Avoid confusion with black mustard (Brassica nigra), brown mustard (Brassica juncea), white mustard (Brassica alba or Sinapis alba), Indian mustard (Brassica juncea), and Chinese mustard (Sinapis juncea).

HEDGE-HYSSOP

This Product is Also Known As
Gratiola, Hedge Hyssop.

Scientific Names
Gratiola officinalis.
Family: Scrophulariaceae.

People Use This For
In folk medicine, people used hedge-hyssop orally for treating the liver, as an emetic, and to induce bowel evacuation. It has also been used in the elimination of intestinal parasites, to increase urination, and has cardiotonic properties (18).

Safety
UNSAFE ...when taken orally (18).
PREGNANCY AND LACTATION: UNSAFE ...due to toxic potential (18).

Effectiveness
There is insufficient reliable information available about the effectiveness of hedge-hyssop.

Possible Mechanism of Action & Active Ingredients
The applicable parts of hedge-hyssop are the above ground parts. Hedge-hyssop contains cucurbitacin glycosides which are released in aqueous environments and are extremely irritating to mucous membranes (18).

Adverse Reactions Including Known Allergies
When taken orally in toxic doses, hedge-hyssop may cause vomiting, bloody diarrhea, colic, and kidney irritation characterized by initial diuresis followed by anuria. When people ingest very high amounts, spasms, paralysis, and circulatory collapse occur. Death occurs rarely (18).

Possible Interactions with Herbs & Other Dietary Supplements
Insufficient reliable information available.

Possible Interactions with Drugs
No interactions are known to occur, and there is no known reason to expect a clinically significant interaction with hedge-hyssop.

Possible Interactions with Foods
No interactions are known to occur, and there is no known reason to expect a clinically significant interaction with hedge-hyssop.

Possible Interactions with Lab Tests
No interactions are known to occur, and there is no known reason to expect a clinically significant interaction with hedge-hyssop.

Possible Interactions with Diseases or Conditions
No interactions are known to occur, and there is no known reason to expect a clinically significant interaction with hedge-hyssop.

Typical Dosages & Routes of Administration that are Commonly Used
No typical dosage.

Comments
Hedge-hyssop is considered unsafe for oral use; avoid using (18).

HEMLOCK SPRUCE

This Product is Also Known As
Balm of Gilead Fir, Balsam Fir, Canada Balsam, Fir Tree, Norway Pine, Norway Spruce, Picea aetheroleum, Picea turiones recentes, Spruce, Spruce Fir.

Scientific Names
Picea excelsa, synonym Picea abies; Abies excelsa.
Family: Coniferae.

People Use This For
Orally, hemlock spruce is used for coughs, the common cold, bronchitis, fevers, inflammation of the mouth and pharynx, muscular and nerve pain, arthritis, and as an antibacterial.
Topically, it is used for inflammation of the respiratory tract, arthritis pain, nerve pain, and for feelings of tension. Hemlock spruce is also used externally as a counterirritant and to improve circulation.
In folk medicine, it was used orally for tuberculosis and topically as a bath additive for individuals who were mentally ill (18).

Safety
There is insufficient reliable information available about the safety of hemlock spruce.
Pregnancy and Lactation: Insufficient reliable information available; avoid using.

Effectiveness

There is insufficient reliable information available about the effectiveness of hemlock spruce.

Possible Mechanism of Action & Active Ingredients

The applicable part of hemlock spruce is the oil obtained by steam distillation from the needles, branch tips or branches and the fresh fir shoots of Picea excelsa (18). There is insufficient reliable information available about the possible mechanism of action and active ingredients.

Adverse Reactions Including Known Allergies

None reported.

Possible Interactions with Herbs & Other Dietary Supplements

Insufficient reliable information available.

Possible Interactions with Drugs

No interactions are known to occur, and there is no known reason to expect a clinically significant interaction with hemlock spruce.

Possible Interactions with Foods

No interactions are known to occur, and there is no known reason to expect a clinically significant interaction with hemlock spruce.

Possible Interactions with Lab Tests

No interactions are known to occur, and there is no known reason to expect a clinically significant interaction with hemlock spruce.

Possible Interactions with Diseases or Conditions

ASTHMA AND WHOOPING COUGH: Hemlock spruce may theoretically worsen asthma and whooping cough.(18).
EXTENSIVE SKIN INJURIES, ACUTE SKIN DISEASES: Hemlock spruce should not be applied to broken skin (18).
CARDIAC INSUFFICIENCY: Avoid use of hemlock spruce (18).

Typical Dosages & Routes of Administration that are Commonly Used

ORAL: The daily dose is 4 drops of oil on a lump of sugar taken three times daily. Alternately, 2 grams oil is added to hot water and inhaled several times daily (18).
TOPICAL: Hemlock spruce is used as a 10-50% semi-solid preparation. Several drops of this oil are rubbed into the affected area (18).

Comments

Hemlock spruce is very similar sounding to water hemlock and European water hemlock, which are entirely different plants. Be careful not to confuse hemlock spruce with either form of water hemlock, because the water hemlocks are very toxic (see separate listings) (18).

HEMP AGRIMONY

This Product is Also Known As

Alpenkraut, Chanvrin, Donnerkraut, Dostenkraut, Drachenkraut, Dutch Agrimony, Dutch Eupatoire Commune, Eupatorium, Gemeiner Wasswedost, Herbe de Sainte Cunegonde, Hirshklee, Holy Rope, Kunigundendraut, Leberkraut, Origan De Marais, St. John's Herb, Sweet Mandulin, Sweet-Smelling Trefoil, Thoroughwort, Wasshanf, Waterhemp, Water Maudlin.

Scientific Names

Eupatorium cannabinum.
Family: Compositae.

People Use This For

Orally, hemp agrimony is used for liver and gallbladder disorders, colds, and fever (18).

Safety

LIKELY UNSAFE …when used orally. Hemp agrimony contains hepatotoxic unsaturated pyrrolizidine alkaloids (UPAs) (12,19). Repeated exposure to low concentrations of UPAs are linked to veno-occlusive disease, a serious condition (4,12). UPAs may also be carcinogenic and mutagenic (12). …when used topically on abraded or broken skin due to potential for systemic absorption (12,19).
PREGNANCY: UNSAFE …contraindicated due to possible menstrual stimulant and abortifacient activities (19).
LACTATION: LIKELY UNSAFE …due to concern that UPAs might be excreted into breast milk (19).

Effectiveness

There is insufficient reliable information available about the effectiveness of hemp agrimony.

Possible Mechanism of Action & Active Ingredients

The applicable part of hemp agrimony is the flowering herb. Some pyrrolizidine alkaloids have shown carcinogenic and mutagenic properties, and there are reports of renal toxicity. However, the primary concern is veno-occlusive disease (12). Unsaturated pyrrolizidine alkaloids are known to be hepatotoxic in animals and humans (4).

Adverse Reactions Including Known Allergies

When used orally, acute toxicity may result in hepatic necrosis; chronic toxicity may cause veno-occlusive liver disease. The potential for hepatotoxicity (due to presence of pyrrolizidine alkaloids) increases with larger doses and longer periods of use (4,12). It can cause an allergic reaction in individuals sensitive to the Asteraceae/Compositae family. Members of this family include ragweed, chrysanthemums, marigolds, daisies, and many other herbs.

Possible Interactions with Herbs & Other Dietary Supplements

EUCALYPTUS: Theoretically, concomitant use might increase the risk of unsaturated pyrrolizidine alkaloid toxicity due to enzyme induction by eucalyptus (19).
PYRROLIZIDINE ALKALOID-CONTAINING HERBS: Concomitant use is contraindicated due to the risk of additive toxicity. Herbs containing unsaturated pyrrolizidine alkaloids include: alkanna (12), borage (271), gravel root (4), hemp agrimony (271), hound's tongue (19), petasites (19), comfrey (271), coltsfoot, and the Senecio species plants; dusty miller (19), alpine ragwort (19), groundsel (271), golden ragwort (19), and tansy ragwort (271).

Possible Interactions with Drugs

No interactions are known to occur, and there is no known reason to expect a clinically significant interaction with hemp agrimony.

Possible Interactions with Foods

No interactions are known to occur, and there is no known reason to expect a clinically significant interaction with hemp agrimony.

Possible Interactions with Lab Tests

No interactions are known to occur, and there is no known reason to expect a clinically significant interaction with hemp agrimony.

Possible Interactions with Diseases or Conditions

CROSS-ALLERGENICITY: Can cause an allergic reaction in individuals sensitive to the Asteraceae/Compositae family. Members of this family include ragweed, chrysanthemums, marigolds, daisies, and many other herbs.

Typical Dosages & Routes of Administration that are Commonly Used

No typical dosage.

Comments

Hemp agrimony is considered likely unsafe for oral use; avoid using (4,12).

HEMPNETTLE

This Product is Also Known As

Galeopsidis Herba.

Scientific Names

Galeopsis segetum, synonym Galeopsis ochroleuca.
Family: Lamiaceae.

People Use This For

Orally, hempnettle is used for mild respiratory tract inflammation (2), cough, and bronchitis (18).
Traditionally, it has been used for pulmonary afflictions and as a diuretic (18).

Safety

POSSIBLY SAFE ...when used orally and appropriately (2).
PREGNANCY AND LACTATION: Insufficient reliable information available; avoid using.

Effectiveness

POSSIBLY EFFECTIVE ...when used orally for mild respiratory tract inflammation (2).
There is insufficient reliable information available about the effectiveness of hempnettle for its other uses.

Possible Mechanism of Action & Active Ingredients

The applicable parts of hempnettle are the above ground parts. Hempnettle can have astringent and expectorant effects (18).

Adverse Reactions Including Known Allergies
None reported.

Possible Interactions with Herbs & Other Dietary Supplements
Insufficient reliable information available.

Possible Interactions with Drugs
No interactions are known to occur, and there is no known reason to expect a clinically significant interaction with hempnettle.

Possible Interactions with Foods
No interactions are known to occur, and there is no known reason to expect a clinically significant interaction with hempnettle.

Possible Interactions with Lab Tests
No interactions are known to occur, and there is no known reason to expect a clinically significant interaction with hempnettle.

Possible Interactions with Diseases or Conditions
No interactions are known to occur, and there is no known reason to expect a clinically significant interaction with hempnettle.

Typical Dosages & Routes of Administration that are Commonly Used
ORAL: The typical dose of hempnettle is 6 grams of the above ground parts per day or one cup of the tea up to three times daily. The tea is prepared by steeping 2 grams of the above ground parts in 150 mL boiling water for 5-10 minutes and then straining (18). The use of hempnettle in children requires a dosing adjustment; however, no additional information is available on the exact dosing adjustments (510).

Comments
None.

HENBANE

This Product is Also Known As
Devil's Eye, Fetid Nightshade, Hen Bell, Hog Bean, Hyoscyami Folium, Jupiter's Bean, Poison Tobacco, Stinking Nightshade.
CAUTION: See separate listing for Belladonna and Bittersweet Nightshade.

Scientific Names
Hyoscyamus niger.
Family: Solanaceae.

People Use This For
Orally, henbane leaf is used for spasms of the gastrointestinal tract (2).
Topically, the leaf oil is used for treating scar tissue (18).

Safety
POSSIBLY SAFE ...when the leaf is used orally and appropriately short-term under medical supervision (2). Contains hyoscyamine and scopolamine alkaloids (2).
LIKELY UNSAFE ...when used orally for self-medication. Hyoscyamine and scopolamine have a narrow range of safe use. Excessive doses can cause poisoning and death (18).
There is insufficient reliable information available about the safety of the topical use of henbane.
PREGNANCY AND LACTATION: LIKELY UNSAFE ...contraindicated for oral use because of its risk of poisoning (18).

Effectiveness
POSSIBLY EFFECTIVE ...when taken orally for spasms of the GI tract (2).
There is insufficient reliable information available about the effectiveness of henbane for its other uses.

Possible Mechanism of Action & Active Ingredients
The applicable part of henbane is the leaf. The alkaloid constituents, which include hyoscyamine and scopolamine, competitively inhibit acetylcholine, causing anticholinergic and parasympathetic effects (18). With storage, hyoscyamine converts to atropine. The inhibition of acetylcholine affects the muscarinic action but not the nicotinic effects of acetylcholine on ganglia and motor endplates. Henbane causes smooth muscle relaxation particularly in the GI tract, relieves muscle tremors of CNS origin, and has a sedative effect (2).

Adverse Reactions Including Known Allergies

Taken orally, henbane can cause dry mouth, red skin, constipation, overheating, reduced sweating, vision disturbances, tachycardia, and difficulty with urinating (2,18). Overdose poisoning symptoms include somnolence followed by CNS stimulation described as restlessness, hallucinations, delirium, and manic episodes followed by exhaustion and sleep. Henbane can cause death by asphyxiation (18).

Possible Interactions with Herbs & Other Dietary Supplements

ANTICHOLINERGIC CONTAINING HERBS: Theoretically, concomitant use of henbane with other anticholinergic alkaloid-containing herbs, including belladonna, deadly nightshade, and jimson weed, can have additive therapeutic and adverse effects.

Possible Interactions with Drugs

ANTICHOLINERGIC DRUGS: Concomitant use of henbane can have additive anticholinergic effects and adverse effects with amantadine, antihistamines, atropine, belladonna alkaloids, hyoscyamine, phenothiazines, procainamide, scopolamine, and tricyclic antidepressants (2).

Possible Interactions with Foods

No interactions are known to occur, and there is no known reason to expect a clinically significant interaction with henbane.

Possible Interactions with Lab Tests

No interactions are known to occur, and there is no known reason to expect a clinically significant interaction with henbane.

Possible Interactions with Diseases or Conditions

CONGESTIVE HEART FAILURE (CHF): Contraindicated; henbane might cause tachycardia and exacerbate CHF due to its hyoscyamine (atropine) and scopolamine content (15).

CONSTIPATION: Contraindicated; henbane might cause constipation due to its hyoscyamine (atropine) and scopolamine content (15).

DOWN SYNDROME: Caution, patients with Down syndrome might be hypersensitive to the antimuscarinic effects (mydriasis, positive chronotropic heart effects, etc.) of hyoscyamine (atropine) and scopolamine contained in henbane (15).

ESOPHAGEAL REFLUX: Contraindicated; henbane might delay gastric emptying and decrease lower esophageal pressure, promoting gastric retention and exacerbating reflux due to its hyoscyamine (atropine) and scopolamine content (15).

FEVER: Contraindicated; henbane might increase the risk of hyperthermia in patients with fever due to its hyoscyamine (atropine) and scopolamine content (15).

GASTRIC ULCER: Contraindicated; henbane might delay gastric emptying and exacerbate gastric ulcers due to its hyoscyamine (atropine) and scopolamine content (15).

GI INFECTIONS: Contraindicated; henbane might suppress GI motility causing retention of infecting organisms or toxins due to its hyoscyamine (atropine) and scopolamine content (15).

HIATAL HERNIA: Contraindicated; henbane might delay gastric emptying and decrease lower esophageal pressure, promoting gastric retention and exacerbating reflux due to its hyoscyamine (atropine) and scopolamine content (15).

TOXIC MEGACOLON: Contraindicated; henbane might suppress intestinal motility, which might produce paralytic ileus and exacerbate toxic megacolon, due to its hyoscyamine (atropine) and scopolamine content (2,15).

NARROW-ANGLE GLAUCOMA: Contraindicated; henbane might increase ocular tension in patients with narrow-angle (angle-closure) glaucoma due to its hyoscyamine (atropine) and scopolamine content (2,15).

OBSTRUCTIVE GI TRACT DISEASE: Contraindicated; henbane might exacerbate obstructive GI tract diseases (including atony, paralytic ileus, and stenosis) due to its hyoscyamine (atropine) and scopolamine content (15).

TACHYARRHYTHMIAS: Contraindicated; henbane might cause tachycardia due to its hyoscyamine (atropine) and scopolamine content (2,15).

URINARY RETENTION: Contraindicated; henbane might increase urinary retention due to its hyoscyamine (atropine) and scopolamine content (2,15).

ULCERATIVE COLITIS: Contraindicated; henbane might suppress intestinal motility, which might produce paralytic ileus and precipitate toxic megacolon, due to its hyoscyamine (atropine) and scopolamine content (15).

Typical Dosages & Routes of Administration that are Commonly Used

ORAL: The average single dose of the standardized henbane powder is 500 mg, which corresponds to 250-350 mg of the total alkaloid (2). The maximum single dose of henbane is 1 gram, which corresponds to 500-700 mg of the total alkaloid (2). The maximum daily dosage is 3 grams, which corresponds to 1.5-2.1 grams of the total alkaloid calculated as hyoscyamine (2).

TOPICAL: No typical dosage.

© Copyright 2000, Natural Medicines Comprehensive Database (209) 472-2244. For updated data, go to www.NaturalDatabase.com

Comments

Avoid confusion with bittersweet nightshade (Solanum dulcamara) and belladonna (deadly nightshade). The flowering branches, dried seeds, and whole, fresh flowering plant of henbane may have medicinal uses (18).

HENNA

This Product is Also Known As

Alcanna, Egyptian Privet, Hennae folium, Henne, Jamaica Mignonette, Mehndi, Mendee, Mignonette Tree, Reseda, Smooth Lawsonia.
CAUTION: See separate listing for Alkanna (Alkanna tinctoria).

Scientific Names

Lawsonia inermis, synonym Lawsonia alba.
Family: Lythraceae.

People Use This For

Orally, henna leaf is used for gastrointestinal ulcers (18).
Topically, it is used for dandruff, eczema, scabies, fungal infections, and ulcers (18). Henna is also used topically for applying decorative henna "tattoos".
Traditionally, henna leaf has been used for amebic dysentery (11,18), cancer, enlarged spleen, headache, jaundice, and skin conditions (11).
In manufacturing, henna is used in cosmetics (18), hair dyes and hair care products (11), and as a dye for nails, hands and clothing (11). Lawsone, a constituent, can be used as an indicator for titration of strong acids with weak bases (11).

Safety

LIKELY SAFE ...when the leaf is used topically. It is approved for topical use as a color additive in hair cosmetics in the US (11). However, contact dermatitis and hypersensitivity reactions have been reported with topical use (1370,4146,4148,6144,6145,6146,6147,6148,6149,6150,6151).
UNSAFE ...when used orally (12).
CHILDREN: POSSIBLY UNSAFE ...when used topically on children, and especially on infants (4147,6144,6149,6150). Use is associated with hemolysis in infants deficient in glucose-6-phosphate dehydrogenase (G6PD) (4147).
UNSAFE ...when used orally (12).
PREGNANCY: UNSAFE ...contraindicated. Henna is believed to have abortifacient properties (12,19).
LACTATION: UNSAFE ...when used orally.

Effectiveness

There is insufficient reliable information available about the effectiveness of henna.

Possible Mechanism of Action & Active Ingredients

The applicable part of henna is the leaf. Henna leaf contains lawsone, gallic acid and 5-10% tannin (11). It is thought to have astringent and diuretic properties (18). Some evidence suggests henna might have activity against Mycobacterium tuberculosis (4150). In female rats, henna leaves inhibit fertility (11). The constituents, lawsone and gallic acid, have antibacterial properties (11). Studies suggest that lawsone might also have antifungal, antitumor, antispasmodic and weak vitamin K activity (11). Evidence shows it might be able to decrease the formation of sickled cells in individuals with sickle cell anemia (4149). An ethanol extract containing luteolin, beta-sitosterol, and lawsone was claimed to have anti-inflammatory, antihyaluronidase, and analgesic activity (11).

Adverse Reactions Including Known Allergies

Taken by mouth, henna can cause an upset stomach, possibly due to tannin content (18). Topical use can cause contact dermatitis, including redness, itching, burning, swelling, scaling, fissuring, papules, blisters, and scarring (1370,4146,6144,6145,6146,6147,6148,6149,6150). There are two reports of occupational exposure associated with immediate-type hypersensitivity involving urticaria, rhinitis, wheezing, and bronchial asthma (4148,6151). In infants with glucose 6-phosphate dehydrogenase (G6PD) deficiency, topical henna use has been associated with hemolysis, anemia, reticulocytosis, and indirect hyperbilirubinemia (4147). Prolonged use on hair may turn the hair orange-red, unless mixed with other dyes to get different shades (11).

Possible Interactions with Herbs & Other Dietary Supplements

Insufficient reliable information available.

Possible Interactions with Drugs

No interactions are known to occur, and there is no known reason to expect a clinically significant interaction with henna.

Possible Interactions with Foods

No interactions are known to occur, and there is no known reason to expect a clinically significant interaction with henna.

Possible Interactions with Lab Tests

No interactions are known to occur, and there is no known reason to expect a clinically significant interaction with henna.

Possible Interactions with Diseases or Conditions

G6PD DEFICIENCY: There are reports of hemolysis in infants with glucose-6-phosphate dehydrogenase deficiency after topical exposure to henna (4147).
HENNA HYPERSENSITIVITY: Avoid topical exposure by individuals with henna hypersensitivity.

Typical Dosages & Routes of Administration that are Commonly Used

No typical dosage.

Comments

Henna is considered unsafe for oral use; avoid using (12). Henna should not be confused with henna root (Alkanna tinctoria), also referred to as alkanna root (6).

HERB PARIS

This Product is Also Known As

Einbeere, Herb-Paris, One Berry, Oneberry, Tilki Uzumu, Uva De Raposa, Wang Sun.

Scientific Names

Paris quadrifolia.
Family: Trilliaceae.

People Use This For

Traditionally, Herb Paris has been used for headache, longevity, neuralgia, rheumatism, genital tumors, palpitation, spasms, and as an emetic, narcotic, poison, and purgative (4017).

Safety

LIKELY UNSAFE ...when taken orally. The plant and berry are poisonous (18).
PREGNANCY AND LACTATION: UNSAFE (18).

Effectiveness

There is insufficient reliable information available about the effectiveness of Herb Paris.

Possible Mechanism of Action & Active Ingredients

The applicable part of Herb Paris is the whole plant with ripe fruit. Herb Paris contains triterpene saponins (pennogenintetra glycosides), also referred to as parissaponins, which cause local irritation, increasing absorption of the toxic constituent, paristyphnin (18). Paristyphnin causes miosis and respiratory paralysis (18).

Adverse Reactions Including Known Allergies

Herb Paris can cause nausea, vomiting, diarrhea, headache, miosis, and respiratory paralysis (18).

Possible Interactions with Herbs & Other Dietary Supplements

Insufficient reliable information available.

Possible Interactions with Drugs

No interactions are known to occur, and there is no known reason to expect a clinically significant interaction with herb Paris.

Possible Interactions with Foods

No interactions are known to occur, and there is no known reason to expect a clinically significant interaction with herb Paris.

Possible Interactions with Lab Tests

No interactions are known to occur, and there is no known reason to expect a clinically significant interaction with herb Paris.

Possible Interactions with Diseases or Conditions

No interactions are known to occur, and there is no known reason to expect a clinically significant interaction with herb Paris.

Typical Dosages & Routes of Administration that are Commonly Used

No typical dosage.

Comments
Herb Paris is considered likely unsafe, poisonous; avoid using.

HERB ROBERT

This Product is Also Known As
Dragon's Blood, Storkbill, Wild Crane's-Bill.
CAUTION: See separate listings for Dragon's Blood (Daemonorops draco) and Sangre de Grado.

Scientific Names
Geranium robertianum.
Family: Geraniaceae.

People Use This For
Orally, Herb Robert is used for diarrhea; to improve functioning of the liver and gallbladder; to reduce inflammation of the kidney, bladder, and gallbladder; and to prevent the formation of calculi (18).
Topically, Herb Robert is used as a mouthwash or gargle and the fresh leaves chewed to relieve inflammation of the mouth and throat (18).

Safety
There is insufficient reliable information available about the safety of Herb Robert. (18).
Pregnancy and Lactation: Insufficient reliable information is available; avoid using.

Effectiveness
There is insufficient reliable information available about the effectiveness of Herb Robert.

Possible Mechanism of Action & Active Ingredients
The applicable parts of Herb Robert are the above ground parts. Herb Robert contains several flavonoids including rutin. Some evidence suggests an ethanolic extract can inhibit the growth of E. coli, P. aeruginosa, and S. aureus. Other evidence indicates the extract of the fresh herb, including the root, has a mild antiviral effect against the vesicular stomatitis virus (18). Although general reviews report Herb Robert has hypotensive effects, no specific information is available (18). Some data show a crystalline fraction can protect the tobacco plant from pathogenic viruses (18).

Adverse Reactions Including Known Allergies
None reported (18).

Possible Interactions with Herbs & Other Dietary Supplements
Insufficient reliable information available.

Possible Interactions with Drugs
No interactions are known to occur, and there is no known reason to expect a clinically significant interaction with Herb Robert.

Possible Interactions with Foods
No interactions are known to occur, and there is no known reason to expect a clinically significant interaction with Herb Robert..

Possible Interactions with Lab Tests
No interactions are known to occur, and there is no known reason to expect a clinically significant interaction with Herb Robert.

Possible Interactions with Diseases or Conditions
No interactions are known to occur, and there is no known reason to expect a clinically significant interaction with Herb Robert.

Typical Dosages & Routes of Administration that are Commonly Used
ORAL: Herb Robert is used as tea, 2 to 3 cups daily between meals (18). To make tea, 1 teaspoon of herb is added to 500 mL of cold water, brought to a boil, allowed to draw, and strained.
TOPICAL: Prepared tea is used as mouthwash or gargle (18). Fresh leaves are chewed to relieve mouth or throat inflammation (18).

Comments
Herb Robert is characterized by an unpleasant smell of goats or bugs (18).

HIBISCUS

This Product is Also Known As
Guinea Sorrel, Jamaica Sorrel, Karkade, Red Tea, Roselle, Sudanese Tea.

Scientific Names
Hibiscus sabdariffa.
Family: Malvaceae.

People Use This For
Orally, hibiscus is used for loss of appetite, colds, upper respiratory tract and stomach mucous membrane inflammation, disorders of circulation, for dissolving phlegm, and as a gentle laxative and diuretic (2).
Historically, the leaves of hibiscus were used for treating heart and nerve diseases (11).
In foods and beverages, hibiscus is used as a flavoring (11). It is also used to improve the odor, flavor, or appearance of tea mixtures (7).

Safety
LIKELY SAFE ...when used orally in amounts found in beverages (maximum use level 0.02%); approved for use in alcoholic beverages in the US (12).
POSSIBLY SAFE ...when used as an oral medicinal (2,12); there are no known risks (2).
PREGNANCY: LIKELY UNSAFE. Hibiscus is thought to be a menstrual stimulant, and might have abortifacient effects (19).
LACTATION: Insufficient reliable information is available; avoid using.

Effectiveness
There is insufficient reliable information available about the effectiveness of hibiscus.

Possible Mechanism of Action & Active Ingredients
The applicable part of hibiscus is the flower. People think the laxative effects of hibiscus are due to high content of poorly absorbable fruit acids (18). Extracts have intestinal and uterine muscle antispasmodic activity (11,18), hypotensive effects (11,18), anthelmintic properties (11), and in vitro antibacterial activity (11).

Adverse Reactions Including Known Allergies
None reported.

Possible Interactions with Herbs & Other Dietary Supplements
Insufficient reliable information available.

Possible Interactions with Drugs
No interactions are known to occur, and there is no known reason to expect a clinically significant interaction with hibiscus.

Possible Interactions with Foods
No interactions are known to occur, and there is no known reason to expect a clinically significant interaction with hibiscus.

Possible Interactions with Lab Tests
No interactions are known to occur, and there is no known reason to expect a clinically significant interaction with hibiscus.

Possible Interactions with Diseases or Conditions
No interactions are known to occur, and there is no known reason to expect a clinically significant interaction with hibiscus.

Typical Dosages & Routes of Administration that are Commonly Used
ORAL: To prepare tea, steep 1.5 grams of flowers in 150 mL boiling water 5-10 minutes, strain (18); no additional dosing or administration information available (18).

Comments
None.

HISTIDINE

This Product is Also Known As
Levo-Histidine, L-Histidine.

Scientific Names
L-2-Amino-3-(1H-imidazol-4-yl) propionic acid; alpha-amino-4-imidazole propanoic acid.

People Use This For

Orally, histidine is used for rheumatoid arthritis, allergic diseases, ulcers, and anemia (2344,2345,2346).

Safety

POSSIBLY SAFE ...when used orally and appropriately. Clinical studies note the absence of side effects at doses up to 4 grams per day (2347,2353).

PREGNANCY AND LACTATION: Insufficient reliable information available; avoid using.

Effectiveness

POSSIBLY INEFFECTIVE ...when taken orally for treating rheumatoid arthritis (2350,2351), anemia of uremia (2352), or anemia associated with chronic dialysis (2352,2353).

There is insufficient reliable information available about the effectiveness of histidine for its other uses.

Possible Mechanism of Action & Active Ingredients

Histidine is an essential amino acid involved in a wide range of metabolic processes (2354).

Adverse Reactions Including Known Allergies

None reported.

Possible Interactions with Herbs & Other Dietary Supplements

Insufficient reliable information available.

Possible Interactions with Drugs

No interactions are known to occur, and there is no known reason to expect a clinically significant interaction with histidine.

Possible Interactions with Foods

No interactions are known to occur, and there is no known reason to expect a clinically significant interaction with histidine.

Possible Interactions with Lab Tests

URINE FORMIMINOGLUTAMIC ACID (FIGLU): Use of histidine in people with folic acid deficiency can cause accumulation of the metabolite formiminoglutamic (2355).

Possible Interactions with Diseases or Conditions

FOLIC ACID DEFICIENCY: Use of histidine in individuals with folic acid deficiency can cause accumulation of the metabolite formiminoglutamic acid (FIGLU) (2355).

Typical Dosages & Routes of Administration that are Commonly Used

ORAL: For rheumatoid arthritis, the usual dose of histidine is 3.7-4.5 grams daily (2347,2350,2351). For anemia of uremia or anemia associated with maintenance dialysis, the typical dose is 1-4 grams daily (2352,2353).

Comments

None.

HOLLY

This Product is Also Known As

Christ's Thorn, Holm, Holme Chase, Holy Tree, Hulm, Hulver Bush, Hulver Tree.

Scientific Names

Ilex aquifolium; Ilex opaca; Ilex vomitoria.
Family: Aquifoliaceae.

People Use This For

Orally, preparations of holly leaf are used as a diuretic, for coughs, digestive disorders, and jaundice (18).
In Chinese medicine, Ilex aquifolium leaves are used for treating intermittent fevers and rheumatism, as an antipyretic, astringent, diuretic, and expectorant (6). Ilex opaca leaves are used as a diuretic, tonic, purgative, and cardiac stimulant (6). Other Ilex species are used for treating coronary heart disease, dizziness, and hypertension (6). Historically, Ilex opaca fruit tea was used as a cardiac stimulant by American Indians (6). Ilex vomitoria was used as an emetic (6), and Youpon tea (mixed leaves of Ilex cassine, Ilex vomitoria, and Ilex dahoon) was used as a ceremonial "cleanser" in South America (6).

Safety

UNSAFE ...when the berries are ingested, poisoning can be fatal (18).
There is insufficient reliable information available about the safety of holly leaves (6,17).
CHILDREN: UNSAFE...when the berries are ingested. Eating berries can be fatal (6).

PREGNANCY AND LACTATION: UNSAFE ...when berries are ingested (6). There is insufficient reliable information available about the safety of holly leaves; avoid using.

Effectiveness
There is insufficient reliable information available about the effectiveness of holly.

Possible Mechanism of Action & Active Ingredients
The applicable parts of holly are the leaf and berry. The constituent saponins are thought to cause GI irritation and emetic effects (6). Holly also contains a cyanogenic glycoside (4).

Adverse Reactions Including Known Allergies
Ingestion of the leaf can cause GI irritation, diarrhea, nausea, and vomiting (6,18). Leaf spines may tear or puncture skin or mucous membranes (6). Ingestion of as few as 2 berries can cause vomiting and diarrhea in small children (6). Ingestion of more than 5 berries can cause nausea, vomiting, diarrhea, and stupor (6,18). Ingestion of 20-30 berries can cause death (18).

Possible Interactions with Herbs & Other Dietary Supplements
Insufficient reliable information available.

Possible Interactions with Drugs
No interactions are known to occur, and there is no known reason to expect a clinically significant interaction with holly.

Possible Interactions with Foods
No interactions are known to occur, and there is no known reason to expect a clinically significant interaction with holly.

Possible Interactions with Lab Tests
No interactions are known to occur, and there is no known reason to expect a clinically significant interaction with holly.

Possible Interactions with Diseases or Conditions
DEHYDRATION: In addition to toxic effects, berry ingestion may cause or exacerbate dehydration by inducing vomiting and diarrhea (6).
ELECTROLYTE IMBALANCE: Berry ingestion may cause or exacerbate electrolyte imbalance by inducing vomiting and diarrhea (6).

Typical Dosages & Routes of Administration that are Commonly Used
ORAL: People typically use 3.9 grams of powdered leaves in a tea, taken to reduce the effects of intermittent fevers. Berries produce emesis in a dose of 10 to 12 berries (5254).

Comments
Many other Ilex species are referred to as holly. English holly, Oregon holly, American holly are used as ornamental Christmas holly (6). Yaupon, Appalachian tea, cassena, deer berry, Indian holly and Indian black drink may be included in discussions of holly (6). Leaf spines may tear or puncture skin or mucous membranes (6).

HOLLYHOCK

This Product is Also Known As
Althea Rose, Hollyhock Flower, Malvae arboreae flos, Malva Flower, Rose Mallow.

Scientific Names
Alcea rosea, synonym Althaea rosea.
Family: Malvaceae.

People Use This For
Orally, the mucilage of hollyhock flower is used for prevention and treatment of diseases and discomforts of the respiratory and gastrointestinal tracts (2).
Topically, it is used for ulcers and inflammation (2).
In herbal teas, hollyhock is used as a brightening agent (2).

Safety
POSSIBLY SAFE ...when used orally. No health hazards are known in conjunction with appropriate use (18). There are no reported safety concerns about the use of hollyhock as a brightening agent in herbal tea mixtures (2).
PREGNANCY AND LACTATION: Insufficient reliable information available.

Effectiveness
There is insufficient reliable information available about the effectiveness of hollyhock.

Possible Mechanism of Action & Active Ingredients

The applicable part of hollyhock is the flower. There is insufficient reliable information available about the possible mechanism of action and active ingredients.

Adverse Reactions Including Known Allergies

None reported.

Possible Interactions with Herbs & Other Dietary Supplements

Insufficient reliable information available.

Possible Interactions with Drugs

No interactions are known to occur, and there is no known reason to expect a clinically significant interaction with hollyhock.

Possible Interactions with Foods

No interactions are known to occur, and there is no known reason to expect a clinically significant interaction with hollyhock.

Possible Interactions with Lab Tests

No interactions are known to occur, and there is no known reason to expect a clinically significant interaction with hollyhock.

Possible Interactions with Diseases or Conditions

No interactions are known to occur, and there is no known reason to expect a clinically significant interaction with hollyhock.

Typical Dosages & Routes of Administration that are Commonly Used

ORAL: People typically use hollyhock flower as a tea (5263).

Comments

There is very little scientific information about this product. Our staff is continually analyzing the available information on natural medicines and will add data here as it becomes available.

HONEY

This Product is Also Known As

Clarified Honey, Honig, Mel, Miel Blanc, Purified Honey, Strained Honey.
CAUTION: See separate listings for Bee Pollen, Honey Bee Venom, and Royal Jelly.

Scientific Names

Apis mellifera (honey bee).
Family: Apidae.

People Use This For

Orally, honey is used for cough, as an expectorant, and for gastric ulcer associated with Helicobacter pylori (6). Topically, honey is used to speed healing in mild sores, wounds, skin ulcerations, burns, treating cataracts, and postherpetic corneal opacities (6).
In foods and manufacturing, honey is also used as a sweetening agent, as a fragrance, and sometimes as a moisturizer in soaps and cosmetics (11).

Safety

LIKELY SAFE ...when used orally in amounts typically found in foods. Honey has Generally Recognized as Safe (GRAS) status in the US (11).
POSSIBLY SAFE ...when honey is used topically (395,396,397,398,399).
CHILDREN: POSSIBLY UNSAFE ...when honey contaminated with Clostridium botulinum spores is ingested by infants posing the risk of botulism poisoning (6,11). This is not a danger for older children or adults.
PREGNANCY AND LACTATION: LIKELY SAFE ...when used orally in amounts typically found in foods.

Effectiveness

POSSIBLY EFFECTIVE ...when used topically for improving healing of mild sores, wounds, burns and skin ulcerations (6,395,396,397,398,399).
There is insufficient reliable information available about the effectiveness of honey for its other uses.

Possible Mechanism of Action & Active Ingredients

Recent research suggests that honey has antibacterial and antifungal activity (6). Antibacterial and antifungal compounds have been isolated from honey, and antibacterial peptides (apidaecins and abaecin) have been isolated in honeybees (6). Researchers think that release of hydrogen peroxide contained in honey, high sugar content of honey, and/or phytochemicals contained in honey might play a role in the antimicrobial activity (1261,1428). Honey and solutions with similar sugar content (15% w/v) demonstrate similar effectiveness at inhibiting Helicobacter pylori (1428) and 2-4% v/v dilutions of various types of honey inhibit the growth of coagulase positive Staphylococcus aureus isolated from infected wounds (1261). Some honey is contaminated with Clostridium botulinum spores, which poses a risk to infants, but not older children or adults (6,11). Botulinum spores can proliferate in the intestines of infants causing botulism poisoning, but older children and adults develop botulism poisoning by a different mechanism (6,11).

Adverse Reactions Including Known Allergies
Oral use can cause allergic reactions. Botulism poisoning can occur in infants (6).

Possible Interactions with Herbs & Other Dietary Supplements
Insufficient reliable information available.

Possible Interactions with Drugs
No interactions are known to occur, and there is no known reason to expect a clinically significant interaction with honey.

Possible Interactions with Foods
No interactions are known to occur, and there is no known reason to expect a clinically significant interaction with honey.

Possible Interactions with Lab Tests
No interactions are known to occur, and there is no known reason to expect a clinically significant interaction with honey.

Possible Interactions with Diseases or Conditions
POLLEN ALLERGIES: Honey may cause allergic reactions (6).

Typical Dosages & Routes of Administration that are Commonly Used
ORAL: Liberal amounts are taken orally.
TOPICAL: Liberal amounts are applied topically.

Comments
Avoid confusion with bee pollen, honey bee venom, and royal jelly.

HONEY BEE venom

This Product is Also Known As
Apis mellifera venom, Apitoxin, Bee Sting Venom, Bee Venom.
CAUTION: See separate listings for Bee Pollen, Honey, and Royal Jelly.

Scientific Names
Apis mellifera.
Family: Apidae.

People Use This For
Honey bee venom is used as a treatment for rheumatoid arthritis, cervicobrachial neuralgia, fibromyositis, myogeloses (areas of abnormal hardening in a muscle), enthesitis (a disease at the insertion of a muscle where recurring muscle stress provokes inflammation leading to fibrosis and calcification), tendonitis and tendosynovitis, multiple sclerosis, and desensitization to bee stings (6,507).

Safety
POSSIBLY SAFE ...when honey bee venom is injected. Keep injectable epinephrine nearby for immediate use if severe allergic reaction occurs (507).
There is insufficient reliable information available about the safety of honey bee venom when given in tablets, capsules, or drops (507).
PREGNANCY AND LACTATION: Insufficient reliable information available; avoid using.

Effectiveness
POSSIBLY EFFECTIVE ...when injected for rheumatoid arthritis, cervicobrachial neuralgia, fibromyositis, myogeloses, enthesitis, tendonitis, and tendosynovitis (507).
POSSIBLY INEFFECTIVE ...when used for treating multiple sclerosis (507).
LIKELY INEFFECTIVE ...when used for desensitization to bee stings (507).

Possible Mechanism of Action & Active Ingredients
Bee venom constituents include the enzymes hyaluronidase and phospholipase A; peptides melittin, apamin, and adolapin. Melittin, a phospholipase-activating protein, stimulates neutriphil degranulation. Adolapin inhibits

inflammation and the prostaglandin-synthase system. Melittin and apamin stimulate the adrenal and pituitary systems to produce cortisol (6,507).

Adverse Reactions Including Known Allergies

Honey bee venom injections can lead to inflammation, swelling, itching, pain, anaphylaxis (507), fatigue, congestion, headache, nausea, vomiting, hypotension, fever, and chills (507).

Possible Interactions with Herbs & Other Dietary Supplements

Insufficient reliable information available.

Possible Interactions with Drugs

HYDROCORTISONE: Co-administration may enhance effects in arthritis (507).

Possible Interactions with Foods

No interactions are known to occur, and there is no known reason to expect a clinically significant interaction with honey bee venom.

Possible Interactions with Lab Tests

No interactions are known to occur, and there is no known reason to expect a clinically significant interaction with honey bee venom.

Possible Interactions with Diseases or Conditions

No interactions are known to occur, and there is no known reason to expect a clinically significant interaction with honey bee venom.

Typical Dosages & Routes of Administration that are Commonly Used

SUBCUTANEOUS (SC), INTRADERMAL (ID), INTRA-ARTICULAR (IA) INJECTION: Purified, sterile bee toxin (apitoxin 2mg/mL) used in one arthritis clinical trial; dose was started at 0.05-0.1 mL; increased at intervals of 5-7 days to 0.25 mL, 0.5 mL, and 1 mL. NOTE: Alcohol and tincture of iodine rapidly destroy the activity of bee venom and should not be applied at the site of injection (507). In China, bee venom is administered by electrophoresis, ultrasonophoresis, and acupuncture.

Comments

Avoid confusion with bee pollen, honey, and royal jelly. Other venoms are derived from related members of the insect order, Hymenoptera (6).

HONEYSUCKLE

This Product is Also Known As

Goat's Leaf, Jinyinhua, Woodbine.
CAUTION: See separate listings for American Ivy, Gelsemium, and Woodbine.

Scientific Names

Lonicera caprifolium; Lonicera japonica; and other Lonicera sp.
Family: Caprifoliaceae.

People Use This For

Orally, honeysuckle is used for digestive disorders, malignant tumors, and to promote sweating. It is also used orally as a laxative (18).
Topically, it is used for inflammation, itching, and as an astringent and antimicrobial (11).
In traditional Chinese medicine, honeysuckle is used orally for colds, fever, inflammation, swelling, boils, sores, and viral and bacterial infections.

Safety

There is insufficient reliable information available about the safety of honeysuckle.
Pregnancy and Lactation: Insufficient reliable information available; avoid using.

Effectiveness

There is insufficient reliable information available about the effectiveness of honeysuckle.

Possible Mechanism of Action & Active Ingredients

The applicable parts of honeysuckle are the flower, seed, and leaf. In vitro data suggests antimicrobial activity against Staphylococcus aureus, Salmonella typhi, Mycobacterium tuberculosis, and bacilli which cause dysentery. It may also have antiviral activity against HIV and influenza virus. It is active, but less so, against dermatophytes. Animal data suggest anti-inflammatory effects, with possible increased resistance to infection, inhibited tumor formation, and decreased intestinal cholesterol absorption. Animal data also suggest that honeysuckle has stimulant effects at about 1/6 the activity of caffeine. Some of these biological activities are attributed to the saponin and chlorogenic acid content of honeysuckle. The LD50 of honeysuckle is low, approximately 53 g/kg when given subcutaneously to mice (11).

Adverse Reactions Including Known Allergies
People who take honeysuckle orally may experience irritation of the gastrointestinal tract, kidneys, and urinary tract (18).

Possible Interactions with Herbs & Other Dietary Supplements
Insufficient reliable information available.

Possible Interactions with Drugs
No interactions are known to occur, and there is no known reason to expect a clinically significant interaction with honeysuckle.

Possible Interactions with Foods
No interactions are known to occur, and there is no known reason to expect a clinically significant interaction with honeysuckle.

Possible Interactions with Lab Tests
No interactions are known to occur, and there is no known reason to expect a clinically significant interaction with honeysuckle.

Possible Interactions with Diseases or Conditions
No interactions are known to occur, and there is no known reason to expect a clinically significant interaction with honeysuckle.

Typical Dosages & Routes of Administration that are Commonly Used
No typical dosage.

Comments
Honeysuckle is considered obsolete as a medicinal herb (18). Avoid confusion with woodbine (Clematis virginiana). Also, avoid confusing honeysuckle with American ivy or gelsemium, which are also known as woodbine.

HOPS

This Product is Also Known As
Common Hops, European Hops, Hopfenzapfen, Hop Strobiles, Houblon, Lupuli Strobulus.

Scientific Names
Humulus lupulus.
Family: Cannabinaceae or Moraceae.

People Use This For
Orally, hops are used for restlessness, anxiety, sleep disorders, tension, excitability (1,2,3), nervousness, and irritability (6121). They are also used as an appetite stimulant (1), a bitter tonic, and for indigestion (6121).
Topically, hops are used as an anti-bacterial (4).
In Chinese medicine, hops are used for tuberculosis and cystitis (11). Traditionally, they have been taken orally as a diuretic (11), for intestinal cramps, mucous colitis, neuralgia, and priapism (4,11). Also, hops have been used topically for leg ulcers.
In foods and beverages, the extracts and oil are used as flavor components (11). The strobile is often used for brewing beer (11).
In manufacturing, the extract is used in skin creams and lotions (11).

Safety
LIKELY SAFE ...when consumed in amounts commonly found in foods and beverages. Hops are Generally Recognized as Safe (GRAS) for food use in the US with a maximum level of 0.072% (11).
POSSIBLY SAFE ...when used orally and appropriately for medicinal purposes (12).
PREGNANCY AND LACTATION: Insufficient reliable information available; avoid using (1).

Effectiveness
POSSIBLY EFFECTIVE ...when taken orally for tenseness, restlessness, anxiety, and sleep disorders (1,2).
There is insufficient reliable information available about the effectiveness of hops for its other uses.

Possible Mechanism of Action & Active Ingredients
The applicable part of hops is the dried, fruiting part. Hops can have sedative, hypnotic, anticonvulsant, antimicrobial, and pain and fever-reducing properties (1,4,11). Its antimicrobial properties are due to the bitter acid constituents, lupulone and humulone (11). The constituent 2-methyl-3-butene-2-ol can have sedative effects in

rats (11). The alcoholic extracts have been used to treat acute bacterial dysentery, leprosy, and pulmonary tuberculosis in humans with varying success (11). An extract of hops competitively inhibits estradiol binding to estrogen receptors and induces transcription activity in estrogen-responsive cells (6180). It also decreases LH (luteinizing hormone) levels in female rats with their ovaries removed (6180).

Adverse Reactions Including Known Allergies
Allergic reactions are possible through contact with the fresh plant and plant dust. Contact dermatitis is attributed to the pollen (4).

Possible Interactions with Herbs & Other Dietary Supplements
HERBS WITH SEDATIVE PROPERTIES: Theoretically, concomitant use with herbs that have sedative properties might enhance therapeutic and adverse effects. These include calamus, calendula, California poppy, catnip, capsicum, celery, couch grass, elecampane, Siberian ginseng, German chamomile, goldenseal, gotu kola, Jamaican dogwood, kava, lemon balm, sage, St. John's wort, sassafras, scullcap, shepherd's purse, stinging nettle, valerian, wild carrot, wild lettuce, withania, and yerba mansa (4,19).

Possible Interactions with Drugs
ALCOHOL, SEDATIVE DRUGS: Concomitant use of hops can potentiate the sedative effects of these drugs (4).
BARBITURATES: Theoretically, concomitant use of hops with barbiturates can cause additive therapeutic and adverse effects (19).
OTHER DRUGS WITH SEDATIVE PROPERTIES: Theoretically, concomitant use with drugs having sedative properties can cause additive therapeutic and adverse effects (19).

Possible Interactions with Foods
ALCOHOL: Concomitant use of hops with alcohol can potentiate the sedative effects (4).

Possible Interactions with Lab Tests
No interactions are known to occur, and there is no known reason to expect a clinically significant interaction with hops.

Possible Interactions with Diseases or Conditions
DEPRESSION: Hops may contribute to depression (12).

Typical Dosages & Routes of Administration that are Commonly Used
ORAL: The typical dose of hops is 0.5-1 grams of the strobile as a single dose (4) or one cup of the tea (4). The tea is prepared by steeping 0.5-1 grams of the strobile in 150 mL boiling water for 5-10 minutes and then straining (4). The usual dose of the liquid extract (1:1, 45% alcohol) is 0.5-2 mL (4). The common dose of the tincture (1:5, 60% alcohol) is 1-2 mL (4). For sleep, 1-2 grams of the strobile are typically used (4), and combination of hops with other plant sedatives can be beneficial (1,2).

Comments
The hops themselves are not reported to interfere with the ability to drive and operate machines (1).

HORSE CHESTNUT branch bark

This Product is Also Known As
Buckeye, Hippocastani Cortex (bark), Hippocastani Semen, Marron Europeen, Spanish Chestnut.
CAUTION: See separate listings for Horse Chestnut flower, Horse Chestnut leaf, and Horse Chestnut seed.

Scientific Names
Aesculus hippocastanum.
Family: Hippocastanaceae.

People Use This For
Orally, horse chestnut bark is used for malaria and dysentery (11).
Topically, horse chestnut bark is used for lupus and skin ulcers (11).
In combination with other herbs, horse chestnut bark together with the flower is used for treating varicose veins, strengthening veins, promoting and supporting cardiac function, treating hemorrhoids and rectal problems, prevention of embolism, improving circulation, ringing in the ears, low and high blood pressure, dizziness, stimulant effect, tendency towards uric acid disturbances, kidney or bladder disease, edema associated with weak heart function, dropsy, liver congestion, bile flow disturbances, and pancreatitis (2).

Safety
There is insufficient reliable information available about the safety of horse chestnut branch bark.
CHILDREN: LIKELY UNSAFE. Poisoning reported from children drinking tea made with twigs (6).
PREGNANCY AND LACTATION: Insufficient reliable information available; avoid using.

Effectiveness
There is insufficient reliable information available about the effectiveness of horse chestnut branch bark (2).

Possible Mechanism of Action & Active Ingredients
Horse chestnut bark contains aescin (11). This is a mixture of triperpene saponins. Aescin seems to have a weak diuretic activity (6). In some countries, intravenous aescin is used after surgery (6). Horse chestnut bark also contains sterols, stigmasterol, alpha-spinasterol, and beta-sitosterol (11). These constituents seem to have anti-inflammatory activity (6). Horse chestnut bark and twigs contain the toxic glycoside aesculin (6,4017). Aesculin is a hydroxycoumarin with potential antithrombin activity (19).

Adverse Reactions Including Known Allergies
There is also the possibility of severe bleeding or bruising due to the antithrombotic activity of horse chestnut bark (19). Children have been poisoned by drinking tea made from horse chestnut leaves and twigs (6).

Possible Interactions with Herbs & Other Dietary Supplements
HERBS WITH ANTICOAGULANT/ANTIPLATELET POTENTIAL: Concomitant use of herbs that have coumarin constituents or affect platelet aggregation could theoretically increase the risk of bleeding in some people. These herbs include: angelica, anise, arnica, asafoetida, bogbean, boldo, capsicum, celery, chamomile, clove, danshen, fenugreek, feverfew, garlic, ginger, ginkgo, ginseng (Panax), horseradish, licorice, meadowsweet, prickly ash, onion, papain, passionflower, poplar, quassia, red clover, turmeric, wild carrot, wild lettuce, willow, and others (4,19).

Possible Interactions with Drugs
ANTICOAGULANTS: Theoretically, the aesculin constituent in horse chestnut bark might increase the effect or adverse effects of anticoagulant drugs (19).
ASPIRIN: Theoretically, concomitant use should be avoided due to the antithrombin effects of aesculin (19).
DIABETES THERAPY: Monitor blood glucose level closely due to claims that horse chestnut bark has hypoglycemic effects (19).

Possible Interactions with Foods
No interactions are known to occur, and there is no known reason to expect a clinically significant interaction with horse chestnut branch bark.

Possible Interactions with Lab Tests
No interactions are known to occur, and there is no known reason to expect a clinically significant interaction with horse chestnut branch bark.

Possible Interactions with Diseases or Conditions
BLEEDING DISORDERS: The antithrombin activity of aesculin can theoretically increase bleeding time (19).
GI CONDITIONS: Can irritate gastrointestinal tract. Contraindicated in individuals with infectious or inflammatory gastrointestinal conditions (19).

Typical Dosages & Routes of Administration that are Commonly Used
Tincture (1:5, 50% alcohol), 3-10 drops, use with care (886).

Comments
Horse chestnut seed is used to manufacture Venastat, which appears to be effective against varicose veins. Sometimes buckeye is referred to as horse chestnut bark. Do not confuse horse chestnut bark with buckeye.

HORSE CHESTNUT flower

This Product is Also Known As
Buckeye, Hippocastani Flos (flower), Marron Europeen, Spanish Chestnut.
CAUTION: See separate listings for Horse Chestnut branch bark, Horse Chestnut leaf, and Horse Chestnut seed.

Scientific Names
Aesculus hippocastanum.
Family: Hippocastanaceae.

People Use This For
Orally, horse chestnut flower, in various combinations with horse chestnut bark and other herbs, is used for hemorrhoids and rectal problems, prevention of embolism, improving circulation, strengthening veins, promoting and supporting cardiac function, ringing in the ears, low and high blood pressure, dizziness, stimulant, uric acid diathesis, kidney or bladder disease, edema due to weak heart function, dropsy, liver congestion, bile flow disturbances, and pancreatitis (2).

Safety

LIKELY UNSAFE ...when used orally (2,11).
There is insufficient reliable information available about the safety of the topical use of horse chestnut flower.
PREGNANCY AND LACTATION: LIKELY UNSAFE; avoid using (11).

Effectiveness

There is insufficient reliable information available about the effectiveness of horse chestnut flower (2).

Possible Mechanism of Action & Active Ingredients

Horse chestnut flower contains aescin (11). This is a mixture of triperpene saponins. Horse chestnut flower also contains sterols, stigmasterol, alpha-spinasterol, and beta-sitosterol. These constituents seem to have anti-inflammatory activity (6). Aescin is a hydroxycoumarin and can lead to increased bleeding. In some countries, an intravenous mixture containing horse chestnut flower is used after surgery. It seems to have a weak diuretic activity.

Adverse Reactions Including Known Allergies

POISONING: Symptoms include nervous muscle twitching, weakness, dilated pupils, vomiting, diarrhea, depression, paralysis, and stupor (11).

Possible Interactions with Herbs & Other Dietary Supplements

HERBS WITH ANTICOAGULANT/ANTIPLATELET POTENTIAL: Concomitant use of herbs that have coumarin constituents or affect platelet aggregation could theoretically increase the risk of bleeding in some people. These herbs include: angelica, anise, arnica, asafoetida, bogbean, boldo, capsicum, celery, chamomile, clove, danshen, fenugreek, feverfew, garlic, ginger, ginkgo, ginseng (Panax), horseradish, licorice, meadowsweet, prickly ash, onion, papain, passionflower, poplar, quassia, red clover, turmeric, wild carrot, wild lettuce, willow, and others (4,19).

Possible Interactions with Drugs

No interactions are known to occur, and there is no known reason to expect a clinically significant interaction with horse chestnut flower.

Possible Interactions with Foods

No interactions are known to occur, and there is no known reason to expect a clinically significant interaction with horse chestnut flower.

Possible Interactions with Lab Tests

No interactions are known to occur, and there is no known reason to expect a clinically significant interaction with horse chestnut flower.

Possible Interactions with Diseases or Conditions

No interactions are known to occur, and there is no known reason to expect a clinically significant interaction with horse chestnut flower.

Typical Dosages & Routes of Administration that are Commonly Used

No typical dosage.

Comments

The horse chestnut flower can be toxic and should not be used. Avoid confusion with horse chestnut branch bark, leaf, and seed. Sometimes buckeye is referred to as horse chestnut. Do not confuse horse chestnut with buckeye. Horse chestnut seed is used to manufacture Venastat which is being shown to be likely effective against varicose veins.

HORSE CHESTNUT leaf

This Product is Also Known As

Buckeye, Hippocastani folium, Marron Europeen, Spanish Chestnut.
CAUTION: See separate listings for Horse Chestnut bark, Horse Chestnut flower, and Horse Chestnut seed.

Scientific Names

Aesculus hippocastanum.
Family: Hippocastanaceae.

People Use This For

Orally, the horse chestnut leaf is used for eczema, varicose veins, discomfort due to varicose veins, supportive treatment of varicose ulcers, treating phlebitis, thrombophlebitis, hemorrhoids, menstrual spastic pain, soft tissue swelling from bone fracture and sprains, and complaints after concussion (2,11).
In combination with other herbs, the horse chestnut leaf is used for discomfort due to hemorrhoids, anal fissures,

and rhagades (linear cracks or fissures in the skin occurring especially at the angles of the mouth or about the anus). Also, the horse chestnut leaf is used in herbal combination products for follow-up treatment of hemorrhoid surgery, for colon stasis, preventing vein weakness, strengthening vein walls, maintaining normal blood supply in tissues, strengthening venous blood circulation, preventing leg and foot fatigue, and for severe disorders of the venous system. Combination products also use horse chestnut for preventing thromboembolism, arteriosclerosis, arthrosis deformans, arthritis, sciatica, rheumatism, lumbago, neuralgia, hematoma, bruises, brachialgia, and as a diuretic and purifying remedy (2).

In folk medicine, it has been used as a cough remedy and for arthritis and rheumatism (18).

Safety

LIKELY UNSAFE ...when taken orally.

There is insufficient reliable information available about the safety of the topical use of horse chestnut leaf.

CHILDREN: UNSAFE...The horse chestnut leaf is toxic (11) and should not be used in children due to the potential for poisoning (6).

PREGNANCY AND LACTATION: UNSAFE ...contraindicated because the horse chestnut leaf can be toxic (11).

Effectiveness

There is insufficient reliable information available about the effectiveness of the horse chestnut leaf for its other uses.

Possible Mechanism of Action & Active Ingredients

The horse chestnut leaf contains the toxic glycoside aesculin (esculin)(6). Aesculin is a hydroxycoumarin with potential antithrombin activity (19).

Adverse Reactions Including Known Allergies

There is one case report of cholestatic liver damage associated with intramuscular injection of a horse chestnut leaf extract (2). Symptoms of horse chestnut leaf poisoning include nervous muscle twitching, weakness, dilated pupils, vomiting, diarrhea, depression, paralysis, and stupor (11). There is also the possibility of severe bleeding or bruising due to the antithrombotic activity of aesculin contained in horse chestnut leaf (19). Children have been poisoned by drinking the tea made from horse chestnut leaves and twigs (6).

Possible Interactions with Herbs & Other Dietary Supplements

HERBS WITH ANTICOAGULANT/ANTIPLATELET POTENTIAL: Concomitant use of herbs that have coumarin constituents or affect platelet aggregation could theoretically increase the risk of bleeding in some people. These herbs include: angelica, anise, arnica, asafoetida, bogbean, boldo, capsicum, celery, chamomile, clove, danshen, fenugreek, feverfew, garlic, ginger, ginkgo, ginseng (Panax), horseradish, licorice, meadowsweet, prickly ash, onion, papain, passionflower, poplar, quassia, red clover, turmeric, wild carrot, wild lettuce, willow, and others (4,19).

Possible Interactions with Drugs

ANTICOAGULANTS AND ASPIRIN: Theoretically, the aesculin component in horse chestnut leaf might increase the effect or adverse effects of anticoagulant drugs or aspirin (19).

Possible Interactions with Foods

No interactions are known to occur, and there is no known reason to expect a clinically significant interaction with horse chestnut leaf.

Possible Interactions with Lab Tests

No interactions are known to occur, and there is no known reason to expect a clinically significant interaction with horse chestnut leaf.

Possible Interactions with Diseases or Conditions

No interactions are known to occur, and there is no known reason to expect a clinically significant interaction with horse chestnut leaf.

Typical Dosages & Routes of Administration that are Commonly Used

No typical dosage.

Comments

The horse chestnut leaf can be toxic and should not be used. Avoid confusion with the horse chestnut bark, flower, and seed. Sometimes buckeye is referred to as horse chestnut. Do not confuse horse chestnut with buckeye.

HORSE CHESTNUT seed

This Product is Also Known As

Chestnut, Escine, Hippocastani Semen, Horse Chestnut, Marron Europeen, Venastat, Venostat, Venostasin Retard.

CAUTION: See separate listings for Horse Chestnut leaf, Horse Chestnut flower, and Horse Chestnut branch bark.

Scientific Names

Aesculus hippocastanum.
Family: Hippocastanaceae.

People Use This For

Orally, horse chestnut seed has been used for the treatment of varicose veins, hemorrhoids, phlebitis, diarrhea, fever, and enlarged prostate (4). Standardized horse chestnut seed extract products are taken orally for the treatment of chronic venous insufficiency (2,7). A specially prepared product made from horse chestnut seed is taken orally for the treatment of varicose veins, hemorrhoids, phlebitis, diarrhea, fever, and enlarged prostate (4).

Safety

POSSIBLY SAFE ...when used orally as the standardized extract product. European preparations of horse chestnut extracts have removed the primary toxic constituent, esculin, and are generally considered safe (2,11,6420). However, this preparation is not available in the US.
UNSAFE ...when used orally as the raw seed. Raw horse chestnut seed preparations contain significant amounts of the toxin esculin and can be lethal (6).
PREGNANCY AND LACTATION: UNSAFE ...when used orally as the raw seed. Raw horse chestnut preparations can be lethal (6); contraindicated.
There is insufficient reliable information available about the safety of horse chestnut seed extract when used during pregnancy and lactation; avoid using.

Effectiveness

LIKELY EFFECTIVE ...when used orally for symptomatic treatment of chronic venous insufficiency, such as varicose veins, and relieving pain, tiredness, tension, swelling in the legs, itching, and edema (281,282,283,284,285). Clinical studies showing the effectiveness of horse chestnut seed have used extracts standardized to 16-20% aescin. There is insufficient reliable information available about the effectiveness of horse chestnut seed for its other uses.

Possible Mechanism of Action & Active Ingredients

Horse chestnut seed contains triterpene saponins referred to as aescin (escin) and the toxic glycoside aesculin (esculin) (11). Aesculin is a hydroxycoumarin which may increase bleeding time due to antithrombin activity (19). Aescin decreases the permeability of venous capillaries. In vitro, aescin, constricts veins and reduces the capillary permeability induced by histamine or serotonin (6). These properties of the saponin components are the basis for the cosmetic applications of horse chestnut seed extract (4). In some countries, an intravenous mixture containing aescin is used after surgery (6). It seems to have a weak diuretic activity (6). Aescin binds to plasma proteins (4).

Adverse Reactions Including Known Allergies

Horse chestnut can cause GI irritation and toxic nephropathy (4). The symptoms of chestnut poisoning include muscle twitching, weakness, loss of coordination, dilated pupils, vomiting, diarrhea, depression, paralysis, and stupor (6). Horse chestnut seed extract taken orally can cause itching and gastric complaints (2). Isolated cases of kidney and liver toxicity have occurred after intravenous administration (512). Intravenous administration of aescin can cause anaphylaxis (18).

Possible Interactions with Herbs & Other Dietary Supplements

HERBS WITH ANTICOAGULANT/ANTIPLATELET POTENTIAL: Concomitant use of herbs that have coumarin constituents or affect platelet aggregation could theoretically increase the risk of bleeding in some people. These herbs include: angelica, anise, arnica, asafoetida, bogbean, boldo, capsicum, celery, chamomile, clove, danshen, fenugreek, feverfew, garlic, ginger, ginkgo, ginseng (Panax), horseradish, licorice, meadowsweet, prickly ash, onion, papain, passionflower, poplar, quassia, red clover, turmeric, wild carrot, wild lettuce, willow, and others (4,19).
HERBS WITH HYPOGLYCEMIC ACTIVITY: Theoretically, concomitant use with herbs having hypoglycemic activity could have additive effects and adverse effects (19).

Possible Interactions with Drugs

ANTICOAGULANTS: Theoretically, horse chestnut can have additive effects and adverse effects with anticoagulants (4).
PROTEIN-BINDING DRUGS: Theoretically, the saponin constituent of horse chestnut seed or extract, aescin, might interfere with the binding of protein binding of drugs (4).
DIABETES THERAPY: Monitor blood glucose level closely due to claims that horse chestnut seeds can have hypoglycemic effects (19).

Possible Interactions with Foods

No interactions are known to occur, and there is no known reason to expect a clinically significant interaction with horse chestnut seed.

Possible Interactions with Lab Tests

No interactions are known to occur, and there is no known reason to expect a clinically significant interaction with horse chestnut seed.

Possible Interactions with Diseases or Conditions

GI IRRITATION: Can irritate gastrointestinal tract. Contraindicated in individuals with infectious or inflammatory gastrointestinal conditions (19).

RENAL IMPAIRMENT: Avoid, toxic nephropathy has been reported as an adverse effect (4).

HEPATIC IMPAIRMENT: Avoid, a report of liver injury associated with horse chestnut (4).

DIABETES: Monitor blood glucose level closely due to claims that horse chestnut seeds can have hypoglycemic effects (19).

Typical Dosages & Routes of Administration that are Commonly Used

ORAL: Typical preparations of horse chestnut capsules contain about 250 mg horse chestnut extract. The usual dose is 1 to 3 capsules daily in divided doses. Some preparations are labeled for aescin content (usually 16 to 21%). Some sources recommend taking an initial dose of 90 – 150 mg of aescin (about 450 to 750 mg horse chestnut extract), and decreasing the maintenance dose to 35 to 70 mg aescin (about 175 to 350 mg extract). A tincture formulation of horse chestnut extract is used in a dose of 1 to 4 mL three times per day (5261,6006).

Comments

Do not confuse the horse chestnut seed with the related species, Aesculus californica and Aesculus glabra, known respectively as the California and Ohio buckeye. Sometimes buckeye is referred to as horse chestnut. Do not confuse horse chestnut with buckeye.

HORSEMINT

This Product is Also Known As

Monarda Lutea, Spotted Monarda, Wild Bergamot.

Scientific Names

Monarda punctata.
Family: Labitae or Lamiaceae.

People Use This For

Orally, horsemint is used for digestive disorders, flatulence, and dysmenorrhea. It is also used orally to promote menstruation and as a stimulant (18).

Safety

There is insufficient reliable information available about the safety of horsemint.

PREGNANCY: UNSAFE …contraindicated due to menstruation promoting and uterine stimulant effects (12).

LACTATION: Insufficient reliable information available; avoid using.

Effectiveness

There is insufficient reliable information available about the effectiveness of horsemint.

Possible Mechanism of Action & Active Ingredients

Insufficient reliable information available.

Adverse Reactions Including Known Allergies

None reported.

Possible Interactions with Herbs & Other Dietary Supplements

Insufficient reliable information available.

Possible Interactions with Drugs

No interactions are known to occur, and there is no known reason to expect a clinically significant interaction with horsemint.

Possible Interactions with Foods

No interactions are known to occur, and there is no known reason to expect a clinically significant interaction with horsemint.

Possible Interactions with Lab Tests

No interactions are known to occur, and there is no known reason to expect a clinically significant interaction with horsemint.

Possible Interactions with Diseases or Conditions

No interactions are known to occur, and there is no known reason to expect a clinically significant interaction with horsemint.

Typical Dosages & Routes of Administration that are Commonly Used

ORAL: The average daily dose is 2-4 mL of syrup prepared from the herb (18).

Comments

Horsemint has a pungent, bitter taste, and has a scent reminiscent of thyme (18).

HORSERADISH

This Product is Also Known As

Amoraciae Rusticanae Radix, Great Raifort, Meerrettich, Mountain Radish, Pepperrot, Red Cole.

Scientific Names

Armoracia rusticana, synonym Armoracia lopathifolia; Cochlearia armoracia; Nasturtium armoracia; Roripa armoracia.
Family: Brassicaceae/Cruciferae.

People Use This For

Orally, horseradish is used for urinary tract infection, urinary stones, edematous conditions, cough, and bronchitis (2,4,18).
Topically, it is used for inflamed joints or tissues and minor muscle aches (2,4).
Traditionally, horseradish has been used for expelling afterbirth, treating gout, rheumatism, gallbladder disorders, sciatica pain, relief of colic, increasing urination, and intestinal worms in children (6,18).
In foods, it is used as a flavoring agent (4).

Safety

LIKELY SAFE ...when the root is used orally in food amounts. It has Generally Recognized as Safe (GRAS) status in the US (4).
POSSIBLY SAFE ...when used orally and appropriately in larger amounts (2,4,6,12,18). ...when topical preparations containing 2% mustard oil, or less are used (2). Mustard oil is a constituent of horseradish.
CHILDREN: POSSIBLY SAFE ...when used as a spice. LIKELY UNSAFE ...when used orally in children less than 4 years of age because it can cause gastrointestinal problems (2,12,19).
PREGNANCY AND LACTATION: LIKELY SAFE ...when used orally in food amounts. LIKELY UNSAFE ...contraindicated for oral use in larger amounts because horseradish contains toxic and irritating mustard oil constituents (4). ...when the tincture is taken regularly and in large amounts, it is considered an abortifacient (19).

Effectiveness

POSSIBLY EFFECTIVE ...when taken orally for inflammation of respiratory tract mucous membranes and as supportive therapy for urinary tract infection (2). ...when used topically for inflammation of respiratory tract mucous membranes and as a counterirritant for minor muscle aches (2).
There is insufficient reliable information available about the effectiveness of horseradish for its other uses.

Possible Mechanism of Action & Active Ingredients

The applicable part of horseradish is the root. Researchers state horseradish has antimicrobial efficacy against gram negative and gram positive bacteria. It also has antispasmodic properties. Horseradish shows evidence that it can stimulate local blood flow; it might also be carcinostatic (2,18). The toxic mustard oil constituents of horseradish are extremely irritating to mucous membranes (2,4) and the urinary tract (19).

Adverse Reactions Including Known Allergies

Consuming large amounts of horseradish can cause gastrointestinal upset, bloody vomiting and diarrhea (2,6), and irritation of mucous membranes (2,4) and the urinary tract (19). Horseradish, and other members of the cabbage and mustard family are associated with depressed thyroid function (4). Skin contact with fresh horseradish can cause irritation (4,19) or allergic reaction (4).

Possible Interactions with Herbs & Other Dietary Supplements

HERBS WITH ANTICOAGULANT/ANTIPLATELET POTENTIAL: Concomitant use of herbs that have coumarin constituents or affect platelet aggregation could theoretically increase the risk of bleeding in some people. These herbs include: angelica, anise, arnica, asafoetida, bogbean, boldo, capsicum, celery, chamomile, clove, danshen, fenugreek, feverfew, garlic, ginger, ginkgo, ginseng (Panax), horse chestnut, licorice, meadowsweet, prickly ash, onion, papain, passionflower, poplar, quassia, red clover, turmeric, wild carrot, wild lettuce, willow, and others (4,19).

Possible Interactions with Drugs

LEVOTHYROXINE: Theoretically, concomitant use of horseradish can interfere with levothyroxine or hypothyroid therapy (4).

Possible Interactions with Foods

No interactions are known to occur, and there is no known reason to expect a clinically significant interaction with horseradish.

Possible Interactions with Lab Tests

No interactions are known to occur, and there is no known reason to expect a clinically significant interaction with horseradish.

Possible Interactions with Diseases or Conditions

KIDNEY DISORDERS: Theoretically, because it has a strong diuretic effect (19), horseradish is contraindicated in individuals with kidney inflammation (2,18,19).
HYPOTHYROIDISM: Theoretically, horseradish might exacerbate hypothyroidism or interfere with therapy (19).
GI CONDITIONS: Horseradish can irritate gastrointestinal tract. Contraindicated in individuals with infectious or inflammatory gastrointestinal conditions, or stomach or intestinal ulcers (19).

Typical Dosages & Routes of Administration that are Commonly Used

ORAL: The typical dose of horseradish is 6-20 grams per day of the root or equivalent preparations (4,6,18).
TOPICAL: Ointments with a maximum of 2% mustard oil content are commonly used (6,18).

Comments

Horseradish has been cultivated for more than two thousand years (6) and is sometimes added to toxic substances as a taste repellent for animals (6002).

HORSETAIL

This Product is Also Known As

Bottle Brush, Corn Horsetail, Dutch Rushes, Field Horsetail, Horsetail Grass, Horsetail Rush, Horse Willow, Paddock-Pipes, Pewterwort, Prele, Scouring Rush, Souring Rush, Shave Grass, Toadpipe.

Scientific Names

Equisetum arvense; Equisetum telmateia.
Family: Equisetaceae.

People Use This For

Orally, the horsetail stem is used for diuresis, edema, kidney and bladder stones, urinary tract infections, and general disturbances of the kidney and bladder (2,6,7,18).
Topically, it is used for supportive treatment of wounds and burns (2,6,18).
In folk medicine, horsetail has been used for alopecia, tuberculosis, brittle fingernails, nasal, pulmonary and gastric hemorrhage, rheumatic diseases, gout, frostbite, and to halt profuse menstruation (18).

Safety

POSSIBLY UNSAFE ...when used orally and appropriately short-term (2,6,12).
LIKELY UNSAFE ...when used orally long-term. It can cause thiamine deficiency. The inorganic silica content can cause toxicity similar to nicotine poisoning. ...when used by individuals with edema due to impaired heart or kidney function (2,12,18).
CHILDREN: LIKELY UNSAFE. Horsetail contains inorganic silica and the powdered herb can cause toxicity similar to nicotine poisonings. Poisoning has been reported in children who chewed on the stem (12).
PREGNANCY AND LACTATION: Insufficient reliable information available; avoid using.

Effectiveness

POSSIBLY EFFECTIVE ...when taken orally for post-traumatic and static edema, for "irrigation therapy" when used as a mild diuretic with copious fluid intake to increase urine flow, for bacterial and inflammatory disease of the lower urinary tract, and renal gravel (2). ...when used topically for supportive treatment of poorly healing wounds (2).
There is insufficient reliable information available about the effectiveness of horsetail for its other uses.

Possible Mechanism of Action & Active Ingredients

Evidence suggests horsetail has a mild diuretic action (18), which is likely due to the constituents, equisetonin and flavone glycosides (6). It also contains minute amounts of nicotine (6).

Adverse Reactions Including Known Allergies

The use of horsetail can cause seborrheic dermatitis (6). Potentially, the use of horsetail can lead to thiamine deficiency, and Canadian products are required to be certified as free from thiaminase-like effect (12). Toxicity has occurred in children who chewed the stems and is similar to nicotine poisoning (12).

Possible Interactions with Herbs & Other Dietary Supplements

CARDIAC GLYCOSIDE-CONTAINING HERBS: Contraindicated; concomitant use may increase the risk of cardiac glycoside toxicity. Cardiac glycoside-containing herbs, include black hellebore, Canadian hemp roots, digitalis leaf, hedge mustard, figwort, lily of the valley roots, motherwort, oleander leaf, pheasant's eye plant, pleurisy root, squill bulb leaf scales, and strophanthus seeds (2,18,19,500).

STIMULANT LAXATIVE HERBS: Theoretically, concomitant use increases the risk of potassium depletion. Stimulant laxative herbs include: aloe dried leaf sap, blue flag rhizome, alder buckthorn, European buckthorn, butternut bark, cascara bark, castor oil, colocynth fruit pulp, gamboge bark exudate, jalap root, black root, manna bark exudate, podophyllum root, rhubarb root, senna leaves and pods, wild cucumber fruit (Ecballium elaterium), and yellow dock root (19).

LICORICE: Theoretically, overuse/misuse of licorice rhizome increases the risk of cardiac toxicity due to potassium depletion. (19).

Possible Interactions with Drugs

DIGITALIS GLYCOSIDE: Increased digitalis toxicity might occur due to the loss of potassium associated with the diuretic effect of horsetail (19).

POTASSIUM-DEPLETING DRUGS: Theoretically, concomitant use with potassium-depleting diuretics or corticosteroids with mineral corticoid activity increases the risk of reduced potassium levels or hypokalemia (4,13).

Possible Interactions with Foods

REGULAR DIET: Horsetail can breakdown thiamine and theoretically increases the risk of thiamine deficiency (19).

Possible Interactions with Lab Tests

No interactions are known to occur, and there is no known reason to expect a clinically significant interaction with horsetail.

Possible Interactions with Diseases or Conditions

THIAMINE DEFICIENCY: Theoretically, the horsetail stem can cause or exacerbate thiamine deficiency (12).

IMPAIRED HEART OR KIDNEY FUNCTION: Contraindicated. The diuretic effect of horsetail can cause an increased excretion of potassium (19).

Typical Dosages & Routes of Administration that are Commonly Used

ORAL: The typical dose of horsetail is 6 grams of the dried stem per day with ample fluid intake (2,18). One cup of the tea is commonly taken several times per day between meals. The tea is prepared by steeping 1.5 grams of the dried stem in 150 mL boiling water for 10-15 minutes and then straining (18). The powdered stem should be used only on a short-term basis in adults. Avoid the use of the powdered stem in children due to its inorganic silica content (12). The usual dose of the liquid extract (1:1 in 25% alcohol) is 1-4 mL three times per day (18). Do not exceed 2 grams of the powdered extract per day (12).

TOPICAL: Horsetail is commonly used as a compress containing 10 grams of the dried stem per L of water (2,18).

Comments

Adulteration with Equisetum palustre, which contains the toxic alkaloid palustrine, has occurred. Palustrine can be toxic in cattle, but toxicity in humans has not yet been established (12).

HOUND'S TONGUE

This Product is Also Known As

Cynoglossi herba, Cynoglossi radix, Dog-Bur, Dog's Tongue, Dogs Tongue, Gypsy Flower, Hounds Tongue, Sheep-Lice, Woolmat.
CAUTION: See separate listing for Deertongue (Trilisa odoratissima).

Scientific Names

Cynoglossum officinale.
Family: Boraginaceae.

People Use This For

Orally, hound's tongue is used for diarrhea and other GI tract complaints, infections, skin diseases, and bronchitis. It is also used as an analgesic, expectorant, and cough sedative (2,18,400).

Topically, hound's tongue is used for painful discomfort of extremities, myalgia, neuralgia, trauma, nervous diseases, wound healing, and for care of scar tissue (2,18).

Safety

LIKELY UNSAFE ...when taken orally; contraindicated (2,18,400), due to significant amounts of unsaturated pyrrolizidine alkaloids (UPAs) (2,19). Repeated exposure to low concentrations of UPAs has been linked to serious liver toxicity (4,12). UPAs may also be carcinogenic and mutagenic (12).

There is insufficient reliable information available about the safety of hound's tongue for topical use; avoid using.

PREGNANCY AND LACTATION: LIKELY UNSAFE ...contraindicated, due to UPA content (2,18).

Effectiveness

There is insufficient reliable information available about the effectiveness of hound's tongue.

Possible Mechanism of Action & Active Ingredients

Researchers think the constituent cynoglossin paralyzes peripheral nerve endings (18). Hound's tongue contains significant amounts of hepatotoxic and hepatocarcinogenic pyrrolizidine alkaloids (2,18). Unsaturated pyrrolizidine alkaloids are known to be hepatotoxic in animals and humans (4).

Adverse Reactions Including Known Allergies

Chronic exposure to plants containing UPA constituents has been associated with veno-occlusive disease (4021). Symptoms of acute veno-occlusive disease are characterized by a dull, dragging ache in the right upper abdomen and marked distention of the abdomen. These symptoms are sometimes accompanied by reduced urine output. Subacute veno-occlusive disease is associated with vague symptoms and persistent liver enlargement (4021).

Possible Interactions with Herbs & Other Dietary Supplements

EUCALYPTUS: Theoretically, concomitant use may increase the risk of unsaturated pyrrolizidine alkaloid toxicity due to enzyme induction by eucalyptus (19).
PYRROLIZIDINE ALKALOID-CONTAINING HERBS: Concomitant use is contraindicated due to the risk of additive toxicity. Herbs containing unsaturated pyrrolizidine alkaloids include: alkanna (12), borage (271), gravel root (4), hemp agrimony (271), hound's tongue (19), petasites (19), comfrey (271), coltsfoot, and the Senecio species plants; dusty miller (19), alpine ragwort (19), groundsel (271), golden ragwort (19), and tansy ragwort (271).

Possible Interactions with Drugs

No interactions are known to occur, and there is no known reason to expect a clinically significant interaction with hound's tongue.

Possible Interactions with Foods

No interactions are known to occur, and there is no known reason to expect a clinically significant interaction with hound's tongue.

Possible Interactions with Lab Tests

No interactions are known to occur, and there is no known reason to expect a clinically significant interaction with hound's tongue.

Possible Interactions with Diseases or Conditions

LIVER DISEASE: Contraindicated due to hepatotoxic potential (19).

Typical Dosages & Routes of Administration that are Commonly Used

No typical dosage.

Comments

Avoid oral or topical use of hound's tongue. It is without documented effectiveness and is likely to be unsafe.

HOUSELEEK

This Product is Also Known As

Aaron's Rod, Ayegreen, Ayron, Bullock's Eye, Hens and Chickens, Jupiter's Beard, Jupiter's Eye, Liveforever, Sengreen, Thor's Beard, Thunder Plant.

Scientific Names

Sempervivum tectorum.
Family: Crassulaceae.

People Use This For

Orally, houseleek is used for severe diarrhea.
Topically, it is used for burns, ulcers, warts, and itchy, burning skin and swelling associated with insect bites. The diluted juice is used as a gargle for stomatitis (18).

Safety

There is insufficient reliable information available about safety of houseleek.
Pregnancy and Lactation: Insufficient reliable information available; avoid using.

Effectiveness

There is insufficient reliable information available about the effectiveness of houseleek.

Possible Mechanism of Action & Active Ingredients

The applicable part of houseleek is the leaf of the nonflowering plant. There is insufficient reliable information available about the possible mechanism of action and active ingredients.

Adverse Reactions Including Known Allergies

None reported.

Possible Interactions with Herbs & Other Dietary Supplements

Insufficient reliable information available.

Possible Interactions with Drugs

No interactions are known to occur, and there is no known reason to expect a clinically significant interaction with houseleek.

Possible Interactions with Foods

No interactions are known to occur, and there is no known reason to expect a clinically significant interaction with houseleek.

Possible Interactions with Lab Tests

No interactions are known to occur, and there is no known reason to expect a clinically significant interaction with houseleek.

Possible Interactions with Diseases or Conditions

No interactions are known to occur, and there is no known reason to expect a clinically significant interaction with houseleek.

Typical Dosages & Routes of Administration that are Commonly Used

ORAL: Houseleek is used as a tea (18).
TOPICAL: Houseleek is used as freshly pressed leaves and juice (18).

Comments

None.

HUPERZINE A

This Product is Also Known As

HupA, Huperzine, Huperzine-A, Selagine.
CAUTION: See separate listing for Chinese Club Moss.

Scientific Names

Huperzine A.

People Use This For

Orally, huperzine A is used for Alzheimer's disease (3138,3140,3171,4624), memory and learning enhancement (4626), age-related memory impairment (3561), increasing alertness and energy (3130), protection from neurotoxic agents including organophosphate nerve gases (3137,3139,3561), glutamate toxicity (3561), and for treating myasthenia gravis (3140,3561).

Safety

POSSIBLY SAFE ...when used orally and appropriately, short-term. Huperzine A has been used safely in clinical trials lasting from 1-3 months (3138,3140,3171,3561,4624,4626).
PREGNANCY AND LACTATION: Insufficient reliable information available; avoid using.

Effectiveness

POSSIBLY EFFECTIVE ...when used orally for improving memory, cognitive function, and behavioral function in Alzheimer's, multi-infarct, and senile dementia (3138,3140,3171,4624). In one clinical trial, patients with Alzheimer's disease treated with huperzine A had significant improvement in memory, cognitive, and behavioral function scales compared to placebo after 8 weeks of treatment (3138). In a small-scale, placebo-controlled trial, multi-infarct and senile dementia patients treated with huperzine A had significant improvement in memory function after 2-4 weeks of treatment (3140). Long-term, large scale trials are necessary to confirm these findings and determine huperzine A's potential role in dementia. ...when used intramuscularly for preventing muscle weakness in patients with myasthenia gravis. In a short-term, small-scale open-label trial, stabilized patients with myasthenia gravis given huperzine A intramuscularly for 10 days maintained muscle strength as well as patients treated with intramuscular neostigmine alternating with intramuscular huperzine A. Huperzine A was reported to have a 7 hour duration of effect compared to 4 hours for neostigmine (3561). Well-controlled, large-scale trials are necessary to confirm huperzine A's potential benefit in myasthenia gravis. ...when used orally in healthy adolescents for improving memory function. In a small-scale, placebo controlled trial, Chinese middle school children complaining of poor memory had significant improvement in memory quotient scores after taking huperzine A for 4 weeks compared to placebo (4626).
There is insufficient reliable information available about the effectiveness of huperzine A for its other uses.

Possible Mechanism of Action & Active Ingredients

Huperzine A is an alkaloid isolated from Chinese club moss, Huperzia serrata and from Lycopodium selago (3082,3130). It is an optically active stereoisomer. Only the levorotatory-isomer is pharmacologically active (3561). Huperzine A is thought to be beneficial in dementia, memory impairment, and myasthenia gravis due to its effects on acetylcholine levels (3133,3134,3135,3136,3172). It is a reversible inhibitor of acetylcholinesterase (AChE) and crosses the blood-brain barrier (3082). Huperzine A inhibits AChE activity in the brain for up to three hours. It produces a variable degree of acetylcholine elevation in different areas of the brain, with maximal values in the frontal and parietal cortex (125% and 105% respectively), and 22-65% in other brain regions (3141). It might be more specific for AChE and have a longer duration of action than AChE inhibitors such as tacrine (Cognex) or donepezil (Aricept), which are marketed as prescription drugs for Alzheimer's disease (3131,3132). In animal studies, huperzine A was found to be 64 times more potent than tacrine. It also is more bioavailable and penetrates the blood-brain barrier better than tacrine (3561). Huperzine A protects neurons against toxic levels of glutamate by blocking glutamate-induce neuronal calcium influx and cell death (3131,3561). Although it has low affinity, huperzine A is also a cerebral cortex N-methyl-D-aspartate (NMDA) receptor antagonist (3129,3137). It might also protect against seizures and neuropathological changes caused by exposure to organophosphate nerve agents such as soman, by protecting peripheral and central stores of acetylcholine (3137,3139).

Adverse Reactions Including Known Allergies

Orally, huperzine A can cause nausea, sweating, blurred vision, hyperactivity, anorexia, decreased heart rate, and fasciculations (3140,3143,3172,3561,4625). It has been suggested that huperzine A might have fewer cholinergic side effects than tacrine (Cognex) and donepezil (Aricept), but this has not been confirmed in human trials (3131). Adverse effects that have been reported with other AChE inhibitors, and theoretically might occur with huperzine A, include vomiting, diarrhea, cramping, hypersalivation, increased urination/incontinence, and bradycardia (14).

Possible Interactions with Herbs & Other Dietary Supplements

Insufficient reliable information available.

Possible Interactions with Drugs

ANTICHOLINERGIC DRUGS: Theoretically, concurrent use of anticholinergic drugs and huperzine A might decrease the effectiveness of huperzine A or the anticholinergic agent. In an animal model, huperzine A reversed cognitive deficits induced by scopolamine (5537). Other anticholinergic drugs include atropine, benztropine (Cogentin), biperiden (Akineton), procyclidine (Kemadrin), and trihexyphenidyl (Artane) (15).
CHOLINERGIC DRUGS, ACETYLCHOLINESTERASE (AChE) INHIBITORS: Theoretically, concurrent use might have additive effects with drugs that promote acetylcholine activity because huperzine A has AChE inhibitor properties (14). AChE inhibitors and cholinergic drugs include bethanechol (Urecholine), donepezil (Aricept), echothiophate (Phospholine Iodide), edrophonium (Enoln, Reversol, Tensilon), neostigmine (Prostigmin), physostigmine (Antilirium), pyridostigmine (Mestinon, Regonol), succinylcholine (Anectine, Quelicin), and tacrine (Cognex) (14).

Possible Interactions with Foods

No interactions are known to occur, and there is no known reason to expect a clinically significant interaction with huperzine A.

Possible Interactions with Lab Tests

No interactions are known to occur, and there is no known reason to expect a clinically significant interaction with huperzine A.

Possible Interactions with Diseases or Conditions

BRADYCARDIA/CARDIOVASCULAR DISEASE: Huperzine A can cause decreased heart rate and might exacerbate bradycardia and other cardiac conditions sensitive to decreased heart rate (3561); use with caution.
EPILEPSY: Theoretically, huperzine A might exacerbate seizure disorders (14); use with caution.
GASTROINTESTINAL TRACT OBSTRUCTION: Theoretically, huperzine A might exacerbate gastrointestinal obstruction due to its pro-secretory effects (14); use with caution.
PEPTIC ULCER DISEASE: Theoretically, huperzine A might exacerbate peptic ulcer disease due to its pro-secretory effects (14); use with caution.
PULMONARY CONDITIONS: Theoretically, huperzine A might exacerbate pulmonary conditions such as asthma and chronic obstructive pulmonary disease due to its pro-secretory effects (14); use with caution.
UROGENITAL TRACT OBSTRUCTION: Theoretically, huperzine A might exacerbate urogenital tract obstruction due to its pro-secretory effects (14); use with caution.

Typical Dosages & Routes of Administration that are Commonly Used

ORAL: For Alzheimer's disease and multi-infarct dementia, doses of 50-200 mcg twice daily have been used (3138,3140,4625). For senile or presenile dementia, doses of 30 mcg twice daily have been used (3140). For improving memory in adolescents, doses of 100 mcg twice daily have been used (4626).
INTRAMUSCULAR: For prevention of muscle weakness in myasthenia gravis, doses of 400 mcg daily have been used (3561).

Comments

The Cerebra brand name used for huperzine A has been confused with the prescription drugs Celebrex, Celexa, and Cerebyx (3142). Huperzine A is also referred to as selagine. Avoid confusion with the prescription drug selegiline (Eldepryl). Huperzine A is a drug that stretches the guidelines of the Dietary Supplement Health and Education Act (DSHEA). Although derived from a plant, huperzine A is a laboratory-manipulated, highly purified drug, unlike herbs which typically contain hundreds of constituents. Caution people that the moss from which huperzine A is derived is an expensive, rare Chinese herb (3143). To date, most clinical studies have been published in the Chinese literature. Synthetic derivatives of huperzine A are now being studied for Alzheimer's disease (3143). Chemical hybrids of huperzine A plus tacrine and huperzine A plus donepezil are being investigated (3143,4625). The hybrid of huperzine A plus donepezil has been referred to as huprine X (4625). Laboratory studies indicate that these hybrids have substantially greater affinity for AChE than tacrine or donepezil and show potential for enhanced efficacy at lower doses, with fewer side effects (3143,4625).

HYDRANGEA

This Product is Also Known As
Mountain Hydrangea, Seven Barks, Smooth Hydrangea, Wild Hydrangea.

Scientific Names
Hydrangea arborescens.
Family: Hydrangeaceae or Saxifragaceae.

People Use This For
Orally, hydrangea is used for conditions of the urinary tract, such as cystitis, urethritis, prostatitis, enlarged prostate, and urinary calculi (4,5,18).

Safety
POSSIBLY SAFE ...when used orally and appropriately, short-term (12).
LIKELY UNSAFE ...when used in excessive amounts (over 2 grams of dried rhizome/root per dose) (4,12). ...when used long-term (4,12).
PREGNANCY AND LACTATION: There is insufficient reliable information available about the safety of oral use during pregnancy and lactation; avoid using (4).

Effectiveness
There is insufficient reliable information available about the effectiveness of hydrangea.

Possible Mechanism of Action & Active Ingredients
The applicable parts of hydrangea are the rhizome/root. Researchers think hydrangea possesses mild diuretic activity and properties which prevent the formation of stones or calculus (4). The cyanogenic glycoside constituent, hydrangin, may be responsible for some of the potential adverse effects (12).

Adverse Reactions Including Known Allergies
Oral use can cause gastroenteritis (4). Overdose symptoms include: vertigo and a feeling of tightness in the chest (4). There is one case report of cholestatic hepatitis associated with Prostata, a multi-ingredient product containing hydrangea (598).

Possible Interactions with Herbs & Other Dietary Supplements
Insufficient reliable information available

Possible Interactions with Drugs
No interactions are known to occur, and there is no known reason to expect a clinically significant interaction with hydrangea.

Possible Interactions with Foods
No interactions are known to occur, and there is no known reason to expect a clinically significant interaction with hydrangea.

Possible Interactions with Lab Tests
No interactions are known to occur, and there is no known reason to expect a clinically significant interaction with hydrangea.

Possible Interactions with Diseases or Conditions
No interactions are known to occur, and there is no known reason to expect a clinically significant interaction with hydrangea.

Typical Dosages & Routes of Administration that are Commonly Used
ORAL: 2-4 grams dried rhizome/root three times daily, or, one cup tea (steep 2-4 grams dried rhizome/root in 150 mL boiling water 5-10 minutes, strain) three times daily (4,12). Liquid extract (1:1 in 25% alcohol), 2-4 mL

three times daily (4,12). Tincture (1:5 in 45% alcohol), 2-10 mL three times daily (4). One reference states not to exceed 2 grams dried rhizome/root per dose (12).

Comments
None.

HYDRAZINE SULFATE

This Product is Also Known As
Hydrazine, Sehydrin.

Scientific Names
Hydrazine sulfate.

People Use This For
Orally, hydrazine sulfate is used for treating cancer and the general weight loss and wasting associated with it (8000,14).

Safety
POSSIBLY SAFE ...when used orally and appropriately (8004,8005).
UNSAFE ...when used topically or by inhalation; avoid using (14).
PREGNANCY: UNSAFE ...when used orally, topically, or by inhalation. Some evidence suggests hydrazine is embryotoxic, fetotoxic, genotoxic, and carcinogenic (14).
LACTATION: Insufficient reliable information available; avoid using.

Effectiveness
POSSIBLY INEFFECTIVE ...when used as a single agent for treating metastatic colorectal cancer (8002).
LIKELY INEFFECTIVE ...when used as an adjunct to chemotherapy for treating non-small cell lung cancer (8001,8003).
There is insufficient reliable information available about the effectiveness of hydrazine sulfate for its other uses.

Possible Mechanism of Action & Active Ingredients
Hydrazine sulfate is an organic compound used in various industrial processes (14). Hydrazine, itself, can be inhaled or absorbed through the skin causing toxicity (14). As a sulfate salt, hydrazine inhibits phosphoenolpyruvate kinase (8000), an enzyme involved in gluconeogenesis. Scientists theorize that excessive gluconeogenesis might be partially responsible for the cachexia that occurs in people with cancer (8000,8005). By blocking gluconeogenesis, hydrazine sulfate might reduce cachexia (8000). Use of hydrazine sulfate has been associated with increased body weight in people with diverse cancers treated with varied chemotherapy regimens (8004). However, when compared to placebo, hydrazine sulfate failed to improve survival or anorexia, it was associated with greater sensory and motor neuropathy, and a poorer quality of life in people with non-small cell lung cancer treated with cisplatin and vinblastine (8003).

Adverse Reactions Including Known Allergies
Hydrazine sulfate can cause nausea, vomiting, dizziness, drowsiness, peripheral neuropathies (8005), weakness, and irregular breathing, confusion, hypoglycemia or hyperglycemia, lethargy, violent behavior, restlessness, seizures, coma, renal toxicity, and hepatotoxicity (14). If hydrazine comes in contact with the skin, eyes, or mucous membranes, it can cause irritation, burns, permanent damage to the eyes, bronchial mucus destruction, pulmonary edema, and death (14). Hydrazine is a sensitizer and can cause an allergic reaction (14).

Possible Interactions with Herbs & Other Dietary Supplements
Insufficient reliable information available.

Possible Interactions with Drugs
CNS DEPRESSANTS: Concomitant use with alcohol, barbiturates, benzodiazepines can increase the toxicity and decrease the effectiveness of hydrazine (8005).
MAOIs: Theoretically, concomitant use might increase the effects and adverse effects associated with monoamine oxidase inhibitors (8005).

Possible Interactions with Foods
TYRAMINE-CONTAINING FOODS: Avoid concomitant use, hydrazine sulfate may have monoamine oxidase inhibiting activity (8005). Tyramine-containing foods, include avocado, banana, brewer's yeast, broad beans, caviar, aged cheese, aged red wine, herring, liver, pickled meats (151).

Possible Interactions with Lab Tests
ALANINE AMINOTRANSFERASE (ALT): Can increase serum levels and test results secondary to hepatotoxicity (275).
ALKALINE PHOSPHATASE (Alk Phos): Can increase serum levels and test results secondary to

hepatotoxicity (275).
ASPARTATE AMINOTRANSFERASE: Can increase serum levels and test results secondary to hepatotoxicity (275).
BILE: Can increase urine levels and test results secondary to hepatotoxicity (275).
BILIRUBIN: Can increase serum levels and test results secondary to hepatotoxicity (275).
BSP RETENTION: Can increase serum levels and test results secondary to hepatotoxicity (275).
ERYTHROCYTE SEDIMENTATION RATE (sed rate): Can increase sed rate results secondary to an SLE-type syndrome (275).
GLUCOSE: Can decrease serum glucose and test results by potentiating insulin effects (275).
5-HYDROXYINDOLACETIC ADIC (5-HIAA): Can decrease urine levels and test results (275).
LE CELLS: Can cause a positive blood test result by activating lupus erythematosus (275).
LYMPHOCYTES: Can decrease blood levels and test results with megadose supplementation (275).
METANEPHRINES (total): Can increase urine levels and test results (275).
NORMETANEPHRINE: Can increase urine levels and test results (275).
VANILLYLMANDELIC ACID: Can increase urine levels and test results (275).

Possible Interactions with Diseases or Conditions

DIABETES: Might interfere with blood glucose control due to effects on gluconeogenesis (14,8000).
KIDNEY DISORDERS: Theoretically, might worsen kidney disorders (14).
LIVER DISORDERS: Theoretically, might worsen liver disorders (14).
PSYCHOSIS: Theoretically, might worsen psychoses (14).
SEIZURE DISORDERS: Can increase incidence of seizures (14).

Typical Dosages & Routes of Administration that are Commonly Used

ORAL: A typical dose used for cachexia in people with cancer on a chemotherapy regimen is 60 mg three times daily for a cycle of 30-45 days followed by a rest period of 2-6 weeks (8004,8005).

Comments

Although some information shows hydrazine sulfate might be useful in the general weight loss and wasting associated with cancer, information is very limited and inconclusive.

HYDROXYMETHYLBUTYRATE (HMB)

This Product is Also Known As
HMB.

Scientific Names
Beta-hydroxy-beta-methylbutyrate.

People Use This For
Orally, HMB is used for increasing the benefits from weight training, exercise, and for promoting healthy arteries (2167,2168).

Safety
POSSIBLY SAFE ...when taken orally for short-term use in amounts of 3 grams or less per day (2168).
PREGNANCY AND LACTATION: Insufficient reliable information available; avoid using.

Effectiveness
POSSIBLY EFFECTIVE ...when taken orally for increasing the benefits from weight training (2168).
There is insufficient reliable information available about the effectiveness of HMB for its other uses.

Possible Mechanism of Action & Active Ingredients
Beta-hydroxy-beta-methylbutyrate is a byproduct of metabolism of the amino acid leucine (2168). It can reduce catabolism of muscle protein and promote muscle growth (2168).

Adverse Reactions Including Known Allergies
No adverse reactions were reported in two clinical studies of HMB (2168).

Possible Interactions with Herbs & Other Dietary Supplements
Insufficient reliable information available.

Possible Interactions with Drugs
No interactions are known to occur, and there is no known reason to expect a clinically significant interaction with HMB.

Possible Interactions with Foods
No interactions are known to occur, and there is no known reason to expect a clinically significant interaction with HMB.

Possible Interactions with Lab Tests

No interactions are known to occur, and there is no known reason to expect a clinically significant interaction with HMB.

Possible Interactions with Diseases or Conditions

No interactions are known to occur, and there is no known reason to expect a clinically significant interaction with HMB.

Typical Dosages & Routes of Administration that are Commonly Used

ORAL: The dose of HMB used in clinical trials evaluating muscle building during weight training is 1.5 grams once or twice daily (2168).

Comments

None.

HYSSOP

This Product is Also Known As

None.

Scientific Names

Hyssopus officinalis.
Family: Labiatae or Lamiaceae.

People Use This For

Orally, hyssop is used for liver and gallbladder complaints, intestinal inflammation (2,18), colds, respiratory and chest ailments (2,6,18), sore throats, asthma, urinary tract inflammation, gas and colic, to stimulate appetite and circulation (2,18), and as an expectorant (6).

Topically, hyssop is used as a gargle, in baths to induce sweating, and for treating skin irritations, burns, bruises and frostbite (11).

Historically, hyssop was used for coughs, colds, breast and lung problems, menstrual complaints (11), and digestive and intestinal problems (11,18).

In foods, hyssop oil and extract are used as a flavoring (11).

In manufacturing, hyssop oil is used as a fragrance in soaps and cosmetics (11).

Safety

LIKELY SAFE ...when hyssop above ground parts are used orally in amounts found in foods (11). It has Generally Recognized as Safe (GRAS) status in the US (11). The maximum level of hyssop herb is 0.06% in alcoholic beverages. The maximum for the extract is 0.03%. The maximum for hyssop oil is 0.004% in alcoholic beverages (11).

POSSIBLY SAFE ...when the above ground parts are used orally and appropriately for medicinal purposes (12).

POSSIBLY UNSAFE ...when hyssop oil is used orally for medicinal purposes. There are reports that associate ingestion of the oil with tonic-clonic convulsions (2,18).

There is insufficient reliable information available about the safety of the topical use of hyssop.

CHILDREN: LIKELY UNSAFE ...hyssop oil is contraindicated because of a report that 2-3 drops over several days caused tonic-clonic convulsions (2,18).

PREGNANCY: LIKELY UNSAFE ...hyssop above ground parts and oil are contraindicated because they might cause uterine stimulant and menstrual stimulant effects (12).

LACTATION: Insufficient reliable information available; avoid using.

Effectiveness

There is insufficient reliable information available about the effectiveness of hyssop.

Possible Mechanism of Action & Active Ingredients

The applicable parts of hyssop are the above ground parts. Constituent marrubiin (11) has cardioactive effects and stimulates bronchial secretions (4). Caffeic acid and tannins may be responsible for effect of extracts of dried leaves. Extracts show antiviral activity against herpes simplex virus and HIV in vitro (6,11). Hyssop oil causes convulsions (of CNS origin) and death in experimental rats (6), thought due to constituents pincamphone and isopincamphone (6). Hyssop oil is associated with tonic-clonic convulsions in adults and children (2,18).

Adverse Reactions Including Known Allergies

Oral use of hyssop oil was associated with tonic-clonic convulsions in two adults (10-30 drops) and in one child (2-3 drops for several days) (2,18).

Possible Interactions with Herbs & Other Dietary Supplements

Insufficient reliable information available.

Possible Interactions with Drugs

No interactions are known to occur, and there is no known reason to expect a clinically significant interaction with hyssop.

Possible Interactions with Foods

No interactions are known to occur, and there is no known reason to expect a clinically significant interaction with hyssop.

Possible Interactions with Lab Tests

No interactions are known to occur, and there is no known reason to expect a clinically significant interaction with hyssop.

Possible Interactions with Diseases or Conditions

SEIZURE DISORDERS: Theoretically, hyssop oil may exacerbate seizure disorders.

Typical Dosages & Routes of Administration that are Commonly Used

ORAL: People take two 445 mg capsules containing the hyssop herb three times daily (5019). Some people take 10-15 drops of the hyssop extract (12-14% by volume) in water two to three times daily (5023). People also consume or gargle the hyssop tea three times daily (5008). The tea is prepared by steeping 1-2 teaspoons of the dried hyssop flower tops in 150 mL boiling water for 10-15 minutes and then straining. Avoid internal use of hyssop oil due to possible neurotoxicity.

Comments

None.

IBOGA

This Product is Also Known As

None.

Scientific Names

Tabernanthe iboga.
Family: Apocyanaceae.

People Use This For

Orally, iboga is used as an aperitif, aphrodisiac, tonic, for convalescence, debility, fever, flu, hypertension, neurasthenia (3919), and preventing fatigue and drowsiness (514).

Safety

There is insufficient reliable information available about the safety of iboga.
Pregnancy and Lactation: Insufficient reliable information available; avoid using.

Effectiveness

There is insufficient reliable information available about the effectiveness of iboga.

Possible Mechanism of Action & Active Ingredients

The applicable part of iboga is the root. The hallucinogenic properties of iboga are due to the indole alkaloids, ibogaine, ibogamone, iboluteine, and tabernanthine (6,514). Ibogaine inhibits cholinesterase, leading to synaptic acetylcholine accumulation (6). The associated dose-dependent CNS stimulation ranges from mild excitation and euphoria to visual and auditory hallucinations (6,514). Ibogaine has kappa agonist effects; it is serotonergic; and it exhibits nicotinic and N-methyl-D-aspartate (NMDA) antagonism (813). Animal experiments suggest these effects may have value in treating human addictions to alcohol, nicotine, opioids, cocaine, and other stimulants (812,813). The constituent tabernanthine demonstrates cardiac conduction effects similar to those of calcium channel antagonists (6).

Adverse Reactions Including Known Allergies

Iboga taken orally may cause bradycardia, hypotension, convulsions, paralysis, and respiratory arrest (6). Amounts large enough to induce hallucinations may also cause anxiety, apprehension, and death (6).

Possible Interactions with Herbs & Other Dietary Supplements

Insufficient reliable information available.

Possible Interactions with Drugs

ANTICHOLINERGIC DRUGS: Theoretically, concomitant use can antagonize anticholinergic effects.
CHOLINERGIC DRUGS: Theoretically, concomitant use may enhance effects and adverse effects.

Possible Interactions with Foods
No interactions are known to occur, and there is no known reason to expect a clinically significant interaction with iboga.

Possible Interactions with Lab Tests
No interactions are known to occur, and there is no known reason to expect a clinically significant interaction with iboga.

Possible Interactions with Diseases or Conditions
No interactions are known to occur, and there is no known reason to expect a clinically significant interaction with iboga.

Typical Dosages & Routes of Administration that are Commonly Used
ORAL: Dry root bark powder or root is chewed (6).

Comments
Iboga is used for ritual and ceremonial purposes in some African cultures (6,514,812).

ICELAND MOSS

This Product is Also Known As
Centraria, Eryngo-leaved Liverwort, Iceland Lichen, Lichen Islandicus.

Scientific Names
Cetraria islandica.
Family: Parmeliaceae.

People Use This For
Orally, Iceland moss is used for irritation of the oral and pharyngeal mucous membranes and associated dry cough, for loss of appetite (2), common cold, cough and bronchitis, dyspeptic complaints, fevers, and the tendency toward infection (18).
In folk medicine, Iceland moss has been used for lung disease, kidney and bladder complaints, and topically for poorly healing wounds (18).
For food uses, it is utilized as an emergency food source in Iceland (3).
In manufacturing, the moss is utilized as a flavoring agent in alcoholic beverages (12).

Safety
POSSIBLY SAFE ...when the dried plant is used orally, short-term for medicinal use (3,12). The dried plant can be contaminated with lead (3).
POSSIBLY UNSAFE ...when used in larger amounts as a food source because lead contamination can occur in amounts of up to 30 mg/kg of its dry weight (3). It is regulated in the US and allowable only as a flavoring agent in alcoholic beverages (12).
PREGNANCY AND LACTATION: POSSIBLY UNSAFE ...when used orally; avoid Iceland moss due to the potential for lead contamination (3).

Effectiveness
POSSIBLY EFFECTIVE ...when taken orally for irritation or inflammation of oral and pharyngeal mucous membranes and the associated dry cough and for the loss of appetite (2).
There is insufficient reliable information available about the effectiveness of Iceland moss for its other uses.

Possible Mechanism of Action & Active Ingredients
The applicable part of Iceland moss is the dried plant body. Iceland moss has soothing and mild antimicrobial action (2). The mucilage constituents, lichenin and isolichenin, and the bitter principles can be responsible for its effects (2,3). The bitter organic acid constituents can be responsible for an antibiotic effect (18).

Adverse Reactions Including Known Allergies
Taken orally, Iceland moss can cause GI irritation (12). Sensitization to Iceland moss is rare (18). It can be contaminated with lead up to 30 mg/kg of its dry weight (3).

Possible Interactions with Herbs & Other Dietary Supplements
Insufficient reliable information available.

Possible Interactions with Drugs
ORAL DRUGS: The fiber in Iceland moss can impair absorption of oral drugs (19).

Possible Interactions with Foods
No interactions are known to occur, and there is no known reason to expect a clinically significant interaction with Iceland moss.

Possible Interactions with Lab Tests

No interactions are known to occur, and there is no known reason to expect a clinically significant interaction with Iceland moss.

Possible Interactions with Diseases or Conditions

GASTRODUODENAL ULCERS: The alcohol extract and powder of Iceland moss is contraindicated due to the potential for mucosal irritation (12).

Typical Dosages & Routes of Administration that are Commonly Used

ORAL: The typical dose of Iceland moss is one cup of the tea several times daily. The tea is prepared by steeping or simmering 1.5-3 grams of the dried plant in 150 mL boiling water for 5-10 minutes and then straining (3,7). The maximum dose of the moss is 4-6 grams per day of the dried plant or equivalent preparations (2).

Comments

Iceland moss is a lichen, or an algae and a fungus growing together in a symbiotic relationship (3). Iceland is one the least polluted countries in the world, which is important for lichens. Lichens derive their nutrients from the environment and are easily contaminated with radioactive or heavy metals. Most of the lichens in Europe were contaminated by the fallout from the Chernobyl accident, but Iceland only received negligible radioactive levels (6002).

IGNATIUS BEAN

This Product is Also Known As

None.

Scientific Names

Strychnos ignatii.
Family: Loganiaceae.

People Use This For

Orally, ignatius bean is used for faintness, as a bitter or tonic, and as an agent to invigorate, refresh or restore body function (18).

Safety

UNSAFE ...when used orally due to its strychnine content (18). FDA banned strychnine from nonprescription drug products in 1989 (14).
PREGNANCY AND LACTATION: UNSAFE ...contraindicated due to toxic effects (18).

Effectiveness

LIKELY INEFFECTIVE ...for any medical use (14).

Possible Mechanism of Action & Active Ingredients

Ignatius bean contains the centrally-acting neurotoxins strychnine and brucine (18). Strychnine competitively antagonizes post-synaptic binding of the inhibitory transmitter glycine, leading to heightened reflex excitability of muscles. External irritations or centrally-acting stimulants can trigger convulsions (2,14,505). Strychnine can selectively inhibit the spinal cord in subconvulsive amounts (2). However, strychnine accumulates with extended administration, particularly in individuals with liver damage. Chronic use of subconvulsive amounts can cause death after a period of weeks (18).

Adverse Reactions Including Known Allergies

ORAL: 30-50 mg ignatius bean (5 mg strychnine) can cause restlessness, feelings of anxiety, heightening of sense perception, enhanced reflexes, equilibrium disorders, painful neck and back stiffness, followed later by twitching, tonic spasms of jaw and neck muscles, painful convulsions of the entire body triggered by visual or tactile stimulation with possible opisthotonos, muscle hypertonicity, and agitation. Dyspnea may follow spasm of respiratory muscles (14,18). Seizures occur within 15 minutes of ingestion (or 5 minutes of inhalation) and may result in hyperthermia, metabolic and respiratory acidosis, rhabdomyolysis, and myoglobinuric renal failure (14,17). 1-2 grams ignatius bean (50 mg strychnine) can be fatal (18); most deaths occur 3-6 hours post-ingestion from respiratory and subsequent cardiac arrest, anoxic brain damage, or multiple organ failure secondary to hyperthermia (14,18,505). Strychnine accumulates with extended administration, particularly in individuals with liver damage. Chronic use of subconvulsive amounts can cause death after a period of weeks (18).

Possible Interactions with Herbs & Other Dietary Supplements

Insufficient reliable information available.

Possible Interactions with Drugs

ANALEPTICS, PHENOTHIAZINES: Contraindicated in individuals with symptoms of poisoning (18).

Possible Interactions with Foods
No interactions are known to occur, and there is no known reason to expect a clinically significant interaction with ignatius bean.

Possible Interactions with Lab Tests
No interactions are known to occur, and there is no known reason to expect a clinically significant interaction with ignatius bean.

Possible Interactions with Diseases or Conditions
LIVER DISEASE: Contraindicated. Strychnine accumulates in individuals with liver damage. Also, strychnine accumulation can cause liver damage (18).

Typical Dosages & Routes of Administration that are Commonly Used
ORAL: TOXIC, avoid using (18).

Comments
Strychnine may be detected by thin-layer chromatography (qualitative analysis) and high performance liquid chromatography (quantitative analysis). Urine and gastric aspirate are most useful in confirming poisoning (17). Strychnine pills are no longer marketed (14). Strychnos ianata and strychnos multiflora seeds were once treated in the same way as ignatius beans (18).

IMMORTELLE

This Product is Also Known As
Common Shrubby Everlasting, Eternal Flower, Goldilocks, Yellow Chaste Weed.
CAUTION: See separate listing for Sandy Everlasting.

Scientific Names
Helichrysum arenarium.
Family: Compositae/Asteraceae.

People Use This For
Orally, immortelle is used for liver and gallbladder disorders, including chronic gallstones with accompanying cramps. It is also used orally for dyspepsia, loss of appetite, to stimulate bile flow, and as an antimicrobial.
In folk medicine, it is used orally as a diuretic (18).

Safety
There is insufficient reliable information available about the safety of immortelle.
Pregnancy and Lactation: Insufficient reliable information available; avoid using.

Effectiveness
There is insufficient reliable information available about the effectiveness of immortelle.

Possible Mechanism of Action & Active Ingredients
The applicable part of immortelle is the dried flower. There is insufficient reliable information available about the possible mechanism of action and active ingredients.

Adverse Reactions Including Known Allergies
When immortelle is used in people with gallstones, it may cause colic (18). Immortelle can cause an allergic reaction in individuals sensitive to the Asteraceae/Compositae family. Members of this family include ragweed, chrysanthemums, marigolds, daisies, and many other herbs.

Possible Interactions with Herbs & Other Dietary Supplements
Insufficient reliable information available.

Possible Interactions with Drugs
No interactions are known to occur, and there is no known reason to expect a clinically significant interaction with immortelle.

Possible Interactions with Foods
No interactions are known to occur, and there is no known reason to expect a clinically significant interaction with immortelle.

Possible Interactions with Lab Tests
No interactions are known to occur, and there is no known reason to expect a clinically significant interaction with immortelle.

Possible Interactions with Diseases or Conditions

BILIARY OBSTRUCTION: Immortelle is contraindicated during biliary obstruction secondary to its possible stimulation of biliary flow.

CROSS-ALLERGENICITY: Can cause an allergic reaction in individuals sensitive to the Asteraceae/Compositae family. Members of this family include ragweed, chrysanthemums, marigolds, daisies, and many other herbs.

Typical Dosages & Routes of Administration that are Commonly Used

ORAL: One cup of tea daily. The tea is prepared by steeping 3-4 grams dried flower in 150 mL of boiling water for 10 minutes and straining. The tea is sometimes drunk throughout the day, but must be made fresh each time. The average daily dose is 3 grams of immortelle (18).

Comments

Immortelle is a protected species. It can easily be confused with sandy everlasting (Helichrysum augustifolium, synonym Helichrysum italicum), or Helichrysum stoechas (18). Avoid confusion with immortal (Asclepias asperula) (11).

INDIAN FRANKINCENSE

This Product is Also Known As

Indian Olibanum, Salai Guggal.
CAUTION: See separate listings for Frankincense and Guggul.

Scientific Names

Boswellia serrata.
Family: Burseraceae.

People Use This For

Orally, Indian frankincense is used for arthritis, as an anti-inflammatory agent (11), and for ulcerative colitis (6). Historically, it has been used for rheumatism, syphilis, painful menstruation, pimples, sores, tumors, cancers, asthma, sore throat, abdominal pain, stomach troubles, nervous problems, as a stimulant, respiratory antiseptic, diuretic, and for stimulating menstrual flow (11).

Other uses include the utilization of the resin oil and extracts in soaps, cosmetics, foods, and beverages. (11)

Safety

LIKELY SAFE ...when consumed in amounts found in foods (maximum use level 0.001% in meat products) (11); approved for food use in the US (11).
POSSIBLY SAFE ...when used appropriately as an oral medicinal agent (6,12).
There is insufficient reliable information available about the topical use of Indian frankincense.
PREGNANCY AND LACTATION: Insufficient reliable information available.

Effectiveness

POSSIBLY EFFECTIVE ...when used orally for arthritis (11), and ulcerative colitis symptoms (6).
There is insufficient reliable information available about the effectiveness of Indian frankincense for its other uses.

Possible Mechanism of Action & Active Ingredients

The applicable part of Indian frankincense is the resin. The principle constituents of Indian frankincense are boswellic acid and alpha-boswellic acid, which have anti-inflammatory properties (6,11,1706). In preliminary research, Indian frankincense extracts show anti-inflammatory and antiarthritis effects, but various Indian frankincense-containing products fail to show antiarthritis, anti-inflammatory, or antipyretic effects (6131). However, an Indian frankincense resin-containing herb/mineral combination product reduces pain and disability in people with arthritis symptoms (6). Indian frankincense resin might improve ulcerative colitis (1708), bronchial asthma symptoms, and indices of respiratory function (1709).

Adverse Reactions Including Known Allergies

None reported.

Possible Interactions with Herbs & Other Dietary Supplements

Insufficient reliable information available.

Possible Interactions with Drugs

No interactions are known to occur, and there is no known reason to expect a clinically significant interaction with Indian frankincense.

Possible Interactions with Foods

No interactions are known to occur, and there is no known reason to expect a clinically significant interaction with Indian frankincense.

Possible Interactions with Lab Tests

No interactions are known to occur, and there is no known reason to expect a clinically significant interaction with Indian frankincense.

Possible Interactions with Diseases or Conditions

No interactions are known to occur, and there is no known reason to expect a clinically significant interaction with Indian frankincense.

Typical Dosages & Routes of Administration that are Commonly Used

ORAL (gum resin preparation): Ulcerative colitis, 350 mg three times daily, reported in one clinical trial (1708). Bronchial asthma, 300 mg three times daily, reported in one clinical trial (1709).
TOPICAL: No typical dosage.

Comments

Olibanum is a term which refers to the oleogum resin exuded from incisions in the bark of several Boswellia species, including Boswellia serrata (Indian frankincense), Boswellia carterii (Bible frankincense), Boswellia frereana (African elemi), and Boswellia bhau-dajiana (11).

INDIAN GOOSEBERRY

This Product is Also Known As

Aamalaki, Amalaki, Amblabaum, Amla, Aonla, Emblic, Emblica, Emblic Myrobalan, Groseillier de Ceylan, Indian-Gooseberry, Mirobalano, Myrobalan Emblic, Neli.

Scientific Names

Emblica officinalis, synonyms Mirobalanus embilica, Phyllanthus emblica.
Family: Euphorbiaceae.

People Use This For

Orally, Indian gooseberry is used for lowering cholesterol, treating atherosclerosis, treating cancer, dyspepsia, eye problems, joint pain, diarrhea, dysentery, "organ restoration", and as an anti-inflammatory and antimicrobial (6). It is also used orally for obesity (2075).
In Ayurvedic medicine, Indian gooseberry fruit juice has been used orally for treating diabetes and pancreatitis (6).
In India, Indian gooseberry fruit is consumed as part of the diet (6).

Safety

LIKELY SAFE ...when consumed in amounts found in foods (6,2076).
There is insufficient reliable information available about the safety of Indian gooseberry when used in amounts greater than those found in foods.
PREGNANCY AND LACTATION: Insufficient reliable information available; avoid using.

Effectiveness

There is insufficient reliable information available about the effectiveness of Indian gooseberry.

Possible Mechanism of Action & Active Ingredients

The applicable part of Indian gooseberry is primarily the fruit (2075), but extracts from the leaves have also been used (6,2078,2079). Indian gooseberry fruit and juice have been shown to lower total serum cholesterol, low-density lipoprotein (LDL), triglycerides, and phospholipids and to have positive effects on atherosclerosis in animals (6). Preliminary evidence suggests Indian gooseberry might also lower total serum cholesterol levels in humans, without affecting high-density lipoprotein (HDL) levels (2077). Indian gooseberry fruit juice also has antimicrobial, antimutagenic and antioxidant activity in animals (6,2080,2081). Indian gooseberry leaf extract has been shown to have anti-inflammatory activity (6,2078,2079).

Adverse Reactions Including Known Allergies

None reported.

Possible Interactions with Herbs & Other Dietary Supplements

Insufficient reliable information available.

Possible Interactions with Drugs

No interactions are known to occur, and there is no known reason to expect a clinically significant interaction with Indian gooseberry.

Possible Interactions with Foods

No interactions are known to occur, and there is no known reason to expect a clinically significant interaction with Indian gooseberry.

Possible Interactions with Lab Tests

No interactions are known to occur, and there is no known reason to expect a clinically significant interaction with Indian gooseberry.

Possible Interactions with Diseases or Conditions

No interactions are known to occur, and there is no known reason to expect a clinically significant interaction with Indian gooseberry.

Typical Dosages & Routes of Administration that are Commonly Used

No typical dosage.

Comments

Indian gooseberry is a native deciduous tree in India and the Middle East (6). Indian gooseberry has been used in Ayurvedic medicine for thousands of years. Reference to Indian gooseberry appeared in an Ayurvedic medicine text in the seventh century (3563).

INDIAN LONG PEPPER

This Product is Also Known As

Jaborandi Pepper, Langer Pfeffer, Long Pepper, Pimenta-Longa, Poivre Long.

Scientific Names

Piper longum.
Family: Piperaceae.

People Use This For

In folk medicine, Indian long pepper is used orally to treat headache, toothache, asthma, beri-beri, bronchitis, mucous membrane inflammation, cholera, coma, cough, diarrhea, dysentery, epilepsy, fever, frigidity, stomachache, stroke, heartburn, indigestion, insomnia, leprosy, lethargy, enlarged spleen, muscle pain, nasal discharge, painful menses, paralysis, psoriasis, sterility in women, snake bites, tetanus, thirst, tuberculosis, and tumors. In folk medicine, it is used during childbirth, and during the 3-6 weeks following childbirth while the uterus returns to normal size. In folk medicine, Indian long pepper fruit is used to stimulate menstrual flow, appetite, and bile flow, to improve digestion, induce sweating, as an abortifacient, analgesic, antiflatulent, aphrodisiac, astringent, bactericide, diuretic, larvicide, sedative, stimulant, tonic, and vermifuge (4017).
In Ayurvedic medicine, piper longum fruit is used in combination herbal preparations (3755).
For food uses, Indian long pepper fruit has a role in cooking, both as an ingredient and a spice. It is used in fresh or dried form.

Safety

LIKELY SAFE …when used orally in amounts found in foods.
There is insufficient reliable information available about the safety of Indian long pepper in larger oral amounts or for topical use.
PREGNANCY AND LACTATION: Insufficient reliable information is available; avoid amounts greater than found in foods.

Effectiveness

There is insufficient reliable information available about the effectiveness of Indian long pepper.

Possible Mechanism of Action & Active Ingredients

The applicable part of Indian long pepper is the fruit. Piper longum contains piperine which can increase oral absorption of drugs and other substances, possibly by modulating intestinal membrane dynamics (3757). Some evidence suggests an ethanolic extract and isolated piperine might have amoebicidal activity (3758). An Ayurvedic herbal preparation containing piper longum (Pippali rasayana) shows evidence that it is useful for managing giardiasis (3754,3755). In mice, an ethanolic extract of piper longum administered chronically increased weights of lung, spleen, and reproductive organs. It also increased sperm count and motility without demonstrating acute or chronic toxicity (3756).

Adverse Reactions Including Known Allergies

None reported.

Possible Interactions with Herbs & Other Dietary Supplements

SPARTEINE: Piperine increases the bioavailability of sparteine, a constituent of scotch broom (19).

Possible Interactions with Drugs

PHENYTOIN: Concomitant administration speeds absorption and slows elimination of phenytoin (Dilantin) (537).
PROPRANOLOL: Concomitant administration speeds and increases absorption, and increases serum concentrations of propranolol (Inderal) (538).

THEOPHYLLINE: Concomitant administration increases absorption and serum concentrations of theophylline (Theo-Dur) (538).

Possible Interactions with Foods
No interactions are known to occur, and there is no known reason to expect a clinically significant interaction with Indian long pepper.

Possible Interactions with Lab Tests
SERUM DRUG ASSAYS: Can increase phenytoin, propranolol, and theophylline serum concentrations and test results (537,538).

Possible Interactions with Diseases or Conditions
No interactions are known to occur, and there is no known reason to expect a clinically significant interaction with Indian long pepper.

Typical Dosages & Routes of Administration that are Commonly Used
No typical dosage.

Comments
Piper nigrum, the source of black pepper and white pepper, also contains the constituent piperine. However, red pepper and cayenne do not.

INDIAN PHYSIC

This Product is Also Known As
American Ipecacuanha, Bowman's Root, Gillenia, Indian Hippo.
CAUTION: See separate listings for Black Root and Canadian Hemp.

Scientific Names
Gillenia trifoliata.

People Use This For
Orally, Indian physic is used for digestive disorders and emetic (18).

Safety
There is insufficient reliable information available about the safety of Indian physic.
Pregnancy and Lactation: Insufficient reliable information available; avoid using.

Effectiveness
There is insufficient reliable information about the effectiveness of Indian physic.

Possible Mechanism of Action & Active Ingredients
The applicable parts of Indian physic are the dried root and root bark. Indian physic is stated to have expectorant, emetic, and "blood purification" properties (18).

Adverse Reactions Including Known Allergies
None reported.

Possible Interactions with Herbs & Other Dietary Supplements
Insufficient reliable information available.

Possible Interactions with Drugs
No interactions are known to occur, and there is no known reason to expect a clinically significant interaction with Indian physic.

Possible Interactions with Foods
No interactions are known to occur, and there is no known reason to expect a clinically significant interaction with Indian physic.

Possible Interactions with Lab Tests
No interactions are known to occur, and there is no known reason to expect a clinically significant interaction with Indian physic.

Possible Interactions with Diseases or Conditions
No interactions are known to occur, and there is no known reason to expect a clinically significant interaction with Indian physic.

Typical Dosages & Routes of Administration that are Commonly Used
ORAL: Used as a powder in tea or tonic (18).

Comments

Avoid confusion with Canadian hemp (Apocynum cannabinum), also known as Indian physic (12). Avoid confusion with black root (Leptandra virginica), also known as bowman's root.

INDIAN SNAKEROOT

This Product is Also Known As

Chandrika, Chota-Chand, Covanamilpori, Dhanburua, Pagla-Ka-Dawa, Patalagandhi, Rauwolfae radix, Rauwolfia, Rauwolfia Serpentina, Rauwolfiawurzel, Sarpagandha.

Scientific Names

Rauvolfia serpentina.
Family: Apocynaceae.

People Use This For

Orally, Indian snakeroot is used for mild essential hypertension (2,18), symptomatic relief in individuals with agitated psychosis unable to tolerate other agents (13), for nervousness, and insomnia (18). As a prescription product, it is used to treat mild to moderate hypertension (15), schizophrenia, and vasospastic attacks due to peripheral vascular disorders (15).

Traditionally, Indian snakeroot has been used for snake and reptile bites, insanity, fever, constipation, feverish intestinal diseases, liver ailments, rheumatism, dropsy (edema), as a tonic for general debilities (18), for mental illness, and epilepsy (514).

Safety

POSSIBLY SAFE ...when the prescription product is used. ...when the standardized extract is used under the supervision of a medical professional trained in the use of Indian snakeroot.
POSSIBLY UNSAFE ...when taken orally for self-medication. Appropriate use of Indian snakeroot requires medical diagnosis and treatment. Large amounts or overdose can lead to CNS depression, convulsions, extrapyramidal effects, and coma (15). ...when used by individuals operating motor vehicles or machinery; Indian snakeroot can alter reaction time (2,15).
PREGNANCY: LIKELY UNSAFE ...contraindicated for oral use (2,18) because the reserpine alkaloid constituents cross the placenta and can be potentially teratogenic (15,4260).
LACTATION: POSSIBLY UNSAFE ...because the reserpine alkaloids are excreted in breast milk although there are no reports of toxicity (4260); avoid using.

Effectiveness

POSSIBLY EFFECTIVE ...when taken orally for treating mild (borderline) essential hypertension when dietary measures are inadequate (2). ...when the prescription product is used.
There is insufficient reliable information available about the effectiveness of Indian snakeroot for its other uses.

Possible Mechanism of Action & Active Ingredients

The applicable part of Indian snakeroot is the root. The properties of the whole root of rauwolfia serpentina differ from those of reserpine. The whole root contains over 50 alkaloids (13). Rauwolfia serpentina demonstrates hypotensive, sedative, and tranquilizing effects (15). It also reduces heart rate (13), has anti-arrhythmic effects (18), and causes a general sense of euphoria (13). The principle constituents of the whole root include the rauwolfia alkaloids, reserpine, rescinnamine, and deserpidine (11-desmethoxyreseroine) (13). Hypotensive effects are believed to be due to the depletion of both catecholamine and serotonin stores and to the prevention of reabsorption (13,18). The greater the proportion of alkaloids present, the greater the hypotensive activity (13). The sedative effects of Indian snakeroot can result from the depletion of amine stores in the central nervous system (13).

Adverse Reactions Including Known Allergies

When used medicinally in low amounts, Indian snakeroot can have adverse reactions including nasal congestion, abdominal cramps, diarrhea, nausea, vomiting, anorexia, increased gastric acid secretion, drowsiness, fatigue, lethargy, slowed reflexes, sexual dysfunction, and bradycardia (15). Cardiac and vascular effects begin with tachycardia and hypertension, and usually within 24 hours progress to bradycardia and hypotension (14). In larger amounts, mental depression can slowly develop. After discontinuation of Indian snakeroot, mental depression can persist for several months (15). In extremely large amounts, Parkinson-like symptoms, extrapyramidal reactions, and convulsions can occur (15). Allergic reactions from the use of Indian snakeroot are rare (15), and it can precipitate asthma (15).

Possible Interactions with Herbs & Other Dietary Supplements

EPHEDRA: Theoretically, concomitant use of Indian snakeroot can decrease ephedrine effects (15).
CARDIOACTIVE GLYCOSIDE-CONTAINING HERBS: Theoretically, concomitant use can increase the risk of bradycardia (2,18), angina-like symptoms, and arrhythmias (15). Cardioactive glycoside containing herbs include black hellebore, digitalis, lily of the valley, oleander leaf, pheasant's eye, and squill (19).

Possible Interactions with Drugs

ALCOHOL (ethanol): Use Indian snakeroot with caution, because concomitant use increases the risk of additive CNS-depressant effects (15).

ANTIHYPERTENSIVE, DIURETICS: Concomitant use of Indian snakeroot can potentiate the hypotensive effects of rauwolfia alkaloids (15).

BARBITURATES: Concomitant use can potentiate the effects of these drugs and the rauwolfia alkaloids (2,18).

DIGOXIN (Lanoxin): Concomitant use with Indian snakeroot can cause bradycardia (2,18), angina-like symptoms, and arrhythmias (15). Avoid large amounts of the rauwolfia alkaloids together with digitalis glycosides (15).

EPHEDRINE: Concomitant use can reduce indirect-sympathomimetic drug activity (15).

LEVODOPA: Avoid the use of Indian snakeroot (15) because concomitant use can reduce drug effectiveness and increase extrapyramidal motor symptoms (2,18,15).

MONOAMINE OXIDASE INHIBITORS (MAOIs): Avoid concomitant or overlapping use of Indian snakeroot within several days, which can increase the risk of excitation and hypertension (15).

NEUROLEPTICS: Concomitant use can potentiate the effects of these drugs and the rauwolfia alkaloids (2,18).

PROPRANOLOL (Inderal): Concomitant use can enhance beta-blockade due to the rauwolfia alkaloid Catecholamine-depleting effects (15).

SYMPATHOMIMETIC DRUGS: Concomitant use can cause an initial increase in blood pressure and enhance or prolong the pressor effects (2,18,15).

TRICYCLIC ANTIDEPRESSANTS can decrease the effectiveness of rauwolfia alkaloids (15).

Possible Interactions with Foods

ALCOHOL (ethanol): Indian snakeroot should be taken with caution, because concomitant use with alcohol increases the risk of additive CNS-depressant effects (15).

Possible Interactions with Lab Tests

BLOOD PRESSURE: Indian snakeroot might lower blood pressure and blood pressure readings in patients with mild to moderate hypertension, due to its rauwolfia alkaloid content (2,15).

BILIRUBIN: Theoretically, large doses of Indian snakeroot might cause falsely high serum bilirubin test results, due to its reserpine content. Reserpine concentrations greater than 61 mg/L can cause falsely high serum bilirubin test results when measured by the Jendrassik and Grof method (275).

CATECHOLAMINES: Overdose of Indian snakeroot might initially increase urinary catecholamine excretion and test results. Rauwolfia alkaloids (contained in Indian snakeroot) release stored norepinephrine, resulting in increased urinary catecholamine excretion. Chronic use of Indian snakeroot might decrease urinary catecholamine excretion, due to its rauwolfia alkaloid content. Chronic use of rauwolfia alkaloids decreases urinary catecholamine excretion (15,275).

GLUCOSE: Theoretically, Indian snakeroot might increase blood glucose concentrations and test results, due to its reserpine content. Reserpine might increase blood glucose concentrations following administration (275).

GUAIACOLS SPOT TEST: Theoretically, Indian snakeroot might cause false-positive urine guaiacols spot test results, due to its reserpine content. Reserpine can cause a false-positive reaction for urinary guaiacols with the screening test of Rogers (275).

17-HYDROXYCORTICOSTEROIDS: Indian snakeroot might reduce urinary 17-hydroxycorticosteroid concentrations and test results, possibly due to suppression of central 17-hydroxycorticosteroid synthesis by its rauwolfia alkaloid content. Indian snakeroot might interfere with colorimetric assays of urinary 17-hydroxycorticosteroid concentrations by the Glenn-Nelson technique, due to its rauwolfia alkaloid content. Theoretically, Indian snakeroot might interfere with colorimetric assays of urinary 17-hydroxycorticosteroid concentrations which rely on the Porter-Silber reaction, due to its reserpine content (15,275).

5-HYDROXYINDOLEACETIC ACID (5-HIAA): Large doses of Indian snakeroot might increase urinary 5-HIAA excretion and test results. Large doses of rauwolfia alkaloids, which are contained in Indian snakeroot, can release serotonin (5-HT) from brain tissues, resulting in increased urinary 5-HIAA excretion (15,275).

4-HYDROXY-3-METHOXY PHENYLETHYLENE GLYCOL (HMPG): Theoretically, Indian snakeroot might increase or decrease urinary HMPG concentrations and test results, due to its reserpine content. Reserpine can increase urinary HMPG concentrations by causing release of stored norepinephrine. Long-term reserpine administration can decrease urinary HMPG concentrations (275).

17-KETOSTEROIDS: Indian snakeroot might interfere with colorimetric assays of urinary 17-ketosteroids by the Holtorff Koch modification of the Zimmerman reaction, due to its rauwolfia alkaloid content (15).

LUPUS ERYTHEMATOSUS (LE) CELLS: Theoretically, Indian snakeroot might trigger the presence of LE cells in the blood and positive LE cell test results, due its reserpine content. Reserpine might cause systemic lupus erythematosus (SLE) and the presence LE cells in the blood. However, this usually normalizes when reserpine is discontinued (275).

NOREPINEPHRINE: Theoretically, Indian snakeroot might decrease urinary norepinephrine concentrations due to its reserpine content. Reserpine can decrease urinary norepinephrine concentration (275).

OCCULT BLOOD: Theoretically, Indian snakeroot might activate peptic ulcers, resulting in bleeding and positive fecal occult blood tests, due to its reserpine content. Reserpine might activate peptic ulcers, resulting in bleeding and occult blood (275).

PLATELETS: Theoretically, Indian snakeroot might cause thrombocytopenia, decreasing blood platelets and platelet counts. Reserpine might cause thrombocytopenia (275).

PROLACTIN: Theoretically, large doses of Indian snakeroot might increase plasma prolactin levels and test results in patients with hypertension, due to its reserpine content. Reserpine, in daily doses greater than 0.25 mg, can increase plasma prolactin levels in patients with hypertension (275).

THYROXINE (T4): Theoretically, Indian snakeroot might decrease serum T4 concentrations and test results, due to its reserpine content. Reserpine can decrease serum T4 concentrations by increasing hepatic T4 metabolism (275).

TYRAMINE: Theoretically, Indian snakeroot might cause false-negative tyramine test results, due to its reserpine content. Reserpine can inhibit patient responsiveness to tyramine tests (275).

VANILLYLMANDELIC ACID (VMA): Overdose of Indian snakeroot might initially increase urinary VMA excretion and test results. Rauwolfia alkaloids (contained in Indian snakeroot) release stored norepinephrine, resulting in increased urinary VMA excretion. Chronic use of Indian snakeroot might decrease urinary VMA excretion, due to its rauwolfia alkaloid content. Chronic use of rauwolfia alkaloids decreases urinary VMA excretion (15,275).

Possible Interactions with Diseases or Conditions

GI CONDITIONS: Indian snakeroot is contraindicated in individuals with active peptic ulcer disease or ulcerative colitis (15). Use cautiously in individuals with a history of these diseases.

GALLBLADDER DISEASE: Use cautiously in individuals with a history of gallstones, because Indian snakeroot could precipitate biliary colic (15).

ELECTROCONVULSIVE THERAPY (ECT): Indian snakeroot is contraindicated during ECT (15), and one week should elapse between cessation of rauwolfia alkaloids and initiation of ECT (15).

HYPERSENSITIVITY: Contraindicated in individuals hypersensitive to rauwolfia alkaloids (15).

MENTAL DEPRESSION: Indian snakeroot is contraindicated, especially in individuals with a past history of depression or suicidal tendencies (15).

PHEOCHROMOCYTOMA: Contraindicated (18).

Typical Dosages & Routes of Administration that are Commonly Used

ORAL: The average daily amount of Indian snakeroot is 600 mg of the powdered whole root, which is equivalent to 6 mg total alkaloids (2,18).

RX PRODUCTS: Rauwolfia serpentina, deserpidine, and reserpine are available as FDA approved prescription drugs (15).

Comments

Reserpine is commercially obtained from Rauvolfia serpentina and the related species, Rauvolfia micrantha, Rauvolfia tetraphylla, and Rauvolfia vomitoria (13). Spelling note: The genus, Rauvolfia, is correctly spelled with a "v", while Rauwolfia or Rauwolfia serpentina (names for the dried root of Rauvolfia serpentina) are correctly spelled with a "w" (2,13).

INOSINE

This Product is Also Known As
Hypoxanthine Riboside, Hypoxanthosine.

Scientific Names
2,3-Diphosphoglycerate; 6,9-Dihydro-9-B-D-ribofuranosyl-1H-puin-6-one; 9-B-D-ribofuranosylhypoxanthine.

People Use This For
Orally, inosine is used for enhancing athletic performance (1900).

Safety
There is insufficient reliable information available about the safety of inosine.
Pregnancy And Lactation: Insufficient reliable information available; avoid using.

Effectiveness
LIKELY INEFFECTIVE ...when taken orally for improving athletic performance (2369,2370).

Possible Mechanism of Action & Active Ingredients
Preliminary evidence suggests inosine might stimulate axon growth from uninjured nerve cells to injured nerve cells of the central nervous system. Further studies in humans are needed to establish whether this finding has significance in restoring function after spinal cord injuries (370).

Adverse Reactions Including Known Allergies
None reported.

Possible Interactions with Herbs & Other Dietary Supplements
Insufficient reliable information available.

Possible Interactions with Drugs

PROBENECID, ALLOPURINOL: Because inosine can make gout worse, concomitant use is not recommended. There is not a direct interaction between these drugs and inosine (217).

Possible Interactions with Foods

No interactions are known to occur, and there is no known reason to expect a clinically significant interaction with inosine.

Possible Interactions with Lab Tests

No interactions are known to occur, and there is no known reason to expect a clinically significant interaction with inosine.

Possible Interactions with Diseases or Conditions

GOUT: Inosine can aggravate gout (217).

Typical Dosages & Routes of Administration that are Commonly Used

ORAL: 5 to 6 grams per day used in clinical studies of effects on athletic performance (2369,2370).

Comments

None.

INOSITOL

This Product is Also Known As

Antialopecia Factor, Cyclohexitol, D-chiro-inositol, Dambrose, Inose, Inosite, Inositol Monophosphate, Lipositol, Meso-inositol, Mouse Antialopecia Factor, Myo-inositol, Vitamin B8.
CAUTION: See separate listings for Inositol Nicotinate and IP-6.

Scientific Names

Hexahydroxycyclohexane, synonym 1,2,3,4,5,6-Cyclohexanehexol, synonym cis-1,2,3,5-trans-4,6-Cyclohexanehexol; D-chiro-inositol, synonym (+)-chiroinositol, synonym 1,2,5/3,4,6-inositol, synonym (1S)-inositol, (1S)-1,2,4/3,5,6-inositol.

People Use This For

Orally, inositol is used for diabetic neuropathy, conditions associated with disorders of fat transport and metabolism (14,2138), panic disorder, high cholesterol, insomnia (2180), cancer (2181), depression (2183), schizophrenia, Alzheimer's disease, attention deficit disorder, autism (2187), treating lithium-induced side effects (2027), and promoting hair growth (2182). Inositol is also used orally for treating conditions associated with polycystic ovary syndrome, including anovulation, hypertension, hypertriglyceridemia, and elevated serum concentrations of testosterone (2028).
Parenterally, inositol is used for treating respiratory distress syndrome in premature infants (14).

Safety

POSSIBLY SAFE ...when used orally and appropriately. Inositol has been used in amounts up to 12 grams per day for up to 4 weeks with no significant adverse effects (2184,2185,2187).
CHILDREN: POSSIBLY SAFE ...when used parenterally and appropriately for treating respiratory distress syndrome in premature infants (2191,2192).
PREGNANCY: Insufficient reliable information available; avoid using.
LACTATION: Insufficient reliable information available; avoid using. Breast milk is rich in endogenous inositol (14,16,2138); however, the effects of exogenously administered inositol are not known.

Effectiveness

POSSIBLY EFFECTIVE ...when used orally for treating panic disorder with or without agoraphobia. In one small-scale, placebo-controlled trial, inositol significantly reduced the severity and rate of panic attacks and severity of agoraphobia compared to placebo over 4 weeks of treatment (2184). Large scale, long-term trials are needed to confirm inositol's potential benefit in panic disorders. ...when used orally for treating depression. In one small-scale, placebo-controlled trial, depressed patients receiving inositol for 4 weeks had significant improvement, based on Hamilton Depression Rating Scale scores, compared to placebo (2185). In a follow-up study, patients initially responding to inositol rapidly relapse upon discontinuation of treatment (2026). Large scale, long-term trials are necessary to confirm inositol's potential benefit in depression. ...when used orally for treating obsessive-compulsive disorder (OCD). In one small-scale, placebo-controlled trial, OCD patients receiving inositol for 6 weeks had significant improvement, based on Yale-Brown Obsessive Compulsive Scale scores, compared to placebo (2186). ...when used parenterally as a nutritional supplement for improving survival and symptoms in premature infants with respiratory distress syndrome. Clinical trials have shown that inositol significantly lowered inspiratory oxygen requirements, mean airway pressure, and the incidence of bronchopulmonary dysplasia in premature infants not receiving surfactant compared to placebo and glucose (2191,2192). ...when used orally for treating symptoms associated with polycystic ovary syndrome. In one clinical trial, the inositol isomer D-chiro-inositol significantly decreased serum triglyceride and testosterone levels, modestly decreased blood pressure, and induced ovulation in obese women with polycystic ovary syndrome (2028).

POSSIBLY INEFFECTIVE ...when used orally for treating schizophrenia (2188). ...when used orally for treating Alzheimer's disease. Inositol was no more effective than placebo for improving symptoms of Alzheimer's disease in one clinical trial (2189). ...when used orally for treating autism. One clinical trial has shown inositol to be no better than placebo (2190). ...when used orally for treating attention deficit disorder. One clinical trial has shown inositol to be no better than placebo (2187). ...when used orally for enhancing the antidepressant effects of selective serotonin reuptake inhibitors (SSRIs). One small-scale clinical trial showed inositol to be no better than placebo when combined with an SSRI as measured by the Hamilton Depression Rating Scale after 4 weeks of combination therapy (2025). ...when used orally for reducing lithium-induced side effects. One uncontrolled trial has shown that inositol has no effect on the occurrence of lithium-induced adverse effects, including tremor, thirst, and thyroid and adrenal function (2027).

LIKELY INEFFECTIVE ...when used orally for reducing symptoms of diabetic neuropathy. Clinical trials suggest that inositol is incapable of significantly improving the symptoms of diabetic neuropathy (2193,2194,2195). There is insufficient reliable information available about the effectiveness of inositol for its other uses.

Possible Mechanism of Action & Active Ingredients

Endogenous inositol is an essential component of cell membrane phospholipids. It has weak lipotropic activity, and can move fat out of liver and intestine cells (2187). Inositol has a variety of stereoisomers, including myo-inositol and D-chiro-inositol. Myo-inositol is the most abundant form in the central nervous system (CNS). Biological function varies among the isomers (2047,2048). Inositol might reverse desensitization of serotonin receptors (2187). Limited clinical evidence suggests exogenous inositol may have similar benefits as the selective-serotonin-reuptake inhibitors (SSRIs) in conditions such as panic disorder, depression, and obsessive-compulsive disorder. Limited evidence suggests that inositol might reverse desensitization of serotonin receptors (2187). Researchers think that D-chiro-inositol isomer induces ovulation in women with polycystic ovary syndrome by improving insulin sensitivity. Reduced insulin resistance is also thought responsible for improving other symptoms associated with polycystic ovary syndrome, including hypertension, hyperlipidemia, type 2 diabetes, obesity, and increased serum testosterone concentrations (2028). Previous research suggests that patients with insulin resistance, including those with impaired glucose intolerance and type 2 diabetes, might have D-chiro-inositol deficiency (2028).

Adverse Reactions Including Known Allergies

None reported.

Possible Interactions with Herbs & Other Dietary Supplements

Insufficient reliable information available.

Possible Interactions with Drugs

No interactions are known to occur, and there is no known reason to expect a clinically significant interaction with inositol.

Possible Interactions with Foods

MINERALS (especially calcium, zinc and iron): Phytic acid, the form of inositol found in foods, may interfere with absorption of minerals (16).

Possible Interactions with Lab Tests

No interactions are known to occur, and there is no known reason to expect a clinically significant interaction with inositol.

Possible Interactions with Diseases or Conditions

No interactions are known to occur, and there is no known reason to expect a clinically significant interaction with inositol.`

Typical Dosages & Routes of Administration that are Commonly Used

ORAL: For panic disorder and depression, inositol 12 grams per day has been used (2184,2185). For obsessive-compulsive disorder, inositol 18 grams per day has been used (2186). For treating symptoms associated with polycystic ovary syndrome, D-chiro-inositol 12 grams per day has been used (2028).

PARENTERAL: For respiratory distress syndrome in premature infants, inositol 80 mg/kg parenterally per day has been used (2191).

Comments

None.

INOSITOL NICOTINATE

This Product is Also Known As
Hexanicotinoyl Inositol, Inositol Hexaniacinate, Inositol Hexanicotinate, Inositol Niacinate, Meso-Inositol Hexanicotinate, No-Flush Niacin.
CAUTION: See separate listings for Inositol and Niacin and Niacinamide (Vitamin B3).

Scientific Names
Hexanicotinyl cis-1,2,3-5-trans-4,6-cyclohexane; Myo-inositol hexa-3-pyridine-carboxylate.

People Use This For
Orally, inositol nicotinate is used for improving circulation (491) and for treating peripheral vascular disease, cerebral vascular disease (9), intermittent claudication, stasis dermatitis, and Raynaud's disease (493,495,496). It is also used for hypercholesterolemia (9), atherosclerosis-related migraines, scleroderma (496), supporting nervous system and brain function, improving sleep, lowering blood pressure, calming effects (491), restless leg syndrome, acne, dermatitis herpetiformis, exfoliative glossitis, psoriasis (496), and schizophrenia and other mental illnesses (494).

Safety
POSSIBLY SAFE ...when used orally and appropriately (496).
PREGNANCY AND LACTATION: Insufficient reliable information available; avoid using.

Effectiveness
POSSIBLY EFFECTIVE ...when used orally for improving symptoms of peripheral vascular disorders, including intermittent claudication and Raynaud's disease (496,498,1544,1545). Several weeks of treatment may be necessary before the full beneficial effects are seen (1544,1545). ...when used orally for treating hyperlipidemia, especially in combination with clofibrate (496,499,1546).
There is insufficient reliable information available about inositol nicotinate for its other uses.

Possible Mechanism of Action & Active Ingredients
Inositol nicotinate consists of six molecules of niacin (nicotinic acid) chemically linked to an inositol molecule. It is hydrolyzed in the body to free niacin and inositol, although this occurs slowly, with peak serum levels not occurring until approximately 10 hours after ingestion (496). It is theoretically possible that this slow conversion might reduce peak plasma levels and thereby reduce the incidence of side effects that have been associated with niacin such as flushing. Inositol nicotinate is reported to have vasodilatory, lipid lowering, and fibrinolytic actions (9,496). The mechanism of action of inositol nicotinate is believed to be the same as that of niacin (496). Several weeks of treatment may be necessary before the full beneficial effects of inositol nicotinate are seen in peripheral vascular disorders such as Raynaud's disease, suggesting that fibrinolysis, lipid lowering, and vasodilatory action contribute to its beneficial effects (1544,1545).

Adverse Reactions Including Known Allergies
Adverse effects from the use of inositol nicotinate in usual doses appear to be rare (496). However, inositol nicotinate is metabolized to niacin which is associated with numerous side effects including flushing, pruritus, GI complaints, hepatotoxicity, hyperuricemia, and impaired glucose tolerance (496).

Possible Interactions with Herbs & Other Dietary Supplements
Insufficient reliable information available.

Possible Interactions with Drugs
ANTICOAGULANTS/FIBRINOLYTIC AGENTS: Theoretically, concomitant use might increase the risk of bleeding, due to the fibrinolytic effects of inositol nicotinate (496).
ANTIDIABETES DRUGS: Theoretically, concomitant use might interfere with blood glucose control, requiring drug dosing adjustment. Niacin can interfere with blood glucose control (15). Inositol nicotinate is metabolized to niacin in the body (496). More frequent blood glucose monitoring may be necessary, particularly early in the course of treatment (15).
GANGLIONIC BLOCKING DRUGS: Theoretically, concomitant use might potentiate the hypotensive effects of ganglionic blocking drugs (15). Niacin can potentiate the hypotensive effects of these drugs (15). Inositol nicotinate is metabolized to niacin in the body (496).
HMG-CoA REDUCTASE INHIBITORS: Concomitant use of niacin and HMG-CoA reductase inhibitors increase the risk of myopathy (14,15). Inositol nicotinate is metabolized to niacin in the body (496). HMG-CoA reductase inhibitors include cerivastatin (Baycol), atorvastatin (Lipitor), lovastatin (Mevacor), pravastatin (Pravachol), and simvastatin (Zocor).
TRANSDERMAL NICOTINE (Nicoderm, Nicotrol): Concomitant use of niacin and transdermal nicotine increases the risk of flushing and dizziness (14). Inositol nicotinate is metabolized to niacin in the body (496).

Possible Interactions with Foods
ETHANOL: Theoretically, inositol nicotinate should be used with caution in heavy ethanol drinkers. Both niacin and ethanol can increase the risk of hepatotoxicity. Niacin-induced flushing can be magnified by concomitant

ingestion of ethanol. Inositol nicotinate is metabolized to niacin (14,15,1289).

HOT DRINKS: Niacin-induced flushing can be magnified by concomitant ingestion of niacin. Inositol nicotinate is metabolized to niacin (14,15,1289).

Possible Interactions with Lab Tests

LIVER FUNCTION TESTS: Inositol nicotinate may increase levels of liver enzymes. Liver function should be monitored periodically when using doses of 2000 mg per day or more (496).

URINARY CATECHOLAMINES: Niacin, a metabolite of inositol nicotinate, can produce fluorescent substances in the urine, which cause false elevations in some fluorometric tests of urinary catecholamines (15).

URINE GLUCOSE: Niacin, a metabolite of inositol nicotinate, can give false-positive reactions with cupric sulfate solution (Benedict's reagent) for urine glucose tests (15).

Possible Interactions with Diseases or Conditions

ALLERGIES: Niacin, a metabolite of inositol nicotinate, might exacerbate allergies by causing histamine release (14,15,496).

ARTERIAL HEMORRHAGE: Contraindicated; niacin, a metabolite of inositol nicotinate, can cause hypotension and might exacerbate hypotension associated with arterial hemorrhage (15,496).

CORONARY ARTERY DISEASE/UNSTABLE ANGINA: Large amounts of niacin, a metabolite of inositol nicotinate, can increase the risk of cardiac arrhythmias (15,496). One study showed an increased incidence of cardiac arrhythmias when niacin was used in patients with coronary artery disease (15); use with caution.

DIABETES: Niacin, a metabolite of inositol nicotinate, can interfere with blood glucose control requiring dosing adjustment of antidiabetic agents (15,496). Niacin and niacinamide can cause hyperglycemia, abnormal glucose tolerance, and glycosuria. Increased blood glucose monitoring might be necessary, particularly early in the course of treatment (15).

GALLBLADDER DISEASE: Niacin, a metabolite of inositol nicotinate, might exacerbate gallbladder disease (14,15,496); use with caution.

GOUT: Caution, large amounts of niacin might precipitate gout. Niacin can cause hyperuricemia. Inositol nicotinate is metabolized to niacin (14,15,496).

SEVERE HYPOTENSION: Contraindicated; niacin, a metabolite of inositol nicotinate, can cause hypotension (15,496).

KIDNEY DISEASE: Niacin, a metabolite of inositol nicotinate, is excreted unchanged in the urine and might accumulate in patients with kidney disease (14,15,496); use with caution.

LIVER DISEASE: Inositol nicotinate should be avoided in people with liver disease. Niacin has been associated with liver damage, and inositol nicotinate is metabolized to niacin (15,496).

NIACIN HYPERSENSITIVITY: Contraindicated; inositol nicotinate is metabolized to niacin (15,496).

PEPTIC ULCER DISEASE: Contraindicated in patients with active peptic ulcer disease. Large amounts of niacin, a metabolite of inositol nicotinate, might activate peptic ulcer disease (14,15,496).

Typical Dosages & Routes of Administration that are Commonly Used

ORAL: For hyperlipoproteinemia, the typical dosing range is 1500-4000 mg daily given in 2-4 divided doses (496,497). For peripheral vascular disorders, the typical dosing range is 1500-4000 mg daily given in 2-4 divided doses (496,497).

Comments

Inositol nicotinate has been used in conventional medical practice in Great Britain for improving symptoms of peripheral vascular disorders and treating hyperlipidemia for many years, although it is not considered an agent of first choice (9,497).

IODINE

This Product is Also Known As

Potassium Iodide, Povidone Iodine.

Scientific Names

Iodine; I; atomic number 53.

People Use This For

Orally, iodine is used as an expectorant, and for treating endemic goiter, thyroid storm, hyperthyroidism, treatment of radiation emergency associated with radioactive iodides, cutaneous sporotrichosis (14,16), and fibrocystic breast disease (2196).

Topically it is used as an antiseptic (14,15), for preventing mucositis from chemotherapy (2198,2199), and treating diabetic ulcers (14).

Iodine is also used for water purification (14).

Safety
LIKELY SAFE ...when taken orally in appropriate amounts (14). ...when used topically as a 2% solution (15). Iodine is a FDA-approved prescription product.
PREGNANCY: POSSIBLY UNSAFE. Iodine crosses the placenta and can cause abnormal fetal thyroid function. Use of iodine is associated with risk to baby but in some situations the benefit to mother might outweigh the risk to baby (14,15). LIKELY UNSAFE ...when iodine is used as an expectorant; contraindicated (4260).
LACTATION: POSSIBLY UNSAFE ...when used orally, vaginally, or topically. Iodine is concentrated in breast milk; avoid using (14,4260).

Effectiveness
EFFECTIVE ...when used orally for treating thyroid storm, radiation emergency associated with radioactive iodides, cutaneous sporotrichosis, hyperthyroidism, and endemic goiter (15). ...when used topically as an antiseptic. ...when used for water purification (14,15,16). Iodine is an FDA-approved prescription product.
POSSIBLY EFFECTIVE ...when used orally for treating fibrocystic breast disease (2197), for preventing mucositis from chemotherapy (2198,2199), and treating diabetic foot ulcers (2200).
There is insufficient reliable information available about the effectiveness of iodine for its other uses.

Possible Mechanism of Action & Active Ingredients
Iodine oxidizes organic substrates, killing microorganisms (15). It inhibits the release of thyroid hormone (14,2138) and may also increase respiratory secretions (15).

Adverse Reactions Including Known Allergies
Marked sensitivity to iodides manifests as angioedema, cutaneous and mucosal hemorrhage, fever, arthralgia, lymph node enlargement, eosinophilia, urticaria, thrombotic thrombocytopenic purpura, and fatal periarteritis (15). Large amounts or chronic use of iodine can cause metallic taste, soreness in teeth and gums, burning in mouth and throat, increased salivation, coryza, sneezing, eye irritation and eyelid swelling, headache, cough, pulmonary edema, swelling of parotid and submaxillary glands, inflammation of the pharynx, larynx and tonsils; acneform skin lesions, gastric upset, diarrhea, anorexia, and depression (14,15,2138). Prolonged use of iodides can cause thyroid gland hyperplasia, thyroid adenoma, goiter, and severe hypothyroidism (15). Applied topically, iodine may stain skin, irritate tissues, and cause sensitization in some individuals (15). Iodine burns are associated with application of 7% hydroalcoholic solution (15).

Possible Interactions with Herbs & Other Dietary Supplements
Insufficient reliable information available.

Possible Interactions with Drugs
ANTITHYROID DRUGS: Concomitant use may result in additive hypothyroid activity, may cause hypothyroidism (14,15,2138).
LITHIUM: Concomitant use may have additive or synergistic hypothyroid effects (15).
POTASSIUM IODIDE: Concomitant use with potassium-containing products, potassium-sparing diuretics, or ACE inhibitors may cause hyperkalemia (15).

Possible Interactions with Foods
No interactions are known to occur, and there is no known reason to expect a clinically significant interaction with iodine.

Possible Interactions with Lab Tests
THYROID VOLUME: The di-iodotyrosine form of iodine can reduce thyroid volume in patients with goiter due to iodine deficiency (14).
THYROID HORMONES: Short term use of potassium iodide can reduce serum thyroid hormone concentrations and test results (14,15).

Possible Interactions with Diseases or Conditions
THYROID DYSFUNCTION: Prolonged use or excessive amounts of iodides may cause or exacerbate thyroid gland hyperplasia, thyroid adenoma, goiter, and hypothyroidism (14,15).

Typical Dosages & Routes of Administration that are Commonly Used
ORAL: Fibrocystic breast disease, 0.08 mg/kg molecular iodine per day reported from human studies (2197).
TOPICAL: Antiseptic, 2% aqueous solution applied to affected skin areas (15). Preventing mucositis from chemotherapy, rinse mouth with povidone iodine solution 4 times daily (2198,2199). Treating diabetic foot ulcers, 0.9% iodine ointment (2200). CAUTION: Avoid occluding skin areas treated with iodine to reduce risk of iodine burn (15).
OTHER: Water purification, 3-10 drops tincture of iodine added to water (14).

Comments
None.

© Copyright 2000, Natural Medicines Comprehensive Database (209) 472-2244. For updated data, go to www.NaturalDatabase.com • 599

IP-6

This Product is Also Known As

Fytic Acid, Inositol Hexaphosphate, IP6, Phytic Acid.
Caution: See separate listings for Inositol, Inositol Nicotinate, and Vitamin B3.

Scientific Names

Inositol hexaphosphate.

People Use This For

Orally, IP-6 is used to treat and prevent cancer, increase white blood cell production, prevent heart attacks, prevent and treat kidney stones, enhance the immune system, and as an antioxidant (1851,1852,1853).

Safety

LIKELY SAFE ...when used in amounts contained in foods (1854).
There is insufficient reliable information available about the safety of IP-6 when used in supplemental doses in amounts greater than those found in foods.
PREGNANCY AND LACTATION: LIKELY SAFE ...when used in amounts contained in foods (1854). There is insufficient reliable information available about the safety of IP-6 when used in amounts greater than those found in foods; avoid using.

Effectiveness

There is insufficient reliable information available about the effectiveness of IP-6.

Possible Mechanism of Action & Active Ingredients

Inositol hexaphosphate (IP-6), the hexaphosphate ester of inositol, is the major phosphorus storage compound of plants, comprising about 1 to 7% of the dry weight of most cereals, nuts, and legumes (1855,1858). Inositol hexaphosphate and its less phosphorylated forms (e.g., inositol triphosphate) are also endogenous to most mammalian cells in much smaller amounts (1857). Cellular functions include signal transduction and cellular proliferation and differentiation (1857). Inositol hexaphosphate chelates multivalent metal ions (particularly zinc, calcium, and iron) forming insoluble salts in the gastrointestinal tract and decreasing mineral bioavailability (1858,1869,1870). Preliminary evidence suggests that the ability of inositol hexaphosphate to chelate minerals might decrease iron-mediated colon cancer risk, and lower serum cholesterol and triglycerides (1858). As a natural antioxidant, inositol hexaphosphate added to food reduces lipid peroxidation and retards spoilage (1855,1858). In preliminary research, inositol hexaphosphate inhibits cancer cell proliferation and increases cancer cell differentiation, sometimes resulting in reversion to a normal phenotype (1859). Inositol hexaphosphate has shown anticancer activity in breast, colon, liver, and prostate cells and experimental tumors (1860,1861,1862,1863,1864,1865). Inositol hexaphosphate might also inhibit platelet aggregation and lower serum cholesterol and triglycerides, according to preliminary studies (1867,1868).

Adverse Reactions Including Known Allergies

None reported.

Possible Interactions with Herbs & Other Dietary Supplements

CALCIUM, IRON, ZINC: Concurrent use can decrease mineral absorption. IP-6 can chelate multivalent metal ions in the gastrointestinal tract, forming insoluble salts and decreasing mineral absorption (1858).
HERBS WITH ANTICOAGULANT/ANTIPLATELET POTENTIAL: Theoretically, concomitant use of IP-6 with herbs that affect platelet aggregation might increase the risk of bleeding. In vitro IP-6 can inhibit platelet aggregation (1867). This effect has not been demonstrated in humans. Herbs with anticoagulant or antiplatelet properties include: angelica, anise, arnica, asafoetida, bogbean, boldo, capsicum, celery, chamomile, clove, danshen, fenugreek, feverfew, garlic, ginger, ginkgo, Panax ginseng, horse chestnut, horseradish, licorice, meadowsweet, prickly ash, onion, papain, passionflower, poplar, quassia, red clover, turmeric, wild carrot, wild lettuce, willow, and others (4,19).

Possible Interactions with Drugs

ANTICOAGULANT/ANTIPLATELET AGENTS: Theoretically, concomitant use of IP-6 with drugs that affect platelet aggregation may increase the risk of bleeding. In vitro IP-6 can inhibit platelet aggregation (1867). This effect has not been demonstrated in humans.

Possible Interactions with Foods

No interactions are known to occur, and there is no known reason to expect a clinically significant interaction with IP-6.

Possible Interactions with Lab Tests

CHOLESTEROL/TRIGLYCERIDES: Theoretically, may reduce serum cholesterol and triglyceride levels. Preliminary research suggests that IP-6 can lower cholesterol and triglyceride levels (1868). This effect has not been demonstrated in humans.

Possible Interactions with Diseases or Conditions
IRON-DEFICIENCY ANEMIA: IP-6 might decrease dietary and supplemental iron absorption. IP-6 chelates multivalent metal ions in the gastrointestinal tract, preventing absorption (1858).
OSTEOPOROSIS/OSTEOPENIA (Paget's Disease): IP-6 may decrease dietary and supplemental calcium absorption. IP-6 chelates multivalent metal ions in the gastrointestinal tract, preventing absorption (1858).
CLOTTING DISORDERS: Theoretically, may increase risk of bleeding (1867). In vitro, IP-6 can inhibit platelet aggregation (1867). This effect has not been demonstrated in humans.

Typical Dosages & Routes of Administration that are Commonly Used
ORAL: For cancer and cardiovascular disease prevention 500 mg to 2 grams twice daily has been used (1852). For those with existing cancer, 5 to 8 grams per day has been used (1852).

Comments
Preliminary studies of inositol hexaphosphate in cancer have been ongoing since 1988; however, to date, no studies in humans with cancer have been performed (1866). "IP-6, Nature's Revolutionary Cancer-Fighter," a book by prominent inositol hexaphosphate researcher, Abulkalam M. Shamsuddin, MD, PhD, has popularized inositol hexaphosphate (1851,1852,1853,1854).

IPECAC

This Product is Also Known As
Brazilian Ipecac, Brazil Root, Cartagena Ipecac, Ipecacuanha, Matto Grosso Ipecac, Nicaragua Ipecac, Panama Ipecac, Rio Ipecac.

Scientific Names
Cephaelis ipecacuanha, synonyms Uragoga ipecacuanha, Psychotria ipecacuanha; Cephaelis acuminata, synonym Uragoga granatensis.
Family: Rubiaceae.

People Use This For
Orally, ipecac is used as an expectorant and emetic (12,13), and for croupous bronchitis in children (18).
Intravenously, it is used for amebic abscesses and hepatitis (6).
Historically, ipecac has been used for amebic dysentery, as an appetite stimulant (small doses), and for treating cancer (11).

Safety
POSSIBLY SAFE ...when the rhizome or syrup of ipecac is used orally and appropriately short-term (12).
POSSIBLY UNSAFE ...when used orally long-term. Theoretically, prolonged use might blunt the emetic reflex (19). ...when in contact with skin or when inhaled. The constituent, emetine is a skin irritant. Ipecac powder is a respiratory irritant (6,18).
LIKELY UNSAFE ...if used in large amounts. Misuse can lead to serious toxicity or death (6,12). ...when a total dose of more than 1 gram is injected, it can cause nervous system symptoms, blood in the urine, and circulatory collapse (6).
CHILDREN: LIKELY SAFE ...when used orally and appropriately to treat poisoning (272). LIKELY UNSAFE ...for other uses. Contraindicated in infants under 1 year old (12,19). Children are more sensitive to large doses and effects on the nervous system than adults (19).
PREGNANCY: LIKELY UNSAFE ...contraindicated because it is a potential uterine stimulant (12,19).
LACTATION: Insufficient reliable information available; avoid using.

Effectiveness
EFFECTIVE ...when used as an emetic (15). Ipecac is an FDA-approved prescription product.
There is insufficient reliable information available about the effectiveness of ipecac for its other uses.

Possible Mechanism of Action & Active Ingredients
Ipecac contains the alkaloids, emetine and cephaeline (13). Ipecac produces emesis by irritating the GI mucosa and by stimulating the chemoreceptor trigger zone in the brain (6,13).

Adverse Reactions Including Known Allergies
Taken orally, ipecac causes nausea, vomiting (3,6,13,15,18), GI irritation, dizziness, hypotension, dyspnea, and tachycardia (11). Chronic use is associated with myopathies and death (6,18). Overdose is associated with erosion of GI tract mucous membranes, cardiac arrhythmias, disorders of respiratory function, convulsions, shock, and coma (18). Topically, emetine is a skin irritant (6). Ipecac powder is a respiratory irritant. When used intravenously, emetine may cause inflammation of the muscle tissue at the injection site with chronic administration. In total doses over 1 gram, it can lead to gastrointestinal and nervous system symptoms, hematuria and circulatory collapse (6).

© Copyright 2000, Natural Medicines Comprehensive Database (209) 472-2244. For updated data, go to www.NaturalDatabase.com • 601

Possible Interactions with Herbs & Other Dietary Supplements
PODOPHYLLUM: Ipecac reduces the intensity of the cathartic effect of podophyllum (19).

Possible Interactions with Drugs
ORAL DRUGS: Emetics can prevent the absorption of oral doses of other drugs.

Possible Interactions with Foods
No interactions are known to occur, and there is no known reason to expect a clinically significant interaction with ipecac.

Possible Interactions with Lab Tests
No interactions are known to occur, and there is no known reason to expect a clinically significant interaction with ipecac.

Possible Interactions with Diseases or Conditions
HEART DISEASES: Contraindicated (12), due to cardiotoxic potential of emetine (6), and its depressive effect on the heart (19).
UNCONSCIOUSNESS: Contraindicated (12).
GI CONDITIONS: Can irritate gastrointestinal tract. Contraindicated in individuals with infectious or inflammatory gastrointestinal conditions (19).
POISONINGS: Contraindicated in individuals poisoned with corrosives (risks re-exposure of esophageal tissue), petroleum distillates (risks aspiration pneumonia), strychnine (risk of convulsions) (12,19).

Typical Dosages & Routes of Administration that are Commonly Used
ORAL: Expectorant (adults), 0.4-1.4 mL ipecac syrup (USP) (12). Emetic, 15 mL ipecac syrup (USP) followed by 1-2 glasses of water (12); may repeat once in 20 minutes if no results (12,13). Before using ipecac syrup to treat poisoning, call poison control for recommendation. Ipecac syrup is available both as a nonprescription product and as a FDA-approved prescription product.

Comments
None.

IPORURU

This Product is Also Known As
Iporoni, Iporuro, Ipurosa, Ipururo, Macochihua, Niando.

Scientific Names
Alchornea castaneifolia.
Family: Euphorbiaceae.

People Use This For
Orally, iporuru is used for coughs, rheumatism (517), impotence, lowering blood sugar levels in individuals with diabetes (3918), diarrhea (517), headache, toothache, snakebite, bronchitis, chancre, chills, conjunctivitis, dysentery, dysmenorrhea, gonorrhea, hemorrhoids, jaundice, leprosy, malaria, ophthalmia, ringworm, stimulating digestion, thrush, urethritis, and as a cathartic, diuretic, emetic (513), and aphrodisiac (517).
Topically, iporuru is used for arthritis, colds, muscle pain, rheumatism (517), and for stingray wounds (3918).

Safety
There is insufficient reliable information available about the safety of iporuru.
Pregnancy and Lactation: Insufficient reliable information available; avoid using.

Effectiveness
There is insufficient reliable information available about the effectiveness of iporuru.

Possible Mechanism of Action & Active Ingredients
The applicable parts of iporuru are the bark, leaf, and root. There is insufficient reliable information available about the possible mechanism of action and active ingredients.

Adverse Reactions Including Known Allergies
None reported.

Possible Interactions with Herbs & Other Dietary Supplements
Insufficient reliable information available.

Possible Interactions with Drugs
No interactions are known to occur, and there is no known reason to expect a clinically significant interaction with iporuru.

Possible Interactions with Foods
No interactions are known to occur, and there is no known reason to expect a clinically significant interaction with iporuru.

Possible Interactions with Lab Tests
No interactions are known to occur, and there is no known reason to expect a clinically significant interaction with iporuru.

Possible Interactions with Diseases or Conditions
No interactions are known to occur, and there is no known reason to expect a clinically significant interaction with iporuru.

Typical Dosages & Routes of Administration that are Commonly Used
ORAL: Iporuru is typically prepared as a tea with 1 teaspoon of dried leaf added to 4 ounces of boiling water and taken 1 to 3 times daily. A 4:1 tincture is taken in a dose of 2 to 3 mL twice daily (5255).

Comments
None.

IPRIFLAVONE

This Product is Also Known As
7-Isopropoxy-Isoflavone, 7-Isopropoxy Isoflavone, FL-113, Phytoestrogen, TC-80.

Scientific Names
7-isopropoxyisoflavone.

People Use This For
Orally, ipriflavone is used for preventing and treating postmenopausal and senile osteoporosis, preventing drug-induced osteoporosis (4746), relieving osteoporotic pain, treating Paget's disease and renal osteodystrophy (14), and for reducing bone loss in hemiplegic stroke patients (429). Ipriflavone is also used by bodybuilders as an anabolic agent (4745).

Safety
POSSIBLY SAFE ...when used orally and appropriately (14). Ipriflavone caused no serious adverse effects in postmenopausal women and elderly women who took the drug for 2 years (432,4756).
PREGNANCY AND LACTATION: Insufficient reliable information available; avoid using.

Effectiveness
LIKELY EFFECTIVE ...when used orally for preventing and treating osteoporosis in postmenopausal women (as a single agent) or in conjunction with low dose estrogen, calcium, or vitamin D (427,428,430,431,432,433,2169,2170,2171,2172,2173,2174,2175,4748,4749). Ipriflavone, alone or in combination with estrogen, calcium, or vitamin D, has been more effective than placebo in increasing bone mineral density in women with natural and surgical menopause (427,428,430,431,432,433,2169,2170,2171,2172,2173,2174,2175,4749). Compared with calcitonin in an open trial, ipriflavone was superior in increasing bone mineral density and improving biochemical markers of bone loss (4748).
POSSIBLY EFFECTIVE ...when used orally for treating osteoporotic pain (2175,4757). Ipriflavone was superior to placebo and at least as effective as inhaled calcitonin for osteoporotic vertebral pain (2175,4757). ...when used orally for Paget's disease (2176). In a small open study, ipriflavone 600 mg and 1200 mg given for 30 days to patients with Paget's disease resulted in a reduction in serum alkaline phosphatase and hydroxyproline/creatinine excretion and less bone pain (2176). ... when used orally for renal osteodystrophy (2177). ...when used orally to prevent bone loss in hemiplegic stroke patients (429). In combination with vitamin D, ipriflavone prevented decreased bone mineral density and increased vitamin D levels superior to placebo or vitamin D alone (429). ...when used orally to treat senile osteoporosis (4756). In a well-designed study lasting 2 years, ipriflavone was superior to placebo in increasing bone mineral density, decreasing pain and analgesic use, and improving bone metabolism parameters in women greater than 65 years of age (4756). ...when used orally to prevent drug-induced osteoporosis (4746). In a double-blind, placebo controlled study, ipriflavone given with calcium prevented loss of bone density induced by the gonadotropin hormone-releasing hormone agonist, leuprolide (Lupron) (4746). Laboratory evidence suggests that ipriflavone may prevent glucocorticoid-induced osteoporosis (4747).
There is insufficient reliable information available about the effectiveness of ipriflavone for other uses.

Possible Mechanism of Action & Active Ingredients
Ipriflavone is a semisynthetic isoflavone manufactured in the laboratory from daidzein, a compound derived from soy (431). Ipriflavone enhances osteoblast function and inhibits bone resorption, mainly by inhibiting recruitment of osteoclasts (14,2173,2176,2179). Preliminary evidence suggests that ipriflavone prevents bone density loss without suppressing the rate of bone formation (unlike 17-beta-estradiol which suppresses the rate of bone formation) (426). Ipriflavone has no direct estrogenic activity in postmenopausal women, but might potentiate the effects of estrogen

on bone, increase uterotropic activity of estrogen, and stimulate estrogen-induced calcitonin secretion (14,434,2179). Clinical evidence suggests that using ipriflavone in combination with conjugated estrogens for postmenopausal osteoporosis might allow for use of a lower estrogen dose (427,2171,2172). Ipriflavone is metabolized extensively by the liver; some metabolites appear to possess pharmacologic activity (14). Ipriflavone, or its metabolite 7-hydroxy-isoflavone, might inhibit cytochrome P450 enzymes CYP1A2 and CYP2C9 (14,2178). Laboratory evidence suggests that isoflavones can inhibit oxidative and conjugative metabolism (4736). Isoflavones might also affect drug absorption and biliary excretion by interacting with drug transporters such as P-glycoprotein and the canalicular multispecific organic anion transporter (4736). Whether ipriflavone has similar activity is unknown.

Adverse Reactions Including Known Allergies
Epigastric pain, diarrhea, and dizziness may occur (14). Gastrointestinal side effects are the most common complaint (432).

Possible Interactions with Herbs & Other Dietary Supplements
VITAMIN D: Concomitant use may enhance effects in preventing osteoporosis (2174).
CALCIUM: Concomitant use may enhance effects in preventing osteoporosis (14,2169,2170,2171,2173,2175).

Possible Interactions with Drugs
CALCITONIN: Ipriflavone may enhance effects of calcitonin (14).
DRUGS METABOLIZED BY CYP1A2, CYP2C9: Theoretically, concomitant use may result in drug accumulation, increased effects and risk of adverse effects (2178).
ESTROGEN: May enhance effects of estrogen (14).
THEOPHYLLINE: Concomitant use reported to decrease theophylline metabolism and elimination (2178).

Possible Interactions with Foods
FOOD: Increases ipriflavone bioavailability (14).

Possible Interactions with Lab Tests
No interactions are known to occur, and there is no known reason to expect a clinically significant interaction with ipriflavone.

Possible Interactions with Diseases or Conditions
LIVER DYSFUNCTION: Ipriflavone is extensively metabolized in the liver and might accumulate in people with liver dysfunction.
RENAL INSUFFICIENCY: Ipriflavone might accumulate in moderate to severe renal impairment (creatinine clearance less than 40 ml/minute) (14).
HISTORY OF BREAST CANCER: Ipriflavone has been reported to potentiate some effects of estrogen (14,434,2179), although its effects on breast tissue have not been investigated.

Typical Dosages & Routes of Administration that are Commonly Used
ORAL: The typical dose for postmenopausal osteoporosis is 200 mg three times daily (14,2169,2170,2171,2172,2173,2175). Senile osteoporosis, 600 mg daily (14). Paget's disease, 600-1200 mg daily (14,2176). Renal osteodystrophy, 400-600 mg daily (14). These conditions should not be self-medicated.

Comments
Ipriflavone is used in Italy and Japan for the treatment of osteoporosis (9).

IRON

This Product is Also Known As
Elemental Iron, Fer, Ferrous Carbonate Anhydrous, Ferrous Fumarate, Ferrous Gluconate, Ferrous Pyrophosphate, Ferrous Sulfate.

Scientific Names
Iron; Fe; atomic number 26.

People Use This For
Orally, iron salts are used for preventing and treating iron deficiency (15) and iron deficiency anemia (9), for attention deficit disorder (1093), improving athletic performance, treating oral canker sores, Crohn's disease, depression, female infertility, and menorrhagia (1900).

Safety
SAFE ...when used orally and appropriately as an FDA-approved prescription product (15).
LIKELY SAFE ...when used as a dietary supplement.
CHILDREN: LIKELY SAFE ...when used orally and appropriately (15). UNSAFE ...if excessive amounts are ingested. Iron is the most common cause of pediatric poisoning deaths (doses as low as 60 mg/kg can be fatal) (15).
PREGNANCY AND LACTATION: LIKELY SAFE ...when used orally and appropriately (15).

Effectiveness

EFFECTIVE ...when used orally for treating iron deficiency anemia (9,945).
POSSIBLY EFFECTIVE ...when used orally for preventing iron deficiency in menstruating women with previous Rouxen Y gastric bypass (1089), improving cognitive function in iron-deficient children and adolescents (1104,1095). ...when given pre-operatively for reducing a drop in hemoglobin during immediate post-operative period in nonanemic patients undergoing major joint replacement (1092).
There is insufficient reliable information available about the effectiveness of iron for its other uses.

Possible Mechanism of Action & Active Ingredients

Iron is required for oxygen and carbon dioxide transport in hemoglobin. It functions as an electron carrier in cytochromes, is found in the functional groups of most enzymes in the Krebs cycle (945), and plays a role in regulating dopamine activity (1093). Iron demand is increased by blood loss and rapid growth (1101).

Adverse Reactions Including Known Allergies

Iron can cause gastrointestinal irritation, abdominal pain, constipation or diarrhea, nausea, and vomiting (9). Liquid oral preparations can blacken teeth (9). Acute overdosage (60 mg/kg and more) can cause gastrointestinal, cardiovascular, or metabolic toxicity, and death (9). Long-term use of high doses of iron can cause hemosiderosis that clinically resembles hemochromatosis (15). There is conflicting data regarding high levels of iron stores and increased cancer risk (1098,1099,1100,1102). High levels of iron stores do not appear to increase the risk of coronary artery disease (1097,1099).

Possible Interactions with Herbs & Other Dietary Supplements

ACACIA: The ferric salt of iron can gelatinize acacia (19).
ANTACIDS: Concomitant administration may decrease iron absorption (15).
CALCIUM: Supplements taken with meals decrease absorption of iron supplements; however, supplements taken on an empty stomach do not interfere with iron supplement absorption (945).
OAK (Quercus species): Can precipitate iron salts (19).
SOY: Soy protein isolate reduces the absorption of non-heme iron from foods (5053). Non-heme iron is found in plant-based foods.
VITAMIN C: Concomitant administration of more than 200 mg of ascorbic acid increases iron supplement absorption (15).
VITAMIN E: Concomitant administration may interfere with vitamin E absorption (15).

Possible Interactions with Drugs

ANTACIDS: Concomitant administration may decrease iron absorption; separate these agents by as much time as possible (15).
ASCORBIC ACID (VITAMIN C): Concomitant administration increases absorption of iron (15).
CHLORAMPHENICOL: Response to iron therapy may be delayed (15).
ERYTHROPOIETIN: Concomitant use with oral iron enhances effect in increasing hemoglobin (1087,1091).
FLUOROQUINOLONES (ciprofloxacin, levofloxacin, ofloxacin, etc.): Concomitant administration decreases the absorption of the fluoroquinolone (15). Administer fluoroquinolones at least two hours before or after iron-containing supplements.
H2-BLOCKERS Cimetidine (Tagamet), Ranitidine (Zantac), Famotidine (Pepcid), and others: Long-term use of high-dose H2-blockers may lead to iron and vitamin B12 malabsorption (4539,4540,4541). The mechanism of this is thought to be through inhibition of gastric acid secretion necessary for absorption of iron and vitamin B12. Monitor for signs or symptoms of anemia. This interaction is theoretically possible with proton pump inhibitors.
TERACYCLINES: Concomitant administration results in lower absorption of iron and tetracyclines (15).
OTHER DRUGS: Concomitant use of iron decreases absorption of ciprofloxacin, methyldopa, norfloxacin, ofloxacin, penicillamine, tetracyclines, and thyroxine replacement therapy (15).

Drug Influences on Nutrient Levels and Depletion

SOME DRUGS CAN AFFECT IRON LEVELS:
H2-BLOCKERS; Cimetidine (Tagamet), ranitidine (Zantac), famotidine (Pepcid), and others: Long-term use of high-dose H2-blockers may lead to iron and B12 malabsorption (4539,4540,4541). The mechanism of this is thought to be through inhibition of gastric acid secretion necessary for absorption of iron and B12. Monitor for signs or symptoms of anemia. This interaction is theoretically possible with proton pump inhibitors.
PROTON PUMP INHIBITORS (Lansoprazole (Prevacid), Omeprazole (Prilosec), Rabeprazole (Aciphex), Pantoprazole (Protonix, Pantoloc)): Concomitant use can decrease absorption of iron in gastrointestinal tract due to elevated pH. The need for supplementation has not been adequately studied. Consider supplementation only if clinical judgment warrants it (31,4483,4484,4485,4486,4539,4540,4541).
TETRACYCLINES: Concomitant administration can decrease iron absorption due to binding in the gastrointestinal tract. Administration should be separated by at least 2 hours (4412,4453,4531,4549,4550).

Possible Interactions with Foods

COFFEE: Coffee inhibits absorption of iron and might lead to iron-deficiency anemia (19).
SOY: Soy protein isolate reduces the absorption of non-heme iron from foods (5053). Non-heme iron is found in plant-based foods.

© Copyright 2000, Natural Medicines Comprehensive Database (209) 472-2244. For updated data, go to www.NaturalDatabase.com

Possible Interactions with Lab Tests

GUAIAC TEST: In individuals taking iron, the guiac test result for occult fecal blood may have false-positive reading (benzidine test for occult fecal blood not likely to be affected) (15).

Possible Interactions with Diseases or Conditions

MALABSORPTION SYNDROMES: Oral iron therapy may be ineffective in individuals with diarrhea, post-gastrectomy, or other malabsorption syndromes (945).

HEMODIALYSIS: Supplemental iron absorption is decreased in people requiring chronic hemodialysis (1088,1090).

IRON DEFICIENCY: Iron absorption is increased (945).

PREMATURE INFANTS: Use of oral iron preparations in premature infants with low serum vitamin E levels may cause hemolysis and hemolytic anemia (15); vitamin E deficiency should be corrected before administering supplemental iron (15).

OTHER HEMOGLOBIN DISEASES: Iron overload is likely to occur in people with hemoglobinopathies or other refractory anemias erroneously diagnosed as iron deficiency anemia (15).

PEPTIC ULCER DISEASE, REGIONAL ENTERITIES, ULCERATIVE COLITIS: Contraindicated (15).

Typical Dosages & Routes of Administration that are Commonly Used

ORAL: Iron Deficiency Anemia: Adults, 50-100 mg elemental iron three times daily; Children, 4-6 mg/kg per day divided into three doses (15); usually continued 6 months to replenish iron stores (15), two to three months treatment may reverse anemia without replenishing iron stores (945). Iron deficiency due to chronic, uncontrolled bleeding requires continuous iron therapy (945). Recommended Daily Allowances (RDAs) for iron are: Infants (0-0.5 year) 6 mg and (0.5-1 year) 10 mg; Children (1-10 years) 10 mg; Males (11-18 years) 12 mg, (19+ years) 10 mg; Females (11-50 years) 15 mg, (51+ years) 10 mg; Pregnancy 30 mg; Lactation 15 mg (1103). NOTE: All forms of iron not equivalent; 1 gram of ferrous gluconate =120 mg elemental iron (12% iron); 1 gram of ferrous sulfate =200 mg (20% iron) elemental iron; 1 gram of ferrous fumarate =330 mg (33% iron) elemental iron (15).

Comments

Plants rich in iron include anise seed, basil leaves, celery seed, coriander, cumin seed, dill leaves, flax seed, lungwort leaves, marjoram leaves, parsley leaves, Laminaria thyme leaves, tumeric root, and yellow dock root and leaves (19).

Boiling, steaming or stir-frying significantly enhances the bioavailability of iron contained in many vegetables, including asparagus, broccoli, cabbage, red and green peppers, and tomatoes. In addition, cold storage of cooked vegetables greatly reduces the increases in iron bioavailability gained from cooking and vegetables should be consumed the same day they are cooked. The results of this unpublished study were presented at the 219th national meeting of the American Chemical Society (5044).

Some researchers think that consuming dietary heme iron in large quantities might increase the risk of myocardial infarction in people with other risk factors for MI, but clinical trial results are inconclusive. Meat is the major source of heme iron (1492).

JABORANDI

This Product is Also Known As

Arruda Bravam, Arruda Do Mato, Jamguarandi, Juarandi, Maranhao Jaborandi.

Scientific Names

Pilocarpus microphyllus.
Family: Rutaceae.

People Use This For

Topically, jaborandi is used for glaucoma.
In folk medicine, it is used orally for diarrhea and to promote sweating (18).

Safety

UNSAFE ...when the leaf is used orally or topically, because it contains pilocarpine. The lethal dose of jaborandi is estimated to be 5-10 grams of leaf (18).

PREGNANCY: UNSAFE ...contraindicated for oral use because it has teratogenic and uterine stimulant effects (19).

LACTATION: UNSAFE (18).

Effectiveness

EFFECTIVE ...when jaborandi component pilocarpine is used for the treatment of glaucoma. Pilocarpine is FDA approved for this indication (15).

There is insufficient reliable information available about the effectiveness of jaborandi for its other uses.

Possible Mechanism of Action & Active Ingredients

The applicable part of jaborandi is the leaf. Jaborandi contains the parasympathetic system stimulant pilocarpine. Among its cholinergic effects are the stimulation of saliva secretion, sweat, and smooth muscle contraction in the gastrointestinal tract (18). It also causes ocular miosis (15).

Adverse Reactions Including Known Allergies

The lethal oral dose of jaborandi is approximately 60 mg, which roughly corresponds to 5-10 mg pilocarpine. Symptoms of poisoning include bradycardia, bronchospasm, colic, cardiac collapse and possible arrest, convulsions, hypotension, dyspnea, nausea, severe salivation, strong secretion of sweat, and vomiting (18).

Possible Interactions with Herbs & Other Dietary Supplements

Insufficient reliable information available.

Possible Interactions with Drugs

No interactions are known to occur, and there is no known reason to expect a clinically significant interaction with jaborandi.

Possible Interactions with Foods

No interactions are known to occur, and there is no known reason to expect a clinically significant interaction with jaborandi.

Possible Interactions with Lab Tests

INTRAOCULAR PRESSURE: Jaborandi might reduce intraocular pressure due to its pilocarpine content (15,18).

Possible Interactions with Diseases or Conditions

No interactions are known to occur, and there is no known reason to expect a clinically significant interaction with jaborandi.

Typical Dosages & Routes of Administration that are Commonly Used

TOPICAL: Pharmaceutical pilocarpine eye drops are a prescription only medication (15,18).

Comments

Jaborandi is considered unsafe for oral use; avoid using. Jaborandi itself is obsolete as a medicinal herb, but it is used in the production of pilocarpine (18). Avoid confusing jaborandi with Pilocarpus jaborandi (Pernambuco jaborandi) (19) and Pilocarpus pennatifolius (Paraguay jaborandi).

JACOB'S LADDER

This Product is Also Known As

Charity, English Green Valerian, Jacobs Ladder.
CAUTION: See separate listings for Abscess Root and Lily of the Valley.

Scientific Names

Polemonium coeruleum.
Family: Polemoniaceae.

People Use This For

Orally, Jacob's ladder is used for fever and inflammation. It is also used orally as an astringent, hemolytic, and to promote sweating (18).

Safety

There is insufficient reliable information available about the safety of Jacob's ladder.
Pregnancy and Lactation: Insufficient reliable information available; avoid using.

Effectiveness

There is insufficient reliable information available about the effectiveness of Jacob's ladder.

Possible Mechanism of Action & Active Ingredients

The applicable parts of Jacob's ladder are the above ground parts. There is insufficient reliable information available about the possible mechanism of action and active ingredients.

Adverse Reactions Including Known Allergies

None reported.

Possible Interactions with Herbs & Other Dietary Supplements

Insufficient reliable information available.

Possible Interactions with Drugs

No interactions are known to occur, and there is no known reason to expect a clinically significant interaction with Jacob's ladder.

Possible Interactions with Foods

No interactions are known to occur, and there is no known reason to expect a clinically significant interaction with Jacob's ladder.

Possible Interactions with Lab Tests

No interactions are known to occur, and there is no known reason to expect a clinically significant interaction with Jacob's ladder.

Possible Interactions with Diseases or Conditions

No interactions are known to occur, and there is no known reason to expect a clinically significant interaction with Jacob's ladder.

Typical Dosages & Routes of Administration that are Commonly Used

ORAL: Jacob's ladder is used as a tea (18).

Comments

There is very little scientific information about this product. Our staff is continually analyzing the available information on natural medicines and will add data here as it becomes available.

JALAP

This Product is Also Known As

Jalapa, Jalape, Mechoacán.
CAUTION: See separate listings for Pokeweed berry, Pokeweed root, and Mexican Scammony Root.

Scientific Names

Ipomoea purga, synonym Exogonium purga; Convolvulus purga.
Family: Convolvulaceae.

People Use This For

Traditionally, jalap has been used as a cathartic, purgative, and diuretic (4017).

Safety

UNSAFE ...when taken orally. Jalap has potent purgative effects (12).
PREGNANCY AND LACTATION: UNSAFE. Jalap can be a menstrual stimulant (19); avoid using.

Effectiveness

There is insufficient reliable information available about the effectiveness of jalap.

Possible Mechanism of Action & Active Ingredients

The applicable part of jalap is the root. Parts of the jalap (ipomoea purga) plant that are under the ground contain gluco-resins that act as a cathartic. They increase water elimination and cause peristalsis (514).

Adverse Reactions Including Known Allergies

Jalap has potent purgative effects (12).

Possible Interactions with Herbs & Other Dietary Supplements

STIMULANT LAXATIVE HERBS: Theoretically, concomitant use with other stimulant laxative herbs may increase the risk of potassium depletion. Stimulant laxative herbs include: aloe dried leaf sap, blue flag rhizome, alder buckthorn, European buckthorn, butternut bark, cascara bark, castor oil, colocynth fruit pulp, gamboge bark exudate, black root, manna bark exudate, podophyllum root, rhubarb root, senna leaves and pods, wild cucumber fruit (Ecballium elaterium), and yellow dock root (19).
HORSETAIL/LICORICE: Theoretically, concomitant use with horsetail plant or licorice rhizome increases the risk of potassium depletion (19).
CARDIAC GLYCOSIDE-CONTAINING HERBS: Overuse/abuse of jalap may increase the risk of cardiac glycoside toxicity. Cardiac glycoside-containing herbs include black hellebore, Canadian hemp roots, digitalis leaf, hedge mustard, figwort, lily of the valley roots, motherwort, oleander leaf, pheasant's eye plant, pleurisy root, squill bulb leaf scales, and strophanthus seeds (2,18,19,500). Jalap may increase risk of cardioglycoside toxicity due to increase risk of potassium loss.

Possible Interactions with Drugs

CARDIAC GLYCOSIDE DRUGS: Theoretically, overuse/abuse of this product increases the risk of adverse effects of cardiac glycoside drugs, e.g. digoxin (Lanoxin). Increases risk of adverse effects of cardiac glycosides due to possible potassium loss.

Possible Interactions with Foods

No interactions are known to occur, and there is no known reason to expect a clinically significant interaction with jalap.

Possible Interactions with Lab Tests

No interactions are known to occur, and there is no known reason to expect a clinically significant interaction with jalap.

Possible Interactions with Diseases or Conditions

GI CONDITIONS: Contraindicated; may have GI irritant effects (19). Contraindicated in individuals with infectious or inflammatory gastrointestinal conditions (19). Stimulant laxatives are contraindicated in individuals with symptoms of appendicitis (abdominal pain, nausea and vomiting) (272).

Typical Dosages & Routes of Administration that are Commonly Used

ORAL: Jalap is prepared as a liquid, using 1 teaspoon root to 1 cup of water. The dose is 1 cup daily, a mouthful at a time (5263). The usual dose of the powdered root is 3 to 20 grains (195 to 1300 mg) (5267). The resin from the root is dosed 60 to 300 mg, and the tincture is taken 2 to 4 mL (5264).

Comments

Avoid confusion with pokeweed (Phytolacca americana), Mexican scammony root (Ipomoea orizabensis), also known as jalap.

JAMAICAN DOGWOOD

This Product is Also Known As

Fishfudle, Fish Poison Bark, Fish-Poison Tree, Jamaica Dogwood, West Indian Dogwood.
CAUTION: See separate listing for American Dogwood.

Scientific Names

Piscidia piscipula, synonym Piscidia communis; Piscidia erythrina; Ichthyomethia piscipula.
Family: Leguminosae or Fabaceae.

People Use This For

Orally, Jamaican dogwood is used for anxiety and fear, and as a daytime sedative (18).
Historically, it has been used for neuralgia, migraine, insomnia (especially sleeplessness due to nervous tension), and dysmenorrhea (4).

Safety

LIKELY UNSAFE ...when the root bark is used orally for self-medication. Considered toxic (4). The elderly are particularly sensitive to potent neuro-muscular depressant effects (19).
CHILDREN: LIKELY UNSAFE ...contraindicated for oral use. Children are particularly sensitive to potent, neuro-muscular depressant effects (19).
PREGNANCY: LIKELY UNSAFE ...contraindicated for oral use, due to possible uterine depressant effects (4).
LACTATION: LIKELY UNSAFE; avoid using.

Effectiveness

There is insufficient reliable information available about the effectiveness of Jamaican dogwood.

Possible Mechanism of Action & Active Ingredients

The applicable part of Jamaican dogwood is the root bark. Animal studies have shown that an extract of Jamaican dogwood has sedative effects, marked antitussive and antipyretic activities, and also anti-inflammatory and antispasmodic action on smooth muscles (4,11). In some in-vitro tests, the extract's antispasmodic effects have been at least as strong as papaverine's (4). The constituent rotenone has shown some anticancer activity towards lymphocytic leukemia and human epidermoid carcinoma of the nasopharynx; yet, paradoxically, rotenone is also documented to be carcinogenic (4). Rotenone is toxic to fish and insects, and to animals when administered parenterally, but non-toxic when administered orally (4). Another constituent, ichtynone, is toxic to fish (4).

Adverse Reactions Including Known Allergies

Jamaican dogwood is an irritant and toxic to humans (4). Overdose symptoms include numbness, tremors, salivation, and sweating (4).

Possible Interactions with Herbs & Other Dietary Supplements

HERBS WITH SEDATIVE PROPERTIES: Theoretically, concomitant use with herbs that have sedative properties might enhance therapeutic and adverse effects. These include calamus, calendula, California poppy, catnip, capsicum, celery, couch grass, elecampane, Siberian ginseng, German chamomile, goldenseal, gotu kola, hops, kava, lemon balm, sage, St. John's wort, sassafras, scullcap, shepherd's purse, stinging nettle, valerian, wild carrot, wild lettuce, withania, and yerba mansa (4,19).

Possible Interactions with Drugs
DRUGS WITH SEDATIVE ACTION: Jamaican dogwood may potentiate sedative effects (4).

Possible Interactions with Foods
No interactions are known to occur, and there is no known reason to expect a clinically significant interaction with Jamaican dogwood.

Possible Interactions with Lab Tests
No interactions are known to occur, and there is no known reason to expect a clinically significant interaction with Jamaican dogwood.

Possible Interactions with Diseases or Conditions
No interactions are known to occur, and there is no known reason to expect a clinically significant interaction with Jamaican dogwood.

Typical Dosages & Routes of Administration that are Commonly Used
No typical dosage.

Comments
Jamaican dogwood is likely unsafe and without any documented effectiveness; avoid using. Root bark and liquid extract are reportedly no longer used (18). Avoid confusion with American dogwood (Cornus florida).

JAMBOLAN bark

This Product is Also Known As
Jambul, Jamum, Java Plum, Jumbul, Rose Apple, Syxygii cumini cortex.
CAUTION: See separate listing for Jambolan seed.

Scientific Names
Syzugium cumini, synonym Syzugium jambolana.
Family: Mytraceae.

People Use This For
Orally, jambolan bark is used for nonspecific, acute diarrhea (2).
Topically, it is used for mild inflammation of the oral-pharyngeal mucosa (2) and of the skin (2).
In folk medicine, jambolan has been used orally for bronchitis, asthma, and dysentery, and topically for ulcers (18).

Safety
POSSIBLY SAFE ...when used appropriately for oral or topical medicinal purposes (2,12).
PREGNANCY AND LACTATION: Insufficient reliable information available; avoid using.

Effectiveness
POSSIBLY EFFECTIVE ...when taken orally for nonspecific, acute diarrhea (2). ...when applied topically for mild inflammation of the oral-pharyngeal mucosa, or mild, superficial inflammation of the skin.
There is insufficient reliable information available about the effectiveness of jambolan bark for its other uses.

Possible Mechanism of Action & Active Ingredients
The astringent effects of jambolan bark can result from the tannin constituents (2). Jambolan bark also possesses antibacterial, hypoglycemic, and CNS-depressant activities (4).

Adverse Reactions Including Known Allergies
None reported (2).

Possible Interactions with Herbs & Other Dietary Supplements
Insufficient reliable information available.

Possible Interactions with Drugs
No interactions are known to occur, and there is no known reason to expect a clinically significant interaction with jambolan bark.

Possible Interactions with Foods
No interactions are known to occur, and there is no known reason to expect a clinically significant interaction with jambolan bark.

Possible Interactions with Lab Tests
No interactions are known to occur, and there is no known reason to expect a clinically significant interaction with jambolan bark.

Possible Interactions with Diseases or Conditions

No interactions are known to occur, and there is no known reason to expect a clinically significant interaction with jambolan bark.

Typical Dosages & Routes of Administration that are Commonly Used

ORAL: The typical dose of jambolan is 3-6 grams of the dried bark per day (2,18). It can also be taken as a tea, which is prepared by simmering 1-2 teaspoons of the dried bark in 150 mL boiling water for 5-10 minutes and then straining (18).
TOPICAL: Jambolan bark is commonly used as a compress made from the tea (18).

Comments

Avoid confusion with jambolan seed.

JAMBOLAN seed

This Product is Also Known As

Jambul, Jamum, Java Plum, Jumbul, Rose Apple, Syxygii cumini semen.
CAUTION: See separate listing for Jambolan bark.

Scientific Names

Syzygium cumini, synonym Syzygium cumini jambolana.
Family: Myrtaceae.

People Use This For

Orally, jambolan seed is used for diabetes (2), flatulence, antispasmodic, stimulating stomach function, as an aphrodisiac, and tonic (2).
In herbal combinations, it is used for atonic and spastic constipation, diseases of the pancreas, gastric and pancreatic complaints, nervous disorders, depression, and exhaustion (2).

Safety

There is insufficient reliable information available about the safety of jambolan seed.
Pregnancy and Lactation: Insufficient reliable information available; avoid using.

Effectiveness

There is insufficient reliable information available about the effectiveness of jambolan seed (2).

Possible Mechanism of Action & Active Ingredients

Insufficient reliable information available.

Adverse Reactions Including Known Allergies

None reported.

Possible Interactions with Herbs & Other Dietary Supplements

Insufficient reliable information available.

Possible Interactions with Drugs

No interactions are known to occur, and there is no known reason to expect a clinically significant interaction with jambolan seed.

Possible Interactions with Foods

No interactions are known to occur, and there is no known reason to expect a clinically significant interaction with jambolan seed.

Possible Interactions with Lab Tests

No interactions are known to occur, and there is no known reason to expect a clinically significant interaction with jambolan seed.

Possible Interactions with Diseases or Conditions

DIABETES THERAPY: Monitor blood glucose levels closely due to claims that jambolan seed has hypoglycemic effects (19).

Typical Dosages & Routes of Administration that are Commonly Used

ORAL: People typically use 0.3 to 2 grams of the powdered seeds. As a liquid extract, the dose is 4 to 8 mL (5264).

Comments

Avoid confusion with jambolan bark. There is very little scientific information about this product. Our staff is continually analyzing the available information on natural medicines and will add data here as it becomes available.

JAPANESE MINT

This Product is Also Known As
Brook mint, Chinese Mint Oil, Cornmint Oil, Field Mint Oil, Mentha arvensis aetheroleum, Mint Oil, Minzol, Poleo.

Scientific Names
Mentha arvensis var. piperascens, synonym Mentha canadensis.
Family: Lamiaceae.

People Use This For
Orally, Japanese mint oil is used for flatulence, improving gastrointestinal and gallbladder function (2), for gallstones, or irritable bowel syndrome (11).

Topically, it is used for myalgia, neuralgic ailments (2), pruritus, urticaria, oral mucosal inflammation, and rheumatic conditions (11).

When inhaled, Japanese mint oil is used for mucous membrane inflammation of the upper respiratory tract (11).

In Chinese medicine, Japanese mint oil is used for the common cold, cough, bronchitis, fever, mouth and pharynx inflammation, pain, liver and gallbladder complaints, tendency to infection (18), for improving appetite and digestion, indigestion, nausea, sore throat, diarrhea, headaches, toothaches, cramps, earache, tumors, sores, cancer, as an aromatic, a stimulant, an antiseptic, a local anesthetic, and an antispasmodic (11).

In folk medicine, Japanese mint oil has been used for functional cardiac complaints, breathing difficulties, and sensitivity to weather changes (18).

In manufacturing, Japanese mint oil is also used as a fragrance in toothpaste, mouthwash, gargles, soaps, detergents, creams, lotions, and perfumes. Commercially it is used as a source of menthol (11).

Safety
POSSIBLY SAFE ...when the oil is used orally and appropriately (2). ...when used topically and appropriately (2). There is insufficient reliable information available about the safety of the inhalation use of Japanese mint.

CHILDREN: LIKELY UNSAFE ...when mint oil is used topically on the faces of infants and children, particularly in the nasal area, it can trigger glottal or bronchial spasm, asthma-like attacks, or even respiratory failure (2). There is insufficient reliable information about Japanese mint oil used for medicinal purposes; avoid using.

PREGNANCY AND LACTATION: Insufficient reliable information available; avoid using.

Effectiveness
POSSIBLY EFFECTIVE ...when used orally to improve gastrointestinal and gall bladder function or for flatulence (2). ...when used as an inhalation for upper respiratory tract mucous membrane inflammation (2). ...when used topically for myalgia and neuralgic ailments (2).

There is insufficient reliable information available about the effectiveness of Japanese mint oil for its other uses.

Possible Mechanism of Action & Active Ingredients
Japanese mint oil is thought to have antiflatulent and cooling effects (2). It might also stimulate bile flow (2). Some evidence demonstrates that Japanese mint oil has cytotoxic properties. Other evidence suggests it might have antimicrobial activity (11). Japanese mint oil contains up to 95% menthol (11). Used topically it has the potential to cause sensitization (18). Processing removes some of the menthol in the Japanese mint oil that is commercially available (2,11).

Adverse Reactions Including Known Allergies
Japanese mint oil can cause stomach upset when taken orally (2). Contact dermatitis can result from topical use (11). In children, topical use on the face can trigger glottal or bronchial spasm, asthma-like attacks, or even respiratory failure (18). If inhaled, the menthol content of Japanese mint oil can worsen bronchial asthma spasms (18). Menthol can also cause allergic reactions including flushing or headache (11).

Possible Interactions with Herbs & Other Dietary Supplements
Insufficient reliable information available.

Possible Interactions with Drugs
No interactions are known to occur, and there is no known reason to expect a clinically significant interaction with Japanese mint.

Possible Interactions with Foods
No interactions are known to occur, and there is no known reason to expect a clinically significant interaction with Japanese mint.

Possible Interactions with Lab Tests
No interactions are known to occur, and there is no known reason to expect a clinically significant interaction with Japanese mint.

Possible Interactions with Diseases or Conditions

GALLBLADDER CONDITIONS: Contraindicated in individuals with bile duct obstruction or gallbladder inflammation (2). Individuals with gallstones may experience pain and spasms (18).

LIVER DISEASE: Contraindicated in individuals with severe liver damage (2).

BRONCHIAL SPASMS: Theoretically, menthol content of Japanese mint oil might worsen bronchial asthma spasms (18).

Typical Dosages & Routes of Administration that are Commonly Used

ORAL: A typical dose is 3-6 drops of oil daily (2).

INHALATION: A typical dose is 3-4 drops of oil in hot water (2).

TOPICAL: Rub several drops of oil or equivalent preparations into affected areas of skin (2). Japanese mint oil is also available as 5-20% oil and semi-solid preparations, in hydroalcoholic preparations of 5-10%, and as 1-5% essential oil in nasal ointments (2).

Comments

Japanese mint oil is the partially dementholated, distilled oil of the above ground parts of Japanese mint (Mentha arvensis var. piperascens) (2,11). There are 20 different species of Mentha with as many as 2300 named variations. Of these half are true names and half are synonyms. Commercial varieties of mint oil can be distinguished by their relative contents of menthol and carvone (11).

JASMINE

This Product is Also Known As

Catalonina Jasmine, Common Jasmine, Italian Jasmine, Poet's Jessamine, Royal Jasmine, Spanish Jasmine.
CAUTION: See separate listing for Gelsemium.

Scientific Names

Jasminium grandiflorum, synonym Jasminium officinale (11).
Family: Oleaceae.

People Use This For

Historically, jasmine has been used for pepatitis, hepatic pain due to cirrhosis, and abdominal pain due to dysentery (11). Many Jasminum species have been used as a sedative, aphrodisiac, or in cancer treatment (11). For food uses, jasmine is utilized to flavor beverages, frozen dairy desserts, candy, baked goods, gelatins, and puddings (11).

In manufacturing, jasmine is used to add fragrance to creams, lotions, and perfumes (11).

Safety

LIKELY SAFE ...when used orally in the amount found in food (12); Generally Recognized as Safe (GRAS) status in the US (11). Maximum use level 0.001% (11).

There is insufficient reliable information available about the safety of the oral medicinal use of jasmine.

PREGNANCY AND LACTATION: Insufficient reliable information available; avoid using in amounts greater than those found in food.

Effectiveness

There is insufficient reliable information available about the effectiveness of jasmine.

Possible Mechanism of Action & Active Ingredients

The applicable part of jasmine is the flower. There is insufficient reliable information available about the possible mechanism of action and active ingredients.

Adverse Reactions Including Known Allergies

Jasmine may possibly cause hypersensitivity (11).

Possible Interactions with Herbs & Other Dietary Supplements

Insufficient reliable information available.

Possible Interactions with Drugs

No interactions are known to occur, and there is no known reason to expect a clinically significant interaction with jasmine.

Possible Interactions with Foods

No interactions are known to occur, and there is no known reason to expect a clinically significant interaction with jasmine.

Possible Interactions with Lab Tests

No interactions are known to occur, and there is no known reason to expect a clinically significant interaction with jasmine.

Possible Interactions with Diseases or Conditions

No interactions are known to occur, and there is no known reason to expect a clinically significant interaction with jasmine.

Typical Dosages & Routes of Administration that are Commonly Used

ORAL: People typically prepare jasmine as a tea, adding 1 to 2 teaspoons of jasmine flowers to 1 cup of water. The dose is 1 cup daily (5263).

Comments

Concrétes are the fat-soluble abstracts of the flower. Absolutes, the alcoholic extracts of concrétes, are more commonly used as a fragrance (11).

JAVA TEA

This Product is Also Known As

Orthosiphon, Orthosiphonis folium.

Scientific Names

Orthosiphon spicatus, synonym Orthosiphon stamineus.
Family: Lamiaceae.

People Use This For

Orally, java tea is taken as "irrigation therapy" (where it is used as a mild diuretic along with copious fluid intake to increase urine flow), for bacterial and inflammatory diseases of the lower urinary tract, renal gravel (2), and liver and gallbladder complaints (18).
In folk medicine, java tea is used for bladder and kidney disorders, gallstones, gout, and rheumatism (18).

Safety

POSSIBLY SAFE ...when taken orally and used appropriately (2).
PREGNANCY AND LACTATION: Insufficient reliable information available; avoid using.

Effectiveness

POSSIBLY EFFECTIVE ...when taken orally as "irrigation therapy," for bacterial and inflammatory diseases of the lower urinary tract and renal gravel (2).
There is insufficient reliable information available about the effectiveness of java tea for its other uses.

Possible Mechanism of Action & Active Ingredients

The applicable parts of java tea are the leaf and stem tip. Java tea is stated to have diuretic, weak antispasmodic, and antimicrobial effects (2,18).

Adverse Reactions Including Known Allergies

None reported.

Possible Interactions with Herbs & Other Dietary Supplements

Insufficient reliable information available.

Possible Interactions with Drugs

No interactions are known to occur, and there is no known reason to expect a clinically significant interaction with java tea.

Possible Interactions with Foods

No interactions are known to occur, and there is no known reason to expect a clinically significant interaction with java tea.

Possible Interactions with Lab Tests

No interactions are known to occur, and there is no known reason to expect a clinically significant interaction with java tea.

Possible Interactions with Diseases or Conditions

EDEMA: Java tea is contraindicated for use as "irrigation therapy" in cases of edema due to limited heart or kidney function (2).

Typical Dosages & Routes of Administration that are Commonly Used
ORAL: The typical dose of java tea is 6-12 grams of the dried leaf or stem tips per day or equivalent preparations, including the prepared tea (2,18). Adequate fluid intake is essential, at least 2 L per day (18).

Comments
None.

JAVANESE TURMERIC

This Product is Also Known As
Curcuma, Curcumae xanthorrhizae rhizoma, Temu Lawak, Temu Lawas, Tewon Lawa.
CAUTION: See separate listings for Goldenseal, Zedoary, and Turmeric.

Scientific Names
Curcuma xanthorrhiza.
Family: Zingiberaceae.

People Use This For
Orally, Javanese turmeric is used for indigestion, feelings of fullness, bloating after meals (18), flatulence (8), peptic disorders (2), and for improving appetite and digestion (8).
In folk medicine, Javanese turmeric has been used for liver and gallbladder complaints (18).

Safety
POSSIBLY SAFE …when the dried rhizome is used orally and appropriately for short periods of time (2,8).
POSSIBLY UNSAFE …when used in large amounts or for prolonged use. Can cause gastric irritation and nausea (2,8).
PREGNANCY AND LACTATION: Insufficient reliable information available; avoid using.

Effectiveness
POSSIBLY EFFECTIVE …when taken orally for "peptic disorders" (2).
There is insufficient reliable information available about the effectiveness of Javanese turmeric for its other uses.

Possible Mechanism of Action & Active Ingredients
The applicable part of Javanese turmeric is the root. Javanese turmeric root contains a volatile oil with the chief components of alpha-curcumene, xanthorrhizole, beta-curcumene, germacrene, furanodien, and furanodienone. The root also contains curcumin, demethoxycurcumin, and non-phenolic diarylheptanoids (18). Javanese turmeric is thought to stimulate bile production (2). It might also have antitumor effects (18).

Adverse Reactions Including Known Allergies
Oral use of large amounts or for prolonged periods of time can cause gastric irritation and nausea (2,8).

Possible Interactions with Herbs & Other Dietary Supplements
Insufficient reliable information available.

Possible Interactions with Drugs
No interactions are known to occur, and there is no known reason to expect a clinically significant interaction with Javanese turmeric.

Possible Interactions with Foods
No interactions are known to occur, and there is no known reason to expect a clinically significant interaction with Javanese turmeric.

Possible Interactions with Lab Tests
No interactions are known to occur, and there is no known reason to expect a clinically significant interaction with Javanese turmeric.

Possible Interactions with Diseases or Conditions
LIVER OR GALLBLADDER DISEASE: Contraindicated in people with acute bile duct inflammation, biliary tree inflammation (8), bile duct obstruction (2,8), or jaundice (8) due to bile stimulating effects (2). Individuals with gallstones should have medical evaluation before using (2).

Typical Dosages & Routes of Administration that are Commonly Used
ORAL: To stimulate bile production, a typical oral dose is one cup tea several times daily between meals. To make tea, steep 0.5-1 grams coarsely powdered root in 150 mL boiling water for 5-10 minutes, and strain. The average daily amount used is 2 grams root or equivalent preparations (2). For improving appetite, digestion, or for flatulence, a typical dose is one cup tea before or during meals. To make tea, steep 0.5-1 grams coarsely powdered root in 150 mL boiling water for 5-10 minutes, and strain (8). The average daily amount used is 2 grams root or equivalent preparations (2).

Comments

Javanese turmeric is indigenous to the forests of Indonesia and the Malaysian peninsula (18).

JEWELWEED

This Product is Also Known As

Balsam-Weed, Garden Balsam, Jewel Balsam Weed, Jewel Weed, Quick-In-The-Hand, Silverweed, Slipper Weed, Speckled Jewels, Spotted Touch-Me-Not, Touch-Me-Not, Wild Balsam, Wild Celandine, Wild Lady's Slipper. CAUTION: See separate listings for Potentilla, Greater Celandine above ground parts, Greater Celandine rhizome/root, and Lesser Celandine.

Scientific Names

Impatiens biflora; Impatiens pallida; Impatiens balsamina; Impatiens capensis.
Family: Balsaminaceae.

People Use This For

Orally, jewelweed is used for mild digestive disorders (18).
Orally and topically, jewelweed is used for poison ivy dermatitis (3).

Safety

POSSIBLY SAFE ...when used orally. ...when used topically. There are no published reports of significant toxicity for either route of administration (18).
PREGNANCY AND LACTATION: Insufficient reliable information available; avoid using.

Effectiveness

There is insufficient reliable information available about the effectiveness of jewelweed.

Possible Mechanism of Action & Active Ingredients

The applicable parts of jewelweed are the above ground parts. Impatiens balsamina has digestive and diuretic effects (18). One constituent, 2-methoxynaphthoquinone, has antifungal activity (6).

Adverse Reactions Including Known Allergies

None reported.

Possible Interactions with Herbs & Other Dietary Supplements

Insufficient reliable information available.

Possible Interactions with Drugs

No interactions are known to occur, and there is no known reason to expect a clinically significant interaction with jewelweed.

Possible Interactions with Foods

No interactions are known to occur, and there is no known reason to expect a clinically significant interaction with jewelweed.

Possible Interactions with Lab Tests

No interactions are known to occur, and there is no known reason to expect a clinically significant interaction with jewelweed.

Possible Interactions with Diseases or Conditions

No interactions are known to occur, and there is no known reason to expect a clinically significant interaction with jewelweed.

Typical Dosages & Routes of Administration that are Commonly Used

No typical dosage.

Comments

Avoid confusion with potentilla (Potentillae anserinae), also known as silverweed.

JIAOGULAN

This Product is Also Known As

Amachazuru, Dungkulcha, Fairy Herb, Miracle Grass, Penta Tea, Southern Ginseng.
CAUTION: See separate listing for Panax Ginseng.

Scientific Names
Gynostemma pentaphyllum, synonym Gynostemma pedatum, Vitis pentaphylla. Family: Cucurbitaceae.

People Use This For
Orally, jiaogulan is used for lowering cholesterol levels (6,319), regulating blood pressure (6), strengthening the immune system (6), increasing stamina and endurance (6), for appetite stimulation, for chronic bronchitis, chronic gastritis, ulcers, constipation, gallstones, obesity, cancer, diabetes, insomnia, backache, and pain. It is also used for improving memory, for improving coronary and cardiovascular functions, for releasing stress, preventing hair loss, and as an anti-aging agent. It is used as an anti-inflammatory agent, antioxidant, detoxifying agent, decongestant and cough suppressant, and as an adaptogen for restoring homeostasis to the body's systems (319).

Safety
There is insufficient reliable information available about the safety of jiaogulan.
Pregnancy and Lactation: Insufficient reliable information available; avoid using.

Effectiveness
POSSIBLY EFFECTIVE ...when used orally to reduce cholesterol and improve HDL/total cholesterol ratio in individuals with hyperlipoproteinemia (6).
There is insufficient reliable information available about the effectiveness of jiaogulan for its other uses.

Possible Mechanism of Action & Active Ingredients
Early research suggests jiaogulan has antioxidant activity (6). Some evidence also suggests it might increase tolerance to fatigue and lack of oxygen (6). The above ground parts of jiaogulan contain a large number of triterpene saponins referred to as gypenosides (6). Some gypenosides are identical to ginsenosides found in Panax ginseng. Many others are similar, although jiaogulan does not contain all of ginseng's biologically active compounds (6). Preliminary evidence suggests that the gypenoside constituents might lower blood pressure, heart rate, blood vessel resistance, increase coronary blood flow, and protect against cerebral ischemic damage (6). A crude saponin extract reduced total cholesterol and increased the HDL/total cholesterol ratio in individuals with hyperlipoproteinemia (6). Preliminary research suggests jiaogulan has immune enhancement and anti-cancer activity (6). In one study, jiaogulan was also beneficial in enhancing the immune function of individuals who had cancer chemotherapy (6).

Adverse Reactions Including Known Allergies
Taken orally, jiaogulan might cause severe nausea and increased bowel movements (6).

Possible Interactions with Herbs & Other Dietary Supplements
Insufficient reliable information available.

Possible Interactions with Drugs
ANTICOAGULANTS: Theoretically, excessive use of jiaogulan might interfere with anticoagulant therapy (6).
ANTIPLATELET DRUGS: Theoretically, excessive use of jiaogulan might interfere with antiplatelet therapy (6).
BARBITURATES: Theoretically, concomitant use can potentiate the effects and adverse effects of barbiturates (6).

Possible Interactions with Foods
No interactions are known to occur, and there is no reason to expect a clinically significant interaction with jiaogulan.

Possible Interactions with Lab Tests
BLOOD PRESSURE: Theoretically, jiaogulan might reduce blood pressure and blood pressure readings (6).
CHOLESTEROL: Jiaogulan might reduce serum total cholesterol concentrations and test results (6).
PLATELET ACTIVITY: Theoretically, excessive use of jiaogulan might interfere the results of platelet activity tests (6).
TRIGLYCERIDES: Theoretically, jiaogulan might reduce triglyceride concentrations and test results (6).

Possible Interactions with Diseases or Conditions
No interactions are known to occur, and there is no reason to expect a clinically significant interaction with jiaogulan.

Typical Dosages & Routes of Administration that are Commonly Used
ORAL: A typical dose for hyperlipidemia is 2 jiaogulan extract capsules twice daily, before breakfast and dinner (320).

Comments
Jiaogulan is a newcomer to traditional Chinese Medicine (6). Jiaogulan's sweetening effect was investigated by the Japanese (6). Jiaogulan has reportedly been adulterated with Cayratia japonica.

JIMSON WEED

This Product is Also Known As
Angel Tulip, Datura, Devil's Apple, Devil's Trumpet, Jamestown Weed, Locoweed, Mad-apple, Nightshade, Peru-apple, Stinkweed, Stinkwort, Stramonium, Thorn-apple.

Scientific Names
Datura stramonium.
Family: Solanaceae.

People Use This For
Orally, jimson weed is used to treat asthma, spastic or convulsive cough, pertussis during bronchitis and influenza, and as basic therapy for diseases of the autonomic nervous system (2,18).
Other uses include ingestion of the seeds or tea prepared from seeds to induce hallucinations and euphoria (5622,5623).

Safety
UNSAFE ...when the leaf or seed are taken orally, inhaled (2,13) or prepared as a tea (5622). Although all parts of the plant contain belladonna alkaloids and are poisonous, the seeds contain the most (5623). Ingestion of jimson weed can cause acute anticholinergic poisoning (17,5621,5622) and death (2,5622). The lethal dose for adults is 15-100 grams of leaf, 15-25 grams of the seeds (equivalent to 100 mg atropine) (18).
CHILDREN: UNSAFE ...when the seed or leaf are taken orally or inhaled. Children are more sensitive to the effects than adults, and the lethal dose is less (18).
PREGNANCY AND LACTATION: UNSAFE ...contraindicated (2).

Effectiveness
There is insufficient reliable information available about the effectiveness of jimson weed.

Possible Mechanism of Action & Active Ingredients
The applicable parts of jimson weed are the leaf and seed. Jimson weed contains 0.1-0.6% alkaloids including atropine, l-hyoscyamine and l-scopolamine which are responsible for anticholinergic action and toxicity (2).

Adverse Reactions Including Known Allergies
Ingestion of jimson weed can cause dilated pupils, dry mouth, dry skin, extreme thirst (13,18), dry mucous membranes, tachycardia, blurred vision, nausea and vomiting, decreased bowel sounds, difficulty swallowing and speaking, auditory and visual hallucinations, hyperthermia, hypertension, seizure (5623), loss of consciousness (13,18) and coma (5623). Potential adverse effects also include confusion, emotional lability, reduced coordination, and headache (636). Death may result from central nervous system depression, circulatory collapse, and hypotension (18). Edema of the lungs and pectichial hemorrhages of the endocardium have been reported at autopsy (5622).

Possible Interactions with Herbs & Other Dietary Supplements
Insufficient reliable information available.

Possible Interactions with Drugs
ANTICHOLINERGIC DRUGS: Avoid; concomitant use may increase anticholinergic effects and adverse effects; drugs include: amantadine, atropine, belladonna alkaloids, phenothiazines, scopolamine, tricyclic antidepressants (506).

Possible Interactions with Foods
No interactions are known to occur, and there is no known reason to expect a clinically significant interaction with jimson weed.

Possible Interactions with Lab Tests
No interactions are known to occur, and there is no known reason to expect a clinically significant interaction with jimson weed.

Possible Interactions with Diseases or Conditions
CONGESTIVE HEART FAILURE (CHF): Contraindicated; jimson weed might cause tachycardia and exacerbate CHF due to its hyoscyamine (atropine) and scopolamine content (15).
CONSTIPATION: Contraindicated; jimson weed might cause constipation due to its hyoscyamine (atropine) and scopolamine content (15).
DOWN SYNDROME: Caution, patients with Down syndrome might be hypersensitive to the antimuscarinic effects (mydriasis, positive chronotropic heart effects, etc.) of hyoscyamine (atropine) and scopolamine contained in jimson weed (15).
ESOPHAGEAL REFLUX: Contraindicated; jimson weed might delay gastric emptying and decrease lower esophageal pressure, promoting gastric retention and exacerbating reflux due to its hyoscyamine (atropine) and scopolamine content (15).
FEVER: Contraindicated; jimson weed might increase the risk of hyperthermia in patients with fever due to its

hyoscyamine (atropine) and scopolamine content (15).

GASTRIC ULCER: Contraindicated; jimson weed might delay gastric emptying and exacerbate gastric ulcers due to its hyoscyamine (atropine) and scopolamine content (15).

GI INFECTIONS: Contraindicated; jimson weed might suppress GI motility causing retention of infecting organisms or toxins due to its hyoscyamine (atropine) and scopolamine content (15).

HIATAL HERNIA: Contraindicated; jimson weed might delay gastric emptying and decrease lower esophageal pressure, promoting gastric retention and exacerbating reflux due to its hyoscyamine (atropine) and scopolamine content (15).

TOXIC MEGACOLON: Contraindicated; jimson weed might suppress intestinal motility, which might produce paralytic ileus and exacerbate toxic megacolon, due to its hyoscyamine (atropine) and scopolamine content (2,15).

NARROW-ANGLE GLAUCOMA: Contraindicated; jimson weed might increase ocular tension in patients with narrow-angle (angle-closure) glaucoma due to its hyoscyamine (atropine) and scopolamine content (2,15).

OBSTRUCTIVE GI TRACT DISEASE: Contraindicated; jimson weed might exacerbate obstructive GI tract diseases (including atony, paralytic ileus, and stenosis) due to its hyoscyamine (atropine) and scopolamine content (15).

TACHYARRHYTHMIAS: Contraindicated; jimson weed might cause tachycardia due to its hyoscyamine (atropine) and scopolamine content (2,15).

URINARY RETENTION: Contraindicated; jimson weed might increase urinary retention due to its hyoscyamine (atropine) and scopolamine content (2,15).

ULCERATIVE COLITIS: Contraindicated; jimson weed might suppress intestinal motility, which might produce paralytic ileus and precipitate toxic megacolon, due to its hyoscyamine (atropine) and scopolamine content (15).

Typical Dosages & Routes of Administration that are Commonly Used
No typical dosage.

Comments
Jimson weed is considered unsafe to use, due to high potential for toxicity.

JOJOBA

This Product is Also Known As
Deernut, Goatnut, Pignut.

Scientific Names
Simmondsia chinensis, synonym Buxus chinensis.
Family: Simmondsiaceae or Buxaceae.

People Use This For
Topically, jojoba oil is used in the management of acne, psoriasis, sunburn, and chapped skin (11). It has been used as a hair restorer (11).

In manufacturing, it is included as a component in shampoo, lipstick, makeup, cleansing products, and in face, hand and body lotions (11).

For food uses, roasted jojoba seeds are used as a coffee substitute (11).

Safety
LIKELY SAFE ...when used topically (6).

LIKELY UNSAFE ...if taken orally; avoid ingestion since it contains 14% erucic acid, which can cause myocardial fibrosis (6).

PREGNANCY AND LACTATION: LIKELY SAFE ...when used topically for hygienic uses.

Effectiveness
There is insufficient reliable information available about the effectiveness of jojoba.

Possible Mechanism of Action & Active Ingredients
Jojoba seeds yield a colorless, odorless oil that is an emollient (11). Jojoba oil penetrates skin and skin oils easily, unclogging hair follicles and preventing sebum build up, which could lead to hair loss (6). Taken by mouth, jojoba wax passes through the body without being digested, but is stored in intestinal cells and the liver (18).

Adverse Reactions Including Known Allergies
The applicable parts of jojoba are the oil and wax. Contact dermatitis occurs with use of shampoos and hair conditioners containing jojoba oil (6). Hypoallergenic sensitivity to jojoba wax may occur (6).

Possible Interactions with Herbs & Other Dietary Supplements
Insufficient reliable information available.

Possible Interactions with Drugs
No interactions are known to occur, and there is no known reason to expect a clinically significant interaction with jojoba.

Possible Interactions with Foods
No interactions are known to occur, and there is no known reason to expect a clinically significant interaction with jojoba.

Possible Interactions with Lab Tests
No interactions are known to occur, and there is no known reason to expect a clinically significant interaction with jojoba.

Possible Interactions with Diseases or Conditions
No interactions are known to occur, and there is no known reason to expect a clinically significant interaction with jojoba.

Typical Dosages & Routes of Administration that are Commonly Used
TOPICAL: Jojoba oil ingredient levels vary. In skin care products 5-10%; shampoos and conditioners 1-2%; bar soaps 0.5-3% (6).

Comments
Jojoba oil and wax are produced from the seeds of jojoba, a shrub native to arid regions of northern Mexico and the southwestern US. (3901).
Jojoba wax is unsuitable for food use (18).

JUJUBE

This Product is Also Known As
Black Date, Chinese Jujube, Da Zao, Hei Zao, Hong Zao, Jujube Plum, Red Date, Zao.

Scientific Names
Zyzyphus jujube.
Family: Rhamnaceae.

People Use This For
Orally, jujube is used for improving muscular strength and to prophylax against liver diseases and stress ulcers. It is also used as a sedative (18).
In Chinese medicine, it is used for dry, itchy skin, neutralizing drug toxicities, lack of appetite, fatigue, diarrhea, hysteria, anemia, hypertension, purpura, and as a sedative.
In Arabic medicine, jujube is used orally for fever wounds, ulcers, inflammation, asthma, and eye diseases (11). Jujube is eaten as a food.
In manufacturing, extracts are used in skin care products for anti-inflammatory, antiwrinkle, moisturizing, and relief from sunburn.

Safety
There is insufficient reliable information available on the oral or topical safety of jujube.
Pregnancy and Lactation: Insufficient reliable information available; avoid using.

Effectiveness
There is insufficient reliable information available about the effectiveness of jujube.

Possible Mechanism of Action & Active Ingredients
The applicable part of jujube is the fruit. Animal data suggests that jujube increases body weight, increases swimming endurance and protects against carbon tetrachloride-induced liver damage. Animal data also suggests anti-inflammatory effects and growth inhibition of Bacillus subtilis with an ethanolic extract. A methanolic extract containing oleanolic acid and ursolic acid inhibits the in vitro dental cavity-producing activity of Streptococcus mutans (11).

Adverse Reactions Including Known Allergies
None reported.

Possible Interactions with Herbs & Other Dietary Supplements
Insufficient reliable information available.

Possible Interactions with Drugs
No interactions are known to occur, and there is no known reason to expect a clinically significant interaction with jujube.

Possible Interactions with Foods

No interactions are known to occur, and there is no known reason to expect a clinically significant interaction with jujube.

Possible Interactions with Lab Tests

No interactions are known to occur, and there is no known reason to expect a clinically significant interaction with jujube.

Possible Interactions with Diseases or Conditions

No interactions are known to occur, and there is no known reason to expect a clinically significant interaction with jujube.

Typical Dosages & Routes of Administration that are Commonly Used

No typical dosage.

Comments

Jujube is no longer used medicinally (18).

JUNIPER

This Product is Also Known As

Common Juniper Berry, Enebro, Geniévre, Ginepro, Juniperi fructus, Wacholderbeeren, Zimbro.
CAUTION: See separate listing for Cade Oil.

Scientific Names

Juniperus communis.
Family: Cupressaceae or Pinaceae.

People Use This For

Orally, the juniper berry is used orally for dyspepsia (2), heartburn, bloating, loss of appetite, urinary tract infections, and kidney and bladder stones (18).
Topically, juniper has been used for rheumatic pains in joints and muscles (4), inflammatory diseases, wounds (6), and bronchitis as a inhaled vapor (11).
Traditionally, it has been used for flatulence, colic (4), snakebite, intestinal worms, gastrointestinal infections, and cancers (11).
For food uses, the berry is often used as a culinary condiment (6). The berry is also utilized as a flavor component in gin and bitter preparations, and the extract and oil are used as a flavoring agent in foods and beverages (11).
In manufacturing, the oil is used as a fragrance component in soaps and cosmetics (11).

Safety

LIKELY SAFE ...when the berry is consumed in amounts commonly found in foods and beverages. The juniper berry has Generally Recognized as Safe (GRAS) status in the US. The maximum level used in food is 0.006% for the oil and 0.01% for the extracts (11). Canadian regulations prohibit juniper as a non-medicinal ingredient in oral use products (12).
POSSIBLY SAFE ...when used orally and appropriately short-term (12). ...when used topically on limited areas of skin (12,18).
LIKELY UNSAFE ...when used orally longer than 4 weeks. Prolonged use increases the potential for kidney damage (8,19). ...when large amounts of juniper are repeatedly used orally, convulsions and kidney damage can result (6,19). ...when used topically on large skin wounds or in individuals with acute skin conditions (18).
PREGNANCY: UNSAFE. Juniper shows evidence that it can increase uterine tone, interfere with fertility, implantation, and cause abortion (4,19).
LACTATION: Insufficient reliable information available; avoid using.

Effectiveness

There is insufficient reliable information available about the effectiveness of juniper.

Possible Mechanism of Action & Active Ingredients

The applicable part of juniper is the berry. Juniper berry has aquaretic, antiseptic, antiflatulent, and antirheumatic effects. It also stimulates stomach function (4,512). Aquaretics increase urine volume (water loss) but not sodium excretion (512). The constituent terpinen-4-ol increases the glomerular filtration rate, but it can also irritate the kidneys (4). In vitro, juniper berry exhibits antiviral activity against the herpes simplex virus and has antifungal activity (4). In experimental animals, the juniper berry extract shows abortifacient, antifertility, anti-inflammatory, anti-implantation, hypotensive, hypertensive, and hypoglycemic effects (4). The juniper berry oil stimulates uterine activity (4). It has diuretic, GI antiseptic, and irritant effects (11). The oil prevents antispasmodic effects in smooth muscle (11).

Adverse Reactions Including Known Allergies

When taken orally, excessive amounts of the juniper berry oil can cause kidney irritation (4). Overdose symptoms include kidney pain, diuresis, albuminuria, hematuria, purplish urine, tachycardia, hypertension, convulsions, metrorrhagia, and abortion (4). The topical use of juniper can cause skin irritation (4). Signs of topical poisoning include burning, erythema, inflammation with blisters, and edema (4). Repeated exposure to the juniper pollen can cause occupational allergies that affect the skin and respiratory tract (6).

Possible Interactions with Herbs & Other Dietary Supplements

Insufficient reliable information available.

Possible Interactions with Drugs

DIURETICS: Theoretically, juniper berry might interfere with diuretic therapy (4,512).
DIABETES: Theoretically, juniper berry might potentiate diabetes therapy (4).

Possible Interactions with Foods

No interactions are known to occur, and there is no known reason to expect a clinically significant interaction with juniper.

Possible Interactions with Lab Tests

URINE TESTS: The juniper berry can interfere with urine assays, and large amounts can cause purplish urine (4).

Possible Interactions with Diseases or Conditions

DIABETES: Monitor blood glucose level closely due to claims that juniper has hypoglycemic effects (4,19).
HYPERTENSION, HYPOTENSION: Theoretically, juniper berry might interfere with blood pressure control (4,512).
KIDNEY DISEASE: Contraindicated (4,12).
SEIZURE DISORDERS: Theoretically, the juniper berry might exacerbate these conditions.
GI CONDITIONS: Juniper berry can irritate the gastrointestinal tract (19). It is contraindicated in individuals with infectious or inflammatory gastrointestinal conditions (19).
OTHER: Individuals with cardiac insufficiency, hypertonia, fever, acute skin disease, or large skin wounds should not use juniper berry (18).

Typical Dosages & Routes of Administration that are Commonly Used

ORAL: The typical dose of juniper is 1-2 grams of the berry three times daily (4) or one cup of the tea three to four times daily (8). The tea is prepared by steeping 1 teaspoon of the crushed juniper berry, about 2-3 grams, in 150 mL boiling water for 10 minutes and then straining. Juniper should be used up to a maximum of 10 grams of the dried berry per day, corresponding to 20-100 mg of the essential oil (2). This dose should not be used longer than four weeks without physician consultation (8). The usual dose of the liquid extract (1:1 in 25% alcohol) is 2-4 mL three times daily (4). The common dose of the tincture (1:5 in 45% alcohol) is 1-2 mL three times daily (4). The berry oil (1:5 in 45% alcohol) is typically taken as 0.03-0.2 mL three times daily (4). CAUTION: The juniper berry oil should only be used under supervision (4).
TOPICAL: The juniper berry is commonly used in bath salts for treating rheumatism (18).

Comments

Avoid confusion with cade oil, which is distilled from juniper wood (Juniperus oxycedrus). Turpentine oil has been used to adulterate juniper berry oil (512).

KAMALA

This Product is Also Known As

Kamcela, Kameela, Rottlera Tinctoria, Spoonwood.

Scientific Names

Mallotus philippinensis.

People Use This For

Orally, kamala is used for treating tape worm infestation (18).

Safety

There is insufficient reliable information available about the safety of kamala.
Pregnancy and Lactation: Insufficient reliable information available; avoid using.

Effectiveness

There is insufficient reliable information available about the effectiveness of kamala.

Possible Mechanism of Action & Active Ingredients

The applicable parts of kamala are the gland and hair of the fruit. Kamala contains berginin and tannins. It is reported to have anthelmintic and purgative effects (18).

Adverse Reactions Including Known Allergies

None reported.

Possible Interactions with Herbs & Other Dietary Supplements

STIMULANT LAXATIVE HERBS: Theoretically, concomitant use with other stimulant laxative herbs may increase effects and adverse effects. Stimulant laxative herbs include: aloe dried leaf sap, blue flag rhizome, alder buckthorn, European buckthorn, butternut bark, cascara bark, castor oil, colocynth fruit pulp, gamboge bark exudate, jalap root, black root, manna bark exudate, podophyllum root, rhubarb root, senna leaves and pods, wild cucumber fruit (Ecballium elaterium), and yellow dock root (19).

Possible Interactions with Drugs

No interactions are known to occur, and there is no known reason to expect a clinically significant interaction with kamala.

Possible Interactions with Foods

No interactions are known to occur, and there is no known reason to expect a clinically significant interaction with kamala.

Possible Interactions with Lab Tests

No interactions are known to occur, and there is no known reason to expect a clinically significant interaction with kamala.

Possible Interactions with Diseases or Conditions

GI CONDITIONS: Stimulant laxatives are contraindicated in individuals with symptoms of appendicitis (abdominal pain, nausea and vomiting) (272).

Typical Dosages & Routes of Administration that are Commonly Used

ORAL: People typically use 2 to 10 grams of kamala powder and 8 to 14 mL of the liquid extract (5264).

Comments

There is very little scientific information about this product. Our staff is continually analyzing the available information on natural medicines and will add data here as it becomes available.

KAOLIN

This Product is Also Known As

Argilla, Bolus Alba, China Clay, Heavy Kaolin, Light Kaolin, Porcelain Clay, White Bole.

Scientific Names

Hydrated aluminum silicate (6).

People Use This For

Orally, kaolin is used for mild to moderate acute diarrhea, cholera, enteritis, and dysentery (6).
Topically, it is used as a poultice, dusting powder, drying agent, and emollient (6,9,16,188,189).
In combination products, kaolin is used for symptomatic diarrhea control (6,9,14,16), in relief of radiation-induced mucositis (14,186,187), in the treatment of chronic ulcerative colitis (16), and to treat spontaneous pneumothorax (9).
Diagnostic uses include as a contrast media agent (C,D), (6,16), automated testing for activated coagulation time (ACT) (6,192), serodiagnosis of tuberculosis (193), and the kaolin agglutination test (KAT) (254).
In manufacturing, kaolin is used as a diluent in tablet preparation (6,194), and a filtering or decolorizing agent (6,16). It is also a food additive (9).

Safety

LIKELY SAFE ...when taken orally in appropriate amounts (6,14). Kaolin is not absorbed systemically and is generally nontoxic (6)...when used topically with appropriate use of sterile products (9,16). Kaolin is an FDA-approved prescription product.
PREGNANCY AND LACTATION: POSSIBLY UNSAFE ...in large amounts because of iron deficiency anemia and hypokalemia secondary to clay ingestion (14).

Effectiveness

POSSIBLY EFFECTIVE ...when taken alone or in combination with pectin and other drugs for the symptomatic control of mild to moderate acute diarrhea (excluding pseudomembranous enterocolitis) (14,15). Kaolin is an FDA-approved prescription product. ...when taken orally in combination with other drugs for relief of pain and to decrease the severity of radiation-induced mucositis (14,186,187). ...when used topically as a drying agent in dusting

© Copyright 2000, Natural Medicines Comprehensive Database (209) 472-2244. For updated data, go to www.NaturalDatabase.com

powder (6,9,16,188).
There is insufficient reliable information available about the effectiveness of kaolin for its other uses.

Possible Mechanism of Action & Active Ingredients

Kaolin may absorb bacteria and toxins in the GI tract, increase fecal bulk and restore stool consistency (6,914,15,16). In radiation-induced mucositis, kaolin may act as a protective coating to decrease the severity of pain (14,186). Topically, kaolin acts as a drying agent adsorbing a wide variety of substances (6,9,16).

Adverse Reactions Including Known Allergies

Taken orally, kaolin can cause constipation, particularly in children and the elderly (14). Occupational kalinosis (pulmonary disease) is reported in miners following inhalation (6,195,196,197).

Possible Interactions with Herbs & Other Dietary Supplements

Insufficient reliable information available.

Possible Interactions with Drugs

NUMEROUS DRUGS: Kaolin actively adsorbs a wide variety of substances (6,9). Concomitant use of kaolin or kaolin/pectin could decrease systemic absorption of digoxin, quinidine, lincomycin, clindamycin, phenothiazines, chloroquine, and trimethoprim (6,14,198,199,250,251,252,253). Separate doses of chloroquine and kaolin by at least four hours (14).

Possible Interactions with Foods

No interactions are known to occur, and there is no known reason to expect a clinically significant interaction with kaolin.

Possible Interactions with Lab Tests

No interactions are known to occur, and there is no known reason to expect a clinically significant interaction with kaolin.

Possible Interactions with Diseases or Conditions

PSEUDOMEMBRANOUS ENTEROCOLITIS: Kaolin/pectin combination is contraindicated in the treatment of diarrhea from pseudomembranous enterocolitis or toxigenic bacteria (14).

Typical Dosages & Routes of Administration that are Commonly Used

ORAL: In diarrhea dose varies ranging between 15-60 grams (6,9) and 50-100 grams at three hour intervals (16). Kaolin is usually taken at first sign of diarrhea and after each loose bowel movement (14). Doses of 15-60 grams (6,9) and doses of 50-100 grams at 3 hours intervals reported (16). For relief of radiation-induced mucositis, 15 ml (50% kaolin/pectin, 50% diphenhydramine) solution, rinse four times a day (14,186). Kaolin is an FDA-approved prescription product.

Comments

Kaolin is hydrated aluminum silicate (16) purified for pharmaceutical use by treatment with hydrochloric acid or sulfuric acid, or both, then washed with water (6,9,16). Heavy kaolin (Kaolinum ponderosum) is the purified natural form of variable composition (9,16), and light kaolin is prepared from heavy kaolin by elutriation (separation of finer from coarser particles by suspension in water) (9,16).

KARAYA GUM

This Product is Also Known As

Bassora Tragacanth, Indian Tragacanth, Kadaya, Kadira, Karaya, Katila, Kullo, Mucara, Sterculia Gum.

Scientific Names

Sterculia urens; Sterculia villosa; Sterculia tragacanth; other Sterculia species.
Family: Sterculiaceae.

People Use This For

Orally, karaya gum is used as a bulk laxative (6).
Historically, it has been used as an aphrodisiac (11).
In manufacturing, karaya gum is used as a thickener in pharmaceuticals and cosmetics (6,11); denture and ostomy adhesives (6,400); and a binder and stabilizer in foods and beverages (6,11).

Safety

LIKELY SAFE ...when taken in amounts found in foods (maximum use level 0.805% in candy) (11); it has Generally Recognized as Safe (GRAS) status in the US (11). ...when used as an oral medicinal (6).
PREGNANCY AND LACTATION: Insufficient information available.

Effectiveness

POSSIBLY EFFECTIVE ...when used as a bulk forming laxative (6,11).
There is insufficient reliable information available about the effectiveness of karaya gum for its other uses.

Possible Mechanism of Action & Active Ingredients

Karaya gum is not digested or absorbed but swells in the presence of water, forming a viscous colloidal solution that stimulates peristalsis in the GI tract (6,11).

Adverse Reactions Including Known Allergies

None reported.

Possible Interactions with Herbs & Other Dietary Supplements

Insufficient reliable information available.

Possible Interactions with Drugs

ORAL DRUGS: Co-administration of oral drugs with bulk forming laxatives may decrease the absorption of the drugs (12).

Possible Interactions with Foods

No interactions are known to occur, and there is no known reason to expect a clinically significant interaction with karaya gum.

Possible Interactions with Lab Tests

No interactions are known to occur, and there is no known reason to expect a clinically significant interaction with karaya gum.

Possible Interactions with Diseases or Conditions

BOWEL OBSTRUCTION: In general, bulk laxatives are contraindicated in individuals with bowel obstruction (12).

Typical Dosages & Routes of Administration that are Commonly Used

No typical dosage.

Comments

Karaya gum is exuded from Sterculia species trees, that are native to India, when charred or scarred (6,3901).
Adequate fluid intake is important with bulk forming laxatives.

KAVA

This Product is Also Known As

Ava, Awa, Intoxicating Pepper, Kava Kava, Kava-kava, Kava Pepper, Kava Root, Kawa, Kawa Kawa, Kawa-Kawa, Kew, Rauschpfeffer, Sakau, Tonga, Wurzelstock, Yagona.

Scientific Names

Piper methysticum.
Family: Piperaceae.

People Use This For

Orally, kava is used to treat anxiety disorders, stress, insomnia, and restlessness (2,214). It is also used for epilepsy, psychosis, and depression (214).
In folk medicine, kava is used orally as a sedative, to promote wound healing, to treat headaches (6) including migraines (11), colds (6) and respiratory tract infections, tuberculosis (11), and rheumatism (6). It is used to treat urogenital infections including chronic cystitis (11), venereal disease, uterine inflammation, menstrual problems (11), and vaginal prolapse (11). Some consider kava an aphrodisiac (6). In folk medicine, kava juice is used topically to treat skin diseases including leprosy (11). It has been used as a poultice for intestinal problems, otitis, and abscesses (11).
Kava is used as a ceremonial beverage to induce relaxation in the South Pacific (6,11).

Safety

LIKELY SAFE ...when used orally and appropriately, short-term (7,12). Standardized kava extracts have been used safely with minimal side effects in studies lasting up to 6 months (7). However, it is generally recommended that use for greater then 3 months should only be conducted under the supervision of a healthcare provider (2,12,19).
POSSIBLY UNSAFE ...when used orally in high doses or long-term. High doses of kava have been associated with severe adverse effects. Prolonged use of kava might lead to habituation (19) and has also been associated with a kava dermopathy when used from 3 months to a year (see Adverse Reactions) (19,1740,6401).
PREGNANCY: POSSIBLY UNSAFE ...when used orally (2,12,19). Theoretically, the pyrone constituents can cause

loss of uterine tone (19); contraindicated.
LACTATION: POSSIBLY UNSAFE …when used orally (2,19). There is concern that the toxic pyrone constituents might pass into breast milk (19); contraindicated.

Effectiveness

LIKELY EFFECTIVE …when used orally for short-term treatment of anxiety disorders. Multiple clinical trials have shown that kava extracts standardized to 70% kava-lactones are superior to placebo (2093,2094,2095), and possibly comparable to low-dose benzodiazepines (2092) for short-term treatment of anxiety. Treatment for 1-8 weeks may be necessary for significant improvement (2094,2095).

Most clinical studies on the effectiveness of kava for anxiety disorders have used the standardized extract WS 1490 (W. Schwabe). This extract is standardized to contain 70% kava-lactones (also known as kavapyrones) (7). It is important to note that this extract is more than twice as concentrated as most products commercially available.

POSSIBLY EFFECTIVE …when used orally for reducing symptoms of anxiety related to climacteric in menopausal women. Two small trials have shown that kava standardized to 15% or 70% kava-lactones is superior to placebo for short-term treatment of neurovegetative and anxiety symptoms related to climacteric. Significant improvement occurred after 1 week of treatment (7,2096). …when used orally for nervous anxiety, stress, and restlessness (2).

There is insufficient reliable information available about the effectiveness of kava for its other uses.

Possible Mechanism of Action & Active Ingredients

The applicable part of kava is the rhizome/root. Pharmacological activity has largely been attributed to the kava-lactones (also known as kavapyrones), kawain, dihydrokawain, methysticin, dihydromethysticin, and others. The dried herb typically provides 3.5% kava-lactones (7), but kava extracts commercially available are generally formulated to provide from 30-70% kava-lactones. Kava has been found to have a variety of central nervous system effects, including anxiolytic, sedative, anticonvulsant, local anesthetic, spasmolytic, and analgesic activities; however, the exact mechanism for these effects is not known. Kava is not thought to affect benzodiazepine or GABA receptors (6401). Analgesia is not believed to occur by the opiate pathway because naloxone will not reverse it (6). Furthermore, kava is thought to produce motor sedation without affecting respiratory processes (2095). Some evidence suggests kava may affect the limbic system (214). When chewed kava root reportedly numbs the mouth similar to cocaine (1740). People consuming kava have reported feeling more sociable, tranquil, and generally happy (1740). The kavapyrones desmethoxyyangonin and methysticin can competitive inhibit monoamine oxidase B (MAO-B) (2500). Kava compounds can also be potent strychnine antagonists (6). The kavapyrone (+)-kawain can have antithrombic action on platelets, probably due to inhibition of cyclo-oxygenase and decreased thromboxane 2 (TXA2) production (2501).

Adverse Reactions Including Known Allergies

The oral use of kava can cause gastrointestinal complaints, headache, dizziness (7), enlarged pupils and disturbances of oculomotor equilibrium and accommodation (2,6), and rarely, allergic skin reactions (2,7). Unlike benzodiazepines, kava is not thought to be associated with impaired cognitive function (7,2097,2098). However, use of normal doses of kava may affect the ability to drive or operate machinery. Driving under the influence (DUI) citations have been issued to individuals observed driving erratically after drinking large amounts of kava tea (535,5079). Kava can cause drowsiness and might impair motor reflexes (2,19). Chewing kava can cause mouth numbness (6). Chronic use of high doses of kava has been associated with kava dermopathy, a pellagra-like syndrome unresponsive to niacinamide treatment (2,6,7,6240). The cause is unknown but may relate to interference with cholesterol metabolism (6240). This syndrome is characterized by dry, flaking skin and reddened eyes, as well as temporary yellow discoloration of the skin, hair, and nails (7,6401). It usually occurs within 3 months to 1 year of kava use and resolves when the kava dose is decreased or discontinued (6401). Kava dose should be decreased or discontinued if kava dermopathy occurs (2,6,7,6401). The long-term use of very large amounts of kava is associated with poor health, including being significantly under weight, reduced protein levels, puffy faces, scaly rashes, hematuria, increased red blood cell volume, decreased platelets and lymphocytes, and possibly pulmonary hypertension (6402). There is one case report of generalized abnormal movements of the body associated with high-dose, chronic kava consumption (534). One report associates the use of kava with a case of recurrent, acute hepatitis (390).

Possible Interactions with Herbs & Other Dietary Supplements

HERBS WITH SEDATIVE PROPERTIES: Theoretically, concomitant use with herbs that have sedative properties might enhance therapeutic and adverse effects. These include calamus, calendula, California poppy, catnip, capsicum, celery, couch grass, elecampane, Siberian ginseng, German chamomile, goldenseal, gotu kola, hops, Jamaican dogwood, lemon balm, sage, St. John's wort, sassafras, scullcap, shepherd's purse, stinging nettle, valerian, wild carrot, wild lettuce, withania, and yerba mansa (4,19).

Possible Interactions with Drugs

ALPRAZOLAM: There is one report of an individual who was hospitalized due to lethargy and disorientation that occurred when alprazolam and kava were used concomitantly (536).
CNS DEPRESSANTS: Concomitant use of alcohol, barbiturates, or benzodiazepines can increase drug effects and risk of adverse effects (2,6).
BARBITURATES: Theoretically, concomitant use with barbiturates might cause additive effects and adverse

effects (19).

DRUGS WITH SEDATIVE PROPERTIES: Theoretically, concomitant use with drugs with sedative properties might cause additive effects and side effects (19).

LEVODOPA (Larodopa, Dopar): There is one report of reduced efficacy of levodopa when an individual used kava and levodopa concomitantly, possibly due to dopamine antagonism (19).

Possible Interactions with Foods

ALCOHOL: Concomitant use with alcohol can increase kava toxicity (2,6). Hypnotic effect of alcohol is increased with the lipid soluble extract (19).

Possible Interactions with Lab Tests

No interactions are known to occur, and there is no known reason to expect a clinically significant interaction with kava.

Possible Interactions with Diseases or Conditions

DEPRESSION: Kava is contraindicated in endogenous depression (2,12), due to the theoretical sedative activity (19).

Typical Dosages & Routes of Administration that are Commonly Used

ORAL: For anxiety disorders, most clinical trials have used kava extract standardized to 70% kava-lactone content. Doses of the kava extract were most commonly 100 mg (70 mg kava-lactones) three times daily (7,2092,2093,2094, 2095,2096). For nervous anxiety, stress, and restlessness, a dose of 60-120 mg kava-lactones daily has been used (2). Kava is also taken as 1 cup of the tea up to 3 times per day. The tea is prepared by simmering 2-4 grams of the root in 150 mL boiling water for 5-10 minutes and then straining (12). Because kava-lactone content varies substantially among products, appropriate dosing will also vary.

Comments

Kava was discovered by Captain Cook who named the plant, "intoxicating pepper" (4208,6240). In the South Pacific, kava is a popular social drink, similar to alcohol in Western societies (6). Kava is also prepared in a defined ritual manner and used for ceremonial purposes and has been used for thousands of years by Pacific Islanders (782,6240). Commercially available kava extracts are prepared from the dried root of Piper methysticum with an ethanol-water mixture (for extracts containing 30% kavapyrones) and with an acetone-water mixture (for extracts containing 70% kavapyrones; one extract is designated WS 1490) (7).

KHAT

This Product is Also Known As

Abyssinian Tea, Chaat, Gat, Kat, Kus es Salahin, Qut, Tchaad, Tohai, Tohat, Tschut.

Scientific Names

Catha edulis.
Family: Celastraceae.

People Use This For

Orally, khat leaf is used for depression, fatigue, obesity, and gastric ulcers (6). The leaf and stem are chewed by people in East Africa and the Arabian countries as a euphoriant (6).

Safety

POSSIBLY UNSAFE ...when used orally. Khat leaf is not physically addicting but is associated with psychological dependence (6).

PREGNANCY: POSSIBLY UNSAFE …when used orally. Khat may reduce birth weight of baby (6).

LACTATION: POSSIBLY UNSAFE …when used orally. Khat contains norpseudoephedrine, which passes into mother's milk (6); avoid using.

Effectiveness

There is insufficient reliable information available about the effectiveness of khat.

Possible Mechanism of Action & Active Ingredients

The applicable parts of khat are the leaf and stem. Contains cathine, which has 1/10 the stimulant effect of d-amphetamine, and cathinone, a more powerful stimulant than cathine. Both decrease food intake and increase locomotor activity (6).

Adverse Reactions Including Known Allergies

Oral consumption results in central stimulation including euphoria, increased alertness, garrulousness, hyperactivity, excitement, aggressiveness, anxiety, elevated blood pressure, and manic behavior. Insomnia, malaise, and lack of concentration usually follow. True psychotic reactions occur much less often than with amphetamines. Cardiovascular effects include tachycardia, palpitations, and increased blood pressure. Other effects include increased respiratory rate, hyperthermia, sweating, pupil dilation, and decreased intraocular pressure, stomatitis, esophagitis, gastritis, periodontal disease, temporomandibular joint dysfunction and keratosis of buccal mucosa, and constipation (6). Chronic use in young people is linked to hypertension. Severe adverse effects include migraine, cerebral hemorrhage, myocardial infarction, pulmonary edema, hepatic cirrhosis, initial increase in men's libido followed by loss of sexual drive, spermatorrhea, and impotence (6). Females report increased sexual desire and improved performance (6).

Possible Interactions with Herbs & Other Dietary Supplements
Insufficient reliable information available.

Possible Interactions with Drugs
No interactions are known to occur, and there is no known reason to expect a clinically significant interaction with khat.

Possible Interactions with Foods
No interactions are known to occur, and there is no known reason to expect a clinically significant interaction with khat.

Possible Interactions with Lab Tests
No interactions are known to occur, and there is no known reason to expect a clinically significant interaction with khat.

Possible Interactions with Diseases or Conditions
DIABETES: Khat use suppresses appetite, causing people to skip meals, decrease adherence to dietary advice, and increase consumption of sweetened beverages aggravating hyperglycemia (6).

Typical Dosages & Routes of Administration that are Commonly Used
No typical dosage.

Comments
None.

KINETIN

This Product is Also Known As
Kinerase, Kinetase.

Scientific Names
N-(2-furanylmethyl)-1H-purin-6-amine; N(6)furfuryladenine; 6-furfurylaminopurine.

People Use This For
Topically, kinetin is used to reduce the effects of skin aging, to reduce skin roughness, fine wrinkles, telangiectasias, and mottled, excessive pigmentation (4276).
In combination, kinetin is also used topically with retinol palmitate to treat signs of aging (4286).

Safety
POSSIBLY SAFE …when kinetin is used topically and appropriately (4276).
There is insufficient reliable information about the safety of kinetin and retinol palmitate used in combination.
PREGNANCY AND LACTATION: Insufficient reliable information available; avoid using.

Effectiveness
There is insufficient reliable information available about the effectiveness of the topical use of kinetin or kinetin used in combination with retinol palmitate.

Possible Mechanism of Action & Active Ingredients
Kinetin is a cytokinin, a potent plant growth factor (4277,4279). Kinetin prevents the aging of leaves; a green leaf dipped in kinetin will not turn brown. Some evidence suggests kinetin might also prevent age-related changes in human skin (4277). Although kinetin's mechanism of action is unknown, limited information suggests it acts as an antioxidant protecting DNA from oxidative damage (4278). Other evidence suggests that it also decreases skin water loss across the epidermis (4276). Unlike other growth agents, kinetin does not increase the maximum lifespan or ability of human skin cells to multiply in culture, suggesting it does not promote skin cancer (4277).

Adverse Reactions Including Known Allergies
Used topically, kinetin 0.1% sometimes initially causes dry skin (4285).

Possible Interactions with Herbs & Other Dietary Supplements
Insufficient reliable information available.

Possible Interactions with Drugs

No interactions are known to occur, and there is no known reason to expect a clinically significant interaction with kinetin.

Possible Interactions with Foods

No interactions are known to occur, and there is no known reason to expect a clinically significant interaction with kinetin.

Possible Interactions with Lab Tests

No interactions are known to occur, and there is no known reason to expect a clinically significant interaction with kinetin.

Possible Interactions with Diseases or Conditions

No interactions are known to occur, and there is no known reason to expect a clinically significant interaction with kinetin.

Typical Dosages & Routes of Administration that are Commonly Used

TOPICAL: A typical dose is 0.05% cream or lotion or 0.1% cream or lotion applied twice daily (4280,4284). Although kinetin does not cause photosensitivity, using a sunscreen with SPF 15 is recommended as the basis of any skin care program (4281,4285).

Comments

To date, no controlled trials in humans have been published in peer-reviewed journals. A study financed by a manufacturer evaluated 64 subjects who used 0.005% kinetin lotion or cream or placebo along with a mild facial cleanser and sunscreen (SPF 15). All study participants showed global improvement, 33-36% using kinetin showed good to excellent improvement compared to 12-21% in the placebo group (4276).

KIWI

This Product is Also Known As

China Gooseberry, Chinese Gooseberry, Kiwi Fruit.

Scientific Names

Actinidia chinensis.
Family: Actinidiaceae.

People Use This For

Kiwi is used as a food, a meat tenderizer, and a component in some sports drinks (6).

Safety

LIKELY SAFE ...when used as a food (6).
PREGNANCY AND LACTATION: LIKELY SAFE ...when used in food amounts (6).

Effectiveness

There is insufficient reliable information available about the effectiveness of kiwi.

Possible Mechanism of Action & Active Ingredients

The applicable part of kiwi is the fruit. Kiwi fruit contains high concentrations of vitamin C and serotonin (6). Enzymatic components may be responsible for adverse effects (6). The constituent, actinidin, is an enzyme with proteolytic activity similar to papain (6).

Adverse Reactions Including Known Allergies

Eating kiwi fruit or drinking the juice can lead to hypersensitivity reactions of the mouth, including dysphagia, urticaria, and vomiting immediately following ingestion (6). Topical use can cause contact urticaria (6).

Possible Interactions with Herbs & Other Dietary Supplements

Insufficient reliable information available.

Possible Interactions with Drugs

No interactions are known to occur, and there is no known reason to expect a clinically significant interaction with kiwi.

Possible Interactions with Foods

No interactions are known to occur, and there is no known reason to expect a clinically significant interaction with kiwi.

Possible Interactions with Lab Tests

URINE TESTS: Kiwi may elevate urine levels of 5-hydroxyindoleacetic acid and interfere with lab tests for this serotonin metabolite (6).

Possible Interactions with Diseases or Conditions

No interactions are known to occur, and there is no known reason to expect a clinically significant interaction with kiwi.

Typical Dosages & Routes of Administration that are Commonly Used

No typical dosage.

Comments

None.

KNOTWEED HERB

This Product is Also Known As

Allseed Nine-Joints, Armstrong, Beggarweed, Bird's Tongue, Birdweed, Centinode, Cow Grass, Crawlgrass, Doorweed, Hogweed, Knotgrass, Ninety-Knot, Pigrush, Pigweed, Polygoni Avicularis Herba, Red Robin, Sparrow Tongue, Swine's Grass, Swynel Grass, Vogelknoeterichkraut.

Scientific Names

Polygonum aviculare.
Family: Polygonaceae.

People Use This For

Knotweed is used for bronchitis, cough, and inflammation of the mouth and pharynx.
In folk medicine, it is used orally for supportive treatment of pulmonary diseases, skin disorders, to suppress perspiration associated with tuberculosis, as a diuretic, and as a hemostatic in cases of hemorrhage (18).

Safety

POSSIBLY SAFE ...for oral or topical use (2,18).
PREGNANCY AND LACTATION: Insufficient reliable information available; avoid using.

Effectiveness

POSSIBLY EFFECTIVE ...when used to treat inflammation of the mouth or pharynx (2).
There is insufficient reliable information available about the effectiveness of knotweed for its other uses.

Possible Mechanism of Action & Active Ingredients

The applicable part of knotweed herb is the whole flowering plant. Knotweed is suggested to have astringent and anticholinergic activity (2,18). There is insufficient reliable information to suggest active ingredients or a mechanism of action for knotweed.

Adverse Reactions Including Known Allergies

None reported.

Possible Interactions with Herbs & Other Dietary Supplements

Insufficient reliable information available.

Possible Interactions with Drugs

No interactions are known to occur, and there is no known reason to expect a clinically significant interaction with knotweed herb.

Possible Interactions with Foods

No interactions are known to occur, and there is no known reason to expect a clinically significant interaction with knotweed herb.

Possible Interactions with Lab Tests

No interactions are known to occur, and there is no known reason to expect a clinically significant interaction with knotweed herb.

Possible Interactions with Diseases or Conditions

No interactions are known to occur, and there is no known reason to expect a clinically significant interaction with knotweed herb.

Typical Dosages & Routes of Administration that are Commonly Used

ORAL: One cup of tea (simmer 1.4 grams dried ground herb in 150 mL of boiling water for 10-15 minutes, strain) is taken orally 3 to 5 times daily. The daily oral dose is 4-6 grams dried ground herb (2,18).

Comments

None.

KOMBUCHA TEA

This Product is Also Known As

Champagne Of Life, Combucha Tea, Dr. Sklenar's Kombucha Mushroom Infusion, Fungus Japonicus, Kargasok Tea, Kombucha Mushroom Tea, Kwassan, Manchurian Fungus, Manchurian Mushroom Tea, Spumonto, T'Chai from the Sea, Tschambucco.

Scientific Names

None.

People Use This For

Orally, kombucha tea is used for memory loss, premenstrual syndrome, rheumatism, aging, anorexia (6), AIDS, cancer (2650), hypertension, increasing T-cell counts (2652), strengthening the immune system and metabolism (2653), constipation, arthritis (2654), and hair regrowth (2655).
Topically, it is used for analgesia (2651).

Safety

POSSIBLY UNSAFE (2650) ...when taken orally because non-sterile home preparations have a high risk of contamination (2651,2652,2653).
LIKELY UNSAFE ...when used orally by individuals with compromised immunity, including HIV/AIDS, due to the risk of transmission of opportunistic pathogens (2652,2653), including Aspergillus (2652,2653) and anthrax (Bacillus anthracis) (2651). ...when kombucha tea prepared in a lead-glazed ceramic container is used orally. Lead poisoning was reported in two people who consumed kombucha tea prepared in a lead-glazed ceramic pot for six months (1366).
PREGNANCY AND LACTATION: POSSIBLY UNSAFE; avoid using.

Effectiveness

There is insufficient reliable information available about the effectiveness of kombucha tea.

Possible Mechanism of Action & Active Ingredients

Kombucha tea can contain up to 1.5% alcohol, vinegar (acetic acid), and a variety of other metabolites (2655). The product contains high levels of B vitamins (2653). No clinically relevant pharmacology has been defined for the kombucha symbiot or its products (6). Caffeine (black tea) and sugar are theorized to account for the increased energy claimed by some tea users (2654). Kombucha tea has the potential to incubate pathogenic organisms, including Aspergillus and anthrax, during its preparation, which is commonly ten days of fermentation at room temperature (2651,2652,2653). Due to the vinegar and ethanol content, it also has the potential to leach lead and other toxic chemicals from the walls of the preparation and storage containers (2650).

Adverse Reactions Including Known Allergies

The oral use of kombucha tea can cause stomach problems, yeast infections (2652), allergic reactions, jaundice, nausea, vomiting, head and neck pain (2656), anthrax (2651), and possibly death (2655). Symptomatic lead poisoning requiring chelation decontamination therapy was reported in two people who consumed kombucha tea prepared in a lead-glazed ceramic pot for six months (1366).

Possible Interactions with Herbs & Other Dietary Supplements

Insufficient reliable information available.

Possible Interactions with Drugs

ACID-SENSITIVE DRUGS: Theoretically, concomitant use of kombucha tea with acid-sensitive oral drugs can interfere with drug therapy due to the acidity of kombucha tea.
DISULFIRAM (Antabuse): Theoretically, concomitant use can cause a disulfiram reaction due to the alcohol contained in the fermented tea (2650).

Possible Interactions with Foods

No interactions are known to occur, and there is no known reason to expect a clinically significant interaction with kombucha tea.

Possible Interactions with Lab Tests

LIVER FUNCTION TESTS: There is one report of increased liver function tests after three weeks of consumption of kombucha tea (6).

Possible Interactions with Diseases or Conditions

ALCOHOLISM: Kombucha tea is contraindicated in people with stabilized or therapeutically-controlled alcoholism, because the alcohol content of the tea can aggravate this condition (2650).

COMPROMISED IMMUNITY: Contraindicated because kombucha tea can harbor or culture organisms that cause opportunistic infections (2652,2653).

Typical Dosages & Routes of Administration that are Commonly Used

No typical dosage.

Comments

The kombucha "mushroom" is a yeast or bacteria fungal symbiot and not an actual mushroom. It is derived from the fermentation of yeasts and bacteria with black tea, sugar, and other ingredients (6,2650). The resulting liquid is called kombucha tea. Although advocates of kombucha tea have attributed many therapeutic effects to the drink in the popular press, there is no scientific evidence to support any therapeutic claims (6,2650,2652,2654,2655). An outbreak of anthrax in twenty people in Iran confirmed the tea is a good culture medium for Bacillus anthracis (2651).

KOUSSO

This Product is Also Known As

Cossoo, Kooso, Kosso.

Scientific Names

Hagenia abyssinica.
Family: Rosaceae.

People Use This For

Orally, kousso was used for tapeworm infestations (18).

Safety

LIKELY UNSAFE ...when used orally (18).
PREGNANCY: UNSAFE ...contraindicated due to abortifacient activity (19).
LACTATION: UNSAFE ...due to its potential for toxicity (18).

Effectiveness

There is insufficient reliable information available about the effectiveness of kousso.

Possible Mechanism of Action & Active Ingredients

There is insufficient reliable information available about the possible mechanism of action or active ingredients.

Adverse Reactions Including Known Allergies

The side effects of kousso include gastrointestinal irritation, with accompanying salivation, headache, and general weakness. With overdose, people experience syncope and vision disorders. It can also cause colic, spasms, acidosis, and shock (18).

Possible Interactions with Herbs & Other Dietary Supplements

Insufficient reliable information available.

Possible Interactions with Drugs

No interactions are known to occur, and there is no known reason to expect a clinically significant interaction with kousso.

Possible Interactions with Foods

No interactions are known to occur, and there is no known reason to expect a clinically significant interaction with kousso.

Possible Interactions with Lab Tests

No interactions are known to occur, and there is no known reason to expect a clinically significant interaction with kousso.

Possible Interactions with Diseases or Conditions

GI CONDITIONS: Can irritate the gastrointestinal tract. Contraindicated in individuals with infectious or inflammatory gastrointestinal conditions (19).

Typical Dosages & Routes of Administration that are Commonly Used

No typical dosage.

Comments

Kousso is considered unsafe for oral use; avoid using. Kousso use is obsolete (18).

KUDZU

This Product is Also Known As
Fen Ke, Fenge, Gange, Ge Gen, Gegen, Japanese Arrowroot, Kudsu, Kudzu Vine, Kwaao Khruea, Mealy Kudzu, Pueraria Root, Radix Peurariae, Yege.

Scientific Names
Pueraria montana var. lobata, synonyms Pueraria lobata, Pueraria thunbergiana, Pueraria pseudohirsuta, Dolichos lobatus; Pueraria montana var. thomsonii, synonym Pueraria thomsonii; Pueraria mirifica, Pueraria tuberosa. Family: Leguminosae.

People Use This For
Orally, kudzu is used alone or in combination with other products for symptoms of alcohol hangover, such as headache, upset stomach, dizziness, and vomiting (11,766).

In traditional Chinese medicine, kudzu has been used for managing alcoholism and drunkenness, myalgia, measles (6,11), dysentery, gastritis (6), fever, diarrhea, thirst, cold, flu, neck stiffness, and as a diaphoretic (11). In recent years, kudzu has been used for hypertension, angina pectoris, arrhythmia, migraine (6,11), deafness, diabetes, traumatic injuries, sinusitis, urticaria, pruritus, and psoriasis (11).

Kudzu root is also consumed as food (11).

Safety
POSSIBLY SAFE ...when taken orally and appropriately (11,12). Daily doses of 50-100 grams kudzu root does not produce adverse effects in humans (11).
PREGNANCY AND LACTATION: Insufficient reliable information available; avoid using.

Effectiveness
There is insufficient reliable information available about the effectiveness of kudzu.

Possible Mechanism of Action & Active Ingredients
The applicable parts of kudzu are the root and flower. Isoflavone constituents (daidzin, daidzein, and puerarin) and their derivatives are thought to be reversible inhibitors of alcohol and aldehyde dehydrogenase (6). However, recent studies dispute this finding (1523,1524). Kudzu extract, daidzein, and daidzin decrease alcohol consumption and peak blood alcohol levels, and shorten alcohol-induced sleep in alcohol-craving animals (6,1523). Decreased peak blood alcohol levels might be due to delayed gastric emptying (1523). Preliminary evidence suggests that puerarin might decrease heart rate, plasma renin activity, capillary permeability, platelet aggregation (11). Puerarin demonstrates hypoglycemic, hypocholesterolemic, antiarrhythmic, antipyretic, and antioxidant activity (11). Kudzu root extracts dilate coronary and cerebral blood vessels and increase myocardial and cerebral blood flow, decrease vascular resistance, myocardial oxygen demand, and lactic acid production in anaerobic myocardial tissues; and increase the blood oxygen supply (11). Studies are needed to investigate the effect(s) of kudzu in humans.

Adverse Reactions Including Known Allergies
None reported.

Possible Interactions with Herbs & Other Dietary Supplements
Insufficient reliable information available.

Possible Interactions with Drugs
ANTICOAGULANTS: Theoretically, kudzu might potentiate the effects of anticoagulants. A constituent of kudzu inhibits platelet activating factor (11).
ASPIRIN: Theoretically, concomitant use might increase the potential for hypoglycemic effects with kudzu. Aspirin increases the hypoglycemic effects of a kudzu constituent in diabetic mice (11).
HYPOGLYCEMIC AGENTS: Theoretically, concomitant use might have additive hypoglycemic effects. A constituent of kudzu has hypoglycemic activity in animals (11).
CARDIOVASCULAR AGENTS: Theoretically, kudzu might interfere with cardiovascular therapies. Kudzu extracts decrease heart rate and have vasodilatory and antiarrhythmic effects in animals (11).

Possible Interactions with Foods
No interactions are known to occur, and there is no known reason to expect a clinically significant interaction with kudzu.

Possible Interactions with Lab Tests
BLOOD GLUCOSE: Theoretically, kudzu might decrease blood glucose levels and test results. A constituent of kudzu has hypoglycemic activity in animals (11).
SERUM CHOLESTEROL: Theoretically, kudzu might decrease serum cholesterol levels and test results. A constituent of kudzu reduces serum cholesterol levels in animals (11).

Possible Interactions with Diseases or Conditions

DIABETES: Theoretically, kudzu might interfere with blood glucose control requiring dosing adjustment of diabetes drug therapy. A constituent of kudzu has hypoglycemic activity in animals (11).

CARDIOVASCULAR CONDITIONS: Theoretically, kudzu might interfere with cardiovascular treatments. Kudzu extracts decrease heart rate and have vasodilatory and antiarrhythmic effects in animals (11).

CLOTTING DISORDERS: Theoretically, kudzu might interfere with anticoagulant therapies. A constituent of kudzu inhibits platelet activating factor (11).

Typical Dosages & Routes of Administration that are Commonly Used

ORAL: People take kudzu root extract 150-300 mg three times daily (5019). Kudzu root extract 300 mg once daily has also been used (3539). In China, people take kudzu root 9-15 grams daily (5011). Kudzu root tablets 30-120 mg (each 10 mg is equivalent to 1.5 grams of crude kudzu root) have also been used (5011).

Comments

Some commercial kudzu products are standardized for daidzin content (3538) (see Mechanism of Action).

L-ARGININE

This Product is Also Known As

Arg, Arginine, Arginine HCl, Arginine Hydrocholoride, L-Arginine HCl, L-Arginine Hydrochloride.

Scientific Names

2-Amino-5-guanidinopentanoic acid.

People Use This For

Orally, L-arginine is used for cardiovascular conditions, including congestive heart failure (6028), angina pectoris (3593) and coronary atherosclerosis (3594), intermittent claudication (3592), and erectile dysfunction (222). L-arginine is also used for prevention of the common cold, male infertility (3592), interstitial cystitis (107,114,3460), treating cyclosporine nephrotoxicity (112), and improving athletic performance (217). It is also used in combination with ibuprofen for migraine headaches (109).

Topically, L-arginine is used as an aid in wound healing, for treating cold hands and feet, and for male and female sexual dysfunction (3213,3258,3259,3260,3591).

Intravenously, L-arginine is use for intermittent claudication associated with peripheral arterial occlusive disease (3465), for detecting growth hormone deficiency, nutritional supplementation for the critically ill (111,113,115), metabolic acidosis (15), and persistent pulmonary hypertension in newborns (120).

Safety

POSSIBLY SAFE …when used orally and appropriately. L-arginine is generally considered safe and has only been associated with minor side effects in clinical studies lasting a few days to 6 months (114,3460,3593,3595,3596,6028).

…when used intravenously and appropriately as an infusion. Parenteral L-arginine is an FDA approved prescription product (15).

There is insufficient information available about the safety L-arginine for its other uses.

PREGNANCY AND LACTATION: Insufficient reliable information available; avoid using.

Effectiveness

POSSIBLY EFFECTIVE …when used orally to improve functional status and peripheral blood flow in patients with congestive heart failure (CHF). Three small-scale studies have evaluated L-arginine in CHF. In one study, supplemental L-arginine significantly improved quality of life based on questionnaire and total walking distance in 6 minutes (3595). Two studies found significantly improved peripheral vasodilation, peripheral blood flow, and arterial compliance (3595,6028). One study also found significantly improved glomerular filtration rate, creatinine clearance, and sodium and water elimination after saline loading in CHF patients receiving L-arginine (3596).

…when used orally for intractable angina pectoris associated with coronary artery disease. In one small-scale study, patients with class IV angina and frequent attacks at rest, despite treatment with standard antianginal agents, were given L-arginine orally over 3 months. Seven out of 10 patients improved from class IV to class II; one person improved to class III and two patients had no improvement. Rapid return to class IV angina occurred when L-arginine was discontinued (3593). …when taken orally for erectile dysfunction (222). In one study, oral L-arginine improved subjective assessment of sexual function in men with organic erectile dysfunction (222). …when taken orally for improving renal vasodilation and sodium excretion in renal transplant patients treated with cyclosporin (112). …when used orally for symptoms (especially pain) associated with interstitial cystitis (107,114,3460). …when used orally in combination with ibuprofen for migraine headache (109). …when used intravenously for improving clinical symptoms of intermittent claudication associated with peripheral arterial occlusive disease (3465). …when used orally for interstitial cystitis. Evidence suggests that patients with interstitial cystitis having a bladder capacity greater than 800 mL and/or a history of recurrent genitourinary infections might respond more favorably to L-arginine than patients with bladder capacity less than 800 mL and/or no history of recurrent genitourinary infections. Three months of treatment may be necessary before significant improvement occurs (3460). There is insufficient reliable information available about the effectiveness of L-arginine for its other uses.

Possible Mechanism of Action & Active Ingredients

L-arginine is an essential amino acid necessary for protein synthesis (15). It is found natural in foods such as red meat, poultry, fish and in dairy products (3592). L-arginine stimulates the release of growth hormone, prolactin, glucagon and insulin, increases gastrin concentrations, and inhibits tubular reabsorption of protein. L-arginine is also a substrate for nitric oxide synthase and increases the body's production of the vasodilator, nitric oxide (3460). The vasodilatory effects of L-arginine are thought to be useful in cardiovascular conditions, including congestive heart failure, coronary heart disease and angina, and erectile dysfunction. Oral L-arginine has been shown to improve coronary small-vessel endothelial function (110), improve brachial artery endothelium-dependent dilation and reduce monocyte/endothelial cell adhesion in coronary artery disease (116). Oral or intravenous L-arginine also improves brachial artery endothelium-dependent dilation in hypercholesterolemia (1362,1363). However, in one study, oral L-arginine did not increase serum nitric oxide levels, enhance brachial artery endothelium-dependent dilation, or effect serum levels of cell adhesion molecules in a group of healthy postmenopausal women (1361). Nitric oxide increases the relaxation of urinary tract smooth muscle (3259,3460) and is involved in erectile function. Although L-arginine appears to be helpful for erectile dysfunction, the hemodynamics of the corpus cavernosum were not affected in one study (222). When used topically for sexual dysfunction in females, L-arginine is purported to increase blood flow to the clitoris and increase sensitivity (3591); however, this effect has not been demonstrated in humans. Evidence suggests nitric oxide might be involved in host inflammatory and microbial killing responses (3460). L-arginine is a precursor for collagen synthesis and, together with fibroblast nitric oxide production, might be important for wound healing (3259,3260). L-arginine has an oral bioavailability of 68% and an elimination half-life of approximately 80 minutes (108).

Adverse Reactions Including Known Allergies

L-arginine can cause abdominal pain and bloating (15); diarrhea; gout (3595); decreased platelet count; elevations of BUN; serum creatine, and creatinine (15); allergic response or airway inflammation (15,117); and exacerbation of airway inflammation in asthma (121). Allergic reactions, including macular rash with hand and facial swelling and redness, nasal obstruction, increased pulse, sweating, and choking, have occurred. Excessively rapid infusion of L-arginine has caused flushing, nausea and vomiting, local venous irritation, numbness and headache. Extravasation has caused necrosis and superficial phlebitis (15).

Possible Interactions with Herbs & Other Dietary Supplements

Insufficient reliable information available.

Possible Interactions with Drugs

CYCLOSPORIN: L-arginine can counteract the anti-natriuretic effect of this drug (112).
ESTROGENS AND ORAL CONTRACEPTIVES elevate the growth hormone response to arginine, and reduce the glucagon and insulin response to L-arginine (15).
XYLITOL, AMINOPHYLLINE reduce the glucagon response to L-arginine (15).
MEDROXYPROGESTERONE/NORETHINDRONE reduce the L-arginine-induced growth hormone response (15).
POTASSIUM INCREASING DRUGS (ACE inhibitors, potassium-sparing diuretics): These drugs can increase the risk of L-arginine-induced hyperkalemia (15).

Possible Interactions with Foods

No interactions are known to occur, and there is no known reason to expect a clinically significant interaction with L-arginine.

Possible Interactions with Lab Tests

BLOOD UREA NITROGEN (BUN): L-arginine has been reported to increase BUN (15).
PLATELET COUNT: In one case, L-arginine has been reported to decrease platelet count (15).
SERUM CREATINE/CREATININE: L-arginine has been reported to increase serum creatine and creatinine (15).

Possible Interactions with Diseases or Conditions

ACROCYANOSIS: L-arginine can exacerbate this condition (15).
ALLERGIC TENDENCIES/ASTHMA: L-arginine can cause an allergic response or aggravate airway inflammation (15,117), and inhaled L-arginine can amplify the inflammatory airway response in people with asthma (121); use with caution.
CIRRHOSIS OF THE LIVER: L-arginine-containing infusions can lead to a hyperdynamic circulatory state related to an elevation of the plasma level of nitrous oxide by L-arginine (123); use with caution.
HERPES VIRUS: Theoretically, L-arginine might exacerbate this condition. Preliminary evidence suggests that L-arginine may be necessary for viral replication (118,119).
HYPERCHLOREMIC ACIDOSIS: The injection of L-arginine can affect the intracellular or extracellular potassium balance (15); avoid using.

RENAL FAILURE: Intravenous administration of L-arginine has been associated with life-threatening hyperkalemia and a high nitrogen load (15); contraindicated.

SICKLE CELL ANEMIA: L-arginine might exacerbate this condition (15); use with caution.

Typical Dosages & Routes of Administration that are Commonly Used

ORAL: For congestive heart failure, doses ranging from 2-5 grams three times per day has been used in clinical studies (3595,3596,6028). For angina pectoris associated with coronary artery disease, 3 grams three times per day has been used (110,3593). For interstitial cystitis, 500 mg per day has been used (114,3460). For organic erectile dysfunction, 5 grams per day has been used (222).

INTRAVENOUS: For intermittent claudication associated with peripheral arterial occlusive disease, 8 grams two times a day for 3 weeks has been used (3465).

Comments

Arginine butyrate has orphan drug status for beta-hemoglobinopathy, beta-thalassemia, and sickle cell disease (10).

L-CARNITINE

This Product is Also Known As

B(t) Factor, Carnitine, Carnitor, D-Carnitine, DL-Carnitine, Levocarnitine, Vitacarn, Vitamin B(t).
CAUTION: See separate listings for Acetyl-L-Carnitine and Propionyl-L-Carnitine.

Scientific Names

3-carboxy-2-hydroxy-N,N,N-trimethyl-1-propanaminium inner salt; (3-carboxy2-hydroxypropyl)trimethylammonium hydroxide inner salt; B-hydroxy-N-trimethyl aminobutyric acid; beta-hydroxy-gamma-trimethylammonium butyrate; L-3-hydroxy-4-(trimethylammonium)-butyrate; (R)-(3-carboxy-2-hydroxypropyl) trimethylammonium hydroxide; (R)-3-hydroxy-4-trimethylammonio-butyrate; 3-hydroxy-4-N-trimethylaminobutyrate.

People Use This For

Orally, L-carnitine is used to treat primary L-carnitine deficiency, secondary L-carnitine deficiency due to inborn errors of metabolism, and L-carnitine deficiency in people requiring hemodialysis (14,3616). It has also been used to treat L-carnitine deficiency associated with valproate toxicity (14), myopathies associated with zidovudine (14,3617,3618), and isotretinoin (3619), myocarditis associated with diphtheria (14,3620,3621), Rett Syndrome (1433,3622), chronic stable angina pectoris (9,1900,3614,3623,3624), congestive heart failure (1900,3625,3626), and myocardial infarction (9,14,3627,3628,3629). It is used as a supplement in low birthweight and preterm infants (9,1930), in strict vegetarians or vegans and in dieters (3615). L-carnitine has also been used for anorexia (1930), chronic fatigue syndrome (1930,3630), diabetes, hyperlipidemias (1900,1930,3613), peripheral vascular disease and intermittent claudication (9,3614,3631), leg ulcers (9), and to enhance athletic performance and endurance (1900,3613).

In combination, L-carnitine is used orally with acetyl-L-carnitine, fructose, and citric acid (in ProXeed) to improve sperm quality and motility in male infertility (1587).

Intravenously, L-carnitine is used to treat secondary L-carnitine deficiencies in people with inborn errors of metabolism, or who require hemodialysis (3616). It has also been used to reduce apoptosis (inappropriate programmed cell death) and increase CD4 cell counts in people with HIV infection (14,798,3632), for acute myocardial infarction (14), and as a supplement in people receiving total parenteral nutrition (14).

Safety

LIKELY SAFE ...when L-carnitine is used orally and appropriately. ...when L-carnitine injection is used as an FDA-approved prescription medicine.

Avoid using D-carnitine and DL-carnitine, because they can act as competitive inhibitors of L-carnitine and cause symptoms of L-carnitine deficiency (9,1946).

PREGNANCY: Insufficient reliable information available; avoid using.

LACTATION: POSSIBLY SAFE ...supplemental doses of L-carnitine have been given to infants in breast milk and formula with no reported adverse effects (9). The effects of large doses taken by a breastfeeding mother are unknown, but L-carnitine is secreted in the breast milk (3616).

Effectiveness

EFFECTIVE ...when L-carnitine is taken orally for acute or chronic treatment of primary L-carnitine deficiency or secondary L-carnitine deficiency due to inborn errors of metabolism (FDA-approved indications) (3616). ...when L-carnitine is given intravenously for acute and chronic treatment of people with an inborn error of metabolism which results in secondary L-carnitine deficiency (FDA-approved) (3616). ...when L-carnitine is given intravenously for prevention and treatment of L-carnitine deficiency in people with end-stage renal disease who are undergoing hemodialysis (FDA-approved) (3616).

POSSIBLY EFFECTIVE ...when L-carnitine is used intravenously or orally to improve fat utilization in preterm infants on total parenteral nutrition (9,3633,3634,3635,3636,3637). ...when L-carnitine is used intravenously for valproate-induced toxicities associated with L-carnitine deficiency (3638). ...when L-carnitine is taken orally for symptomatic

L-carnitine deficiency secondary to valproic acid (9,14). ...when L-carnitine is taken orally to improve exercise tolerance in people with chronic stable angina (9,3623,3624), to improve symptoms in people with congestive heart failure (3625,3626), or after myocardial infarction to reduce complications and mortality (9,3627,3628,3629). ...when DL-carnitine is taken orally for reducing the morbidity and mortality of myocarditis associated with diphtheria (3620,3621).
LIKELY INEFFECTIVE ...when L-carnitine is taken orally for enhancing athletic performance or endurance (1947,3639).
There is insufficient reliable information available about the effectiveness of L-carnitine for its other uses, and insufficient evidence of benefit when used as a nutritional supplement in healthy individuals (14).

Possible Mechanism of Action & Active Ingredients

L-carnitine is found in all mammalian tissue, especially striated muscle and is synthesized in the liver, kidneys and brain from the amino acids lysine and methionine (14). Approximately 98% of L-carnitine in the body is found in cardiac and skeletal muscle, with the remaining 2% being stored in the brain, kidney, and liver (14). It plays important roles in the transport of free fatty acids across the mitochondrial membrane for energy production, in the beta oxidation of fatty acids, and in maintaining an adequate ratio of fatty acyl-CoA compounds to free CoA inside the mitochondria (14). Primary tissue deficiency of L-carnitine may arise from failure of hepatic synthesis, failure of membrane transport, or disorders of reabsorption by the kidney (9,14). It is characterized by low concentrations of L-carnitine in plasma, red blood cells and/or tissues (3616). It may be present with hypoglycemia, encephalopathy, skeletal myopathy, cardiomyopathy, hepatotoxicity, and multiple organ dysfunction (9,14). L-carnitine deficiency can also occur secondary to other disorders, such as inborn errors of metabolism, cirrhosis, and hypopituitarism (9,14). Muscle L-carnitine deficiency has been reported in children with Duchenne muscular dystrophy (3640), and in people with myopathies due to zidovudine (3618) or isotretinoin (3619). Increased urinary losses of L-carnitine have been reported with ifosfamide and cisplatin therapy (3641,3642). Low serum L-carnitine levels have been reported in people receiving valproic acid therapy (14), in pregnant women (14,3643), in people with chronic fatigue syndrome (3630), and in people with HIV infection (3617). However, the relationship between serum and tissue L-carnitine levels is not fully understood and it is not known whether low serum levels necessarily lead to symptomatic deficiency (14). Symptomatic deficiency is unlikely to arise from insufficient dietary intake since the body is usually able to synthesize adequate quantities (9). However, preterm neonates have a reduced capacity to synthesize L-carnitine and they may become deficient, especially if receiving total parenteral nutrition without L-carnitine supplements (3633). Breast milk and some formulas contain L-carnitine; those that do not, generally do not induce symptomatic deficiencies in healthy, full-term infants unless a metabolic disorder is also present, although utilization of fats may be impaired (3644).
Hemodialysis is associated with significant losses of L-carnitine (3616,3645), which may contribute to malaise, muscle weakness, cardiomyopathy and cardiac arrhythmias (3616). L-carnitine supplements, usually given intravenously after dialysis, may improve exercise performance, reduce muscle cramps and hypotension, improve erythrocyte survival time, and decrease dose requirements for erythropoietin used to treat anemia (3645,3646,3647). In people with angina, a reduction in tissue L-carnitine levels has been observed during myocardial ischemia (14), and L-carnitine supplementation may improve exercise performance, reduce angina attacks, and reduce ST segment depression (9,3623,3624). In congestive heart failure, L-carnitine supplementation may improve symptoms and possibly survival (3625,3626). When taken for one to twelve months after a myocardial infarction, L-carnitine has been reported to decrease infarct size, left ventricular dilation, angina attacks, heart failure, arrhythmias, and cardiac deaths (9,3627,3628,3629). Preliminary evidence suggests that L-carnitine may improve walking distances in people with peripheral vascular disease (9,3631). Maximal exercise in trained athletes has been associated with a fall in plasma L-carnitine levels (3648), but although increases in maximum oxygen uptake and power output have been reported with L-carnitine supplements in some studies (3649,3650), there is no evidence that L-carnitine supplementation will improve exercise performance in normal individuals or trained athletes (1947,3639).
Preliminary studies have reported that daily infusions of L-carnitine may improve CD4 cell counts in people with HIV infection and reduce the percentage of CD4 and CD8 cells undergoing apoptosis (798,3632). Preliminary studies also suggest that intravenous infusions of L-carnitine may produce short-term improvements in insulin sensitivity in people with type 2 diabetes (3651,3652). Some experts think that L-carnitine supplementation improves some of the symptoms of Rett syndrome (1433); recent evidence indicates that L-carnitine improves well-being and motor skills, but more studies are needed (1433,3622).
L-carnitine and acetyl-L-carnitine are present in human sperm and seminal fluid (3607). Their levels increase in sperm during the maturation process in the epididymis and coincide with the acquisition of progressive motility (3608,3609). An increase in sperm motility is seen in vitro when L-carnitine or acetyl-L-carnitine is added to the semen sample (3612).

Adverse Reactions Including Known Allergies

L-Carnitine used orally or intravenously has been associated with nausea, vomiting, abdominal cramps, heartburn, gastritis, diarrhea, body odor, and seizures (9,14,3616).
DL-carnitine, but not L-carnitine, has been associated with myasthenia syndrome with severe weakness, muscle wasting, and discolored urine possibly due to myoglobinuria (9,14). This may be due to competitive inhibition of L-carnitine by D-carnitine, leading to symptoms of L-carnitine deficiency (14,1946).

Possible Interactions with Herbs & Other Dietary Supplements

LYSINE, METHIONINE, VITAMIN C, IRON, NIACIN, VITAMIN B6 are all required for L-carnitine production in the body (1900). Inadequate intake of these nutrients can lead to L-carnitine deficiency (1900).

D-CARNITINE: Avoid using; may cause symptoms of L-carnitine deficiency (1946).

COENZYME Q10 may have synergistic effects with L-carnitine (3653).

Possible Interactions with Drugs

HEPARIN: When used as an anticoagulant for whole plasma, heparin interferes with free and total L-carnitine radioenzyme assays, leading to inaccurate results (14).

ACENOCOUMAROL: L-carnitine may potentiate the anticoagulant effects of acenocoumarol (14).

VALPROIC ACID: L-carnitine deficiency may cause or potentiate valproic acid toxicity (14).

Drug Influences on Nutrient Levels and Depletion

SOME DRUGS CAN AFFECT L-CARNITINE LEVELS:

VALPROIC ACID (Depakene, Depakote, VPA): Valproic acid inhibits biosynthesis of carnitine and might decrease tissue uptake of carnitine. Oral L-carnitine supplementation is strongly suggested for symptomatic VPA-associated hyperammonemia, patients with multiple risk factors for VPA-associated hepatotoxicity and infants and young children taking VPA. An oral L-carnitine dosage of 100 mg/kg/day, up to a maximum of 2 g/day has been recommended (4523,4524,4525,4526,4527,4528,4529).

Possible Interactions with Foods

No interactions are known to occur, and there is no known reason to expect a clinically significant interaction with L-carnitine.

Possible Interactions with Lab Tests

CD4/CD8 COUNTS: L-carnitine infusions can increase CD4 and CD8 lymphocyte counts in some individuals with HIV-1 infection who have not been treated with antiretroviral therapy (798).

CHOLESTEROL: Intravenous L-carnitine supplementation can increase serum HDL cholesterol concentrations and test results in children on hemodialysis with type IV hyperlipoproteinemia (275).

L-CARNITINE RADIOENZYME ASSAY: Heparin, when used as an anticoagulant for whole plasma, interferes with free and total L-carnitine assays, leading to inaccurate results (14).

TRIGLYCERIDES: Intravenous L-carnitine supplementation can decrease serum triglyceride concentrations and test results in children on hemodialysis with type IV hyperlipoproteinemia (275).

Possible Interactions with Diseases or Conditions

HEMODIALYSIS/ANURIA/UREMIA: Avoid DL-carnitine; reported to cause myasthenia-like symptoms when administered by IV after dialysis (L-carnitine not reported to have this effect) (9,14).

CHRONIC LIVER DISEASE: Avoid due to impaired L-carnitine metabolism or increased L-carnitine biosynthesis, and potential for intrinsically high L-carnitine levels (1931,1948).

SEIZURES: An increase in seizure frequency or severity has been reported in people with a history of seizures who have taken L-carnitine orally or intravenously (3616).

Typical Dosages & Routes of Administration that are Commonly Used

ORAL: The recommended dose of L-carnitine for adults with primary or secondary deficiencies is 990 mg taken as tablets 2 to 3 times a day, or 1 to 3 grams of oral solution daily in divided doses (3616). The oral solution can also be used for infants or children with these conditions, and the recommended dose is 50 to 100 mg/kg/day in divided doses, to a maximum of 3 grams/day (3616). People with L-carnitine deficiencies should be under medical supervision to ensure that their dose of L-carnitine is appropriate.

As a general dietary supplement 1 to 3 grams per day L-carnitine has been used (3614,3615). For chronic stable angina and congestive heart failure 1 gram twice daily has been used (14,3623,3624,3625,3626), and doses of 2 to 6 grams daily have been used after myocardial infarction (3627,3628,3629). For peripheral vascular disease 2 grams L-carnitine twice daily has been used (14). People on hemodialysis have used 2 to 4 grams per day in divided doses (1933). For Rett syndrome, 100 mg/kg/day L-carnitine in three divided doses has been used (1433).

An oral dose of DL-carnitine of 100 mg/kg/day for 4 days has been used for myocarditis associated with diphtheria (3620,3621).

INTRAVENOUS: The recommended dose of L-carnitine for people with an inborn error of metabolism resulting in secondary L-carnitine deficiency is 50 mg/kg given as a slow (2 to 3 minute) bolus injection or by infusion followed by 50 mg/kg administered in divided doses every 3 to 4 hours over the next 24 hours. Subsequent daily maintenance doses are usually in the range of 50 mg/kg (3616). The recommended starting dose for people with L-carnitine deficiency secondary to hemodialysis is 10 to 20 mg/kg, adjusted according to plasma L-carnitine levels (3616). A dose of 10 mg/kg has been used to improve fat utilization in premature infants on total parenteral nutrition (3637), and 1 to 8 grams per day has been used as a supplement in adults on total parenteral nutrition (14). After acute myocardial infarction, doses of 100 mg/kg every 12 hours for 36 hours have been used (14).

Comments

L-carnitine is found in the diet in meat and dairy products (3613). It is FDA-approved for primary or secondary L-carnitine deficiencies (14). Only FDA approved, prescription L-carnitine should be used for these indications.

Avoid D-carnitine and DL-carnitine which are often present in over-the-counter preparations and dietary supplements. Low serum L-carnitine levels are reported to be less than 20 micromoles/L in term infants and less than 40 to 50 micromoles/L in adults on dialysis (3616).

L-TRYPTOPHAN

This Product is Also Known As
L-trypt, Tryptophan.
CAUTION: See separate listing for 5-HTP.

Scientific Names
L-2-amino-3-(indole-3-yl) propionic acid.

People Use This For
Orally, L-tryptophan is used for insomnia, depression, myofascial pain (512), premenstrual syndrome, as a treatment for smoking cessation, bruxism, grinding teeth during sleep, and to improve athletic performance.

Safety
UNSAFE ...when taken orally due to the risk of eosinophilia myalgia syndrome and death (9,512). The FDA recalled all over-the-counter L-tryptophan in 1990 (512).
PREGNANCY: UNSAFE ...contraindicated because it can cause respiratory depression in utero (14,1142).
LACTATION: UNSAFE; avoid using (14).

Effectiveness
POSSIBLY EFFECTIVE ...when taken orally for treating sleep disorders (512,1144,1146). ...when taken orally for depression (9,512,6245). In a double-blind, placebo-controlled study of 24 depressed patients receiving clomipramine, supplementation with L-tryptophan resulted in more rapid response to treatment (6245). ...when taken orally for premenstrual syndrome (6246). In a randomized controlled, 37 patients with premenstrual dysphoric disorder treated with L-tryptophan 6 g per day had greater symptomatic improvement of dysphoria, mood swings, tension and irritability than 34 women receiving placebo (6246). ...when taken orally as an adjunct treatment for smoking cessation (1138).
POSSIBLY INEFFECTIVE ...when taken orally for treating bruxism (1139), myofascial pain (1140,1145), and improving athletic performance (1135).

Possible Mechanism of Action & Active Ingredients
L-tryptophan is an essential amino acid present in concentrations of 1-2% in many plant and animal proteins (5). L-tryptophan is a precursor of serotonin and is also converted to nicotinic acid and nicotinamide (9). L-tryptophan has sedative effects in humans (1143). Dietary tryptophan depletion has been associated with bulimia relapse (1133) and deterioration of schizophrenia symptoms (1134), but it does not seem to worsen symptoms in people with untreated depression (1136). Preliminary clinical evidence suggests L-tryptophan might be helpful in seasonal affective disorder (6247).

Adverse Reactions Including Known Allergies
Taken orally, L-tryptophan can cause nausea, headache, lightheadedness, and drowsiness (9). Occasionally, sexual disinhibition, reversible dyskinesias, and reversible Parkinsonian-like rigidity can occur in people taking L-tryptophan with or after phenothiazines or benzodiazepines (9). Euphoria can happen with doses of 30-90 mg per kg body weight (14). Symptoms of eosinophilia myalgia syndrome include eosinophilia, fatigue, myalgias, multisystem organ involvement, and inflammatory disorders affecting the joints, skin, connective tissue, lungs, heart, and liver (9). More than 1500 cases of eosinophilia-myalgia syndrome and 37 deaths were associated with L-tryptophan use in the US (9,512), which led to the FDA recall of L-tryptophan in 1990 (512). All L-tryptophan-containing products that were suspected of causing EMS were traced to a single manufacturer in Japan (9). Seventeen contaminants, including 1,1'-ethylidenebis(L-tryptophan) and 3-(phenylamino)-L-alanine, were identified in a batch of L-tryptophan implicated in cases of eosinophilia myalgia syndrome; however, no causative agent was confirmed. Up to 5% of the cases were not linked to contaminated batches of L-tryptophan, suggesting that L-tryptophan can also cause eosinophilia myalgia syndrome (512).

Possible Interactions with Herbs & Other Dietary Supplements
HERBS WITH SEDATIVE PROPERTIES: Theoretically, concomitant use with herbs that have sedative properties might enhance therapeutic and adverse effects. These include calamus, calendula, California poppy, catnip, capsicum, celery, couch grass, elecampane, Siberian ginseng , German chamomile, goldenseal, gotu kola, hops, Jamaican dogwood, kava, lemon balm, sage, St. John's wort, sassafras, scullcap, shepherd's purse, stinging nettle, valerian, wild carrot, wild lettuce, withania, and yerba mansa (4,19).
SEDATIVE SUPPLEMENTS: Theoretically, it can cause additive effects when taken with supplements having sedative activity, including melatonin.

Possible Interactions with Drugs

SELECTIVE SEROTONIN REUPTAKE INHIBITORS (SSRIs): Concomitant use of L-tryptophan can result in serotonin syndrome (1141).

TRAZODONE, MONOAMINE OXIDASE INHIBITORS (MAOIs): Concomitant use of L-tryptophan can exacerbate conditions of psychosis or hypomania (14).

BENZODIAZEPINES, PHENOTHIAZINES: Concomitant use can cause sexual disinhibition, reversible dyskinesias, and reversible Parkinsonian-like rigidity (9).

SEDATIVE DRUGS: Theoretically, it can have additive effects when taken with sedative drugs.

Possible Interactions with Foods

No interactions are known to occur, and there is no known reason to expect a clinically significant interaction with L-tryptophan.

Possible Interactions with Lab Tests

EOSINOPHIL COUNT: In cases of eosinophilia myalgia syndrome, L-tryptophan can increase serum eosinophil counts and test results (9).

LIVER FUNCTION TESTS: In cases of eosinophilia myalgia syndrome, L-tryptophan can increase serum liver enzyme levels and test results (14).

Possible Interactions with Diseases or Conditions

EOSINOPHILIA: L-tryptophan is contraindicated because it can exacerbate this condition.

KIDNEY OR LIVER DYSFUNCTION: Lower amounts of L-tryptophan can be required (9).

Typical Dosages & Routes of Administration that are Commonly Used

Clinical studies for sleep disorders have used oral doses from 1 to 2.5 grams (1144,1146). For depression, 300 mg daily in combination with antidepressants has been used (6245). For premenstrual syndrome, 6 grams daily was used in one study (6246). High dose L-tryptophan (50 mg/kg/day) has been used as adjunct therapy for smoking cessation (1138).

Comments

L-tryptophan is considered unsafe for oral use due to risk of eosinophilia myalsia syndrome. It is not available as a dietary supplement in the US (14). It is unclear whether supplement manufacturers are able to produce contaminant-free, pure L-tryptophan products (512). While L-tryptophan continues to be unavailable in the US, it was reintroduced in 1994 in the UK for restricted use under carefully monitored conditions (9). Older people may require lower amounts (9).

LABDANUM

This Product is Also Known As

Ambreine, Ciste, Cyste, Rockrose.

Scientific Names

Cistus ladanifer, synonym Cistus ladaniferus; Cistus incanus, synonym Cistus villosus; Cistus polymorphus; and other Cistus species.
Family: Cistaceae.

People Use This For

Orally, labdanum is used for inflammation of the respiratory tract mucous membrane (11), bronchitis (4017), diarrhea (11), edema, hernia, tumors, leprosy, and spleen sclerosis (4017). Labdanum is also used orally for its expectorant, stimulant, purgative, and cleansing properties (11,4017).

Topically, labdanum is used for its astringent and hemostatic properties.

In foods and beverages, the absolute, oleoresin, and oil are used as flavoring agents (11).

In cosmetics, labdanum absolute and oil are used as fixative and fragrance components (11). In addition, people use labdanum as a fumigant (11) and insecticide (4017).

Safety

LIKELY SAFE ...when used orally in amounts found in foods (11). Approved for food use in the US, the oil is used at a level less than 0.001%, the absolute is used at a level less than 0.002% (11). ...when used topically in small amounts. In cosmetics, the maximum level used is 0.8% for the oil and 0.04% for the absolute (11).

POSSIBLY SAFE ...when used topically for medicinal purposes. It is nontoxic and nonirritating to human skin (11).

There is insufficient reliable information available about the safety of labdanum for oral medicinal uses.

PREGNANCY AND LACTATION: Insufficient reliable information available; avoid using.

Effectiveness

There is insufficient reliable information available about the effectiveness of labdanum.

Possible Mechanism of Action & Active Ingredients

The applicable parts of labdanum are the above ground parts. Beta-pinene, eugenol, eucalyptol (cineole), and benzaldehyde are thought to be the most active constituents of labdanum (11). Some evidence suggests the essential oil of labdanum and resin might have antibacterial and antifungal activity (11). Other evidence indicates an aqueous extract of Cistus incanus might protect against gastric lesions (4050). One study in experimental animals found that a non-alkaloid substance extracted by alcohol but not water caused liver changes (11), which might indicate some safety risks.

Adverse Reactions Including Known Allergies

There are no reports of adverse reactions associated with the oral or topical use of labdanum (11).

Possible Interactions with Herbs & Other Dietary Supplements

Insufficient reliable information available.

Possible Interactions with Drugs

No interactions are known to occur, and there is no known reason to expect a clinically significant interaction with labdanum.

Possible Interactions with Foods

No interactions are known to occur, and there is no known reason to expect a clinically significant interaction with labdanum.

Possible Interactions with Lab Tests

No interactions are known to occur, and there is no known reason to expect a clinically significant interaction with labdanum.

Possible Interactions with Diseases or Conditions

No interactions are known to occur, and there is no known reason to expect a clinically significant interaction with labdanum.

Typical Dosages & Routes of Administration that are Commonly Used

No typical dosage.

Comments

Labdanum oleoresin (gum, gum cistus) is obtained by boiling the above ground parts of labdanum (Cistus ladanifer) in water and separating the resin layer (11). Labdanum oil is distilled from the above ground parts of labdanum (Cistus ladanifer). Labdanum absolute (cyste absolute) is obtained by evaporation of the alcohol extract of fat soluble portions of labdanum (Cistus ladanifer) after removal of alcohol insoluble substances (11).

LABRADOR TEA

This Product is Also Known As

Continental Tea, Marsh Rosemary, Marsh Tea, St. James's Tea, Wild Rosemary.
CAUTION: See separate listing for Marsh Tea.

Scientific Names

Ledum groenlandicum; Ledum latifolium; Ledum palustre.
Family: Ericaceae or Laminaceae.

People Use This For

Orally, labrador tea is used as an expectorant (18).
In folk medicine, it has been used orally as an abortifacient (18), for "female disorders," sore throat, cough, pulmonary infections and other chest ailments, dysentery, diarrhea, kidney problems, rheumatism, headache, and cancer (6). Topically or in a bath, it has been used for skin problems (6,18). It was used as a substitute for more traditional tea. Some people even added the leaves to beer to make it more intoxicating (6).

Safety

POSSIBLY SAFE ...when the leaves or flowering shoots are used orally as weak tea or in small amounts (6).
LIKELY UNSAFE ...when taken orally in concentrated solutions or in large amounts. It can cause delirium, paralysis, and death (6).
PREGNANCY: UNSAFE ...contraindicated; might induce abortion (18).
LACTATION: Insufficient reliable information available; avoid using.

Effectiveness

There is insufficient reliable information available about the effectiveness of labrador tea.

Possible Mechanism of Action & Active Ingredients

The applicable parts of labrador tea are the leaf and flowering shoot. Labrador tea has expectorant activity (18) and

© Copyright 2000, Natural Medicines Comprehensive Database (209) 472-2244. For updated data, go to www.NaturalDatabase.com • 641

narcotic properties (6). The constituent ledol (ledum camphor) can cause gastrointestinal irritation (vomiting, gastroenteritis, diarrhea), central nervous system excitation, spasms and paralysis (18). The constituent grayanotoxin (andromedotoxin), can cause bradycardia, hypotension, loss of coordination, convulsions, paralysis, and death (6).

Adverse Reactions Including Known Allergies
Labrador tea can cause gastrointestinal irritation (vomiting, gastroenteritis, diarrhea), central nervous system excitation, spasms, paralysis, and death (6,18).

Possible Interactions with Herbs & Other Dietary Supplements
Insufficient reliable information available.

Possible Interactions with Drugs
No interactions are known to occur, and there is no known reason to expect a clinically significant interaction with labrador tea.

Possible Interactions with Foods
No interactions are known to occur, and there is no known reason to expect a clinically significant interaction with labrador tea.

Possible Interactions with Lab Tests
No interactions are known to occur, and there is no known reason to expect a clinically significant interaction with labrador tea.

Possible Interactions with Diseases or Conditions
No interactions are known to occur, and there is no known reason to expect a clinically significant interaction with labrador tea.

Typical Dosages & Routes of Administration that are Commonly Used
No typical dosage.

Comments
Medicinal uses of Labrador tea are now largely obsolete (18).

LABURNUM

This Product is Also Known As
Bean Trifoil, Golden Chain, Pea Tree.

Scientific Names
Cystisus laburnum.
Family: Leguminosae.

People Use This For
Laburnum is used as a pesticide. (18).

Safety
UNSAFE ...for any use (18).
PREGNANCY AND LACTATION: UNSAFE. Laburnum is contraindicated due to its toxic potential (18).

Effectiveness
There is insufficient reliable information available about the effectiveness of laburnum.

Possible Mechanism of Action & Active Ingredients
The applicable part of laburnum is the seed. There is insufficient reliable information available about the possible mechanism of action and active ingredients.

Adverse Reactions Including Known Allergies
The fatal adult dose of laburnum is 20 seeds or 3-4 unripe berries. Symptoms of laburnum poisoning include nausea, dizziness, salivation, and pain in the mouth, throat and stomach. This is accompanied by sweating, headaches, and extended, severe, and occasionally bloody vomiting. The centrally-stimulating effects of laburnum lead to tonic-clonic spasms followed by paralysis. Some patients experience anuria or uremia. Death occurs by asphyxiation (18).

Possible Interactions with Herbs & Other Dietary Supplements
Insufficient reliable information available.

Possible Interactions with Drugs
No interactions are known to occur, and there is no known reason to expect a clinically significant interaction with laburnum.

Possible Interactions with Foods

No interactions are known to occur, and there is no known reason to expect a clinically significant interaction with laburnum.

Possible Interactions with Lab Tests

No interactions are known to occur, and there is no known reason to expect a clinically significant interaction with laburnum.

Possible Interactions with Diseases or Conditions

No interactions are known to occur, and there is no known reason to expect a clinically significant interaction with laburnum.

Typical Dosages & Routes of Administration that are Commonly Used

No typical dosage.

Comments

Laburnum is considered unsafe; avoid using. Laburnum is spelled very similarly to labdanum. They are very different plants. The similar spelling could cause confusion.

LACTASE

This Product is Also Known As

None.

Scientific Names

Beta-galactosidase.

People Use This For

Orally, lactase is used for preventing symptoms of lactose intolerance, of which symptoms include cramps, diarrhea, and gas (1900).

Safety

LIKELY SAFE ...when taken orally in appropriate amounts. There is an absence of adverse effects up to 9,900 IU of lactase (2371,2372,2373). It is a FDA-approved, nonprescription product available in the US.
PREGNANCY AND LACTATION: Insufficient reliable information available; avoid using.

Effectiveness

LIKELY EFFECTIVE ...when taken orally in lactose-intolerant people for reducing GI symptoms and when used before the consumption of lactose or when added to milk prior to consumption (2371,2372,2373).

Possible Mechanism of Action & Active Ingredients

Lactase is a sugar-splitting enzyme that hydrolyzes lactose, a milk sugar, to produce glucose and galactose (9,511).

Adverse Reactions Including Known Allergies

None reported.

Possible Interactions with Herbs & Other Dietary Supplements

Insufficient reliable information available.

Possible Interactions with Drugs

No interactions are known to occur, and there is no known reason to expect a clinically significant interaction with lactase.

Possible Interactions with Foods

No interactions are known to occur, and there is no known reason to expect a clinically significant interaction with lactase.

Possible Interactions with Lab Tests

No interactions are known to occur, and there is no known reason to expect a clinically significant interaction with lactase.

Possible Interactions with Diseases or Conditions

No interactions are known to occur, and there is no known reason to expect a clinically significant interaction with lactase.

Typical Dosages & Routes of Administration that are Commonly Used

ORAL: The typical dose of lactase is 6,000-9,000 IU tablets chewed and swallowed at the start of a lactose-containing meal (2374) or 2000 IU of the solution added to 500 mL of milk immediately before consumption (2375).

Comments

Lactase deficiency can be one of several factors that predispose an individual to the development of osteoporosis, possibly through diminished calcium intake (2376,2377).

LACTOBACILLUS ACIDOPHILUS

This Product is Also Known As

Acidophilus, Probiotic.
CAUTION: See separate listings for Bifidobacterium Bifidum, Brewer's Yeast (Hansen CBS 5926), Lactobacillus GG, Saccharomyces Boulardii, and Yogurt.

Scientific Names

Lactobacillus acidophilus.
Family: Lactobacillaceae.

People Use This For

Orally, lactobacillus acidophilus is used for improving lactose tolerance, for treating vaginal and urinary tract infections, antibiotic-induced diarrhea, oral Candida infections (thrush), reducing high cholesterol levels (6), digestion problems, irritable bowel syndrome (IBS), inflammatory bowel syndrome (IBD), hives, fever blisters, canker sores, and adolescent acne (15).

Safety

LIKELY SAFE ...when used orally and appropriately (6).
CHILDREN: POSSIBLY SAFE ...when used orally for diarrhea.
PREGNANCY AND LACTATION: Insufficient reliable information available; avoid using.

Effectiveness

LIKELY EFFECTIVE ...when used orally for restoring intestinal flora (6).
POSSIBLY EFFECTIVE ...when taken orally for antibiotic-induced diarrhea, reducing recurrence of vaginal and urinary tract infections (6), relief of hives, fever blisters, canker sores, and adolescent acne (15).
LIKELY INEFFECTIVE ...when taken orally for irritable bowel syndrome (IBS) (123).
There is insufficient reliable information available about the effectiveness of lactobacillus acidophilus for its other uses (6,15).

Possible Mechanism of Action & Active Ingredients

Lactobacillus acidophilus is a native inhabitant of the human GI tract. It produces lactic acid and hydrogen peroxide, which can suppress pathogenic bacteria (6). Lactobacillus acidophilus does not appear to attach to the intestinal tissue as well as another Lactobacillus species, Lactobacillus rhamnosis (Lactobacillus GG) (4373).

Adverse Reactions Including Known Allergies

Flatulence can occur with the initial use of Lactobacillus acidophilus. It usually subsides as therapy continues (15).

Possible Interactions with Herbs & Other Dietary Supplements

Insufficient reliable information available.

Possible Interactions with Drugs

AMPICILLIN, AMOXICILLIN: Lactobacillus acidophilus can reduce or prevent antibiotic-induced diarrhea (124,125).

Possible Interactions with Foods

No interactions are known to occur, and there is no known reason to expect a clinically significant interaction with lactobacillus acidophilus.

Possible Interactions with Lab Tests

No interactions are known to occur, and there is no known reason to expect a clinically significant interaction with lactobacillus acidophilus.

Possible Interactions with Diseases or Conditions

LACTOSE INTOLERANCE: Avoid Lactobacillus acidophilus products which contain lactose as an ingredient (15).

Typical Dosages & Routes of Administration that are Commonly Used

ORAL: The typical dose of Lactobacillus acidophilus varies. The strength is sometimes quantified by the number of living organisms per capsule. People usually take 1 to 10 billion viable organisms in three or four divided doses daily (5008). Its potency can be reduced by storage conditions and the length of storage time. Refrigeration in its original container is recommended.

Comments

Lactobacillus acidophilus is also referred to as a "probiotic" agent. Lactobacillus acidophilus is found in dairy products, especially in milk and yogurt (6002). Some products labeled to contain Lactobacillus acidophilus actually contain little, or no Lactobacillus acidophilus. Products may also contain other strains of Lactobacillus, including Lactobacillus bulgaricus. Other products can contain contaminants, including Enterococcus faecium, Clostridium sporogenes, and Pseudomonas species (6). People with lactose intolerance are cautioned to avoid Lactobacillus acidophilus products which contain lactose as an ingredient.

LACTOBACILLUS GG

This Product is Also Known As
Lactobacillus Casei Strain GG, Lactobacillus Rhamnosus, Lactobacillus Rhamnosus GG, Probiotic.

Scientific Names
Lactobacillus casei sp. rhamnosus.

People Use This For
Orally, Lactobacillus GG is used in infants and young children to shorten the severity and duration of diarrhea (4369,4377). It is used orally to prevent diarrhea (4369), to prevent traveler's diarrhea, to prevent and treat diarrhea associated with antibiotics, including relapsing Clostridium difficile colitis (4367,4394), to treat Crohn's disease (4368,4381), and bacterial overgrowth in short bowel syndrome (4375). It is also used orally to prevent cancer or the formation of carcinogens, to stimulate the immune system (4369), to treat Candida-related infections (4385), and as a vaccine adjuvant (4367,4393).
Vaginally, Lactobacillus GG is used to treat persistent vaginitis symptoms (4397).

Safety
LIKELY SAFE ...when Lactobacillus GG is used orally and appropriately (4367,4380).
POSSIBLY SAFE ...when women use Lactobacillus GG vaginally (4397).
CHILDREN: LIKELY SAFE ...when used orally and appropriately (4369,4373,4377,4383).
PREGNANCY AND LACTATION: LIKELY SAFE ...when used orally and appropriately. There is insufficient reliable information about the safety of Lactobacillus GG for vaginal use during pregnancy and lactation; avoid using.

Effectiveness
LIKELY EFFECTIVE ...when Lactobacillus GG is used orally to shorten the diarrheal phase of rotavirus infection in infants and young children (4369,4377).
POSSIBLY EFFECTIVE ...when used orally to prevent antibiotic-associated diarrhea in children (4371,4372). ...when used to prevent diarrhea in undernourished children at increased risk of diarrhea (4373,4383). ...when used to prevent traveler's diarrhea (4374). ...when used along with antibiotics or following antibiotic therapy to treat recurrent Clostridium difficile diarrhea (4392,4394). ...when used in relieving symptoms of atopic eczema in infants allergic to cow's milk (4369).

Possible Mechanism of Action & Active Ingredients
When taken orally, Lactobacillus GG passes through the body and attaches to the human intestinal mucosa. There it persists for at least a week after ingestion (5500). Lactobacillus GG has several effects that can prevent or alleviate diarrhea. It shows evidence that it can affect the immune system, and perhaps promote the gut immunological barrier (4368,4369). It competes with pathogenic viruses for binding sites on epithelial cells (4369), and it can increase the intestinal mucus to prevent organisms from attaching to intestinal cells (4388). Some evidence suggests Lactobacillus GG might be effective in removing the food toxin aflatoxin B1 (4376). Other information suggests Lactobacillus GG might enhance resistance to Salmonella typhimurium C5 infection (4378), colon cancer (4382,4387), and act as a vaccine adjuvant (4393). Preliminary research suggests Lactobacillus GG might be beneficial in protecting young children from developing milk allergy (4379) as well as preventing immune response in individuals who are hypersensitive to milk (4399).

Adverse Reactions Including Known Allergies
Lactobacillus GG is very rarely associated with infection. It can cause bacteremia in severely ill or immunocompromised individuals (4380,4393). There is one report of the organism being isolated from a pericardial infusion following a bone marrow transplant in a child (4391) and another of a liver abscess in an elderly woman (4398). Lactobacillus GG was not being used therapeutically in either case.

Possible Interactions with Herbs & Other Dietary Supplements
Insufficient reliable information available.

Possible Interactions with Drugs
ANTIFUNGALS: Antifungals inactivate Lactobacillus GG.

Possible Interactions with Foods

No interactions are known to occur, and there is no known reason to expect a clinically significant interaction with Lactobacillus GG.

Possible Interactions with Lab Tests

No interactions are known to occur, and there is no known reason to expect a clinically significant interaction with Lactobacillus GG.

Possible Interactions with Diseases or Conditions

SEVERE IMMUNOCOMPROMISE: Rarely, Lactobacillus can cause bacteremia in severely immunocompromised individuals (4393).

Typical Dosages & Routes of Administration that are Commonly Used

ORAL: For infants or toddlers with diarrhea, 5-10 billion live Lactobacillus GG used in rehydrating solution (4369,4370). To prevent antibiotic-associated diarrhea in young children, two doses of 10 billion live Lactobacillus GG in capsules were used during antimicrobial treatment (4372). For recurrent Clostridium difficile, 125 mg was given twice daily for 2 weeks. Each gram contained 5 billion viable Lactobacillus GG organisms (4394). For milk hypersensitivity in adults, 2600 million Lactobacillus GG were used per day (4399). VAGINAL: For vaginitis 1 billion Lactobacillus GG in glycerol suppositories used twice daily for 7 days (4397).

Comments

Although there is at least one case of vancomycin-resistant Lactobacillus GG infection (4390), the resistance factor from Lactobacillus GG is not closely related to the type that causes resistance in enterococcal organisms (4389).

LACTOFERRIN

This Product is Also Known As

Bovine lactoferrin.

Scientific Names

Lactoferrin.

People Use This For

Orally, lactoferrin is used for stimulating the immune system, preventing tissue damage related to aging, promoting healthy intestinal flora, regulating iron metabolism, and as an antioxidant, antibacterial, and antiviral agent (2489).

Safety

There is insufficient reliable information available about the safety of lactoferrin.
Pregnancy and Lactation: Insufficient reliable information available; avoid using.

Effectiveness

There is insufficient reliable information available about the effectiveness of lactoferrin.

Possible Mechanism of Action & Active Ingredients

Lactoferrin is an iron binding protein (a transferrin) found in the milk of several mammalian species, including humans (511). In experimental animals, it appears to offer protection from bacterial infection (2490). Preliminary evidence in healthy males suggests supplementation may increase the phagocytic activity of polymorphonuclear leukocytes and the proportion of natural killer cells in the host defense system (2490). In vitro, lactoferrin B, a peptide derived from lactoferrin, has antibacterial activity against a wide range of gram positive and gram negative bacteria (2491).

Adverse Reactions Including Known Allergies

None reported.

Possible Interactions with Herbs & Other Dietary Supplements

Insufficient reliable information available.

Possible Interactions with Drugs

No interactions are known to occur, and there is no known reason to expect a clinically significant interaction with lactoferrin.

Possible Interactions with Foods

No interactions are known to occur, and there is no known reason to expect a clinically significant interaction with lactoferrin.

Possible Interactions with Lab Tests

No interactions are known to occur, and there is no known reason to expect a clinically significant interaction with lactoferrin.

Possible Interactions with Diseases or Conditions

No interactions are known to occur, and there is no known reason to expect a clinically significant interaction with lactoferrin.

Typical Dosages & Routes of Administration that are Commonly Used

ORAL: People typically take 250 mg daily (5272).

Comments

There is very little scientific information about this product. Our staff is continually analyzing the available information on natural medicines and will add data here as it becomes available.

LADY FERN

This Product is Also Known As

Brake Root, Common Polypod, Oak Fern, Rock Brake, Rock of Polypody.

Scientific Names

Athyrium filix-femina.
Family: Dryopteridaceae.

People Use This For

Orally, lady fern is used for respiratory and gastrointestinal illnesses. It is also used orally as an expectorant (18).

Safety

There is insufficient reliable information available about the safety of lady fern.
Pregnancy and Lactation: Insufficient reliable information available; avoid using.

Effectiveness

There is insufficient reliable information available about the effectiveness of lady fern.

Possible Mechanism of Action & Active Ingredients

The applicable part of lady fern is the root/rhizome. There is insufficient reliable information available about the possible mechanism of action and active ingredients.

Adverse Reactions Including Known Allergies

None reported.

Possible Interactions with Herbs & Other Dietary Supplements

Insufficient reliable information available.

Possible Interactions with Drugs

No interactions are known to occur, and there is no known reason to expect a clinically significant interaction with lady fern.

Possible Interactions with Foods

No interactions are known to occur, and there is no known reason to expect a clinically significant interaction with lady fern.

Possible Interactions with Lab Tests

No interactions are known to occur, and there is no known reason to expect a clinically significant interaction with lady fern.

Possible Interactions with Diseases or Conditions

No interactions are known to occur, and there is no known reason to expect a clinically significant interaction with lady fern.

Typical Dosages & Routes of Administration that are Commonly Used

ORAL: 1-2 tablets or 10-20 drops of a liquid preparation are taken 3 times daily when it is used for functional gastrointestinal illnesses or as a digestive (18).

Comments

There is very little scientific information about this product. Our staff is continually analyzing the available information on natural medicines and will add data here as it becomes available.

LADY'S BEDSTRAW

This Product is Also Known As
Cheese Rennet, Cheese Renning, Curdwort, Ladys Bedstraw, Maid's Hair, Petty Mugget, Yellow Cleavers, Yellow Galium.

Scientific Names
Galium verum.
Family: Rubiaceae.

People Use This For
In folk medicine, lady's bedstraw has been used orally for treating swollen ankles, as a diuretic for bladder and kidney mucous discharge (18), for cancer, epilepsy, hysteria, spasms, tumors, and for relief of chest and lung ailments. It is also used orally to induce sweating, as a tonic, to stimulate appetite, as an aphrodisiac, and for astringent, cleansing, and purgative effects (4017). In folk medicine, lady's bedstraw has been used topically for poorly healing wounds (18), and to stop bleeding (4017).

Safety
There is insufficient reliable information available about the safety of lady's bedstraw.
Pregnancy and Lactation: Insufficient reliable information available; avoid using.

Effectiveness
There is insufficient reliable information available about the effectiveness of lady's bedstraw.

Possible Mechanism of Action & Active Ingredients
The applicable parts of lady's bedstraw are the above ground parts. There is insufficient reliable information available about the possible mechanism of action and active ingredients.

Adverse Reactions Including Known Allergies
None reported.

Possible Interactions with Herbs & Other Dietary Supplements
Insufficient reliable information available.

Possible Interactions with Drugs
No interactions are known to occur, and there is no known reason to expect a clinically significant interaction with lady's bedstraw.

Possible Interactions with Foods
No interactions are known to occur, and there is no known reason to expect a clinically significant interaction with lady's bedstraw.

Possible Interactions with Lab Tests
No interactions are known to occur, and there is no known reason to expect a clinically significant interaction with lady's bedstraw.

Possible Interactions with Diseases or Conditions
No interactions are known to occur, and there is no known reason to expect a clinically significant interaction with lady's bedstraw.

Typical Dosages & Routes of Administration that are Commonly Used
ORAL: Typically, lady's bedstraw is used as a tea (18).
TOPICAL: Lady's bedstraw is used as a poultice. To prepare, pour 250 mL cold water over 2 heaping teaspoons of above ground parts, bring to simmer, and allow to steep (18).

Comments
Lady's bedstraw is considered obsolete for medicinal use (18).

LAMINARIA

This Product is Also Known As
Brown Algae, Horsetail, Kelp, Makombu Thallus, Sea Girdles, Seagirdle Thallus.
CAUTION: See separate listings for Algin and Bladderwrack.

Scientific Names
Laminaria digitata; Laminaria japonica.
Family: Laminariaceae.

People Use This For

Orally, the whole plant of laminaria is used as a bulk laxative and for treating radioactive intoxication (6). Topically, it is used as "a tent" placed into the cervix to cause cervical dilation prior to D & C, for removal of intrauterine devices, for diagnostic procedures, for relief of cervical stenosis, and to facilitate uterine placement of therapeutic radium (6). Laminaria tents are also used in pregnancy for near-term or term cervical ripening particularly for a first pregnancy, to facilitate labor, alone or as adjunct to prostaglandins, and for inducing first-trimester abortions (6).

Sodium alginate, a derivative of laminaria, is used orally as a bulk laxative and in combination with antacids for gastroesophageal reflux (272).

In folk medicine, laminaria has been used orally as a hypotensive agent (6).

Safety

POSSIBLY SAFE ...when the derivative, sodium alginate, is used as a bulk laxative or in combination with an antacid for gastro-esophageal reflux (272).

There is insufficient reliable information available about the safety of the other uses of laminaria.

PREGNANCY: POSSIBLY UNSAFE ...when the plant is used locally for cervical ripening because there is an increased risk of infection and the cervical wall could rupture (6). LIKELY UNSAFE ...when used topically to induce labor because use is associated with maternal endometriosis, neonatal sepsis, fetal hypoxia, and intrauterine death (6). UNSAFE ...when used orally; contraindicated because of potential hormonal effects (19).

LACTATION: LIKELY UNSAFE ...contraindicated for oral use because of potential toxicity (19).

Effectiveness

POSSIBLY EFFECTIVE ...when the derivative, sodium alginate, is used as a bulk laxative (6,11,272). ...when laminaria is used orally for absorption of strontium (11). ...when laminaria is used topically for cervical ripening (6). There is insufficient reliable information available about the effectiveness of laminaria for its other uses.

Possible Mechanism of Action & Active Ingredients

Laminaria contains iodine, and is considered to be a rich source of iron and potassium (19). The constituents of laminaria include alginate, lamine, and laminarin (6). Much of the utility of laminaria relates to its ability to form a viscous colloidal solution of gel in water. This allows laminaria to function as a bulk laxative (6). It also allows laminaria to be used to dilate the cervix for procedures or to ripen the cervix and hasten the onset of labor. For these uses, laminaria "tents" are inserted cervically. They absorb ambient moisture, gradually swelling to a diameter of 1/2 inch over 4-6 hours. This swelling causes cervical dilation that can induce labor (6). The mechanism of cervical "ripening" might be similar to that of a foreign body that disrupts the normal chorioamniotic balance and initiates prostaglandin synthesis. That, in turn, causes myometrial contractions and cervical ripening. An alternative theory is that laminaria causes ripening because it contains high levels of the prostaglandin precursor, arachidonic acid. Still another theory is that laminaria causes partial detachment of the placenta and induces cervical dilation (6). Although laminaria can reduce the duration of labor induction, it is associated with an increased risk for maternal endometritis and neonatal sepsis (6). Some laminaria constituents might also have medical uses. The polysaccharide constituent of laminaria, laminarin, has antilipemic activity when partially sulfated and anticoagulant activity similar to heparin when more extensively sulfated (6). The basal portion of laminaria blades are used as a hypotensive agent; the constituents histamine and lamine may be responsible for hypotensive effects (6). Alginate-containing kelp reduces absorption of radioactive strontium in animals and humans (6) and it has been used for managing radioactive intoxication (6). However, the risk of adverse effects resulting from laminaria's iodide content may outweigh the benefits of its use as a routine preventative measure (515).

Adverse Reactions Including Known Allergies

Use for cervical ripening is associated with neonatal and maternal infection (6). Uterine contractions associated with laminaria use have been implicated in fetal hypoxia and subsequent intrauterine death (6). Tent use is also associated with possible rupture of the cervical wall and subsequent infection (6).

Possible Interactions with Herbs & Other Dietary Supplements

POTASSIUM SUPPLEMENTS: Theoretically, concomitant use can increase the risk of hypokalemia (19).

Possible Interactions with Drugs

POTASSIUM SUPPLEMENTS: Theoretically, concomitant use can increase the risk of hypokalemia (19).

POTASSIUM-SPARING DIURETICS: Contraindicated. Theoretically concomitant use may cause hyperkalemia (19).

ACE INHIBITORS: Use of angiotensin converting enzyme inhibitors is contraindicated. Theoretically, concomitant use might increase the risk of hyperkalemia (19).

DIGOXIN: Caution; theoretically, laminaria may cause hyperkalemia in susceptible individuals, potentiating digoxin effects and adverse effects (19).

Possible Interactions with Foods

No interactions are known to occur, and there is no known reason to expect a clinically significant interaction with laminaria.

Possible Interactions with Lab Tests

POTASSIUM: Theoretically, may increase serum levels and test results (19).

Possible Interactions with Diseases or Conditions

RENAL INSUFFICIENCY: CAUTION; theoretically, laminaria may induce hyperkalemia in people with renal insufficiency on a potassium restricted diet (19).

Typical Dosages & Routes of Administration that are Commonly Used

ORAL: People use capsules or tablets containing 500 to 650 mg of ground laminaria once daily (5008).

Comments

In a small study of "tent" use (see People Use This For) with manufacturer recommended procedures, no infection occurred. Manufacturer recommendation included prior swabbing of the cervical canal with a suitable lubricant and antibacterial agent, then packing the canal with antibacterial gel (6).

LARCH ARABINOGALACTAN

This Product is Also Known As

AG, Ara-6, Larch, Larch Gum, Larix, Mongolian Larch, Mongolian Larchwood, Stractan, Western Larch, Wood Gum, Wood Sugar.
CAUTION: See separate listing for Larch Turpentine.

Scientific Names

Larix dahurica; Larix occidentalis.
Family: Pinaceae.

People Use This For

Orally, larch arabinogalactan is used for the common cold, flu, metastatic liver disease, pediatric otitis media, HIV/AIDS, adjunctive therapy during cancer chemotherapy, and as a dietary fiber supplement, immunostimulant, anti-inflammatory agent, and for hepatic encephalopathy (6,3529,3530,3531).
In food products, Larch arabinogalactan is used as a stabilizer, emulsifier, binder, and sweetener (3529).

Safety

LIKELY SAFE ...when used in amounts found in foods. Larch arabinogalactan is approved by the FDA for use in foods (3529).
POSSIBLY SAFE ...when used orally, appropriately, and short-term in therapeutic amounts (6,3529,3530).
There is insufficient reliable information available about the safety of the long-term use of larch arabinogalactan.
PREGNANCY AND LACTATION: Insufficient reliable information available; avoid using.

Effectiveness

There is insufficient reliable information available about the effectiveness of larch arabinogalactan.

Possible Mechanism of Action & Active Ingredients

Larch arabinogalactan is a polysaccharide produced from the bark of the Larch tree. Arabinogalactans are found throughout nature and are found in other plants with immunostimulatory activity, including echinacea. Larch arabinogalactan is thought to have immunostimulatory effects by increasing release of interferon gamma, tumor necrosis fact alpha, interleukin-1 and interleukin-6 and stimulating phagocytosis and natural killer cell activity. Larch arabinogalactan is a fibrous product which ferments in the gut. It increases gut microflora, e.g., Lactobacillus, increases short-chain fatty acid production, and minimizes ammonia production and absorption. These effects suggest it may be beneficial as a dietary fiber supplement for improving gastrointestinal health and as an adjunct for treating hepatic encephalopathy. Larch arabinogalactan has been shown to concentrate in the liver. Some people think it might block hepatic receptors for metastatic cells and decrease liver metastases (3529,3530).

Adverse Reactions Including Known Allergies

When taken orally, bloating and flatulence have been reported (3530).

Possible Interactions with Herbs & Other Dietary Supplements

Insufficient reliable information available.

Possible Interactions with Drugs

ORAL DRUGS: Theoretically, concurrent administration might decrease the absorption of some oral drugs due to the fibrous nature of larch arabinogalactan.
IMMUNOSUPPRESSANTS: Theoretically, larch arabinogalactan might interfere with immunosuppression therapy due its immunostimulatory activity.

Possible Interactions with Foods

No interactions are known to occur, and there is no known reason to expect a clinically significant interaction with larch arabinogalactan.

Possible Interactions with Lab Tests

No interactions are known to occur, and there is no known reason to expect a clinically significant interaction with larch arabinogalactan.

Possible Interactions with Diseases or Conditions

TRANSPLANT RECIPIENTS: Theoretically, larch arabinogalactan might interfere with immunosuppression therapy.

Typical Dosages & Routes of Administration that are Commonly Used

ORAL: For colds and the flu, mix one teaspoon of larch arabinogalactan powder in juice or water and take 2-3 times daily until symptoms are relieved. Best if used when symptoms first appear (3531).

Comments

Larch arabinogalactan specifically concentrates in hepatocytes and might have future application as a diagnostic tool or as a vehicle for delivering drugs to the liver (3529,3530).

LARCH TURPENTINE

This Product is Also Known As

Terebinthina Laricina, Terebinthina Veneta, Venetian Turpentine.
CAUTION: See separate listing for Larch Arabinogalactan.

Scientific Names

Larix decidua.
Family: Pinaceae.

People Use This For

Topically, larch turpentine is used for treating neuralgia, rheumatic discomfort, furuncles (2), fevers, colds, cough, bronchitis, tendency toward infection, blood pressure problems, and inflammation of the mouth and pharynx (18).

Safety

POSSIBLY SAFE ...when larch turpentine preparations are used topically and appropriately on intact skin (2).
POSSIBLY UNSAFE ...when larch turpentine is used orally (18). ...when larch turpentine is used topically on damaged skin, particularly if used on large areas (18). Skin damage allows systemic absorption, which can cause kidney and central nervous system toxicity (18). ...when larch turpentine is inhaled, because it can cause acute airway inflammation (18).
PREGNANCY AND LACTATION: Insufficient reliable information available; avoid using.

Effectiveness

POSSIBLY EFFECTIVE ...when larch turpentine is used topically for treating neuralgia (2). ...when larch turpentine is used topically for treating rheumatic discomfort (2). ...when larch turpentine is used topically for treating bronchitis (2). ...when larch turpentine is used topically for treating furuncles (2).
There is insufficient reliable information available about the effectiveness of larch turpentine for its other uses.

Possible Mechanism of Action & Active Ingredients

Larch turpentine is an oily exudate obtained by drilling into the trunks of Larix decidua trees. It contains up to 20% volatile oil (2). When topically applied, it increases local blood flow and can have an antiseptic effect (2).

Adverse Reactions Including Known Allergies

When used topically, larch turpentine can cause allergic skin reactions (2). When taken orally or applied to large areas of skin or damaged skin, it can cause kidney and central nervous system damage (18). Inhalation can cause acute respiratory tract inflammation (18).

Possible Interactions with Herbs & Other Dietary Supplements

Insufficient reliable information available.

Possible Interactions with Drugs

No interactions are known to occur, and there is no known reason to expect a clinically significant interaction with larch turpentine.

Possible Interactions with Foods

No interactions are known to occur, and there is no known reason to expect a clinically significant interaction with larch turpentine.

Possible Interactions with Lab Tests
No interactions are known to occur, and there is no known reason to expect a clinically significant interaction with larch turpentine.

Possible Interactions with Diseases or Conditions
BRONCHITIS: Inhalation of larch turpentine is contraindicated; may worsen respiratory tract inflammation (2).

Typical Dosages & Routes of Administration that are Commonly Used
TOPICAL: The ointments, gels, emulsions, and oils commonly contain 10 to 20 percent larch turpentine as liniments for external application (2).

Comments
None.

LARKSPUR

This Product is Also Known As
Knight's Spur, Lark Heel, Lark's Claw, Lark's Toe, Staggerweed.

Scientific Names
Delphinium consolida.
Family: Ranunculaceae.

People Use This For
Orally, larkspur is used as an anthelmintic, diuretic, sedative, and appetite stimulant (18).

Safety
There is insufficient reliable information available about the safety of larkspur.
Pregnancy and Lactation: Insufficient reliable information available; avoid using.

Effectiveness
There is insufficient reliable information available about the effectiveness of larkspur.

Possible Mechanism of Action & Active Ingredients
The applicable part of larkspur is the flower. Animal data suggests that larkspur may have a paralyzing effect on peripheral and motor nerve endings and the central nervous system. Fatal animal poisonings due to asphyxiation have been reported with larkspur (18).

Adverse Reactions Including Known Allergies
None reported.

Possible Interactions with Herbs & Other Dietary Supplements
Insufficient reliable information available.

Possible Interactions with Drugs
No interactions are known to occur, and there is no known reason to expect a clinically significant interaction with larkspur.

Possible Interactions with Foods
No interactions are known to occur, and there is no known reason to expect a clinically significant interaction with larkspur.

Possible Interactions with Lab Tests
No interactions are known to occur, and there is no known reason to expect a clinically significant interaction with larkspur.

Possible Interactions with Diseases or Conditions
No interactions are known to occur, and there is no known reason to expect a clinically significant interaction with larkspur.

Typical Dosages & Routes of Administration that are Commonly Used
No typical dosage.

Comments
Use of larkspur should probably be avoided (18). Avoid confusing larkspur with Delphinium orientale (18).

LATHYRUS

This Product is Also Known As
Caley Pea , Chickling Vetch and Chick-Pea, Everlasting Pea, Flat-Podded Vetch, Singletary Pea, Spanish Vetchling, Sweet Pea, Wild Pea.

Scientific Names
Lathyrus cicera; Lathyrus clymenu; Lathyrus hirsutus; Lathyrus incanus; Lathyrus odoratus; Lathyrus pusillus; Lathyrus sativus; Lathyrus sylvestris.
Family: Leguminosae.

People Use This For
As a food, Lathyrus sativus is used in unleavened Indian bread (6). Lathyrus seeds are eaten as food and used as animal fodder throughout the world (6).
The flowers of sweet pea (Lathyrus odoratus) are cultivated for their color and fragrance (6).

Safety
LIKELY UNSAFE ...when used orally. The seeds of Lathyrus sativus, Lathyrus cicera, and Lathyrus clymenum can be neurotoxic (6).
PREGNANCY AND LACTATION: LIKELY UNSAFE; avoid using.

Effectiveness
There is insufficient reliable information available about the effectiveness of lathyrus.

Possible Mechanism of Action & Active Ingredients
Lathyrus seeds contain multiple constituents including phytates, divicine, and a mixture of alkaloids (6). The toxicity of lathyrus results from several compounds. The neurotoxic effects are linked to constituent beta-N-oxalyl-L-alpha, beta-diaminopropionic acid (ODAP). Constituent beta-aminopropionitrile (BAPN) causes skeletal abnormalities and damage to blood vessels (6).

Adverse Reactions Including Known Allergies
Lathyrus can cause neurotoxic manifestations including muscular rigidity, spasticity, weakness, paralysis of leg muscles, weak pulse, shallow breathing, convulsions, or death (6). Prolonged neurotoxicity is characterized by poor central motor coordination and reduced nerve conduction in the lower limbs (6).

Possible Interactions with Herbs & Other Dietary Supplements
Insufficient reliable information available.

Possible Interactions with Drugs
No interactions are known to occur, and there is no known reason to expect a clinically significant interaction with lathyrus.

Possible Interactions with Foods
No interactions are known to occur, and there is no known reason to expect a clinically significant interaction with lathyrus.

Possible Interactions with Lab Tests
No interactions are known to occur, and there is no known reason to expect a clinically significant interaction with lathyrus.

Possible Interactions with Diseases or Conditions
No interactions are known to occur, and there is no known reason to expect a clinically significant interaction with lathyrus.

Typical Dosages & Routes of Administration that are Commonly Used
Avoid use of certain Lathyrus species (Lathyrus sativus, Lathyrus cicera, and Lathyrus clymenum).

Comments
Neurolathyrism and its complications are rare in western countries, yet they have been documented for more than a century in Europe, Africa, and Asia. Despite the attempt to ban the sale of Lathyrus sativus in several states of India, distribution continues. To deactivate the toxin, several methods have been tried. Typically they involve soaking the seeds in water followed by steaming or sun drying. Roasting the seeds at high temperatures for twenty minutes also helps to destroy the neurotoxic constituent. However, these methods are only 80-85% effective (6).

© Copyright 2000, Natural Medicines Comprehensive Database (209) 472-2244. For updated data, go to www.NaturalDatabase.com

LAURELWOOD

This Product is Also Known As
Alexandrian-laurel, Alexandrinischer Lorbeer, Borneo-mahogany, Caulophyllum Tree, Indian-laurel, Kamani Punna, Palo de Santa Maria, Palo Maria, Punnanga, Undi.

Scientific Names
Calophyllum inophyllum.
Family: Clusiaceae, Guttiferae.

People Use This For
Orally, the laurelwood constituent (+)-calanolide A is used for HIV infection (4290).
Topically, tamanu oil from the nut of the laurelwood is used for skin ailments (4287) including sunburn, rashes, burns, psoriasis, dermatitis, scratches, skin blemishes, acne, skin allergies, bedsores, rosacea, and hemorrhoids; and for infant skin care.
In folk medicine, laurelwood is used for leprosy, piles, scabies, gonorrhea, vaginitis, and chicken pox (4287).

Safety
POSSIBLY SAFE ...when the laurelwood constituent (+)-calanolide A is used orally by HIV-negative individuals (4290).
There is insufficient reliable information available about the safety of laurelwood for its other uses.
PREGNANCY AND LACTATION: Insufficient reliable information available; avoid using.

Effectiveness
There is insufficient reliable information about the effectiveness of laurelwood.

Possible Mechanism of Action & Active Ingredients
Laurelwood is one of many species of Calophyllum. Each species contains somewhat different constituents but many species including Calophyllum cordato-oblongum, Calophyllum lanigerum, Calophyllum teysmannii (synonym Calophyllum miqueli), and Calophyllum cerasiferum as well as the laurelwood contain constituents that seem to have activity against the HIV virus. Recent interest has centered on the calanolide compounds, particularly (+)-calanolide A. This constituent, now in phase I testing, appears to be a unique and specific non-nucleoside inhibitor of the reverse transcriptase of the HIV-1 virus (4292,4293). It does not appear to have activity against HIV-2 (4295). Some evidence suggests calanolide A might have synergistic effects with zidovudine (Retrovir), lamivudine (Epivir), nelfinavir (Viracept) (4290), and nevirapine (Viramune) (4294). At least two isomers of calanolide A known as costatolide and dihydrocostatolide possess similar properties (4291,4292). Calanolide A also shows evidence of antituberculosis effects (4290).

Adverse Reactions Including Known Allergies
The oral use of the laurelwood constituent, (+)- calanolide A, by healthy individuals can cause dizziness, oily aftertaste, headache, and nausea (4290). There are no reported adverse reactions when tamanu oil from the nut of laurelwood is used topically.

Possible Interactions with Herbs & Other Dietary Supplements
Insufficient reliable information available.

Possible Interactions with Drugs
AIDS DRUGS: Some evidence suggests the laurelwood (+)-calanolide A constituent might have synergistic effects with zidovudine (Retrovir), lamivudine (Epivir), nelfinavir (Viracept), and nevirapine (Viramune) (4290,4294).

Possible Interactions with Foods
No interactions are known to occur, and there is no known reason to expect a clinically significant interaction with laurelwood.

Possible Interactions with Lab Tests
No interactions are known to occur, and there is no known reason to expect a clinically significant interaction with laurelwood.

Possible Interactions with Diseases or Conditions
No interactions are known to occur, and there is no known reason to expect a clinically significant interaction with laurelwood.

Typical Dosages & Routes of Administration that are Commonly Used
No typical dosage.

Comments
The laurelwood constituent (+)-canolide A is in Phase IB testing as an anti-HIV agent. The purpose of the current study is to determine its safety and its effect on development of resistance, CD4 count and viral load (4289).

Phase IA testing in 94 healthy HIV-negative individuals showed it was well tolerated (4290). Sarawak MediChem Pharmaceuticals Inc. (Lemont, Illinois) is the agency supporting testing (4289). Avoid confusing laurelwood (Caulophyllum inophyllum) with blue cohosh (Caulophyllum thalictroides).

LAVENDER

This Product is Also Known As

Alhucema, Common Lavender, English Lavender, French Lavender, Garden Lavender, Spanish Lavender, Spike Lavender, True Lavender.
CAUTION: See separate listing for Lavender Cotton.

Scientific Names

Lavandula angustifolia, synonyms Lavandula officinalis, Lavandula vera, Lavandula spica; Lavandula stoechas; Lavandula latifolia; Lavandula dentata; Lavandula pubescens.
Family: Lamiaceae.

People Use This For

Orally, lavender flower and oil are used for restlessness, insomnia, nervous stomach, meteorism (abdominal swelling from gas in the intestinal or peritoneal cavity) (2,18), and loss of appetite (18).
Topically, it is used in baths for functional circulatory disorders (18).
As an inhalant, lavender is used to treat insomnia (6).
Traditionally, the flower and oil have been used for flatulence, colic spasms, giddiness, nervous headaches, migraines, toothaches, sprains, neuralgia, rheumatism, acne, pimples, sores, nausea, and vomiting (11). Spike lavender was used in Europe to promote menstruation and treat cancer (11).
In foods and beverages, lavender products are used as flavor components (11).
In manufacturing, lavender products are utilized in pharmaceutical products (11) and as fragrance ingredients in soaps and cosmetics (11). Another use of lavender is as an insect repellent (6).

Safety

LIKELY SAFE ...when consumed in amounts commonly found in foods and beverages (11), and lavender is Generally Recognized as Safe (GRAS) for food use in the US (11).
POSSIBLY SAFE ...when appropriately used for oral or topical medicinal purposes (2,12).
There is insufficient reliable information available about the safety of inhaling lavender.
PREGNANCY AND LACTATION: Insufficient reliable information available; avoid using.

Effectiveness

POSSIBLY EFFECTIVE ...when taken orally for restlessness, insomnia, nervous stomach irritations, Roehmheld syndrome, nervous internal discomfort, and meteorism (abdominal swelling from gas in the intestinal or peritoneal cavity) (2). ...when applied topically as a bath additive for treating functional circulatory disorders (2). ...when used as aromatherapy for insomnia (6).
There is insufficient reliable information available about the effectiveness of lavender for its other uses.

Possible Mechanism of Action & Active Ingredients

The applicable parts of lavender are the flower and oil. The lavender constituent perillyl alcohol is reported to have anticancer activity in vitro and in experimental animals. It is being investigated for treating human breast, ovarian, and prostate cancers (6). It also reduces vein graft intimal hyperplasia in rabbits and reduces hepatic HMG-CoA reductase activity (6). The lavender volatile oil, which is obtained by steam distillation of lavender flowers, has anticonvulsant effects against electroshock, potentiates chloral hydrate, and has pentobarbital effects in experimental rodents (6,7). As a bath additive, lavender oil reduces postpartum perineal discomfort in humans (6). The decline in selective EEG potentials induced by lavender oil correlate with vigilance, expectancy, and alertness in humans, suggesting sedative and relaxing effects (7). Spike lavender oil has spasmolytic effects on animal smooth muscle (6). Preparations of Lavandula stoechas cause hypoglycemia in normoglycemic rats (6).

Adverse Reactions Including Known Allergies

When taken orally in appropriate amounts, lavender does not commonly cause adverse effects, but the topical use of lavender rarely can cause contact dermatitis (6).

Possible Interactions with Herbs & Other Dietary Supplements

HERBS WITH SEDATIVE OR ANTIFLATULENT EFFECTS: The use of combination products with other sedative and/or antiflatulent herbs can be beneficial (2).

Possible Interactions with Drugs

BARBITURATES, CHLORAL HYDRATE: Theoretically, lavender can potentiate these drug effects (6,7).
CNS DEPRESSANTS: Theoretically, lavender can enhance the therapeutic and adverse effects of CNS depressants.

HMG-CoA REDUCTASE INHIBITORS: Theoretically, it can potentiate the effects of these drugs due to the perillyl alcohol content (6).

Possible Interactions with Foods
No interactions are known to occur, and there is no known reason to expect a clinically significant interaction with lavender.

Possible Interactions with Lab Tests
SERUM CHOLESTEROL: Theoretically, lavender can decrease serum levels and test results (6).

Possible Interactions with Diseases or Conditions
No interactions are known to occur, and there is no known reason to expect a clinically significant interaction with lavender.

Typical Dosages & Routes of Administration that are Commonly Used
ORAL: The typical dose of lavender is one cup of the tea several times a day, especially before bedtime (8). The tea is prepared by steeping 1.5 grams of the flowers in 150 mL boiling water for 5-10 minutes and then straining. The usual dose of the lavender oil is 1-4 drops (20-80 mg) on a sugar cube (2).
TOPICAL: For bath therapy, 20-100 grams of the lavender flowers are commonly steeped in 2 L boiling water, strained, and then added to a bath (2,18).

Comments
Lavender is a popular component for perfumes, potpourri, and decorations (6002). Lavender is commonly adulterated with related species, including Lavandula hybrida, which is a cross between Lavandula angustifolia and Lavandula latifolia, from which lavandin oil is obtained (8).

LAVENDER COTTON

This Product is Also Known As
Santolina.
CAUTION: See separate listing for Lavender.

Scientific Names
Santolina chamaecyparissias.
Family: Asteraceae.

People Use This For
Orally, lavender cotton is used for digestive disorders, premenstrual syndrome, worm infestations, jaundice, and as a spasmolytic. It is also used as an anti-inflammatory (18).
Topically, lavender cotton is used as an insect repellent (4017).

Safety
There is insufficient reliable information available about the safety of lavender cotton.
Pregnancy and Lactation: Insufficient reliable information available; avoid using.

Effectiveness
There is insufficient reliable information available about the effectiveness of lavender cotton.

Possible Mechanism of Action & Active Ingredients
The applicable parts of lavender cotton are the above ground parts. There is insufficient reliable information available about the possible mechanism of action and active ingredients.

Adverse Reactions Including Known Allergies
Lavender cotton can cause an allergic reaction in individuals sensitive to the Asteraceae/Compositae family. Members of this family include ragweed, chrysanthemums, marigolds, daisies, and many other herbs.

Possible Interactions with Herbs & Other Dietary Supplements
Insufficient reliable information available.

Possible Interactions with Drugs
No interactions are known to occur, and there is no known reason to expect a clinically significant interaction with lavender cotton.

Possible Interactions with Foods
No interactions are known to occur, and there is no known reason to expect a clinically significant interaction with lavender cotton.

Possible Interactions with Lab Tests

No interactions are known to occur, and there is no known reason to expect a clinically significant interaction with lavender cotton.

Possible Interactions with Diseases or Conditions

CROSS-ALLERGENICITY: Can cause an allergic reaction in individuals sensitive to the Asteraceae/Compositae family. Members of this family include ragweed, chrysanthemums, marigolds, daisies, and many other herbs.

Typical Dosages & Routes of Administration that are Commonly Used

ORAL: People typically prepare cotton root bark using one teaspoon boiled in a covered container with 3 cups of water for 30 minutes. The liquid is cooled slowly in the closed container and taken cold, 1 to 2 cups per day (5254).

Comments

The whole lavender cotton plant is used externally as a moth and insect repellent due to its strong smell (18). Lavender cotton is unrelated to lavender and its scent is distinctly different from that of lavender (513).

LECITHIN

This Product is Also Known As

Egg Lecithin, Ovolecithin, Soybean Lecithin, Vegilecithin, Vitellin.
CAUTION: See separate listings for Choline and Phosphatidylcholine.

Scientific Names

None.

People Use This For

Orally, lecithin is used for treating dementia and Alzheimer's disease (5135,5136,5137,5149,5150,5151,5152), for extrapyramidal disorders (5138,5139), reducing hepatic steatosis (fat accumulation) in long-term parenteral nutrition patients (5140), treating gallbladder disease (5141,5142,5155), aiding ultrafiltration in peritoneal dialysis (5143), treating liver disease (5144), treating manic-depressive illness (5145), improving memory (5146), treating hypercholesterolemia (5147,5148), for anxiety (5154), and eczema (5154). It is also used as a source of choline, inositol, phosphorus, and linoleic and linolenic acids (5153).
Topically, lecithin is used as a moisturizing agent for dermatitis and dry skin (4921).
As a pharmaceutical and food additive, lecithin is used for emulsifying and stabilizing water-based products, (9), and as an antioxidant in foods and pharmaceutical preparations (16). In the manufacture of preparations for intravenous and subcutaneous use, lecithin is used both as an emulsifying agent and a stabilizing agent (15,19).

Safety

LIKELY SAFE …when used orally in amounts found in foods. It has Generally Recognized as Safe (GRAS) status in the US (4912). …when used orally for medicinal purposes in amounts up to 80 mg day (4914). …when used topically (4914). …when used in an injection intravenously or subcutaneously (16,4914).
PREGNANCY AND LACTATION: Insufficient reliable information available; avoid using in amounts greater than found in foods.

Effectiveness

LIKELY EFFECTIVE …when used intravenously for reducing hepatic steatosis in long-term parenteral nutrition patients (14,5140). …when used topically for dermatitis and dry skin (4921).
POSSIBLY INEFFECTIVE …when used orally for treating gallbladder disease (5141,5142,5155). …when used orally for treating hypercholesterolemia (5147,5148).
LIKELY INEFFECTIVE …when used orally for dementia and Alzheimer's disease (5135,5136,5149,5150,5151,5152). …when used orally for extrapyramidal disorders (5138,5139).
There is insufficient reliable information available about the effectiveness of lecithin for its other uses.

Possible Mechanism of Action & Active Ingredients

Lecithin is a phospholipid composed of phosphatidyl esters (phosphatides), chiefly consisting of phosphatidylcholine, phosphatidylethanolamine, phosphatidylserine and phosphatidylinositol, and varying amounts of other substances such as triglycerides, fatty acids, and carbohydrates, depending on source (9). For example, egg lecithin contains 69% phosphatidylcholine and 24% phosphatidylethanolamine, while soybean lecithin contains 24% phosphatidylcholine, 22% phosphatidylethanolamine, and 19% phosphatidylinositol. Lecithin is a precursor to acetylcholine (5156).

Adverse Reactions Including Known Allergies

Oral lecithin can cause diarrhea, nausea, abdominal pain, or fullness (5136,5138,5140).

Possible Interactions with Herbs & Other Dietary Supplements

Insufficient reliable information available.

Possible Interactions with Drugs

No interactions are known to occur, and there is no known reason to expect a clinically significant interaction with lecithin.

Possible Interactions with Foods

No interactions are known to occur, and there is no known reason to expect a clinically significant interaction with lecithin.

Possible Interactions with Lab Tests

No interactions are known to occur, and there is no known reason to expect a clinically significant interaction with lecithin.

Possible Interactions with Diseases or Conditions

No interactions are known to occur, and there is no known reason to expect a clinically significant interaction with lecithin.

Typical Dosages & Routes of Administration that are Commonly Used

ORAL: A typical oral dose is 1.2–2.4 grams/day (5153).

Comments

Unlike choline, lecithin does not cause unpleasant body and breath odor (5153). Lecithin contains phosphatidylcholine, which contains choline (16). Although closely related, these terms are not synonymous.

LEECH

This Product is Also Known As

Fresh Water Leech, Leeches, Medicinal Leech.

Scientific Names

Hirudo medicinalis.

People Use This For

Topically, leeches are used for stimulating blood flow and relieving venous congestion at postoperative surgical flap sites (2971,2972,2974,2978,2979,2989,2990,2991) and at sites of surgical reattachment, such as fingers, toes, or ears (2971,2978,2990). They are also used for hematoma drainage (2985), varicose veins (2973), purpura fulminans (2975), macroglossia (2976), bladder extrophy (2977), infectious myocarditis (2992), and ear diseases including tinnitus, otitis media, and acute external otitis (2981).

Safety

LIKELY SAFE ...when used topically to aid in blood flow and for venous congestion in post-surgical wound management of flaps and after surgical reattachment (6). Leeches should not be used for self-treatment.
PREGNANCY AND LACTATION: Insufficient reliable information available; avoid using.

Effectiveness

POSSIBLY EFFECTIVE ...when used topically for stimulating blood flow and treating venous congestion at postoperative surgical flap sites (2971,2972,2974,2978,2979,2989,2990,2991) and after surgical reattachment (2971,2978,2990). There is insufficient reliable information available about the effectiveness of leeches for other uses.

Possible Mechanism of Action & Active Ingredients

In vitro, leech saliva inhibits platelet aggregation induced by thrombin, collagen, adenosine diphosphate (ADP), epinephrine, platelet activating factor, and arachidonic acid (2993,2994). No effects on coagulation time or prothrombin time were noted in one study (2962). Leech saliva contains a variety of substances including hirudin, which has anticoagulant properties (see Comments) (6). Hirudin inhibits thrombin when it is bound to a fibrin clot (2995). Other constituents of leech saliva include a vasodilator, a hyaluronidase that aids in the spread of the anticoagulant through the tissue, a collagenase, two fibrinases, and callin, and a platelet adhesion inhibitor (6,2963,2996). There is conflicting evidence whether a constituent with anesthetic activity is present (2997,2998).

Adverse Reactions Including Known Allergies

The use of leeches can cause infections, including those caused by Aeromonas (2964,2965,2968,2970), and Vibrio (2966). Excessive blood loss, anemia (2967,2963), contact dermatitis (2969), allergic reactions (2969), loss of leeches in body orifices (2967), and adverse psychological responses can also occur (2967). In addition, the topical use of leeches can cause epistaxis (2980,2986), tracheal obstruction (2982), hematemesis (2984), and bleeding (2987,2988) due to unrecognized nasal, throat, and vaginal leech infestation.

Possible Interactions with Herbs & Other Dietary Supplements

Insufficient reliable information available.

Possible Interactions with Drugs

ASPIRIN, WARFARIN, NONSTEROIDAL ANTI-INFLAMMATORY DRUGS (NSAIDs): Theoretically, leeches can increase the risk of bleeding in people using these drugs.

Possible Interactions with Foods

No interactions are known to occur, and there is no known reason to expect a clinically significant interaction with leeches.

Possible Interactions with Lab Tests

HEMOGLOBIN, HEMATOCRIT: Leeches can decrease hemoglobin, hematocrit, and test results.

Possible Interactions with Diseases or Conditions

ARTERIAL INSUFFICIENCY: Leeches are contraindicated due to an increased risk of infection (2983).
IMMUNOCOMPROMISED PATIENTS: Theoretically, there can be a risk of overwhelming sepsis with the use of leeches in these patients (2963).
CLOTTING ABNORMALITIES: Theoretically, leeches can increase the risk of excessive bleeding.

Typical Dosages & Routes of Administration that are Commonly Used

TOPICAL: One leech is typically applied two to four times a day for up to one week (6). Leeches are for one-time use and never to be reused (2989). Dispose of used leeches properly per facility guidelines.

Comments

Leeches are unsafe for self-medication. Lepirudin (rDNA), a recombinant hirudin analog, is an FDA-approved prescription drug with specific, direct thrombin-inhibiting activity. Lepirudin is available as an injectable product.

LEMON

This Product is Also Known As

Limon.

Scientific Names

Citrus limon.
Family: Rutaceae.

People Use This For

Orally, lemon is used as a source of vitamin C in the treatment of scurvy, low resistance, and colds. It is also used as an anti-inflammatory, diuretic, and to improve vascular permeability.
Lemon is also used as a food and flavoring agent (18).

Safety

LIKELY SAFE ...when used in amounts found in foods (12).
POSSIBLY SAFE ...when used orally for medicinal purposes in amounts similar to those found in foods (12).
PREGNANCY AND LACTATION: Avoid using in amounts greater than those typically found in foods.

Effectiveness

There is insufficient reliable information available about the effectiveness of lemon.

Possible Mechanism of Action & Active Ingredients

The applicable parts of lemon are the fruit and peel. There is insufficient reliable information to suggest active ingredients or a mechanism of action for lemon. It does contain vitamin C (18).

Adverse Reactions Including Known Allergies

None reported.

Possible Interactions with Herbs & Other Dietary Supplements

Insufficient reliable information available.

Possible Interactions with Drugs

No interactions are known to occur, and there is no known reason to expect a clinically significant interaction with lemon.

Possible Interactions with Foods

No interactions are known to occur, and there is no known reason to expect a clinically significant interaction with lemon.

Possible Interactions with Lab Tests

No interactions are known to occur, and there is no known reason to expect a clinically significant interaction with lemon.

Possible Interactions with Diseases or Conditions

No interactions are known to occur, and there is no known reason to expect a clinically significant interaction with lemon.

Typical Dosages & Routes of Administration that are Commonly Used

ORAL: Lemon is taken as an oil, tincture or fresh fruit (18).

Comments

None.

LEMON BALM

This Product is Also Known As

Balm, Cure-All, Dropsy Plant, Honey Plant, Melissa, Melissae folium, Melissenblatt, Sweet Balm, Sweet Mary.

Scientific Names

Melissa officinalis.
Family: Lamiaceae or Labiatae.

People Use This For

Orally, lemon balm is used for promoting digestion, as a mild tranquilizer, for stimulating appetite (11), as an antispasmodic, for Graves' disease (6), and for functional gastrointestinal disorders with distention and gas (2,18). Topically, it is used for cold sores (herpes labialis) (1,6).
Traditionally, lemon balm has been used for promoting sweating, promoting menstrual flow, for female discomforts, nervous problems, insomnia, cramps, headache, toothache, sores, tumors, insect bites (11), nervous stomach, hysteria and melancholia, chronic bronchial mucous membrane inflammation, nervous palpitations, vomiting, and high blood pressure (18).
In foods and beverages, the extract and oil are utilized (11).

Safety

LIKELY SAFE ...when consumed in amounts found in foods (11). Lemon balm is Generally Recognized as Safe (GRAS) in the US for food use with a maximum level of 0.5% in baked goods (11).
POSSIBLY SAFE ...when used appropriately for oral or topical medicinal purposes on a short-term basis (1,2). The maximum length of use is 14 days (1).
PREGNANCY AND LACTATION: Insufficient reliable information available; avoid using.

Effectiveness

POSSIBLY EFFECTIVE ...when used orally for nervous sleeping disorders and functional gastrointestinal complaints (2). ...when used topically for treating herpes labialis (cold sores) (1,790).
There is insufficient reliable information available about the effectiveness of lemon balm for its other uses.

Possible Mechanism of Action & Active Ingredients

The applicable part of lemon balm is the leaf. Lemon balm has sedative, antiflatulent, spasmolytic, antibacterial, and antiviral activities (2). Activities were formerly attributed to volatile oil; however, a volatile oil free hydroalcoholic extract shows sedative activity in mice (6). Hot water extracts have antiviral effects in egg and cell cultures against herpes simplex virus (6,11) mumps, vaccinia, Newcastle disease (11), and HIV-1 (6). Lemon balm's antiviral activity is due to the tannin and polyphenol constituents (6,11). Freeze-dried extracts containing the constituents, rosmarinic acid and lithospermic acid, bind thyrotropin and block activation of thyrotropin receptor sites (6).

Adverse Reactions Including Known Allergies

Hypersensitivity reactions have been reported (9). There is one report of irritation and one report of exacerbation of herpes symptoms when lemon balm was applied topically (790).

Possible Interactions with Herbs & Other Dietary Supplements

HERBS WITH SEDATIVE PROPERTIES: Theoretically, concomitant use with herbs that have sedative properties might enhance therapeutic and adverse effects. These include calamus, calendula, California poppy, catnip, capsicum, celery, couch grass, elecampane, ginseng Siberian, German chamomile, goldenseal, gotu kola, hops, Jamaican dogwood, kava, sage, St. John's wort, sassafras, scullcap, shepherd's purse, stinging nettle, valerian, wild carrot, wild lettuce, withania root, and yerba mansa (4,19).

Possible Interactions with Drugs

THYROID HORMONE: Theoretically, may interfere with replacement therapy (6).
BARBITURATES: Theoretically, concomitant use with barbiturates may cause additive effects and side effects (19).

OTHER DRUGS WITH SEDATIVE PROPERTIES: Theoretically, concomitant use with drugs with sedative properties may cause additive effects and side effects (19).

Possible Interactions with Foods
No interactions are known to occur, and there is no known reason to expect a clinically significant interaction with lemon balm.

Possible Interactions with Lab Tests
No interactions are known to occur, and there is no known reason to expect a clinically significant interaction with lemon balm.

Possible Interactions with Diseases or Conditions
HYPOTHYROID CONDITIONS: Contraindicated because lemon balm can exacerbate or interfere with treatment (500).

Typical Dosages & Routes of Administration that are Commonly Used
ORAL: The typical dose of lemon balm is one cup of tea several times daily as needed (2,18). The tea is prepared by steeping 1.5-4.5 grams of the leaf in 150 mL boiling water for 10 minutes and then straining. The average amount of lemon balm is 8-10 grams of the leaves per day (18). Used as a combination product with other sedative or antiflatulent herbs can be beneficial (2). The common dose of the tincture (1:5 in 45% alcohol) is 2-6 mL three times daily (1).
TOPICAL: For herpes labialis (cold sores), the cream or ointment containing 1% of a 70:1 lyophilized aqueous extract is usually applied two to four times daily from first sign of prodrome to a few days after the lesions have healed (1). The maximum length of use is 14 days (1). Alternatively, a tea is applied to the lesions with a saturated cotton ball several times daily (3). The tea is prepared by steeping 2-3 teaspoons (2-3 grams) of the finely cut leaf in 150 mL boiling water for 5-10 minutes and then straining.

Comments
None.

LEMON VERBENA

This Product is Also Known As
Herb Louisa, Lemon-Scented Verbena, Louisa.
CAUTION: See separate listing for Verbena.

Scientific Names
Aloysia triphylla, synonyms Aloysia citriodora, Lippia citriodora, Verbena citriodora, Verbena triphylla.
Family: Verbenaceae.

People Use This For
Orally, lemon verbena is used for digestive disorders, agitation, and insomnia (18).
Historically, it has been used for asthma, cold, fever, flatulence, colic, diarrhea, indigestion (4), febrile hemorrhoids, varicose veins, skin conditions, chills, and constipation (18).
In foods and manufacturing, lemon verbena is used as an ingredient in herbal teas (4), as a fragrance component in perfumes (6), and also as an ingredient in alcoholic beverages (4).

Safety
LIKELY SAFE ...when consumed in amounts found in alcoholic beverages since it has Generally Recognized as Safe (GRAS) status in the US for human consumption in alcoholic beverages (4).
POSSIBLY SAFE ...when taken in appropriate amounts as an oral medicinal agent (12).
There is insufficient reliable information available about the safety of the topical use of lemon verbena.
PREGNANCY AND LACTATION: Insufficient reliable information available; avoid excessive amounts (4).

Effectiveness
There is insufficient reliable information available about the effectiveness of lemon verbena.

Possible Mechanism of Action & Active Ingredients
The applicable parts of lemon verbena are the leaf and flower top. Oil of verbena (the essential oil distilled from lemon verbena leaf) may be acaricidal and bactericidal (6). Terpene-rich volatile oils in the plant are considered irritants (4).

Adverse Reactions Including Known Allergies
During excretion, volatile oils may irritate the kidneys (4). Topically, contact dermatitis is possible (6).

Possible Interactions with Herbs & Other Dietary Supplements
Insufficient reliable information available.

Possible Interactions with Drugs
No interactions are known to occur, and there is no known reason to expect a clinically significant interaction with lemon verbena.

Possible Interactions with Foods
No interactions are known to occur, and there is no known reason to expect a clinically significant interaction with lemon verbena.

Possible Interactions with Lab Tests
No interactions are known to occur, and there is no known reason to expect a clinically significant interaction with lemon verbena.

Possible Interactions with Diseases or Conditions
KIDNEY DISEASE: Avoid excessive amounts due to possible kidney irritation (4).

Typical Dosages & Routes of Administration that are Commonly Used
ORAL: One cup tea (steep 5-29 grams leaf in 1 L boiling water 10-15 minutes, strain) two to five times daily (18).
TOPICAL: No typical dosage.

Comments
None.

LEMONGRASS

This Product is Also Known As
British Indian Lemongrass, Capim-Cidrao, Ceylon Citronella Grass, Citronella, Cochin Lemongrass, East Indian Lemongrass, Fever Grass, Guatemala Lemongrass, Lemon Grass, Madagascar Lemongrass, West Indian Lemongrass.
CAUTION: See separate listings for Citronella Oil and Stone Root.

Scientific Names
Cymbopogon citratus, synonym Andropogon citratus; Cymbopogon flexuosus; Cymbopogon nardis.
Family: Gramineae or Poaceae.

People Use This For
Orally, lemongrass is used for treating intestinal spasms, gastrointestinal disorders, hypertension, convulsions, pain and neuralgia, vomiting, cough, rheumatism, fever (6), common cold, exhaustion, as an antiseptic (2), and as a mild astringent and stomach tonic (18).
Topically, lemon grass is used for headache, stomachache, abdominal pain, and rheumatic pain (11).
In Chinese medicine, lemongrass is used for headache, stomachache, abdominal pain, and rheumatic pain (11).
In food and beverages, lemongrass is used as a flavoring (6,11).
In manufacturing, lemongrass is used as a fragrance in soaps and cosmetics. Lemongrass is also used in synthesizing vitamin A and natural citral (11).

Safety
LIKELY SAFE ...when used orally in amounts found in foods (maximum use level 0.004% in baked goods) (11). It has Generally Recognized as Safe (GRAS) status in the US (11).
POSSIBLY SAFE ...when lemongrass is used as an oral or topical medicinal agent (6,12); no adverse reactions were reported during two weeks of daily human use (2612).
PREGNANCY: LIKELY UNSAFE ...contraindicated, due to uterine and menstrual flow stimulation (12).
LACTATION: Insufficient reliable information available; avoid using.

Effectiveness
There is insufficient reliable information available about the effectiveness of lemongrass.

Possible Mechanism of Action & Active Ingredients
The applicable part of lemongrass is the leaf. West Indian lemongrass seems to have antimicrobial properties especially against gram-positive bacteria and fungi. It is a CNS depressant (11), though one human trial found lemongrass lacks central nervous system effects (2612). West Indian lemongrass is also said to have analgesic, antipyretic, and antioxidant properties (11), as well as uterine and menstrual flow stimulating effects (12).

Adverse Reactions Including Known Allergies
Rare allergic reactions have occurred following topical use (2,18). There have been two cases of toxic alveolitis associated with inhalation of an unknown quantity of lemongrass oil (2). There is a single report of fatal poisoning after a child ingested a lemongrass oil-based insect repellent (2).

Possible Interactions with Herbs & Other Dietary Supplements
Insufficient reliable information available.

Possible Interactions with Drugs
No interactions are known to occur, and there is no known reason to expect a clinically significant interaction with lemongrass.

Possible Interactions with Foods
No interactions are known to occur, and there is no known reason to expect a clinically significant interaction with lemongrass.

Possible Interactions with Lab Tests
AMYLASE, BILIRUBIN: Lemongrass may cause elevations in serum bilirubin (direct) and amylase levels (2612).

Possible Interactions with Diseases or Conditions
No interactions are known to occur, and there is no known reason to expect a clinically significant interaction with lemongrass.

Typical Dosages & Routes of Administration that are Commonly Used
ORAL: People typically use 1 to 2 teaspoons of lemongrass in 6 oz boiling water as a tea (6006).
TOPICAL: No typical dosage.

Comments
Avoid confusion with citronella oil.

LENTINAN

This Product is Also Known As
None.
CAUTION: See separate listing for Shiitake Mushroom.

Scientific Names
Polysaccharide derived from Lentinus edodes, synonyms Lenticus edodes, Lentinan edodes, Lentinula edodes, Tricholomopsis edodes.
Family: Polyporaceae.

People Use This For
Lentinan is given by intravenous, intramuscular, and intraperitoneal injection as an adjunctive treatment for cancer (6) and HIV infection (1107).

Safety
There is insufficient reliable information available about the safety of lentinan.
Pregnancy and Lactation: Insufficient reliable information available; avoid using.

Effectiveness
POSSIBLY EFFECTIVE ...when given by injection as adjunctive treatment for breast, gastric, and prostate cancer (6,1108,1109,1112,1113) and as adjunctive treatment with didanosine (ddI) in HIV infection (1107).

Possible Mechanism of Action & Active Ingredients
Lentinan is not directly cytotoxic, but may augment natural killer cell activity, activate macrophages and may enhance T-helper cell function (6). It may enhance the anti-HIV effects of zidovudine (6).

Adverse Reactions Including Known Allergies
Mild thrombocytopenia (6); minor adverse effects (unspecified) were reported in clinical trials (one case report) (6). Rapid intravenous infusion of lentinan is reported to cause "oppression" of the anterior chest and dryness of the throat; these symptoms disappeared with slow drip infusion (1111).

Possible Interactions with Herbs & Other Dietary Supplements
Insufficient reliable information available.

Possible Interactions with Drugs
DIDANOSINE (ddI, Videx): Concomitant use of the nucleoside reverse transcriptase inhibitor (NRTI)-type antiretroviral drug didanosine with lentinan might enhance drug-induced increases in CD4 levels in HIV+ patients (1107).

Possible Interactions with Foods
No interactions are known to occur, and there is no known reason to expect a clinically significant interaction with lentinan.

Possible Interactions with Lab Tests

CD4 COUNTS: Intravenously administered lentinan, combined with didanosine (ddI, Videx), might enhance drug-induced increases in CD4 concentrations and test results in some HIV+ patients with low CD4 counts (1107).

Possible Interactions with Diseases or Conditions

MALNUTRITION: In one clinical trial, gastric cancer patients with low serum protein levels (consistent with poor nutritional status) did not respond to lentinan therapy, while patients with normal serum protein levels (consistent with adequate nutritional status) had favorable responses to lentinan (1110).

Typical Dosages & Routes of Administration that are Commonly Used

ORAL: No typical dosage.
INJECTION: 1-4 mg per week have been used in clinical trials (6,1108,1111).

Comments

Lentinan is a polysaccharide derived from shiitake mushroom (Lenticus edode).

LESSER CELANDINE

This Product is Also Known As

Ficaria, Figwort, Pilewort, Ranunculus, Smallwort.
CAUTION: See separate listings for Greater Celandine, Amaranth, Bulbous Buttercup, and Jewelweed.

Scientific Names

Ranunculus ficaria.
Family: Ranunculaceae.

People Use This For

Orally, lesser celandine is used for scurvy (18).
Topically, it is used for bleeding wounds and gums, swollen joints, warts, scratches (18), and hemorrhoids (internal or prolapsed piles, with or without hemorrhage) (4,18).
For food uses, fresh leaf sheaths are sometimes used in salads (18).

Safety

POSSIBLY SAFE ...when small amounts of fresh leaf sheaths are eaten (18).
POSSIBLY UNSAFE ...when used topically (4,18). Extended contact with the fresh, bruised plant can cause blisters (18).
LIKELY UNSAFE ...when used as an oral medicinal; avoid (4,18).
PREGNANCY AND LACTATION: LIKELY UNSAFE ...contraindicated; avoid using (4).

Effectiveness

There is insufficient reliable information available about the effectiveness of lesser celandine.

Possible Mechanism of Action & Active Ingredients

The applicable parts of lesser celandine are the above ground parts. Lesser celandine contains large amounts of vitamin C (18). It also has astringent and demulcent effects (4). Protoanemonin, a constituent, is believed to be an acrid skin irritant (4). However, when the above ground parts are dried or prepared, protoanemonin changes into a pungent, volatile intermediate that quickly dimerizes to a form that does not irritate the mucous membrane (18). Some studies suggest the constituents, anemonin and protoanemonin, might have antibacterial and antifungal activity (4). The saponin constituents show some evidence of antihemorrhoidal activity (4). Large amounts of protoanemonin-forming plants have caused death of experimental animals by asphyxiation (18).

Adverse Reactions Including Known Allergies

Oral use is associated with severe GI irritation, colic, diarrhea, and irritation of the urinary tract (18). One report associates the use of lesser celandine with a case of recurrent, acute hepatitis (390). Topical use can cause mucous membrane and skin irritation (18). Extended contact with fresh, bruised plant can cause blisters (18). Some Ranunculus species also cause photodermatitis (19).

Possible Interactions with Herbs & Other Dietary Supplements

Insufficient reliable information available.

Possible Interactions with Drugs

No interactions are known to occur, and there is no known reason to expect a clinically significant interaction with lesser celandine.

Possible Interactions with Foods

No interactions are known to occur, and there is no known reason to expect a clinically significant interaction with lesser celandine.

Possible Interactions with Lab Tests

No interactions are known to occur, and there is no known reason to expect a clinically significant interaction with lesser celandine.

Possible Interactions with Diseases or Conditions

GI CONDITIONS: Can irritate gastrointestinal tract. Contraindicated in individuals with infectious or inflammatory gastrointestinal conditions (19).

Typical Dosages & Routes of Administration that are Commonly Used

ORAL: No typical dosage.
TOPICAL: Liquid extract (1:1 in 25% alcohol), 2-5 mL 3 times daily (4). Ointment (3%) or Pilewort Ointment (30% fresh herb in benzoinated lard) (4). Liquid extract can be added to baths for hemorrhoids, warts or scratches (18).

Comments

Avoid confusion with greater celandine (Chelidonium majus). Scrophularia nodosa (Family: Scrophulariaceae) is also referred to as figwort (4). Amaranth and bulbous buttercup are also referred to as pilewort.

LEVANT BERRY

This Product is Also Known As

Cocculus Indicus, Coculus Fructus, Fish Berries, Fish Killer, Hockle Elderberry, Indian Berry, Levant Nut, Louseberry, Poisonberry.

Scientific Names

Anamirta cocculus, synonyms Anamirta paniculata, Menispermum cocculus, Menispermum Lacunosum; Cocculus suberosus; Cocculus lacunosus.
Family: Menispermaceae.

People Use This For

Orally, levant berry is used for peripheral and vestibular nystagmus and peripherally-based dizziness (18).
Topically, it is used as a powder to treat scabies (6).
Historically, the constituent, picrotoxin, was used for treating epilepsy, night sweats, and as a stimulant for barbituric acid poisoning (6,18).
In India, the leaves are inhaled as snuff to relieve malaria (6); whole fruits are used for paralyzing fish and killing birds or dogs (6); picrotoxin is applied to arrow tips for hunting by jungle tribes (6), and was formerly used to paralyze fish in the fishing industry (18); extracts are applied topically for lice (6).

Safety

POSSIBLY UNSAFE ...when applied topically; avoid application to broken skin (6).
LIKELY UNSAFE ...when used orally; avoid due to toxic potential (6). Picrotoxin 30 mg/kg or 2-3 cocculus kernels can cause death (6,18).
PREGNANCY AND LACTATION: LIKELY UNSAFE; avoid using.

Effectiveness

There is insufficient reliable information available about the effectiveness of levant berry.

Possible Mechanism of Action & Active Ingredients

The applicable parts of levant berry are the dried fruit and seed. The seed contains highly toxic picrotoxin (6,18), which stimulates the central nervous system via parasympathetic nerves, is a GI irritant, stimulates the medulla oblongata resulting in changes in respiration rate, slows heart rate due to vagal nerve stimulation, and increases blood pressure (6,18).

Adverse Reactions Including Known Allergies

Picrotoxin is a GI irritant and central nervous system stimulant (6). Mild poisoning can lead to headache, dizziness, nausea, coordination disturbances, depression and spasms or twitching (18). Larger amounts can cause salivation, vomiting, purging, rapid shallow breathing, drowsiness, palpitations or bradycardia, tonic-clonic spasms, stupor, loss of consciousness, and death (6). The lethal dose is stated to be 30 mg/kg (6) or 2-3 Cocculus kernels (seeds) (18).

Possible Interactions with Herbs & Other Dietary Supplements

Insufficient reliable information available.

Possible Interactions with Drugs

No interactions are known to occur, and there is no known reason to expect a clinically significant interaction with levant berry.

Possible Interactions with Foods

No interactions are known to occur, and there is no known reason to expect a clinically significant interaction with levant berry.

Possible Interactions with Lab Tests

No interactions are known to occur, and there is no known reason to expect a clinically significant interaction with levant berry.

Possible Interactions with Diseases or Conditions

No interactions are known to occur, and there is no known reason to expect a clinically significant interaction with levant berry.

Typical Dosages & Routes of Administration that are Commonly Used

Avoid using.

Comments

Although picrotoxin is used experimentally, medicinal use has been abandoned in the US and Europe (6).

LICORICE

This Product is Also Known As

Alcacuz, Alcazuz, Chinese Licorice, Gan Cao, Gan Zao, Glycyrrhiza, Lakritze, Licorice Root, Liquiritiae radix, Liquirizia, Liquorice, Orozuz, Phytoestrogen, Reglisse, Regliz, Russian Licorice, Spanish Licorice, Subholz, Sweet Root.

Scientific Names

Glycyrrhiza glabra; Glycyrrhiza glabra typica; Glycyrrhiza glabra violacea; Glycyrrhiza glabra glandulifera; Glycyrrhiza uralensis, Reglisse.
Family: Fabaceae or Leguminaceae.

People Use This For

Orally, licorice is used for inflammation of the upper respiratory tract mucous membranes, gastric and duodenal ulcers (2), bronchitis, chronic gastritis, colic, primary adrenocortical insufficiency (4), dry cough, arthritis, lupus, and as an antibacterial and antiviral agent (4). It is also used to treat cholestatic liver disorders, hypokalemia, and hypertonia (6121).

Topically, licorice is used as a shampoo to reduce sebum secretion (6).

Intravenously, licorice components are used for treating hepatitis B and C (3247,3248,3249,3250,3251).

In combination with Panax ginseng and Bupleurum falcatum, licorice is used orally to help stimulate adrenal gland function, particularly in patients with a history of long-term corticosteroid use (3234). As a component of the herbal formula, Shakuyaku-Kanzo-To, licorice is used to increase fertility in women with polycystic ovary syndrome (3245). In combination with seven other herbs, licorice is used in PC-SPES to treat prostate cancer (5548). In Chinese medicine, licorice is used for sore throats, abdominal pain, infectious hepatitis, malaria, tuberculosis, sores, abscesses, food poisoning, diabetes insipidus, and contact dermatitis (11).

Licorice is used as a flavoring in foods, beverages (4,11), and tobacco (4,6).

Safety

LIKELY SAFE ...when used orally in amounts commonly found in foods. Foods generally contain less than 0.25% licorice and 0.01% of the constituent ammoniated glycyrrhizin (11). The maximum safe daily intake of licorice is equivalent to 100 mg glycyrrhizin (2). Licorice, glycyrrhiza, and ammoniated glycyrrhizin are Generally Recognized as Safe (GRAS) for food use in the US (11).

POSSIBLY SAFE ...when used orally and appropriately, short-term, for medicinal purposes. Prolonged use of licorice longer than four to six weeks or in large amounts should be supervised (2,12). ...when used orally in a specific herbal combination (PC-SPES) (5548).

PREGNANCY: UNSAFE ...when used orally. Licorice can have abortifacient, estrogenic, and steroid effects and can cause uterine stimulation (4); contraindicated.

LACTATION: Insufficient reliable information available; avoid using.

Effectiveness

POSSIBLY EFFECTIVE ...when taken orally for upper respiratory tract mucous membrane inflammation and gastric or duodenal ulcers (2). .. ...when used orally in a specific herbal combination for prostate cancer. Studies using licorice in combination with seven other herbs (PC-SPES) in prostate cancer patients, found that it significantly decreases prostate-specific antigen (PSA) levels (5548,5122,5913), causes tumor cell death (5913), and causes clinically significant reductions in testosterone (5548). In two reports, PSA levels fell significantly within 1 month of treatment (5548,5122).

There is insufficient reliable information available about the effectiveness of licorice for its other uses.

Possible Mechanism of Action & Active Ingredients

The applicable part of licorice is the root. Licorice has antispasmodic, anti-inflammatory, expectorant, laxative, and soothing properties (4). The constituents, glycyrrhizin and glycyrrhetinic acid, inhibit 11-beta-hydroxysteroid dehydrogenase (4). This inhibition blocks metabolism of prostaglandins E and F2 alpha and may be responsible for peptic ulcer healing observed with these products (3). Glycyrrhizin may contribute to licorice-associated mineralocorticoid side effects including hypertension and hypokalemia both by binding directly to mineralocorticoid receptors and by decreasing the conversion of active cortisol to inactive cortisone (3252,3253). Panax ginseng appears to complement licorice by increasing serum cortisol concentrations (3257). However, no clinical reports support the combination of licorice, Panax ginseng and Bupleurum falcatum for stimulating adrenal function in corticosteroid-dependent patients. Licorice decreases testosterone production, which might account for the decreased serum testosterone concentrations in young healthy men who eat licorice (3246). The glycyrrhizin constituent acts as an expectorant by increasing the bronchial secretion and transport of mucus by a reflex pathway, which originates in the stomach (3). Glycyrrhizin has antitussive activity, perhaps due to its sweetness, which is fifty times sweeter than sugar (3,7). Licorice has both anti-estrogenic and estrogenic action. The anti-estrogenic action, attributed to isoflavone constituents, occurs at relatively high concentrations and is associated with the blocking of estrogen receptors. Licorice also affects estrogen metabolism by decreasing the metabolism when estrogen concentrations are high and potentiating metabolism when concentrations are low (4). A licorice root extract enhances estradiol binding to estrogen receptors, induces transcription activity in estrogen-responsive cells, and enhances estradiol-induced transcription activity in estrogen-responsive cells in vitro (6180). It also increases serum ceruloplasmin oxidase activity (a measure of estrogenic activity in the liver) in female rats with their ovaries removed (6180). In vitro, a coumarin constituent of licorice has antiplatelet activity. Isoliquiritigenin, a constituent, reportedly inhibits aldose reductase and the resultant sorbitol accumulation (4). Liquiritigenin and isoliquiritigenin have MAO-inhibitory activities (11). Glycyrrhetinic acid exhibits anti-inflammatory action against UV erythema and is known to inhibit the Epstein-Barr virus activation by tumor promotors. The isoflavonoid constituents, glabridin, glabrol, and derivatives, show antimicrobial activity against S. aureus, M. smegmatis, and C. albicans. Glycyrrhetinic acid has shown antiviral activity against vaccinia, herpes simplex 1, Newcastle disease, and vesicular stomatitis viruses (4). Glycyrrhizin- and glycyrrhizic acid-containing intravenous preparations (Stronger Neominophagen C and Remefa S) show activity against hepatitis B and C in humans, but the trials are too small to draw any definitive conclusions (3247,3250,3251). In vitro data suggests that glycyrrhizin suppresses the production and expression of hepatitis B surface antigen (HbS-Ag) (3248,3249). Glycyrrhizic acid and the aglycone of glycyrrhizic acid can exert anti-inflammatory and anti-allergenic properties (3). In controlled, clinical trials, they accelerated the healing of gastric ulcers (2,4). Licorice reduces body fat but accompanying fluid retention offsets any change in body weight (6196). When seven healthy adults consumed 3.5 grams of licorice candy (7.6% glycyrrhizic acid) per day for two months, body fat as a percent of total body weight decreased, extracellular water as a percent of body weight increased, the renin aldosterone system was suppressed, and there was no change in body mass index. The results of this unpublished study were presented at the Endocrine society's 82nd annual meeting (6196).

Adverse Reactions Including Known Allergies

The use of licorice can cause amenorrhea. Large amounts of licorice, more than 50 grams per day, or chronic use longer than six weeks can cause pseudoaldosteronism, of which symptoms include hypertension, lethargy, headache, sodium and water retention, and edema. Pseudoaldosteronism can lead to increased blood pressure, hypokalemia, hypokalemic myopathy, rhabdomyolysis, myoglobinuria, severe congestive heart failure with pulmonary edema, lower extremity weakness, hypertensive encephalopathy, and quadriplegia (2,3,4,6). The chronic consumption of large amounts of licorice candy has caused hypermineralocorticoidism (781). Because licorice can decrease serum testosterone and increase 17-hydroxyprogesterone it might cause decreased libido and sexual dysfunction in men (3246). Chewing tobacco flavored with licorice has also been associated with toxicity (6).

Possible Interactions with Herbs & Other Dietary Supplements

HERBS WITH CARDIAC ACTIVITY: Theoretically, the overuse or misuse of licorice can increase the risk of cardiotoxicity due to potassium depletion. Cardioactive herbs include digitalis, lily-of-the-valley, pheasant's eye, and squill.

STIMULANT LAXATIVE HERBS: Theoretically, concomitant overuse or misuse of licorice can increase the risk of potassium depletion. Stimulant laxative herbs include aloe vera, alder buckthorn, European buckthorn, cascara sagrada, castor oil, rhubarb, and senna.

HERBS WITH ANTICOAGULANT/ANTIPLATELET POTENTIAL: Concomitant use of herbs that have coumarin constituents or affect platelet aggregation could theoretically increase the risk of bleeding in some people. These herbs include: angelica, anise, arnica, asafoetida, bogbean, boldo, capsicum, celery, chamomile, clove, danshen, fenugreek, feverfew, garlic, ginger, ginkgo, ginseng Panax, horse chestnut, horseradish, meadowsweet, prickly ash, onion, papain, passionflower, poplar, quassia, red clover, turmeric, wild carrot, wild lettuce, willow, and others (4,19).

Possible Interactions with Drugs

ANTIHYPERTENSIVE DRUGS: Theoretically, licorice might reduce the effect of antihypertensive drug therapy. Large amounts of licorice can cause sodium and water retention, and hypertension (4,515).

© Copyright 2000, Natural Medicines Comprehensive Database (209) 472-2244. For updated data, go to www.NaturalDatabase.com

ASPIRIN: Theoretically, concomitant use might protect against aspirin-induced damage to the gastrointestinal mucosa (19).

CORTICOSTEROIDS: Theoretically, concomitant use might potentiate the duration of activity of corticosteroids, e.g., hydrocortisone (19).

CARDIAC GLYCOSIDES: Overuse or misuse of licorice with cardiac glycoside therapy, e.g., digoxin (Lanoxin), might increase the risk of cardiac toxicity due to potassium loss (2).

CIMETIDINE (Tagamet): Theoretically, concomitant use might provide additive protection from gastrointestinal ulcers (19).

FUROSEMIDE (Lasix), ETHACRYNIC ACID (Edecrin): Theoretically, furosemide and ethacrynic acid might enhance the mineralocorticoid effects of licorice by inhibiting the enzyme that converts cortisol to cortisone; however, bumetanide (Bumex) does not appear to have this effect (3255).

HORMONES: Theoretically, licorice might interfere with estrogen or anti-estrogen therapy due to estrogenic and anti-estrogenic effects (4).

INSULIN: Theoretically, concomitant use might cause hypokalemia and sodium retention (19).

INTERFERON: The licorice component glycyrrhizin, as part of the Japanese intravenous preparation Stronger Neominophagen C (SNMC), might enhance the effectiveness of interferon for treating hepatitis C (3247).

MONOAMINE OXIDASE INHIBITORS (MAOIs): Theoretically, concomitant use might increase the effects of MAOI drugs due to the MAO-inhibiting effects of some licorice constituents (11).

NONSTEROIDAL ANTI-INFLAMMATORY DRUGS (NSAIDs): Theoretically, concomitant use can compound NSAID sodium and water retention (504) and protect against NSAID-induced damage to the gastrointestinal mucosa (19).

POTASSIUM-DEPLETING DRUGS: Concomitant use of licorice and potassium-depleting drugs might increase potassium loss and the risk of potassium depletion. Overuse or misuse of licorice can cause potassium depletion (2,12).

Possible Interactions with Foods

GRAPEFRUIT JUICE: Theoretically, grapefruit juice and its component naringenin might enhance the mineralocorticoid activities of licorice, by blocking the conversion of cortisol to cortisone (3254,3255).

Possible Interactions with Lab Tests

BLOOD PRESSURE: Excessive use of licorice can increase blood pressure and blood pressure readings. Excessive licorice intake can cause hypertension (1372).

17-HYDROXYPROGESTERONE: Licorice can increase serum 17-hydroxyprogesterone concentrations and test results (3246).

POTASSIUM: Excessive use of licorice can cause hypokalemia, reducing serum potassium levels and test results (4).

TESTOSTERONE: Licorice can decrease serum testosterone concentrations and test results (3246).

Possible Interactions with Diseases or Conditions

DIABETES: Contraindicated; licorice can interfere with blood glucose control (4,12).

HEART DISEASE: Licorice is contraindicated in congestive heart disease (4).

HYPERTENSION: Contraindicated; licorice can cause hypertension (1372).

HYPERTONIA: Contraindicated in individuals with hypertonia (2).

LIVER DISEASE: Licorice is contraindicated in cholestatic liver disorders and liver cirrhosis (2). Patients with liver disease might be more sensitive to the mineralocorticoid effects of licorice (4).

HYPOKALEMIA: Contraindicated; licorice use can cause hypokalemia (2).

KIDNEY INSUFFICIENCY: Contraindicated in patients with severe renal insufficiency (2).

LICORICE HYPERSENSITIVITY: Contraindicated in individuals hypersensitive to licorice (14).

SEXUAL DYSFUNCTION: Theoretically, licorice might decrease libido and worsen erectile dysfunction by decreasing testosterone and increasing 17-hydroxyprogesterone serum concentrations (3246).

Typical Dosages & Routes of Administration that are Commonly Used

ORAL: The typical dose of licorice is 1-4 grams of the powdered root or one cup of the tea three times daily (4). The tea is prepared by simmering 1-4 grams of the powdered root in 150 mL boiling water for 5-10 minutes and then straining. The usual dose of Succus liquiritiae is 0.5-1 gram for upper respiratory tract mucous membrane inflammation and 1.5-3 grams for gastric and duodenal ulcers.

Comments

Deglycyrrizinated licorice (DGL) is usually free of adverse effects (12). Studies using DGL for ulcer treatment have been inconclusive (6). Carbenoxolone is a semisynthetic derivative of the licorice constituent, glycyrrhetic acid, which is used outside the US for treating gastric and duodenal disease (6). Many "licorice" products manufactured in the US actually contain no licorice, and instead, they contain anise oil that smells and tastes like licorice (3). Authentic licorice is more commonly used in products manufactured in Europe (5).

LILY-OF-THE-VALLEY

This Product is Also Known As
Constancy, Convallaria, Convallaria herba, Convall-Lily, Jacob's Ladder, Ladder-To-Heaven, Lily, Lily of the Valley, May Bells, May Lily, Muguet, Our Lady's Tears.
CAUTION: See separate listings for Abscess Root and Jacob's Ladder.

Scientific Names
Convallaria majalis.
Family: Liliaceae or Convallariaceae.

People Use This For
Orally, lily-of-the-valley is used for mild cardiac insufficiency, heart insufficiency due to old age, chronic cor pulmonale (2,18), arrhythmias, urinary tract infections, and kidney stones (18).
In folk medicine, it is used for weak contractions in labor, epilepsy, edema, strokes and ensuing paralysis, conjunctivitis, and leprosy.

Safety
POSSIBLY SAFE ...when the standardized extract is used orally under supervision (2,12). Poor oral absorption of its cardiac glycosides can reduce the risk of poisoning (18), but the number of glycosides and their varied properties makes controlled use difficult (7).
LIKELY UNSAFE ...when the standardized extract is used orally for self-medication (12).
PREGNANCY AND LACTATION: UNSAFE ...when used orally for self-medication.

Effectiveness
POSSIBLY EFFECTIVE ...when taken orally for mild cardiac insufficiency, heart insufficiency due to old age, and chronic cor pulmonale (2).
There is insufficient reliable information available about the effectiveness of lily-of-the-valley for its other uses.

Possible Mechanism of Action & Active Ingredients
The applicable parts of lily-of-the-valley are the root, rhizome, and dried flower tips. Lily-of-the-valley contains over 40 cardioactive glycosides, principally convallatoxin, and other minor glycosides, including canvallatoxol and convalloside (13). The cardiac glycosides exert positive inotropic, negative chronotropic, negative dromotropic (conduction), and positive bathmotropic (excitability) effects (7). They can lower the elevated left-ventricular diastolic pressure as well as the pathologically elevated venous pressure (2). Diuretic, natriuretic, and dose-dependent vasoconstrictive effects have been observed in experimental animals (18).

Adverse Reactions Including Known Allergies
Taken orally, lily-of-the-valley can cause nausea, vomiting, cardiac arrhythmias (2), headache, and stupor (18). Visual color disturbances can also occur (18).

Possible Interactions with Herbs & Other Dietary Supplements
CARDIAC GLYCOSIDE-CONTAINING HERBS: Contraindicated. Concomitant use can increase the risk of cardiac glycoside toxicity. Cardiac glycoside-containing herbs include black hellebore, Canadian hemp root, digitalis leaf, hedge mustard, figwort, motherwort, oleander leaf, pheasant's eye plant, pleurisy root, squill bulb leaf scales, strophanthus seeds, and uzara (2,18,19,500).
OTHER CARDIOACTIVE HERBS: Avoid concomitant use with other cardioactive herbs due to the unpredictability of therapeutic and adverse effects. Other cardioactive herbs include calamus, cereus, cola, coltsfoot, devil's claw, European mistletoe, fenugreek, fumitory, ginger, ginseng Panax, hawthorn, white horehound, mate, parsley, quassia, scotch broom flower, shepherd's purse, and wild carrot (4).
STIMULANT LAXATIVE HERBS: Theoretically, the overuse or misuse of stimulant laxatives with cardiac glycoside-containing herbs increases the risk of cardiac toxicity due to potassium depletion. Stimulant laxative herbs include aloe dried leaf sap, blue flag rhizome, alder buckthorn, European buckthorn, butternut bark, cascara bark, castor oil, colocynth fruit pulp, gamboge bark exudate, jalap root, black root, manna bark exudate, podophyllum root, rhubarb root, senna leaves and pods, wild cucumber fruit (Ecballium elaterium), and yellow dock root (19).
LICORICE/HORSETAIL: Theoretically, the overuse or misuse of licorice rhizomes or horsetail plant with cardiac glycoside-containing herbs increases the risk of cardiac toxicity due to potassium depletion (19).

Possible Interactions with Drugs
CALCIUM: Calcium salts can enhance the therapeutic and adverse effects of lily-of-the-valley (18).
CARDIAC DRUGS: Theoretically, concomitant use can increase the risk of cardiac toxicity (152).
DIGOXIN: Contraindicated because therapeutic duplication increases the risk of cardiac glycoside toxicity (2).
GLUCOCORTICOIDS: Theoretically, concomitant, long-term glucocorticoid use can increase the risk of cardiac glycoside toxicity due to potassium depletion (2).
POTASSIUM-DEPLETING DIURETICS: Theoretically, concomitant use can increase the risk of cardiac glycoside toxicity due to potassium depletion (2,506).

QUININE: Theoretically, concomitant use can increase the risk of cardiac toxicity (2,506).

STIMULANT LAXATIVES: Theoretically, the overuse or misuse of stimulant laxatives can increase the risk of cardiac glycoside toxicity due to potassium depletion (2).

TETRACYCLINES and MACROLIDE ANTIBIOTICS (erythromycin-like drugs): Theoretically, concomitant use can increase the risk of cardiac glycoside toxicity (152,17).

Possible Interactions with Foods
No interactions are known to occur, and there is no known reason to expect a clinically significant interaction with lily-of-the-valley.

Possible Interactions with Lab Tests
No interactions are known to occur, and there is no known reason to expect a clinically significant interaction with lily-of-the-valley.

Possible Interactions with Diseases or Conditions
HEART DISEASE: Self-medication of lily-of-the-valley is contraindicated; requires diagnosis, treatment, and monitoring (515).

POTASSIUM DEFICIENCY: Contraindicated (2).

Typical Dosages & Routes of Administration that are Commonly Used
ORAL: The average daily amount is 600 mg of the standardized lily-of-the-valley powder (0.2-0.3% cardioactive glycosides) or equivalent preparations (2).

Comments
It is unsafe for self-use. The large number of cardiac glycosides in lily-of-the-valley makes monitoring and therapeutic control more difficult than digitalis or digoxin therapy (7). Lily-of-the-valley has a short duration of action. This correlates with lower absorption rates and makes treatment more difficult to control than with isolated cardiac glycosides, especially due to the narrow therapeutic range of these constituents (7). When indicated, digoxin of standard potency and purity is a safer alternative than nonstandardized lily-of-the-valley (7). Store lily-of-the-valley in well-sealed containers and protect from light (18).

LIME fruit, peel

This Product is Also Known As
Adam's Apple, Italian Limetta, Limette.
CAUTION: See separate listing for Lime oil.

Scientific Names
Citrus aurantifolia.
Family: Rutaceae.

People Use This For
Orally, lime is used as a source of vitamin C for treating scurvy and low resistance (18).

Safety
LIKELY SAFE …when used in food amounts (12).
POSSIBLY SAFE …when used orally (12).
PREGNANCY AND LACTATION: Avoid using in amounts greater than those typically found in foods.

Effectiveness
There is insufficient reliable information available about the effectiveness of lime.

Possible Mechanism of Action & Active Ingredients
Insufficient reliable information available. Lime does contain vitamin C (18).

Adverse Reactions Including Known Allergies
None reported.

Possible Interactions with Herbs & Other Dietary Supplements
Insufficient reliable information available.

Possible Interactions with Drugs
No interactions are known to occur, and there is no known reason to expect a clinically significant interaction with lime.

Possible Interactions with Foods
No interactions are known to occur, and there is no known reason to expect a clinically significant interaction with lime.

Possible Interactions with Lab Tests
No interactions are known to occur, and there is no known reason to expect a clinically significant interaction with lime.

Possible Interactions with Diseases or Conditions
No interactions are known to occur, and there is no known reason to expect a clinically significant interaction with lime.

Typical Dosages & Routes of Administration that are Commonly Used
ORAL: Lime is taken as a liquid extract or as the fresh fruit (18).

Comments
Lime flower is obtained from a species distinct from lime.

LIME oil

This Product is Also Known As
Adam's Apple, Italian Limetta, Key Lime, Limette.
CAUTION: See separate listing for Lime fruit, peel.

Scientific Names
Citrus aurantifolia, synonym Citrus medica var. acida.
Family: Rutaceae.

People Use This For
In cosmetics, expressed lime oil is used as a fragrance component. Distilled lime oil is used as a fixative in cosmetics and as flavor component in foods and beverages (11).

Safety
LIKELY SAFE ...when lime oil is used orally in amounts found in foods. It has Generally Recognized as Safe (GRAS) status in the US. The maximum level used is 0.078% (11).
POSSIBLY SAFE ...when used topically in amounts found in cosmetics. Maximum use level for expressed and distilled oils is 1.5%.
POSSIBLY UNSAFE ...when used topically in larger amounts than those found in cosmetics. Lime oil can be associated with phototoxic skin reactions (11,19) and should not be used during periods of excessive exposure to sunlight.
PREGNANCY AND LACTATION: LIKELY SAFE ...when used orally in food amounts. There is insufficient reliable information available about the safety of the topical use of lime oil; avoid using.

Effectiveness
There is insufficient reliable information available about the effectiveness of lime oil.

Possible Mechanism of Action & Active Ingredients
Expressed oil contains phototoxic furocoumarins, including bergapten (11). Some evidence suggests expressed and distilled lime oils might promote tumors in the presence of carcinogenic chemicals (11).

Adverse Reactions Including Known Allergies
Topical use is associated with hypersensitivity (4058). Although distilled lime oil is reported to be nonirritating, non-sensitizing, and non-phototoxic to human skin (11), expressed lime oil and lime peel can cause phototoxic skin reactions (11,19).

Possible Interactions with Herbs & Other Dietary Supplements
PHOTOSENSITIZING HERBS: Theoretically, concomitant use with other photosensitizing herbs may increase the risk of phototoxicity (19).

Possible Interactions with Drugs
PSORALENS: Contraindicated. Theoretically, concomitant use might potentiate effects and adverse effects (19).

Possible Interactions with Foods
No interactions are known to occur, and there is no known reason to expect a clinically significant interaction with lime oil.

Possible Interactions with Lab Tests
No interactions are known to occur, and there is no known reason to expect a clinically significant interaction with lime oil.

© Copyright 2000, Natural Medicines Comprehensive Database (209) 472-2244. For updated data, go to www.NaturalDatabase.com

Possible Interactions with Diseases or Conditions

No interactions are known to occur, and there is no known reason to expect a clinically significant interaction with lime oil.

Typical Dosages & Routes of Administration that are Commonly Used

No typical dosage.

Comments

Distilled lime oil is the distilled essential oil of the whole crushed fruit of the lime tree. Expressed lime oil is obtained from unripe lime peel. Expressed lime oil is not as important economically as distilled lime oil [11].

LINDEN CHARCOAL

This Product is Also Known As

Basswood, European Linden, Lime Tree, Tiliae carbo.
CAUTION: See separate listings for Linden dried flower, Linden dried leaf, Linden dried sapwood, and Silver Linden.

Scientific Names

Tilia cordata; Tilia platyphyllos.
Family: Tiliaceae.

People Use This For

Orally, linden charcoal is used for intestinal disorders [2,18].
Topically, linden charcoal is used for lower leg abscesses (ulcus cruris) [2,18].

Safety

There is insufficient reliable information available about the safety of linden charcoal.
Pregnancy and Lactation: Insufficient reliable information available; avoid using.

Effectiveness

There is insufficient reliable information available to evaluate the effectiveness of linden charcoal.

Possible Mechanism of Action & Active Ingredients

Linden charcoal is described as an extremely absorbent charcoal [18].

Adverse Reactions Including Known Allergies

None reported.

Possible Interactions with Herbs & Other Dietary Supplements

Insufficient reliable information available.

Possible Interactions with Drugs

No interactions are known to occur, and there is no known reason to expect a clinically significant interaction with linden charcoal.

Possible Interactions with Foods

No interactions are known to occur, and there is no known reason to expect a clinically significant interaction with linden charcoal.

Possible Interactions with Lab Tests

No interactions are known to occur, and there is no known reason to expect a clinically significant interaction with linden charcoal.

Possible Interactions with Diseases or Conditions

No interactions are known to occur, and there is no known reason to expect a clinically significant interaction with linden charcoal.

Typical Dosages & Routes of Administration that are Commonly Used

No typical dosage.

Comments

Linden charcoal is the charcoal obtained from the wood of the linden tree (Tilia cordata and Tilia platyphyllos). There is very little scientific information about this product. Our staff is continually analyzing the available information on natural medicines and will add data here as it becomes available.

LINDEN dried flower

This Product is Also Known As
Basswood, European Linden, Lime Flower, Lime Tree, Linden Tree, Tiliae flos.
CAUTION: See separate listings for Linden Charcoal, Linden dried leaf, Linden dried sapwood, and Silver Linden.

Scientific Names
Tilia cordata; Tilia platyphyllos.
Family: Tiliaceae.

People Use This For
Orally, the dried flower of linden is used for coughs, cold (2), dry coughs (7), nasal congestion, throat irritation, nervous palpitations, hypertension, headaches, insomnia, sinus headache, migraines, incontinence, and hemorrhage (6).
Topically, it is used for itchy skin and rheumatism (6).
Traditionally, linden has been used for migraines, hysteria, arteriosclerotic hypertension, feverish colds and nervous tension (4), and as a diuretic (6).

Safety
POSSIBLY SAFE ...when taken orally and used appropriately (12).
PREGNANCY AND LACTATION: Insufficient reliable information available; avoid using.

Effectiveness
POSSIBLY EFFECTIVE ...when taken orally for treating colds and cold-related coughs (2).
There is insufficient reliable information available about the effectiveness of linden dried flower for its other uses.

Possible Mechanism of Action & Active Ingredients
The linden dried flower has antispasmodic, diaphoretic, diuretic, sedative, and mild astringent properties (4), and antifungal activity (6). In vitro, its antispasmodic activity is attributed to p-coumaric acid and the flavonoid constituents (4). Diaphoretic effects can be due to kaempferol, p-coumaric acid, and quercetin (6), or perhaps due to the heat of the liquid as a tea combined with warm bed rest (7). The volatile oils, including citral, citronellal, citronellol, eugenol, and limonene, exert sedative and antispasmodic effects (4,6). A diuretic effect can be due to the irritant action of terpenoid on the kidneys (4).

Adverse Reactions Including Known Allergies
Frequent oral use of the linden dried flower tea is associated with cardiac damage, but this is rare (6). Topically, linden can cause contact urticaria (6).

Possible Interactions with Herbs & Other Dietary Supplements
Insufficient reliable information available.

Possible Interactions with Drugs
No interactions are known to occur, and there is no known reason to expect a clinically significant interaction with linden dried flower.

Possible Interactions with Foods
No interactions are known to occur, and there is no known reason to expect a clinically significant interaction with linden dried flower.

Possible Interactions with Lab Tests
No interactions are known to occur, and there is no known reason to expect a clinically significant interaction with linden dried flower.

Possible Interactions with Diseases or Conditions
HEART DISEASE: Frequent use of the linden dried flower tea is associated with cardiac damage and should be used with caution in individuals with heart disease (6).

Typical Dosages & Routes of Administration that are Commonly Used
ORAL: The typical dose of the linden dried flower is one to two cups of the tea used as hot as possible during the second half of the day (8). The tea is prepared by steeping 2 grams of the flowers in 150 mL boiling water for 5-10 minutes and then straining. The linden dried flower should only be used up to 2-4 grams daily (2). The usual dose of the tincture (1:5 in 45% alcohol) is 2-4 mL (4). The common dose of the liquid extract (1:1 in 25% alcohol) is 1-2 mL (4).

Comments
Tilia sylvestris, a related species, has been reported to possess anti-inflammatory and wound healing effects (6).

LINDEN dried leaf

This Product is Also Known As
Basswood, European Linden, Lime Tree, Tiliae folium.
CAUTION: See separate listings for Linden Charcoal, Linden dried flower, Linden dried sapwood, and Silver Linden.

Scientific Names
Tilia cordata; Tilia platyphyllos.
Family: Tiliaceae.

People Use This For
Orally, dried linden leaf is used as a diaphoretic [2,18].

Safety
There is insufficient reliable information available about the safety of linden dried leaf.
Pregnancy and Lactation: Insufficient reliable information available; avoid using.

Effectiveness
There is insufficient reliable information available about the effectiveness of linden dried leaf.

Possible Mechanism of Action & Active Ingredients
Insufficient reliable information available.

Adverse Reactions Including Known Allergies
None reported.

Possible Interactions with Herbs & Other Dietary Supplements
Insufficient reliable information available.

Possible Interactions with Drugs
No interactions are known to occur, and there is no known reason to expect a clinically significant interaction with linden dried leaf.

Possible Interactions with Foods
No interactions are known to occur, and there is no known reason to expect a clinically significant interaction with linden dried leaf.

Possible Interactions with Lab Tests
No interactions are known to occur, and there is no known reason to expect a clinically significant interaction with linden dried leaf.

Possible Interactions with Diseases or Conditions
No interactions are known to occur, and there is no known reason to expect a clinically significant interaction with linden dried leaf.

Typical Dosages & Routes of Administration that are Commonly Used
No typical dosage.

Comments
There is very little scientific information about this product. Our staff is continually analyzing the available information on natural medicines and will add data here as it becomes available.

LINDEN dried sapwood

This Product is Also Known As
Basswood, European Linden, Lime Tree, Linden Wood, Tiliae lignum.
CAUTION: See separate listings for Linden Charcoal, Linden dried flower, Linden dried leaf, and Silver Linden.

Scientific Names
Tilia cordata; Tilia platyphyllos.
Family: Tiliaceae.

People Use This For
Linden dried sapwood is used for liver disease, gallbladder disease, and cellulitis [2,18].

Safety

There is insufficient reliable information available about the safety of linden dried sapwood.
Pregnancy and Lactation: Insufficient reliable information available; avoid using.

Effectiveness

There is insufficient reliable information available about the effectiveness of linden dried sapwood.

Possible Mechanism of Action & Active Ingredients

Insufficient reliable information available.

Adverse Reactions Including Known Allergies

None reported.

Possible Interactions with Herbs & Other Dietary Supplements

Insufficient reliable information available.

Possible Interactions with Drugs

No interactions are known to occur, and there is no known reason to expect a clinically significant interaction with linden dried sapwood.

Possible Interactions with Foods

No interactions are known to occur, and there is no known reason to expect a clinically significant interaction with linden dried sapwood.

Possible Interactions with Lab Tests

No interactions are known to occur, and there is no known reason to expect a clinically significant interaction with linden dried sapwood.

Possible Interactions with Diseases or Conditions

No interactions are known to occur, and there is no known reason to expect a clinically significant interaction with linden dried sapwood.

Typical Dosages & Routes of Administration that are Commonly Used

No typical dosage.

Comments

There is very little scientific information about this product. Our staff is continually analyzing the available information on natural medicines and will add data here as it becomes available.

LIPASE

This Product is Also Known As

None.

Scientific Names

Triacylglycerol lipase.

People Use This For

Orally, lipase is used for indigestion, heartburn, celiac disease, Crohn's disease, and cystic fibrosis (2378).

Safety

LIKELY SAFE ...when used orally (15).
PREGNANCY AND LACTATION: Insufficient reliable information available; avoid using.

Effectiveness

There is insufficient reliable information available about the effectiveness of lipase.

Possible Mechanism of Action & Active Ingredients

Lipase aids in fat digestion by hydrolyzing fat to yield fatty acids and glycerol (9).

Adverse Reactions Including Known Allergies

Taking large amounts of lipase orally can cause nausea, cramping, and/or diarrhea. Extremely large amounts of exogenous pancreatic enzymes (containing lipase) may be associated with hyperuricosuria and hyperuricemia (14).

Possible Interactions with Herbs & Other Dietary Supplements

Insufficient reliable information available.

Possible Interactions with Drugs

No interactions are known to occur, and there is no known reason to expect a clinically significant interaction with lipase.

Possible Interactions with Foods

No interactions are known to occur, and there is no known reason to expect a clinically significant interaction with lipase.

Possible Interactions with Lab Tests

No interactions are known to occur, and there is no known reason to expect a clinically significant interaction with lipase.

Possible Interactions with Diseases or Conditions

GOUT: Excessive ingestion of lipase may exacerbate gout [14].
CYSTIC FIBROSIS: High doses of lipase appear to increase the risk of fibrosing colonopathy and colonic strictures in individuals with cystic fibrosis [2379,2380,2381,2382].

Typical Dosages & Routes of Administration that are Commonly Used

No typical dosage.

Comments

Lipase is a digestive enzyme that is widely distributed in the plant world, in milk, milk products, bacteria, molds, and animal tissues [2383]. Castor beans and dehulled oats are also plant sources of acid-stable lipases [2383]. Lipase is included in many prescription and OTC combination pancreatic enzyme products. Most clinical studies use combination pancreatic enzyme products, rather than lipase-only products, although pancreatic enzyme dosing is often expressed in units of lipase [2384].

LIVERWORT

This Product is Also Known As

American Liverleaf, Anémone à Lobes Aigus, Anémone d'Amérique, Hepatici noblis herba, Hépatique à Lobes Aigus, Hépatique d'Amérique, Herb Trinity, Kidney Wort, Leberbluemchenkraut, Liverleaf, Liverweed, Liverwort-Leaf, Round-Leaved Hepatica, Round-Lobe Hepatica, Sharp-Lobe Hepatica, Trefoil.

Scientific Names

Anemone acutiloba, synonym Hepatica nobilis var. acuta; Anemone americana, synomym Hepatica nobilis var. obtusa; Anemone hepatica.
Family: Ranunculaceae.

People Use This For

Orally, liverwort is used for liver diseases, jaundice, liver enlargement, congestion, portal vein problems, hepatitis, and liver cirrhosis. It is also used orally for gastric and digestive discomfort, stimulating appetite, relieving sensation of fullness, for treating gallstones and gravel, for regulating bowel function, stimulating pancreatic function, regulating blood lipid levels, for varicose veins, stimulating systemic and cardiac circulation, increasing myocardium blood supply, strengthening nerves, "purifying" blood, stimulating metabolism, relief of menopausal symptoms, and as a general tonic or sedative [2].
Topically, liverwort is used for hemorrhoids [2] or as an external rinse [18].

Safety

LIKELY UNSAFE ...when the fresh above ground parts are used orally or topically.
There is insufficient reliable information available about the safety of dried liverwort.
PREGNANCY: LIKELY UNSAFE ...when used orally or topically [2].
LACTATION: LIKELY UNSAFE ...when the fresh above ground parts are used orally or topically. There is insufficient reliable information available about the safety of dried liverwort; avoid using.

Effectiveness

There is insufficient reliable information available about the effectiveness of liverwort.

Possible Mechanism of Action & Active Ingredients

The applicable parts of liverwort are the fresh or dried above ground parts [2]. Liverwort contains ranunculin [18], which hydrolyzes to toxic, unstable protoanemonin, which readily dimerizes to nontoxic anemonin [4]. Some evidence suggests anemonin might be cytotoxic [4]. Other evidence indicates anemonin and protoanemonin might have sedative and antipyretic activity [4]. Protoanemonin has antimicrobial activity [2]. It causes central nervous system stimulation, then paralysis in experimental animals [2]. Kidney and urinary tract irritation might be due to the alkylating action of protoanemonin [2].

Adverse Reactions Including Known Allergies

Ingested orally, fresh liverwort can cause colic, diarrhea, gastrointestinal irritation (18), kidney and urinary tract irritation (2). Skin contact with fresh liverwort can cause irritation, mucous membrane irritation, itching and pustule formation known a ranunculus dermatitis (2). Inhalation of protoanemonin-containing volatile oil can cause nasal mucosal and conjunctival irritation (4).

Possible Interactions with Herbs & Other Dietary Supplements

Insufficient reliable information available.

Possible Interactions with Drugs

No interactions are known to occur, and there is no known reason to expect a clinically significant interaction with liverwort.

Possible Interactions with Foods

No interactions are known to occur, and there is no known reason to expect a clinically significant interaction with liverwort.

Possible Interactions with Lab Tests

No interactions are known to occur, and there is no known reason to expect a clinically significant interaction with liverwort.

Possible Interactions with Diseases or Conditions

No interactions are known to occur, and there is no known reason to expect a clinically significant interaction with liverwort.

Typical Dosages & Routes of Administration that are Commonly Used

No typical dosage.

Comments

None.

LOBELIA

This Product is Also Known As

Asthma Weed, Bladderpod, Emetic Herb, Gagroot, Indian Tobacco, Pukeweed, Vomit Wort, Wild Tobacco.

Scientific Names

Lobelia inflata.
Family: Lobeliaceae or Campanulaceae.

People Use This For

Orally, lobelia is used for asthma and bronchitis (4).
Topically, it's used for muscle inflammation, rheumatic nodules (4), bruises, sprains, insect bites, poison ivy, and ringworm (11).
Historically, it has been used orally for whooping cough, for inducing sweating, and as a sedative (4,11). Lobelia was used as an ingredient in smoking cessation products (11,514) and for treating apnea in newborn infants (514).
Lobelia and lobelia extracts are used in cough preparations and in counterirritant products (11).

Safety

LIKELY UNSAFE ...when preparations of the above ground parts are used orally (3,11). 0.6-1 gram of the leaf is said to be toxic and 4 grams may be fatal (18).
There is insufficient reliable information available about the safety of the topical use of lobelia.
PREGNANCY AND LACTATION: LIKELY UNSAFE ...contraindicated for oral use, because it has emetic effects (4,12). There is insufficient reliable information available about the safety of lobelia for topical use during pregnancy and lactation.

Effectiveness

LIKELY INEFFECTIVE ...when lobeline is used orally for smoking cessation (13).
There is insufficient reliable information available about the effectiveness of lobelia for its other uses.

Possible Mechanism of Action & Active Ingredients

The applicable parts of lobelia are the above ground parts. Lobelia has some anti-asthmatic, antispasmodic, emetic, expectorant and respiratory stimulant effects (4,13). The primary constituent, (-)-lobeline, is known as alpha lobeline, to distinguish it from the mixture of lobelia alkaloids formerly called lobeline. Like nicotine but weaker, alpha lobeline exhibits effects on the peripheral circulation, neuromuscular system and central nervous system (CNS) (4,13). Small amounts of lobeline stimulate respiration and have expectorant activity (11,18). Larger amounts have emetic, purgative, and diuretic effects (11). Lobeline first causes CNS stimulation then CNS and respiratory depression (505). Overdose may cause convulsions, collapse, and possibly death (4,11).

Adverse Reactions Including Known Allergies

Oral use of lobelia can cause nausea, vomiting, diarrhea, coughing, dizziness, and tremors (4). Overdose can lead to sweating, tachycardia, convulsions, hypothermia, hypotension, coma, and possibly death (4,11).

Possible Interactions with Herbs & Other Dietary Supplements

TOBACCO: Concomitant use may enhance nicotine effects and adverse effects (505).

Possible Interactions with Drugs

No interactions are known to occur, and there is no known reason to expect a clinically significant interaction with lobelia.

Possible Interactions with Foods

No interactions are known to occur, and there is no known reason to expect a clinically significant interaction with lobelia.

Possible Interactions with Lab Tests

No interactions are known to occur, and there is no known reason to expect a clinically significant interaction with lobelia.

Possible Interactions with Diseases or Conditions

HEART DISEASE: CAUTION, dose-dependent cardiac activity is reported with lobelia (12).
GI CONDITIONS: Can irritate the gastrointestinal tract. Contraindicated in individuals with infectious or inflammatory gastrointestinal conditions (19).

Typical Dosages & Routes of Administration that are Commonly Used

ORAL: A typical dose as an expectorant is 100 mg of leaf, 0.6-2.0 mL of the tincture (12). The dosage of specific products varies widely from 375 mg once daily to 820 mg three times daily. One supplier warns not to exceed 50 mg of the dried lobelia. An extract of lobelia is used in a dose of 2 to 5 drops three to four times daily. The extract contains alcohol (6006).

Comments

Clinical research was unable to demonstrate lobeline efficacy greater than placebo in smoking cessation (13) and it was disallowed as an ingredient in anti-smoking products in the US in 1993 (11).

LOGWOOD

This Product is Also Known As

Bloodwood, Peachwood.

Scientific Names

Haematoxylon campechianum; Haematoxylon lignum.
Family: Leguminosae.

People Use This For

Orally, logwood is used for diarrhea, hemorrhages and as an astringent (18).

Safety

There is insufficient reliable information available about the safety of logwood.
Pregnancy and Lactation: Insufficient reliable information available; avoid using.

Effectiveness

There is insufficient reliable information available about the effectiveness of logwood.

Possible Mechanism of Action & Active Ingredients

Insufficient reliable information available.

Adverse Reactions Including Known Allergies

None reported.

Possible Interactions with Herbs & Other Dietary Supplements

Insufficient reliable information available.

Possible Interactions with Drugs

No interactions are known to occur, and there is no known reason to expect a clinically significant interaction with logwood.

Possible Interactions with Foods
No interactions are known to occur, and there is no known reason to expect a clinically significant interaction with logwood.

Possible Interactions with Lab Tests
No interactions are known to occur, and there is no known reason to expect a clinically significant interaction with logwood.

Possible Interactions with Diseases or Conditions
No interactions are known to occur, and there is no known reason to expect a clinically significant interaction with logwood.

Typical Dosages & Routes of Administration that are Commonly Used
ORAL: Logwood is used as a tea or liquid extract (18).

Comments
There is very little scientific information about this product. Our staff is continually analyzing the available information on natural medicines and will add data here as it becomes available.

LOOSESTRIFE

This Product is Also Known As
Yellow Willowherb.
CAUTION: See separate listing for Purple Loosestrife.

Scientific Names
Lysimachia vulgaris.
Family: Primulaceae.

People Use This For
Orally, loosestrife is used for scurvy, diarrhea, dysentery, and as an astringent. It is also used for hemorrhages, including nose bleeds and heavy menstrual flow.
Topically, loosestrife is used for wounds (18).

Safety
There is insufficient reliable information available about the safety of loosestrife.
Pregnancy and Lactation: Insufficient reliable information available; avoid using.

Effectiveness
There is insufficient reliable information available about the effectiveness of loosestrife.

Possible Mechanism of Action & Active Ingredients
Insufficient reliable information available.

Adverse Reactions Including Known Allergies
None reported.

Possible Interactions with Herbs & Other Dietary Supplements
Insufficient reliable information available.

Possible Interactions with Drugs
No interactions are known to occur, and there is no known reason to expect a clinically significant interaction with loosestrife.

Possible Interactions with Foods
No interactions are known to occur, and there is no known reason to expect a clinically significant interaction with loosestrife.

Possible Interactions with Lab Tests
No interactions are known to occur, and there is no known reason to expect a clinically significant interaction with loosestrife.

Possible Interactions with Diseases or Conditions
No interactions are known to occur, and there is no known reason to expect a clinically significant interaction with loosestrife.

Typical Dosages & Routes of Administration that are Commonly Used
ORAL: No typical dosage.
TOPICAL: Loosestrife is used as a powder (18).

Comments

Both purple loosestrife (Lythrum salicaria) and Lysimachia vulgaris are known as loosestrife and can be confused for each other.

There is very little scientific information about this product. Our staff is continually analyzing the available information on natural medicines and will add data here as it becomes available.

LORENZO'S OIL

This Product is Also Known As

Lorenzos Oil, Glycerol Trierucate Oil, Glycerol Trioleate Oil.

Scientific Names

13-Docosenoic acid (erucic acid); cis-9-Octadecenoic acid (oleic acid).

People Use This For

Orally, Lorenzo's oil is used as a treatment for two related genetic neurological syndromes: adrenoleukodystrophy, which occurs in children, and adrenomyeloneuropathy, which occurs in adults (6).

Safety

There is insufficient reliable information available about the safety of Lorenzo's oil.
Pregnancy and Lactation: Insufficient reliable information available; avoid using.

Effectiveness

POSSIBLY EFFECTIVE ...when taken orally in slightly slowing clinical progression of adrenoleukodystrophy when given to asymptomatic patients (928).
LIKELY INEFFECTIVE ...when taken orally for treating adrenoleukodystrophy and adrenomyeloneuropathy (920,921,922,923,924,930). There was one case report of modest clinical benefit in a child with symptomatic adrenoleukodystrophy (929).

Possible Mechanism of Action & Active Ingredients

Adrenoleukodystrophy and adrenomyeloneuropathy are rare genetic disorders that result in an impaired ability to oxidize saturated, very-long chain fatty acids. Buildup of these acids is thought to cause neurologic symptoms associated with the disorder (6). Monounsaturated fatty acids have been shown to inhibit production of very-long-chain fatty acids (6). However, when Lorenzo's oil is given to patients with adrenoleukodystrophy, eruric acid does not enter the brain in a significant quantity, which may be a factor in the negative results (931).

Adverse Reactions Including Known Allergies

Asymptomatic thrombocytopenia (927,924), asymptomatic neutropenia (6). One case report of purpura, petechia, and bleeding (926). May cause decrease in plasma docosahexanoic acid levels without essential fatty acid deficiency (individuals studied were also taking supplemental safflower and fish oils) (6).

Possible Interactions with Herbs & Other Dietary Supplements

ESSENTIAL FATTY ACIDS: Supplemental essential fatty acids taken concomitantly may not prevent decreased plasma levels of docosahexaenoic acid (6).

Possible Interactions with Drugs

No interactions are known to occur, and there is no known reason to expect a clinically significant interaction with Lorenzo's oil.

Possible Interactions with Foods

No interactions are known to occur, and there is no known reason to expect a clinically significant interaction with Lorenzo's oil.

Possible Interactions with Lab Tests

PLATELET COUNTS: May cause false low platelet counts (927). High monounsaturated fat diets may cause true thrombocytopenia (925,927). A hand-count of platelets is recommended in individuals taking Lorenzo's oil (927).

Possible Interactions with Diseases or Conditions

Theoretically, may worsen existing thrombocytopenia or neutropenia.

Typical Dosages & Routes of Administration that are Commonly Used

ORAL: People typically use a mixture of approximately 20% erucic acid and 80% oleic acid (5278). One clinical study used 0.3 gram per kg per day of erucic acid and 1.7 grams per kg of oleic acid per day (5277).

Comments

Lorenzo's oil is a combination of erucic acid and oleic acid in a 1:4 ratio.

LOTUS flower

This Product is Also Known As
Lian Fang, Lian Xu.
CAUTION: See separate listing for Lotus seed.

Scientific Names
Nelumbo nucifera.
Family: Nymphaeaceae.

People Use This For
Orally, lotus flowers are used as an astringent for bleeding [18].

Safety
There is insufficient reliable information available about the safety of lotus flower.
Pregnancy and Lactation: Insufficient reliable information available; avoid using.

Effectiveness
There is insufficient reliable information available about the effectiveness of lotus flower.

Possible Mechanism of Action & Active Ingredients
Insufficient reliable information available.

Adverse Reactions Including Known Allergies
None reported.

Possible Interactions with Herbs & Other Dietary Supplements
Insufficient reliable information available.

Possible Interactions with Drugs
No interactions are known to occur, and there is no known reason to expect a clinically significant interaction with lotus flower.

Possible Interactions with Foods
No interactions are known to occur, and there is no known reason to expect a clinically significant interaction with lotus flower.

Possible Interactions with Lab Tests
No interactions are known to occur, and there is no known reason to expect a clinically significant interaction with lotus flower.

Possible Interactions with Diseases or Conditions
No interactions are known to occur, and there is no known reason to expect a clinically significant interaction with lotus flower.

Typical Dosages & Routes of Administration that are Commonly Used
ORAL: Lotus flower is used as a powder or liquid extract [18].

Comments
There is very little scientific information about this product. Our staff is continually analyzing the available information on natural medicines and will add data here as it becomes available.

LOTUS seed

This Product is Also Known As
Lian Zi.
CAUTION: See separate listing for Lotus flower.

Scientific Names
Nelumbo nucifera.
Family: Nymphaeaceae.

People Use This For
Orally, lotus seed is used for digestive disorders and diarrhea [18].

Safety
POSSIBLY SAFE ...when used orally [12].
PREGNANCY AND LACTATION: Insufficient reliable information available; avoid using.

© Copyright 2000, Natural Medicines Comprehensive Database (209) 472-2244. For updated data, go to www.NaturalDatabase.com • 681

Effectiveness

There is insufficient reliable information available about the effectiveness of lotus seed.

Possible Mechanism of Action & Active Ingredients

Insufficient reliable information available.

Adverse Reactions Including Known Allergies

None reported.

Possible Interactions with Herbs & Other Dietary Supplements

Insufficient reliable information available.

Possible Interactions with Drugs

No interactions are known to occur, and there is no known reason to expect a clinically significant interaction with lotus seed.

Possible Interactions with Foods

No interactions are known to occur, and there is no known reason to expect a clinically significant interaction with lotus seed.

Possible Interactions with Lab Tests

No interactions are known to occur, and there is no known reason to expect a clinically significant interaction with lotus seed.

Possible Interactions with Diseases or Conditions

GASTROINTESTINAL DISORDERS: Lotus seed is contraindicated in patients with constipation and stomach distention (12).

Typical Dosages & Routes of Administration that are Commonly Used

ORAL: Lotus seed is used as a powder or liquid extract (18).

Comments

There is very little scientific information about this product. Our staff is continually analyzing the available information on natural medicines and will add data here as it becomes available.

LOVAGE

This Product is Also Known As

Lavose, Levistici radix, Love Parsley, Maggi Plant, Sea Parsley, Smallage, Smellage.

Scientific Names

Levisticum officinale, synonyms Angelica levisticum, Hipposelinum levisticum, Ligusticum levisticum.
Family: Apiaceae or Umbelliferae.

People Use This For

Orally, lovage is used as "irrigation therapy" for inflammation of the lower urinary tract, for prevention of kidney gravel (2,5,7,18), and as a diuretic for urinary tract infections (18) or pedal edema (6,8).
In folk medicine, lovage has been used for indigestion, heartburn, stomach distention, and flatulence (5,6,8,11,18). It has also been used as an expectorant (11), to loosen secretions in respiratory conditions (6,8,18), for menstrual irregularities (5,8,11,12,18), sore throat (5,6), boils (5,6), jaundice, malaria, pleurisy, gout, rheumatism, and migraines (5).
In foods and beverages, the root, oil, and extracts are used as flavor components (11).
In manufacturing, the oil is used as a fragrance component in soaps and cosmetics (11).

Safety

LIKELY SAFE ...when used orally in amounts commonly found in food (11). Lovage is approved for food use in the US (11).
POSSIBLY SAFE ...when the rhizome and root preparations are used orally and appropriately (2,12).
PREGNANCY: LIKELY UNSAFE ...the root and rhizome preparations are contraindicated for oral use because of the possibility of uterine or menstrual stimulation (12).
LACTATION: Insufficient reliable information available; avoid using.

Effectiveness

POSSIBLY EFFECTIVE ...when taken orally as "irrigation therapy" for inflammation of the lower urinary tract and prevention of kidney gravel (2,5,6,8,11). In "irrigation therapy," it is used as a mild diuretic along with copious fluid intake to increase urine flow.
There is insufficient reliable information available about the effectiveness of lovage for its other uses.

Possible Mechanism of Action & Active Ingredients

The applicable parts of lovage are the rhizome and root. Lovage contains 0.2-2% volatile oil (5,6,8,11,18). Its principal constituents are lactone derivatives known as phthalides. Of these, ligustilide has sedative (6,8,11,18), antispasmodic (2,6,8,11,18), and aquaretic (5,6,8,11,18,512), effects in experimental animals. Aquaretics increase urine volume (water loss) but not sodium excretion (512). It can also have varied actions including cholinergic and antimicrobial activity (18), increasing uterine tone (12), and increased gastrointestinal blood flow (6). The bitter taste and aroma of lovage can increase the production of saliva and gastric juices (6,8,18). Theoretically, the coumarin constituents can cause phototoxic reactions including photosensitivity dermatitis (2,5,6,8,11,12).

Adverse Reactions Including Known Allergies

Theoretically, long term use of lovage could result in an increased risk of phototoxic reactions, including photosensitivity dermatitis (2,5,6,8,11,12). Avoid excessive exposure to the sun or UV light if using lovage (2,12).

Possible Interactions with Herbs & Other Dietary Supplements

Insufficient reliable information available.

Possible Interactions with Drugs

DIURETICS: Theoretically, lovage root might increase sodium retention and interfere with diuretic therapy (512).

Possible Interactions with Foods

No interactions are known to occur, and there is no known reason to expect a clinically significant interaction with lovage.

Possible Interactions with Lab Tests

No interactions are known to occur, and there is no known reason to expect a clinically significant interaction with lovage.

Possible Interactions with Diseases or Conditions

HYPERTENSION: Theoretically, lovage root might increase sodium retention and worsen hypertension (512).
EDEMA: "Irrigation therapy," which is the use of a mild diuretic and copious fluid intake to increase urine flow, is contraindicated in cases of edema that are due to limited heart or kidney function (2).
RENAL DISEASE: Lovage is contraindicated in acute kidney inflammation (2,8,12) or impaired kidney function (2,12).

Typical Dosages & Routes of Administration that are Commonly Used

ORAL: The typical dose of lovage is one cup of the tea two to three times per day (8). The tea is prepared by steeping 1.5-3 grams of the dried root in 150 mL boiling water for 10-15 minutes and then straining. Lovage should only be used up to 4-8 grams of the dried root per day (2,7). Ample fluid intake is essential when used for "irrigation therapy" (18). For stomach complaints, one cup of the tea is commonly taken 30 minutes before meals (8). Avoid excessive sun or UV light exposure with prolonged use of lovage due to its phototoxic adverse effects.

Comments

None.

LUFFA

This Product is Also Known As

Angled Loofah, Dishcloth Sponge, Loofa, Loofah, Luffaschwamm, Sigualuo, Silky Loofah, Smooth Loofah, Sponge Cucumber, Vegetable Sponge, Water Gourd.

Scientific Names

Luffa aegyptiaca; Luffa acutangula; Luffa cylindrica.
Family: Cucurbitaceae.

People Use This For

Orally, luffa is used for treating and preventing colds, nasal inflammation, sinusitis, and suppuration of the sinuses (2,18).
Topically, luffa sponge is used to remove dead skin and stimulate the skin. Luffa charcoal is used topically for shingles in the face and eye region.
In Chinese medicine, luffa is used orally for arthritis and associated pain, muscle pain, chest pain, amenorrhea, and to promote lactation.
For food uses, young luffa fruits are eaten as vegetables (11).
In cosmetics, powdered luffa is used in skin care products as an anti-inflammatory and detoxicant.

Safety

LIKELY SAFE ...when used as a sponge for exfoliation.
POSSIBLY SAFE ...in amounts found in foods (11).

There is insufficient reliable information available about the safety of luffa for medicinal use.
PREGNANCY AND LACTATION: POSSIBLY SAFE ...when used orally in amounts found in foods (11).
POSSIBLY UNSAFE ...when used orally n amounts greater than those typically found in foods

Effectiveness
There is insufficient reliable information available about the effectiveness of luffa.

Possible Mechanism of Action & Active Ingredients
The applicable part of luffa is the dried fiber structure from the ripe fruit. The toxicity of luffa is low.

Adverse Reactions Including Known Allergies
None reported.

Possible Interactions with Herbs & Other Dietary Supplements
Insufficient reliable information available.

Possible Interactions with Drugs
No interactions are known to occur, and there is no known reason to expect a clinically significant interaction with luffa.

Possible Interactions with Foods
No interactions are known to occur, and there is no known reason to expect a clinically significant interaction with luffa.

Possible Interactions with Lab Tests
No interactions are known to occur, and there is no known reason to expect a clinically significant interaction with luffa.

Possible Interactions with Diseases or Conditions
No interactions are known to occur, and there is no known reason to expect a clinically significant interaction with luffa.

Typical Dosages & Routes of Administration that are Commonly Used
ORAL: No typical dosage.
TOPICAL: Luffa is powdered and used in skin care products. The intact sponge is also used to remove dead skin (11).

Comments
None.

LUNGMOSS

This Product is Also Known As
Lungwort, Oak Lungs.
CAUTION: See separate listing for Lungwort.

Scientific Names
Lobaria pulmonaria.
Family: Lobariaceae.

People Use This For
Orally, lungmoss is used for bronchitis, asthma, and coughs, including irritable cough and smoker's cough. It is also used orally as an expectorant, anti-inflammatory, antimicrobial and to promote sweating (18).

Safety
There is insufficient reliable information available about the safety of lungmoss.
Pregnancy and Lactation: Insufficient reliable information available; avoid using.

Effectiveness
There is insufficient reliable information available about the effectiveness of lungmoss.

Possible Mechanism of Action & Active Ingredients
Insufficient reliable information available.

Adverse Reactions Including Known Allergies
None reported.

Possible Interactions with Herbs & Other Dietary Supplements
Insufficient reliable information available.

Possible Interactions with Drugs

No interactions are known to occur, and there is no known reason to expect a clinically significant interaction with lungmoss.

Possible Interactions with Foods

No interactions are known to occur, and there is no known reason to expect a clinically significant interaction with lungmoss.

Possible Interactions with Lab Tests

No interactions are known to occur, and there is no known reason to expect a clinically significant interaction with lungmoss.

Possible Interactions with Diseases or Conditions

No interactions are known to occur, and there is no known reason to expect a clinically significant interaction with lungmoss.

Typical Dosages & Routes of Administration that are Commonly Used

ORAL: Lungmoss is used as a powder or a liquid extract (18).

Comments

Lungmoss and Pulmonaria officinalis are both known as lungwort, but are physically distinct. Lungmoss is a lichen; Pulmonaria officinalis is a plant. See separate listing for lungwort (18).

There is very little scientific information about this product. Our staff is continually analyzing the available information on natural medicines and will add data here as it becomes available.

LUNGWORT

This Product is Also Known As

Dage of Jerusalem, Lungenkraut, Pulmonariae herba.
CAUTION: See separate listing for Lungmoss.

Scientific Names

Pulmonaria officinalis.
Family: Boraginaceae.

People Use This For

Orally, lungwort is used for the treatment of conditions of the respiratory tract, gastrointestinal tract, the kidney and urinary tract.

Topically, it is used as an astringent and for wound treatment (2).

In folk medicine, it is used orally in irritant-relieving cough medicine, as a diuretic, and to treat lung diseases such as tuberculosis (18).

Safety

There is insufficient reliable information available about the safety of lungwort.
Pregnancy and Lactation: Insufficient reliable information available; avoid using.

Effectiveness

There is insufficient reliable information available about the effectiveness of lungwort.

Possible Mechanism of Action & Active Ingredients

The applicable parts of lungwort are the above ground parts. Lungwort was thought to contain hepatotoxic pyrrolizidine alkaloids, but gas chromatography analysis of multiple samples failed to detect these compounds (12).

Adverse Reactions Including Known Allergies

None reported.

Possible Interactions with Herbs & Other Dietary Supplements

Insufficient reliable information available.

Possible Interactions with Drugs

No interactions are known to occur, and there is no known reason to expect a clinically significant interaction with lungwort.

Possible Interactions with Foods

No interactions are known to occur, and there is no known reason to expect a clinically significant interaction with lungwort.

© Copyright 2000, Natural Medicines Comprehensive Database (209) 472-2244. For updated data, go to www.NaturalDatabase.com • 685

Possible Interactions with Lab Tests

No interactions are known to occur, and there is no known reason to expect a clinically significant interaction with lungwort.

Possible Interactions with Diseases or Conditions

No interactions are known to occur, and there is no known reason to expect a clinically significant interaction with lungwort.

Typical Dosages & Routes of Administration that are Commonly Used

ORAL: One cup of tea taken as sips repeatedly with honey throughout the day. The tea is prepared by heating or scalding 1.5 grams dried herb rapidly in 150 mL of boiling water, then straining for 5-10 minutes (18).

Comments

The taste of lungwort is described as dry and slimy. Pulmonaria officinalis and lungmoss are both known as lungwort. However, they are physically distinct because Pulmonaria officinalis is a plant and lungmoss is a lichen (see separate listing). In addition, lungwort can easily be mistaken for other Pulmoniaria species, particularly Pulmonaria mollis (18).

LUTEIN

This Product is Also Known As

Xanthophyll, Zeaxanthin.

Scientific Names

Beta, Epsilon-Carotene-3, 31-diol.

People Use This For

Orally, lutein is used for preventing age-related macular degeneration (2394), cataracts (2386,2394), and colon cancer (3962).

Safety

LIKELY SAFE ...when used orally (219,3219,3220).
PREGNANCY AND LACTATION: LIKELY SAFE ...when used orally (219,3219,3220).

Effectiveness

POSSIBLY EFFECTIVE ...when dietary lutein is consumed for reducing the risk of age-related macular degeneration (219,2394). This is based on epidemiological data that identified an association between high dietary lutein intake and reduced risk of age-related macular degeneration. ...when dietary lutein is consumed for reducing the risk of developing cataracts severe enough to require surgical removal (2395,3219,3220). This is based on epidemiological data that identified an association between high dietary lutein intake and reduced risk of cataracts requiring surgery. ...when dietary lutein is consumed for reducing the risk of developing colon cancer (3962). This is based on epidemiological data that identified an association between high dietary lutein intake and reduced risk of colon cancer.

Possible Mechanism of Action & Active Ingredients

Lutein is a carotenoid that is typically found in combination with its stereoisomer, zeaxanthin. They are the two major carotenoids found as a pigment in the human macula and retina (2388,3225). They are thought to function as antioxidants and as a blue light filter protecting underlying ocular tissues from photodamage. Epidemiological evidence associates high dietary lutein intake with reduced risk of developing age-related macular degeneration and cataracts (2394,2395,3219,3220). Increasing dietary lutein intake increases serum lutein levels and macular pigment density (2389). Low dietary lutein intake is associated with males, smokers, and people who drink alcohol (more than 2 drinks per week), while higher dietary lutein intake is associated with females, increasing age, and people with hypertension (2398). Foods containing high concentrations of lutein such as broccoli, spinach, and kale, are associated with the greatest eye health benefits (3219,3220). Other carotenoids and antioxidants such as vitamin A, lycopene, alpha- or beta-carotene, vitamin C, and vitamin E have not been associated with this benefit (3219,3220,3221,3222,3223). Epidemiologic studies have shown that carotenoids might be inversely associated with cancer (3963,3964). Supplemental esterified lutein is better absorbed when taken with high fat (36 grams fat) meals compared to low-fat (3 grams fat) meals (6133).

Adverse Reactions Including Known Allergies

None reported.

Possible Interactions with Herbs & Other Dietary Supplements

BETA-CAROTENE: Concomitant administration may reduce bioavailability of lutein and may reduce or increase bioavailability of beta-carotene (2390,2391).

Possible Interactions with Drugs

No interactions are known to occur, and there is no known reason to expect a clinically significant interaction with lutein.

Possible Interactions with Foods

OLESTRA: Theoretically, may interfere with supplemental lutein activity. Olestra (fat substitute) lowers serum lutein concentrations in healthy people (2392).

Possible Interactions with Lab Tests

No interactions are known to occur, and there is no known reason to expect a clinically significant interaction with lutein.

Possible Interactions with Diseases or Conditions

No interactions are known to occur, and there is no known reason to expect a clinically significant interaction with lutein.

Typical Dosages & Routes of Administration that are Commonly Used

ORAL: For reducing the risk of cataracts and macular degeneration, 6 mg of lutein per day, either through diet or supplementation has been suggested. People consuming 6.9-11.7 mg of lutein per day through diet had the lowest risk of developing age-related macular degeneration and cataracts (3219,3220). There is 44 mg of lutein per cup of cooked kale, 26 mg/cup of cooked spinach, and 3 mg/cup of broccoli (219,3219,3220). Commercial products containing 6 mg or 20 mg of lutein are available (5020). Supplemental esterified lutein is better absorbed when taken with high fat (36 grams fat) meals compared to low-fat (3 grams fat) meals (6133).

Comments

Centrum and Centrum Silver now contain lutein 0.25 mg per tablet, but probably not enough to provide much benefit (219,3219,3220). Avoid confusion with lutein extract (dried powdered hog corpora lutea) formerly used as a source of progesterone (511). Although dark green leafy vegetables contain 15-47% lutein, they have a very low zeaxanthin content (0-3%). Corn is richest in lutein (60% of total carotenoids), and orange pepper is richest in zeaxanthin (37% of total). Substantial amounts of lutein and zeaxanthin (30-50%) are also present in kiwi fruit, grapes, spinach, orange juice, zucchini, and different kinds of squash (3224).

LYCOPENE

This Product is Also Known As

All-Trans Lycopene.

Scientific Names

Psi, psi-carotene.

People Use This For

Orally, lycopene is used for preventing atherosclerosis and cancer (1446,2400).

Safety

LIKELY SAFE ...when consumed in amounts found in foods.
There is insufficient reliable information available about the safety of lycopene supplements.
PREGNANCY AND LACTATION: LIKELY SAFE ...when consumed in amounts found in foods. There is insufficient reliable information available about the safety of lycopene supplements; avoid using lycopene in amounts greater than those typically found in foods.

Effectiveness

POSSIBLY EFFECTIVE ...when lycopene is consumed in the form of tomato products for reducing the risk of prostate cancer. An epidemiological study found an association between dietary consumption of greater than 6 mg per day of lycopene (in the form of tomato products, including tomatoes, tomato sauce, pizza and tomato juice) and a reduced risk of prostate cancer (2406).
POSSIBLY INEFFECTIVE ...when dietary lycopene is consumed for reducing the risk of bladder cancer. Epidemiological studies find no association between dietary lycopene intake or serum lycopene levels, and the risk of bladder cancer (2407).
There is insufficient reliable information available about the effectiveness of lycopene for its other uses. Epidemiological studies of serum lycopene concentrations and the risk of cancers of the breast, cervix, esophagus, larynx, lungs, ovaries, and pancreas have been inconclusive (1444,2407). Epidemiological studies of dietary lycopene intake and prevention of atherosclerosis are inconclusive (1446,1449).

Possible Mechanism of Action & Active Ingredients

Lycopene is the pigment that gives tomatoes their red color. It has antioxidant activity, scavenging free radicals and quenching singlet oxygen (2401). Decreased serum or tissue lycopene concentrations are associated with an increased risk of prostate cancer (1447,1496,2405,2406,2407). Lycopene is better absorbed from tomato products, such as tomato paste, than from fresh tomatoes (1497). Similar serum lycopene levels are achieved when equivalent amounts of lycopene are ingested in the form of tomato juice or lycopene supplements (1498).

Adverse Reactions Including Known Allergies

None reported.

Possible Interactions with Herbs & Other Dietary Supplements

BETA-CAROTENE: Concomitant ingestion may increase lycopene absorption (2403).

Possible Interactions with Drugs

No interactions are known to occur, and there is no known reason to expect a clinically significant interaction with lycopene.

Possible Interactions with Foods

No interactions are known to occur, and there is no known reason to expect a clinically significant interaction with lycopene.

Possible Interactions with Lab Tests

No interactions are known to occur, and there is no known reason to expect a clinically significant interaction with lycopene.

Possible Interactions with Diseases or Conditions

No interactions are known to occur, and there is no known reason to expect a clinically significant interaction with lycopene.

Typical Dosages & Routes of Administration that are Commonly Used

ORAL: People typically use 5 to 10 mg of lycopene daily (6006).

Comments

One cup (240 mL) of tomato juice contains approximately 23 mg lycopene, depending on the brand (1499).
April 12, 1999 (Associated Press)- Researchers from the Karmanos Cancer Institute in Detroit reported that 30 mg lycopene per day, given to men with prostate cancer for one month before surgery, was associated with cancer tissue that was less likely to extend to the edges of the prostate and pre-cancerous prostate cells that were less abnormal in appearance (789). The researchers announced their results at a meeting of the American Association for Cancer Research in Philadelphia.

LYSINE

This Product is Also Known As

L-Lysine, Lys, Lysine Hydrochloride, Lysine Monohydrochloride.

Scientific Names

L-2,6-diaminohexanoic acid.

People Use This For

Orally, lysine is used for preventing and treating clinical symptoms of recurrent herpes simplex labialis (1114). It is also used as an aid to improving athletic performance (217).
Lysine monohydrochloride is used to treat metabolic alkalosis (14).

Safety

POSSIBLY SAFE ...when used orally and appropriately for up to one year (1114,1120).
PREGNANCY AND LACTATION: Insufficient reliable information available; avoid using.

Effectiveness

POSSIBLY EFFECTIVE ...when used orally for reducing recurrences of herpes simplex labialis infections (1114,1115,1116,1118,1120) and for reducing severity and healing time of herpes simplex labialis infections (1119,1120). ...when lysine monohydrochloride is used for treating metabolic alkalosis (14).

Possible Mechanism of Action & Active Ingredients

Lysine is required for collagen synthesis and it may be important to bone health (1124,1130). Lysine antagonizes herpes simplex virus (HSV) growth in vitro and this effect may be important clinically (1117).

Adverse Reactions Including Known Allergies

Diarrhea and abdominal pain occur with use of 10 grams per day for five days (14). There is one case report of supplemental lysine use associated with tubulointerstitial nephritis progressing to chronic renal failure (1121).

Possible Interactions with Herbs & Other Dietary Supplements
CALCIUM SUPPLEMENTS: Concomitant use may increase supplemental calcium absorption and decrease urine calcium loss (1131).

Possible Interactions with Drugs
CALCIUM: Concomitant use may increase supplemental calcium absorption and decrease urine calcium loss (1131).

Possible Interactions with Foods
No interactions are known to occur, and there is no known reason to expect a clinically significant interaction with lysine.

Possible Interactions with Lab Tests
No interactions are known to occur, and there is no known reason to expect a clinically significant interaction with lysine.

Possible Interactions with Diseases or Conditions
KIDNEY DISEASES: There is one case report of supplemental lysine associated with tubulointerstitial nephritis progressing to chronic renal failure (1121).
OSTEOPOROSIS: Concomitant use of lysine and calcium supplements may increase supplemental calcium absorption and decrease urine calcium loss (1131).

Typical Dosages & Routes of Administration that are Commonly Used
ORAL: Recurrent herpes simplex labialis infections, 1000 mg daily for twelve months and 1000 mg three times daily for six months reported in clinical trials (1114,1120). Metabolic alkalosis, 10 grams per day in divided doses for up to five days (14).

Comments
None.

MACA

This Product is Also Known As
Ayak Chichira, Ayuk Willku, Maca Maca, Maino, Maka, Peruvian Ginseng.

Scientific Names
Lepidium meyenii.
Family: Brassicaceae.

People Use This For
Orally, maca root is used for anemia, chronic fatigue syndrome, enhancing energy, stamina, athletic performance and memory, female hormone imbalance, menstrual irregularities, enhancing fertility, menopause symptoms, stomach cancer, tuberculosis, as an aphrodisiac, for impotence, and as an immunostimulant (3918).
For food uses, maca root is eaten baked or roasted, prepared as a porridge, and used for making a fermented drink (3918).

Safety
LIKELY SAFE ...when maca root is consumed in food amounts (6).
There is insufficient information available about the safety of maca root when used orally in therapeutic amounts.
PREGNANCY AND LACTATION: LIKELY SAFE ...when consumed in food amounts (6). There is insufficient reliable information available about the safety of maca in amounts greater than used as food; avoid using amounts greater than found in food.

Effectiveness
There is insufficient reliable information available about the effectiveness of maca root.

Possible Mechanism of Action & Active Ingredients
The applicable part of maca is the root which contains fatty acids and essential amino acids (6).

Adverse Reactions Including Known Allergies
None reported.

Possible Interactions with Herbs & Other Dietary Supplements
Insufficient reliable information available.

Possible Interactions with Drugs
No interactions are known to occur, and there is no known reason to expect a clinically significant interaction with maca.

Possible Interactions with Foods
No interactions are known to occur, and there is no known reason to expect a clinically significant interaction with maca.

Possible Interactions with Lab Tests
No interactions are known to occur, and there is no known reason to expect a clinically significant interaction with maca.

Possible Interactions with Diseases or Conditions
No interactions are known to occur, and there is no known reason to expect a clinically significant interaction with maca.

Typical Dosages & Routes of Administration that are Commonly Used
ORAL: People typically use 1500 to 6000 mg or more per day in three divided doses. A teaspoon of root powder, containing 2800 mg of maca root, is used in 8 ounces of water three times daily (5154).

Comments
Maca root has been cultivated as a vegetable crop in the Andes Mountains of Peru for at least 2000 years (6).

MADAGASCAR PERIWINKLE

This Product is Also Known As
Cape Periwinkle, Catharanthus, Church-Flower, Magdalena, Myrtle, Old Maid, Periwinkle, Ram-Goat Rose, Red Periwinkle.
CAUTION: See separate listing for Periwinkle.

Scientific Names
Catharanthus roseus, synonym Vinca rosea; Lochnera rosea, synonym Ammocallis rosea.
Family: Apocynaceae.

People Use This For
Orally, Madagascar periwinkle is used for diabetes, cancer (6), as a cough remedy, for easing lung congestion, throat inflammation, and as a diuretic (3820).
Topically, it is used as a hemostatic (3820), for insect bites (6), wasp stings, eye irritation, infection (3820), and inflammation (6).

Safety
LIKELY UNSAFE ...when the plant or root are used orally. Madagascar periwinkle contains vinca alkaloids which can cause death (6,3820).
There is insufficient reliable information available about the safety of the topical use of Madagascar periwinkle.
PREGNANCY: LIKELY UNSAFE ...contraindicated because it has abortifacient and teratogenic properties (19).
LACTATION: LIKELY UNSAFE; avoid using.

Effectiveness
There is insufficient reliable information about the effectiveness of Madagascar periwinkle.

Possible Mechanism of Action & Active Ingredients
The applicable parts of Madagascar periwinkle are the above ground parts. The constituent vinca alkaloids, vincristine and vinblastine, block cell mitosis, have immunosuppressive effects, and in high concentrations, exert effects on nucleic acid and protein synthesis (6,15). The constituent, catharanthine, demonstrates diuretic properties (6). Hypotensive constituents, reserpine and alstonine, have been isolated from Madagascar periwinkle root (6). The constituent, ajmalicine, may improve cerebral blood flow, and has been combined with rauwolfia alkaloids for treating high blood pressure (6). Concentrated extracts are reported to lower blood glucose (6), but studies by one pharmaceutical company found the plant had no effect on blood glucose levels (6).

Adverse Reactions Including Known Allergies
Taken orally, the plant is an hallucinogen, and has caused seizures, GI upset, hepatotoxicity, and alopecia (17). Adverse effects of Vinca alkaloids include nausea, vomiting, alopecia, dizziness, nystagmus, vertigo, hearing impairment, leukopenia, thrombocytopenia, bleeding, hyperuricemia, neurotoxicity, (15), and possibly death (6).

Possible Interactions with Herbs & Other Dietary Supplements
Insufficient reliable information available.

Possible Interactions with Drugs
ANTIDIABETES DRUGS: Madagascar periwinkle may cause hypoglycemia (6,19); monitor blood glucose control closely.

Possible Interactions with Foods
No interactions are known to occur, and there is no known reason to expect a clinically significant interaction with Madagascar periwinkle.

Possible Interactions with Lab Tests
BLOOD GLUCOSE: Conflicting information about possible hypoglycemic activity (6,19); may lower blood glucose.

Possible Interactions with Diseases or Conditions
DIABETES: May cause hypoglycemia (6,19).

Typical Dosages & Routes of Administration that are Commonly Used
No typical dosage.

Comments
Madagascar periwinkle is considered likely unsafe; avoid, due to presence of toxic vinca alkaloids. The vinca alkaloids, vinblastine and vincristine, isolated from Madagascar periwinkle, are FDA approved for use as chemotherapeutic agents to treat cancers, including Hodgkin's disease, leukemia, Kaposi's sarcoma, malignant lymphomas, mycosis fungoides neuroblastoma, and Wilm's tumor (6).

MADDER

This Product is Also Known As
Dyer's Madder, Farberrote, Garance, Robbia, Rubiae tinctorum radix.

Scientific Names
Rubia tinctorum.
Family: Rubiaceae.

People Use This For
Orally, madder is used for preventing kidney stones and for disintegrating kidney stones (2,18).
Historically, it has been used for menstrual and urinary disorders (18).

Safety
LIKELY UNSAFE ...when used orally. It is potentially carcinogenic and mutagenic (2,18,19).
PREGNANCY: UNSAFE ...contraindicated in pregnancy because it may be a potential menstrual stimulant and a genotoxin (2,19).
LACTATION: UNSAFE ...contraindicated during lactation because it is a potential genotoxin (2,19). It also can cause red-colored breast milk (2).

Effectiveness
There is insufficient reliable information available about the effectiveness of madder.

Possible Mechanism of Action & Active Ingredients
The applicable part of madder is the root. Madder contains lucidin, which is an anthracene derivative. The Ames test shows that anthracene has genotoxic activity, and causes dose-dependent increases in benign and malignant liver and kidney tumors in experimental rats (3718). Madder also seems to decrease calcium oxalate crystallization in the kidney, which potentially could induce kidney or bladder stones (2).

Adverse Reactions Including Known Allergies
When taken orally, madder can cause red colored urine, saliva, perspiration, and breast milk (2). There is some concern that madder can stain contact lenses. Advise patients to be cautious (7003).

Possible Interactions with Herbs & Other Dietary Supplements
Insufficient reliable information available.

Possible Interactions with Drugs
No interactions are known to occur, and there is no known reason to expect a clinically significant interaction with madder.

Possible Interactions with Foods
No interactions are known to occur, and there is no known reason to expect a clinically significant interaction with madder.

Possible Interactions with Lab Tests
COLORIMETRIC TESTS: Theoretically, madder might interfere with colorimetric tests involving urine, saliva, perspiration, and breast milk due to red coloring of these body fluids (2).

Possible Interactions with Diseases or Conditions

No interactions are known to occur, and there is no known reason to expect a clinically significant interaction with madder.

Typical Dosages & Routes of Administration that are Commonly Used

ORAL: People typically prepare madder bark using one teaspoon boiled in a covered container with 3 cups of water for 30 minutes. The liquid is cooled slowly in the closed container and taken cold, 1 to 2 cups per day (5254).

Comments

None.

MAGGOTS

This Product is Also Known As

Botfly Maggot, Fly Larva, Grub, Living Antiseptic, Surgical Maggot, Viable Antiseptic.

Scientific Names

Lucilia sericata; Phormia regina; and other Calliphoridae family of flies.
Family: Calliphoridae.

People Use This For

Topically, maggots are used for treating infected or necrotic skin wounds including pressure ulcers (14,4946,4949,4994,4995,4996,4997), diabetic foot ulcers (14,4948), venous stasis ulcers (14,4994,4945,4996,4997), abscesses (14,4946,4947,4996,4997,4998), osteomyelitis (14,4989,4990,4991,4992,4993,4994,4995,4996,4997,4998), mastoiditis (4996,4999), empyema (4996), carbuncles (4995,4997), soft tissue wounds (4995,4996,4997,4998), burns (4996), and otitis media (14).

Safety

LIKELY SAFE ...when used topically and when sterile, laboratory-produced larvae are used (14,4986,4951).
LIKELY UNSAFE ...when used topically for self-treatment.
PREGNANCY AND LACTATION: Insufficient reliable information available; avoid using.

Effectiveness

POSSIBLY EFFECTIVE ...when used topically for treating infected or necrotic skin wounds including pressure ulcers (14,4946,4949,4994,4995,4996,4997), diabetic foot ulcers (14,4948), venous stasis ulcers (14,4994,4945,4996,4997), abscesses (14,4946,4947,4996,4997,4998), osteomyelitis (14,4989,4990,4991,4992,4993,4994,4995,4996,4997,4998), mastoiditis (4996,4999), empyema (4996), carbuncles (4995,4997), soft tissue wounds (4995,4996,4997,4998), burns (4996), and otitis media (14).

Possible Mechanism of Action & Active Ingredients

Maggots can improve wound-healing by various mechanisms. They can kill bacteria by producing natural antibiotic-like substances, by raising wound pH, and by ingesting and destroying bacteria through normal feeding behavior (14,4950,4946,4948,4943,5100). They can promote regrowth of healthy granulation tissue by secreting proteolytic enzymes that liquefy necrotic tissue, such as collagenase. They consume necrotic tissue as food. Maggots are irritating to the wound, which can induce serous exudate to mechanically wash out the bacteria. Substances with healing actions such as allantoin, urea, calcium carbonate, and ammonium bicarbonate can be secreted by maggots. The larvae also excrete growth-stimulating factors. In addition, the continuous crawling of the larvae mechanically stimulates viable tissue (14,4950,4946,4948,4943,5101,5102). Maggots do not attack healthy tissue (4946) and cannot multiply within the wound, and the mature breeding insect cannot develop in the wound (4946).

Adverse Reactions Including Known Allergies

When used topically, maggots can cause pain and intense local pruritus, which can require analgesics or sedation (14,4950,4946,4948,4986). If non-sterile larvae are used, wounds can become contaminated with pathogenic organisms, although bacteria cultured from leprous ulcers infected with maggots did not differ from uninfected ulcers (4946,4952). Rarely, a large number of larvae in a granulating wound have caused bleeding, possibly as a result of proteolytic enzymes produced by larvae (4946). Although allergic reactions have not been reported, theoretically they are possible due to the foreign protein of the larvae (4946).

Possible Interactions with Herbs & Other Dietary Supplements

Insufficient reliable information available.

Possible Interactions with Drugs

No interactions are known to occur, and there is no known reason to expect a clinically significant interaction with maggots.

Possible Interactions with Foods

No interactions are known to occur, and there is no known reason to expect a clinically significant interaction with maggots.

Possible Interactions with Lab Tests

No interactions are known to occur, and there is no known reason to expect a clinically significant interaction with maggots.

Possible Interactions with Diseases or Conditions

No interactions are known to occur, and there is no known reason to expect a clinically significant interaction with maggots.

Typical Dosages & Routes of Administration that are Commonly Used

TOPICAL: Depending on the size and depth of the wound, between 50 to 1000 maggots are typically applied to the skin two to five times weekly and left in place usually for 72 hours (14,4946,4948). No more than 10 larvae per square cm should be placed in a wound, and fewer should be used if the wound contains a limited amount of necrotic tissue (4986). About 200 to 600 maggots will consume 10 to 15 grams of necrotic tissue per day (4946). After 72 hours, the larvae will be about one-half inch long, readily visible, and actively crawling (4946). At this time, they should be removed with forceps and a saline lavage (14,4946,4986) and then destroyed (4946,4986). Repeat treatments might be required (4948,4946). Specialized dressings have been developed to prevent larval escape and to absorb exudate or liquefied necrotic tissue (4953,4986).

Comments

Maggots are the larvae of flies. For therapeutic purposes, the most commonly used are the larvae of the green bottle fly or green blow fly (Lucilia sericata) (14,4986) and the black blow fly or black bottle blow fly (Phormia regina) (14,4999). Maggots were commonly used by surgeons to treat skin and bone infections in the US and Europe during the 1930s and early 1940s (4945,4948). Lucilia sericata larva were produced commercially by Lederle (4988). With the advent of antibiotics and surgical debridement, the use of maggots was largely abandoned until the late 1980s (4948). Prior to therapy, patients should be counseled about efficacy and the possible adverse reactions. They should be reassured that maggots do not attack healthy tissue, do not multiply within the wound, and will be removed and killed before the larvae develop into mature insects (4986). Maggot treatment is also called biosurgery (4986).

MAGNESIUM

This Product is Also Known As

Chelated Magnesium, Magnesium Aspartate, Magnesium Carbonate, Magnesium Chloride, Magnesium Citrate, Magnesium Gluconate, Magnesium Hydroxide, Magnesium Lactate, Magnesium Orotate, Magnesium Oxide, Magnesium Sulfate, Magnesium Trisilicate.
CAUTION: See separate listings for Chelated Minerals and Dolomite.

Scientific Names

Magnesium; Mg; atomic number 12.

People Use This For

Orally, magnesium is used for treating and preventing hypomagnesemia (9). It is also used as a laxative for constipation and for preparation of the bowel for surgical or diagnostic procedures. It is used as an antacid for symptoms of gastric hyperacidity (9,15). Magnesium is used orally for treating symptoms of asthma (1169) and for cardiovascular diseases including angina, atrial fibrillation, cardiomyopathy, congestive heart failure, hypertension, intermittent claudication, low high-density lipoprotein (HDL) levels, mitral valve prolapse, myocardial infarction, and stroke. It is also used for treating diabetes, eosinophilia myalgia syndrome, fatigue, fibromyalgia, glaucoma, hearing loss, hypoglycemia, kidney stones, migraine, osteoporosis, premenstrual syndrome, and preventing hearing loss (2000). Magnesium has also been used by athletes to increase energy and endurance (2742,2825,2826,2827,2828,2829,2830).
In combination with malic acid, magnesium has been used orally for decreasing pain and tenderness associated with fibromyalgia (3262).
Topically, magnesium is used for treating infected skin ulcers, boils, and carbuncles (9); and for speeding wound healing (14). It is also used as a cold compress in the treatment of erysipelas, and as a hot compress for deep-seated skin infections (16).
Intravenously, magnesium is used for acute hypomagnesemia occurring in conditions such as pancreatitis, malabsorption disorders, cirrhosis, and as an additive to total parenteral nutrition (TPN) for prevention of hypomagnesemia (14). It is also used intravenously for controlling seizures in patients with epilepsy, glomerulonephritis and uremia, hypothyroidism, and eclampsia in patients with hypomagnesemia (9,14). It has also been used for the treatment of life-threatening arrhythmias such as torsade de pointes, cardiac arrest, and for preventing arrhythmias after myocardial infarction (9,14). Magnesium is also used intravenously for treating acute exacerbations of asthma (14), chronic obstructive pulmonary disease (COPD) (9), as an osmotic agent for cerebral edema, and for tetanus (14).

© Copyright 2000, Natural Medicines Comprehensive Database (209) 472-2244. For updated data, go to www.NaturalDatabase.com

Safety

LIKELY SAFE ...when used orally and appropriately (9,15,3566). ...when used parenterally and appropriately. Parenteral magnesium sulfate is an FDA-approved prescription product (15).

POSSIBLY SAFE ...when used orally and appropriately in combination with malic acid. In one study, magnesium hydroxide and malic acid were used safely in a trial lasting 6 months (3262).

POSSIBLY UNSAFE ...when used orally in high doses. High doses can cause loose stool and diarrhea. Although symptomatic hypermagnesemia, including hypotension, nausea, vomiting, and bradycardia, is rare in patients with normal renal function, it has occurred in patients ingesting magnesium sulfate 30 grams every 4 hours for 3 doses (14). Safe upper limit doses for magnesium have not been established (3566). ...when magnesium sulfate is used topically for prolonged periods or repeatedly, since it may damage the skin (9).

CHILDREN: LIKELY SAFE ...when used orally or parenterally and appropriately (15).

LIKELY UNSAFE ...when used orally in large doses or for an extended period of time. There is one report of fatal hypermagnesemia in a 28-month old boy treated for constipation with oral magnesium oxide 800 mg per day, then 2400 mg per day for several days (see Adverse Reactions)(1360).

PREGNANCY AND LACTATION: LIKELY SAFE ...when used orally in amounts not exceeding the recommended dietary allowance (RDA)(15). POSSIBLY SAFE ...when given intramuscularly prior to delivery. Intramuscular magnesium sulfate is not thought to cause hypermagnesemia in the neonate when administered to toxemic mothers (15). LIKELY UNSAFE ...when given by intravenous infusion less than two hours before delivery. Intravenous infusions of magnesium sulfate can cause neonatal respiratory depression when given to toxemic mothers (14,15).

There is insufficient reliable information available about the safety of oral use of magnesium in pregnancy and lactation when doses exceed the recommended daily allowance; avoid using.

Effectiveness

EFFECTIVE ...when used orally or parenterally for treating and preventing hypomagnesemia (15). There is some controversy regarding whether parenteral or oral magnesium replacement is better. Because higher oral doses of magnesium might result in diarrhea, some suggest parenteral administration is better. However, careful use of oral magnesium can be used in adequate doses for replacement without causing diarrhea. Magnesium gluconate may be preferred for oral replacement because it does not cause as much diarrhea. Magnesium oxide should be avoided due to greater risk for diarrhea. Magnesium carbonate may not be soluble enough to adequately replace magnesium levels and should also be avoided (14). ...when used orally as a laxative for constipation and for preparation of the bowel for surgical or diagnostic procedures (15). Magnesium citrate, sulfate, and hydroxide salts are typically used for this indication (14). ...when used orally as an antacid for symptoms of gastric hyperacidity. Typically, magnesium carbonate, hydroxide, oxide, or trisilicate salts are used (15).

LIKELY EFFECTIVE ...when used intravenously for preventing and managing pre-eclampsia and eclampsia (9,15). Magnesium sulfate is considered the agent of choice for pre-eclampsia and eclampsia (15). ...when used intravenously for acute prevention of uterine contractions in preterm labor (9). Magnesium sulfate is considered a first-line therapy for preterm labor prior to 34 weeks gestation. Magnesium sulfate can delay labor from 24-48 hours. Once premature contractions have ceased for 12-48 hours, intravenous magnesium sulfate is often discontinued and oral maintenance therapy with a beta-adrenergic agonist is initiated. Although oral magnesium therapy has been used in patients who cannot tolerate beta-adrenergic agonists, its effectiveness has not been clearly demonstrated (15).

POSSIBLY EFFECTIVE ...when magnesium is used orally for preventing premenstrual migraine (1186). ...when used orally for relieving premenstrual mood changes (1187) and fluid retention (1188). ...when used orally for reducing activity level in children with attention deficit hyperactivity disorder (1189). ...when used orally for treating pregnancy-induced leg cramps (1194). ...when used orally for reducing symptoms of mitral valve prolapse in people with low serum magnesium levels (1191). ...when used orally for reducing anginal attacks in people with coronary artery disease (1181). ...when used orally for treating mild to moderate hypertension. Supplemental doses from 600-1000 mg per day have been beneficial (1192,1199); however, significantly lower doses have shown no benefit (1180,1195,1197). ...when used orally for preventing calcium oxalate renal stones (1201). ...when used orally for preventing hearing loss in individuals exposed to loud noise (1205). ...when used topically for treating skin ulcers and inflammatory conditions including boils and carbuncles (9). ...when used topically for speeding wound healing (14). ...when used intravenously for treating cluster headaches (1184,1185). ...when used intravenously as adjunctive therapy to reduce morbidity and mortality associated with an acute myocardial infarction. Although some studies have been contradictory, some evidence suggests that early intravenous high-dose magnesium sulfate can reduce post-myocardial infarction ventricular arrhythmias and all-cause mortality (14). ...when used intravenously for treating atrial fibrillation (1202). ...when used intravenously for treating acute exacerbation of chronic obstructive pulmonary disease (1208). ...when magnesium hydroxide is used orally in combination with malic acid (Super Malic tablets) for decreasing fibromyalgia-related pain and tenderness (3262).

POSSIBLY INEFFECTIVE ...when used orally for reducing the risk of cardiac events in survivors of acute myocardial infarction (1198). ...when used orally for improving FEV1 or reducing bronchodilator use in asthma patients (1173). ...when used orally for reducing symptoms of repetitive tachyarrhythmias in people with frequent ventricular arrhythmias (1174). ...when used orally for reducing elevated lipoprotein (a) levels in people with hypercholesterolemia (1193). ...when used orally for improving glycemic control in insulin-dependent type 2 diabetes (1171,1172). ...when used intravenously for improving successful resuscitation in people with cardiac arrest (1190). ...when used to increase energy and endurance in athletic activity, although one study found that magnesium orotate reduced stress response in triathletes (2742,2825,2826,2827,2828,2829,2830).

Possible Mechanism of Action & Active Ingredients

Magnesium is the second most plentiful cation in the intracellular fluid and the most plentiful cation in the body. Up to 50% of the magnesium in the body is present in bone. Magnesium is important to the normal bone structure (272) and it plays an essential role in more than 300 fundamental cellular reactions (945). Magnesium is required for the formation of cyclic AMP (cAMP) and is involved in ion movements across cell membranes (945). It is involved in protein synthesis and carbohydrate metabolism (272). Extracellular magnesium is critical to both maintaining nerve and muscle electrical potentials and transmitting impulses across neuromuscular junctions (272). For cardiovascular conditions and eclampsia, magnesium is thought to act as a physiologic calcium channel blocker (2004). Some evidence suggests it is important in regulating blood pressure (1170,1182). Some evidence also suggests low magnesium levels in the blood might play a role in insulin resistance (1168) and in migraine headaches (1183), which has led to magnesium being used for diabetes and migraines. Uncontrolled clinical trials suggest that magnesium metabolism is a factor in renal stone formation and prevention (2006,2007). In asthma, intravenous administration of magnesium might cause bronchodilation (2003). The mechanism of magnesium for pain of fibromyalgia is not known (3262).

Adverse Reactions Including Known Allergies

Orally, magnesium can cause gastrointestinal irritation, nausea, vomiting, and diarrhea (9,14,15). Although rare, larger amounts may cause hypermagnesemia (9) with symptoms including thirst, hypotension, drowsiness, confusion, loss of tendon reflexes, muscle weakness, respiratory depression, cardiac arrhythmias, coma, cardiac arrest, and death (9). Magnesium sulfate 30 grams every 4 hours for 3 doses has been associated with severe hypermagnesemia (14). A tolerable upper limited has not yet been determined (14). There is one report of fatal hypermagnesemia (serum magnesium 20.3 mg/dL) involving a child treated with oral magnesium oxide, calcium carbonate, multivitamins, essential fatty acids, lactobacillus and bifidobacterium. The 28-month-old boy, with a history of severe mental retardation, spastic quadriplegia and seizure disorder, was treated for constipation with 800 mg magnesium oxide per day, then 2400 mg magnesium oxide for several days before hospital admission (1360). Urticaria has been reported with IV administration (9). Chronic use of magnesium-containing antacids, especially those which do not contain aluminum, can cause diarrhea leading to fluid and electrolyte imbalances (15). Topically, prolonged use of magnesium sulfate in the treatment of boils and carbuncles can cause damage to the surrounding skin (9).

Possible Interactions with Herbs & Other Dietary Supplements

BORON: Can increase serum magnesium levels (940).
MALIC ACID: Malic acid is used with magnesium hydroxide for reducing pain and tenderness associated with fibromyalgia (3262).

Possible Interactions with Drugs

FLUOROQUINOLONES (ciprofloxacin, levofloxacin, ofloxacin, etc.): Concomitant administration decreases the absorption of the fluoroquinolone (15). Administer fluoroquinolones at least two hours before or four hours after magnesium-containing supplements or antacids.
NIFEDIPINE: Profound hypotension or neuromuscular blockade can occur in individuals using oral nifedipine concomitantly with intravenous magnesium sulfate (9).
SKELETAL MUSCLE RELAXANTS: Parenteral magnesium might potentiate the effects of skeletal muscle relaxants, e.g., tubocurarine chloride (9).
EXCRETION-ENHANCING DRUGS: Concomitant use can reduce the effects of supplemental magnesium. Urinary excretion-enhancing drugs include amphotericin B, cisplatin, aminoglycoside antibiotics, cyclosporine, thiazide and loop diuretics, mannitol, and intravenous glucose (945).
EXCRETION-REDUCING DRUGS: Concomitant use can increase the effects of supplemental magnesium and magnesium serum levels. Urinary excretion-reducing drugs include calcitonin, glucagon, and potassium-sparing diuretics (945).

Drug Influences on Nutrient Levels and Depletion

SOME DRUGS CAN AFFECT MAGNESIUM LEVELS:
DIGOXIN (Lanoxin, Lanoxicaps): Digoxin can decrease renal tubule reabsorption and increase excretion of magnesium. The need for supplementation has not been adequately studied. Consider supplementation only if clinical judgment warrants it (4556).
LOOP DIURETICS and THIAZIDE DIURETICS: Use of loop diuretics and thiazide diuretics can increase urinary magnesium loss and reduce serum levels. This is more likely with higher doses or when used in combination with diuretics of another class (4412).
ESTROGENS and ESTROGEN-CONTAINING ORAL CONTRACEPTIVES: Use of estrogens and estrogen-containing oral contraceptives might shift magnesium from the serum to storage in other tissues, decreasing serum magnesium levels. The need for supplementation has not been adequately studied (4470).
PENICILLAMINE (Cuprimine): Penicillamine can reduce serum magnesium levels (4534).

© Copyright 2000, Natural Medicines Comprehensive Database (209) 472-2244. For updated data, go to www.NaturalDatabase.com • 695

Possible Interactions with Foods

No interactions are known to occur, and there is no known reason to expect a clinically significant interaction with magnesium.

Possible Interactions with Lab Tests

ALKALINE PHOSPHATASE (ALK PHOS): Magnesium salts can cause a false increase in serum alkaline phosphatase test results due to the activation of enzymes used in lab procedures (275).

ANGIOTENSIN-CONVERTING ENZYME (ACE): Magnesium sulfate can reduce serum ACE concentrations and test results (275).

CALCIUM: Magnesium salts can cause a false increase in serum calcium test results in some procedures using edetate disodium (EDTA) (275).

CORTISOL: Intravenous magnesium sulfate can decrease plasma cortisol concentrations and test results (275).

DIAGNEX BLUE: Magnesium salts can increase urine diagnex blue concentrations and test results by heavy metal displacement of diagnex blue (275).

PARATHYROID HORMONE: Intravenous magnesium sulfate can reduce plasma parathyroid hormone concentrations and test results (275).

TESTOSTERONE: Intravenous magnesium sulfate can reduce serum testosterone concentrations and test results (275).

BLOOD PRESSURE: Taken orally, magnesium can lower blood pressure and reduce blood pressure readings in patients with mild to moderate hypertension (1192,1199).

ELECTROCARDIOGRAM (ECG): Taken orally, magnesium can normalize arrhythmias and ECG readings in some patients with angina (1181). Intravenous magnesium can normalize arrhythmias and ECG readings in some people with atrial fibrillation or ventricular tachydysrhythmias (1202,3314).

Possible Interactions with Diseases or Conditions

ELDERLY: The elderly have an increased risk for hypomagnesemia (1167).

HEART BLOCK: Contraindicated in people with heart block (9).

RENAL DISEASE: Use cautiously in individuals with reduced kidney function due to increased risk of hypermagnesemia (9).

MALABSORPTION SYNDROMES: Intestinal magnesium absorption can be decreased in bile insufficiency states, gastrointestinal infections, gluten enteropathy, immune diseases with villous atrophy, inflammatory bowel disease, intestinal fistulas, lymphectasia, primary idiopathic hypomagnesemia, radiation enteritis, and sprue (945).

Typical Dosages & Routes of Administration that are Commonly Used

ORAL: Magnesium gluconate is preferred for oral use because it is highly soluble and is less likely to cause diarrhea (14). A typical dose used in hypomagnesemia is empirical, and then the dose is adjusted to maintain normal serum levels (15). Normal serum levels of magnesium are 1.5-2.5 mEq/L (14,15). A typical dose used as a laxative in an adult is magnesium citrate 11-25 grams, or magnesium hydroxide 1.2-4.8 grams or 15-60 mL of milk of magnesia, or magnesium sulfate 10-30 grams (14,15). Magnesium used as a laxative should be used as single doses at infrequent intervals (15). A typical adult dose used as an antacid is magnesium hydroxide 400-1300 mg up to four times daily, or magnesium oxide 400-840 mg per day in divided doses (14). For prophylaxis of migraine headache, 600 mg daily of trimagnesium dicitrate has been used (not available in the US) (4891,4895). To improve glycemic control in type 2 diabetes (NIDDM), 1000 mg elemental magnesium per day has been used (14,1172). For mild to moderate hypertension, 600-1000 mg elemental magnesium per day has been used (1192,1199). For reducing pain and tenderness associated with fibromyalgia, magnesium hydroxide 200-300 mg is taken orally with malic acid 800-1200 mg twice daily, equivalent to 4-6 Super Malic tablets twice daily (3262). The recommended amount of elemental magnesium as a dietary supplement is 54-483 mg daily in divided doses (14). The Adequate Intakes (AI) of magnesium for infants are: 0-6 months, 30 mg; and 7-12 months, 75 mg (3094). The RDAs for magnesium are: Children 1-3 years, 80 mg; Children 4-8 years, 130 mg; Children 9-13 years, 240 mg; Males 14-18 years, 410 mg; Males 19-30 years, 400 mg; Men 31 years and older, 420 mg; Females 14-18 years, 360 mg; Females 19-30 years, 310 mg; Women 31 years and older, 320 mg; Pregnant women up to 18 years, 400 mg; Pregnant women 19-30 years, 350 mg; Pregnant women over 30 years, 360 mg; Lactating women up to 18 years, 360 mg; Lactating women 19-30 years, 310 mg; and Lactating women over 30 years, 320 mg (3094). The maximum daily amount not likely to pose a risk of adverse effects from magnesium is 65 mg for children ages 1-3 years, 110 mg for children ages 4-8 years, and 350 mg for everyone over 8 years of age (3094).

INTRAVENOUS (IV): Intravenous magnesium is available as a prescription product.

Comments

None.

MAGNOLIA bark

This Product is Also Known As
Beaver Tree, Holly Bay, Indian Bark, Red Bay, Swamp Laurel, Swamp Sassafras, Sweet Bay, White Bay, White Laurel.
CAUTION: See separate listing for Magnolia flower bud.

Scientific Names
Magnolia glauca.
Family: Magnoliaceae.

People Use This For
Orally, magnolia bark is used for digestive disorders, as an anti-inflammatory, a stimulant, and to promote sweating. It is also used orally as a tonic, which is an agent used to invigorate, refresh or restore body function (18).

Safety
There is insufficient reliable information available about the safety of magnolia bark.
Pregnancy and Lactation: Insufficient reliable information available; avoid using.

Effectiveness
There is insufficient reliable information available about the effectiveness of magnolia bark.

Possible Mechanism of Action & Active Ingredients
Insufficient reliable information available.

Adverse Reactions Including Known Allergies
None reported.

Possible Interactions with Herbs & Other Dietary Supplements
Insufficient reliable information available.

Possible Interactions with Drugs
No interactions are known to occur, and there is no known reason to expect a clinically significant interaction with magnolia bark.

Possible Interactions with Foods
No interactions are known to occur, and there is no known reason to expect a clinically significant interaction with magnolia bark.

Possible Interactions with Lab Tests
No interactions are known to occur, and there is no known reason to expect a clinically significant interaction with magnolia bark.

Possible Interactions with Diseases or Conditions
No interactions are known to occur, and there is no known reason to expect a clinically significant interaction with magnolia bark.

Typical Dosages & Routes of Administration that are Commonly Used
ORAL: Magnolia bark is used as a powder or liquid extract (18).

Comments
There is very little scientific information about this product. Our staff is continually analyzing the available information on natural medicines and will add data here as it becomes available.

MAGNOLIA flower bud

This Product is Also Known As
Flos Magnoliae, Magnolia Flower Bud.
CAUTION: See separate listing for Magnolia bark.

Scientific Names
Magnolia biondii, synonym Magnolia fargesii; Magnolia denudata, synonym Magnolia heptaperta; Magnolia sprengeri; Magnolia sargentiana, synonym Magnolia emargenata; Magnolia wilsonii; Magnolia salicifolia; other Magnolia species.
Family: Magnoliaceae.

People Use This For

In Chinese medicine, people use magnolia flower bud both orally and topically for nasal congestion, runny nose, common cold, headache and facial dark spots. It is also used topically for toothaches.

In skin care products, magnolia flower bud extract is used topically as a skin whitener and to minimize or counteract irritant effects of other ingredients (11).

Safety

There is insufficient reliable information available about safety of magnolia flower bud. Its regulatory status in the US has not been determined (11).

PREGNANCY: UNSAFE ...contraindicated due to empiric uterine stimulating activity (11).

LACTATION: Insufficient reliable information available; avoid using.

Effectiveness

There is insufficient reliable information available about the effectiveness of magnolia flower bud.

Possible Mechanism of Action & Active Ingredients

Magnolia flower bud has antihistaminic activity and protective activity against asthma in animals. In vitro animal data also suggests anti-inflammatory, hypotensive, uterine stimulating, antifungal, antibacterial, and antiviral effects. It may also have skeletal muscle blocking and muscle relaxant properties. Magnolia flower bud may have activity against allergic and chronic rhinitis as well as some forms of sinusitis (11).

Adverse Reactions Including Known Allergies

None reported.

Possible Interactions with Herbs & Other Dietary Supplements

Insufficient reliable information available.

Possible Interactions with Drugs

No interactions are known to occur, and there is no known reason to expect a clinically significant interaction with magnolia flower bud.

Possible Interactions with Foods

No interactions are known to occur, and there is no known reason to expect a clinically significant interaction with magnolia flower bud.

Possible Interactions with Lab Tests

No interactions are known to occur, and there is no known reason to expect a clinically significant interaction with magnolia flower bud.

Possible Interactions with Diseases or Conditions

No interactions are known to occur, and there is no known reason to expect a clinically significant interaction with magnolia flower bud.

Typical Dosages & Routes of Administration that are Commonly Used

ORAL: Magnolia flower bud is used as a powder or liquid extract (18).

Comments

Magnolia flower bud emits a strong eucalyptus scent when crushed (11).

MAIDENHAIR FERN

This Product is Also Known As

Five-Finger Fern, Hair of Venus, Maiden Fern, Rock Fern, Venus Hair.

Scientific Names

Adiantum pedatum, synonym Adiantum capillus-veneris.
Family: Adiantiaceae.

People Use This For

Orally, maidenhair fern is used for bronchitis, coughs, whooping cough, and painful and excessive menstruation. It is also used orally as an expectorant and demulcent.

In the Middle Ages, it was used orally for various respiratory tract illnesses and severe coughs. It was also used topically for hair loss and to promote dark hair color (18).

Safety

POSSIBLY SAFE ...in amounts found in foods.

There is insufficient reliable information available about the safety of maidenhair fern for medicinal purposes.

PREGNANCY: UNSAFE ...contraindicated, most likely due to its emetic effects at higher doses (12).
LACTATION: Insufficient reliable information available; avoid using.

Effectiveness
There is insufficient reliable information available about the effectiveness of maidenhair fern.

Possible Mechanism of Action & Active Ingredients
Insufficient reliable information available.

Adverse Reactions Including Known Allergies
People who use large amounts may experience emesis (12).

Possible Interactions with Herbs & Other Dietary Supplements
Insufficient reliable information available.

Possible Interactions with Drugs
No interactions are known to occur, and there is no known reason to expect a clinically significant interaction with maidenhair fern.

Possible Interactions with Foods
No interactions are known to occur, and there is no known reason to expect a clinically significant interaction with maidenhair fern.

Possible Interactions with Lab Tests
No interactions are known to occur, and there is no known reason to expect a clinically significant interaction with maidenhair fern.

Possible Interactions with Diseases or Conditions
No interactions are known to occur, and there is no known reason to expect a clinically significant interaction with maidenhair fern.

Typical Dosages & Routes of Administration that are Commonly Used
ORAL: Maidenhair fern is taken as a tea. A single dose is equivalent to 1.5 grams ground or powdered herb. The tea is prepared by steeping 1.5 grams dried herb in 150 mL of boiling water for 10-15 minutes and straining (18).
TOPICAL: No typical dosage.

Comments
Maidenhair tree is another name for Ginkgo biloba, and is distinct from maidenhair fern (18).

MAITAKE

This Product is Also Known As
Dancing Mushroom, Grifola, Hen Of The Woods, King Of Mushrooms, Maitake Mushroom, Monkey's Bench, Shelf Fungi.

Scientific Names
Grifola frondosa.
Family: Polyporaceae.

People Use This For
Orally, maitake is used for cancer, HIV/AIDS, chronic fatigue syndrome (CFS), hepatitis, hay fever, diabetes, high blood pressure, hyperlipidemia, weight loss or control (2008), and chemotherapy support (1900).
For food uses, it is an edible mushroom (1210), and maitake has been consumed in Asia for thousands of years (6).

Safety
POSSIBLY SAFE ...when taken orally and used appropriately (12).
PREGNANCY AND LACTATION: Insufficient reliable information available; avoid using.

Effectiveness
There is insufficient reliable information available about the effectiveness of maitake.

Possible Mechanism of Action & Active Ingredients
The applicable parts of maitake are the fruiting body and mycelium. Maitake contains beta-glucan, which has been shown to possess antitumor activity. The "D-fraction" of betaglucan appears to be the most active and potent form (6). Maitake has immunostimulant effects and activates natural killer cells, cytotoxic T-cells, interleukin-1, and superoxide anions (6). Experiments have shown varied effects. In hypertensive rats, it lowers blood pressure (1213,1214), and it improves the lipid profile in hyperlipidemic rats (1209,1211). In genetically-induced diabetic mice, it lowers blood glucose (1212), and in overweight rats, it reduces weight (6). Maitake might improve

the quality of life of people with cancer by improving cancer symptoms and reducing pain, and it can aid in weight loss in overweight people (6). However, controlled studies are needed to confirm these effects (6).

Adverse Reactions Including Known Allergies
No adverse reactions have been reported with the oral use of maitake. Little or no information is available regarding maitake toxicity (6).

Possible Interactions with Herbs & Other Dietary Supplements
Insufficient reliable information available.

Possible Interactions with Drugs
DIABETES THERAPY: Monitor blood glucose levels closely due to claims that maitake has hypoglycemic effects (19).

Possible Interactions with Foods
No interactions are known to occur, and there is no known reason to expect a clinically significant interaction with maitake.

Possible Interactions with Lab Tests
No interactions are known to occur, and there is no known reason to expect a clinically significant interaction with maitake.

Possible Interactions with Diseases or Conditions
No interactions are known to occur, and there is no known reason to expect a clinically significant interaction with maitake.

Typical Dosages & Routes of Administration that are Commonly Used
ORAL: People typically take 500 to 1000 mg of maitake with water 2 or 3 times daily between meals. Maitake "D fraction" is typically dosed 6 mg twice daily between meals. The "D fraction" is also available as a liquid, approximately 1 mg/mL. For general use as a dietary supplement, the dose is 5 to 6 drops 3 times daily between meals. Health care professionals are directed to prescribe 0.5 to 1 mg/kg of body weight. If maitake causes stomach upset, the supplement is taken with food. Sometimes the dose is doubled or tripled (5273).

Comments
The potential for toxicity exists when other mushrooms are mistaken for maitake (6).

MALABAR NUT

This Product is Also Known As
Adulsa, Arusa.
CAUTION: See separate listing for Garcinia.

Scientific Names
Justicia Adhatoda.
Family: Acanthaceae.

People Use This For
In Indian medicine, people use malabar nut orally as an expectorant and secretory agent. It is also used as a bronchodilatory agent and mild spasmolytic (18).

Safety
There is insufficient reliable information available about the safety of malabar nut.
PREGNANCY: UNSAFE ...contraindicated for oral use (18).
LACTATION: Insufficient reliable information available; avoid using.

Effectiveness
There is insufficient reliable information available about the effectiveness of malabar nut.

Possible Mechanism of Action & Active Ingredients
The applicable part of malabar nut is the leaf. The quinazoline alkaloid vasicine has excitatory activity when taken in large amounts (18).

Adverse Reactions Including Known Allergies
None reported.

Possible Interactions with Herbs & Other Dietary Supplements
Insufficient reliable information available.

Possible Interactions with Drugs

No interactions are known to occur, and there is no known reason to expect a clinically significant interaction with malabar nut.

Possible Interactions with Foods

No interactions are known to occur, and there is no known reason to expect a clinically significant interaction with malabar nut.

Possible Interactions with Lab Tests

No interactions are known to occur, and there is no known reason to expect a clinically significant interaction with malabar nut.

Possible Interactions with Diseases or Conditions

No interactions are known to occur, and there is no known reason to expect a clinically significant interaction with malabar nut.

Typical Dosages & Routes of Administration that are Commonly Used

No typical dosage.

Comments

Vasicine was formerly used as the starting substance for production of mucolytics Bromhexin and Ambroxol. Neither of these products are available in the United States (18).

MALE FERN

This Product is Also Known As

American Aspidium, Bear's Paw, European Aspidium, Knotty Brake, Marginal Fern, Shield Fern.

Scientific Names

Dryopteris Filix-Mas.
Family: Aspleniaceae or Polypodiaceae.

People Use This For

In Chinese medicine, male fern has been used to treat recurrent nose bleeds, heavy menstrual bleeding, and wounds (6).
In veterinary medicine, male fern is used as an antihelmintic to treat worms (6).
Historically, male fern has been used orally for tumors and as an antihelmintic for treating worms (6).

Safety

LIKELY UNSAFE ...when used orally. Male fern can be a violent poison if absorbed (2,11). For this reason, it should no longer be used internally (2). Canada requires that it be labeled "For external use only" (12).
There is insufficient reliable information available about the safety of male fern for its other uses.
PREGNANCY AND LACTATION: LIKELY UNSAFE ...contraindicated (12). Insufficient reliable information available about the safety of topical use; avoid using.

Effectiveness

LIKELY EFFECTIVE ...when used orally for treating tapeworm infestation (2,6).
LIKELY INEFFECTIVE ...when used orally for rheumatism, neuralgia, muscle pain, earache, teething, and sleep disorders (2).
There is insufficient reliable information available about the effectiveness of male fern for its other uses.

Possible Mechanism of Action & Active Ingredients

The applicable parts of male fern are the above ground parts, leaf and rhizome. Male fern contains filicin and filmarone. These are active anthelmintics and act as a vermifuge to kill worms. Active constituents are soluble derivatives of phloroglucinol. These constituents are inactivated in an alkaline environment. Male fern also contains volatile oils, tannin, albaspidin and desaspidin. All these compounds together are called filicin, and work together to kill tapeworms. It is important to remember that once the tapeworm has been killed, a simultaneously administered saline laxative is used expel the worm (6).

Adverse Reactions Including Known Allergies

Male fern taken orally may cause headaches, dyspnea, nausea, diarrhea, vertigo, tremors, convulsions, cardiac and respiratory failure, and optic neuritis (6). Death has occurred with severe poisoning. Symptoms of toxicity include muscular weakness, coma, temporary or permanent blindness (11).

Possible Interactions with Herbs & Other Dietary Supplements

Insufficient reliable information available.

Possible Interactions with Drugs
CASTOR OIL: Enhances absorption and toxic potential of the male fern (6).

Possible Interactions with Foods
FATS, OILS AND ALCOHOL: Increases absorption and side effects (2).

Possible Interactions with Lab Tests
No interactions are known to occur, and there is no known reason to expect a clinically significant interaction with male fern.

Possible Interactions with Diseases or Conditions
Theoretically, in damaged GI mucosa or conditions which prolong GI transit, absorption and risk of side effects may be increased.

Typical Dosages & Routes of Administration that are Commonly Used
ORAL: Adults in a fasting state usually receive 3-6 mL orally. Children up to age two receive up to 2 mL orally in divided doses. Or, children over age two are given 0.25-0.5 mL orally per year of age up to a total of 4 mL orally in divided doses. The dose is typically given with a purgative (saline laxative) to aid expulsion of tapeworms (6,11). Co-administration with castor oil, which can increase absorption, is contraindicated (11).

Comments
High toxic potential precludes use (2,6). Treatment of overdose consists of giving saline cathartic followed by demulcent fluids. It is important to avoid fats and oils. If seizures occur, benzodiazepines may be used, and assisting respiration may be required. Since there are other products available that are effective and safer than male fern, it should not be used (7003).

MALLOW flower

This Product is Also Known As
Blue Mallow Flower, Cheeseflower, High Mallow, Malvae flos, Mauls.
CAUTION: See separate listings for Mallow leaf, Country Mallow, and Marshmallow.

Scientific Names
Malva sylvestris.
Family: Malvaceae.

People Use This For
Orally, mallow flower is used for irritation of the mucosa of the mouth and throat and the associated dry cough (2,8,18).
In folk medicine, it has been used for bronchitis (18), as a mild astringent for gastroenteritis, and for bladder complaints (8,18). Topically, mallow has been used as a poultice or bath additive for wounds (8,18).
It is also a food-coloring agent (8).

Safety
POSSIBLY SAFE ...when taken orally and used appropriately (2,12).
PREGNANCY AND LACTATION: Insufficient reliable information available; avoid using.

Effectiveness
POSSIBLY EFFECTIVE ...when taken orally for irritation of the mouth and throat and the associated dry cough (2). There is insufficient reliable information available about the effectiveness of mallow flower for its other uses.

Possible Mechanism of Action & Active Ingredients
Mallow flower contains mucilage, which protects and soothes mucous membranes (2,18). The anthocyanins constituents are a source of color (8).

Adverse Reactions Including Known Allergies
None reported.

Possible Interactions with Herbs & Other Dietary Supplements
Insufficient reliable information available.

Possible Interactions with Drugs
No interactions are known to occur, and there is no known reason to expect a clinically significant interaction with mallow flower.

Possible Interactions with Foods
No interactions are known to occur, and there is no known reason to expect a clinically significant interaction with mallow flower.

Possible Interactions with Lab Tests

No interactions are known to occur, and there is no known reason to expect a clinically significant interaction with mallow flower.

Possible Interactions with Diseases or Conditions

No interactions are known to occur, and there is no known reason to expect a clinically significant interaction with mallow flower.

Typical Dosages & Routes of Administration that are Commonly Used

ORAL: The typical dose of mallow is one cup of the tea several times daily (6,18). The tea is prepared by steeping 1.5-2 grams of the dried flowers in 150 mL boiling water for 10 minutes and then straining. Up to 5 grams of the dried flowers should be ingested per day (2,8,18).

Comments

Avoid confusion with mallow leaf, other malvae varieties, and marshmallow (Althaea officinalis).

MALLOW leaf

This Product is Also Known As

Blue Mallow, Dwarf Mallow, High Mallow, Malvae folium.
CAUTION: See separate listings for Mallow flower, Country Mallow, and Marshmallow.

Scientific Names

Malva sylvestris; Malva neglecta.
Family: Malvaceae.

People Use This For

Orally, mallow leaf is used for irritation of the mucosa of the mouth and throat and the associated dry cough (2,8). In folk medicine, it has been used for colds and upper respiratory mucous membrane inflammation (8), as a mild astringent for gastroenteritis (8), and topically as a poultice for wounds (8).

Safety

POSSIBLY SAFE ...when taken orally and used appropriately (2).
PREGNANCY AND LACTATION: Insufficient reliable information available; avoid using.

Effectiveness

POSSIBLY EFFECTIVE ...when taken orally for irritation of the mouth and throat and the associated dry cough (2). There is insufficient reliable information available about the effectiveness of mallow leaf for its other uses.

Possible Mechanism of Action & Active Ingredients

Mallow leaf contains mucilage which protects and soothes mucous membranes (2,18). The mucilage has been shown in vitro to inactivate the serum complement, which is a component in the host defense system (1526).

Adverse Reactions Including Known Allergies

None reported.

Possible Interactions with Herbs & Other Dietary Supplements

Insufficient reliable information available.

Possible Interactions with Drugs

No interactions are known to occur, and there is no known reason to expect a clinically significant interaction with mallow leaf.

Possible Interactions with Foods

No interactions are known to occur, and there is no known reason to expect a clinically significant interaction with mallow leaf.

Possible Interactions with Lab Tests

No interactions are known to occur, and there is no known reason to expect a clinically significant interaction with mallow leaf.

Possible Interactions with Diseases or Conditions

No interactions are known to occur, and there is no known reason to expect a clinically significant interaction with mallow leaf.

Typical Dosages & Routes of Administration that are Commonly Used

ORAL: The typical dose of mallow is one cup of the tea several times per day and in the evening before going to sleep (6). It can be sweetened with honey (6). The tea is prepared by steeping 3-5 grams of the dried leaves in 150 mL boiling water for 10-15 minutes and then straining (6). The maximum use of mallow is 5 grams of the dried leaves per day (2).

Comments
Mallow leaf is a rich plant source of vitamin C (19).

MANACA

This Product is Also Known As
Pohl, Vegetable Mercury.

Scientific Names
Brunfelsia hopeana.
Family: Solanaceae.

People Use This For
Orally, manaca is used for arthritis, and as a diuretic (18).

Safety
There is insufficient reliable information available about the safety of manaca.
Pregnancy and Lactation: Insufficient reliable information available; avoid using.

Effectiveness
There is insufficient reliable information available about the effectiveness of manaca.

Possible Mechanism of Action & Active Ingredients
The applicable part of manaca is the root. Animal data suggests that manaca may cause symptoms of anxiety, restlessness, increases in heart and respiratory rates, increased salivation, vomiting, muscle tremors, and may result in death (18).

Adverse Reactions Including Known Allergies
None reported.

Possible Interactions with Herbs & Other Dietary Supplements
Insufficient reliable information available.

Possible Interactions with Drugs
No interactions are known to occur, and there is no known reason to expect a clinically significant interaction with manaca.

Possible Interactions with Foods
No interactions are known to occur, and there is no known reason to expect a clinically significant interaction with manaca.

Possible Interactions with Lab Tests
No interactions are known to occur, and there is no known reason to expect a clinically significant interaction with manaca.

Possible Interactions with Diseases or Conditions
No interactions are known to occur, and there is no known reason to expect a clinically significant interaction with manaca.

Typical Dosages & Routes of Administration that are Commonly Used
ORAL: Manaca is taken as a liquid extract (18).

Comments
There is very little scientific information about this product. Our staff is continually analyzing the available information on natural medicines and will add data here as it becomes available.

MANGANESE

This Product is Also Known As
Manganese Amino Acid Chelate, Manganese Aminoate, Manganese Ascorbate, Manganese Aspartate Complex, Manganese Chloride, Manganese Chloridetetrahydrate, Manganese Dioxide, Manganese Gluconate, Manganese Sulfate, Manganese Sulfate Monohydrate, Manganese Sulfate Tetrahydrate, Manganum.

Scientific Names

Manganese; Mn; atomic number 25.

People Use This For

Orally, manganese is used for osteoporosis (1993), microcytic anemia (9), premenstrual symptoms (2004), and to prevent and treat manganese deficiency (9).

The combination of manganese ascorbate, chondroitin sulfate, and glucosamine hydrochloride is used orally for osteoarthritis (4237). Intravenously, manganese is used as a trace element for supplementation in parenteral nutrition (9,14).

Safety

LIKELY SAFE ...when used orally and appropriately. Adverse effects have not been reported when doses of less than 4.2 mg per day are used (1991). Safety has not been evaluated in the elderly (14,1992). ...when used intravenously and appropriately as a trace element for supplementation in parenteral nutrition (14).

POSSIBLY SAFE ...when manganese ascorbate is used orally and appropriately in combination with chondroitin sulfate and glucosamine hydrochloride for up to 16 weeks (4237). The cited study used 30 mg of elemental manganese per day for 16 weeks, an amount significantly greater than the estimated safe dose of 2-5 mg per day, with no significant adverse effects reported.

CHILDREN: Insufficient reliable information available (14,1992).

PREGNANCY AND LACTATION: Insufficient reliable information available; avoid using.

Effectiveness

EFFECTIVE ...when used orally for preventing or treating manganese deficiency (14). ...when the FDA-approved prescription drug is used intravenously.

POSSIBLY EFFECTIVE ...when used orally in combination with calcium, zinc, and copper for osteoporosis (1994). ...when used orally for premenstrual symptoms including crying, loneliness, anxiety, restlessness, irritability, mood swings, depression, and tension (2004). ...when the combination of manganese ascorbate, chondroitin sulfate, and glucosamine hydrochloride (Cosamin-DS) is used orally for treating knee osteoarthritis pain (4237).

There is insufficient reliable information available about the effectiveness of manganese for its other uses.

Possible Mechanism of Action & Active Ingredients

Manganese acts as a cofactor in metabolic and enzymatic reactions (14,2003). Researchers think manganese enhances bone turnover (1993) and cartilage synthesis (2003). It might also increase the hematinic action of iron in the treatment of microcytic anemia (9). Manganese is normally cleared hepatically and chronic liver disease can cause manganese accumulation and toxicity (1992). Manganese accumulation is thought to be responsible for Parkinsonian symptoms and encephalopathy associated with chronic liver disease (1992). One human trial found a decrease in knee osteoarthritis pain with the combination of manganese ascorbate, chondroitin sulfate, and glucosamine hydrochloride (Cosamin-DS) (4237). Because the study compared the combination to placebo, it is not known if the combination has greater benefit than chondroitin sulfate alone, which demonstrates effectiveness in people with osteoarthritis (see separate listing for chondroitin sulfate). There is currently no clinical evidence that glucosamine hydrochloride alone provides benefit for people with osteoarthritis (see separate listing for glucosamine hydrochloride).

Adverse Reactions Including Known Allergies

Ingesting manganese can cause a hypersensitivity reaction (14) or dark mucosal pigmentation (14). Chronic occupational exposure to manganese dust or fumes is associated with orthostatic hypotension, decreased heart rate, mood disturbance, and dementia (1990). Manganese accumulation might be the cause of Parkinsonian-like extrapyramidal symptoms, encephalopathy and psychosis that occurs in people with chronic liver disease (9,1992).

Possible Interactions with Herbs & Other Dietary Supplements

CALCIUM: Concomitant administration can decrease manganese absorption (2000).

IRON: Concomitant administration can decrease manganese absorption (2004).

ZINC: Concomitant administration can increase manganese absorption and plasma levels (2000).

Possible Interactions with Drugs

No interactions are known to occur, and there is no known reason to expect a clinically significant interaction with manganese.

Possible Interactions with Foods

No interactions are known to occur, and there is no known reason to expect a clinically significant interaction with manganese.

Possible Interactions with Lab Tests

ALKALINE PHOSPHATASE: Magnesium salts can cause a false increase in serum alkaline phosphatase test results due to enzyme activation in the laboratory procedure (275).

BONE MINERAL DENSITY (BMD): Manganese (in combination with calcium, zinc, and copper) might improve BMD and BMD test results in patients with osteoporosis (1994).

STOOL COLOR: Manganese dioxide might cause stool to turn dark brown to black (275).

Possible Interactions with Diseases or Conditions

CHRONIC LIVER DISEASE: Use manganese cautiously. Chronic liver disease can lead to manganese accumulation and toxicity (9,14,1992,2001).

IRON-DEFICIENCY ANEMIA: Individuals with iron-deficiency anemia might have enhanced manganese absorption (2002).

Typical Dosages & Routes of Administration that are Commonly Used

ORAL: No recommended dietary allowances (RDA) for manganese have been established. Estimated safe and adequate daily dietary intake is 2-5 mg per day (9,1991,2005). For osteoporosis, 5 mg per day combined with 1000 mg elemental calcium, 15 mg zinc, and 2.5 mg copper has been used (1994). For decreasing knee osteoarthritis pain, a combination of chondroitin sulfate (1200 mg/day), glucosamine hydrochloride (1500 mg/day), and manganese ascorbate (228 mg/day) (4237), the equivalent to one Cosamin-DS tablet three times daily has been used (3278,4237). The manufacturer recommends one tablet three times daily in people under 200 lbs., and two tablets twice daily in people over 200 lbs (3278).

INTRAVENOUS: Intravenous manganese is available as a FDA-approved prescription product.

Comments

Manganese is found in leafy green vegetables, nuts, seeds, tea, and whole grains (2005,2008).

MANNA

This Product is Also Known As

Flake Manna, Flowering Ash, Manna Ash.

Scientific Names

Fraxinus ornus.
Family: Oleaceae.

People Use This For

Orally, the dried sap of manna is used as a laxative for constipation (2,9,18) and a stool softener for anal fissure, hemorrhoids, and after anorectal surgery (2,18).

Safety

POSSIBLY SAFE ...when used orally and appropriately on a short-term basis (2); avoid extended use of manna (2,18).

PREGNANCY AND LACTATION: Insufficient reliable information available; avoid using.

Effectiveness

POSSIBLY EFFECTIVE ...when taken orally for constipation and as a stool softener for anal fissure, hemorrhoids, and after anorectal surgery (2).

Possible Mechanism of Action & Active Ingredients

Manna contains 40-90% mannitol (9,18), which acts as an osmotic laxative (2,18).

Adverse Reactions Including Known Allergies

Manna can cause nausea or flatulence (2,18).

Possible Interactions with Herbs & Other Dietary Supplements

STIMULANT LAXATIVE HERBS: Theoretically, concomitant use of manna with other stimulant laxative herbs can increase the risk of potassium depletion. Stimulant laxative herbs include aloe dried leaf sap, wild cucumber fruit (Ecballium elaterium), blue flag rhizome, alder buckthorn, European buckthorn, butternut bark, cascara bark, castor oil, colocynth fruit pulp, gamboge bark exudate, jalap root, black root, podophyllum root, rhubarb root, senna leaves and pods, and yellow dock root (19).

POTASSIUM DEPLETING HERBS: Theoretically, concomitant use of manna with horsetail plant or the licorice rhizome increases the risk of potassium depletion.

Possible Interactions with Drugs

CARDIAC GLYCOSIDES: Theoretically, the overuse or abuse of this product increases the risk of adverse effects of cardiac glycoside drugs, e.g. digoxin (Lanoxin).

Possible Interactions with Foods

No interactions are known to occur, and there is no known reason to expect a clinically significant interaction with manna.

Possible Interactions with Lab Tests
No interactions are known to occur, and there is no known reason to expect a clinically significant interaction with manna.

Possible Interactions with Diseases or Conditions
OBSTRUCTION: Manna is contraindicated in cases of bowel obstruction or ileus (2,18).

Typical Dosages & Routes of Administration that are Commonly Used
ORAL: For adults, the typical dose of manna is 20-30 grams per day or equivalent preparations (2,18). For children, the common dose is 2-16 grams per day (2,18). Manna should not be taken for prolonged use (2,18).

Comments
Manna consists of the dried sap collected from the splits in branches and trunk of Fraxinus ornus. The manna bark contains coumarins which can inactivate the serum complement, a component in the host defense system (1527).

MARIJUANA

This Product is Also Known As
Anashca, Banji, Bhang, Cannabis, Charas, Esrar, Gaga, Ganga, Grass, Hash, Hashish, Hemp, Kif, Mariguana, Marihuana, Pot, Sawi, Sinsemilla, Weed.

Scientific Names
Cannabis sativa.
Family: Cannabaceae.

People Use This For
Orally, marijuana is used for euphoria (18). The prescription-only, synthetic dronabinol (Marinol) product is used orally for the treatment of anorexia or appetite loss associated with AIDS and for cancer chemotherapy induced nausea and vomiting unresponsive to traditional medications.
As an inhalant, marijuana is used for treating nausea, reducing intraocular pressure, stimulation of appetite, altering senses (psychoactivity), euphoria (18), mucous membrane inflammation, leprosy, fever, dandruff, hemorrhoids, obesity, asthma, urinary tract infections, cough (6), and treating anorexia associated with weight loss in AIDS patients (2619).

Safety
POSSIBLY UNSAFE ...when marijuana is used orally or inhaled (6).
PREGNANCY: UNSAFE ...when used orally or inhaled; marijuana passes through the placenta and can reduce fetal growth. Marijuana use during pregnancy is also associated with childhood leukemia (4260).
LACTATION: LIKELY UNSAFE ...when used orally or inhaled because dronabinol (THC) is concentrated and excreted in breast milk (6,2619,2620).

Effectiveness
LIKELY EFFECTIVE ...when marijuana is taken orally or smoked as an euphoriant (6,13,18).
POSSIBLY EFFECTIVE ...when marijuana is smoked as an antiemetic (2621,2622). ...when smoked as an appetite stimulant (6,13,18). ...when smoked for reducing intraocular pressure in patients with glaucoma (1268). While studies indicate that marijuana lowers intraocular pressure, well designed trials are needed to determine whether it preserves visual function in patients with glaucoma (6,1268). Questions remain concerning the adverse effect profile associated with therapeutic use of smoked marijuana (1268).
There is insufficient reliable information available about the effectiveness of marijuana for its other uses.

Possible Mechanism of Action & Active Ingredients
The applicable parts of marijuana are the flower and leaf. Marijuana contains cannabinoids, including tetrahydrocannabinol (THC, dronabinol), that act on the central nervous system (CNS) (6,13). The THC concentration is highest in the flowers and leaves and lowest in the stems, roots, and seeds (6). THC can interact with cell-wall lipids or affect prostaglandin biosynthesis (18). It can act via cannabinoid receptors in neural tissues (2619) or opiate receptors in the forebrain, leading to indirect inhibition of the emetic center in the medulla oblongata (13). Marijuana suppresses the immune system in experimental animals (18). While short-term inhalation increases bronchodilation and reduces bronchospasm, long-term use impairs lung function, which can result in constrictive lung disease. Marijuana can cause tachycardia and transient hypertension (6). The cannabinoids in marijuana are allergenic in animal models (6). THC is absorbed orally or by inhalation, is rapidly distributed throughout the body, and has a high affinity for fat tissues (6). The metabolites appear in the urine for ten days or more after a single exposure and for several weeks after chronic exposure (6).

Adverse Reactions Including Known Allergies
The use of marijuana can cause xerostomia, nausea, and vomiting (6). Intoxicating doses of marijuana impairs reaction time, motor coordination, and visual perceptions (6). An individual's driving ability can be impaired up to

eight hours (18). The chronic use of marijuana can cause laryngitis, bronchitis, apathy, psychic decline, sexual dysfunctions (18), and has been associated with several cases of an unusual pattern of bullous emphysema (1395). Signs of acute poisoning from marijuana include nausea, vomiting, lacrimation, hacking cough, disturbed cardiac function, and limb numbness (18). Marijuana has a high abuse potential (6). Regular smoking of 3-4 marijuana cigarettes per day is reported to produce as many symptoms as an average of 22 tobacco cigarettes per day, and comparable airway histological effects as 20 tobacco cigarettes per day (1395).

Regular use of marijuana in middle-aged persons has been associated with an increased risk of myocardial infarction. In an unpublished study, announced at the American Heart Association's 40th Annual Conference on Cardiovascular Disease Epidemiology and Prevention, there was a 4.8 fold increase in relative risk of myocardial infarction within the first hour following smoking marijuana. Regular marijuana smoking was defined as smoking marijuana less than once a month to daily (1356). Further study is needed to confirm these findings.

Possible Interactions with Herbs & Other Dietary Supplements

Theoretically, marijuana can have additive or synergistic effects when used with herbs that possess CNS depressant or stimulant effects.

Possible Interactions with Drugs

BARBITURATES: Marijuana can decrease barbiturate clearance rate (2619).
FLUOXETINE, DISULFIRAM: Concomitant use of marijuana can cause transient hypomanic episodes (2619).
THEOPHYLLINE: Concomitant use can increase theophylline metabolism (2619).
OTHER DRUGS: Use of dronabinol can have additive or synergistic effects with amphetamines, anticholinergics, antihistamines, cocaine, hypnotics, psychomimetics, sedatives, and sympathomimetics (2619).

Possible Interactions with Foods

ALCOHOL: Concomitant use of alcohol with dronabinol can have additive or synergistic CNS effects (2619).

Possible Interactions with Lab Tests

INTRAOCULAR PRESSURE: Marijuana smoking reduces intraocular pressure and test results in some patients with glaucoma (1268).

Possible Interactions with Diseases or Conditions

CARDIOVASCULAR DISEASES: Avoid; marijuana has the potential to cause tachycardia and transient hypertension (6).
COMPROMISED IMMUNE FUNCTION: Theoretically, inhalation of marijuana smoke containing Aspergillus spores increases the risk of fungal infections and sensitization in individuals with compromised immune function (6).
RESPIRATORY DISEASES: Long-term use of marijuana can exacerbate respiratory conditions (6). Chronic marijuana use has been associated with several cases of an unusual pattern of bullous emphysema (1395).
SEIZURE DISORDERS: Marijuana might exacerbate, or help control, seizure disorders in some individuals (6).

Typical Dosages & Routes of Administration that are Commonly Used

ORAL: People typically use 5 to 15 drops of marijuana tincture or 1 to 3 drops of fluid extract.
INHALATION: People typically use 1 to 3 grains (65 to 195 mg) of cannabis for smoking. Hashish, the plant resin, is smoked in a dose of up to 1 grain (16 to 65 mg). Potency may vary. The drug deteriorates rapidly, requiring ascending doses to produce its effect (5267).

Comments

Avoid confusion with hemp, a distinct variety of Cannabis sativa cultivated for its fiber and seeds, which contains less than 1% THC. In March 1999, the Institute of Medicine released a report, titled "Marijuana and Medicine: Assessing the Science Base," which concludes: "Until a non-smoked, rapid-onset cannabinoid drug delivery system becomes available, we acknowledge that there is no clear alternative for people suffering from chronic conditions that might be relieved by smoking marijuana, such as pain or AIDS wasting. One possible approach is to treat patients as n-of-1 clinical trials, in which patients are fully informed of their status as experimental subjects using a harmful drug delivery system, and in which their condition is closely monitored and documented under medical supervision, thereby increasing the knowledge base of the risks and benefits of marijuana use under such conditions."

British health authorities authorized clinical trials of marijuana-based drugs for patients with multiple sclerosis (MS) and severe pain. Participants in these studies will use sublingual formulations manufactured by GW Pharmaceuticals, designed to maximize pain relief. The manufacturer claims that the results of these studies might influence the future legal status of marijuana in Britain (5046).

MARJORAM

This Product is Also Known As

Garden Marjoram, Gartenmajoran, Knotted Marjoram, Majoran, Majorana aetheroleum oil, Majorana herb, Marjolaine, Mejorana, Sweet Marjoram.
CAUTION: See separate listing for Oregano.

Scientific Names

Origanum majorana, synonym Majorana hortensis.
Family: Lamiaceae or Labiatae.

People Use This For

Orally, marjoram is used for rhinitis and colds in infants, rhinitis in toddlers, and gastritis (2,18). Marjoram oil is used for coughs, gall bladder complaints, and gastrointestinal cramps (18).

In combination products, marjoram leaf, flower, or oil are used for stimulating appetite, as a digestive aid, antispasmodic, antiflatulent, astringent, for "strengthening of the stomach," acute and chronic gastritis, ulcus ventriculi, colic-like nervous gastrointestinal disorders, and diathermic effect for circulatory deficiencies in the abdominal regions. Marjoram is also used in combination products as a support of intestinal activity, purification of the system, supportive for acute inflammatory liver diseases, managing gallstones, dry, irritating coughs, swellings of the nasal and pharyngeal mucosa, inflammation of the ears, headaches, reducing blood glucose levels, promoting milk secretion, and as a nerve, heart, and circulation system tonic. Combination products with marjoram are used for promoting healthy sleep, treating mood swings, a tonic during convalescence, a blood builder, anorexia, sprains, bruises, lumbago, dysmenorrhea, climacteric complaints, strengthening of the female organs, an adjuvant for vaginal discharge, adnexitis, menstrual disturbances, urogenital bleeding, and as a diuretic (2).

In folk medicine, the marjoram leaf and flower are used for cramps, depression, dizziness, gastrointestinal disorders, migraines, nervous headaches, neurasthenia, paralysis, paroxysmal coughs, rhinitis, and as a diuretic (18). For food uses, marjoram is a culinary spice and commonly used in foods (11). The oil and oleoresin are used as flavor ingredients in foods and beverages (11).

In manufacturing, the oil is used as a fragrance component in soaps and cosmetics (11).

Safety

LIKELY SAFE ...when the flower, leaf, and oil are consumed in amounts commonly found in food (11). Marjoram has Generally Recognized as Safe (GRAS) status in the US (11).
POSSIBLY SAFE ...when the leaf is used orally for medicinal purposes (12) on a short-term basis (2). ...when marjoram oil is used orally and appropriately (11).
POSSIBLY UNSAFE ...when the flower, leaf, and oil are used long-term because marjoram contains arbutin and hydroxyquinone. Some information suggests hydroxyquinone might cause cancer (2). ...when using fresh marjoram topically because it can cause eye and skin inflammation (11).
CHILDREN: LIKELY SAFE ...when the flower, leaf, and oil are used orally in food amounts. POSSIBLY UNSAFE ...when larger amounts are used in children; avoid using (2).
PREGNANCY: LIKELY SAFE ...when used orally in food amounts (11,12). POSSIBLY UNSAFE ...when used in greater amounts because it has the potential for stimulating menstruation (19).
LACTATION: Insufficient reliable information available; avoid using in amounts larger than those found in foods.

Effectiveness

There is insufficient reliable information available about the effectiveness of marjoram.

Possible Mechanism of Action & Active Ingredients

The applicable parts of marjoram are the flower, leaf and oil. Marjoram has antiflatulent, antispasmodic, diaphoretic, and diuretic properties (11). The volatile oil demonstrates antimicrobial and insecticidal activity (18). There is some evidence that marjoram has antibacterial activity and antiviral activity against the herpes simplex virus (11). The constituents of marjoram include small amounts of arbutin and hydroxyquinone (2). Arbutin, an antibacterial principle, is poorly absorbed from the gastrointestinal tract (7). Marjoram is a rich source of calcium and iron (19).

Adverse Reactions Including Known Allergies

When applied topically, the fresh marjoram can cause eye and skin inflammation (11). Hydroxyquinone can cause skin depigmentation (2); however, this adverse effect has not been reported with the use of the marjoram ointment (2).

Possible Interactions with Herbs & Other Dietary Supplements

Insufficient reliable information available.

Possible Interactions with Drugs

No interactions are known to occur, and there is no known reason to expect a clinically significant interaction with marjoram.

Possible Interactions with Foods

No interactions are known to occur, and there is no known reason to expect a clinically significant interaction with marjoram.

Possible Interactions with Lab Tests

No interactions are known to occur, and there is no known reason to expect a clinically significant interaction with marjoram.

Possible Interactions with Diseases or Conditions

CROSS-ALLERGENICITY: Marjoram can cause allergic reactions in people allergic to the Lamiaceae family plants, which include basil, hyssop, lavender, mint, oregano, and sage (3705).

Typical Dosages & Routes of Administration that are Commonly Used

ORAL: The typical dose of marjoram is one to two cups of the tea throughout the day (18). The tea is prepared by steeping 1-2 teaspoons of the flower or leaf in 250 mL boiling water for 5 minutes and then straining.
TOPICAL: Marjoram is commonly used as a poultice or mouthwash (18).

Comments

In early Greek mythology, the goddess of love, Aphrodite, was believed to have grown marjoram, and marjoram has since been used in various love potions (6002). Avoid confusion with oregano (Origanum vulgare), also referred to as wild marjoram and winter marjoram (2,18).

MARSH BLAZING STAR

This Product is Also Known As

Backache Root, Blazing-Star, Button Snakeroot, Colic Root, Devil's Bite Prairie-Pine, Gayfeather, Gay-Feather.

Scientific Names

Liatris spicata, synonym Laciniaria spicata; Liatris callilepis; Serratula spicata.
Family: Compositae or Asteraceae.

People Use This For

Orally, marsh blazing star root is used for kidney disorders, dysmenorrhea, gonorrhea, and as a diuretic (18).

Safety

There is insufficient reliable information available about the safety of marsh blazing star.
Pregnancy and Lactation: Insufficient reliable information available; avoid using.

Effectiveness

There is insufficient reliable information available about the effectiveness of marsh blazing star.

Possible Mechanism of Action & Active Ingredients

The applicable part of marsh blazing star is the root. Marsh blazing star contains coumarin as its active principle (18). However, coumarin itself is not an anticoagulant. It has only 0.1%-0.02% of the anticoagulant effect of bishydroxy-coumarin (295). Some studies suggest coumarin might be effective in reducing edemas and inflammations by increasing venous and lymphatic return (295).

Adverse Reactions Including Known Allergies

The oral use of marsh blazing star which contains coumarin, can be associated with nausea and vomiting (286), diarrhea, dizziness, insomnia (287), asymptomatic SGOT elevations (286), and liver toxicity (6,18,4501). Handling the plant can cause contact dermatitis (3837). Marsh blazing star can cause an allergic reaction in individuals sensitive to the Asteraceae/Compositae family. Members of this family include ragweed, chrysanthemums, marigolds, daisies, and many other herbs.

Possible Interactions with Herbs & Other Dietary Supplements

Insufficient reliable information available.

Possible Interactions with Drugs

No interactions are known to occur, and there is no known reason to expect a clinically significant interaction with marsh blazing star.

Possible Interactions with Foods

No interactions are known to occur, and there is no known reason to expect a clinically significant interaction with marsh blazing star.

Possible Interactions with Lab Tests

No interactions are known to occur, and there is no known reason to expect a clinically significant interaction with marsh blazing star.

Possible Interactions with Diseases or Conditions

CROSS-ALLERGENICITY: Can cause an allergic reaction in individuals sensitive to the Asteraceae/Compositae family. Members of this family include ragweed, chrysanthemums, marigolds, daisies, and many other herbs.

Typical Dosages & Routes of Administration that are Commonly Used

ORAL: No typical dosage.

Comments

The ground root is used as tea. Warfarin, a closely related compound to coumarin, is a potent anticoagulant and rat poison (6).

MARSH MARIGOLD

This Product is Also Known As

Bull's Eyes, Cowslip, Horse Blobs, Kingcups, Leopard's Foot, Meadow Routs, Palsy Root, Solsequia, Sponsa Solis, Verrucaria, Water Blobs, Water Dragon.

Scientific Names

Caltha palustris.
Family: Ranunculaceae.

People Use This For

Orally, marsh marigold is used to stop pain and cramps, for menstrual disorders and bronchial inflammation. Historically, it was used orally for jaundice, liver and biliary disorders. Marsh marigold was also used as a laxative, diuretic, lower cholesterol levels and raise blood sugar.
Some Native Americans and Russians used marsh marigold topically for cleaning skin lesions and sores (18).

Safety

LIKELY UNSAFE …when the fresh above ground parts are used orally or topically because they cause severe local irritation (18).
There is insufficient reliable information about the safety of the medicinal use of the dried above ground parts.
PREGNANCY AND LACTATION: LIKELY UNSAFE …when the fresh above ground parts are used orally or topically. There is insufficient reliable information available about the safety of the dried above ground parts during pregnancy and lactation (18).

Effectiveness

There is insufficient reliable information available about the effectiveness of marsh marigold.

Possible Mechanism of Action & Active Ingredients

The applicable parts of marsh marigold are the above ground parts of the flowering plant. When the fresh plant is crushed or cut into small pieces, the glycoside ranunculin is enzymatically changed into a severely irritating protoanemonin, which, in turn, rapidly degrades into the less toxic anemonin (18). Both protoanemonin and ranunculin are destroyed to an unknown extent during the drying process (2).

Adverse Reactions Including Known Allergies

Ingestion of marsh marigold can cause severe irritation of the gastrointestinal tract, with colic and diarrhea. Irritation of the urinary tract can also occur. Skin contact with the fresh plant can cause blisters and burns that are difficult to heal (18).

Possible Interactions with Herbs & Other Dietary Supplements

Insufficient reliable information available.

Possible Interactions with Drugs

No interactions are known to occur, and there is no known reason to expect a clinically significant interaction with marsh marigold.

Possible Interactions with Foods

No interactions are known to occur, and there is no known reason to expect a clinically significant interaction with marsh marigold.

Possible Interactions with Lab Tests

No interactions are known to occur, and there is no known reason to expect a clinically significant interaction with marsh marigold.

Possible Interactions with Diseases or Conditions

No interactions are known to occur, and there is no known reason to expect a clinically significant interaction with marsh marigold.

Typical Dosages & Routes of Administration that are Commonly Used
No typical dosage.

Comments
None.

MARSH TEA

This Product is Also Known As
James' Tea, Labrador Tea, Ledi palustris herba, Marsh Citrus, Moth Herb, Romarin Sauvage, Sumpfporst, Swamp Tea, Wild Rosemary.
CAUTION: See separate listing for Labrador Tea.

Scientific Names
Ledum palustre.
Family: Lamiaceae.

People Use This For
Orally, marsh tea is used for rheumatic discomforts, whooping cough [2], for bronchitis, cold, cough, whitlow (herpes infection of the finger), relieving chest and lung ailments, stimulating milk flow, as a diaphoretic, diuretic, abortifacient [2], expectorant, and narcotic [4017].

Safety
LIKELY UNSAFE …when large amounts are used orally to try to cause abortion [2]. The essential oil of marsh tea causes severe gastrointestinal tract irritation, kidneys and urinary tract damage, and central nervous system excitation followed by paralysis [2].
There is insufficient reliable information available about the safety of the oral use of small amounts of the above ground parts of marsh tea [2].
PREGNANCY: LIKELY UNSAFE …contraindicated for oral use [2,19]. Marsh tea is considered to be a potential uterine stimulant [19].
LACTATION: There is insufficient reliable information available about the safety of small amounts used orally during lactation; avoid using.

Effectiveness
There is insufficient reliable information available about the effectiveness of marsh tea.

Possible Mechanism of Action & Active Ingredients
Some evidence suggests marsh tea might have antitussive and anti-inflammatory activity. It might also inhibit motility [2], and stimulate uterine activity [19].

Adverse Reactions Including Known Allergies
Ingestion of large amounts of marsh tea can cause poisoning [2]. The essential oil of marsh tea can cause severe irritation of the gastrointestinal tract, vomiting, diarrhea, irritation and damage to the kidneys and urinary tract, heavy perspiration, myalgias, arthralgias, central nervous system excitation with narcotic intoxication, followed by paralysis [2].

Possible Interactions with Herbs & Other Dietary Supplements
Insufficient reliable information available.

Possible Interactions with Drugs
CNS DEPRESSANTS: Marsh tea can potentiate effects of barbiturates and alcohol [2].

Possible Interactions with Foods
No interactions are known to occur, and there is no known reason to expect a clinically significant interaction with marsh tea.

Possible Interactions with Lab Tests
No interactions are known to occur, and there is no known reason to expect a clinically significant interaction with marsh tea.

Possible Interactions with Diseases or Conditions
KIDNEY DYSFUNCTION: Contraindicated in individuals with kidney dysfunction [2].
GI IRRITATION: Theoretically, might exacerbate gastrointestinal tract inflammation or irritation [2].
URINARY TRACT IRRITATION: Theoretically, might exacerbate urinary tract irritation and inflammation [2].

Typical Dosages & Routes of Administration that are Commonly Used
ORAL: No typical dosage.

Comments
Marsh tea essential oil is unsafe: avoid using.

MARSHMALLOW

This Product is Also Known As
Alteia, Althaeae folium, Althaeae radi, Althea, Herba Malvae , Mallards, Mortification Root, Racine De Guimauve, Sweet Weed, Wymote.
CAUTION: See separate listings for Mallow flower and Mallow leaf.

Scientific Names
Althaea officinalis.
Family: Malvaceae.

People Use This For
Orally, marshmallow leaf and root are used for irritation or inflammation of the mouth and oral pharynx and the associated dry cough (1,2,4,5,6,8,9,11,18), and for inflammation of the gastric mucosa (1,2,4,8,11,18).
Topically, marshmallow leaf and root are used for abscesses (4,18), for varicose and thrombotic ulcers (4), as a poultice for skin inflammation or burns (8,18), and for other wounds (4,18). Marshmallow leaf is used topically as a poultice for insect bites (8). Marshmallow root is used topically in ointments for chapped skin (6,11) and chilblains (11).
In folk medicine, the marshmallow leaf and root have been used for respiratory tract mucous membrane inflammation (4,18), diarrhea (18), peptic ulcers (4), constipation (18), urinary tract inflammation (4,18), and urinary calculus (4).
For food uses, marshmallow leaf is used as a flavoring agent (4).
In manufacturing, the marshmallow root is used in foods and beverages (4,6,11).

Safety
LIKELY SAFE ...when consumed in amounts commonly found in foods (4,11). The leaf and root are approved for use in foods in the US (11). ...when taken orally for medicinal purposes (2,4,12).
POSSIBLY SAFE ...when used topically (4).
PREGNANCY AND LACTATION: Insufficient reliable information available.

Effectiveness
POSSIBLY EFFECTIVE ...when marshmallow leaf or root is taken orally for soothing irritation of the mouth and pharynx (1,2,4,5,6,7,8,9,11), for dry cough (1,2,8), and for irritation of the gastric mucosa (2).
There is insufficient reliable information available about the effectiveness of marshmallow leaf or root for its other uses.

Possible Mechanism of Action & Active Ingredients
The applicable parts of marshmallow are the leaves and the root. Marshmallow leaf and root contain mucilage polysaccharides (1,4,6,7,11,18) that can soothe and protect mucous membranes from local irritation by forming a protective layer (1,2,4,6,7,9,18). The mucilage can inhibit mucociliary transport (1,2,6,18), stimulate phagocytosis (1,2,18) and other immune system activities (1,18), suppress cough (1,6,8,11), increase the anti-inflammatory effects of topical dexamethasone (1,6,18), and have hypoglycemic activity (1,4). The mucilage can also have antimicrobial (4,6), spasmolytic, antisecretory (6), diuretic, antilithic, and wound-healing (4) effects.

Adverse Reactions Including Known Allergies
Marshmallow can cause hypoglycemia (4,11,18).

Possible Interactions with Herbs & Other Dietary Supplements
HERBS AND SUPPLEMENTS: Concomitant use of marshmallow can retard the absorption of other herbs or supplements (1,2,11,12).

Possible Interactions with Drugs
DEXAMETHASONE: Theoretically, marshmallow can increase the topical anti-inflammatory effects of dexamethasone (6,118).
HYPOGLYCEMIC DRUGS: Theoretically, due to claims of hypoglycemic effects, marshmallow might interfere with hypoglycemic therapy (4).
ORAL DRUGS: The fiber in marshmallow might impair absorption of oral drugs (1,2,11,12,19).

Possible Interactions with Foods
No interactions are known to occur, and there is no known reason to expect a clinically significant interaction with marshmallow.

Possible Interactions with Lab Tests

BLOOD GLUCOSE: Theoretically, marshmallow could lower blood glucose and test results (4,11,18).

Possible Interactions with Diseases or Conditions

DIABETES: Theoretically, marshmallow could interfere with blood sugar control (4). Marshmallow syrup also contains sugar (2).

Typical Dosages & Routes of Administration that are Commonly Used

ORAL: For irritation of the mouth or pharynx and associated dry cough, the typical dose of marshmallow is 2-5 grams of the dried leaf, 5 grams of the dried root or one cup of either leaf or root tea three times daily (4). The leaf tea is prepared by steeping 2-5 grams of the dried leaf in 150 mL boiling water for 5-10 minutes and then straining. The root tea is prepared by steeping 2-5 grams of the dried root in 150 mL cold water for 1-1.5 hours, straining, and then warming before consumption. The maximum dose of marshmallow is 5 grams of the dried leaf or 6 grams to 15 grams of the dried root daily (1,2,4,11). The usual dose of the liquid leaf or root extract (1:1 in 25% alcohol) is 2-5 mL three times daily (4). For irritation of oral or pharyngeal mucosa and the associated cough, the common dose of the marshmallow root syrup is 2-10 mL up to three times daily. The root syrup should not be used for any other indication (1,2,4). The syrup does contain sugar (2).

TOPICAL: The 5% powdered leaf in an ointment base is commonly applied three times daily (4).

Comments

Avoid confusion with the mallow (Malva sylvestris) flower and leaf.

MARTAGON

This Product is Also Known As

Purple Turk's Cap Lily, Turk's Cap.

Scientific Names

Lilium martagon.

People Use This For

Orally, martagon is used as a diuretic, and for dysmenorrhea (18).
Topically, it is used for ulcers (18).

Safety

There is insufficient reliable information available about the safety of martagon.
Pregnancy and Lactation: Insufficient reliable information available; avoid using.

Effectiveness

There is insufficient reliable information available about the effectiveness of martagon.

Possible Mechanism of Action & Active Ingredients

The applicable parts of martagon are the leaf, stem, and flower. Lilium martagon contains varied constituents including starch, soluble polysaccharides, gamma-methylene glutamic acid, and tuliposide (18).

Adverse Reactions Including Known Allergies

None reported.

Possible Interactions with Herbs & Other Dietary Supplements

Insufficient reliable information available.

Possible Interactions with Drugs

No interactions are known to occur, and there is no known reason to expect a clinically significant interaction with martagon.

Possible Interactions with Foods

No interactions are known to occur, and there is no known reason to expect a clinically significant interaction with martagon.

Possible Interactions with Lab Tests

No interactions are known to occur, and there is no known reason to expect a clinically significant interaction with martagon.

Possible Interactions with Diseases or Conditions

No interactions are known to occur, and there is no known reason to expect a clinically significant interaction with martagon.

Typical Dosages & Routes of Administration that are Commonly Used

Martagon is used in powdered form for tea and for poultices (18).

Comments

There is very little scientific information about this product. Our staff is continually analyzing the available information on natural medicines and will add data here as it becomes available.

MASTERWORT

This Product is Also Known As

Cow Cabbage, Cow Parsnip, Hogweed, Madnep, Radix Pimpinelle Franconiae, Woolly Parsnip, Youthwort. CAUTION: See separate listing for Goutweed (Aegopodium podagraria), also known as Masterwort.

Scientific Names

Heracleum sphondylium, synonym Heracleum lanatum.
Family: Apiaceae.

People Use This For

In folk medicine, masterwort is used orally for relief of muscle cramps, stomach disorders, digestive problems, diarrhea, and mucous membrane inflammation of the GI tract (18).

Safety

POSSIBLY UNSAFE ...when plant parts are used orally. Masterwort can cause phototoxicity (19) and some of the furocoumarin constituents can be carcinogenic (4).
PREGNANCY: LIKELY UNSAFE ...contraindicated for oral use in early pregnancy, due to the reported ability to stimulate menstruation (19).
LACTATION: POSSIBLY UNSAFE; avoid using.

Effectiveness

There is insufficient reliable information available about the effectiveness of masterwort.

Possible Mechanism of Action & Active Ingredients

Masterwort is considered to be a mild expectorant, although this effect remains unproven (18). It contains furocoumarins (bergapten, isopimpinellin, pimpinellin, isoberapten, spondin) and a volatile oil containing n-octylacetate (18). Bergapten, also known as 5-methoxypysoralen, is phototoxic and may also be carcinogenic (4).

Adverse Reactions Including Known Allergies

Oral use increases skin sensitivity to UV light and can lead to phototoxicity (19). Topical application of the fresh plant can cause photodermatitis (3835). Masterwort may also be carcinogenic.

Possible Interactions with Herbs & Other Dietary Supplements

Insufficient reliable information available.

Possible Interactions with Drugs

PSORALEN THERAPY: Contraindicated due to additive photosensitizing effect (19).

Possible Interactions with Foods

No interactions are known to occur, and there is no known reason to expect a clinically significant interaction with masterwort.

Possible Interactions with Lab Tests

No interactions are known to occur, and there is no known reason to expect a clinically significant interaction with masterwort.

Possible Interactions with Diseases or Conditions

ULTRAVIOLET LIGHT THERAPY: Contraindicated due to photosensitizing effect (19); avoid excessive periods in sun (19).

Typical Dosages & Routes of Administration that are Commonly Used

No typical dosage.

Comments

Masterwort is reportedly used as a replacement/adulterant for greater burnet-saxifrage (Pimpinella major) (7).

© Copyright 2000, Natural Medicines Comprehensive Database (209) 472-2244. For updated data, go to www.NaturalDatabase.com

MASTIC

This Product is Also Known As
Lentisk.

Scientific Names
Pistacia lentiscus.

People Use This For
In dentistry, mastic resin is used as a material for fillings (18). The masticated resin releases substances that freshen the breath and tighten the gums (18).
In manufacturing, mastic resin is used in the food and drink industries (18) and in the production of chewing gum (18).

Safety
POSSIBLY SAFE ...when used orally (18).
PREGNANCY AND LACTATION: Insufficient reliable information available; avoid using.

Effectiveness
There is insufficient reliable information available about the effectiveness of mastic resin.

Possible Mechanism of Action & Active Ingredients
The applicable part of mastic is the resin. Mastic tree contains resins including the triterpenes mastic acid, isomastic acid, oleanlic acid, and tirucallol. It also contains a volatile oil with alpha-pinene as a constituent. The volatile oil and the resin are thought to have astringent and aromatic effects (18). An extract shows evidence that mastic resin might also have antimicrobial and fungal activity (4141). Preliminary evidence suggests that mastic resin might be beneficial in protecting the gastric mucosa when during aspirin, phenylbutazone, or reserpine therapy (4142).

Adverse Reactions Including Known Allergies
Children who ingest mastic tree resin might develop diarrhea (18). The pollen of mastic tree is allergenic (4140). Exposure to mastic tree can cause allergic reactions in individuals allergic to Schinus terebintifolious and other Pistacia species (4140).

Possible Interactions with Herbs & Other Dietary Supplements
CROSS-ALLERGENICITY: Individuals allergic to mastic tree might also have an allergic reaction to Schinus terebintifolious and other Pistacia species (4140).

Possible Interactions with Drugs
No interactions are known to occur, and there is no known reason to expect a clinically significant interaction with mastic.

Possible Interactions with Foods
No interactions are known to occur, and there is no known reason to expect a clinically significant interaction with mastic.

Possible Interactions with Lab Tests
No interactions are known to occur, and there is no known reason to expect a clinically significant interaction with mastic.

Possible Interactions with Diseases or Conditions
No interactions are known to occur, and there is no known reason to expect a clinically significant interaction with mastic.

Typical Dosages & Routes of Administration that are Commonly Used
No typical dosage.

Comments
Mastic resin is the resin from the trunk of Pistacia lentiscus.

MATE

This Product is Also Known As
Hervea, Ilex, Jesuit's Brazil Tea, Jesuit's Tea, Maté Folium, Paraguay Tea, St. Bartholemew's Tea, Yerba Maté, Yerba Mate.
CAUTION: See separate listing for Caffeine.

Scientific Names

Ilex paraguariensis.
Family: Aquifoliaceae.

People Use This For

Orally, maté is used as a stimulant to relieve mental and physical fatigue (2,6,8).

In folk medicine, it has been used as a diuretic (4,6,8), for modifying mood or affective disorders, as a mild analgesic for headache and rheumatic pains (4), and as a laxative in large amounts (13). It has also been used for depression (4), weight loss (8), urinary tract infection, cardiac insufficiency, arrhythmias, nervous heart complaints, kidney and bladder stones (18), and to promote cleansing and excretion of waste (6).

In foods, the use of maté includes a tea-like beverage (5,6,9,13).

Safety

POSSIBLY SAFE ...when taken orally and appropriately on a short-term basis (2,12).

POSSIBLY UNSAFE ...when maté is used orally in large amounts or for prolonged periods of time. Chronic use of the caffeine contained in maté can sometimes produce tolerance, habituation, and psychological dependence (15). The abrupt discontinuation can sometimes result in physical withdrawal symptoms (15).

CHILDREN: POSSIBLY UNSAFE ...when taken orally. The adverse effects of caffeine can be more severe in children than adults (15).

PREGNANCY: There is insufficient reliable information available about the safety of maté during pregnancy. Although the caffeine content of a typical dose should not cause concern, other constituents could be unsafe.

LACTATION: POSSIBLY UNSAFE; avoid using. The caffeine is secreted in breast milk and can cause sleep disturbances in breast-fed infants (18).

Effectiveness

POSSIBLY EFFECTIVE ...when taken orally for relief of mental and physical fatigue (2), as a central nervous system stimulant (12,15,18), as a diuretic (15,18), for headache (15), for increasing blood pressure in hypotension (15), and for weight loss (caffeine/ephedrine) (695,696,1704).

There is insufficient reliable information available about the effectiveness of maté for its other uses.

Possible Mechanism of Action & Active Ingredients

The applicable parts of maté are the leaf and leaf stem. Maté is thought to have appetite suppressant (4), lipolytic, and glycogenolytic activity (2,18). It contains 0.2-2% caffeine (compared to 1-2% in coffee) (4,5,6,7,9,12,13,18) which acts as a central nervous system stimulant (12,15,18), increases heart rate and contractility (7,18), inhibits platelet aggregation (6,18), stimulates gastric acid secretion, causes diuresis (15,18), relaxes extracerebral vascular and bronchial smooth muscle, stimulates the release of catecholamines (18), and might indirectly inhibit histamine release (6130). It also contains theophylline and theobromine, which have actions similar to caffeine (4,6). Maté contains 4-16% tannins (4,12) with possible carcinogenic and hepatotoxic properties (12).

Adverse Reactions Including Known Allergies

Large amounts, or the prolonged use, of maté is associated with an increased risk of cancers of the esophagus (4,6), mouth, larynx (1528), kidney (1529), bladder (1530), and lung (1531). There is one report of venous occlusive disease associated with excessive, long-term maté consumption (4,5614). The caffeine constituent of maté can cause insomnia, nervousness, restlessness, agitation (7,15), gastric irritation (7), nausea, vomiting, diuresis (15), fast heartbeat, arrhythmias, increased respiratory rate, muscle spasms, ringing in the ears, headache, delirium, and convulsions (15,505). The adverse effects of caffeine are usually more severe in children than adults (15). Some evidence shows caffeine is associated with fibrocystic breast disease in women; other evidence disputes this (14,15). The chronic use of caffeine, especially in large amounts, can produce tolerance, habituation, and psychological dependence (15). The abrupt discontinuation of caffeine can result in physical withdrawal symptoms, including irritability, anxiety, headaches, and dizziness (15).

Combining ephedra with maté increases the risk of adverse effects, due to the caffeine contained in maté (2729). One unpublished report associated jitteriness, hypertension, seizures, temporary loss of consciousness, and hospitalization requiring life support with the use of a combination ephedra and guarana (caffeine) product (1380). There is one report of ischemic stroke in an athlete who consumed ephedra 40-60 mg, creatine monohydrate 6 grams, caffeine 400-600 mg, and a variety of other supplements daily for six weeks (1275).

Possible Interactions with Herbs & Other Dietary Supplements

CAFFEINE CONTAINING HERBS/SUPPLEMENTS: Concomitant use of maté and caffeine-containing herbs/supplements constitutes therapeutic duplication (due to the caffeine contained in maté) which increases the risk of caffeine-related adverse effects. Other natural products which contain caffeine include black tea, cocoa, coffee, cola nut, green tea, and guarana.

EPHEDRA (Ma Huang): Concomitant use can increase the risk of stimulatory adverse effects, due to the caffeine contained in maté (7). One unpublished report associated jitteriness, hypertension, seizures, temporary loss of consciousness, and hospitalization requiring life support with the use of a combination ephedra and guarana (caffeine) product (1380).

Possible Interactions with Drugs

ACETAMINOPHEN (Tylenol): Theoretically, concomitant use might increase the pain-relieving activity of acetaminophen, due to the caffeine contained in maté. Caffeine increases the pain-relieving activity of acetaminophen by up to 40% (512).

ASPIRIN: Theoretically, concomitant use might increase the pain-relieving activity of aspirin, due to the caffeine contained in maté. Caffeine increases the pain-relieving activity of aspirin by up to 40% (512).

BENZODIAZEPINES: Theoretically, concomitant use might reduce the sedative and anxiolytic effects of benzodiazepines, due to the caffeine contained in maté (14).

BETA-ADRENERGIC AGONISTS: Theoretically, concomitant use might increase the cardiac inotropic effects of beta agonists, due to the caffeine contained in maté (15). Beta-adrenergic agonists include albuterol (Proventil, Ventolin), metaproterenol (Alupent), terbutaline (Brethine), and isoproterenol (Isuprel).

CIMETIDINE (Tagamet) Theoretically, concomitant use might increase serum caffeine concentrations and the risk of adverse effects, due to the caffeine contained in maté. Cimetidine decreases the rate of caffeine clearance by 30-50% (14).

CLOZAPINE (Clozaril): Theoretically, co-administration might acutely exacerbate psychotic symptoms, due to the caffeine contained in maté. Caffeine can increase the effects and toxicity of clozapine (151). Caffeine doses of 400-1000 mg per day inhibit clozapine metabolism (5051).

CNS STIMULANTS: Concomitant use might increase the risk of stimulant adverse effects, due to the caffeine contained in maté (151,2719). CNS stimulants include nicotine, cocaine, sympathomimetic amines, and amphetamines.

DIABETES THERAPY: Theoretically, concomitant use of maté and diabetes drugs might interfere with blood glucose control, due to the caffeine contained in coffee. This is based in the claim that caffeine might have hyperglycemic effects (19).

DISULFIRAM (Antabuse): Theoretically, concomitant use might increase serum caffeine concentrations and the risk of adverse effects, due to the caffeine contained in maté. Disulfiram decreases the rate of caffeine clearance (15).

EPHEDRINE: Concomitant use might increase the risk of stimulatory adverse effects, due to the caffeine contained in maté (7,19). An unpublished report associated jitteriness, hypertension, seizures, temporary loss of consciousness, and hospitalization requiring life support with the use of a combination ephedra (ephedrine) and guarana (caffeine) product (1380).

ESTROGEN (Estrace): Theoretically, concomitant use might increase serum caffeine concentrations and the risk of adverse effects, due to the caffeine contained in maté. Estrogen inhibits caffeine metabolism (2714).

ERGOTAMINE: Theoretically, concomitant use might increase the GI absorption of ergotamine, due to the caffeine contained in maté. Caffeine increases the GI absorption of ergotamine (15).

LITHIUM (Eskalith, Lithobid): Theoretically, abrupt maté withdrawal might increase serum lithium levels, due to the caffeine contained in maté. There are two case reports of lithium tremor that worsened upon abrupt coffee withdrawal (609,610).

MEXILETINE (Mexitil): Theoretically, concomitant use might increase serum caffeine concentrations and the risk of adverse effects, due to the caffeine contained in maté. Mexiletine reduces caffeine metabolism (14).

MONOAMINE OXIDASE INHIBITORS (MAOIs): Theoretically, concomitant intake of large amounts of maté with MAOIs might precipitate a hypertensive crisis, due to the caffeine contained in maté. This is based on the claim that intake of large amounts of caffeine with MAOIs might precipitate a hypertensive crisis (19).

ORAL CONTRACEPTIVES (OCs): Theoretically, concomitant use might increase serum caffeine concentrations and the risk adverse effects, due to the caffeine contained in maté. OCs decrease the rate of caffeine clearance by 40-65% (14).

PHENYLPROPANOLAMINE (Dexatrim, Propagest): Theoretically, concomitant use might cause an additive increase in blood pressure and serum caffeine concentrations, due to the caffeine contained in maté (14). Concomitant use of caffeine and phenylpropanolamine can cause an additive increase in blood pressure, and increase serum caffeine concentrations (14).

QUINOLONES: Theoretically, concomitant use might increase serum caffeine concentrations and the risk of adverse effects, due to the caffeine contained in maté. Quinolones decrease caffeine clearance (606,607,608). Quinolones (also referred to as fluoroquinolones) include ciprofloxacin (Cipro), enoxacin (Penetrex), gatifloxacin (Tequin), levofloxacin (Levaquin), lomefloxacin (Maxaquin), moxifloxacin (Avelox), norfloxacin (Noroxin), ofloxacin (Floxin), sparfloxacin (Zagam), and trovafloxacin (Trovan).

RILUZOLE (Rilutek): Theoretically, concomitant use might increase serum caffeine and riluzole concentrations and the risk of adverse effects of both caffeine and riluzole, due to the caffeine contained in maté. Caffeine and riluzole are both metabolized by cytochrome P450 1A2 and concomitant use might reduce metabolism of one or both agents (14).

TERBINAFINE (Lamisil): Theoretically, concomitant use might increase serum caffeine concentrations and the risk of adverse effects, due to the caffeine contained in maté. Terbinafine decreases the rate of caffeine clearance (14).

THEOPHYLLINE (Theo-Dur): Theoretically, concomitant use might increase serum theophylline concentrations and the risk of adverse effects, due to the caffeine contained in maté. Large amounts of caffeine might inhibit theophylline metabolism (14).

VERAPAMIL (Calan, Isoptin, Verelan): Theoretically, concomitant use might increase plasma caffeine concentrations and the risk of adverse effects, due to the caffeine contained in maté. Verapamil increases plasma caffeine concentrations by 25% (14).

Possible Interactions with Foods
GRAPEFRUIT JUICE interacts with the caffeine in maté and can increase caffeine levels, its effects, and the risk of adverse effects (504).

Possible Interactions with Lab Tests
BLEEDING TIME: Maté might prolong bleeding time and increase test results, due to its caffeine content (1701).
BLOOD PRESSURE: Maté might increase blood pressure and blood pressure readings, due to its caffeine content (4).
URATE: Maté might falsely increase serum urate test results determined by the Bittner method, due to its caffeine content. Caffeine causes false elevations in serum urate test results determined by the Bittner method (15).
CATECHOLAMINES: Maté might increase urine catecholamine concentrations and test results, due to its caffeine content. Caffeine can increase urine catecholamine concentrations (15).
CREATINE: Maté might increase urine creatine concentrations and test results, due to its caffeine content (1701).
DIPYRIDAMOLE THALLIUM IMAGING: Maté might interfere with dipyridamole thallium imaging studies, due to its caffeine content. Caffeine attenuates the characteristic cardiovascular responses to dipyridamole and has altered test results (14).
5-HYDROXYINDOLEACETIC ACID: Maté might increase urine 5-hydroxyindoleacetic acid concentrations and test results, due to its caffeine content. Caffeine can increase urine catecholamine concentrations (15).
VANILLYLMANDELIC ACID (VMA): Maté might increase urine VMA concentrations and test results, due to its caffeine content. Caffeine can increase urine VMA concentrations (15).
TESTS FOR NEUROBLASTOMA: Maté (due to its caffeine content) might cause false-positive diagnosis of neuroblastoma, when diagnosis is based on tests of urine vanillylmandelic acid (VMA) or catecholamine concentrations. Caffeine can increase urine catecholamine and VMA concentrations (15).
TESTS FOR PHEOCHROMOCYTOMA: Maté (due to its caffeine content) might cause false-positive diagnosis of pheochromocytoma, when diagnosis is based on tests of urine vanillylmandelic acid (VMA) or catecholamine concentrations. Caffeine can increase urine catecholamine and VMA concentrations (15).

Possible Interactions with Diseases or Conditions
ULCERS: The caffeine in maté can aggravate gastric and peptic ulcers; avoid using (14,16).
HEART CONDITIONS: The caffeine in maté might induce cardiac arrhythmias in sensitive individuals (14,16).
DEPRESSION, ANXIETY DISORDERS: The caffeine in maté might aggravate these conditions (14).
KIDNEY DISEASE: The diuretic effect of the caffeine in maté can aggravate certain kidney disorders (19).

Typical Dosages & Routes of Administration that are Commonly Used
ORAL: The typical dose of maté is 2-4 grams of the dried leaf or one cup of the tea three times daily (4,18). The tea is prepared by steeping 2-4 grams of the dried leaf in 150 mL boiling water for 5-10 minutes and then straining. Some authorities suggest a maximum of 3 grams of the dried leaf per day (2,18). The usual dose of the liquid extract (1:1 in 25% alcohol) is 2-4 mL three times per day (4).

Comments
Maté, also known as Yerba Maté, is a popular beverage, much like coffee or tea, in Brazil, Paraguay, and Argentina (6002). The beverage is often prepared from leaves of Ilex paraguariensis, also referred to as Jesuit's tea, Jesuit's Brazil tea, Paraguay tea, and St. Bartholemew's tea. The herbal tea has caused multiple anticholinergic poisonings. However, belladonna alkaloids were identified and the poisonings were traced to a single contaminated lot of imported herbs (785).

MEADOWSWEET

This Product is Also Known As
Bridewort, Dolloff, Dropwort, Filipendula, Lady Of The Meadow, Meadow Queen, Meadow-Wart, Queen Of The Meadow, Spiraeae flos, Spireae herba, Ulmaria.

Scientific Names
Filipendula ulmaria, synonym Spiraea ulmaria.
Family: Rosaceae.

People Use This For
Orally, meadowsweet is used as supportive therapy for colds (2,7,8,18).
In folk medicine, it is used for cough, bronchitis (18), dyspepsia, heartburn, peptic ulcer disease (4), and rheumatic disorders including gout (4,8,9,18). It is also used in folk medicine as a diuretic (8,9,18) and urinary antiseptic for acute cystitis (4).

Safety

POSSIBLY SAFE ...when the above ground parts and flower are used orally and appropriately (2,12).

POSSIBLY UNSAFE ...when an aqueous extract (tea) is used in large amounts or for prolonged periods of time because it contains high amounts of tannins (4).

PREGNANCY: LIKELY UNSAFE ...contraindicated. Some evidence suggests meadowsweet might stimulate uterine activity (4).

LACTATION: Insufficient reliable information available.

Effectiveness

POSSIBLY EFFECTIVE ...when taken orally as supportive therapy for colds (2).

There is insufficient reliable information available about the effectiveness of meadowsweet for its other uses.

Possible Mechanism of Action & Active Ingredients

The applicable parts of meadowsweet are the above ground parts and flower. Meadowsweet has stomachic, mild urinary antiseptic, antirheumatic, astringent, and antacid activities (4). It contains tannins, and the volatile oil contains low concentrations of salicylates (2,7,18). In animals, the above ground parts of meadowsweet decrease motor activity, lower temperature, induce muscle relaxation, and potentiate the effect of narcotics (4). In animals, the flower extract increases life expectancy, decreases vascular permeability, increases bronchial, intestinal, and uterine tone, and promotes uric acid excretion. In vitro, it has bacteriostatic activity (4). Meadowsweet aqueous extracts contain high concentrations of tannins (4) with strong astringent effects and potential adverse effects.

Adverse Reactions Including Known Allergies

Meadowsweet can cause nausea and other stomach complaints (18). Bronchospastic activity has occurred with its use (4). Meadowsweet contains a salicylate constituent. There is insufficient reliable information available to know if the side effects and toxicity normally associated with salicylates could occur. The adverse reactions associated with salicylates include gastric and renal irritation, hypersensitivity, blood in stool, tinnitus, nausea, and vomiting. Salicin has been associated with skin rashes (4).

Possible Interactions with Herbs & Other Dietary Supplements

SALICYLATE-CONTAINING HERBS: Theoretically, concomitant use of meadowsweet could potentiate the therapeutic and adverse effects of other herbs containing salicylate constituents. These herbs include black cohosh, poplar, sweet birch, white willow, and wintergreen (19).

Possible Interactions with Drugs

NARCOTICS: Theoretically, meadowsweet can potentiate the narcotic effects (4).

SALICYLATE INTERACTIONS: Meadowsweet contains a salicylate constituent. There is insufficient reliable information available to determine if enough salicylate is present to cause drug interactions common to salicylates or aspirin. Aspirin can impair the effectiveness of beta-adrenergic blockers, probenecid, and sulfinpyrazone. It can increase the effects, side effects, or toxicity of alcohol, anticoagulants, carbonic anhydrase inhibitors, heparin, methotrexate, sulfonylureas, and valproic acid (151).

Possible Interactions with Foods

No interactions are known to occur, and there is no known reason to expect a clinically significant interaction with meadowsweet.

Possible Interactions with Lab Tests

There are no reports of lab interactions with this product. However, because it contains salicylates, use caution in interpreting test results known to be affected by salicylates.

Possible Interactions with Diseases or Conditions

ASTHMA: Meadowsweet can exacerbate asthma and can have bronchospastic effects. Use cautiously in individuals with asthma (4).

ASPIRIN ALLERGY: Use cautiously in individuals with aspirin allergy; contains salicylate constituent.

Typical Dosages & Routes of Administration that are Commonly Used

ORAL: For adults, the typical dose is one cup of the tea several times per day (2,8,18). The tea is prepared by steeping 2.5-3.5 grams of the dried flower or 4-5 grams of the above ground parts in 150 mL boiling water for 10 minutes and then straining. The usual dose of the liquid extract (1:1 in 25% alcohol) is 1.5-6 mL three times per day (4). The common dose of the tincture (1:5 in 45% alcohol) is 2-4 mL three times per day (4).

Comments

None.

MEDIUM CHAIN TRIGLYCERIDES (MCT)

This Product is Also Known As
MCT.

Scientific Names
Medium chain triglycerides.

People Use This For
Orally, medium chain triglycerides (MCTs) are taken for nutritional support of athletic training (1900), as adjunctive therapy for malabsorption syndromes including diarrhea, steatorrhea (fat indigestion), gastrectomy, and abdominal surgery, and for steatorrhea resulting from pancreas disorders, dilatation of intestinal lymphatic system, and intestinal resections. They are also used for congenital lymphatic anomalies, for chyluria and chylothorax, for akinetic, clonic, and petit mal seizures in children (14), and for decreasing body fat and increasing lean muscle mass (2272).

Intravenously, MCT is used as a source of fat in total parenteral nutrition (14).

Safety
LIKELY SAFE ...when taken orally and used appropriately (14).

There is insufficient reliable information available about the safety of the intravenous use of MCT.

PREGNANCY AND LACTATION: LIKELY SAFE ...when used orally and appropriately (14).

Effectiveness
EFFECTIVE ...when taken orally for malabsorption syndromes including diarrhea, steatorrhea, gastrectomy, abdominal surgery, steatorrhea resulting from pancreas disorder, dilatation of intestinal lymphatic system, and intestinal resections (14).

POSSIBLY EFFECTIVE ...when used orally for treating chyluria, chylothorax (14), and akinetic, clonic, and petit mal seizures in children (14,2273,2274). ...when used as an intravenous (IV) fat source in total parenteral nutrition preparations (2275,2276,2277,2278).

There is insufficient reliable information available about the effectiveness of MCTs for other uses.

Possible Mechanism of Action & Active Ingredients
Medium chain triglycerides (MCTs) are semi-synthetic lipids composed of fatty acids with a chain length of six to twelve carbon atoms (14). They are normally substituted for only 50 to 70% of dietary fat since MCTs do not contain essential fatty acids (14). MCTs improve symptoms associated with malabsorption syndromes. They decrease diarrhea, protein loss, fecal fat, nitrogen excretion, steatorrhea (fat indigestion), and creatorrhea (14). They also increase fat absorption, body weight, and serum albumin and promote a return to normal levels of calcium, phosphorus, and uric acid (14). In healthy individuals, single doses of MCT oil can reduce blood triglyceride levels (834).

Adverse Reactions Including Known Allergies
MCTs can cause diarrhea, vomiting, irritability (2274), nausea, abdominal discomfort, intestinal gas noises, and essential fatty acid deficiency (14).

Possible Interactions with Herbs & Other Dietary Supplements
Insufficient reliable information available.

Possible Interactions with Drugs
No interactions are known to occur, and there is no known reason to expect a clinically significant interaction with MCT.

Possible Interactions with Foods
FOOD: Concomitant administration of MCTs with food can reduce the adverse effects associated with MCT (2273).

Possible Interactions with Lab Tests
TRIGLYCERIDES: MCT can lower blood triglyceride levels and test results (834).

Possible Interactions with Diseases or Conditions
HEPATIC ENCEPHALOPATHY: Contraindicated (14).

CIRRHOSIS: The use of MCTs in individuals with cirrhosis can cause narcosis and coma. Use cautiously (14).

DIABETES: The use of MCTs can cause hyperketonemia (14).

STEATORRHEA: The use of MCTs can cause increased calcium absorption and decreased fecal water, sodium, and potassium excretion (14).

MECHANICAL VENTILATION: The use of MCTs can cause increased oxygen consumption (14).

Typical Dosages & Routes of Administration that are Commonly Used
ORAL: MCT oil contains 8.3 calories per gram, and one tablespoon provides 115 calories and weighs 14 grams (14). For malabsorption syndromes, initially 1 tablespoon is typically taken three to four times per day mixed

with fruit juices, salads, and vegetables, incorporated into sauces for use on fish, chicken, or lean meats, or use in cooking or baking (14). For improving seizure control in children, 60% of the caloric intake is from MCT oil (2274). INTRAVENOUS (IV): As a fat source in total parenteral nutrition formulations, a fat mixture containing 50% MCT and 50% long chain triglycerides is commonly used (2275,2276,2278).

Comments

MCTs ingested with food reduces the adverse effects (2273). Essential fatty acids must be also included in the diet to avoid essential fatty acid deficiency (14).

MELANOTAN-II

This Product is Also Known As

Melanotan II, MT-II.

Scientific Names

Melanotan-II.

People Use This For

Subcutaneously, melanotan-II has been used to evaluate its effects on psychogenic erectile dysfunction (5687,5689), organic erectile dysfunction (5688,5689), and its effects after unilateral nerve-sparing radical prostatectomy (5689). It has also been used subcutaneously to evaluate its effects on tanning of the skin and for the prevention of sunlight-induced skin cancers (5683).

Safety

POSSIBLY SAFE ...when used subcutaneously to initiate penile erections in men with psychogenic or organic erectile dysfunction (5687,5688). Controlled clinical studies suggest mild to moderate adverse effects such as decreased appetite, facial flushing and nausea might occur with a dosage of 0.025 mg/kg (5685,5687,5688). There is insufficient reliable information available about the safety of melanotan-II for its other uses or at other dosages.
PREGNANCY AND LACTATION: Insufficient reliable information available; avoid using.

Effectiveness

POSSIBLY EFFECTIVE ...when used subcutaneously to initiate penile erections in men with psychogenic or organic erectile dysfunction (5687,5688). Preliminary clinical trials have shown melanotan-II is superior to placebo for initiating spontaneous sustained penile erections (5685,5687,5688). ...when used subcutaneously for visible tanning of the skin (5685). A controlled clinical pilot study demonstrated melanotan-II caused increased pigmentation in the face, upper body, and buttocks. (5685).
There is insufficient reliable information available about the effectiveness of melanotan-II for its other uses.

Possible Mechanism of Action & Active Ingredients

Melanotan-I and Melanotan-II are two alpha-melanocyte-stimulating-hormone analogues currently being extensively studied (5686). Both analogues have the ability to darken and tan the skin (5686) and were developed to not only promote skin pigmentation but also to possibly prevent sunlight-induced skin cancers (5683,5686). Compared to alpha-melanocyte-stimulating-hormone, melanotan-I and melanotan-II have increased melanotropic potency (26-100-fold) and increased resistance to degradation by plasma enzymes due to two amino acid substitutions (norleucine for methionine at position 4 and racemization of D-phenylalanine at position 7) in the alpha-melanocyte-stimulating-hormone peptide sequence (5685,5686). Melanotan-II is a cyclic heptapeptide containing a lactam bridge between the amino acids lysine and aspartic acid, enabling it to have even greater melanotropic potency than melanotan-I, a linear tridecapeptide (5685,5686). During a pilot phase-I clinical study, it was discovered by observers that melanotan-II not only caused increased visible tanning but also spontaneous penile erections with use (5685). Subsequent controlled clinical trials have shown melanotan-II initiates erections in men with psychogenic and organic dysfunction (5687,5688). The exact mechanism of action is unknown, but it is hypothesized that melanotan-II acts on pro-erectile pathways at the level of the central nervous system (5687). There are distinct melanocortin receptors found primarily in the brain (5686) and animal data suggests melanotropic peptides act in the hypothalamic regions surrounding the third ventricle (5687). Since dopamine agonists also induce penile erections (and yawning), evidence suggests the central mechanism involves a dopamine-oxytocin pathway (5687). Further clinical trials are in progress evaluating the pharmacokinetics, safety, and efficacy of melanotan-II (5689).

Adverse Reactions Including Known Allergies

Subcutaneously, melanotan-II can cause gastrointestinal cramping (5685), nausea (5685,5687,5688), decreased appetite (5687), facial flushing (5685,5688), fatigue, somnolence (5685), yawning, stretching and spontaneous penile erections (5685,5687,5688). It can also cause increased pigmentation of the face, upper body, and buttocks (5685).

Possible Interactions with Herbs & Other Dietary Supplements

Insufficient reliable information available.

Possible Interactions with Drugs

No interactions are known to occur, and there is no known reason to expect a clinically significant interaction with melanotan-II.

Possible Interactions with Foods

No interactions are known to occur, and there is no known reason to expect a clinically significant interaction with melanotan-II.

Possible Interactions with Lab Tests

No interactions are known to occur, and there is no known reason to expect a clinically significant interaction with melanotan-II.

Possible Interactions with Diseases or Conditions

No interactions are known to occur, and there is no known reason to expect a clinically significant interaction with melanotan-II.

Typical Dosages & Routes of Administration that are Commonly Used

SUBCUTANEOUS: The typical dosage is 0.025 mg/kg (5685,5687,5688). There is no frequency or other dosage information available.

Comments

Melanotan-II is not yet commercially available and is presently being studied in phase-II clinical trials (5689). Commercial dosage forms of melanotan-II such as a nasal spray or as an eyedrop are being investigated (5684,5687,5690).

MELATONIN

This Product is Also Known As

MEL.

Scientific Names

N-acetyl-5-methoxytryptamine.

People Use This For

Orally, people use melatonin for treating jet lag, sleep disorders, sleep disorders in handicapped children and adults (9,14), shift-work disorder (14), circadian rhythm sleep disorders in blind children and adults with minimal or no light perception (6,14), and benzodiazepine withdrawal in people with insomnia (349,1751). People also use melatonin orally for treating and preventing Alzheimer's disease (1728), tinnitus (14), depressive disorders (9,14), migraine and cluster headache (14), hypertension (1724), hyperpigmentation (14), preventing osteoporosis (1687), preventing cancer of the breast, brain, lung and prostate (1687), treating thrombocytopenia or preventing chemotherapy-induced thrombocytopenia (14), and for treating cachexia in people with cancer (14). Melatonin is also used orally as an anti-aging agent (507,1687), for primary and adjunctive cancer treatment (9,14), as an immune system enhancer (1048), antioxidant (1687), adjunctive treatment for epilepsy and non-epileptic myoclonus in children (1699), preanesthetic medication (1770), and contraceptive agent (6,14).
Transbuccal and sublingual forms of melatonin have been used for treating insomnia (1735) and shift-work disorder (1721).
Topically, melatonin is used as a skin protectant against erythema induced by ultraviolet light (sunburn) (1051).
Intramuscularly, melatonin has been used as an adjunct for cancer treatment (1688).
Intravenously, melatonin has been used for treating persistent migraine headaches (1689) and for treating subnormal endogenous melatonin secretion (1690).

Safety

POSSIBLY SAFE ...when used orally or parenterally and appropriately short-term (6,14,507). Several studies have safely used melatonin from 7 days up to 2 months (14,1049,1068,1072,1077,1085,1738,5854,5855,5857).
There is insufficient reliable information available about the safety of melatonin when used for longer periods.
CHILDREN: POSSIBLY UNSAFE ...when used orally or parenterally. Melatonin supplementation might adversely effect children. Young people, up to the age of 20 years produce melatonin endogenously in high levels (1740) and melatonin levels are inversely related to gonadal development (1739,1742,1743). Theoretically, exogenously administered melatonin might adversely effect gonadal development; however this effect has never been demonstrated. Use with caution.
PREGNANCY: POSSIBLY UNSAFE: ...when used orally or parenterally. High doses have been associated with a contraceptive effect (214,1740); avoid use.
LACTATION: Insufficient reliable information available; avoid use (1737).

© Copyright 2000, Natural Medicines Comprehensive Database (209) 472-2244. For updated data, go to www.NaturalDatabase.com

Effectiveness

LIKELY EFFECTIVE ...when used orally for reducing the symptoms of jet lag (9,14,1049,1077,1079,1085,1722). ...when used orally for circadian rhythm sleep disorders in blind children and adults with minimal or no light perception (6,14,1082,1691,1744,1749). The FDA has classified melatonin as an orphan drug for this indication (6). ...when used orally for sleep disorders associated with sleep-wake cycle disturbance in children and adolescents with mental retardation, autism, and other central nervous system disorders (9,14,1056,1745,1746,1747,1771). ...when used orally for treating insomnia. This benefit has primarily been demonstrated in elderly people with decreased melatonin levels (9,14,1072,1729,1738,1754). Findings have not been so clear in non-elderly insomniacs and insomniacs with depression or dementia. Although some studies have demonstrated benefit in these groups (1053,1068,1729), others have reported no effect (1070,1083).

POSSIBLY EFFECTIVE ...when used orally for treating thrombocytopenia associated with cancer, cancer treatment, or certain other disorders, or for preventing thrombocytopenia induced by chemotherapy or interleukin-2 (14,1694,1695,1696,1697). ...when used orally to improve performance status and stabilize disease in some adults with solid tumors who have failed, or cannot receive, other treatments (14,1080,1688,1693). ...when used orally in combination with interleukin-2 to improve response rates and survival for advanced solid tumors of the lung, gastrointestinal tract, liver, kidney, and breast, and melanoma (14,1692,5854,5855). ...when used orally in combination with radiotherapy to prolong survival with glioblastoma (14). ...when used orally in combination with triptorelin for prostate cancer (14). ...when used orally in combination with interferon for renal cell carcinoma (14). ...when used orally to facilitate benzodiazepine withdrawal in elderly people with insomnia. This benefit has only been demonstrated with a controlled-release formulation of melatonin (349,1751). ...when melatonin is used topically as a skin protectant, to prevent erythema when applied prior to exposure to UV light (14,1051,1066,1768,1769).

POSSIBLY INEFFECTIVE ...when used orally to improve sleep and adjustment to rotating shift work (14,507,1052,1054,1721).

LIKELY INEFFECTIVE ...when used orally for depression (9,14,1053,1764,1766).

There is insufficient reliable information available about the effectiveness of melatonin for its other uses.

Possible Mechanism of Action & Active Ingredients

Melatonin is synthesized endogenously in the pineal gland. It is produced from tryptophan, which is converted to 5-hydroxytryptophan then serotonin then N-acetylserotonin and finally melatonin (1773). Light inhibits melatonin secretion and darkness stimulates secretion (1773). Melatonin release peaks between the ages of one to three years of age (507). Contrary to earlier reports, recent reports suggest melatonin secretion does not decline with age after adolescence, and melatonin suppression by light is not affected by age (1775,1781). However, decreased melatonin has been found in insomniacs of all ages (6). Low-dose exogenous melatonin has rapid, transient, and mild sleep-inducing effects. It lowers alertness, body temperature, and performance for three to four hours after oral administration without a "hangover" effect the following day (14,1068,1753,1756,1757,1758,1759,1760,1774). Melatonin can regulate the body's circadian rhythm and sleep patterns by interacting with melatonin receptors in the brain (1773). Melatonin can also act as an antioxidant, protecting cells from oxidative damage from free-radicals (6). Preliminary evidence suggests that melatonin affects immune function, activates monocytes, has oncostatic actions on estrogen sensitive MCF-7 human breast cancer cells, and promotes osteoblast differentiation and matrix mineralization (6,3265). A number of mechanisms have been proposed for the potential effects of melatonin against solid tumors. It may have direct cytostatic activity against some cancers, antagonize macrophage-mediated immunosuppression, amplify host antitumor reactions induced by interleukin-2, increase cancer cell sensitivity to interleukin-2, increase sensitivity to tamoxifen by increasing endocrine receptor expression on cancer cells, and inhibit production of tumor growth factors (1064,5854,5855,5857). Melatonin has been reported to inhibit melanoma cell growth in vitro and in rodents (1064,5856). It has been suggested that melatonin has greatest activity against cancer when given once daily in the evening (1064). Melatonin is involved in the inhibition of gonadal development and in seasonal breeding patterns in animals (9). Melatonin and norethisterone can have additive or synergistic inhibiting effects on the ovarian function in women and possibly act as a contraceptive (769,1740). Some evidence suggests melatonin might enhance the effects of isoniazid (INH) against some Mycobacterium species (330). Preliminary evidence suggests melatonin might be involved in human balance, growth hormone secretion, and pain control (1776,1777,1778). Melatonin undergoes extensive first pass metabolism and is rapidly metabolized, primarily by conjugation and hydroxylation (14,1773). Exogenous melatonin has a half-life of 30-60 minutes in humans (14,1385,1772). Orally administered melatonin undergoes first-pass metabolism, with bioavailability ranging between 3% and 76%. Therapeutic serum levels of melatonin have not been established (14). The timing of melatonin administration appears to be important; however, the optimal timing for jet lag and insomnia has not been established (1772). Transdermal administration of melatonin can result in delayed drug levels (1058).

Adverse Reactions Including Known Allergies

The oral use of melatonin can cause headache, transient depressive symptoms, daytime fatigue and drowsiness, dizziness, abdominal cramps and irritability (14,169), and reduced alertness (14,1078). People should not drive or use machinery for 4 to 5 hours after taking melatonin (1772). Aircraft crew undergoing multiple time zone might experience further disruption in circadian rhythms (1722). Melatonin has exacerbated dysphoria in depressed patients (1764). Whether chronic administration of melatonin suppresses endogenous production of melatonin by the pineal gland is unknown (1772).

Possible Interactions with Herbs & Other Dietary Supplements

HERBS/SUPPLEMENTS WITH SEDATIVE PROPERTIES: Theoretically, concomitant use with herbs that have sedative properties might enhance therapeutic and adverse effects. These include 5-HT, calamus, calendula, California poppy, catnip, capsicum, celery, couch grass, elecampane, ginseng Siberian, German chamomile, goldenseal, gotu kola, hops, Jamaican dogwood, kava, lemon balm, sage, sassafras, scullcap, shepherd's purse, stinging nettle, valerian, wild carrot, wild lettuce, withania root, and yerba mansa (4,19) and others.

Possible Interactions with Drugs

BENZODIAZEPINES: A controlled-release melatonin preparation demonstrates effectiveness for benzodiazepine withdrawal in elderly people with insomnia (349). However, benzodiazepine withdrawal should only be done under the supervision of a health care provider.

BETA BLOCKERS: Melatonin can reverse the negative effects of propranolol (Inderal) and atenolol (Tenormin), but not carvedilol (Coreg), on nocturnal sleep (1062,1780).

CNS DEPRESSANTS: Theoretically, concomitant use of melatonin with alcohol, benzodiazepines, or other sedative drugs might cause additive sedation.

FLUOXETINE (Prozac): Concomitant use with melatonin is reported to improve the sleep of some patients with major depressive disorder taking fluoxetine (1053).

FLUVOXAMINE (Luvox): Concomitant use might increase melatonin's therapeutic and adverse effects. In a single dose study of healthy men, 50 mg fluvoxamine significantly increased the oral bioavailability of 5 mg melatonin (5038).

IMMUNOSUPPRESSIVE DRUGS: Melatonin can affect immune function and might interfere with immunosuppressive therapy (507); avoid use.

ISONIAZID (INH): Theoretically, melatonin might enhance the effects of isoniazid against some Mycobacterium species (330).

VERAPAMIL (Calan, Isoptin, Verelan): Concomitant use can increase melatonin excretion (1063).

Possible Interactions with Foods

No interactions are known to occur, and there is no known reason to expect a clinically significant interaction with melatonin.

Possible Interactions with Lab Tests

HUMAN GROWTH HORMONE: Melatonin supplementation can increase human growth hormone serum levels and test results (1076,1779).

LUTEINIZING HORMONE: Melatonin supplementation can decrease serum luteinizing hormone levels and test results (1741).

MELATONIN: Concomitant use of melatonin and fluvoxamine (Luvox) can significantly increase serum melatonin concentrations and test results. In a single dose study of healthy men, 50 mg fluvoxamine plus 5 mg melatonin increased melatonin AUC 800% to 3125% and Cmax 503% to 1772%, compared to 5 mg melatonin alone (5038).

OXYTOCIN: Melatonin can produce dose-dependent changes in plasma oxytocin concentrations and test results. A 500 mcg melatonin dose increases oxytocin levels, a 5 mg melatonin dose reduces oxytocin levels (1779).

VASOPRESSIN: Melatonin can produce dose-dependent changes in plasma vasopressin concentrations and test results. A 500 mcg melatonin dose increases vasopressin levels, a 5 mg melatonin dose reduces vasopressin levels (1779).

Possible Interactions with Diseases or Conditions

CANCER: Melatonin can decrease the incidence of cytokine (interleukin II and tumor necrosis factor) induced hypotension in cancer patients (1069).

CEREBAL PALSY: There is one case of dyskineais and akathisia in a cerebral palsy patient who abruptly discontinued nightly use of melatonin (14).

DEPRESSION: Melatonin can worsen dysphoria in some people with depression (1764).

LIVER DISEASE: Melatonin is metabolized by the liver. Use in lever disease might increase plasma melatonin concentrations and lead to adverse effects. There is one report of autoimmune hepatitis (14); use with caution.

SEIZURE DISORDERS: Melatonin increased the incidence of seizures in one study (14); use with caution.

Typical Dosages & Routes of Administration that are Commonly Used

ORAL: The optimal oral dose of melatonin has not been established (1772,1774). For sleep disturbance, the typical dose is 0.3-5 mg at bedtime (507). For jet lag, 5 mg is taken at bedtime for one week beginning three days before the flight (9). As adjunctive treatment for cancer, 20-50 mg in combination with radiotherapy or chemotherapy has been used (14,1773). For benzodiazepine withdrawal in elderly people with insomnia, 2 mg of controlled-release melatonin taken bedtime for 6 weeks (the benzodiazepine dosage is reduced 50% during the second week, 75% during weeks 3 and 4, and stopped during weeks 5 and 6) and continued up to 6 months for insomnia, has been used (349).

TOPICAL: For ultraviolet light protection, melatonin 0.6 mg/cM2 is applied 15 minutes before exposure (1768,1769).

Comments

The controlled-released product, Circadin (not available in the U.S.), is undergoing a multi-center Phase III clinical study in France for the indication of sleep. The manufacturer, Neurim Pharmaceutical Labs (Israel), is preparing to apply for approval of Circadin as a prescription drug in Canada and Europe (364). Most commercial melatonin is synthesized in the laboratory. Melatonin from animal sources should be avoided due to the possibility of contamination (1772).

MENTZELIA

This Product is Also Known As
None.

Scientific Names
Mentzelia cordifolia.
Family: Loasaceae.

People Use This For
Traditionally, mentzelia branch tips, stems, and roots have been used orally for gastritis, gastrointestinal mucous membrane inflammation, nervous gastric disorders and digestive symptoms, hyperacidity, gastric spasms, feeling of fullness, pressure on the stomach, upset stomach, gastric irritation due to alcohol abuse, innate digestive weakness, and gastric pain (2).

Safety
There is insufficient reliable information available about the safety of mentzelia.
Pregnancy and Lactation: Insufficient reliable information available; avoid using.

Effectiveness
There is insufficient reliable information available about the effectiveness of mentzelia.

Possible Mechanism of Action & Active Ingredients
The applicable parts of mentzelia are the branch tips, stems and roots. There is insufficient reliable information available about the possible mechanism of action and active ingredients of mentzelia.

Adverse Reactions Including Known Allergies
None reported.

Possible Interactions with Herbs & Other Dietary Supplements
Insufficient reliable information available.

Possible Interactions with Drugs
No interactions are known to occur, and there is no known reason to expect a clinically significant interaction with mentzelia.

Possible Interactions with Foods
No interactions are known to occur, and there is no known reason to expect a clinically significant interaction with mentzelia.

Possible Interactions with Lab Tests
No interactions are known to occur, and there is no known reason to expect a clinically significant interaction with mentzelia.

Possible Interactions with Diseases or Conditions
No interactions are known to occur, and there is no known reason to expect a clinically significant interaction with mentzelia.

Typical Dosages & Routes of Administration that are Commonly Used
No typical dosage.

Comments
There is very little scientific information about this product. Our staff is continually analyzing the available information on natural medicines and will add data here as it becomes available.

MERCURY HERB

This Product is Also Known As
None.

Scientific Names
Mercurialis annua.
Family: Euphorbiaceae.

People Use This For
Orally, the flowering plant of mercury herb is used for inflammation with pus, as a laxative, a diuretic, and as an adjuvant treatment for gastrointestinal and urinary tract disease (18).

Safety
LIKELY UNSAFE ...when the fresh plant, particularly the root and rhizome are used orally (18). Small amounts might cause symptoms no worse than diarrhea.
PREGNANCY AND LACTATION: LIKELY UNSAFE ...insufficient reliable information available; avoid using.

Effectiveness
There is insufficient reliable information available about the effectiveness of mercury herb.

Possible Mechanism of Action & Active Ingredients
Mercury herb contains saponins, a small amount of cyanogenic glycosides, pyridone derivatives including hermidin, amines including methylamine, and flavonoids including rutin, narcissin, and isorhamnetin (18). The root and stock of mercury herb act as strong laxatives (18). There is no information regarding the toxic compound in the plant (18). The insignificant amount of cyanogenic glycosides cannot account for the plant's toxicity (18).

Adverse Reactions Including Known Allergies
Oral ingestion might cause diarrhea and overactive bladder (18). Symptoms of poisoning might include nerve paralysis, liver and kidney failure, as well as death (18). The pollen has shown to be allergenic (4143,4144), and may be responsible for rhinitis and asthmatic symptoms (4143). Mercury herb might also cause allergic reactions in individuals allergic to Olea europaea, Fraxinus elatior, Ricinus communis, Salsola kali, Parietaria judaica, and Artemisia vulgaris (4143).

Possible Interactions with Herbs & Other Dietary Supplements
CROSS-ALLERGENICITY: Individuals allergic to mercury herb might also be allergic to Mercurialis annua and Olea europaea, Fraxinus elatior, Ricinus communis, Salsola kali, Parietaria judaica, and Artemisia vulgaris (4143).

Possible Interactions with Drugs
No interactions are known to occur, and there is no known reason to expect a clinically significant interaction with mercury herb.

Possible Interactions with Foods
No interactions are known to occur, and there is no known reason to expect a clinically significant interaction with mercury herb.

Possible Interactions with Lab Tests
No interactions are known to occur, and there is no known reason to expect a clinically significant interaction with mercury herb.

Possible Interactions with Diseases or Conditions
No interactions are known to occur, and there is no known reason to expect a clinically significant interaction with mercury herb.

Typical Dosages & Routes of Administration that are Commonly Used
The mercury herb is administered as an extract or in juice (18).

Comments
None.

METHIONINE

This Product is Also Known As
L-Methionine.

Scientific Names
L-2-amino-4-(methylthio)butyric acid.

People Use This For
Orally, methionine is used for liver function support (2408) and preventing liver damage in acetaminophen poisoning (2413).

Safety
POSSIBLY SAFE ...when used to treat acetaminophen poisoning (2413).
POSSIBLY UNSAFE ...when used orally for self-medication in amounts greater than those found in foods (2409,2410,2411).

PREGNANCY AND LACTATION: POSSIBLY UNSAFE ...when used for self-medication in amounts greater than found in food.

Effectiveness
POSSIBLY EFFECTIVE ...when taken orally for preventing liver damage in cases of acetaminophen poisoning and when administered within ten hours of acetaminophen ingestion (2413).

Possible Mechanism of Action & Active Ingredients
Methionine is a sulfur-containing essential amino acid (9) found in meat, fish, and dairy products (2408). In children of short stature, methionine can potentiate growth hormone and its releasing hormone secretion (2412). In humans, it can increase serum homocysteine levels (2410,2411). To detoxify, excessive methionine requires glycine; thus, methionine supplementation can compete with the glycine needed for other metabolic processes (2415). In humans, supplementing with methionine prior to nitrous oxide anesthesia can counter the anesthesia-induced reduction in methionine-synthase enzyme activity (2414); however, the clinical significance for this is unknown.

Adverse Reactions Including Known Allergies
Methionine increases plasma homocysteine levels and can promote atherosclerosis (2410,2411).

Possible Interactions with Herbs & Other Dietary Supplements
Insufficient reliable information available.

Possible Interactions with Drugs
ACETAMINOPHEN: Methionine can decrease liver damage in cases of acetaminophen poisoning (2413).

Possible Interactions with Foods
SALT AND NITRITE: A diet rich in methionine, salt, and nitrite can increase the risk of gastric cancer (2409).
GLYCINE: Excess methionine intake can place a competitive demand on the body's availability of glycine (2415).

Possible Interactions with Lab Tests
HOMOCYSTEINE: Methionine can increase plasma homocysteine levels and test results (2410,2411).

Possible Interactions with Diseases or Conditions
ACETAMINOPHEN POISONING: Methionine can decrease liver damage in cases of acetaminophen poisoning (2413).
ATHEROSCLEROSIS: Theoretically, methionine supplementation can promote or exacerbate atherosclerosis by increasing homocysteine levels (2410).

Typical Dosages & Routes of Administration that are Commonly Used
ORAL: People also typically take a 500 mg capsule containing the free form of L-methionine with a meal or glass of water (5026).

Comments
Methionine is possibly unsafe, and should only be used by emergency room personnel for medical emergencies.

MEXICAN SCAMMONY ROOT

This Product is Also Known As
Ipomoea, Orizaba Jalap.
CAUTION: See separate listings for Pokeweed berry, Pokeweed root, and Jalap.

Scientific Names
Ipomoea orizabensis.
Family: Convolvulaceae.

People Use This For
Orally, Mexican scammony root is used as a purgative (18).

Safety
There is insufficient reliable information available about the safety of the dried roots or the steamed, ethanol root extract of Mexican scammony root.
PREGNANCY: LIKELY UNSAFE ...contraindicated for oral use (18).
LACTATION: Insufficient reliable information available; avoid using.

Effectiveness
POSSIBLY EFFECTIVE ...when taken orally as a purgative (18).

Possible Mechanism of Action & Active Ingredients
Mexican scammony root exerts a potent stimulant laxative effect on the intestines. It contains 12-15% resinous polymeric ester glycosides (18).

Adverse Reactions Including Known Allergies

Taken orally, it can cause intestinal colic, and in large amounts, vomiting (18).

Possible Interactions with Herbs & Other Dietary Supplements

STIMULANT LAXATIVE HERBS: Theoretically, concomitant use with other stimulant laxative herbs may increase the risk of potassium depletion. (19).

HORSETAIL/LICORICE: Theoretically, concomitant use with horsetail plant or licorice rhizome increases the risk of potassium depletion (19).

CARDIAC GLYCOSIDE-CONTAINING HERBS: Overuse/abuse may increase the risk of cardiac glycoside toxicity (2,18,19,500).

Possible Interactions with Drugs

CARDIAC GLYCOSIDE DRUGS: Theoretically, overuse/abuse of this product increases the risk of adverse effects of cardiac glycoside drugs, e.g. digoxin.

Possible Interactions with Foods

No interactions are known to occur, and there is no known reason to expect a clinically significant interaction with Mexican scammony root.

Possible Interactions with Lab Tests

No interactions are known to occur, and there is no known reason to expect a clinically significant interaction with Mexican scammony root.

Possible Interactions with Diseases or Conditions

GI CONDITIONS: Contraindicated; may have GI irritant effects (19). Stimulant laxatives are contraindicated in individuals with symptoms of appendicitis (abdominal pain, nausea and vomiting) (272).

Typical Dosages & Routes of Administration that are Commonly Used

ORAL: People typically take 3 to 12 grains (195 to 780 mg) of the powdered root. The powdered resin from the root is dosed 3 to 8 grains (195 to 520 mg) (5267).

Comments

Ipomoea orizabensis is no longer used as a purgative because of the adverse effect of vomiting.

MEZEREON

This Product is Also Known As

Camolea, Daphne, Dwarf Bay, Spurge Flax, Spurge Laurel, Spurge Olive, Wild Pepper.

Scientific Names

Daphne mezereum.
Family: Thymelaeaceae.

People Use This For

Traditionally, the mezereon root has been used orally to relieve headaches and toothaches (18). It has also been used topically for joint pains, and to increase circulation in rheumatic conditions (18).

Safety

POSSIBLY UNSAFE ...when used topically (18). Prolonged skin contact can lead to necrosis (18).

LIKELY UNSAFE ...when used orally. The plant is poisonous and can cause death (18).

PREGNANCY AND LACTATION: LIKELY UNSAFE ...insufficient reliable information; avoid using.

Effectiveness

There is insufficient reliable information available about the effectiveness of mezereon.

Possible Mechanism of Action & Active Ingredients

The applicable part of mezereon is the bark. Mezereon contains diterpenes including mezerein and daphnetoxin. It possesses powerful skin stimulating effects and can be hallucinogenic (18).

Adverse Reactions Including Known Allergies

Ingesting mezereon can cause reddening and swelling of the oral mucous membranes, salivation, thirst, stomach pains, vomiting (18), severe diarrhea (18,4145), and blood in the urine (4145). Symptoms can also include headache, dizziness, stupor, tachycardia, spasms, and death through circulatory collapse (18). Skin contact with mezereon can cause red, painful swelling of the skin, blister formation, and shedding of the epidermis (18). Extended exposure can cause necrosis (18). Contact with the eyes can cause severe conjunctivitis (18).

Possible Interactions with Herbs & Other Dietary Supplements

Insufficient reliable information available.

Possible Interactions with Drugs

No interactions are known to occur, and there is no known reason to expect a clinically significant interaction with mezereon.

Possible Interactions with Foods

No interactions are known to occur, and there is no known reason to expect a clinically significant interaction with mezereon.

Possible Interactions with Lab Tests

No interactions are known to occur, and there is no known reason to expect a clinically significant interaction with mezereon.

Possible Interactions with Diseases or Conditions

No interactions are known to occur, and there is no known reason to expect a clinically significant interaction with mezereon.

Typical Dosages & Routes of Administration that are Commonly Used

TOPICAL: Used as a 20% ointment (18).

Comments

Mezereon is a protected species (18). It is seldom used medicinally today (18).

MGN-3

This Product is Also Known As

Biobran, Hemicellulose Complex with Arabinoxylane.

Scientific Names

None.

People Use This For

Orally, MGN-3 is used for boosting immune function, preventing and treating cancer, treating AIDS, hepatitis, diabetes, chronic fatigue syndrome and other immunodeficiency disorders (3114,3115).

Safety

There is insufficient reliable information available about the safety of MGN-3.
PREGNANCY AND LACTATION: Insufficient reliable information available; avoid using.

Effectiveness

There is insufficient reliable information available about the effectiveness of MGN-3.

Possible Mechanism of Action & Active Ingredients

MGN-3 is a hemicellulose complex containing arabinoxylane as a major component. It is produced by hydrolyzing rice bran using enzymes from mycelia of Shiitake, Kawaratake, and Suehirotake mushrooms (3114). Some studies suggest it might improve immunity by enhancing natural killer cell activity, increasing interferon-gamma production by peripheral blood mononuclear cells, and acting synergistically with interleukin-2 (aldesleukin) to increase natural killer cell activity and production of tumor necrosis factor alpha (3116,3117). Other evidence suggests that MGN-3 has activity against HIV (3113). Results from three small studies of healthy individuals and individuals with cancer suggest that MGN-3 also enhances natural killer cell activity (3118,3119,3120).

Adverse Reactions Including Known Allergies

None reported.

Possible Interactions with Herbs & Other Dietary Supplements

Insufficient reliable information available.

Possible Interactions with Drugs

No interactions known to occur, and there is no known reason to expect a clinically significant interaction with MGN-3.

Possible Interactions with Foods

No interactions known to occur, and there is no known reason to expect a clinically significant interaction with MGN-3.

Possible Interactions with Lab Tests

No interactions known to occur, and there is no known reason to expect a clinically significant interaction with MGN-3.

Possible Interactions with Diseases or Conditions

No interactions known to occur, and there is no known reason to expect a clinically significant interaction with MGN-3.

Typical Dosages & Routes of Administration that are Commonly Used

ORAL: A dose of 3 grams per day has been used in cancer patients (3119,3120).

Comments

The FDA is seeking a permanent injunction against the marketing of MGN-3 by Lane Labs. The complaint charges that MGN-3 is an unapproved drug product promoted as treatment for cancer and HIV infection (387).

MICROALGAE

This Product is Also Known As

Astaxanthin.
CAUTION: See separate listing for Beta-Carotene.

Scientific Names

3,3'-dihydroxy-4,4'-diketo-beta-carotene, 3S, 3'S-astaxanthin; 3R, 3'R-astaxanthin; 3R,3'S-astaxanthin.

People Use This For

Orally, the microalgae constituent astaxanthin is used to treat or prevent macular degeneration in the eyes, for Alzheimer's and Parkinson's disease, to aid in stroke recovery, to protect against cancer, and to reduce LDL cholesterol (4322). It is also used to reduce skin damage from ultraviolet light (4334).
Orally as a nutritional supplement, the microalgae constituent astaxanthin is used to cause coloration in farm-raised fish (4326,4328) and as a nutritional supplement for poultry (4329).

Safety

LIKELY SAFE ...when the microalgae constituent astaxanthin is used orally in food amounts.
POSSIBLY SAFE ...when the microalgae constituent astaxanthin is used orally in medicinal amounts up to 14.4 mg/day for two weeks (4322).
There is insufficient reliable information available about the safety of the microalgae constituent astaxanthin orally in amounts greater than 14.4 mg/day or for longer than two weeks.
PREGNANCY AND LACTATION: LIKELY SAFE ...when the microalgae constituent astaxanthin is used orally in food amounts.
There is insufficient reliable information about the safety of using the microalgae constituent in larger amounts.

Effectiveness

There is insufficient reliable information about the effectiveness of the microalgae constituent astaxanthin.

Possible Mechanism of Action & Active Ingredients

The microalgae constituent astaxanthin is a reddish carotenoid pigment that is a powerful antioxidant (4322,4326,4332). The richest natural source of the microalgae constituent astaxanthin is Haematococcus pluvialis; but salmon, trout, red seabream, shrimp, lobster, fish eggs, and many bird species also contain substantial amounts (4322). Although plants contain astaxanthin, it is usually in the form of the 3S,3'S isomer. In contrast, the astaxanthin found in Atlantic or Pacific salmon consists of three isomeric forms (4326). Some evidence suggests the microalgae constituent astaxanthin might stimulate immunity (4335,4336) or reduce age-related macular degeneration (4330). Other evidence suggests it might protect against mammary, liver, bladder, or oral cancers (4337,4338,4339,4340). It also might have gastroprotective effects against Helicobacter pylori (4341). In farm-raised fish, supplementation can produce pigmentation that cannot be distinguished from that of ocean fish on a natural diet (4331).

Adverse Reactions Including Known Allergies

None reported.

Possible Interactions with Herbs & Other Dietary Supplements

Insufficient reliable information available.

Possible Interactions with Drugs

No interactions are known to occur, and there is no known reason to expect a clinically significant interaction with the microalgae constituent astaxanthin.

Possible Interactions with Foods

No interactions are known to occur, and there is no known reason to expect a clinically significant interaction with the microalgae constituent astaxanthin.

Possible Interactions with Lab Tests
No interactions are known to occur, and there is no known reason to expect a clinically significant interaction with the microalgae constituent astaxanthin.

Possible Interactions with Diseases or Conditions
No interactions are known to occur, and there is no known reason to expect a clinically significant interaction with the microalgae constituent astaxanthin.

Typical Dosages & Routes of Administration that are Commonly Used
ORAL: A typical dose is 2 capsules Haematococcus microalgae per day. Each capsule contains 2.5 mg astaxanthin (4395).

Comments
The Aquasearch company patented a novel process for cultivating microalgae and has been successful in defending that patent. A recent court decision affirmed that the Cyanotech company's method for cultivating microalgae infringed on the patent and that Cyanotech violated the Uniform Trade Secrets Act (4396).

MILK THISTLE above ground parts

This Product is Also Known As
Cardui mariae herba, Holy Thistle, Lady's Thistle, Marian Thistle, Mary Thistle, St. Mary Thistle, Silymarin. CAUTION: See separate listings for Milk Thistle seed and Blessed Thistle.

Scientific Names
Silybum marianum, synonym Carduus marainum.
Family: Asteraceae or Compositae.

People Use This For
Orally, the above ground parts of the milk thistle plant are used for maintaining health, stimulating and treating dysfunction of the gallbladder and liver, and for treating jaundice, pleurisy, and diseases of the spleen (2). Historically, the parts have been used for treating malaria, uterine complaints, and stimulating menstrual flow (18). For food use, the plant is grown in Europe as a vegetable for salads and as a substitute for spinach (6).

Safety
LIKELY SAFE ...when consumed in amounts commonly found in food (11).
There is insufficient reliable information available about the oral medicinal use of the milk thistle above ground parts.
PREGNANCY AND LACTATION: Insufficient reliable information available; avoid using.

Effectiveness
There is insufficient reliable information available about the effectiveness of the above ground parts of the milk thistle plant (2).

Possible Mechanism of Action & Active Ingredients
A milk thistle plant extract enhances estradiol binding to estrogen receptors, induces transcription activity in estrogen-responsive cells, and enhances estradiol-induced transcription activity in estrogen-responsive cells (6180).

Adverse Reactions Including Known Allergies
Milk thistle can cause an allergic reaction in individuals sensitive to the Asteraceae/Compositae family. Members of this family include ragweed, chrysanthemums, marigolds, daisies, and many other herbs.

Possible Interactions with Herbs & Other Dietary Supplements
Insufficient reliable information available.

Possible Interactions with Drugs
No interactions are known to occur, and there is no known reason to expect a clinically significant interaction with milk thistle above ground parts.

Possible Interactions with Foods
No interactions are known to occur, and there is no known reason to expect a clinically significant interaction with milk thistle above ground parts.

Possible Interactions with Lab Tests
No interactions are known to occur, and there is no known reason to expect a clinically significant interaction with milk thistle above ground parts.

Possible Interactions with Diseases or Conditions

CROSS-ALLERGENICITY: Can cause an allergic reaction in individuals sensitive to the Asteraceae/Compositae family. Members of this family include ragweed, chrysanthemums, marigolds, daisies, and many other herbs.

Typical Dosages & Routes of Administration that are Commonly Used

ORAL: The typical dose of milk thistle is one cup of the tea two to three times daily (18). The tea is prepared by steeping 1/2 teaspoon of the above ground parts in 150 mL boiling water for 5-10 minutes and then straining.

Comments

The broken leaves of the milk thistle plant exude a milky sap. Avoid confusion with milk thistle seed. There is limited information available about the above ground parts of the milk thistle plant.

MILK THISTLE fruit, seed

This Product is Also Known As

Cardui mariae fructus, Holy Thistle, Lady's Thistle, Marian Thistle, Mary Thistle, Our Lady's Thistle, St. Mary Thistle, Silybum, Silymarin.
CAUTION: See separate listings for Milk Thistle above ground parts and Blessed Thistle.

Scientific Names

Silybum marianum, synonym Carduus marainum.
Family: Asteraceae or Compositae.

People Use This For

Orally, the fruit and seed of milk thistle are used for dyspeptic complaints (2), as a liver protectant (6,2613), treating toxic liver damage caused by chemicals (6,2614), Amanita mushroom poisoning (6,2615), supportive therapy for chronic inflammatory liver disease and hepatic cirrhosis (2,2616), chronic hepatitis (795), loss of appetite, liver and gallbladder complaints, and diseases of the spleen (8,18).
Intravenously, the seed and fruit are used as a supportive treatment for Amanita phalloides mushroom poisoning (795).
Historically, the fruit and seed are roasted for use as a coffee substitute (11).

Safety

POSSIBLY SAFE ...when used appropriately (2,12,512,795).
PREGNANCY AND LACTACTION: Insufficient reliable information available; avoid using.

Effectiveness

POSSIBLY EFFECTIVE ...when used orally for dyspeptic complaints (2), treating toxic liver damage, supportive treatment of chronic inflammatory liver disease and hepatic cirrhosis (2), alcoholic liver disease (6,795,2618), drug-induced liver disease, bile duct inflammation, and chronic hepatitis (6,795). ...when used intravenously (IV) as supportive treatment for liver damage due to Amanita phalloides mushroom poisoning (6,7,795). Clinical studies of milk thistle's effectiveness have used formulations standardized to 70% silymarin and used an average dose of 200-400 mg daily.
There is insufficient reliable information available about the effectiveness of milk thistle fruit and seed for their other uses.

Possible Mechanism of Action & Active Ingredients

The milk thistle fruit is also referred to as the seed. Silymarin, a milk thistle fruit and seed extract complex, consists of four flavanolignans, silibinin (silybin), isosilybinin, silichristin (silychristin), and silidianin. These exhibit liver-protective and antioxidant effects (6). The therapeutic activity of silymarin is based on two mechanisms of action. The first is an alteration of the outer hepatocyte cell membrane that prevents toxin penetration, and the second involves the stimulation of nucleolar polymerase A resulting in increased ribosomal protein synthesis, which can stimulate liver regeneration and the formation of new hepatocytes (2). Silymarin undergoes enterohepatic recirculation and has higher concentrations in liver cells (6). In vitro, Silymarin inhibits liver damage from chemicals, drugs, alcohol, viruses, and the Amanita phalloides mushroom toxin (6,795). Silymarin can have benefits in alcohol-induced liver disease and in acute viral and chronic hepatitis (6,795). Silymarin decreases insulin resistance in people with alcoholic cirrhosis (2617). Intravenous silibinin greatly improves human survival in cases of Amanita phalloides mushroom poisoning (6,7,795).

Adverse Reactions Including Known Allergies

The fruit and seed of milk thistle taken orally can cause an occasional laxative effect (2,795). There is one reported case of a woman who experienced intermittent episodes of sweating, nausea, abdominal pain, vomiting, diarrhea, weakness and collapse, requiring hospitalization (3525). Mild allergic reactions can occur with milk thistle use (6). It can cause an allergic reaction in individuals sensitive to the Asteraceae/Compositae family. Members of this family include ragweed, chrysanthemums, marigolds, daisies, and many other herbs.

Possible Interactions with Herbs & Other Dietary Supplements
Insufficient reliable information available.

Possible Interactions with Drugs
ASPIRIN: Theoretically, altered aspirin metabolism in individuals with liver cirrhosis might be improved with concomitant use of milk thistle [19].
HEPATOTOXIC DRUGS: Silymarin can help prevent liver damage caused by drugs, including butyrophenones, phenothiazines, phenytoin, acetaminophen, alcohol, and halothane [19].
CISPLATIN: Theoretically, concomitant administration of the constituent, silibinin, might help prevent kidney damage [19].

Possible Interactions with Foods
No interactions are known to occur, and there is no known reason to expect a clinically significant interaction with milk thistle fruit and seed.

Possible Interactions with Lab Tests
LIVER ENZYMES: Silymarin decreases elevated serum transaminase levels and test results [2618].

Possible Interactions with Diseases or Conditions
CROSS-ALLERGENICITY: Can cause an allergic reaction in individuals sensitive to the Asteraceae/Compositae family. Members of this family include ragweed, chrysanthemums, marigolds, daisies, and many other herbs.

Typical Dosages & Routes of Administration that are Commonly Used
ORAL: Clinical studies of milk thistle's effectiveness have used the standardized 70% silymarin extract at a daily dose of 200-400 mg calculated as silibinin [2,7,8]. Alternatively, the typical dose is 12-15 grams of the dried fruit or seed per day [8]. Some people make a milk thistle tea, but the active ingredients are not very soluble in water [8,515].
INTRAVENOUS: For Amanita phalloides mushroom poisoning, the common dose is 20-50 mg/kg over 24 hours, divided into four infusions, each administered over a two hour period. This is usually started within 48 hours after mushroom ingestion [6,7]. Intravenous silibinin is unavailable in the US.

Comments
The broken leaves of the milk thistle plant exude of milky sap, and the plant was once grown in Europe as a vegetable for salads and as a substitute for spinach [6]. Avoid confusion of the seed and fruit with blessed thistle (Cnicus benedictus) or the other parts of milk thistle.

MONEYWORT

This Product is Also Known As
Creeping Jenny, Creeping Joan, Herb Two-Pence, Meadow Runagates, Running Jenny, Serpentaria, String Of Sovereigns, Twopenny Grass, Wandering Jenny, Wandering Tailor.

Scientific Names
Lysimachia nummularia.
Family: Primulaceae.

People Use This For
Topically, moneywort is used for acute and chronic eczema and as a constituent of dermatologic gels, ointments and drops.
Historically, it was used orally for diarrhea, to increase salivation, and as a cough expectorant.
Moneywort is also used as an astringent and antibacterial agent [18].

Safety
There is insufficient reliable information available about the safety of moneywort.
Pregnancy and Lactation: Insufficient reliable information available; avoid using.

Effectiveness
There is insufficient reliable information available about the effectiveness of moneywort.

Possible Mechanism of Action & Active Ingredients
Insufficient reliable information available.

Adverse Reactions Including Known Allergies
None reported.

Possible Interactions with Herbs & Other Dietary Supplements
Insufficient reliable information available.

Possible Interactions with Drugs
No interactions are known to occur, and there is no known reason to expect a clinically significant interaction with moneywort.

Possible Interactions with Foods
No interactions are known to occur, and there is no known reason to expect a clinically significant interaction with moneywort.

Possible Interactions with Lab Tests
No interactions are known to occur, and there is no known reason to expect a clinically significant interaction with moneywort.

Possible Interactions with Diseases or Conditions
No interactions are known to occur, and there is no known reason to expect a clinically significant interaction with moneywort.

Typical Dosages & Routes of Administration that are Commonly Used
ORAL: One cup of tea is taken 2-3 times daily with honey for cough. The tea is prepared by steeping 2 heaping teaspoons of dried herb in 250 mL of boiling water for 5 minutes and straining (18).
TOPICAL: No typical dosage.

Comments
There is very little scientific information about this product. Our staff is continually analyzing the available information on natural medicines and will add data here as it becomes available.

MORINDA

This Product is Also Known As
Indian Mulberry, Noni, Hog Apple, Menkoedoe, Ruibarbo Caribe, Wild Pine, Tahitian Noni Juice, Bois Douleur, Pau-Azeitona, Mora De La India, Mengkudu, Nhau, Nonu, Nono.
CAUTION: See separate listing for Ba Ji Tian.

Scientific Names
Morinda citrifolia.
Family: Rubiaceae.

People Use This For
Orally, morinda is used for berberi, colic, convulsions, cough, diabetes, dysuria, stimulating menstrual flow (emmenagogue), fever, hepatosis, constipation (laxative), leukorrhea (whitish vaginal discharge), malarial fever, nausea, sapraemia (general reaction to circulating toxins from saprophytic, non-pathogenic, organisms), smallpox, splenomegaly, swelling (513), asthma, bone and joint problems, cancer, cataracts, colds, depression, digestive problems, gastric ulcers, heart trouble, high blood pressure, infections, kidney disorders, migraine, premenstrual syndrome, stroke (439), analgesia and sedation (4119).
Topically, morinda is used as an emollient, to reduce signs of aging (437).
Traditionally in Polynesia and the Pacific Islands, the fruit is used for aging, diabetes, bad breath, mouth ulcers, hemorrhoids, tumors, tuberculosis, ciguatera fish poisoning, and high blood pressure (6,438). The leaves have been used in medicines for rheumatic aches and swelling of the joints, stomachache, dysentery, and swelling caused by the parasitic disease filariasis (6,438). The bark has been used in a preparation to aid childbirth (6,435,438). The leaves are used topically for arthritis by wrapping around the affected joint, for headache by applying to the forehead, and for direct application to burns, sores and leprotic lesions (6,438). A mixture of leaves and fruit is applied to abscesses, and preparations of the root are used on stonefish and sting-ray wounds, and as a smallpox salve (438).
The fruit, leaf, root, seed, and bark are also used as food (6,435,438).

Safety
POSSIBLY SAFE ...when used orally or topically and appropriately for medicinal purposes (6). ...when the fruit is used as food (6).
PREGNANCY AND LACTATION: Insufficient reliable information available; avoid using.

Effectiveness
There is insufficient reliable information available about the effectiveness of morinda.

Possible Mechanism of Action & Active Ingredients
The applicable parts of morinda are the fruits, leaves, and roots. The fruit of Morinda citrifolia contains essential oils, hexoic and octoic acids, paraffin, and esters of ethyl and methyl alcohols (6). Ripe fruit contains n-caproic acid (6). Anthraquinones, morindone, alizarin, xeronine, and damnacanthal have also been isolated from various parts of morinda (6). Xeronine is claimed to work at a molecular level to repair damaged cells and regulate their

function (6). Xeronine is mainly present in the plant as an inactive precursor called proxeronine, together with an inactive form of the enzyme required to convert it to xeronine. This conversion takes place in the intestines provided the proenzyme is not destroyed by stomach acid (440). The fruit juice contains a polysaccharide-rich substance which increases survival in mice with Lewis lung carcinoma, possibly by activating the host immune system (441). Damnacanthal, an anthraquinone isolated from the roots of morinda inhibits tyrosine kinase, has a stimulatory effect on ultraviolet-induced apoptosis, and induces normal morphology in ras-transformed cells (442,443). The fruit juice also contains a significant amount of potassium, approximately 56 mEq/L (1298). In mice, lyophilized aqueous extracts of morinda roots have sedative and central analgesic effects, the latter blocked by naloxone (444). Alcoholic extracts of the leaves have anthelmintic activity in vitro (6). Capsules containing morinda extract are reported to contain proteins, fats, carbohydrates, vitamin A, vitamin C, niacin, calcium, iron, sodium and potassium (440).

Adverse Reactions Including Known Allergies
None reported.

Possible Interactions with Herbs & Other Dietary Supplements
Insufficient reliable information is available.

Possible Interactions with Drugs
POTASSIUM-SPARING DIURETICS (Spironolactone, Triamterene): Theoretically, concomitant use of morinda fruit juice (noni juice) and potassium sparing diuretics might increase the risk of hyperkalemia. Morinda fruit juice contains approximately 56 mEq/L of potassium (1298).

Possible Interactions with Foods
FOOD: It is claimed that the increase in stomach acid caused by food ingestion will cause destruction of the enzyme required for formation of the active ingredient xeronine in the intestine (440).

Possible Interactions with Lab Tests
URINE COLOR: The anthraquinone constituents can discolor urine from pink to rust and interfere with diagnostic tests, due to anthraquinone content (275).

Possible Interactions with Diseases or Conditions
CHRONIC RENAL INSUFFICIENCY: Use of morinda fruit juice (noni juice) can increase the risk of hyperkalemia; use with caution. One reported case associates the use on morinda fruit juice with hyperkalemia in a patient with chronic renal insufficiency (1298). Morinda fruit juice contains approximately 56 mEq/L of potassium (1298).
HYPERKALEMIA: Caution, use of morinda fruit juice (noni juice) can contribute to elevated potassium levels; contraindicated. Morinda fruit juice contains approximately 56 mEq/L of potassium (1298).

Typical Dosages & Routes of Administration that are Commonly Used
ORAL: One to 10 ounces daily of juice prepared from the fruit has been used (436,439). Capsules containing 200 to 620 mg of Morinda citrifolia extract are also marketed. It is claimed that 1200 mg from capsules is equivalent to one ounce of juice (439).

Comments
The smell and taste of Morinda citrifolia fruit juice (noni juice) are unpleasant (440). Capsules containing dried plant extracts are marketed to overcome this, but it is not known what effect the drying process has on the constituents. Morinda juice is imported to the US from the islands of French Polynesia. It is very expensive, about $100 a bottle.

MORMON TEA

This Product is Also Known As
Brigham Tea, Desert Tea, Popotillo, Teamster's Tea, Squaw Tea.
CAUTION: See separate listing for Ephedra.

Scientific Names
Ephedra nevadensis.
Family: Ephedraceae.

People Use This For
Historically, Mormon tea has been used for syphilis, gonorrhea, colds, kidney disorders, and as a "spring" tonic (515). It has also been used as a beverage (6).

Safety
LIKELY SAFE ...when consumed in food amounts (12).
There is insufficient reliable information about the safety of Mormon tea for medicinal uses.

PREGNANCY AND LACTATION: Insufficient reliable information available; avoid consuming amounts greater than in food.

Effectiveness
There is insufficient reliable information available about the effectiveness of Mormon tea.

Possible Mechanism of Action & Active Ingredients
Mormon tea contains large amounts of tannins (515). Tannin constituents exert an astringent effect on the mucosal tissue. This effect dehydrates the tissue, reducing internal secretions, and forming external cells into a protective layer (12). Plants with at least 10% tannins can cause gastrointestinal disturbances, kidney damage, and necrotic conditions of the liver (12). Some animal experiments show that tannins might cause cancer. Others show they might prevent it (12). Regular consumption of herbs with high tannin concentrations correlates to an increase in esophageal or nasal cancer (12). Despite the "ephedra" in the scientific name, Mormon tea contains no ephedrine or other alkaloids (515). An aqueous extract demonstrates mild diuresis and constipation (515).

Adverse Reactions Including Known Allergies
None reported.

Possible Interactions with Herbs & Other Dietary Supplements
TANNIN-CONTAINING HERBS: Theoretically, herbs that contain high percentages of tannins might cause precipitation of constituents of other herbs (19).

Possible Interactions with Drugs
ORAL DRUGS: Theoretically, concomitant oral administration may cause precipitation of some drugs due to the high tannin content of Mormon tea (19). Separate administration of oral drugs and tannin-containing herbs by the longest period of time practical (19).

Possible Interactions with Foods
No interactions are known to occur, and there is no known reason to expect a clinically significant interaction with Mormon tea.

Possible Interactions with Lab Tests
No interactions are known to occur, and there is no known reason to expect a clinically significant interaction with Mormon tea.

Possible Interactions with Diseases or Conditions
No interactions are known to occur, and there is no known reason to expect a clinically significant interaction with Mormon tea.

Typical Dosages & Routes of Administration that are Commonly Used
People prepare and consume Mormon tea by steeping the dried branches in 150 mL boiling water for five to ten minutes and then straining (5008).

Comments
None.

MOTHERWORT

This Product is Also Known As
Leonuri cardiacae herba, Leonurus, Lion's Ear, Lion's Tail, Roman Motherwort, Throw-Wort.

Scientific Names
Leonurus cardiaca and other Leonurus species.
Family: Laminaceae or Labiatae.

People Use This For
Orally, the above ground parts of motherwort are taken for cardiac symptoms of neurosis (2,4,9,18), cardiac insufficiency (4,18), fast heart rate or other arrhythmias (4,18), and hyperthyroidism (2,9,18).
In Chinese medicine, the leafy shoots are used topically for itching and shingles. The seeds of Leonurus artemisia or Leonurus heterophyllus are used to improve eyesight and as a general tonic (1532).
In folk medicine, uses of motherwort include treating amenorrhea (4) and flatulence (18).

Safety
POSSIBLY SAFE ...when preparations of above ground parts are used orally and appropriately (2,12).
PREGNANCY: LIKELY UNSAFE ...contraindicated for oral use because it might have uterine-stimulating effects (4,12,19).
LACTATION: Insufficient reliable information available; avoid using.

Effectiveness

POSSIBLY EFFECTIVE ...when taken orally for nervous cardiac disorders and as an adjuvant treatment for hyperthyroidism (2).
There is insufficient reliable information available about the effectiveness of motherwort for its other uses.

Possible Mechanism of Action & Active Ingredients

The applicable parts of motherwort are the above ground parts. Motherwort has sedative (4,18), negative chronotropic, hypotonic (18), cardiac-inhibitory, and antispasmodic effects (4). Constituents include leonurine and stachydrine, which can stimulate uterine tone and blood flow (4,12,19). Ursolic acid can have antiviral, tumor-inhibiting, and cytotoxic activity (4). The intravenous administration of a Leonurus heterophyllus extract can decrease blood viscosity by decreasing platelet aggregation, decreasing fibrinogen, and increasing erythrocyte deformability (1533).

Adverse Reactions Including Known Allergies

Using motherwort in amounts greater than 3 grams can cause diarrhea, stomach irritation, and uterine bleeding (12). The leaves can cause contact dermatitis, and the oil can cause photosensitivity (4). Motherwort can also cause allergic reactions in sensitive individuals (4).

Possible Interactions with Herbs & Other Dietary Supplements

CARDIAC GLYCOSIDE-CONTAINING HERBS: Contraindicated, and concomitant use can increase the risk of cardiac glycoside toxicity. Cardiac glycoside-containing herbs include black hellebore, Canadian hemp roots, digitalis leaf, hedge mustard, figwort, lily of the valley roots, oleander leaf, pheasant's eye plant, pleurisy root, squill bulb leaf scales, strophanthus seeds, and uzara (2,18,19,500).

Possible Interactions with Drugs

CNS DEPRESSANTS: Concomitant use of motherwort can potentiate the sedative and tranquilizing effects of these drugs, including the sedative effects of antihistamines (19).

Possible Interactions with Foods

No interactions are known to occur, and there is no known reason to expect a clinically significant interaction with motherwort.

Possible Interactions with Lab Tests

THYROID FUNCTION: Motherwort might improve thyroid function and thyroid function test results in patients with thyroid hyperfunction (2).

Possible Interactions with Diseases or Conditions

CARDIAC DISORDERS: Excessive use of motherwort can interfere with the treatment of cardiac disorders (4).
UTERINE BLEEDING CONDITIONS: Theoretically, it can exacerbate uterine bleeding due to its possible stimulation of uterine blood flow (4,12,19).

Typical Dosages & Routes of Administration that are Commonly Used

ORAL: The typical dose of motherwort is 2 grams of the dried above ground parts or 1 cup of the tea 3 times per day (4). To prepare tea steep 2 grams of the dried above ground parts in 150 mL boiling water for 5-10 minutes, then strain. The average amount used is 4.5 grams per day (2).

Comments

None.

MOUNTAIN ASH

This Product is Also Known As

Eberesche, Ebereschenbeeren, European Mountain-Ash, Quickbeam, Rowan Tree, Sorb Apple, Sorbi acupariae fructus, Witchen.

Scientific Names

Sorbus aucuparia.
Family: Rosaceae.

People Use This For

Orally, mountain ash berries are used for kidney diseases, diabetes, arthritis, disorders of uric acid metabolism, dissolution of uric acid deposits, mucous membrane inflammation, internal inflammations, vitamin C deficiency, alkalizing the blood, increasing metabolism, purifying the blood (2,18) and for menstrual complaints (18). A berry puree is used for diarrhea (18). Fresh squeezed berry juice is used for lung conditions, especially those associated with fever (18).

In manufacturing, fresh berries are used as an ingredient in marmalade, stewed fruit, juice, liqueur and vinegar. Dried fruit is used in tea mixtures (18).

Safety

POSSIBLY UNSAFE ...when large amounts of fresh berries are ingested. The constituent, parasorbic acid is an irritant and large amounts can cause gastric irritation and kidney damage (18).

There is insufficient reliable information available about the safety of the oral use of dried or cooked berries.

PREGNANCY AND LACTATION: POSSIBLY UNSAFE ...when large amounts of fresh berries are ingested.

There is insufficient reliable information available about the safety of dried or cooked berries; avoid using.

Effectiveness

There is insufficient reliable information available about the effectiveness of mountain ash.

Possible Mechanism of Action & Active Ingredients

The applicable part of mountain ash is the berry used fresh, dried, or cooked then dried. Mountain ash berry contains parasorbic acid, cyanogenic glycosides, fruit acids (malic acid, tartaric acid), tannins, and vitamin C (18). The parasorbic acid that is contained in the fresh berry can cause local irritation. However, the compound is partially degraded by drying and completely destroyed by cooking (2).

Adverse Reactions Including Known Allergies

Ingestion of large amounts of fresh berries may cause gastroenteritis, vomiting, queasiness, gastric pain, diarrhea, kidney damage (albuminuria, glycosuria), and polymorphic xanthomas due to parasorbic acid (18).

Possible Interactions with Herbs & Other Dietary Supplements

Insufficient reliable information available.

Possible Interactions with Drugs

No interactions are known to occur, and there is no known reason to expect a clinically significant interaction with mountain ash.

Possible Interactions with Foods

No interactions are known to occur, and there is no known reason to expect a clinically significant interaction with mountain ash.

Possible Interactions with Lab Tests

No interactions are known to occur, and there is no known reason to expect a clinically significant interaction with mountain ash.

Possible Interactions with Diseases or Conditions

No interactions are known to occur, and there is no known reason to expect a clinically significant interaction with mountain ash.

Typical Dosages & Routes of Administration that are Commonly Used

No typical dosage.

Comments

None.

MOUNTAIN FLAX

This Product is Also Known As

Dwarf Flax, Fairy Flax, Mill Mountain, Purging Flax.

Scientific Names

Linum catharticum.
Family: Linaceae.

People Use This For

Orally, mountain flax is used as an emetic and purgative to cause bowel elimination (18).

Safety

POSSIBLY UNSAFE ...when used orally, particularly with long term use (18).
PREGNANCY AND LACTATION: UNSAFE ...contraindicated due to possible emetic effects (18).

Effectiveness

There is insufficient reliable information available about the effectiveness of mountain flax.

Possible Mechanism of Action & Active Ingredients

The applicable parts of mountain flax are the above ground flowering parts. Mountain flax is thought to have laxative effects at 0.5 grams. It contains the lignan achromatin, tannins and a volatile oil (18).

Adverse Reactions Including Known Allergies
Mountain flax can cause vomiting, gastrointestinal tract inflammation and diarrhea (18).

Possible Interactions with Herbs & Other Dietary Supplements
Insufficient reliable information available.

Possible Interactions with Drugs
No interactions are known to occur, and there is no known reason to expect a clinically significant interaction with mountain flax.

Possible Interactions with Foods
No interactions are known to occur, and there is no known reason to expect a clinically significant interaction with mountain flax.

Possible Interactions with Lab Tests
No interactions are known to occur, and there is no known reason to expect a clinically significant interaction with mountain flax.

Possible Interactions with Diseases or Conditions
No interactions are known to occur, and there is no known reason to expect a clinically significant interaction with mountain flax.

Typical Dosages & Routes of Administration that are Commonly Used
No typical dosage.

Comments
Mountain flax is considered possibly unsafe, avoid using (18).

MOUNTAIN LAUREL

This Product is Also Known As
Broad-Leafed Laurel, Calico Bush, Lambkill, Laurel, Mountain Ivy, Rose Laurel, Sheep Laurel, Spoon Laurel.

Scientific Names
Kalmia latifolia.

People Use This For
Historically, mountain laurel has been used topically for tinea capitis, psoriasis, herpes, and secondary syphilis (18).

Safety
UNSAFE ...when taken orally. Mountain laurel leaf is not only an irritant, but can also lead to cardiac arrest, respiratory failure and death (18).
There is insufficient reliable information available about safety of the topical use of mountain laurel.
PREGNANCY AND LACTATION: UNSAFE ...when taken orally. There is insufficient reliable information available about safety of mountain laurel for topical use; avoid using.

Effectiveness
There is insufficient reliable information available about the effectiveness of mountain laurel.

Possible Mechanism of Action & Active Ingredients
The applicable part of mountain laurel is the fresh or dried leaf. Mountain laurel contains andromedan derivatives, flavonoids, and acylphloroglucinols (18). Andromedan derivatives act on the sodium channels, inhibiting conduction by preventing closure of the excitable cells (18). The andromedan derivative Grayanotoxin I and the acylphloroglucinol constituents can be cytotoxic (4145).

Adverse Reactions Including Known Allergies
Taken orally, mountain laurel can result in painful oral and gastric mucous membranes, increased salivation, cold sweat, nausea, vomiting, diarrhea, and paresthesias (18). Dizziness, headache, fever attacks, and intoxicated states with temporary loss of vision, muscle weakness, coordination disorders, and spasms can also develop. Bradycardia, cardiac arrhythmias, drop in blood pressure, eventual cardiac arrest and respiratory failure can lead to death (18).

Possible Interactions with Herbs & Other Dietary Supplements
Insufficient reliable information available.

Possible Interactions with Drugs
No interactions are known to occur, and there is no known reason to expect a clinically significant interaction with mountain laurel.

Possible Interactions with Foods
No interactions are known to occur, and there is no known reason to expect a clinically significant interaction with mountain laurel.

Possible Interactions with Lab Tests
No interactions are known to occur, and there is no known reason to expect a clinically significant interaction with mountain laurel.

Possible Interactions with Diseases or Conditions
No interactions are known to occur, and there is no known reason to expect a clinically significant interaction with mountain laurel.

Typical Dosages & Routes of Administration that are Commonly Used
Mountain laurel is only available in homeopathic preparations (18).

Comments
None.

MOUSE EAR

This Product is Also Known As
None.
CAUTION: See separate listing for Cudweed.

Scientific Names
Pilosella officinarum.
Family: Asteraceae.

People Use This For
Orally, mouse ear is used for asthma, bronchitis, coughs and whooping cough. It is also used orally as a diuretic, to promote sweating, and to relieve flatulence and colic.
Topically, mouse ear is used for wounds (18).

Safety
There is insufficient reliable information available about the safety of mouse ear.
Pregnancy and Lactation: Insufficient reliable information available; avoid using.

Effectiveness
There is insufficient reliable information available about the effectiveness of mouse ear.

Possible Mechanism of Action & Active Ingredients
The applicable parts of mouse ear are the above ground flowering plant parts. There is insufficient reliable information available about the possible mechanism of action and active ingredients.

Adverse Reactions Including Known Allergies
Mouse ear can cause an allergic reaction in individuals sensitive to the Asteraceae/Compositae family. Members of this family include ragweed, chrysanthemums, marigolds, daisies, and many other herbs.

Possible Interactions with Herbs & Other Dietary Supplements
Insufficient reliable information available.

Possible Interactions with Drugs
No interactions are known to occur, and there is no known reason to expect a clinically significant interaction with mouse ear.

Possible Interactions with Foods
No interactions are known to occur, and there is no known reason to expect a clinically significant interaction with mouse ear.

Possible Interactions with Lab Tests
No interactions are known to occur, and there is no known reason to expect a clinically significant interaction with mouse ear.

Possible Interactions with Diseases or Conditions
CROSS-ALLERGENICITY: Can cause an allergic reaction in individuals sensitive to the Asteraceae/Compositae family. Members of this family include ragweed, chrysanthemums, marigolds, daisies, and many other herbs.

Typical Dosages & Routes of Administration that are Commonly Used
ORAL AND TOPICAL: Mouse ear is used orally and topically as a liquid extract (18).

Comments
None.

MSM (METHYLSULFONYLMETHANE)

This Product is Also Known As
Crystalline DMSO, Dimethyl Sulfone, DMSO2, Methyl Sulfonyl Methane, Sulfonyl Sulfur.

Scientific Names
Methylsulfonylmethane; Dimethylsulfone.

People Use This For
Orally and topically, MSM is used for chronic pain, arthritis, joint inflammation, rheumatoid arthritis, osteoporosis, bursitis, tendinitis, tenosynovitis, musculoskeletal pain, muscle cramps, scleroderma, scar tissue, stretch marks, wrinkles, protection against sun/wind burn, eye inflammation, oral hygiene, periodontal disease, wounds, cuts, and abrasions/accelerated wound healing (3500).

Orally, MSM is also used for relief of allergies (allergic rhinitis, allergic sinusitis, allergy-induced asthma, inhalent allergens, environmental allergens), drug hypersensitivity, gastrointestinal upset, chronic constipation, gastric hyperacidity, ulcers, diverticulosis, premenstrual syndrome, mood elevation, obesity, poor circulation, hypertension, and elevated serum cholesterol. It is also used orally for diabetes mellitus type 2 (NIDDM), interstitial cystitis, hepatic dysfunction, Alzheimer's disease, snoring, lung dysfunction/emphysema, pneumonia, chronic fatigue syndrome, autoimmune disorders (systemic lupus erythematous), HIV infection/AIDS, and cancer (breast cancer, colon cancer). Other oral uses of MSM include eye inflammation, mucous membrane inflammation, myositis ossificans generalis, temporomandibular joint dysfunction, leg cramps, connective tissue disorders, migraine, headaches, hangover, parasitic infections of the intestinal and urogenital tracts including Trichomonas vaginalis and Giardia, Candida albicans and other yeast infections, insect bites, radiation poisoning (3500), and as an immunostimulant (6).

Safety
POSSIBLY SAFE ...when used orally or topically (221).
PREGNANCY AND LACTATION: Insufficient reliable information available; avoid using.

Effectiveness
There is insufficient reliable information available about the effectiveness of MSM.

Possible Mechanism of Action & Active Ingredients
MSM is a precursor source of sulfur for cysteine and methionine. Incorporation of MSM-derived sulfur into methionine is regulated by a limiting step involving micro-organisms in the intestinal lumen (3501). It is an odorless breakdown product of dimethyl sulfoxide (DMSO) (6). MSM delays chemically-induced colon cancer tumor onset in animals (3502). A four percent (4%) MSM solution delays the latency period between induction and onset of chemically induced mammary tumors or cancers in rats (3503). MSM does not affect expression of autoimmune diabetes in spontaneously diabetic mice (3504).

Adverse Reactions Including Known Allergies
MSM can cause nausea, diarrhea, and headache (221).

Possible Interactions with Herbs & Other Dietary Supplements
Insufficient reliable information available.

Possible Interactions with Drugs
No interactions are known to occur, and there is no known reason to expect a clinically significant interaction with MSM.

Possible Interactions with Foods
No interactions are known to occur, and there is no known reason to expect a clinically significant interaction with MSM.

Possible Interactions with Lab Tests
No interactions are known to occur, and there is no known reason to expect a clinically significant interaction with MSM.

Possible Interactions with Diseases or Conditions
No interactions are known to occur, and there is no known reason to expect a clinically significant interaction with MSM.

Typical Dosages & Routes of Administration that are Commonly Used

ORAL: People typically use 1000 to 3000 mg daily with meals. One product suggests 400 mg per 50 pounds of body weight daily (6006). Some people take 250-500 mg per day for adult dietary supplementation (3500).
TOPICAL: No typical dosage.

Comments

MSM occurs naturally in green plants such as field horsetail (Equisetum arvense), certain species of algae, fruits, vegetables, grains, and both bovine and human adrenal glands, milk and urine. It is destroyed with heat or dehydration (6).

MUGWORT

This Product is Also Known As

Armoise Commune, Artemisia, Artemisiae vulgaris herba, Artemisiae vulgaris radix, Carline Thistle, Felon Herb, Gemeiner Beifuss, Hierba de San Juan, Sailor's Tobacco, St. John's Plant, Wild Wormwood.
CAUTION: See separate listings for Tarragon, Wormseed, and Wormwood.

Scientific Names

Artemisia vulgaris.
Family: Asteraceae or Compositae.

People Use This For

Orally, mugwort above ground parts are used for gastrointestinal problems, such as colic, diarrhea, constipation, cramps, weak digestion, stimulation of gastric juice and bile secretion, as a laxative in cases of obesity and "for the liver," for worm infestations, for hysteria, epilepsy, persistent vomiting, convulsions in children, menstrual problems and irregular periods, promoting circulation, and as a sedative (2).
Orally, mugwort root is used as a tonic in individuals with diminished strength and energy (2).
In combination with other ingredients, mugwort root is used for psychoneuroses, neurasthenia, depression, hypochondria, autonomic neuroses, general irritability, restlessness, insomnia, and anxiety (2).

Safety

There is insufficient reliable information available about the safety of mugwort.
PREGNANCY: LIKELY UNSAFE ...use is contraindicated. Mugwort is said to be an abortifacient, and a menstrual and uterine stimulant (2,12).
LACTATION: Insufficient reliable information available; avoid using.

Effectiveness

There is insufficient reliable information available about the effectiveness of mugwort.

Possible Mechanism of Action & Active Ingredients

The applicable parts of mugwort are the above ground parts and root. Mugwort contains sesquiterpene lactones, lipophilic flavonoids, polyenes, umbelliferone and aesculetin. It also contains a complex volatile oil with constituents of 1,8 cineole, camphor, linalool or thujone (18). Some evidence suggests mugwort can stimulate uterine activity (19), possibly due to the thujone content (19). Other evidence suggests the aqueous extract and the volatile oil have antimicrobial properties (18).

Adverse Reactions Including Known Allergies

Mugwort can cause an allergic reaction in individuals sensitive to the Asteraceae/Compositae family. Members of this family include ragweed, chrysanthemums, marigolds, daisies, and many other herbs. Mugwort pollen can cause reactions in people who are allergic to tobacco (3716). Theoretically, mugwort might cause allergic reaction in people allergic to honey or royal jelly (3717).

Possible Interactions with Herbs & Other Dietary Supplements

Insufficient reliable information available.

Possible Interactions with Drugs

No interactions are known to occur, and there is no known reason to expect a clinically significant interaction with mugwort.

Possible Interactions with Foods

No interactions are known to occur, and there is no known reason to expect a clinically significant interaction with mugwort.

Possible Interactions with Lab Tests

No interactions are known to occur, and there is no known reason to expect a clinically significant interaction with mugwort.

Possible Interactions with Diseases or Conditions

CROSS-ALLERGENICITY: Can cause an allergic reaction in individuals sensitive to the Asteraceae/Compositae family. Members of this family include ragweed, chrysanthemums, marigolds, daisies, and many other herbs. Theoretically, mugwort might cause allergic reactions in individuals with allergies to honey or royal jelly (3717). Mugwort pollen might cause reactions in people allergic to tobacco (3716).

Typical Dosages & Routes of Administration that are Commonly Used

People use 5 mL of mugwort tincture 30 minutes before bedtime or 1-4 mL of the tincture up to three times daily (5008). Some people use 10 to 25 drops per dose of mugwort tincture (1:5, 50% alcohol) (5013) or prepare and consume mugwort tea by steeping 15 grams of the dried herb in 500 mL of boiling water and straining (5008). Two to three cups of tea is consumed daily before meals (5008).

Comments

Mugwort has a pleasant, tangy taste. The plant is indigenous to Asia, North America, and Northern Europe (18).

MUIRA PUAMA

This Product is Also Known As

Muira-Puama, Potency Wood, Ptychopetali lignum.

Scientific Names

Ptychopetalum olacoides; Ptychopetalum unicatum.
Family: Olacaeae.

People Use This For

Orally, muira puama is used for preventing sexual disorders, and as an aphrodisiac (2,5,18). It is also used as a nerve stimulant, for dyspepsia, menstrual irregularities, rheumatism, paralysis caused by poliomyelitis, a general tonic, and as an appetite stimulant (5).
Topically, it is used as an aphrodisiac, for rheumatism, and for muscle paralysis (5).
In combination with other herbs, muira puama is used as a remedy for sexual impotence (5).

Safety

There is insufficient reliable information available about the safety of muira puama.
Pregnancy and Lactation: Insufficient reliable information available; avoid using.

Effectiveness

There is insufficient reliable information available about the effectiveness of muira puama.

Possible Mechanism of Action & Active Ingredients

The applicable parts of muira puama are the wood and root. No constituents in muira puama are known to exhibit any pronounced physiological activity (5).

Adverse Reactions Including Known Allergies

None reported.

Possible Interactions with Herbs & Other Dietary Supplements

Insufficient reliable information available.

Possible Interactions with Drugs

No interactions are known to occur, and there is no known reason to expect a clinically significant interaction with muira puama.

Possible Interactions with Foods

No interactions are known to occur, and there is no known reason to expect a clinically significant interaction with muira puama.

Possible Interactions with Lab Tests

No interactions are known to occur, and there is no known reason to expect a clinically significant interaction with muira puama.

Possible Interactions with Diseases or Conditions

No interactions are known to occur, and there is no known reason to expect a clinically significant interaction with muira puama.

Typical Dosages & Routes of Administration that are Commonly Used

ORAL: People typically use 1 to 2 mL of the muira puama extract in water two to three times daily. The number of drops recommended varies among products. The labeling on one product says one dropperful equals 1 mL and

contains 500 mg muira puama. Other products do not specify the concentration of the active ingredient. Shake well before using; contains alcohol (6006).
TOPICAL: No typical dosage.

Comments
Previously, Liriosma ovata and Acanthea virilis were each thought to be the source of muira puama. They continue to be sold as muira puama in the herb trade (5).

MULLEIN

This Product is Also Known As
Aaron's Rod, Adam's Flannel, American Mullein, Beggar's Blanket, Blanket Herb, Blanket Leaf, Bouuillon Blanc, Candleflower, Candlewick, Clot-Bur, Clown's Lungwort, Cuddy's Lungs, Duffle, European Mullein, Feltwort, Flannelflower, Fluffweed, Golden Rod, Hag's Taper, Hare's Beard, Hedge Taper, Higtaper, Jacob's Staff, Longwort, Orange Mullein, Our Lady's Flannel, Rag Paper, Shepherd's Club, Shepherd's Staff, Torches, Torch Weed, Velvet Plant, Verbasci flos, Wild Ice Leaf, Woolen.
CAUTION: See separate listing for Goldenrod.

Scientific Names
Verbascum densiflorum; Verbascum phlomides; Verbascum thapsus; Verbascum thapsiforme.
Family: Scrophulariaceae.

People Use This For
Orally, mullein flower is used for respiratory tract mucous membrane inflammation (2,18) and cough (5,6,7,8,18). Topically, it is used for wounds (8,18), burns, hemorrhoids, bruises (5,6), frostbite, erysipelas (5), and inflamed mucosa (8). The leaves are used topically to soften and protect the skin (6).
In folk medicine, it is taken internally for earaches (5,6), colds, chills and flu (6,7,8), tracheitis (8), asthma (5,6), diarrhea, gastrointestinal bleeding, migraines (5), gout (6), and tuberculosis (5,6). The root is used for croup (6), and the leaf and stem are used for bronchitis (8,18). In folk medicine, mullein is also used as a sedative, narcotic (5), diuretic, and antirheumatic (8,18).
In manufacturing, mullein is used as a flavoring component in alcoholic beverages (12).

Safety
POSSIBLY SAFE ...when used orally and appropriately (2,5,12).
There is insufficient reliable information available about the safety of the topical use of mullein.
PREGNANCY AND LACTATION: Insufficient reliable information available; avoid using.

Effectiveness
POSSIBLY EFFECTIVE ...when used orally for treating respiratory tract mucous membrane inflammation, cough, and sore throat (2,5).
There is insufficient reliable information available about the effectiveness of mullein for its other uses.

Possible Mechanism of Action & Active Ingredients
The applicable part of mullein is the flower. Mullein contains mucilage which alleviates local irritation (2,5,6,18). The saponins in mullein have an expectorant effect (2,5,8,18), and the extract can have activity against influenza and herpes simplex viruses (1534).

Adverse Reactions Including Known Allergies
None reported.

Possible Interactions with Herbs & Other Dietary Supplements
Insufficient reliable information available.

Possible Interactions with Drugs
No interactions are known to occur, and there is no known reason to expect a clinically significant interaction with mullein.

Possible Interactions with Foods
No interactions are known to occur, and there is no known reason to expect a clinically significant interaction with mullein.

Possible Interactions with Lab Tests
No interactions are known to occur, and there is no known reason to expect a clinically significant interaction with mullein.

Possible Interactions with Diseases or Conditions
No interactions are known to occur, and there is no known reason to expect a clinically significant interaction with mullein.

Typical Dosages & Routes of Administration that are Commonly Used

ORAL: The typical dose of mullein is 1.5-2 grams of the dry petals or one cup of tea. up to 3-4 grams dry petals per day (2,7,8,18). The tea is prepared by steeping 1.5-2 grams of the finely chopped, dry petals in 150 mL boiling water for 10-15 minutes and then strain.

Comments

Avoid confusion with goldenrod (Solidago species), also known as Aaron's rod. There is confusion as to which Verbascum species are associated with the name American mullein and which are associated with the name European mullein.

MUSK

This Product is Also Known As

Deer Musk, Tonquin Musk.

Scientific Names

Moschus moschiferus.
Family: Moschidae.

People Use This For

In Chinese medicine, musk is used for stroke, coma, neurasthenia, convulsions, heart pains, and ulcerous sores (11).
For food use, musk is often used with nut, caramel, and fruit-type flavors (11).
In manufacturing, it is also used as a constituent of fragrances and a fixative in perfumes (6).

Safety

LIKELY SAFE ...when taken orally at low concentrations, generally below 0.00001%. It has Generally Recognized as Safe (GRAS) status in the US.
There is insufficient reliable information available about the safety of the oral use of larger amounts of musk.
PREGNANCY AND LACTATION: Insufficient reliable information available; avoid using.

Effectiveness

There is insufficient reliable information available about the effectiveness of musk.

Possible Mechanism of Action & Active Ingredients

Musk contains muscone (0.3%-2%) and normuscone, steroids, paraffins, triglycerides, waxes, mucopyridine, and fatty acids, which may have anti-inflammatory and antihistaminic activity (6).

Adverse Reactions Including Known Allergies

Musk components are known to cause a variety of dermal hypersensitivity reactions (6).

Possible Interactions with Herbs & Other Dietary Supplements

Insufficient reliable information available.

Possible Interactions with Drugs

No interactions are known to occur, and there is no known reason to expect a clinically significant interaction with musk.

Possible Interactions with Foods

No interactions are known to occur, and there is no known reason to expect a clinically significant interaction with musk.

Possible Interactions with Lab Tests

No interactions are known to occur, and there is no known reason to expect a clinically significant interaction with musk.

Possible Interactions with Diseases or Conditions

No interactions are known to occur, and there is no known reason to expect a clinically significant interaction with musk.

Typical Dosages & Routes of Administration that are Commonly Used

No typical dosage.

Comments

Musk is the secretion from the musk gland of the male musk deer. Avoid confusion with sumbul, which is also known as musk root (Ferula sumbul, Family: Apiaceae), which is sometimes substituted for musk (6).

MYRRH

This Product is Also Known As

Abyssinian Myrrh, African Myrrh, Arabian Myrrh, Bal, Balsamodendron Myrrha, Bdellium, Bol, Bola, Commiphora, Didin, Didthin, Guggal Gum and Resin, Gum Myrrh, Heerabol, Opopanax, Somalien Myrrh, Yemen Myrrh.

Scientific Names

Commiphora molmol, synonyms Commiphora abyssinica, Commiphora madagascariensis; Commiphora myrrha; other Commiphora species; Commiphora erythraea.
Family: Burseraceae.

People Use This For

Topically, myrrh resin is used for mild inflammation of the oral and pharyngeal mucosa (2,5,8,9,11,13,18), aphthous ulcers (4), gingivitis (4,8,11), and chapped lips (11).

In folk medicine, it has been used internally, for indigestion (4,5,8,9,11,13,18), ulcers (5), colds (4), cough, asthma (11), bronchial congestion (4,5,8,11,18), arthritic pain (11), cancer, leprosy, and syphilis (5,6). It has also been used as a stimulant (11,13), antispasmodic (11), and to increase menstrual flow (5,6,11). Topically, myrrh has been used in folk medicine for hemorrhoids (5,11), bedsores (5,8,11), wounds (5,11,19), abrasions, furunculosis (4), bad breath, and loose teeth (11). It has also been used in embalming and as incense (5,13).

In foods and beverages, myrrh oil is used as a flavoring component (11).

In manufacturing, myrrh oil is used as a fragrance and fixative in cosmetics (11).

Safety

LIKELY SAFE ...when consumed in amounts commonly found in food (11). Myrrh is approved for use in foods in the US (11).
POSSIBLY SAFE ...when used orally and appropriately (12). ...when used topically and appropriately (2,4,5,11,18).
POSSIBLY UNSAFE ...when used orally in excessive doses (12).
PREGNANCY: LIKELY UNSAFE ...contraindicated for oral use because myrrh stimulates uterine tone and blood flow, and possibly has an abortifacient effect (4,12,19). Insufficient reliable information available about the safety of the topical use of myrrh during pregnancy.
LACTATION: Insufficient reliable information available; avoid using.

Effectiveness

POSSIBLY EFFECTIVE ...when used topically for mild inflammation of the mouth and throat (2).
There is insufficient reliable information available about the effectiveness of myrrh for its other uses.

Possible Mechanism of Action & Active Ingredients

The applicable part of myrrh is resin. Myrrh resin contains a volatile oil and mucilage that have antimicrobial (4,5,6,8,11,18), deodorizing (8), anti-inflammatory (4,8), and antitumor properties (1536). In animals, it exhibits antipyretic (4) and hypoglycemic (4) effects, as well as protects against the development of gastric ulcers (1535). Myrrh can stimulate smooth muscle (6,12) and possibly peristalsis (6). It stimulates uterine tone (6,12) and promotes uterine blood flow (12,19). Most authorities report myrrh has astringent activity (2,4,5,6,9,11,18), although some experts disagree with this (8).

Adverse Reactions Including Known Allergies

Dermatitis has been reported with the use of myrrh (6). Amounts greater than 2-4 grams can cause kidney irritation and diarrhea (12). Large amounts can affect the heart rate (19).

Possible Interactions with Herbs & Other Dietary Supplements

Insufficient reliable information available.

Possible Interactions with Drugs

DIABETES THERAPY: The use of myrrh in diabetics can interfere with their therapy (4).

Possible Interactions with Foods

No interactions are known to occur, and there is no known reason to expect a clinically significant interaction with myrrh.

Possible Interactions with Lab Tests

BLOOD GLUCOSE: Theoretically, myrrh can lower blood glucose and test results.

Possible Interactions with Diseases or Conditions

DIABETES: Theoretically, myrrh can interfere with diabetes therapy (4).
HEART CONDITIONS: Use myrrh with caution in individuals with heart conditions, because large amounts can affect the heart rate (19).
OTHER: Use myrrh with caution because it can exacerbate uterine bleeding (12,19), fever, and systemic inflammation (19).

Typical Dosages & Routes of Administration that are Commonly Used

TOPICAL: For mild mouth and throat irritation, dab the undiluted tincture of myrrh on affected areas two to three times daily. Myrrh is also commonly used as a rinse or gargle with 5-10 drops in a glass of water (2,8). A typical mouthwash can contain 30-60 drops in a glass of water also (8). The tooth powder contains 10% powdered resin (2,18).

Comments

Myrrh is the oelogum resin exuded from fissures or cuts in the bark of Commiphora species trees. While there is confusion about the sources of myrrh, most authorities include Commiphora molmol and other Commiphora species as sources. However, authorities consider Commiphora mukul to be a related species, but not a source of myrrh (8).

MYRTLE

This Product is Also Known As

Myrti aetherolum, Myrti folium.

Scientific Names

Myrtus communis.
Family: Myrtaceae.

People Use This For

Orally, myrtle is used for treating acute and chronic respiratory infections including bronchitis, whooping cough, tuberculosis, bladder conditions, diarrhea, and worm infestation (18).

Safety

LIKELY UNSAFE ...when the undiluted oil is used orally because it contains cineole. Ingesting more than 10 grams of cineole can result in respiratory failure and collapse (18).
There is insufficient reliable information available about the safety of using the leaf and branch.
CHILDREN: LIKELY UNSAFE ...when used orally. Avoid facial contact with myrtle oil preparations which may cause glottal spasm, bronchospasm, asthma-like attacks, or respiratory failure in infants or small children (18).
PREGNANCY AND LACTATION: LIKELY UNSAFE; avoid using.

Effectiveness

There is insufficient reliable information available about the effectiveness of myrtle.

Possible Mechanism of Action & Active Ingredients

The applicable parts of myrtle are the leaf and branch. Myrtle contains a volatile oil, tannins and acylphloroglucinols. Myrtol, a volatile oil, stimulates mucous membranes of the stomach and deodorizes the breath. It might also have fungicidal, disinfectant, and antibacterial properties (18). The volatile oil contains between 15-45% of 1,8-cineole, a constituent responsible for toxicity (18).

Adverse Reactions Including Known Allergies

Used orally, myrtle can cause nausea, vomiting, and diarrhea (18). Consumption of large amounts might lead to low blood pressure, circulatory disorders, respiratory failure and collapse (18). Topically, facial contact with myrtle oil preparations may cause glottal or bronchial spasm, asthma-like attacks or respiratory failure in infants and children (18).

Possible Interactions with Herbs & Other Dietary Supplements

Insufficient reliable information available.

Possible Interactions with Drugs

No interactions are known to occur, and there is no known reason to expect a clinically significant interaction with myrtle.

Possible Interactions with Foods

No interactions are known to occur, and there is no known reason to expect a clinically significant interaction with myrtle.

Possible Interactions with Lab Tests

No interactions are known to occur, and there is no known reason to expect a clinically significant interaction with myrtle.

Possible Interactions with Diseases or Conditions

No interactions are known to occur, and there is no known reason to expect a clinically significant interaction with myrtle.

Typical Dosages & Routes of Administration that are Commonly Used
ORAL: A typical dose is 200 mg one time only (18).

Comments
Myrtle leaves resemble the leaves of Bux semper-virens and Vaccinium vitisidaea (18).

N-ACETYL CYSTEINE

This Product is Also Known As
Acetylcysteine, NAC, N-Acetylcysteine, N-Acetyl-B-Cysteine, N-Acetyl-Cysteine.

Scientific Names
N-acetyl-L-cysteine.

People Use This For
Orally, NAC is used as an antidote for acetaminophen poisoning (14,15), for unstable angina, carbon monoxide poisoning, common bile duct obstruction in infants, lyosomal storage disorders, amyotrophic lateral sclerosis (ALS), phenytoin-induced hypersensitivity, keratoconjunctivitis, reducing lipoprotein (a) levels (14,2244), reducing homocysteine levels (2256), and for chronic bronchitis (6176). NAC is also used orally for myoclonus epilepsy; otitis media (14); for hemodialysis-related pseudoporphyria (5052); Sjogren's syndrome; preventing sports injury complications; radiation therapy; increasing immunity to flu, detoxifying heavy metals such as mercury, lead, and cadmium; preventing alcoholic liver damage; protecting against environmental pollutants, including carbon monoxide, chloroform, urethanes and certain herbicides (2244); reducing toxicity of ifosfamide and doxorubicin (14,2244); and as a hangover remedy (6179).

Safety
LIKELY SAFE ...when used appropriately as an FDA-approved prescription drug for oral, intratracheal and oral inhaled administration (15).
There is insufficient reliable information available about the safety of NAC for its other uses.
PREGNANCY: LIKELY SAFE ...when used appropriately. Pregnancy rating for FDA-approved product is category B.
LACTATION: Insufficient reliable information available; avoid using (15).

Effectiveness
EFFECTIVE ...when used orally for treating acetaminophen poisoning (15). ...when used as an inhalant for a mucolytic adjunctive treatment for acute and chronic bronchopulmonary disorders. ...when used for atelectasis caused by mucus obstruction. ...when used for post-traumatic chest conditions. ...when used for pulmonary complications of surgery and cystic fibrosis (15). ...when used for preparing people for bronchial diagnostic studies (15). ...when used as an adjunct for preventing endotracheal crusting in tracheostomy care (15). ...when used for inhalation injury (15). ...when used intravenously for acrylonitrile poisoning (14).
POSSIBLY EFFECTIVE ...when used orally for treating unstable angina pectoris in combination with nitroglycerin (14,2245). ...when used orally for preventing acute exacerbations in people with chronic bronchitis (6176). A meta-analysis of six double-blind, placebo controlled trials involving 821 patients with chronic bronchitis found that three to six months of various oral doses of N-acetyl cysteine reduced the number of acute exacerbation episodes. ...when used orally for preventing ifosfamide toxicity (14,2250). ...when used orally for reducing homocysteine levels (2256,2258). ...when used orally for treating myoclonus epilepsy (2259). ...when used orally for reducing symptoms of influenza (2260). ...when used topically for reducing dental plaque (14). ...when used rectally for treating meconium ileus (14). ...when used intravenously for treating unstable angina pectoris in combination with nitroglycerin (14,2246) and reducing nitroglycerin tolerance (832,2279).
POSSIBLY INEFFECTIVE ...when used orally for preventing (2252) or reversing (2253) doxorubicin-induced cardiac toxicity. ...when used for treating Sjogren's syndrome (14). ...when used intravenously for treating amyotrophic lateral sclerosis (ALS) (14,2254).
LIKELY INEFFECTIVE ...when used for reducing lipoprotein (a) (2256,2257). ...when used for reducing nitroglycerin tolerance (2281,2282).

Possible Mechanism of Action & Active Ingredients
Acetylcysteine is the N-acetyl (NAC) derivative of the amino acid L-cysteine (15). NAC has mucolytic properties that result from several mechanisms. NAC ruptures mucous disulfide bonds which reduces mucous viscosity. NAC also has an irritating effect on mucosa that stimulates mucociliary clearance (14). NAC maintains or restores glutathione levels in the liver. It acts as an alternative substrate for conjugation of toxic acetaminophen metabolites, thus protecting the liver from acetaminophen damage (15). NAC is an oxygen free-radical scavenger (14). Preliminary evidence suggests that oral NAC might be beneficial in treating cystinosis (2249). Other evidence suggests rectal administration might be beneficial in treating bile duct obstruction (2247,2248). NAC might be useful for lamellar ichthyosis, a congenital skin disease (3974). Preliminary data suggests that NAC has an antiproliferative effect on skin cells, reversibly suppressing fibroblast cell proliferation (3975).

Researchers report that NAC administered to glutathione-deficient, HIV-positive patients improved T-cell function and reduced HIV expression in vitro. Further research is needed to evaluate the clinical effects of NAC in HIV-positive patients and in conjunction with highly active antiretroviral therapy (HAART). The results of this unpublished study were reported at the April 2000 NIAAA conference on Alcohol Use And HIV Pharmacotherapy (5063).

Adverse Reactions Including Known Allergies

NAC can cause nausea, vomiting, generalized urticaria, stomatitis, drowsiness, mild fever, chills, clamminess, severe runny nose, chest tightness, bronchoconstriction, and marked elevations in liver function tests (15). NAC used concomitantly with oral nitroglycerin can cause intolerable headaches (2245,2280), with IV nitroglycerin it can cause severe hypotension (14,2246). Although inhalation therapists report sensitization and dermal eruptions, this has not been confirmed by patch testing (15).

Possible Interactions with Herbs & Other Dietary Supplements

Insufficient reliable information available.

Possible Interactions with Drugs

CARBAMAZEPINE: Concomitant use can reduce carbamazepine (Tegretol) serum levels and therapeutic effects (14).

NITROGLYCERIN: Concomitant administration of NAC and intravenous nitroglycerin use can cause severe hypotension (14,2246); concomitant use of oral NAC and nitroglycerin can cause intolerable headaches (2245,2280).

Possible Interactions with Foods

No interactions are known to occur, and there is no known reason to expect a clinically significant interaction with NAC.

Possible Interactions with Lab Tests

BLOOD PRESSURE: Concomitant administration of intravenous NAC and nitroglycerin can lower blood pressure and reduce blood pressure readings (2246).

CHLORIDE: NAC can cause false-positive serum chloride test results measured with the Beckman Synchron CX3 analyzer (275).

CREATININE: Intravenous NAC can cause falsely low serum creatinine test results when measured by single-slide method on Kodak Ektachem systems (275).

CYSTEINE (FREE): Intravenous NAC can increase free cysteine plasma concentrations and test results (275).

GOLD: Intravenous NAC can increase urinary gold excretion (concentration) and test results in patients previously given gold (275).

KETONES: NAC can cause false-positive urine ketone test results when measured with Chemstrips (Boehringer Mannheim) or Multistix (Miles) (275). NAC can cause false-positive blood or urine ketone test results in procedures using nitroprusside (14).

LIPOPROTEIN A: Used orally, NAC might reduce serum lipoprotein A concentrations and test results in some patients (275).

LITHIUM: Very high serum NAC concentrations might cause falsely low serum lithium test results when measured with Kodak Ektachem systems (275).

LIVER FUNCTION TESTS: NAC might increase liver enzyme (AST, ALT) concentrations and test results. Liver function tests were markedly elevated on two occasions in a child with cystic fibrosis after receiving large NAC doses by rectal and naso-gastric tube administration (15).

PROTHROMBIN TIME (PT): Intravenous NAC can decrease PT and test results (1341).

SALICYLATE: Serum NAC concentrations of 50 mg/dL (occurring with intravenous NAC administration) can cause falsely low serum salicylate test results when measured with Kodak Ektachem systems. Serum NAC concentrations of 10 mg/dL (occurring with oral NAC administration) do not interfere with serum salicylate results measured with Kodak Ektachem systems (275). NAC can interfere with serum salicylate assays measured by colorimetric methods which rely on the reagent 4-aminophenol for the color change (14).

Possible Interactions with Diseases or Conditions

ALLERGY: Contraindicated in individuals with acetylcysteine allergy (15).

ASTHMA: Oral NAC inhalation or intratracheal administration might cause bronchospasm, monitor closely (15).

HEMODIALYSIS-ASSOCIATED PSEUDOPORPHYRIA: NAC might improve pseudoporphyria skin lesions associated with hemodialysis. Two cases are reported in which pseudoporphyria skin lesions healed with oral NAC administration in patients on chronic hemodialysis (5052).

SEPTIC SHOCK: NAC might depress cardiac function (14).

Typical Dosages & Routes of Administration that are Commonly Used

ORAL: A typical dose for unstable angina, 600 mg three times daily with transdermal nitroglycerin; severe headache may limit use (2245). For preventing acute exacerbations of chronic bronchitis, doses of 200 mg twice daily, 200 mg three times daily, 300 mg slow-release twice daily, and 600 mg controlled-release twice daily have been used (6176). For ifosfamide toxicity prophylaxis, 2 grams every 6 hours has been used (2250). For reducing plasma homocysteine levels, 1.2 grams daily has been used (2258). For myoclonus epilepsy, 4-6 grams daily has

been used (2259). For reducing symptoms of influenza, 600 mg twice daily has been used (2260). For hemodialysis-associated pseudoporphyria skin lesions, 200 mg four times daily or 600 mg twice daily has been used (5052).
TOPICAL: For reducing dental plaque, 10% aqueous acetylcysteine solution has been used (14).
RECTAL: For meconium ileus, a typical adult dose is 4-6% acetylcysteine enema every 6 to 12 hours (14); for meconium ileus, a typical pediatric dose is 10% acetylcysteine enema every 3 to 12 hours (14).
INTRAVENOUS: Intravenous acetylcysteine is an FDA designated orphan drug for treating moderate to severe acetaminophen overdose.
ORAL AND INHALED: Acetylcysteine is available as an FDA-approved prescription drug for oral, intratracheal and oral inhaled administration.

Comments
None.

N-ACETYL GLUCOSAMINE

This Product is Also Known As
Acetylglucosamine, N-Acetyl-D-Glucosamine, NAG, Poly-NAG.
CAUTION: See separate listings for Glucosamine Sulfate and Glucosamine Hydrochloride.

Scientific Names
2-acetamido-2-deoxyglucose.

People Use This For
Orally, N-acetyl glucosamine is used for ulcerative colitis, Crohn's disease (2610,2609), and osteoarthritis (2611).

Safety
There is insufficient reliable information available about the safety of N-acetyl glucosamine.
Pregnancy and Lactation: Insufficient reliable information available; avoid using.

Effectiveness
There is insufficient reliable information available about the effectiveness of N-acetyl glucosamine.

Possible Mechanism of Action & Active Ingredients
N-acetyl glucosamine is a glycoprotein derived from marine exoskeletons or produced synthetically (6). In Inflammatory Bowel Disease (IBD), N-acetylation of glucosamine is relatively deficient, possibly reducing the synthesis of the gastric and intestinal mucosa's protective glycoprotein cover (2609). Theoretically, supplementation with N-acetyl glucosamine (IBD) could remedy this deficiency and restore the glycoprotein cover (2609). However, no human studies to date have evaluated this claim. Similarly, no human studies have evaluated N-acetyl glucosamine for treating osteoarthritis. Preliminary evidence suggests glucosamine decreases glucose-induced insulin secretion by inhibiting pancreatic glucokinase in the beta cells of the islet of Langerhans (371,372,3406). Evidence also suggests glucosamine impairs insulin-mediated glucose uptake and metabolism in skeletal muscle. It is hypothesized that glucosamine desensitizes cell membranes to the effects of insulin (372,3406). Evidence suggests that type 2 diabetes and glucosamine induce insulin resistance by acting on a common pathway (3405) and glucosamine-induced insulin resistance might be dose-dependent (3406).

Adverse Reactions Including Known Allergies
There is concern that N-acetyl glucosamine products derived from marine exoskeletons might cause reactions in people allergic to shellfish, although no reactions have been reported. Until more is known, and because the source of N-acetyl glucosamine products is not listed on product labels, use N-acetyl glucosamine with caution in people with shellfish allergy.

Possible Interactions with Herbs & Other Dietary Supplements
Insufficient reliable information available.

Possible Interactions with Drugs
ANTIDIABETES DRUGS: Theoretically, N-acetyl glucosamine might decrease the hypoglycemic effects of insulin and oral antidiabetes agents by increasing insulin resistance and/or decreasing insulin production.

Possible Interactions with Foods
No interactions are known to occur, and there is no known reason to expect a clinically significant interaction with N-acetyl glucosamine.

Possible Interactions with Lab Tests
BLOOD GLUCOSE: Theoretically, N-acetyl glucosamine might increase blood glucose levels and test results, by increasing insulin resistance and/or decreasing insulin production. There are also anecdotal reports of poorer control in people with diabetes who take glucosamine (22,1203,1204,3405,3406).

Possible Interactions with Diseases or Conditions

DIABETES: Theoretically, N-acetyl glucosamine might exacerbate diabetes by increasing insulin resistance and/or decreasing insulin production.

SHELLFISH ALLERGY: There is concern that N-acetyl glucosamine products derived from marine exoskeletons might cause reactions in people allergic to shellfish, although no reactions have been reported. Until more is known, and because the source of N-acetyl glucosamine products is not listed on product labels, use N-acetyl glucosamine with caution in people with shellfish allergy.

Typical Dosages & Routes of Administration that are Commonly Used

ORAL: Most products recommend a daily dosage of 1500 mg, although the suggested dosage ranges from 500 mg to 3000 mg per day in divided doses (5261).

Comments

Avoid confusion with glucosamine sulfate and glucosamine hydrochloride. Read glucosamine product labels carefully for their content. Although glucosamine sulfate or glucosamine hydrochloride are marketed together in combination products with N-acetyl glucosamine, no human studies have evaluated these combinations for treating osteoarthritis. Only glucosamine sulfate has been studied in humans for osteoarthritis. Chitosan is the deacylated polymer of N-acetyl glucosamine (see separate listing for chitosan).

NADH

This Product is Also Known As

B-DPNH, BNADH, Coenzyme 1, Enada, NAD, Reduced DPN, Reduced Nicotinamide Adenine Dinucleotide.

Scientific Names

NADH.

People Use This For

Orally, NADH is used for improving mental clarity, alertness and concentration, improving memory, cellular energy, for antioxidant effects, chronic fatigue syndrome, depression, hypertension, Alzheimer's disease, Parkinson's disease, improving athletic endurance, enhancing energy, improving DNA repair, enhancing immune function, reducing aging, protecting the liver from alcohol damage, preventing alcohol-induced inhibition of testosterone, lowering cholesterol levels, protecting against zidovudine (AZT) toxicity (3075,3076,3077). Intravenously, NADH is used as an IM or IV injection for Parkinson's disease (3085,3086,3089,3090) and depression (3076).

Safety

There is insufficient reliable information available about the safety of NADH.

Pregnancy and Lactation: Insufficient reliable information available; avoid using.

Effectiveness

There is insufficient reliable information available about the effectiveness of NADH.

Possible Mechanism of Action & Active Ingredients

NADH is the reduced form of NAD (nicotinamide adenine dinucleotide), a coenzyme necessary to dehydrogenate primary and secondary alcohols (3082). In dehydrogenation, NAD acts as a hydrogen acceptor, forming NADH. NADH, in turn, serves as a hydrogen donor in the respiratory chain (3082). NADH is an essential intermediate in the cellular processes that generate energy from glucose in the form of ATP (3008). Some evidence suggests oral NADH reduces blood pressure, total cholesterol, and LDL (3083). Preliminary evidence suggests that NADH might help people with chronic fatigue syndrome by triggering energy production through ATP generation (229,3084). Other evidence suggests that NADH might benefit people with Alzheimer's disease (3087). NADH has been proposed as a therapeutic agent for people with Parkinson's disease because evidence suggests it might increase tyrosine hydroxylase activity and dopamine production (3085,3086,3088,3091). However, while two open trials found it was beneficial (3086,3089), one small double-blind study showed it was not (3090).

Adverse Reactions Including Known Allergies

None reported.

Possible Interactions with Herbs & Other Dietary Supplements

Insufficient reliable information available.

Possible Interactions with Drugs

No interactions are known to occur, and there is no known reason to expect a clinically significant interaction with NADH.

Possible Interactions with Foods

No interactions are known to occur, and there is no known reason to expect a clinically significant interaction with NADH.

Possible Interactions with Lab Tests

No interactions are known to occur, and there is no known reason to expect a clinically significant interaction with NADH.

Possible Interactions with Diseases or Conditions

No interactions are known to occur, and there is no known reason to expect a clinically significant interaction with NADH.

Typical Dosages & Routes of Administration that are Commonly Used

ORAL: For nutrition and energy enhancement, a typical dose is 2.5-5 mg daily or every other day (3462). For therapeutic support of Alzheimer's disease, Parkinson's disease and chronic fatigue syndrome, a typical dose is 10-15 mg daily or every other day (3462). Some people recommend the disodium salt form of NADH, taken with water either 30 minutes before or 2 hours after meals (3462).

Comments

None.

NASTURTIUM

This Product is Also Known As

Indian Cress.
CAUTION: See separate listing for Watercress.

Scientific Names

Tropaeolum majus.
Family: Tropaeolaceae.

People Use This For

Orally and in combination with other herbs, nasturtium is used for urinary tract infection, respiratory tract mucous membrane inflammation (2,18), and cough and bronchitis (18).
Topically, it is used in combination with other herbs for mild muscular pain (2).

Safety

POSSIBLY SAFE ...when used topically (2). ...when used orally in combination with other herbs (2).
There is insufficient reliable information available about the safety of nasturtium used orally as a single entity (2,18).
CHILDREN: LIKELY UNSAFE ...when used orally in combination with other herbs. Contraindicated (2,18). There is insufficient reliable information about the safety of the topical use of nasturtium by children.
PREGNANCY AND LACTATION: Insufficient reliable information available; avoid using nasturtium by itself or in combination with other herbs.

Effectiveness

POSSIBLY EFFECTIVE ...when taken orally as a component of herbal combinations for supportive treatment of lower urinary tract infections and respiratory tract mucous membrane inflammation (2). ...when used topically as a component of herbal combinations for treating mild muscular pain (2).
There is insufficient reliable information available about the effectiveness of nasturtium for its other uses.

Possible Mechanism of Action & Active Ingredients

The applicable parts of nasturtium are the above ground parts. Nasturtium contains 300 mg vitamin C per 100 grams of fresh plant (18). Benzyl mustard oil (benzyl isothiocyanate), the principal active constituent of nasturtium, may have bacteriostatic, virustatic, antimycotic (2,18), and antitumor (1537) activity. It is accumulated and excreted mainly in the respiratory and the urinary tracts (2,18). Applied topically, benzyl mustard oil has rubifacient activity (2,18).

Adverse Reactions Including Known Allergies

Large amounts of nasturtium or benzyl mustard oil taken orally can cause GI tract irritation (2,18); one case of urticarial exanthema is reported (2). Large amounts of nasturtium can cause albuminuria due to glomerular and tubular damage (2). Topically, long term intensive contact with the plant can cause skin irritation (18); benzyl mustard oil can cause skin and mucosal irritation (2). Benzyl mustard oil is a contact allergen if applied to the skin (2).

Possible Interactions with Herbs & Other Dietary Supplements
Insufficient reliable information available.

Possible Interactions with Drugs
No interactions are known to occur, and there is no known reason to expect a clinically significant interaction with nasturtium.

Possible Interactions with Foods
No interactions are known to occur, and there is no known reason to expect a clinically significant interaction with nasturtium.

Possible Interactions with Lab Tests
No interactions are known to occur, and there is no known reason to expect a clinically significant interaction with nasturtium.

Possible Interactions with Diseases or Conditions
KIDNEY DISEASE: Contraindicated in individuals with kidney disease.
GI ULCERS: Contraindicated in individuals with gastric or intestinal ulcers (2,18).

Typical Dosages & Routes of Administration that are Commonly Used
ORAL: No typical dosage.
TOPICAL: When used in combination with other herbs, the dose varies according to the combination (2).

Comments
None.

NEEM

This Product is Also Known As
Bead Tree, Holy Tree, Indian Lilac, Margosa, Nim, Nimba, Persian Lilac, Pride of China.

Scientific Names
Azadirachta indica.
Family: Meliaceae.

People Use This For
Intravaginally, neem is used as a contraceptive (6).
In folk medicine, the stem, root bark, and fruit are used as a tonic and astringent; the bark is used for malaria and cutaneous diseases; the leaves are used for worm infections, ulcers, cardiovascular disease, diabetes and gingivitis; all the above ground parts are used as an antipyretic and anti-inflammatory (6).
Neem is also used as an insecticide (6).

Safety
POSSIBLY SAFE ...when the oil is used orally (6).
LIKELY UNSAFE ...when large amounts of seeds are used orally. Can cause poisoning (6).
There is insufficient reliable information available about the safety of the above ground parts of neem.
CHILDREN: LIKELY UNSAFE ...when the oil or seeds are taken orally. There are reports of infants who were severely poisoned and died (3473,3474,3476).
PREGNANCY AND LACTATION: Insufficient reliable information available; avoid using.

Effectiveness
There is insufficient reliable information available about the effectiveness of neem.

Possible Mechanism of Action & Active Ingredients
The applicable parts of neem are the above ground parts. Neem has varied constituents and pharmacological activity. Neem bark and leaves contain tannin and oil (18). Neem seeds yield a fixed oil composed primarily of glycerides and bitter compounds including nimbin, nimbinin and nimbidol (6). A small study in women demonstrated neem oil has spermicidal and contraceptive properties when used intravaginally (6). In animals, oral administration of oil reduced blood glucose levels by up to 48%, which lends some credence to the folk use for diabetes (6). In vitro studies suggest neem oil possesses antibacterial activity against varied organisms (6). A toothpaste containing neem extract exhibited antimicrobial activity and low levels of abrasiveness (6). Leaves of neem may be useful in preventing plaque formation (3). Constituents gedunin and nimbolide show in vitro antimalarial activity (6). Though neem oil is toxic to infants and children, the toxic constituent is unknown (3473,3475). Researchers speculate that a long-chain monounsaturated free acid may be responsible (3475).

Adverse Reactions Including Known Allergies
Severe poisoning in infants and small children characterized by vomiting, loose stools, drowsiness, metabolic

acidosis, anemia, polymorphonuclear leukocytosis, seizure, loss of consciousness, coma, cerebral edema, Reye-like syndrome symptoms and death have been reported to occur within hours after ingestion of neem oil (3473,3474,3476). Liver and renal biopsy reports have revealed pathologic findings seen typically in Reye's syndrome (3473,3474,3475).

Possible Interactions with Herbs & Other Dietary Supplements
Insufficient reliable information available.

Possible Interactions with Drugs
No interactions are known to occur, and there is no known reason to expect a clinically significant interaction with neem.

Possible Interactions with Foods
No interactions are known to occur, and there is no known reason to expect a clinically significant interaction with neem.

Possible Interactions with Lab Tests
No interactions are known to occur, and there is no known reason to expect a clinically significant interaction with neem.

Possible Interactions with Diseases or Conditions
No interactions are known to occur, and there is no known reason to expect a clinically significant interaction with neem.

Typical Dosages & Routes of Administration that are Commonly Used
ORAL: Used as a tincture (18).

Comments
Azadirachtin, the insecticide constituent of seeds, is effective in concentrations as low as 0.1 ppm. It is biodegradable, non-mutagenic and nontoxic to fish, birds and "warm-blooded animals" (6). The Environmental Protection Agency has approved the use of a neem formulation (Margosan-O) as a pesticide for limited use on nonfood crops (6).

NERVE ROOT

This Product is Also Known As
American Valerian, Bleeding Heart, Cypripedium, Lady's Slipper, Moccasin Flower, Monkey Flower, Noah's Ark, Slipper Root, Venus Shoe, Yellows.

Scientific Names
Cypripedium pubescens, synonym Cypripedium calceolus.
Family: Orchidaceae.

People Use This For
Orally, nerve root is used for menorrhagia and diarrhea (18).
Topically, it is used to treat pruritus vulvae (18).
In folk medicine, it has been used for insomnia, emotional tension, hysteria, anxiety states (4), agitation, nervousness (18) and specifically anxiety states associated with insomnia.

Safety
POSSIBLY UNSAFE ...when the root or rhizome are used orally. Nerve root is reported to cause hallucinations (4).
PREGNANCY AND LACTATION: POSSIBLY UNSAFE ...when used orally; avoid using.

Effectiveness
There is insufficient reliable information available about the effectiveness of nerve root.

Possible Mechanism of Action & Active Ingredients
The applicable parts of nerve root are the rhizome and root. Nerve root contains tannins, glycosides, resins, quinones and a volatile oil (4,18), and is said to have astringent and styptic properties (18). The quinone constituent of nerve root is thought to be responsible for its sensitizing properties (4).

Adverse Reactions Including Known Allergies
Taken orally, it can cause hallucinations (4). Large doses are associated with giddiness, restlessness, headache, mental excitement and visual hallucinations (4). Topically, it can cause contact dermatitis (4).

Possible Interactions with Herbs & Other Dietary Supplements
Insufficient reliable information available.

Possible Interactions with Drugs

No interactions are known to occur, and there is no known reason to expect a clinically significant interaction with nerve root.

Possible Interactions with Foods

No interactions are known to occur, and there is no known reason to expect a clinically significant interaction with nerve root.

Possible Interactions with Lab Tests

No interactions are known to occur, and there is no known reason to expect a clinically significant interaction with nerve root.

Possible Interactions with Diseases or Conditions

No interactions are known to occur, and there is no known reason to expect a clinically significant interaction with nerve root.

Typical Dosages & Routes of Administration that are Commonly Used

ORAL: 2-4 grams dried rhizome/root or as tea (steep 2-4 grams dried rhizome/root in 150 mL of boiling water for 5-10 minutes, strain), three times daily (4). Liquid extract (1:1 in 45% alcohol) 2-4 mL three times daily (4).

Comments

Avoid confusion with Calypso bulbosa (Cypripedium bulbosum) and Cypripedium parviflorum, related species also known as lady's slipper.

NEW JERSEY TEA

This Product is Also Known As

Jersey Tea, Mountain-Sweet, Redroot, Red Root, Walpole Tea, Wild Snowball.

Scientific Names

Ceanothus americanus.
Family: Rhamnaeceae.

People Use This For

Historically, New Jersey tea has been used as an expectorant, antispasmodic, clotting agent, and astringent and for gonorrhea, syphilis, colds, fever, and chills (18).

Safety

LIKELY SAFE ...when used as an oral medicinal (12,18).
PREGNANCY AND LACTATION: Insufficient reliable information available; avoid using.

Effectiveness

There is insufficient reliable information available about the effectiveness of New Jersey tea.

Possible Mechanism of Action & Active Ingredients

The applicable parts of New Jersey tea are the root, root bark, and leaf. New Jersey tea contains cyclic peptide alkaloids and triterpenes (18). An aqueous-ethanol extract of New Jersey tea is said to reduce the blood-clotting time by 25% in blood taken from young rats (18).

Adverse Reactions Including Known Allergies

None reported (18).

Possible Interactions with Herbs & Other Dietary Supplements

Insufficient reliable information available.

Possible Interactions with Drugs

No interactions are known to occur, and there is no known reason to expect a clinically significant interaction with New Jersey tea.

Possible Interactions with Foods

No interactions are known to occur, and there is no known reason to expect a clinically significant interaction with New Jersey tea.

Possible Interactions with Lab Tests

No interactions are known to occur, and there is no known reason to expect a clinically significant interaction with New Jersey tea.

Possible Interactions with Diseases or Conditions

No interactions are known to occur, and there is no known reason to expect a clinically significant interaction with New Jersey tea.

Typical Dosages & Routes of Administration that are Commonly Used

ORAL: Used as an extract (18).

Comments

None.

NEW ZEALAND GREEN-LIPPED MUSSEL

This Product is Also Known As

New Zealand Green Lipped Mussel, NZGLM.

Scientific Names

Perna canaliculus.
Family: Mytilidae.

People Use This For

Orally, New Zealand green-lipped mussel is used for symptoms of rheumatoid arthritis and osteoarthritis (6).

Safety

POSSIBLY SAFE ...when used orally, but there is only limited information available (6).
PREGNANCY: POSSIBLY UNSAFE; avoid using. May cause retarded fetal development and delay in parturition (936).
LACTATION: Insufficient reliable information available; avoid using.

Effectiveness

LIKELY INEFFECTIVE ...when taken orally for treating rheumatoid arthritis (6,935); an early report of effectiveness was not reproduced in subsequent studies (6,935).
There is insufficient reliable information available about the effectiveness of New Zealand green-lipped mussel for its other uses.

Possible Mechanism of Action & Active Ingredients

The dried New Zealand green-lipped mussels may contain a prostaglandin inhibitor that exerts an anti-inflammatory effect (932,933).
Researchers report that an extract of green-lipped mussel reduced symptoms in dogs with advanced arthritis. The results of this unpublished study were presented at the Experimental Biology 2000 conference (5055).

Adverse Reactions Including Known Allergies

Taken orally, it can cause diarrhea, nausea, and flatulence (6). One case was reported of reversible, granulomatous hepatitis associated with New Zealand green-lipped mussel (6).

Possible Interactions with Herbs & Other Dietary Supplements

Insufficient reliable information available.

Possible Interactions with Drugs

No interactions are known to occur, and there is no known reason to expect a clinically significant interaction with New Zealand green-lipped mussel.

Possible Interactions with Foods

No interactions are known to occur, and there is no known reason to expect a clinically significant interaction with New Zealand green-lipped mussel.

Possible Interactions with Lab Tests

No interactions are known to occur, and there is no known reason to expect a clinically significant interaction with New Zealand green-lipped mussel.

Possible Interactions with Diseases or Conditions

No interactions are known to occur, and there is no known reason to expect a clinically significant interaction with New Zealand green-lipped mussel.

Typical Dosages & Routes of Administration that are Commonly Used

ORAL: New Zealand green-lipped mussel extract 300-350 mg three times per day was used in human studies for rheumatoid arthritis; except for one early trial, studies found New Zealand green-lipped mussels ineffective (6,935).

Comments

New Zealand green-lipped mussels are available commercially as a freeze dried, ground, and encapsulated product.

NIACIN AND NIACINAMIDE (VITAMIN B3)

This Product is Also Known As

3-Pyridine Carboxamide, Anti-Blacktongue Factor, Antipellagra Factor, Niacin, Niacinamide, Nicamid, Nicosedine, Nicotinamide, Nicotinic Acid, Nicotinic Acid Amide, Nicotylamidum, Pellagra Preventing Factor, Vitamin PP.
CAUTION: See separate listings for Inositol Nicotinate (Inositol Hexaniacinate) and Tryptophan.

Scientific Names

Niacin; Niacinamide; Vitamin B3.

People Use This For

Orally, niacin is used with diet therapy for treating hyperlipoproteinemia. It is also used in conjunction with other therapies for peripheral vascular disease, vascular spasm, migraine headache, Meniere's syndrome, vertigo (15), and to reduce the diarrhea associated with cholera (14).

Orally, niacin or niacinamide is taken for preventing vitamin B3 deficiency, treating pellagra, schizophrenia, drug-induced hallucinations, chronic brain syndrome, hyperkinesis, depression, motion sickness, alcohol dependence, vasculitis associated with skin lesions and edema, acne, leprosy (15), preventing premenstrual headache, improving digestion, protection from toxins and pollutants, for reducing the effects of aging, memory loss, arthritis, lowering blood pressure, improving circulation, promoting relaxation, and improving orgasm (3035,3036,3037).

Orally, niacinamide is used for treating diabetes, and the skin conditions bullous pemphigoid and granuloma annulare (14).

Topically, niacinamide is used for treating inflammatory acne vulgaris (5940).

Safety

LIKELY SAFE ...when used orally and appropriately (15). Niacin and niacinamide are FDA-approved products.
POSSIBLY SAFE ...when niacinamide is used topically and appropriately up to 12 weeks (5940).
PREGNANCY AND LACTATION: LIKELY SAFE ...when used orally in amounts that do not exceed the recommended dietary allowance (3094). There is insufficient reliable information available about the safety of using larger oral amounts of niacin, niacinamide, or topical niacinamide; avoid using.

Effectiveness

EFFECTIVE ...when niacin or niacinamide is used orally for preventing niacin deficiency and treating pellagra. Both niacin and niacinamide are FDA-approved for prevention and treatment of niacin deficiency and pellagra. Niacinamide is sometimes preferred for this indication because it lacks the vasodilating effects of niacin (see Adverse Reactions) (15). ...when niacin is used orally as an adjunct to diet therapy for treating hyperlipoproteinemia (4867,4886,4887,4888,4889,4890). Niacin is FDA-approved for hyperlipoproteinemia not responding to diet therapy alone. The National Cholesterol Education Program (NCEP) recommends niacin as second-line single-drug therapy or in combination with other cholesterol-lowering drugs when diet and single-drug therapy are ineffective (4867). Niacin reduces cholesterol at least as well as statins and bile acid sequestrants in multiple clinical trials, but has a much higher incidence of adverse effects and lower patient tolerance (4867,4886,4887,4888,4889,4890). In a randomized, double-blind, placebo-controlled study, extended-release niacin (Niaspan) 1500 mg and 2000 mg daily raised HDL levels, and reduced apolipoprotein A and fibrinogen levels more effectively than gemfibrozil (Lopid) (4818). In a small study of patients with isolated hypoalphalipoproteinemia (low HDL with other lipid fractions relatively normal), combination therapy with gemfibrozil caused a greater increase in HDL than either agent alone (4817).

POSSIBLY EFFECTIVE ...when niacin is used orally for secondary prevention of myocardial infarction. In a large scale, long-term study, high dose niacin significantly reduced the risk of a second heart attack in men; however, there was not a significant decrease in overall or cause-specific mortality (4847). ...when niacin is used orally in combination with a bile acid sequestrant for atherosclerosis in high-risk men with existing cardiovascular disease. In a large-scale trial, niacin plus colestipol significantly decreased coronary atherosclerosis progression, increased frequency of atherosclerosis regression, and decreased incidence of cardiovascular events, including death, myocardial infarction, and revascularization procedures (4848). ...when niacin is used to control fluid loss due to cholera (4868). In a randomized controlled study divided doses of 2 grams of nicotinic acid daily reduced diarrhea in adults with cholera (4868). Laboratory evidence supports the use of nicotinic acid, but not niacinamide, to reduce intestinal secretion induced by cholera toxin (4869). ...when niacinamide is used to prevent the development of diabetes in high-risk children (4874,4875). High-dose niacinamide was effective in preventing type 1 diabetes in a large trial of high-risk children (4874). Following the success of this trial, a very large, multinational, long-term study was begun to determine whether regular use of niacinamide can prevent diabetes (4876). Preliminary results released by a German group found no protective effect, but the authors cautioned that their findings did not exclude that possibility that niacinamide might be effective (4875). ...when niacinamide is taken to preserve residual beta-cell function in newly diagnosed type 1 diabetes (4877,4878,4879,4880). Clinical trials, including one placebo-controlled trial and one vitamin E-comparison study showed niacinamide might prolong the "honeymoon period" in newly-diagnosed type 1 diabetes when the pancreas is still capable of producing some insulin (4877,4878,4879,4800). The clinical studies to date have been performed by one group of Italian investigators. Concerns about potential concurrent induction of insulin resistance have been raised (4881). ...when niacinamide is taken orally for protecting residual beta-cell function and improving glycemic control in adults with type 2 diabetes (4882). In a small, placebo-controlled, single-blind study, niacinamide increased C-peptide release and improved insulin secretion in lean diabetics who had failed sulfonylurea therapy (4882). ...when niacinamide is taken orally for osteoarthritis (4883). Niacinamide 3 grams daily in divided doses improved joint flexibility and reduced inflammation better than placebo, and allowed for reduction in standard anti-inflammatory drug doses in a double-blind, 12-week study. Adverse effects were mild, but more frequent in the niacinamide group (4883).

LIKELY INEFFECTIVE ...when niacinamide is taken orally for treating schizophrenia (14). ...when niacinamide is taken orally for treating hyperlipidemia (15,4849).

There is insufficient reliable information available about the effectiveness of niacin and niacinamide for its other uses.

Possible Mechanism of Action & Active Ingredients

Vitamin B3 includes niacin (nicotinic acid) and niacinamide (nicotinamide) (4849). The term niacin refers specifically to nicotinic acid, but is also used collectively to refer to both nicotinic acid and nicotinamide (niacinamide). Niacin is converted to niacinamide when ingested in amounts that do not exceed physiological requirements. The pharmacological effects of niacin and niacinamide are indistinguishable. Niacin is a water-soluble vitamin which is well absorbed when taken orally (4849). Dietary sources include meats, beans, and various niacin-fortified foods. In addition, dietary tryptophan is biosynthetically converted to niacin (60 mg tryptophan equals 1 mg of niacin or one niacin equivalent) (4849). Niacinamide is required for lipid metabolism, tissue respiration, and glycogenolysis. Niacinamide is incorporated into the coenzymes, nicotinamide adenine dinucleotide (NAD) and nicotinamide adenine dinucleotide phosphate (NADP). These coenzymes act as hydrogen-carrier molecules. Niacin deficiency causes pellagra, a condition that affects the gastrointestinal tract, skin, and central nervous system (4849). Pellagra was common in the early twentieth century, but niacin-fortified foods have virtually eliminated this deficiency disease except in conditions such as chronic alcoholism (4850). Some researchers think that sleep deprivation-induced dermatitis might be caused by niacin depletion because of similarities between this condition and pellagra (1350). Causes of niacin deficiency include poor diet, isoniazid therapy, carcinoid tumors that decrease endogenous production, and Hartnup disease, an autosomal recessive disorder that interferes with tryptophan absorption (4849). Conditions that increase niacin requirements, such as hyperthyroidism, diabetes mellitus, liver cirrhosis, pregnancy, and lactation, rarely cause deficiency (4969). When doses of niacin or niacinamide greater than 300-800 mg daily are administered different pharmacological effects occur.

Niacin 1000 mg or more per day decreases serum low-density lipoprotein (LDL) by 10 to 25%, increases serum high-density lipoprotein (HDL) concentrations by 15 to 35%, and decreases triglycerides by 20 to 50% (4867). The exact mechanism for the beneficial effects on serum lipids is unknown, but niacin inhibits free fatty acid release from adipose tissue; inhibits cyclic AMP accumulation which controls the activity of triglyceride lipase and hence lipolysis; decreases the rate of liver synthesis of LDL and VLDL; and, increases the rate of chylomicron triglyceride removal from plasma secondary to increased lipoprotein lipase activity (15,4849). Niacin also produces vasodilation of cutaneous blood vessels of the face, neck, and chest, probably mediated by prostaglandins, such as prostacyclin. In most individuals, tolerance to these effects occurs within two weeks (15). Preliminary clinical data suggest that some people with schizophrenia do not experience the characteristic vasodilatory response to niacin, suggesting an impaired response to phospholipid-dependent signaling (4870). Niacin also causes the release of histamine, which increases gastric motility and acid secretion (15). A review of cancer patients taking supplemental multivitamins suggests that niacin in combination with riboflavin might reduce the incidence of cataract development in older people (4885). Preliminary clinical research indicates that niacin reduces the fibrinogen concentration in plasma and stimulates fibrinolysis in hyperlipidemic men (4871). Large amounts of niacin can decrease uric acid excretion and impair glucose tolerance (15). Niacinamide has no beneficial effect on lipids and should not be used for treating hyperlipidemia (4849). Niacinamide does not cause the vasodilation associated with niacin (4849). High-dose niacinamide prevents or delays insulin deficiency in laboratory models of type 1 diabetes and protects islet cells from cytotoxic actions (4872,4873). Niacinamide is a free radical scavenger and might alter the autoimmune processes in type 1 diabetes that cause beta-cell destruction (4872,4873). Niacinamide is hypothesized to inhibit induction of nitric oxide synthase by interleukin 1 in chondrocytes, leading researchers to speculate about its potential use in destructive joint diseases (4884).

Adverse Reactions Including Known Allergies

Naturally occurring niacin in foods causes no known adverse effects (4849). Small amounts of nicotinic acid and niacinamide used for dietary supplementation can cause minor adverse reactions. Flushing, characterized by a burning, tingling, and itching sensation as well as erythema on the face, arms and chest, has been associated with doses as low as 30 mg per day (4849). Flushing may be accompanied by pruritus, headache, increased intracranial blood flow, and occasionally, pain (4849). Onset is highly variable, with 30 minutes to as long as 6 weeks of the initial dose (4849). At higher doses, side effects distinguish nicotinic acid and niacinamide (4849). Large amounts of nicotinic acid are associated with flushing, pruritus, burning sensations, stinging or tingling of the skin, nausea, bloating, flatulence, hunger pains, vomiting, heartburn, diarrhea, increased sebaceous gland activity, hypotension, dizziness, tachycardia, arrhythmias, syncope, vasovagal attacks, headache, and blurred vision (14,15). Dental and gingival pain have also been reported (4862). In most people taking niacin, flushing and other skin sensations, increased sebaceous gland activity, and increased gastrointestinal motility disappear within two weeks; however, adverse effects have been reported to appear up to 2 years after initiation of therapy (4851). Some evidence suggests that extended-release formulations may reduce the occurrence of these side effects (4857). Slow dose titration, pretreatment with 325 mg aspirin, and taking niacin with meals or the sustained release product at bedtime may reduce flushing (4852,4853,4854,4858). Flushing tends to decrease over time, despite dosage elevation (4864). Niacin, particularly at doses of 3 to 9 grams per day, may cause jaundice and elevated serum transaminases (4849). The drug should be discontinued if liver function tests rise to 3 times the upper limit of normal (4863). Severe hepatotoxicity with fulminant hepatitis and subsequent liver transplant has been reported (4849). Whether sustained release niacin is more hepatotoxic than immediate release formulations is controversial (4855,4856). High doses of niacin should not be used without medical supervision. Chronic use of large amounts of niacin have been associated with rash, hyperpigmentation resembling acanthosis nigricans, dry skin, xerostomia, hyperuricemia, gout, peptic ulcer, amblyopia, proptosis, loss of central vision secondary to an atypical form of cystoid macular edema, nervousness, panic, hyperglycemia, abnormal glucose tolerance and glycosuria, hepatotoxicity, abnormal prothrombin times and hypoalbuminemia (14,15). Niacin can significantly raise homocysteine levels at higher doses; a 17% increase with 1000 mg niacin per day and 55% with 3000 mg per day (1733). Elevated homocysteine levels are an independent risk factor for arterial occlusive disease (490); however, the clinical significance of niacin's effects on homocysteine is not yet known. Niacinamide in large amounts is associated with headache, dizziness, nausea and vomiting, diarrhea, blurred vision, hepatotoxicity, hyperglycemia, abnormal prothrombin times, and hypoalbuminemia (14,15).

Possible Interactions with Herbs & Other Dietary Supplements

BORAGE: Theoretically, concomitant use might have additive hepatotoxic effects; avoid concurrent use.
CHAPARRAL: Theoretically, concomitant use might have additive hepatotoxic effects; avoid concurrent use.
VALERIAN: Theoretically, concomitant use might have additive hepatotoxic effects; avoid concurrent use.
UVA URSI: Theoretically, concomitant use might have additive hepatotoxic effects; avoid concurrent use.

Possible Interactions with Drugs

ANTIDIABETES DRUGS: Concomitant use with niacin or niacinamide can interfere with blood glucose control, requiring drug dosing adjustment (15). Monitor blood glucose levels carefully.
CARBAMAZEPINE (Tegretol): Concomitant use with niacinamide can decrease the clearance of carbamazepine and increase the risk of toxicity (14).
GANGLIONIC BLOCKING DRUGS: Concomitant use with niacin can potentiate the hypotensive effects of these drugs (15).
HMG-CoA REDUCTASE INHIBITORS: Concomitant use of niacin with HMG-CoA reductase inhibitors can increase the risk of myopathy. HMG-CoA reductase inhibitors include atorvastatin (Lipitor), cerivastatin (Baycol), fluvastatin (Lescol), lovastatin (Mevacor), pravastatin (Pravachol), and simvastatin (Zocor) (14,15). NCEP guidelines suggest combination therapy only when diet and single drug therapy is not sufficiently effective (4867).
BILE ACID SEQUESTRANTS: Concomitant use of cholestyramine (Questran) or colestipol (Colestid) reduces niacin absorption (14).
ISONIAZID (INH, Laniazid): Isoniazid inhibits the conversion of tryptophan to niacin and might induce pellagra, particularly in poorly nourished patients (4865,4866).
TRANSDERMAL NICOTINE (Nicoderm, Nicotrol): Concomitant use can increase the risk of flushing and dizziness with niacin (14).

Drug Influences on Nutrient Levels and Depletion

SOME DRUGS CAN AFFECT NIACIN AND NIACINAMIDE LEVELS:
ANTIBIOTICS: Destruction of normal gastrointestinal flora by antibiotics can cause decreased production of B vitamins. The clinical significance of this decreased production is not known. Consider supplementation only if clinical judgment warrants it (4434,4435,4436,4437,4438,4439,4440,4441,4442,4443).

Possible Interactions with Foods

ETHANOL: Niacin should be used with caution in heavy alcohol drinkers. Both niacin and ethanol can increase the risk of hepatotoxicity. Niacin-induced flushing can be magnified by concomitant ingestion of ethanol (alcohol) (14,15,1289).
HOT DRINKS: Concomitant ingestion of niacin and hot drinks can magnify niacin-induced flushing (14,15,1289).

Possible Interactions with Lab Tests

CATECHOLAMINES: Niacin can falsely increase some urinary catecholamine fluorometric assay results. Niacin produces fluorescent substances in the urine, which can falsely elevate test results (15).
GLUCOSE: Niacin can increase blood glucose levels and test results. Niacin can also cause false-positive reactions with urine glucose tests which rely on cupric sulfate solution (Benedict's reagent) (15).
CHOLESTEROL: Niacin reduces serum total cholesterol, LDL cholesterol and VLDL cholesterol concentrations and test results. Niacin increases HDL cholesterol concentrations and test results (15).
HOMOCYSTEINE: At higher doses, niacin can increase homocysteine levels. Doses of 1000 mg and 3000 mg per

day reportedly increase homocysteine levels by 17% and 55% respectively (1733).

LIVER FUNCTION TESTS: Both niacin and niacinamide can increase serum bilirubin, alanine aminotransferase (ALT), aspartate aminotransferase (AST), and lactate dehydrogenase (LDH) concentrations and test results. Liver function tests should be monitored regularly, particularly early in the course of therapy and in patients receiving long-term treatment with high doses of niacin or niacinamide (15). Niacin should be discontinued if liver function tests rise to three times the upper limit of normal (4863).

TRIGLYCERIDES: Niacin reduces serum triglyceride concentrations and test results (15).

Possible Interactions with Diseases or Conditions

ALLERGIES: Niacin and niacinamide might exacerbate allergies by causing histamine release (14,15).

CORONARY ARTERY DISEASE/UNSTABLE ANGINA: Large amounts of niacin can increase the risk of cardiac arrhythmias. One study showed an increased incidence of cardiac arrhythmias when niacin was used in patients with coronary artery disease (15); use with caution.

DIABETES: Niacin and niacinamide can interfere with blood glucose control requiring dosing adjustment of antidiabetic agents. Niacin and niacinamide can cause hyperglycemia, abnormal glucose tolerance, and glycosuria. Increased blood glucose monitoring may be necessary, particularly early in the course of treatment (15,4859,4860).

GALLBLADDER DISEASE: Niacin and niacinamide might exacerbate gallbladder disease (14,15); use with caution.

GOUT: Large amounts of niacin or niacinamide might precipitate gout. Niacin and niacinamide can cause hyperuricemia (14,15); use with caution.

ARTERIAL HEMORRHAGE: Contraindicated; niacin can cause hypotension, and might exacerbate hypotension associated with arterial hemorrhage (15).

SEVERE HYPOTENSION: Contraindicated; niacin can cause hypotension (15).

KIDNEY DISEASE: Niacin is excreted unchanged in the urine and might accumulate in patients with kidney disease (14,15); use with caution.

LIVER DISEASE: Contraindicated; niacin and niacinamide have been associated with liver damage. Avoid large amounts in patients with a history of liver disease (15).

PEPTIC ULCER DISEASE: Contraindicated in patients with active peptic ulcer disease. Large amounts of niacin or niacinamide might activate or exacerbate peptic ulcer disease (14,15); use with caution in patients with a history of peptic ulcer disease.

Typical Dosages & Routes of Administration that are Commonly Used

ORAL: The typical dose of niacin as a dietary supplement is 10-20 mg daily (15). Higher doses may be required for liver cirrhosis, carcinoid syndrome, or prolonged isoniazid therapy (4849). Additionally, people with malabsorption syndrome, those undergoing hemodialysis or peritoneal dialysis, pregnant women with multiple fetuses, and women breast-feeding more than one infant may require more niacin (4849). For preventing and treating vitamin B3 deficiency, doses of nicotinic acid and niacinamide are considered equivalent (15). For mild vitamin B3 deficiency, niacin or niacinamide 50-100 mg per day is usually taken (14). For pellagra in adults, niacin or niacinamide 300-500 mg daily is given in divided doses. For pellagra in children, niacin or niacinamide 100-300 mg daily is given in divided doses. For Hartnup disease, niacin or niacinamide 50-200 mg daily is taken. For hyperlipoproteinemia niacin is begun at 125 mg twice daily and gradually titrated to 1.5 to 3 grams per day to minimize side effects (4867). Some people can require up to 9 grams of niacin daily for an adequate response (15). To prevent coronary events in people with hyperlipidemia, niacin 4 grams daily has been used (4848). For reducing fluid loss induced by cholera toxin, niacin 2 grams daily has been used (4868). To prevent type 1 diabetes in high-risk children, sustained-release niacinamide 1.2 grams/m2 (body surface area) per day has been used (4875). To slow disease progression of newly diagnosed type 1 diabetes, niacinamide 25 mg/kg daily has been used (4878). For treating osteoarthritis, niacinamide 3 grams per day in divided doses has been used (4883).

The daily recommended dietary allowances (RDAs) of niacin are: Infants 0-6 months, 2 mg; Infants 7-12 months, 4 mg; Children 1-3 years, 6 mg; Children 4-8 years, 8 mg; Children 9-13 years, 12 mg; Men 14 years and older, 16 mg; Women 14 years and older, 14 mg; Pregnant women, 18 mg; and Lactating women, 17 mg (3094,4849). The maximum daily dose of niacin is: Children 1-3 years, 10 mg; Children 4-8 years, 15 mg; Children 9-13 years, 20 mg; Adults, including Pregnant and Lactating women, 14-18 years, 30 mg; and Adults, including pregnant and lactating women, older than 18 years, 35 mg (3094,4849).

Comments

Vitamin B3 is present in many foods including yeast, meat, fish, milk, eggs, green vegetables, and cereal grains (15). The term niacin is used to refer specifically to nicotinic acid, but is also used collectively to refer to both nicotinic acid and nicotinamide (niacinamide). Niacin and niacinamide are frequently used in combination with other B vitamins in vitamin B complex formulations. Vitamin B complex generally includes vitamin B1 (Thiamine), vitamin B2 (Riboflavin), vitamin B3 (Niacin/Niacinamide), vitamin B5 (pantothenic acid), vitamin B6 (pyridoxine), vitamin B12 (cyanocobalamin), and folic acid. However, some products do not contain all of these ingredients and some may include others, such as biotin, para-aminobenzoic acid (PABA), choline bitartrate, and inositol (3022,3060,3061).

© Copyright 2000, Natural Medicines Comprehensive Database (209) 472-2244. For updated data, go to www.NaturalDatabase.com

NIAULI OIL

This Product is Also Known As
Caje Oil, Niauli Aetheroleum.
CAUTION: See separate listings for Tea Tree Oil and Cajeput Oil.

Scientific Names
Melaleuca viridiflora.
Family: Myrtaceae.

People Use This For
Orally and topically, niauli oil is used for upper respiratory tract mucous membrane inflammation (2,18), cough and bronchitis (18).

Safety
POSSIBLY SAFE ...when the oil is used orally and appropriately (2,18). ...when the oil is used topically and appropriately (12,18).
LIKELY UNSAFE ...when greater than 10 grams of oil is ingested orally. Can cause hypotension, circulatory disorders, and respiratory failure (18).
CHILDREN: LIKELY UNSAFE ...contraindicated for topical use in the nasal and facial areas because it could cause bronchospasm, asthma-like symptoms and respiratory failure (2,18).
PREGNANCY AND LACTATION: Insufficient reliable information available; avoid using.

Effectiveness
POSSIBLY EFFECTIVE ...when used orally or topically for upper respiratory tract mucous membrane inflammation (2).
There is insufficient reliable information available about the effectiveness of niauli oil for its other uses.

Possible Mechanism of Action & Active Ingredients
Contains cineole (7,9), which has in vitro antibacterial activity and stimulates circulation (2,18). Cineole has actions similar to that of eucalyptus oil (9). Cineole induces liver enzymes involved with drug metabolism (18).

Adverse Reactions Including Known Allergies
When taken orally, niauli oil can cause nausea, vomiting, and diarrhea (2). The consumption of amounts greater than 10 grams can cause hypotension, circulatory disorders, collapse, and respiratory failure (18). It can cause glottal spasm, bronchospasm, and respiratory failure when applied to facial and nasal areas of infants and small children (2,18).

Possible Interactions with Herbs & Other Dietary Supplements
Insufficient reliable information available.

Possible Interactions with Drugs
LIVER- METABOLIZED DRUGS: Theoretically, concomitant use of niauli oil can reduce or shorten the effect of some drugs due to induction of hepatic enzymes (2).

Possible Interactions with Foods
No interactions are known to occur, and there is no known reason to expect a clinically significant interaction with niauli oil.

Possible Interactions with Lab Tests
No interactions are known to occur, and there is no known reason to expect a clinically significant interaction with niauli oil.

Possible Interactions with Diseases or Conditions
GI TRACT DISEASE: Niauli oil is contraindicated in individuals with inflammatory diseases of the GI tract.
LIVER DISEASE: Contraindicated in individuals with severe liver disease or bile duct inflammation (2,18).

Typical Dosages & Routes of Administration that are Commonly Used
ORAL: The typical dose of niauli oil is 200 mg per administration, up to 2 grams per day (2,18).
TOPICAL: Niauli oil is commonly used as oily nose drops, consisting of 2-5% niauli oil in vegetable oil (2,18). Other topical preparations contain 10-30% niauli oil in an oil base (2,18).

Comments
Niauli oil consists of the essential oil distilled from leaves of Melaleuca viridiflora. Avoid confusion with tea tree oil (Maleleuca alternifolia) and cajeput oil (Melaleuca leucodendra and Melaleuca quinquenervia).

NORTHERN PRICKLY ASH

This Product is Also Known As
Angelica Tree, Pepper Wood, Prickly Ash, Toothache Bark, Xanthoxylum, Yellow Wood, Zanthoxylum.
CAUTION: See separate listings for Ash and Southern Prickly Ash.

Scientific Names
Zanthoxylum americanum.
Family: Rutaceae.

People Use This For
Orally, northern prickly ash is used for cramps, intermittent claudication, Raynaud's syndrome, chronic rheumatic conditions, peripheral circulatory insufficiency associated with rheumatic symptoms (4), for low blood pressure, fever, and inflammation (18).
Traditionally, it has been used as a tonic, stimulant, for toothache, sores, ulcers, as a diaphoretic in fever, and cancer (as an ingredient in Hoxsey cure) (11).
In manufacturing, northern prickly ash is used as a flavoring agent in foods and beverages (11).

Safety
POSSIBLY SAFE …when the bark or berry are used orally in food flavoring (4). Northern prickly ash is listed by the Council of Europe as a natural source of food flavoring without toxicity assessment. …when the bark is used orally and appropriately in medicinal amounts (12).
There is insufficient reliable information available about the safety of the oral use of northern prickly ash berry.
PREGNANCY: LIKELY UNSAFE …when the bark is used orally; contraindicated (12). There is insufficient reliable information available about the safety of the berry during pregnancy; avoid using.
LACTATION: POSSIBLY UNSAFE ...when used orally; avoid using. There is insufficient reliable information available about the safety of the berry during lactation; avoid using.

Effectiveness
There is insufficient reliable information available about the effectiveness of northern prickly ash (4).

Possible Mechanism of Action & Active Ingredients
The applicable parts of northern prickly ash are the bark and berry. There is insufficient reliable information available about the possible mechanism of action and active ingredients. Contains coumarins and alkaloids which may be pharmacologically active (4).

Adverse Reactions Including Known Allergies
Insufficient reliable information available.

Possible Interactions with Herbs & Other Dietary Supplements
HERBS WITH ANTICOAGULANT/ANTIPLATELET POTENTIAL: Concomitant use of herbs that have coumarin constituents or affect platelet aggregation could theoretically increase the risk of bleeding in some people. These herbs include: angelica, anise, arnica, asafoetida, bogbean, boldo, capsicum, celery, chamomile, clove, danshen, fenugreek, feverfew, garlic, ginger, ginkgo, ginseng Panax, horse chestnut, horseradish, licorice, meadowsweet, onion, papain, passionflower, poplar, quassia, red clover, turmeric, wild carrot, wild lettuce, willow, and others (4,19).

Possible Interactions with Drugs
ACID-INHIBITING DRUGS: Theoretically, due to claims that northern prickly ash increases stomach acid, it might interfere with antacids, sucralfate (Carafate), H-2 antagonists, and proton pump inhibitors (19).
ANTICOAGULANTS: Theoretically, excessive ingestion might interfere with anticoagulant therapy (4).

Possible Interactions with Foods
No interactions are known to occur, and there is no known reason to expect a clinically significant interaction with northern prickly ash.

Possible Interactions with Lab Tests
No interactions are known to occur, and there is no known reason to expect a clinically significant interaction with northern prickly ash.

Possible Interactions with Diseases or Conditions
GASTROINTESTINAL ULCERS: Contraindicated. Northern prickly ash can stimulate gastrointestinal secretions (19).
GI CONDITIONS: Can irritate the gastrointestinal tract. Contraindicated in individuals with infectious or inflammatory gastrointestinal conditions (19).

Typical Dosages & Routes of Administration that are Commonly Used

ORAL, Bark: 1-3 grams dried bark, or drink as decoction (boil 1-3 grams dry bark 10-15 minutes, strain), three times daily; liquid bark extract (1:1 in 45% alcohol) 1-3 mL three times daily; bark tincture (1:5 in 45% alcohol) 2-5 mL three times daily [4].
ORAL, Berry: Liquid berry extract (1:1 in 45% alcohol) 0.5-1.5 mL [4].

Comments

All information is derived from analysis of components. Avoid confusion with ash, southern prickly ash.

NUTMEG AND MACE

This Product is Also Known As

Mace, Macis, Muscadier, Muskatbuam, Muskatnuss, Myristica, Myristicae Aril, Myristicae Semen, Noix Muscade, Nuez Moscada, Nutmeg, Nux Moschata.

Scientific Names

Myristica fragrans, synonym Myristica officinalis.
Family: Myristicaceae.

People Use This For

Orally, nutmeg and mace are used for diarrhea, gastric spasms, flatulence, gastric mucosal inflammation [2], as a tonic [11], and as a hallucinogen [6,13].
Topically, mace and nutmeg are used as an analgesic, especially for rheumatism [11].
Traditionally, nutmeg and mace have been used orally for nausea, stomach complaints, kidney problems, and cancer [11]. Nutmeg has been used for stimulating menstrual flow, insomnia, and as an abortifacient [6]. Topically, nutmeg has been used for mouth sores [6], and mixed with pork fat for paralysis, rheumatism, and as an antiparasitic for mange [11]. Mace has also been used topically for rheumatism [11].
For food uses, nutmeg and mace are used as culinary spices [11]. In foods and beverages, nutmeg, nutmeg oil, mace, and mace oil are used as flavor components [11].
In manufacturing, nutmeg oil is used as a fragrance component in soaps and cosmetics [11].

Safety

LIKELY SAFE ...when used in amounts found in foods. The maximum use level is 0.3% [11]. Nutmeg, mace, nutmeg oil and mace oil have Generally Recognized as Safe (GRAS) status in the US [11].
LIKELY UNSAFE ...when used orally for self-medication in amounts larger than found in foods [12]. Hallucinations, seizures, and death are possible adverse effects of nutmeg [11].
There is insufficient reliable information available about the safety of the topical use of nutmeg and mace.
PREGNANCY: LIKELY SAFE ...when used in amounts found in foods. Contraindicated in larger amounts because it might have abortifacient activity [2] and safrole content might be mutagenic [2,12].
LACTATION: LIKELY SAFE ...when used in amounts found in foods. There is insufficient reliable information available for larger amounts; avoid using.

Effectiveness

There is insufficient reliable information available for the effectiveness of nutmeg and mace.

Possible Mechanism of Action & Active Ingredients

Both nutmeg and mace contain volatile oils with constituents that include myristicin, elemicin, eugenol, isoeugenol, gerinol, and safrole [6,11]. Nutmeg, mace and their oils have antioxidant activity unrelated to the essential oil content [11]. Mace demonstrates antibacterial and antifungal properties [6]. Nutmeg has antispasmodic activity [2,6]. It also has psychoactive properties. Nutmeg can cause hallucinations, feelings of unreality, euphoria, and delusions [11]. Although psychoactivity is attributed to myristicin, a constituent of the volatile oil, synthetic myristicin by itself does not induce hallucinations [14]. Some experiments suggest that other volatile oil constituents, possibly eugenol and gerinol, enhance psychotomimetic effects [14]. Another theory is that the constituents, myristicin and elemicin, are metabolized to amphetamine-related compounds [6] that have activity similar to lysergic acid diethylamide (LSD) [14]. Nutmeg and mace oils have larvicidal properties [11]. A preliminary study suggests hexane-soluble nutmeg extract might inhibit secretory activity of E. coli toxin [6]. Nutmeg has been used to decrease calcium levels in individuals with diarrhea and chronic hypercalcemia secondary to thyroid medullary tumors [6]. Nutmeg extracts, eugenol and isoeugenol exhibit anti-prostaglandin activity [6]. Some evidence suggests myristicin has anti-inflammatory properties, decreases renal prostaglandin production [14], and inhibits platelet aggregation [2]. Gerinol, a constituent of the volatile oil, is a more potent emetic than ipecac [6]. Safrole found in nutmeg oil promotes liver carcinoma in mice [6]. Animal studies suggest myristicin acts as an inducer of cytochrome P-450 enzyme systems [3492,3493] and may inhibit tumor formation [3492].

Adverse Reactions Including Known Allergies

Ingestion of 5 grams or more of powdered nutmeg or mace can cause thirst, weak pulse, hypothermia, disorientation, giddiness, euphoria, nausea and vomiting, feeling of pressure in the chest or lower abdomen, burning epigastric pain, stupor, tachycardia, dryness of mouth, dizziness, anxiety, panic, double vision, headache (6,11,12,18,3492), seizures (9), agitation, hyperactivity, aimless wandering, incoherent and irrelevant speech, combativeness (3494), flushing, miosis, urgency, altered consciousness that ranges from mild to intensive visual hallucinations, often with sensation of limb loss and fear of impending death (6,14,3492,3494). Symptoms occur 2-6 hours after ingestion; recovery usually occurs within 24 hours, but might take several days, depending on the dose (14,3492). An atropine-like effect is reported with ingestion of nine teaspoons of nutmeg powder per day (2), with symptoms including flushing, tachycardia and dry mouth (14). Large amounts can cause abortion (2), shock, coma (3492) or death (12). Topically, nutmeg can cause allergic dermatitis (6,18).

Possible Interactions with Herbs & Other Dietary Supplements

SAFROLE-CONTAINING HERBS: Avoid concomitant use with other safrole-containing herbs due to potential for additive toxicity (12). Other herbs that contain safrole include basil, camphor, and cinnamon (12).

Possible Interactions with Drugs

MAOIs: Theoretically, concomitant use might potentiate monoamine oxidase inhibitor activity (12,19).
PHENOBARBITAL: Theoretically, concomitant use may decrease the therapeutic effects of phenobarbital (3492). Studies suggest myristicin acts as an inducer of cytochrome P-450 enzyme systems (3492,3493).
OTHER DRUGS: Theoretically, concomitant use may affect drugs metabolized by cytochrome P450 enzyme systems (3493). Use caution when considering concomitant use of nutmeg or mace with other drugs affected by cytochrome P450 enzyme systems.

Possible Interactions with Foods

No interactions are known to occur, and there is no known reason to expect a clinically significant interaction with nutmeg and mace.

Possible Interactions with Lab Tests

No interactions are known to occur, and there is no known reason to expect a clinically significant interaction with nutmeg and mace.

Possible Interactions with Diseases or Conditions

No interactions are known to occur, and there is no known reason to expect a clinically significant interaction with nutmeg and mace.

Typical Dosages & Routes of Administration that are Commonly Used

ORAL: Typical dose for antiflatulent effect is 0.03 mL nutmeg oil (17). For nausea, gastric upset, or chronic diarrhea, the common dose is 3-5 drops of the essential oil on a sugar lump or in honey (6002). For diarrhea, 4-6 tablespoons of the powder are also taken daily (6002).
TOPICAL: No typical dosage.

Comments

Nutmeg and mace are likely unsafe for self-medication (12); use should be monitored (12). Nutmeg is the shelled, dried seed of Myristica fragrans (11). Nutmeg oil is distilled from worm-eaten nutmeg seeds; the worms remove much of the starch and fat leaving portions of the seed rich in volatile oil (11). Mace is the dried aril (netlike covering) surrounding the shell of the seed of Myristica fragrans (11). Ingestion of 5-20 grams of nutmeg powder (1-3 whole seeds) might cause psychoactive effects (6). Because nutmeg and mace are so similar, high doses of mace might also have psychoactive effects but as yet this has not been proven (6).

NUX VOMICA

This Product is Also Known As

Brechnusssamen, Poison Nut, Quaker Buttons, Strychni Semen, Strychnos Seed.

Scientific Names

Strychnos nux-vomica.
Family: Loganiaceae.

People Use This For

Nux vomica is used for impotence and for glycine encephalopathy (14). It is also used in combination for diseases of the gastrointestinal tract, organic and functional disorders of the heart and circulatory system, diseases of the eye, nervous conditions, depression, migraine, climacteric complaints, facial neuralgias (Sympatalgien), and Raynaud's disease (2).

Historically, it has been thought of as an oral tonic, and used as an appetite-stimulant. It has also been used for diseases of the respiratory tract, anemia, and geriatric complaints (18). Nux vomica contains strychnine and brucine (13) and has, therefore, been used in manufacturing. It is used as a rodenticide (505).

Safety

UNSAFE ...when used orally (2,13,14,18,505). The FDA banned nux vomica from use in nonprescription drugs in 1989 (14). 30-50 mg of nux vomica contains approximately 5 mg of strychnine, and can cause severe adverse effects. 1-2 grams of nux vomica contains 60-90 mg of strychnine, and can be fatal (13,18). Chronic ingestion of lesser amounts can cause death after a period of weeks (18).
PREGNANCY AND LACTATION: UNSAFE ...contraindicated (2,13,14,18,505).

Effectiveness

LIKELY INEFFECTIVE ...when used orally for any therapeutic effect (14).

Possible Mechanism of Action & Active Ingredients

The applicable part of nux vomica is the seed. Nux vomica contains strychnine and brucine (13). These are centrally-acting neurotoxins. Strychnine competitively antagonizes post-synaptic binding of the inhibitory transmitter glycine, which leads to heightened reflex excitability of muscles. External irritations or centrally-acting stimulants can trigger convulsions (2,14,505). Nux vomica can selectively inhibit the spinal cord in subconvulsive amounts (2). However, strychnine accumulates with extended administration, particularly in individuals with liver damage (2). Chronic use of subconvulsive amounts can cause death after a period of weeks (18). Strychnine causes convulsions by leading to a full contraction of all voluntary muscles. Death is secondary to impaired respiration or exhaustion (13,14,18,505).

Adverse Reactions Including Known Allergies

When taken orally 30-50 mg nux vomica (5 mg strychnine) can cause restlessness, feelings of anxiety, heightening of sense perception, enhanced reflexes, equilibrium disorders, painful neck and back stiffness, followed later by twitching, tonic spasms of jaw and neck muscles, painful convulsions of the entire body triggered by visual or tactile stimulation with possible opisthotonos, muscle hypertonicity and agitation. Dyspnea may follow spasm of the respiratory muscles (14,18). Seizures occur within 15 minutes of ingestion (or 5 minutes of inhalation) and may result in hyperthermia, metabolic and respiratory acidosis, rhabdomyolysis, and myoglobinuric renal failure (14,17). 1-2 grams of nux vomica (60-90 mg strychnine) can be fatal (13,505); most deaths occur 3-6 hours post-ingestion from respiratory and subsequent cardiac arrest, anoxic brain damage, or multiple organ failure secondary to hyperthermia (14,18,505). Strychnine accumulates with extended administration, particularly in individuals with liver damage (2). Chronic use of subconvulsive amounts can cause death after a period of weeks (18).

Possible Interactions with Herbs & Other Dietary Supplements

Insufficient reliable information available.

Possible Interactions with Drugs

ANALEPTICS, PHENOTHIAZINES: Contraindicated in individuals with symptoms of poisoning (18).

Possible Interactions with Foods

No interactions are known to occur, and there is no known reason to expect a clinically significant interaction with nux vomica.

Possible Interactions with Lab Tests

No interactions are known to occur, and there is no known reason to expect a clinically significant interaction with nux vomica.

Possible Interactions with Diseases or Conditions

LIVER DISEASE: Contraindicated. Strychnine accumulates in individuals with liver damage (2). Also, strychnine accumulation can cause liver damage (18).

Typical Dosages & Routes of Administration that are Commonly Used

Toxic, avoid using.

Comments

Strychnine may be detected by thin-layer chromatography (qualitative analysis) and high performance liquid chromatography (quantitative analysis). Urine and gastric aspirate are most useful in confirming poisoning (17). Strychnine pills are no longer marketed (14). Nux vomica powder may be confused with the powder of date nuts, olive stones, and by-products of stone-nut processing (18).

OAK bark

This Product is Also Known As
Common Oak, Durmast Oak, Eichenrinde, English Oak, Pedunculate Oak, Quercus cortex, Sessile Oak, Stave Oak, Stone Oak, Tanner's Bark, Tanner's Oak.

Scientific Names
Quercus robur; Quercus petraea; Quercus alba.
Family: Fagaceae.

People Use This For
Orally, oak bark is used for diarrhea (2), colds, fever, cough and bronchitis, and for stimulating appetite and improving digestion (18).
Topically, oak bark is used for inflammatory skin conditions, mild inflammation of the mouth, throat, genital and anal region (2,7), and for chilblains (8).

Safety
POSSIBLY SAFE ...when used orally (2,12) for up to 3-4 days for treating diarrhea (7). ...when used topically up to 2-3 weeks on intact skin (2).
LIKELY UNSAFE ...when used topically on extensive areas of damaged skin or for longer than 2-3 weeks (2).
PREGNANCY AND LACTATION: Insufficient reliable information available; avoid using.

Effectiveness
POSSIBLY EFFECTIVE ...when used orally for nonspecific acute diarrhea (2). ...when used topically for inflammatory skin diseases, mild inflammation of the mouth, throat, genital and anal region (2,7).
There is insufficient reliable information available about the effectiveness of oak bark for its other uses.

Possible Mechanism of Action & Active Ingredients
Oak bark contains 8-20% tannins, including gallotannins (7,8). Gallotannins are extensively hydrolyzed in the upper small intestine and are unlikely to produce astringent activity in the colon (7,3901). Some studies suggest tannins might have antiviral and antimicrobial effects, CNS depressant and cariostatic effects (11). Other studies suggest they can depress growth. Tannins exert an astringent effect on mucosal tissue. This effect dehydrates the tissue, internally reducing secretions, and externally forming a protective layer of harder, constricted cells (12). Plants with at least 10% tannins can cause gastrointestinal disturbances, kidney damage, and necrotic conditions of the liver (12). Some evidence suggests that tannins might cause cancer. Others information suggests they might prevent it (12). Regular consumption of herbs with high tannin concentrations correlates to an increased incidence of esophageal or nasal cancer (12).

Adverse Reactions Including Known Allergies
Oak bark can cause gastrointestinal disturbances, kidney damage, and necrotic conditions of the liver (12).

Possible Interactions with Herbs & Other Dietary Supplements
ALKALINE CONSTITUENTS: Theoretically, herbs that contain high percentages of tannins such as oak bark may precipitate alkaloids and alkaline constituents of herbs (19).
IRON: Theoretically, concomitant administration might precipitate iron salts due to tannin content (19).

Possible Interactions with Drugs
ALKALOID DRUGS: Theoretically, avoid concomitant administration due to potential of oak bark's tannin content to precipitate alkaloids and other alkaline drugs (19). Separate administration of oral drugs and tannin-containing herbs by the longest period of time practical (19).
IRON: Theoretically, concomitant administration may precipitate iron salts due to tannin content (19).

Possible Interactions with Foods
No interactions are known to occur, and there is no known reason to expect a clinically significant interaction with oak bark.

Possible Interactions with Lab Tests
No interactions are known to occur, and there is no known reason to expect a clinically significant interaction with oak bark.

Possible Interactions with Diseases or Conditions
KIDNEY DYSFUNCTION: Theoretically, oral use of oak bark might worsen kidney dysfunction (12).
LIVER DYSFUNCTION: Theoretically, oral use of oak bark might worsen liver dysfunction (12).
ECZEMA: Oak bark baths are contraindicated in individuals with weeping eczema or large areas of skin damage (2).
INFECTION: Oak bark baths are contraindicated in individuals with febrile or infectious diseases (2).
CARDIAC CONDITIONS: Oak bark baths are contraindicated in individuals with cardiac insufficiency (2).
HYPERTONIA: Oak bark baths are contraindicated in individuals with hypertonia (2).

Typical Dosages & Routes of Administration that are Commonly Used

ORAL: A typical dose of oak bark for diarrhea is one cup tea up to three times a day for up to 3-4 days. To make tea, add 1 gram coarsely powdered bark to 150 mL cold water, boil for a short period of time, strain (8).

TOPICAL: For rinses, compresses, poultices, and gargles, prepare with 20 grams bark in 1 L of water (18). For baths, prepare with 5 grams of bark in 1 L of water, added to bath water (18). Oak bark should not be used topically longer than 2-3 weeks (2).

Comments

None.

OAK MOSS

This Product is Also Known As

Lichen Oak Moss, Tree Moss.
CAUTION: See separate listing for Usnea.

Scientific Names

Evernia prunastri.
Family: Usneaceae.

People Use This For

In folk medicine, oak moss is used as an intestinal tonic (4017).
In manufacturing, it is used as a fragrance component in perfumes (4023).

Safety

POSSIBLY SAFE ...when used orally in prepared teas or aqueous forms for short periods of time (12). Although water extracts of oak moss contain the constituent thujone that is known to cause adverse effects, the amount of thujone is low (2).
LIKELY UNSAFE ...when used orally long-term, in large amounts of tea, or as a hot alcoholic extract (12) because enough thujone might be consumed to cause renal damage (4,12).
There is insufficient reliable information available about the safety of oak moss for topical use.
PREGNANCY AND LACTATION: POSSIBLY UNSAFE ...the constituent thujone shows evidence of uterine stimulant activity (19).

Effectiveness

There is insufficient reliable information available about the effectiveness of oak moss.

Possible Mechanism of Action & Active Ingredients

Oak moss contains thujone, a ketone that shows evidence of neurotoxicity. Thujone intoxication causes psychoactivity resembling that of cannabinoid intoxication (12). Some data suggest thujone-containing volatile oils have uterine stimulant effects (19). Other information suggests thujone might exacerbate liver conditions, e.g. porphyria (12).

Adverse Reactions Including Known Allergies

Large amounts or long-term use of thujone-containing products can cause restlessness, vomiting, vertigo, tremors, renal damage, and convulsions (12). Topical use can cause contact sensitivity (4034,4039) and allergic reaction in people with lichen and moss allergy (4023,4033).

Possible Interactions with Herbs & Other Dietary Supplements

THUJONE CONTAINING HERBS: Avoid; concomitant use may increase the risk of thujone toxicity. Thujone-containing herbs include: oriental arborvitae (12), sage (2,4,12), tansy (2,4,12), thuja (cedar) (11,12), tree moss (12), and wormwood (2,12).

Possible Interactions with Drugs

No interactions are known to occur, and there is no known reason to expect a clinically significant interaction with oak moss.

Possible Interactions with Foods

No interactions are known to occur, and there is no known reason to expect a clinically significant interaction with oak moss.

Possible Interactions with Lab Tests

No interactions are known to occur, and there is no known reason to expect a clinically significant interaction with oak moss.

 © Copyright 2000, Natural Medicines Comprehensive Database (209) 472-2244. For updated data, go to www.NaturalDatabase.com

Possible Interactions with Diseases or Conditions
PORPHYRIA: Can exacerbate porphyria in patients with underlying defects in hepatic heme synthesis (12).
RENAL DYSFUNCTION: Can exacerbate this condition (12).
CROSS-ALLERGENICITY: Can cause reaction in people allergic to lichens and mosses (4023,4033).

Typical Dosages & Routes of Administration that are Commonly Used
No typical dosage.

Comments
Avoid confusing oak moss (Evernia prunastri) with other usnea species. Many, including oak moss, are referred to as tree moss.

OAT above ground parts

This Product is Also Known As
Avenae herba, Oat Herb, Wild Oat Herb.
CAUTION: See separate listings for Oat Bran, Oat Straw, and Oats.

Scientific Names
Avena sativa.
Family: Gramineae or Poaceae.

People Use This For
Orally, the above ground parts of oats are used for acute or chronic anxiety, excitation and stress, neurasthenia and pseudoneurasthenia syndromes, weak bladder, connective tissue disorders (2), for gout, kidney ailments, old age syndromes, opium and nicotine withdrawal, rheumatism, skin diseases (18), and as a tonic (2).
In combination with other herbs, oat above ground parts are used orally for cardiovascular, respiratory, and metabolic diseases, diseases and discomforts of old age, anemia, hypothyroidism, neuralgias and neuritis, hematoma, pulled muscles, sexual disorders, tobacco abuse, spasms, increasing milk production, and for increasing performance capacity (2).

Safety
POSSIBLY SAFE ...when the spikelet, the top of the herb, is used orally or topically (12).
PREGNANCY AND LACTATION: Insufficient reliable information available; avoid using.

Effectiveness
There is insufficient reliable information available about effectiveness of oat above ground parts.

Possible Mechanism of Action & Active Ingredients
The above ground parts of oat contain soluble oligosaccharides and polysaccharides including saccharose, kestose, neokestose, beta-glucans, galactoarabinoxylans, silicic acid, steroid saponins, avenic acid A and B and flavonoids (18).

Adverse Reactions Including Known Allergies
None reported.

Possible Interactions with Herbs & Other Dietary Supplements
Insufficient reliable information available.

Possible Interactions with Drugs
MORPHINE: Theoretically, concomitant use might antagonize morphine (19).
NICOTINE: Theoretically, concomitant use might reduce the hypertensive response from nicotine (19).

Possible Interactions with Foods
No interactions are known to occur, and there is no known reason to expect a clinically significant interaction with oat above ground parts.

Possible Interactions with Lab Tests
No interactions are known to occur, and there is no known reason to expect a clinically significant interaction with oat above ground parts.

Possible Interactions with Diseases or Conditions
No interactions are known to occur, and there is no known reason to expect a clinically significant interaction with oat above ground parts.

Typical Dosages & Routes of Administration that are Commonly Used

ORAL: A typical oral dose is 1 cup tea used repeatedly throughout the day and shortly before bedtime. To make tea, boil 3 grams above ground parts in 250 mL water, and strain (18).

Comments

None.

OAT BRAN

This Product is Also Known As

None.
CAUTION: See separate listings for Oat above ground parts, Oat Straw, Oats, and Wheat Bran.

Scientific Names

Avena sativa.
Family: Poaceae.

People Use This For

Orally, oat bran is used for reducing the risk of heart disease, as part of a diet low in saturated fat and cholesterol(4960,4962,4963,4964,4965,4966,4967,4968), lowering blood cholesterol (4960,4961,4963,4965,4971,4972,4973,4975, 4976,4977,4978), reducing postprandial blood glucose in people with diabetes (4961,4980,4981,4982,4983), blocking fat absorption (4970), preventing gallstones (4984), reducing risk of colon cancer, treating irritable bowel syndrome, diverticulosis, and inflammatory bowel disease (5103,5105,5106).

Safety

LIKELY SAFE ...when used orally and appropriately (4960,4969). Oat bran has Generally Recognized as Safe (GRAS) status in the US (4912).
PREGNANCY AND LACTATION: Insufficient reliable information available; avoid using in amounts greater than found in foods.

Effectiveness

EFFECTIVE ...when used orally as part of a diet low in saturated fat and cholesterol for reducing the risk of heart disease and lowering total and LDL blood cholesterol (4960,4961,4962,4963,4964,4965,4966,4967,4968,4971,4972,4973,4974,4975, 4976,4977,4978,6188). Oat bran products (oat bran muffins, oat bran flakes, oat bran Os, etc.) may vary in their ability to lower cholesterol, depending on the total soluble fiber content and other dietary variables (6188).
POSSIBLY EFFECTIVE ...when used orally for reducing postprandial blood glucose in people with diabetes (4960,4980,4982,6266). In a randomized crossover study of 13 people with type 2 diabetes, a high fiber diet that included oat bran was more effective in lowering preprandial blood glucose and the area under the curve for 24-hour plasma glucose and glucose (measured every 2 hours), and improving cholesterol and triglyceride levels than the standard ADA diet (6266). ...when used orally as part of a high fiber diet for reducing risk factors associated with cardiovascular disease. In a large-scale epidemiological study, consumption of large amounts of dietary fiber was associated with reduction of cardiovascular disease risk factors including reduction in body weight, fasting and postprandial insulin secretion, blood pressure, and improved lipid profile (2737).
LIKELY INEFFECTIVE ...when used orally for reducing risk of colon cancer (5104,6267). A large well-designed study showed that fiber, including oat-bran fiber, does not prevent the recurrence of colorectal adenomas. There is insufficient reliable information available about the effectiveness of oat bran for its other uses.

Possible Mechanism of Action & Active Ingredients

Oat bran decreases serum cholesterol and dependent cardiovascular risk by decreasing absorption of cholesterol or fatty acids and decreasing absorption of biliary cholesterol or bile acids (4974,4960,4963). Dietary fiber, including oat bran, is also thought to decrease the risk of cardiovascular disease by decreasing fasting insulin levels, resulting in decreased obesity, hypertension, and improved lipid profile (2737). Beta-glucan (oat gum), a constituent of oat bran, increases the viscosity of food in the small intestine and delays absorption, thereby reducing peak postprandial plasma glucose and insulin levels both in people with diabetes and normal people (4961,4980,4981,4982,4983). Oat bran combines with intestinal water which forms a gum (4961), increases stool weight, and stool fat excretion (4970). Beta-glucan may help control appetite by slowing stomach emptying, prolonging the feeling of fullness and stabilizing blood sugar (5078). Oat bran alters the metabolism of bile acids (4984). Although earlier studies did not differentiate between types of fiber (5105,5106,5108), later studies indicate that oat bran, unlike wheat bran, does not protect against colon cancer (5104,5107).

Adverse Reactions Including Known Allergies

Oat bran may cause bezoars (concretions) and intestinal obstruction, especially in people who have difficulty chewing or swallowing food, or have conditions that decrease small bowel motility (4979,4985). Oat bran can cause reactions in people with gluten allergy, due to its gluten content (2).

Possible Interactions with Herbs & Other Dietary Supplements

CHOLESTEROL-REDUCING HERBS: Theoretically, concomitant use might cause additive cholesterol-lowering effects.

Possible Interactions with Drugs

CHOLESTEROL-REDUCING DRUGS: Theoretically, concomitant use might cause additive cholesterol-lowering effects.

Possible Interactions with Foods

FATTY FOODS: Concomitant use of foods high in saturated fats or cholesterol can interfere with the cholesterol-lowering effect of oat bran (4960).

Possible Interactions with Lab Tests

CHOLESTEROL: Oat bran lowers blood levels total and low density lipoprotein (LDL) cholesterol and test results (4971).
BLOOD GLUCOSE: Oat bran lowers postprandial blood glucose and test results (4961).
INSULIN: Oat bran lowers postprandial insulin levels and test results (4961).

Possible Interactions with Diseases or Conditions

CELIAC DISEASE: Contraindicated in individuals with celiac disease due to gluten content (6).
GI CONDITIONS: Contraindicated in people with intestinal ulcerations, stenosis, disabling adhesions, cathartic colon or other conditions that may result in intestinal or esophageal obstruction (4921). Use with caution or avoid in people with difficulty chewing or swallowing food, or conditions that decrease small bowel motility (4921).

Typical Dosages & Routes of Administration that are Commonly Used

ORAL: A typical dose for lowering plasma cholesterol, cardiovascular risk and post-prandial glucose is 3 grams of soluble fiber per day (4960). 38 grams of oat bran or 75 grams of dry oatmeal contains about 3 grams of beta-glucan (4961,4971).

Comments

Oat bran is milled from the outer layer of hulled whole oats and is made up of both soluble and insoluble fiber (4960,4961,4970). Oat bran contains oat gum or beta-glucan, a soluble polysaccharide (4961,4981). The FDA allows medical claims for foods containing over 51% whole grains. Therefore, certain breads and cereals, etc., can claim to reduce the risk of certain medical conditions such as heart disease.

OAT STRAW

This Product is Also Known As

Avenae stramentum, Straw.
CAUTION: See separate listings for Oat Bran, Oats, and Oat above ground parts.

Scientific Names

Avena sativa.
Family: Gramineae or Poaceae.

People Use This For

Topically, oat straw is used for skin inflammation, irritation, injury, pruritus, seborrhea (2), warts (18), arthritis, paralysis, and liver disorders (6).
In folk medicine, oat straw has been used as a tea for flu and coughs, abdominal fatigue, bladder and rheumatic disorders, eye ailments, frostbite, gout, impetigo, and metabolic diseases. It has also been used in foot baths for chronically cold or tired feet (18).

Safety

POSSIBLY SAFE ...when used topically and appropriately (2).
There is insufficient reliable information available about the safety of the oral use of oat straw.
PREGNANCY AND LACTATION: Insufficient reliable information available.

Effectiveness

POSSIBLY EFFECTIVE ...when used topically for inflammatory skin conditions and seborrhea (2).
There is insufficient reliable information available about the effectiveness of oat straw for its other uses.

Possible Mechanism of Action & Active Ingredients

Insufficient reliable information available.

Adverse Reactions Including Known Allergies

None reported.

Possible Interactions with Herbs & Other Dietary Supplements

Insufficient reliable information available.

Possible Interactions with Drugs

No interactions are known to occur, and there is no known reason to expect a clinically significant interaction with oat straw.

Possible Interactions with Foods

No interactions are known to occur, and there is no known reason to expect a clinically significant interaction with oat straw.

Possible Interactions with Lab Tests

No interactions are known to occur, and there is no known reason to expect a clinically significant interaction with oat straw.

Possible Interactions with Diseases or Conditions

No interactions are known to occur, and there is no known reason to expect a clinically significant interaction with oat straw.

Typical Dosages & Routes of Administration that are Commonly Used

TOPICAL: To use as a bath additive, simmer 100 grams of chopped straw in 3 liters of water for 20 minutes, strain, and add to bath water (2,18).

Comments

Oat straw consists of the dried threshed, leaf and stem of the oat plant (Avena sativa).

OATS

This Product is Also Known As

Avena Fructus, Groats, Oat Fruit, Oat Grain, Oatmeal.
CAUTION: See separate listings for Oat Bran, Oat above ground parts, and Oat Straw.

Scientific Names

Avena sativa.
Family: Gramineae or Poaceae.

People Use This For

Orally, oat fruit is used for disorders of the gastrointestinal tract (2,18), gallbladder, kidney, and cardiovascular systems (18). It is used for constipation, diarrhea, rheumatism, throat and chest complaints (18), physical fatigue, diabetes (2,18), hypercholesterolemia (6), neurasthenia and neurasthenia syndrome (2), colon cancer prevention (6267), nicotine withdrawal (2,6), and in tonics (2).
Topically, oats are used for managing dry, itchy skin (6), weeping eczema, contact dermatitis, chickenpox, and to enhance skin hydration (272).
In folk medicine, the oat fruit has been used as a sedative, for lowering uric acid levels, and as a diuretic (6).
In traditional Ayurvedic medicine, oats are used for opium withdrawal (6).
For food uses, they are used as a grain or cereal (6).
In manufacturing, oats are a component of bath products and soaps (6).

Safety

LIKELY SAFE …when used orally in food or medicinal amounts (6).
PREGNANCY AND LACTATION: LIKELY SAFE …when used orally.

Effectiveness

POSSIBLY EFFECTIVE …when used orally for reducing postprandial blood glucose in people with diabetes (6266). In a randomized crossover study of 13 people with type 2 diabetes, a high fiber diet that included oatmeal was more effective in lowering preprandial blood glucose and the area under the curve for 24-hour plasma glucose and glucose (measured every 2 hours), and improving cholesterol and triglyceride levels than the standard ADA diet (6266).
POSSIBLY INEFFECTIVE …when used orally for reducing risk of colon cancer (6267). A large well-designed study showed that fiber does not prevent the recurrence of colorectal adenomas (6267).
There is insufficient reliable information available about the effectiveness of oats for other uses (2,272). However, oatmeal might enhance the cholesterol lowering effect of a low-fat diet. In an unpublished study, oatmeal increased the cholesterol lowering effect of an American Heart Association's Step 1 diet in a group of post-menopausal women with initial cholesterol levels above 200 mg/dl. After three weeks of the low-fat diet, cholesterol was lowered by 12 mg/dl. When 1 1/2 cups of cooked oatmeal daily was added to the low fat diet, cholesterol levels were reduced by an additional 8-9 mg/dl (6100).

Preliminary clinical evidence suggests that oatmeal containing 3.5 grams of beta-glucan consumed with a high fat meal might prevent acute fat-induced endothelial dysfunction and benefit cardiovascular health (318). Researchers report that a group of people who ate a high soluble-fiber oatmeal breakfast experienced a greater feeling of fullness and consumed 30% fewer calories at lunch, compared with a group who ate nonfiber sugared corn flakes for breakfast. The results of this unpublished study were presented at the Experimental Biology 2000 meeting (5078).

Possible Mechanism of Action & Active Ingredients

Oats contain oat gluten (6), gel-forming dietary fiber (7), and beta-glucans (18). The dietary fiber found in oat bran acts as a bulk-forming laxative. By stretching the intestinal wall it stimulates increased peristalsis (6). Researchers think that the beta-glucan contained in oats helps control appetite by slowing stomach emptying, prolonging the feeling of fullness, and stabilizing blood sugar (5078). Beta-glucans increase bile acid secretion and some evidence suggests they reduce serum lipids (6). Preliminary information suggests oat tea might aid in opium withdrawal (6). Some information also suggests that an alcoholic oat extract might reduce cigarette use, but a second study failed to reproduce this result (6). Oat bran, milled from the outer layer of hulled whole oats, reduces serum cholesterol (6).

Adverse Reactions Including Known Allergies

Allergic reactions to oat gluten are rare (2). The fiber content in large amounts of oats can cause flatulence, and anal irritation (6).

Possible Interactions with Herbs & Other Dietary Supplements

Insufficient reliable information available.

Possible Interactions with Drugs

ORAL DRUGS: Theoretically, large amounts of oatmeal might interfere with drug absorption (19).
MORPHINE: Theoretically, a green seed extract of oat might antagonize the analgesic effect of morphine (19).
NICOTINE: Theoretically, a green seed extract of oat might antagonize the hypertensive effect of nicotine (19).

Possible Interactions with Foods

No interactions are known to occur, and there is no known reason to expect a clinically significant interaction with oat fruit.

Possible Interactions with Lab Tests

No interactions are known to occur, and there is no known reason to expect a clinically significant interaction with oat fruit.

Possible Interactions with Diseases or Conditions

CELIAC DISEASE: Contraindicated due to gluten content (6).

Typical Dosages & Routes of Administration that are Commonly Used

ORAL: No typical dosage.
TOPICAL: The oat fruit is commonly applied once or twice daily (6002).

Comments

None.

OCTACOSANOL

This Product is Also Known As

Hexacosanol (26-C), Tetracosanol (24-C), Triacontanol (30-C).
CAUTION: See separate listing for Policosanol.

Scientific Names

1-Octacosanol; N-octacosanol; Octacosyl alcohol.

People Use This For

Orally, octacosanol is used for improving strength, stamina, and reaction times (17,2922,2926), for herpes infections (6), for treating inflammatory skin diseases (6), for Parkinson's disease (2920), for amyotrophic lateral sclerosis (ALS) (2921), for hyperlipidemia (2923), and for atherosclerosis (2923).

Safety

There is insufficient reliable information available about the safety of octacosanol.
Pregnancy and Lactation: Insufficient reliable information available; avoid using.

Effectiveness

POSSIBLY INEFFECTIVE ...when taken orally for treating amyotrophic lateral sclerosis (ALS) (2922).
There is insufficient reliable information available about the effectiveness of octacosanol for its other uses.

Possible Mechanism of Action & Active Ingredients

Octacosanol is a 28-carbon waxy alcohol, related to vitamin E (2922). It is hypothesized that octacosanol could improve oxygen utilization during anaerobic glycolysis and aid in lactic acid removal by increasing the efficiency of the tricarboxylic acid cycle (17). In rats, octacosanol suppresses lipid accumulation in adipose tissue and increases the mobilization of free fatty acids from the fat cells in muscle (2924,2925).

Adverse Reactions Including Known Allergies

The use of octacosanol can cause position-related or nonrotational dizziness, increased nervous tension, and worsening of dyskinesias caused by levodopa or carbidopa (6).

Possible Interactions with Herbs & Other Dietary Supplements

Insufficient reliable information available.

Possible Interactions with Drugs

LEVODOPA/CARBIDOPA: Octacosanol can worsen dyskinesias associated with the use of levodopa or carbidopa (6).

Possible Interactions with Foods

No interactions are known to occur, and there is no known reason to expect a clinically significant interaction with octacosanol.

Possible Interactions with Lab Tests

No interactions are known to occur, and there is no known reason to expect a clinically significant interaction with octacosanol.

Possible Interactions with Diseases or Conditions

PARKINSON'S DISEASE: Octacosanol can worsen dyskinesias associated with the levodopa or carbidopa treatment of Parkinson's disease (6).

Typical Dosages & Routes of Administration that are Commonly Used

ORAL: For Parkinson's disease, the typical dose of octacosanol is 5 mg three times a day with meals (6,17). For amyotrophic lateral sclerosis (ALS), the usual dose is 40 mg per day (2921).

Comments

Octacosanol refers specifically to a 28-carbon alcohol, but it is commonly used to denote a mixture of 24- to 36-carbon alcohols, including tetracosanol (24-C), hexacosanol (26-C), and triacontanol (30-C) (6,268,269,270). It is found in a variety of plant sources, including sugar cane (Saccharum officinarum) (6,2923) and wheat germ oil (2922). Avoid confusion with policosanol.

OLEANDER

This Product is Also Known As

Common Oleander, Oleanderblatter, Oleandri folium, Rose Bay, Rose Laurel, Yellow Oleander.

Scientific Names

Nerium oleander; Thevetia peruviana
Family: Apocynaceae.

People Use This For

Orally, oleander is used for cardiac conditions (2,18), asthma, epilepsy, cancer, and dysmenorrhea (214). A fixed combination of oleander leaf powdered extract, pheasant's eye fluid extract, lily-of-the-valley fluid extract and squill powdered extract has been used for treating mild limited heart failure with circulatory instability (2,7).
Topically, it is used to treat skin eruptions (2,18,214) and warts (214).
Traditionally, oleander has been used to treat leprosy, malaria, ringworm, indigestion, venereal disease, and as an abortifacient (5000). In Sri Lanka, yellow oleander seeds have been used orally for deliberate self-poisoning and suicide, particularly in women and children (2532).

Safety

LIKELY UNSAFE ...when taken orally. Ingestion of oleander leaf, oleander leaf tea and oleander seeds has led to fatal poisonings (2,9,3495).
There is insufficient reliable information available about the safety of the topical use of oleander.
PREGNANCY AND LACTATION: LIKELY UNSAFE ...when taken orally; contraindicated. Oleander has been reported to have abortifacient properties (5000). There is insufficient reliable information available about the safety of topical use of oleander during pregnancy and lactation; avoid using.

Effectiveness

There is insufficient reliable information available about the effectiveness of oleander.

Possible Mechanism of Action & Active Ingredients

All parts of the oleander plant contain the cardiac glycosides oleandrin, oleandroside, nerioside, digitoxigenin, which have positive inotropic and negative chronotropic actions (2,3495). They bind to sodium- and potassium-sensitive membrane-bound enzymes called ATPases and inhibit enzyme activities, resulting in increased intracellular sodium ions and calcium ions and increased extracellular potassium levels (3477,5000). At toxic levels, the sodium and calcium ions depolarize the cell after repolarization, causing late afterdepolarization and increased automaticity. Severe toxicity produces bradycardia and heart block (3477). Oleander leaf also contains other biologically active constituents that have antimitotic and insecticidal properties (5000). In folk medicine, oleander is also reported to have emetogenic, cathartic, insecticidic, parasiticidic, antihelmintic, menstrual stimulant, and abortifacient activities (214).

Adverse Reactions Including Known Allergies

Orally, oleander can cause bitter taste, burning sensation in mouth, nausea, vomiting, diarrhea, weakness, headache, stupor (17,18,3495), mucus membrane irritation, increased salivation, abdominal pain, buccal erythema, visual disturbances, mydriasis, peripheral neuritis (3495,5000), malignant dysrhythmias, ventricular ectopy, cardiovascular collapse, cardiac arrest (17), hyperkalemia (2532,3495) and death (3495). Oleander poisoning resembles digitoxin poisoning. Predominant symptoms are nausea and vomiting (onset in several hours), and cardiac toxicity, with conduction delays lasting for 3-6 days (17). Yellow oleander toxicity has been reported to be reversed with anti-digoxin Fab fragments. The majority of patients with yellow oleander toxicity who received anti-digoxin Fab fragments converted from an oleander-induced arrhythmia to normal sinus rhythm within 8 hours. A dose of 800 mg anti-digoxin Fab fragments was used intravenously. Associated hyperkalemia reversed within the first two hours (2532). A recurrence of arrhythmia can occur 48 hours post-exposure from any seed fragments remaining in the gastrointestinal tract (2532).

Possible Interactions with Herbs & Other Dietary Supplements

CALCIUM: Contraindicated (18).
CARDIAC GLYCOSIDE-CONTAINING HERBS: Contraindicated, and concomitant use can increase the risk of cardiac glycoside toxicity. Cardiac glycoside-containing herbs include black hellebore, Canadian hemp roots, digitalis leaf, hedge mustard, figwort, lily of the valley roots, motherwort, pheasant's eye plant, pleurisy root, squill bulb leaf scales, strophanthus seeds, and uzara (2,18,19,500).
OTHER CARDIOACTIVE HERBS: Avoid concomitant use with other cardioactive herbs due to unpredictability of effects (4).
STIMULANT LAXATIVE HERBS: Theoretically, overuse or misuse of stimulant laxatives with cardiac glycoside-containing herbs increases the risk of cardiac toxicity due to potassium depletion (19).
LICORICE/HORSETAIL: Theoretically, overuse/misuse of licorice rhizome or horsetail plant with cardiac glycoside-containing herbs increases the risk of cardiac toxicity due to potassium depletion (19).

Possible Interactions with Drugs

DIGOXIN: Contraindicated; therapeutic duplication increases risk of cardiac glycoside toxicity (2).
CARDIAC DRUGS: Theoretically, concomitant use may increase risk of cardiac toxicity (152).
STIMULANT LAXATIVES: Theoretically, overuse/misuse may increase risk of cardiac glycoside toxicity due to potassium depletion (2).
POTASSIUM-DEPLETING DIURETICS: Theoretically, concomitant use may increase risk of cardiac glycoside toxicity due to potassium depletion (2,506).
QUININE: Theoretically, concomitant use may increase risk of cardiac toxicity (2,506).
TETRACYCLINES AND MACROLIDE ANTIBIOTICS: Theoretically, concomitant use may increase risk of cardiac glycoside toxicity (152,17).
CALCIUM: Calcium salts may enhance effects (18).

Possible Interactions with Foods

No interactions are known to occur, and there is no known reason to expect a clinically significant interaction with oleander.

Possible Interactions with Lab Tests

No interactions are known to occur, and there is no known reason to expect a clinically significant interaction with oleander.

Possible Interactions with Diseases or Conditions

HEART DISEASE: Self-use contraindicated; requires diagnosis, treatment, and monitoring (515).
ELECTROLYTE IMBALANCE: Theoretically, based on digitalis glycosides (15), contraindicated in individuals with potassium deficiency states and hypercalcemia.

Typical Dosages & Routes of Administration that are Commonly Used

No typical dosage.

Comments

The annual incidence of oleander poisoning in Sri Lanka exceeds 150 per 100,000. Approximately 10% of these ingestions are fatal (2532). Abbott TDx Digoxin II assay can be used for rapid confirmation of the ingestion of oleander (17).

OLIVE leaf

This Product is Also Known As

Oleae folium, Olivier.
CAUTION: See separate listing for Olive Oil.

Scientific Names

Olea europea.
Family: Oleaceae.

People Use This For

Orally, olive leaf extract is used for treatment of conditions caused by, or associated with, a virus, retrovirus, bacterium, or protozoan including influenza, the common cold, meningitis, Epstein-Barr Virus (EBV), encephalitis, herpes I and II, human herpes virus 6 and 7, shingles, HIV/ARC/AIDS, chronic fatigue, hepatitis B, pneumonia, tuberculosis, gonorrhea, malaria, dengue, bacteremia, severe diarrhea, blood poisoning, and dental, ear, urinary tract and surgical infections (290).

In folk medicine, olive leaf is used for lowering high blood pressure (2,7,18), treating diabetes (810), to enhance renal and digestive function (514), and as a diuretic (2,18) antipyretic (514).

Safety

There is insufficient reliable information available about the safety of olive leaf.
Pregnancy and Lactation: Insufficient reliable information available; avoid using.

Effectiveness

POSSIBLY EFFECTIVE ...when used orally for lowering blood pressure in people with hypertension (1540).
There is insufficient reliable information available about the effectiveness of olive leaf for its other uses.

Possible Mechanism of Action & Active Ingredients

In animal experiments, olive leaf preparations demonstrate multiple properties including antispasmodic, hypotensive, antiarrhythmic and arrhythmogenic (2,18), hypoglycemic (810), bronchodilator, coronary dilator, antipyretic, and diuretic (2). The constituent, oleuropein, has bacteriostatic (1541) and antioxidant (514) activity. Constituent flavonoids have serum complement-inactivating activity (1542). An aqueous olive leaf extract reduced blood pressure in one small, uncontrolled trial of people with hypertension (1540).

Adverse Reactions Including Known Allergies

Olive tree pollen causes seasonal respiratory allergy (1543).

Possible Interactions with Herbs & Other Dietary Supplements

Insufficient reliable information available.

Possible Interactions with Drugs

DRUGS AFFECTING BLOOD PRESSURE: Theoretically, concomitant use may enhance blood pressure-lowering effects (1540) and may interfere with blood pressure-increasing effects (1540).

Possible Interactions with Foods

No interactions are known to occur, and there is no known reason to expect a clinically significant interaction with olive leaf.

Possible Interactions with Lab Tests

BLOOD PRESSURE: Olive leaf might reduce blood pressure and blood pressure readings (1540).

Possible Interactions with Diseases or Conditions

HYPOTENSION: Theoretically, may exacerbate this condition due to blood pressure-reducing effects (1540).

Typical Dosages & Routes of Administration that are Commonly Used

ORAL: One cup tea (steep 2 teaspoons dried leaf in 150 mL boiling water 30 minutes, strain) three to four times per day (18).

Comments

None.

OLIVE OIL

This Product is Also Known As
Sweet Oil, Salad Oil, Olivae oleum.
CAUTION: See separate listing for Olive leaf.

Scientific Names
Olea europaea.
Family: Oleaceae.

People Use This For
Orally, olive oil is commonly used for preventing cardiovascular disease (14), breast cancer (2222), and rheumatoid arthritis (3454). It is also used orally for migraine headache in adolescents (5097); firming the breasts; treating bile duct and gallbladder inflammation, gallstones, jaundice, flatulence, and meteorism (swelling of the abdomen due to intestinal or peritoneal gas); as a cleanser, purifier, and mild laxative; for lack of bacteria in the intestines, and Roemheld syndrome (2,14,16).
Topically, olive oil is used for softening ear wax (14), treating ringing and pain in the ears (2), as nose drops, for wound dressing, treating minor burns and psoriasis, and preventing and treating stretch marks due to pregnancy (2). For food use, olive oil is used widely as a cooking and salad oil (13).
In manufacturing, olive oil is used to make soaps (13), commercial plasters and liniments, and as a setting-retardant in dental cements (13).

Safety
LIKELY SAFE ...when used orally in the amounts found in foods.
There is insufficient reliable information available about the safety of olive oil used in amounts greater than those used in food preparation.
PREGNANCY AND LACTATION: LIKELY SAFE ...when consumed in food amounts; avoid amounts greater than found in foods (18).

Effectiveness
EFFECTIVE ...when olive oil is used orally as a mild laxative (14,16).
POSSIBLY EFFECTIVE ...when olive oil is used for reducing the risk of coronary artery disease (2219,2220). ...when used orally for reducing the risk of breast cancer (2221,2222,2223). ...when used orally for reducing the risk of rheumatoid arthritis (3454). The risk reduction data come from retrospective studies of dietary olive oil consumption. Such studies can only identify associations between olive oil consumption and disease occurrence. The effects of olive oil on the human cholesterol profile are currently unclear; the available studies differ in their designs and results (3285,3286,3287,3288,3289,3290). ...when used orally as adjunctive therapy in hypertension. In a small-scale, double-blind, crossover trial, patients with mild to moderately-high blood pressure modified diets to include either high amounts of extra virgin olive oil or sunflower oil in combination with conventional antihypertensive medications, including either the beta blocker atenolol (Tenormin), the calcium channel blocker nifedipine (Adalat, Procardia), the angiotensin-converting enzyme (ACE) inhibitor lisinopril (Prinivil, Zestril), the alpha blocker doxazosin (Cardura), or the thiazide diuretic hydrochlorothiazide (HCTZ). After 6-months blood pressure was significantly lower in patients receiving olive oil compared to sunflower oil. Significantly more patients receiving olive oil were able to discontinue antihypertensive medications or decrease the dose. An average antihypertensive dose reduction of approximately 50% was achieved in patients consuming olive oil (5091). ...when used orally for migraine headache prophylaxis in adolescents. In an unpublished small-scale, crossover study announced at the Advancing Children's Health 2000 meeting, adolescent migraineurs receiving olive oil preparations containing oleic acid 1,382 mg daily for 2 months had reduced frequency, duration, and severity of migraine headaches (5097).
POSSIBLY INEFFECTIVE ...when used topically for softening ear wax (3274). ...when used topically for treating ear pain in children with acute otitis media (3276).
There is insufficient reliable information available about the effectiveness of olive oil for its other uses.

Possible Mechanism of Action & Active Ingredients
Olive oil contains unsaturated fatty acids and may reduce cholesterol levels when used to replace saturated fat in the diet (2224). Compounds in olive oil called secoiridoides (oleuropein and derivatives) have broad spectrum in vitro antimicrobial activity (3284). Researchers think that metabolites of oleic acid, an omega-9 monounsaturated fatty acid found in olive oil, might competitively inhibit omega-6 (n-6) fatty acid metabolites (prostaglandins and leukotrienes) and suppress production of inflammatory cytokines (3454). Evidence suggests that olive oil might lower blood pressure, decrease inflammatory n-6 fatty acid concentrations, and increase beneficial n-3 fatty acid concentrations in women with hypertension (3289).

Adverse Reactions Including Known Allergies
Ingestion of olive oil may cause biliary colic in people with gallstones (2,18,19). Topical application may cause allergic reactions (rare) (2). May irritate eyes; avoid eye contact (19). Delayed hypersensitivity and contact dermatitis are reported with topical use (289,3275).

Possible Interactions with Herbs & Other Dietary Supplements
Insufficient reliable information available.

Possible Interactions with Drugs
ANTIHYPERTENSIVE DRUGS: Consumption of olive oil might allow for a reduction in antihypertensive drug doses in people treated for hypertension. In a double-blind, crossover trial, 30-40 grams of olive oil per day for six months lowered blood pressure and allowed for a 50% reduction in antihypertensive medication doses in a group of patients with mild to moderate high blood pressure. The antihypertensive drugs involved in the trial included the beta blocker atenolol (Tenormin), the calcium channel blocker nifedipine (Adalat, Procardia), the angiotensin-converting enzyme (ACE) inhibitor lisinopril (Prinivil, Zestril), the alpha blocker doxazosin (Cardura), and the thiazide diuretic hydrochlorothiazide (HCTZ) (5091).
DIABETES THERAPY: Monitor blood glucose levels closely due to claims that olive oil has hypoglycemic effects (19).

Possible Interactions with Foods
No interactions are known to occur, and there is no known reason to expect a clinically significant interaction with olive oil.

Possible Interactions with Lab Tests
No interactions are known to occur, and there is no known reason to expect a clinically significant interaction with olive oil.

Possible Interactions with Diseases or Conditions
GALLSTONES: Contraindicated; may trigger gallbladder colic (2,18,19).

Typical Dosages & Routes of Administration that are Commonly Used
ORAL: As adjunctive therapy in hypertension, 30-40 grams per day of extra-virgin olive oil has been used as part of the diet (5091). As a laxative, 30 mL has been used (16).

Comments
Olive oil consists of the fatty oil pressed from the drupes (fruit) of olive trees (Olea europaea). It is classified, in part, according to oleic acid content. Extra virgin olive oil contains a maximum of 1% free oleic acid, virgin olive oil contains 2% and ordinary olive oil contains 3.3%. Unrefined olive oils with more than 3.3% free oleic acid are considered "unfit for human consumption" (3273). The American Heart Association recommends a maximum 30% of dietary calories from fat (2224). Some studies show beneficial effects when olive oil is the main source of dietary fat intake (2224).

OMEGA-6 FATTY ACIDS

This Product is Also Known As
N-6, N-6 EFAs, N-6 Essential Fatty Acids, Omega 6 Fatty Acids, Omega-6 Oils, Omega 6 Oils, Polyunsaturated Fatty Acids, PUFAs.
CAUTION: See separate listings for Gamma Linolenic Acid, Evening Primrose Oil, Borage Seed Oil, and Black Currant Seed Oil.

Scientific Names
Omega-6 polyunsaturated fatty acids.

People Use This For
Orally, omega-6 fatty acids are used for reducing the risk of coronary heart disease, lowering total cholesterol and LDL cholesterol levels, increasing HDL cholesterol levels, and reducing cancer risk (3507).
Arachidonic acid, an omega-6 fatty acid, is used as a supplement in infant formulas (424).

Safety
There is insufficient reliable information available about the safety of omega-6 fatty acids for therapeutic purposes.
Pregnancy and Lactation: Insufficient reliable information available; avoid using for therapeutic purposes.

Effectiveness
POSSIBLY INEFFECTIVE ...when arachidonic acid (an omega-6 fatty acid) is used as a supplement in infant formula for improving cognitive and mental development or growth up to 18 months of age (424).
There is insufficient reliable information available about the effectiveness of omega-6 fatty acids for its other uses.

Possible Mechanism of Action & Active Ingredients
Preliminary studies suggest that omega-6 fatty acids might play a role in breast cancer development (3508); however, it is unclear whether omega-6 fatty acids are associated with breast cancer in humans (3508,3511). A low-fat diet with reduced omega-6 fatty acid content can decrease sex steroid hormone levels, alter eicosanoid biosynthesis, and play a role in preventing and treating breast and prostate cancers (3510). Long-chain polyunsaturated fatty acids, such as

arachidonic acid (an omega-6 fatty acid) make up a third of all lipids in the brain's grey matter (425). Arachidonic acid is a membrane component in the central nervous system, and may have a role as a neurotransmitter (424,425). Arachidonic acid is present in human breast milk but not in standard infant formulas. Formula-fed infants have lower plasma arachidonic acid levels than breast milk-fed infants; the clinical significance of this, if any, is unknown (424).

Adverse Reactions Including Known Allergies
The oral use of the omega-6 fatty acids can elevate triglycerides (3509).

Possible Interactions with Herbs & Other Dietary Supplements
Insufficient reliable information available.

Possible Interactions with Drugs
No interactions are known to occur, and there is no known reason to expect a clinically significant interaction with omega-6 fatty acids.

Possible Interactions with Foods
No interactions are known to occur, and there is no known reason to expect a clinically significant interaction with omega-6 fatty acids.

Possible Interactions with Lab Tests
No interactions are known to occur, and there is no known reason to expect a clinically significant interaction with omega-6 fatty acids.

Possible Interactions with Diseases or Conditions
HYPERTRIGLYCERIDEMIA: Avoid the use of the omega-6 fatty acids, because they can elevate triglyceride levels (3509).

Typical Dosages & Routes of Administration that are Commonly Used
ORAL: As a supplement in infant formula, 0.3% of arachidonic acid (an omega-6 fatty acid) has been used (424).

Comments
Omega-6 fatty acids include linoleic acid (LA), gamma-linolenic acid (GLA), and arachidonic acid. Linoleic acid is found in vegetable oils, including corn, evening primrose seed, safflower, and soybean oils (512,3507). Gamma-linolenic acid is found in black currant seed, borage seed, and evening primrose oils (512). Information on omega-6 fatty acid dietary supplementation derives from studies using specific omega-6 fatty acids or plant oils containing omega-6 fatty acids. See separate listings for black currant seed oil, borage seed oil, and evening primrose oil.

ONION

This Product is Also Known As
Allii cepae bulbus, Green Onion.

Scientific Names
Allium cepa.
Family: Alliaceae, Amaryllidaceae or Liliaceae.

People Use This For
Orally, onion is used for loss of appetite, preventing atherosclerosis (2), for treating dyspepsia, fever, colds, cough, bronchitis, hypertension, tendency toward infection, and inflammation of the mouth and pharynx (18).
In folk medicine, it has been used for cough, whooping cough, bronchitis, asthma, angina, stimulation of gallbladder, dehydration, and as a menstruation aid. Onion has also been used for hypertension, diabetes, insect bites, wounds, light burns, furuncles, warts, bruises (18), as an antiflatulent (11), anthelmintic (11,18), and diuretic (6,11). For food uses, onion is considered a culinary food and condiment (11).
In manufacturing, the oil is used as a flavoring agent in foods (11).

Safety
LIKELY SAFE ...when consumed in amounts commonly found in food and has Generally Recognized as Safe (GRAS) status for food use in the US (11).
POSSIBLY SAFE ...when used orally and appropriately (2). A maximum of 35 mg of the diphenylamine constituent is recommended per day if onion preparations are used over several months (2).
There is insufficient reliable information available about the safety of onion for its other uses.
PREGNANCY AND LACTATION: Insufficient reliable information available; avoid amounts greater than used in foods.

Effectiveness
POSSIBLY EFFECTIVE ...when taken orally for appetite stimulation and preventing atherosclerosis (2).
There is insufficient reliable information available about the effectiveness of onion for its other uses.

Possible Mechanism of Action & Active Ingredients

The applicable part of the onion is the bulb. Onion contains essential oils (2), sulfur compounds, and cysteine sulfoxide compounds. One of the sulfur compounds, thiosulphinate, exhibits antimicrobial effects (18). The methyl and propyl compounds of cysteine sulfoxide are primarily responsible for onion flavor and lacrimation (7,11). Diphenylamine is also a constituent of onion (513). Diphenylamine is referred to as a dose standard (2). The mechanism of the diuretic effect of onion is unknown. In people with asthma, an ethanolic onion extract significantly reduced bronchial constriction (18). In sensitized guinea pigs, onion juice provided protection from asthma attacks (18). In humans, eating onions reversed the effect of a fatty meal, restoring fibrinolytic activity (7). In humans, onion also inhibits platelet aggregation (7). Onions show hypoglycemic actions, and in animals, both cholesterol lowering effects and antifungal activities have been noted (11).

Adverse Reactions Including Known Allergies

The consumption of large quantities of onions can cause stomach distress (18). Hand eczema can occur with frequent contact (18).

Possible Interactions with Herbs & Other Dietary Supplements

HERBS WITH ANTICOAGULANT/ANTIPLATELET POTENTIAL: Concomitant use of herbs that have coumarin constituents or affect platelet aggregation could theoretically increase the risk of bleeding in some people. These herbs include: angelica, anise, arnica, asafoetida, bogbean, boldo, capsicum, celery, chamomile, clove, danshen, fenugreek, feverfew, garlic, ginger, ginkgo, ginseng (Panax), horse chestnut, horseradish, licorice, meadowsweet, prickly ash, papain, passionflower, poplar, quassia, red clover, turmeric, wild carrot, wild lettuce, willow, and others (4,19).

Possible Interactions with Drugs

ANTIDIABETES DRUGS: Theoretically, concomitant use might enhance antidiabetes drug effects and alter blood sugar control (19).
ANTIPLATELET DRUGS: Theoretically, concomitant use might enhance antiplatelet drug activity and increase bleeding risk (19).
ASPIRIN: Concomitant intake might augment onion allergy. One case is reported of severe urticaria and swelling in a person with a known mild onion allergy after consuming onion and aspirin (5054).

Possible Interactions with Foods

No interactions are known to occur, and there is no known reason to expect a clinically significant interaction with onion.

Possible Interactions with Lab Tests

BLOOD GLUCOSE: Onions can decrease blood glucose levels and test results (19).

Possible Interactions with Diseases or Conditions

DIABETES: Theoretically, therapeutic amounts of onions can interfere with blood sugar control. Monitor blood sugar carefully when using onion for medicinal purposes (19).

Typical Dosages & Routes of Administration that are Commonly Used

ORAL: The typical dose is 50 grams of fresh onion per day. The juice of 50 grams fresh onion or 20 grams dried onion is also used per day (2). A maximum of 35 mg diphenylamine per day is recommended if onion preparations are used over several months (2).
TOPICAL: An onion slice is typically placed on the skin, or the juice is used as a poultice (18).

Comments

Onions are rich in vitamin C (19) and in folk medicine, were cooked in milk and used as a mucolytic to clear congested airways (7).

OPIUM ANTIDOTE

This Product is Also Known As

Combretum, Jungle Weed.

Scientific Names

Combretum micranthum.
Family: Combretaceae.

People Use This For

Historically, opium antidote has been used orally for gallbladder disease, dyspepsia, and liver disease. It is no longer used as a single entity, only in combination preparations (18).

© Copyright 2000, Natural Medicines Comprehensive Database (209) 472-2244. For updated data, go to www.NaturalDatabase.com

Safety

There is insufficient reliable information available about the safety of opium antidote. (18).
Pregnancy and Lactation: Insufficient reliable information available; avoid using.

Effectiveness

There is insufficient reliable information available about the effectiveness of opium antidote.

Possible Mechanism of Action & Active Ingredients

The applicable parts of opium antidote are the leaf and stem. Opium antidote is said to possess mild bile-stimulating properties and astringent effects. It contains catechin tannins, flavonoids, and pyrrolidine alkaloid betaines. A methanolic extract shows some evidence of activity against HSV-1 and HSV-2 (18). Activity was present only in the extract dissolved 7 days before assay, but not in the freshly prepared extract (5001).

Adverse Reactions Including Known Allergies

None reported.

Possible Interactions with Herbs & Other Dietary Supplements

Insufficient reliable information available.

Possible Interactions with Drugs

No interactions are known to occur, and there is no known reason to expect a clinically significant interaction with opium antidote.

Possible Interactions with Foods

No interactions are known to occur, and there is no known reason to expect a clinically significant interaction with opium antidote.

Possible Interactions with Lab Tests

No interactions are known to occur, and there is no known reason to expect a clinically significant interaction with opium antidote.

Possible Interactions with Diseases or Conditions

No interactions are known to occur, and there is no known reason to expect a clinically significant interaction with opium antidote.

Typical Dosages & Routes of Administration that are Commonly Used

No typical dosage.

Comments

There is very little scientific information about this product. Our staff is continually analyzing the available information on natural medicines and will add data here as it becomes available.

OREGANO

This Product is Also Known As

Dostenkraut, European Oregano, Mountain Mint, Organy, Origani vulgaris herba, Origano, Origanum, Wild Marjoram, Winter Marjoram, Wintersweet.
CAUTION: See separate listing for Marjoram.

Scientific Names

Origanum vulgare.
Family: Lamiaceae or Labiatae.

People Use This For

Orally, oregano leaf is used for respiratory tract disorders, coughs, bronchial mucous membrane inflammation, and as an expectorant (2,18).
In combination with mistletoe berry, mistletoe herb, valerian root, silver weed, rosemary, wormwood, cleavers, and wood betony, oregano is used as a sedative, anti-epileptic, and antispasmodic (2).
In folk medicine, it has been used for gastrointestinal disorders, such as dyspepsia, bloating, stimulating bile excretion and digestion, painful menstruation, rheumatoid arthritis, scrofulosis, urinary tract disorders (2,18), as a nerve tonic, cure for asthma, toothaches, headaches, spider bites, and heart conditions (11). It is used for diaphoretic, appetite stimulant, and antispasmodic properties (2,18).
In foods and beverages, oregano is used as a culinary spice (11).

Safety

LIKELY SAFE ...when used orally in amounts found in foods (11). It has Generally Recognized as Safe (GRAS) status in the US (11).
POSSIBLY SAFE ...when used orally and appropriately in larger amounts (2,12,14). ...when used topically and

© Copyright 2000, Natural Medicines Comprehensive Database (209) 472-2244. For updated data, go to www.NaturalDatabase.com

appropriately (2,18).
PREGNANCY: LIKELY SAFE ...when used in food amounts. POSSIBLY UNSAFE ...when used in excessive amounts (19).
LACTATION: Insufficient reliable information available; avoid using amounts in excess of foods.

Effectiveness

There is insufficient reliable information available about the effectiveness of oregano.

Possible Mechanism of Action & Active Ingredients

The applicable part of oregano is the leaf. Oregano contains the constituents carvacrol and thymol which have antihelmintic, fungicidal, and irritant properties (11). The essential oil has diuretic, expectorant, and antispasmodic properties. It is also a bile stimulant (11). Evidence suggests oregano and its essential oil have antibacterial (3703,6113) and antifungal activity (3704). Other evidence suggests oregano might inhibit the growth of salmonella and yeast (3702). Preliminary evidence suggests oregano binds to progesterone receptors and might be useful against breast cancer (3701).

Adverse Reactions Including Known Allergies

Ingesting large amounts of oregano can cause gastrointestinal upset (14). It might also cause systemic allergic reaction (3705). Individuals allergic to Lamiaceae family plants, including: basil, hyssop, lavender, marjoram, mint, and sage, might also demonstrate an allergic reaction to oregano (3705).

Possible Interactions with Herbs & Other Dietary Supplements

Insufficient reliable information available.

Possible Interactions with Drugs

No interactions are known to occur, and there is no known reason to expect a clinically significant interaction with oregano.

Possible Interactions with Foods

No interactions are known to occur, and there is no known reason to expect a clinically significant interaction with oregano.

Possible Interactions with Lab Tests

No interactions are known to occur, and there is no known reason to expect a clinically significant interaction with oregano.

Possible Interactions with Diseases or Conditions

CROSS-ALLERGENICITY: Oregano can cause reactions in people allergic to Lamiaceae family plants, including: basil, hyssop, lavender, marjoram, mint, and sage (3705).

Typical Dosages & Routes of Administration that are Commonly Used

ORAL: A typical dose is one cup of tea. To make tea, steep 1 heaping teaspoon of leaf in 250 mL boiling water 10 minutes, strain. Tea may be sweetened with honey (18).
TOPICAL: Unsweetened tea is used as a gargle or mouthwash (18). To use oregano as a bath additive, steep 100 grams dried leaf in 1 L water for 10 minutes, strain, and add to full a bath (18).

Comments

None.

OREGON FIR BALSAM

This Product is Also Known As

Balsam Fir Oregon, Balsam Oregon, Coastal Douglas Fir, Douglas Fir, Douglas Spruce, Oregon Balsam, Red Fir.

Scientific Names

Pseudotsuga menziesii, synonym Pseudotsuga douglasii; Pseudotsuga mucronata; Pseudotsuga taxifolia.
Family: Pinaceae.

People Use This For

In traditional medicine, Oregon fir balsam has been used for burns, sores, cuts, relieving heart and chest pain, and for treating tumors (11).

Safety

There is insufficient reliable information available about the safety of Oregon fir balsam.
Pregnancy and Lactation: Insufficient reliable information available; avoid using.

Effectiveness

There is insufficient reliable information available about the effectiveness of Oregon fir balsam.

Possible Mechanism of Action & Active Ingredients

Insufficient reliable information available.

Adverse Reactions Including Known Allergies

None reported.

Possible Interactions with Herbs & Other Dietary Supplements

Insufficient reliable information available.

Possible Interactions with Drugs

No interactions are known to occur, and there is no known reason to expect a clinically significant interaction with Oregon fir balsam.

Possible Interactions with Foods

No interactions are known to occur, and there is no known reason to expect a clinically significant interaction with Oregon fir balsam.

Possible Interactions with Lab Tests

No interactions are known to occur, and there is no known reason to expect a clinically significant interaction with Oregon fir balsam.

Possible Interactions with Diseases or Conditions

No interactions are known to occur, and there is no known reason to expect a clinically significant interaction with Oregon fir balsam.

Typical Dosages & Routes of Administration that are Commonly Used

No typical dosage.

Comments

Oregon fir balsam is an oleoresin (rather than a true balsam) collected from the trunk of the Oregon fir tree. Oregon fir balsam has been detected as an adulterant in Canada balsam (Abies balsamea) (11).

There is very little scientific information about this product. Our staff is continually analyzing the available information on natural medicines and will add data here as it becomes available.

OREGON GRAPE

This Product is Also Known As

Barberry, Blue Barberry, Creeping Barberry, Holly Barberry, Holly-Leaved Berberis, Holly Mahonia, Mountain-Grape, Oregon Barberry, Oregon-Grape, Oregon Grape-Holly, Trailing Mahonia, Water-Holly.
CAUTION: See separate listing for European Barberry.

Scientific Names

Mahonia aquifolium, synonym Berberis aquifolium; Mahonia nervosa, synonym Berberis nervosa; Mahonia repens, synonyms Berberis repens, Berberis sonnei.
Family: Beberidaceae.

People Use This For

Topically, Oregon grape root and rhizome is used for psoriasis (515).
In folk medicine the root and rhizome have been used for ulcers, heartburn, stomach problems, as a bitter tonic, and as a cathartic (515). The American Indians used Oregon grape root and rhizome for general debility and as an appetite stimulant (515).

Safety

POSSIBLY SAFE ...when used topically and appropriately (854,857). Canada has approved a Mahonia aquifolium product for topical use based on safety data (855,856). ...when the root and rhizome are used orally. Amounts of less than 500 mg per day of berberine, a constituent of Oregon grape, are usually considered safe (2,12).
LIKELY UNSAFE ...when more than 500 mg per day berberine is consumed (2,12). Berberine is considered moderately toxic (12). The human LD50 for berberine is reported to be 27.5 mg/kg (12).
PREGNANCY: LIKELY UNSAFE ...contraindicated (12) due to potential uterine stimulant activity of berberine (11,19).
LACTATION: Insufficient reliable information available; avoid using.

Effectiveness

There is insufficient reliable information available about the effectiveness of Oregon grape.

Possible Mechanism of Action & Active Ingredients

The applicable parts of Oregon grape are the rhizome and root. Oregon grape root contains 2.4-4.5% of isoquinoline alkaloid constituents including berberine, berbamine, and oxyacanthine (18,515). Berberine and oxyacanthine show evidence of antibacterial activity (11). Berberine has anticonvulsant, sedative, hypotensive, antifibrillatory, and bile-stimulating effects. In low doses, it is a cardiac and respiratory stimulant. In high doses it is a depressant (11,12,515). Some evidence suggests berberine sulfate might be amebicidal and trypanocidal (11). Other information suggests the constituent berbamine might have anti-arrhythmic, hypotensive, spasmolytic, and immunostimulating activity (11,515). In an open clinical trial, an extract of dried stem, branch bark, and branch tips of Mahonia aquifolium in an ointment base improved psoriasis symptoms and quality of life (857). In another trial, some patients treated with Mahonia aquifolium bark extract in an ointment base found it more useful than placebo for treating mild to moderate psoriasis (854). However, more than half of the other participants and their physicians rated the treatment as ineffective (854).

Adverse Reactions Including Known Allergies

No reports of adverse effects associated with Oregon grape. Ingesting more than 500 mg berberine, a constituent of Oregon grape, can cause lethargy, nosebleed, skin and eye irritation, kidney irritation (12), hemorrhagic nephritis (2), dyspnea, hypotension, cardiac damage (12), nausea, vomiting, diarrhea, respiratory spasms and arrest, and death (2). When used topically, Oregon grape can cause itching, burning, skin irritation, and allergic reactions (854).

Possible Interactions with Herbs & Other Dietary Supplements

BERBERINE-CONTAINING HERBS: Concomitant use can increase the risk of berberine toxicity. Berberine-containing herbs include bloodroot, goldenseal, celandine, Chinese goldthread, goldthread, Oregon grape (Mahonia species), amur cork tree, Chinese corktree (12).

Possible Interactions with Drugs

No interactions are known to occur, and there is no known reason to expect a clinically significant interaction with Oregon grape.

Possible Interactions with Foods

No interactions are known to occur, and there is no known reason to expect a clinically significant interaction with Oregon grape.

Possible Interactions with Lab Tests

No interactions are known to occur, and there is no known reason to expect a clinically significant interaction with Oregon grape.

Possible Interactions with Diseases or Conditions

KIDNEY IRRITATION: CAUTION, berberine may exacerbate kidney irritation. It can cause kidney irritation and nephritis (2).

Typical Dosages & Routes of Administration that are Commonly Used

TOPICAL: Psoriasis, 10% Mahonia aquifolium bark extract ointment applied to affected areas two to three times daily (854). Mahonia aquifolium 10% root extract cream massaged into affected areas three times daily or as directed by physician (855).
ORAL: The common dose of the tincture is 2-4 mL three times daily, and the usual dose of the powder is 0.5 to 1 gram three times daily (6002).

Comments

A Mahonia aquifolium root extract product, Prime Relief, received a Drug Identification Number (DIN) from Health Canada (855). The DIN allows this product to be labeled and marketed for treating psoriasis in Canada (855,856).

ORIENTAL ARBORVITAE

This Product is Also Known As

Chinese Arborvitae.

Scientific Names

Platycladus orientalis, synonyms Biota orientalis, Thuja orientalis.
Family: Cupressaceae.

People Use This For

Orally, Oriental arborvitae is used orally for headache, apprehension, calming nervous disorders and excitement, for cancer, constipation, convulsions, dysmenorrhea, ejaculation problems, narrowing of intestine, fever, vomiting blood, bloody stools, blood in urine, hemorrhage, insomnia, painful menses, heavy menstrual flow, irregular and variable menstrual bleeding, nausea, neurasthenia, palpitation, perspiration, rheumatism, tumors, and as a tonic. It is also used for diuretic, laxative, menstrual-stimulant, pain-reliever, parasiticide, and sedative effects (4017). Topically, it is used for nosebleed, piles, for burns and scalds, and as a hair tonic. It is also used for its astringent and antiperspirant properties (4017).

Safety

POSSIBLY SAFE ...when the seed is used orally (12) ...when the leafy twigs are used orally in tea. It is important to use it short-term and not to exceed the usual dose (12).

PREGNANCY AND LACTATION: POSSIBLY UNSAFE ...contains thujone (12) which shows some evidence of uterine stimulant activity (19); avoid using.

Effectiveness

There is insufficient reliable information is available about the effectiveness of oriental arborvitae.

Possible Mechanism of Action & Active Ingredients

The applicable parts of oriental arborvitae are the seed and the cacumen (leafy twigs) (12). Oriental arborvitae contains thujone in the volatile oil. Alcoholic extracts and essential oils containing thujone can cause neurotoxicity including convulsions and hallucinations (12). Some evidence suggests Thuja orientalis might have antibacterial activity (4041).

Adverse Reactions Including Known Allergies

Thujone intoxication can cause psychoactivity similar to tetrahydrocannibinol, the active constituent in marijuana. Long-term or high dosages of plants containing thujone can cause restlessness, vomiting, dizziness, tremors, renal damage, and convulsions (12).

Possible Interactions with Herbs & Other Dietary Supplements

THUJONE CONTAINING HERBS: Avoid; concomitant use may increase the risk of thujone toxicity. Thujone-containing herbs include: oak moss (12), sage (2,4,12), tansy (2,4,12), thuja (cedar) (11,12), tree moss (12), and wormwood (2,12).

Possible Interactions with Drugs

No interactions are known to occur, and there is no known reason to expect a clinically significant interaction with oriental arborvitae.

Possible Interactions with Foods

No interactions are known to occur, and there is no known reason to expect a clinically significant interaction with oriental arborvitae.

Possible Interactions with Lab Tests

No interactions are known to occur, and there is no known reason to expect a clinically significant interaction with oriental arborvitae.

Possible Interactions with Diseases or Conditions

PORPHYRIA: Can exacerbate porphyria in patients with underlying defects in hepatic heme synthesis (12).
RENAL DYSFUNCTION: Can exacerbate this condition (12).

Typical Dosages & Routes of Administration that are Commonly Used

ORAL: A standard dose for the leafy twigs is 5-15 grams of raw or charred, daily as tea (12). No typical dosage for the seed.

Comments

None.

ORNITHINE

This Product is Also Known As

L-Ornithine.
CAUTION: See separate listing for Ornithine Ketoglutarate.

Scientific Names

L-5-aminorvaline; L-2,5-diaminovaleric acid.

People Use This For

Orally, ornithine is used for improving athletic performance and for wound healing (2416).

Safety

There is insufficient reliable information available about the safety of ornithine used medicinally.
Pregnancy and Lactation: Insufficient reliable information available; avoid using.

Effectiveness

POSSIBLY INEFFECTIVE ...when taken orally for enhancing athletic performance (2417,2418).
There is insufficient reliable information available for the effectiveness of ornithine for wound healing.

Possible Mechanism of Action & Active Ingredients

Ornithine is a non-essential amino acid produced in the body by hydrolysis of arginine (9,511). By supplementing ornithine, people believe they can increase their anabolic hormone levels, reducing skeletal muscle hypertrophy (2147). However, supplemental ornithine has no effect on insulin secretion (2147,2148) or serum human growth hormone (hGH) levels in bodybuilders (2148).

Adverse Reactions Including Known Allergies

None reported.

Possible Interactions with Herbs & Other Dietary Supplements

Insufficient reliable information available.

Possible Interactions with Drugs

No interactions are known to occur, and there is no known reason to expect a clinically significant interaction with ornithine.

Possible Interactions with Foods

No interactions are known to occur, and there is no known reason to expect a clinically significant interaction with ornithine.

Possible Interactions with Lab Tests

No interactions are known to occur, and there is no known reason to expect a clinically significant interaction with ornithine.

Possible Interactions with Diseases or Conditions

No interactions are known to occur, and there is no known reason to expect a clinically significant interaction with ornithine.

Typical Dosages & Routes of Administration that are Commonly Used

ORAL: Take one 500 mg capsule containing L-ornithine daily on an empty stomach before bedtime (5020).

Comments

Avoid confusion with ornithine alpha-ketoglutarate (OKG).
There is very little scientific information about this product. Our staff is continually analyzing the available information on natural medicines and will add data here as it becomes available.

ORNITHINE KETOGLUTARATE

This Product is Also Known As

OKG, Ornicetil, Ornithine Alphaketoglutarate.
CAUTION: See separate listing for Ornithine.

Scientific Names

L(+)-ornithine alpha-ketoglutarate.

People Use This For

Orally, ornithine ketoglutarate is used for enhancing athletic performance and wound healing (2442). Intravenously, it is used as a component in total parenteral nutrition for preventing growth retardation in children receiving long-term total parenteral nutrition (2444). It is also used intravenously for improving skeletal muscle protein synthesis after surgery (2446), preventing decreases in muscle free glutamine concentrations, and preserving protein synthesis after total hip replacement (2448) or stroke (2447).

Safety

POSSIBLY SAFE ...when use intravenously and appropriately (2444,2445,2446,2448).
There is insufficient reliable information available about the safety of the oral use of ornithine ketoglutarate.
PREGNANCY AND LACTATION: Insufficient reliable information available; avoid using.

Effectiveness

POSSIBLY EFFECTIVE ...when taken orally for wound healing in burn patients (2443). ...when used intravenously for preventing growth retardation in children receiving long-term total parenteral nutrition (2444), reducing loss of muscle glutamine after surgical trauma (2445), improving skeletal muscle protein synthesis after surgery (2446), preventing a decrease in the muscle free glutamine concentration, and preservation of protein synthesis after total hip replacement (2448).
POSSIBLY INEFFECTIVE ...when taken orally for enhancing athletic performance (2452).

LIKELY INEFFECTIVE ...when given intravenously for treating encephalopathy in patients with acute and chronic liver disease (2449,2450).

There is insufficient reliable information available about the effectiveness of ornithine ketoglutarate for its other uses.

Possible Mechanism of Action & Active Ingredients

Ornithine ketoglutarate modifies amino acid metabolism and increases blood insulin and glucagon levels in healthy people (2415).

Adverse Reactions Including Known Allergies

None reported.

Possible Interactions with Herbs & Other Dietary Supplements

Insufficient reliable information available.

Possible Interactions with Drugs

No interactions are known to occur, and there is no known reason to expect a clinically significant interaction with ornithine ketoglutarate.

Possible Interactions with Foods

No interactions are known to occur, and there is no known reason to expect a clinically significant interaction with ornithine ketoglutarate.

Possible Interactions with Lab Tests

No interactions are known to occur, and there is no known reason to expect a clinically significant interaction with ornithine ketoglutarate.

Possible Interactions with Diseases or Conditions

No interactions are known to occur, and there is no known reason to expect a clinically significant interaction with ornithine ketoglutarate.

Typical Dosages & Routes of Administration that are Commonly Used

ORAL: For athletic support, 2-4 grams of ornithine ketoglutarate is commonly taken three times per day with meals (2442). For the healing of burn wounds, 30 grams is taken daily as an enteral bolus (2443).

INTRAVENOUS: For preventing growth retardation in children receiving long-term total parenteral nutrition (TPN), 15 grams of ornithine ketoglutarate is typically added to the daily TPN (2444). For improving skeletal muscle protein synthesis after surgery, 350 mg/kg per day is added to the TPN (2446). For preventing decreases in muscle free glutamine concentrations and preserving protein synthesis after total hip replacement, 280 mg/kg per day is added to the TPN (2448).

Comments

Avoid confusion with ornithine.

ORRIS

This Product is Also Known As

Blue Flag, Daggers, Flag, Flaggon, Flag Lily, Fliggers, Florentine Iris, Gladyne, Iris, Jacob's Sword, Liver Lily, Myrtle Flower, Poison Flag, Rhizoma iridis, Segg, Sheggs, Snake Lily, Water Flag, White Dragon Flower, Wild Iris, Yellow Flag, Yellow Iris.

CAUTION: See separate listing for Blue Flag.

Scientific Names

Iris germanica; Iris florentina, synonym Iris x germanica var. florentina
Iris pallida, Rhizoma iridis
Family: Iridaceae.

People Use This For

Orally, orris root is used for "blood-purifying", "gland-stimulating", increasing kidney activity, skin diseases (2), bronchitis, cold, cancer, stimulating appetite and digestion, stimulating bile flow, sciatica, sclerosis, splenitis. It is also used for diuretic, emetic, laxative, purgative, and stimulant properties (513).

Topically, orris root is used for halitosis, nasal polyps, teething, and as a dentifrice (513).

In combination with other herbs, orris root is used orally for headache, toothache, muscle and joint pain, migraine, neuralgia, acute and chronic respiratory tract mucous membrane inflammation, bronchitis, bronchial asthma, cough, mucous congestion, nasal mucous membrane inflammation, hoarseness, for improving bronchial and mucous membrane blood supply, interval therapy of asthma, care of heart, nerves, and stomach, for nervous disturbances of cardiovascular function, loss of appetite, gastrointestinal disturbances, bowel sluggishness, feeling of fullness, bloating, ailments of gallbladder, liver and pancreas, diabetes, relief of irritations caused by urinary tract inflammatory diseases, skin diseases, and as a sedative (2).

In combination with other herbs, orris root is used topically for tumors, swelling of the lymph glands, uric acid sedimentation, kyphosis, keloid formation, rheumatic disorders, burns, and cuts (2).

Safety

POSSIBLY SAFE ...when used orally (12). Orris root must be carefully peeled and dried before using (2). Fresh root and juice can cause severe mucosal and skin irritation (12).

There is insufficient reliable information available about the safety of the topical use of orris (18).

PREGNANCY AND LACTATION: Insufficient reliable information available; avoid using.

Effectiveness

There is insufficient reliable information available about the effectiveness of orris.

Possible Mechanism of Action & Active Ingredients

The applicable parts of orris are the rhizome and root. Orris root contains triterpenes, including irigermanal, and isoflavonoids, including irilon, irisolone, irigenine, and tectoridine. It also contains C-glucosylxanthones and a volatile oil. The chief constituents of the volatile oil are irones, particularly alpha-, beta-, and gamma-irone. Some think orris root has mild expectorant effects (18).

Adverse Reactions Including Known Allergies

No adverse effects are reported when orris root has been carefully peeled and dried. However, taken orally the fresh plant juice or root can cause severe mucosal irritation, abdominal pain, vomiting, and bloody diarrhea (18). Used topically, the fresh plant juice or root can cause severe skin and mucosal irritation (12,18).

Possible Interactions with Herbs & Other Dietary Supplements

Insufficient reliable information available.

Possible Interactions with Drugs

No interactions are known to occur, and there is no known reason to expect a clinically significant interaction with orris.

Possible Interactions with Foods

No interactions are known to occur, and there is no known reason to expect a clinically significant interaction with orris.

Possible Interactions with Lab Tests

No interactions are known to occur, and there is no known reason to expect a clinically significant interaction with orris.

Possible Interactions with Diseases or Conditions

No interactions are known to occur, and there is no known reason to expect a clinically significant interaction with orris.

Typical Dosages & Routes of Administration that are Commonly Used

No typical dosage.

Comments

Orris root is generally used in combination with other herbs and can be found in homeopathic dilutions and tea preparations (18). Historically, orris root was highly prized in the perfume industry. Upon drying, the root develops a pleasant violet-like scent. This scent continues to improve in storage, reaching its peak in about three years. Orris root was widely used in face powders and other cosmetics until it was determined to cause allergic reactions. Orris root powder is still used extensively in potpourris, sachets, and pomanders. It is one of the most effective fixatives and it prolongs the scent of the more transient volatile oils. Of the two orris species, Iris x germanica var. florentina root is considered superior to Iris pallida (4081).

OSTRICH FERN

This Product is Also Known As

None.

Scientific Names

Matteucccia struthiopteris.
Family: Aspleniaceae.

People Use This For

Ostrich fern is used for food. It is regarded as a seasonal delicacy (6).

Safety

LIKELY SAFE ...when used as a food if prepared appropriately (6,5002).
LIKELY UNSAFE ...when not cooked properly (6). May cause severe food poisoning.
PREGNANCY AND LACTATION: Insufficient reliable information available; avoid using.

Effectiveness

There is insufficient reliable information available about the effectiveness of ostrich fern (6).

Possible Mechanism of Action & Active Ingredients

The applicable part of ostrich fern is the young shoot top. One field guide states wild ostrich fern greens have laxative properties (6). Toxins responsible for poisonings have not been identified, but they are believed deactivated by boiling. The CDC recommends thorough cooking (e.g. boiling for 10 minutes) before eating (5002).

Adverse Reactions Including Known Allergies

Centers for Disease Control and Prevention (CDC) links outbreaks of severe food poisoning to consumption of raw or lightly cooked fiddlehead ferns (6,5002). Ostrich fern can cause nausea, vomiting, abdominal cramping (6), diarrhea, and headaches after ingestion (5002).

Possible Interactions with Herbs & Other Dietary Supplements

Insufficient reliable information available.

Possible Interactions with Drugs

No interactions are known to occur, and there is no known reason to expect a clinically significant interaction with ostrich fern.

Possible Interactions with Foods

No interactions are known to occur, and there is no known reason to expect a clinically significant interaction with ostrich fern.

Possible Interactions with Lab Tests

No interactions are known to occur, and there is no known reason to expect a clinically significant interaction with ostrich fern.

Possible Interactions with Diseases or Conditions

No interactions are known to occur, and there is no known reason to expect a clinically significant interaction with ostrich fern.

Typical Dosages & Routes of Administration that are Commonly Used

ORAL: Cook young shoots of ostrich fern (fiddleheads) thoroughly (e.g. boiling for 10 minutes) before eating (5002).

Comments

The tops of the young shoots of ostrich fern, known as fiddleheads, are regarded as a seasonal delicacy. They are available canned, frozen or fresh (6). Boil at least 10 minutes before eating.

OSWEGO TEA

This Product is Also Known As

Bee Balm, Bergamot, Blue Balm, High Balm, Low Balm, Monarda, Mountain Balm, Mountain Mint, Scarlet Monarda.
CAUTION: See separate listings for Bergamot Oil, Bitter Orange peel, Sweet Orange, and Bitter Orange flower.

Scientific Names

Monarda didyma.
Family: Labitae or Lamiaceae.

People Use This For

Orally, oswego tea is used for digestive disorders including flatulence and premenstrual syndrome. It is also used as an antispasmodic and diuretic.
In Europe, oswego tea is used for decreasing fever and as a fragrance (18).

Safety

There is insufficient reliable information available about the safety of the oral use of oswego tea.
PREGNANCY: UNSAFE ...contraindicated because it may possibly promote menstruation and stimulate menstrual flow (12).
LACTATION: Insufficient reliable information available; avoid using.

Effectiveness

There is insufficient reliable information available about the effectiveness of oswego tea.

Possible Mechanism of Action & Active Ingredients

Insufficient reliable information available.

Adverse Reactions Including Known Allergies

None reported.

Possible Interactions with Herbs & Other Dietary Supplements

Insufficient reliable information available.

Possible Interactions with Drugs

No interactions are known to occur, and there is no known reason to expect a clinically significant interaction with oswego tea.

Possible Interactions with Foods

No interactions are known to occur, and there is no known reason to expect a clinically significant interaction with oswego tea.

Possible Interactions with Lab Tests

No interactions are known to occur, and there is no known reason to expect a clinically significant interaction with oswego tea.

Possible Interactions with Diseases or Conditions

No interactions are known to occur, and there is no known reason to expect a clinically significant interaction with oswego tea.

Typical Dosages & Routes of Administration that are Commonly Used

ORAL: Oswego tea is taken as tea prepared from the powdered herb (18).

Comments

Oswego tea got the alternate name bergamot because of the similarity of its pleasant scent to that of the oil of bergamot oranges (see separate listing). During the period of the Boston tea party, it was drunk in place of black tea. Lemon balm is also known as bee balm, a common name for oswego tea, and may be confused with it.

OX-EYE DAISY

This Product is Also Known As

Butter Daisy, Dun Daisy, Golden Daisy, Goldenseal, Great Ox-Eye, Herb Margaret, Horse Daisy, Horse Gowan, Marguerite, Maudlin Daisy, Maudlinwort, Moon Daisy, Moon Flower, Moon Penny, Ox Eye Daisy, Poverty Weed, White Daisy, White Weed.
CAUTION: See separate listing for Goldenseal (Hydrastis canadensis).

Scientific Names

Chrysanthemum leucanthemum.
Family: Compositae.

People Use This For

Orally, ox-eye daisy is used for indications similar to German chamomile. These uses include the common cold, cough, bronchitis, fever, mouth and pharynx inflammation, liver and gallbladder complaints, loss of appetite, and susceptibility to infection. It is also used as an antispasmodic, diuretic, and tonic (18).
Topically, uses include skin inflammation, wounds and burns.

Safety

There is insufficient reliable information available about the safety of ox-eye daisy.
Pregnancy and Lactation: Insufficient reliable information available; avoid using.

Effectiveness

There is insufficient reliable information available about the effectiveness of ox-eye daisy.

Possible Mechanism of Action & Active Ingredients

The applicable parts of ox-eye daisy are the above ground flowering parts. There is insufficient reliable information available about the possible mechanism of action and active ingredients.

Adverse Reactions Including Known Allergies

Ox-eye daisy can cause an allergic reaction in individuals sensitive to the Asteraceae/Compositae family. Members of this family include ragweed, chrysanthemums, marigolds, daisies, and many other herbs.

Possible Interactions with Herbs & Other Dietary Supplements
Insufficient reliable information available.

Possible Interactions with Drugs
No interactions are known to occur, and there is no known reason to expect a clinically significant interaction with ox-eye daisy.

Possible Interactions with Foods
No interactions are known to occur, and there is no known reason to expect a clinically significant interaction with ox-eye daisy.

Possible Interactions with Lab Tests
No interactions are known to occur, and there is no known reason to expect a clinically significant interaction with ox-eye daisy.

Possible Interactions with Diseases or Conditions
CROSS-ALLERGENICITY: Can cause an allergic reaction in individuals sensitive to the Asteraceae/Compositae family. Members of this family include ragweed, chrysanthemums, marigolds, daisies, and many other herbs.

Typical Dosages & Routes of Administration that are Commonly Used
ORAL: The daily dose is equivalent to 10-15 grams dried herb, taken as tea. The tea is prepared by steeping 3 grams dried leaf in 150 mL of boiling water for 10-15 minutes and straining (18).
TOPICAL: A tea is prepared by steeping 2 teaspoons of dried leaf in 1 cup of boiling water for 15 minutes, straining and applied topically. As a bath additive, 50 grams of dried herb is added to 1 L bath water (18).

Comments
Ox-eye daisy is alternately known as goldenseal, but it is unrelated to the more commonly known goldenseal (Hydrastis canadensis).

PAGODA TREE

This Product is Also Known As
None.

Scientific Names
Sophora japonica.
Family: Fabaceae.

People Use This For
Orally, pagoda tree is used in dilutions for dysentery (18).

Safety
POSSIBLY UNSAFE ...when the seeds are used orally (18). Regular use of seed meal can cause facial edema or even death. High doses could cause cystine poisoning (18).
PREGNANCY AND LACTATION: POSSIBLY UNSAFE ...when used orally; avoid using.

Effectiveness
There is insufficient reliable information available about the effectiveness of pagoda tree.

Possible Mechanism of Action & Active Ingredients
The applicable parts of the pagoda tree are the seeds. Cystine poisoning may occur with high dosages (18).

Adverse Reactions Including Known Allergies
None reported with short term use. Using pagoda tree seed long term may cause edema and death (18).

Possible Interactions with Herbs & Other Dietary Supplements
Insufficient reliable information available.

Possible Interactions with Drugs
No interactions are known to occur, and there is no known reason to expect a clinically significant interaction with pagoda tree.

Possible Interactions with Foods
No interactions are known to occur, and there is no known reason to expect a clinically significant interaction with pagoda tree.

Possible Interactions with Lab Tests
No interactions are known to occur, and there is no known reason to expect a clinically significant interaction with pagoda tree.

Possible Interactions with Diseases or Conditions

No interactions are known to occur, and there is no known reason to expect a clinically significant interaction with pagoda tree.

Typical Dosages & Routes of Administration that are Commonly Used

ORAL: Avoid using (18).

Comments

None.

PANAX PSEUDOGINSENG

This Product is Also Known As

Field Seven, Pseudoginseng Root, Samch'il, San Qi, San Qui, Sanshichi, Three Seven, Tian Qi.
CAUTION: See separate listing for Panax ginseng.

Scientific Names

Panax pseudodinseng; Panax notoginseng; Panax zingiberensis.

People Use This For

In Chinese medicine, Panax pseudoginseng root is used orally to stop bleeding, i.e., vomiting blood, coughing up blood, blood in the urine or stool, or nosebleed. It is also used to treat blood stasis, to relieve pain and reduce swelling, and to reduce blood cholesterol level. It is also used for angina and hemorrhagic disease (5558,5559). The flower of Panax pseudoginseng is sometimes used to reduce blood pressure, for dizziness, and acute sore throat (5559).
Topically, Panax pseudoginseng is used to stop bleeding (5559).
In combination with seven other herbs (PC-SPES), Panax pseudoginseng is used to treat prostate cancer (5548).

Safety

POSSIBLY SAFE ...when used orally in a specific herbal combination (PC-SPES) (5548).
There is insufficient reliable information available about the safety of Panax pseudoginseng for its other uses.
PREGNANCY AND LACTATION: LIKELY UNSAFE ...when used orally; contraindicated (5559).

Effectiveness

POSSIBLY EFFECTIVE ...when used orally in a specific herbal combination for prostate cancer. Studies using Panax pseudoginseng in combination with seven other herbs (PC-SPES) in prostate cancer patients, found that it significantly decreases prostate-specific antigen (PSA) levels (5548,5122,5913), causes tumor cell death (5913), and causes clinically significant reductions in testosterone (5548). In two reports, PSA levels fell significantly within 1 month of treatment (5548,5122).
There is insufficient reliable information available about the effectiveness of Panax pseudoginseng for its other uses.

Possible Mechanism of Action & Active Ingredients

The Panax pseudoginseng root contains 12% saponins. Water hydrolysis of the saponins produces panaxadiol and panaxatriol that are the genins of arasaponin. Panax pseudoginseng is believed to dilate the coronary vessels, reduce vascular resistance, and improve the coronary collateral circulation. This could increase blood flow while reducing blood pressure. It would also reduce the heart metabolic rate and oxygen consumption. Some evidence suggests Panax pseudoginseng also has an antiarrhythmic effect (5558).

Adverse Reactions Including Known Allergies

Oral doses of Panax pseudoginseng can cause dry mouth, flushed skin, nervousness, insomnia, nausea, and vomiting (5558).

Possible Interactions with Herbs & Other Dietary Supplements

CARDIOACTIVE HERBS: Avoid concomitant use with other cardioactive herbs due to unpredictability of effects and adverse effects. Cardioactive herbs include: calamus, cereus, cola, coltsfoot, devil's claw, European mistletoe, fenugreek, fumitory, ginger, Panax ginseng, hawthorn, white horehound, mate, parsley, quassia, Scotch broom flower, shepherd's purse, and wild carrot (4). Cardiac glycoside containing herbs, include black hellebore, Canadian hemp roots, digitalis leaf, hedge mustard, figwort, lily of the valley roots, motherwort, oleander leaf, pheasant's eye plant, pleurisy root, squill bulb leaf scales, and strophanthus seeds (2,18,19,500).

Possible Interactions with Drugs

CARDIOACTIVE DRUGS: Theoretically, Panax pseudoginseng could interfere with cardiovascular therapy; avoid using.

Possible Interactions with Foods

No interactions are known to occur, and there is no known reason to expect a clinically significant interaction with Panax pseudoginseng.

Possible Interactions with Lab Tests

CARDIAC FUNCTION: Panax pseudoginseng might improve tests of cardiovascular function.

Possible Interactions with Diseases or Conditions

No interactions are known to occur, and there is no known reason to expect a clinically significant interaction with Panax pseudoginseng.

Typical Dosages & Routes of Administration that are Commonly Used

ORAL: A typical dose is 1-1.5 grams divided into three doses per day (5558).
TOPICAL: No typical dosage.

Comments

None.

PANCREATIN

This Product is Also Known As

Pancreatinum, Pancreatis pulvis.

Scientific Names

Pancreatin.

People Use This For

Orally, pancreatin is used to treat malabsorption syndromes associated with pancreatic insufficiency in cystic fibrosis, chronic pancreatitis, or pancreas removal (15). It is also used for flatulence (14) or as a digestive aid (305,306).

Safety

LIKELY SAFE ...when used orally and appropriately for replacement therapy by individuals with pancreatic insufficiency (15). Some pancreatin products contaminated by Salmonella have caused illness (14). Use only products from reputable manufacturers.
PREGNANCY: Insufficient reliable information available; avoid using unless essential for replacement therapy (15).
LACTATION: Insufficient reliable information available; avoid using unless essential for replacement therapy (15).

Effectiveness

EFFECTIVE ...when used orally as replacement therapy in pancreatic insufficiency due to cystic fibrosis, chronic pancreatitis, or pancreas removal (14,15).
INEFFECTIVE ...when used to treat digestive disorders not related to pancreatic insufficiency, including flatulence (15,16).

Possible Mechanism of Action & Active Ingredients

Pancreatin contains digestive enzymes, principally lipase, protease, and amylase obtained from pork or beef pancreas (14,15). These enzymes catalyze the hydrolysis of fat into glycerol and fatty acids; peptides into proteoses, peptides, and derived substances; and starches into dextrins and sugars (14). They act principally in the duodenum and small intestine (14). Pancreatin is inactivated when acid, including gastric acid, is present in more than trace amounts (15).

Adverse Reactions Including Known Allergies

Excessive doses of pancreatin can cause nausea, vomiting, diarrhea or other transient intestinal upset, and perianal soreness (14,15). Extremely high doses have been associated with high uric acid level in blood and urine, and colon strictures (14,15). Pancreatin preparations that are held in the mouth prior to swallowing can cause irritation of the mucosa, including ulceration and stomatitis (15). Pancreatin powder is irritating to the skin, eyes, mucus membranes, and respiratory tract. Skin contact with or inhalation of the powder should be avoided (14). Hypersensitivity reactions, e.g. sneezing, lacrimation, skin rash, have been reported (14,15). Inhalation of dust containing pancreatin has been associated with pulmonary hypersensitivity reactions, allergic rhinitis, bronchospasm, and asthma (14).

Possible Interactions with Herbs & Other Dietary Supplements

FOLIC ACID: Pancreatin can decrease absorption of folic acid (14).

Possible Interactions with Drugs

ACARBOSE (Precose): Enzymes present in pancreatin can decrease the efficacy of acarbose (14).
GASTRIC ACID INHIBITORS: Pancreatin activity ceases in gastric acid. For this reason, concomitant use of antacids, H-2 receptor antagonists, or other drugs that reduce stomach acidity can increase pancreatin activity (14).

Possible Interactions with Foods

ACIDIC FOODS: Concomitant intake of acidic foods or fruit juices can break down pancreatin enzymes, reducing the activity of pancreatin preparations that are not enteric-coated (14).
ALKALINE FOODS: Mixing enteric-coated granules into alkaline foods, e.g. chicken, veal, green beans, might destroy the coating (14).

Possible Interactions with Lab Tests

URIC ACID: Pancreatin can cause an increase in serum and urine uric acid levels (14).

Possible Interactions with Diseases or Conditions

No interactions are known to occur, and there is no known reason to expect a clinically significant interaction with pancreatin.

Typical Dosages & Routes of Administration that are Commonly Used

ORAL: For pancreatic replacement therapy, the initial dose of pancreatin is usually 8,000 to 24,000 USP units of lipase activity taken before or with each meal or snack. To control steatorrhea, dose can be increased as needed or until nausea, vomiting or diarrhea occurs (15). Pancreatin is available as enteric-coated tablets; powder; or capsules containing powder or enteric-coated granules (14). The powder or contents of the capsules can be mixed with food prior to administration, but should not be allowed to stand for more than an hour (14).

Comments

Each mg of pancreatin contains not less than 25 USP units of amylase activity, not less than 2 USP units of lipase activity, and not less than 25 USP units of protease activity (15,16). Pancreatin that is more potent is labeled as a multiple of these three minimum activities, e.g. pancreatin 4X (10,16).

PANGAMIC ACID

This Product is Also Known As

Calcium Chloride, Calcium Gluconate, Calcium Pangamate, Dicalcium Phosphate, Di-isopropylamine Dichloroacetate, Dimethyl Glycine, Dimethylglycine, DMG, Gluconic Acid, Glycine, Pangamate, Russian Formula, Sodium Gluconate, Vitamin B15.
CAUTION: See separate listing for Dimethylglycine.

Scientific Names

None.

People Use This For

Orally, pangamic acid is used for detoxifying the body, treating asthma and allied diseases, conditions of the skin and respiratory tract, painful nerve and joint afflictions, cell proliferation like cancer, eczema, arthritis, neuritis, and improving the oxygenation of the heart, brain, and other vital organs (5). It is also used for alcoholism, hangovers, fatigue, protecting against urban air pollutants, extending cell life, stimulating increased immune system response, lowering blood cholesterol levels, and assisting in hormone regulation (2643).

Safety

POSSIBLY UNSAFE ...when taken orally (5,2623). There is no standard chemical identity for pangamic acid. Dichloroacetate, present in some formulations, is mutagenic, possibly carcinogenic. Dimethylglycine, present in some formulations, can react with nitrites in the intestines to form the potent carcinogen, dimethylnitrosamine (5).
PREGNANCY AND LACTATION: POSSIBLY UNSAFE; avoid using because it is difficult to know what constituents are present. Dichloroacetate, present in some formulations, is mutagenic according to the Ames test (5).

Effectiveness

POSSIBLY INEFFECTIVE ...when taken orally for improving exercise endurance (2645).
There is insufficient reliable information available about the effectiveness of pangamic acid for its other uses.

Possible Mechanism of Action & Active Ingredients

There is no standard chemical identity for pangamic acid. Formulations can include one or more of the following: sodium gluconate, calcium gluconate, glycine, diisopropylamine dichloroacetate, dimethylglycine, calcium chloride, dicalcium phosphate, stearic acid, cellulose, or other constituents (5). Diisopropylamine acts on the smooth muscle to reduce blood pressure (5). In the intestines, dimethylglycine reacts with nitrates to form the potent carcinogen, dimethylnitrosamine (5). The high phosphate content of dicalcium phosphate has been blamed for upper gastrointestinal lesions and deaths in experimental animals (2644).

Adverse Reactions Including Known Allergies

Pangamic acid can be potentially carcinogenic (2622).

Possible Interactions with Herbs & Other Dietary Supplements

CARDIAC GLYCOSIDE-CONTAINING HERBS: Theoretically, concomitant use of these herbs with large amounts of calcium salts, including calcium chloride and dicalcium phosphate, can increase the inotropic effects of cardiac glycosides and the risk of arrhythmias. Cardiac glycoside-containing herbs include black hellebore (19), Canadian hemp roots (19), digitalis leaf (500), figwort (4), lily of the valley roots (19,500), motherwort (4) oleander leaf (19), pheasant's eye plant (2,19), pleurisy root (19), squill bulb leaf scales (19,500), and strophanthus seeds (19).

Possible Interactions with Drugs

DIGOXIN: Theoretically, concomitant use of digoxin with large amounts of calcium salts, such as calcium chloride and dicalcium phosphate, can increase the inotropic effects of digoxin and the risk of arrhythmias (15).
THIAZIDE DIURETICS: Theoretically, concomitant use of these diuretics with calcium salts like calcium chloride and dicalcium phosphate can result in hypercalcemia (15).
VERAPAMIL: Theoretically, concomitant use of verapamil with calcium salts, including calcium chloride and dicalcium phosphate, can decrease the drug's effects (506).

Possible Interactions with Foods

No interactions are known to occur, and there is no known reason to expect a clinically significant interaction with pangamic acid.

Possible Interactions with Lab Tests

No interactions are known to occur, and there is no known reason to expect a clinically significant interaction with pangamic acid.

Possible Interactions with Diseases or Conditions

KIDNEY DYSFUNCTION: Use pangamic acid with caution, because it can cause oxalate stones and other kidney problems (5).

Typical Dosages & Routes of Administration that are Commonly Used

No typical dosage.

Comments

Avoid the use of pangamic acid because it is possibly unsafe. There is no standard chemical identity for pangamic acid. Pangamic acid is the name given to a product originally claimed to contain D-gluconodimethyl aminoacetic acid, which was obtained from apricot kernels and later from rice bran (5,14). The name pangamic acid comes from the Greek: pan = universal, and gamic = seed, due to its presence in almost all seeds (14). It is also referred to as vitamin B15, but pangamic acid is not generally recognized as a vitamin (2623). Research by Soviet sports scientists focused attention on pangamic acid (2643), but little, if any, research has been conducted in the US (2643). The claims of pangamic acid's effectiveness are controversial (5). Natural sources for D-gluconodimethyl aminoacetic acid include brewer's yeast, whole brown rice, sesame seeds, and pumpkin seeds (2643).

PANTOTHENIC ACID (VITAMIN B5)

This Product is Also Known As

Calcii Pantothenas, Calcium Pantothenate, D-Calcium Pantothenate, Dexpanthenol, Dexpanthenolum, D-Panthenol, D-Pantothenyl Alcohol, Pantothenol, Pantothenylol.

Scientific Names

Pantothenic acid; D-pantothenic acid.

People Use This For

Orally, pantothenic acid and calcium pantothenate are used for treating dietary deficiencies, acne, alcoholism, allergies, alopecia, asthma, autism, burning feet syndrome, candidiasis, cardiac failure, carpal tunnel syndrome, catarrhal respiratory disorders, celiac disease, colitis, conjunctivitis, convulsions, and cystitis. They are used for dandruff, depression, diabetic neuropathy, enhancing immune function, glossitis, gray hair, headache, hyperactivity, hypoglycemia, insomnia, irritability, low blood pressure, multiple sclerosis, muscular dystrophy, muscular cramps in the legs associated with pregnancy or alcoholism, neuralgia, and obesity. They are used for osteoarthritis, rheumatoid arthritis, Parkinson's Disease, peripheral neuritis, premenstrual syndrome, prostatitis, protection against mental and physical stress, psychiatric states, reducing adverse effects of thyroid therapy in congenital hypothyroidism, reducing aging, reducing susceptibility to colds and other infections, retarded growth, shingles, skin disorders, stimulating adrenal glands, stomatitis, chronic fatigue, salicylate toxicity, streptomycin neurotoxicity, vertigo, and wound healing (14,15,3079,3080,3081).
Topically, dexpanthenol, the alcohol analog of pantothenic acid, is used for itching, promoting healing of mild eczemas and dermatoses, insect stings, bites, poison ivy, diaper rash, and acne (14,15).

Intramuscularly or by intravenous infusion, dexpanthenol is used for stimulating intestinal peristalsis, to minimize the possibility of paralytic ileus after major abdominal surgery, for intestinal atony causing abdominal distension, postoperative or postpartum flatus, for postoperative delay in resumption of intestinal motility, and for treating paralytic ileus (14,15).

Safety

LIKELY SAFE ...when used orally and appropriately. Amounts up to 10 grams have been ingested without adverse effects (14,15). ...when used topically and appropriately short-term (14). Dexpanthenol (alcohol analog of pantothenic acid) injection is a FDA-approved prescription drug.
PREGNANCY: LIKELY SAFE ...when used orally at the recommended daily intake of 6 mg (3094). Avoid larger amounts, although no maternal or fetal complications associated with pantothenic acid have been reported (3071).
LACTATION: LIKELY SAFE ...when used orally at the recommended daily intake of 7 mg (3094); avoid larger amounts.

Effectiveness

EFFECTIVE ...when used orally to treat vitamin B5 deficiency (14). Dexpanthenol (alcohol analog of pantothenic acid) injection is a FDA-approved prescription drug.
There is insufficient reliable information available about the effectiveness of pantothenic acid for its other uses.

Possible Mechanism of Action & Active Ingredients

Pantothenic acid is required for intermediary metabolism of carbohydrates, proteins and lipids (15). It is a precursor of coenzyme A which is required for acetylation reactions in gluconeogenesis, in the release of energy from carbohydrates, the synthesis and degradation of fatty acids, and the synthesis of sterols, steroid hormones, porphyrins, acetylcholine and other compounds (15). Pantothenic acid also appears to be essential to normal epithelial function (15). Dietary deficiency of pantothenic acid has not been identified, but experimentally-induced deficiency has been associated with somnolence, fatigue, headache, paresthesia of the hands and feet followed by hyperreflexia and muscle weakness in the legs, cardiovascular instability, GI complaints, changes in disposition, and increased susceptibility to infections (15). Dexpanthenol is converted in the body to pantothenic acid, then coenzyme A which is a cofactor in acetylcholine synthesis. In large parenteral doses, dexpanthenol has been reported to increase gastrointestinal peristalsis by stimulating acetylation of choline to acetylcholine, but efficacy has not been proven (14,15). Some evidence suggests that dexpanthenol stimulates fibroblast proliferation and epithelialization (14).

Adverse Reactions Including Known Allergies

Large amounts of oral pantothenic acid can cause diarrhea (14). Topical use of the alcohol analog, dexpanthenol can cause chronic dermatitis (14).

Possible Interactions with Herbs & Other Dietary Supplements

Insufficient reliable information available.

Possible Interactions with Drugs

PARASYMPATHOMIMETICS: Theoretically, administration of dexpanthenol, the alcohol analog of pantothenic acid, within 12 hours after administration of parasympathomimetics, e.g. neostigmine, might cause additive effects (15). Theoretically, this interaction might also occur with pantothenic acid and calcium pantothenate.
ANTICHOLINESTERASE EYE DROPS: Dexpanthenol, might potentiate the miotic effects of echothiophate iodide or isoflurophate eye drops but the clinical significance is not known (15).

Drug Influences on Nutrient Levels and Depletion

SOME DRUGS CAN AFFECT PANTOTHENIC ACID LEVELS:
ANTIBIOTICS: Destruction of normal gastrointestinal flora by antibiotics can cause decreased production of B vitamins. The clinical significance of this decreased production is not known. Consider supplementation only if clinical judgment warrants it (4434,4435,4436,4437,4438,4439,4440,4441,4442,4443).

Possible Interactions with Foods

No interactions are known to occur, and there is no known reason to expect a clinically significant interaction with pantothenic acid.

Possible Interactions with Lab Tests

No interactions are known to occur, and there is no known reason to expect a clinically significant interaction with pantothenic acid.

Possible Interactions with Diseases or Conditions

HEMOPHILIA: CAUTION, dexpanthenol (alcohol analog of pantothenic acid) may prolong bleeding time (15).
GI OBSTRUCTION: Dexpanthenol (alcohol analog of pantothenic acid) injection is contraindicated in individuals with gastrointestinal obstruction (15).

Typical Dosages & Routes of Administration that are Commonly Used

ORAL: As a dietary supplement, 5-10 mg pantothenic acid (15). Recommended daily intakes for vitamin B5 are as follows; Infants 0-6 months, 1.7 mg; Infants 7-12 months, 1.8 mg; Children 1-3 years, 2 mg; Children 4-8

years, 3 mg; Children 9-13 years, 4 mg; Men and women 14 years and older, 5 mg (3094); Pregnant women, 6 mg; and Lactating women, 7 mg (3094).
TOPICAL: Dexpanthenol 2% cream applied to the affected areas once or twice daily (15). Dexpanthenol is the alcohol analog of pantothenic acid.
INJECTION: Dexpanthenol for injection is a FDA-approved prescription drug.

Comments
Only the dextrorotatory isomer of pantothenic acid has biologic activity (15). Vitamin B5 is commercially available as D-pantothenic acid and the synthetic derivatives, dexpanthenol and calcium pantothenate (15). Pantothenic acid is widely distributed in plant and animal tissues; rich sources include meat, vegetables, cereal grains, legumes, eggs, and milk (15). Calcium pantothenate 10 mg is equivalent to pantothenic acid 9.2 mg (15). Pantothenic acid is frequently used in combination with other B vitamins in vitamin B complex formulations. Vitamin B complex generally includes vitamin B1 (thiamine), vitamin B2 (riboflavin), vitamin B3 (niacin/niacinamide), vitamin B5 (pantothenic acid), vitamin B6 (pyridoxine), vitamin B12 (cyanocobalamin), and folic acid. However, some products do not contain all of these ingredients and some may include others, such as biotin, para-aminobenzoic acid (PABA), choline bitartrate, and inositol (3022,3060,3061).

PAPAIN

This Product is Also Known As
Papainum Crudum, Plant Protease Concentrate, Vegetable Pepsin.
CAUTION: See separate listings for Bromelain, Papaya, and American Pawpaw.

Scientific Names
Carica papaya.
Family: Caricacea.

People Use This For
Orally, papain is used as a digestive aid, for controlling edema and inflammation following trauma and surgery, for treating parasitic worms (2), inflammation of the throat and pharynx (964,968,969), herpes zoster symptoms (965), chronic diarrhea, tumors, hay fever, nasal drainage, and psoriasis.
Topically, it is used to treat infected wounds, sores, and ulcers (11).
In manufacturing, papain is a component of cosmetics, dentifrices, enzymatic soft contact lens cleaners, meat tenderizers, and meat products. It is also used for stabilizing and chillproofing beer (11).

Safety
LIKELY SAFE ...when consumed in amounts commonly found in foods (11). Papain has Generally Recognized as Safe (GRAS) status in the US (11).
POSSIBLY SAFE ...when used orally and appropriately for medicinal purposes (6).
POSSIBLY UNSAFE ...when used orally in large amounts; it may cause esophageal perforation (6) ...when used topically; papaya latex (raw papain) is a severe irritant and vesicant (6).
PREGNANCY: POSSIBLY UNSAFE; avoid using. Crude papain is teratogenic and embryotoxic in rats (6); however, this may be due to extraneous substances rather than the papain (11).
LACTATION: Insufficient reliable information available; avoid using.

Effectiveness
POSSIBLY EFFECTIVE ...when used orally in combination with other agents for treating inflammation and swelling in pharyngitis (964,968,969), and for treating symptoms of herpes zoster (965).
LIKELY INEFFECTIVE ...when used as a vermifuge (2).
There is insufficient reliable information available about the effectiveness of papain for its other uses.

Possible Mechanism of Action & Active Ingredients
Papain is a mixture of the proteolytic enzymes papain, chymopapain A, chymopapain B, papaya peptidase A. Chymopapain A and B have a similar proteolytic spectrum to papain but are less potent (6). A poly-enzyme preparation containing papain was found to increase release of reactive oxygen species by polymorphonuclear cells in healthy people (962).

Adverse Reactions Including Known Allergies
Taken orally, large amounts of papain can cause esophageal perforation (6). Ingestion of papaya latex can cause severe gastritis (6). Topical use of papain can cause itching (966). Papaya latex can cause severe irritation and blisters (6). Severe allergic reactions have been reported in sensitive individuals (6,967). One case report suggests cross-sensitivity between papain, fig, and kiwi (963).

Possible Interactions with Herbs & Other Dietary Supplements
HERBS WITH ANTICOAGULANT/ANTIPLATELET POTENTIAL: Concomitant use of herbs that have coumarin constituents or affect platelet aggregation could theoretically increase the risk of bleeding in some

people. These herbs include: angelica, anise, arnica, asafoetida, bogbean, boldo, capsicum, celery, chamomile, clove, danshen, fenugreek, feverfew, garlic, ginger, ginkgo, ginseng (Panax), horse chestnut, horseradish, licorice, meadowsweet, prickly ash, onion, passionflower, poplar, quassia, red clover, turmeric, wild carrot, wild lettuce, willow, and others (4,19).

Possible Interactions with Drugs

ANTICOAGULANT, ANTIPLATELET DRUGS: Theoretically, concomitant use may increase risk of bleeding. There is one case report of increased International Normalization Ratio (INR) associated with concomitant use of warfarin and papaya extract (papain) (613).

Possible Interactions with Foods

POTATO PROTEIN: May inhibit papain proteolytic activity (958).
FIG, KIWI: Cross sensitivity to papain may occur in individuals sensitive to fig and kiwi (963).

Possible Interactions with Lab Tests

INTERNATIONAL NORMALIZATION RATIO (INR): Concomitant use of papaya extract (papain) and warfarin may increase INR (613).

Possible Interactions with Diseases or Conditions

CLOTTING DISORDERS: Avoid; theoretically, may increase bleeding risk (2).

Typical Dosages & Routes of Administration that are Commonly Used

ORAL: 1500 mg (2520 FIP units) per day used in clinical trials to treat inflammation and swelling following trauma and surgery (2). No typical dosage for the other uses.
TOPICAL: No typical dosage.

Comments

Proteolytic enzyme mixture (papain, chymopapain A, chymopapain B, papaya peptidase A) isolated from the latex of the unripe fruit of Carica papaya.

PAPAYA

This Product is Also Known As

Caricae papayae folium, Mamaerie, Melonenbaumblaetter, Melon Tree, Papaw.
CAUTION: See separate listings for Papain and American Pawpaw.

Scientific Names

Carica papaya.
Family: Caricaceae.

People Use This For

In folk medicine, papaya leaf is used orally for preventing and treating gastrointestinal tract disorders, intestinal parasite infections, and as sedative and diuretic (2). In folk medicine, papaya leaf is used topically for nervous pains and elephantoid growths (4009).

Safety

LIKELY SAFE ...when consumed in amounts commonly found in foods (11). Papaya has Generally Recognized as Safe (GRAS) status in the US (11).
POSSIBLY SAFE ...when used orally and appropriately (6).
POSSIBLY UNSAFE ...when large amounts are ingested orally. Can cause esophageal perforation (6). ...when used topically because papaya latex (raw papain) is a severe irritant and vesicant (6).
PREGNANCY: POSSIBLY UNSAFE ...when used orally; avoid using. Crude papain shows evidence that it is teratogenic and embryotoxic (6); however, this might be due to extraneous substances rather than papain (11).
LACTATION: Insufficient reliable information available; avoid using.

Effectiveness

There is insufficient reliable information available about the effectiveness of papaya leaf.

Possible Mechanism of Action & Active Ingredients

The applicable part of papaya is the leaf. Papaya leaf contains 2% papain and carpain (6). Papain is a mixture of enzymes that degrade protein, carbohydrates, and fats (515). Papain is unstable in digestive juices, which raises questions about whether it can be effective when used orally (515). Carpain is thought to be amebicidal. It might cause bradycardia (4009) or have central nervous system depressant or paralytic effects (4017).

Adverse Reactions Including Known Allergies

Ingestion of large amounts of papain might cause esophageal perforation. Severe allergic reactions can occur in individuals sensitive to papain (6,515).

Possible Interactions with Herbs & Other Dietary Supplements
PAPAIN: Concomitant use of papain and papaya can increase the effects and adverse effects of papain.

Possible Interactions with Drugs
WARFARIN: Concomitant use might potentiate the effects of warfarin (Coumadin) increasing the international normalization ratio (INR) (613).

Possible Interactions with Foods
No interactions are known to occur, and there is no known reason to expect a clinically significant interaction with papaya.

Possible Interactions with Lab Tests
INTERNATIONAL NORMALIZATION RATIO (INR): Papain, which is in papaya leaf, can increase INR in people maintained on warfarin (Coumadin) (613).

Possible Interactions with Diseases or Conditions
No interactions are known to occur, and there is no known reason to expect a clinically significant interaction with papaya.

Typical Dosages & Routes of Administration that are Commonly Used
ORAL: People typically use papaya with enzyme chewable tablets which contain 250 mg of papaya powder, 150 mg of dried pineapple juice powder, and 10 mg of papain (5024). One tablet is chewed up to three times daily, preferably after a meal (5024).

Comments
Fermenting papaya leaves may make more potent, richer brewed teas (515).

PAREIRA

This Product is Also Known As
Ice Vine, Pereira Brava, Velvet Leaf.
CAUTION: See separate listing for Abuta.

Scientific Names
Chondrodendron tomentosum.
Family: Menispermaceae.

People Use This For
Orally, pareira is used as a diuretic and to promote menstruation (18).
Parenterally, the component tubocurarine is used as a neuromuscular blocking agent (18,505).

Safety
There is insufficient reliable information available about the safety of pareira.
PREGNANCY: UNSAFE ...contraindicated because it may promote menstruation (19).
LACTATION: Insufficient reliable information available; avoid using.

Effectiveness
There is insufficient reliable information available about the effectiveness of pareira.

Possible Mechanism of Action & Active Ingredients
The applicable part of pareira is the root. Pareira contains tubocurarine, which is used in modern anesthetics. It competitively inhibits acetylcholine binding at the nicotinic receptors at the neuromuscular junction, resulting in skeletal muscle paralysis. Tubocurarine and the other curare-like alkaloids contained in pareira are quaternary alkaloids and carry a positive charge that is not altered by pH. For this reason, they are poorly absorbed when taken orally and therefore have little neuromuscular blocking activity (505).

Adverse Reactions Including Known Allergies
None reported when pareira is used orally (18). Tubocurarine can cause hypotension due to histamine release and ganglionic blockade if IV administrations is too rapid. The histamine release can also cause increased salivation, and bronchospasm. The ganglionic blockade can cause decreased GI motility and tone. Tubocurarine can also cause allergic reactions in susceptible patients (15).

Possible Interactions with Herbs & Other Dietary Supplements
Insufficient reliable information available.

Possible Interactions with Drugs
No interactions are known to occur, and there is no known reason to expect a clinically significant interaction with pareira.

Possible Interactions with Foods

No interactions are known to occur, and there is no known reason to expect a clinically significant interaction with pareira.

Possible Interactions with Lab Tests

No interactions are known to occur, and there is no known reason to expect a clinically significant interaction with pareira.

Possible Interactions with Diseases or Conditions

No interactions are known to occur, and there is no known reason to expect a clinically significant interaction with pareira.

Typical Dosages & Routes of Administration that are Commonly Used

ORAL: No typical dosage.
PARENTERAL: No typical dosage.

Comments

Tubocurarine, a constituent of pareira, is unsafe for parenteral self-medication (15,505).

PARSLEY leaf, root

This Product is Also Known As

Common Parsley, Garden Parsley, Hamburg Parsley, Persely, Persil, Petersylinge, Petroselini herba, Petrosilini radix, Rock Parsley.
CAUTION: See separate listings for Fool's Parsley, Parsley Piert, and Parsley seed.

Scientific Names

Petroselinum crispum, synonym Apium petroselinum; Carum petroselinum; Petroselinum hortense; Petroselinum sativum.
Family: Apiaceae or Umbelliferae.

People Use This For

Orally, parsley is used as a breath freshener, for urinary tract infections, and kidney or bladder stones (2,11,18). Topically, parsley is used for cracked or chapped skin (11), bruises, tumors, insect bites, lice, parasites, and to stimulate hair growth (6).
Traditionally, parsley has been used for gastrointestinal disorders (6,18), constipation (6), jaundice (6,18), flatulence, indigestion, colic, bronchitic cough (4,6,11), asthma, general edema, rheumatism (11), anemia, hypotension, diseases of the prostate, liver and spleen, and to promote menstrual flow (4,6,11,18). It has also been used as an aphrodisiac (6). In foods and beverages, parsley is widely used as a garnish, condiment, food, and as a flavoring (11).

Safety

LIKELY SAFE ...when used orally in amounts used in foods. Parsley has Generally Recognized as Safe (GRAS) status in the US (11).
POSSIBLY SAFE ...when parsley is used orally and appropriately in amounts larger than those found in foods (2,12).
LIKELY UNSAFE ...when parsley is used orally in very large amounts (i.e. 200 grams) the apiole constituent could cause toxicity. Apiole can cause blood dyscrasias, kidney and liver toxicity (4). ...when parsley oil is ingested orally due to the amount of the potentially toxic constituents apiole and myristicin in oil (2,11). Myristicin can cause giddiness and hallucinations (4).
There is insufficient reliable information available about the safety of the topical use of parsley.
PREGNANCY: LIKELY SAFE ...when parsley is used in food amounts. LIKELY UNSAFE ...when larger amounts are used due to potential abortifacient, uterine or menstrual flow stimulant effects (4,12,515).
LACTATION: Insufficient reliable information available; avoid using.

Effectiveness

POSSIBLY EFFECTIVE ...when used orally for preventing and treating kidney stones (2).
There is insufficient reliable information available about the effectiveness of parsley leaf and root for other uses.

Possible Mechanism of Action & Active Ingredients

Parsley contains a volatile oil, carotene, vitamin B1, vitamin B2, and vitamin C (515). The volatile oil contains apiole, myristicin, and photosensitizing furanocoumarins (psoralens) (512); however, the amounts vary significantly among varieties of parsley (512). Parsley has antiflatulent, antispasmodic, antirheumatic, expectorant, antimicrobial (4), and aquaretic effects (6,18,512). Aquaretics increase urine volume (water loss) but not sodium excretion (512). The constituent apiole appears to be associated with antispasmodic, vasodilator, and menstrual flow-stimulant effects. Apiole can also increase smooth muscle contractibility in the bladder and intestines (11). Both the apiole and myristicin constituents are believed to have aquaretic and uterine stimulant effects (512). The mechanism of aquaresis is that parsley irritates the kidney epithelium which increases renal blood flow and glomerular filtration rate (512). Apiole and myristicin have a structure similar to safrole. Safrole is considered carcinogenic and hepatotoxic (4).

Adverse Reactions Including Known Allergies

Parsley can occasionally cause allergic skin or mucous membrane reactions (2). Adverse effects specifically associated with more than 10 grams of the constituent, apiole, include hemolytic anemia, thrombocytopenia purpura, nephrosis, hepatic dysfunction, and kidney irritation (4). Adverse effects specifically associated with the constituent, myristicin, include giddiness, deafness, hallucinations, hypotension, bradycardia, paralysis, fatty degeneration of the liver and kidneys (4). Parsley oil can cause contact photodermatitis with sun exposure (4).

Possible Interactions with Herbs & Other Dietary Supplements

Insufficient reliable information available.

Possible Interactions with Drugs

ANTICOAGULANTS: Theoretically, large amounts of parsley might interfere with oral anticoagulant therapy, due to the vitamin K contained in parsley (19).
ASPIRIN: Concomitant intake might augment parsley allergy. One case is reported of severe urticaria and swelling in a person with a known mild parsley allergy after consuming parsley and aspirin (5054).
DIURETICS: Theoretically, parsley might interfere with diuretic therapy by enhancing sodium retention (512).
MAOIs: Theoretically, concomitant use of large amounts of parsley or parsley oil might potentiate monoamine oxidase inhibitor drug therapy, due to the myristicin contained in parsley (4).

Possible Interactions with Foods

No interactions are known to occur, and there is no known reason to expect a clinically significant interaction with parsley leaf and root.

Possible Interactions with Lab Tests

No interactions are known to occur, and there is no known reason to expect a clinically significant interaction with parsley leaf and root.

Possible Interactions with Diseases or Conditions

EDEMA: Theoretically, parsley might increase sodium retention and worsen edema (512).
HYPERTENSION: Theoretically, parsley might increase sodium retention and worsen hypertension (512).
KIDNEY DISEASE: Contraindicated in individuals with kidney disease or inflammation. Parsley can aggravate these conditions (4,19).

Typical Dosages & Routes of Administration that are Commonly Used

ORAL: A typical dose for use as a mild diuretic is one cup tea two to three times daily. To make tea, steep 2 grams finely chopped dried root in 150 mL boiling water 10-15 minutes, strain (8). Maximum daily dose is 6 grams root/leaf (2). When used to flush the kidneys, large amounts of water should be consumed (2).

Comments

None.

PARSLEY PIERT

This Product is Also Known As

Field Lady's Mantle, Parsley Breakstone, Parsley Piercestone.
CAUTION: See separate listings for Fool's Parsley, Parsley leaf, root and Parsley seed.

Scientific Names

Aphanes arvensis.
Family: Rosaceae.

People Use This For

Orally, parsley piert is used for reducing fever, urinary tract disorders such as kidney and bladder stones, and as a diuretic (18).

Safety

There is insufficient reliable information available about the safety of parsley piert.
Pregnancy and Lactation: Insufficient reliable information available; avoid using.

Effectiveness

There is insufficient reliable information available about the effectiveness of parsley piert.

Possible Mechanism of Action & Active Ingredients

The applicable parts of parsley piert are the above ground parts. There is insufficient reliable information available about the possible mechanism of action and active ingredients of parsley piert.

Adverse Reactions Including Known Allergies

None reported.

Possible Interactions with Herbs & Other Dietary Supplements

Insufficient reliable information available.

Possible Interactions with Drugs

No interactions are known to occur, and there is no known reason to expect a clinically significant interaction with parsley piert.

Possible Interactions with Foods

No interactions are known to occur, and there is no known reason to expect a clinically significant interaction with parsley piert.

Possible Interactions with Lab Tests

No interactions are known to occur, and there is no known reason to expect a clinically significant interaction with parsley piert.

Possible Interactions with Diseases or Conditions

No interactions are known to occur, and there is no known reason to expect a clinically significant interaction with parsley piert.

Typical Dosages & Routes of Administration that are Commonly Used

ORAL: People typically prepare parsley piert as a tea with 1 to 2 teaspoons of the dried herb added to 1 cup boiling water. The usual dose is 3 cups per day. In tincture form, the usual dose is 2 to 4 mL three times daily (5253).

Comments

Avoid confusion with parsley (Petroselinum crispum) and fool's parsley (Aethusa cynapium).
There is very little scientific information about this product. Our staff is continually analyzing the available information on natural medicines and will add data here as it becomes available.

PARSLEY seed

This Product is Also Known As

Common Parsley, Garden Parsley, Parsley Fruit, Persil, Petroselini fructus.
CAUTION: See separate listing for Fool's Parsley, Parsley leaf, root and Parsley Piert.

Scientific Names

Petroselinum crispum, synonym Apium petroselinum; Carum petroselinum; Petroselinum hortense; Petroselinum sativum.
Family: Apiaceae or Umbelliferae.

People Use This For

Orally, parsley seed is used for ailments of the gastrointestinal tract and urinary tract (2,18), stimulating appetite and improving digestion, treating flatulence, and stimulating menstrual flow (515).
Traditionally, parsley seed has been used orally for inducing abortion (11,515), treating jaundice, menstrual difficulties, asthma, coughs, indigestion, and edema (11).
In foods, parsley seed oil is used as a flavoring (11).
In manufacturing, parsley seed oil is used as a fragrance in soaps, cosmetics, and perfumes (11).

Safety

LIKELY SAFE ...when used orally in amounts found in foods.
POSSIBLY UNSAFE ...when parsley seed is used in tea. The volatile oil of parsley has toxic constituents, and the tea might have a low volatile oil content (2).
LIKELY UNSAFE ...when parsley seed or seed oil is used in amounts greater than found in foods. The volatile oil constituent has been associated with renal epithelium irritation and cardiac arrhythmias (2). ...when parsley seed oil is used topically, it can cause photodermatitis upon sun exposure (4).
PREGNANCY: LIKELY UNSAFE ...contraindicated (2,19). Might have abortifacient, uterine, and menstrual flow-stimulating effects (4,515).
LACTATION: Insufficient reliable information available; avoid using.

Effectiveness

There is insufficient reliable information available about the effectiveness of parsley seed.

Possible Mechanism of Action & Active Ingredients

It is thought that parsley seed's effects can cause mild aquaresis, stimulate appetite, and improve digestion, as a result of the volatile oil content (515). Aquaretics increase urine volume (water loss) but not sodium excretion (512). The constituent apiole is thought to be responsible for antispasmodic, vasodilator, and menstrual flow-stimulant effects. Apiole can increase smooth muscle contractibility in the bladder and intestines (11). Both the apiole and myristicin constituents are believed to have aquaretic and uterine stimulant effects (512). Researchers think aquaretic effects of parsley result from irritation of the kidney epithelium that increases renal blood flow and glomerular filtration rate (512). Apiole and myristicin are documented to have a structure similar to safrole which is known to be carcinogenic and hepatotoxic (4). Parsley seed oil is reported to stimulate hepatic regeneration (4).

Adverse Reactions Including Known Allergies

Oral ingestion of parsley seed oil can cause renal damage and cardiac arrhythmias (2). Adverse effects specifically associated greater than 10 grams of the constituent apiole include hemolytic anemia, thrombocytopenia purpura, nephrosis, hepatic dysfunction, and kidney irritation (4). Adverse effects specifically associated with the constituent myristicin include giddiness, deafness, hallucinations, hypotension, bradycardia, paralysis, fatty degeneration of the liver and kidneys (4). External use of parsley seed oil can cause contact photodermatitis upon exposure to the sun (4).

Possible Interactions with Herbs & Other Dietary Supplements

Insufficient reliable information available.

Possible Interactions with Drugs

DIURETICS: Theoretically, parsley seed might increase sodium retention and interfere with diuretic therapy (512). MAOIs: Theoretically, concomitant use of large amounts of parsley seed or seed oil can potentiate monoamine oxidase inhibitor drug therapy due to the constituent myristicin (4).

Possible Interactions with Foods

No interactions are known to occur, and there is no known reason to expect a clinically significant interaction with parsley seed.

Possible Interactions with Lab Tests

No interactions are known to occur, and there is no known reason to expect a clinically significant interaction with parsley seed.

Possible Interactions with Diseases or Conditions

EDEMA: Theoretically, parsley seed might increase sodium retention and worsen edema (512). HYPERTENSION: Theoretically, parsley seed might increase sodium retention and worsen hypertension (512). KIDNEY DISEASE: Contraindicated in individuals with kidney disease or inflammation. Parsley can aggravate these conditions (4,19).

Typical Dosages & Routes of Administration that are Commonly Used

ORAL: A typical oral dose is one cup tea up to 2-3 times per day. To make tea, steep 1 gram of fresh crushed seed in 150 mL boiling water for 10 minutes, strain (18).

Comments

Parsley seed oil is distilled from the seeds of parsley (Petroselinum crispum).

PARSNIP above ground parts

This Product is Also Known As

Pastinacae herba.
CAUTION: See separate listing for Parsnip root.

Scientific Names

Pastinaca sativa.
Family: Apiaceae.

People Use This For

Orally, parsnip is used for digestive and kidney disorders (18).

Safety

There is insufficient reliable information available about the safety of the above ground parts of parsnip.
Pregnancy and Lactation: Insufficient reliable information available; avoid using.

Effectiveness

There is insufficient reliable information available about the effectiveness of the above ground parts of parsnip.

Possible Mechanism of Action & Active Ingredients

Parsnip contains furocoumarins angelicin, bergapten, xanthotoxin and psoralen. Furocoumarins are phototoxic and mutagenic (2), photosensitizing and are responsible for adverse dermatological reactions (6,11,19,515).

Adverse Reactions Including Known Allergies

Contact dermatitis and phototoxic reactions (including skin blisters) are possible following topical exposure to fresh parsnip plant and exposure to sunlight (6). Light-skinned people may be particularly susceptible to these reactions (18).

Possible Interactions with Herbs & Other Dietary Supplements

Insufficient reliable information available.

Possible Interactions with Drugs

No interactions are known to occur, and there is no known reason to expect a clinically significant interaction with parsnip above ground parts.

Possible Interactions with Foods

No interactions are known to occur, and there is no known reason to expect a clinically significant interaction with parsnip above ground parts.

Possible Interactions with Lab Tests

No interactions are known to occur, and there is no known reason to expect a clinically significant interaction with parsnip above ground parts.

Possible Interactions with Diseases or Conditions

No interactions are known to occur, and there is no known reason to expect a clinically significant interaction with parsnip above ground parts.

Typical Dosages & Routes of Administration that are Commonly Used

ORAL: Eight ounces (240 mL) of tea taken orally three times daily for the first 8 days, and then 360 mL is taken orally daily. The daily dose may be increased to as much as 2 L daily, and is taken for a total of 4-6 weeks. The tea is prepared by simmering one handful of dried herb in 1 L of boiling water for 10 minutes and straining (18).

Comments

There is very little scientific information about this product. Our staff is continually analyzing the available information on natural medicines and will add data here as it becomes available.

PARSNIP root

This Product is Also Known As

Pastinacae Radix.
CAUTION: See separate listings for Parsnip above ground parts.

Scientific Names

Pastinaca sativa.
Family: Apiaceae.

People Use This For

Orally, parsnip root is used for kidney complaints, fever, and as an analgesic and a diuretic (18).

Safety

LIKELY SAFE ... when used orally and appropriately in food amounts (18).
There is insufficient reliable information available about the safety of parsnip root when using greater than food amounts.
PREGNANCY AND LACTATION: LIKELY SAFE ...in food amounts. There is insufficient reliable information available for the safety of using larger amounts; avoid using.

Effectiveness

There is insufficient reliable information available about the effectiveness of parsnip.

Possible Mechanism of Action & Active Ingredients

Parsnip contains furocoumarins angelicin, bergapten, xanthotoxin and psoralen. Furocoumarins are phototoxic and mutagenic (2), photosensitizing and are responsible for adverse dermatological reactions (6,11,19,515).

Adverse Reactions Including Known Allergies

Contact dermatitis and phototoxic reactions (including skin blisters) are possible following topical exposure to fresh parsnip plant and exposure to sunlight (6). Light-skinned people may be particularly susceptible to these reactions (18).

Possible Interactions with Herbs & Other Dietary Supplements
Insufficient reliable information available.

Possible Interactions with Drugs
No interactions are known to occur, and there is no known reason to expect a clinically significant interaction with parsnip root.

Possible Interactions with Foods
No interactions are known to occur, and there is no known reason to expect a clinically significant interaction with parsnip root.

Possible Interactions with Lab Tests
No interactions are known to occur, and there is no known reason to expect a clinically significant interaction with parsnip root.

Possible Interactions with Diseases or Conditions
No interactions are known to occur, and there is no known reason to expect a clinically significant interaction with parsnip root.

Typical Dosages & Routes of Administration that are Commonly Used
ORAL: One teaspoon of freshly grated parsnip taken three times daily (18).

Comments
Parsnip root closely resembles and can be confused with the parsley root. Avoid confusing parsnip root with similar appearing hemlock and bear's breech (or hogweed) root, both of which are toxic (18).

PASSIONFLOWER

This Product is Also Known As
Apricot Vine, Corona De Cristo, Fleischfarbige, Fleur De La Passion, Flor De Passion, Madre Selva, Maypop, Maypop Passion Flower, Passiflora, Passiflorae herba, Passiflore, Passiflorina, Passion Flower, Passion Vine, Passionaria, Passionblume, Passionflower Herb, Passionsblumenkraut, Purple Passion Flower, Water Lemon, Wild Passion Flower.

Scientific Names
Passiflora incarnata.
Family: Passifloraceae.

People Use This For
Orally, the above ground parts of the passionflower are used for nervous restlessness (2), mild insomnia (1,18), and nervous GI complaints (18).
Topically, passionflower is used in bath preparations (11), for hemorrhoids, burns, and inflammation (6).
Traditionally, passionflower has been used orally for neuralgia, generalized seizures, hysteria, spasmodic asthma (4), climacteric symptoms, pediatric attention disorders, pediatric nervousness and excitability, palpitations, cardiac rhythm abnormalities, high blood pressure, and for pain relief.
In foods and beverages, the extract is used as a flavoring (11).

Safety
LIKELY SAFE ...when used orally in food amounts. Passionflower is approved for food use in the US. The maximum level of the extract used is 0.32% in nonalcoholic beverages (11).
POSSIBLY SAFE ...when used orally and appropriately for medicinal purposes (1,2,4,12).
POSSIBLY UNSAFE ...when used orally in excessive amounts (4).
There is insufficient reliable information available about the safety of the topical use of passionflower (4).
PREGNANCY: UNSAFE ...harman alkaloid constituents show evidence of uterine stimulation (4,6).
LACTATION: Insufficient reliable information available; avoid using.

Effectiveness
POSSIBLY EFFECTIVE...when taken orally for nervous restlessness (2). In a double-blind, placebo-controlled trial of 182 outpatients, a 6-ingredient combination product that included passionflower was statistically superior for relieving symptoms of adjustment disorder with anxious mood, as scored on the Hamilton Anxiety Rating Scale (6250). Other herbs in the product were crataegus, ballota, valerian, which have mild sedative effects, and cola and paullinia with stimulant properties (6250). ...when taken orally for mild insomnia (1).
There is insufficient reliable information available about the effectiveness of passionflower for its other uses.

Possible Mechanism of Action & Active Ingredients
The applicable parts of passionflower are the above ground parts. Passionflower has sedative, hypnotic (4,5), and antispasmodic effects (4,11). It also relieves pain (4). Some evidence suggests the passionflower constituent apigenin

© Copyright 2000, Natural Medicines Comprehensive Database (209) 472-2244. For updated data, go to www.NaturalDatabase.com • 805

binds to central benzodiazepine receptors (4001), possibly causing anxiolytic effects without impairing memory or motor skills (4001). Other evidence suggests passionflower extracts might reduce amphetamine-induced hypermotility, aggressiveness, and restlessness, and raise the pain threshold (1,4,11). Although animal data suggest the constituents maltol and ethylmaltol can reduce spontaneous motor activity, prolong barbiturate-induced sleep time, and show anticonvulsant activity (1,4), not enough maltol is found in passionflower preparations to cause these effects (1). The harman (harmala) alkaloids identified in passionflower include harmine, harmaline, harmalol, harman, and harmin (6). Some evidence suggests the harman alkaloids have central stimulant activity via a monoamine oxidase mechanism (4,4002); however, the sedative effects of maltol and ethylmaltol can mask these effects (4). The constituent passicol shows some evidence of antibacterial and antifungal activity (4). The experts do not agree about whether passionflower contains the cyanogenic glycoside gynocardine (3,11,19).

Adverse Reactions Including Known Allergies

Taken orally, passionflower can cause vasculitis and altered consciousness. This has been reported with use of an herbal product (Relaxir) produced mainly from the fruits of passionflower (6). A case report was recently published of toxicity in a 34-year-old woman following passionflower use at therapeutic doses (6251). The patient developed severe nausea, vomiting, drowsiness, prolonged QT interval, and episodes of nonsustained ventricular tachycardia, requiring hospitalization for IV hydration and cardiac monitoring (6251). Although there is disagreement about whether passionflower contains cyanogenic glycosides, several related Passiflora species do contain them (3), including Passiflora edulis, which is associated with liver and pancreas toxicity (7).

Possible Interactions with Herbs & Other Dietary Supplements

HERBS WITH SEDATIVE PROPERTIES: Theoretically, concomitant use with herbs that have sedative properties might enhance therapeutic and adverse effects. These include calamus, calendula, California poppy, catnip, capsicum, celery, couch grass, elecampane, Siberian ginseng , German chamomile, goldenseal, gotu kola, hops, Jamaican dogwood, kava, lemon balm, sage, St. John's wort, sassafras, scullcap, shepherd's purse, stinging nettle, valerian, wild carrot, wild lettuce, withania root, and yerba mansa (4,19).
HERBS WITH ANTICOAGULANT/ANTIPLATELET POTENTIAL: Concomitant use of herbs that have coumarin constituents or affect platelet aggregation could theoretically increase the risk of bleeding in some people. These herbs include: angelica, anise, arnica, asafoetida, bogbean, boldo, capsicum, celery, chamomile, clove, danshen, fenugreek, feverfew, garlic, ginger, ginkgo, ginseng (Panax), horse chestnut, horseradish, licorice, meadowsweet, prickly ash, onion, papain, poplar, quassia, red clover, turmeric, wild carrot, wild lettuce, willow, and others (4,19).

Possible Interactions with Drugs

MONOAMINE OXIDASE INHIBITORS (MAOIs): Theoretically, concomitant use of passionflower can potentiate MAOI activity (4).
BARBITURATES: Theoretically, concomitant use can increase drug-induced sleep time (1).
SEDATIVES, TRANQUILIZERS: Theoretically, concomitant use can potentiate the effects of these drugs, including the sedative effects of antihistamines (19).

Possible Interactions with Foods

No interactions are known to occur, and there is no known reason to expect a clinically significant interaction with passionflower.

Possible Interactions with Lab Tests

No interactions are known to occur, and there is no known reason to expect a clinically significant interaction with passionflower.

Possible Interactions with Diseases or Conditions

No interactions are known to occur, and there is no known reason to expect a clinically significant interaction with passionflower.

Typical Dosages & Routes of Administration that are Commonly Used

ORAL: The typical dose of passionflower is 0.25-2 grams of the dried above ground parts three times daily or one cup of the tea two to three times daily and 30 minutes before bedtime (1,4,18). The tea is prepared by steeping 0.25-2 grams of the dried above ground parts in 150 mL boiling water for 10-15 minutes and then straining. The average amount of passionflower is 4-8 grams per day. The usual dose of the liquid extract (1:1 in 25% alcohol) is 0.5-1.0 mL three times daily. The common dose of the tincture (1:8 in 45% alcohol) is 0.5-2 mL three times daily (4).
TOPICAL: Passionflower is typically used as a hemorrhoid rinse, which is prepared by simmering 20 grams of the dried above ground parts in 200 mL water, straining, and cooling before use (18).

Comments

In 1569, Spanish explorers discovered passionflower in Peru. They believed the flowers symbolized Christ's passion and indicated his approval for their exploration (6). Passionflower is found in combination herbal sedative products, some of which include German chamomile, hops, kava, scullcap, and valerian. Passionflower was formerly approved as an OTC sedative and sleep aid in the US, but it was taken off the market in 1978 because safety and effectiveness had not been proven (11,515).

PATCHOULY OIL

This Product is Also Known As
Patchouli, Patchouly, Putcha-Pat, Huo xiang.

Scientific Names
Pogostemon cablin, synonyms Pogostemon heyneanus, Pogostemon patchouly.
Family: Labiatae or Lamiaceae.

People Use This For
In Chinese medicine, patchouly oil is used orally for colds, headaches, nausea, vomiting, diarrhea, and abdominal pain. It is also used to treat bad breath, particularly when it is associated with alcohol ingestion. The leaf, fruit and flower are used to treat tumors (11).
In foods and beverages, patchouly oil is used as a flavor ingredient (11).
In manufacturing, patchouly oil is used in perfumes and cosmetics (18).

Safety
LIKELY SAFE ...in amounts found in foods. It is approved for use in foods, and the maximum use is 0.0002% (11). There is insufficient reliable information available about the safety of patchouly oil for its other uses.
PREGNANCY AND LACTATION: Insufficient reliable information available; avoid using in amounts greater than those typically found in foods.

Effectiveness
There is insufficient reliable information available about the effectiveness of patchouly oil.

Possible Mechanism of Action & Active Ingredients
Patchouly oil is the oil distilled from the dried leaf, young leaves and shoots of the Pogostemon cablin plant. Animal data suggests that patchouly oil is nontoxic with short term oral use. Patchouly oil may have bactericidal activity, and the component pogostone appears to have antibacterial and antifungal activities. The components eugenol, cinnamaldehyde and benzaldehyde may have insecticidal activity against insects in stored grain (11).

Adverse Reactions Including Known Allergies
None reported.

Possible Interactions with Herbs & Other Dietary Supplements
Insufficient reliable information available.

Possible Interactions with Drugs
No interactions are known to occur, and there is no known reason to expect a clinically significant interaction with patchouly oil.

Possible Interactions with Foods
No interactions are known to occur, and there is no known reason to expect a clinically significant interaction with patchouly oil.

Possible Interactions with Lab Tests
No interactions are known to occur, and there is no known reason to expect a clinically significant interaction with patchouly oil.

Possible Interactions with Diseases or Conditions
No interactions are known to occur, and there is no known reason to expect a clinically significant interaction with patchouly oil.

Typical Dosages & Routes of Administration that are Commonly Used
No typical dosage.

Comments
Patchouly oil can be adulterated with other oils, including gurjun balsam oil, copaiba balsam oil, and cedarwood oil (11).

PAU D'ARCO

This Product is Also Known As
Ipe, Ipe Roxo, Ipes, Lapacho, Lapacho Colorado, Lapacho Morado, Pau dArco, Pau de Arco, Purple Lapacho, Red Lapacho, Taheebo, Taheebo Tea, Trumpet Bush.

Scientific Names

Tabebuia impetiginosa, synonym Tabebuia avellanedae; Tabebuia heptaphylla.
Family: Bignoniaceae.

People Use This For

Orally, pau d'arco is used for Candida yeast infections, viral respiratory infections, including the common cold and flu, infectious diarrhea, bladder infections, and parasitic infections (3564,6006). It has also been used orally for cancer (6,515,6006).

Topically, pau d'arco is used for Candida infections (6).

In folk medicine, pau d'arco has been used orally for cancer, diabetes, ulcers, gastritis, liver ailments, asthma, bronchitis, cystitis, prostatitis, ringworm, rheumatism, hernias, gonorrhea (515), syphilis, chlorosis, boils, wounds, Candida infections, and as a "tonic and blood builder" (6).

Safety

POSSIBLY UNSAFE ...when used orally in typical doses. Significant evaluation of the safety of pau d'arco in typical doses has not been conducted; however, serious toxicities have been found with higher doses (6,515,3564). Pau d'arco should be used with caution.

LIKELY UNSAFE ...when used orally in large doses. In studies in cancer patients, when doses were elevated to provide therapeutic plasma levels of the active constituent lapachol, patients experienced significant toxicities, including increased risk of bleeding (6,515). Doses of pau d'arco providing greater than 1.5 grams per day of the lapachol constituent have been associated with the most risk (6).

There is insufficient reliable information available about the safety of pau d'arco for its other uses.

PREGNANCY: POSSIBLY UNSAFE ...when used orally in typical doses; avoid using. LIKELY UNSAFE ...when used orally in large doses; contraindicated. Significant evaluation of the safety of pau d'arco in typically doses has not been conducted; however, serious toxicities have been found with higher doses (6,515,3564). There is insufficient reliable information available about the safety of pau d'arco used topically in pregnancy.

LACTATION: Insufficient reliable information; avoid using.

Effectiveness

There is insufficient reliable information available about the effectiveness of pau d'arco.

Possible Mechanism of Action & Active Ingredients

The applicable parts of pau d'arco are the bark and the wood. The active constituents are thought to be a naphthoquinone derivative, lapachol, and its derivatives. The wood contains lapachol and the bark contains mostly lapachol derivatives. Lapachol and its derivatives are thought to have similar pharmacological activities (515). Lapachol is thought to be responsible for increasing the risk of bleeding by prolonging prothrombin time. Its effects on clotting are reversible by vitamin K (6). Preliminary data suggests that lapachol also has anti-inflammatory, antimalarial, antibacterial, antifungal, antiparasitic, and immunomodulatory activity (6,515). Some evidence suggests that lapachol is active against sarcomas, but at potentially effective levels, adverse effects are severe enough to prevent its used for that indication (515).

Adverse Reactions Including Known Allergies

In high doses, pau d'arco cause severe nausea, vomiting, diarrhea, dizziness, anemia, and increase the risk of bleeding (515). Doses of pau d'arco providing greater than 1.5 grams per day of the lapachol constituent have been associated with the most risk (6).

Possible Interactions with Herbs & Other Dietary Supplements

HERBS WITH ANTICOAGULANT/ANTIPLATELET POTENTIAL: Certain herbs have the potential to contribute to bleeding because they have coumarin constituents, or they affect platelet aggregation, or they have high vitamin K content. Theoretically, concomitant use of more than one of these herbs could increase the chance of bleeding in susceptible individuals. These herbs include: alfalfa, angelica, anise, arnica, asafoetida, bogbean, boldo, capsicum, celery, Roman and German chamomile, clove, danshen, fenugreek, feverfew, garlic, ginger, ginkgo, ginseng Panax, horse chestnut, horseradish, licorice, meadowsweet, nettle, northern and southern prickly ash, onion, papain, parsley, passionflower, poplar, quassia, red clover, turmeric, wild carrot, wild lettuce, and willow (4,19).

Possible Interactions with Drugs

ANTICOAGULANT, ANTIPLATELET DRUGS: Theoretically, concomitant use with pau d'arco might increase clotting time and increase the risk for bleeding (515).

Possible Interactions with Foods

No interactions are known to occur, and there is no known reason to expect a clinically significant interaction with pau d'arco.

Possible Interactions with Lab Tests

PROTHROMBIN TIME (PT)/INTERNATIONAL NORMALIZED RATION (INR): Pau d'arco can increase PT and INR test results and increase the risk of bleeding (6,515).

Possible Interactions with Diseases or Conditions
COAGULATION DISORDERS: Pau d'arco can increase bleeding time and might interfere with therapy in patients with coagulation disorders (6,515); use with caution.

Typical Dosages & Routes of Administration that are Commonly Used
ORAL: People typically use 1 to 4 grams daily in 2 to 3 divided doses. One manufacturer warns that the product should not be used for more than 7 days; however, the reason for this warning is not known. The contents of pau d'arco capsules may also be emptied and prepared as a tea. A tincture in the amount of 0.5 to 1 mL and a glycerin-based liquid in the amount of 1 to 3 mL, are used 3 times daily (6006).

Comments
Pau d'arco wood is extremely hard and almost indestructible (515). In South America, the Indians used the tree to make bows for hunting. Pau d'arco is the Spanish name for "bow stick" (6002). Teas, labeled as pau d'arco or lapacho, do not always contain the Tabebuia species; in some cases they have contained the related species, Tecoma curialis (515). Some report that the inner-bark preparations of pau d'arco are preferred because they are the most effective. Some products may use the outer-bark and mislabel the product as true inner-bark pau d'arco (3564). The anticancer activity of the pau d'arco constituent lapachol was extensively researched in the 1960s. The research was abandoned due to its toxicity (6).

PEANUT OIL

This Product is Also Known As
Arachis, Earth-Nut, Groundnuts, Monkey Nuts.

Scientific Names
Arachis hypogaea.
Family: Fabaceae.

People Use This For
Orally, peanut oil is used to lower cholesterol and prevent heart disease (18,3295).
It is also used orally to aid in weight loss and decrease appetite, and to help prevent cancer (4262).
Topically, it is used for arthritis and joint pain (3295), scalp crusting and scaling without hair loss, baby care products, dry skin, eczema and ichthyosis (noninflammatory skin disorders that cause scaling) (18).
Rectally, peanut oil is used in ointments and medicinal oils for treating constipation.
It is also used as a vehicle for external, enteral and parenteral pharmaceutical formulations (16,18).
In manufacturing, peanut oil is used in skin care products (18).

Safety
LIKELY SAFE ...when used orally in amounts found in foods. ...when used orally, topically, or rectally in medicinal amounts.
PREGNANCY AND LACTATION: LIKELY SAFE ...when used orally in amounts found in foods.

Effectiveness
There is insufficient reliable information available about the effectiveness of peanut oil (10).

Possible Mechanism of Action & Active Ingredients
Peanuts contain beta-sitosterol and resveratrol, which may contribute to cardioprotective and cancer protective activity (4262,4267,4263). The high monounsaturated, low saturated fat content of peanut oil is thought to prevent heart disease and lower cholesterol (4262). Population studies suggest people who eat nuts have a lower risk of developing heart disease (4264). This benefit must be weighed against animal evidence that suggests peanut oil is atherogenic, perhaps due to the triglyceride content or the presence of a lectin (4265,4266).

Adverse Reactions Including Known Allergies
FABACEAE HERBS: Peanut oil can cause a severe allergic reaction in individuals allergic to the Fabaceae family. Members of this family include peanuts and soybeans (4079,4080).

Possible Interactions with Herbs & Other Dietary Supplements
Insufficient reliable information available.

Possible Interactions with Drugs
No interactions are known to occur, and there is no known reason to expect a clinically significant interaction with peanut oil.

Possible Interactions with Foods
No interactions are known to occur, and there is no known reason to expect a clinically significant interaction with peanut oil.

Possible Interactions with Lab Tests

No interactions are known to occur, and there is no known reason to expect a clinically significant interaction with peanut oil.

Possible Interactions with Diseases or Conditions

CROSS-ALLERGENICITY: Peanut oil can cause a severe allergic reaction in individuals sensitive to the Fabaceae family. Members of this family include peanuts and soybeans (4079,4080).

Typical Dosages & Routes of Administration that are Commonly Used

ORAL: No typical dosage.
TOPICAL: As an enema, 130 mL of room temperature peanut oil is administered rectally. For bath use, 4 mL peanut oil is added to 10 L water. Adults bathe for 15-20 minutes 2-3 times daily. Children bathe for a few minutes 2-3 times weekly (18).

Comments

Sometimes the less expensive soya oil is added to peanut oil (18).

PEAR

This Product is Also Known As

None.

Scientific Names

Pyrus communis.
Family: Rosaceae.

People Use This For

Orally, pear fruit is used for mild digestive disorders (18), for cholera, colic, diarrhea, nausea, liver sclerosis, spasms, tumors (4017), and reducing fevers (18). It is used for laxative, bactericidal, calmative, and diuretic properties (18).
Topically, pear fruit is used as an astringent (4017).
For food use, pears are eaten as fresh fruit, preserved fruit, and used in cooking.

Safety

LIKELY SAFE …when consumed orally (18).
There is insufficient reliable information available about the safety of the topical use of pear fruit.
PREGNANCY AND LACTATION: LIKELY SAFE …when used in food amounts.

Effectiveness

There is insufficient reliable information available about the effectiveness of pear fruit.

Possible Mechanism of Action & Active Ingredients

The applicable part of the pear is the fruit. Pear fruit contains pectin (18) that might contribute to antidiarrheal activity (7).

Adverse Reactions Including Known Allergies

None reported.

Possible Interactions with Herbs & Other Dietary Supplements

Insufficient reliable information available.

Possible Interactions with Drugs

No interactions are known to occur, and there is no known reason to expect a clinically significant interaction with pear fruit.

Possible Interactions with Foods

No interactions are known to occur, and there is no known reason to expect a clinically significant interaction with pear fruit.

Possible Interactions with Lab Tests

No interactions are known to occur, and there is no known reason to expect a clinically significant interaction with pear fruit.

Possible Interactions with Diseases or Conditions

No interactions are known to occur, and there is no known reason to expect a clinically significant interaction with pear fruit.

Typical Dosages & Routes of Administration that are Commonly Used
No typical dosage.

Comments
None.

PECTIN

This Product is Also Known As
Pectinic Acid.

Scientific Names
Pectin.

People Use This For
Orally, pectin is used as an adsorbent (6,14,15,16), for reducing high cholesterol and triglycerides, for reducing the risk of colon cancer, for reducing damage from radiation (6), for treating diabetes (1900), and as an antibacterial (2211). Topically, it used for protecting raw or ulcerated mouth and throat sores (2218).
In combination with kaolin (Kaopectate) (13) and with paregoric (Parepectolin) (15), pectin is used to treat diarrhea.
Pectin is used in food manufacturing (11). It is used as a thickening agent in cooking and baking.
In manufacturing, pectin is used as a denture adhesive component (272).

Safety
LIKELY SAFE ...when consumed in amounts commonly found in foods (11), and pectin has Generally Recognized as Safe (GRAS) status for food use in the US (11). ...when taken for oral medicinal purposes in 10% concentration mixtures with kaolin (16).
PREGNANCY AND LACTATION: LIKELY SAFE ...when consumed in amounts found in foods (11).

Effectiveness
EFFECTIVE ...when taken orally as an adsorbent for treating diarrhea, usually in combination with kaolin or other ingredients (6,14,15).
POSSIBLY EFFECTIVE ...when taken orally as a cholesterol-lowering agent (2214,2215,2216,2217).
There is insufficient reliable information available about the effectiveness of pectin for its other uses.

Possible Mechanism of Action & Active Ingredients
Pectin is a soluble fiber (polysaccharide) obtained from the inner portion of the rind of citrus fruits and apple pomace (14). It is found in the cell walls of plant tissue and helps give plants rigidity (6). Pectin acts as an adsorbent and bulk-forming agent (14) and can interfere with drug and nutrient absorption (6,14,19).

Adverse Reactions Including Known Allergies
The occupational inhalation of pectin dust can cause asthma (580,581,582,583,584).

Possible Interactions with Herbs & Other Dietary Supplements
NUTRITIONAL SUPPLEMENTS: Concomitant use of pectin can interfere with the absorption of nutritional supplements (6).
BETA-CAROTENE: Concomitant use of pectin can significantly reduce beta-carotene absorption (2225).

Possible Interactions with Drugs
BETA-CAROTENE (Solatene): Concomitant use of pectin can significantly reduce beta-carotene absorption (2225).
DIGOXIN (Lanoxin), LOVASTATIN (Mevacor), TETRACYCLINE (Achromycin, Sumycin): Concomitant use of pectin can interfere with the intestinal absorption of these drugs (14,615,2212,2213).
ORAL DRUGS: Concomitant use of pectin can interfere with the absorption of other oral drugs (14).

Possible Interactions with Foods
NUTRIENTS: Pectin can interfere with the absorption of dietary nutrients (6).

Possible Interactions with Lab Tests
CHOLESTEROL: Pectin can decrease serum cholesterol and test results (275).

Possible Interactions with Diseases or Conditions
PECTIN HYPERSENSITIVITY: Contraindicated.

Typical Dosages & Routes of Administration that are Commonly Used
ORAL: As an adsorbent, 30 mL of 10% pectin in a mixture with kaolin is taken as needed (16). As an antihyperlipidemic, 15 grams per day was used in one study (2214).

Comments

Commercial pectin can contain sugars of organic acids and other additives, but pharmaceutical grade pectin contains no impurities or additives (13). The FDA is currently reevaluating the effectiveness of pectin combinations for diarrhea (272).

PELLITORY

This Product is Also Known As

None.
CAUTION: See separate listing for Pellitory-of-the-Wall.

Scientific Names

Anacyclus pyrethrum.
Family: Asteraceae.

People Use This For

Orally, pellitory is used for arthritis and as a digestive aid.
Topically, it is used for toothaches and as an insecticide (18).

Safety

There is insufficient reliable information available about the safety of pellitory.
Pregnancy and Lactation: Insufficient reliable information available; avoid using.

Effectiveness

There is insufficient reliable information available about the effectiveness of pellitory.

Possible Mechanism of Action & Active Ingredients

The applicable part of pellitory is the root. Application of pellitory to skin may stimulate nerve endings and result in redness and irritation, which is felt as a hot, burning sensation. Alkylamines may possibly contribute, since they may stimulate mucous membranes (18).

Adverse Reactions Including Known Allergies

Signs of skin irritation may occur with overuse (18). Pellitory can cause an allergic reaction in individuals sensitive to the Asteraceae/Compositae family. Members of this family include ragweed, chrysanthemums, marigolds, daisies, and many other herbs.

Possible Interactions with Herbs & Other Dietary Supplements

Insufficient reliable information available.

Possible Interactions with Drugs

No interactions are known to occur, and there is no known reason to expect a clinically significant interaction with pellitory.

Possible Interactions with Foods

No interactions are known to occur, and there is no known reason to expect a clinically significant interaction with pellitory.

Possible Interactions with Lab Tests

No interactions are known to occur, and there is no known reason to expect a clinically significant interaction with pellitory.

Possible Interactions with Diseases or Conditions

CROSS-ALLERGENICITY: Can cause an allergic reaction in individuals sensitive to the Asteraceae/Compositae family. Members of this family include ragweed, chrysanthemums, marigolds, daisies, and many other herbs.

Typical Dosages & Routes of Administration that are Commonly Used

No typical dosage.

Comments

Avoid confusing with the similar sounding pellitory-of-the-wall.

PELLITORY-OF-THE-WALL

This Product is Also Known As

Lichwort.
CAUTION: See separate listing for Pellitory.

Scientific Names

Parietaria officinalis.
Family: Urticaceae.

People Use This For

Orally, pellitory-of-the-wall is used for urinary tract diseases and as a diuretic (18).

Safety

POSSIBLY SAFE ...when it is used orally (12).
PREGNANCY AND LACTATION: Insufficient reliable information available; avoid using.

Effectiveness

There is insufficient reliable information available about the effectiveness of pellitory-of-the-wall.

Possible Mechanism of Action & Active Ingredients

Insufficient reliable information available.

Adverse Reactions Including Known Allergies

None reported.

Possible Interactions with Herbs & Other Dietary Supplements

Insufficient reliable information available.

Possible Interactions with Drugs

No interactions are known to occur, and there is no known reason to expect a clinically significant interaction with pellitory-of-the-wall.

Possible Interactions with Foods

No interactions are known to occur, and there is no known reason to expect a clinically significant interaction with pellitory-of-the-wall.

Possible Interactions with Lab Tests

No interactions are known to occur, and there is no known reason to expect a clinically significant interaction with pellitory-of-the-wall.

Possible Interactions with Diseases or Conditions

No interactions are known to occur, and there is no known reason to expect a clinically significant interaction with pellitory-of-the-wall.

Typical Dosages & Routes of Administration that are Commonly Used

No typical dosage.

Comments

Pellitory-of-the-wall is obsolete as a medicinal herb (18). Avoid confusion between pellitory-of-the-wall and the similar sounding pellitory.

PENNYROYAL leaf

This Product is Also Known As

American Pennyroyal, European Pennyroyal, Lurk-In-The-Ditch, Mosquito Plant, Piliolerial, Pudding Grass, Pulegium, Run-By-The-Ground, Squaw Balm, Squawmint, Stinking Balm, Tickweed.
CAUTION: See separate listing for Pennyroyal oil.

Scientific Names

Hedeoma pulegioides, synonym Melissa pulegioides; Mentha pulegium, synonym Pulegium vulgare.
Family: Lamiaceae or Labiatae.

People Use This For

Orally, pennyroyal is used as an antispasmodic, antiflatulent, diaphoretic (4), stimulant, for bowel disorders, pneumonia, stomach pains, weakness (6), and as a diuretic (14). It has been used orally as an abortifacient (4,5,6,9,12), menstrual stimulant or regulator (4,6,14), for intestinal disorders, colds (4,6,18), digestive disorders, liver and gall bladder disorders (18), and respiratory ailments (6).

Safety

LIKELY UNSAFE ...when the alcoholic extract is used orally. Repeated use of the alcoholic extract over a period of two weeks was linked to a death (650).
There is insufficient reliable information available about the safety of the oral use of pennyroyal leaf as tea (4,650).

CHILDREN: UNSAFE …when used orally. Two infants developed severe hepatic and neurologic injuries and one infant died (4,291).

PREGNANCY: LIKELY UNSAFE …when used orally as pennyroyal leaf tea. Reported to cause onset of menses (650). UNSAFE …when used as oil, considered to be an abortifacient and can cause death (4).

LACTATION: LIKELY UNSAFE ...when used orally as an alcoholic extract or oil (650). There is insufficient reliable information available for oral use of pennyroyal leaf tea; avoid using (4,6).

Effectiveness
There is insufficient reliable information available about the effectiveness of pennyroyal leaf.

Possible Mechanism of Action & Active Ingredients
Both American and European pennyroyal leaf contain 1-2% of essential oils (12,14), tannins and flavonoids (18). The volatile oil, pulegone and its metabolite, menthofuran, or methofuran's metabolites might be responsible for hepatotoxicity, neurotoxicity, and bronchiolar epithelial cell destruction (6,650). The oxidative metabolites of pulegone and menthofuran are thought to cause cell damage by binding to target proteins (650). Some metabolites of pulgegone also extensively deplete hepatic glutathione levels (650,291), which allows metabolite accumulation and direct cellular damage similar to acetaminophen toxicity (291). In addition, pulgegone is isomerized to isopulegone, which can be toxic to the lungs and liver (14). Pulegone is less concentrated in the American species (30%) than in European species (62-97%) (12,14).

Adverse Reactions Including Known Allergies
Taken orally, pennyroyal leaf can cause abdominal cramping and pain, fever, nausea (4,6,650), vomiting (possibly bloody), lethargy alternating with agitation, confusion, delirium, restlessness, seizures, dizziness (14), weakness, syncope (650), auditory and visual hallucinations (6), elevated blood pressure and pulse rate, bilateral lung congestion, hepatic failure, renal failure, acidosis, disseminated intravascular coagulation (DIC) (14), abortion (14,18), respiratory failure (18), shock (6), and death (14,650). Topically, it can cause an urticarial rash (4) and dermatitis (6).

Possible Interactions with Herbs & Other Dietary Supplements
Insufficient reliable information available.

Possible Interactions with Drugs
No interactions are known to occur, and there is no known reason to expect a clinically significant interaction with pennyroyal leaf.

Possible Interactions with Foods
No interactions are known to occur, and there is no known reason to expect a clinically significant interaction with pennyroyal leaf.

Possible Interactions with Lab Tests
No interactions are known to occur, and there is no known reason to expect a clinically significant interaction with pennyroyal leaf.

Possible Interactions with Diseases or Conditions
KIDNEY DISEASE: The volatile oil can cause kidney irritation (19).

Typical Dosages & Routes of Administration that are Commonly Used
No typical dosage.

Comments
Pennyroyal leaf is considered likely unsafe; avoid using. American pennyroyal and European pennyroyal are historically interchangeable as a source of pennyroyal oil (12). About 50-100 grams of leaves are required to produce 1 ml of pennyroyal oil (4).

PENNYROYAL oil

This Product is Also Known As
American Pennyroyal, European Pennyroyal, Lurk-In-The-Ditch, Mosquito Plant, Piliolerial, Pudding Grass, Pulegium, Squaw Balm, Squawmint, Stinking Balm, Run-By-The-Ground, Tickweed.
CAUTION: See separate listing for Pennyroyal leaf.

Scientific Names
Hedeoma pulegioides, synonym Melissa pulegioides; Mentha pulegium, synonym Pulegium vulgare.
Family: Lamiaceae or Labiatae.

People Use This For
Orally, pennyroyal oil is used as an antispasmodic, antiflatulent, diaphoretic (4), stimulant, pneumonia, for stomach pains, weakness (6), and as a diuretic (14).
Topically, it is used as an antiseptic, insect repellent (4,6), and for skin diseases (18).

Historically, it has been used orally as an abortifacient (4,5,6,9,12), menstrual stimulant or regulator (4,6,14), for intestinal disorders, colds, respiratory ailments (4,6,18), digestive disorders, and liver and gallbladder disorders (18). Historically, it has been used topically for tactile hallucinations, gout (4), venomous bites, mouth sores, as a flea-killing bath, and counterirritant (6).

In foods and manufacturing, it is used as a flavoring agent (4,6), as a dog and cat flea repellent (6,515), and a fragrance for detergents, perfumes and soaps (6).

Safety

POSSIBLY SAFE ...when used orally as food flavoring. Pulegone-free American pennyroyal is allowed only in alcoholic beverages in Canada (4). The Council of Europe lists pennyroyal as a natural source of food flavoring, without assessment of toxicity (4).

LIKELY UNSAFE ...when used orally or topically. Contraindicated (4). Neurologic injury reported in adults consuming 2.5-5.0 mL of pennyroyal oil (5,6,9). Nephrotoxicity, hepatotoxicity, and death reported after ingestion of 15-30 mL (4,5,6,12,5601). Some evidence suggests oil can be absorbed systemically (6,14,292).

PREGNANCY: LIKELY UNSAFE. Pennyroyal oil is an abortifacient (4).

LACTATION: LIKELY UNSAFE ...contraindicated.

Effectiveness

LIKELY EFFECTIVE ...when taken orally as abortifacient only when lethal or near-lethal amounts (15-30 ml) are ingested (4,5,6,18).

There is insufficient reliable information available about the effectiveness of pennyroyal oil for its other uses.

Possible Mechanism of Action & Active Ingredients

Pennyroyal oil contains pulegone, which may cause hepatotoxicity, neurotoxicity, and bronchiolar epithelial cell destruction (6). The oxidative metabolites of pulegone and its metabolite menthofuran may cause cell damage by binding to target proteins (650), depleting hepatic glutathione levels (650,292), and direct cellular damage similar to acetaminophen toxicity (291). In addition, pulegone is isomerized to isopulegone, which can be toxic to the lungs and liver (14). Its abortifacient effect might be due to uterine contractions triggered by genito-urinary tract irritation (4,6,19). In the American species, pulegone is less concentrated (30%) than in European species (62-97%) (12,14).

Adverse Reactions Including Known Allergies

Taken orally, pennyroyal oil can cause abdominal pain and tenderness (5601), nausea (4,6), vomiting (possibly bloody) (14,5601), burning of the throat (17), fever (4,6), lethargy alternating with agitation, confusion, delirium, restlessness, seizures, dizziness (14,5601), auditory and visual hallucinations (6), elevated blood pressure and pulse rate, bilateral lung congestion, acidosis, disseminated intravascular coagulation (DIC) (14,5601), abortion (14,18), hepatic failure, renal failure (14,5601), respiratory failure (18,5601), shock (6), and death (14,5601). Topically, it can cause a urticarial rash (4,5601) and dermatitis (6).

Possible Interactions with Herbs & Other Dietary Supplements

Insufficient reliable information available.

Possible Interactions with Drugs

No interactions are known to occur, and there is no known reason to expect a clinically significant interaction with pennyroyal oil.

Possible Interactions with Foods

No interactions are known to occur, and there is no known reason to expect a clinically significant interaction with pennyroyal oil.

Possible Interactions with Lab Tests

No interactions are known to occur, and there is no known reason to expect a clinically significant interaction with pennyroyal oil.

Possible Interactions with Diseases or Conditions

KIDNEY DISEASE: The volatile oil can cause kidney irritation (19).

Typical Dosages & Routes of Administration that are Commonly Used

No typical dosage.

Comments

Historically, American pennyroyal and European pennyroyal are interchangeable as sources of pennyroyal oil. (12).

PEONY flower

This Product is Also Known As
European Peony, Paeoniae flos, Piney.
CAUTION: See separate listing for Peony root.

Scientific Names
Paeonia mascula; Paeonia officinalis.
Family: Paeoniaceae.

People Use This For
Orally, peony flowers are used for gout, arthritis, respiratory tract ailments (2,18), and as a cough remedy (8).
Topically, peony flowers are used for skin and mucous membrane diseases, and for healing fissures, especially anal fissures associated with hemorrhoids (2,18)
In herb combinations, peony flowers are used orally for heart trouble and gastritis (2).
In folk medicine, peony flowers were used for epilepsy, bowel complaints, as an emetic, and for inducing menstruation or miscarriage (18).
In manufacturing, peony flowers are also used commercially to color cough syrups (18). It is used in herbal teas to improve their appearance (2,8).

Safety
There is insufficient reliable information available about the safety of peony flower.
PREGNANCY: LIKELY UNSAFE ...contraindicated, due to historical use as an abortifacient and menstruation-inducing agent (18).
LACTATION: Insufficient reliable information available; avoid using.

Effectiveness
There is insufficient reliable information available about the effectiveness of peony flower.

Possible Mechanism of Action & Active Ingredients
Hypertonia has been reported in animal tests, but the peony part(s)/product used were not specified (18).

Adverse Reactions Including Known Allergies
Overdose has reportedly led to gastroenteritis with vomiting, colic, and diarrhea (8,18).

Possible Interactions with Herbs & Other Dietary Supplements
Insufficient reliable information available.

Possible Interactions with Drugs
No interactions are known to occur, and there is no known reason to expect a clinically significant interaction with peony flower.

Possible Interactions with Foods
No interactions are known to occur, and there is no known reason to expect a clinically significant interaction with peony flower.

Possible Interactions with Lab Tests
No interactions are known to occur, and there is no known reason to expect a clinically significant interaction with peony flower.

Possible Interactions with Diseases or Conditions
No interactions are known to occur, and there is no known reason to expect a clinically significant interaction with peony flower.

Typical Dosages & Routes of Administration that are Commonly Used
ORAL: One cup tea (steep 1 gram flowers in 150 mL boiling water 5-10 minutes, strain) daily (8,18).
TOPICAL: No typical dosage.

Comments
Avoid confusion with peony root.

PEONY root

This Product is Also Known As
European Peony, Paeoniae Radix, Piney.
CAUTION: See separate listing for Peony flower.

Scientific Names
Paeonia mascula; Paeonia officinalis.
Family: Paeoniaceae.

People Use This For
Orally, peony is used for spasms (2).
In herbal combinations, peony root is used for arthritis, GI tract diseases, the heart and circulatory system, neuralgia, migraines, as a tonic, and for neurasthenia (characterized by vague fatigue accompanying or following depression, believed to be brought about by psychological factors) (2,18).
In folk medicine, peony is used for epilepsy, excitability, whooping cough, arthritis, bowel complaints, as an emetic, and for inducing menstruation (8).

Safety
There is insufficient reliable information available about the safety of peony root.
PREGNANCY: LIKELY UNSAFE ...historically, used to induce menstruation (18,19).
LACTATION: Insufficient reliable information available; avoid using.

Effectiveness
There is insufficient reliable information available about the effectiveness of peony.

Possible Mechanism of Action & Active Ingredients
Peony root extract exhibits neuroprotective activity and prevents experimentally induced brain neuron spike discharges in rats (3818). Researchers attribute neuroprotection to the constituent gallotannins and paeoniflorin (3818). Hypertonia reported in animal tests (peony part(s)/product used not specified) (18).

Adverse Reactions Including Known Allergies
Peony overdose can result in gastroenteritis with vomiting, colic, and diarrhea (8,18).

Possible Interactions with Herbs & Other Dietary Supplements
Insufficient reliable information.

Possible Interactions with Drugs
No interactions are known to occur, and there is no known reason to expect a clinically significant interaction with peony root.

Possible Interactions with Foods
No interactions are known to occur, and there is no known reason to expect a clinically significant interaction with peony root.

Possible Interactions with Lab Tests
No interactions are known to occur, and there is no known reason to expect a clinically significant interaction with peony root.

Possible Interactions with Diseases or Conditions
No interactions are known to occur, and there is no known reason to expect a clinically significant interaction with peony root.

Typical Dosages & Routes of Administration that are Commonly Used
ORAL: People typically use 1 ounce of the powdered root added to two cups of boiling water. The dose is a cup three or four times daily (5267). One source advises against the use of peony root without medical supervision (5263).

Comments
Avoid confusion with peony flower.

PEPPERMINT leaf

This Product is Also Known As
Brandy Mint, Lamb Mint, Menthae piperitae folium, Menthe poivree.
CAUTION: See separate listing for Peppermint Oil.

Scientific Names
Mentha piperita.
Family: Labiatae.

People Use This For
Orally, peppermint leaf is used for loss of appetite (18), spasms of the gastrointestinal tract, gallbladder, and bile ducts (2), for flatulence, gastritis, and enteritis (1).
In folk medicine, it has been used to treat nausea, vomiting, morning sickness, respiratory infections, and

© Copyright 2000, Natural Medicines Comprehensive Database (209) 472-2244. For updated data, go to www.NaturalDatabase.com

dysmenorrhea (18).

In foods and in herbal teas, peppermint is used as a culinary spice (11).

Safety

LIKELY SAFE ...when consumed in amounts commonly found in foods. Peppermint has Generally Recognized as Safe (GRAS) status for food use in the US (11).

POSSIBLY SAFE ...when taken orally for medicinal purposes and used appropriately (1,12).

CHILDREN: POSSIBLY UNSAFE ...when used in infants and small children because its menthol content can cause unpleasant choking sensations (512).

PREGNANCY: LIKELY SAFE ...when used in food amounts. POSSIBLY UNSAFE ...when used in larger amounts due to its potential to induce menstrual bleeding (19).

LACTATION: Insufficient reliable information available; avoid using amounts greater than found in foods.

Effectiveness

POSSIBLY EFFECTIVE ...when taken orally for gastrointestinal, gallbladder, and bile duct spasms (2).

There is insufficient reliable information available about the effectiveness of peppermint leaf for its other uses.

Possible Mechanism of Action & Active Ingredients

Peppermint has spasmolytic and antiflatulent activities. It also stimulates bile production (2,18). The constituents include the volatile oil menthol (7,11,18), flavonoids (11,18), and azulene (11). In vitro and in animals, menthol's antispasmodic effects result from a direct action on the digestive tract smooth muscle that is characteristic of calcium antagonist activity (1,7). Flavonoids have bile-stimulating effects. In animals, azulene has anti-inflammatory and anti-ulcer effects (11). Peppermint's soothing effect in coughs or colds results from the stimulation of salivation, which increases the swallowing reflex and suppresses cough (3).

Adverse Reactions Including Known Allergies

The peppermint leaf taken orally can increase colic in people with gallstones (2,18,19). It can also cause an unpleasant choking sensation in infants and small children (512).

Possible Interactions with Herbs & Other Dietary Supplements

Insufficient reliable information available.

Possible Interactions with Drugs

No interactions are known to occur, and there is no known reason to expect a clinically significant interaction with peppermint leaf.

Possible Interactions with Foods

No interactions are known to occur, and there is no known reason to expect a clinically significant interaction with peppermint leaf.

Possible Interactions with Lab Tests

No interactions are known to occur, and there is no known reason to expect a clinically significant interaction with peppermint leaf.

Possible Interactions with Diseases or Conditions

GALLSTONES: Physician consultation is advised before the use of the peppermint leaf in individuals with gallstones (2), because it can increase symptoms of colic (18).

HIATAL HERNIA: Theoretically, peppermint can exacerbate hernia symptoms due to its relaxation of the lower esophageal sphincter (500).

Typical Dosages & Routes of Administration that are Commonly Used

ORAL: For upset stomach, the typical dose of peppermint is one cup of the tea three to four times daily between meals (1,512). The tea is prepared by steeping 1 tablespoon of the dried leaf in 150 mL boiling water for 10 minutes and the straining. It can also be consumed at meal times or as needed (7). The average daily amount of the peppermint leaf is 3-6 grams (18). Peppermint tea is contraindicated in infants and small children because its menthol content can cause an unpleasant choking sensation (512). The usual dose of the tincture (1:5 in 45% ethanol) is 2-3 mL three times daily (1).

Comments

None.

PEPPERMINT OIL

This Product is Also Known As

Menthae piperitae aetheroleum, Menthe Poivree.

CAUTION: See separate listing for Peppermint leaf.

Scientific Names
Mentha piperita.
Family: Labiatae.

People Use This For
Orally, peppermint oil is used for colds, coughs, inflammation of the mouth and pharynx, liver and gallbladder complaints, irritable bowel syndrome, cramps of the upper gastrointestinal tract and bile ducts, as an antipyretic and antiflatulent (1,6,7,11,18), and for tension headache (6121).

Topically, the oil is used for headache (6121), myalgias, neuralgias (18,11), toothache (6), oral mucosa inflammation, rheumatic conditions, pruritus, urticaria, as an antibacterial and antiviral agent (1,6,11), and for repelling mosquitos (1263).

As an inhalant, the oil is used as an aromatic (6,7) and for symptomatic treatment of cough and colds (7).

In folk medicine, it has been used for nausea, vomiting, morning sickness, respiratory infections, dysmenorrhea (18), indigestion, nausea, diarrhea, cramps, and as a stimulant (11).

In foods and beverages, peppermint oil is a common flavoring agent (11).

In manufacturing, it is used as a fragrance component in soaps and cosmetics (11) and as a flavoring agent in pharmaceuticals (11).

Safety
LIKELY SAFE ...when consumed in amounts commonly found in foods. Peppermint oil has Generally Recognized as Safe (GRAS) status in the US. The maximum level is 0.104% in candy (11).

POSSIBLY SAFE ...when used orally and appropriately for medicinal purposes (1,2).

LIKELY UNSAFE ...when used orally in large amounts. It has been associated with interstitial nephritis and acute renal failure (7). Menthol, a major constituent, is considered lethal at a dose of 2-9 grams (7). ...when used topically by adults (2).

CHILDREN: LIKELY UNSAFE ...when applied topically to the facial, nasal, and chest areas of infants and small children. The oil can cause bronchospasm (2,6,11). ...when inhaled for medicinal purposes by small children (502).

PREGNANCY: LIKELY SAFE ...when used in food amounts. LIKELY UNSAFE ...when used in larger amounts because it can induce menstruation (19).

LACTATION: Insufficient reliable information available; avoid using.

Effectiveness
POSSIBLY EFFECTIVE ...when taken orally for treating irritable bowel (1,6,3802,3803). ...when taken orally for postoperative nausea (3804). ...when taken orally for spastic discomfort of the upper GI tract and bile ducts (2). ...when applied topically for respiratory tract mucous membrane inflammation (2). ...when applied topically for inflammation of oral mucosa (2). ...when applied topically for myalgias and neuralgias (11). ...when applied topically for relief of coughs and colds (1). ...when applied topically for treating tension headaches (3801,6190). There is insufficient reliable information available about the effectiveness of peppermint oil for its other uses.

Possible Mechanism of Action & Active Ingredients
Peppermint oil is a complex mixture of compounds, including the main constituent menthol, which is a volatile oil (1,6,11,7,18). Peppermint oil demonstrates antimicrobial and antiviral activities in vitro (11). The respiratory tract symptoms are relieved by increased salivation that increases the swallowing reflex and suppresses the cough reflex (3,7), reduced bronchial secretions, and nasal decongestant activity (1). The antispasmodic activity demonstrated in vitro and in animals results from the direct action on GI tract smooth muscle, characteristic of calcium antagonist action (1,7). Peppermint oil relaxes the lower esophageal sphincter, equalizing the intraluminal pressures between the stomach and esophagus (7). Peppermint oil capsules can decrease symptoms in some people with irritable bowel syndrome (1,3803). An aqueous suspension of peppermint oil prevents colonic spasms in people undergoing endoscopic examination (7). Peppermint oil applied to the forehead and temple can reduce sensitivity to experimentally-induced headaches in healthy people (3801). Inhaled menthol increases subjective but not objective measures of increased nasal air flow in people with common colds (1). Unpublished research suggests that peppermint oil might be an effective mosquito repellant with potential for reducing transmission of malaria and other mosquito-borne diseases, and might be useful for killing mosquito larva (1263).

Adverse Reactions Including Known Allergies
When taken orally, peppermint oil can cause heartburn (1) and allergic reactions including flushing and headache (6). Theoretically, the oil can worsen the symptoms of a hiatal hernia due to its relaxation of GI smooth muscle (6). When applied externally, the oil can cause skin irritation (1) and contact dermatitis (6). Application of the oil to facial, nasal or chest areas of babies and small children can cause laryngeal and bronchial spasms and instant collapse (1,6,11). When inhaled, peppermint oil can cause allergic reactions including flushing and headache (6).

Possible Interactions with Herbs & Other Dietary Supplements
Insufficient reliable information available.

Possible Interactions with Drugs

GASTRIC ACID BLOCKING DRUGS (H2 antagonists, prostaglandins, proton pump inhibitors): Use peppermint oil with caution. It is contraindicated in cases of achlorhydria, (787) which may occur with these drugs. Achlorhydria is the absence of hydrochloric acid from the gastric juice.

Possible Interactions with Foods

FOOD: Enteric-coated peppermint oil capsules used for treating irritable bowel syndrome are contraindicated with food, and should be taken between meals (787).

Possible Interactions with Lab Tests

No interactions are known to occur, and there is no known reason to expect a clinically significant interaction with peppermint oil.

Possible Interactions with Diseases or Conditions

ACHLORHYDRIA: Contraindicated when the stomach is not producing hydrochloric acid (787).
GALLSTONES: Peppermint oil should not be used by individuals with gallstones except with medical evaluation and monitoring (2). Use can increase the symptoms of colic (18).
HIATAL HERNIA: Theoretically, the oil can exacerbate symptoms due to its relaxation of GI smooth muscle (6).
HYPERSENSITIVE INDIVIDUALS: Contraindicated (1).
BILE DUCT OBSTRUCTION, SEVERE LIVER DISEASE AND GALLBLADDER INFLAMMATION: Contraindicated (2).

Typical Dosages & Routes of Administration that are Commonly Used

ORAL: The typical dose of peppermint oil for digestive disorders is 0.2-0.4 mL diluted in liquid three times daily (1), and the average daily amount is 6-12 drops (2). For irritable bowel syndrome, the usual dose is 0.2-0.4 mL three times daily in enteric-coated capsules (1), taken between meals (787), and the average daily amount is 0.6 mL (2).
TOPICAL: Peppermint oil is commonly applied as 5-20% semi-solid and oily preparations, 5-10% aqueous-ethanol preparations, and 1-5% nasal ointments. Rub a small amount into affected skin (2). For tension headaches, a 10% peppermint oil in ethanol solution applied across forehead and temples, repeated after 15 and 30 minutes, has been used (6190).
INHALATION: For inhalation, 3-4 drops of the oil are used in hot water. A lozenge containing 2-10 mg is also used (1,2).

Comments

Peppermint oil is distilled from the fresh overground parts of the flowering peppermint plant (Mentha piperita). Avoid confusion with peppermint leaf and rectified mint oil (18).

PERILLA

This Product is Also Known As

Beefsteak Plant, Wild Coleus.

Scientific Names

Perilla frutescens.
Family: Lamiaceae.

People Use This For

In folk medicine, perilla is used as an antispasmodic, for treating asthma, nausea, sunstroke, and inducing sweating (6).
For food use, it is utilized as a food source and flavoring (6).
In manufacturing, perilla seed oil is used commercially in the manufacture of varnishes, dyes, and inks (6).

Safety

There is insufficient reliable information available about the safety of perilla.
Pregnancy and Lactation: Insufficient reliable information available; avoid using.

Effectiveness

There is insufficient reliable information available about the effectiveness of perilla.

Possible Mechanism of Action & Active Ingredients

The applicable parts of perilla are the leaf and seed. Perilla contains multiple flavones. Apigenin and luteolin are the major ones found in seeds; they are also present in the leaves, along with other flavones including shishonin (6). Perilla oil is high in alpha-linolenate. In animal studies, alpha linolenate is associated with decreased serum cholesterol and triglyceride levels and beneficial changes in eicosapentaenoic acid and arachidonic acid levels (6). Animal and in-vitro studies suggest Perilla oil may have antitumor effects (6). Perilla extract may have an immunosuppressant effect by preferentially attenuating IgE production (6). Patch testing suggests 1-perillaldehyde and perillalcohol contained in perilla oil are responsible for the occurrence of dermatitis (6). Cell studies have shown luteolin to have anti-proliferative activity (5003). Animals grazing on perilla have developed pulmonary edema and respiratory distress (6). Animal studies show the oil constituent, perilla ketone induces pulmonary edema (6). Aldehyde antioxide contained in perilla oil may be toxic (6).

Adverse Reactions Including Known Allergies
Perilla used topically may cause contact dermatitis (6).

Possible Interactions with Herbs & Other Dietary Supplements
Insufficient reliable information available.

Possible Interactions with Drugs
No interactions are known to occur, and there is no known reason to expect a clinically significant interaction with perilla.

Possible Interactions with Foods
No interactions are known to occur, and there is no known reason to expect a clinically significant interaction with perilla.

Possible Interactions with Lab Tests
No interactions are known to occur, and there is no known reason to expect a clinically significant interaction with perilla.

Possible Interactions with Diseases or Conditions
No interactions are known to occur, and there is no known reason to expect a clinically significant interaction with perilla.

Typical Dosages & Routes of Administration that are Commonly Used
No typical dosage.

Comments
None.

PERIWINKLE

This Product is Also Known As
Common Periwinkle, Earlyflowering, Evergreen, Lesser Periwinkle, Myrtle, Periwinkle, Small Periwinkle, Vincae minoris herba, Wintergreen.
CAUTION: See separate listing for Madagascar Periwinkle.

Scientific Names
Vinca minor.
Family: Apocynaceae.

People Use This For
Orally, periwinkle is used for "brain health" (increasing cerebral circulation, supporting brain metabolism, increasing mental productivity, preventing memory and concentration impairment and feebleness, improving memory and thinking capacity, preventing premature aging of brain cells and geriatric support). It also is used for mucous membrane inflammation, diarrhea, vaginal discharge, "blood-purification," throat ailments, tonsillitis, angina, sore throat, intestinal inflammation, toothache, edema, promoting wound healing, improving immune function, and as a diuretic, sedative, antihypertensive, hemostatic remedy, and a bitter (2).

Safety
UNSAFE ...when taken orally (2,17). Contains pharmacologically active toxic alkaloids that can cause nerve, liver, and kidney damage (17).
PREGNANCY AND LACTATION: UNSAFE; avoid using.

Effectiveness
There is insufficient reliable information available about the effectiveness of periwinkle.

Possible Mechanism of Action & Active Ingredients
The applicable parts of periwinkle are the above ground parts. Periwinkle contains pharmacologically active, toxic alkaloids including vincristine which have cytotoxic and neurological actions and can injure liver and kidneys (513). Periwinkle may have astringent activity (19). Constituent, vincamine, has hypotensive activity (19). In animals, periwinkle causes leukocytopenia, lymphocytopenia, and lowers alpha-1, alpha-2, and gamma-globulin levels presumably due to immune suppression (2).

Adverse Reactions Including Known Allergies

Cytotoxic, neurologic, liver and kidney damage are possible due to vinca alkaloid constituents [17]. Periwinkle may also potentially cause GI complaints and skin flushing [18]. Consuming large amounts may cause severe drop in blood pressure [18].

Possible Interactions with Herbs & Other Dietary Supplements

Insufficient reliable information available.

Possible Interactions with Drugs

ANTIHYPERTENSIVE, ANTIHYPOTENSIVE DRUGS: Theoretically, concomitant use may interfere with blood pressure control [12,19].

Possible Interactions with Foods

No interactions are known to occur, and there is no known reason to expect a clinically significant interaction with periwinkle.

Possible Interactions with Lab Tests

No interactions are known to occur, and there is no known reason to expect a clinically significant interaction with periwinkle.

Possible Interactions with Diseases or Conditions

HYPOTENSION: Contraindicated, due to potential hypotensive effects [12,19].
CONSTIPATION: Contraindicated, due to astringent activity [12,19].

Typical Dosages & Routes of Administration that are Commonly Used

ORAL: People typically add 3 to 10 drops of the extract to water and use two to three times daily. Periwinkle extract contains glycerin and alcohol [6006].

Comments

Periwinkle has been declared unsafe for human consumption by the FDA [6] due to the toxic alkaloids it contains; avoid using. The periwinkle constituent, vincamine, can be converted in the laboratory to the compound vinpocetine which is marketed as a dietary supplement [14,1799] (see separate listing for Vinpocetine). Avoid confusing periwinkle with Madagascar periwinkle (Catharanthus roseus).

PERU BALSAM

This Product is Also Known As

Balsam of Peru, Balsam Peru, Balsamum Peruvianum, Black Balsam, Indian Balsam, Peruvian Balsam.
CAUTION: See separate listing for Tolu Balsam.

Scientific Names

Myroxylon pereirae, synonym Myroxylon balsamum pereirae.
Family: Leguminosae or Fabaceae.

People Use This For

Topically, Peru balsam is used for infected and poorly healing wounds, burns, decubitus ulcers (bed sores), frost bite, ulcus cruris, bruises caused by prosthetics, hemorrhoids, anal pruritus, diaper rash, and intertrigo [2,11].
In dentistry, peru balsam is a component of dental preparations for treating dry socket and as an ingredient in some dental impression materials. It is also used in toothpaste and toothpowder [11].
In traditional medicine, it has been used for cancer [11], to stop bleeding, promoting wound healing, as a diuretic, and to expel worms [6].
In manufacturing, Peru balsam is utilized as a fixative or fragrance in soaps and cosmetics [11] and as a food flavoring agent [11].

Safety

POSSIBLY SAFE ...when balsam preparations are applied topically and used for less than 1 week [2]. In some individuals, peru balsam is a contact allergen [11].
LIKELY UNSAFE ...when taken orally and should be avoided. Peru balsam is for external use only [2,6]. Kidney damage can occur with internal consumption of large doses [18].
PREGNANCY: Insufficient reliable information available; avoid using.
LACTATION: POSSIBLY UNSAFE ...because systemic toxicity to babies can occur following application of Peru balsam to the nipples of nursing mothers [6].

Effectiveness

POSSIBLY EFFECTIVE ...when used topically for healing wounds, burns, decubitus ulcers (bed sores), frost bite, ulcus cruris, bruises caused by prosthetics, hemorrhoids, and scabies [2].
There is insufficient reliable information available about the effectiveness of Peru balsam for its other uses.

Possible Mechanism of Action & Active Ingredients

The applicable part of peru balsam is the oleo resin. Peru balsam's volatile oil consists mainly of benzoic and cinnamic acid esters, including benzyl benzoate (11). Benzyl benzoate is an effective scabicide (19). Peru balsam also has mild antiseptic and antibacterial properties and is believed to promote epithelial cell growth (11).

Adverse Reactions Including Known Allergies

Taken orally, Peru balsam can cause kidney damage with consumption of large amounts (18). Topically, it can cause allergic skin reactions and contact dermatitis, including urticaria, recurring aphthoid oral ulcers, Quincke's disease, and diffuse purpurea (2,18). It has the potential to cause photodermatitis and phototoxicity (18). Kidney damage can also occur with the external use of large amounts (18).

Possible Interactions with Herbs & Other Dietary Supplements

Insufficient reliable information available.

Possible Interactions with Drugs

No interactions are known to occur, and there is no known reason to expect a clinically significant interaction with Peru balsam.

Possible Interactions with Foods

No interactions are known to occur, and there is no known reason to expect a clinically significant interaction with Peru balsam.

Possible Interactions with Lab Tests

No interactions are known to occur, and there is no known reason to expect a clinically significant interaction with Peru balsam.

Possible Interactions with Diseases or Conditions

PERU BALSAM ALLERGY: Avoid (2).
KIDNEY DISEASE: Use with caution or avoid due to its potential to cause kidney damage.

Typical Dosages & Routes of Administration that are Commonly Used

TOPICAL: Preparations of Peru balsam usually contain 5-20% Peruvian balsam (2). The maximum concentration for extensive surface application is 10% Peruvian balsam (2).

Comments

Peru balsam is the oleo resin exuded from scorched tree stems of Myroxylon balsamum.

PETASITES leaf

This Product is Also Known As

Blatterdock, Bog Rhubarb, Bogshorns, Butter Bur, Butter-Dock, Butterfly Dock, Capdockin, Flapperdock, Langwort, Petasitidis folium, Petasitidis hybridus, Umbrella Leaves.
CAUTION: See separate listing for Petasites root.

Scientific Names

Petasites spp.
Family: Asteraceae or Compositae.

People Use This For

Orally, petasites leaf is used for tension associated with pain, for colic, and headaches. It is also used orally as a sedative or appetite stimulant (2).
Topically, petasites has been used as an aid to wound healing (18).
In folk medicine, petasites has been used orally for respiratory tract disorders, biliary and pancreatic disorders (2,18), for chills, anxiety, and as a sleep aid (2).

Safety

LIKELY UNSAFE ...when used orally due to hepatotoxic unsaturated pyrrolizidine alkaloid (UPA)
constituents (2,18,19). Repeated exposure to low concentrations of UPAs linked to veno-occlusive disease (4,12). UPAs might also be carcinogenic and mutagenic (12). ...when used topically on abraded or broken skin due to potential for systemic absorption (12).
PREGNANCY: LIKELY UNSAFE ...contraindicated due to the possibility UPAs might be teratogenic and hepatotoxic (2,18,19).
LACTATION: POSSIBLY UNSAFE ...contraindicated due to concern that UPA constituents might be excreted in milk (2,18,19).

Effectiveness

POSSIBLY INEFFECTIVE ...when used orally (2).
There is insufficient reliable information available about the effectiveness of petasites leaf for its other uses.

Possible Mechanism of Action & Active Ingredients

Petasites leaf is thought to have antispasmodic effects on smooth muscle (18) possibly due to petasin and sesquiterpene constituents (7). Pyrrolizidine alkaloids with an unsaturated pyrrolizidine nucleus can be hepatotoxic in animals and humans (4). Herbs containing UPAs have shown carcinogenic, mutagenic, and renal toxic effects. However, the primary concern is veno-occlusive disease (12).

Adverse Reactions Including Known Allergies

Chronic exposure to other plants containing UPA constituents has been associated with veno-occlusive disease (4021). Symptoms of acute veno-occlusive disease are characterized by a dull, dragging ache in the right upper abdomen and marked distention of the abdomen. These symptoms are sometimes accompanied by reduced urine output. Subacute veno-occlusive disease is associated with vague symptoms and persistent liver enlargement (4021). Petasites leaf can cause an allergic reaction in individuals sensitive to the Asteraceae/Compositae family. Members of this family include ragweed, chrysanthemums, marigolds, daisies, and many other herbs.

Possible Interactions with Herbs & Other Dietary Supplements

EUCALYPTUS: Theoretically, concomitant use might increase the risk of unsaturated pyrrolizidine alkaloid toxicity due to enzyme induction by eucalyptus (19).
PYRROLIZIDINE ALKALOID-CONTAINING HERBS: Concomitant use is contraindicated due to the risk of additive toxicity. Herbs containing unsaturated pyrrolizidine alkaloids include: alkanna (12), borage (271), gravel root (4), hemp agrimony (271), hound's tongue (19), petasites (19), comfrey (271), coltsfoot, and the Senecio species plants; dusty miller (19), alpine ragwort (19), groundsel (271), golden ragwort (19), and tansy ragwort (271).

Possible Interactions with Drugs

No interactions are known to occur, and there is no known reason to expect a clinically significant interaction with petasites leaf.

Possible Interactions with Foods

No interactions are known to occur, and there is no known reason to expect a clinically significant interaction with petasites leaf.

Possible Interactions with Lab Tests

No interactions are known to occur, and there is no known reason to expect a clinically significant interaction with petasites leaf.

Possible Interactions with Diseases or Conditions

LIVER DISEASE: Contraindicated due to hepatotoxic potential (19).
CROSS-ALLERGENICITY: Can cause an allergic reaction in individuals sensitive to the Asteraceae/Compositae family. Members of this family include ragweed, chrysanthemums, marigolds, daisies, and many other herbs.

Typical Dosages & Routes of Administration that are Commonly Used

No typical dosage.

Comments

Petasites leaf is considered unsafe for oral use; avoid due to hepatotoxic unsaturated pyrrolizidine alkaloid content.

PETASITES root

This Product is Also Known As

Blatterdock, Bog Rhubarb, Bogshorns, Butter Bur, Butter-Dock, Butterfly Dock, Capdockin, Flapperdock, Langwort, Petasitidis rhizoma.
CAUTION: See separate listing for Petasites leaf.

Scientific Names

Petasites hybridus; Petasites officinalis.
Family: Asteraceae or Compositae.

People Use This For

Orally, petasites root is used for spastic pain of the urinary tract especially if stones are present (2,7), kidney and bladder stones, gastrointestinal disorders, coughs, whooping cough, bronchial asthma, and migraine and tension headaches (18).

Safety

POSSIBLY UNSAFE ...when taken orally. Contains hepatotoxic unsaturated pyrrolizidine alkaloid (UPAs) constituents (2,18,19). Repeated exposure to low concentrations of UPAs linked to veno-occlusive disease, a serious condition (4,12). UPAs might also be carcinogenic and mutagenic (12).

If petasites root is used orally, not more than 1 mcg of pyrrolizine alkaloids should be consumed per day for a maximum of 4 to 6 weeks per year (7).

PREGNANCY: LIKELY UNSAFE ...contraindicated due to the possibility UPAs might be teratogenic and hepatotoxic (2,18,19).

LACTATION: POSSIBLY UNSAFE ...contraindicated due to concern that UPA constituents might be excreted in milk (2,18,19).

Effectiveness

POSSIBLY EFFECTIVE ...when taken orally as supportive therapy for acute spastic pain of the urinary tract, particularly if stones are present (2,7).

There is insufficient reliable information available about the effectiveness of petasites root for its other uses.

Possible Mechanism of Action & Active Ingredients

The petasins and sesquiterpene compounds can be responsible for its antispasmodic and analgesic effects on smooth muscle (2,7,18). However, the beneficial effects of urologic teas in urinary tract inflammation can be due to the effect of increased water intake (7). The pyrrolizidine alkaloid constituents have hepatotoxic, mutagenic, teratogenic, and carcinogenic effects (18).

Adverse Reactions Including Known Allergies

Chronic exposure to plants containing UPA constituents has been associated with veno-occlusive disease (4021). Symptoms of acute veno-occlusive disease are characterized by a dull, dragging ache in the right upper abdomen and marked distention of the abdomen. These symptoms are sometimes accompanied by reduced urine output. Subacute veno-occlusive disease is associated with vague symptoms and persistent liver enlargement (4021). It can cause an allergic reaction in individuals sensitive to the Asteraceae/Compositae family. Members of this family include ragweed, chrysanthemums, marigolds, daisies, and many other herbs.

Possible Interactions with Herbs & Other Dietary Supplements

EUCALYPTUS: Theoretically, concomitant use might increase the risk of unsaturated pyrrolizidine alkaloid toxicity due to enzyme induction by eucalyptus (19).

PYRROLIZIDINE ALKALOID-CONTAINING HERBS: Concomitant use is contraindicated due to the risk of additive toxicity. Herbs containing unsaturated pyrrolizidine alkaloids include: alkanna (12), borage (271), gravel root (4), hemp agrimony (271), hound's tongue (19), petasites (19), comfrey (271), coltsfoot, and the Senecio species plants; dusty miller (19), alpine ragwort (19), groundsel (271), golden ragwort (19), and tansy ragwort (271).

Possible Interactions with Drugs

No interactions are known to occur, and there is no known reason to expect a clinically significant interaction with petasites root.

Possible Interactions with Foods

No interactions are known to occur, and there is no known reason to expect a clinically significant interaction with petasites root.

Possible Interactions with Lab Tests

No interactions are known to occur, and there is no known reason to expect a clinically significant interaction with petasites root.

Possible Interactions with Diseases or Conditions

CROSS-ALLERGENICITY: Can cause an allergic reaction in individuals sensitive to the Asteraceae/Compositae family. Members of this family include ragweed, chrysanthemums, marigolds, daisies, and many other herbs.

Typical Dosages & Routes of Administration that are Commonly Used

ORAL: The typical dose of petasites is 4.5-7 grams per day of the root or equivalent preparation (2). The daily intake should not exceed 1 mcg of the pyrrolizine alkaloids (2), and the maximum duration of use should be four to six weeks per year (7).

Comments

Avoid confusion with petasites leaf. Use only the pyrrolizidine alkaloid-free products.

PEYOTE

This Product is Also Known As

Devil's Root, Dumpling Cactus, Mescal Buttons, Mescaline, Pellote, Sacred Mushroom.

Scientific Names

Lophophora williamsii.
Family: Cactaceae.

People Use This For

Orally, peyote is used as a hallucinogen. It does not have known medicinal uses (14).

Safety

UNSAFE ...and illegal in the US. It is a FDA schedule I controlled substance (14).
PREGNANCY AND LACTATION: UNSAFE ...contraindicated due to potential for adverse effects (14).

Effectiveness

There is insufficient reliable information available about the effectiveness of peyote.

Possible Mechanism of Action & Active Ingredients

The applicable parts of peyote are the above ground parts after the hair tufts are removed. The clinical effects of peyote are due to mescaline. It is structurally similar to amphetamines, and similar in activity to LSD, and the mushroom hallucinogens psilocybin and psilocin. In fact, people who take mescaline have a cross-tolerance to these other hallucinogens. Mescaline causes central nervous system and sympathetic stimulation and hallucinations. It's not clear exactly how mescaline causes hallucinations. However, its effects can be blocked by either serotonin antagonist methysergide or dopamine antagonist haloperidol. The hallucinogenic dose of peyote is about 5 mg/kg (14), or 4-12 3-4.5 cm diameter slices of the sprout. Amphetamine-like or sympathomimetic effects are more common with higher doses (18).

Adverse Reactions Including Known Allergies

Nausea and vomiting are usually the first symptoms to occur after peyote ingestion. They usually resolve 2 hours after ingestion. Hallucinogenic effects peak at 3.5 to 4 hours, and resolve 15 hours post-ingestion. The hallucinations include visual, aural, taste, smell, touch, and abnormal perception of time and space. Anxiety, paranoia, fear and emotional instability may also occur. Common physiologic effects include mild elevations in heart rate, blood pressure and respiration rate. Sometimes slow heart beat occurs instead in response to elevated blood pressure. Mydriasis, blurred vision, palpitations, salivation, headache, dizziness, difficulty with walking, and drowsiness may also occur. Ingestion of peyote is rarely fatal. However, people can die as a result of homicidal, psychotic or suicidal behavior associated with their hallucinations. Flashbacks may also occur (14).

Possible Interactions with Herbs & Other Dietary Supplements

Insufficient reliable information available.

Possible Interactions with Drugs

INSULIN: Mescaline can increase the toxic effects of an insulin overdose.
PHYSOSTIGMINE: If given with mescaline, it can increase the risk of death.
METHYSERGIDE, HALOPERIDOL: Block mescaline's hallucinogenic effects.
VERAPAMIL: Can counteract mescaline-induced cerebral vasospasm.
METHADONE, ALCOHOL: Concomitant administration with mescaline can lead to seizures, kidney damage due to protein overload from the seizures (rhabdomyolysis), and prolonged coma (14).

Possible Interactions with Foods

No interactions are known to occur, and there is no known reason to expect a clinically significant interaction with peyote.

Possible Interactions with Lab Tests

No interactions are known to occur, and there is no known reason to expect a clinically significant interaction with peyote.

Possible Interactions with Diseases or Conditions

No interactions are known to occur, and there is no known reason to expect a clinically significant interaction with peyote.

Typical Dosages & Routes of Administration that are Commonly Used

No typical dosage.

Comments

Peyote is considered unsafe and illegal. It should not be used (see Safety) (14). Mescaline is also available as a crystalline powder, tablets, and powder. However, tablets which are perceived as mescaline often contain LSD, PCP, amphetamines, aspirin, STP, and/or strychnine instead. A previous 10 year survey found that 76% of "mescaline" tablets were altered in this manner (14).

PHEASANT'S EYE

This Product is Also Known As
Adonis herba, False Hellebore, Oxeye, Pheasants Eye, Red Morocco, Rose-A-Rubie, Sweet Vernal, Yellow Pheasants Eye, Yellow Pheasant's Eye.
CAUTION: See separate listings for Black Hellebore, White Hellebore, and American Hellebore.

Scientific Names
Adonis vernalis.
Family: Ranunculaceae.

People Use This For
Orally, the above ground parts of pheasant's eye are used for mild heart failure (2,7,18), arrhythmia (18), and nervous heart complaints (18).
In folk medicine, pheasant's eye has been used for dehydration, cramps, fever, and menstrual disorders (18).

Safety
POSSIBLY SAFE ...when the standardized extract is used orally under the supervision of a medical professional trained in the appropriate use of pheasant's eye (2).
LIKELY UNSAFE ...when the standardized extract is used without appropriate medical supervision (18,512). Pheasant's eye contains cardiac glycosides and monitoring is required to minimize serious adverse effects.
UNSAFE ...when the plant is ingested. Pheasant's eye is highly poisonous (18).
PREGNANCY AND LACTATION: LIKELY UNSAFE ...when the standardized extract is taken orally for self-medication (512).

Effectiveness
POSSIBLY EFFECTIVE ...when used orally for mild heart failure (New York Heart Association stage I and II), especially when accompanied by nervous symptoms (2). New York Heart Association (NYHA) stage I and II refers to individuals with heart disease who do not have resulting limitations of physical activity. They are comfortable at rest but ordinary physical activity results in fatigue, palpitation, trouble breathing, or anginal pain (2).
There is insufficient reliable information available about the effectiveness of pheasant's eye for the other uses.

Possible Mechanism of Action & Active Ingredients
The applicable parts of pheasant's eye are the above ground parts. Pheasant's eye contains cardioactive glycosides (2,7,18). It has cardiac effects similar to digoxin, including positive inotropic and negative chronotropic effects (7). In experimental animals, pheasant's eye demonstrates a tonic effect on veins (2).

Adverse Reactions Including Known Allergies
Symptoms of pheasant's eye overdose include nausea, vomiting, and arrhythmias (2).

Possible Interactions with Herbs & Other Dietary Supplements
CALCIUM: Concomitant use with calcium can increase the risk of cardiac toxicity (2,3805).
CARDIAC GLYCOSIDE-CONTAINING HERBS: Contraindicated. Concomitant use can increase the risk of cardiac glycoside toxicity. Cardiac glycoside-containing herbs include black hellebore, Canadian hemp roots, digitalis leaf, hedge mustard, figwort, lily of the valley roots, motherwort, oleander leaf, pleurisy root, squill bulb leaf scales, strophanthus seeds, and uzara (2,18,19,500).
CARDIOACTIVE HERBS: Avoid concomitant use with cardioactive herbs due to unpredictability of effects and adverse effects. These include: calamus, cereus, cola, coltsfoot, devil's claw, European mistletoe, fenugreek, fumitory, ginger, ginseng Panax, hawthorn, white horehound, maté, parsley, quassia, scotch broom flower, shepherd's purse, and wild carrot (4).
LICORICE/HORSETAIL: The overuse or misuse of licorice rhizome or horsetail plant increases the risk of cardiac toxicity due to potassium depletion. (19).
STIMULANT LAXATIVE HERBS: The overuse or misuse of stimulant laxatives increases the risk of cardiac toxicity due to potassium depletion. Stimulant laxative herbs include: aloe dried leaf sap, blue flag rhizome, alder buckthorn, European buckthorn, butternut bark, cascara bark, castor oil, colocynth fruit pulp, gamboge bark exudate, jalap root, black root, manna bark exudate, podophyllum root, rhubarb root, senna leaves and pods, wild cucumber fruit (Ecballium elaterium), and yellow dock root (19).

Possible Interactions with Drugs
CALCIUM: Concomitant use of pheasant's eye with calcium can increase the risk of cardiac glycoside arrhythmias (2,3805).
CORTICOSTEROIDS: Concomitant use of pheasant's eye can increase the therapeutic and adverse effects of long-term corticosteroid use (2).
DIGOXIN: Concomitant use is contraindicated due to an increased risk of cardiac glycoside toxicity (2,4).
POTASIUM DEPLETING DIURETICS, STIMULANT LAXATIVES: Concomitant use of pheasant's eye can increase the risk of cardiac glycoside toxicity due to potassium loss (2).
QUINIDINE: Concomitant use can increase cardiac effects and adverse effects (2).

Possible Interactions with Foods

No interactions are known to occur, and there is no known reason to expect a clinically significant interaction with pheasant's eye.

Possible Interactions with Lab Tests

No interactions are known to occur, and there is no known reason to expect a clinically significant interaction with pheasant's eye.

Possible Interactions with Diseases or Conditions

HYPOKALEMIA: Contraindicated (2,3805).
HYPERCALCEMIA: Contraindicated (2,3805).

Typical Dosages & Routes of Administration that are Commonly Used

ORAL: The average amount of pheasant's eye is 600 mg of the standardized adonis powder (DAB9) per day (2). The maximum single dose is 1 gram (2), and the maximum daily amount is 3 grams (2).

Comments

Pheasant's eye is considered a poisonous plant (18).

PHENYLALANINE

This Product is Also Known As

D-Phenylalanine, DL-Phenylalanine, L-Phenylalanine.

Scientific Names

Beta-phenyl-alanine; Alpha-aminohydrocinnamic acid.

People Use This For

Orally, phenylalanine is used for depression, Parkinson's disease, chronic pain, osteoarthritis, rheumatoid arthritis, alcohol withdrawal symptoms, and vitiligo (2453).
Topically, it is used for vitiligo (2461).

Safety

LIKELY SAFE ...when L-phenylalanine is consumed orally in amounts typically found in foods (2022).
POSSIBLY SAFE ...when L-phenylalanine is used orally for therapeutic purposes (2455,2456,2461,2463,2465,2466, 2467,2468,2469).
There is insufficient reliable information available about the oral safety of D-phenylalanine.
There is insufficient reliable information available about the topical safety of phenylalanine.
PREGNANCY: LIKELY SAFE ...when L-phenylalanine is consumed in amounts typically found in foods by pregnant women with normal phenylalanine metabolism and serum levels (2020,2022). UNSAFE ...when L-phenylalanine is consumed in amounts typically found in foods by pregnant women with serum phenylalanine concentrations greater than 360 micromol/L, which increases the risk of birth defects (1402). The risk for facial defects is highest at gestation weeks 10-14, neurological and growth abnormalities between 3-16 weeks, and cardiovascular defects at 3-8 weeks. Experts recommend that women with high phenylalanine serum concentrations follow a low phenylalanine diet for at least 20 weeks prior to conception to decrease the risk for birth defects (1402). In addition, some experts recommend screening in women not tested for phenylketonuria (PKU) at birth (1401).
There is insufficient reliable information available about the safety of oral, therapeutic amounts of L-phenylalanine in pregnant women with normal phenylalanine metabolism and serum concentrations; avoid using.
There is insufficient reliable information available about the safety of oral D-phenylalanine in pregnant women; avoid using.
LACTATION: LIKELY SAFE ...when L-phenylalanine is consumed in amounts typically found in foods by lactating women with normal phenylalanine metabolism (2020,2022).
There is insufficient reliable information available about the safety of oral, therapeutic amounts of L-phenylalanine in lactating women with normal phenylalanine metabolism; avoid using.
There is insufficient reliable information available about the safety of oral D-phenylalanine in lactating women; avoid using.

Effectiveness

POSSIBLY EFFECTIVE ...when D-phenylalanine is taken orally for treating the symptoms of Parkinson's disease (2455) and for enhancing acupuncture anesthesia for tooth extraction (2456). ...when DL-phenylalanine is taken orally for treating depression (2468). ...when L-phenylalanine is used orally and combined with UVA exposure for treating vitiligo in adults (2461,2463,2464,2466) and in children (2467). ...when used orally for unipolar depression combined with selegiline (Eldepryl) (2469). ...when L-phenylalanine is applied topically and combined with UVA exposure for treating vitiligo (2461).
POSSIBLY INEFFECTIVE ...when D-phenylalanine is taken orally for enhancing acupuncture analgesia for

chronic low back pain (2456) and as analgesia for chronic pain of varied etiology (2459). ...when DL-phenylalanine is taken orally for treating Parkinson's disease (2454).

There is insufficient reliable information available about the effectiveness of phenylalanine for its other uses.

Possible Mechanism of Action & Active Ingredients

Phenylalanine exists as two enantiomers, D-phenylalanine and L-phenylalanine. DL-phenylalanine is a mixture of these two forms. D-phenylalanine is non-nutritive (not an essential human amino acid) and its role in humans is not currently understood. L-phenylalanine is an essential human amino acid, and is the only form of phenylalanine found in proteins. L-phenylalanine is normally metabolized to tyrosine (9). Human data suggests that about one-third of a D-phenylalanine dose is converted to L-phenylalanine (2051,2052). L-phenylalanine exacerbates tardive dyskinesia in people with schizophrenia (2457) and can contribute to the development and severity of tardive dyskinesia in people with unipolar depression treated with neuroleptics (2458). Phenylalanine (enantiomer unspecified) does not alter pain tolerance to burns in healthy people (2460). L-phenylalanine does not alter pain tolerance to burns in healthy people (2460). D-phenylalanine increases the pain threshold in animals, inducing a naloxone-reversible analgesia by blocking enzymatic degradation of enkephalin (2459). Large neutral amino acids (LNAAs) including DL-phenylalanine, leucine, and isoleucine can exacerbate tremor, rigidity, and the "on-off" syndrome in people with Parkinson's disease who have taken levodopa for more than 5-10 years (2454,3291). The amount of dietary LNAAs appears to affect the severity of "on-off" symptoms and may be independent of dietary protein-induced alterations in oral levodopa bioavailability (3291,3292,3293,3294). DL-phenylalanine and other LNAAs might worsen symptoms by decreasing the amount of levodopa that crosses the blood-brain barrier (3291,3294). Preliminary evidence suggests that L-phenylalanine, given with the non-selective monoamine oxidase (MAO-A/MOA-B) inhibitor pargyline, might prevent the elimination of tyramine, increasing the risk of hypertensive crisis (2021). However, hypertensive crisis was not reported in a small number of patients who used L-phenylalanine with the partially selective monoamine oxidase B (MAO-B) inhibitor, selegeline (Eldepryl) (2469).

Adverse Reactions Including Known Allergies

L-phenylalanine used orally can exacerbate tardive dyskinesia in people with schizophrenia (2457). Large neutral amino acids (LNAAs) including DL-phenylalanine, leucine and isoleucine, exacerbate tremor, rigidity, and the "on-off" syndrome in patient's with Parkinson's disease taking levodopa (2454,3291,3292,3293,3294). Birth defects associated with elevated maternal phenylalanine concentrations include severe mental retardation, microcephaly (a smaller than normal head), abnormal facial features and congenital heart disease (1401,1402). The risk of birth defects during pregnancy increases when maternal phenylalanine serum concentrations exceed 360 micromol/L (1402). Preliminary data suggest that L-phenylalanine supplements might cause hypertension or increase the risk of stroke in certain genetically predisposed people (2084).

Possible Interactions with Herbs & Other Dietary Supplements

Insufficient reliable information available.

Possible Interactions with Drugs

NON-SELECTIVE MONOAMINE OXIDASE INIHIBTORS (MAOIs): Theoretically, concomitant use of L-phenylalanine and non-selective MAOI drugs might increase the risk of hypertensive crisis. Some evidence suggests that L-phenylalanine, given with the non-selective MAOI drug pargyline, might prevent the elimination of tyramine, increasing the risk of hypertensive crisis (2021).

SELEGILINE (Eldepryl): Concomitant use of L-phenylalanine with selegiline (selective monoamine oxidase type-B inhibitor) might be effective for treating unipolar depression (2469).

LEVODOPA: Concomitant use of DL-phenylalanine and levodopa can exacerbate tremor, rigidity, and the "on-off" syndrome in patients with Parkinson's disease (2454,3291,3292,3293,3294).

NEUROLEPTIC DRUGS: Concomitant use of L-phenylalanine and neuroleptics can contribute to the development and severity of tardive dyskinesia in patients with neuroleptic-treated unipolar depression (2458).

Possible Interactions with Foods

No interactions are known to occur, and there is no known reason to expect a clinically significant interaction with phenylalanine.

Possible Interactions with Lab Tests

No interactions are known to occur, and there is no known reason to expect a clinically significant interaction with phenylalanine.

Possible Interactions with Diseases or Conditions

ALKAPTONURIA: Contraindicated (2470). Alkaptonuria is an inherited disorder involving the inability to metabolize phenylalanine and tyrosine, leading to ochre pigment deposits in the connective tissues. There are no clinical manifestations until mid-adulthood, when the pigment deposits lead to progressive degenerative joint diseases (2050,2053,2055).

HYPERTENSION: Use with caution in patients at risk for hypertension. Some evidence suggests that L-phenylalanine might cause hypertension in genetically predisposed patients (2084).

PHENYLKETONURIA (PKU): Contraindicated (2470). Phenylketonuria is an inherited disorder involving the inability to metabolize phenylalanine, leading to toxic serum levels of phenylalanine and its metabolites (2050,2053).

SCHIZOPHRENIA: Use with caution. L-Phenylalanine can exacerbate tardive dyskinesia in people with schizophrenia (2457).

STROKE: Use with caution in patients at risk for stroke. Some evidence suggests that L-phenylalanine might increase the risk of stroke in genetically predisposed patients (2084).

TYROSINEMIA/TYROSINURIA: Contraindicated (2470). Tyrosinemia is an inherited disorder involving the inability to metabolize tyrosine leading to toxic serum levels of tyrosine and its metabolites. Because phenylalanine is metabolized to tyrosine, it can also cause toxic tyrosine levels in people with tyrosinemia (2053,2054).

Typical Dosages & Routes of Administration that are Commonly Used

ORAL: For Parkinson's disease, the dose of D-phenylalanine is typically 200 to 500 mg per day (2455). As an adjunct to acupuncture anesthesia or analgesia in tooth extraction: 4 grams of D-phenylalanine is taken 30 minutes before acupuncture (2456). For depression, the usual dose of L-phenylalanine is 250 mg with 5-10 mg L-deprenyl per day (2469), and the common dose of DL-phenylalanine is 150 to 200 mg per day (2468). For vitiligo in adults, 50-100 mg/kg of L-phenylalanine is taken per day along with UVA exposure (2461,2463,2464,2465,2466).

TOPICAL: A 10% L-phenylalanine cream along with UVA exposure is commonly used for vitiligo (2461).

Comments

Phenylalanine exists as two enantiomers, D and L. These molecules are mirror images of each other. The racemic mix DL-phenylalanine (50% D-, 50% L-phenylalanine) is produced by laboratory synthesis. Phenylalanine products are available which contain pure L-phenylalanine (an essential amino acid), pure D-phenylalanine (biological activity unknown), or DL-phenylalanine (2050,2051). Major dietary sources of L-phenylalanine include meat, fish, eggs, cheese, and milk (2023).

PHOSPHATE SALTS

This Product is Also Known As

Aluminum Phosphate;

Calcium Phosphate: Bone Ash, Bone Phosphate, Calcium Orthophosphate, Calcium Phosphate Dibasic Anhydrous, Calcium Phosphate Dibasic Dihydrate, Calcium Phosphate Tribasic, Dicalcium Phosphate, Dicalcium Phosphates, Neutral Calcium Phosphate, Precipitated Calcium Phosphate, Tertiary Calcium Phosphate, Tricalcium Phosphate, Whitlockite;

Potassium Phosphate: Dibasic Potassium Phosphate, Dipotassium Hydrogen Orthophosphate, Dipotassium Monophosphate, Dipotassium Phosphate, Monobasic Potassium Phosphate, Potassium Acid Phosphate, Potassium Biphosphate, Potassium Dihydrogen Orthophosphate;

Sodium Phosphate: Anhydrous Sodium Phosphate, Dibasic Sodium Phosphate, Disodium Hydrogen Orthophosphate, Disodium Hydrogen Orthophosphate Dodecahydrate, Disodium Hydrogen Phosphate, Disodium Phosphate, Phosphate of Soda, Sodium Orthophosphate.

CAUTION: Do not confuse Phosphate Salts with toxic substances such as Organophosphates, or with Tribasic Sodium Phosphates and Tribasic Potassium Phosphates which are strongly alkaline (14).

Scientific Names

Calcium phosphate; Potassium phosphate; Sodium phosphate; Aluminum phosphate.

People Use This For

Orally, calcium, potassium, and sodium phosphates are used for enhancing exercise performance (2499,8300,8301). Sodium and potassium phosphate are used orally for treating hypophosphatemia and hypercalcemia, hypophosphatemic rickets or osteomalacia, and as an urinary acidifier for prevention of recurrent renal calculi (14).

Intravenously, potassium phosphate is used for hypophosphatemia and hypokalemia, preventing hypophosphatemia in people receiving parenteral nutrition, and treating hypercalcemia (9,14,15).

Sodium phosphate is used orally and rectally as a laxative and pre-surgical bowel prep (15).

Calcium phosphate is used orally as a calcium supplement (15).

Aluminum phosphate is used orally as an antacid (15).

Safety

LIKELY SAFE ...when sodium, potassium, aluminum, and calcium phosphates are used orally and appropriately short-term (15). ...when sodium phosphate is used rectally and appropriately short-term (14,15). Long-term use or high doses used orally or rectally require monitoring of serum electrolytes (14,2494,2495,2496,2497,2498,3092). ...when used intravenously, potassium phosphate is an FDA-approved prescription drug.

PREGNANCY AND LACTATION: LIKELY SAFE ...when used at recommended dietary allowances (RDAs) of 1250 mg daily for mothers between 14-18 years of age and 700 mg daily for those over 18 years of age (3094).

Effectiveness

EFFECTIVE ...when sodium and potassium phosphates are used orally for preventing and treating hypophosphatemia, and for prevention of calcium oxalate renal stones (14). ...when sodium phosphates are used orally and appropriately as a laxative and bowel prep for surgery, x-ray, or endoscopy (15). ...when calcium

phosphate is used orally as a calcium supplement (14,15). ...when sodium phosphates are used rectally as a laxative and bowel prep for surgery, x-ray, or endoscopy (14,15). ...when the FDA-approved IV product is used for the correction of hypophosphatemia (8302,8303).
LIKELY EFFECTIVE ...when sodium and potassium phosphates are used orally for treating hypercalcemia (14).
POSSIBLY EFFECTIVE ...when used orally to improve aerobic exercise performance by increasing capacity to use oxygen (V02 max) (217).
LIKELY INEFFECTIVE ...when sodium, potassium, and calcium phosphates are used orally for enhancing anaerobic exercise performance (2499,8300,8301).

Possible Mechanism of Action & Active Ingredients

Phosphate is the most abundant intracellular anion in the body. It is critical for membrane structure, transport and energy storage (3092). Normal plasma concentrations range from 0.8-1.6 mmol/L, or 2.5-5 mg/dL (0.032 mmol phosphate = 1 mg) (14). Phosphate plays an important role in buffering body fluids, and plays a primary role in the renal excretion of hydrogen ions (14). It is present in carbohydrates, proteins, lipids and various enzymes involved in energy transfer (14). It is required for utilization of many B vitamins (14). Serum phosphate levels are inversely related to serum calcium levels (14). Reduced plasma phosphate levels allow more calcium to be present in the blood and inhibit formation of new bone (14). Vitamin D3 and its metabolites influence phosphate absorption from the gut and also affect renal tubular reabsorption of phosphate (14,3092). Hyperphosphatemia can occur with excessive use of phosphate salts by any route, and with excessive intake of vitamin D (3092). Sodium phosphates are saline laxatives. They cause retention of fluids in the intestine by an osmotic action and thereby increase peristalsis (14). Aluminum phosphate taken orally neutralizes gastric acid (15). Oral ingestion of large amounts of sodium dihydrogen phosphate can lower urine pH (14).

Adverse Reactions Including Known Allergies

All phosphate salts, taken orally can cause gastrointestinal irritation, fluid and electrolyte disturbances including hyperphosphatemia and hypocalcemia, and extraskeletal calcification (14). Potassium phosphates can cause hyperkalemia (14). Sodium phosphates can cause hypernatremia and hypokalemia (14,2494,2495,2496,2497). Sodium and potassium phosphates can cause diarrhea (14). Aluminum phosphate can cause constipation (14). Phosphate salts used rectally can cause fluid and electrolyte disturbances including hyperphosphatemia and hypocalcemia, gastrointestinal irritation, and perforation of the rectum (14).

Possible Interactions with Herbs & Other Dietary Supplements

Insufficient reliable information available.

Possible Interactions with Drugs

ANTACIDS: Antacids containing aluminum, calcium, or magnesium can bind phosphate in the gut and prevent its absorption (14).
COLESTIPOL (Colestid) can decrease oral absorption of phosphate (14).

Drug Influences on Nutrient Levels and Depletion

SOME DRUGS CAN AFFECT PHOSPHATE LEVELS:
ALUMINUM SALTS: Use of aluminum salts can bind phosphate in the gut and reduce serum phosphate levels. Avoid prolonged administration of large doses of aluminum-containing drugs which might lead to hypophosphatemia (4400).
MAGNESIUM SALTS: Use of magnesium salts can bind phosphate in the gut and reduce serum phosphate levels. Avoid prolonged administration of large doses of magnesium-containing drugs which might lead to hypophosphatemia (4400).

Possible Interactions with Foods

No interactions are known to occur, and there is no known reason to expect a clinically significant interaction with phosphate salts.

Possible Interactions with Lab Tests

ACID PHOSPHATASE: Phosphates can cause a false-decrease in serum test results. High substrate concentrations can inhibit the analytic reaction (275).
ALKALINE PHOSPHATASE: Phosphates can cause a false-decrease in serum test results. High substrate concentrations can inhibit the analytic reaction (275).
AMMONIA: Phosphates can cause a false-decrease in plasma test results by inhibiting formation of indophenol color in Berthelot reaction (275).
CALCIUM: Phosphates can increase fecal levels and test results (275). Phosphates can cause a false-decrease in serum and urine test results by inhibiting emission in some flame methods and by competing with EDTA for calcium (275).
LIPID GLYCEROL: Phosphates can cause a false-decrease in serum test results by inhibiting phospholipase with method of Horney (275).
MAGNESIUM: Phosphates can decrease urine levels and test results by reducing increased excretion with bed rest (275).
PARATHYROID HORMONE: Phosphates can increase plasma levels and test results (275).

PHOSPHATE: Phosphates increase fecal, serum, and urine levels and test results (275).
POTASSIUM: Phosphates (except potassium phosphate) can decrease serum levels and test results (275).
PYRUVATE KINASE: Phosphates can cause a false-increase in red blood cell test results by activating analytic enzyme (275).

Possible Interactions with Diseases or Conditions

HYPOPHOSPHATEMIA: Low phosphate levels can be associated with many conditions, including poor oral intake or absorption, reduced renal tubular reabsorption, respiratory alkalosis, excessive insulin use, certain malignancies, diabetic ketoacidosis, and chronic alcoholism (14,3092).
HYPERPHOSPHATEMIA: People with Addison's disease, severe cardiopulmonary, renal, or hepatic disease are at risk for hyperphosphatemia and hypocalcemia when phosphates are used (14,2497). Hyperphosphatemia might also occur in people with renal insufficiency, hypoparathyroidism, severe hyperthyroidism, untreated adrenal insufficiency (due to volume contraction, metabolic acidosis and reduced glomerular permeability), metabolic, lactic or respiratory acidosis, rhabdomyolysis, infarction, hemolysis, or tumor lysis syndrome (3092).
EDEMA: Use phosphates with caution in people with cirrhosis, heart failure, or other edematous conditions (14).
KIDNEY DYSFUNCTION: Closely monitor serum electrolytes when phosphates are used by people with mild to moderate renal impairment (14).

Typical Dosages & Routes of Administration that are Commonly Used

ORAL: For bowel preparation for diagnostic tests, a typical dose is dibasic sodium phosphate 3.42 to 7.56 grams and monobasic sodium phosphate 9.1-20.2 grams daily given as a single dose (15). Phosphate laxative preparations should be taken on an empty stomach and with plenty of water (14). For use as an antacid, a typical dose of aluminum phosphate gel is 10-30 mL every 2 hours (14). As a calcium supplement the usual dose of dibasic calcium phosphate is 4.4 grams daily in divided doses (14). The usual dose of tribasic calcium phosphate as a calcium supplement is 1.6 grams twice daily (14). Treating hypophosphatemia or hypercalcemia with oral phosphates requires monitoring of serum electrolyte levels and medical supervision (14). As a supplement, the recommended daily dietary allowances (RDAs) of phosphate (expressed as phosphorus) are: Children 1-3 years, 460 mg; Children 4-8 years, 500 mg; Males and females 9-18 years, 1250 mg; Males and females over 18 years, 700 mg (3094). The adequate intakes (AI) for infants are: 100 mg for infants 0-6 months old and 275 mg for infants 7-12 months of age (3094).
RECTAL: For bowel preparation for diagnostic tests, a typical dose is dibasic sodium phosphate 6.84-7.56 grams and monobasic sodium phosphate 18.24-20.16 grams daily, administered as a single dose (15). Treating hypophosphatemia with rectal phosphates requires monitoring of serum electrolyte levels (14).
INTRAVENOUS: Injectable potassium phosphate is a FDA-approved prescription product.

Comments

Foods high in phosphate include milk, whole grain cereals, nuts, dried fruits and vegetables, and some meats (14). Phosphates present in dairy products and meats are soluble and readily absorbed, whereas those in cereal grains are bound and insoluble, and may be poorly absorbed (3092). Cola drinks contain significant amounts of phosphate and excessive intake can result in hyperphosphatemia and hypocalcemia (14).

PHOSPHATIDYLCHOLINE

This Product is Also Known As

Phosphatidyl Choline.
CAUTION: See separate listings for Lecithin and Choline.

Scientific Names

None.

People Use This For

Orally, phosphatidylcholine is used for treating anxiety (5154), eczema (5154), gallbladder disease (5154,5227), hepatitis (5154,5224,5225,5226,5227), manic-depressive illness (5154), peripheral vascular disorders (9), hyperlipidemias (9,5227), improving ultrafiltration in peritoneal dialysis (5222), tardive dyskinesia (5223), premenstrual syndrome (5227), memory loss (5227,5228), Alzheimer's disease (5227), immunodepression (5227), and preventing aging (5227).

Safety

LIKELY SAFE ...when used orally and appropriately (4914). Even large amounts, 30 grams per day for 6 weeks, has been well tolerated (5223). Lecithin, which contains a substantial amount of phosphatidylcholine, has Generally Recognized as Safe (GRAS) status in the US (4912).
PREGNANCY AND LACTATION: Insufficient reliable information available; avoid using.

Effectiveness

POSSIBLY EFFECTIVE ...when the polyunsaturated form is used orally in combination with interferon for chronic hepatitis C (5226).

POSSIBLY INEFFECTIVE ...when used orally for hepatitis A (5225). Studies regarding hepatitis B show conflicting results (5224,5226). ...when used orally for improving ultrafiltration in peritoneal dialysis (5222). ...when used orally for treating tardive dyskinesia (5223).

There is insufficient reliable information available about the effectiveness of phosphatidylcholine for its other uses.

Possible Mechanism of Action & Active Ingredients

Phosphatidylcholine is a phospholipid and a major constituent of lecithin (9). Egg lecithin contains 69% phosphatidylcholine, while soybean lecithin contains 24% phosphatidylcholine (4914). Phosphatidylcholine is a precursor to acetylcholine (5228). In a clinical trial, a single dose of 25 grams improved explicit memory 90 minutes later (5228).

Adverse Reactions Including Known Allergies

Oral use of phosphatidylcholine can increase sweating (5229). Ingesting large amounts (30 grams per day) can cause gastrointestinal upset and diarrhea (5223).

Possible Interactions with Herbs & Other Dietary Supplements

Insufficient reliable information available.

Possible Interactions with Drugs

No interactions are known to occur, and there is no known reason to expect a clinically significant interaction with phosphatidylcholine.

Possible Interactions with Foods

No interactions are known to occur, and there is no known reason to expect a clinically significant interaction with phosphatidylcholine.

Possible Interactions with Lab Tests

No interactions are known to occur, and there is no known reason to expect a clinically significant interaction with phosphatidylcholine.

Possible Interactions with Diseases or Conditions

No interactions are known to occur, and there is no known reason to expect a clinically significant interaction with phosphatidylcholine.

Typical Dosages & Routes of Administration that are Commonly Used

ORAL: For hepatitis C, 1.8 grams of lecithin used daily with hepatitis C interferon (5226).

Comments

The term "phosphatidylcholine" is sometimes used interchangeably with "lecithin" although the two are different. Choline is a component of phosphatidylcholine, which is a component of lecithin (16). Although closely related, these terms are not synonymous. However, in the clinical literature, they are often confused. Brand names are PhosChol (9,5153,5230), Ultracholine (9).

PHOSPHATIDYLSERINE

This Product is Also Known As

Cephalin, Kephalin, Phosphatidyl Serine, PtdSer.

Scientific Names

Phosphatidylserine.

People Use This For

Orally, phosphatidylserine is used for Alzheimer's disease, depression, and age-related decline in mental function (2436).

Safety

POSSIBLY SAFE ...when taken orally for short-term use. There have been no significant adverse effects reported with 300 mg per day for up to six months (2437,2438,2439,2440,2441).

PREGNANCY AND LACTATION: Insufficient reliable information available; avoid using.

Effectiveness

POSSIBLY EFFECTIVE ...when taken orally for improving cognitive function and other symptoms of Alzheimer's disease (2437,2439). ...when taken orally for improving behavioral symptoms of senile dementia (2438). ...when taken orally for improving age-related cognitive and memory impairment (2440,2441).

There is insufficient reliable information available about the effectiveness of phosphatidylserine for its other uses.

Possible Mechanism of Action & Active Ingredients
Insufficient reliable information available.

Adverse Reactions Including Known Allergies
None reported.

Possible Interactions with Herbs & Other Dietary Supplements
Insufficient reliable information available.

Possible Interactions with Drugs
No interactions are known to occur, and there is no known reason to expect a clinically significant interaction with phosphatidylserine.

Possible Interactions with Foods
No interactions are known to occur, and there is no known reason to expect a clinically significant interaction with phosphatidylserine.

Possible Interactions with Lab Tests
No interactions are known to occur, and there is no known reason to expect a clinically significant interaction with phosphatidylserine.

Possible Interactions with Diseases or Conditions
No interactions are known to occur, and there is no known reason to expect a clinically significant interaction with phosphatidylserine.

Typical Dosages & Routes of Administration that are Commonly Used
ORAL: The typical dose of phosphatidylserine used in clinical studies of Alzheimer's disease, senile dementia, and age-related cognitive or memory impairment is 100 mg three times daily [2437,2438,2440,2441].

Comments
Cephalin (synonym kephalin) is the term formerly used to refer to what are now known as phosphatidylserine and phosphatidylethanolamine [511].

PIMPINELLA above ground parts

This Product is Also Known As
Bibernellkraut, Burnet Saxifrage, Pimpernell, Pimpinellae herba, Saxifrage.
CAUTION: See separate listing for Pimpinella root.

Scientific Names
Pimpinella saxifraga, synonym Pimpinella major.
Family: Apiaceae.

People Use This For
Orally, pimpinella is used for lung ailments and stimulating gastrointestinal activity [2].
Topically, pimpinella above ground parts are used for varicose veins [2].

Safety
There is insufficient reliable information available about the safety of pimpinella above ground parts.
Pregnancy and Lactation: Insufficient reliable information available; avoid using.

Effectiveness
There is insufficient reliable information about the effectiveness of pimpinella above ground parts.

Possible Mechanism of Action & Active Ingredients
Insufficient reliable information available.

Adverse Reactions Including Known Allergies
None reported.

Possible Interactions with Herbs & Other Dietary Supplements
Insufficient reliable information available.

Possible Interactions with Drugs
No interactions are known to occur, and there is no known reason to expect a clinically significant interaction with pimpinella above ground parts.

Possible Interactions with Foods

No interactions are known to occur, and there is no known reason to expect a clinically significant interaction with pimpinella above ground parts.

Possible Interactions with Lab Tests

No interactions are known to occur, and there is no known reason to expect a clinically significant interaction with pimpinella above ground parts.

Possible Interactions with Diseases or Conditions

No interactions are known to occur, and there is no known reason to expect a clinically significant interaction with pimpinella above ground parts.

Typical Dosages & Routes of Administration that are Commonly Used

No typical dosage.

Comments

There is very little scientific information about this product. Our staff is continually analyzing the available information on natural medicines and will add data here as it becomes available.

PIMPINELLA root

This Product is Also Known As

Burnet Saxifrage, Greater Burnet-Saxifrage, Pimpernell, Pimpinellae radix, Saxifrage.
CAUTION: See separate listing for Pimpinella above ground parts.

Scientific Names

Pimpinella major; Pimpinella saxifraga.
Family: Apiaceae.

People Use This For

Orally, pimpinella root is used for upper respiratory tract mucous membrane inflammation [2].
Topically, it is used for inflammation of the oral and pharyngeal mucous membranes, and as a bath additive for poorly healing wounds [18].
In folk medicine, pimpinella is used for urinary tract disorders and inflammation, bladder and kidney stones and edema, and "flushing out" therapy for urinary tract bacterial inflammation [18].

Safety

POSSIBLY SAFE ...when used orally and appropriately [2].
There is insufficient reliable information available about the safety of the topical use of pimpinella root.
PREGNANCY AND LACTATION: Insufficient reliable information available; avoid using.

Effectiveness

POSSIBLY EFFECTIVE ...when used orally for treating upper respiratory tract mucous membrane inflammation [2].
There is insufficient reliable information available about the effectiveness of pimpinella root for its other uses.

Possible Mechanism of Action & Active Ingredients

Pimpinella root is reported to loosen and aid in moving bronchial secretions [18].

Adverse Reactions Including Known Allergies

None reported. However, may cause photosensitivity in fair-skinned individuals [18].

Possible Interactions with Herbs & Other Dietary Supplements

Insufficient reliable information available.

Possible Interactions with Drugs

No interactions are known to occur, and there is no known reason to expect a clinically significant interaction with pimpinella root.

Possible Interactions with Foods

No interactions are known to occur, and there is no known reason to expect a clinically significant interaction with pimpinella root.

Possible Interactions with Lab Tests

No interactions are known to occur, and there is no known reason to expect a clinically significant interaction with pimpinella root.

Possible Interactions with Diseases or Conditions

No interactions are known to occur, and there is no known reason to expect a clinically significant interaction with pimpinella root.

Typical Dosages & Routes of Administration that are Commonly Used

ORAL: One cup tea (briefly steep 3 grams finely cut root in 150 mL boiling water, strain) three to four times daily (8); up to 6-12 grams root per day (2). Tincture (1:5), 6-15 mL per day (8).
TOPICAL: No typical dosage.

Comments

Pimpinella root is often adulterated with other herbs including Hercaleum sphondylium, Heracleum mantegazianum, and Pastinaca sativa (8,18).

PINE

This Product is Also Known As

Dwarf-Pine, Pini Turiones, Pix Liquida, Pumilio Pine, Scotch Fir, Scotch Pine, Swiss Mountain Pine.
CAUTION: See separate listings for Dwarf Pine Needle, Fir Needle Oil, Fir, Poplar, and Scotch Pine Needle.

Scientific Names

Pinus sylvestris.
Family: Pinaceae.

People Use This For

Orally, pine sprout is used for upper and lower respiratory tract mucous membrane inflammation (2), blood pressure problems, common cold, cough or bronchitis, fevers, and a tendency towards infection (18).
Topically, it is used for mild muscular pain and neuralgia (2,18).
In folk medicine, pine sprout has been used to treat uncomplicated coughs and acute bronchial disease, nasal congestion, and hoarseness (18).

Safety

POSSIBLY SAFE ...when used orally and appropriately (2). ...when used topically and appropriately (2).
PREGNANCY AND LACTATION: Insufficient reliable information available; avoid using.

Effectiveness

POSSIBLY EFFECTIVE ...when taken orally for upper and lower respiratory tract mucous membrane inflammation (2). ...when applied topically for mild muscle pain and neuralgias (2).
There is insufficient reliable information available about the effectiveness of pine sprout for its other uses.

Possible Mechanism of Action & Active Ingredients

The applicable part of pine is the sprout. Pine sprouts can dry secretions. They demonstrate mild antiseptic effects and stimulate peripheral circulation (2,18). Pine sprouts contain an essential oil that can stimulate serous bronchial gland function, suppress mucous gland function (7), and aid with expectoration (7).

Adverse Reactions Including Known Allergies

None reported.

Possible Interactions with Herbs & Other Dietary Supplements

Insufficient reliable information available.

Possible Interactions with Drugs

No interactions are known to occur, and there is no known reason to expect a clinically significant interaction with pine.

Possible Interactions with Foods

No interactions are known to occur, and there is no known reason to expect a clinically significant interaction with pine.

Possible Interactions with Lab Tests

No interactions are known to occur, and there is no known reason to expect a clinically significant interaction with pine.

Possible Interactions with Diseases or Conditions

RESPIRATORY CONDITIONS: Pine sprout is contraindicated for oral use in individuals with bronchial asthma or whooping cough (18).
SKIN CONDITIONS: It is contraindicated as a bath additive in individuals with extensive skin injury or acute skin diseases.

FEVER, INFECTIOUS DISEASE, CARDIAC INSUFFICIENCY, OR HYPERTONIA: Contraindicated as a bath additive (18).

Typical Dosages & Routes of Administration that are Commonly Used
ORAL: The average daily amount of pine sprout is 2-9 grams (2,18) as teas, syrups, or tinctures.
TOPICAL: It is applied topically as a 20-50% pine sprout extract in an alcoholic solution, oil, ointment, liquid, or semi-solid preparation (2,18). As a bath, 100 grams of the alcoholic extract is usually added to the bath water (18).

Comments
Avoid confusion with fir shoots (Picea bies or Abies alba) or pine oil.

PINK ROOT

This Product is Also Known As
American Wormgrass, Carolina Pink, Indian Pink, Maryland Pink, Pinkroot, Starbloom, Wormgrass.

Scientific Names
Spigelia marilandica.
Family: Loganiaceae.

People Use This For
Orally, pink root is used to treat worm infestation (18).

Safety
POSSIBLY SAFE …when used orally and appropriately, short-term (12).
POSSIBLY UNSAFE …when fresh root is used or when use is not accompanied by catharsis (12).
PREGNANCY: LIKELY UNSAFE. For pink root to be effective, it must be used along with a purgative laxative. However, purgative laxative use is contraindicated during pregnancy (272). For this reason, pink root should not be used in pregnancy.
LACTATION: Insufficient reliable information available (12,18,272); avoid using.

Effectiveness
There is insufficient reliable information available about the effectiveness of pink root.

Possible Mechanism of Action & Active Ingredients
The applicable parts of pink root are the dried rhizome and root. Pink root has anthelmintic actions (18). Although there has been no recent research involving pink root, older sources, identify the chief constituents as acidic resins, volatile oil, tannins, waxes, and a volatile base (presumably identical to isoquinoline) (18).

Adverse Reactions Including Known Allergies
Pink root allegedly contains a toxin that can paralyze the spinal marrow and lead to death by asphyxiation (18). Theoretically, prolonged use of pink root can cause depressive effects on the heart (19).

Possible Interactions with Herbs & Other Dietary Supplements
Insufficient reliable information available.

Possible Interactions with Drugs
No interactions are known to occur, and there is no known reason to expect a clinically significant interaction with pink root.

Possible Interactions with Foods
No interactions are known to occur, and there is no known reason to expect a clinically significant interaction with pink root.

Possible Interactions with Lab Tests
No interactions are known to occur, and there is no known reason to expect a clinically significant interaction with pink root.

Possible Interactions with Diseases or Conditions
No interactions are known to occur, and there is no known reason to expect a clinically significant interaction with pink root.

Typical Dosages & Routes of Administration that are Commonly Used
ORAL: Adults: 2-5 grams twice daily (12). Children over 4 years: 0.5-4 grams twice daily (12). A strong purgative laxative (e.g. senna) should always be used with pink root (12).

Comments
As late as 1955, pink root was commonly used throughout the country as an antihelmintic. Various unpleasant symptoms have been reported from use of the fresh root or when use is not accompanied by catharsis (12).

© Copyright 2000, Natural Medicines Comprehensive Database (209) 472-2244. For updated data, go to www.NaturalDatabase.com • 837

PINUS BARK

This Product is Also Known As
Canadian Hemlock, Canada Pitch, Eastern Hemlock, Hemlock Bark, Hemlock Gum, Hemlock Spruce, Hemlocktanne, Pruche de l'Est.

Scientific Names
Tsuga canadensis.
Family: Pinaceae or Abietaceae.

People Use This For
Orally, pinus bark is used for digestive disorders, diarrhea, and diseases of the mouth and throat. Historically, it was used to treat scurvy (18).

Safety
There is insufficient reliable information available about the safety of pinus bark.
Pregnancy and Lactation: Insufficient reliable information available; avoid using.

Effectiveness
There is insufficient reliable information available about the effectiveness of pinus bark.

Possible Mechanism of Action & Active Ingredients
Pinus bark is reputed to have astringent, anti-inflammatory, and diuretic properties. It is also thought to induce sweating. The astringent effects of pinus bark are attributed to its tannin content (18). Tannins dehydrate the mucous membrane tissue, reducing internal secretions and causing external cells to form a protective layer. Plants with at least 10% tannins may cause gastrointestinal disturbances, kidney damage, and necrotic conditions of the liver. Some animal experiments show that tannins may cause cancer; others show they may prevent it. Regular consumption of herbs with high tannin concentrations correlates with increased incidence of esophageal or nasal cancer (12).

Adverse Reactions Including Known Allergies
None reported.

Possible Interactions with Herbs & Other Dietary Supplements
TANNIN-CONTAINING HERBS: Theoretically, herbs that contain high percentages of tannins (such as pinus bark) may cause precipitation of constituents of other herbs (19).

Possible Interactions with Drugs
ORAL DRUGS: Theoretically, concomitant oral administration may cause precipitation of some drugs due to the high tannin content of pinus bark (19). Separate administration of oral drugs and tannin-containing herbs by the longest period of time practical (19).

Possible Interactions with Foods
No interactions are known to occur, and there is no known reason to expect a clinically significant interaction with pinus bark.

Possible Interactions with Lab Tests
No interactions are known to occur, and there is no known reason to expect a clinically significant interaction with pinus bark.

Possible Interactions with Diseases or Conditions
No interactions are known to occur, and there is no known reason to expect a clinically significant interaction with pinus bark.

Typical Dosages & Routes of Administration that are Commonly Used
No typical dosage.

Comments
Pinus bark is seldom used (18).

PIPSISSEWA

This Product is Also Known As
Bitter Winter, Bitter Wintergreen, Chimaphila, Ground Holly, Holly, King's Cure, King's Cureall, Love in Winter, Prince's Pine, Rheumatism Weed, Spotted Wintergreen, Umbellate Wintergreen.

Scientific Names

Chimaphila umbellata synonym Chimaphila corymbosa.
Family: Ericaceae.

People Use This For

Orally, pipsissewa is used as a urinary antiseptic (18). It is also used orally as a diuretic, astringent, mild disinfectant, antispasmodic, for bladder stones, epilepsy, nervous disorders, and cancer.
Topically, pipsissewa is used for treating ulcerous sores and blisters.
In food and beverages, pipsissewa extracts are used as flavor components (11).

Safety

LIKELY SAFE ...when the above ground parts are used in amounts found in foods. It has Generally Recognized as Safe (GRAS) status in the US; maximum use is 0.03% (11).
POSSIBLY SAFE ...when used orally short-term (12).
POSSIBLY UNSAFE ...for prolonged oral use because it can cause hydroquinone toxicity (18).
There is insufficient reliable information available about the topical use of pipsissewa.
PREGNANCY AND LACTATION: POSSIBLY SAFE ...when used in food amounts; avoid using larger amounts.

Effectiveness

There is insufficient reliable information available about the effectiveness of pipsissewa.

Possible Mechanism of Action & Active Ingredients

The applicable parts of pipsissewa are the above ground plant parts. The component chimaphilin has a weak sensitizing effect. It is not suitable for long term use due to its hydroquinone glycoside content (18). Chimaphilin may have urinary antiseptic, bacteriostatic, and astringent activity (11). Animal data suggests pipsissewa may elicit hypoglycemia. Arbutin may have urinary antiseptic properties due to hydrolysis to its hydroquinone by the intestinal flora (7,11).

Adverse Reactions Including Known Allergies

Chronic use may lead to hydroquinone toxicity. Symptoms of toxicity include tinnitus, vomiting, delirium, convulsions, and collapse (11).

Possible Interactions with Herbs & Other Dietary Supplements

Insufficient reliable information available.

Possible Interactions with Drugs

No interactions are known to occur, and there is no known reason to expect a clinically significant interaction with pipsissewa.

Possible Interactions with Foods

No interactions are known to occur, and there is no known reason to expect a clinically significant interaction with pipsissewa.

Possible Interactions with Lab Tests

No interactions are known to occur, and there is no known reason to expect a clinically significant interaction with pipsissewa.

Possible Interactions with Diseases or Conditions

No interactions are known to occur, and there is no known reason to expect a clinically significant interaction with pipsissewa.

Typical Dosages & Routes of Administration that are Commonly Used

No typical dosage.

Comments

Pipsissewa is used similarly to uva ursi (18).

PITCHER PLANT

This Product is Also Known As

Eve's Cups, Fly-Catcher, Fly-Trap, Huntsman's Cup, Pitcher Plant, Purple Pitcher Plant, Purple Side-Saddle Flower, Sarapin, Side-Saddle Plant, Smallpox Plant, Water-cup.

Scientific Names

Sarracenia purpurea
Family: Sarraceniaceae.

People Use This For

Orally, pitcher plant is used for digestive disorders, particularly constipation, urinary tract diseases, as a diuretic, as a cure for smallpox, and to prevent scar formation (5050).

By injection, pitcher plant extract (Sarapin) is used as a trigger point injection to treat pain including sciatic pain, intercostal pain, alcoholic or occipital neuritis, brachial plexus neuralgia, meralgia paresthetica, and lumbar or trigeminal neuralgia (5971). Pitcher plant extract (Sarapin) has been used by injection in combination with bupivacaine hydrochloride 0.5% (Marcaine) and gamma globulin to treat the omohyoideus myofascial pain syndrome (5972). It has been used in combinations by injection (extract triamcinolone and lidocaine with adrenalin) to treat migraine cephalagia (5973), for diagnosis and treatment of forms of sciatic pain including piriformis syndrome (extract and lidocaine), quadratus lumborum syndrome (extract and corticosteroid) (5974), and in combination with physiotherapy and an intraoral splint to treat the Ernest Syndrome that is often mistaken for temporomandibular joint problems (5978). It is also used in prolotherapy (phenol and extract) to cause inflammation at the site where the ligaments and tendons attach to the bone to stimulate the body to proliferate stronger, shorter, and less painful ligaments and/or tendons (5977).

Safety

LIKELY SAFE ...when the extract of pitcher plant, Sarapin (a prescription product), is used appropriately by injection by a qualified health professional (5971).

There is insufficient reliable information available about the safety of the oral use of pitcher plant.

POSSIBLY UNSAFE ...when the extract of pitcher plant, Sarapin (a prescription product), is injected in areas of inflammation (5971).

PREGNANCY AND LACTATION: Insufficient reliable information available; avoid using.

Effectiveness

There is insufficient reliable information available about the effectiveness of the extract of pitcher plant (Sarapin) injection (5971). Sarapin was "grandfathered" to prescription drug status in the United States from the time when it was not necessary to prove effectiveness.

There is insufficient reliable information available about the effectiveness of the pitcher plant for its other uses..

Possible Mechanism of Action & Active Ingredients

The pitcher plant leaf and root contain sarracenia acid, tannin, resin, and the alkaloid sarracenin (5950). The extract has an effect on sensory nerves without changing skin sensation or affecting motor nerves. Some evidence suggests that pitcher plant extract affects only C nerve fibers, perhaps containing a biological antagonist that potentiates the action of the ammonium ion (5975). This could be beneficial in chronic neuropathic pain.

Adverse Reactions Including Known Allergies

Used by injection, pitcher plant extract can cause a local sensation of heaviness. Some individuals experience a local sensation of heat or aggravation of symptoms.

Possible Interactions with Herbs & Other Dietary Supplements

Insufficient reliable information available.

Possible Interactions with Drugs

No interactions are known to occur, and there is no known reason to expect a clinically significant interaction with pitcher plant.

Possible Interactions with Foods

No interactions are known to occur, and there is no known reason to expect a clinically significant interaction with pitcher plant.

Possible Interactions with Lab Tests

No interactions are known to occur, and there is no known reason to expect a clinically significant interaction with pitcher plant.

Possible Interactions with Diseases or Conditions

No interactions are known to occur, and there is no known reason to expect a clinically significant interaction with pitcher plant.

Typical Dosages & Routes of Administration that are Commonly Used

INJECTION: Pitcher plant extract (Sarapin) is given by nerve block or local infiltration. Doses are as follows: 2-3 mL cervical, 5-10 mL dorsal, 5-10 mL lumbar, 3-5 mL sacral, 10 mL caudal canal, 10 mL sciatic nerve, 5-10 mL local infiltration. Following injection, patients should be maintained in recumbent position for 15 minutes (5971). For use in migraine, 4 mg triamcinolone, 0.75 mL Sarapin and 0.15 mL lidocaine with adrenalin drawn into a syringe in that order have been administered at the trigger points in both temples using a 28 gauge, 5/8 inch needle (5973).

Sarapin is an FDA approved prescription product. For additional information, contact the manufacturer, High Chemical Company, 1-800-447-8792.

Comments
None.

PLEURISY ROOT

This Product is Also Known As
Butterfly Weed, Canada Root, Flux Root, Orange Milkweed, Orange Swallow-Wort, Swallow-Wort, Tuber Root, White Root, Wind Root.

Scientific Names
Asclepias tuberosa.
Family: Asclepiadaceae.

People Use This For
Orally, pleurisy root is used for coughs, pleurisy, uterine disorders, to ease breathing, and as an analgesic, expectorant, antispasmodic, and to promote sweating [18]. It is also used orally for bronchitis, pneumonitis, and influenza [4].

Safety
POSSIBLY UNSAFE …when the root is used orally because it contains digitalis-like cardenolide glycosides[4]. Can cause vomiting [12]. Canadian regulations do not allow pleurisy root as a non-medicinal ingredient for oral use products [12].
PREGNANCY: UNSAFE ...contraindicated [12] because it might have uterine stimulant and estrogenic activity [19].
LACTATION: POSSIBLY UNSAFE; avoid using.

Effectiveness
There is insufficient reliable information available about the effectiveness of pleurisy root.

Possible Mechanism of Action & Active Ingredients
Pleurisy root contains digitalis-like cardenolide glycosides [18]. Animal data suggest that pleurisy root does not affect blood pressure, respiration, or heart muscle. [4].

Adverse Reactions Including Known Allergies
Pleurisy root may cause dermatitis. It is also a gastrointestinal irritant and emetic, and can cause nausea and vomiting [19]. At higher doses, it may cause digitalis-like poisoning symptoms [18].

Possible Interactions with Herbs & Other Dietary Supplements
CARDIAC GLYCOSIDE-CONTAINING HERBS: Contraindicated, and concomitant use can increase the risk of cardiac glycoside toxicity. Cardiac glycoside-containing herbs include black hellebore, Canadian hemp roots, digitalis leaf, hedge mustard, figwort, lily of the valley roots, motherwort, oleander leaf, pheasant's eye plant, squill bulb leaf scales, strophanthus seeds, and uzara [2,18,19,500].

Possible Interactions with Drugs
DIGOXIN: Because pleurisy root contains cardenolide glycosides, it could have additive effects with digoxin [19].
ANTIDEPRESSANTS: Theoretically, excessive amounts of pleurisy root might interfere with antidepressant therapy [4].
HORMONES: Theoretically, excessive amounts of pleurisy root might interfere with hormone drug therapy [4].

Possible Interactions with Foods
No interactions are known to occur, and there is no known reason to expect a clinically significant interaction with pleurisy root.

Possible Interactions with Lab Tests
No interactions are known to occur, and there is no known reason to expect a clinically significant interaction with pleurisy root.

Possible Interactions with Diseases or Conditions
CARDIAC CONDITIONS: CAUTION; pleurisy root may worsen or interfere with cardiac drug therapy [4].

Typical Dosages & Routes of Administration that are Commonly Used
No typical dosage.

Comments
Pleurisy root is considered possibly unsafe; avoid using.

PODOPHYLLUM

This Product is Also Known As

American Mandrake, Devil's Apple, Duck's Foot, Ground Lemon, Himalayan Mayapple, Hog Apple, Indian Apple, Indian Podophyllum, Mandrake, Mayapple, Podophylli pelati rhizoma/resina, Podophyllum peltatum, Raccoon Berry, Vegetable Mercury, Wild Lemon, Wild Mandrake.
CAUTION: See separate listings for Bryonia (English Mandrake) and European Mandrake.

Scientific Names

Podophyllum peltatum; Podophyllum hexandrum, synonym Podophyllum emodi.
Family: Berberidaceae.

People Use This For

Topically, podophyllum resin is used for removal of topical warts (6,5617), including plantar warts (9), condyloma acuminata (venereal warts) (2,6,7,9,11,5617), and other papillomas (11).
Historically, podophyllum resin has been taken orally as a cathartic, for jaundice and liver ailments, fever, syphilis, and cancer (11,5617). The resin has also been taken orally as an antihelmintic and an antidote for snake bites (6). It has also been used as an abortifacient (5618).

Safety

POSSIBLY SAFE ...when used topically and appropriately (9,12). Podophyllum must be applied in low concentration solutions (0.5% podophyllotoxin) (6,9) to small surface areas (25 square cm or less) (2,7,18) with protection of adjacent skin (2,7) and washed off within 1-4 hours (6,9). Contact with skin should not exceed 6 hours (6). Risk of systemic toxicity increases if applied to large areas, open lesions, normal skin or mucous membranes, with prolonged use (9) and use of ointment form (6).
LIKELY UNSAFE ...when used orally; potentially lethal. ...when used topically for self-medication (2,6,9,5617). ...when used near eyes (19), on cervical or urethral warts (9). Contraindicated for use on moles, birthmarks, or inflamed warts because it can cause permanent skin damage (19). Fatalities have been reported from oral ingestion and topical application (6,9,5617).
PREGNANCY: LIKELY UNSAFE ...when used orally or topically for self-medication; contraindicated. Considered potentially embryotoxic and teratogenic (2,7,9,11,12,5618). Fetal intrauterine death and multiple birth deformities associated with oral and topical podophyllum use have been reported (5618).
LACTATION: LIKELY UNSAFE ...when used for self-medication; contraindicated.

Effectiveness

LIKELY EFFECTIVE ...when used topically for removal of benign epithelial growths, including warts, fibroids, papillomas (15), and anogenital condylomata acuminata (2). ...when used orally as a laxative (6,7,9,11,13,15), but it is unsafe for oral ingestion (2,6,9).
There is insufficient reliable information available about the effectiveness of podophyllum for its other uses.

Possible Mechanism of Action & Active Ingredients

The applicable parts of podophyllum are the root, rhizome, and resin. The major active constituents in podophyllum are lignan derivatives (6,9,11), including podophyllotoxin (2,6,7,9,11), which is antimitotic (9,11,13,18) and antineoplastic (6,11). It induces catharsis through irritation of the intestinal mucosa (6,9), it induces lymphocyte activating factor/interleukin 1, it stimulates macrophage proliferation, and it modulates other cytokines (11). Significant absorption occurs through the skin (6) and the gastrointestinal tract (5617). Etoposide and teniposide, semisynthetic analogs of podophyllotoxin, are active against testicular cancer, small cell lung cancer, leukemia, lymphoma (6,11,13), Kaposi's sarcoma, neuroblastoma (13), rheumatoid arthritis (6,11), and psoriasis (11). Podophyllotoxin exposure during pregnancy is considered to be highly embryotoxic (6,7,11,5618); teratogenicity has been reported (6,5618) but not confirmed by studies in experimental animals (7,11).

Adverse Reactions Including Known Allergies

Oral ingestion and topical application can cause severe abdominal pain (18), nausea, vomiting (6,5617), bloody-watery diarrhea, vomiting of bile, dizziness, headache, coordination disorders, spasms, nephritis (18), fever, altered mental status, visual hallucinations, confusion, tachypnea, peripheral neuropathy, muscle paralysis, hypotension, bone marrow suppression, renal failure (6,5617), coma, respiratory failure, and death (6,18,5617). Chronic use as a cathartic can cause hypokalemia and metabolic alkalosis (6,5617). Oral or topical use of podophyllum in pregnant women can cause fetal congenital malformations and death (6,5618). Podophyllum can cause severe local irritation, especially to eyes and mucous membranes (9,11,18). It might also cause transformation of condyloma to squamous cell carcinoma (9). Symptoms of toxicity usually do not appear for a period of time, ranging from a few to 13 hours after ingestion or absorption (5617). Neurologic changes may progress rapidly after onset of symptoms (6).

Possible Interactions with Herbs & Other Dietary Supplements

CARDIAC GLYCOSIDE-CONTAINING HERBS: Contraindicated; concomitant use may increase the risk of cardiac glycoside toxicity. Cardiac glycoside-containing herbs include: black hellebore, Canadian hemp roots, digitalis leaf, hedge mustard, figwort, lily of the valley roots, motherwort, oleander leaf, pheasant's eye plant, pleurisy root, squill bulb leaf scales, and strophanthus seeds (2,18,19,500).

STIMULANT LAXATIVE HERBS: Theoretically, concomitant use with other stimulant laxative herbs may increase the risk of potassium depletion. Stimulant laxative herbs include: aloe dried leaf sap, wild cucumber fruit (Ecballium elaterium), blue flag rhizome, alder buckthorn, European buckthorn, butternut bark, cascara bark, castor oil, colocynth fruit pulp, gamboge bark exudate, jalap root, black root, manna bark exudate, rhubarb root, senna leaves and pods, and yellow dock root (19).

POTASSIUM-DEPLETING HERBS: Theoretically, concomitant use with horsetail plant or licorice rhizome increases the risk of potassium depletion.

Possible Interactions with Drugs
No interactions are known to occur, and there is no known reason to expect a clinically significant interaction with podophyllum.

Possible Interactions with Foods
No interactions are known to occur, and there is no known reason to expect a clinically significant interaction with podophyllum.

Possible Interactions with Lab Tests
No interactions are known to occur, and there is no known reason to expect a clinically significant interaction with podophyllum.

Possible Interactions with Diseases or Conditions
GALLSTONES: Contraindicated. Theoretically, podophyllum can stimulate bile secretion (19).
GI CONDITIONS: Contraindicated. Podophyllum can irritate the gastrointestinal tract, exacerbating infectious or inflammatory conditions (19).

Typical Dosages & Routes of Administration that are Commonly Used
ORAL: No typical dosage.
TOPICAL: 1.5-3 grams root or fluid extract, or 2.5-7.5 grams tincture (5-25% in benzoin), applied once or twice per week to an area no more than 25 square cm, with protection of surrounding skin (2,6,7,13,18). Alternatively, 0.5% solution applied twice per day for three days, washed off after 1-6 hours (6-9), or 0.15% cream applied twice per day for three days (9). Lower concentrations applied twice per day are at least as effective as higher concentrations applied twice per week (6,7,9). Should not be used for self-treatment; requires supervision.

Comments
Podophyllum is considered unsafe and potentially lethal (see Safety). Podophyllum resin is prepared from the root and rhizome of the plant. Podophyllum toxicity has been successfully treated using charcoal hemoperfusion (6,5617).

POINSETTIA

This Product is Also Known As
Christmas Flower, Easter Flower, Lobster Flower Plant, Lobsterplant, Mexican Flame Leaf, Mexican Flameleaf, Paintedleaf, Papagallo.

Scientific Names
Euphorbia pulcherrima; Euphorbia poinsettia; Poinsettia pulcherrima.
Family: Euphorbiaceae.

People Use This For
Orally, poinsettia is used as an antipyretic, to stimulate milk production, and as an abortifacient (6). The latex is taken orally as an analgesic, antibacterial, and emetic (6).
Topically, the latex is used as a depilatory, (6).
In folk medicine, it has been used as a skin remedy, for warts, and toothaches (6).

Safety
POSSIBLY UNSAFE ...when the plant or latex are used orally or topically, but toxicity is limited to local irritation, contact dermatitis, mucosal burns, and keratoconjunctivitis (17).
CHILDREN: POSSIBLY UNSAFE. Poinsettia was implicated in the poisoning death of a 2 year old child (6).
PREGNANCY AND LACTATION: POSSIBLY UNSAFE ...when used orally or topically; avoid using.

Effectiveness
There is insufficient reliable information available about the effectiveness of poinsettia.

Possible Mechanism of Action & Active Ingredients
The applicable parts of poinsettia are the whole plant and latex. There is insufficient reliable information available about the possible mechanism of action and active ingredients of poinsettia.

Adverse Reactions Including Known Allergies
Toxicity is limited to local irritation, contact dermatitis, mucosal burns, and keratoconjunctivitis (17).

Possible Interactions with Herbs & Other Dietary Supplements
Insufficient reliable information available.

Possible Interactions with Drugs
No interactions are known to occur, and there is no known reason to expect a clinically significant interaction with poinsettia.

Possible Interactions with Foods
No interactions are known to occur, and there is no known reason to expect a clinically significant interaction with poinsettia.

Possible Interactions with Lab Tests
No interactions are known to occur, and there is no known reason to expect a clinically significant interaction with poinsettia.

Possible Interactions with Diseases or Conditions
GI IRRITATION, INFLAMMATION: Euphorbia species are said to have GI irritant effects (19); avoid using.

Typical Dosages & Routes of Administration that are Commonly Used
No typical dosage.

Comments
Recent studies indicate that the plant is less toxic than once believed (6). American Association of Poison Control Centers reported 22,793 cases of poisoning with no fatalities and 92.4% with no toxicity (3838).

POISON IVY

This Product is Also Known As
Markweed, Poison Vine, Three-Leafed Ivy.

Scientific Names
Toxicodendron radicans; Rhus Toxicodendron (Rhus radicans).
Family: Anacardiaceae.

People Use This For
In folk medicine, poison ivy has been used as a narcotic (18).

Safety
LIKELY UNSAFE ...when used orally or topically (6).
PREGNANCY AND LACTATION: LIKELY UNSAFE ...when used orally or topically.

Effectiveness
There is insufficient reliable information available about the effectiveness of poison ivy.

Possible Mechanism of Action & Active Ingredients
Poison ivy is a severe skin irritant that stimulates the immune system (18). Contact sensitivity is due to the urushiols, which bind to skin proteins, sensitizing the individual (6). Once sensitized, re-exposure leads to allergic reactions (6).

Adverse Reactions Including Known Allergies
Taken orally, the plant can cause severe mucous membrane irritation, nausea, vomiting, intestinal colic, diarrhea, dizziness, stupor, nephritis, hematuria, fever, and unconsciousness (18). Inhalation due to burning of the plant can result in fever, major lung infection, and death from throat swelling (6). Topically, the plant can cause contact dermatitis, reddening, swelling, herpes-like blisters (18), and erythema multiforme (3839). Eye contact can cause severe conjunctivitis, corneal inflammations, or loss of sight (18).

Possible Interactions with Herbs & Other Dietary Supplements
GINKGO BILOBA: Fruit pulp can cause cross-reactivity in people allergic to poison ivy (6).
JEWELWEED: Topical application of a 1:4 preparation may relieve symptoms of poison ivy dermatitis in humans (512).

Possible Interactions with Drugs
No interactions are known to occur, and there is no known reason to expect a clinically significant interaction with poison ivy.

Possible Interactions with Foods
MANGO: Fruit skin can cause cross-reactivity in people allergic to poison ivy (6,735). CASHEW: Nut shell oil can cause cross-reactivity in people allergic to poison ivy (6,735).

Possible Interactions with Lab Tests
No interactions are known to occur, and there is no known reason to expect a clinically significant interaction with poison ivy.

Possible Interactions with Diseases or Conditions
No interactions are known to occur, and there is no known reason to expect a clinically significant interaction with poison ivy.

Typical Dosages & Routes of Administration that are Commonly Used
No typical dosage.

Comments
Poison ivy is likely unsafe; avoid using. To prevent poison ivy from causing skin irritation, wash exposed area with water within 5 to 10 minutes (6). Use soap and water first, then ether or alcohol (18).

POISONOUS BUTTERCUP

This Product is Also Known As
Celery-Leafed Crowfoot, Cursed Crowfoot.
CAUTION: See separate listings for Buttercup and Bulbous Buttercup.

Scientific Names
Ranunculus sceleratus.
Family: Ranunculaceae.

People Use This For
Topically, poisonous buttercup is used as a stimulant for skin diseases (e.g. scabies) and leucoderma (18).

Safety
LIKELY UNSAFE ...when the above ground parts are used orally or topically. The fresh plant causes severe local irritation (18).
There is insufficient reliable information about the safety of the oral or topical use of the dried, cut leaf.
PREGNANCY: LIKELY UNSAFE ...contraindicated for oral or topical use. Oral use might possibly stimulate uterine activity (19).
LACTATION: LIKELY UNSAFE ...contraindicated for oral or topical use (18).

Effectiveness
There is insufficient reliable information available about the effectiveness of poisonous buttercup.

Possible Mechanism of Action & Active Ingredients
The applicable parts of poisonous buttercup are the above ground parts. Poisonous buttercup contains ranunculin, anemonin, and protoanemonin. Protoanemonin is a potent topical irritant (18). It causes pain and burning sensations, severe tongue inflammation, and increases salivation. When the freshly harvested plant is cut into small pieces or perhaps when it is dried, protoanemonin changes into a pungent, volatile intermediate that quickly dimerizes to a form that does not irritate the mucous membrane. In vitro, leaf extracts have shown a wide fungicidal spectrum of activity (3836).

Adverse Reactions Including Known Allergies
Extended contact with fresh or bruised plant can lead to blisters and burns that are difficult to heal (18). Some species of Ranunculus can cause photodermatitis. Avoid excessive sunlight or ultraviolet light exposure while using this product (19).

Possible Interactions with Herbs & Other Dietary Supplements
Insufficient reliable information available.

Possible Interactions with Drugs
No interactions are known to occur, and there is no known reason to expect a clinically significant interaction with poisonous buttercup.

Possible Interactions with Foods
No interactions are known to occur, and there is no known reason to expect a clinically significant interaction with poisonous buttercup.

Possible Interactions with Lab Tests
No interactions are known to occur, and there is no known reason to expect a clinically significant interaction with poisonous buttercup.

Possible Interactions with Diseases or Conditions
No interactions are known to occur, and there is no known reason to expect a clinically significant interaction with poisonous buttercup.

Typical Dosages & Routes of Administration that are Commonly Used
No typical dosage.

Comments
Poisonous buttercup is used as a tincture (18).

POKEWEED berry

This Product is Also Known As
American Nightshade, American Spinach, Bear's Grape, Branching Phytolacca, Cancer Jalap, Chongras, Coakum, Coakum-Chorngras, Cokan, Crowberry, Fitolaca, Garget, Hierba Carmín, Inkberry, Jalap, Kermesbeere, Phytolacca Berry, Pigeonberry, Pocan, Poke, Pokeberry, Raisin d'Amérique, Red-Ink Plant, Red Plant, Red Weed, Scoke, Skoke, Teinturière, Virginian Poke.
CAUTION: See separate listings for Jalap, Mexican Scammony Root, and Pokeweed root.

Scientific Names
Phytolacca americana, synonym Phytolacca decandra.
Family: Phytolaccaceae.

People Use This For
Pokeweed is used as a food, red food coloring (18), and wine coloring agent (6).
In manufacturing, it is used to make ink and dye (6).

Safety
LIKELY UNSAFE ...when the fresh berry is ingested. One berry can be toxic to a child; 10 berries to an adult (6,18). Green berries are considered more toxic than mature, red berries (4). ...when pokeweed berry and juice comes in contact with broken skin or is ingested, it can cause hematological changes (4,3477,3481,3482). Protective gloves should be used to handle the plant (6,3477). All parts of the pokeweed plant, especially the root, are considered to be toxic (3477,3479,3483). Severe poisoning has been reported from ingesting tea brewed from pokeweed root (6,3478) and pokeweed leaves (3480). Poisoning also has resulted from ingestion of pokeberry wine and pokeberry pancakes (3479).
CHILDREN: UNSAFE ...consumption of even one berry can be toxic. Children have died after ingesting pokeweed berries (3479,3483).
PREGNANCY AND LACTATION: LIKELY UNSAFE; avoid using. Evidence suggests the berry has uterine stimulant and abortifacient effects (4,19).

Effectiveness
There is insufficient reliable information about the effectiveness of pokeweed berry.

Possible Mechanism of Action & Active Ingredients
Pokeweed contains saponin glycosides, proteinaceous mitogens (3477,3478), tannin, and resin (6). The toxicity of pokeweed is attributed to proteinaceous mitogens and the saponin glycosides which include phytolaccatoxin and phytolaccagenin. The saponin glycosides cause gastrointestinal irritation and the proteinaceous mitogens are thought to affect thymus-dependent (T) cells and thymus-independent (B) lymphocytes (3477,3478).

Adverse Reactions Including Known Allergies
Taken orally, all parts of the pokeweed plant can cause nausea, vomiting, cramping, abdominal pain, diarrhea, burning sensation in mouth and throat, weakness, bloody emesis, hypotension, bloody diarrhea, tachycardia, difficulty in breathing, salivation, urinary incontinence, spasm, convulsion (4,3477,3478,3479), severe thirst, somnolence, transient blindness, respiratory failure (18,3477,3479), and death (4,18,3477,3483). Plasmacytosis, mitotic changes in peripheral blood cells, eosinophilia, thrombocytopenia, abnormal platelet morphology and other hematologic abnormalities may result from topical exposure (especially in individuals with cuts or abrasions on hands or other extremities) and ingestion of pokeweed plant, berries or root (3477,3478,3481,3482).

Possible Interactions with Herbs & Other Dietary Supplements
Insufficient reliable information available.

Possible Interactions with Drugs
No interactions are known to occur, and there is no known reason to expect a clinically significant interaction with pokeweed berry.

Possible Interactions with Foods
No interactions are known to occur, and there is no known reason to expect a clinically significant interaction with pokeweed berry.

Possible Interactions with Lab Tests

No interactions are known to occur, and there is no known reason to expect a clinically significant interaction with pokeweed berry.

Possible Interactions with Diseases or Conditions

No interactions are known to occur, and there is no known reason to expect a clinically significant interaction with pokeweed berry.

Typical Dosages & Routes of Administration that are Commonly Used

No typical dosage.

Comments

Avoid confusion with jalap (Ipomoea orizabensis). All parts of the pokeweed plant are considered toxic except the above ground leaves grown in early spring (6). The immature leaves are canned and marketed as the food product, "poke salad" (6). In folk medicine, the leaves have been used for rheumatism, arthritis, emesis, and purging (6). Ongoing research is investigating the use of pokeweed in flu, HSV-1, and polio (4,18). The United Kingdom allows pokeweed in medicinal products provided toxic constituents are absent and the product adheres to mandated limits (4).

POKEWEED root

This Product is Also Known As

American Nightshade, American Spinach, Bear's Grape, Branching Phytolacca, Cancer Jalap, Chongras, Coakum, Coakum-Chorngras, Cokan, Crowberry, Fitolaca, Garget, Hierba Carmín, Inkberry, Jalap, Kermesbeere, Phytolacca Berry, Pigeonberry, Pocan, Poke, Pokeberry, Raisin d'Amérique, Red-Ink Plant, Red Plant, Red Weed, Scoke, Skoke, Teinturière, Virginian Poke.
CAUTION: See separate listings for Jalap, Mexican Scammony Root, and Pokewood berry.

Scientific Names

Phytolacca americana, synonym Phytolacca decandra.
Family: Phytolaccaceae.

People Use This For

Orally, pokeweed root is used as an emetic (18).
Historically, it has been used for rheumatism, mucous membrane inflammation of upper and lower respiratory tract, tonsillitis, laryngitis, adenitis, mastitis, mumps, skin infections (scabies, tinea, sycosis, ringworm, acne), mammary abscesses (4), edema, skin cancers, dysmenorrhea, mumps, tonsillitis, and syphilis (6).

Safety

LIKELY UNSAFE ...when taken orally. All parts of the pokeweed plant, especially the root, are considered to be toxic (3477,3479,3483). The Herb Trade Association recommends against selling pokeweed root as an herbal beverage or food (4,3478). Severe poisoning has been reported from ingesting tea brewed from pokeweed root (6,3478) and pokeweed leaves (3480). ...when root comes in contact with broken skin or is ingested, it can cause hematological changes (3477,3481,3482). Protective gloves should be used to handle the plant (6,3477).
PREGNANCY AND LACTATION: LIKELY UNSAFE; avoid using. Evidence suggests it might have uterine stimulant and abortifacient effects (4,19).

Effectiveness

There is insufficient reliable information available about the effectiveness of pokeweed root.

Possible Mechanism of Action & Active Ingredients

Pokeweed contains saponin glycosides, proteinaceous mitogens (3477,3478), tannin, and resin (6). The toxicity of pokeweed is attributed to proteinaceous mitogens and the saponin glycosides which include phytolaccatoxin and phytolaccagenin. The saponin glycosides cause gastrointestinal irritation and the proteinaceous mitogens are thought to affect thymus-dependent (T) cells and thymus-independent (B) lymphocytes (3477,3478).

Adverse Reactions Including Known Allergies

Taken orally, all parts of the pokeweed plant can cause nausea, vomiting, cramping, abdominal pain, diarrhea, burning sensation in mouth and throat, weakness, bloody emesis, hypotension, bloody diarrhea, tachycardia, difficulty in breathing, salivation, urinary incontinence, spasm, convulsion (4,3477,3478,3479), severe thirst, somnolence, transient blindness, respiratory failure (18,3477,3479), and death (4,18,3477,3483). Plasmacytosis, mitotic changes in peripheral blood cells, eosinophilia, thrombocytopenia, abnormal platelet morphology and other hematologic abnormalities may result from topical exposure (especially in individuals with cuts or abrasions on hands or other extremities) and ingestion of pokeweed plant, berries or root (3477,3478,3481,3482).

Possible Interactions with Herbs & Other Dietary Supplements
Insufficient reliable information available.

Possible Interactions with Drugs
No interactions are known to occur, and there is no known reason to expect a clinically significant interaction with pokeweed root.

Possible Interactions with Foods
No interactions are known to occur, and there is no known reason to expect a clinically significant interaction with pokeweed root.

Possible Interactions with Lab Tests
No interactions are known to occur, and there is no known reason to expect a clinically significant interaction with pokeweed root.

Possible Interactions with Diseases or Conditions
No interactions are known to occur, and there is no known reason to expect a clinically significant interaction with pokeweed root.

Typical Dosages & Routes of Administration that are Commonly Used
No typical dosage.

Comments
Avoid confusion with jalap (Ipomoea orizabensis). All parts of the pokeweed plant are considered toxic except the above ground leaves grown in early spring [6]. The immature leaves are canned and marketed as the food product, "poke salad" [6]. In folk medicine, the leaves have been used for rheumatism, arthritis, emesis, and purging [6]. Ongoing research is investigating the use of pokeweed in flu, HSV-1, and polio [4,18]. The United Kingdom allows pokeweed in medicinal products provided toxic constituents are absent and the product adheres to mandated limits [4].

POLICOSANOL

This Product is Also Known As
None.
CAUTION: See separate listing for Octacosanol.

Scientific Names
Policosanol.

People Use This For
Orally, policosanol is used for hyperlipidemia [2923,2942], for intermittent claudication [2931], for decreasing myocardial ischemia in patients with coronary heart disease [2941], and as an anti-plaque agent [2942].

Safety
POSSIBLY SAFE ...when taken orally in amounts of 10 mg per day and used for up to 24 months [2927].
PREGNANCY AND LACTATION: Insufficient reliable information available; avoid using.

Effectiveness
POSSIBLY EFFECTIVE ...when taken orally for treating hypercholesterolemia [2927,2928,2929,2930,2943,2944] and intermittent claudication [2931].
There is insufficient reliable information about the effectiveness of policosanol for its other uses.

Possible Mechanism of Action & Active Ingredients
Policosanol shows evidence that it might inhibit hepatic cholesterol synthesis [2934,2939] and increase the degradation of LDL cholesterol [2939]. Policosanol reduces total and LDL cholesterol and increases HDL cholesterol in people with hypercholesterolemia [2927,2928,2943] or hypercholesterolemia with type 2 (NIDDM) diabetes [2929]. It also reduces total and LDL cholesterol in people with coronary heart disease (CHD) and high cholesterol [2930], and in people with hypertension and high cholesterol [2944]. Policosanol decreases arachidonic acid and the collagen-induced platelet aggregation in healthy people [2936,2937,2938], and in people with high cholesterol [2933,2935]. It does this without affecting coagulation time [2935,2937]. In healthy people, 20 mg per day of policosanol can be as effective as 100 mg per day of aspirin for decreasing experimentally-induced platelet aggregation [2937]. Policosanol improves walking distance in individuals with intermittent claudication [2931].

Adverse Reactions Including Known Allergies
Taken orally, policosanol can cause erythema [2929], migraines, insomnia, somnolence, irritability, dizziness, upset stomach, polyphagia, dysuria, weight loss, skin rash, and nose bleeds [786].

Possible Interactions with Herbs & Other Dietary Supplements
Insufficient reliable information available.

Possible Interactions with Drugs
ASPIRIN, WARFARIN, NONSTEROIDAL ANTI-INFLAMMATORY DRUGS (NSAIDs): Theoretically, due to the antiplatelet effects of policosanol [2936,2937,2938] concomitant use might increase the risk of bleeding.

Possible Interactions with Foods
No interactions are known to occur, and there is no known reason to expect a clinically significant interaction with policosanol.

Possible Interactions with Lab Tests
CHOLESTEROL: Evidence suggests policosanol can decrease serum total cholesterol and LDL cholesterol levels and increase HDL cholesterol level [2927,2928,2943], and it can affect these lab tests results.

Possible Interactions with Diseases or Conditions
CARDIOVASCULAR DISEASE: Theoretically, policosanol might decrease the risk of stroke or heart attack due to its antiplatelet activity.
CORONARY ARTERY DISEASE: Theoretically, policosanol might slow the progression of coronary artery disease due to its cholesterol-lowering effects.

Typical Dosages & Routes of Administration that are Commonly Used
ORAL: For hypercholesterolemia, the typical dose of policosanol is 5-10 mg twice daily [2927,2928,2929,2930]. For intermittent claudication, 10 mg is usually taken twice daily [2931].

Comments
Policosanol is derived from sugar cane [2942] and refers to a mixture of 24-34 carbon alcohols comprised primarily of octacosanol (28-C) and including tetracosanol (24-C), hexacosanol (26-C), heptacosanol (27-C), nonacosanol (29-C), triacontanol (30-C), dotriacontanol (32-C), and tetratriacontanol [268,269,270,2942]. Avoid confusion with octacosanol.

POMEGRANATE

This Product is Also Known As
Granada, Grenadier, Shi Liu Gen Pi, Shi Liu Pi.

Scientific Names
Punica granatum.
Family: Punicaceae.

People Use This For
Orally, pomegranate is used for tapeworm infestations, and opportunistic intestinal worms. It is also used as an astringent, for diarrhea and dysentery, and as an abortive.
Topically, it is used as a gargle for sore throat and to treat hemorrhoids [18].

Safety
POSSIBLY SAFE ...when the fruit rind is used orally [12].
UNSAFE ...when the root is taken orally because it contains the toxic alkaloid pelletierine. The FDA recommends that pomegranate root be prohibited for use in foods as a flavoring agent [12]. ...when the fruit rind is used in individuals with diarrhea [12].
There is insufficient reliable information available about the topical safety of pomegranate bark and root.
PREGNANCY: UNSAFE. The bark, root, and fruit rind could stimulate menstruation or uterine contractions [12,19].
LACTATION: UNSAFE ...when the bark or root is used orally. There is insufficient reliable information available about the safety of pomegranate for using the bark or root topically, or using the fruit rind; avoid using.

Effectiveness
There is insufficient reliable information available about the effectiveness of pomegranate.

Possible Mechanism of Action & Active Ingredients
The applicable parts of the pomegranate are the bark, rind, root, seed, and stem [18,1287]. The seed oil contains polyphenols and fatty acids, including punicic acid, palmitic acid, stearic acid, oleic acid, and linoleic acid [1287]. Fermented pomegranate juice and cold pressed seed oil demonstrate antioxidant activity, possibly due to their flavonoid content [1287]. Pomegranate root and stem contain the piperidine alkaloids isopelletierine, N-methyliospelletierine, and pseudopelletierin. The root contains up to 25% tannins, the fruit rind contains up to 28% tannins [18]. Tannins can exert an astringent effect on mucosal tissues, dehydrating the tissue, reducing internal secretions and forming a hardened, external protective layer of cells. Plants with at least 10% tannins can cause

gastrointestinal disturbances, kidney damage, and necrotic conditions of the liver. Some preliminary data suggest that tannins might cause cancer; other data suggest tannins may prevent it. Regular consumption of herbs with high tannin concentrations correlates with increased incidence of esophageal or nasal cancer (12).

Adverse Reactions Including Known Allergies

Overdoses can cause strychnine-like effects in the form of heightened reflex arousal that can escalate to paralysis. At amounts greater than 80 grams, people experience vomiting, including bloody emesis, followed by dizziness, chills, vision disorders, collapse, and possibly death due to respiratory failure. Total blindness can occur within a few hours to a few days after ingestion, and resolves after several weeks (18).

Possible Interactions with Herbs & Other Dietary Supplements

TANNIN-CONTAINING HERBS: Theoretically, herbs that contain high percentages of tannins (such as pomegranate) may cause precipitation of constituents of other herbs (19).

Possible Interactions with Drugs

ORAL DRUGS: Theoretically, concomitant oral administration may cause precipitation of some drugs due to the high tannin content of pomegranate (19). Separate administration of oral drugs and tannin-containing herbs by the longest period of time practical (19).

Possible Interactions with Foods

No interactions are known to occur, and there is no known reason to expect a clinically significant interaction with pomegranate.

Possible Interactions with Lab Tests

No interactions are known to occur, and there is no known reason to expect a clinically significant interaction with pomegranate.

Possible Interactions with Diseases or Conditions

No interactions are known to occur, and there is no known reason to expect a clinically significant interaction with pomegranate.

Typical Dosages & Routes of Administration that are Commonly Used

No typical dosage.

Comments

The root and stem bark are unsafe for self-medication (12). When used to treat parasites, the fruit rind should not be taken with fats or oils (12).

POPLAR

This Product is Also Known As

Balm of Gilead, Balsam Poplar Buds, Pappelknospen, Populi Gemma.
CAUTION: See separate listings for Dwarf Pine Needle, Fir Needle Oil, Fir, Pine, and Scotch Pine Needle.

Scientific Names

Populus tacamahacca; Populus balsamifera; Populus candicans.
Family: Salicaceae.

People Use This For

Orally, poplar is used as an ingredient in herbal cough preparations. It is also used as a stimulant and expectorant (11).
Topically, it is used for sores, bruises, cuts, pimples (11), external hemorrhoids, frostbite, and sunburn (2).

Safety

LIKELY SAFE ...when applied topically and used appropriately (2,12). ...when used in alcoholic beverages in amounts that have been approved in the US (11).
POSSIBLY SAFE ...when used topically in individuals with aspirin allergy. Poplar contains salicylates but is not usually cross-reactive (12).
There is insufficient reliable information available about the safety of the oral use of poplar.
PREGNANCY AND LACTATION: Insufficient reliable information available; avoid using.

Effectiveness

POSSIBLY EFFECTIVE ...when used for the topical treatment of superficial skin injuries, external hemorrhoids, frostbite, and sunburn (2).
There is insufficient reliable information available about the effectiveness of poplar for its other uses.

Possible Mechanism of Action & Active Ingredients

The applicable parts of the poplar are the dried unopened leaf buds. Poplar contains salicin (11).

Adverse Reactions Including Known Allergies
Occasional allergic skin reactions can occur with the topical use of poplar (2). There are no reports of aspirin-type allergic reactions with the use of salicin-rich plants (12).

Possible Interactions with Herbs & Other Dietary Supplements
No interactions are known to occur, and there is no known reason to expect a clinically significant interaction with poplar.

Possible Interactions with Drugs
ANTICOAGULANTS: Preliminary data suggests that salicin does not potentiate the effects of anticoagulant drugs (12).

Possible Interactions with Foods
No interactions are known to occur, and there is no known reason to expect a clinically significant interaction with poplar.

Possible Interactions with Lab Tests
No interactions are known to occur, and there is no known reason to expect a clinically significant interaction with poplar.

Possible Interactions with Diseases or Conditions
ALLERGIES: Contraindicated in people allergic to poplar buds, propolis, Peru balsam, or salicylates (2,18).

Typical Dosages & Routes of Administration that are Commonly Used
TOPICAL: The common application of poplar is 5 grams of the dried buds per day or semi-solid preparations equivalent to 20-30% dried buds per day (2,18).

Comments
CAUTION: Available information supports only the external use of poplar. Avoid confusion with spruce (Picea excelsa) and Canada balsam (Abies balsamea), also known as balm of Gilead.

PORIA MUSHROOM

This Product is Also Known As
Fu Ling, FuShen, Hoelen, Indian Bread, Matsuhodo, Polyporus, Poria, Tuckahoe.

Scientific Names
Wolfiporia cocos, synonym Poria cocos.
Family: Polyporaceae.

People Use This For
Traditionally, poria filaments have been used for amnesia, anxiety, restlessness, fatigue, tension, nervousness, dizziness, dysuria and urination problems, edema, insomnia, splenitis, stomach problems, diarrhea, tumors, and as an antitussive (847,4017). Poria filaments have been used as a component of various herbal combinations for treating diarrhea (3731,3732), chronic glomerulonephritis (3733), tinnitus (3734), and for decreasing upper gastrointestinal tract bleeding (3735).

Safety
POSSIBLY SAFE …when used orally (12).
PREGNANCY AND LACTATION: Insufficient reliable information available; avoid using.

Effectiveness
There is insufficient reliable information available about the effectiveness of poria mushroom.

Possible Mechanism of Action & Active Ingredients
The applicable part is the sclerotium (filaments) of the poria fungus. Poria contains pachyman which prevents urinary protein excretion, serum cholesterol elevation, and reduces the degree of histopathological changes in nephritic rats (3727). Some evidence suggests a hydroalcoholic extract (3728) and isolated triterpene constituents (3729,3736,3737) might have anti-inflammatory activity. Other evidence suggests poria extracts might also have immunosuppressive effects (3726). In addition, isolated triterpene constituents show evidence that they might have antitumor (3729) and anti-emetic effects (3730).

Adverse Reactions Including Known Allergies
None reported.

Possible Interactions with Herbs & Other Dietary Supplements
Insufficient reliable information available.

Possible Interactions with Drugs

No interactions are known to occur, and there is no known reason to expect a clinically significant interaction with poria mushroom.

Possible Interactions with Foods

No interactions are known to occur, and there is no known reason to expect a clinically significant interaction with poria mushroom.

Possible Interactions with Lab Tests

No interactions are known to occur, and there is no known reason to expect a clinically significant interaction with poria mushroom.

Possible Interactions with Diseases or Conditions

No interactions are known to occur, and there is no known reason to expect a clinically significant interaction with poria mushroom.

Typical Dosages & Routes of Administration that are Commonly Used

ORAL: People typically use 10 to 15 grams per day (1663).

Comments

Various combination herbal mixtures containing poria are reported to be effective for treating diarrhea (3731,3732), chronic glomerulonephritis (3733), tinnitus (3734), and decreasing upper gastrointestinal tract bleeding (3735). Further studies are needed to verify these results.

POTASSIUM

This Product is Also Known As

Potassium Acetate, Potassium Bicarbonate, Potassium Chloride, Potassium Citrate, Potassium Gluconate, Potassium Phosphate.

Scientific Names

Potassium; K; atomic number 19.

People Use This For

Orally, potassium is used for treating hypokalemia (14,15,16), preventing potassium depletion (14,15,16), preventing hypertension (14,15), treating Menière's disease (16), thallium poisoning (15), hypercalciuria (14), urinary alkalinization (14), insulin resistance (14), myocardial infarction (14), stroke prevention (2201), fatigue and mood swing in early menopause (2201), and infant colic (2201). It is also used orally for allergies (2201,2202), headaches (2201,2202), acne, alcoholism, Alzheimer's disease, arthritis, blurred vision, cancer, chronic fatigue syndrome, colitis, confusion, constipation, dermatitis, edema, fever, gout, insomnia, irritability, mononucleosis, muscle weakness, muscular dystrophy, stress (2202), and as an adjunct for treating myasthenia gravis (15).
Intravenously, potassium is used for treating and preventing hypokalemia when oral replacement is not possible (14,15), for arrhythmias (14,15), including atrial tachycardia and ventricular arrhythmias (14,2207), and for myocardial infarction (14,2210).

Safety

LIKELY SAFE ...when consumed orally in amounts up to 80-90 mEq total potassium (supplements and diet) per day by individuals with normal renal function (14,15,16). Larger amounts increase the risk of hyperkalemia (15). ...when used intravenously (IV). Parental potassium is a FDA-approved prescription product.
UNSAFE ...when use results in blood levels above 7 mEq/L. This is potentially life-threatening (14).
PREGNANCY AND LACTATION: LIKELY SAFE ...at the normal dietary intake of 40-80 mEq per day, which is adequate to maintain the mother's serum potassium between 3.5-5 mEq/L (14). When the mother's serum potassium levels are in the normal range, levels in breast milk are generally low (14).

Effectiveness

EFFECTIVE ...when taken orally for treating and preventing hypokalemia (14,15) and for producing urinary alkalinization (14). ...when the FDA-approved, intravenous (IV) prescription product is used.
LIKELY EFFECTIVE ...when taken orally for treating hypertension (14) and hypercalciuria (14,2208,2209).
There is insufficient reliable information available about the effectiveness of potassium for its other uses.

Possible Mechanism of Action & Active Ingredients

The potassium mineral plays a role in many body functions including acid-base balance, electrodynamic characteristics of the cell, isotonicity, and various enzymatic reactions (15). It is essential in physiological processes including nerve impulse transmission, cardiac, smooth, and skeletal muscle contraction, gastric secretion, renal function, tissue synthesis, and carbohydrate synthesis (15). Evidence suggests that inadequate dietary intake of potassium can play a role in the development of hypertension. A potassium intake of 48-90 mEq/day can benefit people with hypertension (14,15).

Adverse Reactions Including Known Allergies

The oral or IV use of potassium can cause stomach upset, nausea, diarrhea, vomiting, flatulence, ulcerations, and hyperkalemia (14,15,16). Large amounts of potassium can cause paresthesias, generalized weakness, flaccid paralysis, listlessness, vertigo, mental confusion, hypotension, cardiac arrhythmias, heart block, and death (14,15,16).

Possible Interactions with Herbs & Other Dietary Supplements

Insufficient reliable information available.

Possible Interactions with Drugs

ACE INHIBITORS, POTASSIUM-SPARING DIURETICS: Concomitant use with these drugs can increase potassium levels and the risk of hyperkalemia adverse effects (15).

Drug Influences on Nutrient Levels and Depletion

SOME DRUGS CAN AFFECT POTASSIUM LEVELS:
AMPHOTERICIN B: Hypokalemia may develop in patients receiving amphotericin B (2529).
LOOP DIURETICS and THIAZIDE DIURETICS: Use of loop diuretics and thiazide diuretics increases urine potassium excretion and can cause hypokalemia. Monitor potassium serum levels and give potassium supplements when appropriate (15,4412,4425,4449).
BISACODYL (Dulcolax): Bisacodyl can cause potassium loss in patients undergoing bowel-cleansing regimens. Use caution in patients who are predisposed to hypokalemia (i.e., diuretic therapy), monitor potassium serum levels, and give potassium supplements when appropriate (4411,4412).
STIMULANT LAXATIVES: Excessive use of stimulant laxatives can result in potassium loss and hypokalemia. Limit stimulant laxatives to short-term use (4411,4412,4425,4453).

Possible Interactions with Foods

POTASSIUM-CONTAINING FOODS: Theoretically, concomitant use can increase potassium levels and the risk of adverse effects, especially in individuals with renal dysfunction, ACE inhibitor or potassium-sparing diuretic therapy. Potassium-containing foods include fruits (especially dried), cereals, beans, milk, and vegetables (16).
POTASSIUM-CONTAINING SALT SUBSTITUTES: Theoretically, concomitant use can increase potassium levels and the risk of adverse effects, especially in individuals with renal dysfunction, ACE inhibitor or potassium-sparing diuretic therapy.

Possible Interactions with Lab Tests

POTASSIUM: Potassium supplementation increases serum and urine potassium concentrations and test results (15).
BLOOD PRESSURE: Potassium taken orally can reduce blood pressure and blood pressure readings (14).

Possible Interactions with Diseases or Conditions

ELECTROLYTE IMBALANCES: Potassium is contraindicated in individuals with untreated Addison's disease, heat cramps, acute dehydration, hyperkalemia from any cause (14,15,16), adynamia episodica hereditaria (14,16), severe renal impairment with oliguria, anuria, or azotemia (14,15), or who have extensive tissue breakdown, e.g. severe burns (15). Use potassium with caution in people with heart and kidney disease (15,16), GI disease with risk of bleeding (14,15), and sickle cell anemia (14).
GI MOTILITY CONDITIONS: Oral potassium tablets and capsules are contraindicated in individuals with gastrointestinal motility conditions (15).
ASPIRIN OR TARTRAZINE SENSITIVITY: Avoid oral potassium products that contain tartrazine (15).

Typical Dosages & Routes of Administration that are Commonly Used

ORAL: Potassium supplementation must be individualized and based on the person's serum potassium level, which should be maintained between 3.5-5 mEq/L (14). The normal adult daily requirement and usual dietary intake is 40-80 mEq daily (15). For preventing hypokalemia, 20 mEq is typically taken daily (15). The common dose of potassium for treating hypokalemia is 40-100 mEq or more daily, in two to four divided amounts (15). For hypercalciuria, 1 mEq/kg is taken daily (14) or four tablets of Urophos-K are taken twice a day (2209). The typical dose for hypertension is 48-90 mEq daily (14,15). The common dose of potassium citrate for urinary alkalinization is 20-30 mEq four times daily (14).
INTRAVENOUS (IV): IV potassium products are prescription products.

Comments

Potassium tablets or capsules are available as food supplements and are not required to meet the rigorous standards for prescription medications.

POTATO

This Product is Also Known As

Irish Potato, White Potato.
CAUTION: See separate listing for African Wild Potato.

Scientific Names

Solanum tuberosum.
Family: Solanaceae.

People Use This For

Orally, raw potato juice is used for gastritis and stomach disorders (6). A purified protein extract from potato is used as an appetite suppressant for weight loss (473).
Topically, raw potato is used as a poultice for arthritis, infections, boils, burns, and sore eyes (6).
Traditionally, brewed potato peel tea is used orally for edema and to soothe bodily swelling (6).
Potato is eaten as a food, used as a source of starch, and fermented into alcohol (6).

Safety

LIKELY SAFE ...when unblemished, ripe potatoes are used as food (6).
POSSIBLY SAFE ...when the purified protein extract from potato is used orally and appropriately (473). ...when unblemished, ripe potatoes are used orally for medicinal purposes (6).
LIKELY UNSAFE ...when damaged, green potatoes and sprouts are consumed. These contain toxic solanum alkaloids that cannot be destroyed by cooking and can cause serious adverse effects (See Adverse Reactions). There is insufficient reliable information available about the safety of topical use of potato.
PREGNANCY AND LACTATION: LIKELY SAFE ...when unblemished, ripe potatoes are used orally in food amounts. There is insufficient information available about the safety of oral or topical use of potato in pregnancy and lactation for medicinal purposes.

Effectiveness

There is insufficient reliable information available about the effectiveness of potato.

Possible Mechanism of Action & Active Ingredients

The applicable part of the potato is the tuber. Potatoes are a source of vitamin C, iron, riboflavin, and are rich in carbohydrates (6). A proteinase inhibitor isolated from potatoes is claimed to increase the effects of cholecystokinin (CCK), by blocking the effects of the enzymes chymotrypsin and trypsin, which break down CCK (473). CCK produces satiety and has been shown to play a role in the short-term inhibition of food intake (476,477,6255). It has been reported by the manufacturer of a purified protein extract from potato (Satietrol), which contains this proteinase inhibitor and other nutrients and minerals claimed to affect CCK, that the product reduced feelings of hunger by 30-32% 3.5 hours after a fixed calorie meal. These effects were also found in a group of people who lost weight on a calorie-controlled diet (473). Damaged, green potatoes, and sprouts contain toxic solanum alkaloids that cannot be destroyed by cooking (see Adverse Reactions). Researchers report that a potato peel extract inhibited bacterial adhesion to host cells without killing the bacteria. They believe this activity might be due to polyphenol oxidase, a compound known to have anti-adhesive properties. This unpublished research was presented at the 2000 Annual Meeting of the American Society for Microbiology (6107).

Adverse Reactions Including Known Allergies

Adverse reactions have not been reported with unblemished, ripe potatoes. Solanum glycosides found in damaged, green potatoes and sprouts can cause headache, flushing, nausea, vomiting, diarrhea, abdominal pain, thirst, and restlessness. Deaths have been reported in malnourished individuals who may not have received adequate medical care (17). Twenty mg solanine per 100 grams potato is the maximum concentration considered safe. Solanum glycosides cannot be destroyed by cooking (6). Exposure to potato dust is associated with a high-incidence of respiratory symptoms due to bacterial and fungal contaminants (6).

Possible Interactions with Herbs & Other Dietary Supplements

Insufficient reliable information available.

Possible Interactions with Drugs

DIABETES THERAPY: Concomitant use of potato may interfere with blood sugar control and insulin levels (6).
THROMBOLYTICS (tPA, Alterplase): Theoretically, concomitant use of potato may enhance thrombolytic effects. A carboxypeptidase inhibitor isolated from potato tubers may have inhibitory effects on thrombin-activatable thrombolysis inhibitor, and thereby enhance the activity of thrombolytic agents (474,475).

Possible Interactions with Foods

No interactions are known to occur, and there is no known reason to expect a clinically significant interaction with potato.

Possible Interactions with Lab Tests
No interactions are known to occur, and there is no known reason to expect a clinically significant interaction with potato.

Possible Interactions with Diseases or Conditions
DIABETES: Potatoes can affect blood sugar control. They should be consumed as appropriate carbohydrate equivalents (6).

Typical Dosages & Routes of Administration that are Commonly Used
ORAL: For appetite suppression and weight loss, a purified protein extract from potato (Satietrol) containing a proteinase inhibitor, is marketed as a powder to be mixed with 8 ounces of water and taken 15 minutes before meals (473). There is no typical dosage of potato juice.
TOPICAL: Raw potato is used as a poultice (6).

Comments
The potato is one of the main food crops of the world (6).

POTENTILLA

This Product is Also Known As
Crampweed, Goosegrass, Goose Tansy, Goosewort, Moor Grass, Prince's Feathers, Silverweed, Trailing Tansy, Wild Agrimony.
CAUTION: See separate listings for Agrimony, Tormentil, and Jewelweed.

Scientific Names
Potentilla anserina.
Family: Rosacea.

People Use This For
Orally, potentilla flower and leaf are used for premenstrual syndrome, mild dysmenorrhea, diarrhea (2,18),
Topically, potentilla flower and leaf are used for the local treatment of oropharyngeal inflammation (2,7,18).

Safety
POSSIBLY SAFE ...when used orally and appropriately (2).
PREGNANCY AND LACTATION: Insufficient reliable information available; avoid using.

Effectiveness
POSSIBLY EFFECTIVE ...when taken orally for premenstrual syndrome, mild dysmenorrhea, and acute, nonspecific diarrhea (2). ...when applied topically for local treatment of oropharyngeal inflammation (7).

Possible Mechanism of Action & Active Ingredients
The applicable parts of the potentilla are the flower and leaf. The tannin constituents of potentilla have astringent effects (2) and are likely responsible for antidiarrheal and local anti-inflammatory activity. Potentilla also increases tonus and the contraction frequency of isolated animal uterus (2,7).

Adverse Reactions Including Known Allergies
Taken orally, potentilla can cause stomach irritation (7,12).

Possible Interactions with Herbs & Other Dietary Supplements
Insufficient reliable information available.

Possible Interactions with Drugs
No interactions are known to occur, and there is no known reason to expect a clinically significant interaction with potentilla.

Possible Interactions with Foods
No interactions are known to occur, and there is no known reason to expect a clinically significant interaction with potentilla.

Possible Interactions with Lab Tests
No interactions are known to occur, and there is no known reason to expect a clinically significant interaction with potentilla.

Possible Interactions with Diseases or Conditions
No interactions are known to occur, and there is no known reason to expect a clinically significant interaction with potentilla.

Typical Dosages & Routes of Administration that are Commonly Used

ORAL: The typical dose of potentilla is one cup of the tea two to three times daily (18). The tea is prepare by steeping 2 grams of the finely cut flower or leaf in 150 mL boiling water for 10 minutes and then straining. Up to 4-6 grams of the flower or leaf should be used per day (2).

Comments

Avoid confusion with agrimony (Agrimonia eupratoria) and tormentil (Potentilla erecta), also referred to as potentilla. Avoid confusion with jewelweed, also known as silverweed.

PRECATORY BEAN

This Product is Also Known As

Bead Vine, Black-Eyed Susan, Buddhist Rosary Bead, Crab's Eye, Indian Bead, Jequirity Bean, Jequirity Seed, Love Bean, Lucky Bean, Ojo De Pajaro, Prayer Beads, Prayer Head, Rosary Pea, Seminole Bead, Weather Plant.

Scientific Names

Abrus pecatorius.
Family: Leguminosae or Fabacae.

People Use This For

In folk medicine, precatory bean has been used to quicken labor, as an abortifacient, oral contraceptive, and as analgesic in terminally-ill patients (6). The whole plant has been used for ophthalmic inflammations (6).

Safety

LIKELY UNSAFE ...when taken orally; 5 mg of abrin, a constituent of precatory bean, is considered toxic to humans (6). Significant precatory bean ingestion causes severe gastroenteritis, followed by diarrhea and vomiting that can become bloody. Symptoms may not appear for several days (3499). Fatalities can occur after 3-4 days of persistent gastroenteritis (17,3499).
CHILDREN: UNSAFE ...when taken orally. Ingestion of one seed in young children can be fatal (6,3499,5607). Older children (ages 9-12) have been reported to experience severe abdominal pain, vomiting and bloody stools after ingestion of one or more seeds (5607).
PREGNANCY AND LACTATION: LIKELY UNSAFE ...contraindicated.

Effectiveness

There is insufficient reliable information available about the effectiveness of precatory bean.

Possible Mechanism of Action & Active Ingredients

The plant contains the indole alkaloids abrine, abrus agglutinin, hyaphorine, and precatorine (6). Abrin, isolated from the seeds, is a potent inhibitor of protein synthesis and moderate inhibitor of DNA synthesis. In vitro, ethanol extracts of the seeds caused irreversible impairment in human sperm motility (3842). Some isoflavanquinone constituents isolated from the root inhibit platelet aggregation; others possess potent anti-inflammatory and anti-allergic effects (3841).

Adverse Reactions Including Known Allergies

Taken orally, the seeds that are chewed or with cracked shells can cause stomach cramping, nausea (6), vomiting, severe diarrhea (possibly bloody) (3499), cold sweat (6), fever, weakness (3499), tachycardia, coma, circulatory collapse (6,3499), cerebral edema (3499), and death (17,3499,5608). Topically, the seeds when used as a necklace can cause dermatitis (6). Eye contact with the seed's contents can cause necrotizing conjunctivitis (3499).

Possible Interactions with Herbs & Other Dietary Supplements

Insufficient reliable information available.

Possible Interactions with Drugs

No interactions are known to occur, and there is no known reason to expect a clinically significant interaction with precatory bean.

Possible Interactions with Foods

No interactions are known to occur, and there is no known reason to expect a clinically significant interaction with precatory bean.

Possible Interactions with Lab Tests

No interactions are known to occur, and there is no known reason to expect a clinically significant interaction with precatory bean.

Possible Interactions with Diseases or Conditions

No interactions are known to occur, and there is no known reason to expect a clinically significant interaction with precatory bean.

Typical Dosages & Routes of Administration that are Commonly Used
No typical dosage.

Comments
Precatory bean is considered unsafe for oral use. Children are attracted to the bright colors of the seed (17). The hard coat of a mature seed may resist digestion when swallowed but treatment for suspected poisoning should begin as soon as possible (3499). Abrin, a constituent of precatory bean, is being investigated for the treatment of experimental cancers and is used as a "molecular probe" to investigate cell function (6).

PREGNENOLONE

This Product is Also Known As
None.
CAUTION: See separate listings for Progesterone and Wild Yam.

Scientific Names
Pregnenolone; (3 beta)-3-hydroxypregn-5-en-20-one; delta 5-pregnen-3 beta-ol-20-one; 17 beta-(1-ketoethyl)-delta 5-androsten-3 beta-ol.

People Use This For
Orally, pregnenolone is used for slowing or reversing aging, for arthritis, depression, endometriosis, fatigue, fibrocystic breast disease, memory enhancement, menopause, premenstrual syndrome (PMS), stress, increasing energy, and improving immunity. It is also used for strengthening the heart, Alzheimer's disease, allergic reactions, detoxification, lupus, multiple sclerosis, prostate disorders, psoriasis, scleroderma, seizures, trauma, and injuries (3000-3004).

Safety
There is insufficient reliable information available about the safety of pregnenolone.
Pregnancy and Lactation: Insufficient reliable information available; avoid using.

Effectiveness
There is insufficient reliable information available about the effectiveness of pregnenolone.

Possible Mechanism of Action & Active Ingredients
Pregnenolone is produced by the body from cholesterol and is the precursor for all the steroid hormones, including progesterone, aldosterone, cortisol, dehydroepiandrosterone (DHEA), testosterone, and estrogens (3008). Lower cerebrospinal fluid (CSF) levels of pregnenolone are reported in people with affective disorders, particularly during episodes of active depression (3005). Pregnenolone has antagonist activity at GABA-A receptors in the brain and induces changes in the sleep EEG by increasing the time spent in slow wave sleep (3007). Higher pregnenolone concentrations in the luteal phase serum are associated with more severe PMS symptoms (3006). Reliable information on the effects of exogenously administered pregnenolone is not available (3005).

Adverse Reactions Including Known Allergies
Theoretically, supplemental pregnenolone can cause steroid-related adverse effects. There have been warnings of overstimulation, insomnia, irritability, anger, anxiety, acne, headache, negative mood changes, facial hair growth, hair loss, and arrhythmias (3004).

Possible Interactions with Herbs & Other Dietary Supplements
Insufficient reliable information available.

Possible Interactions with Drugs
STEROID HORMONE DRUGS: Theoretically, pregnenolone can enhance the effects of steroid hormone drugs (see Mechanism of Action).

Possible Interactions with Foods
No interactions are known to occur, and there is no known reason to expect a clinically significant interaction with pregnenolone.

Possible Interactions with Lab Tests
No interactions are known to occur, and there is no known reason to expect a clinically significant interaction with pregnenolone.

Possible Interactions with Diseases or Conditions
No interactions are known to occur, and there is no known reason to expect a clinically significant interaction with pregnenolone.

Typical Dosages & Routes of Administration that are Commonly Used
No typical dosage.

Comments
Pregnenolone was studied for stress, fatigue, and arthritis in the 1940s before synthetic hormones became available (3000).

PREMORSE

This Product is Also Known As
Devil's Bit, Ofbit, Premorse Scaboius.

Scientific Names
Scabiosa succisa.
Family: Dipsacaceae.

People Use This For
Orally, premorse is used for febrile colds and coughs. It is also used to promote sweating (18).

Safety
There is insufficient reliable information available about the safety of the oral use of premorse.
Pregnancy and Lactation: Insufficient reliable information available; avoid using.

Effectiveness
There is insufficient reliable information available about the effectiveness of premorse.

Possible Mechanism of Action & Active Ingredients
The applicable parts of the premorse are the above ground parts. There is insufficient reliable information available about the possible mechanism of action and active ingredients of premorse.

Adverse Reactions Including Known Allergies
None reported.

Possible Interactions with Herbs & Other Dietary Supplements
Insufficient reliable information available.

Possible Interactions with Drugs
No interactions are known to occur, and there is no known reason to expect a clinically significant interaction with premorse.

Possible Interactions with Foods
No interactions are known to occur, and there is no known reason to expect a clinically significant interaction with premorse.

Possible Interactions with Lab Tests
No interactions are known to occur, and there is no known reason to expect a clinically significant interaction with premorse.

Possible Interactions with Diseases or Conditions
No interactions are known to occur, and there is no known reason to expect a clinically significant interaction with premorse.

Typical Dosages & Routes of Administration that are Commonly Used
ORAL: Premorse is used as a tea (18).

Comments
There is very little scientific information about this product. Our staff is continually analyzing the available information on natural medicines and will add data here as it becomes available.

PRICKLY PEAR CACTUS

This Product is Also Known As
Cactus Flowers, Gracemere-Pear, Tuna Cardona, Opuntia, Nopol, Westwood-Pear.

Scientific Names
Opuntia streptacantha.
Family: Cactaceae.

People Use This For

Orally, the young leaves and stems of the prickly pear cactus are used to treat diabetes (5951), high cholesterol levels (5952), for weight reduction, and as an antiviral (5952).

Orally, the cactus flowers of the prickly pear cactus are used for colitis, diarrhea, and prostatic hypertrophy (5953). In foods, the prickly pear juice is used in jellies and candies.

Safety

LIKELY SAFE ...when prickly pear cactus is used orally as a food (5951,5969).

POSSIBLY SAFE ...when the leaves, stems, or standardized product are used short-term (5951,5959,5960,5963).

Although the prickly pear cactus reduces blood sugar it does not appear to cause hypoglycemia.

There is insufficient reliable information available about the safety of prickly pear cactus for its other uses.

PREGNANCY AND LACTATION: Insufficient reliable information available; avoid using.

Effectiveness

POSSIBLY EFFECTIVE ...when used orally to reduce blood glucose. Very small patient populations suggest prickly pear cactus stems can reduce blood glucose 41-46% in individuals with diabetes (5951,5959,5961,5962), and limit increase in blood glucose when normal subjects are made hyperglycemic (5959,5960,5963).

There is insufficient reliable information about the effectiveness of prickly pear cactus for its other uses.

Possible Mechanism of Action & Active Ingredients

The young leaves of prickly pear cactus contain mucopolysaccharide soluble fibers, and phytochemicals. The fiber and pectin content is believed responsible for the activity in reducing blood sugar and lipid levels (5952,5958). Broiling the stems increases the hypoglycemic effect (5961,5964). After ingestion, hypoglycemic activity is progressive, reaching its greatest effect at 3-4 hours after eating and lasting for up to 6 hours. Some evidence suggests the pectin component can alter the liver metabolism of cholesterol (5958). Pectin is also thought to play a role in weight reduction. At least one prickly pear cactus manufacturer standardizes the product to specific phytochemical markers of polysaccharides, mucopolysaccharides, and lignins (5952). The prickly pear cactus shows evidence of antiviral activity against the herpes simplex virus, respiratory syncytial virus, and HIV virus (5956).

Adverse Reactions Including Known Allergies

Oral use of prickly pear cactus leaves and stems can cause an increase in stool volume, frequency, and abdominal fullness (5951).

Possible Interactions with Herbs & Other Dietary Supplements

Insufficient reliable information available.

Possible Interactions with Drugs

DIABETES DRUGS: One case report describes additive effects of chlorpropamide and prickly pear cactus on diabetic symptoms, and insulin and blood glucose levels (5868).

Possible Interactions with Foods

No interactions are known to occur, and there is no known reason to expect a clinically significant interaction with prickly pear cactus.

Possible Interactions with Lab Tests

BLOOD GLUCOSE: Prickly pear cactus stems and leaves can reduce blood glucose level (5957).

CHOLESTEROL LEVEL: Some evidence suggests prickly pear cactus might reduce blood cholesterol level (5958).

Possible Interactions with Diseases or Conditions

DIABETES: Prickly pear cactus stems and leaves can reduce blood glucose (5957).

CHOLESTEROL LEVEL: Some evidence suggests prickly pear cactus might reduce blood cholesterol (5958).

Typical Dosages & Routes of Administration that are Commonly Used

ORAL: A typical dose of the broiled stems for diabetes is 500 grams (5964). A typical dose of the flowers for colitis, diarrhea or prostatic disease is 0.3-1 gram or as a tea. A typical dose of the liquid extract of dried flowers is 0.3-1 mL of 1:1 in 25% alcohol (5953).

Comments

Although multiple species are known as Opuntia, other subspecies have not yet been shown useful in normalizing blood sugars or blood lipid levels (5952). Opuntia megacantha has shown indications it can reduce blood sugar, but preliminary evidence suggests using the leaf extract orally might cause renal damage (5954). Opuntia ficus indica also appears to have some hypoglycemic effects but the dose required is impractical (5970). Preliminary evidence suggests Opuntia fuliginosa might be useful but further testing is needed (5955).

PROCAINE

This Product is Also Known As
Gero-Vita, Gerovital, Gerovital-H3, GH-3, KH-3, Procaine Hydrochloride.

Scientific Names
2-Dietylaminoethyl p-aminobenzoate monohydrochloride.

People Use This For
Orally or parenterally, procaine is used for arthritis, cerebral atherosclerosis, dementia, depression, hair loss, hypertension, sexual dysfunction, and an overall rejuvenating effect (6).
Parenterally, prescription-only procaine is used for local anesthesia (6).

Safety
LIKELY SAFE ...when the prescription-only product is used as a local anesthetic (15).
There is insufficient reliable information available about the safety of the oral use of procaine.
PREGNANCY: LIKELY UNSAFE ...when used for self-medication. Contraindicated (6).
LACTATION: Insufficient reliable information available for self-medication; avoid using.

Effectiveness
EFFECTIVE ...when the parenteral, prescription-only product is used for local anesthesia (15).
LIKELY INEFFECTIVE ...when taken orally (6).

Possible Mechanism of Action & Active Ingredients
Procaine has poor oral absorption, and there is no evidence that pharmacologic levels are achieved with oral administration (6). Hematoporphyrin is added to some oral preparations to increase procaine absorption (6), although no evidence supports this effect.

Adverse Reactions Including Known Allergies
Procaine can cause heartburn, migraines, and systemic lupus erythematosus (SLE) (6).

Possible Interactions with Herbs & Other Dietary Supplements
DIGITALIS: IV procaine hydrochloride is contraindicated with concurrent use of digitalis (15).

Possible Interactions with Drugs
AMINOSALICYLIC ACID, SULFONAMIDES: The procaine metabolite aminobenzoic acid can antagonize activity of these drugs. Avoid concomitant use (15).
ANTICHOLINESTERASE DRUGS, DIGOXIN, SUCCINYLCHOLINE: IV procaine hydrochloride is contraindicated (15).

Possible Interactions with Foods
No interactions are known to occur, and there is no known reason to expect a clinically significant interaction with procaine.

Possible Interactions with Lab Tests
No interactions are known to occur, and there is no known reason to expect a clinically significant interaction with procaine.

Possible Interactions with Diseases or Conditions
MYASTHENIA GRAVIS: The intravenous use of procaine is contraindicated in individuals with myasthenia gravis, which is progressive muscular weakness (15).
SYSTEMIC LUPUS ERYTHEMATOSUS (SLE): Contraindicated. Theoretically, procaine might exacerbate this condition (6).
PSEUDOCHOLINESTERASE DEFICIENCY: Contraindicated (6).

Typical Dosages & Routes of Administration that are Commonly Used
PARENTERAL PRESCRIPTION PRODUCT: For use as an anesthetic.
ORAL: People typically take procaine in a cyclical regimen: 200 mg procaine once or twice daily for 25 days, then no drug for 5 days, then repeat the cycle (5274).

Comments
None.

PROGESTERONE

This Product is Also Known As
Corpus Luteum Hormone, Luteal Hormone, Luteohormone, Lutine, NSC-9704, Pregnancy Hormone, Pregnanedione, Progestational Hormone, Progesteronum.
CAUTION: See separate listings for Pregnenolone and Wild Yam.

Scientific Names
Progesterone; 4-Pregnene-3; 20-Dione.

People Use This For
Orally, progesterone is used for treating secondary amenorrhea (15,226,1215,1217), abnormal uterine bleeding associated with hormonal imbalance (15), treating severe symptoms of premenstrual syndrome (PMS) (1220), and treating benzodiazepine dependence and withdrawal (1221). Oral progesterone preparations are also used in combination with estrogens as part of hormone replacement therapy to prevent irregular bleeding and the increased risk of endometrial carcinoma associated with estrogen monotherapy (15,226,228,1215,1216,1217).

Topically, progesterone is used as an alternative to oral treatment as a component of hormone replacement therapy and for treating menopausal vasomotor symptoms (224,1429,2031). Topical progesterone is also used for treating or preventing hormone-mediated allergies, bloating, breast tenderness, decreased sex drive, depression, fatigue, fibrocystic breasts, headaches, hypoglycemia, increased blood clotting, infertility, irritability, memory loss, miscarriages, osteoporosis, premenopausal bone loss, symptoms of premenstrual syndrome, thyroid dysfunction, unclear thinking, uterine cancer, uterine fibroids, water retention, weight gain (1209), and treating lichen sclerosis (1210).

Intravaginally, progesterone is used for cervical ripening (15), mastodynia in women with benign breast disease (1223), and to prevent and treat endometrial hyperplasia (2031,2033). Progesterone is also used intravaginally or intramuscularly for treating infertility in women (9,2032), anovulatory bleeding, and treating symptoms of premenstrual syndrome (9).

Safety
LIKELY SAFE ...when used orally and appropriately. Micronized progesterone (Prometrium) is an FDA-approved prescription product. Micronized progesterone (Prometrium) has been safely used in multiple clinical trials lasting up to 3 years (15,226,228,1216,1220,1221,1224). ...when used intravaginally and appropriately, short-term (1225,2031,2032,2033,2034). Progesterone intravaginal gel (Crinone) is an FDA-approved prescription product. Progesterone intravaginal gel (Crinone) has been safely used in trials lasting up to 3 months (1225,2031,2033,2034,2041). ...when used intramuscularly and appropriately, short-term (227,1218,1225,2034). Progesterone oil for intramuscular injection is an FDA-approved prescription product (227,1218,1225,2034). ...when used transdermally and appropriately. Transdermal progesterone has been used safely in clinical trials lasting up to a year (224,1229).

There is insufficient reliable information available about the safety of other progesterone preparations.

PREGNANCY: LIKELY SAFE ...when used intravaginally and appropriately as part of infertility treatment. Intravaginal progesterone gel (Crinone 8%) is FDA-approved for use in conjunction with infertility treatment (1225). LIKELY UNSAFE ...when used orally, intramuscularly, intravaginally, or transdermally for purposes other than medically supervised adjunctive treatment for infertility; contraindicated (15).

LACTATION: There is insufficient reliable information available (15); avoid using.

Effectiveness
LIKELY EFFECTIVE ...when used orally in combination with estrogen as a component of hormone replacement therapy in women with a uterus. Micronized progesterone (Prometrium) is FDA-approved for use with estrogen as a component of hormone replacement therapy. Micronized progesterone (Prometrium) has been shown to provide the same protection against the effects of unopposed estrogen therapy as medroxyprogesterone (226,228,1216,1217,1226,1230). In one trial, micronized progesterone (Prometrium) did not reduce the beneficial lipid effects of estrogen therapy as much as medroxyprogesterone (226); however, this effect was not seen in another trial (1216). ...when used orally for secondary amenorrhea in premenopausal women. Micronized progesterone is FDA-approved for the treatment of secondary amenorrhea (15). ...when used intravaginally in infertile women as a component of infertility treatment. Intravaginal progesterone gel (Crinone 8%) is FDA-approved for use as a component of infertility treatment in women. Clinical trials have shown that intravaginal progesterone achieves pregnancy rates comparable to oral progesterone in women infertile due to various etiologies (1225,2032,2087,2088,2091). Clinical trials comparing intravaginal progesterone to intramuscular progesterone have shown varying relative efficacy results (1218,2086,2089). ...when used intravaginally for secondary amenorrhea in premenopausal women. Intravaginal progesterone gel (Crinone 4%) is FDA-approved for the treatment of secondary amenorrhea. Several open-label clinical trials have shown intravaginal progesterone gel (Crinone 4%) to be effective for restoring menses when used in conjunction with estrogen replacement therapy (2041,2088,2091).

POSSIBLY EFFECTIVE ...when used intravaginally to prevent endometrial hyperplasia associated with estrogen replacement therapy. One short-term clinical trial has shown that intravaginal progesterone (Crinone) prevents endometrial hyperplasia in women with an intact uterus taking estrogen replacement therapy (2031). ...when used intravaginally for treating mastodynia. One clinical trial has shown that intravaginal progesterone gel (Crinone) is

© Copyright 2000, Natural Medicines Comprehensive Database (209) 472-2244. For updated data, go to www.NaturalDatabase.com • 861

superior to placebo for reducing breast pain and tenderness in women with benign breast disease (1223). ...when used topically for treating menopausal vasomotor symptoms. One clinical trial has shown that topical progesterone cream (Progest) is superior to placebo for reducing vasomotor symptoms such as hot flashes in menopausal women (224). ...when used intravaginally for treatment of benign endometrial hyperplasia. One short term, open label clinical trial has shown that a specific intravaginal progesterone cream may help reverse endometrial hyperplasia and decrease vaginal bleeding in premenopausal women with benign hyperplasia (2033). ...when used intramuscularly in infertile women as a component of infertility treatment. Clinical trials have shown that intramuscular progesterone achieves pregnancy rates comparable to oral progesterone (227), and with varying efficacy relative to intravaginal progesterone in infertile women (1218,2086).

POSSIBLY INEFFECTIVE ...when used orally for treating symptoms of premenstrual syndrome (PMS). One clinical trial has shown that oral micronized progesterone is comparable to placebo and inferior to alprazolam for relieving symptoms associated with PMS (9,1220). ...when used orally for benzodiazepine dependence and withdrawal. One clinical trial has shown that oral micronized progesterone is comparable to placebo for relieving symptoms of withdrawal and for helping patients remain drug-free from diazepam (1221). ...when used topically for treating vulval lichen sclerosis. One clinical trial has shown that topical progesterone is comparable to placebo and inferior to clobetasol (Temovate) for treating the signs and symptoms of vulval lichen sclerosis (225). ...when used topically for preventing postmenopausal bone loss. One clinical trial has shown that topical progesterone is comparable to placebo for increasing bone mineral density in postmenopausal women (224).

There is insufficient reliable information available about the effectiveness of progesterone for its other uses.

Possible Mechanism of Action & Active Ingredients

Progesterone is an endogenous progestin secreted by the corpus luteum. It is primarily secreted during the luteal phase of the menstrual cycle, but small amounts are also secreted during the follicular phase (15). The normal physiological effects of progesterone are responsible for its therapeutic benefit when administered exogenously. Progesterone transforms proliferative endometrium into a secreting endometrium. This effect is beneficial in preventing and treating endometrial hyperplasia. It may also be beneficial in infertility because progesterone is necessary for implantation of the fertilized ovum and for maintaining pregnancy (15). In premenstrual syndrome (PMS), progesterone has been proposed as a therapy because the symptoms of PMS are thought to correlate with physiological fluctuations in endogenous progesterone (1220). It was thought to be beneficial for preventing benzodiazepine withdrawal because metabolites of progesterone have been found to have sedative-hypnotic properties (1221). Other effects of progesterone include growth of mammary tissue and uterine smooth muscle relaxation. Progesterone also has mild estrogenic and androgenic effects (15). Intravaginal, topical, and intramuscular administration of progesterone may be advantageous over oral dosing because it avoids first-pass effect and may achieve greater concentrations in the uterus (2033,2034).

Adverse Reactions Including Known Allergies

Progesterone can cause gastrointestinal disturbances, changes in appetite, weight gain, fluid retention and edema, fatigue (14,1224), acne, drowsiness or insomnia, allergic skin rashes, hives, fever, headache, depression, breast discomfort or enlargement (14), PMS-like syndrome, altered menstrual cycles, or irregular bleeding (14). Topical progesterone can cause vaginal spotting (224).

Possible Interactions with Herbs & Other Dietary Supplements

Insufficient reliable information available.

Possible Interactions with Drugs

CONJUGATED EQUINE ESTROGENS (Premarin): Concomitant use can cause breast tenderness (228). Use of conjugated equine estrogens with oral micronized progesterone in postmenopausal women may blunt the beneficial effects of estrogen on the lipoprotein profile (1216), although it might not affect estrogen-induced reduction in plasma lipoprotein (a) (1217).

Possible Interactions with Foods

Oral, micronized progesterone is better absorbed when taken with food (1222).

Possible Interactions with Lab Tests

ALANINE AMINOTRANSFERASE (ALT): Can increase serum levels and test results due to hepatotoxicity (275).
ALBUMIN: May increase serum levels and test results (275).
ALKALINE PHOSPHATASE (Alk Phos): Can increase serum levels and test results due to hepatotoxicity (275).
ASPARTATE AMINOTRANSFERASE (AST): Progesterone can decrease serum levels and test results in healthy people or increase serum levels and test results due to hepatotoxicity (275).
BILE: Can increase urine levels and test results due to hepatotoxicity (275).
BILIRUBIN: Can increase serum levels and test results due to hepatotoxicity (275).
CHOLESTEROL: Might decrease serum levels and test results (275).
GLOBULIN: Can decrease serum levels and test results (275).
GAMMA-GLOBULIN: Can increase serum levels and test results (275).
GLUCARIC ACID: Can increase urine level and test results (275).
17-HYDROXYCORTICOSTEROIDS: Can decrease urine level and test results (275).
16-ALPHA-HYDROXYPROGESTERONE: Can cause increase in plasma test results (275).

LUTEINIZING HORMONE (LH): Can decrease peak plasma level and test results (275).
MAGNESIUM: Can increase serum level and test results (275).
PREGNANEDIOL: Can decrease urine level and test results (275).
PROGESTERONE: Can decrease plasma levels and test results (275).
PROSTAGLANDIN: Can decrease urine levels and test results (275).
PROTEIN: Can increase serum levels and test results (275).
SODIUM: Can increase serum and test results due to sodium retention (275). Large doses of progesterone can increase urine levels and test results (275).
THYROXINE (T4) BINDING GLOBULIN: Can increase serum levels and test results due to increased synthesis (275).

Possible Interactions with Diseases or Conditions

ARTERIAL DISEASE: Contraindicated in individuals with high risk arterial disease (9).
BREAST CANCER: Should be avoided except as part of the management of breast cancer (9).
DEPRESSION: Use cautiously in individuals with a history of major depression (9).
FLUID RETENTION PROBLEMS: Use cautiously in individuals with conditions that can be aggravated by fluid retention (14), including cardiovascular or renal impairment, diabetes mellitus, asthma, epilepsy, and migraine.
LIVER DISEASE: Contraindicated. Progesterone has been associated with attacks of acute porphyria (9).
VAGINAL BLEEDING: Contraindicated in women who have undiagnosed vaginal bleeding (9).

Typical Dosages & Routes of Administration that are Commonly Used

ORAL: For hormone replacement therapy, 200 mg micronized progesterone (Prometrium) orally per day is given for 12 days of a 25 day cycle with 0.625 mg conjugated estrogens (1215,1217).
TOPICAL: For menopausal vasomotor symptoms, 20 mg progesterone cream (equivalent to 1/4 teaspoon Progest cream) is applied daily to rotating sites including upper arms, thighs or breasts (224).
INTRAMUSCULAR: As a component of in vitro fertilization, 50 mg is used intramuscularly (227,1218,1225,2034).
INTRAVAGINAL: For mastodynia associated with benign breast disease, a dose of 4 grams of vaginal cream containing 2.5% natural progesterone is placed intravaginally from the 19th to the 25th day of a 28 day cycle (1223). As a component of in vitro fertilization, one applicator (90 mg) of progesterone gel (Crinone 8%) is placed intravaginally 1-2 times daily (2032,2036). For secondary amenorrhea, one applicator (90 mg) of progesterone gel (Crinone 4% or 8%) is placed intravaginally every other day for 6 days per month (2041). For hormone replacement therapy, one applicator (90 mg) of progesterone gel (Crinone 4% or 8%) is placed intravaginally on days 17, 19, 21, 23, 25, and 27 of a 28 day cycle with 0.625 mg conjugated equine estrogens (2031). For reducing intravaginal bleeding and reversal of hyperplasia in premenopausal women with benign endometrial hyperplasia, a dose of 100 mg progesterone cream placed intravaginally daily from day 10 to day 25 of a 28 day cycle has been used (2033).

Comments

The term "Natural Progesterone" is really a misnomer. Products marketed as natural progesterone are those products that are structurally identical to endogenous progesterone. However, these products must be prepared in a laboratory. "Natural progesterones," including the prescription products Crinone and Prometrium, are synthesized from the constituent diosgenin, isolated from wild yam. In the laboratory, this constituent is converted to pregnenolone and then to progesterone. The human body is not capable of synthesizing progesterone from diosgenin in vivo (515).
OTC progesterone products may not contain progesterone concentrations as labeled. According to a British report, two-ounce jars of Progest cream used in a clinical trial contained 100 mg progesterone per ounce rather than the 465 mg claimed by the manufacturer (848,1228,1231). Topical progesterone products marketed as cosmetics require no FDA approval prior to marketing (853). There is currently no limit on the amount of progesterone allowed in cosmetic products. In 1993 the FDA proposed, but never finalized, a rule limiting progesterone-containing cosmetic products to a maximum level of 5 mg/oz with the product label specifying consumer usage not to exceed 2 oz per month (365).

PROPIONYL-L-CARNITINE

This Product is Also Known As

L-carnitine Propionyl, LPC, PLC, Propionylcarnitine.
CAUTION: See separate listings for Acetyl-L-Carnitine and L-Carnitine.

Scientific Names

Propionyl-L-carnitine.

People Use This For

Orally, propionyl-L-carnitine is used for treating peripheral vascular disease (PVD), atherosclerotic and diabetic angiopathies, intermittent claudication, and congestive heart failure (14,1434,1435,1436).
Intravenously, propionyl-L-carnitine has been used for treating peripheral vascular disease and intermittent

claudication (1437); to improve healing of ulcerative lesions in people with peripheral vascular disease (1574); and to treat ischemic heart disease, angina and congestive heart failure (1571,1572,1573,1575).

Safety

LIKELY SAFE ...when propionyl-L-carnitine is used orally and appropriately (1434,1435,1436,1437). ...when single intravenous doses of propionyl-L-carnitine are used under appropriate medical supervision (1571,1572,1573,1575).
PREGNANCY AND LACTATION: Insufficient reliable information available; avoid using.

Effectiveness

POSSIBLY EFFECTIVE ...when propionyl-L-carnitine is taken orally for improving physical functioning and quality of life in people with peripheral vascular disease and intermittent claudication characterized by a maximal walking distance less than 250 meters (14,1434,1435,1436,1576). ...when taken orally to produce small improvements in myocardial ischemia and exercise capacity in people with chronic, stable angina (1579,1580,1581). ...when taken orally to improve left ventricular function and exercise capacity in people with class II or III congestive heart failure (1575,1582,1583). ...when single doses of propionyl-L-carnitine are used intravenously for improving maximal walking capacity in people with peripheral vascular disease (14,1437). ...when single doses are given intravenously to produce short-term increases in left ventricular function and cardiac output, and a reduction in myocardial ischemia in people with chronic ischemic heart disease (1571,1572,1573).
LIKELY INEFFECTIVE ...when propionyl-L-carnitine is taken orally for improving physical functioning in people with peripheral vascular disease (PVD) characterized by a maximal walking distance greater than 250 meters (1434,1435,1436).
There is insufficient reliable information about the effectiveness of propionyl-L-carnitine for its other uses.

Possible Mechanism of Action & Active Ingredients

L-carnitine is an essential cofactor in skeletal muscle and myocardium for transfer of long-chain fatty acids to intramitochondrial beta-oxidation sites where they are transformed into energy. There may be altered homeostasis and reduced levels of L-carnitine in peripheral vascular disease, myocardial ischemia, and heart failure (14,1572). Propionyl-L-carnitine may be hydrolyzed in the blood to L-carnitine and acetyl-L-carnitine, and also converted to L-carnitine and propionyl coenzyme A in the mitochondria of cells (14). Within cells, propionyl-L-carnitine helps to maintain mitochondrial acyl-CoA/CoA ratios which are increased in L-carnitine deficiency states, leading to deficient metabolism of fatty acids and urea synthesis (1439). Propionyl-L-carnitine also increases pyruvate flux into the Krebs cycle, stimulates pyruvate dehydrogenase activity, has free radical scavenging activity, improves homeostasis in the coagulation cascade, and has positive effects on blood viscosity (1578). Compared with L-carnitine, propionyl-L-carnitine may produce greater increases in cellular L-carnitine concentrations, possibly by being transported more easily into muscle fibers, and may provide additional substrates for muscle-cell energy production (14). Heart tissues may be able to utilize exogenous propionyl-L-carnitine to stimulate the tricarboxylic acid cycle and protect against ischemia (1439).

Treatment with intravenous propionyl-L-carnitine has been reported to restore levels of muscle L-carnitine which are deficient in people with peripheral vascular disease (14). Intravenous and oral treatment may improve physical functioning in some people with peripheral vascular disease (1434,1435,1436,1437,1576), but a study suggesting that propionyl-L-carnitine was superior to L-carnitine in this regard used only single intravenous doses, and the clinical significance of the difference was questionable (14,1437).

Propionyl-L-carnitine improves energy metabolism and myocardial contractility in experimental models of heart failure (1577). Small studies suggest that propionyl-L-carnitine may have a positive inotropic effect and improve ventricular function and cardiac output in chronic heart failure (1571,1572,1573). It reduces myocardial ischemia, as measured by ST segment depression, in people with angina (1573,1579).

Adverse Reactions Including Known Allergies

Nausea, vomiting, gastric pain, asthenia, and angina have been reported (14).

Possible Interactions with Herbs & Other Dietary Supplements

No interactions are known to occur, and there is no known reason to expect a clinically significant interaction with propionyl-L-carnitine.

Possible Interactions with Drugs

No interactions are known to occur, and there is no known reason to expect a clinically significant interaction with propionyl-L-carnitine.

Possible Interactions with Foods

No interactions are known to occur, and there is no known reason to expect a clinically significant interaction with propionyl-L-carnitine.

Possible Interactions with Lab Tests

No interactions are known to occur, and there is no known reason to expect a clinically significant interaction with propionyl-L-carnitine.

Possible Interactions with Diseases or Conditions

GASTROINTESTINAL DISORDERS (type unspecified): Might be exacerbated by propionyl-L-carnitine (14).
HYPERSENSITIVITY: Contraindicated in people with known hypersensitivity to propionyl-L-carnitine or L-carnitine (14).

Typical Dosages & Routes of Administration that are Commonly Used

ORAL: For peripheral vascular disease (PVD), atherosclerotic or diabetic arteriopathies, and intermittent claudication, 500-1500 mg propionyl-L-carnitine twice daily has been used (14,1434,1435,1436). One study in peripheral vascular disease used 1000 mg three times daily (1576). A dose of 500 mg three times daily has been used in congestive heart failure and stable angina (1579,1580,1581,1583).
INTRAVENOUS: A 1500 mg bolus followed by 1 mg/kg/minute infused for 30 minutes has been used to restore muscle L-carnitine levels in people with peripheral vascular disease (14). Single 600 mg bolus doses have also been tested in people with peripheral vascular disease (14,1437), and infusions of 2000 mg twice daily have been used to improve healing of ulcerative lesions in people with peripheral vascular disease (1574). Single doses of 15 to 30 mg/kg have been used in people with chronic ischemic heart disease or congestive heart failure (1571,1572,1573,1575).

Comments

None.

PROPOLIS

This Product is Also Known As

Bee Glue, Bee Propolis, Hive Dross, Propolis Balsam, Propolis Resin, Propolis Wax, Russion Penicillin.

Scientific Names

Propolis.

People Use This For

Orally, propolis is used for tuberculosis, bacterial and fungal infections, nasopharyngeal carcinoma, antioxidation, improving immune response, gastric disturbances including duodenal ulcer (5), anti-inflammatory effects (6), and antiprotozoal activity. Propolis is also used orally for eradicating Helicobacter pylori infection in peptic ulcer disease (6109).
Topically, it is used for wound cleansing (5,6), for genital herpes (6), and as a mouth rinse for enhanced healing following sulcoplasty (799).
In manufacturing, it is used as an ingredient in cosmetics (6).

Safety

There is insufficient reliable information available about the safety of propolis.
Pregnancy and Lactation: Insufficient information available; avoid using.

Effectiveness

POSSIBLY EFFECTIVE ...when used as a mouth rinse for healing intra-buccal surgical wounds, analgesia, and controlling inflammation following sulcoplasty (799).
There is insufficient reliable information available about the effectiveness of propolis for its other uses.

Possible Mechanism of Action & Active Ingredients

Propolis is a resinous material from poplar and conifer buds used by bees for maintaining their hives. Because propolis is incorporated into bee hives, harvesting the pure product for human use is difficult. Propolis preparations may frequently be contaminated with bee hive by-products (3574). Propolis contains caffeic acid phenethyl ester (CAPE). In vitro, CAPE demonstrates cancer chemopreventive properties (2629). In vivo, dietary propolis suppresses the lipoxygenase pathway of arachidonic acid metabolism during inflammation (2630). The antimicrobial properties of propolis are attributed to the flavonoid constituents pinocembrin, galangin, pinobanksin, and pinobanksin-3-acetate (5). A propolis extract shows weak free radical-scavenging effects (6). In mice exposed to radiation, propolis is associated with increased longevity (6). In vitro, an ethanolic extract of propolis suppresses prostaglandin and leukotriene generation by murine peritoneal macrophages and during zymosan-induced acute peritoneal inflammation in vivo (2630). Propolis extracts with high pinocembrin and galangin concentrations are associated with the control of oral pathogens in vitro (2631). In rats, topical application of a hydro-alcoholic propolis solution accelerates epithelial repair after tooth extraction but has no effect on socket wound healing (800). Propolis is a potent skin sensitizer (2632). The caffeic acid esters constituents of the poplar species are shown to be contact allergens (2633). Preliminary evidence indicates propolis has activity against Helicobacter pylori (H. pylori). In one report, propolis inhibited the growth of a variety of strains of H. pylori bacteria in the laboratory. The results of this unpublished study were presented at Digestive Disease Week 2000 meeting (6109).

Adverse Reactions Including Known Allergies

Using propolis can cause allergic reactions, including dermatitis with propolis-containing cosmetics (6) and acute oral mucositis with ulceration from the use of the lozenges (2632). Occupational allergic eczematous contact dermatitis is reported among beekeepers (2632).

Possible Interactions with Herbs & Other Dietary Supplements

Insufficient reliable information available.

Possible Interactions with Drugs

No interactions are known to occur, and there is no known reason to expect a clinically significant interaction with propolis.

Possible Interactions with Foods

No interactions are known to occur, and there is no known reason to expect a clinically significant interaction with propolis.

Possible Interactions with Lab Tests

No interactions are known to occur, and there is no known reason to expect a clinically significant interaction with propolis.

Possible Interactions with Diseases or Conditions

ASTHMA: Some sources suggest allergens in propolis may worsen asthma (3574); avoid using.
HYPERSENSITIVITY: Avoid using propolis in people hypersensitive to bee by-products including honey, conifers, poplars, Peruvian balsam, and salicylates (19).

Typical Dosages & Routes of Administration that are Commonly Used

ORAL: No typical dosage.
TOPICAL: As a mouth rinse after sulcoplasty, a 5% aqueous alcohol solution of propolis is commonly used (799).

Comments

Propolis has a long history of medicinal use, dating back to 350 B.C., the time of Aristotle. Greeks have used propolis for abscesses; Assyrians have used it for healing wounds and tumors; and Egyptians have used it for mummification (3574).

PUFF BALL

This Product is Also Known As

Bovista, Deer Balls, Hart's Truffle.

Scientific Names

Lycoperdon spp.
Family: Gasteromycetes.

People Use This For

Orally, puff ball aerial parts and spores are used for nosebleeds and skin disorders (18).
For food uses, young mushrooms are edible (18).

Safety

LIKELY SAFE ...when young mushrooms are consumed orally (18).
There is insufficient reliable information available about the safety of the oral use of puff ball for medicinal purposes.
PREGNANCY AND LACTATION: Insufficient reliable information available; avoid using.

Effectiveness

There is insufficient reliable information available about the effectiveness of puff ball.

Possible Mechanism of Action & Active Ingredients

The applicable parts of puff ball are the aerial parts and spores. Puff ball contains amino acids, glucosamine, sterol, enzymes, and approximately 3% urea (18).

Adverse Reactions Including Known Allergies

Adverse reactions are not reported with oral ingestion of puff ball. Inhaling the spores can cause respiratory illness, pneumonia-like symptoms, and widespread lung densities (3846,3847).

Possible Interactions with Herbs & Other Dietary Supplements

Insufficient reliable information available.

Possible Interactions with Drugs
No interactions are known to occur, and there is no known reason to expect a clinically significant interaction with puff ball.

Possible Interactions with Foods
No interactions are known to occur, and there is no known reason to expect a clinically significant interaction with puff ball.

Possible Interactions with Lab Tests
No interactions are known to occur, and there is no known reason to expect a clinically significant interaction with puff ball.

Possible Interactions with Diseases or Conditions
No interactions are known to occur, and there is no known reason to expect a clinically significant interaction with puff ball.

Typical Dosages & Routes of Administration that are Commonly Used
ORAL: Puff ball is used in pulverized form or in alcoholic extracts (18).

Comments
None.

PULSATILLA

This Product is Also Known As
Easter Flower, European Pasqueflower, Meadow Anenome, Meadow Windflower, Pasque Flower, Pasqueflower, Passe Flower, Wind Flower.

Scientific Names
Anemone pulsatilla, synonym Pulsatilla vulgaris; Anemone pratensis, synonym Anemone nigricans; Pulsatilla nigricans; Pulsatilla pratensis.
Family: Ranunculaceae.

People Use This For
The above ground parts of pulsatilla are used for painful conditions of the male or female reproductive system, such as dysmenorrhea, orchitis, ovaralgia, or epididymitis. Pulsatilla is used for tension headache, hyperactive states, insomnia, boils, skin eruptions associated with bacterial infection, asthma and pulmonary disease, earache (4), migraines, neuralgia, general restlessness, diseases and functional disorders of the GI and urinary tract, inflammatory and infectious diseases of the skin and mucosa (2).

Safety
LIKELY UNSAFE ...when fresh above ground parts are used orally or topically because pulsatilla is a severe local irritant (4).
There is insufficient reliable information available about the safety of the use of dried pulsatilla.
PREGNANCY: LIKELY UNSAFE ...when used orally the fresh or dried above ground parts are contraindicated because they might cause abortifacient and teratogenic effects (2). ...when the fresh above ground parts are used topically. There is insufficient reliable information available about the safety of the topical use of dried pulsatilla during pregnancy.
LACTATION: LIKELY UNSAFE ...when the fresh above ground parts are used for oral or topical use (19). There is insufficient reliable information available about the safety of dried pulsatilla during lactation.

Effectiveness
There is insufficient reliable information available about the effectiveness of pulsatilla.

Possible Mechanism of Action & Active Ingredients
The applicable parts of pulsatilla are the above ground parts. Pulsatilla has analgesic, antispasmodic, sedative, and antibacterial properties. It exhibits both uterine stimulant and depressant activities. Pulsatilla contains ranunculin, which hydrolyzes to toxic, unstable protoanemonin, which readily dimerizes to nontoxic anemonin (4). Protoanemonin causes central nervous system stimulation, then paralysis in experimental animals. It also has antimicrobial activity (2). Both anemonin and protoanemonin show some evidence of sedative and antipyretic activity (4). Irritation of the kidney and urinary tract might be due to the alkylating action of protoanemonin (2). Some evidence suggests anemonin might be cytotoxic (4).

Adverse Reactions Including Known Allergies
Fresh pulsatilla is a toxic gastrointestinal irritant (4,19). It can cause kidney and urinary tract irritation (2). Contact with the fresh plant can cause skin irritation, mucous membrane irritation, itching and pustule formation known as

© Copyright 2000, Natural Medicines Comprehensive Database (209) 472-2244. For updated data, go to www.NaturalDatabase.com

ranunculus dermatitis (2). Inhalation of protoanemonin-containing volatile oil may cause nasal mucosal and conjunctival irritation (4). Allergic reactions have been documented with patch tests (4).

Possible Interactions with Herbs & Other Dietary Supplements
Insufficient reliable information available.

Possible Interactions with Drugs
No interactions are known to occur, and there is no known reason to expect a clinically significant interaction with pulsatilla.

Possible Interactions with Foods
No interactions are known to occur, and there is no known reason to expect a clinically significant interaction with pulsatilla.

Possible Interactions with Lab Tests
No interactions are known to occur, and there is no known reason to expect a clinically significant interaction with pulsatilla.

Possible Interactions with Diseases or Conditions
No interactions are known to occur, and there is no known reason to expect a clinically significant interaction with pulsatilla.

Typical Dosages & Routes of Administration that are Commonly Used
ORAL: A typical oral dose is 120-300 mg dried above ground parts three times daily. Alternatively one cup tea consumed three times daily. To make tea, steep or simmer 120-300 mg dried above ground parts in 150 mL water 5-10 minutes, strain (4). Liquid extract (1:1 in 25% alcohol), 0.12-0.3 mL three times daily (4). Tincture (1:10 in 40% alcohol), 0.3-1 mL three times daily (4).

Comments
None.

PUMPKIN

This Product is Also Known As
Cucurbitea peponis semen, Field Pumpkin, Pepo.

Scientific Names
Cucurbita pepo.
Family: Cucurbitaceae.

People Use This For
Orally, pumpkin seeds are used for dysuria secondary to benign prostatic hyperplasia (BPH), bladder irritation (2,5,7,18), and treating intestinal worms (515).
In combination, pumpkin seed oil extract is used in a herbal combination to treat symptoms of BPH (5093).
In folk medicine, they have been used to treat pyelonephritis (18).
The roasted pumpkins seeds are considered a snack food (6002).

Safety
POSSIBLY SAFE ...when used orally and appropriately (2,7,18).
PREGNANCY AND LACTATION: Insufficient reliable information available; avoid using amounts greater than found in food.

Effectiveness
POSSIBLY EFFECTIVE ...when taken orally for dysuria associated with BPH and bladder irritation (2).
POSSIBLY INEFFECTIVE ...when an herbal blend containing pumpkin seed oil extract is used orally for treating symptoms of BPH. In a double-blind placebo controlled trial, an herbal product containing pumpkin seed oil extract 160 mg, saw palmetto lipodal extract 106 mg, nettle root extract 80 mg, lemon bioflavonoid extract 33 mg, and vitamin A (100% as beta-carotene) 190 IU taken three times daily for six months failed to significantly improve symptoms in a group of men with BPH (5093).
There is insufficient reliable information available about the effectiveness of pumpkin seed for its other uses.

Possible Mechanism of Action & Active Ingredients
The applicable part of pumpkin is the seed. Pumpkin seeds contain as much as 50% fatty oil (515). Pumpkin seeds are also rich in carotenoids, including lutein, carotene and beta carotene (6,515). The seed oil is rich in unsaturated fatty acids, including 55% linoleic acid and 25% oleic acid (6). The oil is also rich in vitamin E, primarily gamma-tocopherol (6). Pumpkin seed oil can exhibit a diuretic effect, which can relieve bladder discomfort, causing the perception of reduced prostate gland swelling without reducing the gland size. The phytosterol constituents are also

believed to affect urine flow. Another constituent, cucurbitin, has antihelmintic effects. Concentration of cucurbitin varies significantly among Cucurbita species (515).

Adverse Reactions Including Known Allergies

One case is reported of decreased ejaculatory volume associated with an herbal blend product containing pumpkin seed oil extract, saw palmetto extract, nettle root extract, lemon bioflavonoid extract, and beta-carotene (5093).

Possible Interactions with Herbs & Other Dietary Supplements

Insufficient reliable information available.

Possible Interactions with Drugs

No interactions are known to occur, and there is no known reason to expect a clinically significant interaction with pumpkin.

Possible Interactions with Foods

No interactions are known to occur, and there is no known reason to expect a clinically significant interaction with pumpkin.

Possible Interactions with Lab Tests

No interactions are known to occur, and there is no known reason to expect a clinically significant interaction with pumpkin.

Possible Interactions with Diseases or Conditions

No interactions are known to occur, and there is no known reason to expect a clinically significant interaction with pumpkin.

Typical Dosages & Routes of Administration that are Commonly Used

ORAL: For dysuria secondary to benign prostatic hyperplasia and bladder irritation, the typical dose is 5 grams of the ground seeds two times daily (2,7,18). As an antihelmintic, 20-167 grams of the seeds are commonly taken three times daily (515).

Comments

Seeds of autumn squash (Cucurbita maxima) and Canadian pumpkin (crooked neck squash, Cucurbita moschata) have properties similar to Cucurbita pepo seed (515).

PUNCTURE VINE

This Product is Also Known As

Abrojos, Caltrop, Cat's-Head, Common Dubbletjie, Devil's-Thorn, Devil's-Weed, Espigón, Goathead, Gokhru, Nature's Viagra, Puncturevine, Tribule terrestre, Tribulus.

Scientific Names

Tribulus terrestris.
Family: Zygophyllaceae.

People Use This For

Orally, puncture vine extract is used for angina pectoris (3931), male impotence, enhancing athletic performance (817), treating anemia, Bright's disease, cancer, coughs, improving digestion, treating flatulence, gonorrhea, headache, hepatitis, inflammation, stomatitis, vertigo, leprosy, nasal tumors, neurasthenia, painful urination, childbirth, psoriasis, rheumatism, scabies, sore throat, and spermatorrhea. It is also used as a gentle laxative, for stimulating appetite, stimulating milk flow, as an abortifacient, aphrodisiac, astringent, diuretic, tonic, and vermifuge (3919).

Safety

LIKELY UNSAFE ...when the spine-covered fruit is ingested orally. There has been one report of a bilateral pneumothorax adverse effect (818).
There is insufficient reliable information available about the safety of the parts of puncture vine other than the fruit.
PREGNANCY: POSSIBLY UNSAFE; avoid using. It has been used as an abortifacient (3919).
LACTATION: Insufficient reliable information available; avoid using.

Effectiveness

There is insufficient reliable information available about effectiveness of puncture vine.

Possible Mechanism of Action & Active Ingredients

Puncture vine contains diosgenin and other saponins (3929). An unidentified saponin of Tribulus terrestris is reported effective for treating angina pectoris in people with coronary heart disease (3931).

Adverse Reactions Including Known Allergies

Taken orally there is one case report of bilateral pneumothorax following the removal of a puncture vine fruit with sharp spines (818).

Possible Interactions with Herbs & Other Dietary Supplements

Insufficient reliable information available.

Possible Interactions with Drugs

No interactions are known to occur, and there is no known reason to expect a clinically significant interaction with puncture vine.

Possible Interactions with Foods

No interactions are known to occur, and there is no known reason to expect a clinically significant interaction with puncture vine.

Possible Interactions with Lab Tests

No interactions are known to occur, and there is no known reason to expect a clinically significant interaction with puncture vine.

Possible Interactions with Diseases or Conditions

No interactions are known to occur, and there is no known reason to expect a clinically significant interaction with puncture vine.

Typical Dosages & Routes of Administration that are Commonly Used

ORAL: Puncture vine is used as an extract (817).

Comments

Puncture vine was so named because its sharp seeds can flatten bicycle tires (817).

PURPLE LOOSESTRIFE

This Product is Also Known As

Blooming Sally, Flowering Sally, Long Purples, Loosestrife, Lythrum, Milk Willow-Herb, Purple Willow-Herb, Rainbow Weed, Salicare, Soldiers, Spiked, Spiked Loosestrife, Willow Sage.
CAUTION: See separate listings for Loosestrife and Sage.

Scientific Names

Lythrum salicaria.
Family: Lythraceae.

People Use This For

Orally, purple loosestrife is used for diarrhea, chronic intestinal inflammation, and menstrual complaints. It is also used as an anti-inflammatory, astringent, and antibiotic.
Topically, it is used for varicose veins, bleeding gums, hemorrhoids, and eczema.

Safety

There is insufficient reliable information available about the safety of purple loosestrife.
Pregnancy and Lactation: Insufficient reliable information available; avoid using.

Effectiveness

There is insufficient reliable information available about the effectiveness of purple loosestrife.

Possible Mechanism of Action & Active Ingredients

The applicable parts of purple loosestrife are the above ground flowering parts. The astringent effects are attributed to tannins and salicarin. Salicarin may also have antimicrobial effects against intestinal bacteria (18).

Adverse Reactions Including Known Allergies

None reported.

Possible Interactions with Herbs & Other Dietary Supplements

Insufficient reliable information available.

Possible Interactions with Drugs

No interactions are known to occur, and there is no known reason to expect a clinically significant interaction with purple loosestrife.

Possible Interactions with Foods

No interactions are known to occur, and there is no known reason to expect a clinically significant interaction with purple loosestrife.

Possible Interactions with Lab Tests
No interactions are known to occur, and there is no known reason to expect a clinically significant interaction with purple loosestrife.

Possible Interactions with Diseases or Conditions
No interactions are known to occur, and there is no known reason to expect a clinically significant interaction with purple loosestrife.

Typical Dosages & Routes of Administration that are Commonly Used
ORAL: The daily dose is 2-3 cups of tea. The tea is prepared by steeping 3 grams dried herb in 100 mL of boiling water for 10-15 minutes and straining. Alternately, 2-3 teaspoons of tincture are taken daily. The tincture is taken by adding 20 grams dried herb to 100 mL of a 20% alcohol solution and straining after 5 days (18).
TOPICAL: No typical dosage.

Comments
There is very little scientific information about this product. Our staff is continually analyzing the available information on natural medicines and will add data here as it becomes available.

PYCNOGENOL

This Product is Also Known As
None.

Scientific Names
Pinus pinaster, synonym Pinus maritima.

People Use This For
Orally, pycnogenol is used to slow the aging process, reduce allergies, for hypertension, preventing circulatory problems including heart disease and varicose veins, muscle soreness, pain relief, treating diabetes and preventing diabetic retinopathy (802), for preventing stroke, vascular and heart diseases, arthritis, and edema, and maintaining skin health (803).
Topically, pycnogenol is used in "antiaging" creams (6).

Safety
There is insufficient reliable information available about the safety of pycnogenol.
Pregnancy and Lactation: Insufficient reliable information available; avoid using.

Effectiveness
There is insufficient reliable information available about the effectiveness of pycnogenol.

Possible Mechanism of Action & Active Ingredients
Pycnogenol is a free radical scavenger, that is, it has antioxidant activity (2636). Scientists theorize that pycnogenol reduces atherogenesis and thrombus formation by increasing nitric oxide levels. An increased nitric oxide level reduces vasoconstriction caused by epinephrine and norepinephrine. It also decreases platelet aggregation and adhesion, and inhibits oxidation of low-density lipoprotein (LDL) cholesterol (2637). In preliminary research, 100-200 mg of orally administered pycnogenol appears to prevent smoking-related increases in platelet activity leading to platelet aggregation (3283). Pycnogenol does not appear to increase bleeding risk or affect smoking-related increases in blood pressure or heart rate (3283). Some evidence suggests that oral pycnogenol might improve the T- and B-cell function as well as augment the capacity of hemopoietic progenitors of bone marrow (2636). Other evidence suggests procyandiol oligomers could play a role in increasing resistance to elastin degradation that occurs in inflammation (2635). Preliminary information suggests pycnogenol used concomitantly with dextroamphetamine might improve target symptoms in individuals with attention deficit hyperactivity disorder (811).

Adverse Reactions Including Known Allergies
None reported.

Possible Interactions with Herbs & Other Dietary Supplements
Insufficient reliable information available.

Possible Interactions with Drugs
DEXTROAMPHETAMINE: There is one case report that concomitant use of pycnogenol and dextroamphetamine (Dexedrine) improved target symptoms in a child with attention deficit hyperactivity disorder (811).

Possible Interactions with Foods
No interactions are known to occur, and there is no known reason to expect a clinically significant interaction with pycnogenol.

Possible Interactions with Lab Tests

No interactions are known to occur, and there is no known reason to expect a clinically significant interaction with pycnogenol.

Possible Interactions with Diseases or Conditions

No interactions are known to occur, and there is no known reason to expect a clinically significant interaction with pycnogenol.

Typical Dosages & Routes of Administration that are Commonly Used

ORAL: People typically take 50 mg per day, although recommended doses range from 25 mg per day to 150 mg per day.

Comments

Pycnogenol is the US registered trademark for a product derived from Pine Bark (Pinus pinaster) which contains proanthocyanadins, a group of bioflavonoids. Originally, the term pycnogenol was used as a generic term for proanthocyanadins. Proanthocyanadins are also referred to as Condensed Tannins, Leucoanthocyanadins, Proanthocyanadins, Procyanadins, Oligomeric Proanthocyanadins (OPCs), Procyandiol Oligomers (PCOs). Proanthocyanadins are derived from various other sources besides pine bark. Other common sources include peanut skins (Arachis hypogaea), grape seed (Vitis vinifera) (515), and witch hazel bark (Hamamelis virginiana) (2641).

PYGEUM

This Product is Also Known As

African Plum Tree.

Scientific Names

Prunus africana, previously referred to as Pygeum africanum.
Family: Rosaceae.

People Use This For

Orally, pygeum bark is used for treating functional symptoms of benign prostatic hyperplasia (nocturia, dysuria, pollakiuria micturitional disorders, and bladder fullness) (6,7,3902,3903).
Traditionally, pygeum bark has been used orally for inflammation, kidney disease, urinary problems, malaria, stomachache, fever, difficult urination, fever, madness, prostate gland inflammation, and as an aphrodisiac (515).

Safety

LIKELY SAFE ...when used orally and appropriately (6,7,3902,3903).
PREGNANCY AND LACTATION: Insufficient reliable information available; avoid using.

Effectiveness

LIKELY EFFECTIVE ...when used for treating functional symptoms of benign prostatic hyperplasia (BPH) (6,7,3902,3903,4302).
POSSIBLY EFFECTIVE ...when used for functional symptoms of prostatic adenoma (3904).
There is insufficient reliable information available about the effectiveness of pygeum for its other uses.

Possible Mechanism of Action & Active Ingredients

The applicable part of pygeum is the bark. Scientists theorize that fibroblast proliferation plays a key role in development of BPH. Some information suggests that pygeum extracts can have antiproliferative effects on fibroblasts (4301). Pygeum bark contains varied constituents that demonstrate benefit in individuals with benign prostatic hyperplasia (BPH) (6,7). Ferulic acid esters of fatty acids reduce prostatic cholesterol levels, limiting synthesis of testosterone (6,7). Theoretically the phytosterols, including beta-sitosterol, beta-sitosterone and campesterol (6,7), compete with androgen precursors and inhibit prostaglandin biosynthesis (7). Some evidence suggests that the triterpenes, including oleanolic, crataegolic and ursolic acid, might have anti-inflammatory activity in prostrate connective tissue (6,7). Pygeum bark extract also increases prostatic secretions and improves seminal fluid composition (6). Multiple clinical trials demonstrate that pygeum bark extract improves symptoms of BPH (6,7). However, not all symptoms are improved in every patient. More trials reported nocturia and maximum flow improved than report reduction in residual volume (4302). Pygeum bark extract also appears to offer similar benefits to individuals with prostatic adenoma (3904).

Adverse Reactions Including Known Allergies

Pygeum bark can cause nausea and abdominal pain (6,7).

Possible Interactions with Herbs & Other Dietary Supplements

Insufficient reliable information available.

Possible Interactions with Drugs
No interactions are known to occur, and there is no known reason to expect a clinically significant interaction with pygeum.

Possible Interactions with Foods
No interactions are known to occur, and there is no known reason to expect a clinically significant interaction with pygeum.

Possible Interactions with Lab Tests
No interactions are known to occur, and there is no known reason to expect a clinically significant interaction with pygeum.

Possible Interactions with Diseases or Conditions
No interactions are known to occur, and there is no known reason to expect a clinically significant interaction with pygeum.

Typical Dosages & Routes of Administration that are Commonly Used
ORAL: A typical dose used for functional symptoms of BPH is 100-200 mg standardized lipophilic extract (14% triterpenes, 0.5 % n-docosanol) per day in 6-8 week cycles (6,7).

Comments
Some think saw palmetto is a better choice for treating BPH than pygeum. In one study it was more effective in treating functional symptoms of BPH and had fewer adverse effects (6). Pygeum is more expensive than saw palmetto. Also, overharvesting of the bark of pygeum is threatening the survival of the species (515).

PYRETHRUM

This Product is Also Known As
Dalmation Insect Flowers, Dalmation Pellitory.

Scientific Names
Chrysanthemum cinerariifolium.
Family: Asteraceae.

People Use This For
Topically, pyrethrum is used as an insecticide, particularly for head lice, crablice and their nits, and as an antiscabies agent (18).

Safety
LIKELY SAFE ...when the commercially available combination of pyrethrins (0.17-0.33%) and piperonyl butoxide (2-4%) are used topically and appropriately in a nonaerosol preparation (272).
POSSIBLY SAFE ...when pyrethrins are used topically in amounts less than 2 grams (18). Contact with eyes and mucous membranes should be avoided (272).
POSSIBLY UNSAFE ...in individuals with allergies to ragweed, chrysanthemums, marigolds, daisies and many herbs due to cross-allergenicity.
There is insufficient reliable information available about the safety of pyrethrum flowerheads for topical use.
CHILDREN: POSSIBLY UNSAFE ...when used in children under the age of 2 years (4084).
PREGNANCY: Insufficient reliable information available; avoid using. Topical use of pyrethrins with piperonyl butoxide has not been proven safe in pregnancy; avoid using (4084).
LACTATION: Insufficient reliable information available; avoid using.

Effectiveness
EFFECTIVE ...when pyrethrins are used topically and appropriately in concentrations of 0.17-.0.33% for 12-24 hours. They are usually combined with piperonyl butoxide (2-4%) (272). Brand names include: A-200 Pyrinate, Barc, Lice-Enz, Licetrol, Pronto, R and C, RID, Tisit, Tisit Blue, Triple X.
There is insufficient reliable information available about the effectiveness of pyrethrum flowers for lice infections.
INEFFECTIVE ...when pyrethrins flowers are used to treat scabies (4084).

Possible Mechanism of Action & Active Ingredients
The applicable part of pyrethrum is the flower head. Pyrethrum is also the name of the crude extract obtained from flowers of Chrysanthemum cinerariifolium. Pyrethrin refers to more refined extract containing several naturally occurring pyrethrins (505). The active constituents, the pyrethrins, are toxic to insect nervous systems (18).

Adverse Reactions Including Known Allergies
Pyrethrum flower has limited toxicity. The symptoms of overdose include headache, tinnitus, nausea, tingling of fingers and toes, respiratory disturbances, and other symptoms of neurotoxicity (18). The pyrethrum flower or

derivatives of it might cause an allergic reaction in individuals sensitive to the Asteraceae/Compositae family. Members of this family include ragweed, chrysanthemums, marigolds, daisies, and many other herbs.

Possible Interactions with Herbs & Other Dietary Supplements

Insufficient reliable information available.

Possible Interactions with Drugs

No interactions are known to occur, and there is no known reason to expect a clinically significant interaction with pyrethrum.

Possible Interactions with Foods

No interactions are known to occur, and there is no known reason to expect a clinically significant interaction with pyrethrum.

Possible Interactions with Lab Tests

No interactions are known to occur, and there is no known reason to expect a clinically significant interaction with pyrethrum.

Possible Interactions with Diseases or Conditions

CROSS-ALLERGENICITY: Can cause an allergic reaction in individuals sensitive to the Asteraceae/Compositae family. Members of this family include ragweed, chrysanthemums, marigolds, daisies, and many other herbs.

Typical Dosages & Routes of Administration that are Commonly Used

TOPICAL: Externally as a liquid extract, rinse after use (18). In general, the OTC combination of pyrethrins (0.17-0.33%) and piperonyl butoxide (2-4%) are applied to the infested area and allowed to remain for not less than 10 minutes. It is then thoroughly washed off with warm water (272).

Comments

To treat lice, the OTC combination products with piperonyl butoxide are preferred for safety and effectiveness (272).

PYRIDOXINE (VITAMIN B6)

This Product is Also Known As

Adermine Hydrochloride, Pyridoxal, Pyridoxamine, Pyridoxine Hydrochloride.

Scientific Names

Pyridoxine; Vitamin B6.

People Use This For

Orally, pyridoxine is used most commonly for treating premenstrual syndrome (3093), vitamin B6 deficiency, "morning sickness" in pregnancy, depression associated with pregnancy or oral contraceptive use, primary homocystinuria, and preventing neuritis associated with isoniazid or penicillamine (15). Pyridoxine is also used orally for boosting immunity, muscle cramps, protection against cancer, diuresis, conjunctivitis, cystitis (3038,3039,3040), primary hyperoxaluria (15), preventing kidney stones, carpal tunnel syndrome, night leg cramps, arthritis, and allergies (3038,3039,3040). It is used for asthma (15), pyridoxine-responsive sideroblastic anemia, xanthurenic aciduria, primary cystathioninuria, acne, various skin conditions, stimulating appetite, hyperlipidemia, heart disease (3038,3039,3040), radiation sickness, menopausal symptoms, infertility (3038,3039,3040), amenorrhea-galactorrhea syndrome, and suppressing postpartum lactation. Pyridoxine is also used for dizziness, motion sickness, psychosis (15), autism (14), hyperkinesis, acute chorea, chronic progressive hereditary chorea, tardive dyskinesia, absence (petit mal) seizures (15), febrile convulsions (14), gyrate atrophy of the choroid and retina (15), diabetes (3038,3039,3040), diabetic neuropathy (14), alcohol intoxication, preventing leukopenia secondary to mitomycin, reversing procarbazine neurotoxicity, preventing anemia due to pyridoxine deficiency, preventing seizures associated with cycloserine (15), fluorouracil-induced erythrodysesthesia, and acute hydrazine toxicity (14). Intravenously, pyridoxine is used for seizures in infants unresponsive to other therapies, acute toxicity due to isoniazid, cycloserine or hydrazine overdose, and acute poisoning from mushrooms of the genus Gyromitra (15).

Safety

LIKELY SAFE ...when used orally and appropriately. ...when used as an injectable. Injectable pyridoxine is a FDA-approved prescription product (15).
POSSIBLY UNSAFE ...when used orally and long-term in large doses (15).
PREGNANCY: LIKELY SAFE ...when used at the recommended dietary allowance (RDA) of 1.9 mg per day (3094) and up to FDA-approved 75 mg per day in a sustained release product. POSSIBLY UNSAFE ...when used in doses greater than the FDA-approved 75 mg per day. Anecdotal reports have linked high-dose maternal pyridoxine to neonatal seizures, although causality has not been established (4608,4609). Prolonged exposure to doses as low as 200 mg per day in the general population has been associated with sensory neuropathy (4610). The effect of prolonged fetal exposure to high-dose maternal pyridoxine is unknown.
LACTATION: LIKELY SAFE ...when used at the recommended dietary allowance (RDA) of 2 mg per day (3094).

Effectiveness

EFFECTIVE ...when taken orally for preventing and treating vitamin B6 deficiency; for hereditary sideroblastic anemia; and treating some people with metabolic disorders, including xanthurenic aciduria, primary cystathioninuria, primary hyperoxaluria, and primary homocystinuria (15). Injectable pyridoxine is a FDA-approved prescription product (15).

POSSIBLY EFFECTIVE ...when used orally for treating pregnancy-induced nausea and vomiting. In one clinical trial, pyridoxine 25 mg every eight hours for 72 hours improved vomiting and severe nausea, but not mild-moderate nausea in a group of pregnant women (6168). In a second trial, pyridoxine 10 mg every eight hours improved nausea but not vomiting in pregnant women (6167). ...when used orally for premenstrual syndrome (3093). ...when used orally in combination with folic acid to prevent the development or progression of subclinical atherosclerosis. Siblings of people with premature atherothrombotic disease treated with folic acid and pyridoxine had reduced levels of homocysteine and decreased rate of abnormal exercise EKG tests, but no change in peripheral arterial indicators (3886). However, EKG changes on an exercise stress test are not very sensitive for detecting disease in people who do not have cardiac symptoms (3887). ...when used for improving biochemical parameters and behavior in conjunction with other therapies in autism, and for partially reversing fluorouracil-induced erythrodysesthesia in metastatic colon cancer patients so that further therapy with fluorouracil is possible (14).

POSSIBLY INEFFECTIVE ...when used orally in combination with magnesium for treating children with autism. Ten weeks of high-dose oral pyridoxine and magnesium failed to ameliorate autistic behaviors in a group of ten children with autism (5049).

LIKELY INEFFECTIVE ...when taken orally for diabetic neuropathy, familial hypercholesterolemia, suppressing lactation, and premenstrual syndrome (14).

There is insufficient reliable information available about the effectiveness of pyridoxine for its other uses.

Possible Mechanism of Action & Active Ingredients

Pyridoxine is required for amino acid metabolism. It is also involved in carbohydrate and lipid metabolism (15). In the body, pyridoxine is converted to pyridoxal phosphate and pyridoxamine phosphate, which are coenzymes in a wide variety of metabolic reactions. These reactions include transamination of amino acids, conversion of tryptophan to niacin, synthesis of gamma-aminobutyric acid (GABA) in the CNS, metabolism of serotonin, norepinephrine and dopamine, metabolism of polyunsaturated fatty acids and phospholipids, and the synthesis of heme, a hemoglobin constituent (14,15). Pyridoxine is involved with several of the reactions important for the overall metabolism of nitrogen; therefore, pyridoxine requirements are related to the total amino acid nitrogen burden to be metabolized (14). Pyridoxine is a cofactor for enzymes involved in the metabolism of homocysteine, and high levels of homocysteine are a risk factor for atherosclerosis (1483,3047). Pyridoxine deficiency has been associated with elevated plasma homocysteine levels, but there is currently insufficient evidence that pyridoxine supplements reduce plasma homocysteine levels or the incidence of atherosclerosis (1483,3047,3048,3049,3050). In preliminary clinical trials, methionine loading acutely elevates plasma homocysteine levels and induces endothelial dysfunction (6235). Pyridoxine in combination with folic acid and cyanocobalamin, has improved endothelial function, as measured by flow-mediated vasodilation, following a methionine load in healthy volunteers (6235). Early clinical data suggests that pyridoxine supplements might be useful for treating hyperhomocysteinuria in people with renal insufficiency (1489). Pyridoxine deficiency in adults principally affects the peripheral nerves, skin, mucous membranes, and hematopoietic system. In children, the CNS is also affected. Deficiency can occur in people with uremia, alcoholism, cirrhosis, hyperthyroidism, malabsorption syndromes, and congestive heart failure; and in those receiving isoniazid, cycloserine, ethionamide, hydralazine, penicillamine, or pyrazinamide (15).

Adverse Reactions Including Known Allergies

Pyridoxine, either orally or by injection, can cause nausea, vomiting, abdominal pain, loss of appetite, headache, paresthesia, somnolence, increased serum AST (SGOT), decreased serum folic acid concentrations, skin reactions and other allergic reactions, breast soreness or enlargement, and photosensitivity (14,15). Long-term use of two months or longer with large amounts of pyridoxine (as little as 50 mg per day, but usually 2 grams or more per day) can cause sensory neuropathy or neuronopathy syndromes (14,15). The mechanism of the neurotoxicity is unknown, but it is characterized by impairment of the sense of position and vibration of the distal limbs and gradual, progressive sensory ataxia. Improvement is gradual when vitamin B6 is stopped (15). Injectable pyridoxine can also cause burning or stinging at the injection site, seizures after the IV administration of large amounts (15), and hypotonia and respiratory distress in infants (14).

Possible Interactions with Herbs & Other Dietary Supplements

Insufficient reliable information available.

Possible Interactions with Drugs

AMIODARONE (Cordarone): Concomitant use can increase the risk of amiodarone-induced photosensitivity (14).

DOXYLAMINE: Concomitant administration of pyridoxine and doxylamine (Diclectin) is approved for treating nausea and vomiting of pregnancy in Canada (24).

LEVODOPA (Larodopa): Concomitant use accelerates peripheral metabolism of levodopa, reversing the therapeutic effects. This interaction does not occur when carbidopa is taken concurrently with levodopa (Sinemet) (15).

PHENYTOIN (Dilantin), PHENOBARBITAL: Concomitant use can decrease the serum concentrations of phenytoin and phenobarbital (15).

Drug Influences on Nutrient Levels and Depletion

SOME DRUGS CAN AFFECT PYRIDOXINE LEVELS:

ANTIBIOTICS: Destruction of normal gastrointestinal flora by antibiotics can cause decreased production of B vitamins. The clinical significance of this decreased production is not known. Consider supplementation only if clinical judgment warrants it (4434,4435,4436,4437,4438,4439,4440,4441,4442,4443).

ESTROGENS and ESTROGEN-CONTAINING ORAL CONTRACEPTIVES: Use of estrogens and estrogen-containing oral contraceptives can interfere with vitamin B6 metabolism, reducing serum vitamin B6 levels. The need for vitamin B6 supplementation has not been adequately studied (4498).

THEOPHYLLINE (Theodur): Theophylline interferes with vitamin B6 metabolism, reducing serum vitamin B6 levels. The need for vitamin B6 supplementation has not been adequately studied (4522).

HYDRALAZINE (Apresoline): Hydralazine can increase vitamin B6 requirements. The need for vitamin B6 supplementation has not been adequately studied (14,4453,4531,4533).

PENICILLAMINE (Cuprimine): Penicillamine can increase vitamin B6 requirements. The need for vitamin B6 supplementation has not been adequately studied (14,4453,4531).

ISONIAZID (INH, Rifamate): Isoniazid can increase pyridoxine requirements. Patients receiving more than 10 mg/kg/day of INH should be supplemented with 50-100 mg of pyridoxine per day (14,4481,4482).

Possible Interactions with Foods

No interactions are known to occur, and there is no known reason to expect a clinically significant interaction with pyridoxine.

Possible Interactions with Lab Tests

UROBILINOGEN: Pyridoxine can cause a false positive result in the spot test with Ehrlich's reagent (15).

Possible Interactions with Diseases or Conditions

No interactions are known to occur, and there is no known reason to expect a clinically significant interaction with pyridoxine.

Typical Dosages & Routes of Administration that are Commonly Used

ORAL: As a dietary supplement, 2 mg per day of pyridoxine is generally considered sufficient in individuals with normal GI absorption (14,15). For vitamin B6 deficiency in adults, the typical dose is 2.5-25 mg daily for three weeks, then 1.5-2.5 mg per day as maintenance therapy (14,15). For vitamin B6 deficiency in women taking oral contraceptives, the dose is 25-30 mg per day (15). For symptoms associated with premenstrual syndrome (PMS), the daily dose is 50-100 mg. Doses as high as 500 mg per day have been used, but daily doses over 100 mg don't appear to have additional benefit, and may increase the risk for adverse effects (3093). For hereditary sideroblastic anemia, initially 200-600 mg per day is taken, decreasing to 30-50 mg daily after an adequate response (15). For metabolic disorders, including xanthurenic aciduria, primary cystathioninuria, primary hyperoxaluria, or primary homocystinuria, 100-500 mg daily is generally effective (15). For preventing anemia due to pyridoxine deficiency or neuritis in people receiving isoniazid or penicillamine, the typical dose is 10-50 mg daily (15). For premenstrual syndrome, 50-100 mg is commonly taken per day (3093). For preventing seizures in people receiving cycloserine, 100-300 mg is taken daily in divided doses (15). For nausea during pregnancy, 10-25 mg pyridoxine every eight hours has been used (6167,6168); alternatively, 75 mg of sustained-release pyridoxine combined with 12 mcg vitamin B12 (cyanocobalamin), 1 mg folic acid, and 200 mg calcium (PremesisRx), is used daily as a FDA-approved prescription supplement for nausea during pregnancy (23). The daily recommended dietary allowances (RDAs) of vitamin B6 are: Infants 0-6 months, 0.1 mg; Infants 7-12 months, 0.3 mg; Children 1-3 years, 0.5 mg; Children 4-8 years, 0.6 mg; Children 9-13 years, 1 mg; Males 14-50 years, 1.3 mg; Men over 50 years, 1.7 mg; Females 14-18 years, 1.2 mg; Women 19-50 years, 1.3 mg; Women over 50 years, 1.5 mg; Pregnant women, 1.9 mg; and Lactating women, 2 mg (3094). The recommended maximum daily intake is: Children 1-3 years, 30 mg; Children 4-8 years, 40 mg; Children 9-13 years, 60 mg; Adults, pregnant and lactating women, 14-18 years, 80 mg; and Adults, pregnant and lactating women, over 18 years, 100 mg (3094).

INJECTION: This is a FDA-approved prescription product that is available as a 100 mg/mL injection.

Comments

Vitamin B6 is present in many foods including cereal grains, legumes, vegetables, liver, meat, and eggs (15). Pyridoxine is frequently used in combination with other B vitamins in vitamin B complex formulations. Vitamin B complex generally includes vitamin B1 (thiamine), vitamin B2 (riboflavin), vitamin B3 (niacin/niacinamide), vitamin B5 (pantothenic acid), vitamin B6 (pyridoxine), vitamin B12 (cyanocobalamin), and folic acid. However, some products do not contain all of these ingredients and some may include others, such as biotin, para-aminobenzoic acid (PABA), choline bitartrate, and inositol (3022,3060,3061).

PYRUVATE

This Product is Also Known As
2-Oxypropanoic Acid, Acetylformic Acid, Alpha-Ketopropionic Acid, Calcium Pyruvate, Magnesium Pyruvate, Potassium Pyruvate, Proacemic Acid, Sodium Pyruvate.

Scientific Names
2-Oxopropanoate (pyruvate); 2-oxopropanoic acid (pyruvic acid).

People Use This For
Orally, pyruvate is used for weight loss, improving exercise endurance, and inhibiting tumor growth (2471).

Safety
There is insufficient reliable information available about the safety of pyruvate.
Pregnancy and Lactation: Insufficient reliable information available; avoid using.

Effectiveness
POSSIBLY EFFECTIVE ...when used orally for enhancing weight loss (2472,2474).
There is insufficient reliable information available about the effectiveness of pyruvate for its other uses.

Possible Mechanism of Action & Active Ingredients
Some evidence suggests that pyruvate reduces free radical production (2487), increases lipid oxidation and decreases carbohydrate oxidation (2488). Very small clinical trials suggest dietary supplementation with dihydroxyacetone and pyruvate increases arm and leg exercise endurance (807,808). Very preliminary evidence also suggests a liquid diet supplemented with pyruvate might inhibit tumor growth (806).

Adverse Reactions Including Known Allergies
Ingesting large amounts of pyruvate can cause GI upset, including gas, bloating, and diarrhea (2471). A death was associated with intravenous use in a child with restrictive cardiomyopathy (2473).

Possible Interactions with Herbs & Other Dietary Supplements
Insufficient reliable information available.

Possible Interactions with Drugs
No interactions are known to occur, and there is no known reason to expect a clinically significant interaction with pyruvate.

Possible Interactions with Foods
No interactions are known to occur, and there is no known reason to expect a clinically significant interaction with pyruvate.

Possible Interactions with Lab Tests
No interactions are known to occur, and there is no known reason to expect a clinically significant interaction with pyruvate.

Possible Interactions with Diseases or Conditions
CARDIOMYOPATHY: A death was associated with intravenous use in a child with restrictive cardiomyopathy (2473).

Typical Dosages & Routes of Administration that are Commonly Used
ORAL: A typical dose used for weight loss is 22 to 44 grams per day, as supplement to a low-cholesterol, low-fat diet (2474).

Comments
None.

QUASSIA

This Product is Also Known As
Amargo, Bitter-Ash, Bitter Wood, Bitterwood, Jamaican Quassia, Picrasma, Quassia Bark, Ruda, Surinam Quassia, Surinam Wood.

Scientific Names
Quassia amara; Picrasma excelsa.
Family: Simaroubaceae.

People Use This For
Orally, quassia is used for anorexia; indigestion; constipation (7); fever (11); as an anthelmintic for thread worms,

© Copyright 2000, Natural Medicines Comprehensive Database (209) 472-2244. For updated data, go to www.NaturalDatabase.com

nematodes, and ascaris (4,18); as a tonic or purgative (18); and as a mouthwash (6).

Topically, quassia is used for pediculosis (4).

Rectally, quassia is used for nematode infestation (4).

In manufacturing, quassia is used as a flavoring agent in foods, beverages, pastilles, lozenges, and laxatives (4,11). The bark and wood have been used as an insecticide (6,11).

Safety

POSSIBLY SAFE ...when consumed in amounts found in foods and beverages. It has Generally Recognized as Safe (GRAS) status in the US (4). Maximum reported use level is 0.007% in nonalcoholic beverages (11).

POSSIBLY UNSAFE ...when used orally in therapeutic amounts. Quassia wood contains cardioactive glycosides (4), but toxicity is likely limited by emetic effects of large doses (4).

There is insufficient reliable information available about the safety of the topical or rectal use of quassia.

PREGNANCY AND LACTATION: LIKELY UNSAFE ...contraindicated for oral use. Quassia has cytotoxic and emetic properties (4,18,19). Insufficient reliable information available about the safety of rectal or topical use; avoid using.

Effectiveness

POSSIBLY EFFECTIVE ...when used in a tincture as a scalp lotion to treat head lice (4).

There is insufficient reliable information available about the effectiveness of quassia for its other uses.

Possible Mechanism of Action & Active Ingredients

The applicable part of quassia is the wood (4,8,11). Quassia leaves are also reportedly used (6). Quassia contains quassinoids that have potent bitter properties (11). Quassia also contains beta-carboline alkaloids, quassin, quassimarin, canthin-6-one (4), and small amounts of the coumarin scopoletin (4). The quassinoid constituents increase gastric acid and bile secretions, perhaps accounting for appetite stimulant and digestive effects (18,19,4). There is evidence that the beta-carboline alkaloids might have positive inotropic activity (4). The constituent canthin-6-one is reported to have antibacterial, antifungal, and cytotoxic activity (4). Quassimarin demonstrates evidence of antileukemic (11) and antitumor effects (18,4). Quassin demonstrates antilarval activity against Culex quinquefasciatus (mosquito) (3302).

Adverse Reactions Including Known Allergies

Quassia can cause mucous membrane irritation, nausea, and vomiting (4,18). Long-term use can cause vision changes and blindness (18).

Possible Interactions with Herbs & Other Dietary Supplements

CARDIOACTIVE GLYCOSIDE-CONTAINING HERBS: Theoretically, concomitant use with other cardiac glycoside-containing herbs might increase risk of cardiac toxicity. Cardiac glycoside containing herbs, including black hellebore, Canadian hemp roots, digitalis leaf, hedge mustard, figwort, lily of the valley roots, motherwort, oleander leaf, pheasant's eye plant, pleurisy root, squill bulb leaf scales, and strophanthus seeds (2,18,19).

CARDIOACTIVE HERBS: Avoid concomitant use with other cardioactive herbs due to unpredictability of effects and adverse effects. Other cardioactive herbs include: calamus, cereus, cola, coltsfoot, devil's claw, European mistletoe, fenugreek, fumitory, ginger, Panax ginseng, hawthorn, white horehound, mate, parsley, scotch broom flower, shepherd's purse, and wild carrot (4).

HORSETAIL/LICORICE: Theoretically, abuse of licorice or horsetail might increase risk of cardiac toxicity due to potassium loss (4).

STIMULANT LAXATIVE HERBS: Theoretically, abuse might increase risk of cardiac toxicity due to potassium depletion. Stimulant laxative herbs include: aloe dried leaf sap, blue flag rhizome, alder buckthorn, European buckthorn, butternut bark, cascara bark, castor oil, colocynth fruit pulp, gamboge bark exudate, jalap root, black root, manna bark exudate, podophyllum root, rhubarb root, senna leaves and pods, wild cucumber fruit (Ecballium elaterium), and yellow dock root (19).

HERBS WITH ANTICOAGULANT/ANTIPLATELET POTENTIAL: Concomitant use of herbs that have coumarin constituents or affect platelet aggregation could theoretically increase the risk of bleeding in some people. These herbs include: angelica, anise, arnica, asafoetida, bogbean, boldo, capsicum, celery, chamomile, clove, danshen, fenugreek, feverfew, garlic, ginger ginkgo, Panax ginseng, horse chestnut, horseradish, licorice, meadowsweet, prickly ash, onion, papain, passionflower, poplar, red clover, turmeric, wild carrot, wild lettuce, willow, and others (4,19).

Possible Interactions with Drugs

ACID INHIBITORS: Theoretically, because quassia stimulates gastric acid, it might oppose effect of antacids and H-2 antagonists (11,19).

CARDIAC THERAPY: Theoretically, concomitant use with cardiac medications increases risk of cardiac effects and adverse effects (4).

POTASSIUM-DEPLETING DRUGS: Theoretically, concomitant use of potassium-depleting diuretics or stimulant laxative abuse might increase risk of cardiac glycoside toxicity due to potassium loss (13).

ANTICOAGULANTS: Theoretically, excessive doses might have additive effects with anticoagulant therapy with warfarin (Coumadin) (4).

Possible Interactions with Foods

No interactions are known to occur, and there is no known reason to expect a clinically significant interaction with quassia.

Possible Interactions with Lab Tests

No interactions are known to occur, and there is no known reason to expect a clinically significant interaction with quassia.

Possible Interactions with Diseases or Conditions

GI IRRITATION/INFLAMMATION: In large amounts quassia can irritate the gastrointestinal tract; avoid using (8).

Typical Dosages & Routes of Administration that are Commonly Used

ORAL: A typical dose is one cup tea 2-3 times daily (12). To make tea, simmer 1-2 grams of wood in 150 mL boiling water 10-15 minutes, strain (12).
RECTAL: As an enema (1:20): 150 mL rectally every morning for 3 days with 16 gram magnesium sulfate orally (4).

Comments

Quassia bark has been used as an insecticide (11).

QUEBRACHO

This Product is Also Known As

Quebracho Blanco, White Quebracho.

Scientific Names

Aspidosperma quebracho-blanco.
Family: Apocynaceae.

People Use This For

Orally, quebracho is used for asthma and conditions of the lower respiratory tract. It is also used as an expectorant and respiratory tract stimulant (18). Sometimes it is used to lower blood pressure (particularly arterial hypertension), as a spasmolytic, diuretic, peripheral vasoconstrictor, uterine sedative and local anesthetic.
In folk medicine, quebracho is used orally to decrease fever and as an aphrodisiac.
In foods and beverages, it is used as a flavoring agent (11).

Safety

LIKELY SAFE …in amounts found in food. It is approved for food use in the US (11).
There is insufficient reliable information available about the oral use of quebracho bark in amounts exceeding those found in foods.
PREGNANCY AND LACTATION: Avoid using in amounts greater than those typically found in foods.

Effectiveness

There is insufficient reliable information available about the effectiveness of quebracho.

Possible Mechanism of Action & Active Ingredients

The applicable part of quebracho is the bark. There is insufficient reliable information available about the possible mechanism of action and active ingredients.

Adverse Reactions Including Known Allergies

People who take quebracho bark orally may experience side effects including salivation, headache, outbreaks of sweating, vertigo, stupor and sleepiness. In large doses, it can cause nausea and vomiting (18).

Possible Interactions with Herbs & Other Dietary Supplements

Insufficient reliable information available.

Possible Interactions with Drugs

No interactions are known to occur, and there is no known reason to expect a clinically significant interaction with quebracho.

Possible Interactions with Foods

No interactions are known to occur, and there is no known reason to expect a clinically significant interaction with quebracho.

Possible Interactions with Lab Tests

No interactions are known to occur, and there is no known reason to expect a clinically significant interaction with quebracho.

Possible Interactions with Diseases or Conditions
No interactions are known to occur, and there is no known reason to expect a clinically significant interaction with quebracho.

Typical Dosages & Routes of Administration that are Commonly Used
ORAL: It is used as an extract or powder and in combination bronchial preparations (18).

Comments
The bark is odorless and has a bitter taste. Quebracho Colorado or red quebracho is also known as quebracho, but is chemically distinct from white quebracho. Be careful not to confuse these two plants (11).

QUEEN'S DELIGHT

This Product is Also Known As
Cockup Hat, Marcory, Queens Delight, Queen's Root, Queens Root, Silver Leaf, Stillingia, Yaw Root.

Scientific Names
Stillingia sylvatica, synonym Stillingia treculeana.
Family: Euphorbiaceae.

People Use This For
Orally, queen's delight is used as a "blood purifier", for digestive disorders, treatment of hepatic, gallbladder and skin diseases, and as an emetic and laxative (18).
Historically, it has been used orally for bronchitis, laryngitis, laryngismus stridulus, and constipation (4). It has also been used topically for cutaneous eruptions, hemorrhoids, and exudative skin eruptions with lymphatic involvement (4).

Safety
POSSIBLY UNSAFE ...when used orally in medicinal amounts because the dried root preparations contain diterpene esters that are highly irritating (4,12). Queen's delight might activate latent viruses, and there is some evidence it might be carcinogenic (18). ...when the dried or fresh root preparations are used topically (4).
LIKELY UNSAFE ...when the fresh root is used orally because it contains caustic white latex that is highly irritating to mucous membranes (12).
PREGNANCY: POSSIBLY UNSAFE ...when the dried root preparations are used orally or when the dried or fresh root are used topically; avoid using (4). LIKELY UNSAFE ...when the fresh root preparations are used orally (12).
LACTATION: POSSIBLY UNSAFE ...when the dried or fresh root are used topically. LIKELY UNSAFE ...contraindicated for oral use (4,12,19).

Effectiveness
There is insufficient reliable information available about the effectiveness of queen's delight.

Possible Mechanism of Action & Active Ingredients
The applicable part of queen's delight is the root. Queen's delight contains a volatile oil and diterpenes including prostatin, gnidilatidin, and others (18). Diterpene esters, isolated in the latex (or milky juice) of the fresh or green root, are potent irritants that cause swelling of the skin and mucous membranes (4,18). Diterpenes may also be carcinogenic agents; they are believed able to activate latent viruses (18).

Adverse Reactions Including Known Allergies
Taken orally, queen's delight can cause vomiting, diarrhea (18), and nausea (19). In large amounts, it may cause a burning sensation of the mouth, throat, diarrhea, nausea, vomiting, dysuria, aches and pains, pruritus, skin eruptions, cough, depression, fatigue, and perspiration (4). Topically, it may cause inflammation, swelling (18), and contact dermatitis (19).

Possible Interactions with Herbs & Other Dietary Supplements
Insufficient reliable information available.

Possible Interactions with Drugs
No interactions are known to occur, and there is no known reason to expect a clinically significant interaction with queen's delight.

Possible Interactions with Foods
No interactions are known to occur, and there is no known reason to expect a clinically significant interaction with queen's delight.

Possible Interactions with Lab Tests

No interactions are known to occur, and there is no known reason to expect a clinically significant interaction with queen's delight.

Possible Interactions with Diseases or Conditions

GI CONDITIONS: Contraindicated in individuals with gastrointestinal irritation, inflammation, nausea or vomiting (19).

Typical Dosages & Routes of Administration that are Commonly Used

ORAL: People typically prepare queen's delight as a liquid, boiling 1 teaspoon of the dried root with one cup of water. The suggested dose is a cup a day, taken a mouthful at a time. As a tincture, queen's delight is taken in a dose of 5 to 20 drops (5263).

Comments

None.

QUERCETIN

This Product is Also Known As

Meletin, Sophretin.

Scientific Names

3,3',4'5,7-Penthydroxyflavone.

People Use This For

Orally, quercetin is used for treating atherosclerosis (1900,2006), hypercholesterolemia (1900), coronary heart disease (1995), diabetes (1995), cataracts (1900.2006), hay fever (1900,2006), peptic ulcer (1900), schizophrenia (1996), inflammation, asthma, gout, viral infections, preventing cancer (483), and for treating chronic, bacterial prostatitis (481).

Intravenously and intraperitoneally, quercetin is used for treating cancer (2006).

Safety

POSSIBLY SAFE ...when used orally in amounts up to 500 mg twice daily for up to one month (481). There is insufficient reliable information available about the safety of larger oral doses or longer periods of oral use. ...when used intravenously in amounts less than 945 mg/m2 (2007).

LIKELY UNSAFE ...when used intravenously in amounts greater that 945 mg/m2 which are reported to cause nephrotoxicity (2007).

There is insufficient reliable information available about the safety of intraperitoneal quercetin.

PREGNANCY AND LACTATION: Insufficient reliable information available; avoid using.

Effectiveness

POSSIBLY EFFECTIVE ...when used orally for treating symptoms of chronic, nonbacterial prostatitis (481). In one clinical trial, quercetin reduced pain and improved quality of life, but had no effect on voiding dysfunction (481). There is insufficient reliable information available about the effectiveness of quercetin for its other uses.

Possible Mechanism of Action & Active Ingredients

Quercetin is a dietary flavonoid found in many plants (481,483,1995). It has antioxidant, anti-inflammatory, nitric oxide inhibitor, and tyrosine kinase inhibitor (leading to inhibition of the division and growth of T cells and some cancer cells) activity (481,1995). The anti-inflammatory effects of quercetin might be due to inhibition of the production and activity of leukotrienes and prostaglandins, and inhibition of histamine release by basophils and mast cells (483). Quercetin appears to reduce capillary fragility and it might offer some protection against diabetic cataracts, possibly by inhibiting aldose reductase in the lens (483,2006). The anti-inflammatory and antioxidant effects might be responsible for the observed benefits in men with chronic, nonbacterial prostatitis (481). Scientists theorize that quercetin might reduce cancer risk by inactivating malignant precursors or by inhibiting carcinogenesis (2006). Preliminary studies suggest it might have inhibitory effects on various cancer types, including breast, leukemia, colon, ovary, oral squamous cell, endometrial, gastric and non-small-cell lung (483,485). Quercetin has antiestrogenic effects in cultures of breast cancer cells (484). It also inhibits estrone sulfatase and estrogen synthesis in liver cells (489). Existing evidence suggests quercetin alters intestinal cell homeostasis of copper, iron, and manganese (1997). Although researchers believe quercetin might protect against heart disease (1995), short term supplementation does not show affect on any of the known risk factors for heart disease (1998,1999). Preliminary evidence suggests that quercetin might inhibit collagen- and ADP-induced platelet aggregation, but at concentrations much higher than those achieved with typical oral dosing (488). Evidence suggests that quercetin might benefit some people with schizophrenia when used in combination with other antioxidants, polysorb, and conventional therapy (1996). Quercetin demonstrates activity against retroviruses, Herpes simplex, polio, parainfluenza and respiratory syncytial viruses (483). The oral absorption of quercetin is highly variable, depending on the source. The degree of glycosylation and plasma protein binding, as well as absorption, affect the activity of quercetin (481,486,487).

Adverse Reactions Including Known Allergies
Orally, quercetin can cause headache and tingling of the extremities (481). Intravenous administration of quercetin is associated with flushing, sweating, dyspnea, nausea, and vomiting (2007). Injection pain can be minimized by premedicating patient with 10 mg of morphine and administering amounts greater than 945 mg/m2 over 5 minutes (2007). Nephrotoxicity has been reported with use of amounts greater than 945 mg/m2 (2006,2007).

Possible Interactions with Herbs & Other Dietary Supplements
VITAMIN C: Concurrent use enhances the antioxidant activity of quercetin (2006).
PAPAIN, BROMELAIN: Concomitant administration of quercetin with papain or bromelain might increase GI absorption of quercetin (481).

Possible Interactions with Drugs
QUINOLONE ANTIBIOTICS: Quercetin might competitively inhibit quinolone antibiotics by binding to the DNA gyrase site on bacteria (481).

Possible Interactions with Foods
No interactions are known to occur, and there is no known reason to expect a clinically significant interaction with quercetin.

Possible Interactions with Lab Tests
No interactions are known to occur, and there is no known reason to expect a clinically significant interaction with quercetin.

Possible Interactions with Diseases or Conditions
KIDNEY DYSFUNCTION: Theoretically, intravenous quercetin may exacerbate kidney dysfunction (2006).

Typical Dosages & Routes of Administration that are Commonly Used
ORAL: 400-500 mg three times daily is a common dose (483). For prostatitis, 500 mg twice daily has been used (481).
INTRAVENOUS: For treating cancer, 420-1400 mg/m2 by IV bolus weekly or in 3-week intervals has been used (2007).
INTRAPERITONEAL: No typical dosage.

Comments
Quercetin is a dietary flavonoid that occurs abundantly in red wine, onions, green tea, apples, berries and brassica vegetables (481,483,1995). Quercetin is found in Ginkgo biloba, St. John's Wort (Hypericum perforatum) and American Elder (Sambucus canadensis) (483).

QUILLAIA

This Product is Also Known As
China Bark, Murillo Bark, Panama Bark, Quillaja, Soapbark, Soap Tree, Soap Tree Bark.

Scientific Names
Quillaja saponaria.
Family: Rosaceae.

People Use This For
Orally, quillaia inner bark is used for cough, bronchitis (6), and pulmonary ailments (11).
Topically, quillaia extract is used to treat skin sores, athletes foot (11), itchy scalp (6), in shampoos for dandruff (6,11), in hair tonic preparations, in douches (11), and for leukorrhea (12).
For food uses, quillaia is used in frozen dairy desserts, candy, baked goods, gelatins, and puddings (11).
In manufacturing, quillaia extracts are used in dermatological creams, as foaming agents in root beer (11), in beverages, and cocktails (6). Quillaia is also used as a foaming agent in fire extinguishers (11).

Safety
LIKELY SAFE ...when used orally and in food amounts. Approved for food use in the US (11). The maximum level used is 0.01% in beverages (11).
POSSIBLY UNSAFE ...when used orally in medicinal amounts. Quillaia is a gastrointestinal tract irritant that contains oxalates and tannins. Large amounts can cause liver damage, respiratory failure, convulsions, and coma (12).
There is insufficient reliable information available about the safety of the topical or vaginal use of quillaia.
PREGNANCY AND LACTATION: LIKELY SAFE ...when used orally in food amounts. POSSIBLY UNSAFE ...when used orally in amounts larger than those found in foods; avoid using.

Effectiveness

There is insufficient reliable information available about the effectiveness of quillaia.

Possible Mechanism of Action & Active Ingredients

The applicable part of quillaia is the inner bark. Quillaia contains tannins, oxalates, and saponins. Tannins possess strong astringent properties (7,12). Upon contact, they dehydrate the external layer of tissue, reducing internal secretions, and forming external cells into a protective layer (12). Plants with at least 10% tannins, like quillaia (19) can cause gastrointestinal disturbances, kidney damage, and necrotic conditions of the liver (12). Some evidence suggests that tannins might cause cancer; other evidence shows they might prevent it (12). Regular consumption of herbs with high tannin concentrations correlates with increased incidence of esophageal or nasal cancer (12). When ingested, oxalates combine with calcium in the blood forming insoluble oxalates and depleting available calcium, potentially to deficiency levels. Insoluble calcium oxalate, deposited in the kidneys can cause mechanical damage. Precipitation of calcium oxalate in renal tubules can result in acute renal failure (12). Some evidence suggests saponins might cause red blood cell hemolysis and GI irritation (11). Other evidence suggests they might have anti-inflammatory, antimicrobial, and cytotoxic effects (11). They also possess expectorant properties, can induce sneezing, and can depress cardiac and respiratory activity (6,11). Preliminary information suggests quillaia saponins can reduce the rate of absorption of bile salts (3850), suggesting they might be effective in reducing cholesterol levels (11). QS-21, an isolated saponin from the bark, appears to be a potent immuno-stimulatory complex adjuvant when administered with vaccines (6). It shows evidence that it might augment both antibody and cell-mediated immune responses (3851), significantly increasing antibody levels (6). For this reason it is being evaluated in HIV patients (11). Another purified saponin, DS-1, is being investigated as a pharmaceutical excipient in nasal and ocular delivery of insulin (3852), and also as a transmucosal delivery agent for the aminoglycoside antibiotics (3853).

Adverse Reactions Including Known Allergies

Large amounts, ingested orally are associated with liver damage, diarrhea, respiratory failure, stomach pain, convulsions, coma (12), red blood cell hemolysis (11), and renal failure (12). If inhaled, the powder can cause sneezing (6). It also can be caustic to mucosa (12).

Possible Interactions with Herbs & Other Dietary Supplements

MINERALS: Theoretically, concomitant use with calcium, magnesium, or iron can decrease mineral absorption due to tannin content (7).

Possible Interactions with Drugs

ORAL MEDICATION: Theoretically, the tannin content might delay absorption of sedatives, hypnotics, antidepressants, and tranquilizers due to tannin content (19,7).
METFORMIN: Quillaia might reduce efficacy of metformin (Glucophage) (7).

Possible Interactions with Foods

No interactions are known to occur, and there is no known reason to expect a clinically significant interaction with quillaia.

Possible Interactions with Lab Tests

No interactions are known to occur, and there is no known reason to expect a clinically significant interaction with quillaia.

Possible Interactions with Diseases or Conditions

KIDNEY DISEASE: Contraindicated in individuals with kidney disease or a history of kidney stones due to oxalate content (12,19).
GI CONDITIONS: Contraindicated in individuals with gastrointestinal inflammation or irritation due to irritant properties (18).

Typical Dosages & Routes of Administration that are Commonly Used

ORAL: A typical dose is 200 mg prepared as tea (12).
TOPICAL: No typical dosage.

Comments

In South America, quillaia bark is used to wash clothes (6).

QUINCE

This Product is Also Known As

None.

Scientific Names

Cydonia oblongata.
Family: Rosaceae.

People Use This For

Orally, quince seed is used for digestive disorders, diarrhea, coughs, and gastrointestinal inflammation. Topically, it is used as a compress or poultice for injuries, inflammation of the joints, injuries of the nipples, and gashed or deeply cut fingers. A topical lotion is used to soothe the eyes (18).

Safety

There is insufficient reliable information available about the safety of quince seed.
Pregnancy and Lactation: Insufficient reliable information available; avoid using.

Effectiveness

There is insufficient reliable information available about the effectiveness of quince.

Possible Mechanism of Action & Active Ingredients

The applicable part of quince is the seed. The seeds contain cyanogenic glycosides as amygdalin at 0.4-1.5%, or 27-75 mg cyanide per 100 grams of seeds, suggesting potential toxicity (18).

Adverse Reactions Including Known Allergies

None reported.

Possible Interactions with Herbs & Other Dietary Supplements

Insufficient reliable information available.

Possible Interactions with Drugs

May impair absorption of concomitantly administered medications due to possible binding by the high water-soluble fiber content of quince seed (19).

Possible Interactions with Foods

May reduce serum nutrient levels due to possible binding by the high water-soluble fiber content of quince seed (19).

Possible Interactions with Lab Tests

No interactions are known to occur, and there is no known reason to expect a clinically significant interaction with quince.

Possible Interactions with Diseases or Conditions

No interactions are known to occur, and there is no known reason to expect a clinically significant interaction with quince.

Typical Dosages & Routes of Administration that are Commonly Used

ORAL: Quince seed is taken as a powder, extract, or tea. The tea is prepared by steeping 1 teaspoon of whole seeds in 150 mL of boiling water for 10-15 minutes and straining (18).
TOPICAL: A viscous poultice is prepared from the ground seeds (18).

Comments

None.

RADISH

This Product is Also Known As

Radis, Raphani sativi radix, Small Radish, Turnip Radish.

Scientific Names

Raphanus sativus.
Family: Brassicaceae.

People Use This For

Orally, radish is used for peptic disorders, dyskinesia of the bile ducts, loss of appetite, inflammation of the mouth and pharynx, tendency towards infections, inflammation or excessive mucus of the respiratory tract, bronchitis, fever, colds, and cough (2,18).

Safety

LIKELY SAFE ...when used orally in moderate amounts (2,18). Large amounts may lead to gastrointestinal irritation (18).
PREGNANCY AND LACTATION: Insufficient reliable information available; avoid very large doses.

Effectiveness

POSSIBLY EFFECTIVE ...when used orally for peptic disorders involving bile duct motility conditions and for respiratory tract mucous membrane inflammation (2).
There is insufficient reliable information available about the effectiveness of radish for its other uses.

Possible Mechanism of Action & Active Ingredients

The applicable part of radish is the root. Radish root stimulates secretions in the upper GI tract, promotes motility, stimulates bile flow, and has antimicrobial effects (2,18).

Adverse Reactions Including Known Allergies

Large amounts may cause irritation of the gastrointestinal mucus membrane (18).

Possible Interactions with Herbs & Other Dietary Supplements

Insufficient reliable information available.

Possible Interactions with Drugs

No interactions are known to occur, and there is no known reason to expect a clinically significant interaction with radish.

Possible Interactions with Foods

No interactions are known to occur, and there is no known reason to expect a clinically significant interaction with radish.

Possible Interactions with Lab Tests

No interactions are known to occur, and there is no known reason to expect a clinically significant interaction with radish.

Possible Interactions with Diseases or Conditions

CHOLELITHIASIS: Contraindicated, might cause biliary colic (2,18).

Typical Dosages & Routes of Administration that are Commonly Used

ORAL: 0.5 tablespoons pressed root juice, several times daily; up to 50-100 mL per day (2,18).

Comments

None.

RASPBERRY

This Product is Also Known As

Framboise, Red Raspberry, Rubi idaei folium, Rubus.
CAUTION: See separate listing for Blackberry leaf.

Scientific Names

Rubus idaeus, synonym Rubus strigosus.
Family: Rosaceae.

People Use This For

Orally, raspberry leaf is used for GI tract disorders, upper and lower respiratory tract disorders, cardiovascular system disorders, influenza, fever, diabetes, vitamin deficiency, as a diaphoretic or diuretic, for stimulating bile production, "purification of skin and blood" (2), diarrhea, dysmenorrhea, menorrhagia, morning sickness associated with pregnancy, preventing miscarriage, and facilitating labor and delivery (3,4,5).
Topically, it is used for inflammation of the mouth and throat (2,8), and skin rash and inflammation (2).
For food uses, the berry is eaten as fruit. In small quantities, the leaf and fruit (berry) serve as sources of natural flavoring for foods in Europe (4).

Safety

LIKELY SAFE ...when the leaf and fruit are consumed in amounts found in foods (4); small quantities of leaf are listed by the Council of Europe as natural sources of flavoring (4).
POSSIBLY SAFE ...when the leaf is used orally in medicinal amounts (12).
There is insufficient reliable information available about the safety of the topical use of raspberry leaf.
PREGNANCY: POSSIBLY SAFE ...when the leaf is used as a food flavoring. LIKELY UNSAFE ...when the leaf is used orally during pregnancy because it can cause uterine contractions (4,19). There is insufficient reliable information available about the safety of topical use of raspberry during pregnancy; avoid using.
LACTATION: Insufficient reliable information available; avoid using in amounts greater than those found in foods.

Effectiveness

There is insufficient reliable information available about the effectiveness of raspberry leaf.

Possible Mechanism of Action & Active Ingredients

The applicable part of raspberry is the leaf. The high (13-15%) tannin content of raspberry leaf is responsible for the astringent properties of the plant (4). Tannins, applied topically to mucous membranes or abraded skin, cause capillary vasoconstriction, a decrease in vascular permeability, and a local anti-inflammatory effect (7). Aqueous leaf extracts reduce and initiate contractions in uterine tissue, and contain constituents with smooth muscle stimulant, anticholinesterase and antispasmodic activities (4). A raspberry leaf extract increases serum ceruloplasmin oxidase activity (a measure of estrogenic activity in the liver) in female rats with their ovaries removed (6180).

Adverse Reactions Including Known Allergies

None reported.

Possible Interactions with Herbs & Other Dietary Supplements

IRON, CALCIUM, MAGNESIUM: Theoretically, concomitant use may decrease mineral absorption due to tannin content (7).

Possible Interactions with Drugs

ORAL MEDICATION: Theoretically, tannin content of raspberry leaf may modify absorption of sedatives, hypnotics, antidepressants, and tranquilizers (7,19).
METFORMIN (GLUCOPHAGE): Theoretically, concomitant use may reduce effectiveness (7).

Possible Interactions with Foods

No interactions are known to occur, and there is no known reason to expect a clinically significant interaction with raspberry.

Possible Interactions with Lab Tests

No interactions are known to occur, and there is no known reason to expect a clinically significant interaction with raspberry.

Possible Interactions with Diseases or Conditions

No interactions are known to occur, and there is no known reason to expect a clinically significant interaction with raspberry.

Typical Dosages & Routes of Administration that are Commonly Used

ORAL: One cup tea; steep 1.5 grams (2 teaspoons) finely cut leaves in 150 mL boiling water 5 minutes, strain (8,18); up to six times per day (3). Alternatively, soak finely cut leaves in cold water for 2 hours, strain (3). Liquid extract (1:1 in 25% alcohol), take 4-8 mL three times daily (4).

Comments

None.

RED BUSH TEA

This Product is Also Known As

Kaffree Tea, Red Bush, Rooibos Tea.

Scientific Names

Aspalathus linearis, synonyms Aspalathus contaminata, Borbonia pinfolia, Psoralea linearis.
Family: Fabaceae or Leguminosae.

People Use This For

Orally, red bush tea is used as a nonstimulating, nonsedating beverage (6).

Safety

LIKELY SAFE ...when used orally as a beverage (6,4120).
PREGNANCY AND LACTATION: Insufficient reliable information available.

Effectiveness

There is insufficient reliable information available for the effectiveness of red bush tea.

Possible Mechanism of Action & Active Ingredients

Red bush tea contains almost no active constituents (5,6). It contains acid polysaccharides (4120,4121), flavonoids (6,4122), a low amount of tannins (less than 5%) (5,6), and a relatively high amount of vitamin C (9.4%) (6). Some evidence suggests daily intake of acid polysaccharides found in the extracts of red bush tea might suppress HIV infection (4120,4121). Other information suggests the tea could prevent age-related changes to the central nervous system (4123) or suppress mutagenic activity (6).

Adverse Reactions Including Known Allergies
One report of salmonella contamination has occurred, possibly from lizard origin (6).

Possible Interactions with Herbs & Other Dietary Supplements
Insufficient reliable information available.

Possible Interactions with Drugs
No interactions are known to occur, and there is no known reason to expect a clinically significant interaction with red bush tea.

Possible Interactions with Foods
No interactions are known to occur, and there is no known reason to expect a clinically significant interaction with red bush tea.

Possible Interactions with Lab Tests
No interactions are known to occur, and there is no known reason to expect a clinically significant interaction with red bush tea.

Possible Interactions with Diseases or Conditions
No interactions are known to occur, and there is no known reason to expect a clinically significant interaction with red bush tea.

Typical Dosages & Routes of Administration that are Commonly Used
Brewed like normal tea (5).

Comments
Tea is made from the branches and twigs of Aspalathus linearis. The fragrant, caffeine-free tea is the national drink of South Africa (5,6,7).

RED CLOVER

This Product is Also Known As
Beebread, Cow Clover, Isoflavone as a constituent, Meadow Clover, Phytoestrogen, Purple Clover, Trefoil, Trifolium, Wild Clover.
CAUTION: See separate listing for Sweet Clover.

Scientific Names
Trifolium pratense.
Family: Leguminosae.

People Use This For
Orally, red clover is used for whooping cough (4,18), cough, asthma, bronchitis (11), sexually transmitted diseases (5), cancer prevention, indigestion, and to reduce menopausal symptoms (4734).
Topically, it is used for cancerous growths (5), skin sores, burns, sore eyes, and chronic skin diseases including eczema and psoriasis (4,18).
In foods and beverages, the solid extract is used as a flavoring ingredient (11).

Safety
POSSIBLY SAFE ...when used orally in the small amounts commonly used in foods. Red clover is listed by the Council of Europe as a natural source of food flavoring (4). ...when the flower tops are used orally in medicinal amounts (12).
There is insufficient reliable information available about the safety of the topical use of red clover.
PREGNANCY AND LACTATION: LIKELY UNSAFE ...contraindicated for oral medicinal use because it has estrogenic activity (4,12). There is insufficient reliable information available about the safety of the topical use of red clover during pregnancy and lactation.

Effectiveness
There is insufficient reliable information available about the effectiveness of red clover. However, 40 mg of red clover isoflavones daily for one year reduced the extent of loss of spinal bone mineral density (BMD) and bone mineral content (BMC) in a group of pre- and perimenopausal women, but not in postmenopausal women. In this placebo-controlled trial, red clover extract had no effect on hip bone density or mineral content in pre-, peri-, or postmenopausal women. The results of this unpublished study were presented at Endo 2000, the 82nd Annual Meeting of the Endocrine Society (6127).
In another unpublished trial, 40-80 mg of red clover isoflavones daily for three months decreased nocturnal frequency and international prostate symptom scores (IPSS), and improved quality of life scores in a group of men

with benign prostatic hyperplasia (BPH). In this trial, red clover extract had no effect on urine flow rate, PSA values, blood biochemistry, hematology, or prostate size. The results of this unpublished study were presented at Endo 2000, the 82nd Annual Meeting of the Endocrine Society (6128).

Possible Mechanism of Action & Active Ingredients

The applicable part of red clover is the flower top, which contains more than 100 different chemicals (4744). Red clover is thought to have antispasmodic and expectorant activities (4,11). The constituent tannins have astringent activity (4), while the isoflavone constituents show evidence of estrogenic activity (4,11). Preliminary evidence suggests that a standardized red clover extract containing the isoflavones genisten, daidzein, biochanin, and formononetin improves systemic arterial compliance in menopausal women. However, it does not seem to improve the plasma lipid profiles (836). Clinical studies indicate that isoflavonoids do not lower serum lipids or blood pressure (4738,4739). An extract of red clover isoflavones demonstrates modest spinal bone-sparing effects in pre- and perimenopausal women, but not in postmenopausal women, possibly as a result of decreased bone resorption (6127). A red clover isoflavone extract shows early evidence of improving symptoms in men with benign prostatic hyperplasia (BPH) (6128). The isoflavone, biochanin A, found in red clover shows some evidence of anticarcinogenic activity (4740,4742). Isoflavones might exert anticancer effects through both estrogenic and nonestrogenic mechanisms (4741). Whether this laboratory evidence will translate into efficacy for oncologic disease in humans is unknown. Red clover also contains coumestrol, which has activity qualitatively similar to diethylstilbestrol (DES) in laboratory studies (4743,4744). The coumarin constituents contained in red clover can cause anticoagulant effects (4). Laboratory evidence suggests that isolfavones can inhibit oxidative and conjugative metabolism (4736). Isoflavones might also affect drug absorption and biliary excretion by interacting with multi-drug transporters such as P-glycoprotein (4736). Given the wide range of drugs and metabolites whose pharmacokinetics depend on these mechanisms, drug interactions with isoflavones might be more common than literature reports suggest.

Adverse Reactions Including Known Allergies

Red clover taken orally can cause rash-like reactions (4). Theoretically, it can cause estrogenic-type activity.

Possible Interactions with Herbs & Other Dietary Supplements

HERBS WITH ANTICOAGULANT/ANTIPLATELET POTENTIAL:
Concomitant use of herbs that have coumarin constituents or affect platelet aggregation could theoretically increase the risk of bleeding in some people. These herbs include: angelica, anise, arnica, asafoetida, bogbean, boldo, capsicum, celery, chamomile, clove, danshen, fenugreek, feverfew, garlic, ginger, ginkgo, ginseng Panax, horse chestnut, horseradish, licorice, meadowsweet, prickly ash, onion, papain, passionflower, poplar, quassia, turmeric, wild carrot, wild lettuce, willow, and others (4,19).
HERBS WITH ESTROGENIC ACTIVITY: Theoretically, red clover could be additive or possibly antagonistic with other herbs with estrogenic activity. These herbs include black cohosh, ipriflavone, and soy.

Possible Interactions with Drugs

ANTICOAGULANT DRUGS: Theoretically, concomitant use of large amounts of red clover can increase the anticoagulant effects and bleeding risk of these drugs due to its coumarin content (4).
ESTROGEN OR ORAL CONTRACEPTIVES: Theoretically, concomitant use of large amounts of red clover might interfere with hormone replacement therapy or oral contraceptives through competition for estrogen receptors (4737,4743).

Possible Interactions with Foods

No interactions are known to occur, and there is no known reason to expect a clinically significant interaction with red clover.

Possible Interactions with Lab Tests

No interactions are known to occur, and there is no known reason to expect a clinically significant interaction with red clover.

Possible Interactions with Diseases or Conditions

COAGULATION DISORDERS: Use red clover with caution and avoid large amounts due to its coumarin content, which might increase the risk of bleeding (4).
ESTROGEN-SENSITIVE CONDITIONS: Red clover contains constituents thought to have estrogenic properties (4). Theoretically, these could interact with diseases or conditions sensitive to such ingredients.

Typical Dosages & Routes of Administration that are Commonly Used

ORAL: The typical dose of red clover is 4 grams of the flower tops three times daily or one cup of the tea three times daily (4). The tea is prepared by steeping 4 grams of the flower tops in 150 mL boiling water for 10-15 minutes, and then straining (4). The liquid extract (1:1 in 25% alcohol) is commonly taken 1.5-3 mL three times per day (4,18). The tincture (1:10 in 45% alcohol) is usually dosed as 1-2 mL three times daily (4).

Comments

Red clover in large quantities induces sterility in livestock (4743). The cheetah population in zoos was threatened by reproductive failure and liver disease, thought to be caused by diets high in isoflavones (4735).

RED MAPLE

This Product is Also Known As
Bird's Eye Maple, Sugar Maple, Swamp Maple.

Scientific Names
Acer rubrum.
Family: Aceraceae.

People Use This For
In Native American folk medicine, red maple was used topically for eye conditions and as an astringent (18).

Safety
There is insufficient reliable information available about the safety of red maple.
Pregnancy and Lactation: Insufficient reliable information available; avoid using.

Effectiveness
There is insufficient reliable information available about the effectiveness of red maple.

Possible Mechanism of Action & Active Ingredients
The applicable part of red maple is the bark. There is insufficient reliable information available about the possible mechanism of action and active ingredients.

Adverse Reactions Including Known Allergies
None reported.

Possible Interactions with Herbs & Other Dietary Supplements
Insufficient reliable information available.

Possible Interactions with Drugs
No interactions are known to occur, and there is no known reason to expect a clinically significant interaction with red maple.

Possible Interactions with Foods
No interactions are known to occur, and there is no known reason to expect a clinically significant interaction with red maple.

Possible Interactions with Lab Tests
No interactions are known to occur, and there is no known reason to expect a clinically significant interaction with red maple.

Possible Interactions with Diseases or Conditions
No interactions are known to occur, and there is no known reason to expect a clinically significant interaction with red maple.

Typical Dosages & Routes of Administration that are Commonly Used
TOPICAL: Red maple is used as dried, powdered herb (18).

Comments
There is very little scientific information about this product. Our staff is continually analyzing the available information on natural medicines and will add data here as it becomes available.

RED SANDALWOOD

This Product is Also Known As
Red Sanderswood, Red Saunders, Rubywood, Sandalwood Padauk, Santali lignum rubrum, Sappan.
CAUTION: See separate listings for White Sandalwood oil and White Sandalwood wood.

Scientific Names
Pterocarpus santalinus.
Family: Fabaceae.

People Use This For
Orally, red sandalwood is used for ailments of the gastrointestinal tract, as a diuretic or astringent, for "blood purification," and coughs (2).
In manufacturing, it is used as a flavoring in alcoholic beverages (12).

Safety

LIKELY SAFE ...when used as flavoring in alcoholic beverages (12).
POSSIBLY SAFE ...when used for oral medicine (12,18).
PREGNANCY AND LACTATION: Insufficient reliable information available; avoid using.

Effectiveness

There is insufficient reliable information available about the effectiveness of red sandalwood.

Possible Mechanism of Action & Active Ingredients

The applicable part of red sandalwood is the heartwood (18). Red sandalwood contains the constituent santalins A and B, neoflavonoids, stilbene derivatives, and a volatile oil with traces of pterocarpol, isopterocarpol, and eudesmol (18). It is said to have diuretic and astringent effects (18).

Adverse Reactions Including Known Allergies

None reported.

Possible Interactions with Herbs & Other Dietary Supplements

Insufficient reliable information available.

Possible Interactions with Drugs

No interactions are known to occur, and there is no known reason to expect a clinically significant interaction with red sandalwood.

Possible Interactions with Foods

No interactions are known to occur, and there is no known reason to expect a clinically significant interaction with red sandalwood.

Possible Interactions with Lab Tests

No interactions are known to occur, and there is no known reason to expect a clinically significant interaction with red sandalwood.

Possible Interactions with Diseases or Conditions

No interactions are known to occur, and there is no known reason to expect a clinically significant interaction with red sandalwood.

Typical Dosages & Routes of Administration that are Commonly Used

No typical dosage.

Comments

Avoid confusion with white sandalwood (Santalum album).
There is very little scientific information about this product. Our staff is continually analyzing the available information on natural medicines and will add data here as it becomes available.

RED SOAPWORT

This Product is Also Known As

Bouncing-Bet, Saponariae rubrae radix, Soapwort.
CAUTION: See separate listing for White Soapwort.

Scientific Names

Saponaria officinalis.
Family: Caryophyllaceae.

People Use This For

Orally, red soapwort is used for inflammation of mucous membranes in the upper and lower respiratory tract (2).
Topically, it is used as a remedy for poison ivy, acne, psoriasis, eczema, and boils (6).
It is used as a foaming agent in beer (6).
In manufacturing, red soapwort is used as an ingredient in soaps, herbal shampoos (6002), and detergents (6).

Safety

LIKELY SAFE ...when used topically. Red soapwort is widely used in soaps and shampoos (6) without reports of adverse effects.
POSSIBLY SAFE ...when used orally (2).
PREGNANCY AND LACTATION: Insufficient reliable information available; avoid using.

Effectiveness

POSSIBLY EFFECTIVE ...when taken orally for inflammation of the mucous membranes in the upper and lower respiratory tract (2).
There is insufficient reliable information available about the effectiveness of red soapwort for its other uses.

Possible Mechanism of Action & Active Ingredients

The applicable part of red soapwort is the root. The root contains saponin constituents that have expectorant effects. Saponins irritate the gastric mucosa, which then stimulate bronchial mucous secretion via the parasympathetic sensory pathways (7). In large amounts, red soapwort is cytotoxic (2).

Adverse Reactions Including Known Allergies

Red soapwort taken orally can cause stomach irritation (2), nausea, and vomiting (7).

Possible Interactions with Herbs & Other Dietary Supplements

Insufficient reliable information available.

Possible Interactions with Drugs

No interactions are known to occur, and there is no known reason to expect a clinically significant interaction with red soapwort.

Possible Interactions with Foods

No interactions are known to occur, and there is no known reason to expect a clinically significant interaction with red soapwort.

Possible Interactions with Lab Tests

No interactions are known to occur, and there is no known reason to expect a clinically significant interaction with red soapwort.

Possible Interactions with Diseases or Conditions

GI MUCOSAL IRRITATION (e.g. ulcers, etc.): Red soapwort is contraindicated, because it can exacerbate existing GI mucosal irritation due to its saponin content (6).

Typical Dosages & Routes of Administration that are Commonly Used

ORAL: The typical dose of red soapwort is 1.5 grams of the dried root per day as a tea or equivalent preparation (2).

Comments

In the Middle Ages, Franciscan and Dominican monks viewed soapwort as a divine gift that was meant to keep them clean (6). Avoid confusion with white soapwort root.

RED YEAST

This Product is Also Known As

Monascus, Red Rice Yeast, XueZhiKang, ZhiTai.

Scientific Names

Monascus purpureus Went; other Monascus species.
Family: Monascaceae.

People Use This For

Orally, red yeast is used for maintaining desirable cholesterol levels in healthy people (796) and reducing cholesterol in people with hypercholesterolemia (6,512,2624).
In Chinese medicine, red yeast is used for indigestion, diarrhea, improving blood circulation, and for spleen and stomach health (6,512).
For food uses, red yeast is used as a food coloring for Peking duck and other foods (512).
In manufacturing, the Monascus yeast is used in making rice wine (512).

Safety

POSSIBLY SAFE ...when red yeast (Cholestin), is used orally and appropriately (512,2624).
CHILDREN: POSSIBLY UNSAFE ...when used orally. Safety has not been established in children under 18 years of age and questions remain about the benefit of lowering cholesterol in children (512).
PREGNANCY: LIKELY UNSAFE ...contraindicated because cholesterol is necessary for fetal development (512) and lovastatin has induced skeletal malformations in animals (2619). Lovastatin has the FDA pregnancy rating of X (266).
LACTATION: Insufficient reliable information available; avoid using.

Effectiveness

LIKELY EFFECTIVE ...when red yeast (Cholestin, see Dosage) is used orally for lowering cholesterol and triglyceride levels (6,15,512,2624).
There is insufficient reliable information available about the effectiveness of red yeast for its other uses.

Possible Mechanism of Action & Active Ingredients

Red yeast is the product of rice fermented with Monascus purpureus yeast (512). Red yeast contains a variety of mevinic acids (statins), primarily lovastatin (also referred to as monacolin K or mevinolin) (512). These compounds competitively inhibit 3-hydroxy-3-methyl-glutaryl-coenzyme A (HMG-CoA) reductase, blocking cholesterol biosynthesis (512). The commercial red yeast product, Cholestin (see Dosage), lowers serum total cholesterol, LDL cholesterol, and triglycerides in healthy patients with hyperlipidemia (2624).

Adverse Reactions Including Known Allergies

Red yeast taken orally can cause gastritis, abdominal discomfort, and elevated liver enzymes (512). Lovastatin can cause destruction of skeletal muscle (rhabdomyolysis) with renal dysfunction that is secondary to the urinary excretion of muscle hemoglobin (myoglobinuria) (15).

Possible Interactions with Herbs & Other Dietary Supplements

Insufficient reliable information available.

Possible Interactions with Drugs

CHOLESTEROL-LOWERING DRUGS: If red yeast is used along with cholesterol-lowering drugs, monitoring is important to determine if there is benefit to the combination and to limit adverse effects.
HMG-CoA REDUCTASE INHIBITORS: Avoid concomitant use. Using red yeast with these drugs might increase the risk of adverse effects without improving therapeutic benefit.
CYTOCHROME P450-3A INHIBITING DRUGS: Concomitant use with lovastatin and other mevinic acid compounds can increase serum levels and the risk of adverse effects. Drugs with this interaction include theophylline, cisapride, astemizole, terfenadine, ketoconazole, itraconazole, and fluconazole (15).
LEVOTHYROXINE: Concomitant use of levothyroxine with lovastatin can cause thyroid function abnormalities (15).

Possible Interactions with Foods

FOOD: Enhances the bioavailability of lovastatin (15), a constituent of red yeast.
GRAPEFRUIT JUICE: Concomitant use of grapefruit juice and lovastatin, a constituent of red yeast, can increase serum lovastatin levels and the risk of adverse effects (794).

Possible Interactions with Lab Tests

LIVER ENZYMES: Red yeast might increase serum liver transaminase concentrations and test results due its lovastatin content. Lovastatin can increase serum liver transaminase concentrations and test results (15).
CREATINE KINASE (CK): Red yeast might increase serum creatine kinase concentrations and test results due its lovastatin content. Lovastatin can increase serum creatine kinase concentrations and test results (15).
SERUM CHOLESTEROL: Red yeast can reduce serum cholesterol concentrations and test results. Red yeast contains a mixture of lovastatin and other HMG-CoA reductase inhibitors (6,15,512,2624).

Possible Interactions with Diseases or Conditions

LIVER DYSFUNCTION: Red yeast is contraindicated in people with liver dysfunction, risk of liver dysfunction, or abnormal liver function test results (512,2619).
THYROID DYSFUNCTION: Concomitant use of lovastatin with levothyroxine can interfere with thyroid therapy (15).

Typical Dosages & Routes of Administration that are Commonly Used

ORAL: For hypercholesterolemia, a typical dose of red yeast is 1200 mg two times daily with food, equivalent to 2 Cholestin capsules twice daily (2624). The Cholestin manufacturer, Pharmanex, cautions not to take more than 4 capsules in any 24-hour period (796). A total daily dose of 2400 mg red yeast contains approximately 9.6 mg total statins, of which 7.2 mg is lovastatin (2624). Cholestin is marketed as a dietary supplement intended for use by healthy adults over the age of 20 as part of a cholesterol maintenance program that includes regular exercise and a healthy diet with reduced saturated fats and high cholesterol foods (796).

Comments

Red yeast is the product of rice fermented with the Monascus purpureus yeast that contains monacolin K (lovastatin, mevinolin) and other HMG-CoA reductase inhibiting compounds (512). Red yeast is marketed as a dietary supplement, Cholestin (Pharmanex). The FDA is currently investigating whether red yeast should be classified as a drug or a dietary supplement. In June 1998, the FDA banned the sale of Cholestin in the US, claiming it was an unregulated drug (2625). In February 1999, a US Federal judge overrode the FDA decision, saying Cholestin could be sold as a food supplement (2626). Until more clinical information is available, red yeast should be treated as a HMG-CoA reductase inhibitor, with all the possible side effects, drug interactions, and precautions associated with this drug class. Hypercholesterolemia is a medical condition requiring appropriate intervention, and the pharmacologic treatment, including with red yeast, requires monitoring by a qualified medical professional. There is no evidence that healthy people with normal cholesterol benefit from cholesterol-lowering agents, including red yeast.

RED-SPUR VALERIAN

This Product is Also Known As
Bouncing Bess, Bovis and Soldier, Delicate Bess, Drunken Sailor, Pretty Betsy, Red Spur Valerian.

Scientific Names
Centranthus ruber.

People Use This For
In traditional medicine, red-spur valerian is used as a sedative (18).

Safety
There is insufficient reliable information available about the safety of red-spur valerian.
Pregnancy and Lactation: Insufficient reliable information available; avoid using.

Effectiveness
There is insufficient reliable information available about the effectiveness of red-spur valerian.

Possible Mechanism of Action & Active Ingredients
The applicable part of red-spur valerian is the root. Red-spur valerian contains valepotriate, that may have sedative and equilibrate properties (18).

Adverse Reactions Including Known Allergies
None reported (18).

Possible Interactions with Herbs & Other Dietary Supplements
Insufficient reliable information available.

Possible Interactions with Drugs
No interactions are known to occur, and there is no known reason to expect a clinically significant interaction with red-spur valerian.

Possible Interactions with Foods
No interactions are known to occur, and there is no known reason to expect a clinically significant interaction with red-spur valerian.

Possible Interactions with Lab Tests
No interactions are known to occur, and there is no known reason to expect a clinically significant interaction with red-spur valerian.

Possible Interactions with Diseases or Conditions
No interactions are known to occur, and there is no known reason to expect a clinically significant interaction with red-spur valerian.

Typical Dosages & Routes of Administration that are Commonly Used
ORAL: People typically use 0.3 to 1 mL valerian liquid extract or 4 to 8 mL valerian tincture (5264).

Comments
There is very little scientific information about this product. Our staff is continually analyzing the available information on natural medicines and will add data here as it becomes available.

REED HERB

This Product is Also Known As
Reed.

Scientific Names
Phragmites communis.

People Use This For
Orally, reed herb stem and rhizome are used for digestive disorders (18).
Topically, the juice of reed herb is used to relieve insect bites (18).
In Oriental medicine, reed herb is used for diabetes, leukemia, and breast cancer (18).

Safety

There is insufficient reliable information available about the safety of reed herb.
Pregnancy and Lactation: Insufficient reliable information available; avoid using.

Effectiveness

There is insufficient reliable information available about the effectiveness of reed herb.

Possible Mechanism of Action & Active Ingredients

The applicable parts of reed herb are the stem and rhizome. Reed herb contains vitamin A, vitamin C, and several vitamins of the B-group (18). It also contains triterpenes (beta-amyrin and taraxerol) and several flavonoids including chrysoeriol, isoquercitrin, luteolin, rutin, and tricin (18). The plant is thought to have diuretic effects and stimulate sweating (18).

Adverse Reactions Including Known Allergies

None reported.

Possible Interactions with Herbs & Other Dietary Supplements

Insufficient reliable information available.

Possible Interactions with Drugs

No interactions are known to occur, and there is no known reason to expect a clinically significant interaction with reed herb.

Possible Interactions with Foods

No interactions are known to occur, and there is no known reason to expect a clinically significant interaction with reed herb.

Possible Interactions with Lab Tests

No interactions are known to occur, and there is no known reason to expect a clinically significant interaction with reed herb.

Possible Interactions with Diseases or Conditions

No interactions are known to occur, and there is no known reason to expect a clinically significant interaction with reed herb.

Typical Dosages & Routes of Administration that are Commonly Used

Reed herb is prepared as a tea for oral or topical use (18).

Comments

None.

REISHI MUSHROOM

This Product is Also Known As

Ling Chih, Ling Zhi, Mannentake, Mushroom Of Immortality, Mushroom of Spiritual Potency, Spirit Plant (12,5474).

Scientific Names

Ganoderma lucidum.
Family: Ganodermataceae.

People Use This For

Orally, reishi mushroom is used for enhancing the immune system, lowering blood pressure and cholesterol, treating and preventing viral infections and tumors, treating inflammatory disease, cardiovascular disease, asthma and bronchial diseases. It is used for reducing stress, providing a kidney tonic, treating hepatitis and liver disease, supporting HIV disease, treating or preventing altitude sickness, and supporting chemotherapy. Other oral uses include preventing fatigue, treating insomnia, gastric ulcers, neurasthenia, poisoning (5472,5473,5474,5475,5493), post-herpeticneuralgia, and herpes zoster pain (5485).
It is also used in combination with seven other herbs (PC-SPES) to treat prostate cancer (5548).

Safety

POSSIBLY SAFE ...when used orally and appropriately (12). ...when used orally in a specific herbal combination (PC-SPES) (5548).
PREGNANCY AND LACTATION: Insufficient reliable information available; avoid using.

Effectiveness

POSSIBLY EFFECTIVE ...when used orally in a specific herbal combination for prostate cancer. Studies using reishi mushroom in combination with seven other herbs (PC-SPES) in prostate cancer patients, found that it significantly decreases prostate-specific antigen (PSA) levels (5548,5122,5913), causes tumor cell death (5913), and causes clinically significant reductions in testosterone (5548). In two reports, PSA levels fell significantly within 1 month of treatment (5548,5122).

There is insufficient reliable information available about the effectiveness of reishi mushroom for its other uses.

Possible Mechanism of Action & Active Ingredients

The applicable parts of reishi mushrooms are the fruiting body and mycelium (12). Reishi mushrooms have a long history in folk medicine, but researchers are just beginning to isolate and identify medicinal substances in reishi that have antitumor, immune modulating, anti-aging, cardiovascular, anticoagulant, cholesterol lowering, hypoglycemic, hepatoprotective, antiviral, and antibacterial effects (5476,5477,5481,5482,5483,5484,5485,5486,5487,5488,5489, 5490,5491,5492). Protease inhibitors and other anti-HIV substances have been found in reishi mushrooms (5479,5480). Studies of these compounds have not been performed in humans. Reishi mushroom extracts contain high levels of adenosine (5478).

Adverse Reactions Including Known Allergies

Reishi mushroom, when taken orally can cause dryness of the mouth, throat, and nasal area, itchiness, stomach upset, nosebleed, and bloody stools which have occurred with extended oral use (3 to 6 months) (12). Also, a rash with the consumption of reishi wine and respiratory allergy to reishi spores can occur (12,5479).

Possible Interactions with Herbs & Other Dietary Supplements

HERBS WITH ANTICOAGULANT/ANTIPLATELET POTENTIAL: Concomitant use of with herbs that have anticoagulant or antiplatelet activity could theoretically increase the risk of bleeding in some people (5476). These herbs include: angelica, anise, arnica, asafoetida, bogbean, boldo, capsicum, celery, chamomile, clove, danshen, fenugreek, feverfew, garlic, ginger, ginkgo, ginseng Panax, horse chestnut, horseradish, licorice, meadowsweet, prickly ash, onion, papain, passionflower, poplar, quassia, red clover, turmeric, wild carrot, wild lettuce, willow, and others (4,19).

HERBS/SUPPLEMENTS WITH HYPOTENSIVE ACTIVITY: Theoretically, concurrent use might increase risk of hypotension with herbs that lower blood pressure (5488), including black cohosh, celery seed, Panax ginseng, and others (4).

Possible Interactions with Drugs

DRUGS WITH ANTIPLATELET ACTIVITY: Theoretically, concurrent use might increase the risk of bleeding with drugs that inhibit platelet aggregation (5476).

ANTICOAGULANTS: Theoretically, concurrent use might increase the risk of bleeding (5476).

ANTIHYPERTENSIVE DRUGS: Theoretically, concurrent use might increase risk of hypotension with drugs that lower blood pressure (5488).

Possible Interactions with Foods

No interactions are known to occur, and there is no known reason to expect a clinically significant interaction with reishi mushroom.

Possible Interactions with Lab Tests

BLEEDING TIME: Theoretically, reishi mushroom use might prolong coagulation and bleeding time results (5476).

Possible Interactions with Diseases or Conditions

THROMBOCYTOPENIA: Theoretically, reishi mushroom use might increase the risk of bleeding in people with thrombocytopenia (5476).

HYPOTENSION: Theoretically, reishi mushroom use might worsen hypotension or interfere with drug therapy to increase blood pressure (5488).

Typical Dosages & Routes of Administration that are Commonly Used

ORAL: People typically use 1.5-9 grams orally per day of the crude dried mushroom, 1-1.5 grams per day of reishi powder, or 1 mL per day of reishi tincture (5473). Reishi tea is also used therapeutically (5473).

Comments

Reishi mushroom is used medicinally but not eaten. The flesh is described as "tough" and "woody" with a bitter taste (353).

RESVERATROL

This Product is Also Known As

Cis-Resveratrol, Kojo-Kon, Phytoestrogen, Trans-Resveratrol.
CAUTION: See separate listings for Grape seed, Grape Skin Extract, Quercetin, and Wine.

Scientific Names

3,4',5-stilbenetriol; 3,5,4' -trihydroxystilbene; 3,4',5-trihydroxystilbene.

People Use This For

Orally, resveratrol is used for atherosclerosis (2945), lowering cholesterol levels (2946,2957), increasing HDL cholesterol levels (2946), and preventing cancer (2945,2947,2956,2957).

In Japanese and Chinese folk medicine, it is used for several disorders, including atherosclerosis (2946).

Safety

LIKELY SAFE ...when consumed in amounts found in foods (2030).

There is insufficient reliable information available about the safety of resveratrol when used in supplemental doses in amounts greater than those found in foods.

PREGNANCY AND LACTATION: LIKELY SAFE ...when used in amounts found in some foods (2030).

Resveratrol is found in grape skins, grape juice, wine, and other food sources. Wine should not be used as a source of resveratrol during pregnancy and lactation.

Effectiveness

There is insufficient reliable information available about the effectiveness of resveratrol.

Possible Mechanism of Action & Active Ingredients

Resveratrol is a polyphenolic compound that exists in nature as cis- and trans- stereoisomers. The biological activity of cis-resveratrol is not entirely known, but preliminary data suggests that it has antiplatelet activity (2030,2950). Preliminary evidence suggests that trans-resveratrol has antioxidant, antimutagenic (2948), antitumor (2958,2959) and phytoestrogenic activity (2960). Preliminary evidence also suggest that trans-resveratrol inhibits cyclooxygenases 1 and 2, hydroperoxidases, 5-lipoxygenase (2030,2948), platelet aggregation (2949,2950,2951,2952,2961), and causes blood vessel dilation (2954,2955). Early research suggests resveratrol might reduce the risk of cancer (2948,2959). Biological activity in humans has not yet been described (2030). Resveratrol is primarily found in red wine, red grape skins, purple grape juice, mulberries, and in smaller amounts in peanuts (513,2030,2956). Other sources include eucalyptus (Eucalyptus wandoo, Eucalyptus sideroxylon), spruce (Picea excelsa), and Bauhinia racemosa (2030). Polygonum cuspidatum, the roots of which are used in Chinese and Japanese traditional medicine, is considered to be one of the richest sources of trans-resveratrol (2030). The trans-resveratrol content of wine is highly dependent on grape type, climate, and practices used to make the wine (9). White wines have very low trans-resveratrol concentrations. Pinot Noir consistently has the highest concentrations of trans-resveratrol, regardless of climate. Other red wines, including Cabernet Sauvignon, produced in cold, humid climates, such as Bordeaux and Canada, have higher trans-resveratrol content than those produced in hot, dry climates (2030).

Adverse Reactions Including Known Allergies

None reported.

Possible Interactions with Herbs & Other Dietary Supplements

Insufficient reliable information available.

Possible Interactions with Drugs

No interactions are known to occur, and there is no known reason to expect a clinically significant interaction with resveratrol.

Possible Interactions with Foods

No interactions are known to occur, and there is no known reason to expect a clinically significant interaction with resveratrol.

Possible Interactions with Lab Tests

No interactions are known to occur, and there is no known reason to expect a clinically significant interaction with resveratrol.

Possible Interactions with Diseases or Conditions

No interactions are known to occur, and there is no known reason to expect a clinically significant interaction with resveratrol.

Typical Dosages & Routes of Administration that are Commonly Used

ORAL: Resveratrol is frequently given in combination with other products, such as grape seed extract. Supplemental doses of resveratrol are typically 200-600 mcg per day and may be divided and given twice daily (2945,5021). One glass of red wine provides approximately 640 mcg and a handful of peanuts provides approximately 73 mcg of resveratrol (2945).

Comments

There is very little scientific information about this product. Our staff is continually analyzing the available information on natural medicines and will add data here as it becomes available.

RHATANY

This Product is Also Known As
Brazilian Rhatany, Krameria, Mapato, Peruvian Rhatany, Pumacuchu, Raiz Para Los Dientes, Ratanhiawurzel, Red Rhatany, Rhatanhia, Rhatania, Ratanhiae radix.

Scientific Names
Krameria triandra; Krameria argentea.
Family: Krameriaceae.

People Use This For
Orally, rhatany is used as an antidiarrheal agent for enteritis (8,18) and angina (8).
Topically, rhatany is used for mild inflammation of the oral and pharyngeal mucosa (2,8,14,18), inflammation of the gums (8,18), fissures of the tongue, stomatitis, pharyngitis (8), non-infectious canker sores (3,18), chilblains, and leg ulcers (8).

Safety
POSSIBLY SAFE ...when used topically for short term use (2,12). Use should be limited to two weeks unless medical evaluation determines that there is no problem and use can continue (2).
There is insufficient reliable information available about the safety of the oral use of rhatany.
PREGNANCY AND LACTATION: Insufficient reliable information available; avoid using.

Effectiveness
POSSIBLY EFFECTIVE ...when used topically for mild inflammation of the oral and pharyngeal mucosa (2).
There is insufficient reliable information available about the effectiveness of rhatany for its other uses.

Possible Mechanism of Action & Active Ingredients
The applicable part of rhatany is the root. Rhatany contains high concentrations of proanthocyanidin tannins (10-15%), which are responsible for the observed astringent properties (2,3,18,4100). The alcohol in the tincture preparation may enhance astringent effects (4102). Astringents precipitate the surface proteins of cells decreasing the cell size (4101) and secretions from the inflamed tissues (4102), diminishing inflammation. Astringents also have the ability to alleviate inflammation by constricting the blood vessels and reducing the supply of blood to the affected area (4102).

Adverse Reactions Including Known Allergies
Rhatany taken orally can cause digestive complaints (18). Rarely, allergic mucous membrane reactions have occurred (2,18).

Possible Interactions with Herbs & Other Dietary Supplements
Insufficient reliable information available.

Possible Interactions with Drugs
No interactions are known to occur, and there is no known reason to expect a clinically significant interaction with rhatany.

Possible Interactions with Foods
No interactions are known to occur, and there is no known reason to expect a clinically significant interaction with rhatany.

Possible Interactions with Lab Tests
No interactions are known to occur, and there is no known reason to expect a clinically significant interaction with rhatany.

Possible Interactions with Diseases or Conditions
ALLERGY: Contraindicated if rhatany allergy.

Typical Dosages & Routes of Administration that are Commonly Used
ORAL: Rhatany is sometimes taken as a decoction of 1 gram of the herb in 1 cup of water or as 5-10 drops of the tincture in one glass of water (6002).
TOPICAL: As mouth wash or gargle (simmer 1-1.5 grams of powdered root in 150 mL boiling water 10-15 minutes, strain) two to three times daily (8). As mouth wash or gargle, 5-10 drops of rhatany tincture in one glass of water two to three times daily (8). Undiluted rhatany tincture (oral paint) used directly on the affected area two to three times daily (2). Limit rhatany use to maximum two weeks without medical evaluation (2).

Comments
Avoid confusion with roots of other Krameria species (18). Rhatany (Krameria triandra) root is difficult to find and adulteration is common with other Krameria species (8).

RHUBARB

This Product is Also Known As
Chinese Rhubarb, Da Huang, Garden Rhubarb, Himalayan Rhubarb, Indian Rhubarb, Medicinal Rhubarb, Rhei radix, Turkey Rhubarb.

Scientific Names
Rheum officinale; Rheum palmatum; Rheum tanguticum; Rheum australe, synonym Rheum emodi; Rheum x cultorum, synonym Rheum rhabarbarum.
Family: Polygonaceae.

People Use This For
Orally, rhubarb root or rhizome is used for constipation (2,4,12,18), diarrhea (4,7), dyspepsia, gastritis (7), preparation for gastrointestinal diagnostic procedures after recto-anal surgery, for bowel movement relief when anal fissures are present, and for hemorrhoids (18).
For food uses, rhubarb stems are edible. Rhubarb is also used as a flavoring agent.

Safety
LIKELY SAFE ...when the root or rhizome are used in food amounts. The maximum use is 0.05% (11). Chinese and garden rhubarb are approved for food use in the US (11).
POSSIBLY SAFE ...when used orally and appropriately in medicinal amounts for less than eight days.
CHILDREN: POSSIBLY UNSAFE. Rhubarb root or rhizome should not be used in children under age 12 (2,12). There is one report of a 4-year-old who ingested rhubarb leaves (containing oxalic acid) and died (17).
PREGNANCY AND LACTATION: LIKELY SAFE ...when used in food amounts. POSSIBLY UNSAFE ...when used in larger amounts because it is a stimulant laxative; avoid using (2,4,12).

Effectiveness
POSSIBLY EFFECTIVE ...when used orally for constipation at high doses (2,4,7,12). ...when used orally for diarrhea at low doses (4,7,12).
There is insufficient reliable information available about the effectiveness of rhubarb for its other uses.

Possible Mechanism of Action & Active Ingredients
The applicable parts of rhubarb are the rhizome and root. Rhubarb contains anthraquinones, tannins and calcium oxalate (4,7,12,18). At low doses, the tannin effects predominate and have an astringent effect on the gastrointestinal tract that relieves diarrhea (4,7). At higher doses, anthraquinone effects seem to predominate, producing a stimulant laxative effect that relieves constipation (4,7). Anthroid laxative use is not associated with an increased risk of developing colorectal ademoma or carcinoma (6138).

Adverse Reactions Including Known Allergies
With short-term use, rhubarb can cause cramp-like or spasmodic gastrointestinal discomforts, watery diarrhea, uterine contractions, and there has been one report of anaphylaxis (2,4,12,18). Chronic use or abuse of rhubarb can cause electrolyte loss (especially potassium), hyperaldosteronism, accelerated bone deterioration, albuminuria, hematuria, dehydration, inhibition of gastric motility, pseudomelanosis coli, arrhythmias, muscular weakness, nephropathies, and edema (2,12). Chronic use of anthroid laxatives can cause pseudomelanosis coli (pigment spots in intestinal mucosa) which is harmless, usually reverses with discontinuation (2), and is not associated with an increased risk of developing colorectal ademoma or carcinoma (6138).

Possible Interactions with Herbs & Other Dietary Supplements
CARDIAC GLYCOSIDE-CONTAINING HERBS: Overuse of rhubarb might cause potassium depletion, increasing the risk of cardiac toxicity. Cardiac glycoside-containing herbs include black hellebore, Canadian hemp root, digitalis leaf, hedge mustard, figwort, lily of the valley roots, motherwort, oleander leaf, pheasant's eye plant, pleurisy root, squill bulb leaf scales, and strophanthus seeds (2,18,19,500).
CARDIOACTIVE HERBS: Overuse of rhubarb might cause potassium depletion increasing risk of toxicity of cardioactive herbs. These include calamus, cereus, cola, coltsfoot, devil's claw, European mistletoe, fenugreek, fumitory, ginger, ginseng Panax, hawthorn, maté, parsley, quassia, scotch broom flower, shepherd's purse, white horehound, and wild carrot (4).
STIMULANT LAXATIVE HERBS: Theoretically, concomitant use with other stimulant laxative herbs may increase the risk of potassium depletion. Stimulant laxative herbs include aloe dried leaf sap, blue flag rhizome, alder buckthorn, European buckthorn, butternut bark, cascara bark, castor oil, colocynth fruit pulp, gamboge bark exudate, jalap root, black root, manna bark exudate, podophyllum root, senna leaves and pods, wild cucumber fruit (Ecballium elaterium), and yellow dock root (19).
LICORICE/HORSETAIL: Theoretically, concomitant use with horsetail plant or licorice rhizome increases the risk of potassium depletion (19).

Possible Interactions with Drugs
ANTIARRHYTHMIC DRUGS: Overuse of rhubarb might cause potassium depletion, increasing the risk of antiarrhythmic drug toxicity (664).

CORTICOSTEROIDS: Overuse of rhubarb might compound corticosteroid-induced potassium loss (2).
DIGOXIN: Overuse of rhubarb might cause potassium depletion, increasing the risk of digoxin toxicity (2).
LAXATIVE DRUGS: Concomitant use might compound fluid and electrolyte loss.
POTASSIUM-DEPLETING DIURETICS: Overuse of rhubarb might compound diuretic-induced potassium loss (2).
ORAL DRUGS: Concomitant use might reduce absorption of drugs due to reduced GI transit time (500).
CARDIAC GLYCOSIDES: Theoretically, overuse of rhubarb increases the risk of adverse effects of cardiac glycoside drugs, e.g. digoxin (Lanoxin).

Possible Interactions with Foods
No interactions are known to occur, and there is no known reason to expect a clinically significant interaction with rhubarb.

Possible Interactions with Lab Tests
URINE TESTS: Rhubarb might discolor urine and interfere with diagnostic tests (2).

Possible Interactions with Diseases or Conditions
CONSTIPATION, DIARRHEA: Can exacerbate diarrhea or constipation (4,12).
KIDNEY STONES: Rhubarb contains calcium oxalate. Use it with caution in people with a history of kidney stones (4,12).
GI CONDITIONS: Contraindicated in cases of intestinal obstruction, appendicitis, abdominal pain of unknown origin, inflammatory conditions of the intestine including Crohn's disease, colitis, and irritable bowel syndrome (2,12).

Typical Dosages & Routes of Administration that are Commonly Used
ORAL: Use is individualized to the smallest amount that is effective to normalize bowel movements (2). Rhubarb is used for short term use only, ideally less than eight days (2,12). When rhubarb is used for constipation, 1-4 grams of the dried root are used per day (7). When rhubarb is used for diarrhea, 100-300 mg of the dried root are used per day (7).

Comments
None.

RIBOFLAVIN (VITAMIN B2)

This Product is Also Known As
Flavin, Flavine, Lactoflavin, Riboflavine, Vitamin G.

Scientific Names
Riboflavin; Vitamin B2.

People Use This For
Orally, riboflavin is used for preventing riboflavin deficiency, treating ariboflavinosis, preventing migraine headaches, treating acne, congenital methemoglobinemia, muscle cramps, burning feet syndrome, carpal tunnel syndrome, red blood cell aplasia, multiple acylcoenzyme A dehydrogenase deficiency (14,15), eye fatigue, cataracts, and glaucoma. It is also used orally for increasing energy levels; boosting immune system function; maintaining healthy hair, skin, mucous membranes, and nails; for slowing aging; canker sores; memory loss including Alzheimer's disease; ulcers; boosting athletic performance; promoting healthy reproductive function; burns; alcoholism; liver disease; sickle cell anemia (3031,3032,3033,3034); and for treating lactic acidosis induced by nucleoside analog reverse transcriptase inhibitor (NRTI) drugs (2024,6132).

Safety
LIKELY SAFE ...when taken orally. No toxic effects have been reported (15,1396,1397,1398).
PREGNANCY: LIKELY SAFE ...when used at the recommended dietary allowance (RDA) of 1.4 mg per day (3094). There is insufficient reliable information about the safety of using larger amounts during pregnancy.
LACTATION: LIKELY SAFE ...when used at the recommended dietary allowance (RDA) of 1.6 mg per day (3094). There is insufficient reliable information about the safety of using larger amounts during lactation.

Effectiveness
EFFECTIVE ...when used orally for preventing riboflavin deficiency (15) and for treating ariboflavinosis (15).
POSSIBLY EFFECTIVE ...when taken orally for preventing migraine headaches (1397,1398). In one human trial, riboflavin reduced headache frequency similar to the beta-blockers, bisoprolol (Zebeta) and metoprolol (Lopressor) (1396).
POSSIBLY INEFFECTIVE ...when use orally for reducing severity or duration of migraine headaches, acute anti-migraine drug consumption, or migraine-associated gastrointestinal symptoms (1398).
There is insufficient reliable information available about the effectiveness of riboflavin for its other uses.

Possible Mechanism of Action & Active Ingredients

Riboflavin is required for tissue respiration (15). It is converted to the coenzyme riboflavin 5-phosphate (flavin mononucleotide, FMN) and then to the coenzyme flavin adenine dinucleotide (FAD) (15). These act as hydrogen carriers for several enzymes known as flavoproteins, which are involved in oxidation-reduction reactions of organic substrates and in intermediary metabolism (15). Riboflavin is a cofactor for various respiratory enzymes such as glutaryl coenzyme A dehydrogenase, erythrocyte glutathione reductase, sarcosine dehydrogenase, electron-transferring flavoprotein, ETF dehydrogenase, and NADH dehydrogenase (14). It is also indirectly involved in maintaining erythrocyte integrity (15). Riboflavin deficiency, or ariboflavinosis, is characterized by cheilosis, angular stomatitis, glossitis, sore throat, keratitis, scrotal skin changes, neuropathy, and seborrheic dermatitis (14,15). In severe cases there is a normocytic and normochromic anemia (15). Riboflavin deficiency can occur in people with long-standing infections such as HIV-1, liver disease, alcoholism, malignancy, and in those taking probenecid (15). Researchers think that riboflavin deficiency might contribute to lactic acidosis that can occur in HIV patients taking stavudine (d4T, Zerit), zidovudine (AZT, Retrovir) and similar nucleoside analog reverse transcriptase inhibitor (NRTI) drugs (2024). Although NRTI-induced lactic acidosis has been considered irreversible and fatal, riboflavin reportedly can reverse this condition in some patients (2024).

Adverse Reactions Including Known Allergies

Large oral doses of riboflavin (400 mg per day) might cause diarrhea and polyuria (1398). Riboflavin can cause a yellow-orange discoloration of the urine (14).

Possible Interactions with Herbs & Other Dietary Supplements

Insufficient reliable information available.

Possible Interactions with Drugs

ASPIRIN: Concomitant use might cause gastric intolerance. One participant taking riboflavin 400 mg/day plus aspirin 75 mg/day withdrew from a study after two weeks due to gastric intolerance (1397).
BETA-BLOCKERS: Theoretically, concomitant use of riboflavin and beta-blockers might enhance migraine prevention without increasing adverse effects. Clinical data suggest that riboflavin and the beta-blockers, bisoprolol and metoprolol, might prevent migraines by two different pathophysiological mechanisms (1396). Beta-blockers include atenolol (Tenormin), bisoprolol (Zebeta), metoprolol (Lopressor), nadolol (Corgard), propranolol (Inderal), and timolol (Blocadren).
LAMIVUDINE (3TC, Epivir), STAVUDINE (d4T, Zerit), ZIDOVUDINE (AZT, Retrovir): Riboflavin is reported to reverse the lactic acidosis caused by nucleoside reverse transcriptase inhibitor (NRTI)-type antiretroviral drugs, including lamivudine, stavudine, and zidovudine (2024,6132).
PROBENECID (Benemid) decreases riboflavin absorption (15).
PROPANTHELINE (Pro-Banthine) delays and increases riboflavin absorption (15).

Drug Influences on Nutrient Levels and Depletion

SOME DRUGS CAN AFFECT RIBOFLAVIN LEVELS:
ANTIBIOTICS: Destruction of normal gastrointestinal flora by antibiotics can cause decreased production of B vitamins. The clinical significance of this decreased production is not know. Consider supplementation only if clinical judgment warrants it (4434,4435,4436,4437,4438,4439,4440,4441,4442,4443).
METOCLOPRAMIDE (Reglan, Maxeran): Concomitant use can decrease riboflavin absorption in the gastrointestinal tract. The need for supplementation has not been adequately studied. Consider supplementation only if clinical judgment warrants it (4561).
ORAL CONTRACEPTIVES: Use of oral contraceptives can reduce serum vitamin B2 levels. The mechanism of this interaction is unknown. The need for supplementation has not been adequately studied (4548).
PHENOTHIAZINES: Use of phenothiazines can increase urinary vitamin B2 excretion and reduce serum vitamin B2 levels. The need for supplementation has not been adequately studied, although doses of 2-5 mg/day of riboflavin have been used (4425).
PROBENECID (Benemid): Probenecid inhibits dietary vitamin B2 absorption. The clinical relevance and the need for supplementation has not been adequately studied (15).
PROPANTHELINE BROMIDE (Pro-Banthine): Propantheline bromide delays and increases supplemental riboflavin absorption (15). The clinical relevance of this interaction has not been adequately studied (15).

Possible Interactions with Foods

FOOD increases riboflavin absorption (15).

Possible Interactions with Lab Tests

ACETOACETATE DECARBOXYLASE: Riboflavin can falsely increase serum acetoacetate decarboxylase test results, due to enzyme activation (275).
CATECHOLAMINES: Riboflavin can falsely elevate plasma and urine fluorometric catecholamine test results, due to fluorescent substances it produces in the plasma and urine (15,275).
COLORIMETRIC TESTS: Large amounts of riboflavin can interfere with urinalysis based on spectrometry or color reactions. Large amounts of riboflavin cause bright yellow urine (15,275).
DIAGNEX BLUE EXCRETION: Riboflavin can falsely increase urine diagnex blue excretion test results, by color interference (275).

DRUGS-OF-ABUSE ASSAYS: Large doses of riboflavin (200 mg twice daily) cause errors in Abbott TDx drugs-of-abuse urine assays. Riboflavin produces a fluorophore that competes with the fluorescein-labeled antibody used in the assay (1266).

UROBILINOGEN: Riboflavin can falsely increase plasma and urine fluorometric urobilinogen test results, due to fluorescent substances it produces in the plasma and urine (15,275).

Possible Interactions with Diseases or Conditions

HEPATITIS, CIRRHOSIS, BILIARY OBSTRUCTION: Riboflavin absorption is decreased in these conditions (15).

Typical Dosages & Routes of Administration that are Commonly Used

ORAL: As a dietary supplement, 1-4 mg a day is generally sufficient (15). For riboflavin deficiency in adults, 5-30 mg is taken daily in divided doses (15). For multiple acylcoenzyme A dehydrogenase deficiency, the usual dose is 100 mg one to three times daily (14). For preventing migraine headaches, a dose of 400 mg per day has been used (1396,1397,1398), and maximum benefit might take up to three months to achieve (1398). The daily recommended dietary allowances (RDAs) of riboflavin are: Infants 0-6 months, 0.3 mg; Infants 7-12 months, 0.4 mg; Children 1-3 years, 0.5 mg; Children 4-8 years, 0.6 mg; Children 9-13 years, 0.9 mg; Males 14 years or older, 1.3 mg; Women 14-18 years, 1 mg; Women over 18 years, 1.1 mg; Pregnant women, 1.4 mg; and Lactating women, 1.6 mg (3094). For treating stavudine or zidovudine-induced lactic acidosis, 50 mg per day has been used (2024,6132).

Comments

Riboflavin is found in many foods including milk, meat, eggs, nuts, enriched flour, and green vegetables (15). Riboflavin is frequently used in combination with other B vitamins in vitamin B complex formulations. Vitamin B complex generally includes vitamin B1 (thiamine), vitamin B2 (riboflavin), vitamin B3 (niacin/niacinamide), vitamin B5 (pantothenic acid), vitamin B6 (pyridoxine), vitamin B12 (cyanocobalamin), and folic acid. However, some products do not contain all of these ingredients and some may include others, such as biotin, para-aminobenzoic acid (PABA), choline bitartrate, and inositol (3022,3060,3061).

RIBOSE

This Product is Also Known As

D-ribose.

Scientific Names

Beta-D-ribofuranose.

People Use This For

Orally, ribose is used to increase muscle function (5673), recovery (5671,5672,5673), athletic performance (5672,5673,5675), boost muscle tissue energy (5670,5671), and enhance effectiveness of creatine, maximize ribose production, replenish ATP stores (5668,5671), and improve or maintain nucleotide salvage and/or synthesis in heart and skeletal muscles following high intensity exercise (5668,5674). It has also been used to improve exercise tolerance (5669), maintain or increase energy stores in the heart or muscle cells (5667), and improve quality of life (5668) in individuals with reduced myocardial blood flow such as improving the heart's tolerance to ischemia in patients with coronary artery disease (5664). Oral ribose has been used to prevent symptoms such as cramping, pain and stiffness after exercise in patients with myoadenylate deaminase deficiency (MAD) (5676,5677,5679,5680), also known as AMP deaminase deficiency (AMPD deficiency) (5681). Ribose has also been used to improve exercise tolerance in patients with McArdle's disease (5678).

Intravenously, ribose has been used to facilitate thallium-201 redistribution and improve imaging of ischemic myocardium in patients with coronary artery disease (5661,5662,5663). It has also been used intravenously in patients with MAD to prevent symptoms such as cramping, pain and stiffness (5676).

Safety

POSSIBLY SAFE ...when used orally or intravenously and appropriately, short-term (5661,5662,5663,5664,5676, 5677,5679,5680).

There is insufficient reliable information available about the safety of long-term use of ribose or the use of ribose in children.

PREGNANCY AND LACTATION: Insufficient reliable information available; avoid using.

Effectiveness

LIKELY EFFECTIVE ...when used intravenously to facilitate thallium-201 redistribution and improve imaging of ischemic myocardium in patients with coronary artery disease. Studies show ribose accelerates clearance of thallium-201 from normal, nonischemic regions of coronary arteries (5661,5662,5663).

POSSIBLY EFFECTIVE ...when used orally to improve the heart's tolerance to ischemia in patients with coronary artery disease. A small randomized and placebo controlled study showed increased time to onset of moderate

© Copyright 2000, Natural Medicines Comprehensive Database (209) 472-2244. For updated data, go to www.NaturalDatabase.com

angina and time to ST depression during treadmill walking exercise testing in patients with coronary artery disease (5664). ...when used orally or intravenously to prevent symptoms such as cramping, pain and stiffness after exercise in patients with myoadenylate deaminase deficiency (MAD), also known as AMP deaminase deficiency (AMPD deficiency). One case report and a small clinical study suggest symptoms can be prevented with administration of ribose before and during exercise (5677,5679).

LIKELY INEFFECTIVE ...when used orally to improve exercise tolerance in patients with McArdle's disease. A double blind placebo controlled crossover trial reported no benefit to patients with McArdle's disease (5678). There is insufficient reliable information available about the effectiveness of ribose for its other uses.

Possible Mechanism of Action & Active Ingredients

Ribose, a pentose sugar which is usually supplied by the oxidative pentose phosphate pathway (PPP) (also known as the hexose monophosphate shunt), is rapidly taken up by cells and phosphorylated to ribose-5-phosphate (5653). Ribose is rate-limiting in the production of phosphoribosyl-pyrophosphate (PRPP) (5652,5653,5682), a precursor for the salvage and de-novo adenine nucleotide synthetic pathways which maintain adenine, ADP, and AMP levels for the resynthesis of ATP (5651,5652,5665,5682). High energy bonds of ATP are the direct source for myocardial contractions (5652). During ischemia, the levels of ATP in the myocardium fall as the rate of oxidative phosphorylation decreases (5651,5653) and do not recover if the period of no perfusion is too long (5651). ADP and AMP levels rise transiently during ischemia but decrease as they are dephosphorylated into metabolites (adenine, inosine and hypoxanthine) which easily diffuse through the cell membrane and are washed out of the myocardium during reperfusion (5652,5653). Since the metabolites which use the salvage synthetic pathway are no longer available as precursors for ATP resynthesis, the de-novo synthetic pathway is activated (5652). Restoration of ATP levels via this pathway is slow in comparison to the salvage pathway (5652,5664) due to the short supply of PRPP which is usually supplied by the oxidative pentose phosphate pathway (5664). Studies suggest that this also occurs during ischemic events after high intensity exercise in skeletal muscle (5656,5657,5658). Evidence suggests exogenous ribose bypasses the PPP when it is converted to ribose-5-phosphate, increasing the amount of PRPP available for the de-novo synthetic pathway and ultimately resulting in the repletion of ATP levels in the myocardium (5652). Animal studies suggest exogenous ribose with adenine improves myocardial ATP, ADP and adenine nucleotide recovery after moderate periods of ischemia and improves recovery of contractile myocardial function (5652,5653). Other animal studies suggest exogenous ribose given during both periods of ischemia and reperfusion significantly increases ATP levels (5659) and may shorten ATP recovery time (5654,5659,5660). There have been no human studies done to confirm these findings. Laboratory evidence also suggests ribose may have a role in preserving hearts for transplantation by maintaining ATP levels (5666). Controlled human studies have established that infusion of ribose facilitates the distribution and accelerates the clearance of thallium-201 from normal (nonischemic) regions of the coronary artery, leaving only thallium-201 in ischemic myocardium (5661,5662,5663). The mechanism of action on how this occurs is unknown (5662). A small, randomized, placebo study controlled reported oral ribose given to patients with coronary artery disease may improve their tolerance to ischemia during exercise (5664). Other studies suggest oral ribose may prevent exercise-induced muscle pain and stiffness in patients with myoadenylate deaminase deficiency (5677,5676,5679,5680). Randomized, prospective controlled human studies are needed to establish the mechanism of action and the effectiveness of exogenous ribose when used to improve tolerance to exercise-induced ischemia in healthy individuals and patients with unstable cardiac condition such as coronary artery disease.

Adverse Reactions Including Known Allergies

Orally, ribose can cause diarrhea (5676), decreased blood glucose levels (5667), gastrointestinal discomfort, nausea and headache (5664). Hypoglycemia (5650,5662,5676), slightly increased serum insulin levels (5663) and decreased serum phosphate (5650) have been reported after infusion of ribose.

Possible Interactions with Herbs & Other Dietary Supplements

Insufficient reliable information available.

Possible Interactions with Drugs

INSULIN: Theoretically, ribose may increase the hypoglycemic effect of insulin and should be avoided by people taking insulin.

ORAL ANTIHYPERGLYCEMIC AGENTS: Theoretically, ribose may increase the hypoglycemic effect of oral antihyperglycemic agents such at the sulfonylureas, biguanides, alfa-glucosidase inhibitors, thiazolidinediones and meglitinides.

SALICYLATES: Theoretically, ribose may enhance the hypoglycemic effects of salicylates.

MAOIs: Theoretically, ribose may enhance the hypoglycemic effects of MAOIs.

OTHER AGENTS WHICH MAY CAUSE HYPOGLYCEMIA: Theoretically, ribose may increase the hypoglycemic effect of other agents such as ethanol and propranolol. Individuals taking any agents which may cause hypoglycemia should avoid taking ribose.

Possible Interactions with Foods

No interactions are known to occur, and there is no known reason to expect a clinically significant interaction with ribose.

Possible Interactions with Lab Tests

GLUCOSE: Ribose may decrease serum glucose levels (5650,5662,5667,5676).
PHOSPHATE: Ribose may decrease serum phosphate levels (5650).
INSULIN: Ribose may increase serum insulin levels (5663).

Possible Interactions with Diseases or Conditions

HYPOGLYCEMIA: Theoretically, ribose should be avoided in patients who have hypoglycemia, or diseases or conditions that may increase their risk for hypoglycemia.
DIABETES: Theoretically, ribose should be avoided in patients with diabetes since it may interfere and enhance the glucose lowering effects of insulin or any oral antihyperglycemic agents.

Typical Dosages & Routes of Administration that are Commonly Used

ORAL: People typically take 2.2 grams per day 30 minutes following exercise or before bedtime on days with no scheduled exercise. Individuals who feel they are overly tired or are concerned about their energy stores typically take 2.2-3.0 grams twice per day or adjust to perceived benefit. A dose typically may be taken before exercise and additional doses of 1.0-2.2 grams may be taken every hour of exercise (5668).
To improve exercise tolerance in patients with coronary artery disease, 15 grams four times per day has been used (5664). Beginning 1 hour before exercise until the end of the exercise session, 3 grams every 10 minutes has been used to reduce exercise-induced symptoms such as muscle stiffness and cramps associated with myoadenylate deaminase deficiency (5679).
INTRAVENOUS: For imaging of coronary arteries using thallium-201, a 30 minute 3.3 mg/kg/minute infusion of ribose as a 10% solution has been used (5662,5663).
No typical dosage information is available for other indications.

Comments

There are some preparations available containing both ribose and creatine (5673).

RICE BRAN

This Product is Also Known As

Stabilized Rice Bran, Rice Bran Oil.
CAUTION: See separate listings for Oat Bran and Wheat Bran.

Scientific Names

Oryza sativa.

People Use This For

Orally, rice bran is used for diabetes, hypertension, hyperlipidemia, alcoholism, weight loss, AIDS, preventing cancer, strengthening the immune system, increasing energy, enhancing athletic performance, aiding and improving liver function, preventing cardiovascular disease, and as an antioxidant (863). Rice bran oil is also used orally for hyperlipidemia (1354).
Topically, rice bran is used for ectopic dermatitis (872).

Safety

LIKELY SAFE ...when used orally in amounts found in foods (6405).
POSSIBLY SAFE ...when used orally and appropriately for medicinal purposes. No serious side effects reported in rice bran studies lasting more than 5 years (876,880).
There is insufficient reliable information available about the safety of rice bran oil used orally or topical use of rice bran.
PREGNANCY AND LACTATION: LIKELY SAFE ...when used orally in amounts found in foods (6405).
POSSIBLY SAFE ...when used orally and appropriately for medicinal purposes (6405). Use of rice bran for medicinal purposes during pregnancy should only be done under close supervision of a health care provider.

Effectiveness

POSSIBLY EFFECTIVE ...when used orally for moderate hypercholesterolemia (865,877). In one study, rice bran was compared to oat and wheat bran for decreasing serum cholesterol. Each fiber was given as part of the diet at 11.8 grams per day for 4 weeks. Only oat bran significantly lowered total cholesterol, but rice bran exerted a mild effect (877). In another study, a higher dose of 84 grams per day was used and full-fat rice bran was compared to oat bran and placebo administered over 6 weeks in combination with a low-fat diet. Rice bran significantly lowered low-density lipoprotein (LDL) and total cholesterol. Triglycerides and high-density lipoprotein (HDL) levels were not affected. Oat bran produced a slightly greater decrease in cholesterol (877). Rice bran oil has also been shown to be beneficial for hypercholesterolemia. In a 1 year clinical trial, rice bran oil non-saponifiables reduced total cholesterol by 14%, LDL cholesterol by 20%, triglycerides by 20%, and increased HDL cholesterol by 41% (1354). Lipid lowering effects have not been demonstrated in men without high lipid levels (873). ...when used orally to reduce urine calcium excretion and stone formation in people with hypercalciuria (876,878,880,881,882). ...when

© Copyright 2000, Natural Medicines Comprehensive Database (209) 472-2244. For updated data, go to www.NaturalDatabase.com

used orally in combination with cholestyramine to increase fecal excretion of polychlorinated biphenyl (PCB) and polychlorinated dibenzofuran (PCDF) in people who have ingested these chemicals (867,870). ...when rice bran broth is used topically to treat symptoms of ectopic dermatitis (872).

There is insufficient reliable information available about the effectiveness of rice bran for its other uses.

Possible Mechanism of Action & Active Ingredients

Rice bran contains 21% fiber, 21% lipids, 13% amino acids, and a wide variety of vitamins and minerals (864,884,885). Rice bran oil contains gamma oryzanol (871,879), tocopherols, tocotrienols, unsaturated fatty acids (877), and other non-saponifiable constituents (1354). The hypercholesterolemic effect of fiber has been attributed primarily to soluble forms of fiber. It is thought that soluble fiber adsorbs bile, preventing bile acid reabsorption, and decreasing cholesterol absorption. This results in upregulation of low-density lipoprotein (LDL) receptors and increased catabolism of LDL cholesterol (877). However, most of the fiber in rice bran is insoluble. Rice bran contains significantly less soluble fiber than oat bran. The unusually high amount of oil contained in rice bran is thought to contribute significantly to its antihypercholesterolemic effects, due to non-saponifiable constituents or the fatty acid content (877). Rice bran can increase stool size by several mechanisms, including water retention (871,879). Scientists think increased fecal bulk reduces risk of cancer because it dilutes carcinogens, especially tumor promoters such as secondary bile acids (871). Diets high in fiber have resulted in lower insulin levels, less weight gain, and a reduction in cardiovascular disease risk factors such as hypertension and adverse cholesterol profile (2737). Rice bran reduces the risk of recurrent urinary stone disease, perhaps because the phytin in rice bran reduces calcium absorption (881). Healthy women on a calcium-rich diet, who added rice bran to their diets decreased renal excretion of calcium and increased renal excretion of oxalic acid (874). A rice bran isolate designated as Compound X shows evidence of antihistamine activity. It also inhibits bacterial growth (884). A modified rice bran isolate, MGN-3 (see separate listing), exhibits anti-HIV activity (866).

Adverse Reactions Including Known Allergies

Increasing the amount of bran in the diet can cause erratic bowel habits, flatulence and abdominal discomfort during the first few weeks (272). Topical use of rice bran broth baths can cause itching, skin redness (872).

Possible Interactions with Herbs & Other Dietary Supplements

HERBS AND SUPPLEMENTS: Theoretically, a diet high in rice bran might slow or reduce the absorption of some herbs and supplements.

Possible Interactions with Drugs

ORAL DRUGS: Theoretically, a diet high in rice bran might slow or reduce the absorption of some oral drugs.

DIGOXIN: Theoretically, rice bran may interfere with digoxin absorption (156).

Possible Interactions with Foods

NUTRIENTS: Theoretically, a diet high in rice bran might slow or reduce the absorption of nutrients in foods.

IRON: Fiber inhibits dietary iron absorption (156).

Possible Interactions with Lab Tests

No interactions are known to occur, and there is no known reason to expect a clinically significant interaction with rice bran.

Possible Interactions with Diseases or Conditions

HYPOCALCEMIA: Rice bran can decrease dietary absorption of calcium (272); avoid concurrent administration of rice bran and calcium replacement therapy.

LOW IRON LEVELS: Rice bran can decrease dietary absorption of iron (272); avoid concurrent administration of rice bran and iron replacement therapy.

GASTROINTESTINAL CONDITIONS: Contraindicated in people with intestinal ulcerations, stenosis, disabling adhesions, cathartic colon or other conditions that may result in intestinal or esophageal obstruction (4921). Use with caution or avoid in people with difficulty chewing or swallowing food, or conditions that decrease small bowel motility (4921).

Typical Dosages & Routes of Administration that are Commonly Used

ORAL: For reducing cholesterol, 12-84 grams rice bran per day (865,877), or 4.8 grams rice bran oil (providing 312 mg tocotrienols, 360 mg tocopherols, and 2.4 grams other non-saponifiables) per day has been used (1354). For reducing the risk of kidney stones, 10 grams rice bran twice daily has been used (881,882). For decontamination of ingested polychlorinated biphenyl (PCB) and polychlorinated dibenzofuran (PCDF), 10 grams rice bran with a dietary fiber content 50% and 4 grams cholestyramine (Questran) three times a dayhas been used (870).

Comments

Rice bran is the outer grain hull of rice (Oryza sativa) (515) and is also referred to as stabilized rice bran.

RNA AND DNA

This Product is Also Known As
Nucleotides, Purines, Pyrimidines.

Scientific Names
Deoxyribonucleic Acid; Ribonucleic Acid.

People Use This For
Orally, RNA/DNA combinations are used to improve memory and mental sharpness (5529), to treat or prevent Alzheimer's disease (5528), to treat depression, increase energy, tighten skin, increase sex drive, and to counteract the effects of aging (5529,5530,5901).

Enterally, RNA is used in nutrition formulations that include omega-3 fatty acids and arginine for reducing the time needed for recovery after surgery (5531,5534), to boost immune response (5532,5533), and to improve outcomes of burn patients (5535) and intensive care patients (5536).

In Chinese medicine, RNA is used as a subcutaneous injection to treat eczema, psoriasis, hives, and shingles (5538).

Safety
LIKELY SAFE ...when RNA and DNA are consumed in food. ...when RNA is used in enteral nutrition along with omega-3 fatty acids and arginine (5531,5533,5534,5535,5536).

POSSIBLY SAFE ...when RNA is injected subcutaneously (5538).

There is insufficient reliable information available about the safety of oral RNA/DNA supplement combinations.

CHILDREN: LIKELY SAFE ...when infant formulas contain nucleotide supplements (5900).

PREGNANCY AND LACTATION: LIKELY SAFE ...when RNA and DNA are consumed in food. POSSIBLY UNSAFE ...when used as supplements. Some evidence suggests some orally ingested DNA might cross the placenta and be mutagenic (5539).

Effectiveness
POSSIBLY EFFECTIVE ...when RNA is used enterally to reduce the recovery time after surgery or serious illness and to boost the immune response (5531,5532,5533). ...when nucleotide supplements are used in infant formula to boost immune response (5900).

POSSIBLY INEFFECTIVE ...in producing better outcome in burn patients than standard nutritional formulas (5535).

Possible Mechanism of Action & Active Ingredients
Although most organisms can synthesize nucleotides (5900), dietary nucleotides (derived from DNA and RNA) appear to be essential under conditions of rapid growth such as intestinal development, liver resection or injury and also during challenges to the immune system. When preformed nucleotides are consumed, they are degraded to free bases in the intestine before absorption. Experimental evidence shows they are incorporated into the hepatic pyrimidine nucleotide pool (5900) and that they affect the hepatic RNA content. The hepatic RNA content, in turn, affects the recovery time from liver injury. In protein-deprived animals, dietary nucleotides appear to benefit the intestinal tract. They can also restore immune function, while restoring the nitrogen balance (protein intake) does not (5543). In the absence of nucleotides, normal T-lymphocyte maturation is blocked (5543). A Crohn's disease model in rats shows RNA has a highly significant effect upon the healing intestinal ulcerations (5900). Supplementing an enteral diet with arginine, RNA, and omega-3 fatty acids can reduce concentrations of tumor necrosis factor alpha, and interleukin-6 and accelerate the recovery in the concentration of interleukin-1 beta and interleukin-2 alpha receptor (5532).

Adverse Reactions Including Known Allergies
A subcutaneous injection of RNA can cause itching, redness, and swelling at the injection site (5538).

Possible Interactions with Herbs & Other Dietary Supplements
Insufficient reliable information available.

Possible Interactions with Drugs
No interactions are known to occur, and there is no known reason to expect a clinically significant interaction with RNA and DNA.

Possible Interactions with Foods
No interactions are known to occur, and there is no known reason to expect a clinically significant interaction with RNA and DNA.

Possible Interactions with Lab Tests
No interactions are known to occur, and there is no known reason to expect a clinically significant interaction with RNA and DNA.

Possible Interactions with Diseases or Conditions
No interactions are known to occur, and there is no known reason to expect a clinically significant interaction with RNA and DNA.

Typical Dosages & Routes of Administration that are Commonly Used

ORAL: A typical oral dose of RNA/DNA is 1-1.5 grams/day (5530).
ENTERAL: A typical enteral dose of RNA is 30 mg/kg/day along with arginine and omega-3 fatty acids (5533,5534).
INJECTION: A typical dose is 10 mg injectable RNA every other day for 2-4 weeks (5538).

Comments

RNA/DNA can be derived from cultivated brewer's yeast (5529) or salmon (5530).

ROMAN CHAMOMILE

This Product is Also Known As

Chamomile, Chamomillae ramane flos, English Chamomile, Fleur De Camomille Romaine, Flores Anthemidis, Garden Chamomile, Grosse Kamille, Ground Apple, Low Chamomile, Manzanilla, Römische Kamille, Sweet Chamomile, Whig Plant.
CAUTION: See separate listing for German Chamomile.

Scientific Names

Chamaemelum nobile, synonym Athemis nobilis.
Family: Asteraceae or Compositae.

People Use This For

Orally, Roman chamomile flowerheads are used for indigestion, nausea and vomiting, anorexia, morning sickness, painful menstrual periods, flatulent indigestion associated with mental stress (4), inflammation of the oral and pharyngeal cavities, nasal mucous membrane inflammation, and sinusitis (2).

Topically, Roman chamomile is used for eczema, wounds, and inflammation (2).

Topically, the extract of Roman chamomile is used in antiseptic ointments, creams, and gels to treat cracked nipples, sore gums, inflammations, and irritation of the skin and mucosa (11).

In oral herbal combinations, Roman chamomile is used for liver and gallbladder disease, gallstones, fatty liver, chronic heartburn, loss of appetite, bloating, upset stomach, digestive disturbances, Roemheld's syndrome, flatulent indigestion, indigestion in infants, and in spastic constipation. It is used as a "blood purification" remedy, a general tonic during puberty and menopause, a preventative for menstrual discomforts, for missed periods, and for insufficient or irregular periods.

In herbal inhalation therapy, Roman chamomile is used as steam baths for frontal sinus mucous membrane inflammation, hay fever, nasal and pharyngeal mucosal swelling, and inflammation of the ears.

In topical herbal combinations, Roman chamomile is used for wounds, burns, frostbite, diaper rash on infants and toddlers, decubitus ulcers, and hemorrhoids (2).

Historically, Roman chamomile has been used to treat digestive and rheumatic disorders. Teas have also been used as a hair tint and conditioner, and to treat parasitic worm infections.

In foods and beverages, the essential oil and extract are used as flavor components (11).

In manufacturing, the volatile oil of Roman chamomile is used as a fragrance component in soaps, cosmetics and perfumes (11), and to flavor cigarette tobacco (6). The extract is also used in cosmetics, soaps, and other personal care products (11).

Safety

LIKELY SAFE ...when used in amounts found in foods. It has Generally Recognized as Safe (GRAS) status in the US (11). The maximum use level is 0.002% for the oil (11).

POSSIBLY SAFE ...when the dried flower preparations are used orally and appropriately in medicinal amounts (2,12).

There is insufficient reliable information available about the safety of the topical use of Roman chamomile.

PREGNANCY: LIKELY UNSAFE ...when used orally in medicinal amounts. Roman chamomile is believed to be an abortifacient (4). There is insufficient reliable information available about the safety of the topical use of Roman chamomile during pregnancy.

LACTATION: Insufficient reliable information available; avoid using (4).

Effectiveness

There is insufficient reliable information available about the effectiveness of Roman chamomile.

Possible Mechanism of Action & Active Ingredients

The applicable part of Roman chamomile is the flowerhead. Roman chamomile possesses antiflatulent, antispasmodic, and sedative properties (4). Large amounts of Roman chamomile can act as an emetic while small amounts act as an anti-emetic (4). In cosmetics, Roman chamomile is considered a deodorant and a stimulant to skin metabolism (11). Roman chamomile contains the coumarin scopoletin-7-glucoside and varied flavonoids, their glycosides (including rutin and volatile oils), as well as other constituents (4). Some evidence suggests azulene constituents contained in volatile oils exert anti-allergy and anti-inflammatory effects by inhibiting histamine release. However, the constituent nobilin, a sesquiterpene lactone, is thought to trigger allergy in sensitive individuals (4). Some evidence suggests Roman chamomile acts on the central nervous system, possibly reducing aggressive behavior (18). Experimental evidence suggests the volatile oil could have anti-inflammatory, antidiuretic, and sedative effects (4). The essential oil is active against gram-positive bacteria and dermatomyces (18). The sesquiterpinoids nobilin, 1,10-epoxynobilin, and 3-dehydronobilin show some evidence of antitumor activity (4). Although the constituents of Roman chamomile are not identical to those of German chamomile both plants are similarly used (512).

Adverse Reactions Including Known Allergies

Ingesting large amounts of Roman chamomile might cause vomiting (11), although this is disputed (12). Topical use can cause contact dermatitis (4,567). Allergic skin reactions occur in up to 20% of individuals (19). It can cause an allergic reaction in individuals sensitive to the Asteraceae/Compositae family. Members of this family include ragweed, chrysanthemums, marigolds, daisies, and many other herbs. It can also cause rhinitis in individuals with atopic allergy to mugwort (2).

Possible Interactions with Herbs & Other Dietary Supplements

HERBS WITH ANTICOAGULANT/ANTIPLATELET POTENTIAL: Concomitant use of herbs that have coumarin constituents or affect platelet aggregation could theoretically increase the risk of bleeding in some people. These herbs include: angelica, anise, arnica, asafoetida, bogbean, boldo, capsicum, celery, clove, danshen, fenugreek, feverfew, garlic, ginger, ginkgo, ginseng (Panax), horse chestnut, horseradish, licorice, meadowsweet, prickly ash, onion, papain, passionflower, poplar, quassia, red clover, turmeric, wild carrot, wild lettuce, willow, and others (4,19).

Possible Interactions with Drugs

ANTICOAGULANTS: Theoretically, concomitant use might potentiate effects and adverse effects of anticoagulants (4).

Possible Interactions with Foods

No interactions are known to occur, and there is no known reason to expect a clinically significant interaction with Roman chamomile.

Possible Interactions with Lab Tests

No interactions are known to occur, and there is no known reason to expect a clinically significant interaction with Roman chamomile.

Possible Interactions with Diseases or Conditions

ASTHMA: May exacerbate asthma (4).
CROSS-ALLERGENICITY: Can cause an allergic reaction in individuals sensitive to the Asteraceae/Compositae family. Members of this family include ragweed, chrysanthemums, marigolds, daisies, and many other herbs. Can cause rhinitis in individuals with atopic allergy to mugwort (2).

Typical Dosages & Routes of Administration that are Commonly Used

ORAL: A typical dose is 1-4 grams dried flowerheads three times daily, or one cup tea. To make tea, steep 1-4 grams dried flowerheads in 150 mL of boiling water for 5-10 minutes, strain (4). Liquid extract (1:1 in 70% alcohol), 1-4 mL three times daily (4).
TOPICAL: A 3% steeped tea is prepared for topical use (8).

Comments

Though widely used, there is very little information about Roman chamomile. Most of the existing information concerns German chamomile (4,7) but it is extrapolated to Roman chamomile.

ROSE GERANIUM

This Product is Also Known As

Aetheroleum Pelargonii, Algerian Geranium Oil, Bourbon Geranium Oil, Moroccan Geranium Oil, Oleum Geranii, Pelargonium Oil.

Scientific Names

Pelargonium graveolens.
Family: Geraniaceae.

People Use This For

In African traditional medicine, the roots of various Pelargoinum species are used as astringents and for diarrhea.
In foods and beverages, rose geranium oil is used as a flavoring agent (11).
In manufacturing, rose geranium oil is used as an inexpensive substitute for rose oil (11). It is also used as a fragrance component in soaps, cosmetics, and perfumes (11).

Safety

LIKELY SAFE ...when used in amounts found in foods (11). It has Generally Recognized as Safe (GRAS) status in the US (11).

PREGNANCY AND LACTATION: Insufficient reliable information; avoid amounts greater than found in foods.

Effectiveness

There is insufficient reliable information about the effectiveness of rose geranium.

Possible Mechanism of Action & Active Ingredients

The applicable part of rose geranium is the oil that is distilled from the stem and leaf. The geranium oil constituents citronellol, citronellyl acetate, citronellyl formate, and geraniol exhibit marginal antitumor activity (3751). The essential oils from Pelargonium species show some indication of antibacterial and antifungal activity (3752,3753).

Adverse Reactions Including Known Allergies

Geranium oil has been associated with dermatitis in hypersensitive individuals (11), however, geranium is generally considered to be nonsensitizing, nonirritating, and nonphototoxic to human skin (11).

Possible Interactions with Herbs & Other Dietary Supplements

Insufficient reliable information available.

Possible Interactions with Drugs

No interactions are known to occur, and there is no known reason to expect a clinically significant interaction with rose geranium.

Possible Interactions with Foods

No interactions are known to occur, and there is no known reason to expect a clinically significant interaction with rose geranium.

Possible Interactions with Lab Tests

No interactions are known to occur, and there is no known reason to expect a clinically significant interaction with rose geranium.

Possible Interactions with Diseases or Conditions

No interactions are known to occur, and there is no known reason to expect a clinically significant interaction with rose geranium.

Typical Dosages & Routes of Administration that are Commonly Used

No typical dosage.

Comments

Avoid confusing rose geranium oil with East Indian or Turkish geranium oil (known as palmorosa oil) that is derived from a different plant (11).

ROSE HIP

This Product is Also Known As

Cynosbatos, Heps, Hip, Hipberry, Hip Fruit, Hip Sweet, Hop Fruit, Rosa de castillo, Rosae pseudofructus cum semen, Rose Hips, Rose Hip with seed, Rosehips, Wild Boar Fruit.

CAUTION: See separate listings for Acerola, Vitamin C, and Cherokee Rosehip.

Scientific Names

Rosa canina; other Rosa species including Rosa alba, Rosa centifolia, Rosa damascena; Rosa gallica; Rosa rugosa; Rosa villosa, synonym Rosa pomifera.

Family: Rosaceae.

People Use This For

Orally, rose hips with the seeds are used as a supplemental source of dietary vitamin C (6,11) and for preventing and treating colds, influenza-like infections, infectious diseases, vitamin C deficiencies, fever, increasing immune function during exhaustion, gastric spasms, gastric acid deficiency, preventing gastric mucosal inflammation and gastric ulcers, and as a "stomach tonic" for intestinal diseases. It is also used orally for diarrhea, gallstones, gallbladder ailments, lower urinary tract and kidney disorders, dropsy (edema), gout, disorders of uric acid metabolism, arthritis, sciatica, diabetes, increasing peripheral circulation, for reducing thirst (6), and as a laxative and diuretic (2).

In folk medicine, rose hip with the seed has been used to treat chest ailments (6).

In foods and in manufacturing, it is used for rose hip tea, jam and soup (5,8), and as a natural source of vitamin C (11).

Safety

LIKELY SAFE ...when consumed in amounts commonly found in foods (11). Rosa alba, Rosa centifiolia, Rosa damascena, and Rosa gallica have Generally Recognized as Safe (GRAS) status for food use in the US (11).
POSSIBLY SAFE ...when used orally and appropriately for medicinal purposes (12).
PREGNANCY AND LACTATION: Insufficient reliable information available; avoid amounts greater than those found in foods.

Effectiveness

POSSIBLY INEFFECTIVE ...when the dry rose hips and powder are taken orally as sources of vitamin C for treating or preventing vitamin C deficiency and other uses (2). Much of the vitamin C is destroyed during drying, processing, and in storage (2,11).
There is insufficient reliable information available about the effectiveness of rose hip for its other uses.

Possible Mechanism of Action & Active Ingredients

Rose hip contains pectin, citric acid, and malic acid, which can have laxative and diuretic activities (5,18). The diuretic activity is controversial (8). Fresh rose hip contains between 0.5-1.7% vitamin C (5,8) and is estimated to contain 1250 mg vitamin C per 100 grams of rose hip (6). However, much of the vitamin C is destroyed during drying and processing (11), and declines rapidly with storage (2). Vitamin C is required for collagen formation and tissue repair (15). It is an enzyme cofactor in the synthesis of collagen, carnitine, norepinephrine, and peptide hormones, and in tyrosine metabolism (3042). Vitamin C is also involved in oxidation-reduction reactions, conversion of folic acid to folinic acid, carbohydrate metabolism, synthesis of lipids and proteins, iron metabolism, resistance to infections, and cellular respiration (15). It acts as an antioxidant, decreasing oxidants in gastric juice, decreasing lipid peroxidation, and decreasing oxidative DNA and protein damage (3042). Vitamin C deficiency that lasts for three to five months results in symptomatic scurvy that affects collagenous structures, bones, and blood vessels (15). Vitamin C enhances the absorption of soluble non-heme iron, either by reducing it (converting ferric to ferrous) or by preventing chelation by phytates or other food ligands (14,3042). The interaction between iron salts and vitamin C can be variable (14).

Adverse Reactions Including Known Allergies

When taken orally, the adverse effects of vitamin C are related to the amount of vitamin C actually contained in the rose hip product (see Effectiveness). The adverse reactions include nausea, vomiting, esophagitis, heartburn, abdominal cramps, GI obstruction, fatigue, flushing, headache, insomnia, sleepiness, diarrhea, hyperoxaluria, precipitation of urate, oxalate, or cysteine stones or drugs in the urinary tract (14,15). Large amounts are associated with deep vein thrombosis (15). The inhalation of the rose hip dust is reportedly a respiratory allergen in production workers. It can cause mild to moderate anaphylaxis (6). Topically, the rose hip dust ("itching powder") can cause itching by mechanical irritation (6).

Possible Interactions with Herbs & Other Dietary Supplements

IRON: Concomitant use interacts with the vitamin C in rose hip; 200 mg of vitamin C per 30 mg of elemental iron increases oral iron absorption, especially ferric iron (14,15,3042).

Possible Interactions with Drugs

Rose hip interactions depend on the amount of vitamin C present (see Effectiveness).
ASPIRIN AND OTHER SALICYLATES: Concomitant use interacts with the vitamin C in rose hip and can increase urinary excretion of ascorbic acid and decrease excretion of salicylates, but this may not have a clinically significant effect on salicylate plasma levels (15,3046).
ALUMINUM-CONTAINING ANTACIDS: Concomitant use interacts with the vitamin C in rose hip and can increase aluminum absorption, but the clinical significance of this is unknown (3046). Administer rose hip with vitamin C two hours before or four hours after antacids (3046).
IRON: Concomitant use interacts with the vitamin C in rose hip; 200 mg of vitamin C per 30 mg of elemental iron increases iron absorption, especially ferric iron (14,15,3042).
WARFARIN: Concomitant use interacts with the vitamin C in rose hip. Large amounts of vitamin C can impair the warfarin response (3046).
INCREASED VITAMIN C REQUIREMENTS: Estrogens, oral contraceptives, barbiturates, tetracyclines, and salicylates increase the vitamin C requirements (15).

Possible Interactions with Foods

Rose hip interactions depend on the amount of vitamin C present (see Effectiveness).
IRON: Concomitant use interacts with the vitamin C in rose hip and can increase the absorption of dietary (ferric) iron (14,3042).

Possible Interactions with Lab Tests

Rose hip interactions depend on the amount of vitamin C present (see Effectiveness).
URIC ACID: Large amounts of the vitamin C in rose hip can cause a true decrease in serum uric acid concentrations and test results with enzymatic method assays (15) and a false increase in test results with assays based on other methods (14).
CALCIUM/SODIUM: 3-6 grams of vitamin C daily can cause a true increase in urinary calcium and test results (15)

and a true decrease in urinary sodium and test results.

ASPARTATE AMINOTRANSFERASE (AST, SGOT): Large amounts of the vitamin C in rose hip can cause a false increase in results of serum tests relying on color reactions (Redox reactions) and Technicon SMA 12/60 (14).

LDH: The vitamin C in rose hip can cause a false decrease measured by Technicon SMA 12/60 and Abbott 100 methods (14).

BILIRUBIN: Large amounts of the vitamin C in rose hip can cause a false increase in serum test results measured by Technicon SMA 12/60 or colorimetric methods (14).

CARBAMAZEPINE (Tegretol): Large amounts of the vitamin C in rose hip can cause falsely increased serum assay results measured by Ames ARIS method (14).

THEOPHYLLINE: Large amounts of the vitamin C in rose hip can cause falsely decreased serum assay results when measured by the ARIS system or Ames Seralyzer photometer (14).

CREATININE: The vitamin C in rose hip can cause a false increase in serum creatinine or urine test results (14).

GLUCOSE: Large amounts of the vitamin C in rose hip can cause false increases in urine test results measured by copper reduction methods (e.g. Clinitest) and false decreases in results measured by glucose oxidase methods (e.g. Clinistix, Tes-Tape) (14,15).

ACETAMINOPHEN: The vitamin C in rose hip can cause false negative urine results with methods based on hydrolysis and formation of an indophenol blue chromagen (14).

OCCULT BLOOD: The vitamin C in rose hip may cause false negative guaiac results to occur with 250 mg or more of vitamin C per day (3042).

Possible Interactions with Diseases or Conditions

DIABETES: The vitamin C in rose hip might affect glycogenolysis and the control of diabetes, but not all experts agree on this (15).

GLUCOSE-6-PHOSPHATE DEHYDROGENASE DEFICIENCY: Large amounts of the vitamin C in rose hip might increase the risk of oxalate stone formation (15).

SICKLE CELL DISEASE: The vitamin C in rose hip rarely can decrease the blood pH, precipitating sickle cell crisis (15).

HEMOCHROMATOSIS, THALASSEMIA, SIDEROBLASTIC ANEMIA: Use rose hip with caution, because the vitamin C content can increase iron absorption, which could worsen this condition (14,15).

INCREASED NEEDS: Vitamin C requirements increase in pregnancy, lactation, hyperthyroidism, stress, fever, infection, trauma, burns, smoking, and cold exposure (15).

Typical Dosages & Routes of Administration that are Commonly Used

ORAL: The typical dose of rose hips is as a tea, which is prepared by steeping 2-2.5 grams of the crushed rose hips in 150 mL boiling water for 10-15 minutes and then straining (8).

Comments

Rose hip with seed is the ripe, dried receptacle (hip) with fruit (seed) of various Rosa species, including dog rose (Rosa canina), white rose (Rosa alba), provence rose (Rosa centifolia), and damask rose (Rosa damascena). Avoid confusion with Cherokee roseship, rose flower, and vitamin C. CAUTION: Sometimes rose hip seeds or plain rose hip receptacles without seeds are sold. These are different than rose hip with seed. Fresh rose hips contain a high concentration of vitamin C; however, much of the vitamin C is destroyed during drying and processing (11) and declines rapidly with storage (2). Many rose hip-derived "natural" vitamin C products are supplemented with synthetic vitamin C (6,11), but may not be clearly labeled accordingly (6).

ROSEMARY

This Product is Also Known As

Compass Plant, Compass-Weed, Old Man, Polar Plant, Rosemary.

Scientific Names

Rosmarinus officinalis.
Family: Labiatae or Lamiaceae.

People Use This For

Orally, rosemary is used for a digestive aid, dyspepsia (2,4,5,18), promotion of menstrual flow, inducing abortion (5,6), headache (4), liver and gallbladder complaints, loss of appetite, and blood pressure problems (18).

Topically, rosemary is used as a hair tonic to prevent baldness (5,6), for circulatory disturbances, supportive therapy for joint or musculoskeletal pain (2,5,18), myalgia, sciatica, intercostal neuralgia (4), balneotherapy (18), and as an insect repellent (6).

Historically, rosemary has also been used for flatulence, gout, toothache, headache, cough (400), eczema, and as a poultice for poorly healing wounds (18). In foods, rosemary is used as a spice (5,6). The leaf and oil are used in foods, and the oil in beverages (11).

In manufacturing, rosemary oil is used as a fragrant component in soaps and perfumes (11).

© Copyright 2000, Natural Medicines Comprehensive Database (209) 472-2244. For updated data, go to www.NaturalDatabase.com

Safety

LIKELY SAFE ...when the leaves or oil are used in amounts that are typically found in foods. Rosemary has Generally Recognized as Safe (GRAS) status in the US (11). The maximum use level of the leaves is 0.41% in baked goods. The maximum level of oil used is 0.003% (4,11).

POSSIBLY SAFE ...when the leaf products are used orally and appropriately in medicinal amounts (18). ...when used topically and appropriately (18).

LIKELY UNSAFE ...when the undiluted essential oil is ingested. Can cause stomach, intestine, and kidney irritation (515).

PREGNANCY: LIKELY SAFE ...when the leaf or oil is used in food amounts. LIKELY UNSAFE ...contraindicated for oral use in larger amounts. Considered to have abortifacient, uterine and menstrual flow stimulant effects (4,12,18). There is insufficient reliable information available about the safety of the topical use of rosemary during pregnancy.

LACTATION: Insufficient reliable information available; avoid using leaf or oil in amounts greater than typically found in foods.

Effectiveness

POSSIBLY EFFECTIVE ...when used orally for dyspepsia (2,5). ...when used topically as supportive therapy for joint or musculoskeletal pain and circulatory problems (2,5).

POSSIBLY INEFFECTIVE ...when used as an abortifacient (5,6).

There is insufficient reliable information available about the effectiveness of rosemary for its other uses.

Possible Mechanism of Action & Active Ingredients

The applicable part of rosemary is the leaf. Dried leaves of rosemary contain from 1-2.5% volatile oil. The volatile oil seems to be responsible for the pharmacological activity (4,5,18). The volatile oil consists primarily of cineole, borneol, camphor, and pinenes (4,6). When rosemary is taken orally, it might relieve dyspeptic complaints due to a spasmolytic effect on smooth muscle of the gastrointestinal tract and in the ducts of the gallbladder (2,4). Rosemary also seems to have positive inotropic effects and increases coronary blood flow (2). When rosemary is used topically, it is a skin irritant which might increase circulation (2). Animal studies show rosemary has an effect on smooth muscle described as contractile, followed by spasmolytic action. Rosemary has antibacterial, antifungal (4) and antioxidant properties (4,6), and possibly anticancer effects (6). It also inhibits endotoxin-induced activation of serum complement (4).

Adverse Reactions Including Known Allergies

Taken orally, large amounts of leaves containing rosemary oil might cause deep coma, spasm, vomiting, gastroenteritis, uterine bleeding, kidney irritation, pulmonary edema, and death (18). Ingestion of undiluted oil might cause stomach and intestinal irritation, kidney damage, and seizures (5,6). The camphor constituent can sometimes lead to seizures (4).

Rosemary used topically can lead to photosensitivity, erythema, and dermatitis in hypersensitive individuals (4,6). Asthma due to repeated occupational exposure (occupational asthma) can occur (783).

Possible Interactions with Herbs & Other Dietary Supplements

Insufficient reliable information available.

Possible Interactions with Drugs

No interactions are known to occur, and there is no known reason to expect a clinically significant interaction with rosemary.

Possible Interactions with Foods

No interactions are known to occur, and there is no known reason to expect a clinically significant interaction with rosemary.

Possible Interactions with Lab Tests

No interactions are known to occur, and there is no known reason to expect a clinically significant interaction with rosemary.

Possible Interactions with Diseases or Conditions

SEIZURE DISORDERS: Theoretically, rosemary might potentiate seizure activity; avoid (4).

Typical Dosages & Routes of Administration that are Commonly Used

ORAL: 1-2 grams leaf three times daily, or, one cup tea (steep 1-2 grams leaf in 150 mL boiling water 5-10 minutes, strain) three times daily (2,4,18); up to 4-6 grams leaf per day (2). Liquid extract (1:1 in 45% alcohol), 2-4 mL three times daily (4). Undiluted oil should not be ingested (5) (see Adverse Reactions).

TOPICAL: Semi-solid or liquid preparations containing 6-10% essential oil (2,18). For a rosemary bath, add 50 grams leaf to 1 L hot water and add to bath water (18).

Comments

None.

© Copyright 2000, Natural Medicines Comprehensive Database (209) 472-2244. For updated data, go to www.NaturalDatabase.com

ROSEROOT

This Product is Also Known As
Arctic Root, Golden Root, King's Crown, Rose Root, Rosenroot.

Scientific Names
Rhodiola rosea, synonyms Sedum rhodiola, Sedum rosea.
Family: Crassulaceae.

People Use This For
Orally, people use roseroot for increasing energy, stamina, strength and mental capacity, and as an adaptogen (to help the body adapt to, and resist physical, chemical and environmental stress). It is used for improving athletic performance, improving sexual function (3186), as an alternative to ginseng, for treating depression, reducing stress-induced cardiac disorders, reducing harmful blood lipids, regulating heartbeat and counteracting arrhythmias. It is used to treat cancer, aging (as an antioxidant), diabetes, in protecting the liver from environmental toxins, improving hearing (3187), strengthening the nervous system, enhancing immunity (3188), and shortening recovery time after prolonged workouts (3189).

In Siberia, roseroot has been used for preventing sickness during the winter, and in Mongolia for treating tuberculosis and cancer (3187).

Safety
There is insufficient reliable information about the safety of roseroot.

Pregnancy and Lactation: Insufficient reliable information available; avoid using.

Effectiveness
There is insufficient reliable information available about the effectiveness of roseroot.

Possible Mechanism of Action & Active Ingredients
The applicable part of roseroot is the root. Roseroot extracts demonstrate antiarrhythmic properties and protection against reperfusion injury after ischemia. These effects can be abolished by naloxone infusion, suggesting that the mechanism might involve an increase in endogenous opioids (3191,3192,3195). Roseroot extracts might also prevent stress-induced cardiac damage by preventing rises in cardiac catecholamines and cyclic-AMP (3193). Roseroot extract reduces experimentally induced mutations, possibly by increasing the efficiency of intracellular DNA repair mechanisms (3190). Roseroot extracts also demonstrate hepatoprotective (3196) and myeloprotective effects (3197). Roseroot extract also demonstrates potential for improving learning and memory (3198). Preliminary research in a small number of patients with superficial bladder cancer suggests that roseroot extract might improve cell characteristics and reduce relapses (3194).

Adverse Reactions Including Known Allergies
None reported.

Possible Interactions with Herbs & Other Dietary Supplements
Insufficient reliable information available.

Possible Interactions with Drugs
No interactions are known to occur, and there is no known reason to expect a clinically significant interaction with roseroot.

Possible Interactions with Foods
No interactions are known to occur, and there is no known reason to expect a clinically significant interaction with roseroot.

Possible Interactions with Lab Tests
No interactions are known to occur, and there is no known reason to expect a clinically significant interaction with roseroot.

Possible Interactions with Diseases or Conditions
No interactions are known to occur, and there is no known reason to expect a clinically significant interaction with roseroot.

Typical Dosages & Routes of Administration that are Commonly Used
Oral: Commonly reported doses vary considerably, from 50-250 mg roseroot extract, one to three times daily (3188,3189).

Comments
Roseroot is native to the arctic regions of eastern Siberia, Scandinavia, Lapland and Alaska (3187,3189). It is reported that Chinese emperors sent expeditions to Siberia to collect the plant in the hope that it would bring long life or immortality (3187). Roseroot has been used as an ingredient in folk medicine love potions (3189).

 © Copyright 2000, Natural Medicines Comprehensive Database (209) 472-2244. For updated data, go to www.NaturalDatabase.com

ROSINWEED

This Product is Also Known As
Compass Weed, Pilot Weed, Polar Plant.
CAUTION: See separate listing for Cup Plant.

Scientific Names
Silphium laciniatum.

People Use This For
Rosinweed is only used in homeopathy for digestive disorders (18).

Safety
There is insufficient reliable information available about the safety of rosinweed.
Pregnancy and Lactation: Insufficient reliable information available; avoid using.

Effectiveness
There is insufficient reliable information available about the effectiveness of rosinweed.

Possible Mechanism of Action & Active Ingredients
The applicable part of rosinweed is the root. Rosinweed root is stated to have antispasmodic, diaphoretic, and diuretic effects (18).

Adverse Reactions Including Known Allergies
None reported.

Possible Interactions with Herbs & Other Dietary Supplements
Insufficient reliable information available.

Possible Interactions with Drugs
No interactions are known to occur, and there is no known reason to expect a clinically significant interaction with rosinweed.

Possible Interactions with Foods
No interactions are known to occur, and there is no known reason to expect a clinically significant interaction with rosinweed.

Possible Interactions with Lab Tests
No interactions are known to occur, and there is no known reason to expect a clinically significant interaction with rosinweed.

Possible Interactions with Diseases or Conditions
No interactions are known to occur, and there is no known reason to expect a clinically significant interaction with rosinweed.

Typical Dosages & Routes of Administration that are Commonly Used
ORAL: People typically use 2 to 4 mL of rosinweed liquid extract (5264).

Comments
Avoid confusion with cup plant (Silphium perfoliatum), also referred to as rosinweed.
There is very little scientific information about this product. Our staff is continually analyzing the available information on natural medicines and will add data here as it becomes available.

ROYAL JELLY

This Product is Also Known As
None.
CAUTION: See separate listings for Bee Pollen, Honey, and Honey Bee venom.

Scientific Names
Apis mellifera.
Family: Apidae.

People Use This For
Orally, royal jelly is used as a health tonic (3513), for rejuvenation (3514), potentiating the immune system (3512), for treating bronchial asthma, liver disease, pancreatitis, insomnia, stomach ulcers, kidney disease, bone fractures, skin disorders (3512), and hyperlipidemia (3515).
Topically, it is used as a skin tonic and hair growth stimulant (6).

Safety

There is insufficient reliable information available about the safety of royal jelly.
Pregnancy and Lactation: Insufficient reliable information available; avoid using.

Effectiveness

POSSIBLY EFFECTIVE ...when taken orally for reducing total serum lipids and cholesterol levels (3515).
There is insufficient reliable information available about the effectiveness of royal jelly for its other uses.

Possible Mechanism of Action & Active Ingredients

Researchers report that royal jelly shows antitumor activity in experimental animals (6). The results of a human study for revitalizing skin were inconclusive (6). In trials in rabbits and humans, royal jelly reduced serum total lipids and cholesterol levels. In rabbits, consuming a hyperlipemic diet, royal jelly delayed the formation of aortic atheromas (3515).

Adverse Reactions Including Known Allergies

There is one case report of hemorrhagic colitis with abdominal pain, bloody diarrhea with concomitant hemorrhagic and edematous mucosa of the sigmoid colon after taking royal jelly orally (3516). Allergy to royal jelly may result in asthma, anaphylaxis, and death (792,3513). When used topically, skin irritation (6), exacerbation of dermatitis, or contact dermatitis may occur (791).

Possible Interactions with Herbs & Other Dietary Supplements

Insufficient reliable information available.

Possible Interactions with Drugs

No interactions are known to occur, and there is no known reason to expect a clinically significant interaction with royal jelly.

Possible Interactions with Foods

No interactions are known to occur, and there is no known reason to expect a clinically significant interaction with royal jelly.

Possible Interactions with Lab Tests

No interactions are known to occur, and there is no known reason to expect a clinically significant interaction with royal jelly.

Possible Interactions with Diseases or Conditions

DERMATITIS: Contraindicated, topical application may exacerbate this condition (791).
HYPERSENSITIVE INDIVIDUALS: Contraindicated.

Typical Dosages & Routes of Administration that are Commonly Used

ORAL: Hyperlipidemia, 50-100 mg once a day reported from human study (3515).

Comments

Royal jelly is a milky secretion produced by worker honey bees (Apis mellifera) for the exclusive development and nurture of queen bees (6). Avoid confusion with bee pollen and honey bee venom.

RUE

This Product is Also Known As

Common Rue, Garden Rue, German Rue, Herb-of-Grace, Herbygrass, Raute, Ruda, Rue Officinale, Rutae folium, Rutae herba.
CAUTION: See separate listing for Goat's Rue.

Scientific Names

Ruta graveolens.
Family: Rutaceae.

People Use This For

Orally, the above-ground parts of rue are used for menstrual disorders and discomforts, as a uterine stimulant and abortifacient, for loss of appetite, dyspepsia, circulatory disorders, arteriosclerosis, heart palpitations, nervousness, hysteria, fever (2), feverish infectious diseases, cramps, hepatitis, diarrhea (18), pleurisy, headaches, neuralgic afflictions, and weakness of the eyes. It is also used orally for respiratory complaints, arthritis (2), intestinal worm infestations, epilepsy, multiple sclerosis, Bell's palsy, and cancer of the mouth (2). It is used as an antispasmodic, diuretic (2), antibacterial, antifungal (6), hemostatic (11), or contraceptive agent (18).
Topically, rue is used for arthritis, dislocations, sprains, injuries of the bone, inflammation of the skin, oral and

pharyngeal cavities, earaches, toothaches (18), headaches (515), tumors and warts, and as an insect repellent (6).
In foods and beverages, rue and its oil are used as flavor components (11).
In manufacturing, rue oil is used as a fragrance ingredient in soaps and cosmetics (11).

Safety

LIKELY SAFE ...when consumed in amounts commonly found in foods. Rue and its oil have Generally Recognized as Safe (GRAS) status for food use in the US. The maximum level is 0.001% for rue and 0.0002% for the oil (11).
LIKELY UNSAFE ...when the fresh rue is taken orally for medicinal purposes (2). Fresh rue can cause severe kidney and liver damage (2). ...when more than 120 grams of leaves or 100 mL oil are ingested. Can cause severe gastrointestinal upset, systemic complications, and death (2,6). Dried rue leaf contains less volatile oil than fresh rue, and it has milder effects (515). Canadian regulations prohibit the use of rue as a non-medicinal ingredient in oral products (12). ...when fresh rue is applied topically (2), because it can cause contact dermatitis and severe photodermatitis (2,6,11,19).
PREGNANCY: LIKELY UNSAFE ...oral use is contraindicated because it might cause uterine stimulant and abortifacient effects (12). Deaths have been reported in women who used rue as an abortifacient (2).
LACTATION: POSSIBLY SAFE ...when consumed in food amounts. LIKELY UNSAFE ...when used in larger amounts than those found in food.

Effectiveness

There is insufficient reliable information available about the effectiveness of rue.

Possible Mechanism of Action & Active Ingredients

The applicable parts of rue are the above-ground parts. Rue contains the alkaloids arborine, arborinine, and gamma-fagarine, and the furocoumarins rutamarin, bergapten, and xanthotoxin. The alkaloids and the furocoumarins show evidence of reversible spasmolytic activity and anti-inflammatory and antihistaminic properties (6,11,515). The furocoumarins also have photosensitizing, phototoxic, and mutagenic effects (2) and they are responsible for adverse skin reactions (6,11,19,515). The constituent, chalepensin, shows some evidence of antifertility and anti-implantation effects. The rutin constituent shows evidence of antispasmodic activity, and it might decrease capillary permeability and fragility. Rue oil has antihelmintic activities, possibly due to the constituent 2-undecanone (11). It can also cause abortions (11). Although rue oil caused fatal adrenal gland, liver, and kidney hemorrhage in animals (11), 30 mg per day for three months did not affect liver function in humans (11). Rue extract's effect on neuromuscular conditions is thought to result from potassium channel-blocking in myelinated nerve cells (6).

Adverse Reactions Including Known Allergies

Used orally, rue can cause GI irritation (12), melancholic mood, sleep disorders, tiredness, dizziness, spasms, and severe kidney and liver damage (2). The fresh leaf juice can cause painful stomach and intestinal irritation, fainting, lethargy, bradycardia, abortion, swelling of the tongue, and clammy skin (2). Rue oil causes severe stomach pain, vomiting, exhaustion, confusion, and convulsions (11). Large amounts, over 100 mL of the oil or 120 grams of the leaf, can cause vomiting, violent gastric pain, systemic complications, and death (2,6). Contact dermatitis (2) and phototoxic reactions including skin blisters have occurred with topical exposure to the fresh plant and rue-containing products followed by exposure to sunlight (2,6). There is one case report of increased phototoxic response to PUVA therapy associated with ingestion of a rue remedy (6177).

Possible Interactions with Herbs & Other Dietary Supplements

GOLDENSEAL: Reports that the effects of large amounts of rue can be overcome by administering goldenseal are unsubstantiated (515).

Possible Interactions with Drugs

PUVA: Rue might increase the phototoxic response to PUVA therapy due to its 5-methoxypsoralen content. There is one case report of increased phototoxic response to PUVA therapy associated with ingestion of a rue remedy (6177). Drugs used in PUVA therapy include, methoxsalen (8-methoxypsoralen, 8-MOP, Oxsoralen) and Trioxsalen (Trisoralen).

Possible Interactions with Foods

No interactions are known to occur, and there is no known reason to expect a clinically significant interaction with rue.

Possible Interactions with Lab Tests

No interactions are known to occur, and there is no known reason to expect a clinically significant interaction with rue.

Possible Interactions with Diseases or Conditions

KIDNEY OR LIVER DYSFUNCTION: Contraindicated (2,12).
GASTROINTESTINAL TRACT PROBLEMS: Rue can exacerbate pre-existing inflammation or irritation of the gastrointestinal tract (19).
URINARY TRACT PROBLEMS: Rue can exacerbate kidney inflammation and urinary tract discomfort (19).

© Copyright 2000, Natural Medicines Comprehensive Database (209) 472-2244. For updated data, go to www.NaturalDatabase.com

Typical Dosages & Routes of Administration that are Commonly Used

ORAL: People typically use 500 mg crushed rue. A maximum dose of 1 gram per day is recommended. As a tea, 1 cup of boiling water is poured over 1 teaspoon of the herb. The tea is taken cold, 1 cup per day (5252,5254).

Comments

Avoid confusion with goat's rue (Galega officinalis) and meadow rue (Thalictrum species).

RUPTUREWORT

This Product is Also Known As

Bruchkraut, Flax weed, Herniariae herba, Herniary.

Scientific Names

Herniaria glabra; Herniaria hirsuta.
Family: Rutaceae.

People Use This For

Orally, rupturewort is used for disorders of the urinary and respiratory tracts, nerve inflammation, gout, arthritis, rheumatism, for "purifying the blood" (2,18), and as a diuretic (8).

Safety

There is insufficient reliable information available about the safety of rupturewort.
Pregnancy and Lactation: Insufficient reliable information available; avoid using.

Effectiveness

There is insufficient reliable information available about the effectiveness of rupturewort.

Possible Mechanism of Action & Active Ingredients

The applicable parts of rupturewort are the above ground parts. The constituents triterpene saponins, flavonoids, coumarins, and tannins seem to have mild spasmolytic and diuretic activity (18), but these effects have not been scientifically proven (18).

Adverse Reactions Including Known Allergies

None reported.

Possible Interactions with Herbs & Other Dietary Supplements

Insufficient reliable information available.

Possible Interactions with Drugs

No interactions are known to occur, and there is no known reason to expect a clinically significant interaction with rupturewort.

Possible Interactions with Foods

No interactions are known to occur, and there is no known reason to expect a clinically significant interaction with rupturewort.

Possible Interactions with Lab Tests

No interactions are known to occur, and there is no known reason to expect a clinically significant interaction with rupturewort.

Possible Interactions with Diseases or Conditions

No interactions are known to occur, and there is no known reason to expect a clinically significant interaction with rupturewort.

Typical Dosages & Routes of Administration that are Commonly Used

ORAL: As a diuretic, take one cup tea (simmer 1.5 grams finely cut above ground parts in 150 mL boiling water for 5 minutes, strain) 2-3 times daily (8).

Comments

None.

RUSTY-LEAVED RHODODENDRON

This Product is Also Known As

Rhododendri Ferruginei Folium, Rosebay, Rust-Red Rhododendron, Rusty Leaved Rhododendron, Snow Rose.

© Copyright 2000, Natural Medicines Comprehensive Database (209) 472-2244. For updated data, go to www.NaturalDatabase.com

Scientific Names
Rhododendron ferrugineum.
Family: Ericaceae.

People Use This For
In combination with other herbs, rusty-leaved rhododendron is used for extreme tension of the muscles or arteries (hypertonia), muscle and joint rheumatism, joint disease, hardening of muscles, muscular pain, weak connective tissue, neuralgia, sensitivity to weather change, sciatica, trigeminal neuralgia, migraine, headaches, intercostal neuralgia, gout, biliary or urinary stones, and geriatric and aging disorders (2).
In folk medicine, rusty-leaved rhododendron has been used for stones, geriatric complaints, gout, hypertension, migraine, muscular pain, and rheumatic complaints (18).

Safety
LIKELY UNSAFE ...when used orally (2). The entire plant is considered poisonous (2,7,18,3477,3496). Hydroquinone toxicity is also a potential risk with long-term use (2). Most poisonings result from the consumption of honey made from rhododendron nectar (3477).
PREGNANCY AND LACTATION: LIKELY UNSAFE ...when used orally.

Effectiveness
There is insufficient reliable information available about the effectiveness of rusty-leaved rhododendron (2).

Possible Mechanism of Action & Active Ingredients
The applicable part of rusty-leaved rhododendron is the leaf. Rusty-leaved rhododendron contains grayanotoxins and arbutin (2). Grayanotoxins lower blood pressure (7). Grayanotoxins also prevent nerve conduction by inhibiting the closure of sodium channels on cell membranes, which increases sodium conductance and causes cellular depolarization (18,3477). Grayanotoxin toxicity includes muscular and respiratory paralysis (7). Arbutin is hydrolyzed to hydroquinone by the intestinal flora (7). As a result, long-term use may to lead to hydroquinone toxicity (2).

Adverse Reactions Including Known Allergies
Adverse effects of ingestion include weakness, dizziness, nausea, vomiting hypotension, bradycardia, transient A-V dissociation (17,3496) and blurred vision (17). Symptoms of poisoning due to the constituent grayanotoxin include sweating, impaired consciousness (2,3496) chills, fainting (2), shock (3496), seizure (3477), cardiac and respiratory arrest (2,3477), severe stupor (18), and possibly death (18,3477). Chronic use may lead to hydroquinone toxicity (2). Hydroquinone toxicity is characterized by a gastroenteritis-like syndrome (17).

Possible Interactions with Herbs & Other Dietary Supplements
Insufficient reliable information available.

Possible Interactions with Drugs
No interactions are known to occur, and there is no known reason to expect a clinically significant interaction with rusty-leaved rhododendron.

Possible Interactions with Foods
No interactions are known to occur, and there is no known reason to expect a clinically significant interaction with rusty-leaved rhododendron.

Possible Interactions with Lab Tests
No interactions are known to occur, and there is no known reason to expect a clinically significant interaction with rusty-leaved rhododendron.

Possible Interactions with Diseases or Conditions
No interactions are known to occur, and there is no known reason to expect a clinically significant interaction with rusty-leaved rhododendron.

Typical Dosages & Routes of Administration that are Commonly Used
No typical dosage.

Comments
Rusty-leaved rhododendron is considered likely unsafe; avoid using. Rusty-leaved rhododendron is considered a poisonous plant (2,7,18). Rhododendron honey is also known as "mad honey" (3477,3496).

RUTIN

This Product is Also Known As
Eldrin, Oxerutin, Quercetin-3-rhamnoglucoside, Quercetin-3-rutinoside, Rutine, Rutinum, Rutosid, Rutoside, Rutosidum, Sclerutin, Sophorin.

Scientific Names
Rutin, rutoside.

People Use This For
Orally, rutin is used as a vascular protectant (14); for reducing capillary permeability, fragility and bleeding (3,9,11,14); for treating varicose vein symptoms (3,14); and prophylaxis of mucositis associated with cancer treatments (210).

In combination with trypsin and bromelain, rutin is used orally for osteoarthritis (6252).

In Chinese medicine, rutin has been used orally to treat internal bleeding and bleeding hemorrhoids, and to prevent strokes (11).

Safety
LIKELY SAFE ...when used orally in amounts present in fruits and vegetables.

POSSIBLY UNSAFE ...when used orally in amounts greater than those found in foods. Although rutin is generally considered nontoxic, there are reports of rutin forming an obstructive mass in the gastrointestinal tract (11). There is also concern that flavonoids, including rutin, could become mutagenic and play a role in the etiology of gastric cancer (3106).

PREGNANCY AND LACTATION: Insufficient reliable information available; avoid using amounts greater than those found in foods.

Effectiveness
POSSIBLY EFFECTIVE ...when taken orally in combination with trypsin and bromelain for treating osteoarthritis (6252). In a double-blind trial, 73 patients with painful osteoarthritis of the knee were randomly assigned the combination enzyme product (Phlogenzym) or diclofenac (Voltaren) 50 mg three times daily during the first week and then twice daily in weeks 2 and 3. The enyzme product was similar to diclofenac in relieving pain and improving knee function (6252).

There is insufficient reliable information about the effectiveness of rutin for its other uses.

Possible Mechanism of Action & Active Ingredients
Rutin is thought to be an antioxidant, a free radical scavenger, and an iron-chelator (209,3100). It has been reported to decrease capillary fragility and permeability, although the existing evidence is inconclusive (11). Some studies suggest rutin might offer protection from damage induced by asbestos (209,3103), cytotoxic effects of oxidized low density lipoproteins (11,3105), and gastric injury from ethanol (3107). Other evidence suggests it might be beneficial in inflammatory bowel disease (3101,3102). When added to the diet, rutin appears to offer some protection against DNA damage caused by hepatocarcinogens (3104). However, limited preliminary evidence suggests rutin might worsen the progression of melanoma (211).

Adverse Reactions Including Known Allergies
Rutin may cause headache, flushing, rashes, or mild gastrointestinal disturbance (313).

Possible Interactions with Herbs & Other Dietary Supplements
IRON: Some information suggests that rutin might have iron-chelating properties (209).

Possible Interactions with Drugs
No interactions are known to occur, and there is no known reason to expect a clinically significant interaction with rutin.

Possible Interactions with Foods
No interactions are known to occur, and there is no known reason to expect a clinically significant interaction with rutin.

Possible Interactions with Lab Tests
No interactions are known to occur, and there is no known reason to expect a clinically significant interaction with rutin.

Possible Interactions with Diseases or Conditions
No interactions are known to occur, and there is no known reason to expect a clinically significant interaction with rutin.

Typical Dosages & Routes of Administration that are Commonly Used
ORAL: As a supplement, a common dose of rutin is 500 mg per day (312). For relief of symptoms of edema associated with chronic venous insufficiency, a typical dose is 500 mg twice daily (313). For osteoarthritis, a combination enzyme product (Phlogenzym), which contains rutin 100 mg, trypsin 48 mg, and bromelain 90mg, was given 2 tablets 3 times daily (6252).

Comments
Rutin (rutoside) is a flavonoid present in numerous plants. The major sources of rutin for medical use include buckwheat, Japanese pagoda tree, and Eucalyptus macrorhyncha (11). Other sources of rutin include the leaves of several species of eucalyptus (9), lime tree flowers, elder flowers (8), hawthorn leaves and flowers (2,3,8), rue (2), St. John's Wort (3), Ginkgo biloba (3), apples (3100), and other fruits and vegetables (3108).

RYE GRASS

This Product is Also Known As
Grass Pollen, Grass Pollen Extract, Rye Grass Pollen, Rye Grass Pollen Extract, Rye Pollen Extract.

Scientific Names
Secale cereale.
Family: Poaceae or Gramineae.

People Use This For
Orally, rye grass pollen extract is used for shrinking prostate size, relieving the symptoms of benign prostatic hyperplasia (BPH), that include frequency, nocturia, urgency, decreased urine flow rate, dribbling, painful urination, and residual volume after voiding (5292,5293,5294,5295). It is also used for chronic prostatitis and prostate pain (5296), promoting men's health and prostate health (5291).

Safety
POSSIBLY SAFE …when products of good quality are used orally. There are no reports of toxicity in clinical trials (5292,5293,5294,5296).
PREGNANCY AND LACTATION: Insufficient reliable information available; avoid using.

Effectiveness
POSSIBLY EFFECTIVE …when rye grass pollen extract is used orally for the management of BPH symptoms that include frequency, nocturia, urgency, decreased urine flow rate, dribbling, painful urination, residual urine volume after voiding. …when used for shrinking prostate size (5292,5293,5294,5295). …when used for prostatitis and prostatodynia (5296). Studies have used Cernilton brand rye grass pollen extract (5292,5293,5294).

Possible Mechanism of Action & Active Ingredients
The applicable part of rye grass is the pollen extract. Rye grass pollen extract is prepared by microbial digestion of the pollen, followed by water and acetone extraction (5290,5295). The extract does not affect luteinizing hormone, follicle-stimulating hormone, testosterone, or dihydrotestosterone (5292). Some evidence suggests that rye grass pollen extract might inhibit prostate cancer cell growth (5297). Other evidence suggests that it might interfere with inflammation by inhibiting the biosynthesis of prostaglandins and leukotrienes (5298).

Adverse Reactions Including Known Allergies
Adverse reactions include abdominal distention, heartburn, and nausea (5293).

Possible Interactions with Herbs & Other Dietary Supplements
Insufficient reliable information available.

Possible Interactions with Drugs
No interactions are known to occur, and there is no known reason to expect a clinically significant interaction with rye grass pollen extract.

Possible Interactions with Foods
No interactions are known to occur, and there is no known reason to expect a clinically significant interaction with rye grass pollen extract.

Possible Interactions with Lab Tests
No interactions are known to occur, and there is no known reason to expect a clinically significant interaction with rye grass pollen extract.

Possible Interactions with Diseases or Conditions
No interactions are known to occur, and there is no known reason to expect a clinically significant interaction with rye grass pollen extract.

Typical Dosages & Routes of Administration that are Commonly Used
ORAL: The typical dose of rye grass pollen is 126 mg three times daily (5294). Clinical studies have used Cerniltin, a brand manufactured by Cernitin.

Comments
Clinical evidence for the effectiveness of rye grass extract is limited. For BPH, there was one double-blind, placebo-controlled study (5292) that showed marginal benefit and two open trials (5293,5294). For treating prostatitis and prostatodynia, the evidence is limited to one open trial (5296).

SACCHAROMYCES BOULARDII

This Product is Also Known As
Probiotic.
CAUTION: See separate listings for Bifidobacterium Bifidum, Brewer's Yeast (Hansen CBS 5926), Lactobacillus Acidophilus, and Lactobacillus GG.

Scientific Names
Saccharomyces boulardii.

People Use This For
Orally, Saccharomyces boulardii is used for preventing and treating diarrhea (4347). It is also used to protect the gut from amebas and cholera, to keep Candida from spreading, to alleviate diarrhea caused by Clostridium difficile, Crohn's disease, diarrhea, and traveler's diarrhea (4364).

Safety
LIKELY SAFE ...when used orally and appropriately (4353).
CHILDREN: POSSIBLY SAFE ...when used orally (4347,4356). There is one report of fungemia associated with use (4357).
PREGNANCY AND LACTATION: Insufficient reliable information available; avoid using.

Effectiveness
POSSIBLY EFFECTIVE ...when used orally to prevent diarrhea associated with use of antibiotics (4353,4355). ...when used in tube feedings to prevent diarrhea (4349). ...when used orally to prevent travelers diarrhea (4356). ...when used orally to treat acute diarrhea in infants (4347). ...when used orally to treat HIV-associated diarrhea (4347). ...when used in combination with vancomycin or metronidazole to treat recurrent Clostridium difficile disease (4352,4354).
There is insufficient reliable information available about the effectiveness of Saccaromyces boulardii for its other uses.

Possible Mechanism of Action & Active Ingredients
When Saccharomyces boulardii is given to healthy volunteers, a maximum steady state is reached in 3 days. It does not multiply in the gut and less than 1% of the ingested dose is recovered from stools (4363). Some evidence suggests that Saccharomyces boulardii protease weakens the toxicity of Clostridium difficile toxins A and B (4348), perhaps by coupling a protein of the yeast to adenylate cyclase (4361). Other evidence suggests Saccharomyces boulardii might cause an increase in the intestinal chloride resorption (4362). Individuals who have low stool concentrations of Clostridium difficile after repeated use of Saccharomyces boulardii, are most likely to have recurrence (4360). In addition to its effect on Clostridium difficile, Saccharomyces boulardii also shows evidence of interaction with cholera toxin (4363).

Adverse Reactions Including Known Allergies
Rarely, oral use is associated with fungemia (4357,4358,4360).

Possible Interactions with Herbs & Other Dietary Supplements
Insufficient reliable information available.

Possible Interactions with Drugs
ANTIFUNGALS: Antifungals can cause Saccharomyces boulardii to be ineffective.
ANTIBIOTICS: Saccharomyces boulardii can prevent diarrhea associated with antibiotic use (4353,4355).

Possible Interactions with Foods
No interactions are known to occur, and there is no known reason to expect a clinically significant interaction with Saccharomyces boulardii.

Possible Interactions with Lab Tests
No interactions are known to occur, and there is no known reason to expect a clinically significant interaction with Saccharomyces boulardii.

Possible Interactions with Diseases or Conditions
IMMUNOSUPPRESSION: Although Saccaromyces boulardii is a nonpathogenic organism, use caution in immunosuppressed individuals because there are reports of fungemia.
YEAST ALLERGY: Likely unsafe when used by individuals with yeast allergy.

Typical Dosages & Routes of Administration that are Commonly Used
ORAL: A typical dose to prevent diarrhea is 250-500 mg two to four times a day (4355). A typical dose to treat recurrent diarrhea in adults is 1 gram daily for four weeks along with antibiotic therapy (4352). To treat AIDS-related diarrhea, people typically begin with a dose of 3 grams per day, reducing dose to 1 gram/day as symptoms lessen (4364,4365). Infants: 250 mg two to four times a day according to age (4356).

To prevent contamination of indwelling catheters, open packets or capsules with glove, outside the individual's room (4359). Refrigerate after opening to preserve potency (4366).

Comments

One study that concluded Saccharomyces boulardii is ineffective in preventing antibiotic-associated diarrhea in the elderly (4350) is criticized because the follow-up period was too short (4351). Another study found Saccharomyces boulardii in combination with vancomycin or metronidazole (Flagyl) no more effective than vancomycin or metronidazole alone for initial episode of Clostridium difficile, but the study may have lacked adequate statistical evidence (4352).

SAFFLOWER

This Product is Also Known As

American Saffron, Bastard Saffron, Dyer's Saffron, Fake Saffron, False Saffron, Hing Hua, Honghua, Zaffer, Zafran.

Scientific Names

Carthamus tinctorius.
Family: Asteraceae or Compositae.

People Use This For

Orally, safflower seed oil is used for reducing the risk of cardiovascular disease (6) and preventing atherosclerosis (18).
In Chinese medicine, safflower flower is used for hyperemia in women (18) and hair growth (11).
In folk medicine, safflower is used orally for fever (6), tumors, coughs, bronchial conditions (18), blood stasis, pain, blood invigoration, amenorrhea, painful menses, stimulating menstruation, coronary heart disease, chest pain, traumatic injuries (11,18), inducing sweating (6), as a laxative (6), purgative, stimulant, antiperspirant, abortifacient, and expectorant (18).
For food uses, safflower seed oil is used as a cooking oil (6).
In manufacturing, safflower flower is used to color cosmetics and dye fabrics. Safflower seed oil is used as a paint solvent (6).

Safety

LIKELY SAFE ...when used orally as safflower seed oil (6).
POSSIBLY SAFE ...when used orally and appropriately as safflower flower (6,12,18).
PREGNANCY: LIKELY SAFE ...when used orally as safflower seed oil in food amounts. LIKELY UNSAFE ...when safflower flower is used because it has abortifacient, menstrual stimulant, and uterine stimulant effects (11,12).
LACTATION: LIKELY SAFE ...when used orally as safflower seed oil in food amounts. There is insufficient reliable information available about the safety of safflower flower during lactation; avoid using.

Effectiveness

POSSIBLY EFFECTIVE ...when safflower oil is used as a dietary supplement to reduce the risk of cardiovascular disease (6).
There is insufficient reliable information available about the effectiveness of safflower for its other uses.

Possible Mechanism of Action & Active Ingredients

The applicable parts of safflower are flower and seed oil. Safflower flower contains a complex mixture of red and yellow pigments (11,18). The constituent, safflower yellow, has immunosuppressive and anticoagulant activity (11). Safflower polysaccharide has immunopotentiating effects (11). Safflower extracts exhibit cardiac stimulant, vasodilating, hypolipemic, hypotensive, and uterine stimulant properties (11). Safflower seed oil is a rich source of the essential unsaturated fatty acid, linoleic acid (6). It also contains linolenic acid (18). Some evidence suggests essential fatty acids are necessary to maintain the integrity of the central nervous system (6). Other evidence suggests that diets high in unsaturated and polyunsaturated fatty acids reduce atherosclerosis and the risk of heart disease (6). A diet rich in safflower oil can increase platelet linoleic acid levels, reduce serum cholesterol particularly low-density lipoprotein (LDL) cholesterol, and apolipoprotein B levels (6) without affecting serum triglyceride, high-density (HDL) lipoprotein cholesterol or apolipoprotein A-1 levels (6). However, recent research suggests the improving the lipid profile might not be as important to reducing the risk of cardiovascular disease as previously suggested (6).

Adverse Reactions Including Known Allergies

Safflower can cause an allergic reaction in individuals sensitive to the Asteraceae/Compositae family. Members of this family include ragweed, chrysanthemums, marigolds, daisies, and many other herbs.

Possible Interactions with Herbs & Other Dietary Supplements

HERBS WITH ANTICOAGULANT/ANTIPLATELET POTENTIAL: Concomitant use of herbs that have coumarin constituents or affect platelet aggregation could theoretically increase the risk of bleeding in some people. These herbs include: angelica, anise, arnica, asafoetida, bogbean, boldo, capsicum, celery, chamomile, clove, danshen, fenugreek, feverfew, garlic, ginger, ginkgo, ginseng (Panax), horse chestnut, horseradish, licorice, meadowsweet, prickly ash, onion, papain, passionflower, poplar, quassia, red clover, turmeric, wild carrot, wild lettuce, willow, and others (4,19).

Possible Interactions with Drugs

ANTICOAGULANTS: Theoretically concomitant use with safflower might increase effects and adverse effects of anticoagulants.

Possible Interactions with Foods

No interactions are known to occur, and there is no known reason to expect a clinically significant interaction with safflower.

Possible Interactions with Lab Tests

No interactions are known to occur, and there is no known reason to expect a clinically significant interaction with safflower.

Possible Interactions with Diseases or Conditions

BLEEDING DISORDERS: Contraindicated in people with hemorrhagic diseases, peptic ulcers, or clotting disorders. Safflower can prolong coagulation time (12).
CROSS-ALLERGENICITY: Can cause an allergic reaction in individuals sensitive to the Asteraceae/Compositae family. Members of this family include ragweed, chrysanthemums, marigolds, daisies, and many other herbs.

Typical Dosages & Routes of Administration that are Commonly Used

ORAL: A typical dose is one cup tea up to three times daily. To make tea, simmer 1 gram dried flower in 150 mL boiling water, 5-10 minutes, strain (18).

Comments

Although safflower seed oil is a rich source of linoleic acid, some experts contend gamma-linolenic acid might be more useful as a physiologic source of essential fatty acids. To be useful in the body, linoleic acid must be converted to dihomo-gamma-linolenic acid (DHGA) and arachidonic acid (6). Gamma-linolenic acid does not require this conversion before it can be used in the body.

SAFFRON

This Product is Also Known As

Autumn Crocus, Azafron, Croci stigma, Indian Saffron, Saffron Crocus, Safran, Spanish Saffron, True Saffron.

Scientific Names

Crocus sativus.
Family: Iridaceae.

People Use This For

Orally, saffron is used for asthma, insomnia, cancer (11), atherosclerosis (6), cough, whooping cough, stomach gas (11), and as a sedative (2).
In combination with opium and quinine, it is used for premature ejaculation (6).
In combination with salicylic acid and vegetable oils, an extract of saffron is used topically for treating baldness (6,11).
In Chinese medicine, saffron is used for depression, fright, shock, spitting up blood, pain and difficulties in menstruation and after childbirth (11).
In folk medicine, saffron is used as a digestive stimulant (11,18), an aphrodisiac (6,11), a pain reliever, and a sedative (2), for stimulating menstruation (11), for dry skin (6), to induce sweating, and as an expectorant.
In food, saffron is used as a culinary spice, yellow food coloring (11), and as a flavoring agent (11).
In manufacturing, saffron extracts are used as fragrance in perfumes (11) and as a dye for cloth (6).

Safety

LIKELY SAFE ...when used orally and appropriately in amounts typically found in foods. Saffron has Generally Recognized as Safe (GRAS) status in the US (11). The maximum use level is 0.1% (11).
POSSIBLY SAFE ...when the pistil and stigmata preparation is used orally in amounts up to 1.5 g per day (11,12).
...when used in excessive amounts, 5 grams can cause severe side effects (2,12); 12-20 grams can be lethal (18). There is insufficient reliable information available about the safety of the topical use of saffron.
PREGNANCY: LIKELY SAFE ...when used orally in amounts typically found in foods. LIKELY UNSAFE ...contraindicated in larger amounts, because it can cause abortion (2,18). There is insufficient reliable

information available about the safety of the topical use of saffron during pregnancy.
LACTATION: Insufficient reliable information available; avoid amounts greater than found in foods.

Effectiveness
There is insufficient reliable information available about the effectiveness of saffron.

Possible Mechanism of Action & Active Ingredients
Saffron constituents include crocin, picrocrocin, and crocetin (6,11). Picrocrocin is responsible for the characteristic bitter taste of saffron and crocin for the yellow-red color used for coloring food and cloth (11). In rabbits, crocetin appears to improve atherosclerosis by increasing plasma oxygen diffusion (6,11,18) and decreasing cholesterol and triglyceride levels (4110). In addition, crocetin binds to albumin (4109), potentially increasing oxygen diffusion and improving atherosclerosis (4109). Small amounts of saffron stimulate gastric secretions (18); larger amounts appear to stimulate uterine smooth muscle, contributing to abortifacient affects (18). Saffron extracts limit the in vitro growth of experimental tumor colony cells by inhibiting cellular nucleic acid synthesis (4104,4105).

Adverse Reactions Including Known Allergies
No adverse effects have been reported with up to 1.5 grams of saffron taken orally per day (2,11,12). Poisoning can occur with 5 grams (2,11,18), symptoms include: yellow appearance of the skin, sclera, and mucous membranes (mimicking icterus), vomiting, vertigo, bloody diarrhea, hematuria, bleeding from the nose, lips, eyelids or uterus, numbness, uremic collapse, and thrombocytopenic purpura leading to severe necrosis of the nose (2,11). 10 grams can induce abortion (2), 12-20 grams is reportedly lethal (2,12,18).
ALLERGY: Rhinoconjunctivitis and allergy induced asthma reported (4106). Anaphylactic reactions can occur within minutes of eating food prepared with saffron (4107).

Possible Interactions with Herbs & Other Dietary Supplements
CROSS-SENSITIVITY: Cross-reactivity exists between saffron and Lolium, Olea (includes olive), and Salsola species plants (4106).

Possible Interactions with Drugs
No interactions are known to occur, and there is no known reason to expect a clinically significant interaction with saffron.

Possible Interactions with Foods
No interactions are known to occur, and there is no known reason to expect a clinically significant interaction with saffron.

Possible Interactions with Lab Tests
No interactions are known to occur, and there is no known reason to expect a clinically significant interaction with saffron.

Possible Interactions with Diseases or Conditions
CROSS-ALLERGENICITY: Cross-reactivity reported between saffron and Lolium, Olea (includes olive), and Salsola species plants (4106).

Typical Dosages & Routes of Administration that are Commonly Used
ORAL: People typically use 12 to 15 stigmas (the thread-like pistils) in a cup of boiling water and drink one cup daily (5250).

Comments
None.

SAGE

This Product is Also Known As
Common Sage, Dalmatian Sage, Garden Sage, Meadow Sage, Sauge, Scarlet Sage, Spanish Sage, True Sage.
CAUTION: See separate listings for Boneset, Clary Sage, Danshen, German Sarsaparilla, Purple Loosestrife, Spearmint, and Wood Sage.

Scientific Names
Salvia officinalis; Salvia lavandulaefolia.
Family: Labiatae or Lamiaceae.

People Use This For
Orally, sage is used for loss of appetite, excessive perspiration (2,6), dysmenorrhea, diarrhea, gastritis (6), galactorrhea, reduction of saliva secretion and digestive problems including flatulence, bloating and dyspepsia (4,7,18).
Topically, sage is used as a gargle for laryngitis, pharyngitis, stomatitis, gingivitis, glossitis, minor oral injuries (4,7,18) and inflammation of the nasal mucosa (2).

As an inhalant, sage is used for asthma (6).
In foods, it is used as a culinary spice (4,5,6).
In manufacturing, sage is used as a fragrance component in soaps and cosmetics (11).

Safety
LIKELY SAFE ...when used orally in amounts typically found in foods (11). Sage is approved for use in foods in the US (11).
POSSIBLY UNSAFE ...when used orally in amounts greater than those found in foods, or when used long-term (4,5,12). Sage contains thujone constituent that can be toxic if enough is consumed (12).
LIKELY UNSAFE ...when used orally as sage oil (2,4).
There is insufficient reliable information about the safety of the topical or inhalant use of sage.
PREGNANCY: LIKELY UNSAFE ...contraindicated (2,4,5,6,12). Thujone, which is a constituent, can have menstrual stimulant and abortifacient effects (19).
LACTATION: POSSIBLY UNSAFE ...thought to reduce mother's milk supply (12,19).

Effectiveness
POSSIBLY EFFECTIVE ...when used orally for flatulence, bloating, dyspepsia, and excessive perspiration (2,6).
...when used topically for nose and throat mucous membrane inflammation (2,5).
There is insufficient reliable information available about the effectiveness of sage for its other uses.

Possible Mechanism of Action & Active Ingredients
The applicable part of sage is the leaf. Sage contains 1-2.8% of volatile oil that may be responsible for pharmacological activity. The volatile oil contains camphor and thujone which are potentially toxic (4,5). Sage seems to have antiflatulent, antispasmodic, astringent (4), antibacterial, fungistatic, virustatic, antiperspirant, secretion promoting (2), and blood sugar lowering (5) activities.

Adverse Reactions Including Known Allergies
Sage taken orally can cause cheilitis, stomatitis, dry mouth, local irritation (6), and mental and physical deterioration (5). Large amounts or prolonged use of sage leaf, or ingestion of sage oil, may cause restlessness, vomiting, vertigo, tachycardia, tremors, seizures, and kidney damage (2,4,5,12,18). Poisoning was reported following ingestion of sage oil (4).

Possible Interactions with Herbs & Other Dietary Supplements
HERBS WITH SEDATIVE PROPERTIES: Theoretically, concomitant use with herbs that have sedative properties might enhance therapeutic and adverse effects. These include calamus, calendula, California poppy, catnip, capsicum, celery, couch grass, elecampane, Siberian ginseng, German chamomile, goldenseal, gotu kola, hops, Jamaican dogwood, kava, lemon balm, St. John's wort, sassafras, scullcap, shepherd's purse, stinging nettle, valerian, wild carrot, wild lettuce, withania root, and yerba mansa (4,19).

Possible Interactions with Drugs
ANTICONVULSANTS: Some species of sage can cause convulsions. Theoretically, this might interfere with anticonvulsant drug therapy (4).
HYPOGLYCEMIC DRUGS: Theoretically, due to claims of hypoglycemic activity, sage might have additive effects and adverse effects with hypoglycemic drugs (4).
DRUGS WITH SEDATIVE PROPERTIES: Theoretically, concomitant use with drugs with sedative properties might cause additive effects and side effects (4).

Possible Interactions with Foods
No interactions are known to occur, and there is no known reason to expect a clinically significant interaction with sage.

Possible Interactions with Lab Tests
No interactions are known to occur, and there is no known reason to expect a clinically significant interaction with sage.

Possible Interactions with Diseases or Conditions
DIABETES: Sage might interfere with blood sugar control (4).
SEIZURE DISORDERS: Avoid, due to the potential for causing seizures (2,4,5,12).

Typical Dosages & Routes of Administration that are Commonly Used
ORAL: 1-2 grams leaf three times daily, or, one cup tea (steep 1-2 grams leaf in 150 mL boiling water 5-10 minutes, strain) three times daily (2,4); up to 4-6 grams leaf per day (2); not for long term use (12). Liquid extract (1:1 in 45% alcohol), 1-4 mL three times daily (4).
TOPICAL: For gargles and rinses, 2.5 grams leaf or 2-3 drops essential oil in 100 mL of water, or 5 grams alcohol extract in 1 glass of water (2).

Comments
Sage is a rich source of beta-carotene (19).

 © Copyright 2000, Natural Medicines Comprehensive Database (209) 472-2244. For updated data, go to www.NaturalDatabase.com

SALEP

This Product is Also Known As
Cuckoo Flower, Levant Salep, Orchid, Sahlep, Saloop, Satyrion.

Scientific Names
Orchis morio.
Family: Orchidaceae.

People Use This For
Orally, salep is used for diarrhea (particularly in children), heartburn, flatulence, and indigestion (18).

Safety
POSSIBLY SAFE ...when the tuber is used orally (18).
CHILDREN: Insufficient reliable information available; avoid using.
PREGNANCY AND LACTATION: Insufficient reliable information available; avoid using.

Effectiveness
There is insufficient reliable information available about the effectiveness of salep.

Possible Mechanism of Action & Active Ingredients
The applicable part of salep is the tuber. Salep contains up to 40% mucilage including glucans, glucomannans, starch, and protein (18).

Adverse Reactions Including Known Allergies
None reported (18).

Possible Interactions with Herbs & Other Dietary Supplements
Insufficient reliable information available.

Possible Interactions with Drugs
No interactions are known to occur, and there is no known reason to expect a clinically significant interaction with salep.

Possible Interactions with Foods
No interactions are known to occur, and there is no known reason to expect a clinically significant interaction with salep.

Possible Interactions with Lab Tests
No interactions are known to occur, and there is no known reason to expect a clinically significant interaction with salep.

Possible Interactions with Diseases or Conditions
No interactions are known to occur, and there is no known reason to expect a clinically significant interaction with salep.

Typical Dosages & Routes of Administration that are Commonly Used
ORAL: Used as a powdered formulation in medicinal preparations. Taken in water before or after meals (18).

Comments
None.

SAMe

This Product is Also Known As
Ademetionine, Adenosylmethionine, S-Adenosyl-L-Methionine, S-Adenosylmethionine, S-Adenosyl-Methionine, S-Adenosyl Methionine, SAM-e, Sammy.

Scientific Names
S-adenosyl-L-methionine.

People Use This For
Orally, SAMe is used for depression, heart disease (5182), fibromyalgia, osteoarthritis, bursitis, tendonitis, chronic low back pain, dementia, Alzheimer's disease, Parkinson's disease, improving intellectual performance, slowing the aging process (5187), multiple sclerosis (5232), spinal cord injury (6), seizures, migraine headache, chronic lead poisoning, disorders of porphyrin, and bilirubin metabolism (5231).
Intravenously, SAMe is used for treating depression (5231), osteoarthritis (5188), AIDS-related myelopathy (5232),

© Copyright 2000, Natural Medicines Comprehensive Database (209) 472-2244. For updated data, go to www.NaturalDatabase.com • 925

fibromyalgia (5221), liver disease, cirrhosis, and intrahepatic cholestasis (5198,5219,5231).
Intramuscularly, SAMe is injected for fibromyalgia (5231), depression (5193), and Alzheimer's disease (5220).

Safety

LIKELY SAFE ...when used orally, intravenously, or intramuscularly and appropriately (5231,5232). Serious toxicity has not been reported in multiple clinical studies involving as many as 22,000 patients and lasting from a few days to 2 years (5189,5201,5202,5209,5219,5231).

PREGNANCY: POSSIBLY SAFE ...when used intravenously short-term during the third trimester of pregnancy. In two small-scale trials, SAMe 800 mg daily was used intravenously for 14-20 days during the third trimester of pregnancy for intrahepatic cholestasis. No adverse effects in the mother or fetus were observed (5219,5231,5240). Large-scale trials are needed to confirm the safety of SAMe use in pregnancy. Use of SAMe in pregnancy should only be considered when benefits clearly outweigh the potential risks. There is insufficient reliable information available about the use of SAMe at higher doses, for extended periods of time, or during the earlier trimesters of pregnancy.

LACTATION: Insufficient reliable information available; avoid using.

Effectiveness

LIKELY EFFECTIVE ...when used orally for relieving symptoms of osteoarthritis. Multiple clinical trials have shown that SAMe is superior to placebo and comparable to NSAIDs for decreasing symptoms associated with osteoarthritis in studies lasting from several weeks to 2 years (5188,5199,5203,5204,5205,5206,5207,5208,5209,5215). Significant symptom relief with SAMe may require up to 30 days of treatment compared to only 15 days with NSAIDs. Some evidence suggests that intravenous loading doses of SAMe given over 5 days, followed by oral treatment, can speed symptom relief to 14 days (5188). ...when used intravenously or intramuscularly for short-term treatment of major depression. Several small-scale clinical trials have shown that parenterally administered SAMe is superior to placebo and possibly as effective as intravenous or oral tricyclic antidepressants in studies lasting up to 30 days (2082,3562,5184,5189,5200,5231). Significantly more studies have been done with parenteral SAMe than oral SAMe. In some trials, the antidepressant effect occurred rapidly, within 1-2 weeks of initiation of treatment (5200); however, this benefit is likely the result of the parenteral route of administration (3562). Parenteral SAMe has been used successfully in combination with an oral tricyclic antidepressant to speed the onset of antidepressant action (5193). Available studies are limited by small numbers of patients, inconsistent diagnostic criteria, and short treatment periods (5189,5231). Further study is needed to clarify benefit of extended treatment with parenteral SAMe compared to conventional antidepressant therapy.

POSSIBLY EFFECTIVE ...when used orally for short-term treatment of major depression. Several studies have shown that orally administered SAMe is superior to placebo and possibly as effective as tricyclic antidepressants in trials lasting up to 42 days (2082,2083,5189,5190,5192,5195,5196,5231). Available studies are limited by small numbers of patients, inconsistent diagnostic criteria, short treatment periods, and flawed study designs (3562,5189,5231). Well designed, large scale studies are needed to clarify the benefit of orally administered SAMe in major depression. ...when used orally for treating fibromyalgia. Two clinical trials demonstrated significant improvement in symptoms of fibromyalgia compared to placebo (5211,5241). ...when used orally or intravenously for treating intrahepatic cholestasis associated with acute or chronic liver disease. Multiple clinical trials have shown that short-term SAMe therapy is superior to placebo in decreasing pruritus, fatigue, alkaline phosphatase levels, and total and conjugated bilirubin (5219,5238,5239,5240). Trials have more frequently used injectable dosage forms than oral formulations (5219). ...when used intravenously for treating intrahepatic cholestasis due to pregnancy (ICP). One clinical trial using intravenous SAMe during the third trimester of pregnancy demonstrated significant benefit compared to placebo for normalizing liver function tests, decreasing associated symptoms, and preventing premature labor and low infant birthweight in pregnant women with ICP (5219,5240). ...when used intravenously for AIDS-related myelopathy. SAMe has investigational orphan drug status for this use (682,5217,5185,5218). ...when used orally to improve mortality and delay liver transplantation in patients with early stages of alcoholic liver cirrhosis. In one study, there was a significant decrease in overall mortality and transplantation rate when only patients with early stages of liver disease were included (1712). ...when used orally or intravenously for decreasing signs and symptoms of chronic liver disease due to medications, alcoholism, or lead poisoning. Multiple clinical trials have shown that SAMe can normalize liver enzymes, decrease bilirubin, and decrease symptoms associated with various forms of chronic liver disease. Most trials have enrolled small numbers of patients and have been short duration (5198,5231,5235,5236,5238). Large-scale studies are needed to confirm SAMe's potential benefit in liver disease.

POSSIBLY INEFFECTIVE ...when used intravenously for treating fibromyalgia (5221). ...when used orally to improve mortality and delay liver transplantation in patients with advanced alcoholic liver cirrhosis. In one trial, there was not a significant difference in mortality and transplantation rate in patients with alcoholic liver cirrhosis compared to placebo when the patient population included patients with advanced liver disease (1712).

There is insufficient reliable information available about the effectiveness of SAMe for its other uses.

Possible Mechanism of Action & Active Ingredients

S-adenosylmethionine (SAMe) is a naturally occurring molecule that is distributed throughout virtually all body tissues and fluids (5231). It plays an essential role in many biochemical reactions involving enzymatic transmethylation. It contributes to the synthesis, activation and/or metabolism of hormones, neurotransmitters, nucleic acids, proteins, phospholipids, and some drugs (5231,5232). SAMe is produced endogenously from methionine and adenosine triphosphate (ATP). SAMe synthesis is closely linked to vitamin B12 and folate metabolism (5231). Deficiencies of these vitamins can result in decreased SAMe concentrations in the central nervous system (5231). SAMe supplementation may be beneficial in osteoarthritis due to analgesic and anti-inflammatory effects. Preliminary evidence suggests SAMe might also stimulate articular cartilage growth and repair (5209). The mechanism of antidepressant effect is unknown, but SAMe is associated with increased serotonin turnover and elevated dopamine and norepinephrine levels (5196,5232). SAMe may also work by altering cellular membrane fluidity. Changes in neuronal membrane fluidity might facilitate signal transduction across membranes and increase the efficiency of receptor-effector coupling (5196). In liver disease, exogenously administered SAMe might act as an essential nutrient by restoring biochemical factors that are depleted in people with liver dysfunction. People with acute or chronic liver disease lose the ability to synthesize SAMe from methionine, which can lead to deficiencies in cysteine and choline. It can also lead to depletion of glutathione, which plays a major role in liver detoxification and antioxidant reactions. This depletion may in turn exacerbate liver disease (5198,5219,5236). SAMe may also be beneficial in AIDS-related myelopathy, by replenishing depleted endogenous SAMe. Epidemiological data suggests that people with AIDS have a deficiency of SAMe in their cerebrospinal fluid, and this may lead to myelopathy by impairing SAMe dependent myelin and oligodendrocyte repair mechanisms (682,5185,5217,5218). Some evidence suggests that SAMe might also have a gastric cytoprotective effect (5213). Exogenously administered SAMe has low oral bioavailability, presumably the result of significant first-pass effect and rapid hepatic metabolism (5231). It achieves peak plasma concentrations 3 to 5 hours after ingestion of an enteric-coated tablet (5231), has a half-life of about 100 minutes and is excreted in urine and feces (5231). SAMe crosses the blood-brain barrier (5231). SAMe is metabolized to s-adenosylhomocysteine, which can be metabolized to homocysteine (5232). Homocysteine is remethylated to form methionine, which can form more SAMe, or converted via transsulfuration to the antioxidant, glutathione (5232). These reactions require folate, cyanocobalamin, and pyridoxine (5231). Elevated levels of homocysteine have been linked to cardiovascular and renal disease (1698). The long-term effect of SAMe administration on atherosclerotic and thrombotic vascular disorders is unknown, although there was no difference in cardiovascular mortality in a study of people with cirrhosis taking SAMe 1200 mg daily for 2 years (1712). Low levels of SAMe have been correlated with coronary artery disease (1714). Administration of SAMe to healthy people has shown a positive effect on 5-methyltetrahydrofolate, a key cofactor in homocysteine metabolism. SAMe supplementation has been suggested as a remedy for elevated homocysteine levels (1713).

Adverse Reactions Including Known Allergies

When taken orally, SAMe can cause flatulence, vomiting, diarrhea, headache (347), and nausea. These side effects are more common with higher doses (5231). Anxiety has occurred in people with depression (5231) and hypomania in people with bipolar disorder (5231). When used as an injection, SAMe has caused mania in people with bipolar disorder (5216,5231).

Possible Interactions with Herbs & Other Dietary Supplements

Insufficient reliable information available.

Possible Interactions with Drugs

ANTIDEPRESSANTS: Concurrent use may cause additive serotonergic effects and serotonin syndrome-like effects, including agitation, tremors, anxiety, tachycardia, tachypnea, diarrhea, hyperreflexia, shivering, and diaphoresis (3521,5193). In a case report, SAMe 100 mg intramuscularly was given daily along with clomipramine (Anafranil) 25 mg per day. The clomipramine dose was later increased to 75 mg per day, and 48-72 hours later the patient experienced side effects similar to serotonin syndrome, requiring hospitalization (3521). Theoretically, this may also occur when SAMe is used with other tricyclic antidepressants and with non-tricyclic antidepressants (5193). Concurrent use of SAMe with imipramine (Tofranil) has resulted in a more rapid onset of antidepressant action (5193,5231). Theoretically, this effect may also occur with other antidepressants.
HEPATOTOXIC DRUGS: SAMe protects against hepatic dysfunction caused by acetaminophen, alcohol, estrogens, monoamine oxidase inhibitors, phenobarbital, phenytoin, and steroids (5231).

Possible Interactions with Foods

No interactions are known to occur, and there is no known reason to expect a clinically significant interaction with SAMe.

Possible Interactions with Lab Tests

No interactions are known to occur, and there is no known reason to expect a clinically significant interaction with SAMe.

Possible Interactions with Diseases or Conditions

BIPOLAR DISORDER: Use of SAMe can cause patients to convert from a depressed state to a hypomanic or manic state (3523).

Typical Dosages & Routes of Administration that are Commonly Used

ORAL: For depression, an oral dose of 400-1600 mg per day has been used (5231). Doses of 1600 mg per day are the most commonly used in clinical trials (5189). For osteoarthritis, an oral dose of 200 mg three times daily is typically used (5188). For alcoholic liver disease or cirrhosis, oral doses of 1200-1600 mg per day have been

© Copyright 2000, Natural Medicines Comprehensive Database (209) 472-2244. For updated data, go to www.NaturalDatabase.com

used (1712,5231,5238,5241). For intrahepatic cholestasis, an oral dose of 800 mg twice daily is typically used (5219,5231,5239). For fibromyalgia, an oral dose of 800 mg per day is typically used (5241).

PARENTERAL: For depression, an intravenous or intramuscular injection of 200-400 mg per day is typically used (5231). For speeding the onset of antidepressant effect in combination with a tricyclic antidepressant, SAMe 200 mg intramuscularly for the first 2 weeks of tricyclic antidepressant therapy has been used (5193). For osteoarthritis, an intravenous dose of 400 mg per day has been used (5188). For intrahepatic cholestasis, an intravenous dose of 800 mg per day is typically used (9,5219,5231). For intrahepatic cholestasis of pregnancy (ICP), an intravenous dose of 800 mg per day has been used (5219,5231,5240). For AIDS-related myelopathy, an intravenous dose of 800 mg daily for 14 days has been used (5217).

Comments

Early studies utilized parenteral SAMe before an oral formulation was available (5231). Currently, several oral salt forms of SAMe are available: sulfate, sulfate-p-toluenesulfonate (also labeled as tosylate), and butanedisulfonate (5231,5444,5447). The tosylate salt has a 1% oral bioavailability and the butanedisulfonate salt has a 5% oral bioavailability, presumably due to a large first pass effect (1896,1897). Concerns about the stability of the tosylate formulation have been expressed (5446), while the butanedisulfonate salt is stable for 2 years at room temperature (1896,5444).

SAMPHIRE

This Product is Also Known As
Crest Marine, Peter's Cress, Pierce-Stone, Sampier, Sea Fennel.

Scientific Names
Crithum maritimum.
Family: Umbelliferae.

People Use This For
Orally, samphire is used for "states of general resistance" and scurvy (18).

Safety
POSSIBLY SAFE ...when used orally (18).
PREGNANCY AND LACTATION: Insufficient reliable information available; avoid using.

Effectiveness
There is insufficient reliable information available about the effectiveness of samphire.

Possible Mechanism of Action & Active Ingredients
The applicable parts of samphire are the above ground parts. Samphire is thought to be a diuretic (18). It contains vitamin C (ascorbic acid) (18), which is used to treat and prevent scurvy (16).

Adverse Reactions Including Known Allergies
No adverse reactions or known allergies are generally known (18).

Possible Interactions with Herbs & Other Dietary Supplements
Insufficient reliable information available.

Possible Interactions with Drugs
No interactions are known to occur, and there is no known reason to expect a clinically significant interaction with samphire.

Possible Interactions with Foods
No interactions are known to occur, and there is no known reason to expect a clinically significant interaction with samphire.

Possible Interactions with Lab Tests
No interactions are known to occur, and there is no known reason to expect a clinically significant interaction with samphire.

Possible Interactions with Diseases or Conditions
No interactions are known to occur, and there is no known reason to expect a clinically significant interaction with samphire.

Typical Dosages & Routes of Administration that are Commonly Used
ORAL: Used as an extract and a food additive (18).

Comments

There is very little scientific information about this product. Our staff is continually analyzing the available information on natural medicines and will add data here as it becomes available.

SANDY EVERLASTING

This Product is Also Known As

Common Shrubby Everlasting, Eternal Flower, Everlasting, Fleur de Pied de Chat, Goldilocks, Harnblumen, Helichrysum, Katzenpfotchenbluten, Yellow Chaste Weed.
CAUTION: See separate listing for Immortelle.

Scientific Names

Helichrysum augustifolium, synonym Helichrysum italicum; Helichrysum stoechas; Helichrysum oriental.
Family: Asteraceae or Compositae.

People Use This For

Orally, sandy everlasting is used for peptic discomforts (2), (e.g. dyspepsia) (18), liver complaints, chronic cholecystitis, and gallbladder complaints with accompanying cramps (18).
Historically, sandy everlasting has been used as a diuretic (18), and for chronic bronchitis, asthma, whooping cough, psoriasis, burns, rheumatism, headache, migraine, allergies, and liver ailments (11).
In foods and beverages, the extract is used as a flavoring component, and in flavoring tobacco (11).
In manufacturing, it is used in perfumes, and before- and after-sun products (11).

Safety

LIKELY SAFE ...when used in amounts typically found in foods (11). Sandy everlasting has Generally Recognized as Safe (GRAS) status in the US (11).
POSSIBLY SAFE ...when used orally and appropriately (2).
PREGNANCY AND LACTATION: Insufficient reliable information available; avoid in amounts greater than amounts generally found in foods and beverages.

Effectiveness

POSSIBLY EFFECTIVE ...when used orally for treating peptic discomforts such as dyspepsia (2,18).
There is insufficient reliable information available about the effectiveness of sandy everlasting for its other uses.

Possible Mechanism of Action & Active Ingredients

The applicable part of sandy everlasting is the dried flower. Sandy everlasting contains flavonoids, quercitrin, kaempferol, naringenin, and isohelichrysin. These components might increase bile secretion. They have been shown to increase bile secretion in animals (11). The flavonoids also absorb UV light (11). Quercitrin increases the detoxifying function of the liver and exhibits anti-inflammatory activity (11). The constituent arenarin has antibacterial activity and promotes gastric and pancreatic secretions (8). The volatile oil of Helichrysum italicum flowers seems to have some antibacterial and antifungal activity (11).

Adverse Reactions Including Known Allergies

Sandy everlasting can cause an allergic reaction in individuals sensitive to the Asteraceae/Compositae family. Members of this family include ragweed, chrysanthemums, marigolds, daisies, and many other herbs.

Possible Interactions with Herbs & Other Dietary Supplements

Insufficient reliable information available.

Possible Interactions with Drugs

No interactions are known to occur, and there is no known reason to expect a clinically significant interaction with sandy everlasting.

Possible Interactions with Foods

No interactions are known to occur, and there is no known reason to expect a clinically significant interaction with sandy everlasting.

Possible Interactions with Lab Tests

No interactions are known to occur, and there is no known reason to expect a clinically significant interaction with sandy everlasting.

Possible Interactions with Diseases or Conditions

BILIARY OBSTRUCTION: Contraindicated, due to bile stimulating effects (2,18).
GALLSTONES: Sandy everlasting might complicate therapy (2,18).
CROSS-ALLERGENICITY: Can cause an allergic reaction in individuals sensitive to the Asteraceae/Compositae family. Members of this family include ragweed, chrysanthemums, marigolds, daisies, and many other herbs.

Typical Dosages & Routes of Administration that are Commonly Used

ORAL: One cup fresh tea (made by steeping 1 gram dried flower in 150 mL boiling water 5-10 minutes, strain) several times per day (8,18); average amount 3 grams of dried flower per day (2).
TOPICAL: No typical dosage.

Comments

None.

SANGRE DE GRADO

This Product is Also Known As

Blood of the Dragon, Drago, Dragon's Blood, Lan-Hiqui, Laniqui, Sangre de Drago, Sangre de Dragon, Sangue de Agua, Sangue de Drago, SP 303, SP-303, Taspine.
CAUTION: See also Dragon's Blood (Draconis resina) and Herb Robert (Geranium robertianum).

Scientific Names

Croton lechleri.
Family: Euphorbiaceae.

People Use This For

Orally, sangre de grado or its constituent, SP-303, is used for treating diarrhea associated with cholera, AIDS, traveling, cancer treatment, Clostridium difficile infection, and irritable bowel syndrome (2784,2785,2801), for supporting the body's tissue repair mechanisms (2800), and treating viral respiratory infection (2789,2804).
Topically, sangre de grado or its constituent, SP-303, is used for treating herpes simplex virus (types 1 and 2) (2787,2788).
Traditionally, sangre de grado has been used for oropharyngeal and gastrointestinal ulcers, fever, hemorrhage, bleeding gums, fractures, wound healing, hemorrhoids, eczema, insect bites and stings, vaginitis, for vaginal baths before childbirth, and as a general tonic (2802,2803,2804).

Safety

POSSIBLY SAFE ...when SP-303, a derivative of sangre de grado, is used orally and appropriately (2784). ...when SP-303, a derivative of sangre de grado, is used topically and appropriately (2787,2788).
There is insufficient reliable information available about the safety of sangre de grado.
PREGNANCY AND LACTATION: Insufficient reliable information available; avoid using.

Effectiveness

POSSIBLY EFFECTIVE ...when a standardized resin extract containing SP-303 (SB-Normal Stool Formula, ShamanBotanicals.com) is taken orally for reducing stool weight and frequency in people with AIDS-related diarrhea (2784). ...when a standardized resin extract containing SP-303 (SB-Normal Stool Formula, ShamanBotanicals.com) is taken orally for symptomatic treatment of traveler's diarrhea (2806). ...when a standardized resin extract containing SP-303 (currently unavailable in the US), is used topically for treating genital and anal herpes simplex lesions in people with AIDS (2788).
POSSIBLY INEFFECTIVE ...when a standardized resin extract containing SP-303 is used topically for treating acyclovir-unresponsive mucocutaneous herpes simplex lesions in people with AIDS (2787).
There is insufficient reliable information available about the effectiveness of sangre de grado for its other uses. However, topically applied sangre de grado resin alleviated the symptoms of insect bites (fire ants, wasps, bees) and plant reactions in a group of pest control workers. The results of this unpublished study were presented at the Pediatric Academic Societies and the American Academy of Pediatrics 2000 Joint Meeting (6114).

Possible Mechanism of Action & Active Ingredients

Sangre de grado is a tree native to the Amazon regions of South America (2805,2784). The resin, a viscous red latex, and bark have a long history of oral and topical medicinal use (2784,2797). Sangre de grado is reported to have anti-inflammatory (2804,6114), antibacterial, anti-hemorrhagic, antiseptic, and anti-tumor properties (2804). Topically, it has been shown to reduce vasodilation, swelling, and secretory response to irritants, promote mucosal healing, and prevent hyperalgesic responses in the laboratory (6114). Several active constituents of sangre de grado have been isolated, including SP-303 and tapsine (2786,2796). All published human experience has been with SP-303 (see Effectiveness). Preliminary evidence suggests that the constituent SP-303 might control diarrhea by inhibiting cyclic adenosine monophosphate (cAMP), which causes chloride and fluid secretion (2786). SP-303 shows activity against types 1 and 2 herpes simplex viruses, respiratory syncytial virus (RSV), and influenza A virus, possibly by inhibiting viral penetration of cells (2790,2791,2792,2793,2794). Tapsine demonstrates anti-inflammatory and wound healing properties when applied topically (2795,2796). Sangre de grado does not stimulate cell proliferation and has not shown carcinogenic activity after 17 months of treatment in experimental models (2796,2797,2798). Preliminary evidence suggests that sangre de grado resin is not cytotoxic, and has antibacterial and pro-oxidant activity (2798,2799).

Adverse Reactions Including Known Allergies

No serious adverse reactions or lab abnormalities have been reported in clinical studies using the sangre de grado derivative, SP-303, when given orally (2784,2806).
Topically, SP-303 can cause local pain and burning (2787). Topical sangre de grado resin can cause scarring (2803).

Possible Interactions with Herbs & Other Dietary Supplements

Insufficient reliable information available.

Possible Interactions with Drugs

No interactions are known to occur, and there is no known reason to expect a clinically significant interaction with sangre de grado.

Possible Interactions with Foods

No interactions are known to occur, and there is no known reason to expect a clinically significant interaction with sangre de grado.

Possible Interactions with Lab Tests

No interactions are known to occur, and there is no known reason to expect a clinically significant interaction with sangre de grado.

Possible Interactions with Diseases or Conditions

No interactions are known to occur, and there is no known reason to expect a clinically significant interaction with sangre de grado.

Typical Dosages & Routes of Administration that are Commonly Used

ORAL: For treating AIDS-related diarrhea, a sangre de grado extract containing 500 mg of SP-303 (SB-Normal Stool Formula, ShamanBotanicals.com) every 6 hours has been used (2784). For treating traveler's diarrhea, a sangre de grado extract containing 125-500 mg SP-303 (SB-Normal Stool Formula, ShamanBotanicals.com) 4 times daily for 2 days has been used (2806).

Comments

SP-303 was in Phase III clinical trials with "fast track" designation for treatment of AIDS-related diarrhea and Phase II trials for traveler's diarrhea (2807). After the FDA rejected a new drug application and requested additional clinical testing, the manufacturer, Shaman Pharmaceuticals, became Shaman Botanicals.com and elected to market SP-303 as a dietary supplement, SB-Normal Stool Formula (2807).

SANICLE

This Product is Also Known As

European Sanicle, Poolroot, Saniculae herba, Self-Heal, Wood Sanicle.

Scientific Names

Sanicula europaea.
Family: Apiaceae.

People Use This For

Orally, sanicle is used for mild respiratory tract mucous membrane inflammation (2), cough, and bronchitis (18).

Safety

POSSIBLY SAFE ...when used orally and appropriately (2,12).
PREGNANCY AND LACTATION: Insufficient reliable information available; avoid using.

Effectiveness

POSSIBLY EFFECTIVE ...when used orally for mild respiratory tract mucous membrane inflammation (2).

Possible Mechanism of Action & Active Ingredients

The applicable parts of sanicle are the above ground parts. Sanicle contains triterpene saponins, caffeine derivatives, and flavonoids such as rutin, isoquercitrin, astragalin. It seems to have astringent and expectorant effects (18). The expectorant effect seems to result from the irritation caused by the saponins on the gastric mucosa that reflexly stimulates the bronchial mucous glands via parasympathetic sensory pathways (7). Large amounts of saponins may cause stomach upset, nausea, and vomiting (7). In animals, sanicle demonstrates edema reduction (18).

Adverse Reactions Including Known Allergies

Theoretically, when taken orally in large amounts, sanicle may cause upset stomach, nausea, and vomiting due to saponin content (7).

Possible Interactions with Herbs & Other Dietary Supplements

Insufficient reliable information available.

Possible Interactions with Drugs
No interactions are known to occur, and there is no known reason to expect a clinically significant interaction with sanicle.

Possible Interactions with Foods
No interactions are known to occur, and there is no known reason to expect a clinically significant interaction with sanicle.

Possible Interactions with Lab Tests
No interactions are known to occur, and there is no known reason to expect a clinically significant interaction with sanicle.

Possible Interactions with Diseases or Conditions
GI MUCOSAL IRRITATION (e.g. ulcers, etc.): Theoretically, contraindicated, may exacerbate existing GI mucosal irritation due to saponin content (6).

Typical Dosages & Routes of Administration that are Commonly Used
ORAL: 4-6 grams dried above ground parts or per day (2).

Comments
Avoid confusion with Prunella vulgaris, also referred to as self-heal. In commerce, sanicle may be mixed with leaves of Cardamine enneaphylos, and Astrantia major is sometimes labeled as sanicle (18).

SARSAPARILLA

This Product is Also Known As
Ecuadorian Sarsaparilla, Honduras Sarsaparilla, Jamaican Sarsaparilla, Mexican Sarsaparilla, Salsaparilha, Salsepareille, Sarsa, Sarsaparillae radix, Sarsaparillewurzel, Smilax.
CAUTION: See separate listings for Couch Grass, German Sarsaparilla, and Tormentil.

Scientific Names
Smilax medica, synonyms Smilax aristolochiifolia, Smilax aristolochiaefolii; Smilax regelii, synonym Smilax officinalis; Smilax febrifuga; Smilax regelii; other Smilax species.
Family: Smilacaceae.

People Use This For
Orally, sarsaparilla root is used for psoriasis (2,4) and other skin diseases (2), rheumatoid arthritis (2,4), kidney disease, as an anabolic for performance enhancement or body-building in athletes (5,11), and as a diuretic and diaphoretic (2). Mexican and Honduran sarsaparilla have been used for treating gonorrhea, fevers, and digestive disorders (11).
Traditionally, sarsaparilla has been used as an adjunct for treating leprosy (4) and for syphilis (3,5,11).
In manufacturing, sarsaparilla is used as a flavoring agent in foods, beverages (2,11), and pharmaceuticals (3,4).

Safety
LIKELY SAFE ...when used in the amounts commonly found in foods (11). It is approved for food use in the US (11).
POSSIBLY SAFE ...when used orally and appropriately for medicinal purposes (12).
POSSIBLY UNSAFE ...when used in excessive amounts and should be avoided due to the possible gastrointestinal irritation of its saponin constituents (4).
PREGNANCY AND LACTATION: Insufficient reliable information available and excessive amounts can have irritant effects; avoid using (4).

Effectiveness
There is insufficient reliable information available about the effectiveness of sarsaparilla.

Possible Mechanism of Action & Active Ingredients
The applicable part of sarsaparilla is the root. Sarsaparilla can have antirheumatic, antiseptic, and antipruritic activity (4). It contains about 2% saponins and other varied constituents, including quercetin and phytosterols (beta-sitosterol, stigmasterol, pollinastanol). The saponins, including sarsasapogenin and smilagenin (3,4,5,11), exhibit diuretic, diaphoretic, expectorant, and laxative effects (5). The sterols contained in sarsaparilla are not anabolic steroids nor are they converted in vivo to anabolic steroids (3,11). Testosterone has never been detected in any plant, including sarsaparilla (3,5). Sarsaparilla also improves appetite and digestion (4), and its extracts can improve psoriasis symptoms (4). Sarsaparilla shows liver-protective and anti-inflammatory activity in rats (4).

Adverse Reactions Including Known Allergies

Sarsaparilla taken orally can cause gastric irritation with excessive amounts or temporary kidney impairment (11). Large doses can lead to European cholera, worsened diuresis, and shock (18). Occupational exposure to sarsaparilla root dust can cause rhinitis and asthma symptoms (4111).

Possible Interactions with Herbs & Other Dietary Supplements

DIGITALIS: Sarsaparilla can increase digitalis glycoside absorption (2,11).
OTHER HERBS: Theoretically, sarsaparilla can alter the absorption or elimination of simultaneously administered herbs, which will effect the herbs' actions (2).

Possible Interactions with Drugs

DIGOXIN: Sarsaparilla can increase digitalis glycoside absorption (2,11).
ORAL DRUGS: Theoretically, sarsaparilla increases the absorption or elimination of simultaneously administered drugs, resulting in unpredictable effects (2).
HYPNOTIC DRUGS: Sarsaparilla can accelerate the elimination of these drugs (2,11).

Possible Interactions with Foods

No interactions are known to occur, and there is no known reason to expect a clinically significant interaction with sarsaparilla.

Possible Interactions with Lab Tests

No interactions are known to occur, and there is no known reason to expect a clinically significant interaction with sarsaparilla.

Possible Interactions with Diseases or Conditions

ASTHMA: Sarsaparilla root dust can cause the symptoms of asthma (4111).
KIDNEY DYSFUNCTION: Theoretically, sarsaparilla can exacerbate kidney impairment (2,11).

Typical Dosages & Routes of Administration that are Commonly Used

ORAL: The typical oral dose of sarsaparilla is 1-4 grams of the dried root or one cup of the tea three times daily. The tea is prepared by simmering 1-4 grams of the dried root in boiling water for 5-10 minutes and then straining (4). The typical dose of the liquid extract (1:1 in 20% alcohol, 10% glycerol) is 8-15 mL (4).

Comments

In the Old West of the United States, sarsaparilla was the most popular drink of the cowboys (6002). Avoid confusion with Indian or false sarsaparilla (Hemidesmus indicus, Family: Asclepiadaceae), reportedly a widespread adulterant of sarsaparilla (3,5,11). False sarsaparilla contains none of the saponins or other principal constituents found in sarsaparilla (5).

SASSAFRAS

This Product is Also Known As

Ague Tree, Cinnamon Wood, Common Sassafras, Kuntze Saloop, Sassafrax, Saxifrax.

Scientific Names

Sassafras ablidum, synonyms Sassafras officinale, Sassafras varifolium.
Family: Lauraceae.

People Use This For

Orally, sassafras root bark is used for urinary tract disorders, mucous membrane inflammation, syphilis (18), and as a tonic and "blood purifier"(3).
Topically, the root bark is used to treat skin eruptions, rheumatism, eye inflammation, sprains, swelling, and for relief of insect bites or stings (6). Topically, sassafras oil is used as an antiseptic and pediculicide (4).
In folk medicine, it has been used for bronchitis, geriatric high blood pressure, gout, arthritis, skin problems, kidney disorders, and cancers (11).
In beverages and candy, a safrole-free bark extract has limited use as a flavoring agent (11).

Safety

POSSIBLY SAFE ...when consumed in amounts found in foods and beverages if safrole-free (11). Safrole-free sassafras is approved for food use in the US (11). The maximum level used is 0.22% extract in nonalcoholic beverages.
POSSIBLY UNSAFE ...when safrole-free sassafras is used in amounts larger than food. Some studies link even safrole-free sassafras extracts to tumors (515).
LIKELY UNSAFE ...when taken as an oral medicinal agent; avoid using (3,4). Sassafras root bark and oil contain safrole and related compounds that are carcinogenic and hepatotoxic in animals (4,12,17). Consumption of 5 mL sassafras oil can be fatal in adults (4). ...when used topically; avoid external use due to toxic safrole content (4).

© Copyright 2000, Natural Medicines Comprehensive Database (209) 472-2244. For updated data, go to www.NaturalDatabase.com • 933

CHILDREN: LIKELY UNSAFE ...a few drops of sassafras oil can be fatal (4).
PREGNANCY AND LACTATION: LIKELY UNSAFE ...contraindicated (12). Sassafras oil has abortifacient effects (4).

Effectiveness
POSSIBLY INEFFECTIVE ...as a tonic and "blood purifier" (3).
There is insufficient reliable information available about the effectiveness of sassafras for its other uses.

Possible Mechanism of Action & Active Ingredients
The applicable part of sassafras is the root bark. The major constituent of the volatile oil, safrole, is carcinogenic (causes malignant liver tumors in experimental animals) (6,11). Safrole and its metabolite, 1-hydroxysafrole, are neurotoxic (6).

Adverse Reactions Including Known Allergies
Taken orally, sassafras can cause diaphoresis and hot flashes (11). Consumption of large amounts of sassafras oil can cause hallucinations lasting for several days (4). In adults, 5 mL sassafras oil can cause shakes, vomiting, dilated pupils, hypertension, tachycardia, stupor, collapse (6), abortion, paralysis, liver cancer, and death (4,6). A few drops of sassafras oil may be fatal in children (4). Topical application can result in contact dermatitis (6).

Possible Interactions with Herbs & Other Dietary Supplements
SAFROLE-CONTAINING HERBS: Avoid concomitant use with other safrole-containing herbs due to potential for additive toxicity (12). Other herbs that contain safrole include basil, camphor, cinnamon, and nutmeg (12).
HERBS WITH SEDATIVE PROPERTIES: Theoretically, concomitant use with herbs that have sedative properties might enhance therapeutic and adverse effects. These include calamus, calendula, California poppy, catnip, capsicum, celery, couch grass, elecampane, Siberian ginseng, German chamomile, goldenseal, gotu kola, hops, Jamaican dogwood, kava, lemon balm, sage, St. John's wort, scullcap, shepherd's purse, stinging nettle, valerian, wild carrot, wild lettuce, withania, and yerba mansa (4,19).

Possible Interactions with Drugs
BARBITURATES: Theoretically, concomitant use with barbiturates may cause additive effects (19).
OTHER DRUGS WITH SEDATIVE PROPERTIES: Theoretically, concomitant use with drugs with sedative properties may cause additive effects (19).

Possible Interactions with Foods
No interactions are known to occur, and there is no known reason to expect a clinically significant interaction with sassafras.

Possible Interactions with Lab Tests
PHENYTOIN: Sassafras oil may cause false-positive blood phenytoin test results (6).

Possible Interactions with Diseases or Conditions
URINARY CONDITIONS: CAUTION; sassafras can aggravate urinary irritation (19).

Typical Dosages & Routes of Administration that are Commonly Used
No typical dosage.

Comments
Sassafras is considered likely unsafe; avoid due to toxic safrole content. Use only safrole-free extract and leaves. Sassafras was used in the past to flavor root beer (11). In 1976, the FDA banned marketing of sassafras for sassafras tea (4). One study estimates that safrole 0.66 mg/kg could be toxic. One cup of tea made with 2.5 grams of sassafras is estimated to contain 200 mg of safrole (approximately 3 mg/kg) (4).

SAVIN TOPS

This Product is Also Known As
Sabina, Savin, Savine.

Scientific Names
Juniperus sabina.

People Use This For
Orally, the branches and leaves of savin tops are used to induce abortions (18).
Topically, they are used as a powder to treat fig warts (18).

Safety
POSSIBLY UNSAFE ...when used topically. Savin tops can cause severe irritation of skin and mucous membranes (18).

UNSAFE ...when used orally. Savin tops may be fatal if ingested as a powder or tea; 6 drops of the volatile oil can cause death (18).
PREGNANCY: UNSAFE ...contraindicated due to overall toxicity as well as ability to induce abortions (19).
LACTATION: Insufficient reliable information available; avoid using.

Effectiveness
There is insufficient reliable information available about the effectiveness of savin tops.

Possible Mechanism of Action & Active Ingredients
The applicable parts of savin tops are the branches and leaves. Savin tops contains ligans (thujone, podophyllotoxin, and others), hydroxycoumarins, and volatile oil (3-5%) including sabinyl acetate and sabinene (18). The ligans may have antineoplastic and antiviral properties (18). Savin tops has powerful irritant properties that can cause inflammation of the skin and mucous membranes (18,19).

Adverse Reactions Including Known Allergies
Symptoms of poisoning include queasiness, cardiac rhythm disorders, spasm, kidney damage, hematuria, central paralysis, unconsciousness and death (18). Ingestion can also cause irritation of the mucous membranes resulting in gastroenteritis, hepatitis, pneumonitis, and nephritis (19). When used topically, the volatile oil can cause skin irritation, blisters, necroses, and resorbent poisoning (18).

Possible Interactions with Herbs & Other Dietary Supplements
Insufficient reliable information available.

Possible Interactions with Drugs
No interactions are known to occur, and there is no known reason to expect a clinically significant interaction with savin tops.

Possible Interactions with Foods
No interactions are known to occur, and there is no known reason to expect a clinically significant interaction with savin tops.

Possible Interactions with Lab Tests
No interactions are known to occur, and there is no known reason to expect a clinically significant interaction with savin tops.

Possible Interactions with Diseases or Conditions
INFLAMMATION: Components of the essential oil (sabinene and sabinyl acetate) may increase irritation of the skin or mucous membranes (19).

Typical Dosages & Routes of Administration that are Commonly Used
ORAL: No typical dosage.
TOPICAL: Powder applied twice daily (amount unspecified); "put bandages into skin folds" (18).

Comments
Savin tops are likely unsafe; avoid due to toxic safrole content. Use only safrole-free extract and leaves. The toxicity of the oil depends on how long it has been stored. Toxicity of oil develops over time through terpene peroxide formation (18). The toxicity of fresh branch tips is apparently low.

SAW PALMETTO

This Product is Also Known As
American Dwarf Palm Tree, Cabbage Palm, Palmier Nain, Sabal, Sabal Fructus, Saw Palmetto Berry.

Scientific Names
Serenoa repens, synonyms Serenoa serrulata, Sabal serrulata.
Family: Arecaceae/Palmaceae.

People Use This For
Orally, saw palmetto is used for symptoms of benign prostatic hyperplasia (BPH) (2,4). It is also used as a mild diuretic (6), a sedative, an anti-inflammatory, and as an antiseptic (4208).
Saw palmetto is also used in combination with seven other herbs (PC-SPES) to treat prostate cancer (5548).
Historically, saw palmetto has been used to increase breast size, to improve sexual vigor, and as an aphrodisiac (6,515). In the past it has also been used orally to stimulate hair growth (515), treat colds, coughs, irritated mucous membranes, sore throat, asthma, chronic bronchitis, migraines, and cancer. The powdered fruit has been used as a uterine and vaginal tonic suppository (11).

© Copyright 2000, Natural Medicines Comprehensive Database (209) 472-2244. For updated data, go to www.NaturalDatabase.com

Safety

LIKELY SAFE ...when used orally and appropriately (2,4,12,2735).

POSSIBLY SAFE ...when used orally in a specific herbal combination (PC-SPES) (5548).

PREGNANCY AND LACTATION: LIKELY UNSAFE ...when used orally. Saw palmetto has antiandrogen and estrogenic activity (4,6,11); contraindicated.

Effectiveness

LIKELY EFFECTIVE ...when used orally for treating symptoms of benign prostatic hyperplasia (BPH) (2,4,7,5094). Clinical studies have used a liposterolic extract of saw palmetto berry containing 80-90% fatty acids. Improvement can take up to two months of treatment (2732).

POSSIBLY EFFECTIVE ...when used orally in a specific herbal combination for prostate cancer. Studies using saw palmetto in combination with seven other herbs (PC-SPES) in prostate cancer patients, found that it significantly decreases prostate-specific antigen (PSA) levels (5548,5122,5913), causes tumor cell death (5913), and causes clinically significant reductions in testosterone (5548). In two reports, PSA levels fell significantly within 1 month of treatment (5548,5122).

POSSIBLY INEFFECTIVE ...when a saw palmetto herbal blend is used orally for treating symptoms of BPH. In a double-blind, placebo controlled trial, an herbal product containing saw palmetto lipoidal extract 106 mg, nettle root extract 80 mg, pumpkin seed oil extract 160 mg, lemon bioflavonoid extract 33 mg, and vitamin A (100% as beta-carotene) 190 IU taken three times daily for six months failed to significantly improve symptoms in a group of men with BPH (5093).

There is insufficient reliable information available about the effectiveness of saw palmetto for its other uses.

Possible Mechanism of Action & Active Ingredients

The applicable part of saw palmetto is the ripe fruit. Saw palmetto is used most commonly for treating the symptoms of benign prostatic hyperplasia (BPH). BPH can result from increased dihydrotestosterone (DHT) synthesis in the prostate and a shift favoring estrogen in the androgen and estrogen ratio (7). It is believed that saw palmetto inhibits dihydrotestosterone binding at androgen receptors and 5-alpha-reductase activity on testosterone, preventing the conversion of testosterone to DHT. However, 5-alpha-reductase levels in prostatic tissue and serum testosterone, DHT, and PSA are not significantly reduced by saw palmetto (4,2735). Besides possible hormonal mechanisms, saw palmetto might inhibit growth factors and exert an anti-inflammatory effect (3,2735). In addition, saw palmetto demonstrates alpha-adrenergic inhibitory properties (5095). Saw palmetto does not affect overall prostate size, but shrinks the inner prostatic epithelium (transition zone) (12,2736,5093). Saw palmetto berry and lipophilic berry extract can improve BPH symptom scores and measurements of urine flow, and reduce frequency of nocturia and ultrasound-determined residual urine volumes (7,2732,2733,2734,2735,2736). The lipid fraction of the volatile oil and fatty oils contains the constituents active in treating BPH (3,6). Water extraction (including brewed tea) might not adequately extract fat-soluble active constituents (2738). The most effective saw palmetto products seem to be whole berries or berry extracts prepared with nonpolar solvents (2738).

Adverse Reactions Including Known Allergies

Saw palmetto can cause headache (6) and rarely stomach problems (2). There is one case report of cholestatic hepatitis associated with the use of the multi-ingredient product, Prostata, that contains saw palmetto (598), and one case reported of decreased ejaculatory volume associated with an herbal blend product containing saw palmetto extract, nettle root extract, pumpkin seed oil extract, lemon bioflavonoid extract, and beta-carotene (5093). Some clinicians are concerned that saw palmetto may cause erectile dysfunction, ejaculatory disturbance, or altered libido because of saw palmetto's potential effects on 5-alpha-reductase. However, this side effect has not been described in the literature.

Possible Interactions with Herbs & Other Dietary Supplements

Insufficient reliable information available.

Possible Interactions with Drugs

ORAL CONTRACEPTIVES, HORMONE THERAPY: Concomitant use with saw palmetto can interfere with oral contraceptives and hormone therapy (4).

Possible Interactions with Foods

No interactions are known to occur, and there is no known reason to expect a clinically significant interaction with saw palmetto.

Possible Interactions with Lab Tests

PROSTATE-SPECIFIC ANTIGEN: Contrary to earlier concerns, saw palmetto extract appears to have no significant effect on serum prostate-specific antigen (PSA) levels (764).

Possible Interactions with Diseases or Conditions

No interactions are known to occur, and there is no known reason to expect a clinically significant interaction with saw palmetto.

Typical Dosages & Routes of Administration that are Commonly Used

ORAL: For treating symptoms of benign prostatic hyperplasia, the recommended daily dose is 1-2 grams of whole berries or 320 mg of a lipophilic extract, prepared with a lipophilic solvent such as hexane or ethanol 90% v/v (2,2738). A liquid extract (concentration unspecified) is commonly dosed as 0.6-1.5 mL (4). A tea prepared by simmering 0.5-1 grams of dried berry in 150 mL boiling water for 5-10 minutes and then straining is taken three times daily (4). However, brewed teas or other hydrophilic preparations might not contain adequate active constituents (see Mechanism of Action) (2738). Clinical studies reporting effectiveness of saw palmetto for BPH have used liposterolic extracts containing 80-90% fatty acids. Products with extracts containing 80-90% fatty acids include Saw Palmetto (Nature's Way), Masculex, ProstaMed, and Saw Palmetto Complex (Enzymatic Therapy). Prostate problems should not be self-treated (12).

Comments

Perhaps even before the time of the Mayan Indians, people were using saw palmetto as a tonic (4208). In the first half of the twentieth century, saw palmetto tea was included in the United States Pharmacopeia and the National Formulary (4229).

SCARLET PIMPERNEL

This Product is Also Known As

Adder's Eyes, Phytoestrogen, Poor Man's Weatherglass, Red Chickweed, Red Pimpernel, Shepherd's Barometer.

Scientific Names

Anagallis arvensis.
Family: Primulaceae.

People Use This For

Orally, scarlet pimpernel is used for depression, mucous membrane disorders, liver disorders, herpes, and as supportive therapy for carcinomas. It is also used orally for painful kidney disorders, particularly those with inflammation and an increase in urination.
Topically, scarlet pimpernel is used for poorly healing wounds and pruritus.
It is used both orally and topically to treat painful joints (18).

Safety

POSSIBLY UNSAFE ...when used orally or topically long-term (18).
There is insufficient reliable information available about the safety of scarlet pimpernel for short-term oral or topical use.
PREGNANCY: LIKELY UNSAFE ... when used orally or topically long-term. Scarlet pimpernel shows evidence of uterine stimulant activity (18).
LACTATION: POSSIBLY UNSAFE ...when used orally or topically long-term; avoid using.

Effectiveness

There is insufficient reliable information available about the effectiveness of scarlet pimpernel.

Possible Mechanism of Action & Active Ingredients

The applicable parts of scarlet pimpernel are the above ground flowering plant parts. In vitro data suggests that the aqueous extract has fungitoxic activity, and the isolated components triterpenglycoside, anagalloside and aglycon anagalligenone have bacteriostatic activity. Animal and human tissue data suggests uterine contracting activity. Triterepene saponins isolated from scarlet pimpernel may have activity against human sperm and may have estrogenic activity. A methanolic extract has hemolytic activity in human blood, and has activity against herpes simplex I, adenovirus type II, and polio type II. The gastroenteritis and nephritis that occurs with large doses or long-term administration is probably due to the cucurbitacins that are present in scarlet pimpernel (18).

Adverse Reactions Including Known Allergies

None reported with short-term use. With large doses or long-term administration, gastroenteritis and nephritis may occur (18).

Possible Interactions with Herbs & Other Dietary Supplements

Insufficient reliable information available.

Possible Interactions with Drugs

No interactions are known to occur, and there is no known reason to expect a clinically significant interaction with scarlet pimpernel.

Possible Interactions with Foods

No interactions are known to occur, and there is no known reason to expect a clinically significant interaction with scarlet pimpernel.

Possible Interactions with Lab Tests

No interactions are known to occur, and there is no known reason to expect a clinically significant interaction with scarlet pimpernel.

Possible Interactions with Diseases or Conditions

No interactions are known to occur, and there is no known reason to expect a clinically significant interaction with scarlet pimpernel.

Typical Dosages & Routes of Administration that are Commonly Used

ORAL: One cup of tea is taken throughout the day. The tea is prepared by steeping teaspoons of dried plant in 150 mL of boiling water for 10 minutes and straining. The usual daily dosage can be up to 1.8 grams 4 times daily (18).
TOPICAL: No typical dosage.

Comments

None.

SCHISANDRA

This Product is Also Known As

Bac Ngu Vi Tu, Beiwuweizi, Bei Wu Wei Zi, Chinesischer Limonenbaum, Chosen-Gomischi, Five-Flavor-Fruit, Five-Flavor-Seed, Gomishi, Hoku-Gomishi, Kita-Gomishi, Limonnik Kitajskij, M Mei Gee, Magnolia Vine, Matsbouza, Nanwuweizi, Ngu Mei Gee, Northern Schisandra, Omicha, Schisandra Berry, Schizandra, Southern Schisandra, Wuweizi, Wu-Wei-Zi, Wu Wei Zi, Western Shisandra, Xiwuweizi.

Scientific Names

Schisandra chinensis; Schisandra splenanthera; other Schisandra species.
Family: Schisandraceae.

People Use This For

Orally, schisandra is used as an adaptogen for increasing resistance to disease and stress, increasing energy (515), and increasing physical performance and endurance (3559). Schisandra is also used orally for improving vision, boosting muscular activity, improving cellular energy, for hepatitis, liver protection, preventing premature aging, increasing lifespan, for premenstrual syndrome, stimulating the immune system, speeding recovery after surgery, protecting against radiation, counteracting the effects of sugar, preventing motion sickness, normalizing blood sugar and blood pressure, reducing high cholesterol, preventing infection, improving adrenal health, and energizing RNA-DNA to rebuild cells (515).

In traditional Chinese medicine, schisandra is used for coughs, asthma, insomnia, neurasthenia, chronic diarrhea, dysentery, night sweats, spontaneous sweating, involuntary seminal discharge, thirst, impotence, physical exhaustion, excessive urination (11), depression, irritability, and memory loss (6).
Schisandra fruit is eaten as a food (11).

Safety

POSSIBLY SAFE ...when used orally and appropriately (12,3559).
PREGNANCY: POSSIBLY UNSAFE; avoid using. Some evidence suggests schisandra fruit is a uterine stimulant (11,3559).
LACTATION: Insufficient reliable information; avoid using.

Effectiveness

POSSIBLY EFFECTIVE ...when schisandra fruit extract is used orally for improving liver function in patients with hepatitis (3559). Schisandra fruit extracts reduce serum glutamic-pyruvic transaminase (SGPT) levels in patients with viral or drug-induced hepatitis (3559). ...when schisandra fruit extract is used orally for improving concentration, coordination, and endurance (3559).
There is insufficient reliable information available about the effectiveness of schisandra for its other uses.

Possible Mechanism of Action & Active Ingredients

The applicable part of schisandra is the fruit. A variety of active constituents including schizandrins, schizandrols, gomisins, schizandrers, schisantherins, wuweizisus, and many others, collectively known as lignans, have been isolated from schisandra (11,3559). Some schisandra extracts are standardized based on specific lignan content (3559). Schisandra improves liver function by increasing hepatic glutathione, glucose-6-phosphate, and glutathione-reductase activity. It might also have a hepatoprotective effect by inhibiting lipid peroxidation, increasing liver glycogen production, inducing the hepatic microsomal cytochrome P-450 system, and promoting hepatocyte growth (11,3559). Schisandra is referred to as an adaptogen; it increases concentration, coordination, and endurance in workers and athletes (3559). The mechanism(s) for these effects is not known. Schisandra also has antioxidant and anti-inflammatory properties (3559). Other reported properties of various schisandra lignans include antitussive (6), anticonvulsant, antidepressant, antifatigue, tranquilizing, respiratory stimulant (11), and platelet activating factor (PAF) inhibition (3767).

Adverse Reactions Including Known Allergies

Schisandra used orally can cause heartburn, acid indigestion, decreased appetite, stomach pain, allergic skin rashes, urticaria (11,3559), and severe CNS depression (6).

Possible Interactions with Herbs & Other Dietary Supplements

Insufficient reliable information available.

Possible Interactions with Drugs

HEPATICALLY METABOLIZED DRUGS: Theoretically, concurrent administration may interfere with metabolism of some drugs, due to the hepatic enzyme-activating effects of schisandra (6).

Possible Interactions with Foods

No interactions are known to occur, and there is no known reason to expect a clinically significant interaction with schisandra.

Possible Interactions with Lab Tests

SERUM GLUTAMIC-PYRUVIC TRANSAMINASE (SGPT)/ALANINE AMINOTRANSFERASE (ALT): Schisandra might lower serum SGPT/ALT levels and test results (11,3559).

Possible Interactions with Diseases or Conditions

GASTROESOPHAGEAL REFLUX DISEASE (GERD), PEPTIC ULCER DISEASE (PUD): Schisandra might exacerbate GERD or PUD by increasing gastric acidity (3559).
EPILEPSY: One source recommends avoiding use in these patients (3559). The reason for this warning is not clear, but it may be due to schisandra's potential CNS stimulating effects (6).
HIGH INTRACRANIAL PRESSURE: One source recommends avoiding use in these patients (3559). The reason for this warning is not clear, but it may be due to schisandra's potential CNS stimulating effects (6).

Typical Dosages & Routes of Administration that are Commonly Used

ORAL: For hepatitis, schisandra extract standardized to 20 mg lignan content (equivalent to 1.5 grams crude schisandra) given daily has been used (3559). For improving mental and physical performance, schisandra extract 500 mg to 2 grams daily or crude schisandra 1.5-6 grams daily have been used (3559); Crude schisandra decoction (boiled tea) 5-15 grams daily has also been used (3559). People have also taken schisandra extract 100 mg twice daily (6002). Appropriate dosing may vary depending on extract type and standardization.

Comments

Some evidence suggests that nigranoic acid, isolated from the stem of Schisandra sphaerandra, might be useful in HIV therapy. In vitro it exhibits anti-HIV reverse transcriptase and polymerase activity (3768). An antihepatotoxic drug known as DBD has been developed in China derived from the schisandra constituent schisandrin C (3559).

SCOPOLIA

This Product is Also Known As

Belladonna, Belladonna Scopola, Glockenbilsenkraut, Japanese Belladonna, Russian Krainer Tollkraut, Scopola, Scopoliae Rhizoma.

Scientific Names

Scopolia carniolica.
Family: Solanaceae.

People Use This For

Orally, scopolia root or rhizome is used for spasms of the gastrointestinal (GI) tract, bile ducts, and urinary tract (2), and for liver and gallbladder complaints (18).
In folk medicine, scopolia is used orally as a diuretic, a sedative, a hypnotic, a narcotic, for dilating pupils, and for pain relief (4017).

Safety

LIKELY UNSAFE ...when used orally for self-medication (12). Use of scopolia requires monitoring (12). The lethal adult dose is considered to be 100 mg of atropine which is approximately 20-50 grams of scopolia root or rhizome depending on its alkaloid content (18).
PREGNANCY AND LACTATION: LIKELY UNSAFE ...when used orally for self-medication (12); avoid using.

Effectiveness

LIKELY EFFECTIVE ...when used for spasms of the gastrointestinal (GI) tract, bile ducts, and urinary tract for adults and children older than 6 years (2).
There is insufficient reliable information available about the effectiveness of scopolia for its other uses.

Possible Mechanism of Action & Active Ingredients

The applicable parts of scopolia are the rhizome and root. Scopolia root or rhizome contains 0.3-0.8% alkaloids, primarily L-hyoscyamine and lesser amounts of atropine and scopolamine (2). L-Hyoscyamine, the levorotatory isomer of atropine, is considered the active principle (2). Scopolia root has parasympatholytic activity. It is a competitive antagonist of acetylcholine, acting preferentially at the muscarinic receptors (2). Scopolia has antispasmodic effects, relaxing the smooth muscle of the gastrointestinal tract and bile ducts (2). Scopolia root can eliminate muscular tremors and muscular rigidity caused by central nervous impulses. It also has positive chronotropic and dromotropic effects (2).

Adverse Reactions Including Known Allergies

Scopolia root can cause dry mouth, dry, reddened skin, hyperthermia, disturbance of ocular accommodation, tachycardia, difficulty urinating, glaucoma attacks (2), and constipation (18). Early symptoms of poisoning include reddened skin, dry mouth, and tachycardiac arrhythmias (18). Ingestion of large amounts can cause central excitation including restlessness, compulsive speech, hallucinations, delirium, manic episodes, followed by exhaustion and sleep, and asphyxiation (18).

Possible Interactions with Herbs & Other Dietary Supplements

ANTICHOLINERGIC HERBS: Can potentiate the effects and adverse effects of other herbs with anticholinergic activity including belladonna, henbane, mandrake, and jimson weed (12).

Possible Interactions with Drugs

ANTICHOLINERGIC DRUGS: The alkaloid constituents, hyoscyamine, scopolamine, and atropine could potentiate the effects and adverse effects of anticholinergic drugs (15).
TRICYCLIC ANTIDEPRESSANTS: Concomitant use can potentiate anticholinergic effects and adverse effects (2).
AMANTADINE: Concomitant use might increase effects (2).
QUINIDINE: Concomitant use might increase effects (2).

Possible Interactions with Foods

No interactions are known to occur, and there is no known reason to expect a clinically significant interaction with scopolia.

Possible Interactions with Lab Tests

No interactions are known to occur, and there is no known reason to expect a clinically significant interaction with scopolia.

Possible Interactions with Diseases or Conditions

CONGESTIVE HEART FAILURE (CHF): Contraindicated; scopolia might cause tachycardia and exacerbate CHF due to its hyoscyamine (atropine) and scopolamine content (15).
CONSTIPATION: Contraindicated; scopolia might cause constipation due to its hyoscyamine (atropine) and scopolamine content (15).
DOWN SYNDROME: Caution, patients with Down syndrome might be hypersensitive to the antimuscarinic effects (mydriasis, positive chronotropic heart effects, etc.) of hyoscyamine (atropine) and scopolamine contained in scopolia (15).
ESOPHAGEAL REFLUX: Contraindicated; scopolia might delay gastric emptying and decrease lower esophageal pressure, promoting gastric retention and exacerbating reflux due to its hyoscyamine (atropine) and scopolamine content (15).
FEVER: Contraindicated; scopolia might increase the risk of hyperthermia in patients with fever due to its hyoscyamine (atropine) and scopolamine content (15).
GASTRIC ULCER: Contraindicated; scopolia might delay gastric emptying and exacerbate gastric ulcers due to its hyoscyamine (atropine) and scopolamine content (15).
GI INFECTIONS: Contraindicated; scopolia might suppress GI motility causing retention of infecting organisms or toxins due to its hyoscyamine (atropine) and scopolamine content (15).
HIATAL HERNIA: Contraindicated; scopolia might delay gastric emptying and decrease lower esophageal pressure, promoting gastric retention and exacerbating reflux due to its hyoscyamine (atropine) and scopolamine content (15).
TOXIC MEGACOLON: Contraindicated; scopolia might suppress intestinal motility, which might produce paralytic ileus and exacerbate toxic megacolon, due to its hyoscyamine (atropine) and scopolamine content (2,15).
NARROW-ANGLE GLAUCOMA: Contraindicated; scopolia might increase ocular tension in patients with narrow-angle (angle-closure) glaucoma due to its hyoscyamine (atropine) and scopolamine content (2,15).
OBSTRUCTIVE GI TRACT DISEASE: Contraindicated; scopolia might exacerbate obstructive GI tract diseases (including atony, paralytic ileus, and stenosis) due to its hyoscyamine (atropine) and scopolamine content (15).
TACHYARRHYTHMIAS: Contraindicated; scopolia might cause tachycardia due to its hyoscyamine (atropine)

and scopolamine content (2,15).
URINARY RETENTION: Contraindicated; scopolia might increase urinary retention due to its hyoscyamine
(atropine) and scopolamine content (2,15).
ULCERATIVE COLITIS: Contraindicated; scopolia might suppress intestinal motility, which might produce
paralytic ileus and precipitate toxic megacolon, due to its hyoscyamine (atropine) and scopolamine content (15).

Typical Dosages & Routes of Administration that are Commonly Used
ORAL: The average daily dose is 0.25 mg total alkaloids calculated as hyoscyamine (2). The maximum single dose
is 1 mg total alkaloids calculated as hyoscyamine (2). The maximum daily dose is 3 mg total alkaloids calculated as
hyoscyamine. Scopolia is administered as pulverized root, powder, or other preparations (2).

Comments
Scopolia is likely unsafe; avoid using (see Safety).

SCOTCH BROOM flower

This Product is Also Known As
Bannal, Besenginaterkraut, Broom Tops, Butcher's-Broom, Cystisi scoparii flos, Genet a Balais, Ginsterkraut,
Herbe de Hogweed, Hogweed, Irish Broom Tops, Scoparius.
CAUTION: See separate listings for Butcher's Broom, Scotch Broom herb, and Spanish Broom.

Scientific Names
Cytisus scoparius, synonyms Sarothamnus scoparius, Sarothamnus vulgaris, Spartium scoparium.
Family: Leguminosae or Fabaceae.

People Use This For
Orally, scotch broom flower is used as a mild diuretic (9), and for improving circulation (6).
Topically, it is used for sore muscles, abscesses, and swelling (11). It is used in hair rinses to lighten and brighten
hair (11).
Historically, it has been used as a cathartic, emetic (6), for cardiac dropsy, tachycardia, and profuse menstruation (4).

Safety
POSSIBLY SAFE ...when consumed in food amounts. It is listed as a flavoring agent by Council of Europe
without safety assessment (4).
LIKELY UNSAFE ...when used orally for self-medication in amounts greater than those found in foods (4,12).
Contains sparteine, an alkaloid with cardiac depressant activities similar to quinidine (4).
There is insufficient reliable information available about the safety of scotch broom flower for topical use.
PREGNANCY: LIKELY UNSAFE ...contraindicated. Appears to be an abortifacient (5,9,12).
LACTATION: POSSIBLY SAFE ...when used orally in food amounts. LIKELY UNSAFE ...when used orally in
amounts larger than found in foods; avoid using (4,12).

Effectiveness
There is insufficient reliable information available about the effectiveness of scotch broom flower.

Possible Mechanism of Action & Active Ingredients
Contains sparteine, an alkaloid, which has a curare-like properties and mimics quinidine's anti-arrhythmic effect (4).
Sparteine extends diastole without a positive inotropic effect (8). Diuretic effect of the herb may be due to the
flavone glycoside, scoparoside (5). Also contains tyramine (4,6,11).

Adverse Reactions Including Known Allergies
Taken orally, it may cause nausea, diarrhea, vertigo, stupor, tachycardia with circulatory collapse, and respiratory
arrest (4). Smoking scotch broom cigarettes may cause headaches and uterine stimulation (6), and may risk
contracting pulmonary aspergillosis (5,6).

Possible Interactions with Herbs & Other Dietary Supplements
Insufficient reliable information available.

Possible Interactions with Drugs
MONOAMINE OXIDASE INHIBITORS (MAOIs): Tyramine content can cause hypertensive crisis (2).

Possible Interactions with Foods
No interactions are known to occur, and there is no known reason to expect a clinically significant interaction with
scotch broom flower.

Possible Interactions with Lab Tests
No interactions are known to occur, and there is no known reason to expect a clinically significant interaction with
scotch broom flower.

Possible Interactions with Diseases or Conditions

HYPERTENSION: Contraindicated due to vasoconstrictive effect (2,4).
CARDIAC DISEASE: Contraindicated due to negative inotropic and negative chronotropic effects (2,4).
KIDNEY DISORDERS: The component, scoparin, might have diuretic activity which could aggravate kidney disorders (19).
SPLEEN AND LIVER DISORDERS: Contraindicated (19).

Typical Dosages & Routes of Administration that are Commonly Used

ORAL: Drink as tea (steep 1-2 grams in boiling water 5-10 minutes, strain) three times daily (4). Liquid extract (1:1 in 25% alcohol), 1-2 mL (4) Tincture: (1:5 in 45% alcohol) 0.5-2 mL (4).

Comments

Avoid confusion with butcher's broom root, scotch broom herb, and Spanish broom flower. Scotch broom seeds used as a coffee substitute are dangerous (6).

SCOTCH BROOM herb

This Product is Also Known As

Bannal, Basam, Besom, Bizzom, Broom, Browme, Breeam, Brum, Cytisi scoparii herba, Hogweed, Irish Broom, Scoparium, Scoparius.
CAUTION: See separate listings for Butcher's Broom, Scotch Broom flower, and Spanish Broom.

Scientific Names

Cytisus scoparius, synonyms Sarothamnus scoparius, Sarothamnus vulgaris, Spartium scoparium.
Family: Leguminosae or Fabaceae.

People Use This For

Orally, scotch broom is used for heart and circulatory disorders (2).
Historically, people used scotch broom for edema, cardiac arrhythmia, racing heartbeat, low blood pressure, heavy menstruation, hemorrhaging after birth, as a contraction stimulant, for bleeding gums, hemophilia, gout, rheumatism, sciatica, gallbladder and kidney stones, enlarged spleen, jaundice, bronchial conditions, and snake bites (18).

Safety

POSSIBLY SAFE ...when the aqueous-ethanolic extract is used orally and appropriately (2).
LIKELY UNSAFE ...when used in excessive amounts. Toxicity has been reported with ingestion of more than 300 mg sparteine (30 grams of above ground parts) (18).
PREGNANCY: POSSIBLY UNSAFE; avoid due to potential for uterine contractions (6,18).
LACTATION: Insufficient reliable information available; avoid using.

Effectiveness

POSSIBLY EFFECTIVE ...when used orally for cardiac and circulatory disorders (2). Functional heart and circulatory disorders require medical management rather than self-medication.
There is insufficient reliable information available about the effectiveness of scotch broom for its other uses.

Possible Mechanism of Action & Active Ingredients

The constituent, sparteine, has negative inotropic and chronotropic effects, which are responsible for its cardiac activity. It also seems to stimulate uterine contractions (6). The constituent tyramine, acts as an indirect vasoconstrictor and hypertensive (18).

Adverse Reactions Including Known Allergies

Sparteine toxicity can occur with doses greater than 300 mg of sparteine, which is roughly equivalent to 30 grams of scotch broom. Symptoms of this toxicity include dizziness, headache, palpitations, prickling in the extremities, feeling of weakness in the legs, sweating, sleepiness, pupil dilation, and ocular palsy (18).

Possible Interactions with Herbs & Other Dietary Supplements

Insufficient reliable information available.

Possible Interactions with Drugs

MONOAMINE OXIDASE INHIBITORS (MAOIs): Scotch broom contains tyramine. It should not be used with monoamine oxidase inhibitors because it might cause a hypertensive crisis (2,18)
METABOLISM INHIBITORS: Quinidine (Quinidex) and haloperidol (Haldol) inhibit sparteine metabolism, which is found in scotch broom herb, increasing the risk of adverse effects including circulatory collapse (17).

Possible Interactions with Foods

No interactions are known to occur, and there is no known reason to expect a clinically significant interaction with scotch broom herb.

Possible Interactions with Lab Tests
No interactions are known to occur, and there is no known reason to expect a clinically significant interaction with scotch broom herb.

Possible Interactions with Diseases or Conditions
A-V BLOCK: Contraindicated (18).
HIGH BLOOD PRESSURE: Contraindicated (18).

Typical Dosages & Routes of Administration that are Commonly Used
ORAL: One cup freshly brewed tea 3-4 times daily. To make tea, steep 1 level teaspoon (1-2 grams) above ground parts in 150 mL boiling water 5-10 minutes , strain (7). Liquid extract: 1-2 mL daily (18). Tincture: 0.5-2 mL daily (18). Aqueous-ethanolic extracts: 1-1.5 grams of above ground parts (7).

Comments
Avoid confusion with butcher's broom, scotch broom flower, and Spanish broom.

SCOTCH PINE NEEDLE

This Product is Also Known As
Pine Oils, Pini Atheroleum.
CAUTION: See separate listings for Dwarf Pine Needle, Fir Needle Oil, Poplar, Fir, and Pine.

Scientific Names
Pinus sylvestris.
Family: Pinaceae.

People Use This For
Orally or by inhalation, scotch pine needle oil is used for the common cold, cough, and bronchitis.
Orally, it is used for fever, inflammation of the mouth and pharynx, and the tendency for infection (18).
Topically, scotch pine needle oil is used for rheumatic and neuralgic ailments (18).

Safety
There is insufficient reliable information available about the safety of scotch pine needle oil.
Pregnancy and Lactation: Insufficient reliable information available; avoid using.

Effectiveness
There is insufficient reliable information available about the effectiveness of scotch pine needle oil.

Possible Mechanism of Action & Active Ingredients
The applicable part of scotch pine needle is the oil. The essential oil includes alpha-pinene, delta3-carene, camphene, beta-pinene, limonene, myrcene, and terpinolene. People think scotch pine needle oil has hyperemic, weak antiseptic, and secretolytic properties (18).

Adverse Reactions Including Known Allergies
Scotch pine needle oil can worsen bronchospasms (18). Used topically, scotch pine needle oil can be irritating to the skin and mucous membranes (18).

Possible Interactions with Herbs & Other Dietary Supplements
Insufficient reliable information available.

Possible Interactions with Drugs
No interactions are known to occur, and there is no known reason to expect a clinically significant interaction with scotch pine needle.

Possible Interactions with Foods
No interactions are known to occur, and there is no known reason to expect a clinically significant interaction with scotch pine needle.

Possible Interactions with Lab Tests
No interactions are known to occur, and there is no known reason to expect a clinically significant interaction with scotch pine needle.

Possible Interactions with Diseases or Conditions
CARDIAC DISORDERS: Avoid using as bath additive in individuals with a history of cardiac insufficiency (18).
INFECTION: Avoid using as bath additive in individuals with fever or infectious diseases (18).
HYPERTONIA: Avoid using as bath additive (18).
RESPIRATORY ILLNESS: Contraindicated in individuals with asthma and whooping cough because scotch pine needle oil might cause or worsen bronchospasms (18).

SKIN CONDITIONS: Avoid using as bath additive when extensive skin injuries or acute skin diseases are present (18).

Typical Dosages & Routes of Administration that are Commonly Used
ORAL: An average daily dose is 5 grams (18).
INHALATION: Place several drops in hot water and breathe in the vapors (18).
TOPICAL: Several drops or semi-solid preparation containing 10-50 % drug may be rubbed onto the affected area (18). As a bath additive 25 mg drug per liter water used in bubble bath or bath salts (18).
The essential oil is administered in alcoholic solutions, ointments, gels, emulsions, oils, or as an inhalant (18).

Comments
Avoid confusion with "pine oils" that are synthetically produced (18).

SCOTCH THISTLE

This Product is Also Known As
Woolly Thistle.

Scientific Names
Onopordum acanthium.
Family: Asteraceae.

People Use This For
Orally, scotch thistle is used as a cardiac stimulant (18).

Safety
There is insufficient reliable information available about the safety of scotch thistle.
Pregnancy and Lactation: Insufficient reliable information available; avoid using.

Effectiveness
There is insufficient reliable information available about the effectiveness of scotch thistle.

Possible Mechanism of Action & Active Ingredients
Insufficient reliable information available.

Adverse Reactions Including Known Allergies
Scotch thistle can cause an allergic reaction in individuals sensitive to the Asteraceae/Compositae family. Members of this family include ragweed, chrysanthemums, marigolds, daisies, and many other herbs.

Possible Interactions with Herbs & Other Dietary Supplements
Insufficient reliable information available.

Possible Interactions with Drugs
No interactions are known to occur, and there is no known reason to expect a clinically significant interaction with scotch thistle.

Possible Interactions with Foods
No interactions are known to occur, and there is no known reason to expect a clinically significant interaction with scotch thistle.

Possible Interactions with Lab Tests
No interactions are known to occur, and there is no known reason to expect a clinically significant interaction with scotch thistle.

Possible Interactions with Diseases or Conditions
CROSS-ALLERGENICITY: Can cause an allergic reaction in individuals sensitive to the Asteraceae/Compositae family. Members of this family include ragweed, chrysanthemums, marigolds, daisies, and many other herbs.

Typical Dosages & Routes of Administration that are Commonly Used
ORAL: Scotch thistle is available in Europe as Cardiodoron (18).

Comments
Scotch thistle sounds and looks similar to milk thistle. Be careful not to confuse the two. There is very little scientific information about this product. Our staff is continually analyzing the available information on natural medicines and will add data here as it becomes available.

SCULLCAP

This Product is Also Known As
Blue Pimpernel, Helmet Flower, Hoodwort, Mad-Dog Herb, Mad-Dog Weed, Mad Weed, Quaker Bonnet, Skullcap.

Scientific Names
Scutellaria lateriflora.
Family: Labiatae or Lamiaceae.

People Use This For
Orally or by injection, scullcap above ground parts are used for cerebral thrombosis, cerebral embolism, and paralysis caused by stroke (4). Scullcap is also used as an antipyretic (18), for "female weakness" (5,6), as a tonic, and for rabies (5,6,18).
Traditionally, scullcap is used orally as a tranquilizer (5,6) for grand mal seizures (4), chorea, epilepsy, hysteria, insomnia, nervous tension, and spasms (4).
In combination with seven other herbs (PC-SPES), skullcap is used to treat prostate cancer (5548).

Safety
POSSIBLY SAFE ...when used orally in a specific herbal combination (PC-SPES) (5548).
There is insufficient reliable information available about the safety of scullcap for its other uses.
PREGNANCY and LACTATION: Insufficient reliable information available; avoid use.

Effectiveness
POSSIBLY EFFECTIVE ...when used orally in a specific herbal combination for prostate cancer. Studies using scullcap in combination with seven other herbs (PC-SPES) in prostate cancer patients, found that it significantly decreases prostate-specific antigen (PSA) levels (5548,5122,5913), causes tumor cell death (5913), and causes clinically significant reductions in testosterone (5548). In two reports, PSA levels fell significantly within 1 month of treatment (5548,5122). ...when the constituent scutellarin is used orally, intravenously, or intramuscularly for cerebral thrombosis, cerebral embolism, and paralysis caused by stroke (4).
There is insufficient reliable information available about the effectiveness of scullcap for its other uses.

Possible Mechanism of Action & Active Ingredients
The applicable parts of scullcap are the above ground parts. Scullcap contains flavonoids including scutellarin, catalpol, lignin, resin, tannin, and volatile oil (4,18). People claim scullcap has anticonvulsant, sedative (4,18), anti-inflammatory, and lipid peroxidation inhibitor effects (18).

Adverse Reactions Including Known Allergies
Ingesting large amounts of scullcap can cause giddiness, stupor, confusion, limb twitching, seizures (4,6), "intermission" of the pulse, and other symptoms consistent with epilepsy (6). There are four reports of hepatotoxicity, one of which led to a fatality. However, it is uncertain whether hepatotoxicity resulted from scullcap, or an adulterant e.g. germander, or a combination of scullcap with valerian (515).

Possible Interactions with Herbs & Other Dietary Supplements
HERBS WITH SEDATIVE PROPERTIES: Theoretically, concomitant use with herbs that have sedative properties might enhance therapeutic and adverse effects. These include calamus, calendula, California poppy, catnip, capsicum, celery, couch grass, elecampane, ginseng Siberian, German chamomile, goldenseal, gotu kola, hops, Jamaican dogwood, kava, lemon balm, sage, St. John's wort, sassafras, shepherd's purse, stinging nettle, valerian, wild carrot, wild lettuce, withania root, and yerba mansa (4,19).

Possible Interactions with Drugs
No interactions are known to occur, and there is no known reason to expect a clinically significant interaction with scullcap.

Possible Interactions with Foods
No interactions are known to occur, and there is no known reason to expect a clinically significant interaction with scullcap.

Possible Interactions with Lab Tests
No interactions are known to occur, and there is no known reason to expect a clinically significant interaction with scullcap.

Possible Interactions with Diseases or Conditions
LIVER DISORDERS: Avoid use in individuals with liver disorders. Scullcap has been associated with some reports of liver toxicity, though adulterants might be responsible (515).

Typical Dosages & Routes of Administration that are Commonly Used

ORAL: A typical dose is 1-2 grams or as a tea three times daily (4). To make tea, steep 1-2 grams above ground parts in 150 mL of boiling water for 5-10 minutes, strain. Extract: 2-4 mL (1:1 in 25% alcohol) three times daily. Tincture: 1-2 mL (1:5 in 45 % alcohol) three times daily (4).

Comments

Scullcap has been commonly adulterated with germander and teucrium (4,5,12).

SCURVY GRASS

This Product is Also Known As

Scrubby Grass, Spoonwort.
CAUTION: See separate listing for Watercress.

Scientific Names

Cochlearia officinalis.
Family: Brassicaceae.

People Use This For

Orally, scurvy grass is used for vitamin C deficiency, gout, arthritis, stomachache, and as a blood purifier (18).
Topically, it is used for skin irritations and gum disease (18).
Historically, it was used to remove undesirable agents from the blood (18).

Safety

There is insufficient reliable information available about the safety of scurvy grass.
Pregnancy and Lactation: Insufficient reliable information available; avoid using.

Effectiveness

There is insufficient reliable information available about the effectiveness of scurvy grass.

Possible Mechanism of Action & Active Ingredients

The applicable parts of scurvy grass are the above ground flowering plant parts. There is insufficient reliable information about the active ingredients or possible mechanism of action for scurvy grass. The mustard oils in scurvy grass can irritate the mucous membranes (18).

Adverse Reactions Including Known Allergies

When large amounts of scurvy grass are taken orally, symptoms of gastrointestinal irritation may occur. Skin irritation may occur with topical application (18).

Possible Interactions with Herbs & Other Dietary Supplements

Insufficient reliable information available.

Possible Interactions with Drugs

No interactions are known to occur, and there is no known reason to expect a clinically significant interaction with scurvy grass.

Possible Interactions with Foods

No interactions are known to occur, and there is no known reason to expect a clinically significant interaction with scurvy grass.

Possible Interactions with Lab Tests

No interactions are known to occur, and there is no known reason to expect a clinically significant interaction with scurvy grass.

Possible Interactions with Diseases or Conditions

No interactions are known to occur, and there is no known reason to expect a clinically significant interaction with scurvy grass.

Typical Dosages & Routes of Administration that are Commonly Used

No typical dosage.

Comments

Some people use the freshly pressed juice orally (18). The alcoholic extracts are used topically (18).
Scurvy grass is also known as watercress (see separate listing). Be careful not to confuse these two plants. The scurvy grass flowers have a strong fragrance and taste when they are rubbed (18).

SEA BUCKTHORN

This Product is Also Known As

Argasse, Argousier, Dhar-Bu, Espino Armarillo, Espino Falso, Finbar,
Seabuckthorn, Sea-Buckthorn, Sea Buckhorn, Sallow Thorn, Grisset, Meerdorn, Oblepikha, Purging Thorn,
Sanddorn, Rokitnik, Sceitbezien, Seedorn, Star-Bu, Tindved.
CAUTION: See separate listing for Alder Buckthorn, European Buckthorn, and Cascara (California Buckthorn).

Scientific Names

Hippophae rhamnoides.
Family: Elaeagnaceae.

People Use This For

Orally, sea buckthorn leaves and flowers are used for treating arthritis, gastrointestinal ulcers, gout, and
exanthemata (4500,4501). A tea containing sea buckthorn leaves is used as a source of vitamins, flavones, amino acids,
fatty acids and minerals; for improving blood pressure and blood lipids; preventing and controlling blood vessel
diseases; removing free radicals; and boosting immunity (461).
Orally, sea buckthorn berries are used for preventing infections, improving sight, and inhibiting sclerosis and
aging (18).
Orally, sea buckthorn seed or berry oil is used as an expectorant, for treating asthma, cardiac disorders including
angina, for lowering cholesterol, preventing atheroma, as an antioxidant, for postponing senility, reducing cancer
morbidity and the toxicity of chemotherapy, for balancing the immune system, for stomach and intestinal diseases
including ulcers and reflux esophagitis (459,462,464,478,479,480), for treating night blindness (463), and as a supplemental
source of vitamins C, A, and E, beta carotene, flavonoids, superoxide dismutase, minerals, amino acids, and fatty
acids (459,460,462).
Topically, sea buckthorn berries, berry concentrate, and berry or seed oil are used as a sunscreen, for treating
radiation damage from x-rays and sunburns (18,458,462,4500), for healing wounds including bedsores, burns,
cuts (18,458,462,4501), in cosmetics and anti-aging preparations (458,465), for acne, dermatitis, dry skin, eczema, skin
ulcers and postpartum pigmentation (458,459), and for protecting mucus membranes (463).
In foods, sea buckthorn berries are used to make jellies, juices, purees, and sauces (4500,4501,4503).

Safety

LIKELY SAFE ...when consumed in amounts found in foods.
POSSIBLY SAFE ...when used orally and appropriately. There are no published reports of toxicity (18,4501).
PREGNANCY AND LACTATION: Insufficient reliable information available; avoid using in amounts greater
than those found in foods.

Effectiveness

There is insufficient reliable information about the effectiveness of sea buckthorn.

Possible Mechanism of Action & Active Ingredients

The applicable parts of sea buckthorn are the flowers, fruit, seeds, and leaves. Sea buckthorn contains ascorbic
acid (vitamin C) (18,4504), fruit acids (malic acid, acetic acid, and quinic acid), flavonoids (kaempferol, isorhamnetin,
quercetin tri- and tetra-glycosides), carotenoids (beta-carotene, gamma-carotene, lycopene), fatty oils (oleic acid,
isolinol acid, linolenic acid, and stearic acid), and sugar alcohols (mannitol and quebrachit) (18). A volatile oil in the
fruit contains vitamins A, B1, B2, B6, in addition to vitamin C (4501). Preliminary evidence suggests that sea
buckthorn extract (plant part not specified) and two constituents of the seed oil (beta-sitosterol-beta-D-glucoside
and its aglycone) might have activity against gastric ulcers (466,472). The fruit juice reduces the incidence and growth
of experimentally-induced tumors (468). The seed oil might protect against carbon tetrachloride, ethyl alcohol and
acetaminophen-induced liver damage (469,470). Some data suggest that sea buckthorn extract (plant part not
specified) might protect cells from lipid peroxidation injury (471) and might increase the rate and extent of wound
tissue epithelialization and granulation (467). Preliminary human evidence indicates that sea buckthorn seed oil
might reduce the toxicity of chemotherapy on the blood, gastrointestinal tract and immune system (478), improve
symptoms of reflux esophagitis (479), and improve the symptoms and cure rate of peptic ulcers (480).

Adverse Reactions Including Known Allergies

None reported.

Possible Interactions with Herbs & Other Dietary Supplements

Insufficient reliable information available.

Possible Interactions with Drugs

No interactions are known to occur, and there is no known reason to expect a clinically significant interaction with
sea buckthorn.

Possible Interactions with Foods

No interactions are known to occur, and there is no known reason to expect a clinically significant interaction with sea buckthorn.

Possible Interactions with Lab Tests

No interactions are known to occur, and there is no known reason to expect a clinically significant interaction with sea buckthorn.

Possible Interactions with Diseases or Conditions

No interactions are known to occur, and there is no known reason to expect a clinically significant interaction with sea buckthorn.

Typical Dosages & Routes of Administration that are Commonly Used

ORAL: 1-2 cups of a tea prepared from the leaves is typically consumed daily (461). 1-3 seed oil capsules (500 mg per capsule) are commonly used three times daily (462,464). 3-5 mL of the seed oil is commonly used three times daily (478,479). Up to 2 dropperfuls of the berry oil is commonly used three times daily (463).
TOPICAL: The berry or seed oil is typically applied three or four times per day (462,463).

Comments

Avoid confusion with alder buckthorn (Rhamnus frangula). The fatty oil of sea buckthorn seeds and berries is harvested from August until the first snow of December (18). The fruit juices and purees are popular due to their flavor (4504).

SECRETIN

This Product is Also Known As

None.

Scientific Names

Secretin; Oxykrinin.

People Use This For

Sublingually, secretin is used for treating autism (2919).
By injection (prescription-only product), secretin is used for diagnosis of Zollinger-Ellison syndrome (14,15), pancreatic dysfunction (14,15), hyperparathyroidism (14), for preventing stress ulcers (2911,2912,2913), for treating duodenal ulcers (2909,2910), gastrointestinal bleeding (2905,2906,2907,2908), pancreatitis (2918), cardiac failure (2903,2904), autism (2900,2901,2902,2915,2917), and pervasive developmental disorder (6136).

Safety

LIKELY SAFE ...when the FDA-approved, prescription-only parenteral product is used for approved indications (15).
There is insufficient reliable information available about the safety of secretin for the other uses, including sublingual.
PREGNANCY AND LACTATION: Insufficient reliable information available; avoid using (14,15).

Effectiveness

LIKELY EFFECTIVE ...when the FDA-approved, prescription-only parenteral product is used for approved indications (15).
POSSIBLY INEFFECTIVE ...when a single infusion of synthetic human secretin is used to treat autism or pervasive developmental disorder. In a double-blind trial, secretin proved no better than placebo in any of 16 outcome measures. However, both secretin and placebo significantly reduced scores in six of the 16 outcome measures (6136). In an open label trial, three children with autism experienced improved social and language skills five weeks after a single dose of secretin was injected to stimulate pancreaticobiliary secretion (2917).
There is insufficient reliable information available about the effectiveness of secretin for its other uses.

Possible Mechanism of Action & Active Ingredients

Secretin increases the volume and bicarbonate content of pancreatic secretions, stimulates excretion of insulin, stimulates gastrin release in people with gastrinoma, increases cardiac output and peripheral blood flow, and inhibits kidney bicarbonate reabsorption (14,15,2916). Secretin is not effective when administered orally due to its inactivation by proteolytic enzymes (15).

Adverse Reactions Including Known Allergies

Usually secretin is well tolerated with no serious side effects. Some side effects that can occur are red lips, vomiting, and flushing on the chest (6007). The use of secretin can also cause diarrhea, fainting, and vein thrombosis (14,15). Allergic reactions can occur with its use, including urticaria, erythema, and anaphylaxis (14).

Possible Interactions with Herbs & Other Dietary Supplements

Insufficient reliable information available.

Possible Interactions with Drugs

ANTICHOLINERGIC MEDICATIONS: Concomitant use with secretin injection can cause hyporesponsiveness to a secretin stimulation test (15,2916).

Possible Interactions with Foods

No interactions are known to occur, and there is no known reason to expect a clinically significant interaction with secretin.

Possible Interactions with Lab Tests

No interactions are known to occur, and there is no known reason to expect a clinically significant interaction with secretin.

Possible Interactions with Diseases or Conditions

No interactions are known to occur, and there is no known reason to expect a clinically significant interaction with secretin.

Typical Dosages & Routes of Administration that are Commonly Used

INTRAVENOUS: The appropriate dose remains unclear for autism. One physician gives each patient one entire vial (75 CU of Secretin-Kabi by Pharmacia). The powder is reconstituted and given by intravenous injection using a butterfly needle. Whether or not the dose will need to be repeated remains unclear. If improvement occurs, it appears to be long lasting. One report suggests repeating the dose in 9 months (6007). IV secretin is available only by prescription.

SUBLINGUAL: Drops containing pancreatic enzymes (secretin content not specified), ginkgo biloba, echinacea, pancreas, Q-10, and homeopathic alcohol 30% [sic], are available. An unspecified dose based on age and weight is given sublingually 3 times per day (5256,5257,5258,5270). Sublingual secretin is considered a dietary supplement and is not subject to FDA regulation as a drug. There is no published clinical data regarding the safety or efficacy of sublingual secretin for any use.

Comments

In some countries, secretin doses are expressed in Crick-Harper-Raper (CHR) units (14). In the United States and other countries, secretin doses are expressed in clinical units (CU) (14), where 4 CHR units = 1 CU (14). Secretin products are available in the forms of purified porcine secretin and synthetic human secretin (6136).

SELENIUM

This Product is Also Known As

None.

Scientific Names

Selenium; Se; atomic number 34.

People Use This For

Orally, selenium is used as an antioxidant and for preventing cancer, treating AIDS, heart disease, arthritis (2661), rheumatoid arthritis (2662), abnormal pap smears, atherosclerosis, macular degeneration, to prevent gray hair, Osgood-Schlatter disease (1900), and Keshan disease (2619,2671).

Safety

LIKELY SAFE ...when taken orally in amounts up to 400 mcg daily (4896).

LIKELY UNSAFE ...when used in doses greater than 400 mcg. Blood selenium levels can be used to assess the degree of toxicity from dietary selenium: levels below 1000 mcg/L are not usually associated with serious damage, whereas levels above 2000 mcg/L are predictive of serious damage (14,4896). Supplemental selenium toxicity is less predictable (4896). The chemical form of selenium, e.g., selenite, selenomethionine, affects blood and tissue levels in varying degrees (4896).

PREGNANCY: LIKELY SAFE ...when used at the recommended dietary allowance (RDA) of 60 mcg per day (4896). Some evidence suggests larger amounts might be teratogenic or associated with miscarriage (14).

LACTATION: LIKELY SAFE ...when used at the recommended dietary allowance (RDA) of 70 mcg per day; avoid using larger amounts (4896).

Effectiveness

POSSIBLY EFFECTIVE ...when taken orally for reducing total cancer mortality, total cancer incidence, and the incidence of lung, colorectal, and prostate cancers (2664,2667,2673).

There is insufficient reliable information available about the effectiveness of selenium for its other uses.

Possible Mechanism of Action & Active Ingredients

Selenium is an antioxidant that regulates the activity of glutathione peroxidase enzymes. These enzymes catalyze the detoxification of hydrogen peroxide and organic hydroperoxides. Selenium deficiency has been implicated in the etiology of Keshan disease, an endemic cardiomyopathy observed in China, and congestive cardiomyopathy in people on artificial nutrition. Selenium's protection against cardiovascular diseases is hypothesized to result from an increased resistance of low-density lipoproteins against oxidative modification, modulation of prostaglandin synthesis and platelet aggregation, and protection against toxic heavy metals (2676). Selenium can also be useful in rheumatoid arthritis. The antioxidants reduce inflammation by reducing the cellular production or concentration of toxic oxygen species (2662). In clinical trials, a combination selenium and vitamin E supplement alleviated articular pain and morning stiffness (2262). Selenium inhibits tumorigenesis via antioxidant pathways. In large amounts, it inhibits tumor growth and stimulates apoptosis, where cells are fragmented and absorbed by other cells (2664).

Adverse Reactions Including Known Allergies

Taken orally, selenium can cause acute toxicity symptoms, which include nausea, vomiting, nail changes, fatigue, and irritability (17). Chronic toxicity resembles arsenic toxicity, with symptoms including hair loss, white horizontal streaking on fingernails, paronychia, fatigue, irritability, hyperreflexia, nausea, vomiting, garlic odor on breath, and a metallic taste. Muscle tenderness, tremor, lightheadedness, and facial flushing are observed in selenium poisoning (17). Selenium can cause thrombocytopenia and moderate hepatorenal dysfunction (17). Blood selenium levels can be used to assess the degree of toxicity: levels below 1000 mcg/L are not usually associated with serious damage, whereas levels above 2000 mcg/L are predictive of serious damage (14).

Possible Interactions with Herbs & Other Dietary Supplements

Insufficient reliable information available.

Possible Interactions with Drugs

CISPLATIN (Platinol-AQ): Concomitant use of selenium can increase the cytotoxic effects of cisplatin in the presence of the chelate ethylenediaminetetraacetic acid (EDTA), in comparison to cisplatin treatment alone (2668).

Possible Interactions with Foods

No interactions are known to occur, and there is no known reason to expect a clinically significant interaction with selenium.

Possible Interactions with Lab Tests

BLOOD SELENIUM ASSAYS: Avoid powdered gloves when drawing blood for selenium and other trace element assays due to the potential for sample contamination (2663).
CREATININE KINASE: Selenium toxicity can elevate serum creatinine kinase levels (17).
EKG: Selenium toxicity can elevate the ST segment and cause T-wave changes characteristic of myocardial infarction (17).

Possible Interactions with Diseases or Conditions

No interactions are known to occur, and there is no known reason to expect a clinically significant interaction with selenium.

Typical Dosages & Routes of Administration that are Commonly Used

ORAL: For cancer prevention, the typical dose of selenium is 200 mcg per day (2664). The daily recommended dietary allowances (RDAs) of selenium, which were revised by the Institute of Medicine in April, 2000, are: Infants 0-12 months, not determined; Children 1-3 years, 20 mcg; Children 4-8 years, 30 mcg; Children 9-13 years, 40 mcg; People over 13 years, 55 mcg; Pregnant women, 60 mcg; and Lactating women, 70 mcg (4896). In humans, 30 mcg per day is considered necessary to prevent Keshan disease, which is associated with selenium deficiency (2671). The tolerable upper limit for adults to avoid selenosis is 400 mcg per day (4896).

Comments

Dietary selenium deficiency has been linked to diseases as diverse as cancer, heart disease, arthritis, and AIDS; epidemiological evidence is now emerging for the beneficial effects of selenium supplementation (2662). Most selenium enters the human body via the diet; therefore, the amount of selenium in food depends on where it is grown or raised (2671). Natural selenium levels in the soil are highly variable throughout the world (2671). In the US, the Eastern Coastal Plain and the Pacific Northwest have the lowest selenium levels, and people in these regions naturally ingest about 60 to 90 mcg per day (2671). The average daily intake in the US is 125 mcg, ranging between 60 to 200 mcg (2671).

SELF-HEAL

This Product is Also Known As

All-Heal, Blue Curls, Brownwort, Carpenter's Herb, Carpenter's Weed, Heal-All, Heart of the Earth, Hercules Woundwort, Hock-Heal, Prunella, Self Heal, Sicklewort, Siclewort, Slough-Heal, Woundwort.

Scientific Names

Prunella vulgaris.
Family: Labiatae or Lamiaceae.

People Use This For

Orally, self-heal is used for inflammatory diseases, mouth and throat ulcers, and gastroenteritis. It is also used for diarrhea, hemorrhaging, and gynecological disorders [18].

Safety

POSSIBLY SAFE ...when self-heal is used orally [12].
PREGNANCY AND LACTATION: Insufficient reliable information available; avoid using.

Effectiveness

There is insufficient reliable information available about the effectiveness of self-heal.

Possible Mechanism of Action & Active Ingredients

Insufficient reliable information available.

Adverse Reactions Including Known Allergies

None reported.

Possible Interactions with Herbs & Other Dietary Supplements

Insufficient reliable information available.

Possible Interactions with Drugs

No interactions are known to occur, and there is no known reason to expect a clinically significant interaction with self-heal.

Possible Interactions with Foods

No interactions are known to occur, and there is no known reason to expect a clinically significant interaction with self-heal.

Possible Interactions with Lab Tests

No interactions are known to occur, and there is no known reason to expect a clinically significant interaction with self-heal.

Possible Interactions with Diseases or Conditions

No interactions are known to occur, and there is no known reason to expect a clinically significant interaction with self-heal.

Typical Dosages & Routes of Administration that are Commonly Used

ORAL: One cup of tea. The tea is prepared by simmering one teaspoon of the dried plant in 150 mL of boiling water for 10-15 minutes and straining. For a gargle, the tea is simmered for 9 minutes [18].

Comments

Sanicle is also known as self-heal. Be careful not to confuse these two plants.

SENEGA

This Product is Also Known As

Chinese Senega, Flax, Klapperschlangen, Milkwort, Mountain Polygala, Polygalae radix, Rattlesnake Root, Senaga Snakeroot, Seneca, Seneca Snakeroot, Senega, Senega Snakeroot, Seneka, Snake Root.
CAUTION: See separate listings for Asarabacca and Bitter Milkwort.

Scientific Names

Polygala senega, synonym Polygala senega latifolia; Polygala tenuifolia; Polygala reinii; Polygala glomerata; Polygala japonica.
Family: Polygalaceae.

People Use This For

Orally, senega root is used for respiratory tract mucous membrane inflammation [2], bronchial asthma, chronic bronchitis [4,515], emphysema [8], for inducing sweating, increasing saliva, as an expectorant, and as an emetic [515]. Topically, senega root is used as a gargle for pharyngitis [4].
Historically, senega root was a cure for rattlesnake bite [515].

Safety

POSSIBLY SAFE ...when used orally and appropriately short-term [12].
LIKELY UNSAFE ...for prolonged use, can cause gastrointestinal irritation [12].

There is insufficient reliable information available about the safety of the topical use of senega.

PREGNANCY: LIKELY UNSAFE ...when used orally. Contraindicated because it appears to have uterine and menstrual flow stimulant effects (12,19). There is insufficient reliable information available about the safety of the topical use of senega during pregnancy.

LACTATION: Insufficient reliable information available; avoid using.

Effectiveness

POSSIBLY EFFECTIVE ...when used orally for inflammation of respiratory tract mucous membrane (2). There is insufficient reliable information available about the effectiveness of senega for its other uses.

Possible Mechanism of Action & Active Ingredients

The applicable part of senega is the root. Senega root contains salicylic acid, methyl salicylate, and a saponin mixture referred to as senegin (4). People claim senega has expectorant and emetic activity, and that it can stimulate sweating and saliva (2,4,515). The active expectorant principles are triterpenoid saponins (515). Researchers think the saponins irritate the gastrointestinal tract mucosa and cause reflex secretion of mucus in the bronchioles (515). A French patent based on human studies states that a triterpenic acid extract has anti-inflammatory activity, and is effective against graft rejection, eczema, psoriasis, and multiple sclerosis (4).

Adverse Reactions Including Known Allergies

Prolonged oral use of senega root can cause gastrointestinal irritation (2). Taken in large amounts it can cause diarrhea, dizziness (8), queasiness (18), vomiting, and purging (4).

Possible Interactions with Herbs & Other Dietary Supplements

Insufficient reliable information available.

Possible Interactions with Drugs

No interactions are known to occur, and there is no known reason to expect a clinically significant interaction with senega.

Possible Interactions with Foods

No interactions are known to occur, and there is no known reason to expect a clinically significant interaction with senega.

Possible Interactions with Lab Tests

No interactions are known to occur, and there is no known reason to expect a clinically significant interaction with senega.

Possible Interactions with Diseases or Conditions

FEVER: Contraindicated due to CNS depressant effects (19).

GI CONDITIONS: Contraindicated in individuals with gastrointestinal conditions including inflammation and gastritis or gastric ulcers (4,12) due to local stimulant activity and intestinal irritant effects (19).

Typical Dosages & Routes of Administration that are Commonly Used

ORAL: A typical oral dose is 0.5-1 grams dried root or 1 cup of tea three times daily. To make tea, steep 0.5-1 grams dried root in 150 mL boiling water 5-10 minutes, and strain (4).

Comments

Avoid confusion with Polygala sibirica, also referred to as polygala.

SENNA

This Product is Also Known As

Alexandrian Senna, Alexandrinische Senna, Casse, Indian Senna, Khartoum Senna, Sena Alejandrina, Séné d'Egypte, Senna Alexandrina, Sennae folium, Sennae fructus, Sennae fructus acutifoliae, Sennae fructus angustifolia, Tinnevelly Senna, True Senna.

Scientific Names

Senna alexandrina, synonyms Cassia acutifolia, Cassia angustifolia, Cassia senna.

People Use This For

Orally, senna leaf and fruit are used as a laxative for constipation (2), for hemorrhoids, after anorectal surgery, for evacuating the GI tract to facilitate diagnostic tests, for evacuation relief in individuals with anal fissures (18), and in "slimming" and "cleansing" teas (8).

Safety

LIKELY SAFE ...when used orally and appropriately short-term (2,12,272).

POSSIBLY UNSAFE ...when used longer than one to two weeks (2,12). Frequent use causes the colon to function poorly, creating laxative dependence (6,272).

CHILDREN: LIKELY SAFE …when the standardized nonprescription products are used orally and appropriately (272). If senna is used to treat constipation, only standardized products should be used.
PREGNANCY: POSSIBLY UNSAFE. Constipation in pregnancy should not be self-medicated (2,6,12).
LACTATION: POSSIBLY UNSAFE. Anthraquinone constituents cross into breast milk and can cause loose stools in some breast-fed infants (272).

Effectiveness
LIKELY EFFECTIVE …when used orally for constipation (2,6). …when used for bowel evacuation regimens (6). There is insufficient reliable information available about the effectiveness of senna for its other uses.

Possible Mechanism of Action & Active Ingredients
The applicable parts of senna are the leaf and fruit. Senna leaf and fruit are stimulant laxatives (272). The cathartic properties of the leaf are greater than the fruit (4). Senna contains anthraquinones including dianthrone that consists mostly of sennosides A and B and minor amounts of sennosides C and D (6,11). Senna also contains small amounts of free anthraquinones. The dianthrone glycosides are not present in the fresh leaf, but appear to form during the drying process (11). Although it is not known exactly how the anthraquinone laxatives work, the cathartic action is limited primarily to the colon (272). Sennosides irritate the lining of the large intestine, causing contraction. Sennosides A and B also seem to induce fluid secretion in the colon. Prostaglandins might be involved in the laxative effect (6). Anthroquinone laxatives produce an effect 8-12 hours after administration, though sometimes up to 24 hours can be required (272). Anthroid laxative use is not associated with an increased risk of developing colorectal ademoma or carcinoma (6138).

Adverse Reactions Including Known Allergies
Oral use of senna can cause abdominal discomfort, colic, and cramps (4). Excessive use or abuse is associated with potassium depletion, finger clubbing, development of cachexia, decreased serum globulin concentrations (4), heart function disorders, muscular weakness (2), osteomalacia, arthropathy, hepatitis, coma, neuropathy, asthma, allergy symptoms, and rhinoconjunctivitis (6). Chronic use can cause pseudomelanosis coli (pigment spots in intestinal mucosa) which is harmless, usually reverses with discontinuation (2), and is not associated with an increased risk of developing colorectal ademoma or carcinoma (6138). Prolonged senna use can cause "laxative-dependency syndrome" characterized by poor gastric motility (6), non-functioning colon (4) and laxative-induced diarrhea (6). Occupational exposure has been linked to asthma and allergy symptoms, including rhinoconjunctivitis (6).

Possible Interactions with Herbs & Other Dietary Supplements
STIMULANT LAXATIVE HERBS: Theoretically, concomitant use with other stimulant laxative herbs increases the risk of potassium depletion. Stimulant laxative herbs include aloe dried leaf sap, wild cucumber fruit (Ecballium elaterium), blue flag rhizome, alder buckthorn, European buckthorn, butternut bark, cascara bark, castor oil, colocynth fruit pulp, gamboge bark exudate, jalap root, black root, manna bark exudate, podophyllum root, rhubarb root, and yellow dock root (19).
HORSETAIL/LICORICE: Theoretically, concomitant use with horsetail plant or licorice rhizome increases the risk of potassium depletion (19).

Possible Interactions with Drugs
CARDIAC GLYCOSIDE DRUGS: Theoretically, overuse/abuse of this product increases the risk of adverse effects of cardiac glycoside drugs, e.g. digoxin (Lanoxin).

Possible Interactions with Foods
No interactions are known to occur, and there is no known reason to expect a clinically significant interaction with senna.

Possible Interactions with Lab Tests
COLORIMETRIC TESTS: Senna can discolor urine (pink, red, purple, orange, rust), interfering with diagnostic tests that depend on a color change, due to its anthraquinone content (1,4,12,275).
POTASSIUM: Excessive use of senna can cause potassium depletion, reducing serum potassium concentrations and test results (1,2,4,12,19).

Possible Interactions with Diseases or Conditions
GI CONDITIONS: Contraindicated in people with abdominal pain, intestinal obstruction, and acute intestinal inflammation including Crohn's disease, ulcerative colitis, appendicitis (2), stomach inflammation, anal prolapse, hemorrhoids (19), or undiagnosed abdominal pain (2,4).
HEART DISEASE: CAUTION; overuse can cause electrolyte disturbances and exacerbate these conditions.
ELECTROLYTE DISTURBANCES, POTASSIUM DEFICIENCY: Overuse can exacerbate these conditions (2).
FLUID DEPLETION: Contraindicated in individuals with dehydration, diarrhea or loose stools. Senna use can exacerbate these conditions.

Typical Dosages & Routes of Administration that are Commonly Used
ORAL: A typical dose is 15-30 mg hydroxyanthracene derivatives daily, calculated as sennoside B (1,2). Senna leaf is used as a tea, one cup in the morning and/or at bedtime. To make tea, steep 0.5-2 grams finely chopped leaf in warm but not boiling water for 10 minutes, and strain (8). Alternatively, a cold water tea might have less adverse GI

effects. To make cold water tea, steep 0.5-2 grams finely chopped leaf in cold water for 10-12 hours, and strain (8). Liquid leaf extract (1:1 in 25% alcohol), 0.5-2.0 mL (frequency unspecified) (4). One cup of fruit tea is taken in the morning and/or at bedtime. To make tea, steep 1/2 flat teaspoon of senna fruit in 150 mL warm, but not boiling water, for ten minutes, and strain (8). Individualize senna dosing to the smallest amount necessary to maintain a soft stool (2). Senna leaf should not be used continuously for more than one to two weeks (2). Use of standardized OTC senna leaf preparations reduces variability and improves dosing control (4,515).

Comments

Because senna fruit is gentler than senna leaf, the American Herbal Products Association only warns against long-term use for senna leaf, not senna fruit (12). The AHPA recommends that senna leaf products be labeled "Do not use this product if you have abdominal pain or diarrhea. Consult a health care provider prior to use if you are pregnant or nursing. Discontinue use in the event of diarrhea or watery stools. Do not exceed recommended dose. Not for long-term use." (12).

SHARK CARTILAGE

This Product is Also Known As
None.

Scientific Names
Squalus acanthias.

People Use This For
Orally, shark cartilage is used for cancer (2013,2014,2015,2019), arthritis (2014,2019), psoriasis (2014,2019), enteritis (2014), diabetic retinopathy (2014), and wound-healing (2015,2019).
Topically, it is used for arthritis (2014,2019) and rectally for cancer (2013,2014).
Shark cartilage also is used in investigational studies for advanced stage breast cancer, advanced stage colon cancer, advanced stage primary intercranial tumor, and spinal axis tumor (840).

Safety
There is insufficient reliable information available about the safety of shark cartilage.
Pregnancy and Lactation: Insufficient reliable information available; avoid using.

Effectiveness
LIKELY INEFFECTIVE ...when used orally or rectally for treating cancer (2013,2015).
There is insufficient reliable information available about the effectiveness of shark cartilage for its other uses.

Possible Mechanism of Action & Active Ingredients
Researchers theorize that shark cartilage might inhibit angiogenesis, preventing new vessel growth required for solid tumor proliferation (2013). Shark cartilage is about 40% proteins, 5-20% glycosaminoglycans, and calcium salts (2019).

Adverse Reactions Including Known Allergies
Oral use of shark cartilage can cause a bad taste in the mouth, nausea, vomiting, dyspepsia, constipation, hypotension, dizziness, hyperglycemia, hypercalcemia, altered consciousness, decreased motor strength, decreased sensation, generalized weakness, fatigue, and decreased performance (2014,2015,2019). It can also cause signs of acute hepatitis, including low-grade fever, jaundice, yellowing of eyes, right upper quadrant tenderness, and elevated liver enzymes (2012).

Possible Interactions with Herbs & Other Dietary Supplements
CALCIUM: CAUTION, shark cartilage can cause hypercalcemia (2019); concomitant use with supplemental calcium can exacerbate this adverse effect.

Possible Interactions with Drugs
No interactions are known to occur, and there is no known reason to expect a clinically significant interaction with shark cartilage.

Possible Interactions with Foods
FRUIT JUICE: Over time, the acidity of fruit juice can reduce potency. When adding shark cartilage to fruit juice (orange, apple, grape or tomato), mix immediately prior to drinking (2014).

Possible Interactions with Lab Tests
CALCIUM: Might increase serum calcium levels and test results (2019).

Possible Interactions with Diseases or Conditions
HYPERCALCEMIA: Shark cartilage is reported to cause hypercalcemia (2019) and might exacerbate this condition; avoid using.

Typical Dosages & Routes of Administration that are Commonly Used

ORAL: The typical doses found in commercially available products vary and can have daily doses from 500 mg to 4500 mg (6002). The dosing intervals can range from two to six times daily (6002). The concentrates of shark cartilage are usually taken as 1 to 2 tablespoons daily (6002). Administer with meals (2015).

Comments

Shark cartilage is obtained from sharks caught in the Pacific Ocean (6). Some shark cartilage products have an offensive odor and taste (2014). Phase II clinical trials of shark cartilage for use in prostate cancer and AIDS-related Kaposi's sarcoma (KS) reported in 1995 (2013) were not completed (840). Squalus acanthias is known as spiny dogfish shark, Sphyrna lewini is known as hammerhead shark.

Proponents of shark cartilage as a cancer therapy claim that sharks do not get cancer. However, researchers report that renal cell carcinoma, lymphoma and cartilage tumors have been identified in sharks. The National Cancer Institute Registry of Tumors in Lower Animals has also identified various cancers in other cartilaginous fish. Results of this unpublished research were reported at the 91st annual meeting of the American Association for Cancer Research (5045).

The FDA is seeking a permanent injunction against the marketing of BeneFin brand shark cartilage by Lane Labs. The complaint charges that BeneFin is an unapproved drug promoted as a treatment for cancer and other diseases. The action against the BeneFin brand of shark cartilage does not affect brands of shark cartilage that are not intended for use in the treatment of disease and that are otherwise lawfully marketed as dietary supplements (387).

SHARK LIVER OIL

This Product is Also Known As

Basking Shark Liver Oil, Deep Sea Shark Liver Oil, Dog Fish Liver Oil, Shark Liver, Shark Oil.
CAUTION: See separate listings for Shark Cartilage and Squalamine.

Scientific Names

Cetorhinus maximus; Centroporus squamosus; Sqaulus acanthias.

People Use This For

Orally, shark liver oil is used as adjunctive treatment of leukemia and other cancers (6,2552), to prevent radiation illness from cancer X-ray therapy, to prevent the common cold and flu, and for general immunostimulation. It is also used orally for increasing leukocyte and thrombocyte counts during chemotherapy (6,2552).
Topically, shark liver oil is used for skin conditions, skin cancer, and as a topical protectant (6,2551).

Safety

There is insufficient reliable information available about the safety of shark liver oil.
PREGNANCY AND LACTATION: Insufficient reliable information available; avoid use.

Effectiveness

There is insufficient reliable information available about the effectiveness of shark liver oil.

Possible Mechanism of Action & Active Ingredients

Shark liver oil is a major source of squalene and alkylglycerols (6). Shark liver oil is classified as a topical protectant (6,2551). Alkoxyglycerol derived from shark liver oil may decrease irradiation damage in patients undergoing treatment of uterine cancer (2552). It is thought that the radioprotective properties of alkoxyglycerol may stem from its incorporation into a pool of platelet-activating factors, and resulting in biosynthesis (2550). Alkoxyglycerol may also increase leukocyte and thrombocyte counts within specific dose ranges (2552). Shark liver oil has been shown in animals to have antiangiogenesis properties in certain cancers, including cutaneous lesions, kidney cancer and urinary bladder cancer including L-1 syngeneic (2549). However, other findings are contradictory (2552).

Adverse Reactions Including Known Allergies

Both shark liver oil and the constituent squalene have been associated with cases of aspiration and subsequent lipoid pneumonia (2546,2547,2548).

Possible Interactions with Herbs & Other Dietary Supplements

Insufficient reliable information available.

Possible Interactions with Drugs

No interactions are known to occur, and there is no known reason to expect a clinically significant interaction with shark liver oil.

Possible Interactions with Foods

No interactions are known to occur, and there is no known reason to expect a clinically significant interaction with shark liver oil.

Possible Interactions with Lab Tests

No interactions are known to occur, and there is no known reason to expect a clinically significant interaction with shark liver oil.

Possible Interactions with Diseases or Conditions

No interactions are known to occur, and there is no known reason to expect a clinically significant interaction with shark liver oil.

Typical Dosages & Routes of Administration that are Commonly Used

No typical dosage.

Comments

Shark liver oil is commercially derived from the livers of three species of shark: the deep sea shark (Centrophorus squamosus), the dogfish (Sqaulus acanthias) and the basking shark (Cetorhinus maximus) (6). The liver constitutes 25% of the total shark body weight (6).

SHELLAC

This Product is Also Known As

Gommelaque, Lac, Lacca.

Scientific Names

Laccifer.
Family: Coccidae.

People Use This For

In dentistry, shellac is used as a binding agent for dentures, restorations, moldings, and as a constituent in "artificial calculus" in dental schools (6).
In the pharmaceutical industry, shellac is used in tablet coating formulations, enteric coating, microencapsulation, matrix formulation, humidity tolerance, and for its binding ability (6).
In manufacturing, shellac is used as a finish for furniture, an ingredient in hair spray and in other cosmetics (6).

Safety

LIKELY SAFE ...when used orally. It has Generally Recognized as Safe (GRAS) status in the US (6).
PREGNANCY AND LACTATION: Insufficient reliable information available.

Effectiveness

There is insufficient information available about the effectiveness of shellac.

Possible Mechanism of Action & Active Ingredients

Aleuretic acid, r-butolic acid, shellolic acid, and jalaric acid are the major constituents of shellac (6).

Adverse Reactions Including Known Allergies

There is one report of contact cheilitis associated with shellac (6).

Possible Interactions with Herbs & Other Dietary Supplements

Insufficient reliable information available.

Possible Interactions with Drugs

No interactions are known to occur, and there is no known reason to expect a clinically significant interaction with shellac.

Possible Interactions with Foods

No interactions are known to occur, and there is no known reason to expect a clinically significant interaction with shellac.

Possible Interactions with Lab Tests

No interactions are known to occur, and there is no known reason to expect a clinically significant interaction with shellac.

Possible Interactions with Diseases or Conditions

SHELLAC ALLERGY: Contraindicated.

Typical Dosages & Routes of Administration that are Commonly Used

No typical dosage.

Comments

Shellac is derived from the secretions of the insect Laccifer. Although shellac has been used for years in pharmacy, dentistry, and as a finish for furniture, it has fallen into disfavor for some products because it ages over time (6).

SHEPHERD'S PURSE

This Product is Also Known As
Blind Weed, Bursae Pastoris Herba, Capsella, Caseweed, Cocowort, Lady's Purse, Mother's-Heart, Pepper-And-Salt, Pick-Pocket, Poor Man's Parmacettie, Rattle Pouches, Sanguinary, Shepherd's Heart, Shepherds Purse, Shepherd's Purse Herb, Shepherd's Scrip, Shepherd's Sprout, Shovelweed, St. James' Weed, Toywort, Witches' Pouches.

Scientific Names
Capsella bursa-pastoris.
Family: Brassicaceae.

People Use This For
Orally, shepherd's purse is used for headache, mild cardiac insufficiency, hypotension, nervous heart complaints, premenstrual complaints (18), prolonged or painful menstrual periods (2,4), vomiting blood, blood in urine, diarrhea, and acute catarrhal cystitis (4).
Topically, it is used for nosebleeds, superficial burns, and bleeding skin injuries (2,18).

Safety
POSSIBLY SAFE ...when preparations of the above ground parts are used orally and appropriately (2,4,12). ...when used topically (2,4).
POSSIBLY UNSAFE ...when large amounts of shepherd's purse are ingested, it can cause heart palpitations (12).
PREGNANCY: LIKELY UNSAFE ...contraindicated because it seems to cause uterine stimulation, menstrual flow stimulation, and might cause miscarriage (12).
LACTATION: Insufficient reliable information available; avoid excessive use (4).

Effectiveness
POSSIBLY EFFECTIVE ...when used for mildly prolonged or painful menstrual periods (2). ...when used topically for nosebleeds and superficial bleeding from skin injuries (2).
There is insufficient reliable information available about the effectiveness of shepherd's purse for its other uses.

Possible Mechanism of Action & Active Ingredients
The applicable parts of shepherd's purse are the above ground parts. Shepherd's purse has constituents that cause positive and negative inotropic effects, and positive and negative chronotropic effects. It also seems to cause hypertensive and sometimes antihypertensive effects. It stimulates smooth muscle and increases uterine contraction. It also has abortifacient effects, and antihemorrhagic and urinary antiseptic effects (2,4,18). One constituent in shepherd's purse is sinigrin, which can be broken down to allyl isothiocyanate. Allyl isothiocyanate is associated with abnormal thyroid function and goiter (4).

Adverse Reactions Including Known Allergies
Sedation, hypertension, hypotension, abnormal thyroid function, abnormal menstruation (4), palpitations (12). Toxic doses in animals have caused sedation, paralysis, respiratory depression, and death (4).

Possible Interactions with Herbs & Other Dietary Supplements
HERBS WITH SEDATIVE PROPERTIES: Theoretically, concomitant use with herbs that have sedative properties might enhance therapeutic and adverse effects. These include calamus, calendula, California poppy, catnip, capsicum, celery, couch grass, elecampane, Siberian ginseng, German chamomile, goldenseal, gotu kola, hops, Jamaican dogwood, kava, lemon balm, sage, St. John's wort, sassafras, scullcap, stinging nettle, valerian, wild carrot, wild lettuce, withania root, and yerba mansa (4,19).

Possible Interactions with Drugs
ANTIHYPERTENSIVE, ANTIHYPOTENSIVE DRUGS: Theoretically, concomitant use may interfere with blood pressure control (4).
CARDIOVASCULAR DRUGS: Theoretically, concomitant use may interfere with cardiovascular therapy (4).
THYROID THERAPY: Theoretically, concomitant use may interfere with thyroid dysfunction therapy (4).
DRUGS WITH SEDATIVE PROPERTIES: Theoretically, concomitant use with drugs with sedative properties may cause additive effects and side effects (4).

Possible Interactions with Foods
No interactions are known to occur, and there is no known reason to expect a clinically significant interaction with shepherd's purse.

Possible Interactions with Lab Tests
No interactions are known to occur, and there is no known reason to expect a clinically significant interaction with shepherd's purse.

© Copyright 2000, Natural Medicines Comprehensive Database (209) 472-2244. For updated data, go to www.NaturalDatabase.com • 957

Possible Interactions with Diseases or Conditions

KIDNEY STONES: Contains oxalate, use with caution in people with a history of kidney stones (12).
CARDIOVASCULAR CONDITIONS: Use with caution, may interfere with therapy (4).
THYROID CONDITIONS: Use with caution, may interfere with therapy (4).

Typical Dosages & Routes of Administration that are Commonly Used

ORAL: 1-4 grams dried above ground parts three times daily, or one cup tea (steep 1-4 grams dried above ground parts in 150 mL boiling water 10-15 minutes, strain) three times daily (4); up to 10-15 grams dried above ground parts per day (2). Liquid extract (1:1 in 25% alcohol), 1-4 mL three times daily (4). Avoid excessive amounts (12).
TOPICAL: Apply tea (steep 3-5 grams dried above ground parts in 180 mL boiling water 10-15 minutes, strain) topically (2).

Comments

None.

SHIITAKE MUSHROOM

This Product is Also Known As

Forest Mushroom, Hua Gu, Lentinula, Pasania Fungus, Shitake, Snake Butter.
CAUTION: See separate listing for Lentinan.

Scientific Names

Lentinus edodes, synonyms Lenticus edodes, Lentinan edodes, Lentinula edodes, Tricholomopsis edodes.
Family: Polyporaceae.

People Use This For

Orally, shiitake mushrooms are used for boosting the immune system, reducing serum cholesterol levels, and as an anti-aging agent (1156).
For food uses, the edible mushroom is used in Japanese cooking (6).

Safety

LIKELY SAFE ...when consumed in food amounts (6).
POSSIBLY UNSAFE ...when taken as an oral medicinal; ingestion of 4 grams shiitake powder daily for 10 weeks can cause eosinophilia (1149).
PREGNANCY AND LACTATION: Insufficient reliable information available; avoid consuming greater than food amounts.

Effectiveness

There is insufficient reliable information available about the effectiveness of shiitake mushroom.

Possible Mechanism of Action & Active Ingredients

Shiitake contains very low concentrations of lentinan (0.02%), which has antitumor effects (6). Shiitake may reduce plasma levels of free cholesterol, triglycerides, and phospholipids. (1155).

Adverse Reactions Including Known Allergies

Taken orally, shiitake mushrooms can cause abdominal discomfort, eosinophilia (1149), "shiitake" dermatitis (1148,1152), and possibly photosensitivity (1148). There is one report of abdominal obstruction and death due to ingestion of a whole shiitake mushroom (1147). Ingestion of 4 grams shiitake powder daily for 10 weeks caused eosinophilia in 5 of 10 healthy humans (1149). An allergic contact dermatitis can be induced by shiitake hyphae (filaments) (1153). In mushroom workers, hypersensitivity pneumonitis due to shiitake spore inhalation has occurred (1150,1151).

Possible Interactions with Herbs & Other Dietary Supplements

Insufficient reliable information available.

Possible Interactions with Drugs

No interactions are known to occur, and there is no known reason to expect a clinically significant interaction with shiitake mushrooms.

Possible Interactions with Foods

No interactions are known to occur, and there is no known reason to expect a clinically significant interaction with shiitake mushrooms.

Possible Interactions with Lab Tests

No interactions are known to occur, and there is no known reason to expect a clinically significant interaction with shiitake mushrooms.

Possible Interactions with Diseases or Conditions
EOSINOPHILIA: Contraindicated, may exacerbate condition (1149).

Typical Dosages & Routes of Administration that are Commonly Used
No typical dosage.

Comments
None.

SILVER LINDEN

This Product is Also Known As
Tiliae tormentosae flos.
CAUTION: See separate listings for Linden Charcoal, Linden dried flower, Linden dried leaf, and Linden dried sapwood.

Scientific Names
Tilia tormentosa, synonym Tilia argentea.
Family: Tiliaceae.

People Use This For
Orally, silver linden is used for respiratory tract mucous membrane inflammation, for its antispasmodic effects, as an expectorant, a diaphoretic, and for its diuretic effects (2).

Safety
There is insufficient reliable information available about the safety of silver linden.
Pregnancy and Lactation: Insufficient reliable information available; avoid using.

Effectiveness
There is insufficient reliable information available about the effectiveness of silver linden.

Possible Mechanism of Action & Active Ingredients
The applicable part of silver linden is the dried flower. Pharmacologically active benzodiazepine receptor ligands have been isolated from silver linden (6).

Adverse Reactions Including Known Allergies
None reported.

Possible Interactions with Herbs & Other Dietary Supplements
Insufficient reliable information available.

Possible Interactions with Drugs
No interactions are known to occur, and there is no known reason to expect a clinically significant interaction with silver linden.

Possible Interactions with Foods
No interactions are known to occur, and there is no known reason to expect a clinically significant interaction with silver linden.

Possible Interactions with Lab Tests
No interactions are known to occur, and there is no known reason to expect a clinically significant interaction with silver linden.

Possible Interactions with Diseases or Conditions
CARDIAC CONDITIONS: Avoid with existing cardiac conditions (4,6).

Typical Dosages & Routes of Administration that are Commonly Used
ORAL: 2 grams of flowertops as tea (steeped in boiling water for 5 to 10 minutes) (18). 2-4 grams daily dose (2,4,18)
Tincture (1:5 in 45% alcohol) 2-4 mL or liquid extract (1:1 in 25% alcohol) 1-2 mL (4).
TOPICAL: No typical dosage.

Comments
Avoid confusion with linden charcoal, linden flower, linden leaf and linden wood.
There is very little scientific information about this product. Our staff is continually analyzing the available information on natural medicines and will add data here as it becomes available.

SIMARUBA

This Product is Also Known As
Bitter Damson, Dysentery Bark, Mountain Damson, Slave Wood, Stave Wood, Sumaruba.

Scientific Names
Simaruba amara.

People Use This For
Orally, simaruba bark is used to treat diarrhea, dysentery, malaria, water-retention, fever, unspecified gastrointestinal upset, as a tonic, and to cause abortion (18,4500).

Safety
There is insufficient reliable information available about the safety of simaruba.
PREGNANCY AND LACTATION: LIKELY UNSAFE; avoid due to apparent abortifacient effects (18,4500).

Effectiveness
There is insufficient reliable information available about the effectiveness of simaruba.

Possible Mechanism of Action & Active Ingredients
The applicable part of simaruba is the bark. Simaruba contains the following active ingredients: 20-27% tannins, simarubin, essential oil, and fat (18,4500). It also contains the following bitter substances: quassinoids including simarolide, simarubidin, 13,18-dehydro-glaucarubinone; 0.1-0.2% 5-hydroxy-canthin-6-one a volatile oil; and unspecified alkaloids (18).

Adverse Reactions Including Known Allergies
Ingesting large amounts can cause vomiting (18).

Possible Interactions with Herbs & Other Dietary Supplements
Insufficient reliable information available.

Possible Interactions with Drugs
No interactions are known to occur, and there is no known reason to expect a clinically significant interaction with simaruba.

Possible Interactions with Foods
No interactions are known to occur, and there is no known reason to expect a clinically significant interaction with simaruba.

Possible Interactions with Lab Tests
No interactions are known to occur, and there is no known reason to expect a clinically significant interaction with simaruba.

Possible Interactions with Diseases or Conditions
No interactions are known to occur, and there is no known reason to expect a clinically significant interaction with simaruba.

Typical Dosages & Routes of Administration that are Commonly Used
ORAL: A typical dose is 1 gram (18).

Comments
Simaruba amara grows in the Caribbean islands and in the northern parts of South America (18).

SITOSTANOL

This Product is Also Known As
Beta-sitostanol, Dihydro-beta-sitosterol, Fucostanol, Phytostanol, Plant Stanol, Stigmastanol, 24-alpha-ethylcholestanol.
CAUTION: See separate listing for Beta-sitosterol.

Scientific Names
3-beta,5-alpha-stigmastan-3-ol.

People Use This For
Orally, sitostanol is used for lowering total and LDL serum cholesterol in adults (1886,3888,5429,5430,5431,5432,5433, 5434,5435,5437,5438,5439,5441,5442,5443) and reducing cholesterol absorption and lowering LDL in children with familial hypercholesterolemia (3888,3889,5436).

Safety

LIKELY SAFE ...when used orally and appropriately (5429,5430,5431,5432,5433,5434,5435,5436,5437,5438,5439,5441,5442,5443).
PREGNANCY AND LACTATION: Insufficient reliable information available.

Effectiveness

LIKELY EFFECTIVE ...when used orally for lowering total and LDL serum cholesterol (1886,3888,5429,5430,5431,5432, 5433,5434,5435,5437,5438,5439,5441,5442,5443). Sitostanol can lower total and LDL cholesterol levels by 10 to 15 percent (5443). A dose of 1.6 grams of sitostanol per day provides the maximum cholesterol lowering benefit. Larger doses do not provide additional cholesterol lowering benefit (6185).
POSSIBLY EFFECTIVE ...when used orally for reducing cholesterol absorption and lowering LDL serum cholesterol in children with familial hypercholesterolemia (3888,3889,5436).

Possible Mechanism of Action & Active Ingredients

Sitostanol is a saturated form of plant sterols, prepared commercially from vegetable oils or the oil from pine tree wood pulp and rendered fat-soluble with canola oil (5435,5430,5814). Sitostanol is essentially unabsorbable and tasteless, structurally resembles cholesterol, and competitively inhibits both dietary and biliary cholesterol absorption by competing for the limited space for cholesterol in mixed micelles (5435,5439,5443,5814). Sitostanol can lower total and LDL cholesterol levels by 10 to 15 percent (5443). In some patients, hepatic cholesterol synthesis might increase in response to decreased availability of cholesterol, resulting in no change in cholesterol levels (5430,5443). Preliminary human evidence suggests that sitostanol in lecithin micelles might reduce cholesterol absorption to a greater extent than sitostanol alone (1888). Sitostanol can reduce the absorption of dietary beta-carotene, but has no effect on retinol and vitamin D (5434).

Adverse Reactions Including Known Allergies

No adverse effects have been reported in clinical trials (5429,5430,5431,5432,5433,5434,5435,5436,5437,5438,5439,5441,5442,5443).

Possible Interactions with Herbs & Other Dietary Supplements

CHOLESTEROL LOWERING HERBS/SUPPLEMENTS: Theoretically, sitostanol might enhance the effects of herbs and supplements that also lower cholesterol.
CAROTENE, VITAMIN E: Beta-sitostanol may reduce absorption and blood levels of alpha and beta-carotene and vitamin E (3888,5434,5814).

Possible Interactions with Drugs

CHOLESTEROL LOWERING DRUGS: Sitostanol might enhance the effects of cholesterol lowering drugs. Sitostanol in combination with pravastatin lowers total and LDL cholesterol better than either treatment alone (5433). Sitostanol given concurrently with simvastatin might result in additional lowering of LDL cholesterol (3888,5431).

Possible Interactions with Foods

CAROTENE, VITAMIN E: Beta-sitostanol may reduce absorption and blood levels of alpha and beta-carotene and vitamin E (3888,5434,5814).

Possible Interactions with Lab Tests

SERUM CHOLESTEROL: Sitostanol decreases total and LDL cholesterol and test results (5429,5431,5432,5433,5435, 5437,5438,5439,5441,5442).

Possible Interactions with Diseases or Conditions

No interactions are known to occur, and there is no known reason to predict an interaction with sitostanol. Unlike products containing sitosterol, sitostanol can be safely taken by people with sitosterolemia (phytosterolemia) (5440).

Typical Dosages & Routes of Administration that are Commonly Used

ORAL: Sitostanol is an ingredient in Benecol margarine and salad dressings. There are 1.5 grams of sitostanol per serving (1-1/2 teaspoon) of Benecol margarine (5443). The recommended oral dose is 3 servings per day (5443), although a human dose-response study shows that 1.6 grams of sitostanol per day provides the maximum cholesterol lowering benefit in hypercholesterolemic adults. Larger doses do not provide additional cholesterol lowering benefit (6185).

Comments

Avoid confusing sitostanol with beta-sitosterol, an unsaturated plant sterol in the cholesterol-lowering margarine Take Control (5443). Sitostanol may produce slightly greater reductions in total and LDL cholesterol than beta-sitosterol, and it may also raise HDL "good" cholesterol levels (3665,3666,5814).

SKIRRET

This Product is Also Known As

None.

Scientific Names
Sium sisarum.
Family: Apiaceae.

People Use This For
Orally, skirret is used for digestive disorders and loss of appetite.
Historically, it was used orally for chest complaints (18).

Safety
There is insufficient reliable information available about the safety of skirret.
Pregnancy and Lactation: Insufficient reliable information available; avoid using.

Effectiveness
There is insufficient reliable information available about the effectiveness of skirret.

Possible Mechanism of Action & Active Ingredients
The applicable part of skirret is the root. There is insufficient reliable information available about the possible mechanism of action and active ingredients of skirret.

Adverse Reactions Including Known Allergies
None reported.

Possible Interactions with Herbs & Other Dietary Supplements
Insufficient reliable information available.

Possible Interactions with Drugs
No interactions are known to occur, and there is no known reason to expect a clinically significant interaction with skirret.

Possible Interactions with Foods
No interactions are known to occur, and there is no known reason to expect a clinically significant interaction with skirret.

Possible Interactions with Lab Tests
No interactions are known to occur, and there is no known reason to expect a clinically significant interaction with skirret.

Possible Interactions with Diseases or Conditions
No interactions are known to occur, and there is no known reason to expect a clinically significant interaction with skirret.

Typical Dosages & Routes of Administration that are Commonly Used
ORAL: Skirret is used in powdered form (18).

Comments
There is very little scientific information about this product. Our staff is continually analyzing the available information on natural medicines and will add data here as it becomes available.

SKUNK CABBAGE

This Product is Also Known As
Dracontium, Meadow Cabbage, Polecatweed, Skunkweed, Spathyema Foetida, Swamp Cabbage.

Scientific Names
Symplocarpus foetidus, synonym Dracontium foetidum.
Family: Araceae.

People Use This For
Orally, skunk cabbage is used to treat bronchitis, asthma (18), and whooping cough (4).
In folk medicine, it was used as a gastrointestinal stimulant (12), and to treat catarrh, cancer, chorea, convulsions, cough, edema, epilepsy (4500,4502), headache, hemorrhage, hysteria, pregnancy, labor, treating worms (4500,4502), rheumatism, ringworm, scabies, snakebite, skin sores, spasms, splinters, swellings, toothache, and wounds (4500,4502).
As a food, American Indians boil and eat young leaves, roots, and stalks (4500,4501,4502).

Safety
POSSIBLY SAFE ...when used orally and appropriately; the boiled leaves, roots, and stalks are used as food (4500,4501,4502) without reports of serious adverse effects (4).

PREGNANCY AND LACTATION: POSSIBLY UNSAFE; avoid using. May affect the menstrual cycle (4), and irritant properties may stimulate uterine contractions (4,12).

Effectiveness
There is insufficient reliable information available about the effectiveness of skunk cabbage.

Possible Mechanism of Action & Active Ingredients
Skunk cabbage contains a variety of constituents, including an acrid principle, unspecified alkaloids, an essential oil, a fatty oil, phenolic compounds, and tannin (4,4502). The seeds are reported to contain a narcotic (4502). The root contains calcium oxalate which could irritate the kidney or promote kidney stones in sensitive individuals (12,4502). The leaves contain n-hydroxytryptamine (4).

Adverse Reactions Including Known Allergies
Large amounts taken orally are reported to cause nausea, vomiting, headache, vertigo, and dimness of vision (18,4502). Excessive use of gastrointestinal irritants can cause abdominal cramps, burning, blistering in the mouth and throat, nausea, colic, and watery or bloody diarrhea (12). Topically, fresh plant can cause severe itching, inflammation, and blistering (4,4502).

Possible Interactions with Herbs & Other Dietary Supplements
Insufficient reliable information available.

Possible Interactions with Drugs
No interactions are known to occur, and there is no known reason to expect a clinically significant interaction with skunk cabbage.

Possible Interactions with Foods
No interactions are known to occur, and there is no known reason to expect a clinically significant interaction with skunk cabbage.

Possible Interactions with Lab Tests
No interactions are known to occur, and there is no known reason to expect a clinically significant interaction with skunk cabbage.

Possible Interactions with Diseases or Conditions
KIDNEY STONES: Individuals with a history of oxalate kidney stones should avoid or use cautiously (12,4502).
GI CONDITIONS: May aggravate GI ulcers, GI inflammation or irritation (12,19).

Typical Dosages & Routes of Administration that are Commonly Used
ORAL: Powdered rhizome/root: 0.5-1 mg three times daily mixed with honey or by infusion or decoction. Liquid extract: (1:1 in 25% alcohol) 0.5-1 mL three times daily. Tincture: (1:10 in 45% alcohol) 2-4 mL three times daily (4).

Comments
Skunk cabbage is a common name for members of the toxic Veratrum family (4501). Skunk cabbage gets it name from a volatile oil emitted by the plant that has a disagreeable odor (18).

SLIPPERY ELM

This Product is Also Known As
Indian Elm, Moose Elm, Red Elm, Sweet Elm.

Scientific Names
Ulmus rubra; Ulmus fulva.
Family: Ulmaceae.

People Use This For
Orally, slippery elm is used for coughs, sore throat, colic, diarrhea, constipation, hemorrhoids, irritable bowel syndrome, cystitis, urinary inflammation, urinary tract infections, syphilis, herpes, and for expelling tapeworms. It is also used orally for protecting against stomach and duodenal ulcers, for colitis, diverticulitis, GI inflammation, and acidity. The whole bark (probably not the inner bark) of slippery elm is an abortifacient (4,6121).
Topically, slippery elm is used for wounds, burns (18), gout, rheumatism, cold sores, boils, abscesses, ulcers, toothaches, sore throat, and as a lubricant to ease labor (6).
Slippery elm is found in some baby foods and adult nutritionals, and in some oral lozenges used for soothing throat pain (6).

Safety
LIKELY SAFE ...when the inner bark is used in amounts found in food. ...when used orally and appropriately for medicinal purposes (4,12,512).

PREGNANCY: POSSIBLY SAFE ...when the inner bark is used orally in amounts used in foods (4). LIKELY UNSAFE ...when the whole bark is used. Use of the whole bark is contraindicated because it is an abortifacient (4,6).

LACTATION: Insufficient reliable information available; avoid using.

Effectiveness

EFFECTIVE ...when used topically as an oral demulcent (agent capable of soothing mucous membranes) for sore throat, according to the FDA (512).

There is insufficient reliable information available about the effectiveness of slippery elm for its other uses.

Possible Mechanism of Action & Active Ingredients

The applicable part of slippery elm is the inner bark rind. The mucilages are considered the principal constituent. They are responsible for slippery elm's demulcent and emollient effects (4,18). Taken internally, slippery elm preparations cause reflex stimulation of nerve endings in the GI tract, leading to mucus secretion (6). This induced mucus may protect the GI tract against ulcers, excess acidity, etc. Tannin constituents have astringent properties (4). Oleoresins of some species are responsible for contact dermatitis (6).

Adverse Reactions Including Known Allergies

The whole bark, when taken orally, is an abortifacient (4). Extracts of slippery elm used topically can cause contract dermatitis (6). The pollen is an allergen (6).

Possible Interactions with Herbs & Other Dietary Supplements

Insufficient reliable information available.

Possible Interactions with Drugs

ORAL DRUGS: Theoretically, may slow the absorption and reduce serum levels of orally administered drugs due to mucilage content (19).

Possible Interactions with Foods

No interactions are known to occur, and there is no known reason to expect a clinically significant interaction with slippery elm.

Possible Interactions with Lab Tests

No interactions are known to occur, and there is no known reason to expect a clinically significant interaction with slippery elm.

Possible Interactions with Diseases or Conditions

No interactions are known to occur, and there is no known reason to expect a clinically significant interaction with slippery elm.

Typical Dosages & Routes of Administration that are Commonly Used

ORAL: Powdered inner bark (1:8 as a decoction) 4-16 mL three times daily (4). Nutritional supplement, 4 grams powdered inner bark in 500 mL boiling water, three times daily (4). Alcohol extract (1:1 in 60% alcohol), 5 mL three times daily (4).

TOPICAL: As a poultice, coarse powdered inner bark mixed with boiling water (4).

Comments

Avoid confusing whole bark with inner bark. Commercial lozenges containing slippery elm are preferred to the native herb when used for cough and sore throat, because they provide sustained release of mucilage to the throat (3).

SMARTWEED

This Product is Also Known As

Arsesmart, Water Pepper.

Scientific Names

Polygonum hydropiper.

People Use This For

Orally, smartweed is used to treat bleeding of the womb, menstrual bleeding, bleeding hemorrhoids, and diarrhea (18).

Topically, smartweed is used to wash bloody wounds (18).

Safety

There is insufficient reliable information available about the safety of smartweed.

Pregnancy and Lactation: Insufficient reliable information available; avoid using.

Effectiveness
There is insufficient reliable information available about the effectiveness of smartweed.

Possible Mechanism of Action & Active Ingredients
The applicable parts of smartweed are the leaf, and the entire plant during flowering season. Smartweed contains tannins, hydropiperoside, sesquiterpenealdehydes, and flavonoids (18). Smartweed is reported to stop bleeding. It is also thought to influence the elimination of urine and to have some effect on rheumatic pain (18).

Adverse Reactions Including Known Allergies
Smartweed can cause gastrointestinal irritation (19). Handling the fresh plant can cause inflammatory reactions due to chemical irritation (18).

Possible Interactions with Herbs & Other Dietary Supplements
Insufficient reliable information available.

Possible Interactions with Drugs
WARFARIN: Concomitant use can decrease the anticoagulant effects of warfarin (Coumadin), possibly increasing the risk of clotting (19).

Possible Interactions with Foods
No interactions are known to occur, and there is no known reason to expect a clinically significant interaction with smartweed.

Possible Interactions with Lab Tests
No interactions are known to occur, and there is no known reason to expect a clinically significant interaction with smartweed.

Possible Interactions with Diseases or Conditions
GASTROINTESTINAL DISORDERS: Smartweed can exacerbate inflammatory conditions by irritating the mucus membranes (19).

Typical Dosages & Routes of Administration that are Commonly Used
ORAL: A small amount of the powdered drug three times a day or one cup tea (one teaspoon of the drug per cup, boil) three times per day (18).

Comments
Smartweed has an extraordinary hot pepper-like taste (18).

SMOKELESS TOBACCO

This Product is Also Known As
Chaw, Chew, Chewing Tobacco, Dip, Snuff, Tobacco.

Scientific Names
Nicotiana tabacum.

People Use This For
Smokeless tobacco is used recreationally as "snuff" by buccal and nasal routes (6).

Safety
LIKELY UNSAFE ...when used recreationally (6). Nicotine, a constituent is lethal at 40-100 mg, though the lethal level might be elevated through habituation (18). Nicotine is associated with increased risk of cancer and cardiovascular complications (6).
PREGNANCY: LIKELY UNSAFE (19,4125). Nicotine is a teratogen and it is likely to reduce infant birth weight and size as well as increasing the risk of miscarriage, prematurity, and neurologic impairment of baby (19).
LACTATION: LIKELY UNSAFE (19,4125); avoid using.

Effectiveness
There is no medicinal use for smokeless tobacco.

Possible Mechanism of Action & Active Ingredients
The main active constituent of smokeless tobacco is nicotine (18). Small doses increase blood pressure (6,18) and gastric mucosal activity (18). Larger doses can reduce blood pressure, lower gastrointestinal muscle tone (18), produce tachycardia, and may be vasoconstrictive (6). Tobacco stimulates respiratory and tremor centers (18). In human studies, tobacco is known to decrease the level of high-density lipoproteins (HDLs) (19). Evidence suggests that nitrosamines found in tobacco might cause tumors (6).

Adverse Reactions Including Known Allergies

Nausea and dizziness are common with initial recreational use (6). Use of "snuff" affects blood pressure and heart rate (6,18), causes loss of taste and smell, gingival recession, periodontal tissue destruction, tooth loss, soft tissue erythema, oral leukoplakia, epidermoid carcinoma, oropharyngeal cancer (6). A single case of thromboangiitis obliterans has been linked to chronic use (6). The saccharin found in flavored tobacco might increase the risk of bladder cancer (6). Bad breath and discolored teeth are common problems associated with smokeless tobacco (6). The symptoms of nicotine poisoning are dizziness, salivation, vomiting, diarrhea, trembling, weak legs, spasms, unconsciousness, cardiac arrest, and respiratory failure (18,4125).

Possible Interactions with Herbs & Other Dietary Supplements

OATS: Theoretically, oats might decrease the hypertensive response to nicotine (19).

Possible Interactions with Drugs

ACETAMINOPHEN: Interacts with the nicotine in smokeless tobacco and decreases the blood levels of acetaminophen (Tylenol) (19).
ADENOSINE: Interacts with the nicotine in smokeless tobacco and increases the circulatory effects of adenosine (19).
AMOBARBITOL: Interacts with the nicotine in smokeless tobacco and increases the elimination of amobarbital (Amytal) (19).
BENZODIAZEPINES: Interact with the nicotine in smokeless tobacco and increases the elimination of benzodiazepines (19).
BETA-BLOCKERS: Interact with the nicotine in smokeless tobacco and decreases the effectiveness of beta-blockers (19).
CAFFEINE: Interacts with the nicotine in smokeless tobacco and increases the elimination of caffeine (19).
CIMETIDINE: Interacts with the nicotine in smokeless tobacco and decreases the blood levels of cimetidine (Tagamet). Cimetidine reduces the metabolic breakdown of nicotine (19).
DIFLUNISAL: Interacts with the nicotine in smokeless tobacco and increases the elimination of diflunisal (Dolobid) (19).
ESTROGEN: Interacts with the nicotine in smokeless tobacco and increases the metabolism of estrogen (19).
FUROSEMIDE: Interacts with the nicotine in smokeless tobacco and decreases the effectiveness of furosemide (Lasix) (19).
GLUTETHIMIDE: Interacts with the nicotine in smokeless tobacco and enhances the effects of glutethimide (19).
HALOPERIDOL: Interacts with the nicotine in smokeless tobacco and increases the metabolism of haloperidol (Haldol) (19).
HEPARIN: Interacts with the nicotine in smokeless tobacco and increases the elimination of heparin (19).
INSULIN: Interacts with the nicotine in smokeless tobacco and decreases the effectiveness of insulin (19).
ORAL CONTRACEPTIVES: Interact with the nicotine in smokeless tobacco and increases the risk of blood clots in women over age 30 using oral contraceptives (19).
PHENOTHIAZINES: Interact with the nicotine in smokeless tobacco and increases the metabolism of phenothiazines (19).
PENTAZOCINE: Interacts with the nicotine in smokeless tobacco and increases the elimination of pentazocine (Talwin) (19).
PHENYLBUTAZONE: Interacts with the nicotine in smokeless tobacco; nicotine increases the metabolism of phenylbutazone (19).
PROPOXYPHENE: Interacts with the nicotine in smokeless tobacco and decreases the effectiveness of propoxyphene (Darvon) (19).
QUININE: Interacts with the nicotine in smokeless tobacco and increases the metabolism of quinine (19).
RANITIDINE: Ranitidine (Zantac) reduces the metabolic breakdown of nicotine, a constituent of smokeless tobacco (19).
TACRINE: Interacts with the nicotine in smokeless tobacco and increases the metabolism of tacrine (Cognex) (19).
THEOPYLLINE: Interacts with the nicotine in smokeless tobacco and increases the metabolism of theophylline (19).
THIOTHIXENE: Interacts with the nicotine in smokeless tobacco and increases the metabolism of thiothixene (Navane) (19).
TRICYCLIC ANTIDEPRESSANTS: Interact with the nicotine in smokeless tobacco and increases the elimination of tricyclic antidepressants (19).
VITAMIN B12: Interacts with the nicotine in smokeless tobacco and decreases the blood levels of vitamin B12 (19).
VITAMIN C: Interacts with the nicotine in smokeless tobacco and increases the elimination of vitamin C (19).
ZOLPIDEM: Interacts with the nicotine in smokeless tobacco and increases the metabolism of zolpidem (Ambien) (19).

Possible Interactions with Foods

No interactions are known to occur, and there is no known reason to expect a clinically significant interaction with smokeless tobacco.

Possible Interactions with Lab Tests
No interactions are known to occur, and there is no known reason to expect a clinically significant interaction with smokeless tobacco.

Possible Interactions with Diseases or Conditions
DIABETES: Persistent hyperglycemia has been observed in diabetic patients who use "candified" chewing tobacco and regularly swallow the salivary juices (6). Long term nicotine use leads to insulin resistance (4133).
GASTROINTESTINAL ULCERS: The nicotine in smokeless tobacco stimulates gastric acid secretion, causing ulcer exacerbation (19).
HEART DISEASE: The nicotine in smokeless tobacco decreases HDL level and increases blood pressure (19). High doses of nicotine can increase heart rate and potentiate cardiac arrhythmia or ischemia (4132).
OSTEOPOROSIS: The nicotine in smokeless tobacco causes further deterioration of bone disease (19,4126).

Typical Dosages & Routes of Administration that are Commonly Used
No typical dosage.

Comments
Smokeless tobacco is considered likely unsafe.

SNEEZEWORT

This Product is Also Known As
None.

Scientific Names
Achillea ptarmica.

People Use This For
Orally, sneezewort root is used for rheumatic and painful disorders, toothache, diarrhea, nausea, vomiting, and flatulence (18).
Topically, sneezewort is used for toothache (18).
In folk medicine, sneezewort has been used for tiredness, urinary tract complaints, and as an appetite stimulant (18).

Safety
There is insufficient reliable information available about the safety of sneezewort.
Pregnancy and Lactation: Insufficient reliable information available; avoid using.

Effectiveness
There is insufficient reliable information available about the effectiveness of sneezewort.

Possible Mechanism of Action & Active Ingredients
The applicable part of sneezewort is the dried root. Sneezewort contains alkamides, polyynes, and volatile oil (18).

Adverse Reactions Including Known Allergies
Allergic reaction can occur (18).

Possible Interactions with Herbs & Other Dietary Supplements
Insufficient reliable information is available.

Possible Interactions with Drugs
No interactions are known to occur, and there is no known reason to expect a clinically significant interaction with sneezewort.

Possible Interactions with Foods
No interactions are known to occur, and there is no known reason to expect a clinically significant interaction with sneezewort.

Possible Interactions with Lab Tests
No interactions are known to occur, and there is no known reason to expect a clinically significant interaction with sneezewort.

Possible Interactions with Diseases or Conditions
SNEEZEWORT ALLERGY: Contraindicated.

Typical Dosages & Routes of Administration that are Commonly Used

ORAL: A typical dose is two cups of tea daily. To make tea, simmer 2 teaspoons of the cut root in two 2 cups of water (18).

TOPICAL: The fresh root can be chewed (18).

Comments

None.

SOLOMON'S SEAL

This Product is Also Known As

Dropberry, Ladys Seals, Lady's Seals, Sealroot, Sealwort, Solomons Seal, St Marys Seal, St. Mary's Seal.

Scientific Names

Polygonatum multiflorum.
Family: Liliaceae.

People Use This For

Historically, Solomon's seal was used for respiratory and lung disorders, and as an astringent and anti-inflammatory. It has also been used topically for bruises, furuncles, ulcers or boils on the fingers, hemorrhoids, skin redness, edema, and hematoma (18).

Safety

POSSIBLY SAFE ...when taken orally for short duration (12).
PREGNANCY AND LACTATION: Insufficient reliable information available; avoid using.

Effectiveness

There is insufficient reliable information available about the effectiveness of Solomon's seal.

Possible Mechanism of Action & Active Ingredients

There is insufficient reliable information available about the active ingredients or possible mechanism of action for Solomon's seal. Solomon's seal may cause hypoglycemia (19).

Adverse Reactions Including Known Allergies

Long-term use may cause gastrointestinal irritation. Use of large doses or overdoses may cause nausea, diarrhea, gastric complaints, and nausea (18).

Possible Interactions with Herbs & Other Dietary Supplements

HYPOGLYCEMIC HERBS: Theoretically, concomitant use with other hypoglycemic herbs may have additive effects (19).

Possible Interactions with Drugs

DIABETES THERAPY: Theoretically, concomitant use may enhance hypoglycemic drug effects and alter blood glucose control (19). Monitor blood glucose.
INSULIN: Insulin dosage adjustments may be necessary, due to the possible hypoglycemic effects of Solomon's seal (19).
CHLORPROPAMIDE (Diabinese): Concomitant use may cause additive hypoglycemic effects (19).

Possible Interactions with Foods

No interactions are known to occur, and there is no known reason to expect a clinically significant interaction with Solomon's seal.

Possible Interactions with Lab Tests

No interactions are known to occur, and there is no known reason to expect a clinically significant interaction with Solomon's seal.

Possible Interactions with Diseases or Conditions

DIABETES: Theoretically may interfere with blood glucose control (19).

Typical Dosages & Routes of Administration that are Commonly Used

No typical dosage.

Comments

Solomon's seal is obsolete as a medicinal herb.

SORREL

This Product is Also Known As
Acedera Común, Azeda-Brava, Garden Sorrel, Sorrel Dock, Sour Dock, Wiesensauerampfer.

Scientific Names
Rumex acetosa.
Family: Polygonaceae.

People Use This For
Orally, sorrel is used for acute and chronic inflammation of the nasal passages and respiratory tract, and as an adjunct to antibacterial therapy. It is also used as a diuretic and to stimulate secretions (18).
In combination with gentian root, European elder flower, verbena, and cowslip flower, sorrel is used orally for maintaining healthy sinuses (373) and treating sinusitis (7,374,379).

Safety
POSSIBLY SAFE ...when leaves are used as food in limited amounts (4247). ...when sorrel is taken orally with gentian root, European elder flower, verbena, and cowslip flower (Quanterra Sinus Defense, Sinupret) (7,374,379).
LIKELY UNSAFE ...when used in large amounts. A 53 year old who ingested 500 grams of sorrel in soup died (17). There is insufficient reliable information available about the safety of sorrel used in medicinal amounts.
CHILDREN: POSSIBLY UNSAFE ...because it contains oxalic acid. A four-year old child died after consuming rhubarb leaves, which is also a source of oxalic acid (17).
PREGNANCY AND LACTATION: LIKELY SAFE ...when used orally in food amounts. There is insufficient reliable information available about the safety of sorrel in amounts larger than those found in foods during pregnancy and lactation; avoid using.

Effectiveness
POSSIBLY EFFECTIVE ...when sorrel is taken orally with gentian root, European elder flower, verbena, and cowslip flower (Quanterra Sinus Defense, Sinupret) for treating acute or chronic sinusitis (7,374,379).
There is insufficient reliable information available about the effectiveness of sorrel for its other uses.

Possible Mechanism of Action & Active Ingredients
Sorrel contains 7-15% tannins (11), which exert an astringent effect on the mucosal tissue. This effect dehydrates the tissue, reducing internal secretions and forming the external cells into a protective layer. Plants with at least 10% tannins may cause gastrointestinal disturbances, kidney damage, and necrotic conditions of the liver. Some animal data show that tannins may cause cancer; other data show they may prevent it. Regular consumption of herbs with high tannin concentrations correlates with increased incidence of esophageal or nasal cancer (12). Sorrel leaf has a 0.3% oxalate content (12). Once absorbed, the oxalic acid reacts with calcium in plasma and resulting insoluble calcium oxalate may precipitate in the kidneys, blood vessels, heart, lungs, and liver. This may also cause hypocalcemia (12,17). Oxalate crystals damage mucosal tissue, resulting in severe irritation and possible damage. The systemic absorption of oxalates may result in kidney damage, both in people with pre-existing kidney disease and in healthy kidneys (19).

Adverse Reactions Including Known Allergies
Consuming excessive amounts of sorrel can cause diarrhea, nausea, polyuria (6), dermatitis (4) and gastrointestinal symptoms. Oxalic acid (constituent) poisoning affects skin, eyes, respiratory system, and kidneys. Oral symptoms of oxalate irritation include swelling of the mouth, tongue, and throat, with difficulty in speaking and suffocation. It has a corrosive effect on the digestive tract and can lead to oxalic acid crystals in the kidneys, blood vessels, heart, lungs, liver, and/or hypocalcemia (17).

Possible Interactions with Herbs & Other Dietary Supplements
TANNIN-CONTAINING HERBS: Theoretically, herbs that contain high percentages of tannins (such as sorrel) may cause precipitation of constituents of other herbs (19).

Possible Interactions with Drugs
ORAL DRUGS: Theoretically, concomitant oral administration may cause precipitation of some drugs due to the high tannin content of sorrel (19). Separate administration of oral drugs and tannin-containing herbs by the longest period of time practical (19).
DOXYCYCLINE (Vibramycin): Concurrent use of sorrel, gentian root, European elder flower, verbena, and cowslip flower (Quanterra Sinus Defense, Sinupret) with doxycycline and a topical decongestant might improve the outcome of conventional (antibiotic/decongestant) therapy for acute bacterial sinusitis (374).

Possible Interactions with Foods
No interactions are known to occur, and there is no known reason to expect a clinically significant interaction with sorrel.

Possible Interactions with Lab Tests

No interactions are known to occur, and there is no known reason to expect a clinically significant interaction with sorrel.

Possible Interactions with Diseases or Conditions

COAGULATION DISORDERS: Oxalate constituents can alter the calcium concentrations and decrease coagulation time (4,12).

GI CONDITIONS: Theoretically, sorrel can exacerbate stomach and intestinal ulcers due to mucosal irritant effect (19).

KIDNEY DISEASE: Can damage kidneys with formation of insoluble oxalate; use with caution or avoid in individuals with history of kidney stones (12,19).

Typical Dosages & Routes of Administration that are Commonly Used

ORAL: For acute or chronic sinusitis, two Sinupret tablets three times daily for up to two weeks has been used in clinical trials (7,374,379), equivalent to gentian root 12 mg, European elder flower 36 mg, verbena 36 mg cowslip flower 36 mg and sorrel 36 mg three times daily. For maintaining healthy sinuses, a typical dose is one tablet of Quanterra Sinus Defense three times daily with water, equivalent to gentian root 9 mg, European elder flower 29 mg, verbena 29 mg, cowslip flower 29 mg, and sorrel 29 mg three times daily (373). Each tablet of Quanterra Sinus Defense contains 125 mg of the herbal combination found in Sinupret (373).

Comments

Roselle (Hibiscus sabdariffa) is also known as Jamaica sorrel or Guinea sorrel. It could be confused with sorrel (11,18).

SOUR CHERRY

This Product is Also Known As

Cerezo Acido, Cerisier Acide, English Morello, Ginjeira, Griottier, Guindo, Montmorency Cherry, Morello Cherry, Pie Cherry, Red Cherry, Richmond, Sauerkirsche, Sauerkirschenbaum, Tart Cherry.

Scientific Names

Prunus Cerasus, synonyms Cerasus vulgaris, Prunus vulgaris.
Family: Rosaceae.

People Use This For

In traditional medicine, the fruit of sour cherry has been used orally for arthritis and gout (6).
In folk medicine, the stem of the sour cherry is used to cause diuresis and facilitate digestion (4284).
In food use, sour cherries are eaten as a food or flavoring, and used in pies and other baked goods (6).
In manufacturing, sour cherry fruit is used to make cherry syrup USP, a vehicle for drugs with unpleasant taste (6).

Safety

LIKELY SAFE …when the fruit is used orally for food or medicinal use.
There is insufficient reliable information available about the safety of the oral use of sour cherry stem.
PREGNANCY AND LACTATION: LIKELY SAFE …when the fruit is consumed in typical food amounts. There is insufficient reliable information available about the safety of sour cherry stem use during pregnancy or lactation.

Effectiveness

There is insufficient reliable information about the effectiveness of sour cherry.

Possible Mechanism of Action & Active Ingredients

Sour cherry fruit contains vitamin C, vitamin A, alpha-linolenic acid, and traces of vitamin E, beta-carotene, folacin thiamine, as well as other constituents (4282). It contains varied antioxidants including kaempferol and quercetin (4282,4283). A preliminary study at Michigan State University suggests compounds found in the sour cherry have anti-inflammatory effects that are ten times stronger than aspirin but without aspirin's side effects (6). The stem of the sour cherry contains an isoflavone constituent, prunetin 5-O-beta-D-glycopyranoside (4284).

Adverse Reactions Including Known Allergies

None reported.

Possible Interactions with Herbs & Other Dietary Supplements

Insufficient reliable information available.

Possible Interactions with Drugs

No interactions are known to occur, and there is no known reason to expect a clinically significant interaction with sour cherry.

Possible Interactions with Foods

No interactions are known to occur, and there is no known reason to expect a clinically significant interaction with sour cherry.

Possible Interactions with Lab Tests

No interactions are known to occur, and there is no known reason to expect a clinically significant interaction with sour cherry.

Possible Interactions with Diseases or Conditions

No interactions are known to occur, and there is no known reason to expect a clinically significant interaction with sour cherry.

Typical Dosages & Routes of Administration that are Commonly Used

No typical dosage.

Comments

Of the more than 270 varieties of sour cherry, only a few are important commercially. These include the Montmorency, Richmond, and English morello [6].

SOUTHERN PRICKLY ASH

This Product is Also Known As

Prickly Ash, Prickly Yellow Wood, Sea Ash, Toothache Tree, Xanthoxylum, Zanthoxylum.
CAUTION: See separate listings for Ash and Northern Prickly Ash.

Scientific Names

Zanthoxylum clava-herculis.
Family: Rutaceae.

People Use This For

Orally, southern prickly ash bark and berry are used for cramps, intermittent claudication, Raynaud's syndrome, chronic rheumatic conditions, and peripheral circulatory insufficiency associated with rheumatic symptoms [4]. In folk medicine, southern prickly ash has been used as a tonic, stimulant, for toothache, sores, ulcers, as a diaphoretic in fever, and for cancer (as an ingredient in Hoxsey cure) [11].

Safety

POSSIBLY SAFE ...when used orally and appropriately in food flavoring [4]. It is listed by the Council of Europe as a natural source of food flavoring. ...when the bark is used orally in medicinal amounts [12].
There is insufficient reliable information about the safety of the oral use of the berry.
PREGNANCY: LIKELY UNSAFE ...the bark is contraindicated for oral use [12] because it might have menstrual stimulant effects [19]. There is insufficient reliable information about the safety of the berry during pregnancy; avoid using.
LACTATION: LIKELY UNSAFE ...contraindicated for oral use because it might cause colic in the breast-fed infant [19]. There is insufficient reliable information about the safety of the berry during lactation; avoid using.

Effectiveness

There is insufficient reliable information available about the effectiveness of southern prickly ash.

Possible Mechanism of Action & Active Ingredients

The applicable parts of southern prickly ash are the bark and berry. Southern prickly ash contains nitidine (hypotensive, antileukemic, hepatic enzyme inhibitor), chelerythrine (anti-inflammatory, antibiotic against gram positive bacteria, potentiates barbiturate induced sleep, hepatic enzyme inhibitor), asarinin (antitubercular), and neoherculin (insecticidal, salivation stimulant) [4]. Reports of death after ingestion by cattle, chickens, and fish attributed to the neuromuscular blocking properties of the bark [4].

Adverse Reactions Including Known Allergies

None reported.

Possible Interactions with Herbs & Other Dietary Supplements

DIGITALIS: May interfere with cardiac glycoside therapy [4].
HERBS WITH ANTICOAGULANT/ANTIPLATELET POTENTIAL: Certain herbs have the potential to contribute to bleeding because they have coumarin constituents, or they affect platelet aggregation, or they have high vitamin K content. Theoretically, concomitant use of more than one of these herbs could increase the chance of bleeding in susceptible individuals. These herbs include: alfalfa, angelica, anise, arnica, asafoetida, bogbean, boldo, capsicum, celery, Roman and German chamomile, clove, danshen, fenugreek, feverfew, garlic, ginger, ginkgo, ginseng (Panax), horse chestnut, horseradish, licorice, meadowsweet, nettle, onion, papain, parsley, passionflower, poplar, quassia, red clover, turmeric, wild carrot, wild lettuce, and willow [4,19].

Possible Interactions with Drugs

ACID-INHIBITING DRUGS: Theoretically, due to claims that southern prickly ash increases stomach acid, it might interfere with antacids, sucralfate (Carafate), H-2 antagonists, and proton pump inhibitors (19).

Possible Interactions with Foods

No interactions are known to occur, and there is no known reason to expect a clinically significant interaction with southern prickly ash.

Possible Interactions with Lab Tests

No interactions are known to occur, and there is no known reason to expect a clinically significant interaction with southern prickly ash.

Possible Interactions with Diseases or Conditions

LIVER DISEASE: Theoretically, may inhibit hepatic enzymes.

Typical Dosages & Routes of Administration that are Commonly Used

ORAL (Bark): 1-3 grams dried bark, or drink as decoction (boil 1-3 grams dry bark 10-15 minutes, strain), three times daily; liquid bark extract (1:1 in 45% alcohol) 1-3 mL three times daily; bark tincture (1:5 in 45% alcohol) 2-5 mL three times daily (4).
ORAL (Berry): 0.5-1.5 grams dried berry; liquid berry extract (1:1 in 45% alcohol) 0.5-1.5 mL (4).

Comments

None.

SOY

This Product is Also Known As

Frijol de Soya, Haba Soya, Isoflavone, Phytoestrogen, Plant Estrogen, Shoyu, Soja, Sojabohne, Soya, Soybean, Soybean Curd, Soy Fiber, Soy Milk, Soy Protein, Soy-Protein, Tofu.

Scientific Names

Glycine max, synonym Glycine soja.
Family: Fabaceae.

People Use This For

Orally, soy is used for menopausal symptoms (2296,2297), preventing hot flashes in breast cancer survivors (3991), and for preventing osteoporosis and cardiovascular disease in postmenopausal women (3978,3979,3986). Soy is also used for hypertension (2296); hyperlipidemia (2296,3402,6412); constipation; diarrhea (6);slowing the progression of kidney disease (2286) and decreasing urine protein excretion (2287); and for preventing breast, endometrial, and prostate cancer (3978,3979).
Intravenously, soy is used as a source of calories and fatty acids in fat emulsions (14,15).
As a food, soy is also used as a milk substitute for infant feeding formulas and as an alternative to cow's milk in vegetarian diets (6,3400,6413). Soybeans are eaten boiled or roasted. Soy flour and soy oil are used as ingredients in foods, beverages, and condiments (6).

Safety

LIKELY SAFE ...when used orally in amounts found in foods (6). ...when used orally and appropriately for medicinal purposes (6). ...when soy protein is used intravenously as an emulsion (15).
CHILDREN: LIKELY SAFE ...when used orally in amounts found in food or as a component of infant formula (3400). POSSIBLY UNSAFE ...when used as an alternative to cow's milk in children with severe milk allergy. Although soy-protein based infant formulas are often promoted for children with milk allergy, children with a severe allergy to cow's milk are also frequently sensitive to soy protein (14). LIKELY UNSAFE ...when soy milk is used orally as a substitute for infant formula. Soy milk products carry the warning, "Not for use as infant formula."
PREGNANCY: LIKELY SAFE ...when used in amounts found in foods (6,14). POSSIBLY UNSAFE ...when used orally in medicinal amounts, due to the hormonal effects of soy preparations (6,14). Theoretically, therapeutic use of soy might adversely effect fetal development; avoid using.
LACTATION: LIKELY SAFE ...when used in amounts found in foods. In one study, a single dose of 20 grams of roasted soybeans containing 37 mg of the active isoflavones produced 4-6 times less isoflavones in breast milk than would be provided in a soy-based infant formula (2290). There is insufficient reliable information available about the safety of long-term use of therapeutic amounts of soy during lactation.

Effectiveness

EFFECTIVE ...when used orally in combination with a low fat diet for hyperlipidemia. The FDA has approved labeling soy products for cholesterol reduction when used in combination with a diet low in saturated fat and cholesterol. To be eligible for this labeling, soy products must provide at least 6.25 grams of soy protein per serving, which is 25% of the effective amount of 25 grams per day (3977). The FDA-authorized soy health claim refers only to adult nutrition and is not applicable to soy-based infant formulas (6139). In studies, soy protein preparations have reduced total cholesterol and low-density lipoprotein (LDL) levels in hyper- and normocholesterolemic men (2293,2294,3402,4755,6412), normocholesterolemic perimenopausal women, and hypercholesterolemic postmenopausal women (842,2296,3402,4755). In normocholesterolemic premenopausal women soy protein providing a high amount of isoflavones (129 mg/day) significantly lowered LDL cholesterol only during the middle of the menstrual cycle (6413). Meta-analysis of controlled clinical studies indicates that replacement of dietary animal protein with soy protein significantly decreases serum total cholesterol by 9.3%, LDL cholesterol by 12.9%, and triglycerides by 10.5%, without affecting serum HDL cholesterol (3401). In most studies, treatment duration was from 1-2 months. Some studies indicate that beneficial effects might be attributed to the isoflavone content of soy protein, with preparations providing higher concentrations of isoflavones producing more significant effects (3402,6413). ...when used intravenously as a soy fat emulsion as a source of calories and fatty acids (14,15). ...when taken orally as an isolated soy protein-based formula as an alternative for providing nutrition in term infants (3400).

POSSIBLY EFFECTIVE ...when used orally for relief of hot flashes due to menopause. Epidemiological studies show that Asian women who eat a high-soy diet have fewer hot flashes. Clinical studies have shown modest, but significant improvement (2296,2297,3978,3986,3987). In one study lasting 12 weeks, a soy extract significantly reduced the number of hot flashes when given alone, but had an even greater effect when given concurrently with conjugated estrogens (4751). ...when used orally to reduce the risk of osteoporosis in postmenopausal women (386,842). Soy protein containing higher amounts of constituent isoflavones might have a greater effect. In one controlled study, postmenopausal women received 40 grams of soy protein containing either 1.39 mg or 2.25 mg isoflavones per gram. After 6 months, there were significant increases in spinal bone mineral content and density in the women who consumed the high-isoflavone content soy protein, but not in the women receiving the low-isoflavone content soy protein (842). ...when soy fiber is used orally for reducing the duration of diarrhea in infants (2291,2292). ...when isolated soy protein-based formula is used orally in infants with galactosemia, hereditary lactase deficiency, or lactose intolerance (3400)....when soy protein is used orally for reducing proteinuria in people with kidney disease (2286,2287,2288). ...when soy milk is used orally for reducing the risk of prostate cancer in men (2298). ...when soy protein is used to lower blood pressure in perimenopausal women (2296).

POSSIBLY INEFFECTIVE ...when used to prevent hot flashes in breast cancer survivors (3991).

There is insufficient reliable information available about the effectiveness of soy for its other uses.

Possible Mechanism of Action & Active Ingredients

Soybeans are legumes which contain up to 25% oil, 24% carbohydrates, and 50% protein, as well as stearic, linoleic, and palmitic acids. They are also rich in calcium, iron, potassium, amino acids, vitamins, and fiber (6). Non-fortified soy beverages, also known as soy milk, contain only about 10 mg of calcium per serving. Calcium-fortified soy milk can contain from 80-500 mg of calcium per serving in the form of tricalcium phosphate (6414). However, calcium from cow's milk is significantly better absorbed than calcium from fortified soy milk (6414). Soybeans and soy foods contain the most significant dietary source of isoflavones (3978,4753,6029). The isoflavones are hydrolyzed by beta-glucosidases in the jejunum, releasing the phytoestrogens genistein and daidzein (3982). These are widely distributed in the body with peak concentrations at 4 to 8 hours after dietary intake and excretion within 24 hours (3982). The absorption of isoflavones from food may be saturable, suggesting improved effect if ingested throughout the day (3982). Isoflavone bioavailability does not seem to be affected by food source of isoflavones or other foods in the diet (4750). Phytoestrogens might act as selective estrogen-receptor modulators (SERMs) (3990). This means that in premenopausal women with normal endogenous estrogen levels, soy phytoestrogens may have an anti-estrogen effect. In postmenopausal women with low endogenous estrogens, soy phytoestrogens are likely to act as weak estrogens (3988,3989,3990,3994,6029). Phytoestrogens have a higher affinity for the beta estrogen receptor than the classical alpha estrogen receptor (3983,3992,6029). The beta estrogen receptor predominates in the heart, vasculature, bone, and bladder, which may account for some of soy's beneficial effects. Soy may also have nonestrogenic mechanisms (3990). The mechanism for reducing cholesterol in hyperlipidemia is not clear. However, it is thought that the estrogenic effects of soy isoflavones play a role in modulating lipid metabolism. Soy can also increase bile acid excretion and might upregulate low-density lipoprotein (LDL) receptors (6029,6030). Soy might also have other activities that might be beneficial in cardiovascular disease (6029). For example, soy is thought to have weak antioxidant effects (6029) and might improve arterial compliance (851) and possibly inhibit platelet aggregation (3992). Osteoporosis in postmenopausal women is related to declining estrogen levels. Soy is thought to be beneficial for preventing osteoporosis due to its weak estrogenic effects, although the precise mechanism is not known (6029). Estrogenic effects of soy have also been attributed to benefit in menopausal symptoms such as hot flashes. However, the incidence of hot flashes does not seem correlate with serum levels of the phytoestrogens genistein, diadzein, and equol. Components of soy other than phytoestrogens may be responsible for reduction in hot flashes (4752). In cancer soy is thought to be beneficial due to preliminary evidence that suggests isoflavones in soy have antioxidant, antiproliferative, and antiangiogenic activity (2296,3983). However, due to the estrogenic effects of soy, there is some concern that it may increase the risk of breast cancer (6030). In prostatic diseases, preliminary evidence suggests that soy phytoestrogens may be beneficial due to estrogenic mechanisms as well as inhibition of 5 alpha-reductase and 17 beta-hydroxysteroid dehydrogenase (3984,3985). Laboratory evidence suggests that isoflavones can inhibit oxidative and conjugative metabolism of drugs (4736). Isoflavones might also affect drug absorption and biliary excretion by interacting with drug transporters such as P-glycoprotein and the canalicular multispecific organic anion transporter (4736). Given the wide range of drugs and metabolites whose pharmacokinetics depends on these mechanisms, drug interactions with isoflavones might be more common than literature reports suggest.

Adverse Reactions Including Known Allergies

Oral ingestion of soy has primarily been associated with gastrointestinal side effects, such as constipation, bloating, and nausea (2297). Soy has also caused allergic reactions (14,2280), such as skin rash and itching (6412). Inhaled soy dust and soy hull aeroallergen can trigger symptoms of asthma. The risk and severity increase with exposure (5084). Inhaled soy dust was reported as the cause of an asthma epidemic in Spain (5084,5085,5086).

There may be a link between tofu ingestion and cognitive functioning. Data collected from the Honolulu-Asia Aging Study and the Honolulu Heart Program shows a possible association of high midlife tofu consumption (two or more servings per week) with cognitive impairment in late life (6415). Of the 3,734 Japanese-American men participating, cognitive impairment was identified in 19% of the high tofu users versus 4% of the low tofu users approximately 30 years later when the men were between 71-93 years of age. Some suggest that this relationship is questionable. Other factors, such as lifestyle and health of the participants, may be involved. A larger percentage of the high tofu users were immigrants from Japan, had fewer years of education, and had worked at low complexity jobs. The high tofu users had also experienced a greater incidence of strokes. The results are considered too preliminary for any recommendations to be made at this time (6416).

Possible Interactions with Herbs & Other Dietary Supplements

Insufficient reliable information available.

Possible Interactions with Drugs

ESTROGEN: Theoretically, soy might competitively inhibit the effects of estrogen replacement therapy (3860).

Possible Interactions with Foods

PLANT-BASED FOODS: Soy protein isolate reduces the absorption of non-heme iron from foods (5053). Non-heme iron is found in plant-based foods.

Possible Interactions with Lab Tests

No interactions are known to occur, and there is no known reason to expect a clinically significant interaction with soy.

Possible Interactions with Diseases or Conditions

ASTHMA: People with asthma are at increased risk for soy hull allergy. The risk and severity of symptoms increase with increased exposure (5084).

ALLERGIC RHINITIS: People with allergic rhinitis are at increased risk for soy hull allergy. The risk and severity of symptoms increase with increased exposure (5084).

BREAST CANCER: Soy isoflavones have estrogenic properties. Some experts are concerned about the use of soy in women with breast cancer because estrogens can increase this risk. However, some preclinical studies show that soy may have protective effects for breast cancer (3976) while others suggest soy might increase breast cell proliferation (3980,3981). Because there is insufficient reliable information about the effects of soy preparations in patients with breast cancer, a history of breast cancer, or a family history of breast cancer, therapeutic use of soy should be done with caution in these patients (956).

CYSTIC FIBROSIS: Children with cystic fibrosis may develop hypoproteinemia when fed soy milk (368).

HYPOTHYROID: Soy can inhibit thyroid hormone synthesis (6,14).

HYPERBILIRUBINEMIA: Large amounts of soybean oil (2-3 g/kg) might worsen hyperbilirubinemia in infants (14).

MILK ALLERGY: Children who are severely allergic to cow's milk are frequently sensitive to soy as well (14); Use with caution or avoid.

Typical Dosages & Routes of Administration that are Commonly Used

ORAL: For lowering cholesterol, a typical dose is 20-50 grams per day of soy protein (2293,2295,2296,3401,6412). For preventing osteoporosis, a typical dose is 40 grams per day soy protein containing 2.25 mg isoflavones per gram of protein (842). For reducing the severity and number of hot flashes, a typical dose is 20-60 grams per day of soy protein (2296,2297). For reducing risk of prostate cancer, two or more glasses of soy milk daily has been used (2298). For proteinuria, a diet limited to 700-800 mg/kg soy protein daily has been used (2287). For diarrhea in infants, soy fiber fortified formula containing 18-20 grams of soy protein per liter has been used (2291,2292).

Comments

None.

SOYBEAN OIL

This Product is Also Known As

Intralipid, Soyca, Take Control, Travmulsion.

Scientific Names

Glycine soja.
Family: Fabaceae.

People Use This For

Parenterally, soybean oil is used in nutrient formulas. It is also used as a source of lecithin (4077).
Plant sterols, derived from soybean oil, are used to lower total and LDL cholesterol without affecting HDL (4086).
Soybean oil has been used as a filler in some breast implants (see Comments) (6125).

Safety

LIKELY SAFE ...when soybean oil or the plant sterols from soybean oil are used orally and appropriately in margarine. ...when soybean oil is used in pharmaceutical grade parenteral formulas. Soybean oil is listed in the United States Pharmacopeia (10).
PREGNANCY: LIKELY SAFE ...when used orally in amounts found in foods. Avoid using in amounts greater than those typically found in foods. Theoretically, parenteral use of lipids like soybean oil during pregnancy might lead to hypertriglyceridemia, ketonemia, premature labor, and placental infection. However, women have used parenteral nutrition with lipids to treat severe morning sickness without any adverse effects (4084).
LACTATION: LIKELY SAFE ...when used orally in amounts found in foods. Avoid using in amounts greater than those typically found in foods.

Effectiveness

EFFECTIVE ...when soybean oil is used as a parenteral nutrient (16).
POSSIBLY EFFECTIVE ...when the plant sterols from soybean oil are used in margarine to lower total and LDL cholesterol without affecting HDL (4086). The FDA has approved such labeling for the products Take Control and Benecol as a structure/function claim under the Dietary Supplement Health Education Act, not as a drug (4087).

Possible Mechanism of Action & Active Ingredients

Soybean oil is used in parenteral nutrition as a source of fatty acids (16). In a comparison between diets with 20% fat from butter or soybean oil, people using soybean oil demonstrated a 12% decrease in LDL and a 3% reduction in HDL (4085). People using a margarine containing plant sterols from soybean oil reduced total and LDL cholesterol by 8-13% compared to a control group (4086).

Adverse Reactions Including Known Allergies

FABACEAE HERBS: Soybean oil can cause an allergic reaction in individuals allergic to the Fabaceae family. Members of this family include peanuts and soybeans (4079,4080).

Possible Interactions with Herbs & Other Dietary Supplements

Insufficient reliable information available.

Possible Interactions with Drugs

No interactions are known to occur, and there is no known reason to expect a clinically significant interaction with soybean oil.

Possible Interactions with Foods

No interactions are known to occur, and there is no known reason to expect a clinically significant interaction with soybean oil.

Possible Interactions with Lab Tests

CHOLESTEROL: Soybean oil sterols can reduce serum total cholesterol and LDL cholesterol concentrations, and test results (4086).

Possible Interactions with Diseases or Conditions

CROSS-ALLERGENICITY: Soybean oil can cause an allergic reaction in individuals sensitive to the Fabaceae family. Members of this family include peanuts and soybeans (4079,4080).

Typical Dosages & Routes of Administration that are Commonly Used

ORAL: In the form of a plant sterol-enriched margarine, such as Take Control, a serving size is one tablespoon, or 14 grams.
PARENTERAL: No typical dosage.

Comments

Soybean oil is obtained by cold pressing the seeds of the Glycine soja (18).
The British Health Ministry recommends that women with soybean oil filled (Trilucent) breast implants have them removed as a precautionary measure. While there is currently no evidence of any serious medical problems, tests reveal that the soybean oil filler can break down producing aldehydes which might be toxic to the implant recipient or to a developing fetus (6125).

SPANISH BROOM

This Product is Also Known As
Genet, Weaver's Broom.
CAUTION: See separate listings for Butcher's Broom, Scotch Broom flower, and Scotch Broom herb.

Scientific Names
Spartium junceum, synonym Genista juncea.
Family: Leguminosae or Fabaceae.

People Use This For
Historically, Spanish broom has been used as a laxative and diuretic (11).
In foods and beverages, Spanish broom extracts are used as a flavor component. (11).
In manufacturing, an extract is used as a fragrance in soaps and cosmetics (11).

Safety
LIKELY SAFE ...when used orally in amounts found in foods. Spanish broom is approved for food use in the US (11).
PREGNANCY AND LACTATION: POSSIBLY UNSAFE ...large amounts of the alkaloid constituent sparteine can stimulate menstrual flow (19). The most common Spanish broom extract, Genet absolute, should not contain alkaloids because of the extraction method used, however, other extracts might (11).

Effectiveness
There is insufficient reliable information about the effectiveness of Spanish broom.

Possible Mechanism of Action & Active Ingredients
The applicable part of Spanish broom is the flower. Sparteine seems to hasten childbirth (11). No other data is available on the pharmacology of Spanish broom.

Adverse Reactions Including Known Allergies
None reported.

Possible Interactions with Herbs & Other Dietary Supplements
Insufficient reliable information available.

Possible Interactions with Drugs
No interactions are known to occur, and there is no known reason to expect a clinically significant interaction with Spanish broom.

Possible Interactions with Foods
No interactions are known to occur, and there is no known reason to expect a clinically significant interaction with Spanish broom.

Possible Interactions with Lab Tests
No interactions are known to occur, and there is no known reason to expect a clinically significant interaction with Spanish broom.

Possible Interactions with Diseases or Conditions
No interactions are known to occur, and there is no known reason to expect a clinically significant interaction with Spanish broom.

Typical Dosages & Routes of Administration that are Commonly Used
No typical dosage.

Comments
Avoid confusion with butcher's broom, scotch broom flower, and scotch broom herb. Spanish broom stems have appeared as an adulterant to scotch broom (Cytisus scoparius).

SPANISH ORIGANUM OIL

This Product is Also Known As
Origanum Oil, Sicilian Thyme, Spanish Origanum, Spanish Thyme.
CAUTION: See separate listings for Thyme oil, Thyme, and Wild Thyme.

Scientific Names
Thymus capitatus, synonym Coridothymus capitatus; Satureja capitata; carvacrol-rich Origanum species.
Family: Labiatae or Lamiaceae.

People Use This For

Spanish origanum oil has no reported medicinal uses.

In food and beverages, Spanish origanum oil is used as a flavor component (11).

In manufacturing, it is used as a fragrance component in soaps, cosmetics, and perfumes.

Safety

LIKELY SAFE ...when used in amounts found in foods. Spanish origanum is approved for food use in the US. The maximum use level is 0.01% (11).

PREGNANCY AND LACTATION: Insufficient reliable information available; avoid amounts greater than found in foods.

Effectiveness

There is insufficient reliable information available about the effectiveness of Spanish origanum oil.

Possible Mechanism of Action & Active Ingredients

Spanish origanum oil is characterized by its carvacrol content (11). It contains carvacrol and thymol (11) which show some evidence of anthelmintic (11), antifungal (4059,4060,4062,4063), and antibacterial (4064,4065,4066) activity. These constituents also demonstrate some evidence of antioxidant activity, including decreased Fe (III) catalyzed phospholipid liposome peroxidation and peroxy radical scavenging activity (4067).

Adverse Reactions Including Known Allergies

None reported.

Possible Interactions with Herbs & Other Dietary Supplements

Insufficient reliable information available.

Possible Interactions with Drugs

No interactions are known to occur, and there is no known reason to expect a clinically significant interaction with Spanish origanum oil.

Possible Interactions with Foods

No interactions are known to occur, and there is no known reason to expect a clinically significant interaction with Spanish origanum oil.

Possible Interactions with Lab Tests

No interactions are known to occur, and there is no known reason to expect a clinically significant interaction with Spanish origanum oil.

Possible Interactions with Diseases or Conditions

No interactions are known to occur, and there is no known reason to expect a clinically significant interaction with Spanish origanum oil.

Typical Dosages & Routes of Administration that are Commonly Used

No typical dosage.

Comments

Spanish origanum oil is distilled from the flowering tops of Thymus capitatus and carvacrol-rich Origanum species.

SPEARMINT

This Product is Also Known As

Curled Mint, Fish Mint, Garden Mint, Green Mint, Lamb Mint, Mackerel Mint, Our Lady's Mint, Sage of Bethlehem, Spire Mint, Yerba buena.

CAUTION: See separate listing for Sage.

Scientific Names

Mentha spicata, synonym M. viridis.

Family: Labiatae or Lamiaceae.

People Use This For

Orally, spearmint is used for digestive disorders, including flatulence (18), indigestion, nausea, sore throat, diarrhea, colds, headaches, toothaches, cramps, and cancer.

Topically, it is used for oral mucosal inflammation, arthritis, local muscle and nerve pain, and skin conditions including pruritus and urticaria.

In Europe, it is used orally under the direction of a physician for bile duct and gallbladder inflammation, gallstones, upper gastrointestinal tract spasms, flatulence, irritable bowel syndrome, and inflammation of respiratory tract. It is also used as an aromatic, stimulant, antiseptic, local anesthetic, and antispasmodic.

Spearmint is used as a flavoring agent in foods, beverages and in pharmaceutical and health food products. It is also used in herb teas, and oral hygiene products such as mouthwash and toothpaste, and cosmetics (11).

Safety

LIKELY SAFE ...when used in amounts found in foods and consumed in appropriate amounts. It has Generally Recognized as Safe (GRAS) status in the US and its maximum use is 0.132% (11).

POSSIBLY SAFE ...when used orally and topically for medicinal reasons (11,12).

PREGNANCY AND LACTATION: Avoid using in amounts greater than those typically found in foods.

Effectiveness

There is insufficient reliable information available about the effectiveness of spearmint leaf and oil.

Possible Mechanism of Action & Active Ingredients

The applicable parts of spearmint are the leaf and oil. There is insufficient reliable information available about the possible mechanism of action and active ingredients of spearmint.

Adverse Reactions Including Known Allergies

None reported.

Possible Interactions with Herbs & Other Dietary Supplements

Insufficient reliable information available.

Possible Interactions with Drugs

No interactions are known to occur, and there is no known reason to expect a clinically significant interaction with spearmint.

Possible Interactions with Foods

No interactions are known to occur, and there is no known reason to expect a clinically significant interaction with spearmint.

Possible Interactions with Lab Tests

No interactions are known to occur, and there is no known reason to expect a clinically significant interaction with spearmint.

Possible Interactions with Diseases or Conditions

No interactions are known to occur, and there is no known reason to expect a clinically significant interaction with spearmint.

Typical Dosages & Routes of Administration that are Commonly Used

ORAL: Spearmint is taken in tea, and is also available in tablets, capsules, tinctures and other oral formulations (11).

Comments

None.

SPINACH

This Product is Also Known As

Spinaciae folium, Spinatblatter.

Scientific Names

Spinacia oleracea.
Family: Chenopodiaceae.

People Use This For

Orally, spinach is used for gastrointestinal complaints and fatigue. It is also used as a blood-builder, an appetite stimulant, for stimulating growth in children, and during convalescence (2).

For food uses, spinach is a commonly consumed vegetable.

Safety

LIKELY SAFE ...when consumed in food amounts.

CHILDREN: LIKELY UNSAFE ...when used in infants under 4 months old because the nitrate content can cause methemoglobinemia (18).

PREGNANCY AND LACTATION: LIKELY SAFE ...when consumed in food amounts; avoid amounts greater than those consumed in food.

Effectiveness

There is insufficient reliable information available about the effectiveness of spinach.

Possible Mechanism of Action & Active Ingredients

The applicable part of spinach is the leaf. Spinach contains vitamin C (18), vitamin E, vitamin K, magnesium (19), and nitrates (18). It also contains triterpene saponins including oxalic acid (18). Spinach is thought to have hypoglycemic effects (19). Consumption of fresh spinach is associated with a decreased risk of stomach cancer in humans (4112). Preliminary research suggests that compounds contained in spinach might slow aging effects on the nervous system (1418,1419).

Adverse Reactions Including Known Allergies

May cause methemoglobinemia in infants younger than four months old (18).

Possible Interactions with Herbs & Other Dietary Supplements

Insufficient reliable information available.

Possible Interactions with Drugs

ANTICOAGULANTS: Spinach contains vitamin K. Individuals using anticoagulants should consume a consistent daily amount to maintain the effect of anticoagulant therapy (19).
DIABETES THERAPY: Monitor blood glucose level closely due to claims that spinach leaves have hypoglycemic effects (19).

Possible Interactions with Foods

No interactions are known to occur, and there is no known reason to expect a clinically significant interaction with spinach.

Possible Interactions with Lab Tests

No interactions are known to occur, and there is no known reason to expect a clinically significant interaction with spinach.

Possible Interactions with Diseases or Conditions

KIDNEY DISEASE: May cause formation of insoluble oxalate crystals in the kidneys causing further damage (19).
DIABETES: Theoretically, may interfere with blood glucose control (19).

Typical Dosages & Routes of Administration that are Commonly Used

No typical dosage.

Comments

Spinach is rich in beta-carotene, vitamin E, vitamin K, and magnesium (19).

SPINY RESTHARROW

This Product is Also Known As

Cammock, Ground Furze, Hauhechelwurzel, Land Whin, Ononidis radix, Petty Whin, Restharrow, Stay Plough, Stinking Tommy, Wild Liquorice.

Scientific Names

Ononis spinosa.
Family: Fabacea.

People Use This For

Orally, spiny restharrow root is used for gout, kidney and bladder stones, rheumatic complaints, urinary tract infections (18), irrigation therapy for inflammatory disease of the lower urinary tract, and prevention and treatment of kidney gravel (2,18).

Safety

POSSIBLY SAFE ...when used orally and appropriately for the prevention and treatment of kidney gravel. ...when used orally and appropriately as irrigation therapy for urinary tract inflammatory disorders (2). Copious fluid intake is important to success of irrigation therapy (2).
There is insufficient reliable information available about the safety of spiny restharrow for its other uses.
PREGNANCY AND LACTATION: Insufficient reliable information available; avoid using.

Effectiveness

POSSIBLY EFFECTIVE ...when used for the prevention and treatment of kidney gravel. ...when used as irrigation therapy for inflammatory disorders of the urinary tract (2).
There is insufficient reliable information available about the effectiveness of spiny restharrow for its other uses.

Possible Mechanism of Action & Active Ingredients

The applicable part of spiny restharrow is the root. The drug contains isoflavonoids including ononin (2,18), triterpenes including alphaonoceradiendiol (18), and volatile oil (18). The volatile oil contains anethole, carvone, and menthol (18). Spiny restharrow is reported to have a diuretic effect (2,18).

© Copyright 2000, Natural Medicines Comprehensive Database (209) 472-2244. For updated data, go to www.NaturalDatabase.com • 979

Adverse Reactions Including Known Allergies
None reported.

Possible Interactions with Herbs & Other Dietary Supplements
Insufficient reliable information available.

Possible Interactions with Drugs
No interactions are known to occur, and there is no known reason to expect a clinically significant interaction with spiny restharrow.

Possible Interactions with Foods
No interactions are known to occur, and there is no known reason to expect a clinically significant interaction with spiny restharrow.

Possible Interactions with Lab Tests
No interactions are known to occur, and there is no known reason to expect a clinically significant interaction with spiny restharrow.

Possible Interactions with Diseases or Conditions
EDEMA: Contraindicated in individuals with edema resulting from cardiac or kidney impairment (2,18).

Typical Dosages & Routes of Administration that are Commonly Used
ORAL: A typical oral dose is 6-12 grams daily or as a tea (2,18). To prepare tea, pour boiling water over 2-2.5 grams of ground drug, strain after 20-30 minutes (18). Drink with plenty of liquid (2,18).

Comments
None.

SQUALAMINE

This Product is Also Known As
Spiny Dogfish Shark.

Scientific Names
Squalus acanthias.

People Use This For
Orally, squalamine has been used experimentally as an antibiotic (6).
Topically, synthetic squalamine compounds have been investigated as antibiotics (4138).
In combination with captopril, oral squalamine is being investigated as an anti-angiogenic therapy for diabetic retinopathy (1269).
Squalamine is being investigated as a possible treatment for pediatric solid tumors (5043).

Safety
There is insufficient reliable information available about the safety of squalamine or its derivative SM-7.
Pregnancy and Lactation: Insufficient reliable information available.

Effectiveness
There is insufficient reliable information available about the effectiveness of squalamine or its derivative SM-7.

Possible Mechanism of Action & Active Ingredients
Squalamine was first isolated from the spiny dogfish shark and later synthesized synthetically. It shows evidence that it might have fungicidal and antiprotozoal activity (4139). Squalamine has also demonstrated significant activity against gram (-) and gram (+) bacteria (4139). Some compounds that mimic the structure of squalamine show promise in their activity against gram (-) rods, gram (+) cocci including methicillin-resistant Staphylococcus aureus, vancomycin-resistant Enterococcus faecium, and fungi (4138). In addition to antibiotic activity, squalamine also shows promise in inhibiting angiogenesis, and preventing formation and growth of tumors (4137,5043). Researchers report that squalamine demonstrates activity in breast, lung, and neuroblastoma cancer models. This unpublished research was reported at the American Association for Cancer Research 91st Annual Meeting (5043).

Adverse Reactions Including Known Allergies
None reported.

Possible Interactions with Herbs & Other Dietary Supplements
Insufficient reliable information available.

Possible Interactions with Drugs

CISPLATIN: Theoretically, concomitant use might inhibit growth and promote shrinkage of neuroblastomas. Preclinical data suggest that squalamine used in combination with cisplatin might inhibit tumor growth and promote tumor shrinkage in the treatment of neuroblastomas. This unpublished research was reported at the American Association for Cancer Research 91st Annual Meeting (5043).

Possible Interactions with Foods

No interactions are known to occur, and there is no known reason to expect a clinically significant interaction with squalamine.

Possible Interactions with Lab Tests

No interactions are known to occur, and there is no known reason to expect a clinically significant interaction with squalamine.

Possible Interactions with Diseases or Conditions

No interactions are known to occur, and there is no known reason to expect a clinically significant interaction with squalamine.

Typical Dosages & Routes of Administration that are Commonly Used

No typical dosage.

Comments

Squalamine has been isolated from the stomach and liver tissues of the spiny dogfish shark. Synthetic products that mimic the structure of squalamine appear to be good candidates for further development as topical antimicrobial agents. They have broad spectrum antimicrobial activity, but their potential for systemic toxicity limits their use (4138). Avoid confusion with shark cartilage, which is prepared from the cartilage of spiny dogfish shark, hammerhead shark (Sphyrna lewini), and other shark species (6).

Researchers at Georgetown University Medical Center plan a study of squalamine as an antiangiogenic therapy in combination with captopril for diabetic retinopathy (1269).

Magainin, the manufacturer of an investigational squalamine drug product plans a clinical study of squalamine in the treatment of pediatric solid tumors (5043).

SQUAWVINE

This Product is Also Known As

Checkerberry, Deerberry, Hive Vine, Noon Kie Oo Nah Yeah, One-Berry, Partridgeberry, Running Box, Squaw Berry, Squaw Vine, Twinberry, Two-Eyed Berry, Winter Clover.

Scientific Names

Mitchella repens.
Family: Rubiaceae.

People Use This For

Orally, squawvine is used for amenorrhea (absence of menstruation), anxiety, diarrhea, edema, excessive menstruation, fibrocystic disease of the breast, oliguria (lack of urination), painful menstruation, postpartum depression, varicose veins (3199), pregnancy (to make labor less difficult) (407,3199), improving lactation, insomnia, congestive heart failure, kidney failure, liver failure (407), chronic dysentery, spermatorrhea (involuntary discharge of semen without orgasm), as an emmenagogue (to promote menstruation), as an astringent for treating colitis, and reducing mucous membrane and leukorrheal (whitish vaginal) discharges (411).

Topically, squawvine is used for treating sore nipples (410).

Traditionally, squawvine was used by American Indians for promoting easy childbirth (taken during the last few weeks of pregnancy only), and as an abortifacient (408).

Safety

POSSIBLY SAFE ...when used orally and appropriately (12).
There is insufficient reliable information about the safety of squawvine for its other uses.
PREGNANCY: POSSIBLY UNSAFE ...when used orally due to reported abortifacient properties.
LACTATION: Insufficient reliable information available; avoid using.

Effectiveness

There is insufficient reliable information available about the effectiveness of squawvine.

Possible Mechanism of Action & Active Ingredients

The applicable parts of squawvine are the above ground parts (herb) (12), stem (407), and leaf (408). Squawvine is reported to contain resin, wax, mucilages, dextrin, saponins, and unspecified alkaloids, glycosides and tannins (407,410,411).

Adverse Reactions Including Known Allergies
None reported.

Possible Interactions with Herbs & Other Dietary Supplements
Insufficient reliable information available.

Possible Interactions with Drugs
No interactions are known to occur, and there is no known reason to expect a clinically significant interaction with squawvine.

Possible Interactions with Foods
No interactions are known to occur, and there is no known reason to expect a clinically significant interaction with squawvine.

Possible Interactions with Lab Tests
No interactions are known to occur, and there is no known reason to expect a clinically significant interaction with squawvine.

Possible Interactions with Diseases or Conditions
No interactions are known to occur, and there is no known reason to expect a clinically significant interaction with squawvine.

Typical Dosages & Routes of Administration that are Commonly Used
ORAL: A typical dose is 20-50 mg.

Comments
None.

SQUILL

This Product is Also Known As
European Squill, Indian Squill, Mediterranean Squill, Red Squill, Sea Onion, Sea Squill Bulb, Scilla, White Squill.

Scientific Names
Urginea maritima, synonyms Drimia maritima, Scilla maritima, Urginea scilla; Urginea indica, synonyms Drimia indica, Scilla indica.
Family: Liliaceae.

People Use This For
Orally, squill is used for mild heart failure (2,7,18), arrhythmias, nervous heart complaints, some venous conditions (18), edema, inducing emesis, as an expectorant (6), for chronic bronchitis, asthma with bronchitis, and whooping cough (4).
Historically, squill has been used as a diuretic (6,11,13), expectorant, abortifacient, emetic, heart tonic, and a rat poison (3488,3489).
In manufacturing, squill has been used in pest control as a rodenticide (red squill) (11,13).

Safety
UNSAFE ...when used orally (4,6,18,512). Squill contains cardiac glycosides that can cause adverse effects (512).
PREGNANCY: UNSAFE ...when taken orally. Squill is contraindicated during pregnancy because it can have an abortifacient effect (4).
LACTATION: UNSAFE ...when taken orally (4).

Effectiveness
POSSIBLY EFFECTIVE ...when taken orally. Squill seems to help patients with mild heart failure, even in people with impaired kidney function (2).
There is insufficient reliable information available about the effectiveness of squill for its other uses.

Possible Mechanism of Action & Active Ingredients
Squill contains cardioactive glycosides, including bufadienolides, scillaren A, and proscillaridin A (2,4,6,18). Squill seems to have cardiac effects similar to digoxin, including positive inotropic and negative chronotropic effects (4,7). The aglycones in squill are poorly absorbed from the gastrointestinal tract and are therefore less potent than digitalis cardiac glycosides. Squill has additional cardiovascular properties that include reducing left ventricular diastolic pressure, and reducing pathologically elevated venous pressure (2,18). Large amounts of squill can induce vomiting due to gastric irritation and central action (4). In lesser amounts squill causes an expectorant-like effect (6).

Adverse Reactions Including Known Allergies
Taken orally, squill can cause gastric irritation, loss of appetite, diarrhea, vomiting, stomach disorders, headache, irregular pulse (2,18), and convulsions (6). Skin contact with the fresh bulb can cause dermatitis (18). Signs of

overdose include restlessness, nausea, vomiting, life-threatening arrhythmias (ventricular tachycardia, atrial tachycardia with atrioventricular block, ventricular fibrillation), stupor, vision disorders, depression, confusion, hallucinations, psychosis, seizure, cardiac arrest, asphyxiation and death (18,3488). A fatality has been reported after ingestion of squill bulb (3488).

Possible Interactions with Herbs & Other Dietary Supplements

CALCIUM: Concomitant use of calcium may increase risk of cardiac toxicity (2,3805).

CARDIAC GLYCOSIDE-CONTAINING HERBS: Contraindicated, and concomitant use can increase the risk of cardiac glycoside toxicity. Cardiac glycoside-containing herbs include black hellebore, Canadian hemp roots, digitalis leaf, hedge mustard, figwort, lily of the valley roots, motherwort, oleander leaf, pheasant's eye plant, pleurisy root, strophanthus seeds, and uzara (2,18,19,500).

OTHER CARDIOACTIVE HERBS: Avoid concomitant use with other cardioactive herbs due to unpredictability of effects and adverse effects. Other cardioactive herbs include: calamus, cereus, cola, coltsfoot, devil's claw, European mistletoe, fenugreek, fumitory, ginger, Panax ginseng, hawthorn, white horehound, mate, parsley, quassia, scotch broom flower, shepherd's purse, and wild carrot (4). See individual product listings.

STIMULANT LAXATIVE HERBS: Theoretically, overuse or misuse of stimulant laxatives with cardiac glycoside-containing herbs increases the risk of cardiac toxicity due to potassium depletion. Stimulant laxative herbs include: aloe dried leaf sap, blue flag rhizome, alder buckthorn, European buckthorn, butternut bark, cascara bark, castor oil, colocynth fruit pulp, gamboge bark exudate, jalap root, black root, manna bark exudate, podophyllum root, rhubarb root, senna leaves and pods, wild cucumber fruit (Ecballium elaterium), and yellow dock root (19).

LICORICE/HORSETAIL: Theoretically, overuse/misuse of licorice rhizome or horsetail plant with cardiac glycoside-containing herbs increases the risk of cardiac toxicity due to potassium depletion (19).

Possible Interactions with Drugs

ARRHYTHMOGENIC AGENTS: Increased risk of arrhythmias when used with sympathomimetics, methylxanthines and phosphodiesterase inhibitors (18).

CALCIUM: Concomitant use may increase risk of cardiac toxicity (2,3805).

CORTICOSTEROIDS: Concomitant use may increase effects and adverse effects of long-term corticosteroid use (2).

DIGOXIN: Concomitant use contraindicated, due to increased risk of cardiac glycoside toxicity (2,4).

POTASIUM DEPLETING DIURETICS, STIMULANT LAXATIVES: Concomitant use may increase risk of cardiac glycoside toxicity due to potassium loss (2).

QUINIDINE: Concomitant use may increase cardiac effects and adverse effects (2).

Possible Interactions with Foods

No interactions are known to occur, and there is no known reason to expect a clinically significant interaction with squill.

Possible Interactions with Lab Tests

No interactions are known to occur, and there is no known reason to expect a clinically significant interaction with squill.

Possible Interactions with Diseases or Conditions

ELECTROLYTE IMBALANCE: Contraindicated in individuals with hypokalemia or hypercalcemia.

CARDIAC CONDITIONS: Contraindicated in individuals with second or third degree atrioventricular block, hypertrophic cardiomyopathy, carotid sinus syndrome, ventricular tachycardia, or thoracic aortic aneurysm Wolff-Parkinson-White syndrome (18).

GI CONDITIONS: Can irritate gastrointestinal tract. Contraindicated in individuals with infectious or inflammatory gastrointestinal conditions (19).

Typical Dosages & Routes of Administration that are Commonly Used

ORAL: Mild heart failure (NYHA stage I and II heart disease), 100-500 mg standardized squill bulb powder per day (2,7).

Comments

Unsafe for self-medication (512). New York Heart Association (NYHA) stage I and II heart disease refers to people with heart disease who do not have limitations of physical activity. They are comfortable at rest but ordinary physical activity results in fatigue, palpitation, trouble breathing, or anginal pain (2).

ST. JOHN'S WORT

This Product is Also Known As

Amber, Amber Touch-and-Heal, Demon Chaser, Fuga Daemonum, Goatweed, Hardhay, Hypereikon, Hyperici Herba, Hypericum, Johns Wort, Klamath Weed, Millepertuis, Rosin Rose, Saint Johns Wort, Saint John's Wort, Saynt Johannes Wort, SJW, St Johns Wort, St John's Wort, Tipton Weed.

Scientific Names

Hypericum perforatum.
Family: Hypericaceae.

People Use This For

Orally, St. John's wort is used for depression and dysthymic disorder (5087); secondary symptoms associated with depression such as fatigue, loss of appetite, insomnia (376,377), anxiety, or nervous unrest (2); obsessive-compulsive disorder (OCD) (5075); mood disturbances associated with menopause (4); migraine headache (3572); neuralgia; excitability; fibrositis; sciatica (4); lack of drive; palpitations; exhaustion; headache; and muscle pain (376). It is also used orally for treating cancer, vitiligo, and as a diuretic (6). Oily St. John's wort preparations are used orally for gastric indigestion (2).

Topically, oily St. John's wort preparations are used for treating bruises and abrasions, muscle pain, first degree burns (2), hemorrhoids (6), relieving inflammation, promoting healing (6), treating vitiligo (6), and neuralgia (6121). In manufacturing, the hypericin-free extract is used in the making of alcoholic beverages (11).

Safety

LIKELY SAFE ...when used orally and appropriately, short-term for medicinal purposes (4,5,6,7,12,3547,3548,3549, 3550,5087). St. John's wort extracts have been shown to be safe in clinical trials lasting up to 8 weeks (7,3548,3549, 3551,6400). Extensive use in Germany has not resulted in reports of serious toxicities (3549,3552). ...when used orally and appropriately as the hypericin-free extract in amounts commonly found in beverages. It has Generally Recognized as Safe (GRAS) status in the US for use in alcoholic beverages (11).

POSSIBLY UNSAFE ...when used orally in large doses (1800 mg or more of hypericum extract per day) because of the risk of severe phototoxic skin reactions (7,758). People with severe depression, HIV, or AIDS are more likely to use larger doses (758).

PREGNANCY: POSSIBLY UNSAFE ...when used orally. St. John's wort is thought to increase muscle tone of the uterus (4); avoid using.

LACTATION: POSSIBLY UNSAFE ...when used orally. In one study, colic, drowsiness, and lethargy were reported in infants whose mothers used St. John's wort while breast feeding. In this study, more adverse effects were reported in breast-fed infants whose mothers took St. John's wort while breast feeding than in breast-fed infants whose mothers did not use St. John's wort (1377); avoid using.

Effectiveness

LIKELY EFFECTIVE ...when used orally for treating mild to moderate major depression (2,4,166,168,202,203, 204,205,3548,3549,3551,3552,5087). Current guidelines for the pharmacological management of acute major depression suggest St. John's wort as an option for the short-term treatment of mild acute major depression (5087). Multiple clinical trials have shown that St. John's wort extracts, standardized based on hypericin content, are superior to placebo (7,203,204,205,3548,3549,3551,3552), are likely as effective as low-dose tricyclic antidepressants (7,3548,3549,3551), and possibly as effective as fluoxetine (3550) for short-term treatment of mild to moderate major depression.

Standardized extracts based on constituents other than hypericin have not been as extensively studied. One clinical trial using a standardized extract based on hyperforin content showed significant improvement in patients with mild to moderate major depression (761). In another study, the same St. John's wort extract, standardized based on hyperforin, was compared to the selective-serotonin reuptake inhibitor, sertraline (Zoloft). Patients with a diagnosis of mild to moderate major depression were included. Patients were titrated to a dose of 900 mg daily for St. John's wort and 75 mg daily for sertraline (Zoloft) following the first week of treatment. After 7 weeks of treatment, there was significant improvement for both treatment groups. The effectiveness was similar between St. John's wort and sertraline (Zoloft) treated patients (6400). Although most studies point to beneficial effects, one report has found conflicting results. In an unpublished study announced at the 2000 American Psychiatric Association annual meeting, St. John's wort 900-1200 mg daily was no better than placebo after 8 weeks of treatment in patients with major depression (5096).

Most clinical studies on the effectiveness of St. John's wort have used preparations containing the following specific standardized extracts: Lichtwer LI 160- each 300 mg contains 92 mcg hypericin, 262 mcg pseudohypericin, and 18.37 mg hyperforin (382). LI 160 is contained in the product Kira (Lichtwer Pharma US, Inc.). Lichtwer LI 160 WS is the hyperforin stabilized version of LI 160. LI 160 WS is contained in the product Quanterra Emotional Balance (Warner-Lambert).

POSSIBLY EFFECTIVE ...when used orally for treating somatic symptoms associated with mild depression (376). A small-scale clinical trial using a standardized extract based on hypericin content demonstrated significant improvement in somatic symptoms in patients with mild depression (376). ...when used orally for treating anxiety or nervous unrest (2). ...when oily St. John's wort preparations are used orally for dyspepsia (2). ...when oily St. John's wort preparations are used topically for treating bruises and abrasions, myalgia, and first degree burns (2).

POSSIBLY INEFFECTIVE ...when taken orally as an antiretroviral agent in HIV-infected adults (206).

There is insufficient reliable information available about the effectiveness of St. John's wort for its other uses. However, in one unpublished open-label study, announced at the 1999 New Clinical Drug Evaluation Unit annual meeting, a small group of patients with obsessive-compulsive disorder (OCD) had significantly improved symptoms after treatment with St. John's wort for 9 weeks (5075). Although these initial findings look promising, further research is necessary to rate the effectiveness of St. John's wort for OCD.

 © Copyright 2000, Natural Medicines Comprehensive Database (209) 472-2244. For updated data, go to www.NaturalDatabase.com

Possible Mechanism of Action & Active Ingredients

The applicable parts of St. John's wort are the dried, above ground parts. Several active constituents have been isolated from St. John's wort preparations, all of which may contribute to its pharmacological effects (761). The precise mechanism of action in depression and the constituents responsible have not been clearly identified. Two constituents that may play a significant role are hypericin and hyperforin. Hypericin has been shown to inhibit catechol-O-methyl transferase (COMT) and monoamine oxidase (MAO) in vitro. However, hypericin may not reach adequate concentrations in human tissue to achieve these effects (167,759). Hypericin also has affinity for sigma receptors and acts as a receptor antagonist at adenosine, benzodiazepine, GABA-A, GABA-B, and inositol triphosphate receptors (759). Recently hyperforin has been identified as a probable major player in St. John's wort's antidepressant activity (762,763). Hyperforin has been shown to modulate the effects of serotonin, possibly through serotonin reuptake inhibition (763,3553) and 5-HT3 and 5-HT4 receptor antagonism (762). Hyperforin has also been shown to inhibit synaptosomal uptake of gamma-butyric acid (GABA) and L-glutamate (3553). Extracts of St. John's wort have been shown to inhibit reuptake of serotonin, norepinephrine and dopamine in vitro and to down-regulate beta-adrenergic and 5-HT2 receptors when used chronically in animals (763). It is likely that constituents other than hypericin and hyperforin also contribute to the antidepressant action of St. John's wort preparations (762). St. John's wort extracts have also been shown to prolong narcotic-induced sleep time, decrease barbiturate-induced sleep time, and antagonize the effects of reserpine (758). St. John's wort and its constituents, hypericin and pseudohypericin, have been shown to have activity against viruses and bacteria including influenza virus, herpes simplex virus types I and II, Sindbis virus, poliovirus, retrovirus, murine cytomegalovirus, hepatitis C, and Gram negative and Gram positive bacteria (6). Hyperforin has been shown to inhibit growth of penicillin- and methicillin-resistant Staphylococcus aureus and other Gram positive organisms, but not Gram negative organisms (3554). Hypericin is photodynamically active and is thought to be the constituent responsible for phototoxicity reactions (3547). The polar fraction of a methanolic St. John's wort extract, but not isolated hypericin, inhibits cytochrome P450 3A4 (CYP3A4) activity in human liver microsomes (1379). However, in vivo, St. John's wort extract does not appear to significantly inhibit CYP3A4 or CYP2D6 (3570,3588). Clinical evidence suggests that St. John's wort actually induces these enzymes (1291,1292,1293). Evidence suggests that St. John's wort might also affect the activity of P-glycoprotein which mediates the absorption and elimination of digoxin and other drugs (382,1293). St. John's wort does not appear to affect CYP1A2 or N-acetyltransferase (NAT2) (3571).

Adverse Reactions Including Known Allergies

St. John's wort taken orally can cause insomnia, vivid dreams, restlessness, anxiety, agitation, irritability (3569), gastrointestinal discomfort, fatigue, dry mouth, dizziness (394,758,3547), headache (3547), paresthesias (5073), delayed hypersensitivity (4), and can induce hypomania in depressed patients (325,3524,3568) and mania in depressed patients with occult bipolar disorder (3555). In one report, insomnia was the most common side effect. In some cases, insomnia was alleviated by decreasing the dose or taking St. John's wort in the morning (3569). Colic, drowsiness, and lethargy have been reported in breast-fed infants whose mothers used St. John's wort while breast feeding (1377). St. John's wort use has been associated with reports of intermenstrual bleeding and one report of changed menstrual bleeding (1292). Most of the women in these reports were taking an oral contraceptive and the changes in menstrual bleeding may be the result of a drug interaction (see Interactions with Drugs) (1292). Overall, St. John's wort extracts have been better tolerated than tricyclic antidepressants in comparative trials (3548,3549), but similarly well tolerated as fluoxetine in one comparative trial (3550). In one trial, St. John's wort extracts did not adversely affect cardiac conduction measures on ECG, as has been found with tricyclic antidepressants (3552). Photodermatitis was reported in a patient after using St. John's wort extract for more than three years (620). Photosensitivity has also been reported with the ingestion of St. John's wort extract 1800 mg per day for 15 days (758) and phototoxicity has been reported with ingestion of hypericin 0.5 mg/kg per day (206). Lower doses may not cause this effect. For example, a single dose of St. John's wort extract 1800 mg (5.4 mg hypericin) followed by 900 mg (2.7 mg hypericin) daily does not produce skin hypericin concentrations thought to be high enough to cause phototoxicity (3539). Light or fair-skinned people should employ protective measures against direct sunlight when using St. John's wort due to its potential photosensitivity effects (2,11,628). Neuropathy after sun exposure has been reported with the use of St. John's wort (621). There is some indication that St. John's wort may be associated with a higher incidence of cataracts (223). The hypericin constituent is photoactive and, in the presence of light, may damage lens proteins, leading to cataracts (1296); however, studies evaluating this association are not available. Some evidence suggests that high doses of St. John's wort might reduce male and female fertility (4239,4240), but this effect has not been demonstrated in humans. St. John's wort might lead to withdrawal effects similar to those found with conventional antidepressants, including headache, nausea, dizziness, insomnia, paresthesias, confusion, and fatigue. In one report, withdrawal effects were most likely to occur within 2 days after discontinuation, but in some cases didn't occur for more than 1 week after stopping treatment. Occurrence of withdrawal symptoms did not appear to relate to dose or duration of use (3569). Topically, St. John's wort oil may irritate the skin (4).

Possible Interactions with Herbs & Other Dietary Supplements

HERBS WITH SEDATIVE PROPERTIES: Theoretically, concomitant use with herbs that have sedative properties might enhance therapeutic and adverse effects. These include calamus, calendula, California poppy, catnip, capsicum, celery, couch grass, elecampane, ginseng Siberian, German chamomile, goldenseal, gotu kola, hops, Jamaican dogwood, kava, lemon balm, sage, sassafras, scullcap, shepherd's purse, stinging nettle, valerian, wild carrot, wild lettuce, withania root, and yerba mansa (4,19).

© Copyright 2000, Natural Medicines Comprehensive Database (209) 472-2244. For updated data, go to www.NaturalDatabase.com • 985

DIGITALIS: Concomitant use might reduce the therapeutic effects of digitalis. St. John's wort extract (LI 160) decreases digoxin serum levels in healthy people. St. John's wort seems to lower digoxin serum concentrations about 25% (382).

Possible Interactions with Drugs

5-HT1 AGONISTS (Triptans): Theoretically, concomitant use of St. John's wort with selective serotonin agonists increases the risk of serotonergic adverse effects and serotonin syndrome. Concomitant use should be avoided (3572). The "triptans" include frovatriptan (Miguard), naratriptan (Amerge), rizatriptan (Maxalt), sumatriptan (Imitrex), and zolmitriptan (Zomig).

AMITRIPTYLINE (Elavil): Concomitant use reduces serum amitriptyline concentrations. In a 14 day human study, concomitant use of St. John's wort and amitriptyline reduced serum concentrations of amitriptyline and its metabolite, nortriptyline (1378).

ANTIDEPRESSANTS: Concomitant use can lead to increased adverse effects (4,12,16,166) and increase the risk of serotonergic side effects, including serotonin syndrome (166,542,3569). Although this effect has only been reported with nefazodone (Serzone), paroxetine (Paxil), and sertraline (Zoloft) (see Nafazodone, Paroxetine, and Sertraline below), it may theoretically also occur with other antidepressants. Use of St. John's wort with other antidepressants should only be done with close supervision of a healthcare provider.

BARBITURATES: St. John's wort can decrease barbiturate-induced sleep time (6,758).

CYCLOSPORINE (Neoral, Sandimmune): Concomitant use may decrease plasma cyclosporine levels. There are multiple case reports of patients with heart, kidney, or liver transplants treated with cyclosporine, in whom use of St. John's wort was associated with a drop in plasma cyclosporine to subtherapeutic levels and in some cases resulted in acute transplant rejection (1293,6112). This interaction might be due to induction of cytochrome P450 3A4 enzymes and modulation of the multidrug transporter, P-glycoprotein, by St. John's wort (1291,1293).

DIGOXIN (Lanoxin): Concomitant use might reduce serum levels and the therapeutic effects of digoxin, requiring dosing adjustments when St. John's wort is started or stopped. St. John's wort extract 900 mg daily has been shown to reduce serum digoxin levels by 25% after 10 days in healthy people (382). St. John's wort is thought to affect the multidrug transporter, P-glycoprotein, which mediates digoxin and other drugs' absorption and elimination (382).

FENFLURAMINE (Pondimin): Concomitant use with St. John's wort may increase the risk of serotonergic side effects and serotonin syndrome-like symptoms. In one report, a woman experienced nausea, headache, and anxiety after taking St. John's wort 600 mg per day with fenfluramine (3569).

NARCOTICS: St. John's wort can increase narcotic-induced sleep time (6,758).

NEFAZODONE (Serzone): Concomitant use has been associated with serotonergic side effects, including nausea, vomiting, and restlessness (5074).

NONNUCLEOSIDE REVERSE TRANSCRIPTASE INHIBITORS (NNRTIs): Concomitant use might decrease serum levels of NNRTIs. In a study in healthy volunteers, concomitant administration of St. John's wort and the protease inhibitor indinavir (Crixivan) substantially decreased indinavir plasma concentrations (1290). Since NNRTIs and protease inhibitors are metabolized through similar routes, NNRTIs may also be affected. Subtherapeutic concentrations are associated with therapeutic failure, development of viral resistance, and development of drug class resistance. St. John's wort is thought to induce cytochrome P450 enzymes (1290,1291). NNRTI-type antiretroviral drugs include nevirapine (Viramune), delavirdine (Rescriptor), and efavirenz (Sustiva).

NORTRIPTYLINE (Pamelor, Aventyl): Concomitant use might reduce serum nortriptyline concentrations. In a 14 day human study, concomitant use of St. John's wort and amitriptyline reduced serum concentrations of amitriptyline and its metabolite, nortriptyline (1378).

ORAL CONTRACEPTIVES: Concomitant use may decrease steroid concentrations resulting in breakthrough bleeding and irregular menstrual bleeding. There are multiple reports of breakthrough bleeding and irregular menstrual bleeding in women concomitantly taking oral contraceptives and St. John's wort. Bleeding irregularities usually occurred after one week of starting St. John's wort and regular cycles returned when St. John's wort was discontinued. St. John's wort is thought to induce the cytochrome P450 3A4 enzymes, which are responsible for steroid metabolism (1292). Women taking St. John's wort and oral contraceptives concurrently should use an alternative form of birth control.

PAROXETINE (Paxil): Concomitant use with St. John's wort may increase the risk of adverse effects and serotonin syndrome-like symptoms. There is one case report of nausea, weakness, fatigue, lethargy, inability to arise from bed, and incoherence with the combined use of St. John's wort and paroxetine (542). In another report a patient experienced nervousness, hyperactivity, and diaphoresis after taking St. John's wort 900 mg per day with paroxetine (3569).

PHOTOSENSITIZING DRUGS: Theoretically, concomitant use might result in increased photosensitivity (166). Some drugs that cause photosensitivity include amitriptyline, quinolones, sulfa drugs, and tetracycline.

PROTEASE INHIBITORS (PIs): Concomitant use might reduce serum concentrations of protease inhibitors. In a study of healthy volunteers, concomitant administration of St. John's wort and the protease inhibitor indinavir (Crixivan) reduced the serum indinavir area under the curve (AUC) by 57% and the extrapolated trough by 81%. Subtherapeutic concentrations are associated with therapeutic failure, development of viral resistance, and development of drug class resistance. St. John's wort is thought to induce cytochrome P450 enzymes and might also affect other protease inhibitor-type antiretroviral drugs (1290,1291), including amprenavir (Angenerase), nelfinavir (Viracept), ritonavir (Norvir), and saquinavir (Fortovase, Invirase).

RESERPINE: St. John's wort can antagonize the effects of reserpine (758).

SERTRALINE (Zoloft): Concomitant use has been associated with serotonergic side effects, including dizziness, nausea, vomiting, epigastric pain, headache, anxiety, confusion, and feelings of restlessness and irritability (5074).

THEOPHYLLINE: Concomitant use might decrease serum levels and the therapeutic effects of theophylline, requiring dose adjustment. One case report describes a clinically significant decrease in serum theophylline levels after St. John's wort extract 300 mg daily was started. Discontinuation of St. John's wort resulted in increased serum levels of theophylline (3556).

WARFARIN (Coumadin): Concomitant use might decrease the therapeutic effects of warfarin (1292). Multiple cases of decreased International Normalized Ratio (INR) have been reported, although none have involved thromboembolic complications (1292). St. John's wort is thought to induce the cytochrome P450 2C9 enzyme, which is involved in warfarin's metabolism (1292).

OTHER DRUGS: Based on documented interactions with St. John's wort and drugs metabolized by cytochrome P450 3A4, 2C9, and 2D6 enzymes and St. John's wort's affects on P-glycoprotein (1290,1292,1293), use caution when considering concomitant use of St. John's wort and other drugs affected by these systems. Drugs which might be affected include some calcium channel blockers (diltiazem, nicardipine, verapamil), chemotherapeutic agents (etoposide, paclitaxel, vinblastine, vincristine, vindesine), antifungals (ketoconazole, itraconazole), glucocorticoids, cisapride (Propulsid), losartan (Cozaar), fluoxetine (Prozac), omeprazole (Prilosec), fexofenadine (Allegra), and others.

Possible Interactions with Foods

TYRAMINE-CONTAINING FOODS: Theoretically, concomitant use of large amounts of St. John's wort and tyramine-containing foods might cause a hypertensive crisis (166). St. John's wort has weak monoamine oxidase inhibitory activity. This interaction has not been described in the literature.

Possible Interactions with Lab Tests

PROTHROMBIN TIME (PT), INTERNATIONAL NORMALIZED RATIO (INR): St. John's wort can decrease PT/INR test results in patients treated with warfarin (Coumadin) (1292).

Possible Interactions with Diseases or Conditions

UNIPOLAR DEPRESSION: St. John's wort can induce hypomania with typical doses in patients with major depression (325,3524,3568). In one case hypomania occurred after four to eight weeks of treatment with St. John's wort and was effectively managed by decreasing the dose and initiating valproic acid (3568).

BIPOLAR DISORDER: St. John's wort can induce hypomania or mania when used in patients with bipolar disorder or depressed patients with occult bipolar disorder (3555,3568). In some cases, mania occurred after 2-8 weeks of treatment with St. John's wort and was effectively managed by decreasing the dose of St. John's wort and increasing the dose of mood stabilizers such as lithium (3568). Theoretically, like other antidepressants, St. John's wort may also induce rapid cycling between depression and mania in patients with bipolar disorder (3555).

INFERTILITY: Preliminary evidence suggests that St. John's wort might inhibit oocyte fertilization and alter sperm DNA (4239,4240). This effect has not yet been demonstrated in humans; however, until more is known, use with caution in couples attempting to conceive and avoid use in couples having difficulty conceiving.

Typical Dosages & Routes of Administration that are Commonly Used

ORAL: For mild to moderate major depression, most clinical trials have used St. John's wort extract standardized to 0.3% hypericin content. Doses were most commonly 300 mg three times daily (7,3548,3549). Doses of 1200 mg daily have also been used (5096). A St. John's wort extract standardized to 5% hyperforin and dosed at 300 mg three times daily has also been used (761,6400). In cases of long-term maintenance therapy, daily doses of 300-600 mg have been used (7). For obsessive-compulsive disorder, one study used an extended-release preparation of St. John's wort extract standardized to 0.3% hypericin content, dosed at 450 mg twice daily (5075). For somatic symptoms associated with depression, 300 mg three times daily of the standardized hypericin extract has been used (376). The typical daily dose of the crude drug is 2-4 grams of the above-ground parts per day or 0.2-1 mg of total hypericin in other forms (2). One cup of the tea is usually taken one to three times per day and is prepared by steeping 2-4 grams of the dried herb in 150 mL of boiling water for 5-10 minutes and then straining (4). The liquid extract (1:1 in 25% alcohol) is typically taken as 2-4 mL three times daily (4). The tincture (1:10 in 45% alcohol) is commonly dosed 2-4 mL three times daily (4). Patients should be advised to avoid abrupt discontinuation of St. John's wort due to the risk of adverse withdrawal effects (see Adverse Reactions) (3569).

Comments

St. John's wort is a natural source of food flavoring in Europe, limited to a final concentration of 0.1 mg/kg hypericin in the finished product, except in pastilles or lozenges (1 mg/kg hypericin) and alcoholic beverages (2 mg/kg hypericin) (4). St. John's wort is native to Europe but is commonly found in the US and Canada in the dry ground of roadsides, meadows, and woods (6). Its flowers can have the brightest appearance on June 24th, the birthday of John the Baptist (6). Hypericin, a constituent of St. John's wort, has been identified by the FDA as an investigational new drug, now being studied and developed by VIMRx Pharmaceuticals for the treatment of HIV (6). The Federal Institute for Drugs and Medical Products in Germany no longer bases dose recommendations on the hypericin content of St. John's wort products (7).

STAR ANISE

This Product is Also Known As
Aniseed Stars, Anisi stellati fructus, Badiana, Chinese Anise, Chinese Star Anise, Eight-Horned Anise, Eight Horns, Illicium.
CAUTION: See separate listing for Anise.

Scientific Names
Illicium verum.
Family: Illiciacae.

People Use This For
Orally, star anise seed is used for respiratory tract mucous membrane inflammation, peptic discomfort (2,18), flatulence (11), loss of appetite, cough, and bronchitis (18).
As an inhalant, it is used for respiratory tract congestion (11).
In Chinese medicine, star anise is used for increasing milk secretion, promoting menstruation, facilitating childbirth, increasing libido, and treating symptoms of male climacteric (11).
In foods and beverages, star anise is considered a culinary spice; both the seed and oil are used as flavor ingredients (11).
In manufacturing, the oil is used as a fragrance component in soaps, cosmetics, perfumes, and toothpaste, and to mask undesirable odors in drug products (11).

Safety
LIKELY SAFE ...when consumed in amounts commonly found in foods (11), and has Generally Recognized as Safe (GRAS) status in the US for food use (11).
POSSIBLY SAFE ...when taken orally for medicinal purposes and used appropriately (12).
There is insufficient reliable information available about the safety of star anise as an inhalant.
PREGNANCY AND LACTATION: Insufficient reliable information available; avoid using.

Effectiveness
POSSIBLY EFFECTIVE ...when taken orally for respiratory tract mucous membrane inflammation and peptic discomfort (2).
There is insufficient reliable information available about the effectiveness of star anise for its other uses.

Possible Mechanism of Action & Active Ingredients
The applicable part of star anise is the seed. Star anise seed contains a volatile oil (11,18), of which the chief constituent is anethole (80-90%). Anethole has antiflatulent and expectorant effects. It also can have insecticidal and antifungal activity (11). At one time anethole was considered the active estrogenic agent in the essential oil. However, more recent information suggests the active estrogenic compounds are the anethole polymers, dianethole and photoanethole (11). Anethole might be mutagenic (11).

Adverse Reactions Including Known Allergies
When taken orally and appropriately, star anise does not appear to have adverse effects, but the topical use of the constituent anethole can cause dermatitis, including erythema, scaling, and vesiculation (11). Sensitization rarely occurs (18).

Possible Interactions with Herbs & Other Dietary Supplements
Insufficient reliable information available.

Possible Interactions with Drugs
No interactions are known to occur, and there is no known reason to expect a clinically significant interaction with star anise.

Possible Interactions with Foods
No interactions are known to occur, and there is no known reason to expect a clinically significant interaction with star anise.

Possible Interactions with Lab Tests
No interactions are known to occur, and there is no known reason to expect a clinically significant interaction with star anise.

Possible Interactions with Diseases or Conditions
No interactions are known to occur, and there is no known reason to expect a clinically significant interaction with star anise.

Typical Dosages & Routes of Administration that are Commonly Used
ORAL: The typical dose of star anise is one cup of the tea (8). The tea is prepared by steeping 0.5-1 grams of the coarsely powdered seed in 150 mL boiling water for 10 minutes and then straining. The average amount of star

anise is 3 grams of the seed or 300 mg of the essential oil per day (2,8).
INHALED: Products containing 5-10% essential oil are commonly used for inhalation of star anise (11).

Comments
Star anise oil is the distilled oil of the seed (fruit) of star anise (Illicium verum). Avoid confusing star anise with Japanese star anise (Illicium lanceolatum), a highly poisonous species (11). In the US, star anise oil (derived from Illicium verum) and anise oil (derived from Pimpinella anisum) are used interchangeably and both are recognized as "anise oil" in the USP (11).

STAVESACRE

This Product is Also Known As
Lousewort.

Scientific Names
Delphinium staphisagria.

People Use This For
Topically, stavesacre seeds are used to treat lice infestation (18).
Historically, the stavesacre plant was used for neuralgia (18).

Safety
LIKELY UNSAFE ...when used orally. The seeds are poisonous (18).
There is insufficient reliable information available about the safety of the topical use of stavesacre and the use of stavesacre extracts.
PREGNANCY AND LACTATION: LIKELY UNSAFE ...when used orally.

Effectiveness
There is insufficient reliable information available about the effectiveness of stavesacre (18).

Possible Mechanism of Action & Active Ingredients
Stavesacre contains diterpene alkaloids including delphinine, staphisine, and staphisagroine, which are reported to have effects similar to aconitine (18). Aconitine is a nor-diterpene alkaloid found in Monkshood, a highly toxic plant.

Adverse Reactions Including Known Allergies
Ingesting a stavesacre extract can cause inflammation of the alimentary tract (18,19), nausea, pruritus, urinary and stool urgency (18). Ingesting 2 teaspoons of seeds can cause weakened pulse, stomach pain, labored breathing, and collapse (18). Topical use of stavesacre can cause inflammation, eczema, and reddening of the skin (18).

Possible Interactions with Herbs & Other Dietary Supplements
Insufficient reliable information available.

Possible Interactions with Drugs
No interactions are known to occur, and there is no known reason to expect a clinically significant interaction with stavesacre.

Possible Interactions with Foods
No interactions are known to occur, and there is no known reason to expect a clinically significant interaction with stavesacre.

Possible Interactions with Lab Tests
No interactions are known to occur, and there is no known reason to expect a clinically significant interaction with stavesacre.

Possible Interactions with Diseases or Conditions
GASTROINTESTINAL IRRITATION: Can aggravate inflammation of the alimentary tract by irritating mucosal membranes (19).

Typical Dosages & Routes of Administration that are Commonly Used
ORAL: No typical dosage.
TOPICAL: Washes and ointments are used to treat lice.

Comments
Stavesacre is considered likely unsafe when used orally; avoid using (18).

STEVIA

This Product is Also Known As

Azucacaa, Caa-He-É, Ca-A-Jhei, Ca-A-Yupi, Capim Doce, Eira-Caa, Erva Doce, Kaa Jhee, Paraguayan Sweet Herb, Sweetleaf, Sweet Leaf of Paraguay, Yerba Dulce.

Scientific Names

Stevia rebaudiana, synonym Stevia eupatorium.
Family: Asteraceae/Compositae.

People Use This For

Stevia leaf is used as a weight loss aid [6].

Traditionally, stevia leaf has been used for treating diabetes, as a contraceptive [11], for hypertension, heartburn, lowering uric acid levels, as a cardiotonic and diuretic [3918].

For food uses, stevia leaf has a centuries-long history of use as a sweetener in Paraguay and is used as a non-caloric sweetener in South America and Asia [6,11].

Safety

POSSIBLY SAFE ...when used orally in small amounts as an occasional food or beverage sweetener [12].

There is insufficient reliable information about the safety of stevia used in larger amounts or long-term. The FDA, regulatory agencies in Europe, and the World Health Organization have not approved stevia due to unanswered questions regarding chronic use and toxicity [5037].

PREGNANCY AND LACTATION: Insufficient reliable information available; avoid using.

Effectiveness

There is insufficient reliable information available about the effectiveness of stevia leaf.

Possible Mechanism of Action & Active Ingredients

The applicable part of stevia is the leaf. Stevia leaf contains the glycoside stevioside which is non-caloric, heat and acid stable, and 100 times sweeter than sucrose at 10% sucrose concentration [11]. Stevioside increases hepatic glycogen synthesis in animal experiments [3750]. It might also have androgenic activity, perhaps without effect on male fertility [14]. Stevia extract and stevioside decrease blood pressure [3745,3747], and stevia extract has vasodilating and diuretic activity in rats [3746,3747]. Preliminary evidence suggests that the stevia constituents, stevioside and steviol, might stimulate insulin secretion via a direct action on beta cells [5032]. Additional evidence suggests that steviol might inhibit GI glucose absorption [5035]. An aqueous stevia leaf extract increased glucose tolerance and reduced plasma glucose levels in a small group of healthy people [3301], but has not been studied in people with diabetes. A fermented aqueous extract of stevia is bactericidal against many food-borne pathogenic bacteria in vitro, including E. coli 0157:H7, the enterohemorrhagic E. coli responsible for outbreaks of severe food poisoning in recent years [3300]. Stevioside shows no evidence of mutagenic, genotoxic, antifertility, or teratogenic effects [11]. However, the stevia constituent steviol, and metabolized steviol, are mutagenic in vitro [3748,3749]. Some evidence suggests that stevia might adversely affect reproduction. An aqueous stevia extract reduced sperm production and testis weight in male rats [5033]. Steviol fed to female hamsters reduced the number and birth weight of offspring [5036].

Adverse Reactions Including Known Allergies

Theoretically, stevia might cause allergic reactions in individuals sensitive to Asteraceae/Compositae family plants. Members of this family include ragweed, chrysanthemums, marigolds, daisies, and many other herbs.

Possible Interactions with Herbs & Other Dietary Supplements

Insufficient reliable information available.

Possible Interactions with Drugs

DIABETES DRUGS: Theoretically, stevia might enhance blood glucose control requiring dosing adjustment of diabetes drug therapy in patients with type 2 diabetes [3301,5032,5035].

VERAPAMIL (Calan, Isoptin, Verelan): Theoretically, stevia and verapamil might have additive antihypertensive activity. Preliminary evidence suggests that concomitant use might have additive blood pressure lowering effects, due to the stevioside contained in stevia [5031].

Possible Interactions with Foods

No interactions are known to occur, and there is no known reason to expect a clinically significant interaction with stevia.

Possible Interactions with Lab Tests

BLOOD PRESSURE: Theoretically, stevia might reduce blood pressure and blood pressure readings. Preliminary evidence suggests that stevia extract and stevioside, contained in stevia, might lower blood pressure [3745,3747,5031].

GLUCOSE: Theoretically, stevia might decrease blood glucose concentrations and test results [3301,5032,5035].

Possible Interactions with Diseases or Conditions

CROSS-ALLERGENICITY: Theoretically, stevia might cause allergic reactions in individuals sensitive to Asteraceae/Compositae family plants. Members of this family include ragweed, chrysanthemums, marigolds, daisies, and many other herbs.

DIABETES: Theoretically, stevia might reduce blood glucose and alter blood glucose control in patients with type 2 diabetes (3301,5032,5035).

KIDNEY DISEASE: Theoretically, stevia might cause kidney damage. Preliminary evidence suggests that large amounts of steviol, contained in stevia, might cause acute renal damage (5034).

Typical Dosages & Routes of Administration that are Commonly Used

ORAL: A typical dose of powdered stevia leaf is 1000 mg per day (342,343).

Comments

Avoid confusion with Stevia salifolia, commonly referred to as ronion or roninowa, which contains the bitter glycoside stevisalioside (14).

In a 1991 import alert, the FDA identified stevia as an "unsafe food additive" (12) and banned importation (11). The alert was revised in 1995 to allow stevia to be imported "explicitly labeled as a dietary supplement or for use as a dietary ingredient of a dietary supplement" (12). Canada and the European Community prohibit stevia as a food additive (5030). The FDA, regulatory agencies in Europe, and the World Health Organization have not approved stevia due to unanswered safety questions (5037).

STINGING NETTLE above ground parts

This Product is Also Known As

Common Nettle, Great Stinging Nettle, Nettle, Nettles, Ortie, Small Nettle, Urtica, Urticae herba et folium.
CAUTION: See separate listings for Stinging Nettle root and White Dead Nettle Flower.

Scientific Names

Urtica dioica; Urtica urens; and hybrid species.
Family: Urticaceae.

People Use This For

Orally, stinging nettle is used for inflammation or infection of the lower urinary tract (1,2,5,6,9,11,18), kidney and bladder stones (2,6,11,18), as "irrigation therapy" (use of a mild diuretic and copious fluid intake to increase urine flow), or for rheumatic complaints (1,2,5,6,8,9,11,18).

Topically, stinging nettle is used for rheumatic ailments (2,5,6,18).

Historically, people used stinging nettle orally for internal bleeding (including uterine bleeding, epistaxis, and melena) (4,11), anemia (8,11,18), poor circulation, enlargement of the spleen (11), diabetes (4,6,8,18), glandular diseases (11), hypersecretion of gastric juices (6,8), biliary complaints (8), diarrhea and dysentery (11), asthma (5,6), allergies (6,11), pulmonary congestion (5,6,11), rashes, eczema (4,6), cancer, aging (6), as an antispasmodic (5,6,11), blood purifier (11), astringent (5,11), tonic (5), and wound-healing agent (6,8). Historically, stinging nettle was used topically for scalp seborrhea, oily hair (6,8,18), and hair loss (5,6).

For food uses, young stinging nettle is eaten as a cooked vegetable (11).

In manufacturing, the extract is used as an ingredient in hair and skin care products (11).

Safety

POSSIBLY SAFE ...when preparations of the above ground parts are used orally and appropriately (1,2,12).

PREGNANCY: LIKELY UNSAFE ...contraindicated for oral use during pregnancy due to possible abortifacient and uterine-stimulant effects (4,6,19).

LACTATION: There is insufficient reliable information available about the safety of oral use during lactation; avoid using.

Effectiveness

POSSIBLY EFFECTIVE ...when used orally as "irrigation therapy" (use of a mild diuretic and copious fluid intake to increase urine flow) for inflammation of the lower urinary tract and preventing and treating urinary calculus (1,2,8), for supportive therapy for rheumatic ailments (1,2), and for allergic rhinitis (11). ...when the freeze-dried nettle is used orally for treating allergic rhinitis (11). ...when used topically as supportive therapy for rheumatic ailments (2).

There is insufficient reliable information available about the effectiveness of stinging nettle for its other uses.

Possible Mechanism of Action & Active Ingredients

Stinging nettle leaf hairs (stings) contain histamine, acetylcholine (1,4,5,8,11,18), and serotonin (1,4,8,11,18), which can cause local irritation. The plant contains significant amounts of vitamin C (11), vitamin K (19), potassium (2,8,11,18), and calcium (2,11). The components in stinging nettle seem to cause anti-inflammatory, local anesthetic (1), hemostatic (4), antibacterial (11), antiviral (6), and hyperglycemic effects (4). They may inhibit adrenergic stimulation,

© Copyright 2000, Natural Medicines Comprehensive Database (209) 472-2244. For updated data, go to www.NaturalDatabase.com

tumor necrosis factor, and platelet activation factor (1). Nettle juice increases urine output and slightly decreases systolic blood pressure and body weight in people with myocardial or chronic venous insufficiency (1,11). Some studies of experimental animals have shown diuretic activity (1,11). Some studies show oral administration of nettle causes analgesic effects (1,4). The leaf extract enhances anti-inflammatory effects of low doses of diclofenac (Cataflam, Voltaren) (19). Nettle extract provides subjective improvement in individuals with rheumatic complaints (1). There is some evidence to suggest that stinging nettle can decrease blood pressure and heart rate when given intravenously (1,4). It can cause CNS depression (4,6,11), anti-seizure activity, and decreased temperature (4).

Adverse Reactions Including Known Allergies
When taken orally, stinging nettle juice may cause diarrhea (1). Fresh nettle applied topically (or touched accidentally) can cause local irritation (4,19).

Possible Interactions with Herbs & Other Dietary Supplements
HERBS WITH SEDATIVE PROPERTIES: Theoretically, concomitant use with herbs that have sedative properties might enhance therapeutic and adverse effects. These include calamus, calendula, California poppy, catnip, capsicum, celery, couch grass, elecampane, ginseng Siberian, German chamomile, goldenseal, gotu kola, hops, Jamaican dogwood, kava, lemon balm, sage, St. John's wort, sassafras, scullcap, shepherd's purse, valerian, wild carrot, wild lettuce, withania, and yerba mansa (4,19).
HERBS WITH CLOTTING POTENTIAL: Excessive use of herbs that contain vitamin K, an essential coagulation factor, can increase the risk of clotting in people using anticoagulants. These herbs include: alfalfa, parsley, nettle, plantain, and others.

Possible Interactions with Drugs
ANTICOAGULANTS: Concomitant use can decrease drug effectiveness and increase risk of clotting, due to vitamin K content of nettle (19).
ANTIDIABETES DRUGS: Theoretically, concomitant use of excessive amounts of nettle can interfere with blood glucose control (4).
ANTIHYPERTENSIVE, ANTIHYPOTENSIVE DRUGS: Theoretically, concomitant use of excessive amounts of nettle can interfere with blood pressure control (4); monitor.
CNS DEPRESSANTS: Theoretically, concomitant use of excessive amounts of nettle can potentiate depressant effects of drugs (4).
DICLOFENAC (Cataflam, Voltaren): Concomitant use of leaf extract enhances diclofenac anti-inflammatory effect (19).

Possible Interactions with Foods
No interactions are known to occur, and there is no known reason to expect a clinically significant interaction with stinging nettle.

Possible Interactions with Lab Tests
No interactions are known to occur, and there is no known reason to expect a clinically significant interaction with stinging nettle.

Possible Interactions with Diseases or Conditions
HEART OR KIDNEY INSUFFICIENCY: Contraindicated for "irrigation therapy" (use of a mild diuretic and copious fluid intake to increase urine flow) in the presence of edema (2,18).
DIABETES, HYPERTENSION, HYPOTENSION: Theoretically, excessive intake of nettle can interfere with treatment of these conditions (4).

Typical Dosages & Routes of Administration that are Commonly Used
ORAL: One cup tea (made by steeping 1.5-5 grams above ground parts in 150 mL boiling water 10 minutes, strain) up to three times per day with ample fluid intake (1,2,4,8), especially when used for "irrigation therapy"; average amount 8-12 grams per day (2,8). Fresh juice, 10-15 mL three times per day (1). Dried extract (7:1), 770 mg twice per day (1). Liquid extract (1:1 in 25% alcohol), 3-4 mL three times per day (4). Tincture (1:5 in 25% alcohol), 2-6 mL three times daily (1,4).
TOPICAL: Tincture/spirit (1:10) for external use (18).

Comments
Avoid confusion with stinging nettle root. Stinging nettle fruit and seed have also been used orally and externally in folk medicine (8).

STINGING NETTLE root

This Product is Also Known As
Common Nettle, Great Stinging Nettle, Nettle, Nettles, Small Nettle, Urtica, Urticae Radix.
CAUTION: See separate listing for Stinging Nettle above ground parts and White Dead Nettle Flower.

Scientific Names
Urtica dioica; Urtica urens; hybrid species.
Family: Urticaceae.

People Use This For
Orally, stinging nettle root is used for urination disorders associated with benign prostatic hyperplasia (BPH), including nocturia, frequency, dysuria, urinary retention, and irritable bladder (1,2,5,6,7,8,18).
In folk medicine, stinging nettle root has been used for joint ailments (6,7), as a diuretic (6,7,8), and an astringent (8).

Safety
POSSIBLY SAFE ...when used orally and appropriately (1,2).
PREGNANCY AND LACTATION: Insufficient reliable information available; avoid using.

Effectiveness
POSSIBLY EFFECTIVE ...when used orally for symptoms associated with benign prostatic hyperplasia (BPH) Stages I and II (1,2).
POSSIBLY INEFFECTIVE ...when an herbal blend containing nettle root extract is used orally for treating symptoms of BPH. In a double-blind, placebo controlled trial, an herbal product containing nettle root extract 80 mg, saw palmetto lipoidal extract 106 mg, pumpkin seed oil extract 160 mg, lemon bioflavonoid extract 33 mg, and vitamin A (100% as beta-carotene) 190 IU taken three times daily for six months failed to significantly improve symptoms in a group of men with BPH (5093).
There is insufficient reliable information available about the effectiveness of stinging nettle root for its other uses.

Possible Mechanism of Action & Active Ingredients
Stinging nettle root contains polysaccharides with immunomodulating (1,18) and weak anti-inflammatory (1,7) effects. Hydroalcoholic extracts decrease binding capacity of sex hormone binding globulin (1,7,8) and might suppress prostatic cell metabolism (1,7). In several clinical trials of varying design quality, hydroalcoholic root extracts increased urine output (1,2,7), decreased nocturia (1,6,11), and decreased urinary frequency (1). In some clinical trials urine flow increased (1,7), and in other trials residual volume decreased (1,2,7), although in one well-designed study there was no improvement in subjective symptoms, urine flow, or residual volume (7). Studies investigating the effect of nettle root on prostate size have produced contradictory results (1,2,18).

Adverse Reactions Including Known Allergies
Oral use of stinging nettle root can cause gastrointestinal complaints (1,2,7,18), sweating (7), and allergic skin reactions (1,7). One case is reported of decreased ejaculatory volume associated with an herbal blend product containing nettle root extract, saw palmetto extract, pumpkin seed oil extract, lemon bioflavonoid extract, and beta-carotene (5093).

Possible Interactions with Herbs & Other Dietary Supplements
Insufficient reliable information available.

Possible Interactions with Drugs
No interactions are known to occur, and there is no known reason to expect a clinically significant interaction with stinging nettle root.

Possible Interactions with Foods
No interactions are known to occur, and there is no known reason to expect a clinically significant interaction with stinging nettle root.

Possible Interactions with Lab Tests
No interactions are known to occur, and there is no known reason to expect a clinically significant interaction with stinging nettle root.

Possible Interactions with Diseases or Conditions
No interactions are known to occur, and there is no known reason to expect a clinically significant interaction with stinging nettle root.

Typical Dosages & Routes of Administration that are Commonly Used
ORAL: Symptomatic treatment of benign prostatic hyperplasia (BPH): Dried hydroalcoholic extract (5:1, extracted with 20% methanol), 600-1200 mg per day (1). Liquid extract (1:1 in 45% alcohol), 1.5-7.5 mL three times per day (1). Ethanolic extract (1:5 in 40% alcohol), 5 mL per day (1). Tea, one cup tea (steep 1.5 grams dried, powdered root in 150 mL boiling water 5-10 minutes, strain) up to 4-6 grams per day (1,2,8,18).

Comments
Avoid confusing stinging nettle with white dead nettle. Stinging nettle root is used predominantly for urinary disorders, including BPH. White dead nettle herb is used for gastrointestinal complaints. White dead nettle flower is used for inflammation of the mucous membranes of the upper respiratory tract and vaginal discharge.

STONE ROOT

This Product is Also Known As

Citronella, Hardback, Hardhack, Heal-all, Horse Balm, Horseweed, Knob Grass, Knob Root, Knobweed, Richleaf, Rich Weed.
CAUTION: See separate listings for Citronella Oil and Lemongrass.

Scientific Names

Collinsonia canadensis.
Family: Labiatae.

People Use This For

Orally stone root rhizome and root are used to treat bladder inflammation (18), edema (18), gastrointestinal disorders (18), headaches (4501), hyperuricuria (4), indigestion (4501), kidney stones (4,18), urea "bladder semolina" (18), urinary calculus (4,18), water retention (4501), and as a tonic (18,4501).

Safety

POSSIBLY SAFE ...when used orally and appropriately. There are no reports of serious adverse effects (4,12,18).
PREGNANCY AND LACTATION: Insufficient reliable information available; avoid using (4).

Effectiveness

There is insufficient reliable information available about the effectiveness of stone root.

Possible Mechanism of Action & Active Ingredients

The applicable parts of stone root are the rhizome and root. Stone root rhizome or root contains a volatile oil, caffeic acid derivatives including rosmaric acid (18), saponins, tannin, mucilage, and resin (4,4501). Constituents of the volatile oil include caryophyllene, germacrene D, limonene, alpha- and beta-pinenes (18). Although no pharmacologic data is documented (4), stone root is said to have antifungal effects (4501), diuretic effects (4,6,18,4501), stimulate stomach function (18), cause sweating (4), and reduce occurrence of urinary stones and help rid the body of stones (4).

Adverse Reactions Including Known Allergies

Ingesting large amounts of stone root can cause intestinal tract irritation and colic-like pain, dizziness, nausea, and painful urination (18).

Possible Interactions with Herbs & Other Dietary Supplements

HERBS WITH DIURETIC PROPERTIES: Theoretically, due to the diuretic effects of stone root (4,6,18,4501), there may be additive effects and side effects with herbs having diuretic activity.

Possible Interactions with Drugs

DIURETICS: Theoretically, due to the diuretic effects of stone root (4,6,18,4501), there may be additive effects and side effects with drugs having diuretic activity.

Possible Interactions with Foods

No interactions are known to occur, and there is no known reason to expect a clinically significant interaction with stone root.

Possible Interactions with Lab Tests

No interactions are known to occur, and there is no known reason to expect a clinically significant interaction with stone root.

Possible Interactions with Diseases or Conditions

No interactions are known to occur, and there is no known reason to expect a clinically significant interaction with stone root.

Typical Dosages & Routes of Administration that are Commonly Used

ORAL: A typical dose of dried root is 1-4 grams or as tea three times daily (4). To make tea, simmer 1-4 grams root or rhizome in 150 mL of boiling water for 5-10 minutes, strain. As liquid extract: (1:1 in 25% alcohol) 1-4 mL three times daily (4). Tincture, (1:5 in 40% alcohol) 2-8 mL three times daily (4); tincture of Collinsonia, 2-8 mL (4).

Comments

This aromatic perennial herb has a strong, unpleasant smell that is reported to be numbing in large amounts (18).

STORAX

This Product is Also Known As
American Storax, Balsam Styracis, Balsamum Styrax Liquidus, Copalm, Estoraque Liquido, Gum Tree, Levant Storax, Liquid Amber, Liquid Storax, Opossum Tree, Red Gum, Styrax, Sweet Gum, White Gum.

Scientific Names
Liquidamber orientalis; Liquidambar styraciflua.
Family: Hamamelidaceae or Atlingiaceae.

People Use This For
Orally, storax balsam is used for cancer (11), coughs (11), colds (11), diarrhea (6), epilepsy (11), sore throats (6), and parasitic infections (6).
Topically, storax balsam is used to protect wounds (6,11), for ulcers (18), and scabies. Storax balsam is an ingredient in Compound Benzoin Tincture (6,11).
As an inhalant, it is placed in a vaporizer and used to treat coughs (6) and bronchitis (18).
Historically, storax balsam was used for parasitic skin diseases (9).
For food uses, it is used as a flavor component or fixative (6,11).
In manufacturing, storax is used as a fragrance component or fixative in soaps and perfumes (6,11).
Storax balsam has also been used as a fumigant and imbedding material in microscopy (4501).

Safety
LIKELY SAFE ...when the balsam is used in food amounts. Storax is approved for food use and the maximum level used is 0.002% (11).
POSSIBLY SAFE ...when used orally. There are no published reports of toxicity from oral use (6,18,4501). ...when used topically. Storax should not be used topically on large, open wounds (18).
POSSIBLY UNSAFE ...when large amounts are ingested. ...when applied to large open wounds. Systemic absorption can cause poisoning including kidney damage, e.g., albuminuria and hemorrhagic nephritis (18).
PREGNANCY AND LACTATION: Insufficient reliable information available; avoid using.

Effectiveness
There is insufficient reliable information available about the effectiveness of storax.

Possible Mechanism of Action & Active Ingredients
The applicable part of storax is the balsam. American storax balsam and Levant storax balsam are very similar chemically. Both contain aromatic alcohols (18), cinnamic acid (18,4503), cinnamic acid esters (6,18), storesins (13,4501), styrene (6,18,4503), a volatile oil (11,13), vanillin (6,11,18) and triterpenes (18). However, the amount of constituents varies between the species. In Levant storax, the volatile oil is usually less than 1%. In American storax, it ranges from 7 to over 20% (11). Storax has stimulant, antiseptic, and expectorant properties (11,13). It is also reported to have antimicrobial and anti-inflammatory properties (11).

Adverse Reactions Including Known Allergies
Oral use of storax balsam can cause diarrhea (18). Topical use can cause skin sensitization and contact allergies (9,18). When applied to large, open wounds, systemic absorption can cause kidney damage, e.g. albuminuria and hemorrhagic nephritis (18).

Possible Interactions with Herbs & Other Dietary Supplements
Insufficient reliable information available.

Possible Interactions with Drugs
No interactions are known to occur, and there is no known reason to expect a clinically significant interaction with storax.

Possible Interactions with Foods
No interactions are known to occur, and there is no known reason to expect a clinically significant interaction with storax.

Possible Interactions with Lab Tests
No interactions are known to occur, and there is no known reason to expect a clinically significant interaction with storax.

Possible Interactions with Diseases or Conditions
No interactions are known to occur, and there is no known reason to expect a clinically significant interaction with storax.

© Copyright 2000, Natural Medicines Comprehensive Database (209) 472-2244. For updated data, go to www.NaturalDatabase.com

Typical Dosages & Routes of Administration that are Commonly Used

ORAL: No typical dosage.
TOPICAL/INHALATION: Storax is applied topically and administered by inhalation via a vaporizer (6,18). It is available commercially in combination products.

Comments

Storax is a medicinal balsam obtained from the tree trunks of Liquidambar orientalis (Levant storax) or Liquidambar styraciflua (American storax) (13,4503). It is obtained by traumatizing the bark of the tree in early summer and stripping the bark later, perhaps as late as autumn. The bark is pressed in cold water, alternating with boiling water, and the crude liquid storax is collected (6). Storax is considered to be similar to Peru balsam in its effects (9,4501).

STRAWBERRY

This Product is Also Known As

Alpine Strawberry, Fragariae folium, Mountain Strawberry, Virginian Strawberry, Wild Strawberry, Wood Strawberry.

Scientific Names

Fragaria vesca; Fragaria virginiana; Fragaria viridis.
Family: Rosaceae.

People Use This For

Orally, strawberry is used for GI tract mucous membrane inflammation, diarrhea, intestinal sluggishness, liver disease, jaundice, upper and lower respiratory tract mucous membrane inflammation, gout, arthritis, nervous tension, kidney ailments involving gravel and stones, diuretic, supportive for heart and circulatory ailments, fever, night sweats, blood purification, for stimulating metabolism, anemia, as a tonic, for inhibiting menstruation, and supporting "natural weight loss" (2).
Topically, strawberry is used as a compress for rashes (2).

Safety

POSSIBLY SAFE ...when used orally and appropriately (12).
PREGNANCY AND LACTATION: Insufficient reliable information available; avoid using.

Effectiveness

There is insufficient reliable information available about the effectiveness of strawberry.

Possible Mechanism of Action & Active Ingredients

The applicable part of strawberry is the leaf and fruit. Strawberry leaf contains ellagic acid tannins, oligomeric proanthocyanidins, and flavonoids including rutin and quercetin. People claim that strawberry leaf has astringent and diuretic activity (18); however, there are no data to support these claims (18). Strawberry leaves are rich in vitamin C (19). Preliminary research suggests that compounds contained in strawberry fruit might slow aging effects on the nervous system (1418,1419).

Adverse Reactions Including Known Allergies

May cause allergic reaction in people sensitive to strawberries (2).

Possible Interactions with Herbs & Other Dietary Supplements

Insufficient reliable information available.

Possible Interactions with Drugs

No interactions are known to occur, and there is no known reason to expect a clinically significant interaction with strawberry.

Possible Interactions with Foods

No interactions are known to occur, and there is no known reason to expect a clinically significant interaction with strawberry.

Possible Interactions with Lab Tests

No interactions are known to occur, and there is no known reason to expect a clinically significant interaction with strawberry.

Possible Interactions with Diseases or Conditions

STRAWBERRY HYPERSENSITIVITY: Contraindicated (18).

Typical Dosages & Routes of Administration that are Commonly Used

ORAL: Diarrhea, one cup tea (steep 1 gram dried leaf in 250 mL boiling water 5-10 minutes, strain); several cups daily (18).

Comments

None.

STROPHANTHUS

This Product is Also Known As

Kombe, Kombe-Strophanthus Seeds, Strophanthi Grati Semen, Strophanthi Kombe Semen, Strophanthus Seeds.

Scientific Names

Strophanthus gratus; Strophanthus kombe.
Family: Apocynaceae.

People Use This For

Orally, strophanthus seeds are used for arteriosclerosis, cardiac insufficiency, gastrocardial symptoms, hypertension, and neurodystonia (18).

Safety

UNSAFE ...for oral self-medication (12,4077).
PREGNANCY: UNSAFE ...contraindicated due to possible uterine stimulating effects (19).
LACTATION: UNSAFE; avoid using (4077).

Effectiveness

There is insufficient reliable information available about the effectiveness of strophanthus.

Possible Mechanism of Action & Active Ingredients

The applicable part of strophanthus is the seed. Strophanthus gratus contains a cardiac glycoside strophanthin-G (ouabain) which has digitalis-like effects, but milder. The cardiac glycoside in Strophanthus kombe, strophanthin-K (strophoside), has milder effects than strophanthin-G (18,4077).

Adverse Reactions Including Known Allergies

Side effects include nausea, vomiting, headache, stupor, disturbance of color vision, and cardiac arrhythmias, particularly when strophanthin-G is administered parenterally and during overdose (18).

Possible Interactions with Herbs & Other Dietary Supplements

ANTHROQUINONE-CONTAINING HERBS AND LAXATIVE HERBS: Anthroquinone-containing herbs such as aloe, alder buckthorn, European buckthorn, cascara sagrada, frangula, rhubarb, and senna; laxative herbs such as castor bean can worsen strophanthus seed toxicity, particularly with long-term use, due to electrolyte loss (19).
LICORICE: Can worsen effects of strophanthus seed due to hypokalemia (19).
CARDIAC GLYCOSIDE-CONTAINING HERBS: Contraindicated, and concomitant use can increase the risk of cardiac glycoside toxicity. Cardiac glycoside-containing herbs include black hellebore, Canadian hemp roots, digitalis leaf, hedge mustard, figwort, lily of the valley roots, motherwort, oleander leaf, pheasant's eye plant, pleurisy root, squill bulb leaf scales, and uzara (2,18,19,500).
CINCHONA, EPHEDRA: Use with strophanthus seed may increase risk of toxicity (18,19).

Possible Interactions with Drugs

CARDIAC MEDICATIONS: Cardiac medications, including quinidine (and related noncardiac medication quinine) may increase risk of toxicity; contraindicated (18).
DIGOXIN: Therapeutic duplication, avoid using (2).
LAXATIVES: Overuse/misuse may cause electrolyte depletion and increase risk of strophanthus seed toxicity (18,19).
POTASSIUM DEPLETING DIURETICS, GLUCOCORTICOIDS: May cause electrolyte depletion and increase risk of strophanthus seed toxicity (18,19).
CALCIUM SALTS: Contraindicated (18).

Possible Interactions with Foods

No interactions are known to occur, and there is no known reason to expect a clinically significant interaction with strophanthus.

Possible Interactions with Lab Tests

No interactions are known to occur, and there is no known reason to expect a clinically significant interaction with strophanthus.

Possible Interactions with Diseases or Conditions
CARDIAC CONDITIONS: CAUTION, strophanthus seed may cause arrhythmias (18).

Typical Dosages & Routes of Administration that are Commonly Used
No typical dosage.

Comments
Strophanthus is considered unsafe for self medication (18,19,4077). Strophanthus seeds can be confused with other African Strophanthus species (18). Strophanthus is used as an arrow poison in Africa (4077).

SUMA

This Product is Also Known As
Brazilian Ginseng, Pfaffia.

Scientific Names
Pfaffia paniculata.
Family: Amaranthaceae.

People Use This For
Orally, suma is used as an immune enhancer or adaptogen, which is a substance that is thought to help the body adapt to all types of stress by enhancing or restoring the immune system.

In the Amazon, people use it orally for cancer, diabetes, tumors, and as a tonic, which is an agent used to invigorate, refresh or restore body function. They also use it topically for wounds and skin problems (515).

Safety
POSSIBLY SAFE …when used orally short-term (12).
There is insufficient reliable information available about the safety of the topical use of suma.
PREGNANCY AND LACTATION: Insufficient reliable information available; avoid using.

Effectiveness
There is insufficient reliable information available about the effectiveness of suma.

Possible Mechanism of Action & Active Ingredients
The applicable part of suma is the root. Cell culture data suggests that isolated constituents pfaffic acid, a nortriterpene, and saponin derivatives pfaffosiges A through F inhibit melanoma growth. An ethanolic extract had mild anti-inflammatory and analgesic effect, but did not relieve noninflammatory pain (515). At present, we don't know how these components relate to the uses of suma.

Adverse Reactions Including Known Allergies
Powdered suma root can cause occupational asthma during industrial exposure to the root powder (515).

Possible Interactions with Herbs & Other Dietary Supplements
Insufficient reliable information available.

Possible Interactions with Drugs
No interactions are known to occur, and there is no known reason to expect a clinically significant interaction with suma.

Possible Interactions with Foods
No interactions are known to occur, and there is no known reason to expect a clinically significant interaction with suma.

Possible Interactions with Lab Tests
No interactions are known to occur, and there is no known reason to expect a clinically significant interaction with suma.

Possible Interactions with Diseases or Conditions
No interactions are known to occur, and there is no known reason to expect a clinically significant interaction with suma.

Typical Dosages & Routes of Administration that are Commonly Used
No typical dosage.

© Copyright 2000, Natural Medicines Comprehensive Database (209) 472-2244. For updated data, go to www.NaturalDatabase.com

Comments

Suma is called Brazilian ginseng, presumably to present the herb in terms that consumers understand. It is unrelated to the ginsengs (American ginseng and Panax Ginseng) or other plants which use ginseng as an alternate common name (Blue Cohosh, Canaigre, Codonopsis, Siberian Ginseng, Withania), but may be confused with them (515).

SUMBUL

This Product is Also Known As

Ferrula, Musk Root.

Scientific Names

Ferula sumbul.
Family: Apiaceae.

People Use This For

Orally, sumbul is used for asthma and bronchitis. It is also used as an antispasmodic and sedative (18).

Safety

There is insufficient reliable information available about the safety of sumbul.
Pregnancy and Lactation: Insufficient reliable information available; avoid using.

Effectiveness

There is insufficient reliable information available about the effectiveness of sumbul.

Possible Mechanism of Action & Active Ingredients

The applicable part of sumbul is the root/rhizome. There is insufficient reliable information available about the possible mechanism of action and active ingredients.

Adverse Reactions Including Known Allergies

None reported.

Possible Interactions with Herbs & Other Dietary Supplements

Insufficient reliable information available.

Possible Interactions with Drugs

No interactions are known to occur, and there is no known reason to expect a clinically significant interaction with sumbul.

Possible Interactions with Foods

No interactions are known to occur, and there is no known reason to expect a clinically significant interaction with sumbul.

Possible Interactions with Lab Tests

No interactions are known to occur, and there is no known reason to expect a clinically significant interaction with sumbul.

Possible Interactions with Diseases or Conditions

No interactions are known to occur, and there is no known reason to expect a clinically significant interaction with sumbul.

Typical Dosages & Routes of Administration that are Commonly Used

ORAL: Sumbul is used as a liquid extract or tincture (18).

Comments

There is very little scientific information about this product. Our staff is continually analyzing the available information on natural medicines and will add data here as it becomes available.

SUMMER SAVORY

This Product is Also Known As

Bean Herb, Bohnenkraut, Savory.
CAUTION: See separate listing for Winter Savory.

Scientific Names

Satureja hortensis, synonym Calamintha hortensis.
Family: Labiatae or Lamiaceae.

People Use This For

Orally, summer savory leaves and stem are used as an appetite stimulant or expectorant, for coughs, flatulence (5), intestinal disorders including cramps, indigestion, diarrhea, nausea (5,6,11,18), and to relieve frequent thirst in people with diabetes (5).

Topically, summer savory is used topically for insect bites (11). Traditionally, summer savory has been used as a tea for sore throats (11), as a tonic, astringent (6,11), antiflatulent (5,6,11), and as an aphrodisiac (6,11).

For food uses, summer savory is used in cooking as a culinary spice (5,6). The oil is used as a flavoring agent (5,6,11).

Safety

LIKELY SAFE ...when used in amounts found in food (6,11). The maximum use level is 0.519 % for summer savory spice and 0.036 % for the oil (11). Summer savory has Generally Recognized as Safe (GRAS) status in the US (11).
POSSIBLY SAFE ...when used orally and appropriately in medicinal amounts (5,6,18). ...when used topically as dilute oil (6,11), summer savory is nonirritating and nonsensitizing (11). Undiluted oil is a severe topical irritant (6).
PREGNANCY AND LACTATION: Insufficient reliable information available; avoid using amounts in excess of foods.

Effectiveness

There is insufficient reliable information available about the effectiveness of summer savory.

Possible Mechanism of Action & Active Ingredients

The applicable parts of summer savory are the leaves and stem. Summer savory contains tannins (18), and a volatile oil (0.2-3.0 %) including thymol, carvacrol, p-cymene, limonene, and camphene (5,6,11,18). Other constituents also present include vitamin A, calcium, potassium, and proteins (11). Summer savory oil has antifungal, antibacterial, and spasmolytic properties (6,11). The mild antiseptic activity is due to cymene and carvacrol (5,18). A mild antidiarrheal effect is reportedly due to the astringent activity of the tannins (5,6,18).

Adverse Reactions Including Known Allergies

Summer savory can cause skin eruptions (12). The concentrated oil of summer savory is strongly irritating (6).

Possible Interactions with Herbs & Other Dietary Supplements

Insufficient reliable information available.

Possible Interactions with Drugs

No interactions are known to occur, and there is no known reason to expect a clinically significant interaction with summer savory.

Possible Interactions with Foods

No interactions are known to occur, and there is no known reason to expect a clinically significant interaction with summer savory.

Possible Interactions with Lab Tests

No interactions are known to occur, and there is no known reason to expect a clinically significant interaction with summer savory.

Possible Interactions with Diseases or Conditions

No interactions are known to occur, and there is no known reason to expect a clinically significant interaction with summer savory.

Typical Dosages & Routes of Administration that are Commonly Used

ORAL: A typical dose is 3 teaspoons. In making the drink, do not boil, allow plant to soak (18).
TOPICAL: No typical dosage.

Comments

Summer savory is prized both for its value as a spice and in folk medicine as an aphrodisiac. Many sources agree that it adds flavor to beans and other legumes (5), but there is no information to support other uses.

SUNDEW

This Product is Also Known As

Dew Plant, Drosera, Lustwort, Red Rot, Round-Leafed Sundew, Youthwort.

Scientific Names

Drosera rotundifolia; Drosera Ramentacea; Drosera longifolia; Drosera intermedia.
Family: Droseraeae

People Use This For

Orally, sundew is used for bronchitis, asthma, pertussis, tracheitis, gastric ulceration (4), coughing fits, and dry cough (2).

Safety

POSSIBLY SAFE ...when used orally and appropriately (2,4).
PREGNANCY AND LACTATION: Insufficient reliable information available; avoid using (4).

Effectiveness

POSSIBLY EFFECTIVE ...when used orally for coughing fits and dry coughs (2).
There is insufficient reliable information available about the effectiveness of sundew for its other uses.

Possible Mechanism of Action & Active Ingredients

Sundew seems to cause antispasmodic, demulcent, and expectorant effects (4). Researchers wonder if the antitussive effect demonstrated in animals is due to naphthoquinone constituents (4). Antimicrobial activity reported in vitro for naphthaquinone constituents (4).

Adverse Reactions Including Known Allergies

None reported.

Possible Interactions with Herbs & Other Dietary Supplements

Insufficient reliable information available.

Possible Interactions with Drugs

No interactions are known to occur, and there is no known reason to expect a clinically significant interaction with sundew.

Possible Interactions with Foods

No interactions are known to occur, and there is no known reason to expect a clinically significant interaction with sundew.

Possible Interactions with Lab Tests

No interactions are known to occur, and there is no known reason to expect a clinically significant interaction with sundew.

Possible Interactions with Diseases or Conditions

No interactions are known to occur, and there is no known reason to expect a clinically significant interaction with sundew.

Typical Dosages & Routes of Administration that are Commonly Used

ORAL: 1-2 grams dried plant three times daily, or one cup tea (made by steeping 1-2 grams dried plant in 150 mL boiling water 5-10 minutes, strain) three times daily (4); 3 grams dried plant is the average daily dose (2). Liquid extract (1:1 in 25% alcohol), 0.5-2 mL three times daily (4). Tincture (1:5 in 60% alcohol), 0.5-1 mL three times daily (4).

Comments

None.

SUNFLOWER OIL

This Product is Also Known As

Corona Solis, Helianthi Annui Oleum, Marigold of Peru.

Scientific Names

Helianthus annuus.
Family: Asteraceae.

People Use This For

Orally, it is used for constipation.
Topically, it is used for poorly healing wounds, skin lesions, psoriasis, arthritis, and as a massage oil (18). People use sunflower oil as a cooking oil.

Safety

LIKELY SAFE ...when used in amounts found in foods.
There is insufficient reliable information available about the safety of oral or topical medicinal uses for sunflower oil.
PREGNANCY AND LACTATION: Insufficient reliable information available.

Effectiveness

There is insufficient reliable information available about the effectiveness of sunflower oil.

Possible Mechanism of Action & Active Ingredients

Sunflower oil is cold pressed from the seeds of Helianthus annuus (18). There is insufficient reliable information available about the possible mechanism of action and active ingredients.

Adverse Reactions Including Known Allergies

Sunflower oil can cause an allergic reaction in individuals sensitive to the Asteraceae/Compositae family. Members of this family include ragweed, chrysanthemums, marigolds, daisies, and many other herbs.

Possible Interactions with Herbs & Other Dietary Supplements

Insufficient reliable information available.

Possible Interactions with Drugs

No interactions are known to occur, and there is no known reason to expect a clinically significant interaction with sunflower oil.

Possible Interactions with Foods

No interactions are known to occur, and there is no known reason to expect a clinically significant interaction with sunflower oil.

Possible Interactions with Lab Tests

No interactions are known to occur, and there is no known reason to expect a clinically significant interaction with sunflower oil.

Possible Interactions with Diseases or Conditions

CROSS-ALLERGENICITY: Can cause an allergic reaction in individuals sensitive to the Asteraceae/Compositae family. Members of this family include ragweed, chrysanthemums, marigolds, daisies, and many other herbs.

Typical Dosages & Routes of Administration that are Commonly Used

No typical dosage.

Comments

None.

SUPEROXIDE DISMUTASE

This Product is Also Known As

Orgotein, SOD.

Scientific Names

Superoxide dismutase.

People Use This For

Orally, superoxide dismutase is used for removing wrinkles (6), regenerating tissue (2227), and extending the length of life (6).

As an injection, superoxide dismutase is used for inflammatory diseases including osteoarthritis, sports injuries, rheumatoid arthritis (6), radiation-induced or interstitial cystitis (6), hyperuricemic syndromes (6), acute paraquat poisoning (6), for improving tolerance to radiation therapy (6), treating cancer (2226), improving rejection rates in kidney transplantation (6), managing reperfusion injury in acute myocardial infarction (6), and treating respiratory distress syndrome (6).

Safety

There is insufficient reliable information available about the safety of superoxide dismutase. However, there have been no reports of toxicity. Some evidence suggests SOD is not teratogenic (6).

Pregnancy and Lactation: Insufficient reliable information available; avoid using.

Effectiveness

POSSIBLY EFFECTIVE ...when used as an injection for treating osteoarthritis (2228,2229) or rheumatoid arthritis (2230,2231,2232). ...when used as an injection for reducing bronchopulmonary dysplasia in neonates with respiratory distress syndrome (2242). ...when used as an injection for interstitial cystitis (2233).

LIKELY INEFFECTIVE ...when used orally (6). ...when used as an injection for managing reperfusion injury in acute myocardial infarction (2241,2243).

There is insufficient reliable information available about the effectiveness of superoxide dismutase for its other uses.

Possible Mechanism of Action & Active Ingredients

Superoxide dismutase is an essential enzyme found in all living cells. It catalyzes the conversion of toxic superoxide to oxygen and hydrogen peroxide (6,511). The action of SOD is believed to prevent oxygen-related damage to body tissues (6). SOD isoenzymes contain copper and zinc, or manganese (511). They are acid-labile and appear to have no oral bioavailability even when administered as enteric coated capsules (6). SOD deficiency is associated with amyotrophic lateral sclerosis (511). Results of two clinical trials suggest SOD can prevent or reduce radiation-induced cystitis (2234,2236), but a third trial suggests SOD is ineffective and allergenic (2235). Results of two clinical trials suggest SOD can improve rejection rates as adjunct therapy in kidney transplantation (2239,2240), but a third trial suggests it has no significant effect (2238).

Adverse Reactions Including Known Allergies

SOD used orally has no reported adverse reactions. Given as an injection, SOD can cause pain or allergic reactions at injection site (6).

Possible Interactions with Herbs & Other Dietary Supplements

Insufficient reliable information available.

Possible Interactions with Drugs

No interactions are known to occur, and there is no known reason to expect a clinically significant interaction with superoxide dismutase.

Possible Interactions with Foods

No interactions are known to occur, and there is no known reason to expect a clinically significant interaction with superoxide dismutase.

Possible Interactions with Lab Tests

No interactions are known to occur, and there is no known reason to expect a clinically significant interaction with superoxide dismutase.

Possible Interactions with Diseases or Conditions

No interactions are known to occur, and there is no known reason to expect a clinically significant interaction with superoxide dismutase.

Typical Dosages & Routes of Administration that are Commonly Used

ORAL: No typical dosage.
INJECTION: For osteoarthritis, 16 mg as an intra-articular injection is used twice (2228,2229). For rheumatoid arthritis a typical dose is 4 mg as an intra-articular injection per week (2230,2232). A typical dose for interstitial or radiation-induced cystitis is 12 mg injected into the bladder wall, up to 6 times (2233). For radiation-induced cystitis, a typical dose is 8 mg injected intramuscularly per day (2234). For reducing rejection risk in kidney transplantation, a typical dose is 200 mg intravenously during surgery (2239). For reducing bronchopulmonary dysplasia in neonatal respiratory distress syndrome, 0.25 mg/kg subcutaneously twice daily until ventilator support is no longer required (2242).

Comments

Oral SOD products purchased in health food stores might not have any of the activity stated on the label because they are acid labile and break down before absorption (6). However, bovine or recombinant (rh-SOD) source parenteral SOD products are available (2238).

SWAMP MILKWEED

This Product is Also Known As

Rose-Colored Silkweed, Swamp Silkweed.

Scientific Names

Asclepias incarnata.
Family: Asclepiadaceae.

People Use This For

Orally, swamp milkweed root and rhizome is used for digestive disorders (18).

Safety

LIKELY UNSAFE ...when used orally. Contains cardenolides, a type of cardioactive steroid. Digitalis-like poisonings are possible (18).
PREGNANCY AND LACTATION: LIKELY UNSAFE ...when used orally due to presence of cardioactive steroid; avoid using.

© Copyright 2000, Natural Medicines Comprehensive Database (209) 472-2244. For updated data, go to www.NaturalDatabase.com

Effectiveness

There is insufficient reliable information available about the effectiveness of swamp milkweed.

Possible Mechanism of Action & Active Ingredients

The applicable parts of swamp milkweed are the root and rhizome. Swamp milkweed contains cardioactive steroids known as cardenolides. In swamp milkweed, they have little therapeutic significance (18), but the concentration of the specific cardenolide present is not reported. In large amounts, swamp milkweed has an emetic effect (18).

Adverse Reactions Including Known Allergies

Ingesting large amounts of swamp milkweed can cause vomiting (18). Handling the plant can cause local inflammation (19).

Possible Interactions with Herbs & Other Dietary Supplements

CARDIAC GLYCOSIDE-CONTAINING HERBS: Contraindicated; concomitant use increases the risk of cardiac glycoside toxicity. Cardiac glycoside-containing herbs, include black hellebore, Canadian hemp roots, digitalis leaf, hedge mustard, figwort, lily of the valley roots, motherwort, oleander leaf, pheasant's eye plant, pleurisy root, squill bulb leaf scales, and strophanthus seeds (2,18,19,500).
OTHER CARDIOACTIVE HERBS: Avoid concomitant use with other cardioactive herbs due to unpredictability of effects and adverse effects. Other cardioactive herbs include calamus, cereus, cola, coltsfoot, devil's claw, European mistletoe, fenugreek, fumitory, ginger, Panax ginseng, hawthorn, white horehound, mate, parsley, quassia, scotch broom flower, shepherd's purse, and wild carrot (4).
STIMULANT LAXATIVE HERBS: Theoretically, overuse or misuse of stimulant laxatives with cardiac glycoside-containing herbs increases the risk of cardiac toxicity due to potassium depletion. Stimulant laxative herbs include: aloe dried leaf sap, blue flag rhizome, alder buckthorn, European buckthorn, butternut bark, cascara bark, castor oil, colocynth fruit pulp, gamboge bark exudate, jalap root, black root, manna bark exudate, podophyllum root, rhubarb root, senna leaves and pods, wild cucumber fruit (Ecballium elaterium), and yellow dock root (19).
LICORICE/HORSETAIL: Theoretically, overuse/misuse of licorice rhizome or horsetail plant with cardiac glycoside-containing herbs increases the risk of cardiac toxicity due to potassium depletion (19).

Possible Interactions with Drugs

DIGOXIN: Contraindicated; therapeutic duplication increases risk of cardiac glycoside toxicity (2).
CARDIAC DRUGS: Theoretically, concomitant may increase risk of cardiac toxicity (152).
STIMULANT LAXATIVES: Theoretically, overuse/misuse may increase risk of cardiac glycoside toxicity due to potassium depletion (2).
POTASSIUM-DEPLETING DIURETICS: Theoretically, concomitant use might increase risk of cardiac glycoside toxicity due to potassium depletion (2,506).
QUININE: Theoretically, concomitant use might increase risk of cardiac toxicity (2,506).
TETRACYCLINES AND MACROLIDE ANTIBIOTICS (erythromycin-like drugs): Theoretically, concomitant use might increase risk of cardiac glycoside toxicity (152,17).

Possible Interactions with Foods

No interactions are known to occur, and there is no known reason to expect a clinically significant interaction with swamp milkweed.

Possible Interactions with Lab Tests

No interactions are known to occur, and there is no known reason to expect a clinically significant interaction with swamp milkweed.

Possible Interactions with Diseases or Conditions

HEART DISEASE: Contraindicated; theoretically the cardiac glycosides contained in swamp milkweed (18) might exacerbate the condition or interfere with existing drug therapy.

Typical Dosages & Routes of Administration that are Commonly Used

No typical dosage.

Comments

None.

SWEET ALMOND

This Product is Also Known As

Almond Oil, Amygdala Dulcis, Expressed Almond Oil, Fixed Almond Oil, Sweet Almond Oil.
CAUTION: See separate listing for Bitter Almond.

Scientific Names

Prunus amygdalus dulcis.
Family: Rosaceae.

People Use This For

Orally, sweet almond oil is used as a mild laxative (11).

Topically, it is used as an emollient for chapped skin, to soothe mucous membranes (as a demulcent), and as a weak antibacterial (11).

Parenterally, sweet almond oil is also used as a solvent for injectable drugs (11).

In folk medicine, sweet almond has been used as a remedy for cancer of the bladder, breast, mouth, spleen, and uterus (11).

Sweet almonds, themselves, are a familiar food.

In manufacturing, sweet almond oil is used widely in cosmetics.

Safety

LIKELY SAFE ...when used orally (11). Unlike bitter almond oil, sweet almond oil contains no benzaldehyde and no (or only trace) poisonous hydrocyanic acid HCN (11,12). ...when used topically. Almond oil is nonirritating and nonsensitizing to skin (11).

PREGNANCY AND LACTATION: Insufficient reliable information available; avoid using.

Effectiveness

POSSIBLY EFFECTIVE ...when used orally as a laxative (11). ...when used topically as an emollient and demulcent (11).

Possible Mechanism of Action & Active Ingredients

The applicable part of sweet almond is the fixed oil. Researchers believe the effects of sweet almond oil are due to the presence of many triglycerides (largely triolein and dioleolinolein) and fatty acids (oleic, linoleic, palmitic, stearic, lauric, myristic and palmitoleic acids) (11). A Japanese patent claims isolation of low molecular weight peptides with analgesic and anti-inflammatory properties (11).

Adverse Reactions Including Known Allergies

None reported.

Possible Interactions with Herbs & Other Dietary Supplements

Insufficient reliable information available.

Possible Interactions with Drugs

No interactions are known to occur, and there is no known reason to expect a clinically significant interaction with sweet almond.

Possible Interactions with Foods

No interactions are known to occur, and there is no known reason to expect a clinically significant interaction with sweet almond.

Possible Interactions with Lab Tests

No interactions are known to occur, and there is no known reason to expect a clinically significant interaction with sweet almond.

Possible Interactions with Diseases or Conditions

No interactions are known to occur, and there is no known reason to expect a clinically significant interaction with sweet almond.

Typical Dosages & Routes of Administration that are Commonly Used

ORAL: As a laxative in doses up to 30 mL (11).

Comments

Avoid confusion between volatile almond oil and fixed almond oil. Fixed almond oil (sweet almond oil) is prepared by pressing the kernels of both sweet almond and bitter almond. It does not contain benzaldehyde or hydrocyanic acid (HCN). Sweet almond does not yield a volatile oil. Volatile almond oil (bitter almond oil) contains 95% benzaldehyde and 2-4% poisonous HCN. It is made by water maceration and steam distillation of partially defatted bitter almond (Prunus dulcis amara), apricot (Prunus armeniaca), peach (Prunus persica), and plum (Prunus domestica) kernels (11).

SWEET ANNIE

This Product is Also Known As

Annual Mugwort, Annual Wormwood, Artemisinin, Chinese Wormwood, Ching-hao, Qing Hao, Qinghao, Qinghaosu, Sweet Wormwood.

Scientific Names

Artemisia annua.
Family: Asteraceae or Compositae.

People Use This For

Orally, sweet Annie is used for dysentery, dyspepsia, fever (antipyretic), jaundice, night-sweats, scabies, tuberculosis (1277), cryptosporidiosis in people with AIDS (3173), preventing pneumocystis carinii infections in people with AIDS (3177), psoriasis, systemic lupus erythematosus and other autoimmune disorders (3175), bacterial and fungal infections, malaria, inflammatory conditions (3176), anorexia, circulatory disorders, common cold, constipation, gallbladder disorders, gastritis, nematode infestation, painful menstruation, and rheumatism (3179). Topically, sweet Annie is used for bacterial and fungal infections (3176), arthritis, rheumatism, bruises, neuralgia, and sprains (3179).

In Chinese medicine, sweet Annie is used orally for infections, fever, and malaria (3177,3178).

Safety

POSSIBLY SAFE ...when used orally and appropriately (12).
There is insufficient reliable information available about the safety of sweet Annie for its other uses.
PREGNANCY: LIKELY UNSAFE ...contraindicated (12,19).
LACTATION: Insufficient reliable information available; avoid using.

Effectiveness

EFFECTIVE ...when the sweet Annie extract, artemisinin, is used orally and by injection for treating malaria (14,3180).
There is insufficient reliable information available about the effectiveness of sweet Annie for its other uses.

Possible Mechanism of Action & Active Ingredients

The above ground parts (herb) of sweet Annie are used (12). The constituent, artemisinin (qinghaosu), is a sesquiterpene lactone with antimalarial activity (14,3178). Preliminary evidence suggests that artemisinin and quercetagetin 6,7,3',4'-tetramethyl ether might have cytotoxic effects against some types of tumor cells (3183). Extracts of sweet Annie are reported to have antipyretic, anti-inflammatory, and bacteriostatic properties (3184). Evidence suggests that sweet Annie promotes cell-mediated immunity and inhibits antibody responses (3177). Preliminary research suggests that capsules containing sweet Annie herb might have antimalarial activity (3185).

Adverse Reactions Including Known Allergies

The use of artemether, the semisynthetic derivative of artemisinin, which is a constituent of sweet Annie, has been associated with hypoglycemia, prolongation of the QT interval on the electrocardiogram, abdominal pain, and local injection site pain (3180). Artesunate has been associated with prolonged ataxic gait and slurred speech (450).
Sweet Annie might cause an allergic reaction in people sensitive to the Asteraceae/Compositae family. Members of this family include ragweed, chrysanthemums, marigolds, daisies, and many other herbs.

Possible Interactions with Herbs & Other Dietary Supplements

Insufficient reliable information available.

Possible Interactions with Drugs

No interactions are known to occur, and there is no known reason to expect a clinically significant interaction with sweet Annie.

Possible Interactions with Foods

No interactions are known to occur, and there is no known reason to expect a clinically significant interaction with sweet Annie.

Possible Interactions with Lab Tests

No interactions are known to occur, and there is no known reason to expect a clinically significant interaction with sweet Annie.

Possible Interactions with Diseases or Conditions

CROSS-ALLERGENICITY: Sweet Annie might cause an allergic reaction in people sensitive to the Asteraceae/Compositae family. Members of this family include ragweed, chrysanthemums, marigolds, daisies, and many other herbs.

Typical Dosages & Routes of Administration that are Commonly Used

ORAL: Daily doses of 3-9 grams of sweet Annie above ground parts have been used (3176,3177).

Comments
The semisynthetic derivatives of artemisinin (a constituent of sweet Annie); artemether, arteether, and artesunate, are used as prescription antimalarial drugs in Asia, Africa, and Europe (14,3178,3181,3182).

SWEET BAY

This Product is Also Known As
Bay, Bay Laurel, Bay Tree, Daphne, Grecian Laurel, Laurel, Mediterranean Bay, Noble Laurel, Roman Laurel, Sweet Bay, True Bay.
CAUTION: See separate listing for Allspice (West Indian Bay).

Scientific Names
Laurus nobilis.
Family: Lauraceae; other botanicals also referred to as bay, including: Pimenta racemosa (West Indian Bay); Umbellularia californica (California Bay) (11).

People Use This For
Orally, sweet bay leaf and oil are used to treat cancer, and as a bile and general stimulant, antiflatulent, diaphoretic (11), and herb for foods (11).
Topically, sweet bay is used as an anti-dandruff agent (11), as a counterirritant, and to treat rheumatic conditions (18). In veterinary medicine, sweet bay is used as an udder ointment (18).
Historically, the fruit essential and fatty oils of sweet bay have been used for treating furuncles, a localized infection of hair follicles (18).
For food uses, sweet bay is used as a seasoning, and extensively in manufacturing as an herb and oil in processed foods (11).
In manufacturing, the oil is used in cosmetics, soaps, and detergents (11).

Safety
LIKELY SAFE ...when taken orally (12); although, the whole, intact leaf is indigestible and can become lodged in the esophagus and hypopharynx (132,133,134,137) and perforate the intestinal lining (135,136). The highest levels of sweet bay used in food are 0.1% as a herb and a 0.02% oil (11).
PREGNANCY AND LACTATION: Insufficient reliable information available; avoid using in amounts exceeding those commonly found in foods.

Effectiveness
There is insufficient reliable information available about the effectiveness of sweet bay.

Possible Mechanism of Action & Active Ingredients
The applicable part of sweet bay is the dried leaf. The sweet bay constituent, methyl eugenol, has sedative and narcotic properties in mice. The essential oil has bactericidal and fungicidal properties (11). The other constituents of sweet bay include proanthocyanidins, alkaloids, and plant acids (11).

Adverse Reactions Including Known Allergies
Sweet bay can cause allergic reactions, including contact dermatitis (11). The whole, intact leaf is indigestible and can become lodged in the esophagus and hypopharynx (132,133,134,137) and perforate the intestinal lining (135,136).

Possible Interactions with Herbs & Other Dietary Supplements
Insufficient reliable information available.

Possible Interactions with Drugs
SEDATIVE DRUGS AND NARCOTIC ANALGESICS: Because sweet bay theoretically can enhance the therapeutic and adverse effects of sedatives and narcotics, concomitant use should be avoided.

Possible Interactions with Foods
No interactions are known to occur, and there is no known reason to expect a clinically significant interaction with sweet bay.

Possible Interactions with Lab Tests
No interactions are known to occur, and there is no known reason to expect a clinically significant interaction with sweet bay.

Possible Interactions with Diseases or Conditions
SWEET BAY ALLERGY: Because of contact dermatitis, sweet bay should be avoided in those having sensitivity to it.

© Copyright 2000, Natural Medicines Comprehensive Database (209) 472-2244. For updated data, go to www.NaturalDatabase.com • 1007

Typical Dosages & Routes of Administration that are Commonly Used

TOPICAL: An extract of sweet bay is typically used in baths and soaks (5008).
ORAL: No typical dosage.

Comments

The ancient Greeks and Romans crowned their victors with the leafy branches of sweet bay (11). Avoid confusion with West Indian bay.

SWEET CICELY

This Product is Also Known As

British Myrrh, Shepherd's Needle, Sweet Bracken, Sweet Chervil, Sweet-Cus, Sweet-Fern, Sweet-Humlock, Sweets, The Roman Plant.

Scientific Names

Myrrhis odorata.
Family: Apiaceae.

People Use This For

Orally, sweet cicely is used for breathing difficulties, asthma, as an expectorant, digestive aid, and blood purifier. It is also used orally for chest and throat complaints, and for urinary tract complaints (18).
Topically, the fresh herb is used for gout swelling and indurations.

Safety

There is insufficient reliable information available about the safety of sweet cicely.
Pregnancy and Lactation: Insufficient reliable information available; avoid using.

Effectiveness

There is insufficient reliable information available about the effectiveness of sweet cicely.

Possible Mechanism of Action & Active Ingredients

Insufficient reliable information available.

Adverse Reactions Including Known Allergies

None reported.

Possible Interactions with Herbs & Other Dietary Supplements

Insufficient reliable information available.

Possible Interactions with Drugs

No interactions are known to occur, and there is no known reason to expect a clinically significant interaction with sweet cicely.

Possible Interactions with Foods

No interactions are known to occur, and there is no known reason to expect a clinically significant interaction with sweet cicely.

Possible Interactions with Lab Tests

No interactions are known to occur, and there is no known reason to expect a clinically significant interaction with sweet cicely.

Possible Interactions with Diseases or Conditions

No interactions are known to occur, and there is no known reason to expect a clinically significant interaction with sweet cicely.

Typical Dosages & Routes of Administration that are Commonly Used

Sweet cicely is used as a tea or tonic (18).

Comments

There is very little scientific information about this product. Our staff is continually analyzing the available information on natural medicines and will add data here as it becomes available.

SWEET CLOVER

This Product is Also Known As
Common Melilot, Field Melilot, Hart's Tree, Hay Flower, King's Clover, Melilot, Meliloti herba, Melilotus, Sweet Lucerne, Sweet Melilot, Tall Melilot, Wild Laburnum, Yellow Melilot, Yellow Sweet Clover.
CAUTION: See separate listings for Red Clover and Hay Flower.

Scientific Names
Melilotus officinalis; Melilotus altissimus.
Family: Fabaceae.

People Use This For
Orally, sweet clover is used for symptoms of chronic venous insufficiency and varicose veins, including leg pain and heaviness, night cramps, pruritus and edema (1,2,18), supportive treatment of thrombophlebitis (2,8,18), hemorrhoids (2,18), post-thrombotic syndromes, and lymphatic congestion (2).
Topically, sweet clover is used for contusions and ecchymoses (2,18).
Historically, sweet clover has been used as a diuretic (8,18).

Safety
LIKELY SAFE ...when preparations of the flowering branch and leaf are used orally in moderate amounts (1,2,18).
LIKELY UNSAFE ...when large amounts are used orally because it can cause transient liver injury (18).
PREGNANCY: Insufficient reliable information available. A study of 30 second and third trimester pregnant women did not report any adverse effects (1).
LACTATION: Insufficient reliable information available; avoid using.

Effectiveness
POSSIBLY EFFECTIVE ...when used orally for problems associated with chronic venous insufficiency (1,2), including leg pain and heaviness, nighttime leg cramps, itching and swelling, for supportive treatment of thrombophlebitis, lymphatic congestion, post-thrombotic syndromes, and hemorrhoids (2). ...when used for contusions and ecchymoses (2). ...when used intravenously for treating symptoms of phlebitis, chronic thrombophlebitis, and varicose veins (1).
There is insufficient reliable information available about the effectiveness of sweet clover for its other uses.

Possible Mechanism of Action & Active Ingredients
The applicable parts of sweet clover are the flowering branch and leaf. Fresh herb contains coumarinic acids (18), which are converted to free coumarins during drying (1,8,18). Dicoumarol, which has anticoagulant activity, can be formed if the fresh herb is allowed to spoil (1). There is some evidence to suggest that sweet clover aids wound healing (2,8), and a locally perfused sweet clover extract might eliminate adrenaline-induced vasoconstriction. This would indicate peripheral vasodilation (1). Coumarin isolated from sweet clover reduces experimentally-induced paw inflammation in rats (1). Intravenous administration decreases pain, edema, and improves wound healing in people with phlebitis, and relieves symptoms of varicose veins (1). Sweet clover seems to increase venous reflux and improve lymphatic kinetics, and therefore reduces edema (2).

Adverse Reactions Including Known Allergies
Taken orally, headaches are rare (1,2,18), and large amounts can cause stupor and transient liver injury in susceptible individuals (18). There was one case report of bleeding diathesis following two months ingestion of large amounts of a multi-herb, "seasonal tonic" tea containing melilot, sweet woodruff, and tonka bean (all coumarin-containing herbs) (809).

Possible Interactions with Herbs & Other Dietary Supplements
HERBS WITH ANTICOAGULANT/ANTIPLATELET POTENTIAL: Concomitant use of herbs that have coumarin constituents or affect platelet aggregation could theoretically increase the risk of bleeding in some people. These herbs include: angelica, anise, arnica, asafoetida, bogbean, boldo, capsicum, celery, chamomile, clove, danshen, fenugreek, feverfew, garlic, ginger, ginkgo, ginseng Panax, horse chestnut, horseradish, licorice, meadowsweet, prickly ash, onion, papain, passionflower, poplar, quassia, red clover, turmeric, wild carrot, wild lettuce, willow, and others (4,19).

Possible Interactions with Drugs
ANTICOAGULANT, ANTIPLATELET DRUGS: Theoretically, concomitant use might increase bleeding risk (19).
HEPATOTOXIC DRUGS: Theoretically, concomitant use might increase risk of hepatotoxicity (see Adverse Reactions).

Possible Interactions with Foods
No interactions are known to occur, and there is no known reason to expect a clinically significant interaction with sweet clover.

Possible Interactions with Lab Tests

LIVER ENZYMES: Sweet clover might cause an increase in liver enzymes and test results, indicating liver damage; monitor (18).

Possible Interactions with Diseases or Conditions

LIVER DISEASE: Theoretically, sweet clover might exacerbate liver disease (see Adverse Reactions) (18); avoid using.

Typical Dosages & Routes of Administration that are Commonly Used

ORAL: Average amount, sweet clover preparations equivalent to 3-30 mg coumarin per day (1,2). Phlebitis or varicose veins, one cup (made by steeping 1-2 teaspoons finely chopped sweet clover in 150 mL boiling water 5-10 minutes, strain) two to three cups per day (8,18); 6 mL Melilotus/rutin preparation (600 mg Melilotus extract containing 3 mg coumarin and 150 mg rutin) per day reported in one clinical trial (1). CAUTION: Monitor liver enzymes with oral use (18), especially in people at risk for liver damage.
TOPICAL: Sweet clover extract in semi-solid preparations containing 3-5 mg/g coumarin (2,8,18). As a poultice for sores and hemorrhoids, wrap sweet clover in linen, thoroughly soak with hot water, place on the affected area (8).
INJECTION: Liquid forms for parenteral use corresponding to 1-7.5 mg coumarin per day (2,8).

Comments

Avoid confusion with red clover (Trifolium pratense) and hay flower, the sieved flower and fruit from cut hay grass (Poaceae family) plants.

SWEET GALE

This Product is Also Known As

Bayberry, Bog Myrtle, Dutch Myrtle.
CAUTION: See separate listing for Bayberry.

Scientific Names

Myrica gale.
Family: Myricaceae.

People Use This For

Orally, sweet gale leaf, branch, and wax from catkin are used for digestive disorders.
In Sweden, a strong brew of dried bark is used as an antihelmintic and to cure itching (18).

Safety

There is insufficient reliable information available about the safety of sweet gale. The volatile oil of sweet gale is considered toxic (18).
Pregnancy and Lactation: Insufficient reliable information available; avoid using.

Effectiveness

There is insufficient reliable information available about the effectiveness of sweet gale.

Possible Mechanism of Action & Active Ingredients

The applicable parts of sweet gale are the leaf, branch, and wax from catkin. Sweet gale contains 0.4-0.7% of a volatile oil that contains alpha-pinene, delta-cadinene, gamma-cadinene, limonene, beta-myrcene, beta-phellandrene, and 1,8 cineole. It also contains flavonoids including myricitrin (18). Sweet gale is thought to have astringent and aromatic properties (18).

Adverse Reactions Including Known Allergies

None reported although the volatile oil is considered toxic.

Possible Interactions with Herbs & Other Dietary Supplements

Insufficient reliable information available.

Possible Interactions with Drugs

No interactions are known to occur, and there is no known reason to expect a clinically significant interaction with sweet gale.

Possible Interactions with Foods

No interactions are known to occur, and there is no known reason to expect a clinically significant interaction with sweet gale.

Possible Interactions with Lab Tests

No interactions are known to occur, and there is no known reason to expect a clinically significant interaction with sweet gale.

Possible Interactions with Diseases or Conditions

No interactions are known to occur, and there is no known reason to expect a clinically significant interaction with sweet gale.

Typical Dosages & Routes of Administration that are Commonly Used

No typical dosage.

Comments

In the Middle ages, sweet gale was mixed with beer, and is said to have led to periods of extreme excitation [18].

SWEET ORANGE

This Product is Also Known As

Citri Sinensis, Jaffa Orange, Navel Orange, Pericarpium, Valencia Orange.
CAUTION: See separate listings for Bergamot Oil, Oswego Tea, Bitter Orange flower, and Bitter Orange peel.

Scientific Names

Citrus sinensis, synonyms Citrus aurantium sinensis, Citrus aurantium dulcis.
Family: Rutaceae.

People Use This For

Orally, sweet orange peel is used as an appetite stimulant [2].
In Chinese medicine, sweet orange peel is used to reduce phlegm, treat coughs, colds, anorexia, and malignant breast sores [11].
Historically, it has been used as a tonic, antiflatulent, and for dyspepsia [11].

Safety

LIKELY SAFE ...when used orally. ... when used topically. The volatile oil of sweet orange peel has a low potential for sensitizing skin [18].
CHILDREN: LIKELY UNSAFE ...when taken orally in large amounts; avoid using. There are reports of intestinal colic, convulsions, and death [11].
PREGNANCY AND LACTATION: Insufficient reliable information available; avoid using.

Effectiveness

POSSIBLY EFFECTIVE ...when taken orally as an appetite stimulant and for dyspeptic ailments [2].
There is insufficient reliable information available about the effectiveness of sweet orange for its other uses.

Possible Mechanism of Action & Active Ingredients

The applicable parts of sweet orange are the peel and juice. Orange peel contains essential oil and bitter principles [11]. The constituents naringin and nobiletin might have anti-inflammatory activity [11,1281]. The flavonoid and pectin constituents have antibacterial and antifungal activities. Pectin also seems to lower cholesterol in the blood [11].
Researchers report that flavonoids contained in orange juice might inhibit growth of human prostate, lung, melanoma and colon cancer cells. Results of this unpublished research were presented at the 219th American Chemical Society National Meeting [5042].

Adverse Reactions Including Known Allergies

There have been reports of intestinal colic, convulsions, and death in children following ingestion of large amounts of sweet orange peel [11].

Possible Interactions with Herbs & Other Dietary Supplements

Insufficient reliable information available.

Possible Interactions with Drugs

No interactions are known to occur, and there is no known reason to expect a clinically significant interaction with sweet orange.

Possible Interactions with Foods

No interactions are known to occur, and there is no known reason to expect a clinically significant interaction with sweet orange.

Possible Interactions with Lab Tests

No interactions are known to occur, and there is no known reason to expect a clinically significant interaction with sweet orange.

Possible Interactions with Diseases or Conditions

No interactions are known to occur, and there is no known reason to expect a clinically significant interaction with sweet orange.

Typical Dosages & Routes of Administration that are Commonly Used
ORAL: 10-15 grams fresh or dry peel (free of white pulp layer) per day as a digestive aid (2). Peel may be used to prepare a tea (steep peel in boiling water 10-15 minutes, strain) or in other herbal preparations (2). Store peel away from children, due to reported death after ingestion of large amounts (11).

Comments
Researchers report that drinking three glasses of orange juice daily might increase HDL cholesterol in people with high cholesterol (346). Further research is needed to verify this finding. Avoid confusion with bergamot oil, oswego tea, bitter orange flower, and bitter orange peel.

SWEET SUMACH

This Product is Also Known As
None.

Scientific Names
Rhus aromatica.
Family: Anacardiaceae.

People Use This For
Orally, sweet sumach is used for irritable bladder, urinary incontinence, bed-wetting, kidney and bladder disorders, and uterine hemorrhages (18).

Safety
There is insufficient reliable information available about the safety of sweet sumach.
Pregnancy and Lactation: Insufficient reliable information available; avoid using.

Effectiveness
There is insufficient reliable information available about the effectiveness of sweet sumach.

Possible Mechanism of Action & Active Ingredients
The applicable part of sweet sumach is the root bark. There is insufficient reliable information available about the possible mechanism of action and active ingredients of sweet sumach.

Adverse Reactions Including Known Allergies
Sweet sumach can cause contact allergic dermatitis in susceptible individuals (4078).

Possible Interactions with Herbs & Other Dietary Supplements
Insufficient reliable information available.

Possible Interactions with Drugs
No interactions are known to occur, and there is no known reason to expect a clinically significant interaction with sweet sumach.

Possible Interactions with Foods
No interactions are known to occur, and there is no known reason to expect a clinically significant interaction with sweet sumach.

Possible Interactions with Lab Tests
No interactions are known to occur, and there is no known reason to expect a clinically significant interaction with sweet sumach.

Possible Interactions with Diseases or Conditions
No interactions are known to occur, and there is no known reason to expect a clinically significant interaction with sweet sumach.

Typical Dosages & Routes of Administration that are Commonly Used
No typical dosage.

Comments
Sweet sumach belongs to the same family as poison ivy, and can cause similar dermal reactions (4078).
There is very little scientific information about this product. Our staff is continually analyzing the available information on natural medicines and will add data here as it becomes available.

SWEET VERNAL GRASS

This Product is Also Known As
Grass, Spring Grass.

Scientific Names
Anthoxanthum odoratum.

People Use This For
Orally, the whole plant of sweet vernal grass is used for headache (18), nausea (18), sleeplessness (18), and conditions of the urinary tract (route unspecified).
In Russia, sweet vernal grass was used as an ingredient in certain brandies (6).
For food uses, sweet vernal grass has been used as a flavoring agent.

Safety
LIKELY UNSAFE ...when used orally for medicinal use. ...when the whole plant is used orally as a flavoring or in larger amounts. Sweet vernal grass contains the constituent, dicumarol that has anticoagulant properties (6,18). It also contains the constituent coumarin, which the FDA has banned for flavoring purposes. Coumarin has been associated with hepatotoxicity ranging from elevated liver enzymes to severe hepatic damage (6,18,297,4501). There is insufficient reliable information available about the safety of the topical use of sweet vernal grass.
PREGNANCY AND LACTATION: LIKELY UNSAFE ...contraindicated for oral use.

Effectiveness
There is insufficient reliable information available about the effectiveness of sweet vernal grass (18).

Possible Mechanism of Action & Active Ingredients
Sweet vernal grass contains hydroxycinnamic acid glycosides that form coumarin (up to 1.5%) when the harvested plant is dehydrated (18). After an outbreak of hemorrhagic diathesis in cattle fed sweet vernal grass hay, veterinary experiments identified dicumarol, a known anticoagulant, in the hay (6). There is some evidence that coumarin can reduce edema and inflammation by increasing venous and lymphatic return (295).

Adverse Reactions Including Known Allergies
Use of high levels of sweet vernal grass can cause headaches and dizziness (18). The oral use of sweet vernal grass when the harvested plant is dehydrated can be associated with nausea and vomiting (286), diarrhea, dizziness, insomnia (287), asymptomatic SGOT elevations (286), and rarely, liver toxicity (6,18,297,4501). Cattle poisoned by sweet vernal hay showed characteristically rapid onset of symptoms including progressive weakness, mucosal pallor, stiff gait, tachypnea, tachycardia, and hematomata, quickly resulting in death (6).

Possible Interactions with Herbs & Other Dietary Supplements
HERBS WITH ANTICOAGULANT/ANTIPLATELET POTENTIAL: Concomitant use of herbs that have coumarin constituents or affect platelet aggregation could theoretically increase the risk of bleeding in some people. These herbs include: angelica, anise, arnica, asafoetida, bogbean, boldo, capsicum, celery, chamomile, clove, danshen, fenugreek, feverfew, garlic, ginger, ginkgo, ginseng Panax, horse chestnut, horseradish, licorice, meadowsweet, prickly ash, onion, papain, passionflower, poplar, quassia, red clover, turmeric, wild carrot, wild lettuce, willow, and others (4,19).

Possible Interactions with Drugs
ANTICOAGULANTS/ANTIPLATELETS: Theoretically, sweet vernal grass might cause additive effects and side effects with drugs having anticoagulant or antiplatelet properties (19).

Possible Interactions with Foods
No interactions are known to occur, and there is no known reason to expect a clinically significant interaction with sweet vernal grass.

Possible Interactions with Lab Tests
No interactions are known to occur, and there is no known reason to expect a clinically significant interaction with sweet vernal grass.

Possible Interactions with Diseases or Conditions
LIVER DISEASE: Although it is rare, coumarin can cause liver toxicity (298).

Typical Dosages & Routes of Administration that are Commonly Used
ORAL: No typical dosage.
TOPICAL: Used as an extract (18).

Comments
Sweet vernal grass is likely unsafe for oral use; avoid using. This aromatic plant has been used as a flavoring agent due to its vanilla-like aroma (6).

SWEET VIOLET

This Product is Also Known As
Garden Violet, Sweet Violet Herb, Sweet Violet Root, Violae Odoratae Rhizoma, Herba, Violet.
CAUTION: See separate listing for Garden Violet.

Scientific Names
Viola odorata.
Family: Violaceae.

People Use This For
In herbal combinations, sweet violet is used for acute and chronic bronchitis, bronchial asthma, acute and chronic mucous inflammations of the upper and lower respiratory tract, cold symptoms of the upper respiratory tract, hoarseness, cough, mucous congestion, bronchial inflammation, and late "flu" symptoms. It is also used for chesty, spastic and whooping coughs, emphysema, "dust-damaged" lung (2), urinary incontinence due to senility, irritable bladder, enuresis nocturna or prostate condition (2), insomnia, and improving deep sleep.

Orally, sweet violet is also used for calming and relaxing nerves (2), physical and mental exhaustion (2), physical and psychological symptoms associated with menopause (hot flashes), metabolic imbalances, to "detoxify blood," for depression, irritability, anxiety (2), GI complaints, abdominal pain, gallbladder complaints, mucous membrane inflammation of the stomach and intestines, enteritis, duodenitis, digestion problems caused by improper diet, flatulence, heartburn, and loss of appetite (2).

Topically, it is used for skin impurities and disorders (2), and as a skin cleanser (18).

In folk medicine, the root has been used for respiratory tract conditions, particularly dry mucous membrane inflammation, rheumatism of the minor joints, fever, skin diseases, inflammation of the oral mucosa, nervous strain, headache, and insomnia (18). In folk medicine, the herb has been used for coughs, hoarseness, tuberculosis, throat inflammation, bronchitis accompanied by fixed mucous, nervous strain, insomnia, and hysteria (18).

Safety
POSSIBLY SAFE ...when taken orally in appropriate amounts (2,18).
There is insufficient reliable information available about the safety of the topical use of sweet violet.
PREGNANCY AND LACTATION: Insufficient reliable information available; avoid using.

Effectiveness
There is insufficient reliable information available about the effectiveness of sweet violet.

Possible Mechanism of Action & Active Ingredients
The applicable parts of sweet violet are the root and above ground parts. Sweet violet contains saponins (2), which have expectorant properties, and in high doses irritate mucous membranes (2).

Adverse Reactions Including Known Allergies
None reported.

Possible Interactions with Herbs & Other Dietary Supplements
Insufficient reliable information available.

Possible Interactions with Drugs
No interactions are known to occur, and there is no known reason to expect a clinically significant interaction with sweet violet.

Possible Interactions with Foods
No interactions are known to occur, and there is no known reason to expect a clinically significant interaction with sweet violet.

Possible Interactions with Lab Tests
No interactions are known to occur, and there is no known reason to expect a clinically significant interaction with sweet violet.

Possible Interactions with Diseases or Conditions
No interactions are known to occur, and there is no known reason to expect a clinically significant interaction with sweet violet.

Typical Dosages & Routes of Administration that are Commonly Used
ORAL: The typical dose of sweet violet as an herb is one cup tea (steep 2 teaspoons herb in 250 mL boiling water 10-15 minutes, strain) 2-3 times daily (18). As a root (5% w/v), take 1 tablespoon 5-6 times daily (simmer 20 grams (18) in boiling water for 10-15 minutes, and strain). The daily average amount of root used is 1 gram (18).

Comments
None.

 © Copyright 2000, Natural Medicines Comprehensive Database (209) 472-2244. For updated data, go to www.NaturalDatabase.com

SWEET WOODRUFF

This Product is Also Known As
Galii odorati herba, Master of the Wood, Waldmeister, Woodruff, Wordward.

Scientific Names
Galium odorata, synonym Asperula odorata.
Family: Rubiaceae.

People Use This For
Orally, sweet woodruff above ground parts are used for preventing and treating respiratory tract, gastrointestinal tract, liver, gallbladder, and urinary tract disorders; for blood purification, venous complaints, weak veins, hemorrhoids, vasodilation; spasms, abdominal discomforts; strengthening the nervous system (2), agitation, hysteria, nervous menstrual disorders (18), restlessness, insomnia, neuralgia (11); strengthening heart function (2), cardiac irregularity (18); stomachache, migraine, and bladder stones (11). Sweet woodruff is also used orally for inducing sweating, as an antispasmodic, diuretic (11), or expectorant (6).
Topically, sweet woodruff is used for skin diseases, treating wounds (2), venous conditions, hemorrhoids, and for reducing inflammation (11).
In foods and beverages, sweet woodruff is used as a flavoring component (11).
In manufacturing, the extracts of sweet woodruff above ground parts are used as fragrance components in perfumes (11).

Safety
LIKELY SAFE ...when used orally in amounts found in alcoholic beverages (11). Approved only for use in alcoholic beverages in the US (11).
POSSIBLY SAFE ...when used orally and appropriately for medicinal uses on a short-term basis (12,18).
There is insufficient reliable information available about the safety of the topical use of sweet woodruff.
PREGNANCY AND LACTATION: Insufficient reliable information available; avoid using.

Effectiveness
There is insufficient reliable information available about the effectiveness of sweet woodruff.

Possible Mechanism of Action & Active Ingredients
The applicable parts of sweet woodruff are the above ground parts. Sweet woodruff leaves and the constituent asperuloside show evidence of anti-inflammatory activity (11). Sweet woodruff also demonstrates antibacterial activity (4009). The fresh plant contains up to 1% coumarin as a bound glycoside. Coumarin is supposedly enzymatically released during dehydration (11). Interestingly, one investigation failed to detect any coumarins in sweet woodruff (11). The coumarin constituent is thought to have anti-inflammatory, anti-edema, spasmolytic, and lymphokinetic effects, but the levels found in sweet woodruff are so low that therapeutic effects are doubtful (18). Other constituents present in sweet woodruff include monotopein, tannins, anthracene and naphthalene derivatives, plus traces of nicotinic acid, a fixed oil, and a bitter principle (11).

Adverse Reactions Including Known Allergies
Oral use of sweet woodruff above ground parts can be associated with headache (12), and in larger amounts, stupor (18). Long-term usage can cause liver damage (18).

Possible Interactions with Herbs & Other Dietary Supplements
Insufficient reliable information available.

Possible Interactions with Drugs
No interactions are known to occur, and there is no known reason to expect a clinically significant interaction with sweet woodruff.

Possible Interactions with Foods
No interactions are known to occur, and there is no known reason to expect a clinically significant interaction with sweet woodruff.

Possible Interactions with Lab Tests
No interactions are known to occur, and there is no known reason to expect a clinically significant interaction with sweet woodruff.

Possible Interactions with Diseases or Conditions
No interactions are known to occur, and there is no known reason to expect a clinically significant interaction with sweet woodruff.

Typical Dosages & Routes of Administration that are Commonly Used
ORAL: A typical dose is one cup tea. To make tea, use 2 teaspoons (1.8 grams) in a glass of water (18). The average single dose is 1 gram during the day or shortly before bedtime (18).

© Copyright 2000, Natural Medicines Comprehensive Database (209) 472-2244. For updated data, go to www.NaturalDatabase.com • 1015

Comments
Sweet woodruff root contains a red dye (6). Sweet woodruff is considered obsolete for medicinal use in many countries (18). Avoid confusing sweet woodruff, Galium odoratum, with Asperula odorata which is also referred to as woodruff.

TAGETES

This Product is Also Known As
African Marigold, Aztec Marigold, Big Marigold, Chinchilla Enana, Dwarf Marigold, French Marigold, Huacatay, Mexican Marigold, Muster John Henry, Saffron Marigold, Stinking-Roger, Tagetes.

Scientific Names
Tagetes erecta; Tagetes patula; Tagetes minuta , synonym Tagetes glandulifera.
Family: Asteraceae or Compositae.

People Use This For
Orally, the flowerheads and foliage of African marigold have been used as an antihelmintic, a menstrual flow stimulant, and for treating colic (11). The flowerheads of African marigold have been used orally in treating whooping cough, cough, colds, mumps, mastitis, and sore eyes (11).

The Mexican marigold has been used orally for improving digestion, stimulating appetite, inducing sweating, as an antihelmintic, as a bile flow stimulant, as a sedative in gastric pain, as an antiflatulent, as a diuretic, and antiabortifacient (11).

The French marigold is used orally for coughs and dysentery (11).

Topically, the African marigold leaf is used for treating sores and ulcers (11). The juice of the leaf is used topically for eczema (11). The oil of the Mexican marigold is used for treating wound maggots (11).

In manufacturing, oil from the Mexican marigold is used as fragrance in perfumes (11) and a flavor component in foods and beverages (11). The flowers of the African marigold are useful as mosquito repellent (11). The dried, ground flowers of marigolds are used as chicken feed to enhance the characteristic yellow color of chicken skin and egg yolk (11).

Safety
LIKELY SAFE ...when used orally in amounts found in foods. Tagetes oil has Generally Recognized as Safe (GRAS) status in the US (11). The maximum use level of the oil in foods is 0.003% (11).

There is insufficient reliable information available about the safety of tagetes used in amounts greater than those found in foods.

PREGNANCY AND LACTATION: Insufficient reliable information available; avoid amounts greater than found in foods.

Effectiveness
There is insufficient reliable information available about the effectiveness of tagetes.

Possible Mechanism of Action & Active Ingredients
The applicable parts of tagetes are the above ground parts. Some evidence suggests tagetes oil might have tranquilizing, hypotensive, bronchodilatory, spasmolytic, and anti-inflammatory properties (11). The constituent ocimenone demonstrates cidal activity against mosquito larvae (11). Alpha-terthienyl, isolated from the African marigold, exhibits nematocidal and larvicidal activity (11). Patulin, isolated from the French marigold is antispasmodic, reduces capillary permeability, and increases blood pressure (11).

Adverse Reactions Including Known Allergies
Tagetes can cause contact dermatitis (11). Tagetes can also cause an allergic reaction in individuals sensitive to the Asteraceae/Compositae family. Members of this family include ragweed, chrysanthemums, marigolds, daisies, and many other herbs.

Possible Interactions with Herbs & Other Dietary Supplements
Insufficient reliable information available.

Possible Interactions with Drugs
No interactions are known to occur, and there is no known reason to expect a clinically significant interaction with tagetes.

Possible Interactions with Foods
No interactions are known to occur, and there is no known reason to expect a clinically significant interaction with tagetes.

Possible Interactions with Lab Tests

No interactions are known to occur, and there is no known reason to expect a clinically significant interaction with tagetes.

Possible Interactions with Diseases or Conditions

CROSS-ALLERGENICITY: Can cause an allergic reaction in individuals sensitive to the Asteraceae/Compositae family. Members of this family include ragweed, chrysanthemums, marigolds, daisies, and many other herbs.

Typical Dosages & Routes of Administration that are Commonly Used

No typical dosage.

Comments

Tagetes oil is distilled from the above ground parts of Tagetes erecta, minuta, and patula [11].

TAMARIND

This Product is Also Known As

Imlee, Tamarindo.
CAUTION: See separate listing for Garcinia.

Scientific Names

Tamarindus indica.
Family: Leguminosae or Fabaceae.

People Use This For

Orally, tamarind is used for chronic or acute constipation, liver and gallbladder disorders, and to decrease fever [18]. Topically, a thick paste of the seeds is used as a cast for broken bones.
In China, it is also used to treat pregnancy-related nausea and as an anthelmintic in children.
In Arabia, it is used for stomach disorders, colds, and fevers.
In foods and beverages, tamarind is used as a flavoring agent . It is also widely used in Asian cuisine for chutneys and curries [11].

Safety

LIKELY SAFE ...when used orally and appropriately in amounts found in foods. It has Generally Recognized as Safe (GRAS) status in the US, and its maximum use is 0.81% [11].
There is insufficient reliable information available about the safety of tamarind used in amounts greater than those found in food.
PREGNANCY AND LACTATION: Insufficient reliable information available; avoid using in amounts greater than found in foods.

Effectiveness

There is insufficient reliable information available about the effectiveness of tamarind.

Possible Mechanism of Action & Active Ingredients

The partially dried, fruit/pod of tamarind is used medicinally. It contains plant acids, largely d-tartaric acid, sugars, pectin, protein, vitamins, and minerals. The volatile oil contains over 60 compounds including methyl salicylate and safrole. The fruit pulp has mild laxative properties, but heat causes loss of this effect. Some evidence suggests an aqueous extract is highly toxic to the trematode Schistosoma mansoni, and the parasite-carrying snail Bulinus trucatus. Other evidence suggests that the tamarind constituent, tamarindienal might have antifungal activity against Aspergillus niger and Candida albicans, and antibacterial activity against Bacillus subtilis, Staphylococcus aureus, Escherichia coli, and Pseudomonas aeruginosa [11].

Adverse Reactions Including Known Allergies

None reported.

Possible Interactions with Herbs & Other Dietary Supplements

Insufficient reliable information available.

Possible Interactions with Drugs

No interactions are known to occur, and there is no known reason to expect a clinically significant interaction with tamarind.

Possible Interactions with Foods

No interactions are known to occur, and there is no known reason to expect a clinically significant interaction with tamarind.

Possible Interactions with Lab Tests

No interactions are known to occur, and there is no known reason to expect a clinically significant interaction with tamarind.

Possible Interactions with Diseases or Conditions

No interactions are known to occur, and there is no known reason to expect a clinically significant interaction with tamarind.

Typical Dosages & Routes of Administration that are Commonly Used

ORAL: As a laxative, 10-50 grams of tamarind paste is taken orally as fruit cubes (18). This is a paste prepared from the fermented fruit of Tamarindus indica (18).

Comments

None.

TANNIC ACID

This Product is Also Known As

None.

Scientific Names

Tannic acid.

People Use This For

Topically, tannic acid is used for cold sores and fever blisters (272), diaper rash and prickly heat (272), poison ivy (272), ingrown toenails (272), sore throat, inflamed tonsils, spongy or receding gums, acute dermatitis, and as a styptic.

Vaginally, tannic acid is used as a douche for leukorrhea (12).

In Chinese medicine, nutgalls that contain a high concentration of tannic acid have been used to treat cancer.

In folk medicine, tannic acid has been used orally and topically for bleeding, chronic diarrhea, dysentery, bloody urine, painful joints, persistent coughs, and cancer (11).

In foods and beverages, tannic acid is used as a flavoring agent (11).

In manufacturing, it has been used in hemorrhoidal ointments and suppositories (11), for tanning hides and manufacturing ink (11), and to kill dust mites on furniture (272).

Safety

LIKELY SAFE ...when used orally in amounts found in foods. Tannic acid has Generally Recognized as Safe (GRAS) status in the US. The maximum use level is 0.018% (11).

POSSIBLY UNSAFE ...when used topically to treat diaper rash and prickly heat (272), and minor burn or sunburn (272).

There is insufficient reliable information available about the safety of the topical use of tannic acid to treat cold sores and fever blisters. The FDA's concern about potential oral absorption and toxicity has prompted requests for further data (272).

PREGNANCY AND LACTATION: LIKELY UNSAFE ...when used topically on damaged skin or large areas of skin (2). There is insufficient reliable information available about the safety of the oral use of tannic acid during pregnancy and lactation; avoid using amounts greater than found in foods.

Effectiveness

POSSIBLY INEFFECTIVE ...when used topically to treat cold sores and fever blisters (272). ...when used topically to treat diaper rash or prickly heat (272). ...when used topically to treat minor burn or sunburn (272).

There is insufficient reliable information available about the effectiveness of tannic acid for its other uses.

Possible Mechanism of Action & Active Ingredients

Tannic acid is a mixture of glycosides of phenolics, mainly gallic acid (11). Pharmaceutical grade tannic acid is generally considered to be pentadigalloylglucose (11). Tannic acid has astringent effects (11,12). It dehydrates tissue, internally reducing secretions, and externally forming a protective layer of harder, constricted cells (12). Tannins show some evidence of antiviral, antimicrobial, CNS depressant, and cariostatic effects (11). Some evidence suggests that tannins might cause cancer, but other evidence shows tannins might prevent it (12). Regular consumption of herbs with high tannin concentrations correlates with increased incidence of esophageal or nasal cancer (12).

Adverse Reactions Including Known Allergies

Ingesting large amounts of tannic acid can cause gastric irritation, nausea, and vomiting (11). Tannins have been associated with fatal liver damage from extensive use on burns or in enemas (11). However, the toxicity may be due to an impurity, digallic acid, rather than the tannins themselves (11).

Possible Interactions with Herbs & Other Dietary Supplements

ORAL HERBS: Theoretically, herbs that contain high percentages of tannins (such as oak bark) might precipitate alkaloids and other alkaline constituents of herbs (19).

Possible Interactions with Drugs

ORAL DRUGS: Theoretically, avoid concomitant administration due to potential of tannic acid to precipitate alkaloids and other basic drugs (19). Separate administration of oral drugs and tannic acid by the longest period of time practical (19).

Possible Interactions with Foods

No interactions are known to occur, and there is no known reason to expect a clinically significant interaction with tannic acid.

Possible Interactions with Lab Tests

No interactions are known to occur, and there is no known reason to expect a clinically significant interaction with tannic acid.

Possible Interactions with Diseases or Conditions

KIDNEY DYSFUNCTION: Theoretically, oral use of tannic acid is contraindicated in individuals with kidney dysfunction. Tannic acid can cause kidney damage, potentially exacerbating a pre-existing condition (12).
LIVER DYSFUNCTION: Theoretically, oral use of tannic acid is contraindicated in individuals with liver dysfunction. Tannic acid can cause liver damage, potentially exacerbating a pre-existing condition (12).
SKIN CONDITIONS: Full baths with tannic acid tea are contraindicated in individuals with weeping eczema and extensive skin damage (12).
PRE-EXISTING CONDITIONS: Theoretically, full baths are contraindicated in individuals with fever or infectious diseases, NYHA III and IV heart failure, or hypertonia stage IV (WHO) (2).

Typical Dosages & Routes of Administration that are Commonly Used

No typical dosage.

Comments

New York Heart Association (NYHA) stage I and II heart disease refers to people with heart disease without resulting limitations of physical activity and who are comfortable at rest and in whom ordinary physical activity results in fatigue, palpitation, trouble breathing, or anginal pain (2). Tannic acid is extracted from the nutgalls formed on twigs of certain oak trees by insects (Quercus infectoria and other Quercus species). The "universal antidote," formerly used for poisoning, contained tannic acid, activated charcoal, and magnesium oxide. These three ingredients in combination were believed to synergistically reduce the absorption of poisons. Unfortunately, tannic acid was instead adsorbed by activated charcoal, which diminished the benefit of the combination (272).

TANSY

This Product is Also Known As

Bitter Buttons, Buttons, Chrysanthemi vulgaris flos, Chrysanthemi vulgaris herba, Daisy, Hindheal, Parsley Fern, Tansy Flower, Tansy Herb, Scented Fern, Stinking Willie.

Scientific Names

Tanacetum vulgare, synonym Chrysanthemum vulgare.
Family: Asteraceae or Compositae.

People Use This For

Traditionally, tansy above ground parts are used orally for stimulating menstrual flow (5,6), as an abortifacient (2), an antihelmintic (2,18,515), for roundworm or threadworm infestation in children (4), for migraines, neuralgia (4,6), epilepsy (4009), rheumatism, improving digestion and stimulating appetite (4009), as an antispasmodic (4,6), for flatulence (4), bloating due to intestinal or peritoneal gas (2,18), stomach and duodenal ulcers, noninflammatory gallbladder conditions, palpitation, sciatica, stomachache (4009), edema associated with weak heart, colds, fever, inducing sweating, hysteria, calming nerves, gout, kidney problems, or tuberculosis. Tansy above ground parts have also been used as an antioxidant, antiseptic, bactericide, cordial, narcotic, pediculicide, tonic, and stimulant (4009).
Topically, tansy above ground parts have been used for scabies, pruritus ani (4), bruises, sores, sprains, swelling, freckles, inflammation, leukorrhea, sunburn, swelling, toothache, tumors, and as an insect repellent (515,4009).
In foods and manufacturing, the extracts are used in perfume (6), as a flavoring agent in foods and beverages (4,515), and a source of green dye (6).

Safety

POSSIBLY UNSAFE ...when used topically. Can cause severe contact dermatitis (6,18,19).
LIKELY UNSAFE ...when varieties containing the toxic constituent thujone are used orally (2,6,515). Fatalities

© Copyright 2000, Natural Medicines Comprehensive Database (209) 472-2244. For updated data, go to www.NaturalDatabase.com • 1019

have been associated with ingestion of as little as 10 drops tansy oil, although one individual recovered after ingesting 15 mL (6). Fatalities have also been reported from prepared teas or powdered forms (4,6). However, thujone concentration varies widely amongst tansy species (4,6,515).

PREGNANCY: LIKELY UNSAFE ...contraindicated due to potential abortifacient, menstrual flow, and uterine stimulant effects (12,19).

LACTATION: POSSIBLY UNSAFE; avoid using due to thujone content.

Effectiveness

There is insufficient reliable information available about the effectiveness of tansy.

Possible Mechanism of Action & Active Ingredients

The applicable parts of tansy are the above ground parts. The activity and toxicity of the above ground parts of tansy vary greatly according to the subspecies (515). Thujone, a constituent with both activity and toxicity ranging from a concentration of 0-95% in the volatile oil (4,515). The thujone constituent causes an increase in salivation and an increase in blood flow to the mucous membranes and pelvic viscera (7). Researchers think thujone has a mind-altering effect similar to tetrahydrocannabinol, the active principle in marijuana (515). Thujone also shows evidence of neurotoxicity (2), hepatotoxicity, and it might be harmful to individuals with defects in hepatic heme synthesis (4,12). Chronic thujone poisoning leads to seizures, delirium, and hallucinations (7). Tansy extracts have demonstrated effects in alleviating pain, stimulating bile, and increasing appetite in individuals with liver and gallbladder disorders (4). Some evidence suggests tansy extracts might also have antispasmodic activity (4). Other evidence suggests the constituent, caffeic acid, might have a role in the bile-stimulating effects (4). Tansy shows evidence that it might reduce serum lipid levels and has some hypoglycemic effects (4). Tansy demonstrates antifungal activity (4). Some evidence suggests tansy oil has antibacterial activity (6). In addition, tansy oil, ether extract, and the constituent beta-thujone show evidence of antihelmintic activity (4). Aqueous extracts of tansy can partially inactivate tick-borne encephalitis in vitro. They also induce resistance in experimental animals (6). Preliminary studies suggest tansy has some antitumor effects (4). The constituents believed to be responsible for allergic contact dermatitis are the sesquiterpene lactones (4,6,19).

Adverse Reactions Including Known Allergies

Ingesting large amounts of thujone or using thujone-containing products long-term can cause restlessness, vomiting, vertigo, tremors, renal damage, and convulsions (12). Symptoms of toxicity include rapid, feeble pulse (4,6), severe gastroenteritis (2), severe spasms (4), convulsions (2,4), rapid breathing (2), vomiting, abdominal pain, facial flushing, loss of consciousness, irregular heartbeat, dilated pupils, pupillary rigidity, uterine bleeding, abortion, kidney damage, and liver damage (2,18). Death can occur 1-3.5 hours after ingestion (18). Topical use is associated with severe contact dermatitis (6,19) and local mucosal membrane irritation (19). It can cause an allergic reaction in individuals sensitive to the Asteraceae/Compositae family. Members of this family include ragweed, chrysanthemums, marigolds, daisies, and many other herbs.

Possible Interactions with Herbs & Other Dietary Supplements

THUJONE-CONTAINING HERBS: Concomitant use of herbs containing thujone can increase the risk of thujone toxicity. Thujone-containing herbs include oak moss, oriental arborvitae, sage, wormwood, thuja (cedar), and tree moss (12); avoid using.

Possible Interactions with Drugs

ALCOHOL: The constituent, thujone, heightens and alters the effect of alcohol (7).

HYPOGLYCEMIC DRUGS: Theoretically, might interfere with hypoglycemic therapy and blood sugar control (4).

Possible Interactions with Foods

No interactions are known to occur, and there is no known reason to expect a clinically significant interaction with tansy.

Possible Interactions with Lab Tests

No interactions are known to occur, and there is no known reason to expect a clinically significant interaction with tansy.

Possible Interactions with Diseases or Conditions

PORPHYRIA: Theoretically, can exacerbate porphyria in people with underlying defects in hepatic heme synthesis (12).

CROSS-ALLERGENICITY: Can cause an allergic reaction in individuals sensitive to the Asteraceae/Compositae family. Members of this family include ragweed, chrysanthemums, marigolds, daisies, and many other herbs.

Typical Dosages & Routes of Administration that are Commonly Used

No typical dosage.

Comments

Tansy is considered unsafe; avoid using. The name tansy is derived from the Greek word, athanasia, for immortality. Tansy was thought to impart mortality and it was used for embalming (6). Avoid confusion with tansy ragwort (Senecio species) and other plants generically referred to as "tansy."

TANSY RAGWORT

This Product is Also Known As

Cankerwort, Common Ragwort, Dog Standard, European Ragwort, Ragweed, Ragwort, Staggerwort, Stammerwort, St. James Wort, Stinking Nanny.
CAUTION: See separate listing for Golden Ragwort.

Scientific Names

Senecio jacoboea.
Family: Asteraceae/Compositae.

People Use This For

Tansy ragwort is used for cancer, colic, wound-healing, spasms, as a laxative, to induce sweating, to induce menstruation, and for "cleansing and purification" (4017).

Safety

UNSAFE …when used orally. Tansy ragwort contains hepatotoxic unsaturated pyrrolizidine alkaloids (UPAs) (12,19). Repeated exposure to low concentrations of UPAs linked to veno-occlusive disease, a serious condition (4,12). UPAs may also be carcinogenic and mutagenic (12). Topical use on abraded or broken skin might be unsafe due to potential for systemic absorption (12,19).
PREGNANCY: UNSAFE …tansy ragwort is contraindicated because of possible menstruation promoting and oxytocic activity, and teratogenic effects (19).
LACTATION: UNSAFE …tansy ragwort is contraindicated due to pyrrolizidine alkaloid (19).

Effectiveness

There is insufficient reliable information available about the effectiveness of tansy ragwort.

Possible Mechanism of Action & Active Ingredients

The applicable parts of tansy ragwort are the above-ground flowering parts. Some pyrrolizidine alkaloids have shown carcinogenic and mutagenic properties, and there are reports of renal toxicity. However, the primary concern is veno-occlusive disease (12). Unsaturated pyrrolizidine alkaloids are known to be hepatotoxic in animals and humans (4).

Adverse Reactions Including Known Allergies

Chronic exposure to plants containing UPA constituents has been associated with veno-occlusive disease (4021). Symptoms of acute veno-occlusive disease are characterized by a dull, dragging ache in the right upper abdomen and marked distention of the abdomen. These symptoms are sometimes accompanied by reduced urine output. Subacute veno-occlusive disease is associated with vague symptoms and persistent liver enlargement (4021). Tansy ragwort can cause an allergic reaction in individuals sensitive to the Asteraceae/Compositae family. Members of this family include ragweed, chrysanthemums, marigolds, daisies, and many other herbs.

Possible Interactions with Herbs & Other Dietary Supplements

EUCALYPTUS: Theoretically, concomitant use might increase the risk of unsaturated pyrrolizidine alkaloid toxicity due to enzyme induction by eucalyptus (19).
PYRROLIZIDINE ALKALOID-CONTAINING HERBS: Concomitant use is contraindicated due to the risk of additive toxicity. Herbs containing unsaturated pyrrolizidine alkaloids include: alkanna (12), borage (271), gravel root (4), hemp agrimony (271), hound's tongue (19), petasites (19), comfrey (271), coltsfoot, and the Senecio species plants; dusty miller (19), alpine ragwort (19), groundsel (271), golden ragwort (19), and tansy ragwort (271).

Possible Interactions with Drugs

No interactions are known to occur, and there is no known reason to expect a clinically significant interaction with tansy ragwort.

Possible Interactions with Foods

No interactions are known to occur, and there is no known reason to expect a clinically significant interaction with tansy ragwort.

Possible Interactions with Lab Tests

No interactions are known to occur, and there is no known reason to expect a clinically significant interaction with tansy ragwort.

Possible Interactions with Diseases or Conditions

LIVER DISEASE: Contraindicated.
CROSS-ALLERGENICITY: Can cause an allergic reaction in individuals sensitive to the Asteraceae/Compositae family. Members of this family include ragweed, chrysanthemums, marigolds, daisies, and many other herbs.

Typical Dosages & Routes of Administration that are Commonly Used

No typical dosage.

© Copyright 2000, Natural Medicines Comprehensive Database (209) 472-2244. For updated data, go to www.NaturalDatabase.com • 1021

Comments

Tansy ragwort is considered unsafe; avoid using (12,18). Both tansy ragwort and golden ragwort are known as ragweed and can therefore be confused (see separate listing). American Herbal Products Association recommends labeling all botanical products that contain toxic pyrrolizidine alkaloids "For external use only. Do not apply to broken or abraded skin; do not use when nursing" (12).

TARRAGON

This Product is Also Known As
Estragon, Little Dragon, Mugwort.
CAUTION: See separate listing for Mugwort (Artemisia vulgaris).

Scientific Names
Artemisia dracunculus.
Family: Asteraceae or Compositae.

People Use This For
Orally, tarragon is used for digestive disorders, toothache, to promote menstruation, as a diuretic, appetite stimulant, and hypnotic.
In foods and beverages, it is used as a culinary herb and a flavor component .
In manufacturing, tarragon is used as a fragrance component in soaps and cosmetics (11).

Safety
LIKELY SAFE ...when used in amounts found in foods. It has Generally Recognized as Safe (GRAS) status in the US. The maximum use level is 0.27% (11).
POSSIBLY SAFE ...when used orally short-term in medicinal amounts (12).
POSSIBLY UNSAFE ...for extended oral use due to estragole, which can be carcinogenic (12).
PREGNANCY AND LACTATION: LIKELY SAFE ...when used in food amounts. LIKELY UNSAFE ...contraindicated in larger amounts due to possible menstrual promoting effects (11).

Effectiveness
There is insufficient reliable information available about the effectiveness of tarragon.

Possible Mechanism of Action & Active Ingredients
The applicable parts of tarragon are the above ground parts. Estragole is the main constituent of tarragon's essential oil (81%). The constituent estragole is a procarcinogen but the carcinogenic risk is minimal. It is not directly hepatotoxic or hepatocarcinogenic but requires activation by liver enzymes to reach full toxicity. In the liver other enzymes inactivate the carcinogenic metabolites, limiting possible damage to the liver (12). Tarragon shows evidence of antibacterial activity, but estragole does not appear to be responsible. Some information suggests undiluted tarragon oil can irritate the skin, but a concentration of 4% in petrolatum appears to be nonirritating and nonsensitizing (11).

Adverse Reactions Including Known Allergies
Tarragon can cause an allergic reaction in individuals sensitive to the Asteraceae/Compositae family. Members of this family include ragweed, chrysanthemums, marigolds, daisies, and many other herbs.

Possible Interactions with Herbs & Other Dietary Supplements
Insufficient reliable information available.

Possible Interactions with Drugs
No interactions are known to occur, and there is no known reason to expect a clinically significant interaction with tarragon.

Possible Interactions with Foods
No interactions are known to occur, and there is no known reason to expect a clinically significant interaction with tarragon.

Possible Interactions with Lab Tests
No interactions are known to occur, and there is no known reason to expect a clinically significant interaction with tarragon.

Possible Interactions with Diseases or Conditions
CROSS-ALLERGENICITY: Can cause an allergic reaction in individuals sensitive to the Asteraceae/Compositae family. Members of this family include ragweed, chrysanthemums, marigolds, daisies, and many other herbs.

Typical Dosages & Routes of Administration that are Commonly Used
No typical dosage.

Comments

Tarragon is also known as mugwort. Be careful not confuse it with mugwort (Artemisia vulgaris). Tarragon is a rich plant source of potassium (19). Adulteration of tarragon oil is common (11).

TAUMELLOOLCH

This Product is Also Known As
Bearded Darnel, Cheat, Darnel, Drake, Ray-Grass, Tare.

Scientific Names
Lolium temulentum.
Family: Poaceae.

People Use This For
Orally, taumelloolch seed is used for blood poisoning (4502), cancer (4502), cysts (4502), dizziness (18), eczema (4502), hemorrhage (4502), idiocy (4502), indurations (4502), "knots" (4502), leprosy (4502), migraine (4502), nerve pain (18), nose bleeds (18), putrid flesh (4502), sleeplessness (18), stomach cramps (18), involuntary dyskinetic movements (4502), toothache (4502), tumors (4502), and urinary incontinence (4502).
In children, taumelloolch is used orally for colic (4502).
Topically, taumelloolch seed is used as a poultice for skin diseases, to draw out splinters, and for broken bones (4502).
In folk medicine taumelloolch is used orally for gangrene (4502), headache (4502), meningitis (4502), neuralgia (4502), rheumatism (4502), and sciatica (4502).

Safety
LIKELY UNSAFE …when used orally. Symptoms of toxicity range from confusion and giddiness to weakness and death from respiratory failure (18,4502).
There is insufficient reliable information available about the safety of the topical use of taumelloolch.
PREGNANCY AND LACTATION: LIKELY UNSAFE (18,4502).

Effectiveness
There is insufficient reliable information available about the effectiveness of taumelloolch.

Possible Mechanism of Action & Active Ingredients
The applicable part of taumelloolch is the seed. The active agents of taumelloolch are temulentin, temultin acid, tannin, and glycoside (18). It has analgesic and narcotic properties, as well as toxicity (4502). Much of what is known about the toxicity of taumelloolch is anecdotal. Poisoning has been reported from ingestion of the grain, ingestion of the berries mixed with grains, and ingestion of the seed infected with a bacterial toxin (18,4502). To date, the toxic principle has not been identified (18,4502). No cases of poisonings have been reported in recent times, although the plant has become extremely rare through intensive seed-corn purification (18).

Adverse Reactions Including Known Allergies
Symptoms of taumelloolch toxicity include colic, confusion, giddiness, weakness, dizziness, dilated pupils, headache, confusion, staggering, somnolence, trembling, vision and speech disorders, vomiting, delirium, and death from respiratory failure (18,4502).

Possible Interactions with Herbs & Other Dietary Supplements
Insufficient reliable information available.

Possible Interactions with Drugs
No interactions are known to occur, and there is no known reason to expect a clinically significant interaction with taumelloolch.

Possible Interactions with Foods
No interactions are known to occur, and there is no known reason to expect a clinically significant interaction with taumelloolch.

Possible Interactions with Lab Tests
No interactions are known to occur, and there is no known reason to expect a clinically significant interaction with taumelloolch.

Possible Interactions with Diseases or Conditions
No interactions are known to occur, and there is no known reason to expect a clinically significant interaction with taumelloolch.

Typical Dosages & Routes of Administration that are Commonly Used
No typical dosage.

© Copyright 2000, Natural Medicines Comprehensive Database (209) 472-2244. For updated data, go to www.NaturalDatabase.com • 1023

Comments

Taumelloolch is considered likely unsafe; avoid using. Taumelloolch is believed to be the tares of the biblical parable of the wheat and the tares (4502). Some information suggests that an ergot component extracted from the grass and seeds of taumelloolch is used by a mystic cult to induce religious ecstasy (4502).

TEA TREE OIL

This Product is Also Known As

Australian Tea Tree Oil, Oleum Melaleucae.
CAUTION: See separate listings for Cajeput Oil and Niauli Oil.

Scientific Names

Melaleuca alternifolia.
Family: Myrtaceae.

People Use This For

In folk medicine, tea tree oil is used as a local antiseptic for cuts, abrasions, burns, lice, scabies, insect bites, stings, acne, boils, athlete's foot, ringworm, vaginal infections, infections of the mouth and nose, and sore throat (6,9,11,515). Topically, it is also used as a bath additive to treat cough, bronchial congestion, and pulmonary inflammation (6,11).

Safety

POSSIBLY SAFE ... when used topically and appropriately (11,512).
LIKELY UNSAFE ...when ingested orally. Contains terpin-4-ol which is chemically-related to cineole (6,515).
CHILDREN: LIKELY UNSAFE ...when ingested orally (6).
PREGNANCY AND LACTATION: POSSIBLY SAFE ...when used topically. POSSIBLY UNSAFE ...when used orally.

Effectiveness

POSSIBLY EFFECTIVE ...when used topically for treating acne vulgaris (11,515), for symptomatic treatment of fungal skin infections (6), and for treating onychomycosis (515).
There is insufficient reliable information available about the effectiveness of tea tree oil for its other uses.

Possible Mechanism of Action & Active Ingredients

Tea tree oil contains terpinen-4-ol (11,515), which is active against numerous pathogenic bacteria (5,6,9,11) and fungi (6,9) but can spare normal skin flora (6). The constituents, alpha-terpineol and linalool, can also contribute to its antimicrobial activity (515). The constituent alpha-limonene can be responsible for the adverse effect of contact eczema (6). In humans, 10% tea tree oil cream can be as effective as 1% tolnaftate cream for reducing symptoms of tinea pedis (6). Compared to 5% benzoyl peroxide lotion for treating acne vulgaris, 5% tea tree oil gel is better tolerated, but it is less effective and has a slower onset of action (11). Applied topically, 100% tea tree oil can be as effective as 1% clotrimazole in improving nail appearance and symptoms (1538); however, both treatments can have high rates of recurrence (1538).

Adverse Reactions Including Known Allergies

There is one case report of an adult with petechial body rash (minute spots) and marked neutrophil leukocytosis after ingestion of 2.5 mL tea tree oil (6). There is also a case report of an infant with ataxia and drowsiness after ingestion of less than 10 mL tea tree oil (6). Topically, tea tree oil can cause local irritation (5), allergic contact eczema, and dermatitis (6,658).

Possible Interactions with Herbs & Other Dietary Supplements

Insufficient reliable information available.

Possible Interactions with Drugs

No interactions are known to occur, and there is no known reason to expect a clinically significant interaction with tea tree oil.

Possible Interactions with Foods

No interactions are known to occur, and there is no known reason to expect a clinically significant interaction with tea tree oil.

Possible Interactions with Lab Tests

No interactions are known to occur, and there is no known reason to expect a clinically significant interaction with tea tree oil.

Possible Interactions with Diseases or Conditions

No interactions are known to occur, and there is no known reason to expect a clinically significant interaction with tea tree oil.

 © Copyright 2000, Natural Medicines Comprehensive Database (209) 472-2244. For updated data, go to www.NaturalDatabase.com

Typical Dosages & Routes of Administration that are Commonly Used
TOPICAL: People typically use 70 to 100% tea tree oil, applied to the affected areas twice daily. For treatment of acne, the concentration is 5 to 15%. For vaginal douches, concentrations as strong as 40% are used. Higher concentrations for douches should be used with caution and medical advice (6006).
ORAL: The oil should never be taken internally (6006).

Comments
Tea tree oil is obtained by the distillation of the leaves of the tea tree (teatree, Melaleuca alternifolia). Tea tree oil was used during World War II to treat skin injuries of workers in munition factories and was commonly used in surgery and dentistry in the mid 1920s (6). Avoid confusion with cajeput oil and niauli oil.

TEAZLE

This Product is Also Known As
Barber's Brush, Brushes and Combs, Card Thistle, Church Broom, Teasel, Venus' Basin.

Scientific Names
Dipsacus silvestris.
Family: Dipsacaceae.

People Use This For
Topically, teazle is used for small wounds, fistulae, psoriasis, and as a rub for arthritis (18).

Safety
There is insufficient reliable information available about the safety of teazle.
Pregnancy and Lactation: Insufficient reliable information available; avoid using.

Effectiveness
There is insufficient reliable information available about the effectiveness of teazle.

Possible Mechanism of Action & Active Ingredients
The applicable part of teazle is the root. There is insufficient reliable information available about the possible mechanism of action and active ingredients.

Adverse Reactions Including Known Allergies
None reported.

Possible Interactions with Herbs & Other Dietary Supplements
Insufficient reliable information available.

Possible Interactions with Drugs
No interactions are known to occur, and there is no known reason to expect a clinically significant interaction with teazle.

Possible Interactions with Foods
No interactions are known to occur, and there is no known reason to expect a clinically significant interaction with teazle.

Possible Interactions with Lab Tests
No interactions are known to occur, and there is no known reason to expect a clinically significant interaction with teazle.

Possible Interactions with Diseases or Conditions
No interactions are known to occur, and there is no known reason to expect a clinically significant interaction with teazle

Typical Dosages & Routes of Administration that are Commonly Used
TOPICAL: Teazle is used as an alcoholic extract (18).

Comments
Avoid confusing teazle with boneset, which is also called teasel. (18).
There is very little scientific information about this product. Our staff is continually analyzing the available information on natural medicines and will add data here as it becomes available.

TERMINALIA

This Product is Also Known As

Arjuna, Axjun Argun, Bahera, Bahira, Bala Harade, Balera, Behada, Beleric Myrobalan, Chebulic Myrobalan, Hara, Harada, Haritaki, He Zi, Hirala, Indian Almond, Myrobalan.

Scientific Names

Terminalia arjuna; Terminalia bellirica, synonym Terminalia belerica; Terminalia chebula.
Family: Combretaceae.

People Use This For

Orally, Terminalia arjuna is used for cardiovascular conditions, including ischemic heart disease and angina, hypertension, and hyperlipidemia (6,33). It is also used orally as a diuretic, for earaches, dysentery, venereal and urogenital diseases, and as an aphrodisiac (6,33,3565).

Orally, Terminalia belerica and Terminalia chebula are used for hyperlipidemia (2527,2519) and digestive disorders, including both diarrhea and constipation, and indigestion (6,33). They have also been used for HIV infection (2518). Terminalia belerica is also used orally as a hepatoprotectant and for respiratory conditions, including respiratory tract infections, cough, and sore throat (6,33). Terminalia chebula is also used orally for dysentery (33).

Topically, Terminalia belerica and Terminalia chebula are used as a lotion for sore eyes. Terminalia chebula is also used topically as a mouthwash and gargle (6,33).

Intravaginally, Terminalia chebula is used as a douche for treating vaginitis (6,33).

In traditional Ayurvedic medicine, Terminalia belerica has been used as a "health-harmonizer" in combination with Terminalia chebula and Emblica officinalis (6). This combination is also used to lower cholesterol and to prevent necrosis of cardiac tissue (6). In traditional Ayurvedic medicine, Terminalia arjuna has been used to balance the three humors, kapha, pitta, and vata (6,33). It has also been used for asthma, bile duct disorders, scorpion stings, and for poisonings (33).

Safety

POSSIBLY SAFE ...when used orally and appropriately, short term. Several small studies have used the powdered bark of Terminalia arjuna safely in cardiac patients in trials lasting from 2 weeks to 3 months (2502,2503,2504); however, patients should avoid self-treatment with this product, due to the potentially significant cardiovascular effects. Further study is needed to determine the safety of Terminalia arjuna for long-term use.

There is insufficient reliable information available about the safety of Terminalia belerica and Terminalia chebula (6).

PREGNANCY: POSSIBLY UNSAFE ...when used orally. One source warns against using Terminalia belerica and Terminalia chebula during pregnancy; however, the reason for this warning is not described (33); avoid using.

There is insufficient reliable information available about the safety of Terminalia arjuna in pregnancy; avoid using.

LACTATION: Insufficient reliable information available; avoid using.

Effectiveness

POSSIBLY EFFECTIVE ...when used orally as a short-term adjunct to conventional therapy for treating postmyocardial infarction angina. In one small clinical trial, postmyocardial infarction patients with angina received the standard therapy of nitrates, aspirin, and/or a calcium channel blocker plus the powdered bark of Terminalia arjuna or the standard therapy alone for 3 months. Patients receiving Terminalia arjuna experienced significantly less angina, improved left ventricular ejection fractions, and decreased left ventricular mass compared to patients receiving the standard therapy alone (2502,2503). ...when Terminalia arjuna is used as a short-term adjunct to conventional therapy for treating severe congestive heart failure. In a small cross-over trial, patients with severe, refractory congestive heart failure had significant reductions in symptoms and improved left ventricular function after 2 weeks of treatment (2504).

Large-scale, long-term trials are necessary to clarify Terminalia arjunas' potential role in the treatment of cardiovascular conditions.

There is insufficient reliable information available for the effectiveness of Terminalia belerica and Terminalia cebula for any medicinal use.

Possible Mechanism of Action & Active Ingredients

There are three species of terminalia of medicinal interest: Terminalia arjuna, Terminalia belerica and Terminalia chebula (6,33). The applicable part of Terminalia arjuna is the bark. The bark contains several active constituents, including Terminalia arjuna gallic acid, ethyl gallate, and the flavone luteolin. Luteolin may have anticancer properties (2506). The bark of Terminalia arjuna is reported to be beneficial in cardiovascular conditions; however, the exact mechanism is not known. Terminalia arjuna is reported to lower serum cholesterol and low-density lipoprotein (LDL) levels (2505,2517,2519). It is also thought to have an antihypertensive effect and act as a cardiac stimulant. However, studies have been conflicting; some indicating that it may actually increase blood pressure (33). The applicable part of Terminalia belerica and Terminalia chebula is the fruit (6). These species also have been reported to improve lipid profiles, but to a lesser degree than Terminalia arjuna. Terminalia chebula is reported to have a greater effect on lipids than Terminalia belerica (2517,2519). The astringent properties of Terminalia belerica and Terminalia chebula are attributed to their beneficial effects in bowel irregularity and indigestion (33).

Terminalia belerica also contains gallic acid, and is thought to have hepatoprotective properties (2507). An ethanolic extract of Terminalia chebula containing gallic acid and its ethyl ester may have activity against methicillin-resistant Staphylococcus aureus (2508). Terminalia chebula may also have activity against cytomegalovirus, herpes simplex I, Streptococcus mutans, Salmonella sp., Shigella, and retroviral reverse transcriptase (2509,2510,2511,2512,2513,2514). Both Terminalia belerica and Terminalia chebula may have activity against HIV (2518). The gallic acid and chebulagic acid in Terminalia chebula may have immunosuppressive effects against cytotoxic T lymphocytes (2515).

Adverse Reactions Including Known Allergies
None reported in humans. In animal studies, Terminalia chebula has caused hepatic and renal lesions (2516).

Possible Interactions with Herbs & Other Dietary Supplements
Insufficient reliable information available.

Possible Interactions with Drugs
No interactions are known to occur, and there is no known reason to expect a clinically significant interaction with terminalia.

Possible Interactions with Foods
No interactions are known to occur, and there is no known reason to expect a clinically significant interaction with terminalia.

Possible Interactions with Lab Tests
No interactions are known to occur, and there is no known reason to expect a clinically significant interaction with terminalia.

Possible Interactions with Diseases or Conditions
No interactions are known to occur, and there is no known reason to expect a clinically significant interaction with terminalia.

Typical Dosages & Routes of Administration that are Commonly Used
ORAL: For improving left ventricular function and treating postmyocardial infarction anginal pain as an adjunct to conventional therapy, a dose of the powdered bark of Terminalia arjuna 500 mg every 8 hours has been used (2502,2503). For improving left ventricular function and symptoms in congestive heart failure, a dose of the powdered bark of Terminalia arjuna 500 mg every 8 hours has been used (2502,2504).

Comments
The bark of Terminalia arjuna has been used in India for more than 3000 years, primarily as a heart remedy. An Indian physician named Vagbhata has been credited as the first to use this product for heart conditions in the seventh century A.D. Research on Terminalia has been going on since the 1930s, but pharmacological studies have provided mixed results. Its role in heart disease remains unclear.

THIAMINE (VITAMIN B1)

This Product is Also Known As
Antiberiberi Factor, Antiberiberi Vitamin, Antineuritic Factor, Antineuritic Vitamin, Anurine, Aneurine Hydrochloride, Thiamin Chloride, Thiamin Hydrochloride, Thiamine Chloride, Thiamine Hydrochloride, Thiaminium Chloride Hydrochloride.

Scientific Names
Thiamine; Thiamin; Vitamin B1; Vitamin B-1.

People Use This For
Orally, thiamine is used for thiamine deficiency syndromes, including beriberi, peripheral neuritis associated with pellagra, and neuritis of pregnancy. It is used for poor appetite, ulcerative colitis, chronic diarrhea, GI disorders, cerebellar syndrome, an insect repellent (15), diabetic neuropathy, AIDS (14), maintaining a positive mental attitude, enhancing learning abilities, heart disease, alcoholism, stress, and aging. Thiamine is also taken for canker sores, immunodepression, memory loss including Alzheimer's disease, vision problems such as cataracts and glaucoma, motion sickness, and increasing energy (3027,3028,3029,3030).
The injection (IM, IV) of thiamine is used for Wernicke's encephalopathy syndrome, other thiamine deficiency syndromes in critically ill people, acute alcohol withdrawal, and coma or hypothermia of unknown origin (14,15).

Safety
LIKELY SAFE ...when taken orally and is generally considered nontoxic; although, rare hypersensitivity reactions have occurred (15). ...when used appropriately as the injectable product (IM, IV). It is a FDA-approved prescription product.
PREGNANCY AND LACTATION: LIKELY SAFE ...when used at the recommended dietary allowance (RDA)

© Copyright 2000, Natural Medicines Comprehensive Database (209) 472-2244. For updated data, go to www.NaturalDatabase.com • 1027

of 1.4 mg per day (3094). There is insufficient reliable information available about the safety of using larger amounts during pregnancy or lactation.

Effectiveness

EFFECTIVE ...when taken orally for the treatment of thiamine deficiency syndromes including beriberi and peripheral neuritis associated with pellagra or neuritis of pregnancy. ...when taken orally as a dietary supplement to prevent deficiency in people with malabsorption conditions such as alcoholism, cirrhosis, and GI diseases, in those with inadequate intake due to severe anorexia, nausea, or vomiting, and in those with increased requirements due to pregnancy, increased carbohydrate intake, increased physical activity, hyperthyroidism, infection, and hepatic disease, although deficiency is rare with these conditions. ...when taken orally for temporary correction of metabolic disorders associated with genetic diseases such as subacute necrotizing encephalopathy (SNE, Leigh's disease), maple syrup urine disease (branched-chain aminoacidopathy), and lactic acidosis associated with pyruvate carboxylase deficiency and hyperalaninemia (15). ...when used as the FDA-approved, prescription-only, injectable (IM, IV) product.

POSSIBLY EFFECTIVE ...when taken orally for diabetic neuropathy (14).

There is insufficient reliable information available about the effectiveness of thiamine for its other uses.

Possible Mechanism of Action & Active Ingredients

Thiamine is required for carbohydrate metabolism (15). It combines with adenosine triphosphate (ATP) to form thiamine diphosphate, a coenzyme in carbohydrate metabolism, wherein the decarboxylation of pyruvic acid and alpha-ketoglutaric acids occurs. This coenzyme is also a part of transketolation reactions (15). Thiamine is also a coenzyme in the utilization of pentose in the hexose monophosphate shunt (15). Thiamine deficiency leads to decreased transketolase activity in erythrocytes and to increased pyruvic acid concentration in the blood, both of which can be used to diagnose deficiency (15). Pyruvic acid is converted to lactic acid, and lactic acidosis can therefore occur in vitamin B1 deficiency (15). Syndromes associated with vitamin B1 deficiency are beriberi and Wernicke-Korsakoff syndrome (3041). Beriberi is characterized by anorexia, abdominal discomfort, constipation, peripheral neurologic changes, sleep disturbance, poor memory, and sometimes cardiovascular symptoms, including dyspnea, edema, palpitations, vasodilation, warm extremities, and high output cardiac failure. Wernicke-Korsakoff syndrome is characterized by confusion, aphonia, confabulation, nystagmus, ophthalmoplegia, and coma.

Adverse Reactions Including Known Allergies

Taken orally, thiamine rarely can cause dermatitis and other hypersensitivity reactions (14). Injection of thiamine can cause feelings of warmth, tingling, pruritus, pain, urticaria, weakness, sweating, nausea, restlessness, tightness of the throat, angioedema, respiratory distress, cyanosis, pulmonary edema, GI bleeding, transient vasodilation and hypotension, vascular collapse, and death. Tenderness and induration can occur at IM injection sites (15).

Possible Interactions with Herbs & Other Dietary Supplements

HORSETAIL: Theoretically, it might cause the breakdown of thiamine (19).

Possible Interactions with Drugs

NEUROMUSCULAR BLOCKING AGENTS: Concomitant use of thiamine can enhance the effects of neuromuscular blocking agents (15).

Drug Influences on Nutrient Levels and Depletion

SOME DRUGS CAN AFFECT THIAMINE LEVELS:

ANTIBIOTICS: Destruction of normal gastrointestinal flora by antibiotics can cause decreased production of B vitamins. The clinical significance of this decreased production is not known. Consider supplementation only if clinical judgment warrants it (4434,4435,4436,4437,4438,4439,4440,4441,4442,4443).

LOOP DIURETICS: Use of loop diuretics can increase urinary thiamine excretion resulting in thiamine depletion. Thiamine depletion might contribute to impaired heart function in some patients with congestive heart failure (CHF) treated long-term with furosemide. Supplementation with 200 mg thiamine (orally or intravenously) per day can replete thiamine, and in some cases, improve left ventricular function in patients with congestive heart failure (CHF) treated with furosemide. Consider thiamine supplementation in patients using loop diuretics, especially long-term (1282,1283,1284,1284,1285,1286).

Possible Interactions with Foods

No interactions are known to occur, and there is no known reason to expect a clinically significant interaction with thiamine.

Possible Interactions with Lab Tests

URIC ACID: Thiamine can cause false positive results in the phosphotungstate method for uric acid determination (15).

UROBILINOGEN: Thiamine can cause false positive results in the urine spot test with Ehrlich's reagent for urobilinogen (15).

SERUM THEOPHYLLINE: Large amounts of thiamine can interfere with Schack and Waxler spectrophotometric determination of serum theophylline concentrations (15).

Possible Interactions with Diseases or Conditions
ALCOHOLISM, CIRRHOSIS, MALABSORPTION SYNDROMES: Thiamine absorption is decreased in these conditions (15).

Typical Dosages & Routes of Administration that are Commonly Used
ORAL: As a dietary supplement in adults, 1-2 mg per day is commonly taken. For mild thiamine deficiency syndromes in adults, the usual dose of thiamine is 5-30 mg daily in either a single dose or divided doses for one month (14,15). The typical dose for severe deficiency can be up to 300 mg per day (14). Parenteral thiamine is recommended for critically ill people (15). For genetic enzyme deficiency disorders, 10-20 mg daily is recommended, although 600-4000 mg daily in divided doses may be needed for Leigh's disease (14,15). For maple syrup urine disease, 100-200 mg daily is recommended, although up to 1000 mg has been used (14). The daily recommended dietary allowances (RDAs) of thiamine are: Infants 0-6 months, 0.2 mg; Infants 7-12 months, 0.3 mg; Children 1-3 years, 0.5 mg; Children 4-8 years, 0.6 mg; Males 9-13 years, 0.9 mg; Males 14 years and older, 1.2 mg; Females 9-13 years, 0.9 mg; Women 14-18 years, 1 mg; Women over 18 years, 1.1 mg; Pregnant women, 1.4 mg; and Lactating women, 1.5 mg (3094).
INJECTION: IM or slow IV.

Comments
Thiamine is present in many foods including yeast, cereal grains, legumes, nuts, and meat (15). Thiamine is frequently used in combination with other B vitamins in vitamin B complex formulations. Vitamin B complex generally includes vitamin B1 (thiamine), vitamin B2 (riboflavin), vitamin B3 (niacin/niacinamide), vitamin B5 (pantothenic acid), vitamin B6 (pyridoxine), vitamin B12 (cyanocobalamin), and folic acid. However, some products do not contain all of these ingredients and some may include others, such as biotin, para-aminobenzoic acid (PABA), choline bitartrate, and inositol (3022,3060,3061).

THUNDER GOD VINE

This Product is Also Known As
Huang-T'eng Ken, Lei Gong Teng, Lei-Kung T'eng, Taso-Ho-Hua, Threewingnut, Yellow Vine.

Scientific Names
Tripterygium wilfordii.
Family: Celastraceae.

People Use This For
Orally, thunder god vine leaf and root are used as a male antifertility agent, for rheumatoid arthritis, heavy menstrual periods, and multiple sclerosis (6).
In Chinese medicine, it is used for abscesses, boils, fever, and inflammation (6).
Other uses include utilization as an insecticide for killing maggots or larvae, and as a rat and bird poison (6).

Safety
LIKELY UNSAFE ...when the vine leaf and root are used orally. Can have immunosuppressant effects, possibly including reduced lymphocyte levels (6).
PREGNANCY: LIKELY UNSAFE ...contraindicated for oral use because thunder god vine leaf and root are thought to be teratogens (6,4047).
LACTATION: LIKELY UNSAFE ...when used orally; avoid using.

Effectiveness
POSSIBLY EFFECTIVE ...when used orally as a male antifertility agent (6,4046). ...when used orally for treating rheumatoid arthritis (6,4046).
There is insufficient reliable information available about the effectiveness of thunder god vine for its other uses.

Possible Mechanism of Action & Active Ingredients
The applicable parts of thunder god vine are the leaf and root. Thunder god vine leaf and root are reported to have antifertility effects in males, and immunosuppressive, antiviral, and antitumor activities (6). Thunder god vine appears to inhibit spermatogenesis and reduce sperm motility, without affecting testosterone levels. These activities are attributed triptolide and tripdiolide, and possibly four other compounds (6). Male fertility appears to return to normal 6 weeks after discontinuation (6). The immunosuppressive effects of thunder god vine are attributed to the constituents tripchlorolide, tribromolide, and demethylzeylasteral (6). Thunder god vine shows evidence of multiple mechanisms of immunosuppression. It inhibits production of cytokine IL2 and gamma interferon; it inhibits response of human mononuclear cells; and it inhibits generation of cytotoxic T-cells (6). T-2, an alcoholic extract that contains triptolide and tripdiolide, inhibits T-cell and B-cell proliferation, as well as B-cells production of immunoglobulin production (6). Several diterpenes, including triptolide and tripdiolide show evidence of anti-inflammatory and immunosuppressive effects (6). In one clinical study, thunder god vine extract improved the symptoms of rheumatoid arthritis in individuals taking concomitant nonsteroidal anti-inflammatory drugs (4046).

Low doses of triptolide show evidence of antitumor and antileukemic effects (6). The isolated constituent, triterene, inhibits antibody response and granuloma growth in rats (6). Demethylzeylasteral has anti-angiogenic effects (6). Neotripterifordin, tripteriforrdin, and salaspermic acid exhibit potent anti-HIV replication activity in vitro (6,4048,4049).

Adverse Reactions Including Known Allergies

Oral use of thunder god vine is associated with gastrointestinal upset, infertility, lymphocytes suppression (6), and skin reactions (4046). Women using the extract "T2" developed amenorrhea (6). Adverse effects appear to be more prevalent with immediate-release products than with sustained release products (6). There is one report of a young male with some evidence of pre-existing heart damage who developed vomiting, diarrhea, leukopenia, renal failure, hypotension, shock, and died three days after ingestion (6). There is also one report of an infant born with meningoencephalocele after the mother used thunder god vine for rheumatoid arthritis during pregnancy (4047).

Possible Interactions with Herbs & Other Dietary Supplements

Insufficient reliable information available.

Possible Interactions with Drugs

IMMUNOSUPPRESSIVE DRUGS: Theoretically, concomitant use might enhance drug effects.

Possible Interactions with Foods

No interactions are known to occur, and there is no known reason to expect a clinically significant interaction with thunder god vine.

Possible Interactions with Lab Tests

No interactions are known to occur, and there is no known reason to expect a clinically significant interaction with thunder god vine.

Possible Interactions with Diseases or Conditions

IMMUNE SYSTEM COMPROMISE: Theoretically, thunder god vine might exacerbate these conditions (6).

Typical Dosages & Routes of Administration that are Commonly Used

ORAL: Rheumatoid arthritis, 30 mg thunder god vine polyglycoside extract per day was used in one study (6).

Comments

None.

THYME flower, leaf

This Product is Also Known As

Common Thyme, French Thyme, Garden Thyme, Rubbed Thyme, Spanish Thyme, Thymi herba.
CAUTION: See separate listings for Thyme Oil and Wild Thyme.

Scientific Names

Thymus vulgaris; Thymus zygis.
Family: Lamiaceae.

People Use This For

Orally, thyme is used for bronchitis, pertussis (2,18), sore throat, colic, and dyspnea (6121).
Topically, thyme is used for upper respiratory tract mucous membrane inflammation, laryngitis, tonsillitis (2,18), stomatitis, and halitosis (1).
In folk medicine, thyme was used as an appetite stimulant (11), for dyspepsia, chronic gastritis, diarrhea in children, enuresis in children (4), as an antiflatulent, diuretic, urinary disinfectant, antihelmintic (18), and for rheumatic and skin disorders (11).
In foods, thyme is used as a culinary herb (4,11).

Safety

LIKELY SAFE ...when used in the amounts found in foods (11). Thyme has Generally Recognized as Safe (GRAS) status in the US (11). Maximum use of thyme in foods is 0.172%. Maximum use of thyme oil is 0.003% (11).
POSSIBLY SAFE ...when used orally and appropriately (1,2,12). ...when used topically and appropriately (18). There is insufficient reliable information available for larger amounts; avoid using (4).
PREGNANCY: LIKELY SAFE ...when taken in food amounts. UNSAFE ...when used in larger amounts because it might induce menstruation (4,19).
LACTATION: LIKELY SAFE ...when taken in food amounts.

Effectiveness

POSSIBLY EFFECTIVE ...when used for symptoms of bronchitis and pertussis (1,2). ...when used topically for upper respiratory tract mucous inflammation (2), stomatitis, and halitosis (1).
There is insufficient reliable information available about the effectiveness of thyme for its other uses.

Possible Mechanism of Action & Active Ingredients

Thyme contains thymol, carvacrol, and flavonoid constituents, which are responsible for the antispasmodic, antitussive, and expectorant effects [4]. This explains why thyme is used as an antiflatulent, antispasmodic, antitussive, astringent, expectorant, antibacterial, antihelmintic, and to stimulate saliva [2,4,18]. There may also be phenolic compounds of the volatile oil and flavonoids associated with antispasmodic activity. This mechanism may involve calcium channel blockade. However, some scientists question whether the phenolic components are involved [4]. The antibacterial and antifungal activity is associated with the thymol and carvacrol [1]. Thymol also demonstrates antihelmintic activity [4]. The constituent, rosmarinic acid, reduces experimentally-induced edema, inhibits passive cutaneous anaphylaxis, and impairs experimental activation of macrophages in vivo [1]. In animals, the thyme extract seems to have analgesic and antipyretic effects [4]. The thymus vulgaris also has antithyrotropic activity [11]. The fluid extracts show antispasmodic activity in smooth muscle, but the active constituents causing this activity have not been identified [11].

Adverse Reactions Including Known Allergies

Topically thyme oil can lead to irritation [4]. There is a low potential for sensitization [18].

Possible Interactions with Herbs & Other Dietary Supplements

Insufficient reliable information available.

Possible Interactions with Drugs

No interactions are known to occur, and there is no known reason to expect a clinically significant interaction with thyme.

Possible Interactions with Foods

No interactions are known to occur, and there is no known reason to expect a clinically significant interaction with thyme.

Possible Interactions with Lab Tests

No interactions are known to occur, and there is no known reason to expect a clinically significant interaction with thyme.

Possible Interactions with Diseases or Conditions

URINARY TRACT INFLAMMATION: CAUTION, use might exacerbate inflammation [19].
GI IRRITATION (e.g., ulcers, etc.): CAUTION, use can exacerbate inflammation [19].
CROSS-ALLERGENICITY: CAUTION, cross-reactivity to oregano and other Labiatae species reported in an individual allergic to thyme [3808].
OTHER: When used as a bath, be cautious in cases of extensive skin injuries or disease, or in cases involving high fever or infectious disease, cardiac insufficiency or hypertonia [18].

Typical Dosages & Routes of Administration that are Commonly Used

ORAL: 1-2 grams dried leaf/flower several times daily, or one cup tea (steep 1-2 grams dried leaf/flower in 150 mL boiling water for 10 minutes, strain) several times daily as needed [1,2,18]; not to exceed 10 grams dried leaf with 0.03% phenol (calculated as thymol) per day [18]. Fluid extract, 1-2 grams up to three times daily [2].
TOPICAL: Gargle [1] or compress [2,18], steep 5 grams dried leaf per 100 mL boiling water 10 minutes, strain [1,2,18].

Comments

Thyme is a plant rich in iron [19].

THYME OIL

This Product is Also Known As

Common Thyme, Red Thyme Oil, Spanish Thyme, Thyme Aetheroleum, Thyme Oil, White Thyme Oil.
CAUTION: See separate listings for Thyme, Spanish Origanum oil, and Wild Thyme.

Scientific Names

Thymus vulgaris; Thymus zygis.
Family: Lamiaceae.

People Use This For

Orally, thyme oil is used to prevent bedwetting in children [4], and as an antispasmodic and antiflatulent [11].
Topically, it is a counterirritant, an antiseptic in mouthwashes and liniments [11], and is used as a counterirritant in douche products [272].
Otically, it is an antibacterial and antifungal ingredient [272].
In manufacturing, red thyme oil is used in perfumes [11]. Thyme oil is also used in soaps, cosmetics, toothpastes, and as a flavor component in foods [11].

Safety

LIKELY SAFE ...when taken in amounts found in foods (11). It has Generally Recognized as Safe (GRAS) status in the US. The maximum use levels are less than 0.003% (11).
LIKELY UNSAFE ...when taken as an oral medicinal because thyme oil is considered toxic (4). ...when used topically unless it is diluted (4).
PREGNANCY: LIKELY SAFE ...when used orally in food amounts. LIKELY UNSAFE ...contraindicated in larger amounts because it might induce menstruation (4,12).
LACTATION: LIKELY SAFE ...when used orally in food amounts. There is insufficient reliable information available about the safety of thyme oil for larger amounts; avoid using.

Effectiveness

There is insufficient reliable information available about the effectiveness of thyme oil.

Possible Mechanism of Action & Active Ingredients

The thymol and carvacrol constituents of the volatile oil may have antispasmodic, antitussive, and expectorant effects (4). Thymol has fungicidal, antibacterial, anthelmintic (especially hookworms), and counterirritant properties (4,11).

Adverse Reactions Including Known Allergies

Taken orally, thyme oil can cause nausea, vomiting, gastric pain, headache, dizziness, convulsions, coma, and cardiac and respiratory arrest (4). Topically, it can cause skin or mucous membrane irritation, cheilitis, and glossitis (4).

Possible Interactions with Herbs & Other Dietary Supplements

Insufficient reliable information available.

Possible Interactions with Drugs

No interactions are known to occur, and there is no known reason to expect a clinically significant interaction with thyme oil.

Possible Interactions with Foods

No interactions are known to occur, and there is no known reason to expect a clinically significant interaction with thyme oil.

Possible Interactions with Lab Tests

No interactions are known to occur, and there is no known reason to expect a clinically significant interaction with thyme oil.

Possible Interactions with Diseases or Conditions

SKIN INJURIES: Medical consultation needed before use in individuals with extensive skin injuries/disease (18).
INFECTION: Medical consultation needed before use in individuals with high fever or infectious disease.
CARDIAC INSUFFICIENCY AND HYPERTONIA: Medical consultation needed before use in individuals with cardiac insufficiency or hypertonia (18).

Typical Dosages & Routes of Administration that are Commonly Used

ORAL: People typically take 2 to 3 drops on a sugar cube, 2 or 3 times a day (5263).
TOPICAL: Must be diluted (4). Thyme oil is commonly applied as needed in 1% to 2% ointments (6002).

Comments

Thyme oil is obtained by distillation of the leaves and flowering tops of thyme (Thymus vulgaris and/or Thymus zygis). White thyme oil (redistilled red thyme oil) is often adulterated (11).

TIRATRICOL

This Product is Also Known As

Triac, triiodothyroacetic acid.

Scientific Names

3,3',5-triiodothyroacetic acid.

People Use This For

Orally, tiratricol is used for treating pituitary resistance to thyroid hormone (PRTH) (1607,1608,1609,1610,1615), treating thyroid cancer (orphan drug designation) (1604,1616,1617,1618), treating fetal hypothyroidism (1613,1614), increasing metabolic rate for weight loss, and reducing cellulite (1601,1602,1606,1611,1612).

Safety

LIKELY SAFE ...when used orally under medical supervision for treating thyroid cancer (1604,1616,1617,1618). ...when used orally under medical supervision for treating pituitary resistance to thyroid hormone (PRTH) (1607,1608,1609, 1610,1615).
POSSIBLY SAFE ...when used orally under medical supervision for treating fetal hypothyroidism (1613,1614).
POSSIBLY UNSAFE ...when used orally in the elderly, tiratricol might aggravate occult cardiac disease (15); avoid using.
LIKELY UNSAFE ...when used orally for increasing metabolic rate for weight loss or reducing cellulite (1620,1621,1622,1623,1624,1625). The FDA has issued a warning against tiratricol use for weight loss (1605).
PREGNANCY: POSSIBLY SAFE ...when used orally under medical supervision for treating fetal hypothyroidism (1613,1614).
LIKELY UNSAFE ...when used orally for other purposes during pregnancy due to possible risk of fetal heart damage (1627,1628); avoid using.
LACTATION: Insufficient reliable information available; avoid using.

Effectiveness

LIKELY EFFECTIVE ...when taken orally for treating pituitary resistance to thyroid hormone (PRTH) (1607,1608, 1609,1610,1615).
POSSIBLY EFFECTIVE ...when taken orally for treating fetal hypothyroidism (1613,1614). ...when taken orally for thyroid cancer in combination with levo-thyroxine (1616,1617,1618). Tiratricol is an FDA designated orphan drug under study for use in combination with levo-thyroxine to suppress thyroid stimulating hormone (TSH) in patients with well-differentiated thyroid cancer who are intolerant to adequate doses of levo-thyroxine alone (1604).
LIKELY INEFFECTIVE ...when taken orally for increasing metabolic rate for weight loss in people with normal thyroid function (1611,1612).
There is insufficient reliable information available about the effectiveness of tiratricol for its other uses.

Possible Mechanism of Action & Active Ingredients

Tiratricol is a naturally occurring metabolite of T4 (thyroxine) and a structural analog of T3 (triiodothyronine) (1633,1634). Low concentrations of tiratricol are found in plasma, but tiratricol has no known role in thyroid physiology (1633). Tiratricol has a high affinity for T3 receptors and suppresses thyroid stimulating hormone (TSH) secretion at therapeutic doses without causing significant peripheral effects, such as increased basal metabolism rate and heart rate (1634). Tiratricol might lower total and LDL cholesterol, and stimulate bone formation (1632). About 67% of an oral dose of tiratricol is absorbed; the half-life is 6 hours (1631).

Adverse Reactions Including Known Allergies

Tiratricol taken orally can cause severe diarrhea, fatigue, lethargy, and profound weight loss (1605). Heart attacks and strokes are possible, as well as symptoms of hyperthyroidism, including increased appetite, abdominal cramps, tremors, menstrual irregularities, nervousness, insomnia, sweating, intolerance to heat, fever, palpitations, tachycardia, increased pulse and blood pressure, chest pain, and cardiac arrhythmias (15,1605). Case reports have implicated tiratricol in centrally-mediated hypothyroidism, pseudohypothyroidism, internuclear ophthalmoplegia, and hepatotoxicity (1621,1623,1624,1625).

Possible Interactions with Herbs & Other Dietary Supplements

HERBS WITH THYROID ACTIVITY: Theoretically, tiratricol might enhance the effects and adverse effects of herbs that affect thyroid function, including bugleweed, balm leaf, and wild thyme.
HERBS & SUPPLEMENTS WITH SYMPATHOMIMETIC ACTIVITY: Theoretically, large doses of tiratricol might enhance the effects and adverse effects of herbs and supplements that have sympathomimetic activity, including caffeine, guarana, and ephedra (15).
VITAMIN K: Theoretically, tiratricol might antagonize the prothrombinemic effects of vitamin K by increasing catabolism of vitamin K-dependent clotting factors (15).

Possible Interactions with Drugs

ANTICOAGULANTS: Theoretically, tiratricol might potentiate the hypoprothrombinemic effects of oral anticoagulants, including warfarin (Coumadin), by increasing catabolism of vitamin K-dependent clotting factors (15).
ANTI-DIABETES DRUGS: Theoretically, tiratricol might interfere with blood glucose control requiring adjustment of diabetes drug therapy (15); monitor closely.
CHOLESTYRAMINE (Questran): Theoretically, cholestyramine might decrease tiratricol absorption (15).
SYMPATHOMIMETIC DRUGS: Theoretically, large doses of tiratricol might enhance the effects and adverse effects of sympathomimetic drugs (15).
THYROID HORMONES: Concurrent use can have additive effects (1617); use only under medical supervision.
VITAMIN K: Theoretically, tiratricol might antagonize the prothrombinemic effects of vitamin K by increasing catabolism of vitamin K-dependent clotting factors (15).

Possible Interactions with Foods

No interactions are known to occur, and there is no known reason to expect a clinically significant interaction with tiratricol.

Possible Interactions with Lab Tests

THYROID FUNCTION TESTS: Abnormalities have been reported in people taking tiratricol (1604).
THYROID-STIMULATING HORMONE (TSH): Tiratricol reduces serum TSH levels, and test results (1631).
THYROTRPIN-RELEASING HORMONE (TRH) STIMULATION: Tiratricol reduces TSH secretion, serum levels and test results, to exogenous TRH stimulation (1609,1611,1617,1623,1633).
PROTHROMBIN TIME (PT), INTERNATIONAL NORMALIZATION RATIO (INR): Theoretically, tiratricol might increase prothrombin time, increasing PT and INR test results, by increasing catabolism of vitamin K-dependent clotting factors (15).

Possible Interactions with Diseases or Conditions

ADRENAL INSUFFICIENCY, DIABETES, HYPOPITUITARISM: Theoretically, tiratricol might unmask symptoms of these conditions in patients with untreated hypothyroidism (15).
ANGINA, CARDIOVASCULAR DISEASE, HYPERTENSION: Theoretically, tiratricol might aggravate symptoms of these conditions (15); avoid using.
PROLONGED CLOTTING TIME: Theoretically, tiratricol might increase the risk of bleeding in people with prolonged clotting time by increasing catabolism of vitamin K-dependent clotting factors (15).
DIABETES: Theoretically, tiratricol might interfere with blood glucose control requiring adjustment of diabetes drug therapy (15), monitor closely.
MYXEDEMA: Patients with myxedema might be particularly sensitive to thyroid agents, including tiratricol (15).
LIVER DISEASE: Tiratricol is potentially hepatotoxic and might worsen liver disease (1624); avoid using.

Typical Dosages & Routes of Administration that are Commonly Used

ORAL: The oral dose for TSH suppression tests used in clinical trials is 10-24 mcg twice daily initially, titrated to a TSH concentration of less than 0.1 mU/L (1632,1633). The oral dose typically used for weight loss is 1 mg twice daily (1601).

Comments

Tiratricol is a thyroid supplement and should not be taken by anyone with normal thyroid function (1605). The drug, which is available by prescription in France, has been studied since the fifties, mostly for thyroid disease (9,1629,1630). The FDA has determined that the product Triax (TRIAC, tiratricol) is not a dietary supplement but an unapproved new drug containing a potent thyroid hormone, which may cause serious health consequences. The State of Missouri embargoed the product at its distributor (Syntrax) and the Utah-based manufacturer (Pharmatech) has agreed to stop distributing any product containing the ingredient TRIAC. Further action by the US Food and Drug Administration is being considered.

TOLU BALSAM

This Product is Also Known As

Balsam of Tolu, Balsam Tolu, Balsamum Tolutanum, Opobalsam, Resina Tolutana, Resin Tolu, Thomas Balsam, Tolu, Toluiferum Balsamum.
CAUTION: See separate listing for Peru Balsam.

Scientific Names

Myroxylon balsamum, synonym Myroxylon balsamum genuinum; Toliufera balsamum, synonyms Myroxylan balsamum, Myroxylan toluiferum.
Family: Leguminosae or Fabaceae.

People Use This For

Orally, tolu balsam is used for cough, bronchitis (18), inflammation of respiratory tract mucous membranes (2), and as a flavoring and expectorant ingredient in cough medicines (11).
Topically, it is used as an ingredient in Compound Benzoin Tincture, for treatment of bedsores, cracked nipples, lips, and minor skin cuts.
As an inhalant, tolu balsam is used to treat laryngitis and croup (11).
Historically, tolu balsam has been used for cancer (11).
For food uses, tolu balsam is also used to flavor chewing gum, foods, and beverages (11).
In manufacturing, balsam and balsam oil are used as fixatives or as fragrances in soaps and cosmetics (11).

Safety

LIKELY SAFE ...when the oleo resin is used orally in the very low amounts found in foods. Tolu balsam has been approved for food use in the US (11).
POSSIBLY SAFE ...when used orally and appropriately for medicinal purposes (2).
There is insufficient reliable information available about the safety of the topical use of tolu balsam.
PREGNANCY AND LACTATION: Insufficient reliable information available; avoid using.

Effectiveness

POSSIBLY EFFECTIVE ...for oral use in treating inflammation of respiratory tract mucous membranes (2).
There is insufficient reliable information available about the effectiveness of tolu balsam for its other uses.

Possible Mechanism of Action & Active Ingredients

The applicable part of tolu balsam is the oleo resin. Tolu balsam has mild antiseptic action and expectorant properties (11).

Adverse Reactions Including Known Allergies

May cause allergic reactions (11), kidney irritation (12).

Possible Interactions with Herbs & Other Dietary Supplements

Insufficient reliable information available.

Possible Interactions with Drugs

No interactions are known to occur, and there is no known reason to expect a clinically significant interaction with tolu balsam.

Possible Interactions with Foods

No interactions are known to occur, and there is no known reason to expect a clinically significant interaction with tolu balsam.

Possible Interactions with Lab Tests

No interactions are known to occur, and there is no known reason to expect a clinically significant interaction with tolu balsam.

Possible Interactions with Diseases or Conditions

FEVER: Theoretically, contraindicated in individuals with fever or inflammation (12,19).
KIDNEY DISEASE: Theoretically, might exacerbate kidney disease.
TOLU BALSAM ALLERGY: Avoid use of tolu balsam (11).

Typical Dosages & Routes of Administration that are Commonly Used

ORAL: 500-600 mg per day (2,18).
TOPICAL: No typical dosage.

Comments

Avoid confusion with Peru balsam. Tolu balsam is the oleo resin exuded from slits cut in the trunk Myroxylon balsamum.

TOMATO

This Product is Also Known As

Love Apple.
CAUTION: See Lycopene for the active ingredient in the tomato fruit.

Scientific Names

Lycopersicon esculentum.
Family: Solanaceae.

People Use This For

Orally, tomato fruit is used orally for reducing the risk of cancer (2404,2405,2406,2407).
Orally, tomato plant leaf and vine are used for treating arthritis, colds, chills and digestive disorders (18).

Safety

LIKELY SAFE ...when tomato fruit or its products are consumed in amounts found in foods (2406).
POSSIBLY UNSAFE ...when the leaf is used orally (18).
There is insufficient reliable information about the safety of the tomato vine.
PREGNANCY AND LACTATION: LIKELY SAFE ...when tomato fruit or its products are consumed in typical food amounts. Avoid using amounts greater than those typically consumed as foods.

Effectiveness

POSSIBLY EFFECTIVE...when tomato fruit products are consumed for reducing the risk of prostate cancer. Epidemiological studies suggest that the risk of prostate cancer is decreased in men who consume four or more weekly servings of tomato products, including tomatoes, tomato sauce, pizza and tomato juice (2406).
POSSIBLY INEFFECTIVE ...when tomato fruit products are consumed for reducing the risk of bladder cancer. Epidemiological studies find no association between consumption of tomatoes and tomato-based products, and the risk of bladder cancer (2407).
There is insufficient reliable information available about the effectiveness of tomato fruit for its other uses.

Epidemiological studies of consumption of tomatoes and tomato-based products, and the risk of cancers of the breast, cervix, colon, esophagus, larynx, lungs, oral cavity, ovaries, pancreas, pleura, rectum, and stomach, are inconclusive (1444,2404,2407).

There is insufficient reliable information available about the effectiveness of tomato leaf and vine.

Possible Mechanism of Action & Active Ingredients

The applicable parts are the tomato fruit, leaf, and vine. Tomatoes are the major dietary source of the carotenoid, lycopene. Decreased serum or tissue lycopene concentrations are associated with an increased risk of prostate cancer (1447,1496,2405,2406,2407). Lycopene is better absorbed from tomato products, such as tomato paste, than from fresh tomatoes (1497). Consumption of tomato juice significantly increases serum lycopene levels (1498).

Adverse Reactions Including Known Allergies

Signs of oral poisoning are not expected with ingestion of less than 100 grams of tomato leaves. Symptoms of toxicity may include severe mucous membrane irritation, including vomiting, diarrhea, and colic. This is followed by dizziness, stupor, headache, bradycardia, respiratory disturbances, and mild spasms. In very severe cases, death by respiratory failure might occur (18).

No adverse reactions are reported with ingestion of ripe tomatoes. Adverse reactions are not expected with ingestion of less than 100 grams of green (unripe) tomatoes.

Possible Interactions with Herbs & Other Dietary Supplements

Insufficient reliable information available.

Possible Interactions with Drugs

No interactions are known to occur, and there is no known reason to expect a clinically significant interaction with tomato.

Possible Interactions with Foods

No interactions are known to occur, and there is no known reason to expect a clinically significant interaction with tomato.

Possible Interactions with Lab Tests

No interactions are known to occur, and there is no known reason to expect a clinically significant interaction with tomato.

Possible Interactions with Diseases or Conditions

No interactions are known to occur, and there is no known reason to expect a clinically significant interaction with tomato.

Typical Dosages & Routes of Administration that are Commonly Used

ORAL: For preventing prostate cancer, four or more servings of tomato products per week (equivalent to a dietary lycopene intake of greater than 6 mg daily) has been proposed (2406).

Comments

Use of other parts of the tomato plant, particularly the leaf or vine, is possibly unsafe (18). One cup (240 mL) of tomato juice contains approximately 23 mg lycopene, depending on the brand (1499).

TONKA BEAN

This Product is Also Known As

Coumarouna Odorata, Cumaru, Dutch Tonka, English Tonka, Tonka, Tonka Seed, Tonquin Bean, Torquin Bean.

Scientific Names

Dipteryx odorata.
Family: Leguminosae.

People Use This For

Orally, tonka bean fruit and seed is used as a tonic (6,4500), to treat cachexia (4502), cramps (4502,4507), lymphedema (4507), nausea (4502,4507), cough (4500), schistosomiasis (6,4502), spasms (4502), and tuberculosis (4500). Topically, it is used for mouth ulcers (4500,4502), earache (4502), and sore throat (4502).

In manufacturing, coumarin, one of the active constituents is used as a flavoring and fragrance in various products in the food, liquor, tobacco, soap, and cosmetic industries (6,13,4502,4507).

In other uses, the fruit is used as an aphrodisiac (4502,4507) and the seeds are used to make a nutty-flavored beverage (6,4502).

Safety

LIKELY UNSAFE ...contraindicated for oral use. The FDA deems any food containing tonka bean or tonka bean extract to be impure (6). Rarely, coumarin, a constituent, has been associated with hepatotoxicity ranging from elevated liver enzymes to severe hepatic damage (6,18,297,4501). In a number of countries, coumarin-containing products have been removed from the market (4501).

There is insufficient reliable information available about the safety of the topical use of tonka bean.

PREGNANCY AND LACTATION: LIKELY UNSAFE …contraindicated for oral use; avoid using.

Effectiveness

There is insufficient reliable information available about the effectiveness of tonka bean.

Possible Mechanism of Action & Active Ingredients

The applicable parts of tonka bean are the fruit and seed. Tonka bean seeds usually contain 1-3% coumarin but may contain up to 10% (6,4501,4502). Tonka bean seeds also contain coumaric-acid-beta-glucoside, o-coumaric acid, linoleic acid, oleic-acid, sitosterol, stearic acid, stigmasterol, and umbelliferone (296). The fruit contains melilotoside-1-p-coumaryl-beta-d-glucose (296). There is some evidence that coumarin can reduce edema and inflammation by increasing venous and lymphatic return (295). Other information suggests tonka bean might have narcotic and spasmolytic properties (4502,18).

Adverse Reactions Including Known Allergies

The oral use of coumarin can be associated with nausea, vomiting (286), diarrhea, dizziness, insomnia (287), asymptomatic SGOT elevations (286), and rarely, liver toxicity (6,18,297,4501). Large doses of the extract can paralyze the heart (4502).

Possible Interactions with Herbs & Other Dietary Supplements

HERBS WITH ANTICOAGULANT/ANTIPLATELET POTENTIAL: Concomitant use of herbs that have coumarin constituents or affect platelet aggregation could theoretically increase the risk of bleeding in some people. These herbs include: angelica, anise, arnica, asafoetida, bogbean, boldo, capsicum, celery, chamomile, clove, danshen, fenugreek, feverfew, garlic, ginger, ginkgo, ginseng Panax, horse chestnut, horseradish, licorice, meadowsweet, prickly ash, onion, papain, passionflower, poplar, quassia, red clover, turmeric, wild carrot, wild lettuce, willow, and others (4,19).

Possible Interactions with Drugs

ANTICOAGULANTS/ANTIPLATELETS: Theoretically, tonka bean might cause additive effects and side effects with drugs having anticoagulant or antiplatelet properties (19).

Possible Interactions with Foods

No interactions are known to occur, and there is no known reason to expect a clinically significant interaction with tonka bean.

Possible Interactions with Lab Tests

No interactions are known to occur, and there is no known reason to expect a clinically significant interaction with tonka bean.

Possible Interactions with Diseases or Conditions

LIVER DISEASE: Although it is rare, coumarin can cause liver toxicity (298).

Typical Dosages & Routes of Administration that are Commonly Used

ORAL: Some people use an amount of tonka bean based on its coumarin content, and the typical dose of coumarin used is 60 mg daily (5008).

Comments

Tonka bean is likely unsafe, and in a number of countries, coumarin-containing products have been removed from the market (4501). The term coumarin is derived from Coumarou, the Caribbean name for the tonka tree (13). In plants, more than 700 different coumarins have been identified. Coumarin, itself, is widely distributed and has the characteristic odor of new-mown hay (13). Do not confuse coumarin with the potent anticoagulants bishydroxycoumarin or dicumarol (13,295) or warfarin which is a derivative of 4-hydroxycoumarin (16).

TORMENTIL

This Product is Also Known As

Biscuits, Bloodroot, Cinquefoil, Earthbank, English Sarsaparilla, Ewe Daisy, Flesh and Blood, Potentilla, Septfoil, Shepherd's Knapperty, Shepherd's Knot, Thormantle, Tormentilla, Tormentillae rhizoma.

CAUTION: See separate listings for Couch Grass, Potentilla, German Sarsaparilla, and Sarsaparilla.

Scientific Names

Potentilla erecta.

Family: Rosaceae.

People Use This For

Orally, tormentil is used to treat diarrhea (2,18), acute and subacute gastroenteritis (18), and fever (400). Topically, it is used for reducing superficial bleeding (400) and treating mild inflammation of the oral and pharyngeal mucus membranes (2,18).

Safety

POSSIBLY SAFE ...when used orally or topically and appropriately (2,12).
PREGNANCY AND LACTATION: Insufficient reliable information available; avoid using.

Effectiveness

POSSIBLY EFFECTIVE ...when taken orally for diarrhea (2,7,12,18). ...when applied topically for mild oral and pharyngeal mucus membrane inflammation (2,7,12,18).
There is insufficient reliable information available about the effectiveness of tormentil root for its other uses.

Possible Mechanism of Action & Active Ingredients

The applicable part of tormentil is the root. It contains 17-22% tannins, proanthocyanidins, flavonoids, and triterpenes (18). The astringent effect of tannins relieves diarrhea and soothes mucus membrane inflammation. Tannins reduce superficial bleeding by causing skin and superficial capillary contraction (400). Tannins also show some evidence of antiviral, antimicrobial, CNS depressant, and cariostatic effects (11). Some evidence suggests that tannins might cause cancer but other evidence shows tannins might prevent it (12). Regular consumption of herbs with high tannin concentrations correlates with increased incidence of esophageal or nasal cancer (12).

Adverse Reactions Including Known Allergies

The oral use of tormentil can cause nausea, vomiting (7,12,18), and stomach complaints (2). Because tormentil contains more than 10% tannins, theoretically it also has the potential to cause kidney damage and necrotic conditions of the liver (12). No adverse reactions have been reported with the topical use of the tormentil root.

Possible Interactions with Herbs & Other Dietary Supplements

Insufficient reliable information available.

Possible Interactions with Drugs

No interactions are known to occur, and there is no known reason to expect a clinically significant interaction with tormentil.

Possible Interactions with Foods

MILK: When added to tormentil tea, milk can bind to the tannins and decrease their astringent and adverse effects (12).

Possible Interactions with Lab Tests

No interactions are known to occur, and there is no known reason to expect a clinically significant interaction with tormentil.

Possible Interactions with Diseases or Conditions

No interactions are known to occur, and there is no known reason to expect a clinically significant interaction with tormentil.

Typical Dosages & Routes of Administration that are Commonly Used

ORAL: For diarrhea, a typical dose is one cup of the tea 2 to 4 times daily between meals, up to 4-6 grams of root per day. The tea is prepared by steeping 2-3 grams of the finely cut or powdered root in 150 mL boiling water for 10-15 minutes and then straining (2,7,18). Diarrhea lasting longer than 3 to 4 days should be medically evaluated (2).
TOPICAL: The usual daily dose of the tincture (1:10) is 10-20 drops in one glass of water used as a mouth or throat rinse (2,18).

Comments

Avoid confusion with potentilla (Potentilla anserina).

TRAGACANTH

This Product is Also Known As

Goat's Thorn, Green Dragon, Gum Dragon, Gummi Tragacanthae, Gum Tragacanth, Hog Gum, Syrian Tragacanth, Tragacanth Gum.
CAUTION: See separate listing for Astragalus.

Scientific Names

Astragalus gummifera; other Astragalus species.
Family: Leguminosae or Fabaceae.

People Use This For
Orally, tragacanth is used both for diarrhea (6) and as a laxative (18).

Topically, it is an ingredient in toothpastes, hand lotions, and vaginal creams and jellies (11).

For food uses, it is important for stabilizing, thickening, and suspending ingredients in salad dressings, foods, and beverages (11).

In pharmaceutical preparations, it is used as an emulsifier, binding agent, and demulcent (11). Tragacanth is also a component of denture adhesives (6).

Safety
LIKELY SAFE ...when used orally in amounts found in foods. It has Generally Recognized as Safe (GRAS) status in the US. The maximum level used is 1.3% (11). ...when used topically, in the amounts found in cosmetics. Tragacanth is not considered to be irritating, sensitizing, or phototoxic (4072).

POSSIBLY SAFE ...when used orally in greater amounts for medicinal purposes (4068). However, insufficient fluid intake with tragacanth might lead to esophageal closure or obstruction ileus (18).

PREGNANCY AND LACTATION: Insufficient reliable information available; avoid using amounts greater than found in foods.

Effectiveness
There is insufficient reliable information available about the effectiveness of tragacanth.

Possible Mechanism of Action & Active Ingredients
Tragacanth contains water-soluble tragacanthin and water-insoluble bassorin (11). When added to water, tragacanthin dissolves to form a viscous colloidal solution; bassorin swells to form a thick gel (11). Among plant gums, tragacanth produces the most viscous solution (11). When ingested, the bulk of tragacanth stretches the intestinal wall, increasing peristalsis (18). Although tragacanth increases stool weight and decreases GI transit time, it does not appear to affect cholesterol, triglyceride, or phospholipid levels as do other soluble fibers (6). Some preliminary data indicate that people with diabetes who ingest tragacanth along with a high sugar load have lower peak serum glucose and insulin levels (4069). However this effect has not been consistent (6). The mucilaginous, adhesive properties of tragacanth justify its use as a component in denture adhesives (6). Tragacanth appears to inhibit growth of cancer cells (11). Preliminary evidence suggests tragacanthin polysaccharides might offer some protection from hantavirus infections (4070). Tragacanth is highly susceptible to bacterial digestion, even in the presence of preservatives (11).

Adverse Reactions Including Known Allergies
When used orally, insufficient fluid intake can lead to obstruction ileus and esophageal closure (18). Tragacanth can cause asthma symptoms in people who are sensitive to quillaia bark (6).

Possible Interactions with Herbs & Other Dietary Supplements
HERBS AND SUPPLEMENTS: Theoretically, concomitant administration might reduce absorption of supplements and/or herbs due to hydrocolloidal fiber content of tragacanth (19).

Possible Interactions with Drugs
ORAL DRUGS: Theoretically, concomitant administration of oral drugs might reduce drug absorption due to hydrocolloidal fiber content of tragacanth (19).

Possible Interactions with Foods
NUTRIENTS: Theoretically, concomitant administration might impair nutrient absorption from foods due to hydrocolloidal fiber content of tragacanth (19).

Possible Interactions with Lab Tests
No interactions are known to occur, and there is no known reason to expect a clinically significant interaction with tragacanth.

Possible Interactions with Diseases or Conditions
QUILLAIA ALLERGY: Tragacanth can cause asthma symptoms in individuals sensitive to quillaia bark (19).

Typical Dosages & Routes of Administration that are Commonly Used
ORAL: No typical dosage.

Comments
Karaya gum is a common adulterant in tragacanth (16). It is important to use any amount with adequate fluid intake to prevent esophageal closure or obstruction of the ileus (18).

TRAILING ARBUTUS

This Product is Also Known As
Gravel Plant, Ground Laurel, Mountain Pink, Water Pink, Winter Pink.

Scientific Names
Epigaea repens.
Family: Ericaceae.

People Use This For
Orally, trailing arbutus is used for urinary tract conditions, as an astringent, and a diuretic (18).

Safety
POSSIBLY SAFE …when the leaves are used orally short-term (12).
UNSAFE …when the fresh or dried leaves are used orally long-term because they could cause hydroquinone toxicity (18).
PREGNANCY AND LACTATION: Insufficient reliable information available for oral use; avoid using.

Effectiveness
There is insufficient reliable information available about the effectiveness of trailing arbutus.

Possible Mechanism of Action & Active Ingredients
The applicable parts of trailing arbutus are the above ground parts. Trailing arbutus is not suitable for long term use due to its hydroquinone glycoside content (18). Arbutin may have urinary antiseptic properties due to hydrolysis to its hydroquinone by the intestinal flora (7,11). As a result, long term use is stated to lead to hydroquinone toxicity (18).

Adverse Reactions Including Known Allergies
Chronic use of trailing arbutus may lead to hydroquinone toxicity. Symptoms of toxicity include tinnitus, vomiting, delirium, convulsions, and collapse (11). Liver damage, cachexia, hemolytic anemia, and hair depigmentation may also occur with long term use (18). Overdosage could lead to inflammation of the mucous membranes of the bladder and urinary tract, and may be accompanied by bloody urine, difficulty with urination, and painful urination (18).

Possible Interactions with Herbs & Other Dietary Supplements
Insufficient reliable information available.

Possible Interactions with Drugs
No interactions are known to occur, and there is no known reason to expect a clinically significant interaction with trailing arbutus.

Possible Interactions with Foods
No interactions are known to occur, and there is no known reason to expect a clinically significant interaction with trailing arbutus.

Possible Interactions with Lab Tests
No interactions are known to occur, and there is no known reason to expect a clinically significant interaction with trailing arbutus.

Possible Interactions with Diseases or Conditions
No interactions are known to occur, and there is no known reason to expect a clinically significant interaction with trailing arbutus.

Typical Dosages & Routes of Administration that are Commonly Used
ORAL: Trailing arbutus is taken as a tea or extract (18).

Comments
Trailing arbutus's alternate name of gravel plant is similar to that of gravel root. Be careful not to confuse the two.

TRAVELER'S JOY

This Product is Also Known As
Travelers Joy.
CAUTION: See separate listings for Clematis and Woodbine.

Scientific Names
Clematis vitalba.
Family: Ranunculaceae.

People Use This For
Orally, traveler's joy was formerly used for diseases of the male genitals.
Topically, it is used for poorly healing wounds.
Orally and topically, it is used in small doses for migraine headaches (18).

Safety

LIKELY UNSAFE ...when used orally or topically for any reason due to protoanemonin, a severe local irritant (18).
PREGNANCY AND LACTATION: LIKELY UNSAFE ...contraindicated for oral or topical use (18).

Effectiveness

There is insufficient reliable information available about the effectiveness of traveler's joy.

Possible Mechanism of Action & Active Ingredients

The applicable part of traveler's joy is the fresh leaf. When the fresh plant is crushed or cut into small pieces, the glycoside ranunculin is enzymatically changed into a severely irritating protoanemonin, which, in turn, rapidly degrades into the less toxic anemonin (18). Both protoanemonin and ranunculin are destroyed to an unknown extent during the drying process (2).

Adverse Reactions Including Known Allergies

Ingestion of traveler's joy can cause severe irritation of the gastrointestinal tract, including colic and diarrhea. Irritation of the urinary tract can also occur. Skin contact can cause blisters and burns that are difficult to heal (18).

Possible Interactions with Herbs & Other Dietary Supplements

Insufficient reliable information available.

Possible Interactions with Drugs

No interactions are known to occur, and there is no known reason to expect a clinically significant interaction with traveler's joy.

Possible Interactions with Foods

No interactions are known to occur, and there is no known reason to expect a clinically significant interaction with traveler's joy

Possible Interactions with Lab Tests

No interactions are known to occur, and there is no known reason to expect a clinically significant interaction with traveler's joy.

Possible Interactions with Diseases or Conditions

No interactions are known to occur, and there is no known reason to expect a clinically significant interaction with traveler's joy.

Typical Dosages & Routes of Administration that are Commonly Used

No typical dosage.

Comments

Traveler's joy is considered likely unsafe; avoid using (18).

TREE OF HEAVEN

This Product is Also Known As

Ailanthus Glandulosa, Ailanto, A-Lan-Thus, Chinese Sumach, Copal Tree, Heaven Tree, Paradise Tree, Varnish Tree, Vernis de Japon.

Scientific Names

Ailanthus altissima.
Family: Simaroubaceae.

People Use This For

In Chinese medicine, dried bark of the tree of heaven is used for pathological leukorrhea, diarrhea, chronic diarrhea, chronic dysentery, and dysmenorrhea (18).
In Africa, it has been used to treat asthma, cramps, epilepsy, fast heart rate, gonorrhea, malaria, and tapeworms (18). It has also been used as a bitter and a tonic (4500).
For food uses, the young leaves of the tree are eaten (4500).
In manufacturing, the quassinoid constituents of the tree of heaven are used as insecticide (4500,4501).

Safety

There is insufficient reliable information available about the safety of tree of heaven. However, fatal poisonings have been reported in animal experiments (18).
Pregnancy and Lactation: Insufficient reliable information available; avoid using.

Effectiveness

There is insufficient reliable information about the effectiveness of tree of heaven.

Possible Mechanism of Action & Active Ingredients

The applicable parts of tree of heaven are the dried trunk and root bark. The bark of the tree of heaven is said to have astringent, antipyretic, and antispasmodic properties (18). Some evidence suggests the quassionoid constituents, including ailanthone and quassin, have antiprotozoan, antihelminthic, antileukemic, and cytotoxic properties (18,4501). The bark also contains tannins and indole alkaloids of the beta-carbolic type (18).

Adverse Reactions Including Known Allergies

Ingesting large amounts of the tree of heaven bark can cause queasiness, dizziness, headache, limb tingling, and diarrhea (18). Skin contact with the leaves can cause dermatitis (4501).

Possible Interactions with Herbs & Other Dietary Supplements

Insufficient reliable information available.

Possible Interactions with Drugs

No interactions are known to occur, and there is no known reason to expect a clinically significant interaction with tree of heaven.

Possible Interactions with Foods

No interactions are known to occur, and there is no known reason to expect a clinically significant interaction with tree of heaven.

Possible Interactions with Lab Tests

No interactions are known to occur, and there is no known reason to expect a clinically significant interaction with tree of heaven.

Possible Interactions with Diseases or Conditions

No interactions are known to occur, and there is no known reason to expect a clinically significant interaction with tree of heaven.

Typical Dosages & Routes of Administration that are Commonly Used

Daily dose is 6-9 grams (18). No further information available.

Comments

Although native to China, the tree of heaven has been naturalized to the United States (4501). Until recently, it was used only in folk medicine. Currently, it is being investigated as a potential drug (18).

TRYPSIN

This Product is Also Known As

Proteinase, Proteolytic Enzyme, Tripsin.

Scientific Names

Trypsin.

People Use This For

Orally, trypsin is used for digestive enzyme supplementation in conjunction with lipase, amylase, and other proteases (801,2647).

In combination with bromelain and rutin, trypsin is used for osteoarthritis (6252).

Topically, it is used for wound and ulcer cleansing to remove necrotic tissue and debris (13). Also, the prescription aerosol products containing trypsin, Peru balsam, and castor oil are applied topically for enzymatic debridement, promotion of normal wound healing (506), and promoting the healing of necrotic oral mucosa ulcers (2644).

Safety

POSSIBLY SAFE ...when used topically by health care professionals trained in wound debridement (506). The topical combination containing trypsin, Peru balsam, and castor oil is a FDA-approved prescription aerosol product.

There is insufficient reliable information available about the safety of trypsin for its other uses.

PREGNANCY AND LACTATION: Insufficient reliable information available; avoid using.

Effectiveness

POSSIBLY EFFECTIVE ...when taken orally in combination with bromelain and rutin for treating osteoarthritis (6252). In a double-blind trial, 73 patients with painful osteoarthritis of the knee were randomly assigned the combination enzyme product (Phlogenzym) or diclofenac (Voltaren) 50 mg three times daily during the first week and then twice daily in weeks 2 and 3. The enzyme product was similar to diclofenac in relieving pain and improving knee function (6252). ...when used topically for cleansing wounds of necrotic material and enhancing wound healing (2643,2645).

There is insufficient reliable information available about the effectiveness of trypsin for its other uses.

Possible Mechanism of Action & Active Ingredients

Trypsin is a proteolytic enzyme formed in the small intestines by the action of enteropeptidase on trypsinogen (511). It is used to remove dead tissue that remains after trauma, infections such as decubitus ulcers, and surgical procedures. The removal of dead cells allows the growth of healthy tissues (13). Some topical preparations that are available contain balsam of Peru and castor oil to protect the skin and prevent premature epithelial destruction (13). Evidence from in vitro studies of necroses and purulent exudates (2648) and a human study (2649) shows streptokinase-streptodornase can have better proteolytic activity than trypsin alone.

Adverse Reactions Including Known Allergies

When applied topically, trypsin can cause localized pain (2643) and transient burning (506).

Possible Interactions with Herbs & Other Dietary Supplements

There is insufficient reliable information available.

Possible Interactions with Drugs

No interactions are known to occur, and there is no known reason to expect a clinically significant interaction with trypsin.

Possible Interactions with Foods

No interactions are known to occur, and there is no known reason to expect a clinically significant interaction with trypsin.

Possible Interactions with Lab Tests

No interactions are known to occur, and there is no known reason to expect a clinically significant interaction with trypsin.

Possible Interactions with Diseases or Conditions

No interactions are known to occur, and there is no known reason to expect a clinically significant interaction with trypsin.

Typical Dosages & Routes of Administration that are Commonly Used

ORAL: For osteoarthritis, a combination enzyme product (Phlogenzym), which contains rutin 100 mg, trypsin 48 mg, and bromelain 90 mg, was given 2 tablets 3 times daily (6252).
TOPICAL: Wound debridement products (Dermuspray, Granulderm, Granulex, and GranuMed) containing trypsin, Peru balsam, and castor oil (506) are FDA-approved prescription products.

Comments

Commercial trypsin is prepared from animal sources, such as ox pancreas (13).

TUNG SEED

This Product is Also Known As

Balucanat, Candleberry, Candle-berry Tree, Candlenut, China-Wood Oil, Country Walnut, Indian Walnut, Kukui, Otaheite Walnut, Tung, Varnish Tree.

Scientific Names

Aleurites moluccana or Aleurites cordata.
Family: Euphorbiaceae.

People Use This For

Orally, tung seed is used for asthma (6), bloody diarrhea (4502), dysentery (4502), sprue (4502), and as a bowel stimulant (6,4502).
Topically, tung seed is used to stimulate hair growth and for constipation (4502).
In manufacturing, the oil of tung seed is used in soaps, rubber substitutes, linoleum, and insulation (6,4502). The seed cake of tung seed is used as a fertilizer (6). The seed is also the source of the oil that is widely used as a wood preservative and varnish (6,4502).

Safety

LIKELY UNSAFE ...when used orally (6,4501). Tung seed is believed to contain toxalbumin and hydrogen cyanide (6). Toxicity ranges from severe gastrointestinal irritation to death (6,4501,4502). Even a single seed might cause severe poisoning (4502).
There is insufficient reliable information available about the safety of the topical use of tung seed.
PREGNANCY AND LACTATION: LIKELY UNSAFE ...when used orally (6,4501).

Effectiveness

There is insufficient reliable information available about the effectiveness of tung seed.

Possible Mechanism of Action & Active Ingredients

Tung seed contains an oil that consists of eleostearic acid, linolenic, linoleic and oleic acid. It is also thought to contain a toxalbumin and hydrogen cyanide (6). Taken internally, tung oil has cathartic effects (6,4502). The kernels have laxative and stimulant effects. They also promote sweating (4502).

Adverse Reactions Including Known Allergies

Ingestion of the raw seed of tung seed can cause severe stomach pain, violent vomiting, debility, diarrhea, slowed reflexes, slowed breathing, and possibly death (6,4501,4502). Skin contact with tung seed can cause acute dermatitis (4501,4502).

Possible Interactions with Herbs & Other Dietary Supplements

Insufficient reliable information available.

Possible Interactions with Drugs

No interactions are known to occur, and there is no known reason to expect a clinically significant interaction with tung seed.

Possible Interactions with Foods

No interactions are known to occur, and there is no known reason to expect a clinically significant interaction with tung seed

Possible Interactions with Lab Tests

No interactions are known to occur, and there is no known reason to expect a clinically significant interaction with tung seed.

Possible Interactions with Diseases or Conditions

No interactions are known to occur, and there is no known reason to expect a clinically significant interaction with tung seed.

Typical Dosages & Routes of Administration that are Commonly Used

No typical dosage.

Comments

Tung seed is considered likely unsafe; avoid using. The seeds of the fruit from this plant resemble a walnut, and the term walnut is applied to this species (4501). Tung seed should never be confused with the common walnut. Unlike the walnut, if tung seeds are eaten raw they are toxic. When roasted, the kernels are reported to be edible (6,4501). It is said that fishermen throw tung seeds into the water to stupefy the fish (6,4502).

TURKEY CORN

This Product is Also Known As

Bleeding Heart, Corydalis, Dutchman's Breeches, Squirrel Corn, Staggerweed.
CAUTION: See separate listing for Corydalis.

Scientific Names

Dicentra cucullaria.
Family: Furnariaceae.

People Use This For

Orally, the tuber of turkey corn is used for digestive and menstrual disorders, urinary tract diseases, and skin rashes (18).

Safety

POSSIBLY UNSAFE …when the dried tuber is used orally. Theoretically, the constituent bicuculline, an antagonist of gamma-aminobutyric acid (GABA), could cause poisoning (18).
PREGNANCY AND LACTATION: POSSIBLY UNSAFE; avoid using.

Effectiveness

There is insufficient reliable information available about the effectiveness of turkey corn.

Possible Mechanism of Action & Active Ingredients

The applicable part of turkey corn is the dried tuber. Turkey corn is thought to have diuretic and tonic properties (18). It contains various isoquinoline alkaloids, including bicuculline, corlumine, protopine, cryptopine, and cularine. Bicuculline is a centrally-acting, spasmogenic antagonist of GABA (18).

Adverse Reactions Including Known Allergies

None reported.

Possible Interactions with Herbs & Other Dietary Supplements
Insufficient reliable information available.

Possible Interactions with Drugs
No interactions are known to occur, and there is no known reason to expect a clinically significant interaction with turkey corn.

Possible Interactions with Foods
No interactions are known to occur, and there is no known reason to expect a clinically significant interaction with turkey corn

Possible Interactions with Lab Tests
No interactions are known to occur, and there is no known reason to expect a clinically significant interaction with turkey corn.

Possible Interactions with Diseases or Conditions
No interactions are known to occur, and there is no known reason to expect a clinically significant interaction with turkey corn.

Typical Dosages & Routes of Administration that are Commonly Used
ORAL: No typical dosage.

Comments
Turkey corn is used as a liquid extract (18).

TURMERIC

This Product is Also Known As
Curcuma, Curcumae longae rhizoma, Curcumin, Indian Saffron, Tumeric, Turmeric, Turmeric Root.
CAUTION: See separate listings for Javanese Turmeric, Zedoary, and Goldenseal.

Scientific Names
Curcuma longa, synonyms Curcuma domestica, Curcuma aromatica.
Family: Zingiberaceae.

People Use This For
Orally, turmeric root is used for dyspepsia (2,18), hemorrhage, jaundice, hepatitis (6), flatulence (6,18), abdominal bloating, feelings of fullness after meals, loss of appetite, liver and gallbladder complaints, headaches, abdominal pains, chest infections, fever, diarrhea, amenorrhea, and "blood rushes" (18).
Topically, turmeric is used for analgesia, ringworm (6), bruising, leech bites, festering eye infections, inflammatory skin conditions, inflammation of the oral mucosa, and infected wounds (18).
In folk medicine, turmeric root is used for diarrhea, intermittent fever, edema, bronchitis, colds, worms, leprosy, kidney inflammation, cystitis (18), and as an anticancer treatment (6).
In food and manufacturing, the essential oil is used in perfumes (11), and turmeric and its resin are used as a flavor and color component in foods (11). Turmeric is a culinary spice and a major ingredient in curry powder (6).

Safety
LIKELY SAFE ...in amounts commonly found in foods (11). It has Generally Recognized as Safe (GRAS) status in the US as a food product (11). Maximum amount used in food is 22%, maximum amount used as a is spice 0.883%.
POSSIBLY SAFE ...when used orally or topically in medicinal amounts (2,12).
PREGNANCY: LIKELY SAFE ...when used as a spice. LIKELY UNSAFE ...when used in larger amounts because it might stimulate menstrual flow and the uterus (12).
LACTATION: LIKELY SAFE ...when used in amounts in food as a spice. There is insufficient reliable information available about the safety of larger amounts of turmeric during lactation.

Effectiveness
POSSIBLY EFFECTIVE ...when taken orally for dyspepsia (2).
There is insufficient reliable information available about the effectiveness of turmeric for its other uses.

Possible Mechanism of Action & Active Ingredients
The applicable part of turmeric is the root. Turmeric is rich in potassium and iron (19). Turmeric root contains volatile oil and diarylheptanoids, including curcumin. The constituents of the oil show evidence of anti-inflammatory and antiarthritic activity (11). In preliminary research, turmeric-containing products demonstrate anti-inflammatory effects, but fail to show antipyretic activity (6131). Curcumin can have bile-stimulating, liver-protectant, antioxidant, and anticancer effects (6,18). Aqueous extracts also show some evidence of hypotensive effects and antispasmodic activity (11). Some evidence suggests they might also lower serum cholesterol and triglycerides. Curcuminoid constituents are responsible for the yellow color of turmeric (512).

Adverse Reactions Including Known Allergies
Overuse or long-term use of turmeric orally can cause GI disturbances and complaints (18,512).

Possible Interactions with Herbs & Other Dietary Supplements
HERBS WITH ANTICOAGULANT/ANTIPLATELET POTENTIAL: Concomitant use of herbs that have coumarin constituents or affect platelet aggregation could theoretically increase the risk of bleeding in some people. These herbs include: angelica, anise, arnica, asafoetida, bogbean, boldo, capsicum, celery, chamomile, clove, danshen, fenugreek, feverfew, garlic, ginger, ginkgo, ginseng (Panax), horse chestnut, horseradish, licorice, meadowsweet, prickly ash, onion, papain, passionflower, poplar, quassia, red clover, wild carrot, wild lettuce, willow, and others (4,19).

Possible Interactions with Drugs
ANTIPLATELET DRUGS: Theoretically, turmeric might increase the effects and adverse effects of antiplatelet drugs (19).
RESERPINE AND INDOMETHACIN: Theoretically, turmeric root might reduce the frequency of reserpine and indomethacin induced gastric/duodenal ulcers (19).

Possible Interactions with Foods
No interactions are known to occur, and there is no known reason to expect a clinically significant interaction with turmeric.

Possible Interactions with Lab Tests
No interactions are known to occur, and there is no known reason to expect a clinically significant interaction with turmeric

Possible Interactions with Diseases or Conditions
OBSTRUCTION/GALLSTONES: Turmeric is contraindicated in individuals with bile duct obstruction (2,12) or gallstones.
GI DISORDERS: Turmeric is contraindicated in individuals with stomach ulcers or hyperacidity disorders (12).

Typical Dosages & Routes of Administration that are Commonly Used
ORAL: The typical dose of turmeric is 0.5-1 grams of the powdered root several times daily between meals (8) up to 1.5-3 grams per day (2). Standardized preparations are preferred to tea preparations due to the low aqueous solubility of the volatile oil and the other active constituents (8). The tincture (1:10) is commonly dosed as 10-15 drops two to three times daily (18).
TOPICAL: No typical dosage.

Comments
Turmeric has a warm, bitter taste and a yellow color, and it is frequently used to flavor or color curry powders, mustards, butters, and cheeses (6,6002). Avoid confusion with Javanese tumeric root.

TURPENTINE OIL

This Product is Also Known As
Purified Turpentine Oil, Spirits Of Turpentine, Terebinthinae aetheroleum, Turpentine.

Scientific Names
Pinus palustris, synonym Pinus australis; Pinus pinaster; other Pinus species.
Family: Pinaceae.

People Use This For
Topically, turpentine oil is used for rheumatic and neuralgic ailments (2), muscle pain, toothaches, and disseminated sclerosis (6).
By inhalation, the vapors of turpentine oil are used to reduce the thickened secretions associated with chronic diseases of the bronchi (2).
In foods and beverages, distilled turpentine oil is used as a flavoring ingredient (11).
In manufacturing, the turpentine resin is often used as an ingredient in soap and cosmetics (11). Turpentine oil is also utilized as a paint solvent (6).

Safety
LIKELY SAFE ...when used in the very small amounts used in foods. In the US, turpentine oil is approved for food use, and the maximum level is 0.002% (11).
POSSIBLY SAFE ...when used topically and appropriately (2). ...when the vapors are inhaled appropriately (2).
POSSIBLY UNSAFE ...when applied topically to large areas (2).
LIKELY UNSAFE ...when taken orally for medicinal purposes. 2 mL/kg of turpentine oil is considered

toxic (17). 120-180 mL is potentially lethal in adults (17). Pulmonary aspiration can cause hemorrhagic pulmonary edema (17).

CHILDREN: LIKELY UNSAFE ...when used orally, 15 mL is potentially lethal (17). There is insufficient reliable information available about the safety of turpentine oil applied topically or inhaled as vapors in children.

PREGNANCY AND LACTATION: LIKELY UNSAFE ...contraindicated for oral use. It might be an abortifacient (19). There is insufficient reliable information available about the safety of turpentine oil applied topically or inhaled as vapors during pregnancy and lactation.

Effectiveness

POSSIBLY EFFECTIVE ...when used as inhalation therapy for chronic diseases of the bronchi with heavy secretion (2). ...when used topically for rheumatic and neuralgic ailments (2).

There is insufficient reliable information available about the effectiveness of turpentine oil for its other uses.

Possible Mechanism of Action & Active Ingredients

Turpentine oil is a central nervous system depressant and a pulmonary aspiration hazard. When applied topically, turpentine oil is irritating and exhibits rubefacient and counterirritant effects (6,11). When inhaled, turpentine oil can have a decongestant effect, possibly by stimulating the cold receptors, which results in reflex vasoconstriction (7).

Adverse Reactions Including Known Allergies

Turpentine oil used orally can cause headache, insomnia, coughing, vomiting, hematuria, albuminuria (6), urinary tract inflammation (17), coma (6), and death (17). Pulmonary aspiration produces hemorrhagic pulmonary edema (17). When used as an inhalation therapy, it can cause mild respiratory tract inflammation (17). Turpentine can exacerbate bronchial spasms in people with asthma and whooping cough (7). Topically, it can cause skin irritation, contact allergies, and hypersensitivity (6). Symptoms of poisoning can occur when turpentine oil is applied extensively, including kidney and central nervous system damage (2).

Possible Interactions with Herbs & Other Dietary Supplements

Insufficient reliable information available.

Possible Interactions with Drugs

No interactions are known to occur, and there is no known reason to expect a clinically significant interaction with turpentine oil.

Possible Interactions with Foods

No interactions are known to occur, and there is no known reason to expect a clinically significant interaction with turpentine oil.

Possible Interactions with Lab Tests

No interactions are known to occur, and there is no known reason to expect a clinically significant interaction with turpentine oil.

Possible Interactions with Diseases or Conditions

ACUTE RESPIRATORY TRACT INFLAMMATION: Inhalation of turpentine is contraindicated (2).
ASTHMA, WHOOPING COUGH: Turpentine can exacerbate bronchial spasms (7).
HYPERSENSITIVITY: Contraindicated (2).

Typical Dosages & Routes of Administration that are Commonly Used

INHALATION: The vapors of turpentine are often inhaled as several drops of the oil in hot water (2).
TOPICAL: Several drops of the oil are typically rubbed onto the affected area. The liquid and semi-solid preparations are commonly made in concentrations of 10-50% (2). Application of turpentine should not exceed three to four times per day (3).

Comments

Turpentine oil is obtained by the distillation of the oleoresin (gum turpentine) of longleaf pine (Pinus palustris) and other Pinus species. Terpin hydrate is a semi-synthetic derivative of turpentine (6). Turpentine oil has been used to adulterate juniper berry oil (512). Avoid confusion with gum turpentine, which is the oleoresin (6).

TURTLE HEAD

This Product is Also Known As

Balmony, Bitter Herb, Chelone, Hummingbird Tree, Salt-rheum Weed, Shellflower, Snakehead, Turtlebloom.

Scientific Names

Chelone glabra.
Family: Scrophulariaceae.

People Use This For

Orally, turtle head above ground parts and roots are used as a cathartic tonic (4500).

Safety

POSSIBLY SAFE ...when used orally(12,18).
PREGNANCY AND LACTATION: Insufficient reliable information available; avoid using.

Effectiveness

There is insufficient reliable information available about the effectiveness of turtle head (18).

Possible Mechanism of Action & Active Ingredients

The applicable parts of turtle head are the above ground parts and root. Contains iridoide monoterpenes including catalpol and a bitter-tasting resin (18).

Adverse Reactions Including Known Allergies

None reported.

Possible Interactions with Herbs & Other Dietary Supplements

Insufficient reliable information available.

Possible Interactions with Drugs

No interactions are known to occur, and there is no known reason to expect a clinically significant interaction with turtle head.

Possible Interactions with Foods

No interactions are known to occur, and there is no known reason to expect a clinically significant interaction with turtle head.

Possible Interactions with Lab Tests

No interactions are known to occur, and there is no known reason to expect a clinically significant interaction with turtle head.

Possible Interactions with Diseases or Conditions

No interactions are known to occur, and there is no known reason to expect a clinically significant interaction with turtle head.

Typical Dosages & Routes of Administration that are Commonly Used

No typical dosage.

Comments

Avoid confusion with Chelone obliqua commonly known as red turtle head (4500).

USNEA

This Product is Also Known As

Beard Moss, Old Man's Beard, Tree Moss, Tree's Dandruff, Usnea Lichen, Woman's Long Hair.
CAUTION: See separate listing for Oak Moss.

Scientific Names

Usnea species, including Usnea barbata, Usnea florida, Usnea hirta, Usnea plicata.
Family: Usneaceae.

People Use This For

Topically, usnea is used for mild inflammation of the mouth and pharynx (2,18).

Safety

POSSIBLY SAFE ...when applied topically and used appropriately (2,12).
PREGNANCY AND LACTATION: Insufficient reliable information available; avoid using.

Effectiveness

POSSIBLY EFFECTIVE ...when used topically for mild inflammation of the oral and pharyngeal mucosa (2).

Possible Mechanism of Action & Active Ingredients

The applicable part of usnea is the plant body. Usnea contains a variety of lichen acids including usnic acid, thamnolic acid, lobaric acid, stictinic acid, evernic acid, barbatic acid, diffractaic acid, protocetraric acid. However, the exact composition varies significantly amongst species. Usnea is considered to have antimicrobial activity (2). The hydroalcoholic extracts of Usnea barbata and Usnea hirta have anti-inflammatory, analgesic, and antipyretic activity (852).

Adverse Reactions Including Known Allergies

Adverse reactions are uncommon in appropriate amounts. Poisoning can be possible, although signs of poisoning have not yet been described (18).

Possible Interactions with Herbs & Other Dietary Supplements
Insufficient reliable information available.

Possible Interactions with Drugs
No interactions are known to occur, and there is no known reason to expect a clinically significant interaction with usnea.

Possible Interactions with Foods
No interactions are known to occur, and there is no known reason to expect a clinically significant interaction with usnea.

Possible Interactions with Lab Tests
No interactions are known to occur, and there is no known reason to expect a clinically significant interaction with usnea.

Possible Interactions with Diseases or Conditions
No interactions are known to occur, and there is no known reason to expect a clinically significant interaction with usnea.

Typical Dosages & Routes of Administration that are Commonly Used
TOPICAL: The typical dose of usnea is one lozenge three to six times per day. Each lozenge usual contains the equivalent of 100 mg dried usnea (2).

Comments
Usnea species are whitish, reddish, or black lichens that grow on a variety of trees. Avoid confusion with oak moss (Evernia prunastri), also referred to as tree moss.

UVA URSI

This Product is Also Known As
Arberry, Arcostaphylos, Bearberry, Beargrape, Bearsgrape, Bear's Grape, Common Bearberry, Hogberry, Kinnikinnik, Manzanita, Mountain Box, Mountain Cranberry, Ptarmigan Berry, Raisin D'Ours, Red Bearberry, Redberry, Rockberry, Sagackhomi, Sandberry, Uvae ursi folium, Uva-ursi.
CAUTION: See separate listings for Alpine Cranberry, Cramp Bark, and Cranberry.

Scientific Names
Arctostaphylos uva-ursi, synonym Arbutus uva-ursi.
Family: Ericacea.

People Use This For
Orally, uva ursi is taken for urinary tract infections (4,5,6,18), inflammatory conditions of the efferent urinary tract (2,5,18), cystitis, urethritis, diuresis, constipation (4,5,6), lithuria, dysuria, acidic urine, pyelonephritis (4), and bronchitis (11).
In combination, an herbal preparation containing uva ursi, hops, and peppermint is used to treat people with compulsive, strangury enuresis and painful urination (4).

Safety
POSSIBLY SAFE ...when the leaf is used orally and appropriately on a short-term basis (2,4,12). Urinary tract symptoms persisting longer than 48 hours should be medically evaluated (4).
POSSIBLY UNSAFE ...when used orally longer than 1 week or more than 5 times per year. It should be monitored because the constituent, hydroquinone, can have mutagenic and carcinogenic effects. Over extended periods of time, hydroquinone can also lead to hepatotoxicity (2,7,18).
CHILDREN: LIKELY UNSAFE ... contraindicated for use due to the risk of hepatotoxicity in children less than 12 years old (2,7,18).
PREGNANCY: LIKELY UNSAFE ...contraindicated for use (2,4,6,7,12,18) because it can be oxytocic (increases the rapidity of labor) (19).
LACTATION: Insufficient reliable information available; avoid using (2).

Effectiveness
POSSIBLY EFFECTIVE ...when used orally for inflammatory disorders of the efferent urinary tract (2). Clinical studies on the effectiveness of uva ursi have used extracts standardized to 20% arbutin.
There is insufficient reliable information available about the effectiveness of uva ursi for its other uses.

Possible Mechanism of Action & Active Ingredients
The applicable part of uva ursi is the leaf. Uva ursi can have urinary antiseptic and astringent effects (4). Some references report diuretic activity, but others disagree (6,8). Its constituents include arbutin (a phenol), tannins, and hydroquinone (4,6,7). The tannins can be responsible for adverse gastrointestinal tract effects (5) and limit the

duration of use (4). Uva ursi and the constituent, arbutin, exhibit antimicrobial activity in vitro (2,4). Arbutin is absorbed from the gastrointestinal tract unchanged and is hydrolyzed to hydroquinone in alkaline urine. There it can exert antiseptic and astringent effects (4,5,7). Hydroquinone is cytotoxic in vitro (4). Crude uva ursi extract can be more effective than the constituent arbutin as an astringent and antiseptic (4). In rats, uva ursi shows anti-inflammatory activity against experimentally-induced inflammation (4). Large amounts of uva ursi are reported to be oxytocic, although in vitro studies show no uteroactivity (4).

Adverse Reactions Including Known Allergies

Uva ursi taken orally can cause nausea, vomiting (2), gastrointestinal discomfort, and a greenish-brown discoloration of the urine (4). Large amounts can be oxytocic, increasing the rapidity of labor (4). One gram of hydroquinone, equivalent to 6-20 grams of uva ursi, can cause tinnitus, nausea, vomiting, shortness of breath, cyanosis, convulsions, delirium, and collapse (4). Five grams of hydroquinone, equivalent to 30-100 grams of uva ursi, can cause death (4). Other adverse effects due to uva ursi include hepatotoxicity and irritation and inflammation of the urinary tract mucous membranes (18). Chronic use, especially in children (18), can cause liver impairment due to its tannin content (4).

Possible Interactions with Herbs & Other Dietary Supplements

URINE-ACIDIFIERS: Theoretically, concomitant use of uva ursi with products that acidify the urine, including vitamin C, can reduce the antibacterial activity of uva ursi (2,12,19).
URINE-ALKALINIZERS: Theoretically, concomitant use of uva ursi with products that alkalinize the urine, including sodium bicarbonate, can enhance the antibacterial activity of uva ursi (8).

Possible Interactions with Drugs

URINE-ACIDIFYING DRUGS: Concomitant use with drugs that acidify the urine can reduce the antibacterial efficacy of uva ursi (2,19).
URINE-ALKALINIZING DRUGS: Theoretically, concomitant use with drugs that alkalinize the urine can enhance the antibacterial activity of uva ursi (2,19).

Possible Interactions with Foods

URINE-ACIDIFYING FOODS: Foods that acidify urine, including acidic fruits and juices, can reduce the antibacterial activity of uva ursi (2,5,19).
URINE-ALKALINIZING FOODS: Foods that alkalinize urine can enhance the antibacterial activity of uva ursi (7,8).

Possible Interactions with Lab Tests

COLORIMETRIC URINE TESTS: Theoretically, uva ursi can interfere with colorimetric urine tests and can turn urine greenish-brown (4).

Possible Interactions with Diseases or Conditions

KIDNEY DISORDERS: Contraindicated (12,19).
GI IRRITATION: Because excessive use of uva ursi can lead to stomach distress due to its tannin content, its use is contraindicated in patients with GI irritation (12,19).

Typical Dosages & Routes of Administration that are Commonly Used

ORAL: The typical dose is one cup of the tea taken up to four times daily. The tea is prepared by steeping 3 grams of the dried leaf in 150 mL cold water for 12-24 hours and then straining (2,7,515). Uva ursi leaf teas should be prepared with cold water to minimize the tannin content (515). The hydroquinone derivative, calculated as water-free arbutin, is commonly dosed as 100-210 mg up to four times daily (2,7,515). Clinical studies on the effectiveness of uva ursi have used extracts standardized to 20% arbutin. The fluid extract (1:1 in 25% alcohol) is given 1.5-4 mL three times daily (4). Medical consultation is needed for urinary tract symptoms persisting longer than 48 hours (4). Uva ursi should not be used longer than one week without monitoring due to its potential risks (7). Limit its use to less than five times per year (7).

Comments

Bears are particularly fond of the fruit, which is implied in the Latin name "uva ursi", which means "bear's grape" (6). Most authorities refer to Arctostaphylos uva-ursi as uva ursi. However, the related plants, Arctostaphylos adentricha and Arctostaphylos coactylis, have also been termed uva ursi by some authors (6). Although the chemistry of uva ursi and the pharmacologic activity of arbutin and hydroquinone are well-documented (4), clinical studies are needed to evaluate uva ursi treatment in urinary tract infections (4,7).

UZARA

This Product is Also Known As

Uzara, Uzarae radix.

Scientific Names
Xysmalobium undulatum.
Family: Asclepiadaceae.

People Use This For
Orally, uzara root is used for diarrhea (2,18).

Safety
POSSIBLY SAFE ...when taken orally for short-term use (2). Medical consultation is needed for diarrhea persisting more than three to four days (2).
LIKELY UNSAFE ...Deaths have occurred after parenteral administration of uzara products (18).
PREGNANCY AND LACTATION: Insufficient reliable information available; avoid using.

Effectiveness
POSSIBLY EFFECTIVE ...when taken orally for nonspecific, acute diarrhea (2).

Possible Mechanism of Action & Active Ingredients
The applicable part of uzara is the root. It inhibits intestinal motility (2), and in larger amounts, it can have digitalis-like effects on the heart (2). Uzara contains a cardiac glycoside mixture of cardenolides, which include uzarone, xysmalobin, and uzarin. The glycosides can be poorly absorbed (2,18).

Adverse Reactions Including Known Allergies
There have been no reports of adverse reactions associated with white uzara, but it is theoretically possible due to the cardiac glycoside content (2,18). Deaths have occurred after parenteral administration of uzara products (18).

Possible Interactions with Herbs & Other Dietary Supplements
CARDIAC GLYCOSIDE-CONTAINING HERBS: Uzara is contraindicated with these herbs, and concomitant use can increase the risk of cardiac glycoside toxicity. Cardiac glycoside containing herbs include black hellebore, Canadian hemp roots, digitalis leaf, hedge mustard, figwort, lily of the valley roots, motherwort, oleander leaf, pheasant's eye plant, pleurisy root, squill bulb leaf scales, and strophanthus seeds (2,18,19,500).
OTHER CARDIOACTIVE HERBS: Avoid concomitant use with other cardioactive herbs due to the unpredictability of therapeutic and adverse effects. Other cardioactive herbs include calamus, cereus, cola, coltsfoot, devil's claw, European mistletoe, fenugreek, fumitory, ginger, ginseng Panax, hawthorn, white horehound, mate, parsley, quassia, scotch broom flower, shepherd's purse, and wild carrot (4).
STIMULANT LAXATIVE HERBS: Theoretically, overuse or misuse of stimulant laxatives with cardiac glycoside-containing herbs increases the risk of cardiac toxicity due to potassium depletion. Stimulant laxative herbs include the dried leaf sap of aloe, blue flag rhizome, alder buckthorn, European buckthorn, butternut bark, cascara bark, castor oil, colocynth fruit pulp, gamboge bark exudate, jalap root, black root, manna bark exudate, podophyllum root, rhubarb root, senna leaves and pods, wild cucumber fruit (Ecballium elaterium), and yellow dock root (19).
LICORICE/HORSETAIL: Theoretically, overuse or misuse of the licorice rhizome or horsetail plant with cardiac glycoside-containing herbs increases the risk of cardiac toxicity due to potassium depletion (19).

Possible Interactions with Drugs
DIGOXIN: Uzara is contraindicated with digoxin because therapeutic duplication increases the risk of cardiac glycoside toxicity (2).
CARDIAC DRUGS: Theoretically, concomitant use with uzara can increase the risk of cardiac toxicity (152).
STIMULANT LAXATIVES: Theoretically, overuse or misuse can increase the risk of cardiac glycoside toxicity due to potassium depletion (2).
POTASSIUM-DEPLETING DIURETICS: Theoretically, concomitant use with uzara can increase the risk of cardiac glycoside toxicity due to potassium depletion (2,506).
QUININE: Theoretically, concomitant use can increase the risk of cardiac toxicity (2,506).
TETRACYCLINES and MACROLIDE ANTIBIOTICS (erythromycin-like drugs): Theoretically, concomitant use with uzara can increase the risk of cardiac glycoside toxicity (152,17).

Possible Interactions with Foods
No interactions are known to occur, and there is no known reason to expect a clinically significant interaction with uzara.

Possible Interactions with Lab Tests
No interactions are known to occur, and there is no known reason to expect a clinically significant interaction with uzara.

Possible Interactions with Diseases or Conditions
HEART DISEASE: Uzara is contraindicated in individuals with heart disease (2,18). Theoretically, the cardiac glycosides contained in uzara can exacerbate this condition or interfere with existing drug therapy.
HYPOKALEMIA: Theoretically, the use of uzara can increase the risk of cardiac toxicity in hypokalemic patients.

© Copyright 2000, Natural Medicines Comprehensive Database (209) 472-2244. For updated data, go to www.NaturalDatabase.com

Typical Dosages & Routes of Administration that are Commonly Used

ORAL: Uzara is commonly taken as liquid ethanol-water extracts or dry extracts obtained from methanol-water extractions (2). The initial dose is 75 mg of the total glycosides calculated as uzarin or the equivalent to 1 gram of the dried root (2). Then the dose is 45-90 mg per day of the total glycosides calculated as uzarin (2). Seek medical consultation for diarrhea persisting more than three to four days (2).

Comments

None.

VALERIAN

This Product is Also Known As

Amantilla, All-Heal, Baldrian, Baldrianwurzel, Belgium Valerian, Common Valerian, Fragrant Valerian, Garden Heliotrope, Garden Valerian, Indian Valerian, Mexican Valerian, Pacific Valerian, Valeriana, Valerianae radix, Valeriana rhizome, Valeriane.

Scientific Names

Valeriana officinalis; Valeriana jatamansii, synonym Valeriana wallichii; Valeriana edulis; Valeriana sitchensis. Family: Valerianaceae.

People Use This For

Orally, valerian is used as a sedative-hypnotic and anxiolytic for restlessness and sleeping disorders associated with nervous conditions (2). It is also used for mood disorders such as depression (7), infantile convulsions, mild tremors, epilepsy, and attention deficit hyperactivity disorder (ADHD). It is used for rheumatic pain (6121), conditions associated with psychological stress including anxiety, nervous asthma, nervous headaches, gastric spasms, colic, and menstrual cramps, as well as nervous complaints caused by menopause and hot flashes (304,3484).

Topically, valerian is used as a bath additive for restlessness and sleep disorders (2,18).

Traditionally, valerian has been used for hysterical states, excitability, hypochondria, migraine, and rheumatic pains (4).

In manufacturing, the extracts and essential oil are used as flavoring in foods and beverages (11).

Safety

LIKELY SAFE ...when used in amounts found in foods. The maximum use level in foods is 0.01% for the extract and 0.002% for the essential oil. Valeriana officinalis is approved for food use in the US and has Generally Recognized as Safe (GRAS) status in the US (11,3484).

POSSIBLY SAFE ...when used orally and appropriately, short-term for medicinal purposes (12). Clinical studies have reported safe use of valerian in over 12,000 patients in trials lasting up to 14 days (304,2074,3484,3485).

POSSIBLY UNSAFE ...when used orally long term or in high doses. Extended use has been associated with a benzodiazepine-like withdrawal syndrome when discontinued. Long-term use of valerian has been associated with hepatotoxicity in four cases (304); however, some suggest that hepatotoxicity may be an idiosyncratic reaction to valerian rather than dose-related (304).

PREGNANCY AND LACTATION: Insufficient reliable information available; avoid using (4).

Effectiveness

POSSIBLY EFFECTIVE ...when used orally for decreasing sleep latency and subjectively improving the quality of sleep (7,304,3484,3485,6248,6249). Several small-scale studies have shown consistent benefit in reducing the time to sleep onset in patients using valerian compared to placebo. Some of these studies also found subjective improvement in sleep quality. However, the reliability of these positive findings is difficult to assess due to variable doses and extracts of valerian used, subject characteristics, and inconsistent methodologies (3484). A recent randomized, double-blind, placebo-controlled, cross-over study used polysomnography to determine the short-term (single dose) and long-term (14 days with multiple dosage) effects of a valerian extract versus placebo on objective sleep parameters in patients with insomnia (6249). Subjective parameters such as sleep quality, morning feeling, daytime performance, subjectively perceived duration of sleep latency, and sleep period time were assessed by means of questionnaires. No effect was observed after a single dose; however, on multiple dosing, valerian had modest positive effects on sleep structure, particularly reduction of slow-wave sleep latency, and sleep perception (6249). ...when used orally for subjective improvement in restlessness and sleep disorders associated with behavioral disorders and anxiety (2,7,304). ...when used orally for improving mood (7). Studies indicate that significant improvement may require 2-4 weeks of treatment (7). ...when used orally for subjective improvement in ability to concentrate (304,2074).

Clinical studies have used a variety of valerian root extracts (7,304,3484,3485), including some that were standardized to contain 0.4-0.6% valerenic acid (7).

There is insufficient reliable information available about the effectiveness of valerian for its other uses.

Possible Mechanism of Action & Active Ingredients

The applicable part of valerian is the root. Valerian is reported to have sedative-hypnotic, anxiolytic, antidepressant, anticonvulsant, and antispasmodic effects (7,3484,3485). Valerian might also have hypotensive and mild analgesic properties (4). The pharmacological effects of valerian have primarily been attributed to constituents known as valepotriates and volatile oils, including monoterpenes and sesquiterpenes. The primary monoterpene is berneol and the primary sesquiterpenes are valerenic acid, valerenone, and kessyl glycol (4,7,3484,3486). However, because valerian extracts without some of these constituents have similar effects, it is likely that multiple constituents are responsible for its pharmacological effects (304). Valepotriate constituents are known to have sedative-hypnotic and spasmolytic effects. Valepotriates have also been shown to decrease benzodiazepine withdrawal in an animal model and to bind dopamine receptors (3484,3486). The valepotriates might possibly act as prodrugs. They are thought to rapidly decompose to homobaldrinal in the intestine after ingestion (3486). Valepotriates are highly unstable and rapidly decompose in acid or alkaline environments and at high temperatures. Although there are published reports of toxicity due to the valepotriate constituents, because these constituents are poorly absorbed and quickly degraded to less toxic metabolites, they are not likely to cause acute adverse reactions (12). Commercial preparations are thought to rarely contain valepotriates (2,7,304). The presence of an epoxide group on the valepotriates has raised concern about possible cytotoxicity and carcinogenicity (7,3485,3486); however, in-vivo studies to date have failed to show any carcinogenic effects (3486). The sesquiterpenes, valerenic acid and kessyl glycol have been shown to cause sedation in animals (3486). Valerenic acid also appears to inhibit the enzyme system responsible for the central catabolism of GABA, increasing GABA concentrations and decreasing CNS activity (4,3486). There is some evidence that valerian might also contain other constituents such as lignans and GABA which may also be responsible for the sedative effects of valerian (304,3486).

Adverse Reactions Including Known Allergies

Valerian taken orally can cause headache, excitability, uneasiness, cardiac disturbances, and insomnia (6,12,3484). Occasionally, valerian causes morning drowsiness (2074). Although most reports describe a lack of residual morning effects on alertness and concentration, a few reports suggest that impaired alertness and information processing does occur (12,2074). Impairment is dose-dependent and peaks within the first few hours after an oral valerian dose (304,2074). Patients should be warned against driving or operating dangerous machinery after taking valerian (304). Signs of valerian toxicity include trouble walking, hypothermia, and increased muscle relaxation (6). Side effects are rare in products without valepotriate constituents (7). In one individual, 20 times the normal dose caused fatigue, tight chest, abdominal cramping, and tremor of the hand and foot (659). Extended use can cause benzodiazepine-like withdrawal symptoms when treatment is discontinued (304,3487). Patients should taper doses slowly after extended use. There have been several case reports of hepatotoxicity associated with use of multi-ingredient preparations containing valerian. In these cases, it is thought that the preparations may have been adulterated with hepatotoxic agents (304). Four other cases of hepatotoxicity involving long-term use of single-ingredient valerian preparations have also been reported (304,3484). Because a variety of doses were used in the cases reported and many people have used higher doses safely, some suggest these hepatotoxic reactions might have been idiosyncratic (304).

Possible Interactions with Herbs & Other Dietary Supplements

HERBS WITH SEDATIVE PROPERTIES: Theoretically, concomitant use with herbs that have sedative properties might enhance therapeutic and adverse effects. These include calamus, calendula, California poppy, catnip, capsicum, celery, couch grass, elecampane, ginseng Siberian, German chamomile, goldenseal, gotu kola, hops, Jamaican dogwood, kava, lemon balm, sage, St. John's wort, sassafras, scullcap, shepherd's purse, stinging nettle, wild carrot, wild lettuce, withania root, and yerba mansa (4,19).

Possible Interactions with Drugs

ALCOHOL: Theoretically, valerian can potentiate the sedative effects of alcohol (4).
BARBITURATES: Theoretically, concomitant use of valerian with barbiturates can cause additive therapeutic and adverse effects (19).
BENZODIAZEPINES: Theoretically, concomitant use with benzodiazepines can cause additive therapeutic and adverse effects (19).
OTHER DRUGS WITH SEDATIVE PROPERTIES: Theoretically, concomitant use of valerian and drugs with sedative properties can cause additive therapeutic and adverse effects (4,19).

Possible Interactions with Foods

ALCOHOL: Theoretically, valerian can potentiate the sedative effects of alcohol (4).

Possible Interactions with Lab Tests

No interactions are known to occur, and there is no known reason to expect a clinically significant interaction with valerian.

Possible Interactions with Diseases or Conditions

No interactions are known to occur, and there is no known reason to expect a clinically significant interaction with valerian.

Typical Dosages & Routes of Administration that are Commonly Used

ORAL: The typical dose of valerian is one cup of the tea taken one to several times per day. The tea is prepared by steeping 2-3 grams of the root in 150 mL of boiling water for 5-10 minutes and then straining (2). The maximum dose of valerian is 15 grams of the root per day (18). The simple tincture is commonly taken as 1-3 mL once to several times per day (2,18). The tincture (1:5) is typically dosed as 15-20 drops in water several times per day (18). Extracts in amounts equivalent to 2-3 grams of the root have been taken several times per day (2). For decreasing sleep latency and improving sleep quality, some studies have used 400-900 mg valerian extract up to 2 hours before bedtime for as long as 14 days (7,304,2074,3484). Other studies have used valerian extract 45 mg given 3 to 9 times daily or 450 mg three times daily (304,3484).

TOPICAL: Usually made by mixing 100 grams of the root with 2 L of hot water, and adding to one full bath (2,18).

Comments

In Germany, one specific tincture is required to carry a label warning of reduced ability to drive or operate machinery (12). Even though there is some evidence that valepotriate constituents might be mutagenic, they are rarely found in commercial products because they are unstable and heat labile (304).

VANADIUM

This Product is Also Known As

Metavanadate, Orthovanadate, Vanadate, Vanadium Pentoxide, Vanadyl, Vanadyl Sulfate.

Scientific Names

Vanadium;V; atomic number 23.

People Use This For

Orally, vanadium is used for diabetes, hypoglycemia, lowering serum cholesterol, heart disease, edema, improving athlete's performance in weight training (3052,3053), and protecting against cancer (14,3009,3010). Historically, in the 19th century vanadium was used for treating tuberculosis, diabetes, syphilis, and a form of microcytic anemia (chlorosis) (14).

Safety

POSSIBLY SAFE ...when taken orally in microgram amounts for short-term use. Vanadium and its salts appear to have low oral toxicity (14).

POSSIBLY UNSAFE ...when taken in larger amounts and/or for prolonged use (14).

PREGNANCY AND LACTATION: POSSIBLY UNSAFE; avoid using.

Effectiveness

POSSIBLY EFFECTIVE ...when the vanadyl sulfate form of vanadium is used orally for improving hepatic and peripheral insulin sensitivity in individuals with type 2 diabetes (3055,3056,3057). In a single-blind study, the vanadyl sulfate form of vanadium reduced blood glucose in eight people with type 2 diabetes (3057). Well designed human studies are needed to assess the effect of the vanadyl sulfate form of vanadium on blood glucose control in type 2 diabetes.

There is insufficient reliable information available about the effectiveness of vanadium for its other uses.

Possible Mechanism of Action & Active Ingredients

Vanadium is a biologically important element (511). Several forms of vanadium are available, including vanadium pentoxide, vanadyl sulfate, and salts of metavanadate and orthovanadate. Vanadium appears to be important in normal bone growth (511) and as a cofactor for varied enzyme reactions. Preliminary data show prolonged administration could be associated with dose-dependent increases in blood pressure (3012). Vanadium has digitalis-like effects on heart muscle, producing positive inotropic effects, diuresis, and natriuresis (14). It can reduce plasma cholesterol levels by inhibiting cholesterol synthesis from mevalonic acid (14). In healthy young men, vanadium decreased plasma phospholipid and cholesterol levels; however, it was not effective in older people or in those with hypercholesterolemia and ischemic heart disease (3012). Some evidence suggests that vanadium can mimic the actions of insulin, possibly by causing phosphorylation of insulin receptor proteins. Vanadium activates the receptor (3012,3013), stimulates glucose oxidation and transport, inhibits lipolysis in adipose tissue, stimulates glycogen synthesis in the liver, inhibits hepatic gluconeogenesis, inhibits intestinal glucose transport, and increases glucose uptake, utilization, and glycogen synthesis in skeletal muscle (3012,3013). It appears to augment the effects of insulin in insulin-resistant type 2 diabetes, but might not have an effect in type 1 diabetes (482). Preliminary evidence suggests that L-glutamic acid gamma-monohydroxamate might activate endogenous vanadium, facilitating glucose metabolism through conversion of intracellular vanadium into an active insulinomimetic compound (388). Other evidence suggests vanadium might protect against dental caries (3012). A few studies suggest vanadium might offer protection against hematological toxicity and the development of hepatic carcinoma (3014,3016), but others suggests that vanadium is potentially mutagenic, carcinogenic (3019), and might interfere with mitosis and chromosome distribution (3051).

 © Copyright 2000, Natural Medicines Comprehensive Database (209) 472-2244. For updated data, go to www.NaturalDatabase.com

Adverse Reactions Including Known Allergies

Taken orally, vanadium can cause a green discoloration of tongue (14). Ingestion of vanadium pentoxide has been associated with gastrointestinal disturbances, abnormalities of renal function tests, and nervous system effects (3011). Vanadium taken as 22.5 mg daily for five months is associated with cramps and diarrhea (3012). High body levels of vanadium have been associated with an increased incidence of renal stone disease, distal renal tubular acidosis, hypokalemic periodic paralysis, sudden unexplained nocturnal death, and malnutrition-related diabetes mellitus (3020). Severe and chronic respiratory tract disorders have been reported from occupational exposure to vanadium dusts (17). Toxic effects from systemic exposure to industrial vanadium-containing compounds include peripheral vasoconstriction, arrhythmias, CNS depression, tremors, headaches, neuropathy, abdominal cramping, diarrhea, anemia, and neutropenia (14). Significant toxic effects have been observed in animal studies of vanadium for the treatment of diabetes. These include decreased weight gain, deterioration in health, pro-oxidant effects, alteration in renal function, increased serum urea and creatinine levels, tissue vanadium accumulation, and some deaths (3017,3018,3021).

Possible Interactions with Herbs & Other Dietary Supplements

Insufficient reliable information available.

Possible Interactions with Drugs

ANTICOAGULANTS: Theoretically, the sodium orthovanadate form of vanadium might potentiate anticoagulant therapeutic and adverse effects (3054).
ANTIDIABETES DRUGS: The vanadyl sulfate form of vanadium might have additive effects with diabetes drug therapy. The vanadyl sulfate form of vanadium increases insulin sensitivity (3055,3056,3057) and might lower blood glucose (3057) in individuals with type 2 diabetes. Monitor carefully.
DIGOXIN: Theoretically, concomitant use might increase the therapeutic and adverse effects of digoxin, due to digitalis-like effects of vanadium (14).

Possible Interactions with Foods

No interactions are known to occur, and there is no known reason to expect a clinically significant interaction with vanadium.

Possible Interactions with Lab Tests

BLOOD GLUCOSE: The vanadyl sulfate form of vanadium might lower blood glucose levels and test results in people with type 2 diabetes. In a single-blind study, the vanadyl sulfate form of vanadium reduced fasting blood glucose in eight people with type 2 diabetes (3057).

Possible Interactions with Diseases or Conditions

DIABETES: The vanadyl sulfate form of vanadium might alter blood glucose control in patients with type 2 diabetes. The vanadyl sulfate form of vanadium increases insulin sensitivity (3055,3056,3057) and might lower blood glucose (3057) in individuals with type 2 diabetes. Monitor carefully.

Typical Dosages & Routes of Administration that are Commonly Used

ORAL: People typically take from 10 to 60 mcg per day with food or after meals (5275). Some say the estimated vanadium requirement is less than 10 mcg per day, and an average diet provides 15 to 30 mcg per day (6006).

Comments

Vanadium is a trace element that performs essential functions in the body (17). Food sources include milk, seafood, oils, cereals, and vegetables. Drinking water can contain trace amounts (14,3011). Dental and orthopedic implants can contain vanadium (14).

VANILLA

This Product is Also Known As

Bourbon Vanilla, Common Vanilla, Madagascar Vanilla, Mexican Vanilla, Réunion Vanilla, Tahitian Vanilla, Tahiti Vanilla.

Scientific Names

Vanilla planifolia; Vanilla tahitensis; Vanilla plaifolia, synonym V. fragrans; V. tahitensis.
Family: Orchidaceae.

People Use This For

Traditionally, the vanilla fruit is used orally as an aphrodisiac, an antiflatulent, an antipyretic, and stimulant (6).
In foods and beverages, vanilla is used as a flavoring agent (11). It is added to foods to reduce the amount of sugar needed for sweetening and inhibit the development of dental caries (6).
In manufacturing, vanilla is used as a flavoring agent in syrups for pharmaceutical use (11). It is also used as a fragrance in perfumes (11).

Safety

LIKELY SAFE ...when used orally (12). Has Generally Recognized as Safe (GRAS) status in the US (11). Maximum use level in baked goods is about 0.964% (11).

PREGNANCY AND LACTATION: Insufficient reliable information available; avoid amounts in excess of that contained in food.

Effectiveness

There is insufficient reliable information available about the effectiveness of vanilla.

Possible Mechanism of Action & Active Ingredients

The applicable part of vanilla is the fruit. Although the constituent vanillin is primarily responsible for the flavor of vanilla (11), over 150 aromatic compounds contribute to its fragrance (11,6). The catechin content of vanilla shows evidence of an anti-caries effect (6). In controlled studies, meals flavored with vanilla provided a higher degree of satisfaction than identical meals without vanilla flavoring (6). Contact dermatitis associated with the vanilla plant is thought to be due to the calcium oxalate crystals in the plant (6).

Adverse Reactions Including Known Allergies

Oral and topical use of vanilla has been associated with allergic responses including contact dermatitis (6,11). Workers preparing vanilla have reported headache, dermatitis, and insomnia, characterized as "vanillism."

Possible Interactions with Herbs & Other Dietary Supplements

Insufficient reliable information available.

Possible Interactions with Drugs

No interactions are known to occur, and there is no known reason to expect a clinically significant interaction with vanilla.

Possible Interactions with Foods

No interactions are known to occur, and there is no known reason to expect a clinically significant interaction with vanilla.

Possible Interactions with Lab Tests

No interactions are known to occur, and there is no known reason to expect a clinically significant interaction with vanilla.

Possible Interactions with Diseases or Conditions

No interactions are known to occur, and there is no known reason to expect a clinically significant interaction with vanilla.

Typical Dosages & Routes of Administration that are Commonly Used

No typical dosage.

Comments

Synthetically-produced vanillin is often used as a substitute for vanilla (6), even though the fragrance, rather than the vanillin content, determines the value of vanilla (11). Vanilla extracts have been extensively adulterated (11). Extracts of Mexican origin have been adulterated with coumarin, often due to tonka beans (6). Since 1954, the FDA has prohibited the use of coumarin in food (6).

VERBENA

This Product is Also Known As

Blue Vervain, Common Verbena, Common Vervain, Eisenkraut, Enchanter's Plant, European Vervain, Herb of Grace, Herb of the Cross, Holywort, Juno's Tears, Pigeon's Grass, Pigeonweed, Simpler's Joy, Turkey Grass, Verbenae herba, Vervain.
CAUTION: See separate listing for Lemon Verbena.

Scientific Names

Verbena officinalis.
Family: Verbenaceae.

People Use This For

Orally, the above ground parts of verbena are used for sore throats and other oral and pharyngeal inflammation, respiratory tract diseases such as asthma and whooping cough, and angina (2).
Topically, the above ground parts of verbena are used for poorly healing wounds, abscesses and burns (2), as a gargle for cold symptoms and oral/pharyngeal cavity diseases, arthritis, rheumatism, dislocations, contusions, itching, and minor burns (18).
In combination with gentian root, European elder flower, verbena, cowslip flower, and sorrel, it is used orally for

maintaining healthy sinuses (373) and treating sinusitis (7,374,379).

In folk medicine, verbena is used orally for depression, melancholia, hysteria, generalized seizure, gallbladder pain, fever, debility of convalescence after fevers (4), pains, spasms, exhaustion, angina, nervous conditions, digestive disorders, liver and gallbladder diseases, jaundice, kidney and lower urinary tract ailments and diseases, menopausal complaints, irregular menstruation, for lactation during nursing, arthritic conditions, gout, metabolic disorders, anemia, and edema associated with weak heart (2,18).

In manufacturing, the flowers are used as a flavoring agent in alcoholic beverages (4,12).

Safety

LIKELY SAFE …when used orally in amounts used as flavoring. In the US, the flowers are allowable as a flavoring agent only in alcoholic beverages (12).

POSSIBLY SAFE …when preparations of the above ground parts are used orally and appropriately in therapeutic amounts (12). …when verbena is used orally with gentian root, European elder flower, cowslip flower, and sorrel (Quanterra Sinus Defense, Sinupret) (7,374,379).

LIKELY UNSAFE …when preparations of the above ground parts are used orally in excessive amounts because the constituent, verbenalin, can cause stupor and convulsions (4).

There is insufficient reliable information available about the safety of the topical use of verbena.

PREGNANCY: LIKELY UNSAFE …contraindicated for oral use because verbena is believed to be an abortifacient and oxytocic agent (4). There is insufficient reliable information available about the safety of topical use during pregnancy.

LACTATION: Insufficient reliable information available; avoid using.

Effectiveness

POSSIBLY EFFECTIVE …when verbena is taken orally with gentian root, European elder flower, cowslip flower, and sorrel (Quanterra Sinus Defense, Sinupret) for treating acute or chronic sinusitis (7,374,379).

There is insufficient reliable information available about the effectiveness of verbena for its other uses.

Possible Mechanism of Action & Active Ingredients

The applicable parts of verbena are the above ground parts. They contain the iridoid glycosides verbascoside (acetoside), verbenalin, and verbenin (aucubin) (4). Verbena possesses weak parasympathetic properties and can cause a slight contraction of the uterus. The herb shows evidence of luteinizing activity, perhaps by inhibiting the gonadotrophic activity of the posterior pituitary (4). Some evidence indicates the iridoid glycosides have a mild laxative effect. Small amounts of the constituent, verbenin, appear to stimulate sympathetic activity. Larger amounts of verbenin inhibit sympathetic activity (4). Preliminary evidence suggests verbenin might also stimulate milk secretion (4). The constituent, verbenalin, shows evidence of uterine stimulant activity (4). The constituent verbascoside shows evidence of analgesic and antihypertensive activity. Verbascoside also appears to enhance the antitremor action of levodopa (4).

Adverse Reactions Including Known Allergies

Excessive amounts of the constituent, verbenalin, can cause CNS paralysis, stupor, and convulsions (4).

Possible Interactions with Herbs & Other Dietary Supplements

Insufficient reliable information available.

Possible Interactions with Drugs

DOXYCYCLINE (Vibramycin): Concurrent use of verbena, gentian root, European elder flower, cowslip flower, and sorrel (Quanterra Sinus Defense, Sinupret) with doxycycline and a topical decongestant might improve the outcome of conventional (antibiotic/decongestant) therapy for acute bacterial sinusitis (374).

LEVODOPA: Theoretically, concomitant use might enhance the antitremor effects of levodopa (4).

HYPERTENSIVE, HYPOTENSIVE DRUGS: Theoretically, excessive amounts of verbena can interfere with drug therapy for hypertension or hypotension (4).

HORMONE THERAPY: Theoretically, excessive amounts of verbena can interfere with hormone therapies (4).

Possible Interactions with Foods

No interactions are known to occur, and there is no known reason to expect a clinically significant interaction with verbena.

Possible Interactions with Lab Tests

No interactions are known to occur, and there is no known reason to expect a clinically significant interaction with verbena.

Possible Interactions with Diseases or Conditions

HYPERTENSION: Theoretically, excessive amounts of verbena might reduce blood pressure (4).

HYPOTENSION: Theoretically, excessive amounts of verbena might exacerbate this condition (4).

Typical Dosages & Routes of Administration that are Commonly Used

ORAL: A typical dose is one cup tea three times daily (4). To make tea, steep 2-4 grams dried above ground parts in 150 mL boiling water for 5 10 minutes and strain (4). Liquid extract (1:1 in 25% ethanol), 2-4 mL three times daily (4). Tincture (1:1 in 40% ethanol), 5-10 mL three times daily (4).

For acute or chronic sinusitis, two Sinupret tablets three times daily for up to two weeks has been used in clinical trials (7,374,379), equivalent to gentian root 12 mg, European elder flower 36 mg, verbena 36 mg, cowslip flower 36 mg, and sorrel 36 mg three times daily. For maintaining healthy sinuses, a typical dose is one tablet of Quanterra Sinus Defense three times daily with water, equivalent to gentian root 9 mg, European elder flower 29 mg, verbena 29 mg, cowslip flower 29 mg, and sorrel 29 mg three times daily (373). Each tablet of Quanterra Sinus Defense contains 125 mg of the herbal combination found in Sinupret (373).
TOPICAL: No typical dosage.

Comments

Despite evidence that verbena can stimulate milk production, there are no human studies to validate its safety and effectiveness.

VERONICA

This Product is Also Known As

Ehrenpreiskraut, Gypsyweed, Speedwell, Veronicae herba, Veronica Herb.
CAUTION: See separate listings for Black Root (Leptandra virginica) and Brooklime (Veronica beccabungo) which are both known also as Speedwell.

Scientific Names

Veronica officinalis.
Family: Scrophulariaceae.

People Use This For

Orally, veronica is used for diseases and discomforts of the respiratory tract, gastrointestinal tract, liver, kidney and lower urinary tract, gout, arthritis, rheumatic complaints, diseases of the spleen, scrofulosis, as an appetite stimulant and tonic, and to induce sweating (2).

Topically, it is used as a gargle for inflammation of the oral and pharyngeal mucosa, for perspiration of the feet, stimulation of wound healing, chronic skin conditions, and itching (2).

In folk medicine, it is used orally for nervous irritation, "blood purification," and promotion of metabolism (2,18).

Safety

LIKELY SAFE ...when consumed in amounts found in alcoholic beverages; allowable flavoring agent in alcoholic beverages in the US (12).
POSSIBLY SAFE ...when used appropriately as an oral medicinal agent (12).
There is insufficient reliable information available about the safety of the topical use of veronica.
PREGNANCY AND LACTATION: Insufficient reliable information available; avoid using.

Effectiveness

There is insufficient reliable information available about the effectiveness of veronica.

Possible Mechanism of Action & Active Ingredients

The applicable parts of veronica are the above ground parts. Extracts protected against ulcers induced by indomethacin. May enhance gastric mucosa regeneration (4010).

Adverse Reactions Including Known Allergies

None reported.

Possible Interactions with Herbs & Other Dietary Supplements

Insufficient reliable information available.

Possible Interactions with Drugs

NONSTEROIDAL ANTI-INFLAMMATORY DRUGS (NSAIDs): Theoretically, concomitant use may protect against NSAID-induced ulcerogenic activity (4010).

Possible Interactions with Foods

No interactions are known to occur, and there is no known reason to expect a clinically significant interaction with veronica.

Possible Interactions with Lab Tests

No interactions are known to occur, and there is no known reason to expect a clinically significant interaction with veronica.

Possible Interactions with Diseases or Conditions

GASTRIC ULCERS: Theoretically, may enhance ulcer healing (4010).

Typical Dosages & Routes of Administration that are Commonly Used

ORAL: As an expectorant, 1 cup tea (steep 1.5 grams finely cut above ground parts in 150 mL boiling water 10 minutes, strain) 2-3 times daily (18).

TOPICAL: For lavages and compresses for eczema, ulcers, wounds, boil 1 handful above ground parts in 1 L water for 10 minutes) (18); frequency unspecified (18).

Comments

Avoid confusion with other Veronica species, including Veronica allionii and Veronica chamaedrys (18).

VETIVER

This Product is Also Known As

Chiendent Odorant, Cuscus, Cuscus Grass, Khas-khas, Khus Khus, Khus-khus Grass, Vétiver, Vetivergras, Zacate Violeta.

Scientific Names

Vetiveria zizanoides.
Family: Poaceae.

People Use This For

Orally, vetiver root is used as a uterine stimulant to promote menses and to cause abortion (12). It is also used orally for nervous and circulatory problems (5279).

Topically, it is used for stress relief, recovery from emotional traumas and shocks (5283), treatment of lice (5279), and as an insect repellent (513).

As an inhalant, vetiver is used for "aroma therapy" for nervousness, insomnia, rheumatism, and muscle relaxation (5281,5282).

In manufacturing, vetiver is used as a flavoring in alcoholic beverages (12).

Safety

LIKELY SAFE ...when used in amounts found in alcoholic beverages. It is approved as a flavoring additive in alcoholic beverages in the US (308).

POSSIBLY SAFE ...when used orally (12).

PREGNANCY: LIKELY UNSAFE ...when used orally because it is a potential abortifacient and it has menstrual and uterine stimulant effects (12).

LACTATION: Insufficient reliable information available: avoid using.

Effectiveness

There is insufficient reliable information about the effectiveness of vetiver.

Possible Mechanism of Action & Active Ingredients

The applicable part of vetiver is the root. Vetiver root contains numerous constituents including limonene, p-cymene, palmitic acid, benzoic acid, delta-3-carene (513). Vetiver may contain a volatile oil which accounts for its use as a repellent to flies, cockroaches, bedbugs, and clothes moths (5279).

Adverse Reactions Including Known Allergies

None reported.

Possible Interactions with Herbs & Other Dietary Supplements

Insufficient reliable information available.

Possible Interactions with Drugs

No interactions are known to occur, and there is no known reason to expect a clinically significant interaction with vetiver.

Possible Interactions with Foods

No interactions are known to occur, and there is no known reason to expect a clinically significant interaction with vetiver.

Possible Interactions with Lab Tests

No interactions are known to occur, and there is no known reason to expect a clinically significant interaction with vetiver.

Possible Interactions with Diseases or Conditions

No interactions are known to occur, and there is no known reason to expect a clinically significant interaction with vetiver.

Typical Dosages & Routes of Administration that are Commonly Used

No typical dosage.

Comments

None.

VINPOCETINE

This Product is Also Known As

AY-27255, Cavinton, Ethyl Apovincaminate, Ethylapovincaminoate, RGH-4405, TCV-3b.

Scientific Names

Eburnamenine-14-carboxylic acid, ethyl ester.

People Use This For

Orally, vinpocetine is used for enhancing memory (1782,1783,1796,1797), improving cerebral blood flow, improving cerebral oxygen and glucose utilization (1782,1783), protecting against age-related cognitive decline and Alzheimer's disease (14,1783,1784), treating cerebrovascular disease (14,1789,1793), preventing post-stroke morbidity and mortality (14,1785), treating organic psychosyndromes (1787), treating intractable tumoral calcinosis in people undergoing hemodialysis (14,1788), decreasing stroke risk (14,1790,1791), treating menopausal symptoms (1792), seizure disorders (1795), and preventing motion sickness (1798).

Intravenously, vinpocetine is injected for treating seizure disorders (1794) and stroke (1786).

Safety

POSSIBLY SAFE ...when used orally and appropriately (14,1784). No significant adverse effects were reported in a study of people with Alzheimer's disease treated with large doses of vinpocetine (60 mg per day) for one year (1784).
PREGNANCY AND LACTATION: Insufficient reliable information available; avoid using.

Effectiveness

POSSIBLY EFFECTIVE ...when vinpocetine is used orally for cerebrovascular diseases (14,1787,1789,1793). ...when used orally for enhancing memory (1796,1797).
POSSIBLY INEFFECTIVE ...when used orally for preventing post-stroke morbidity and mortality (14,1785).
There is insufficient reliable information available about the effectiveness of vinpocetine for its other uses.

Possible Mechanism of Action & Active Ingredients

Vinpocetine is a synthetic derivative of vincamine, a compound derived from the periwinkle plant, Vinca minor (see separate listing for Periwinkle) (14). Vinpocetine appears to have many varied pharmacologic effects, but mechanisms of action are unclear, and well-designed clinical studies to substantiate activity have not been published (14). A few studies using vinpocetine for poorly-defined cerebrovascular diseases have indicated some efficacy, but faulty study design limits interpretation (14,1787,1789,1793). Vinpocetine had no effect on dementia progression in 15 people with Alzheimer's disease treated for one year with gradually increasing doses up to 60 mg/day (1784). Vinpocetine does not appear to be effective for preventing post-stroke debility or death (14,1785). Some studies indicate that vinpocetine might enhance cerebral blood flow without affecting peripheral blood flow (14,1786,1793). Preliminary evidence indicates that vinpocetine stimulates cerebral metabolism (14). Vinpocetine improves memory in healthy subjects and healthy volunteers with benzodiazepine-induced memory impairment (1796,1797). Potential mechanisms for the nootropic-like effects of vinpocetine include indirect or direct cholinergic activity, augmented norepinephrine effects on cortical cyclic adenosine monophosphate (AMP), increased turnover of brain catecholamines, and inhibition of adenosine reuptake (14,1800). Other pharmacological effects of vinpocetine include increased cerebral glucose utilization, anticonvulsant activity, neuronal protectant activity, adenosine-like effects, and phosphodiesterase inhibition (14). Vinpocetine inhibits drug-induced platelet aggregation (14,1801). The bioavailability of vinpocetine varies from 7% to 57%, and food significantly enhances absorption (14,1802). Vinpocetine undergoes hepatic metabolism to inactive compounds (14). The elimination half-life of vinpocetine is 1-2.5 hours (14). Vinpocetine has been shown not to interact with desipramine, imipramine, glyburide, and oxazepam (14).

Adverse Reactions Including Known Allergies

Adverse effects include stomach pressure, upper abdominal pain, nausea, facial flushing, slight reductions in systolic and diastolic blood pressure, sleep disturbances, and headache (14).

Possible Interactions with Herbs & Other Dietary Supplements

HERBS WITH ANTICOAGULANT/ANTIPLATELET POTENTIAL: Theoretically, concomitant use of herbs that have coumarin constituents or affect platelet aggregation might increase the risk of bleeding in some people. These herbs include: angelica, anise, arnica, asafoetida, bogbean, boldo, capsicum, celery, chamomile, clove, danshen, fenugreek, feverfew, garlic, ginger, ginkgo, ginseng Panax, horse chestnut, horseradish, licorice, meadowsweet, prickly ash, onion, papain, passionflower, poplar, quassia, red clover, turmeric, wild carrot, wild lettuce, willow, and others (4,19).

Possible Interactions with Drugs

ANTI-PLATELET DRUGS: Theoretically, concomitant use might enhance anti-platelet effects and increase bleeding risk (14,1801).

WARFARIN (Coumadin): Concomitant use might increase anticoagulant effects and increase bleeding risk; monitor INR (14).

BLOOD PRESSURE LOWERING DRUGS: Theoretically, concomitant use might enhance blood pressure lowering effects; monitor blood pressure (14).

Possible Interactions with Foods

Food enhances the absorption of oral vinpocetine (1802).

Possible Interactions with Lab Tests

PROTHROMBIN TIME (PT), INTERNATIONAL NORMALIZATION RATIO (INR): Vinpocetine might increase PT and INR (14). It has been reported to modestly increase warfarin AUC, PT, and factor VII clotting time (14).

BLOOD PRESSURE: Theoretically, vinpocetine might lower blood pressure and blood pressure measurements (14).

BLOOD GLUCOSE: Theoretically, vinpocetine might reduce blood sugar levels and test results (14).

Possible Interactions with Diseases or Conditions

COAGULOPATHIES: Vinpocetine should not be used by people with blood-clotting disorders because it might increase bleeding risk (14,1801).

Typical Dosages & Routes of Administration that are Commonly Used

ORAL: The dose used for cerebrovascular disorders is 5-10 mg three times daily (14). People typically take 10 mg three times daily with food (1799).

Comments

Vinpocetine is a synthetic derivative of apovincamine which is found in periwinkle. Vinpocetine synthesis requires considerable laboratory manipulation, stretching the Dietary Supplement Health and Education Act (DSHEA) definition of a "dietary supplement" (14,1799). Vinpocetine is sold by prescription in Germany under the brand name, Cavinton (9). It has also been referred to generically as cavinton (9). Although website advertising claims that "more than a hundred" safety and effectiveness studies have been funded by the Hungarian manufacturer Gedeon Richter, few double-blind controlled clinical studies have been published (14,1782,1785).

VITAMIN A

This Product is Also Known As

Antixerophthalmic Vitamin, Axerophtholum, Dehydroretinol - 3-dehydroretinol - Vitamin A2, Oleovitamin A, Retinol - Vitamin A1, Retinol Acetate, Retinol Palmitate, Retinyl Acetate, Retinyl Palmitate, Vitaminum A. CAUTION: See separate listing for Beta-Carotene.

Scientific Names

Vitamin A.

People Use This For

Orally, vitamin A is most commonly used to prevent and treat the symptoms of vitamin A deficiency; promote good vision; prevent glaucoma and cataracts; prevent and speed recovery from infections; improve immune function; and for skin conditions including acne, eczema, psoriasis, cold sores, wounds and burns, sunburn, keratosis follicularis (Darier's disease), ichthyosis (noninflammatory skin scaling), lichen planus pigmentosus, and pityriasis rubra pilaris (14,15,3062,3064,3065). Vitamin A is also used orally to prevent and treat vitamin A deficiency due to abnormal storage and transport of vitamin A in people with abetalipoproteinemia, protein deficiency, diabetes mellitus, hyperthyroidism, fever, liver disease, or cystic fibrosis with liver involvement. It is also used for heavy menses, premenstrual syndrome, atrophic vaginitis, candidiasis, fibrocystic breast disease, reduced sperm count, gastrointestinal ulcers, Crohn's disease, periodontal disease, diabetes, Hurler syndrome (mucopolysaccharidosis), sinusitis, urinary tract infections, reducing complications of measles, with antibiotics for hastening clinical shigellosis cure, atrophic rhinitis, loss of sense of smell, asthma, persistent headaches, kidney stones, hyperthyroidism, anemia, deafness, tinnitus, cataracts, glaucoma, leukoplakia, preventing and treating cancer, degenerative diseases of the nervous system, protecting the heart and cardiovascular system (antioxidant effects), and slowing the aging process (14,15,3062,3064,3065). Vitamin A is used orally to decrease morbidity associated with malaria in children (1464), and to reduce morbidity and mortality from pneumonia and HIV in children with vitamin A deficiency (1465,1466).

Topically, Vitamin A is used to improve wound healing, reduce wrinkles, and to protect the skin against UV radiation (14,1468,3063).

As an intramuscular injection, Vitamin A is used for preventing and treating the symptoms of vitamin A deficiency, including xerophthalmia and night blindness; preventing vitamin A deficiency in people with

© Copyright 2000, Natural Medicines Comprehensive Database (209) 472-2244. For updated data, go to www.NaturalDatabase.com

malabsorption; preventing bronchopulmonary dysplasia in premature infants; and preventing stress ulcers in severely ill hospitalized patients (14,15).

Safety

LIKELY SAFE ...when used orally or intramuscularly and appropriately (15).

POSSIBLY UNSAFE ...when used orally in doses exceeding the recommended daily allowance (RDA). Accumulation can occur when vitamin A is taken daily in doses exceeding the RDA for prolonged periods of time. The risk for developing hypervitaminosis A is related to total cumulative dose of vitamin A rather than a specific daily dose (5,1467,1469). However, specific amounts that cause hypervitaminosis A vary considerably among individuals (5).

CHILDREN: LIKELY SAFE ...when used orally or intramuscularly and appropriately (15). POSSIBLY UNSAFE ...when used orally in amounts larger than the RDA. A single dose of 25,000 units/kg can cause signs of toxicity (15).

PREGNANCY: LIKELY SAFE ...when used orally or intramuscularly in amounts not exceeding the recommended dietary allowance (RSA). LIKELY UNSAFE ...when used orally in amounts exceeding the recommended dietary allowance (RDA). Greater than 5000-10,000 units vitamin A1 (retinol) per day are associated with fetal malformations (14,15,3066). The provitamin A carotenoids found in plant sources are believed safer than vitamin A and are preferred during pregnancy (3066). However, supplementation of vitamin A or carotenoids during pregnancy should only be done under the close supervision of a healthcare provider.

LACTATION: LIKELY SAFE ...when used orally in amounts not exceeding the recommended dietary allowance (RDA) (15). There is insufficient reliable information available about the safety of vitamin A in amounts exceeding the RDA during lactation; avoid using.

Effectiveness

EFFECTIVE ...when vitamin A is used orally for preventing and treating the symptoms of vitamin A deficiency, including xerophthalmia and night blindness (15). ...when used orally for preventing and treating vitamin A deficiency due to abnormal storage and transport of vitamin A in people with abetalipoproteinemia, protein deficiency, diabetes mellitus, hyperthyroidism, fever, liver disease, or cystic fibrosis with liver involvement (15).

POSSIBLY EFFECTIVE ...when vitamin A is used orally for reducing the complications of measles in children with vitamin A deficiency (14,15). ...when used orally in large amounts for treating acne vulgaris, though other retinoids have largely replaced retinol for this use (14). ...when used orally for decreasing malaria symptoms in children under 3 years of age living in endemic areas (1464). ...when used orally as an adjunct for decreasing mortality from HIV and diarrhea in children with vitamin A deficiency in developing countries (1465). Epidemilogical data suggests an association between increasing amounts of dietary vitamin A and reduced risk of breast cancer risk among premenopausal women with a positive family history of breast cancer (1444). Well designed clinical trials are needed to determine whether a cause-effect relationship exists between dietary or supplemental vitamin A intake and breast cancer. ...when vitamin A is taken orally by malnourished women to reduce pregnancy-related mortality. In one trial, 23,300 IU retinyl acetate taken weekly before, during and after pregnancy by malnourished women in Nepal reduced pregnancy-related mortality by 40% (6153). ...when vitamin A is taken orally by malnourished women to reduce the occurrence of pregnancy-related night blindness. In one trial, 23,300 IU retinyl acetate taken weekly before, during and after pregnancy by malnourished women in Nepal reduced, but did not eliminate, the occurrence of pregnancy-related night blindness (6154).

POSSIBLY INEFFECTIVE ...when vitamin A is taken orally by malnourished women to reduce fetal and early infant mortality. In one trial, 23,300 IU retinyl acetate weekly taken before, during, and after pregnancy by malnourished women in Nepal failed to reduce fetal and early infant mortality (6152).

LIKELY INEFFECTIVE ...when vitamin A is used orally for decreasing the severity of pneumonia in children living in developing countries (1466).

There is insufficient reliable information available about the effectiveness of vitamin A for its other uses.

Possible Mechanism of Action & Active Ingredients

Vitamin A is a fat-soluble vitamin found in several forms, including retinol, 3-dehydroretinol, and provitamin A carotenoids (15). The body stores vitamin A as retinol predominantly in the liver, but also maintains stores in the retina, kidneys, lungs, adrenals, and intraperitoneal fat (15,1467). Retinol-binding protein is required to transport retinol from the liver. Transport protein levels can be reduced in people with protein malnutrition, causing signs of vitamin A deficiency (15). Vitamin A toxicity can occur when retinol-binding protein capacity is exceeded and unbound retinol enters the circulation resulting in vitamin A excess (hypervitaminosis A) (15). Vitamin A is required for growth and bone development, vision, reproduction, and the integrity of mucosal and epithelial surfaces (14). Retinoic acid is thought to be the active form of vitamin A in processes involving growth and differentiation (14). Vitamin A acts as a cofactor in mucopolysaccharide synthesis, cholesterol synthesis, hydroxysteroid metabolism, and glycoprotein glycosylation (14,15). Some evidence suggests vitamin A might enhance immune system function, and there is limited evidence that it might protect against some cancers (14). An inverse relationship between dietary intake of vitamin A and cancer incidence has been suggested, but it is not known whether supplements have the same effect (14,1444). In the retina, retinol is converted to cis-retinal, which combines with opsin to form rhodopsin, the visual pigment (14). Diets high in the provitaminA carotenoids lutein and zeaxanthin might protect against the risk for developing cataracts severe enough to require surgical removal in both men and women (3219,3220). Preliminary evidence suggests that all-trans-retinoic acid applied topically might help protect the skin against UV radiation-related damage (1468).

Adverse Reactions Including Known Allergies

With chronic use of large amounts, early symptoms of vitamin A overdose include fatigue, malaise, lethargy, irritability, psychiatric changes mimicking severe depression or schizophrenic disorder, anorexia, abdominal discomfort, nausea and vomiting, mild fever, and excessive sweating (14,15). Sometimes children fail to gain weight normally while adults lose weight (14,15). Slow growth, premature epiphyseal closure, painful hyperostosis of the long bones, osteosclerosis, joint pain, muscle pain, hypercalcemia, and hypercalciuria have been reported (14,15). CNS symptoms of hypervitaminosis include increased intracranial pressure, pseudotumor cerebri, bulging fontanelles in infants, headache, swelling of the optic disk, bulging eyeballs, dizziness, and visual disturbances. Other symptoms include dry skin and lips; cracking, scaling, and itchy skin; skin redness, hyperpigmentation, and massive skin peeling. Hypervitaminosis A can cause brittle nails, cheilitis, gingivitis, hair loss, reduced menstrual flow, hepatosplenomegaly, cirrhosis, jaundice, ascites, spider angiomas, elevated serum AST (SGOT) and ALT (SGPT) concentrations, anemia, leukopenia, leukocytosis, and thrombocytopenia (14,15). Toxicity from a single ingestion of a large dose of vitamin A is more common in young children than adults (15). Approximately 25,000 units/kg can cause irritability, drowsiness, dizziness, delirium, coma, vomiting, diarrhea (15), increased intracranial pressure with bulging fontanelles in infants, headache, swelling of the optic disk, bulging eyeballs, and visual disturbances (15). Skin redness and generalized peeling of the skin occur a few days later and may last for several weeks (15).

Possible Interactions with Herbs & Other Dietary Supplements

VITAMIN E: Concomitant use can increase the absorption, utilization, and storage of vitamin A, and may protect against hypervitaminosis A, although these effects are controversial (15).
MINERAL OIL: Concomitant use can decrease oral vitamin A absorption (15).

Possible Interactions with Drugs

CHEMOTHERAPEUTIC AGENTS: Theoretically, concomitant use might decrease the effectiveness of chemotherapy. Preliminary evidence from an unpublished study suggests that antioxidants such as vitamin E and vitamin A may decrease the effectiveness of chemotherapy (14,391).
NEOMYCIN (Neo-Fradin): Concomitant use of neomycin can reduce supplemental vitamin A absorption (14,15).
MINOCYCLINE (Minocin): Concomitant, long-term administration increases the risk of pseudotumor cerebri (benign intracranial hypertension) (14).

Drug Influences on Nutrient Levels and Depletion

SOME DRUGS CAN AFFECT VITAMIN A LEVELS:
CHOLESTYRAMINE (Questran): Cholestyramine can reduce dietary vitamin A absorption and serum levels. Supplementation with water-miscible vitamin A is recommended for patients during long-term cholestyramine therapy (15,4455,4456).
COLESTIPOL (Colestid): Colestipol can reduce dietary vitamin A absorption and serum levels (4460).
MINERAL OIL: Use of mineral oil can reduce dietary vitamin A absorption and serum levels. Avoid long-term use of mineral oil (4495). Vitamin A refers to beta-ionone derivatives, with the biological activity of retinol (511). Vitamin A does not include provitamin A carotenoids.
ORLISTAT (Xenical): Orlistat can reduce vitamin A levels (1725,1726,1727,1730). Consider a multivitamin with fat-soluble vitamins, taken at least 2 hours before or after orlistat, or at bedtime.

Possible Interactions with Foods

No interactions are known to occur, and there is no known reason to expect a clinically significant interaction with vitamin A.

Possible Interactions with Lab Tests

CHOLESTEROL: There are unsubstantiated reports that vitamin A can produce false increases in serum cholesterol test results measured by the Zlatkis-Zak reaction (15).
BILIRUBIN: Vitamin A can cause false increase in bilirubin test results using Ehrlich's reagent (15).

Possible Interactions with Diseases or Conditions

DECREASED ABSORPTION: Oral vitamin A absorption is decreased in the following conditions: fat malabsorption, low protein intake, hepatic or pancreatic disease, ascariasis, giardiasis, hookworm, salmonellosis, and schistosomiasis (14,15).
HYPERVITAMINOSIS: The risk of vitamin A toxicity is increased in individuals with renal or hepatic disease, low body weight, protein malnutrition, hyperlipoproteinemia, alcoholism, and vitamin C deficiency (14).

Typical Dosages & Routes of Administration that are Commonly Used

ORAL: As a dietary supplement the usual recommended dose of vitamin A is 4000-5000 units or 1200-1500 retinol equivalents daily (15). The recommended dose for treatment of deficiency in adults without corneal changes is 10,000 to 25,000 units daily until clinical improvement occurs, usually 1-2 weeks (15). Amounts of more than 25,000 units require monitoring (15). Individuals with fat malabsorption, low protein intake, or hepatic or pancreatic disease might benefit from water-miscible oral preparations. If oral absorption is still insufficient, parenteral administration may be necessary (15).

PARENTERAL: Injectable vitamin A is available as a FDA-approved prescription product.

The daily recommended dietary allowances (RDAs) of vitamin A expressed in RE (retinol equivalents) and unit conversions are: Infants up to 1 year, 375 RE (1250 units); Children 1-3 years, 400 RE (1300 units); Children 4-6 years, 500 RE (1700 units); Children 7-10 years, 700 RE (2300 units); Males 11 years and older, 1000 RE (3300 units); Females 11 years and older, 800 RE (2700 units); Pregnant women, 800 RE (2700 units); Lactating women, first 6 months, 1300 RE (4300 units); Lactating women, second 6 months, 1200 RE (4000 units) (15). Vitamin A refers to beta-ionone derivatives, with the biological activity of retinol (511). Vitamin A does not include provitamin A carotenoids. Vitamin A activity is expressed in retinol equivalents, USP units, International units, or beta carotene equivalents. USP and International units are equivalent; one unit of vitamin A equals the biologic activity of 0.3 mcg all-trans retinol, 0.344 mcg all-trans retinol acetate, or 0.6 mcg beta carotene (14,15). One retinol equivalent equals the activity of 1 mcg all-trans retinol, 6 mcg beta carotene, or 12 mcg of other provitamin A carotenoids (15). Since a normal diet contains both retinol and carotenoids, the calculation of dietary vitamin A combines both sources, e.g., 1000 retinol equivalents corresponds to 3300 units of retinol, but 5000 units of dietary vitamin A (14).

Comments

Vitamin A is found in foods in several forms. Retinol is present in esterified form in eggs, whole milk, butter, fortified margarine, meat, and oily, salt-water fish (15). 3-Dehydroretinol is present in fresh-water fish, but has only 30-40% of the biologic activity of retinol (15). ProvitaminA carotenoid pigments (including alpha-, beta-, and gamma-carotene and cryptoxanthin) are present in green and yellow vegetables and fruits and are converted to retinol in humans (see listing for Beta Carotene) (15).

VITAMIN B12

This Product is Also Known As

Bedumil, Cobamin, Cobalamins, Cyanocobalamin, Cyanocobalaminum, Cycobemin, Hydroxocobalamin, Hydroxocobalaminum, Hydroxocobemine, Idrossocobalamina, Methylcobalamin, Vitadurin.
CAUTION: See separate listing for Dibencozide.

Scientific Names

Vitamin B12; Cyanocobalamin; Hydroxocobalamin; Methylcobalamin.

People Use This For

Orally, vitamin B12 is used for treating circadian rhythm sleep disorders (1344).

It is also used orally for treating primary hyperhomocystinemia (3233), as a component of general multivitamin supplements, psychiatric disorders (15), for aging, allergies, asthma, diabetes, heart disease, immunosuppression, memory loss, improving concentration, Alzheimer's disease, multiple sclerosis, osteoporosis, protection against the toxins and allergens from tobacco smoke, mood elevation, boosting energy, maintaining fertility (3024,3025,3026), treating AIDS, hives, inflammatory bowel disease, seborrheic dermatitis, and tendinitis (3234).

Orally and by injection, vitamin B12 is used for pernicious anemia and vitamin B12 deficiency (15).

Orally and by injection, vitamin B12 prescription products are used for increased vitamin B12 requirements due to pregnancy, thyrotoxicosis, hemorrhage, malignancy, and liver or kidney disease (15).

As a nasal gel, vitamin B12 is applied topically for nutritional B12 deficiency (266).

Hydroxocobalamin is being investigated for treating cyanide toxicity (14).

Safety

LIKELY SAFE ...when taken orally or when the prescription-only, injectable product is used appropriately. Vitamin B12 is generally considered nontoxic, even in large amounts (15); however, rare, fatal anaphylactic reactions have been reported (15).

There is insufficient reliable information available about the safety of vitamin B12 for its other uses.

PREGNANCY: LIKELY SAFE ...when used at the recommended dietary allowance (RDA) of 2.6 mcg per day (3094).

LACTATION: LIKELY SAFE ...when used at the recommended dietary allowance (RDA) of 2.8 mcg per day (3094). There is insufficient reliable information available about the safety of larger amounts of vitamin B12 used during lactation.

Effectiveness

EFFECTIVE ...when taken orally as a dietary supplement for those with a documented dietary deficiency, which is, most frequently, strict vegetarians, and in those with increased vitamin B12 requirements, like deficiencies associated with pregnancy, thyrotoxicosis, hemolytic anemia, hemorrhage, malignancy, and hepatic and renal disease (15). ...when the prescription-only, injectable product is used appropriately.

POSSIBLY EFFECTIVE ...when used orally for treating pernicious anemia and other vitamin B12 deficiency states, but the vitamin B12 injection is preferred.

POSSIBLY INEFFECTIVE ...when the methylcobalamin form of vitamin B12 is used orally for four weeks for

treating patients with delayed sleep phase syndrome. This is based on the results of the only reported double-blind, placebo controlled trial of methylcobalamin for sleep disorders (1346). Case reports and uncontrolled clinical trials report mixed results when the methylcobalamin form of vitamin B12 (with or without bright light therapy) is used orally for treating some patients with various primary circadian rhythm sleep disorders (1344,1345,1347,1348).
LIKELY INEFFECTIVE ...when taken orally for treating psychiatric disorders, unless they are proven to be a consequence of vitamin B12 deficiency (15).
There is insufficient reliable information available about the effectiveness of vitamin B12 for its other uses.

Possible Mechanism of Action & Active Ingredients

Vitamin B12 is required for nucleoprotein and myelin synthesis, cell reproduction, normal growth, and normal erythropoiesis (15). Vitamin B12 can be converted to coenzyme B12 which is essential for the conversion of methylmalonate to succinate, and the synthesis of methionine from homocysteine (15). Vitamin B12 is essential for folate utilization, and its absence results in a functional folate deficiency (15). Vitamin B12 deficiency can take months to years to become symptomatic due to large body stores (3023). Vitamin B12 can be involved in maintaining sulfhydryl groups in the reduced form required by enzymes involved in fat and carbohydrate metabolism and protein synthesis (15). Vitamin B12 deficiency results in megaloblastic anemia, gastrointestinal lesions, and neurologic damage, beginning with an inability to produce myelin and progressing to degeneration of the axon and nerve head (15). Vitamin B12 deficiency is independently associated with elevated homocysteine levels, although not as strongly as folic acid deficiency (see Folic Acid monograph). Elevated homocysteine concentrations are in turn associated with an increased risk of vascular disease (1483,3234). In preliminary clinical trials, methionine loading acutely elevates plasma homocysteine levels and induces endothelial dysfunction (6235). Vitamin B12, in combination with folic acid and pyridoxine, has improved endothelial function, as measured by flow-mediated vasodilation, following a methionine load in healthy volunteers (6235). Elevated methylmalonate levels occur early in vitamin B12 deficiency, and may precede other symptoms (1484,1485). Neurologic symptoms and elevated homocysteine levels can occur without any signs of B12 deficiency anemia (1484,1485,3235). Epidemiological data suggest that the risk for vitamin B12 deficiency increases with age, male gender, and in people of Caucasian and Latin American descent. Research suggests this might be due to vitamin B12 malabsorption (1484,1485). Limited clinical data demonstrate a decrease in hyperhomocystinuria with vitamin B12 and folic acid supplementation in people with renal insufficiency (1489). Other epidemiological data suggest an association between low vitamin B12 serum concentrations and hearing loss in healthy women aged 60-71 (1482). The methylcobalamin form of vitamin B12 improves alertness and reduces sleep time in humans with normal sleep patterns (1349). Some researchers think the cyanocobalamin form of vitamin B12 influences melatonin levels (1349).

Adverse Reactions Including Known Allergies

The oral use of vitamin B12 can cause diarrhea, peripheral vascular thrombosis, itching, transitory exanthema, urticaria, feelings of swelling of the entire body, and anaphylaxis. Treatment of vitamin B12 deficiency can unmask polycythemia vera, which is an increase in blood volume and the number of red blood cells (15).

Possible Interactions with Herbs & Other Dietary Supplements

VITAMIN C: Large amounts of vitamin C can destroy vitamin B12 and should not be taken within an hour of oral vitamin B12 (15).

Possible Interactions with Drugs

REDUCED GI ABSORPTION: Absorption of oral, supplemental vitamin B12 can be decreased by aminoglycoside antibiotics, colchicine, colestipol, extended release potassium preparations, aminosalicylic acid and its salts, anticonvulsants (e.g. phenytoin, phenobarbital, and primidone), cobalt irradiation of the small bowel, and excessive alcohol intake lasting longer than two weeks (14,15).
H2-BLOCKERS Cimetidine (Tagamet), Ranitidine (Zantac), Famotidine (Pepcid), and others: Long-term use of high-dose H2-blockers may lead to iron and vitamin B12 malabsorption (4539,4540,4541). The mechanism of this is thought to be through the inhibition of gastric acid secretion necessary for absorption of iron and vitamin B12. Monitor for signs and symptoms of anemia. This interaction is theoretically possible with proton pump inhibitors.
VITAMIN C: Concomitant administration of large amounts of vitamin C can destroy vitamin B12 and should not be taken within an hour of oral vitamin B12 (15).
CHLORAMPHENICOL (Chloromycetin): Chloramphenicol can impair hematopoietic response to supplemental vitamin B12 (15).
METFORMIN (Glucophage): May reduce serum folic acid and vitamin B12 levels (32,4490). A multivitamin preparation may be valuable in some patients.
ZIDOVUDINE (Retrovir and an ingredient of Combivir): Patients with HIV disease taking zidovudine may have subnormal B12 concentrations, possibly predisposing them to hematologic toxicity, especially anemia (30). Give supplements of B12 only if clinical judgment warrants it.

Drug Influences on Nutrient Levels and Depletion

SOME DRUGS CAN AFFECT VITAMIN B12 LEVELS:
ANTIBIOTICS: Destruction of normal gastrointestinal flora by antibiotics can cause decreased production of B vitamins. The clinical significance of this decreased production is not known. Consider supplementation only if clinical judgment warrants it (4434,4435,4436,4437,4438,4439,4440,4441,4442,4443).
COLCHICINE: Use of colchicine can reduce dietary vitamin B12 absorption. The significance of this and need for

supplementation has not been adequately studied (4543,4544,4545).

METFORMIN (Glucophage): Metformin may reduce serum folic acid and vitamin B12 levels (32,4490). A multivitamin preparation may be valuable in some patients.

H2-BLOCKERS; Cimetidine (Tagamet), Rantidine (Zantac), Famotidine (Pepcid), and others: Long-term use of high-dose H2-blockers may lead to iron and B12 malabsorption (4539,4540,4541). The mechanism of this is thought to be through the inhibition of gastric acid secretion necessary for absorption of iron and B12. Monitor for signs/symptoms of anemia. This interaction is theoretically possible with proton pump inhibitors.

PROTON PUMP INHIBITORS; Lansoprazole (Prevacid), Omeprazole (Prilosec, Losec), Rabeprazole (Aciphex), Pantoprazole (Protonix, Pantoloc): Proton pump inhibitors might decrease dietary, but not supplemental, vitamin B12 absorption and resulting serum levels. The need for vitamin B12 supplementation has not been adequately studied. Vitamin B12 depletion may be particularly important in patients with inadequate diet, poor stores of the vitamin, and in patients receiving continuous, long-term therapy (see H2 Blockers above).

ORAL CONTRACEPTIVES: Use of oral contraceptives can increase vitamin B12 metabolism, decrease binding capacity, and reduce vitamin B12 serum levels. The significance of this and the need for vitamin B12 supplementation has not been adequately studied (4547).

POTASSIUM CHLORIDE (extended release products, K-Dur): Use of potassium chloride can reduce dietary vitamin B12 absorption and serum levels. The need for supplementation has not been adequately studied (4511,4512).

NICOTINE: Nicotine can reduce vitamin B12 blood levels. The need for vitamin B12 supplementation has not been adequately studied (19).

ZIDOVUDINE (Retrovir and an ingredient of Combivir): Patients with HIV disease taking zidovudine may have subnormal B12 concentrations, possibly predisposing them to hematologic toxicity, especially anemia (30). Give supplements of B12 only if clinical judgment warrants it.

Possible Interactions with Foods

No interactions are known to occur, and there is no known reason to expect a clinically significant interaction with vitamin B12.

Possible Interactions with Lab Tests

INTRINSIC FACTOR: Vitamin B12 can cause a false-positive test result for intrinsic factor antibodies (15).

Possible Interactions with Diseases or Conditions

POLYCYTHEMIA VERA: The treatment of vitamin B12 deficiency can unmask the symptoms of polycythemia vera (15).

MEGALOBLASTIC ANEMIA: Use vitamin B12 with caution. The correction of megaloblastic anemia with vitamin B12 can result in fatal hypokalemia and gout in susceptible individuals, and it can obscure folate deficiency in megaloblastic anemia (15); use with caution.

COBALAMIN OR COBALT HYPERSENSITIVITY: Contraindicated (15).

LEBER'S DISEASE: Vitamin B12 is contraindicated in early Leber's disease, which is hereditary optic nerve atrophy. Vitamin B12 can cause severe and swift optic atrophy (15).

OTHER: The therapeutic response to vitamin B12 can be impaired by concurrent infections, uremia, and folic acid or iron deficiency (15).

Typical Dosages & Routes of Administration that are Commonly Used

ORAL: The dietary supplement amount of vitamin B12 is 1-25 mcg per day (15). A supplemental amount of 6 mcg per day is recommended for strict vegetarians (14). The recommended amount for nutritional deficiency is 25-250 mcg per day (3022). Oral administration is markedly inferior to parenteral administration for treating documented vitamin B12 deficiency, but oral amounts up to 1 mg (1000 mcg) daily have been used successfully in people who refused parenteral therapy (15). For primary circadian rhythm sleep disorders, 0.5-1 mg of the methylcobalamin form of vitamin B12 three times daily has been used, with or without bright light therapy (1345,1347).

The daily recommended dietary allowances (RDAs) of vitamin B12 are: Infants 0-6 months, 0.4 mcg; Infants 7-12 months, 0.5 mcg; Children 1-3 years, 0.9 mcg; Children 4-8 years, 1.2 mcg; Children 9-13 years, 1.8 mcg; Older children and adults, 2.4 mcg; Pregnant women 2.6 mcg; and Lactating women, 2.8 mcg (3094). Because 10-30% of older people can malabsorb food-bound vitamin B12, those over 50 years should meet the RDA by eating foods fortified with B12 or take a vitamin B12 supplement (3094).

INJECTION : Prescription only.

Comments

Vitamin B12 is present in meat, fish, and dairy products (14). The intrinsic factor, a glycoprotein secreted by the gastric mucosa, is required for vitamin B12 absorption from the gut (15). Normal serum vitamin B12 levels range between 200-900 pg/mL. Serum concentrations less than 200 pg/mL indicate deficiency, and concentrations less than 100 pg/mL usually result in megaloblastic anemia or neurologic damage (15). The hydroxocobalamin injection is a form of B12 with a hematopoietic effect equivalent to cyanocobalamin but having a longer duration of action (272). Vitamin B12 is frequently used in combination with other B vitamins in vitamin B complex formulations. Vitamin B complex generally includes vitamin B1 (thiamine), vitamin B2 (riboflavin), vitamin B3 (niacin/niacinamide), vitamin B5 (pantothenic acid), vitamin B6 (pyridoxine), vitamin B12 (cyanocobalamin), and folic acid. However, some products do not contain all of these ingredients and some may include others, such as biotin, para-aminobenzoic acid (PABA), choline bitartrate, and inositol (3022,3060,3061).

VITAMIN C (ASCORBIC ACID)

This Product is Also Known As
Ascorbate, Ascorbic Acid, Antiscorbutic Vitamin, Calcium Ascorbate, Cevitamic Acid, Sodium Ascorbate, Vitamin C.
CAUTION: See separate listings for Acerola, Cherokee Rosehip, and Rose Hip.

Scientific Names
Ascorbic acid.

People Use This For
Orally, vitamin C is used for preventing and treating scurvy; preventing deficiency in people with GI diseases and those on chronic total parenteral nutrition or chronic hemodialysis; increasing iron absorption from the GI tract; increasing the healing rate of wounds, burns, fractures, ulcers and pressure sores; and urinary acidification. It is used for treating idiopathic methemoglobinemia, correcting tyrosinemia in premature infants on high-protein diets, increasing iron excretion (in combination with deferoxamine), preventing and treating the common cold and other viral infections, tuberculosis, dysentery, furunculosis, hematuria, retinal hemorrhages, hemorrhagic states, and anemia. Ascorbic acid is taken by mouth for atherosclerosis, preventing vascular thrombosis and myocardial infarction, hypertension, lowering cholesterol, glaucoma, preventing cataracts, dental caries, pyorrhea, gum infections, constipation, peptic ulcer, acne, dermatitis, improving immune function, hay fever, asthma, bronchitis, cystic fibrosis, cystitis, prostatitis, infertility, and diabetes. Vitamin C is also used for mental depression; cognitive impairment; stress; fatigue; attention deficit disorder; autism; collagen disorders; arthritis; bursitis; back pain and disc inflammation; cancer; osteogenesis imperfecta; improving physical endurance; reducing aging; heat prostration; protection against free radicals, heavy metals, and other pollutants; for counteracting the side effects of cortisone and related drugs; aiding drug withdrawal in addiction; and treatment of levodopa, succinylcholine, or arsenic toxicity (14,15,3044,3045).
In combination with vitamin K3, vitamin C is used for treating prostate and breast cancers (1257).
Topically, it is used for improving skin conditions, protecting against free radicals and pollutants (3043), and photoaged skin (6155). It is also applied topically for ulcerative mucositis associated with radiation therapy (6103).
By injection, vitamin C is used for preventing and treating ascorbic acid deficiency and correcting tyrosinemia in premature infants on high-protein diets (15).

Safety
LIKELY SAFE ...when taken orally and appropriately. Vitamin C is generally considered nontoxic even at doses exceeding the recommended dietary allowance; however, side effects are dose-related and may occur with greater frequency at higher doses (see Adverse Reactions) (14,15,3042). ...when the injectable form is given intravenously or intramuscularly and appropriately. Injectable vitamin C is a FDA-approved prescription product (15).
There is insufficient information about the safety of the topical use of vitamin C.
PREGNANCY AND LACTATION: LIKELY SAFE ...when used orally in doses that do not exceed the recommended dietary allowance (14,15). POSSIBLY UNSAFE ...when used orally in doses exceeding the recommended dietary allowance. Large doses of ascorbic acid in pregnancy are associated with newborn scurvy; avoid using (14,15).

Effectiveness
EFFECTIVE ...when taken orally or given intramuscularly for preventing and treating vitamin C deficiency, including scurvy. Vitamin C administration can reverse complications of scurvy within two days to three weeks (15).
LIKELY EFFECTIVE ...when taken orally for improving iron absorption. Concurrent administration of at least 200 mg vitamin C per 30 mg iron can increase iron absorption (14,15,3402).
POSSIBLY EFFECTIVE ...when taken orally from dietary sources for reducing cancer risk. People consuming fruits and vegetables that provide vitamin C 200 mg per day may have a decreased risk of developing cancers of the mouth, esophagus, stomach, colon, and lung (1444,3042). ...when used orally with vitamin E for preventing pre-eclampsia in high-risk pregnancies (3236). ...when used orally as an adjunct to medication to lower blood pressure. In a small study, hypertensive patients had supplemental vitamin C added to their medication regimen and demonstrated a decrease in both systolic and mean blood pressure, but had no decrease in diastolic readings (2044). ...when used orally to protect against vascular dementia (4846). A large epidemiological study associated concurrent use of vitamins C and E with a lower incidence of vascular dementia. No protective effect was found for Alzheimer's dementia (4846). ...when used orally to decrease exercise-induced asthma (1443). ...when used orally to decrease the risk of developing reflex sympathetic dystrophy after wrist fractures. In one placebo-controlled study, patients given vitamin C supplements for 50 days after a wrist fracture were significantly less

likely to develop reflex sympathetic dystrophy (2045). ...when taken orally from dietary sources to lower blood lead levels (3097,3098,3099). ...when taken orally to prevent the development of nitrate tolerance in patients taking sublingual nitroglycerin (1441). ...when L-ascorbic acid is applied topically for improving photoaged facial skin. In one trial, a topical preparation containing L-ascorbic acid 10%, acetyl tyrosine, zinc sulfate, sodium hyaluronate, and bioflavonoids (Cellex-C High Potency Serum) for three months to photoaged facial skin improved fine and coarse wrinkling, yellowing/sallowness, roughness, and skin tone compared to placebo (6155,6166).

POSSIBLY INEFFECTIVE ...when taken orally for preventing and treating the common cold (14,15,3042). ...when used orally as an urinary acidifier (14,15). ...when supplemental vitamin C is used orally to decrease cancer risk (3042).

LIKELY INEFFECTIVE ...when used in high doses to treat cancer (4842,4843). Two double-blind, placebo-controlled trials found no benefit of vitamin C 10 grams daily in patients with advanced cancer, regardless of prior chemotherapy (4842,4843).

There is insufficient reliable information available about the effectiveness of vitamin C for its other uses.

Possible Mechanism of Action & Active Ingredients

Vitamin C is present in fresh fruits and vegetables, especially the citrus fruits. Vitamin C is required for collagen formation and tissue repair (15). It is an enzyme cofactor in the synthesis of collagen, carnitine, norepinephrine, and peptide hormones, and in tyrosine metabolism (3042). Vitamin C is involved in a variety of metabolic processes including oxidation-reduction reactions, the conversion of folic acid to folinic acid, carbohydrate metabolism, synthesis of lipids and proteins, iron metabolism, and cellular respiration (15). Vitamin C also plays a role in immune function and infection resistance (15). It acts as an antioxidant, decreasing oxidants in gastric juice, decreasing lipid peroxidation, and decreasing oxidative DNA and protein damage (3042). Sustained vitamin C deficiency lasting from three to five months results in symptomatic scurvy that affects collagenous structures, bones, and blood vessels (15). Wound healing is also delayed in people with vitamin C deficiency; however, there is no evidence to indicate that vitamin C supplementation improves healing in people with normal nutritional status (14). Vitamin C in combination with vitamin K3 might be useful against prostate and breast cancer. Preliminary research suggests that this combination might cause a unique kind of tumor cell death (1257). Cancer cells have higher concentrations of vitamin C than normal tissue (4838). Colony-stimulating factors appear to stimulate update of vitamin C by host defense cells (4840). Unlike normal cells, cancer cells cannot import ascorbic acid and appear to oxidize ascorbic acid to dehydroascorbic acid, which is moved into the cell by a specialized glucose transport system. Once inside the tumor cell, dehydroascorbic acid is reduced to ascorbic acid for use by the malignant cell. Although vitamin C supplementation in cancer patients has not been beneficial, whether a higher concentration of vitamin C augments growth of cancer cells is unknown (4838,4839,4840,4841,4842). For radiation-induced oral mucositis, the reduced form of vitamin C might be beneficial due to its antioxidant effect and role in maintaining connective tissue integrity. Preliminary evidence using an animal model suggests that topical application of the reduced form of vitamin C, dehydroascorbic acid, can reduce the severity of oral mucositis associated with radiation therapy (6103). Free radicals generated in the skin by exposure to ultraviolet light cause photoaging. Ascorbic acid in the skin is believed to play a key role in neutralizing these free radicals and reducing UV skin damage (6155). A stable topical formulation of L-ascorbic acid, tyrosine, and zinc significantly increases skin ascorbic acid levels and improves the appearance of photoaged facial skin (6155).

Adverse Reactions Including Known Allergies

The adverse effects of vitamin C are dose-related (3042) and include nausea, vomiting, esophagitis, heartburn, abdominal cramps, gastrointestinal obstruction, fatigue, flushing, headache, insomnia, sleepiness, diarrhea, hyperoxaluria, and the precipitation of urate, oxalate, or cysteine stones or drugs in the urinary tract (14,15). Hyperoxaluria, hyperuricosuria, hematuria, and crystalluria have occurred in people taking 1 gram or more per day (14,3042). Large amounts of vitamin C are associated with deep vein thrombosis. Prolonged use of large amounts of vitamin C can also result in increased metabolism of vitamin C and scurvy can occur when vitamin C intake is reduced (15). Oral supplementation with vitamin C has also been associated with an increased rate of carotid inner wall thickening in men. In an unpublished study, announced at the American Heart Association's 40th Annual Conference on Cardiovascular Disease Epidemiology and Prevention, supplemental intake of vitamin C 500 mg daily for 18 months resulted in a 2.5-fold increased rate of carotid inner wall thickening in non-smoking men and a 5-fold increased rate in men who smoked. The men in this study were 40-60 years old. This effect was not associated with vitamin C from dietary sources (1355).

Possible Interactions with Herbs & Other Dietary Supplements

IRON: Concomitant use of 200 mg of vitamin C per 30 mg of elemental iron increases oral iron absorption, especially ferric iron (14,15,3042).

Possible Interactions with Drugs

ASPIRIN AND OTHER SALICYLATES: Concomitant use can increase urinary excretion of ascorbic acid and decrease excretion of salicylates. However, it might not have a clinically significant effect on salicylate plasma levels (15,3046).

ALUMINUM-CONTAINING ANTACIDS: Concomitant use might increase aluminum absorption. Clinical significance is unknown (3046). Administer vitamin C two hours before, or four hours after taking an antacid (3046).

IRON: 200 mg vitamin C per 30 mg of elemental iron increases iron (especially ferric iron) absorption (14,15,3042).

WARFARIN: Concomitant use with large amounts vitamin C might impair response to warfarin (3046).

Drug Influences on Nutrient Levels and Depletion

SOME DRUGS CAN AFFECT VITAMIN C LEVELS.

ASPIRIN AND OTHER SALICYLATES: Concomitant use can increase urinary excretion of vitamin C. However, there is no evidence of vitamin C deficiency associated with use of aspirin and other salicylates. Consider supplementation only in patients on long-term salicylate therapy with signs of vitamin C deficiency (15,3046).

BARBITURATES: Barbiturates can increase elimination of vitamin C (15,19). Consider supplementation only if clinical judgment warrants it.

ESTROGEN and ORAL CONTRACEPTIVES: Estrogens can increase elimination of vitamin C (15,19). Consider supplementation only if clinical judgment warrants it.

NICOTINE: Nicotine can increase elimination of vitamin C (19). Consider supplementation only if clinical judgment warrants it.

TETRACYCLINES: Tetracyclines can increase elimination of vitamin C (15,19). Consider supplementation only if clinical judgment warrants it.

Possible Interactions with Foods

IRON: Vitamin C can increase the absorption of dietary ferric iron (14,3042).

Possible Interactions with Lab Tests

URIC ACID: Large amounts of vitamin C can cause a decrease in serum uric acid concentrations and test results with enzymatic method assays (15), and a false increase in test results with assays based on other methods (14).

CALCIUM/SODIUM: 3-6 grams of vitamin C daily can cause an increase in urinary calcium and test results (15), and a decrease in urinary sodium and test results.

ASPARTATE AMINOTRANSFERASE (AST, SGOT): Large amounts of ascorbic acid can cause a false increase in results of serum tests relying on color reactions (Redox reactions) and Technicon SMA 12/60 (14).

LDH: Vitamin C can cause a false decrease measured by Technicon SMA 12/60 and Abbott 100 methods (14).

BILIRUBIN: Large amounts of vitamin C can cause a false increase in serum test results measured by Technicon SMA 12/60 or colorimetric methods (14).

CARBAMAZEPINE (Tegretol): Large doses of vitamin C can cause falsely increased serum assay results measured by Ames ARIS method (14).

THEOPHYLLINE: Large amounts of vitamin C can cause falsely decreased serum assay results when measured by the ARIS system or Ames Seralyzer photometer (14).

CREATININE: Vitamin C can cause a false increase in serum creatinine or urine test results (14).

GLUCOSE: Large amounts of vitamin C can cause false increases in urine test results measured by copper reduction methods (e.g. Clinitest), and false decreases in results measured by glucose oxidase methods (e.g. Clinistix, Tes-Tape) (14,15).

ACETAMINOPHEN: Vitamin C can cause false-negative urine results with methods based on hydrolysis and formation of an indophenol blue chromagen (14).

OCCULT BLOOD: False-negative guaiac results occur with 250 mg or more of vitamin C per day (3042).

Possible Interactions with Diseases or Conditions

DIABETES: Vitamin C can affect glycogenolysis and increase blood sugar, but this effect remains controversial (15).

GLUCOSE-6-PHOSPHATE DEHYDROGENASE DEFICIENCY: Large amounts of vitamin C can cause hemolysis in individuals with glucose-6-phosphate dehydrogenase deficiency (15).

KIDNEY STONES: Large amounts of vitamin C can increase the risk of oxalate stone formation (15).

SICKLE CELL DISEASE: Vitamin C can decrease blood pH, which rarely precipitates sickle cell crisis (15).

HEMOCHROMATOSIS, THALASSEMIA, SIDEROBLASTIC ANEMIA: Use vitamin C with caution, because it can increase iron absorption, which could worsen this condition (14,15).

INCREASED NEEDS: Vitamin C requirements are increased in pregnancy, lactation, hyperthyroidism, stress, fever, infection, trauma, burns, smoking, and cold exposure (15).

Typical Dosages & Routes of Administration that are Commonly Used

ORAL: As a dietary supplement, 75 to 90 mg of vitamin C is taken per day (4844). Vitamin C can be more beneficial as a dietary supplement when 100-200 mg is taken daily from fruits and vegetables (3042). For chronic hemodialysis in adults, 100-200 mg per day is recommended (15). The usual dose of vitamin C for scurvy is 100-250 mg once or twice daily for several days, although larger amounts are sometimes used (15). Alternatively, vitamin C deficiency is treated with 100 mg three times daily for one week and then once daily until tissue saturation is normal (14). The daily recommended dietary allowances (RDAs) of vitamin C were changed by the Food and Nutrition Board of the National Institute of Medicine in April 2000. The new recommendations are: Infants 0 to 12 months, human milk content (older recommendations specified 30 to 35 mg); Children 1 to 3 years, 15 mg; Children 4 to 8 years, 25 mg; Children 9 to 13 years, 45 mg; Adolescents 14 to 18 years, 75 mg for boys and 65 mg for girls; Adults age 19 and greater, 90 mg for men and 75 mg for women; Pregnancy and Lactation: age 18 or younger, 115 mg; ages 19 to 50 years 120 mg (14,4844). People who use tobacco should take an additional 35 mg per day (4844). The upper limit was set at 2000 mg per day, based on the adverse effect of osmotic diarrhea (4844).

INJECTION (IM, IV or subcutaneous): This is an FDA-approved prescription product.

Comments

The American Heart Association recommends obtaining antioxidants, including vitamin C, from a diet high in fruits, vegetables, and whole grains rather than through supplements until more information is known from randomized trials (1440). Vitamin C is labile, and the amount in foods can decrease significantly with cooking and storage (3042). A recent review by an independent laboratory found that 15% of the vitamin C in products tested did not meet labeled potency, including one product that claimed USP standards (4845).

VITAMIN D

This Product is Also Known As

Calcifediol: 25-hydroxyvitamin D3, 25-hydroxycholecalciferol, 25-HCC, 25-OHCC, 25-OHD3. Calcitriol: 1,25-dihydroxyvitamin D3, 1,25-dihydroxycholecalciferol, 1,25-DHCC, 1,25-diOHC, 1,25(0H)2D3. Cholecalciferol: vitamin D3, activated 7-dehydrocholesterol, colecalciferol. Dihydrotachysterol: DHT, dichysterol, dihydrotachysterol 2. Ergocalciferol: vitamin D2, calciferol, activated ergosterol, viosterol, ergocalciferolum, irradiated ergosterol. Calcipotriene: calcipotriol. Paricalcitol: paracalcin, 19-nor-1,25-dihydroxyvitamin D2.

Scientific Names

Vitamin D; calcifediol; 25-hydroxycholecalciferol; calcitriol; 1,25-dihydroxycholecalciferol; cholecalciferol; dihydrotachysterol; ergocalciferol; calcipotriene; paricalcitol.

People Use This For

Orally, vitamin D is used for building bone mass and preventing bone loss; protecting against muscle weakness; promoting strong teeth (3058,3059); reducing risk of colon, breast, and prostate cancer (15); treating cancer; enhancing immune function; preventing autoimmune diseases (3058,3059); and rheumatoid arthritis (14,15). It is used orally for preventing and treating rickets, postmenopausal osteoporosis, corticosteroid-induced osteoporosis, osteomalacia, anticonvulsant-induced osteomalacia, renal osteodystrophy, osteitis fibrosa in people on dialysis, hepatic osteodystrophy, osteogenesis imperfecta, preventing and treating hypocalcemia and tetany in premature infants, hypocalcemic tetany, bone disorders in people with familial hypophosphatemia, hypophosphatemia associated with Fanconi syndrome, hypocalcemia associated with postoperative or idiopathic hypoparathyroidism or pseudohypoparathyroidism, plaque-type psoriasis, actinic keratoses, lupus vulgaris, squamous cell carcinomas, vitiligo, scleroderma, myelodysplastic syndrome (14,15), and treating multiple sclerosis (5083).

Topically, vitamin D is used as calcitriol or calcipotriene for plaque-type psoriasis (14).

Intravenously, vitamin D, administered as calcitriol, is used for hypocalcemic tetany in premature infants, hypocalcemia and hyperparathyroidism in renal dialysis patients, and osteitis fibrosa (14,15).

Intramuscularly, vitamin D is administered as ergocalciferol for hepatic osteodystrophy, and as an injectable source of vitamin D (14,15).

Safety

LIKELY SAFE ...when used orally and appropriately (15). Therapeutic amounts do not differ much from amounts that can cause hypercalcemia.

PREGNANCY: LIKELY SAFE ...when used at the recommended adequate intake of 200 units daily, and in amounts up to 400 units daily found in many prenatal vitamin supplements (15); avoid larger amounts (15). Hypercalcemia during pregnancy due to vitamin D intake can lead to suppression of parathyroid hormone, hypocalcemia, tetany, seizures, aortic valve stenosis, retinopathy, and mental and/or physical retardation in the infant (15).

LACTATION: LIKELY SAFE ...when used at amounts up to 400 units daily (15); avoid larger amounts.

Effectiveness

EFFECTIVE ...when oral calcifediol is used for treating osteomalacia secondary to liver disease (hepatic osteodystrophy). ...when oral calcifediol is used for managing hypocalcemia and preventing renal osteodystrophy in people with chronic renal failure undergoing dialysis. ...when oral calcifediol is used for preventing corticosteroid-induced osteopenia and osteoporosis (14,15). ...when oral calcitriol is used for preventing tetany in vitamin D-deficient premature infants with hypocalcemia. ...when oral calcitriol is used in conjunction with phosphate supplements for treating bone disorders in people with familial hypophosphatemia. ...when oral calcitriol is used for vitamin D-dependent rickets. ...when oral calcitriol is used for managing hypocalcemia and preventing renal osteodystrophy in people with chronic renal failure undergoing dialysis. ...when oral calcitriol is used for treating osteitis fibrosa. ...when oral calcitriol is used for anticonvulsant-induced rickets. ...when oral calcitriol is used for plaque-type psoriasis. ...when oral calcitriol is used for increasing serum calcium concentrations in people with hypoparathyroidism or pseudohypoparathyroidism (14,15). ...when topical calcitriol is used for treating plaque-type psoriasis (14). ...when oral cholecalciferol is used for treating nutritional rickets and osteomalacia. ...when oral cholecalciferol is used for preventing corticosteroid-induced osteopenia and osteoporosis (15). ...when oral dihydrotachysterol is used in conjunction with phosphate supplements for treating bone disorders in people with familial hypophosphatemia. ...when oral dihydrotachysterol is used for renal osteodystrophy and osteitis fibrosa. ...when oral dihydrotachysterol is used for managing hypocalcemia and preventing renal osteodystrophy in people with chronic renal failure undergoing dialysis. ...when oral dihydrotachysterol is used for increasing serum calcium concentrations in people with hypoparathyroidism or pseudohypoparathyroidism. ...when oral dihydrotachysterol is used for preventing and treating hypocalcemic tetany (14,15). ...when oral ergocalciferol is used for treating nutritional rickets and osteomalacia due to malabsorption syndromes. ...when oral ergocalciferol is used for neonatal rickets. ...when oral ergocalciferol is used in very large doses and in conjunction with phosphate supplements for bone disorders in people with familial hypophosphatemia. ...when oral ergocalciferol is used for hypophosphatemia associated with Fanconi syndrome. ...when oral ergocalciferol is used in large amounts for vitamin D-dependent rickets. ...when oral ergocalciferol is used in high doses for increasing serum calcium concentrations in people with hypoparathyroidism or pseudohypoparathyroidism (14,15). ...when calcipotriene is used topically for treating moderate plaque psoriasis (14).

POSSIBLY EFFECTIVE ...when oral calcifediol is used for anticonvulsant-induced osteomalacia. ...when oral calcifediol is used for postmenopausal osteoporosis (14). ...when oral calcitriol is used with isotretinoin for treating actinic keratoses and early squamous cell carcinomas. ...when oral calcitriol is used for myelodysplastic syndrome. ...when oral calcitriol is used for postmenopausal osteoporosis (14). ...when oral dihydrotachysterol is used in conjunction with calcium supplements and sodium fluoride supplements for treating osteoporosis. ...when oral dihydrotachysterol is used for osteogenesis imperfecta (14,15). ...when oral ergocalciferol is used in conjunction with calcium supplements and sodium fluoride supplements for treating postmenopausal osteoporosis. ...when oral ergocalciferol is used for preventing and treating anticonvulsant-induced rickets and osteomalacia. ...when oral ergocalciferol is used for preventing corticosteroid-induced osteomalacia. ...when oral ergocalciferol is used for hepatic osteodystrophy (14,15). ...when topical calcipotriene is used for treating vitiligo and scleroderma (14). ...when vitamin D3 is used orally for decreasing secondary hyperparathyroidism and bone turnover in black women. In one study, supplementation with vitamin D3 resulted in increased serum levels of 25-hydroxyvitamin D, reduced levels of parathyroid hormone, and decreased production of markers of bone turnover (3463). ...when vitamin D is given orally in breast-fed infants for increasing bone mineral density. In a retrospective study, prepubertal girls who received vitamin D in infancy had significantly greater bone mineral density at some skeletal sites compared to girls that did not receive vitamin D during infancy (3464).

POSSIBLY INEFFECTIVE ...when used orally for preventing bone loss associated with long-term renal transplantation (4823). Calcitriol 0.25 mcg per day in combination with calcium carbonate 500 mg per day did not significantly improve bone loss in renal transplant patients; however, the treatment group had less osteoclast suppression and there was a trend to maintenance of trabecular bone volume and wall thickness, and some improvement in axial bone mineral density (4823).

LIKELY INEFFECTIVE ...when oral calcitriol is used for corticosteroid-induced osteoporosis (14).

Possible Mechanism of Action & Active Ingredients

The principal source of vitamin D is through exposure of the skin to sunlight (15). Cholecalciferol, also known as vitamin D3, is formed from 7-dehydrocholesterol in the skin after exposure to UV light (15). Vitamin D is stored in body fat for use during periods without sun exposure (15). Conversely, excessive sun exposure causes photodegradation of vitamin D produced in the skin, limiting the risk of vitamin D toxicity from such exposure (15). In the body, cholecalciferol is hydroxylated to calcifediol, also known as 25-hydroxyvitamin D, 25-hydroxycholecalciferol, in the liver, and then to calcitriol, also known as 1,25-dihydroxyvitamin D, 1,25-dihydroxycholecaliferol, in the kidneys (14,15). The active forms of vitamin D produced endogenously and from dietary sources (i.e. 1,25-dihydroxyergocalciferol, calcitriol, 25-hydroxydihydrotachysterol and calcifediol) work with parathyroid hormone and calcitonin to regulate serum calcium and phosphorus concentrations, principally by enhancing intestinal absorption of these minerals (15). Vitamin D deficiency causes increased parathyroid hormone activity, which acts to maintain serum calcium and phosphate concentrations, at the expense of skeletal calcium (15). Provided permanent skeletal deformities have not occurred, supplementing vitamin D in the form of ergocalciferol or cholecalciferol will correct deficiency in people who can activate and utilize them. Since part of the activation process , namely the 1-hydroxylation, occurs in the kidneys, people with chronic renal failure might not be able to activate these forms of vitamin D. Instead, they require calcitriol, dihydrotachysterol, or calcifediol (15). Liver disease can prevent 25-hydroxylation of vitamin D. Therefore, people with liver disease might need supplemental 25-hydroxylated vitamin D derivatives, e.g. calcifediol (14). Epidemiologic evidence suggests that vitamin D deficiency may be associated with an increased risk of colon, breast and prostate cancer, but this has not been confirmed (15). Topical calcipotriene and calcitriol inhibit epidermal proliferation and stimulate the differentiation of epidermal cells (14).

Adverse Reactions Including Known Allergies

Early symptoms of vitamin D toxicity are those of hypercalcemia. They include weakness, fatigue, sleepiness, headache, loss of appetite, dry mouth, metallic taste, nausea, vomiting, abdominal cramps, constipation, diarrhea, dizziness, ringing in the ears, trouble walking, skin eruptions, hypotonia in infants, muscle pain, bone pain, and irritability. Advanced symptoms may include runny nose, itching, decreased libido, and kidney insufficiency due to precipitation of calcium phosphate in the tubules. Symptoms of renal impairment include frequency, nighttime awakening to urinate, thirst, inability to concentrate urine, and proteinuria. Other symptoms include osteoporosis in adults, decreased growth in children, weight loss, anemia, calcific conjunctivitis, photophobia, metastatic calcification, pancreatitis, generalized vascular calcification, and seizures. Rarely, people develop hypertension and psychosis. Lab values of urinary calcium, phosphate, albumin, blood urea nitrogen, serum cholesterol, aspartate aminotransferase, and alanine aminotransferase concentrations might increase (15). Serum alkaline phosphatase concentrations can decrease (15). Serum electrolyte imbalances, along with mild acidosis, might result in cardiac arrhythmias (15). Topical use of calcipotriene can cause hypercalcemia, hypercalciuria, burning, itching, skin irritation, erythema, dry skin, peeling, rash, dermatitis, and hyperpigmentation (14).

Possible Interactions with Herbs & Other Dietary Supplements

CARDIAC GLYCOSIDE-CONTAINING HERBS: Vitamin D should be administered with caution to people taking cardiac glycosides, because hypercalcemia can cause cardiac arrhythmias (15). Cardiac glycoside-containing herbs include black hellebore, Canadian hemp, digitalis, hedge mustard, figwort, lily-of-the-valley, motherwort, oleander, pheasant's eye, pleurisy, squill, and strophanthus (2,18,19,500).

MINERAL OIL: Excessive use can interfere with intestinal absorption of vitamin D (15).

Possible Interactions with Drugs

CORTICOSTEROIDS: Corticosteroids increase the need for supplemental vitamin D (15).

DIGOXIN: Vitamin D should be administered with caution to people taking cardiac glycosides, because hypercalcemia can cause cardiac arrhythmias (15).

THIAZIDE DIURETICS: Concomitant use of thiazides and pharmacologic amounts of vitamin D in people with hypoparathyroidism might result in hypercalcemia (15).

PHENYTOIN (Dilantin), PHENOBARBITAL: Concomitant use might reduce plasma concentrations of the active 25-hydroxylated vitamin D analogs and increase metabolism to inactive metabolites. Vitamin D analogs that require 25-hydroxylation in the body for activity might be ineffective when taken with phenobarbital or phenytoin (14,15).

HEPATIC ENZYME INDUCERS: Concomitant use of drugs that induce hepatic enzymes might reduce plasma concentrations of the active 25-hydroxylated vitamin D analogs and increase metabolism to inactive metabolites (15).

MINERAL OIL can reduce supplemental vitamin D absorption. Avoid long-term use of mineral oil (4495).

Drug Influences on Nutrient Levels and Depletion

SOME DRUGS CAN AFFECT VITAMIN D LEVELS:

CHOLESTYRAMINE (Questran, LoCholest, Prevalite): Concomitant use can decrease vitamin D absorption in the gastrointestinal tract. However, there is no clinical evidence that supplementation is necessary (4454,4455,4456,4457, 4458,4459).

COLESTIPOL (Colestid): Concomitant use can decrease vitamin D absorption in the gastrointestinal tract. In some cases, supplementation may be appropriate (4460,4461).

RIFAMPIN (Rimactane): Rifampin increases vitamin D metabolism and reduces vitamin D serum levels. The need for vitamin D supplementation has not been adequately studied (4514).

CARBAMAZEPINE (Tegretol): Carbamazepine increases vitamin D metabolism and reduces vitamin D serum levels. The necessity for supplementation with vitamin D has not been adequately studied (4430,4431).

PHENYTOIN (Dilantin) and FOSPHENYTOIN (Cerebyx): Use of phenytoin and fosphenytoin can cause vitamin D deficiency when used long-term. Some authors suggest that patients receiving long-term phenytoin therapy should receive 400-800 IU/day of vitamin D and maintain a diet rich in calcium (4475).

PHENOBARBITAL (Luminal): Phenobarbital can cause vitamin D deficiency when used long-term. Some authors recommended that patients receiving long-term phenobarbital therapy take 400-800 IU/day of vitamin D and maintain a diet rich in calcium. Other authors suggest that vitamin D should be supplemented only if deficiencies are noted (4453,4531).

MINERAL OIL: Mineral oil can reduce dietary vitamin D absorption. Avoid long-term use of mineral oil (4495).

ORLISTAT (Xenical): Orlistat can reduce vitamin D levels (1725,1726,1727,1730). Consider a multivitamin with fat-soluble vitamins, taken at least 2 hours before or after orlistat, or at bedtime.

STIMULANT LAXATIVES: Excessive use of stimulant laxatives can result in vitamin D depletion. Limit stimulant laxatives to short-term use (4425).

CORTICOSTEROIDS: Use of corticosteroids can cause osteoporosis and calcium depletion with long-term administration. This calcium depletion creates a greater need for both supplemental calcium and vitamin D, which is necessary for calcium absorption. It might be prudent to supplement calcium and vitamin D (calcitriol) before, during, and after long-term and/or high-dose corticosteroid therapy (4462,4463,4464,4465,4466,4467).

Possible Interactions with Foods

No interactions are known to occur, and there is no known reason to expect a clinically significant interaction with vitamin D.

Possible Interactions with Lab Tests

SERUM CHOLESTEROL: Vitamin D might cause false increases in serum cholesterol test results measured by the Zlatkis-Zak reaction (15).

Possible Interactions with Diseases or Conditions

HYPERCALCEMIA: Contraindicated (14,15).

SARCOIDOSIS, HYPOPARATHYROIDISM might predispose individuals to increased sensitivity to vitamin D (15).

RENAL DISEASE: Use ergocalciferol with extreme caution in individuals with renal failure or renal stones, if at all (15).

ARTERIOSCLEROSIS, HEART DISEASE: Use ergocalciferol with extreme caution in individuals with arteriosclerosis (15).

Typical Dosages & Routes of Administration that are Commonly Used

ORAL: A typical dose of calcifediol, calcitriol, cholecalciferol, and ergocalciferol is present in many multivitamin supplements. Amounts used as dietary supplements must not exceed the recommended dietary allowance (RDA) of 400 units daily (14). Larger amounts require supervision, and must be individualized to maintain serum calcium concentrations of 9-10 mg/dL and avoid hypercalcemia (15). Daily recommended dietary allowances (RDAs) of vitamin D are no longer published because both sunlight exposure and dietary intake of vitamin D in the general population vary (15). The National Academy of Sciences now publishes an Adequate Intake (AI) which is an estimate of the amount of vitamin D that appears to sustain normal functioning (15). The current daily AI of vitamin D used as cholecalciferol or ergocalciferol to prevent rickets in healthy children and osteomalacia in adults is based on age. Birth through 50 years of age, 5 mcg (200 units); Adults (ages 51 to 70), 10 mcg (400 units); Adults (greater than 70 years of age), 15 mcg (600 units) daily (15). The upper intake levels (UL) for vitamin D are 25 mcg for infants 0-12 months and 50 mcg for everyone over one year of age (3094).

Other vitamin D analogs and vitamin D products for other routes of administration are available as FDA-approved prescription drugs.

Comments

The main dietary sources of vitamin D are fish liver oils, butter, eggs, and fortified milk and cereals (15). One unit of vitamin D equals the biologic activity of 25 mg of ergocalciferol or cholecalciferol (15).

Researchers report that 4 mcg per day of 19-nor vitamin D for more than 9 months had no effect clinically or on the rate of appearance of new brain lesions in a group of patients with relapsing-remitting multiple sclerosis. The results of this unpublished trial were reported at the American Academy of Neurology's 52nd Annual Meeting (5083).

VITAMIN E

This Product is Also Known As

All Rac-Alpha-Tocopherol, Alpha-Tocopherol, d-Alpha-Tocopherol, d-Alpha-Tocopheryl, d-Alpha-Tocopheryl Acetate, d-Alpha-Tocopheryl Succinate, dl-Alpha-Tocopherol, dl-Alpha-Tocopheryl, dl-Alpha-Tocopheryl Acetate, d-Tocopherol, dl-Tocopherol, d-Beta-Tocopherol, d-Delta-Tocopherol, d-Gamma-Tocopherol, Mixed Tocopherols, RRR-Alpha-Tocopherol, Tocopherol, Tocopheryl Acetate, Tocopheryl Acid Succinate, Tocopheryl Succinate, Tocotrienol, Tocotrienol Concentrate from Vitamin E.

Scientific Names

Alpha-tocopherol; beta-tocopherol; delta-tocopherol; gamma-tocopherol; alpha tocotrienol; beta tocotrienol; delta tocotrienol; gamma tocotrienol.

People Use This For

Orally, vitamin E is used for replacement therapy in vitamin E deficiency, treating and preventing cardiovascular disease, including slowing atherogenesis and preventing heart attacks. It is used for angina, thrombophlebitis, intermittent claudication, and preventing ischemia-reperfusion injury after coronary artery bypass surgery.

Vitamin E is used for preventing cancer, particularly lung and oral cancer in smokers, colorectal cancer and polyps, and gastric, prostate, and pancreatic cancer (14,15). Vitamin E is used for Alzheimer's disease and other dementias, night cramps, and Parkinson's disease (14,15). Vitamin E is also used orally for preventing pre-eclampsia in high-risk women (3236), for improving physical endurance, increasing energy, preventing allergies, for asthma and infections, for protecting against negative effects of air pollution, preventing aging, preventing cataracts, inflammatory skin disorders, burns, cystic fibrosis, oral leukoplakia, premenstrual syndrome, habitual abortion, menopausal syndrome, infertility, impotence, chronic cystic mastitis, mammary dysplasia, peptic ulcers, porphyria, tardive dyskinesia, neuromuscular disorders, Huntington's chorea, chronic progressive hereditary chorea, and myotonic dystrophy. Additionally, vitamin E is used orally for preventing vitamin E deficiency in people with malabsorption syndromes or abetalipoproteinemia, treating hemolytic anemia caused by vitamin E deficiency in premature neonates, preventing retinopathy of prematurity, preventing bronchopulmonary dysplasia secondary to oxygen therapy in neonates, and preventing intraventricular hemorrhage in premature neonates. Vitamin E is used for correcting erythrocyte membrane abnormalities in people with beta-thalassemia, for hereditary spherocytosis, glucose-6-phosphate dehydrogenase deficiency or sickle-cell anemia, treating anemia in conjunction with erythropoietin in people on dialysis, reducing doxorubicin-induced hair loss, reducing amiodarone-induced

© Copyright 2000, Natural Medicines Comprehensive Database (209) 472-2244. For updated data, go to www.NaturalDatabase.com • 1073

pulmonary toxicity (4706,4707), and for radiation-induced fibrosis (14,15,3067,3068).
Topically, vitamin E is used for dermatitis, granuloma annulare, and protecting against skin ulceration caused by extravasation of chemotherapy drugs (14).

Safety

LIKELY SAFE ...when used orally and appropriately (14). Vitamin E is generally considered non-toxic, even at doses exceeding the recommended dietary allowance (RDA); however, adverse effects are more likely to occur with higher doses (see Adverse Reactions) (15). The recommended tolerable upper limit of vitamin E is 1000 mg per day, equivalent to 1100 IU of synthetic vitamin E and 1500 IU of natural vitamin E (4729).
POSSIBLY UNSAFE ...when used orally in excessive amounts (4729). Repeated administration of doses exceeding the recommended tolerable upper limit has been associated with significant side effects (see Adverse Reactions) (3582,4729). The recommended tolerable upper limit of vitamin E is 1000 mg per day, equivalent to 1100 IU of synthetic vitamin E and 1500 IU of natural vitamin E (4729). Mega-dosing should be avoided. ...when used intravenously in large doses. Large repeated intravenous doses of all-rac-vitamin E (synthetic vitamin E) were associated with decreased activity of clotting factors and bleeding in one report (See Adverse Reactions) (3074).
PREGNANCY: LIKELY SAFE ...when used orally in amounts that do not exceed the recommended dietary allowance (RDA) (15); however, maternal supplementation is not generally recommended unless dietary vitamin E falls below the RDA (3071). POSSIBLY SAFE ...when used orally and appropriately in amounts exceeding the recommended dietary allowance (RDA). No adverse effects were reported with oral intake of 400 IU per day starting at weeks 18-22 of pregnancy in women at high risk for pre-eclampsia (3236) or with 600-900 IU daily during the last two months of pregnancy (3071).
LACTATION: LIKELY SAFE ...when used orally in amounts that do not exceed the recommended dietary allowance (RDA) (15). There is insufficient reliable information about the safety of vitamin E supplementation in amounts greater than the RDA during lactation.

Effectiveness

EFFECTIVE ...when used orally for preventing and treating vitamin E deficiency (10,15). However, vitamin E deficiency is rare in humans. It most commonly occurs in people with malabsorption disorders such as abetalipoproteinemia, cystic fibrosis, gastrectomy, heptatic-biliary tract disease including chronic cholestasis, hepatic cirrhosis, biliary atresia, obstructive jaundice, infants receiving formula with insufficient vitamin E, intestinal diseases including celiac and tropical sprue, and regional enteritis (10). Vitamin E supplementation may be of most benefit in this population.
POSSIBLY EFFECTIVE ...when used orally for treating tardive dyskinesia. In several small, but well-designed studies, vitamin E improved the Abnormal Involuntary Movement Scale (AIMS) scores significantly more than placebo (3942,3943,3944,3945,3946,3947,3948). Vitamin E tended to be more effective in people who took higher doses and had experienced tardive dyskinesia symptoms for less than five years (3942,3943,3944,3945,3948). Some conflicting findings have been reported. In the largest study to date, vitamin E was no better than placebo for tardive dyskinesia. However, this study has not yet been published, preventing further evaluation of its findings (3947). Both RRR-alpha-tocopherol (natural vitamin E) and unspecified forms were used in clinical trials (3942,3943,3944,3945,3946,3947,3948). ...when used orally for reducing the incidence of prostate cancer (3959,4643,4644,4645,4646). In one study, 29,133 smokers taking 50 mg per day of all-rac-alpha-tocopherol (synthetic vitamin E), either alone or in combination with beta-carotene, had a significantly lower incidence of prostate cancer and mortality associated with prostate cancer (3959). Epidemiological studies also support an inverse relationship between vitamin E consumption and the risk of prostate cancer. These epidemiological studies did not distinguish between different forms of vitamin E (4644,4645,4646). ...when used orally for slowing cognitive decline in Alzheimer's disease (4635,4636). In one well-designed study, all-rac-alpha-tocopherol (synthetic vitamin E) 2000 IU per day was similar to selegiline (Eldepryl) and superior to placebo in slowing cognitive function decline in patients with moderately severe Alzheimer's disease. There was no additive effect when vitamin E was used in combination with selegiline (Eldepryl) (4635). ...when used orally with vitamin C for protecting against development of vascular and mixed dementias. A longitudinal cohort study of 3,385 elderly men aged 71 to 93 years found that men who consumed supplemental vitamin E and vitamin C had a decreased risk of developing vascular and mixed or other dementias; however, there was no protective effect for Alzheimer's dementia. This study did not distinguish between different forms of vitamin E (4636). ...when used to delay neurologic symptoms in early Huntington's chorea (4686). In a double-blind controlled trial, RRR-alpha-tocopherol (natural vitamin E) significantly improved symptoms in patients with early Huntington's disease. This benefit was not seen in patients with more advanced disease (4686). ...when used orally to reduce pain associated with rheumatoid arthritis (4723). When used as an adjunct to standard therapy, vitamin E was superior to placebo in reducing pain but not inflammation (4723). ...when used orally for improving sperm function and fertilization rates (3583,4693,4695). In one study, males with asthenospermia or oligoasthenospermia receiving vitamin E supplementation achieved impregnation at a rate of 21% compared to none for similar patients receiving placebo (4695). In another study, males enrolled in an in vitro fertilization program who had previously had low fertilization rates were treated with vitamin E 200 mg daily over three months. Fertilization rates increased significantly from 19% to 29% after 1 month of treatment (3583). In a crossover trial, males found to have elevated reactive oxygen species in their semen, which might be associated with infertility, were treated with vitamin E. After treatment, in vitro sperm binding to the zona pellucida was significantly increased (4693). Interestingly, in one study, high-dose vitamin E in combination

with vitamin C appeared to offer no benefit to sperm functionality (4696). In another study, vitamin E in combination with selenium improved measures of sperm functionality, but failed to improve fertilization rates (3585). Although vitamin E preparations used alone appear to offer some benefit in men with asthenospermia or oxidative damage to sperm, combining vitamin E with vitamin C or selenium does not appear to be beneficial. Studies did not differentiate between different forms of vitamin E. ...when used orally to normalize retinal blood flow and improve renal function in type 1 diabetic patients. In a crossover trial, patients with type 1 diabetes of less than ten years were given Vitamin E 1800 IU daily for four months. At the end of the treatment period, retinal blood flow was similar to controls without diabetes and creatinine clearance was significantly decreased (4725). ...when used orally in combination with vitamin C to treat uveitis (4730). In a double-blind, placebo-controlled study, visual acuity improved in patients with acute anterior uveitis who received vitamins E and C, although inflammation measured by laser flare was similar to placebo (4730). ...when used orally to prevent nitrate tolerance in patients with ischemic heart disease (4705). In a small placebo-controlled study, patients with ischemic heart disease and healthy volunteers receiving vitamin E had a decreased attenuation of response to nitroglycerin compared to placebo (4705). ...when used orally in conjunction with erythropoietin for anemia in patients on dialysis. Two small studies in adults and children on chronic hemodialysis showed improved response to erythropoietin with vitamin E supplementation (4640,4647). In one study, children given vitamin E 15 mg/kg in combination with erythropoietin had significantly increased hemoglobin (Hgb) and hematrocrit (Hct) levels after two weeks of combination treatment compared to eight and five weeks in patients without combination treatment (4640). In a study in adults, concurrent supplementation with vitamin E 500 mg daily allowed dose reductions of erythropoietin from an average of 93 U/kg/week to 74 U/kg/week with the same results on Hgb levels (4647). ...when used orally to treat focal segmental glomerulosclerosis in children (4675). A small, open-label study showed vitamin E reduced proteinuria in children refractory to standard medical management (4675). ...when used orally for correcting erythrocyte membrane abnormalities in people with beta-thalassemia and low vitamin E plasma concentrations (4642). ...when used to control hemolysis in adults and children with glucose-6-phosphate dehydrogenase (G6PD) deficiency (4682,4683). There is recent renewed interest in vitamin E for G6PD deficiency (4685). In two open studies, vitamin E 800 IU alone or in combination with selenium reduced hemolysis and reticulocytosis and increased red blood cell (RBC) half-life and vitamin E levels in patients with G6PD deficiency (4682,4683). In one study, vitamin E plus selenium 25 mcg daily offered significantly more improvement compared to vitamin E alone (4683). These findings are contrary to an earlier study that found no effect with vitamin E at 2000 to 2400 IU per day (4684). ...when used orally with vitamin C for preventing pre-eclampsia in high-risk women (3236). Combination vitamin E 400 IU and vitamin C 1000 mg daily significantly reduced the risk of proteinuric hypertension when begun in weeks 16 to 22 of pregnancy (3236). Other researchers using vitamin E in combination with vitamin C and allopurinol beginning at 24 to 32 weeks gestation found the combination similar to placebo (4718). ...when used to reduce the symptoms of premenstrual syndrome (4719,4720). Two double-blind, placebo-controlled studies found vitamin E superior to placebo for reducing anxiety, craving, and depressive symptoms (4719,4720). ...when used orally for retrolental fibroplasia, intracranial hemorrhage, and intraventricular hemorrhage in premature neonates (10,4655,4656). ...when used orally in combination with pentoxifylline (Trental) to treat radiation-induced fibrosis (4672,4673). An open-label study and a case study showed vitamin E 1000 U plus pentoxifylline 800 mg given daily reversed radiation-induced fibrosis (4672,4673). Regression of radiation-induced fibrosis was significant after three months of treatment and improved over the 12-month study period. After 12 months of treatment, mean surface area of fibrosis decreased by 66% (4672). ...when used orally in combination with vitamin C to prevent ultraviolet-induced erythema (sunburn) (4715,4716). High dose oral RRR-alpha-tocopherol (natural vitamin E) in combination with vitamin C protected against skin inflammation after exposure to ultraviolet (UV) radiation in two small, double-blind, placebo-controlled studies (4715,1416). In another study, oral alpha-tocopherol acetate 400 IU alone did not protect from UVB radiation (1417). ...when used topically in combination with vitamin C and melatonin to prevent ultraviolet-induced erythema (sunburn). In one study, topically applied vitamin E in combination with topical vitamin C and melatonin provided modest photoprotective effect when used prior to UV exposure and had no effect when used during or after UV exposure (4713,4714). ...when used topically in combination with dimethyl sulfoxide (DMSO) for treating chemotherapy extravasation (4668). ...when used topically to treat granuloma annulare (14,4681). A small, open study and case study showed topical vitamin E cleared granuloma annulare lesions within one to three weeks (14,4681). ...when used in combination with vitamin C and allopurinol to reduce ischemia reperfusion injury during coronary artery bypass surgery. When vitamin E, vitamin C, and allopurinol were given two days prior to surgery and one day postoperatively, patients had fewer perioperative infarctions and less creatine kinase-MB release (4699). This benefit was not found when using RRR-alpha-tocopherol (natural vitamin E) or all rac-alpha-tocopherol (synthetic vitamin E) only in combination with vitamin C (4697,4698). ...when used orally in combination with beta-carotene, and selenium for prevention of gastroesophageal cancer. In a large-scale study in 29,584 people in China, the combination of vitamin E, beta-carotene, and selenium over 5.25 years significantly reduced total mortality, total cancer mortality, and stomach cancer mortality. However, this population has a high risk of gastric cancer, which is thought to be related to poor vitamin and mineral intake (4679). It is unknown if supplementation with these vitamins and minerals would be beneficial in people with adequate nutrition. This benefit has not been realized with vitamin E alone. Although there has been some conflicting evidence (4677), the only large-scale controlled trial indicates that supplementation with only rac-alpha tocopherol (synthetic vitamin E) 50 mg daily has no effect on the rate of gastric cancer (3960,4676). ...when used orally in combination with vitamin A and vitamin C or multivitamin to prevent colorectal adenoma. Vitamin E in combination with vitamins A and C, has shown a protective effect in patients with previous colorectal adenomas (3954,3956). A retrospective study has also associated vitamin E and multivitamin use with a lower incidence of colorectal cancer (3958). Vitamin E alone has not been shown to be beneficial. Several large-scale studies in smokers and the general population showed no effect of supplemental vitamin E alone in preventing colorectal adenoma (3953,3955,3957). ...when used orally to enhance immune function in elderly people (4687,4689,4690,4691). Vitamin E supplementation 100 to 200 mg daily improved immune system function in elderly people (4687,4689,4690,4691). Lower doses may not provide this benefit (4692).

POSSIBLY INEFFECTIVE ...when used orally for reducing the risk of heart disease and cardiovascular events including myocardial infarction, stroke, and death (3896,3897,3935,3937). The use of vitamin E for heart disease is controversial due to inconsistent findings in studies. The FDA has refused to allow labeling vitamin E supplements for prevention of cardiovascular disease primarily based on recent large-scale controlled studies that found no benefit with vitamin E supplementation (3939). These studies include the Heart Outcomes Prevention Evaluation Study (HOPE) (3896) and the GISSI-Prevenzione study (3897). In the HOPE study, 9,541 men and women aged 55 and older with cardiovascular disease or diabetes were treated with RRR-alpha-tocopherol (natural vitamin E) 400 IU daily for an average of 4.5 years. A similar rate of cardiovascular events including myocardial infarction, stroke, and death occurred in patients receiving vitamin E compared to placebo. There were also no differences in rates of hospitalization for unstable angina or heart failure, revascularization procedures, or amputations (3896). In the GISSI-Prevenzione study, 11,000 patients who had recently survived a myocardial infarction were treated with supplemental all-rac-alpha tocopherol (synthetic vitamin E) 300 mg per day for 3.5 years. Patients taking vitamin E had similar rates of death, non-fatal myocardial infarction, and stroke as patients taking placebo (3897). In another study, the Alpha-Tocopherol, Beta-Carotene Cancer Prevention Study (ATBC), cardiovascular effects were analyzed as a secondary outcome in 27,271 Finnish male smokers. In this study, supplementation with all rac-alpha-tocopherol (synthetic vitamin E) 50 mg per day did not significantly lower fatal or non-fatal cardiovascular events in male smokers with or without a previous myocardial infarction (3935,3937). Some studies have produced conflicting findings. Only one of these studies is a controlled trial. The Cambridge Heart Antioxidant Study (CHAOS) showed that an unspecified form of vitamin E 400 or 800 IU daily in patients with atherosclerosis produced a 77% reduction in nonfatal myocardial infarction. However, there was not a significant effect on mortality (3936). Prospective cohort studies have yielded mixed results. The US Nurses Health Study showed that vitamin E 100 IU daily was associated with a 34% reduction in risk of coronary heart disease after two years of supplementation (3898). In the Iowa Women's Health Study, increased dietary vitamin E, but not supplemental vitamin E, significantly lowered risk of death from coronary heart disease (3934). In the Health Professionals' Follow-Up Study, men without heart disease or diabetes taking vitamin E 100 IU daily for two years or longer resulted in a 39% reduction of ischemic heart disease or coronary surgery (3933). Despite some conflicting findings, the weight of the evidence at this point indicates that supplemental vitamin E alone does not significantly alter cardiovascular outcomes. However, preliminary evidence suggests that combinations of antioxidants may offer some benefits. In an epidemiological study, more than 11,000 elderly people taking both vitamin E and vitamin C had a lower risk of cardiovascular and all-cause mortality (3986). The Antioxidant Supplement Atherosclerosis Prevention (ASAP) Study, a double-blind, placebo-controlled trial reported at the 21st Congress of the European Society of Cardiology, found that high-risk men taking vitamin E 200 mg and vitamin C 500 mg daily for three years had a 45% reduction in progression of atherosclerosis. This benefit was not found in women (6204). ...when used to reduce angina. Although vitamin E may have some effect on endothelial dysfunction, it has not benefited nonsmokers or smokers with angina (3896,4634,4649,4650,4651,4652). ...when used to treat intermittent claudication in male smokers (4732). All rac-alpha-tocopherol (synthetic vitamin E) had no effect when used alone or in combination with beta-carotene on symptoms or disease progression (4732). ...when used orally in combination with vitamin C to prevent development of Alzheimer's disease in elderly men. A longitudinal cohort study of 3,385 elderly men aged 71 to 93 years found that men who consumed supplemental vitamin E and vitamin C developed Alzheimer's dementia at the same rate as those men who did not (4636). ...when used orally to prevent cataracts. Although there is some conflicting evidence, the only controlled trial indicates that that vitamin E does not reduce the risk of cataracts. In a large-scale controlled study of 28,934 male smokers, those taking all rac-alpha-tocopherol (synthetic vitamin E) 50 mg per day had a similar rate of cataract extraction compared to placebo (4666). Epidemiological studies report conflicting findings (2395,4663,4664,4665,4759). ...when used orally for reducing the risk of lung cancer in male smokers (3949). In a large Finnish study, 29,133 male smokers taking all rac-alpha-tocopherol (synthetic vitamin E) 50 mg per day for five to eight years were as likely to be diagnosed with lung cancer as those receiving placebo (3949). ...when used to prevent oral mucosal lesions in smokers. Although there is some conflicting evidence (3951,4708), the largest and most significant controlled trial indicates that supplementation with all rac-alpha-tocopherol (synthetic vitamin E) 50 mg daily for five to seven years has no effect on the incidence of oral lesions in male cigarette smokers (3951). ...when used to prevent carcinoma of the pancreas or reduce mortality associated with pancreatic cancer in male smokers (3961). All rac-alpha-tocopherol (synthetic vitamin E) 50 mg daily supplements taken for five to eight years by male smokers did not affect the incidence or mortality of carcinoma of the pancreas (3961). ...when used to prevent age-related maculopathy in men who smoke (4667). ...when used in combination with penicillamine for slowing progression of Duchenne muscular dystrophy (4703). A double-blind study in 106 boys for 18 months found no difference between placebo and combination vitamin E and penicillamine for slowing disease progression (4703). ...when used orally in combination with selenium for myotonic dystrophy. A small study comparing placebo to combination vitamin E and selenium showed no difference in functional deterioration over two years (4704). ...when used orally for Parkinson's disease (4709,4710,4711). A large double-blind, placebo-controlled study using all rac-alpha-tocopherol (synthetic vitamin E) 2000 IU daily showed no delay in disease progression, benefit to cognitive performance, or amelioration of levodopa side effects (4709,4710,4711). However, preliminary evidence suggests that dietary vitamin E might be useful for preventing Parkinson's disease. In one epidemiological study, high dietary vitamin E intake was associated with a decreased occurrence of Parkinson's disease (4712). ...when used for hemolytic anemia associated with vitamin E deficiency in premature infants. Vitamin E 25 IU per day given to premature infants for six weeks had no beneficial effects on hemolytic anemia (4648). ...when used for bronchopulmonary dysplasia in premature infants. In one study, vitamin E had no benefit in premature infants weighing less than 1500 grams at birth (4657). ...when used topically to reduce surgical wound scarring (4721,4722).

LIKELY INEFFECTIVE ...when used to prevent breast cancer (4658,4659). Neither dietary nor supplemental vitamin E intake has shown any protective effect for breast cancer (4658,4659). ...when used for benign breast disease (4660,4661). Three well-designed studies of supplemental vitamin E 600 mg per day found no effect on mammary dysplasia (4660,4661,4662).

There is insufficient reliable information available to rate the effectiveness of vitamin E for other its other uses. However, limited evidence suggests vitamin E might offer some benefit for nocturnal leg cramps (14,4700,4701). Current studies have been conflicting (4702). Limited evidence also suggests vitamin E might reduce seizure frequency in refractory epilepsy; however, trials have been few and contradictory (4670,4671). Preliminary small-scale clinical studies have also indicated that vitamin E might be beneficial in diabetes and diabetic neuropathy. Some evidence suggests it improves glucose disposal in type 2 diabetics (4726,4727) and can improve nerve conduction in diabetic neuropathy (4724). Further study is needed to rate the effectiveness of vitamin E for these uses.

Possible Mechanism of Action & Active Ingredients

Vitamin E is a fat-soluble vitamin present in many foods including vegetable oils, cereal grains, animal fats, meat, poultry, eggs, fruits, and vegetables. Wheat germ oil is a particularly rich source (15). Vitamin E deficiency is rare and most typically seen in genetic abnormalities that prevent maintenance of normal blood concentrations of vitamin E or conditions that prevent absorption. Vitamin E deficiency does not cause specific disease in adults, although creatinuria, ceroid deposition, muscle weakness, and decreased erythrocyte survival are associated with low serum tocopherol concentrations. In adults, total body stores of vitamin E, found in adipose tissue, have been estimated to be 3-8 grams and are sufficient to meet the body's requirements for four or more years of a deficient diet. In premature infants, vitamin E deficiency can cause irritability, edema, thrombosis, and hemolytic anemia (15). Unlike most nutrients, vitamin E does not appear to have a specific role in a required metabolic process. The major function of vitamin E is probably that of a chain-breaking antioxidant that prevents the formation of free radicals. Vitamin E's therapeutic benefits have primarily been attributed to its antioxidant effects. Vitamin E exists in eight forms, including alpha-, beta-, gamma-, and delta-tocopherols and four tocotrienols. Although vitamin E exists in numerous forms, supplemental vitamin E usually refers to alpha-tocopherol. For biological activity, vitamin E is dependent on hepatic alpha-tocopherol transfer protein (alpha-TTP) for distribution. Although the typical diet contains other forms of vitamin E (beta-, gamma-, and delta- tocopherols), these have very limited systemic bioavailability because they do not bind with alpha-TTP. Supplemental beta-, gamma-, and delta-tocopherols, and tocotrienols appear to have little in vivo activity in humans and do not contribute toward meeting established vitamin E requirements (4844). Only the alpha-tocopherol form of vitamin E is maintained in plasma and thought to be therapeutically useful. Alpha-tocopherol exists as eight stereoisomers. The RRR-alpha-tocopherol isomer, formerly called d-alpha-tocopherol, has the greatest affinity for alpha-TTP and the most biologic activity (4844). RRR-alpha-tocopherol is sometimes called natural vitamin E and occurs naturally in foods (3940,4844). The racemic mixture of all eight alpha-tocopherol isomers, or all rac-alpha-tocopherol, was formerly known as dl-alpha-tocopherol (4844). All rac-alpha-tocopherol, sometimes called synthetic vitamin E, is found in vitamin E-fortified foods. Both forms of vitamin E, natural and synthetic, can be found in vitamin E supplements. All rac-alpha-tocopherol has lower affinity for alpha-TTP and thus has less biologic activity than RRR-alpha-tocopherol (4627,4844). Based on weight, 15 mg of RRR-alpha tocopherol is approximately equivalent in potency to 30 mg of all rac-alpha-tocopherol (4844). Therapeutic benefits of vitamin E have largely been attributed to its role as an antioxidant. Oxidative damage has been attributed to many conditions which vitamin E is used for, including lipid peroxidation in heart disease (6204). In tardive dyskinesia, it is thought that some patients may have increased dopamine turnover resulting in increased production of free radicals and structural damage. Additionally, people with tardive dyskinesia may have decreased levels of vitamin E and vitamin C (3598). Oxidative damage has also been associated with diabetes and complications of diabetes and has long been associated with the development of cancers. In dementia, preliminary data in animals suggest vitamin E might improve cognitive function by decreasing beta-amyloid damage (4637,4638,4639). In addition to its antioxidant function, vitamin E inhibits protein kinase C activity, which is involved in cell proliferation and differentiation in several cell types, including smooth muscle, platelets, and monocytes (4844). Large amounts of vitamin E interfere with vitamin K-dependent clotting factor production, producing hypoprothrombinemic effects, especially in people with vitamin K deficiency or those who are taking oral anticoagulants (14,15,3046,3072,3073,3074). For immune function in the elderly, vitamin E supplementation might replenish an unapparent deficiency. Deficiency of vitamin E and other micronutrients are common in apparently well-nourished people over age 90 and might affect the number and function of natural killer cells in old age (4688). Although biological activity of other forms is significantly less and current guidelines do not include forms of vitamin E other than alpha-tocopherol for meeting dietary requirements (4844), the other forms, such as gamma-tocopherol and the tocotrienols, have been associated with some pharmacological activity. For example, gamma-tocopherol appears to decrease the programmed death of human coronary artery endothelial cells, possibly by decreasing LDL oxidation (4092). Gamma-tocopherol inhibits prostate cancer cell growth in vitro (4089). Gamma-tocopherol also appears to prolong prothrombin and partial thromboplastin times and has caused hemorrhage in experimental animals (4098). Beta- and delta-tocopherol have also been shown to prolong prothrombin and partial thromboplastin times in laboratory animals (4098). The tocotrienols from rice and barley bran might lower total cholesterol and LDL, possibly by decreasing activity of HMG CoA reductase, but in a different way than "statin" drugs (3237,3238,3239,3240,3241). Tocotrienols might also be capable of decreasing carotid artery plaque size in some people, possibly by decreasing platelet aggregation (3239). Natural vitamin E (d-alpha-tocopherol) is similarly absorbed when taken with high-fat (36 grams) or low-fat (3 grams fat) meals (6133).

Adverse Reactions Including Known Allergies

Vitamin E is seldom associated with adverse effects. Rarely, vitamin E causes nausea, diarrhea, intestinal cramps, fatigue, weakness, headache, blurred vision, rash, gonadal dysfunction, and creatinuria. Vitamin E has been associated with the development of thrombophlebitis and pulmonary embolism, but this is controversial (14). It is unclear if vitamin E contributes to increased risk of hemorrhagic stroke. One study suggested a higher incidence of hemorrhagic stroke in male smokers taking all rac-alpha-tocopherol (synthetic vitamin E), but several other studies lasting from 1.4 years to 4.5 years with study participants taking either all rac-alpha-tocopherol (synthetic vitamin E) or RRR-alpha-tocopherol (natural vitamin E) showed no increased risk for stroke (3896,3897,3936,3949,4635). High doses of vitamin E might increase the risk of bleeding due to antagonism of vitamin K-dependent clotting factors and platelet aggregation. Patients with vitamin K deficiencies or taking anticoagulant or antiplatelet drugs are at a greater risk for bleeding (4844). Although only certain isomers of vitamin E are included for determination of dietary requirements, all isomers are considered for determining safe intake levels. All the isomers are thought to potentially contribute to toxicity. Topical application of vitamin E has been associated with contact dermatitis, inflammatory reactions, and eczematous lesions (14,15).

Possible Interactions with Herbs & Other Dietary Supplements

IRON: Concomitant use of vitamin E in amounts greater than 10 units/kg per day can delay the response to iron therapy in children with iron-deficiency anemia (15).
MINERAL OIL: Concomitant use can decrease the absorption of vitamin E and other fat-soluble vitamins (14,15).
OMEGA-6 FATTY ACIDS: Increased intake of omega-6 fatty acids may increase vitamin E requirements, particularly at higher doses (4844).
VITAMIN A: Concomitant use can increase the absorption, utilization and storage of vitamin A. Vitamin E might also protect against hypervitaminosis A (15).
VITAMIN C: Concomitant use helps reduce the risk of pre-eclampsia in high-risk women (3236). Laboratory evidence suggests that vitamin C might help recycle oxidized alpha-tocopherol (4844).
HERBS WITH ANTICOAGULANT/ANTIPLATELET POTENTIAL: Concomitant use of herbs that have coumarin constituents or affect platelet aggregation could theoretically increase the risk of bleeding in some people. These herbs include: angelica, anise, arnica, asafoetida, bogbean, boldo, capsicum, celery, chamomile, clove, danshen, fenugreek, feverfew, garlic, ginger, ginkgo, Panax ginseng, horse chestnut, horseradish, licorice, meadowsweet, prickly ash, onion, papain, passionflower, poplar, quassia, red clover, turmeric, wild carrot, wild lettuce, willow, and others (4,19).

Possible Interactions with Drugs

ANTICOAGULANT/ANTIPLATELET AGENTS: Concomitant use of vitamin E and anticoagulant or antiplatelet agents might increase the risk of bleeding, possibly through inhibition of platelet aggregation and antagonism of vitamin K-dependent clotting factors (4733,4844). These agents include aspirin, clopidogrel (Plavix), dalteparin (Fragmin), enoxaparin (Lovenox), heparin, ticlopidine (Ticlid), warfarin (Coumadin) and others.
CHEMOTHERAPY: Preliminary evidence that suggests that antioxidants such as vitamin E and vitamin A might reduce the effectiveness of cancer chemotherapy (391). Patients undergoing chemotherapy should not use vitamin E and other antioxidants without the supervision of a health care provider.
NITRATES: Vitamin E might prevent tolerance to nitrates (4705).
WARFARIN (Coumadin): Concomitant use of greater than 400 units of vitamin E per day with warfarin might prolong prothrombin time (PT), INR, and increase the risk of bleeding, due to interference with production of vitamin K-dependent factors (14,15,3046,3072).

Drug Influences on Nutrient Levels and Depletion

SOME DRUGS CAN AFFECT VITAMIN E LEVELS.
CHOLESTYRAMINE (Questran): Cholestyramine can reduce dietary vitamin E absorption and serum levels (4455,4456).
COLESTIPOL (Colestid): Colestipol can reduce dietary vitamin E absorption and serum levels (4460,4461).
GEMFIBROZIL (Lopid): Gemfibrozil can decrease serum levels of both alpha- and gamma- tocopherol, but the clinical significance of this is not known (4096).
MINERAL OIL: Mineral oil can reduce dietary vitamin E absorption and serum levels. Avoid long-term use of mineral oil (4495,4496).
ETHANOL: Theoretically, ethanol might decrease serum levels of alpha- and gamma-tocopherol, contributing to liver injury (4097). One unit of vitamin E equals the biologic activity of 1 mg of dl-alpha-tocopheryl acetate, 1.12 mg

 © Copyright 2000, Natural Medicines Comprehensive Database (209) 472-2244. For updated data, go to www.NaturalDatabase.com

of dl-alpha-tocopheryl acid succinate, 0.91 mg of dl-alpha-tocopherol, 0.735 mg of d-alpha-tocopheryl acetate, 0.83 mg of d-alpha-tocopheryl acid succinate, and 0.67 mg of d-alpha-tocopherol (15).
ORLISTAT (Xenical): Orlistat can reduce the absorption of beta-carotene and some fat-soluble vitamins. (1725,1726,1727,1730). Consider a multivitamin with fat-soluble vitamins, taken at least 2 hours before or after orlistat, or at bedtime.

Possible Interactions with Foods
FOODS HIGH IN FAT: High-fat meals might increase vitamin E absorption; however, the amount of fat required to facilitate vitamin E absorption has not been established (4844).

Possible Interactions with Lab Tests
CHOLESTEROL: In rare cases, vitamin E can increase serum cholesterol and triglycerides levels (15).
CREATINE PHOSPHOKINASE (CPK): In rare cases, vitamin E can increase serum creatine phosphokinase (15).
PROTHROMBIN TIME (PT)/INTERNATIONAL NORMALIZED RATIO (INR): High dose vitamin E might increase PT/INR in patients concurrently taking warfarin or other anticoagulant (4844).
URINE HORMONES: In rare cases, vitamin E can increase urinary estrogens and androgens (15).
THYROXINE AND TRIIODOTHYRONINE: In rare cases, vitamin E can decrease serum thyroxine and triiodothyronine (15).

Possible Interactions with Diseases or Conditions
VITAMIN K DEFICIENCY: Vitamin E might worsen coagulation defects in people with vitamin K deficiency (15).
PRE-ECLAMPSIA: Vitamin E with vitamin C helps prevent pre-eclampsia in high-risk women (3236).

Typical Dosages & Routes of Administration that are Commonly Used
ORAL: A typical dose for vitamin E deficiency in adults is RRR-alpha tocopherol (natural vitamin E) 60-75 IU per day (15). For tardive dyskinesia, most studies used RRR-alpha-tocopherol (natural vitamin E)1600 IU daily (3942,3943,3944). For preventing prostate cancer, vitamin E (type unspecified) 59 to 100 IU daily has been used (3959,4646). For improving male fertility, vitamin E (type unspecified) 200 to 600 IU daily has been used (3584,4693). A typical dose for Alzheimer's disease is up to 2000 IU daily (15). For early Huntington's chorea one study used RRR-alpha-tocopherol (natural vitamin E) 3000 IU (4686). Rheumatoid arthritis pain has been treated with vitamin E (type unspecified) 600 IU twice daily (4723). For diabetic neuropathy, vitamin E (type unspecified) 900 mg daily has been used (4724). For improving retinal blood flow and creatinine clearance in Type 1 diabetes, vitamin E (type unspecified) 1800 IU has been used (4725). For enhancing immune function in elderly people vitamin E (type unspecified) 100 to 200 mg daily has been used (4687,4689,4690). For preventing nitrate tolerance, vitamin E (type unspecifed) 200 mg three times daily has been used (4705). For improving response to erythropoietin in people on dialysis, adults have received vitamin E (type unspecified) 300 to 500 mg daily, and children have received 15 mg per kg per day (4640,4641,4647). For children with focal segmental glomerulosclerosis, vitamin E (type unspecified) 200 IU has been used to reduce proteinuria (4675). For G6PD deficiency, vitamin E (type unspecified) 800 IU daily has been used (4682,4683). Premenstrual syndrome has been treated with RRR-alpha-tocopherol (natural vitamin E) 400 IU daily (4719). In premature neonates, oral vitamin E (type unspecified) 15 to 30 IU per kg per day has been used to prevent retinopathy and bronchopulmonary dysplasia (15). For nocturnal leg cramps, vitamin E (type unspecified) 400 IU at bedtime has been used (4701). Radiation-induced fibrosis has been treated with vitamin E (form unspecified) 1000 IU daily in combination with pentoxifylline 800 mg (4672,4673). For beta-thalassemia, vitamin E 750 IU daily has been used (15). For preventing sunburn, RRR-alpha-tocopherol 1000 IU in combination with 2 grams of ascorbic acid has been used (4716). For reducing the risk of cancer, heart disease, and cataracts, people have used multiple forms of vitamin E 200-800 IU per day (839). For sickle cell anemia, 450 IU daily has been used (15). For preventing pre-eclampsia in high risk women, vitamin E 400 IU with vitamin C 1000 mg daily has been used (3236). The oral dose of palm oil tocotrienols (Palmvitee) used to reduce lipids is 200-260 mg per day (3238,3239,3240).
TOPICAL: For treating chemotherapy extravasation, 10% vitamin E (type unspecified) has been used topically in combination with 90% dimethyl sulfoxide (DMSO) (4713).
The recommended daily intake of vitamin E for adults was recently increased. Both women and men should consume 15 milligrams of vitamin E from food (4844). This is equivalent to 22 IU of the RRR-alpha-tocopherol (natural vitamin E) or 33 IU of the all rac-alpha-tocopherol (synthetic vitamin E) (4729). For Infants 7-12 months, 6 mg; Children 1-3 years, 7 mg; Children 4 -8 years, 11 mg; Older children and adults 15 mg; Pregnant women, 15 mg; Lactating women, 19 mg (4844). The recommended upper dosage limit for all forms of supplemental alpha-tocopherol is 1000 mg (4729). Dosing for vitamin E can be confusing. Some sources and clinical studies choose to express vitamin E dosing base on milligrams or International Units (IU). Current guidelines have expressed recommended dietary allowance (RDA) and upper tolerable limits for vitamin E in milligrams. However most products are still labeled in IUs. It becomes important to understand how to convert between IUs and milligrams of vitamin E. The appropriate method for doing this depends of the formulation of vitamin E being considered and whether or not you are determining RDA or tolerable upper limit. For conversions related to RDA and to convert IUs of RRR-alpha-tocopherol (natural vitamin E) to milligrams of alpha-tocopherol, multiply by a factor of 0.67. For example, 30 IU of RRR-alpha-tocopherol is 20 mg RRR-alpha-tocopherol (natural vitamin E). To convert IUs of all-rac-tocopherol (synthetic vitamin E) to milligrams of alpha-tocopherol, multiply by a factor of 0.45. For example, 30 IU all rac-tocopherol equals 13.5 mg of all rac-alpha-tocopherol (synthetic vitamin E).

The tolerable upper limit conversion factor for racemic and RRR-alpha tocopherol assumes that all isomers of vitamin E might contribute to toxicity so the conversion factor for all rac-alpha tocopherol (synthetic vitamin E) is different. For conversions related to upper limit and to convert IUs all rac-alpha tocopherol (synthetic vitamin E), multiply by a factor of 0.91. For example, 2000 IUs all rac-alpha tocopherol (synthetic vitamin E) is equivalent to 1820 mg. The conversion factor of 0.67 is the same for calculating upper limit for RRR-alpha tocopherol (natural vitamin E). The same factors are used for either acetate or succinate salts because the content has been adjusted for the molecular weights of the salts (4844). Natural vitamin E (d-alpha-tocopherol) is similarly absorbed when taken with high-fat (36 grams) or low-fat (3 grams fat) meals (6133).

Comments

The American Heart Association recommends obtaining antioxidants, including vitamin E, from a diet high in fruits, vegetables and whole grains rather than from supplements, until more is known about the risks and benefits of supplementation (1440).

VITAMIN K

This Product is Also Known As

Vitamin K1: Methylphytyl Naphthoquinone, Phylloquinone, Phytomenadione, Phytonadione, 2-Methyl-3-Phytyl-1,4-Naphthoquinone.
Vitamin K2: Menaquinone, Menaquinone-6, Menaquinone-7, Menatetrenone.
Vitamin K3: Menadione, Menadione Sodium Bisulfite, 2-Methyl-1,4-Naphthoquinone.
Vitamin K4: Menadiol Acetate, Menadiol Sodium Diphosphate, Menadiol Sodium Phosphate, Menadiolum Solubile.
Vitamin K5: 4-Amino-2-Methyl-1-Naphthol.

Scientific Names

Phylloquinone (K1); menaquinone (K2); menadione (K3); menadiol acetate (K4); 4-amino-2-methyl-1-naphthol (K5).

People Use This For

Orally, phytonadione, also known as vitamin K1, is used for preventing and treating hypoprothrombinemia caused by vitamin K deficiency; to counteract excessive doses of oral anticoagulants; to prevent hemorrhagic disease of the newborn; to treat hypoprothrombinemia induced by salicylates, sulfonamides, quinine, quinidine, or broad-spectrum antibiotic therapy; to prevent osteoporosis, and relieve itching associated with primary biliary cirrhosis (14,15). Menadiol sodium diphosphate, also known as vitamin K4, is used orally for treating hypoprothrombinemia resulting from impaired absorption or synthesis of vitamin K (14). In combination with vitamin C, vitamin K3 is used for treating prostate and breast cancers (1257).
Topically, phytonadione, also known as vitamin K1, is used for eliminating spider veins, bruises, scars, stretch marks and burns, treating rosacea, speeding healing, and reducing postoperative bruising and swelling (3069).
By injection, phytonadione, also known as vitamin K1, is given to prevent and treat hypoprothrombinemia caused by vitamin K deficiency, especially that associated with malabsorption syndromes or prolonged parenteral nutrition, to counteract excessive doses of oral anticoagulants, to prevent and treat hemorrhagic disease of the newborn, treat hypoprothrombinemia induced by salicylates, sulfonamides, quinine, quinidine, or broad-spectrum antibiotic therapy (15). Menadiol sodium diphosphate, also known as vitamin K4, is injected for treating hypoprothrombinemia resulting from impaired absorption or synthesis of vitamin K (14).

Safety

LIKELY SAFE …when used orally and appropriately (14,15).
Vitamin K injections are available as FDA-approved drugs.
There is insufficient reliable information available about the safety of the topical use of vitamin K.
CHILDREN: LIKELY UNSAFE …when menadiol sodium diphosphate is administered to neonates due to a higher incidence of hyperbilirubinemia and kernicterus than with phytonadione (14).
PREGNANCY: LIKELY SAFE ...when used at the recommended dietary allowance (RDA) of 65 mcg daily (15); avoid larger amounts. Large amounts of vitamin K, particularly as menadiol, that are administered to mothers near term are associated with hyperbilirubinemia and kernicterus in newborn infants (14).
LACTATION: LIKELY SAFE …when used at the recommended dietary allowance (RDA) of 65 mcg daily (15); avoid larger amounts.

Effectiveness

EFFECTIVE …when phytonadione, also known as vitamin K1, is used orally for preventing and treating hypoprothrombinemia caused by vitamin K deficiency. …when phytonadione is used orally to counteract excessive amounts of oral anticoagulants. …when phytonadione is used orally for preventing hemorrhagic disease of newborns. …when phytonadione is used orally for treating hypoprothrombinemia induced by salicylates, sulfonamides, quinine, quinidine, or broad-spectrum antibiotic therapy (15). …when menadiol sodium diphosphate is used orally for treating hypoprothrombinemia resulting from impaired absorption or synthesis of vitamin K (14).

Possible Mechanism of Action & Active Ingredients

Vitamin K is required for the synthesis of blood coagulation factors II (prothrombin), VII (proconvertin), IX (Christmas factor or plasma thromboplastin component), and X (Stuart-Prower factor) in the liver. It is involved in carboxylation of the inactive precursors of these factors (15). In adequate doses, vitamin K reverses the inhibitory effects of coumarin and warfarin derivatives on the synthesis of clotting factors (15). Phytonadione, vitamin K1, is the most potent form of vitamin K, and is the form found in foods (14). Menadiol sodium diphosphate is a synthetic, water-soluble salt of menadione and is converted to menadione in the liver (14). Menaquinone, vitamin K2, is synthesized by bacteria in the intestines (14). Bile salts are required for oral absorption of phytonadione and menaquinone, but not menadiol sodium diphosphate (14,15). Only small amounts of vitamin K are stored in body tissues (15). Low dietary intake of vitamin K is associated with increased risk of hip fracture, but not bone mineral density, in women and men (837,6193). Eating one or more servings per day of lettuce or other vitamin K containing foods is inversely correlated with risk of hip fracture (837).

Adverse Reactions Including Known Allergies

Few adverse effects are reported from oral vitamin K (14,15). Menadiol sodium diphosphate has been associated with gastrointestinal irritation (14). There have been very rare cases of hemolytic anemia and thrombocytopenia, usually in neonates. The rare cases of thrombosis usually occur in people with other predisposing factors (14). Contact dermatitis has been reported with occupational exposure to menadione and menadiol (14).

Possible Interactions with Herbs & Other Dietary Supplements

Insufficient reliable information available.

Possible Interactions with Drugs

WARFARIN: Vitamin K antagonizes the effects of oral anticoagulants such as warfarin (Coumadin) (15). Excessive vitamin K intake, either from supplements or from changes in the diet, can reduce anticoagulation effect (15).

Drug Influences on Nutrient Levels and Depletion

SOME DRUGS CAN AFFECT VITAMIN K LEVELS:

CHOLESTYRAMINE (Questran): Cholestyramine might reduce dietary vitamin K absorption and serum levels (15,4455).

CHOLESTIPOL (Colestid): Colestipol might reduce dietary vitamin K absorption and serum levels (15,4460,4461).

ORAL ANTIBIOTICS: Various beneficial intestinal bacteria are eliminated when oral antibiotics are taken. Some of these intestinal bacteria are responsible for producing vitamin K. The nutritional importance of the quantity of vitamin K produced by these organisms can vary between individuals (4439).

MINERAL OIL: Mineral oil reduces gastrointestinal absorption of vitamin K (14). Avoid prolonged use.

ORLISTAT (Xenical): Orlistat can reduce the absorption of some fat-soluble vitamins, although the effect of orlistat on nutritionally derived vitamin K is unknown (1725,1726,1727,1730). Consider a multivitamin with fat-soluble vitamins, taken at least 2 hours before or after orlistat, or at bedtime.

Possible Interactions with Foods

No interactions are known to occur, and there is no known reason to expect a clinically significant interaction with vitamin K.

Possible Interactions with Lab Tests

BILIRUBIN: Large amounts of vitamin K can increase serum bilirubin and test results in neonates or people with G-6-PD deficiency (275).

CALCIUM: Can reduce urinary calcium excretion and test results (275).

ERYTHROCYTES: Can decrease blood erythrocyte levels and test results (275).

HEMATOCRIT: Vitamin K3 and vitamin K4 might decrease hematocrit and test results, especially in people with G-6-PD deficiency (275).

HEMOGLOBIN: Vitamin K3 and vitamin K4 might decrease blood hemoglobin level and test results, especially in people with G-6-PD deficiency (275).

HEMOGLOBIN: Can increase urine hemoglobin levels and test results (275).

17-HYDROXYCORTICOSTEROIDS: Might cause false increase in urine test results due to in vitro interference with Reddy method (275).

HYDROXYPROLINE: Can decrease urine levels and test results (275).

LEUKOCYTES, PLATELETS: Vitamin K3 and vitamin K4 can decrease blood levels and test results due to pancytopenia (275).

OSTEOCALCIN: Can increase serum levels and test results in postmenopausal women (275).

PORPHYRINS: Can increase urine levels and test results (275).

PROTEIN: Can increase urine levels and test results (275).

PROTHROMBIN TIME (PT): Can decrease PT due to procoagulation effects of vitamin K (275).

UROBILINOGEN: May increase urine levels and test results due to hemolytic anemia in G-6-PD deficiency (275).

Possible Interactions with Diseases or Conditions

BILIARY FISTULA, OBSTRUCTIVE JAUNDICE: Menadiol sodium diphosphate should be used with caution (14).

REDUCED BILE SECRETION: People with decreased bile secretion may require coadministration of supplemental bile salts to ensure adequate vitamin K absorption (15).

G6-PD DEFICIENCY: Menadiol sodium diphosphate should be used with caution in individuals with glucose-6-phosphate dehydrogenase deficiency due to an increased risk of hemolysis (14).

HEMODIALYSIS: Excessive vitamin K intake has been associated with soft tissue calcification (14).

LIVER DISEASE: Vitamin K should be discontinued promptly in people with liver disease and hypoprothrombinemia who do not respond to initial treatment with vitamin K; continued treatment may further decrease prothrombin concentrations (14).

VITAMIN K HYPERSENSITIVITY: Contraindicated (14).

Typical Dosages & Routes of Administration that are Commonly Used

ORAL: There is no typical dose for vitamin K. Doses should be individualized and medically supervised (15). People with decreased bile secretion might require co-administration of supplemental bile salts to ensure adequate vitamin K absorption (15). The daily recommended dietary allowances (RDAs) for vitamin K are: Infants 0-6 months, 5 mcg; Infants 6-12 months, 10 mcg; Children 1-3 years, 15 mcg; Children 4-6 years, 20 mcg; Children 7-10 years, 30 mcg; Males 11-14 years, 45 mcg; Males 15-18 years, 65 mcg; Men 19-24 years, 70 mcg; Men 25 years and older, 80 mcg; Females 11-14 years, 45 mcg; Females 15-18 years, 55 mcg; Women 19-24 years, 60 mcg; Women 25 years and older, pregnant and lactating women, 65 mcg (15).

INJECTION: Injectable vitamin K is a FDA-approved prescription product.

Comments

Vitamin K is a generic term for compounds with the biological activity of phylloquinone, also referred to as antihemorrhagic factor and antihemorrhagic vitamin. Vitamin K is present in many foods including leafy green vegetables, meat, cow's milk, vegetable oils, egg yolks, and tomatoes (15). Phytonadione is generally the preferred form of vitamin K, due to lower toxicity, rapid effects, greater potency, and superior efficacy in some indications, such as oral anticoagulant-induced hypoprothrombinemia (14). New research suggests that a combination of vitamin K3 and vitamin C might be useful for treating prostate and breast cancers. The vitamin combination appears to cause a unique type of tumor cell death (1257).

VITAMIN O

This Product is Also Known As

Liquid Oxygen, Stabilized Liquid Oxygen, Stabilized Oxygen.

Scientific Names

None.

People Use This For

Orally, vitamin O is used for increasing energy; improving immune function; eliminating bacteria, viruses, fungi and parasites; treating yeast infections; eliminating toxins and poisons from the body; and healing mouth sores. Vitamin O is also used for improving concentration, memory and alertness; calming the nervous system; easing depression, irritability, unexplained hostility and dizziness; relieving arthritis, muscle aches and pains, asthma, bronchial problems, emphysema and lung disease, sinus infection, diabetes, body weakness, chronic fatigue, and heart and circulation problems. Vitamin O has been used for obesity; constipation; gas and bloating; loss of appetite; poor digestion; stomach acid; premenstrual syndrome (PMS); menopause; sexual dysfunction; headaches; migraines; premature aging; rashes; skin problems; itchy ears, nose and anus; and tumors and deposit buildup (5316,5317,5318,5319).

Topically, it is used as an antiseptic (5316).

Safety

There is insufficient reliable information available about the safety of vitamin O.

Pregnancy and Lactation: Insufficient reliable information available; avoid using.

Effectiveness

There is insufficient reliable information available about the effectiveness of vitamin O.

Possible Mechanism of Action & Active Ingredients

The chemical formula of the oxygen compound in vitamin O is not disclosed in promotional information. One supplier describes its product as a mildly buffered solution of deionized water and sodium chloride with a pH of 7.2 (5318). Another supplier lists magnesium peroxide as the active ingredient (5320). Still another claims the ingredients are secret (5321).

Adverse Reactions Including Known Allergies

None reported.

Possible Interactions with Herbs & Other Dietary Supplements
Insufficient reliable information available.

Possible Interactions with Drugs
No interactions are known to occur, and there is no known reason to expect a clinically significant interaction with vitamin O.

Possible Interactions with Foods
No interactions are known to occur, and there is no known reason to expect a clinically significant interaction with vitamin O.

Possible Interactions with Lab Tests
No interactions are known to occur, and there is no known reason to expect a clinically significant interaction with vitamin O.

Possible Interactions with Diseases or Conditions
No interactions are known to occur, and there is no known reason to expect a clinically significant interaction with vitamin O.

Typical Dosages & Routes of Administration that are Commonly Used
ORAL: In capsule form of unspecified strength, the dose is typically two capsules three times per day with water (5320). Various quantities, usually measured in drops, of solutions are recommended (e.g., 6 drops in 8 ounces of water, juice, milk, etc; 20 drops 3 times a day in a glass of water; 20 drops per gallon of water) (5321).

Comments
Although vitamin O is called liquid oxygen, remember that oxygen only exists in a liquid form at temperatures below -183 degrees C and that water, by weight, is about 88% oxygen (16). The FTC states that Vitamin O appears to be nothing more than saltwater (311).

In May 2000, Rose Creek Health Products agreed to pay $375,000 to settle Federal Trade Commission charges that they made false and unsubstantiated health claims in their advertising for "Vitamin O". The settlement prohibits the company from making unsupported representations that "Vitamin O" is an effective treatment for any life-threatening diseases, or that the effectiveness of "Vitamin O" is established by medical or scientific research or studies (5076).

WAFER ASH

This Product is Also Known As
Pickaway Anise, Prairie Grub, Scubby Trefoil, Stinking Prairie Bush, Swamp Dogwood, Three-Leaved Hop Tree, Wingseed.

Scientific Names
Ptelea trifoliata.
Family: Rutaceae.

People Use This For
Orally, wafer ash root bark is used for stomach complaints, gallstones, rheumatism, as an appetite stimulant or tonic (18).
Topically, wafer ash is used as a wound dressing (18).

Safety
There is insufficient reliable information available about the safety of wafer ash.
Pregnancy and Lactation: Insufficient reliable information is available; avoid using.

Effectiveness
There is insufficient reliable information available about the effectiveness or wafer ash.

Possible Mechanism of Action & Active Ingredients
The applicable part of wafer ash is the root bark. Wafer ash contains furoquinoline alkaloids including kokusaginin, skimmianine, ptelein, and dictamnine. It also contains furocoumarins (18). Scientists think the alkaloid, pteleatinium chloride, is the active constituent of wafer ash. Pteleatinium chloride shows evidence of antimicrobial activity (3854), particularly against mycobacterium tuberculosis and yeast fungus (18).

Adverse Reactions Including Known Allergies
Skin contact with the wafer ash plant can trigger phototoxic reactions (18).

Possible Interactions with Herbs & Other Dietary Supplements
Insufficient reliable information available.

Possible Interactions with Drugs

No interactions are known to occur, and there is no known reason to expect a clinically significant interaction with wafer ash.

Possible Interactions with Foods

No interactions are known to occur, and there is no known reason to expect a clinically significant interaction with wafer ash.

Possible Interactions with Lab Tests

No interactions are known to occur, and there is no known reason to expect a clinically significant interaction with wafer ash.

Possible Interactions with Diseases or Conditions

No interactions are known to occur, and there is no known reason to expect a clinically significant interaction with wafer ash.

Typical Dosages & Routes of Administration that are Commonly Used

No typical dosage.

Comments

Wafer ash is used as an extract. There is very little scientific information about this product. Our staff is continually analyzing the available information on natural medicines and will add data here as it becomes available.

WAHOO

This Product is Also Known As

Arrowwood, Bitter Ash, Bleeding Heart, Burning Bush, Bursting Heart, Eastern Burning Bush, Fish Wood, Fusanum, Fusoria, Gadrose, Gatten, Gatter, Indian Arrowroot, Indian Arrowwood, Pegwood, Pigwood, Prickwood, Skewerwood, Spindle Tree, Strawberry Bush, Strawberry Tree.

Scientific Names

Euonymus atropurpureus.
Family: Celastraceae.

People Use This For

Orally, wahoo root bark is used orally for indigestion, to stimulate bile production, and as a laxative, diuretic, or tonic (18).

Safety

LIKELY UNSAFE ...when the bark, seeds or berries are used orally. Ingesting 36 berries can be fatal (18). The poisonous principle has not been identified (17).
PREGNANCY AND LACTATION: LIKELY UNSAFE (18).

Effectiveness

There is insufficient reliable information available about the effectiveness of wahoo.

Possible Mechanism of Action & Active Ingredients

The applicable parts of wahoo are the trunk, root bark, and fruit. The seeds contain cardioactive steroids known as cardenolides. The trunk, root bark, and fruit also contain varied alkaloids, caffeine, and theobromine (18). Wahoo is thought to stimulate bile flow and have laxative effects. In larger amounts, it can affect the heart (18).

Adverse Reactions Including Known Allergies

Wahoo is considered poisonous (17). Several hours after ingesting wahoo seeds, people experience severe upset stomach, sometimes with bloody diarrhea, fever, shortness of breath, circulatory problems, signs of collapse, stupor increasing to unconsciousness, alternating with motor restlessness, severe tonic-clonic spasms with locked jaw muscles and coma.

Possible Interactions with Herbs & Other Dietary Supplements

CARDIAC GLYCOSIDE-CONTAINING HERBS: Contraindicated; concomitant use increases the risk of cardiac glycoside toxicity. Cardiac glycoside containing herbs include black hellebore, Canadian hemp roots, digitalis leaf, hedge mustard, figwort, lily of the valley roots, motherwort, oleander leaf, pheasant's eye plant, pleurisy root, squill bulb leaf scales, and strophanthus seeds (2,18,19,500).
OTHER CARDIOACTIVE HERBS: Avoid concomitant use with other cardioactive herbs due to unpredictability of effects and adverse effects. Other cardioactive herbs include: calamus, cereus, cola, coltsfoot, devil's claw, European mistletoe, fenugreek, fumitory, ginger, Panax ginseng, hawthorn, white horehound, mate, parsley, quassia, scotch broom flower, shepherd's purse, and wild carrot (4).
STIMULANT LAXATIVE HERBS: Theoretically, use of stimulant laxatives can have additive effects and adverse

effects. Use also increases the risk of cardiac toxicity due to potassium depletion. Stimulant laxative herbs include: aloe dried leaf sap, blue flag rhizome, alder buckthorn, European buckthorn, butternut bark, cascara bark, castor oil, colocynth fruit pulp, gamboge bark exudate, jalap root, black root, manna bark exudate, podophyllum root, rhubarb root, senna leaves and pods, wild cucumber fruit (Ecballium elaterium), and yellow dock root (19).
LICORICE/HORSETAIL: Theoretically, overuse/misuse of licorice rhizome or horsetail plant with wahoo increases the risk of cardiac toxicity due to potassium depletion (19).

Possible Interactions with Drugs

DIGOXIN: Contraindicated. Using cardenolide constituents with digoxin increases risk of cardiac glycoside toxicity (2).
CARDIAC DRUGS: Theoretically, concomitant might increase risk of cardiac toxicity (152).
STIMULANT LAXATIVES: Theoretically, use of stimulant laxatives can have additive effects and adverse effects. It can also increase risk of cardiac glycoside toxicity due to potassium depletion (2).
POTASSIUM-DEPLETING DIURETICS: Theoretically, concomitant use increases risk of cardiac glycoside toxicity due to potassium depletion (2,506).
QUININE: Theoretically, concomitant use might increase risk of cardiac toxicity (2,506).
TETRACYCLINES and MACROLIDE ANTIBIOTICS (erythromycin-like drugs): Theoretically, concomitant use can increase risk of cardiac glycoside toxicity (152,17).

Possible Interactions with Foods

No interactions are known to occur, and there is no known reason to expect a clinically significant interaction with wahoo.

Possible Interactions with Lab Tests

No interactions are known to occur, and there is no known reason to expect a clinically significant interaction with wahoo.

Possible Interactions with Diseases or Conditions

GI CONDITIONS: Theoretically, wahoo can increase gastric secretions and stimulate peristalsis. These effects might exacerbate gastrointestinal irritation or inflammation (18).
HEART DISEASE: Contraindicated; theoretically cardiac glycosides contained in wahoo seed can exacerbate the condition or interfere with existing drug therapy.

Typical Dosages & Routes of Administration that are Commonly Used

No typical dosage.

Comments

Wahoo is considered unsafe (18); avoid using. Avoid confusion with Euonymus europaeus (18).

WALLFLOWER

This Product is Also Known As

Beeflower, Gillyflower, Giroflier, Handflower, Keiri, Wallstock-Gillofer.

Scientific Names

Cheiranthus cheiri.
Family: Brassicaceae.

People Use This For

Orally, wallflower is used for cardiac insufficiency, to encourage menstruation, and as a laxative. It was also used for liver and gallbladder diseases because of its bitter taste.

Safety

POSSIBLY UNSAFE …when it is taken orally (18).
PREGNANCY AND LACTATION: POSSIBLY UNSAFE …due to its possible toxic effects; avoid using (18).

Effectiveness

There is insufficient reliable information available about the effectiveness of wallflower.

Possible Mechanism of Action & Active Ingredients

The applicable parts of wallflower are the above ground parts. It does contain cardiac glycosides, but they may be poorly absorbed when wallflower is taken orally (18).

Adverse Reactions Including Known Allergies

Poisoning may occur with parenteral administration, but is expected to be low with oral administration due to poor absorption of the cardiac glycosides (18).

Possible Interactions with Herbs & Other Dietary Supplements

STIMULANT LAXATIVE HERBS: Theoretically, overuse or misuse of stimulant laxatives with cardiac glycoside-containing herbs increases the risk of cardiac toxicity due to potassium depletion. Stimulant laxative herbs include: aloe dried leaf sap, blue flag rhizome, alder buckthorn, European buckthorn, butternut bark, cascara bark, castor oil, colocynth fruit pulp, gamboge bark exudate, jalap root, black root, manna bark exudate, podophyllum root, rhubarb root, senna leaves and pods, wild cucumber fruit (Ecballium elaterium), and yellow dock root (19).

LICORICE/HORSETAIL: Theoretically, overuse/misuse of licorice rhizome or horsetail plant with cardiac glycoside-containing herbs increases the risk of cardiac toxicity due to potassium depletion (19).

CARDIAC GLYCOSIDE-CONTAINING HERBS: Contraindicated, concomitant use may increase the risk of cardiac glycoside toxicity. Cardiac glycoside-containing herbs include: black hellebore, Canadian hemp roots, digitalis leaf, hedge mustard, figwort, lily-of-the-valley roots, motherwort, oleander leaf, pheasant's eye plant, pleurisy root, squill bulb leaf scales, and strophanthus seeds (2,18,19,500).

OTHER CARDIOACTIVE HERBS: Avoid concomitant use with other cardioactive herbs due to unpredictability of effects and adverse effects. Other cardioactive herbs include: calamus, cereus, cola, coltsfoot, devil's claw, European mistletoe, fenugreek, fumitory, ginger, ginseng Panax, hawthorn, white horehound, mate, parsley, quassia, scotch broom flower, shepherd's purse, and wild carrot (4). See individual product listings.

CHINCHONA, EPHEDRA: Use with wallflower seed may increase risk of toxicity (18,19).

Possible Interactions with Drugs

CARDIAC MEDICATIONS: Cardiac medications, including quinidine (and related noncardiac medication quinine) may increase risk of toxicity; contraindicated (18).

DIGOXIN: Therapeutic duplication, avoid (2).

LAXATIVES: Overuse/misuse may cause electrolyte depletion and increase risk of wallflower seed toxicity (18,19).

POTASSIUM DEPLETING DIURETICS, GLUCOCORTICOIDS: May cause electrolyte depletion and increase risk of wallflower seed toxicity (18,19).

CALCIUM SALTS: Contraindicated (18).

Possible Interactions with Foods

No interactions are known to occur, and there is no known reason to expect a clinically significant interaction with wallflower.

Possible Interactions with Lab Tests

No interactions are known to occur, and there is no known reason to expect a clinically significant interaction with wallflower

Possible Interactions with Diseases or Conditions

CARDIAC CONDITIONS: CAUTION, wallflower seed may cause arrhythmias (18).

Typical Dosages & Routes of Administration that are Commonly Used

No typical dosage.

Comments

Wallflower is considered unsafe for self medication, requires monitoring (18). Canadian hemp is also known as wallflower (Cheiranthus cheiri). Wallflower is considered obsolete as a medicinal herb (18).

WATER AVENS

This Product is Also Known As

Chocolate Root, Cure All, Indian Chocolate, Throat Root, Water Chisch, Water Flower.

Scientific Names

Geum rivale.
Family: Rosaceae.

People Use This For

Orally, water avens underground parts, and the fresh, flowering plant are used orally for diarrhea (4), catarrhal colitis (4), passive uterine hemorrhage (4), intermittent fevers (4), and ulcerative colitis (4).

Safety

There is insufficient reliable information is available about the safety of water avens.
Pregnancy and Lactation: Insufficient reliable information is available; avoid using.

Effectiveness

There is insufficient reliable information available about the effectiveness of water avens.

Possible Mechanism of Action & Active Ingredients

The applicable parts of water avens are the underground parts, fresh flowering plant, and root. High tannin content of water avens is probably responsible for astringent action. The freshly harvested rhizome and root contain trace amounts of the volatile oil eugenol (18).

Adverse Reactions Including Known Allergies

None reported.

Possible Interactions with Herbs & Other Dietary Supplements

MINERALS: Theoretically, can decrease absorption of iron, calcium, and magnesium, due to tannin content (7).

Possible Interactions with Drugs

ORAL MEDICATION: Theoretically, the tannin content might delay absorption of sedatives, hypnotics, antidepressants, and tranquilizers (19,7).
METFORMIN: Theoretically, water avens might reduce the efficacy of metformin (7).

Possible Interactions with Foods

No interactions are known to occur, and there is no known reason to expect a clinically significant interaction with water avens.

Possible Interactions with Lab Tests

No interactions are known to occur, and there is no known reason to expect a clinically significant interaction with water avens.

Possible Interactions with Diseases or Conditions

No interactions are known to occur, and there is no known reason to expect a clinically significant interaction with water avens.

Typical Dosages & Routes of Administration that are Commonly Used

No typical dosage.

Comments

There is very little scientific information about this product. Our staff is continually analyzing the available information on natural medicines and will add data here as it becomes available.

WATER DOCK

This Product is Also Known As

None.

Scientific Names

Rumex aquaticus.
Family: Polygaceae.

People Use This For

Orally, water dock is used for "blood purification" and constipation (18).
Topically, it is used for mouth ulcers, skin sores, scorbutic conditions, and for cleaning the teeth (18).
For food uses, the leaves are used in salads (18).

Safety

There is insufficient reliable information available about the safety of water dock.
Pregnancy and Lactation: Insufficient reliable information is available; avoid using.

Effectiveness

There is insufficient reliable information available about the effectiveness of water dock.

Possible Mechanism of Action & Active Ingredients

The applicable part of water dock is the dried root. Water dock contains anthracene derivatives, oxalic acid and calcium oxalate, and tannins (18), an essential oil, fat, protein, quercitrin, starch, and tannin. Water dock is considered to have digestive properties (18).

Adverse Reactions Including Known Allergies

None reported (18).

Possible Interactions with Herbs & Other Dietary Supplements

Insufficient reliable information available.

Possible Interactions with Drugs
No interactions are known to occur, and there is no known reason to expect a clinically significant interaction with water dock.

Possible Interactions with Foods
No interactions are known to occur, and there is no known reason to expect a clinically significant interaction with water dock.

Possible Interactions with Lab Tests
No interactions are known to occur, and there is no known reason to expect a clinically significant interaction with water dock.

Possible Interactions with Diseases or Conditions
COAGULATION DISORDERS: Oxalate constituents can alter serum calcium concentrations, possibly decreasing coagulation time (12).
KIDNEY DISEASE: Use with caution in individuals with a history of kidney stones. Insoluble oxalate crystals may form in the kidneys, causing further damage (12).

Typical Dosages & Routes of Administration that are Commonly Used
Water dock is used orally or topically as a liquid extract or as a powder.

Comments
None.

WATER FENNEL

This Product is Also Known As
Horsebane, Water Dropwort.

Scientific Names
Oenanthe aquatica.

People Use This For
Orally, the ripe seeds of water fennel are used orally as an expectorant, for the relief of coughs, as a diuretic, and as an antiflatulent (18).

Safety
There is insufficient reliable information available about the safety of water fennel.
Pregnancy and Lactation: Insufficient reliable information is available; avoid using.

Effectiveness
There is insufficient reliable information available about the effectiveness of water fennel.

Possible Mechanism of Action & Active Ingredients
The applicable part of water fennel is the ripe seed. The active agents include fatty oil, volatile oil (including (+)-beta-phellandrene, dillapiol, myristicin, androle), resin, wax, galacton, mannan, and rubber substances (18).

Adverse Reactions Including Known Allergies
None reported.

Possible Interactions with Herbs & Other Dietary Supplements
Insufficient reliable information available.

Possible Interactions with Drugs
No interactions are known to occur, and there is no known reason to expect a clinically significant interaction with water fennel.

Possible Interactions with Foods
No interactions are known to occur, and there is no known reason to expect a clinically significant interaction with water fennel.

Possible Interactions with Lab Tests
No interactions are known to occur, and there is no known reason to expect a clinically significant interaction with water fennel.

Possible Interactions with Diseases or Conditions
No interactions are known to occur, and there is no known reason to expect a clinically significant interaction with water fennel.

Typical Dosages & Routes of Administration that are Commonly Used

ORAL: A typical dose of water fennel is 1 gram as a tea or extract (18).

Comments

There is very little scientific information about this product. Our staff is continually analyzing the available information on natural medicines and will add data here as it becomes available.

WATER GERMANDER

This Product is Also Known As

None.

Scientific Names

Teucrium scordium.
Family: Lamiaceae.

People Use This For

Water germander is used for bronchial asthma, diarrhea, fever, intestinal parasites, hemorrhoids, and festering and inflamed wounds (18).

Safety

There is insufficient reliable information available about the safety of water germander.
Pregnancy and Lactation: Insufficient reliable information is available; avoid using.

Effectiveness

There is insufficient reliable information available about the effectiveness of water germander.

Possible Mechanism of Action & Active Ingredients

The applicable parts of water germander are the above ground parts. There is insufficient reliable information available about the possible mechanism of action and active ingredients.

Adverse Reactions Including Known Allergies

None reported.

Possible Interactions with Herbs & Other Dietary Supplements

Insufficient reliable information available.

Possible Interactions with Drugs

No interactions are known to occur, and there is no known reason to expect a clinically significant interaction with water germander.

Possible Interactions with Foods

No interactions are known to occur, and there is no known reason to expect a clinically significant interaction with water germander.

Possible Interactions with Lab Tests

No interactions are known to occur, and there is no known reason to expect a clinically significant interaction with water germander.

Possible Interactions with Diseases or Conditions

No interactions are known to occur, and there is no known reason to expect a clinically significant interaction with water germander.

Typical Dosages & Routes of Administration that are Commonly Used

ORAL OR TOPICAL: A typical dose is four teaspoonfuls (7.2 grams) above ground parts per day, as a prepared tea (18). The same preparation can be used internally or externally (18).

Comments

There is very little scientific information about this product. Our staff is continually analyzing the available information on natural medicines and will add data here as it becomes available.

WATER PLANTAIN

This Product is Also Known As

Mad-Dog Weed.
CAUTION: See separate listings for Great Plantain, Buckhorn Plantain, Blond Psyllium, Black Psyllium.

Scientific Names
Alisma plantago-aquatica.
Family: Alismataceae.

People Use This For
Orally, water plantain is used for bladder and urinary tract diseases (18).

Safety
POSSIBLY UNSAFE ...for oral use (18).
PREGNANCY AND LACTATION: POSSIBLY UNSAFE ...due to its toxic potential; avoid using (18).

Effectiveness
There is insufficient reliable information available about the effectiveness of water plantain.

Possible Mechanism of Action & Active Ingredients
The applicable part of water plantain is the root/rhizome. The fresh rootstock is thought to be poisonous. It contains the cyanogenic chlorogenic acid sulfate (18).

Adverse Reactions Including Known Allergies
None reported.

Possible Interactions with Herbs & Other Dietary Supplements
Insufficient reliable information available.

Possible Interactions with Drugs
No interactions are known to occur, and there is no known reason to expect a clinically significant interaction with water plantain.

Possible Interactions with Foods
No interactions are known to occur, and there is no known reason to expect a clinically significant interaction with water plantain.

Possible Interactions with Lab Tests
No interactions are known to occur, and there is no known reason to expect a clinically significant interaction with water plantain.

Possible Interactions with Diseases or Conditions
No interactions are known to occur, and there is no known reason to expect a clinically significant interaction with water plantain.

Typical Dosages & Routes of Administration that are Commonly Used
No typical dosage.

Comments
Water plantain is considered possibly unsafe; avoid using (18). Water plantain rootstock is said to be bitter in taste (18). It sounds similar to either the common or species names of great plantain, and buckhorn plantain. Be careful not to confuse them.

WATERCRESS

This Product is Also Known As
Agrião, Berro, Berro Di Agua, Brunnenkresse, Crescione Di Fonte, Cresson au Poulet, Cresson D'eau, Cresson De Fontaine, Indian Cress, Mizu-Garashi, Nasilord, Nasturtii herba, Oranda-Garashi, Scurvy Grass, Selada-Air, Tall Nasturtium, Wasserkresse, Waterkres.
CAUTION: See separate listings for Nasturtium and Scurvy Grass.

Scientific Names
Nasturtium officinale.
Family: Brassicaceae.

People Use This For
Orally, watercress above ground parts are used for respiratory tract mucous membrane inflammation (2).
Topically, watercress is used for arthritis, rheumatoid arthritis (18), earache, eczema, scabies, and warts (4017).
In folk medicine, watercress is used orally for coughs, bronchitis, as a spring tonic, an appetite stimulant (18), improving digestion and stimulating appetite (8), alopecia, cancer, flu, goiter, polyps, scurvy, tuberculosis, gland tumors, as an abortifacient, aphrodisiac, bactericide, laxative, restorative, stimulant, antihelmintic (4017).
For food uses, watercress is widely used in leaf salads and as a culinary spice (12).

 © Copyright 2000, Natural Medicines Comprehensive Database (209) 472-2244. For updated data, go to www.NaturalDatabase.com

Safety

LIKELY SAFE …when the above ground parts are used orally in food amounts (18).

POSSIBLY SAFE …when used short-term for oral medicinal use (2,8,12).

POSSIBLY UNSAFE ...when used in large amounts or for extended use. Can cause gastric mucosal irritation (8,12) or damage (19).

LIKELY UNSAFE ...contraindicated for use by individuals with gastric or duodenal ulcers, or inflammatory kidney diseases (2,12,19).

CHILDREN: LIKELY SAFE ...when used in amounts commonly found in food. LIKELY UNSAFE ...when used in larger amounts. Contraindicated in children younger than 4 years old (2,12,19).

PREGNANCY: LIKELY SAFE ...when used orally in amounts commonly found in foods. LIKELY UNSAFE ...when used in larger amounts. Might stimulate menstruation or have abortifacient effects (19).

LACTATION: Insufficient reliable information available; avoid using.

Effectiveness

POSSIBLY EFFECTIVE …when used orally for respiratory tract mucous membrane inflammation (2).

There is insufficient reliable information available about the effectiveness of watercress for its other uses.

Possible Mechanism of Action & Active Ingredients

The applicable parts of watercress are the above ground parts. Watercress is thought to have antibiotic and diuretic activity (18). The above ground parts contain mustard oil (18), vitamin C, and beta-carotene, and vitamin K (19). Mustard oil is believed responsible for diuretic effects and gastrointestinal irritation after consumption of large amounts of watercress (18). The constituent, phenethyl isothiocyanate, released by chewing watercress, inhibits metabolic activation of a lung carcinogen (4019).

Adverse Reactions Including Known Allergies

Consuming large amounts of watercress can cause gastrointestinal irritation (18). Theoretically, excessive or prolonged use might cause kidney damage (19). No adverse effects are reported from topical use.

Possible Interactions with Herbs & Other Dietary Supplements

Insufficient reliable information available.

Possible Interactions with Drugs

CHLORZOXAZONE: Concomitant use may potentiate effects of chlorzoxazone (Paraflex) due to reduced metabolism and elimination (4018).

WARFARIN: Theoretically, consuming large amount amounts of watercress with its high vitamin K content might antagonize the anticoagulant effects of warfarin (Coumadin) (19).

Possible Interactions with Foods

No interactions are known to occur, and there is no known reason to expect a clinically significant interaction with watercress.

Possible Interactions with Lab Tests

COAGULATION TESTS: Might decrease prothrombin time, INR, and test results due to high vitamin K content (19).

Possible Interactions with Diseases or Conditions

No interactions are known to occur, and there is no known reason to expect a clinically significant interaction with watercress.

Typical Dosages & Routes of Administration that are Commonly Used

ORAL: A typical dose is one cup of tea before meals, 2-3 times daily. To make tea, pour 150 mL boiling water over 2 grams above ground parts, cover for 10 minutes, strain (18). A daily dose ranges to 4-6 grams dried herb, 20-30 grams fresh herb, or 60-150 grams freshly pressed juice (2).

TOPICAL: Watercress is used topically as a poultice or compress (18).

Comments

Avoid confusing watercress with nasturtium (Tropaeolum majus).

WHEAT BRAN

This Product is Also Known As

Bran.

CAUTION: See separate listings for Oat Bran and Rice Bran.

Scientific Names

Triticum aestrivum.

Family: Poaceae.

© Copyright 2000, Natural Medicines Comprehensive Database (209) 472-2244. For updated data, go to www.NaturalDatabase.com

People Use This For

Orally, wheat bran is used as a supplemental source of dietary fiber for preventing colon diseases (including cancer); reducing the risk of hemorrhoids and hiatus hernia; reducing cholesterol and blood sugar levels (5); reducing the risk of breast cancer (160) and gallbladder disease (162); and to improve glycemic control in type 2 diabetes (6266).

Safety

LIKELY SAFE ...when used orally (5).
PREGNANCY AND LACTATION: LIKELY SAFE (5).

Effectiveness

LIKELY EFFECTIVE ...when taken orally as a source of fiber (163).
POSSIBLY EFFECTIVE ...when used for treating constipation and restoring normal bowel function, reducing risk of hemorrhoids or hiatus hernia, preventing GI diseases (5,162,163), lowering blood pressure (157), and reducing plasma estradiol level when used in conjunction with a low fat diet (160). ...when used to improve glycemic control in type 2 diabetes (6266). In a randomized crossover study of 13 people with type 2 diabetes, a high fiber diet that included wheat bran was more effective in lowering preprandial blood glucose and the area under the curve for 24-hour plasma glucose and glucose (measured every 2 hours), and improving cholesterol and triglyeride levels than the standard ADA diet (6266).
POSSIBLY INEFFECTIVE ... when used to reduce the risk of colorectal cancer (4819,4820,4821). Several large well-designed studies showed that fiber, including wheat-bran fiber, does not prevent the recurrence of colorectal adenomas, despite earlier evidence that suggested a beneficial effect (160,4819,4820,4821).
There is insufficient reliable information available about the effectiveness of wheat bran for its other uses.

Possible Mechanism of Action & Active Ingredients

The applicable part of wheat bran is the outer hull of the grain, which is largely composed of insoluble fiber (157). The laxative effect of wheat bran is dependent on particle size; larger particles have a greater laxative effect than smaller particles (6265). Wheat bran has negligible water-holding capacity and no stool softening effect in people with normal stools (6265). Wheat bran increases colonic transit time, stool output, and bowel movement frequency (6265). It might reduce breast cancer risk by lowering plasma estrogen levels by interfering with enterohepatic circulation and increasing the rate of fecal estrogen excretion (162). Wheat bran might be beneficial in controlling insulin-resistance syndrome (162). Preliminary evidence suggests consumption of wheat bran might move the digestion site of foods from the proximal to distal portion of the colon (375). In the distal colon, butyrate produced from digestion of grains and starches reduces ammonia produced by fermentation of foods high in fat and sugar, possibly preventing cell damage and reducing the risk of colon cancer (375).

Adverse Reactions Including Known Allergies

Theoretically, may cause flatulence and GI discomfort, especially with initial use. One carefully controlled study designed to look at side effects noted no increase in GI symptoms in subjects taking 20 to 40 grams of wheat bran per day (6265).

Possible Interactions with Herbs & Other Dietary Supplements

Insufficient reliable information available.

Possible Interactions with Drugs

DIGOXIN: Theoretically, may interfere with absorption (156).

Possible Interactions with Foods

IRON: Wheat fiber inhibits dietary iron absorption (156).

Possible Interactions with Lab Tests

BLOOD PRESSURE: Wheat bran might lower blood pressure and blood pressure readings in individuals with hypertension (157).

Possible Interactions with Diseases or Conditions

No interactions are known to occur, and there is no known reason to expect a clinically significant interaction with wheat bran.

Typical Dosages & Routes of Administration that are Commonly Used

ORAL: Adults: 20-35 grams per day or 10-13 grams dietary fiber per 1000 kcal. In one study, 40 grams per day was no more effective than 20 grams for laxative effect (6265). Children 2 years of age and older: fiber intake equal to their age plus 5 grams (163). For best results, slowly increase fiber intake while reducing intake of foods high in fat, salt and sugar (5).

Comments

Wheat bran is the outer grain hull of wheat (Triticum aestrivum).

WHEATGRASS

This Product is Also Known As
Wheat Grass.

Scientific Names
None.

People Use This For
Orally, wheatgrass is used for increasing hemoglobin production, improving blood sugar disorders, for preventing tooth decay, improving wound healing, and preventing bacteria colonization (5285). It is also used orally for removing deposits of drugs, heavy metals, and carcinogens from the body, neutralizing toxins, removing toxins from the liver, removing toxins from the blood stream (5285).

Historically, wheatgrass has been used for preventing gray hair, reducing high blood pressure, aiding in the prevention and cure of cancer, improving digestion (5285), and blocking intestinal cholesterol absorption (5281).

Safety
LIKELY SAFE ...when consumed in food amounts (5286).
There is insufficient reliable information available about the safety of wheatgrass used in larger amounts.
PREGNANCY AND LACTATION: Insufficient reliable information available; avoid using.

Effectiveness
There is insufficient reliable information available about the effectiveness of wheatgrass.

Possible Mechanism of Action & Active Ingredients
The above ground parts are the applicable parts. There is insufficient reliable information available about the possible mechanism of action and active ingredients.

Adverse Reactions Including Known Allergies
None reported.

Possible Interactions with Herbs & Other Dietary Supplements
Insufficient reliable information available.

Possible Interactions with Drugs
WARFARIN: Theoretically, due to the vitamin K content, wheatgrass might decrease the anticoagulant effect of warfarin (Coumadin) (15). A 3.5 gram dose of wheatgrass contains 35 mcg vitamin K, according to supplier labeling (5287).

Possible Interactions with Foods
No interactions are known to occur, and there is no known reason to expect a clinically significant interaction with wheatgrass.

Possible Interactions with Lab Tests
No interactions are known to occur, and there is no known reason to expect a clinically significant interaction with wheatgrass.

Possible Interactions with Diseases or Conditions
No interactions are known to occur, and there is no known reason to expect a clinically significant interaction with wheatgrass.

Typical Dosages & Routes of Administration that are Commonly Used
ORAL: A typical oral wheatgrass dose is 3.5 grams, 1 teaspoon or 7 tablets (5281,5287). It might also be 2-4 ounces of wheatgrass juice (5289).

Comments
There are at least 25 varieties of wheatgrass in the following plant families: Agropyron, Elytrigia, Eremopyrum, Pascopyrum, Pseudoroegneria (5284). Wheatgrass juice or tablets are used as a part of an uncooked vegan diet, also known as a "living food" diet (5286). Wheatgrass products claim nutritional benefits similar to dark green salad (5281), e.g., seven 500 mg tablets or 1 teaspoonful powder wheatgrass to a serving of a 1/3 to 1 cup leafy dark green salad (5287,5288).

WHEY PROTEIN

This Product is Also Known As
Bovine Whey Protein Concentrate.

Scientific Names
None.

People Use This For
Orally, whey protein is used as a food supplement, for promoting positive nitrogen balance (4924,4941), as an alternative to milk for people with lactose intolerance, for protein allergy, asthma, high cholesterol, obesity (4925), replacing or supplementing milk-based infant formulas (4921), decreasing the risk of developing atopic disease in infants genetically predisposed to allergy (4927,4929), treating metastatic carcinoma (4930,4933), preventing colon cancer (4928), and reversing weight loss and increasing glutathione (GSH) in people with HIV disease (4926,4932,4935,4936).

Safety
LIKELY SAFE ...when quality products are used orally and appropriately. There are no reports of toxicity in clinical trials (4926,4927,4929,4930,4932,4935,4936,4941).
PREGNANCY: LIKELY SAFE ...when quality products are used appropriately (4921).
LACTATION: LIKELY SAFE ...when quality products are used appropriately (4929).

Effectiveness
EFFECTIVE ...when used orally as a replacement for, or in addition to, milk-based infant formulas (4921).
POSSIBLY EFFECTIVE ...when used orally for reversing weight loss and increasing glutathione (GSH) in people with HIV disease (4926,4932,4935,4936). ...when used orally to decrease the risk of developing atopic disease in infants genetically predisposed to allergy (4927,4929). ...when used for treating metastatic carcinoma (4930).
There is insufficient reliable information available about the effectiveness of whey protein for its other uses.

Possible Mechanism of Action & Active Ingredients
Whey is a by-product of cheese making which contains carbohydrates including lactose; minerals including calcium (4923); proteins including alpha-lactalbumin, beta-lactoglobulin, lactoferrin, serum albumin, lysozyme and immunoglobulins A, G, and M (4921); and cysteine (4937). The concentrations of whey protein, lactose, and minerals can be increased or reduced as required for the intended use of the product (4923). Whey protein is added to infant formula to more closely imitate human milk (4921). In people with HIV disease, whey protein increases body weight (4926,4935,4936), elevates glutathione (GSH) in mononuclear cells (4926), increases albumin, CD8 and CD4 counts (4935), and reduces diarrhea (4932,4936). Whey protein shows evidence of immunomodulating activity (4939,4940). Preliminary evidence suggests that whey protein (Immunocal) might enhance the reduced-to-oxidized glutathione ratio (GSH/GSSG) in lymphocytes, a marker of oxidative stress in reactive oxygen species (ROS)-mediated diseases, including AIDS-related wasting (1382). Whey protein (Immunocal) has anti-HIV and anti-apoptotic effects in vitro (4937). Whey protein reduces gastrointestinal Cryptosporidium parvum infection in mice (4934). Whey protein might prevent cancer by providing GSH substrates, increasing tissue GSH levels (4943). Whey protein (Immunocal) might exert antitumor effects by depleting tumor cells, that typically have increased amounts of GSH, making them more vulnerable to chemotherapy (4930). Preliminary evidence suggests whey protein might protect against breast cancer (3976). Some evidence suggests that whey protein might protect against colon cancer (4928) and reduce the tumor burden (4933). Preliminary research suggests that a unique combination of hydrolyzed whey protein isolates inhibits angiotensin converting enzyme (ACE), leading researchers to wonder whether it might be useful for treating high blood pressure (6171).

Adverse Reactions Including Known Allergies
None reported.

Possible Interactions with Herbs & Other Dietary Supplements
Insufficient reliable information available.

Possible Interactions with Drugs
LEVODOPA: Theoretically, concomitant use might decrease levodopa (Laradopa) absorption (10,4944).
MINERAL/DRUG INTERACTIONS: Theoretically, concomitant use of fluoride (Fluoritab), fluoroquinolones, tetracyclines, and alendronate (Fosamax) can decrease absorption of these drugs, due to whey protein mineral content (9). To avoid interaction, separate administration by at least two hours.

Possible Interactions with Foods
No interactions are known to occur, and there is no known reason to expect a clinically significant interaction with whey protein.

Possible Interactions with Lab Tests
No interactions are known to occur, and there is no known reason to expect a clinically significant interaction with whey protein.

Possible Interactions with Diseases or Conditions
MILK ALLERGY: Individuals allergic to bovine milk products should avoid using whey protein (4942).

Typical Dosages & Routes of Administration that are Commonly Used
ORAL: A typical dose as a dietary supplement in people with HIV disease is 8.4-84 grams per day (4926,4935), or 2.4 g/kg per day in a calorie-enriched formula (4941), or 42-84 grams per day in a glutamine enriched formula (4935). A dose for treating metastatic carcinoma is 30 grams per day (4930).

Comments
Whey protein is the soluble protein contained in whey, the watery portion of milk that separates from the curds in the process of cheese making (516,5121). A bovine whey protein concentrate product (Immuno-C) was investigated for treating Cryptosporidium infection in immunocompromised or immunocompetent people (FDA orphan drug status) (14); the product has not been approved for this use and no published clinical data are available.

WHITE COHOSH

This Product is Also Known As
Baneberry, Coralberry, Doll's Eye, Snakeberry, White Baneberry.
CAUTION: See separate listings for Black Cohosh, Blue Cohosh, and European Baneberry.

Scientific Names
Actaea alba, synonym Actaea pachypoda; Actaea rubra.
Family: Ranunculaceae.

People Use This For
Historically, white cohosh has been used to stimulate menstruation and to treat other female disorders. The root has been used for colds and cough, urogenital disorders, stomach disorders, reviving those near death, as a purgative, in childbirth, and for curing itching (6).

Safety
LIKELY UNSAFE ...when used orally. All plant parts are toxic (6,14).
PREGNANCY AND LACTATION: LIKELY UNSAFE ...contraindicated for oral use due to toxicity (6).

Effectiveness
There is insufficient reliable information available about the effectiveness of white cohosh.

Possible Mechanism of Action & Active Ingredients
The constituent protoanemonin is believed to cause irritant effects (6). The fruit and berries are especially toxic. They contain toxic glycosides and an essential oil (6).

Adverse Reactions Including Known Allergies
When used orally white cohosh can cause gastrointestinal irritation (19), acute stomach cramping, headache, tachycardia, vomiting, delirium, circulatory failure (6), bloody diarrhea, dysuria, hematuria, visual hallucinations, and incoherence (14). Topical application can lead to inflammation and skin blistering (6).

Possible Interactions with Herbs & Other Dietary Supplements
Insufficient reliable information available.

Possible Interactions with Drugs
No interactions are known to occur, and there is no known reason to expect a clinically significant interaction with white cohosh.

Possible Interactions with Foods
No interactions are known to occur, and there is no known reason to expect a clinically significant interaction with white cohosh.

Possible Interactions with Lab Tests
No interactions are known to occur, and there is no known reason to expect a clinically significant interaction with white cohosh.

Possible Interactions with Diseases or Conditions
GI CONDITIONS: Can irritate the gastrointestinal tract. Contraindicated in individuals with infectious or inflammatory gastrointestinal conditions (19).

Typical Dosages & Routes of Administration that are Commonly Used
No typical dosage.

Comments

White cohosh appears to be a substance with no reliable evidence to support its use, yet with documented toxicity. It should not be confused with black cohosh, used for symptoms of menopause, nor with blue cohosh, a substance used as a uterine stimulant and antispasmodic (6). White cohosh is also known as baneberry but it should not be confused with European baneberry.

WHITE DEAD NETTLE FLOWER

This Product is Also Known As

Archangel, Bee Nettle, Blind Nettle, Deaf Nettle, Dumb Nettle, Lamii Albi Flos, Stingless Nettle, White Archangel.
CAUTION: See separate listings for Stinging Nettle above ground parts and Stinging Nettle root.

Scientific Names

Lamium album.
Family: Lamiaceae.

People Use This For

Orally, white dead nettle is used for simple inflammation of mucous membranes in the upper respiratory tract (2,8). Topically, it is used for mild inflammation of the mouth, throat, and skin (2,18), and for non-specific vaginal discharge (2,18).
In folk medicine, white dead nettle has been used as an ingredient in sedative herbal teas (8).

Safety

LIKELY SAFE ...when taken orally and used appropriately (2,18).
PREGNANCY AND LACTATION: Insufficient reliable information available; avoid using.

Effectiveness

POSSIBLY EFFECTIVE ...when taken orally for simple inflammation of mucous membranes in the upper respiratory tract (2). ...when used topically for mild inflammation of the oropharynx and skin and for non-specific vaginal discharge (2).
There is insufficient reliable information available about the effectiveness of white dead nettle flower for its other uses.

Possible Mechanism of Action & Active Ingredients

Nettle flowers contain tannin, mucilage, and saponins (2). These give nettle expectorant and astringent effects.

Adverse Reactions Including Known Allergies

None reported (2).

Possible Interactions with Herbs & Other Dietary Supplements

Insufficient reliable information available.

Possible Interactions with Drugs

No interactions are known to occur, and there is no known reason to expect a clinically significant interaction with white dead nettle flower.

Possible Interactions with Foods

No interactions are known to occur, and there is no known reason to expect a clinically significant interaction with white dead nettle flower.

Possible Interactions with Lab Tests

No interactions are known to occur, and there is no known reason to expect a clinically significant interaction with white dead nettle flower.

Possible Interactions with Diseases or Conditions

No interactions are known to occur, and there is no known reason to expect a clinically significant interaction with white dead nettle flower.

Typical Dosages & Routes of Administration that are Commonly Used

ORAL: The average daily dose is 3 grams (2).
TOPICAL: 5 grams of the white dead nettle flower is commonly added to a sitz bath (2).

Comments

Avoid confusion with stinging nettle herb and stinging nettle root.

WHITE HELLEBORE

This Product is Also Known As
European Hellebore, European White Hellebore, Langwort.
CAUTION: See separate listings for Black Hellebore, American Hellebore, Pheasant's Eye (false hellebore).

Scientific Names
Veratrum album.
Family: Liliaceae.

People Use This For
Orally, white hellebore is used to treat cholera, gout, and hypertension (6).
Topically, it is used for herpetic lesions (6).
In Roman times, it was used as a poison; an extract has been used as an arrow tip poison (6).
It has also been used as an insecticide against flies and mosquitoes (6).

Safety
LIKELY UNSAFE ...when taken orally since all plant parts are considered toxic (6). Between 10-20 mg of alkaloids (1-2 grams of rhizome/root) are lethal (18,6). ...when used topically since toxic alkaloids can be absorbed through intact skin (18,6).
PREGNANCY: LIKELY UNSAFE ...when used orally or topically. Contraindicated because it could be teratogenic (6).
LACTATION: LIKELY UNSAFE ...when used orally or topically; avoid using.

Effectiveness
There is insufficient reliable information available about the effectiveness of white hellebore.

Possible Mechanism of Action & Active Ingredients
The applicable parts of white hellebore are the rhizome and root. White Hellebore contains the toxic ester-alkaloids protoveratrine A and B (13), which are sensory nerve irritants (18). These alkaloids inhibit the inactivation of the sodium ion channels and thus have a paralyzing effect on many excitable cells, including those of the heart (18).

Adverse Reactions Including Known Allergies
Taken orally, white hellebore can cause mucous membrane irritation (18), a burning sensation in upper abdomen, salivation, vomiting, gastric erosion, severe hypotension, bradycardia, and shock (6,553). Large doses may cause central respiratory depression, blindness, paralysis, convulsions, cardiac arrhythmias, and death (6). The powdered root, taken by inhalation, induces violent sneezing and runny nose (6). Topically, it can cause skin irritation (18); and the toxic alkaloids could be absorbed.

Possible Interactions with Herbs & Other Dietary Supplements
Insufficient reliable information available.

Possible Interactions with Drugs
No interactions are known to occur, and there is no known reason to expect a clinically significant interaction with white hellebore.

Possible Interactions with Foods
No interactions are known to occur, and there is no known reason to expect a clinically significant interaction with white hellebore.

Possible Interactions with Lab Tests
No interactions are known to occur, and there is no known reason to expect a clinically significant interaction with white hellebore.

Possible Interactions with Diseases or Conditions
No interactions are known to occur, and there is no known reason to expect a clinically significant interaction with white hellebore.

Typical Dosages & Routes of Administration that are Commonly Used
No typical dosage.

Comments
White hellebore is considered likely unsafe; avoid due to toxic alkaloid content (18). Crude white hellebore is not used therapeutically (13), though it is sometimes used in homeopathic dilutions (18).

WHITE HOREHOUND

This Product is Also Known As
Common Hoarhound, Hoarhound, Horehound, Houndsbane, Marrubii herba, Marrubium, Mastranzo.
CAUTION: See separate listing for Black Horehound.

Scientific Names
Marrubium vulgare.
Family: Lamiaceae.

People Use This For
Orally, the above ground parts of white horehound are used for loss of appetite (2), cough/bronchitis, respiratory tract mucous membrane inflammation, indigestion, bloating and flatulence, liver and gallbladder complaints (4,18,512).
Topically, white horehound is used for skin damage, ulcers, and wounds (18).
In traditional medicine, the above ground parts of white horehound are used orally for whooping cough, asthma, tuberculosis, diarrhea, jaundice, debility, painful menstruation, as a laxative (18), an antihelmintic (515), as a diuretic, and to induce sweating (6).
In manufacturing, the extracts of white horehound are used as flavoring in foods and beverages (11), and as an expectorant in cough syrups and lozenges (515).

Safety
LIKELY SAFE …when used orally in amounts found in foods. It has Generally Recognized as Safe (GRAS) status in the US (11). The maximum use level is 0.073% for the extract.
POSSIBLY SAFE …when the above ground parts are used orally and appropriately (2,12).
POSSIBLY UNSAFE …when used orally in excessive amounts because it can have a purgative effect (4,12).
There is insufficient reliable information available about the safety of the topical use of white horehound.
PREGNANCY: LIKELY UNSAFE …contraindicated for oral use. Might have abortifacient effect (19), or stimulate menstrual flow and the uterus (12). Insufficient reliable information available about the topical use; avoid using.
LACTATION: Insufficient reliable information available for oral use; avoid amounts greater than found in foods. Insufficient reliable information available about topical use; avoid using.

Effectiveness
POSSIBLY EFFECTIVE …when used orally to stimulate appetite. …when used orally for indigestion, bloating, and flatulence (2). …when used orally for coughs and colds (8,11,515).
There is insufficient reliable information available about the effectiveness of white horehound for its other uses.

Possible Mechanism of Action & Active Ingredients
The applicable parts of white horehound are the above ground parts. White horehound contains marrubiin, bitter ingredients, volatile oil, and tannins (515). The constituent, marrubiin does not exist in the fresh plant; it is formed from premarrubiin during processing (515). The volatile oil of white horehound exhibits vasodilation, expectorant (11), and antischistosomal activity (4). Some evidence suggests the hydroxycinnamic derivatives might have weak antioxidant activity (11). Other evidence suggests marrubinic acid stimulates bile secretion (515). Marrubiin's expectorant effect results from direct stimulation of bronchial mucosal secretions (512). Marrubiin shows some evidence it can normalize extrasystolic arrhythmias (4,11), but large amounts might cause arrhythmias (4). An alcoholic extract reduces spasms of gastrointestinal tract (515). An aqueous extract demonstrates evidence that it can antagonize serotonin (11) and exerts anti-inflammatory activity (4,11).

Adverse Reactions Including Known Allergies
Ingesting large amounts of white horehound can cause purgative effects (4,12). Skin contact with the irritant in plant juice can cause contact dermatitis (4).

Possible Interactions with Herbs & Other Dietary Supplements
Insufficient reliable information available.

Possible Interactions with Drugs
No interactions are known to occur, and there is no known reason to expect a clinically significant interaction with white horehound.

Possible Interactions with Foods
No interactions are known to occur, and there is no known reason to expect a clinically significant interaction with white horehound

Possible Interactions with Lab Tests
No interactions are known to occur, and there is no known reason to expect a clinically significant interaction with white horehound.

Possible Interactions with Diseases or Conditions
HEART CONDITIONS: Theoretically, large amounts of white horehound might cause arrhythmias (4).

Typical Dosages & Routes of Administration that are Commonly Used
ORAL: A typical dose is 1-2 grams dried above ground parts or one cup tea three times daily before meals to stimulate bile secretion or during the day as an expectorant (8). To make tea, steep 1-2 grams dried above ground parts in 150 mL boiling water 5-10 minutes, and strain (4,8). Up to 4.5 grams dried above ground parts or 2-6 tablespoons of pressed juice (or equivalent preparations) are used per day (2). A typical dose of pressed juice is 30-60 mL daily (18). Liquid extract (1:1 in 25% ethanol), 1-3 mL three times daily (4). Tincture (1:10 in 45% alcohol), 1-2 mL three times daily (4).
TOPICAL: No typical dosage.

Comments
White horehound derives its name from ancient Greece where it was used for treating mad-dog bites (515).

WHITE LILY

This Product is Also Known As
Baurenlilien, Farmer's Lily, Madonna Lily, Meadow Lily.

Scientific Names
Lilium candidium.
Family: Liliaceae.

People Use This For
Orally, white lily is used for gynecological disorders.
Topically, it is used for ulcers, inflammation, furuncles, finger ulcers, reddened skin, burns, and injuries.
Historically, it has been used as an astringent, anti-inflammatory, softener, pain reliever, diuretic, antihemorrhagic, and expectorant (18).

Safety
There is insufficient reliable information available about the safety of white lily.
Pregnancy and Lactation: Insufficient reliable information available; avoid using.

Effectiveness
There is insufficient reliable information available about the effectiveness of white lily.

Possible Mechanism of Action & Active Ingredients
The applicable part of white lily is the root/bulb. There is insufficient reliable information available about the possible mechanism of action and active ingredients.

Adverse Reactions Including Known Allergies
None reported.

Possible Interactions with Herbs & Other Dietary Supplements
Insufficient reliable information available.

Possible Interactions with Drugs
No interactions are known to occur, and there is no known reason to expect a clinically significant interaction with white lily.

Possible Interactions with Foods
No interactions are known to occur, and there is no known reason to expect a clinically significant interaction with white lily.

Possible Interactions with Lab Tests
No interactions are known to occur, and there is no known reason to expect a clinically significant interaction with white lily.

Possible Interactions with Diseases or Conditions
No interactions are known to occur, and there is no known reason to expect a clinically significant interaction with white lily.

Typical Dosages & Routes of Administration that are Commonly Used
ORAL: No typical dosage.
TOPICAL: A thick paste made from the fresh or cooked root is placed in the middle of a compress or poultice and applied to the affected area several times throughout the day (18).

© Copyright 2000, Natural Medicines Comprehensive Database (209) 472-2244. For updated data, go to www.NaturalDatabase.com • 1099

Comments

There is very little scientific information about this product. Our staff is continually analyzing the available information on natural medicines and will add data here as it becomes available.

WHITE MUSTARD

This Product is Also Known As

Sinapis albae semen, Weibe Senfsamen.
CAUTION: See separate listings for Black Mustard, Black Mustard Oil, and Hedge Mustard.

Scientific Names

Sinapis alba; Brassica alba.
Family: Cruciferae or Brassicaceae.

People Use This For

Orally, white mustard is used "to brighten and clear" the voice and for those with a tendency for infection (18). Topically, white mustard is used for cough and colds (11,18), pulmonary congestion (2,11), bronchitis (18), joint and soft tissue inflammation, rheumatism (2,18), arthritis (2,11,18), lumbago (11), inflammation of the mouth and pharynx, and hyperemization of the skin (18).

Traditionally, it has been used orally as an emetic, diuretic, and appetite stimulant (6,11) and topically as a counterirritant (6) and a bath to treat paralytic symptoms (18).

In foods and condiments, white mustard is a common flavoring agent (11), and is considered a culinary spice (11).

Safety

LIKELY SAFE ...in the amounts commonly found in foods (11,12). White mustard has Generally Recognized as Safe (GRAS) status in the US. The maximum level used is 12.4% (11).

POSSIBLY SAFE ...when used orally and appropriately for medicinal purposes (12). ...when used topically and appropriately (12,19).

LIKELY UNSAFE ...when taken orally as an emetic because mustard is an irritant. Used as an emetic, the esophageal tissue is twice exposed to the corrosive effects of white mustard (19). Ingestion of a large quantity can cause irritant poisoning (12,19). ...when used topically for more than 15-30 minutes because severe burns can occur (12,19). ...when used topically on a regular basis for more than 2 weeks (2,12,19).

CHILDREN: LIKELY SAFE...when used orally in food amounts.

LIKELY UNSAFE ...in larger amounts...when used topically in children under 6 years of age (2,12,19).

PREGNANCY: LIKELY SAFE ...when used orally in food amounts. LIKELY UNSAFE ...when used in larger amounts because white mustard can have abortifacient and menstrual-stimulant properties (19).

LACTATION: Insufficient reliable information available; avoid using.

Effectiveness

POSSIBLY EFFECTIVE ...when used topically for pulmonary congestion and for inflammation of the joints and soft tissue (2).

There is insufficient reliable information available about the effectiveness of white mustard for its other uses.

Possible Mechanism of Action & Active Ingredients

The applicable part of white mustard is the seed. White mustard seeds contain mustard oil glycosides and mustard oils (2). White mustard contains the glucosinolate sinalbin, which on hydrolysis yields p-hydroxybenzyl isothiocyanate, p-hydroxybenzylamine, and other constituents, such as proteins, fatty oil, and sinapine (11,18). These products of hydrolysis possess irritant and bacteriostatic properties (18). Mustard's pungent taste comes from p-hydroxybenzyl isothiocyanate (11). Some evidence suggests the glucosinolate products can have protective effects against carcinogens (11).

Adverse Reactions Including Known Allergies

Long-term oral use of white mustard can increase the risk of nerve damage (2,18). Isothiocyanates, such as those in mustard, can cause endemic goiters (6,11). Topically, white mustard can cause blistering and skin ulceration, as well as nerve damage (2,12,18,19).

Possible Interactions with Herbs & Other Dietary Supplements

Insufficient reliable information available.

Possible Interactions with Drugs

No interactions are known to occur, and there is no known reason to expect a clinically significant interaction with white mustard.

Possible Interactions with Foods

No interactions are known to occur, and there is no known reason to expect a clinically significant interaction with white mustard.

Possible Interactions with Lab Tests

No interactions are known to occur, and there is no known reason to expect a clinically significant interaction with white mustard.

Possible Interactions with Diseases or Conditions

KIDNEY DISEASE: Irritant poisoning from white mustard can occur in people with kidney disorders (12,19).

Typical Dosages & Routes of Administration that are Commonly Used

ORAL: The average amount of white mustard is 60-150 grams daily (18). To "brighten and clear" the voice, mustard flour, or powdered mustard, is stirred with honey to form balls (18). One or two of these honey balls are taken on an empty stomach (18).

TOPICAL: As a foot bath, 20 to 30 grams of mustard flour is typically mixed in 1 liter of water (18). For a mustard bath, 150 grams of mustard flour in a pouch is commonly placed in the bath (18). For local application, 4 tablespoons (50-70 grams) of the powdered seeds are usually mixed with warm water to form a soft material, which is applied for 10-15 minutes for adults and 5-10 minutes for children older than 6 years of age (2,18). Decrease the application time in individuals with sensitive skin (2). Treatment should not exceed two weeks (2,12,18,19).

Comments

Avoid confusion with other Sinapis or Brassica species (black mustard, Brassica nigra; brown mustard, Brassica juncea).

WHITE SANDALWOOD oil

This Product is Also Known As

East Indian Sandalwood Oil, Sanderswood, Santal Oil, White Saunders Oil, Yellow Sandalwood Oil, Yellow Saunders Oil.
CAUTION: See separate listings for Red Sandalwood and White Sandalwood wood.

Scientific Names

Santalum album.
Family: Santalaceae.

People Use This For

White sandalwood oil is used as adjuvant therapy for lower urinary tract infection (2), common cold, cough/bronchitis, fevers, urinary tract inflammatory conditions, mouth and pharynx inflammation, liver and gallbladder complaints, and infection (18).
In folk medicine, white sandalwood is used orally, for stomachache, vomiting, gonorrhea, pains, "strengthening the heart" (11), headache, urogenital disorders (6), to reduce libido, for heatstroke, sunstroke, and resulting fever (18).
In food and beverages, it is used as a flavor component (11).
In manufacturing, white sandalwood oil is used as a fragrance ingredient in soaps, cosmetics, and perfumes (11).

Safety

LIKELY SAFE …when used orally in amounts found in food. Approved for food use in the US. The average level used is less than 0.001% (11). …when used topically in amounts found in cosmetics unless allergic to sandalwood oil. The maximum use level is 1% in perfumes (11).
POSSIBLY SAFE …when used orally for short-term medicinal use as enteric-coated products (2).
POSSIBLY UNSAFE …when used orally for longer than 6 weeks, condition should be medically evaluated (2,19). There is insufficient reliable information available about the safety of the topical use of white sandalwood in amounts greater than found in cosmetics.
PREGNANCY: POSSIBLY SAFE …when used as a flavoring. LIKELY UNSAFE …contraindicated for oral use in medicinal amounts because it might have abortifacient effect (19). There is insufficient reliable information available about the safety of topical use during pregnancy.
LACTATION: Insufficient reliable information available; avoid using amounts greater than found in foods.

Effectiveness

POSSIBLY EFFECTIVE …when used orally as an adjuvant therapy for lower urinary tract infections (2). There is insufficient reliable information available about the effectiveness of white sandalwood oil for its other uses.

Possible Mechanism of Action & Active Ingredients

White sandalwood oil is reported to have antifungal, antiseptic, diuretic (11), antibacterial, and spasmolytic activity (2). It is considered to be a kidney irritant (19). Although some evidence suggests it is not irritating, sensitizing, or phototoxic when applied to the skin, the constituent, santolol, can cause contact dermatitis (11).

Adverse Reactions Including Known Allergies

Oral use of white sandalwood oil can cause itching, nausea, gastrointestinal complaints, and blood in the urine (18). Topical use can cause contact dermatitis in sensitive individuals (11).

Possible Interactions with Herbs & Other Dietary Supplements

Insufficient reliable information available.

Possible Interactions with Drugs

No interactions are known to occur, and there is no known reason to expect a clinically significant interaction with white sandalwood oil.

Possible Interactions with Foods

No interactions are known to occur, and there is no known reason to expect a clinically significant interaction with white sandalwood oil

Possible Interactions with Lab Tests

No interactions are known to occur, and there is no known reason to expect a clinically significant interaction with white sandalwood oil.

Possible Interactions with Diseases or Conditions

KIDNEY DISEASE: Contraindicated in kidney disease, particularly in individuals with diseases of the kidney parenchyma (2,19).

Typical Dosages & Routes of Administration that are Commonly Used

ORAL: A typical oral dose is 1-1.5 grams of oil per day in an enteric-coated form, maximum use 6 weeks without medical evaluation (2).

Comments

None.

WHITE SANDALWOOD wood

This Product is Also Known As

East Indian Sandalwood, Sandalwood, Santali Lignum Albi, Tan Xiang,
White Saunders, Yellow
Sandalwood, Yellow Saunders.
CAUTION: See separate listings for Red Sandalwood and White Sandalwood oil.

Scientific Names

Santalum album.
Family: Santalaceae.

People Use This For

Orally, white sandalwood is used as an adjunct therapy for lower urinary tract infections (2,18), treating colds, cough, bronchitis, fevers, inflammatory conditions of the mouth, pharynx, or efferent urinary tract, and for liver and gallbladder complaints (18).
In folk medicine, it has been used for heat stroke, sun stroke and associated fever, gonorrhea, and as an anti-aphrodisiac (18).

Safety

POSSIBLY SAFE ...when the wood is used orally and appropriately short-term, for less than 6 weeks (2,12).
POSSIBLY UNSAFE ...when used orally longer than 6 weeks (2,12,18).
PREGNANCY: LIKELY UNSAFE …when used orally. Contraindicated because it is believed to have abortifacient effects (19).
LACTATION: Insufficient reliable information available; avoid using.

Effectiveness

POSSIBLY EFFECTIVE ...when taken orally as adjunctive therapy for lower urinary tract infections (2).
There is insufficient reliable information available about the effectiveness of white sandalwood for its other uses.

Possible Mechanism of Action & Active Ingredients

Sandalwood has antibacterial, spasmolytic, and urinary disinfectant activities (2,18).

Adverse Reactions Including Known Allergies

White sandalwood taken orally can cause nausea, gastrointestinal complaints, itching, and hematuria (blood in the urine) (2,18). High doses or use longer than six weeks can cause kidney toxicity (2,12,18). White sandalwood has minimal potential for sensitization (18).

Possible Interactions with Herbs & Other Dietary Supplements
Insufficient reliable information available.

Possible Interactions with Drugs
No interactions are known to occur, and there is no known reason to expect a clinically significant interaction with white sandalwood.

Possible Interactions with Foods
No interactions are known to occur, and there is no known reason to expect a clinically significant interaction with white sandalwood.

Possible Interactions with Lab Tests
No interactions are known to occur, and there is no known reason to expect a clinically significant interaction with white sandalwood.

Possible Interactions with Diseases or Conditions
KIDNEY DISEASE: White sandalwood is contraindicated in diseases of kidney parenchyma (2,12,18).

Typical Dosages & Routes of Administration that are Commonly Used
ORAL: The typical dose is 10-20 grams of the wood per day, brewed as a tea or other preparations (2). White sandalwood should not be used for more than a six-week duration (2,12).

Comments
Sandalwood has a very dense composition and is valued as a wood for carving (6). Avoid confusion with red sandalwood (Pterocarpus santalinus) and white sandalwood oil.

WHITE SOAPWORT

This Product is Also Known As
Gypsophilae radix, Soapwort.
CAUTION: See separate listing for Red Soapwort.

Scientific Names
Gypsophila paniculata and other Gypsophila species.
Family: Caryophyllaceae.

People Use This For
Orally, white soapwort is used for cough, bronchitis (18), and inflammation of the mucous membrane in the upper and lower respiratory tract (2).
In folk medicine, it has been used topically for chronic skin disorders and eczema (18).

Safety
POSSIBLY SAFE ...when used orally and appropriately (2).
PREGNANCY AND LACTATION: Insufficient reliable information; avoid using.

Effectiveness
POSSIBLY EFFECTIVE ...when taken orally for upper and lower respiratory tract mucous membrane inflammation (2).
There is insufficient reliable information available about the effectiveness of white soapwort for its other uses.

Possible Mechanism of Action & Active Ingredients
The applicable part of white soapwort is the root. White soapwort has expectorant, emetic, antibiotic, and insecticidal effects (18). In large amounts, it is cytotoxic (2). The saponin constituents exhibit expectorant effects (2), and they irritate the gastric mucosa to stimulate the bronchial mucous glands via parasympathetic sensory pathways (7). Saponins can cause stomach upset, nausea, and vomiting (7).

Adverse Reactions Including Known Allergies
White soapwort taken orally can cause stomach irritation (2), nausea, and vomiting (7).

Possible Interactions with Herbs & Other Dietary Supplements
Insufficient reliable information available.

Possible Interactions with Drugs
No interactions are known to occur, and there is no known reason to expect a clinically significant interaction with white soapwort.

Possible Interactions with Foods

No interactions are known to occur, and there is no known reason to expect a clinically significant interaction with white soapwort.

Possible Interactions with Lab Tests

No interactions are known to occur, and there is no known reason to expect a clinically significant interaction with white soapwort.

Possible Interactions with Diseases or Conditions

GI IRRITATION: Theoretically, the saponin content of white soapwort can exacerbate existing gastrointestinal mucosal irritation (6).

Typical Dosages & Routes of Administration that are Commonly Used

ORAL: The typical dose of white soapwort is 30-150 mg per day of the dried root or 3-15 mg per day of the gysophila saponin or equivalent preparations (2).

Comments

In the Middle Ages, Franciscan and Dominican monks viewed soapwort as a divine gift that was meant to keep them clean (6). Avoid confusion with the red soapwort root.

WILD CARROT

This Product is Also Known As

Beesnest Plant, Bird's Nest Root, Daucus, Queen Anne's Lace.

Scientific Names

Daucus carota L. subspecies carota.
Family: Apiaceae or Umbelliferae.

People Use This For

Orally, the above ground parts of wild carrot have been used for urinary calculus or stones, high uric acid in urine, cystitis, and gout (4).

Traditionally, carrot seed oil has been used for dysentery, indigestion, uterine pain, gout, heart disease, cancer, kidney problems, as a nerve tonic, as a diuretic, an antiflatulent, as an aphrodisiac, to induce menstruation, and as an anthelmintic (6,11).

For food uses, it is used as a flavoring agent in alcoholic and non-alcoholic beverages, frozen dairy desserts, candy, baked goods, gelatins, puddings, meat and meat products, condiments relishes, and soups (4,11).

In manufacturing, carrot seed oil is used as a fragrance in soaps, detergents, creams lotions, and perfumes (11).

Safety

LIKELY SAFE ...when carrot seed oil is used in food. It has Generally Recognized as Safe (GRAS) status in the US (11). Maximum amount found in foods is less than 0.003% (11).

POSSIBLY SAFE ...when carrot seed oil is used orally and appropriately in medicinal amounts (4,11).

LIKELY UNSAFE ...when an excessive amount of carrot seed oil is used orally, it can cause renal irritation (4). Because the seed contains the psychoactive agent myristicin, theoretically high doses of oil could cause neurological effects (6).

There is insufficient reliable information available about the safety of the oral use of the above ground parts of wild carrot.

PREGNANCY: LIKELY UNSAFE ...the seeds, oil, and above ground parts are contraindicated for oral use because they can cause uterine stimulant, abortifacient, and menstrual stimulant effects (19).

LACTATION: POSSIBLY UNSAFE. Carrot seed oil has mild estrogenic activity and irritant effects (4). There is insufficient reliable information available about the safety of the oral use of the seeds or above ground parts during lactation.

Effectiveness

There is insufficient reliable information available about the effectiveness of wild carrot.

Possible Mechanism of Action & Active Ingredients

Carrot fruit/seed contains flavones including apigenin, chrysin, luteolin; flavonols including kaempferol and quercetin and various glycosides. The amount and composition of the volatile oil contained in the fruit/seed varies between different cultivars. The furanocoumarins, 8-methoxypsoralen and 5 methoxypsoralen are found in the plant (4). Some evidence suggests that wild carrot might have significant antifertility activity (4,3858). Other evidence suggests that wild carrot has cholinergic-type actions, perhaps due to the choline constituents (4). Carrot seed oil shows some evidence of vasodilation, cardiac depressant, and smooth muscle relaxation effects (11). Terpinen-4-ol, a component of the seed oil, is a renal irritant and believed to cause a diuretic effect (4). A tertiary base isolated from wild carrot seed appears to have papaverine-like antispasmodic activity.

Adverse Reactions Including Known Allergies
Ingesting excessive doses can cause renal irritation or neurological effects. Hypersensitivity reactions and increased sensitivity to UV light and sunburn might occur (19,4). Contact with the plant can cause dermatitis (4).

Possible Interactions with Herbs & Other Dietary Supplements
HERBS WITH SEDATIVE PROPERTIES: Theoretically, concomitant use with herbs that have sedative properties might enhance therapeutic and adverse effects. These include calamus, calendula, California poppy, catnip, capsicum, celery, couch grass, elecampane, Siberian ginseng, German chamomile, goldenseal, gotu kola, hops, Jamaican dogwood, kava, lemon balm, sage, St. John's wort, sassafras, scullcap, shepherd's purse, stinging nettle, valerian, wild lettuce, withania root, and yerba mansa (4,19).
HERBS WITH ANTICOAGULANT/ANTIPLATELET POTENTIAL: Concomitant use of herbs that have coumarin constituents or affect platelet aggregation could theoretically increase the risk of bleeding in some people. These herbs include: angelica, anise, arnica, asafoetida, bogbean, boldo, capsicum, celery, chamomile, clove, danshen, fenugreek, feverfew, garlic, ginger, ginkgo, Panax ginseng, horse chestnut, horseradish, licorice, meadowsweet, prickly ash, onion, papain, passionflower, poplar, quassia, red clover, turmeric, wild lettuce, willow, and others (4,19).

Possible Interactions with Drugs
HORMONES: Theoretically, excessive use of the above ground parts of wild carrot might interfere with hormonal therapy (4).
CARDIAC OR BLOOD PRESSURE MEDICATIONS: Theoretically, excessive doses of carrot seed oil might affect therapy (4).
PSORLENS: Concomitant use of psoralens is contraindicated due to the potential of an additive, photosensitizing effect (19).

Possible Interactions with Foods
No interactions are known to occur, and there is no known reason to expect a clinically significant interaction with wild carrot.

Possible Interactions with Lab Tests
No interactions are known to occur, and there is no known reason to expect a clinically significant interaction with wild carrot.

Possible Interactions with Diseases or Conditions
UV LIGHT THERAPY: Contraindicated due to photosensitizing effect; avoid excessive periods in the sun (19).
RENAL INFLAMMATION/IRRITATION: Contraindicated due to renal irritant properties (4,19).

Typical Dosages & Routes of Administration that are Commonly Used
ORAL: Dried above ground parts: 2-4 grams or as tea three times daily. To make tea, steep 2-4 grams of above ground parts in boiling water for 5-10 minutes, strain (4). Liquid extract (1:1 in 25% alcohol) 2-4 mL three times daily (4).

Comments
Carrot seed oil is steam-distilled from the dried root of both the familiar vegetable known as carrot, and the wild carrot. Avoid confusing wild carrot (which has an inedible white tap root) with the common carrot (Daucus carota subspecies sativus) (4).

WILD CHERRY

This Product is Also Known As
Black Cherry, Black Choke, Choke Cherry, Rum Cherry Bark, Virginian Prune, Wild Black Cherry.
CAUTION: See separate listing for Cherry Laurel Water.

Scientific Names
Prunus serotina; Prunus virginiana.
Family: Rosaceae.

People Use This For
Orally, wild cherry is widely used in cough syrups because of its sedative, expectorant, astringent, and antitussive effects (9,11,13,18).
In folk medicine, it was used for colds, whooping cough, bronchitis and other lung problems, diarrhea, nervous digestive disorders, pain, and cancer (11,18).
In foods and beverages, wild cherry is used as a flavoring agent (11).

Safety

LIKELY SAFE ...when the stem bark is used orally in amounts found in foods and beverages. It has Generally Recognized as Safe (GRAS) status in the US (11).

POSSIBLY SAFE ...when used orally and appropriately short-term, in limited amounts (12).

POSSIBLY UNSAFE ...when used orally and long-term or in excessive amounts (12,19). The constituent, prunasin, hydrolyzes to hydrocyanic acid (HCN) (11,12,13,18).

PREGNANCY: LIKELY UNSAFE ...contraindicated because prunasin is potentially teratogenic (19).

LACTATION: Insufficient reliable information available; avoid using.

Effectiveness

There is insufficient reliable information available about the effectiveness of wild cherry.

Possible Mechanism of Action & Active Ingredients

The applicable part of wild cherry is the stem bark. Wild cherry bark has astringent, antitussive, and sedative effects (18). It contains prunasin, a cyanogenic glycoside that is hydrolyzed to toxic hydrocyanic acid (HCN) and benzaldehyde (11). Bark collected in the fall has a higher HCN yield (approximately 0.15%) than bark collected in the spring (approximately 0.05%). Leaves collected in the spring have the highest HCN yield (approximately 0.25%) (11).

Adverse Reactions Including Known Allergies

Ingestion of large amounts can lead to fatal poisonings (18).

Possible Interactions with Herbs & Other Dietary Supplements

Insufficient reliable information available.

Possible Interactions with Drugs

No interactions are known to occur, and there is no known reason to expect a clinically significant interaction with wild cherry.

Possible Interactions with Foods

No interactions are known to occur, and there is no known reason to expect a clinically significant interaction with wild cherry.

Possible Interactions with Lab Tests

No interactions are known to occur, and there is no known reason to expect a clinically significant interaction with wild cherry.

Possible Interactions with Diseases or Conditions

No interactions are known to occur, and there is no known reason to expect a clinically significant interaction with wild cherry.

Typical Dosages & Routes of Administration that are Commonly Used

ORAL: People use 5 to 12 drops of the liquid extract containing wild cherry bark (12-14% by volume) in water two to three times daily (5023).

Comments

Avoid confusion with cherry laurel water. In Chinese medicine, the stem and bark of related species (Prunus armeniaca) may be effective as an antidote for apricot kernel poisoning (18).

WILD DAISY

This Product is Also Known As

Bruisewort.

Scientific Names

Bellis perennis.
Family: Asteraceae.

People Use This For

In folk medicine, wild daisy is used orally for coughs, bronchitis, disorders of the liver and kidneys, inflammation, and as an expectorant and astringent. It is used topically for wounds and skin diseases. It was historically used as a "blood purifier" (18).

Safety

There is insufficient reliable information available about the safety of wild daisy.
Pregnancy and Lactation: Insufficient reliable information available; avoid using.

Effectiveness

There is insufficient reliable information available about the effectiveness of wild daisy.

Possible Mechanism of Action & Active Ingredients

Insufficient reliable information available.

Adverse Reactions Including Known Allergies

Wild daisy can cause an allergic reaction in individuals sensitive to the Asteraceae/Compositae family. Members of this family include ragweed, chrysanthemums, marigolds, daisies, and many other herbs.

Possible Interactions with Herbs & Other Dietary Supplements

Insufficient reliable information available.

Possible Interactions with Drugs

No interactions are known to occur, and there is no known reason to expect a clinically significant interaction with wild daisy.

Possible Interactions with Foods

No interactions are known to occur, and there is no known reason to expect a clinically significant interaction with wild daisy.

Possible Interactions with Lab Tests

No interactions are known to occur, and there is no known reason to expect a clinically significant interaction with wild daisy.

Possible Interactions with Diseases or Conditions

CROSS-ALLERGENICITY: Can cause an allergic reaction in individuals sensitive to the Asteraceae/Compositae family. Members of this family include ragweed, chrysanthemums, marigolds, daisies, and many other herbs.

Typical Dosages & Routes of Administration that are Commonly Used

ORAL: One cup of tea taken orally 2-4 times daily. The tea is prepared by steeping 2 teaspoons of dried herb in 300 mL of boiling water for 20 minutes and straining (18).

Comments

There is very little scientific information about this product. Our staff is continually analyzing the available information on natural medicines and will add data here as it becomes available.

WILD INDIGO

This Product is Also Known As

American Indigo, False Indigo, Horsefly Weed, Indigo Broom, Rattlebush, Yellow Broom, Yellow Indigo.

Scientific Names

Baptista tinctoria.
Family: Fabaceae.

People Use This For

Orally, wild indigo is used for diphtheria, influenza, malaria, septic angina, typhoid fever with prostration, and fever. It is also used for upper respiratory tract infections, common head cold, tonsillitis, stomatitis, inflammation of the mouth and throat mucous membranes, fever, lymphadenitis, furunculosis (18), and Crohn's disease (392). Topically, wild indigo is used for painless ulcers, inflamed nipples, and as a douche for leukorrhea. Historically, the root has been used as an oral tea for fever, scarlet fever, typhoid, and pharyngitis in North America. It was used topically for cleaning open and inflamed wounds (18).

Safety

UNSAFE ...long term oral or topical use is contraindicated due to potential toxicity (12,19).
PREGNANCY: UNSAFE ...wild indigo is contraindicated due to its toxic potential (12,19).
LACTATION: UNSAFE ...wild indigo is contraindicated due to its toxic potential (12,19).

Effectiveness

There is insufficient reliable information available about the effectiveness of wild indigo.

Possible Mechanism of Action & Active Ingredients

The applicable part of wild indigo is the root. Preliminary evidence suggests that glycoprotein constituents might have lymphocyte stimulating activity (393). Quinolizidine alkaloids cause gastrointestinal symptoms with high doses (18).

Adverse Reactions Including Known Allergies

Large doses can cause vomiting, diarrhea, gastrointestinal complaints, and spasms (12).

Possible Interactions with Herbs & Other Dietary Supplements

Insufficient reliable information available.

Possible Interactions with Drugs

No interactions are known to occur, and there is no known reason to expect a clinically significant interaction with wild indigo.

Possible Interactions with Foods

No interactions are known to occur, and there is no known reason to expect a clinically significant interaction with wild indigo.

Possible Interactions with Lab Tests

No interactions are known to occur, and there is no known reason to expect a clinically significant interaction with wild indigo.

Possible Interactions with Diseases or Conditions

GASTRIC DISORDERS: Use of wild indigo is contraindicated in patients with inflammatory gastrointestinal conditions, particularly with accompanying capillary congestion (19).

Typical Dosages & Routes of Administration that are Commonly Used

ORAL: One cup of tea taken orally 3 times daily. The tea is prepared by simmering 0.5-1 grams dried root in 150 mL of boiling water for 10-15 minutes and straining (18).
TOPICAL: An ointment is prepared using one part of liquid extract to 8 parts of ointment base and applied to the affected area (18).

Comments

None.

WILD LETTUCE

This Product is Also Known As

Acrid Lettuce, Bitter Lettuce, German Lactucarium, Green Endive, Lactucarium, Lettuce Opium, Poison Lettuce, Strong-Scented Lettuce.

Scientific Names

Lactuca virosa.
Family: Asteraceae or Compositae.

People Use This For

Orally, wild lettuce is used for whooping cough, mucous inflammations of the bronchial tract, asthma, urinary tract diseases (18), and irritable cough (4). The seed oil is used orally for arteriosclerosis and as a substitute for wheat germ oil (18).
Topically, wild lettuce latex is used as an antiseptic.
Traditionally, wild lettuce latex and leaf has been used for insomnia, restlessness and excitability in children, priapism, painful menses, nymphomania, muscular or joint pains (4), for aiding circulation, swollen genitals, and opium substitute in cough preparations (6).
Wild lettuce latex is also smoked for a recreational "high" or hallucinogenic effect (6).

Safety

POSSIBLY SAFE …when the latex and leaf are used orally and appropriately (12,4).
LIKELY UNSAFE …when large doses are used because they can cause stupor, depressed respiration, and even death (4).
PREGNANCY AND LACTATION: Insufficient reliable information available; avoid using (4).

Effectiveness

There is insufficient reliable information available about the effectiveness of wild lettuce for its other uses.

Possible Mechanism of Action & Active Ingredients

The applicable parts of wild lettuce are the latex and leaf. Wild lettuce is thought to have mild sedative, analgesic and hypnotic or tranquilizing effects (4,18). Wild lettuce contains lactucin and lactupicrin (4). The milky latex, known as lactucarium, can cause mydriasis (4). This effect is theorized to be due to the presence of hyoscyamine (4); however, the dried sap contains no hyoscyamine (4). Wild lettuce has sedative activity (4). Lactucin, lactupicrin, and hyoscyamine have all been proposed responsible for this activity, but the active constituent(s) has not been identified (4). Low concentrations (nanogram amounts) of morphine have been found in Lactuca species and are considered too low to have a pharmacological effect (4).

Adverse Reactions Including Known Allergies

Ingesting large amounts can cause sweating, increased respiration, tachycardia, pupil dilation, dizziness, ringing in the ears, vision disorders, pressure in the head, somnolence, excitatory states (18), respiratory depression, coma, and death (4). Topical use of wild lettuce latex can cause contact dermatitis (4). It can cause an allergic reaction in individuals sensitive to the Asteraceae/Compositae family. Members of this family include ragweed, chrysanthemums, marigolds, daisies, and many other herbs.

Possible Interactions with Herbs & Other Dietary Supplements

HERBS WITH SEDATIVE PROPERTIES: Theoretically, concomitant use with herbs that have sedative properties might enhance therapeutic and adverse effects. These include: calamus, calendula flowers, California poppy plant, catnip leaves, capsicum fruit, celery, couch grass, elecampane, Siberian ginseng, German chamomile, goldenseal, gotu kola, hops, Jamaican dogwood bark, kava root, lemon balm, passionflower, sage, St. John's wort, sassafras bark, scullcap plant, shepherd's purse, stinging nettle, valerian root/rhizome, wild carrot, withania root, and yerba mansa (4,19).

HERBS WITH ANTICOAGULANT/ANTIPLATELET POTENTIAL: Concomitant use of herbs that have coumarin constituents or affect platelet aggregation could theoretically increase the risk of bleeding in some people. These herbs include: angelica, anise, arnica, asafoetida, bogbean, boldo, capsicum, celery, chamomile, clove, danshen, fenugreek, feverfew, garlic, ginger, ginkgo, ginseng (Panax), horse chestnut, horseradish, licorice, meadowsweet, prickly ash, onion, papain, passionflower, poplar, quassia, red clover, turmeric, wild carrot, willow, and others (4,19).

Possible Interactions with Drugs

DRUGS WITH SEDATIVE PROPERTIES: Theoretically, concomitant use with drugs with sedative effects might cause additive effects and adverse effects (19).

Possible Interactions with Foods

No interactions are known to occur, and there is no known reason to expect a clinically significant interaction with wild lettuce.

Possible Interactions with Lab Tests

No interactions are known to occur, and there is no known reason to expect a clinically significant interaction with wild lettuce.

Possible Interactions with Diseases or Conditions

BENIGN PROSTATIC HYPERPLASIA (BPH): Contraindicated in prostate enlargement (12). Wild lettuce might contain hyoscyamine (4) which is contraindicated in conditions involving urinary retention, including BPH (15). CROSS-ALLERGENICITY: Wild lettuce can cause an allergic reaction in individuals sensitive to members of the Asteraceae/Compositae plant family. Members of this family include ragweed, chrysanthemums, marigolds, daisies, and many other herbs. NARROW-ANGLE GLAUCOMA: Contraindicated (12). Wild lettuce might contain hyoscyamine (4) which can exacerbate narrow-angle (closed-angle) glaucoma (15).

Typical Dosages & Routes of Administration that are Commonly Used

ORAL: A typical dose is 0.5-3 grams dried leaves or as tea three times daily. To make tea, steep 0.5 - 3 grams dried leaves in 150 mL of boiling water, and strained (4). As the liquid extract (1:1 in 25% alcohol), 0.5 - 3 mL three times daily (4). For the dried latex extract, lactucarium, 0.3 -1 grams three times daily (4). Also available as a soft extract, with the usual dose of 0.3 - 1 grams three times daily (4).

Comments

None.

WILD MINT

This Product is Also Known As

Hairy Mint, Marsh Mint, Water Mint.

Scientific Names

Mentha aquatica.
Family: Labiatae or Lamiaceae.

People Use This For

Orally, water mint is used for diarrhea and painful menstruation. It is also used as an astringent and stimulant (18).

Safety
There is insufficient reliable information available about the safety of wild mint.
Pregnancy and Lactation: Insufficient reliable information available; avoid using.

Effectiveness
There is insufficient reliable information available about the effectiveness of wild mint.

Possible Mechanism of Action & Active Ingredients
The applicable part of wild mint is the leaf. There is insufficient reliable information available about the possible mechanism of action and active ingredients.

Adverse Reactions Including Known Allergies
None reported.

Possible Interactions with Herbs & Other Dietary Supplements
Insufficient reliable information available.

Possible Interactions with Drugs
No interactions are known to occur, and there is no known reason to expect a clinically significant interaction with wild mint.

Possible Interactions with Foods
No interactions are known to occur, and there is no known reason to expect a clinically significant interaction with wild mint.

Possible Interactions with Lab Tests
No interactions are known to occur, and there is no known reason to expect a clinically significant interaction with wild mint.

Possible Interactions with Diseases or Conditions
No interactions are known to occur, and there is no known reason to expect a clinically significant interaction with wild mint.

Typical Dosages & Routes of Administration that are Commonly Used
ORAL: One small cup of tea is taken orally throughout the day.

Comments
There is very little scientific information about this product. Our staff is continually analyzing the available information on natural medicines and will add data here as it becomes available.

WILD RADISH

This Product is Also Known As
Joint-Podded Charlock.

Scientific Names
Raphanus raphanistrum.
Family: Brassicaceae.

People Use This For
Orally, wild radish is used for skin conditions and stomach disorders [18].

Safety
There is insufficient reliable information available about the safety of wild radish.
Pregnancy and Lactation: Insufficient reliable information available; avoid using.

Effectiveness
There is insufficient reliable information available about the effectiveness of wild radish.

Possible Mechanism of Action & Active Ingredients
The applicable part of wild radish is the fresh plant before flowering. Wild radish contains glucosinolates (glucopurtranjivine) in freshly harvested, unbruised plants that produce isopropyl mustard oil upon aging [18].

Adverse Reactions Including Known Allergies
At high doses, oral use of the wild radish plant can cause mucous membrane irritation of the GI tract [18].

Possible Interactions with Herbs & Other Dietary Supplements
Insufficient reliable information available.

Possible Interactions with Drugs

No interactions are known to occur, and there is no known reason to expect a clinically significant interaction with wild radish.

Possible Interactions with Foods

No interactions are known to occur, and there is no known reason to expect a clinically significant interaction with wild radish.

Possible Interactions with Lab Tests

No interactions are known to occur, and there is no known reason to expect a clinically significant interaction with wild radish.

Possible Interactions with Diseases or Conditions

No interactions are known to occur, and there is no known reason to expect a clinically significant interaction with wild radish.

Typical Dosages & Routes of Administration that are Commonly Used

ORAL: Wild radish plant is used ground or as an alcoholic extract (18).

Comments

There is very little scientific information about this product. Our staff is continually analyzing the available information on natural medicines and will add data here as it becomes available.

WILD THYME

This Product is Also Known As

Mother of Thyme, Serpyllum, Shepherd's Thyme.
CAUTION: See separate listings for Thyme, Spanish Origanum oil, and Thyme Oil.

Scientific Names

Thymus serpyllum.
Family: Labiatae or Lamiaceae.

People Use This For

Orally, wild thyme is used for cough, bronchitis, and inflammation of the respiratory tract.
In folk medicine, it is used orally for kidney and bladder disorders, to relieve flatulence and colic, as a digestive aid, expectorant, aromatic, and antimicrobial. It is used topically in folk medicine for arthritis and sprains (18).

Safety

LIKELY SAFE ...when used in amounts found in foods. Wild thyme has Generally Recognized as Safe (GRAS) status in the US (4083).
POSSIBLY SAFE ...when preparations of the above ground flowering parts are used orally and appropriately (12).
PREGNANCY AND LACTATION: LIKELY SAFE ...when used orally in food amounts; avoid amounts greater than those typically found in foods.

Effectiveness

There is insufficient reliable information available about the effectiveness of wild thyme.

Possible Mechanism of Action & Active Ingredients

The applicable parts of wild thyme are the above ground, flowering parts. There is insufficient reliable information available about the possible mechanism of action and active ingredients.

Adverse Reactions Including Known Allergies

None reported.

Possible Interactions with Herbs & Other Dietary Supplements

Insufficient reliable information available.

Possible Interactions with Drugs

No interactions are known to occur, and there is no known reason to expect a clinically significant interaction with wild thyme.

Possible Interactions with Foods

No interactions are known to occur, and there is no known reason to expect a clinically significant interaction with wild thyme.

Possible Interactions with Lab Tests

No interactions are known to occur, and there is no known reason to expect a clinically significant interaction with wild thyme

Possible Interactions with Diseases or Conditions

THYROID DISORDERS: Can suppress thyroid function by decreasing hormone production and/or release (19).

Typical Dosages & Routes of Administration that are Commonly Used

ORAL: One cup of tea taken orally before meals. The tea is prepared by steeping 1.5-2 grams dried plant in 150 mL of boiling water for 10 minutes and straining. The daily dose is equivalent to 4-6 grams dried herb (18).

Comments

None.

WILD YAM

This Product is Also Known As

Atlantic Yam, Barbasco, China Root, Colic Root, Devil's Bones, Mexican Yam, Phytoestrogen, Rheumatism Root, Wild Mexican Yam, Yuma.
CAUTION: See separate listings for Pregnenolone and Progesterone.

Scientific Names

Discorea villosa; Discorea floribunda; Discorea composita; Discorea mexicana, synonym Dioscorea macrostachya. Family: Dioscoreaceae.

People Use This For

Orally, wild yam root or rhizome is used as a "natural alternative" for estrogen replacement therapy (515), postmenopausal vaginal dryness (5121), premenstrual syndrome, osteoporosis (5125), increasing energy and libido in men and women (5127), and for breast enlargement (5121). Wild yam root and rhizome are used orally for treating diverticulosis (5121), gallbladder colic, painful menstruation, cramps (18), rheumatoid arthritis (5124), and for increasing energy (5126).

The constituent of wild yam root, diosgenin, is used as a precursor for commercial chemical synthesis of human steroidal hormones (515,816).

Safety

POSSIBLY SAFE ...when used orally (12).
There is insufficient reliable information available about the safety of the topical use of wild yam.
PREGNANCY AND LACTATION: Insufficient reliable information available; avoid using.

Effectiveness

There is insufficient reliable information available about the effectiveness of wild yam.

Possible Mechanism of Action & Active Ingredients

The applicable part of wild yam is the root/rhizome. The tubers of Dioscorea species contain the glycoside diosgenin, a steroid precursor that was used in the first commercial production of oral contraceptives, topical hormones, systemic corticosteroids, androgens, estrogens, progestogens, and other sex hormones (515). Dioscorea continues to be used as the precursor for manufacturing progesterone contained in some "natural progesterone" cosmetic products. The chemical transformation of diosgenin to estrogen, progesterone, or any other steroidal compound does not occur in the human body (515). Diosgenin prevents estrogen-induced bile flow suppression (5129). It shows some evidence that it might stimulate growth of mammary tissue (5130), and attenuate indomethacin-induced intestinal inflammation (5131). A wild yam extract enhances estradiol binding to estrogen receptors and induces transcription activity in estrogen-responsive cells (6180).

Adverse Reactions Including Known Allergies

Oral ingestion of large amounts of wild yam tincture has caused emesis (12).

Possible Interactions with Herbs & Other Dietary Supplements

Insufficient reliable information is available.

Possible Interactions with Drugs

No interactions are known to occur, and there is no known reason to expect a clinically significant interaction with wild yam.

Possible Interactions with Foods

No interactions are known to occur, and there is no known reason to expect a clinically significant interaction with wild yam.

© Copyright 2000, Natural Medicines Comprehensive Database (209) 472-2244. For updated data, go to www.NaturalDatabase.com

Possible Interactions with Lab Tests

No interactions are known to occur, and there is no known reason to expect a clinically significant interaction with wild yam.

Possible Interactions with Diseases or Conditions

No interactions are known to occur, and there is no known reason to expect a clinically significant interaction with wild yam.

Typical Dosages & Routes of Administration that are Commonly Used

No typical dosage.

Comments

Diosogen, a component of wild yam, is promoted as a natural precursor to dehydroepiandrosterone (DHEA) to increase athletic performance and slow the aging process. Although diosogen can be converted to steroidal compounds in the laboratory, this chemical synthesis does not occur in the human body (515).

WILLARD WATER

This Product is Also Known As

Biowater, Carbonaceous Activated Water, Catalyst Altered Water, Williard's Water.

Scientific Names

None.

People Use This For

Orally, Willard water is used for arthritis, acne, anxiety, nervous stomach, hypertension, ulcers, and hair growth. In manufacturing, it has been used as a food preserver, laundry aid, and a treatment for bovine and feline leukemia (6).

Safety

There is insufficient reliable information available about the safety of Willard water.
Pregnancy and Lactation: Insufficient reliable information available; avoid using.

Effectiveness

There is insufficient reliable information available about the effectiveness of Willard water.

Possible Mechanism of Action & Active Ingredients

The formula for Willard water has changed over time. Some of the ingredients found in products analyzed by the FDA included rock salt in various combinations, lignite, sodium metasilicate, sulfated castor oil, calcium chloride, and magnesium sulfate (18).

Adverse Reactions Including Known Allergies

None reported.

Possible Interactions with Herbs & Other Dietary Supplements

Insufficient reliable information available.

Possible Interactions with Drugs

No interactions are known to occur, and there is no known reason to expect a clinically significant interaction with Willard water.

Possible Interactions with Foods

No interactions are known to occur, and there is no known reason to expect a clinically significant interaction with Willard water

Possible Interactions with Lab Tests

No interactions are known to occur, and there is no known reason to expect a clinically significant interaction with Willard water.

Possible Interactions with Diseases or Conditions

No interactions are known to occur, and there is no known reason to expect a clinically significant interaction with Willard water.

Typical Dosages & Routes of Administration that are Commonly Used

No typical dosage.

Comments

Willard water was developed in the early twentieth century at the South Dakota School of Mines by a chemistry professor named John Wesley Willard, Ph.D. It was developed and patented as an industrial cleanser to clean and degrease train parts. However, it became legendary among townsfolk who used Williard water to treat almost every disease known to humans and animals, and as a plant fertilizer. It is not recognized as safe or effective by the FDA (6).

WILLOW BARK

This Product is Also Known As
Basket Willow, Bay Willow, Brittle Willow, Crack Willow, Daphne Willow, Knackweide, Laurel Willow, Lorbeerweide, Osier Rouge, Purple Osier, Purple Osier Willow, Pupurweide, Reifweide, Salicis cortex, Silberweide, Violet Willow, Weidenrinde, White Willow.

Scientific Names
Salix alba; Salix daphnoides; Salix fragilis; Salix pentandra; Salix purpurea; other Salix species. Family: Salicaeae.

People Use This For
Orally, willow bark is used for mild feverish colds and infections, headaches (8), pain (512), pain caused by inflammation (8), muscle and joint aches, influenza, respiratory tract mucous membrane inflammation, gouty arthritis, ankylosing spondylitis, rheumatoid arthritis, and other systemic connective tissue disorders characterized by inflammatory changes (4), and diseases accompanied by fever, and rheumatic ailments (2).
Historically, willow bark has been used for gout and inflammatory joint disease (7).

Safety
POSSIBLY SAFE …when the bark is used orally and appropriately (2,12).
CHILDREN: POSSIBLY UNSAFE …when used orally for viral infections. Although Reyes syndrome has not been reported (12), similarity of constituents of willow bark to aspirin prompt concern (15).
PREGNANCY: Insufficient reliable information available; avoid using. Willow bark contains salicylates (4).
LACTATION: POSSIBLY UNSAFE. …Willow bark contains salicylates which are excreted in breast milk and have been linked to macular rashes in breast-fed infants (4).

Effectiveness
POSSIBLY EFFECTIVE …when used orally for conditions accompanied by fever, rheumatic ailments, and headaches (2), although the effectiveness of specific products depends on the actual salicin content (8,18).
There is insufficient reliable information available about the effectiveness of willow bark for its other uses.

Possible Mechanism of Action & Active Ingredients
Willow constituents include flavonoids, tannins, and salicylates. Most of the information about willow is based on documented pharmacology for salicylates. These actions include anti-inflammatory, antipyretic, dose-dependent hyperglycemic/hypoglycemic, uricosuric/antiuricosuric activities, increase in blood clotting time and plasma-albumin binding (4). Though researchers long believed salicin was the active principle, studies have shown that a series of phenolic glycosides designated salicortin, fragilin, tremulacin, and others are present, some in larger amounts than true salicin (512). These phenolic glycosides are heat labile and they convert to salicin if willow bark is dried (512). Salicin is a prodrug that is metabolized to saligenin in the gastrointestinal tract and to salicylic acid after absorption (4). Because time is required for the prodrugs to convert to salicylic acid, the properties of willow bark have a slower onset and a longer effectiveness than salicylate itself (3). In vitro tests show that salicin and salicortin inhibit cyclooxygenase. This means irreversible inhibition of thrombocytes is unlikely and there should be no increased interaction with blood coagulants (8). The tannins constituents have astringent properties (4). Tannins also show some evidence of antiviral, antimicrobial, non-specific CNS depressant and cariostatic effects (11). Tannins exert an astringent effect on mucosal tissue. This effect dehydrates the tissue, internally reducing secretions, and externally forming a protective layer of harder, constricted cells (12). Plants with at least 10% tannins can cause gastrointestinal disturbances, kidney damage, and necrotic conditions of the liver (12). Some evidence suggests that tannins might cause cancer. Other evidence shows they may prevent it (12). Regular consumption of herbs with high tannin concentrations correlates with increased incidence of esophageal or nasal cancer (12).

Adverse Reactions Including Known Allergies
No adverse reactions are reported from the oral use of willow bark. Theoretically, gastrointestinal disturbances, kidney damage, and necrotic conditions of the liver are possible due to the tannin content (12). Theoretically, adverse reactions associated with salicylates are possible including gastric and renal irritation, hypersensitivity, blood in stool, tinnitus, nausea, and vomiting. Salicin has been associated with skin rashes (4).

Possible Interactions with Herbs & Other Dietary Supplements
SALICYLATE-CONTAINING HERBS: Theoretically, concomitant use may potentiate salicylate effects and adverse effects. Salicylate-containing herbs include aspen bark, black cohosh, poplar, sweet birch, and wintergreen (19).
HERBS WITH ANTICOAGULANT/ANTIPLATELET POTENTIAL: Concomitant use of herbs that have coumarin constituents or affect platelet aggregation could theoretically increase the risk of bleeding in some

people. These herbs include: angelica, anise, arnica, asafoetida, bogbean, boldo, capsicum, celery, chamomile, clove, danshen, fenugreek, feverfew, garlic, ginger, ginkgo, ginseng (Panax), horse chestnut, horseradish, licorice, meadowsweet, prickly ash, onion, papain, passionflower, poplar, quassia, red clover, turmeric, wild carrot, wild lettuce, and others (4,19).

ORAL HERBS: Theoretically, herbs that contain high percentages of tannins such as willow bark might precipitate alkaloids and other alkaline constituents of other herbs.

Possible Interactions with Drugs

ANTICOAGULANTS/ANTIPLATELETS: Theoretically, data suggests irreversible inhibition of thrombocytes is unlikely and there should be no increased interaction with blood coagulants (8).

SALICYLATE INTERACTIONS: There is insufficient reliable information available to determine if enough salicylate is present in willow bark to cause drug interactions common to salicylates or aspirin. Aspirin can impair the effectiveness of beta-adrenergic blockers, probenecid, and sulfinpyrazone. It can increase the effects, side effects, or toxicity of alcohol, anticoagulants, carbonic anhydrase inhibitors, heparin, methotrexate, NSAIDS, sulfonylureas, and valproic acid (151).

ORAL DRUGS: Theoretically, avoid concomitant administration of oral drugs due to potential of willow bark's tannin content to precipitate alkaloids and other basic drugs (19). Separate administration of oral drugs and tannin-containing herbs by the longest period of time practical (19).

Possible Interactions with Foods

No interactions are known to occur, and there is no known reason to expect a clinically significant interaction with willow bark.

Possible Interactions with Lab Tests

There are no lab interactions reported with willow bark. However, due to the variable salicylate content, use caution in interpreting test results known to be affected by salicylates.

Possible Interactions with Diseases or Conditions

SALICYLATE PRECAUTIONS: Avoid or use cautiously in individuals with aspirin hypersensitivity, asthma, active peptic ulcer disease, diabetes, gout, hemophilia, hypoprothrombinemia, kidney or liver disease (4).

KIDNEY OR LIVER DYSFUNCTION: Theoretically, oral use of willow bark is contraindicated in people with kidney or liver dysfunction because it might exacerbate these conditions. Plants with at least 10% tannins are reported to have the potential to cause kidney damage and liver necrosis (12).

Typical Dosages & Routes of Administration that are Commonly Used

ORAL: A typical dose is 1-3 grams dried bark three to four times daily, or one cup tea. To make tea, steep 1-3 grams bark in 150 mL of boiling water for 5 minutes, and strain (4,8). Liquid extract (1:1 in 25% alcohol), 1-3 mL three times daily (4). The average daily dosage equivalent to 60-120 mg total salicin (2), although the effectiveness of this amount is questioned (512).

Comments

Salicylate concentrations vary greatly among Salix species (4,12,512). Salix alba bark is reported to contain 0.49-0.98% salicin (4); Salix purpurea bark contains 3-9%; Salix daphnoides 4.9-5.6%; Salix fragilis 3.9-10.2% (8).

Based on a willow bark content of 7% salicin (superior quality willow bark), 1.5 gallons of willow bark tea per day would have to be consumed to obtain the pain relief of 4.5 grams of aspirin, the average daily dose used to treat arthritic-rheumatic disorders (512).

WINE

This Product is Also Known As

None.
CAUTION: See separate listing for Resveratrol.

Scientific Names

Vitis vinifera.
Family: Vitaceae.

People Use This For

Orally, wine is used for anxiety, achlorhydria, malabsorption syndromes, reducing the risk of heart disease and stroke, and as an appetite stimulant (6).

Topically, wine is used to stimulate wound healing and improve rheumatoid skin ulcerations (6).

Safety

LIKELY SAFE ...when up to two 120 mL drinks are used orally per day (6,14).
POSSIBLY UNSAFE ...when used orally in amounts greater than two 120 mL drinks per day, as larger amounts

can cause minimal to significant adverse effects (6,14).

PREGNANCY: LIKELY UNSAFE ...contraindicated for oral use; alcohol is a teratogen. Use during pregnancy, especially during the first two months after conception, is associated with significant risk of spontaneous abortion, as well as fetal alcohol syndrome, and developmental and behavioral dysfunction in infants and children exposed to alcohol in utero (2264).

LACTATION: LIKELY UNSAFE ...contraindicated for oral use; alcohol is secreted in breast milk. It can cause abnormal psychomotor development, pseudo-Cushing syndrome, alcohol poisoning, and potentiate severe hypoprothrombic bleeding in infants (2264).

Effectiveness

POSSIBLY EFFECTIVE ...when used orally for preventing cardiovascular disease (2058,2060,2261,2267,2268, 2269,2270,2271). The benefit of wine in the prevention of heart disease is controversial. Epidemiological research suggests that people who consume red wine have a lower rate of heart disease. Human studies have yielded mixed results. Different study outcomes might be attributable primarily to differences in study design. Several human studies suggest that alcohol, regardless of the source, is protective against cardiovascular disease in amounts of one drink/day or less (841,2060,2268). However, a recent, well-designed human trial suggests that moderate wine, but not beer, consumption decreases relative mortality from all causes without increased risk from alcohol-related deaths (2058). ...when used orally in moderation for reducing the risk of type 2 diabetes in healthy men (6172). Light to moderate alcohol consumption (2-7 or more drinks per week) is associated with a reduced risk of type 2 diabetes in healthy male physicians. This study investigated alcohol consumed from various sources, including wine (6172). ...when used orally for preventing stroke (2271,2279). ...when used orally for treating anxiety (2265,2266).

POSSIBLY INEFFECTIVE ...when used orally for reducing morbidity and mortality in men with established coronary heart disease (CHD) (6173). Consumption of 1-14 drinks per week has no effect on CHD, cardiovascular disease or all cause mortality compared to drinking less than 1 drink per week. More than 3 drinks per day is associated with increased mortality in men with a history of heart attacks. This study investigated alcohol consumed from various sources, including wine (6173).

There is insufficient reliable information available about the effectiveness of wine for its other uses.

Possible Mechanism of Action & Active Ingredients

Wine is the natural yeast fermentation product of the juice of sun-ripened grapes, the fruit of Vitis vinifera. Wine normally contains 10-14% alcohol, predominantly as ethanol, which is a central nervous system depressant (6,2263). Numerous polyphenolic compounds in red wine exhibit antioxidant properties, including trans-resveratrol, proanthocyanidins, and flavonoids such as quercetin, kaempferol, and catechins (6,1262,2057). The polyphenol content of wine is highly dependent on grape type, climate, and practices used to make the wine (9,2057). Unlike red wines, white wines have very low polyphenol concentrations (2030). Wine is theorized to lower incidence of coronary heart disease by increasing HDL and reducing oxidation of LDL cholesterol (6,1262). New research suggests that polyphenols in red wine do not acutely influence lipoprotein oxidation (1262), but may have benefits with long-term consumption (2059). Several red wine components also exhibit in vitro antiplatelet effects, including trans-resveratrol, quercetin, and catechin (6,2057). Human studies have failed to demonstrate any additional antiplatelet activity of red wine over white wine (2057,2949). Human data also suggest rebound hypercoagulability that can occur when acute or chronic alcohol consumption stops, but that red wine attenuates this effect (2060,2061). Human studies also suggest that red wine reduces mutagenic DNA damage and improves endothelial function when added to a high fat diet, and has additive vasorelaxing benefits with a low-fat, high plant material diet (2059).

Adverse Reactions Including Known Allergies

Adverse reactions to drinking ethanol vary with individuals and the amount ingested. They include flushing, confusion, emotional liability, perceptual and sensation disturbances, possible blackout spells, incoordination, trouble walking, central nervous system depression, seizures, drowsiness, respiratory depression, hypothermia, hypoglycemia, lactic or ketoacidosis, hypokalemia, anemia, thrombocytopenia, nausea, vomiting, diarrhea, abdominal pain and bleeding, arrhythmias, and cancers of the esophagus and liver (14). Chronic ethanol ingestion adverse reactions vary with individuals, including physical dependence, malnutrition, amnesia, dementia, somnolence, cardiac myopathy, hepatotoxicity, pancreatitis, hypomagnesemia, acute and chronic skeletal myopathies, Wernicke's encephalopathy, Korsakoff's psychosis, and chronic cerebellar syndrome (14). Repeated topical use of wine can dry the skin (14). Wine is associated with triggering asthma reactions in people with a history of asthma, possibly due to salicylates and/or added sulfites contained in wines (6174). People who are allergic to sulfites and/or yeast might react to wine (6).

Possible Interactions with Herbs & Other Dietary Supplements

KAVA: Concomitant use with alcohol may cause additive adverse effects (2).

Possible Interactions with Drugs

ASPIRIN/NSAIDs: Concomitant use of aspirin or nonsteroidal anti-inflammatory drugs with alcohol can increase the risk of gastrointestinal bleeding (2262).

BENZODIAZEPINES, BARBITURATES, NARCOTICS: Concomitant consumption of large amounts of alcohol may decrease metabolism of narcotics, barbiturates, and benzodiazepines (15,2262).

CISAPRIDE: Concomitant use of cisapride (Propulsid) might increase blood alcohol levels and effects, due to the alcohol in wine (2262). Red wine increases plasma cisapride concentrations, possibly by reducing metabolism (1383).

CNS DEPRESSANTS: Concomitant use of antihistamines, barbiturates, benzodiazepines, and tricyclic antidepressants with alcohol may increase sedative and other adverse effects (2262).

CYCLOSPORINE: Red wine reduces plasma cyclosporine concentrations, possibly by reducing cyclosporine absorption. In one study, red wine reduced cyclosporine AUC by 36% in caucasian males and 8% in Asian males (1384,1387).

DRUGS THAT CAUSE DISULFIRAM-LIKE REACTIONS: Disulfiram-like reactions can occur when alcohol is used concomitantly with chlorpropamide (Diabinese) (506), disulfiram (Antabuse), tolbutamide (Orinase), metronidazole (Flagyl), sulfonamides, griseofulvin (Fulvicin), cefoperazone (Cefobid), and cefamandole (Mandol) (2262).

ERYTHROMYCIN: Concomitant use with alcohol can increase blood alcohol levels and effect (2262).

H2-RECEPTOR ANTAGONISTS: Concomitant use of cimetidine (Tagamet) and ranitidine (Zantac) with alcohol may increase blood alcohol levels and adverse effects (2262).

HEPATOTOXIC DRUGS: Concomitant use with acetaminophen, isoniazid, and phenylbutazone alcohol can increase the risk of hepatotoxicity (2262).

HYPOGLYCEMIC DRUGS: Alcohol may cause hypoglycemia secondary to decreased gluconeogenesis (2263), and concomitant use may increase the risk of hypoglycemia with long-acting sulfonylureas such as chlorpropamide (Diabinese) (2262).

MONOAMINE OXIDASE INHIBITORS (MAOIs): CAUTION; concomitant use of monoamine oxidase inhibitors with red wine can cause hypertensive crisis due to tyramine content (506).

METFORMIN: Concomitant consumption of large amounts of alcohol may increase the risk of lactic acidosis with metformin (Glucophage) (2262).

PHENYTOIN: Concomitant consumption of large amounts of alcohol may induce metabolism, reducing therapeutic effectiveness of phenytoin (Dilantin) (15,2262).

WARFARIN: Acute alcohol intoxication can decrease metabolism and increase effects of warfarin (Coumadin) (15,2262). In contrast, chronic intoxication can induce metabolism of warfarin, reducing therapeutic effectiveness (15,2262).

Possible Interactions with Foods

FOOD: Concomitant chronic use of alcohol might interfere with absorption of B vitamins and other nutrients (2263).

Possible Interactions with Lab Tests

INCREASE RESULTS: Chronic alcohol ingestion can increase mean corpuscular volume (MCV), triglycerides, alkaline phosphatase (Alk phos), alanine aminotransferase (ALT), aspartate aminotransferase (AST), gamma-glutamyltransferase (GGT), and bilirubin test results (2263).

DECREASE RESULTS: Chronic alcohol ingestion may decrease folate levels and test results (2263).

Possible Interactions with Diseases or Conditions

ASTHMA: Wine is associated with triggering asthma reactions, possibly due to salicylates and/or added sulfites contained in wines (6174).

GOUT: Alcohol ingestion can exacerbate gout (2263).

HEART CONDITIONS: Alcohol use can exacerbate variant angina (14) and congestive heart failure (2261,2263).

HIGH BLOOD PRESSURE: Consuming three or more alcoholic drinks a day can increase blood pressure and exacerbate hypertension (2261).

HYPERTRIGLYCERIDEMIA: Alcohol ingestion can exacerbate hypertriglyceridemia (2261,2263).

INSOMNIA: Alcohol use can exacerbate insomnia (2263).

LIVER DISEASE: Ingesting alcohol can exacerbate liver disease (2261).

PANCREATITIS: Alcohol ingestion can exacerbate pancreatitis (2261).

PEPTIC ULCER DISEASE (PUD)/GASTROESOPHAGEAL REFLUX DISEASE (GERD): Ingesting alcohol can exacerbate peptic ulcer disease and gastroesophageal reflux disease (2261,2263).

PORPHYRIA: Alcohol can exacerbate porphyria (2261).

PSYCHIATRIC DISORDERS: Consuming three or more drinks of alcohol a day can also exacerbate psychiatric disorders and increase cognitive impairment (2261).

Typical Dosages & Routes of Administration that are Commonly Used

ORAL: For reducing risk of cardiovascular disease and stroke, 1-2 glasses (120-240 mL) of wine per day (2261).

Comments

A recent report disputes the "French paradox" and suggests that reduced risk of heart disease in the French population is not due to red wine consumption, but due to the traditional French diet, which is low in animal fat (835).

WINTER CHERRY

This Product is Also Known As
Cape Gooseberry, Coqueret, Strawberry Tomato.
CAUTION: See separate listing for Withania.

Scientific Names
Physalis alkekengi.
Family: Solanaceae.

People Use This For
Orally, winter cherry is used for arthritis, gout, and as a diuretic in kidney and bladder conditions [18].

Safety
There is insufficient reliable information available about the safety of winter cherry.
Pregnancy and Lactation: Insufficient reliable information available; avoid using.

Effectiveness
There is insufficient reliable information available about the effectiveness of winter cherry.

Possible Mechanism of Action & Active Ingredients
The applicable part of winter cherry is the ripe fruit. There is insufficient reliable information available about the possible mechanism of action and active ingredients.

Adverse Reactions Including Known Allergies
The unripe fruit has caused poisoning in animals [18].

Possible Interactions with Herbs & Other Dietary Supplements
Insufficient reliable information available.

Possible Interactions with Drugs
No interactions are known to occur, and there is no known reason to expect a clinically significant interaction with winter cherry.

Possible Interactions with Foods
No interactions are known to occur, and there is no known reason to expect a clinically significant interaction with winter cherry.

Possible Interactions with Lab Tests
No interactions are known to occur, and there is no known reason to expect a clinically significant interaction with winter cherry.

Possible Interactions with Diseases or Conditions
No interactions are known to occur, and there is no known reason to expect a clinically significant interaction with winter cherry.

Typical Dosages & Routes of Administration that are Commonly Used
ORAL: Winter cherry is used either in ground form or as an extract [18].

Comments
Avoid confusing this product with withania, which is also known as winter cherry. There is very little scientific information about this product. Our staff is continually analyzing the available information on natural medicines and will add data here as it becomes available.

WINTER SAVORY

This Product is Also Known As
Savory.
CAUTION: See separate listing for Summer Savory.

Scientific Names
Satureja montana, synonyms Satureja obovata, Calamintha montana.
Family: Labiatae or Lamiaceae.

People Use This For
Orally, winter savory is used for intestinal disorders including cramps, indigestion, diarrhea, nausea, flatulence [11], sore throat, as a tonic, and as an expectorant.

In folk medicine, winter savory was used to decrease libido (5).
In manufacturing, the oleoresin of winter savory oil is used as a flavoring agent (11).

Safety
LIKELY SAFE …when used appropriately as food. Maximum level used in food is 0.013 % for winter savory oleoresin (11).
There is insufficient reliable information available about the safety of the medicinal use of winter savory.
PREGNANCY AND LACTATION: Insufficient reliable information available; avoid using.

Effectiveness
There is insufficient reliable information available about the effectiveness of winter savory.

Possible Mechanism of Action & Active Ingredients
The applicable parts of winter savory are the leaf and stem. Winter savory contains flavonoids (11), ursolic and oleanolic acids, and 1.6% volatile oil. Constituents of the volatile oil include carvacrol, p-cymene, and thymol (6,11). Some evidence suggests the flavonoid, eriodictyol, might have a vasodilator effect (4124). Other information indicates carvacrol, found in both savories, might have diuretic effects (6,11).

Adverse Reactions Including Known Allergies
None reported.

Possible Interactions with Herbs & Other Dietary Supplements
Insufficient reliable information available.

Possible Interactions with Drugs
No interactions are known to occur, and there is no known reason to expect a clinically significant interaction with winter savory.

Possible Interactions with Foods
No interactions are known to occur, and there is no known reason to expect a clinically significant interaction with winter savory.

Possible Interactions with Lab Tests
No interactions are known to occur, and there is no known reason to expect a clinically significant interaction with winter savory.

Possible Interactions with Diseases or Conditions
No interactions are known to occur, and there is no known reason to expect a clinically significant interaction with winter savory.

Typical Dosages & Routes of Administration that are Commonly Used
No typical dosage.

Comments
Although summer savory and winter savory are both used as spices, in the United States summer savory is the most common (6).

WINTER'S BARK

This Product is Also Known As
Pepper Bark, Wintera, Wintera Aromatica, Winters Bark, Winters Cinnamon, Winter's Cinnamon.

Scientific Names
Drimys winteri.

People Use This For
Orally, winter's bark is used for digestive disorders, flatulence, colic, and stomach ache (18).
Topically, it is used for toothaches, and dermatitis (18).

Safety
There is insufficient reliable information available about the safety of winter's bark.
Pregnancy and Lactation: Insufficient reliable information available; avoid using.

Effectiveness
There is insufficient reliable information available about the effectiveness of winter's bark.

Possible Mechanism of Action & Active Ingredients
Winter's bark contains sesquiterpenes and volatile oils (eugenol, caryophyllene, 1,8-cineole, and pines), which have carminative, stomachic, and tonic properties (18).

Adverse Reactions Including Known Allergies

None reported.

Possible Interactions with Herbs & Other Dietary Supplements

Insufficient reliable information available.

Possible Interactions with Drugs

No interactions are known to occur, and there is no known reason to expect a clinically significant interaction with winter's bark.

Possible Interactions with Foods

No interactions are known to occur, and there is no known reason to expect a clinically significant interaction with winter's bark.

Possible Interactions with Lab Tests

No interactions are known to occur, and there is no known reason to expect a clinically significant interaction with winter's bark.

Possible Interactions with Diseases or Conditions

No interactions are known to occur, and there is no known reason to expect a clinically significant interaction with winter's bark.

Typical Dosages & Routes of Administration that are Commonly Used

ORAL: People typically use 30 grains (1950 mg) of the powdered bark (5267).

Comments

There is very little scientific information about this product. Our staff is continually analyzing the available information on natural medicines and will add data here as it becomes available.

WINTERGREEN leaf

This Product is Also Known As

Boxberry, Canada Tea, Checkerberry, Deerberry, Ground Berry, Hilberry, Mountain Tea, Partridge Berry, Spiceberry, Teaberry, Wax Cluster.
CAUTION: See separate listing for Wintergreen oil.

Scientific Names

Gaultheria procumbens.
Family: Ericaceae.

People Use This For

In folk medicine, wintergreen leaf has been used orally for headache, stomachache, flatulence, fever, kidney disorders (11), asthma (18), neuralgia (particularly sciatica), pleurisy (and pain associated with), ovarian pain, inflammation of the testis, epididymis, or diaphragm; gouty arthritis, and dysmenorrhea (18). Topically, wintergreen leaf has been used as a wash for rheumatism, sore muscles, and lumbago (11).
In manufacturing, wintergreen leaf is used as a flavoring agent in food, candies (6), teas (11) and pharmaceutical products (3800).

Safety

LIKELY SAFE ...when used orally and appropriately in medicinal amounts (12). ...when consumed as a flavoring agent in amounts found in foods (12).
CHILDREN: POSSIBLY UNSAFE ...potentially toxic to small children (19).
PREGNANCY: Insufficient reliable information; avoid amounts greater than those found in foods.
LACTATION: POSSIBLY UNSAFE ...potentially toxic to infants (19).

Effectiveness

There is insufficient reliable information available about the effectiveness of wintergreen leaf.

Possible Mechanism of Action & Active Ingredients

When freshly harvested, the plant contains gaultherin that changes into methyl salicylate as the plant is dried (18). The leaves contain 0.5-0.8% wintergreen oil (6).

Adverse Reactions Including Known Allergies

Topical use can cause contact dermatitis due to the essential oils (18). Symptoms of toxicity (salicylism) include tinnitus, nausea, vomiting (6), diarrhea, headache, stomach pain, and confusion (3805).

Possible Interactions with Herbs & Other Dietary Supplements

Insufficient reliable information available.

© Copyright 2000, Natural Medicines Comprehensive Database (209) 472-2244. For updated data, go to www.NaturalDatabase.com

Possible Interactions with Drugs

No interactions are known to occur, and there is no known reason to expect a clinically significant interaction with wintergreen leaf.

Possible Interactions with Foods

No interactions are known to occur, and there is no known reason to expect a clinically significant interaction with wintergreen leaf.

Possible Interactions with Lab Tests

No interactions are known to occur, and there is no known reason to expect a clinically significant interaction with wintergreen leaf.

Possible Interactions with Diseases or Conditions

GI CONDITIONS: Contraindicated; may aggravate gastrointestinal irritation or inflammation (19).

Typical Dosages & Routes of Administration that are Commonly Used

ORAL: People typically prepare wintergreen leaf as a tea with 1 teaspoon of the dried leaves added to 1 cup boiling water. The tea is taken cold, 1 cup per day (5253,5254).

Comments

None.

WINTERGREEN oil

This Product is Also Known As

Boxberry, Canada Tea, Checkerberry, Deerberry, Gaultheria Oil, Ground Berry, Hilberry, Mountain Tea, Partridge Berry, Spiceberry, Teaberry, Wax Cluster.
CAUTION: See separate listing for Wintergreen leaf.

Scientific Names

Gaultheria procumbens.
Family: Ericaceae.

People Use This For

Orally, small doses of wintergreen oil have been used to stimulate gastric secretion and aid digestion (6).
Topically, wintergreen oil is used as a counterirritant (272), for musculoskeletal pain, and as an antiseptic (3800).
In manufacturing, the oil is used as a flavoring agent in food, candies (6), teas (11), and in pharmaceutical products (3800).

Safety

LIKELY SAFE ...when consumed as a flavoring agent in amounts commonly found in foods (12). The maximum level of methyl salicylate is 0.04% in candy flavoring (6). ...when used topically and appropriately (272).
LIKELY UNSAFE ...when taken orally as a medicinal, unless the methyl salicylate content is highly diluted (6,272).
CHILDREN: LIKELY UNSAFE ...when used orally. 4-10 mL can be lethal (159). ...when used topically in children less than 2 years old (272). Children can be poisoned by ingesting topical liniment. 1 teaspoon of topical liniment contains 7 grams salicylates or approximately 22 adult aspirin tablets (159). Child-resistant containers are required for topical liquid preparations containing more than 5% methyl salicylate (6,272).
PREGNANCY: LIKELY SAFE ...when used in amounts commonly found in foods. There is insufficient reliable information available about the safety of wintergreen oil in large amounts; avoid amounts greater than found in foods.
LACTATION: LIKELY UNSAFE ...when used orally. It might be toxic to nursing infants (19).

Effectiveness

LIKELY EFFECTIVE ...when used as a counterirritant in adults and children older than 2 years of age, according to an FDA Advisory Panel (272).
There is insufficient reliable information available about the effectiveness of wintergreen oil for its other uses.

Possible Mechanism of Action & Active Ingredients

Wintergreen oil contains 98% methyl salicylate (6). It has antipyretic, anti-inflammatory, and analgesic properties (11), possibly due to its counterirritant effect (6).

Adverse Reactions Including Known Allergies

When used topically, contact dermatitis can occur due to the essential oils (18). Other symptoms of toxicity (salicylism) include tinnitus, nausea, vomiting (6), diarrhea, headache, stomach pain, and confusion (3805).
When applied topically and covered with an occlusive dressing, 12-20% of methyl salicylate was absorbed systemically over ten hours (272).

Possible Interactions with Herbs & Other Dietary Supplements

Insufficient reliable information available.

Possible Interactions with Drugs

WARFARIN: Concomitant use of topical wintergreen oil-containing products and warfarin can increase INR and bleeding risk due to systemic absorption of the methyl salicylate contained in wintergreen oil (3811,6181). Topical analgesic gels, lotions, creams, ointments, liniments, and sprays can contain up to 55% methyl salicylate (6181).
ASPIRIN: Topical use of wintergreen oil in large amounts, with occlusive dressings, or for prolonged periods of time, can cause additive salicylate toxicity (159,272).

Possible Interactions with Foods

No interactions are known to occur, and there is no known reason to expect a clinically significant interaction with wintergreen oil.

Possible Interactions with Lab Tests

No interactions are known to occur, and there is no known reason to expect a clinically significant interaction with wintergreen oil.

Possible Interactions with Diseases or Conditions

GASTROINTESTINAL INFLAMMATION: Oral use is contraindicated because it can aggravate inflammation (19).
SALICYLATE ALLERGY/ASTHMA: Individuals with salicylate allergy, asthma, or nasal polyps should use cautiously due to its potential for allergic reaction (272).

Typical Dosages & Routes of Administration that are Commonly Used

TOPICAL: Apply as gels, lotion, ointments, or liniments (containing 10-60% methyl salicylate) 3-4 times daily (3). Heat can increase skin absorption; do not apply after strenuous exercise or use a heating pad after application (3).

Comments

Wintergreen oil is obtained by steam distillation of warmed, water-macerated leaves.

WITCH HAZEL

This Product is Also Known As

Hamamelis, Hazel, Snapping Tobacco Wood, Spotted Elder, Winter Bloom, Witchazel.

Scientific Names

Hamamelis virginiana.
Family: Hamamelidaceae.

People Use This For

Orally, witch hazel is used for diarrhea, mucus colitis, vomiting blood, coughing up blood (4,6), tuberculosis, colds, and fevers (6).
Topically, witch hazel is used for itching, skin inflammation, eye inflammation (6), skin injury, mucus membrane inflammation, varicose veins (2), hemorrhoids, and bruises (4).
Rectally, witch hazel is used as an enema for bleeding "piles" (6).
Traditionally, witch hazel is used orally for tumors (6) and cancer (11). Traditionally, witch hazel is used topically for insect bites, minor burns and other skin irritations (11).
In manufacturing, witch hazel leaf extract, bark extract, and witch hazel water are used as astringents and hemostatics in preparations for insect bites, stings, teething (13), hemorrhoids, itching, irritations, and minor pain (11).

Safety

LIKELY SAFE ...when witch hazel water is used externally and appropriately (6,272).
POSSIBLY SAFE ...when leaf or bark is used orally and appropriately (2,12). In high doses, tannins in bark can cause liver damage (8). The volatile oil contains safrole, a known carcinogen, but in amounts too small for concern (4).
PREGNANCY AND LACTATION: Insufficient reliable information available; avoid using.

Effectiveness

LIKELY EFFECTIVE ...when witch hazel water is used topically for temporary relief of itching, discomfort, irritation, and burning associated with anorectal disorders (272).
POSSIBLY EFFECTIVE ...when bark, leaf or witch hazel water is used for treating mild skin injury, local skin and mucous membrane inflammation, varicose veins (2), or as a styptic (7,8).
There is insufficient reliable information available about the effectiveness of witch hazel for its other uses.

Possible Mechanism of Action & Active Ingredients

The applicable parts of witch hazel are the leaf and bark. Witch hazel leaf and bark possess astringent, styptic, and anti-inflammatory properties (4). Researchers attribute astringent and hemostatic properties to the tannin constituents (4). The leaf contains 8-10% tannins (512). The bark contains up to 12% tannins (7). Tannins, applied topically to broken skin or mucous membranes induce protein precipitation. They tighten up superficial cell layers and shrink colloidal structures thereby causing capillaries to constrict. The decrease in vascular permeability approximates an anti-inflammatory effect. The astringent activity of tannins also causes an indirect antibacterial effect (7). Tannins are not without adverse effects. Plants with at least 10% tannins can cause gastrointestinal disturbances, kidney damage, and necrotic conditions of the liver (12). Some evidences suggests that tannins might cause cancer. Other evidence shows tannins may prevent it (12). Regular consumption of herbs with high tannin concentrations correlates with increased incidence of esophageal or nasal cancer (12). Steam distillation used for producing Hamamelis water removes the tannins (13). Thus, the astringent properties of Hamamelis water result from its 14-15% alcohol content (13).

Adverse Reactions Including Known Allergies

Oral use of witch hazel might infrequently cause stomach irritation. Rarely, it might cause liver damage (8). Because of the tannins, ingestion of 1 gram witch hazel can cause nausea, vomiting, and possibly impactions (6). Topical use can cause contact dermatitis (6).

Possible Interactions with Herbs & Other Dietary Supplements

Insufficient reliable information is available.

Possible Interactions with Drugs

No interactions are known to occur, and there is no known reason to expect a clinically significant interaction with witch hazel.

Possible Interactions with Foods

No interactions are known to occur, and there is no known reason to expect a clinically significant interaction with witch hazel.

Possible Interactions with Lab Tests

No interactions are known to occur, and there is no known reason to expect a clinically significant interaction with witch hazel.

Possible Interactions with Diseases or Conditions

No interactions are known to occur, and there is no known reason to expect a clinically significant interaction with witch hazel.

Typical Dosages & Routes of Administration that are Commonly Used

ORAL: A typical dose is 2 grams of dried leaves three times daily or as tea. To make tea, steep 2 grams in 150 mL of boiling water for 5-10 minutes, and strain (4). Hamamelis Liquid Extract (1:1 in 45% alcohol), 2-4 mL three times daily (4).
TOPICAL: For compresses and irrigations, simmer 5-10 grams leaf and bark per 250 mL of water (2). For poultice, use witch hazel water (Hamamelis water) undiluted or diluted 1:3 with water. Semi-solid preparations 20-30% (2). Extracts, semi solid and liquid preparations corresponding to 5-10% leaf and bark (2).
RECTAL: Suppositories, corresponding to 0.1-1 grams leaf and bark applied 1-3 times daily (2). Anorectal disorders, Hamamelis water applied externally up to six times a day or after each bowel movement (272).

Comments

Witch hazel water (Hamamelis water, distilled witch hazel extract) is distilled from dried leaves, bark and partially dormant twigs of Hamamelis virginiana (11).

WITHANIA

This Product is Also Known As

Ashwaganda, Ashwagandha, Aswagandha, Avarada, Indian Ginseng, Turangi-Ghanda, Winter Cherry.
CAUTION: See separate listings for Ginseng American, Blue Cohosh, Canaigre, Codonopsis, Ginseng Siberian, Ginseng Panax, and Winter Cherry.

Scientific Names

Withania somnifera; Withania coagulans.
Family: Solanaceae.

People Use This For

Orally, withania root and berries have been used for tumors, tuberculosis (6), and chronic liver complications (6). The root is used orally as a tonic (3), and the berries have been used orally as an emetic (6).

Topically, the plant has been used for treating swelling and ulcerations (6).

In Ayurvedic, Indian, and Unani medicine, withania is used to "balance life forces" (6), and for its anti-stress, immunomodulatory, cognition-facilitating, anti-inflammatory and anti-aging effects (4116).

Safety

There is insufficient reliable information available about the safety of withania.

PREGNANCY: LIKELY UNSAFE ...abortifacient (12,19).

LACTATION: Insufficient reliable information available; avoid using.

Effectiveness

There is insufficient reliable information available about the effectiveness of withania.

Possible Mechanism of Action & Active Ingredients

The applicable parts of withania are the root and berry. Withania contains withanolides (6,18,4116), the essential oil known as ipuranol, and withaniol (6). Although it is reputed to have sedative, diuretic, and anti-inflammatory activity, animal studies do not support its use as a diuretic (6). Some studies suggest withania may have antistressor (6,4113,4116) and antioxidant (4116) effects. A total extract of the fruit shows evidence of CNS depression, blood pressure reduction, respiratory stimulation, and smooth muscle relaxation (6). An alcoholic extract exhibits anti-inflammatory effects (6) and preliminary studies suggest it might reduce cyclophosphamide-induced leukopenia (4114). The constituents withaferin-A and withanolide-D show evidence of significant immunosuppressant properties (6).

Adverse Reactions Including Known Allergies

None reported.

Possible Interactions with Herbs & Other Dietary Supplements

HERBS WITH SEDATIVE PROPERTIES: Theoretically, concomitant use with herbs that have sedative properties might enhance therapeutic and adverse effects. These include calamus, calendula, California poppy, catnip, capsicum, celery, couch grass, elecampane, Siberian ginseng, German chamomile, goldenseal, gotu kola, hops, Jamaican dogwood, kava, lemon balm, sage, St. John's wort, sassafras, scullcap, shepherd's purse, stinging nettle, valerian, wild carrot, wild lettuce, and yerba mansa (4,19).

Possible Interactions with Drugs

AMPHETAMINE: Theoretically, concomitant use of withania extracts might increase the effects of amphetamine which can be lethal (6).

BARBITURATES, AND OTHER SEDATIVES AND ANXIOLYTICS: Theoretically, withania's sedative effect can potentiate the effects of barbiturates, other sedatives, and anxiolytics (19).

Possible Interactions with Foods

No interactions are known to occur, and there is no known reason to expect a clinically significant interaction with withania.

Possible Interactions with Lab Tests

No interactions are known to occur, and there is no known reason to expect a clinically significant interaction with withania.

Possible Interactions with Diseases or Conditions

No interactions are known to occur, and there is no known reason to expect a clinically significant interaction with withania.

Typical Dosages & Routes of Administration that are Commonly Used

ORAL: People typically use 1 to 2 grams of the whole herb, taken each day in capsule or tea form. The tea is prepared by boiling withania roots in water for 15 minutes and cooled. The usual dose is 3 cups daily. Tincture or fluid extracts are dosed 2 to 4 mL 3 times per day (6006).

Comments

In Ayurvedic, Indian, and Unani medicine, withania is described as "Indian ginseng" (6). Avoid confusing withania with Physalis alkekengi, also known as winter cherry.

WOOD ANEMONE

This Product is Also Known As

Crowfoot, Smell Fox, Wind Flower.

Scientific Names

Anemone nemorosa.

Family: Ranunculaceae.

People Use This For

In Russian folk medicine, the aerial parts of wood anemone are used orally for stomach pains, delayed menstruation, gout, whooping cough, and asthma (18).

Safety

LIKELY UNSAFE ...when the fresh plant is used orally. Freshly harvested wood anemone can cause severe irritation to the gastrointestinal tract. Ingesting 30 freshly harvested plants is believed to be fatal (18).
There is insufficient reliable information available about the safety of the dried, cut above ground parts.
PREGNANCY AND LACTATION: LIKELY UNSAFE ...when the fresh plant is used orally or topically (18).
There is insufficient reliable information available about the safety of the oral or topical use of the dried, cut plant during pregnancy and lactation.

Effectiveness

There is insufficient reliable information available about the effectiveness of wood anemone.

Possible Mechanism of Action & Active Ingredients

The applicable parts of wood anemone are the above ground parts. When the fresh plant is crushed or cut into small pieces, the glycoside ranunculin is enzymatically changed into a severely irritating protoanemonin, which, in turn, rapidly degrades into the less toxic anemonin (18). Both protoanemonin and ranunculin are destroyed to an unknown extent during the drying process (2).

Adverse Reactions Including Known Allergies

Ingestion of freshly harvested wood anemone can cause colic, diarrhea, and severe irritation to the gastrointestinal tract and the urinary drainage passages (18). After prolonged skin contact, wood anemone can cause slow healing blisters and burns (18).

Possible Interactions with Herbs & Other Dietary Supplements

Insufficient reliable information is available.

Possible Interactions with Drugs

No interactions are known to occur, and there is no known reason to expect a clinically significant interaction with wood anemone.

Possible Interactions with Foods

No interactions are known to occur, and there is no known reason to expect a clinically significant interaction with wood anemone.

Possible Interactions with Lab Tests

No interactions are known to occur, and there is no known reason to expect a clinically significant interaction with wood anemone.

Possible Interactions with Diseases or Conditions

No interactions are known to occur, and there is no known reason to expect a clinically significant interaction with wood anemone.

Typical Dosages & Routes of Administration that are Commonly Used

No typical dosage.

Comments

Avoid confusion with the poisonous plant, pasque flower (Pulsatilla pratensis). Although the two plants are from the same botanical family and have similar pharmacological compounds, they are not synonymous (2,18).

WOOD SAGE

This Product is Also Known As

Ambroise, Garlic Sage, Hind Heal, Large-Leaved Germander.
CAUTION: See separate listing for Sage.

Scientific Names

Teucrium scorodonia.
Family: Lamiaceae.

People Use This For

Orally, wood sage is used for gastrointestinal tract disorders, tuberculosis, mucous membrane inflammation of the bronchi and nose, throat spasms, hypertension, healing wounds, and liver disorders (18).

Safety

There is insufficient reliable information available about the safety of wood sage.
Pregnancy and Lactation: Insufficient reliable information is available; avoid using.

Effectiveness

There is insufficient reliable information available about the effectiveness of wood sage.

Possible Mechanism of Action & Active Ingredients

The applicable parts of wood sage are the above ground parts. Wood sage is thought to have spasmolytic and expectorant properties (18). It contains flavonoids, a volatile oil, diterpenes, and iridoide monoterpenes (18).

Adverse Reactions Including Known Allergies

None reported.

Possible Interactions with Herbs & Other Dietary Supplements

There is insufficient reliable information available.

Possible Interactions with Drugs

No interactions are known to occur, and there is no known reason to expect a clinically significant interaction with wood sage.

Possible Interactions with Foods

No interactions are known to occur, and there is no known reason to expect a clinically significant interaction with wood sage.

Possible Interactions with Lab Tests

No interactions are known to occur, and there is no known reason to expect a clinically significant interaction with wood sage.

Possible Interactions with Diseases or Conditions

No interactions are known to occur, and there is no known reason to expect a clinically significant interaction with wood sage.

Typical Dosages & Routes of Administration that are Commonly Used

ORAL: A typical dose for bronchitis is one cup of tea. To make tea, steep 2 teaspoons of dried herb in 150 mL water for 10-15 minutes, and strain.

Comments

Wood sage smells faintly of leeks when being dried. In most countries, wood sage is obsolete as a drug (18).

WOOD SORREL

This Product is Also Known As

Common Sorrel, Cuckoo Bread, Cuckowes Meat, Fairy Bells, Green Sauce, Hallelujah, Mountain Sorrel, Shamrock, Sour Trefoil, Stickwort, Stubwort, Surelle, Three-Leaved Grass, White Sorrel, Wood Sour.

Scientific Names

Oxalis acetosella.
Family: Oxalidaceae.

People Use This For

Orally, wood sorrel is used for liver and digestive disorders.
Historically, it was used to treat scurvy, wounds, and inflammation of the gums (18).

Safety

POSSIBLY UNSAFE …when the flowering plant is used orally, particularly in large amounts.
CHILDREN: POSSIBLY UNSAFE …when used orally. One four-year old child died after consuming rhubarb leaves, which is also a source of oxalic acid (17).
PREGNANCY: LIKELY UNSAFE …when used orally. Contraindicated because it might stimulate menses (19).
LACTATION: POSSIBLY UNSAFE; avoid using.

Effectiveness

There is insufficient reliable information available about the effectiveness of wood sorrel.

Possible Mechanism of Action & Active Ingredients

The applicable part of wood sorrel is the whole flowering plant. It contains 0.3-1.25% oxalic acid (18). Oxalate content is high in fresh leaves and roots (17,19). Once absorbed, the oxalic acid reacts with calcium in plasma and resulting insoluble calcium oxalate may precipitate in the kidneys, blood vessels, heart, lungs, and liver. This may also cause hypocalcemia (12,17). Oxalate crystals damage mucosal tissue, resulting in severe irritation and possible damage. The systemic absorption of oxalates may result in kidney damage, both in people with pre-existing kidney disease and in healthy kidneys (19).

Adverse Reactions Including Known Allergies

Consuming excessive amounts of wood sorrel can cause diarrhea, nausea, polyuria (6), dermatitis (4) and gastrointestinal symptoms due to its oxalic acid content. Oxalic acid poisoning affects skin, eyes, respiratory system and kidneys. Oral symptoms of oxalate irritation include swelling of the mouth, tongue and throat, with difficulty in speaking and suffocation. It has a corrosive effect on the digestive tract. It can lead to oxalic acid crystals in the kidneys, blood vessels, heart, lungs, liver, and/or hypocalcemia (17).

Possible Interactions with Herbs & Other Dietary Supplements

Insufficient reliable information available.

Possible Interactions with Drugs

No interactions are known to occur, and there is no known reason to expect a clinically significant interaction with wood sorrel.

Possible Interactions with Foods

No interactions are known to occur, and there is no known reason to expect a clinically significant interaction with wood sorrel.

Possible Interactions with Lab Tests

No interactions are known to occur, and there is no known reason to expect a clinically significant interaction with wood sorrel.

Possible Interactions with Diseases or Conditions

COAGULATION DISORDERS: Oxalate constituents can alter the calcium concentrations and decrease coagulation time (4,12).
GI CONDITIONS: Theoretically can exacerbate stomach and intestinal ulcers due to mucosal irritant effect (19).
KIDNEY DISEASE: Can damage kidneys with formation of insoluble oxalate; use with caution or avoid in individuals with history of kidney stones (12,19).

Typical Dosages & Routes of Administration that are Commonly Used

No typical dosage.

Comments

Wood sorrel is considered possibly unsafe, avoid using (12,19). Wood sorrel is also called common sorrel, and could be confused for sorrel.

WOODBINE

This Product is Also Known As

Clematis, Devil's-Darning-Needle, Old-Man's Beard, Traveler's-Joy, Vine Bower, Virgin's Bower.
CAUTION: See separate listing for Clematis and Traveler's Joy.

Scientific Names

Clematis virginiana.
Family: Rananculaceae.

People Use This For

Historically, woodbine leaf has been used orally for skin sores, cuts, itching, venereal disorders, cancer, tumors, itching, fever, nephrosis, ulcers, diuretic, purgative, tuberculosis, and cervical lymphadenitis (6).

Safety

LIKELY UNSAFE ...when the leaf is used orally or topically because it is a powerful irritant (6).
PREGNANCY AND LACTATION: LIKELY UNSAFE; avoid using.

Effectiveness

There is insufficient reliable information available about the effectiveness of woodbine.

Possible Mechanism of Action & Active Ingredients

The applicable part of woodbine is the leaf. There is insufficient reliable information available about the possible mechanism of action and active ingredients.

Adverse Reactions Including Known Allergies

The juice derived from the woodbine leaf is said to be a powerful local irritant (6).

Possible Interactions with Herbs & Other Dietary Supplements
Insufficient reliable information available.

Possible Interactions with Drugs
No interactions are known to occur, and there is no known reason to expect a clinically significant interaction with woodbine.

Possible Interactions with Foods
No interactions are known to occur, and there is no known reason to expect a clinically significant interaction with woodbine.

Possible Interactions with Lab Tests
No interactions are known to occur, and there is no known reason to expect a clinically significant interaction with woodbine.

Possible Interactions with Diseases or Conditions
No interactions are known to occur, and there is no known reason to expect a clinically significant interaction with woodbine.

Typical Dosages & Routes of Administration that are Commonly Used
ORAL: People typically make a liquid preparation of woodbine, combining one heaping teaspoon of leaves and flowers with one cup of water and allowing the mixture to stand for 30 minutes. The dose is one tablespoon 4 to 6 times daily (5263).

Comments
Avoid confusion with American ivy, gelsemium or honeysuckle, which are also known as woodbine.

WORMSEED

This Product is Also Known As
Levant, Santonica, Sea Wormwood.
CAUTION: See separate listings for Chenopodium oil, Wormwood Oil, Mugwort, and Wormwood.

Scientific Names
Artemisia cina.
Family: Asteraceae.

People Use This For
Orally, wormseed is used for ascaris and oxyuris infestations (18).

Safety
UNSAFE ...when used orally due to its highly toxic adverse effects (18).
PREGNANCY AND LACTATION: UNSAFE ...contraindicated due to potential for toxicity (18).

Effectiveness
There is insufficient reliable information available about the effectiveness of wormseed.

Possible Mechanism of Action & Active Ingredients
The antihelmintic activity is attributed to the sesquiterpene lactone beta-santonin. When wormseed is used with a laxative, it appears to paralyze the muscles of ascarids and facilitate their elimination from the body . Some data suggest wormseed lowers body temperature when a fever is present (18).

Adverse Reactions Including Known Allergies
Death has been reported with less than 10 grams of herb. Symptoms of poisoning are possible in amounts used to treat parasitic infestations. Symptoms may include kidney irritation, gastroenteritis, stupor, visual disorders, muscle twitching, and epileptiform spasms (18). It can cause an allergic reaction in individuals sensitive to the Asteraceae/Compositae family. Members of this family include ragweed, chrysanthemums, marigolds, daisies, and many other herbs.

Possible Interactions with Herbs & Other Dietary Supplements
Insufficient reliable information available.

Possible Interactions with Drugs
No interactions are known to occur, and there is no known reason to expect a clinically significant interaction with wormseed.

Possible Interactions with Foods
No interactions are known to occur, and there is no known reason to expect a clinically significant interaction with wormseed.

Possible Interactions with Lab Tests
No interactions are known to occur, and there is no known reason to expect a clinically significant interaction with wormseed.

Possible Interactions with Diseases or Conditions
CROSS-ALLERGENICITY: Can cause an allergic reaction in individuals sensitive to the Asteraceae/Compositae family. Members of this family include ragweed, chrysanthemums, marigolds, daisies, and many other herbs.

Typical Dosages & Routes of Administration that are Commonly Used
No typical dosage.

Comments
Wormseed is considered unsafe for oral use; avoid using (18). Wormseed is considered obsolete as a medicinal herb. Avoid confusing wormseed with chenopodium oil (or wormseed oil), wormwood oil, or wormwood. Avoid confusing wormseed, also referred to as levant, with levant berry.

WORMWOOD above ground parts

This Product is Also Known As
Absinth, Absinthe, Absinthii Herba, Absinthites, Absinthium, Ajenjo, Armoise, Artesian Absinthium, Common Wormwood, Green Ginger, Herbe d'Absinthe, Wermut, Wermutkraut, Wurmkraut.
CAUTION: See separate listings for Wormwood oil and Mugwort.

Scientific Names
Artemisia absinthium.
Family: Asteraceae or Compositae.

People Use This For
Orally, wormwood is used for loss of appetite, indigestion, biliary dyskinesia (2), and gastrointestinal complaints such as low acidity gastritis (8).
Topically, wormwood is used for healing wounds and insect bites (18).
In combination with other herbs, wormwood is used for indigestion, particularly functional disorders of the gallbladder drainage system, loss of appetite, and discomfort due to fullness and flatulence (2).
Historically, wormwood was used as an antihelmintic, aphrodisiac, tonic (515), antispasmodic (8), and to stimulate sweating.
In manufacturing, wormwood is used for flavoring alcoholic bitters and vermouth (11).

Safety
LIKELY SAFE ...when used orally in the amount found in bitters and vermouth. Approved for food use in the US provided finished products are thujone-free (11). The maximum use level is 0.024% (11).
POSSIBLY SAFE ...when used orally and appropriately short-term (12). Although aqueous extracts or brewed teas are reported to contain the toxic constituent thujone, the amount is low (12).
LIKELY UNSAFE ...when wormwood is used orally long-term or in excessive amounts.
There is insufficient reliable information available about the safety of the topical use of wormwood.
PREGNANCY: UNSAFE ...contraindicated. Thujone has potential uterine and menstrual stimulant effects (12).
LACTATION: Insufficient reliable information available; avoid using.

Effectiveness
POSSIBLY EFFECTIVE ...when used orally for loss of appetite, indigestion, and biliary dyskinesia (2).
There is insufficient reliable information available about the effectiveness of wormwood for its other uses.

Possible Mechanism of Action & Active Ingredients
Wormwood contains bitter principles (absinthin and anabsinthin) and a volatile oil composed of up to 70% thujone (7). In small doses, wormwood acts as an aromatic bitter (7). As the amount ingested increases, the toxic effects of thujone become more pronounced leading to increased salivation and increased blood flow to mucous membranes and pelvic viscera (7). Thujone heightens and alters the effect of alcohol (7). Chronic thujone poisoning leads to seizures, delirium and hallucinations (7). Researchers think thujone has a mind-altering effect similar to tetrahydrocannabinol, the active principle in marijuana (515). Some evidence suggests that thujone exposure might be harmful to individuals with underlying defects in hepatic heme synthesis (12). Thujone also induces synthesis of a rate-controlling enzyme for the 5-aminolevulinic acid synthase pathway. This effect is similar to that of phenobarbital and glutethimide, drugs with known porphyrinogenic activity (12). Thujone shows evidence of antioxidant, antimicrobial and antifungal activity (12).

Adverse Reactions Including Known Allergies

Habitual use of large amounts of wormwood can cause restlessness, insomnia, nightmares, vomiting, stomach and intestinal cramps (8), dizziness, tremors (11,12), urine retention (8), renal damage, and convulsions (11,12). Absinthism, a group of neurological symptoms, is characterized by digestive disorders, thirst, restlessness, vertigo, tremor, numbness of extremities, diminished intellect, delirium, paralysis, and death (17). Skin contact with fresh wormwood can cause contact dermatitis (19). Wormwood can also cause an allergic reaction in people sensitive to the Asteraceae/Compositae family. Members of this family include ragweed, chrysanthemums, marigolds, daisies, and many other herbs.

Possible Interactions with Herbs & Other Dietary Supplements

THUJONE-CONTAINING HERBS: Avoid concomitant use with other herbs that contain thujone to avoid increased risk of thujone toxicity. Thujone-containing herbs include: oak moss, oriental arborvitae, sage, tansy, thuja (cedar), and tree moss (12).

Possible Interactions with Drugs

ACID-INHIBITING DRUGS: Theoretically, due to claims that wormwood increases stomach acid, it might interfere with antacids, sucralfate (Carafate), H-2 antagonists, or proton pump inhibitors (19).
ANTICONVULSANTS: Theoretically, concomitant use might interfere with the effectiveness of anticonvulsant drugs due to wormwood's potential to cause seizures (8,11,12).

Possible Interactions with Foods

No interactions are known to occur, and there is no known reason to expect a clinically significant interaction with wormwood.

Possible Interactions with Lab Tests

No interactions are known to occur, and there is no known reason to expect a clinically significant interaction with wormwood.

Possible Interactions with Diseases or Conditions

ULCERS: Contraindicated in individuals with gastric or duodenal ulcers due to potential for stomach irritation and intestinal tract stimulation (8,19).
CROSS-ALLERGENICITY: Wormwood can cause an allergic reaction in people sensitive to the Asteraceae/Compositae family. Members of this family include ragweed, chrysanthemums, marigolds, daisies, and many other herbs (4).

Typical Dosages & Routes of Administration that are Commonly Used

ORAL: A typical dose is one cup tea before eating as an appetite stimulant or after meals as a bile flow stimulant (8). To make tea, steep 1-1.5 grams (1 teaspoon) finely chopped above ground parts in 150 mL boiling water 10 minutes, and strain. Total daily dose is up to 3 grams per day (2). Do not exceed 1.5 grams above ground parts per dose (8).

Comments

Wormwood is the principal flavor ingredient in absinthe, a 136-proof alcoholic beverage popular at the turn of the century (515). Absinthe is historically associated with addiction, acts of violence (515), damage to the nervous system and mental deterioration (17). Vincent van Gogh's self-amputation of his left ear is attributed to his absinthe addiction (11,515). Absinthe was banned in many countries by 1915, including the US (11).

WORMWOOD oil

This Product is Also Known As

None.
CAUTION: See separate listing for Wormwood above ground parts.

Scientific Names

Artemisia absinthium.
Family: Asteraceae/Compositae.

People Use This For

Topically, wormwood oil is used as a counterirritant (11).
In manufacturing, it is used as a fragrance component in soaps, cosmetics and perfumes and as a flavoring agent in foods (11).

Safety

LIKELY SAFE ...when used topically in amounts found in cosmetics, it is considered nontoxic. The maximum level used is 0.25% in perfumes (11).
POSSIBLY SAFE ...when used orally in very small, thujone-free amounts. Thujone-free wormwood oil is

approved for use in foods in the US (11). The maximum use level for the thujone-free oil is 0.0006% (11).

LIKELY UNSAFE ...when thujone-containing wormwood oil is used orally. One-half ounce of thujone-containing volatile oil can cause convulsions and unconsciousness (17,515).

There is insufficient reliable information available about the safety of wormwood oil when used topically in amounts greater than those found in cosmetics.

PREGNANCY: LIKELY UNSAFE ...contraindicated. Wormwood oil might have uterine and menstrual stimulant effects (12,19) and thujone could be toxic.

LACTATION: LIKELY UNSAFE ...contraindicated. There is concern about the toxic potential of thujone.

Effectiveness

There is insufficient reliable information available about the effectiveness of wormwood oil.

Possible Mechanism of Action & Active Ingredients

The volatile oil of wormwood is considered an active narcotic poison (17). The major constituents of the oil are azulenes (11,515) but it also contains 3-12% thujone (11,515). The azulene constituents have anti-inflammatory and antipyretic activity (11). They also have antibacterial effects against Staphylococcus aureus, the penicillin-resistant strain S. aureus, Klebsiella pneumoniae and Pseudomonas aeruginosa (11). The constituent, thujone is chemically related to camphor (12). As the amount of thujone ingested is increased, the toxic effect becomes pronounced, leading to increased salivation and erythema of the mucous membranes and pelvic viscera. Thujone heightens and alters the effect of alcohol. Researchers think thujone has a mind-altering effect similar to tetrahydrocannabinol, the active constituent marijuana (4). Chronic thujone poisoning leads to epileptic seizures, delirium and hallucinations (7). Some evidence suggests thujone might be harmful to individuals with underlying defects in hepatic heme synthesis. Other evidence suggests thujone induces synthesis of a rate-controlling enzyme for the 5-aminolevulinic acid synthase pathway. Phenobarbital and glutethimide have similar effects, suggesting thujone might have porphyrinogenic activity (12).

Adverse Reactions Including Known Allergies

Ingesting wormwood oil can cause nausea, vomiting, diffuse muscle aches, acute renal toxicity, seizures, rhabdomyolysis and acute renal failure (661,662). Wormwood oil can cause an allergic reaction in people sensitive to the Asteraceae/Compositae family. Members of this family include ragweed, chrysanthemums, marigolds, daisies, and many other herbs.

Possible Interactions with Herbs & Other Dietary Supplements

THUJONE-CONTAINING HERBS: Avoid; concomitant use might increase the risk of thujone toxicity. Thujone-containing herbs include: oak moss, oriental arborvitae, sage, tansy, thuja (cedar), and tree moss (12).

Possible Interactions with Drugs

No interactions are known to occur, and there is no known reason to expect a clinically significant interaction with wormwood oil.

Possible Interactions with Foods

No interactions are known to occur, and there is no known reason to expect a clinically significant interaction with wormwood oil.

Possible Interactions with Lab Tests

No interactions are known to occur, and there is no known reason to expect a clinically significant interaction with wormwood oil.

Possible Interactions with Diseases or Conditions

CROSS-ALLERGENICITY: Can cause an allergic reaction in individuals sensitive to the Asteraceae/Compositae family. Members of this family include ragweed, chrysanthemums, marigolds, daisies, and many other herbs.

Typical Dosages & Routes of Administration that are Commonly Used

No typical dosage.

Comments

Wormwood oil is distilled from leaves and flowers of Artemisia absinthium just before or during flowering. Thujone-containing wormwood oil is highly toxic.

XANTHAN GUM

This Product is Also Known As

Corn Sugar Gum.

Scientific Names

Xanthomonas campestris.

People Use This For

Orally, xanthan gum is used for lowering blood glucose and total plasma cholesterol in people with diabetes (4916). It is also used as a laxative (4917,4918).

Topically, xanthan gum is used as a saliva substitute in people with Sjogren's syndrome (4915).

In manufacturing, xanthan gum is used as a thickening, suspending, emulsifying, and stabilizing agent in foods, toothpastes, and pharmaceutical products (13,16).

Safety

LIKELY SAFE ...when used in amounts found in foods, up to 10 mg/kg per day (4914). Has Generally Recognized as Safe (GRAS) status in the US (4912). ...when used orally for medicinal use in amounts up to 15 grams per day (4914,4916,4917,4918). ...when used topically and appropriately (4914).

PREGNANCY AND LACTATION: Insufficient reliable information is available; avoid in amounts greater than found in foods.

Effectiveness

POSSIBLY EFFECTIVE ...when used orally as a bulk-forming laxative (4917,4918). ...when used for lowering blood glucose and cholesterol in people with diabetes (4916). ...when used topically as a saliva substitute in people with Sjogren's syndrome (4915).

Possible Mechanism of Action & Active Ingredients

Xanthan gum is a bulk-forming laxative. In the body it forms an emollient gel that stimulates peristalsis and passage of intestinal contents (4917,4921). Xanthan gum slows gastric emptying and intestinal absorption of glucose (4916). It mimics saliva as a lubricating and wetting agent in humans (4915), and shows evidence that it might reduce demineralization of tooth enamel (4920). Xanthan gum demonstrates antitumor activity, and shows evidence of synergism with 5-fluorouracil and bleomycin (11).

Adverse Reactions Including Known Allergies

Oral use of xanthan gum can cause flatulence and abdominal distention (4916,4918). Occupational exposure in workers handling xanthan gum powder can cause flu-like symptoms, nose and throat irritation without acute or chronic loss of pulmonary function (4913).

Possible Interactions with Herbs & Other Dietary Supplements

BULK-FORMING LAXATIVE HERBS AND SUPPLEMENTS: Theoretically, concomitant use may increase likelihood of flatulence and abdominal distention.

HERBS THAT CAN CAUSE HYPOGLYCEMIA: Theoretically, concomitant use with pharmacologically active amounts of xanthan gum could result in excessive lowering of blood glucose.

Possible Interactions with Drugs

BULK-FORMING LAXATIVES: Theoretically, concomitant use may increase likelihood of flatulence and abdominal distension.

DRUGS THAT CAN CAUSE HYPOGLYCEMIA: Theoretically, concomitant use with pharmacologically active amounts of xanthan gum could result in excessive lowering of blood glucose.

Possible Interactions with Foods

No interactions are known to occur, and there is no known reason to expect a clinically significant interaction with xanthan gum.

Possible Interactions with Lab Tests

BLOOD GLUCOSE: Might lower blood glucose and test results (4916).
CHOLESTEROL: Might lower serum cholesterol and test results (4916).

Possible Interactions with Diseases or Conditions

CONTRAINDICATIONS: Bulk forming laxative are contraindicated in individuals with nausea, vomiting, or other symptoms of appendicitis, acute surgical abdomen, fecal impaction, intestinal obstruction, or undiagnosed abdominal pain (506,4921).

INTESTINAL STENOSIS: Avoid xanthan gum in amounts greater than found in foods (4921).

Typical Dosages & Routes of Administration that are Commonly Used

ORAL: The World Health Organization (WHO) has set the maximum acceptable intake for xanthan gum as a food additive at 10 mg/kg per day (4914), and as a laxative at 15 grams per day (4918). For safety and effectiveness, bulk laxatives require adequate fluid intake (4921). For diabetes a typical dose is 12 grams per day as an ingredient in muffins (4916).

TOPICAL: Saliva substitutes, 0.018% or 0.092% aqueous solutions with added electrolytes and peppermint flavoring (4915).

Comments

Xanthan gum is a polysaccharide produced by fermenting carbohydrate with the bacterium Xanthomonas campestris (13,16). Xanthan gum is an ingredient in some sustained release matrix tablets (4914).

YARROW

This Product is Also Known As

Achilee, Achillea, Acuilee, Band Man's Plaything, Bauchweh, Birangasifa, Bloodwort, Carpenter's Weed, Civan Percemi, Common Yarrow, Devil's Nettle, Devil's Plaything, Erba Da Cartentieri, Erba Da Falegname, Gemeine Schafgarbe, Green Arrow, Herbe Aux Charpentiers, Katzenkrat, Milefolio, Milfoil, Millefeuille, Millefolii flos, Millefolii herba, Millefolium, Millegoglie, Noble Yarrow, Nosebleed, Old Man's Pepper, Roga Mari, Sanguinary, Soldier's Wound Wort, Staunchweed, Tausendaugbram, Thousand-Leaf, Wound Wort.

Scientific Names

Achillea millefolium.
Family: Asteraceae/Compositae.

People Use This For

Orally, yarrow is used for fever, common cold, amenorrhea, dysentery, diarrhea (4,8), loss of appetite, mild or spastic gastrointestinal tract discomfort (2), inducing sweating (6), and specifically for thrombotic conditions with hypertension, including cerebral and coronary thromboses (4).

Fresh leaves of yarrow are chewed to relieve toothache (6).

Topically, yarrow is used as a styptic (4), for wounds (7), and as a sitz bath for painful, lower pelvic, cramp-like conditions of psychosomatic origin in women (2).

In combination with other herbs, yarrow is used for bloating, flatulence, mild gastrointestinal cramping, and nervous gastrointestinal complaints (7).

In folk medicine, yarrow is used as a styptic for bleeding hemorrhoids (18).

For food uses, the young leaves and flowers of yarrow are used in salads.

In manufacturing, yarrow is also used as a cosmetic cleanser (6) and in snuff (6). Yarrow oil is used in shampoos (6).

Safety

LIKELY SAFE ...when used orally in typical food amounts (11). Approved for use only in alcoholic beverages in the US (11). Finished products must be thujone-free (11), although the volatile oil of yarrow is believe to contain only a trace of thujone (11).

POSSIBLY SAFE ...when used orally and appropriately for medicinal purposes (2,12).

PREGNANCY: LIKELY UNSAFE ...contraindicated for oral use because it is believed to be an abortifacient and affect the menstrual cycle (12).

LACTATION: Insufficient reliable information available; avoid excessive amounts during lactation (4).

Effectiveness

POSSIBLY EFFECTIVE ...when used orally for the loss of appetite and mild indigestion and spastic gastrointestinal discomfort (2). ...when used as a sitz bath for painful, lower pelvic, cramp-like conditions of psychosomatic origin in women (2).

There is insufficient reliable information available about the effectiveness of yarrow for its other uses.

Possible Mechanism of Action & Active Ingredients

The applicable parts of yarrow are the above ground parts. Yarrow has diaphoretic, antipyretic, hypotensive, astringent, diuretic, urinary antiseptic, spasmolytic, and antiflatulent effects (4). Yarrow contains amino acids, fatty acids, ascorbic acid, caffeic acid, folic acid, salicylic acid and succinic acid; alkaloids; flavonoids including rutin; tannins; a volatile oil, an unknown cyanogenetic compound, and sugars (4). The volatile oil contains chamazulene, other azulenes (11), and trace amounts of thujone (4,11) The volatile oil content, and especially the azulene content, varies considerably depending on the source (11). Some evidence suggests that achilleine, an alkaloid constituent, might decrease clotting time (4). The alkaloid fraction has shown evidence of antipyretic and hypotensive effects (4). An aqueous extract shows some evidence of anti-inflammatory and diuretic activity (4). Researchers think that anti-inflammatory and anti-allergy activities are associated with the constituent chamazulene (6). Not all species contain azulene constituents (6). An ethanolic extract shows moderate antibacterial activity against Staphylococcus aureus, Bacillus subtilis, Mycobacterium smegmatis, Escherichia coli, Shigella sonnei, and Shigella flexneri (4). Some evidence suggests that the volatile oil of yarrow might have CNS depressant activity (4).

Adverse Reactions Including Known Allergies

Ingesting large amounts of yarrow might cause sedative and diuretic effects (4,5). Topical use can cause dermatitis (4). It can cause an allergic reaction in individuals sensitive to the Asteraceae/Compositae family. Members of this family include ragweed, chrysanthemums, marigolds, daisies, and many other herbs.

Possible Interactions with Herbs & Other Dietary Supplements

SEDATIVE HERBS: Theoretically, concomitant use might enhance sedative effects of other herbs with sedative properties, including German chamomile, hops, kava, scullcap, and valerian (19).

THUJONE CONTAINING HERBS: Avoid; concomitant use can increase the risk of thujone toxicity. Thujone-containing herbs include: oak moss, oriental arborvitae, sage, tansy, thuja (cedar), tree moss, and wormwood (2,4,11,12).

© Copyright 2000, Natural Medicines Comprehensive Database (209) 472-2244. For updated data, go to www.NaturalDatabase.com • 1133

Possible Interactions with Drugs

ACID-INHIBITING DRUGS: Theoretically, due to claims that yarrow increases stomach acid, it might interfere with antacids, sucralfate (Carafate), H-2 antagonists, or proton pump inhibitors (19).
ANTICOAGULANTS: Theoretically, concomitant use might cause increased effects and adverse effects (4).
BARBITURATES: Theoretically, concomitant use might prolong barbiturate-induced sleep time (4).
HYPERTENSIVE or HYPOTENSIVE DRUG THERAPY: Theoretically, concomitant use might interfere with drug therapy (4).

Possible Interactions with Foods

No interactions are known to occur, and there is no known reason to expect a clinically significant interaction with yarrow.

Possible Interactions with Lab Tests

No interactions are known to occur, and there is no known reason to expect a clinically significant interaction with yarrow.

Possible Interactions with Diseases or Conditions

CROSS-ALLERGENICITY: Can cause an allergic reaction in individuals sensitive to the Asteraceae/Compositae family. Members of this family include ragweed, chrysanthemums, marigolds, daisies, and many other herbs.

Typical Dosages & Routes of Administration that are Commonly Used

ORAL: A typical oral dose is 2-4 grams dried flowerheads or one cup tea three times daily. To make tea, steep 2-4 grams dried flowerhead or 2 grams finely cut above ground parts in 150 mL of boiling water for 10-15 minutes, and strain (4). A daily dose is up to 4.5 grams above ground parts, 3 grams flowerheads, 3 teaspoons pressed juice from fresh plants, or equivalent preparations per day. Liquid extract (1:1 in 25% alcohol), 2-4 mL three times daily (4). Tincture (1:5 in 45% alcohol), 2-4 mL three times daily (4).
TOPICAL: As a sitz bath, add 100 grams above ground parts per 20 L of water (2).

Comments

None.

YELLOW DOCK

This Product is Also Known As

Broad-Leaved Dock, Curled Dock, Curly Dock, Field Sorrel, Narrow Dock, Rumex, Sheep Sorrel, Sorrel, Sour Dock.

Scientific Names

Rumex crispus; Rumex obtusifolius.
Family: Polygonaceae.

People Use This For

Orally, yellow dock is used for acute and chronic inflammation of nasal passages and the respiratory tract, as an adjunct to antibacterial therapy (18), as a laxative (4,5,6), tonic (6), and for treating venereal diseases (5,6).
Yellow dock is used as a dentifrice (6).
Historically, it has been used for chronic skin diseases (4,6,18), dermatitis, rashes (6), scurvy (18), obstructive jaundice, and psoriasis with constipation (4).
For food uses, the leaf stalks are used in salads (6).

Safety

POSSIBLY SAFE ...when consumed in amounts commonly found in foods. Young leaves must be boiled to remove the oxalate content; death has occurred after consuming uncooked leaves (6,18). ...when used orally and appropriately for medical purposes.
PREGNANCY: POSSIBLY UNSAFE; avoid using. Contains anthraquinone glycosides, and unstandardized laxatives are not desirable during pregnancy (4).
LACTATION: POSSIBLY UNSAFE; avoid using. Anthraquinones are secreted into breast milk (4,5).

Effectiveness

LIKELY EFFECTIVE ...when used as a laxative (5,6,12).
LIKELY INEFFECTIVE ...when used for venereal and skin diseases (5,6).
There is insufficient reliable information available about the effectiveness of yellow dock for its other uses.

Possible Mechanism of Action & Active Ingredients

The applicable parts of yellow dock are the root and rhizome. Yellow dock contains anthroquinone glycosides (chrysophanic acid, emodin, physcion), oxalates (oxalic acid and calcium oxalate), and tannins (4,5,6,12). Oxalate content is high in the leaves and low in the stalks (17). The anthroquinones (2-4%) have a mild stimulant laxative effect (4,6,12). Anthroid laxative use is not associated with an increased risk of developing colorectal ademoma or carcinoma (6138). The tannins (12-20%) (12,19) are responsible for the astringent effect (5). Yellow dock is reported to stimulate bile production (4). The leaves of yellow dock contain provitamin A (beta-carotene) and iron (19).

Adverse Reactions Including Known Allergies
Vomiting may occur after ingestion of fresh rhizome (18). Consuming excessive amounts can cause diarrhea, nausea, polyuria (6), or dermatitis (4). Excessive use can cause abdominal cramps, hypokalemia, and intestinal atrophy (4). There is one report of a death, preceded by vomiting, diarrhea, coma, respiratory depression, liver and kidney failure, severe metabolic acidosis, and ventricular fibrillation, after ingestion of 500 g of yellow dock (17). Oxalic acid reacts with calcium in plasma, forming insoluble calcium oxalate, which can cause hypocalcemia; the crystals may precipitate in the kidneys, blood vessels, heart, lungs, and liver. Individuals with a history of kidney stones should use yellow dock cautiously (12). Sensitive people can develop dermatitis after contact with the plant (6). Older or uncooked leaves should be avoided (6).
CROSS-ALLERGENICITY: Can cause allergic reaction in individuals allergic to ragweed (4117).

Possible Interactions with Herbs & Other Dietary Supplements
CARDIAC-GLYCOSIDE-CONTAINING HERBS: Theoretically, concomitant use may increase the risk of cardiac glycoside toxicity because of the presence of stimulant laxatives in yellow dock, which can decrease serum potassium (19).
STIMULANT LAXATIVE HERBS: Theoretically, concomitant use of yellow dock with other stimulant laxative herbs can increase the risk of potassium depletion. Stimulant laxative herbs include aloe dried leaf sap, blue flag rhizome, alder buckthorn, European buckthorn, butternut bark, cascara bark, castor oil, colocynth fruit pulp, gamboge bark exudate, jalap root, black root, manna bark exudate, podophyllum root, rhubarb root, senna leaves and pods, and wild cucumber fruit (19).

Possible Interactions with Drugs
DIGOXIN: Toxic effects due to hypokalemia (4) are possible when yellow dock is used chronically or in large amounts (19).

Possible Interactions with Foods
No interactions are known to occur, and there is no known reason to expect a clinically significant interaction with yellow dock.

Possible Interactions with Lab Tests
COLORIMETRIC TESTS: Yellow dock might discolor urine (pink, red, purple, orange, rust), interfering with diagnostic tests that depend on a color change, due to its anthraquinone content (12,275).
SERUM POTASSIUM: Excessive use of yellow dock might cause potassium depletion, reducing serum potassium concentrations and test results (4,19).

Possible Interactions with Diseases or Conditions
COAGULATION DISORDERS: Oxalate constituents can alter calcium concentrations and decrease coagulation time (4,12).
GI CONDITIONS: Avoid use in individuals with intestinal obstruction (4). Theoretically, yellow dock can exacerbate stomach and intestinal ulcers due to its mucosal irritant effect (19).
KIDNEY DISEASE: Yellow dock can damage kidneys with formation of insoluble oxalate; use with caution or avoid in individuals with a history of kidney stones (12,19). Yellow dock contains oxalates, and thus should be avoided in individuals with kidney disease (12).

Typical Dosages & Routes of Administration that are Commonly Used
ORAL: Dried root: 2-4 grams or as a tea (Simmer 2-4 grams root in 150 mL of boiling water for 5-10 minutes, strain) 3 times daily (4). Liquid extract: 2-4 mL (1:1 in 25% alcohol) 3 times daily (4). Tincture: 1-2 mL (1:5 in 45% alcohol) (4).

Comments
None.

YELLOW LUPIN

This Product is Also Known As
None.

Scientific Names
Lupinus luteus.
Family: Leguminosae.

People Use This For

Orally, yellow lupin is used for urinary tract disorders, as an anthelmintic for worm infestations and as a diuretic. Topically, it is used for ulcers.

Safety

POSSIBLY UNSAFE ...when the seeds or above ground parts are taken orally (18).
There is insufficient reliable information available about the topical safety of yellow lupin.
PREGNANCY AND LACTATION: POSSIBLY UNSAFE; avoid using.

Effectiveness

There is insufficient reliable information available about the effectiveness of yellow lupin.

Possible Mechanism of Action & Active Ingredients

Yellow lupin contains 0.6-1.6% quinolizidine alkaloids in the above ground plant parts, including sparteine, 13-hydroxylupanine, lupinines and p-cumaroyllupinine. The seed contain 0.4-3.3% quinolizidine alkaloids, including lupinines, sparteine, and in some cultivated strains, gramine. At present, we don't know how these components relate to the uses of lupin. Poisoning has been seen in animals, and is known as "lupinosis." It is due to the presence of mycotoxins that are produced by the fugus Phomopsis leptostromiformis, which sometimes lives in lupins (18).

Adverse Reactions Including Known Allergies

Symptoms of poisoning following ingestion include salivation, vomiting, dysphagia, cardiac arrhythmias, ascending paralysis and possibly death due to respiratory failure (18).

Possible Interactions with Herbs & Other Dietary Supplements

Insufficient reliable information available.

Possible Interactions with Drugs

No interactions are known to occur, and there is no known reason to expect a clinically significant interaction with yellow lupin.

Possible Interactions with Foods

No interactions are known to occur, and there is no known reason to expect a clinically significant interaction with yellow lupin.

Possible Interactions with Lab Tests

No interactions are known to occur, and there is no known reason to expect a clinically significant interaction with yellow lupin.

Possible Interactions with Diseases or Conditions

No interactions are known to occur, and there is no known reason to expect a clinically significant interaction with yellow lupin.

Typical Dosages & Routes of Administration that are Commonly Used

No typical dosage.

Comments

Yellow lupin is considered unsafe; avoid using (18).

YELLOW TOADFLAX

This Product is Also Known As

Brideweed, Butter and Eggs, Buttered Hayhocks, Calves' Snout, Churnstaff, Devil's Head, Devil's Ribbon, Doggies, Dragon-Bushes, Eggs and Bacon, Eggs and Collops, Flaxweed, Fluelli, Gallwort, Larkspur Lion's Mouth, Monkey Flower, Pattens and Clogs, Pedlar's Basket, Pennywort, Rabbits, Ramsted, Snapdragon, Toadpipe, Yellow Rod.

Scientific Names

Linaria vulgaris.
Family: Scrophulariaceae.

People Use This For

Orally, yellow toadflax is used for digestive and urinary tract disorders. It is also used as an anti-inflammatory, diuretic, and to stimulate sweating (18).
Topically, yellow toadflax is used for hemorrhoids, festering wounds, skin rashes, and ulcus cruris (18).

Safety

There is insufficient reliable information available about the safety of yellow toadflax.
Pregnancy and Lactation: Insufficient reliable information available; avoid using.

Effectiveness
There is insufficient reliable information available about the effectiveness of yellow toadflax.

Possible Mechanism of Action & Active Ingredients
The applicable part of yellow toadflax is the whole flowering plant. There is insufficient reliable information available about the possible mechanism of action and active ingredients.

Adverse Reactions Including Known Allergies
None reported.

Possible Interactions with Herbs & Other Dietary Supplements
Insufficient reliable information available.

Possible Interactions with Drugs
No interactions are known to occur, and there is no known reason to expect a clinically significant interaction with yellow toadflax.

Possible Interactions with Foods
No interactions are known to occur, and there is no known reason to expect a clinically significant interaction with yellow toadflax.

Possible Interactions with Lab Tests
No interactions are known to occur, and there is no known reason to expect a clinically significant interaction with yellow toadflax.

Possible Interactions with Diseases or Conditions
No interactions are known to occur, and there is no known reason to expect a clinically significant interaction with yellow toadflax.

Typical Dosages & Routes of Administration that are Commonly Used
ORAL: One batch of tea taken over the course of one day. The tea is prepared by steeping 2 teaspoons dried herb in 300-600 mL of boiling water for 18 minutes and straining (18).
TOPICAL: Yellow toadflax is used in a poultice (18).

Comments
There is very little scientific information about this product. Our staff is continually analyzing the available information on natural medicines and will add data here as it becomes available.

YERBA MANSA

This Product is Also Known As
Lizard's Tail, Swamp Root.

Scientific Names
Anemopsis californica.
Family: Saururaceae.

People Use This For
Orally, yerba mansa is used for cancer, catarrh, common cold, cough, gastrointestinal disturbances; orthopedic, skin, and throat ailments; tuberculosis, venereal diseases, and women's ailments. It is used as an analgesic, disinfectant, emetic, laxative, tonic, and to induce sweating (4206).

Safety
There is insufficient reliable information available about the safety of yerba mansa.
Pregnancy and Lactation: Insufficient reliable information is available; avoid using.

Effectiveness
There is insufficient reliable information available about the effectiveness of yerba mansa.

Possible Mechanism of Action & Active Ingredients
The applicable parts of yerba mansa are the root and rhizome. Yerba mansa is believed to have sedative effects. It is also a urinary irritant (19). In animals, methyleugenol, a constituent of the volatile oil, prolongs the hypnotic effect of barbiturates and CNS depressant effects of chlorpromazine (19).

Adverse Reactions Including Known Allergies
None reported.

Possible Interactions with Herbs & Other Dietary Supplements

HERBS WITH SEDATIVE PROPERTIES: Theoretically, concomitant use with herbs that have sedative properties might enhance therapeutic and adverse effects. These include calamus, calendula, California poppy, catnip, capsicum, celery, couch grass, elecampane, ginseng Siberian, German chamomile, goldenseal, gotu kola, hops, Jamaican dogwood, kava, lemon balm, sage, St. John's wort, sassafras, scullcap, shepherd's purse, stinging nettle, valerian, wild carrot, wild lettuce, and withania root (4,19).

Possible Interactions with Drugs

DRUGS WITH SEDATIVE PROPERTIES: Theoretically, concomitant use might cause additive or prolonged sedative effects (19).
BARBITURATES: Theoretically, methyleugenol, a constituent of the volatile oil might prolong the hypnotic effect of barbiturates (19).
CHLORPROMAZINE: Theoretically, methyleugenol, a constituent of the volatile oil might prolong the CNS depressant effects of chlorpromazine (Thorazine) (19).

Possible Interactions with Foods

No interactions are known to occur, and there is no known reason to expect a clinically significant interaction with yerba mansa.

Possible Interactions with Lab Tests

No interactions are known to occur, and there is no known reason to expect a clinically significant interaction with yerba mansa.

Possible Interactions with Diseases or Conditions

URINARY TRACT INFLAMMATION: Contraindicated due to urinary irritant effects (19).

Typical Dosages & Routes of Administration that are Commonly Used

No typical dosage.

Comments

There is very little scientific information about this product. Our staff is continually analyzing the available information on natural medicines and will add data here as it becomes available.

YERBA SANTA

This Product is Also Known As

Bear's Weed, Consumptive's Weed, Eriodictyon, Gum Bush, Gum Plant, Hierba Santa, Holy Herb, Holy Weed, Mountain Balm, Sacred Herb, Tarweed.

Scientific Names

Eriodictyon californicum; Eriodictyon glutinosum; Wigandia californicum.
Family: Hydrophyllaceae.

People Use This For

Orally, yerba santa is used for coughs, colds, tuberculosis (6), asthma (6,11,18), and chronic bronchitis (11).
Topically, the herb is used as a poultice to treat bruises (6,11), sprains, wounds, insect bites (11), and to relieve rheumatism (6).
In folk medicine, it has been used as an antispasmodic, a tonic (11), an antipyretic, and an expectorant (6,11).
In foods and beverages, a fluid extract of yerba santa is used as a flavoring component (6,11).
In manufacturing, the herb is also used as a pharmaceutical flavoring agent to mask the bitter taste of other drugs (6,11,18).

Safety

LIKELY SAFE ...when consumed in food amounts (11). ...when used as an oral medicinal (6,12,18).
There is insufficient reliable information about the safety of the topical use of yerba santa.
PREGNANCY AND LACTATION: Insufficient reliable information available.

Effectiveness

There is insufficient reliable information available about the effectiveness of yerba santa.

Possible Mechanism of Action & Active Ingredients

The applicable part of yerba santa is the leaf. Yerba santa contains several flavonoids including eriodictyonine (6%), eriodictyol (0.5%) (6,11,18), chrysoeriol, and cirsimaritin (4118); tannins (11,18), and a trace amount of volatile oil (6,11,18). Yerba santa may have a mild diuretic effect (18). Eriodictyol is reported to exert an expectorant effect (6,11).

Adverse Reactions Including Known Allergies
None reported.

Possible Interactions with Herbs & Other Dietary Supplements
Insufficient reliable information available.

Possible Interactions with Drugs
No interactions are known to occur, and there is no known reason to expect a clinically significant interaction with yerba santa.

Possible Interactions with Foods
No interactions are known to occur, and there is no known reason to expect a clinically significant interaction with yerba santa.

Possible Interactions with Lab Tests
No interactions are known to occur, and there is no known reason to expect a clinically significant interaction with yerba santa.

Possible Interactions with Diseases or Conditions
No interactions are known to occur, and there is no known reason to expect a clinically significant interaction with yerba santa.

Typical Dosages & Routes of Administration that are Commonly Used
ORAL: People typically prepare yerba santa using 1 teaspoon of the leaves added to 1 cup boiling water. The liquid is taken warm, 30 minutes before bedtime or a mouthful taken 3 times a day (5254).

Comments
None.

YEW

This Product is Also Known As
Chinwood, Common Yew, English Yew, Pacific Yew, Western Yew.

Scientific Names
Taxus bacatta; Taxus brevifolia; and other Taxus species.
Family: Taxaceae.

People Use This For
Pacific yew bark is the source of the drug paclitaxel (Taxol) (13,512), which is FDA-approved for the treatment of breast and ovarian cancer.
In folk medicine, yew has been used for promoting menstruation, inducing abortion, treating diphtheria, tapeworm infestation, tonsillitis, epilepsy (18), rheumatism, urinary tract conditions, and liver conditions (6).

Safety
LIKELY UNSAFE ...when taken orally (6,18). All parts of the yew plant are considered poisonous (5604). Ingestion of 50-100 grams of yew needles can cause death (18,5604). Yew can cause severe gastrointestinal irritation and can cause heart rate to slow dangerously (17,159). Many of the reported fatalities have occurred after ingestion of large amounts of plant material, especially yew needles (5603,5604,5605).
CHILDREN: UNSAFE ...when yew berry is ingested orally. One chewed berry is potentially lethal (159).
PREGNANCY AND LACTATION: UNSAFE ...when the needles or berries are ingested. Yew needles have been used as an abortifacient (16,18).

Effectiveness
There is insufficient reliable information available about the effectiveness of yew.

Possible Mechanism of Action & Active Ingredients
The applicable parts of yew are the bark, branch tip, and needle. The yew bark is reported to have antispasmodic, nerve toxicant and cardiac metabolism effects (6,18). It contains many alkaloids of which taxine A and B are considered to be cardiotoxic (5603,5604). Taxine B affects myocardial cells of the heart by inhibiting both calcium and sodium transport across cell membranes (5604). Yew also contains flavonoids (18). Old growth Pacific yew bark contains 0.01% paclitaxel (13,512). Initially, the small yield from the bark limited the amount of drug that could be produced. Efforts to increase the drug without decimating the supply of the Pacific yew resulted in a semi-synthetic process that produces larger yields (512). English yew needles can be used to isolate 10 desacetylbaccatin III which is converted to paclitaxel (13,512). Paclitaxel is available as the prescription drug, Taxol, for treating advanced ovarian cancer, non-small cell lung cancer, metastatic breast cancer, esophageal cancer, bladder cancer, head and neck cancer, and AIDS-related Kaposi's sarcoma (15).

Adverse Reactions Including Known Allergies

Death has occurred with ingestion of 50-100 grams of yew needles (18,5604). Symptoms of poisoning include queasiness, dry mouth, (18) vomiting, vertigo, severe abdominal pain, weakness (5604), nervousness, trembling, dyspnea, incoordination (5603), tachycardia, bradycardia, arrhythmias, hypotension, unconsciousness, coma (5604), mydriasis, reddening of the lips, pale and cyanotic skin (6,18), and death secondary to cardiac arrest (5604).

Possible Interactions with Herbs & Other Dietary Supplements

Insufficient reliable information available.

Possible Interactions with Drugs

No interactions are known to occur, and there is no known reason to expect a clinically significant interaction with yew.

Possible Interactions with Foods

No interactions are known to occur, and there is no known reason to expect a clinically significant interaction with yew.

Possible Interactions with Lab Tests

No interactions are known to occur, and there is no known reason to expect a clinically significant interaction with yew.

Possible Interactions with Diseases or Conditions

No interactions are known to occur, and there is no known reason to expect a clinically significant interaction with yew.

Typical Dosages & Routes of Administration that are Commonly Used

No typical dosage.

Comments

Yew is considered likely unsafe; avoid using.

YIN CHEN

This Product is Also Known As

Armoise Capillaire, Capillary Wormwood, Chiu, In Chen, Inchin-Ko-To, Inchinko, Kawara-Yomogi, Kyunchinho, Rumput Roman, Shih Yin Ch'en, Yin Ch'en, Yin Ch'en Hao, Yin Chen Hao.

Scientific Names

Artemisia capillaris; Artemisia scoparia.
Family: Asteraceae or Compositae.

People Use This For

In Chinese and Japanese medicine, yin chen above ground parts are used orally to treat hepatitis, infectious cholecystitis, and hyperlipidemia (4343). Yin chen is used to stimulate the bile flow, the liver, and gallbladder (4342,4343). Yin chen is also used orally for newborn kernicterus (4343), for symptoms of intermittent fever and chills, bitter taste in the mouth, chest constriction, flank pain, dizziness, nausea, and loss of appetite (4342,4343). In addition, it is used for headache, constipation, painful urination, fever (4327), itching, tumors, catarrh, rheumatism, painful menses, malaria, and spasms (4327).
In Chinese and Japanese herbal combinations, yin chen is used orally for jaundice with fever, urinary dysfunction, constipation, and abdominal distention (4242).
Yin chen is contained in inchin-ko-to, a Kampo (Chinese/Japanese) medicine (4343) used to treat hepatitis C (4333).

Safety

POSSIBLY SAFE ...when the above ground parts are used orally and appropriately (12,4342). However, serious conditions such as hepatitis require medical management by a physician and should not be self-treated.
CHILDREN: POSSIBLY UNSAFE ...children under the age of 12 years should not use except under care of physician (4344).
PREGNANCY AND LACTATION: LIKELY UNSAFE; avoid using (12).

Effectiveness

POSSIBLY EFFECTIVE ...when used orally to treat acute hepatitis, jaundice, and gallstone-related illness (4342,4343).
There is insufficient reliable information available about the effectiveness of yin chen for its other uses.

Possible Mechanism of Action & Active Ingredients

Yin chen above ground parts contains varied constituents. Scoparone, chlorogenic acid and caffeic acid have demonstrated effects in stimulating bile secretion and protecting the liver against carbon tetrachloride injury (4343).

The essential oils cause yin chen to have antipyretic (4343) and antifungal properties (4344). Yin chen is also believed to have bactericide, anti-inflammatory, and diuretic properties (4342,4343,4344). Some evidence suggests yin chen can reduce blood pressure, cholesterol levels, and act as an antiasthmatic agent (4342,4243). Inchin-ko-to, a medicine that contains yin chen, shows evidence that it can prevent apoptosis that is believed to be the mechanism of cell death in viral and fulminant hepatitis (4345). Genepin, a metabolite of inchin-ko-to, appears to be responsible for therapeutic effects (4346).

Adverse Reactions Including Known Allergies
Oral use of yin chen is associated with nausea, abdominal distention, and dizziness (4343). One study using yin chen and da zao (Fructus Zizyphi Jujubae) orally to treat infectious hepatitis reported 2 women developed Adams-Stokes syndrome. This syndrome is usually associated with heart block (4342). Yin chen can cause an allergic reaction in individuals sensitive to the Asteraceae/Compositae family. Members of this family include ragweed, chrysanthemums, marigolds, daisies, and many other herbs.

Possible Interactions with Herbs & Other Dietary Supplements
Insufficient reliable information available.

Possible Interactions with Drugs
No interactions are known to occur, and there is no known reason to expect a clinically significant interaction with yin chen.

Possible Interactions with Foods
No interactions are known to occur, and there is no known reason to expect a clinically significant interaction with yin chen.

Possible Interactions with Lab Tests
No interactions are known to occur, and there is no known reason to expect a clinically significant interaction with yin chen.

Possible Interactions with Diseases or Conditions
No interactions are known to occur, and there is no known reason to expect a clinically significant interaction with yin chen.

Typical Dosages & Routes of Administration that are Commonly Used
ORAL: A typical dose of yin chen is 9-15 grams. In very serious conditions up to 30 g might be used three times daily (4342). Yin chen is most often used in herbal combinations.

Comments
Traditional Chinese medicine nearly always uses herbal combinations. A well accepted motto in herbal medicine translates as "One ruler, two ministers, three aides, and four guides." In this expression, the active principle is the ruler and the other nine are helpers with different degrees of strength (4343).

YLANG YLANG OIL

This Product is Also Known As
None.
CAUTION: See separate listing for Cananga Oil (Cananga odorata macrophylla).

Scientific Names
Cangana odorata genuina, synonym Canangium odoratum genuina.
Family: Annonaceae.

People Use This For
There are no medicinal uses described for ylang ylang oil (11).
In manufacturing, it is used as a fragrance for cosmetics (maximum levels 1% in perfumes) and soaps (11); and as a flavoring agent in foods and beverages (11).

Safety
LIKELY SAFE ...when consumed in amounts found in foods (11); It has Generally Recognized as Safe (GRAS) status in the US. ...when applied topically in amounts found in cosmetics and soaps (11) it is nonirritating and nonsensitizing to skin, and no phototoxicity is reported (11).
PREGNANCY AND LACTATION: Insufficient reliable information available; avoid using.

Effectiveness
There is insufficient reliable information available about the effectiveness of ylang ylang oil.

Possible Mechanism of Action & Active Ingredients
Insufficient reliable information available.

Adverse Reactions Including Known Allergies
None reported.

Possible Interactions with Herbs & Other Dietary Supplements
Insufficient reliable information available.

Possible Interactions with Drugs
No interactions are known to occur, and there is no known reason to expect a clinically significant interaction with ylang ylang oil.

Possible Interactions with Foods
No interactions are known to occur, and there is no known reason to expect a clinically significant interaction with ylang ylang oil.

Possible Interactions with Lab Tests
No interactions are known to occur, and there is no known reason to expect a clinically significant interaction with ylang ylang oil.

Possible Interactions with Diseases or Conditions
No interactions are known to occur, and there is no known reason to expect a clinically significant interaction with ylang ylang oil.

Typical Dosages & Routes of Administration that are Commonly Used
No typical dosage.

Comments
Ylang ylang oil is the distilled oil from freshly harvested Cangana odorata genuina flower.

YOGURT

This Product is Also Known As
Acidophilus Milk, Bulgarian Yogurt, Live Culture Yogurt, Probiotic, Yoghurt.
CAUTION: See separate listings for Bifidobacterium Bifidum, Brewer's Yeast (Hansen CBS 5926), Lactobacillus Acidophilus, Lactobacillus GG, and Saccharomyces Boulardii.

Scientific Names
None.

People Use This For
Orally, yogurt is used for restoring gastrointestinal normal flora after antibiotic therapy (6,3589), reducing antibiotic-associated diarrhea (1255,3589), acute diarrhea in children (1253), and treating and preventing vaginal candidiasis and bacterial vaginosis (6,1245). Yogurt is also used orally for reducing the risk of colorectal cancer , treating hyperlipidemia (6,3590), eradicating Helicobacter pylori infection in peptic ulcer disease (6110), and preventing sunburns (6141).
Intravaginally, yogurt is used in women for treating vaginal candidiasis (6), and bacterial vaginosis in pregnancy (1248).
Yogurt is also eaten as a food and used as an alternative to milk in lactose-intolerant individuals (6).

Safety
LIKELY SAFE ...when used in food amounts. ...when used orally for medicinal purposes (6).
POSSIBLY SAFE ...when used intravaginally. There are no adverse reactions reported in a small clinical study (1248).
PREGNANCY: LIKELY SAFE ...when used orally in food amounts (6). There is insufficient reliable information available about the safety of the intravaginal use of yogurt (6), although no adverse reactions were reported in a small clinical study of pregnant women with bacterial vaginosis (1248).
LACTATION: LIKELY SAFE ...when used orally in food amounts (6). There is insufficient reliable information available about the safety of the intravaginal use of yogurt.

Effectiveness
POSSIBLY EFFECTIVE ...when used orally as a component of nutritional support for children with acute diarrheal illnesses (1242,1246,1253). ...when used orally for promoting recovery from persistent diarrhea in children (1250,1254). ...when used orally for borderline to moderate hyperlipidemia (1240,1241,3590). Fermented milk or yogurt products fermented with specific organisms including Lactobacillus acidophilus and a combination of Enterococcus faecium and Streptococcus thermophilus have been shown to produce mild to moderate reductions in serum cholesterol (1240,1241,3590). In one crossover study, four weeks of treatment with a human strain of Lactobacillus acidophilus resulted in a significant 3.2% reduction in total serum cholesterol (1240). In another small crossover study, a milk preparation fermented with Lactobacillus acidophilus plus added fructo-oligosaccharides

was tested in men. After three weeks of treatment, there was a significant decrease in total cholesterol (4.4%), low-density lipoprotein (LDL) levels (5.4%), and the LDL/high-density lipoprotein (HDL) ratio (5.3%). There were not significant changes in triglyceride or HDL levels (1241). In a larger study, borderline hyperlipidemic men and women taking a specific yogurt fermented with a strain of Enterococcus faecium and two strains of Streptococcus thermophilus (CAUSIDO culture) for eight weeks had a significant average LDL reduction of 8.4% after adjusting for changes in body mass. Yogurts in this study fermented with a Streptococcus thermophilus/Lactobacillus acidophilus combination and a Streptococcus thermophilus/lactobacillus rhamnosus combination did not significantly reduce LDL cholesterol (3590). ...when used orally for reducing symptoms of antibiotic-associated diarrhea. Studies have evaluated yogurt in cases of erythromycin-induced diarrhea (1255,3589). In one small study, healthy volunteers taking erythromycin plus a yogurt fermented with Lactobacillus rhamnosus GG had less diarrhea, abdominal distress, stomach pain, and flatulence compared to placebo (1255). ...when used orally as an alternative to milk for lactose-intolerant individuals (6). ...when used orally for preventing vaginal candidiasis (1245,1249). ...when used orally for bacterial vaginosis (1245). ...when used intravaginally for treating bacterial vaginosis in pregnancy (1248).

POSSIBLY INEFFECTIVE ...when used orally as an adjunctive treatment for asthma (1244,3589).

There is insufficient reliable information available about the effectiveness of yogurt for its other uses.

Possible Mechanism of Action & Active Ingredients

Yogurt is a dairy preparation produced by fermenting milk using one or more of a variety of specific organisms such as Lactobacillus acidophilus, Lactobacillus rhamnosus, Lactobacillus bulgaricus, Enterococcus faecium, Streptococcus thermophilus, and others (1240,1241,3586,3589,3590). Yogurt is a good dietary source of calcium (6,3586), protein, phosphorus, and riboflavin (3586). However, yogurt's medicinal benefit has primarily been attributed to the live cultures it contains as a source of probiotics. Probiotics are symbiotic bacteria similar to the human gastrointestinal normal flora that, when ingested, can pass through the stomach and potentially colonize the lower gastrointestinal tract. It is thought that this colonization might restore the normal flora after antibiotic therapy and maintain the balance of flora to prevent or minimize antibiotic-associated diarrhea (3587,3589). Probiotics contained in yogurt are also thought to help restore normal flora and normal bowel function in other cases of diarrhea (3587). For candidal vaginal infections, probiotics, particularly Lactobacillus acidophilus strains, are thought to be beneficial by helping to restore the normal flora of the vagina. Lactobacillus strains are normal flora in the vagina. Lactobacillus acidophilus has also been found to inhibit growth of Candida albicans. Presence of Lactobacillus species in the rectum has been associated with Lactobacillus colonization in the vagina (3588). For lowering cholesterol in hyperlipidemia, it is thought that certain culture strains found in yogurt might deconjugate bile salts (3590). People with lactase deficiency sometimes tolerate pasteurized yogurt or live culture yogurt better than milk (6). However, lactose absorption is probably greater with live culture yogurt than pasteurized yogurt (1256). Enzymes contained in live culture yogurt are thought to help in the breakdown and absorption of lactose (3586). The lactic acid bacteria found in yogurt can also suppress growth of pathogenic bacteria (3589) such as Salmonella typhimurium (6). Bulgaricum, a compound produced by some Lactobacillus bulgaricus strains, has also been shown to inhibit Gram positive and Gram negative bacteria (6). Preliminary evidence indicates that a yogurt-like fermented milk has activity against Helicobacter pylori (H. pylori). In one report, a liquid fraction of milk fermented overnight with Lactobacillus casei killed H. pylori bacteria. Although this mixture is essentially yogurt, commercial yogurt preparations did not demonstrate the same anti-H. pylori activity. The results of this unpublished study were reported at the 2000 annual meeting of the American Society for Microbiology (6110). Yogurt also shows some evidence that it might stimulate the immune system (6,3589). In vitro studies have produced an increase of immune related substances after yogurt consumption or exposure to lactic acid bacteria (3589). Other components of yogurt, such as whey protein, short peptides, and conjugated linoleic acid, may contribute to its proposed immune effects (3589). Yogurt may have an effect on IgE-mediated diseases such as asthma by decreasing IgE production, but human studies have produced conflicting results (3589). Yogurt may reduce nitrite concentrations in the gastrointestinal tract (3589). In animals, nitrites lead to the formation of carcinogenic compounds. In healthy infants, milk fermented with Lactobacillus casei increases fecal lactobacilli and decreases potentially harmful beta-glucosidase enzyme activity. Beta-glucosidase is a bacterial enzyme that has been associated with enterohepatic circulation of toxins and carcinogens. Beta-glucosidase has been shown to be elevated in diets high in meat (1243).

Adverse Reactions Including Known Allergies

Contamination of yogurt can cause adverse effects. A batch of yogurt contaminated with a toxic strain of E. coli caused hemolytic uremic syndrome (6).

Possible Interactions with Herbs & Other Dietary Supplements

Insufficient reliable information is available.

Possible Interactions with Drugs

CIPROFLOXACIN: Concomitant administration can significantly reduce absorption of ciprofloxacin (Cipro) (1252).
ERYTHROMYCIN: Concomitant use might reduce erythromycin-associated diarrhea (1255,3589).
TETRACYCLINES: Concomitant administration can reduce the absorption of tetracyclines (15).

Possible Interactions with Foods
No interactions are known to occur, and there is no known reason to expect a clinically significant interaction with yogurt.

Possible Interactions with Lab Tests
No interactions are known to occur, and there is no known reason to expect a clinically significant interaction with yogurt.

Possible Interactions with Diseases or Conditions
SHORT BOWEL SYNDROME: People with short bowel syndrome absorb lactose from yogurt better than from milk (6).

Typical Dosages & Routes of Administration that are Commonly Used
ORAL: Yogurt should be labeled with a "Live and Active Cultures" seal from the National Yogurt Association, indicating the product reliably contains at least 100 million active cultures per gram of yogurt (e.g., Dannon, Yoplait). Some researchers recommend 8 ounces of yogurt twice daily for eight days taken concurrently with antibiotics to prevent diarrhea (1736). Separate antibiotic administration and yogurt by at least two hours (1740). Children with acute diarrhea used 125 grams Lactobacillus casei yogurt twice a day in one clinical trial (1253). For reducing cholesterol, a typical dose is 200 mL Lactobacillus acidophilus yogurt per day (1240), 125 mL Lactobacillus acidophilus yogurt with 2.5% fructo-oligosaccharides three times daily (1241), or 450 ml daily of yogurt containing the CAUSIDO culture (3590). For preventing vaginal candidiasis and bacterial vaginosis, a typical dose is 150 mL Lactobacillus acidophilus yogurt per day (1245).
INTRAVAGINAL: No typical dosage.

Comments
Yogurt is milk that has been fermented with Lactobacillus acidophilus, Lactobacillus bulgaricus, Streptococcus lactis, Streptococcus thermophilus, or other bacteria (6,511). Bulgarian yogurt is concentrated by a factor of 1.5 and contains the highest amount of lactose (6).

YOHIMBE

This Product is Also Known As
Johimbi, Yohimbehe, Yohimbehe cortex.

Scientific Names
Pausinystalia yohimbe, synonyms Pausinystalia johimbe, Corynanthe johimbi, Corynanthe yohimbi.
Family: Rubiaceae.

People Use This For
Orally, yohimbe is used for impotence, as an aphrodisiac, for exhaustion (2), angina, hypertension (19), diabetic neuropathy, and postural hypotension (505). Yohimbine, the active constituent of yohimbe, has been used for sexual dysfunction caused by selective serotonin reuptake inhibitors (SSRI) (3970,3971).
Yohimbe bark is also smoked or snuffed for its hallucinogenic effects (6,515).

Safety
LIKELY UNSAFE ...when yohimbe bark is used orally (6,515). The FDA considers the primary active ingredient, yohimbine, to be unsafe and ineffective for nonprescription use (515). Large doses can cause toxicity that includes severe hypotension, heart conduction disorders, and death (18).
There is insufficient reliable information available about the safety of inhaling yohimbe bark.
CHILDREN: LIKELY UNSAFE ...when used orally. Children are more sensitive to the effects of yohimbe on the nervous system than adults (19).
PREGNANCY: LIKELY UNSAFE ...when yohimbe bark is used orally; contraindicated due to its potential as a uterine relaxant and fetal toxin (19). The safety of the prescription product, yohimbine (Yocon), in pregnancy is not certain.
LACTATION: LIKELY UNSAFE; avoid using.

Effectiveness
POSSIBLY EFFECTIVE ...when taken orally for impotence (6,11).
There is insufficient reliable information available about the effectiveness of yohimbe for its other uses.

Possible Mechanism of Action & Active Ingredients
The applicable part of yohimbe is the bark. Yohimbe bark contains approximately 6% yohimbine (6), the constituent alkaloid considered responsible for the pharmacological effects (11). Aphrodisiac activity is attributed to genital blood vessel dilation, nerve impulse transmission to genital tissue, and increased reflex excitability in the sacral region of the spinal cord (11). Yohimbine readily penetrates the CNS and works primarily through alpha 2-adrenergic receptor blockade (6,11). It also has monoamine oxidase inhibiting, calcium channel blocking, and

peripheral serotonin receptor blocking effects (6,11). The effect of yohimbine on impotence can be mediated through increased penile blood flow and increased central excitatory impulses to the genital tissue (11). It can be most effective for men with organic vascular dysfunction (6,11). Yohimbine can be useful for treating diabetic neuropathy and postural hypotension (505). Yohimbine has been successfully used for sexual dysfunction induced by selective serotonin reuptake inhibitors (SSRI) (3970,3971,3972,3973).

Adverse Reactions Including Known Allergies

Taking yohimbe orally can cause excitation, tremor, insomnia, anxiety, hypertension, tachycardia, nausea, and vomiting (11). The constituent, yohimbine, is associated with salivation, irritability, and fluid retention (2,11). Respiration is stimulated by relatively low amounts of yohimbine and depressed by larger amounts (11). There is one case report of fever, chills, malaise, itchy, scaly skin, progressive renal failure and lupus-like syndrome associated with ingestion of a one-day dose of yohimbine (6169). Yohimbine is reported to trigger psychosis in people predisposed to it (2,11). Symptoms of yohimbine toxicity include paralysis, severe hypotension, cardiac conduction disorders, cardiac failure, and death (6,18).

Possible Interactions with Herbs & Other Dietary Supplements

CAFFEINE-CONTAINING HERBS: Theoretically, concomitant use of yohimbe with large amounts of caffeine-containing herbs or products can increase the risk of hypertensive crisis (12). Caffeine-containing herbs include coffee, cola, guarana, mate, and tea.
EPHEDRA: Theoretically, concomitant use of large amounts of ephedra can increase the risk of hypertensive crisis due to ephedrine content (12).
HERBS WITH MONOAMINE OXIDASE INHIBITING (MAOI) ACTIVITY: Theoretically, concomitant use of these herbs with yohimbe can have additive therapeutic and adverse effects (12). Herbs with MAOI activity include California poppy, ginkgo, mace, and St. John's wort (12).

Possible Interactions with Drugs

ALPHA 2-ADRENERGIC-BLOCKING DRUGS: Yohimbe is contraindicated due to the risk of increased alpha-adrenergic blockade (19).
ANTIDIABETES DRUGS: Theoretically, concomitant use of yohimbe can interfere with antidiabetes drugs due to MAOI activity (15,515).
ANTIHYPERTENSIVE DRUGS: Concomitant use of yohimbe can interfere with blood pressure control and should be used with caution (6,11).
BETA-BLOCKING DRUGS: Theoretically, these drugs can protect against yohimbine toxicity (19).
CLONIDINE (Catapres), GUANABENZ (Wytensin): Avoid concomitant use of these drugs because yohimbine antagonizes their effects (11,19).
MONOAMINE OXIDASE INHIBITORS (MAOIs): Concomitant use with yohimbe can result in additive effects (6,11,12).
NALOXONE (Narcan): Concomitant use can have additive therapeutic and adverse effects (19).
PHENOTHIAZINES: Yohimbe is contraindicated with phenothiazines due to the risk of increased alpha 2-adrenergic antagonism (19).
SYMPATHOMIMETIC DRUGS: Yohimbe is contraindicated because concomitant use increases the risk of hypertensive crisis due to yohimbe MAOI activity (5,6).
TRICYCLIC ANTIDEPRESSANTS: Yohimbe is contraindicated due to its potential to increase or decrease blood pressure (19).

Possible Interactions with Foods

TYRAMINE-CONTAINING FOODS: Avoid concomitant consumption of large amounts of tyramine-containing foods, due to the risk of hypertensive crisis (5,6,11). Tyramine-containing foods include aged cheeses, fermented meats, red wines, and others (506).
VASOPRESSOR-CONTAINING FOODS: Avoid concomitant consumption of large amounts of vasopressor-containing foods due to the risk of hypertensive crisis (5,6,11). Vasopressor-containing foods include overripe fava beans, coffee, tea, colas, and chocolate (506).

Possible Interactions with Lab Tests

No interactions are known to occur, and there is no known reason to expect a clinically significant interaction with yohimbe.

Possible Interactions with Diseases or Conditions

ANGINA, HEART DISEASE: Contraindicated, due to the cardiovascular effects of the yohimbe constituent, yohimbine (6,11,19,515).
ANXIETY: Avoid; the yohimbe constituent, yohimbine, might cause anxiety (19,515).
BENIGN PROSTATIC HYPERPLASIA (BPH): Contraindicated. Theoretically, yohimbe might exacerbate symptoms of BPH due to the presynaptic alpha-2 blocking activity of the constituent yohimbine (14).
DIABETES: Avoid, due to the monoamine oxidase inhibiting (MAOI) activity of yohimbe (15,515). Use of MAO inhibitors in patients receiving insulin or oral antidiabetes drugs has been associated with hypoglycemic episodes (15).
DEPRESSION: Contraindicated. The constituent yohimbine might elicit manic-like symptoms in individuals with

bipolar depression or suicidal tendencies in individuals with endogenous depression (19).
HYPERTENSION: Avoid; small amounts of yohimbine can increase blood pressure (6,19).
HYPOTENSION: Contraindicated; large amounts of yohimbine can cause hypotension (6,515).
KIDNEY DISEASE: Contraindicated (2,6,11,12,18,19,515). Theoretically, yohimbine might have antidiuretic effects (19).
LIVER DISEASE: Contraindicated (2,6,11,12,19,515). Theoretically, liver disease might alter metabolism of the constituent yohimbine (19).
POST-TRAUMATIC STRESS DISORDER (PTSD): Avoid; the constituent yohimbine has been associated with triggering acute symptoms in four individuals with PTSD (1294).
PROSTATE INFLAMMATION: Contraindicated (11,12). Theoretically, yohimbe might exacerbate symptoms of prostate inflammation due to the presynaptic alpha-2 blocking activity of the constituent yohimbine (14).
SCHIZOPHRENIA: Caution, the constituent yohimbine might activate psychoses in patients with schizophrenia (19,515).
YOHIMBE HYPERSENSITIVITY: Contraindicated (19).

Typical Dosages & Routes of Administration that are Commonly Used

People typically use yohimbe products that are labeled with a standardized 15 mg yohimbine content (3895). A tincture (concentration not specified) of the bark is sometimes used in the amount of 5-10 drops three times per day (3895). Yohimbine in 5.4 mg tablets is available as a prescription drug with no FDA-approved indications.

Comments

Yohimbe is the name of an evergreen tree that is native to Zaire, Cameroon, and Gabon. The bark of the yohimbe tree contains the alkaloid, yohimbine (6,4201).

YUCCA

This Product is Also Known As

Adam's Needle, Aloe Yucca, Bear Grass, Dagger Plant, Joshua Tree, Mohave Yucca, Our-Lord's-Candle, Soapweed, Spanish Bayonet.

Scientific Names

Yucca schidigera, synonym Yucca mohavensis; Yucca brevifolia, synonym Yucca arborescens; Yucca aloifolia; Yucca filamentosa; Yucca glauca; Yucca whipplei; and other Yucca species.
Family: Liliaceae or Agavaceae.

People Use This For

Orally, yucca is used to treat arthritis (4,5,6,11), hypertension, migraine headaches, colitis, hypercholesterolemia (6), stomach disorders, diabetes, poor circulation (4), and liver and gallbladder disorders (Yucca filamentosa) (18). Topically, it is used for sores, skin diseases, inflammation, preventing bleeding, sprains, broken limbs, dandruff, baldness (11), joint pain, and as a hair wash (4). Yucca is a traditional foodstuff of American Indians (4).
In manufacturing, an extract (especially Mojave yucca) is used as a foaming and flavoring agent in carbonated beverages (6,11); and compounds within the plant have been used in the synthesis of new drugs (6).

Safety

LIKELY SAFE ...when consumed in amounts commonly found in foods (11); Mojave yucca and Joshua tree are both approved for food use in the US (11).
POSSIBLY SAFE ...when used orally and appropriately, short term (12).
Insufficient reliable information available about the safety of the topical or long-term use of yucca (6,11).
PREGNANCY AND LACTATION: POSSIBLY SAFE in amounts found in foods (yucca saponins are thought not to be absorbed from the GI tract) (4); avoid amounts greater than in foods (4).

Effectiveness

POSSIBLY EFFECTIVE ...when used orally for lowering high blood pressure and correcting abnormal triglycerides and high cholesterol when combined with diet and exercise (4,6).
There is insufficient reliable information available about the effectiveness of yucca for its other uses.

Possible Mechanism of Action & Active Ingredients

Yucca contains saponins that are believed responsible for the pharmacologic activity of the plant (4,6,11). In experimental animals, yucca extracts exhibit anti-inflammatory, antitumor and antiviral activity (4,6,11). A twelve-week study of Mohave yucca extract in rats showed no evidence of toxicity (11). In vitro, the extract had hemolytic activity (6,11). A human study of "saponin extract" of the "desert yucca plant" provides inconclusive evidence that it may reduce arthritic symptoms of pain, swelling and stiffness (4,6). It may also reduce high blood pressure, high triglyceride and cholesterol levels, and incidence of migraine headaches (4,6). The mechanism for these effects is unknown because researchers do not believe yucca saponins are absorbed from the gastrointestinal tract (4).

Adverse Reactions Including Known Allergies
Taken orally, yucca can cause stomach upset (7,18), mucous membrane irritation, bitter taste, nausea, and vomiting (7). Intravenous administration may result in hemolysis (6).

Possible Interactions with Herbs & Other Dietary Supplements
Insufficient reliable information available.

Possible Interactions with Drugs
No interactions are known to occur, and there is no known reason to expect a clinically significant interaction with yucca.

Possible Interactions with Foods
No interactions are known to occur, and there is no known reason to expect a clinically significant interaction with yucca.

Possible Interactions with Lab Tests
No interactions are known to occur, and there is no known reason to expect a clinically significant interaction with yucca.

Possible Interactions with Diseases or Conditions
No interactions are known to occur, and there is no known reason to expect a clinically significant interaction with yucca.

Typical Dosages & Routes of Administration that are Commonly Used
ORAL: People typically use 380 to 490 mg of the powdered yucca stalk or root two to three times daily. One yucca supplier suggests three daily doses based on body weight: under 100 pounds, 380 mg per dose; 100 to 175 pounds, 760 mg; and over 175 pounds, 1140 mg. Yucca can be prepared as a liquid by boiling one-fourth ounce of the root in 16 ounces of water for 15 minutes. People typically drink 3 to 5 cups of the liquid per day (6006).
TOPICAL: No typical dosage.

Comments
None.

ZEDOARY

This Product is Also Known As
Cedoaria, Cetoal, E Zhu, E-Zhu, Indian Arrowroot, Kua, Shoti, Temu Kuning, Temu Putih, Turmeric, Zedoaire, Zedoária, Zedoarie rhizoma, Zitwer, Zitwerwirtzelstock.
CAUTION: See separate listings for Turmeric, Goldenseal, and Javanese Turmeric.

Scientific Names
Curcuma zedoaria.
Family; Zingiberaceae.

People Use This For
Orally, zedoary rhizome is used for colic, spasms, stimulating appetite, and improving digestion (2), stimulating bile flow, and as an anti-inflammatory (512).
In combination herbal products, zedoary rhizome extracts are used for gastrointestinal complaints and stimulating bile flow (18).
In folk medicine, zedoary rhizome is used for nervous diseases (18).

Safety
POSSIBLY SAFE ...when used orally and appropriately (12).
PREGNANCY: LIKELY UNSAFE ...contraindicated for oral use (12) due to potential abortifacient effects (19).
LACTATION: Insufficient reliable information available; avoid using.

Effectiveness
There is insufficient reliable information available about the effectiveness of zedoary.

Possible Mechanism of Action & Active Ingredients
The applicable part of zedoary is the rhizome. Zedoary contains a volatile oil and curcuminoids (18). Zedoary is thought to stimulate bile production and gallbladder emptying (512). The volatile oil contains sesquiterpene ketones known as turmerones that are believed responsible for increasing bile production (512). The curcuminoid constituents are believed to be responsible for gallbladder emptying effects (512). The isolated sesquiterpene constituent dehydrocurdione shows some evidence of anti-inflammatory activity (4011). Experimental evidence suggests other sesquiterpenes isolated from zedoary might be hepatoprotective (4012). Compounds isolated from zedoary demonstrate some evidence of antifungal (4013) and cytotoxic (4014) activity.

Adverse Reactions Including Known Allergies
None reported.

Possible Interactions with Herbs & Other Dietary Supplements
Insufficient reliable information is available.

Possible Interactions with Drugs
No interactions are known to occur, and there is no known reason to expect a clinically significant interaction with zedoary.

Possible Interactions with Foods
No interactions are known to occur, and there is no known reason to expect a clinically significant interaction with zedoary.

Possible Interactions with Lab Tests
No interactions are known to occur, and there is no known reason to expect a clinically significant interaction with zedoary.

Possible Interactions with Diseases or Conditions
HEAVY MENSES: Some experts suggest that zedoary should not be used by women who have heavy menstrual periods (12).

Typical Dosages & Routes of Administration that are Commonly Used
ORAL: One cup of tea three times daily at meals. To make tea, steep 1-1.5 grams powdered dried rhizome in 150 mL boiling water, 5-10 minutes, and strain (18).

Comments
Traditional methods for preparing zedoary involve prolonged washing with water changes to remove most of the protein, water-soluble nutrients, and presumably, an unidentified toxic constituent (4015).

ZINC

This Product is Also Known As
Zinc Acetate, Zinc Aspartate, Zinc Gluconate, Zinc Methionine, Zinc Monomethionine, Zinc Oxide, Zinc Sulfate.

Scientific Names
Zinc; Zn; atomic number 30.

People Use This For
Orally, zinc is used as a dietary supplement, as a prenatal supplement, and as replacement therapy for treatment and prevention of zinc deficiency. It is also used for treating the common cold (2619), anorexia nervosa, improving athletic performance and strength, benign prostatic hyperplasia (BPH), Crohn's disease, diabetes, Down's syndrome, improving immune function, male infertility, macular degeneration, night blindness, osteoporosis, peptic ulcers, recurrent ear infections, rheumatoid arthritis, sickle cell anemia (1900), Alzheimer's disease, Wilson's disease (2619,2662,2678,2679,2742,2808,2824), acrodermatitis enteropathica, and delayed wound healing associated with zinc deficiency (2619). Zinc is also used for acute diarrhea in children with zinc deficiency (825,826,827,2680,3455,3456), improving growth and health in zinc-deficient stunted children (6191), severe head injuries (2696), hypertension (3581), and muscle cramps in patients with cirrhosis (1352).
Topically, zinc is used for treating acne (2619) and speeding wound healing (2694). Zinc is used intranasally for treating the common cold (385).
Intravenously, zinc is used as a component of total parenteral nutrition (14).

Safety
LIKELY SAFE ...when used orally in amounts that do not exceed the recommended dietary allowance (RDA) (14).
...when used topically and appropriately on intact skin (14). Although topical absorption can occur, as much as 2g/kg of topical zinc oxide has been tolerated (14).
POSSIBLY SAFE ...when used orally and appropriately in amounts greater than the recommended dietary allowance (RDA) (14).
LIKELY UNSAFE ...when taken orally in excessive amounts. Chronic intake of 450-1600 mg daily of supplemental zinc is associated with sideroblastic anemia (14). Ingestion of 10-30 grams of zinc sulfate can be lethal in adults, the amount of zinc that causes acute toxicity varies with the salt form (14).
PREGNANCY: LIKELY SAFE ...when used orally in amounts that do not exceed the recommended dietary allowance (RDA) (14,2674). POSSIBLY SAFE ...when used orally and appropriately in amounts slightly exceeding the recommended daily allowance (RDA). In one study, pregnant women received zinc supplements of 25 mg daily throughout pregnancy without reported adverse effects on the fetus (301). Zinc supplementation above the RDA during pregnancy should only be done under the close supervision of a health care professional.

 © Copyright 2000, Natural Medicines Comprehensive Database (209) 472-2244. For updated data, go to www.NaturalDatabase.com

LIKELY UNSAFE ...when used orally in large amounts. Premature births and stillbirth have been reported when 100 mg three times daily was consumed during the third trimester (332).

LACTATION: LIKELY SAFE ...when used orally in amounts that do not exceed the recommended dietary allowance (RDA) (2674). POSSIBLY UNSAFE ...when used orally in amounts exceeding the recommended dietary allowance (RDA). Zinc appears in breast milk and can cause zinc-induced copper deficiency in nursing infants (14).

Effectiveness

EFFECTIVE ...when used orally or intravenously for preventing and treating zinc deficiency (14,15,2619). However, routine zinc supplementation is not recommended (403). Zinc deficiency requiring supplementation may occur in severe diarrhea, malabsorption syndromes, liver cirrhosis and alcoholism, after major surgery, and during long-term administration of total parenteral nutrition (3539).

LIKELY EFFECTIVE ...when used orally for reducing the duration and severity of acute diarrhea in malnourished or zinc-deficient young children (825,826,827,3455,3456).

POSSIBLY EFFECTIVE ...when used as a lozenge for decreasing the duration of the common cold in adults. Multiple studies have shown a significant decrease in the duration of symptoms of the common cold when zinc gluconate lozenges containing 13.3-23 mg zinc were taken every 2 hours while awake in adults (333,334,335); however, zinc gluconate lozenges containing only 4.5 mg of zinc have not been effective (339). In children, zinc gluconate lozenges have also not been shown to be effective (341). Preliminary evidence suggests that a new zinc gel nasal spray (Zicam Cold Remedy, Gel Tech) can shorten the duration of a cold when administered starting within 24 hours of onset of symptoms; however, the results of this pilot study have not been published (1278). ...when used orally for Wilson's disease (822,823,2693). ...when used orally for acrodermatitis enteropathica (821,2689,2690,2691). ...when used orally for increasing birth weight and head circumference by pregnant women with mildly low plasma zinc levels (301). ...when given orally for improving growth and overall health in zinc-deficient stunted infants (6191). In one study, 10 mg zinc sulfate daily for six months improved growth, increased body weight, and reduced the incidence of anorexia, cough, diarrhea, fever, and vomiting in a group of stunted, zinc-deficient infants in Ethiopia (6191). ...when used orally for treating muscle cramps in zinc-deficient patients with cirrhosis (1352). ...when used topically with erythromycin for treating acne (819,820,2687,2688). ...when used parenterally immediately post-head trauma for improving rate of neurological recovery (2696).

POSSIBLY INEFFECTIVE ...when used orally for improving iron status in pregnant women taking supplemental iron and folic acid (6104).

There is insufficient reliable information available about the effectiveness of zinc for its other uses.

Possible Mechanism of Action & Active Ingredients

Zinc is a biologically essential trace element (511). It is a co-factor in many biological processes, including DNA, RNA, and protein synthesis. Zinc also plays a role in immune function and wound healing, reproduction, growth and development, behavior and learning, taste and smell, blood clotting, thyroid hormone function, and is associated with insulin action (331,403). Meat, seafood, dairy products, nuts, legumes, and whole grains contain relatively high concentrations of zinc (331). Zinc is absorbed from foods at a rate of 15-40%. Bioavailability is influenced by zinc status. More zinc is absorbed in states of zinc deficiency. Zinc deficiency is characterized by growth retardation, low insulin levels, anorexia, mental lethargy, irritability, low sperm count, generalized hair loss, rough and dry skin, skin lesions, slow wound healing, decreased thyroid function, delayed onset of puberty, poor sense of smell and taste, diarrhea, and nausea. Deficiency is rare in the United States; most diets provide more than the recommended dietary allowance (RDA) (3539). For the common cold, zinc supplementation is theorized to be beneficial by inhibiting viral replication and boosting immune function (3581). In one study, supplemental zinc improved cell-mediated immune response in older people (824). It is believed that the amount of available ionized zinc determines the effectiveness of zinc in treating the common cold (336). The extent of zinc ionization varies with different lozenge formulations (340). Preliminary evidence suggests that addition of citric acid, mannitol or sorbitol to zinc gluconate lozenge preparations decreases the extent of zinc ionization, while the addition of glycine to zinc gluconate lozenges does not (300). For wound healing, topical zinc might enhance re-epithelialization, decrease inflammation, and inhibit bacterial growth, thus enhancing wound healing (2699). Topical zinc might be effective for treating acne (819,820,2687,2688) due to anti-inflammatory activity resulting from inhibition of polymorphonuclear leukocyte chemotaxis induced by decreased granulocyte zinc levels (2686). Zinc may also inhibit conversion of testosterone to dihydrotestosterone (DHT), which has been associated with acne (3581). Zinc blocks copper absorption and increases copper elimination in the stool of people with Wilson's disease (2692). Evidence suggests that zinc regulates linoleic acid and serum lipoprotein metabolism in acrodermatitis enteropathica (2689). A combination zinc monomethionine/aspartate, magnesium aspartate, and pyridoxine product reportedly increased zinc and magnesium levels, anabolic hormone levels, and strength in athletes (2742). Zinc sulfate ophthalmic solution acts as a mild astringent, precipitating protein and clearing mucus from the outer surface of the eye (15). Zinc oxide absorption is best in an acidic environment (2809). Zinc acetate is absorbed over a wide pH range and might be a better choice in people with reduced stomach acid (2809). An enteric-coated zinc aspartate preparation (Taurizine) showed no absorption (2740). Zinc uptake in human intestinal epithelial cells was similar with zinc chloride, zinc methionine, or zinc propionate (2739). Preliminary evidence also suggests that zinc aspartate might have antioxidant properties (2741).

Adverse Reactions Including Known Allergies

Zinc taken orally can cause nausea and vomiting (2619), watery diarrhea (1352), irritation and corrosion of the gastrointestinal tract, acute renal tubular necrosis, and interstitial nephritis (331). Symptoms of toxicity include flu-like and central nervous system symptoms, fever, coughing, nausea, vomiting, diarrhea, epigastric pain, lethargy, fatigue and neuropathy (2663,2681), dehydration, severe vomiting, and zinc-induced copper deficiency with symptoms including sideroblastic anemia, neutropenia, impaired immune function and an increase in the ratio of low-density-lipoprotein to high-density-lipoprotein (LDL/HDL) cholesterol (2619,2681). Chronic intake of 450-1600 mg daily of a zinc supplement has been associated with sideroblastic anemia (14). Occupational inhalation of zinc oxide fumes can cause metal fume fever with symptoms including: fatigue, chills, fever, myalgias, cough, dyspnea, leukocytosis, thirst, metallic taste, and salivation (331).

Possible Interactions with Herbs & Other Dietary Supplements

COPPER: Concomitant use may impair copper absorption (2693).
COFFEE: Concomitant use may decrease zinc absorption up to 50% (14).

Possible Interactions with Drugs

CAPTOPRIL (Capoten): Concomitant use can interfere with zinc supplementation by increasing urinary zinc elimination (25,26). There is no data on other ACEIs. The clinical consequence of urinary zinc loss in hypertensive patients is unknown (25,26). Give supplements of zinc only if clinical judgment warrants it.
CHLORTHALIDONE (Hygroton): Concomitant use might increase serum and hair zinc levels, and also increase urinary zinc elimination (275).
CISPLATIN (Platinol-AQ): Concomitant use with zinc might increase the cytotoxicity of cisplatin when in the presence of the chelate ethylenediaminetetraacetic acid (EDTA), as compared to cisplatin treatment alone (2668).
TETRACYCLINES: Concomitant use decreases absorption and serum levels of demeclocycline (Declomycin), minocycline (Minocin), and tetracycline (Achromycin) due to zinc binding (15,506). Concomitant use can also reduce the effects of zinc supplementation due to reduced zinc absorption. Doxycycline (Vibramycin) does not interact with zinc (15,506).
FLUOROQUINOLONES: Concomitant use reduces drug absorption and serum levels of fluoroquinolones due to zinc binding (506,828,2682). Concomitant use can also reduce the effects of zinc supplementation due to reduced zinc absorption.
INTERFERON ALFA-2B (Intron A): Concomitant use might be effective for treating necrolytic acral erythema associated with hepatitis C (6192). There is one case report of oral zinc sulfate 225 mg twice daily plus interferon alfa-2b for six months resolving all lesions in a woman with necrolytic acral erythema and hepatitis C (6192). Necrolytic acral erythema is categorized in the family of necrolytic erythemas which includes acrodermatitis enteropathica (see Effectiveness) (6192).
PENICILLAMINE (Cuprimine): Concomitant use can reduce the effects of supplemental zinc (2678).
POTASSIUM-SPARING DIURETICS: Concomitant use can lead to zinc accumulation and increase risk of adverse effects (830).
THIAZIDE DIURETICS: Concomitant use can interfere with zinc supplementation by increasing urinary zinc elimination (830,831).

Drug Influences on Nutrient Levels and Depletion

SOME DRUGS CAN AFFECT ZINC LEVELS:
CAPTOPRIL (Capoten): Captopril may increase urinary zinc excretion in patients with hypertension. There is no data on other ACEIs. The clinical consequence of urinary zinc loss in hypertensive patients is unknown (25,26).
FLUOROQUINOLONES: Treatment with fluoroquinolones can reduce dietary zinc absorption. The clinical significance is yet to be determined, and the need for supplementation has not been adequately studied. Consider zinc supplementation in patients on long-term fluoroquinolone therapy (506,828,2682).
PENICILLAMINE (Cuprimine): Penicillamine can reduce serum zinc levels and might cause zinc depletion in some patients (4453,4531,4534).
LOOP DIURETICS and THIAZIDE DIURETICS: Use of loop diuretics and thiazide diuretics can increase urinary zinc loss and reduce serum levels. This is more likely with higher doses or when used in combination with diuretics of another class (4412,4425).
TETRACYCLINES: Tetracyclines except doxycycline (Vibramycin) can reduce dietary zinc absorption and serum levels due to zinc binding. The clinical significance is yet to be determined, and the need for supplementation has not been adequately studied. Consider zinc supplementation in patients on long-term tetracycline therapy (15,506).

Possible Interactions with Foods

FOODS: Concomitant administration with foods containing bran, protein, phytates, calcium, or phosphorus may decrease supplemental zinc absorption (506).
COFFEE: Concomitant use might decrease zinc absorption up to 50% (14).

Possible Interactions with Lab Tests

BLOOD ZINC ASSAYS: Avoid using powdered gloves when drawing blood for zinc assays, due to potential for sample contamination (2663).

LIPID PROFILES: Zinc supplementation might reduce high-density lipoprotein (HDL) cholesterol levels and test results (2681). Zinc supplementation might increase the ratio of low-density-lipoprotein to high-density-lipoprotein (LDL/HDL) cholesterol and test results (2681).

Possible Interactions with Diseases or Conditions

ALLERGY: Contraindicated in people with known hypersensitivity to zinc compounds (14).

HEMOCHROMATOSIS: Use caution in people who are homozygous for hemochromatosis (14).

HIV: Contraindicated in people with human immunodeficiency virus infection. Some evidence suggests association between higher intakes of zinc and reduced survival time (14).

GLAUCOMA: Avoid, or use zinc-containing ophthalmic solutions with caution (14).

RHEUMATOID ARTHRITIS: Zinc absorption is reduced in people with rheumatoid arthritis (2823).

Typical Dosages & Routes of Administration that are Commonly Used

ORAL: The typical adult dose for treating the common cold is one zinc gluconate-glycine lozenge (containing 13.3-23 mg zinc) dissolved in the mouth every 2 hours while awake when cold symptoms are present (333,335,336). For acute diarrhea in malnourished or zinc-deficient children, 10-40 mg elemental zinc is given daily (825,826,827,3455,3456). For improving growth and health in zinc-deficient stunted children, 10 mg zinc sulfate daily has been used (6191). For muscle cramps in zinc deficient patients with cirrhosis, zinc sulfate 220 mg twice daily has been used (1352). The daily recommended dietary allowances of zinc are: Infants under 1 year of age, 5 mg; Children 1-10 years, 10 mg; Males 11 years and older, 15 mg; Females 11 years and older, 12 mg; Pregnant women, 15 mg; Lactating women (during first 6 months), 19 mg; Lactating women (during second 6 months), 16 mg (2674).

Different salt forms provide different amounts of elemental zinc: Zinc sulfate contains 23% elemental zinc (220 mg zinc sulfate contains 50 mg zinc). Zinc gluconate contains 14.3% elemental zinc (10 mg zinc gluconate contains 1.43 mg zinc) (506).

TOPICAL: For acne vulgaris, zinc acetate 1.2% with erythromycin 4% as a lotion has been applied twice daily (819).

Comments

Zinc acetate (Galzin) is a FDA-approved orphan drug for treating Wilson's disease.

REFERENCE CITATIONS

1 Monographs on the Medicinal Uses of Plant Drugs. Exeter, UK: European Scientific Cooperative on Phytotherapy, 1997.

2 Blumenthal M, et al. ed. The Complete German Commission E Monographs: Therapeutic Guide to Herbal Medicines. Trans. S. Klein. Boston, MA: American Botanical Council, 1998.

3 Tyler VE. Herbs of Choice. Binghamton, NY: Pharmaceutical Products Press, 1994.

4 Newall CA, Anderson LA, Philpson JD. Herbal Medicine: A Guide for Healthcare Professionals. London, UK: The Pharmaceutical Press, 1996.

5 Foster S, Tyler VE. Tyler's Honest Herbal: A Sensible Guide to the Use of Herbs and Related Remedies. 3rd ed., Binghamton, NY: Haworth Herbal Press, 1993.

6 The Review of Natural Products by Facts and Comparisons. St. Louis, MO: Wolters Kluwer Co., 1999.

7 Schulz V, Hansel R, Tyler VE. Rational Phytotherapy: A Physician's Guide to Herbal Medicine. Trans. Terry C. Telger. 3rd ed. Berlin, Germany: Springer, 1998.

8 Wichtl MW. Herbal Drugs and Phytopharmaceuticals. Ed. N.M. Bisset. Stuttgart: Medpharm GmbH Scientific Publishers, 1994.

9 Martindale W. Martindale the Extra Pharmacopoeia. Pharmaceutical Press, 1999.

10 United States Pharmacopeial Convention, Inc., ed. Drug Information for the Health Care Professional. 19th ed. Englewood, CO: Micromedex Inc., 1999.

11 Leung AY, Foster S. Encyclopedia of Common Natural Ingredients Used in Food, Drugs and Cosmetics. 2nd ed. New York, NY: John Wiley & Sons, 1996.

12 McGuffin M, et al., ed. American Herbal Products Association's Botanical Safety Handbook. Boca Raton, FL: CRC Press, 1997.

13 Robbers JE, Speedie MK, Tyler VE. Pharmacognosy and Pharmacobiotechnology. Baltimore, MD: Williams & Wilkins, 1996.

14 Micromedex(R) Healthcare Series: Micromedex Inc., Englewood, Colorado. (Vol.101, expires 9/1999).

15 McKevoy GK, ed. AHFS Drug Information. Bethesda, MD: American Society of Health-System Pharmacists, 1998.

16 Gennaro A. Remington: The Science and Practice of Pharmacy. 19th ed. Lippincott: Williams & Wilkins, 1996.

17 Ellenhorn MJ, et al. Ellenhorn's Medical Toxicology: Diagnoses and Treatment of Human Poisoning. 2nd ed. Baltimore, MD: Williams & Wilkins, 1997.

18 Gruenwald J, et. al. PDR for Herbal Medicines. 1st ed. Montvale, NJ: Medical Economics Company, Inc., 1998.

19 Brinker F. Herb Contraindications and Drug Interactions. 2nd ed. Sandy, OR: Eclectic Medical Publications, 1998.

21 Miller LG. Herbal medicinals: selected clinical considerations focusing on known or potential drug-herb interactions. *Arch Int Med* 1998;158(20):2200-11.

22 Adams ME. Hype about glucosamine. *Lancet* 1999;354(9176):353.

23 O'Mara NB. PremesisRx. Therapeutic Research Faculty. *Pharmacist's Letter/Prescriber's Letter* 1999;15(12):151206.

24 Cheung D. Is Diclectin safe for morning sickness? Therapeutic Research Faculty. *Pharmacist's Letter/ Prescriber's Letter* 2000;16(3):160316.

25 Golik A, Zaidensttein R, Dishi V, et al. Effects of captopril and enalapril on zinc metabolism in hypertensive patients. *J Am Coll Nutr* 1998;17:75-8.

26 Golik A, Modai D, Averbukh Z, et al. Zinc metabolism in patients treated with captopril versus enalapril. *Metabolism* 199;39:665-7.

27 Kung AWC, Pun KK. Bone mineral density in premenopausal women receiving long-term physiological doses of levothyroxine. *JAMA* 1991;265:2688-91.

28 Schneider DL, Barrett-Connor EL, Morton DJ. Thyroid hormone use and bone mineral density in elderly men. *Arch Intern Med* 1995;155:2005-7.

29 Franklyn AJ, Betteridge J, Daykin J, et al. Long-term thyroxine treatment and bone mineral density. *Lancet* 1992;340:9-13.

30 Paltiel O, Falutz J, Veilleux M, et al. Clinical correlates of subnormal vitamin B12 levels in patients infected with the human immunodeficiency virus. *Am J Hematol* 1995;49:318-22.

31 Tang G, Serfaty-Lacrosniere C, Camilo ME, et al. Gastric acidity influences the blood response to a beta-carotene dose in humans. *Am J Clin Nutr* 1996;64:622-6.

32 Carlsen SM, Folling I, Grill V, et al. Metformin increases total homocysteine levels in non-diabetic male patients with coronary heart disease. *Scand J Clin Lab Invest* 1997;57:521-7.

33 Chevallier A. Encyclopedia of Medicinal Plants. New York, NY: DK Publishing, 1996;141, 273.

34 Leatherdale B, et al. Improvement in glucose tolerance due to Momordica charantia. *Br Med J* 1981;282:1823-4.

35 Welihinda J, et al. Effect of Momordica charantia on the glucose tolerance in maturity onset diabetes. *J Ethnopharmacology* 1986;17:277-82.

36 Srivastava Y, et al. Antidiabetic and adaptogenic properties of Momordica charantia extract: An experimental and clinical evaluation. *Phytother Res* 1993;7:285-9.

37 Raman A, et al. Anti-diabetic properties and phytochemistry of Momordica charantia L. (Cucurbitaceae). *Phytomedicine* 1996;294.

38 Baldwa VS, Bhandari CM, Pangaria A, Goyal RK. Clinical trial in patients with diabetes mellitus of an insulin-like compound obtained from plant sources. *Upsala J Med Sci* 1977;82:39-41.

39 Perossini M, et al. Diabetic and hypertensive retinopathy therapy with Vaccinium myrtillus anthocyanosides (Tegens). Double blind placebo-controlled clinical trial. *Ann Ottalmol Clin Ocul* 1987;113:1173.

40 Scharrer A, Ober M. Anthocyanosides in the treatment of retinopathies. *Kiln Monastbl Augenheilk* 1981;178:386-9.

42 Cucinotta D, Passeri M, Ventura S, et al. Multicenter clinical placebo-controlled study with acetyl-L-carnitine (ALC) in the treatment of mildly demented elderly patients *Drug Development Res* 1988;14:213-6.

43 Kidd PM. A review of nutrients and botanicals in the integrative management of cognitive dysfunction. *Alternative Medicine Review* 1999;4(3):144-61.

44 Mayeux R, Sano M. Treatment of Alzheimer's Disease. *NEJM* 1999;341(22):1670-9.

45 Shanmugasundaram ER, rajeswari G, Baskaran K, et al. Use of Gymnema sylvestre leaf extract in the control of blood glucose in insulin-dependent diabetes mellitus. *J Ethnopharmacol* 1990;30:281-94.

REFERENCES

46   Baskaran K, Kizar-Ahamath B, Shanmugasundaram MR, Shanmugasundaram ERB. Antidiabetic effect of leaf extract from Gymnema sylvestre in non-insulin-dependent diabetes mellitus patients. *J Ethnopharmacol* 1990;30:295-300.

47   Head KA. Type 1 diabetes: prevention of the disease and its complications. *Townsend Letter for Doctors & Patients* 1998;180:72-84.

48   Sinsheimer JE, Subba-Rao G, McIlhenny HM. Constitents from G sylvestre leaves: isolation and preliminary characterization of the gymnemic acids. *J Pharmacol* 1970;59:622-8.

101 Klein AD, Penneys NS. Aloe Vera. *J Am Acad Dermatol* 1988; 714-9.

102 Lyss G, et al. "Helenalin, an antiinflammatory sesquiterpene lactone from Arnica, selectively inhibits transcription factor NF-kappa B." *Biol Chem* 1997; 378(9):951-61.

103 Baillargeon L, et al. "The effects of Arnica montana on blood coagulation. Radomized controlled trial." *Can Fam Physician* 1993; 2362-7.

104 Schroder H, et al. "Helenalin and 11 alpha, 13-dihydrohelenalin, two constituents from Arnica montana L., inhibit human platelet function via thiol-dependent pathways." *Thromb Res* 1990; 57(6):829-45.

105 Sabeel AI, Kurkus J, Lindholm T. "Intensive Hemodialysis and Hemoperfusion Treatment of Amanita Mushroom Poisoning." *Mycopathologica* 1995;131(2):107-114.

106 Bustamante J, et al. "Alpha-lipoic acid in Liver Metabolism and Disease." *Free Radic Biol Med* 1998; 24(6):1023-39.

107 Ehren I, et al. "Effects of L-arginine treatment on symptoms and bladder nitric oxide levels in patients with interstitial cystitis." *Urology* 1998; 52(6):1026-9.

108 Bode-Boger SM, et al. "L-arginine-induced vasodilation in healthy humans: pharmacokinetic-pharmacodynamic relationship." *Br J Clin Pharmacol* 1998; 46(5):489-97.

109 Sandrini G, et al. "Effectiveness of ibuprofen-arginine in the Treatment of Acute Migraine Attacks." *Int J Clin Pharmacol Res* 1998; 18(3):145-50.

110 Lerman A, et al. Long-term L-arginine supplementation improves small-vessel coronary endothelial function in humans. *Circulation* 1998;97(21):2123-8.

111 Chuntrasakul C, et al. Metabolic and immune effects of dietary arginine, glutamine, and omega-3 fatty acids supplementation in immunocompromised patients. *J Med Assoc Thai* 1998;81(5):334-43.

112 Andres A, et al. "L-arginine reverses the antinatriuretic effect of cyclosporin in renal transplant patients." *Nephrol Dial Transplant* 1997 Jul;12(7):1437-40.

113 Pichard C, et al. A randomized double-blind controlled study of 6 months of oral nutritional supplementation with arginine and omega-3 fatty acids in HIV-infected patients. Swiss HIV Cohort Study. *AIDS* 1998;12(1):53-63.

114 Wheeler MA, et al. "Effect of long-term oral L-arginine on the nitric oxide synthase pathway in the urine from patients with interstitial cystitis." *J Urol* 1997;158(6):2045-50.

115 Saffle JR, et al. "Randomized trial of immune-enhancing enteral nutrition in burn patients." *J Trauma* 1997;42(5):793-800, discussion 800-2.

116 Adams MR, et al. "Oral L-arginine improves endothelium-dependent dilatation and reduces monocyte adhesion to endothelial cells in young men with coronary artery disease." *Atherosclerosis* 1997;129(2):261-9.

117 Takano H, et al. "Oral administration of L-arginine potentiates allergen-induced airway inflammation and expression of interleukin-5 in mice." *J Pharmacol Exp Ther* 1998;286(2):767-71.

118 Hibbard MK, Sandri-Goldin, RM. "Arginine-rich regions succeeding the nuclear localization region of the herpes simplex virus type 1 regulatory protein ICP27 are required for efficient nuclear localization and late gene expression." *J Virol* 1995;69(8):4656-7.

119 Griffith RS, DeLong DC, Nelson JD. "Relation of arginine-lysine antagonism to herpes simplex growth in tissue culture." *Chemotherapy* 1981; 27(3):209-13.

120 McCaffrey MJ, et al. "Effect of L-arginine infusion on infants with persistent pulmonary hypertension of the newborn." *Biol Neonate* 1995;67(4):240-3.

121 Sapienza MA, et al. "Effect of inhaled L-arginine on exhaled nitric oxide in normal and asthmatic subjects." *Thorax* 1998 Mar;53(3):172-5.

122 Saijyo T, et al. "Autonomic nervous system activity during infusion of L-arginine in patients with liver cirrhosis." *Liver* 1998 Feb;18(1):27-31.

123 Newcomer AD, et al. "Response of patients with irritable bowel syndrome and lactase deficiency using unfermented acidophilus milk." *Am J Clin Nutr* 1983 Aug;38(2):257-63.

124 Gotz V, et al. "Prophylaxis against ampicillin-associated diarrhea with a lactobacillus preparation." *Am J Hosp Pharm* 1979 Jun;36(6):754-7.

125 Contardi I. "Oral bacterial therapy in prevention of antibiotic-induced diarrhea in childhood." *Clin Ter* 1991 Mar 31;136(6):409-13. [Article in Italian]

126 Kaaja RJ, et al. "Treatment of cholestasis of pregnancy with peroral activated charcoal. A preliminary study." *Scand J Gastroenterol* 1994 Feb;29(2):178-81.

127 Bowry VW, Ingold KU, Stocker R. "Vitamin E in human density lipoprotein. When and how this antioxidant becomes a pro-oxidant." *Biochem J* 1992; 288(Pt 2):341-4.

128 Kagan VE, et al. "Recycling of vitamin E in human low density lipoproteins." *J Lipid Res* 1992;22(3):385-97.

129 Back DJ, et al. "Interaction of ethinyloestradiol with ascorbic acid in man." *Br Med J* 1981;282:1516.

130 Morris JC, et al. [Letter] *Br Med J* 1981;283:503.

131 Levine M, et al. "Vitamin C pharmacokinetics in healthy volunteers: evidence for recommended dietary allowance." *Proc Natl Acad Sci USA* 1996;93(8):3704-9.

132 Buto SK, et al. "Bay Leaf Impaction in the Esophagus and Hypopharynx." *Annals of Internal Medicine* 1990;113(1):82-3.

133 Johns AN. "Beware of the Bay Leaf." *British Medical Journal* 1980;281:1682.

134 Belitsos NJ. "Bay Leaf Impaction." *Annals of Internal Medicine* 1990;113(6): 483-4.

135 Bell CD, Mustar, RA. "Bay Leaf Perforation of Meckel's Diverticulum." *JCC* 1997;40(2):146.

136 Palin WE, Richardson JD. "Complications From Bay Leaf Ingestions." *JAMA* 1983;289(6):729-30.

137 Brokaw SA. "Complications of Bay Leaf Ingestion" [letter]. *JAMA* 1983;250(6):729.

138 Price JF. "Antioxidant vitamins in the prevention of cardiovascular disease. The epidemiological evidence." *European Heart Journal* 1997;18:719-27.

139 Omenn GS. "Chemoprevention of Lung Cancer: The

Rise and Demise of Beta-Carotene." *Annu Rev Public Health* 1998;19:73-99.

140 Giuliano AR, Gapstur S. "Can Cervical Dysplasia and Cancer Be Prevented with Nutrients?" *Nutrition Reviews* 1998;56(1):9-16.

141 Lieberman S. "A Review of the Effectiveness of Cimicifuga racemosa (Black Cohosh) for the Symptoms of Menopause." *Journal of Women's Health* 1998;7(5):525-9.

142 Jarboe CH, et al. "Uterine Relaxant Properties of Viburnium." *Nature* 1966;212:837.

143 Soderling E, et al. "Betaine-containing toothpaste relieves subjective symptoms of dry mouth." *Acta Odontol Scand* 1998;56(2):65-9.

144 Barak AJ, Beckenhauer HC, Tuma DJ. "Betaine, ethanol, and the liver, a review." *Alcohol* 1996;13(4):395-8.

145 Wilcken DE, et al. "Homocystinuria-the effects of betaine in the treatment of patients not responsive to pyridoxine." *N Engl J Med* 1983;309(8):448-53.

146 Duell PG, Malinow MR. "Homocysteine: An important risk factor for atherosclerotic vascular disease." *Curr Opin Lipidol* 1997; 8(1);28-34.

147 Bakker RC, Brandjes DP. "Hyperhomocysteinaemia and associated disease." *Pharm World Sci* 1997; 19(3):126-32.

148 Daviglus ML, et al. "Dietary beta-carotene, vitamin C, and risk of prostate cancer: results from the Western Electric Study." *Epidemiology* 1996;7(5):472-7.

149 Giovannucci E. et al. "Intake of carotenoids and retinol in relation to risk of prostate cancer." *J Natl Cancer Inst* 1995 87(23):1767-76.

150 Johnson JA, Lalonde RL. "Congestive Heart Failure." Eds. DiPiro JT, et al. Pharmacotherapy, third ed. Stamford: Appleton and Lange, 1997.

151 Sklar S. et al. Drug Therapy Screening System. Indianapolis: First Data Bank 99.1-99.2 editions.

152 Bourgoin BP, et al. Lead content in 70 brands of dietary calcium supplements. *Am J Public Health* 1993;83(8):1155-60.

153 Elmer GW, Surawicz CM, McFarland LV. "Biotherapeutic Agents, A Neglected Modality for the Treatment and Prevention of Selected Intestinal and Vaginal Infections." *JAMA* 1996;275(11): 870-5.

154 Renk BZ. Wisconsin Alumni Research Foundation. Probiotic Bifidobacterium Strains, URL: www.wisc.edu/warf.boi/p98062us.html (Accessed 29 January 1999).

155 Scarpignato C, Rampal P. Prevention and Treatment of Traveler's Diarrhea: A Clinical Pharmacological Approach. *Chemotherapy* 1995;41(suppl 1)48-81.

156 Chiesara E, Borghini R, Marabini. "Dietary fibre and drug interactions." *European Journal of Clinical Nutrition* 1995;49(suppl 3):S123-8.

157 VanHorn L. "Fiber, Lipids and Coronary Heart Disease. A Statement for Healthcare Professionals From the Nutrition Committee, American Heart Association." *Circulation* 95(12):2701-4.

158 Pandya DP "Nutrition and Coronary Heart Disease." *Comp Ther* 1998;24(4):198-204.

159 Gossel TA, Bricker JD. *Principles of Clinical Toxicology*. New York: Raven Press, 1994.

160 ECP Consensus Panel on Cereals and Cancer. *European Journal of Cancer Prevention* 1998;7(suppl 2)S1-S2.

161 Saavedra JM, et al. "Feeding of Bifidobacterium bifidum and Streptococcus thermophilus to infants in hospital for prevention of diarrhea and shedding of rotavirus." *Lancet* 1994;344:1046-9.

162 Bouhnik Y, et al. "Fecal Recovery in Humans of Viable Bifidobacterium Ingested in Fermented Milk." *Gastroenterology* 1992;102:875-8.

163 Sauvaire Y, et al. "4-hydroxyisoleucine. A novel amino acid potentiator of insulin secretion." *Diabetes* 1998;47:206-10.

164 Madar A, Thorne R. Dietary fiber. *Prog Food Nutr Sci* 1987;11:153-74.

165 Melchart D, et al. "Echinacea root extracts for the prevention of upper respiratory tract infections: a double-blind, placebo-controlled randomized trial." *Archives of Family Medicine* 1998;7(6):541-5.

166 Miller LG. "Herbal Medicinals. Selected Clinical Considerations Focusing on Known or Potential Drug-Herb Interactions." *Arch Intern Med* 1998;158:2200-11.

167 Bennett DA Jr, Phun L, Polk JF, et al. "Neuropharmacology of St. John's Wort (Hypericum)." *Ann Pharmacother* 1998 Nov;32(11):1201-8.

168 Hippius H. "St. John's Wort (Hypericum perforatum)-a herbal antidepressant." *Curr Med Res Opin* 1998;14(3):171-84.

169 Wagner J, Wagner ML, Hening WA. "Beyond Benzodiazepines: Alternative Pharmacologic Agents for the Treatment of Insomnia." *Ann Pharmacother* 1998;32(6):680-91.

170 Henry JG, Sobki S, Afafat N. "Interference by biotin therapy on measurement of TSH and FT4 by enzyme immunoassay on Boehringer Mannheim ES 700 analyzer. " *Ann Clin Biochem* 1996;33:162-3.

171 Hochman LG, Scher RK, Meyerson MS. "Brittle nails: response to daily biotin supplementation." *Cutis* 1993;51:303-5.

172 Said HM, Redha R, Nylander W. "Biotin transport in the human intestine: inhibition by anticonvulsant drugs." *Am J Clin Nutr* 1989;49:127-31.

173 Bonjour JP. "Biotin in human nutrition." *Annals New York Academy of Sciences* 1985;447:97-104.

174 Nyhan WL. "Clinical problems relating to biotin." *Annals New York Academy of Sciences* 1985;447:222-4.

175 Krause KH, et al. "Biotin Status of Epileptics." *Annals New York Academy of Sciences* 1985;447:297-313.

176 Mock DM, et al. "Disturbances in biotin Metabolism in children undergoing long-term anticonvulsant therapy." *Journal of Pediatric and Gastroentereology & Nutrition* 1998;26(3):245-50.

177 Coggeshall JC, et al. "Biotin status and plasma glucose in diabetics." *Annals New York Academy of Sciences* 1985;447:389-92.

178 Arvill A, Bodin L. "Effect of short-term ingestion of konjac glucomannan on serum cholesterol in healthy men." *Am J Clin Nutr* 1995;61(3):585-9.

179 Vido L, et al. "Childhood obesity treatment: double blinded trial on dietary fibres (glucomannan) versus placebo." *Padiatr Padol* 1993;28(5):133-6.

180 Livieri C, Novazi F, Lorini R. "The use of highly purified glucomannan-based fibers in childhood obesity." [Article in Italian] *Pediatr Med Chir* 1992;14(2):195-8.

181 Vita PM, et al. "Chronic use of glucomannan in the dietary treatment of severe obesity." [Article in Italian] *Minerv Med* 1992;83(3):135-9.

182 Walsh DE, Yaghoubian V, Behforooz A. "Effect of glucomannan on obese patients: a clinical study." *Int J Obes* 1984;8(4):289-93.

183 Cairella M, Marchini GAD. "Evaluation of the action of

glucomannan on metabolic parameters and on the sensation of satiation in overweight and obese patients". [Article in Italian] *Clin Ter*, 1995; 146:269-74.

184 Koshy KM, Griswold E, Schneeberger EE. "Interstitial Nephritis in a Patient Taking Creatine." *NEJM* 1999;340(10):814-5.

185 Kubota K, et al. "Effect of green tea on iron absorption in elderly patients with iron deficiency anemia." [Article in Japanese] *Nippon Ronen Igakkai Zasshi* 1990;27(5):555-8.

186 Barker G, et al. "The effects of sucralfate suspension and diphenhydramine syrup plus kaolin-pectin on radiotherapy-induced mucositis." *Oral Surg Oral Med Oral Pathol* 1991;71(3):288-93.

187 Carnel SB, et al. "Treatment of radiation- and chemotherapy-induced stomatitis." *Otolaryngol Head Neck Surg* 1990;102(4):326-30.

188 Epstein WL ."Topical prevention of poison ivy/oak dermatitis." *Arch Dermatol* 1989;125(4):499-501.

189 Juch RD, et al. "Pharmazeutische Praparate, Egerkingen, Schweiz. Pastes: what do they contain? How do they work?" *Dermatology* 1994;189(4):373-7.

190 Tart RP, et al. "Enteric MRI contrast agents: comparative study of five potential agents in humans." *Magn Reson Imaging* 1991;9(4):559-68.

191 Mitchell DG, et al. "Comparison of Kaopectate with barium for negative and positive enteric contrast at MR imaging." *Radiology* 1991;181(2):475-80.

192 Despotis GJ, et al. "DG Response of kaolin ACT to heparin: evaluation with an automated assay and higher heparin doses." *Ann Thorac Surg* 1996;61(3):795-9.

193 Paquet C. "Assessment of kaolin agglutination test." *Tuber Lung Dis* 1994; 75(5):397.

194 Sarnaik RM, et al. Serodiagnosis of tuberculosis: assessment of kaolin agglutination test. *Tuber Lung Dis* 1993;74(6):405-6.

195 Levin JL, et al. "Kaolinosis in a cotton mill worker." *Am J Ind Med* 1996;29(2):215-21.

196 Chaudhary BA, Kanes GJ, Pool WH. "Pleural thickening in mild kaolinosis." *South Med J* 1997; 90(11):1106-9.

197 Altekruse EB, et al. "Kaolin dust concentrations and pneumoconiosis at a kaolin mine." *Thorax* 1984;39(6):436-41.

198 Rodin SM, Johnson BF. "Pharmacokinetic interactions with digoxin." *Clin Pharmacokinet* 1988;15(4):227-44.

199 Babhair SA, Tariq M. "Effect of magnesium trisilicate and kaolin-pectin on the bioavailability of trimethoprim." *Res Commun Chem Pathol Pharmacol* 1983;40(1):165-8.

201 Dobelis IN, Dwyer J, Rattray D, Ferguson G, et.al.(Editors). Magic and Medicine of Plants. Pleasantville, NY: The Reader's Digest Association, Inc. 1986.

202 Laakmann G, Schule C, Baghai T, Kieser M. St. John's wort in mild to moderate depression: the relevance of hyperforin for the clinical efficacy *Pharmacopsychiatry* 1998;31(Suppl 1):54-9.

203 Vorbach EU, Arnoldt KH, Hubner. Efficacy and tolerability of St. John's wort extract LI 160 versus imipramine in patients with severe depressive episodes according to ICD- 10. *Pharmacopsychiatry* 1997;30(Suppl 2):81-5.

204 Wheatley D. LI 160, an extract of St. John's wort, versus amitriptyline in mildly to moderately depressed outpatients—a controlled 6-week clinical trial. *Pharmacopsychiatry* 1997;30 Suppl 2:77-80.

205 Volz HP. Controlled clinical trials of hypericum extracts in depressed patients— an overview. *Pharmacopsychiatry* 1997;30 Suppl 2:72-6.

206 Gulick RM, McAuliffe V, Holden-Wiltse J, et al. Phase I studies of hypericin, the active compound in St. John's Wort, as an antiretroviral agent in HIV-infected adults. AIDS Clinical Trials Group Protocols 150 and 258. *Ann Intern Med* 1999;130(6):510-4.

207 http://www.flash.net/%7Edrj2142/beatals.html (Accessed 6 November 1999).

208 http://www.flash.net/%7Edrj2142/files/creatine.txt (Accessed 6 November 1999).

209 Kostyuk VA, Potapovich AI. Antiradical and chelating effects in flavonoid protection against silica-induced cell injury. *Arch Biochem Biophys* 1998;355(1):43-8.

210 Rahn R, Adamietz IA, Boettcher HD, et al. Povidone-iodine to prevent mucositis in patients during antineoplastic radiochemotherapy. *Dermatology* 1997;195(Suppl 2):57-61.

211 Drewa G, Schachtschabel DO, Palgan K, et al. The influence of rutin on the weight, metastasis and melanin content of B16 melanotic melanoma in C57BL/6 mice. *Neoplasma* 1998;45(4):266-71.

212 Kehoe, WA. Ginkgo biloba for SSRI-induced sexual dysfunction. Therapeutic Research Center. *Pharmacist's Letter* 1997;13(9):130916.

213 Paick J, Lee J. An experimental study of the effect of ginkgo biloba extract on the human and rabbit corpus cavernosum tissue. *J Urol* 1996;156:1876-80.

214 Fetrow CW, Avala JR. Professional's Handbook of Complementary and Alternative Medicines. Springhouse Corporation, 1999.

215 Osol and Farar. The Dispensatory of the United States of America, 25th ed. JB Lippincott Company, 1955.

216 Dorland's Illustrated Medical Dictionary, 25th ed. WB Saunders Company, 1974.

217 Pheatt N, ed. *Sports Supplements. Pharmacist's Letter* Continuing Education Booklet 1999;99(2):1-56.

219 Pratt S. Dietary prevention of age-related macular degeneration. *J Am Optom Assoc* 1999;70:39-47.

220 Hertog MGL, Sweetnam PM, Fehily AM, et al. Antioxidant flavonols and ischemic heart disease in a Welsh population of men: the Caerphilly Study. *Am J Clin Nutr* 1997;65:1489-94.

221 Jacob SW, Lawrence RM, Zucker M, Regelson W. The Miracle of MSM: The Natural Solution for Pain. Penquin USA, February 1999.

222 Chen J, Wollman Y, Chernichovsky T, et al. Effect of oral administration of high-dose nitric oxide donor L-arginine in men with organic erectile dysfunction: results of a double-blind, randomized, placebo-controlled study. *BJU Int* 1999;83:269-73.

223 Johnson N. Sun trap. 24 July 1999. URL: http://www.newscientist.com/ns/1990724/newsstory9.html (Accessed 20 August 1999).

224 Leonetti HB, Longo S, Anasti JN. Transdermal progesterone cream for vasomotor symptoms and postmenopausal bone loss. *Obstet Gynecol* 1999;94:225-8.

225 Bracco GL, Carli P, Sonni L, et al. Clinical and histologic effects of topical treatments of vulval lichen sclerosus. A critical evaluation. *J Reprod Med* 1993;38(1):37-40.

226 Langer RD. Micronized progesterone: a new therapeutic option. *Int J Fertil Womens Med* 1999;44(2):67-73.

227 Licciardi FL, Kwiatkoski A, Noyes NL, et al. Oral

1156 • © Copyright 2000, Natural Medicines Comprehensive Database (209) 472-2244. For updated data, go to www.NaturalDatabase.com.

REFERENCES

versus intramuscular progesterone for in vitro fertilization: a prospective randomized study. *Fertil Steril* 1999;71(4):614-8.

228 Greendale GA, Reboussin BA, Hogan P, et al. Symptom relief and side effects of postmenopausal hormones: results from the Postmenopausal Interventions Trial. *Obstet Gynecol* 1998;92(6):982-8.

229 Jellin J, ed. Dietary Supplements. *Pharmacist's Letter* 1999;14(4):22.

230 Sloane P. Advances in the treatment of Alzheimer's disease. *An Fam Physician* 1998;58:1577-86, 1589-90.

231 Morris M, Beckett L, Scherr P, et al. Vitamin E and vitamin C supplement use and risk of incident Alzheimer's disease. *Alzheimer's Dis Assoc Disord* 1998;12:121-6.

232 Sano M, Ernesto C, Thomas R, et al. A controlled trial of selegiline, alpha-tocopherol, or both as treatment for Alzheimer's disease. The Alzheimer's Disease Cooperative Study. *N Engl J Med* 1997;336:1216-22.

233 Chakravarty N. Inhibition of histamine release from mast cells by nigellone. *Ann Allergy* 1993;70(3):237-42.

234 Haq A, Abdullatif M, Lobo PI, et al. Black seed: effect on human lymphocytes and polymorphonuclear leukocyte phagocytic activity. *Immunopharmacology* 1995;30(2):147-55.

235 Houghton PJ, Zarka R, de las Heras B, Hoult JR. Fixed oil of Black seed and derived thymoquinone inhibit eicosanoid generation in leukocytes and membrane lipid peroxidation. *Planta Med* 1995;61(1):33-6.

236 Salomi NJ, Nair SC, Jayawardhanan KK, et al. Antitumour principles from Black seed seeds. *Cancer Lett* 1992;63(1):41-6.

237 Daba MH, Abdel-Rahman MS. Hepatoprotective activity of thymoquinone in isolated rat hepatocytes. *Toxicol Lett* 1998;95(1):23-9.

238 Worthen DR, Ghosheh OA, Crooks PA. The in vitro anti-tumor activity of some crude and purified components of blackseed, Black seed L. *Anticancer Res* 1998;18(3A):1527-32.

239 Badary OA, Al-Shabanah OA, Nagi MN, et al. Inhibition of benzo(a)pyrene-induced forestomach carcinogenesis in mice by thymoquinone. *Eur J Cancer Prev* 1999;8(5):435-40.

240 Nagi MN, Alam K, Badary OA, et al. Thymoquinone protects against carbon tetrachloride hepatotoxicity in mice via an antioxidant mechanism. *Biochem Mol Biol Int* 1999;47(1):153-9.

241 Aqel M, Shaheen R. Effects of the volatile oil of Black seed seeds on the uterine smooth muscle of rat and guinea pig. *J Ethnopharmacol* 1996;52(1):23-6.

242 Keshri G, Singh MM, Lakshmi V, Kamboj VP. Post-coital contraceptive efficacy of the seeds of Black seed in rats. *Indian J Physiol Pharmacol* 1995;39(1):59-62.

243 Hanafy MS, Hatem ME. Studies on the antimicrobial activity of Black seed seed (black cumin). *J Ethnopharmacol* 1991;34(2-3):275-8.

244 Akhtar MS, Riffat S. Field trial of Saussurea lappa roots against nematodes and Black seed seeds against cestodes in children. *J Pak Med Assoc* 1991;41(8):185-7.

245 Tennekoon KH, Jeevathayaparan S, Kurukulasooriya AP, Karunanayake EH. Possible hepatotoxicity of Black seed seeds and Dregea volubilis leaves. *J Ethnopharmacol* 1991;31(3):283-9.

246 Medenica RD. Use of Black seed to increase immune function. U.S. Patent 5,482,711, issued January 9, 1996. Obtained from The United States Patent and Trademark Office on April 12, 2000 http://www.uspto.gov/patft/index.htm.

250 Bucci AJ, et al. In vitro interaction of quinidine with kaolin and pectin. *Pharm Sci* 1981;70(9):999-1002.

251 Allen MD, et al. "Effect of magnesium-aluminum hydroxide and kaolin-pectin on absorption of digoxin from tablets and capsules." *J Clin Pharmacol* 1981;21(1):26-30.

252 Albert KS, et al. "Influence of kaolin-pectin suspension on digoxin bioavailability." *J Pharm Sc* 1978;67(11):1582-6.

253 Albert KS, et al. "Pharmacokinetic evaluation of a drug interaction between kaolin-pectin and clindamycin." *J Pharm Sci* 1978 67(11):1579-82.

254 Huyzen RJ, et al. "Alternative perioperative anticoagulation monitoring during cardiopulmonary bypass in aprotinin-treated patients." *J Cardiothorac Vasc Anesth* 1994;8(2):153-6.

255 Grim W, Muller H. "A Randomized Controlled Trial of the Effect of Fluid Extract of Echinacea Purpurea on the Incidence and Severity of Colds and Respiratory Infections." *The American Journal of Medicine* 106:138-143.

256 He K, et al. "Additional bioactive annonaceous acetogenins from Asminia triloba (Annonaceae)." *Bioorg Med Chem* 1997;5(3):501-6.

257 Ratnayake S, et al. "Evaluation of various parts of the paw paw tree, Asmina triloba (Annonaceae), as commercial sources for the pesticidal annonaceous acetogenins." *J Econ Entomol* 1992;85(6):2353-6.

258 Zhao GX, et al. "Asimin, asimininacin, and asiminecin: novel highly cytotoxic asimicin isomers from Asiminia triloba." *J Med Chem* 1994;37(13):1971-6.

259 Johnson JA, Lalonde R. "Congestive Heart Failure." Eds. Dipiro JT, et al. Pharmacotherapy, A Pathophysiologic Approach 3rd ed., 1997;232.

260 Cone EH, Lange R, Darwin WD. "In vivo adulteration: excess fluid ingestion causes false-negative marijuana and cocaine urine test results." *J Anal Toxicol* 1998;22(6):460-73.

261 Wu AH, et al. "CEDIA for screening drugs of abuse in urine and the effect of adulterants." *J Forensic Sci* 1995;40(4):614-8.

262 Rabbani GH, et al. "Randomized controlled trial of berberine sulfate therapy for diarrhea due to enterotoxigenic Escherichia coli and Vibrio cholerae." *J Infect Dis* 1987;155(5):979-84.

263 Sheng WD, et al. "Treatment of chloroquine-resistant malaria using pyrimethamine in combination with berberine, tetracycline, or cotrimoxazole." *East Afr Med J* 1997;74(5):283-4.

264 Khosla PG, et al. "Berberine, a potential drug for trachoma." *Rev Int Trach Pathol Ocul Trop Subtrop Sante Publique* 1992;69:147-65.

265 Tamminga C, et al. "Depression associated with oral choline." [letter] *Lancet* 1976;2(7991):905.

266 Facts and Comparisons staff. *Drug Facts and Comparisons*. St Louis: Wolters Kluwer Company (updated monthly).

267 *Pharmacist's Letter* "Chaparral." February, 1999.

268 Merck Index, 12th ed. Whitehouse Station: Merck Research Laboratories, 1996.

269 Neal H. Dictionary of Chemical Names and Synonyms. Chelsea: Lewis Publishers, 1992.

270 Parker SP. ed. McGraw Hill Dictionary of Chemistry. New York: McGraw-Hill Book Company 1984.

REFERENCES

271 Bruneton J. Pharmacognosy, Phytochemistry, Medicinal Plants. Paris: Lavoisier Publishing, 1995.

272 Covington TR, et al. Handbook of Nonprescription Drugs. Washington, D.C.: the American Pharmaceutical Association, 1996.

273 FDA. "FDA warns about GBL-related products." *FDA Talk Paper.* vm.cfsan.fda.gov/~1rd/ (Accessed 11 May 1999).

274 Chenoy R, et al. "Effect of oral gamolenic acid from evening primrose oil on menopausal flushing." *BMJ* 19 Feb 1994; 308(6927):501-3.

275 Young DS. Effects of Drugs on Clinical Laboratory Tests 4th ed. Washington: AACC Press, 1995.

276 Balch JF, Balch PA. Prescription for Nutritional Healing. Garden City Park: Avery Publishing Group, 1997.

277 Silagy CA, Neil HA. "A meta-analysis of the effect of garlic on blood pressure." *J Hypertension* 1994;12(4):463-8.

278 McMahon FG, Vargas R. "Can garlic lower blood pressure? A pilot study." *Pharmacotherapy* 1993;13(4):406-7.

279 Auer W, Eiber A, Hertkorn E, et al. Hypertension and hyperlipidaemia: garlic helps in mild cases. *Br J Clin Pract Symp Suppl* 1990;69:3-6.

280 Hentschel C, Dressler S, Hahn EG. "Fumaria officinalis (fumitory)-clinical applications." *Fortschr Med* 1995;113(19):291-2.

281 Pittler MH, Ernst E. "Horse-chestnut seed extract for chronic venous insufficiency. A criteria-based systematic review." *Arch Dermatol* 1998;134(11):1356-60.

282 Greeske K, Pohlmann BK. "Horse chestnut seed extract-an effective therapy principle in general practice. Drug therapy of chronic venous insufficiency." *Fortschr Med* 1996;14(15):196-200.

283 Diehm C, et al. "Comparison of leg compression stocking and oral horse-chestnut seed extract in patients with chronic venous insufficiency." *Lancet* 1996;347(8997):292-4.

284 Diehm C, et al. "Medical edema protection-clinical benefit in patients with chronic deep vein incompetence." *Vassa* 1992;21(2):188-92.

285 Bisler H, et al. "Effects of horse-chestnut seed on transcapillary filtration in chronic venous insufficiency." *Dtsch Med Wochenschr* 1986;111(35):1321-9.

286 Mohler JL, et al. Phase II evaluation of coumarin (1,2-benzopyrone) in metastatic prostatic carcinoma. *Prostate* 1992;20(2):123-31.

287 Marshall ME, Butler K, Fried A. *Mol Biother* 1991;3(3):170-8.

288 Howanitz JH, Howanitz PJ, eds. "Renal Function" by D.O. Rogerson Laboratory Medicine Test Selection and Interpretation. New York: Churchill Livingstone, 1991.

289 van Joost T, Smitt JH, van Ketel WG. "Sensitization to olive oil (olea europeae)." *Contact Dermatitis* 1981;7(6):309-10.

290 Privitera JR. "Olive Leaf Extract : A New/Old Healing Bonanza for Mankind." URL: www.oliveleafextract.com/contents.html (23 Jun 1999).

291 Bakerink JA, Gospe SM Jr, Dimand RJ, Eldridge MW. Multiple organ failure after ingestion of pennyroyal oil from herbal tea in two infants. *Pediatrics* 1996;98(5):944-7.

292 Sudekum M, Poppenga RH, Raju N, Braselton WE Jr. Pennyroyal oil toxicosis in a dog. *J Am Vet Med Assoc* 1992;200(6):817-8.

293 Gittleman AL. Eat Fat, Lose Weight. Los Angeles: Keat's Publishing 1999.

294 Werbach M. Healing Through Nutrition. A Natural Approach to Treating 50 Common Illnesses with Diet and Nutrients. New York: Harper Collins 1993.

295 Ritschel WA, Brady ME, Tan HIS, et al. Pharmacokinetics of Coumarin and its 7-hyroxy-metabolites upon intravenous and peroral administration of coumarin in man. *European Journal of Clinical Pharmacology* 1997;12:457-61.

296 Website URL: www.ars-grin.gov/duke/ (Accessed 7 July 1999).

297 Cox D, O'Kennedy R, Thornes RD. "The rarity of toxicity in patients treated with coumarin (1,2-benzopyrone)." *Hum Toxicol* 1989;(6):501-6.

298 Mann J, Truswell AS, eds. Essentials of Human Nutrition. Oxford: Oxford University Press 1998.

299 Rozanova IA, et al. "Effect of antiatherosclerotic diet, containing polyunsaturated fatty acids of the omega-3 family from flax oil, on fatty acid composition of cell membranes of patients with ischemic heart disease. Hypertensive disease and hyperlipoproteinemia." *Vopr Pitan* 1997;(5):15-7.

300 Zarembo JE, Godfrey JC, Godfrey NJ. Zinc(II) in saliva: determination of concentrations produced by different formulations of zinc gluconate lozenges containing common excipients. *J Pharm Sci* 1992;81(2):128-30.

301 Goldenberg RL, Tamura T, Neggers Y, et al. The effect of zinc supplementation on pregnancy outcome." *JAMA* 1995;274(6):463-8.

302 Upton R, ed. Hawthorn Berry: analytical, quality control, and therapeutic monograph. Santa Cruz, CA: *American Herbal Pharmacopoeia* 1999;1-19.

303 Upton R (ed). Astragalus Root: analytical, quality control, and therapeutic monograph. Santa Cruz, CA: *American Herbal Pharmacopoeia*; 1999;1-25.

304 Upton R, ed. Valerian Root: analytical, quality control, and therapeutic monograph. Santa Cruz, CA: *American Herbal Pharmacopoeia*; 1999;1-25.

305 Life Extension Foundation web site. URL http://lef.org/prod_desc/item132.html (Accessed 7 September 1999).

306 Nature's Life web site, URL http://www.natlife.com/pancreat.htm (Accessed 7 September 1999).

307 Huggins C. Calcium-rich food at each meal ensures intake. New York, Reuters Health, Oct. 1, 1999, www.reutershealth.com/eline/open/1999100109.html (Accessed 4 October 1999).

308 FDA. Office of Regulatory Affairs Food Additive Status List, URL: www.fda.gov/ora/inspect-ref/iom/exhibits/ApA2.html (Accessed 5 October 1999).

309 Fatty acid may be key to new treatment for cystic fibrosis. Reuters Health website, URL:www.reutershealth.com/eline/open/1999100810.html (Accessed 10 October 1999).

310 Penzak SR, Gubbins PO, Gurley BJ, et al. Grapefruit juice decreases the systemic availability of itraconazole capsules in healthy volunteers. *Ther Drug Monit* 1999;21(3):304-9.

311 FTC Charges Marketer of "Vitamin O" with Making False Health Claims. Federal Trade Commission website, URL: www.ftc.gov/opa/1999/9903/rosecreek.htm (Accessed 12 October 1999).

312 MedicineShoppe.com website, URL: www.medicineshoppe.com (Accessed 14 October 1999).

313 Mehta DK (Ex Ed). British National Formulary, Number 37. British Medical Association and Royal Pharmaceutical Society of Great Britain: London,

England, March 1999.

314 Breastfeeding/Nursing/Parenting, Herbs for Milk Production. URL:www.gentlebirth.org/archives/ bestfeed.html#Herbs (Accessed 18 October 1999).

317 Fernandez-Anaya S, Crespo JF, Rodriguez JR, et al. Beer anaphylaxis. *J Allergy Clin Immunol* 1999;103(5 Pt 1):959-60.

318 Katz DL. Acute nutrient effects in endothelial function: a randomized, single-blind crossover trial in healthy adults. American College of Nutrition 40th Annual Meeting, October 1999, Washington, DC.

319 Watson Nutritional Products Group website, URL:www.yuanlin.com.tw/e/efunction.html (Accessed 8 September 1999).

320 Watson Nutritional Products Group website, URL:www.yuanlin.com.tw/e/eorder.html (Accessed 8 September 1999).

321 Traditional Uses for Medicinal Mushrooms, Garuda International website, URL: garudaint.com/ amush.htm#cordyceps (Accessed 9 September 1999).

322 Morreale P, Manopulo R, Galati M, et al. Comparison of the anti-inflammatory efficacy of chondroitin sulfate and diclofenac sodium in patients with knee osteoarthritis. *J Rheumatol* 1996;23(8):1385-91.

323 Conrozier T. [Anti-arthrosis treatments: efficacy and tolerance of chondroitin sulfates]. [Article in French] *Presse Med* 1998;27(36):1862-5.

324 Mazieres B, Loyau G, Menkes CJ, et al. [Chondroitin sulfate in the treatment of gonarthrosis and coxarthrosis. 5-months result of a multicenter double-blind controlled prospective study using placebo]. [Article in French] *Rev Rhum Mal Osteoartic* 1992;59(7-8):466-72.

325 O'Breasail AM, Argouarch S. Hypomania and St John's wort. *Can J Psychiatry* 1998;43(7):746-7.

326 Trivedy C, Warnakulasuriya S, Peters TJ. Areca nuts can have deleterious effects. *BMJ* 1999;318(7193):1287.

327 Cox SC, Walker DM. Oral submucous fibrosis. A review. *Aust Dent J* 1996;41(5):294-9.

328 Gupta PC, Sinor PN, Bhonsle RB, et al. Oral submucous fibrosis in India: a new epidemic? *Natl Med J India* 1998;11(3):113-6.

329 VanWyk CW. Oral submucous fibrosis. The South African experience. *Indian J Dent Res* 1997 8(2):39-45.

330 Wiid I, Hoal-van Helden E, Hon D, et al. Potentiation of isoniazid activity against Mycobacterium tuberculosis by melatonin. *Antimicrob Agents Chemother* 1999;43(4):975-7.

331 Barceloux DG. Zinc. *J Toxicol Clin Toxicol* 1999;37(2):279-92.

332 (no authors listed). Zinc for the common cold. *Med Lett Drugs Ther* 1997;39(993):9-10.

333 Mossad SB, Macknin ML, Medendorp SV, Mason P. Zinc gluconate lozenges for treating the common cold. A randomized, double-blind, placebo-controlled study. *Ann Intern Med* 1996;125(2):81-8.

334 Godfrey JC, Conant Sloane B, Smith DS, et al. Zinc gluconate and the common cold: a controlled clinical study. *J Int Med Res* 1992;20(3):234-6.

335 Al-Nakib W, Higgins PG, Barrow I, et al. Prophylaxis and treatment of rhinovirus colds with zinc gluconate lozenges. *J Antimicrob Chemother* 1987;20(6):893-901.

336 Eby GA, Davis DR, Halcomb WW. Reduction in duration of common colds by zinc gluconate lozenges in a double-blind study. *Antimicrob Agents Chemother* 1984;25(1):20-4.

337 Farr BM, Conner EM, Betts RF, et al. Two randomized controlled trials of zinc gluconate lozenge therapy of experimentally induced rhinovirus colds. *Antimicrob Agents Chemother* 1987;31(8):1183-7.

338 Smith DS, Helzner EC, Nuttall CE Jr, et al. Failure of zinc gluconate in treatment of acute upper respiratory tract infections. *Antimicrob Agents Chemother* 1989;33(5):646-8.

339 Weismann K, Jakobsen JP, Weismann JE, et al. Zinc gluconate lozenges for common cold. A double-blind clinical trial. *Dan Med Bull* 1990;37(3):279-81.

340 Eby GA. Zinc ion availability—the determinant of efficacy in zinc lozenge treatment of common colds. *J Antimicrob Chemother* 1997;40(4):483-93.

341 Macknin ML, Piedmonte M, Calendine C, et al. Zinc gluconate lozenges for treating the common cold in children: a randomized controlled trial. *JAMA* 1998;279(24):1962-7.

342 VitaminShoppe.com website, URL: www.vitaminshoppe.com/ product.asp?dispmode=quick&tab=1&sku=ON-1028 (Accessed 3 November 1999).

343 Stevia. MotherNature.com website, URL: www.mothernature.com/ency/Herb/Stevia.asp (Accessed 3 November 1999).

344 Mother's intake of soy may affect development of fetus. Reuters website, URL: www.reutershealth.com/ frame_eline.html (Accessed 5 November 1999).

345 Carta A, Calvani M, Bravi D, Bhuachalla SN. "Acetyl-L-carnitine and Alzheimer's disease: pharmacological considerations beyond the cholinergic sphere." *Ann N Y Acad Sci* 1993;695:324-6.

346 Orange juice raises "good" cholesterol. Reuters Health, URL: www.reutershealth.com/frame_elinehtml (Accessed 9 November 1999).

347 SAMe for depression. *Medical Letter* 1999;41:107-8.

348 CBS HealthWatch by Medscape, URL: healthwatch.medscape.com/medscape/p/gcommunity/ ghome2.asp (Accessed 16 November 1999).

349 Garfinkel D, Zisapel N, Wainstein J, Laudon M. Facilitation of benzodiazepine discontinuation by melatonin, a new clinical approach. *Arch Intern Med* 1999;159(20):2456-60.

350 Glucosamine reduces knee osteoarthritis. Reuters Health Nov. 15, 1999. Reuters Health, URL: www.reutershealth.com/frame_eline.html (Accessed 16 November 1999).

351 Black walnut hull capsules, VitaminShoppe.com website, URL: www.vitaminshoppe.com/ product.asp?dispmode=quick&tab=1&sku=NW-1035(Accessed 16 November 1999).

352 Black walnut hull liquid extract, VitaminShoppe.com website, URL: www.vitaminshoppe.com/ product.asp?dispmode=quick&tab=1&sku=NW-2263 (Accessed 16 November 1999).

353 Reishi: Ancient medicine is modern hope. URL: home.pacific.net.hk/~gng/reishi.html (Accessed 20 November 1999).

354 Kobashi Y, Nakajima M, Niki Y, Matsushima T. [A case of acute eosinophilic pneumonia due to Sho-saiko-to]. [Article in Japanese] *Nippon Kyobu Shikkan Gakkai Zasshi* 1997;35(12):1372-7.

355 Wada Y, Kubo M. [Acute lymphoblastic leukemia complicated by type C hepatitis during treatment and further by acute interstitial pneumonia due to sho-saiko-to in 7-year-old]. [Article in Japanese] *Arerugi* 1997;46(11):1148-55.

REFERENCES

356 Sato A, Toyoshima M, Kondo A, et al. [Pneumonitis induced by the herbal medicine Sho-saiko-to in Japan]. [Article in Japanese] *Nippon Kyobu Shikkan Gakkai Zasshi* 1997;35(4):391-5.

357 Daibo A, Yoshida Y, Kitazawa S, et al. [A case of pneumonitis and hepatic injury caused by a herbal drug (sho-saiko-to)]. [Article in Japanese] *Nippon Kyobu Shikkan Gakkai Zasshi* 1992;30(8):1583-8.

358 Sugiyama H, Nagai M, Kotajima F, et al. [A case of interstitial pneumonia with chronic hepatitis C following interferon-alfa and sho-saiko-to therapy]. [Article in Japanese] *Arerugi* 1995;44(7):711-4.

359 Ishizaki T, Sasaki F, Ameshima S, et al. Pneumonitis during interferon and/or herbal drug therapy in patients with chronic active hepatitis. *Eur Respir J* 1996;9(12):2691-6.

360 Nakagawa A, Yamaguchi T, Takao T, Amano H. [Five cases of drug induced pneumonitis due to Sho-saiko-to or interferon-alpha or both]. [Article in Japanese] *Nippon Kyobu Shikkan Gakkai Zasshi* 1995;33(12):1361-6.

361 Miyazaki E, Ando M, Ih K, et al. [Pulmonary edema associated with the Chinese medicine shosaikoto]. [Article in Japanese] *Nihon Kokyuki Gakkai Zasshi* 1998;36(9):776-80.

362 Piras G, Makino M, Baba M. Sho-saiko-to, a traditional Kampo medicine, enhances the anti-HIV-1 activity of lamivudine (3TC) in vitro. *Microbiol Immunol* 1997;41(10):835-9.

363 Benninger J, Schneider HT, Schuppan D, et al. Acute Hepatitis Induced by Greater Celandine (Chelidonium majus). *Gastroenterology* 1999;117(5):1234-7.

364 Pipeline. Paladin Labs, Inc. website, URL: www.pharmanex.com/e/index.html (Accessed 21 November 1999).

365 FDA. Guide to inspections of cosmetic product manufacturers: Products containing estrogenic hormones, placental extract or vitamins. FDA website, URL: www.fda.gov/ora/inspect_ref/igs/cosmet.html (Accessed 22 November 1999).

366 Nityanand S, Srivastava JS, Asthana OP. Clinical trials with gugulipid. A new hypolipidaemic agent. *J Assoc Physicians India* 1989;37(5):323-8.

367 Arandjelovic C. Canadian Health Officials Pull Chinese Herbal Drugs. (Reprinted from Reuters). *Richters HerbLetter*, 23 November 1999.

368 Skopnik H, Heimann G. [Manifestation of intolerance to cow's milk protein in mucoviscidosis with the symptom triad of hypoproteinemia, edema and anemia]. [Article in German] *Klin Padiatr* 1987;199(6):453-6.

369 "New health claim proposed for relationship of soy protein and coronary heart disease". Food and Drug Administration. URL: http://www.fda.gov/bbs/topics/ANSWERS/ANS00923.html (Accessed 16 November 1999).

370 Benowitz LI, Goldberg DE, Madsen JR, et al. Inosine stimulates extensive axon collateral growth in the rat corticospinal tract after injury. *Proc Natl Acad Sci* 1999;96(23):13486-90.

371 Balkan B, Dunning BE. Glucosamine inhibits glucokinase in vitro and produces a glucose-specific impairment of in vivo insulin secretion in rats. *Diabetes* 1994;43(10):1173-9.

372 Giaccari A, Morviducci L, Zorretta D, et al. In vivo effects of glucosamine on insulin secretion and insulin sensitivity in the rat: possible relevance to the maladaptive responses to chronic hyperglycaemia. *Diabetologia* 1995;38(5):518-24.

373 Sinupret, URL: www.takeyourq.com/secondary/sinus_copy.html (Accessed 29 November 1999).

374 Neubauer N, Marz RW. Placebo-controlled, randomized double-blind clincal trial with Sinupret® sugar coated tablets on the basis of a therapy with antibiotics and decongestant nasal drops in acute sinusitis. *Phytomedicine* 1994;1:177-81.

375 Govers MJ, Gannon NJ, Dunshea FR, et al. Wheat bran affects the site of fermentation of resistant starch and luminal indexes related to colon cancer risk: a study in pigs. *Gut* 1999;45:840-7.

376 Hubner WD, Lande S, Podzuweit H. Hypericum treatment of mild depressions with somatic symptoms. *Geriatr Psychiatry Neurol* 1994;7 Suppl 1:S12-4.

377 Stevinson C, Dixon M, Ernst E. Hypericum for fatigue. *Phytomedicine* 1998;5(6):443-7.

378 Heavy cocaine use puts rate of coronary aneurysms at 30%. Reuters Health, Nov. 29, 1999, URL: www.reutershealth.com/frame_mednews.html (Accessed 29 November 1999).

379 Marz RW, Ismail C, Popp MA. Action profile and efficacy of a herbal combination preparation for the treatment of sinusitis. *Wien Med Wochenschr* 1999;149(8-10):202-8.

380 Dupuis, C. Poison ivy. Pharmacy Practice, 1995;11(5):51-2,54-5.

381 Malinow MR, Bardana EJ Jr, Goodnight SH Jr. Pancytopenia during ingestion of alfalfa seeds. *Lancet* 14 March 1981;1(8220 Pt 1):615.

382 Johne A, Brockmoller J, Bauer S, et al. Pharmacokinetic interaction of digoxin with an herbal extract from St John's wort (Hypericum perforatum). *Clin Pharmacol Ther* 1999;66(4):338-45.

383 Dalvi SS, Nayak VK, Pohujani SM, et al. Effect of gugulipid on bioavailability of diltiazem and propranolol. *J Assoc Physicians India* 1994;42(6):454-5.

384 JointFlex website, URL: www.jointflex.com/products.html (Accessed 4 December 1999).

385 Zicam. URL:www.zicam.com/home.html (Accessed 9 December 1999).

386 Soy Isoflavones Strengthen Bone Mass in Women, Chinese Study Reports; 'Encouraging News' on Fractures. PR Newswire website, URL: www.prnewswire.com (Accessed 12 December 1999).

387 FDA Talk Paper: FDA Takes Action Against Firm Marketing Unapproved Drugs. FDA website. URL: www.fda.gov/bbs/topics/ANSWERS/ANS00988.html (Accessed 14 December 1999).

388 Goldwaser I, Li J, Gershonov E, Armoni M, et al. L-Glutamic acid gamma-monohydroxamate. A potentiator of vanadium-evoked glucose Metabolism in vitro and in vivo. *J Biol Chem* 1999;274(37):26617-24.

389 Duda RB, Zhong Y, Navas V, et al. American ginseng and breast cancer therapeutic agents synergistically inhibit MCF-7 breast cancer cell growth. *J Surg Oncol* 1999;72(4):230-9.

390 Strahl S, Ehret V, Dahm HH, Maier KP. [Necrotizing hepatitis after taking herbal medication]. [Article in German] *Dtsch Med Wochenschr* 1998;123(47):1410-4.

391 Vitamins may interfere with cancer chemotherapy. Reuters Health website, URL: www.reutershealth.com/frame_eline.html (Accessed 15 December 1999).

392 Wild Indigo, MotherNature.com website, URL:www.mothernature.com/ency/Herb/

Wild_Indigo.asp (Accessed 18 December 1999).

393 Beuscher N, Scheit KH, Bodinet C, Kopanski L. [Immunologically active glycoproteins of Baptisia tinctoria]. [Article in German] *Planta Med* 1989;55(4):358-63.

394 Anon. A better treatment for depression? University of California at Berkeley *Wellness Letter* 1997;13(12):1-2.

395 Subrahmanyam M. A prospective randomized clinical and histological study of superficial burn wound healing with honey and silver sulfadiazine. *Burns* 1998;24(2):157-61.

396 Subrahmanyam M. Honey dressing versus boiled potato peel in the treatment of burns: a prospective randomized study. *Burns* 1996;22(6):491-3.

397 Subrahmanyam M. Honey-impregnated gauze versus amniotic membrane in the treatment of burns. *Burns* 1994;20(4):331-3.

398 Subrahmanyam M. Honey impregnated gauze versus polyurethane film (OpSite) in the treatment of burns—a prospective randomized study. *Br J Plast Surg* 1993;46(4):322-3.

399 Subrahmanyam M. Topical application of honey in treatment of burns. *Br J Surg* 1991;78(4):497-8.

400 Magic and Medicine of Plants. 7th ed. New York: Readers Digest Association, 1993.

402 Covington TR, ed. The Handbook of Non-Prescription Drugs. Washington, DC: APhA, 1996.

403 Whitney E, Cataldo CB, Rolfes SR, eds. Understanding Normal and Clinical Nutrition. Belmont, CA: Wadsworth, 1998.

404 Kehoe WA. "Grapefruit juice and lovastatin: Is this an important interaction?" *Pharmacist's Letter*, Dec. 1998:Detail Document #141204.

405 Cook IJ, et al. "Effect of dietary fiber on rectosigmoid motility in patients with irritable bowel syndrome: A controlled, crossover study." *Gastroenterology* 1990;98:66-72.

406 Upton R, ed. Hawthorn Leaf with Flower: quality control, analytical and therapeutic monograph. Santa Cruz, CA: American Herbal Pharmacopoeia; 1999;1-29.

407 Thrive Online website. URL http://thriveonline.com/health/Library/vitamins/vitamin215.html (Accessed 22 November 1999).

408 Native American Indian Resources website. URL http://indy4.fdl.cc.mn.us/~isk/food/parttrib.html (Accessed 22 November 1999).

410 A Modern Herbal (Mrs.M.Grieve) website. URL http://botanical.com/botanical/mgmh/s/squawv85.html (Accessed 25 November 1999).

411 HolisticOnLine website. URL http://holisticonline.com/Herbal-Med/_scripts/getHerb_Dir.idc?Herb_Names=275 (Accessed 25 November 1999).

412 Woo KS, Chook P, Lolin YI, et al. Folic acid improves arterial endothelial function in adults with hyperhomocysteinemia. *J Am Coll Cardiol* 1999;34:2002-6.

413 Horticopia plant information website. URL www.horticopia.com/p&a.htm (Accessed 5 December 1999).

414 Common poisonous or irritating plants. Star Nursery website. URL www.starnursery.com/005.htm (Accessed 18 December 1999).

415 MotherNature.com Health Encyclopedia. URL www.mothernature.com/ency/Herb/Ligustrum.asp (Accessed 5 December 1999).

416 Pajaron MJ, Vila L, Prieto I, et al. Cross-reactivity of Olea europaea with other Oleaceae species in allergic rhinitis and bronchial asthma. *Allergy* 1997;52(8):829-35.

417 Batanero E, Gonzalez De La Pena MA, Villalba M, et al. Isolation, cDNA cloning and expression of Lig v 1, the major allergen from privet pollen. *Clin Exp Allergy* 1996;26(12):1401-10.

418 Khoo KS, Ang PT. Extract of astragalus membranaceus and ligustrum lucidum does not prevent cyclophosphamide-induced myelosuppression. *Singapore Med J* 1995;36(4):387-90.

419 Lau BH, Ruckle HC, Botolazzo T, Lui PD. Chinese medicinal herbs inhibit growth of murine renal cell carcinoma. *Cancer Biother* 1994;9(2):153-61.

420 Niikawa M, Hayashi H, Sato T, et al. Isolation of substances from glossy privet (Ligustrum lucidum Ait.) inhibiting the mutagenicity of benzo[a]pyrene in bacteria. *Mutat Res* 1993;319(1):1-9.

421 Rittenhouse JR, Lui PD, Lau BH. Chinese medicinal herbs reverse macrophage suppression induced by urological tumors. *J Urol* 1991;146(2):486-90.

423 Sun Y, Hersh EM, Talpaz M, et al. Immune restoration and/or augmentation of local graft versus host reaction by traditional Chinese medicinal herbs. *Cancer* 1983;52(1):70-3.

424 Lucas A, Stafford M, Morley R, et al. Efficacy and safety of long-chain polyunsaturated fatty acid supplementation of infant-formula milk: a randomised trial. *Lancet* 1999;354(9194):1948-54.

425 Gibson RA. Long-chain polyunsaturated fatty acids and infant development (editorial). *Lancet* 1999;354(9194):1919.

426 Arjmandi BH, Birnbaum RS, Juma S, et al. The synthetic phytoestrogen, ipriflavone, and estrogen prevent bone loss by different mechanisms. *Calcif Tissue Int* 2000;66(1):61-5.

427 Melis GB, Paoletti AM, Bartolini R, et al. Ipriflavone and low doses of estrogens in the prevention of bone mineral loss in climacterium. *Bone Miner* 1992;19,Suppl 1:S49-56.

428 Agnusdei D, Adami S, Cervetti R, et al. Effects of ipriflavone on bone mass and calcium Metabolism in postmenopausal osteoporosis. *Bone Miner* 1992;19,Suppl 1:S43-8.

430 Ohta H, Komukai S, Makita K, et al. Effects of 1-year ipriflavone treatment on lumbar bone mineral density and bone metabolic markers in postmenopausal women with low bone mass. *Horm Res* 1999;51(4):178-83.

431 Head KA. Ipriflavone: an important bone-building isoflavone. *Altern Med Rev* 1999;4(1):10-22.

432 Agnusdei D, Bufalino L. Efficacy of ipriflavone in established osteoporosis and long-term safety. *Calcif Tissue Int* 1997;61,Suppl 1:S23-7.

433 Gennari C, Adami S, Agnusdei D, et al. Effect of chronic treatment with ipriflavone in postmenopausal women with low bone mass. *Calcif Tissue Int* 1997;61,Suppl 1:S19-22.

434 Petilli M, Fiorelli G, Benvenuti S, et al. Interactions between ipriflavone and the estrogen receptor. *Calcif Tissue Int* 1995;56(2):160-5.

435 History and tradition of Morinda Citrifolia. URL: www.freeyellow.com/members2/rsscomp/morindacitrifoliastory.htm (Accessed 6 December 1999).

436 Brunner Professional Services Tahitian Noni product overview. URL www.brunnerbiz.com/noni/fact3.html (Accessed 6 December 1999).

REFERENCES

437 Brunner Professional Services Tahitian Noni skin supplement information URL: www.brunnerbiz.com/noni/skinsupp.html (Accessed 6 December 1999).

438 Herbex Ltd. Website: Use of Noni in the Pacific Islands. URL http://4-u-veges.com/noni_use.html (Accessed 6 December 1999).

439 Maui Noni website. URL: www.timewealth.com/story.htm (Accessed 6 December 1999).

440 Herb's herbs website, Noni information. URL: www.hookele.com/noni/ (Accessed 1 January 2000).

441 Hirazumi A, Furusawa E. An immunomodulatory polysaccharide-rich substance from the fruit juice of Morinda citrifolia (noni) with antitumour activity. *Phytother Res* 1999;13(5):380-7.

442 Hiwasa T, Arase Y, Chen Z, Kita K, et al. Stimulation of ultraviolet-induced apoptosis of human fibroblast UVr-1 cells by tyrosine kinase inhibitors. *FEBS Lett* 1999;444(2-3):173-6.

443 Hiramatsu T, Imoto M, Koyano T, Umezawa K. Induction of normal phenotypes in ras-transformed cells by damnacanthal from Morinda citrifolia. *Cancer Lett* 1993;73(2-3):161-6.

444 Younos C, Rolland A, Fleurentin J, Lanhers MC, et al. Analgesic and behavioural effects of Morinda citrifolia. *Planta Med* 1990;56(5):430-4.

445 Nature's Sunshine website. URL: www.parentzone.com/sunshine/morinda.htm (Accessed 6 December 1999).

446 Samra Health and Beauty website. URL: www.samra.com/herb.htm (Accessed 6 December 1999).

447 The Herbal Marketplace website. URL: http://members.aol.com/genery/morinda.htm (Accessed 6 December 1999).

448 Yoshikawa M, Yamaguchi S, Nishisaka H, et al. Chemical constituents of Chinese natural medicine, morindae radix, the dried roots of morinda officinalis how: structures of morindolide and morofficinaloside. *Chem Pharm Bull* (Tokyo) 1995;43(9):1462-5.

449 Cui C, Yang M, Yao Z, et al. Antidepressant active constituents in the roots of Morinda officinalis how. [Article in Chinese]. *Chung Kuo Chung Yao Tsa Chih* 1995;20(1):36-9, 62-3.

450 Miller LG, Panosian CB. Ataxia and slurred speech after artesunate treatment for falciparum malaria (letter). *N Engl J Med* 1997;336(18):1328.

451 Yang YJ, Shu HY, Min ZD. Anthraquinones isolated from Morinda officinalis and Damnacanthus indicus. [Article in Chinese]. *Yao Hsueh Hsueh Pao* 1992;27(5):358-64.

452 Li S, Ouyang Q, Tan X, et al. Chemical constituents of Morinda officinalis how [Article in Chinese]. *Chung Kuo Chung Yao Tsa Chih* 1991;16(11):675-6, 703.

453 Qiao ZS, Wu H, Su ZW. Comparison with the pharmacological actions of Morinda officinalis, Damnacanthus officinarum and Schisandra propinqua. [Article in Chinese]. *Chung Hsi I Chieh Ho Tsa Chih* 1991;11(7):390,415-7.

458 Canada Seabuckthorn Enterprises Ltd. Website. URL: www.seabuckthorn.com (Accessed 10 January 2000).

459 Seabuckthorn Seminar news release from Okanagan University College, 3333 College Way, Kelowna, British Columbia, Canada V1V 1V7. Dec. 29, 1998. URL: www.ouc.bc.ca/update/news82.htm (Accessed 10 January 2000).

460 Sneddon Enterprises website. URL: www.sneddonenterprises.com/Seabuckthornhome.html (Accessed 10 January 2000).

461 KeDi High-Tech Industrial Co (Xiamen Office) website. URL: www.eckorea.net/co/kedi/3.asp (Accessed 10 January 2000).

462 Seabuckthorn seed oil. RichNature Incorporated website. URL: www.richnature.com/products/herbal/seaseed.htm (Accessed 10 January 2000).

463 Seabuckthorn berry oil. RichNature Incorporated website. URL www.richnature.com/products/herbal/seaberry.htm (Accessed 10 January 2000).

464 Shineway website. URL: www.shineway.com/seabuckt.htm (Accessed 10 January 2000).

465 Floraleads GR website. URL: http://floraleads.com/OILSEA.HTM (Accessed 10 January 2000).

466 Amosova EN, Zueva EP, Razina TG, et al. The search for new anti-ulcer agents from plants in Siberia and the Far East [Article in Russian]. *Eksp Klin Farmakol* 1998;61(6):31-5.

467 Ianev E, Radev S, Balutsov M, et al. The effect of an extract of sea buckthorn (Hippophae rhamnoides L.) on the healing of experimental skin wounds in rats [Article in Bulgarian]. *Khirurgiia* (Sofiia) 1995;48(3):30-3.

468 Li Y, Liu H. Prevention of tumour production in rats fed aminopyrine plus nitrite by sea buckthorn juice. *IARC Sci Publ* 1991;(105):568-70.

469 Cheng TJ, Pu JK, Wu LW, et al. An preliminary study on hepato-protective action of seed oil of Hippophae rhamnoides L. (HR) and mechanism of the action [Article in Chinese]. *Chung Kuo Chung Yao Tsa Chih* 1994;19(6):367-70, 384.

470 Cheng TJ. Protective action of seed oil of Hippophae rhamnoides L. (HR) against experimental *Liver* injury in mice [Article in Chinese]. *Chung Hua Yu Fang I Hsueh Tsa Chih* 1992;26(4):227-9.

471 Wang Y, Lu Y, Liu X, et al. The protective effect of Hippophae rhamnoides L. on hyperlipidemic serum cultured smooth muscle cells in vitro [Article in Chinese]. *Chung Kuo Chung Yao Tsa Chih* 1992;17(10):601, 624-6, inside back cover.

472 Xiao M, Yang Z, Jiu M, et al. The antigastroulcerative activity of beta-sitosterol-beta-D-glucoside and its aglycone in rats [Article in Chinese]. *Hua Hsi I Ko Ta Hsueh Hsueh Pao* 1992;23(1):98-101.

473 Satietrol press releases. PacificHealth Laboratories, Inc., Woodbridge, NJ. URL: www.satietrol.com/press.htm and www.satietrol.com/press1.htm (Accessed 10 January 2000).

474 Klement P, Liao P, Bajzar L. A novel approach to arterial thrombolysis. *Blood* 1999;94(8):2735-43.

475 Redlitz A, Nicolini FA, Malycky JL, et al. Inducible carboxypeptidase activity. A role in clot lysis in vivo. *Circulation* 1996;93(7):1328-30.

476 Kopin AS, Mathes WF, McBride EW, et al. The cholecystokinin-A receptor mediates inhibition of food intake yet is not essential for the maintenance of body weight. *J Clin Invest* 1999;103(3):383-91.

477 Lam WF, Gielkens HA, de Boer SY, et al. Influence of hyperglycemia on the satiating effect of CCK in humans. *Physiol Behav* 1998;65(3):505-11.

478 Zhongrui L, Shuzhen T. Clinical observation on curative effect of oral seabuckthorn seed oil on cancers under chemotherapy. *Hippophae* 1993;6(4):39-41. (Translation from Chinese provided by Flocare Medical.)

479 Changshun L, Xinming C, Fenrong W, et al. Clinical observation on reflux esophagitis treated with seabuckthorn seed oil. *Hippophae* 1996;9(4):40-1. (Translation from Chinese provided by Flocare Medical.)

480 Gengquan Q, Xiang Q. A clinical report on the therapeutics of seabuckthorn oil softgels on peptic ulcer in 30 cases. *Hippophae* 1997;10(4):39-41. (Translation from Chinese provided by Flocare Medical.)

481 Shoskes DA, Zeitlin SI, Shahed A, Rajfer J. Quercetin in men with category III chronic prostatitis: A preliminary prospective, double-blind, placebo-controlled trial. *Urology* 1999;54:960-3.

482 Aharon Y, Mevorach M, Shamoon H. Vanadyl sulfate does not enhance insulin action in patients with type 1 diabetes. *Diabetes Care* 1998;21(12):2194-5.

483 Anon. Quercetin. Alt Med Rev 1998;3(2):140-3.

484 Miodini P, Fioravanti L, Di Fronzo G, Cappelletti V. The two phyto-oestrogens genistein and quercetin exert different effects on oestrogen receptor function. *Br J Cancer* 1999;80(8):1150-5.

485 El Attar TM, Virji AS. Modulating effect of resveratrol and quercetin on oral Cancer cell growth and proliferation. *AntiCancer Drugs* 1999;10(2):187-93.

486 Wiseman H. The bioavailability of non-nutrient plant factors: dietary flavonoids and phyto-oestrogens. *Proc Nutr Soc* 1999;58(1):139-46.

487 McAnlis GT, McEneny J, Pearce J, Young IS. Absorption and antioxidant effects of quercetin from onions, in man. *Eur J Clin Nutr* 1999;53(2):92-6.

488 Janssen K, Mensink RP, Cox FJ, et al. Effects of the flavonoids quercetin and apigenin on hemostasis in healthy volunteers: results from an in vitro and a dietary supplement study. *Am J Clin Nutr* 1998;67(2):255-62.

489 Huang Z, Fasco MJ, Kaminsky LS. Inhibition of estrone sulfatase in human *Liver* microsomes by quercetin and other flavonoids. *J Steroid Biochem Mol Biol* 1997;63(1-3):9-15.

490 Garg R, Malinow MR, Pettinger M, et al. Niacin treatment increases plasma homocysteine levels. *Am Heart J* 1999;138:1082-7.

491 The Way Up website. URL: www.thewayup.com/products/0187.htm (Accessed 3 February 2000).

493 Intermittent claudication information from MotherNature.com website. URL: www.mothernature.com/ency/Concern/Intermittent_Claudication.asp (Accessed 3 February 2000).

494 Alternatives Natural Products website. URL: www.alternativesnatural.com/vs/ (Accessed 3 February 2000).

495 Prevention.com homepage. URL: www.prevention.com/healing/vitamin/ail/raynauds/more2.html (Accessed 3 February 2000).

496 Anon. Inositol hexaniacinate. *Altern Med Rev*, 1998;3(3):222-3.

497 Mehta DK (Executive Editor). *British National Formulary 38*. British Medical Association and Royal Pharmaceutical Society of Great Britain, London, UK. 1999. pg.104.

498 Sunderland GT, Belch JJ, Sturrock RD, et al. A double blind randomized placebo controlled trial of hexopal in primary Raynaud's disease. *Clin Rheumatol* 1988;7(1):46-9.

499 Hutt V, Wechsler JG, Klor HU, Ditschuneit H. [Effect of a clofibrate-inositol nicotinate combination on lipids and lipoproteins in primary hyperlipoproteinemia of types IIa, IV and V]. [Article in German]. *Arzneimittelforschung* 1983;33(5):776-9.

500 Brinker F. Herb Contraindications and Drug Interactions. Sandy, Oregon: Eclectic Medical Publications, 1997.

501 De Smet PAGM, Keller K, Hansel R, Chandler RF, eds. Adverse Effects of Herbal Drugs 1. -Verlag Berlin: Springer, 1992.

502 De Smet PAGM, Keller K, Hansel R, Chandler RF, eds. Adverse Effects of Herbal Drugs 2. -Verlag, Berlin: Springer, 1993.

504 Holt GA. Food & Possible Interactions with Drugs: Revised and Expanded Edition. Chicago, IL: Precept Press; 1998.

505 Hardman JG, Limbird LL, eds. Goodman and Gillman's The Pharmacological Basis of Therapeutics, ninth edition, New York: McGraw-Hill, 1996.

506 Burnham TH, ed. *Drug Facts and Comparisons*, Updated Monthly. Facts and Comparisons, St. Louis, MO.

507 Pheatt N, ed. *Nonherbal Dietary Supplements. Pharmacist's Letter* Continuing Education Booklet 1998;98(4):1-51.

508 Lieberman S. The Real Vitamin and Mineral Book. Honesdale, PA: Paragon Press, 1997.

509 Dukes, MNG. Meyler's Side Effects of Drugs. 13th ed. Elsevier, Amsterdam, 1997.

510 Meuss, AR, trans. Phytotherapy in Paediatrics-Handbook for Physicians and Pharmacists by H. Schilcher. 2nd edition. Stuttgart, Germany: Medpharm GmbH Scientific Publishers, 1997.

511 Spraycar M, ed. Stedman's Medical Dictionary. 26th ed. Baltimore, MD: Williams & Wilkins, 1995.

512 Robbers JE, Tyler VE. Tyler's Herbs of Choice. Binghamton, NY: Haworth Herbal Press, 1999.

513 Agricultural Research Service: Dr. Duke's Phytochemical and Ethnobotanical Databases. URL: www.ars-grin.gov/duke (Accessed 3 November 1999).

514 Bruneton J. Pharmacognosy, Phytochemistry, Medicinal Plants. Paris: Lavoisier Publishing, 1995.

515 Foster S, Tyler VE. Tyler's Honest Herbal, fourth ed., Binghamton, NY: Haworth Herbal Press, 1999.

516 Morrix W, ed. The American Heritage Dictionary of the English Language. New York: American Heritage Publishing, 1969.

517 Duke JA, Vasquez R. Amazonian Ethnobotanical Dictionary. Boca Raton, FL: CRC Press, 1994.

518 Schultes RE, Raffauf RF. The Healing Forest, Medicinal and Toxic Plants of the Northwest Amazonia. Portland, OR: Dioscorides Press, 1990.

520 Richter W, et al. "Interaction between fibre and lovastatin." *Lancet* 1991;338:706.

521 Kantola T, et al. "Grapefruit juice greatly increases serum concentrations of lovastatin and lovastatin acid." *Clin Pharmacol Ther* 1998;63:397-402.

522 Ioannides-Demos, LL, et al. "Dosing implications of a clinical interaction between grapefruit juice and cyclosporine and metabolite concentrations in patients with autoimmune diseases." *J Rheumatol* 1997;24:49-54.

523 Josefsson M, et al. "Effect of grapefruit juice on the pharmacokinetics of amlodipine in healthy volunteers." *Eur J Clin Pharmacol* 1996;51:189-93.

524 Garg SK, et al. "Effect of grapefruit juice on carbamazepine bioavailability in patients with epilepsy." *Clin Pharmacol Ther* 1998;64:286-8.

525 Weber A, et al. "Can grapefruit juice influence ethinylestradiol bioavailability? " *Contraception* 1996;53:41-7.

526 Schubert W, et al. "Inhibition of 17 beta-estradiol Metabolism by grapefruit juice in ovariectomized women." *Maturitas* 1994;20:155-63.

527 Kantola T, et al. "Grapefruit juice greatly increases

© Copyright 2000, Natural Medicines Comprehensive Database (209) 472-2244. For updated data, go to www.NaturalDatabase.com. • 1163

R
E
F
E
R
E
N
C
E
S

serum concentrations of lovastatin and lovastatin acid." *Clin Pharmacol Ther* 1998 63:397-402.

528   Bailey DG, et al. "Interaction of citrus juices with felodipine and nifedipine." *Lancet* 1991;337:268-9.

529   Bailey DG, et al. "Effect of grapefruit juice and naringin on nisoldipine pharmacokinetics." *Clin Pharmacol Ther* 1993;54:589-94.

530   Rau SE, et al. "Grapefruit juice-terfenadine single-dose interaction: magnitude, mechanism, and relevance." *Clin Pharmacol Ther* 1997 61:401-9.

531   Robbins RC, et al. "Ingestion of grapefruit lowers elevated hematocrits in human subjects." *Int J Vitam Nutr Res* 1988;58:414-7.

532   Gin H, et al. "The influence of Guar gum on absorption of metformin from the Gut in healthy volunteers." *Horm Metab Res* 1989;21:81-3.

533   Huupponen R, et al. "Effect of guar gum, a fibre preparation, on digoxin and penicillin absorption in man." *Eur J Clin Pharmacol* 1984;26:279-81.

534   Spillane PK, et al. "Neurological manifestations of kava intoxication." *Med J Aust* 1997;167:172-3.

535   Swensen JN. "Man convicted of driving under the influence of kava." *Deseret News*, Salt Lake City, UT, 5 Aug. 96.

536   Almeida JC, et al. "Coma from the health food store: interaction between kava and alprazolam." *Ann Intern Med* 1996;125:940-1.

537   Bano G, et al. "The effect of piperine on pharmacokinetics of phenytoin in healthy volunteers." *Planta Med* 1987;53:568-9.

538   Bano G, et al. "Effect of piperine on bioavailability and pharmacokinetics of propranolol and theophylline in healthy volunteers." *Eur J Clin Pharmacol* 1991;41;615-7.

539   Etman M. "Effect of a bulk forming laxative on the bioavailablility of caramazepine in man." *Drug Devel Indus Pharm* 1995;21:1901-6.

540   Perlman BB. "Interaction between lithium salts and ispaghula husk." *Lancet* 1990; 35:416.

541   Amabeoku, GJ, et al. "Pharmacokinetic interaction of single doses of quinine and carbamazepine, phenobarbitone and phenytoin in healthy volunteers." *East Afr Med J* 1993;70:90-3.

542   Gordon JB. "SSRIs and St. John's Wort: possible toxicity?" *Am Fam Physician* 1998;57(5):950,953.

543   McRae S. "Elevated serum digoxin levels in a patient taking digoxin and Siberian ginseng." *Can Med Assoc J* 1996;155:293-5.

544   Tatro D, ed. Anticoagulants-Vitamin E; in Drug Interaction Facts, Facts and Comparisons. St. Louis, MO, January 1997.

545   Dunbain DW, et al. "Lead poisoning from Indian herbal medicine (Ayurveda)." *Med J Aust* 1992;157:835-6.

546   Sheerin NS, et al. "Simultaneous exposure to lead, arsenic and mercury from Indian ethnic remedies." *Br J Clin Pract* 1994;48:332-3.

547   Markowitz SB, et al. "Lead poisoning due to Hai Ge Fan, the porphyrin content of individual erythrocytes." *JAMA* 1994;271:932-4.

548   Tay CH, et al. "Arsenic Poisoning from anti-asthmatic herbal preparations." *Med J Aust* 1975;2:424-8.

549   Colgrove ML, et al. "Lead poisoning-associated death from Asian Indian folk remedies—Florida." *MMWR* 1984;33:642-5.

550   Schaumburg HH, et al. "Alopecia and sensory polyneuropathy from thallium in a Chinese herbal

551   Espinoza EO, et al. "Toxic metals in selected traditional Chinese medicinals." *Journal of Forensic Sciences* 1996;41:453-6.

552   Takegoshi K, et al. "A case of Venoplant-induced hepatic injury." *Gastroenterol Jpn* 1986;21:62-5.

553   Jaspersen-Schib R, et al. [Serious plant poisonings in Switzerland 1966-1994. Case analysis from the Swiss Toxicology Information Center].[German] *Schweiz Med Wochenschr* 1996;126:1085-98. (English abstract)

554   Cerulli J, et al. "Chromium picolinate toxicity." *Ann Pharmacother* 1998;32:428-31.

555   Lin JL, et al. "Flavonoid-induced acute nephropathy." *Am J Kidney Dis* 1994;23:433-40.

556   Becker BN. "Ginseng-induced diuretic resistance." *JAMA* 1996 276:606-7.

557   Tao SH, Bolger, PM. "Hazard assessment of germanium supplements." *Regul Toxicol Pharmacol* 1997;25:211-9.

558   Tai YT. "Adverse effects from traditional Chinese medicine." *Lancet* 1993;341:892.

559   Tai YT, et al. "Cardiotoxicity after accidental herb-induced aconite poisoning." *Lancet* 1992;340:1254-6.

560   Tai YT. "Adverse effects from traditional Chinese medicine." *Lancet* 1993;341:892.

561   Fatovich DM. "Aconite: a lethal Chinese herb." *Ann Emerg Med* 1992;21:309-11

562   Tomlinson B, et al. "Herb-induced aconite poisoning." *Lancet* 1993;341:370-1.

563   Chan TYK, et al. "Aconitine poisoning following the ingestion of Chinese herbal medicines: a report of eight cases." *Aust NZ J Med* 1993;23:268-71.

564   van Ypersele de Strihou, C, et al. "The tragic paradigm of Chinese herbs nephropathy." *Nephrol Dial Transplant* 1995;10:157-60.

565   Blumenthal, HJ, et al. "Chewing gum headaches." *Headache* 1997;37:665-6.

566   Jones TK, et al. "Profound neonatal congestive heart failure caused by maternal consumption of blue cohosh herbal medication." *J Pediatr* 1998;132:550-2.

567   Subiza J, et al. "Anaphylactic reaction after the ingestion of chamomile tea; a study of cross-reactivity with other composite pollens." *J Allergy Clin Immunol* 1989;84:353-8.

568   Smith BC, et al. "Acute hepatitis induced by ingestion of the herbal medication chaparral." *Aust NZ Med J* 1993;23:526.

569   Gordon DW, et al. "Chaparral ingestion: the broadening spectrum of Liver injury caused by herbal medications. *JAMA* 1995;273:489-90.

570   Batchelor WB, et al. "Chaparral-induced hepatic injury." *Am J Gastroenterol* 1995;90:831-3.

571   Katz M, et al. "Herbal hepatitis: subacute hepatic necrosis secondary to chaparral leaf." *J Clin Gastroenterol* 1990;12:203-6.

572   Ko RJ, et al. "Lethal ingestion of Chinese herbal tea containing ch'an su." *West J Med* 1996; 64:71-5.

573   Chan JCN, et al. "Anticholinergic poisoning from Chinese herbal medciines." *Aust NZ J Med* 1994;24:317-8.

574   Sperl W, et al. "Reversible hepatic veno-occlusive disease in an infant after consumption of pyrrolizidine-containing herbal tea." *Eur J Pediatr* 1995;154:112-6.

575   Roulet M, et al. "Hepatic veno-occlusive disease in newborn infant of a woman drinking herbal tea." *J Pediatr* 1988;112:433-4.

576   Mathews, MK. "Association of Ginkgo biloba with

intracerebral hemorrhage." *Neurology* 1998;50:1934.

577 Gilbert GJ. "Ginkgo biloba." *Neurology* 1997;48:1137.

578 Rowin J, Lewis SL. "Spontaneous bilateral subdural hemotomas with chronic Gingko biloba ingestion." *Neurology* 1996;46:1775-6.

579 Rosenblatt M, Mindel T. "Spontaneous hyphema associated with ingestion of Gingko biloba extract." *N Engl J Med* 1997;336:1108.

580 Jaakkola MS, et al. "Asthma caused by occupational exposure to pectin." *J Allergy Clin Immunol* 1997;100:575-6.

581 Westphal W, et al. [Exogenous allergic asthma following pectin exposure-a new occupational allergen].[German] *Pneumologie* 1990;44(Suppl 1):337-8. (English abstract)

582 Baldwin JL, et al. "Pectin-induced occupational asthma." *Chest* 1993;104:1936-7.

583 Cohen AJ, et al. "Occupational asthma caused by pectin inhalation during the manufacture of jam." *Chest* 1993;103:309-11.

584 Kraut A, et al. "Christmas candy maker's asthma. IgG4-mediated pectin allergy." *Chest* 1992;102:1605-7.

585 Garty BZ. "Garlic burns." *Pediatrics* 1993 91:658-9.

586 Rose KD, et al. "Spontaneous spinal epidural hematoma with associated platelet dysfunction from excessive garlic ingestion: a case report." *Neurosurgery* 1990 2:880-2.

587 Burnham BE. "Garlic as a possible risk for postoperative bleeding." *Plast-Reconstr-Surg* 1995;95:213.

588 Shuster J. "Black cohosh root? Chasteberry Tree? Seizures!" *Hospital Pharmacy* 1996;31:1553-4.

589 Scaglione F, et al. "Efficacy and safety of the standardized Ginseng extract G115 for potentiating vaccination against the influenza syndrome and protection against the common cold." *Drugs Exp Clin Res* 1996;22:65-72.

590 Palmer BV, et al. "Gin Seng and mastalgia." *BMJ* 1978;1:1284.

591 Hopkins MP, et al. "Ginseng face cream and unexplained vaginal bleeding." *Am J Obstet Gynecol* 1988;159:1121-2.

592 Greenspan EM. "Ginseng and vaginal bleeding." *JAMA* 1983;249:2018.

593 Koren G, et al. "Maternal ginseng use associated with neonatal androgenization." *JAMA* 1990;264:2866.

594 Gonzalez-Seijo JC, et al. Manic episode and ginseng: Report of a possible case. *J Clin Psychopharmcol* 1995;15:447-8.

595 Ryu S, Chien Y. Ginseng-associated cerebral arteritis. *Neurology* 1995;45:829-30.

596 Dega H, et al. "Ginseng as a cause of Stevens-Johnson syndrome." *Lancet* 1996;313:756.

597 Brown R. "Potential interactions of herbal medicines with antipsychotics, antidepressants and hypnotics." *European Journal of Herbal Medicine* 1997;3:25-8.

598 Hamid S, et al. "Protracted cholestatic hepatitis after the use of Prostata." *Ann Intern Med* 1997;127:169-70.

599 Cohen AJ. "Long term safety and efficacy of ginkgo biloba extract in the treatment of anti-depressant-induced sexual dysfunction." Psychiatry On-Line Website URL: www.priory.com/pharmol/gingko.htm. (Accessed 24 July 1999).

600 Malo JL, et al. "Prevalence of occupational asthma and immunologic sensitization to guar gum among employees at a carpet-manufacturing plant." *J Allergy Clin Immunol* 1990;86(4 Pt 1):562-9.

601 Lagier F, et al. "Occupational asthma caused by guar gum." *J Allergy Clin Immunol* 1990;85:785-90.

602 Lewis JH. "Esophageal and small bowel obstruction from guar gum-containing "diet pills": analysis of 26 cases reported to the Food and Drug Administration." *Am J Gastroenterol* 1992;87:1424-8.

603 Norton SA, et al. "Kava dermopathy." *J Am Acad Dermatol* 1994;31(1):89-97.

604 Agha FP, et al. ""Giant colonic bezoar:" a medication bezoar due to psyllium seed husks." *Am J Gastroenterol* 1984;79:319-21.

605 Brown R. Potential interactions of herbal medicines with antipsychotics, antidepressants and hypnotics. *European Journal of Herbal Medicine* 1997;3:25-8.

606 Harder S, et al. "Ciprofloxacin-caffeine: a drug interaction established using in vivo and in vitro investigations." *Am J Med* 1989;87(Suppl 5A):89S-91S.

607 Carbo M, et al. "Effect of quinolones on caffeine disposition." *Clin Pharmacol Ther* 1989;45:234-40.

608 Healy DP, et al. "Interaction between oral ciprofloxacin and caffeine in normal volunteers." *Antimicrob Agents Chemother* 1989;33:474-8.

609 Mester R, et al. "Caffeine withdrawal increases lithium Blood levels." *Biol Psychiatry* 1995;37:348-50.

610 Jefferson JW. "Lithium tremor and caffeine intake: two cases of drinking less and shaking more." *J Clin Psychiatry* 1988;49 72-3.

611 Yu CM, et al. "Chinese herbs and warfarin potentiation by 'Danshen'." *J Intern Med* 1997;241:337-9.

612 Tam LS, et al. "Warfarin interacions with Chinese traditional medicines: danshen and methyl salicylate medicated oil." *Aust NZ J Med* 1995;25:258.

613 Shaw D, et al. "Traditional remedies and food supplements: a 5-year toxicological study (1991-1995)." *Drug Safety* 1997;17:342-56.

614 Personal correspondence. Efamol Nutraceuticals, Boston, MA, 22 January 1998.

615 Richter WO, Jacob BG, Schwandt P. "Interaction between fibre and lovastatin." *Lancet* 1991;338:706.

616 Sunter WH "Warfarin and garlic." *Pharm J*, 1991; 246:722.

617 Shader RI, Greenblatt DJ. "Phenylzine and the dream machine-ramblings and reflections." *J Clin Psychopharmcol* 1985;5:65.

618 Jones BD, Runikis AM. "Interaction of ginseng with phenelzine." *J Clin Psychopharmcol* 1987;7:201-2.

619 Janetzky K, et al. "Probable interaction between warfarin and ginseng." *Am J Health-Syst Pharm* 1997;54:692-3.

620 Golsch S, et al. [Reversible increase in photosensitivity to UV-B caused by St. John's wort extract]. [German] *Hautarzt* 1997;48:249-52. (English abstract)

621 Bove GM. "Acute neuropathy after exposure to sun in a patient treated with St. John's Wort." *Lancet* 1998;352:1121-2.

622 Sharma RD, et al. "Effect of fenugreek seeds on *Blood* glucose and serum lipids in type I diabetes." *Eur J Clin Nutr* 1990;44:301-6.

623 Thys-Jacobs S, et al. "Calcium carbonate and the premenstrual syndrome: Effects on premenstrual and menstrual symptoms." *Am J Obstet Gynecol* 1998;179:444-52.

624 Chang T, et al. "The effect of water-soluble vitamin E on cyclosporine pharmacokinetics in healthy volunteers." *Clin Pharmacol Ther* 1996;59:297-303.

625 Pan SH, et al. "Enhanced oral cyclosporine absorption with water-soluble vitamin E early after Liver transplantation." *Pharmacotherapy* 1996;16:59-65.

REFERENCES

R E F E R E N C E S

626 Lasswell WL Jr., et al. "In vitro interaction of neuroleptics and tricylic antidepressants with coffee, tea, and gallotannic acid." *J Pharm Sci* 1984; 73:1056-8.

627 Kulhanek F, et al. "Precipitation of Antipsychotic drugs in interaction with coffee or tea." *Lancet* 1979;2:1130.

628 Brockmoller J, et al. "Hypericin and pseudohypericin: pharmacokinetics and effects on photosensitivity in humans." *Pharmacopsychiatry* 1997;30(Suppl 2):94-101.

629 Kang-yum E, et al. "Chinese patent Medicine as a potential source of mercury poisoning." *Vet Hum Toxicol* 1992;34:235-8.

630 Prussick R, et al. "The protective effect of vitamin E on the hemolysis associated with Dapsone treatment in patients with dermatitis herpetiformis." *Arch Dermatol* 1992;128:210-3.

631 Merhav H, et al. "Tea drinking and microcytic anemia in infants." *Am J Clin Nutr* 1985;41:1210-3.

632 Ridker PM, et al. "Comfrey herb tea and hepatic veno-occlusive disease." *Lancet* 1989;2:657-8.

633 Weston CFM, et al. "Veno-occlusive disease of the *Liver* secondary to ingestion of comfrey." *BMJ* 1987;295:183.

634 Bach N, et al. "Comfrey herb tea-induced heapatic veno-occlusive disesae." *Am J Med* 1989;87:97-9.

635 Yeong ML, et al. "Hepatic veno-occlusive disease associated with comfrey ingestion." *J Gastroenterol Hepatol* 1990;5:211-4.

636 Hassell LH, et al. "Acute anticholinergic syndrome following ingestion of Angel's trumpet tea." *Hawaii Medical Journal* 1995;54:669-70.

637 Kamiyama T, et al. "Autoimmune hepatitis triggered by administration of an herbal medicine." *Am J Gastroenterol* 1997;92:703-4.

638 Mullins RJ. "Echinacea-associated anaphylaxis." *Med J Aust* 1998;168:170-1.

639 Doyle H, et al. "Herbal stimulant containing ephedrine has also caused psychosis." *BMJ* 1996;313:756.

640 Castot A, et al. [Pharmacovigilance off the beaten track: herbal surveillance or pharmacovigilance of medicinal plants]. [French] *Therapie* 1997;52:97-103. (English abstract)

641 Mostefa-Kara N, et al. "Fatal hepatitis after herbal tea." *Lancet* 1992;340:674.

642 Larrey D, et al. "Hepatitis after germander (Teucrium chamaedrys) administration: another instance of herbal medicine hepatotoxicity." *Ann Intern Med* 1992;117:129-32.

643 Woolf, GM. "Jin Bu Huan toxicity in adults- Los Angeles, 1993." *MMWR* 1993;42:920-2.

644 Horowitz RS, et al. "Jin Bu Huan toxicity in children- Colorado, 1993." *MMWR* 1993;42:633-5.

645 Pye KG, et al. "Severe dyserythropoeisis and autoimmune thrombocytopenia associated with ingestion of kelp supplement." *Lancet* 1992;339:1540.

646 Spiller HA, et al. "Retrospective study of mistletoe ingestion." *Clinical Toxicology* 1996;34:405-8.

647 Harvey J, et al. "Mistletoe hepatitis." *Br Med J* 1981;282:186-7.

648 Krenzelok EP, et al. "American mistletoe exposures." *Am J Emerg Med* 1997;15:516-20.

649 Solbakken AM, et al. [Nature Medicine as intoxicant]. [Norwegian] *Tidsskr Nor Laegeforen* 1997;117:1140-1. (English abstract)

650 Anderson IB, et al. Pennyroyal Toxicity: Measurement of toxic metabolite levels in two cases and review of the literature. *Ann Intern Med* 1996;124:726-34.

651 Takahashi M, et al. "Contact Dermatitis due to honeybee royal jelly." *Contact Dermatitis* 1983;9:452-5.

652 Bullock RJ, et al. "Fatal royal jelly-induced asthma." *Med J Aust* 1994;160:44.

653 Thien FCK, et al. "Royal jelly-induced asthma." *Med J Aust* 1993;159:639.

654 Beuers U. "Hepatitis after chronic abuse of senna." *Lancet* 1991;337:372-3.

655 Ortiz Cansado A, et al. [Veno-occlusive *Liver* disease due to intake of Senecio vulgaris tea]. [Spanish] *Gastroenterol Hepatol* 1995;18:413-6. (English abstract)

656 Tomioka M, et al. [Hepatic veno-occlusive disease associated with ingestion of Senecio tephrosioides]. [Spanish] *Rev Gastroenterol Peru* 1995;15:299-302. (English abstract)

657 But PHP, et al. "Hepatitis related to the Chinese Medicine Shou-wu-pian manufactured from Polygonum multiflorum." *Vet Hum Toxicol* 1996;38:280-2.

658 De Groot AC. "Airborn allergic Contact Dermatitis from tea tree oil." *Contact Dermatitis* 1996;35:304-5.

659 Willey LB, et al. "Valerian overdose: a case report." *Vet Hum Toxicol* 1995;37:364-5.

660 Cahill DJ, et al. "Multiple follicular development associated with herbal medicine." *Hum Reprod* 1994;9:1469-70.

661 Berlin R, et al. Wormwood: Oregon Poison Center. Portland, OR: Oregon Health Sciences University 1996.

662 Weisbord SD, Soule JB, Kimmel PL. "Poison on line-acute renal failure caused by oil of wormwood purchased through the Internet." *N Engl J Med* 1997;337:825-7.

663 Graedon J, Graedon T. The People's Guide to Deadly Possible Interactions with Drugs. New York: St. Martin's Press, 1995.

664 Blumenthal M. Herb and conventional Possible Interactions with Drugs. Austin, TX: American Botanical Council, 1997.

665 LoVecchio F, Curry SC, Bagnasco T. Butyrolactone-induced central nervous system depression after ingestion of RenewTrient, a dietary supplement. *N Engl J Med* 1998;339(12):847-8.

666 Personal correspondence. Dave Kanyer, Asst. Director of Pharmacy, Community Hospital of the Monterey Peninsula, Dec 1998.

667 Blickstein D, et al. "Warfarin antagonism by avocado." *Lancet* 1991;337(8746):914-5.

668 Colquhoun DM, et al. "Comparison of the effects on lipoproteins and apolipoproteins of a diet high in monounsaturated fatty acids, enriched with avocado, and a high-carbohydrate diet." *Am J Clin Nutr* 1992;56(4):671-77.

669 Lopez Ledesma R, et al. "Monounsaturated fatty acid (avocado) rich diet for mild hypercholesterolemia." *Arch Med Res* 1996;27(4):519-23.

670 Carranza J, et al. "Effects of avocado on the level of *Blood* lipids in patients with phenotype II and IV dyslipidemias." [Spanish] *Arch Inst Cardiol Mex* 1995;65(4):342-8.

671 Lerman-Garber I, et al. "Effect of a high-monounsaturated fat diet enriched with avocado in NIDDM patients." *Diabetes Care* 1994;17(4):311-5.

672 van Weerden WM, et al. "Effects of adrenal androgens on the transplantable human prostate tumor PC-82." *Endocrinology* 1992;131(6):2909-13.

673 Mecenas CA, et al. "Production of premature delivery in pregnant rhesus monkeys by androstenedione infusion." *Nat Med* 1996;2(4):443-8.

674 "Creatine and androstenedione-two "dietary supplements." *Med Lett Drugs Ther* 1998;40(1039):105-6.

675 Alvizouri-Munoz M, et al. "Effects of avocado as a source of monounsaturated fatty acids on plasma lipid levels." *Arch Med Res* 1992;23(4):163-7.

676 Chen Z, et al. "Identification of hevein (Hev b 6.02) in Hevea latex as a major cross- reacting allergen with avocado fruit in patients with latex allergy." *J Allergy Clin Immunol* 1998;102(3):476-81.

677 Diehl HW, May EL. "Cetyl myristoleate isolated from Swiss albino mice: an apparent protective agent against adjuvant arthritis in rats." *J Pharm Sci* 1994;83(3):296-9.

678 Plaitakis A, et al. "Pilot trial of branched-chain aminoacids in amyotrophic lateral sclerosis." *Lancet* 1988;1(8593):1015-8.

679 "Branched-chain amino acids and amyotrophic lateral sclerosis: a treatment failure? The Italian ALS Study Group." *Neurology* 1993;43(12):2466-70.

680 Testa D, Caraceni T, Fetoni V. "Branched-chain amino acids in the treatment of amyotrophic lateral sclerosis." *J Neurol* 1989;236(8):445-7.

681 Tandan R, et al. "A controlled trial of amino acid therapy in amyotrophic lateral sclerosis: I. Clinical, functional, and maximum isometric torque data." *Neurology* 1996;47(5):1220-6.

682 *FDA*. "FDA warns about products containing gamma butyrolactone or GBL and asks companies to issue a recall." Talk Paper, 21 January 1999.

683 Leclercq I, Desager JP, Horsmans Y. "Inhibition of chlorzoxazone metabolism, a clinical probe for CYP2E1, by a single ingestion of watercress." *Clin Pharmacol Ther* 1998 64(2):144-9.

684 Plauth M, et al. "Long-term treatment of latent portosystemic encephalopathy with branched-chain amino acids. A double-blind placebo-controlled crossover study." *J Hepatol* 1993;17(3):308-14.

685 Egberts EH, et al. "Branched chain amino acids in the treatment of latent portosystemic encephalopathy. A double-blind placebo-controlled crossover study." *Gastroenterology* 1985;88(4):887-95

686 Rossi Fanelli, F, et al. "Use of branched chain amino acids for treating hepatic encephalopathy: clinical experiences." *Gut* 1986; 27(Suppl 1):111-5.

687 Wahren J, et al. "Is intravenous administration of branched chain amino acids effective in the treatment of hepatic encephalopathy? A multicenter study." *Hepatology* 1983;3(4):475-80.

688 Michel H, et al. "Treatment of acute hepatic encephalopathy in cirrhotics with a branched-chain amino acids enriched versus a conventional amino acids mixture. A controlled study of 70 patients." *Liver* 1985 5(5):282-9.

689 Vilstrup H, et al. "Branched chain enriched amino acid versus glucose treatment of hepatic encephalopathy. A double-blind study of 65 patients with cirrhosis." *J Hepatol* 1990;10(3):291-6.

690 Marchesini G, et al. "Long-term oral branched-chain amino acid treatment in chronic hepatic encephalopathy. A randomized double-blind casein-controlled trial. The Italian Multicenter Study Group." *J Hepatol* 1990;11(1):92-101.

691 Chuah SY, Ellis BJ, Mayberry JF. "Exacerbation of hepatic encephalopathy by branched-chain amino acids-a case report." *J Hum Nutr Diet* 1992;5(1):53-6.

692 Blomstrand E, et al. "Influence of ingesting a solution of branched-chain amino acids on perceived exertion during exercise." *Acta Physiol Scand* 1997;159(1):41-9.

693 MacLean DA, Graham TE. "Branched-chain amino acid supplementation augments plasma ammonia responses during exercise in humans." *J Appl Physiol* 1993;74(6):2711-7.

694 MacLean DA, Graham TE, Saltin B. "Branched-chain amino acids augment ammonia metabolism while attenuating protein breakdown during exercise." *Am J Physiol* 1994;267(6 Pt 1):E1010-22.

695 Breum L, et al. "Comparison of an ephedrine/caffeine combination and dexfenfluramine in the treatment of obesity. A double-blind multi-centre trial in general practice." *Int J Obes Relat Metab Disord* 1994;18(2):99-103.

696 Toubro S, et al. "The acute and chronic effects of ephedrine/caffeine mixtures on energy expenditure and glucose *Metabolism* in humans." *Int J Obes Relat Metab Disord* 1993;17(Suppl 3):S73-7.

697 Toubro S, et al. "Safety and efficacy of long-term treatment with ephedrine, caffeine and an ephedrine/ caffeine mixture." *Int J Obes Relat Metab Disord* 1993;17(Suppl 1):S69-72.

698 Cystadane (betaine anhydrous for oral solution) Package Insert, Orphan Medical, revised 10/96.

699 Feldman J, et al. [Double-blind study of the treatment of disc lumbosciatica by chemonucleolysis.] [Article in French]. *Rev Rhum Mal Osteoartic* 1986; 53(3):147-52.

700 Nordby EJ. "A comparison of discectomy and chemonucleolysis." *Clin Orthop* 1985;(200):279-83.

701 Javid MJ. "Chemonucleolysis versus laminectomy. A cohort comparison of effectiveness and charges." *Spine* 1995;20(18):2016-22.

702 Kuthan F. [Bee Venom Treatment of Rheumatic Disorders. (Summary of paper presented concerning apitherapy at the International Apicultural Congress of Apimondia in Bucharest, Romania).] [Article in German]. URL: www.beesting.com/kuthan.html. May 1999. (Accessed 23 July 1999)

703 Clarkson PM, Haymes EM. "Trace mineral requirements for athletes." *Int J Sport Nutr* 1994;4(2):104-19.

704 Clarkson PM. "Minerals: exercise performance and supplementation in athletes." *J Sports Sci* 1991;9:91-116.

705 Campbell WW, Anderson RA. "Effects of aerobic exercise and training on the trace minerals chromium, zinc and copper." *Sports Med* 1987 4(1):9-18.

706 Broun ER, et al. "Excessive zinc ingestion. A reversible cause of sideroblastic anemia and bone marrow depression." *JAMA* 1990;264(11):1441-3.

707 Sandstead HH. "Requirements and toxicity of essential trace elements, illustrated by zinc and copper." *Am J Clin Nutr* 1995 61(3 Suppl):621S-4S.

708 Brewer GJ, et al. "Treatment of Wilson's disease with zinc: XV long-term follow-up studies." *J Lab Clin Med* 1998;132(4):264-78.

709 Weight LM, et al. "Vitamin and mineral status of trained athletes including the effects of supplementation." *Am J Clin Nutr* 1988;47(2):186-91.

710 Finley EB, Cerklewski FL. "Influence of ascorbic acid supplementation on copper status in young adult men *Am J Clin Nutr* 1983;37(4):553-6.

711 Scharf MB, et al. "Effect of gamma-hydroxybutyrate on pain, fatigue, and the alpha sleep anomaly in patients with fibromyalgia. Preliminary report." *J Rheumatol* 1998;25(10):1986-90.

REFERENCES

R E F E R E N C E S

712 Chin RL, et al. "Clinical course of gamma-hydroxybutyrate overdose." *Ann Emerg Med* 1998;31(6):716-22.

713 Tunnicliff, G. Sites of action of gamma-hydroxybutyrate (GHB)-a neuroactive drug with abuse potential. *J Toxicol Clin Toxicol* 1997;35(6):581-90.

714 *FDA Talk Paper*. FDA re-issues warning on GHB. 18 February 1997.

715 Latha B, et al. "The efficacy of trypsin: chymotrypsin preparation in the reduction of oxidative damage during burn injury." *Burns* 1998;24(6):532-8.

716 Latha B, et al. "Serum enzymatic changes modulated using trypsin: chymotrypsin preparation during burn wounds in humans." *Burns* 1997;23(7-8):560-4.

717 Shaw PC. "The use of a trypsin-chymotrypsin formulation in fractures of the hand." *Br J Clin Pract* 1969;23(1):25-6.

718 McCue FC, Webster TM, Gieck J. "Clinical effects of proteolytic enzymes after reconstructive hand surgery." *Int Surg* 1972;57(6):479-82.

719 Patil SP, Niphadkar PV, Bapat MM. "Allergy to fenugreek (Trigonella foenum graecum)." *Ann Allergy Asthma Immunol* 1997;78(3):297-300.

720 Ahsan SK, et al. "Effect of Trigonella foenum-graecum and Ammi majus on calcium oxalate urolithiasis in rats." *J Ethnopharmacol* 1989;26(3):249-54.

721 Fischer-Rasmussen W, Kjaer SK, Dahl C, Asping U. Ginger treatment of hyperemesis gravidarum. *Eur J Obstet Gynecol Reprod Biol* 1991;38(1):19-24.

722 Phillips S, Ruggier R, Hutchinson SE. "Zingiber officinale (ginger)-an antiemetic for day case surgery." *Anaesthesia* 1993;48(8):715-7.

723 Bone ME, et al. "Ginger root-a new antiemetic. The effect of ginger root on postoperative nausea and vomiting after major gynaecological surgery." *Anaesthesia* 1990;45(8):669-71.

724 Foster S. *Feverfew, Tanacetum parthenium, Botanical Series No. 310*. Austin, TX: American Botanical Council, 1996.

725 Awang, DVC. "Feverfew effective in Migraine prevention." *HerbalGram* 1998;42:18.

726 Awang, DVC. "Feverfew trials: The promise of- and the problem with- standardized extracts." *HerbalGram* 1997;41:16-7.

727 Kuritsky A, et al. "Feverfew in the treatment of migraine: its effect on serotonin uptake and platelet activity." *Neurology* 1994:44(Suppl 2):A201. (Abstract 293P)

728 Heymsfield SB, et al. "Garcinia cambogia (hydroxycitric acid) as a potential antiobesity agent: a randomized controlled trial." *JAMA* 1998;280(18):1596-600.

729 "Natural Remedies, Garcinia cambogia." Natural Remedies Pvt. Ltd. URL: www.indianherbs.com/gar_cal.htm. (Accessed 16 July 1999)

730 "Latest Research Reveals New Native Asian Fruit Has the Ability to Reduce Body-Fat Production by 40-70%. Recent Studies Have Discovered An All Natural Substance Derived from a Native Asian Fruit Plant Decreases Appetite, Speeds up Calorie Burning and Inhibits Your Body's Ability to Store Fat!" URL: www.quickresults.com.au/weightloss/asianf.htm. (Accessed 16 July 1999)

731 Isaacsohn JL, et al. Garlic powder and plasma lipids and lipoproteins, a multicenter, randomized, placebo-controlled trial. *Arch Intern Med* 1998;158:1189-94.

732 Berthold HK, Sudhop T, von Bergmann K. "Effect of a garlic oil preparation on serum lipoproteins and cholesterol metabolism." *JAMA* 1998;279(23):1900-2.

733 Mitscher LA, et al. "Chemoprotection: a review of the potential therapeutic antioxidant properties of green tea (Camellia sinensis) and certain of its constituents." *Med Res Rev* 1997;17(4):327-65.

734 Kono S, et al. "Green tea consumption and serum lipid profiles: a cross-sectional study in northern Kyushu, Japan." *Prev Med* 1992;21(4):526-31.

735 Kingsbury JM. "Poison ivy, poison sumac, and other rash-producing plants." York State College of Agriculture and Life Sciences, *Information Bulletin 105*, 1976.

736 Liu JH, et al. "Angelol-type coumarins from Angelica pubescence F. biserrata and their inhibitory effect on platelet aggregation." *Phytochemistry* 1995;39(5):1099-101.

737 Lo ACT, et al. "Danggui (Angelica sinensis) affects the pharmacodynamics but not the pharmacokinetics of warfarin in rabbits." *Eur J Drug Metab Pharmacokinet* 1995;20:55-60.

738 Hirata JD, et al. "Does dong quai have estrogenic effects in postmenopausal women? A double-blind, placebo-controlled trial." *Fertil Steril* 1997;68(6):981-6.

739 Cooper RL, Cooper MM. "Red pepper-induced dermatitis in breast-fed infants." *Dermatology* 1996;93(1):61-2.

740 Stone-Dorshow T, Levitt MD. "Gaseous response to ingestion of a poorly absorbed fructo-oligosaccharide sweetener." *Am J Clin Nutr* 1987;46:61-5.

741 Bornet FR. "Undigestible sugars in food products." *Am J Clin Nutr* 1994;59(Suppl):763S-9S.

742 Roberfroid MB. "Prebiotics and synbiotics: concepts and nutritional properties." *Br J Nutr* 1998;80:S197-202.

743 Schaafsma G, et al. "Effects of a milk product, fermented by Lactobacillus acidophilus and with fructo-oligosaccharides added, on blood lipids in male volunteers." *Eur J Clin Nutr* 1998;52:436-40.

744 Roberfroid M. "Dietary fiber, inulin, and oligofructose: a review comparing their physiological effects." *Crit Rev Food Sci Nutr* 1993;33:103-48.

745 Briet F, et al. "Symptomatic response to varying levels of fructo-oligosaccharides consumed occasionally or regularly." *Eur J Clin Nutr* 1995;49:501-7.

746 Mitsuoka T, Hidaka H, Eida T. "Effect of fructo-oligosaccharides on intestinal microflora." *Nahrung* 1987;31:427-36.

747 Alles MS, et al. "Fate of fructo-oligosaccharides in the human intestine." *Br J Nutr* 1996;76:211-21.

748 Pierre F, et al. "Short-chain fructo-oligosaccharides reduced the occurrence of colon tumors and develop gut-associated lymphoid tissue in Min mice." *Br J Nutr* 1997;57:225-8.

749 Gibson GR. "Dietary modulation of the human *Gut* microflora using prebiotics." *Br J Nutr* 1998;80:S209-12.

750 Bouhnik Y, et al. "Short-chain fructo-oligosaccharide administration dose-dependently increases fecal bifidobacteria in healthy humans." *J Nutr* 1999;129:113-6.

751 Fry AC, et al. "The effects of gamma-oryzanol supplementation during resistance exercise training." *Int J Sport Nutr* 1997;7:318-29.

752 Sasaki J, et al. "Effects of gamma-oryzanol on serum lipids and apolipoproteins in dyslipidemic schizophrenics receiving major tranquilizers." *Clin Ther*

1990;12:263-8.

753 Shimomura Y, et al. "Effect of gamma-oryzanol on serum TSH concentrations in primary hypothyroidism." *Endocrinol Jpn* 1980;27:83-6.

754 Sugano M, Tsuji E. "Rice bran oil and human health." *Biomed Environ Sci* 1996;9:242-6.

755 Wheeler KB, Garleb KA. "Gamma oryzanol-plant sterol supplementation: metabolic, endocrine, and physiologic effects." *Int J Sports Nutr* 1991;1:170-7.

756 Seetharamaiah GS, Chandrasekhara N. "Effect of oryzanol on cholesterol absorption and biliary and fecal bile acids in rats." *Indian J Med Res* 1990;92:471-5.

757 Ishihara M, et al. [Clinical effect of gamma-oryzanol on climacteric disturbance- on serum lipid peroxides.] [Article in Japanese] *Nippon Sanka Fujinka Gakkai Zasshi* 1982;34:243-51.

758 Upton R, ed. St. John's wort, Hypericum perforatum: quality control,analytical and therapeutic monograph. Santa Cruz, CA: *American Herbal Pharmacopoeia*; 1997;1-32.

759 Chavez ML,Chavez PI. "Saint John's wort." *Hospital Pharmacy*, 1997; 32(12):1621-32.

760 Chavez ML. Glucosamine sulfate and chondroitin sulfates. *Hospital Pharmacy*, 1997;32(9):1275-85.

761 Laakmann G, et al. "St. John's wort in mild to moderate depression: the relevance of hyperforin for the clinical efficacy." *Pharmacopsychiatry* 1998;31(Suppl 1):54-9.

762 Chatterjee SS, et al. "Antidepressant activity of hypericum perforatum and hyperforin: the neglected possibility." *Pharmacopsychiatry* 1998;31(Suppl 1):7-15.

763 Muller WE, et al. "Hyperforin represents the neurotransmitter reuptake inhibiting constituent of hypericum extract." *Pharmacopsychiatry* 1998;31(Suppl 1):16-21.

764 Gerber GS, et al. "Saw palmetto (Serenoa repens) in men with lower urinary tract symptoms: effects on urodynamic parameters and voiding symptoms." *Urology* 1998;51(6):1003-7.

765 *FDA*. "Unapproved Over-the-Counter (OTC) Drugs Still Marketed?" FDA Medical Bulletin, 1996;26(1). URL: www.fda.gov/medbull/january96/otc.html (Accessed 23 July 1999).

766 Young at Heart. AL-CO-EZE Website. URL: www.yatheartmktg.com/yath8.html (Accessed 16 July 1999).

767 Shiroky JB, et al. "Low-dose methotrexate with leucovorin (folinic acid) in the management of rheumatoid arthritis. Results of a multicenter randomized, double-blind, placebo-controlled trial." *Arthritis Rheum* 1993;36(6):795-803.

768 Duhra P. "Treatment of gastrointestinal symptoms associated with methotrexate therapy for psoriasis." *J Am Acad Dermatol* 1993;28(3):466-9.

769 Voordouw BC, et al. "Melatonin and melatonin-progestin combinations alter pituitary-ovarian function in women and can inhibit ovulation." *J Clin Endocrinol Metab* 1992;74(1):108-17.

770 Becker BN. "Ginseng-induced diuretic resistance." *JAMA* 1996;276(8):606-7.

771 Walaszek Z. "Potential use of D-glucarate derivatives in Cancer prevention." *Cancer Letters* 1990;54:1-8.

772 Dwivedi C, et al. "Effect of calcium glucarate on B-glucuronidase activity and glucarate content on certain vegetables and fruits." *Biochemical Med and Metab Bio* 1990;43:83-92.

773 Heerdt AS, Young CW, Borgen PI. "Calcium glucarate as a chemopreventive agent in breast cancer." *Isr J Med Sci* 1995;31:101-5.

774 Walaszek Z, et al. "Metabolism, uptake and excretion of D-glucaric acid salt and its potential use in Cancer prevention." *Cancer Detect Prev* 1997;21(2):178-90.

775 Walaszek Z, et al. "Dietary glucarate as anti-promter of 7,12-dimethylbenz(a)anthracene-induced mammary tumorigenesis." *Carcinogenesis* 1986;7(9):1463-6.

776 Curley RW Jr., et al. "Activity of D-glucarate analogues: synergistic antiproliferative effects with retinoid in cultured human mammary tumor cells appear to specifically require the D-glucarate structure." *Life Sci* 1994;54(18):1299-303.

777 Furuno K, et al. "Preventive effect of D-glucarate against renal damage induced by kanamycin." *Antibiot* (Tokyo) 1976;29(9):950-3.

778 Kampf D, Roots I, Hildenbrandt AG. "Urinary excretion of D-glucarate, an indicator of drug metabolizing enzyme activity, in patients with impaired renal function." *Eur J Clin Pharmacol* 1980;18(3):255-61.

779 Mezey E. "Increased urinary excretion of D-glucarate acid in alcoholism." *Res Commun Chem Pathol Pharmacol* 1976;15(4);735-42.

780 Pointel JP, et al. "Titrated extract of Centella asiatica (TECA) in the treatment of venous insufficiency of the lower limbs." *Angiology* 1987;38(1 Pt 1):46-50.

781 Farese RV Jr., et al. "Licorice-induced hypermineralocorticoidism." *N Engl J Med* 1991;325(17):1223-7.

782 Singh YN, Blumenthal M. "Kava an overview." *HerbalGram* 1997;39:33-44, 46-55.

783 Cartier LC, Lehrer A, Malo JL. "Occupational asthma caused by aromatic herbs." *Allergy* 1996;51:647-9.

784 Joy JE, Watson SJ Jr., Benson JA Jr., eds. "Marijuana and Medicine, Assessing the Science Base." Division of Neuroscience and Behavioral Health, Institute Of Medicine, National Academy Press, Washington, D.C. 1999. URL: www.nap.edu/readingroom/books/marimed/ (Accessed 23 July 1999).

785 Hsu CK, et al. "Anticholinergic poisoning associated with herbal tea." *Arch Intern Med* 1995;155(20):2245-8.

786 GVI Sourcing webpage: URL: www.gvisourcing.com/ pharmaceuticals/ppg/default.html (Accessed 16 July 1999).

787 Foster S. Peppermint, Menta x piperita, Botanical Series No. 306. Austin, TX: American Botanical Council, 1990.

788 Kapil A, Moza N. "Anticomplementary activity of boswellic acids-an inhibitor of C3-convertase of the classical complement pathway." *Int J Immunopharmacol* 1992;14(7):1139-43.

789 Haney DQ. "Tomato nutrient is found to fight Prostate cancer. " Associated Press, Philadelphia, 12 April 1999.

790 W_lbling RH, Leonhardt K. "Local therapy of herpes simplex with dried extract from Melissa officinalis." *PhytoMedicine* 1994;1:25-31.

791 Takahashi M, Matsuo I, Ohkido M. "Contact Dermatitis due to honeybee royal jelly." *Contact Dermatitis* 1983 9:452-5.

792 Bullock RJ, et al. "Fatal royal jelly-induced asthma." *Med J Aust* 1994;160:44.

793 Reiter WJ, et al. "Dehydroepiandrosterone in the treatment of erectile dysfunction: A prospective, double-blind, randomized, placebo-controlled study." *Urology* 1999;53(3):590-5.

794 Kantola T, Kivisto KT, Neuvonen PJ. "Grapefruit juice

REFERENCES

REFERENCES

greatly increases serum concentrations of lovastatin and lovastatin acid." *Clin Pharmacol Ther* 1998;63(4):397-402.

795 Foster S. Milk Thistle, Silybum marianum, Botanical Series No. 305. Austin, TX: American Botanical Council, 1996.

796 Cholestin webpage, URL: www.pharmanex.com/products/heart_health/cholestin.html (Accessed 21 November 1999).

797 Awang DVC. "Siberian ginseng toxicity may be case of mistaken identity." [Letter]. *Can Med Assoc J* 1996;155(9):1237.

798 Moretti S. "Effect of L-carnitine on human immunodeficiency virus-1 infection-associated apoptosis: a pilot study." *Blood* 1998;91(10):3817-24.

799 Magro-Filho O, de Carvalho AC. "Topical effect of propolis in the repair of sulcoplasties by the modified Kazanjian technique. Cytological and clinical evaluation." *J Nihon Univ Sch Dent* 1994;36(2):102-11.

800 Magro Filho O, de Carvalho AC. "Application of propolis to dental sockets and skin wounds." *J Nihon Univ Sch Dent* 1990;32(1):4-13.

801 Emerson Ecologics "New Products" Website: URL: www.emersonecologics.com/homepage/Promotions/Hot1.html (Accessed 19 July 1999).

802 "Pycnogenol." Robar Health Resources Website. URL: cybermontana.com/robar/pycnogenol.html.

803 "What is Pycnogenol." HealthTrak Website. URL: www.healthtrak.com/whatispyc.html.

805 Bartram T. Encyclopedia of Herbal Medicine. Dorset, UK :Grace Publishers; 1995.

806 Stanko RT, Mullick P, Clarke MR, et al. "Pyruvate inhibits growth of mammary adenocarcinoma 13762 in rats." *Br J Nutr* 1994;54(4):1004-7.

807 Stanko RT, Robertson RJ, Galbreath RW, et al. "Enhanced leg exercise endurance with a high-carbohydrate diet and dihydroxyacetone and pyruvate." *J Appl Physiol* 1990;69(5):1651-6.

808 Stanko RT, Robertson RJ, Spina RJ, et al. "Enhancement of arm exercise endurance capacity with dihydroxyacetone and pyruvate." *J Appl Physiol* 1990;68(1):119-24.

809 Hogan III RP. "Hemorrhagic diathesis caused by drinking an herbal tea." *JAMA* 1983;249:2679-80.

810 Gonzalez M, Zarzuelo A, Gamez MJ, et al. "Hypoglycemic Activity of Olive Leaf." *Planta Medica* 1992;58(6):513-5.

811 Heimann SW. "Pycnogenol for ADHD?" *J Am Acad Child Adolesc Psychiatry* 1999;38(4):357-8.

812 Mash DC, Kovera CA, Buck BE, et al. "Medication development of ibogaine as a Pharmacotherapy for drug dependence." *Ann N Y Acad Sci* 1998;844:274-92.

813 Glick SD, Maisonneuve IS. "Mechanisms of antiaddictive actions of ibogaine." *Ann N Y Acad Sci* 1998;844:214-26.

815 Royal Botanical Gardens Kew Online Databases, URL: www.rbgkew.org.uk/web.dbs/webdbsintro.html.

816 Germplasm Resources Information Network Website, URL: www.ars-grin.gov/npgs (Accessed 3 November 1999).

817 Harrington C. Plant Dubbed 'Nature's Viagra'. Calgary, Ca: Canadian Press; 15 Nov. 1998.

818 Dudley JP. "Bilateral pneumothorax resulting from the bronchoscopic removal of a puncture vine fruit." *Ann Otol Rhinol Laryngol* 1983;92(4 Pt 1):396-7.

819 Pierard-Franchimont C, Goffin V, Visser JN, et al. A double-blind controlled evaluation of the sebosuppressive activity of topical erythromycin-zinc complex. *Eur J Clin Pharmacol* 1995;49(1-2):57-60.

820 Feucht CL, Allen BS, Chalker DK, et al. Topical erythromycin with zinc in acne. A double-blind controlled study. *J Am Acad Dermatol* 1980;3(5):483-91.

821 Mostafa WZ, al-Zayer AA. Acrodermatitis enteropathica in Saudi Arabia. *Int J Dermatol* 1990;29(2):134-8.

822 Hoogenraad TU, Van Hattum J, Van den Hamer CJ. Management of Wilson's disease with zinc sulphate. Experience in a series of 27 patients. *J Neurol Sci* 1987;77(2-3):137-46.

823 Anderson LA, Hakojarvi SL, Boudreaux SK. Zinc acetate treatment in Wilson's disease. *Ann Pharmacother* 1998;32(1):78-87.

824 Fortes C, Forastiere F, Agabiti N, et al. The effect of zinc and vitamin A supplementation on immune response in an older population. *J Am Geriatr Soc* 1998;46(1):19-26.

825 Faruque AS, Mahalanabis D, Haque SS, et al. Double-blind, randomized, controlled trial of zinc or vitamin A supplementation in young children with acute diarrhea. *Acta Pediatr* 1999;88(2):154-60.

826 Roy SK, Tomkins AM, Akramuzzaman SM, et al. Randomized controlled trial of zinc supplementation in malnourished Bangladeshi children with acute diarrhea. *Arch Dis Child* 1997;77(3):196-200.

827 Sazawal S, Black RE, Bhan MK, et al. Zinc supplementation in young children with acute diarrhea in India. *N Engl J Med* 1995;333(13):839-44.

828 Blondeau JM. Expanded activity and utility of the new fluoroquinolones: a review. *Clin Ther* 1999;21(1):3-40.

829 Mountokalakis T, Dourakis S, Karatzas N, et al. Zinc deficiency in mild hypertensive patients treated with diuretics. *J Hypertens Suppl* 1984;2(3):S571-2.

830 Reyes AJ, Olhaberry JV, Leary WP, et al. Urinary zinc excretion, diuretics, zinc deficiency and some side-effects of diuretics. *S Afr Med J* 1983;64(24):936-41.

831 Cohanim M, Yendt ER. The effects of thiazides on serum and urinary zinc in patients with renal calculi. *Johns Hopkins Med J* 1975;136(3):137-44.

832 Ghio S, de Servi S, Perotti R, et al. "Different susceptibility to the development of nitroglycerin tolerance in the arterial and venous *Circulation* in humans-Effects of N-acetylcysteine administration." *Circulation* 1992;86:798-802.

834 Calabrese C, Myer S, Munson S, et al. "A cross-over study of the effect of a single oral feeding of medium chain triglyceride oil vs. canola oil on post-ingestion plasma triglyceride levels in healthy men." *Altern Med Rev* 1999;4(1):23-8.

835 Law M, Wald N. Why heart disease mortality is low in France: the time lag explanation. *BMJ* 1999;318(7196):1471-80.

836 Nestel PJ, Pomeroy S, Kay S, et al. Isoflavones from red clover improve systemic arterial compliance but not plasma lipids in menopausal women. *J Clin Endocrinol Metab* 1999;84(3):895-8.

837 Feskanich D, Weber P, Willett WC, et al. "Vitamin K intake and hip fractures in women: a prospective study." *Am J Clin Nutr* 1999;69(1):74-9.

838 Zheng GQ, Kenney PM, Lam LK. "Sesquiterpenes from clove (Eugenia caryophyllata) as potential anticarcinogenic agents." *J Nat Prod* 1992;55(7):999-1003.

839 Anon. "The wellness guide to dietary supplements." *UC Berkeley Wellness Letter* 1998;14(11):WNL SUPP.

840 Personal correspondence. Lane Labs, Inc. Allendale, NJ, June 28, 1999.

841 Hart CL, Smith GD, Hole DJ, Hawthorne VM. Alcohol consumption and mortality from all causes, coronary heart disease, and stroke: results from a prospective cohort study of Scottish men with 21 years of follow up. *BMJ* 1999;318(7200):1725-9.

842 Potter SM, Baum JA, Teng H, et al. "Soy protein and isoflavones: their effects on blood lipids and bone density in postmenopausal women. *Am J Clin Nutr* 1998;68(6 Suppl):1375S-9S.

843 "Flaxseed Oil: Filling A Vital Need," Barleans Organic Oils Website. URL: barleans.com/vital.html (Accessed 23 July 1999).

844 "Flaxseed oil," MotherNature.com Website. URL: www.mothernature.com/ency/Supp/Flaxseed.asp (Accessed 23 July 1999).

845 Allman MA, Pena MM, Pang D. "Supplementation with flaxseed oil versus sunflower seed oil in healthy young men consuming a low fat diet: effects on platelet composition and function." *Eur J Clin Nutr* 1995;49(3):169-78.

846 Personal correspondence: Paddock Laboratories, Inc., Minneapolis, MN, July 6, 1999.

847 Poria Cocos - Fu Ling, URL: www.go-symmetry.com/poria-cocos.html (Accessed 16 July 1999).

848 Personal correspondence: Transitions for Health, Inc., Portland, OR, June 5, 1999.

850 Waller DP, et al. "Lack of androgenicity of Siberian ginseng." *JAMA* 1992;267(17):2329.

851 Nestel PJ, Yamashita T, Sasahara T, et al. "Soy isoflavones improve systemic arterial compliance but not plasma lipids in menopausal and perimenopausal women." *Arterioscler Thromb Vasc Biol* 1997;17(12):3392-8.

852 Dobrescu D, Tanasescu M, Mezdrea A, et al. "Contributions to the complex study of some lichens-Usnea genus. Pharmacological studies on Usnea barbata and Usnea hirta species." *Rom J Physiol* 1993;30(1-2):101-7.

853 US Food and Drug Administration, Center for Food Safety and Applied Nutrition, Office of Cosmetics Fact Sheet, February 23, 1995. URL: vm.cfsan.fda.gov/~dms/cos-210.html (Accessed 14 July 1999).

854 Wiesenauer M, LŸdtke R. "Mahonia aquifolium in patients with Psoriasis vulgaris- an intraindividual study." *PhytoMedicine* 1996;3(3):231-5.

855 Personal correspondence. Prime Pharmaceutical Corporation, Toronto, Ontario, Canada, June 28, 1999.

856 Natural Health Remedies, Health Canada Website. URL: hc-sc.gc.ca/english/archives/96-97/herbnae.html (Accessed 16 July 1999).

857 Gieler U, von der Weth A, Heger M. "Mahonia aquifolium- a new type of topical treatment for psoriasis." *Journal of Dermatological Treatment* 1995;6:31-4.

858 Hiermann A, Bucar F. "Studies of Epilobium angustifolium extracts on growth of accessory sexual organs in rats." *J Ethnopharmacol* 1997;55(3):179-83.

859 Hiermann A, Reidlinger M, Juan H, Sametz W. [Isolation of the antiphlogistic principle from Epilobium angustifolium]. [Article in German] *Planta Med* 1991;57(4):357-60.

860 Hiermann A, Juan H, Sametz W. "Influence of Epilobium extracts on prostaglandin biosynthesis and carrageenin induced edema of the rat paw." *J Ethnopharmacol* 1986;17(2):161-9.

861 AA. Cramp bark, Myst Herb & Tea Website, URL: www.mystherb.com (Accessed 19 July 1999).

862 United States Food and Drug Administration, List of Orphan Designations and Approvals. URL: www.fda.gov/orphan/designat/list.html (Accessed 20 July 1999).

863 Via-Bran Website. URL: www.viabran.com (Accessed 20 July 1999).

864 USDA Nutrient Database for Standard Reference, Release 12 (March 1998), Crude rice bran. URL: www.nal.usda.gov/fnic/cgi-bin/list_nut.pl (Accessed 20 July 1999).

865 Gerhardt AL, Gallo NB. "Full-fat rice bran and oat bran similarly reduce hypercholesterolemia in humans." *J Nutr* 1998;128(5):865-9.

866 Ghoneum M. "Anti-HIV activity in vitro of MGN-3, an activated arabinoxylane from rice bran." *Biochem Biophys Res Commun* 1998;243(1):25-9.

867 Iida T, Nakagawa R, Hirakawa H, et al. "Clinical trial of a combination of rice bran fiber and cholestyramine for promotion of fecal excretion of retained polychlorinated dibenzofuran and polychlorinated biphenyl in Yu-Cheng patients." *Fukuoka Igaku Zasshi* 1995;86(5):226-33.

870 Iida T, Hirakawa H, Matsueda T, et al. [Therapeutic trials for promotion of faecal excretion of PCDFs by the administration of rice bran fiber and cholestyramine in Yusho patients]. [Article in Japanese] *Fukuoka Igaku Zasshi* 1993;84(5):257-62.

871 Weisburger JH, Reddy BS, Rose DP, et al. "Protective mechanisms of dietary fibers in nutritional carcinogenesis." *Basic Life Sci* 1993;61:45-63.

872 Fujiwaki T, Furusho K. "The effects of rice bran broth bathing in patients with atopic dermatitis." *Acta Paediatr Jpn* 1992;34(5):505-10.

873 Sanders TA, Reddy S. "The influence of rice bran on plasma lipids and lipoproteins in human volunteers." *Eur J Clin Nutr* 1992;46(3):167-72.

874 Jahnen A, Heynck H, Gertz B, et al. "Dietary fibre: the effectiveness of a high bran intake in reducing renal calcium excretion." *Urol Res* 1992;20(1):3-6.

875 Cara L, Dubois C, Borel P, et al. "Effects of oat bran, rice bran, wheat fiber, and wheat germ on postprandial lipemia in healthy adults. *Am J Clin Nutr* 1992;55(1):81-8.

876 Ebisuno S, Morimoto S, Yasukawa S, Ohkawa T. "Results of long-term rice bran treatment on stone recurrence in hypercalciuric patients." *Br J Urol* 1991;67(3):237-40.

877 Kestin M, Moss R, Clifton PM, Nestel PJ. "Comparative effects of three cereal brans on plasma lipids, blood pressure, and glucose metabolism in mildly hypercholesterolemic men." *Am J Clin Nutr* 1990;52(4):661-6.

878 Noronha IL, Andriolo A, Lucon AM, et al. [Rice bran in the treatment of idiopathic hypercalciuria in patients with urinary calculosis]. [Article in Portugese] *Rev Paul Med* 1989;107(1):19-24.

879 Tomlin J, Read NW. "Comparison of the effects on colonic function caused by feeding rice bran and wheat bran." *Eur J Clin Nutr* 1988;42(10):857-61.

880 Ebisuno S, Morimoto S, Yoshida T, et al. "Rice-bran treatment for calcium stone formers with idiopathic hypercalciuria." *Br J Urol* 1986;58(6):592-5.

© Copyright 2000, Natural Medicines Comprehensive Database (209) 472-2244. For updated data, go to www.NaturalDatabase.com. • 1171

REFERENCES

881 Ohkawa T, Ebisuno S, Kitagawa M, et al. Rice bran treatment for patients with hypercalciuric stones: experimental and clinical studies. *J Urol* 1984;132(6):1140-5.

882 Ohkawa T, Ebisuno S, Kitagawa M, et al. "Rice bran treatment for hypercalciuric patients with urinary calculous disease." *J Urol* 1983;129(5):1009-11.

883 Tsuda M. "Purification and characterization of a lectin from rice bran." *J Biochem* (Tokyo) 1979;86(5):1451-61.

884 Kumar B, Chaudhuri DK. "Isolation, partial characterization of antithiamine factor present in rice-bran and its effect on TPP-transketolase system and Staphylococcus aureus." *Int J Vitam Nutr Res* 1976;46(2):154-9.

885 Guerra MJ, Jaffe WG [Nutritional studies with rice bran]. [Article in Spanish] *Arch Latinoam Nutr* 1975;25(4):401-17.

886 Herb Website, URL: www.herb.com/materia.htm (Accessed 30 July 99).

901 Birdsall TC. "5-Hydroxytryptophan: A Clinically-Effective Serotonin Precursor." *Altern Med Rev* 1998;3(4):271-80.

902 Michelson D, Page SW, Casey R, et al. "An eosinophilia-myalgia syndrome related disorder associated with exposure to L-5-hydroxytryptophan." *J Rheumatol* 1994;21(12):2261-5.

903 Nakajima T, Kudo Y, Kaneko Z. "Clinical evaluation of 5-hydroxy-L-tryptophan as an antidepressant drug." *Folia Psychiatr Neurol Jpn* 1978;32(2):223-30.

904 Coppen A. Whybrow PC. Noguera R. et al. "The comparative antidepressant value of L-tryptophan and imipramine with and without attempted potentiation by liothyronine." *Arch Gen Psychiatry* 1972;26(3):234-41.

906 Rao B, Broadhurst AD. "Tryptophan and depression." [letter] *Br Med J* 1976; 1(6007):460.

912 Van Hiele LJ. "L-5-hydroxytryptophan in depression: the first substitution therapy in psychiatry: the treatment of 99-out-patients with "therapy-resistant" depressions. *Neuropsychobiology* 1980;6:230-40.

913 Puttini PS, Caruso I. "Primary fibromyalgia syndrome and 5-hydroxy-L-tryptophan: a 90-day open study." *J Int Med Res* 1992;20(2):182-9.

914 Cangiano C, Ceci F, Cancino A, et al. "Eating behavior and adherence to dietary prescriptions in obese adult subjects treated with 5-hydroxytryptophan." *Am J Clin Nutr* 1992;56(5):863-7.

915 Kahn RS, Westenberg HGM. "L-5-hydroxytryptophan in the treatment of anxiety disorders." *J Affective Disorders* 1985;8:197-200.

916 Trouillas P, Brudon F, Adeleine P. "Improvement of cerebellar ataxia with levorotatory form of 5-hydroxytryptophan: a double-blind study with quantified data processing." *Arch Neurol* 1988;45:1217-22.

917 Williams A, Goodenberger D, Caline DB, et al. "Palatal myclonus following herpes zoster amellorated by 5-hydroxytryptophan and carbidopa." *Neurology* 1978;28:358-9.

918 Meyer JS, Welch KM, Deshmukh VD, et al. "Neurotransmitter precursor amino acids in the treatment of multi-infarct dementia and Alzheimer's disease." *J Amer Geriat Soc* 1977;25:289-98.

919 FDA Talk Paper. Impurities confirmed in dietary supplement 5-hydroxy-L-tryptophan. August 31, 1998. http://vm.cfsan.fda.gov/~lrd/tp5htp.html (Accessed 17 September 1999).

920 Kaplan PW, Tusa RJ, Shankroff J, et al. "Visual evoked potentials in adrenoleukodystrophy: a trial with glycerol trioleate and Lorenzo oil." *Ann Neurol* 1993;34(2):169-74.

921 Poulos A, Gibson R, Sharp P, et al. Very long chain fatty acids in X-linked adrenoleukodystrophy brain after treatment with Lorenzo's oil. *Ann Neurol* 1994;36(5):741-6.

922 Duchesne N, Dufour M, Bouchard G, et al. "Adrenoleukodystrophy: magnetic resonance follow-up after Lorenzo's oil therapy." *Can Assoc Radiol J* 1995;46(5):386-91.

923 Moser HW. Clinical and therapeutic aspects of adrenoleukodystrophy and adrenomyeloneuropathy. *J Neuropathol Exp Neurol* 1995;54(5):740-5.

924 Aubourg P, Adamsbaum C, Lavallard-Rousseau MC, et al. "A two-year trial of oleic and erucic acids ("Lorenzo's oil") as treatment for adrenomyeloneuropathy." *N Engl J Med* 1993;329(11):745-52.

925 Kickler TS, Zinkham WH, Moser A, et al. "Effect of erucic acid on platelets in patients with adrenoleukodystrophy." *Biochem Mol Med* 1996;57(2):125-33.

926 Chai BC, Etches WS, Stewart MW, Siminoski K. "Bleeding in a patient taking Lorenzo's oil: evidence for a vascular defect." *Postgrad Med J* 1996;72(844):113-4.

927 Revell P, Green A, Green S. "Platelets in treated adrenoleukodystrophy: a brief report." *J Inherit Metab Dis* 1995;18(5):635-7.

928 Moser HW. Komrower Lecture. Adrenoleukodystrophy: natural history, treatment and outcome. *J Inherit Metab Dis* 1995;18(4):435-47.

929 Maeda K, Suzuki Y, Yajima S, et al. "Improvement of clinical and MRI findings in a boy with adrenoleukodystrophy by dietary erucic acid therapy." *Brain Dev* 1992;14(6):409-12.

930 Wong V. Adrenoleukodystrophy in a Chinese boy. *Brain Dev* 1992;4(4):276-7.

931 Rasmussen M, Moser AB, Borel J, et al. "Brain, liver, and adipose tissue erucic and very long chain fatty acid levels in adrenoleukodystrophy patients treated with glyceryl trierucate and trioleate oils (Lorenzo's oil)." *Neurochem Res* 1994;19(8):1073-82.

932 Miller TE, Dodd J, Ormrod DJ, Geddes R. "Anti-inflammatory activity of glycogen extracted from Perna canaliculus (NZ green-lipped mussel)." *Agents Actions* 1993;38 Spec No:C139-42.

933 Couch RA, Ormrod DJ, Miller TE, Watkins WB. "Anti-inflammatory activity in fractionated extracts of the green-lipped mussel." *N Z Med J* 1982;95(720):803-6.

934 Miller TE, Ormrod D. "The anti-inflammatory activity of Perna canaliculus (NZ green lipped mussel)." *N Z Med J* 1980;92(667):187-93.

935 Larkin JG, Capell HA, Sturrock RD. "Seatone in rheumatoid arthritis: a six-month placebo-controlled study." *Ann Rheum Dis* 1985;44(3):199-201.

936 Miller T, Wu H. "In vivo evidence for prostaglandin inhibitory activity in New Zealand green-lipped mussel extract." *N Z Med J* 1984;97(757):355-7.

937 Naghii MR, Samman S. The effect of boron supplementation on its urinary excretion and selected cardiovascular risk factors in healthy male subjects. *Biol Trace Elem Res* 1997;56(3):273-86.

939 Usuda K, Kono K, Iguchi K, et al. "Hemodialysis effect on serum boron level in the patients with long term hemodialysis." *Sci Total Environ* 1996;191(3):283-90.

940 Meacham SL, Taper LJ, Volpe SL. "Effect of boron supplementation on blood and urinary calcium, magnesium, and phosphorus, and urinary boron in athletic and sedentary women." *Am J Clin Nutr* 1995;61(2):341-5.

941 Newnham RE. "Essentiality of boron for healthy bones and joints." *Environ Health Perspect* 1994;102(Suppl 7):83-5.

942 Meacham SL, Taper LJ, Volpe SL. "Effects of boron supplementation on bone mineral density and dietary, blood, and urinary calcium, phosphorus, magnesium, and boron in female athletes." *Environ Health Perspect* 1994;102(Suppl 7):79-82.

943 Penland JG. "Dietary boron, brain function, and cognitive performance." *Environ Health Perspect* 1994;102(Suppl 7):65-72.

944 Green NR, Ferrando AA. "Plasma boron and the effects of boron supplementation in males." *Environ Health Perspect* 1994;102(Suppl 7):73-7.

945 Shils M, Olson A, Shike M. *Modern Nutrition in Health and Disease*. 8th ed. Philadelphia, PA: Lea and Febiger, 1994.

946 Wyatt RJ, Engelman K, Kupfer DJ, et al. "Effects of L-tryptophan (a natural sedative) on human sleep." *Lancet* 1970;2(7678):842-6.

947 Hunt MJ, Barnetson R. "A comparative study of gluconolactone versus benzoyl peroxide in the treatment of acne." *Australas J Dermatol* 1992;33(3):131-4.

948 Thueson DO, Chan EK, Oechsli LM, Hahn GS. "The roles of pH and concentration in lactic acid-induced stimulation of epidermal turnover." *Dermatol Surg Jun* 1998;24(6):641-5.

949 Kempers S, Katz HI, Wildnauer R, Green B. "An evaluation of the effect of an alpha hydroxy acid-blend skin cream in the cosmetic improvement of symptoms of moderate to severe xerosis, epidermolytic hyperkeratosis, and ichthyosis." *Cutis* 1998;61(5):347-50.

950 Berardesca E, Distante F, Vignoli GP, et al. "Alpha hydroxyacids modulate stratum corneum barrier function." *Br J Dermatol* 1997;137(6):934-8.

951 Rawlings AV, Davies A, Carlomusto M, et al. "Effect of lactic acid isomers on keratinocyte ceramide synthesis, stratum corneum lipid levels and stratum corneum barrier function." *Arch Dermatol* Res 1996;288(7):383-90.

952 Stiller MJ, Bartolone J, Stern R, et al. "Topical 8% glycolic acid and 8% L-lactic acid creams for the treatment of photodamaged skin. A double-blind vehicle-controlled clinical trial." *Arch Dermatol* 1996;132(6):631-6.

953 Piacquadio D, Dobry M, Hunt S, et al. "Short contact 70% glycolic acid peels as a treatment for photodamaged skin. A pilot study." *Dermatol Surg* 1996;22(5):449-52.

954 Ditre CM, Griffin TD, Murphy GF, et al. "Effects of alpha-hydroxy acids on photoaged skin: a pilot clinical, histologic, and ultrastructural study [see comments]." *J Am Acad Dermatol* 1996;34(2 Pt 1):187-95.

955 Wehr R, Krochmal L, Bagatell F, Ragsdale W. "A controlled two-center study of lactate 12 percent lotion and a petrolatum-based creme in patients with xerosis." *Cutis* 1986;37(3):205-7, 209.

956 Barnes S. "Phytoestrogens and breast cancer." *Baillieres Clin Endocrinol Metab December* 1998;12(4):559-79.

957 Hotz G, Frank T, Zoller J, Wiebelt H. "Antiphlogistic effect of bromelaine following third molar removal." [article in German]. *Dtsch Zahnarztl Z* 1989;44(11):830-2.

958 Valueva TA, Revina TA, Mosolov VV. "Potato tuber protein proteinase inhibitors belonging to the Kunitz soybean inhibitor family." *Biochemistry* (Mosc) 1997;62(12):1367-74.

959 Tanabe S, Tesaki S, Watanabe M, Yanagihara Y. "Cross-reactivity between bromelain and soluble fraction from wheat flour"." [Article in Japanese] *Arerugi* 1997;46(11):1170-3.

960 Masson M. "Bromelain in blunt injuries of the locomotor system. A study of observed applications in general practice." [Article in German] *Fortschr Med* 1995;113(19):303-6.

961 Zimacheva AV, Mosolov VV. "Cysteine proteinase inhibitors from soy seeds." [Article in Russian] *Biokhimiia* 1995;60(1):118-23.

962 Zavadova E, Desser L, Mohr T. "Stimulation of reactive oxygen species production and cytotoxicity in human neutrophils in vitro and after oral administration of a polyenzyme preparation." *Cancer Biother* 1995;10(2):147-52.

963 Diez-Gomez ML, Quirce S, Aragoneses E, Cuevas M. "Asthma caused by Ficus benjamina latex: evidence of cross-reactivity with fig fruit and papain." *Ann Allergy Asthma Immunol* 1998;80(1):24-30.

964 Raus I. "Clinical studies on Frubienzyme in a controlled double-blindtrial." [Article in German]. *Fortschr Med* 1976;94(28):1579-82.

965 Billigmann P. "Enzyme therapy-an alternative in treatment of herpes zoster. A controlled study of 192 patients." [Article in German]. *Fortschr Med* 1995;113(4):43-8.

966 Shuttleworth D, Hill S, Marks R, Connelly DM. "Relief of experimentally induced pruritus with a novel eutectic mixture of local anaesthetic agents." *Br J Dermatol* 1988;119(4):535-40.

967 Mansfield LE, Ting S, Haverly RW, Yoo TJ. "The incidence and clinical implications of hypersensitivity to papain in an allergic population, confirmed by blinded oral challenge." *Ann Allergy* 1985;55(4):541-3.

968 Bienen H, Raus I. "Therapeutic comparison of throat lozenges (author's transl)." [Article in German]. *MMW Munch Med Wochenschr* 1981;123(18):745-7.

969 Reinecke M. "Treatment of inflammatory diseases of the mouth and throat with Larypront in ENT practice (author's transl)." [Article in German]. *MMW Munch Med Wochenschr* 1976;118(39):1253-4.

970 Baron JA, Beach M, Mandel JS, et al. "Calcium supplements for the prevention of colorectal adenomas. Calcium Polyp Prevention Study Group." *N Engl J Med* 1999;340(2):101-7.

971 Levine RJ, Hauth JC, Curet LB, et al. "Trial of calcium to prevent preeclampsia." *N Engl J Med* 1997;337(2):69-76.

972 Whelton PK, Kumanyika SK, Cook NR, et al. "Efficacy of nonpharmacologic interventions in adults with high-normal blood pressure: results from phase 1 of the Trials of Hypertension Prevention. Trials of Hypertension Prevention Collaborative Research Group." *Am J Clin Nutr* 1997;65(2 Suppl):652S-60S.

973 Purwar M, Kulkarni H, Motghare V, Dhole S. "Calcium supplementation and prevention of pregnancy induced hypertension." *J Obstet Gynaecol Res* 1996;22(5):425-30.

© Copyright 2000, Natural Medicines Comprehensive Database (209) 472-2244. For updated data, go to www.NaturalDatabase.com. • 1173

REFERENCES

974   Yamamoto ME, Applegate WB. Klag MJ, et al. "Lack of *Blood* pressure effect with calcium and magnesium supplementation in adults with high-normal blood pressure. Results from Phase I of the Trials of Hypertension Prevention (TOHP). Trials of Hypertension Prevention (TOHP) Collaborative Research Group." *Ann Epidemiol* 1995;5(2):96-107.

975   Petersen LJ, Rudnicki M, Hojsted J. "Long-term oral calcium supplementation reduces diastolic blood pressure in end stage renal disease. A randomized, double-blind, placebo controlled study." *Int J Artif Organs* 1994;17(1):37-40.

976   Weinberger MH, Wagner UL, Fineberg NS. "The blood pressure effects of calcium supplementation in humans of known sodium responsiveness." *Am J Hypertens* 1993;6(9):799-805.

977   Storm D, Eslin R, Porter ES, et al. "Calcium supplementation prevents seasonal bone loss and changes in biochemical markers of bone turnover in elderly new england women: a randomized placebo-controlled trial." *J Clin Endocrinol Metab* 1998;83(11):3817-25.

978   Baeksgaard L, Andersen KP, Hyldstrup L. "Calcium and vitamin D supplementation increases spinal BMD in healthy, postmenopausal women." *Osteoporos Int* 1998;8(3):255-60.

979   Riggs BL, et al. "Long-term effects of calcium supplementation on serum parathyroid hormone level, bone turnover, and bone loss in elderly women." *J Bone Miner Res* 1998;13(2):168-74.

980   Dawson-Hughes B, et al. "Effect of calcium and vitamin D supplementation on bone density in men and women 65 years of age or older." *N Engl J Med* 1997;337(10):670-6.

981   Devine A, et al. "A 4-year follow-up study of the effects of calcium supplementation on bone density in elderly postmenopausal women." *Osteoporos Int* 1997;7(1):23-8.

982   Bernstein CN, et al. "A randomized, placebo-controlled trial of calcium supplementation for decreased bone density in corticosteroid-using patients with inflammatory bowel disease: a pilot study." *Aliment Pharmacol Ther Oct.* 1996;10(5):777-86.

983   Ilich-Ernst JZ, et al. "Iron status, menarche, and calcium supplementation in adolescent girls." *Am J Clin Nutr* Oct. 1998;68(4):880-7.

984   Dwyer JH, et al. "Dietary calcium, calcium supplementation, and blood pressure in African American adolescents." *Am J Clin Nutr* Sep. 1998;68(3):648-55.

985   Thys-Jacobs S, et al. "Calcium carbonate and the premenstrual syndrome: effects on premenstrual and menstrual symptoms. Premenstrual Syndrome Study Group." *Am J Obstet Gynecol* Aug.1998;179(2):444-52.

986   Reid IR. "The roles of calcium and vitamin D in the prevention of osteoporosis." *Endocrinol Metab Clin North Am* 1998;27(2):389-98.

987   Ricci TA, et al. "Calcium supplementation suppresses bone turnover during weight reduction in postmenopausal women." *J Bone Miner Res* 1998;13(6):1045-50.

988   Kalkwarf HJ, et al. "The effect of calcium supplementation on bone density during lactation and after weaning." *N Engl J Med* 1997;337(8):523-8.

989   McKenna AA, et al. "Zinc balance in adolescent females." *Am J Clin Nutr* 1997;65(5):1460-4.

990   Gupta SK, et al. "Reversal of fluorosis in children." *Acta Paediatr Jpn* 1996;38(5):513-9.

991   Steinbach G, et al. "Calcium carbonate treatment of diarrhea in intestinal bypass patients." *Eur J Gastroenterol Hepatol* 1996;8(6):559-62.

992   Lupton JR, et al. "Calcium supplementation modifies the relative amounts of bile acids in bile and affects key aspects of human colon physiology*J Nutr* 1996;126(5):1421-8.

993   Alberts DS, et al. "Randomized, double-blinded, placebo-controlled study of effect of wheat bran fiber and calcium on fecal bile acids in patients with resected adenomatous colon polyps." *J Natl Cancer Inst* 1996;88(2):81-92.

994   Baron JA, et al. "Calcium supplementation and rectal mucosal proliferation: a randomized controlled trial." *J Natl Cancer Inst* 1995;87(17):1303-7.

995   Gallagher JC, Riggs BL, DeLuca. "Effect of estrogen on calcium absorption and serum vitamin D metabolites in postmenopausal osteoporosis." *J Clin Endocrinol Metab* 1980;51(6):1359-64.

996   Whiting SJ. "Safety of some calcium supplements questioned." *Nutr Rev* 1994;52(3):95-7.

997   Roberts HJ. "Potential toxicity due to dolomite and bonemeal." *South Med J* 1983;76(5):556-9.

998   Dietary Reference Intakes (DRI's), Institute of Medicine of the National Academy of Sciences, 1997.

999   Akedo I, et al. "Three cases with familial adenomatous polyposis diagnosed as having malignant lesions in the course of a long-term trial using docosahexanoic acid (DHA)-concentrated fish oil capsules." *Jpn J Clin Oncol* 1998;28(12):762-5.

1000   Danno K, Sugie N. "Combination therapy with low-dose etretinate and eicosapentaenoic acid for psoriasis vulgaris." *J Dermatol* 1998;25(11):703-5.

1001   Prisco D, et al. "Effect of medium-term supplementation with a moderate dose of n-3 polyunsaturated fatty acids on blood pressure in mild hypertensive patients." *Thromb Res* 1998;1(3):105-12.

1002   Gans RO, et al. "Fish oil supplementation in patients with stable claudication." *Am J Surg* 1990;160(5):490-5.

1003   Vognild E, et al. "Effects of dietary marine oils and olive oil on fatty acid composition, platelet membrane fluidity, platelet responses, and serum lipids in healthy humans." *Lipids* 1998;33(4):427-36.

1004   Mayser P, Mrowietz U, Arenberger P, et al. "Omega-3 fatty acid-based lipid infusion in patients with chronic plaque psoriasis: results of a double-blind, randomized, placebo-controlled, multicenter trial [published erratum appears in *J Am Acad Dermatol*, 1998;39(3):421]." *J Am Acad Dermatol* 1998;38(4):539-47.

1005   Campan P, Planchand PO, Duran D. "Pilot study on n-3 polyunsaturated fatty acids in the treatment of human experimental gingivitis." *J Clin Periodontol* 1997;24(12):907-13.

1006   Thies N. "The effect of 12 months' treatment with eicosapentaenoic acid in five children with cystic fibrosis." *J Paediatr Child Health* 1997;33(4):349-51.

1007   Singh RB, et al. "Randomized, double-blind, placebo-controlled trial of fish oil and mustard oil in patients with suspected acute myocardial infarction: the Indian experiment of infarct survival-4. *Cardiovasc Drugs Ther* 1997;11(3):485-91.

1008   Sagar PS, et al. "Cytotoxic action of cis-unsaturated fatty acids on human cervical carcinoma (HeLa) cells: relationship to free radicals and lipid peroxidation and its modulation by calmodulin antagonists." *Cancer Lett* 1992;63(3):189-98.

1009 Grimsgaard S, et al. "Highly purified eicosapentaenoic acid and docosahexaenoic acid in humans have similar triacylglycerol-lowering effects but divergent effects on serum fatty acids." *Am J Clin Nutr* 1997;66(3):649-59.

1011 Allard JP, et al. "Lipid peroxidation during n-3 fatty acid and vitamin E supplementation in humans." *Lipids* 1997;32(5):535-41.

1012 Andreassen AK, et al. "Hypertension prophylaxis with omega-3 fatty acids in heart transplant recipients." *J Am Coll Cardiol* 1997;29:1324-31.

1013 Badalamenti S, et al. "Lack of renal effects of fish oil administration in patients with advanced cirrhosis and impaired glomerular filtration." *Hepatology* 1997;25(2):313-6.

1014 Agren JJ, et al. "Fish diet, fish oil and docosahexaenoic acid rich oil lower fasting and postprandial plasma lipid levels." *Eur J Clin Nutr* 1996;50(11):765-71.

1016 Saynor R, Gillott T. "Changes in blood lipids and fibrinogen with a note on safety in a long term study on the effects of n-3 fatty acids in subjects receiving fish oil supplements and followed for seven years." *Lipids* 1992;27(7):533-8.

1017 van der Tempel H, et al. "Effects of fish oil supplementation in rheumatoid arthritis." *Ann Rheum Dis* 1990;49(2):76-80.

1018 Rambjor GS, et al. "Eicosapentaenoic acid is primarily responsible for hypotriglyceridemic effect of fish oil in humans." *Lipids* 1996;31(Suppl:S45-9).

1019 Behan PO, Behan WM, Horrobin D. "Effect of high doses of essential fatty acids on the postviral fatigue syndrome." *Acta Neurol Scand* 1990;82(3):209-216.

1020 Toft I, et al. "Effects of n-3 polyunsaturated fatty acids on glucose homeostasis and blood pressure in essential hypertension. A randomized, controlled trial." *Ann Intern Med* 1995;123(12):911-8.

1021 Badalamenti S, Salerno F, Lorenzano E. "Renal effects of dietary supplementation with fish oil in cyclosporine-treated *Liver* transplant recipients." *Hepatology* 1995;22(6):1695-71.

1022 Sacks FM, et al. "Controlled trial of fish oil for regression of human coronary atherosclerosis. HARP Research Group." *J Am Coll Cardiol* 1995;25(7):1492-8.

1023 Sakakibara H, et al. "Effect of supplementation with eicosapentaenoic acid ethylster MND- 21, on generation of leukotrienes by calcium ionophore-activated leukocytes in bronchial asthma." *Nihon Kyobu Shikkan Gakkai Zasshi* 1995;33(4):395-402.

1024 Eritsland J, et al. "Long-term metabolic effects of n-3 polyunsaturated fatty acids in patients with coronary artery disease." *Am J Clin Nutr* 1995;61(4):831-6.

1025 Shimizu H, et al. "Long-term effect of eicosapentaenoic acid ethyl (EPA-E) on albuminuria of non-insulin dependent diabetic patients." *Diabetes Res Clin Pract* 1995;28(1):35-40.

1026 Onwude JL, et al. "A randomised double blind placebo controlled trial of fish oil in high risk pregnancy." *Br J Obstet Gynaecol* 1995;102(2):95-100.

1027 Bulstra-Ramakers, MT, et al. "The effects of 3g eicosapentaenoic acid daily on recurrence of intrauterine growth retardation and pregnancy induced hypertension." *Br J Obstet Gynaecol* 1995;102(2):123-6.

1028 Leaf A, et al. "Do fish oils prevent restenosis after coronary angioplasty?" *Circulation* 1994;90(5):2248-57.

1029 McVeigh GE, et al. "Fish oil improves arterial compliance in non-insulin-dependent Diabetes mellitus." *Arterioscler Thromb* 1994;14(9):1425-9.

1030 Sacks FM, et al. "Short report: the effect of fish oil on blood pressure and high-density lipoprotein-cholesterol levels in phase I of the Trials of Hypertension Prevention." *J Hypertens* 1994;12(2):209-13.

1031 Lau CS, Morley KD, Belch JJ. "Effects of fish oil supplementation on non-steroidal anti-inflammatory drug requirement in patients with mild rheumatoid arthritis- a double blind placebo controlled study." *Br J Rheumatol* 1993;32:982-9.

1032 Rossi, E, Costa M. "Fish oil derivatives as a prophylaxis of recurrent miscarriage associated with antiphospholipid antibodies (APL): a pilot study." *Lupus* 1993;2(5):319-23.

1033 Vandongen R, Mori TA, Burke V, et al. "Effects on blood pressure of omega 3 fats in subjects at increased risk of cardiovascular disease." *Hypertension* 1993;22(3):371-9.

1034 Grimminger F, et al. "A double-blind, randomized, placebo-controlled trial of n-3 fatty acid based lipid infusion in acute, extended guttate psoriasis. Rapid improvement of clinical manifestations an changes in neutrophil leukotriene profile." *Clin Investig* 1993;71(8):634-43.

1035 Soyland E, et al. "Effect of dietary supplementation with very-long-chain n-3 fatty acids in patients with psoriasis." *N Engl J Med* 1993;328(25):1812-6.

1036 Thien FC, Mencia-Huerta J, Lee TH. "Dietary fish oil effects on seasonal hay fever and asthma in pollen-sensitive subjects." *Am Rev Respir Dis* 1993;147(5):1138-43.

1037 Greenfield SM, et al. "A randomized controlled study of evening primrose oil and fish oil in ulcerative colitis." *Aliment Pharmacol Ther* 1993;7(2):159-66.

1038 Bellamy CM, et al. "Can supplementation of diet with omega-3 polyunsaturated fatty acids reduce coronary angioplasty restenosis." *Eur Heart J* 1992;13(12):1626-31.

1039 Kjeldsen-Kragh J, et al. "Dietary omega-3 fatty acid supplementation and naproxen treatment in patients with rheumatoid arthritis." *J Rheumatol* 1992;19(10):1531-6.

1040 Hawthorne AB, et al. "Treatment of ulcerative colitis with fish oil supplementation: a prospective 12 month randomised controlled trial." *Gut* 1992;33(7):922-8.

1041 Astorga G, et al. "Active rheumatoid arthritis: effect of dietary supplementation with omega-3 oils. A controlled double-blind trial." *Rev Med Chil* 1991;119(3):267-72.

1042 D'Almeida A, et al. "Effects of a combination of evening primrose oil (gamma linolenic acid) and fish oil (eicosapentaenoic + docahexaenoic acid) versus magnesium, and versus placebo in preventing pre-eclampsia." *Women Health* 1992;19(2-3):117-31.

1043 Hamazaki T, et al. "The effect of docosahexaenoic acid on aggression in young adults. A placebo-controlled double-blind study. *J Clin Invest* 1996;97(4):1129-33.

1044 Conquer JA, Holub BJ. "Supplementation with an algae source of docosahexaenoic acid increases (n-3) fatty acid status and alters selected risk factors for heart disease in vegetarian subjects." *J Nutr* 1996;126(12):3032-9.

1045 Carlson SE, Werkman SH. "A randomized trial of visual attention of preterm infants fed docosahexaenoic acid until two months." *Lipids* 1996;31(1):85-90.

1046 Buckley LM, et al. "Calcium and vitamin D3 supplementation prevents bone loss in the spine secondary to low-dose corticosteroids in patients with rheumatoid arthritis. A randomized double-blind, placebo-controlled trial." *Ann Intern Med* 1996;125(12):961-8.

1047 White E, Shannon JS, Patterson RE. "Relationship between vitamin and calcium supplement use and colon cancer." *Cancer Epidemiol Biomarkers Prev* 1997;6(10):769-74.

1048 Mindell, Earl. *Earl Mindell's Supplement Bible*. Simon and Schuster: NY, NY, 1998.

1049 Suhner A, et al. "Comparative study to determine the optimal melatonin dosage form for the alleviation of jet lag." *Chronobiol Int* 1998;15(6):655-6.

1050 Suhner A, et al. "Impact of melatonin on driving performance." *J Travel Med* 1998;5(1):7-13.

1051 Dreher F, et al. "Topical melatonin in combination with vitamins E and C protects skin from ultraviolet-induced erythema: a human study in vivo." *Br J Dermatol* 1998;139(2):332-9.

1052 Wright SW, et al. "Randomized clinical trial of melatonin after night-shift work: efficacy and neuropsychologic effects." *Ann Emerg Med* 1998 32(3 Pt 1):334-40.

1053 Dolberg OT, Hirschmann S, Grunhaus L. "Melatonin for the treatment of sleep disturbances in major depressive disorder." *Am J Psychiatry* 1998;55(8):1119-21.

1054 James M, et al. "Can melatonin improve adaptation to night shift?" *Am J Emerg Med* 1998;16(4):367-70.

1055 Nagtegaal JE, et al. "Melatonin-responsive headache in delayed sleep phase syndrome: preliminary observations." *Headache* 1998;38(4):303-7.

1056 McArthur AJ, Budden S. "Sleep dysfunction in Rett syndrome: a trial of exogenous melatonin treatment." *Dev Med Child Neurol* 1998;40(3):186-92.

1057 Rosenberg SI, et al. "Effect of melatonin on tinnitus." *Laryngoscope* 1998;108(3):305-10.

1058 Benes L, et al. "Transmucosal, oral controlled-release, and transdermal drug administration in human subjects: a crossover study with melatonin." *J Pharm Sci* 1997;86(10):1115-9.

1059 Leibenluft E, et al. "Effects of exogenous melatonin administration and withdrawal in five patients with rapid-cycling bipolar disorder." *J Clin Psychiatry* 1997;58(9):383-8.

1060 Lissoni P, et al. "A randomized study of chemotherapy with cisplatin plus etoposide versus chemoendocrine therapy with cisplatin, etoposide and the pineal hormone melatonin as a first-line treatment of advanced non-small cell lung cancer patients in a poor clinical state." *J Pineal Res* 1997;23(1):15-9.

1061 Lissoni P, et al. "Biotherapy with the pineal immunomodulating hormone melatonin versus melatonin plus aloe vera in untreatable advanced solid neoplasms." *Nat Immun* 1998;16(1):27-33.

1062 Van Den Heuvel CJ, Reid KJ, Dawson D. "Effect of atenolol on nocturnal sleep and temperature in young men: reversal by pharmacological doses of melatonin." *Physiol Behav* 1997;61(6):795-802.

1063 Wikner J, Wetterberg L, Rojdmark S. "Does hypercalcaemia or calcium antagonism affect human melatonin secretion or renal excretion?" *Eur J Clin Invest* 1997;27(5):374-9.

1064 Lissoni P, et al. "Adjuvant therapy with the pineal hormone melatonin in patients with lymph node relapse due to malignant melanoma." *J Pineal Res* 1996;21(4):239-42.

1065 Leone M, Amico D, Moschiano F. "Melatonin versus placebo in the prophylaxis of cluster headache: a double-blind pilot study with parallel groups." *Cephalalgia* 1996;16(7):494-6.

1066 Bangha E, Elsner P, Kistler GS. "Suppression of UV-induced erythema by topical treatment with melatonin (N-acetyl-5-methoxytryptamine). A dose response study." *Arch Dermatol Res* 1996;288(9):522-6.

1067 Lissoni P, et al. "Is there a role for melatonin in the treatment of neoplastic cachexia?" *Eur J Cancer* 1996;2A(8):1340-3.

1068 Attenburrow ME, Cowen PJ, Sharpley AL. "Low dose melatonin improves sleep in healthy middle-aged subjects." *Psychopharmacology* (Berl) 1996;126(2):179-81.

1069 Lissoni P, et al. "Prevention of cytokine-induced hypotension in cancer patients by the pineal hormone melatonin." *Support Care Cancer* 1996;4(4):313-6.

1070 Ellis CM, Lemmens G, Parkes JD. "Melatonin and insomnia." *J Sleep Res* 1996;5(1):61-5.

1071 Lissoni P, et al. "Increased survival time in brain glioblastomas by a radioneuroendocrine strategy with radiotherapy plus melatonin compared to radiotherapy alone." *Oncology* 1996;53(1):43-6.

1072 Garfinkel D, et al. "Improvement of sleep quality in elderly people by controlled-release melatonin." *Lancet* 1995;346(8974):541-4.

1073 Barni S, et al. "A randomized study of low-dose subcutaneous interleukin-2 plus melatonin versus supportive care alone in metastatic colorectal cancer patients progressing under 5-fluorouracil and folates." *Oncology* 1995;52(3):243-5.

1074 Lissoni P, et al. "A randomized study of immunotherapy with low-dose subcutaneous interleukin-2 plus melatonin vs chemotherapy with cisplatin and etoposide as first-line therapy for advanced non-small cell lung cancer." *Tumori*, 1994;80(6):464-7.

1075 Jan JE, Espezel H, Appleton RE. "The treatment of sleep disorders with melatonin." *Dev Med Child Neurol* 1994;36(2):97-107.

1076 Valcavi R, et al. "Melatonin stimulates growth hormone secretion through pathways other than the growth hormone-releasing hormone." *Clin Endocrinol* (Oxf) 1993;39(2):193-9.

1077 Petrie K, et al. "A double-blind trial of melatonin as a treatment for jet lag in international cabin crew." *Biol Psychiatry* 1993;33(7):526-30.

1078 Dollins AB, et al. "Effect of pharmacological daytime doses of melatonin on human mood and performance." *Psychopharmacology* (Berl) 1993;112(4):490-6.

1079 Claustrat B, et al. "Melatonin and jet lag: confirmatory result using a simplified protocol." *Biol Psychiatry* 1992;32(8):705-11.

1080 Lissoni P, et al. "Randomized study with the pineal hormone melatonin versus supportive care alone in advanced nonsmall cell lung cancer resistant to a first-line chemotherapy containing cisplatin." *Oncology* 1992;49(5):336-9.

1081 Dahlitz M, et al. "Delayed sleep phase syndrome response to melatonin." *Lancet* 1991;337(8750):1121-4.

1082 Sack RL, et al. "Melatonin administration to blind people: phase advances and entrainment." *J Biol Rhythms* 1991;6(3):249-61.

1083 James SP, et al. "Melatonin administration in insomnia." *Neuropsychopharmacology* 1990;3(1):19-23.

1084 Wirz-Justice A, et al. "Morning or night-time melatonin is ineffective in seasonal affective disorder." *J Psychiatr Res* 1990;24(2):129-37.

1085 Petrie K, et al. "Effect of melatonin on jet lag after long haul flights." *BMJ* 1989;298(6675):705-7.

1086 Guardiola-Lemaitre B. "Toxicology of melatonin." *J Biol Rhythms* 1997;12(6):697-706.

1087 Carnielli VP, Da Riol R, Montini G. "Iron supplementation enhances response to high doses of recombinant human erythropoietin in preterm infants." *Arch Dis Child Fetal Neonatal Ed* 1998;79(1):F44-8.

1088 Silva J, et al. Iron supplementation in haemodialysis-practical clinical guidelines. *Nephrol Dial Transplant* 1998;13(10):2572-7.

1089 Brolin RE, et al. Prophylactic iron supplementation after Roux-en-Y gastric bypass: a prospective, double-blind, randomized study. *Arch Surg* 1998;133(7):740-4.

1090 Fudin R, et al. "Correction of uremic iron deficiency anemia in hemodialyzed patients: a prospective study." *Nephron* 1998;79(3):299-305.

1091 Sowade O, et al. "The estimation of efficacy of oral iron supplementation during treatment with epoetin beta (recombinant human erythropoietin) in patients undergoing cardiac surgery." *Eur J Haematol* 1998;60(4):252-9.

1092 Andrews CM, Lane DW, Bradley JG. "Iron pre-load for major joint replacement." *Transfus Med* 1997;7(4):281-6.

1093 Sever Y, et al. "Iron treatment in children with attention deficit hyperactivity disorder. A preliminary report." *Neuropsychobiology* 1997;35(4):178-80.

1094 Cook JD, Skikne BS, Baynes RD. Iron deficiency: the global perspective. *Adv Exp Med Biol* 1994;356:219-28.

1095 Bruner AB, et al. "Randomized study of cognitive effects of iron supplementation in non- anaemic iron-deficient adolescent girls." *Lancet* 1996;348(9033):992-6.

1096 Pool GF, van Jaarsveld H. Dietary iron elevates LDL-cholesterol and decreases plasma antioxidant levels: influence of antioxidants. *Res Commun Mol Pathol Pharmacol* 1998;100(2):139-50.

1097 Corti MC, et al. Serum iron level, coronary artery disease, and all-cause mortality in older men and women. *Am J Cardiol* 1997;79(2):120-7.

1098 Ullen H, et al. Supplementary iron intake and risk of cancer: reversed causality? *Cancer Lett* 1997;114(1-2):215-6.

1099 Reunanen A, et al. Body iron stores, dietary iron intake and coronary heart disease mortality. *J Intern Med* 1995;238(3):223-30.

1100 Lund EK, et al. "Oral ferrous sulfate supplements increase the free radical-generating capacity of feces from healthy volunteers." *Am J Clin Nutr* 1999;69(2):250-5.

1101 Schumann K, Elsenhans, Maurer A. "Iron supplementation." *J Trace Elem Med Biol* 1998;12(3):129-40.

1102 Rehman A, et al. The effects of iron and vitamin C co-supplementation on oxidative damage to DNA in healthy volunteers. *Biochem Biophys Res Commun* 1998;246(1):293-8.

1103 *Recommended Dietary Allowances*. Institute of Medicine of the National Academy of Sciences, 1989.

1104 Soewondo S. The effect of iron deficiency and mental stimulation on Indonesian children's cognitive performance and development. *Kobe J Med Sci* 1995;41(1-2):1-17.

1105 Budeiri D, Li Wan Po A, Dornan JC. Is evening primrose oil of value in the treatment of premenstrual syndrome? *Control Clin Trials* 1996;17(1):60-8.

1106 Khoo SK, Munro C, Battistutta D. Evening primrose oil and treatment of premenstrual syndrome. *Med J Aust* 1990;153(4):189-92.

1107 Gordon M, et al. "A phase II controlled study of a combination of the immune modulator, lentinan, with didanosine (ddI) in HIV patients with CD4 cells of 200-500/mm3." *J Med* 1995;26(5-6):193-207.

1108 Yoshiyuki T, et al. "Treatment for peritoneal dissemination of gastric cancer by intraperitoneal administration of CDDP through Infuse-a-Port." *Gan To Kagaku Ryoho* 1994;21(13):2323-5.

1109 Tari K, et al. "Effect of lentinan for advanced prostate carcinoma." *Hinyokika Kiyo* 1994;40(2):119-23. *Endocrinol Metab* 1998;83(11):3817-25.

1110 Nishihira T, Akimoto M, Mori S. "Anti-cancer effects of BRMs associated with nutrition in cancer patients." *Gan To Kagaku Ryoho*,1988;15(4 Pt 2-3):1615-20.

1111 Wada T, et al. "A comparative clinical trial with tegafur plus lentinan treatment at two different doses in advanced cancer." *Gan To Kagaku Ryoho* 1987;14(8):2509-11.

1112 Kosaka A, et al. "Synergistic action of lentinan (LNT) with endocrine therapy of breast cancer in rats and humans."*Gan To Kagaku Ryoho* 1987;14(2):516-22.

1113 Taguchi T. "Clinical efficacy of lentinan on patients with stomach cancer: end point results of a four-year follow-up survey." *Cancer Detect Prev Suppl* 1987;1:333-49.

1114 Thein DJ, Hurt WC. "Lysine as a prophylactic agent in the treatment of recurrent herpes simplex labialis." *Oral Surg Oral Med Oral Pathol* 1984;58(6):659-66.

1115 McCune MA, et al. "Treatment of recurrent herpes simplex infections with L-lysine monohydrochloride." *Cutis* 1984;34(4):366-73.

1116 DiGiovanna JJ, Blank H. "Failure of lysine in frequently recurrent herpes simplex infection. Treatment and prophylaxis." *Arch Dermatol* 1984;120(1):48-51.

1117 Griffith RS, DeLong DC, Nelson JD. "Relation of arginine-lysine antagonism to herpes simplex growth in tissue culture." *Chemotherapy* 1981;27(3):209-13.

1118 Milman N, Scheibel J, Jessen O. "Lysine prophylaxis in recurrent herpes simplex labialis: a double-blind, controlled crossover study." *Acta Derm Venereol* 1980;60(1):85-7.

1119 Griffith RS, Norins A, Kagan C. "A multicentered study of lysine therapy in Herpes simplex infection." *Dermatologica* 1978;156(5):257-67.

1120 Griffith RS, et al. "Success of L-lysine therapy in frequently recurrent herpes simplex infection. Treatment and prophylaxis." *Dermatologica* 1987;175(4):183-90.

1121 Lo JC, et al. "Fanconi's syndrome and tubulointerstitial nephritis in association with L-lysine ingestion." *Am J Kidney Dis* 1996;28(4):614-7.

1122 Yamori Y, et al. "Prophylactic trials for stroke in stroke-prone SHR. (3) Amino acid analysis of various diets and their prophylactic effect." *Jpn Heart J* 1978;19(4):624-6.

1123 Wu G. "Intestinal mucosal amino acid catabolism." *J Nutr* 1998;128(8):1249-52.

1124 Flodin NW. "The metabolic roles, pharmacology, and toxicology of lysine." *J Am Coll Nutr* 1997;16(1):7-12.

1125 Millward J. "Can we define indispensable amino acid requirements and assess protein quality in adults?" *J Nutr* 1994;124(8 Suppl):1509S-16S.

1126 Phillips RD. "Starchy legumes in human nutrition, health and culture." *Plant Foods Hum Nutr* 1993;44(3):195-211.

1127 Sanchez A, Hubbard RW. "Plasma amino acids and the

insulin/glucagon ratio as an explanation for the dietary protein modulation of atherosclerosis." *Med Hypotheses* 1991;36(1):27-32.

1128 Kurpad AV, et al. "An initial assessment, using 24-h [13C]leucinekinetics, of the lysine requirement of healthy adult Indian subjects." *Am J Clin Nutr* 1998;67(1):58-66.

1129 Duncan AM, Ball RO, Pencharz PB. "Lysine requirement of adult males is not affected by decreasing dietary protein." *Am J Clin Nutr* 1996;64(5):718-25.

1130 Hall SL, Greendale GA. "The relation of dietary vitamin C intake to bone mineral density: results from the PEPI study." *Calcif Tissue Int* 1998;63(3):183-9.

1131 Civitelli R, et al. "Dietary L-lysine and calcium metabolism in humans." *Nutrition* 1992;8(6):400-5.

1132 Kritchevsky D. "Protein and atherosclerosis." *J Nutr Sci Vitaminol* (Tokyo) 1990;36(Suppl 2):S81-6.

1133 Smith KA, Fairburn CG, Cowen PJ. "Symptomatic relapse in bulimia nervosa following acute tryptophan depletion." *Arch Gen Psychiatry* 1999;56(2):171-6.

1134 Sharma RP, Shapiro LE, Kamath SK. "Acute dietary tryptophan depletion: effects on schizophrenic positive and negative symptoms." *Neuropsychobiology* 1997;35(1):5-10.

1135 van Hall G, Raaymakers JS, Saris WH. "Ingestion of branched-chain amino acids and tryptophan during sustained exercise in man: failure to affect performance." *J Physiol* (Lond) 1995;486(Pt 3):789-94.

1136 Delgado PL, Price LH, Miller HL. "Serotonin and the neurobiology of depression. Effects of tryptophan depletion in drug-free depressed patients." *Arch Gen Psychiatry* 1994;51(11):865-74.

1137 Menkes DB, Coates DC, Fawcett JP. "Acute tryptophan depletion aggravates premenstrual syndrome." *J Affect Disord* 1994;32(1):37-44.

1138 Bowen DJ, Spring B, Fox E. "Tryptophan and high-carbohydrate diets as adjuncts to smoking cessation therapy." *J Behav Med* 1991;14(2):97-110.

1139 Etzel KR, Stockstill JW, Rugh JD. "Tryptophan supplementation for nocturnal bruxism: report of negative results." *Rugh JDJ Craniomandib Disord* 1991;5(2):115-20.

1140 Stockstill JW, McCall D Jr., Gross AJ. "The effect of L-tryptophan supplementation and dietary instruction on chronic myofascial pain." *J Am Dent Assoc* 1989;118(4):457-60.

1141 Messiha FS. "Fluoxetine: adverse effects and drug-drug interactions." *J Toxicol Clin Toxicol* 1993;31(4):603-30.

1142 Devoe LD, Castillo RA, Searle NS. "Maternal dietary substrates and human fetal biophysical activity. The effects of tryptophan and glucose on fetal breathing movements." *Am J Obstet Gynecol* 1986;155(1):135-9.

1143 Lieberman HR, Corkin S, Spring BJ. "The effects of dietary neurotransmitter precursors on human behavior." *Am J Clin Nutr* 1985;42(2):366-70.

1144 Schmidt HS. "L-tryptophan in the treatment of impaired respiration in sleep." *Bull Eur Physiopathol Respir* 1983;19(6):625-9.

1145 Seltzer S, Dewart D, Pollack R. "The effects of dietary tryptophan on chronic maxillofacial pain and experimental pain tolerance." *J Psychiatr Res* 1982-83;17(2):181-6.

1146 Hartmann E, Spinweber CL. "Sleep induced by L-tryptophan. Effect of dosages within the normal dietary intake." *J Nerv Ment Dis* 1979;167(8):497-9.

1147 Hitosugi M, et al. "Autopsy case of duodenal obstruction from impacted mushroom." *J Gastroenterol* 1998;33(4):562-5.

1148 Hanada K, Hashimoto I. "Flagellate mushroom (Shiitake) dermatitis and photosensitivity." *Dermatology* 1998;197(3):255-7.

1149 Levy AM, et al. "Eosinophilia and gastrointestinal symptoms after ingestion of shiitake mushrooms." *J Allergy Clin Immunol* 1998;101(5):613-20.

1150 Murakami M, et al. "Decreased pulmonary perfusion in hypersensitivity pneumonitis caused by Shiitake mushroom spores." *J Intern Med* 1997;241(1):85-8.

1151 Matsui S, et al. "Hypersensitivity pneumonitis induced by Shiitake mushroom spores." *Intern Med* 1992;31(10):1204-6.

1152 Nakamura T. "Shiitake (Lentinus edodes) dermatitis." *Contact Dermatitis* 1992;27(2):65-70.

1153 Ueda A, et al. "Allergic contact dermatitis in shiitake (Lentinus edodes (Berk) Sing) growers." *Contact Dermatitis* 1992;26(4):228-33.

1154 Kabir Y, Kimura S. "Dietary mushrooms reduce *Blood* pressure in spontaneously hypertensive rats (SHR)." *J Nutr Sci Vitaminol* (Tokyo) 1989;35(1):91-4.

1155 Otsuka M, et al. "Influences of a shiitake (Lentinus edodes)-fructo-oligosaccharide mixture (SK-204) on experimental pulmonary thrombosis in rats." *Yakugaku Zasshi* 1996;116(2):169-73.

1156 Shitake Components, Website, URL: www.rainforest-mushrooms.com/ShitakeComponents.html (Accessed (23 July 1999).

1157 Colloidal Minerals in Brief Website, URL: www.colloidal.com.au/ (Accessed 23 July 1999).

1158 Wallach J. "Dr. Joel Wallach's Colloidal Minerals" Website, URL: www.elementsofhealth.com/b1.html (Accessed 23 July 1999).

1159 Schauss A. "Colloidal minerals: Clinical implications of clay suspension products sold as dietary supplements." *Amer J of Nat Med* 1997;4(1):5-10.

1160 Sposito G, Skipper NT, Sutton R, et al. "Surface geochemistry of the clay minerals." *Proc Natl Acad Sci USA* 1999;96(7):3358-64.

1161 Schrauzer G. "An overview of liquid mineral supplements." *International J of Integrative Med* 1999;1(2):18-22.

1162 Branton SL, Lott BD, Maslin WR, et al. "Fatty liver-hemorrhagic syndrome observed in commercial layers fed diets containing chelated minerals." *Avian Dis* 1995;39(3):631-5.

1163 Infinity2 Product Question and Answers Website, URL: www.infinity2.net/ChelatedMineralsQuestionF.html (Accessed 23 July 1999).

1164 Chelated Minerals Website, URL: www.netmins.com/chelndx.html (Accessed 23 July 1999).

1165 Youngevity Website, URL: www.ciya.com/13.html (Accessed 23 July 1999).

1166 Reach for Life Quality Products Website, URL: www.reach4life.com/1111.html (Accessed 23 July 1999).

1167 Durlach J, Bac P, Durlach V, et al. "Magnesium status and ageing: an update." *Magnes Res* 1998;11(1):25-42.

1168 Scheen AJ. "Perspective in the treatment of insulin resistance." Hum Reprod 1997;12(Suppl 1):63-71.

1169 Ziment I. "Alternative therapies for asthma." *Curr Opin Pulm Med* 1997;3(1):61-7.

1170 Preuss HG, Gondal JA, Lieberman S. "Association of macronutrients and energy intake with hypertension." *J Am Coll Nutr* 1996;15(1):21-35.

1171 de Valk HW, Verkaaik R, van Rijn HJ, et al. "Oral

magnesium supplementation in insulin-requiring Type 2 diabetic patients." *Diabet Med* 1998;15(6):503-7.

1172 Lima M de L, Cruz T, Pousada JC, et al. "The effect of magnesium supplementation in increasing doses on the control of type 2 diabetes." *Diabetes Care* 1998;21(5):682-6.

1173 Hill J, Micklewright A, Lewis S, et al. "Investigation of the effect of short-term change in dietary magnesium intake in asthma." *Eur Respir J* 1997;10(10):2225-9.

1174 Zehender M, Meinertz T, Faber T, et al. "Antiarrhythmic effects of increasing the daily intake of magnesium and potassium in patients with frequent ventricular arrhythmias. Magnesium in Cardiac Arrhythmias (MAGICA)Investigators." *J Am Coll Cardiol* 1997;29(5):1028-34.

1180 Witteman JC, Grobbee DE, Derkx FH, et al. "Reduction of blood pressure with oral magnesium supplementation in women with mild to moderate hypertension." *Am J Clin Nutr* 1994 60(1):129-35.

1181 Lasserre B, Spoerri M, Moullet V, et al. "Should magnesium therapy be considered for the treatment of coronary heart disease? II. Epidemiological evidence in outpatients with and without coronary heart disease." *Magnes Res* 1994;7(2):145-53.

1182 Yamori Y, Nara Y, Mizushima S, et al. "Nutritional factors for stroke and major cardiovascular diseases: international epidemiological comparison of dietary prevention." *Health Rep* 1994;6(1):22-7.

1183 Mauskop A, Altura BT, Cracco RQ, et al. "Deficiency in serum ionized magnesium but not total magnesium in patients with migraines. Possible role of ICa2+/IMg2+ ratio." *Headache* 1993;33(3):135-8.

1184 Mauskop A, Altura BT, Cracco RQ, et al. "Intravenous magnesium sulfate relieves cluster headaches in patients with low serum ionized magnesium levels." *Headache* 1995;35(10):597-600.

1185 Mauskop A, Altura BT, Cracco RQ, Altura BM. "Intravenous magnesium sulphate relieves migraine attacks in patients with low serum ionized magnesium levels: a pilot study." *Clin Sci* (Colch) 1995;89(6):633-6.

1186 Facchinetti F, Sances G, Borella P, et al. "Magnesium prophylaxis of menstrual migraine: effects on intracellular magnesium." *Headache*, 1991; 31(5):298-301.

1187 Facchinetti F, Borella P, Sances G, et al. "Oral magnesium successfully relieves premenstrual mood changes." *Obstet Gynecol* 1991;78(2):177-81.

1188 Walker AF, De Souza MC, Vickers MF, et al. "Magnesium supplementation alleviates premenstrual symptoms of fluid retention." *J Womens Health* 1998;7(9):1157-65.

1189 Starobrat-Hermelin B, Kozielec T. "The effects of magnesium physiological supplementation on hyperactivity in children with attention deficit hyperactivity disorder (ADHD). Positive response to magnesium oral loading test." *Magnes Res* 1997;10(2):149-56.

1190 Thel MC, Armstrong AL, McNulty SE, et al. "Randomised trial of magnesium in in-hospital cardiac arrest. Duke Internal Medicine Housestaff." *Lancet* 1997;350(9087):1272-6.

1191 Lichodziejewska B, Klos J, Rezler J, et al. "Clinical symptoms of mitral valve prolapse are related to hypomagnesemia and attenuated by magnesium supplementation." *Am J Cardiol* 1997;79(6):768-72.

1192 Sanjuliani AF, de Abreu Fagundes VG, Francischetti EA. "Effects of magnesium on blood pressure and intracellular ion levels of Brazilian hypertensive patients." *Int J Cardiol* 1996;56(2):177-83.

1193 Hoogerbrugge N, Cobbaert C, de Heide L, et al. "Oral physiological magnesium supplementation for 6 weeks with 1 g/d magnesium oxide does not affect increased Lp(a) levels in hypercholesterolaemic subjects." *Magnes Res* 1996;9(2):129-32.

1194 Dahle LO, Berg G, Hammar M, Hurtig M, et al. "The effect of oral magnesium substitution on pregnancy-induced leg cramps." *Am J Obstet Gynecol* 1995;173(1):175-80.

1195 Plum-Wirell M, Stegmayr BG, Wester PO. "Nutritional magnesium supplementation does not change blood pressure nor serum or muscle potassium and magnesium in untreated hypertension. A double-blind crossover study." *Magnes Res* 1994;7(3-4):277-83

1197 Purvis JR, Cummings DM, Landsman P, et al. "Effect of oral magnesium supplementation on selected cardiovascular risk factors in non-insulin-dependent diabetics." *Arch Fam Med* 1994;3(6):503-8.

1198 Galloe AM, Rasmussen HS, Jorgensen LN, et al. "Influence of oral magnesium supplementation on cardiac events among survivors of an acute myocardial infarction." *BMJ* 1993;307(6904):585-7.

1199 Widman L, Wester PO, Stegmayr BK, et al. "The dose-dependent reduction in blood pressure through administration of magnesium. A double blind placebo controlled cross-over study." *Am J Hypertens* 1993;6(1):41-5.

1201 Rattan V, Sidhu H, Vaidyanathan S. "Effect of combined supplementation of magnesium oxide and pyridoxine in calcium-oxalate stone formers." *Urol Res* 1994;22(3):161-5.

1202 Brodsky MA, Orlov MV, Capparelli EV, et al. "Magnesium therapy in new-onset atrial fibrillation." *Am J Cardiol* 1994;73(16):1227-9.

1203 Holmang A, Nilsson C, Niklasson M, et al. Induction of insulin resistance by glucosamine reduces blood flow but not interstitial levels of either glucose or insulin. *Diabetes* 1999;48:106-11.

1204 Kim YB, Zhu JS, Zierath JR, et al. Glucosamine infusion in rats rapidly impairs insulin stimulation of phosphoinositide 3-kinase but does not alter activation of Akt/protein kinase B in skeletal muscle. *Diabetes* 1999;48:310-20.

1205 Attias J, Weisz G, Almog S, et al. "Oral magnesium intake reduces permanent hearing loss induced by noise exposure." *Am J Otolaryngol* 994;15(1):26-32.

1208 Skorodin MS, Tenholder MF, Yetter B, et al. "Magnesium sulfate in exacerbations of chronic obstructive pulmonary disease." *Arch Intern Med* 1995;155(5):496-500.

1209 Menopause Help Online, Natural Progesterone for Hormonal Balance in Women Website, URL: www.menopause-help-online.com (Accessed 23 July 1999).

1210 Chang R. "Functional properties of edible mushrooms." *Nutr Rev* 1996;54(11 Pt 2):S91-3.

1211 Kubo K, Nanba H. "The effect of maitake mushrooms on liver and serum lipids." *Altern Ther Health Med* 1996;2(5):62-6.

1212 Kubo K, Aoki H, Nanba H. "Anti-diabetic activity present in the fruit body of Grifola frondosa (Maitake)." *I. Biol Pharm Bull* 1994;17(8):1106-10.

1213 Kabir Y, Kimura S. "Dietary mushrooms reduce blood

pressure in spontaneously hypertensive rats (SHR)." *J Nutr Sci Vitaminol* (Tokyo) 1989;35(1):91-4.

1214 Kabir Y, Yamaguchi M, Kimura S. "Effect of shiitake (Lentinus edodes) and maitake (Grifola frondosa) mushrooms on blood pressure and plasma lipids of spontaneously hypertensive rats." *J Nutr Sci Vitaminol* (Tokyo) 1987;33(5):341-6.

1215 Espeland MA, Hogan PE, Fineberg SE, et al. "Effect of postmenopausal hormone therapy on glucose and insulin concentrations. PEPI Investigators. Postmenopausal Estrogen/Progestin Interventions." *Diabetes Care* 1998;21(10):1589-95.

1216 Chen FP, Lee N, Soong YK. "Changes in the lipoprotein profile in postmenopausal women receiving hormone replacement therapy. Effects of natural and synthetic progesterone." *J Reprod Med* 1998;43(7):568-74.

1217 Espeland MA, Marcovina SM, Miller V, et al. "Effect of postmenopausal hormone therapy on lipoprotein(a) concentration. PEPI Investigators. Postmenopausal Estrogen/Progestin Interventions." *Circulation* 1998;97(10):979-86.

1218 Perino M, Brigandi FG, Abate FG, et al. "Intramuscular versus vaginal progesterone in assisted reproduction: a comparative study." *Clin Exp Obstet Gynecol* 1997;24(4):228-31.

1219 Benifla JL, Dumont M, Levardon M, et al. "Effects of micronized natural progesterone on the liver during the third trimester of pregnancy." [Article in French] *Contracept Fertil Sex* 1997;25(2):165-9.

1220 Freeman EW, Rickels K, Sondheimer SJ, et al. "A double-blind trial of oral progesterone, alprazolam, and placebo in treatment of severe premenstrual syndrome." *JAMA* 1995;274(1):51-7.

1221 Schweizer E, Case WG, Garcia-Espana F, et al. "Progesterone co-administration in patients discontinuing long-term benzodiazepine therapy: effects on withdrawal severity and taper outcome." *Psychopharmacology* (Berl) 1995;117(4):424-9.

1222 Simon JA, Robinson DE, Andrews MC, et al. "The absorption of oral micronized progesterone: the effect of food, dose proportionality, and comparison with intramuscular progesterone." *Fertil Steril* 1993;60(1):26-33.

1223 Nappi C, Affinito P, Di Carlo C, et al. "Double-blind controlled trial of progesterone vaginal cream treatment for cyclical mastodynia in women with benign breast disease." *J Endocrinol Invest* 1992;15(11):801-6.

1224 Freeman EW, Weinstock L, Rickels K, et al. "A placebo-controlled study of effects of oral progesterone on performance and mood." *Br J Clin Pharmacol* 1992;33(3):293-8.

1225 Smitz J, Devroey P, Faguer B, et al. "A prospective randomized comparison of intramuscular or intravaginal natural progesterone as a luteal phase and early pregnancy supplement." *Hum Reprod* 1992;7(2):168-75.

1226 Darj E, Nilsson S, Axelsson O, et al. "Clinical and endometrial effects of oestradiol and progesterone in post-menopausal women." *Maturitas* 1991;13(2):109-15.

1227 Saarikoski S, Yliskoski M, Penttila I. "Sequential administration of norethisterone and natural oral progesterone during premenopausal menstrual cycle disorders." [Article in French] *Rev Fr Gynecol Obstet* 1991;86(6):475-80.

1228 Cooper A, Spencer, Whitehead MI et al. "Systemic absorption of progesterone cream from Progest cream in postmenopausal women." *Lancet* 1998;351:1255-6.

1229 Burry KA, Paton PE, Hermsmeyer K. "Percutaneous absorption of progesterone in postmenopausal women treated with transdermal estrogen." *Am J Obstet Gynecol* 1999;180(6Part 1):1504-11.

1230 Website, URL: www.verity.fda.gov/default.html.

1231 Cooper AJ, Whitehead MI. "Correspondence." *Lancet* 1998;352:906.

1232 Grifon Maitake Caplet Website, URL: www.maitake.com/qm caplet.html (Accessed 23 July 1999).

1240 Anderson JW, Gilliland SE. "Effect of fermented milk (yogurt) containing Lactobacillus acidophilus L1 on serum cholesterol in hypercholesterolemic humans." *J Am Coll Nutr* 1999;18(1):43-50.

1241 Schaafsma G, Meuling WJ, van Dokkum W L, et al. "Effects of a milk product, fermented by Lactobacillus acidophilus and with fructo-oligosaccharides added, on blood lipids in male volunteers." *Eur J Clin Nutr* 1998;52(6):436-40.

1242 Bhatnagar S, Singh KD, Sazawal S, et al. "Efficacy of milk versus yogurt offered as part of a mixed diet in acute noncholera diarrhea among malnourished children." *J Pediatr* 1998;132(6):999-1003.

1243 Guerin-Danan C, Chabanet C, Pedone C, et al. "Milk fermented with yogurt cultures and Lactobacillus casei compared with yogurt and gelled milk: influence on intestinal microflora in healthy infants." *Am J Clin Nutr* 1998;67(1):111-7.

1244 Wheeler JG, Shema SJ, Bogle ML, et al. "Immune and clinical impact of Lactobacillus acidophilus on asthma." *Ann Allergy Asthma Immunol* 1997;79(3):229-33.

1245 Shalev E, Battino S, Weiner E, et al. "Ingestion of yogurt containing Lactobacillus acidophilus compared with pasteurized yogurt as prophylaxis for recurrent candidal vaginitis and bacterial vaginosis." *Arch Fam Med* 1996;5(10):593-6.

1246 Nizami SQ, Bhutta ZA, Molla AM. "Efficacy of traditional rice-lentil-yogurt diet, lactose free milk protein-based formula and soy protein formula in management of secondary lactose intolerance with acute childhood diarrhea." *J Trop Pediatr* 1996;42(3):133-7.

1247 Shermak MA, Saavedra JM, Jackson TL, et al. "Effect of yogurt on symptoms and kinetics of hydrogen production in lactose-malabsorbing children." *Am J Clin Nutr* 1995;62(5):1003-6.

1248 Neri A, Sabah G, Samra Z. "Bacterial vaginosis in pregnancy treated with yogurt." *Acta Obstet Gynecol Scand* 1993;72(1):17-9.

1249 Hilton E, Isenberg HD, Alperstein P, et al. "Ingestion of yogurt containing Lactobacillus acidophilus as prophylaxis for candidal vaginitis. *Ann Intern Med* 1992;116(5):353-7.

1250 Touhami M, Boudraa G, Mary JY, et al. "Clinical consequences of replacing milk with yogurt in persistent infantile diarrhea." *Ann Pediatr* (Paris) 1992;39(2):79-86.

1251 Neuvonen PJ, Kivisto KT. "Milk and yogurt do not impair the absorption of ofloxacin." *Br J Clin Pharmacol* 1992;33(3):346-8.

1252 Neuvonen PJ, Kivisto KT, Lehto P. "Interference of dairy products with the absorption of ciprofloxacin." *Clin Pharmacol Ther* 1991;50(5 Pt 1):498-502.

1253 Isolauri E, Juntunen M, Rautanen T, et al. "A human Lactobacillus strain (Lactobacillus casei sp strain GG) promotes recovery from acute diarrhea in children." *Pediatrics* 1991;88(1):90-7.

1254 Boudraa G, Touhami M, Pochart P, et al. "Effect of feeding yogurt versus milk in children with persistent diarrhea." *J Pediatr Gastroenterol Nutr* 1990;11(4):509-12.

1255 Siitonen S, Vapaatalo H, Salminen S, et al. "Effect of Lactobacillus GG yogurt in prevention of antibiotic associated diarrhea." *Ann Med* 1990;22(1):57-9.

1256 Lerebours E, N'Djitoyap NC, Lavoine A, et al. "Yogurt and fermented-then-pasteurized milk: effects of short-term and long-term ingestion on lactose absorption and mucosal lactase activity in lactase-deficient subjects." *Am J Clin Nutr* 1989;49(5):823-7.

1257 Vitamins C plus K3 cause unique type of tumor apoptosis. Reuters Health website, URL:www.reutershealth.com/cgi-bin/ssi/framethis?catalog=mednews&file=1991227scc.html (Accessed 27 December 1999).

1258 Alexandrakis G, Tse DT, Rosa RH Jr, Johnson TE. Nasolacrimal duct obstruction and orbital cellulitis associated with chronic intranasal cocaine abuse. *Arch Ophthalmol* 1999;117(12):1617-22.

1259 Ros JJ, Pelders MG, De Smet PA. A case of positive doping associated with a botanical food supplement. *Pharm World Sci* 1999;21(1):44-6.

1260 Joeres R, Klinker H, Heusler H, et al. Influence of mexiletine on caffeine elimination. *Pharmacol Ther* 1987;33(1):163-9.

1261 Cooper RA, Molan PC, Harding KG. Antibacterial activity of honey against strains of Staphylococcus aureus from infected wounds. *J R Soc Med* 1999;92(6):283-5.

1262 Caccetta RA, Croft KD, Beilin LJ, Puddey IB. Ingestion of red wine significantly increases plasma phenolic acid concentrations but does not acutely affect ex vivo lipoprotein oxidizability. *Am J Clin Nutr* 2000;71:67-74.

1263 *Richters HerbLetter*, 99/12/31. URL: www.richters.com/newdisplay.cgi?page=./HL/HerbLett.html&cart_id=3085578.5928 (Accessed 31 December 1999).

1264 Cignarella A, Nastasi M, Cavalli E, Puglisi L. Novel lipid-lowering properties of Vaccinium myrtillus L. leaves, a traditional antidiabetic treatment, in several models of rat dyslipidaemia: a comparison with ciprofibrate. *Thromb Res* 1996;84(5):311-22.

1265 Fraisse D, Carnat A, Lamaison JL. [Polyphenolic composition of the leaf of bilberry]. *Ann Pharm Fr* 1996;54(6):280-3.

1266 Kunsman GW, Levine B, Smith ML. Vitamin B2 interference with TDx drugs-of-abuse assays. *J Forensic Sci* 1998;43(6):1225-7.

1267 Personal correspondence. David Winston, Herbalist AHG. Herbal Therapeutics Inc. Research Library Washington, NJ. January 2000.

1268 Merritt JC, Crawford WJ, Alexander PC, et al. Effect of marihuana on intraocular and blood pressure in glaucoma. *Ophthalmology* 1980;87(3):222-8.

1269 Magainin Pharmaceuticals Announces New Research Program for Anti-Angiogenesis Agent — Squalamine — at Georgetown University Medical Center. PRNewswire, URL: www.prnewswire.com (Accessed 22 January 2000).

1270 Okada S, Rohan PJ, Miller FW, et al. Myopathies following ingestion of special nutritional products. *Arthritis Rheum* 1996;39(9):349.

1271 Zaacks SM, Klein L, Tan CD, et al. Hypersensitivity myocarditis associated with ephedra use. *J Toxicol Clin Toxicol* 1999;37(4):485-9.

1272 Powell T, Hsu FF, Turk J, Hruska K. Ma-huang strikes again: ephedrine nephrolithiasis. *Am J Kidney Dis* 1998;32(1):153-9.

1273 Nadir A, Agrawal S, King PD, Marshall JB. Acute hepatitis associated with the use of a Chinese herbal product, ma-huang. *Am J Gastroenterol* 1996;91(7):1436-8.

1274 Theoharides TC. Sudden death of a healthy college student related to ephedrine toxicity from a ma huang-containing drink. *J Clin Psychopharmacol* 1997;17(5):437-9.

1275 Vahedi K, Domingo V, Amarenco P, Bousser MG. Ischemic stroke in a sportsman who consumed MaHuang extract and creatine monohydrate for bodybuilding. *J Neurol Neurosurg Psychiatry* 2000;68:112-3.

1276 Doyle H, Kargin M. Herbal stimulant containing ephedrine has also caused psychosis. *BMJ* 1996;313(7059):756.

1277 Agricultural Research Service: Dr.Duke's Phytochemical and Ethnobotanical Databases. URL www.ars-grin.gov/duke (Accessed 25 January 2000).

1278 Zicam Reduces Length of Common Cold. Medscape website, URL: www.medscape.com/reuters/eline/wed/t0201-1f.html (Accessed 02 February 2000).

1280 Baur A, Harrer T, Peukert M, et al. Alpha-lipoic acid is an effective inhibitor of human immuno-deficiency virus (HIV-1) replication. *Klin Wochenschr* 1991;69(15):722-4.

1281 Ishiwa J, Sato T, Mimaki Y, et al. A citrus flavonoid, nobiletin, suppresses production and gene expression of matrix metalloproteinase 9/gelatinase B in rabbit synovial fibroblasts. *J Rheumatol* 2000;27(1):20-5.

1282 Rieck J, Halkin H, Almog S, et al. Urinary loss of thiamine is increased by low doses of furosemide in healthy volunteers. *J Lab Clin Med* 1999;134(3):238-43.

1283 Brady JA, Rock CL, Horneffer MR. Thiamin status, diuretic medications, and the management of congestive heart failure. *J Am Diet Assoc* 1995;95(5):541-4.

1284 Shimon I, Almog S, Vered Z, et al. Improved left ventricular function after thiamine supplementation in patients with congestive heart failure receiving long-term furosemide therapy. *Am J Med* 1995;98(5):485-90.

1285 Pfitzenmeyer P, Guilland JC, d'Athis P, et al. Thiamine status of elderly patients with cardiac failure including the effects of supplementation. *Int J Vitam Nutr Res* 1994;64(2):113-8.

1286 Seligmann H, Halkin H, Rauchfleisch S, et al. Thiamine deficiency in patients with congestive heart failure receiving long-term furosemide therapy: a pilot study. *Am J Med* 1991;91(2):151-5.

1287 Schubert SY, Lansky EP, Neeman I. Antioxidant and eicosanoid enzyme inhibition properties of pomegranate seed oil and fermented juice flavonoids. *J Ethnopharmacol* 1999;66(1):11-7.

1288 Cheng TO. Ginseng-warfarin interaction. *ACC Current Journal Review* 2000;9(1):84.

1289 DiPiro JT, Talbert RL, Yee GC, et al, eds. Pharmacotherapy: A Pathophysiologic Approach. 4th edition. Appleton & Lange: Stamford, CT 1999.

1290 Piscitelli SC, Burstein AH, Chaitt D, et al. Indinavir concentrations and St. John's wort. *Lancet* 2000;355(9203):547-8.

1291 Risk of drug interactions with St. John's wort and indinavir and other drugs. URL: www.fda.gov/cder/drug/advisory/stjwort.html (Accessed 11 February 2000).

© Copyright 2000, Natural Medicines Comprehensive Database (209) 472-2244. For updated data, go to www.NaturalDatabase.com. • 1181

REFERENCES

1292 Yue QY, Bergquist C, Gerden B. Safety of St John's wort (Hypericum perforatum). *Lancet* 2000;355(9203):576-7.

1293 Ruschitzka F, Meier PJ, Turina M, et al. Acute heart transplant rejection due to Saint John's wort. *Lancet* 2000;355(9203):548-9.

1294 Southwick SM, Morgan CA 3rd, Charney DS, High JR. Yohimbine use in a natural setting: effects on post-traumatic stress disorder. *Biol Psychiatry* 1999;46(3):442-4.

1295 Androgenic Hormone Improves Symptoms, Improves Bone Density in Lupus. www.medscape.com/reuters/prof/2000/02/02.15/cl02150p.html (Accessed 15 February 2000).

1296 Roberts JE, Wang RH, Tan IP, et al. Hypericin (active ingredient in St. John's wort) photo-oxidation of lens proteins. *Photochem Photobiol* 1999;69(S):42S.

1297 Frieling UM, Schaumberg DA, Kupper TS, et al. A randomized, 12-year primary-prevention trial of beta carotene supplementation for nonmelanoma skin cancer in the physicians' health study. *Arch Dermatol* 2000;136(2):179-184.

1298 Mueller BA, Scott MK, Sowinski KM, Prag KA. Noni juice (Morinda citrifolia): hidden potential for hyperkalemia? *Am J Kidney Dis* 2000;35(2):310-2.

1299 Speetjens JK, Collins RA, Vincent JB, Woski SA. The nutritional supplement chromium(III) tris(picolinate) cleaves DNA. *Chem Res Toxicol* 1999;12(6):483-7.

1300 Weiss W, Huber G, Engel KH, et al. Identification and characterization of wheat grain albumin/globulin allergens. *Electrophoresis* 1997;18(5):826-33.

1302 Singh AK, Granley K, Misrha U, et al. Screening and confirmation of drugs in urine: interference of hordenine with the immunoassays and thin layer chromatography methods. *Forensic Sci Int* 1992; 54(1):9-22.

1304 Millet Y, Jouglard J, Steinmetz MD, et al. "Toxicity of some essential plant oils. Clinical and experimental study." *Clin Toxicol* 1981;18(12):1485-98.

1305 Gohla SH, Haubeck HD, Neth RD. "Mitogenic activity of high molecular polysaccharide fractions isolated from the Cupressaceae Thuja occidentale L. I. Macrophage-dependent injuction of CD-4-positive T-helper (Th+) lymphocytes." *Leukemia* 1988;2(8):528-33.

1306 Offergeld R, Reinecker C, Gumz E, et al. "Mitogenic activity of high molecular polysaccharide fractions isolated from the cuppressaceae Thuja occidentalis L. enhanced cytokine-production by thyapolysaccharide, g-fraction (TPSg)." *Leukemia* 1992;6(Suppl 3):189S-91S.

1307 Wu ZL, Chen JK, Ong T, et al. "Antitransforming activity of chlorophyllin against selected carcinogens and complex mixtures." *Teratog Carcinog Mutagen* 1994;14(2):75-81.

1309 Dashwood RH, Breinholt V, Bailey GS. "Chemopreventive properties of chlorophyllin: Inhibition of aflatoxin B1 (AFB1)-DNA binding in vivo and anti-mutagenic activity against AFB1 and two heterocyclic amines in the Salmonella mutagenicity assay." *Carcinogenesis* 1991;12(5):939-42.

1311 Sarkar D, Sharma A, Talukder G. "Clastogenic activity of pure chlorophyll and anticlastogenic effects of equivalent amounts of crude extract of Indian spinach leaf and chlorophyllin following dietary supplementation to mice." *Environ Mol Mutagen*, 1996; 28(2):121-6.

1312 Amara-Mokrane YA, Lehucher-Michel MP, Balansard G, et al. "Protective effects of alpha-hederin, chlorophyllin and ascorbic acid towards the induction of micronuclei

by doxorubicin in cultured human lymphocytes." *Mutagenesis*, 1996; 11(2):161-7.

1314 Dai R, Shoemaker R, Farrens D, et al. "Characterization of silkworm chlorophyll metabolites as an active photosensitizer for photodynamic therapy." *J Nat Prod*, 1992; 55(9):1241-51.

1315 Lee WY, Park JH, Kim BS, et al. "Chlorophyll derivatives (CpD) extracted from silk worm excreta are specifically cytotoxic to tumor cells in vitro." *Yonsei Med J*, 1990; 31(3):225-33.

1321 Young RW, Beregi JS Jr. "Use of chlorophyllin in the care of geriatric patients." *J Am Geriatr Soc*, 1980; 28(1):46-7.

1322 Christiansen SB, Byel SR, Stromsted H, et al. "Can chlorophyll reduce fecal odor in colostomy patients?" [Article in Danish]. *Ugeskr Laeger*, 1989; 151(27):1753-4.

1323 Nahata MC, Slencsak CA, Kamp J. "Effect of chlorophyllin on urinary odor in incontinent geriatric patients." *Drug Intell Clin Pharm*, 1983; 17(10):732-4.

1324 Yoshida A, Yokono O, Oda T. "Therapeutic effect of chlorophyll-a in the treatment of patients with chronic pancreatitis." *Gastroenterol Jpn*, 1980; 15(1):49-61.

1326 Mathews-Roth MM. "Carotenoids in erythropoietic protoporphyria and other photosensitivity diseases." *Ann NY Acad Sci*, 1993; 691:127-38.

1329 Cardiovascular Benefits Claimed For Cocoa Flavonoids. www.medscape.com/reuters/prof/2000/02/02.21/dd02210b.html (Accessed 21 February 2000).

1330 Rindone JP, Hiller D, Collacott E, et al. Randomized, controlled trial of glucosamine for treating osteoarthritis of the knee. *West J Med*, 2000;172(2):91-94.

1331 Düker EM, Kopanski L, Jarry H, Wuttke W. Effects of extracts from Cimicifuga racemosa on gonadotropin release in menopausal women and ovariectomized rats. *Planta Med* 1991;57(5):420-424.

1341 Jepsen S, Hansen AB. The influence of N-acetylcysteine on the measurement of prothrombin time and activated partial thromboplastin time in healthy subjects. *Scand J Clin Lab Invest* 1994;54(7):543-547.

1342 Leeb BF, Schweitzer H, Montag K, Smolen JS. A meta-analysis of chondroitin sulfate in the treatment of osteoarthritis. *J Rheumatol* 2000;27(1):205-211.

1344 Yamadera W, Sasaki M, Itoh H, et al. Clinical features of circadian rhythm sleep disorders in outpatients. *Psychiatry Clin Neurosci* 1998;52(3):311-316.

1345 Okawa M, Uchiyama M, Ozaki S, et al. Circadian rhythm sleep disorders in adolescents: clinical trials of combined treatments based on chronobiology. *Psychiatry Clin Neurosci* 1998;52(5):483-490.

1346 Okawa M, Takahashi K, Egashira K, et al. Vitamin B12 treatment for delayed sleep phase syndrome: a multi-center double-blind study. *Psychiatry Clin Neurosci* 1997;51(5):275-279.

1347 Yamadera H, Takahashi K, Okawa M. A multicenter study of sleep-wake rhythm disorders: therapeutic effects of vitamin B12, bright light therapy, chronotherapy and hypnotics. *Psychiatry Clin Neurosci* 1996;50(4):203-209.

1348 Ohta T, Ando K, Iwata T, et al. Treatment of persistent sleep-wake schedule disorders in adolescents with methylcobalamin (vitamin B12). *Sleep* 1991;14(5):414-418.

1349 Mayer G, Kroger M, Meier-Ewert K. Effects of vitamin B12 on performance and circadian rhythm in normal subjects. *Neuropsychopharmacology* 1996;15(5):456-

464.

1350 Reimund E. Sleep deprivation-induced dermatitis: further support of nicotinic acid depletion in sleep deprivation. *Med Hypotheses* 1991;36(4):371-373.

1351 Shad JA, Chinn CG, Brann OS. Acute hepatitis after ingestion of herbs. *South Med J* 1999;92(11):1095-1097.

1352 Kugelmas M. Preliminary observation: oral zinc sulfate replacement is effective in treating muscle cramps in cirrhotic patients. *J Am Coll Nutr* 2000;19(1):13-15.

1353 Grubben MJ, Boers GH, Blom HJ, et al. Unfiltered coffee increases plasma homocysteine concentrations in healthy volunteers: a randomized trial. *Am J Clin Nutr* 2000;71(2):480-484.

1354 Watkins TR, Geller M, Kooyenga DK, Bierenbaum ML. Hypocholesterolemic and antioxidant effect of rice bran oil non-saponifiables in hypercholesterolemic subjects. *Environmental & Nutritional Interactions* 1999;3:115-122.

1355 Vitamin C Supplements May Promote Atherosclerosis. www.medscape.com/reuters/prof/2000/03.03.03/ep03030a.html (Accessed 03 March 2000).

1356 Marijuana Use by Middle-Aged Adults Linked to Increased Risk of MI. www.medscape.com/reuters/prof/2000/03.03.03/ep03030b.html (Accessed 03 March 2000).

1357 Feigin A, Kieburtz K, Como P, et al. Assessment of coenzyme Q10 tolerability in Huntington's disease. *Mov Disord* 1996;11(3):321-323.

1358 Today's findings from the AAAAI Annual Meeting unveil new research on alternative therapies and food allergy: Echinacea can cause allergic reactions. American Academy of Allergy, Asthma and Immunology, URL: www.aaaai.org/media/pressreleases/2000/03/000307.html (Accessed 08 March 2000).

1360 McGuire JK, Kulkarni MS, Baden HP. Fatal hypermagnesemia in a child treated with megavitamin/megamineral therapy. *Pediatrics* 2000;105(2):e18 (electronic article). URL: www.pediatrics.org/cgi/content/abstract/105/2/e18 (Accessed 8 March 2000).

1361 Blum A, Hathaway L, Mincemoyer R, et al. Effects of oral L-arginine on endothelium-dependent vasodilation and markers of inflammation in healthy postmenopausal women. *J Am Coll Cardiol* 2000;35(2):271-6.

1362 Creager MA, Gallagher SJ, Girerd XJ, et al. L-arginine improves endothelium-dependent vasodilation in hypercholesterolemic humans. *J Clin Invest* 1992;90(4):1248-53.

1363 Clarkson P, Adams MR, Powe AJ, et al. Oral L-arginine improves endothelium-dependent dilation in hypercholesterolemic young adults. *J Clin Invest* 1996;97(8):1989-94.

1366 Phan TG, Estell J, Duggin G, et al. Lead poisoning from drinking Kombucha tea brewed in a ceramic pot. *Med J Aust* 1998;169(11-12):644-646.

1370 Lyon MJ, Shaw JC. Allergic Contact Dermatitis Reaction to Henna. *Arch Dermatol* 2000;136(1):124-125.

1371 Leppala JM, Virtamo J, Fogelholm R, et al. Controlled trial of alpha-tocopherol and beta-carotene supplements on stroke incidence and mortality in male smokers. *Arterioscler Thromb Vasc Biol.* 2000;20(1):230-235.

1372 Sigurjonsdottir HA, Ragnarsson J, Franzson L, Sigurdsson G. Is blood pressure commonly raised by moderate consumption of liquorice? *J Hum Hypertens*, May 1995;9(5):345-348.

1373 Baron AM, Donnerstein RL, Samson RA, et al. Hemodynamic and electrophysiologic effects of acute chocolate ingestion in young adults. *Am J Cardiol* 1999;84(3):370-373.

1374 Friedman G. Diet and the irritable bowel syndrome. *Gastroenterol Clin North Am* 1991;20(2):313-324.

1375 Blue-Green Algae Protein Is a Promising Anti-HIV Microbicide Candidate. URL: www.medscape.com/reuters/prof/2000/03/03.16/dd03160g.html (Accessed 16 March 2000).

1376 Anderson JW, Allgood LD, Lawrence A, et al. Cholesterol-lowering effects of psyllium intake adjunctive to diet therapy in men and women with hypercholesterolemia: meta-analysis of 8 controlled trials. *Am J Clin Nutr* 2000;71(2):472-479.

1377 Lee A, Minhas R, Ito S, et al. Safety of St. John's wort during breastfeeding. *Clin Pharmacol Ther* 2000;67(2):130 (abstract PII-64).

1378 Roots I, Johne A, Schmider, Brockmoller J, et al. Interaction of a herbal extract from St. John's wort with amitriptyline and its metabolites. *Clin Pharmacol Ther* 2000;67(2):159 (abstract PIII-69).

1379 Carson SW, Hill-Zabala CE, Roberts SH, Hawke RL. Inhibitory effect of methanolic solution of St. John's wort (hypericum perforatum) on cytochrome p450 3A4 activity in human liver microsomes. *Clin Pharmacol Ther* 2000;67(2):99 (abstract PI-39).

1380 For Dieter, Nearly the Ultimate Loss. URL: www.washingtonpost.com/wp-dyn/articles/A33421-2000Mar17.html (Accessed 19 March 2000).

1381 FDA Takes Aim at Ephedra. URL: www.washingtonpost.com/wp-dyn/articles/A33439-2000Mar17.html (Accessed 19 March 2000).

1382 Dallas S, Stempak D, Koren G, et al. Whey protein concentrate (WPC) modulation of lymphocyte glutathione levels in vitro. *Clin Pharmacol Ther* 2000;67(2):156 (abstract PIII-56).

1383 Offman EM, Freeman DJ, Dresser GK, et al. Cisapride interaction with grapefruit juice and red wine. *Clin Pharmacol Ther* 2000;67(2):110 (abstract PI-83).

1384 Tsunoda SM, Christians U, Velez RL, et al. Red wine (RW) effects on cyclosporine (CyA) metabolites. *Clin Pharmacol Ther*, 2000;67(2):150 (abstract PIII-35).

1385 Bertino JS, Demuro RL, Blask DE, et al. Absolute bioavailability (F) of oral melatonin (M). *Clin Pharmacol Ther* 2000;67(2):106 (abstract PI-72).

1386 Veronese M, Burke J, Dorval E, et al. Grapefruit juice (GFJ) inhibits hepatic and intestinal CYP3A4 dose-dependently. *Clin Pharmacol Ther* 2000;67(2):151 (abstract PIII-37).

1387 Tsunoda SM, Harris RZ, Velez RL, et al. Red wine (RW) effects on cyclosporine (CyA) Pharmacokinetics. *Clin Pharmacol Ther*, 1998;65(2):159 (abstract PII-51).

1388 Bailey DG, Dresser GK, Kreeft JH, et al. Grapefruit juice-felodipine interaction: Effect of segments and an extract from unprocessed fruit. *Clin Pharmacol Ther* 2000;67(2):107 (abstract PI-71).

1389 Frye RF, Kroboth PD, Folan MM, et al. Effect of DHEA on CYP3A-mediated metabolism of triazolam. *Clin Pharmacol Ther* 2000;67(2):109 (abstract PI-82).

1390 Soldner A, Christians U, Susanto M, et al. Grapefruit juice exerts stimulatory effects on p-glycoprotein. *Clin Pharmacol Ther* 1998;65(2): (abstract OIII-B-4).

1391 Zaidenstein R, Avni B, Dishi V, et al. Effect of grapefruit juice on the pharmacokinetics of losartan in healthy volunteers. *Clin Pharmacol Ther*, 1998;65(2): (abstract PI-60).

© Copyright 2000, Natural Medicines Comprehensive Database (209) 472-2244. For updated data, go to www.NaturalDatabase.com.

REFERENCES

1392 Dresser GK, Bailey DG, Carruthers SG. Grapefruit juice-felodipine interaction in healthy seniors. *Clin Pharmacol Ther* 1998;65(2): (abstract PIII-63).

1394 John Mendelson J, TolLiver B, Delucchi K, Berger P. Capsaicin increases the lethality of cocaine. *Clin Pharmacol Ther*, 1998;65(2): (abstract PII-27).

1395 Johnson MA, Robin P Smith RP, Morrisona D, et al. Large lung bullae in marijuana smokers. *Thorax*, 2000;55(4):340-342.

1396 Sandor PS, Afra J, Ambrosini A, Schoenen J. Prophylactic treatment of migraine with beta-blockers and riboflavin: differential effects on the intensity dependence of auditory evoked cortical potentials. *Headache*, 2000;40:30-35.

1397 Schoenen J, Lenaerts M, Bastings E. High-dose riboflavin as a prophylactic treatment of migraine: results of an open pilot study. *Cephalalgia*, 1994;14(5):328-329.

1398 Schoenen J, Jacquy J, Lenaerts M. Effectiveness of high-dose riboflavin in migraine prophylaxis. A randomized controlled trial. *Neurology*, 1998;50(2):466-470.

1399 Synthetic DHEA Enhances Post-Burn Skin Graft Re-Epithelialization Rate. URL: www.medscape.com/reuters/prof/2000/03/03.27/cl03270m.html (Accessed 27 March 2000).

1400 Vatassery GT, Bauer T, Dysken M. High doses of vitamin E in the treatment of disorders of the central nervous system in the aged. *Am J Clin Nutr* 1999;70(5):793-801.

1401 Jardim LB, Palma-Dias R, Silva LC, et al. Maternal hyperphenylalaninaemia as a cause of microcephaly and mental retardation. *Acta Paediatr* 1996;85(8):943-946.

1402 Rouse B, Azen C, Koch R, et al. Maternal phenylketonuria collaborative Study (MPKUCS) offspring: facial anomalies, malformations, and early neurological sequelae. *Am J Med Genet*, 1997;69:89-95.

1403 Sternberg EM, Van Woert MH, Young SN, et al. Development of a scleroderma-like illness during therapy with L-5-hydroxytryptophan and carbidopa. *N Engl J Med* 1980;303:782-7.

1404 Joly P, Lampert A, Thomine E, et al. Development of pseudobullous morphea and scleroderma-like illness during therapy with L-5-hydroxytryptophan and carbidopa. *J Am Acad Dermatol* 1991;25(2 Pt 1):332-3.

1405 Anderson JW, Allgood LD, Turner J, et al. Effects of psyllium on glucose and serum lipid responses in men with type 2 *Diabetes* and hypercholesterolemia. *Am J Clin Nutr* 1999;70:466-73.

1407 O'Brien PM, Pipkin FB. The effect of essential fatty acid and specific vitamin supplements on vascular sensitivity in the mid trimester of human pregnancy. *Clin Exp Hypertens* 1983;2:247-54.

1408 O'Brien PM, Morrison R, Pipken FB. Effect of dietary supplementation with linoleic and gammalinolenic acids on the pressor response to angiotensin II—possible role in pregnancy induced hypertension? *Br J Clin Pharmacol* 1985;19:335-342.

1409 Laivuori H, Hovatta O, Viinikka L, et al. Dietary supplementation with primrose oil or fish oil does not change urinary excretion of prostacyclin and thromboxane metabolites in pre-eclamptic women. *Prostaglandins Leukot Essent Fatty Acids* 1993;49:691-4.

1410 Bruemmer B, White E, Vaughan TL, Cheney CL. Fluid intake and the incidence of bladder cancer among middle-aged men and women in a three-county area of western Washington. *Nutr Cancer* 1997;29(2):163-8.

1411 Dove D, Johnson P. Oral evening primrose oil: its effect on length of pregnancy and selected intrapartum outcomes in low-risk nulliparous women. *J Nurse Midwifery* 1999;44:320-4.

1412 Brinkeborn RM, Shah DV, Degenring FH. Echinaforce and other Echinacea fresh plant preparations in the treatment of the common cold. A randomized, placebo controlled, double-blind clinical trial. *PhytoMedicine* 1999;6:1-6.

1413 Mengs U, Clare CB, Poiley JA. Toxicity of Echinacea purpurea. Acute, subacute and genotoxicity studies. *Arzneimittelforschung* 1991;41:1076-81.

1414 Awang DVC, Kindack DG. Echinacea. *Can Pharm J* November 1999:512-16.

1415 D'Avanzo B, La Vecchia C, Franceschi S, et al. Coffee consumption and bladder cancer risk. *Eur J Cancer* 1992;28A(8-9):1480-1484.

1416 Pannelli F, La Rosa F, Saltalamacchia G, et al. Tobacco smoking, coffee, cocoa and tea consumption in relation to mortality from urinary bladder cancer in Italy. *Eur J Epidemiol* 1989;5(6):392-397.

1417 Slattery ML, West DW, Robison LM. Fluid intake and bladder cancer in Utah. *Int J Cancer* 1988;42(1):7-22.

1418 Joseph JA, Shukitt-Hale B, Denisova NA, et al. Long-term dietary strawberry, spinach, or vitamin E supplementation retards the onset of age-related neuronal signal-transduction and cognitive behavioral deficits. *J Neurosci* 1998;18(19):8047-55.

1419 Joseph JA, Shukitt-Hale B, Denisova NA, et al. Reversals of age-related declines in neuronal signal transduction, cognitive, and motor behavioral deficits with blueberry, spinach, or strawberry dietary supplementation. *J Neurosci* 1999;19(18):8114-21.

1420 Cao G, Shukitt-Hale B, Bickford PC, et al. Hyperoxia-induced changes in antioxidant capacity and the effect of dietary antioxidants. *J Appl Physiol*, 1999;86:1817-1822.

1421 Gebhardt R. Hepatoprotection with artichoke extract. *Pharm Ztg* 1995;140:34-37.

1422 Gebhardt R. Antioxidative and protective properties of extracts from leaves of the artichoke (Cynara scolymus L.) against hydroperoxide-induced oxidative stress in cultured rat hepatocytes. *Toxicol Appl Pharmacol* 1997;144:279-86.

1423 Hammerl WH, Kindler K, Kranzl C, et al. Effect of cynarin (cynarine) on hyperlipidemia, especially on hypercholesterolemia. *Wien Med Wochenschr* 1973;123:601-605.

1424 Heckers H, Dittmar K, Schmahl FW, et al. Inefficiency of cynarin as therapeutic regimen in familial type II hyperlipoproteinaemia. *Atherosclerosis* 1977;26:249-53.

1425 Gebhardt R. Inhibition of cholesterol biosynthesis in primary cultured rat hepatocytes by artichoke (Cynara scolymus L.) extracts. *J Pharmacol Exp Therap* 1998;386:1122-1128.

1426 Brown JE, Rice-Evans CA. Luteolin-rich artichoke extract protects low density lipoprotein from oxidation in vitro. *Free Radic Res* 1998;29:247-55.

1427 Vogler BK, Pittler MH, Ernst E. The efficacy of ginseng. A systemic review of randomized clinical trials. *Eur J Clin Pharmacol* 1999;55:567-575.

1428 Osato MS, Reddy SG, Graham DY. Osmotic effect of honey on growth and viability of Helicobacter pylori. *Dig Dis Sci* 1999;44(3):462-4.

1429 Leonetti HB, Longo S, Anasti JN. Transdermal progesterone cream for vasomotor symptoms and postmenopausal bone loss. *Obstet Gynecol*, 1999;94: 225-228.

1430 Anon. Adverse events associated with ingestion of gamma-butyrolactone—Minnesota, New Mexico, and Texas, 1998-1999. *MMWR Morb Mortal Wkly Rep* 1999;48(7):137-40.

1431 Harrington RD, Woodward JA, Hooton TM, et al. Life-threatening interactions between HIV-1 protease inhibitors and the illicit drugs MDMA and gamma-hydroxybutyrate. *Arch Intern Med* 1999;159:2221-4.

1433 Ellaway CM, Williams K, Leonard H, et al. Rett syndrome: randomized controlled trial of L-carnitine. *J Child Neurol*, 1999;14:162-167.

1434 Brevetti G, Diehm C, Lambert D, et al. European multicenter study on propionyl-L-carnitine in intermittent claudication. *J Am Coll Cardiol*, 1999;34:1618-1624.

1435 Brevetti G, Perna S, Sabba C, et al. Propionyl-L-carnitine in intermittent claudication: double-blind, placebo-controlled, dose titration, multicenter study. *J Am Coll Cardiol*, 1995;26:1411-1416.

1436 Brevetti G, Perna S, Sabba C, et al. Effect of propionyl-L-carnitine on quality of life in intermittent claudication. *Am J Cardiol*, 1997;79:777-780.

1437 Brevetti G, Perna S, Sabba C, et al. Superiority of L-propionylcarnitine vs L-carnitine in improving walking capacity in patients with peripheral vascular disease: an acute, intravenous, double-blind, cross-over study. *Eur Heart J*, 1992;13(2):251-255.

1439 Siliprandi N, Di Lisa F, Menabo R. Propionyl-L-carnitine: biochemical significance and possible role in cardiac metabolism. *Cardiovasc Drugs Ther*, 1991;5 Suppl 1:11-15.

1440 Tribble DL. AHA Science Advisory. Antioxidant consumption and risk of coronary heart disease: emphasis on vitamin C, vitamin E, and beta-carotene: A statement for healthcare professionals from the American Heart Association. *Circulation* 1999;99:591-595.

1441 Watanabe H, Masaaki K, Ohtsuka S, et al. Randomized, double-blind, placebo-controlled study of the preventative effect of supplemental oral vitamin C on attenuation of development of nitrate tolerance. *J Am Coll Cardiol* 1998;31:1323-1329.

1442 Kugiyama K, Motoyama T, Hirashima O, et al. Vitamin C attenuates abnormal vasomotor reactivity in spasm coronary spastic angina. *J Am Coll Cardiol* 1999;32:103-109.

1443 Cohen HA, Neuman I, Nahum H. Blocking effect of vitamin C in exercise-induced asthma. *Arch Pediatr Adolesc Med* 1997;151(32):103-109.

1444 Zhang S, Hunter DJ, Forman MR, et al. Dietary carotenoids and vitamins A, C, and E and risk of breast cancer. *J Natl Cancer Inst* 1999;91(6):547-556.

1445 Taddei S, Virdis A, Ghiadoni L, et al. Vitamin C improves endothelium-dependent vasodilation by restoring nitric oxide activity in essential hypertension. *Circulation* 1998;97:2222-2229.

1446 Klipstein-Grobusch K, Launer LJ, Geleijnse JM, et al. Serum carotenoids and atherosclerosis. The Rotterdam Study. *Atherosclerosis* 2000;148:49-56.

1447 Gann PH, Ma J, Giovannucci E, Willett W, et al. Lower prostate cancer risk in men with elevated plasma lycopene levels: results of a prospective analysis. *Cancer Research* 1999;59:1225-230.

1448 Lee IM, Cook NR, Manson JE, et al. Beta-carotene supplementation and incidence of cancer and cardiovascular disease: the Women's Health Study. *J Natl Cancer Inst* 1999;91(24):2102-2106.

1449 Ascherio A, Rimm EB, Hernan MA, et al. Relation of consumption of vitamin E, vitamin C, and carotenoids to risk for stroke among men in the United States. *Ann Intern Med*, 1999;130:963-970.

1450 Caffeine Content of Foods and Drugs. Center for Science in the Public Interest, URL: www.cspinet.org/new/cafchart.htm (Accessed 9 December 1999).

1451 Wakabayashi K, Kono S, Shinchi K, et al. Habitual coffee consumption and blood pressure: A study of self-defense officials in Japan. *Eur J Epidemiol* 1998;14(7):669-73.

1452 Hodgson JM, Puddey IB, Burke V, et al. Effects on blood pressure of drinking green and black tea. *J Hypertens* 1999;17(4):457-63.

1453 Dulloo AG, Duret C, Rohrer D, et al. Efficacy of a green tea extract rich in catechin polyphenols and caffeine in increasing 24-h energy expenditure and fat oxidation in humans. *Am J Clin Nutr* 1999;70:1040-5.

1454 Garbisa S, Biggin S, Cavallarin N, et al. Tumor invasion: molecular shears blunted by green tea. *Nat Med* 1999;5:1216.

1455 Cao Y and Cao R. Angiogenesis inhibited by drinking tea. *Nature* 1999;398:381.

1456 L'Allemain G. Multiple actions of EGCG, the main component of green tea. *Bull Cancer* 1999;86:721-4. [Article in French]

1457 Bushman JL. Green tea and cancer in humans: a review of the literature. *Nutr Cancer* 1998;31(3):151-159.

1458 Wakai K, Ohno Y, Obata K. Prognostic significance of selected lifestyle factors in urinary bladder cancer. *Jpn J Br J Nutr* 1993;84(12):1223-1229.

1459 Ohno Y, Aoki K, Obata K, et al. Case-control study of urinary bladder cancer in metropolitan Nagoya. *Natl Cancer Inst Monogr* 1985;69:229-34.

1460 Booth SL, Madabushi HT, Davidson KW, et al. Tea and coffee brews are not dietary sources of vitamin K-1 (phylloquinone). *J Am Diet Assoc* 1995;95:82-3.

1461 Lou FQ, Zhang MF, Zhang XG, et al. A study on tea-pigment in prevention of atherosclerosis. *Chin Med J (Engl)* 1989;102:579-83.

1462 Ali M, Afzal M. A potent inhibitor of thrombin stimulated platelet thromboxane formation from unprocessed tea. *Prostaglandins Leukot Med* 1987;27:9-13.

1463 Graham HN. Green tea composition, consumption, and polyphenol chemistry. *Prev Med* 1992;21:334-50.

1464 Shankar AH, Genton B, Semba RD, et al. Effect of vitamin A supplementation on morbidity due to Plasmodium falciparum in young children in Papua New Guinea: a randomised trial. *Lancet* 1999;354(9174):203-209.

1465 Fawzi WW, Mbise RL, Hertzmark E, et al. A randomized trial of vitamin A supplements in relation to mortality among human immunodeficiency virus-infected and uninfected children in Tanzania. *Pediatr Infect Dis J* 1999;18(2):127-133.

1466 Fawzi WW, Mbise RL, Fataki MR, et al. Vitamin A supplementation and severity of pneumonia in children admitted to the hospital in Dar es Salaam, Tanzania. *Am J Clin Nutr* 1998;68(1):187-192.

1467 Kowalski TE, Falestiny M, Furth E, Malet PF. Vitamin A hepatotoxicity: a cautionary note regarding 25,000 IU

© Copyright 2000, Natural Medicines Comprehensive Database (209) 472-2244. For updated data, go to www.NaturalDatabase.com. • 1185

REFERENCES

REFERENCES

supplements. *Am J Med* 1994;97(6):523-528.

1468 Wang Z, Boudjelal M, Kang S, et al. Ultraviolet irradiation of human skin causes functional vitamin A deficiency, preventable by all-trans retinoic acid pretreatment. *Nat Med* 1999;5(4):418-422.

1469 Meyers DG, Maloley PA, Weeks D. Safety of antioxidant vitamins. *Arch Intern Med* 1996;156(9):925-935.

1470 Cooper DA, Eldridge AL, Peters JC. Dietary carotenoids and certain cancers, heart disease, and age-related macular degeneration: a review of recent research. *Nutr Rev* 1999;57(7):201-214.

1471 Cooper DA, Eldridge AL, Peters JC. Dietary carotenoids and lung cancer: a review of recent research. *Nutr Rev* 1999;57(5 Pt 1):133-145.

1472 Garewal HS, Katz RV, Meyskens F, et al. Beta-carotene produces sustained remissions in patients with oral leukoplakia: results of a multicenter prospective trial. *Arch Otolaryngol Head Neck Surg* 1999;125(12):1305-1310.

1473 Cook NR, Stampfer MJ, Ma J, et al. Beta-carotene supplementation for patients with low baseline levels and decreased risks of total and *Prostate* carcinoma. *Cancer* 1999;86(9):1783-1792.

1474 Neuman I, Nahum H, Ben-Amotz A. Prevention of exercise-induced asthma by a natural isomer mixture of beta-carotene. *Ann Allergy Asthma Immunol* 1999;82(6):549-553.

1475 Pallast EG, Schouten EG, de Waart FG, et al. Effect of 50- and 100-mg vitamin E supplements on cellular immune function in noninstitutionalized elderly persons. *Am J Clin Nutr* 1999;69(6):1273-1281.

1476 Woodson K, Tangrea JA, Barrett MJ, et al. Serum alpha-tocopherol and subsequent risk of lung cancer among male smokers. *J Natl Cancer Inst* 1999;91(20):1738-1743.

1477 Perkins AJ, Hendrie HC, Callahan CM, et al. Association of antioxidants with memory in a multiethnic elderly sample using the Third National Health and Nutrition Examination Survey. *Am J Epidemiol* 1999;150(1):37-44.

1478 Bursell SE, Clermont AC, Aiello LP, et al. High-dose vitamin E supplementation normalizes retinal blood flow and creatinine clearance in patients with type 1 diabetes. *Diabetes Care* 1999;22(8):1245-1251.

1479 Devaraj S, Jialal I. Alpha-tocopherol decreases interleukin-1 beta release from activated human monocytes by inhibition of 5-lipoxygenase. *Arterioscler Thromb Vasc Biol* 1999;19(4):1125-1133.

1480 Meydani SN, Meydani M, Blumberg JB, et al. Vitamin E supplementation and in vivo immune response in healthy elderly subjects. A randomized controlled trial. *JAMA* 1997;277(17):1380-1386.

1482 Houston DK, Johnson MA, Nozza RJ, et al. Age-related hearing loss, vitamin B-12, and folate in elderly women. *Am J Clin Nutr* 1999;69(3):564-71.

1483 Selhub J, Jacques PF, Wilson PW, et al. Vitamin status and intake as primary determinants of homocysteinemia in an elderly population. *JAMA* 1993;270(22):2693-2698.

1484 Carmel R, Green R, Jacobsen DW, et al. Serum cobalamin, homocysteine, and methylmalonic acid concentrations in a multiethnic elderly population: ethnic and sex differences in cobalamin and metabolite abnormalities. *Am J Clin Nutr* 1999;70(5):904-10.

1485 Stabler SP, Allen RH, Fried LP, et al. Racial differences

in prevalence of cobalamin and folate deficiencies in disabled elderly women. *Am J Clin Nutr* 1999;70(5):911-919.

1489 Bostom AG, Gohh RY, Beaulieu AJ, et al. Treatment of hyperhomocysteinemia in renal transplant recipients. A randomized, placebo-controlled trial. *Ann Intern Med* 1997;127(12):1089-1092.

1492 Klipstein-Grobusch K, Grobbee DE, den Breeijen JH, et al. Dietary iron and risk of myocardial infarction in the Rottersam Study. *Am J Epidemiol* 1999;149:421-28.

1493 Slattery ML, Schumacher MC, West DW, Robinson LM. Smoking and bladder cancer. The modifying effect of cigarettes on other factors. *Cancer* 1988;61(2):402-8.

1494 Jensen OM, Wahrendorf J, Knudsen JB, Sorenson BL. The Copenhagen case-control study of bladder cancer. II. Effect of coffee and other beverages. *Int J Cancer* 1986;37(5):651-7.

1495 Nomura AM, Kolonel LN, Hankin JH, Yoshizawa CN. Dietary factors in cancer of the lower urinary tract. *Int J Cancer* 1991;48(2):199-205.

1496 Clinton SK, Emenhiser C, Schwartz SJ, et al. cis-trans lycopene isomers, carotenoids, and retinol in the human prostate. *Cancer Epidemiol Biomarkers Prev* 1996;5(10):823-33.

1497 Gartner C, Stahl W, Sies H. Lycopene is more bioavaiable from tomato paste than from fresh tomatoes. *Am J Clin Nutr,* 1997;66(1):116-122.

1498 Paetau I, Khachik F, Brown ED, et al. Chronic ingestion of lycopene-rich tomato juice or lycopene supplements significantly increases plasma concentrations of lycopene and related tomato carotenoids in humans. *Am J Clin Nutr* 1998;68(6):1187-195.

1500 Rueff F, Schoepf P, Pfuetzner W, Przybilla B. "Sensitization to condurango bark is frequent in patients with *Allergy* to natural rubber latex." *J Allergy Clin Immunol,* 1998; 101(1 Pt 2):S207.

1501 Pfutzner W, Thomas P, Rueff F, Przybilla B. "Anaphylactic reaction elicited by condurango bark in a patient allergic to natural rubber latex." *J Allergy Clin Immunol,* 1998; 101(2 Pt 1):281-2.

1502 *Medicinal Plants.* Springer Verlag: Lavoisier, NY, 1995.

1503 Reichert R. "Sedative Effects of California Poppy and Corydalis." *Quarterly Review of Natural Medicine,* Winter 1996:256.

1504 Brown D, Gaby A, Reichert R. *Quarterly Review of Natural Medicine,* Winter 1997:337.

1505 Trivedi CP, et al. "Bronchodilator and anti-inflammatory effect of glycosidal fraction of Acacia farnesiana." *Indian J Physiol Pharmacol,* 1986; 30(3):267-8.

1506 Leung A. "Better Health with (Mostly) Chinese Herbs and Foods." AYSL, Glen Rock, NJ, 1995.

1507 Liu ZY, et al. [Effect of improving memory and inhibiting acetylcholinesterase activity by invigorating-qi and warming-yang recipe]. *Chung Kuo Chung Hsi I Chieh Ho Tsa Chih* 1993 Nov; 13(11):675-6, 164.

1508 Zhang H, et al. [Preliminary study of traditional Chinese *Medicine* treatment of minimal brain dysfunction: analysis of 100 cases]. *Chung Hsi I Chieh Ho Tsa Chih* 1990 May;10(5):278-9, 260.

1509 Zneg XL, et al. [Immunological and hematopoietic effect of Codonopsis pilosula on cancer patients during radiotherapy]. Chung Kuo *Chung Hsi I Chieh Ho Tsa Chih* 1992 Oct;12(10):607-8, 581.

1510 O'Brien LW. "Interactions and Toxicities of Drugs for HIV Disease." *Arch Intern Med,* 1991; 151:2281-2288.

1512 Anonymous. "In vitro screening of traditional medicines for anti-HIV activity: memorandum from a WHO meeting." *Bull World Health Organ* 1989;67(6):613-8.

1513 Zhu SC. [Clinical observations on 36 cases of viral myocarditis treated with Epimedium grandiflorum Moor and vitamin C]. *Chung Hsi I Chieh Ho Tsa Chih* 1984 Sep;4(9):523-4, 514.

1514 Le Bars PL, et al. "A placebo-controlled, double-blind, randomized trial of an extract of Ginkgo biloba for dementia. North American EGb Study Group." *JAMA* 1997 Oct 22; 278:1327-1332.

1515 Oken BS, et al. "The efficacy of Ginkgo biloba on cognitive function in Alzheimer disease." *Arch Neurol.* 1998 Nov;55(11):1409-15.

1516 Akhtar MS, et al. "Field trial of Saussurea lappa roots against nematodes and Nigella sativa seeds against cestodes in children." *JPMA J Pak Med Assoc* 1991 Aug; 41(8) 185-7.

1517 Froohlich HH, et al. [Physical investigations into the thermotherapeutic action of the Kneipp hay flower sack]. *MMW Munch Med Wochenschr* 1975 Mar 14; 117(11):443-8.

1518 Frohlich HH, et al. [The sedative effect of the Kneipp hay sack and balneological preparations of hay (author's transl)]. *MMW Munch Med Wochenschr* 1976 Mar 12;118(11):317-20.

1519 Tona L, et al. "Antiamoebic and phytochemical screening of some Congolese medicinal plants." *Ethnopharmacol* 1998 May, 61(1):57-65.

1520 Allen JD, et al. "Ginseng supplementation does not enhance healthy young adults' peak aerobic exercise performance." *J Am Coll Nutr* 1998 Oct;17(5):462-6.

1521 Engels HJ, et al. "No ergogenic effects of ginseng (Panax ginseng C.A. Meyer) during graded maximal aerobic exercise." *J Am Diet Assoc.* 1997 Oct;97(10):1110-5.

1522 Park HJ, et al. "Effects of dietary supplementation of lipophilic fraction from Panax ginseng on cGMP and cAMP in rat platelets and on blood coagulation." *Biol Pharm Bull.* 1996 Nov;19(11):1434-9.

1523 Lin RC, et al. "Effects of isoflavones on *Alcohol* pharmacokinetics and alcohol-drinking behavior in rats." *Am J Clin Nutr* 1998 Dec;68(6 Suppl):1512S-1515S.

1524 Xie CI, et al. "Daidzin, an antioxidant isoflavonoid, decreases blood Alcohol levels and shortens sleep time induced by ethanol intoxication." *Alcohol Clin Exp Res* 1994 Dec;18(6):1443-7.

1525 Avalos J, et al. "Guinea pig maximization test of the bark extract from pawpaw, Asimina triloba (Annonaceae)." *Contact Dermatitis* 1993 Jul;29(1):33-5.

1526 Tomoda M, et al. "Plant mucilages. XLII. An anti-complementary mucilage from the leaves of Malva sylvestris var. mauritiana." *Chem Pharm Bull* (Tokyo) 1989 Nov;37(11):3029-32.

1527 Stefanova Z, et al. Effect of a total extract from Fraxinus ornus stem bark and esculin on zymosan- and carrageenan-induced paw oedema in mice. *J Ethnopharmacol* 1995 May;46(2):101-6.

1528 Pintos J, et al. "Mate, coffee, and tea consumption and risk of cancers of the upper aerodigestive tract in southern Brazil." *Epidemiology* 1994 Nov;5(6):583-90.

1529 De Stefani E, et al. "Meat intake, 'mate' drinking and renal cell cancer in Uruguay: a case-control study." *Br J Cancer* 1998 Nov;78(9):1239-43.

1530 De Stefani E, et al. "Black tobacco, mate, and bladder cancer. A case-control study from Uruguay." *Cancer* 1991 Jan 15;67(2):536-40.

1531 De Stefani E, et al. "Mate drinking and risk of lung cancer in males: a case-control study from Uruguay." *Cancer Epidemiol Biomarkers* Prev 1996 Jul;5(7):515-9.

1532 Kong YC, et al. "Isolation of the uterotonic principle from Leonurus artemisia, the Chinese motherwort." *Am J Chin Med* 1976 Winter;4(4):373-82.

1533 Zou QZ, et al. "Effect of motherwort on blood hyperviscosity." *Am J Chin Med* 1989;17(1-2):65-70.

1534 Zgorniak-Nowosielska I, et al. "Antiviral activity of Flos verbasci infusion against influenza and Herpes simplex viruses." *Arch Immunol Ther Exp* (Warsz) 1991;39(1-2):103-8.

1535 al-Harbi MM, et al. "Gastric antiulcer and cytoprotective effect of Commiphora molmol in rats." *J Ethnopharmacol* 1997 Jan;55(2):141-50.

1536 al-Harbi MM, et al. "Anticarcinogenic effect of Commiphora molmol on solid tumors induced by Ehrlich carcinoma cells in mice." *Chemotherapy* 1994 Sep-Oct;40(5):337-47.

1537 Pintao AM, et al. "In vitro and in vivo antitumor activity of benzyl isothiocyanate: a natural product from Tropaeolum majus." *Planta Med* 1995 Jun;61(3):233-6.

1538 Buck DS, et al. "Comparison of two topical preparations for the treatment of onychomycosis: Melaleuca alternifolia (tea tree) oil and clotrimazole." *J Fam Pract* 1994 Jun;38(6):601-5.

1539 Mahabir D, et al. "Use of medicinal plants for diabetes in Trinidad and Tobago." *Rev Panam Salud Publica* 1997 Mar;1(3):174-9.

1540 Cherif S, et al. [A clinical trial of a titrated Olea extract in the treatment of essential arterial hypertension]. *J Pharm Belg* 1996 Mar-Apr;51(2):69-71.

1541 Aziz NH, et al. "Comparative antibacterial and antifungal effects of some phenolic compounds." *Microbios* 1998;93(374):43-54.

1542 Pieroni A, et al. "In vitro anti-complementary activity of flavonoids from olive (Olea europaea L.) leaves." *Pharmazie* 1996 Oct;51(10):765-8.

1543 Liccardi G, et al. "Oleaceae pollinosis: a review." *Int Arch Allergy Immunol* 1996 Nov;111(3):210-7.

1544 Holti G. An experimentally controlled evaluation of the effect of inositol nicotinate upon the digital blood flow in patients with Raynaud's phenomenon. *J Int Med Res* 1979;7(6):473-483.

1545 Ring EF, Bacon PA. Quantitative thermographic assessment of inositol nicotinate therapy in Raynaud's phenomena. *J Int Med Res* 1977;5(4):217-222.

1546 Wilke H, Frahm H. [Treatment of hyperlipoproteinaemia types IIa, IIb, IV and V with a combination of clofibrate and inositol nicotinate]. [Article in German]. *Dtsch Med Wochenschr* 1976;101(11):401-405.

1547 Anon. Alpha-lipoic acid. *Altern Med Rev* 1998;3(4):308-310.

1548 Berkson BM. Thioctic acid in treatment of hepatotoxic mushroom (Phalloides) poisoning (letter). *N Engl J Med* 1979;300(7):371.

1549 Roldan EJ, Perez Lloret A. Thioctic acid in Amanita poisoning (letter). *Crit Care Med* 1986;14(8):753-754.

1550 Biewenga GP, Haenen GR, Bast A. The pharmacology of the antioxidant lipoic acid. *Gen Pharmacol* 1997;29(3):315-331.

1551 Filina AA, Davydova NG, Endrikhovskii SN, Shamshinova AM. Lipoic acid as a means of metabolic therapy of open-angle glaucoma [Article in Russian]. *Vestn Oftalmol* 1995;111(4):6-8.

REFERENCES

1552 Filina AA, Davydova NG, Kolomoitseva EM. The effect of lipoic acid on the components of the glutathione system in the lacrimal fluid of patients with open angle glaucoma [Article in Russian]. *Vestn Oftalmol* 1993;109(5):5-7.

1554 Matalon R, Stumpf DA, Michals K, et al. Lipoamide dehydrogenase deficiency with primary lactic acidosis: favorable response to treatment with oral lipoic acid. *J Pediatr* 1984;104:65-69.

1555 Yoshida I, Sweetman L, Kulovich S, et al. Effect of lipoic acid in patient with defective activity of pyruvate dehydrogenase, 2-oxoglutarate dehydrogenase, and branched-chain keto acid dehydrogenase. *Pediatr Res* 1990;27:75-79.

1556 Dana Consortium on the therapy of HIV dementia and related cognitive disorders. A randomized, double-blind, placebo-controlled trial of deprenyl and thioctic acid in human immunodeficiency virus-associated cognitive impairment. *Neurology* 1998;50:645-651.

1557 Maesaka H, Komiya K, Misugi K, Tada K. Hyperalaninemia hyperpyruvicemia and lactic acidosis due to pyruvate carboxylase deficiency of the liver; treatment with thiamine and lipoic acid. *Eur J Pediatr* 1976;122(2):159-168.

1561 Packer L, Tritschler HJ, Wessel K. Neuroprotection by the metabolic antioxidant alpha-lipoic acid. *Free Radic Biol Med* 1997;22(1-2):359-378.

1562 Merin JP, Matsuyama M, Kira T, et al. Alpha-lipoic acid blocks HIV-1 LTR-dependent expression of hygromycin resistance in THP-1 stable transformants. *FEBS Lett* 1996;394(1):9-13.

1563 Suzuki YJ, Aggarwal BB, Packer L. Alpha-lipoic acid is a potent inhibitor of NF-kappa B activation in human T cells. *Biochem Biophys Res Commun* 1992;189(3):1709-1715.

1570 Lipoic acid. The Natural Pharmacist website. URL: www.tnp.com/substance.asp?ID=149. (Accessed 17 February 2000).

1571 Chiddo A, Gaglione A, Musci S, et al. Hemodynamic study of intravenous propionyl-L-carnitine in patients with ischemic heart disease and normal left ventricular function. *Cardiovasc Drugs Ther*, 1991;5 Suppl 1:107-111.

1572 Bartels GL, Remme WJ, Pillay M, et al. Acute improvement of cardiac function with intravenous L-propionylcarnitine in humans. *J Cardiovasc Pharmacol*, 1992;20(1):157-164.

1573 Bartels GL, Remme WJ, Pillay M, et al. Effects of L-propionylcarnitine on ischemia-induced myocardial dysfunction in men with angina pectoris. *Am J Cardiol*, 1994;74(2):125-130.

1574 Persico G, Amato B, Aprea G, et al. The early effects of intravenous L-propionyl carnitine on ulcerative trophic lesions of the lower limbs in arteriopathic patients: a controlled randomized study. *Drugs Exp Clin Res*, 1995;21(5):187-198.

1575 Anand I, Chandrashekhan Y, De Giuli F, et al. Acute and chronic effects of propionyl-L-carnitine on the hemodynamics, exercise capacity, and hormones in patients with congestive heart failure. *Cardiovasc Drugs Ther*, 1998;12(3):291-299.

1576 Dal Lago A, De Martini D, Flore R, et al. Effects of propionyl-L-carnitine on peripheral arterial obliterative disease of the lower limbs: a double-blind clinical trial. *Drugs Exp Clin Res*, 1999;25(1):29-36.

1577 Ferrari R, De Giuli F. The propionyl-L-carnitine hypothesis: an alternative approach to treating heart failure. *J Card Fail*, 1997;3(3):217-224.

1578 Wiseman LR, Brogden RN. Propionyl-L-carnitine. *Drugs Aging*, 1998;12(3):243-248; discussion 249-250.

1579 Cherchi A, Lai C, Onnis E, et al. Propionyl carnitine in stable effort angina. *Cardiovasc Drugs Ther*, 1990;4(2):481-486.

1580 Bartels GL, Remme WJ, den Hartog FR, et al. Additional anti-ischemic effects of long-term L-propionylcarnitine in anginal patients treated with conventional antianginal therapy. *Cardiovasc Drugs Ther*, 1995;9(6):749-753.

1581 Bartels GL, Remme WJ, Holwerda KJ, Kruijssen DA. Anti-ischaemic efficacy of L-propionylcarnitine - a promising novel metabolic approach to ischaemia? *Eur Heart J*, 1996;17(3):414-420.

1582 Caponnetto S, Canale C, Masperone MA, et al. Efficacy of L-propionylcarnitine treatment in patients with left ventricular dysfunction. *Eur Heart J*, 1994;15(9):1267-1273.

1583 Mancini M, Rengo F, Lingetti M, et al. Controlled study on the therapeutic efficacy of propionyl-L-carnitine in patients with congestive heart failure. *Arzneimittelforschung*, 1992;42(9):1101-1104.

1584 Anon. Acetyl-L-Carnitine. MotherNature.com website. URL: www.mothernature.com/ency/Supp/Acetyl-L-Carnitine.asp (Accessed 27 February 2000).

1585 James JS. *AIDS* treatment news archives. URL: http://aids.org/immunet/atn.nsf/page/a-267-(Accessed 27 February 2000).

1586 Anon. Acetylcarnitine. iHerb Ltd website. URL / www.iherb.com/acetyl1.html (Accessed 27 February 2000).

1587 Anon. ProXeed Fact Sheet. URL www.proxeed.com/physicians/studies/abstract.asp (Accessed 27 February 2000).

1588 De Falco FA, D'Angelo E, Grimaldi G, et al. [Effect of the chronic treatment with L-acetylcarnitine in Down's syndrome]. [Italian] *Clinica Terapeutica*, 1994;144(2):123-127.

1589 Tempesta E, Troncon R, Janiri L, et al. Role of acetyl-L-carnitine in the treatment of cognitive deficit in chronic alcoholism. *Int J Clin Pharmacol Res*, 1990;10(1-2):101-107.

1590 Mezzina C, De Grandis D, Calvani M, et al. Idiopathic facial paralysis: new therapeutic prospects with acetyl-L-carnitine. *Int J Clin Pharmacol Res*, 1992;12(5-6):299-304.

1591 Postiglione A, Soricelli A, Cicerano U, et al. Effect of acute administration of L-acetyl carnitine on cerebral blood flow in patients with chronic cerebral infarct. *Pharmacol Res*, 1991;23(3):241-246.

1592 Rosadini G, Marenco S, Nobili F, et al. Acute effects of acetyl-L-carnitine on regional cerebral blood flow in patients with brain ischaemia. *Int J Clin Pharmacol Res*, 1990;10(1-2):123-8.

1593 Onofrj M, Fulgente T, Melchionda D, et al. L-acetylcarnitine as a new therapeutic approach for peripheral neuropathies with pain. *Int J Clin Pharmacol Res*, 1995;15(1):9-15.

1594 Thal LJ, Carta A, Clarke WR, et al. A 1-year multicenter placebo-controlled study of acetyl-L-carnitine in patients with Alzheimer's Disease. *Neurology*, 1996;47:705-711.

1595 Sano M, Bell K, Cote L, et al. Double-blind parallel design pilot study of acetyl levocarnitine in patients with Alzheimer's Disease. *Arch Neurol*, 1992;49:1137-1141.

1596 Spagnoli A, Lucca U, Menasce G, et al. Long-term acetyl-L-carnitine treatment in Alzheimer's Disease. *Neurology*, 1991;41:1726-1732.

1597 Brooks JO, Yesavage JA, Carta A, Bravi D. Acetyl L-carnitine slows decline in younger patients with Alzheimer's disease: a reanalysis of a double-blind, placebo-controlled study using the trilinear approach. *Int Psychoger*, 1998;10(2):193-203.

1598 Pettegrew JW, Klunk WE, Panchalingam K, et al. Clinical and neurochemical effects of acetyl-L-carnitine in Alzheimer's disease. *Neurobiol Aging*, 1995;16(1):1-4.

1599 Rai G, Wright G, Scott L, et al. Double-blind, placebo controlled study of acetyl-l-carnitine in patients with Alzheimer's dementia. *Curr Med Res Opin*, 1990;11(10):638-647.

1600 Dong Y, Yang MM, Kwan CY. In vitro inhibition of proliferation of HL-60 cells by tetrandrine and coriolus versicolor peptide derived from Chinese medicinal herbs. *Life Sci*, 1997;60(8):PL135-140.

1601 Netrition. "Triax" website: www.netrition.com/ triax_page.html (Accessed 14 November 1999).

1602 Get Huge. "The Triac Story" website: www.gethuge.net/ triac (Accessed 14 November 1999).

1604 FDA Orphan Drug List. http://www.fda.gov/orphan/ designat/list.htm (Accessed 14 November 1999).

1605 FDA warns against consuming triax metabolic accelerator. FDA website, URL: www.fda.gov/bbs/ topics/ANSWERS/ANS00984.html (Accessed 15 November 1999).

1606 Precision Athletics. "Triarcanna" website: www.precisionathletics.com/triac.html (Accessed 15 November 1999).

1607 McDermott MT, Ridgway EC. Central hyperthyroidism. *Endocrinol Metab Clin North Am* 1998;27(1):187-203.

1608 Takeda T, Suzuki S, Liu RT, et al. Triiodothyroacetic acid has unique potential for therapy of resistance to thyroid hormone. *J Clin Endocrinol Metab* 1995;80(7):2033-2040.

1609 Kunitake JM, Hartman N, Henson LC, et al. 3,5,3'-triiodothyroacetic acid therapy for thyroid hormone resistance. *Clin Endocrinol Metab* 1989;69(2):461-466.

1610 Dulgeroff AJ, Geffner ME, Koyal SN, et al. Bromocriptine and Triac therapy for hyperthyroidism due to pituitary resistance to thyroid hormone. *J Clin Endocrinol Metab* 1992;75(4):1071-1075.

1611 Beck-Peccoz P, Sartorio A, De Medici C, et al. Dissociated thyromimetic effects of 3, 5, 3'-triiodothyroacetic acid (TRIAC) at the pituitary and peripheral tissue levels. *J Endocrinol Invest* 1988;11(2):113-118.

1612 Lind P, Langsteger W, Koltringer P, et al. 3,5,3'-Triiodothyroacetic acid (TRIAC) effects on pituitary thyroid regulation and on peripheral tissue parameters. *Nuklearmedizin* 1989;28(6):217-220.

1613 Nicolini U, Venegoni E, Acaia B, et al. Prenatal treatment of fetal hypothyroidism: is there more than one option? *Prenat Diagn* 1996;16(5):443-448.

1614 Asteria C, Rajanayagam O, Collingwood TN, et al. Prenatal diagnosis of thyroid hormone resistance. *J Clin Endocrinol Metab* 1999;84(2):405-410.

1615 Radetti G, Persani L, Molinaro G, et al. Clinical and hormonal outcome after two years of triiodothyroacetic acid treatment in a child with thyroid hormone resistance. *Thyroid* 1997;7(5):775-778.

1616 Jaffiol C, Daures JP, Nsakala N, et al. [Long term follow up of medical treatment of differentiated thyroid cancer]. [Article in French] *Ann Endocrinol* (Paris) 1995;56(2):119-126.

1617 Mueller-Gaertner HW, Schneider C. 3,5,3'-Triiodothyroacetic acid minimizes the pituitary thyrotrophin secretion in patients on levo-thyroxine therapy after ablative therapy for differentiated thyroid carcinoma. *Clin Endocrinol* (Oxf) 1988;28(4):345-351.

1618 Mechelany C, Schlumberger M, Challeton C, et al. TRIAC (3,5,3'-triiodothyroacetic acid) has parallel effects at the pituitary and peripheral tissue levels in thyroid cancer patients treated with L-thyroxine. *Clin Endocrinol* (Oxf) 1991;35(2):123-128.

1620 Chow WS; Lam KS. An overweight woman with galactorrhoea. *Postgrad Med J* 1998;74:121-122.

1621 Lledo Carreres M, Lajo Garrido JL, Gonzalez Rico M, et al. Toxic internuclear ophthalmoplegia related to antiobesity treatment. *Ann Pharmacother* 1992;26(11):1457-8.

1622 Ferner RE; Burnett A; Rawlins MD. Triiodothyroacetic acid abuse in a female body builder. *Lancet* 1986;1:383.

1623 Heim J. [Hypothyroidism of central origin corrected by the cessation of Triac therapy]. [Article in French]. *Ann Med Interne* (Paris) 1982;133(8):588-589.

1624 Jean-Pastor MJ, Jean P, Biour M, et al. [Hepatopathies from treatment with a specialty drug combination of tiratricol-cyclovalone-retinol]. [Article in French]. *J Toxicol Clin Exp* 1986;6(2):115-121.

1625 Bentin J, Desir D, Mockel J. Triac (3,5,3'-triiodo-thyroacetic acid) induced "pseudohypothyroidism". *Acta Clin Belg* 1984;39(5):285-289.

1627 Hawkey CM, Olsen EG, Symons C. Production of cardiac muscle abnormalities in offspring of rats receiving triiodothyroacetic acid (triac) and the effect of beta adrenergic blockade. *Cardiovasc Res* 1981;15(4):196-205.

1628 Olsen EG, Symons C, Hawkey C. Effect of triac on the developing heart. *Lancet* 1977;2(8031):221-223.

1629 Pitt-Rivers R. Physiological activity of the acetic acid analogues of some iodinated thyronines. *Lancet* 1953;2:234.

1630 Lerman JL, Pitt-rivers R. Physiological activity of triiodo and tetraiodothyroacetic acid on blood-cholesterol levels. *Lancet* 1956;1:885-9.

1631 Menegay C, Juge C, Burger AG. Pharmacokinetics of 3,5,3'-triiodothyroacetic acid and its effects on serum TSH levels. *Acta Endocrinol* (Copenh) 1989;121(5):651-658.

1632 Sherman SI, Ringel MD, Smith MJ, et al. Augmented hepatic and skeletal thyromimetic effects of tiratricol in comparison with levothyroxine. *J Clin Endocrinol Metab* 1997;82(7):2153-2158.

1633 Sherman SI, Ladenson PW. Organ-specific effects of tiratricol: a thyroid hormone analog with hepatic, not pituitary, superagonist effects. *J Clin Endocrinol Metab* 1992;75(3):901-905.

1634 Bracco D, Morin O, Schutz Y, et al. Comparison of the metabolic and endocrine effects of 3,5,3'-triiodothyroacetic acid and thyroxine. *J Clin Endocrinol Metab* 1993;77(1):221-228.

1635 Ng TB. A review of research on the protein-bound polysaccharide (polysaccharopeptide, PSP) from the mushroom Coriolus versicolor (Basidiomycetes: Polyporaceae). *Gen Pharmacol*, 1998;30(1):1-4.

1636 Mizutani Y, Yoshida O. Activation by the protein-bound polysaccharide PSK (krestin) of cytotoxic lymphocytes

REFERENCES

REFERENCES

that act on fresh autologous tumor cells and T24 human urinary bladder transitional carcinoma cell line in patients with urinary bladder cancer. *J Urol*, 1991;145(5):1082-1087.

1637 Kobayashi H, Matsunaga K, Oguchi Y. Antimetastatic effects of PSK (Krestin), a protein-bound polysaccharide obtained from basidiomycetes: an overview. *Cancer Epidemiol Biomarkers* Prev, 1995;4(3):275-281.

1638 Dong Y, Kwan CY, Chen ZN, et al. Antitumor effects of a refined polysaccharide peptide fraction isolated from Coriolus versicolor: in vitro and in vivo studies. *Res Commun Mol Pathol Pharmacol*, 1996;92(2):140-148.

1639 Kanoh T, Saito K, Matsunaga K, et al. Enhancement of the antitumor effect by the concurrent use of a monoclonal antibody and the protein bound polysaccharide PSK in mice bearing a human cancer cell line. *In Vivo*, 1994;8(2):241-245.

1640 Maehara Y, Inutsuka S, Takeuchi H, et al. Postoperative PSK and OK-432 immunochemotherapy for patients with gastric cancer. *Cancer Chemother Pharmacol*, 1993;33(2):171-175.

1641 Harada M, Matsunaga K, Oguchi Y, et al. Oral administration of PSK can improve the impaired anti-tumor CD4+ T-cell response in gut associated lymphoid tissue (GALT) of specific-pathogen-free mice. *Int J Cancer*, 1997;70(3):362-372.

1642 Tsukagoshi S, Hashimoto Y, Fujii G, et al. Krestin (PSK). *Cancer Treat Rev*, 1984;11(2):131-155.

1643 Collins RA, Ng TB. Polysaccharopeptide from Coriolus versicolor has potential for use against human immunodeficiency virus type 1 infection. *Life Sci*, 1997;60(25):PL383-387.

1644 Tochikura TS, Nakashima H, Hirose K, et al. A biological response modifier, PSK, inhibits human immunodeficiency virus infection in vitro. *Biochem Biophys Res Commun*, 1987;148(2):726-733.

1645 Gong S, Zhang HQ, Yin WP, et al. Involvement of interleukin-2 in analgesia produced by Coriolus versicolor polysaccharide peptides. *Chung Kuo Yao Li Hsueh Pao*, 1998;19(1):67-70.

1646 Ng TB, Chan WY. Polysaccharopeptide from the mushroom Coriolus versicolor possesses analgesic activity but does not produce adverse effects on female reproductive or embryonic development in mice. *Gen Pharmacol*, 1997;29(2):269-273.

1647 Yeung JH, Chiu LC, Ooi VE. Effect of polysaccharide peptide (PSP) on glutathione and protection against paracetamol-induced hepatotoxicity in the rat. *Methods Find Exp Clin Pharmacol*, 1994;16(10):723-729.

1648 Iino Y, Yokoe T, Maemura M, et al. Immunochemotherapies versus chemotherapy as adjuvant treatment after curative resection of operable breast cancer. *AntiCancer Res*, 1995;15(6B):2907-2911.

1649 Ogoshi K, Satou H, Isono K, et al. Immunotherapy for esophageal cancer. A randomized trial in combination with radiotherapy and radiochemotherapy. Cooperative Study Group for Esophageal cancer in Japan. *Am J Clin Oncol*, 1995;18(3):216-222.

1650 Yokoe T, Iino Y, Takei H, et al. HLA antigen as predictive index for the outcome of breast cancer patients with adjuvant immunochemotherapy with PSK. *AntiCancer Res*, 1997;17(4A):2815-2818.

1651 Nakazato H, Koike A, Saji S, et al. Efficacy of immunochemotherapy as adjuvant treatment after curative resection of gastric cancer. Study Group of Immunochemotherapy with PSK for Gastric Cancer.

Lancet , 1994;343(8906):1122-1126.

1652 Sugimachi K, Maehara Y, Ogawa M, et al. Dose intensity of uracil and tegafur in postoperative chemotherapy for patients with poorly differentiated gastric cancer. *Cancer Chemother Pharmacol*, 1997;40(3):233-238.

1653 Hayakawa K, Mitsuhashi N, Saito Y, et al. Effect of Krestin as adjuvant treatment following radical radiotherapy in non-small cell lung cancer patients. *Cancer Detect Prev*, 1997;21(1):71-77.

1654 Morimoto T, Ogawa M, Orita K, et al. Postoperative adjuvant randomised trial comparing chemoendocrine therapy, chemotherapy and immunotherapy for patients with stage II breast cancer: 5-year results from the Nishinihon Cooperative Study Group of Adjuvant Chemoendocrine Therapy for Breast cancer (ACETBC) of Japan. *Eur J Cancer*, 1996;32A(2):235-242.

1655 Suto T, Fukuda S, Moriya N, et al. Clinical study of biological response modifiers as maintenance therapy for hepatocellular carcinoma. *Cancer Chemother Pharmacol*, 1994;33 Suppl:S145-148.

1656 Toi M, Hattori T, Akagi M et al. Randomized adjuvant trial to evaluate the addition of tamoxifen and PSK to *Chemotherapy* in patients with primary breast cancer. 5-Year results from the Nishi-Nippon Group of the Adjuvant Chemoendocrine Therapy for Breast Cancer Organization. *Cancer*, 1992;70(10):2475-2483.

1657 Mitomi T, Tsuchiya S, Iijima N, et al. Randomized, controlled study on adjuvant immunochemotherapy with PSK in curatively resected colorectal cancer. The Cooperative Study Group of Surgical Adjuvant Immunochemotherapy for cancer of Colon and Rectum (Kanagawa). *Dis Colon Rectum*, 1992;35(2):123-130.

1658 Nio Y, Tsubono M, Tseng CC, et al. Immunomodulation by orally administered protein-bound polysaccharide PSK in patients with gastrointestinal cancer. *Biotherapy*, 1992;4(2):117-128.

1659 Kondo T, Sakamoto J, Nakazato H. Alternating immunochemotherapy of advanced gastric carcinoma: a randomized comparison of carbazilquinone and PSK to carbazilquinone in patients with curative gastric resection. *Biotherapy*, 1991;3(4):287-295.

1660 Torisu M, Hayashi Y, Ishimitsu T, et al. Significant prolongation of disease-free period gained by oral polysaccharide K (PSK) administration after curative surgical operation of colorectal cancer. *Cancer Immunol Immunother*, 1990;31(5):261-268.

1661 Go P, Chung CH. Adjuvant PSK immunotherapy in patients with carcinoma of the nasopharynx. *J Int Med Res*, 1989;17(2):141-149.

1662 Fukushima M. Adjuvant therapy of gastric cancer: the Japanese experience. *Semin Oncol*, 1996;23(3):369-378.

1663 Healthlink. "Monograph: Poria", URL: www.healthlink.us-inc.com/publiclibrary/htm-data/htm-herb/bhp985.htm (Accessed 22 November 1999).

1664 Life Extension Vitamin Supplies, Inc. "DMAE" website: www.lifeextensionvitamins.com/lifeextensionvitamins/dmae.html (Accessed 23 November 1999).

1665 Mothernature.com Health Encyclopedia. "DMAE" website: www.mothernature.com/ency/supp/dmae.asp (Accessed 23 November 1999).

1666 Smart Basic. "Glossary: DMAE" website: www.smartbasic.com/glos.nutrients/dmae.glos.html. (Accessed 23 November 1999).

1667 Life Link. "DMAE" website: www.west.net/~lifelink/dmae2.htm (Accessed 23 November 1999).

1668 Davies C, Maidment S, Hanley P, et al. Dimethylaminoethanol (DMAE). HSE. Risk assessment document; EH72/2;1997. (TOXLINE).

1669 Re' O. 2-Dimethylaminoethanol (deanol): a brief review of its clinical efficacy and postulated mechanism of action. *Curr Ther Res Clin Exp* 1974;16(11):1238-1242.

1670 Rimland B. Controversies in the treatment of autistic children: vitamin and drug therapy. *J Child Neurol* 1988;3 Suppl:S68-72.

1671 Pieralisi G, Ripari P, Vecchiet L. Effects of a standardized ginseng extract combined with dimethylaminoethanol bitartrate, vitamins, minerals, and trace elements on physical performance during exercise. *Clin Ther* 1991;13(3):373-382.

1672 George J, Pridmore S, Aldous D. Double blind controlled trial of deanol in tardive dyskinesia. *Aust N Z J Psychiatry* 1981;15(1):68-71.

1673 Penovich P, Morgan JP, Kerzner B, et al. Double-blind evaluation of deanol in tardive dyskinesia. *JAMA* 1978;239(19):1997-1998.

1674 de Montigny C, Chouinard G, Annable L. Ineffectiveness of deanol in tardive dyskinesia: a placebo controlled study. *Psychopharmacology* (Berl) 1979;65(3):219-223.

1675 Lindeboom SF, Lakke JP. Deanol and physostigmine in the treatment of L-dopa-induced dyskinesias. *Acta Neurol Scand* 1978;58(2):134-138.

1676 Jus A, Villeneuve A, Gautier J, et al. Deanol, lithium and placebo in the treatment of tardive dyskinesia. A double-blind crossover study. *Neuropsychobiology* 1978;4(3):140-149.

1677 Oettinger L Jr. Pediatric psychopharmacology. A review with special reference to deanol. *Dis Nerv Syst* 1977;38(12 Pt 2):25-31.

1678 Lewis JA, Lewis BS. Deanol in minimal brain dysfunction. *Dis Nerv Syst* 1977;38(12 Pt 2):21-24.

1679 Lewis JA, Young R. Deanol and methylphenidate in minimal brain dysfunction. *Clin Pharmacol Ther* 1975;17(5):534-540.

1680 Fisman M, Mersky H, Helmes. Double-blind trial of 2-dimethylaminoethanol in Alzheimer's disease. *Am J Psychiatry* 1981;138(7):970-972.

1681 Ferris SH, Sathananthan G, Gershon S, et al. Senile dementia: treatment with deanol. *J Am Geriatr Soc* 1977;25(6):241-244.

1682 Cherkin A, Exkardt MJ. Effects of dimethylaminoethanol upon life-span and behavior of aged Japanese quail. *J Gerontol* 1977;32(1):38-45.

1683 Stenback F, Weisburger JH, Williams GM. Effect of lifetime administration of dimethylaminoethanol on longevity, aging changes, and cryptogenic neoplasms in C3H mice. *Mech Ageing Dev* 1988;42(2):129-138.

1684 Haug BA, Holzgraefe M. Orofacial and respiratory tardive dyskinesia: potential side effects of 2-dimethylaminoethanol (deanol)? *Eur Neurol* 1991;31(6):423-425.

1685 Casey DE. Mood alterations during deanol therapy. *Psychopharmacology* (Berl) 1979;62(2):187-191.

1686 Sergio W. Use of DMAE (2-dimethylaminoethanol) in the induction of lucid dreams. *Med Hypotheses* 1988;26(4):255-257.

1687 Consumer Guide to Melatonin. MotherNature.com website, URL: www.mothernature.com/cg/melatonin.asp (Accessed 29 November 1999).

1688 Lissoni P, Barni S, Cattaneo G, et al. Clinical results with the pineal hormone melatonin in advanced cancer resistant to standard antitumor therapies. *Oncology* 1991;48(6):448-450.

1689 Claustrat B, Brun J, Geoffriau M, et al. Nocturnal plasma melatonin profile and melatonin kinetics during infusion in status migrainosus. *Cephalalgia* 1997;17(4):511-517; discussion 487.

1690 Mallo C, Zaidan R, Galy G, et al. Pharmacokinetics of melatonin in man after intravenous infusion and bolus injection. *Eur J Clin Pharmacol* 1990;38(3):297-301.

1691 List of Orphan Designations and Approvals. FDA Office of Orphan Product Development website, URL: www.fda.gov/orphan/designat/list.htm (Accessed 29 November 1999).

1692 Lissoni P, Tisi E, Barni S, et al. Biological and clinical results of a neuroimmunotherapy with interleukin-2 and the pineal hormone melatonin as a first line treatment in advanced non-small cell lung cancer. *Br J Cancer* 1992;66(1):155-158.

1693 Lissoni P, Barni S, Ardizzoia A, et al. A randomized study with the pineal hormone melatonin versus supportive care alone in patients with brain metastases due to solid neoplasms. *Cancer* 1994;73(3):699-701.

1694 Lissoni P, Tancini G, Paolorossi F, et al. Chemoneuroendocrine therapy of metastatic breast *Cancer* with persistent thrombocytopenia with weekly low-dose epirubicin plus melatonin: a phase II study. *J Pineal Res* 1999;26(3):169-173.

1695 Lissoni P, Tancini G, Barni S, et al. The pineal hormone melatonin in hematology and its potential efficacy in the treatment of thrombocytopenia. *Recenti Prog Med* 1996;87(12):582-585.

1696 Lissoni P, Barni S, Brivio F, et al. A biological study on the efficacy of low-dose subcutaneous interleukin-2 plus melatonin in the treatment of cancer-related thrombocytopenia. *Oncology* 1995;52(5):360-362.

1697 Bregani ER, Lissoni P, Rossini F, et al. Prevention of interleukin-2-induced thrombocytopenia during the immunotherapy of cancer by a concomitant administration of the pineal hormone melatonin. *Recenti Prog Med* 1995;86(6):231-233.

1698 Perna AF, Castaldo P, Ingrosso D, et al. Homocysteine, a new cardiovascular risk factor, is also a powerful uremic toxin. *J Nephrol* 1999;12(4):230-240.

1699 Fauteck J, Schmidt H, Lerchl A, et al. Melatonin in epilepsy: first results of replacement therapy and first clinical results. *Biol Signals Recept* 1999;8(1-2):105-110.

1700 Brendler T. "Herbal Remedies;" Disk. First Edition; Berlin; 1996.

1701 Wallach J. Interpretation of Diagnostic Tests. A synopsis of Laboratory Medicine, Fifth ed; Boston, MA: Little Brown, 1992.

1704 Toubro S, Astrup A. "Randomised comparison of diets for maintaining obese subjects' weight after major weight loss: ad lib, low fat, high carbohydrate diet v fixed energy intake." *BMJ*, 1997; 314(7073):2934.

1705 Heymsfield SB, Allison DB, Vasselli JR, et al. "Garcinia cambogia (Hydroxycitric acid) as a potential antiobesity agent: a randomized controlled trial." *JAMA*, 1998; 280(18):1596-1600.

1706 Ammon HP, Safayhi H, Mack T, Sabieraj J. Mechanism of antiinflammatory actions of curcumine and boswellic acids. *Journal of Ethnopharmacol*ogy 1993;38(23):1139.

1707 De Smet PAGM, Keller K, Hansel R, Chandler RF. Adverse Effects of Herbal Drugs Vol. 3, Springer-Verlag,

Berlin, 1997.

1708 Gupta I, Gupta V, Parihar A, et al. Effects of Boswellia serrata gum resin in patients with bronchial asthma: results of a double-blind, placebo-controlled, 6-week clinical study. *Eur J Med Res* 1998;3(11):511-4.

1709 Gupta I, Parihar A, Malhotra P, et al. Effects of Boswellia serrata gum resin in patients with ulcerative colitis. *Eur J Med Res* 1997;2(1):37-43.

1710 Smith WM. "Treatment of mild hypertension: results of a ten-year intervention trial." *Circulation Research*, 1977; 40(5 Suppl 1):I98-105.

1711 "Low doses v standard dose of reserpine. A randomized, doubleblind, multiclinic trial in patients taking chlorthalidone." *JAMA*, 1982; 248(19):2471-7.

1712 Mato JM, Camara J, Fernandez de Paz J, et al. S-adenosylmethionine in alcoholic liver cirrhosis: a randomized, placebo-controlled, double-blind, multicenter clinical trial. *J Hepatol* 1999;30(6):1081-1089.

1713 Loehrer FM, Schwab R, Angst CP, et al. Influence of oral S-adenosylmethionine on plasma 5-methyltetrahydrofolate, S-adenosylhomocysteine, homocysteine and methionine in healthy humans. *J Pharcol Exp Ther* 1997;22(2):845-850.

1714 Loehrer FM, Angst CP, Haefeli WE, et al. Low whole-blood S-adenosylmethionine and correlation between 5-methyltetrahydrofolate and homocysteine in coronary artery disease. *Arterioscler Thromb Vasc Biol* 1996;16(6):727-733.

1715 Louis E. Tremor disorders: identification and treatment. Medical Update for Psychiatrists 1997;2:172-176.

1716 Leeb BF, Witzmann G, Ogris E, et al. Folic acid cyanocobalamin levels in serum and erythrocytes during low-dose methotrexate therapy n rheumatoid arthritis and psoriatic arthritis patients. *Clin Exp Rheumatol* 1995;13:459-463.

1717 Morgan SL, Baggott JE, Lee JY, et al. Folic acid supplementation prevents deficient blood folate levels and hyperhomocysteinemia during long-term, low dose methotrexate therapy for rheumatoid arthritis: Implications for cardiovascular disease prevention. *J Rheumatol* 1999;25:441-446.

1718 Dijkmans BA. Folate supplementation and methotrexate. *Br J Rheumatol* 1995;34:1172-1174.

1719 American College of Rheumatology ad hoc committee on clinicial guidelines. Guidelines for monitoring drug therapy in rheumatoid arthritis. *Arthritis & Rheumatism* 1996;39:723-731.

1720 Spitzer RL, Terman M, Williams JB, et al. Jet lag: clinical features, validation of a new syndrome-specific scale, and lack of response to melatonin in a randomized, double-blind trial. *Am J Psychiatry* 1999;156(9):1392-1396.

1721 Jorgensen KM, Witting MD. Does exogenous melatonin improve day sleep or night alertness in emergency physicians working night shifts? *Ann Emerg Med* 1998;31(6):699-704.

1722 Sanders DC, Chaturvedi AK, Hordinsky JR. Melatonin: aeromedical, toxicopharmacological, and analytical aspects. *J Anal Toxicol* 1999;23(3):159-167.

1723 Ghielmini M, Pagani O, de Jong J, et al. Double-blind randomized study on the myeloprotective effect of melatonin in combination with carboplatin and etoposide in advanced lung cancer. *Br J Cancer* 1999;80(7):1058-1061.

1724 Arangino S, Cagnacci A, Angiolucci M, et al. Effects of

melatonin on vascular reactivity, catecholamine levels, and blood pressure in healthy men. *Am J Cardiol* 1999;83(9):1417-1419.

1725 Zhi J, Jelia AT, Koss-Twardy SG, et al. The effect of orlistat, an inhibitor of dietary fat absorption, on the pharmacokinetics of beta-carotene in healthy volunteers. *J Clin Pharmacol* 1996;36:152-159.

1726 James WP, Avenell A, Broom J, et al. A one-year trial to assess the value of orlistat in the management of obesity. *Int J Obes Relat Metab Disord* 1997;21:S24-S30.

1727 Melia AT, Loss-Twardy SG, Zhi J. The effect of orlistat, an inhibitor of dietary fat absorption, on the absorption of vitamins A and E in healthy volunteers. *J Clin Pharmacol* 1996;36:647-653.

1728 Brusco LI, Marquez M, Cardinali DP. Monozygotic twins with Alzheimer's disease treated with melatonin: Case report. *J Pineal Res* 1998;25(4):260-263.

1729 Brusco LI, Fainstein I, Marquez M, et al. Effect of melatonin in selected populations of sleep-disturbed patients. *Biol Signals Recept* 1999;8(1-2):126-131.

1730 Roche, Inc. *Xenical* package insert. Nutley, NJ:1999 May.

1731 Chen RM, Wu JJ, Lee SC, et al. Increase of intestinal Bifidobacterium and suppression of coliform bacteria with short-term yogurt ingestion. *J Dairy Sci* 1999:82:2308-2314.

1733 Garg R, Malinow M, Pettinger M. Niacin treatment increases plasma homocyst(e)ine levels. *Am Heart J* 1999;138:1082-1087.

1734 Evaluation of an unconventional cancer treatment (the Di Bella multitherapy): results of phase II trials in Italy. Italian Study Group for the Di Bella Multitherapy Trials. *BMJ* 1999;318(7178):224-248.

1735 Dawson D, Rogers NL, van den Heuvel CJ, et al. Effect of sustained nocturnal transbuccal melatonin administration on sleep and temperature in elderly insomniacs. *Rhythms* 1998;13(6):532-538.

1736 Anon. Yogurt cuts down diarrhea. *HealthNews*, November 1999.

1737 Weaver DR. Reproductive safety of melatonin: a "wonder drug" to wonder about. *J Biol Rhythms* 1997;12(6):682-689.

1738 Haimov I, Lavie P, Laudon M, et al. Melatonin replacement therapy of elderly insomniacs. *Sleep* 1995;18(7):598-603.

1739 Luboshitzky R, Wagner O, Lavi S, et al. Abnormal melatonin secretion in hypogonadal men: the effect of testosterone treatment. *Clin Endocrinol* (Oxf) 1997;47(4):463-469.

1740 Pierce A. The American Pharmaceutical Association Practical Guide to Natural Medicines. New York: The Stonesong Press, 1999:19.

1741 Nordlund JJ, Lerner AB. The effects of oral melatonin on skin color and on the release of pituitary hormones. *J Clin Endocrinol Metab* 1977;45(4):768-774.

1742 Cavallo A, Ritschel WA. Pharmacokinetics of melatonin in human sexual maturation. *J Clin Endocrinol Metab* 1996;81(5):1882-1886.

1743 Commentz JC, Uhlig H, Henke A, et al. Melatonin and 6-hydroxymelatonin sulfate excretion is inversely correlated with gonadal development in children. *Horm Res* 1997;47(3):97-101.

1744 Palm L, Blennow G, Wetterberg L. Long-term melatonin treatment in blind children and young adults with circadian sleep-wake disturbances. *Dev Med Child Neurol* 1997;39(5):319-325.

1745   Lancioni GE, O'Reilly MF, Basili G. Review of strategies for treating sleep problems in persons with severe or profound mental retardation or multiple handicaps. *Am J Ment Retard* 1999;104(2):170-186.

1746   Jan JE, O'Donnell ME. Use of melatonin in the treatment of paediatric sleep disorders. *J Pineal Res* 1996;21(4):193-199.

1747   O'Callaghan FJ, Clarke AA, Hancock E, et al. Use of melatonin to treat sleep disorders in tuberous sclerosis. *Dev Med Child Neurol* 1999;41(2):123-126.

1748   Miyamoto A, Oki J, Takahashi S, et al. Serum melatonin kinetics and long-term melatonin treatment for sleep disorders in Rett syndrome. *Brain Dev* 1999;21(1):59-62.

1749   Skene DJ, Lockley SW, Arendt J. Melatonin in circadian sleep disorders in the blind. *Biol Signals Recept* 1999;8(1-2):90-95.

1750   MacFarlane JG, Cleghorn JM, Brown GM, et al. The effects of exogenous melatonin on the total sleep time and daytime alertness of chronic insomniacs: a preliminary study. *Biol Psychiatry* 1991;30(4):371-376.

1751   Dagan Y, Zisapel N, Nof D, et al. Rapid reversal of tolerance to benzodiazepine hypnotics by treatment with oral melatonin: a case report. *Neuropsychopharmacol* 1997;7(2):157-160.

1752   Saavedra JM. Probiotics plus antibiotics: Regulating our bacterial environment. *J Pediatr* 1999;135:535-537.

1753   Waldhauser F, Saletu B, Trinchard-Lugan I. Sleep laboratory investigations on hypnotic properties of melatonin. *Psychopharmacology* (Berl) 1990;100(2):222-226.

1754   Garfinkel D, Laudon M, Nof D, et al. Improvement of sleep quality in elderly people by controlled-release melatonin. *Lancet* 1995;346(8974):541-544.

1755   James SP, Sack DA, Rosenthal NE, et al. Melatonin administration in insomnia. *Neuropsychopharmacology* 1990;3(1):19-23.

1756   Dollins AB, Zhdanova IV, Wurtman RJ, et al. Effect of inducing nocturnal serum melatonin concentrations in daytime on sleep, mood, body temperature, and performance. *Proc Natl Acad Sci USA* 1994;91(5):1824-1828.

1757   Zhdanova IV, Wurtman RJ, Lynch HJ, et al. Sleep-inducing effects of low doses of melatonin ingested in the evening. *Clin Pharmacol Ther* 1995;57(5):552-558.

1758   Nave R, Peled R, Lavie P. Melatonin improves evening napping. *Eur J Pharmacol* 1995;275(2):213-216.

1759   Zhdanova IV, Wurtman RJ, Morabito C, et al. Effects of low oral doses of melatonin, given 2-4 hours before habitual bedtime, on sleep in normal young humans. *Sleep* 1996;19(5):423-431.

1760   Attenburrow ME, Cowen PJ, Sharpley AL. Low dose melatonin improves sleep in healthy middle-aged subjects. *Psychopharmacology* (Berl) 1996;126(2):179-181.

1761   Dahlitz M, Alvarez B, Vignau J, et al. Delayed sleep phase syndrome response to melatonin. *Lancet* 1991;337(8750):1121-1124.

1762   Oldani A, Ferini-Strambi L, Zucconi M, et al. Melatonin and delayed sleep phase syndrome: ambulatory polygraphic evaluation. Neuroreport 1994;6(1):132-134.

1763   Wurtman RJ, Zhdanova I. Improvement of sleep quality by melatonin. *Lancet* 1995;346(8988):1491.

1764   Carman JS, Post RM, Buswell R, et al. Negative effects of melatonin on depression. *Am J Psychiatry* 1976;33(10):1181-1186.

1765   Dolberg OT, Hirschmann S, Grunhaus L. Melatonin for the treatment of sleep disturbances in major depressive disorder. *Am J Psychiatry* 1998;155(8):1119-11121.

1766   Leibenluft E, Feldman-Naim S, Turner EH, et al. Effects of exogenous melatonin administration and withdrawal in five patients with rapid-cycling bipolar disorder. *J Clin Psychiatry* 1997;58(9):383-388.

1767   Gismondo MR, Drago L, Lombardi A. Review of probiotics available to modify gastrointestinal flora. *Int J Antimicrob Agents* 1999;12:287-292.

1768   Bangha E, Elsner P, Kistler GS. Suppression of UV-induced erythema by topical treatment with melatonin (N-acetyl-5-methoxytryptamine). Influence of the application time point. *Dermatology* 1997;195(3):248-252.

1769   Fischer T, Bangha E, Elsner P, et al. Suppression of UV-induced erythema by topical treatment with melatonin. Influence of the application time point. *Biol Signals Recept* 1999;8(1-2):132-135.

1770   Naguib M, Samarkandi AH. Premedication with melatonin: a double-blind, placebo-controlled comparison with midazolam. *Br J Anaesth* 1999;82(6):875-880.

1771   Jan JE, Freeman RD, Fast DK. Melatonin treatment of sleep-wake cycle disorders in children and adolescents. *Dev Med Child Neurol* 1999;41(7):491-500.

1772   Avery D, Lenz M, Landis C. Guidelines for prescribing melatonin. *Ann Med* 1998;30(1):122-130.

1773   Brzezinski A. Melatonin in humans. *N Engl J Med* 1997; 336(3):186-195.

1774   Arendt J. Melatonin. *BMJ* 1996;312(7041):1242-1243.

1775   Nathan PJ, Burrows GD, Norman TR. The effect of age and pre-light melatonin concentration on the melatonin sensitivity to dim light. *Int Clin Psychopharmacol* 1999;14(3):189-192.

1776   Fraschini F, Cesarani A, Alpini D, et al. Melatonin influences human balance. *Biol Signals Recept* 1999;8(1-2):111-119.

1777   Meeking DR, Wallace JD, Cuneo RC, et al. Exercise-induced GH secretion is enhanced by the oral ingestion of melatonin in healthy adult male subjects. *Eur J Endocrinol* 1999;141(1):22-26.

1778   Ebadi M, Govitrapong P, Phansuwan-Pujito P, et al. Pineal opioid receptors and analgesic action of melatonin. *J Pineal Res* 1998;24(4):193-200.

1779   Forsling ML, Wheeler MJ, Williams AJ. The effect of melatonin administration on pituitary hormone secretion in man. *Clin Endocrinol* (Oxf) 1999;51(5):637-642.

1780   Stoschitzky K, Sakotnik A, Lercher P, et al. Influence of beta-blockers on melatonin release. *Eur J Clin Pharmacol* 1999;55(2):111-115.

1781   Zeitzer JM, Daniels JE, Duffy JF, et al. Do plasma melatonin concentrations decline with age? *Am J Med* 1999;107(5):432-436.

1782   Smartbasic.com. "Glossary" website: www.smartbasic.com/glos.drugs/vinpocetine.glos.html (Accessed 16 December 1999).

1783   Life-enhancement.com. "VincaClear" website. www.life-enhancement.com/vinca.html (Accessed 16 December 1999).

1784   Thal LJ, Salmon DP, Lasker B, et al. The safety and lack of efficacy of vinpocetine in Alzheimer's disease. *J Am Geriatr Soc* 1989;37(6):515-520.

1785   Bereczki D, Fekete I. A systematic review of vinpocetine therapy in acute ischaemic stroke. *Eur J Clin Pharmacol* 1999;55(5):349-352.

REFERENCES

R E F E R E N C E S

1786 Szakall S, Boros I, Balkay L, et al. Cerebral effects of a single dose of intravenous vinpocetine in chronic stroke patients: a PET study. *J Neuroimaging* 1998;8(4):197-204.

1787 Hindmarch I, Fuchs HH, Erzigkeit H. Efficacy and tolerance of vinpocetine in ambulant patients suffering from mild to moderate organic psychosyndromes. *Int Clin Psychopharmacol* 1991;6(1):31-43.

1788 Ueyoshi A, Ota K. Clinical appraisal of vinpocetine for the removal of intractable tumoral calcinosis in haemodialysis patients with renal failure. *J Int Med Res* 1992;20(5):435-443.

1789 Balestreri R, Fontana L, Astengo F. A double-blind placebo controlled evaluation of the safety and efficacy of vinpocetine in the treatment of patients with chronic vascular senile cerebral dysfunction. *J Am Geriatr Soc* 1987;35(5):425-430.

1790 Hayakawa M. Effect of vinpocetine on red blood cell deformability in stroke patients. *Arzneimittelforschung* 1992;42(4):425-427.

1791 Hayakawa M. Comparative efficacy of vinpocetine, pentoxifylline and nicergoline on red blood cell deformability. *Arzneimittelforschung* 1992;42(2):108-110.

1792 Kiss E. Adjuvant effect of cavinton in the treatment of climacteric symptoms. *Ther Hung* 1990;38(4):170-173.

1793 Miyazaki M. The effect of a cerebral vasodilator, vinpocetine, on cerebral vascular resistance evaluated by the Doppler ultrasonic technique in patients with cerebrovascular diseases. *Angiology* 1995;46(1):53-58.

1794 Dutov AA, Gal'tvanitsa GA, Volkova VA, et al. [Cavinton in the prevention of the convulsive syndrome in children after birth injury]. [Article in Russian] *Zh Nevropatol Psikhiatr Im S S Korsakova* 1991;91(8):21-22.

1795 Dutov AA, Tolpyshev BA, Petrov AP, et al. [Use of cavinton in epilepsy]. [Article in Russian] *Zh Nevropatol Psikhiatr Im S S Korsakova* 1986;86(6):850-855.

1796 Bhatti JZ, Hindmarch I. Vinpocetine effects on cognitive impairments produced by flunitrazepam. *Int Clin Psychopharmacol* 1987;2(4):325-331.

1797 Subhan Z, Hindmarch I. Psychopharmacological effects of vinpocetine in normal healthy volunteers. *Eur J Clin Pharmacol* 1985;28(5):567-571.

1798 Bodo D, Kotovskaia AR, Galle RR, et al. [Effectiveness of the preparation Gavinton in preventing motion sickness]. [Article in Russian] *Kosm Biol Aviakosm Med* 1982;16(3):49-51.

1799 The Natural Pharmacist. "Vinpocetine" website: www.tnp.com/substance.asp?ID=573. (Accessed 16 December 1999).

1800 Nicholson CD. Pharmacology of nootropics and metabolically active compounds in relation to their use in dementia. *Psychopharmacology* (Berl) 1990;101(2):147-159.

1801 Akopov SE, Gabrielian ES. Effects of aspirin, dipyridamole, nifedipine and cavinton which act on platelet aggregation induced by different aggregating agents alone and in combination. *Eur J Clin Pharmacol* 1992;42(3):257-259.

1802 Lohmann A, Dingler E, Sommer W, et al. Bioavailability of vinpocetine and interference of the time of application with food intake. *Arzneimittelforschung* 1992;42(7):914-917.

1803 McGrath JJ, Soares KVS. Cholinergic medication for neuroleptic-induced tardive dyskinesia (Cochrane Review). In: The Cochrane Library, Issue 4, 1999. Oxford: Update Software. www.imbi.uni-freiburg.de/mirrors/som.flinders.edu.au/FUSA/COCHRANE/cochrane/revabstr/ab000207.htm. (Accessed 4 January 2000).

1804 Soares KV, McGrath JJ. The treatment of tardive dyskinesia—a systematic review and meta-analysis. *Schizophr Res* 1999;39:1-16; discussion 17-18.

1805 Life Enhancement. DMAE: the Mood-Elevating Smart Nutrient website, URL: www.life-enhancement.com/n37/n37dmae.html (Accessed 4 January 2000).

1816 Allen LV. Nutritional Products. In: Covington TR, Ed. *Handbook of Nonprescription Drugs.* Washington, DC: American Pharmaceutical Association;1996:361-392.

1817 Valimaki MJ, Kinnunen K, Volin L, et al. A prospective study of bone loss and turnover after allogeneic bone marrow transplantation: effect of calcium supplementation with or without calcitonin. *Bone Marrow Transplant* 1999;23:355-361.

1818 Allender PS, Cutler JA, Follmann D, et al. Dietary calcium and blood pressure: a meta-analysis of randomized clinical trials. *Ann Intern Med* 1996;124:825-831.

1819 Bucher HC, Cook RJ, Guyatt GH, et al. Effects of dietary calcium supplementation on blood pressure. A meta-analysis of randomized controlled trials. *JAMA* 1996; 275:1016-1022.

1820 Kawano Y, Yoshimi H, Matsuoka H, et al. Calcium supplementation in patients with essential hypertension: assessment by office, home and ambulatory blood pressure. *J Hypertens* 1998;16:1693-1699.

1821 Griffith LE, Guyatt GH, Cook RJ, et al. The influence of dietary and nondietary calcium supplementation on blood pressure: an updated meta-analysis of randomized controlled trials. *Am J Hypertens* 1999;12:84-92.

1822 Thys-Jacobs S, Starkey P, Bernstein D, Tian J. Calcium carbonate and the premenstrual syndrome: effects on premenstrual and menstrual symptoms. Premenstrual Syndrome Study Group. *Am J Obstet Gynecol*, 1998;179:444-452.

1823 Alvir JM, Thys-Jacobs S. Premenstrual and menstrual symptom clusters and response to calcium treatment. *Psychopharmacol Bull*, 1991;27:145-148.

1824 Thys-Jacobs S, Ceccarelli S, Bierman A, et al. Calcium supplementation in premenstrual syndrome: a randomized crossover trial. *J Gen Intern Med* 1989;4:183-189.

1825 Steinbach G, Lupton J, Reddy BS, et al. Calcium carbonate treatment of diarrhoea in intestinal bypass patients. *Eur J Gastroenterol Hepatol* 1996;8:559-562.

1826 Steinbach G, Lupton J, Reddy BS, et al. Effect of calcium supplementation on rectal epithelial hyperproliferation in intestinal bypass subjects. *Gastroenterology* 1994;106:1162-1167.

1827 Barsotti G, Cupisti A, Morelli E, et al. Secondary hyperparathyroidism in severe chronic renal failure is corrected by very-low dietary phosphate intake and calcium carbonate supplementation. *Nephron* 1998;79:137-141.

1828 Tsukamoto Y, Moriya R, Nagaba Y, et al. Effect of administering calcium carbonate to treat secondary hyperparathyroidism in nondialyzed patients with chronic renal failure. *Am J Kidney Dis* 1995;25:879-886.

1829 Rudnicki M, Hojsted J, Petersen LJ, et al. Oral calcium effectively reduces parathyroid hormone levels in hemodialysis patients: a randomized double-blind placebo-controlled study. *Nephron* 1993;65:369-374.

1830 Adachi JD, Ioannidis G. Calcium and vitamin D therapy in corticosteroid-induced bone loss: what is the evidence? *Calcif Tissue Int* 1999;65:332-336.

1831 Adachi JD, Bensen WG, Bianchi F, et al. Vitamin D and calcium in the prevention of corticosteroid induced osteoporosis: a 3 year followup. *J Rheumatol* 1996;23:995-1000.

1832 Recommendations for the prevention and treatment of glucocorticoid-induced osteoporosis. American College of Rheumatology Task Force on Osteoporosis Guidelines. *Arthritis Rheum* 1996;39:1791-801.

1833 Crowther CA, Hiller JE, Pridmore B, et al. Calcium supplementation in nulliparous women for the prevention of pregnancy-induced hypertension, preeclampsia and preterm birth: an Australian randomized trial. FRACOG and the ACT Study Group. *Aust N Z J Obstet Gynaecol*, 1999;39:12-18.

1834 Power ML, Heaney RP, Kalkwarf HJ, et al. The role of calcium in health and disease. *Am J Obstet Gynecol* 1999;181:1560-1569.

1835 Dawson-Hughes B, Harris SS, Krall EA, Dallal GE. Effect of calcium and vitamin D supplementation on bone density in men and women 65 years of age or older. *N Engl J Med* 1997;337:670-676.

1836 Chapuy MC, Arlot ME, Duboeuf F, et al. Vitamin D3 and calcium to prevent hip fractures in the elderly women. *N Engl J Med* 1992;327(23):1637-1642.

1837 Celotti F, Bignamini A. Dietary calcium and mineral/ vitamin supplementation: a controversial problem. *J Int Med Res* 1999;27:1-14.

1838 Heller HJ, Stewart A, Haynes S, Pak CY. Pharmacokinetics of calcium absorption from two commercial calcium supplements. *J Clin Pharmacol* 1999;39:1151-1154.

1839 Fujita T, Ohue T, Fujii Y, et al. Heated oyster shell-seaweed calcium (AAA Ca) on osteoporosis. *Calcif Tissue Int* 1996;58:226-230.

1840 Fujita T, Ohue T, Fujii Y, et al. Effect of calcium supplementation on bone density and parathyroid function in elderly subjects. *Miner Electrolyte Metab* 1995;21:229-231.

1841 Talbot JR, Guardo P, Seccia S, etal. Calcium bioavailability and parathyroid hormone acute changes after oral intake of dairy and nondairy products in healthy volunteers. *Osteoporos Int* 1999;10:137-142.

1842 Heaney RP, Dowell MS, Barger-Lux MJ. Absorption of calcium as the carbonate and citrate salts, with some observations on method. *Osteoporos Int* 1999;9:19-23.

1843 Maton PN, Burton ME. Antacids revisited: a review of their clinical pharmacology and recommended therapeutic use. *Drugs* 1999;57:855-870.

1844 Clemens JD, Feinstein AR. Calcium carbonate and constipation: a historical review of medical mythopoeia. *Gastroenterology* 1977;72:957-961.

1845 Saunders D, Sillery J, Chapman R. Effect of calcium carbonate and aluminum hydroxide on human intestinal function. *Dig Dis Sci* 1988;33:409-413.

1846 Krall EA, Dawson-Hughes B. Smoking increases bone loss and decreases intestinal calcium absorption. *J Bone Miner Res* 1999;14:215-220.

1847 Praet JP, Peretz A, Mets T, Rozenberg S. Comparative study of the intestinal absorption of three salts of calcium in young and elderly women. *J Endocrinol Invest* 1998;21:263-267.

1848 Minihane AM, Fairweather-Tait SJ. Effect of calcium supplementation on daily nonheme-iron absorption and long-term iron status. *Am J Clin Nutr* 1998;68:96-102.

1849 Sokoll LJ, Dawson-Hughes B. Calcium supplementation and plasma ferritin concentrations in premenopausal women. *Am J Clin Nutr* 1992;56:1045-1048.

1850 Kalkwarf HJ, Harrast SD. Effects of calcium supplementation and lactation on iron status. *Am J Clin Nutr* 1998;67:1244-1249.

1851 Sam's General Store. "IP-6 (Inositol Hexaphosphate)" website: www.samsstore.com/samsgeneralstore/ip6.html. (Accessed 11 January 2000).

1852 MotherNature.com. "IP-6: New Nutraceutical from Fiber Fights Cancer" website: www.mothernature.com/news/ 1998_09_10/research_update.stm. (Accessed 11 January 2000).

1853 University of Maryland. "Natural Sugar-Phosphate Compound Shows Promise as cancer Treatment" website: www.oea.umaryland.edu/Media/NewsSum/ NewsDetail/archive/1998_03/IP.htm. (Accessed 11 January 2000).

1854 Steinmetz KA, Potter JD. Vegetables, fruit, and *Cancer* prevention: a review. *J Am Diet Assoc* 1996;96:1027-1039.

1855 Graf E, Eaton JW. Antioxidant functions of phytic acid. *Free Radic Biol Med* 1990;8:61-69.

1857 Shamsuddin AM, Vucenik I, Cole KE. IP6: a novel anti-cancer agent. *Life Sci* 1997;61:343-354.

1858 Zhou JR, Erdman JW Jr. Phytic acid in health and disease. *Crit Rev Food Sci Nutr*, 1995;35:495-508.

1859 Shamsuddin AM. Metabolism and cellular functions of IP6: a review. *AntiBr J Nutr* 1999;19:3733-3736.

1860 Shamsuddin AM, Vucenik I. Mammary tumor inhibition by IP6: a review. *AntiBr J Nutr* 1999;19:3671-3674.

1861 Challa A, Rao DR, Reddy BS. Interactive suppression of aberrant crypt foci induced by azoxymethane in rat colon by phytic acid and green tea. *Carcinogenesis* 1997;18:2023-2026.

1862 Saied IT, Shamsuddin AM. Up-regulation of the tumor suppressor gene p53 and WAF1 gene expression by IP6 in HT-29 human colon carcinoma cell line. *AntiBr J Nutr* 1998;18:1479-1484.

1863 Thompson LU, Zhang L. Phytic acid and minerals: effect on early markers of risk for mammary and colon Carcinogenesis. *Carcinogenesis* 1991;12:2041-2045.

1864 Vucenik I, Zhang ZS, Shamsuddin AM. IP6 in treatment of liver cancer. II. Intra-tumoral injection of IP6 regresses pre-existing human liver cancer xenotransplanted in nude mice. *AntiBr J Nutr* 1998;18:4091-4096.

1865 Shamsuddin AM, Yang GY. Inositol hexaphosphate inhibits growth and induces differentiation of PC-3 human prostate cancer cells. *Carcinogenesis* 1995;16:1975-1979.

1866 Shamsuddin AM, Elsayed AM, Ullah A. Suppression of large intestinal cancer in F344 rats by inositol hexaphosphate. *Carcinogenesis* 1988;9:577-580.

1867 Vucenik I, Podczasy JJ, Shamsuddin AM. Antiplatelet activity of inositol hexaphosphate. *AntiBr J Nutr* 1999;19:3689-3693.

1868 Jariwalla RJ. Inositol hexaphosphate (IP6) as an anti-neoplastic and lipid-lowering agent. *AntiBr J Nutr* 1999;19:3699-3702.

1869 Sandberg AS, Brune M, Carlsson NG, et al. Inositol phosphates with different numbers of phosphate groups

REFERENCES

influence iron absorption in humans. *Am J Clin Nutr* 1999;70:240-246.

1870 Sandstrom B, Sandberg AS. Inhibitory effects of isolated inositol phosphates on zinc absorption in humans. *J Trace Elem Electrolytes Health Dis* 1992;6:99-103.

1871 Ide N, Lau BH. Garlic compounds protect vascular endothelial cells from oxidized low density lipoprotein-induced injury. *J Pharm Pharmacol* 1997;49:908-911.

1872 Wakunaga Products. "Wakunga Products" Webpage: www.kyolic.com/green.htm. (Accessed 17 January 2000).

1873 Steiner M, Khan AH, Holbert D, Lin RI. A double-blind crossover study in moderately hypercholesterolemic men that compared the effect of aged garlic extract and placebo administration on blood lipids. *Am J Clin Nutr* 1996;64:866-870.

1874 Steiner M, Lin RS. Changes in platelet function and susceptibility of lipoproteins to oxidation associated with administration of aged garlic extract. *J Cardiovasc Pharmacol* 1998;31:904-908.

1875 Lau BHS, Lam F, Wang-Cheng R. Effect of an odor-modified garlic preparation on blood lipids. *Nutrition Research* 1987;7:139-149.

1876 Munday JS, James KA, Fray LM, et al. Daily supplementation with aged garlic extract, but not raw garlic, protects low density lipoprotein against in vitro oxidation. *Atherosclerosis* 1999;143:399-404.

1877 Imai J, Ide N, Nagae S, et al. Antioxidant and radical scavenging effects of aged garlic extract and its constituents. *Planta Med* 1994;60:417-420.

1878 Moriguchi T, Saito H, Nishiyama N. Aged garlic extract prolongs longevity and improves spatial memory deficit in senescence-accelerated mouse. *Biol Pharm Bull* 1996;19:305-307.

1879 Efendy JL, Simmons DL, Campbell GR, Campbell JH. The effect of the aged garlic extract, 'Kyolic', on the development of experimental atherosclerosis. *Atherosclerosis* 199711;132:37-42.

1880 Ide N, Lau BH. Aged garlic extract attenuates intracellular oxidative stress. *PhytoMedicine* 1999;6:125-131.

1881 Sigounas G, Hooker J, Anagnostou A, Steiner M. S-allylmercaptocysteine inhibits cell proliferation and reduces the viability of erythroleukemia, breast, and prostate cancer cell lines. *Nutr Cancer* 1997;27:186-191.

1882 Zhang Y, Moriguchi T, Saito H, Nishiyama N. Functional relationship between age-related immunodeficiency and learning deterioration. *N Eur J Neurosci* 1998;10:3869-3875.

1883 Wang BH, Zuzel KA, Rahman K, Billington D. Treatment with aged garlic extract protects against bromobenzene toxicity to precision cut rat liver slices. *Toxicology* 1999;132:215-225.

1884 Gwilt PR, Lear CL, Tempero MA, et al. The effect of garlic extract on human metabolism of acetaminophen. *Cancer Epidemiol Biomarkers Prev* 1994;3:155-160.

1885 Horie T, Matsumoto H, Kasagi M, et al. Protective effect of aged garlic extract on the small intestinal damage of rats induced by methotrexate administration. *Planta Med* 1999;65:545-548.

1886 Nguyen TT, Dale LC, von Bergmann K, Croghan IT. Cholesterol-lowering effect of stanol ester in a US population of mildly hypercholesterolemic men and women: a randomized controlled trial. *Mayo Clin Proc* 1999;74:1198-1206.

1887 Plat J, Mensink RP. Vegetable oil based versus wood based stanol ester mixtures: effects on serum lipids and hemostatic factors in non-hypercholesterolemic subjects. *Atherosclerosis* 2000;148:101-112.

1888 Ostlund RE Jr, Spilburg CA, Stenson WF. Sitostanol administered in lecithin micelles potently reduces cholesterol absorption in humans. *Am J Clin Nutr* 1999;70:826-831.

1889 Mook-Jung I, Shin JE, Yun SH, et al. Protective effects of asiaticoside derivatives against beta-amyloid neurotoxicity. *J Neurosci Res* 1999;58:417-425.

1890 Maquart FX, Chastang F, Simeon A, et al. Triterpenes from Centella asiatica stimulate extracellular matrix accumulation in rat experimental wounds. *Eur J Dermatol* 1999;9:289-296.

1891 Refsum H, Ueland PM, Nygard O, Vollset SE. Homocysteine and cardiovascular disease. *Annu Rev Med* 1998;49:31-62.

1892 Malinow MR, Bostom AG, Krauss RM. Homocyst(e)ine, diet, and cardiovascular diseases: a statement for healthcare professionals from the Nutrition Committee, American Heart Association. *Circulation* 1999;99:178-182.

1893 Boushey CJ, Beresford SA, Omenn GS, Motulsky AG. A quantitative assessment of plasma homocysteine as a risk factor for vascular disease. Probable benefits of increasing folic acid intakes. *JAMA* 1995;274(13):1049-1057.

1894 Personal Communication: Edwin W. Grimsley, MD. Savanah, GA. January, 2000.

1895 Personal correspondence, 3M Pharmaceuticals, Drug Surveillance and Information; January, 2000.

1896 Investigator's Brochure: Ademetionine 1,4-butanedisulfonate. Knoll Pharmaceuticals.

1897 Stramentinoli G, Gualano M, Galli-Kienle M. Intestinal absorption of S-adenosyl-L-methionine. *J Pharmacol Exp Ther* 1979;209(3):323-6.

1898 Morrow LE, Grimsley EW. Long-term diuretic therapy in hypertensive patients: effects on serum homocysteine, vitamin B6, vitamin B12, and red blood cell folate concentrations. *South Med J* 1999;92(9):866-870.

1899 Christensen B, Landaas S, Stensvold I, et al. Whole blood folate, homocysteine in serum, and risk of first acute myocardial infarction. *Atherosclerosis* 1999;147(2):317-326.

1900 Lininger SW. The Natural Pharmacy. 1st ed. Rocklin, CA: Prima Publishing; 1998.

1901 Brewster MA, Schedewie H. "Trimethylaminuria." *Ann Clin Lab Sci*, Jan.-Feb. 1983; 13(1):20-4.

1902 *Meyler's Side Effects of Drugs*.

1903 Burnham T (ed). *Facts and Comparisons Drug Information* (loose leaf edition). St. Louis, MO : Facts and Comparisons; (updated monthly).

1930 Kelly GS. "L-carnitine: therapeutic applications of a conditionally-essential amino acid." *Altern Med Rev*, 1998;3(5):345-60.

1931 Krahenbuhl S. Carnitine metabolism in chronic liver disease. *Life Sci*, 1996;59(19):1579-99.

1932 Krahenbuhl S. "Carnitine metabolism in chronic liver disease." *Life Sci*, 1996; 59(19):1579-99.

1933 Brass E. "Pharmacokinetic considerations for the therapeutic use of carnitine in hemodialysis patients." *Clin Ther*, Mar.-Apr. 1995; 17(2):176-85; discussion 175.

1934 Lee NA, Reasner CA. "Beneficial effect of chromium

supplementation on serum triglyceride levels in NIDDM." *Diabetes Care*, 1994;17(12):1449-52.

1935 Fox GN, Sabovic Z. "Chromium picolinate supplementation for Diabetes mellitus." *J Fam Pract*, Jan. 1998; 46(1):83-6.

1936 Reading SA. "Chromium picolinate." *J Fla Med Assoc*, Jan. 1996; 83(1):29-31.

1937 Urberg M, Zemel MB. "Evidence for synergism between chromium and nicotinic acid in the control of glucose tolerance in elderly humans." *Metabolism*, Sep. 1987; 36(9):896-9.

1938 Mohamedshah FY, Moser-Veillon PB, Yamini S, Douglass LW, Anderson RA, Veillon C. "Distribution of a stable isotope of chromium (53Cr) in serum, urine, and breast milk in lactating women." *Am J Clin Nutr*, Jun. 1998; 67(6):1250-5.

1939 Grant KE, Chandler RM, Castle AL, Ivy JL. "Chromium and exercise training: effect on obese women." *Med Sci Sports Exerc*, Aug. 1997; 29(8):992-8.

1940 Felt O, Buri P, Gurny R. Chitosan: a unique polysaccharide for drug delivery. *Drug Dev Ind Pharm*, 1998;24(11)979-93.

1941 Illum L. Chitosan and its use as a pharmaceutical excipient. *Pharm Res*, 1998;15(9):1326-1331.

1942 Jing SB, Li L, Ji D, Takiguchi Y, Yamaguchi T. "Effect of chitosan on renal function in patients with chronic renal failure." *J Pharm Pharmacol*, 1997; 49(7):721-3.

1943 Rao SB, Sharma CP. Use of chitosan as a biomaterial: studies on its safety and hemostatic potential. *J Biomed Mater Res*, 1997;34(1):21-28.

1944 Biagini G, Bertani A, Muzzarelli R, et al. "Wound management with N-carboxybutyl chitosan." *Biomaterials*, 1991; 12(3):281-6.

1945 Muzzarelli R, Biagini G, Pugnaloni A, et al. "Reconstruction of parodontal tissue with chitosan." *Biomaterials*, 1989; 10(9):598-603.

1946 Tsoko M, Beauseigneur F, Gresti J, et al. Enhancement of activities relative to fatty acid oxidation in the liver of rats depleted of L-carnitine by D-carnitine and a gamma-butyrobetaine hydroxylase inhibitor. *Biochem Pharmacol*, 17 May 1995;49(10):1403-10.

1947 Colombani P, Wenk C, Kunz I, et al. Effects of L-carnitine supplementation on physical performance and energy metabolism of endurance-trained athletes: a double-blind crossover field study. *Eur J Appl Physiol*, 1996;73(5):434-439.

1948 Krahenbuhl S, Reichen J. Carnitine metabolism in patients with chronic liver disease. *Hepatology*, January 1997;25(1):148-153.

1949 Gauthier S, Bouchard R, Bacher Y, et al. Progress report on the Canadian Multicentre Trial of tetrahydroaminoacridine with lecithin in Alzheimer's disease. *Can J Neurol Sci*, November 1989;16(4 Suppl):543-546.

1950 Hahn CJ, Evans GW. "Absorption of trace metals in the zinc-deficient rat." *Am J Physiol*, 1975; 228(4):1020-3

1951 Wasser WG, Feldman NS, D'Agati VD. "Chronic renal failure after ingestion of over-the-counter chromium picolinate." [letter] *Ann Intern Med*, 1 Mar 1997; 126(5):410.

1952 Mertz W. "Interaction of chromium with insulin: a progress report." *Nutr Rev*, Jun. 1998; 56(6):174-7.

1953 Anderson RA. "Chromium, glucose intolerance and diabetes." *J Am Coll Nutr*, Dec. 1998; 17(6):548-55.

1954 Levin HS. "Treatment of postconcussional symptoms with CDP-choline." *J Neurol Sci*, Jul. 1991; 103

Suppl:S39-42.

1955 Gauthier S, Bouchard R, Lamontagne A. "Tetrahydroaminoacridine-lecithin combination treatment in patients with intermediate-stage Alzheimer's disease. Results of a Canadian double-blind, crossover, multicenter study." *N Engl J Med*, 3 May 1990; 322(18):1272-6.

1956 Chatellier G, Lacomblez L. "Tacrine (tetrahydroaminoacridine; THA) and lecithin in senile dementia of the Alzheimer type: a multicentre trial. Groupe Francais d'Etude de la Tetrahydroaminoacridine." *BMJ*, 24 Feb. 1990; 300(6723):495-9.

1957 Chan H, Abraham G, Oreopoulos DG. "Oral lecithin improves ultrafiltration in patients on peritoneal dialysis." *Perit Dial Int*, 1989; 9(3):203-5.

1958 Mohs RC, Davis KL. "Interaction of choline and scopolamine in human memory." *Life Sci*, 15 Jul. 1985; 37(2):193-7.

1959 Lozano FR. "Efficacy and safety of oral CDP-choline. Drug surveillance study in 2817 cases." *Arzneimittelforschung*, 1983; 33(7A):1073-80.

1960 Dinsdale JR, Griffiths GK, Castello J, Maddock J, Ortiz JA, Aylward M. "CDP-choline: repeated oral dose tolerance studies in adult healthy volunteers." *Arzneimittelforschung*, 1983 ;33(7A):1061-5.

1961 Niederau C, Strohmeyer G, Heintges T, Peter K, Gopfert E. "Polyunsaturated phosphatidyl-choline and interferon alpha for treatment of chronic hepatitis B and C: a multi-center, randomized, double-blind, placebo-controlled trial. Leich Study Group." *Hepatogastroenterology*, May-Jun. 1998; 45(21):797-804.

1962 Shronts EP. "Essential Nature of choline with implications for total parenteral nutrition." *J Am Diet Assoc*, Jun. 1997; 97(6):639-49.

1963 Secades JJ, Frontera G. "CDP-choline: pharmacological and clinical review." *Clin Pharmacol*, Oct. 1995; 17 Suppl B:2-54.

1964 Melancon SB, Vanasse M, Geoffroy G, et al. "Oral lecithin and linoleic acid in Friedreich's ataxia:" *Can J Neurol Sci*. May 1982; 9(2):155-64.

1965 McNamara JO, Carwile S, Hope V, Luther J, Miller P. "Effects of oral choline on human complex partial seizures." *Neurology*, Dec. 1980; 30(12):1334-6.

1966 Sehested P, Lund HI, Kristensen O. "Oral choline in cerebellar ataxia." *Acta Neurol Scand*, Aug. 1980; 62(2):124-6.

1967 Simons LA, Hickie JB, Ruys J. "Treatment of hypercholesterolaemia with oral lecithin." *Aust N Z J Med*, Jun. 1977; 7(3):262-6.

1968 Growdon JH, Cohen EL, Wurtman RJ. "Huntington's disease: clinical and chemical effects of choline administration." *Ann Neurol*, May. 1977; 1(5):418-22.

1969 Toouli J, Jablonski P, Watts JM. "Gallstone dissolution in man using cholic acid and lecithin." *Lancet* , 6 Dec. 1975; 2(7945):1124-6.

1970 Uebelhart D, Thonar EJ, Delmas PD, Chantraine A, Vignon E. "Effects of oral chondroitin sulfate on the progression of knee osteoarthritis: a pilot study." *Osteoarthritis Cartilage*, May. 1998; 6 Suppl A:39-46.

1971 Bourgeois P, Chales G, Dehais J, Delcambre B, Kuntz JL, Rozenberg S. "Efficacy and tolerability of chondroitin sulfate 1200 mg/day vs chondroitin sulfate 3 x 400 mg/day vs placebo." *Osteoarthritis Cartilage*, May 1998; 6 Suppl A:25-30.

1972 Bucsi L, Poor G. "Efficacy and tolerability of oral

© Copyright 2000, Natural Medicines Comprehensive Database (209) 472-2244. For updated data, go to www.NaturalDatabase.com. • 1197

REFERENCES

R
E
F
E
R
E
N
C
E
S

chondroitin sulfate as a symptomatic slow-acting drug for osteoarthritis (SYSADOA) in the treatment of knee osteoarthritis." *Osteoarthritis Cartilage*, May 1998; 6 Suppl A:31-6.

1973 Kelly GS. "The role of glucosamine sulfate and chondroitin sulfates in the treatment of degenerative joint disease." *Altern Med Rev*, Feb. 1998; 3(1):27-39.

1974 Limberg MB, McCaa C, Kissling GE, Kaufman HE. "Topical application of hyaluronic acid and chondroitin sulfate in the treatment of dry eyes." *Am J Ophthalmol*, 15 Feb. 1987; 103(2):194-7.

1975 Fan YY, Chapkin RS. "Importance of dietary gamma-linolenic acid in human health and nutrition." *J Nutr*, Sep. 1998; 128(9):1411-4.

1976 Johnson MM, Swan DD, Surette ME. "Dietary supplementation with gamma-linolenic acid alters fatty acid content and eicosanoid production in healthy humans." *J Nutr*, Aug. 1997; 127(8):1435-44.

1977 Stainforth JM, Layton AM, Goodfield MJ. "Clinical aspects of the use of gamma linolenic acid in systemic sclerosis." *Acta Derm Venereol*, Mar. 1996; 76(2):144-6.

1978 McCaul JA, Lamey PJ. "Multiple oral mucoceles treated with gamma-linolenic acid: report of a case." *Br J Oral Maxillofac Surg*, Dec. 1994; 32(6):392-3.

1979 Guivernau M, Meza N, Barja P, Roman O. "Clinical and experimental study on the long-term effect of dietary gamma-linolenic acid on plasma lipids, platelet aggregation, thromboxane formation, and prostacyclin production." *Prostaglandins Leukot Essent Fatty Acids*, Nov. 1994; 51(5):311-6.

1980 Jamal GA. "The use of gamma linolenic acid in the prevention and treatment of diabetic neuropathy." *Diabet Med*, Mar. 1994; 11(2):145-9.

1981 Horrobin DF. "The use of gamma-linolenic acid in diabetic neuropathy." *Agents Actions Suppl*, 1992; 37:120-44.

1982 Cant A, Shay J, Horrobin DF. "The effect of maternal supplementation with linoleic and gamma- linolenic acids on the fat composition and content of human milk: a placebo-controlled trial." *J Nutr Sci Vitaminol* (Tokyo), Dec. 1991; 37(6):573-9.

1983 van der Merwe CF, Booyens J, Joubert HF, van der Merwe CA. "The effect of gamma-linolenic acid, an in vitro cytostatic substance contained in evening primrose oil, on primary liver cancer. A double- blind placebo controlled trial." *Prostaglandins Leukot Essent Fatty Acids*, Jul. 1990; 40(3):199-202.

1984 Jamal GA, Carmichael H. "The effect of gamma-linolenic acid on human diabetic peripheral neuropathy: a double-blind placebo-controlled trial." *Diabet Med*, May 1990; 7(4):319-23.

1985 Pullman-Mooar S, Laposata M, Lem D. "Alteration of the cellular fatty acid profile and the production of eicosanoids in human monocytes by gamma-linolenic acid." *Arthritis Rheum*, Oct. 1990; 33(10):1526-33.

1986 Carella F, Girotti F, Scigliano G, Caraceni T, Joder-Ohlenbusch AM, Schechter PJ. "Double-blind study of oral gamma-vinyl GABA in the treatment of dystonia." *Neurology*, Jan. 1986; 36(1):98-100.

1987 Lambert PA, Cantiniaux P, Chabannes JP, Tell GP, Schechter PJ, Koch-Weser J. [Therapeutic trial of gamma-vinyl GABA, an inhibitor of GABA transaminase, in tardive dyskinesias induced by neuroleptics.] "Essai therapeutique du gamma-vinyl GABA, un inhibiteur de la GABA- transaminase, dans les dyskinesies tardives induites par les neuroleptiques."

Encephale, 1982; 8(3):371-6.

1988 Cavagnini F, Invitti C, Pinto M. "Effect of acute and repeated administration of gamma aminobutyric acid (GABA) on growth hormone and prolactin secretion in man." *Acta Endocrinol* (Copenh), Feb. 1980; 93(2):149-54.

1989 Felt O, Buri P, Gurny R. "Chitosan: a unique polysaccharide for drug delivery." *Drug Dev Ind Pharm*, 1998; 24(11):979-93.

1990 Barrington WW, Angle CR, Willcockson NK, Padula MA, Korn T. "Autonomic function in manganese alloy workers." *Environ Res*, Jul. 1998; 78(1):50-8.

1991 Greger JL. "Dietary standards for manganese: overlap between nutritional and toxicological studies." *J Nutr*, Feb. 1998; 128(2 Suppl):368S-371S.

1992 Hauser RA, Zesiewicz TA, Martinez C, Rosemurgy AS, Olanow CW. "blood manganese correlates with brain magnetic resonance imaging changes in patients with *Liver* disease." *Can J Neurol Sci*, May 1996; 23(2):95-8.

1993 Okano T. "Effects of essential trace elements on bone turnover-in relation to the osteoporosis." *Nippon Rinsho*, Jan. 1996; 54(1):148-54.

1994 Strause L, Saltman P, Smith KT, Bracker M, Andon MB. "Spinal bone loss in postmenopausal women supplemented with calcium and trace minerals." *J Nutr*, Jul. 1994; 124(7):1060-4.

1995 Lean ME, Noroozi M, Kelly I. "Dietary flavonols protect diabetic human lymphocytes against oxidative damage to DNA." *Diabetes*, Jan. 1999; 48(1):176-81.

1996 Rachkauskas GS. "The efficacy of enterosorption and a combination of antioxidants in schizophrenics." *Lik Sprava*, Jun. 1998; (4):122-4.

1997 Kuo SM, Leavitt PS, Lin CP. "Dietary flavonoids interact with trace metals and affect metallothionein level in human intestinal cells." *Biol Trace Elem Res*, Jun. 1998; 62(3):135-53.

1998 Conquer JA, Maiani G, Azzini E, Raguzzini A, Holub BJ. "Supplementation with quercetin markedly increases plasma quercetin concentration without effect on selected risk factors for heart disease in healthy subjects." *J Nutr*, Mar. 1998; 128(3):593-7.

1999 Janssen K, Mensink RP, Cox FJ, et al. "Effects of the flavonoids quercetin and apigenin on hemostasis in healthy volunteers: results from an in vitro and a dietary supplement study." *Am J Clin Nutr*, Feb. 1998; 67(2):255-62.

2000 Freeland-Graves JH, Lin PH. "Plasma uptake of manganese as affected by oral loads of manganese, calcium, milk, phosphorus, copper, and zinc." *J Am Coll Nutr*, Feb. 1991; 10(1):38-43.

2001 Krieger D, Krieger S, Jansen O, Gass P, Theilmann L, Lichtnecker H. "Manganese and chronic hepatic encephalopathy." *Lancet* , 29 Jul. 1995; 346(8970):270-4.

2002 O'Dell BL. "Mineral interactions relevant to nutrient requirements." *J Nutr*, Dec. 1989; 119(12 Suppl):1832-8.

2003 Moghissi KS. "Risks and benefits of nutritional supplements during pregnancy." *Obstet Gynecol*, Nov. 1981; 58(5 Suppl):68S-78S.

2004 Penland JG, Johnson PE. "Dietary calcium and manganese effects on menstrual cycle symptoms." *Am J Obstet Gynecol*, May 1993; 168(5):1417-23.

2005 Freeland-Graves JH, Turnlund JR. "Deliberations and evaluations of the approaches, endpoints and paradigms for manganese and molybdenum dietary recommendations." *J Nutr*, Sep. 1996; 126(9

Suppl):2435S-2440S.

2006 Stavric B. "Quercetin in our diet: from potent mutagen to probable anticarcinogen." *Clin Biochem*, Aug. 1994; 27(4):245-8.

2007 Ferry DR, Smith A, Malkhandi J, et al. "Phase I clinical trial of the flavonoid quercetin: pharmacokinetics and evidence for in vivo tyrosine kinase inhibition." *Clin Cancer Res*, Apr. 1996; 2(4):659-68.

2008 Freeland-Graves JH. "Manganese: an essential nutrient for humans." *Nutr Today*, 1988; 23:13-9.

2009 Prudden JF, Balassa LL. "The biological activity of bovine cartilage preparations. Clinical demonstration of their potent anti-inflammatory capacity with supplementary notes on certain relevant fundamental supportive studies." *Semin Arthritis Rheum*, Summer 1974; 3(4):287-321.

2010 Prudden JF. "The treatment of human *Cancer* with agents prepared from bovine cartilage." *J Biol Response Mod*, Dec. 1985; 4(6):551-84.

2011 Durk H, Haase K, Saal J, Becker W, Berg PA. "Nephrotic syndrome after injections of bovine cartilage and marrow extract." [letter] *Lancet* , 18 Mar. 1989; 1(8638):614.

2012 Ashar B, Vargo E. "Shark cartilage-induced hepatitis." [letter] *Ann Intern Med*, 1 Nov. 1996; 125(9):780-1.

2013 Hunt TJ, Connelly JF. "Shark cartilage for cancer treatment." *Am J Health Syst Pharm*, 15 Aug. 1995; 52(16):1756-60.

2014 Lane IW, Comac L. Sharks don't get cancer. Garden City, NY: Avery Publishing Group; 1992.

2015 Miller DR, Anderson GT, Stark JJ, Granick JL, Richardson D. "Phase I/II trial of the safety and efficacy of shark cartilage in the treatment of advanced cancer." *J Clin Oncol*, Nov. 1998; 16(11):3649-55.

2016 Bovine cartilage, Vitamin Connection Website, URL: www.vitaminconnect.com (24 June 1999)

2017 Bovine cartilage, ecoNugenics Website, URL: www.econugenics.com (24 June 1999)

2018 Trial information, CenterWatch Website, URL: www.centerwatch.com (24 June 1999)

2019 CancerNet, National Cancer Institute Website; URL: cancernet.nci.nih.gov (28 June 1999)

2020 Sturtevant FM. Use of aspartame in pregnancy. *Int J Fertil* 1985;30(1):85-87.

2021 Silkaitis RP, Mosnaim AD. Pathways linking L-phenylalanine and 2-phenylethylamine with p-tyramine in rabbit brain. *Brain Res* 1976;114(1):105-115.

2022 Recommended Daily Allowances. USDA website, URL: www.nal.usda.gov/fnic/dga/rda.pdf (Accessed 8 March 2000).

2023 PKU - Dietary Treatment of the Untreated Adult PKU. National Society for Phenylketonuria (NSPKU) website, URL: web.ukonline.co.uk/nspku/untreatd.htm (Accessed 8 March 2000).

2024 Fouty B, Frerman F, Reves R. Riboflavin to treat nucleoside analogue-induced lactic acidosis. *Lancet* 1998;352(9124):291-2.

2025 Levine J, Mishori A, Susnosky M, et al. Combination of inositol and serotonin reuptake inhibitors in the treatment of depression. *Biol Psychiatry*, 1999;45(3):270-273.

2026 Levine J, Barak Y, Kofman O, Belmaker RH. Follow-up and relapse analysis of an inositol study of depression. *Isr J Psychiatry Relat Sci*, 1995;32(1):14-21.

2027 Souza FG, Mander AJ, Foggo M, et al. The effects of lithium discontinuation and the non-effect of oral inositol upon thyroid hormones and cortisol in patients with bipolar affective disorder. *J Affect Disord*, 1991;22(3):165-170.

2028 Nestler JE, Jakubowicz DJ, Reamer P, et al. Ovulatory and metabolic effects of D-chiro-inositol in the polycystic ovary syndrome. *N Engl J Med*, 1999;340(17):1314-1320.

2030 Soleas GJ, Diamandis EP, Goldberg DM. Resveratrol: a molecule whose time has come? And gone? *Clin Biochem* 1997;30(2):91-113.

2031 Ross D, Cooper AJ, Pryse-Davies J, et al. Randomized, double-blind, dose-ranging study of the endometrial effects of a vaginal progesterone gel in estrogen-treated postmenopausal women. *Am J Obstet Gynecol* 1997;177(4):937-941.

2032 Pouly JL, Bassil S, Frydman R, et al. Luteal support after in-vitro fertilization: Crinone 8%, a sustained release vaginal progesterone gel, versus Utrogestan, an oral micronized progesterone. *Hum Reprod* 1996;11(10):2085-2089.

2033 Affinito P, Di Carlo C, Di Mauro P, et al. Endometrial hyperplasia: efficacy of a new treatment with a vaginal cream containing natural micronized progesterone. *Maturitas* 1994;20(2-3):191-198.

2034 Miles RA, Paulson RJ, Lobo RA, et al. Pharmacokinetics and endometrial tissue levels of progesterone after administration by intramuscular and vaginal routes: a comparative study. *Fertil Steril* 1994;62(3):485-490.

2037 The Heart Outcomes Prevention Evaluation Study Investigators. Vitamin E Supplementation and Cardiovascular Events in High-Risk Patients. *N Engl J Med* 2000;342(3):154-160.

2038 Gruppo Italiano per lo Studio della Sopravvivenza nell'Infarto miocardico. Dietary supplementation with n-3 polyunsaturated fatty acids and vitamin E after myocardial infarction: results of the GISSI-Prevenzione trial. *Lancet* 1999;354(9177):447-455.

2041 Warren MP, Biller BMK, Shangold MM. A new clinical option for hormone replacement therapy in women with secondary amenorrhea: effects of cyclic administration of progesterone from the sustained-release vaginal gel Crinone (4% and 8%) on endometrial morphologic features and withdrawal bleeding. *Am J Obstet Gynecol* 1999;180(1 Pt 1):42-48.

2042 van den Berg H. Carotenoid interactions. *Nutr Rev* 1999;57(1):1-10.

2043 Mazzotta G, Sarchielli P, Alberti A, Gallai V. Intracellular Mg++ concentration and electromyographical ischemic test in juvenile headache. *Cephalalgia* 1999;19(9):802-809.

2044 Duffy SJ, Gokce N, Holbrook M, et al. Treatment of hypertension with ascorbic acid. *Lancet* 1999;354(9195):2048-2049.

2045 Zollinger PE, Tuinebreijer WE, Kreis RW, Breederveld RS. Effect of vitamin C on frequency of reflex sympathetic dystrophy in wrist fractures: a randomized trial. *Lancet* 1999;354(9195):2025-2028.

2046 Gorton HC, Jarvis K. The effectiveness of vitamin C in preventing and relieving the symptoms of virus-induced respiratory infections. *J Manipulative Physiol Ther* 1999;22(8):530-533.

2047 Colodny L, Hoffman RL. Inositol—clinical applications for exogenous use. *Altern Med Rev*, 1998;3(6):432-447.

2048 Nomenclature of Cyclitols. IUPAC Commission on the Nomenclature of Organic Chemistry (CNOC) and

REFERENCES

R
E
F
E
R
E
N
C
E
S

IUPAC-IUB Commission on Biochemical Nomenclature (CBN). URL: http://www.chem.qmw.ac.uk/iupac/cyclitol/ (Accessed 28 January 2000).

2049 Mori TA, Bao DQ, Burke V, et al. Dietary fish as a major component of a weight-loss diet: effect on serum lipids, glucose, and insulin metabolism in overweight hypertensive subjects. *Am J Clin Nutr* 1999;70(5):817-825.

2050 Stryer L. Biochemistry, third edition. W.H. Freeman and Co., New York, 1988.

2051 www.quest-iv-health.com/articles/amino.html (Accessed 2 February 2000).

2052 Lehmann WD, Theobald N, Fischer R, Heinrich HC. Stereospecificity of phenylalanine plasma kinetics and hydroxylation in man following oral application of a stable isotope-labelled pseudo-racemic mixture of L- and D-phenylalanine. *Clin Chim Acta* 1983;128(2-3):181-198.

2053 Disorders of amino-acid metabolism. Encyclopaedia Britannica website: www.britannica.com/bcom/eb/article/5/0,5716,118195+10,00.html (Accessed 3 February 2000).

2054 Tyrosinemia. Encyclopaedia Britannica website: www.britannica.com/bcom/eb/article/idxref/5/0,5716,507499,00.html (Accessed 3 February 2000).

2055 Alkaptonuria. Encyclopaedia Britannica website: www.britannica.com/bcom/eb/article/idxref/5/0,5716,507502,00.html (Accessed 3 February 2000).

2056 Kraft K. Artichoke leaf extract- recent findings reflecting effects on lipid metabolism, liver and gastrointestinal tracts. *PhytoMedicine* 1997;4(4):369-78.

2057 Soleas GJ, Diamandis EP, Goldberg DM. Wine as a biological fluid: history, production, and role in disease prevention. *J Clin Lab Anal* 1997;11(5):287-313.

2058 Renaud SC, Gueguen R, Siest G, Salamon R. Wine, beer, and mortality in middle-aged men from eastern France. *Arch Intern Med* 1999;159(16):1865-1870.

2059 Leighton F, Cuevas A, Guasch V, et al. Plasma polyphenols and antioxidants, oxidative DNA damage and endothelial function in a diet and wine intervention study in humans. *Drugs Exp Clin Res* 1999;25(2-3):133-141.

2060 Criqui MH. Alcohol and coronary heart disease: consistent relationship and public health implications. *Clin Chim Acta* 1996;246(1-2):51-57.

2061 Renaud SC, Ruf JC. Effects of Alcohol on platelet functions. *Clin Chim Acta* 1996;246(1-2):77-89.

2062 Renaud SC, Beswick AD, Fehily AM, et al. Alcohol and platelet aggregation: the Caerphilly Prospective Heart Disease Study. *Am J Clin Nutr* May 1992;55(5):1012-1017.

2063 Yun TK, Choi SY. Non-organ specific cancer prevention of ginseng: a prospective study in Korea. *Int J Epidemiol* 1998;27(3):359-364.

2064 Sorensen H, Sonne J. A double-masked study of the effects of ginseng on cognitive functions. *Curr Ther Res* 1996;57(12):959-968.

2065 Bitzan MM, Gold BD, Philpott DJ, et al. Inhibition of Helicobacter pylori and Helicobacter mustelae binding to lipid receptors by bovine colostrum. *J Infect Dis* 1998;177(4):955-61.

2066 Lissner R, Schmidit H, Karch H. A standard immunoglobulin preparation produced from bovine colostra shows antibody reactivity and neutralization activity against Shiga-like toxins and EHEC-hemolysin of Escherichia coli O157:H7. *Infection* 1996;24(5):378-

83.

2067 Huppertz HI, Rutkowski S, Busch DH, et al. Bovine colostrum ameliorates diarrhea in infection with diarrheogenic Escherichia coli, shiga toxin-producing E. Coli, and E. coli expressing intimin and hemolysin. *J Pediatr Gastroenterol Nutr* 1999;29(4):452-6.

2068 Freedman DJ, Tacket CO, Delehanty A, et al. Milk immunoglobulin with specific activity against purified colonization factor antigens can protect against oral challenge with enterotoxigenic Escherichia coli. *J Infect Dis* 1998;177(3):662-7.

2069 Tacket CO, Losonsky G, Link H, et al. Protection by milk immunoglobulin concentrate against oral challenge with enterotoxigenic Escherichia coli. *N Engl J Med* 1988;318(19):1240-3.

2070 Tacket CO, Binion SB, Bostwick E, et al. Efficacy of bovine milk immunoglobulin concentrate in preventing illness after Shigella flexneri challenge. *Am J Trop Med Hyg* 1992;47(3):276-283.

2071 Tacket CO, Losonsky G, Livio S, et al. Lack of prophylactic efficacy of an enteric-coated bovine hyperimmune milk product against enterotoxigenic Escherichia coli challenge administered during a standard meal. *J Infect Dis* 1999 Dec;180(6):2056-9.

2072 Petschow BW, Talbott RD. Reduction in virus-neutralizing activity of a bovine colostrum immunoglobulin concentrate by gastric acid and digestive enzymes. *J Pediatr Gastroenterol Nutr* 1994;19(2):228-35.

2073 Lissner R, Thurmann PA, Merz G, Karch H. Antibody reactivity and fecal recovery of bovine immunoglobulins following oral administration of a colostrum concentrate from cows (Lactobin) to healthy volunteers. *Int J Clin Pharmacol Ther* 1998;36(5):239-45.

2074 Kuhlmann J, Berger W, Podzuweit H, Schmidt U. The influence of valerian treatment on "reaction time, alertness and concentration" in volunteers. *Pharmacopsychiatry* 1999;32(6):235-241.

2075 Dev S. Ancient-modern concordance in Ayurvedic plants: some examples. *Environ Health Perspect* 1999;107(10):783-789.

2076 GRIN Taxonomy search page http://www.ars-grin.gov/cgi-bin/npgs/html/tax_search.pl? (Accessed 27 February 2000).

2077 Jacob A, Pandey M, Kapoor S, Saroja R. Effect of the Indian gooseberry (amla) on serum cholesterol levels in men aged 35-55 years. *Eur J Clin Nutr* 1988;42(11):939-944.

2078 Asmawi MZ, Kankaanranta H, Moilanen E, Vapaatalo H. Anti-inflammatory activities of Emblica officinalis Gaertn leaf extracts. *J Pharm Pharmacol* 1993;45(6):581-584.

2079 Ihantola-Vormisto A, Summanen J, Kankaanranta H, et al. Anti-inflammatory activity of extracts from leaves of Phyllanthus emblica. *Planta Med* 1997;63(6):518-524.

2080 Hu JF. [Inhibitory effects of Phyllanthus emblica juice on formation of N-nitrosomorpholine in vitro and N-nitrosoproline in rat and human]. [Article in Chinese] *Chung Hua Yu Fang I Hsueh Tsa Chih* 1990;24(3):132-135.

2081 Bhattacharya A, Chatterjee A, Ghosal S, Bhattacharya SK. Antioxidant activity of active tannoid principles of Emblica officinalis (amla). *Indian J Exp Biol* 1999;37(7):676-680.

2082 Janicak PG, Lipinski J, Davis JM, et al. S-adenosylmethionine in depression. A literature review and preliminary report. *Ala J Med Sci* 1988;25(3):306-313.

2083 De Vanna M, Rigamonti R. Oral S-adenosyl-L-methionine in depression. *Curr Ther Res* 1992;52(3):478-485.

2084 Zhao G. [Inherited metabolic aberration of phenylalanine in the family members of patients with essential hypertension and stroke][Article in Chinese]. *Chung Hua I Hsueh Tsa Chih* (Taipei) 1991;71(7):28, 388-90.

2085 Dr. Duke's Phytochemical and Ethnobotanical Databases; URL: www.ars-grin.gov/duke/ (Accessed 24 March 2000).

2086 Damario MA, Goudas VT, Session DR, et al. Crinone 8% vaginal progesterone gel results in lower embryonic implantation efficiency after in vitro fertilization-embryo transfer. *Fertil Steril*, 1999;72(5):830-836.

2087 Columbia Labs. HYPERLINK URL: http://www.columbialabs.com/html/crinhealth/progesterone/dosage.htm (Accessed 9 March 2000).

2088 Clinical Pharmacology. HYPERLINK URL: http://www.imc.gsm.com/scripts/frameset.asp (Accessed 9 March 2000).

2089 Gibbons WE, Toner JP, Hamacher P, Kolm P. Experience with a novel vaginal progesterone preparation in a donor oocyte program. *Fertil Steril*, 1998;69(1):96-101.

2090 Bals-Pratsch M, Al-Hasani S, Schopper B, et al. A simple, inexpensive and effective artificial cycle with exogenous transdermal oestradiol and vaginal progesterone for the transfer of cryopreserved pronucleated human oocytes in women with normal cycles. *Hum Reprod*. 1999;14 Suppl 1:222-230.

2091 HYPERLINK URL: http://www.fda.gov/medwatch/safety/1998/may98.htm#crinon (Accessed 9 March 2000).

2092 Woelk H, Kapoula O, S. Lehrl S, et al. Comparison of Kava Special Extract WS 1490 and Benzodiazepines in Patients with Anxiety. [English translation from German]. *Z Allg Med* 1993;69:271–277.

2093 Pittler MH, Ernst E. Efficacy of kava extract for treating anxiety: systematic review and meta-analysis. *J Clin Psychopharmacol* 2000;20(1):84-89.

2094 Volz HP, Kieser M. Kava-kava extract WS 1490 versus placebo in anxiety disorders—a randomized placebo-controlled 25-week outpatient trial. *Pharmacopsychiatry* 1997;30(1):1-5.

2095 Lehmann E, Kinzler E, Friedemann J. Efficacy of a special Kava extract (Piper methysticum) in patients with states of anxiety, tension and excitedness of non-mental origin- a double-blind placebo-controlled study of four weeks treatment. *PhytoMedicine* 1996;3(2):113-9.

2096 Warnecke G. [Psychosomatic dysfunctions in the female climacteric. Clinical effectiveness and tolerance of Kava Extract WS 1490]. [Article in German]. *Fortschr Med* 1991;109(4):119-22.

2097 Heinze HJ, Munthe TF, Steitz J, Matzke M. Pharmacopsychological effects of oxazepam and kava-extract in a visual search paradigm assessed with event-related potentials. *Pharmacopsychiatry* 1994;27(6):224-30.

2098 Munte TF, Heinze HJ, Matzke M, Steitz J. Effects of oxazepam and an extract of kava roots (Piper methysticum) on event-related potentials in a word recognition task. *Neuropsychobiology* 1993;27(1):46-53.

2099 "Folic acid." SupraHealth, Inc. Website. URL: www.suprahealth.com/folic.htm. (Accessed 7 July 1999).

2100 Kreider RB, Ferreira M, Wilson M, et al. "Effects of creatine supplementation on body composition, strength, and sprint performance." *Med Sci Sports Exerc* 1998;30(1):73-82.

2101 Vandenberghe K, Goris M, Van Hecke P, et al. "Long-term creatine intake is beneficial to muscle performance during resistance training." *J Appl Physiol* 1997;83(6):2055-2063.

2102 Earnest CP, Snell PG, Rodriguez R, et al. "The effect of creatine monohydrate ingestion on anerobic power indices, muscular strength and body composition." *Acta Physiol Scand* 1995;153:207-209.

2103 Balsom PD, Soderland K, Ekblom B. "Creatine in humans with special reference to creatine supplementation." *Sports Med* 1994;18(4):268-280.

2104 Hultman E, Soderlund K, Timmons JA, et al. Muscle creatine loading in men. *J Appl Physiol* 1996;81:232-237.

2105 Burke LM, Pyne DB, Telford RD. "Oral creatine supplementation does not improve sprint performance in elite swimmers." *Med Sci Sports Exerc* 1995;27:S146.

2106 Mujika I, Chatard J, Lacoste L, et al. "Creatine supplementation does not improve sprint performance in competitive swimmers." *Med Sci Sports Exerc* 1996;28(11):1435-41.

2107 Hanioka T, Tanaka M, Ojima M, et al. "Effect of topical application of coenzyme Q10 on adult periodontitis." *Molec Aspects Med* 1994;15 (Suppl): S241-8.

2108 Watts TLP. "Coenzyme Q10 and periodontal treatment: is there any beneficial effect?" *Br Dent J* 1995;178:209-13.

2109 Malm C, Svensson M, Ekblom B, et al. "Effects of ubiquinone-10 supplementation and high intensity training on physical performance in humans." *Acta Physiol Scand* 1997;161:379-84.

2110 Weston SB, Zhou S, Weatherby RP, et al. "Does exogenous coenzyme Q10 affect aerobic capacity in endurance athletes?" *Int J Sport Nutr* 1997;7:197-206.

2111 Kuritzky L. "DHEA: Science or Wishful Thinking?" *Hosp Pract* 1998; 33(5):85-86.

2112 Skolnick AA. "Scientific Verdict Still Out on DHEA." *JAMA* 1996; 276(17): 1365-67.

2113 Van Vollenhoven RF, Morabito LM, Engleman EG, et al. "Treatment of Systemic Lupus Erythematosus with Dehydroepiandrosterone: 50 Patients Treated up to 12 Months." *J Rheumatol* 1998; 25:285-9.

2114 Van Vollenhoven RF, Engleman EG, McGurie JL. "Dehydroepiandrosterone in Systemic Lupus Erythematosus." *Arthr Rheum* 1995; 38(12):1826-31.

2115 Ebeling P, Koivisto VA. "Physiological Importance of dehydroepiandrosterone." *Lancet* 1994; 343:1479-81.

2116 "Dehydroepiandrosterone (DHEA)." *Med Lett Drugs Ther* 1996; 38:91-2.

2117 Vandeberghe K, Gillis N, Van Leemputte M, et al. "Caffeine counteracts the ergogenic action of muscle creatine loading." *J Appl Physiol* 1996;80(2):452-7.

2118 Pritchard NR, Kalra PA. "Renal dysfunction accompanying oral creatine supplements." *Lancet* 1998;351(9111):1252-3.

2119 Poortmans JR, Francaux M. "Renal dysfunction accompanying oral creatine supplements." *Lancet* 1998;352(9123):234.

2120 Poortmans JR, Auquier H, Renaut V, et al. "Effect of short-term creatine supplementation on renal responses in men." *Eur J Appl Physiol* 1997;76:566-67.

2121 Kamikawa T, Kobayashi A, Yamashita T, et al. "Effects of coenzyme Q10 on exercise tolerance in chronic stable angina pectoris." *Am J Cardiol* 1985;56(4):247-51.

2122 Langsjoen P, Willis R, Folkers K. "Treatment of essential hypertension with coenzyme Q10." *Mol Aspects Med* 1994;15 Suppl:S265-72.

2123 Folkers K, Hanioka T, Xia LJ, et al. "Coenzyme Q10 increases T4/T8 ratios of lymphocytes in ordinary subjects and relevance to patients having the AIDS related complex." *Biochem Biophys Res Commun* 1991;176(2):786-91.

2124 Folkers K, Langsjoen P, Nara Y, et al. "Biochemical deficiencies of coenzyme Q10 in HIV-infection and exploratory treatment." *Biochem Biophys Res Commun.* 1988;153(2):888-96.

2125 Suzuki S, Hinokio Y, Ohtomo M, et al. "The effects of coenzyme Q10 treatment on maternally inherited *Diabetes* mellitus and deafness, and mitochondrial DNA 3243 (A to G) mutation." *Diabetologia.* 1998;41(5):584-8.

2126 Andersen CB, Henriksen JE, Hother-Nielsen O, et al. "The effect of coenzyme Q10 on blood glucose and insulin requirement in patients with insulin dependent *Diabetes* mellitus." *Mol Aspects Med.* 1997;18 Suppl:S307-9.

2127 Folkers K, Simonsen R. "Two successful double-blind trials with coenzyme Q10 (vitamin Q10) on muscular dystrophies and neurogenic atrophies." *Biochem Biophys Acta.* 1995;1271(1):281-6.

2128 Spigset O. "Reduced effect of warfarin caused by ubidecarenone." *Lancet* 1994;334:1372-1373.

2129 Morales AJ, Nolan JJ, Nelson JC, et al. "Effects of replacement Dose of Dehydroepiandrosterone in Men and Women of Advancing Age." *J Clin Endocrinol Metab* 1994;78(6):1360-1367.

2130 Wolf OT, Neumann O, Hellhammer DH, et al. "Effects of a Two-Week Physiological Dehydroepiandrosterone Substitution on Cognitive Performance and Well-Being in Healthy Elderly Women and Men." *J Clin Endocrinol Metab* 1997;82(7):2363-2367.

2131 Danenberg HD, Ben-Yehuda A, Zakay-Rones Z, et al. "Dehydroepiandrosterone treatment is not beneficial to the immune response to influenza in elderly subjects." *J Clin Endocrinol Metab.* 1997;82(9):2911-4.

2132 Degelau J, Guay D, Hallgren H. "The effect of DHEAS on influenza vaccination in aging adults." *J Am Geriatr Soc* 1997;45(7):747-51.

2133 Yen SS, Morales AJ, Khorram O. "Replacement of DHEA in aging men and women. Potential remedial effects." *Ann N Y Acad Sci* 1995;774:128-42.

2134 Greenberg S, Fishman WH. "Coenzyme Q10: A New Drug for Cardiovascular Disease." *J Clin Pharmacol* 1990;30:596-608.

2135 Lewin A, Lavon H. "The effect of coenzyme Q10 on sperm motility and function." *Mol Aspects Med* 1997;18 Suppl:S213-9.

2136 Vollenhoven RF, Engleman EG, McGuire JL. "Dehydroepiandrosterone in Systemic Lupus Erythematosus." *Arthritis Rheum* 1994;37(9):1305-1310.

2137 "Coenzyme Q10." Go-Symmetry Website URL: www.go-symmetry.com. (7 July 1999).

2138 Goodman GA, Rall TW, Nies AS, Taylor P. The Pharmacological Basis of Therapeutics 9th edition.

2139 Ma J, Stampfer MJ, Giovannucci E, et al. "Methylenetetrahydrofolate reductase polymorphism, dietary interactions, and risk of colorectal cancer." *Br J Nutr* 1997;57(6):1098-102

2140 Lashner GA, Provencher KS, Seidner DL, Knesebeck A, Brzezinski A. "The effect of folic acid supplementation on the risk for cancer or dysplasia in ulcerative colitis." *Gastroenterol* 1997;112(1):29-32.

2141 La Vecchia C, Braga C, Negri E et al. "Intake of selected micronutrients and risk of colorectal cancer." *Int J Cancer* 1997;73:525-30.

2142 Tseng M, Murray SC, Kupper LL, Sandler RS. "Micronutrients and the risk of colorectal adenomas." *Am J Epidemiol* 1996;144(11):1005-14.

2143 Baron JA, Sandler RS, Haile RW, et al. "Folate intake, *Alcohol* consumption, cigarette smoking, and risk of colorectal adenomas." *J Natl Cancer Inst* 1998;90(1):57-62.

2144 Slattery ML, Schaffer D, Edwards SL, Ma KN, et al. "Are dietary factors involved in DNA methylation associated with colon cancer?" *Nutr Cancer* 1997;28(1):52-62.

2145 Freudenheim JL, Graham S, Marshall JR, et al. "Folate intake and *Carcinogenesis* of the colon and rectum." *Int J Epidemiol* 1991;20(2):368-74.

2146 Brouwer IA, van Dusseldorp M, Thomas CM, et al. "Low-dose folic acid supplementation decreases plasma homocysteine concentrations: a randomized trial." *Am J Clin Nutr* 1999;69(1):99-104.

2147 Landgren F, Israelsson B, Lindgren A, et al. "Plasma homocysteine in acute myocardial infarction: homocysteine-lowering effect of folic acid." *J Intern Med* 1995;237(4):381-8.

2148 Woodside JV, Yarnell JW, McMaster D, et al. "Effect of B-group vitamins and antioxidant vitamins on hyperhomocysteinemia: a double-blind, randomized, factorial-design, controlled trial." *Am J Clin Nutr* 1998;67(5):858-66.

2149 Brattstrom LE, Israelsson B, Jeppsson JO, et al. "Folic acid-an innocuous means to reduce plasma homocysteine." *Scand J Clin Lab Invest* 1988;48(3):215-21.

2150 Brown RS, Di Stanislao PT, Beaver WT, et al. "The administration of folic acid to institutionalized epileptic adults with phenytoin-induced gingival hyperplasia. A double-blind, placebo-controlled, parallel study." *Oral Surg Oral Med Oral Pathol* 1991;71(5): 565-8.

2151 Drew HJ, Vogel RI, Molofsky W, et al. "Effect of folate on phenytoin hyperplasia." *J Clin Periodontol* 1987;14(6):350-6.

2152 Pack AR, Thomson ME. "Effects of topical and systemic folic acid supplementation on gingivitis in pregnancy." *J Clin Periodontol* 1980;7(5):402-14.

2153 Juhlin L, Olsson MJ. "Improvement of vitiligo after oral treatment with vitamin B12 and folic acid and the importance of sun exposure." *Acta Derm Venereol* 1997;77(6):460-2 .

2154 Montes LF, Diaz ML, Lajous J, et al. "Folic acid and vitamin B12 in vitiligo: a nutritional approach." *Cutis* 1992;50(1):39-42.

2155 Strom CM, Brusca RM, Pizzi WJ "Double-blind, placebo-controlled crossover study of folinic acid Leucovorin for the treatment of fragile X syndrome." *Am J Med Genet* 1992;44(5):676-82.

2156 Fisch GS, Cohen IL, Gross AC, et al. "Folic acid treatment of fragile X males: a further study." *Am J Med Genet* 1988;30(1-2):393-9.

2157 Gillberg C, Wahlstrom J, Johansson R, et al. "Folic acid as an adjunct in the treatment of children with the autism fragile-X syndrome (AFRAX)." *Dev Med Child Neurol* 1986;28(5):624-7.

2158 Rosenblatt DS, Duschenes EA, Hellstrom FV, et al. "Folic acid blinded trial in identical twins with fragile X syndrome." *Am J Hum Genet* 1985;37(3):543-52.

2159 Hagerman RJ, Jackson AW, Levitas A, et al. "Oral folic acid versus placebo in the treatment of males with the fragile X syndrome." *Am J Med Genet* 1986;23(1-2):241-62.

2160 Brown WT, Cohen IL, Fisch GS, et al. "High dose folic acid treatment of fragile (X) males." *Am J Med Genet* 1986;23(1-2):263-71.

2161 Muggia FM, Synold TW, Newman EM, et al. "Failure of pretreatment with intravenous folic acid to alter the cumulative hematologic toxicity of lometrexol." *J Natl Cancer Inst* 1996;88(20):1495-1496.

2162 Morgan SL, Baggott JE, Vaughn WH, et al. "Supplementation with folic acid during methotrexate therapy for rheumatoid arthritis. A double-blind, placebo-controlled trial." *Ann Intern Med* 1994;121(11):833-41.

2163 Morgan SL, Baggott JE, Vaughn WH, et al. "The effect of folic acid supplementation on the toxicity of low-dose methotrexate in patients with rheumatoid arthritis." *Arthritis Rheum* 1990;33(1):9-18.

2164 Ortiz Z, Shea B, Suarez-Almazor ME, Moher D, et al. "The efficacy of folic acid and folinic acid in reducing methotrexate gastrointestinal toxicity in rheumatoid arthritis. A metaanalysis of randomized controlled trials." *J Rheumatol* 1998;25(1):36-43.

2165 Kelly GS. "Folates: supplemental forms and therapeutic applications." *Altern Med Rev* 1998;3(3):208-20.

2166 Pack AR . "Effects of folate mouthwash on experimental gingivitis in man." *J Clin Periodontol* 1986;13(7):671-6.

2167 "HMB" Musclesoft Website. URL: musclesoft.com/ hmb.htm (24 July 1999).

2168 Nissen S, Sharp R, Ray M, et al. "Effect of leucine metabolite beta-hydroxy-beta-methylbutyrate on muscle *Metabolism* during resistance-exercise training." *J Appl Physiol* 1996;81(5):2095-104.

2169 Gennari C, Agnusdei D, Crepaldi G, et al. "Effect of ipriflavone-a synthetic derivative of natural isoflavones-on bone mass loss in the early years after menopause." *Menopause* 1998;5(1):9-15.

2170 Agnusdei D, Crepaldi G, Isaia G, et al. "A double blind, placebo-controlled trial of ipriflavone for prevention of postmenopausal spinal bone loss." *Calcif Tissue Int* 1997;61(2):142-7.

2171 Gambacciani M, Ciaponi M, Cappagli B, et al. "Effects of combined low dose of the isoflavone derivative ipriflavone and estrogen replacement on bone mineral density and metabolism in postmenopausal women." *Maturitas* 1997;28(1):75-81.

2172 Agnusdei D, Gennari C, Bufalino L. "Prevention of early postmenopausal bone loss using low doses of conjugated estrogens and the non-hormonal, bone-active drug ipriflavone." *Osteoporos Int* 1995;5(6):462-6.

2173 Valente M, Bufalino L, Castiglione GN, et al. "Effects of 1-year treatment with ipriflavone on bone in postmenopausal women with low bone mass." *Calcif Tissue Int* 1994;54(5):377-80.

2174 Ushiroyama T, Okamura S, Ikeda A, et al. "Efficacy of ipriflavone and 1 alpha vitamin D therapy for the cessation of vertebral bone loss." *Int J Gynaecol Obstet* 1995;48(3):283-8.

2175 Agnusdei D, Zacchei F, Bigazzi S, et al. "Metabolic and clinical effects of ipriflavone in established post-menopausal osteoporosis." *Drugs Exp Clin Res* 1989;15(2):97-104.

2176 Agnusdei D, Camporeale A, Gonnelli S, et al. "Short-term treatment of Paget's disease of bone with ipriflavone." *Bone Miner* 1992;19 Suppl 1:S35-42.

2177 Hyodo T, Ono K, Koumi T, et al. "A study of the effects of ipriflavone administration on hemodialysis patients with renal osteodystrophy: preliminary report." *Nephron* 1991;58(1):114-5.

2178 Monostory K, Vereczkey L, Levai F, et al. "Ipriflavone as an inhibitor of human cytochrome P450 enzymes." *Br J Pharmacol* 1998;123(4):605-10.

2179 Melis GB, Paoletti AM, Cagnacci A, et al. "Lack of any estrogenic effect of ipriflavone in postmenopausal women." *J Endocrinol Invest* 1992;15(10):755-61.

2180 "Inositol." Mmead Website. URL: www.mmeade.com/ cheat/inositol.html (Accessed 24 July 1999).

2181 "Inositol." CW Institute Website. URL: www.cwinstitute.com/cp/_disc16/00000009.htm (Accessed 24 July 1999).

2182 "Inositol." Tell A Friend Website. URL: tellafriend.net/ inositol.htm (Accessed 24 July 1999).

2183 "Inositol." Mother Nature's Encyclopedia. URL: www.mothernature.com/ency/Supp/Inositol.asp (24 July 1999).

2184 Benjamin J, Levine J, Fux M, et al. "Double-blind, placebo-controlled, crossover trial of inositol treatment for panic disorder." *Am J Psychiatry* 1995;152(7):1084-6.

2185 Levine J, et al. "Double-blind, controlled trial of inositol treatment of depression." *Am J Psychiatry*, 1995; 152(5):792-94.

2186 Fux M, et al. "Inositol treatment of obsessive-compulsive disorder." *Am J Psychiatry*, 1996; 153(9):1219-221.

2187 Levine J "Controlled trials of inositol in psychiatry." *Eur Neuropsychopharmacol*, 1997; 7(2):147-55.

2188 Levine J, et al. "CSF inositol in schizophrenia and high-dose inositol treatment of schizophrenia." *Eur Neuropsychopharmacol*, 1994; 4(4):487-90.

2189 Barak Y, et al. "Inositol treatment of Alzheimer's disease: a double blind, cross-over placebo controlled trial." *Prog Neuropsychopharmacol Biol Psychiatry*, 1996; 20(4):729-35.

2190 Levine J, et al. "Inositol treatment of autism." *J Neural Transm*, 1997; 104(2-3):307-310.

2191 Hallman M, et al. "Inositol supplementation in premature infants with respiratory distress syndrome." *N Engl J Med*, 1992; 326(19):1233-239.

2192 Hallman M, Pohjavuori M, Bry K. "Inositol supplementation in respiratory distress syndrome." *Lung*, 1990; 168 Suppl:877-82.

2193 Gregersen G, et al. "Oral supplementation of myoinositol: effects on peripheral nerve function in human diabetics and on the concentration in plasma, erythrocytes, urine and muscle tissue in human diabetics and normals." *Acta Neurol Scand*, 1983; 67(3):164-72.

2194 Salway JG, Whitehead L, Finnegan JA. "Effect of myo-inositol on peripheral-nerve function in diabetes." *Lancet*

REFERENCES

R E F E R E N C E S

1978; 2(8103):1282-284.

2195 Gregersen G, et al. "Myoinositol and function of peripheral nerves in human diabetics. A controlled clinical trial." *Acta Neurol Scand*, 1978; 58(4):241-48.

2196 "Iodine." URL: www.suprahealth.com/iodine.htm (19 July 1999).

2197 Ghent WR, et al. "Iodine replacement in fibrocystic disease of the breast." *Can J Surg*, 1993; 36(5):453-60.

2198 Adamietz IA, et al. "Prophylaxis with povidone-iodine against induction of oral mucositis by radiochemotherapy." *Support Care Cancer*, 1998; 6(4):373-77.

2199 Rahn R, et al. "Povidone-iodine to prevent mucositis in patients during antineoplastic radiochemotherapy." *Dermatology*, 1997; 195 Suppl 2:57-61.

2200 Apelqvist J, Ragnarson Tennvall G. "Cavity foot ulcers in diabetic patients: a comparative study of cadexomer iodine ointment and standard treatment. An economic analysis alongside a clinical trial." *Acta Derm Venereol*, 1996; 76(3):231-35.

2201 Vitamins etc. "Potassium." URL: bookman.com.au/vitamins/potassium.html (19 July 1999).

2202 Sequential Healing Health Services. "Potassium." URL: www.sequentialhealing.com/vit-min-nutrients/potassium.html (19 July 1999).

2203 Langsjoen PH, et al. "Treatment of hypertrophic cardiomyopathy with coenzyme Q10." *Mol Aspects Med*, 1997; 18 Suppl:S145-51.

2204 Folkers K, et al. "Lovastatin decreases coenzyme Q levels in humans." *Proc Natl Acad Sci* USA, 1990; 87(22):8931-934.

2205 Facts and Comparisons. *Drug Facts and Comparisons*. St. Louis: Wolters Kluwer Co., 1998.

2206 Maloney JD, et al. "Potassium loading as adjunct treatment of repetitive ventricular arrhythmias." *Cleve Clin J Med*, 1990; 57(3):223-31.

2207 Ovrum E, et al. "Conversion of postischemic ventricular fibrillation with intraaortic infusion of potassium chloride." *Ann Thorac Surg*, 1995; 60(1):156-59.

2208 Breslau NA, et al. "Physiological effects of slow release potassium phosphate for absorptive hypercalciuria: a randomized double-blind trial." *J Urol*, 1998; 160(3 Pt 1):664-68.

2209 Heller HJ, et al. "Sustained reduction in urinary calcium during long-term treatment with slow release neutral potassium phosphate in absorptive hypercalciuria." *Urol*, 1998; 159(5):1451-455; discussion 1455-456.

2210 Singh RB, et al. "Effect of treatment with magnesium and potassium on mortality and reinfarction rate of patients with suspected acute myocardial infarction." *Int J Clin Pharmacol Ther*, 1996; 34(5):219-25.

2211 "Pectin." Vitawise Inc Website, URL: vitawise.com/apcc.htm

2212 Albert KS, Ayres JW, DiSanto AR, et al. "Influence of kaolin-pectin suspension on digoxin bioavailability." *J Pharm Sci*, 1978;67(11):1582-6.

2213 Albert KS, Welch RD, DeSante KA, et al. "Decreased tetracycline bioavailability caused by a bismuth subsalicylate antidiarrheal mixture." *J Pharm Sci*, 1979;68(5):586-8.

2214 Veldman FJ, Nair CH, Vorster HH, et al. "Dietary pectin influences fibrin network structure in hypercholesterolaemic subjects." *Thromb Res*, 1997;86(3):183-96.

2215 Davidson MH, Dugan LD, Stocki J, et al. "A low-viscosity soluble-fiber fruit juice supplement fails to lower cholesterol in hypercholesterolemic men and women." *J Nutr*, 1998;128(11):1927-32.

2216 Cerda JJ, Robbins FL, Burgin CW,et al. "The effects of grapefruit pectin on patients at risk for coronary heart disease without altering diet or lifestyle." *Clin Cardiol*, 1988;11(9):589-94.

2217 Hillman LC, Peters SG, Fisher CA, et al. "The effects of the fiber components pectin, cellulose and lignin on serum cholesterol levels." *Am J Clin Nutr*, 1985;42(2):207-13.

2218 Marti J. *The Alternative Health & Medicine Encyclopedia*. 2nd ed. Detroit, MI: Gale Research International Limited; 1998.

2219 Trevisan M, Krogh V, Freudenheim J, et al. "Consumption of olive oil, butter, and vegetable oils and coronary heart disease risk factors. The Research Group ATS-RF2 of the Italian National Research Council." *JAMA* , 1990;263(5):688-92.

2220 Keys A, Menotti A, Karvonen MJ , et al. "The diet and 15-year death rate in the seven countries study." *Am J Epidemiol*, 1986;124(6):903-15.

2221 Martin-Moreno JM, Willett WC, Gorgojo L, et al. "Dietary fat, olive oil intake and breast cancer risk." *Int J Cancer*, 1994;58(6):774-80.

2222 la Vecchia C, Negri E, Franceschi S, et al. "Olive oil, other dietary fats, and the risk of breast cancer (Italy)." *Cancer Causes Control*, 1995;6(6):545-50.

2223 Trichopoulou A, Katsouyanni K, Stuver S, et al. "Consumption of olive oil and specific food groups in relation to breast cancer risk in Greece." *Natl Cancer Inst*, 1995;87(2):110-6.

2224 Katan MB, Zock PL, Mensink RP. "Dietary oils, serum lipoproteins, and coronary heart disease." *Am J Clin Nutr*, 1995;61(6 Suppl):1368S-1373S.

2225 Rock CL, Swendseid ME. "Plasma beta-carotene response in humans after meals supplemented with dietary pectin." *Am J Clin Nutr*, 1992;55(1):96-9.

2226 "Superoxide dismutase (SOD)." BC Cancer Agency. URL: www.bccancer.bc.ca/uctm/36.html.

2227 "Superoxide dismutase." Medquest Pharmacy. URL: www.medquestpharmacy.com/store/prodtemplate.asp?product_id=76.

2228 McIlwain H, Silverfield JC, Cheatum DE, et al. "Intra-articular orgotein in osteoarthritis of the knee: a placebo-controlled efficacy, safety, and dosage comparison." *Am J Med*, 1989;87(3):295-300.

2229 Gammer W, Broback LG. "Clinical comparison of orgotein and methylprednisolone acetate in the treatment of osteoarthrosis of the knee joint." *Scand J Rheumatol*, 1984;13(2):108-12.

2230 Goebel KM, Storck U, Neurath F. "Intrasynovial orgotein therapy in rheumatoid arthritis." *Lancet* 1981;1(8228):1015-7.

2231 Walravens M, Dequeker J. "Comparison of gold and orgotein treatment in rheumatoid arthritis." *Curr Ther Res Clin Exp*, 1976; 20(1):62-9.

2232 Goebel KM, Storck U. "Effect of intra-articular orgotein versus a corticosteroid on rheumatoid arthritis of the knees." *Am J Med*, 1983;74(1):124-8.

2233 Kadrnka F. "Results of a multicenter orgotein study in radiation induced and interstitial cystitis." [Article in German] *Eur J Rheumatol Inflamm*, 1981;4(2):237-43.

2234 Sanchiz F, Milla A, Artola N, et al. "Prevention of radioinduced cystitis by orgotein: a randomized study." *AntiCancer Res*, 1996;16(4A):2025-8.

2235 Nielsen OS, Overgaard J, Overgaard M, et al. "Orgotein

in radiation treatment of bladder cancer. A report on allergic reactions and lack of radioprotective effect." *Acta Oncol*, 1987;26(2):101-4.

2236 Marberger H, Bartsch G, Huber W, et al. "Orgotein: a new drug for the treatment of radiation cystitis." *Curr Ther Res Clin Exp*, 1975;18(3):466-75

2238 Pollak R, Andrisevic JH, Maddux MS, et al. "A randomized double-blind trial of the use of human recombinant superoxide dismutase in renal transplantation." *Transplantation*, 1993 Jan;55(1):57-60.

2239 Land W, Schneeberger H, Schleibner S, et al. The beneficial effect of human recombinant superoxide dismutase on acute and chronic rejection events in recipients of cadaveric renal transplants. *Transplantation*, 1994;57(2):211-7.

2240 Schneeberger H, Schleibner S, Illner WD, et al. "The impact of free radical-mediated reperfusion injury on acute and chronic rejection events following cadaveric renal transplantation." *Clin Transpl* 1993;:219-32.

2241 Flaherty JT, Pitt B, Gruber JW, et al. "Recombinant human superoxide dismutase (h-SOD) fails to improve recovery of ventricular function in patients undergoing coronary angioplasty for acute myocardial infarction." *Circulation*, 1994;89(5):1982-91.

2242 Rosenfeld W, Evans H, Concepcion L, et al. "Prevention of bronchopulmonary dysplasia by administration of bovine superoxide dismutase in preterm infants with respiratory distress syndrome." *J Pediatr*, 1984;105(5):781-5.

2243 Murohara Y, Yui Y, Hattori R, et al. "Effects of superoxide dismutase on reperfusion arrhythmias and left ventricular function in patients undergoing thrombolysis for anterior wall acute myocardial infarction." *Am J Cardiol*, 1991;67(8):765-7.

2244 "N-acetylcysteine." Smart Basics Inc. Website, URL: webu5156.ntx.net/glos.news/feb_march1999/ immunityagainstflu.htm

2245 Ardissino D, Merlini PA, Savonitto S, et al. "Effect of transdermal nitroglycerin or N-acetylcysteine, or both, in the long-term treatment of unstable angina pectoris." *J Am Coll Cardiol*, 1997;29(5):941-7.

2246 Horowitz JD, Henry CA, Syrjanen ML, et al. "Nitroglycerine/N-acetylcysteine in the management of unstable angina pectoris." *Eur Heart J*, 1988;9 Suppl A:95-100.

2247 Brown DM. "Bile plug syndrome: successful management with a mucolytic agent." *Pediatr Surg* 1990;25(3):351-2.

2248 Evans JS, George DE, Mollit D. "Biliary infusion therapy in the inspissated bile syndrome of cystic fibrosis." *J Pediatr Gastroenterol Nutr* 1991;12(1):131-5.

2249 Mulvaney WP, Quilter T, Mortera A. "Experiences with acetylcysteine in cystinuric patients." *J Urol* 1975;114(1):107-8.

2250 Giovannucci E, et al. "Multivitamin use, folate, and colon cancer in women in the Nurses' Health Study. *Ann Intern Med*, 1998; 129 (7):517-24.

2251 Drew HJ, Vogel RI, Molofsky W, et al. "Effect of folate on phenytoin hyperplasia." *J Clin Periodontol*, 1987;14(6):350-6

2252 Unverferth DV, Jagadeesh JM, Unverferth Bj, et al. "Attempt to prevent doxorubicin-induced acute human myocardial morphologic damage with acetylcysteine." *J Natl Cancer Inst*, 1983;71(5):917-20.

2253 Dresdale AR, Barr LH, Bonow RO, et al. "Prospective randomized study of the role of N-acetyl cysteine in reversing doxorubicin-induced cardiomyopathy." *Am J Clin Oncol*, 1982;5(6):657-63.

2254 Louwerse ES, Weverling GJ, Bossuyt PM, et al. "Randomized, double-blind, controlled trial of acetylcysteine in amyotrophic lateral sclerosis." *Arch Neurol*, 1995;52(6):559-64.

2256 Wiklund O, Fager G, Andersson A, et al. "N-acetylcysteine treatment lowers plasma homocysteine but not serum lipoprotein(a) levels." *Atherosclerosis*, 1996;119(1):99-106.

2257 Kroon AA, Demacker PN, Stalenhoef AF. "N-acetylcysteine and serum concentrations of lipoprotein(a)." *J Intern Med*, 1991;230(6):519-26.

2258 Bostom AG, Shemin D, Yoburn D, et al. "Lack of effect of oral N-acetylcysteine on the acute dialysis-related lowering of total plasma homocysteine in hemodialysis patients." *Atherosclerosis*, 1996;120(1-2):241-4.

2259 Hurd RW, Wilder BJ, Helveston WR, et al. "Treatment of four siblings with progressive myoclonus epilepsy of the Unverricht-Lundborg type with N-acetylcysteine." *Neurology*, 1996;47(5):1264-8.

2260 De Flora S, Grassi C, Carati L. "Attenuation of influenza-like symptomatology and improvement of cell-mediated immunity with long-term N-acetylcysteine treatment." *Eur Respir J*, 1997;10(7):1535-41.

2261 Pearson TA. Alcohol and Heart Disease. American Heart Association Medical/Scientific Statement. URL: www.americanheart.org/Scientific/statements/1996/ 1116.html.

2262 Fraser AG. Pharmacokinetic interactions between alcohol and other drugs. *Clin Pharmacokinet*, 1997;33(2):79-90.

2263 Isselbacher KJ, Braunwald E, Wilson JD, et al. *Harrison's Principles of Internal Medicine*. 13th Ed. New York, NY: McGraw-Hill; 1994.

2264 Briggs GG. Drugs in pregnancy and lactation. 5th edition. Baltimore, MD: Williams & Wilkins; 1998.

2265 Kushner MG, Mackenzie TB, Fiszdon J, et al. The effects of alcohol consumption on laboratory-induced panic and state anxiety. *Arch Gen Psychiatry*, 1996;53(3):264-270.

2266 de Boer MC, Schippers GM, van der Staak. Alcohol and social anxiety in women and men: pharmacological and expectancy effects. *Addict Behav*, 1993;18(2):117-26.

2267 Kiechl S, Willeit J, Rungger G, et al. Alcohol consumption and Atherosclerosis: what is the relation? Prospective results from the Bruneck Study. *Stroke*, 1998;29(5):900-907.

2268 Klatsky AL, Armstrong MA, Friedman GD. Red wine, white wine, liquor, beer, and risk for coronary artery disease hospitalization. *Am J Cardiol*, 1997;80(4):416-420.

2269 Siscovick DS, Weiss NS, Fox N. Moderate Alcohol consumption and primary cardiac arrest. *Am J Epidemiol*, 1986;123(3):499-503.

2270 Hennekens CH, Willett W, Rosner B, et al. Effects of beer, wine, and liquor in coronary deaths. *JAMA* 1979;242(18):1973-1974.

2271 Stampfer MJ, Colditz GA, Willett WC, et al. A prospective study of moderate alcohol consumption and the risk of coronary disease and stroke in women. *N Engl J Med*, 1988;319(5):267-273.

2272 "Advanced Medium Chain Triglycerides." Prolithic Sports website, URL: www.prolithic.com/hpages/efoods/ mct.html.

© Copyright 2000, Natural Medicines Comprehensive Database (209) 472-2244. For updated data, go to www.NaturalDatabase.com. • 1205

2273 Sills MA, Forsythe WI, Haidukewych D, et al. "The medium chain triglyceride diet and intractable epilepsy." *Arch Dis Child*, 1986;61(12):1168-72.

2274 Trauner DA. "Medium-chain triglyceride (MCT) diet in intractable seizure disorders." *Neurology*, 1985;35(2):237-8.

2275 Nijveldt RJ, Tan AM, Prins HA, et al. "Use of a mixture of medium-chain triglycerides and longchain triglycerides versus long-chain triglycerides in critically ill surgical patients: a randomized prospective double-blind study." *Clin Nutr*, 1998;17(1):23-9.

2276 Ball MJ. "Parenteral nutrition in the critically ill: use of a medium chain triglyceride emulsion." *Intensive Care Med*, 1993;19(2):89-95.

2277 Jiang ZM, Zhang SY, Wang XR, et al. "A comparison of medium-chain and long-chain triglycerides in surgical patients." *Ann Surg*, 1993;217(2):175-84.

2278 Clarke PJ, Ball MJ, Hands LJ, et al. "Use of a lipid containing medium chain triglycerides in patients receiving TPN: a randomized prospective trial." *Br J Surg*, 1987;74(8):701-4.

2279 Truelsen T, Gronbaek M, Schnohr P, et al. Intake of beer, wine, and spirits and risk of stroke: the copenhagen city heart study. *Stroke*, 1998;29(12):2467-2472.

2280 Iversen HK. "N-acetylcysteine enhances nitroglycerin-induced headache and cranial arterial responses." *Clin Pharmacol, Ther* 1992;52(2):125-33.

2281 Hogan JC, Lewis MJ, Henderson AH. "N-acetylcysteine fails to attenuate haemodynamic tolerance to glyceryl trinitrate in healthy volunteers." *Br J Clin Pharmacol*, 1989;28(4):421-6.

2282 Hogan JC, Lewis MJ, Henderson AH. "Chronic administration of N-acetylcysteine fails to prevent nitrate tolerance in patients with stable angina pectoris." *Br J Clin Pharmacol*, 1990;30(4):573-7.

2283 American Pharmaceutical Association. Handbook of Nonprescription Drugs. 11th Ed. Washington, DC: American Pharmaceutical Association; 1996.

2285 "Phyto-soy." 1001Herbs. URL: www.1001herbs.com/phyto-soy/index.html

2286 Soroka N, Silverberg DS, Greemland M, et al. "Comparison of a vegetable-based (soya) and an animal-based low-protein diet in predialysis chronic renal failure patients." *Nephron*, 1998;79(2):173-80.

2287 Gentile MG, Fellin G, Cofano F, et al. "Treatment of proteinuric patients with a vegetarian soy diet and fish oil." *Clin Nephrol*, 1993 Dec;40(6):315-20.

2288 D'Amico G, Gentile MG. "Effect of dietary manipulation on the lipid abnormalities and urinary protein loss in nephrotic patients." *Miner Electrolyte Metab*, 1992;18(2-5):203-6.

2289 Anderson JW, Blake JE, Turner J, et al. "Effects of soy protein on renal function and proteinuria in patients with type 2 diabetes." *Am J Clin Nutr*, 1998;68(6 Suppl):1347S-1353S.

2290 Franke AA, Custer LJ, Tanaka Y. "Isoflavones in human breast milk and other biological fluids." *Am J Clin Nutr*, 1998;68(6 Suppl):1466S-1473S.

2291 Brown KH, Perez F, Peerson JM, et al. "Effect of dietary fiber (soy polysaccharide) on the severity, duration, and nutritional outcome of acute, watery diarrhea in children." *Pediatrics* 1993;92(2):241-7.

2292 Vanderhoof JA, Murray ND, Paule CL, et al. "Use of soy fiber in acute diarrhea in infants and toddlers." *Clin Pediatr* (Phila), 1997;36(3):135-9.

2293 Wong WW, Smith EO, Stuff JE, et al. "Cholesterol-lowering effect of soy protein in normocholesterolemic and hypercholesterolemic men." *Am J Clin Nutr*, 1998;68(6 Suppl):1385S-1389S.

2294 Nilausen K, Meinertz H. "Variable lipemic response to dietary soy protein in healthy, normolipemic men." *Am J Clin Nutr*, 1998;68(6 Suppl):1380S-1384S.

2295 Bakhit RM, Klein BP, Essex-Sorlie D, et al. "Intake of 25 g of soybean protein with or without soybean fiber alters plasma lipids in men with elevated cholesterol concentrations." *J Nutr*, 1994;124(2):213-22.

2296 Washburn S, Burke GL, Morgan T, et al. "Effect of soy protein supplementation on serum lipoproteins, blood pressure, and menopausal symptoms in perimenopausal women." *Menopause*, 1999;6(1):7-13.

2297 Albertazzi P, Pansini F, Bonaccorsi G, et al. "The effect of dietary soy supplementation on hot flushes." *Obstet Gynecol*, 1998;91(1):6-11.

2298 Jacobsen BK, Knutsen SF, Fraser GE. "Does high soy milk intake reduce prostate cancer incidence? The Adventist Health Study." *Cancer Causes Control*, 1998;9(6):553-7.

2331 Burton Goldberg Group. Alternative Medicine: The Definitive Guide. Puyallup, WA: Burton Goldberg Group, 1994.

2332 Cambridge Nutraceuticals, "Glutamine." URL: www.cambridgenutra.com. (19 July 1999).

2333 Balch JF, Balch PA. Prescription for Nutritional Healing. 2nd ed., Garden City Park, NY: Avery Publishing Group, 1997.

2334 Scolapio JS, et al. "Effect of growth hormone, glutamine, and diet on adaptation in short-bowel syndrome: a randomized, controlled study." *Gastroenterology*, 1997; 113(4):1074-1081.

2335 Shabert J, et al. "Glutamine/antioxidant supplementation promotes gain in body cell mass in HIV patients with weight loss." *Int Conf AIDS*, 1998; 12:841(abstract no 42336).

2336 Anderson PM, Schroeder G, Skubitz KM. "Oral glutamine reduces the duration and severity of stomatitis after cytotoxic cancer chemotherapy." *Cancer*, 1998; 83(7):1433-439.

2337 Noyer CM, et al. "A double-blind placebo-controlled pilot study of glutamine therapy for abnormal intestinal permeability in patients with AIDS." *Am J Gastroenterol*, 1998; 93(6):972-75.

2338 Den Hond E, et al. "Effect of long-term oral glutamine supplements on small intestinal permeability in patients with Crohn's disease." *J Parenter Enteral Nutr*, 1999; 23(1):7-11.

2339 Van Den Berg CJ, et al. "Glutamine therapy of cystinuria." *Invest Urol*, 1980; 18(2):155-57.

2341 Haub MD, et al. "Acute L-glutamine ingestion does not improve maximal effort exercise." *J Sports Med Phys Fitness*, 1998; 38(3):240-44.

2342 Castell LM, Newsholme EA. "The effects of oral glutamine supplementation on athletes after prolonged, exhaustive exercise." *Nutrition*, 1997; 13(7-8):738-42.

2343 Shils ME, Young VR, eds. *Modern Nutrition in Health and Disease*. 7th ed., Philadelphia: Lea and Febiger, 1988.

2344 Alternative Medicines, "Histidine."URL: www.alternative-medicines.com/herbdesc2/1histidi.htm (19 July 1999).

2345 Staying Healthy With Nutrition, URL: www.healthy.net (19 July 1999).

2346 "Reference Guide for Amino Acids." URL:

www.realtime.net/anr/aminoacd.html#hisidine (19 July 1999).

2347 Gerber DA, Tanenbaum L, Ahrens M. "Free serum histidine levels in patients with rheumatoid arthritis and control subjects following an oral load of free L-histidine." *Metabolism*, 1976; 25(6):655-57.

2348 Discontinued citation (see Ref 2352).

2349 Dixon JS, et al. "The effect of drugs on serum histidine levels in rheumatoid arthritis." *Rheumatol Int*, 1983; 3(4):145-49.

2350 Pinals RS, et al. "Treatment of rheumatoid arthritis with L-histidine: a randomized, placebo-controlled, double-blind trial." *J Rheumatol*, 1977; 4(4):414-19.

2351 Gerber DA, Tanenbaum L, Ahrens M. "Free serum histidine levels in patients with rheumatoid arthritis and control subjects following an oral load of free L-histidine." *Metabolism*, 1976; 25(6):655-57.

2352 Blumenkrantz MJ, et al. "Histidine supplementation for treatment of anaemia of uraemia." *Br Med J* 1975;2(5970):530-33.

2353 Reeves RD, et al. "Failure of histidine supplementation to improve anemia in chronic dialysis patients." *Am J Clin Nutr*, 1977; 30(4):579-81.

2354 Bigwood EJ, ed. Protein and amino acid functions. Oxford, NY: Pergamon Press, 1972.

2355 Sacher RA, McPherson RA, eds. Widdmann's Clinical Interpretation of Laboratory Tests. 10th ed., Philadelphia: FA Davis Company, 1991.

2356 Asai K. Miracle Cure: Organic Germanium. New York: Japan Publications, 1980.

2357 "Germanium." URL: www.tasqbase.com:80/german.htm (19 July 1999).

2358 "Germanium." URL: www.tellafriend.net/germanium.htm (19 July 1999).

2359 Nutri-Mart Cyber Store, "Organic Germanium Info." URL: www.nutrimart.com/ge-132.htm (19 July 1999).

2360 Tao SH, Bolger PM. "Hazard assessment of germanium supplements." Regul Toxicol Pharmacol, 1997; 25(3):211-19.

2361 Byrne TA, et al. "A new treatment for patients with short-bowel syndrome. Growth hormone, glutamine, and a modified diet." *Ann Surg*, 1995; 222(3):243-54.

2362 Byrne TA, et al. "Growth hormone, glutamine, and a modified diet enhance nutrient absorption in patients with severe short bowel syndrome." *JPEN J Parenter Enteral Nutr*, 1995; 19(4):296-302.

2363 Morlion BJ, et al. "Total parenteral nutrition with glutamine dipeptide after major abdominal surgery: a randomized, double-blind, controlled study." *Ann Surg*, 1998; 227(2):302-308.

2364 Skubitz KM, Anderson PM. "Oral glutamine to prevent chemotherapy induced stomatitis: a pilot study." *J Lab Clin Med*, 1996; 127(2):223-28.

2365 Jebb SA, et al. "5-fluorouracil and folinic acid-induced mucositis: no effect of oral glutamine supplementation." *Br J Cancer*, 1994; 70(4):732-35.

2366 Ziegler TR, et al. "Clinical and metabolic efficacy of glutamine-supplemented parenteral nutrition after bone marrow transplantation. A randomized, double-blind, controlled study." *Ann Intern Med*, 1992; 116(10):821-28.

2367 Jebb SA, et al. "5-fluorouracil and folinic acid-induced mucositis: no effect of oral glutamine supplementation." *Br J Cancer*, 1994; 70(4):732-35.

2368 Anderson PM, et al. "Effect of low-dose oral glutamine on painful stomatitis during bone marrow transplantation." *Bone Marrow Transplant*, 1998; 22(4):339-44.

2369 Starling RD, et al. "Effect of inosine supplementation on aerobic and anaerobic cycling performance." *Med Sci Sports Exerc*, 1996; 28(9):1193-198.

2370 Williams MH, et al. "Effect of inosine supplementation on 3-mile treadmill run performance and VO2 peak." *Med Sci Sports Exerc*, 1990; 22(4):517-22.

2371 Ramirez FC, Lee K, Graham DY. "All lactase preparations are not the same: results of a prospective, randomized, placebo-controlled trial." *Am J Gastroenterol*, 1994; 89(4):566-70.

2372 Sanders SW, Tolman KG, Reitberg DP. "Effect of a single dose of lactase on symptoms and expired hydrogen after lactose challenge in lactose-intolerant subjects." *Clin Pharm*, 1992; 11(6):533-38.

2373 Lin MY, et al. "Comparative effects of exogenous lactase (beta-galactosidase) preparations on in vivo lactose digestion." *Dig Dis Sci*, 1993; 38(11):2022-2027.

2374 DairyEase product information. McNeil-PPC Inc. Fort Washington, PA 19034.

2375 Lami F, et al. "Efficacy of addition of exogenous lactase to milk in adult lactase deficiency." *Am J Gastroenterol*, 1988; 83(10):1145-149.

2376 Horowitz M, et al. "Lactose and calcium absorption in postmenopausal osteoporosis." *Arch Intern Med*, 1987; 147(3):534-36.

2377 Newcomer AD, et al. "Lactase deficiency: prevalence in osteoporosis." *Ann Intern Med*, 1978; 89(2):218-20.

2378 Mother Nature's Encyclopedia, "Lipase." URL: www.mothernature.com/ency/Supp/Lipase.asp (19 July 1999).

2379 Lloyd-Still JD. "Cystic fibrosis and colonic strictures. A new "iatrogenic" disease." *J Clin Gastroenterol*, 1995; 21(1):2-5.

2380 Croft NM, Marshall TG, Ferguson A. "Gut inflammation in children with cystic fibrosis on high-dose enzyme supplements." *Lancet* , 1995; 346(8985):1265-267.

2381 Smyth RL, et al. "Fibrosing colonopathy in cystic fibrosis: results of a case-control study." *Lancet* , 1995; 346(8985):1247-251.

2382 Smyth RL, et al. "Strictures of ascending colon in cystic fibrosis and high-strength pancreatic enzymes." *Lancet* , 1994; 343(8889):85-86.

2383 Tursi JM, Phair PG, Barnes GL. "Plant sources of acid stable lipases: potential therapy for cystic fibrosis." *J Paediatr Child Health*, 1994; 30(6):539-43.

2384 Malesci A, "New enteric-coated high-lipase pancreatic extract in the treatment of pancreatic steatorrhea." *J Clin Gastroenterol*, 1994; 18(1):32-35.

2386 Mother Nature's Encyclopedia, "Macular Degeneration." URL: www.mothernature.com/ency/CONCERN/Macular_Degeneration.asp (19 July 1999).

2387 Sies H, Stahl W, Sundquist AR. "Antioxidant functions of vitamins. Vitamins E and C, beta-carotene, and other carotenoids." *Ann N Y Acad Sci*, 1992; 669:7-20.

2388 Snodderly DM. "Evidence for protection against age-related macular degeneration by carotenoids and antioxidant vitamins." *Am J Clin Nutr*, 1995; 62(6 Suppl):1448S-461S.

2389 Landrum JT, Bone RA, Joa H, et al. "A one year study of the macular pigment: the effect of 140 days of a lutein supplement." *Exp Eye Res*, 1997; 65(1):57-62.

2390 van den Berg H, van Vliet T. "Effect of simultaneous, single oral doses of beta-carotene with lutein or lycopene on the beta-carotene and retinyl ester responses in the

REFERENCES

triacylglycerol-rich lipoprotein fraction of men." *Am J Clin Nutr*, 1998; 68(1):82-89.

2391 Kostic D, White WS, Olson JA. "Intestinal absorption, serum clearance, and interactions between lutein and beta-carotene when administered to human adults in separate or combined oral doses." *Am J Clin Nutr*, 1995; 62(3):604-610.

2392 Koonsvitsky BP, et al. "Olestra affects serum concentrations of alpha-tocopherol and carotenoids but not vitamin D or vitamin K status in free-living subjects. *J Nutr*, 1997; 127(8 Suppl):1636S-645S.

2393 Street DA, et al. "Serum antioxidants and myocardial infarction. Are low levels of carotenoids and alpha-tocopherol risk factors for myocardial infarction?" *Circulation*, 1994; 90(3):1154-161.

2394 Seddon JM, et al. "Dietary carotenoids, vitamins A, C, and E, and advanced age-related macular degeneration. Eye Disease Case-Control Study Group." *JAMA* , 1994; 272(18):1413-420.

2395 Hankinson SE, et al. "Nutrient intake and cataract extraction in women: a prospective study." *BMJ*, 1992; 305(6849):335-39.

2396 Zhang S, et al. "Dietary carotenoids and vitamins A, C, and E and risk of breast cancer." *J Natl Cancer Inst*, 1999; 91(6):547-56.

2397 Le Marchand L, et al. "Intake of specific carotenoids and lung cancer risk." *Cancer Epidemiol Biomarkers Prev*, 1993; 2(3):183-87.

2398 Lyle BJ, Mares-Perlman JA, Klein BE, et al. Antioxidant intake and risk of incident age-related nuclear cataracts in the Beaver Dam Eye Study. *Am J Epidemiol* 1999;149:801-809.

2399 Olmedilla B, et al. "Seasonal and sex-related variations in six serum carotenoids, retinol, and alpha-tocopherol." *Am J Clin Nutr*, 1994; 60(1):106-110.

2400 Mother Nature's Encyclopedia. Lycopene. URL: www.mothernature.com/ency/Supp/Lycopene.asp. (Accessed16 July 1999).

2401 Rao AV, Agarwal S. "Bioavailability and in vivo antioxidant properties of lycopene from tomato products and their possible role in the prevention of cancer." *Nutr Cancer*, 1998; 31(3): 199-203.

2402 Paetau I, et al. "Chronic ingestion of lycopene-rich tomato juice or lycopene supplements significantly increases plasma concentrations of lycopene and related tomato carotenoids in humans." *Am J Clin Nut*, 1998; 68(6): 1187-195.

2403 Johnson EJ, et al. "Ingestion by men of a combined dose of beta-carotene and lycopene does not affect the absorption of beta-carotene but improves that of lycopene." *J Nutr*, 1997; 127(9): 1833-837.

2404 La Vecchia C. Mediterranean epidemiological evidence on tomatoes and the prevention of digestive-tract cancers. *Proc Soc Exp Biol Med* 1998;218(2):125-28.

2405 Tzonou A, Signorello LB, Lagiou P, et al. Diet and cancer of the prostate: a case-control study in Greece. *Int J Cancer* 1999;80(5):704-708.

2406 Giovannucci E, Ascherio A, Rimm EB, et al. Intake of carotenoids and retinol in relation to risk of *Prostate* cancer. *J Natl Cancer Inst* 1995;87(23):1767-776.

2407 Giovannucci E. Tomatoes, tomato-based products, lycopene, and cancer: review of the epidemiologic literature. *J Natl Cancer Inst*, 1999;91(4):317-31.

2408 Mother Nature's Encyclopedia. "Methionine." URL: www.mothernature.com/ency/Supp/Methionine.asp (16 July 1999).

2409 La Vecchia C, et al. "Case-control study on influence of methionine, nitrite, and salt on gastric *Carcinogenesis* in northern Italy." *Nutr Cancer*, 1997; 27(1): 65-68.

2410 Bellamy MF, et al. "Hyperhomocysteinemia after an oral methionine load acutely impairs endothelial function in healthy adults." *Circulation*, 1998; 98(18): 1848-852.

2411 Hladovec, J, Sommerova Z, Pisarikova A. "Homocysteinemia and endothelial damage after methionine load." *Thromb Res*, 1997; 88(4): 361-64.

2412 Bellone J, et al. "Methionine potentiates both basal and GHRH-induced GH secretion in children." *Clin Endocrinol*, 1997; 47(1): 61-64.

2413 Vale JA, Meredith TJ, Goulding R. "Treatment of acetaminophen poisoning. The use of oral methionine." *Arch Intern Med*, 1981;141(3 Spec No): 394-396.

2414 Christensen B, et al. "Preoperative methionine loading enhances restoration of the cobalamin-dependent enzyme methionine synthase after nitrous oxide anesthesia." *Anesthesiology*, 1994; 80(5): 1046-056.

2415 Meakins TS, Persaud C, Jackson AA. "Dietary supplementation with L-methionine impairs the utilization of urea-nitrogen and increases 5-L-oxoprolinuria in normal women consuming a low protein diet." *J Nutr*, 1998; 128(4): 720-27.

2416 Mother Nature's Encyclopedia. "Ornithine." URL: www.mothernature.com/ency/Supp/Ornithine.asp. (16 July 1999).

2417 Bucci LR, et al. "Ornithine supplementation and insulin release in bodybuilders." *Int J Sport Nutr*, 1992; 2(3): 287-91.

2418 Fogelholm GM, et al. "Low-dose amino acid supplementation: no effects on serum human growth hormone and insulin in male weightlifters." *Int J Sport Nutr*, 1993; 3(3): 290-97.

2419 Mother Nature's Encyclopedia. "Lecithin." URL: www.mothernature.com/ency/Supp/Lecithin.asp (16 July 1999).

2420 Toouli J, P Jablonski, Watts JM. "Gallstone dissolution in man using cholic acid and lecithin." *Lancet* , 1975; 2(7945): 1124-126.

2421 Tuzhilin SA, et al. "The treatment of patients with gallstones by lecithin." *Am J Gastroenterol*, 1976; 165: 231-35.

2422 Holan KR, et al. "Effect of oral administration of 'essential' phospholipid, beta-glycerophosphate, and linoleic acid on biliary lipids in patients with cholelithiasis." *Digestion*, 1979; 19(4): 251-58.

2423 Jenkins PJ, et al. "Use of polyunsaturated phosphatidyl choline in HBsAg negative chronic active hepatitis: results of prospective double-blind controlled trial." *Liver*, 1982; 2(2): 77-81.

2424 Niederau C, et al. "Polyunsaturated phosphatidyl-choline and interferon alpha for treatment of chronic hepatitis B and C: a multi-center, randomized, double-blind, placebo-controlled trial." *Hepatogastroenterology*, 1998; 45(21): 797-804.

2425 Glenberg AJ, et al. "Lithium and lecithin in tardive dyskinesia: an update." *Psychiatry Res*, 1986; 19(2): 101-04.

2426 Volavka J, et al. "Lithium and lecithin in tardive dyskinesia: an update." *Psychiatry Res*, 1986; 19(2): 101-04.

2427 Domino EF, et al. "Lack of clinically significant improvement of patients with tardive dyskinesia following phosphatidylcholine therapy." *Biol Psychiatry*, 1985; 20(11): 1189-196.

2428 Thal LJ, et al. "Oral physostigmine and lecithin improve memory in Alzheimer disease." *Ann Neurol*, 1983; 13(5): 491-96.

2429 Little A, et al. "A double-blind, placebo controlled trial of high-dose lecithin in Alzheimer's disease." *J Neurol Neurosurg Psychiatry*, 1985; 48(8): 736-42.

2430 Jenike MA, et al. "Combination therapy with lecithin and ergoloid mesylates for Alzheimer's disease." *J Clin Psychiatry*, 1986; 47(5): 249-51.

2431 Foster NL, et al. "An enriched-population, double-blind, placebo-controlled, crossover study of tacrine and lecithin in Alzheimer's disease." The Tacrine 970-6 Study Group. *Dementia*, 1996; 7(5): 260-66.

2432 Heyman A, et al. "Failure of long term high-dose lecithin to retard progression of early- onset Alzheimer's disease." *J Neural Transm Suppl*, 1987; 24: 279-86.

2433 Cohen BM, et al. "Lecithin in the treatment of mania: double-blind, placebo-controlled trials." *Am J Psychiatry*, 1982; 139(9): 1162-164.

2434 Ladd SL, et al. "Effect of phosphatidylcholine on explicit memory." *Clin Neuropharmacol*, 1993; 16(6): 540-49.

2435 Harris CM, et al. "Effect of lecithin on memory in normal adults." *Am J Psychiatry*, 1983; 140(8): 1010-012.

2436 Mother Nature's Encyclopedia. "Phosphatidylserine." URL: www.mothernature.com/ency/Supp/ Phosphatidylserine.asp. (16 July 1999).

2437 Crook T, et al. "Effects of phosphatidylserine in Alzheimer's disease." *Psychopharmacol Bull*, 1992; 28(1): 61-66.

2438 Delwaide PJ, et al. "Double-blind randomized controlled study of phosphatidylserine in senile demented patients." *Acta Neurol Scand*, 1986; 73(2): 136-40.

2439 Engel RR, et al. "Double-blind cross-over study of phosphatidylserine vs. placebo in patients with early dementia of the Alzheimer type." *Eur Neuropsychopharmacol*, 1992; 2(2): 149-55.

2440 Cenacchi T, et al. "Cognitive decline in the elderly: a double-blind, placebo-controlled multicenter study on efficacy of phosphatidylserine administration." *Aging* (Milano), 1993; 5(2): 123-33.

2441 Crook TH, et al. "Effects of phosphatidylserine in age-associated memory impairment." *Neurology*, 1991; 41(5): 644-49.

2442 Mother Nature's Encyclopedia. "OKG." URL: www.mothernature.com/ency/Supp/OKG.asp. (16 July 1999).

2443 De Bandt JP, et al. "A randomized controlled trial of the influence of the mode of enteral ornithine alpha-ketoglutarate administration in burn patients." *J Nutr*, 1998; 128(3): 563-69.

2444 Moukarzel AA, et al. "Growth retardation in children receiving long-term total parenteral nutrition: effects of ornithine alpha-ketoglutarate." *Am J Clin Nutr*, 1994; 60(3): 408-13.

2445 Wernerman J, et al. "Glutamine and ornithine-alpha-ketoglutarate but not branched-chain amino acids reduce the loss of muscle glutamine after surgical trauma." *Metabolism*, 1989; 38(8 Suppl 1): 63-66.

2446 Wernerman J, et al. "Ornithine-alpha-ketoglutarate improves skeletal muscle protein synthesis as assessed by ribosome analysis and nitrogen use after surgery." *Ann Surg*, 1987; 206(5): 674-78.

2447 Woollard ML, et al. "Controlled trial of ornithine alpha ketoglutarate (OAKG) in patients with stroke." *Stroke*, 1978; 9(3): 218-22.

2448 Blomqvist BI, et al. "Glutamine and alpha-ketoglutarate prevent the decrease in muscle free glutamine concentration and influence protein synthesis after total hip replacement." *Metabolism*, 1995; 44(9): 1215-222.

2449 Chainuvati T, Plengvanit U, Viranuvatti V. "Ornicetil on encephalopathy. Effect of ornicetil (ornithine alpha-ketoglutarate) on encephalopathy in patients with acute and chronic liver disease." *Acta HepatoGastroenterol* (Stuttg), 1977; 24(6): 434-39.

2450 Gay G, et al. "Effects of ornithine alphaketoglutarate on blood insulin, glucagon and aminoacids in alcoholic cirrhosis." *Biomedicine*, 1979; 30(3): 173-77.

2451 Cynober L, et al. "Action of ornithine alpha-ketoglutarate, ornithine hydrochloride, and calcium alpha-ketoglutarate on plasma amino acid and hormonal patterns in healthy subjects." *J Am Coll Nutr*, 1990; 9(1): 2-12.

2452 Marconi C, Sassi G, Cerretelli P. "The effect of an alpha-ketoglutarate-pyridoxine complex on human maximal aerobic and anaerobic performance." *Eur J Appl Physiol*, 1982; 49(3): 307-17.

2453 Mother Nature's Enculclopedia. "Phenylalanine." URL: www.mothernature.com/ency/Supp/Phenylalanine.asp (Accessed 16 July 1999).

2454 Cotzias GC, Van Woert MH, Schiffer LM. "Aromatic amino acids and modification of parkinsonism." *N Engl J Med*, 1967;276(7): 374-79.

2455 Heller, Fischer BE, Martin R. "Therapeutic action of D-phenylalanine in Parkinson's disease." *Arzneimittelforschung*, 1976;26(4):577-579.

2456 Kitade T, et al. "Studies on the enhanced effect of acupuncture analgesia and acupuncture anesthesia by D-phenylalanine (2nd report)- schedule of administration and clinical effects in low back pain and tooth extraction." *Acupunct Electrother Res*, 1990;15(2): 121-135.

2457 Mosnik DM, et al. "Tardive dyskinesia exacerbated after ingestion of phenylalanine by schizophrenic patients." *Neuropsychopharmacology*, 1997;16(2):136-146.

2458 Gardos G, et al. "The acute effects of a loading dose of phenylalanine in unipolar depressed patients with and without tardive dyskinesia." *Neuropsychopharmacology*, 1992;6(4):241-247.

2459 Walsh NE, Ramamurthy S, Schoenfeld L, Hoffman J. Analgesic effectiveness of D-phenylalanine in chronic pain patients. *Arch Phys Med Rehabil* 1986;67(7):436-439.

2460 Mitchell MJ, Daines GE, Thomas BL. "Effect of L-tryptophan and phenylalanine on burning pain threshold." *Phys Ther*, 1987;67(2):203-205.

2461 Antoniou C, et al. "Vitiligo therapy with oral and topical phenylalanine with UVA exposure." *Int J Dermatol*, 1989;28(8):545-547.

2462 Greiner D, Ochsendorf F, Milbradt R. [Vitiligo therapy with phenylalanine/UV A. Catamnestic studies after five years]. [Article in German]. *Hautarzt*, 1994;45(7):460-463.

2463 Siddiqui AH, et al. "L-phenylalanine and UVA irradiation in the treatment of vitiligo." *Dermatology*, 1994; 188(3): 215-18.

2464 Thiele B, Steigleder GK. [Repigmentation treatment of vitiligo with L-phenylalanine and UVA irradiation]. [Article in German]. *Z Hautkr*, 1987; 62(7): 519-23.

2465 Cormane RH, et al. "Phenylalanine and UVA light for the treatment of vitiligo." *Arch Dermatol Res*, 1985;

REFERENCES

R
E
F
E
R
E
N
C
E
S

277(2): 126-30.

2466 Kuiters GR, et al. "Oral phenylalanine loading and sunlight as source of UVA irradiation in vitiligo on the Caribbean island of Curacao NA." *J Trop Med Hyg*, 1986; 89(3): 149-55.

2467 Schulpis CH, et al. "Phenylalanine plus ultraviolet light: preliminary report of a promising treatment for childhood vitiligo." *Pediatr Dermatol*, 1989; 6(4): 332-35.

2468 Beckmann H, et al. "DL-phenylalanine versus imipramine: a double-blind controlled study." *Arch Psychiatr Nervenkr*, 1979; 227(1): 49-58.

2469 Birkmayer W, et al. "L-deprenyl plus L-phenylalanine in the treatment of depression." *J Neural Transm*, 1984; 59(1): 81-87.

2470 Henry JB, ed. Clinical Diagnosis and Management by Laboratory Methods. 19th ed. Philadelphia,PA: W.B. Saunders, 1996.

2471 Mother Nature Website, Pyruvate. URL: www.mothernature.com/ency/Supp/Pyruvate.asp.

2472 Stanko RT, Tietze DL, Arch JE. "Body composition, energy utilization, and nitrogen Metabolism with a 4.25-MJ/d low-energy diet supplemented with pyruvate." *Am J Clin Nutr*, 1992; 56(4): 630-35.

2473 Matthys D, Van Coster R, Verhaaren H. "Fatal outcome of pyruvate loading test in child with restrictive cardiomyopathy." *Lancet* , 1991; 338(8773): 1020-021.

2474 Stanko RT, et al. "Pyruvate supplementation of a low-cholesterol, low-fat diet: effects on plasma lipid concentrations and body composition in hyperlipidemic patients." *Am J Clin Nutr*, 1994; 59(2): 423-27.

2475 Wagner DR "Hyperhydrating with glycerol: implications for athletic performance." *J Am Diet Assoc*, 1999; 99(2): 207-12.

2476 Murray R, et al. "Physiological responses to glycerol ingestion during exercise." *J Appl Physiol*, 1991; 71(1): 144-49.

2477 Robergs RA, Griffin SE. "Glycerol. Biochemistry, pharmacokinetics and clinical and practical applications." *Sports Med*, 1998; 26(3): 145-67.

2478 Arnall DA, Goforth HW. "Failure to reduce body water loss in cold-water immersion by glycerol ingestion." *Undersea Hyperb Med*, 1993; 20(4): 309-20.

2479 Montner P, et al. "Pre-exercise glycerol hydration improves cycling endurance time." *Int J Sports Med*, 1996; 17(1): 27-33.

2480 Yu YL, et al. "Treatment of acute cortical infarct with intravenous glycerol. A double-blind, placebo-controlled randomized trial." *Stroke*, 1993; 24(8): 1119-124.

2481 Yu YL, et al. "Treatment of acute cerebral hemorrhage with intravenous glycerol. A double-blind, placebo-controlled, randomized trial." *Stroke*, 1992; 23(7): 967-71.

2482 Frei A, et al. "Glycerol and dextran combined in the therapy of acute stroke. A placebo-controlled, double-blind trial with a planned interim analysis." *Stroke*, 1987; 18(2): 373-79.

2483 Bayer AJ, Pathy MS, Newcombe R. "Double-blind randomised trial of intravenous glycerol in acute *s*troke." *Lancet* 1987; 1(8530): 405-08.

2484 Friedli W, et al. [Treatment with 10% glycerin in acute ischemic cerebral infarct. Doubleblind study]. [Article in German]. *Schweiz Med Wochenschr*, 1979; 109(20): 737-42.

2485 Bjorvell H, Hylander B, Rossner S. "Effects of glycerol addition to diet in weight-reducing clubs." *Int J Obes*,

1984; 8(2): 129-33.

2486 Fawer R, et al. "Intravenous glycerol in cerebral infarction: a controlled 4-month trial." *Stroke*, 1978; 9(5): 484-86.

2487 Ivy JL, et al. "Effects of pyruvate on the Metabolism and insulin resistance of obese Zucker rats." *Am J Clin Nutr*, 1994; 59(2): 331-37.

2488 DeBoer LW, et al. "Pyruvate enhances recovery of rat hearts after ischemia and reperfusion by preventing free radical generation." *Am J Physiol*, 1993; 265(5 Pt 2): H1571-576.

2489 DMV International Nutritionals. "Health Benifits of Lactoferrin." URL: www.lfplus.com/s2/2.html. (16 July 1999).

2490 Yamauchi K, et al. "Effects of orally administered bovine lactoferrin on the immune system of healthy volunteers." *Adv Exp Med Biol*, 1998; 443: 261-65.

2491 Bellamy W, et al. "Antibacterial spectrum of lactoferricin B, a potent bactericidal peptide derived from the N-terminal region of bovine lactoferrin." *J Appl Bacteriol*, 1992; 73(6): 472-79.

2492 Inder WJ, et al. "The effect of glycerol and desmopressin on exercise performance and hydration in triathletes." *Med Sci Sports Exerc*, 1998; 30(8): 1263-269.

2493 Tremblay MS, Galloway SD, Sexsmith JR. "Ergogenic effects of phosphate loading: physiological fact or methodological fiction?" *Physiol*, 1994; 19(1): 1-11.

2494 Hill AG, et al. "Cellular potassium depletion predisposes to hypokalaemia after oral sodium phosphate." *Aust N Z J Surg*, 1998; 68(12): 856-58.

2495 Clarkston WK, et al. "Oral sodium phosphate versus sulfate-free polyethylene glycol electrolyte lavage solution in outpatient preparation for colonoscopy: a prospective comparison." *Gastrointest Endosc*, 1996; 43(1): 42-48.

2496 Fine A, Patterson J. "Severe hyperphosphatemia following phosphate administration for bowel preparation in patients with renal failure: two cases and a review of the literature." *Am J Kidney Dis*, 1997; 29(1): 103-05.

2497 DiPalma JA, et al. "Biochemical effects of oral sodium phosphate." *Dig Dis Sci*, 1996; 41(4): 749-53.

2498 Helikson MA, Parham WA, Tobias JD. "Hypocalcemia and hyperphosphatemia after phosphate enema use in a child." *J Pediatr* Surg, 1997; 32(8): 1244-246.

2499 Galloway SD, et al. "The effects of acute phosphate supplementation in subjects of different aerobic fitness levels." *Eur J Appl Physiol*, 1996; 72(3): 224-30.

2500 Uebelhack R, Franke L, Schewe HJ. Inhibition of platelet MAO-B by kava pyrone-enriched extract from Piper methysticum Forster (kava-kava). *Pharmacopsychiatry* 1998;31(5):187-92.

2501 Gleitz J, Beile A, Wilkens P, et al. Antithrombotic action of the kava pyrone (+)-kavain prepared from Piper methysticum on human platelets. *Planta Med* 1997;63(1):27-30.

2502 Dwivedi S, Jauhari R . Beneficial effects of Terminalia arjuna in coronary artery disease. *Indian Heart J* 1997;49(5):507-510.

2503 Dwivedi S, Agarwal MP. Antianginal and cardioprotective effects of Terminalia arjuna, an indigenous drug, in coronary artery disease. *J Assoc Physicians India* 1994;42(4):287-289.

2504 Bharani A, Ganguly A, Bhargava KD. Salutary effect of Terminalia Arjuna in patients with severe refractory heart failure. *Int J Cardiol* 1995;49(3):191-199.

2505 Ram A, Lauria P, Gupta R, et al. Hypocholesterolaemic effects of Terminalia arjuna tree bark. *J Ethnopharmacol* 1997;55(3):165-169.

2506 Pettit GR, Hoard MS, Doubek DL, et al. Antineoplastic agents 338. The cancer cell growth inhibitory. Constituents of Terminalia arjuna (Combretaceae). *J Ethnopharmacol* 1996;53(2):57-63.

2507 Anand KK, Singh B, Saxena AK, et al. 3,4,5-Trihydroxy benzoic acid (gallic acid), the hepatoprotective principle in the fruits of Terminalia belerica-bioassay guided activity. *Pharmacol Res* 1997;36(4):315-321.

2508 Sato Y, Oketani H, Singyouchi K, et al. Extraction and purification of effective antimicrobial constituents of Terminalia chebula RETS. against methicillin-resistant Staphylococcus aureus. *Biol Pharm Bull* 1997 Apr;20(4):401-404.

2509 Yukawa TA, Kurokawa M, Sato H, et al. Prophylactic treatment of cytomegalovirus infection with traditional herbs. *Antiviral Res* 1996;32(2):63-70.

2510 Shiraki K, Yukawa T, Kurokawa M, Kageyama S. Cytomegalovirus infection and its possible treatment with herbal medicines. [Article in Japanese] *Nippon Rinsho* 1998;56(1):156-160.

2511 Suthienkul O, Miyazaki O, Chulasiri M, et al. Retroviral reverse transcriptase inhibitory activity in Thai herbs and spices: screening with Moloney murine leukemia viral enzyme. *Southeast Asian J Trop Med Public Health* 1993;24(4):751-755.

2512 Kurokawa M, Nagasaka K, Hirabayashi T, et al. Efficacy of traditional herbal medicines in combination with acyclovir against herpes simplex virus type 1 infection in vitro and in vivo. *Antiviral Res* 1995;27(1-2):19-37.

2513 Jagtap AG, Karkera SG. Potential of the aqueous extract of Terminalia chebula as an anticaries agent. *J Ethnopharmacol* 1999 Dec 15;68(1-3):299-306.

2514 Phadke SA, Kulkarni SD. Screening of in vitro antibacterial activity of Terminalia chebula, Eclapta alba and Ocimum sanctum. *Indian J Med Sci* 1989;43(5):113-117.

2515 Hamada S, Kataoka T, Woo JT, et al. Immunosuppressive effects of gallic acid and chebulagic acid on CTL-mediated cytotoxicity. *Biol Pharm Bull* 1997;20(9):1017-1019.

2516 Arseculeratne SN, Gunatilaka AA, Panabokke RG. Studies of medicinal plants of Sri Lanka. Part 14: Toxicity of some traditional medicinal herbs. *J Ethnopharmacol* 1985;13(3):323-335.

2517 Shaila HP, Udupa SL, Udupa AL. Hypolipidemic activity of three indigenous drugs in experimentally induced Atherosclerosis. *Int J Cardiol* 1998;67(2):119-214.

2518 el-Mekkawy S, Meselhy MR, Kusumoto IT, et al. Inhibitory effects of Egyptian folk medicines on human immunodeficiency virus (HIV) reverse transcriptase. *Chem Pharm Bull* (Tokyo) 1995;43(4):641-648.

2519 Thakur CP, Thakur B, Singh S, et al. The Ayurvedic medicines Haritaki, Amala and Bahira reduce cholesterol-induced atherosclerosis in rabbits. *Int J Cardiol* 1988;21(2):167-175.

2520 Kiistala R, Makinen-Kiljunen S, Heikkinen K, et al. Occupational allergic rhinitis and contact urticaria caused by bishop's weed (Ammi majus). *Allergy* 1999;54(6):635-639.

2521 Ossenkoppele PM, van der Sluis WG, van Vloten WA. [Phototoxic dermatitis following the use of Ammi majus fruit for vitiligo]. [Article in Dutch] *Ned Tijdschr Geneeskd* 1991;135(11):478-480.

2522 Harvengt C, Desager JP. HDL-cholesterol increase in normolipaemic subjects on khellin: a pilot study. *Int J Clin Pharmacol Res* 1983;3(5):363-366.

2523 Durate J, Vallejo I, Perez-Vizcaino F, et al. Effects of visnadine on rat isolated vascular smooth muscles. *Planta Med* 1997;63(3):233-236.

2524 Duarte J, Perez-Vizcaino F, Torres AI, et al. Vasodilator effects of visnagin in isolated rat vascular smooth muscle. *Eur J Pharmacol* 1995;286(2):115-122.

2525 Rauwald HW, Brehm O, Odenthal KP. The involvement of a Ca2+ channel blocking mode of action in the pharmacology of Ammi visnaga fruits. *Planta Med* 1994;60(2):101-105.

2526 Ahsan SK, Tariq M, Ageel AM, et al. Effect of Trigonella foenum-graecum and Ammi majus on calcium oxalate urolithiasis in rats. *J Ethnopharmacol* 1989;26(3):249-254.

2527 Shlosberg A, Egyed MN. Examples of poisonous plants in Israel of importance to animals and man. *Arch Toxicol Suppl* 1983;6:194-196.

2528 Bethea D, Fullmer B, Syed S, et al. Psoralen photobiology and photochemotherapy: 50 years of science and medicine. *J Dermatol Sci*, 1999;19(2):78-88.

2529 McKevoy GK, ed. AHFS Drug Information. Bethesda, MD: American Society of Health-System Pharmacists, 2000.

2530 Rehman J, Dillow JM, Carter SM, et al. Increased production of antigen-specific immunoglobulins G and M following in vivo treatment with the medicinal plants Echinacea angustifolia and Hydrastis canadensis. *Immunol Lett* 1999;68(2-3):391-5.

2532 Eddleston M, S Rajapakse S, Rajakanthan K, et al. Anti-digoxin Fab fragments in cardiotoxicity induced by ingestion of yellow oleander: a randomized controlled trial. *Lancet* , 2000; 355(9208):967-972.

2533 McAlindon TE, LaValley MP, Gulin JP, Felson DT. Glucosamine and Chondroitin for Treatment of Osteoarthritis A Systematic Quality Assessment and Meta-analysis. *JAMA* 2000;283:1469-1475.

2534 Jensen GS, Ginsberg DJ, Huerta P, et al. Consumption of Aphanizomenon flos-aquae has rapid effects on the circulation and function of immune cells in humans. A novel approach to nutritional mobilization of the immune system. *JANA*, 2000;2(3):50;50-56.

2535 Kushak RI, Drapeau C, Van Cott EM, Winter HH. Favorable effects of blue-green algae Aphanizomenon flos-aquae on rat plasma lipids. *JANA*, 2000;2(3):50;59-65.

2537 Choi HK, Jung GW, Moon KH, et al. Clinical study of SS-Cream in patients with lifelong premature ejaculation. *Urology*, 2000;55(2):257-261.

2538 Kiesewetter H, Koscielny J, Kalus U, et al. Efficacy of orally administered extract of red vine leaf AS 195 (folia vitis viniferae) in chronic venous insufficiency (stages I-II). A randomized, double-blind, placebo-controlled trial. *Arzneimittelforschung* 2000;50(2):109-17.

2539 Xiao Dong S, Zhi Ping Z, Zhong Xiao W, et al. Possible enhancement of the first-pass metabolism of phenacetin by ingestion of grape juice in Chinese subjects. *Br J Clin Pharmacol* 1999;48(4):638-40.

2540 Ozturk HS, Kacmaz M, Cimen MY, Durak I. Red wine and black grape strengthen blood antioxidant potential. *Nutrition* 1999;15(11-12):954-5.

2541 Bombardelli E and Morazzoni P. *Vitis vinifera L.*

REFERENCES

Fitoterapia 1995; LXVI(4):291-317.

2546 Lee JY, Lee KS, Kim TS, et al. Squalene-induced extrinsic lipoid pneumonia: serial radiologic findings in nine patients. *J Comput Assist Tomogr* 1999;23(5):730-5.

2547 Lee JS, Im JG, Song KS, et al. Exogenous lipoid pneumonia: high-resolution CT findings. *Eur Radiol* 1999;9(2):287-91.

2548 Asnis DS, Saltzman HP, Melchert A. Shark oil pneumonia. An overlooked entity. *Chest* 1993,103(3):976-7.

2549 Skopinska-Rozewska E, Krotkiewski M, Sommer E, et al. Inhibitory effect of shark liver oil on cutaneous angiogenesis induced in Balb/c mice by syngeneic sarcoma L-1, human urinary bladder and human kidney tumour cells. *Oncol Rep* 1999;6(6):1341-4.

2550 Hichami A, Duroudier V, Leblais V, et al. Modulation of platelet-activating-factor production by incorporation of naturally occurring 1-O-alkylglycerols in phospholipids of human leukemic monocyte-like THP-1 cells. *Eur J Biochem* 1997;250(2):242-8.

2551 Loftsson T, Petersen DS, Le Goffic F, Olafsson JH. Unsaturated glycerol monoethers as novel skin penetration enhancers. *Pharmazie* 1997;52(6):463-5.

2552 Hasle H, Rose C. [Shark liver oil (alkoxyglycerol) and cancer treatment]. *Ugeskr Laeger* 1991;153(5):343-6. [Article in Danish]

2583 Sun D, Abraham SN, Beachey EH. Influence of berberine sulfate on synthesis and expression of Pap fimbrial adhesin in uropathogenic Escherichia coli. *Antimicrob Agents Chemother* 1988;32(8):1274-7.

2584 Sun D, Courtney HS, Beachey EH. Berberine sulfate blocks adherence of Streptococcus pyogenes to epithelial cells, fibronectin, and hexadecane. *Antimicrob Agents Chemother* 1988;32(9):1370-4.

2585 Amin AH, Subbaiah TV, Abbasi KM. Berberine sulfate: antimicrobial activity, bioassay, and mode of action. *Can J Microbiol.* 1969 Sep;15(9):1067-76.

2586 Khin-Maung-U, Myo-Khin, Nyunt-Nyunt-Wai, Clinical trial of berberine in acute watery diarrhoea. *Br Med J* (Clin Res Ed) 1985;291(6509):1601-5.

2587 Kaneda Y, Torii M, Tanaka T, Aikawa M. In vitro effects of berberine sulphate on the growth and structure of Entamoeba histolytica, Giardia lamblia and Trichomonas vaginalis. *Ann Trop Med Parasitol* 1991;85(4):417-25.

2588 Gupte S. Use of berberine in treatment of giardiasis. *Am J Dis Child* 1975; 129:866.

2589 Chan E. Displacement of bilirubin from albumin by berberine. *Biol Neonate* 1993;63(4):201-8.

2590 Winek CL, Elzein EO, Wahba WW, Feldman JA. Interference of herbal drinks with urinalysis for drugs of abuse. *J Anal Toxicol* 1993;17(4):246-7.

2591 Bhide MB, Shaven SR, Dutta NK. Absorption, distribution, and excretion of berberine. *Indian J Med Res* 1969;57(11):2128-31.

2596 Osterhoudt KC, Lee SK, Callahan JM, Henretig FM. Catnip and the alteration of human consciousness. *Vet Hum Toxicol* 1997 Dec;39(6):373-5.

2597 Just MJ, Recio MC, Giner RM, et al. Anti-inflammatory activity of unusual lupane saponins from Bupleurum fruticescens. *Planta Med* 1998;64(5):404-7.

2598 Matsumoto T, Yamada H. Regulation of immune complexes binding of macrophages by pectic polysaccharide from Bupleurum falcatum L.: pharmacological evidence for the requirement of intracellular calcium/calmodulin on Fc receptor up-regulation by bupleuran 2IIb. *J Pharm Pharmacol*

1995;47(2):152-6.

2599 Gil ML, Jimenez J, Ocete MA, et al. Comparative study of different essential oils of Bupleurum gibraltaricum Lamarck. *Pharmazie* 1989;44(4):284-7.

2600 Drovanti A, Bignamini AA, Rovati AA. Therapeutic activity of oral glucosamine sulfate in osteoarthrosis: a placebo-controlled double-blind investigation. *Clin Ther*, 1980;3:260-272.

2601 da Camara CC, Dowless GV. Glucosamine sulfate for osteoarthritis. *Ann Pharmacother*, 1998;32:580-587.

2602 Vaz AL. Double-blind clinical evaluation of the relative efficacy of ibuprofen and glucosamine sulphate in the management of osteoarthrosis of the knee in out-patients. *Curr Med Res Opin*, 1982;8:145-149.

2603 Pugalte JM, Llavore EP, Ylescupidez FR. Double-blind clinical evaluation of oral glucosamine sulphate in the basic treatment of osteoarthrosis. *Curr Med Res Opin*, 1980;7:110-114.

2604 Qiu GX, et al. Efficacy and safety of glucosamine sulfate versus ibuprofen in patients with knee osteoarthritis. *Arzneimittelforschung*, 1998;48:469-474.

2605 Reichelt A. Efficacy and safety of intramuscular glucosamine sulfate in osteoarthritis of the knee. A randomised, placebo-controlled, double-blind study. *Arzneimittelforschung*, 1994;44:75-80.

2606 Forster KK, et al. Longer-term treatment of mild-to-moderate osteoarthritis of the knee with glucosamine sulfate - a randomized, controlled, double-blind clinical study. *Euro J Clin Pharmacol*, 1996;50:542.

2607 Setnikar I, et al. Pharmacokinetics of glucosamine in man. *Arzneimittelforschung*, 1993;43:1109-1113.

2608 Barclay TS, Tsourounis C, McCart GM. Glucosamine. *Ann Pharmacother*, 1998;32:574-579.

2609 Burton AF, Anderson FH. "Decreased incorporation of 14C-glucosamine relative to 3H-N-acetyl glucosamine in the intestinal mucosa of patients with inflammatory bowel disease." *Am J Gastroenterol*, 1983; 78: 19-22.

2610 Goodman MJ, Kent PW, Truelove SC. "Glucosamine synthetase activity of the colonic mucosa in ulcerative colitis and Crohn's disease." *Gut*, 1977; 18: 219-28.

2611 Talent JM, Gracy RW. "Pilot study of oral polymeric N-acetyl-D-glucosamine as a potential treatment for patients with osteoarthritis." *Clin Ther*, 1996; 18: 1184-190.

2612 Leite JR, et al. "Pharmacology of lemongrass (Cymbopogon citratus Stapf). III. Assessment of eventual toxic, hypnotic and anxiolytic effects on humans." *J Ethnopharmacol*, 1986; 17: 75-83.

2613 Feher J, et al. [Liver-protective action of silymarin therapy in chronic alcoholic liver diseases]. *Orv Hetil*, 1989; 130: 2723-727.

2614 Szilard S, Szentgyorgyi D, Demeter I. "Protective effect of Legalon in workers exposed to organic solvents." *Acta Med Hung*, 1988; 45: 249-56.

2615 Hruby, et al. "Chemotherapy of Amanita phalloides poisoning with intravenous silibinin." *Hum Toxicol*, 1983; 2: 183-95.

2616 Ferenci P, et al. "Randomized controlled trial of silymarin treatment in patients with cirrhosis of the liver." *J Hepatol*, 1989; 9: 105-13.

2617 Velussi M, et al. "Long-term (12 months) treatment with an anti-oxidant drug (silymarin) is effective on hyperinsulinemia, exogenous insulin need and malondialdehyde levels in cirrhotic diabetic patients." *J Hepatol*, 1997; 26: 871-79.

2618 Salmi HA, Sarna S. "Effect of silymarin on chemical,

functional, and morphological alterations of the liver. A double-blind controlled study." *Scand J Gastroenterol*, 1982; 17: 517-21.

2619 Hebel SK, ed. Drug Facts and Comparisons. 52nd ed. St. Louis: Facts and Comparisons, 1998.

2620 Tyrey. "Delta 9-Tetrahydrocannabinol: a potent inhibitor of episodic luteinizing hormone secretion." *J Pharmacol Exp Ther*, 1980; 213: 306-08.

2621 Sallan SE, Zinberg NE, Frei E 3d. "Antiemetic effect of delta-9-tetrahydrocannabinol in patients receiving cancer chemotherapy." *N Engl J Med*, 1975;293:795-797.

2622 Schwartz RH, Beveridge RA. "Marijuana as an antiemetic drug: how useful is it today? Opinions from clinical oncologists." *J Addict Dis*, 1994; 13: 53-65.

2623 FDA/ORA CPG 7121.01. Sec. 457.100 "Pangamic Acid and Pangamic Acid Products Unsafe for Food and Drug Use." (CPG 7121.01) URL: www.fda.gov/ora/compliance_ref/cpg/cpgdrg/cpg457-100.html (16 July 1999).

2624 Heber D, et al. "Cholesterol-lowering effects of a proprietary Chinese red-yeast-rice dietary supplement." *Am J Clin Nutr*, 1999; 69: 231-36.

2625 Food and Drug Administration web site. "FDA Talk Paper: FDA determines Cholestin to be unapproved drug." URL: www.fda.gov/bbs/topics/ANSWERS/ANS00871.html (3 May 1999).

2626 Nando Media Web site. "Judge rules against FDA in Cholestin challenge." URL: www.nandotimes.com/healthscience/story/body/0,1079,19548-32099-232485-0,00.html (Accessed 3 May 1999).

2627 Puente S, et al. "Eosinophilic gastroenteritis caused by bee pollen sensitization." *Med Clin (Barc)*, 10 May 1997; 108(18): 698-700.

2628 Fleche C, et al. "Contamination of bee products and risk for human health: situation in France." *Rev Sci Tech*, 1997; 16: 609-19.

2629 Lee SK, et al. "Modulation of in vitro biomarkers of the carcinogenic process by chemopreventive agents." *AntiCancer Res*. 1999; 19(1A): 35-44.

2630 Mirzoeva OK, Calder PC. "The effect of propolis and its components on eicosanoid production during the inflammatory response." *Prostaglandins Leukot Essent Fatty Acids*, 1996; 55: 441-49.

2631 Park YK, et al. "Antimicrobial activity of propolis on oral microorganisms." *Curr Microbiol*, 1998; 36: 24-28.

2632 Hay KD, Greig DE. "Propolis allergy: a cause of oral mucositis with ulceration." *Oral Surg Oral Med Oral Pathol*, 1990; 70: 584-86.

2633 Hashimoto T, et al. "Synthesis of two allergenic constituents of propolis and poplar bud excretion." *Z Naturforsch [C]*, 1988; 43: 470-72.

2634 Brumfitt W, Hamilton-Miller JM, Franklin I. "Antibiotic activity of natural products: 1. Propolis." *Microbios*, 1990; 62: 19-22.

2635 Tixier JM, et al. "Evidence by in vivo and in vitro studies that binding of pycnogenols to elastin affects its rate of degradation by elastases." *Biochem Pharmacol*. 1984; 33: 3933-939.

2636 Liu FJ, Zhang YX, Lau BH. "Pycnogenol enhances immune and haemopoietic functions in senescence-accelerated mice." *Cell Mol Life Sci*, 1998; 54: 1168-172.

2637 Fitzpatrick DF, Bing, Rohdewald P. "Endothelium-dependent vascular effects of Pycnogenol." *J Cardiovasc Pharmacol*, 1998; 32: 509-15.

2638 Practical Health web site. "Pycnogenol." URL: www.practicalhealth.com/pagebetweeneducationalandorder.htm (16 July 1999).

2639 Nuttall SL, et al. "An evaluation of the antioxidant activity of a standardized grape seed extract, Leucoselect." *J Clin Pharm Ther*, 1998; 23: 385-89.

2640 Yamakoshi J, et al. "Proanthocyanidin-rich extract from grape seeds attenuates the development of aortic Atherosclerosis in cholesterol-fed rabbits." *Atherosclerosis*, 1999; 142: 139-49.

2641 Dauer A, Metzner P, Schimmer O. "Proanthocyanidins from the bark of Hamamelis virginiana exhibit antimutagenic properties against nitroaromatic compounds." *Planta Med*, 1998; 64: 324-27.

2642 Miura S, et al. "The inhibitory effects of tea polyphenols (flavan-3-ol derivatives) on Cu2+ mediated oxidative modification of low density lipoprotein." *Biol Pharm Bull*, 1994; 17: 1567-572.

2643 SmartBasics Web site. "Vitamin B15 or pangamic acid." webu5156.ntx.net/glos.vitamins/vit.b15.glos.html (18 May 1999).

2644 Wallner-Pendleton EA, et al. "Toxicity of excess dicalcium phosphate in the diet of turkey poults." *Avian Dis*, 1989; 33: 375-78.

2645 Gray ME, Titlow LW. "The effect of pangamic acid on maximal treadmill performance." *Med Sci Sports Exerc*, 1982; 14(6): 424-27.

2646 Ziemlanski S, Puzynska L, Panczenko-Kresowska B. "The effect of long-term enrichment of diet with selenium, vitamin E and B15 on the activity of certain enzymes in rat brain." *Acta Physiol Pol*, 1987; 38: 323-30.

2647 "Prolyt formula." The Apothecary Website. URL: www.intr.net/apothecary/lyt.html. (24 May 1999).

2648 Hellgren L, Vincent J. "Degradation and liquefication effect of streptokinase-streptodornase and stabilised trypsin on tissue necroses, crusts of fibrinoid, purulent exudate and clotted blood from leg ulcers." *J Int Med Res*, 1977;5:334-337.

2649 Suomalainen O. "Evaluation of two enzyme preparations-Trypure and Varidase in traumatic ulcers." *Ann Chir Gynaecol*, 1983;72:62-65.

2650 FDA. "FDA Talk Paper." Food and Drug Administration Website. URL: www.vm.cfsan.fda.gov/~lrd/TPMUSHRM.html (Accessed 24 May 1999).

2651 Sadjadi J. "Anthrax associated with the Kombucha "mushroom" in Iran." *JAMA*, 1998;280:1567-1568.

2652 "Kombucha-toxicity alert." *Crit Path AIDS Proj*, 1994;30:31-32 1994-95.

2653 Gamundi R; Valdivia M. "The Kombucha mushroom: two different opinions." *Sidahora*, 1995;90:34-35.

2654 Majchrowicz M. "Kombucha: a dubious "cure"." *GMHC Treat Issues*, 1995;9:10.

2655 "CDC. Unexplained severe illness possibly associated with consumption of Kombucha tea-Iowa, 1995." *MMWR* 1995;44:892-893,899-900.

2656 Srinivasan R, Smolinske S, Greenbaum DJ. "Probable gastrointestinal toxicity of Kombucha tea: is this beverage healthy or harmful?" *Gen Intern Med*. 1997;12:643-644.

2661 May SW, Pollock SH. Selenium-based antihypertensives. Rationale and potential. *Drugs*, 1998;56(6):959-964.

2662 Aaseth J, Haugen M, Forre O. "Rheumatoid arthritis and metal compounds-perspectives on the role of oxygen radical detoxification." *Analyst*, 1998; 123:3-6.

2663 Chan S, Gerson B, Subramaniam S. "The role of copper,

© Copyright 2000, Natural Medicines Comprehensive Database (209) 472-2244. For updated data, go to www.NaturalDatabase.com. • 1213

REFERENCES

molybdenum, selenium, and zinc in nutrition and health." *Clin Lab Med* 1998;18:673-685.

2664 Clark LC, Combs GF Jr, Turnbull BW, et al. "Effects of selenium supplementation for cancer prevention in patients with carcinoma of the skin. A randomized controlled trial." *JAMA* , 1996;276:1957-1963.

2667 Clark LC, Dalkin B, Krongrad A, et al. "Decreased incidence of prostate cancer with selenium supplementation: results of a double-blind cancer prevention trial." *Br J Urol*, 1998;81:730-734.

2668 Maier RH, Purser SM, Nicholson DL, Pories WJ. "The cytotoxic interaction of inorganic trace elements with EDTA and cisplatin in sensitive and resistant human ovarian cancer cells." *In Vitro Cell Dev Biol Anim*, 1997;33:218-221.

2671 Koller LD, Exon JH. "The two faces of selenium-deficiency and toxicity-are similar in animals and man." *Can J Vet Res*, 1986;50(3):297-306.

2673 Mark SD, Wang W, Fraumeni JF Jr, et al. "Do nutritional supplements lower the risk of stroke or hypertension?" *Epidemiology*, 1998;9:9-15.

2674 Knoben JE, Anderson PO. *Handbook of Clinical Drug Data*. 7th edition. Hamilton, IL: Drug Intelligence Publications, Inc.; 1993.

2676 Neve J. "Selenium as a risk factor for cardiovascular diseases." *J Cardiovasc Risk*, 1996;3(1):42-7.

2678 Brewer GJ, Yuzbasiyan-Gurkan V, Johnson V, et al. "Treatment of Wilson's disease with zinc: XI. Interaction with other anticopper agents." *J Am Coll Nutr*, 1993;12(1):26-30.

2679 Brewer GJ, Johnson V, Kaplan J. "Treatment of Wilson's disease with zinc: XIV. Studies of the effect of zinc on lymphocyte function." *J Lab Clin Med*, 1997;129(6):649-52.

2680 Fuchs GJ. "Possibilities for zinc in the treatment of acute diarrhea." *Am J Clin Nutr*, 1998;68(2 Suppl):480S-483S.

2681 Fosmire GJ. "Zinc toxicity." *Am J Clin Nutr*, 1990;51:225-227.

2682 Lomaestro BM, Bailie GR. "Absorption interactions with fluoroquinolones. 1995 update." *Drug Saf*, 1995;12(5):314-33.

2686 Dreno B, Trossaert M, Boiteau HL, Litoux P. "Zinc salts effects on granulocyte zinc concentration and chemotaxis in acne patients." *Acta Derm Venereol*, 1992;72(4):250-2.

2687 Schachner L, Eaglstein W, Kittles C, Mertz P. "Topical erythromycin and zinc therapy for acne." *J Am Acad Dermatol*, 1990;22(2 Pt 1):253-60.

2688 Habbema L, Koopmans B, Menke HE, et al. "A 4% erythromycin and zinc combination (Zineryt) versus 2% erythromycin (Eryderm) in acne vulgaris: a randomized, double-blind comparative study." *Br J Dermatol* 1989;121(4):497-502.

2689 Walldius G, Michaelsson G, Hardell LI, Aberg H. "The effects of diet and zinc treatment on the fatty acid composition of serum lipids and adipose tissue and on serum lipoproteins in two adolescent patients with acrodermatitis enteropathica." *Am J Clin Nutr*, 1983;38(4):512-22.

2690 Koletzko B, Bretschneider A, Bremer HJ. "Fatty acid composition of plasma lipids in acrodermatitis enteropathica before and after zinc supplementation." *Eur J Pediatr*, 1985;143(4):310-314.

2691 Borroni G, Brazzelli V, Vignati G, et al. "Bullous lesions in acrodermatitis enteropathica. Histopathologic findings regarding two patients." *Am J Dermatopathol*,

1992;14(4):304-9.

2692 Sturniolo GC, Mestriner C, Irato P, et al. "Zinc therapy increases duodenal concentrations of metallothionein and iron in Wilson's disease patients." *Am J Gastroenterol*, 1999;94(2):334-8.

2693 Brewer GJ, Dick RD, Johnson VD, et al. "Treatment of Wilson's disease with zinc: XV long-term follow-up studies." *J Lab Clin Med*, 1998;132(4):264-78.

2694 Rittenhouse T. The management of lower-extremity ulcers with zinc-saline wet dressings versus normal saline wet dressings. *Adv Ther*, 1996;13(2):88-94.

2696 Young B, Ott L, Kasarskis E, et al. Zinc supplementation is associated with improved neurologic recovery rate and visceral protein levels of patients with severe closed head injury. *J Neurotrauma*, 1996; 13(1):25-34.

2699 Agren MS. "Studies on zinc in wound healing." *Acta Derm Venereol Suppl* (Stockh), 1990;154:1-36.

2700 Shukla A, Rasik AM, Jain GK, et al. In vitro and in vivo wound healing activity of asiaticoside isolated from Centella asiatica. *J Ethnopharmacol* 1999;65:1-11.

2701 FDA Orphan Drugs. "List of Orphan Designations and Approvals" website: http://www.fda.gov/orphan/DESIGNAT/list.htm (Accessed 19 January 2000).

2702 Shabert JK, Winslow C, Lacey JM, Wilmore DW. Glutamine-antioxidant supplementation increases body cell mass in AIDS patients with weight loss: a randomized, double-blind controlled trial. *Nutrition* 1999;15:860-864.

2703 Scolapio JS. Effect of growth hormone, glutamine, and diet on body composition in short bowel syndrome: a randomized, controlled study. *JPEN J Parenter Enteral Nutr* 1999;23:309-312.

2704 Rubio IT, Cao Y, Hutchins LF, et al. Effect of glutamine on methotrexate efficacy and toxicity. *Ann Surg* 1998;227:772-778.

2705 Yoshida S, Matsui M, Shirouzu Y, et al. Effects of glutamine supplements and radiochemotherapy on systemic immune and gut barrier function in patients with advanced esophageal cancer. *Ann Surg* 1998;227:485-491.

2706 Osol A, Hoover JE, eds. Remington's Pharmaceutical Science, 15th ed. Easton, PA: Mack Publishing Company, 1975.

2707 Zahn KA, Li RL, Purssell RA. Cardiovascular toxicity after ingestion of "herbal ecstacy". *J Emerg Med* 1999;17:289-291.

2708 Center for the Evaluation of Risks to Human Reproduction (CERHR). "Caffeine" website: URL: http://cerhr.niehs.nih.gov/genpub/topics/caffeine.html (Accessed 19 January 2000).

2709 Klebanoff MA, Levine RJ, DerSimonian R, et al. Maternal serum paraxanthine, a caffeine metabolite, and the risk of spontaneous abortion. *N Engl J Med* 1999;341:1639-1644.

2710 Eskenazi B. Caffeine—filtering the facts. *NEJM* 1999;341:1688-1689.

2711 Fernandes O, Sabharwal M, Smiley T, et al. Moderate to heavy caffeine consumption during pregnancy and relationship to spontaneous abortion and abnormal fetal growth: a meta-analysis. *Reprod Toxicol* 1998;12:435-444.

2712 Stookey JD. The diuretic effects of alcohol and caffeine and total water intake misclassification. *Eur J Epidemiol* 1999;15:181-188.

2713 Wemple RD, Lamb DR, McKeever KH. Caffeine vs caffeine-free sports drinks: effects on urine production at rest and during prolonged exercise. *Int J Sports Med* 1997;18:40-46.

2714 Pollock BG, Wylie M, Stack JA, et al. Inhibition of caffeine metabolism by estrogen replacement therapy in postmenopausal women. *J Clin Pharmacol* 1999;39:936-940.

2715 Goldstein J, Hoffman HD, Armellino JJ, et al. Treatment of severe, disabling migraine attacks in an over-the-counter population of migraine sufferers: results from three randomized, placebo-controlled studies of the combination of acetaminophen, aspirin, and caffeine. *Cephalalgia* 1999;19:684-691.

2716 Lipton RB, Stewart WF, Ryan RE Jr, et al. Efficacy and safety of acetaminophen, aspirin, and caffeine in alleviating migraine headache pain: three double-blind, randomized, placebo-controlled trials. *Arch Neurol* 1998;55:210-217.

2717 Silberstein SD, Armellino JJ, Hoffman HD, et al. Treatment of menstruation-associated migraine with the nonprescription combination of acetaminophen, aspirin, and caffeine: results from three randomized, placebo-controlled studies. *Clin Ther* 1999;21:475-491.

2718 Migliardi JR, Armellino JJ, Friedman M, et al. Caffeine as an analgesic adjuvant in tension headache. *Clin Pharmacol Ther* 1994;56:576-586.

2719 DiPiro JT, Talbert RL, Yee GC, et al. Pharmacotherapy: A Pathophysiologic Approach, fourth edition. Appleton & Lange: Stamford, CT, 1999.

2720 Rees K, Allen D, Lader M. The influences of age and caffeine on psychomotor and cognitive function. *Psychopharmacology* (Berl) 1999;145:181-188.

2721 Hogervorst E, Riedel WJ, Kovacs E, et al. Caffeine improves cognitive performance after strenuous physical exercise. *Int J Sports Med* 1999;20:354-361.

2722 Nurminen ML, Niittynen L, Korpela R, Vapaatalo H. Coffee, caffeine and blood pressure: a critical review. *Eur J Clin Nutr* 1999;53:831-839.

2723 Dews PB, Curtis GL, Hanford KJ, O'Brien CP. The frequency of caffeine withdrawal in a population-based survey and in a controlled, blinded pilot experiment. *J Clin Pharmacol* 1999;39:1221-1232.

2724 Akhtar S, Wood G, Rubin JS, et al. Effect of caffeine on the vocal folds: a pilot study. *J Laryngol Otol* 1999;113:341-345.

2725 Weber JG, Klindworth JT, Arnold JJ, et al. Prophylactic intravenous administration of caffeine and recovery after ambulatory surgical procedures. *Mayo Clin Proc* 1997;72:621-626.

2726 Hampl KF, Schneider MC, Ruttimann U, et al. Perioperative administration of caffeine tablets for prevention of postoperative headaches. *Can J Anaesth* 1995;42:789-792.

2727 Yucel A, Ozyalcin S, Talu GK, et al. Intravenous administration of caffeine sodium benzoate for postdural puncture headache. *Reg Anesth Pain Med* 1999;24:51-54.

2728 Camann WR, Murray RS, Mushlin PS, Lambert DH. Effects of oral caffeine on postdural puncture headache. A double-blind, placebo-controlled trial. *Anesth Analg* 1990;70:181-184.

2729 FDA. "Proposed Rule: Dietary Supplements Containing Ephedrine Alkaloids." website: http://www.verity.fda.gov/ (Accessed 25 January 2000).

2732 Wilt TJ, Ishani A, Stark G, et al. Saw palmetto extracts for treatment of benign prostatic hyperplasia: a systematic review. *JAMA* 1998;280:1604-1609.

2733 Gerber GS, Zagaja GP, Bales GT, et al. Saw palmetto (Serenoa repens) in men with lower urinary tract symptoms: effects on urodynamic parameters and voiding symptoms. *Urology* 1998;51:1003-1007.

2734 Lowe FC, Fagelman E. Phytotherapy in the treatment of benign prostatic hyperplasia: an update. *Urology* 1999;53:671-678.

2735 Marks LS, Tyler VE. Saw palmetto extract: newest (and oldest) treatment alternative for men with symptomatic benign prostatic hyperplasia. *Urology* 1999;53:457-461.

2736 USRF Research. "Clinical Effects of Saw Palmetto Extract in Men with Symptomatic BPH" webpage: www.usrf.org/spepapers.html (Accessed 26 January 2000).

2737 Ludwig DS, Pereira MA, Kroenke CH, et al. Dietary fiber, weight gain, and cardiovascular disease risk factors in young adults. *JAMA* , 1999;282:1539-1546.

2738 Robbers JE, Tyler VE. Tyler's Herbs of Choice. Haworth Press, New York, 1999.

2739 Beutler KT, Pankewycz O, Brautigan DL. Equivalent uptake of organic and inorganic zinc by monkey kidney fibroblasts, human intestinal epithelial cells, or perfused mouse intestine. *Biol Trace Elem Res* 1998;61:19-31.

2740 Duisterwinkel FJ, Wolthers BG, Koopman BJ, et al. Bioavailability of orally administered zinc, using Taurizine. *Pharm Weekbl [Sci]* 1986;8:85-88.

2741 Bagchi D, Bagchi M, Stohs SJ. Comparative in vitro oxygen radical scavenging ability of zinc methionine and selected zinc salts and antioxidants. *Gen Pharmacol* 1997;28:85-91.

2742 Muscle Photos. "ZMA for Athletes" website: www.musclephotos.com/zma.html (Accessed 26 January 2000).

2743 Dr. Duke's Phytochemical and Ethnobotanical Databases. "Ethnobotanical uses: Andrographis paniculata" website: www.ars-grin.gov/cgi-bin/duke/ethnobot.pl?andrographis%20pnaiculata (Accessed 27 January 2000).

2744 Caceres DD, Hancke JL, Burgos RA, et al. Use of visual analogue scale measurements (VAS) to asses the effectiveness of standardized Andrographis paniculata extract SHA-10 in reducing the symptoms of common cold. A randomized double blind-placebo study. *PhytoMedicine* 1999;6:217-223.

2745 Ambrosia Herbals. "Herbal Extracts of Therapuetic Use" website: www.ambrosiaherbals.com/acorus_calamus.html (accessed 1/27/00).

2746 Indian Herbs. "Andrographis paniculata" website: www.indianherbs.com/andro.htm (accessed 1/27/00).

2747 Kan Jang. "Kang Jang Herbal Remedy for Colds,Flu, Sinusitis, Allergies from [sic] Swedish Herbal Institute" website: www.kanjang.com (accessed 1/27/00).

2748 Thamlikitkul V, Dechatiwongse T, Theerapong S, et al. Efficacy of Andrographis paniculata, Nees for pharyngotonsillitis in adults. *J Med Assoc Thai* 1991;74:437-442.

2749 Martz W. Plants with a reputation against snakebite. *Toxicon* 1992;30:1131-1142.

2750 Madav S, Tripathi HC, Tandan SK, et al. Antiallergic activity of andrographolide. *Indian J Pharm Sci* 1998;60:176-178.

2751 Gupta PP, Tandon JS, Patnaik GK. Antiallergic activity of andrographolides isolated from Andrographis paniculata (Burm. F) Wall. *Pharm Biol* 1998;36:72-74.

2752 Kumar S, Gopal K. Screening of plant species for inhibition of bacterial population of raw water. *Journal*

Of Environmental Science And Health (Part A Toxic-Hazardous Substances & Environmental Engineering) 1999;34:975-987.

2753 Madav S, Tripathi HC, Tandan Mishra SK. Analgesic, antipyretic and antiulcerogenic effects of andrographolide. *Indian J Pharm Sci* 1995;57:121-125.

2754 Vedavathy S, Rao KN. Antipyretic activity of six indigenous medicinal plants of Tirumala Hills, Andhra Pradesh, India. *J Ethnopharmacol* 1991;33:193-196.

2755 Zhang CY, Tan BK. Mechanisms of cardiovascular activity of Andrographis paniculata in the anaesthetized rat. *J Ethnopharmacol* 1997;56:97-101.

2756 Guo ZL, Zhao HY, Zheng XH. The effect of andrographis paniculata nees (APN) in alleviating the myocardial ischemic reperfusion injury. *J Tongji Med Univ* 1994;14:49-51.

2757 Guo Z, Zhao H, Fu L. Protective effects of API0134 on myocardial ischemia and reperfusion injury. *J Tongji Med Univ* 1996;16:193-197.

2758 Zhao HY, Fang WY. Antithrombotic effects of Andrographis paniculata nees in preventing myocardial infarction. *Chin Med J* (Engl) 1991;104:770-775.

2759 Amroyan E, Gabrielian E, Panossian A, et al. Inhibitory effect of andrographolide from Andrographis paniculata on PAF-induced platelet aggregation. *PhytoMedicine* 1999;6:27-31.

2760 Zhang C, Kuroyangi M, Tan BK. Cardiovascular activity of 14-deoxy-11,12-didehydroandrographolide in the anaesthetised rat and isolated right atria. *Pharmacol Res* 1998;38:413-417.

2761 Shukla B, Visen PK, Patnaik GK, Dhawan BN. Choleretic effect of andrographolide in rats and guinea pigs. *Planta Med* 1992;58:146-149.

2762 Visen PK, Shukla B, Patnaik GK, Dhawan BN. Andrographolide protects rat hepatocytes against paracetamol-induced damage. *J Ethnopharmacol* 1993;40:131-136.

2763 Rana AC, Avadhoot Y. Hepatoprotective effects of Andrographis paniculata against carbon tetrachloride-induced *Liver* damage. *Arch Pharm Res* 1991;14:93-95.

2764 Leelarasamee A, Trakulsomboon S, Sittisomwong N. Undetectable anti-bacterial activity of Andrographis paniculata (Burma) wall. ex ness. *J Med Assoc Thai* 1990;73:299-304.

2765 Chang RS, Ding L, Chen GQ, et al. Dehydroandrographolide succinic acid monoester as an inhibitor against the human immunodeficiency virus. *Proc Soc Exp Biol Med* 1991;197:59-66.

2766 Puri A, Saxena R, Saxena RP, et al. Immunostimulant agents from Andrographis paniculata. *J Nat Prod* 1993;56:995-999.

2767 Raj RK. Screening of indigenous plants for anthelmintic action against human Ascaris lumbricoides: Part II. *Ind J Physiol Pharmacol* 1975;19(1);47-49.

2768 Matsuda T, Kuroyanagi M, Sugiyama S, et al. Cell differentiation-inducing diterpenes from Andrographis paniculata Nees. *Chem Pharm Bull* (Tokyo)1994;42:1216-1225.

2769 Akbarsha MA, Manivannan B, Hamid KS, Vijayan B. Antifertility effect of Andrographis paniculata (Nees) in male albino rat. *Indian J Exp Biol* 1990;28:421-426.

2770 Burgos RA, Caballero EE, Sanchez NS, et al. Testicular toxicity assessment of Andrographis paniculata dried extract in rats. *J Ethnopharmacol* 1997;58:219-224.

2771 Panossian A, Kochikian A, Gabrielian E, et al. Effect of Andrographis paniculata extract on progesterone in blood plasma of pregnant rats. *PhytoMedicine* 1999;6:157-161.

2772 Caceres DD, Hancke JL, Burgos RA, Wikman GK. Prevention of common colds with Andrographis Paniculata dried extract: a pilot double blind trial. *PhytoMedicine* 1997;4:101-104.

2773 Melchior J, Palm S, Wikman G. Controlled clinical study of standardized Androgrpahis paniculata in common cold – a pilot trial. *Phytomedicine* 1996/97;3:315-318.

2774 Hancke J, Burgos R, Caceres D, Wikman G. A double-blind study with a new monodrug kan jang: decrease of symptoms and improvement in the recovery from common colds. *Phytotherapy Res* 1995; 9:559-562.

2775 GRIN/NPGS Taxonomy Information. "Taxon: Andrographis paniculata (Burm. f.) Well. Ex Nees" website: www.ars-grin.gov/cgi-bin/npgs/html/taxon.pl?414228 (accessed 1/27/00).

2776 Zoha MS, Hussain AH, Choudhury SA. Antifertility effect of andrographis paniculata in mice. *Bangladesh Med Res Counc Bull* 1989;15:34-37.

2777 Gozalbes R, Galvez J, Garcia-Domenech R, Derouin F. Molecular search of new active drugs against Toxoplasma gondii. *SAR QSAR Environ Res* 1999;10:47-60.

2778 Kapil A, Koul IB, Banerjee SK, Gupta BD. Antihepatotoxic effects of major diterpenoid constituents of Andrographis paniculata. *Biochem Pharmacol* 1993;46:182-185.

2779 Gupta S, Yadava JN, Tandon JS. Antisecretory (antidiarrheal) activity of Indian medicinal plants against Escherichia coli enterotoxin-induced secretion in rabbit and guinea pig ileal loop models. *Int J Pharmacogn* 1993;31:198-204.

2780 Najib NA, Rahman N, Furuta T et al. Antimalarial activity of extracts of Malaysian medicinal plants. *J Ethnopharmacol* 1999;64:249-254.

2781 Misra P, Pal NL, Guru PY, et al. Antimalarial activity of Andrographis paniculata (Kalmegh) against Plasmodium berghei NK 65 in Mastomys natalensis. *Int J Pharmacogn* 1992;30:263-274.

2782 Wang DW, Zhao HY. Prevention of atherosclerotic arterial stenosis and restenosis after angioplasty with Andrographis paniculata nees and fish oil. Experimental studies of effects and mechanisms. *Chin Med J* (Engl) 1994;107:464-470.

2783 Wang DW, Zhao HY. Experimental studies on prevention of atherosclerotic arterial stenosis and restenosis after angioplasty with Andrographis Paniculata Nees and fish oil. *J Tongji Med Univ* 1993;13:193-198.

2784 Holodniy M, Koch J, Mistal M, et al. A double blind, randomized, placebo-controlled phase II study to assess the safety and efficacy of orally administered SP-303 for the symptomatic treatment of diarrhea in patients with AIDS. *Am J Gastroenterol* 1999;94:3267-3273.

2785 Shaman Botanicals. "The Ethnobotanical Story Behind ShamanBotanicals.com SB Normal Stool Formula" website: URL: www.shamanbotanicals.com/traditionaluse.htm (Accessed 31 January 2000).

2786 Gabriel SE, Davenport SE, Steagall RJ, et al. A novel plant-derived inhibitor of cAMP-mediated fluid and chloride secretion. *Am J Physiol* 1999;276:G58-G63.

2787 Safrin S, McKinley G, McKeough M, et al. Treatment of acyclovir-unresponsive cutaneous herpes simplex virus infection with topically applied SP-303. *Antiviral*

Res 1994;25:185-192.

2788 Orozco-Topete R, Sierra-Madero J, Cano-Dominguez C, et al. Safety and efficacy of Virend for topical treatment of genital and anal herpes simplex lesions in patients with AIDS. *Antiviral Res* 1997;35:91-103.

2789 King SR, Tempesta MS. From shaman to human clinical trials: the role of industry in ethnobotany, conservation and community reciprocity. *Ciba Found Symp* 1994;185:197-206.

2790 Barnard DL, Smee DF, Huffman JH, et al. Antiherpesvirus activity and mode of action of SP-303, a novel plant flavonoid. *Chemotherapy* 1993;39:203-211.

2791 Wyde PR, Ambrose MW, Meyerson LR, Gilbert BE. The antiviral activity of SP-303, a natural polyphenolic polymer, against respiratory syncytial and parainfluenza type 3 viruses in cotton rats. *Antiviral Res* 1993;20:145-154.

2792 Barnard DL, Huffman JH, Meyerson LR, Sidwell RW. Mode of inhibition of respiratory syncytial virus by a plant flavonoid, SP-303. *Chemotherapy* 1993;39:212-217.

2793 Sidwell RW, Huffman JH, Moscon BJ, Warren RP. Influenza virus-inhibitory effects of intraperitoneally and aerosol-administered SP-303, a plant flavonoid. *Chemotherapy* 1994;40:42-50.

2794 Gilbert BE, Wyde PR, Wilson SZ, Meyerson LR. SP-303 small-particle aerosol treatment of influenza A virus infection in mice and respiratory syncytial virus infection in cotton rats. *Antiviral Res* 1993;21:37-45.

2795 Perdue GP, Blomster RN, Blake DA, Farnsworth NR. South American plants II: taspine isolation and anti-inflammatory activity. *J Pharm Sci* 1979;68:124-126.

2796 Vaisberg AJ, Milla M, Planas MC, et al. Taspine is the cicatrizant principle in Sangre de Grado extracted from Croton lechleri. *Planta Med* 1989;55:140-143.

2797 Pieters L, de Bruyne T, Claeys M, et al. Isolation of a dihydrobenzofuran lignan from South American dragon's blood (Croton spp.) as an inhibitor of cell proliferation. *J Nat Prod* 1993;56:899-906.

2798 Chen ZP, Cai Y, Phillipson JD. Studies on the anti-tumour, anti-bacterial, and wound-healing properties of dragon's blood. *Planta Med* 1994;60:541-545.

2799 Desmarchelier C, Witting Schaus F, Coussio J, Cicca G. Effects of Sangre de Drago from Croton lechleri Muell.-Arg. on the production of active oxygen radicals. *J Ethnopharmacol* 1997;58:103-108.

2800 Ashaninka Imports, Inc. "Sangre de Drago" website: URL: http://www.ashaninka.com/sangre.htm (Accessed 31 January 2000).

2801 Shaman Botanicals. "Types of Diarrhea and ShamanBotanicals.com SB Normal Stool Formula" website: http://www.shamanbotanicals.com/dcmaster.htm (Accessed 31 January 2000).

2802 Dr. Duke's Syllabus. "Module 8: Amazonian (Iberoamerican)" website: www.ars-grin.gov/duke/syllabus/module8.htm (Accessed 31 January 2000).

2803 Iowa State University. "Medicinal Plants of EcuadorMedicinal Plants of the Quijos - Quichua Shamen, Ecuador" website: www.public.iastate.edu/~cbutter/ethnobot.htm (Accessed 31 January 2000).

2804 Raintree Nutrition. "Sangre de Grado" website: www.rain-tree.com/sangre.htm (Accessed 31 January 2000).

2805 USDA, ARS, National Genetic Resources Program. Germplasm Resources Information Network - (GRIN). "Taxon: Croton lechleri Mull. Arg" website: www.ars-grin.gov/cgi-bin/npgs/html/tax_search.pl?croton+lechleri (Accessed 31 January 2000).

2806 Dicesare D, Dupont HL, Mathewson JJ, et al. A double-blind randomized, placebo-controlled study of SP-303 (Provir) in the symptomatic treatment of acute diarrhea among travelers to Mexico and Jamaica. Infectious Diseases Society of America Annual Meeting, 1998 (abstract).

2807 BioWorld Today. "Shaman Will Sidestep FDA By Selling Product Over Internet" website: http://www.bioworld.com/index.html (Accessed 6 January 2000).

2808 FDA. "List of Orphan Designations and Approvals" website: http://www.fda.gov/orphan/DESIGNAT/list.htm (Accessed 6 February 2000).

2809 Henderson LM, Brewer GJ, Dressman JB, et al. Effect of intragastric pH on the absorption of oral zinc acetate and zinc oxide in young healthy volunteers. *J Parenter Enteral Nutr* 1995;19:393-397.

2810 Dr. Duke's Phytochemical and Ethnobotanical Databases. website: www.ars-grin.gov/cgi-bin/duke/ethnobot.pl (Accessed 7 February 2000).

2811 Schlager TA, Anderson S, Trudell J, Hendley JO. Effect of cranberry juice on bacteriuria in children with neurogenic bladder receiving intermittent catheterization. *J Pediatr* 1999;135:698-702.

2812 Sobota AE. Inhibition of bacterial adherence by cranberry juice: potential use for the treatment of urinary tract infections. *J Urol* 1984;131:1013-1016.

2813 Howell AB, Vorsa N, Foo LY, et al. Inhibition of the Adherence of P-Fimbriated Escherichia coli to Uroepithelial-Cell Surfaces by Proanthocyanidin Extracts from Cranberries (letter). *NEJM* 1998;339:1085-1086.

2814 Ahuja S, Kaack B, Roberts J. Loss of fimbrial adhesion with the addition of Vaccinum macrocarpon to the growth medium of P-fimbriated Escherichia coli. *J Urol* 1998;159:559-562.

2815 Habash MB, Van der Mei HC, Busscher HJ, Reid G. The effect of water, ascorbic acid, and cranberry derived supplementation on human urine and uropathogen adhesion to silicone rubber. *Can J Microbiol* 1999;45:691-694.

2816 Weiss EI, Lev-Dor R, Kashamn Y, et al. Inhibiting interspecies coaggregation of plaque bacteria with a cranberry juice constituent. *J Am Dent Assoc* 1998;129:1719-1723.

2817 Saltzman JR, Kemp JA, Golner BB, et al. Effect of hypochlorhydria due to omeprazole treatment or atrophic gastritis on protein-bound vitamin B12 absorption. *J Am Coll Nutr* 1994;13:584-591.

2818 USDA, ARS, National Genetic Resources Program. "Germplasm Resources Information Network - (GRIN) Online Database" website: www.ars-grin.gov/cgi-bin/npgs/html/taxon.pl?41030 (Accessed 7 February 2000).

2819 USDA, ARS, National Genetic Resources Program. "Germplasm Resources Information Network - (GRIN). Online Database" website: www.ars-grin.gov/cgi-bin/npgs/html/taxon.pl?41047 (Accessed 7 February 2000).

2820 The Natural History of the Northwoods. "Small Cranberry Vaccinium oxycoccus" website: www.rook.org/earl/bwca/nature/shrubs/vacciniumoxy.html (Accessed 4 February 2000).

2821 Wisconsin State Cranberry Growers Association. "A History of Cranberry Growing" website: www.wiscran.org/history.html (Accessed 7 February

© Copyright 2000, Natural Medicines Comprehensive Database (209) 472-2244. For updated data, go to www.NaturalDatabase.com. • 1217

**R
E
F
E
R
E
N
C
E
S**

2000).

2822 www.healthlink.com.au/nat_lib/htm-data/htm-herb/
bhp770.htm (Accessed 8 February 2000).

2823 Naveh Y, Schapira D, Ravel Y, et al. Zinc metabolism in
rheumatoid arthritis: plasma and urinary zinc and
relationship to disease activity. *J Rheumatol*
1997;24:643-646.

2824 Potocnik FC, van Rensburg SJ, Park C, et al. Zinc and
platelet membrane microviscosity in Alzheimer's
disease. The in vivo effect of zinc on platelet
membranes and cognition. *S Afr Med J* 1997;87:1116-
1119.

2825 de Haan A, van Doorn JE, Westra HG. Effects of
potassium plus magnesium aspartate on muscle
Metabolism and force development during short
intensive static exercise. *Int J Sports Med* 1985;6:44-9.

2826 Golf SW, Bender S, Gruttner J. On the significance of
magnesium in extreme physical stress. *Cardiovasc
Drugs Ther* 1998;12:197-202.

2827 Golf SW, Happel O, Graef V, Seim KE. Plasma
aldosterone, cortisol and electrolyte concentrations in
physical exercise after magnesium supplementation. *J
Clin Chem Clin Biochem* 1984;22:717-721.

2828 Hagan RD, Upton SJ, Duncan JJ, et al. Absence of
effect of potassium-magnesium aspartate on physiologic
responses to prolonged work in aerobically trained men.
Int J Sports Med 1982;3:177-81.

2829 Maughan RJ, Sadler DJ. The effects of oral
administration of salts of aspartic acid on the metabolic
response to prolonged exhausting exercise in man. *Int J
Sports Med* 1983;4:119-23.

2830 Weller E, Bachert P, Meinck HM, et al. Lack of effect of
oral Mg-supplementation on Mg in serum, blood cells,
and calf muscle. *Med Sci Sports Exerc* 1998;30:1584-
91.

2900 Autism Society of America Website: URL:
www.autism-society.org. (16 July 1999).

2901 Autism Research Institute Website: URL:
www.autism.com/ari (16 July 1999).

2902 Baker SM. Website: URL: www.sbakermd.com/info/
autism/Secretin.htm (16 July 1999).

2903 Gunnes P, Rasmussen K. "Haemodynamic effects of
pharmacological doses of secretin in patients with
impaired left ventricular function." *Eur Heart J*, 1986;
7(2): 146-49.

2904 Gunnes P, et al. "Cardiovascular effects of secretin
infusion in man." *Scand J Clin Lab* Invest, 1983; 43(7):
637-42.

2905 Tulassay Z, et al. [Secretin versus cimetidine in the
therapy of active bleeding from peptic gastroduodenal
lesions. A prospective, randomized, double-blind,
multicentric study]. [Article in German]. *Wien Med
Wochenschr*, 1990; 140(13): 361-64.

2906 Wagner PK, Rothmund M. [Effect of cimetidine and
synthetic secretin as treatment of acute upper
gastrointestinal bleeding-a prospective alternate trial].
[Article in German]. *Z Gastroenterol*, 1980; 18(6): 337-
41.

2907 Berg P, et al. [Comparative treatment of gastroduodenal
haemorrhage with secretin and cimetidine]. [Article in
German]. *Dtsch Med Wochenschr*, 1982; 107(48): 1831-
36.

2908 Rothmund M, Wagner PK. [Effect of cimetidine and
secretin on acute bleedings from gastroduodenal ulcers
and erosions: a prospective study]. [Article in German].
Dtsch Med Wochenschr, 1982; 107(7): 245-48.

2909 Scholten T, et al. [Treatment of duodenal ulcer with
synthetic depot secretin - a double-blind study]. [Article
in German]. *Z Gastroenterol*, 1983; 21(5): 212-19.

2910 Demling L, et al. "Treatment of duodenal ulcer with a
long-acting synthetic secretin: a pilot trial." *Acta
HepatoGastroenterol* (Stuttg), 1975; 22(5): 310-13.

2911 Lehmann, et al. "pH-control via secretin or antacid:
prophylaxia of stress ulcers in high-risk surgical
patients." *Intensive Care Med*, 1984; 10(5): 239-43.

2912 Spilker G, et al. [Long-acting secretin for the prevention
of stress ulcers in surgery]. [Article in French]. *Nouv
Presse Med*, 1982; 11(4): 267-69.

2913 Theisinger W, Spilker G, Bader M . [Prevention of stress
ulcers with synthetic depot secretin]. [Article in
German]. *Med Klin*, 1981; 76(10): 291-93.

2914 Piubello W, et al. "Effect of graded doses of secretin on
parathormone serum levels in man." *Digestion*, 1981;
22(6): 321-23.

2915 Center for the Study of Autism: URL: www.autism.org/
secretin.html. (16 July 1999).

2916 Product information. "Secretin." Ferring Pharmaceticals,
Tarrytown, NY; 6/88.

2917 Horvath K, Stefatos G, Sokolski KN. "Improved social
and language skills after secretin administration."
*Journal of the Association for Academic Minority
Physicians*, 1998; 9(1): 9-15.

2918 Tympner F, Rosch W. "The treatment of chronic
recurrent pancreatitis with depot secretin-a preliminary
report." *Hepatogastroenterology*, 1986; 33(4): 159-62.

2919 Autism Research Unit Web site:
osiris.sunderland.ac.uk.autism/sec.htm (16 July 1999).

2920 Snider SR. "Octacosanol in parkinsonism." *Ann Neurol*,
1984; 16(6): 723.

2921 Norris FH, Denys EH, Fallat RJ. "Trial of octacosanol in
amyotrophic lateral sclerosis." *Neurology*, 1986; 36(9):
1263-264.

2922 Nutrimart, "Octacosonol" Website: URL:
www.nutrimart.com/Bulk/Description/octacosonol.htm
(18 July 1999).

2923 Mother Nature's Encyclopedia, "Octacosonol" Website:
URL: www.mothernature.com/ency/supp/
octacosanol.asp (18 July 1999).

2924 Kato S, et al. "Octacosanol affects lipid metabolism in
rats fed on a high-fat diet." *Br J Nutr*, 1995; 73(3): 433-
41.

2925 Kabir Y, Kimura S. "Distribution of radioactive
octacosanol in response to exercise in rats." *Nahrung*,
1994; 38(4): 373-77.

2926 Beltz SD, Doering PL. "Efficacy of nutritional
supplements used by athletes." *Clin Pharm*, 1993;
12(12): 900-08.

2927 Canetti M, et al. "A two-year study on the efficacy and
tolerability of policosanol in patients with type II
hyperlipoproteinaemia." *Int J Clin Pharmacol Res*,
1995; 15(4): 159-65.

2928 Pons P, et al. "Effects of successive dose increases of
policosanol on the lipid profile of patients with type II
hypercholesterolaemia and tolerability to treatment." *Int
J Clin Pharmacol Res*, 1994; 14(1): 27-33.

2929 Torres O, et al. "Treatment of hypercholesterolemia in
NIDDM with policosanol." *Diabetes Care*, 1995; 18(3):
393-97.

2930 Batista J, et al. "Effect of policosanol on hyperlipidemia
and coronary heart disease in middle-aged patients. A
14-month pilot study." *Int J Clin Pharmacol Ther*, 1996;
34(3): 134-37.

2931 Castano G, et al. "A double-blind, placebo-controlled study of the effects of policosanol in patients with intermittent claudication." *Angiology*, 1999; 50(2): 123-30.

2932 Mesa AR, et al. "Toxicity of policosanol in beagle dogs: one-year study." *Toxicol Lett*, 1994; 73(2): 81-90.

2933 Arruzazabala ML, et al. "Effect of policosanol on platelet aggregation in type II hypercholesterolemic patients." *Int J Tissue React*, 1998; 20(4): 119-24.

2934 Menendez R, et al. "Cholesterol-lowering effect of policosanol on rabbits with hypercholesterolaemia induced by a wheat starch-casein diet." *Br J Nutr*, 1997; 77(6): 923-32.

2935 Arruzazabala ML, et al. "Effect of policosanol successive dose increases on platelet aggregation in healthy volunteers." *Pharmacol Res*, 1996; 34(5-6): 181-85.

2936 Carbajal D, et al. "Effect of policosanol on platelet aggregation and serum levels of arachidonic acid metabolites in healthy volunteers." *Prostaglandins Leukot Essent Fatty Acids*, 1998; 58(1): 61-64.

2937 Arruzazabala ML, et al. "Comparative study of policosanol, aspirin and the combination therapy policosanol-aspirin on platelet aggregation in healthy volunteers." *Pharmacol Res*, 1997; 36(4): 293-97.

2938 Valdes S, Arruzazabala ML, Fernandez L. "Effect of policosanol on platelet aggregation in healthy volunteers." *Int J Clin Pharmacol Res*, 1996; 16(2-3): 67-72.

2939 Menendez R, et al. "Policosanol inhibits cholesterol biosynthesis and enhances low density lipoprotein processing in cultured human fibroblasts." *Biol Res*, 1994; 27(3-4): 199-203.

2940 Aleman CL, et al. "A 12-month study of policosanol oral toxicity in Sprague Dawley rats." *Toxicol Lett*, 1994; 70(1): 77-87.

2941 Stusser R, et al. "Long-term therapy with policosanol improves treadmill exercise-ECG testing performance of coronary heart disease patients." *Int J Clin Pharmacol Ther*, 1998; 36(9): 469-73.

2942 From GVI Sourcing Website: URL: www.gvisourcing.com/pharmaceuticals/ppg/specs.html (16 July 1999).

2943 Castano G, et al. "Efficacy and tolerability of policosanol in elderly patients with type II hypercholesterolemia: A 12-month study." *Curr Ther Res*, 1995; 56(8): 819-23.

2944 Castano G, et al. "Effects of policosanol in hypertensive patients with type II hypercholesterolemia." *Curr Ther Res*, 1996; 57(9): 691-95.

2945 Mother Nature's Encyclopedia Website, "Resveratrol." URL: www.mothernature.com/ency/supp/resveratrol.asp (16 July 1999).

2946 Resveratrol Website: URL: www.resveratrol.com/lib7.html (16 July 1999).

2947 PanoLife Products, Inc. Website: URL: www.pano.com/science.html (16 July 1999).

2948 Jang M, et al. "Cancer chemopreventive activity of resveratrol, a natural product derived from grapes." *Science*, 1997; 275(5297): 218-20.

2949 Pace-Asciak CR, Rounova O, Hahn SE, Diamandis P, et al. Wines and grape juices as modulators of platelet aggregation in healthy human subjects. *Clin Chim Acta*, 1996;246(1-2):163-182.

2950 Bertelli AA, et al. "Antiplatelet activity of cis-resveratrol." *Drugs Exp Clin Res*, 1996; 22(2): 61-63.

2951 Pace-Asciak CR, et al. "The red wine phenolics trans-resveratrol and quercetin block human platelet aggregation and eicosanoid synthesis: implications for protection against coronary heart disease." *Clin Chim Acta*, 1995; 235(2): 207-19.

2952 Bertelli A, et al. "Plasma and tissue resveratrol concentrations and pharmacological activity." *Drugs Exp Clin Res*, 1998; 24(3): 133-38.

2953 Belguendouz L, Fremont L, Gozzelino MT. "Interaction of transresveratrol with plasma lipoproteins." *Biochem Pharmacol*, 1998; 55(6): 811-16.

2954 Chen CK, Pace-Asciak CR. "Vasorelaxing activity of resveratrol and quercetin in isolated rat aorta." *Gen Pharmacol*, 1996; 27(2): 363-66.

2956 Tyler VE. "Grape expectations: Compound in grapes may fight cancer." Purdue Website. URL: www.purdue.edu/UNS/Clips/clips.7.97/9706.Prevention.html. (16 July 1999).

2957 Hewitt D. "Resveratrol." From Immortality Website: URL: www.immortality.org/resveratrol.html (16 July 1999).

2958 Huang C, et al. "Resveratrol suppresses cell transformation and induces apoptosis through a p53-dependent pathway." *Carcinogenesis*, 1999; 20(2): 237-42.

2959 Carbo N, et al. Resveratrol, a natural product present in wine, decreases tumour growth in a rat tumour model. *Biochem Biophys Res Commun*, 1999;254(3):739-743.

2960 Gehm BD, et al. "Resveratrol, a polyphenolic compound found in grapes and wine, is an agonist for the estrogen receptor." *Proc Natl Acad Sci U S A*, 1997; 94(25): 14138-4143.

2961 Bertelli AA, et al. "Antiplatelet activity of synthetic and natural resveratrol in red wine." *Int J Tissue React*, 1995; 17(1): 1-3.

2962 Blackshear J, Ebener MK. "Leeching, hirudin, and coagulation tests." *Ann Intern Med*, 1994; 121(2): 151-52.

2963 Haycox CL, et al. "Indications and complications of medicinal leech therapy." *J Am Acad Dermatol*, 1995; 33(6): 1053-055.

2964 Fenollar F, Fournier PE, Legre R. "Unusual case of Aeromonas sobria cellulitis associated with the use of leeches." *Eur J Clin Microbiol Infect Dis*, 1999; 18(1): 72-73.

2965 Mackay DR, et al. "Aeromonas species isolated from medicinal leeches." *Ann Plast Surg*, 1999; 42(3): 275-79.

2966 Varghese MR, et al. "Vibrio fluvialis wound infection associated with medicinal leech therapy." *Clin Infect Dis*, 1996; 22(4): 709-10.

2967 de Chalain TM. "Exploring the use of the medicinal leech: a clinical risk-benefit analysis." *J Reconstr Microsurg*, 1996; 12(3): 165-72.

2968 Lineaweaver WC, et al. "Aeromonas hydrophila infections following use of medicinal leeches in replantation and flap surgery." *Ann Plast Surg*, 1992; 29(3): 238-44.

2969 Dejobert Y, et al. "Contact Dermatitis from topical leech extract." *Contact Dermatitis*, 1991; 24(5): 366-67.

2970 Lineaweaver WC. "Aeromonas hydrophila infections following clinical use of medicinal leeches: a review of published cases." *Blood Coagul Fibrinolysis*, 1991; 2(1): 201-03.

2971 Concannon MJ, Puckett CL. "Microsurgical replantation of an ear in a child without venous repair." *Plast Reconstr Surg*, 1998; 102(6): 2088-093; discussion

2094-096.

2972 Utley DS, Koch RJ, Goode RL. "The failing flap in facial plastic and reconstructive surgery: role of the medicinal leech." *Laryngoscope*, 1998; 108(8 Pt 1): 1129-135.

2973 Bapat RD, et al. "Leech therapy for complicated varicose veins." *Indian J Med Res*, 1998; 107: 281-84.

2974 Daane S, Zamora S, Rockwell WB. "Clinical use of leeches in reconstructive surgery." *Am J Orthop*, 1997; 26(8): 528-32.

2975 de Chalain T, Cohen SR, Burstein FD. "Successful use of leeches in the treatment of purpura fulminans." *Ann Plast Surg*, 1995; 35(3): 300-04; discussion 304-06.

2976 Smeets IM, Engelberts I. "The use of leeches in a case of post-operative life-threatening macroglossia." *J Laryngol Otol*, 1995; 109(5): 442-44.

2977 Iafolla AK. "Medicinal leeches in the postoperative care of bladder exstrophy." *J Perinatol*, 1995; 15(2): 135-38.

2978 Soucacos PN, et al. "The use of medicinal leeches, Hirudo medicinalis, to restore venous circulation in trauma and reconstructive microsurgery." *Int Angiol*, 1994; 13(3): 251-58.

2979 Soucacos PN, et al. "Successful treatment of venous congestion in free skin flaps using medical leeches." *Microsurgery*, 1994; 15(7): 496-501.

2980 Bergua A, et al. [Unavoidable epistaxis in the nasal infestation of leeches]. Acta Otorrinolaringol Esp, 1993; 44(5): 391-93.

2981 Seleznev KG, et al. "Use of the medicinal leech in the treatment of ear diseases." *ORL J Otorhinolaryngol Relat Spec*, 1992; 54(1): 1-4.

2982 Solomon E. "Leech-an unusual cause of (laryngo-tracheal) obstruction." *Ethiop Med J*, 1991; 29(3): 141-42.

2983 Wade JW, Brabham RF, Allen RJ. "Medicinal leeches: once again at the forefront of medicine." *South Med J*, 1990; 83(10): 1168-173.

2984 el-Awad ME, Patil K. "Haematemesis due to leech infestation." *Ann Trop Paediatr*, 1990; 10(1): 61-62.

2985 Isgar B, Turner AG. "Large scrotal haematoma treated with medicinal leeches." *Br J Urol*, 1989; 64(5): 549-50.

2986 Golz A, et al. [Epistaxis caused by leeches]. [Article in Hebrew] *Harefuah*, 1989; 117(5-6): 141-43.

2987 Prasad SB, Sinha MR. "Vaginal bleeding due to leech." *Postgrad Med J*, 1983; 59(690): 272.

2988 Hernandez M, Ramirez Gutierrez RE. [Internal hirudiniasis: vaginal bleeding resulting from leech bite]. *Ginecol Obstet Mex*, 1998; 66: 284-86.

2989 Leeches USA Website, "Leeches." URL: www.accurate-assi-leeches.com/leeches/leeches2.html (16 July 1999).

2990 Biopharm Website, "Leeches." URL: www.biopharm-leeches.com/uses.htm (16 July 1999).

2991 Mortenson BW, Dawson KH, Murakami C. "Medicinal leeches used to salvage a traumatic nasal flap." *Br J Oral Maxillofac Surg*, 1998; 36(6): 462-64.

2992 Nazar PS, Doroshenko BH. [The leech therapy of infectious myocarditis]. [Article in Ukrainian]. *Lik Sprava*, 1998; 6(6): 146-48.

2993 Rigbi M, Orevi M, Eldor A. "Platelet aggregation and coagulation inhibitors in leech saliva and their roles in leech therapy." *Semin Thromb Hemost*, 1996; 22(3): 273-78.

2994 Orevi M, et al. "A potent inhibitor of platelet activating factor from the saliva of the leech Hirudo medicinalis." *Prostaglandins*, 1992; 43(5): 483-95.

2995 Wallis RB. "Hirudins: from leeches to man." Semin Thromb Hemost, 1996; 22(2): 185-96.

2996 Munro R, Jones CP, Sawyer RT. "Calin-a platelet adhesion inhibitor from the saliva of the medicinal leech." *Blood Coagul Fibrinolysis*, 1991; 2(1): 179-84.

2997 Baskova IP. "Inhibition of plasma kallikrein. Kininase and kinin-like activities of preparations from the medicinal leeches." *Thromb Res*, 1992; 67(6): 721-30.

2998 Rigbi M, et al. "The saliva of the medicinal leech Hirudo medicinalis-II. Inhibition of platelet aggregation and of leukocyte activity and examination of reputed anaesthetic effects." *Comp Biochem Physiol C*, 1987; 88(1): 95-98.

3000 Higher Ideals Website URL: www.healthy-u.com/17895/promise.html (10 April 1999).

3001 Life Enhancement Website URL: www.life-enhancement.com/pregnenolone.html (10 April 1999).

3002 Medquest Pharmacy Website URL: www.medquest-pharmacy.com/store /prodtemplate. asp?product_id=59 (10 April 1999).

3003 Resource Development Specialists Website URL: www.intellex.com/~gilbert/pregmeta.html (Accessed 10 April 1999).

3004 Sahelian R. Pregnenolone: Natureõs Feel Good Hormone Website URL: www.raysahelian.com/pregnenolone.html (10 April 1999).

3005 George MS, et al. "CSF neuroactive steroids in affective disorders: pregnenolone, progesterone, and DBI." *Biol Psych*, 1994; 35(10): 775-80.

3006 Wang M, et al. *J Clin Endocrinol Metab*, 1996; 81(3): 1076-082.

3007 Steiger A, et al. "Neurosteroid pregnenolone induces sleep-EEG changes in man compatible with inverse agonistic GABAA-receptor modulation." *Brain Research*, 1993; 615(2): 267-74.

3008 Devlin TM, ed. Textbook of Biochemistry With Clinical Correlations. third ed. New York: Wiley-Liss Inc., 1992.

3009 Wallach J "Nutritional help for diabetes" Website URL: www.costarr.com/eze.htm (10 April 1999).

3010 Kombucha Power Products Website URL: www.kombuchapower.com/diabetes.htm (10 April 1999).

3011 Klaassen CD, ed. Casarett and Doull's Toxicology: The Basic Science of Poisons. fifth ed. New York: McGraw-Hill, 1996.

3012 Harland BF, Harden-Williams BA. "Is vanadium of human nutritional importance yet?" *J Am Diet Assoc*, 1994; 94(8): 891-94.

3013 Malabu UH, et al. "Effects of chronic vanadate administration in the STZ-induced diabetic rat." *Diabetes*, 1994; 43: 9-15.

3014 Bishayee A, et al. "Vanadium mediated chemoprotection against chemical hepatocarcinogenesis in rats: haematological and histological characteristics." *Eur J Cancer* Prev, 1997; 6(1): 58-70.

3015 Domingo JL. "Vanadium: a review of the reproductive and developmental toxicity." *Reprod Toxicol*, 1996; 10(3): 175-82.

3016 Chakraborty A, Chatterjee M. "Enhanced erythropoietin and suppression of gamma-glutamyl-transpeptidase (GGT) activity in murine lymphoma following administration of vanadium." *Neoplasma*, 1994; 41(5): 291-96.

3017 Domingo JL, et al. "Oral vanadate and Tiron in treatment of diabetes mellitus in rats: improvement of glucose homeostasis and negative side effects." *Vet Human*

R E F E R E N C E S

Toxicol, 1993; 35(6): 495-500.

3018 Oster MH, et al. "Vanadium treatment of diabetic Sprague-Dawley rats results in tissue vanadium accumulation and pro-oxidant effects." *Toxicology*, 1993; 83(1-3): 115-30.

3019 Stern A, et al. "Vanadium as a modulator of cellular regulatory cascades and oncogene expression." *Biochem Cell Biol*, 1993; 71(3-4): 103-12.

3020 Sitprija V, et al. "Metabolic problems in northeastern Thailand: possible role of vanadium." *Ineral Electrolyte MetabMineral Electrolyte Metab*, 1998; 19(1): 51-56.

3021 Domingo JL, et al. "Oral vanadium administration to streptozocin-diabetic rats has marked negative side-effects which are independent of the form of vanadium used." *Toxicology*, 1991; 66(3): 279-87.

3022 Kastrup EK. Drug Facts and Comparisons. 1998 ed. St. Louis, MO: Facts and Comparisons, 1998.

3023 Lacy C, et al. Drug Information Handbook. fifth ed. Hudson, OH: Lexi-Comp Inc., 1997.

3024 SupraHealth Inc. Website URL: www.suprahealth.com/ vitb12.htm (26 April 1999).

3025 WellBeings Website URL: www.americahealth.com/ B12.html (26 April 1999).

3026 Nutra-Chem Inc. Website URL: www.nutrachem.com/ b12.html (26 April 1999).

3027 BioSynergy Health Alternatives Website URL: www.biosynergy.com/b1.htm (26 April 1999).

3028 WellBeings Website URL: www.americahealth.com/ B1.html (26 April 1999).

3029 SupraHealth Inc. Website URL: www.suprahealth.com/ vit-b1.htm (26 April 1999).

3030 Fresh Samantha Inc. Website URL: www.freshsamantha.com/vitamin_b1.htm (26 April 1999).

3031 BioSynergy Health Alternatives Website URL: www.biosynergy.com/b2.htm (Accessed 26 April 1999).

3032 SupraHealth Inc. Website URL: www.suprahealth.com/ vit-b2.htm (Accessed 26 April 1999).

3033 WellBeings Website URL: www.americahealth.com/ B2.html (Accessed 26 April 1999).

3034 Vitamins Plus Website URL: www.vitaminsplus.com/ library/vitamins/vitaminb2.htm#BENEFITS (Accessed 26 April 1999).

3035 Cybervitamins USA Website URL: www.cybervitamins.com/niacin.htm (Accessed 3 May 1999).

3036 SupraHealth Inc. Website URL: www.suprahealth.com/ vit-b3.htm (Accessed 3 May 1999).

3037 Life Extension Foundation Website URL lef.org/ prod_desc/item412.html (Accessed 3 May 1999).

3038 WellBeings Website URL: www.americahealth.com/ B6.html (Accessed 9 May 1999).

3039 BioSynergy Health Alternatves Website URL: www.biosynergy.com/b6.htm (Accessed 9 May 1999).

3040 Life Extension Foundation Website URL: lef.org/ prod_desc/item417.html (9 May 1999).

3041 Beers MH, Berkow R. *The Merck Manual of Diagnosis and Therapy*. 17th ed. West Point, PA: Merck and Co., Inc., 1999.

3042 Levine M, et al. "Criteria and recommendations for vitamin C intake." *JAMA*, 1999; 281: 1415-423.

3043 Monarch-One Website URL: www.monarch-one.com/ reviva.html (13 May 1999).

3044 Enlightened Associates Website URL: enlightassoc.com/ antioxidants.html (13 May 1999).

3045 Haas EM. "Staying healthy with nutrition: vitamin C."

HealthWorld Online Website. URL: www.healthy.net/ library/books/haas/vitamins/cvit.htm (13 May 1999).

3046 Hansten PD, Horn JR. *Drug Interactions Analysis and Management*. Vancouver, WA: Applied Therapeutics Inc., 1997 and updates.

3047 Mayer EL, Jacobsen DW, Robinson K. "Homocysteine and coronary Atherosclerosis." *J Am Coll Cardiol*, 1996; 27: 517-27.

3048 Robinson K, et al. "Low circulating folate and vitamin B6 concentrations: Risk factors for stroke, peripheral vascular disease, and coronary artery disease." *Circulation*, 1998; 97: 437-43.

3049 Omenn GS, Beresford SAA, Motulsky AG. "Preventing coronary heart disease: B vitamins and homocysteine." *Circulation*, 1998; 97: 421-24.

3050 Rimm EB, et al. "Folate and vitamin B6 from diet and supplements in relation to risk of coronary heart disease among women." *JAMA*, 1998; 279: 359-64.

3051 Leonard A, Gerber GB. "Mutagenicity, carcinogenicity and teratogenicity of vanadium Compounds." *Mutation Research*, 1994; 317(1): 81-88.

3052 Fawcett JP, et al. "Oral vanadyl sulphate does not affect blood cells, viscosity or biochemistry in humans." *Pharmacol Toxicol*, 1997; 80(4): 202-06.

3053 Fawcett JP, et al. "The effect of oral vanadyl sulfate on body composition and performance in weight-training athletes." *Int J Sport Nutr*, 1996; 6(4): 382-90.

3054 Funakoshi T, et al. "Anticoagulant action of vanadate." *Chem Pharmaceut Bull*, 1992; 40(1): 174-76.

3055 Halberstam M, et al. "Oral vanadyl sulfate improves insulin sensitivity in NIDDM but not in obese nondiabetic subjects." *Diabetes*, 1996; 45(5): 659-66.

3056 Cohen N, et al. "Oral vanadyl sulfate improves hepatic and peripheral insulin sensitivity in patients with non-insulin-dependent diabetes mellitus." *J Clin Invest*, 1995; 95: 2501-509.

3057 Boden G, et al. "Effects of vanadyl sulfate on carbohydrate and lipid metabolism in patients with non-insulin-dependent diabetes mellitus." *Metabolism*, 1996; 45(9): 1130-135.

3058 KCWeb Website URL: www.kcweb.com/herb/vit_d.htm (30 May 1999).

3059 Smart Basics Inc Website URL: www.smartbasic.com/ glos.vitamins/vit.d.glos.html (30 May 1999).

3060 Quest Vitamins Website URL: www.questvitmains.co.uk/vitb.htm (30 May 1999).

3061 Herbs 4 Us Website URL: www.herbs4us.com/ vitaminb.htm (30 May 1999).

3062 Smart Basics Inc. Website URL: www.smartbasic.com/ glos.vitamins/vit.a.glos.html (Accessed 10 June 1999).

3063 Wells International Derma-E Natural Skin Care Website URL: www.derma-e/com/vitamina.html (Accessed 10 June 1999).

3064 SupraHealth Inc. Website URL: www.suprahealth.com/ vit-a.htm (Accessed 10 June 1999).

3065 WellBeings Website URL: www.americahealth.com/ A.html (Accessed 10 June 1999).

3066 FDA Talk Paper: Vitamin A and birth defects (T95-56). Food and Drug Administration, U.S.Department of Health and Human Services, Rockville, MD. 6 October 1995.

3067 Life Plus Website URL: enlightassoc.com/ antioxidants.html (Accessed 20 June 1999).

3068 HerbsNow Website URL: www.herbsnow.com/ vitamins.htm (Accessed 20 June 1999).

3069 Nature's Wonders Website URL:

www.natureswonders.com/dermalk.html (Accessed 21 June 1999).

3070 Verhoef P, Stampfer MJ, Buring JE, et al. "Homocysteine Metabolism and risk of myocardial infarction: relation with vitamin B6, B12 and folate." *Am J Epidemiol*, 1996; 143:845-859.

3071 Briggs GG, Freeman RK, Yaffe SJ. Drugs in Pregnancy and Lactation, fifth edition. Williams and Wilkins, Baltimore, MD. 1998.

3072 Tatro DS, ed. *Drug Interactions Facts*. Facts and Comparisons Inc., St.Louis, MO. 1999.

3073 Frank J, Weiser H, Biesalski HK. "Interaction of vitamins E and K: effect of high dietary vitamin E on phylloquinone activity in chicks." *Int J Vit Nutr Res*, 1997; 67(4):242-247.

3074 Helson L. "The effect of intravenous vitamin E and menadiol sodium diphosphate on vitamin K dependent clotting factors." *Thromb Res*, 1984; 35(1):11-18.

3075 Netrition Website URL: www.netrition.com/enada_page.html (21 June 1999).

3076 Renascent Systems Inc. Website URL: www.nadh.com/index.html (21 June 1999).

3077 The Healing Network Website URL: www.thehealingnetwork.com/nadh.htm (21 June 1999).

3078 Hardman JG, Limbird LE, ed. Goodman and Gilman's The Pharmacological Basis of Therapeutics, ninth edition. McGraw-Hill, New York, NY, 1996.

3079 Totally Natural Website URL: www.quickresults.com.au/foodsupps.b5.htm (29 June 1999).

3080 Herbal Hope Website URL: www.herbalhope.com/ing/vitamin_b5.html (29 June 1999).

3081 Sequential Healing Health Services Website URL: www.sequentialhealing.com/vit-min-nutrients/vit-b5.html (29 June 1999).

3082 Budavari S, ed. The Merck Index, 12th edition. Merck & Co., Inc. Whitehouse Station, NJ, 1996.

3083 Bushehri N, Jarrell ST, Lieberman S, et al. "Oral reduced B-nicotinamide adenine dinucleotide (NADH) affects blood pressure, lipid peroxidation, and lipid profile in hypertensive rats (SHR)." *Geriatr Nephrol Urol*, 1998; 8(2):95-100.

3084 Forsyth LM, Preuss HG, MacDowell AL, et al. "Therapeutic effects of oral NADH on the symptoms of patients with chronic fatigue syndrome." *Ann All Asthma Immunol*, 1999; 82(2):185-191.

3085 Swerdlow RH. "Is NADH effective in the treatment of Parkinson's disease?." *Drugs & Aging*, 1998; 13(4):263-268.

3086 Kuhn W, Muller T, Winkel R, et al. "Parenteral application of NADH in Parkinson's disease: clinical improvement partially due to stimulation of endogenous levodopa biosynthesis." *J Neural Transmiss* (Budapest), 1996; 103(10):1187-1193.

3087 Birkmayer JG. "Coenzyme nicotinamide adenine dinucleotide: new therapeutic approach for improving dementia of the Alzheimer type." *Ann Clin Lab Sci*, 1996; 26(1):1-9.

3088 Vrecko K, Birkmayer JG, Krainz J. "Stimulation of dopamine biosynthesis in cultured PC 12 phaeochromocytoma cells by the coenzyme nicotinamide adeninedinucleotide (NADH)." *J Neural Transmiss* (Parkinsons Disease & Dementia Section), 1993; 5(2):147-156.

3089 Birkmayer JG, Vrecko C, Volc D, Birkmayer W. "Nicotinamide adenine dinucleotide (NADH)—a new therapeutic approach to Parkinson's disease. Comparison

of oral and parenteral application." *Acta Neurol Scand Suppl*, 1993; 146:32-35.

3090 Dizdar N, Kagedal B, Lindvall B. "Treatment of Parkinson's disease with NADH." *Acta Neurol Scand*, 1994; 90(5):345-347.

3091 Vrecko K, Storga D, Birkmayer JG, et al. "NADH stimulates endogenous dopamine biosynthesis by enhancing the recycling of tetrahydrobiopterin in rat phaeochromocytoma cells." *Biochim Biophys Acta*, 1997; 1361(1):59-65.

3092 Fauci AS, Braunwald E, Isselbacher KJ, et al. Harrison's Principles of Internal Medicine, 14th edition. McGraw-Hill, New York, NY, 1998.

3093 Wyatt KM, Dimmock PW, Jones PW, O'Brien PM. "Efficacy of vitamin B6 in the treatment of premenstrual syndrome." *BMJ* 1999; 318:1375-1381.

3094 Yates AA, Schlicker SA, Suitor CW. "Dietary reference intakes: The new basis for recommendations for calcium and related nutrients, B vitamins, and choline." *J Am Diet Assoc*, 1998; 98:699-706.

3097 Simon JA, Hudes ES. Relationship of ascorbic acid to blood lead levels. *JAMA* , 1999; 281(24):2289-2293.

3098 Dawson EB, Evans DR, Harris WA, et al. The effect of ascorbic acid supplementation on the blood lead levels of smokers. *J Am Coll Nutr*, 1999; 18(2):166-170.

3099 Cheng Y, Willett WC, Schwartz J, et al. Relation of nutrition to bone lead and blood lead levels in middle-aged to elderly men. The Normative Aging Study. *Am J Epidemiol*, 1998; 147(12):1162-1174.

3100 Escarpa A, Gonzalez MC. High-performance liquid chromatography with diode-array detection for the determination of phenolic compounds in peel and pulp from different apple varieties. *J Chromatog A* 1998;823(1-2):331-337.

3101 Cruz T, Galvez J, Ocete MA, et al. Oral administration of rutoside can ameliorate inflammatory bowel disease in rats. *Life Sci* 1998;62(7):687-695.

3102 Galvez J, Cruz T, Crespo E, et al. Rutoside as mucosal protective in acetic acid-induced rat colitis. *Planta Med* 1997;63(5):409-414.

3103 Kostyuk VA, Potapovich AI, Speransky SD, Maslova GT. Protective effect of natural flavonoids on rat peritoneal macrophages injury caused by asbestos fibers. *Free Radical Biol Med* 1996;21(4):487-493.

3104 Webster RP, Gawde MD, Bhattacharya RK. Protective effect of rutin, a flavonol glycoside, on the carcinogen-induced DNA damage and repair enzymes in rats. *Cancer Lett*, 1996;109(1-2):185-191.

3105 Schmitt A, Salvayre R, Delchambre J, Negre-Salvayre A. Prevention by alpha-tocopherol and rutin of glutathione and ATP depletion induced by oxidized LDL in cultured endothelial cells. *Br J Pharmacol* 1995;116(3):1985-1990.

3106 Rueff J, Gaspar J, Laires A. Structural requirements for mutagenicity of flavonoids upon nitrosation. A structure-activity study. *Mutagenesis* 1995;10(4):325-328.

3107 Perez Guerrero C, Martin MJ, Marhuenda E. Prevention by rutin of gastric lesions induced by ethanol in rats: role of endogenous prostaglandins. *Gen Pharmacol* 1994;25(3):575-580.

3108 Deschner EE, Ruperto J, Wong G, Newmark HL. Quercetin and rutin as inhibitors of azoxymethanol-induced colonic neoplasia. *Carcinogenesis* 1991;12(7):1193-1196.

3110 Health Quest website URL www.healthquest4u.com/jcp/blindstudy.htm (Accessed 2 September 1999).

REFERENCES

3111 Barnett ML, Kremer JM, St.Clair W, et al. Treatment of rheumatoid arthritis with oral type II collagen. *Arthr Rheum*, 1998; 41(2):290-297.

3112 Barnett ML, Combitchi D, Trentham DE. A pilot trial of oral type II collagen in the treatment of juvenile rheumatoid arthritis. *Arthr Rheum*, 1996; 39(4):623-628.

3113 Ghoneum M. Anti-HIV activity in vitro of MGN-3, an activated arabinoxylane from rice bran. *Biochem Biophys Res Commun* 1998;243(1):25-9.

3114 The Healing Network website URL: www.anaturalchoice.com/is.htm (Accessed 22 September 1999).

3115 CompassioNet Online website URL www.compassionet.com/mgn3.htm (Accessed 22 September 1999).

3116 Ghoneum M, Namatalla G, Kim C. Effect of MGN-3 on human natural killer cell activity and interferon-gamma synthesis in vitro. Abstract. *Federation of American Societies for Experimental Biology Journal*, 1996;10(6):26-32.

3117 Ghoneum M, Jewett A. Synergistic effect of modified arabinoxylane (MGN-3) and low dose of recombinant IL-2 on human NK cell activity and TNF production. Abstract. *American Acadamy of Anti-Aging Medicine Educational Conference*, August 15-16, 1998.

3118 Ghoneum M. Enhancement of human natural killer cell activity by modified arabinoxylane from rice bran (MGN-3). *Int J Immunotherapy*, 1998;14(2):89-99.

3119 Ghoneum M, Namatalla G. NK immunomodulatory function in 27 *Cancer* patients by MGN-3, a modified arabinoxylane from rice bran. Abstract. *87th Annual Meeting of the American Association for Cancer Research*. April 20-24, 1996.

3120 Ghoneum M. Immunomodulatory and anti-cancer properties of MGN-3, a modified xylose from rice bran, in 5 patients with breast cancer. Abstract. American Association for Cancer Research Special Conference. November 5-8, 1995.

3125 Kalden JR, Sieper J. Oral collagen in the treatment of rheumatoid arthritis [editorial]. *Arthr Rheum*, 1998;41(2):191-194.

3126 Trentham DE. Oral tolerization as a treatment of rheumatoid arthritis. *Rheum Dis Clin North Am*, 1998; 24(3):525-536.

3127 Mullins RJ, Richards C, Walker T. Allergic reactions to oral, surgical and topical bovine collagen. Anaphylactic risk for surgeons. *Aust N Z J Ophthalmol*, 1996; 24(3):257-260.

3128 AutoImmune Inc. announces phase III trial results for Colloral. URL http://www.autoimmune.com/clinic/coll.html (Accessed 24 October 1999).

3129 Wang XD, Zhang JM, Yang HH, Hu GY. Modulation of NMDA receptor by huperzine A in rat cerebral cortex. *Chung Kuo Yao Li Hsueh Pao*, 1999;20(1):31-35.

3130 DHM Inc. website. URL http://www.huperzine.net (Accessed 26 October 1999).

3131 Skolnick AA. Old Chinese herbal Medicine used for fever yields possible new Alzheimer Disease therapy. *JAMA* 1997;277:776.

3132 Wang H, Tang XC. Anticholinesterase effects of huperzine A, E2020, and tacrine in rats. *Chung Kuo Li Hsueh Pao*, 1998;19(1):27-30.

3133 Xiong ZQ, Cheng DH, Tang XC. Effects of huperzine A on nucleus basalis magnocellularis lesion-induced spatial working memory deficit. *Chung Kuo Yao Li Hsueh Pao*, 1998;19(2):128-132.

3134 Ye JW, Cai JX, Wang LM, Tang XC. Improving effects of huperzine A on spatial working memory in aged monkeys and young adult monkeys with experimental cognitive impairment. *J Pharmacol Exp Ther*, 1999;288(2):814-819.

3135 Wang T, Tang XC. Reversal of scopolamine-induced deficits in radial maze performance by (-)-huperzine A: comparison with E2020 and tacrine. *Eur J Pharmacol*, 1998;349(2-3):137-142.

3136 Cheng DH, Tang XC. Comparative studies of huperzine A, E2020, and tacrine on behavior and cholinesterase activities. *Pharmacol Biochem Behav*, 1998;60(2):377-386.

3137 Lallement G, Veyret J, Masqueliez C, et al. Efficacy of huperzine in preventing soman-induced seizures, neuropathological changes and lethality. *Fundam Clin Pharmacol*, 1997;11(5):387-394.

3138 Xu SS, Gao ZX, Weng Z, et al. Efficacy of tablet huperzine-A on memory, cognition, and behavior in Alzheimer's disease. *Chung Kuo Yao Li Hsueh Pao*, 1995;16(5):391-395.

3139 Grunwald J, Raveh L, Doctor BP, Ashani Y. Huperzine A as a pretreatment candidate drug against nerve agent toxicity. *Life Sci*, 1994;54(14):991-997.

3140 Zhang RW, Tang XC, Han YY, et al. [Drug evaluation of huperzine A in the treatment of senile memory disorders]. *Chung Kuo Yao Li Hsueh Pao*, 1991;12(3):250-252.

3141 Tang XC, De Sarno P, Sugaya K, Giacobini E. Effect of huperzine A, a new cholinesterase inhibitor, on the central cholinergic system of the rat. *J Neurosci Res*, 1989;24(2):276-285.

3142 Safety Briefs, ISMP Medication Safety Alert, vol.4, #4. Institute for Safe Medication Practices, Warminster, PA. February 24, 1999.

3143 Potential new East-West combination drug for Alzheimer's shows promise. Reuters Health, URL: www.reutershealth.com/frame_eline.html (Accessed 2 November 1999).

3144 A Modern Herbal website. URL www.botanical.com/botanical/mgmh/m/mandra10.html (Accessed 9 November 1999).

3145 Health 4 Free web site. URL http://health4free.com/Product%20List/Bupleurum.htm (Accessed 26 October 1999).

3146 Yu D, et al. Treatment of primary thrombocytopenic purpura by modified minor decoction of bupleurum. Journal of Traditional Chinese Medicine, 1995;15(2):96-98. URL http://www.itppeople.com/articles/Bupleurum.htm (Acceessed 26 October 1999).

3147 Miller L, Murray WJ, eds. *Herbal Medicinals: A Clinician's Guide*. Pharmaceutical Products Press, Binghamton, NY, 1998.

3148 Bupleurum falcatum Bitter & cool. The Australian Naturopath Network web site. URL: www.comcen.com.au/~sburgess/herbs/Monographs/bupleuru.htm (Accessed 13 November 1999).

3149 Sequential Healing Health Services web site. URL http://www.sequentialhealing.com/herbs/bupleurum.html (Accessed 13 November 1999).

3150 PanoLife Products Inc. website. URL http://www.pano.com/huperzia.html (Accessed 26 October 1999).

3151 Jing H, Jiang Y, Luo S. [Chemical constituents of the roots of Bupleurum longicaule Wall. ex DC. var. franchetii de Boiss and B. chaishoui Shan et Sheh].

REFERENCES

[Article in Chinese] *Chung Kuo Chung Yao Tsa Chih*, 1996;21(12):739-741,762.

3152 Yen MH, Lin CC, Chuang CH, Liu SY. Evaluation of root quality of Bupleurum species by TLC scanner and the liver protective effects of "xiao-chai-hu-tang" prepared using three different Bupleurum species. *J Ethnopharmacol*, 1991;34(2-3):155-165.

3153 Sakurai MH, Matsumoto T, Kiyohara H, Yamada H. B-cell proliferation activity of pectic polysaccharide from a medicinal herb, the roots of Bupleurum falcatum L. and its structural requirement. *Immunology*, 1999;97(3):540-547.

3154 Yamada H. [Structure and pharmacological activity of pectic polysaccharides from the roots of Bupleurum falcatum L]. [Article in Japanese] *Nippon Yakurigaku Zasshi,* 1995;106(3):229-237.

3155 Matsumoto T, Moriguchi R, Yamada H. Role of polymorphonuclear leucocytes and oxygen-derived free radicals in the formation of gastric lesions induced by HCl/ethanol, and a possible mechanism of protection by anti-ulcer polysaccharide. *J Pharm Pharmacol*, 1993;45(6):535-539.

3156 Hattori T, Ito M, Suzuki Y. [Studies on antinephritic effects of plant components in rats (1). Effects of saikosaponins original-type anti-GBM nephritis in rats and its mechanisms]. [Article in Japanese] *Nippon Yakurigaku Zasshi*, 1991;97(1):13-21.

3157 Ahn BZ, Yoon YD, Lee YH, et al. Inhibitory effect of bupleuri radix saponins on adhesion of some solid tumor cells and relation to hemolytic action: screening of 232 herbal drugs for anti-cell adhesion. *Planta Med*, 1998;64(3):220-224.

3158 Nose M, Amagaya S, Ogihara Y. Corticosterone secretion-inducing activity of saikosaponin metabolites formed in the alimentary tract. *Chem Pharm Bull* (Tokyo), 1989;37(10):2736-2740.

3159 Chang WC, Hsu FL. Inhibition of platelet activation and endothelial cell injury by flavan-3-ol and saikosaponin compounds. *Prostaglandins Leukot Essent Fatty Acids*, 1991;44(1):51-56.

3160 Kato M, Pu MY, Isobe K, et al. Characterization of the immunoregulatory action of saikosaponin-d. *Cell Immunol*, 1994;159(1):15-25.

3161 Ushio Y, Oda Y, Abe H. Effect of saikosaponin on the immune responses in mice. *Int J Immunopharmacol*, 1991;13(5):501-508.

3162 Abe H, Sakaguchi M, Odashima S, Arichi S. Protective effect of saikosaponin-d isolated from Bupleurum falcatum L. on CCl4-induced liver injury in the rat. *Int J Immunopharmacol*, 1982;320(3):266-271.

3163 Chiu HF, Lin CC, Yen MH, et al. Pharmacological and pathological studies on hepatic protective crude drugs from Taiwan (V): The effects of Bombax malabarica and Scutellaria rivularis. *Am J Chin Med*, 1992;20(3-4):257-264.

3164 Izumi S, Ohno N, Kawakita T, et al. Wide range of molecular weight distribution of mitogenic substance(s) in the hot water extract of a Chinese herbal medicine, Bupleurum chinense. *Biol Pharm Bull*, 1997;20(7):759-764.

3165 Guinea MC, Parellada J, Lacaille-Dubois MA, Wagner H. Biologically active triterpene saponins from Bupleurum fruticosum. *Planta Med*, 1994;60(2):163-167.

3166 Martin S, Padilla E, Ocete MA, et al. Anti-inflammatory activity of the essential oil of Bupleurum fruticescens.

Planta Med, 1993;59(6):533-536.

3167 Lorente I, Ocete MA, Zarzuelo A, et al. Bioactivity of the essential oil of Bupleurum fruticosum. *J Nat Prod*, 1989;52(2):267-272.

3168 Bermejo Benito P, Abad Martinez MJ, Silvan Sen AM, et al. In vivo and in vitro antiinflammatory activity of saikosaponins. *Life Sci*, 1998;63(13):1147-1156.

3169 Nakano Y, Matsunaga H, Saita T, et al. Antiproliferative constituents in Umbelliferae plants II. Screening for polyacetylenes in some Umbelliferae plants, and isolation of panaxynol and falcarindiol from the root of Heracleum moellendorffii. *Biol Pharm Bull*, 1998;21(3):257-261.

3170 Estevez-Braun A, Estevez-Reyes R, Moujir LM, et al. Antibiotic activity and absolute configuation of 8S-heptadeca-2(Z),9(Z)-diene-4,6-diyne-1,8-diol from Bupleurum salicifolium. *J Nat Prod*, 1994;57(8):1178-1182.

3171 Zhang SL. Therapeutic effects of huperzine A on the aged with memory impairment. [article in Chinese] New Drugs and Clinical Remedies 1986;5(5):260-262.

3172 Cheng YS, Lu CZ, Ying ZL, et al. 128 cases of myasthenia gravis treated with huperzine A. [article in Chinese] *New Drugs and Clinical Remedies* 1986;5(4):197-199.

3173 *AIDS* Treatment News Archive. URL: 4.17.177.49/ immunet/atn.nsf/page/a-049-01 (Accessed 25 November 1999).

3174 Strictly Medicinal Herb Seeds website. URL: www.budget.net/~herbseed/sweetann.htm (Accessed 25 November 1999).

3175 Herb facts of the month. Herbal Connections website. URL: www.herbworld.com/snst/arc8-8.htm (Accessed 25 November 1999).

3176 HolisticOnLine website. URL: holisticonline.com/ Herbal-Med/_scripts/getHerb_Dir.idc?Herb_Names=365 (Accessed 25 November 1999).

3177 Dharmananda S. PCP prophylaxis with drugs and herbs. Institute for Traditional Medicine Online. URL: www.rdi.gpo.or.th/NetZine/V3N42/pcp.htm (Accessed 25 November 1999).

3178 Artemether/Artenam website. URL: www.arenco.be/ (Accessed 25 November 1999).

3179 Herbal Review, Sequential Healing Health Services website. URL: www.sequentialhealing.com/herbs/sweet-Annie.html (Accessed 25 November 1999).

3180 Pittler MH, Ernst E. Artemether for severe malaria: a meta-analysis of randomized clinical trials. *Clin Infect Dis* 1999;28(3):597-601.

3181 van Agtmael MA, Eggelte TA, van Boxtel CJ. Artemisinin drugs in the treatment of malaria: from medicinal herb to registered medication. *Trends Pharmacol Sci* 1999;20(5):199-205.

3182 Moneton P, Ducret JP. Positioning, labeling and control of medical information: artesunate strategy and Arsumax development story. *Med Trop* (Mars) 1998;58(3 Suppl):70-72.

3183 Zheng GQ. Cytotoxic terpenoids and flavonoids from Artemisia annua. *Planta Med* 1994;60(1):54-57.

3184 Huang L, Liu JF, Liu LX, et al. [Antipyretic and anti-inflammatory effects of Artemisia annua L]. *Chung Kuo Chung Yao Tsa Chih* 1993;18(1):44-48,63-64.

3185 Wan YD, Zang QZ, Wang JS. [Studies on the antimalarial action of gelatin capsule of Artemisia annua]. *Chung Kuo Chi Sheng Chung Hsueh Yu Chi Sheng Chung Ping Tsa Chih* 1992;10(4):290-294.

3186 Swedish Herbal Institute website. URL http://www.adaptogen.com/shi_np2.html (Accessed 22 November 1999).

3187 PlanetHerbs Online website. URL http://www.planetherbs.com/articles/rhodiola%20rosea.htm (Accessed 22 November 1999).

3188 Mother Nature's General Store, Inc. website. URL http://www.herbalphen.com/rhod.htm (Accessed 22 November 1999).

3189 Nutri-Mart Cyberstore. URL http://www.nutrimart.com/Bulk/Description/rhodiola_rosea.htm (Accessed 22 November 1999).

3190 Salikhova RA, Aleksandrova IV, Mazurik VK, et al. [Effect of Rhodiola rosea on the yield of mutation alterations and DNA repair in bone marrow cells]. *Patol Fiziol Eksp Ter* 1997;(4):22-24.

3191 Lishmanov IuB, Naumova AV, Afanas'ev SA, Maslov LN. [Contribution of the opioid system to realization of inotropic effects of Rhodiola rosea extracts in ischemic and reperfusion heart damage in vitro]. *Eksp Klin Farmakol* 1997;60(3):34-36.

3192 Maimeskulova LA, Maslov LN, Lishmanov IuB, Krasnov EA. [The participation of the mu-, delta- and kappa-opioid receptors in the realization of the anti-arrhythmia effect of Rhodiola rosea]. *Eksp Klin Farmakol* 1997;60(1):38-39.

3193 Maslova LV, Kondrat'ev BIu, Maslov LN, Lishmanov IuB. [The cardioprotective and antiadrenergic activity of an extract of Rhodiola rosea in stress]. *Eksp Klin Farmakol* 1994;57(6):61-63.

3194 Bocharova OA, Matveev BP, Baryshnikov AIu, et al. [The effect of a Rhodiola rosea extract on the incidence of recurrences of a superficial bladder cancer]. *Urol Nefrol* (Mosk) 1995;(2):46-47.

3195 Lishmanov IuB, Maslova LV, Maslov LN, Dan'shina EN. [The anti-arrhythmia effect of Rhodiola rosea and its possible mechanism]. *Biull Eksp Biol Med* 1993;116(8):175-176.

3196 Udintsev SN, Krylova SG, Fomina TI. [The enhancement of the efficacy of adriamycin by using hepatoprotectors of plant origin in metastases of Ehrlich's adenocarcinoma to the Liver in mice]. *Vopr Onkol* 1992;38(10):1217-1222.

3197 Udintsev SN, Shakhov VP. [Changes in clonogenic properties of bone marrow and transplantable mice tumor cells during combined use of cyclophosphane and biological response modifiers of adaptogenic origin]. *New Drugs and Clinical Remedies* 1990;12(6):55-56.

3198 Petkov VD, Yonkov D, Mosharoff A, et al. Effects of alcohol aqueous extract from Rhodiola rosea L. roots on learning and memory. *Acta Physiol Pharmacol Bulg* 1986;12(1):3-16.

3199 Sequential Healing Health Services website. URL www.sequentialhealing.com/herbs/squawvine.html (Accessed 22 November 1999).

3219 Brown L, Rimm EB, Seddon JM, et al. A prospective study of carotenoid intake and risk of cataract extraction in US men. *Am J Clin Nutr* 1999;70:517-24.

3220 Chasan-Taber L, Willett WC, Seddon JM, et al. A prospective study of carotenoid and vitamin A intakes and risk of cataract extraction in US women. *Am J Clin Nutr* 1999;70:509-16.

3221 Lyle BJ, Mares-Perlman JA, Klein BE, et al. Antioxidant intake and risk of incident age-related nuclear cataracts in the Beaver Dam Eye Study. *Am J Epidemiol* 1999;149:801-9.

3222 Teikari JM, Rautalahti M, Haukka J, et al. Incidence of cataract operations in Finnish male smokers unaffected by alpha tocopherol or beta carotene supplements. *J Epidemiol Community Health* 1998;52:468-72.

3223 Teikari JM, Virtamo J, Rautalahti M, et al. Long-term supplementation with alpha-tocopherol and beta-carotene and age-related cataract. *Acta Ophthalmol Scand* 1997;75:634-40.

3224 Sommerburg O, Keunen JE, Bird AC, et al. Fruits and vegetables that are sources for lutein and zeaxanthin: the macular pigment in human eyes. *Br J Ophthalmol* 1998;82:907-10.

3225 Hammond BR Jr, Wooten BR, Snodderly DM, et al. Density of the human crystalline lens is related to the macular pigment carotenoids, lutein and zeaxanthin. *Optom Vis Sci* 1997;74:499-504.

3226 Gross AS, Goh YD, Addison RS, et al. Influence of grapefruit juice on cisapride pharmacokinetics. *Clin Pharmacol Ther* 1999; 65:395-401.

3227 Lilja JJ, Kivisto KT, Neuvonen PJ. Grapefruit juice increases serum concentrations of atorvastatin and has no effect on pravastatin. *Clin Pharmacol Ther* 1999; 66:118-27.

3228 Ozdemir M, Aktan Y, Boydag BS. Interaction between grapefruit juice and diazepam in humans. *Eur J Drug Metab Pharmacokinet* 1998; 23:55-9.

3229 Grapefruit-drug interactions. URL: powernetdesign.com/grapefruit (Accessed 26 September 1999).

3230 Zaidenstein R, Dishi V, Gips M, et al. The effect of grapefruit juice on the pharmacokinetics of orally administered verapamil. *Eur J Clin Pharmacol* 1998; 54:337-40.

3231 Arlt W, Callies F, van Vlijmen JC, et al. Dehydroepiandrosterone replacement in women with adrenal insufficiency. *N Engl J Med* 1999;341:1013-20.

3232 Oelkers W. Dehydroepiandrosterone for adrenal insufficiency (editorial). *New Eng J Med* 1999;341:1073-4.

3233 Selhub J, Jacques PF, Rosenberg IH, et al. Serum total homocysteine concentrations in the Third National Health and Nutrition Examination Survey (1991-1994): population reference ranges and contribution of vitamin status to high serum concentrations. *Ann Intern Med* 1999;131(5):331-9.

3234 Murray M, Pizzorno J. Encyclopedia of Natural Medicine, second edition. Rocklin, CA: Prima Health, 1998.

3235 Lindenbaum J, Healton EB, Savage DG, et al. Neuropsychiatric disorders caused by cobalamin deficiency in the absence of anemia or macrocytosis. *N Engl J Med*, 1988;318:1720-1728.

3236 Chappell LC, Seed PT, Briley AL, et al. Effect of antioxidants on the occurrence of pre-eclampsia in women at increased risk: a randomized trial. *Lancet* 1999;354:810-816.

3237 Mensink RP, van Houwelingen AC, Kromhout D, Hornstra G. A vitamin E concentrate rich in tocotrienols had no effect on serum lipids, lipoproteins, or platelet function in men with mildly elevated serum lipid concentrations. *Am J Clin Nutr* 1999;69:213-9.

3238 Qureshi AA, Qureshi N, Wright JJ, et al. Lowering of serum cholesterol in hypercholesterolemic humans by tocotrienols (palmvitee). *Am J Clin Nutr* 1991;53(4 Suppl):1021S-1026S.

3239 Tomeo AC, Geller M, Watkins TR, et al. Antioxidant effects of tocotrienols in patients with hyperlipidemia

REFERENCES

and carotid stenosis. *Lipids* 1995;30:1179-83.

3240 Qureshi AA, Bradlow BA, Brace L, et al. Response of hypercholesterolemic subjects to administration of tocotrienols. *Lipids* 1995;30:1171-7.

3241 Qureshi AA, Bradlow BA, Slaser WA, et al. Novel tocotrienols of rice bran modulate cardiovascular disease risk parameters of hypercholesterolemic humans. *Nutritional Biochemistry* 1997;8:290-98.

3242 Conte A, de Bernardi M, Palmieri L, et al. Metabolic fate of exogenous chondroitin sulfate in man. *Arzneimittelforschung* 1991; 4:768-72.

3243 Pittler MH, Abbot NC, Harkness EF, et al. Randomized, double-blind trial of chitosan for body weight reduction. *Eur J Clin Nutr* 1999;53:379-81.

3244 Wuolijoki E, Hirvela T, Ylitalo P. Decrease in serum LDL cholesterol with microcrystalline chitosan. Methods Find Exp *Clin Pharmacol* 1999;21:357-61.

3245 Takahashi K, Yoshino K, Shirai T, et al. Effect of a traditional herbal *Medicine* (shakuyaku-kanzo-to) on testosterone secretion in patients with polycystic ovary syndrome detected by ultrasound. *Nippon Sanka Fujinka Gakkai Zasshi* 1988;40:789-92.

3246 Armanini D, Bonanni G, Palermo M, et al. Reduction of serum testosterone in men by licorice. *New Eng J Med* 1999;341:1158.

3247 Abe Y, Ueda T, Kato T, Kohli Y. [Effectiveness of interferon, glycyrrhizin combination therapy in patients with chronic hepatitis C].[Article in Japanese]. *Nippon Rinsho* 1994 Jul;52(7):1817-22.

3248 Sato H, Goto W, Yamamura J, et al. Therapeutic basis of glycyrrhizin on chronic hepatitis B. *Antiviral Res* 1996;30:171-7.

3249 Takahara T, Watanabe A, Shiraki K. Effects of glycyrrhizin on hepatitis B surface antigen: a biochemical and morphological study. *J Hepatol* 1994;21:601-9.

3250 Acharya SK, Dasarathy S, Tandon A, et al. A preliminary open trial on interferon stimulator (SNMC) derived from Glycyrrhiza glabra in the treatment of subacute hepatic failure. *Indian J Med Res* 1993;98:69-74.

3251 Eisenburg J. [Treatment of chronic hepatitis B. Part 2: Effect of glycyrrhizic acid on the course of illness]. [Article in German]. *Fortschr Med* 1992;110(21):395-8.

3252 Armanini D, Lewicka S, Pratesi C, et al. Further studies on the mechanism of the mineralocorticoid action of licorice in humans. *J Endocrinol Invest* 1996;19:624-9.

3253 Krahenbuhl S, Hasler F, Frey BM, et al. Kinetics and dynamics of orally administered 18 beta-glycyrrhetinic acid in humans. *J Clin Endocrinol Metab* 1994;78:581-5.

3254 Lee YS, Lorenzo BJ, Koufis T, et al. Grapefruit juice and its flavonoids inhibit 11 beta-hydroxysteroid dehydrogenase. *Clin Pharmacol Ther* 1996;59:62-71.

3255 Zhang YD, Lorenzo B, Reidenberg MM. Inhibition of 11 beta hydroxysteroid dehydrogenase obtained from guinea pig kidney by furosemide, naringenin and some other compounds. *J Steroid Biochem Mol Biol* 1994;49:81-5.

3256 Hiai S, Yokoyama H, Oura H, et al. Stimulation of pituitary-adrenocortical system by ginseng saponin. *Endocrinol Jpn* 1979;26:661-5.

3257 Kase Y, Saitoh K, Ishige A, et al. Mechanisms by which Hange-shashin-to reduces prostaglandin E2 levels. *Biol Pharm Bull* 1998;21:1277-81.

3258 Natural Pleasure website, URL: www.netoz.au.com/np/larginin.htm (Accessed 15 October 1999).

3259 Peters H, Noble NA. Dietary L-arginine in renal disease.

Semin Nephrol 1996;16(6):567-75.

3260 Wang R, Ghahary A, Shen YJ, et al. Human dermal fibroblasts produce nitric oxide and express both constitutive and inducible nitric oxide synthase isoforms. *J Invest Dermatol* 1996;106:419-27.

3261 Moody JA, Vernet D, Laidlaw S, et al. Effects of long-term oral administration of L-arginine on the rat erectile response. *J Urol* 1997;158(3 Pt 1):942-7.

3262 Russell IJ, Michalek JE, Flechas JD, et al. Treatment of fibromyalgia syndrome with Super Malic: a randomized, double blind, placebo controlled, crossover pilot study. *J Rheumatol* 1995;22:953-8.

3263 Koo WK, Walters JC, Esterlitz J, et al. Maternal calcium supplementation and fetal bone mineralization. *Obstet Gynecol* 1999; 94:577-82.

3264 Raman L, Rajalakshmi K, Krishnamachari KAVR, et al. Effect of calcium supplementation to undernourished mothers during pregnancy on the bone density of the neonates. *Am J Clin Nutr* 1978; 31:466-9.

3265 Roth JA, Kim B-G, Lin W-L, et al. Melatonin promotes osteoblast differentiation and bone formation. *J Biol Chem* 1999; 31:22041-7

3267 Singh RB, Niaz MA, Ghosh S. Hypolipidemic and antioxidant effects of Commiphora mukul as an adjunct to dietary therapy in patients with hypercholesterolemia. *Cardiovasc Drugs Ther* 1994;8:659-64.

3268 Thappa DM, Dogra J. Nodulocystic acne: oral gugulipid versus tetracycline. *J Dermatol* 1994;21(10):729-31.

3269 Adzet T, Camarasa J, Laguna JC. Hepatoprotective activity of polyphenolic compounds from Cynara scolymus against CCl4 toxicity in isolated rat hepatocytes. *J Nat Prod* 1987;50:612-7.

3270 Wolkowitz OM, Reus VI, Keebler A, et al. Double-blind treatment of major depression with dehydroepiandrosterone. *Am J Psychiat* 1999;156:646-9.

3271 Gokce N, Keaney JF, Frei B, et al. Long-term ascorbic acid administration reverses endothelial vasomotor dysfunction in patients with coronary artery disease. *Circulation* 1999;99:3234-3240.

3272 Raintree Nutrition, Inc. URL http://www.rain-tree.com/index.html (Accessed 27 November 1999).

3273 The IOOC's Trade Standard Applying to Olive Oil and Olive Pomace Oil. URL: sovrana.com/ioocdef.htm (Accessed 20 November 1999).

3274 Kamien M. Practice tip. Which cerumenolytic? *Aust Fam Physician* 1999;28:817,828.

3275 Isaksson M, Bruze M. Occupational allergic contact dermatitis from olive oil in a masseur. *J Am Acad Dermatol* 1999;41(2 Pt 2):312-5.

3276 Hoberman A, Paradise JL, Reynolds EA, et al. Efficacy of Auralgan for treating ear pain in children with acute otitis media. *Arch Pediatr Adolesc Med*, July 1997;151(7):675-8.

3278 Nutrimax Labs website, URL: www.nutramaxlabs.com/human/cosamin.htm (Accessed 19 November 1999).

3279 Chavez MI, Chavez PI. Echinacea. *Hospital Pharmacy* 1998;33(2):180-188.

3280 Gunning K. Echinacea in the treatment and prevention of upper respiratory tract infections. *West J Med* 1999;171:198-200.

3281 Barrett B, Vohmann M, Calabrese C. Echinacea for upper respiratory infection. *J Fam Pract* 1999;48:628-35.

3282 Grimm W, Muller HH. A randomized controlled trial of the effect of fluid extract of Echinacea purpurea on the incidence and severity of colds and respiratory infections. *Am J Med* 1999;106:138-43.

3283 Putter M, Grotemeyer KH, Wurthwein G, et al. Inhibition of smoking-induced platelet aggregation by aspirin and pycnogenol. *Thromb Res* 1999;95(4):155-61.

3284 Bisignano G, Tomaino A, Lo Cascio R, et al. On the in-vitro antimicrobial activity of oleuropein and hydroxytyrosol. *J Pharm Pharmacol* 1999;51:971-4.

3285 Mensink RP, Katan MB. An epidemiological and an experimental study on the effect of olive oil on total serum and HDL cholesterol in healthy volunteers. *Eur J Clin Nutr* 1989;43 Suppl 2:43-8.

3286 Mata P, Alvarez-Sala LA, Rubio MJ, et al. Effects of long-term monounsaturated- vs polyunsaturated-enriched diets on lipoproteins in healthy men and women. *Am J Clin Nutr* 1992;55:846-50.

3287 Lichtenstein AH, Ausman LM, Carrasco W, et al. Effects of canola, corn, and olive oils on fasting and postprandial plasma lipoproteins in humans as part of a National Cholesterol Education Program Step 2 diet. *Arterioscler Thromb* 1993;13:1533-42.

3288 Zambon A, Sartore G, Passera D, et al. Effects of hypocaloric dietary treatment enriched in oleic acid on LDL and HDL subclass distribution in mildly obese women. *J Intern Med* 1999;246:191-201.

3289 Ruiz-Gutierrez V, Muriana FJ, Guerrero A, et al. Plasma lipids, erythrocyte membrane lipids and blood pressure of hypertensive women after ingestion of dietary oleic acid from two different sources. *J Hypertens* 1996;14:1483-90.

3290 Tsimikas S, Philis-Tsimikas A, Alexopoulos S, et al. LDL isolated from Greek subjects on a typical diet or from American subjects on an oleate-supplemented diet induces less monocyte chemotaxis and adhesion when exposed to oxidative stress. *Arterioscler Thromb Vasc Biol* 1999;19:122-30.

3291 Nutt JG, Woodward WR, Hammerstad JP, et al. The "on-off" phenomenon in Parkinson's disease. Relation to levodopa absorption and transport. *N Engl J Med* 1984;310:483-8.

3292 Baruzzi A, Contin M, Riva R, et al. Influence of meal ingestion time on pharmacokinetics of orally administered levodopa in parkinsonian patients. *Clin Neuropharmacol* 1987;10(6):527-37.

3293 Juncos JL, Fabbrini G, Mouradian MM, et al. Dietary influences on the antiparkinsonian response to levodopa. *Arch Neurol* 1987;44:1003-5.

3294 Eriksson T, Granerus AK, Linde A et al: 'On-off' phenomenon in Parkinson's disease: relationship between dopa and other large neutral amino acids in plasma. *Neurology* 1988;38:1245-1248.

3295 Prevention magazine Online. http://www.healthyideas.com (Accessed 20 September 1999).

3300 Tomita T, Sato N, Arai T, et al. Bactericidal activity of a fermented hot-water extract from Stevia rebaudiana Bertoni towards enterohemorrhagic Escherichia coli O157:H7 and other food-borne pathogenic bacteria. *Microbiol Immunol* 1997;41(12):1005-9.

3301 Curi R, Alvarez M, Bazotte RB, et al. "Effect of Stevia rebaudiana on glucose tolerance in normal adult humans." *Braz J Med Biol Res*, 1986;19(6):771-4.

3302 Evans DA, Raj RK. Larvicidal efficacy of Quassin against Culex quinquefasciatus. *Indian J Med Res* 1991;93:324-7.

3314 Anderson PO, Knoben JE, Troutman WG. Handbook of Clinical Drug Data. 9th edition. Stamford, CT: Appleton & Lange, 1999.

3400 Committee on Nutrition, American Academy of Pediatrics. Soy Protein-based Formulas: Recommendations for Use in Infant Feeding. *Pediatrics* 1998;101(1):148-153.

3401 Anderson JW, Johnstone BM, Cook-Newell ME. Meta-analysis of the effects of soy protein intake on serum lipids. *N Engl J Med* 1995;333(5):276-82.

3402 Crouse JR 3rd, Morgan T, Terry JG, et al. A randomized trial comparing the effect of casein with that of soy protein containing varying amounts of isoflavones on plasma concentrations of lipids and lipoproteins. *Arch Intern Med* 1999;159(17):2070-2076.

3403 Zhu JS, Halpern GM, Jones K. The scientific rediscovery of an ancient Chinese herbal medicine: Cordyceps sinensis: part I. *J Altern Complement Med* 1998;4(3):289-303.

3404 Zhu JS, Halpern GM, Jones K. The scientific rediscovery of a precious ancient Chinese herbal regimen: Cordyceps sinensis: part II. *J Altern Complement Med* 1998;4(4):429-57.

3405 Rossetti L, Hawkins M, Chen W, et al. In vivo glucosamine infusion induces insulin resistance in normoglycemic but not in hyperglycemic conscious rats. *J Clin Invest* 1995;96(1):132-40.

3406 Shankar RR, Zhu JS, Baron AD. Glucosamine infusion in rats mimics the beta-cell dysfunction of non-insulin-dependent diabetes mellitus. *Metabolism* 1998;47(5):573-7.

3407 Nakamura K, Yamaguchi Y, Kagota S, et al. Inhibitory effect of Cordyceps sinensis on spontaneous liver metastasis of Lewis lung carcinoma and B16 melanoma cells in syngeneic mice. *Jpn J Pharmacol* 1999;79(3):335-41.

3408 Zhang ZJ, Luo HL, Li JS. [Clinical and experimental studies on elimination of oxygen free radical of jinshuibao capsule in treating senile deficiency syndrome and its deoxyribonucleic acid damage repairing effects]. [Article in Chinese] *Chung Kuo Chung Hsi I Chieh Ho Tsa Chih* 1997;17(1):35-8.

3409 Chiu JH, Ju CH, Wu LH, et al. Cordyceps sinensis increases the expression of major histocompatibility complex class II antigens on human hepatoma cell line HA22T/VGH cells. *Am J Chin Med* 1998;26(2):159-70.

3410 Bok JW, Lermer L, Chilton J, et al. Antitumor sterols from the mycelia of Cordyceps sinensis. *Phytochemistry* 1999;51(7):891-8.

3411 Li LS, Zheng F, Liu ZH. [Experimental study on effect of Cordyceps sinensis in ameliorating aminoglycoside induced nephrotoxicity]. [Article in Chinese] Chung Kuo Chung Hsi I Chieh Ho Tsa Chih 1996;16(12):733-7.

3412 Wang SM, Lee LJ, Lin WW, Chang CM. Effects of a water-soluble extract of Cordyceps sinensis on steroidogenesis and capsular morphology of lipid droplets in cultured rat adrenocortical cells. *J Cell Biochem* 1998;69(4):483-9.

3414 Chen YJ, Shiao MS, Lee SS, Wang SY. Effect of Cordyceps sinensis on the proliferation and differentiation of human leukemic U937 cells. *Life Sci* 1997;60(25):2349-59.

3415 Kiho T, Yamane A, Hui J, et al. Polysaccharides in fungi. XXXVI. Hypoglycemic activity of a polysaccharide (CS-F30) from the cultural mycelium of Cordyceps sinensis and its effect on glucose metabolism in mouse liver. *Biol Pharm Bull* 1996;19(2):294-6.

3416 Kuo YC, Tsai WJ, Shiao MS, et al. Cordyceps sinensis as an immunomodulatory agent. *Am J Chin Med*

© Copyright 2000, Natural Medicines Comprehensive Database (209) 472-2244. For updated data, go to www.NaturalDatabase.com. • 1227

REFERENCES

1996;24(2):111-25.

3417 Zhou DH, Lin LZ. [Effect of Jinshuibao capsule on the immunological function of 36 patients with advanced cancer]. [Article in Chinese] *Chung Kuo Chung Hsi I Chieh Ho Tsa Chih* 1995;15(8):476-8.

3418 Xu F, Huang JB, Jiang L, et al. Amelioration of cyclosporin nephrotoxicity by Cordyceps sinensis in kidney-transplanted recipients. *Nephrol Dial Transplant* 1995;10(1):142-3.

3419 Bao ZD, Wu ZG, Zheng F. [Amelioration of aminoglycoside nephrotoxicity by Cordyceps sinensis in old patients]. [Article in Chinese] *Chung Kuo Chung Hsi I Chieh Ho Tsa Chih* 1994;14(5):271-3, 259.

3420 Kuo YC, Lin CY, Tsai WJ, et al. Growth inhibitors against tumor cells in Cordyceps sinensis other than cordycepin and polysaccharides. *Cancer Invest* 1994;12(6):611-5.

3421 Kiho T, Hui J, Yamane A, Ukai S. Polysaccharides in fungi. XXXII. Hypoglycemic activity and chemical properties of a polysaccharide from the cultural mycelium of Cordyceps sinensis. *Biol Pharm Bull* 1993;16(12):1291-3.

3424 Chen JR, Yen JH, Lin CC, et al. The effects of Chinese herbs on improving survival and inhibiting anti-ds DNA antibody production in lupus mice. *Am J Chin Med* 1993;21(3-4):257-62.

3425 Liu C, Lu S, Ji MR. [Effects of Cordyceps sinensis (CS) on in vitro natural killer cells]. [Article in Chinese] Chung Kuo *Chung Hsi I Chieh Ho Tsa Chih* 1992;12(5):267-9, 259.

3427 Xu RH, Peng XE, Chen GZ, Chen GL. Effects of cordyceps sinensis on natural killer activity and colony formation of B16 melanoma. *Chin Med J* (English) 1992;105(2):97-101.

3428 Cheng Q. [Effect of cordyceps sinensis on cellular immunity in rats with chronic renal insufficiency]. [Article in Chinese] *Chung Hua I Hsueh Tsa Chih* (Taipei) 1992;72(1):27-9, 63.

3429 Zhao Y. [Inhibitory effects of alcoholic extract of Cordyceps sinensis on abdominal aortic thrombus formation in rabbits].[Article in Chinese] *Chung Hua I Hsueh Tsa Chih* (Taipei) 1991; 71(11):612-5, 42.

3431 Chen GZ, Chen GL, Sun T, et al. Effects of Cordyceps sinensis on murine T lymphocyte subsets. *Chin Med J* (English) 1991; 104(1):4-8.

3432 Zhu XY, Yu HY. [Immunosuppressive effect of cultured Cordyceps sinensis on cellular immune response]. [Article in Chinese] *Chung Hsi I Chieh Ho Tsa Chih* 1990; 10(8):485-7, 454.

3434 Yamaguchi N, Yoshida J, Ren LJ, et al. Augmentation of various immune reactivities of tumor-bearing hosts with an extract of Cordyceps sinensis. *Biotherapy* 1990;2(3):199-205.

3435 Zhou L, Yang W, Xu Y, et la. [Short-term curative effect of cultured Cordyceps sinensis (Berk.) Sacc. Mycelia in chronic hepatitis B]. [Article in Chinese] *Chung Kuo Chung Yao Tsa Chih* 1990;15(1):53-5, 65.

3436 Mei QB, Tao JY, Gao SB, et al. [Antiarrhythmic effects of Cordyceps sinensis (Berk.) Sacc]. [Article in Chinese] *Chung Kuo Chung Yao Tsa Chih* 1989;14(10):616-8, 640.

3437 Yoshida J, Takamura S, Yamaguchi N, et al. Antitumor activity of an extract of Cordyceps sinensis (Berk.) Sacc. against murine tumor cell lines. *Jpn J Exp Med* 1989;59(4):157-61.

3450 Geleijnse JM, Launer LJ, Hofman A, et al. Tea flavonoids may protect against *Atherosclerosis*: the Rotterdam Study. *Arch Intern Med* 1999;159(18):2170-2174.

3451 Schechter JO. Treatment of disequilibrium and nausea in the SRI discontinuation syndrome. *J Clin Psychiatry* 1998;59(8):431-2.

3452 Arfeen Z, Owen H, Plummer JL, et al. A double-blind randomized controlled trial of ginger for the prevention of postoperative nausea and vomiting. *Anaesth Intensive Care* 1995;23(4):449-52.

3453 Visalyaputra S, Petchpaisit N, Somcharoen K, Choavaratana R. The efficacy of ginger root in the prevention of postoperative nausea and vomiting after outpatient gynaecological laparoscopy. *Anaesthesia* 1998;53(5):506-10.

3454 Linos A, Kaklamani VG, Kaklamani E, et al. Dietary factors in relation to rheumatoid arthritis: a role for olive oil and cooked vegetables? *Am J Clin Nutr* 1999;70(6):1077-82.

3455 Penny ME, Peerson JM, Marin RM, et al. Randomized, community-based trial of the effect of zinc supplementation, with and without other micronutrients, on the duration of persistent childhood diarrhea in Lima, Peru. *J Pediatr* 1999;135(2 Pt 1):208-17.

3456 Bhutta ZA, Black RE, Brown KH, et al. Prevention of diarrhea and pneumonia by zinc supplementation in children in developing countries: Pooled analysis of randomized controlled trials. *J Pediatr* 1999;135:689-97.

3457 Bostick RM, Kushi LH, Wu Y, et al. Relation of calcium, vitamin D, and dairy food intake to ischemic heart disease mortality among postmenopausal women. *Am J Epidemiol* 1999;149(2):151-61.

3458 Steinbach G, Lupton J, Reddy BS, et al. Calcium carbonate treatment of diarrhea in intestinal bypass patients. *Eur J Gastroenterol Hepatol* 1996;8(6):559-562.

3459 Thys-Jacobs S, Starkey P, Bernstein D, Tian J. Calcium carbonate and the premenstrual syndrome: effects on premenstrual and menstrual symptoms. Premenstrual Syndrome Study Group. *Am J Obstet Gynecol* 1998;179(2):444-452.

3460 Korting GE, Smith SD, Wheeler MA, et al. A randomized double-blind trial of oral L-arginine for treatment of interstitial cystitis. *J Urol* 1999;161(2):558-65.

3461 Schweizer J, Hautmann C. Comparison of two dosages of Ginkgo biloba Extract Egb 761 in patients with peripheral arterial occlusive disease Fontain's stage llb / A randomised, double-blind, multicentric clinical Trial. *Arzneimittelforschung* 1999;49(11):900-904.

3462 Hawkins EB. NADH: Advanced supplementation for more energy and slower aging. *Natural Pharmacy* July 1998;2(7):10.

3463 Kyriakidou-Himonas M, Aloia JF, Yeh JK. Vitamin D supplementation in postmenopausal black women. *J Clin Endocrinol Metab* 1999;84(11):3988-3990.

3464 Zamora SA, Rizzoli R, Belli DC, Slosman DO, Bonjour JP. Vitamin D supplementation during infancy is associated with higher bone mineral mass in prepubertal girls. *J Clin Endocrinol Metab* 1999;84(12):4541-4544.

3465 Boger RH, Bode-Boger SM, Thiele W, et al. Restoring vascular nitric oxide formation by L-arginine improves the symptoms of intermittent claudication in patients with peripheral arterial occlusive disease. *J Am Coll Cardiol* 1998;32(5):1336-1344.

3466 Boger RH, Bode-Boger SM, Thiele W, et al. Biochemical evidence for impaired nitric oxide synthesis in patients with peripheral arterial occlusive disease. *Circulation* 1997;95f(8):2068-2074.

3467 Nittynen L, Nurminen ML, Korpela R, et al. Role of arginine, taurine and homocysteine in cardiovascular diseases. *Ann Med* 1999;31(5):318-326.

3468 Beaumier L, Castillo L, Yu YM, et al. Arginine; new and exciting developments for an "old" amino acid. *Biomed Environ Sci* 1996;9(2-3):296-315.

3469 Butland BK, Fehily AM, Elwood PC. Diet and lung function decline in a cohort of 2512 middle aged men. *Thorax*, 2000;55(2):102-108.

3470 Le Marchand L, Murphy SP, Hankin JH, et al. Intake of flavonoids and lung cancer. *J Natl Cancer Inst* 2000;92(2):154-160.

3471 Gulyas A, Repges R, Dethlefsen U. Therapy of chronic obstructive pulmonary diseases in children. *Atemvegs und Lungenkrankheiten* 1997;23:291-294.

3472 Dekkers R. Apple juice and the chemical-contact softening of gallstones. *Lancet* , 1999;354(9196):2171.

3473 Sinniah D, Baskaran G. Margosa oil poisoning as a cause of Reye's syndrome. *Lancet* 1981;1(8218):487-489.

3474 Sinniah D, Baskaran G, Looi LM, Leong KL. Reye-like syndrome due to margosa oil poisoning: report of a case with postmortem findings. *Am J Gastroenterol* 1982;77(3):158-161.

3475 Sinniah R, Sinniah D, Chia LS, Baskaran G. Animal model of margosa oil ingestion with Reye-like syndrome. Pathogenesis of microvesicular fatty liver. *J Pathol* 1989;159(3):255-264.

3476 Lai SM, Lim KW, Cheng HK. Margosa oil poisoning as a cause of toxic encephalopathy. *Singapore Med J* 1990;31(5):463-465.

3477 Furbee B, Wermuth M. Life-threatening plant poisoning. *Crit Care Clin*, 1997;13(4):849-888.

3478 Lewis WH, Smith PR. Poke root herbal tea poisoning. *JAMA* , 1979;242(25):2759-2760.

3479 Roberge R, Brader E, Martin ML, Jehle D, et al. The root of evil-pokeweed intoxication. *Ann Emerg Med*, 1986;15(4):470-473.

3480 Jaeckle KA, Freemon FR. Pokeweed poisoning. *South Med J*, 1981;74(5):639-640.

3481 Barker BE, Farnes P, LaMarche PH. Haematological effects of pokeweed. *Lancet* , 1967;1:437.

3482 Kell SO, Rosenberg SA, Conlon TJ, Spyker DA. A peek at poke: mitogenicity and epidemiology. *Vet Hum Toxicol* 1982;24(4):36.

3483 Anon. Toxic reactions to plant products sold in health food stores. *Med Lett Drugs Ther*, 1979;21:29-32.

3484 Klepser TB, Klepser ME. Unsafe and potentially safe herbal therapies. *Am J Health Syst Pharm* 1999;56:125-138.

3485 Plushner SL. Valerian: Valerian officinalis. *Am J Health Syst Pharm* 2000;57:328, 333, 335.

3486 Houghton PJ. The scientific basis for the reputed activity of Valerian. *J Pharm Pharmacol* 1999;51(5):505-512.

3487 Garges HP, Varia I, Doraiswamy PM. Cardiac complications and delirium associated with Valerian root withdrawal. [Letter to the Editor] *JAMA* 1998;280(18):1566-1567.

3488 Tuncok Y, Kozan O, Cavdar C, et al. Urginea maritima (squill) toxicity. *J Toxicol Clin Toxicol*, 1995;33(1):83-86.

3489 Wax PM. Squill through the ages. *J Toxicol Clin Toxicol*, 1995;33(1):86.

3490 But PP, Tai YT, Young K. Three fatal cases of herbal aconite poisoning. *Vet Hum Toxicol* 1994;36(3):212-215.

3491 Feldkamp A, Koster B, Weber HP. [Fatal poisoning caused by aconite monk's hood]. [Article in German] *Monatsschr Kinderheilkd* 1991;139(6):366-367.

3492 Hallstrom H, Thuvander A. Toxicological evaluation of myristicin. *Nat Toxins* 1997;5(5):186-192.

3493 Jeong HG, Yun CH. Induction of rat hepatic cytochrome P450 enzymes by myristicin. *Biochem Biophys Res Commun* 1995;217(3):966-971.

3494 3494. Dinakar HS. Acute psychosis associated with nutmeg toxicity. *Med Times* 1977;105(12):63-64.

3495 Haynes BE, Bessen HA, Wightman WD. Oleander tea: herbal draught of death. *Ann Emerg Med* 1985;14(4):350-353.

3496 Biberoglu S, Biberoglu K, Komsuoglu B. Mad honey. [Letter to the Editor] *JAMA* , 1988;259(13):1943.

3497 Sheikh NM, Philen RM, Love LA. Chaparral-associated hepatotoxicity. *Arch Intern Med* 1997;157(8):913-919.

3498 Mrvos RM, Reilly PE, Dean BS, Krenzelok EP. Massive caffeine ingestion resulting in death. *Vet Hum Toxicol* 1989;31(6):571-572.

3499 Davies JH. Abrus precatorius (rosary pea). The most common lethal plant poison. *J Fla Med Assoc* 1978;65(3):188-191.

3500 Herschler R. Methylsulfonylmethane in dietary products. United States Patent number 4,616,039; 1986.

3501 Richmond VL. "Incorporation of methylsulfonylmethane sulfur into guinea pig serum proteins." *Life Sci*, 1986; 39(3): 263-68.

3502 O'Dwyer PJ, et al. "Use of polar solvents in chemoprevention of 1,2-dimethylhydrazine-induced colon cancer." *Cancer*, 1988; 62(5): 944-48.

3503 McCabe D, et al. "Polar solvents in the chemoprevention of dimethylbenzanthracene-induced rat mammary cancer." *Arch Surg*, 1986; 62(12): 1455-459.

3504 Klandorf H, et al. "Dimethyl sulfoxide modulation of diabetes onset in NOD mice." *Diabetes*, 1998; 62(2): 194-97.

3507 IFIC Review: "Sorting Out the Facts About Fat" Website: ificinfo.health.org/review/ir-fat.htm (16 July 1999).

3508 Godley PA. "Essential fatty acid consumption and risk of breast cancer." *Breast Br J Nutr Treat*, Jul 1995; 35(1): 91-95.

3509 Malloy MJ, Kane JP. *Agents used in hyperlipidemia. In: Basic and Clinical Pharmacology.* Fourth ed. B. Katzung, ed. Norwald, CT/San Mateo, CA: Appleton and Lange, 1989.

3510 Rose DP. "The mechanistic rationale in support of dietary cancer prevention." *Prev Med*, 1996; 25(1): 34-37.

3511 Noguchi M, et al. "The role of fatty acids and eicosanoid synthesis inhibitors in breast carcinoma." *Oncology*, 1995; 52(4): 265-71.

3512 Balch, JF; Balch, PA. *Prescription for Nutritional Healing.* Garden City Park, NY: Avery Publishing Group.

3513 Thien FC, Leung R, Baldo BA, et al. "Asthma and anaphylaxis induced by royal jelly." *Clin Exp Allergy*, 1996;26(2):216-22.

3514 Roger A, Rubira N, Nogueiras C, et al. "Anaphylaxis caused by royal jelly." [Article in Spanish] *Allergol*

R
E
F
E
R
E
N
C
E
S

Immunopathol, (Madr) 1995;23(3):133-5.

3515 Vittek J. "Effect of royal jelly on serum lipids in experimental animals and humans with Atherosclerosis." *Experientia* 1995;51(9-10):927-35.

3516 Yonei Y, Shibagaki K, Tsukada N, et al. "Case report: haemorrhagic colitis associated with royal jelly intake." *J Gastroenterol Hepatol*, 1997;12(7):495-9

3521 Iruela LM, et al. Toxic interaction of S-adenosylmethionine and clomipramine. *Am J Psych* 1993; 150:522.

3523 Carney MW, et al. The switch mechanism and the bipolar/unipolar dichotomy. *Br J Psychiatry* 1989; 154:48-51.

3524 Schneck C. St. John's wort and hypomania. *J Clin Psychiatry* 1998; 59:689.

3525 An adverse reaction to the herbal medication milk thistle (Silybum marianum). Adverse Drug Reactions Advisory Committee. *Med J Aust* 1999;170:218-19.

3526 Page RL 2nd, Lawrence JD. Potentiation of warfarin by dong quai. *Pharmacotherapy* 1999;19(7):870-6.

3527 Amaranthine Aromatics. Essential Oil Safety. http://www.amaranthine.com/product/esssafe.html (Accessed 6 November 1999).

3529 D'Adamo P. Larch arabinogalactan. *J Naturopath Med* 1996;6:33-37.

3530 Kelly GS. Larch arabinogalactan: Clinical relevance of a novel immune-enhancing polysaccharide. *Alt Med Rev* 1999;4:96-103.

3531 Anon. Best herb for fighting off colds. *Bottom Line* 1999;20:1.

3532 Priesnitz M. Blue green algae – superfood or pond scum? Natural Life, June 28, 1999; URL: www.life.ca/nl/68/algae.html (Accessed 5 December 1999).

3533 Anon. Spirulina. URL: www.go-symmetry.com/spirulina.htm (Accessed 5 December 1999).

3534 Anon. Earthrise Farms spirulina safety assurance. Earthrise Farms 1998; URL: www.spirulina.com/SPLSAssurance.html (Accessed 5 December 1999).

3535 Anon. Toxic algae in lake Sammamish. King County, WA. October 28, 1998; URL: splash.metrokc.gov/wlr/waterres/lakes/bloom.htm (Accessed 5 December 1999).

3536 Anon. Health Canada announces results of blue-green algal products testing – only Spirulina found Microcystin-free. Health Canada, September 27, 1999; URL: www.hc-sc.gc.ca/english/archives/releases/99_114e.htm (Accessed 27 October 1999).

3537 Anon. Butternut. Sequential Healing Health Services. http://www.sequentialhealing.com/herbs/butternut.html (Accessed 15 December 1999).

3538 Anon. Butternut. http://www.comcen.com.au~sburgess/herbs/Monographs/Juglans.htm. (Accessed 15 December 1999).

3539 Peirce A. The American Pharmaceutical Association Practical Guide to Natural Medicines. New York: The Stonesong Press, 1999.

3540 Ziegler D, Hanefeld M, Ruhnau K, et al. Treatment of symptomatic diabetic polyneuropathy with the antioxidant alpha-lipoic acid: A 7-month multicenter randomized controlled trial (ALADIN III Study). *Diabetes Care* 1999;22:1296-1301.

3541 Reljanovic M, Reichel G, Rett K, et al. Treatment of diabetic polyneuropathy with the antioxidant thioctic acid (alpha-lipoic acid): A two year multicenter randomized double-blind placebo controlled tiral (ALADIN II). Alpha Lipoic Acid in Diabetic Neuropathy [abstract]. *Free Radic Res* 1999;31:171-77.

3542 Ziegler D, Schatz H, Conrad F, et al. Effects of treatment with the antioxidant alpha-lipoic acid on cardiac autonomic neuropathy in NIDDM patients. *Diabetes Care* 1997;20:369-373.

3543 Obrosova I, Cao X, Greene DA, et al. Diabetes-induced changes in lens antioxidant status, glucose utilization and energy metabolism: Effect of DL-alpha-lipoic acid. *Diabetologia* 1998;41:1442-450.

3544 Streeper RS, Henriksen EJ, Jacob S, et al. Differential effects of lipoic acid stereoisomers on glucose metabolism in insulin-resistant skeletal muscle. *Am J Physiol* 1997;273:E185-E191.

3545 Konrad T, Vicini P, Kusterer K, et al. Alpha-lipoic acid treatment decreases serum lactate and pyruvate concentrations and improves glucose effectiveness in lean and obese patients with Type 2 diabetes. *Diabetes Care* 1999;22:280-287.

3546 Packer L. Antioxidant properties of lipoic acid and its therapeutic effects in prevention of diabetes complications and cataracts. *Ann NY Acad Sci* 1994;738:257-64.

3547 Schempp CM, Winghofer B, Langheinrich M, et al. Hypericin levels in human serum and interstitial skin blister fluid after oral single-dose and steady state administration of Hypericum perforatum extract (St. John's Wort). *Skin Pharmacol Appl Skin Physiol* 1999;12:299-304.

3548 Kim HL, Streltzer J, Goebert D. St. John's wort for depression: A meta analysis of well-defined clinical trials. *J Nerv Ment Dis* 1999;187:532-39.

3549 Linde K, Ramirez G, Mulrow CD, et al. St. John's wort for depression: an overview and meta-analysis of randomized clinical trials. *Br Med J* 1996;313:253-258.

3550 Harrer G, et al. Comparison of equivalence between the St. John's wort extract LoHyp-57 and fluoxetine. *Arzneimittelforschung* 1999;49:289-296.

3551 Philipp M, Kohnen R, Hiller KO. Hypericum extract versus imipramine or placebo in patients with moderate depression: randomized mulicentre study of treatment for eight weeks. *Br Med J* 1999;319:1534-539.

3552 Gaster B, Holroyd J. St John's wort for depression. *Arch Intern Med* 2000;160:152-56.

3553 Singer A, Wonnemann M, Muller WE. Hyperforin, a major antidepressant constituent of St. John's wort, inhibits serotonin uptake by elevating free intracellular Na+11. *J Pharmacol Exp Ther* 1999;290:1363-368.

3554 Schempp C, Pelz K, Wittmer A, et al. Antibacterial activity of hyperforin from St. John's wort, against multiresistant Stapylococcus aureus and gram-positive bacteria. *Lancet* 1999;353:2129.

3555 Nierenberg AA, Burt T, Matthews J, et al. Mania associated with St. John's wort. *Biol Psychiatry* 1999;46:1707-708.

3556 Nebel A, Schneider BJ, Baker RA, et al. Potential metabolic interaction between St. John's wort and theophylline. *Ann Pharmacother* 1999;33:502.

3557 Ziegler D, Hanefeld M, Ruhnau KJ, et al. Treatment of symptomatic diabetic peripheral neuropathy with the antioxidant alpha-lipoic acid: A 3-week multicenter randomized controlled trial (ALADIN Study). *Diabetologia* 1995;38:1425-1433.

3558 Huang KC. *The Pharmacology of Chinese Herbs*. 2nd Ed. Boca Raton:CRC Press, 1999:267.

3559 Upton R, ed. Schisandra Berry: Analytical, Quality Control, and Therapeutic Monograph. Santa Cruz, CA: *American Herbal Pharmacopoeia* 1999;1-25

3561 Pepping J. Huperzine A. *Am J Health-Syst Pharm* 2000;57:530-534.

3562 Gaster B. S-adenosylmethionine (SAMe) for treatment of depression. *Alternative Medicine Alert*, 1999;12:133-135.

3563 Chevallier A. *Encyclopedia of Medicinal Plants*. New York, NY: DK Publishing 1996;202.

3564 Anon. Lapacho. The Natural Pharmacist 2000. http://www.tnp.com/substance.asp?ID=67 (Accessed 7 April 2000).

3565 Kumar DS, Prabhakar YS. On the ethnomedical significance of the Arjun tree, Terminalia arjuna (Roxb.) Wight & Arnot. *J Ethnopharmacol* 1987;20:173-190.

3566 Anon. Magnesium. The Natural Pharmacist. Prima Communications; 2000. http://www.tnp.com/substance.asp?ID=161#P5 (Accessed 4 May 2000).

3567 Anon. Colostrum. The Natural Pharmacist. Prima Communications, Inc., 2000. http://www.tnp.com/substance.asp?ID=121 (Accessed 5 May 2000).

3568 Moses EL, Mallinger AG. St. John's wort: Three cases of possible mania induction. *J Clin Psychopharmacol* 2000;20:115-117.

3569 Beckman SE, Sommi RW, Switzer J. Consumer use of St. John's wort: A survey of effectiveness, safety, and tolerability. *Pharmacotherapy* 2000;20:568-574.

3570 Ereshefsky B, Gewertz N, Lam YMF, et al. Determination of SJW differential metabolism at CYP2D6 and CYP3A4, using dextromethorphan probe methodology. Abstract Poster Presentations, 39th NCDEU Annual Meeting, 1999:Poster 130 128.

3571 Gewertz N, Ereshefsky B, Lam YWF, et al. Determination of the differential effects of St. John's wort on the CYP1A2 and NAT2 metabolic pathways using caffeine probe methodology. Abstract Poster Presentations, *39th NCDEU Annual Meeting*, 1999:Poster 131.

3572 Brandes JL, Edvinsson L, Marcus D, et al. New treatment options for migraine. Medscape Neurology Treatment Updates 2000. http://www.medscape.com/medscape/Neurology/TreatmentUpdate/2000/tu05/TU05-05.html (Accessed 18 May 2000).

3573 Towheed TE, Anastassiades TP. Glucosamine and Chondriotin for treating symptoms of osteoarthritis. Evidence is widely touted but incomplete. *JAMA* 2000;238(11):1483-4.

3574 Anon. Bee Propolis. MotherNature.com 1999. http://www.mothernature.com/library/books/natmed/bee_propolis.asp (Accessed 28 May 2000).

3575 US Food and Drug Administration. Special Nutritional Adverse Event Monitoring System. US FDA 1998. http://vm.cfsan.fda.gov/~dms/aems.html (Accessed 12 June 2000).

3576 Ault A. Chinese herbal remedy holds promise for prostate cancer. Reuters Health May 23, 2000. http://www.medscape.com/reuters/prof/2000/05/05.23/20000523clin013.html (accessed 2 June 2000).

3577 Anon. PC-SPES. UCSF Cancer Center Communications 2000. URL: http://cc.ucsf.edu/clinical/uro_pc-spes.html (Accessed 2 June 2000).

3578 Dillard J. Grape leaf for ADHD? OnHealth, March 19, 1999. http://onhealth.com/alternative/columnist/item,49799.asp (Accessed 3 June 2000).

3580 Anon. OPCs (Oligomeric Proanthocyanidins). The Natural Pharmacist 2000. http://www.tnp.com/substance.asp?ID=181 (Accessed 3 June 2000).

3581 Murray MT. Natural Alternatives to Over-the-Counter and Prescription Drugs. New York: Quill, 1994.

3582 Murray MT, Pizzorno JE. Vitamin toxicities and therapeutic monitoring. In: Pizzorno JE, Murray MT, eds. Textbook of Natural Medicine. 2nd ed. New York: Chuchill Livingstone 1999; p. 1015-8.

3583 Geva E, Bartoov B, Zabludovsky N, et al. The effect of antioxidant treatment on human spermatozoa and fertilization rate in an in vitro fertilization program. *Fertil Steril* 1996;66:430-4.

3585 Vezina D, Mauffette F, Roberts KD, et al. Selenium-vitamin E supplementation in infertile men. Effects on semen parameters and micronutrient levels and distribution. *Biol Trace Elem Res* 1996;53:65-83.

3586 Anon. Health benefits of yogurt. National Yogurt Association 1999. http://www.yaourt.org/healthbenefits.html (Accessed 6 June 2000).

3587 Gregory PJ. Probiotics for antibiotic-associated diarrhea. *Pharmacist's Letter* 2000;16(1):160103.

3588 Murray MT, Pizzorno JE. Probiotics. In: Pizzorno JE, Murray MT, eds. *Textbook of Natural Medicine*. 2nd ed. Edinburgh:Churchill Livingstone, 1999:893-7.

3589 Meydani SN, Ha WK. Immunologic effects of yogurt. *Am J Clin Nutr* 2000;71:861-72.

3590 Agerholm-Larsen L, Raben A, Haulrik N, et al. Effect of 8 week intake of probiotic milk products on risk factors for cardiovascular diseases. *European Journal of Clinical Nutrition* 2000;54:288-7.

3591 Anon. Female Viagra equivalent now available – Topical Natural Sensation from Strategic Science and Technologies, Inc. *PRNewswire* May 25, 2000.

3592 Anon. Arginine. The Natural Pharmacist 2000. http://www.tnp.com/substance.asp?ID=106. (accessed 14 June 2000).

3593 Blum A, Porat R, Rosenschein U, et al. Clinical and inflammatory effects of dietary L-arginine in patients with intractable angina pectoris. *Am J Cardiol* 1999;15:1488-90.

3594 Tentolouris C, Tousoulis D, Toutouzas P, et al. Effects of acute L-arginine administration in coronary *Atherosclerosis* [letter]. *Circulation* 1999;99:1648.

3595 Rector TS, Bank AJ, Mullen KA, et al. Randomized, double-blind, placebo-controlled study of supplemental oral L-arginine in patients with heart failue. *Circulation* 1996;93:2135-41.

3596 Watanabe G, Tomiyama H, Doba N. Effects of oral administration of L-arginine on renal function in patients with heart failure. *J Hypertens* 2000;18:229-34.

3598 Kehoe WA. Vitamin E for neuroleptic-induced tardive dyskinesia. *Pharmacist's Letter* 1999;15(1):150105.

3599 Markowitz JS, DeVane CL, Boulton DW, et al. Effect of St. John's wort (Hypericum Perforatum) on cytochrome P-450 2D6 and 3A4 activity in healthy volunteers. *Life Sciences* 2000;66:PL 133-9.

3600 Salvioli G, Neri M. L-acetylcarnitine treatment of mental decline in the elderly. *Drugs Exp Clin Res*, 1994;20(4):169-176.

3601 Passeri M, Cucinotta D, Bonati PA, et al. Acetyl-L-carnitine in the treatment of mildly demented elderly patients. *Int J Clin Pharmacol Res*, 1990;10(1-2):75-79.

3602 Bella R, Biondi R, Raffaele R, Pennisi G. Effect of acetyl-L-carnitine on geriatric patients suffering from dysthymic disorders. *Int J Clin Pharmacol Res* 1990;10(6):355-360.

3603 Garzya G, Corallo D, Fiore A, et al. Evaluation of the effects of L-acetylcarnitine on senile patients suffering from depression. *Drugs Exp Clin Res*, 1990;16(2):101-

REFERENCES

106.

3604 Tempesta E, Casella L, Pirrongelli C, et al. L-acetylcarnitine in depressed elderly subjects. A cross-over study vs placebo. *Drugs Exp Clin Res* 1987;13(7):417-423.

3605 Di Marzio L, Moretti S, D'Alo S, et al. Acetyl-L-carnitine administration increases insulin-like growth factor 1 levels in asymptomatic HIV-1-infected subjects: correlation with its suppressive effect on lymphocyte apoptosis and ceramide generation. *Clin Immunol*, 1999;92(1):103-110.

3606 Famularo G, Moretti S, Marcellini S, et al. Acetyl-carnitine deficiency in AIDS patients with neurotoxicity on treatment with antiretroviral nucleoside analogues. *AIDS*, 1997;11(2):185-190.

3607 Moncada ML, Vicari E, Cimino C, et al. Effect of acetylcarnitine treatment in oligoasthenospermic patients. *Acta Europ Fertil* 1992;23(5):221-224.

3608 Jeulin C, Lewin LM. Role of free L-carnitine and acetyl-L-carnitine in post-gonadal maturation of mammalian spermatozoa. *Human Reprod Update*, 1996;2(2):87-102.

3609 Jeulin C, Soufir JC, Marson J, et al. [Acetylcarnitine and spermatozoa: relationship with epididymal maturation and motility in the boar and man.] [French]. *Reprod Nutr Develop*, 1988;28(5):1317-1327.

3610 Golan R, Weissenberg R, Lewin LM. Carnitine and acetylcarnitine in motile and immotile human spermatozoa. *Int J Androl* 1984;7(6):484-494.

3611 Kohengkul S, Tanphaichitr V, Muangmun V, Tanphaichitr N. Levels of L-carnitine and L-O-acetylcarnitine in normal and infertile human semen: a lower level of L-O-acetycarnitine in infertile semen. *Fertil Steril*, 1977;28(12):1333-1336.

3612 Tanphaichitr N. In vitro stimulation of human sperm motility by acetylcarnitine. *Int J Fertil*, 1977;22(2):85-91.

3613 Anon. Carnitine. Supplementwatch.com. URL www.supplementwatch.com/sup-atoz/c/carnitine.html (Accessed 22 February 2000).

3614 Anon. L-carnitine. Vitaminbuzz, sponsored by the Vitamin Shoppe. URL: www.vitaminbuzz.com/Supp/Carnitine-F.htm (Accessed 27 February 2000).

3615 Anon. L-carnitine. Whole Health Discount Center. URL: www.wholehealthdiscountcenter.com/lc/ (Accessed 27 February 2000).

3616 Anon. Carnitor (levocarnitine) package insert. Sigma-Tau Pharmaceuticals Inc, Gaithersburg, MD. December 1999.

3617 Mintz M. Carnitine in human immunodeficiency virus type 1 infection/acquired immune deficiency syndrome. J Child Neurol, 1995;10 Suppl 2:S40-S44.

3618 Dalakas MC, Leon-Monzon ME, Bernardini I, et al. Zidovudine-induced mitochondrial myopathy is associated with muscle carnitine deficiency and lipid storage. *Ann Neurol* 1994;35(4):482-487.

3619 Georgala S, Schulpis KH, Georgala C, Michas T. L-carnitine supplementation in patients with cystic acne on isotretinoin therapy. *J Eur Acad Dermatol Venereol*, 1999;13(3):205-209.

3620 Ramos AC, Barrucand L, Elias PR, et al. Carnitine supplementation in diphtheria. *Indian Pediatr*, 1992;29(12):1501-1505.

3621 Ramos AC, Elias PR, Barrucand L, Da Silva JA. The protective effect of carnitine in human diphtheric myocarditis. *Pediatr Res*, 1984;18(9):815-819.

3622 Plioplys AV, Kasnicka I. L-carnitine as a treatment for Rett syndrome. *South Med J*, 1993;86(12):1411-1412.

3623 Cacciatore L, Cerio R, Ciarimboli M, et al. The therapeutic effect of L-carnitine in patients with exercise-induced stable angina: a controlled study. *Drugs Exp Clin Res*, 1991;17(4):225-235.

3624 Cherchi A, Lai C, Angelino F, et al. Effects of L-carnitine on exercise tolerance in chronic stable angina: a multicenter, double-blind, randomized, placebo controlled crossover study. *Int J Clin Pharmacol Ther Toxicol*, 1985;23(10):569-572.

3625 Rizos I. Three-year survival of patients with heart failure caused by dilated cardiomyopathy and L-carnitine administration. *Am Heart J*, 2000;139(2 Pt 3):S120-S123.

3626 Ghidini O, Azzurro M, Vita G, Sartori G. Evaluation of the therapeutic efficacy of L-carnitine in congestive heart failure. *Int J Clin Pharmacol Ther Toxicol*, 1988;26(4):217-220.

3627 Singh RB, Niaz MA, Agarwal P, et al. A randomized, double-blind, placebo-controlled trial of L-carnitine in suspected acute myocardial infarction. *Postgrad Med J* 1996;72(843):45-50.

3628 Iliceto S, Scrutinio D, Bruzzi P, et al. Effects of L-carnitine administration on left ventricular remodeling after acute anterior myocardial infarction: the L-Carnitine Ecocardiografia Digitalizzata Infarto Miocardico (CEDIM) Trial. *J Am Coll Cardiol*, 1995;26(2):380-387.

3629 Davini P, Bigalli A, Lamanna F, Boem A. Controlled study on L-carnitine therapeutic efficacy in post-infarction. *Drugs Exp Clin Res* 1992;18(8):355-365.

3630 Plioplys AV, Plioplys S. Amantadine and L-carnitine treatment of Chronic Fatigue Syndrome. *Neuropsychobiology*, 1997;35(1):16-23.

3631 Brevetti G, Chiariello M, Ferulano G, et al. Increases in walking distance in patients with peripheral vascular disease treated with L-carnitine: a double-blind, cross-over study. *Circulation*, 1988;77(4):767-773.

3632 Cifone MG, Alesse E, Di Marzio L, et al. Effect of L-carnitine treatment in vivo on apoptosis and ceramide generation in peripheral blood lymphocytes from AIDS patients. *Proc Assoc Am Physicians*, 1997;109(2):146-153.

3633 Scaglia F, Longo N. Primary and secondary alterations of neonatal carnitine metabolism. *Semin Perinatol*, 1999;23(2):152-161.

3634 Bonner CM, DeBrie KL, Hug G, et al. Effects of parenteral L-carnitine supplementation on fat metabolism and nutrition in premature neonates. *J Pediatr*, 1995;126(2):287-292.

3635 Schmidt-Sommerfeld E, Penn D. Carnitine and total parenteral nutrition of the neonate. *Biol Neonate* 1990;58 Suppl 1:81-88.

3636 Melegh B, Kerner J, Sandor A, et al. Oral L-carnitine supplementation in low-birth-weight newborns: a study on neonates requiring combined parenteral and enteral nutrition. *Acta Paediatr Hung*, 1986;27(3):253-258.

3637 Schmidt-Sommerfeld E, Penn D, Wolf H. Carnitine deficiency in premature infants receiving total parenteral nutrition: effect of L-carnitine supplementation. *J Pediatr* 1983;102(6):931-935.

3638 De Vivo DC, Bohan TP, Coulter DL, et al. L-carnitine supplementation in childhood epilepsy: current perspectives. *Epilepsia*, 1998;39(11):1216-1225.

3639 Heinonen OJ. Carnitine and physical exercise. Sports

Med, 1996;22(2):109-132.

3640 Berthillier G, Eichenberger D, Carrier HN, et al. Carnitine metabolism in early stages of Duchenne muscular dystrophy. *Clin Chim Actam*, 1982;122(3):369-375.

3641 Marthaler NP, Visarius T, Kupfer A, Lauterburg BH. Increased urinary losses of carnitine during ifosfamide chemotherapy. *Cancer Chemother Pharmacol*, 1999;44(2):170-172.

3642 Heuberger W, Berardi S, Jacky E, Pey P, Krahenbuhl S. Increased urinary excretion of carnitine in patients treated with cisplatin. *Eur J Clin Pharmacol*, 1998;54(7):503-508.

3643 Schoderbeck M, Auer B, Legenstein E, et al. Pregnancy-related changes of carnitine and acylcarnitine concentrations of plasma and erythrocytes. *J Perinat Med*, 1995;23(6):477-485.

3644 Novak M. Carnitine supplementation in soy-based formula-fed infants. *Biol Neonate*, 1990;58 Suppl 1:89-92

3645 Goral S. Levocarnitine and muscle metabolism in patients with end-stage renal disease. *J Ren Nutr*, 1998;8(3):118-121.

3646 Kletzmayr J, Mayer G, Legenstein E, et al. Anemia and carnitine supplementation in hemodialyzed patients. *Kidney Int Suppl*, 1999;69:S93-106.

3647 Ahmad S, Robertson HT, Golper TA, et al. Multicenter trial of L-carnitine in maintenance hemodialysis patients. II. Clinical and biochemical effects. *Kidney Int*, 1990;38(5):912-918.

3648 Nuesch R, Rossetto M, Martina B. Plasma and urine carnitine concentrations in well-trained athletes at rest and after exercise. Influence of L-carnitine intake. *Drugs Exp Clin Res*, 1999;25(4):167-171.

3649 Vecchiet L, Di Lisa F, Pieralisi G, et al. Influence of L-carnitine administration on maximal physical exercise. *Eur J Appl Physiol*, 1990;61(5-6):486-490.

3650 Marconi C, Sassi G, Carpinelli A, Cerretelli P. Effects of L-carnitine loading on the aerobic and anaerobic performance of endurance athletes. *Eur J Appl Physiol*, 1985;54(2):131-135.

3651 Mingrone G, Greco AV, Capristo E, et al. L-carnitine improves glucose disposal in type 2 diabetic patients. *J Am Coll Nutr*, 1999;18(1):77-82.

3652 Capaldo B, Napoli R, Di Bonito P, et al. Carnitine improves peripheral glucose disposal in non-insulin-dependent diabetic patients. *Diabetes Res Clin Pract*, 1991;14(3):191-195.

3653 Bertelli A, Ronca G. Carnitine and coenzyme Q10: biochemical properties and functions, synergism and complementary action. *Int J Tissue React*, 1990;12(3):183-186.

3654 Anon. Moducare website. URL http://www.moducare.com/ (Accessed 30 March 2000).

3655 Anon. Seacoast Vitamins website. URL http://www.seacoastvitamins.com/NaturalBalance/Sterinol.html (Accessed 30 March 2000).

3656 Anon. Carmichael Wellness Products website. URL http://www.cwproducts.com/newpg/44490.asp (Accessed 30 March 2000).

3657 Anon. Natur Leaf website. URL http://www.naturleaf.com/introduction.asp (Accessed 30 March 2000).

3658 Anon. W&B Associates Inc. website. URL http://www.wandb.com/cholesterol.6.htm (Accessed 30 March 2000).

3659 Anon. 2000+ Nutrition Center website. URL http://store.yahoo.com/rcnc2000/metasitosterol.html (Accessed 30 March 2000).

3661 Patel SB, Honda A, Salen G. Sitosterolemia: exclusion of genes involved in reduced cholesterol biosynthesis. *J Lipid Res* 1998;39(5):1055-61.

3662 Salen G, Shore V, Tint GS, et al. Increased sitosterol absorption, decreased removal, and expanded body pools compensate for reduced cholesterol synthesis in sitosterolemia with xanthomatosis. *J Lipid Res* 1989;30(9):1319-30.

3663 Nguyen LB, Shefer S, Salen G, et al. Competitive inhibition of hepatic sterol 27-hydroxylase by sitosterol: decreased activity in sitosterolemia. *Proc Assoc Am Physicians* 1998;110(1):32-9.

3665 Jones PJ, MacDougall DE, Ntanios F, Vanstone CA. Dietary phytosterols as cholesterol-lowering agents in humans. *Can J Physiol Pharmacol* 1997;75(3):217-27.

3666 Heinemann T, Kullak-Ublick GA, Pietruck B, von Bergmann K. Mechanisms of action of plant sterols on inhibition of cholesterol absorption. Comparison of sitosterol and sitostanol. *Eur J Clin Pharmacol* 1991;40 Suppl 1:S59-63.

3667 Awad AB, von Holtz RL, Cone JP, et al. Beta-sitosterol inhibits growth of HT-29 human colon cancer cells by activating the sphingomyelin cycle. *AntiBr J Nutr* 1998;18(1A):471-3.

3668 Awad AB, Chen YC, Fink CS, Hennessey T. Beta-sitosterol inhibits HT-29 human colon cancer cell growth and alters membrane lipids. *AntiBr J Nutr* 1996;16(5A):2797-804.

3669 Bouic PJ, Etsebeth S, Liebenberg RW, et al. Beta-sitosterol and beta-sitosterol glucoside stimulate human peripheral blood lymphocyte proliferation: implications for their use as an immunomodulatory vitamin combination. *Int J Immunopharmacol* 1996;18(12):693-700.

3672 Hidaka H, Kojima H, Kawabata T, et al. Effects of an HMG-CoA reductase inhibitor, pravastatin, and bile sequestering resin, cholestyramine, on plasma plant sterol levels in hypercholesterolemic subjects. *J Atheroscler Thromb* 1995;2(1):60-5.

3673 Ntanios FY, Jones PJ, Frohlich JJ. Effect of 3-hydroxy-3-methylglutaryl coenzyme A reductase inhibitor on sterol absorption in hypercholesterolemic subjects. *Metabolism* 1999;48(1):68-73.

3677 Anon. LifeLink Products - Ultradiol website. URL www.lifelinknet.com/Ultra.htm (Accessed 9 April 2000).

3678 Anon. FDA alert on misuse of consumer products containing GHB, GBL and BD. Issued June 15,1999. Food and Drug Administration, Rockville, MD. URL www.fda.gov/cder/graphics/ghb.gif (Accessed 9 April 2000).

3679 Anon. Important message for health professionals: Report serious adverse events associated with dietary supplements containing GBL, GHB or BD. Food and Drug Administration, Rockville, MD. August 25, 1999. URL http://vm.cfsan.fda.gov/~dms/mwgblghb.html (Accessed 9 April 2000).

3680 Otto A. Acquaintance rape drug may one day help instead of hurt (news). *Pharmacy Today*. American Pharmaceutical Association, Washington, DC. April 2000:17.

3681 Hillory J. Farias and Samantha Reid Date-Rape Drug Prohibition Act of 2000. One Hundred Sixth Congress of the United States of America. HR 2130.

R
E
F
E
R
E
N
C
E
S

3682 Anon. Multistate Outbreak of poisonings associated with illicit use of gamma hydroxy butyrate. *J Am Med Assoc* 1991;265(4):447-8.

3683 Kalra MA, Hart LL. Gammahydroxybutyrate in narcolepsy. *Ann Pharmacother* 1992;26:647-48.

3684 Addolorato G, Cibin M, Caprista E, et al. Maintaining abstinence from alcohol with gamma hydroxybutyric acid. [Letter] *Lancet* 1998;351:38.

3685 Strong AJ. Gamma hydroxybutyric acid and intracranial pressure. [Letter] *Lancet* 1984;1(8389):1304.

3686 Gallimberti L, Canton G, Gentile N, et al. Gamma-hydroxybutyric acid for treatment of *Alcohol* withdrawal syndrome. *Lancet* 1989;2(8666):787-9.

3687 Smith KM. Drugs used in acquaintance rape. J Am Pharm Assoc 1999;39:519-25.

3688 Dyer JE. Gamma-Hydroxybutyrate: a health-food product producing coma and seizure-like activity. *Am J Emerg Med* 1991;9(4):321-4.

3689 Scrima L, Hartman PG, Johnson FH Jr, et al. The effects of gamma-hydroxybutyrate on the sleep of narcolepsy patients: a double-blind study. *Sleep* 1990;13(6):479-90.

3690 Scrima L, Hartman PG, Johnson FH Jr, Hiller FC. Efficacy of gamma-hydroxybutyrate versus placebo in treating narcolepsy-cataplexy: double-blind subjective measures. *Biol Psychiatry* 1989;26(4):331-43.

3691 Scharf MB, Brown D, Woods M, et al. The effects and effectiveness of gamma-hydroxybutyrate in patients with narcolepsy. *J Clin Psychiatry* 1985;46(6):222-5.

3692 Broughton R, Mamelak M. The treatment of narcolepsy-cataplexy with nocturnal gamma-hydroxybutyrate. *Can J Neurol Sci* 1979;6(1):1-6.

3693 Hoes MJ, Vree TB, Guelen PJ. Gamma-hydroxybutyric acid as hypnotic. Clinical and pharmacokinetic evaluation of gamma-hydroxybutyric acid as hypnotic in man. *Encephale* 1980;6(1):93-9.

3694 Gallimberti L, Schifano F, Forza G, et al. Clinical efficacy of gamma-hydroxybutyric acid in treatment of opiate withdrawal. Eur Arch *Psychiatry Clin Neurosci* 1994;244(3):113-4.

3695 Gallimberti L, Cibin M, Pagnin P, et al. Gamma-hydroxybutyric acid for treatment of opiate withdrawal syndrome. *Neuropsychopharmacology* 1993;9(1):77-81.

3696 Gallimberti L, Ferri M, Ferrara SD, et al. Gamma-Hydroxybutyric acid in the treatment of alcohol dependence: a double-blind study. *Alcohol Clin Exp Res* 1992;16(4):673-6.

3697 Kleinschmidt S, Schellhase C, Mertzlufft F. Continuous sedation during spinal anaesthesia: gamma-hydroxybutyrate vs. propofol. Eur J Anaesthesiol 1999;16(1):23-30.

3698 Kleinschmidt S, Grundmann U, Knocke T, et al. Total intravenous anaesthesia with gamma-hydroxybutyrate (GHB) and sufentanil in patients undergoing coronary artery bypass graft surgery: a comparison in patients with unimpaired and impaired left ventricular function. *Eur J Anaesthesiol* 1998;15(5):559-64.

3699 Tunnicliff G. Significance of gamma-hydroxybutyric acid in the brain. *Gen Pharmacol* 1992;23(6):1027-34.

3700 Goodman LS, Gilan A. The Pharmacological Basis of Therapeutics. fifth ed. New York: Macmillan Publishing Co., Inc., 1975.

3701 Zava DT, Dollbaum CM, Blen M. Estrogen and progestin bioactivity of foods, herbs, and spices. *Proc Soc Exp Biol Med*, 1998;217(3):369-78.

3702 Rodriguez M, Alvarez M, Zayas M. [Microbiological quality of spices consumed in Cuba]. [Article in Spanish]. *Rev Latinoam Microbiol*, 1991;33(2-3):149-151.

3703 Kivanc M, Akgul A, Dogan A. Inhibitory and stimulatory effects of cumin, oregano and their essential oils on growth and acid production of Lactobacillus plantarum and Leuconostoc mesenteroides. *Int J Food Microbiol*, 1991;13(1):81-85.

3704 Akgul A, Kivanc M. Inhibitory effects of selected Turkish spices and oregano components on some foodborne fungi. *Int J Food Microbiol*, 1988;6(3):263-268.

3705 Benito M, et al. "Labiatae allergy: systemic reactions due to ingestion of oregano and thyme." *Ann Allergy Asthma Immunol*, 1996; 76(5): 416-18.

3706 Krenzelok EP, Jacobsen TD, Aronis J. American mistletoe exposures. *Am J Emerg Med*, 1997;15(5):516-520.

3707 Friess H, et al. Treatment of advanced pancreatic cancer with mistletoe: results of a pilot trial. *AntiCancer Res*, Mar-Apr 1996;16(2):915-920.

3708 Kunze E. Lack of an antitumoral effect of immunomodulatory galactoside-specific mistletoe lectin on N-methyl-N-nitrosourea-induced urinary bladder carcinogenesis in rats. *Exp Toxicol Pathol*, 1997;49(3-4):167-180.

3709 Kuttan G, et al. "Anticarcinogenic and antimetastatic activity of Iscador." *AntiCancer Drugs*, 1997; 8 Suppl 1: S15-16.

3710 Lenartz D, et al. "Efficiency of treatment with galactoside-specific lectin from mistletoe against rat glioma." *AntiCancer Res*, 1998; 18(2A): 1011-014.

3711 Weber K, et al. "Effects of a standardized mistletoe preparation on metastatic B16 melanoma colonization in murine lungs." *Arzneimittelforschung*, 1998; 48(5): 497-502.

3712 Bussing A, Schaller G, Pfuller U. "Generation of reactive oxygen intermediates (ROI) by the thionins from Viscum album L." *AntiCancer Res*, 1998; 18(6A): 4291-296.

3713 Heiny BM, Albrecht V, Beuth J. "Correlation of immune cell activities and beta-endorphin release in breast carcinoma patients treated with galactose-specific lectin standardized mistletoe extract." *AntiCancer Res*, 1998;18(1B): 583-86.

3714 Nikolai G, et al. "Effect of a mistletoe extract (Iscador QuFrF) on viability and migratory behavior of human peripheral CD4+ and CD8+ T lymphocytes in three-dimensional collagen lattices." *In Vitro Cell Dev Biol Anim*, 1997; 33(9): 710-16.

3715 Vehmeyer K, et al. "Lectin-induced increase in clonogenic growth of haematopoietic progenitor cells." *Eur J Haematol*, Jan. 1998; 60(1): 16-20.

3716 Ortega N, et al. "Tobacco allergy: demonstration of cross-reactivity with other members of Solanaceae family and mugwort pollen." *Ann Allergy Asthma Immunol*, Feb. 1999; 82(2): 194-97.

3717 Lombardi C, et al. "Allergic reactions to honey and royal jelly and their relationship with sensitization to compositae." *Allergol Immunopathol (Madr)*, 1998; 26(6): 288-90 .

3718 Westendorf J, Pfau W, Schulte A. "Carcinogenicity and DNA adduct formation observed in ACI rats after long-term treatment with madder root, Rubia tinctorum L." *Carcinogenesis*, 1998; 19(12): 2163-168.

3719 Friese KH, et al. "The homoeopathic treatment of otitis media in children-comparisons with conventional therapy." *Int J Clin Pharmacol Ther*, 1997; 35(7): 296-301.

3720 Bourinbaiar AS, Lee-Huang S. "Potentiation of anti-HIV activity of anti-inflammatory drugs, dexamethasone and indomethacin, by MAP30, the antiviral agent from bitter melon." *Biochem Biophys Res Commun*, 1995;208(2):779-85.

3721 Lee-Huang S, Huang PL, Chen HC, et al. "Anti-HIV and anti-tumor activities of recombinant MAP30 from bitter melon." *Gene*, 1995;161(2):151-6.

3722 Cunnick JE, Sakamoto K, Chapes SK, et al. "Induction of tumor cytotoxic immune cells using a protein from the bitter melon (Momordica charantia)." *Cell Immunol*, 1990;126(2):278-89.

3723 Jilka C, Strifler B, Fortner GW, et al. "In vivo antitumor activity of the bitter melon (Momordica charantia)." *Cancer Res*, 1983;43(11):5151-5.

3724 Leung SO, Yeung HW, Leung KN. "The immunosuppressive activities of two abortifacient proteins isolated from the seeds of bitter melon (Momordica charantia)." *Immunopharmacology*, 1987;13(3):159-71.

3726 Tseng J, Chang JG. "Suppression of tumor necrosis factor-alpha, interleukin-1 beta, interleukin-6 and granulocyte-monocyte colony stimulating factor secretion from human monocytes by an extract of Poria cocos." *Chung Hua Min Kuo Wei Sheng Wu Chi Mien I Hsueh Tsa Chih*, 1992;25(1):1-11.

3727 Hattori T, Hayashi K, Nagao T, et al. "Studies on antinephritic effects of plant components (3): Effect of pachyman, a main component of Poria cocos Wolf on original-type anti-GBM nephritis in rats and its mechanisms." Jpn J Pharmacol, 1992;59(1):89-96.

3728 Cuellar MJ, Giner RM, Recio MC, et al. "Effect of the basidiomycete Poria cocos on experimental dermatitis and other inflammatory conditions." *Chem Pharm Bull* (Tokyo), 1997;45(3):492-4.

3729 Kaminaga T, Yasukawa K, Kanno H, et al. "Inhibitory effects of lanostane-type triterpene acids, the components of Poria cocos, on tumor promotion by 12-O tetradecanoylphorbol-13-acetate in two-stage carcinogenesis in mouse skin." *Oncology*, 1996;53(5):382-5.

3730 Tai T, Akita Y, Kinoshita K, et al. "Anti-emetic principles of Poria cocos." *Planta Med*, 1995;61(6):527-30.

3731 Wang SS, Yang S, Ma Y. "Efficacy of poria-polyporus anti-diarrhea oral liquor in treating infantile rotavirus diarrhea: a controlled study with smicta." [Article in Chinese] *Chung Kuo Chung Hsi I Chieh Ho Tsa Chih*, 1995;15(5):284-6.

3732 Li YL. "Clinical and experimental study on the treatment of children diarrhea by granule of children-diarrhea fast-stopping." [Article in Chinese]. *Chung Hsi I Chieh Ho Tsa Chih*, 1991;11(2):79-82,67.

3733 Wang SQ, Du XR, Lu HW, et al. "Experimental and clinical studies of "Shen Yan Ling" in treatment of chronic glomerulonephritis." J Tradit Chin Med, 1989;9(2):132-4.

3734 Yang DJ. "Tinnitus treated with combined traditional Chinese *Medicine* and Western medicine." [Article in Chinese] *Chung Hsi I Chieh Ho Tsa Chih*, 1989;9(5):270-1,259-60.

3735 Gong QM, Wang SL, Gan C. "A clinical study on the treatment of acute upper digestive tract hemorrhage with wen-she decoction." [Article in Chinese] *Chung Hsi I Chieh Ho Tsa Chih*, 1989;9(5):272-3,260.

3736 Yasukawa K, Kaminaga T, Kitanaka S, et al. "3 beta-p-hydroxybenzoyldehydrotumulosic acid from Poria cocos, and its anti-inflammatory effect." *Phytochemistry*, 1998;48(8):1357-60.

3737 Nukaya H, Yamashiro H, Fukazawa H, et al. "Isolation of inhibitors of TPA-induced mouse ear edema from Hoelen, Poria cocos." *Chem Pharm Bull* (Tokyo), 1996;44(4):847-9.

3740 Kouzi SA, McMurtry RJ, Nelson SD. "Hepatotoxicity of germander (Teucrium chamaedrys L.) and one of its constituent neoclerodane diterpenes teucrin A in the mouse." *Chem Res Toxicol*, 1994;7(6):850-6.

3741 Larrey D, Vial T, Pauwels A, et al. "Hepatitis after germander (Teucrium chamaedrys) administration: another instance of herbal medicine hepatotoxicity." *Ann Intern Med*, 1992;117(2):129-32.

3742 Pauwels A, Thierman-Duffaud D, Azanowsky JM, et al. "Acute hepatitis caused by wild germander. Hepatotoxicity of herbal remedies. Two cases." [Article in French] *Gastroenterol Clin Biol*, 1992;16(1):92-5.

3743 Castot A, Djezzar S, Deleau N, et al. "Pharmacovigilance off the beaten track: herbal surveillance or pharmacovigilance of medicinal plants." [Article in French] *Therapie*, 1997;52(2):97-103.

3744 Mostefa-Kara N, Pauwels A, Pines E, et al. "Fatal hepatitis after herbal tea." *Lancet*, 1992;340(8820):674.

3745 Chan P, Xu DY, Liu JC, et al. "The effect of stevioside on blood pressure and plasma catecholamines in spontaneously hypertensive rats." *Life Sci*, 1998;63(19):1679-84.

3746 Melis MS. "A crude extract of Stevia rebaudiana increases the renal plasma flow of normal and hypertensive rats." *Braz J Med Biol Res*, 1996;29(5):669-75.

3747 Melis MS. "Chronic administration of aqueous extract of Stevia rebaudiana in rats: renal effects." *J Ethnopharmacol*, 1995;47(3):129-34.

3748 Matsui M, Matsui K, Kawasaki Y, et al. "Evaluation of the genotoxicity of stevioside and steviol using six in vitro and one in vivo mutagenicity assays." *Mutagenesis*, 1996;11(6):573-9.

3749 Pezzuto JM, Compadre CM, Swanson SM, et al. "Metabolically activated steviol, the aglycone of stevioside, is mutagenic." *Proc Natl Acad Sci USA*, 1985;82(8):2478-82.

3750 Hubler MO, Bracht A, Kelmer-Bracht AM. "Influence of stevioside on hepatic glycogen levels in fasted rats." *Res Commun Chem Pathol Pharmacol*, 1994;84(1):111-8.

3751 Fang HJ, Su XL, Liu HY, Cet al. "Studies on the chemical components and anti-tumour action of the volatile oils from Pelargonium graveoleus." [Article in Chinese] *Yao Hsueh Hsueh Pao*, 1989;24(5):366-71.

3752 Lis-Balchin M, Buchbauer G, Hirtenlehner T, Resch M. "Antimicrobial activity of Pelargonium essential oils added to a quiche filling as a model food system." *Lett Appl Microbiol*, 1998;27(4):207-10.

3753 Pattnaik S, Subramanyam VR, Kole C. "Antibacterial and antifungal activity of ten essential oils in vitro." *Microbios*, 1996;86(349):237-46.

3754 Agarwal AK, Singh M, Gupta N, et al. "Management of giardiasis by an immuno-modulatory herbal drug Pippali rasayana." *J Ethnopharmacol*, 1994;44493):143-6.

3755 Agarwal AK, Tripathi DM, Sahai R, et al. "Management of giardiasis by a herbal drug 'Pippali Rasayana': a clinical study." *J Ethnopharmacol*, 1997;56(3):233-6.

REFERENCES

3756 Shah AH, Al-Shareef AH, Ageel AM, Qureshi S. "Toxicity studies in mice of common spices, Cinnamomum zeylanicum bark and Piper longum fruits." *Plant Foods Hum Nutr*, 1998;52(3):231-9.

3757 Khajuria A, Zutshi U, Bedi KL. "Permeability characteristics of piperine on oral absorption-an active alkaloid from peppers and a bioavailability enhancer." *Indian J Exp Biol*, 1998;36(1):46-50.

3758 Ghoshal S, Prasad BN, Lakshmi V. "Antiamoebic activity of Piper longum fruits against Entamoeba histolytica in vitro and in vivo." *J Ethnopharmacol*, 1996;50(3):167-70.

3759 el-Mofty MM, Khudoley VV, Shwaireb MH. "Carcinogenic effect of force-feeding an extract of black pepper (Piper nigrum) in Egyptian toads (Bufo regularis)." *Oncology*, 1991;48(4):347-50.

3760 Singh A, Rao AR. Evaluation of the modulatory influence of black pepper (Piper nigrum, L.) on the hepatic detoxication system." *Cancer Lett*, 1993; 72(1-2):5-9.

3761 Nalini N, Sabitha K, Viswanathan P, Menon VP. "Influence of spices on the bacterial (enzyme) activity in experimental colon cancer." *J Ethnopharmacol*, 1998;62(1):15-24.

3762 Day C, Cartwright T, Provost J, Bailey CJ. "Hypoglycaemic effect of Momordica charantia extracts." *Planta Med*, 1990;56(5):426-9.

3763 Ali L, Khan AK, Mamun MI, et al. "Studies on hypoglycemic effects of fruit pulp, seed, and whole plant of Momordica charantia on normal and diabetic model rats." *Planta Med*, 1993;59(5):408-12.

3764 Cakici I, Hurmoglu C, Tunctan B, et al. "Hypoglycaemic effect of Momordica charantia extracts in normoglycaemic or cyproheptadine-induced hyperglycaemic mice." *J Ethnopharmacol*, 1994;44(2):117-21.

3765 Sarkar S, Pranava M, Marita R. "Demonstration of the hypoglycemic action of Momordica charantia in a validated animal model of diabetes." *Pharmacol Res*, 1996;33(1):1-4.

3766 Hansson A, Veliz G, Naquira C, et al. "Preclinical and clinical studies with latex from Ficus glabrata HBK, a traditional intestinal anthelminthic in the Amazonian area." *J Ethnopharmacol*, 1986;17(2):105-38.

3767 Lee IS, Jung KY, Oh SR, et al. "Structure-activity relationships of lignans from Schisandra chinensis as platelet activating antagonists." *Biol Pharm Bull*, 1999 ;22(3): 265-7.

3768 Sun HD, Qiu SX, Lin LZ, Wang ZY, Lin ZW, Pengsuparp T, et al. "Nigranoic acid, a triterpenoid from Schisandra sphaerandra that inhibits HIV-1 reverse transcriptase." *J Nat Prod*, 1996; 59(5):525-7.

3769 Fukuda K, Ohta T, Oshima Y, Ohashi N, Yoshikawa M, Yamazoe Y. "Specific CYP3A4 inhibitors in grapefruit juice: furocoumarin dimers as components of drug interaction." *Pharmacogenetics*, 1997; 7(5):391-6.

3770 Fukuda K, Ohta T, Yamazoe Y. "Grapefruit component interacting with rat and human P450 CYP3A: possible involvement of non-flavonoid components in drug interaction." *Biol Pharm Bull*, 1997; 20(5):560-4.

3771 Lilja JJ, Kivisto KT, Backman JT, Lamberg TS, Neuvonen PJ. "Grapefruit juice substantially increases plasma concentrations of buspirone." *Clin Pharmacol Ther*, 1998; 64(6):655-60.

3772 Penzak SR, Gubbins PO, Gurley BJ, Wang PL, Saccente M. "Grapefruit juice decreases the systemic availability of itraconazole capsules in healthy volunteers." *Ther Drug Monit*, 1999; 21(3):304-9.

3773 Kupferschmidt HH, Fattinger KE, Ha HR, Follath F, Krahenbuhl S. "Grapefruit juice decreases the systemic availability of itraconazole capsules in healthy volunteers." *Br J Clin Pharmacol*, 1998; 45(4):355-9.

3774 Lilja JJ, Kivisto KT, Neuvonen PJ. "Grapefruit juice-simvastatin interaction: effect on serum concentrations of simvastatin, simvastatin acid, and HMG-CoA reductase inhibitors." *Clin Pharmacol Ther*, 1998 ; 64(5):477-83.

3775 Ameer B, Weintraub RA. "Drug interactions with grapefruit juice." *Clin Pharmacokinet*, 1997; 33(2):103-21.

3800 Tyler VE, Brady LR, Robbers JE. Pharmacognosy, 7th Edition. Lea & Febiger, Philadelphia, PA, 1976.

3801 Gobel H, Schmidt G, Soyka D. Effect of peppermint and eucalyptus oil preparations on neurophysiological and experimental algesimetric headache parameters. *Cephalalgia* 1994;14(3):228-34; discussion 182.

3802 Liu JH, Chen GH, Yeh HZ, et al. Enteric-coated peppermint-oil capsules in the treatment of irritable bowel syndrome: a prospective, randomized trial. J *Gastroenterol* 1997;32(6):765-8.

3803 Pittler MH, Ernst E. Peppermint oil for irritable bowel syndrome: a critical review and metaanalysis. *Am J Gastroenterol* 1998;93(7):1131-5.

3804 Tate S. Peppermint oil: a treatment for postoperative nausea. *J Adv Nurs* 1997;26(3):543-9.

3805 United States Pharmacopeial Convention I, editor. *Drug Information for the Health Care Professional*. 19th Edition. Micromedex, 1999.

3807 Correa CM, Tibana A, Gontijo Filho PP. Vegetables as a source of infection with Pseudomonas aeruginosa in a University and Oncology Hospital of Rio de Janeiro. *J Hosp Infect* 1991;18(4):301-6.

3808 Benito M, Jorro G, Morales C, et al. Labiatae allergy: systemic reactions due to ingestion of oregano and thyme. *Ann Allergy Asthma Immunol*, 1996; 76(5):416-8.

3811 Chan TY. Potential dangers from topical preparations containing methyl salicylate. *Hum Exp Toxicol* 1996;15(9):747-50.

3818 Tsuda T, Sugaya A, Ohguchi H, et al. Protective effects of peony root extract and its components on neuron damage in the hippocampus induced by the cobalt focus epilepsy model. *Exp Neurol* 1997; 146(2):518-25.

3819 Croton, Botanical.com A Modern Herbal website. URL: www.botanical.com/botanical/mgmh/c/croto118.html. Access Date: May 12, 1999.

3820 Description and Natural History of the Periwinkle. URL: biotech.icmb.utexas.edu/botany/perihist.html

3821 Coolwort, Botanical.com A Modern Herbal website. URL: www.botanical.com/botanical/mgmh/c/coolwo97.html. Access Date: May 12, 1999.

3822 Mossa JS, Tariq M, Mohsin A, et al. Pharmacological studies on aerial parts of Calotropis procera. *Am J Chin Med* 1991;19(3-4):223-31.

3823 Kumar VL, Basu N. Anti-inflammatory activity of the latex of Calotropis procera. *J Ethnopharmacol* 1994;44(2):123-5.

3824 Mascolo N, Sharma R, Jain SC, et al. Ethnopharmacology of Calotropis procera flowers. *J Ethnopharmacol* 1988;22(2):211-21.

3825 Sen T, Basu A, Chaudhuri AK. Studies on the possible mechanism of the gastric mucosal protection by Calotropis procera—involvement of 5-lipoxygenase pathway. *Fundam Clin Pharmacol* 1998;12(1):82-7.

3826　Levy L. The activity of chaulmoogra acids against Mycobacterium leprae. *Am Rev Respir Dis* 1975;111(5):703-5.

3827　Cowhage, Botanical.com A Modern Herbal website. URL: www.botanical.com/botanical/mgmh/c/cowha111.html. Access Date: May 12, 1999.

3828　Mascolo N, Autore G, Capasso F. Local anti-inflammatory activity of Tamus communis. *J Ethnopharmacol* 1987;19(1):81-4.

3829　Schmidt RJ, Moult SP. The dermatitic properties of black bryony (Tamus communis L.). *Contact Dermatitis* 1983;9(5):390-6.

3830　Carotenuto A, De Feo V, Fattorusso E, et al. The flavonoids of Allium ursinum. *Phytochemistry* 1996;41(2):531-6.

3831　Rietz B, Isensee H, Strobach H, et al. Cardioprotective actions of wild garlic (allium ursinum) in ischemia and reperfusion. *Mol Cell Biochem* 1993;119(1-2):143-50.

3832　Rana BK, Singh UP, Taneja V. Antifungal activity and kinetics of inhibition by essential oil isolated from leaves of Aegle marmelos. *J Ethnopharmacol* 1997;57(1):29-34.

3833　Prakash D, Joshi BD, Pal M. Vitamin C in leaves and seed oil composition of the Amaranthus species. *Int J Food Sci Nutr* 1995;46(1):47-51.

3834　Sharma SR, Dwivedi SK, Swarup D. Hypoglycaemic, antihyperglycaemic and hypolipidemic activities of Caesalpinia bonducella seeds in rats. *J Ethnopharmacol* 1997;58(1):39-44.

3835　Ippen H. [Phytophotodermatitis caused by plant trimming (edger's rash)]. *Derm Beruf Umwelt* 1990;38(6):190-2.

3836　Misra SB, Dixit SN. Antifungal properties of leaf extract of Ranunculus sceleratus L. *Experientia* 1978;34(11):1442-1443.

3837　Goerz G, Wirth G, Maas B, et al. [Allergic Contact Dermatitis due to Asteraceae (Compositae). Cross reaction with Liatris spicata]. *Derm Beruf Umwelt* 1985;33(3):95-8.

3838　Krenzelok EP, Jacobsen TD, Aronis JM. Poinsettia exposures have good outcomes...just as we thought. *Am J Emerg Med* 1996;14(7):671-4.

3839　Cohen LM, Cohen JL. Erythema multiforme associated with Contact Dermatitis to poison ivy: three cases and a review of the literature. *Cutis*, 1998; 62(3):139-42.

3841　Kuo SC, Chen SC, Chen LH, et al. Potent antiplatelet, anti-inflammatory and antiallergic isoflavanquinones from the roots of Abrus precatorius. *Planta Med* 1995;61(4):307-12.

3842　Wang JP, Hsu MF, Chang LC, et al. Inhibition of plasma extravasation by abruquinone A, a natural isoflavanquinone isolated from Abrus precatorius. *Eur J Pharmacol* 1995;273(1-2):73-81.

3846　Henriksen NT. Lycoperdonosis. Acta Paediatr Scand 1976;65(5):643-5.

3847　Respiratory illness associated with inhalation of mushroom spores— Wisconsin, 1994. *MMWR* Morb Mortal Wkly Rep 1994;43(29):525-6.

3850　Sidhu GS, Oakenfull DG. A mechanism for the hypocholesterolaemic activity of saponins. *Br J Nutr* 1986;55(3):643-9.

3851　Wu JY, Gardner BH, Murphy CI, et al. Saponin adjuvant enhancement of antigen-specific immune responses to an experimental HIV-1 vaccine. *J Immunol* 1992;148(5):1519-25.

3852　Pillion DJ, Amsden JA, Kensil CR, et al. Structure-function relationship among Quillaja saponins serving as excipients for nasal and ocular delivery of insulin. *J Pharm Sci* 1996;85(5):518-24.

3853　Recchia J, Lurantos MH, Amsden JA, et al. A semisynthetic Quillajasaponin as a drug delivery agent for aminoglycoside antibiotics. *Pharm Res* 1995;12(12):1917-23.

3854　Mitscher LA, Bathala MS, Clark GW, et al. Antimicrobial agents from higher plants. The quaternary alkaloids of Ptelea trifoliata. *Lloydia* 1975;38(2):109-16.

3858　Majumder PK, Dasgupta S, Mukhopadhaya RK, et al. Anti-steroidogenic activity of the petroleum ether extract and fraction 5 (fatty acids) of carrot (Daucus carota L.) seeds in mouse ovary. *J Ethnopharmacol* 1997;57(3):209-12.

3859　Maher TJ. Chromium and other minerals in diabetes mellitus. *US Pharm* November 1999:66-76.

3860　Nisley N, Klepser T. Phytoestrogens for the prevention and treatment of osteoporosis. *Alternative Medicine Alert* 1999;December:138-142.

3861　Leder BZ, Longcope C, Catlin DH, et al. Oral androstenedione administration and serum testosterone concentrations in young men. *JAMA* 2000;283:779-782.

3862　Rasmussen BB, Volpi E, Gore DC, Wolfe RR. Androstenedione does not stimulate muscle anabolism in young healthy men. *J Clin Endocinol Metab* 2000;55-59.

3863　Tode T, Kikuchi Y, Hirata J, et al. Effect of Korean red ginseng on psychological functions in patients with severe climacteric syndromes. *Int J Gynaecol Obstet* 1999;67:169-174.

3864　Rabkin JG, Ferrando SJ, Wagner GJ, Rabkin R. DHEA treatment for HIV positive patients: effects on mood, androgenic and anabolic parameters. *Psychoneuroendocrinology* 2000;25:53-68.

3865　Dyner TS, Lang W, Geaga J et al. An open-label dose-escalation trial of oral dehydroepiandrosterone tolerance and pharmacokinetics in patients with HIV disease. *J Acquir Immune Defic Syndr* 1993;6:459-465.

3866　Henderson E, Yang JY, Schwartz A. Dehydroepiandrosterone (DHEA) and synthetic DHEA analogs are modest inhibitors of HIV-1 IIIB replication. *AIDS Res Hum Retroviruses* 1992;8:625-631.

3867　Christeff N, Gherbi N, Mammes O, et al. Serum cortisol and DHEA concentrations during HIV infection. *Psychoneuroendocrinology* 1997;22:S11-18.

3868　Ruhnau KJ, Meissner HP, Finn JR, et al. Effects of 3-week oral treatment with the antioxidant thioctic acid (alpha-lipoic acid) in symptomatic diabetic polyneuropathy. *Diabet Med* 1999;16:1040-1043.

3869　Sachse G, Willms B. Efficacy of thioctic acid in the therapy of peripheral diabetic neuropathy. *Horm Metab Res Suppl* 1980;9:105-107.

3870　Gleiter CH, Schreeb KH, Freudenthaler S, et al. Lack of interaction between thioctic acid, glibenclamide and acarbose. *Br J Clin Pharmacol* 1999;48:819-825.

3871　Packer L, Witt EH, Tritschler HJ. alpha-Lipoic acid as a biological antioxidant. *Free Radic Biol Med* 1995;19:227-250.

3872　Teichert J, Kern J, Tritschler HJ. Investigations on the pharmacokinetics of alpha-lipoic acid in healthy volunteers. *Int J Clin Pharmacol Ther* 1998;36:625-628.

3873　Nagamatsu M, Nickander KK, Schmelzer JD, et al. Lipoic acid improves nerve blood flow, reduces

© Copyright 2000, Natural Medicines Comprehensive Database (209) 472-2244. For updated data, go to www.NaturalDatabase.com.

Reference Citations

oxidative stress, and improves distal nerve conduction in experimental diabetic neuropathy. *Diabetes Care* 1995;18:1160-1167.

3874 Jacob S, Henriksen EJ, Tritschler HJ, et al. Improvement of insulin-stimulated glucose-disposal in type 2 diabetes after repeated parenteral administration of thioctic acid. *Exp Clin Endocrinol Diabetes* 1996;104:284-288.

3875 Jacob S, Henriksen EJ, Schiemann AL, et al. Enhancement of glucose disposal in patients with type 2 diabetes by alpha-lipoic acid. *Arzneimittelforschung* 1995;45:872-874.

3876 Jacob S, Ruus P, Hermann R, et al. Oral administration of RAC-alpha-lipoic acid modulates insulin sensitivity in patients with type-2 diabetes mellitus: a placebo-controlled pilot trial. *Free Radic Biol Med* 1999;27:309-314.

3877 Haramaki N, Assadnazari H, Zimmer G, et al. The influence of vitamin E and dihydrolipoic acid on cardiac energy and glutathione status under hypoxia-reoxygenation. *Biochem Mol Biol Int* 1995;37:591-597.

3878 Kishi Y, Schmelzer JD, Yao JK, et al. Alpha-lipoic acid: effect on glucose uptake, sorbitol pathway, and energy metabolism in experimental diabetic neuropathy. *Diabetes* 1999;48:2045-2051.

3879 Bustamante J, Lodge JK, Marcocci L, et al. Alpha-lipoic acid in liver metabolism and disease. *Free Radic Biol Med* 1998;24:1023-1039.

3880 Marshall AW, Graul RS, Morgan MY, Sherlock S. Treatment of alcohol-related liver disease with thioctic acid: a six month randomized double-blind trial. *Gut* 1982;23:1088-1093.

3881 Conlon BJ, Aran JM, Erre JP, Smith DW. Attenuation of aminoglycoside-induced cochlear damage with the metabolic antioxidant alpha-lipoic acid. *Hear Res* 1999;128:40-44.

3882 Vilas GL, Aldonatti C, San Martin de Viale LC, Rios de Molina MC. Effect of Alpha-lipoic acid amide on hexachlorobenzene porphyria. *Biochem Mol Biol Int* 1999;47:815-823.

3883 Gurer H, Ozgunes H, Oztezcan S, Ercal N. Antioxidant role of alpha-lipoic acid in lead toxicity. *Free Radic Biol Med* 1999;27:75-81.

3884 Altenkirch H, Stoltenburg-Didinger G, Wagner HM, et al. Effects of lipoic acid in hexacarbon-induced neuropathy. *Neurotoxicol Teratol* 1990;12:619-622.

3885 Fuchs J, Schofer H, Milbradt R, et al. Studies on lipoate effects on blood redox state in human immunodeficiency virus infected patients. *Arzneimittelforschung* 1993;43:1359-1362.

3886 Vermeulen EG, Stehouwer CD, Twisk JW, et al. Effect of homocysteine-lowering treatment with folic acid plus vitamin B6 on progression of subclinical Atherosclerosis: a randomised, placebo-controlled trial. *Lancet* 2000;355:517-522.

3887 Bostom AG, Garber C. Endpoints for homocysteine-lowering trials. *Lancet* 2000;355:511-512.

3888 Vuorio AF, Gylling H, Turtola H, et al. Stanol ester margarine alone and with simvastatin lowers serum cholesterol in families with familial hypercholesterolemia caused by the FH-north karelia mutation. *Arterioscler Thromb Vasc Biol* 2000;20:500-506.

3889 Becker M, Staab D, Von Bergmann K. Treatment of severe familial hypercholesterolemia in childhood with sitosterol and sitostanol. *J Pediatr* 1993;122:292-296.

3890 American Diabetes Association. Nutrition and principles for people with diabetes mellitus. *Diabetes Care* 2000;23 (suppl 1). http://journal.diabetes.org/fulltext/ supplements/diabetescare/supplement/243.html (Accessed 20 January 2000).

3891 Paice JA, Ferrans CE, Lashley FR, et al. Topical capsaicin in the management of HIV-associated peripheral neuropathy. *J Pain Symptom Manage* 2000;19:45-52.

3892 Bloch M, Schmidt PJ, Danaceau MA, et al. Dehydroepiandrosterone treatment of midlife dysthymia. *Biol Psychiatry* 1999;45:1533-1541.

3893 Wolf OT, Neumann O, Hellhammer DH, et al. Effects of a two-week physiological dehydroepiandrosterone substitution on cognitive performance and well-being in healthy elderly women and men. *J Clin Endocrinol Metab* 1997;82:2363-2367.

3894 MotherNature Encyclopedia. "Alpha-lipoic Acid" website: www.mothernature.com (Accessed 29 February 2000).

3895 MotherNature. "Yohimbe Products" website: www.mothernature.com (Accessed 29 February 2000).

3896 Yusuf S, Dagenais G, Pogue J, et al. Vitamin E supplementation and cardiovascular events in high-risk patients. The Heart Outcomes Prevention Evaluation Study Investigators. *N Engl J Med* 2000;342:154-160.

3897 GISSI-Prevenzione Investigators. Dietary supplementation with n-3 polyunsaturated fatty acids and vitamin E after myocardial infarction: results of the GISSI-Prevenzione trial. *Lancet* 1999;354:447-455.

3898 Stampfer MJ, Hennekens CH, Manson JE, et al. Vitamin E consumption and the risk of coronary disease in women. *N Engl J Med* 1993;328:1444-1449.

3899 Malinow MR, Bostom AG, Kraus RM. Homocyst(e)ine, diet, and cardiovascular diseases: a statement for healthcare professionals from the Nutrition Committee, American Heart Association. *Circulation* 1999;99:178-182.

3900 Peirce A. The American Pharmaceutical Association Practical Guide to Natural Medicines. New York: William Morrow and Company, 1999.

3901 Tyler VE, Brady LR, Robbers JB. Pharmacognosy. Philadelphia: Lea and Fibiger, 1981.

3902 Barlet A, et al. "Efficacy of Pygeum africanum extract in the medical therapy of urination disorders due to benign prostatic hyperplasia: evaluation of objective and subjective parameters. A placebo-controlled double-blind multicenter study." *Wien Klin Wochenschr*, 1990; 102(22):667-73.

3903 Breza J, et al. "Efficacy and acceptability of tadenan (Pygeum africanum extract) in the treatment of benign prostatic hyperplasia (BPH): a multicentre trial in central Europe." *Curr Med Res Opin*, 1998; 14(3):127-39.

3904 Dufour B, et al. "Controlled study of the effects of Pygeum africanum extract on the functional symptoms of prostatic adenoma." *Ann Urol (Paris)*, 1984; 18(3):193-95.

3905 Whitmore A. "FDA warns consumers against dietary supplement products that may contain Digitalis mislabeled as "Plantain"." Food and Drug Administration, U.S. Department of the Interior, Washington, DC, 1997.

3906 Garcia-Gonzalez JJ, et al. "Prevalence of atopy in students from Malaga, Spain." *Ann Allergy Asthma Immunol*, 1998; 80(3):237-44.

3907 Sugano M, Tsuji E. "Rice bran oil and cholesterol metabolism. *J Nutr*, 1997; 127(3):521S-24S.

3908 Rukmini C, Raghuram TC. "Nutritional and biochemical aspects of the hypolipidemic action of rice bran oil: a review. *J Am Coll Nutr*, 1991; 10(6):593-601.

3909 Grunewald KK, Bailey RS. "Commercially marketed supplements for bodybuilding athletes." *Sports Med*, 1993; 15(2):90-103.

3910 Fry AC, et al. "The effects of gamma-oryzanol supplementation during resistance exercise training." *Int J Sport Nutr*, 1997; 7(4):318-29.

3911 Singer P, Wirth M, Berger I. "A possible contribution of decrease in free fatty acids to low serum triglyceride levels after diets supplemented with n-6 and n-3 polyunsaturated fatty acids." *Atherosclerosis* 1990; 83(2-3):167-75.

3912 Fischer S, et al. "Results of linseed oil and olive oil therapy in hyperlipoproteinemia patients." *Dtsch Z Verdau Stoffwechselkr*, 1984; 44(5):245-51.

3913 Castner JL, Timme SL, Duke JA. A Field Guide to Medicinal and Useful Plants of the Upper Amazon. Gainesville, FL: Feline Press, 1998.

3914 Mongelli E, et al. "Antimicrobial activity and interaction with DNA of medicinal plants from the Peruvian Amazon region." *Rev Argent Microbiol*, 1995; 27(4):199-203.

3915 Bisset NG. "War and hunting poisons of the New World. Part 1. Notes on the early history of curare." *J Ethnopharmacol*, 1992; 36(1):1-26.

3916 Manabe H, et al. "Effects of Catuaba extracts on microbial and HIV infection." *In Vivo*, 1992; 6(2):161-65.

3917 Rain Tree Website, URL: www.rain-tree.com/catuaba.htm. (23 July 1999).

3918 Taylor L. Herbal Secrets of the Rainforest. Rocklin, CA: Prima Publishing, 1998.

3919 Agricultural Research Service. Dr. Duke's Phytochemical and Ethnobotanical Databases. URL: www.ars-grin.gov/duke/.

3920 Burkill JD. A Dictionary of the Economic Products of the Malay Peninsula. Kuala Lumpur: Art Printing Works, 1966.

3921 Calixto JB. "Antispasmodic effects of an alkaloid extracted from Phyllanthus sellowianus: A comparative study with papaverine." *Braz J Med Biol Res*, 1984; 17:313-321. [primary reference in Taylor].

3922 Syamasundar KV. "Antihepatotoxic principles of Phyllanthus niruri herbs. *J Ethnopharmacol*, 1985; 14:41-44. [primary reference in Taylor].

3923 Calixto JB, et al. "A review of the plants of the genus Phyllanthus: their chemistry, pharmacology, and therapeutic potential." *Med Res Rev*, 1998; 18(4):225-58.

3924 Milne A, et al. "Failure of New Zealand hepatitis B carriers to respond to Phyllanthus amarus." *N Z Med J*, 1994; 107(980):243.

3925 Wang M, et al. "Herbs of the genus Phyllanthus in the treatment of chronic hepatitis B: observations with three preparations from different geographic sites." *J Lab Clin Med*, 1995; 126(4):350-52.

3926 Berk L, et al. "Beneficial effects of Phyllanthus amarus for chronic hepatitis B, not confirmed [letter]." *J Hepatol*, 1991; 12(3):405-406.

3927 Qian-Cutrone J, et al. "Niruriside, a new HIV REV/RRE binding inhibitor from Phyllanthus niruri." *J Nat Prod*, 1996; 59(2):196-99.

3928 Srividya N, Periwal S. "Diuretic, hypotensive and hypoglycaemic effect of Phyllanthus amarus." *Indian J Exp Biol*, 1995; 33:861-64.

3929 Wilkins AL, et al. "Photosensitivity in South Africa. IX. Structure elucidation of a beta-glucosidase-treated saponin from Tribulus terrestris, and the identification of saponin chemotypes of South African T. terrestris." Onderstepoort Journal Veterinary Res, 1996; 63:327-34.

3930 De Toro AA. "Blackcurrants as an energy crop and for production of essential oils: A review of the literature." *Biomass Bioenergy*, 1994; 6:261-68.

3931 Wang B, Ma L, Liu T. "406 cases of angina pectoris in coronary heart disease treated with saponin of Tribulus terrestris." *Chung Hsi I Chieh Ho Tsa Chih*, 1990; 10(2):85-87, 68.

3932 Harvey J, Colin-Jones DG. "Mistletoe hepatitis." *Br Med J*, 1981; 282:186-87.

3933 Rimm EB, Stampfer MJ, Ascherio A, et al. Vitamin E consumption and the risk of coronary heart disease in men. *N Engl J Med* 1993;328:1450-1456.

3934 Kushi LH, Folsom AR, Prineas RJ, et al. Dietary antioxidant vitamins and death from coronary heart disease in postmenopausal women. *N Engl J Med* 1996;334:1156-1162.

3935 Virtamo J, Rapola JM, Ripatti S, et al. Effect of vitamin E and beta carotene on the incidence of primary nonfatal myocardial infarction and fatal coronary heart disease. *Arch Intern Med* 1998;158:668-675.

3936 Stephens NG, Parsons A, Schofield PM, et al. Randomised controlled trial of vitamin E in patients with coronary disease: Cambridge Heart Antioxidant Study. *Lancet* 1996;347:781-786.

3937 Rapola JM, Virtamo J, Ripatti S, et al. Randomised trial of alpha-tocopherol and beta-carotene supplements on incidence of major coronary events in men with previous myocardial infraction. *Lancet* 1997;349:1715-1720.

3938 Losonczy KG, Harris TB, Havlik RJ. Vitamin E and vitamin C supplement use and risk of all-cause and coronary heart disease mortality in older persons: the Established Populations for Epidemiologic Studies of the Elderly. *Am J Clin Nutr* 1996;64:190-196.

3939 Anon. Vitamin E health claim falls short of significant scientific agreement - FDA. FDC Reports: "The Tan Sheet." January 24, 2000;10.

3940 Emmert DH, Kirchner JT. The role of vitamin E in the prevention of heart disease. *Arch Fam Med* 1999;8:537-542.

3941 Christen S, Woodall AA, Shigenaga MK, et al. Gamma-tocopherol traps mutagenic electrophiles such as NO(X) and complements alpha-tocopherol: physiological implications. *Proc Natl Acad Sci* U S A 1997;94:3217-3222.

3942 Adler LA, Edson R, Lavori P, et al. Long-term treatment effects of vitamin E for tardive dyskinesia. *Biol Psychiatry* 1998;43:868-872.

3943 Sajjad SH. Vitamin E in the treatment of tardive dyskinesia: a preliminary study over 7 months at different doses. *Int Clin Psychopharmacol* 1998;13:147-155.

3944 Lohr JB, Caligiuri MP. A double-blind placebo-controlled study of vitamin E treatment of tardive dyskinesia. *J Clin Psychiatry* 1996;57:167-173.

3945 Shriqui CL, Bradwejn J, Annable L, Jones BD. Vitamin E in the treatment of tardive dyskinesia: a double-blind placebo-controlled study. *Am J Psychiatry* 1992;149:391-393.

3946 Dorfman-Etrog P, Hermesh H, Prilipko L, et al. The

REFERENCES

effect of vitamin E addition to acute neuroleptic treatment on the emergence of extrapyramidal side effects in schizophrenic patients: an open label study. *Eur Neuropsychopharmacol* 1999;9:475-477.

3947 Boomershine KH, Shelton PS, Boomershine JE. Vitamin E in the treatment of tardive dyskinesia. *Ann Pharmacother* 1999;33:1195-1202.

3948 Dabiri LM, Pasta D, Darby JK, Mosbacher D. Effectiveness of vitamin E for treatment of long-term tardive dyskinesia. *Am J Psychiatry* 1994;151:925-926.

3949 The Alpha-Tocopherol, Beta Carotene *Cancer* Prevention Study Group. The effect of vitamin E and beta carotene on the incidence of lung *Cancer* and other cancers in male smokers. *N Engl J Med* 1994;330:1029-1035.

3951 Liede K, Hietanen J, Saxen L, et al. Long-term supplementation with alpha-tocopherol and beta-carotene and prevalence of oral mucosal lesions in smokers. *Oral Dis* 1998;4:78-83.

3952 Hofstad B, Almendingen K, Vatn M, et al. Growth and recurrence of colorectal polyps: a double-blind 3-year intervention with calcium and antioxidants. *Digestion* 1998;59:148-156.

3953 Malila N, Virtamo J, Virtanen M, et al. The effect of alpha-tocopherol and beta-carotene supplementation on colorectal adenomas in middle-aged male smokers. *Cancer Epidemiol Biomarkers Prev* 1999;8:489-493.

3954 Roncucci L, Di Donato P, Carati L, et al. Antioxidant vitamins or lactulose for the prevention of the recurrence of colorectal adenomas. Colorectal *Cancer* Study Group of the University of Modena and the Health Care District 16. *Dis Colon Rectum* 1993;36:227-234.

3955 Greenberg ER, Baron JA, Tosteson TD, et al. A clinical trial of antioxidant vitamins to prevent colorectal adenoma. Polyp Prevention Study Group. *N Engl J Med* 1994;331:141-147.

3956 Paganelli GM, Biasco G, Brandi G, et al. Effect of vitamin A, C, and E supplementation on rectal cell proliferation in patients with colorectal adenomas. *J Natl Cancer Inst* 1992;84:47-51.

3957 McKeown-Eyssen G, Holloway C, Jazmaji V, et al. A randomized trial of vitamins C and E in the prevention of recurrence of colorectal polyps. *Br J Nutr* 1988;48:4701-4705.

3958 White E, Shannon JS, Patterson RE. Relationship between vitamin and calcium supplement use and colon cancer. *Cancer Epidemiol Biomarkers Prev* 1997;6:769-774.

3959 Heinonen OP, Albanes D, Virtamo J, et al. Prostate cancer and supplementation with alpha-tocopherol and beta-carotene: incidence and mortality in a controlled trial. *J Natl Cancer Inst* 1998;90:440-446.

3960 Varis K, Taylor PR, Sipponen P, et al. Gastric cancer and premalignant lesions in atrophic gastritis: a controlled trial on the effect of supplementation with alpha-tocopherol and beta-carotene. The Helsinki Gastritis Study Group. *Scand J Gastroenterol* 1998;33:294-300.

3961 Rautalahti MT, Virtamo JR, Taylor PR, et al. The effects of supplementation with alpha-tocopherol and beta-carotene on the incidence and mortality of carcinoma of the pancreas in a randomized, controlled trial. *Cancer* 1999;86:37-42.

3962 Slattery ML, Benson J, Curtin K, et al. Carotenoids and colon cancer. *Am J Clin Nutr* 2000;71:575-582.

3963 Steinmetz KA, Potter JD. Vegetables, fruit, and cancer. I. Epidemiology. *Cancer Causes Control* 1991;2:325-357.

3964 Slattery ML, Potter JD, Coates A, et al. Plant foods and colon cancer: an assessment of specific foods and their related nutrients (United States). *Cancer Causes Control* 1997;8:575-590.

3965 Cohen AJ, Bartlik B. Ginkgo biloba for antidepressant-induced sexual dysfunction. *J Sex Marital Ther* 1998;24:139-143.

3966 Balon R. Ginkgo biloba for antidepressant-induced sexual dysfunction? J Sex Marital Ther 1999;25:1-2.

3967 Ellison JM, DeLuca P. Fluoxetine-induced genital anesthesia relieved by Ginkgo biloba extract. *J Clin Psychiatry* 1998;59:199-200.

3968 Balon R. The effects of antidepressants on human sexuality: diagnosis and management update 1999. *Primary Psychiatry* 1999;6:40-54.

3969 Levine SB. Caution Recommended. J Sex Marital Ther 1999;25:2-5.

3970 Jacobsen FM. Fluoxetine-induced sexual dysfunction and an open trial of yohimbine. *J Clin Psychiatry* 1992;53:119-122.

3971 Hollander E, McCarley A. Yohimbine treatment of sexual side effects induced by serotonin reuptake blockers. *J Clin Psychiatry* 1992;53:207-209.

3972 Harvey KV, Balon R. Clinical implications of antidepressant drug effects on sexual function. *Ann Clin Psychiatry* 1995;7:189-201.

3973 Balon R. The effects of anitdepressants on human sexuality: diagnosis and management update 1999. *Primary Psychiatry* 1999;6:40-54.

3974 Redondo P, Bauza A. Topical N-acetylcysteine for lamellar ichthyosis. *Lancet* 1999;354:1880.

3975 Sekharam M, Trotti A, Cunnick JM, Wu J. Suppression of fibroblast cell cycle progression in G1 phase by N-acetylcysteine. *Toxicol Appl Pharmacol* 1998;149:210-216.

3976 Hakkak R, Korourian S, Shelnutt SR, et al. Diets containing whey proteins or soy protein isolate protect against 7,12-dimethylbenz(a)anthracene-induced mammary tumors in female rats. *Cancer Epidemiol Biomarkers Prev* 2000;9:113-117.

3977 FDA. Federal Register website: http://www.accessdata.fda.gov/scripts/oc/ohrms/index.cfm (Accessed 9 March 2000).

3978 Tham DM, Gardner CD, Haskell WL. Clinical review 97: Potential health benefits of dietary phytoestrogens: a review of the clinical, epidemiological, and mechanistic evidence. *J Clin Endocrinol Metab* 1998;83:2223-2235.

3979 Setchell KD. Phytoestrogens: the biochemistry, physiology, and implications for human health of soy isoflavones. *Am J Clin Nutr* 1998;68:1333S-1346S.

3980 McMichael-Phillips DF, Harding C, Morton M, et al. Effects of soy-protein supplementation on epithelial proliferation in the histologically normal human breast. *Am J Clin Nutr* 1998;68:1431S-1435S.

3981 Petrakis NL, Barnes S, King EB, et al. Stimulatory influence of soy protein isolate on breast secretion in pre- and postmenopausal women. *Cancer Epidemiol Biomarkers Prev* 1996;5:785-794.

3982 Setchell KD. Absorption and metabolism of soy isoflavones-from food to dietary supplements and adults to infants. *J Nutr* 2000;130:654S-655S.

3983 Barnes S, Kim H, Darley-Usmar V, et al. Beyond ERalpha and ERbeta: Estrogen receptor binding is only part of the isoflavone story. *J Nutr* 2000;130:656S-657S.

3984 Evans BA, Griffiths K, Morton MS. Inhibition of 5 alpha-reductase in genital skin fibroblasts and prostate tissue by dietary lignans and isoflavonoids. *J Endocrinol* 1995;147:295-302.

3985 Adlercreutz H, Mazur W, Bartels P, et al. Phytoestrogens and prostate disease. *J Nutr* 2000;130:658S-659S.

3986 Brzezinski A, Adlercreutz H, Sheoul R, et al. Short-term effects of phytoestrogen-rich diet on postmenopausal women. *Menopause* 1997;4:89-94.

3987 Kurzer M. Hormonal effects of soy isoflavones: Studies in premenopausal and postmenopausal women. *J Nutr* 2000;130:660S-661S.

3988 Baird DD, Umbach DM, Lansdell L, et al. Dietary intervention study to assess estrogenicity of dietary soy among postmenopausal women. *J Clin Endocrinol Metab* 1995;80:1685-1690.

3989 Duncan AM, Underhill KE, Xu X, et al. Modest hormonal effects of soy isoflavones in postmenopausal women. *J Clin Endocrinol Metab* 1999;84:3479-3484.

3990 Ginsburg J, Prelevic GM. Lack of significant hormonal effects and controlled trials of phyto-oestrogens. *Lancet* 2000;355:163-164.

3991 Quella SK, Loprinzi CL, Barton DL, et al. Evaluation of Soy Phytoestrogens for the Treatment of Hot Flashes in Breast Cancer Survivors: A North Central Cancer Treatment Group Trial. *J Clin Oncol* 2000;18:1068.

3992 Anthony MS. Soy and cardiovascular disease: Cholesterol lowering and beyond. *J Nutr* 2000;130:662S-663S.

3993 Ingram D, Sanders K, Kolybaba M, Lopez D. Case-control study of phyto-oestrogens and breast cancer. *Lancet* 1997;350:990-994.

3994 Hargreaves DF, Potten CS, Harding C, et al. Two-week dietary soy supplementation has an estrogenic effect on normal premenopausal breast. *J Clin Endocrinol Metab* 1999;84:4017-4024.

3995 Martini MC, Dancisak BB, Haggans CJ, et al. Effects of soy intake on sex hormone metabolism in premenopausal women. *Nutr Cancer* 1999;34:133-139.

3996 Poortmans JR, Francaux M. Long-term oral creatine supplementation does not impair renal function in healthy athletes. *Med Sci Sports Exerc* 1999;31:1108-1110.

3997 Juhn MS, Tarnopolsky M. Potential side effects of oral creatine supplementation: a critical review. *Clin J Sport Med* 1998;8:298-304.

3998 Graham AS, Hatton RC. Creatine: a review of efficacy and safety. *J Am Pharm Assoc* (Wash) 1999;39:803-810.

3999 Pepping J. Creatine. *Am J Health Syst Pharm* 1999;56:1608-1610.

4000 Medina JH, et al. "Overview-flavonoids: a new family of benzodiazepine receptor ligands." *Neurochem Res*, 1997; 22(4): 419-25.

4001 Salgueiro JB, et al. "Anxiolytic natural and synthetic flavonoid ligands of the central benzodiazepine receptor have no effect on memory tasks in rats." *Pharmacol Biochem Behav*, 1997; 58(4): 887-91.

4002 Rommelspacher H, et al. "(1-methyl-beta-carboline) is a natural inhibitor of monoamine oxidase type A in rats." *Eur J Pharmacol*, 24 Jan. 1994; 252(1): 51-59.

4003 Moon JY, Lee DW, Park KH. "Inhibition of 7-ethoxycoumarin O-deethylase activity in rat *Liver* microsomes by naturally occurring flavonoids: structure-activity relationships." *Xenobiotica*, 1998; 28(2): 117-26.

4004 Siess MH, et al. "Heterogenous effects of natural flavonoids on monooxygenase activities in human and rat liver microsomes." *Toxicol Appl Pharmacol*, 1995; 130(1): 73-78.

4005 Grases F, et al. "Effect of Herniaria hirsuta and Agropyron repens on calcium oxalate urolithiasis risk in rats." *J Ethnopharmacol*, 1995; 45(3): 211-14.

4006 Neef H, et al. "Inhibitory effects of Galega officinalis on glucose transport across monolayers of human intestinal epithelial cells (Caco-2)." *Pharm Pharmacol Lett*, 1996; 6(2): 86-89.

4007 Atanasov AT. "Effect of Galega officinalis L. extract on platelet aggregation in rats." *J. Herbs Spices Med. Plants*, 1995; 3(3): 71-76.

4008 Huxtable CR, Dorling RR, Colegate SM. "Identification of galegine, an isoprenyl guanidine, as the toxic principle of Schoenus asperocarpus (poison sedge)." *Aust Vet J*, 1993; 70(5): 169-71.

4009 Dukes JA. *CRC* Handbook of Medicinal Herbs. first ed. Boca Raton, FL: CRC Press, Inc., 1985.

4010 Scarlat M, et al. "Experimental anti-ulcer activity of Veronica officinalis L. extracts." *J Ethnopharmacol*, 1985; 13(2): 157-63.

4011 Yoshioka T, Fujii E, Endo M, et al. "Antiinflammatory potency of dehydrocurdione, a zedoary-derived sesquiterpene." *Inflamm Res*, 1998; 47(12):476-481.

4012 Matsuda H, Ninomiya K, Morikawa T, et al. "Inhibitory effect and action mechanism of sesquiterpenes from Zedoariae Rhizoma on D-galactosamine/lipopolysaccharide-induced *Liver* injury." *Bioorg Med Chem Lett*, 1998; 8(4):339-344.

4013 Gupta SK, Banerjee AB, Achari B. "Isolation of Ethyl p-methoxycinnamate, the major antifungal principle of Curcumba zedoaria." *Lloydia*, 1976; 39(4):218-222.

4014 Syu WJ, Shen CC, Don MJ, et al. "Cytotoxicity of curcuminoids and some novel compounds from Curcuma zedoaria." *J Nat Prod*, 1998; 61(12):1531-1534.

4015 Latif MA, Morris TR, Miah AH, et al. "Toxicity of shoti (Indian arrowroot: Curcuma zedoaria) for rats and chicks." *Br J Nutr*, 1979; 41(1):57-63.

4016 Wu D, Meydani M, Leka LS, et al. Effect of dietary supplementation with black currant seed oil on the immune response of healthy elderly subjects. *Am J Clin Nutr* 1999;70:536-43.

4017 Agricultural Research Service. Dr. Duke's Phytochemical and Ethnobotanical Databases. URL: www.ars-grin.gov/duke (Accessed 23 July 1999).

4018 Leclercq I, Desager JP, Horsmans Y. "Inhibition of chlorzoxazone metabolism, a clinical probe for CYP2E1, by a single ingestion of watercress". *Clin Pharmacol Ther*, 1998; 64:144-149.

4019 Hecht SS, Chung FL, Richie JP Jr., et al. "Effects of watercress consumption on metabolism of a tobacco-specific lung carcinogen in smokers." *Cancer Epidemiol Biomarkers Prev*, 1995; 4:877-884.

4020 Habtemariam S. "Cistifolin, an integrin-dependent cell adhesion blocker from the anti- rheumatic herbal drug, gravel root (rhizome of Eupatorium purpureum)." *Planta Med* 1998 Dec;64(8):683-5.

4021 WHO working group. Pyrrolizidine alkaloids. Environmental Health Criteria, 80. *WHO: Geneva*, 1988.

4022 Cardarelli M, Serino G, Campanella L, et al. "Antimitotic effects of usnic acid on different biological systems." *Cell Mol Life Sci*, 1997; 53:667-672.

4023 Dahlquist I, Fregert S. "Contact allergy to atranorin in lichens and perfumes." *Contact Dermatitis*, 1980;

© Copyright 2000, Natural Medicines Comprehensive Database (209) 472-2244. For updated data, go to www.NaturalDatabase.com. • 1241

6:111-119.

4024   Lauterwein M, Oethinger M, Belsner K, et al. "In vitro activities of the lichen secondary metabolites vulpinic acid, (+)-usnic acid, and (-)-usnic acid against aerobic and anaerobic microorganisms." *Antimicrob Agents Chemother*, 1995; 39:2541-2543.

4025   Ghione M, Parrello D, Grasso L. "Usnic acid revisited, its activity on oral flora." *Chemioterapia*, 1988; 7:302-5.

4026   Ingolfsdottir K, Chung GA, Skulason VG, et al. "Antimycobacterial activity of lichen metabolites in vitro." *Eur J Pharm Sci*, 1998 Apr;6(2):141-4.

4027   Krishna DR, Ramana DV, Mamidi NV. "In vitro protein binding and tissue distribution of D(+) usnic acid." *Drug Metabol Drug Interact*, 1995;12(1):53-63.

4028   Proksa B, Sturdikova M, Pronayova N, et al. "Usnic acid and its derivatives: their inhibition of fungal growth and enzyme activity." *Pharmazie*, 1996; 51: 195-196.

4029   Fournet A, Ferreira ME, Rojas de Arias A, et al. "Activity of compounds isolated from Chilean lichens against experimental cutaneous leishmaniasis." *Comp Biochem Physiol C Pharmacol Toxicol Endocrinol*; 1997; 116:51-54.

4030   Yamamoto Y, Miura Y, Kinoshita Y, et al. "Screening of tissue cultures and thalli of lichens and some of their active constituents for inhibition of tumor promoter-induced Epstein- Barr virus activation." *Chem Pharm Bull* (Tokyo), 1995; 43:1388-1390.

4031   Okuyama E, Umeyama K, Yamazaki M, et al. "Usnic acid and diffractaic acid as analgesic and antipyretic components of Usnea diffracta." *Planta Med*, 1995; 61:113-115.

4032   Goncalves J, Proenca J, Paiva MQ. "Study of the activity of usnic acid on H1 and H2 receptors." *Rev. Port. Farm.*, 1987; 37: 23-26.

4033   Goncalo S. "Contact sensitivity to lichens and compositae in Frullania dermatitis." *Contact Dermatitis* 1987 Feb;16(2):84-86.

4034   Goncalo S, Cabral F, Goncalo M. "Contact sensitivity to oak moss." *Contact Dermatitis*, 1988; 19:355-357.

4035   Thune PO, Solberg YJ. "Photosensitivity and allergy to aromatic lichen acids, Compositae oleoresins and other plant substances." *Contact Dermatitis*, 1980; 6: 81-87.

4036   Thune PO, Solberg YJ. "Photosensitivity and allergy to aromatic lichen acids, Compositae oleoresins and other plant substances." *Contact Dermatitis*, 1980; 6: 64-71.

4037   Thune P. "Contact allergy due to lichens in patients with a history of photosensitivity." *Contact Dermatitis* 1977 Oct;3(5):267-272.

4038   Sandberg M, Thune P. "The sensitizing capacity of atranorin." *Contact Dermatitis*, 1984;11:168-173.

4039   Thune P, Solberg Y, McFadden N, et al. "Perfume allergy due to oak moss and other lichens." *Contact Dermatitis*, 1982; 8: 396-400.

4040   al-Bekairi AM, Qureshi S, Chaudhry MA, et al. "Mitodepressive, clastogenic and biochemical effects of (+)-usnic acid in mice." *J Ethnopharmacol* 1991 Jul;33(3):217-20.

4041   Chen CP, Lin CC, Namba T. "Screening of Taiwanese crude drugs for antibacterial activity against Streptococcus mutans." *J Ethnopharmacol*, 1989;27:285-295.

4042   Akihisa T, Yasukawa K, Kimura Y, et al. "Five D:C-friedo-oleanane triterpenes from the seeds of Trichosanthes kirilowii Maxim. and their anti-inflammatory effects." *Chem Pharm Bull* (Tokyo), 1994; 42:1101-1105.

4043   Ozaki Y, Xing L, Satake M. "Anti-inflammatory effect of Trichosanthes kirilowii Maxim, and its effective parts." *Biol Pharm Bull*, 1996; 19:1046-1048.

4044   Takano F, Yoshizaki F, Suzuki K, et al. "Anti-ulcer effects of Trichosanthes fruits." *Chem Pharm Bull* (Tokyo), 1990; 38:1313-1316.

4045   Hikino H, Yoshizawa M, Suzuki Y, et al. "Isolation and hypoglycemic activity of trichosans A, B, C, D, and E: glycans of Trichosanthes kirilowii roots." *Planta Med*, 1989; 55: 349-350.

4046   Tao XL, Sun Y, Dong Y, et al. "A prospective, controlled, double-blind, cross-over study of tripterygium wilfodii hook F in treatment of rheumatoid arthritis." *Chin Med J* (Engl), 1989; 102:327-332.

4047   Nagashima G, Suzuki R, et al. "Meningoencephalocele associated with Tripterygium wilfordii treatment." *Pediatr Neurosurg*, 1997; 27:45-48.

4048   Chen K, Shi QA, Fujioka T, et al. "Anti-AIDS agents, 4. Tripterifordin, a novel anti-HIV principle from Tripterygium wilfordii: isolation and structural elucidation." *J Nat Prod*, 1992;55:88-92.

4049   Chen K, Shi Q, Kashiwada Y, et al. "Anti-AIDS agents, 6. Salaspermic acid, an anti-HIV principle from Tripterygium wilfordii, and the structure-activity correlation with its related compounds." *J Nat Prod*, 1992; 55:340-346.

4050   Attaguile G, Caruso A, Pennisi G, et al. "Gastroprotective effect of aqueous extract of Cistus incanus L. in rats." *Pharmacol Res*, 1995; 3: 29-32.

4051   Liu FJ, Sun DM. "Studies on the active constituents lowering blood lipid in beeswax." *J. Chin. Mater. Med.* (Zhongguo Zhongyao Zazhi), 1996; 21: 553-554.

4052   Carbajal D, Molina V, Valdes S, et al. "Anti-inflammatory activity of D-002: an active product isolated from beeswax." *Prostaglandins Leukot Essent Fatty Acids*, 1998;59: 235-238.

4053   Carbajal D, Molina V, Valdes S, et al. "Possible cytoprotective mechanism in rats of D-002, an anti-ulcerogenic product isolated from beeswax." *J Pharm Pharmacol*, 1996; 48: 858-860.

4054   Carbajal D, Molina V, Valdes S, et al. "Anti-ulcer activity of higher primary alcohols of beeswax." *J Pharm Pharmacol*, 1995;47: 731-733.

4055   Shilo S, Hirsch HJ. "Iodine-induced hyperthyroidism in a patient with a normal thyroid gland." *Postgrad Med J*, 1986; 62: 661-662.

4056   Ripsin CM, Keenan JM, Jacobs DR Jr, et al. "Oat products and lipid lowering. A meta-analysis." *JAMA*, 1992; 267:3317-3325.

4057   Davidson MH, Dugan LD, *Burns JH*, et al. "The hypocholesterolemic effects of beta-glucan in oatmeal and oat bran. A dose-controlled study." *JAMA* 1991 Apr 10;265(14):1833-9.

4058   Roesyanto-Mahadi ID, Geursen-Reitsma AM, van Joost T, et al. "Sensitization to fragrance materials in Indonesian cosmetics." *Contact Dermatitis*, 1990; 22: 212-217.

4059   Arras G, Grella GE. "Wild thyme, Thymus capitatus, essential oil seasonal changes and antimycotic activity." *J Hortic Sci*; 1992; 67: 197-202.

4060   Thompson DP. "Effect of phenolic compounds on mycelial growth of Fusarium and Penicillium species." *J Food Protection*; 60 (10). 1997. 1262-1264.

4061   Akgul A, Kivanc M, Sert S. "Effect of carvacrol on growth and toxin production by Aspergillus flavus and Aspergillus parasiticus." *Sci Aliments*, 1991; 11: 361-

370.

4062 Stiles JC, Sparks W, Ronzio RA "The inhibition of Candida albicans by Oregano." *J Appl Nutrition*, 1995; 47: 96-102.

4063 Viollon C, Chaumont JP. "Antifungal properties of essential oils and their main components upon Cryptococcus neoformans." *Mycopathologia*, 1994; 128: 151-153.

4064 Osawa K, Matsumoto T, Maruyama T, et al. "Studies of the antibacterial activity of plant extracts and their constituents against periodontopathic bacteria." *Bull Tokyo Dent Coll*, 1990; 31:17-21.

4065 Ultee A, Gorris LG, Smid EJ. "Bactericidal activity of carvacrol towards the food-borne pathogen Bacillus cereus." *J Appl Microbiol*, 1998; 85:211-218.

4066 Helander IM, Alakomi H-L, Latva-Kala K, et al. "Characterization of the action of selected essential oil components on gram-negative bacteria." *J Agricultural and Food Chemistry*, 1998; 46: 3590-3595.

4067 Aeschbach R, Loliger J, Scott BC. "Antioxidant actions of thymol, carvacrol, 6-gingerol, zingerone and hydroxytyrosol." *Food Chem Toxicol*, 1994; 32: 31-36.

4068 Eastwood MA, Brydon WG, Anderson DM, et al. "The effects of dietary gum tragacanth in man." *Toxicol Lett*, 1984; 21: 73-81.

4069 Jenkins DJ, Wolever TM, Leeds AR, et al. "Dietary fibres, fibre analogues, and glucose tolerance: importance of viscosity." *Br Med J*, 1978; 1: 1392-1394.

4070 Smee DF, Sidwell RW, Huffman JH, et al. "Antiviral activities of tragacanthin polysaccharides on Punta Toro virus infections in mice." *Chemotherapy*, 1996;42:286-293.

4071 FAO and WHO working groups. Tragacanth gum. WHO Food additives series, 1985; 20: 253-262.

4072 Anonymous. "Final report on the safety assessment of Tragacanth Gum." *J Am Coll Toxicol*, 1987; 6: 1-22.

4073 Vaswani SK, Hamilton RG, Carey RN, et al. "Anaphylaxis recurrent urticaria and angioedema from grape hypersensitivity." *J All Clin Immunol* 1998; 101 (1 Part 2): S31.

4074 BIBRA working group. Anthocyanins. Toxicity profile. BIBRA *Toxicology International*, 1991; 6.

4075 Garcia Ortiz JC, Cosmes Martin P, Lopez-Asunsolo A. "Melon sensitivity shares allergens with Plantago and grass pollens." *Allergy (Copenhagen)*, 1995; 50: 269-273.

4076 Hollis S. The Country Diary Herbal. Henry Holt and Company, New York, 1990.

4077 Tyler VE, Brady LR, Robbers JE. Pharmacognosy, 9th edition. Lea & Febiger, Philadelphia, 1988.

4078 Foster S, Duke JA. The Peterson Field Guide to Medicinal Plants: Eastern and Central North America. Houghton Mifflin Company, Boston, 1990.

4079 Eigenmann PA, Burks AW, Bannon GA, et al. "Identification of unique peanut and soy allergens in sera adsorbed with cross-reacting antibodies." *J Allergy Clin Immunol*, 1996; 98(5 Pt 1): 969-978.

4080 Bardare M, Magnolfi C, Zani G. "Soy sensitivity: personal observation on 71 children with food intolerance." *Allerg Immunol* (Paris), 1988; 20:63-66.

4081 Van Hevelingen A. "The orris iris." The Herb Companion, 1992; 4: 32-35.

4082 Schmidt GD, Roberts LS. "Foundations of Parasitology." Times Mirror/Mosby College Publishing, St. Louis, 1985.

4083 21 CFR 182.10. Obtained from Website, URL: www.access.gpo.gov/nara/cfr/ (1 August 1999).

4084 *Drugs in Pregnancy and Lactation*, 4th edition. Baltimore: Williams & Wilkens, 1994.

4085 Lichtenstein AH, Ausman LM, Jalbert SM, et al. "Effects of different forms of dietary hydrogenated fats on serum lipoprotein cholesterol levels." *N Engl J Med*, 1999;340: 1933-1940.

4086 Weststrate JA, Meijer GW. "Plant sterol-enriched margarines and reduction of plasma total- and LDL-cholesterol concentrations in normocholesterolaemic and mildly hypercholesterolaemic subjects." *Eur J Clin Nutr*, 1998; 52:334-343.

4087 FDA. Center for Science in the Public Interest. News Release: "Statement on FDA Review of Take Control Margarine." May 5, 1999. Retrieved from URL: www.fda.gov. (Accessed 5 May 1999).

4088 Ingles SA, Bird C, Shikany J, et al. Plasma tocopherol and prevalence of colorectal adenomas in a multiethnic population. *Cancer Res.* 1998;58:661-666.

4089 Moyad MA, Brumfield SK, Pienta KJ. Vitamin E, alpha- and gamma-tocopherol, and prostate cancer. *Semin Urol Oncol* 1999;17:85-90.

4090 Kontush A, Spranger T, Reich A et al. Lipophilic antioxidants in blood plasma as markers of Atherosclerosis: the role of alpha-carotene and gamma-tocopherol. *Atherosclerosis* 1999;144:117-122.

4091 Ziouzenkova O, Winklhofer-Roob BM, Puhl H, et al. Lack of correlation between the alpha-tocopherol content of plasma and LDL, but high correlations for gamma-tocopherol and carotenoids. *J Lipid Res* 1996;37(9):1936-46.

4092 Li D, Saldeen T, Mehta JL. Gamma-tocopherol decreases ox-LDL-mediated activation of nuclear factor-kappaB and apoptosis in human coronary artery endothelial cells. *Biochem Biophys Res Commun* 1999;259:157-161.

4093 Dillard CJ, Gavino VC, Tappel AL. Relative antioxidant effectiveness of alpha-tocopherol and gamma-tocopherol in iron-loaded rats. *J Nutr* 1983;113:2266-2273.

4094 Cooney RV, Franke AA, Harwoood PJ, et al. Gamma-Tocopherol detoxification of nitrogen dioxide: Superiority to alpha-tocopherol. *Proc Natl Acad Sci USA.* 1993;90;1771-1775.

4095 Christen S, Woodall AA, Shigenaga MK, et al. Gamma-tocopherol traps mutagenic electrophiles such as NO(X) and complements alpha-tocopherol: physiological implications. *Proc Natl Acad Sci U S A* 1997;94(7):3217-3222.

4096 Aberg F, Appelkvist EL, Broijersen A et al. Gemfibrozil-induced decrease in serum ubiquinone and alpha- and gamma- tocopherol levels in men with combined hyperlipidaemia. *Eur J Clin Invest* 1998;28:235-242.

4097 Sadrzadeh SM, Nanji AA, Meydani M. Effect of chronic ethanol feeding on plasma and *Liver* alpha- and gamma-tocopherol levels in normal and vitamin E-deficient rats. Relationship to lipid peroxidation. *Biochem Pharmacol* 1994;47(11):2005-10.

4098 Takahashi O. Haemorrhagic toxicity of a large dose of alpha-, beta-, gamma- and delta-tocopherols, ubiquinone, beta-carotene, retinol acetate and L-ascorbic acid in the rat. *Food and Chemical Toxicology.* 1995;33:121-128.

4099 Murray ED Jr, Wechter WJ, Kantoci D, et al. Endogenous natriuretic factors 7: biospecificity of a natriuretic gamma- tocopherol metabolite LLU-alpha. *J Pharmacol Exp Ther* 1997;282(2):657-62.

REFERENCES

4100 Scholz E, Rimpler R. "Proanthocyanidins from Krameria triandra root." *Planta Med*, 1989; 55(4): 379-84.

4101 The Bantam Medical Dictionary. revised ed. New York: Bantam Books, 1990.

4102 Covington TR, Berardi RR, Young LL. Handbook of Nonprescription Drugs. 11th ed. Washington, DC: American Pharmaceutical Association, 1996.

4104 Abdullaev FI, Gonzalez de Mejia E. "Antitumor activity of natural substances: lectins and saffron." *Arch Latinoam Nutr*, 1997; 47(3): 195-202.

4105 Nair SC, Pannikar B, Panikkar KR. "Antitumor activity of Saffron (Crocus sativus)." *Cancer Lett*, 1991; 57(2): 109-14.

4106 Feo F, et al. "Occupational Allergy to Saffron Workers." *Allergy*, 1997; 52(6): 633-41.

4107 Wuthrich B, Schmid-Grendelmeyer P, Lundberg M. "Anaphylaxis to saffron." *Allergy*, 1997; 52(4): 476-77.

4108 Gainer JL. "Hypoxia and Atherosclerosis: re-evaluation of an old hypothesis." *Atherosclerosis*, 1987; 68(3): 263-66.

4109 Miller TL, et al. "Binding of crocetin to plasma albumin." *J Pharm Sci*, 1982; 71(2): 173-77.

4110 Grainer JL, Jones JR. "The Use of Crocetin in Experimental Atherosclerosis." *Experientia*, 1975; 31: 548-49.

4111 Vandenplas O, Depelchin S, Toussaint G, et al. "Occupational asthma caused by sarsaparilla root dust." *J Allergy Clin Immunol*, 1996;97(6):1416-8.

4112 Ahn YO. "Diet and stomach cancer in Korea." *Int J Cancer*, 1997;10:7-9.

4113 Archana R, Namasivayam A. "Antistressor effect of Withania somnifera." *J Ethnopharmacol*, 1999;64(1):91-3.

4114 Davis L, Kuttan G. "Suppressive effect of cyclophosphamide-induced toxicity by Withania somnifera extract in mice." *J Ethnopharmacol*, 1998;62(3):209-14.

4116 Bhattacharya SK, Satyan KS, Ghosal S. Antioxidant activity of glycowithanolides from Withania somnifera. *Indian J Exp Biol*, 1997; 35(3):236-9.

4117 Shen HD, Chang LY, Gong YJ, et al. "A monoclonal antibody against ragweed pollen cross-reacting with yellow dock pollen." *Chung Hua Min Kuo Wei Sheng Wu Chi Mien I Hsueh Tsa Chih*, 1985;18(4):232-9.

4118 Liu YL, Ho DK, Cassady JM, et al. "Isolation of potential cancer chemopreventive agents from Eriodictyon californicum." *J Nat Prod*, 1992;55(3):357-63.

4119 Younos C, Rolland A, Fleurentin J, et al. "Analgesic and behavioural effects of Morinda citrifolia." *Planta Med*, 1990;56(5):430-4.

4120 Nakano M, Nakashima H, Itoh Y. "Anti-human immunodeficiency virus activity of oligosaccharides from rooibos tea (Aspalathus linearis) extracts in vitro." *Leukemia*, 1997;11(3):128-30.

4121 Nakano M, Itoh Y, Mizuno T, Nakashima H. "Polysaccharide from Aspalathus linearis with strong anti-HIV activity." *Biosci Biotechnol Biochem*, 1997;61(2):267-71.

4122 Shimoi K, Masuda S, Shen B, et al. "Radioprotective effects of antioxidative plant flavonoids in mice." *Mutat Res*, 1996;350(1):153-61.

4123 Inanami O, Asanuma T, Inukai N, et al. "The suppression of age-related accumulation of lipid peroxides in rat brain by administration of Rooibos tea (Aspalathus linearis)." *Neurosci Lett*, 1995;196(1-2):85-8.

4124 Sanchez de Rojas VR, Somoza B, Ortega T, et al.

"Vasodilatory effect in rat aorta of eriodictyol obtained from Satureja obovata." *Planta Med*, 1999;65(3):234-8.

4125 Lacy CF, Armstrong LL, Ingrim NB, Lance LL. Drug Information Handbook. Hudson, Ohio: Lexi Comp Inc; 1998-1999.

4126 Wolinsky-Friedland M. "Drug-induced metabolic bone disease." *Endocrinol Metab Clin North Am*, 1995; 24(2):395-420.

4132 Tzivoni D, Keren A, Meyler S, et al. "Cardiovascular safety of transdermal nicotine patches in patients with coronary artery disease who try to quit smoking." *Cardiovasc Drugs Ther*, 1998; 12(3):239-44.

4133 Eliasson B, Taskinen MR, Smith U. "Long-term use of nicotine gum is associated with hyperinsulinemia and insulin resistance." *Circulation*, 1996; 94(5):878-81.

4137 Sills AK Jr, Williams JI, Tyler BM, et al. "Squalamine inhibits angiogenesis and solid tumor growth in vivo and perturbs embryonic vasculature." *Cancer Res*, 1998;58(13):2784-92.

4138 Kikuchi K, Bernard EM, Sadownik A, et al. "Antimicrobial activities of squalamine mimics." *Antimicrob Agents Chemother*, 1997;41(7):1433-8.

4139 Moore KS, Wehrli S, Roder H, et al. "Squalamine: an aminosterol antibiotic from the shark." *Proc Natl Acad Sci U S A*, 1993;90(4):1354-8.

4140 Keynan N, Tamir R, Waisel Y, et al. "Allergenicity of the pollen of Pistacia." *Allergy*, 1997;52(3):323-30.

4141 Iauk L, Ragusa S, Rapisarda A, et al. "In vitro antimicrobial activity of Pistacia lentiscus L. extracts: preliminary report." *J Chemother*, 1996; 8(3):207-9.

4142 Al-Said MS, Ageel AM, Parmar NS, Tariq M. "Evaluation of mastic, a crude drug obtained from Pistacia lentiscus for gastric and duodenal anti-ulcer activity." *J Ethnopharmacol*, 1986; 15(3):271-8.

4143 Vallverdu A, Garcia-Ortega P, Martinez J, et al. "Mercurialis annua: characterization of main allergens and cross- reactivity with other species." *Int Arch Allergy Immunol*, 1997;112(4):356-64.

4144 Garcia-Ortega P, Martinez J, Martinez A, et al. "Mercurialis annua pollen: a new source of allergic sensitization and respiratory disease." *J Allergy Clin Immunol*, 1992;89(5):987-93.

4145 Mancini SD, Edwards JM. "Cytotoxic principles from the sap of Kalmia latifolia." *J Nat Prod*. 1979;42(5):483-8.

4146 Garcia Ortiz JC, Terron M, Bellido J. "Contact allergy to henna." *Int Arch Allergy Immunol*, 1997;114(3):298-9.

4147 Kandil HH, al-Ghanem MM, Sarwat MA, al-Thallab FS. "Henna (Lawsonia inermis Linn.) inducing haemolysis among G6PD-deficient newborns. A new clinical observation." *Ann Trop Paediatr*, 1996;16(4):287-91.

4148 Majoie IM, Bruynzeel DP. "Occupational immediate-type hypersensitivity to henna in a hairdresser." *Am J Contact Dermat*, 1996;7(1):38-40.

4149 Clarke DT, Jones GR, Martin MM. "The anti-sickling drug lawsone (2-OH-1,4-naphthoquinone) protects sickled cells against membrane damage." *Biochem Biophys Res Commun*, 1986;139(2):780-6.

4150 Sharma VK. "Tuberculostatic activity of henna (Lawsonia inermis Linn.)." *Tubercle*, 1990;71(4):293-5.

4151 Van Damme EJ, Roy S, Barre A, et al. "The major elderberry (Sambucus nigra) fruit protein is a lectin derived from a truncated type 2 ribosome-inactivating protein." *Plant J* 1997;12(6):1251-60.

4152 Todorov S, Philianos S, Petkov V, et al. "Experimental pharmacological study of three species from genus

REFERENCES

Salvia." *Acta Physiol Pharmacol Bulg*, 1984;10(2):13-20.

4200 Bak AAA, Grobbee DE. The effect of serum cholesterol levels of coffee brewed by filtering or boiling. *N Engl J Med* 1989;321(21):1432-37.

4201 Chevallier A. The Encyclopedia of Medicinal Plants. London: Dorling Kindersley, Limited; 1996.

4202 Andermann G, Dietz M. The influence of the route of administration on the bioavailability of an endogenous macromolecule: chondroitin sulphate (CSA). *Eur J Drug Metab Pharmacokinet* 1982;7:11-6.

4203 Ronca F, Palmieri L, Panicucci P, et al. Anti-inflammatory activity of chondroitin sulfate. *Osteoarthritis Cartilage* 1998;6 Suppl A:14-21.

4204 Conte A, Volpi N, Palmieri L, et al. Biochemical and pharmacokinetic aspects of oral treatment with chondroitin sulfate. *Arzneimittelforschung* 1995;45:918-925.

4205 Silvestro L, Lanzarotti E, Marchi E, et al. Human pharmacokinetics of glycosaminoglycans using deuterium-labeled and unlabeled substances: evidence for oral absorption. *Semin Thromb Hemost* 1994;20(3):281-92.

4206 (http://www.herbweb.com/herbage/80.htm in CRC Ethnobotany Desk Reference, CRC Press, 1999).

4207 Vale S. "Subarachnoid haemorrhage associated with Ginkgo biloba." *The Lancet* , 1998; (352):36.

4208 Ritchason J. The Little Herb Encyclopedia. Pleasant Grove, Utah, Woodland Health Books, 1995.

4209 Alic M. Green Tea for remission maintenance in Crohn's disease. *Am J Gastroenterol* 1999; 94(6):1710-1.

4210 Gupta S, Ahmad N, Mukhtar H. Prostate chemoprevention by green tea. *Semin Urol Oncol* 1999; 17(2):70-6.

4211 Taylor JR, Wilt VM. Probable antagonism of warfarin by green tea. *Ann Pharmacother* 1999; 33(4):426-8.

4212 Klaunig JE, Xu Y, Han C, et al. The effect of tea consumption on oxidative stress in smokers and nonsmokers. *Proc Soc Exp Biol Med* 1999;220(4):249-54.

4213 Li N, Sun Z, Han C, Chen J. The chemopreventive effects of tea on human oral precancerous mucosa lesions. *Proc Soc Exp Biol Med* 1999;220(4):218-24.

4214 Rasheed A, Haider M. Antibacterial activity of Camellia sinensis extracts against dental caries. *Arch Pharm Res* 1998; 21(3):348-52.

4215 Viereck EG. Alaska's Wilderness Medicines Healthful Plants of the Far North. Anchorage: Alaska Northwest Books, 1998.

4216 Curhan GC, Willett WC, Speizer FE, Stamfer MJ. Beverage use and risk of kidney stones in women. *Ann Intern Med* 1998; 128(7):534-40.

4217 Lee IP, Kim YH, Kang MH, et al. Chemopreventive effect of green tea (Camellia sinensis) against cigarette smoke induced mutations in humans. *J Cell Biochem* Suppl 1997;27:68-75.

4218 Kaegi E. Unconventional therapies for cancer:2. Green tea. The Task Force on Alternative Therapies of the Canadian Breast Cancer Research Initiative. *CMAJ* 1998;158(8):1033-5.

4219 Hollman PC, Feskens EJ, Katan MB. Tea flavonols in cardiovascular disease and cancer epidemiology. *Proc Soc Exp Biol Med* 1999;220(4):198-202.

4221 Durlach PJ. The effects of a low dose of caffeine on cognitive performance. *Psychopharmacology* 1998;140(1):116-119.

4222 Sesso HD, Gaziano JM, Buring JE, et al. Coffee and tea intake and the risk of myocardial infarction. *Am J Epidemiol* 1999;149:162-167.

4223 Weisburger JH. Tea and health: the underlying mechanisms. *Proc Soc Exp Biol Med* 1999;220(4):271-275.

4224 Hindmarch I, Quinlan PT, Moore KL, Parkin C. The effects of black tea and other beverages on aspects of cognition and psychomotor performance. *Psychopharmacology* 1998; 139(3):230-8.

4225 Sotaniemi EA, Haapakoski E, Rautio A. Ginseng therapy in non-insulin dependent diabetic patients. *Diabetes Care* 1995;18(10):1373-1375.

4226 http://www.uwcm.ac.uk/uwcm/dm/BoDD/ BotDermFolder/BotDermR/RANU.html (Accessed 6 October 1999).

4227 Lee BM, Lee SK, Kim HS. Inhibition of oxidative DNA damage, 8-OHdG, and carbonyl contents in smokers treated with antioxidants (vitamin E, vitamin C, beta-carotene and red ginseng.) *Cancer Lett* 1998;132(1-2):219-27.

4228 Oh M, Choi YH, Choi S, et al. Anti-proliferating effects of ginsenosider Rh2 on MCF-7 human breast cancer cells. *Int J Oncol* 1999; 14(5):869-75.

4229 Fetrow CW, Avila JR. *Professional's Handbook of Complementary and Alternative Medicines*. Springhouse, PA: Springhouse Corporation, 1999.

4230 Allen JD, McLung J, Nelson AG, Welsch M. Ginseng supplementation does not enhance healthy young adult's peak aerobic exercise performance. *J Am Coll Nutr* 1998; 17(5):462-6.

4231 Engels HJ, Wirth JC. No ergogenic effects of ginseng (Panax ginseng C.A. Meyer) during grades maximal aerobic exercise. *J Am Diet Assoc* 1997;97(10):1110-5.

4233 Wolkowitz OM, Reus VI, Manfredi F, et al. Dehydroepiandrosterone (DHEA) Treatment of Depression. *Biol Psychiatry* 1997;41:311-318.

4234 Salvati G, Genovesi G, Marcellini L, et al. Effects of Panax ginseng C.A. Meyer saponins on male fertility. *Panminerva Med* 1996; 38(4):249-54.

4235 Yun TK. Experimental and epidemiological evidence of the cancer-preventive effects of Panax ginseng C.A. Meyer. *Nutr Rev* 1996;54(11 Pt2): S71-81.

4236 Morris AC, Jacobs I, McLellan TM, et al. No ergogenic effect of ginseng ingestion. *Int J Sport Nutr* 1996;6(3):263-71.

4237 Leffler CT, Philippi AF, Leffler SG, et al. Glucosamine, chondroitin, and manganese ascorbate for degenerative joint disease of the knee or low back: a randomized, double-blind, placebo-controlled pilot study. *Mil Med* 1999;164:85-91.

4239 Ondrizek RR, Chan PJ, Patton WC, King A. Inhibition of human sperm motility by specific herbs used in alternative medicine[Abstract]. *J Assist Reprod Genet* 1999;16:87-91.

4240 Ondrizek RR, Chan PJ, Patton WC, King A. An alternative medicine study of herbal effects on the penetration of zona-free hamster oocytes and the integrity of sperm deoxyribonucleic acid. *Fert Steril* 1999;71:517-22.

4242 Labrie F, Diamond P, Cusan L, et al. Effect of 12 month dehydroepiandrosterone replacement therapy on bone, vagina, and endometrium in postmenopausal women. *J Clin Endocrinol Metab* 1997;82(10):3498-3505.

4243 Ding DZ, Shen TK, Cui YZ. Effects of red ginseng on the congestive heart failure and its mechanism. *Chung*

Kuo Chung His I Chieh Ho Tsa Chih 1995; 15(6Z):325-7.

4244 Bahrke MS, Morgan WP. Evaluation of the ergogenic properties of ginseng. *Sports Med* 1994; 18(4):229-48.

4245 Tyler, V. Herb News. *Prevention* 1999; (9): 105.

4248 Kroboth PD, Salek FS, Pittenger AL, et al. DHEA and DHEA-S: A review. *J Clin Pharmacol* 1999;39:327-348.

4249 Casson PR, Faquin LC, Stentz FB. Replacement of dehydroepiandrosterone enhances T-lymphocyte insulin binding in postmenopausal women. *Fertility and Sterility* 1995;63(5):1027-1031.

4250 Bates GW, Egerman RS, Umstot ES, Buster JE, Casson PR. Dehydroepiandrosterone attenuates study-induced declines in insulin sensitivity in postmenopausal women. *Ann NY Acad Sci* 1995;774:291-293.

4251 Morales AJ, Haubrich RH, Hwang JY, et al. The effect of six months treatment with 100 mg daily dose of dehydroepiandrosterone (DHEA) on circulating sex steroids, body composition and muscle strength in age-advanced men and women. *Clinical Endocrinol* 1998;49:421-32.

4252 Casson PR, Andersen RN, Herrod HG, et al. Oral dehyroepiandrosterone in physiologic doses modulates immune function in postmenopausal women. *Am J Obstet Gynecol* 1995;1536-1539.

4253 Arlt W, Justl H, Callies F, et al. Oral dehydroepiandrosterone for adrenal androgen replacement: pharmacokinetics and peripheral conversion to androgens and estrogens in young healthy females after dexamethasone suppression. *J Clin Endocrinol Metab* 1998; 83:1928-1934.

4254 Kudielka B, Hellhammer J, Hellhammer D, et al. Sex differences in endocrine and psychological responses to psychosocial stress in healthy elderly subjects and the impact of a 2 week dehydroepiandrosterone treatment. *J Clin Endocrinol Metab*, 1998;83:1756-1761.

4255 Flynn MA, Weaver-Osterholtz D, Sharpe-Timms KL, et al. Dehydroepiandrosterone replacement in aging humans. *J Clin Endocrinol Metab*, 1999;84:1527-1533.

4256 Wolkowitz O. Personal memo to Karen Davidson 10/18/99.

4257 Heinonen OP, Albanes D, Virtamo J, et al. prostate cancer and supplementation with alpha-tocopherol and beta-carotene: incidence and mortality in a controlled trial. *J Natl Cancer Inst* 1998; 90(6):440-6.

4258 Young LY, Koda-Kimble MA. Applied Therapeutics: The Clinical Use of Drugs, *6th ed.* Vancouver: Applied Therapeutics, Inc. 1995.

4259 FDA Press Release. FDA Warns About GBL-Related Products. FDA website, URL: vm.cfsan.fda.gov/~lrd/tpgbl2.html (Accessed 11 May 1999).

4260 Briggs GB, Freeman RK, Yaffe SJ. Drugs in Pregnancy and Lactation: A Reference Guide to Fetal and Neonatal Risk, 5th ed. Philadelphia: Lippincott, Williams, and Wilkins; 1998.

4261 FDA. http://www.fda.gov/orphan/designat/list.htm (Accessed 11 November 1999).

4262 http://www.peanut-institute.org/Equal_Olive_Oil_PR.html (Accessed 19 September 1999).

4263 Sobolev VS, Cole RJ, Dorner JW, et al. Isolation, Purification, and Liquid Chromatographic Determination of Stilbene Phytoalexins in Peanuts. *J AOAC International*, 1995;78:1177-1182.

4264 Stampfer J, Manson JE, Rimm EB, et al. Frequent nut consumption and risk of coronary heart disease study.

BMJ 1998; 17:1341-1345.

4265 Kritchevsky D, Tepper SA, Klurfeld DM. Lectin may contribute to the atherogenicity of peanut oil. *Lipids* 1998;33:821-823.

4266 Kritchevsky D. Cholesterol vehicle in experimental Atherosclerosis. A brief review with special reference to peanut oil. *Arch Pathol Lab Med* 1988; 112:1041-1044.

4267 la Vecchia C, Negri E, Franceschi S, Decarli A, Giacosa A, Lipworth L. Olive oil, other dietary fats, and the risk of breast cancer. (Italy) *Cancer Causes Control* November, 1995;6(6):545-50.

4269 Muzzarelli RA, Biagini G, Bellardini, et al. Osteoconduction exterted by methylpyrrolidinone chitosan used in dental surgery. *Biomaterials* 1993;14(1):39-43.

4270 Muzzarelli R, Tarsi R, Fillippini O, et al. Antimicrobial properties of N-carboxybutyl chitosan. *Antimicrob Agents Chemother* 1990;34(10):2019-23.

4271 Fischer T, Wigger-Alberti W, Elsner P. Melatonin in dermatology. Experimental and clinical aspects. *Hautarzt* 199 50(1):5-11.

4272 Lee BJ, Cui JH, Parrott KA, Ayres JW, Sack RL. Percutaneous absorption and model membrane variations of melatonin in aqueous-based propylene glycol and 2-hydroxypropyl-beta-cyclodextran vehicles. *Arch Pharm Res* 1998;21(5):503-7.

4273 Prevention. http://www.prevention.com/healing/living/980929.lvg4.html. (Accessed 23 November 1999).

4274 Riordan SM, Williams R. Treatment of Hepatic Encephalopathy 1997; *NEJM* 337(7):473-479.

4275 Shipochliev T. Uterotonic action of extracts from a group of medicinal plants. *Vet Med Nauki* 1981;18(4):94-8.

4276 http://www.pharmacotherapy.medscape.com/IMNG/SkinAllergyN<sum>/san2810.28.01.htm (Accessed 23 February 2000).

4277 http://www.senetekplc.com/sci-kinetin.html (Accessed 23 February 2000).

4278 Olsen A, Siboska GE, Clark BF, Rattan SI. N(6)-Furfuryladenine, kinetin, protects against Fenton reaction-mediated oxidative damage to DNA. *Biochem Biophys Res Commun* 1999;265(2):499-502.

4279 http://www.senetekplc.com/amhealth.html (Accessed 23 February 2000).

4280 http://www.keechstudio.com/osm/PRODUCTS/KINETIN/kinetin.html (Accessed 24 February 2000).

4281 http://www.icnpharm.com/kinerase/facts.html (Accessed 24 February 2000).

4282 National Genetics Resources Program. The Germplasm Resources Information Network http://www.ars-grin.gov/ (Accessed 24 February 2000).

4283 Wang H, Nair MG, Strasburg GM, et al. Novel antioxidant compounds from tart cherries (Prunus cerasus). *J Nat Prod* 1999;62(1):86-88.

4284 Bruneton J. Pharmacognosy Phytochemistry Medicinal Plants, 2nd ed. Paris: Lavoisier, 1999:142

4285 Phone conversation with Michelle, ICN Pharmaceuticals. 4:20 pm, 24 February 2000.

4286 http://www.youngagain2000.com/marcella75/kinetin.html (Accessed 25 February 2000).

4287 http://www.amfoundation.org/herbs/calophyllum.htm (Accessed 23 February 2000).

4289 Protocol Title: A Phase 1B Dose-Range Study to Evaluate the Safety, Pharmacokinetics, and Effects of (+)-calaonlide A on surrogate markers in HIV-positive patients with no previous antiretroviral therapy. Protocol ID numbers: FDA 297A.

4290   Reuters Health. Anti-HIV herbal product shows therapeutic potential in phase I trial. November 1, 1999.

4291   Newman RA, Chen W, Madden TL. Pharmaceutical properties of related calanolide compounds with activity against human immunodeficiency virus. *J Pharm Sci* 1998;87:1077-1080.

4292   Buckheit RW, White EL, Fliakas-Boltz V, et al. Unique anti-human immunodeficiency virus activities of the nonnucleoside reverse transcriptase inhibitors calanolide A, costatolide, and dihydrocostatolide. *Antimicrob Agents Chemother* 1999;43(8):1827-1834.

4293   Boyer PL, Currens MH, McMahon JB. Analysis of nonnucleoside drug-resistant variants of human immunodeficiency virus type 1 reverse transcriptase. *J Virol* 1993;67(4):2412-1201.

4294   Currens MJ, Nariner JM, McMahon JB, Boyd MR. Kinetic analysis of inhibition of human immunodeficiency virus type-a reverse transcriptase by calanolide A. *J Pharmacol Exp Ther* 1996;279(2):652-661.

4295   Currens MJ, Gulakowski RJ, Mariner JM, et al. Antiviral activity and mechanism of action of calanolide A against the human immunodeficiency virus type-1. *J Pharmacol Exp Ther* 1996;279(2):645-651.

4299   Kanth VR, Diwan PV. Analgesic, anti-inflammatory and hypoglycaemic activities of Sida cordifolia. *Phytother Res* February 1999;13(1):75-77.

4300   Fuhr U. "Drug Interactions with Grapefruit Juice." *Drug Safety* 1998;(4):251-272.

4301   Yablonsky F, et al. "Antiproliferative effect of Pygeum africanum extract on rat prostatic fibroblasts." *J Urol* 1997; 157:2881-7.

4302   Andro MC, Riffaud JP. "Pygeum africanum extract for the treatment of patients with benign prostatic hyperplasia. A review of 25 years of published experience." *Curr Ther Res*, 1995;56:796-817.

4303   Homer KA, Manji F, Beighton D. Inhibition of peptidase and glycosidase activities of Porphyromonas gingivalis, Bacteroides intermedius and Treponema denticola by plant extracts. *J Clin Periodontol* May 1992;19(5):305-310.

4304   Anon. Sida Cordifolia. http://metromkt.net/viable/1sidacor.shtml. (Accessed 9 March 2000).

4305   Anon. SinuS? For Soothing Sinus Support. http://www.djtrading.com/sinus.htm. (Accessed 9 March 2000).

4306   W&B Associates, Inc. Dr. Harris' Original Allergy Formula. http://www.wandb.com/sinus.htm. (Accessed 9 March 2000).

4307   Anon. Extreme Sports Nutrition. http://www.extremesn.com/sports/prolab/provate1.htm. (Accessed 9 March 2000).

4308   Anon. Spectrum Nutrition the Leader in Pro-hormonal supplementation. http://www.spectrumnutrition.com/spectrumnutrition/prolther60ca.html. (Accessed 9 March 2000).

4309   Anon. Concentrated Natural Supplement with Sida Cordifolia. http://www.customdirecttoyou.com/katieseyes/ther50.html. (Accessed 9 March 2000).

4310   Anon. Sida Cordifolia Linn. http://www.modern-natural.com/sida_cordifolia.htm. (Accessed 9 March 2000).

4311   International Cyberbusiness Services, Inc. Herb Information; 1999. http://www.holisticonline.com/Herbal-Med/w_herb_dir.htm. (Accessed 9 March 2000).

4312   Silesia Group, Inc. The oldest and most effective herbal mixtures from India. http://www.biznet1.com/herbs/india/index.htm. (Accessed 9 March 2000).

4313   Anon. Go with herbs. http://www.gowithherbs.com/1297-2.htm. (Accessed 9 March 2000).

4314   Anon. Strictly Medicinal Herb Seeds. http://www.chatlink.com/~herbseed/sida.html. (Accessed 9 March 2000).

4315   Anon. Ayurvedic Rasayanas. http://www.ayurveda-herbs.com/Aphrodisiac-Sex-Impotency.htm. (Accessed 9 March 2000).

4316   Dharma Group. Herbal Accelerator. http://www.dharmagroup.com/web/herbal.htm. (Accessed 9 March 2000).

4317   Anon. JNT-AV (100). http://www.herbwise.com:8001/encyclo/products/1296-1.htf. (Accessed 9 March 2000).

4318   Anon. Fastrak. http://members.tripod.com/~Roe/fastrak. (Accessed 9 March 2000).

4319   Prime Nutrition. Pyroclen Thermo Burn 100's. http://www.primenutrition.com/primen/sanpyrtherbu.html. (Accessed 9 March 2000).

4320   Anon. Pyruvate Formulas. http://www.undergroundsports.com/pyruvate.htm. (Accessed 9 March 2000).

4321   Maharishi Ayur-Ved Products Inc. 1998; Ayurvedic Herbs: Bala. http://www.mapi.com/cgi-local/shop.pl/page=herbbala.html/SID=1877132249. (Accessed 9 March 2000).

4322   4322 Aquasearch Incorporated. Aquasearch Technology and Markets. 1999. URL. http://www.aqse.com/astax.htm. (Accessed 14 March 2000).

4323   Anon. Eat and lose weight. http://www.pricespower.com/eat&lose.htm. (Accessed 9 March 2000).

4324   Diet Gems. Fantastic products for weight loss. http://store.yahoo.net/dietgems/. (Accessed 9 March 2000).

4325   Anon. Ayurvedic Rasanas. http://www.ayurveda-herbs.com/Narayana-Massage-Oil-Pain.htm. (Accessed 9 March 2000).

4326   Goodwin TW. Metabolism, nutrition, and function of carotenoids. *Ann Rev Nutr* 1986;6:273-297.

4327   Duke J. ETHNOBOT. http://www.ars-grin.gov/duke (Accessed 14 March 2000).

4328   Igene Biotechnology Incorporated. Product Information. 2000. URL. http://www.igene.com/products.htm. (Accessed 14 March 2000).

4329   Cyanotech corporation. Natur Rose. 1999. URL. http://www.cyanotech.com. (Accessed 14 March 2000).

4330   Cyanotech. Cyanotech Launches Natural Astaxanthin as Human Dietary Supplement; Powerful Antioxidant Promises Key Benefits 2000. URL. http://www.npicenter.com/dailynewswire/archive/19990311/9/comt x-13365M3b921 161962.asp. (Accessed 14 March 2000).

4331   Storebakken, T. Utilization of astaxanthin from red yeast (Phaffia rhodozyma) in comparison with synthetic astaxanthin by Atlantic salmon. 1998. URL. http://www.igene.com/norway.html. (Accessed 14 March 2000).

4332   Kobayashi M, Kakizono T, Nishio N, et al. Antioxidant role of astaxanthin in the green alga Haematococcus pluvialis. *Applied Microbiology and Biotechnology*, 1997;48(3):351-356.

4333   Dolan M. Hepatitis C-clinical background and treatment options. http://www.positivehealth.com/permit/Articles/Nutrition/hepc.htm. (Accessed 12 March 2000).

4334   Anon. Astaxanthin promoted as dietary supplement.

1999. URL. http://www.nzhealth.co.nz/nutrition/
nutnews199903172.html. (Accessed 14 March 2000).

4335 Jyonouchi H, Sun S, Tomita Y, et al. Astaxathin, a
carotenoid without vitamin A activity augments antibody
responses in cultures including T-helpe cell clones and
suboptimal doses of antigen. *J Nutr* 1995;125(10):2483-
2492.

4336 Chew BP, Wong MW, Park JS, et al. Dietary beta-
carotene and astaxanthin but not canthaxanthin stimulate
splenocyte function in mice. *AntiCancer Research*
1999;19;5223-5228.

4337 Chew BP, Park JS, Wong MW, et al. A comparison of
the anticancer activities of dietary beta-carotene,
canthaxanthin and astaxanthin in mice in vivo.
AntiCancer Research 1999;19:1849-1854.

4338 Tanaka T, Morishita Y, Suzui M, et al. Chemoprevention
of mouse urinary bladder Carcinogenesis by the
naturally occurring carotenoid astaxanthin.
Carcinogenesis 1994;15(1):15-19.

4339 Tanaka T, Makita H, Oshnishi M, et al.
Chemoprevention of rat oral Carcinogenesis by naturally
occurring xanthophylls, astaxanthin, and canthaxanthin.
Cancer Research 1995;55:4059-4064.

4340 Gradelet S, Le Bon AM, Berges R, et al. Dietary
carotenoids inhibit aflatoxin B1-induced liver
preneoplastic foci and DNA damage in the rat: role of
the modulation of aflatoxin B1 metabolism.
Carcinogenesis 1998; 19(3):403-411.

4341 Bennedsen M, Wang X, Willen R, et al. Treatment of H.
pylori infected mice with antioxidant astaxanthin
reduces gastric inflammation, bacterial load and
modulates cytokine release by splenocytes. *Immunol
Lett*, 1999;70(3):185-189.

4342 Bensky D, Gamble A, Kaptchuk T. Chinese Herbal
Medicine Materia Medica. Seattle: Eastland Press.
1996:214-216.

4343 Huang KC. The Pharmacology of Chinese Herbs, 2nd
ed. Boca Raton: CRC Press LLC. 1999:258.

4344 Chevallier A. The Encyclopedia of Medicinal Plants.
New York: DK Publishing. 1996:170.

4345 Yamamoto M, Ogawa K, Morita M, et al. The herbal
medicine Inchin-ko-to inhibits liver cell apoptosis
induced by transforming growth factor beta 1.
Hepatology 1996;32(3):552-559.

4346 Yamamoto M, Miura N, Ohtake N, et al. Genipin, a
metabolite derived from the herbal medicine Inchin-ko-
to, and suppression of fas-induced lethal liver apoptosis
in mice. *Gastroenterology* 2000;118:380-389.

4347 Saavedra J. Probiotics and infectious diarrhea. The
American Journal of *Gastroenterology* 2000;95(1
Suppl):S16-S18.

4348 Castagliuolo I, Riegler MF, Valenick L, et al.
Saccharomyces boulardii protease inhibits the effects of
clostridium difficile toxins A and B in human colonic
mucosa. *Infection and Immunity* 1999;67(1):302-307.

4349 Bleichner G, Blehaut H, Mentec H, et al.
Saccharomyces boulardii prevents diarrhea in critically
ill tube-fed patients. *Intensive Care Med* 1997;23:517-
523.

4350 Lewis SJ, Potts LF, Barry RE. The lack of therapeutic
effect of Saccharomyces boulardii in the prevention of
antibiotic-related diarrhea in elderly patients. *J Infect*
1998;36:171-174.

4351 Elmer GW, McFarland LV. Comment on the lack of
therapeutic effect of Saccharomyces boulardii in the
prevention of antibiotic-related diarrhea in elderly

patients. *J Infect*, 1998;36(2):171-174.

4352 McFarland LV, Surawicz CM, Greenberg RN, et al. A
randomized placebo-controlled trial of Saccharomyces
boulardii in combination with standard antibiotics for
Clostridium difficile disease. *JAMA*
1994;271(24):1913-1918.

4353 McFarland LV, Surawicz, Greenberg RN, et al.
Prevention of beta-lactam associated diarrhea by
Saccharomyces boulardii compared with placebo. *The
American Journal of Gastroenterology* 1995;90(3):439-
448.

4354 Surawicz CM, McFarland LV, Elmer G, et al. Treatment
of recurrent clostridium difficile colitis with vancomycin
and Saccharomyces boulardii. *The American Journal of
Gastroenterology* 1989;84(10):1285-1287.

4355 Surawicz CM, Elmer GW, Speelman P, et al. Prevention
of antibiotic-associated diarrhea by Saccharomyces
boulardii: a prospective study. *Gastroenterology*
1989;96:981-988.

4356 Buts JP, Corthier G, Delmee M. Saccharomyces
boulardii for Clostridium difficile-associated
enteropathies in infants. *J of Pediatr Gastroenterol and
Nutr* 1993;16(4):419-425.

4357 Pletinex M, Legein J, Vandenplas Y. Fungemia with
Saccharomyces boulardii in a 1-year-old girl with
protracted diarrhea. *Journal of Pediatric
Gastroenterology and Nutrition* 1995;21:113-115.

4358 Fredenucci I, Chomarat M, Boucaud C, et al.
Saccharomyces boulardii fungemia in a patient receiving
ultra-levure therapy. *CID* 1998;27:222-223.

4359 Hennequin C, Kauffmann-Lacroix C, Jobert A, et al.
Possible role of catheters in Saccharomyces boulardii
fungemia. *Eur J Clin Microbiol Infect Dis*
2000;19(1):16-20.

4360 Elmer GW, McFarland LV, Surawicz CM, et al.
Behaviour of Saccharomyces boulardii in recurrent
Clostridium difficile disease patients. *Alimen Pharmacol
Ther* 1999;13(12):1663-1668.

4361 Czerucka D, Roux I, Rampal P. Saccharomyces
boulardii inhibits secretagogue-mediated adenosine 3',5'-
cyclic monophosphate induction in intestinal cells.
Gastroenterology 1994;106(1):65-72.

4362 Krammer M, Karbach U. Antidiarrheal action of the
yeast Saccharomyces boulardii in the rat small and large
intestine by stimulating chloride absorption. Z
Gastroenterol, 1993;31:73-77.

4363 Lewis SJ, Freedman AR. Review article: the use of
biotherapeutic agents in the prevention and treatment of
gastrointestinal disease. *Aliment Pharmacol Ther*
1998;12:807-822.

4364 PWA Health Group. SACCHAROMYCES
BOULARDII INFO SHEET http://208.178.40.64/
pwahg/info/sacc.html. (Accessed 16 March 2000).

4365 James JS. *AIDS* Treatment Archives. http://aids.org/
immunet/atn.nsf/page/x-Saccharomyces-boulardii.
(Accessed 16 March 2000).

4367 Gorbach SL. Probiotics and gastrointestinal health. *Am J
Gastroenterol* 2000;95(1 Suppl):S2-S4.

4368 Schultz M, Sartor RB. Probiotics and inflammatory
bowel diseases. *The Am J of Gastroenterol*
2000;95(1):S19-S21.

4369 deRoos NM, Katan MB. Effects of probiotic bacteria on
diarrhea, lipid metabolism, and *Carcinogenesis*: a review
of papers published between 1988 and 1998. *Am J Clin
Nutr* 2000; 71:405-1411.

4370 Guandalini S, Pensabene L, Zikri MA, et al.

Lactobacillus GG administered in oral rehydration solution to children with acute diarrhea: a multicenter European trial. *J of Ped Gastroenterol Nutr* 2000;30:54.

4371 Vanderhoof JA, Whitney DB, Antonson DL, et al. Lactobacillus GG in the prevention of antibiotic-associated diarrhea in children. *J Pediatr* 1999;135(5):564-568.

4372 Arvola T, Laiho K, Torkkeli S, et al. Prophylactic Lactobacillus GG reduces antibiotic-associated diarrhea in children with respiratory infections: a randomized study. *Pediatrics* 1999;104(5):e64.

4373 Oberhelman RA, Gilman RH, Sheen P, et al. A placebo-controlled trial of Lactobacillus GG to prevent diarrhea in undernourished Peruvian children. *J Pediatr*, 1999;134(1):15-20.

4374 Hilton E, Kolakowski P, Singer C, et al. Efficacy of Lactobacillus GG as a Diarrheal Preventative in Travelers. *J Travel Med* 1997;4(1):41-43.

4375 Vanderhoof JA, Young RJ, Murray N, et al. Treatment strategies for small bowel bacterial overgrowth in short bowel syndrome. *J Pediatr Gastroenterol Nutr* 1998;27(2):155-160.

4376 El-Nezami H, Kankaanpaa P, Salminen S, et al. Ability of dairy strains of lactic acid bacteria to bind a common food carcinogen, aflatoxin B1. *Food Chem Toxicol* 1998;36(4):321-326.

4377 Guarino A, Canani RB, Spagnuolo MI, et al. Oral bacterial therapy reduces the duration of symptoms and of viral excretion in children with mild diarrhea. *J Pediatr Gastroenterol Nutr* 1997;25(5):516-519.

4378 Hudault S, Lievin V, Bernet-Camard MF, et al. Antagonistic activity exerted in vitro and in vivo by Lactobacillus casei (strain GG) against Salmonella typhimurium C5 infection. *Appl Environ Microbiol* 1997;63(2):513-518.

4379 Sutas Y, Hurme M, Isolauri E. Down-regulations of anti-CD3 antibody-induced IL-4 production by bovine caseins hydrolyzed with Lactobacillus GG-derived enzymes. *Scand J Immunol* 1996;43(6):687-689.

4380 Saxelin M, Chuang NH, Chassy B, et al. Lactobacilli and bacteremia in southern Finland 1989-1992. *Clin Infect Dis* 1996;22(3):564-566.

4381 Malin M, Suomalainen H, Saxelin M, et al. Promotion of IgA immune response in patients with Crohn's disease by oral bacteriotherapy with Lactobacillus GG. *Ann Nutr Metab* 1996;40(3):137-145.

4382 Goldin BR, Gualtieri LJ, Moore RP. The effect of Lactobacillus GG on the initiation and promotion of DMH-induced intestinal tumors in the rat. *Nutr Cancer* 1996;25(2):197-204.

4383 Adis Editors. http://aids.medscape.com/adis/IP/1999/1179/ip1179.01.html (Accessed 18 March 2000).

4384 Anon. New dietary supplement with research-proven intestinal health benefits now available. 2000. URL. http://www.conagra.com/092398_2.html. (Accessed 18 March 2000).

4385 Anon. Lactobacillus GG and CRC. 2000. URL. http://www.geocities.com/HotSprings/Falls/4425/lgg.html (Accessed 18 March 2000).

4386 Valio. Valio Products. 2000. URL. http://www.valio.fi/english/products.html. (Accessed 18 March 2000).

4387 McIntosh GH, Royle PJ, Playne MJ. A probiotic strain of L. acidophilus reduces DMH-induced large intestinal tumors in male Sprague-Dawley rats. *Nutr Cancer* 1999;35(2):153-159.

4388 Mack DR, Michail S, Shu W, et al. Probiotics inhibit enteropathogenic E. coli adherence in vitro by inducing intestinal mucin gene expression. *Clin Exp Immunol* 1999;116(2):276-282.

4389 Tynkkynen S, Singh KV, Varmanen P. Vancomycin resistance factor of Lactobacillus rhamnosus GG in relation to enterococcal vancomycin resistance (van) genes. *Int J Food Microbiol* 1998; 41(3):195-204.

4390 Klein G, Zill E, Schindler R, et al. Peritonitis associated with vancomycin-resistant Lactobacillus rhamnosus in a continuous ambulatory peritoneal dialysis patient; organism identification, antibiotic therapy, and case report. *J Clin Microbiol* 1998;36(6):1781-1783.

4391 Kalima P, Masterton RG, Roddie PH, et al. Lactobacillus rhamnosus infection in a child following bone marrow transplant. *J Infect* 1996;32(2):165-167.

4392 Pochapin M. The effect of probiotics on Clostridium difficile diarrhea. *The American Journal of Gastroenterology* 2000;95(1 Suppl 1):S11-S13.

4393 Goldin BR. Health Benefits of probiotics. *Br J Nutr* 1998;80(4):S203-S207.

4394 Biller JA, Katz AJ, Flores AF, et al. Treatment of recurrent Clostridium difficile colitis with Lactobacillus GG. *J Pediatr Gastroenterol Nutr* 1995;21(2):224-226.

4395 Anon. Aquasearch Announces Launch of The AstaFactor(TM).2000.URL. http://www.aquasearch.com/whatsnew.htm (Accessed 20 March 2000).

4396 Anon. U.S. district court grants Aquasearch's motion for summary judgement. Court rules that Cyanotech infringed key Aquasearch patent, misappropriated Aquasearch trade secrets, and breached its contract with Aquasearch. 2000. URL. http://www.aquasearch.com/whatsnew.htm. (Accessed 20 March 2000).

4397 Hilton E, Rindos P, Isenberg HD. Lactobacillus GG Vaginal Suppositories and Vaginitis. *Journal of Clinical Microbiology* 1995;33(5):1433.

4398 Rautio M, Jousimies-Somer H, Kauma H, et al. Liver abscess due to Lactobacillus rhamnosus strain indistinguishable from L. rhamnosus strain GG. *Clinical Infectious Diseases* 199;28:1159-1160.

4399 Pelto L, Ioslauri E, Lilius EM, et al. Probiotic bacteria down-regulate the milk-induced inflammatory response in milk-hypersensitive subjects but have an immunostimulatory effect in healthy subjects. *Clinical and Experimental Allergy* 1998;28:1474-1479.

4400 Spencer H, Menaham L. Adverse effects of aluminum-containing antacids on mineral metabolism. *Gastroenterology*, 1979;76:603-606.

4401 Balasa RW, Murray RL, Kondelis NP, et al. Phosphate binding properties and electrolyte content of aluminum hydroxide antacids. *Nephron*, 1987;45(1):16-21.

4402 Baker LR, Ackrill P, Cattell WR, et al. Iatrogenic osteomalacia and myopathy due to phosphate depletion. *Br Med J*, 1974;3(924):150-152.

4403 Insogna KL, Bordley DR, Caro JF, Lockwood DH. Osteomalacia and weakness from excessive antacid ingestion. *JAMA*, 1980;244:2544-2546.

4404 Folkers K, Langsjoen P, Willis R, et al. Lovastatin decreases coenzyme Q levels in humans. *Proc Natl Acad Sci USA*, 1990;87(22):8931.

4405 Mortensen SA, Leth A, Agner E, et al. Dose-related decrease of serum coenzyme Q10 during treatment with HMG-CoA reductase inhibitors. *Mol Aspects Med*, 1997;18(Suppl):S137-S144.

4406 Ghirlanda G, Oradei A, Manto A, et al. Evidence of plasma CoQ10-lowering effect by HMG-CoA reductase

REFERENCES

inhibitors: A double blind, placebo-controlled study. *J Clin Pharmacol*, 1993;33(3):226-229.

4407 De Pinieux G, Chariot P, Ammi-Said M, et al. Lipid-lowering drugs and mitochondrial function: Effects of HMG-CoA Reductase inhibitors on serum ubiquinone and blood lactate/pyruvate ratio. *Br J Clin Pharmacol*, 1996;42(3):333-337.

4408 Bargossi AM, Grossi G, Fiorella PL, et al. Exogenous CoQ10 supplementation prevents plasma ubiquinone reduction induced by HMG-CoA reductase inhibitors. *Mol Aspects Med*, 1994;15(Suppl):187-193.

4409 Watts GF, Castelluccio C, Rice-Evans C, et al. Plasma coenzyme Q (ubiquinone) concentrations in patients treated with simvastatin. *J Clin Pathol*, 1993;46(11):1055-1057.

4410 Hanaki Y, Sugiyama S, Ozawa, et al. Coenzyme Q10 and coronary artery disease. *Clin Investig*, 1993;71(8 Suppl):S97-S102.

4411 Ritsema GH, Ellers G. Potassium supplements prevent serious hypokalemia in colon cleansing. *Clin Radiol*, 1994;49(12):874-876.

4412 Murry JJ, Healy MD. Drug-mineral interactions: a new responsibility for the hospital dietician. *J Am Diet Assoc*, 1991;91(1):66-73.

4413 Suki WN, Yium JJ, Von Minden M, et al. Acute treatment of hypercalcemia with furosemide. *N Engl J Med*, 1970;283(16):836-840.

4414 Quamme GA. Renal magnesium handling: New insights in understanding old problems. *Kidney Int*, 1997;52(5):1180-1195.

4415 Schwinger RH, Erdman E. Heart failure and electrolyte disturbances. Methods Find Exp *Clin Pharmacol*, 1992;14(4):315-325.

4416 Al-Ghamdi SM, Cameron EC, Sutton RA. Magnesium deficiency: Pathophysiologic and clinical overview. *Am J Kidney Dis*, 1994;24(5):737-752.

4417 Iseri LT, Freed J, Bures AR. Magnesium deficiency and cardiac disorders. *Am J Med*, 1975;58(6):837-846.

4418 Lucker PW, Witzmann HK. Influence of magnesium and potassium deficiency on renal elimination and cardiovascular function demonstrated by impedence cardiography. *Magnesium*, 1984;3(4-6):265-273.

4419 Ryan MP, Devane J, Ryan MF, et al. Effects of diuretics on the renal handling of magnesium. *Drugs*, 1984;28 (Suppl 1):167-181.

4420 Cohen N, Golik A, Dishi V, et al. Effect of furosemide oral solution versus furosemide tablets on diuresis and electrolytes in patients with moderate congestive heart failure. *Ineral Electrolyte MetabMineral Electrolyte Metab*, 1996;22(4):248-252.

4421 Lindeman RD. Hypokalemia: causes, consequences, and correction. *Am J Med* Sci, 1976;272(1):5-17.

4422 Nuutinen LS. The effect of furosemide on potassium balance in open heart surgery. *Ann Chir Gynaecol*, 1976;65(4):277-281.

4423 Valmin K, Hansen T, Ronsted P. Treatment of benign essential hypertension with frusemide in different doses. *Pharmacotherapeutica*, 1980;2(5):541-544.

4424 Wester PO. Urinary zinc excretion during treatment with different diuretics. *Acta Med Scand*, 1980;208(3)209-212.

4425 Garabedian-Ruffalo SM, Ruffalo RL. Drug and nutrient interactions. *AFP*, 1986;33(2):165-174.

4426 Kishi T, Fujita N, Eguchi T, et al. Mechanism for reduction of serum folate by antiepileptic drugs during prolonged therapy. *J Neurol Sci*, 1997;145(1):109-112.

4427 Froscher W, Maier V, Laage M, et al. Folate deficiency, anticonvulsant drugs, and psychiatric morbidity. *Clin Neuropharmacol*, 1995;18(2):165-182.

4428 Hendel J, Dam M, Gram L, et al. The effects of carbamazepine and valproate on folate metabolism in man. *Acta Neurol Scan*, 1984;69(4)-226-231.

4429 Traccis S, Monaco F, Sechi GP, et al. Long-term therapy with carbamazepine: Effects on nerve conduction velocity. *Eur Neurol*, 1983;22(6):410-416.

4430 Hoikka V, Alhava EM, Karjalainen P, et al. Carbamazepine and bone mineral metabolism. *Acta Neurol Scand*, 1984;70(2):77-80.

4431 Rajantie J, Lamberg-Allardt C, Wilska M. Does carbamazepine treatment lead to a need of extra vitamin D in some mentally retarded children? *Acta Pediatr Scand*, 1984;73(3):325-328.

4432 Gough H, Goggin T, Bissessar A, et al. A comparative study of the relative influence of different anticonvulsant drugs, UV exposure and diet on vitamin D and calcium *Metabolism* in outpatients with epilepsy. *Q J Med*, 1986;59(230):569-577.

4433 Vakimaki MJ, Tiihonen M, Laitinen K, et al. Bone mineral density measured by dual-energy x-ray absorptiometry and novel markers of bone formation and resorption in patients on antiepileptic drugs. *J Bone Miner Res*, 1994;9(5):631-637.

4434 Cummings JH, Macfarlane G. Role of intestinal bacteria in nutrient metabolism. *J Parenter Enteral Nutr*, 1997;21(6):357-365.

4435 Honma N. The effect of lactic acid bacteria, Part 1: Biological significance. *New Medicines and Clinics*, 1986;35(12):1-3.

4436 Gorbach SL, Bengt E. Gustafsson memorial lecture. Function of the normal human microflora. *Scand J Infect Dis Suppl*, 1986;49:17-30.

4437 Hill MJ. Intestinal flora and endogenous vitamin synthesis. *Eur J Cancer Prev*, 1997;6(Suppl 1):S43-S45.

4438 Conly J, Stein K. Reduction of vitamin K2 concentrations in human liver associated with the use of broad spectrum antimicrobials. *Clin Invest Med*, 1994;17(6):531-539.

4439 Conly JM, Stein K, Worobetz, et al. The contribution of vitamin K2 (menaquinones) produced by the intestinal microflora to human nutritional requirements for vitamin K. *Am J Gastroenterol*, 1994;89(6):915-923.

4440 Cordes I, Buchmann S, Scheffner D. Vitamin K deficiency with erythromycin. Observation of a boy treated with valproate. *Monatsschr Kinderhdilkd*, 1990;138(2):85-87.

4441 Lipsky JJ. Antibiotic-associated hypoprothrombinemia. *J Antimicrob Chemother*, 1988;21(3):281-300.

4442 Alitalo R, Ruutu M, Valtonen V, et al. Hypoprothrombinemia and bleeding during administration of cefamandole and cefoperazone. Report of three cases. *Ann Clin Res*, 1985;17(3):116-119.

4443 Shimada K, Matsuda T, Inamatsu T, et al. Bleeding secondary to vitamin K deficiency in patients receiving parenteral cephem antibiotics. *J Antimicrob Chemother*, 1984;14(Suppl B):325-220.

4444 Malini PL, Strocchi E, Valtancoli G, et al. Angiotensin-converting enzyme inhibitors, thiazide diuretics and magnesium balance. A preliminary study. *Magnes Res*, 1990;3(3):193-196.

4445 Hollifield JW. Potassium and magnesium abnormalities: Diuretics and arrhythmias in hypertension. *Am J Med*, 1984;77(5A0):28-32.

4446 Dyckner T, Wester PO. Potassium/Magnesium depletion in patients with cardiovascular disease. *Am J Med*, 1987;82(3A):11-17.

4447 Petri M, Cumber P, Grimes L, et al. The metabolic effects of thiazide therapy in the elderly: A population study. *Age Ageing*, 1986;15(3)151-155.

4448 Gettes LS. Electrolyte abnormalities underlying lethal and ventricular arrhythmias. *Circulation*, 1992;85(Suppl 1):170-176.

4449 Robertson JI. Diuretics, potassium depletion and risk of arrhythmias. *Eur Heart J*, 1984;5(Supp A):25-28.

4450 Reyes AJ, Olhaberry JV, Leary WP, et al. Urinary zinc excretion, diuretics, zinc deficiency and some side-effects of diuretics. *S Afr Med J*, 1983;64(24):936-941.

4451 Reyes AJ, Leary WP, Lockett CJ, et al. Diuretics and zinc. *S Afr Med J*, 1982;62(11):373-375.

4452 Mountokalakis T, Dourakis S, Karatzas N, et al. Zinc deficiency in mild hypertensive patients treated with diuretics. *J Hypertens Suppl*, 1984;2(3):S571-S572.

4453 Thomas JA. Drug-nutrient interactions. *Nutrition Rev*, 1995;53(10):271-282.

4454 Hathcock JN. Metabolic mechanisms of drug-nutrient interactions. *Fed Proc*, 1985;44(1 Pt 1):124-129.

4455 West RJ, Lloyd JK. The effect of cholestyramine on intestinal absorption. *Gut*, 1975;16(2):93-98.

4456 Cywes C, Millar AJ. Assessment of the nutritional status of infants and children with biliary atresia. *S Afr Med J*, 1990;77(3):131-135.

4457 Elinder LS, Hadell K, Johansson J, et al. Probucol treatment decreases serum concentrations of diet-derived antioxidants. *Arterioscler Throm Vasc Biol*, 1995;15(8):1057-1063.

4458 Knodel LC, Talbert RL. Adverse effects of hypolipidaemic drugs. *Med Toxicol*, 1987;2(1):10-32.

4459 Matsui MS, Rozovski SJ. Drug-nutrient interaction. *Clin Ther*, 1982;4(6):423-440.

4460 Schwarz KB, Goldstein PD, Witztum JL, et al. Fat-soluble vitamin concentrations in hypercholestrolemic children treated with colestipol. *Pediatrics*, 1980;65(2):243-250.

4461 Tonstad S, Silverstein M, Aksnes L, et al. Low dose colestipol in adolescents with familial hypercholesterolemia. *Arch Dis Child*, 1996;74(2):157-160.

4462 Lems WF, Van Veen GJ, Gerrits MI, et al. Effect of low-dose prednisolone (with calcium and calcitriol supplementation) on calcium and bone metabolism in healthy volunteers. *Br J Rheumatol*, 1998;37(1):27-33.

4463 Reid DM, Kennedy NS, Smith MA, et al. Total body calcium in rheumatoid arthritis: Effects of disease activity and corticosteroid treatment. *Br Med J* (Clin Res Ed), 1982;285(6338):330-332.

4464 Lems WF, Jacobs JW, Netelenbos JC, et al. Pharmacological prevention of osteoporosis in patients on corticosteroid medication, *Ned Tijdschr Geneeskd*, 1998;142(34):1904-1908.

4465 Gennari C. Differential effect of glucocorticoids on calcium absorption and bone mass. *Br J Rheumatol*, 1993;32(Suppl 2):11-14.

4466 Need AG, Philcox JC, Hartley TF, et al. Calcium metabolism and osteoporosis in corticosteroid-treated postmenopausal women. *Aust N Z J Med*, 1986;16(3):341-346.

4467 Reid IR, Ibbertson HK. Calcium supplements in the prevention of steroid-induced osteoporosis. *Am J Clin Nutr*, 1986;44(2):287-290.

4468 Kahn SB, Fein SA, Brodsky I. Effects of trimethoprim on folate metabolism in man. *Clin Pharmacol Ther*, 1968;9(5):550-560.

4469 Haspels AA, Bennink HJ, Schreurs WH. Disturbance of tryptophan metabolism and its correction during oestrogen treatment in postmenopausal women. *Maturitas*, 1978;1(1):15-20.

4470 Blum M, Kitai E, Ariel Y, et al. Oral contraceptive lowers serum magnesium. *Harefuah*, 1991;121(10):363-364.

4471 Lewis DP, Van Dyke DC, Willhite LA, et al. Phenytoin-folic acid interaction. *Ann Pharmacother*, 1995;29(7-8):726-735.

4472 Berg MJ, Stumbo PJ, Chenard CA, et al. Folic acid improves phenytoin pharmacokinetics. *J Am Diet Assoc*, 1995;95(3):352-356.

4473 Berg MJ, Fincham RW, Ebert BE, et al. Phenytoin pharmacokinetics: Before and after folic acid administration. *Epilepsia*, 1992;33(4):712-720.

4474 Zerwekh JE, Homan R, Tindall R, et al. Decreased serum 24,25-dihydroxy vitamin D concentration during long-term anticonvulsant therapy in adult epileptics. *Ann Neurol*, 1982;12(2):184-186.

4475 Bell RD, Pak CY, Zerwekh J, et al. Effect of phenytoin on bone and mineral density in ambulatory epileptic children. *Brain Dev*, 1994;16(5):382-385.

4476 Gascon-Barre M, Villeneuve JP, Lebrun LH. Effect of increasing doses of phenytoin on the plasma 25-hydroxy vitamin D and 1,25-dihydroxy vitamin D concentrations. *J Am Coll Nutr*, 3(1):45-50.

4477 Shafer RB, Nuttall FQ. Calcium and folic acid absorption in patients taking anticonvulsant drugs. *J Clin Endocrinol Metab*, 1975;41(06):1125-1129.

4478 Gough H, Goggin T, Bissessar A, et al. A comparative study of the relative influence of different anticonvulsant drugs, UV exposure and diet on vitamin D and calcium metabolism in outpatients with epilepsy. *Q J Med*, 1986;59(230):569-577.

4479 Kishi T, Kishi H, Watanabe T, et al. Bioenergetics in clinical medicine. XI. Studies on coenzyme Q and diabetes mellitus. *J Med*, 1976;7(3-4):307-321.

4480 Matsui MS, Rozovski SJ. Drug-nutrient interaction. *Clin Ther*, 1982;4(6):423-440.

4481 Pellock JM, Howell J, Kendig EI Jr, et al. Pyridoxine deficiency in children treated with isoniazid. *Chest*, 1985;87(5):658-661.

4482 Snider DE Jr. Pyridoxine supplementation during isoniazid therapy. *Tubercle*, 1980;61(4):191-196.

4483 Termanini B, Gibril F, Sutliff VE, et al. Effect of long-term gastric acid suppressive therapy on serum vitamin B12 levels in patients with Zollinger-Ellison syndrome. *Am J Med*, 1998;104(5):422-430.

4484 Bellou A, Aimone-Gastin I, De Korwin JD, et al. Cobalamin deficiency with megaloblastic anaemia in one patient under long-term omeprazole therapy. *J Intern Med*, 1996;240(3):161-164.

4485 Saltzman JR, Kemp JA, Golner BB, et al. Effect of hypochlorhydria due to omeprazole treatment or atrophic gastritis on protein-bound vitamin B12 absorption. *J Am Coll Nutr*, 1994;13(6):584-91.

4486 Marcuard SP, Albernaz L, Khazaine PG. Omeprazole therapy causes malabsorption of cyanocobalamin. *Ann Intern Med*, 1994;120(3):211-215.

4487 Adams JF, Clark JS, Ireland JT, et al. Malabsorption of vitamin B12 and intrinsic factor secretion during biguanide therapy. *Diabetologia*, 1983;24(1):16-18.

© Copyright 2000, Natural Medicines Comprehensive Database (209) 472-2244. For updated data, go to www.NaturalDatabase.com. • 1251

4488 Berger W. Incidence of severe side effects during treatment with sulfonylureas and biguanides. *Horm Metab Res Suppl*, 1985;15:111-115.

4489 Rieder HP, Berger W, Fridrich R. Vitamin status in diabetic neuropathy. *Z Ernahrungswiss*, 1980;19(1):1-13.

4490 Carpentier JL, Bury J, Luyckx A, et al. Vitamin B12 and folic acid serum levels in diabetics under various therapeutic regimens. *Diabete Metab*, 1976;2(4):187-190.

4491 Bristol-Myers Squibb Company. Glucophage package insert. Princeton, NJ; January 1999.

4492 Leeb BF, Witzmann G, Ogris E, et al. Folic acid cyanocobalamin levels in serum and erythrocytes during low-dose methotrexate therapy in rheumatoid arthritis and psoriatic arthritis patients. *Clin Exp Rheumatol*, 1995;13(4):459-463.

4493 Morgan SL, Baggott JE, Lee JY, et al. Folic acid supplementation prevents deficient blood folate levels and hyperhomocysteinemia during long-term, low dose methotrexate therapy for rheumatoid arthritis: Implications for cardiovascular disease prevention. *J Rheumatol*, 1998;25(3):441-446.

4494 Dijkmans BA. Folate supplementation and methotrexate. *Br J Rheumatol*, 1995;34(12):1172-1174.

4495 Becker GL. The case against mineral oil. *Am J Digestive Dis*, 1953;19:344-347.

4496 Clark JH, Russell GJ, Fitzgerald JF, et al. Serum beta-carotene, retinal, and alpha-tocopherol levels during mineral oil therapy for constipation. *Am J Dis Child*, 1987;141(11):1210-1212.

4497 Webb JL. Nutritional effects of oral contraceptive use: A review. *J Reprod Med*, 1980;25(4):150-156.

4498 Prasad AS, Lei KY, Moghissi KS, et al. Effect of oral contraceptives on nutrients. III. Vitamins B6, B12 and folic acid. *Am J Obstet Gynecol*, 1976;125(8):1063-1069.

4499 Matsui MS, Rozovski SJ. Drug-nutrient interaction. *Clin Ther*, 1982;4(6):423-440.

4500 Hocking GM. A Dictionary of Natural Products. second ed. Medford: Plexus Publishing, 1997.

4501 Micromedex Healthcare Series. Poisindex. Englewood, CO: Micromedex, Inc.

4502 Duke JA. CRC Handbook of Medicinal Herbs. first ed. Boca Raton: CRC Press, 1985.

4503 Bruneton J. Pharmacognosy, Phytochemistry, Medicinal Plants. second ed. Andover: Intercept Ltd, 1995.

4504 Weiss RF. Herbal Medicine. fifth ed. Beaconsfield: Beaconsfield Publishers Ltd, 1998.

4505 DeSmet P, ed. Adverse Effects of Herbal Drugs. first ed. Berlin Heidelberg: Springer-Verlag, 1993.

4506 Miller LG, Wallace JM, eds. Herbal Medicinals, A Clinician's Guide. first ed. New York: Pharmaceutical Products Press, 1998.

4507 Fetrow CW, Avila JR. Professional's Handbook of Complementary and Alternative Medicines. first ed. Springhouse: Springhouse Corporation, 1999.

4510 Ahmed F, Bamji MS, Lyengar L. Effect of oral contraceptive agents on vitamin nutrition status. *Am J Clin Nutr*, 1975;28(6):606-615.

4511 Palva IP, Salokannel SJ, Timonen T, et al. Drug-induced malabsorption of vitamin B12. IV. Malabsorption and deficiency of B12 during treatment with slow-release potassium chloride. *Acta Med Scand*, 1972;191(4):355-357.

4512 Salokannel SJ, Palva IP, Takkunen, et al. Malabsorption of vitamin B12 during treatment with slow-release potassium choloride. Preliminary report. *Acta Med Scand*. 1970;187(5):431-432.

4513 Brodie MJ, Boobis AR, Dollery CT, et al. Rifampicin and vitamin D metabolism. *Clin Pharmacol Ther*, 1980;27(6):810-814.

4514 D'Erasmo E, Ragno A, Raejntroph N, et al. Drug-induced osteomalacia. *Recenti Prog Med*, 1998;89(10):529-533.

4515 Krogh-Jensen M, Ekelund S, Svendsen L. Folate and homocysteine status and haemolysis in patients treated with sulphasalazine for arthritis. *Scand J Clin Lab Invest*, 1996;56(5):421-429.

4516 Logan EC, Williamson LM, Ryrie DR. Sulphasalazine associated pancytopenia may be caused by acute folate deficiency. *Gut*, 1986;27(7):868-872.

4517 Grieco A, Caputo S, Bertoli A, et al. Megaloblastic anemia due to sulphasalazine responding to drug withdrawal alone. *Postgrad Med J*, 1986;62(726):307-308.

4518 Martinez de Haas MG, Poels PJ, de Weert CJ, et al. Subnormal vitamin B6 levels in theophylline users. *Ned Tijdshcr Geneeskd*. 1997;141(45):2176-2179.

4519 Shimizu T, Maeda S, Arakawa H, et al. Relation between theophylline and circulating vitamin levels in children with asthma. *Pharmacology*, 1996;53(6):384-389.

4520 Tanaka I, Ito Y, Hiraga Y, et al. Serum concentrations of the pyridoxal and pyridoxal-5'-phosphate in children during sustained-release theophylline therapy. *Arerugi*, 1996;45(10):1098-105.

4521 Shimizu T, Meada S, Mochizuki H, et al. Theophylline attenuates circulating vitamin B6 levels in children with asthma. *Pharmacology*, 1994;49(6):392-397.

4522 Delport R, Ubbink JB, Serfontein WJ, et al. Vitamin B6 nutritional status in asthma. The effect of theophylline therapy on plasma pyridoxal-5-phosphate and pyridoxal levels. *Int J Vitam Nutr Res*, 1988;58(1):67-72.

4523 Van Wouwe JP. Carnitine deficiency during valproic acid treatment. *Int J Vitam Nutr Res*, 1995;65(3):211-214.

4524 Matsuda I, Ohtani Y, Ninomiya N. Renal handling of carnitine in children with carnitine deficiency and hyperammonemia associated with valproate theapy. *J Pediatr*, 1986;109(1):131-134.

4525 Ohtani Y, Endo F, Matsuda I. Carnitine deficiency and hyperammonemia associated with valproic acid therapy. *J Pediatr*, 1982;101(5):782-785.

4526 Opala G, Winter S, Vance C, et al. The effect of valproic acid on plasma carnitine levels. *Am J Dis Child*, 1991;145(9):999-1001.

4527 Melegh B, Kerner J, Kispal G, et al. Effect of chronic valproic acid treatment on plasma and urine carnitine levels in children: Decreased urinary excretion. *Acta Paediatr Hung* 1987;28(2):137-142.

4528 De Vivo DC, Bohan TP, Coulter DL, et al. L-carnitine supplementation in childhood epilepsy: Current perspectives. *Epilepsia*, 1998;39(11):1216-1225.

4529 Coulter DL. Carnitine, valproate, and toxicity. *J Child Neurol*, 1991;6(1):7-14.

4530 Taliani U, Camellini A, Bernardi P, et al. A clinical case of severe megaloblastic anemia during treatment with primidone. *Acta Biomed Ateneo Parmense*, 1989;60(5-6):245-248.

4531 Segal S, Kaminski S. Drug-nutrient interactions. *American Druggist*, July 1996:42-48.

4532 Glaxo-Wellcome, Inc. Daraprim package insert. Research Triangle Park, NC; August, 1996.

4533 Raskin HN, Fishman RA. Pyridoxine-deficiency neuropathy due to hydralazine. *N Engl J Med*, 1965;273(22):1182-1185.

4534 Seelig MS. Auto-immune complications of D-penicillamine – A possible result of zinc and magnesium depletion and of pyridoxine inactivation. *J Am Coll Nutr*, 1982;1(2):207-214.

4535 Jaffe IA. The antivitamin B6 effect of penicillamine. Clinical and immunological implications. *Adv Biochem Psypharmacol*, 1972;4:217-226.

4536 Lambie DG, Johnson RH. Drugs and folate metabolism. *Drugs*, 1985;30(2):145-155.

4537 Joosten E, Pelemans W. Megaloblastic anaemia in an elderly patient treated with triamterene. *Neth J Med*, 1991; 38(5-6):209-211.

4538 Force RW, Nahata MC. Effect of histamine H2-receptor antagonists on vitamin B12 absorption. *Ann Pharmacother*, 1992;26(10):1283-1286.

4539 Aymard JP, Aymard B, Netter P, et al. Haematological adverse effects of histamine H2-receptor antagonists. *Med Toxicol Adverse Drug Exp*, 1988;3(6):430-448.

4540 Belaiche J, Zittoun J, Marquet J, et al. Effect of ranitidine on secretion of gastric intrinsic factor and absorption of vitamin B12. *Gastroenerol Clin Biol*, 1983;7(4):381-384.

4541 Salom IL, Silvis SE, Doscherholmen A. Effect of cimetidine on the absorption of vitamin B12. *Scand J Gastroenterol*, 1982;17(1):129-131.

4542 Steinberg WM, King CE, Toskes PP. Malabsorption of protein-bound cobalamin, but not unbound cobalamin during cimetidine administration. *Dig Dis Sci*, 1980;25(3):188-191.

4543 Race TF, Paes IC, Faloon WW. Intestinal malabsorption induced by oral colchicine. Comparison with neomycin and cathartic agents. *Am J Med* Sci, 1970;259(1):32-41.

4544 Faloon WW, Chodos RB. Vitamin B12 absorption studies using colchicines, neomycin and continuous 57Co B12 administration. *Gastroenerology*, 1969;56:1251.

4545 Webb DI, Chodos RB, Mahar CQ, et al. Mechanism of vitamin B12 malabsorption in patients receiving colchicine. *N Engl J Med*, 1968;279(16):845-850.

4546 American college of rheumatology ad hoc committee on clinical guidelines. Guidelines for monitoring drug therapy in rheumatoid arthritis. *Arthritis & Rheumatism*, 1996;39(5):723-731.

4547 Hielt K, Brynskov J, Hippe E, et al. Oral contraceptives and the cobalamin (vitamin B12) metabolism. *Acta Obstet Gynecol Scand* 1985;64(1):59-63.

4548 Sanpitak N, Chayutimonkul L. Oral contraceptives and riboflavin nutrition. Lancet 1974;1(7862):836-837.

4562 Andrews R, Greenhaff P, Curtis S, et al. The effect of dietary creatine supplementation on skeletal muscle *Metabolism* in congestive heart failure. *Eur Heart J* 1998;19:617-622.

4563 Gordon A, Hultman E, Kaijser L, et al. Creatine supplementation in chronic heart failure increases skeletal muscle creatine phosphate and muscle performance. *Cardiovasc Res* 1995;30:413-418.

4564 Tarnopolsky M, Martin J. Creatine monohydrate increases strength in patients with neuromuscular disease. *Neurology* 1999;52:854-857.

4565 Tarnopolsky MA, Roy BD, MacDonald JR. A randomized, controlled trial of creatine monohydrate in patients with mitochondrial cytopathies. *Muscle Nerve* 1997;20:1502-1509.

4566 Klivenyi P, Ferrante RJ, Matthews RT, et al. Neuroprotective effects of creatine in a transgenic animal model of amyotrophic lateral sclerosis. *Nat Med* 1999;5:347-350.

4567 Matthews RT, Yang L, Jenkins BG, et al. Neuroprotective effects of creatine and cyclocreatine in animal models of Huntington's disease. *J Neurosci* 1998;18:156-163.

4568 Matthews RT, Ferrante RJ, Klivenyi P, et al. Creatine and cyclocreatine attenuate MPTP neurotoxicity. *Exp Neurol* 1999;157:142-149.

4569 Mihic S, MacDonald JR, McKenzie S, Tarnopolsky MA. Acute creatine loading increases fat-free mass, but does not affect blood pressure, plasma creatinine, or CK activity in men and women. *Med Sci Sports Exerc* 2000;32:291-296.

4570 Rawson ES, Clarkson PM. Acute creatine supplementation in older men. *Int J Sports Med* 2000;21:71-75.

4571 Bermon S, Venembre P, Sachet C, et al. Effects of creatine monohydrate ingestion in sedentary and weight-trained older adults. *Acta Physiol Scand* 1998;164:147-155.

4572 Rawson ES, Wehnert ML, Clarkson PM. Effects of 30 days of creatine ingestion in older men. *Eur J Appl Physiol* 1999;80:139-144.

4573 Earnest CP, Almada AL, Mitchell TL. High-performance capillary electrophoresis-pure creatine monohydrate reduces blood lipids in men and women. *Clin Sci* (Colch) 1996;91:113-118.

4574 Demant TW, Rhodes EC. Effects of creatine supplementation on exercise performance. *Sports Med* 1999;28:49-60.

4575 Williams MH, Branch JD. Creatine supplementation and exercise performance: an update. *J Am Coll Nutr* 1998;17:216-234.

4576 The Physician and Sportsmedicine. "Oral Creatine Supplementation" website: www.physsportsmed.com/issues/1999/05_99/juhn.htm (Accessed 17 March 2000).

4577 Heinanen K, Nanto-Salonen K, Komu M, et al. Creatine corrects muscle 31P spectrum in gyrate atrophy with hyperornithinaemia. *Eur J Clin Invest* 1999;29:1060-1065.

4578 Sipila I, Rapola J, Simell O, Vannas A. Supplementary creatine as a treatment for gyrate atrophy of the choroid and retina. *N Engl J Med* 1981;304:867-870.

4579 Ingwall JS, Morales MF, Stockdale FE, Wildenthal K. Creatine: a possible stimulus skeletal cardiac muscle hypertrophy. *Recent Adv Stud Cardiac Struct Metab* 1975;8:467-481.

4580 Vandenberghe K, Van Hecke P, Van Leemputte M, et al. Phosphocreatine resynthesis is not affected by creatine loading. *Med Sci Sports Exerc* 1999;31:236-242.

4582 Febbraio MA, Flanagan TR, Snow RJ, et al. Effect of creatine supplementation on intramuscular TCr, *Metabolism* and performance during intermittent, supramaximal exercise in humans. *Acta Physiol Scand* 1995;155:387-395.

4583 Harris RC, Soderlund K, Hultman E. Elevation of creatine in resting and exercised muscle of normal subjects by creatine supplementation. *Clin Sci* (Colch) 1992;83:367-374.

4584 Juhn MS, O'Kane JW, Vinci DM. Oral creatine supplementation in male collegiate athletes: a survey of dosing habits and side effects. *J Am Diet Assoc* 1999;99:593-595.

© Copyright 2000, Natural Medicines Comprehensive Database (209) 472-2244. For updated data, go to www.NaturalDatabase.com. • 1253

REFERENCES

REFERENCES

4585 FDA. "Special Nutritionals Adverse Event Monitoring System" website: http://vm.cfsan.fda.gov/cgi-bin/aems.cgi?QUERY=creatine&STYPE=EXACT (Accessed 17 March 2000).

4586 Cisowski M, Bochenek A, Kucewicz E, et al. The use of exogenous creatine phosphate for myocardial protection in patients undergoing coronary artery bypass surgery. *J Cardiovasc Surg* (Torino) 1996;37:75-80.

4587 Chambers DJ, Haire K, Morley N, et al. St. Thomas' Hospital cardioplegia: enhanced protection with exogenous creatine phosphate. *Ann Thorac Surg* 1996;61:67-75.

4588 Francaux M, Poortmans JR. Effects of training and creatine supplement on muscle strength and body mass. *Eur J Appl Physiol* 1999;80:165-168.

4589 Green AL, Hultman E, Macdonald IA, et al. Carbohydrate ingestion augments skeletal muscle creatine accumulation during creatine supplementation in humans. *Am J Physiol* 1996;271:E821-E826.

4591 Balsom PD, Soderlund K, Sjodin B, Ekblom B. Skeletal muscle metabolism during short duration high-intensity exercise: influence of creatine supplementation. *Acta Physiol Scand* 1995;154:303-310.

4592 Birch R, Noble D, Greenhaff PL. The influence of dietary creatine supplementation on performance during repeated bouts of maximal isokinetic cycling in man. *Eur J Appl Physiol* 1994;69:268-276.

4593 Dawson B, Cutler M, Moody A, et al. Effects of oral creatine loading on single and repeated maximal short sprints. *Aust J Sci Med Sport* 1995;27:56-61.

4594 Prevost MC, Nelson AG, Morris GS. Creatine supplementation enhances intermittent work performance. *Res Q Exerc Sport* 1997;68:233-240.

4595 Barnett C, Hinds M, Jenkins DG. Effects of oral creatine supplementation on multiple sprint cycle performance. *Aust J Sci Med Sport* 1996;28:35-39.

4596 Cooke WH, Barnes WS. The influence of recovery duration on high-intensity exercise performance after oral creatine supplementation. *Can J Appl Physiol* 1997;22:454-467.

4597 Vanakoski J, Kosunen V, Meririnne E, Seppala T. Creatine and caffeine in anaerobic and aerobic exercise: effects on physical performance and pharmacokinetic considerations. *Int J Clin Pharmacol Ther* 1998;36:258-262.

4598 Cooke WH, Grandjean PW, Barnes WS. Effect of oral creatine supplementation on power output and fatigue during bicycle ergometry. *J Appl Physiol* 1995;78:670-673.

4599 Odland LM, MacDougall JD, Tarnopolsky MA, et al. Effect of oral creatine supplementation on muscle [PCr] and short-term maximum power output *Med Sci Sports Exerc* 1997;29:216-219.

4600 Snow RJ, McKenna MJ, Selig SE, et al. Effect of creatine supplementation on sprint exercise performance and muscle metabolism. *J Appl Physiol* 1998;84:1667-1673.

4601 Leenders NM, Lamb DR, Nelson TE. Creatine supplementation and swimming performance. *Int J Sport Nutr* 1999;9:251-262.

4602 Jones AM, Atter T, Georg KP. Oral creatine supplementation improves multiple sprint performance in elite ice-hockey players. *J Sports Med Phys Fitness* 1999;39:189-196.

4603 Theodorou AS, Cooke CB, King RF, et al. The effect of longer-term creatine supplementation on elite swimming performance after an acute creatine loading. *J Sports Sci* 1999;17:853-859.

4604 Kamber M, Koster M, Kreis R, et al. Creatine supplementation—part I: performance, clinical chemistry, and muscle volume. *Med Sci Sports Exerc* 1999;31:1763-1769.

4605 McNaughton LR, Dalton B, Tarr J. The effects of creatine supplementation on high-intensity exercise performance in elite performers. *Eur J Appl Physiol* 1998;78:236-240.

4606 McKenna MJ, Morton J, Selig SE, Snow RJ. Creatine supplementation increases muscle total creatine but not maximal intermittent exercise performance. *J Appl Physiol* 1999;87:2244-2252.

4607 Rossiter HB, Cannell ER, Jakeman PM. The effect of oral creatine supplementation on the 1000-m performance of competitive rowers. *J Sports Sci* 1996;14:175-179.

4611 Foster S. Black cohosh (Cimicifuga racemosa): a literature review. *Herbalgram* 1999;45:35-39.

4612 Enzymatic Therapy. "Remifemin" website: http://www.enzy.com/products/individual/eprod141.html (Accesssed 21 March 2000).

4613 Phytopharmica. "Remifemin" website: http://www.phytopharmica.com/consumer/products/1855-BP-remifemin.html (Accesssed 21 March 2000).

4614 Liske E, Wustenberg P. Therapy of climacteric complaints with Cimicifuga racemosa: herbal medicine with clinically proven evidence. *Menopause* 1998;5:250.

4615 Pepping J. Black cohosh: Cimicifuga racemosa. *Am J Health Syst Pharm* 1999;56:1400-1402.

4616 Liske E. Therapeutic efficacy and safety of Cimicifuga racemosa for gynecologic disorders. *Adv Ther* 1998;15:45-53.

4617 Robbers JE, Tyler VE. Tyler's Herbs of Choice: The Therapeutic Use of Phytomedicinals. New York: The Haworth Herbal Press, 1999.

4618 Kruse SO, Lohning A, Pauli GF, et al. Fukiic and piscidic acid esters from the rhizome of Cimicifuga racemosa and the in vitro estrogenic activity of fukinolic acid. *Planta Med* 1999;65:763-764.

4619 Einer-Jensen N, Zhao J, Andersen KP, Kristoffersen K. Cimicifuga and Melbrosia lack oestrogenic effects in mice and rats. *Maturitas* 1996;25:149-153.

4620 Lehmann-Willenbrock E, Riedel HH. [Clinical and endocrinologic studies of the treatment of ovarian insufficiency manifestations following hysterectomy with intact adnexa]. *Zentralbl Gynakol* 1988;110:611-618.

4621 Gruenwald J. Standardized black cohosh (Cimicifuga) extract clinical monograph. *Q Rev Nat Med* 1998;3:117-125.

4622 Huperzine Website. "Huperzine A (Cerebra): Memory and Alertness Enhancing Nutriceutical" website: www.hyperzine.net/about.htm (Accessed 24 March 2000).

4623 Consumer Lab. "Product Review: Glucosamine and Chondroitin" website: http://www.consumerlab.com/results/gluco.html (Accessed 24 March 2000).

4624 Xu SS, Cai ZY, Qu ZW, et al. Huperzine-A in capsules and tablets for treating patients with Alzheimer disease. *Chung Kuo Yao Li Hsueh Pao* 1999;20:486-490.

4625 Camps P, Cusack B, Mallender WD, et al. Huprine X is a novel high-affinity inhibitor of acetylcholinesterase that is of interest for treatment of Alzheimer's disease.

Mol Pharmacol 2000;57:409-417.

4626 Sun QQ, Xu SS, Pan JL, et al. Huperzine-A capsules enhance memory and learning performance in 34 pairs of matched adolescent students. *Chung Kuo Yao Li Hsueh Pao* 1999;20:601-603.

4627 Horwitt MK. My valedictory on the differences in biological potency between RRR-alpha-tocopheryl and all-rac-alpha-tocopheryl acetate. *Am J Clin Nutr* 1999;69:341-342.

4628 Burton GW, Traber MG, Acuff RV, et al. Human plasma and tissue alpha-tocopherol concentrations in response to supplementation with deuterated natural and synthetic vitamin E. *Am J Clin Nutr* 1998;67:669-684.

4629 Cheeseman KH, Holley AE, Kelly FJ, et al. Biokinetics in humans of RRR-alpha-tocopherol: the free phenol, acetate ester, and succinate ester forms of vitamin E. *Free Radic Biol Med* 1995;19:591-598.

4630 Cohn W. Evaluation of vitamin E potency. *Am J Clin Nutr* 1999;69:156-158.

4631 Burton GW, Ingold KU, Traber MG, Kayden HJ. Reply to W Cohn. *Am J Clin Nutr* 1999: 157-158.

4632 Chopra RK, Bhagavan HN. Relative bioavailabilities of natural and synthetic vitamin E formulations containing mixed tocopherols in human subjects. *Int J Vitam Nutr Res* 1999;69:92-95.

4633 Kiyose C, Muramatsu R, Kameyama Y, et al. Biodiscrimination of alpha-tocopherol stereoisomers in humans after oral administration. *Am J Clin Nutr* 1997;65:785-789.

4634 Neunteufl T, Priglinger U, Heher S, et al. Effects of vitamin E on chronic and acute endothelial dysfunction in smokers. *J Am Coll Cardiol* 2000;35:277-283.

4635 Sano M, Ernesto C, Thomas RG, et al. A controlled trial of selegiline, alpha-tocopherol, or both as treatment for Alzheimer's disease. The Alzheimer's Disease Cooperative Study. *N Engl J Med* 1997;336:1216-1222.

4636 Masaki KH, Losonczy KG, Izmirlian G, et al. Association of vitamin E and C supplement use with cognitive function and dementia in elderly men. *Neurology* 2000;54:1265-1272.

4637 Socci DJ, Crandall BM, Arendash GW. Chronic antioxidant treatment improves the cognitive performance of aged rats. *Brain Res* 1995;693:88-94.

4638 Yamada K, Tanaka T, Han D, et al. Protective effects of idebenone and alpha-tocopherol on beta-amyloid-(1-42)-induced learning and memory deficits in rats: implication of oxidative stress in beta-amyloid-induced neurotoxicity in vivo. *Eur J Neurosci* 1999;11:83-90.

4639 Joseph JA, Shukitt-Hale B, Denisova NA, et al. Long-term dietary strawberry, spinach, or vitamin E supplementation retards the onset of age-related neuronal signal-transduction and cognitive behavioral deficits. *J Neurosci* 1998;18:8047-8055.

4640 Nemeth I, Turi S, Haszon I, Bereczki C. Vitamin E alleviates the oxidative stress of erythropoietin in uremic children on hemodialysis. *Pediatr Nephrol* 2000;14:13-17.

4641 Inal M, Kanbak G, Sen S, et al. Antioxidant status and lipid peroxidation in hemodialysis patients undergoing erythropoietin and erythropoietin-vitamin E combined therapy. *Free Radic Res* 1999;31:211-216.

4642 Suthutvoravut U, Hathirat P, Sirichakwal P, et al. Vitamin E status, glutathione peroxidase activity and the effect of vitamin E supplementation in children with thalassemia. *J Med Assoc Thai* 1993;76:146-152.

4643 Hartman TJ, Albanes D, Pietinen P, et al. The association between baseline vitamin E, selenium, and prostate cancer in the alpha-tocopherol, beta-carotene cancer prevention study. *Cancer Epidemiol Biomarkers Prev* 1998;7:335-340.

4644 Deneo-Pellegrini H, De Stefani E, Ronco A, Mendilaharsu M. Foods, nutrients and prostate cancer: a case-control study in Uruguay. *Br J Cancer* 1999;80:591-597.

4645 Kristal AR, Stanford JL, Cohen JH, et al. Vitamin and mineral supplement use is associated with reduced risk of prostate cancer. *Cancer Epidemiol Biomarkers Prev* 1999;8:887-892.

4646 Chan JM, Stampfer MJ, Ma J, et al. Supplemental vitamin E intake and prostate cancer risk in a large cohort of men in the United States. *Cancer Epidemiol Biomarkers Prev* 1999;8:893-899.

4647 Cristol JP, Bosc JY, Badiou S, et al. Erythropoietin and oxidative stress in haemodialysis: beneficial effects of vitamin E supplementation. *Nephrol Dial Transplant* 1997;12:2312-2317.

4648 Zipursky A, Brown EJ, Watts J, et al. Oral vitamin E supplementation for the prevention of anemia in premature infants: a controlled trial. *Pediatrics* 1987;79:61-68.

4649 Ferns G, Williams J, Forster L, et al. Cholesterol standardized plasma vitamin E levels are reduced in patients with severe angina pectoris. *Int J Exp Pathol* 2000;81:57-62.

4650 Motoyama T, Kawano H, Kugiyama K, et al. Vitamin E administration improves impairment of endothelium-dependent vasodilation in patients with coronary spastic angina. *J Am Coll Cardiol* 1998;32:1672-1679.

4651 Rapola JM, Virtamo J, Ripatti S, et al. Effects of alpha tocopherol and beta carotene supplements on symptoms, progression, and prognosis of angina pectoris. *Heart* 1998;79:454-458.

4652 Spencer AP, Carson DS, Crouch MA. Vitamin E and coronary artery disease. *Arch Intern Med* 1999;159:1313-1320.

4653 Mino M. Clinical uses and abuses of vitamin E in children. *Proc Soc Exp Biol Med* 1992;200:266-270.

4654 Phelps DL The role of vitamin E therapy in high-risk neonates. *Clin Perinatol* 1988;15:955-963.

4655 Fish WH, Cohen M, Franzek D, et al. Effect of intramuscular vitamin E on mortality and intracranial hemorrhage in neonates of 1000 grams or less. *Pediatrics* 1990;85:578-584.

4656 Chiswick M, Gladman G, Sinha S, et al. Vitamin E supplementation and periventricular hemorrhage in the newborn. *Am J Clin Nutr* 1991;53:370S-372S.

4657 Watts JL, Milner R, Zipursky A, et al. Failure of supplementation with vitamin E to prevent bronchopulmonary dysplasia in infants less than 1,500 g birth weight. *Eur Respir J* 1991;4:188-190.

4658 Hunter DJ, Manson JE, Colditz GA, et al. A prospective study of the intake of vitamins C, E, and A and the risk of breast cancer. *N Engl J Med* 1993;329:234-240.

4659 Rohan TE, Howe GR, Friedenreich CM, et al. Dietary fiber, vitamins A, C, and E, and risk of breast cancer: a cohort study. *Cancer Causes Control* 1993;4:29-37.

4660 Ernster VL, Goodson WH 3d, Hunt TK, et al. Vitamin E and benign breast "disease": a double-blind, randomized clinical trial. *Surgery* 1985;97:490-494.

4661 Meyer EC, Sommers DK, Reitz CJ, Mentis H. Vitamin E and benign breast disease. *Surgery* 1990 May;107(5):549-51.

REFERENCES

REFERENCES

4662 London RS, Sundaram GS, Murphy L, et al. The effect of vitamin E on mammary dysplasia: a double-blind study. *Obstet Gynecol* 1985;65:104-106.

4663 Leske MC, Chylack LT Jr, He Q, et al. Antioxidant vitamins and nuclear opacities: the longitudinal study of cataract. *Ophthalmology* 1998;105:831-836.

4664 Seddon JM, Christen WG, Manson JE, et al. The use of vitamin supplements and the risk of cataract among US male physicians. *Am J Public Health* 1994;84:788-792.

4665 Tavani A, Negri E, La Vecchia C. Food and nutrient intake and risk of cataract. *Ann Epidemiol* 1996;6:41-46.

4666 Teikari JM, Rautalahti M, Haukka J, et al. Incidence of cataract operations in Finnish male smokers unaffected by alpha tocopherol or beta carotene supplements. *J Epidemiol Community Health* 1998;52:468-472.

4667 Teikari JM, Laatikainen L, Virtamo J, et al. Six-year supplementation with alpha-tocopherol and beta-carotene and age-related maculopathy. *Acta Ophthalmol Scand* 1998;76:224-229.

4668 Ludwig CU, Stoll HR, Obrist R, Obrecht JP. Prevention of cytotoxic drug induced skin ulcers with dimethyl sulfoxide (DMSO) and alpha-tocopherol. *Eur J Cancer Clin Oncol* 1987;23:327-329.

4669 Lucero MJ, Vigo J, Rabasco AM, et al. Protection by alpha-tocopherol against skin necrosis induced by doxorubicin hydrochloride. *Pharmazie* 1993;48:772-775.

4670 Raju GB, Behari M, Prasad K, Ahuja GK. Randomized, double-blind, placebo-controlled, clinical trial of D-alpha-tocopherol (vitamin E) as add-on therapy in uncontrolled epilepsy. *Epilepsia* 1994;35:368-372.

4671 Ogunmekan AO, Hwang PA. A randomized, double-blind, placebo-controlled, clinical trial of D-alpha-tocopheryl acetate (vitamin E), as add-on therapy, for epilepsy in children. *Epilepsia* 1989;30:84-89.

4672 Delanian S, Balla-Mekias S, Lefaix JL. Striking regression of chronic radiotherapy damage in a clinical trial of combined pentoxifylline and tocopherol. *J Clin Oncol* 1999;17:3283-3290.

4673 Delanian S. Striking regression of radiation-induced fibrosis by a combination of pentoxifylline and tocopherol. *Br J Radiol* 1998;71:892-894.

4674 Lefaix JL, Delanian S, Vozenin MC, et al. Striking regression of subcutaneous fibrosis induced by high doses of gamma rays using a combination of pentoxifylline and alpha-tocopherol: an experimental study. *Int J Radiat Oncol Biol Phys* 1999;43:839-847.

4675 Tahzib M, Frank R, Gauthier B, et al. Vitamin E treatment of focal segmental glomerulosclerosis: results of an open-label study. *Pediatr Nephrol* 1999;13:649-652.

4676 Varis K, Taylor PR, Sipponen P, et al. Gastric cancer and premalignant lesions in atrophic gastritis: a controlled trial on the effect of supplementation with alpha-tocopherol and beta-carotene. The Helsinki Gastritis Study Group. *Scand J Gastroenterol* 1998;33:294-300.

4677 Bukin YV, Draudin-Krylenko VA, Kuvshinov YP, et al. Decrease of ornithine decarboxylase activity in premalignant gastric mucosa and regression of small intestinal metaplasia in patients supplemented with high doses of vitamin E. *Cancer Epidemiol Biomarkers Prev* 1997;6:543-546.

4678 Dawsey SM, Wang GQ, Taylor PR, et al. Effects of vitamin/mineral supplementation on the prevalence of histological dysplasia and early cancer of the esophagus and stomach: results from the Dysplasia Trial in Linxian, China. *Cancer Epidemiol Biomarkers Prev* 1994;3:167-172.

4679 Wang GQ, Dawsey SM, Li JY, et al. Effects of vitamin/mineral supplementation on the prevalence of histological dysplasia and early cof the esophagus and stomach: results from the General Population Trial in Linxian, China. *Cancer Epidemiol Biomarkers Prev* 1994;3:161-166.

4681 Goldstein RK, Zillikens D, Miller K, Elsner P, Burg G. Local treatment of disseminated granuloma anulare with a vitamin E emulsion. *Hautarzt* 1991;42:176-178.

4682 Eldamhougy S, Elhelw Z, Yamamah G, et al. The vitamin E status among glucose-6 phosphate dehydrogenase deficient patients and effectiveness of oral vitamin E. *Int J Vitam Nutr Res* 1988;58:184-188.

4683 Hafez M, Amar ES, Zedan M, et al. Improved erythrocyte survival with combined vitamin E and selenium therapy in children with glucose-6-phosphate dehydrogenase deficiency and mild chronic hemolysis. *J Pediatr* 1986;108:558-561.

4684 Johnson GJ, Vatassery GT, Finkel B, Allen DW. High-dose vitamin E does not decrease the rate of chronic hemolysis in glucose-6-phosphate dehydrogenase deficiency. *N Engl J Med* 1983;308:1014-1017.

4685 Chan AC, Chow CK, Chiu D. Interaction of antioxidants and their implication in genetic anemia. *Proc Soc Exp Biol Med* 1999;222:274-282.

4686 Peyser CE, Folstein M, Chase GA, et al. Trial of d-alpha-tocopherol in Huntington's disease. *Am J Psychiatry* 1995;152:1771-1775.

4687 Meydani SN, Meydani M, Blumberg JB, et al. Vitamin E supplementation and in vivo immune response in healthy elderly subjects. A randomized controlled trial. *JAMA* 1997;277:1380-1386.

4688 Ravaglia G, Forti P, Maioli F, et al. Effect of micronutrient status on natural killer cell immune function in healthy free-living subjects aged >/=90 y. *Am J Clin Nutr* 2000;71:590-598.

4689 Pallast EG, Schouten EG, de Waart FG, et al. Effect of 50- and 100-mg vitamin E supplements on cellular immune function in noninstitutionalized elderly persons. *Am J Clin Nutr* 1999;69:1273-1281.

4690 de la Fuente M, Ferrandez MD, Burgos MS, et al. Immune function in aged women is improved by ingestion of vitamins C and E. *Can J Physiol Pharmacol* 1998;76:373-380.

4691 Buzina-Suboticanec K, Buzina R, Stavljenic A, et al. Aging, nutritional status and immune response. *Int J Vitam Nutr Res* 1998;68:133-141.

4692 De Waart FG, Portengen L, Doekes G, et al. Effect of 3 months vitamin E supplementation on indices of the cellular and humoral immune response in elderly subjects. *Br J Nutr* 1997;78:761-774.

4693 Kessopoulou E, Powers HJ, Sharma KK, et al. A double-blind randomized placebo cross-over controlled trial using the antioxidant vitamin E to treat reactive oxygen species associated male infertility. *Fertil Steril* 1995;64:825-831.

4694 Kodama H, Yamaguchi R, Fukuda J, et al. Increased oxidative deoxyribonucleic acid damage in the spermatozoa of infertile male patients. *Fertil Steril* 1997;68:519-524.

4695 Suleiman SA, Ali ME, Zaki ZM, et al. Lipid peroxidation and human sperm motility: protective role of vitamin E. *J Androl* 1996;17:530-537.

4696 Rolf C, Cooper TG, Yeung CH, Nieschlag E.

Antioxidant treatment of patients with asthenozoospermia or moderate oligoasthenozoospermia with high-dose vitamin C and vitamin E: a randomized, placebo-controlled, double-blind study. *Hum Reprod* 1999;14:1028-1033.

4697 Yau TM, Weisel RD, Mickle DA, et al. Vitamin E for coronary bypass operations. A prospective, double-blind, randomized trial. *J Thorac Cardiovasc Surg* 1994;108:302-310.

4698 Westhuyzen J, Cochrane AD, Tesar PJ, et al. Effect of preoperative supplementation with alpha-tocopherol and ascorbic acid on myocardial injury in patients undergoing cardiac operations. *J Thorac Cardiovasc Surg* 1997;113:942-948.

4699 Sisto T, Paajanen H, Metsa-Ketela T, et al. Pretreatment with antioxidants and allopurinol diminishes cardiac onset events in coronary artery bypass grafting. *Ann Thorac Surg* 1995;59:1519-1523.

4700 Riley JD, Antony SJ. Leg cramps: differential diagnosis and management. *Am Fam Physician* 1995;52:1794-1798.

4701 Roca AO, Jarjoura D, Blend D, et al. Dialysis leg cramps. Efficacy of quinine versus vitamin E. *ASAIO J* 1992;38:M481-485.

4702 Connolly PS, Shirley EA, Wasson JH, Nierenberg DW. Treatment of nocturnal leg cramps. A crossover trial of quinine vs vitamin E. *Arch Intern Med* 1992;152:1877-1880.

4703 Fenichel GM, Brooke MH, Griggs RC, et al. Clinical investigation in Duchenne muscular dystrophy: penicillamine and vitamin E. *Muscle Nerve* 1988;11:1164-1118.

4704 Orndahl G, Grimby G, Grimby A, et al. Functional deterioration and selenium-vitamin E treatment in myotonic dystrophy. A placebo-controlled study. *J Intern Med* 1994;235:205-210.

4705 Watanabe H, Kakihana M, Ohtsuka S, Sugishita Y. Randomized, double-blind, placebo-controlled study of supplemental vitamin E on attenuation of the development of nitrate tolerance. *Circulation* 1997;96:2545-2550.

4706 Honegger UE, Scuntaro I, Wiesmann UN. Vitamin E reduces accumulation of amiodarone and desethylamiodarone and inhibits phospholipidosis in cultured human cells. *Biochem Pharmacol* 1995;49:1741-1745.

4707 Kachel DL, Moyer TP, Martin WJ 2d. Amiodarone-induced injury of human pulmonary artery endothelial cells: protection by alpha-tocopherol. *J Pharmacol Exp Ther* 1990;254:1107-1112.

4708 Benner SE, Winn RJ, Lippman SM, et al. Regression of oral leukoplakia with alpha-tocopherol: a community clinical oncology program chemoprevention study. *J Natl Cancer Inst* 1993;85:44-47.

4709 The Parkinson Study Group. Effects of tocopherol and deprenyl on the progression of disability in early Parkinson's disease. *N Engl J Med* 1993;328:176-183.

4710 Kieburtz K, McDermott M, Como P, et al. The effect of deprenyl and tocopherol on cognitive performance in early untreated Parkinson's disease. Parkinson Study Group. *Neurology* 1994;44:1756-1759.

4711 Parkinson Study Group. Impact of deprenyl and tocopherol treatment on Parkinson's disease in DATATOP patients requiring levodopa. *Ann Neurol* 1996;39:37-45.

4712 de Rijk MC, Breteler MM, den Breeijen JH, et al. Dietary antioxidants and Parkinson disease. The Rotterdam Study. *Arch Neurol* 1997;54:762-765.

4713 Dreher F, Gabard B, Schwindt DA, Maibach HI. Topical melatonin in combination with vitamins E and C protects skin from ultraviolet-induced erythema: a human study in vivo. *Br J Dermatol* 1998;139:332-339.

4714 Dreher F, Denig N, Gabard B, et al. Effect of topical antioxidants on UV-induced erythema formation when administered after exposure. *Dermatology* 1999;198:52-55.

4715 Fuchs J, Kern H. Modulation of UV-light-induced skin inflammation by D-alpha-tocopherol and L-ascorbic acid: a clinical study using solar simulated radiation. *Free Radic Biol Med* 1998;25:1006-1012.

4716 Eberlein-Konig B, Placzek M, Przybilla B. Protective effect against sunburn of combined systemic ascorbic acid (vitamin C) and d-alpha-tocopherol (vitamin E). *J Am Acad Dermatol* 1998;38:45-48.

4717 Werninghaus K, Meydani M, Bhawan J, et al. Evaluation of the photoprotective effect of oral vitamin E supplementation. *Arch Dermatol* 1994;130:1257-1261.

4718 Gulmezoglu AM, Hofmeyr GJ, Oosthuisen MM. Antioxidants in the treatment of severe pre-eclampsia: an explanatory randomised controlled trial. *Br J Obstet Gynaecol* 1997;104:689-696.

4719 London RS, Murphy L, Kitlowski KE, Reynolds MA. Efficacy of alpha-tocopherol in the treatment of the premenstrual syndrome. *J Reprod Med* 1987;32:400-404.

4720 London RS, Sundaram GS, Murphy L, Goldstein PJ. The effect of alpha-tocopherol on premenstrual symptomatology: a double-blind study. *J Am Coll Nutr* 1983;2:115-122.

4721 Baumann LS, Spencer JS. The Effects of Topical Vitamin E on the Cosmetic Appearance of Scars. *Dermatol Surg* 1999;25:311-315.

4722 Jenkins M, Alexander JW, MacMillan BG, et al. Failure of topical steroids and vitamin E to reduce postoperative scar formation following reconstructive surgery. *J Burn Care Rehabil* 1986;7:309-312.

4723 Edmonds SE, Winyard PG, Guo R, et al. Putative analgesic activity of repeated oral doses of vitamin E in the treatment of rheumatoid arthritis. Results of a prospective placebo controlled double blind trial. *Ann Rheum Dis* 1997;56:649-655.

4724 Tutuncu NB, Bayraktar M, Varli K. Reversal of defective nerve conduction with vitamin E supplementation in type 2 diabetes: a preliminary study. *Diabetes Care* 1998;21:1915-1918.

4725 Bursell SE, Clermont AC, Aiello LP, et al. High-dose vitamin E supplementation normalizes retinal blood flow and creatinine clearance in patients with type 1 diabetes. *Diabetes Care* 1999;22:1245-1251.

4726 Paolisso G, D'Amore A, Giugliano D, et al. Pharmacologic doses of vitamin E improve insulin action in healthy subjects and non-insulin-dependent diabetic patients. *Am J Clin Nutr* 1993;57:650-656.

4727 Paolisso G, Di Maro G, Galzerano D, et al. Pharmacological doses of vitamin E and insulin action in elderly subjects. *Am J Clin Nutr* 1994;59:1291-1296.

4728 McBride JM, Kraemer WJ, Triplett-McBride T, Sebastianelli W. Effect of resistance exercise on free radical production. *Med Sci Sports Exerc* 1998;30:67-72.

4729 National Academy of Science, Institute of Medicine.

© Copyright 2000, Natural Medicines Comprehensive Database (209) 472-2244. For updated data, go to www.NaturalDatabase.com. • 1257

R
E
F
E
R
E
N
C
E
S

"Dietary Reference Intakes for Vitamin C, Vitamin E, Selenium, and Carotenoids." http://www4.nas.edu/iom/iomhome.nsf/Pages/Recently+Released+Reports (Accessed 20 April 2000).

4730 van Rooij J, Schwartzenberg SG, Mulder PG, Baarsma SG. Oral vitamins C and E as additional treatment in patients with acute anterior uveitis: a randomised double masked study in 145 patients. *Br J Ophthalmol* 1999;83:1277-1282.

4731 Leppala JM, Virtamo J, Fogelholm R, et al. Controlled trial of alpha-tocopherol and beta-carotene supplements on stroke incidence and mortality in male smokers. *Arterioscler Thromb Vasc Biol* 2000;20:230-235.

4732 Tornwall ME, Virtamo J, Haukka JK, et al. The effect of alpha-tocopherol and beta-carotene supplementation on symptoms and progression of intermittent claudication in a controlled trial. *Atherosclerosis* 1999;147:193-197.

4733 Liede KE, Haukka JK, Saxen LM, Heinonen OP. Increased tendency towards gingival bleeding caused by joint effect of alpha-tocopherol supplementation and acetylsalicylic acid. *Ann Med* 1998;30:542-546.

4734 ARS-GRIN. "Herbalist's Desk Reference (HDR)" URL: www.ars-grin.gov (Accessed 25 April 2000).

4735 Setchell KD, Gosselin SJ, Welsh MB, et al. Dietary estrogens—a probable cause of infertility and *Liver* disease in captive cheetahs. *Gastroenterology* 1987;93:225-233.

4736 Evans AM. Influence of dietary components on the gastrointestinal metabolism and transport of drugs. *Ther Drug Monit* 2000;22:131-136.

4737 Anon. Phytoestrogens. *Med Letter* 2000;42:17-18.

4738 Hodgson JM, Puddey IB, Beilin LJ, et al. Supplementation with isoflavonoid phytoestrogens does not alter serum lipid concentrations: a randomized controlled trial in humans. *J Nutr* 1998;128:728-732.

4739 Hodgson JM, Puddey IB, Beilin LJ, et al. Effects of isoflavonoids on blood pressure in subjects with high-normal ambulatory blood pressure levels: a randomized controlled trial. *Am J Hypertens* 1999;12:47-53.

4740 Yanagihara K, Ito A, Toge T, Numoto M. Antiproliferative effects of isoflavones on human *Cancer* cell lines established from the gastrointestinal tract. *Br J Nutr* 1993;53:5815-5821.

4741 Le Bail JC, Champavier Y, Chulia AJ, Habrioux G. Effects of phytoestrogens on aromatase, 3beta and 17beta-hydroxysteroid dehydrogenase activities and human breast cancer cells. *Life Sci* 2000;66:1281-1291.

4742 Cassady JM, Zennie TM, Chae YH, et al. Use of a mammalian cell culture benzo(a)pyrene metabolism assay for the detection of potential anticarcinogens from natural products: inhibition of metabolism by biochanin A, an isoflavone from Trifolium pratense L. *Br J Nutr* 1988;48:6257-6261.

4743 Kurzer MS, Xu X. Dietary phytoestrogens. Annu Rev Nutr 1997;17:353-381.

4744 ARS-GRIN. Dr. Duke's Phytochemical and Ethnobotanical Databases URL: www.ars-grin.gov (Accessed 24 April 2000).

4745 Absolute Truth Hardcore Bodybuilding. "Ipriflavone" website: http://members.tripod.com/~absolutetruth/index2.htm (Accessed 26 April 2000).

4746 Gambacciani M, Cappagli B, Piaggesi L, et al. Ipriflavone prevents the loss of bone mass in pharmacological menopause induced by GnRH-agonists. *Calcif Tissue Int* 1997;61:S15-S18.

4747 Yamazaki I, Shino A, Shimizu Y, et al. Effect of ipriflavone on glucocorticoid-induced osteoporosis in rats. *Life Sci* 1986;38:951-958.

4748 Cecchettin M, Bellometti S, Cremonesi G, et al. Metabolic and bone effects after administration of ipriflavone and salmon calcitonin in postmenopausal osteoporosis. *Biomed Pharmacother* 1995;49:465-468.

4749 Nozaki M, Hashimoto K, Inoue Y, et al. Treatment of bone loss in oophorectomized women with a combination of ipriflavone and conjugated equine estrogen. *Int J Gynaecol Obstet* 1998;62:69-75.

4750 Xu X, Wang HJ, Murphy PA, Hendrich S. Neither background diet nor type of soy food affects short-term isoflavone bioavailability in women. *J Nutr* 2000;130:798-801.

4751 Scambia G, Mango D, Signorile PG, et al. Clinical effects of a standardized soy extract in postmenopausal women: a pilot study. *Menopause* 2000;7:105-111.

4752 Albertazzi P, Pansini F, Bottazzi M, et al. Dietary soy supplementation and phytoestrogen levels. *Obstet Gynecol* 1999;94:229-231.

4753 Kurzer MS, Xu X. Dietary phytoestrogens. *Annu Rev Nutr* 1997;17:353-381.

4754 Jenkins DJ, Kendall CW, Garsetti M, et al. Effect of soy protein foods on low-density lipoprotein oxidation and ex vivo sex hormone receptor activity--a controlled crossover trial. *Metabolism* 2000;49:537-543.

4755 Sirtori CR, Pazzucconi F, Colombo L, et al. Double-blind study of the addition of high-protein soya milk v. cows' milk to the diet of patients with severe hypercholesterolemia and resistance to or intolerance of statins. *Br J Nutr* 1999;82:91-96.

4756 Maugeri D, Panebianco P, Russo MS, et al. Ipriflavone-treatment of senile osteoporosis: results of a multicenter, double-blind clinical trial of 2 years. *Arch Gerontol Geriatr* 1994;19:253-263.

4757 Scali G, Mansanti P, Zurlo A, et al. Analgesic effect of ipriflavone versus sCalcitonin in the treatment of osteoporotic vertebral pain. *Curr Ther Res* 1991;49:1004-1010.

4759 Mares-Perlman JA, Brady WE, Klein BE, et al. Serum carotenoids and tocopherols and severity of nuclear and cortical opacities. *Invest Ophthalmol Vis Sci* 1995;36:276-288.

4760 MotherNature.Com. "The Consumer Guide to Garlic" and "Garlic" website: www.mothernature.com (Accessed 4 May 2000).

4761 Graham DY, Anderson SY, Lang T. Garlic or jalapeno peppers for treatment of Helicobacter pylori infection. *Am J Gastroenterol* 1999;94:1200-2.

4762 Ernst E. Is garlic an effective treatment for Helicobacter pylori infection? *Arch Intern Med* 1999;159:2484-5.

4763 Aydin A, Ersoz G, Tekesin O, et al. Garlic oil and Helicobacter pylori infection. *Am J Gastroenterol* 2000;95:563-4.

4764 O'Gara EA, Hill DJ, Maslin DJ. Activities of Garlic Oil, Garlic Powder, and Their Diallyl Constituents against Helicobacter pylori. *Appl Environ Microbiol* 2000;66:2269-73.

4765 Calvet X, Carod C, Gene E. Re: Peppers at treatment for Helicobacter pylori infection. *Am J Gastroenterol* 2000;95:820-1.

4766 Ledezma E, DeSousa L, Jorquera A, et al. Efficacy of ajoene, an organosulphur derived from garlic, in the short-term therapy of tinea pedis. *Mycoses* 1996;39:393-5.

4767 Ledezma E, Lopez JC, Marin P, et al. Ajoene in the

topical short-term treatment of tinea cruris and tinea corporis in humans. Randomized comparative study with terbinafine. *Arzneimittelforschung* 1999;49:544-7.

4768 Ankri S, Mirelman D. Antimicrobial properties of allicin from garlic. *Microbes Infect* 1999;1:125-9.

4769 Weber ND, Andersen DO, North JA, et al. In vitro virucidal effects of Allium sativum (garlic) extract and compounds. *Planta Med* 1992;58:417-23.

4770 Steinmetz KA, Kushi LH, Bostick RM, et al. Vegetables, fruit, and colon cancer in the Iowa Women's Health Study. *Am J Epidemiol* 1994;139:1-15.

4771 Witte JS, Longnecker MP, Bird CL, et al Relation of vegetable, fruit, and grain consumption to colorectal adenomatous polyps. *Am J Epidemiol* 1996;144:1015-25.

4772 Le Marchand L, Hankin JH, Wilkens LR, et al. Dietary fiber and colorectal cancer risk. *Epidemiology* 1997;8:658-65.

4773 Dorant E, van den Brandt PA, Goldbohm RA. A prospective cohort study on the relationship between onion and leek consumption, garlic supplement use and the risk of colorectal carcinoma in The Netherlands. *Carcinogenesis* 1996;17:477-84.

4774 You WC, Zhang L, Gail MH, et al. Helicobacter pylori infection, garlic intake and precancerous lesions in a Chinese population at low risk of gastric cancer. *Int J Epidemiol* 1998;27:941-4.

4775 You WC, Blot WJ, Chang YS, et al. Allium vegetables and reduced risk of stomach cancer. *J Natl Cancer Inst* 1989;81:162-4.

4776 Takezaki T, Gao CM, Ding JH, et al. Comparative study of lifestyles of residents in high and low risk areas for gastric Cancer in Jiangsu Province, China; with special reference to allium vegetables. *J Epidemiol* 1999;9:297-305.

4777 Key TJ, Silcocks PB, Davey GK, et al. A case-control study of diet and prostate cancer. *Br J Cancer* 1997;76:678-87.

4778 Dorant E, van den Brandt PA, Goldbohm RA. A prospective cohort study on Allium vegetable consumption, garlic supplement use, and the risk of lung carcinoma in The Netherlands. *Br J Nutr* 1994;54:6148-53.

4779 Dorant E, van den Brandt PA, Goldbohm RA. Allium vegetable consumption, garlic supplement intake, and female breast carcinoma incidence. *Breast Br J Nutr Treat* 1995;33:163-70.

4780 Mostafa MG, Mima T, Ohnishi ST, Mori K. S-allylcysteine ameliorates doxorubicin toxicity in the heart and liver in mice. *Planta Med* 2000;66:148-51.

4781 Ali M, Thomson M. Consumption of a garlic clove a day could be beneficial in preventing thrombosis. *Prostaglandins Leukot Essent Fatty Acids* 1995;53:211-2.

4782 Holzgartner H, Schmidt U, Kuhn U. Comparison of the efficacy and tolerance of a garlic preparation vs. bezafibrate. *Arzneimittelforschung* 1992;42:1473-7.

4783 Jain AK, Vargas R, Gotzkowsky S, McMahon FG. Can garlic reduce levels of serum lipids? A controlled clinical study. *Am J Med* 1993;94:632-35.

4784 Mader FH. Treatment of hyperlipidaemia with garlic-powder tablets. Evidence from the German Association of General Practitioners' multicentric placebo-controlled double-blind study. *Arzneimittelforschung* 1990;40:1111-6.

4785 Rotzsch W, Richter V, Rassoul F, Walper A.

[Postprandial lipemia under treatment with Allium sativum. Controlled double-blind study of subjects with reduced HDL2-cholesterol]. [Article in German] *Arzneimittelforschung* 1992;42:1223-7.

4786 Silagy C, Neil A. Garlic as a lipid lowering agent--a meta-analysis. *J R Coll Physicians Lond* 1994;28:39-45.

4787 Vorberg G, Schneider B. Therapy with garlic: results of a placebo-controlled, double-blind study. *Br J Clin Pract Symp Suppl* 1990;69:7-11.

4788 Warshafsky S, Kamer RS, Sivak SL. Effect of garlic on total serum cholesterol. A meta-analysis. *Ann Intern Med* 1993;119:599-605.

4789 Adler AJ, Holub BJ. Effect of garlic and fish-oil supplementation on serum lipid and lipoprotein concentrations in hypercholesterolemic men. *Am J Clin Nutr* 1997;65:445-50.

4790 Morcos NC. Modulation of lipid profile by fish oil and garlic combination. *J Natl Med Assoc* 1997;89:673-8.

4791 Kenzelmann R, Kade F. Limitation of the deterioration of lipid parameters by a standardized garlic-ginkgo combination product. A multicenter placebo-controlled double-blind study. *Arzneimittelforschung* 1993;43:978-81.

4792 Superko HR, Krauss RM. Garlic powder, effect on plasma lipids, postprandial lipemia, low-density lipoprotein particle size, high-density lipoprotein subclass distribution and lipoprotein(a). *J Am Coll Cardiol* 2000;35:321-6.

4793 Simons LA, Balasubramaniam S, von Konigsmark M, et al. On the effect of garlic on plasma lipids and lipoproteins in mild hypercholesterolaemia. *Atherosclerosis* 1995;113:219-25.

4794 Luley C, Lehmann-Leo W, Moller B, et al. Lack of efficacy of dried garlic in patients with hyperlipoproteinemia. *Arzneimittelforschung* 1986;36:766-8.

4795 Neil HA, Silagy CA, Lancaster T, et al. Garlic powder in the treatment of moderate hyperlipidaemia: a controlled trial and meta-analysis. *J R Coll Physicians Lond* 1996;30:329-34.

4796 McCrindle BW, Helden E, Conner WT. Garlic extract therapy in children with hypercholesterolemia. *Arch Pediatr Adolesc Med* 1998;152:1089-94.

4797 Breithaupt-Grogler K, Ling M, Boudoulas H, Belz GG. Protective effect of chronic garlic intake on elastic properties of aorta in the elderly. *Circulation* 1997;96:2649-55.

4798 Koscielny J, Klussendorf D, Latza R, et al. The antiatherosclerotic effect of Allium sativum. *Atherosclerosis* 1999;144:237-49.

4799 Chutani SK, Bordia A. The effect of fried versus raw garlic on fibrinolytic activity in man. *Atherosclerosis* 1981;38:417-21.

4800 Blumenthal M, Goldberg A, Brinckmann J (eds). Herbal Medicine Expanded Commission E Monographs. Newton, MA: Integrative Medicine Communications, 2000.

4801 Kiesewetter H, Jung F, Jung EM, et al. Effects of garlic coated tablets in peripheral arterial occlusive disease. *Clin Investig* 1993;71:383-6.

4802 Kiesewetter H, Jung F, Jung EM, et al. Effect of garlic on platelet aggregation in patients with increased risk of juvenile ischaemic attack. *Eur J Clin Pharmacol* 1993;45:333-6.

4803 Legnani C, Frascaro M, Guazzaloca G, et al. Effects of a dried garlic preparation on fibrinolysis and platelet

REFERENCES

aggregation in healthy subjects. *Arzneimittelforschung* 1993;43:119-22.

4804 Ali M, Bordia T, Mustafa T. Effect of raw versus boiled aqueous extract of garlic and onion on platelet aggregation. *Prostaglandins Leukot Essent Fatty Acids* 1999;60:43-7.

4805 Morris J, Burke V, Mori TA, et al. Effects of garlic extract on platelet aggregation: a randomized placebo-controlled double-blind study. *Clin Exp Pharmacol Physiol* 1995;22:414-7.

4806 Kiesewetter H, Jung F, Pindur G, et al. Effect of garlic on thrombocyte aggregation, microcirculation, and other risk factors. *Int J Clin Pharmacol Ther Toxicol* 1991;29:151-5.

4807 Arora RC, Arora S. Comparative effect of clofibrate, garlic and onion on alimentary hyperlipemia. *Atherosclerosis* 1981;39:447-52.

4808 Sasaki J, Kita T, Ishita K, et al. Antibacterial activity of garlic powder against Escherichia coli O-157. *J Nutr Sci Vitaminol* (Tokyo) 1999;45:785-90.

4809 Jepson RG, Kleijnen J, Leng GC. Garlic for peripheral arterial occlusive disease (Cochrane Review). In: The Cochrane Library, Issue 2, 2000. Oxford: Update Software.

4810 Gebhardt R, Beck H. Differential inhibitory effects of garlic-derived organosulfur compounds on cholesterol biosynthesis in primary rat hepatocyte cultures. *Lipids* 1996;31:1269-76.

4811 Qureshi AA, Din ZZ, Abuirmeileh N, et al. Suppression of avian hepatic lipid metabolism by solvent extracts of garlic: impact on serum lipids. *J Nutr* 1983;113:1746-55.

4812 Pedraza-Chaverri J, Tapia E, Medina-Campos ON, et al. Garlic prevents hypertension induced by chronic inhibition of nitric oxide synthesis. *Life Sci* 1998;62:71-7.

4813 Dirsch VM, Kiemer AK, Wagner H, Vollmar AM. Effect of allicin and ajoene, two compounds of garlic, on inducible nitric oxide synthase. *Atherosclerosis* 1998;139:333-9.

4815 Ip C, Lisk DJ. Efficacy of cancer prevention by high-selenium garlic is primarily dependent on the action of selenium. *Carcinogenesis* 1995;16:2649-52.

4816 Anibarro B, Fontela JL, De La Hoz F. Occupational asthma induced by garlic dust. *J Allergy Clin Immunol* 1997;100:734-8.

4817 Zema MJ. Gemfibrozil, nicotinic acid and combination therapy in patients with isolated hypoalphalipoproteinemia: a randomized, open-label, crossover study. *J Am Coll Cardiol* 2000;35:640-6.

4818 Guyton JR, Blazing MA, Hagar J, et al. Extended-release niacin vs gemfibrozil for the treatment of low levels of high-density lipoprotein cholesterol. Niaspan-Gemfibrozil Study Group. *Arch Intern Med* 2000;160:1177-84.

4819 Alberts DS, Martinez ME, Roe DJ, et al. Lack of effect of a high-fiber cereal supplement on the recurrence of colorectal adenomas. Phoenix Colon cancer Prevention Physicians' Network. *N Engl J Med* 2000;342:1156-1162.

4820 Schatzkin A, Lanza E, Corle D, et al. Lack of effect of a low-fat, high-fiber diet on the recurrence of colorectal adenomas. Polyp Prevention Trial Study Group. *N Engl J Med* 2000;342:1149-1155.

4821 Fuchs CS, Giovannucci EL, Colditz GA, et al. Dietary fiber and the risk of colorectal cancer and adenoma in women. *N Engl J Med* 1999;340:169-176.

4822 Iso H, Stampfer MJ, Manson JE, et al. Prospective study of calcium, potassium, and magnesium intake and risk of stroke in women. *Stroke* 1999;30:1772-1779.

4823 Cueto-Manzano AM, Konel S, Freemont AJ, et al. Effect of 1,25-dihydroxyvitamin D3 and calcium carbonate on bone loss associated with long-term renal transplantation. *Am J Kidney Dis* 2000;35:227-236.

4824 Zittermann A, Bock P, Drummer C, et al. Lactose does not enhance calcium bioavailability in lactose-tolerant, healthy adults. *Am J Clin Nutr* 2000;71:931-936.

4825 Chan JM, Giovannucci E, Andersson SO, et al. Dairy products, calcium, phosphorous, vitamin D, and risk of prostate cancer. *Cancer Causes Control* 1998;9:559-566.

4826 Bounous G, et al. "Whey proteins as a food supplement in HIV-seropositive individuals." *Clin Invest Med*, 1993; 16(3): 204-09.

4827 Harvard School of Public Health Press Releases. "Higher Intake of Dairy Products May Be Linked to prostate cancer Risk" website: www.hsph.harvard.edu/ press/releases/press04042000.html. (Accessed 5 May 2000).

4828 Mennella JA, Johnson A, Beauchamp GK. Garlic ingestion by pregnant women alters the odor of amniotic fluid. *Chem Senses* 1995;20:207-9

4829 Mennella JA, Beauchamp GK. Maternal diet alters the sensory qualities of human milk and the nursling's behavior. *Pediatrics* 1991;88:737-44.

4830 Mennella JA, Beauchamp GK. The effects of repeated exposure to garlic-flavored milk on the nursling's behavior. *Pediatr Res* 1993;34:805-8.

4831 Lee JH, Kang HS, Roh J. Protective effects of garlic juice against embryotoxicity of methylmercuric chloride administered to pregnant Fischer 344 rats. *Yonsei Med J* 1999;40:483-9.

4832 Cronin E. Dermatitis of the hands in caterers. *Contact Dermatitis* 1987;17:265-269.

4833 Lee TY, Lam TH. Contact Dermatitis due to topical treatment with garlic in Hong Kong. *Contact Dermatitis* 1991;24:193-6.

4834 Barton DL, Loprinzi CL, Quella SK, et al. Prospective evaluation of vitamin E for hot flashes in breast cancer survivors. *J Clin Oncol*, 1998;16:495-500.

4835 Raal FJ, Pilcher GJ, Veller MG, et al. Efficacy of vitamin E compared with either simvastatin or atorvastatin in preventing the progression of Atherosclerosis in homozygous familial hypercholesterolemia. *Am J Cardiol* 1999;84:1344-1346.

4836 Jha P, Flather M, Lonn E, et al. The antioxidant vitamins and cardiovascular disease. A critical review of epidemiologic and clinical trial data. *Ann Intern Med* 1995;123:860-872.

4837 Steinberg D. Clinical trials of antioxidants in Atherosclerosis: are we doing the right thing? *Lancet* 1995;346:36-38.

4838 Vera JC, Rivas CI, Zhang RH, et al. Human HL-60 myeloid leukemia cells transport dehydroascorbic acid via the glucose transporters and accumulate reduced ascorbic acid. *Blood* 1994;84:1628-1634.

4839 Spielholz C, Golde DW, Houghton AN, et al. Increased facilitated transport of dehydroascorbic acid without changes in sodium-dependent ascorbate transport in human melanoma cells. *Br J Nutr* 1997;57:2529-2537.

4840 Vera JC, Rivas CI, Zhang RH, Golde DW. Colony-stimulating factors signal for increased transport of vitamin C in human host defense cells. *Blood* 1998;91:2536-2546.

4841 Agus DB, Vera JC, Golde DW. Stromal cell oxidation: a mechanism by which tumors obtain vitamin C. *Br J Nutr* 1999;59:4555-4558.

4842 Moertel CG, Fleming TR, Creagan ET, et al. High-dose vitamin C versus placebo in the treatment of patients with advanced cancer who have had no prior chemotherapy. A randomized double-blind comparison. *N Engl J Med* 1985;312:137-141.

4843 Creagan ET, Moertel CG, O'Fallon JR, et al. Failure of high-dose vitamin C (ascorbic acid) therapy to benefit patients with advanced cancer. A controlled trial. *N Engl J Med* 1979;301:687-690.

4844 Food and Nutrition Board, Institute of Medicine. "Dietary Reference Intakes for Vitamin C, Vitamin E, Selenium, and Carotenoids" website: www.iom.edu/IOM/IOMHome.nsf/Pages/Recently+Released+Reports (Accessed 17 May 2000).

4845 Consumer Lab. "Product Review: Vitamin C" website: http://www.consumerlab.com/results/vitaminc.html (Accessed 17 May 2000).

4846 Masaki KH, Losonczy KG, Izmirlian G, et al. Association of vitamin E and C supplement use with cognitive function and dementia in elderly men. *Neurology* 2000;54:1265-1272.

4847 Canner PL, Berge KG, Wenger NK, et al. Fifteen year mortality in Coronary Drug Project patients: long-term benefit with niacin. *J Am Coll Cardiol* 1986;8:1245-55.

4848 Zhao XQ, Brown BG, Hillger L, et al. Effects of intensive lipid-lowering therapy on the coronary arteries of asymptomatic subjects with elevated apolipoprotein B. *Circulation* 1993;88:2744-53.

4849 Institute of Medicine. Dietary Reference Intakes for Thiamin, Riboflavin, Niacin, Vitamin B6, folate, Vitamin B12, Pantothenic Acid, Biotin, and Choline. website: http://books.nap.edu/books/0309065542/html/123.html#pagetop (Accessed 24 May 2000).

4850 Park YK, Sempos CT, Barton CN, et al. Effectiveness of food fortification in the United States: the case of pellagra. *Am J Public Health* 2000;90:727-38.

4851 Gibbons LW, Gonzalez V, Gordon N, Grundy S. The prevalence of side effects with regular and sustained-release nicotinic acid. *Am J Med* 1995;99:378-85.

4852 Whelan AM, Price SO, Fowler SF, Hainer BL. The effect of aspirin on niacin-induced cutaneous reactions. *J Fam Pract* 1992;34:165-8.

4853 Jungnickel PW, Maloley PA, Vander Tuin EL, et al. Effect of two aspirin pretreatment regimens on niacin-induced cutaneous reactions. *J Gen Intern Med* 1997;12:591-6.

4854 Capuzzi DM, Guyton JR, Morgan JM, et al. Efficacy and safety of an extended-release niacin (Niaspan): a long-term study. *Am J Cardiol* 1998;82:74U-81U;discussion 85U-86U.

4855 Gray DR, Morgan T, Chretien SD, Kashyap ML. Efficacy and safety of controlled-release niacin in dyslipoproteinemic veterans. *Ann Intern Med* 1994;121:252-8.

4856 McKenney JM, Proctor JD, Harris S, Chinchili VM. A comparison of the efficacy and toxic effects of sustained-vs immediate-release niacin in hypercholesterolemic patients. *JAMA* 1994;271:672-7.

4857 Knopp RH, Alagona P, Davidson M, et al. Equivalent efficacy of a time-release form of niacin (Niaspan) given once-a-night versus plain niacin in the management of

hyperlipidemia. *Metabolism* 1998;47:1097-104.

4858 Knopp RH. Clinical profiles of plain versus sustained-release niacin (Niaspan) and the physiologic rationale for nighttime dosing. *Am J Cardiol* 1998;82:24U-28U;discussion 39U-41U.

4859 Crouse JR 3rd. New developments in the use of niacin for treatment of hyperlipidemia: new considerations in the use of an old drug. *Coron Artery Dis* 1996;7:321-6.

4860 Garg A, Grundy SM. Nicotinic acid as therapy for dyslipidemia in non-insulin-dependent Diabetes mellitus. *JAMA* 1990;264:723-6.

4862 Leighton RF, Gordon NF, Small GS, et al. Dental and gingival pain as side effects of niacin therapy. *Chest* 1998;114:1472-4.

4863 American Society of Health-System Pharmacists. ASHP Therapeutic Position Statement on the safe use of niacin in the management of dyslipidemias. *Am J Health Syst Pharm* 1997;54:2815-9.

4864 Goldberg AC. Clinical trial experience with extended-release niacin (Niaspan): dose-escalation study. *Am J Cardiol* 1998;82:35U-38U;discussion 39U-41U.

4865 Ishii N, Nishihara Y. Pellagra encephalopathy among tuberculous patients: its relation to isoniazid therapy. *J Neurol Neurosurg Psychiatry* 1985;48:628-34.

4866 Darvay A, Basarab T, McGregor JM, Russell-Jones R. Isoniazid induced pellagra despite pyridoxine supplementation. *Clin Exp Dermatol* 1999;24:167-9.

4867 National Cholesterol Education Program. Cholesterol Lowering in the Patient with Coronary Heart Disease. website: http://www.nhlbi.nih.gov/health/prof/heart/chol/chol_low.pdf (Accessed 25 May 2000).

4868 Rabbani GH, Butler T, Bardhan PK, Islam A. Reduction of fluid-loss in cholera by nicotinic acid: a randomized controlled trial. *Lancet* 1983;2:1439-42.

4869 Briend A, Nath SK, Heyman M, Desjeux JF. Comparative effects of nicotinic acid and nicotinamide on cholera toxin-induced secretion in rabbit ileum. *J Diarrhoeal Dis Res* 1993;11:97-100.

4870 Hudson CJ, Lin A, Cogan S, et al. The niacin challenge test: clinical manifestation of altered transmembrane signal transduction in schizophrenia? *Biol Psychiatry* 1997;41:507-13.

4871 Johansson JO, Egberg N, Asplund-Carlson A, Carlson LA. Nicotinic acid treatment shifts the fibrinolytic balance favourably and decreases plasma fibrinogen in hypertriglyceridaemic men. *J Cardiovasc Risk* 1997;4:165-71.

4872 Kolb H, Burkart V. Nicotinamide in type 1 diabetes. Mechanism of action revisited. *Diabetes Care* 1999;22:B16-20.

4873 Gale EA. Theory and practice of nicotinamide trials in pre-type 1 diabetes. *J Pediatr Endocrinol Metab* 1996;9:375-9.

4874 Elliott RB, Pilcher CC, Fergusson DM, Stewart AW. A population based strategy to prevent insulin-dependent Diabetes using nicotinamide. *J Pediatr Endocrinol Metab* 1996;9:501-9.

4875 Lampeter EF, Klinghammer A, Scherbaum WA, et al. The Deutsche Nicotinamide Intervention Study: an attempt to prevent type 1 diabetes. DENIS Group. *Diabetes* 1998;47:980-4.

4876 Reimers JI, Andersen HU, Pociot F. [Nicotinamide and prevention of insulin-dependent Diabetes mellitus. Rationale, effects, Toxicology and clinical experiences. ENDIT Group]. *Ugeskr Laeger* 1994;156:461-5.

4877 Pozzilli P, Visalli N, Cavallo MG, et al. Vitamin E and nicotinamide have similar effects in maintaining residual beta cell function in recent onset insulin-dependent diabetes. *Eur J Endocrinol* 1997;137:234-9.

4878 Visalli N, Cavallo MG, Signore A, et al. A multi-centre randomized trial of two different doses of nicotinamide in patients with recent-onset type 1 diabetes (the IMDIAB VI). *Diabetes Metab Res Rev* 1999;15:181-5.

4879 Pozzilli P, Visalli N, Signore A, et al. Double blind trial of nicotinamide in recent-onset IDDM (the IMDIAB III study). *Diabetologia* 1995;38:848-52.

4880 Pozzilli P, Browne PD, Kolb H. Meta-analysis of nicotinamide treatment in patients with recent-onset IDDM. The Nicotinamide Trialists. *Diabetes Care* 1996;19:1357-63.

4881 Greenbaum CJ, Kahn SE, Palmer JP. Nicotinamide's effects on glucose Metabolism in subjects at risk for IDDM. *Diabetes* 1996;45:1631-4.

4882 Polo V, Saibene A, Pontiroli AE. Nicotinamide improves insulin secretion and metabolic control in lean type 2 diabetic patients with secondary failure to sulphonylureas. *Acta Diabetol* 1998;35:61-4.

4883 Jonas WB, Rapoza CP, Blair WF. The effect of niacinamide on osteoarthritis: a pilot study. *Inflamm Res* 1996;45:330-4.

4884 McCarty MF, Russell AL. Niacinamide therapy for osteoarthritis--does it inhibit nitric oxide synthase induction by interleukin 1 in chondrocytes? *Med Hypotheses* 1999;53:350-60.

4885 Sperduto RD, Hu TS, Milton RC, et al. The Linxian cataract studies. Two nutrition intervention trials. *Arch Ophthalmol* 1993;111:1246-53.

4886 Illingworth DR, Stein EA, Mitchel YB, et al. Comparative effects of lovastatin and niacin in primary hypercholesterolemia. A prospective trial. *Arch Intern Med* 1994;154:1586-95.

4887 Vacek JL, Dittmeier G, Chiarelli T, et al. Comparison of lovastatin (20 mg) and nicotinic acid (1.2 g) with either drug alone for type II hyperlipoproteinemia. *Am J Cardiol* 1995;76:182-4.

4888 Vega GL, Grundy SM. Lipoprotein responses to treatment with lovastatin, gemfibrozil, and nicotinic acid in normolipidemic patients with hypoalphalipoproteinemia. *Arch Intern Med* 1994 Jan 10;154(1):73-82.

4889 Guyton JR, Goldberg AC, Kreisberg RA, et al. Effectiveness of once-nightly dosing of extended-release niacin alone and in combination for hypercholesterolemia. *Am J Cardiol* 1998;82:737-43.

4890 Lal SM, Hewett JE, Petroski GF, et al. Effects of nicotinic acid and lovastatin in renal transplant patients: a prospective, randomized, open-labeled crossover trial. *Am J Kidney Dis* 1995;25:616-22.

4891 Peikert A, Wilimzig C, Kohne-Volland R. Prophylaxis of migraine with oral magnesium: results from a prospective, multi-center, placebo-controlled and double-blind randomized study. *Cephalalgia* 1996;16:257-63.

4892 Pfaffenrath V, Wessely P, Meyer C, et al. Magnesium in the prophylaxis of migraine--a double-blind placebo-controlled study. *Cephalalgia* 1996;16:436-40.

4893 Mauskop A, Altura BM. Role of magnesium in the pathogenesis and treatment of migraines. *Clin Neurosci* 1998;5:24-7.

4894 Ginder S, Oatman B, Pollack M. A prospective study of iv magnesium and iv prochlorperazine in the treatment of headaches. *J Emerg Med* 2000;18:311-5.

4895 Taubert K. [Magnesium in migraine. Results of a multicenter pilot study *Fortschr Med* 1994;112:328-30.

4896 National Academy of Science, Institute of Medicine. "Dietary Reference Intakes for Vitamin C, Vitamin E, Selenium, and Carotenoids." http://www.nap.edu/pdf/0309069351/pdf_image/284.pdf. (Accessed 6 June 2000).

4897 Schrader E. Equivalence of St. John's wort extract (Ze 117) and fluoxetine: a randomized, controlled study in mild-moderate depression. *Int Clin Psychopharmacol* 2000;15:61-8.

4899 Linde K, Mulrow CD. St. John's wort for depression. *Cochrane Database Syst Rev* 2000;2:CD000448.

4900 Murch SJ, Simmons CB, Saxena PK. Melatonin in feverfew and other medicinal plants. *Lancet* 1997;350(9091):1598-1599. www.theLancet .com (November 29, 1997) (Accessed 6 June 2000).

4901 Mero A, et al. "Effects of bovine colostrum supplementation on serum IGF-I, IgG, hormone, and saliva IgA during training." *Appl Physiol*, 1997; 83(4): 1144-151.

4902 Alternative Health Care, "Colostrum" Website. URL: www.healthalternative.org/colostrum/ (16 July 1999).

4903 Sarker SA, et al. "Successful treatment of rotavirus diarrhea in children with immunoglobulin from immunized bovine colostrum." *Pediatr Infect Dis J*, 1998; 17(12): 1149-154.

4904 Mitra AK, et al. "Hyperimmune cow colostrum reduces diarrhoea due to rotavirus: a double-blind, controlled clinical trial." *Acta Paediatr*, 1995; 84(9): 996-1001.

4905 Greenberg PD, Cello JP. "Treatment of severe diarrhea caused by Cryptosporidium parvum with oral bovine immunoglobulin concentrate in patients with AIDS." *J Acquir Immune Defic Syndr Hum Retrovirol*, 1996; 13(4): 348-54.

4906 Plettenberg A, et al. "A preparation of bovine colostrum in the treatment of HIV-positive patients with chronic diarrhea." *Clin Investig*, 1993; 71(1): 42-45.

4907 Rump JA, et al. "Treatment of diarrhea in human immunodeficiency virus-infected patients with immunoglobulins from bovine colostrum." *Clin Investig*, 1992; 70(7): 588-94.

4908 Nord J, et al. "Treatment with bovine hyperimmune colostrum of cryptosporidial diarrhea in AIDS patients." *AIDS*, 1990; 4(6): 581-84.

4909 Ylitalo S, et al. "Rotaviral antibodies in the treatment of acute rotaviral gastroenteritis." *Acta Paediatr* , 1998; 87(3): 264-67.

4910 "Mother can transmit Lyme to fetus." Reuters News 8 May 1997.

4911 Playford RJ, et al. "Bovine colostrum is a health food supplement which prevents NSAID induced Gut damage." *Gut*, 1999; 44(5): 653-58.

4912 U. S. Food and Drug Administration, Center for Food Safety and Applied Nutrition, Office of Premarket Approval, "EAFUS: A Food Additive Database" Website: vm.cfsan.fda.gov/~dms/eafus.html (Accessed 20 July 1999).

4913 Sargent EV, Adolph J, Clemmons MK, et al. "Evaluation of flu-like symptoms in workers handling xanthan gum powder." *Occup Med*, 1990;32(7):625-30.

4914 Wade A, Weller PJ, ed. Handbook of Pharmaceutical Excipients. 2nd ed., Washington: American Pharmaceutical Association, 1994.

4915 van der Reijden WA, et al. "Treatment of xerostomia with polymer-based saliva substitutes in patients with

REFERENCES

Sjogren's syndrome." *Arthritis Rheum*, 1996; 39(1): 57-63.

4916 Osilesi O, et al. "Use of xanthan gum in dietary management of Diabetes mellitus." *Am J Clin Nutr*, 1985; 42(4): 597-603.

4917 Eastwood MA, Brydon WG, Anderson DM. "The dietary effects of xanthan gum in man." *Food Addit Contam*, 1987; 4(1): 17-26.

4918 Daly J, Tomlin J, Read NW. "The effect of feeding xanthan gum on colonic function in man: correlation with in vitro determinants of bacterial breakdown." *Br J Nutr*, 1993; 69(3): 897-902.

4920 van der Reijden WA, et al. "Influence of polymers for use in saliva substitutes on de- and remineralization of enamel in vitro." *Caries Res*, 1997; 31(3): 216-23.

4921 Covington TR, ed. Handbook of Nonprescription Drugs. 11th ed. Washington, DC: American Pharmaceutical Association, 1996.

4922 Dairy Managaemnt, Inc. "Whey" Website: URL: www.drymilk.com/infolib/factsht/factwhey.htm (16 July 1999).

4923 Dairy Management, Inc. Website: URL: www.drymilk.com/infolib/order/orderwhey.htm (16 July 1999).

4924 URL: www.creatine-glutamine.com/creatinecentral/whey.html

4925 URL: www.countryfreshfarms.com

4926 Bounous G, Baruchel S, Falutz J, et al. "Whey proteins as a food supplement in HIV-seropositive individuals." *Clin Invest Med* 1993;16(3):204-9.

4927 Vandenplas Y, et al. "Effect of a whey hydrolysate prophylaxis of atopic disease." *Ann Allergy*, 1992; 68(5): 419-24.

4928 McIntosh GH. "Colon cancer: 4743 Kurzer MS, Xu X. Dietary phytoestrogens. *Annu Rev Nutr* 1997;17:353-381.

4929 Fukushima J, et al. "Long-term consumption of whey hydrolysate formula by lactating women reduces the transfer of beta-lactoglobulin into human milk." *Nutr Sci Vitaminol* (Tokyo), 1997; 43(6): 673-78.

4930 Kennedy RS, et al. "The use of a whey protein concentrate in the treatment of patients with metastatic carcinoma: a phase I-II clinical study." *AntiCancer Res*, 1995; 15(6B): 2643-649.

4932 Salomon SB, et al. "An elemental diet containing medium-chain triglycerides and enzymatically hydrolyzed protein can improve gastrointestinal tolerance in people infected with HIV." *J Am Diet Assoc*, 1998; 98(4): 460-62.

4933 Papenburg R, et al. "Dietary milk proteins inhibit the development of dimethylhydrazine-induced malignancy." *Tumour Biol*, 1990; 11(3): 129-36.

4934 Fayer R, Guidry A, Blagburn BL. "Immunotherapeutic efficacy of bovine colostral immunoglobulins from a hyperimmunized cow against cryptosporidiosis in neonatal mice." *Infect Immun*, 1990; 58(9): 2962-965.

4935 Vergel NR, Salvato P, Mooney M. "Anabolic steroids, resistance exercise and protein supplementation effect on lean body mass in HIV+ patients." *Int Conf AIDS*, 1998; 12: 557 (abstract no. 32185).

4936 Voss T, et al. "Management of HIV-related weight loss and diarrhea with an enteral formula containing whey peptides and medium-chain triglycerides." *Int Conf AIDS*, 1991; 7(2): 223 (abstract no. W.B.2165).

4937 Baruchel S, Olivier R, Wainberg M. "Anti-HIV and anti-apoptotic activity of the whey protein concentrate: IMMUNOCAL." *Int Conf AIDS*, 1994; 10(2): 32 (abstract no. 421A).

4938 Wong CW, et al. "Effects of purified bovine whey factors on cellular immune functions in ruminants." *Vet Immunol Immunopathol*, 1997; 56(1-2): 85-96.

4939 Wong CW, et al. "Influence of whey and purified whey proteins on neutrophil functions in sheep." *J Dairy Res*, 1997; 64(2): 281-88.

4940 Wong CW, Watson DL. "Immunomodulatory effects of dietary whey proteins in mice." *J Dairy Res*, 1995; 62(2): 359-68.

4941 Engelson ES, et al. "Effect of a high protein diet upon protein *Metabolism* in HIV-infected men and women." *Int Conf AIDS*, 1998; 12: 553 (abstract no. 32166).

4942 Laoprasert N, et al. "Anaphylaxis in a milk-allergic child following ingestion of lemon sorbet containing trace quantities of milk." *J Food Prot*, 1998; 61(11): 1522-524.

4943 Bounous G, Batist G, Gold P. "Whey proteins in *Cancer* prevention." *Cancer Lett*, 1991; 57(2): 91-94.

4944 Semla TP, Beizer JL, Higbee MD. *Geriatric Dosage Handbook*. fourth ed. Hudson, OH: Lexicomp, 1998.

4945 Sherman RA, Tran JM, Sullivan. "R.Maggot therapy for venous stasis ulcers." *Arch Dermatol*, 1996;132(3):254-256.

4946 Teich S, Myers RA. "Maggot therapy for severe skin infections." *South Med J*, 1986; 79(9): 1153-155.

4947 Reames MK, Christensen C, Luce EA. "The use of maggots in wound debridement." *Ann Plast Surg*, 1988; 21(4): 388-91.

4948 Mumcuoglu KY, et al. "Maggot therapy for the treatment of diabetic foot ulcers." *Diabetes Care*, 1998; 21(11): 2030-031.

4949 Sherman RA, Wyle F, Vulpe M. "Maggot therapy for treating pressure ulcers in spinal cord injury patients." *J Spinal Cord Med*, 1995; 18(2): 71-74.

4950 Thomas S, Andrews A, Jones M, et al. "Maggots are useful in treating infected or necrotic wounds." *BMJ* 1999;318(7186):807-808.

4951 Sherman RA, Wyle FA. "Low-cost, low-maintenance rearing of maggots in hospitals, clinics, and schools." *Am J Trop Med Hyg*, 1996; 54(1): 38-41.

4952 Husain A, Sreevatsa Malaviya GN, Husain S, et al. "Characterization of microbial flora of leprous ulcers infested with maggots." *Acta Leprol*, 1993;8(3):143-147.

4953 Sherman RA. "A new dressing design for use with maggot therapy." *Plast Reconstr Surg*, 1997;100(2):451-456.

4960 *FDA Talk Paper*. "FDA Allows Whole Oat Foods to make Claim on Reducing the Risk of Heart Disease." FDA Website: vm.cfsan.fda.gov/~lrd/tpoats.html (Accessed16 July 1999).

4961 Wursch P, Pi-Sunyer FX. "The role of viscous soluble fiber in the metabolic control of diabetes. A review with special emphasis on cereals rich in beta-glucan." *Diabetes Care*, 1997; 20(11): 1774-780.

4962 Pietinen P, Rimm EB, Korhonen P, et al. "Intake of dietary fiber and risk of coronary heart disease in a cohort of Finnish men. The alpha-tocopherol, beta-carotene cancer prevention study." *Circulation*, 1996;94(11):2720-2727.

4963 Van Horn L. "Fiber, lipids, and coronary heart disease. A statement for healthcare professionals from the Nutrition Committee, American Heart Association." *Circulation*, 1997; 95(12): 2701-704.

4964 Rimm EB, et al. "Vegetable, fruit, and cereal fiber intake

© Copyright 2000, Natural Medicines Comprehensive Database (209) 472-2244. For updated data, go to www.NaturalDatabase.com. • 1263

REFERENCES

REFERENCES

and risk of coronary heart disease among men." *JAMA*, 1996; 275(6): 447-51.

4965 He J, et al. "Oats and buckwheat intakes and cardiovascular disease risk factors in an ethnic minority of China." *Am J Clin Nutr*, 1995; 61(2): 366-72.

4966 Khaw KT, Barrett-Connor E. "Dietary fiber and reduced ischemic heart disease mortality rates in men and women: a 12-year prospective study." *Am J Epidemiol*, 1987; 126(6): 1093- 102.

4967 Morris JN, Marr JW, Clayton DG. "Diet and heart: a postscript." *Br Med J*, 1977; 2(6098): 1307-314.

4968 Kromhout D, de Lezenne C, Coulander C. "Diet, prevalence and 10-year mortality from coronary heart disease in 871 middle-aged men. The Zutphen Study." *Am J Epidemiol*, 1984; 119(5): 733-741.

4969 American Dietetic Association Website: URL: www.eatright.org/adap1097.html (16 July 1999).

4970 Chen HL, et al. "Mechanisms by which wheat bran and oat bran increase stool weight in humans." *Am J Clin Nutr*, 1998; 68(3): 711-19.

4971 Brown L, et al. "Cholesterol-lowering effects of dietary fiber: a meta-analysis." *Am J Clin Nutr*, 1999; 69(1): 30-42.

4972 Kwiterovich PO Jr. "The role of fiber in the treatment of hypercholesterolemia in children and adolescents." *Pediatrics*, 1995; 96(5 Pt 2): 1005-009.

4973 Romero AL, et al. "Cookies enriched with psyllium or oat bran lower plasma LDL cholesterol in normal and hypercholesterolemic men from Northern Mexico." *J Am Coll Nutr*, 1998; 17(6): 601-08.

4974 Marlett JA, et al. "Mechanism of serum cholesterol reduction by oat bran." *Hepatology*, 1994; 20(6): 1450-457.

4975 Poulter N, et al. "Lipid profiles after the daily consumption of an oat-based cereal: a controlled crossover trial." *Am J Clin Nutr*, 1994; 59(1): 66-69.

4976 Braaten JT, et al. "Oat beta-glucan reduces blood cholesterol concentration in hypercholesterolemic subjects." *Eur J Clin Nutr*, 1994; 48(7): 465-74.

4977 Ripsin CM, et al. "Oat products and lipid lowering. A meta-analysis." *JAMA*, 1992; 267(2): 3317-325.

4978 Davidson MH, et al. "The hypocholesterolemic effects of beta-glucan in oatmeal and oat bran. A dose-controlled study." *JAMA*, 1991; 265(14): 1833-839.

4979 Cooper SG, Tracey EJ. "Small-bowel obstruction caused by oat-bran bezoar." *N Engl J Med*, 1989; 320(17): 1148-9.

4980 Pick ME, et al. "Oat bran concentrate bread products improve long-term control of diabetes: a pilot study." *J Am Diet Assoc*, 1996; 96(12): 1254-261.

4981 Wood PJ, et al. "Effect of dose and modification of viscous properties of oat gum on plasma glucose and insulin following an oral glucose load." *Br J Nutr*, 1994; 72(5): 731-43.

4982 Braaten JT, et al. "High beta-glucan oat bran and oat gum reduce postprandial blood glucose and insulin in subjects with and without type 2 diabetes." *Diabet Med*, 1994; 11(3): 312-18.

4983 Braaten JT, et al. "Oat gum lowers glucose and insulin after an oral glucose load." *Am J Clin Nutr*, 1991; 53(6): 1425-430.

4984 Arffmann S, et al. "Effect of oat bran on lithogenic index of bile and bile acid metabolism." *Digestion*, 1983; 28(3): 197-200.

4985 Rosario PG, et al. "Dentureless distention: oat bran bezoars cause obstruction." *J Am Geriatr Soc*, 1990;

38(5): 608.

4986 Surgical Materials Testing Laboratory Website: URL: www.smtl.co.uk/WMPRC/Maggots/maggots.html (22 Mar 1999).

4987 Reames MK, Christensen C, Luce EA. "The use of maggots in wound debridement." *Ann Plast Surg*, 1988; 21(4): 388-91.

4988 Council on Pharmacy and Chemistry. "Surgical Maggots - Lederle." *JAMA*, 1932; 98(5): 401.

4989 Livingston SK. "Maggots in the treatment of chronic osteomyelitis, infected wounds, and compound fractures." *Surg Gynec Obst*, 1932: 54: 702-06.

4990 Buchman J, Blair JE. "Maggots and their use in the treatment of chronic osteomyelitis." *Surg Gynec Obst*, 1932; 55: 177-90.

4991 Buchman J. "The rationale of the treatment of chronic osteomyelitis with special reference to maggot therapy." *Ann Surg*, 1934; 99: 251-59.

4992 Wilson EH, Doan CA, Miller DF. "The Baer maggot treatment of osteomyelitis." *JAMA*, 1932; 98(14): 1149-152.

4993 Baer WS. "The treatment of chronic osteomyelitis with the maggot (larva of the blow fly)." *J Bone Joint Surg*, 1931; 13: 438-75.

4994 Livingston SK. "The therapeutic active principle of maggots." *J Bone Joint Surg*. 1936; 18(3): 751-56.

4995 Fine A, Alexander H. "Maggot therapy - technique and clincial application." *J Bone Joint Surg*, 1934; 16: 572-78.

4996 Robinson W. "Progress of maggot therapy in the United States and Canada in the treatment of suppurative diseases." *Am J Surg*, 1935; 29(1): 67-71.

4997 Ferguson LK, McLaughlin CW. "Maggot therapy - a rapid method of removing necrotic tissues." *Am J Surg*, 1935; 29(1): 72-84.

4998 Weil GS, Simon RJ, Sweadner WR. "A biological, bacteriological and clinical study of larval or maggot therapy in the treatment of acute and chronic pyogenic infections." *Am J Surg*, 1933; 19(1): 36-48.

4999 "Maggot therapy for subacute mastoiditis." *Arch Otolaryngol*, 1976; 102: 377-79.

5000 Langford SD, Boor PJ. "Oleander toxicity: an examination of human and animal toxic exposures." *Toxicology*. 1996; 109(1): 1-13.

5001 Ferrea G, et al. "In vitro activity of a Combretum micranthum extract against herpes simplex virus types 1 and 2." *Antiviral Research*, Aug. 1993; 21(4): 317-25.

5002 Centers for Disease Control and Prevention. "Ostrich fern poisoning-New York and western Canada, 1994." *JAMA* 22-29 Mar. 1995; 273(12): 912-13.

5003 Makino T, et al. "Inhibitory effect of Perilla frutescens and its phenolic constituents on cultured murine mesangial cell proliferation." *Planta Med*, 1998; 64(6): 541-45.

5004 Bruynzeel DP. Bulb dermatitis. "Dermatological problems in the flower bulb industries." *Contact Dermatitis*, 1997 Aug;37(2):70-7.

5005 Bruynzeel DP, de Boer EM, Brouwer EJ, de Wolff FA, de Haan P. "Dermatitis in bulb growers." *Contact Dermatitis*, 1993 Jul;29(1):11-5

5007 Moraes-Cerdeira RM, Burandt CL Jr, Bastos JK, Nanayakkara D, Mikell J, Thurn J, McChesney JD. *Evaluation of four Narcissus.*

5008 Fetrow CW, Avila JR. Professional's Handbook of Complementary and Alternative Medicines, Springhouse Corporation: Springhouse, PA 1999.

5009 Murray M, Pizzorno J. Encyclopedia of Natural Medicine, second ed. Prima Health, Rocklin, CA, 1998.

5010 Murray M. The Healing Power of Herbs, second ed. Prima Health, Rocklin, CA, 1995.

5011 Lininger S. The Natural Pharmacy, Prima Health, Rocklin, CA, 1998.

5012 Mother Nature Website, URL: www.mothernature.com.

5013 Moore M. Herbal Materia Medica fifth edition, Southwest School of Botanical Medicine: Bisbee, AZ 1995.

5014 Manufacturer: Aubrey Organics. Tampa, FL.

5015 Manufacturer: Lily of the Desert. Denton, TX.

5016 Manufacturer: Schiff Pharmaceuticals. Salt Lake City, UT.

5017 Manufacturer: Country Life.

5018 Manufacturer: Kal.

5019 Manufacturer: Nature's Way. Springville, UT.

5020 Manufacturer: Twinlab. Ronkonkoma, NY.

5021 Manufacturer: Vitaline Formulas. Ashland, OR.

5022 Manufacturer: Earthrise. Petaluma, CA.

5023 Manufacturer: Nature's Answer. Hanppange, NY.

5024 Manufacturer: Walgreens. Deerfield, IL.

5025 Manufacturer: Natrol. Chatsworth, CA

5026 Manufacturer: Solaray.

5027 Manufacturer: Atkins Nutritionals.

5028 Personal correspondence. Jaana Leppala, jleppala@ucla.edu (4 March 2000).

5029 Cockerham MB, Weinberger BB, Lerchie SB. Oral glutamine for the prevention of oral mucositis associated with high-dose paclitaxel and melphalan for autologous Bone Marrow Transplantation. *Ann Pharmacother*, 2000;34(3):300-303.

5030 Schardt D. Stevia, A Bittersweet Tale. Nutrition Action Healthletter April 2000- U.S. Edition. URL: www.cspinet.org/nah/4_00/stevia.html (Accessed 28 March 2000).

5031 Melis MS, Sainati AR. Effect of calcium and verapamil on renal function of rats during treatment with stevioside. *J Ethnopharmacol*, 1991;33(3):257-622.

5032 Jeppesen PB, Gregersen S, Poulsen CR, Hermansen K. Stevioside acts directly on pancreatic beta cells to secrete insulin: actions independent of cyclic adenosine monophosphate and adenosine triphosphate-sensitive K+-channel activity. *Metabolism*, 2000;49(2):208-214.

5033 Melis MS. Effects of chronic administration of Stevia rebaudiana on fertility in rats. *J Ethnopharmacol*, 1999;67(2):157-161.

5034 Toskulkao C, Chaturat L, Temcharoen P, Glinsukon T. Acute toxicity of stevioside, a natural sweetener, and its metabolite, steviol, in several animal species. *Drug Chem Toxicol* 1997;20(1-2):31-44.

5035 Toskulkao C, Sutheerawatananon M, Wanichanon C, et al. Effects of stevioside and steviol on intestinal glucose absorption in hamsters. *J Nutr Sci Vitaminol* (Tokyo), 1995;41(1):105-113.

5036 Wasuntarawat C, Temcharoen P, Toskulkao C, et al. Developmental toxicity of steviol, a metabolite of stevioside, in the hamster. *Drug Chem Toxicol*, 1998;21(2):207-222.

5037 Stevia: Not Ready For Prime Time. Center for Science in the Public Interest. URL: www.cspinet.org/additives/stevia (Accessed 28 March 2000).

5038 Hartter S, Grozinger M, Weigmann H, et al. Increased bioavailability of oral melatonin after fluvoxamine coadministration. *Clin Pharmacol Ther*, 2000;67(1):1-6.

5039 Ravina A, Slezak L, Mirsky N, et al. Reversal of corticosteroid-induced diabetes mellitus with supplemental chromium. *Diabet Med*, 1999;16(2):164-167.

5040 Roeback JR Jr, Hla KM, Chambless LE, Fletcher RH. Effects of chromium supplementation on serum high-density lipoprotein cholesterol levels in men taking beta-blockers. A randomized, controlled trial. *Ann Intern Med*, 1991;115(12):917-924.

5041 NBA Bans Androstenedione. URL: nba.com/news/nba_androban_000330.html (Accessed 31 March 2000).

5042 Tangerine, Orange Juice May Inhibit Cancer Cell Growth. URL: www.medscape.com/reuters/eline/mon/t033120f.html (Accessed 3 April 2000).

5043 Magainin Presents Neuroblastoma Data for Squalamine at AACR Meeting. URL: www.prnewswire.com (Accessed 3 April 2000).

5044 Iron Chefs Get Nutritional Boost Cooking Vegetables. American Chemical Society website. URL: center.acs.org/applications/news//story.cfm?story=347 (Accessed 6 April 2000).

5045 Sharks Do Get Cancer, So Shark Cartilage Unlikely to Contain Anticancer Agent. URL: www.medscape.com/reuters/prof/2000/04/04.07/20000407clin011.html (Accessed 7 April 2000).

5046 UK Patients To Test Cannabis Medicines. URL: www.medscape.com/reuters/eline/fri/t040630f.html (Accessed 7 April 2000).

5047 FDA Announces The Availability Of New Ephedrine And "Street Drug Alternative" Documents. URL: www.fda.gov (Accessed 6 April 2000).

5048 Cocaine Use Increases Risk of Hemorrhagic Stroke. URL: www.medscape.com (Accessed 13 April 2000).

5049 Findling RL, Maxwell K, Scotese-Wojtila L, et al. High-dose pyridoxine and magnesium administration in children with autistic disorder: an absence of salutary effects in a double-blind, placebo-controlled study. *J Autism Dev Disord*, 1997;27(4):467-478.

5050 Coleman M. Infantile spasms associated with 5-hydroxytryptophan administration in patients with Down's syndrome. *Neurology* 1971;21(9):911-919.

5051 Hagg S, Spigset O, Mjorndal T, Dahlqvist R. Effect of caffeine on clozapine pharmacokinetics in healthy volunteers. *Br J Clin Pharmacol* 2000;49(1):59-63.

5052 Vadoud-Seyedi J, de Dobbeleer G, Simonart T. Treatment of haemodialysis-associated pseudoporphyria with N-acetylcysteine: report of two cases. *Br J Dermatol* 2000;142(3):580-81.

5053 Lynch SR, Dassenko SA, Cook JD, et al. Inhibitory effect of a soybean-protein—related moiety on iron absorption in humans. *Am J Clin Nutr* 1994;60(4):567-572.

5054 Eberhard P, Gall HM, Muller I, Moller R. Dramatic augmentation of a food allergy by acetylsalicylic acid. *J Allergy Clin Immunol* 2000;105(4):844.

5055 Mundell EJ. Mussel extract helps arthritic dogs. URL: www.reutershealth.com (Accessed 18 April 2000).

5056 Mundell EJ. Trying To Lose Weight? Calcium May Help. URL: www.medscape.com/reuters/eline/tue/t0417-4f.html (Accesed 18 April 2000).

5057 Mundell EJ. Cocoa May Help Fight Cholesterol. URL: www.medscape.com (Accessed 18 April 2000).

5058 Researchers Find Potential Additional Health Benefit of Cranberries. URL: www.prnewswire.com (Accessed 19 April 2000).

5059 Mundell EJ. Glucosamine supplements may raise dDiabetes risk. URL: www.reutershealth.com/

© Copyright 2000, Natural Medicines Comprehensive Database (209) 472-2244. For updated data, go to www.NaturalDatabase.com. • 1265

REFERENCES

REFERENCES

(Accessed 19 April 2000).

5060 Mundell EJ. Bone loss resumes when calcium supplementation stops. URL: www.medscape.com/ reuters/prof/2000/04/04.19/20000419clin002.html (Accessed 19 April 2000).

5061 Antioxidant lozenge could help ward off flu. URL: www.reutershealth.com (Accessed 19 April 2000).

5062 Mundell EJ. Sterol-Enriched Diets Reduce Cholesterol Levels. URL: www.medscape.com/reuters/prof/2000/ 04/04.21/20000421clin012.html (Accessed 21 April 2000).

5063 Medscape. Bussey E. N-Acetylcysteine Boosts T-Cell Function in HIV-Infected Patients. URL: www.medscape.com/reuters/prof/2000/04/04.28/ 20000428clin005.html (Accessed 28 April 2000).

5064 Oesterheld J, Kallepalli BR. Grapefruit juice and clomipramine: shifting metabolitic ratios. *J Clin Psychopharmacol* 1997;17(1):62-63.

5065 van Agtmael MA, Gupta V, van der Wosten TH, et al. Grapefruit juice increases the bioavailability of artemether. *Eur J Clin Pharmacol* 1999;55(5):405-410.

5066 van Agtmael MA, Gupta V, van der Graaf CA, van Boxtel CJ. The effect of grapefruit juice on the time-dependent decline of artemether plasma levels in healthy subjects. *Clin Pharmacol Ther* 1999;66(4):408-414.

5067 Damkier P, Hansen LL, Brosen K. Effect of diclofenac, disulfiram, itraconazole, grapefruit juice and erythromycin on the pharmacokinetics of quinidine. *Br J Clin Pharmacol* 1999;48(6):829-838.

5068 Takanaga H, Ohnishi A, Murakami H, et al. Relationship between time after intake of grapefruit juice and the effect on pharmacokinetics and pharmacodynamics of nisoldipine in healthy subjects. *Clin Pharmacol Ther* 2000;67(3):201-214.

5069 Takanaga H, Ohnishi A, Matsuo H, et al. Pharmacokinetic analysis of felodipine–grapefruit juice interaction based on an irreversible enzyme inhibition model. *Br J Clin Pharmacol* 2000;49(1):49-58.

5070 Dresser GK, Spence JD, Bailey DG. Pharmacokinetic-pharmacodynamic consequences and clinical relevance of cytochrome P450 3A4 inhibition. *Clin Pharmacokinet* 2000;38(1):41-57.

5071 Gillis MC (ed). Coreg monograph, in CPS (Compendium of Pharmaceuticals and Specialities), 34th edition. Ottawa, Ontario, Canada: Canadian Pharmacists Association, 1999: 395.

5072 He K, Iyer KR, Hayes RN, et al. Inactivation of cytochrome P450 3A4 by bergamottin, a component of grapefruit juice. *Chem Res Toxicol* 1998;11(4):252-259.

5073 Ernst E, Rand JI, Barnes J, Stevinson C. Adverse effects profile of the herbal antidepressant St. John's wort (Hypericum perforatum L.). *Eur J Clin Pharmacol* 1998;54(8):589-594.

5074 Lantz MS, Buchalter E, Giambanco V. St. John's wort and antidepressant drug interactions in the elderly. *J Geriatr Psychiatry Neurol* 1999;12(1):7-10.

5075 Taylor LvH, Kobak KA. An open-label trial of St. John's wort in obsessive compulsive disorder. Abstract Poster Presentations, 39th NCDEU Annual Meeting, 1999:Poster.

5076 Federal Trade Commission. Marketers of "Vitamin O" Settles FTC Charges of Making False Health Claims. URL: www.ftc.gov/opa/2000/05/rosecreek2.htm (Accessed 1 May 2000).

5077 Ginkgo May Protect Against Stroke Damage. URL: www.medscape.com/reuters/prof/2000/05/05.03/

20000503scie002.html (Accessed 3 May 2000).

5078 Beta-Glucan Key to Cardiovascular Health Benefits. URL: www.medscape.com/MedscapeWire/2000/0500/ medwire.0502.Beta.html (Accessed 3 May 2000).

5079 Lickteig MA. DUI charge for drinking tea. URL: 209.207.168.170/local/Wnews/ 03kavadui_a3empirea.html (Accessed 4 May 2000).

5080 McCrory DC, Matchar DB, Gray RN, et al. Evidence-Based Guidelines for Migraine Headache: Overview of Program Description and Methodology. US Headache Consortium, April 2000. website www.aan.com/cgi-bin/ whatsnewlink.pl?loc=/public/practiceguidelines (Accessed 3 May 2000).

5081 Butner LE, Fulco PP, Feldman G, et al. Calcium carbonate-induced hypothyroidism. *Ann Intern Med* 2000:132(4):595.

5082 Schneyer CR. Calcium carbonate and reduction of levothyroxine efficacy. *JAMA* 1998;279(10):750.

5083 Vitamin D Does Not Benefit Patients With Relapsing-Remitting MS. URL: www.medscape.com/reuters/prof/ 2000/05/05.08/20000508clin009.html (Accessed 8 May 2000).

5084 Codina R, Ardusso L, Lockey RF, et al. Sensitization to soybean hull allergens in subjects exposed to different levels of soybean dust inhalation in Argentina. *J Allergy Clin Immunol*, 2000;105(3):570-576.

5085 Anto JM, Sunyer J, Rodriguez-Roisin R, et al. Community outbreaks of asthma associated with inhalation of soybean dust. Toxicoepidemiological Committee. *N Engl J Med* 1989;320(17):1097-1102.

5086 White MC, Etzel RA, Olson DR, Goldstein IF. Re-examination of epidemic asthma in New Orleans, Louisianna, in relation to the presence of soy at the harbor. *Am J Epidemiol* 1997;145(5):432-438.

5087 Snow V, Lascher S, Mottur-Pilson C. Pharmacologic treatment of acute major depression and dysthymia. *Ann Intern Med* 2000;132(9):738-742.

5088 Schedules of controlled substances: addition of gamma-hydroxybutyric acid to Schedule I. Federal Register 2000;65(49):13235-13238.

5089 Kachhi PN, Henderson SO. Priapism after androstenedione intake for athletic performance enhancement. *Ann Emerg Med* 2000;35(4):391-393.

5090 Khatta M, Alexander BS, Krichten CM, et al. The effect of coenzyme Q10 in patients with congestive heart failure. *Ann Intern Med* 2000;132(8):636-640.

5091 Ferrara LA, Raimondi AS, d'Episcopo L, et al. Olive oil and reduced need for antihypertensive medications. *Arch Intern Med* 2000;160(6):837-842.

5092 McEvoy AW, Kitchen ND, Thomas DG. Intracerebral haemorrhage in young adults: the emerging importance of drug misuse. *BMJ* 2000;320(7245):1322-1324.

5093 Marks L, Partin AW, Epstein JI, et al. Effects of a saw palmetto herbal blend in men with symptomatic benign prostatic hyperplasia. *J Urol* 2000;163(5):1451-1456.

5094 Gerber GS. Saw palmetto for the treatment of men with lower urinary tract symptoms. *J Urol* 2000;163(5):1408-1412.

5095 Goepel M, Hecker U, Krege S, et al. Saw palmetto extracts potently and noncompetitively inhibit human alpha1-adrenoceptors in vitro. *Prostate* 1999;38(3):208-15.

5096 St. John's Wort Equivalent to Placebo For Treatment of Depression. URL: www.medscape.com/reuters/prof/ 2000/05/05.17/20000517clin015.html (Accessed 17 May 2000).

5097 Harel Z, Gascon G, Riggs S, et al. Fish oil versus olive oil in the management of recurrent headaches in adolescents. Advancing Children's Health 2000, Joint Meeting of the Pediatric Academic Societies and the American Academy of Pediatrics; Abstract 30. URL: www.abstracts-on-line.com/abstracts/pas/aol.asp (Accessed 17 May 2000).

5098 Olsen SF, Secher NJ, Tabor A, et al. Randomized clinical trials of fish oil supplementation in high risk pregnancies. Fish Oil Trials In Pregnancy (FOTIP) Team. *BJOG* 2000;107(3):382-95.

5099 National Organization of Rare Diseases. "Choline" Website: URL: www.stepstn.com/nord/db/dbsearch/search.htm (20 July 1999).

5100 Pavillard ER, Wright EA. "An antibiotic from maggots." Nature, 1957; 180: 916-17.

5101 Robinson W. "Stimulation of healing in non-healing wounds by allantoin occurring in maggot secretions and of wide biological distribution." *J Bone Joint Surg*, 1935; 17(2): 267-71.

5102 Ziefren SW, et al. "The secretion of collagenase by maggots and its implication." *Ann Surg*, 1953; 138(6): 9332-334.

5103 Bennett WG, JJ Cerda. "Benefits of dietary fiber. Myth or medicine?" *Postgrad Med*, 1996; 99(2): 153-56, 166-68, 171-72 passim.

5104 Reddy BS. "Role of dietary fiber in colon cancer: an overview." *Am J Med* , 1999; 106(1A): 16S-19S.

5105 Almy TP. "Fiber and the gut." *Am J Med*, 1981; 71(2): 193-95.

5106 Almy TP, Howell DA. "Medical progress. Diverticular disease of the colon." *N Engl J Med*, 1980; 302(6): 324-31.

5107 Kritchevsky D. "Dietary fibre and cancer." *Eur J Cancer Prev*, 1997; 6(5): 435-41.

5108 Dwyer JT, et al. "Drug therapy reviews: dietary fiber and fiber supplements in the therapy of gastrointestinal disorders." *Am J Hosp Pharm*; 1978; 35(3): 278-87.

5109 Kalant H, Roschlau WHE, eds. Principles of Medical Pharmacology. New York: Oxford University Press, 1998.

5110 Bloom FE, Kupfer DJ. Psychopharmacology: The Fourth Generation of Progress. New York: Raven Press, Ltd, 1995.

5111 Website: URL: www.betterbodz.com.

5112 Website: URL: www.thewayup.com.

5113 Cocito L, et al. "GABA and phosphatidylserine in human photosensitivity: a pilot study." Epilepsy Res, 1994; 17(1): 49-53.

5114 Cavagnin F, et al. "Effects of gamma aminobutyric acid (GABA) and muscimol on endocrine pancreatic function in man." *Metabolism*, 1982; 31(1): 73-77.

5115 Cavagnini F, et al. "Effect of acute and repeated administration of gamma aminobutyric acid (GABA) on growth hormone and prolactin secretion in man." *Acta Endocrinol* (Copenh), 1980; 93(2): 149-54.

5116 Nurnberger JI Jr., et al. "Intravenous GABA administration is anxiogenic in man." *Psychiatry Res*, 1986; 19(2): 113-17.

5117 Gamma-Aminobutyric Acid (GABA) Website: URL: www.axiom.net/conrucopia/gaba.html. (Accessed 15 June 1999).

5118 URL: www.smartbasic.com/glos.aminos/gaba.glos.html. (Accessed 15 June 1999).

5119 Brown D. Encyclopedia of Herbs and Their Uses. first ed. New York: Dorland Kindersley Publishing Inc., 1995.

5120 Mcguffin M, et al, ed. American Herbal Products Association's Botanical Safety Handbook. Boca Raton FL: CRC Press LLC, 1997.

5121 Duke JA. The Green Pharmacy. Emmaus, PA: Rodale Press, 1997.

5122 Moyad MA, Pienta KJ, Montie JE. Use of PC-SPES, a commercially available supplement for prostate cancer, in a patient with hormone-naive disease. *Urology* 54(2):319-28.

5123 "Estronol: Wild Mexican Yam" Website: URL: www.essentialcomputing.com/ams/estronol.htm (16 July 1999).

5124 "Wild Mexican Yam" Website: URL: www.nutrition-warehouse.com/Wild.Mexican.Yam.html (16 July 1999).

5125 1st Choice Products Website: URL: www.owasso.com/1sstchoice/index.htm (16 July 1999).

5126 "Dioscorea: Wild Mexican Yam" Website: URL: www.usvitamin.com/fatigue/diosin.shtml (16 July 1999).

5127 "Men's Wild Yam efx" Website: URL: www.shop4value.com/hormone/manyam.htm (16 July 1999).

5129 Accatino L, Pizarro M, Solis N, Koenig CS. "Effects of diosgenin, a plant-derived steroid, on bile secretion and hepatocellular cholestasis induced by estrogens in the rat." *Hepatology* 1998;28(1):129-140.

5130 Aradhana AR, Rao, Kale RK. "Diosgenin-a growth stimulator of mammary gland of ovariectomized mouse." *Indian J Exp Biol*, 1992; 30(5): 367-70.

5131 Yamada T, et al. "Dietary diosgenin attenuates subacute intestinal inflammation associated with indomethacin in rats." *Am J Physiol*, 1997; 273(2 Pt 1): G355-64.

5132 5Y6 Vitamin Sotres, Inc, "Dibencozide" Website:URL: www.healthdepo.com/healthdepo/1457.htm (20 July 1999).

5133 Beltz SD, Doering PL. "Efficacy of nutritional supplements used by athletes." *Clin Pharm*, 1993; 12(12):900-908.

5134 Health & Scientce Research Institute. "Anemia, Anxiety, & Depression." Website: URL: www.heath-science.com/anemia2.html (20 July 1999).

5135 Life Plus. "Clear Edge." Website: URL: www.staywellvitamins.com/clear.htm (20 July 1999).

5136 Wagner JC. "Use of chromium and cobamamide by athletes." *Clin Pharm*, 1989; 8:832, 834.

5137 Williams MH. "Vitamin and mineral supplements to athletes: do they help?" *Clin Sports Med*, 1984; 3(3):623-37.

5138 National Academy Press. "Vitamin B-12" Website: books.nap.edu/books/0309065542/html/199.html (20 July 1999).

5139 Gilman AG, et al, eds. Goodman and Gilman's The Pharmacological Basis of Therapeutics. eighth ed., New York: Pergamon Press, 1990.

5140 Buchman AL, et al. "Lecithin increases plasma free choline and decreases hepatic steatosis in long-term total parenteral nutrition patients." *Gastroenterology*, 1992; 102(4 Pt 1):1363-370.

5141 Wagenmakers A. "Muscle amino acid metabolism at rest and during exercise: role in human physiology and metabolism." *Exerc Sport Sci Rev*, 1998; 26:287-314.

5142 Tuzhilin SA, et al. "The treatment of patients with gallstones by lecithin." *Am J Gastroenterol*, 1976; 65(3):231-35.

5143 Chan H, Abraham G, Oreopoulos DG. "Oral lecithin improves ultrafiltration in patients on peritoneal

© Copyright 2000, Natural Medicines Comprehensive Database (209) 472-2244. For updated data, go to www.NaturalDatabase.com. • 1267

REFERENCES

dialysis." *Perit Dial Int*, 1989; 9(3):203-205.

5144 Lieber C.S. "Alcohol and the liver: 1994 update." *Gastroenterology*, 1994; 106(4):1085-105.

5145 Cohen BM, Lipinski JF, Altesman RI. "Lecithin in the treatment of mania: double-blind, placebo-controlled trials." *Am J Psychiatry*, 1982; 139(9):1162-164.

5146 Harris CM, et al. "Effect of lecithin on memory in normal adults." *Am J Psychiatry*, 1983; 140(8):1010-1012.

5147 Simons LA, Hickie JB, Ruys J. "Treatment of hypercholesterolaemia with oral lecithin." *Aust N Z J Med*, 1977; 7(3):262-66.

5148 Oosthuizen W, et al. "Lecithin has no effect on serum lipoprotein, plasma fibrinogen and macro molecular protein complex levels in hyperlipidaemic men in a double-blind controlled study." *Eur J Clin Nutr*, 1998; 52(6):419-24.

5149 Brinkman SD, et al. "Lecithin and memory training in suspected Alzheimer's disease." *J Gerontol*, 1982; 37(1):4-9.

5150 Brinkman SD, et al. "A dose-ranging study of lecithin in the treatment of primary degenerative dementia (Alzheimer disease)." *J Clin Psychopharmacol*, 1982; 2(4):281-85.

5151 Pomara N, et al. "Failure of single-dose lecithin to alter aspects of central cholinergic activity in Alzheimer's disease." *J Clin Psychiatry*, 1983; 44(8):293-95.

5152 Etienne P, et al. "Alzheimer disease: lack of effect of lecithin treatment for 3 months." *Neurology*, 1981; 31(12):1552-554.

5153 *Facts and Comparisons*, Loose-leaf edition, 1999.

5154 Mother Nature's Encyclopedia. "Lecithin/ Phosphatidylcholine? Choline" Website: URL: www:mothernature.com/ency/supp/lecithin.asp (20 July 1999).

5155 Holan KR, et al. "Effect of oral administration of 'essential' phospholipid, beta-glycerophosphate, and linoleic acid on biliary lipids in patients with cholelithiasis." *Digestion*, 1979; 19(4):251-58.

5156 Maltby N, et al. "Efficacy of tacrine and lecithin in mild to moderate Alzheimer's disease: double blind trial." *BMJ*, 1994; 308(6933):879-83.

5157 Gilman AG, et al, eds. Goodman and Gilman's Pharmacological Basis of Therapeutics. eighth ed. New York: Pergamon Press, 1990.

5158 Supplements On Line. "Choline" Website: URL: www.supplementatson-line.com/client/ename/ remedies.nsf/allremedies/choline (20 July 1999).

5159 Herbal Information Center. "Choline" Website: URL: www.kcweb.com/herb/vit_cho.htm (20 July 1999).

5160 Grunewald KK, Bailey RS. "Commercially marketed supplements for bodybuilding athletes." *Sports Med*, 1993; 15(2):90-103.

5161 Sehested P, Lund HI, Kristensen O. "Oral choline in cerebellar ataxia." *Acta Neurol Scand*, 1980; 62(2):124-26.

5162 McNamara JO, et al. "Effects of oral choline on human complex partial seizures. *Neurology*, 1980; 30 (12):1334-336.

5163 Shronts EP. "Essential nature of choline with implications for total parenteral nutrition." *J Am Diet Assoc*, 1997; 97(6):639-46, 649.

5164 Spector SA, et al. "Effect of choline supplementation on fatigue in trained cyclists." *Med Sci Sports Exerc*, 1995; 27(5):668-73.

5165 Gupta SK, Gaur SN. "A placebo controlled trial of two dosages of LPC antagonist-choline in the management of bronchial asthma." *Indian J Chet Dis Allied Sci*, 1997; 39(3):149-56.

5166 Gaur SN, Agarwal G, Gupta SK. "Use of LPC antagonist, choline, in the management of bronchial asthma." *Indian J Chest Dis Allied Sci*, 1997; 39(2):107-113.

5167 Growdon JH, Cohen EL, Wurtman RJ. "Huntington's disease: clinical and chemical effects of choline administration." *Ann Neurol*, 1977; 1(5):418-22.

5168 Davis KL, et al. "Cholinomimetics and memory. The effect of choline chloride." *Arch Neurol*, 1980; 37(1):49-52.

5169 Mohs RC, et al. "Choline chloride treatment of memory deficits in the elderly." *Am J Psychiatry*, 1979; 136(10):1275-277.

5170 Mohs RC, et al. "Choline chloride effects on memory in the elderly." *Neurobiol Aging*, 1980; 1(1):21-25.

5171 Davis KL, Berger PA. "Pharmacological investigations of the cholinergic imbalance hypotheses of movement disorders and psychosis." *Biol Psychiatry*, 1978; 13(1):23-49.

5172 Davis KL, Hollister LE, Berger PA. "Choline chloride in schizophrenia." *Am J Psychiatry*, 1979; 136(12):1581-584.

5173 Lawrence CM, et al. "The use of choline chloride in ataxic disorders." *J Neurol Neurosurg Psychiatry*, 1980; 43(5):452-54.

5174 Buchman AL, et al. "Choline deficiency: a cause of hepatic steatosis during parenteral nutrition that can be reversed with intravenous choline supplementation." *Hepatology*, 1995; 22(5):1399-403.

5175 Tan J, et al. "Lack of effect of oral choline supplement on the concentrations of choline metabolites in human brain." *Magn Reson Med*, 1998; 39(6):1005-1010.

5178 Albright CD, et al. "Diet, apoptosis, and Carcinogenesis." *Adv Exp Med Biol*, 1997; 422:97-107.

5179 Yen CL, Mar MH, Zeisel SH. "Choline deficiency-induced apoptosis in PC12 cells is associated with diminished membrane phosphatdylcholine and sphingomyelin, accumulation of ceramide and diacylglycerol, and activiation of a caspase." *FASEB J*, 1999; 13(1):135-42.

5180 Zeisel SH. "Choline: an important nutrient in brain development, liver function and carcinogenesis." *J Am Coll Nutr*, 1992; 11(5):473-81.

5181 Yates AA, Schlicker SA, Suitor CW. "Dietary Reference Intakes: the new basis for recommendations for calcium and related nutrients, B vitamins, and choline." *J Am Diet Assoc*, 1998; 98(6):699-706.

5182 Carmichael Wellness Products. "Depression and Anxiety" Website: URL: www.cwinstitute.com/ diseases3.asp (20 July 1999).

5183 Newsweek. "SAMe" Website: URL: www.newsweekinteractive.net/nw-sv/printed/us/st/ he0112_1.htm (20 July 1999).

5184 Fava M, et al. "Rapidity of onset of the antidepressant effect of parenteral S-adenosyl-L-methionine." *Psychiatry Res*, 1995; 56(3):295-97.

5185 FDA. "Orphan Drug List" Website: URL: www.fda.gov/orphan/designat/list.htm. Orphan Drug Information S-adenosylmethionine Designated:Treatment of *AIDS* myelopathy. (Accessed 20 July 1999).

5186 Internet Grateful Med. "ChemID" Website: igm.nlm.nih.gov (20 July 1999).

5187 The Way UP. "S-adenosyl-methionine" Website: URL: www.theway up.com/products/0235. (20 July 1999).

5188 Bradley JD, et al. "A randomized, double blind, placebo controlled trial of intravenous loading with S-adenosylmethionine (SAM) followed by oral SAM therapy in patients with knee osteoarthritis." *J Rheumatol*, 1994; 21(5):905-11.

5189 Bressa GM. "S-adenosyl-l-methionine (SAMe) as antidepressant: meta-analysis of clinical studies." *Acta Neurol Scans Suppl*, 1994; 154:7-14.

5190 Bell KM, et al. "S-adenosylmethionine blood levels in major depression: changes with drug treatment." *Acta Neurol Scand Suppl*, 1994; 154:15-18.

5191 Bottiglieri T, Hyland K. "S-adenosylmethionine levels in psychiatric and neurological disorders: a review." *Acta Neurol Scand Suppl*, 1994; 154:19-26.

5192 Salmaggi P, et al. "Double-blind, placebo-controlled study of S-adenosyl-L-methionine in depressed postmenopausal women." *Psychother Psychosom*, 1993; 59(1):34-40.

5193 Berlanga C, et al. "Efficacy of S-adenosyl-L-methionine in speeding the onset of action of imipramine." *Psychiatry Res*, 1992; 44(3):257-62.

5194 Bottiglieri T, et al. "Cerebrospinal fluid S-adenosylmethionine in depression and dementia: effects of treatment with parenteral and oral S-adenosylmethionine." J Neurol Neurosurg Psychiatry, 1990; 53(12):1096-1098.

5195 Kagan BL, et al. "Oral S-adenosylmethionine in depression: a randomized, double-blind, placebo-controlled trial." *Am J Psychiatry*, 1990; 147(5):591-95.

5196 Rosenbaum JF, et al. "The antidepressant potential of oral S-adenosyl-l-methionine." *Acta Psychiatr Scand*, 1990; 81(5):432-36.

5197 Fava M, et al. "Neuroendocrine effects of S-adenosyl-L-methionine, a novel putative antidepressant." *J Psychiatr Res*, 1990; 24(2):177-84.

5198 Chawla RK, Bonkovsky HL, Galambos JT. "Biochemistry and pharmacology of S-adenosyl-L-methionine and rationale for its use in liver disease." *Drugs*, 1990; 40 Suppl 3:98-110.

5199 Domljan Z, et al. "A double-blind trial of ademetionine vs naproxen in activated gonarthrosis." *Int J Clin Pharmacol Ther Toxicol*, 1989; 27(7):329-33.

5200 Bell KM, et al. "S-adenosylmethionine treatment of depression: a controlled clinical trial." *Am J Psychiatry*, 1988; 145(9):1110-114.

5201 Vahora SA, Malek-Ahmasi P. "S-adenosylmethionine in the treatment of depression." *Neurosci Biobehav Rev*, 1988; 12(2):139-41.

5202 Baldessarini RJ. "Neuropharmacology of S-adenosyl-L-methionine." *Am J Med*, 1987; 83(5A):95-103.

5203 Konig B. "A long-term (two years) clinical trial with S-adenosylmethionine for the treatment of osteoarthritis." *Am J Med*, 1987; 83(5a):78-80.

5204 Berger R, Nowak H. "A new medical approach to the treatment of osteoarthritis. Report of an open phase IV study with ademetionine (Gumbaral)." *Am J Med*, 1987; 83(5A):84-88.

5205 Muller-Fassbender H. "Double-blind clinical trial of S-adenosylmethionine versus ibuprofen in the treatment of osteoarthritis." *Am J Med*, 1987; 83(5A):81-83.

5206 Vetter G. "Double-blind comparative clinical trial with S-adenosylmethionine and indomethacin in the treatment of osteoarthritis." *Am J Med*, 1987; 83(5A):78-80.

5207 Maccagno A, et al. "Double-blind controlled clinical trial of oral S-adenosylmethionine versus piroxicam in knee osteoarthritis." *Am J Med*, 1987; 83(5A):72-77.

5208 Caruso I, Pietrogrande V. "Italian double-blind multicenter study comparing S-adenosylmethionine, naproxen, and placebo in the treatment of degenerative joint disease." *Am J Med*, 1987; 83(5A):66-71.

5209 di Padova C. "S-adenosylmethionine in the treatment of osteoarthritis. Review of the clinical studies." *Am J Med*, 1987; 83(5A):60-65.

5210 Stramentinoli G. "Pharmacologic aspects of S-adenosylmethionine. Pharmacokinetics and pharmacodynamics." *Am J Med*, 1987; 83(5A):35-42.

5211 Tavoni A, et al. "Evaluation of S-adenosylmethionine in primary fibromyalgia. A double-blind crossover study." *Am J Med*, 1987; 83(5A):107-110.

5212 Carney MW, Toone BK, Reynolds EH. "S-adenosylmethionine and affective disorder." *Am J Med*, 1987; 83(5A):104-106.

5213 Laudanno OM. "Cytoprotective effect of S-adenosylmethionine compared with that of misoprostol against ethanol-, aspirin-, and strees-induced gastric damage." *Am J Med*, 1987; 83(5A):43-47.

5214 Carney MW, et al. "Affective illness and S-adenosyl methionine: a preliminary report." *Clin Neuropharmacol*, 1986; 9(4):379-85.

5215 Glorioso S, et al. "Double-blind multicentre study of the activity of S-adenosylmethionine in hip and knee osteoarthritis." *Int J Clin Pharmacol Res*, 1985; 5(1):39-49.

5216 Lipinski JF, et al. "Open trial of S-adenosylmethionine for treatment of depression." *Am J Psychiatry*, 1984; 141(3):448-50.

5217 Castagna A, et al. "Cerebrospinal fluid S-adenosylmethionine (SAMe) and glutathione concentrations in HIV infection: effect of parenteral treatment with SAMe." *Neurology*, 1995; 45(9):1678-683.

5218 Tan SV, Guiloff RJ. "Hypothesis on the pathogenesis of vacuolar myelopathy, dementia, and peripheral neuropathy in AIDS." *J Neurol Neurosurg Psychiatry*, 1998; 65(1):23-28.

5219 Almasio P, et al. "Role of S-adenosyl-L-methionine in the treatment of intrahepatic cholestasis." *Drugs*, 1990; 40 Suppl 3:111-23.

5220 Cohen BM, Satlin A, Zubenko GS. "S-adenosyl-L-methionine in the treatment of Alzheimer's disease." *J Clin Psychopharmacol*, 1988; 8(1):43-47.

5221 Volkmann H, et al. "Double-blind, placebo-controlled cross-over study of intravenous S-adenosyl-L-methionine in patients with fibromyalgia." *Scand J Rheumatol*, 1997; 26(3):206-11.

5222 Chan PC, et al. "Effect of phosphatidylcholine on ultrafiltration in patients on continuous ambulatory peritoneal dialysis." *Nephron*, 1991; 59(1):100-103.

5223 Domino EF, et al. "Lack of clinically significant improvement of patients with tardive dyskinesia following phosphatidylcholine therapy." *Biol Psychiatry*, 1985; 20(11):1189-196.

5224 Jenkins PJ, et al. "Use of polyunsaturated phosphatidyl choline in HBsAg negative chronic active hepatitis: results of prospective double-blind controlled trial." *Liver*, 1982; 2(2):77-81.

5225 Guan R, et al. "The effect of polyunsaturated phosphatidyl choline in the treatment of acute viral hepatitis." *Aliment Pharmacol Ther*, 1995; 9(6):699-703.

5226 Niederau C, et al. "Polyunsaturated phosphatidyl-choline and interferon alpha for treatment of chronic hepatitis B and C: a multi-center, randomized, double-blind, placebo-controlled trial. Leich Study Group." *Hepatogastroenterology*, 1998; 45(21):797-804.

5227 SupraHealth. "Choline" Website: URL: www.suprahealth.com/choline.htm.

5228 Ladd SL, et al. "Effect of phosphatidylcholine on explicit memory." *Clin Neuropharmacol*, 1993; 16(6):540-49.

5229 Aronson PJ, Lorincz AL. "Promotion of palmar sweating with oral phosphatidylcholine." *Acta Derm Venereol*, 1985; 65(1):19-24.

5230 American Lecithin Co. "PhosChol" Website: members.aol.com/alcolec/phoschol.htm (20 July 1999).

5231 Friedel HA, Goa KL, Benfield P. "S-adenosyl-L-methionine. A review of its pharmacological properties and therapeutic potential in liver dysfunction and affective disorders in relation to its physiological role in cell metabolism." *Drugs*, 1989; 38(3):389-416.

5232 Bottiglieri T, Hyland K, Reynolds EH. "The clinical potential of ademetionine (S-adenosylmethionine) in neurological disorders." *Drugs*, 1994; 4 8(2):137-52.

5233 Moyad MA. Alternative therapies for advanced prostate cancer. What should I tell my patients? *Urologic Clinics of North America* 1999;26:413-7.

5234 Almasio P, et al. "Role of S-adenosyl-L-methionine in the treatment of intrahepatic cholestasis." *Drugs*, 1990; 40 Suppl 3:111-23.

5235 Diaz BA, Dominguez HR, Uribe AF. "Parenteral S-adenosylmethionine compared to placebos in the treatment of alcoholic liver diseases." *An Med Interna*, 1996; 13(1):9-15.

5236 Loguercio C, et al. "Effect of S-adenosyl-L-methionine administration on red blood cell cysteine and glutathione levels in alcoholic patients with and without liver disease." *Alcohol Alcohol*, 1994; 29(5):597-604.

5237 Rafique S, et al. "Reversal of extrahepatic membrane cholesterol deposition in patients with chronic liver diseases by S-adenosyl-L-methionine." *Clin Sci* (Colch), 1992; 83(3):353-56.

5238 Podymova SD, Nadinskaia M. "Clinical trial of heptral in patients with chronic diffuse liver disease with intrahepatic cholestasis syndrome." *Klin Med* (Mosk), 1998; 76(10):45-48.

5239 Frezza M, et al. "Oral S-adenosylmethionine in the symptomatic treatment of intrahepatic cholestasis. A double-blind, placebo-controlled study." *Gastroenterology*, 1990; 99(1):211-15.

5240 Frezza M, et al. "S-adenosylmethionine for the treatment of intrahepatic cholestasis of pregnancy. Results of a controlled clinical trial." *Hepatogastroenterology*, 1990; 37 Suppl 2:122-25.

5241 Jacobsen S, Danneskiold-Samsoe B, Andersen RB. "Oral S-adenosylmethionine in primary fibromyalgia. Double-blind clinical evaluation." *Scand J Rheumatol*, 1991; 20(4):294-302.

5243 Heyman JA, et al. "Failure of long term high-dose lecithin to retard progression of early-onset Alzheimer's disease." *Neural Transm Suppl*, 1987; 24:279-86.

5244 Little A, et al. "A double-blind, placebo controlled trial of high-dose lecithin in Alzheimer's disease." *J Neurol Neurosurg Psychiatry*, 198; 48(8):736-42.

5245 Thal LJ, et al. "Oral physostigmine and lecithin improve memory in Alzheimer disease." *Ann Neurol*, 1983; 13(5):491-96.

5246 Gelenberg AJ, et al. "A crossover study of lecithin

treatment of tardive dyskinesia." *Clin Psychiatry*, 1990; 51(4):149-53.

5247 Volavka J, et al. "Lithium and lecithin in tardive dyskinesia: an update." *Psychiatry Res*, 1986; 19(2):101-104.

5249 Toouli J, Jablonski P, Watts JM. "Gallstone dissolution in man using cholic acid and lecithin." *Lancet* 1975; 2(7945):1124-126.

5250 Castleman M. The Healing Herbs, the Ultimate Guide to the Curative Power of Nature's Medicines, second ed. Bantam Books: New York, NY 1995.

5251 Reid D. A Handbook of Chinese Healing Herbs. Shambhala: Boston, MA 1995.

5252 Sifton D, ed. The PDR Family Guide to Natural Medicines & Healing Therapies. Three Rivers Press: New York, 1999.

5253 Hoffman D. The Herbal Handbook: a User's Guide to Medical Herbalism (revised ed.). Healing Arts Press: Rochester, Vermont, 1998.

5254 Weiner MA, Weiner JA. Herbs that Heal: Prescription for Herbal Healing. Quantum Books: Mill Valley, California, 1999.

5255 Raintree Tropical Plant Database. "Amazon Plants" Website URL: www.rain-tree.com/plants.htm (7/30/99).

5256 Autism Research Institute. "Center for the Study of Autism" Website, URL: www.autism.com/ari/editorials/march99.html (7/31/99).

5257 Autism Research Unit. "Secretin" Website: URL: osiris.sunderland.ac.uk/autism/sec.htm (7/31/99).

5258 S.A.N.D. (Support All Neurological Diseases). "Sublingual Secretin Study" Website: URL: home.pacbell.net/mken (7/31/99).

5259 HealthNotes Online. "Herbal Demo" Website: www.heatlhnotes.com/demopro/herb/elderberry.htm (accessed 7/26/99).

5260 Zakay-Rones Z, Varsano N, Zlotnik M, et al. Inhibition of several strains of influenza virus in vitro and reduction of symptoms by an elderberry extract (Sambucus nigra L.) during an outbreak of influenza B Panama. *J Altern Complement Med* 1995;1(4):361-9.

5261 VitaminShoppe.com. "Herbal Products" Website: URL: www.vitaminshoppe.com/a2z.asp?tab=1 (7/23/99).

5262 Herbs USA. "Aphrodisiacs" Website: URL: www.aphrodisiacs.net (7/23/99).

5263 Lust J. The herb book. Bantam Books, New York, 1999.

5264 Williamson EM, Evans FJ. Potter's New Cyclopaedia of Botanical Drugs and Preparations.CW Daniel Company Limited: Essex, England, 1988.

5265 Vitamin Power. "Products," Website: www.vitaminpower.com (7/23/99).

5266 Health Source. "Bear Paw Garlic" Website: URL: www.health.source.tm/garlic2.htm (7/31/99)

5267 Botanical.Com "A Modern Herbal" Website: URL: www.botanical.com (7/31/99).

5268 HolisticOnLine. "Herb Directory" Website: URL: www.holisticonline.com (8/1/99).

5269 Healthlink. "Herbal Monographs" Website: www.healthline.com (8/1/99)

5270 Healthboards. "Autism" Website: URL: www.healthboards.com/autism/139.html (7/31/99).

5272 Colostrum Lactoferrin Direct. "Lactoferrin" website: www.colostrumdirect.com/lycopene/lactoferrin.html (Accessed 3 August 1999).

5273 Maitake Products Inc. "Grifon Maitake Caplets" website: www.maitake.com (Accessed 3 August 1999).

5274 Gerovital Direct Products. "GHS Gold" website:

www:gerivital.co.uk (Accessed 3 August 1999).

5275 PlanetRX. "Vanadium" website: www.planetrx.com/ product/nonRx (Accessed 4 August 1999).

5276 Herbal Materia Medica 4.0. Website: www.herb.com/ materia.htm (Acessed 6 August 1999).

5277 Aubourg P, Adamsbaum C, Lavallard-Rousseau MC, et al. A two-year trial of oleic and erucic acids ("Lorenzo's oil") as treatment for adrenomyeloneuropathy. *N Engl J Med*, 1993;329(11):745-752.

5278 DiGregoiro VY, Schroeder DJ. Lorenzo's oil therapy of adrenoleukodystrophy. *Ann Pharmacother*, 1995;29(3):312-313.

5279 Brown D. Encyclopedia of Herbs and Their Uses. Dorland Kindersley Publishing, Inc., New York, 1995.

5281 MotherNature.com. website: www.mothernature.com (Accessed 26 September 1999).

5282 BOF's Website. "Aromatherapy" website: www.glink.net.hk/~aromatherapy (Accessed 26 September 1999).

5283 URL: Moonmom Website. "Essential oils" website: www.provalue.net/users/moonmom/essentia.html (Accessed 26 September 1999).

5284 Gardenweb.com. "Plant database" website: www.gardenweb.com/plants/nph/nph-ind.cgi. (Accessed 26 September 1999).

5285 Wheatgrass Express Inc. "Wheatgrass" website: www.wheat-grass.com (Accessed 26 September 1999).

5286 Rauma AL, Nenonen M, Helve T, et al. Effect of a strict vegan diet on energy and nutrient intakes by Finnish rheumatoid patients. *Eur J Clin Nutr* 1993; 47(10):747-749.

5287 Pines Wheat Grass. "Nutrional Analysis" website: www.wheatgrass.com/introtowg/factsheets/ nutritionanalysis.html (Accessed 26 September 1999).

5288 Dole 5-A-Day. "Spinach" website: www.dole5aday.com/nut_center/veg/NUTVEG.html (Accessed 29 September 1999).

5289 Hawkhaven Greenhouse International. "VerdeGrass Nutritional Information" website: www.hawkhaven.com/ nutritionalinfo.html (Accessed 26 September 1999).

5290 Lowe FC, Dreikorn K, Borkowski A, et al. Review of recent placebo-controlled trials utilizing phytotherapeutic agents for treatment of BPH. *Prostate*, 1998;37(3):187-193.

5291 Purple Mountain Products. "AIM ReAssure for men1s Prostate Health" website: www.purplemountainproducts.com/reassurre.htm (Accessed 26 September 1999).

5292 Buck AC, Cox R, Rees RW, et al. Treatment of outflow tract obstruction due to benign prostatic hyperplasia with the pollen extract, cernilton. A double-blind, placebo-controlled study. *Br J Urol*, 1990;66(4):398-404.

5293 Rugendorff EW, Weidner W, Ebeling L, Buck AC. Results of treatment with pollen extract (Cernilton N) in chronic prostatitis and prostatodynia. *Br J Urol*, 1993;71(4):433-438.

5294 Yasumoto R, Kawanishi H, Tsujino T, et al. Clinical evaluation of long-term treatment using cernitin pollen extract in patients with benign prostatic hyperplasia. *Clin Ther*, 1995;17(1):82-87.

5295 Lowe FC, Ku JC. Phytotherapy in treatment of benign prostatic hyperplasia: a critical review. *Urology*, 1996;48(1):12-20.

5296 Buck AC, Rees RW, Ebeling L. Treatment of chronic prostatitis and prostatodynia with pollen extract. *Br J Urol*, 1989;64(5):496-469.

5297 Habib FK, Ross M, Lewenstein A, et al. Identification of a prostate inhibitory substance in a pollen extract. Prostate, 1995;26(3):133-139.

5298 Loschen G, Ebeling L. [Inhibition of arachidonic acid cascade by extract of rye pollen]. [Article in German]. *Arzneimittelforschung*, 1991;41(2):162-167.

5299 Agricultural Research Service: Dr. Duke's Phytochemical and Ethnobotanical Databases. URL: www.ars-grin.gov/duke (27 September 1999).

5300 Peruvian Journey website, URL: www.peruvian-journey.com/BHWS.htm (Accessed 30 September 1999).

5301 Al-Assmar SE. The Seeds of the Hawaiian Baby Woodrose Are a Powerful Hallucinogen. *Arch Intern Med* 1999;159(17):2090. Archives of Internal *Medicine* website, URL: archinte.ama assn.org/issues/current/full/ ilt0999-3.html (Accessed 27 September 1999).

5302 Tabu-smart. "Baby Hawaiian Woodrose" website: www.tabu-smart.com/woodrose.html. (Accessed 4 October 1999).

5303 Nature's Treasures. "The List of Psychoactive Plants" website: www.geocities,com.RainForest/ 3322naturetreasures.html (Accessed 4 October 1999).

5304 Shawcross WE. Recreational use of ergoline alkaloid from Argyreia nervosa. *J Psychoactive Drugs*. 1983;15:251-259.

5305 The Way Up. "Alpha-ketoglutaric Acid" website: www.thewayup.com/products.0048.htm (Accessed 6 October 1999).

5307 Smart Basics "Alpha-Ketoglutaric Acid" website: www.smartbasic.com/cat.supplements/ alpha.ketoglucaric.acid.html (Accessed 5 October 1999).

5308 Jeppsson A, Ekroth R, Friberg P, et al. Renal effects of alpha-ketoglutarate early after coronary operations. *Ann Thorac Surg* 1998;65(3):684-690.

5309 Wernerman J, Hammarqvist F, Vinnars E. Alpha-ketoglutarate and postoperative muscle catabolism. *Lancet* 1990;335(8691):701-703.

5310 Blomqvist BI, Hammarqvist F, von der Decken A, et al. Glutamine and alpha-ketoglutarate prevent the decrease in muscle free glutamine concentration and influence protein synthesis after total hip replacement. *Metabolism* 1995;44(9):1215-1222.

5311 Riedel E, Nundel M, Hampl H. Alpha-Ketoglutarate application in hemodialysis patients improves amino acid metabolism. *Nephron* 1996;74(2):261-265.

5312 Kjellman U, Bjork K, Ekroth R, et al. Alpha-ketoglutarate for myocardial protection in heart surgery. *Lancet* 1995;345(8949):552-553.

5313 Kjellman UW, Bjork K, Ekroth R, et al. Addition of alpha-ketoglutarate to blood cardioplegia improves cardioprotection. *Ann Thorac Surg* 1997;63(6):1625-1633.

5314 Aussel C, Coudray-Lucas C, Lasnier E, et al. Alpha-Ketoglutarate uptake in human fibroblasts. *Cell Biol Int* 1996;20(5):359-363.

5316 HerbsNStuff. "Stabilized Liquid Oxygen" website: www.angelfire.com/biz2/herbsnstuff/oxy.html (Accessed 5 October 1999).

5317 Matrix Health. "Earth's Bounty Oxy-caps" website: www.matrixhealth.com/product1.htm (Accessed 5 October 1999).

5318 Portal Market. "Stabilized Oxygen" webiste: www.portalmarket.com/earthportals/Portal_Market/ eathportals/portal_Ma_/oxygen.htm (Accessed 7 October 1999).

5319 Technical White Paper: "Vitamin O" Fact Sheet website:

© Copyright 2000, Natural Medicines Comprehensive Database (209) 472-2244. For updated data, go to www.NaturalDatabase.com. • 1271

REFERENCES

www.rgarden.com/vitamino.htm (Accessed 16 March 1999).

5320 Lifeplus Vitamins. "Oxygen Caps" website: www.lifeplusvitamins.simpletnet.com/1p27p.html (Accessed 7 October 1999).

5321 O2oxboost. "How to use Oxy Boost" website: www.o2xyboost.com/howto.htm (Accessed 7 October 1999).

5322 Nutrimart. "Beta sitosterol" website: www.nutrimart.com/Bulk/Description/betasist.htm (Accessed 11 October 1999).

5323 Nutrition House. "Damiana" website: www.nutritionhouse.com/page387.html (Accessed 11 October 1999).

5324 Mother Nature. "Beta sitosterol-power" website: www.mothernature.com/asp/product.asp?product+3005401103 (Accessed 11 October 1999).

5325 Mother Nature. "Saw Palmetto & Beta sitosterol-power" website: www.mothernature.com/asp/product.asp?product+3005401285 (Accessed 11 October 1999).

5326 Salen G, Shefer S, Nguyen L, et al. Sisterolemia. *J Lipid Res* 1992;33(7):945-955.

5327 Berges RR, Windeler J, Trampisch HJ, et al. Randomised, placebo-controlled, double-blind clinical trial of beta-sitosterol in patients with benign prostatic hyperplasia. Beta-sitosterol Study Group. *Lancet* 1995;345(8964):1529-1532.

5328 Klippel KF, Hiltl DM, Schipp B. A multicentric, placebo-controlled, double-blind clinical trial of beta-sitosterol (phytosterol) for the treatment of benign prostatic hyperplasia. *Br J Urol* 1997;80(3):427-432.

5329 Wilt TJ, MacDonald R, Ishani A. beta-sitosterol for the treatment of benign prostatic hyperplasia: a systematic review. *BJU Int* 1999;83(9):976-983.

5330 Becker M, Staab D, Von Bergmann K. Treatment of severe familial hypercholesterolemia in childhood with sitosterol and sitostanol. *J Pediatr* 1993;122(2):292-296.

5331 Oster P, Schlierf G, Heuck CC, et al. [Sitosterol in familial hyperlipoproteinemia type II. A randomized double-blind cross-over study]. [Article in German] *Dtsch Med Wochenschr* 1976;101(36):1308-1311.

5332 Schlierf G, Oster P, Heuck CC, et al. Sitosterol in juvenile type II hyperlipoproteinemia. *Atherosclerosis* 1978;30(4):245-248.

5333 Schwartzkopff W, Jantke HJ. [Dose-effect of beta-sitosterin in type IIa and IIb ypercholesterolemias]. [Article in German] *MMW Munch Med Wochenschr* 1978;120(47):1575-1578.

5334 Becker M, Staab D, Von Bergman K. Long-term treatment of severe familial hypercholesterolemia in children: effect of sitosterol and bezafibrate. *Pediatrics* 1992;89(1):138-142.

5335 Bouic PJ, Clark A, Lamprecht J, et al. The effects of B-sitosterol (BSS) and B-sitosterol glucoside (BSSG) mixture on selected immune parameters of marathon runners: inhibition of post marathon immune suppression and inflammation. *Int J Sports Med* 1999;20(4):258-262.

5336 Weststrate JA, Meijer GW. Plant sterol-enriched margarines and reduction of plasma total- and LDL-cholesterol concentrations in normocholesterolaemic and mildly hypercholesterolaemic subjects. *Eur J Clin Nutr* 1998;52(5):334-343.

5337 Donald PR, Lamprecht JH, Freestone M, et al. A randomised placebo-controlled trial of the efficacy of beta-sitosterol and its glucoside as adjuvants in the treatment of pulmonary tuberculosis. *Int J Tuberc Lung Dis* 1997;1(6):518-522.

5338 Gerolami A, Sarles H. Letter: Beta-sitosterol and chenodeoxycholic acid in the treatment of cholesterol gallstones. *Lancet* 1975;2(7937):721.

5339 Tangedahl TN, Thistle JL, Hofmann AF, et al. Effect of beta-sitosterol alone or in combination with chenic acid on cholesterol saturation of bile and cholesterol absorption in gallstone patients. *Gastroenterology* 1979;76(6):1341-1346.

5340 Anon. Cholesterol-lowering Margarines. *Med Lett Drugs Ther* 1999;41(1055):56-8.

5341 Drug Info Line. "Benecol: A Cholesterol Lowering margarine" website: http://www.pharminfo.com/pubs/druginfoline/druginfo1_22.html (Accessed 12 October 1999).

5342 Bouic PJ, Lamprecht JH, Plant sterols and sterolins: a review of their immune-modulating properties. *Altern Med Rev* 1999;4(3):170-177.

5344 Lomaestro BM, Malone M. Glutathione in health and disease: pharmacotherapeutic issues. *Ann Pharmacother* 1995;29(12):1263-1273.

5345 Flagg EW, Coates RJ, Jones DP, et al. Dietary glutathione intake and the risk of oral and pharyngeal cancer. *Am J Epidemiol* 1994;139(5):453-465.

5346 Walsh SW, Wang Y. Deficient glutathione peroxidase activity in preeclampsia is associated with increased placental production of thromboxane and lipid peroxides. *Am J Obstet Gynecol* 1993;169(6):1456-1461.

5347 Knapen MF, Mulder TP, Van Rooij IA, et al. Low whole blood glutathione levels in pregnancies complicated by preeclampsia or the hemolysis, elevated liver enzymes, low platelets syndrome. *Obstet Gynecol* 1998;92(6):1012-1015.

5348 Knapen MF, Peters WH, Mulder TP, et al. Glutathione and glutathione-related enzymes in decidua and placenta of controls and women with pre-eclampsia. *Placenta* 1999;20(7):541-546.

5349 Marshall KA, Reist M, Jenner P, el al. The neuronal toxicity of sulfite plus peroxynitrite is enhanced by glutathione depletion: implications for Parkinson's disease. *Free Radic Biol Med* 1999;27(5-6):515-520.

5350 Jenner P, Olanow CW. Understanding cell death in Parkinson's disease. *Ann Neurol* 1998;44(3 Suppl 1):S72-84.

5351 Jenner P. Oxidative mechanisms in nigral cell death in Parkinson's disease. *Mov Disord* 1998;(13 Suppl)1:24-34.

5352 Pearce RK, Owen A, Daniel S, et al. Alterations in the distribution of glutathione in the substantia nigra in Parkinson's disease. *J Neural Transm* 1997;104(6-7):661-677.

5353 Merad-Boudia M, Nicole A, Santiard-Baron D, et al. Mitochondrial impairment as an early event in the process of apoptosis induced by glutathione depletion in neuronal cells: relevance to Parkinson's disease. *Biochem Pharmacol* 1998;56(5):645-655.

5354 Sechi G, Deledda MG, Bua G, et al. Reduced intravenous glutathione in the treatment of early Parkinson's disease. Prog Neuropsychopharmacol *Biol Psychiatry* 1996;20(7):1159-1170.

5355 Life Extension Foundation. "Mega L-glutathione" website: www.lef.org/prod_des/item56.html (Accessed 18 October 1999).

5356 Suprahealth. "L-Glutathione" website: www.suprahealth.com/gluathi.htm (Accessed 18 October 1999).

5357 De Mattia G, Bravi MC, Laurenti O, et al. Influence of reduced glutathione infusion on glucose metabolism in patients with non-insulin-dependent siabetes mellitus. *Metabolism* 1998;47(8):993-997.

5358 Ciuchi E, Odetti P, Prando R. The effect of acute glutathione treatment on sorbitol level in erythrocytes from diabetic patients. *Diabetes Metab* 1997;23(1):58-60.

5359 Usberti M, Lima G, Arisi M, et al. Effect of exogenous reduced glutathione on the survival of red blood cells in hemodialyzed patients. *J Nephrol* 1997;10(5):261-265.

5360 Amano J, Suzuki A, Sunamori M. Salutary effect of reduced glutathione on renal function in coronary artery bypass operation. *J Am Coll Surg* 1994;179(6):714-720.

5361 Cook GC, Sherlock S. Results of a controlled clinical trial of glutathione in cases of hepatic cirrhosis. *Gut* 1965; 6(5):472-476.

5362 Witschi A, Reddy S, Stofer B, et al. The systemic availability of oral glutathione. *Eur J Clin Pharmacol* 1992;43(6):667-669.

5363 Hagen TM, Wierzbicka GT, Bowman BB, et al. Fate of dietary glutathione: disposition in the gastrointestinal tract. *Am J Physiol* 1990;259(4 Pt 1):G530-535.

5364 Aw TY, Wierzbicka G, Jones DP. Oral glutathione increases tissue glutathione in vivo. *Chem Biol Interact* 1991;80(1):89-97.

5365 Smart Basics. "Glossary – glutathione" website: http://www.smartbasic.com/glos.aminos/glutathione.glos.html (Accessed 19 October 1999).

5366 MotherNature. "Glutathione — Nutricology": http://www.mothernature.com/asp/product.asp?product=1394750140 (Accessed 19 October 1999).

5367 Roum JH, Borok Z, McElvaney NG, et al. Glutathione aerosol suppresses lung epithelial surface inflammatory cell-derived oxidants in cystic fibrosis. *J Appl Physiol* 1999;87(1):438-443.

5368 Holroyd KJ, Buhl R, Borok Z, et al. Correction of glutathione deficiency in the lower respiratory tract of HIV seropositive individuals by glutathione aerosol treatment. *Thorax* 1993;48(10):985-989.

5369 Borok Z, Buhl R, Grimes GJ, et al. Effect of glutathione aerosol on oxidant-antioxidant imbalance in idiopathic pulmonary fibrosis. *Lancet* 1991;338(8761):215-216.

5372 Marrades RM, Roca J, Barbera JA, et al. Nebulized glutathione induces bronchoconstriction in patients with mild asthma. *Am J Respir Crit Care Med* 1997;156(2 Pt 1):425-430.

5373 Smyth JF, Bowman A, Perren T, et al. Glutathione reduces the toxicity and improves quality of life of women diagnosed with ovarian cancer treated with cisplatin: results of a double-blind, randomised trial. *Ann Oncol* 1997;8(6):569-573.

5374 Cascinu S, Cordella L, Del Ferro E, et al. Neuroprotective effect of reduced glutathione on cisplatin-based *Chemotherapy* in advanced gastric cancer: a randomized double-blind placebo-controlled trial. *J Clin Oncol* 1995;13(1):26-32.

5375 Links M, Lewis C. Chemoprotectants: a review of their clinical pharmacology and therapeutic efficacy. *Drugs* 1999;57(3):293-308.

5376 Leone R, Fracasso ME, Soresi E, et al. Influence of glutathione administration on the disposition of free and

5376 total platinum in patients after administration of cisplatin. *Cancer Chemother Pharmacol* 1992;29(5):385-390.

5377 Graziano F, Cardarelli N, Marcellini M, et al. A pilot clinical trial of postoperative intensive weekly Chemotherapy using cisplatin, epi-doxorubicin, 5-fluorouracil, 6S-leucovorin, glutathione and filgrastim in patients with resected gastric cancer. *Tumori* 1998;84(3):368-371.

5378 Plaxe S, Freddo J, Kim S, et al. Phase I trial of cisplatin in combination with glutathione. *Gynecol Oncol* 1994;55(1):82-86.

5379 Locatelli MC, D'Antona A, Labianca R, et al. A phase II study of combination chemotherapy in advanced ovarian carcinoma with cisplatin and cyclophosphamide plus reduced glutathione as potential protective agent against cisplatin toxicity. *Tumori* 1993;79(1):37-39.

5380 Di Re F, Bohm S, Oriana S, et al. High-dose cisplatin and cyclophosphamide with glutathione in the treatment of advanced ovarian cancer. *Ann Oncol* 1993;4(1):55-61.

5381 Parnis FX, Coleman RE, Harper PG, et al. A randomised double-blind placebo controlled clinical trial assessing the tolerability and efficacy of glutathione as an adjuvant to escalating doses of cisplatin in the treatment of advanced ovarian cancer. *Eur J Cancer* 1995;31A(10):1721.

5382 Cascinu S, Frontini L, Comella G, et al. Intensive weekly Chemotherapy is not effective in advanced pancreatic Cancer patients: a report from the Italian Group for the Study of Digestive Tract Cancer (GISCAD). *Br J Cancer* 1999;79(3-4):491-494.

5383 Cascinu S, Labianca R, Alessandroni P, et al. Intensive weekly Chemotherapy for advanced gastric Cancer using fluorouracil, cisplatin, epi-doxorubicin, 6S-leucovorin, glutathione, and filgrastim: a report from the Italian Group for the Study of Digestive Tract Cancer. *J Clin Oncol* 1997;15(11):3313-3319.

5384 Lenzi A, Culasso F, Gandini L, Placebo-controlled, double-blind, cross-over trial of glutathione therapy in male infertility. *Hum Reprod* 1993;8(10):1657-1662.

5385 Coppola L, Grassia A, Giunta R, et al. Glutathione (GSH) improved haemostatic and haemorheological parameters in atherosclerotic subjects. *Drugs Exp Clin Res* 1992;18(11-12):493-498.

5386 Powers SK, Hamilton K. Antioxidants and exercise. *Clin Sports Med* 1999;18(3):525-536.

5387 Anderson ME. Glutathione: an overview of biosynthesis and modulation. *Chem Biol Interact* 1998;24;111-112:1-14.

5388 Lu SC. Regulation of hepatic glutathione synthesis: current concepts and controversies. *FASEB J* 1999;13(10):1169-1183.

5389 Amores-Sanchez MI, Medina MA. Glutamine, as a precursor of glutathione, and oxidative stress. *Mol Genet Metab* 1999;67(2):100-105.

5392 Ruffmann R, Wendel A. GSH rescue by N-acetylcysteine. *Klin Wochenschr* 1991;69(18):857-862.

5393 Droge W, Holm E. Role of cysteine and glutathione in HIV infection and other diseases associated with muscle wasting and immunological dysfunction. *FASEB J* 1997;11(13):1077-1089.

5394 Herzenberg LA, De Rosa SC, Dubs JG, et al. Glutathione deficiency is associated with impaired survival in HIV disease. *Proc Natl Acad Sci USA* 1997;94(5):1967-1972.

5395 Samiec PS, Drews-Botsch C, Flagg EW, et al.

© Copyright 2000, Natural Medicines Comprehensive Database (209) 472-2244. For updated data, go to www.NaturalDatabase.com. • 1273

Glutathione in human plasma: decline in association with aging, age-related macular degeneration, and diabetes. *Free Radic Biol Med* 1998;24(5):699-704.

5396 Bains JS, Shaw CA. Neurodegenerative disorders in humans: the role of glutathione in oxidative stress-mediated neuronal death. *Brain Res Brain Res Rev* 1997;25(3):335-358.

5397 Loguercio C, Di Pierro M. The role of glutathione in the gastrointestinal tract: a review. *Ital J Gastroenterol Hepatol* 1999;31(5):401-407.

5398 Powers SK, Ji LL, Leeuwenburgh C. Exercise training-induced alterations in skeletal muscle antioxidant capacity: a brief review. *Med Sci Sports Exerc* 1999;31(7):987-997.

5399 NuTriVene-D. "What is NuTriVene-D" website: www.nutrivene.com/whatis.html (Accessed 20 October 1999).

5400 Nutrichem. "MSB Plus" website: www.nutrichem.com/custom/index.html (Accessed 21 October 1999).

5401 Warner House. "Trisomy 21" website: www.warnerhouse.com/ (Accessed 21 October 1999).

5402 Trisomy 21 Research Foundation. "Targeted Nutritional Intervention (TNI) in the Treatment of Children and Adults with Down Syndrome" website: www.tri21.org/leictman/ (Accessed 21 October 1999).

5403 Cognitive Enhancement Research Institute. "Smart Drugs and Down's Syndrome" website: www.ceri.com/downs.htm. (Accessed 21 October 1999).

5404 National Down Syndrome Congress. "Position Statement: Nutritional Intervention in Children with Down Syndrome" website: http://members.carol.net/~ndsc/tni.html (Accessed 21 October 1999).

5405 National Down Syndrome Society. "Clinical Information" website: http://www.ndss.org/AboutDS/ClinicalInfo/clinicalinfo.html (Accessed 24 October 1999).

5406 Colombo ML, Girardo E, Incarbone E, et al. [Vitamin C in children with trisomy 21]. [Article in Italian]. *Minerva Pediatr* 1989;41(4):189-192.

5407 Pueschel SM, Hillemeier C, Caldwell M, et al. Vitamin A gastrointestinal absorption in persons with Down's syndrome. *J Ment Defic Res* 1990;34(Pt 3):269-275.

5408 Del Arco C, Riancho JA, Luzuriaga C, et al. Vitamin D status in children with Down's syndrome. *J Intellect Disabil Res* 1992;6(Pt 3):251-257.

5409 Metcalfe T, Bowen DM, Muller DP. Vitamin E concentrations in human brain of patients with Alzheimer's disease, fetuses with Down's syndrome, centenarians, and controls. *Neurochem Res* 1989;14(12):1209-1212.

5410 Menolascino FJ, Donaldson JY, Gallagher TF, et al. Vitamin supplements and purported learning enhancement in mentally retarded children. *J Nutr Sci Vitaminol* (Tokyo) 1989;35(3):181-92.

5411 Harrell RF, Capp RH, Davis DR, et al. Can nutritional supplements help mentally retarded children? an exploratory study. *Proc Natl Acad Sci USA*, 1981;78(1):574-578.

5412 Pruess JB, Fewell RR, Bennett FC. Vitamin therapy and children with Down syndrome: a review of research. *Except Chil* 1989;55(4):336-341.

5413 Weathers C. Effects of nutritional supplementation on IQ and certain other variables associated with Down syndrome. *Am J Ment Defic* 1983;88(2):214-217.

5414 Kleijnen J, Knipschild P. Niacin and vitamin B6 in mental functioning: a review of controlled trials in humans. *Biol Psychiatry* 1991;29(9):931-41.

5415 Smith GF, Spiker D, Peterson CP, et al. Use of megadoses of vitamins with minerals in Down syndrome. *J Pediatr* 1984;105(2):228-234.

5416 Bidder RT, Gray P, Newcombe RG, et al. The effects of multivitamins and minerals on children with Down syndrome. *Dev Med Child Neurol* 1989;31(4):532-537.

5417 Anneren G, Gebre-Medhin M, Gustavson KH. Increased plasma and erythrocyte selenium concentrations but decreased erythrocyte glutathione peroxidase activity after selenium supplementation in children with Down syndrome. *Acta Paediatr Scand* 1989;78(6):879-884.

5418 Anneren G, Magnusson CG, Nordvall SL. Increase in serum concentrations of IgG2 and IgG4 by selenium supplementation in children with Down's syndrome. *Arch Dis Child* 1990;65(12):1353-1355.

5419 Brigino EN, Good RA, Koutsonikolis A, et al. Normalization of cellular zinc levels in patients with Downs syndrome does not always correct low thymulin levels. *Acta Paediatr* 1996;85(11):1370-1372.

5420 Licastro F, Mocchegiani E, Zannotti M, et al. Zinc affects the metabolism of thyroid hormones in children with Down's syndrome: normalization of thyroid stimulating hormone and of reversal triiodothyronine plasmic levels by dietary zinc supplementation. *Int J Neurosci* 1992;65(1-4):259-268.

5421 Antonucci A, Di Baldassarre A, Di Giacomo F, et al. Detection of apoptosis in peripheral blood cells of 31 subjects affected by Down syndrome before and after zinc therapy. *Ultrastruct Pathol* 1997;21(5):449-452.

5422 Bucci I, Napolitano G, Giuliani C, et al. Zinc sulfate supplementation improves thyroid function in hypozincemic Down children. *Biol Trace Elem Res* 1999;67(3):257-268.

5423 Lockitch G, Puterman M, Godolphin W, et al. Infection and immunity in Down syndrome: a trial of long-term low oral doses of zinc. *J Pediatr* 1989;114(5):781-787.

5424 Lejeune J, Rethore MO, de Blois MC, et al. [Amino acids and trisomy 21]. [Article in French] *Ann Genet* 1992;35(1):8-13.

5425 Heggarty HJ, Ball R, Smith M, et al. Amino acid profile in Down's syndrome. *Arch Dis Child* 1996;74(4):347-349.

5426 Busciglio J, Yankner BA. Apoptosis and increased generation of reactive oxygen species in Down's syndrome neurons in vitro. *Nature* 1995;378(6559):776-779.

5427 Quackwatch. "Nutritional Supplements for Down Syndrome" website: www.quackwatch.com/01quackeryrelatedtopics/down.html (Accessed 24 October 1999).

5428 Downsnet. "Multi-nutrient Formulas and Other Substances as Therapies for Down Syndrome" website: www.downsnet.org/library/dsnu/01/2/70 (Accessed 24 October 1999).

5429 Gylling H, Miettinen TA. Cholesterol reduction by different plant stanol mixtures and with variable fat intake. *Metabolism* 1999;48(5):575-580.

5430 Gylling H, Puska P, Vartiainen E, et al. Serum sterols during stanol ester feeding in a mildly hypercholesterolemic population. *J Lipid Res* 1999;40(4):593-600.

5431 Gylling H, Radhakrishnan R, Miettinen TA. Reduction of serum cholesterol in postmenopausal women with previous myocardial infarction and cholesterol malabsorption induced by dietary sitostanol ester margarine: women and dietary sitostanol. *Circulation* 1997;96(12):4226-4231.

5432 Gylling H, Miettinen TA. Serum cholesterol and cholesterol and lipoprotein Metabolism in hypercholesterolaemic NIDDM patients before and during sitostanol ester-margarine treatment. *Diabetologia* 1994;37(8):773-780.

5433 Gylling H, Miettinen TA. Effects of inhibiting cholesterol absorption and synthesis on cholesterol and lipoprotein Metabolism in hypercholesterolemic non-insulin-dependent diabetic men. *J Lipid Res* 1996;37(8):1776-1785.

5434 Gylling H, Puska P, Vartiainen E, et al. Retinol, vitamin D, carotenes and alpha-tocopherol in serum of a moderately hypercholesterolemic population consuming sitostanol ester margarine. *Atherosclerosis* 1999;145(2):279-285.

5435 Hallikainen MA, Uusitupa MI. Effects of 2 low-fat stanol ester-containing margarines on serum cholesterol concentrations as part of a low-fat diet in hypercholesterolemic subjects. *Am J Clin Nutr* 1999;69(3):403-410.

5436 Heinemann T, Kullak-Ublick GA, Pietruck B, et al. Mechanisms of action of plant sterols on inhibition of cholesterol absorption. Comparison of sitosterol and sitostanol. *Eur J Clin Pharmacol* 1991;40 Suppl 1:S59-63.

5437 Jones PJ, Ntanios FY, Raeini-Sarjaz M, et al. Cholesterol-lowering efficacy of a sitostanol-containing phytosterol mixture with a prudent diet in hyperlipidemic men. *Am J Clin Nutr* 1999;69(6):1144-1150.

5438 Gylling H, Siimes MA, Miettinen TA. Sitostanol ester margarine in dietary treatment of children with familial hypercholesterolemia. *J Lipid Res* 1995;36(8):1807-12.

5439 Miettinen TA, Puska P, Gylling H, et al. Reduction of serum cholesterol with sitostanol-ester margarine in a mildly hypercholesterolemic population. *N Engl J Med* 1995;333(20):1308-1312.

5440 Lutjohann D, von Bergmann K. Phytosterolaemia: diagnosis, characterization and therapeutical approaches. *Ann Med* 1997;29(3):181-184.

5441 Vanhanen HT, Kajander J, Lehtovirta H. Serum levels, absorption efficiency, faecal elimination and synthesis of cholesterol during increasing doses of dietary sitostanol esters in hypercholesterolaemic subjects. *Clin Sci (Colch)* 1994;87(1):61-67.

5442 Weststrate JA, Meijer GW. Plant sterol-enriched margarines and reduction of plasma total- and LDL-cholesterol concentrations in normocholesterolaemic and mildly hypercholesterolaemic subjects. *Eur J Clin Nutr* 1998;52(5):334-343.

5443 Cholesterol-lowering margarines. *Medical Letter* 1999;41:56-58.

5444 Cowley G, Underwood A. *Newsweek*. July 5, 1999, 46-50.

5446 Czap A. Beware the son of SAMe. *Altern Med Rev*, 1999;4(2):73.

5447 Natrol. "SAM Sulfate" website: www.natrol.com (Accessed 3 November 1999).

5448 Powell-Tuck J, Jamieson CP, Bettany GE, et al. A double blind, randomised, controlled trial of glutamine supplementation in parenteral nutrition. *Gut* 1999;45(1):82-88.

5449 Houdijk AP, Rijnsburger ER, Jansen J, et al. Randomised trial of glutamine-enriched enteral nutrition on infectious morbidity in patients with multiple trauma. *Lancet* 1998; 352(9130):772-776.

5450 Jones C, Palmer TE, Griffiths RD. Randomized clinical outcome study of critically ill patients given glutamine-supplemented enteral nutrition. *Nutrition* 1999;15(2):108-15.

5451 Schloerb PR, Skikne BS. Oral and parenteral glutamine in Bone Marrow Transplantation: a randomized, double-blind study. *JPEN J Parenter Enteral Nutr* 1999;23(3):117-122.

5452 Brown SA, Goringe A, Fegan C, et al. Parenteral glutamine protects hepatic function during Bone Marrow Transplantation. *Bone Marrow Transplant* 1998;22(3):281-284.

5453 Ziegler TR, Bye RL, Persinger RL, et al. Effects of glutamine supplementation on circulating lymphocytes after Bone Marrow Transplantation: a pilot study. *Am J Med* Sci 1998;315(1):4-10.

5454 Wilmore DW, Schloerb PR, Ziegler TR. Glutamine in the support of patients following Bone Marrow Transplantation. *Curr Opin Clin Nutr Metab Care* 1999;2(4):323-327.

5455 Rohde T, Asp S, MacLean DA, et al. Competitive sustained exercise in humans, lymphokine activated killer cell activity, and glutamine—an intervention study. *Eur J Appl Physiol* 1998;78(5):448-453.

5456 Rohde T, MacLean DA, Pedersen BK. Effect of glutamine supplementation on changes in the immune system induced by repeated exercise. *Med Sci Sports Exerc* 1998;30(6):856-862.

5457 Bowtell JL, Gelly K, Jackman ML, et al. Effect of oral glutamine on whole body carbohydrate storage during recovery from exhaustive exercise. *J Appl Physiol* 1999;86(6):1770-1777.

5458 Decker-Baumann C, Buhl K, Frohmuller S, et al. Reduction of chemotherapy-induced side-effects by parenteral glutamine supplementation in patients with metastatic colorectal cancer. *Eur J Cancer* 1999;35(2):202-207.

5460 Niihara Y, Zerez CR, Akiyama DS, et al. Oral L-glutamine therapy for sickle cell anemia: I. Subjective clinical improvement and favorable change in red cell NAD redox potential. *Am J Hematol* 1998;58(2):117-121.

5461 Noyer CM, Simon D, Borczuk A, et al. A double-blind placebo-controlled pilot study of glutamine therapy for abnormal intestinal permeability in patients with AIDS. *Am J Gastroenterol* 1998;93(6):972-975.

5462 Okuno SH, Woodhouse CO, Loprinzi CL, et al. Phase III controlled evaluation of glutamine for decreasing stomatitis in patients receiving fluorouracil (5-FU)-based chemotherapy. *Am J Clin Oncol* 1999;22(3):258-261.

5464 Castell LM, Newsholme EA. Glutamine and the effects of exhaustive exercise upon the immune response. *Can J Physiol Pharmacol* 1998;76(5):524-532.

5465 Antonio J, Street C. Glutamine: a potentially useful supplement for athletes. Can *J Appl Physiol* 1999;24(1):1-14.

5466 Walsh NP, Blannin AK, Robson PJ, et al. Glutamine, exercise and immune function. Links and possible mechanisms. *Sports Med* 1998;26(3):177-191.

5467 Griffiths RD. Glutamine: establishing clinical indications. *Curr Opin Clin Nutr Metab Care* 1999;2(2):177-182.

5468 Sacks GS. Glutamine supplementation in catabolic patients. *Ann Pharmacother* 1999;33(3):348-354.

REFERENCES

5469 Miller AL. Therapeutic considerations of L-glutamine: a review of the literature. *Altern Med Rev* 1999;4(4):239-248.

5470 Amores-Sanchez MI, Medina MA. Glutamine, as a precursor of glutathione, and oxidative stress. *Mol Genet Metab* 1999;67(2):100-105.

5471 Betterbodz. "FAQs about GABA" website, URL: www.betterbodz.com/library2/gabaquest.html (Accessed 4 November 1999).

5472 Mushroom Nutraceuticals. "Mushrooms, *Nutrition* and Health" website: www.gmushrooms.com/health/nmh.html. (Accessed 7 November 1999).

5473 Mother*Nature* Encyclopedia. "Reishi" website: ww.mothernature.com/ency/herb/reishi.asp. (Accessed 7 November 1999).

5474 Vitamin Planet. "Reishi Mushroom" website: www.vitaminplante.com/nutrition/reishi.htm. (Accessed 7 November 1999).

5475 Health Foods Business. "Reishi: Ancient Medicine is Modern Hope" website: www.home.pacific.net.hk/~gng/reishi.html. (Accessed 7 November 1999).

5476 Tao J, Feng KY. Experimental and clinical studies on inhibitory effect of ganoderma lucidum on platelet aggregation. *J Tongji Med Univ* 1990;10(4):240-243.

5477 Wasser SP, Weis AL. Therapeutic effects of substances occurring in higher Basidiomycetes mushrooms: a modern perspective. *Crit Rev Immunol* 1999;19(1):65-96.

5478 Gau JP, Lin CK, Lee SS, et al. The lack of antiplatelet effect of crude extracts from ganoderma lucidum on HIV-positive hemophiliacs. *Am J Chin Med* 1990;18(3-4):175-179.

5479 Singh AB, Gupta SK, Pereira BM, et al. Sensitization to Ganoderma lucidum in patients with respiratory allergy in India. *Clin Exp Allergy* 1995;25(5):440-447.

5480 Min BS, Nakamura N, Miyashiro H, et al. Triterpenes from the spores of Ganoderma lucidum and their inhibitory activity against HIV-1 protease. *Chem Pharm Bull* (Tokyo) 1998;46(10):1607-1612.

5481 el-Mekkawy S, Meselhy MR, Nakamura N, et al. Anti-HIV-1 and anti-HIV-1-protease substances from Ganoderma lucidum. *Phytochemistry* 1998;49(6):1651-1657.

5482 Kim RS, Kim HW, Kim BK. Suppressive effects of Ganoderma lucidum on proliferation of peripheral blood mononuclear cells. *Mol Cells* 1997;7(1):52-57.

5483 Wang SY, Hsu ML, Hsu HC, et al. The anti-tumor effect of Ganoderma lucidum is mediated by cytokines released from activated macrophages and T lymphocytes. *Int J Cancer* 1997;70(6):699-705.

5484 Kim HS, Kacew S, Lee BM. In vitro chemopreventive effects of plant polysaccharides (Aloe barbadensis miller, Lentinus edodes, Ganoderma lucidum and Coriolus versicolor). *Carcinogenesis* 1999;20(8):1637-1640.

5485 Hijikata Y, Yamada S. Effect of Ganoderma lucidum on postherpetic neuralgia. *Am J Chin Med* 1998;26(3-4):375-381.

5486 Komoda Y, Shimizu M, Sonoda Y, et al. Ganoderic acid and its derivatives as cholesterol synthesis inhibitors. *Chem Pharm Bull* (Tokyo) 1989;37(2):531-533.

5487 Hikino H, Ishiyama M, Suzuki Y, et al. Mechanisms of hypoglycemic activity of ganoderan B: a glycan of Ganoderma lucidum fruit bodies. *Planta Med* 1989;55(5):423-428.

5488 Lee SY, Rhee HM. Cardiovascular effects of mycelium extract of Ganoderma lucidum: inhibition of sympathetic outflow as a mechanism of its hypotensive action. *Chem Pharm Bull* (Tokyo) 1990;38(5):1359-1364.

5489 Kim DH, Shim SB, Kim NJ, et al. Beta-glucuronidase-inhibitory activity and hepatoprotective effect of Ganoderma lucidum. *Biol Pharm Bull* 1999;22(2):162-164.

5490 Yoon SY, Eo SK, Kim YS, et al. Antimicrobial activity of Ganoderma lucidum extract alone and in combination with some antibiotics. *Arch Pharm Res* 1994;17(6):438-442.

5491 Chen K, Li C. Recent advances in studies on traditional Chinese anti-aging materia medica. *J Tradit Chin Med* 1993;13(3):223-226.

5492 van der Hem LG, van der Vliet JA, Bocken CF, et al. Ling Zhi-8: studies of a new immunomodulating agent. *Transplantation* 1995;60(5):438-443.

5493 Wang WK, Chen HL, Hsu TL. Alteration of pulse in human subjects by three Chinese herbs. *Am J Chin Med* 1994;22(2):197-203.

5494 Wang HX, NG TB, Liu WK, et al. Polysaccharide-peptide complexes from the cultured mycelia of the mushroom Coriolus versicolor and their culture medium activate mouse lymphocytes and macrophages. *Int J Biochem Cell Biol*, 1996;28(5):601-607.

5495 Wellness MD Webstore. "Coriolus-MRL" website: www.store.wellnessmd.com/store-welnessmd-com/MP1000chk. (Accessed 10 November 1999).

5496 JHS Natural Products. "Coriolus Versicolor Introduction" website:www.jhsnaturals.com/history.html. (Accessed 10 November 1999).

5497 Mycoinfo. "A Polyspore Named Versicolor" website: www.mycoinfo.com/trametes.html. (Accessed 10 November 1999).

5498 Polysaccharide Peptides, Inc. "Coriolus-PSP" website: www.psp.bc.ca/e-coriolus-psp.htm. (Accessed 10 November 1999).

5499 Chem ID. website http://igm.nlm.nih.gov/cgibin/doler?account=++&password=++&datafile=cheid (Accessed 10 November 1999).

5500 Alander M, Satokari R, Korpela R, et al. Persistence of colonization of human colonic mucosa by a probiotic strain, Lactobacillus rhamnosus GG, after oral consumption. *Applied and Environmental Microbiology* 199;65(1):351-354.

5501 Bensky D, Gamble A, Kaptchuk T. Chinese Herbal Medicine Materia Medica. Seattle: Eastland Press. 1996;483-485.

5502 Huang KC. The Pharmacology of Chinese Herbs. 2nd ed. Boca Raton: CRC Press LLC. 1999;266-267.

5503 Kim HS, Lim HK, Park WK. Antinarcotic effects of the velvet antler water extract on morphine in mice. *J Ethnopharmacol*, 1999;66(1):41-49.

5504 Goldsmith LA. The velvet case. *Arch Dermatol*, 124(5):768.

5505 Anon. Human clinical trials show significant results for New Zealand deer antler velvet's effect on sports performance. 2000. URL: www.prnewswire.com (Accessed 7 March 2000).

5506 Elk Meadows Distributing. Start your family health tradition today with Vital-EX and feel great naturally. July 19, 1998. URL: http://www.idsnowman.com/indexxx.htm. (Accessed 22 March 2000).

5507 Anon. Attributes of velvet deer antler. 2000. URL: http://angelfire.com/oh2/fountainofyouth/velvet.html. (Accessed 22 March 2000).

5508 DeerVelvet. org/GMTC Ltd. 2/21/99. URL: http://deervelvet.org/index.html. (Accessed 22 March 2000).

5509 Hart. January 30, 2000. URL: http://mysite.xtralco.nz/~BRAVEHART/. (Accessed 22 March 2000).

5510 Anon. Improve your health, revitalize your body with CERAVEL Deer Velvet TONIC. 2000. URL. http://www.ceravel.co.nz/. (Accessed 22 March 2000).

5511 Anon. Deer Velvet of New Zealand. 2000. http://www.comcen.com.u/~lawriedunn/deervelvet.html. (Accessed 22 March 2000).

5512 Anon. Immunostimulatory effects. 2000. http://www.countrylodge.co.nz/nutrition.html. (Accessed 22 March 2000).

5513 Anon. Deer Velvet Antler Nature's Superior Health Tonic. 2000. URL. http://www.gold-mountain.co.nz. (Accessed 22 March 2000).

5514 Suttie JM, Fennessy PR, Haines SR, et al. The Velvet Antler Industry: Background Research and Findings. 2000. http://www.healthy.net/library/articles/abdo/antler.htm (Accessed 22 March 2000).

5515 Mascot Enterprise. Super Nutrition Power-Herbal Supplement. 2000. URL: http://www.mascotsnp.com/ (Accessed 22 March 2000).

5516 Anon. 2000. URL. http://www.nutrisana.com/html/deer.velvet antler.html. (Accessed 22 March 2000).

5517 Sim JS, Sunwoo HH. Canadian Scientists Study Velvet Antler for Arthritis Treatment. 1999. URL. http://qeva.com/research/UofA.htm (Accessed 22 March 2000).

5518 Ko KM, Yip TT, Tsao SW, Kong YC, et al. Epidermal growth factor from deer (Cervus elaphus) submaxillary gland and velvet antler. Gen Comp Endocrinol, September 1986;63(3):431-440.

5519 Colloidal Silver Discovery Center. 2000. URL. http://colloidalsilver.net/info.html. (Accessed 24 March 2000).

5520 Anon. What is colloidal silver? 2000. URL. http://apothecary.hypermart.net/what_is_cs.htm. (Accessed 24 March 2000).

5521 Coburn DL. Colloidal Silver-A healthy silver lining. 1999. URL. http://www.colloidal-silver.com/ (Accessed 24 March 2000).

5522 Robey M, Medical and Non-medical uses. 1999. URL. http://www.colloidal-silver.com/ (Accessed 24 March 2000).

5523 Barrett S. Colloidal Silver: risk without benefit. November 5,1999. URL. http://www.quackwatch.com/01QuackeryRelated Topics/PhonyAds/silverad.html (Accessed 24 March 2000).

5524 Department of Health and Human Services. 21 CFR Part 310. Federal Register: August 17, 1999. URL. http://www.verity.fda.gov/search97cgi/s97_cgi.exe?action=View&VdkVgwKey=http (Accessed 21 March 2000).

5525 Fung MC, Bowen DL. Silver products for medical indications: risk-benefit assessment. Clinical Toxicology 1996; 34(1):119-126. Center of Drug Evaluation and Research, Food and Drug Administration, Rockville, Maryland, USA.

5526 Fung MC, Weintraub M, Bowen DL. Colloidal silver proteins marketed as health supplements. JAMA 1995;274(15):1196-1197.

5527 Anon. Life Plus the very finest in health and nutrition supplements. 2000. URL. http://www.lifeplusvitamins.com/colloidl.html. (Accessed 24 March 2000).

5528 Anon. 2000. Supplement explanations. URL: http://alzheimersmemory.com/supplement1.html. (Accessed 21 March 2000).

5529 Anon. 2000 URL: http://www.angelfire.com/co2/slendermummie/madna.html. (Accessed 21 March 2000).

5530 Anon. 2000. URL. http://www.moon-light.com/ (Accessed 21 March 2000).

5531 Daly JM, Lieberman MD, Goldfine J, et al. Enteral nutrition with supplemental arginine, RNA, and omega-3 fatty acids in patients after operation: immunologic, metabolic and clinical outcome. Surgery 1992;112(1):56-67.

5532 Senkal M, Kemen M, Homann HH, et al. Modulation of postoperative immune response by enteral nutrition with a diet enriched with arginine, RNA, and omega-3 fatty acids in patients with upper gastrointestinal cancer. Eur J Surg 1995;161:115-122.

5533 Kemen M, Senkal M, Homann HH, et al. Early postoperative enteral nutrition with arginine-omega-3 fatty acids and ribonucleic acid-supplemented diet versus placebo in cancer patients: an immunologic evaluation of Impact. Critical Care Medicine 1995;23(4):652-659.

5534 Gianotti L, Braga M, Fortis C, et al. A prospective, randomized clinical trial on perioperative feeding with an arginine, omega-3-fatty acid, and RNA-enriched enteral diet: effect on host response and nutritional status. Journal of Parenteral and Enteral Nutrition 1999;23(6):314-20.

5535 Saffle JR, Wiebke G, Jennings K, et al. Randomized trial of immune-enhancing enteral nutrition in burn patients. The Journal of Trauma, Injury, Infection and Critical Care 1997;42(5):793-802.

5536 Bower RH, Cerra FB, Bershadsky B, et al. Early enteral administration of a formula (Impact) supplemented with arginine, nucleotides, and fish oil in intensive care unit patients: results of a multicenter, prospective, randomized, clinical trial. Critical Care Medicine 1995;23(3):436-449.

5537 Wang T, Tang XC. Reversal of scopolamine-induced deficits in radial maze performance by (-)-huperzine A: comparison with E2020 and tacrine. European Journal of Pharmacology, 1998;349(2-3):137-142.

5538 Li L. Erythematous skin reaction to subcutaneous injection of ribonucleic acid. Contact Dermatitis 1999;41:239.

5539 Schubert R, Hohlweg U, Renz D, Doefler W. On the fate of orally ingested foreign DNA in mice: chromosomal association and placental transmission o the fetus. Mole Gen Genet 1998;259:569-576.

5541 Huang KC. The Pharmacology of Chinese Herbs. 2nd ed. New York: CRC Press LLC. 1999;385-386, 400-401.

5542 Bruneton J. Pharmacognosy, Phytochemistry, Medicinal Plants. 2nd ed. Paris: Lavoisier Publishing. 1999;652.

5543 Van Buren CT, Rudolph F. Dietary nucleotides: a conditional requirement. Nutrition 1997;13(5):470-472.

5544 Bensky D, Gamble A, Kaptchuk T. Chinese Herbal Medicine Materia Medica. Eastland Press: Seattle. 1996:107-108.

5545 Huang KC. The Pharmacology of Chinese Herbs. 2nd ed. New York: CRC Press LLC. 1999:113-114, 417.

5546 Chen SH, Yen YP, Chen XS. Effect of jiantangkang on blood glucose, sensitivity of insulin, and blood viscosity in non-insulin dependent Diabetes mellitus. Chung Kuo Chung His I Chieh Ho Tsa Chih 1997;17(11):666-668.

5547 Wang HK, Xia Y, Yang ZY, et al. Recent advances in the

REFERENCES

discovery and development of flavonoids and their analogues as antitumor and anti-HIV agents. *Adv Exp Med Biol*, 1998;439:191-225.

5548 DiPaola RS, Zhang H, Lambert GH, et al. Clinical and biologic activity of an estrogenic herbal combination (PC-SPES) in Prostate cancer. *NEJM*, 1998;339(12):785-91.

5549 Smol'ianinov ES, Gol'dberg VE, Matiash MG, et al. Effect of Scutellaria baicalensis extract on the immunologic status of patients with lung cancer receiving antineoplastic chemotherapy. *Eksp Klin Farmakol*, 1997;60(6):49-51.

5550 Gol'dberg VE, Ryzhakov VM, Matiash MG, et al. Dry extract of Scutellaria baicalensis as a hemostimulant in antineoplastic chemotherapy in patients with lung cancer. *Eksp Klin Farmakol*, 1997;60(6):28-30.

5551 Zhang H, Huang J. Preliminary study of traditional Chinese Medicine treatment of minimal brain dysfunction: analysis of 100 cases. *Chung Hsi I Chieh Ho Tsa Chih*, 1990;10(5):278-279, 260.

5552 Kuno Y, Kawabe Y, Sakakibara S. Allergic Contact Dermatitis associated with photosensitivity, from alantolactone in a chrysanthemum farmer. *Contact Dermatitis*, 1999;40(4):224-225.

5553 Paulsen E, Sogaard J, Andersen KE. Occupational dermatitis in Danish gardeners and greenhouse workers (III). Compositae-related symptoms. *Contact Dermatitis*, 1998;38(3):140-146.

5554 deJong NW, Vermeulen AM, van Wijik RG, deGroot H. Occupational Allergy caused by flowers. *Allergy*, 1998;53(2):204-209.

5555 Yu XY. A prospective clinical study on reversion of 200 precancerous patients with hua-sheng-ping. *Chung Kuo Chung His I Chieh Ho Tsa Chih*, 1993;13(3):147-149.

5556 Camplimi P, Sertoli A, Fabbri P, Panconesi E. Alantolactone sensitivity in chrysanthemum contract dermatitis. *Contact Dermatitis*, 1978;4(2):93-102.

5557 Bleumink E, Mitchell JC, Geismann TA, Towers GH. Contact hypersensitivity to sesquiterpene lactones in Chrysanthemum dermatitis. *Contact Dermatitis*, 1976;2(2):81-88.

5558 Huang KC. The Pharmacology of Chinese Herbs. 2nd ed. New York: CRC Press LLC. 1999:101-102.

5559 Bensky D, Gamble A, Kaptchuk T. Chinese Herbal Medicine Materia Medica. Seattle: Eastland Press. 1996:359-360.

5599 Lutz M, Bonilla S, Concha J, Alvarado J, Barraza P. Effect of dietary oils, cholesterol and antioxidant vitamin supplementation on Liver microsomal fluidity and xenobiotic-metabolizing enzymes in rats. *Annals of Nutrition and Metabolism* 1998;42(6):350-9.

5600 Farber JM, Carter AO, Varughese PV, et al. Listeriosis traced to the consumption of alfalfa tablets and soft cheese. [Letter to the Editor] *NEJM* 1990;322:338.

5601 Sullivan JB Jr, Rumack BH, Thomas H Jr, et al. Pennyroyal oil poisoning and hepatotoxicity. *JAMA* 1979;242(26):2873-2874.

5602 Anon. Toxic hypoglycemic syndrome—Jamaica, 1989-1991. *MMWR Morb Mortal Wkly Rep*,1992;41(4):53-55.

5603 Sinn LE, Porterfield JF. Fatal taxine poisoning from yew leaf ingestion. *J Forensic Sci* 1991;36(2):599-601.

5604 Van IG, Visser R, Peltenburg H, et al. Sudden unexpected death due to Taxus poisoning. A report of five cases, with review of the literature. *Forensic Sci Int* 1992;56(1):81-87.

5605 Krenzelok EP, Jacobsen TD, Aronis J. Is the yew really poisonous to you? *J Toxicol Clin Toxicol* 1998;36(3):219-223.

5606 Fox DW, Hart MC, Bergeson PS, et al. Pyrrolizidine (Senecio) intoxication mimicking Reye syndrome. *J Pediatr* 1978;93(6):980-982.

5607 Sullivan G, Chavez PI. Mexican good-luck charm potentially dangerous. *Vet Hum Toxicol* 1981;23(4):259-260.

5608 Niyogi SK. Deadly crab's eye: Abrus precatorius poisoning. *N Engl J Med* 1969;281(1):51-52.

5609 Sherratt HS, Turnbull DM. Methylene blue and fatal encephalopathy from ackee fruit poisoning. *Lancet* 1999;353(9164):1623-1624.

5610 Lebo DB, Ditto AM, Boxer MB, et al. Anaphylaxis to ackee fruit. *J Allergy Clin Immunol*, 1996;98(5Pt1):997-998.

5611 Challoner KR, McCarron MM. Castor bean intoxication. *Ann Emerg Med* 1990;19(10):1177-1183.

5612 Palatnick W, Tenenbein M. Hepatotoxicity from castor bean ingestion in a child. *J Toxicol Clin Toxicol* 2000;38(1):67-69.

5613 Aplin PJ, Eliseo T. Ingestion of castor oil plant seeds. *Med J Aust* 1997;167(5);260-261.

5614 McGee J, Patrick RS, Wood CB, Blumgart LH. A case of veno-occlusive disease of the *Liver* in Britain associated with herbal tea consumption. *J Clin Pathol* 1976;29(9):788-794.

5615 Jappe U, Franke I, Reinhold D, Gollnck HP. Sebotrophic drug reaction from kava-kava extract therapy: a new entity? *J Am Acad Dermatol* 1998;38(1):104-106.

5616 Schelosky L, Raffauf C, Jendroska K, Poewe W. Kava and dopamine antagonism. *J Neurol Neurosurg Psychiatry* 1995;58(5):639-640.

5617 Cassidy DE, Drewry J, Fanning JP. Podophyllum toxicity: a report of a fatal case and a review of the literature. *J Toxicol Clin Toxicol* 1982;19(1):35-44.

5618 Rosenstein G, Rosenstein H, Freeman M, Weston N. Podophyllum- a dangerous laxative. *Pediatrics* 1976;57(3):419-421.

5619 Cohle SD, Trestrail JD 3d, Graham MA, et al. Fatal pepper aspiration. *Am J Dis Child* 1988;142(6):633-636.

5620 Sheahan K, Page DV, Kemper T, Suarez R. Childhood sudden death secondary to accidental aspiration of black pepper. *Am J Forensic Med Pathol* 1988;9(1):51-53.

5621 Anon. Plant Poisonings-New Jersey. *MMWR Morb Mortal Wkly Rep* 1981;30(6):65-67.

5622 Urich RW, Bowerman DL, Levisky JA, Pflug JL. Datura stramonium: a fatal poisoning. *J Forensic Sci* 1982;27(4):948-954.

5623 Anon. Jimson weed poisoning—Texas, New York, and California, 1994. *MMWR Morb Mortal Wkly Rep* 1995;44(3):41-44.

5624 McHenry LE, Hall RC. Angel's trumpet. Lethal and psychogenic aspects. *J Fla Med Assoc* 1978;65(3):192-196.

5625 Hall RC, Popkin MK, Mchenry LE. Angel's Trumpet psychosis: a central nervous system anticholinergic syndrome. *Am J Psychiatry* 1977;134(3):312-314.

5626 Greene GS, Patterson SG, Warner E. Ingestion of angel's trumpet: an increasingly common source of toxicity. *South Med J* 1996;89(4):365-369.

5627 Francis PD, Clarke CF. Angel trumpet lily poisoning in five adolescents: clinical findings and management. *J Paediatr Child Health* 1999;35(1):93-95.

5628 Anon. FDA Import Alert #53-03 1991.http:// www.verity.fda.gov/search97cgi/s97_cgi.exe?. (Accessed 9 May 2000).

5629 Pine, D. Cool tips for a hot season. FDA/CFSAN Cosmetics 1992. http://vm.cfsan.fda.gov/~dms/cos-815.html. (Accessed 9 May 2000).

5630 Anon. Color additives approved for use in human food. FDA/CFSAN/OPA 1988. http://vm.cfsan.fda.gov/~dms/opa-col2.html. (Accessed 9 May 2000).

5631 Jackson R. Quick "suntan" pills in Canada. *J Am Acad Dermatol* 1981;4(2):233.

5632 Lober CW. Canthaxanthin—the "tanning" pill. *J Am Acad Dermatol* 1985;13(4):660.

5633 Anon. A "suntan" in capsules—orobronze. *Drug Ther Bull* 1983;21(15):57.

5634 Rock GA, Decary F, Cole RS. Orange plasma from tanning capsules. *Lancet* 1981;1(8235):1419-20.

5635 Bluhm R, Branch R, Johnston P, Stein R. Aplastic anemia associated with canthaxanthin ingested for 'tanning' purposes. *JAMA* 1990;264(9):1141-2.

5636 Harnois C, Samson J, Malenfant M, Rousseau A. Canthaxanthin retinopathy. Anatomic and funtional reversibility. *Arch Ophthalmol* 1989;107(4):538-40.

5637 Herbert V. Canthaxanthin toxicity. *Am J Clin Nutr* 1991;53(2):573-4.

5638 White GL Jr, Beesley R, Thiese SM, Murdock RT. Retinal crystals and oral tanning agents. *Am Fam Physician* 1988;37(3):125-6.

5639 Chang TS, Aylward W, Clarkson JG, Gass JD. Asymmetric canthaxanthin retinopathy. *Am J Ophthalmol* 1995;119(6):801-2.

5640 Leyon H, Ros AM, Nyberg S, Algvere P. Reversibility of canthaxanthin deposits within the retina. *Acta Ophthalmol* (Copenh) 1990;68(5):607-11.

5641 Espaillat A, Aiello LP, Arrigg PG, et al. Canthaxanthine retinopathy. *Arch Ophtahalmol* 1999;117:412-3.

5642 Anon. Permitted colouring agents for use in medicinal products - E 161 Canthaxanthine. Health and Consumer Protection - The European Commission 1998. http://europa.eu.int/comm/dg24/health/sc/scmp/out10_en.html. (Accessed 9 May 2000).

5643 Mathews-Roth MM. Beta-carotene thereapy for erythropoietic protoporphyria and other photosensitivity diseases. Biochimie 1986;68(6):875-84.

5644 Anon. Porphyria information for patients and their families. University of Cape Town / Medical Research Council - *Liver* Research Center 2000. www.uct.ac.za/depts/liver/porphpts.htm. (Accessed 9 May 2000).

5645 Mathews-Roth MM. Carotenoids in erythropoietic protoporphyria and other photosensitivity diseases. *Ann N Y Acad Sci* 1993;691:127-38.

5646 Bertram JS. Cancer prevention by carotenoids. Mechanistic studies in cultured cells. *Ann N Y Acad Sci* 1993;691:177-91.

5647 Vainio H, Rautalahti M. An international evaluation of the Cancer preventive potential of carotenoids. *Cancer Epidemiol Biomarkers Prev* 1998;7(8):725-8.

5648 Huang DS, Odeleye OE, Watson RR. Inhibitory effects of canthaxanthin on in vitro growth of murine tumor cells. *Cancer Lett* 1992;65(3):209-13.

5649 Stahl W, Sies H. The role of carotenoids and retinoids in gap junctional communication. *Int J Vitam Nutr Res* 1998;68(6):354-9.

5650 Segal S, Foley J. The Metabolism of D-ribose in man. *J Clin Invest* 1958;37:719-35.

5651 Foker JE, Einzig S, Wang T. Adenosine Metabolism and myocardial preservation. Consequences of adenosine catabolism on myocardial high-energy compounds and tissue blood flow. *J Thorac Cardiovasc Surg* 1980;80(4):506-6.

5652 Pasque MK, Spray TL, Pellom GL, et al. Ribose-enhanced myocardial recovery following ischemia in the isolated working rat heart. *J Thorac Cardiovasc Surg* 1982;83(3):390-8.

5653 Pasque MK, Wechsler AS. Metabolic intervention to affect myocardial recovery following ischemia. *Ann Surg* 1984;200(1):1-12.

5654 Ward HB, St Cyr JA, Cogordan JA. Recovery of adenine nucleotide levels after global myocardial ischemia in dogs. *Surgery* 1984;96(2):248-55.

5655 Jennings RB, Reimer KA. The cell biology of acute myocardial ischemia. *Annu Rev Med* 1991;42:225-46.

5656 Stathis CG, Febbraio MA, Carey MF, et al. Influence of sprint training on human skeletal muscle purine nucleotide metabolism. *J Appl Physiol* 1994;76(4):1802-9.

5657 Tullson PC, Bangsbo J, Hellsten Y, et al. IMP Metabolism in human skeletal after exhaustive exercise. *J Appl Physiol* 1995;78(1):146-52.

5658 Hellsten-Westing Y, Norman B, Balsom PD, et al. Decreased resting levels of adenine nucleotides in human skeletal muscle after high-intensity training. *J Appl Physiol* 1993;74(5):2523-8.

5659 Chatham JC, John Challiss RA, Radda GK, et al. Studies of the protective effect of ribose in myocardial ischaemia by using P31-nuclear-magnetic-resonance spectroscopy. *Biochem Soc Trans* 1985;13:885-6.

5660 St Cyr JA, Bianco RW, Schneider JR, et al. Enhanced high energy phosphate recovery with ribose infusion after global myocardial ischemia in a canine model. *J Surg Res* 1989;46(2):157-62.

5661 Angello DA, Wilson RA, Gee D. Effect of ribose on thallium-201 myocardial redistribution. *J Nucl Med* 1988;29(12):1943-50.

5662 Perlmutter NS, Wilson RA, Angello DA, et al. Ribose facilitates thallium-201 redistribution in patients with coronary artery disease. *J Nucl Med* 1991;32(2):193-200.

5663 Hegewald MG, Palac RT, Angello DA, et al. Ribose infusion accelerates thallium redistribution with early imaging compared with late 24-hour imaging without ribose. *J Am Coll Cardiol* 1991;18(7):1671-81.

5664 Pliml W, von Arnim T, Stalein A, et al. Effects of ribose on excercise-induced ischaemia in stable coronary artery disease. *Lancet* 1992;340(8818):507-10.

5665 Geisbuhler TP, Schwager TL. Ribose-enhanced synthesis of UTP, CTP, and GTP from parent nucleosides in cardiac myocytes. *J Mol Cell Cardiol* 1998;30(4):879-87.

5666 Muller C, Zimmer HG, Gross M, et al. Effect of ribose on cardiac adenine nucleotides in a donor model for heart transplantation. *Eur J Med Res* 1998;3:554-8.

5667 Burke ER. D-Ribose What You Need To Know. Garden City Park, NY:Avery Publishing Group 1999: 1-43.

5668 Anon. Bioenergy Ribose-The Absolute Energy Source 2000. http://www.ribose.com (Accessed 16 May 2000).

5669 Almada AL. D-Ribose: Leave the sugar blues behind! *Alive* 1999;199:74,76.

5670 Anon. It's raining men...supplements, that is. *Nutrition News* September 30, 1999;1.

5671 Anon. Ribose size-the great genetic equalizer 2000. http://www.muscle-link.com/products/ribosesize.html

© Copyright 2000, Natural Medicines Comprehensive Database (209) 472-2244. For updated data, go to www.NaturalDatabase.com. • 1279

REFERENCES

(Accessed 24 May 2000).

5672 Anon. Liquid Ribose 2000. http://www.performancebiolabs.com/liquid_ribose.htm (Accessed 24 May 2000).

5673 Anon. Ribose-C. George Stavrou's Bodysculpting 2000. http://www.bdsclpt.com/itm00003.htm (Accessed 24 May 2000).

5674 Anon. Ribose. Cutting Edge Nutrition 2000. http://www.cuttingedgenutrition.com/cuttingedge/ribose.html (Accessed 16 May 2000).

5675 Blackwood JS. Supplement spotlight: ribose. Nutripeak.com 2000. http://www.nutripeak.com/features/9910_spotlight3.asp (Accessed 16 May 2000).

5676 Gross M, Reiter S, Zollner N. Metabolism of D-ribose administered continuously to healthy persons and to patients with myoadenylate deaminase deficiency. *Klin Wochenschr* 1989;67(23):1205-13.

5677 Zollner N, Reiter S, Gross M, et al. Myoadenylate deaminase deficiency: successful symptomatic therapy by high dose oral administration of ribose. *Klin Wochenscher* 1986;64(24):1281-90.

5678 Steele IC, Patterson VH, Nicholls DP. A double blind, placebo controlled, crossover trial of D-ribose in McArdle's disease. *J Neurol Sci* 1996 136(1-2): 174-7.

5679 Wagner DR, Gresser U, Zollner N. Effects of oral ribose on muscle metabolism during bicycle ergometer in AMPD-deficient patients. *Ann Nutr Metab* 1991;35(5):297-302.

5680 Wagner DR, Felbel J, Gresser U, et al. Muscle Metabolism and red cell ATP/ADP concentration during bicycle ergometer in patients with AMPdeficiency. *Klin Wochnescher* 1991;69(6):251-5.

5681 Gross M. Clinical heterogeneity and molecular mechanisms in inborn muscle AMP deaminase deficiency. *J Inherit Metab Dis* 1997;20(2):186-92.

5682 Fox IH, Kelley WN. Phosphoribosylpyrophosphate in man: biochemical and clinical significance. *Ann Intern Med* 1971;74:424-33.

5683 Lan EL, Ugwu SO, Blanchard J, et al. Preformulation studies with melanotan II: a potential skin Cancer chemopreventive peptide. *J Pharm Sci* 1994;83(8):1081-4.

5684 Pinsuwan S, Myrdal PB, Yalkowsky SH. Systemic delivery of melanotan II through the ocular route in rabbits. *J Pharm Sci* 1997;86(3):396-7.

5685 Dorr RT, Lines R, Levine N, et al. Evaluation of melanotan-II, a superpotent cyclic melanotropic peptide in a pilot phase-I clinical study. *Life Sci* 1996;58(20):1777-84.

5686 Hadley ME, Hruby VJ, Blanchard J, et al. Discoverdevelopment of novel melanogenic drugs. Melanotan-I and -II. *Pharm Biotechnol* 1998;11:575-95.

5687 Wessells H, Fuciarelli K, Hansen J, et al. Synthetic melanotropic peptide initiates erections in men with psychogenic erectile dysfunction; double-blind, placebo controlled crossover study. *J Urol* 1998;160(2):389-93.

5688 Wessells H, Gralnek DR, Dorr RT, et al. Erectogenic properties of melanotan II in men with organic erectile dysfunction. 1999 Abstract Info-American Urological Association, Inc. http://www.auanet.org/meeting/annual_meeting/abstractinfo/AUA99_1603.cfm. (Accessed 5 June 2000).

5689 Wessells H. Hunter Wessells, MD.,FACS. Impotence Specialists 2000. http://www.impotencespecialists.com/drwessells/wessells.html (Accessed 4 June 2000).

5690 Rutz D. Tanning drug my find new life as Viagra alternatives. CNN 1999. http://cnn.com/HEALTH/men/9906/17/viagra.alternative/ (Accessed 2 June 2000).

5701 Barber MD, Ross JA, Voss AC, et al. The effect of an oral nutritional supplement enriched with fish oil on weight-loss in patients with pancreatic cancer. *Br J Cancer* 1999;81(1):80-6.

5702 Goodfellow J, Bellamy MF, Ramsey MW, et al. Dietary supplementation with marine omega-3 fatty acids improve systemic large artery endothelial function in subjects with hypercholesterolemia. *J Am Coll Cardiol* 2000;35(2):265-70.

5703 Fenton WS, Hibbeln J, Knable M. Essential fatty acids, lipid membrane abnormalities, and the diagnosis and treatment of schizophrenia. *Biol Psychiatry* 2000;47(1):8-21.

5704 Nordoy A, Bonaa KH, Sandset PM, et al. Effect of omega-3 fatty acids and simvastatin on hemostatic risk factors and postprandial hyperlipemia in patients with combined hyperlipemia. *Arterioscler Thromb Vasc Biol* 2000;20(1):259-65.

5705 Hsu HC, Lee YT, Chen MF. Effect of n-3 fatty acids on the composition and binding properties of lipoproteins in hypertriglyceridemic patients. *Am J Clin Nutr* 2000 Jan;71(1):28-35.

5706 Roche HM, Gibney MJ. Effect of long-chain n-3 polyunsaturated fatty acids on fasting and postprandial triacylglycerol metabolism. *Am J Clin Nutr* 2000;71(1 Suppl):232S-7S.

5707 Nestel PJ. Fish oil and cardiovascular disease: lipids and arterial function. *Am J Clin Nutr* 2000;71(1 Suppl):228S-31S.

5708 Stordy BJ. Dark adaptation, motor skills, docosahexaenoic acid, and dyslexia. *Am J Clin Nutr* 2000;71(1 Suppl):323S-6S.

5709 Belluzzi A, Boschi S, Brignola C, et al. Polyunsaturated fatty acids and inflammatory bowel disease. *Am J Clin Nutr* 2000 Jan;71(1 Suppl):339S-42S.

5710 Navarro E, Esteve M, Olive A, et al. Abnormal fatty acid pattern in rheumatoid arthritis. A rationale for treatment with marine and botanical lipids. *J Rheumatol* 2000;27(2):298-303.

5711 Burgess JR, Stevens L, Zhang W, Peck L. Long-chain polyunsaturated fatty acids in children with attention-deficit hyperactivity disorder. *Am J Clin Nutr* 2000;71(1 Suppl):327S-30S.

5800 Cash CD. Gamma-hydroxybutyrate: an overview of the pros and cons for it being a neurotransmitter and/or a useful therapeutic agent. *Neurosci Biobehav Rev* 1994;18(2):291-304.

5801 Maitre M. The gamma-hydroxybutyrate signaling system in brain: organization and functional implications. *Prog Neurobiol* 1997;51(3):337-61.

5802 Feigenbaum JJ, Howard SG. Gamma hydroxybutyrate is not a GABA agonist. *Prog Neurobiol* 1996;50(1):1-7.

5803 Mamelak M. Gammahydroxybutyrate: an endogenous regulator of energy metabolism. *Neurosci Biobehav Rev* 1989;13(4):187-98.

5804 Van Cauter E, Plat L, Scharf MB, et al. Simultaneous stimulation of slow-wave sleep and growth hormone secretion by gamma-hydroxybutyrate in normal young Men. *J Clin Invest* 1997;100(3):745-53.

5805 Cash CD. What is the role of the gamma-hydroxybutyrate receptor? *Med Hypotheses* 1996;47(6):455-9.

5806 Gerra G, Caccavari R, Fontanesi B, et al. Naloxone and metergoline effects on growth hormone response to gamma-hydroxybutyric acid. *Int Clin Psychopharmacol* 1995;10(4):245-50.

5807 Ferrara SD, Tedeschi L, Frison G, Rossi A. Fatality due to gamma-hydroxybutyric acid (GHB) and heroin intoxication. *J Forensic Sci* 1995;40(3):501-4.

5808 Galloway GP, Frederick SL, Staggers FE Jr, et al. Gamma-hydroxybutyrate: an emerging drug of abuse that causes physical dependence. *Addiction* 1997;92(1):89-96

5809 Craig K, Gomez HF, McManus JL, Bania TC. Severe gamma-hydroxybutyrate withdrawal: a case report and literature review. *J Emerg Med* 2000;18(1):65-70.

5810 Ellinwood EH Jr, Gonzalez AE, Dougherty GG Jr. Gamma-Butyrolactone effects on behavior induced by dopamine agonists. *Biol Psychiatry* 1983;18(9):1023-32.

5811 Dougherty GG, Ellinwood EH Jr. Influence of gamma-butyrolactone on behavior due to dopaminergic drugs. *Physiol Behav* 1983;30(4):607-12.

5812 Snead OC 3d, Bearden LJ. Naloxone overcomes the dopaminergic, EEG, and behavioral effects of gamma-hydroxybutyrate. *Neurology* 1980;30(8):832-8.

5813 Kohrs FP, Porter WH, et al. Gamma-hydroxybutyrate intoxication and overdose. [Letter and responses]. *Ann Emerg Med* 1999;33(4):475-6.

5814 Law M. Plant sterol and stanol margarines and health. *Br Med J* 2000;320:861-4.

5815 Anon. Healing With Nutrition website. URL: www.healingwithnutrition.com/aminoacid.html#Dimethylglycine(DMG) (Accessed 20 May 2000).

5816 Kendall RV. N,N-Dimethylglycine (DMG): The Metabolic Enhancer that boosts the immune system, enhances performance and improves cardiovascular function. FoodScience of Vermont website. URL: www.fslabs.com/dmg_tb.htm (Accessed 20 May 2000).

5817 Rimland B. Dimethylglycine (DMG), a nontoxic metabolite, and autism. Autism Research Institute website. URL: www.autism.org/dmg.html (Accessed 20 May 2000).

5818 Anon. Natural Health Consultants website. URL: www.naturalhealthconsult.com/Monographs/dmg.html (Accessed 20 May 2000).

5819 Bolman WM, Richmond JA. A double-blind, placebo-controlled, crossover pilot trial of low dose dimethylglycine in patients with autistic disorder. *J Autism Dev Disord* 1999;29(3):191-4.

5820 Reap EA, Lawson JW. Stimulation of the immune response by dimethylglycine, a nontoxic metabolite. *J Lab Clin Med* 1990;115(4):481-6.

5821 Tonda ME, Hart LL. N,N-dimthylglycine and L-carnitine as performance enhancers in athletes. *Ann Pharmacother* 1992;26:935-7.

5822 Weiss RC. Immunologic responses in healthy random-source cats fed N,N-dimethylglycine-supplemented diets. *Am J Vet Res* 1992;53(5):829-33.

5823 Gascon G, Patterson B, Yearwood K, Slotnick H. N,N-dimethylglycine and epilepsy. *Epilepsia* 1989;30(1):90-3.

5824 Freed WJ. Prevention of strychnine-induced seizures and death by the N-methylated glycine derivatives betaine, dimethylglycine and sarcosine. *Phrmacol Biochem Behav* 1985;22(4):641-3.

5825 Graber CD, Goust JM, Glassman AD, et al. Immunomodulating properties of dimethylglycine in humans. *J Inf Dis* 1981;143(1):101-5.

5826 Roach ES, Carlin L. N,N dimethylglycine for epilepsy [letter]. *New Engl J Med* 1982;307:1081-2.

5827 Herbert V. N,N-dimethylglycine for epilepsy [letter]. *New Engl J Med* 1983;308:527-8.

5828 Freed WJ. N,N-dimethylglycine, betaine and seizures [letter]. *Arch Neurol* 1984;41:1129-30.

5829 Ward TN, Smith EB, Reeves AG. Dimethylglycine and reduction of mortality in penicillin-induced seizures [letter]. *Ann Neurol* 1985;17(2):213.

5830 Kendall RV. Comment: N,N-dimethylglycine and L-carnitine as performance enhancers in athletes [letter]. *Ann Pharmacother* 1994;28:973.

5834 Anon. Natural Health Consultants website. URL http://www.naturalhealthconsult.com/Monographs/7Keto.html (Accessed 8 June 2000).

5835 Anon. Humanetics Corporation website. URL http://humaneticscorp.com/7keto.html (Accessed 8 June 2000).

5836 Anon. Chatham Health and Wellness Store website. URL http://www.chathamhealth.com/accord/twin7ketfuel.html (Accessed 8 April 2000).

5837 Lardy H, Partridge B, Kneer N, Wei Y. Ergosteroids: induction of thermogenic enzymes in Liver of rats treated with steroids derived from dehydroepiandrosterone. *Proc Natl Acad Sci USA* 1995;92(14):6617-9. (Medline abstract only).

5838 Henwood SM, Weeks CE, Lardy H. An escalating dose oral gavage study of 3beta-acetoxyandrost-5-ene-7, 17-dione (7-oxo-DHEA-acetate) in rhesus monkeys. *Biochem Biophys Res Commun* 1999;254(1):124-6. (Medline abstract only).

5839 Shi J, Schulze S, Lardy HA. The effect of 7-oxo-DHEA acetate on memory in young and old C57BL/6 mice. *Steroids* 2000;65(3):124-9. (Medline abstract only).

5840 Davidson MH, Weeks C, Lardy H, et al. Clinical Safety and Endocrine Effects of 7-KETO-DHEA. Abstract presented at: Experimental Biology 98, April 19-22, 1998, San Francisco, CA. Abstract obtained from Humanetics Corporation website. URL http://humaneticscorp.com/7ketoabstracts.html (Accessed 8 June 2000).

5841 Nelson R, Herron M, Weeks C, Lardy H. Dehydroepiandrosterone and 7-KETO-DHEA augment Interleukin 2 (IL2) Production by Human Lymphocytes In Vitro. Abstract presented at: The 5th Conference on Retroviruses and Opportunistic Infections, February 1-5, 1998, Chicago, IL. Abstract obtained from Humanetics Corporation website. URL http://humaneticscorp.com/7ketoabstracts.html (Accessed 8 June 2000).

5842 Colker CM, Torina GC, Swain MA, Kalman DS. Double-Blind Study Evaluating the Effects of Exercise Plus 3-Acetyl-7-oxo-dehydroepiandrosterone on Body Composition and the Endocrine System in Overweight Adults. Abstract presented at 2nd ASEP Annual Meeting, October 14-16, 1999, and published in *Journal of Exercise Physiology* online, Volume 2 Number 4 October 1999.

5843 Anon. Natures Herbs website. URL: www.natures-herbs.com/chlorella.htm (Accessed 6 April 2000).

5844 Anon. Mother Nature.com website. URL www.mothernature.com/cg/chlorella.asp (Accessed 6 June 2000).

5845 Anon. Tisco website. URL www.sunchlorella.net/chlorellaindetail.htm (Accessed 6 June 2000).

5846 Peirce A. The American Pharmaceutical Association Practical Guide to Natural Medicines. William Morrow & Co.Inc., New York. 1999.

© Copyright 2000, Natural Medicines Comprehensive Database (209) 472-2244. For updated data, go to www.NaturalDatabase.com. • 1281

REFERENCES

REFERENCES

5847 Ng TP, Tan WC, Lee YK. Occupational asthma in a pharmacist induced by chlorella, a unicellular algae preparation. *Resp Medicine* 1994;88:555-7.

5848 Ruama AL, Torronen R, Hanninen O, Mykkanen H. Vitamin B12 status of long-term adherents of a strict uncooked vegan diet ("living food diet") is compromised. *J Nutr* 1995;125(10):2511-5. (Medline abstract only).

5849 Davis DR. Some algae are potentially adequate sources of vitamin B-12 for vegans (letter, comment). *J Nutr* 1997;127(2):378,380.

5850 Morimoto T, Nagatsu A, Murakami N, et al. Anti-tumor-promoting glyceroglycolipids from the green alga, Chlorella vulgaris. *Phytochemistry* 1995;40(5):1433-7. (Medline abstract only).

5851 Tyml R. Present state and possibilities of the medical use of chlorococcal algae. *Acta Universitatis Palackianae Olomucensis Facultatis Medicae* 1982;103:273-9.

5852 Jitsukawa K, Suizu R, Hidano A. Chlorella photosensitization. New phytophotodermatosis. *Int J Dermatol* 1984;23(4):263-8. (Medline abstract only).

5853 Nelson AM, Neafie RC. Protothecosis. In: Strickland GT. Hunter's Tropical Medicine and Emerging Infectious Disease. 8th edition. WB Saunders Co., Philadelphia, PA. 2000:547.

5854 Lissoni P, Barni S, Cazzaniga M, et al. Efficacy of the concomitant administration of the pineal hormone melatonin in Cancer immunotherapy with low-dose IL-2 in patients with advanced solid tumors who had progressed on Il-2 alone. *Oncology* 1994;51:344-7.

5855 Lissoni P, Barni S, Tancini G, et al. A randomised study with subcutaneous low-dose interleukin 2 alone vs. interleukin 2 plus the pineal neurohormone melatonin in advanced solid neoplasms other than renal Cancer and melanoma. *Br J Cancer* 1994;69(1):196-9.

5856 Bubis M, Zisapel N. Modulation by melatonin of protein secretion from melanoma cells: is cAMP involved? *Molecular and Cellular Endocrinology* 1995;112:169-73.

5857 Lissoni P, Paolorossi F, Tancini G, et al. A phase II study of tamoxifen plus melatonin in metastatic solid tumour patients. *Br J Cancer* 1996;74(9):1466-8.

5900 Rudolph FB, Van Buren CT. The metabolic effects of enterally administered ribonucleic acids. *Current Opinion in Clinical Nutrition and Metabolic Care* 1998;1(6):527-530.

5901 Anon. 2000. Austin Nutritional Research. URL: http://www.realtime.net/anr/nutrient.html#Rnadna. (Accessed 9 May 2000).

5902 Kenny FS, Pinder SE, Ellis IO, et al. Gamma linolenic acid with tamoxifen as primary therapy in breast cancer. *Int J Cancer* 2000; 85:643-648.

5903 Anon. 2000. Herbal Information Center General Store. URL:www.kcweb.com.herb/p_applecider.htm. (Accessed 10 May 2000).

5904 Anon. 2000. The book lovers' community for our community. URL: http://www.thathomesite.com/forums/load/health.msg0322241820838.html. (Accessed 10 May 2000).

5905 Anon. 2000. Apple Cider Vinegar with Centella for weight loss and so much more. URL: http://www.ageless.co.za/applecider.htm. (Accessed 10 May 2000).

5906 Good Health Organization International Ltd 2000. Organic Apple Cider Vinegar. URL: http://www.gho.co.nz/vinegar.html. (Accessed 10 May 2000).

5907 Anon. 2000. Apple Cider Vinegar. URL: http://www.go-symmetry.com/apple-vinegar.htm (Accessed 10 May 2000).

5908 Anon. 2000. Bragg Apple Cider Vinegar. URL:http://www.bragg.com/acvproduct.html. (Accessed 10 May 2000).

5909 Anon. Apple Cider Vinegar. URL:http://www.healthness.com/applecidervinegar.htm. (Accessed 10 May 2000).

5910 Duke J. The Green Pharmacy. Emmaus: Rodale Press. 1997:156, 444.

5911 Lhotta K, Hofle G, Gasser R, Finkenstedt G. Hyperkalemia, hyperreninemia, and osteoporosis in a patient ingesting large amounts of cider vinegar. *Nephron* 1998;80:242-243.

5912 Nutrition Search. Nutrition Almanac, Revised Edition. New York: McGraw-Hill Book Company. 1979.

5913 Burton TM. In trials, potion of herbs slows Prostate cancer. *The Wall Street Journal*, May 17, 2000, p.B-1.

5914 Anonymous. Pure Emu Oil and Emu Oil Products for Natural Healing and Better Health. 1999. URL: http://www.uniquelyemu.com (Accessed 18 May 2000).

5915 Anonymous. 2000. Welcome to Coopers Emu Oil Products. URL: http://www.coppersemuoilproducts.com/ (Accessed 18 May 2000).

5916 Anonymous. 2000. Aussiepol Trading Benefits of Emu Oil. URL. http://homepages.tig.com.au/~asuuipol/emuoil.html (Accessed 18 May 2000).

5917 Anonymous. 2000. Amazing Emu Oil. URL: http://mars.ark.com/~emuzing/emuoil.html (Accessed 19 May 2000).

5918 Anonymous. 2000. Reported Uses of Em Oil. URL: http://www.gentleridge.com/emuoiluses.html (Accessed 19 May 2000).

5919 Anonymous. 1999. Chemical Analysis of Emu Oil. URL: http://www.emu-oil.com/analysis.htm (Accessed 19 May 2000).

5920 Hopkins L. 2000. Would you believe? URL. http://www.pureemuoil.com/pr6.htm (Accessed 19 May 2000).

5921 Anonymous. 2000. URL. http://turnagefarmsinc.com/emu2.htm (Accessed 19 May 2000).

5922 Anonymous. 2000. Moanui Natural Relief and Skin Care Products. URL http://www.moanui.co.nz/benefits.html. (Accessed 19 May 2000).

5923 Lopez A, Sims DE, Ablett RF, et al. Effect of emu oil on auricular inflammation with croton oil in mice. American Journal of Veterinary Research 1999;60(12):1558-61.

5924 Pariza M, Park Y, Cook ME. Conjugated linoleic acid and the control of Cancer and obesity. *Toxicological Sciences* 1999;52 (Supplement) 107-10.

5925 Jiang J, Wolk A, Vessby B. Relation between the intake of milk fat and the occurrence of conjugated linoleic acid in human adipose tissue. *Am J Clin Nutr* 1999;70:21-7.

5926 O'Shea M, Stanton C, Devery R. Antioxidant enzyme defense responses of human MCF-7 and SW480 Cancer cells to conjugated linoleic acid. *AntiCancer Research* 1999;1953-60.

5927 Cesano Al, Visonneau S, Scimeca JA, et al. Opposite effects of linoleic acid and conjugated linoleic acid on human prostatic cancer in SCID mice. *AntiCancer Research* 1998;18:833-8.

5928 West DB, Delany JP, Camet PM, et al. Effects of conjugated linoleic acid on body fat and energy

Metabolism in the mouse. *Am J Physiol* (Regulatory Integrative Comp Physiol) 1998;255:44:R667-72.

5929 DeLany JP, Blohm F, Truett AA, et al. Conjugated linoleic acid rapidly reduced body fat content in mice without affecting energy intake. *Am J Physiol* (Regulatory Integrative Comp Physiol) 1999;276:45:R1172-9.

5930 Clement I, Banni S, Andioni E, et al. Conjugated linoleic acid-enriched butter fat alters mammary gland morphogenesis and reduces Cancer risk in rats. *J Nutr.* 1999;129:2135-42.

5931 Banni S, Angioni E, Casu V, et al. An increase in vitamin A status by the feeding of conjugated linoleic acid. *Nutrition and Cancer* 1999;33(1):53-7.

5932 Kelly ML, Berry JR, Dwyer DA, et al. Dietary fatty acid sources affect conjugated linoleic acid concentrations in milk from lactating dairy cows. *J Nutr* 128:881-5.

5933 Herbel BK, McGuire MK, McGuire MA, Shultz TD. Safflower oil consumption does not increase plasma conjugated linoleic acid concentrations in humans. *Am J Clin Nutr* 1998;67:332-7.

5934 Sebedio JL, Gnaedig S, Chardigny JM. Recent advances in conjugated linoleic acid research. *Current Opinion in Clinical Nutrition and Metabolic Care* 1999;2(6):499-506.

5935 Scimeca JA. Toxicological evaluation of dietary conjugated linoleic acid in male Fischer 344 rats. *Food and Chemical Toxicology* 1998;36(5);391-5.

5936 McCarty MF. Toward a wholly nutritional therapy for type 2 diabetes. *Med Hypothesis* 2000;54(3):483-7.

5937 Anon. Peak Nutrition 2000. URL:http://www.newpeak.com/aapi/cla180cap500.html (Accessed 27 May 2000).

5938 Faloon B. Conjugated linoleic acid-new studies 2000. URL: http:www.dietsexercise.com/CLAText.htm. (Accessed 27 May 2000).

5939 Reiner S. CLA: Does fat have a silver lining? 1996. URL: http://www.acsh.org/Publications/Priorities/0804/cla.html (Accessed 27 May 2000).

5940 Shalita AR, Smith JG, Parish LC, et al. Topical nicotinamide compared with clindamycin gel in the treatment of inflammatory acne vulgaris. *Int J Dermatol* 1995;34:434-7.

5941 Birch EE, Garfield S, Hoffman DR, et al. A randomized controlled trial of early dietary supply of long-chain polyunsaturated fatty acids and mental development in term infants. *Developmental Med and Child Neurol* 2000;42:174-81.

5942 Berges RR, Windeler J, Trampisch HJ, et al. Randomized, placebo-controlled, double-blind clinical trial of beta-sitosterol in patients with benign prostatic hyperplasia. *The Lancet* 1995;345:1529-1532.

5943 Bruneton J. Pharmacognosy Phytochemistry Medicinal Plants. 2nd ed. Paris:Lavoisier Publishing, 1999. p291-292.

5944 Fleming T, ed. PDR for Herbal Medicines, 2nd ed. Montvale: Medical Economics 2000. p7-8.

5945 Anonymous. 2000. The power of healing plants. 2000 URL. http://www.african.savana.co.za/power.htm. (Accessed 30 May 2000).

5946 Anonymous. 2000. Research. 2000 URL. http://www.african-savana.co.za/research.htm (Accessed 30 May 2000).

5951 Frati A. 2000 Medical implications of prickly pear cactus. URL: http:www.tamuk.edu/webuser/cactus/cac_med.html. (Accessed 30 May 2000).

5952 Anonymous. 2000. Opticantha. URL. http://opticantha.com/ataglance.html. (Accessed 30 May 2000).

5953 Anonymous. 2000. Opuntia. URL. http:///www.healthlink.com.au/nat_lib/htm-herb/BPH691.HTM. (Accessed 30 May 2000).

5954 Bwititi P, Musabayane CT, Nhachi CF. Effects of Opuntia megacantha on blood glucose and kidney function in streptozotocin diabetic rats. *J Ethnopharmacol* 2000;69(3):247-52.

5955 Trejo-Gonzalez A, Gabriel-Ortiz G, Puebla-Perez Am, et al. A purified extract from prickly pear cactus (Opuntia fuliginosa) controls experimentally induced Diabetes in rats. *J Ethnopharmacol* 1996;55(1):27-33.

5956 Ahmad A, Davies J, Randall S, Skinner GR. Antiviral properties of extract of Opuntia streptacantha. *Antiviral Res* 1996;30(2-3):75-85.

5957 Roman-Ramos R, Flores-Saenz JL, Alarcon-Aguilar FJ. Anti-hyperglycemic effect of some edible plants. *J Ehtnopharmacol* 1995;48(1):25-32.

5958 Fernandez ML, Lin EC, Trejo A, McNamara DJ. Prickly pear (Opuntia sp.) pectin alters hepatic cholesterol Metabolism without affecting cholesterol absorption in guinea pigs fed a hypercholesterolemic diet. *J Nutr* 1994;124(6):817-24.

5959 Frati AC, Xilotl Diaz N, Altamirano P, et al. The effect of two sequential doses of Opuntia streptacantha upon glycemia. *Arch Invest Med (Mex)* 1991;22(3-4):333-6.

5960 Frati-Munari AC, Licona-Quesada R, Araiza-Andraca CR, et al. Activity of Opuntia streptocantha in healthy individuals with induced hyperglycemia. *Arch Invest Med (Mex)* 1990;21(2):99-102.

5961 Frati-Munari AC, Altamirano-Bustamante E, Rodrigues-Barcenas N, et al. Hypoglycemic action of Opuntia streptacantha Lemaire: study using raw extracts. *Arch Invest Med (Mex)* 1989;20(4):321-5.

5962 Frati-Munari AC, Del Valle-Martinez LM, Ariza-Andraca CR, et al. Hypoglycemic action of different doses of nopol (Opuntia streptacantha) in patients with type II Diabetes mellitus. *Arch Invest Med (Mex)* 1989;20(2):197-201.

5963 Frati Munari AC, Quiroz Lazaro JL, Alramirano Bustamante P, et al. The effect of various doses of nopal (Opuntia streptacantha Lemaire) on the glucose tolerance test in healthy individuals. *Arch Invest Med (Mex)* 1988;19(2):143-8.

5964 Frati-Munari AC, Gordillo BE, Altamirano P, Ariza CR. Hypoglycemic effect of Opuntia streptacantha Lemaire in NIDDM. *Diabetes Care* 1988;11(1):63-6.

5968 Meckes-Lozyoa M, Roman-Ramos R. Opuntia streptacantha; a coadjutor in the treatment of diabetes mellitus. *Am J Chin Med* 1986;14(3-4):116-8.

5969 Munari-Frati AC, Roca-Vides RA, Lopez-Perez RJ, et al. The glycemic index of some foods common in Mexico. *Gac Med Mex* 1991;127(2):163-70.

5970 Frati Munari AC, Vera Lastra O, Ariza Andraca CR. Evaluation of nopol capsules in diabetes mellitus. *Gaeceta Medica de Mexico* 1992;128(4):431-6.

5971 Medical Economic. Physician's Desk Reference. Montvale:Medical Economics, 1999:1289.

5972 Rask MR. The Omohyoideus myofascial pain syndrome: report of four patients. *The Journal of Cranomandibular Practice* 1984;2(3):256-62.

5973 McCalla CX. Instantaneous cure of acute frontal Cephalalgia. Manufacturer information from High Chemical Company; 1995.

5974 Vuturo AE, Executive Editor. Differential diagnosis and treatment of sciatica: the non-diskogenic causes. *Advanced Clinical Updates*; 1985.

5975 Manufacturer Information. Sarapin. Injection technique in pain control. High Chemical Company. Information not dated

5976 Anonymous. Quarter Horse Woes. The Investigators. 2000. URL:http://www.kwtv.com/investigators/horse2.htm. (Accessed 19 June 2000).

5977 Gracer RI. A better method of pain management 2000. URL.http://www.tldp.com/issue/175-6/Prolong.html. (Accessed 19 June 2000).

5978 Wilk SJ. Pain disorders that are confused with TMJ. 2000. URL:http://tmjheadaches.com/conf.htm. (Accessed 19 June 2000).

5979 Harkins JD, Mundy GD, Stanley SD, Sams RA, Tobin T. Lack of local anaesthetic efficacy of Sarapin in the abaxial sesamoid block model. *J Vet Pharmacol Ther* 1997; Jun;20(3):229-32.

5980 National Germplasm Resources Laboratory. National Genetic Resources Program 2000. Pitcher plant. URL:http:www.ars-grin.gov/cgi-bin/npgs/html. (Accessed 19 June 2000).

5991 Asero R. Detection and clinical characterization of patients with oral allergy syndrome caused by stable allergens in Rosaceae and nuts. *Annals of Allergy, Asthma, & Immunology* 1999; 83(5):377-83.

5992 Durak I, Kacmaz M, Buyukkocak S, Cimen BM, Ozturk HS. Hazelnut supplementation enhances plasma antioxidant potential and lowers plasma cholesterol levels [letter]. *Clinica Chimica Acta* 1999; 284(1):113-5.

5993 Caballero T, Pascual C, Garcia-Ara MC, Ojeda JA, Martin-Esteban M. IgE crossreactivity between mugwort pollen (Artemisia vulgaris) and hazelnut (Abellana nux) in sera from patients with sensitivity to both extracts. *Clinical & Experimental Allergy* 1997; 27(10):1203-11.

5994 Pumphrey RS, Wilson PB, Faragher EB, Edwards SR. Specific immunoglobulin E to peanut, hazelnut and brazil nut 731 patients: similar patterns found at all ages. *Clinical & Experimental Allergy* 1999;29(9):1256-9.

5995 Savage GP, McNeil DL. Chemical composition of hazelnuts (Corylus avellana) grown in New Zealand. *International Journal of Food Sciences & Nutrition* 1998;49(3):199-203.

5996 Caballero T, Martin-Esteban M. Association between pollen hypersensitivity and edible vegetable allergy: a review. *Journal of Investigational Allergology & Clinical Immunology* 1998;8(1):6-16.

5997 Sutherland MF, O'Hehir RE, Czarny D, Suphioglu C. Macadamia nut anaphylaxis: demonstration of specific IgE reactivity and partial cross-reactivity with hazelnut. *J Allergy Clin Immunol* 1999; 104 (4 Pt 1):889-90.

5998 Munoz MF, Lopez Cazana JM, Villas F, Contreras JF, Diaz JM, Ojeda JA. Exercise-induced anaphylactic reaction to hazelnut. *Allergy* 1994;49(5):314-6.

5999 O'Mahony M, Mitchell E, Gilbert RJ, Hutchinson DN, Begg NT, Rodhouse JC, Morris JE. *Epidemiol Infect* 1990;104(3):389-95.

6000 King DS, et al. "Effect of oral androstenedione on serum testosterone and adaptations to resistance training in young men. A randomized controlled trial." *JAMA*, 2 Jun. 1999; 281(21): 2020-028.

6001 Roche Laboratories, Inc. Package insert for *Xenical*. April 1999.

6002 Fetrow CW, Avila JR. Professional's Handbook of Complementary & Alternative Medicines. Springhouse,

6003 Pennsylvania: Springhouse Corporation, 1999.

6003 Offenbacher EG, Pi-Sunyer FX. Beneficial effect of chromium-rich yeast on glucose tolerance and blood lipids in elderly subjects. *Diabetes*, Nov. 1980; 29(11): 919-25.

6004 Rabinowitz MB, Gonick HC, Levin SR, Davidson MB. Effects of chromium and yeast supplements on carbohydrate and lipid metabolism in diabetic men. *Diabetes Care*, Jul-Aug 1983; 6(4): 319-27.

6005 *Arch Gen Psychiatry*. 1999;56:380,407,413.

6006 Mother Nature "Products" Website: www.mothernature.com (Accessed 23 July 1999).

6007 Levien T. Midazolam (Versed Syrup) *Pharmacist's Letter* Detail Document #141211. December, 1998.

6008 Gurley BJ, Gardner SF, Hubbard MA. Content versus label claims in ephedra-containing dietary supplements. *Am J Health-Syst Pharm* 2000;57:963-9.

6009 White LM, Gardner SF, Gurley BJ, et al. Pharmacokinetics and Cardiovascular Effects of Ma-Huang (Ephedra sinica) in Normotensive Adults. *J Clin Pharmacol* 1997;37:116-22.

6010 Arlt W, Haas J, Callies F, et al. Biotransformation of Oral Dehydroepiandrosterone in Elderly Men: Significant Increase in Circulating Estrogens. *J Clin Endocrinol Metab* 1999;84(6):2170-6.

6011 Barnhart KT, Freeman E, Grisso JA, et al. The Effect of Dehydroepiandrosterone Supplementation to Symptomatic Perimenopausal Women on Serum Endocrine Profiles, Lipid Parameters, and Health-Related Quality of Life. *J Clin Endocrinol Metab* 1999;84(11):3896-902.

6012 Callies F, Arlt W, Siekmann L, et al. Influence of oral dehydroepiandrosterone (DHEA) on urinary steroid metabolites in males and females. *Steroids* 2000;65:98-102.

6013 Tilvis RS, Kahonen M, Harkonen M. Dehydroepiandrosterone Sulfate, Diseases and Mortality in a General Aged Population. *Aging (Milano)* 1999;11(1):30-4.

6014 Mazza E, Maccario M Ramunni J, et al. Dehydroepiandrosterone Sulfate Levels in Women. Relationships With Age, Body Mass Index and Insulin Levels. *J Endocrinol Invest* 1999;22(9):681-7.

6015 Rossouw F, Kruger PE, Rossouw J. The Effect of Creatine Monohydrate Loading on Maximal Intermittent Exercise and Sport-Specific Strength in Well Trained Power-Lifters. *Nutrition Research* 2000;20(4):505-14.

6016 Timby N, Eriksson A. Gamma-Hydroxybutyrate-Associated Deaths. *Am J Med* 2000;108:518.

6017 Connor WE. Harbingers of coronary heart disease: dietary saturated fatty acids and cholesterol. Is chocolate benign because of its stearic acid content? *Am J Clin Nutr* 1999;70(6):951-2.

6018 Arts IC, Hollman PC, Kromhout D. Chocolate as a source of tea flavonoids (Letter). *Lancet* 1999;354:488.

6019 Bruinsma K, Taren DL. Chocolate: Food or Drug? *J Am Diet Assoc* 1999;99(10):1249-58.

6020 Mustad VA, Kris-Etherton PM, Derr J, et al. Comparison of the effects of diets rich in stearic acid versus myristic acid and lauric acid on platelet fatty acids and excretion of thromboxane A2 and PGI2 metabolites in healthy young men. *Metabolism* 1993;42(4):463-9.

6022 Ross GW, Abbott RD, Petrovitch H, et al. Association of coffee and caffeine intake with the risk of parkinson disease. *JAMA* 2000;283:2674-79.

6023 Tobias JD. Caffeine in the treatment of apnea associated with respiratory syncytial virus infection in neonates and infants. *South Med J* 2000;93(3):297-304.

6024 Watson JM, Jenkins EJ, Hamilton P, et al. Influence of caffeine on the frequency and perception of hypoglycemia in free-living patients with type 1 diabetes. *Diabetes Care* 2000;23(4):455-9.

6025 Lloyd T, Johnson-Rollings N, Eggli DF, et al. Bone status among postmenopausal women with different habitual caffeine intakes: a longitudinal investigation. *J Am Coll Nutr* 2000;19(2):256-61.

6026 American Academy of Pediatrics. "The transfer of drugs and other chemicals into human milk (RE9403)" website: URL: http://www.aap.org/policy/00026.html (Accessed 13 June 2000).

6027 Hu FB, Stampfer MJ, Manson JE, et al. Dietary saturated fats and their food sources in relation to the risk of coronary heart disease in women. *Am J Clin Nutr* 1999;70(6):1001-8.

6028 Hambrecht R, Hilbrich L, Erbs S, et al. Correction of endothelial dysfunction in chronic heart failure: additional effects of exercise training and oral L-arginine supplementation. *J Am Coll Cardiol* 2000;35(3):706-13.

6029 Setchell KD, Cassidy A. Dietary isoflavones: biological effects and relevance to human health. *J Nutr* 1999;129:758S-67S.

6030 Wroblewski Lisson L, Cooke JP. Phytoestrogens and cardiovascular health. *J Am Coll Cardiol* 2000;35:1403-10.

6031 Nemecz G. Green tea. U.S. Pharmacist 2000;May:67-70.

6032 Leenen R, Roodenburg AJ, Tijburg LB, et al. A single dose of tea with or without milk increases plasma antioxidant activity in humans. *Eur J Clin Nutr* 2000;54:87-92.

6033 Hodgson JM, Puddey IB, Croft KD, et al. Acute effects of ingestion of black and green tea on lipoprotein oxidation. *Am J Clin Nutr* 2000;71:1103-7.

6034 Hardy ML. Herbs of special interest to women. *J Am Pharm Assoc* 200;40:234-42.

6035 Bendich A. The potential for dietary supplements to reduce premenstrual syndrome (PMS) symptoms. *J Am Coll Nutr* 2000;19(1):3-12.

6036 Belch J, Hill A. Evening primrose oil and borage oil in rheumatologic conditions. *Am J Clin Nutr* 2000;71(1):352S-356S.

6100 Thumbs Up for Oats, but Not for Soy. URL: www.healthscout.com/cgi-bin/WebObjects/ Af.woa?id=95821&ap=24 (Accessed 19 May 2000).

6101 Jarrar D, Wang P, Cioffi WG, et al. Mechanisms of the salutary effects of dehydroepiandrosterone after trauma-hemorrhage. Direct or indirect effects on cardiac and hepatocellular functions? *Arch Surg* 2000;135(4):416-23.

6102 Markowitz JS, Carson WH, Jackson CW. Possible dihydroepiandrosterone-induced mania. *Biol Psychiatry* 1999;45(2):241-2.

6103 Israel RJ, Sonis ST. Topical dehydroascorbic acid (DHA) reduces moderate to severe mucositis in the hamster acute radiation model. 36th American Society of Clinical Oncology Annual Meeting Program Proceedings/Abstracts: Abstract 2367. URL: www.asco.org/prof/me/html/00abstracts/sm/m_2367.htm (Accessed 22 May 2000).

6104 Zavaleta N, Caulfield LE, Garcia T. Changes in iron status during pregnancy in peruvian women receiving prenatal iron and folic acid supplements with or without

zinc. *Am J Clin Nutr* 2000;71(4):956-61.

6105 Gossage C, Deyhim M, Moser-Veillon PB, et al. Effect of beta-carotene supplementation and lactation on carotenoid Metabolism and mitogenic T lymphocyte proliferation. *Am J Clin Nutr* 2000;71(4):950-955.

6106 Thijs C, van Houwelingen A, Poorterman I, et al. Essential fatty acids in breast milk of atopic mothers: comparison with non-atopic mothers, and effect of borage oil supplementation. *Eur J Clin Nutr* 2000;54(3):234-8.

6107 Agrawal A. Potato Peel Extract Holds Potential as Antiboitic. Reuters Health, May 23, 2000. URL: www.medscape.com/reuters/prof/2000/05/05.23/ 20000523drgd003.html (Accessed 23 May 2000).

6108 Ginseng effective in treating lung infection in mice. Reuters Health, May 24 2000. URL: www.reutershealth.com/frame/eline.html (Accessed 25 May 2000).

6109 Beehive material fights ulcer bacteria. Reuters Health, May 25 2000. URL: www.reutershealth.com/frame/ eline.html (Accessed 26 May 2000).

6110 Fermented milk kills ulcer bug. Reuters Health, May 25 2000. URL: www.reutershealth.com/frame/eline.html (Accessed 26 May 2000).

6111 Ginger reduces motion sickness. Reuters Health, May 26 2000. URL: www.reutershealth.com/frame/ eline.html (Accessed 30 May 2000).

6113 Oregano slows bacterial growth. Reuters Health, May 26 2000. URL: www.reutershealth.com/frame/eline.html (Accessed 30 May 2000).

6114 Miller MJ, Vergnolle N, Wallace JL, et al. Sangre de grado is a potent and unique inhibitor of neurogenic inflammation and promotes healing in experimental necrotizing enterocolitis. Pediatric Academic Societies and the American Academy of Pediatics Joint Meeting, May 12-16, 2000:Abstract 979. www.abstracts-on-line.com/abstracts/PAS (Accessed 30 May 2000).

6115 Bratman S, Kroll D. Natural Health Bible. Rocklin, CA; Prima Publishing, 1999.

6116 Blumenthal M, Goldberg A, Brinckmann J (eds). *Herbal Medicine Expanded Commission E Monographs.* Newton,MA;Integrative Medicine Communications, 2000.

6117 Creatine Generally Considered Safe, but Supplement's Value Still Questioned. Reuters Health, URL: www.medscape.com/reuters/prof/2000/06/06.02/ 20000602clin014.html (Accessed 2 June 2000).

6118 Lewis CJ, Alpert S. Letter to Health Care Professionals on FDA Concerned About Botanical Products, Including Dietary Supplements, Containing Aristolochic Acid. Office of Nutritional Products, Labeling, and Dietary Supplements, Center for Food Safety and Applied Nutrition, U. S. Food and Drug Administration, May 31, 2000. URL: vm.cfsan.fda.gov/~dms/ds-botl2.html (Accessed 1 April 2000).

6119 Lewis CJ. Letter to Industry on FDA Concerned About Botanical Products, Including Dietary Supplements, Containing Aristolochic Acid, Office of Nutritional Products, Labeling, and Dietary Supplements, Center for Food Safety and Applied Nutrition. U.S. Food and Drug Administration, May 30, 2000. URL: vm.cdsan.fda.gov/ ~dms/ds-botl1.html (Accessed 1 June 2000).

6121 Gardiner P, Kemper KJ. Herbs in pediatric and adolescent medicine. *Pediatr Rev* 2000;21(2):44-57.

6122 Calcium supplements. *Med Lett* 2000;42(1075):29-31.

6123 Beall DP, Scofield RH. Milk-alkali syndrome associated

© Copyright 2000, Natural Medicines Comprehensive Database (209) 472-2244. For updated data, go to www.NaturalDatabase.com.

R
E
F
E
R
E
N
C
E
S

with calcium carbonate consumption. Report of 7 patients with parathyroid hormone levels and an estimate of prevalence among patients hospitalized with hypercalcemia. *Medicine* (Baltimore) 1995;74(2):89-96.

6124 Moser LR, Smythe MA, Tisdale JE. The use of calcium salts in the prevention and management of verapamil-induced hypotension. *Ann Pharmacother* 2000;34(5):622-9.

6125 Reaney P. UK women told to have soy breast implants removed. Reuters Health June 06 2000; URL: www.reutershealth.com/frame/eline.html (Accessed 7 June 2000).

6126 Yanagisawa H, Yamazaki N, Sato G, Wada O. L-arginine treatment may prevent tubulointerstitial nephropathy caused by germanium dioxide. *Kidney Int* 2000;57(6):2257-84.

6127 Atkinson C, Compston JE, Robins SP, Bingham SA. The effects of isoflavone phytoestrogens on bone; preliminary results from a large randomized controlled trial. *The Endocrine Society's 82nd Annual Meeting*, Toronto, Canada June 21-24, 2000: Abstract 196.

6128 Gerber G, Lowe FC, Spigelman S. The use of a standardized extract of red clover isoflavones for the alleviation of BPH symptoms. *The Endocrine Society's 82nd Annual Meeting*, Toronto, Canada June 21-24, 2000: Abstract 2359.

6129 Mitchell S. Plant Modification May Enhance Public Consumption of Omega-3 Fatty Acids. Reuters Health, Jun 08 2000. URL: www.medscape.com/reuters/prof/ 2000/06/06.08/20000608publ001.html (Accessed 8 June 2000).

6130 Pearson H. A real lifesaver, Who says there's no cure for the summertime blues? New Scientist, 10 June 2000. URL: www.newscientist.com/nl/0610/coffee.html (Accessed 8 June 2000).

6131 Turmeric has anti-inflammatory effects. Reuters Health, Jun 08 2000. URL: www.reutershealth.com/frame/ eline.html (Accessed 9 June 2000).

6132 Kulkarni PM, Schuman PC, Merlino NS, Kinzie JL. Lactic acidosis and hepatic steatosis in HIV seropositive patients treated with nucleoside analogues. Digestive Disease Week Liver Conference, San Diego, May 21-24, 2000:Report 11. National AIDS Treatment Advocacy Project website. URL: www.natap.org (Accessed 9 June 2000).

6133 Roodenburg AJ, Leenen R, van het Hof KH, et al. Amount of fat in the diet affects bioavailability of lutein esters but not of alpha-carotene, beta-carotene, and vitamin E in humans. *Am J Clin Nutr* 2000;71(5):1187-93.

6134 Stahl W, Heinrich U, Jungmann H, et al. Carotenoids and carotenoids plus vitamin E protect against ultraviolet light-induced erythema in humans. *Am J Clin Nutr* 2000;71(3):795-8.

6135 Zhu M, Wong PY, Li RC. Effect of oral administration of fennel (Foeniculum vulgare) on ciprofloxacin absorption and disposition in the rat. *J Pharm Pharmacol* 1999;51(12):1391-6.

6136 Sandler AD, Sutton KA, DeWeese J, et al. Lack of benefit of a single dose of synthetic human secretin in the treatment of autism and pervasive developmental disorder. *N Engl J Med* 1999;341(24):1801-6.

6138 Nusko G, Schneider B, Schneider I, et al. Anthranoid laxative use is not a risk factor for colorectal neoplasia: results of a prospective case control study. *Gut* 2000;46(5):651-5.

6139 The International Formula Council Clears up Confusion on Soy Health Claim . PRNewswire June 9 2000. URL: www.prnewswire.com (Accessed 12 June 2000).

6140 NCAA Prohibits Schools From Supplying Creatine to Students. Reuters Heath, Jun 13 2000. URL: www.medscape.com/reuters/prof/2000/06/06.13/ 20000613publ004.html (Accessed 13 June 2000).

6141 Yogurt Helps Fight Sunburns, Nutritionist Says. News and Analysis @dairynetwork.com 6/8/2000. URL: www.dairynetwork.com (Accessed 13 June 2000).

6143 Mori TA, Burke V, Puddey IB, et al. Purified eicosapentaenoic and docosahexaenoic acids have differential effects on serum lipids and lipoproteins, LDL particle size, glucose, and insulin in mildly hyperlipidemic men. *Am J Clin Nutr* 2000;71(5):1085-94.

6144 Lewin PK. Temporary henna tattoo with permanent scarification. *CMAJ* 1999;160(3):310.

6145 Lestringant GG, Bener A, Frossard PM. Cutaneous reactions to henna and associated additives. *Br J Dermatol* 1999;141(3):598-600.

6146 Etienne A, Piletta P, Hauser C, Pasche-Koo F. Ectopic Contact Dermatitis from henna. *Contact Dermatitis* 1997;37(4):183.

6147 Wantke F, Gotz M, Jarisch R. Contact Dermatitis due to henna, solvent red 1 and solvent red 3, a case report. *Contact Dermatitis* 1992;27(5):346-7.

6148 Nigam PK, Saxena AK. Allergic Contact Dermatitis from henna. *Contact Dermatitis* 1988;18(1):55-56.

6149 Gupta BN, Mathur AK, Agarwal C, Singh A. Contact sensitivity to henna. *Contact Dermatitis* 1986;15(5):303-4.

6150 Pasricha JS, Gupta R, Panjwani S. Contact Dermatitis to henna (Lawsonia). *Contact Dermatitis* 1980;6(4):288-9.

6151 Cronin E. Immediate type hypersensitivity to henna. *Contact Dermatitis* 1979;5(3):198-9.

6152 Katz J, West, Jr KP, Khatry SK, et al. Maternal low-dose vitamin A or {beta}-carotene supplementation has no effect on fetal loss and early infant mortality: a randomized cluster trial in Nepal. *Am J Clin Nutr* 2000;71(6):1570-6.

6153 West KP Jr, Katz J, Khatry SK, et al. Double blind, cluster randomised trial of low dose supplementation with vitamin A or beta carotene on mortality related to pregnancy in Nepal. The NNIPS-2 Study Group. *BMJ* 1999;318(7183):570-5.

6154 Christian P, West KP Jr, Khatry SK, et al. Vitamin A or beta-carotene supplementation reduces but does not eliminate maternal night blindness in Nepal. *J Nutr* 1998;128(9):1458-63.

6155 Traikovich SS. Use of topical ascorbic acid and its effects on photodamaged skin topography. *Arch Otolaryngol Head Neck Surg* 1999;125(10):1091-8.

6166 Cellex-C Product Information for Professionals. Cellex-C website, URL: www.cellex-c.com/pro_side/ navigator.html (Accessed 14 June 2000).

6167 Vutyavanich T, Wongtra-ngan S, Ruangsri R. Pyridoxine for nausea and vomiting of pregnancy: a randomized, double-blind, placebo-controlled trial. *Am J Obstet Gynecol* 1995;173(3 Pt 1):881-4.

6168 Sahakian V, Rouse D, Sipes S, et al. Vitamin B6 is effective therapy for nausea and vomiting of pregnancy: a randomized, double-blind placebo-controlled study. *Obstet Gynecol* 1991;78(1):33-6.

6169 Sandler B, Aronson P. Yohimbine-induced cutaneous drug eruption, progressive renal failure, and lupus-like syndrome. *Urology* 1993;41(4):343-5.

6170 Wang ZQ, Zhang XH, Baldor LC, et al. Chromium picolinate enhances insulin sensitivity in an animal model for the metabolic syndrome: the obese, insulin resistant JCR:LA-corpulent rat. *American Diabetes Association's 60th Scientific Sessions and Exposition*, San Antonio, Texas, June 9-13, 2000: Abstract 291. URL: www.diabetes.org/am2000/ NumberResults.asp?idAbs=29 (Accessed 15 June 2000).

6171 Nelson L, Rao A, Olson P. Unique hydrolyzed whey protein isolates with antihypertensive activity. Institute of Food Technologistsí 2000 Annual Meeting & Food Expo; Abstract 38-6. URL: ift.confex.com/ift/2000/ techprogram/paper_5129.htm (Accessed 15 June 2000)

6172 Ajani UA, Hennekens CH, Spelsberg, A, et al. Alcohol consumption and risk of type 2 Diabetes mellitus among us male physicians. *Arch Intern Med* 2000;160(7):1025-30.

6173 Shaper AG, Wannamethee SG. Alcohol intake and mortality in middle aged men with diagnosed coronary heart disease. *Heart* 2000;83(4):394-9.

6174 Vally H, de Klerk N, Thompson PJ. Alcoholic drinks: Important triggers for asthma. *J Allergy Clin Immunol* 2000;105(3):462-7.

6175 Lanthony P, Cosson JP. [The course of color vision in early diabetic retinopathy treated with ginkgo biloba extract. A preliminary double-blind versus placebo study.] [Article in French] *J Fr Ophtalmol* 1988;11(10):671-4.

6176 Grandjean EM, Berthet P, Ruffmann R, Leuenberger P. Efficacy of oral long-term N-acetylcysteine in chronic bronchopulmonary disease: a meta-analysis of published double-blind, placebo-controlled clinical trials. *Clin Ther* 2000;22(2):209-21.

6177 Puig L. Pharmacodynamic interaction with phototoxic plants during PUVA therapy. *Br J Dermatol* 1997;136(6):973-4.

6178 Gral N, Beani JC, Bonnot D, et al. [Plasma levels of psoralens after celery ingestion]. [French] *Ann Dermatol Venereol* 1993;120(9):599-603.

6179 Desperate remedies. New Scientist, Nov 27,1999:34-6.

6180 Eagon PK, Elm MS, Hunter DS, et al. Medicinal herbs: modulation of estrogen action. *Era of Hope Meeting for the Department of Defense Breast Cancer Research Program*, Atlanta, Georgia June 8-11, 2000.

6181 Joss JD, LeBlond RF. Potentiation of warfarin anticoagulation associated with topical methyl salicylate. *Ann Pharmacother* 2000;34(6):729-33.

6182 Walter MC, Lochmuller H, Reilich P, et al. Creatine monohydrate in muscular dystrophies: A double-blind, placebo-controlled clinical study. *Neurology* 2000;54(9):1848-50.

6183 Gilliam JD, Hohzorn C, Martin D, Trimble MH. Effect of oral creatine supplementation on isokinetic torque production. *Med Sci Sports Exerc* 2000;32(5):993-6.

6185 Hallikainen MA, Sarkkinen ES, Uusitupa MI. Plant stanol esters affect serum cholesterol concentrations of hypercholesterolemic men and women in a dose-dependent manner. *J Nutr* 2000;130(4):767-76.

6186 Rome LA, Lippmann ML, Dalsey WC, et al. Prevalence of cocaine use and its impact on asthma exacerbation in an urban population. *Chest* 2000;117(5):1324-9.

6187 Potter SM, Zelazo PR, Stack DM, Papageorgiou AN. Adverse effects of fetal cocaine exposure on neonatal auditory information processing. *Pediatrics* 2000;105(3) [cited 2000 Mar 10]. Available from: URL:

6188 Maier SM, Turner ND, Lupton JR. Serum lipids in hypercholesterolemic men and women consuming oat bran and amaranth products. *Cereal Chem* 2000:77(3);297-302.

6189 Pitchford P. *Healing With Whole Foods*. Berkeley, CA; North Atlantic Books, 1993.

6190 Gobel H, Fresenius J, Heinze A, et al. [Effectiveness of Oleum menthae piperitae and paracetamol in therapy of Headache of the tension type]. [Article in German] *Nervenarzt* 1996;67(8):672-81.

6191 Umeta M, West CE, Haidar J, et al. Zinc supplementation and stunted infants in Ethiopia: a randomised controlled trial. *Lancet* 2000;355(9220):2021-6.

6192 Khanna VJ, Shieh S, Benjamin J, et al. Necrolytic acral erythema associated with hepatitis C effective treatment with interferon alfa and zinc. *Arch Dermatol* 2000;136(6):755-7.

6193 Booth SL, Tucker KL, Chen H, et al. Dietary vitamin K intakes are associated with hip fracture but not with bone mineral density in elderly men and women. *Am J Clin Nutr* 2000;71(5):1201-8.

6196 Spinella P, De Palo CB, Scaroni C, et al. Effect of licorice on reduction of body fat mass. The Endocrine Society's 82nd Annual Meeting, Toronto, Canada June 21-24, 2000: Abstract 2065. URL: www.abstracts-on-line.com/abstracts/ENDO/search/results.asp?Num-0%2E2697367.

6200 Rey JM, Walter G. Hypericum perforatum (St. John's wort) in depression: pest or blessing? *Med J Aust* 1998;169:583-6.

6201 Brown TM. Acute St. John's wort toxicity. *Am J Emerg Med* 2000;18:231-2.

6202 Breidenbach T, Hoffman MW, Becker T, et al. Drug interaction of St. John's wort with ciclosporin. *Lancet* 2000;355:1912.

6203 Ohtsuka Y, Nakaya J. Effect of oral administration of L-arginine on senile dementia. *Am J Med* 2000;108:439.

6204 Kehoe WA. Vitamin E and heart disease. *Pharmacist's Letter* 2000;16(3):160307.

6205 Melchart D, Linde K, Fischer P, Kaesmayr J. Echinacea for preventing and treating the common cold. *Cochrane Database Syst Rev* 2000;2:CD000530.

6206 Szolomicki S, Samochowiec L, Wojcicki J, Drozdzik M. The influence of active components of Eleutherococcus senticosus on cellular defense and physical fitness in man. *Phytother Res* 2000;14:30-35.

6207 Turner RB, Riker DK, Gangemi JD. Ineffectiveness of echinacea for prevention of experimental rhinovirus colds. *Antimicrob Agents Chemother* 2000;44:1708-1709.

6208 Diamond BJ, Shiflett SC, Feiwel N, et al. Ginkgo biloba extract: mechanisms and clinical indications. *Arch Phys Med Rehabil* 2000;81:668-78.

6209 Ashton AK, Ahrens K, Gupta S, Masand PS. Antidepressant-induced sexual dysfunction and Ginkgo Biloba. *Am J Psychiatry* 2000;157:836-7.

6210 Evans JR. Ginkgo biloba extract for age-related macular degeneration. *Cochrane Database Syst Rev* 2000;2:CD001775.

6211 Pittler MH, Ernst E. Ginko Biloba extract for the treatment of intermittent claudication: a meta-analysis of randomized trials. *Am J Med* 2000,108:276-81.

6212 Li AL, Shi YD, Landsmann B, et al. Hemorheology and walking of peripheral arterial occlusive diseases patients

© Copyright 2000, Natural Medicines Comprehensive Database (209) 472-2244. For updated data, go to www.NaturalDatabase.com. • 1287

R E F E R E N C E S

during treatment with Ginkgo biloba extract. *Chung Kuo Yao Li Hsueh Pao* 1998;19:417-21.

6213 Peters H, Kieser M, Holscher U. Demonstration of the efficacy of ginkgo biloba special extract EGb 761 on intermittent claudication—a placebo-controlled, double-blind multicenter trial. *Vasa* 1998;27:106-10.

6214 Rigney U, Kimber S, Hindmarch I. The effects of acute doses of standardized Ginkgo biloba extract on memory and psychomotor performance in volunteers. *Phytother Res* 1999;13:408-15.

6215 Subhan Z, Hindmarch I. The psychopharmacological effects of Ginkgo biloba extract in normal healthy volunteers. *Int J Clin Pharmacol Res* 1984;4:89-93.

6216 Rai GS, Shovlin C, Wesnes KA. A double-blind, placebo controlled study of Ginkgo biloba extract ('tanakan') in elderly outpatients with mild to moderate memory impairment. *Curr Med Res Opin* 1991;12:350-5.

6217 Winter E. Effects of an extract of Ginkgo biloba on learning and memory in mice. *Pharmacol Biochem Behav* 1991;38:109-14.

6218 Holgers KM, Axelsson A, Pringle I. Ginkgo biloba extract for the treatment of tinnitus. *Audiology* 1994;33:85-92.

6219 Meyer B. [Multicenter randomized double-blind drug vs. placebo study of the treatment of tinnitus with Ginkgo biloba extract]. *Presse Med* 1986;15:1562-4.

6220 Cesarani A, Meloni F, Alpini D, et al. Ginkgo biloba (EGb 761) in the treatment of equilibrium disorders. *Adv Ther* 1998;15:291-304.

6221 Haguenauer JP, Cantenot F, Koskas H, Pierart H. [Treatment of equilibrium disorders with Ginkgo biloba extract. A multicenter double-blind drug vs. placebo study]. *Presse Med* 1986;15:1569-72.

6222 Hopfenmuller W. [Evidence for a therapeutic effect of Ginkgo biloba special extract. Meta-analysis of 11 clinical studies in patients with cerebrovascular insufficiency in old age]. *Arzneimittelforschung* 1994;44:1005-13.

6223 Kleijnen J, Knipschild P. Ginkgo biloba for cerebral insufficiency. *Br J Clin Pharmacol* 1992;34:352-8.

6224 Wettstein A. Cholinesterase inhibitors and Gingko extracts—are they comparable in the treatment of dementia? Comparison of published placebo-controlled efficacy studies of at least six months' duration. *PhytoMedicine* 2000;6:393-401.

6225 Kanowski S, Herrmann WM, Stephan K, et al. Proof of efficacy of the ginkgo biloba special extract EGb 761 in outpatients suffering from mild to moderate primary degenerative dementia of the Alzheimer type or multi-infarct dementia. *Pharmacopsychiatry* 1996;29:47-56.

6226 National Institute of Health. Clinical Trials.gov website: www.clinicaltrials.gov/ct/gui/c/r (Accessed 15 June 2000).

6227 Lebuisson DA, Leroy L, Rigal G. [Treatment of senile macular degeneration with Ginkgo biloba extract. A preliminary double-blind drug vs. placebo study]. *Presse Med* 1986;15:1556-8.

6228 Evans JR. Ginkgo biloba extract for age-related macular degeneration. *Cochrane Database* Syst Rev 2000;2:CD001775.

6229 Tamborini A, Taurelle R. [Value of standardized Ginkgo biloba extract (EGb 761) in the management of congestive symptoms of premenstrual syndrome]. *Rev Fr Gynecol Obstet* 1993;88:447-57.

6230 Roncin JP, Schwartz F, D'Arbigny P. EGb 761 in Control of Acute Mountain Sickness and Vascular Reactivity to Cold Exposure. *Aviat Space Environ Med* 1996;67:445-52.

6231 Fowler JS, Wang GJ, Volkow ND et al. Evidence that gingko biloba extract does not inhibit MAO A and B in living human brain. *Life Sci* 2000;66:141-6.

6232 Porsolt RD, Roux S, Drieu K. Evaluation of a ginkgo biloba extract (EGb 761) in functional tests for monoamine oxidase inhibition. *Arzneimittelforschung* 2000;50:232-5.

6233 White HL, Scates PW, Cooper BR. Extracts of Ginkgo biloba leaves inhibit monoamine oxidase. *Life Sci* 1996;58:1315-21.

6234 Snowdon DA, Tully CL, Smith CD, et al. Serum folate and the severity of atrophy of the neocortex in Alzheimer disease: findings from the Nun study. *Am J Clin Nutr* 2000;71:993-8.

6235 Chao CL, Chien KL, Lee YT. Effect of short-term vitamin (folic acid, vitamins B6 and B12) administration on endothelial dysfunction induced by post-methionine load hyperhomocysteinemia. *Am J Cardiol* 1999;84:1359-61.

6236 Usui M, Matsuoka H, Miyazaki H, et al. Endothelial dysfunction by acute hyperhomocyst(e)inaemia: restoration by folic acid. *Clin Sci (Colch)* 1999;96:235-9.

6237 Nelen WL, Blom HJ, Steegers EA, et al. Homocysteine and folate levels as risk factors for recurrent early pregnancy loss. *Obstet Gynecol* 2000;95:519-24.

6238 Ortega RM, Manas LR, Andres P, et al. Functional and psychic deterioration in elderly people may be aggravated by folate deficiency. *J Nutr* 1996;126:1992-9.

6239 Fava M, Borus JS, Alpert JE, et al. Folate, vitamin B12, and homocysteine in major depressive disorder. *Am J Psychiatry* 1997;154:426-8.

6240 Brown DJ, et al. Phytotherapeutic and nutritional approaches to Diabetes mellitus. *Quarterly Review of Natural Medicine* Dec. 1998:329-51.

6241 Suitor CW, Bailey LB. Dietary folate equivalents: interpretation and application. *J Am Diet Assoc* 2000;100:88-94.

6242 Suitor CW, Bailey LB. Food folate vs synthetic folic acid: a comparison. *J Am Diet Assoc* 1999;99:285.

6243 Institute of Medicine. Dietary Reference Intakes for Thiamin, Riboflavin, Niacin, Vitamin B6, folate, Vitamin B12, Pantothenic Acid, Biotin, and Cholin. website: http://books.nap.edu/books/0309065542/html/196.html#pagetop (Accessed 17 June 2000).

6244 Winther K, Randlov C, Rein E, Mehlsen J. Effects of ginkgo biloba extract on cognitive function and blood pressure in elderly subjects. *Curr Ther Res* 1998;59:881-8.

6245 Nardini M, De Stefano R, Iannuccelli M, et al. Treatment of depression with L-5-hydroxytryptophan combined with chlorimipramine, a double-blind study. *Int J Clin Pharmacol Res* 1983;3:239-50.

6246 Steinberg S, Annable L, Young SN, Liyanage N. A placebo-controlled study of the effects of L-tryptophan in patients with premenstrual dysphoria. *Adv Exp Med Biol* 1999;467:85-8.

6247 Ghadirian AM, Murphy BE, Gendron MJ. Efficacy of light versus tryptophan therapy in seasonal affective disorder. *J Affect Disord* 1998;50:23-7.

6248 Leathwood PD, Chauffard F, Heck E, Munoz-Box R. Aqueous extract of valerian root (Valeriana officinalis

L.) improves sleep quality in man. *Pharmacol Biochem Behav* 1982;17:65-71.

6249 Donath F, Quispe S, Diefenbach K, et al. Critical evaluation of the effect of valerian extract on sleep structure and sleep quality. *Pharmacopsychiatry* 2000;33:47-53.

6250 Bourin M, Bougerol T, Guitton B, Broutin E. A combination of plant extracts in the treatment of outpatients with adjustment disorder with anxious mood: controlled study versus placebo. *Fundam Clin Pharmacol* 1997;11:127-32.

6251 Fisher AA, Purcell P, Le Couteur DG. Toxicity of Passiflora incarnata L. *J Toxicol Clin Toxicol* 2000;38:63-6.

6252 Klein G, Kullich W. Short-term treatment of painful osteoarthritis of the knee with oral enzymes. *Clin Drug Invest* 2000;19:15-23.

6253 Kane S, Goldberg MJ. Use of bromelain for mild ulcerative colitis. *Ann Intern Med* 2000;132:680.

6254 Caso MA, Vargas RR, Salas VA, Begona IC. Double-blind study of a multivitamin complex supplemented with ginseng extract. *Drugs Exp Clin Res* 1996;22:323-9.

6255 Hill AJ, Peikin SR, Ryan CA, Blundell JE. Oral administration of proteinase inhibitor II from potatoes reduces energy intake in man. *Physiol Behav* 1990;48:241-6.

6256 Akobeng AK, Miller V, Stanton J, et al. Double-blind randomized controlled trial of glutamine-enriched polymeric diet in the treatment of active Crohn's disease. *J Pediatr Gastroenterol Nutr* 2000;30:78-84.

6257 Belluzzi A, Brignola C, Campieri M, et al. Effect of an enteric-coated fish-oil preparation on relapses in Crohn's disease. *N Engl J Med* 1996;334:1557-60.

6258 Belluzzi A, Brignola C, Campieri M, et al. Effects of new fish oil derivative on fatty acid phospholipid-membrane pattern in a group of Crohn's disease patients. *Dig Dis Sci* 1994;39:2589-94.

6259 Lorenz-Meyer H, Bauer P, Nicolay C, et al. Omega-3 fatty acids and low carbohydrate diet for maintenance of remission in Crohn's disease. A randomized controlled multicenter trial. Study Group Members (German Crohn's Disease Study Group). *Scand J Gastroenterol* 1996;31:778-85

6260 Smith W, Mitchell P, Leeder SR. Dietary fat and fish intake and age-related maculopathy. *Arch Ophthalmol* 2000;118:401-4.

6261 Anderson JW, Davidson MH, Blonde L, et al. Long-term cholesterol-lowering effects of psyllium as an adjunct to diet therapy in the treatment of hypercholesterolemia. *Am J Clin Nutr* 2000;71:1433-8.

6262 Davidson MH, Maki KC, Kong JC, et al. Long-term effects of consuming foods containing psyllium seed husk on serum lipids in subjects with hypercholesterolemia. *Am J Clin Nutr* 1998;67:367-76.

6263 Olson BH, Anderson SM, Becker MP, et al. Psyllium-enriched cereals lower blood total cholesterol and LDL cholesterol, but not HDL cholesterol, in hypercholesterolemic adults: results of a meta-analysis. *J Nutr* 1997;127:1973-80.

6264 U. S. Food and Drug Administration, Center for Food Safety and Applied Nutrition. "FDA Allows Foods Containing Psyllium To Make Health Claim On Reducing Risk Of Heart Disease" website: http://vm.cfsan.fda.gov/~lrd/tpsylliu.html (Accessed 19 June 2000).

6265 McRorie J, Kesler J, Bishop L, et al. Effects of wheat bran and Olestra on objective measures of stool and subjective reports of GI symptoms. *Am J Gastroenterol* 2000;95:1244-52.

6266 Chandalia M, Garg A, Lutjohann D, et al. Beneficial effects of high dietary fiber intake in patients with type 2 diabetes mellitus. *N Engl J Med* 2000;342:1392-8.

6267 Schatzkin A, Lanza E, Corle D, et al. Lack of effect of a low-fat, high-fiber diet on the recurrence of colorectal adenomas. Polyp Prevention Trial Study Group. *N Engl J Med* 2000;342:1149-55.

6268 National Academy of Science, Institute of Medicine. "Dietary Reference Intakes for Vitamin C, Vitamin E, Selenium, and Carotenoids http://www.nap.edu/pdf/0309069351/pdf_image/325.pdf (Accessed 21 June 2000).

6269 Kuroki F, Lida M, Tominaga M, et al. Multiple vitamin status in Crohn's disease. Correlation with disease activity. *Dig Dis Sci* 1993;38:1614-8.

6270 Lashner BA, Provencher KS, Seidner DL, et al. The effect of folic acid supplementation on the risk for cancer or dysplasia in ulcerative colitis. *Gastroenterology* 1997;112:29-32.

6271 Lashner BA. Red blood cell folate is associated with the development of dysplasia and cancer in ulcerative colitis. *J Br J Nutr Clin Oncol* 1993;119:549-54.

6400 Brenner R, Azbel V, Madhusoodanan S, et al. Comparison of an extract of Hypericum (LI 160) and sertraline in the treatment of depression: A double-blind, randomized pilot study. *Clin Ther* 2000;22:411-9.

6401 Murray MT, Pizzorno JE. Piper methysticum (Kava). In: Pizzorno JE, Murray MT, eds. *Textbook of Natural Medicine*. 2nd ed. Edinburgh:Churchill Livingstone, 1999:887-92.

6402 Mathews JD, Riley MD, Fejo L, et al. Effects of heavy usage of kava on physical health: Summary of a pilot survey in an aboriginal community. *Med J Aust* 1988;148:548-55.

6403 Imai K. Nakachi K. Cross-sectional study of effects of drinking green tea on cardiovascular and Liver diseases. *BMJ* 1995;310:693-6.

6404 Hegarty VM, May HM, Khaw K. Tea drinking and bone mineral density in older women. *Am J Clin Nutr* 2000;71:1003-7.

6405 Anon. Drugs, vitamins, minerals, in pregnancy: Fiber. MDX Family Health Library 1999. http://healthgate.com/cgi-bin/q-format.cgi?f=G&d=mdx4&m=67 (Accessed 4 June 2000).

6406 Pye JK, Mansel RE, Hughes LE. Clinical experience of drug treatments for mastalgia. *Lancet* 1985;845:373-7.

6407 Morisco C, Trimarco B, Condorelli M. Effect of coenzyme Q10 therapy in patients with congestive heart failure: A long-term multicenter randomized study. *Clin Invest* 1993;71(Suppl. 8): S134–6.

6408 Hofman-Bang C, et al. Coenzyme Q10 as an adjunctive treatment of congestive heart failure. *J Card Fail* 1995;1:101-7.

6409 Baggio E, Gandini R, Plauncher AC, et al. Italian multicenter study on the safety and efficacy of coenzyme Q10 as adjunctive therapy in heart failure. CoQ10 Drug Surveillance Investigators. *Mol Aspects Med* 1994;(15 Suppl):S287-94.

6410 Gaby AR. Coenzyme Q10. In: Pizzorno JE, Murray MT, eds. *Textbook of Natural Medicine*. 2nd Ed. New York: Churchill Livingstone, 1999;663.

© Copyright 2000, Natural Medicines Comprehensive Database (209) 472-2244. For updated data, go to www.NaturalDatabase.com. • 1289

R E F E R E N C E S

6411 Anon. Goldenseal. *The Natural Pharmacist*, 1999. http://www.tnp.com/propages.asp?ID=26. (Accessed 22 June 2000).

6412 Teixeira, SR, Potter SM, Weigel R, et al. Effects of feeding 4 levels of soy protein for 3 and 6 wk on blood lipids and apolipoproteins in moderately hypercholesterolemic men. *Am J Clin Nutr* 2000;71:1077-84.

6413 Merz-Demlow BE, Duncan AM, Wangen KE, et al. Soy isoflavones improve plasma lipids in normocholesterolemic, premenopausal women. *Am J Clin Nutr* 2000;71:1462-9.

6414 Heaney RP, Dowell MS, Rafferty K, et al. Bioavailability of the calcium in fortified soy imitation milk, with some observations on method. *Am J Clin Nutr* 2000;71:1166-9.

6415 White LR, Petrovitch H, Ross GW, et al. Brain aging and midlife tofu consumption. *Journal of the American College of Nutrition* 2000;19:242-55.

6416 Grodstein F, Mayeux R, Stampfer MJ. Tofu and cognitive function: food for thought. *Journal of the American College of Nutrition* 2000;19:207-9.

6420 Anon. Horse Chestnut. The Natural Pharmacist 2000. http://www.tnp.com/substance.asp?ID=62. (Accessed 24 June 2000).

7000 Greenberg S, Frishman WH. Co-enzyme Q10: a new drug for cardiovascular disease. *J Clin Pharmacol* 1990;30:596-608.

7001 Ubiquinone. In: Olin B.R., ed. "The Lawrence review of natural products." St. Louis, MO: *Facts and Comparisons*; 1997.

7002 Stockley. *Drug Interactions*, 4th Edition, 1996.

7003 Fetrow CW, Avila JR. "*Complementary & Alternative Medicines.*" Springhouse Corporation, Springhouse, PA 1999.

7005 Locock RA. Capsicum. *Can Pharm J*, 1985; 118: 517-9.

7006 Visudhiphan S, Poolsuppasit S, Piboonnukarintr O, Timliang S. "The relationship between high fibrinolytic activity and daily capsicum ingestion in Thais." *Am J Clin Nut*, 1982; 35: 1452-8.

7007 Cordell GA, Araujo OE. "Capsaicin: Identification, nomenclature, and Pharmacotherapy." *Ann of Pharmacotherapy*, 1993; 27: 330-336.

7008 Avorn J, Manone M, Gurwitz JH, et al. "Reduction of bacteriuria and pyuria after ingestion of cranberry juice." *JAMA* , 1994; 271:751-54.

7009 Bomser J, Madhavi DL, Singletary K, Smith MAL. "In vitro anticancer activity of fruit extracts from Vaccinium species." *Planta Medica*, 1996; 62: 212-6.

7010 Brown D. Herbal Prescriptions for Better Health. Rocklin, CA: Prima Publishing; 1996.

7011 Amann W. "Akne vulgaris und agnus castus (Agnolyt)." *Z Allgemeinmed*, 1975; 14: 1645-47 [German].

7012 Du Mee C. "Vitex agnus castus." *Aust J Med Herb*, 1993; 5(3): 63-65.

7013 Brown D. "Vitex agnus castus Clinical Monograph." Quarterly Review of Natural Medicine, 1994; 2(2): 111-121.

7014 Wuttke W. Dopaminergic "Action of Extracts of Agnus Castus." *Forschende Komplementarmedizen*, 1996; 3(6): 329-330.

7015 Jarry H, Leonhardt S., Gorkow C, Wuttke W. "In vitro prolactin but not LH and FSH release is inhibited by compounds in extracts of Agnus Castus: direct evidence for a dopaminergic principle by the dopamine receptor assay." *Experimental and Clinical Endocrinology*, 1994;

102:448-454.

7016 Merz P, Gorkow C, Schroder A, et al. "The effects of a special Agnus castus extract (BP1095el) on prolactin secretion in healthy male subjects." *Endocrinology and Diabetes*, 1996; 104: 447-453.

7200 Fetrow CW, Avila JR. Professional's Handbook of Complementary and Alternative Medicines. First ed. Springhouse: Springhouse Corporation, 1999.

7201 Jumaan AO, et al. "Beta-carotene intake and risk of postmenopausal breast cancer." *Epidemiology* 1999 Jan;10(1):49-53.

7202 Stoll AL, Severus WE, Freeman MP, et al. "Omega 3 fatty acids in bipolar disorder: A preliminary double-blind, placebo-controlled trial." *Arch Gen Psychiatry* 1999;56:407-412.

8000 Loprinzi CL, Goldberg RM, Burnham NL. Cancer-associated anorexia and cachexia. Implications for drug therapy. *Drugs* 1992;43(4):499-506.

8001 Loprinzi CL, Goldberg RM, Su JQ, et al. Placebo-controlled trial of hydrazine sulfate in patients with newly diagnosed non-small-cell lung cancer. *J Clin Oncol* 1994;12(6):1126-9.

8002 Loprinzi CL, Kuross SA, O'Fallon JR, et al. Randomized placebo-controlled evaluation of hydrazine sulfate in patients with advanced colorectal cancer. *J Clin Oncol* 1994;12(6):1121-5.

8003 Kosty MP, Fleishman SB, Herndon JE 2nd, et al. Cisplatin, vinblastine, and hydrazine sulfate in advanced, non-small-cell lung cancer: a randomized placebo-controlled, double-blind phase III study of the Cancer and Leukemia Group B. *J Clin Oncol* 1994;12(6):1113-20.

8004 Chlebowski RT, Bulcavage L, Grosvenor M, et al. Hydrazine sulfate in Cancer patients with weight loss. A placebo-controlled clinical experience. *Cancer* 1987;59(3):406-10

8005 Kaegi E. Unconventional therapies for cancer: 4. Hydrazine sulfate. Task Force on Alternative Therapies of the Canadian Breast Cancer *Research* Initiative. *CMAJ* 1998;158(10):1327-30

8006 Blumenthal M, Goldberg A, Brinckmann J. (eds.). Herbal Medicine: Expanded Commission E Monographs. Newton, MA: Integrative Medicine Communications, 2000.

8300 Bredle DL, et al. "Phosphate supplementation, cardiovascular function, and exercise performance in humans." *J Appl Physiol*, 1988; 65(4): 1821-826.

8301 Duffy DJ, Conlee RK. "Effects of phosphate loading on leg power and high intensity treadmill exercise." *Med Sci Sports Exerc*, 1986; 18(6): 674-77.

8302 Perreault MM, Ostrop NJ, Tierney MG. "Efficacy and safety of intravenous phosphate replacement in critically ill patients." *Ann Pharmacother*, 1997; 31(6): 683-88.

8303 Rosen GH, et al. "Intravenous phosphate repletion regimen for critically ill patients with moderate hypophosphatemia." *Crit Care Med*, 1995;23(7):1204-210.

8304 Androstenediol 4AD, Vitanet website. URL: store.yahoo.com/vitanet/vitan.html (Accessed 8 December 1999).

Some Brand Name Natural Products - What they Contain
www.NaturalDatabase.com contains MANY more listings than appear here.

A & D Natural Capsules — Progressive Labs
Each softgel contains: Vitamin A (from fish liver oil, Skip Jack liver oil) 10,000 IU • Vitamin D (from fish liver oil, Skip Jack liver oil) 400 IU.

A Kid's Companion High Potency Chewable Multi-Vitamin Mineral Formula — Natrol
Two wafers contain: Vitamins/Minerals: Vitamin A Activity (Palmitate) 2500 IU • Vitamin A (Beta Carotene) 2500 IU • Vitamin D (Calciferol) 400 IU • Vitamin E (d-Alpha Tocopheryl Succinate) 30 IU • Vitamin C (Ascorbic Acid) 60 mg • Vitamin B1 (Thiamine HCI) 2.5 mg • Vitamin B2 (Riboflavin) 2.5 mg • Vitamin B6 (Pyridoxine HCI) 2.5 mg • Vitamin B12 (Cyanocobalamin) 10 mcg • Niacinamide 20 mg • Calcium (Carbonate) 200 mg • Iron (Gluconate) 5 mg • Folic Acid 400 mcg • Biotin 150 mcg • Pantothenic Acid (Calcium d-Pantothenate) 12.5 mg • Choline (Bitartrate) 10 mg • Inositol 10 mg • PABA (Para Amino Benzoic Acid) 5 mg • Iodine (Kelp) 150 mcg • Magnesium (Oxide) 50 mg • Zinc (Gluconate) 2.5 mg • Copper (Gluconate) 200 mcg • Vitamin K 25 mcg • Selenium, organically bound concentrate 5 mcg • Chromium (ChromeMate) 10 mcg • Manganese (Gluconate) 1 mg • Potassium (Chloride) 1 mg • Silica from standardized Horsetail extract 1.5 mg • Glycine 200 mg • Lemon Bioflavonoids 25 mg • Bee Pollen 25 mg • Acerola 25 mg • Black Currant 25 mg. Flavored with natural fruit extracts (Lemon, Orange) natural flavors (Butterscotch, Vanilla) & sweetened with Fructose.

A.S.A.P. — The Herbalist
Black Cohosh root • Passionflower herb • Scullcap herb • Valerian root • Lobelia leaf • Prickly Ash bark.

A+Zinc — Nutrilite
Each tablet contains: Vitamin A 10000 IU • Zinc Oxide 15 mg • Zinc Gluconate 15 mg.

A-25 Plex — Progressive Labs
Each softgel contains: Vitamin A (Beta Carotene) 15000 IU • Vitamin A (from fish liver oil) 10000 IU • Alfalfa 5 mg • Cranberry juice concentrate 5 mg • Carrot oil 6 mg • Lecithin 5 mg.

Absorbable Iron with Hematinic Factors —
The Vitamin Shoppe
Each tablet provides: Iron 50 mg • Heme Iron 25 mg • Vitamin C 75 mg • Copper 1 mg • Folic Acid 200 mcg • Vitamin B12 12.5 mcg.

AbsorbAid — Nature's Sources
Two capsules contain: Lipase 1145 LU • Amylase • 8316 SKBU • Protease (from Bromelain) 36 GDU • Cellulase 299 CU • Lactase 900 LacU.

Absorbitol Fat Binder — Natrol
Two capsules contain: Chitosan Complex 900 mg. Other ingredients: Magnesium Stearate, Gelatin.

Acceleration — Phytopharmica
Each capsule contains: Cola Nut extract (cola nitida) 250 mg (contains 35 mg of caffeine) • Green Tea extract (Camellia sinensis) 250 mg (contains 15 mg of caffeine) • Ma Huang extract (Ephedra sinensis) 250 mg (contains 15 mg of ephedrine). Contains no sugar, salt, yeast, wheat, corn, soy, dairy products, coloring, flavoring or preservatives.

ACE Antioxidant Complex — Nature's Life
Each tablet contains: Beta Carotene (Vitamin A equivalent to 5000 IU) 3 mg • Vitamin C 500 mg • Vitamin E (d-Alpha Tocopheryl Succinate) 200 IU • Selenium (Selenomax Selenomethionine) 25 mcg. In a natural base of Rose Hips powder & Nature's Life Greens (A proprietary blend of 24 vegetables & herbs, microalgae, sea vegetables & sprouts).

ACE Ultimate Antioxidant Plus — Nature's Life
Two capsules contain: Antioxidant Nutrients: Beta Carotene (Vitamin A equivalent to 25000 IU) 15 mg • Vitamin C 1000 mg • Vitamin E (d-Alpha Tocopheryl Succinate) 300 IU • Vitamin B2 (Riboflavin, Riboflavin-5-phosphate) 10 mg • Selenium (Selenite, Methionine) 200 mcg • Glutathione (Glutamine/Cysteine/Glycine Tripeptide) 100 mg • Superoxide Dismutase inducing Minerals: Zinc (Citrate, Picolinate) 10 mg • Manganese (Citrate) 10 mg • Copper (Citrate, Gluconate) 1 mg • Antioxidant Flavonoids: Lemon Bioflavonoids Complex (TESTLAB 50% total bioflavonoids as Flavanones, Hesperidin, Naringenin & Eriocitrin = 50%) [Carbohydrate, Protein, Moisture & Fiber = 50%] 25 mg • Quercetin (Dimorphandra pod) 25 mg • Rutin (Saphora japonica) 25 mg • Hesperidin (citrus) 25 mg • Proanthocyanidins [(Pinus maritima) Pine bark extract] 5 mg •

Epigallocatechin Gallate [(Camellia sinensis) Green Tea extract] 5 mg.

Acetabolan — Muscletech
Six capsules contain: Acetyl-L-Carnitine 1000 mg • Glutamine 2000 mg • L-Leucine 1000 mg • L-Valine 250 mg • L-Isoleucine 250 mg • OKG 100 mg • Zinc 60 mg • Taurine 1000 mg.

Acetabolan II — Muscletech
Six capsules contain: NAC (as N-Acetyl-Cysteine Hydrochloride) 400 mg. Ingredients: Acetyl-L-Carnitine • Tribulus terrestris • ZincTech (a unique blend of Chelated Zinc, Magnesium, & Vitamin B6).

Acid-A-Cal — Enzymatic Therapy
Each capsule contains: Calcium Chloride 96 mg • Calcium Phosphate 90 mg • Magnesium Glycerophosphate 51 mg • Vitamin C (Ascorbic Acid/Rose Hips) 50 mg • Vitamin B6 (Pyridoxine HCL) 25 mg • Other ingredients: Betaine HCL 96 mg • Ammonium Chloride 96 mg • Raw Kidney Tissue 30 mg • Citrus Bioflavonoids 30 mg. All organs & glands derived from bovine sources.

Acida-Zyme — Progressive Labs
Each capsule contains: Betaine HCl 200 mg • Glutamic Acid HCl 100 mg • Ammonium Chloride 35 mg • Pepsin USP/NF 25 mg • Protease (from plant enzymes) 150 Units.

Acidophilase — Wakunaga of America
Each caspule contains: Lactobacillus acidophilus 1 billion live cells • Food Enzyme complex 155 mg: Protease, Amylase, & Lactase in a vegetable starch complex.

Acidophilis Xtra — Sundown Vitamins
Each caplet contains: Acidophilis • Bulgaricus • Thermophilus • Bifidum.

Acidophilus E.C. — Progressive Labs
Each high potency capsule contains 2.8 billion live organisms from specially selected strains of lactobacillus acidophilus and lactobacillus casei subsp. Rhamnosus in a base of maltodextrin. Hypoallergenic, contains no milk, whey, soy, corn, wheat, yeast or preservatives. Product should be refrigerated to maintain maximum potency.

Acne Support — Amazon Support
Each capsule contains: Abuta • Bitter Melon • Chuchuhuasi • Espinheira Santa • Fedegosa • Sarsaparilla • Tayuya.

Actilife Super Antioxidant — Crystal Springs
Two tablets contain: Red Grape extract seeds 100 mg • Polygonum cuspidatum extract root 100 mg • Trans-Resveratrol 20 mg • Total Resveratrols 24 mg • Emodin 10 mg • Zinc 30 mg.

Actisyn — SportPharma
Each packet contains: Calories 150 • Total Fat 1 g • Total Carbohydrate 8 g • Protein 27 g. Vanilla ingredients: Actipro Protein Substrate (Ion Exchanged Whey Protein Isolate, Whey Protein Concentrate, Enzymatically Hydrolyzed Whey Protein, Pepti-Lean Select Micro-Peptides) • Actiplex (Specific Ratios of L-Glutamine, Taurine, L-Leucine, & N-Acetyl-L-Cysteine) • Anticell Vitamins & Minerals (Ascorbic Acid, DL- Alpha Tocopheryl Acetate, Vitamin A Palmitate, Potassium Chloride, Magnesium Aspartate, Magnesium Fumerate, Magnesium Oxide, Pyridoxine HCL, Niacinamide, Calcium Phosphate, Magnesium Orotate, Sodium Chloride, Alpha Lipoic Acid, Calcium Alpha-Ketoglutarate, Zinc Gluconate, L-Selenomethionine) • Maltodextrin • Actigen (Tri-Methyl Glycine, Specific Nucleotides including: Purine and Pyrimidine Isolates, RNA Hydrolysates) • natural & artificial Vanilla & Cream Flavors • CMC Gum • Aspartame • Sunett Brand Sweetener (Acesulfame K).

Active B-50 — The Vitamin Shoppe
Each capsule contains: Vitamin B1 (Thiamin) 50 mg • Vitamin B2 (Riboflavin) 50 mg • Vitamin B6 (Pyridoxine HCl) 50 mg • Vitamin B12 (Cobalamin Concentrate) 50 mcg • Niacinamide 50 mg • Folic Acid 400 mcg • Pantothenic Acid (d-Calcium Pantothenate) 50 mg • Biotin 50 mcg • Choline 50 mg • Inositol 50 mg • PABA (Para Amino Benzoic Acid) 50 mg. In a base of Alfalfa, Watercress, Parsley, Lecithin, and Rice Concentrate. No Yeast, Corn, Wheat, Soy, Salt, Sugar, Starch, Preservatives, Artificial Colors or Flavors added.

Activin 50 Mg Grape Seed Extract — Natrol
One tablet contains: ActiVin (Grape Seed extract) 50 mg. Other ingredients: Dicalcium Phosphate, Microcrystalline Cellulose, Mono & Di-Glycerides, Stearic Acid, Silicon Dioxide, Magnesium Stearate.

© Copyright 2000, Natural Medicines Comprehensive Database (209) 472-2244. For updated data, go to www.NaturalDatabase.com. • 1291

Some Brand Name Natural Products - What they Contain
www.NaturalDatabase.com contains MANY more listings than appear here.

B
R
A
N
D

N
A
M
E
S

Acti-Zyme — Nature's Plus
Two capsules contain: Live Food Enzymes: Aminogen (Aspergillus niger & Aspergillus oryzae proteolytic enzyme complex) 100 mg • Lugamase (Saccharamyces cerevisae & Aspergillus oryzae oligosaccharide enzyme complex) 100 mg • Amylase (30000 units/gram) 50 mg • Lactase (1000 units/gram) 50 mg • Lipase (5000 units/gram) 50 mg • Cellulase (5000 units/gram) 50 mg • Protease (100000 units/gram) 50 mg • Oxidase (5000 units/gram) 50 mg • Bromelain (2000 GDU/gram) 50 mg • Diastase (1000 units/gram) 5 mg • Maltase (1000 units/gram) 5 mg. Lactic Flora & Growth Accelerants: FOS (Fructooligosaccharides), lactic flora growth accelerant 100 mg • Lactospor, micro-encapsulated pure culture of B.Coagulans, provides 300 million viable cells 50 mg. Bioavailability Enhancing Phytonutrient: Bioperine (Piper nigrum fruit) standardized 95% 1-piperoylpiperidine 5 mg. Contains no yeast, wheat, corn, soy, milk, salt, or starch.

Acutrim 16-Hour Steady Control —
Ciba Self-Medication, Inc.
Each tablet contains: Active Ingredient: Phenylpropanolamine HCl 75 mg. Other Ingredients: Cellulose Acetate, Hydroxypropyl Methylcellulose, Stearic Acid.

Acutrim Maximum Strength — Ciba Self-Medication, Inc.
Each tablet contains: Active Ingredient: Phenylpropanolamine HCl 75 mg. Inactive Ingredients: Acacia • Calcium Carbonate • D&C Yellow #10 Aluminum Lake • FD&C Yellow #6 Aluminum Lake • Guar Gum • Hydroxypropyl Methylcellulose • Microcrystalline Cellulose • Silicon Dioxide • Stearic Acid.

Adaptrin — Pacific BioLogic
Iceland Moss • Red Sandalwood • Hardy Orange • Vetiver • Margosa • Spiral Flag • White Sandalwood • Cloves • Columbine • Wild Lettuce • Marigold • Knotgrass • Licorice • Valerian • Camphor bark • Gypsum • Cardamom • Jamaican Pepper • Ribwort (plantain) • Heartleaved Sida • Myrobalan • Blackthorn • Golden Cinquefoil • Gingerlily • Homeopathic Monkshood.

AD-FX — HerbTech
Each capsule contains: HT-1001 biologically standardized extract (American Ginseng containing >15% ginsenosides) 125 mg • Ginkgo biloba standardized extract 29 mg (containing >4% terpenelactones).

Adipokinetix — Syn Trax
Each capsule or tablet contains: Caffeine 90 mg • 1R, 2S Norephedrine HCL 25 mg • Yohimbine HCL 2.75 mg.

Adrenal Chelate — Atrium
Each tablet contains: Raw Adrenal concentrate (not an extract) 80 mg • L-Leucine 10 mg • L-Isoleucine 20 mg • D-Calcium Pantothenate 60 mg • Sodium Ascorbate 120 mg • Potassium Aspartate 30 mg • Hesperidin Complex 150 mg • Bioflavonoid Complex 75 mg • Chlorophyll 10 mg. In a base of Alfalfa, Celery & Parsley.

Adrenal Plus — Futurebiotics
Raw Adrenal concentrate 80 mg* • Vitamin C (Ascorbic Acid) 150 mg • Pantothenic Acid 60 mg • Zinc (Gluconate) 5 mg • Manganese (Amino Acid Chelate) 1 mg • Schizandra (6:1) 20 mg** • Chinese Licorice (10:1) 12 mg** • Niacinamide 80 mg. *The freeze-dried adrenal concentrate in this product comes from imported range fed cattle growing naturally, unexposed to drugs or chemically influenced foods. **Extracts equivalent to Licorice & Schizandra powders 120 mg.

Adrenal-Cortex Complex — Enzymatic Therapy
Each capsule contains: Adrenal-Cortex Complex 250 mg • Multi-Glandular Complex: Raw Liver, Raw Lung, Raw Pancreas, Raw Heart, Raw Kidney, Raw Spleen, & Raw Brain 100 mg. Contains no sugar, salt, yeast, wheat, corn, soy, dairy products, coloring, flavoring or preservatives.

Adrenal-Cortex Fractions — Phytopharmica
Each capsule contains: Adrenal-Cortex Complex 250 mg • Multi-Glandular Complex 100 mg containing: Raw Liver, Raw Lung, Raw Pancreas, Raw Heart, Raw Kidney, Raw Spleen & Raw Brain. Contains no sugar, salt, yeast, wheat, corn, soy, dairy products, coloring, flavoring or preservatives. All organs & glands derived from bovine sources except raw pancreas (porcine).

Adren-Comp — Enzymatic Therapy
Each capsule contains: Chinese Thoroughwax extract (Bupleurum falcatum) 150 mg • Korean Ginseng root extract 3:1 (Panax ginseng) 100 mg • Siberian Ginseng extract (Eleutherococcus senticosus)

standardized to contain greater than 1% eleutheroside E, 100 mg • Mexican Yam extract 10:1 (Dioscorea spinosa) standardized to contain 10% Diosgenin 100 mg • Licorice root extract (Glycyrrhiza glabra) standardized to contain 5% Glycyrrhizic acid 50 mg • Curcuma root extract 10:1 (Curcuma longa) 50 mg.

Adrenerlin — Bodyonics
Two capsules contain: Maca Pure (Lepidum meyenii)(Standardized to contain 0.6% macamides and macanes) 450 mg • Jeevani Botanical Complex (Tricopus zylanicus, Ashwanga (Withania somnifera), Piper Longum, Vishnukranthi (Evolvus alsinoies) 150 mg • Peptide GPX 250 mg • D-Ribose 10 mg • Acetyl-L-Carnitine 10 mg • Bitter Orange (Standardized 4% synephrine) 83.3 mg • Yerba Mate and Guarana Extract (Standardized 200 mg Methylxanthines/ Caffeine 910 mg • Mucuna pruriens (Standardized 15% L-Dopa) 33.3 mg • Calcium Pyruvate 10 mg. Other Ingredients: Magnesium Stearate, Gelatin.

Adreno Chelate — Progressive Labs
Each capsule contains: Calcium (Proteinate) 27 mg • Chloride (Proteinate) 50 mg • Sodium (Proteinate) 20 mg • Potassium (Proteinate) 20 mg • Raw Bovine Adrenal concentrate 40 mg • L-Isoleucine 10 mg • L-Leucine 10 mg.

Adreno Trophic — Progressive Labs
Each capsule contains: Pantothenic Acid (Calcium Pantothenate) 50 mg • Raw Bovine Adrenal concentrate 80 mg.

Adreno-Cortex — Atrium
Each tablet contains: Adrenal Cortex • Pituitary Anterior 20 mg • Pineal, bovine source 10 mg • Vitamin C (Calcium Ascorbate) 25 mg.

Adreno-Medulla Plus — Atrium
Each tablet contains: Adrenal Medulla 100 mg • Hypothalamus 15 mg • Pituitary Posterior Bovine Source 10 mg • Vitamin C (Calcium Ascorbate) 25 mg.

Adult Echinacea+C+Zinc Cherry Flavor —
LiFizz Effervescent Vitamins
Each tablet contains: Vitamin C 1500 mg • Zinc 15 mg • Echinacea extract (Echinacea purpurea) 100 mg. Other Ingredients: Citric Acid, Sodium Bicarbonate, Sorbitol, Mannitol, Polyethylene Glycol 6000, Cherry Flavor, Povidone, Aspartame, Acesulfame Potassium, Magnesium Stearate, Silicon Dioxide, Simethicone.

Adult Echinacea+C+Zinc Lemon/Lime Flavor — LiFizz Effervescent Vitamins
Each tablet contains: Vitamin C 1500 mg • Zinc 15 mg • Echinacea extract (Echinacea purpurea) 100 mg. Other ingredients: Citric Acid, Sodium Bicarbonate, Sorbitol, Mannitol, Polyethylene Glycol 6000, Lemon Flavor, Povidone, Aspartame, Acesulfame Potassium, Lemon/Lime Flavor, Magnesium Stearate, Silicon Dioxide, Simethicone.

Adult Multi-Vitamin Orange Flavor —
LiFizz Effervescent Vitamins
Each tablet contains: Vitamin A (Palmitate and Beta Carotene) 5000 IU • Vitamin C 60 mg • Vitamin D 400 IU • Vitamin E 15 IU • Thiamin 1.5 mg • Riboflavin 1.7 mg • Niacinamide 20 mg • Vitamin B6 2 mg • Folic Acid 400 mcg • Vitamin B12 6 mcg • Biotin 300 mcg • Pantothenic Acid 10 mg • Calcium 200 mg • Iron 6 mg • Magnesium 80 mg • Zinc 5 mg.

Adult-C-Vitamin Pink Grapefruit Flavor —
LiFizz Effervescent Vitamins
Each tablet contains: Vitamin C (Ascorbic Acid) 500 mg. Other Ingredients: Citric Acid, Sorbitol, Potassium Bicarbonate, Sodium Bicarbonate, mannitol, Grapefruit Flavor, Polyethylene Glycol 6000, Orange Flavor, Aspartame, Acesulfame Potassium, Wild Berry Powder, Silicon Dioxide, Lemon/Lime Flavor, Magnesium Stearate.

Adult-C-Vitamin Raspberry Flavor —
LiFizz Effervescent Vitamins
Each tablet contains: Vitamin C (Ascorbic Acid) 500 mg. Other Ingredients: Citric Acid, Sodium bicarbonate, Potassium bicarbonate, Sorbitol, Raspberry Flavor, Aspartame, Acesulfame Potassium, Magnesium Stearate.

AdvaCal — LaneLabs
Three capsules contain: Elemental Calcium (as calcium hydroxide, calcium oxide, combined with algae amino acid extract) 450 mg. Other Ingredients: Citric Acid, Gelatin, Water, Glycerine.

Advanced CoQ10 — Changes - TwinLab
One capsule contains: Coenzyme Q10 50 mg.

Some Brand Name Natural Products - What they Contain
www.NaturalDatabase.com contains MANY more listings than appear here.

Advanced Formula — Biotech
Each tablet contains: Folate 400 mg • Pantothenic Acid 100 mg • Biotin 700 mcg • Iodine 75 mcg • Zinc 75 mg • Shen Min 225 mg • Shen Min (He Shou Wu root powder) 435 mg • Isoflavones 10 mg • Saw Palmetto berries standardized extract 160 mg • Silica 20 mg • Black Pepper extract 2.5 mg.

Advanced Joint Support — Futurebiotics
Four capsules supply: Glucosamine Sulfate 1000 mg • Vitamin C (Buffered Ascorbate) 750 mg • Vitamin E (natural) 400 IU • Calcium (Ascorbate) 185 mg • Selenium (Amino Acid Chelate) 100 mcg • Zinc (Amino Acid Chelate) 15 mg • Bovine Cartilage 200 mg • Pancreatin 4X (Quadruple Strength) 100 mg containing: (Lipase 1600 USP units, Amylase 10000 USP units, Protease 10000 USP units) • Papain 60 mg • Bromelain 50 mg • Turmeric (standardized Curcumin) 250 mg • Cayenne powder 15 mg • Ginger powder 100 mg • Boswellin (standardized for 65% Boswellic Acid) 100 mg • Devil's Claw 50 mg • Rutin 50 mg.

Advanced Prostate Formula — Rx Vitamins
Three capsules contain: Saw Palmetto fruit 320 mg • Stinging Nettle root 100 mg • African Pygeum bark 50 mg • Zinc 50 mg • Glycine 50 mg • Alanine 50 mg • Glutamic Acid 50 mg • Vitamin B6 50 mg • Vitamin E 100 IU in Borage seed oil.

Aflexa — McNeil Consumer Healthcare
One tablet contains: Glucosamine 340 mg (Glucosamine Sulfate, Glucosamine Hydrochloride). Other ingredients: Cellulose, Hydroxypropyl, Methylcellulose, Polyethylene Glycol, Silicon Dioxide, Propylene Glycol, Crospovidone, Hydroxypropyl Cellulose, Titanium Dioxide, Magnesium Stearate, Polysorbate 80, Povidone.

Age Right Formula — Nature's Way
Four capsules contain: Acetylcarnitine 50 mcg • Acetylcysteine 50 mcg • Betaine Anhydrous 50 mg • Biotin (Biotin Triurate) 500 mcg • Boron (Amino Acid Chelate) 500 mcg • Calcium 43 mg • Calcium Pantethonate 175 mg • Caromix (Mixed Carotenoids) 2000 IU • Chromium Picolinate 100 mcg • Citrus Bioflavonoids 250 mg • Coenzyme Q10 (Ubiquinone) 15 mg • Copper (Amino Acid Chelate) 500 mcg • Fizyme Enzyme Formula 65 mg • Folic Acid (Folate) 250 mcg • Grape seed dried extract 15 mg • Green Tea (Polyphenol Catechin extract) 75 mg • Inositol 15 mg • Kelp (whole Thallus) 25 mcg • Manganese (Amino Acid Chelate) 2.5 mg • Molybdenum Triturate 25 mcg • Niacinamide 47.5 mg • Potassium (Aspartate, Chloride) 25 mg • Riboflavin (Vitamin B2) 25 mg • Selenium (l-Selenomethione) 25 mcg • Thiamine (Vitamin B1) 25 mg • Vitamin A (Retinol Palmitate) 2530 IU • Vitamin B12 (Cyanocobalamin) 250 mcg • Vitamin B6 (Pyridoxine HCL) 25 mg • Vitamin C (Ascorbic Acid) 250 mg • Vitamin D3 (Cholecalciferol) 200 IU • Vitamin E (d-Alpha Tocopheryl) 200 IU • Vitamin K (Phytonadione) 30 mcg • Zinc (Amino Acid Chelate) 5 mg. Other ingredients: Gelatin, Magnesium Stearate, Millet.

AgeErasers SAMe — Bodyonics
Each tablet contains: Vitamin B12 50 mcg • Folic Acid 100 mcg • SAMe 200 mg. Other Ingredients: Calcium Phosphate, Stearic Acid, Croscarmellose, Magnesium Strearate.

Air Power — Enzymatic Therapy
Each tablet contains: Active ingredient: Glycerol Guaiacolate 200 mg. Other ingredients: Fenugreek Powder 4:1 (Trigonella foenum-graecum) 350 mg • Marshmallow extract 4:1 mucilage content 30-40% (Althaea officinalis) 125 mg • PABA (Para-Aminobenzoic Acid) 50 mg • Mullein leaf (Verbascum nigrum) 50 mg. Contains no sugar, salt, yeast, wheat, corn, soy, dairy products, coloring, flavoring or preservatives.

AKG Fuel — TwinLab
Three capsules contain: Alpha-Ketoglutaric Acid (from Magnesium Alpha-Ketoglutarate) 1250 mg • Magnesium (from Magnesium Alpha-Ketoglutarate) 210 mg • L-Glutamine 1000 mg.

AKN Skin Care — Nature's Way
Two capsules contain: Burdock root • Capsicum root • Dandelion root • Echinacea purpurea root • Kelp (whole Thallus) • Licorice root • Plantain leaf • Sarsaparilla root • Yellow Dock root. Other ingredients: Gelatin.

ALC Fuel — TwinLab
Each capsule contains: The highest quality pharmaceutical-grade Acetyl-L-Carnitine (ALC) 1000 mg.

Alert — Phytopharmica
Each capsule contains: Cola Nut extract (Cola nitida) 250 mg (contains 35 mg caffeine) • Green Tea extract (Camellia sinensis) 250 mg (contains 15 mg caffeine) • Oat Straw extract 10:1 (Avena sativa) 50 mg • Schisandra extract 50 mg (standardized to contain 9% schizandrin) • Siberian Ginseng extract (Eleutherococcus senticosus) 50 mg (standardized to contain greater than 1% eleutheroside E) • Ginger root extract 6.5:1 (Zingiber officinale) 25 mg • Korean Ginseng root extract (Panax ginseng) 10 mg (standardized to contain 7% saponis calculated as ginsenoside Rg1) • Chromium (Polynicotinate) 100 mcg.

Alertis Compound — The Herbalist
False Unicorn root • Squaw Vine herb • Cramp bark • Blue Cohosh root • Ginger root.

Alfalfa — Quest
Each tablet contains: Organic Alfalfa 650 mg. Other Ingredients: Terra Alba, Silica, Magnesium Stearate (vegetable source).

Alfalfa-Devil's Claw Formula — Quest
Each caplet contains: Alfalfa leaf powder (Medicago sativa) 70 mg • Alfalfa seed powder 70 mg • Burdock root powder (Arctium lappa) 70 mg • Celery seed powder (Apium graveolens) 70 mg • Devil's Claw root powder (Herpagophytum procumbens) 70 mg • Cayenne powder (Capsicum) 35 mg • Kelp powder (Fucus versiculosis) 35 mg • Queen of the Meadow root powder (Filipendula ulmaria) 5 mg • Sarsaparilla root powder (Smilax officinalis) 5 mg. Other Ingredients: Calcium Phosphate, Microcrystalline Cellulose, Vegetable Stearin, Croscarmellose Sodium, Magnesium Stearate (vegetable source).

Alka-Mine Coral Calcium — Ericssons
Coral Calcium • Magnesium • Ascorbic Acid • Silver.

Aller-B — Progressive Labs
Each capsule contains: Thiamin (Vitamin B1) 50 mg • Riboflavin (Vitamin B2) 50 mg • Niacinamide 50 mg • Vitamin B6 50 mg • Folate (Folic Acid) 400 mcg • Vitamin B12 60 mcg • Biotin 50 mcg • Pantothenic Acid 100 mg • Choline Bitartrate 50 mg • Inositol 25 mg • PABA (Para Aminobenzioc Acid) 50 mg.

Aller-C Support Formula — The Vitamin Factory
Each tablet contains: Vitamin C (Calcium Ascorbate) 500 mg • Calcium (Ascorbate, Citrate, Pantothenate) 100 mg • Vitamin B5 (Calcium Pantothenate) 50 mg • Pycnogenol (Maritime Pine bark extract) 15 mg.

Aller-Cal — Atrium
Each tablet contains: Adrenal 80 mg • Pituitary 10 mg • Liver Substance 6 mg • Parathyroid 5 mg • Calcium 20.4 mg • Pantothenic Acid 26 mg • Folic Acid 130 mcg • Ammonium Chloride 30 mg • Choline Bitartrate 25 mg • Methionine 14 mg • Inositol 12 mg • Glutamic Acid HCL 12 mg • Betaine HCL 3.6 mg • Hydrolized Amino Acids 150 mg • Dulse 50 mg • Persic oil 36 mg • Linseed oil 12 mg.

AllerClear — Enzymatic Therapy
Active ingredient: Pseudophedrine HCl (from Ephedra sinensis) 60 mg. Other ingredients: Vitamin E (DL-Alpha Tocopherol) 75 IU • Vitamin C (Ascorbic Acid) 150 mg • Pantothenic Acid (D-Calcium Pantothenate) 150 mg • Choline (Bitartrate) 150 mg • Macrocystis pyrifera 150 mg • Lung extract 90 mg • Adrenal extract 80 mg • Methionine 75 mg • Pancreatic Enzymes (3X) treated for enteric activity 65 mg • Ammonium Chloride 50 mg • Calcium Chloride 50 mg • Glutamic Acid HCL 50 mg • Betaine HCL 50 mg • Pepsin (1:10000) 49 mg • Magnesium Glycerophosphate 30 mg • Spleen extract 25 mg • Pancreas extract 15 mg • Thymus extract 15 mg • Niacinamide 10 mg • Liver Fractions 10 mg • Vitamin B6 (Pyridoxine HCl) 5 mg. Contains no sugar, salt, yeast, wheat, corn, soy, dairy products, coloring, flavoring or preservatives.

Allergia — HerbaSway
Bitter Orange • Ginger • Panax Ginseng • Blackberry • Kudzu • HerbaSwee (Cucurbitaceae fruit).

Allergy Support — Amazon Support
Each capsule contains: Nettles • Yerba Mate • Jatoba • Gervao • Pau d'arco • Picao Preto • Bitter Melon • Carqueja • Suma.

Allergy Support — Olympia Nutrition
Quercetin • Nettle • Licorice • Vitamin C.

Aller-Max — Biochem
Two capsules contain: Quercetin 250 mg • N-Acetyl Cysteine 200 mg

© Copyright 2000, Natural Medicines Comprehensive Database (209) 472-2244. For updated data, go to www.NaturalDatabase.com. • 1293

• Bromelain 100 mg • L-Histidine 200 mg • Vitamin A (Palmitate) 2500 IU • Vitamin C (Calcium Ascorbate) 250 mg • Pantothenic Acid 200 mg • Zinc 10 mg • Grape seed extract 5 mg • Stinging Nettle 100 mg • Cayenne 20 mg.

AllerPlus — Phytopharmica
Two capsules contain: Active ingredient: Pseudoephedrine HCl (from Ephedra sinensis) 60 mg. Other Ingredients: Vitamin E (DL-Alpha Tocopherol) 75 IU • Vitamin C (Ascorbic Acid) 150 mg • Pantothenic Acid (D-Calcium Pantothenate) 150 mg • Choline (Bitartrate) 150 mg • Macrocystis Pyrifera 150 mg • Lung extract 90 mg • Adrenal extract 80 mg • Methionine 75 mg • Pancreatic Enzymes (3X) 65 mg (Treated for enteric activity) • Ammonium Chloride 50 mg • Calcium Chloride 50 mg • Glutamic Acid HCL 50 mg • Betaine HCL 50 mg • Pepsin (1:10000) 49 mg • Magnesium Glycerophosphate 30 mg • Spleen extract 25 mg • Pancreas extract 15 mg • Thymus extract 15 mg • Niacinamide 10 mg • Liver Fractions 10 mg • Vitamin B6 (Pyridoxine HCl) 5 mg.

Allicin Rich Garlic Powder — Jamieson
Each caplet contains: Garlic bulb powder (containing 750 mcg Allicon and 5000 mcg Alliin) 300 mg.

Aloe & E with Allantoin — Derma E
Aloe Vera gel • Vitamin E.

Aloe Vera Deep Skin Moisturizer Vitamin D Cell Refining Cream — Orjene
85% pure Aloe Vera • Bee Pollen • Vitamin F Complex • PABA-free sunblock.

Alpha betic — Abkit
Each caplet contains: Vitamin A 5000 IU • Vitamin C (as ascorbic acid) 120 mg • Vitamin D (as cholecalciferol) 400 IU • Vitamin E (d-alpha tocopheryl succinate) 60 IU • Thiamin (Vitamin B1) 1.5 mg • Riboflavin (Vitamin B2) 1.7 mg • Niacin (Vitamin B3) 20 mg • Vitamin B6 (as pyroxidine) 2 mg • Folic Acid 400 mcg • Vitamin B12 (as cyanocobalamin) 6 mcg • Biotin 150 mcg • Pantothenic Acid (as d-calcium pantothenate) 10 mg • Magnesium 200 mg • Zinc (as Zinc Citrate) 15 mg • Selenium (Selenite) 50 mcg • Copper (as Copper Gluconate) 2 mg • Manganese (Sulfate) 5 mg • Chromium (as Chromium Picolinate) 200 mcg • Potassium (as Potassium Chloride) 100 mg • Vanadium (as Vanadium Sulfate) 100 mcg • Alpha Lipoic Acid (Imported from Germany) 60 mg. Other Ingredients: Calcium Sulfate, Stearic Acid, Cellulose, Magnesium Stearate. Coating: Beta Carotene, Riboflavin (B2).

Alternecal-Rx — Alternecare Health Products
Each tablet contains: Tri-Calcium Phosphate 1000 mg • Magnesium 500 mg • Zinc 10 mg • Copper 3 mg • Oat Straw 25 mg • Boron 3 mg • Vitamin C 30 mg • Vitamin D 400 IU • Ashwagandha 25 mg • Silica 25 mg.

Alticort — Phytopharmica
Contains: 1.8% Salicylic Acid. Other Ingredients: Purified Water • Organic Fatty Acid Complex (C11-C18), Glyceryl Stearate, Chamomile extract (0.5% Flavonoid Content) • 18-Beta-Glycyrrhetinic Acid (from Licorice root extract) • Allantoin 2.0% from Comfrey root extract • Dimethicone, Vitamin E (Antioxidant). Hypoallergenic Fragrance Cruelty-free-no animal testing. Contains no animal products.

AM Plus (Brain 111 Formula) — Alpha Zebra
AM Super capsule: Two capsules contain: Beta Carotene 25 IU • Thiamine HCl (Vitamin B1) 50 mg • Riboflavin (Vitamin B2) 50 mg • Niacin (Vitamin B3) 20 mg • Pantothenic Acid (Vitamin B5) 75 mg • Pyridoxine HCl (Vitamin B6) 50 mg • Cyanocobalamin concentrate (Vitamin B12/Sorbitol) 500 mcg • Vitamin C 55 mg • Bioflavonoids with Rose Hips 45 mg • Vitamin E Dry (dl-Alpha Tocopherol) 25 IU • Biotin 300 mcg • Choline Bitartrate (Phosphatidyl) 75 mg • Soya Lecithin(Phospholipids) 50 mg • Folic Acid 500 mcg • Inositol 50 mg • Inosine 40 mg • Para-Aminobenzioc Acid (PABA) 30 mg • Calcium Phosphate (Chelated) 40 mg • Chromium Picolinate (Chelated) 200 mcg • Copper (Oxide) (Chelated) 1 mg • Magnesium (Oxide) (Chelated) 25 mg • Manganese (Oxide) (Chelated) 45 mg • Phosphorus (Oxide) (Chelated)12 mg • Potassium (Oxide) (Chelated) 50 mg • Zinc (Oxide) (Chelated) 50 mg • Boron (Chelated) 1 mg • Molybdenum (Oxide) (Chelated) 100 mcg • Selenium (Oxide) (Chelated) 200 mcg • Silicon 400 mcg • L-Aspartic Acid 25 mg • L-Cysteine 15 mg • L-Glutamine 115 mg • L-Glycine 15 mg • L-Leucine 50 mg • L-Lysine 15 mg • L-Methionine 70 mg • L-Tyrosine 70 mg • L-Phenylalanine 100 mg • L-Serine 25 mg • A-Ketoglutaric

Acid 15 mg • Adrenal Raw freeze dried concentrate 25 mg • Gamma Aminobutyric Acid - GABA 25 mg • Glutamic Acid 5 mg • RNA./DNA (Complex) 25 mg • Beta Hydrochloride 5 mg • Bromelain 3 mg • Pancreatin 10 mg • Papain 10 mg • Pepsin 10 mg • Protease Enzyme 3 mg • Bee Pollen 40 mg • Royal Jelly 35 mg • Ginkgo Biloba (50:1) (contains 24% Ginkgolides Heterosides) 50 mg • Ginkgo Biloba (8:1) contains 24% Ginkgolides 160 mg • Heterosides Gotu Kola 128 mg • Panax Korean Ginseng 88 mg • Ginger root 80 mg • Mexican Yam 80 mg • Echinacea augustifolia 76 mg • Spirulina algae 75 mg • Fo-Ti 60 mg • Oat Straw 60 mg • Siberian Ginseng 60 mg • Beet root powder 60 mg • Alfalfa 50 mg • Peppermint leaves 60 mg • Eyebright (Euphrasia herb) 60 mg • Licorice root (De-Glycyrrhiznated) 56 mg • Passionflower 48 mg • Capsicum 40 mg • Dandelion root 40 mg • Hawthorn berry 40 mg • Mexican Damiana leaves 32 mg • Kelp 28 mg • Aloe Vera 28 mg • Fennel 28 mg • Sarsaparilla 28 mg • Cabbage seed 24 mg • Sea Plant concentrate 20 mg • Saw Palmetto berry 20 mg • Burdock root 20 mg • Chamomile 20 mg • Slippery Elm 20 mg • Kava Kava 16 mg • Horseradish 16 mg • Suma 12 mg. Energizer Formula: Each capsule contains: Niacinamide (Vitamin B3) 40 mg • Pyridoxine HCl (Vitamin B6) 25 mg • Cyanocobalamin concentrate (Vitamin B12 w/Sorbitol) 500 mcg • Bioflavonoids (including Rose Hips) 30 mg • L-Glutamine 50 mg • L-Phenylalanine 50 mg • L-Methionine 30 mg • L-Tyrosine 25 mg • L-Aspartic Acid 10 mg • L-Taurine 10 mg • L-Asparigne 10 mg • L-Alanine 10 mg • L-Glycine 10 mg • Pancreatin 20 mg • Gamma Aminobutyric Acid (GABA) 10 mg • Soy Lecithin (Phospholipids) 10 mg • Royal Jelly 25 mg • Beet root powder 80 mg • Cantaloupe 80 mg • Yucca 60 mg • American Cenuary 60 mg • Mexican Yam 60 mg • Bissy Nut 60 mg • Kava Kava root 56 mg • Fo-Ti 48 mg • Oat Straw 48 mg • Capsicum/Cayenne 44 mg • Bee Pollen 40 mg • Dandelion root 40 mg • Brigham Tea 40 mg • Artichoke 40 mg • Wild Lettuce 40 mg • Rosemary leaves 40 mg • Yerba Mate 32 mg • Peppermint leaves 32 mg • Sarsaparilla 25 mg • Ginger root 24 mg • Suma 24 mg • Hawthorn berry 16 mg • American Ginseng 16 mg • Cabbage seed 16 mg • Parsley 16 mg • Fenugreek 16 mg • Gotu Kola 16 mg • Muira Puama 12 mg • Spirulina algae 12 mg.

American Ginzing — Traditional Medicinals
Contains: American Ginseng root • Licorice root • Ginger rhizome • Cinnamon bark • Sarsaparilla root • Dong Quai root.

Amino 2222 Capsules — Optimum Nutrition
Two capsules contain: Pharmaceutical Grade 3Amino Acids2 (derived from Predigested Lactalbumen, Soy Protein Isolate & Whey Protein concentrate) 2222 mg • L-Ornithine • L-Carnitine.

Amino Acid 1000 mg — Nature's Life
Ten capsules contain: Casein Hydrolysate • Glycine • L-Proline • L-Arginine • L-Alanine • Pyridoxine HCl • L-Ornithine • L-Serine • L-Cystine • whole Egg powder. Ten capsules provide, based on a typical analysis: L-Alanine 663 mg • L-Arginine 665 mg • L-Aspartic Acid 447 mg • L-Cystine 4 mg • L-Glutamic Acid 1222 mg • Glycine 1806 mg • L-Histidine 157 mg • L-Isoleucine (Esssential Amino Acid) 313 mg • L-Leucine (Essential Amino Acid) 512 mg • L-Ornithine 250 mg • L-Lysine (Essential Amino Acid) 471 mg • L-Methionine (Essential Amino Acid) 166 mg • L-Phenylalanine (Essential Amino Acid) 313 mg • L-Proline 1640 mg • L-Serine 505 mg • L-Threonine (Essential Amino Acid) 262 mg • L-Tryptophan (Essential Amino Acid) 70 mg • L-Tyrosine 200 mg • L-Valine (Essential Amino Acid) 408 mg.

Amino Blend — Progressive Labs
Three 750 mg capsules contain: L-Alanine 147 mg • L-Arginine 138 mg • L-Cysteine 23 mg • L-Cystine 26 mg • L-Glutamine 28 mg • Glycine 95 mg • L-Histidine 73 mg • L-Isoleucine 71 mg • L-Leucine 203 mg • L-Lysine 203 mg • L-Methionine 55 mg • L-Ornithine 23 mg • L-Proline 77 mg • L-Serine 95 mg • L-Threonine 91 mg • L-Tyrosine 77 mg • L-Valine 120 mg • Taurine 48 mg • L-Aspartic Acid 206 mg • L-Phenylalanine 102 mg • L-Glutamic Acid 349 mg.

Amino Fuel (Anabolic Amino Acid Drink) — TwinLab
Peptide Bonded & Free Amino Acids (derived from the natural Pancreatic digests of Whey Protein & Egg White Protein) 20 g • Protein-sparing Carbohydrates (predominantly from Glucose Polymers) 50 g. Other Ingredients: L-Carnitine, Branched Chain Amino Acids (L-Leucine, L-Isoleucine & L-Valine), Essential Vitamins & Minerals, Zinc Picolinate, Boron, GTF Chromium, Chromium Picolinate & Chromium Polynicotinate.

Amino Fuel (Mega Anabolic Chewable Wafers) 7500 mg — TwinLab
Two wafers contain: Peptide Bonded & Free Amino Acids 7500 mg (7.5 g). Each wafer contains: L-Carnitine • Branched Chain Amino

B
R
A
N
D

N
A
M
E
S

Acids (L-Leucine, L-Isoleucine & L-Valine) • Pharmaceutical Grade Peptide Bonded & Free Amino Acids derived from the natural Pancreatic digests of Whey Protein (Lactalbumin) & Egg White (Albumin).

Amino Fuel (Peptide Bonded Amino Acid Liquid Concentrate) — TwinLab

L-Carnitine • Branched Chain Amino Acids (L-Leucine, L-Isoleucine & L-Valine) • Pharmaceutical Grade, Peptide Bonded & Free Amino Acids • Stress B Complex Vitamins • Lipotropic Factors: (Choline & Inositol) • Complex Carbohydrates (Glucose Polymers) • Pure Crystalline Fructose. Each serving contains: Peptide Bonded & Free Amino Acids [derived from the natural Pancreatic digests of Whey Protein (Lactalbumin), Egg Protein (Albumin), Liver Protein & other Animal Proteins] 15 g.

Amino Fuel (Peptide Bonded Amino Acid Tablets) — TwinLab

L-Carnitine • Branched Chain Amino Acids (L-Leucine, L-Isoleucine & L-Valine) • Peptide Bonded Amino Acids [derived from Pharmaceutical Grade Pancreatic (Enzymatic) digests of Whey Protein (Lactalbumin) & Egg White Protein (Albumin)].

Amino Fuel 1000 Tabs — TwinLab

L-Carnitine • Branched Chain Amino Acids (L-Leucine, L-Isoleucine & L-Valine) • Peptide Bonded Amino Acids [derived from Pharmaceutical Grade Pancreatic (Enzymatic) digests of Whey Protein (Albumin)].

Amino Fuel 1500 Tablets — TwinLab

Each tablet contains: Peptide Bonded Amino Acids & Branched Chain Amino Acids [derived from Pharmaceutical Grade Pancreatic digests of Whey Protein (Lactalbumin) & Egg White Protein (Albumin)] 1500 mg. No lower quality amino acid sources are present, such as soy or casein.

Amino Fuel 2000 (Extra Strength Amino Acid Tablets) — TwinLab

Each tablet contains: Protein (as Peptide Bonded Amino Acids) derived from Pharmaceutical Grade Pancreatic digests of Whey Protein (Lactalbumin) & Egg White Protein 2000 mg.

Amino Fuel Stack — TwinLab

Six capsules contain: B-Hydroxy B-Methylbutyrate Monohydrate (HMB) 3000 mg • L-Glutamine 2000 mg • Acetyl-L-Carnitine 1000 mg • Taurine 200 mg • N-Acetyl-Cysteine (NAC) 200 mg.

Amino-BC — ANS

Branched Chain Amino Acids.

AminoBuild: Chocolate Flavor — Pharmanex

Three scoops (45 g) contain: Vitamin A (as Vitamin A Palmitate) 1000 IU • Vitamin C (as Ascorbic Acid) 60 mg • Vitamin D3 (as Cholecalciferol) 40 IU • Vitamin E (as d-Alpha Tocopheryl Acetate) 30 IU • Thiamin (as Thiamon Mononitrate) 0.3 mg • Riboflavin (as Riboflavin) 0.34 mg • Niacin (as Niacinamide) 4 mg • Vitamin B6 (as Pyridoxine Hydrochloride) 0.4 mg • Folate (as Folic Acid) 80 mcg • Vitamin B12 (as Cyanocobalamin) 1.2 mcg • Biotin (as Biotin) 60 mcg • Pantothenic Acid (as d-Clcium Pantothenate) 2 mg • Calcium (as Dicalcium Phosphate) 540 mg • Phosphorus (as Dicalcium Phosphate) 400 mg • Iodine (as Calcium Iodate) 15 mcg • Magnesium (as Magnesium Citrate) 80 mg • Zinc (as Zinc Gluconate) 3 mg • Selenium (as Sodium Selenate) 14 mcg • Copper (as Copper Gluconate) 0.2 mg • Manganese (as Manganese Gluconate) 0.4 mg • Chromium (as Chromium Polynicotinate 24 mcg • Molybdenum (as Sodium Molybdate) 15 mcg • Sodium (as Sodium Chloride, Soy Protein Isolate) 250 mg • Potassium (from Soy Protein Isolate) 360 mg • Stevia (Stevia Rebaudiana) (Leaves) 50 mg. Other Ingredients: Protein Blend (Supro& Soy Protein Isolate, Cross Flow Microfiltration Whey Protein Isolate, Whey Protein Hydrolysate), Crystalline Fructose, Natural Flavors, Alkalized Cocoa Powder, Magnesium Citrate, Sodium Chloride, Diclcium Phosphate, Ascorbic Acid, dl-Alpha Tocopheryl Acetate, Stevia, Medium Chain Triglycerides, Zinc Gluconate, Chromium Polynicotinate, Biotin, Vitamin A Palmitate, Niacinamide, Manganese Gluconate, Copper Gluconate, d-Calcium Pantothenate, Pyrioxide Hydrochloride, Cholecalciferol, Riboflavin, Thiamin Monoitrate, Cyanocobalamin, Folic Acid, Calcium Iodate, Sodium Molybdate, Sodium Selenate.

AminoBuild: Vanilla Flavor — Pharmanex

Three scoops (45 g) Contain: Vitamin A (as Vitamin A Palmitate) 1000 IU • Vitamin C (as Ascorbic Acid) 60 mg • Vitamin D3 (as Cholecalciferol) 40 IU • Vitamin E (as d-Alpha Tocopheryl Acetate) 30 IU • Thiamin (as Thiamon Mononitrate) 0.3 mg • Riboflavin (as Riboflavin) 0.34 mg • Niacin (as Niacinamide) 4 mg • Vitamin B6 (as Pyridoxine Hydrochloride) 0.4 mg • Folate (as Folic Acid) 80 mcg • Vitamin B12 (as Cyanocobalamin) 1.2 mcg • Biotin (as Biotin) 60 mcg • Pantothenic Acid (as d-Clcium Pantothenate) 2 mg • Calcium (as Dicalcium Phosphate) 540 mg • Phosphorus (as Dicalcium Phosphate) 400 mg • Iodine (as Calcium Iodate) 15 mcg • Magnesium (as Magnesium Citrate) 80 mg • Zinc (as Zinc Gluconate) 3 mg • Selenium (as Sodium Selenate) 14 mcg • Copper (as Copper Gluconate) 0.2 mg • Manganese (as Manganese Gluconate) 0.4 mg • Chromium (as Chromium Polynicotinate 24 mcg • Molybdenum (as Sodium Molybdate) 15 mcg • Sodium (as Sodium Chloride, Soy Protein Isolate) 250 mg • Potassium (from Soy Protein Isolate) 360 mg • Stevia (Stevia Rebaudiana) (Leaves) 50 mg. Other Ingredients: Protein Blend (Supro& Soy Protein Isolate, Cross Flow Microfiltration Whey Protein Isolate, Whey Protein Hydrolysate), Crystalline Fructose, Natural Vanilla Flavors, Magnesium Citrate, Sodium Chloride, Diclcium Phosphate, Ascorbic Acid, Stevia, Medium Chain Triglycerides, dl-Alpha Tocopheryl Acetate, Zinc Gluconate, Chromium Polynicotinate, Biotin, Vitamin A Palmitate, Niacinamide, Manganese Gluconate, Copper Gluconate, d-Calcium Pantothenate, Pyrioxide Hydrochloride, Cholecalciferol, Riboflavin, Thiamin Monoitrate, Cyanocobalamin, Folic Acid, Calcium Iodate, Sodium Molybdate, Sodium Selenate.

Amino-Cartilage — Nutri-Quest

Each tablet contains: Natural Hydrolyzed Protein 1000 mg (minimum 16% Nitrogen content, 92-97% Protein content). Six tablets contain: Natural Laevorotatory Amino Acids (L): Isoleucine 66 mg • Leucine 174 mg • Lysine 216 mg • Methionine 30 mg • Phenylalanine 126 mg • Threonine 120 mg • Valine 168 mg • Arginine 468 mg • Histidine 36 mg • Alanine 546 mg • Tyrosine 24 mg • Serine 198 mg • Aspartic Acid 336 mg • Glutamic Acid 582 mg • Glycine 1362 mg • Hydroxlysine 60 mg • Hydroxyproline 654 mg • Proline 834 mg.

Aminologic — PhysioLogics

Three capsules contain: L-Glutamine 185 mg • L-Aspartic Acid 107 mg • L-Tyrosine 103 mg • L-Leucine 97 mg • L-Valine 97 mg • Taurine 90 mg • L-Phenylalanine 88 mg • L-Proline 82 mg • L-Lysine 77 mg • L-Isoleucine 71 mg • L-Serine 71 mg • L-Alanine 60 mg • L-Threonine 59 mg • L-Methionine 55 mg • L-Arginine 54 mg • Papain NF 50 mg • Bromelain 50 mg • Glycine 48 mg • L-Histidine 41 mg • Pancreatin 4X 25 mg • L-Cystine 23 mg.

AminoZyme — Nature's Plus

Each capsule contains: AMINOGEN (Aspergillus niger & Aspergillus oryzae proteolytic complex) 250 mg • Vitamin B6 (Pyridoxine HCL) 10 mg • CoQ10 (Ubiquinone) 2.5 mg • Chromium (Polynicotinate) 25 mcg • Vanadium (Sulfate) 10 mcg. Contains no yeast, wheat, corn, soy, milk, salt, sugar or starch.

Amore Plus-Rx — H Enterprise

Vitamin E • Calcium • Arginine • Saw Palmetto • Damiana • Celery • Cinnamon (chinese) • Pygeum Africanum bark • Gotu Kola • Rice flour • Magnesium Stearate • Silica.

Anabolic Complex — The Kutting Edge

Two capsules contains: 10-Norandrosenedione 100 mg • 5-Andro-3B-17B Diol 100 mg • Androstenedoine 100 mg • Phosphatidylserine 100 mg • Tribulus 150 mg • Chrysin 50 mg.

Anabolic Fuel — TwinLab

Four capsules contain: L-Leucine 2000 mg • L-Valine 500 mg • L-Isoleucine 500 mg.

Anabolic Max — Biochem

Four tablets contain: L-Glutamine 1000 mg • L-Arginine (Pyroglutamate) 900 mg • Creatine Monohydrate 500 mg • L-Citrulline 300 mg • Taurine 300 mg • Betaine HCL 300 mg • Cinnamon extract 250 mg • Green Tea extract 100mg • DHA (Docosahexaenoic Acid) 100 mg • Ginseng (Panax ginseng) 50 mg • PAK (Pyridoxine, Alpha-Ketoglutarate) 25 mg • Niacin 25 mg • Pantothenic Acid/Pantethine 90/10 25 mg.

Andro Heat — Substrate Solutions

Four capsules contain: Caffeine (naturally occuring in 2000 mg of Kola Nut herb) 200 mg • Ephedrine (naturally occuring in 250 mg of Ma Huang herb) 20 mg • 4-Androstenediol 100 mg.

Andro Stack — Substrate Solutions

Each capsule contains: 4-Androstenediol 100 mg • 4-Androstenedione 100 mg.

© Copyright 2000, Natural Medicines Comprehensive Database (209) 472-2244. For updated data, go to www.NaturalDatabase.com. • 1295

Some Brand Name Natural Products - What they Contain
www.NaturalDatabase.com contains MANY more listings than appear here.

B
R
A
N
D

N
A
M
E
S

Andro Surge — Country Life
Each capsule contains: Tribulus Terrestris 100 mg • Moomiyo 50 mg • Dehydroepiandrosterone 50 mg • Vitamin E 25 IU.

Andro Surge — MRM
Each capsule contains: Androstenedione 100 mg.

Andro-6 — EAS
Four tablets contain: DHEA 50 mg • Androstenedione 100 mg • Tribulus terrestris 250 mg • Chrysin 150 mg • Saw Palmetto extract 180 mg • Indole-3-Carbinol 50 mg • Zinc Glycinate 8 mg.

Androbolic — ProLab
Each two tablets contain: 19-Norandrostenedione 100 mg • 4-Androstene-3,17 Diol 100 mg • 5-Androstene-3,17 Diol 50 mg • Tribulus Terrestris 250 mg • Saw Palmetto 180 mg • Chrysin 150 mg • Indole 3 Carbinol 50 mg.

ANDRO-DIOL — New Hope Health Products
Each capsule contains: 4-androstene-3, 17-diol 100 mg.

Androdyne — Cytodyne Technologies
Three capsules contain: 19-Norandrostenedione 100 mg • 5-Androstene-3B, 17b-Diol 50 mg • 4-Androstene-3, 17-dione 50 mg • AA-t3 Anti-Aromatase Complex 100 mg (proprietary blend of Chrysin, Indole 3-Carbinol & 7-IsoPropoxyIsoflavone) • Zinc Gluconate 20 mg • B3 (Nicotinic Acid) 50 mg.

AndroPlex 700 — AST Sports Science
Two capsules contain: Tribulus Terrestris 500 mg • Androstenedione 100 mg • DHEA 100 mg.

Andro-Stack 850 — Optimum Nutrition
Two capsules contain: pharmaceutical grade Androstenedione (Delta-4-androstene-3-17-dione) 100 mg • pharmaceutical grade DHEA (Dehydroepiandrosterone) 100 mg • Tribulus terrestris 650 mg.

AndrosteDERM — MedLean
2 ml contain: 4-Androstenediol (Androdiol from Pat Arnold's LPJ Research) 90 mg • Androstenedione 30 mg.

ANDRO-SURGE — New Hope Health Products
Each capsule contains: Androstenedione (4-androstene-3, 17-dione) 100 mg.

ANDRO-Xtreme — New Hope Health Products
Each capsule contains: Dehydroepiandrosterone (DHEA) 100 mg • Androstenedione (4-androstene-3, 17-dione) 100 mg • 5-androstenediol (5-androstene-3, 17-diol) 50 mg • Tribulus terrestris 500 mg • Chrysin 250 mg.

Androzyme — Progressive Labs
Each capsule contains: Vitamin E (d-alpha tocopheryl succinate) 50 IU • Zinc (as zinc aspartate) 15 mg • Raw Orchic concentrate (bovine) 100 mg • Siberian Ginseng (Eleutherococcus senticosus) 100 mg • L-Carnitine 30 mg.

Anotesten — Muscletech
Six capsules contain: 4-Androstenediol 150 mg • Androstenedione 250 mg • DHEA 100 mg • Tribulus Terrestris 1000 mg • Chrysin 150 mg • Indole-3-Carbinol (I3C) 50 mg • Saw Palmetto (standardized for 25% fatty acids) 320 mg.

Antacid — Progressive Labs
Each tablet contains Calcium Carbonate 500 mg which supplies: Calcium (from calcium carbonate) 200 mg. Other Ingredients: Dextrose, Mannitol, Cellulose, Magnesium Stearate, Glycine and Spearmint oil. Free of Sodium & Aluminum.

Anti-Aging Breakthrough — Jason
Six antioxidant Vitamin C.

Anti-Anxiety — Phytopharmica
Twenty drops contain: Cicuta virosa 4x • Gaultheria 4x • Ignatia 4x • Staphysagria 4x • Asa foetida 3x • Corydalis formosa 3x • Hyoscyamus 3x • Sumbulus 3x • Valeriana officianalis 3x • Avena sativa 1x • In a base of 40% USP alcohol by volume.
Editor's Comments: This is a homeopathic product. It is so extremely diluted that its activity can not be explained by conventional scientific methods. Therefore this product can not be rated by the scientific criteria used in this Database. A patient receiving the extreme dilution of this product will not receive many, if any, molecules of the original active ingredient. Therefore, there are no harmful pharmacologic effects, and any beneficial effects are controversial and not due to a direct biochemical action of the ingredient on the body. Homeopathic products are allowed for sale in the U.S. due to legislation passed in the 19th century sponsored by a homeopathic physician who was also a Senator. The law still requires that the FDA allow the sale of products listed in this Homeopathic Pharmacopea of the United States.

Anti-Arthritis Glucosamine Chondroitin — Crystal Springs
Each tablet contains: Glucosamine (Sulfate) 600 mg • Chondroitin (Sulfate) 400 mg.

AntiBio 1 — Dial Herbs
Echinacea • Goldenseal • Poke root • Cayenne.

AntiBio 2 — Dial Herbs
Echinacea • Myrrh • Poke root • Cayenne.

Anti-Catabolic Fuel — TwinLab
Four capsules contain: L-Leucine 1000 mg • L-Valine 225 mg • L-Isoleucine 225 mg • Ketoisocaproate (KIC) 100 mg • L-Ornithine Alpha-Ketoglutarate 1000 mg • L-Glutamine 250 mg.

Anti-Depression Support — Amazon Support
Each capsule contains: Tayuya • Damiana • Muira Puama • Passion Flower • Chamomile.

Anti-Fatigue — Phytopharmica
Twenty drops contain: Zincum muriaticum 8x • Gelsemium sempervirens 6x • Picricum acidum 6x • Acidum phosphoricum 3x • Valeriana officinalis 1x • In a base of 45% USP alcohol by volume.
Editor's Comments: This is a homeopathic product. It is so extremely diluted that its activity can not be explained by conventional scientific methods. Therefore this product can not be rated by the scientific criteria used in this Database. A patient receiving the extreme dilution of this product will not receive many, if any, molecules of the original active ingredient. Therefore, there are no harmful pharmacologic effects, and any beneficial effects are controversial and not due to a direct biochemical action of the ingredient on the body. Homeopathic products are allowed for sale in the U.S. due to legislation passed in the 19th century sponsored by a homeopathic physician who was also a Senator. The law still requires that the FDA allow the sale of products listed in this Homeopathic Pharmacopea of the United States.

Anti-Fungal — The Herbalist
Thuja leaf • Usnea lichen • Spilanthes herb • Pau D'Arco inner bark • Echinacea root • Calendula flower • Cayenne pepper.

Anti-Fungal Salve — Blessed Herbs
Jewelweed • Black Walnut hulls • Pau d'Arco bark • Usnea lichen • Calendula flowers • Spilanthes • Echinacea Angustifolia root • Goldenseal root • Myrrh Gum • Organic Cold-Pressed Olive oil • Beeswax • Essential oils of Tea Tree & Thyme linalol.

Anti-Fungal Support — Amazon Support
Each capsule contains: Jatoba • Fedegosa • Brazilian Peppertree • Pau d'Arco.

Anti-Insom — Dial Herbs
Hops • Lobelia • Valerian • Cayenne.

Anti-Ox: Herbal Antioxidant — The Herbalist
Pau D'Arco inner bark • Astralagus root • Ginkgo leaf • Milk Thistle seed • Licorice root • Cayenne pepper.

Antioxidant Caps — Now
Two capsules contain: Vitamin A (from 15 mg Beta-Carotene) 25000 IU • Vitamin C (from Calcium Ascorbate) 500 mg • Vitamin E (natural d-Alpha Succinate) 300 IU • Calcium (Ascorbate) 50 mg • Zinc (Picolinate) 5 mg • Selenium (L-Selenomethionine) 25 mcg • N-Acetyl-Cysteine 100 mg • L-Glutathione 25 mg • Alfalfa juice concentrate (Green Superfood) 250 mg • Wheat Sprout concentrate (Enzyme active) 100 mg.

Antioxidant Cocktail Custom Paks — The Vitamin Shoppe
Each packet contains: Vitamin A (as 100% beta-carotene) 15 mg (25000 IU) • Vitamin C (as ascorbic acid) 2000 mg • Vitamin E (as d-alpha, d-gamma, d-beta, d-delta tocopherol) 400 IU • Selenium (as selenomethionine) 200 mcg • Alpha-carotene 1 mg (833 IU) • Lycopene (LYC-O-MATO) 5 mg • Lutein 5 mg • Zeaxanthin 0.24 mg • Phytoene 0.055 mg • Phytofluene 0.026 mg • Citrus Bioflavonoids 1000 mg • Hesperidin 100 mg • Rutin 100 mg • Rose Hips (Rosa canina) fruit 160 mg • Acerola 20 mg.

Antioxidant Cocktail II — The Vitamin Shoppe
Two capsules contain: Pine bark extract (Pycnogenol) 30 mg • Grape

Some Brand Name Natural Products - What they Contain
www.NaturalDatabase.com contains MANY more listings than appear here.

Seed Extract (Vitis vinifera) (Activin) 50 mg • Alpha Lipoic Acid 50 mg • Green Tea leaves (Camellia sinensis) standardized to 75% polyphenols 50 mg.

Antioxidant Fuel — TwinLab
Three capsules contain: Beta-Carotene (pro-Vitamin A) 25000 IU • Vitamin C 1000 mg • Natural Vitamin E (Succinate) 800 IU • CoQ10 (Coenzyme Q10) 30 mg • N-Acetyl Cysteine (NAC) 200 mg • L-Glutathione 100 mg • Selenium (from Selenomethionine & Selenate 50/50 mixture) 100 mcg • Alpha-Lipoic Acid (reduced) 100 mcg.

Anti-Parasite Support — Amazon Support
Each capsule contains: Macela • Graviola • Quinine Bark • Picao Preto • Carqueja • Papaya • Fedegosa • Simaruba • Epazote • Cat's Claw.

AntiSpasmodic — Dial Herbs
Scullcap • Skunk Cabbage • Black Cohosh • Myrrh • Lobelia • Cayenne.

Anti-Stress Support — Amazon Support
Each capsule contains: Passion Flower • Chamomile • Manaca • Bitter Melon • Suma • Sarsaparilla • Tayuya • Damiana • Mulungu • Muira Puama.

Anti-Viral — Amazon Support
Each capsule contains: Bitter Melon • Brazilian Peppertree • Catuaba • Cha de Bugre • Chanca Piedra • Clavelilla • Macela • Vassourinha.

Anxiety Control — Pain & Stress Center
Four capsules contain: GABA 800 mg • Glycine 200 mg • Glutamine 280 mg • Magnesium 200 mg • Passion Flower 300 mg • Primula officinalis 300 mg • Vitamin B6 20 mg.

Aorta-Glycan — Enzymatic Therapy
Each capsule contains: Aorta-Glycan (Mesoglycan) 50 mg, a mixture of highly-purified bovine-derived glycosaminoglycans (GAGs) naturally present in the aorta including: Dermatan Sulfate, Heparan Sulfate, Hyaluronic Acid, Chondroitin Sulfate, & related Hexosaminoglycans. Contains no sugar, salt, yeast, wheat, corn, soy, dairy products, coloring, flavoring or preservatives.

Appleheart Chondroitin Sulfate — Appleheart
Each capsule contains: Chondroitin Sulfate 300 mg. Other Ingredients: Cellulose, Gelatin, Vegetable Stearate.

Appleheart Echinacea — Appleheart.
Each capsule contains: standardized Echinacea Angustifolia and Echinacea Purpurea 250 mg • Rice Protein • Gelatin • Cellulose • Vegetable Stearate. Contains no Dairy, Yeast, Corn, Sugar, Starch, Soy, Preservatives, Hydrogenated Oils.

Appleheart Glucosamine Sulfate — Appleheart
Each capsule contains: Glucosamine Sulfate (from Glucosamine Sulfate Potassium) 500 mg • Potassium 65 mg. Other Ingredients: Gelatin, Cellulose, Vegetabel Stearate.

Appleheart Melatonin — Appleheart
Each capsule contains: Melatonin 3mg.

Appleheart Saw Palmetto — Appleheart
Each capsule contains: Saw Palmetto berry 160 mg • Olive Oil • Water • Gelatin. Contains no dairy, yeast, corn, sugar, starch, soy, preservatives or hydrogenated oils.

Appleheart St. John's Wort — Appleheart
Each capsule contains: standardized St. John's Wort 250 mg • Gelatin • Rice Protein • Cellulose • Magnesium Stearate (Vegetable Source).

Apple-Honey Lactobacillus Acidophilus — Nature's Life
Two tablespoons (1 fl.oz or 29.6 ml) contain: Calories: 11 • Cholesterol: 0 • Fiber 0.1 g • Protein: 0.7 g • Fat: 0 • Carbohydrates: 2 g. Full disclosure ingredients: Unfiltered Apple juice, Purified Water, Pasteurized Honey, Soy Protein Isolate & Lactobacillus Acidophilus Culture.

AppSignal — Pharmanex
Two wafers contain: Sucrose • Cocoa Powder • Microcrystalline Cellulose • Protein Complex (Hydrolyzed Soy Protein, Soy Protein Isolate, Egg Albumin) • L-Tyrosine • AbsorbaLean Fiber Complex (Apple Pectin, Fructooligosaccharides, Locust Bean Gum, Carrageenan, Microcrystalline Cellulose) • Stearic Acid • Lecithin Powder • Natural and Artificial Flavors • Sorbitol • L-Histidine Hydrochloride • Pyridoxine Hydrochloride • Magnesium Stearate • Folic Acid.

Aqua Ban — Thompson Medical Co.
Each tablet contains: Active Ingredient: Pamabrom 50 mg (Diuretic). Other ingredients: Carnauba Wax • Croscarmellose Sodium • FD&C Blue No. 1 Aluminum Lake • Hydroxypropyl Methylcellulose • Lactose • Magnesium Stearate • Microcrystalline Cellulose • Polyethylene Glycol • Polysorbate 80 • Starch • Titanium Dioxide.

Aqua Greens — Futurebiotics
Twelve tablets contain: Chlorella 1000 mg • Spirulina 2500 mg • Klamath Blue/Green Algae 500 mg • Kelp 250 mg • D. Salina 100 mg.

AquaActin — Nature's Plus
Two capsules contain: Chinese Green Tea [(Camellia sinensis leaf) decaffeinated, standardized 50% Polyphenols] 250 mg • Horsetail [(Equisetum arvense stem) standardized 10% Silicic Acid, 7% Silica] 150 mg • Uva Ursi [(Arctostaphylos uva-ursi leaf) standardized 20-25% Arbutin] 100 mg • Vitamin B6 (Pyridoxine HCI) 75 mg • Goldenseal [(Hydrastis canadensis root & rhizome) standardized 10% Alkaloids, 5% Hydrastine] 50 mg • Artichoke [(Cynara scolymus flower) standardized 2.5-5% Caffeylquinic Acids] 50 mg.

Aqua-Action — Nature's Plus
Each capsule contains: Buchu leaves 125 mg • Couchgrass 100 mg • Juniper berries 100 mg • Parsley leaves 100 mg • Corn Silk 75 mg • Uva Ursi leaves 50 mg • Celery seed 50 mg. Contains no yeast, wheat, soy, milk, salt, sugar or starch.

Aqua-Flow — Enzymatic Therapy
Two capsules contain: Potassium Citrate 200 mg • Magnesium (Oxide) 50 mg • Vitamin B6 (Pyridoxine HCL) 25 mg • Other ingredients: Bearberry extract (Uva Ursi) contains 10% Arbutin 200 mg • Lespedeza extract (Lespedeza capitatae) contains 8% Flavonoids 100 mg • Boldo extract (Peumus boldo) contains 1.52% essential oils 100 mg • Goldenrod extract (Solidago virgaurea) contains 5% flavonoids 100 mg. Contains no sugar, salt, yeast, wheat, corn, soy, dairy products, coloring, flavoring, or preservatives.

Aqua-Lim — Aspen Group, Inc.
Each tablet contains: Buchu leaves 70 mg • Couch Grass 70 mg • Hydrangea root 35 mg • Corn Silk 35 mg • Uva Ursi 10 mg • Hypothalamus 30 mg • Raw Kidney concentrate 30 mg • Vitamin B6 16 mg • Bladder Wrack 100 mg • Magnesium: Protein Chelated 50 mg.

Arbu-Tone — Phytopharmica
Two capsules contain: Potassium Citrate 200 mg • Magnesium (Oxide) 50 mg • Vitamin B6 (Pyridoxine HCL) 25 mg • Other ingredients: Bearberry extract (Uva Ursi) 200 mg standardized to contain 10% arbutin • Lespedeza extract (Lespedeza capitatae) 100 mg standardized to contain 8% flavonoids • Boldo extract (Peumus boldo) 100 mg standardized to contain 1.52% essential oils • Goldenrod extract (Solidago vigaurea) 100 mg standardized to contain 5% flavonoids. Contains no sugar, salt, yeast, wheat, corn, soy, dairy products, coloring, flavoring or preservatives.

Arctic Root — Swedish Herbal Institute
Each tablet contains Rhodiola rosea, extract SHI-Rr5 180 mg.

ArginMax — Unknown
Six capsules contain: Vitamin A palmitate 5,000 IU• L-Arginine 3000 mg • Folate (as Folic Acid) 400 mcg • Biotin 300 mcg 90% • American Ginseng (Panax quinquefolius) standardized (5% Ginsenosides) 100 mg • Korean Ginseng (Panax Ginseng) standardized (30% ginsenosides) 100 mg • Selenium (Sodium Selenate) 70 mcg • Vitamin C (Ascorbic Acid) 60 mg • Ginkgo Biloba standardized (24% Flavone Glycosides, 6% Terpene Lactones) 50 mg • Vitamin E (as d-Alpha-Tocopheryl Acetate) 30 IU • Niacin (as Niacinamide) 20 mg • Zinc (Zinc Gluconate) 15 mg • Vitamin B5 (Pantothenic Acid) (as Calcium Pantothenate) 10 mg • Vitamin B12 (Cyanocobalamin) 6 mcg • Vitamin B6 (Pyridoxine HCl) 2 mg • Vitamin B2 (Riboflavin) • Vitamin B1 (Thiamin) (as Thiamin Mononitrate) 1.5 mg.

Arnica Oil — Blessed Herbs
Arnica flower • leaf & Organic Cold-Pressed Olive oil.

ArteClear — Pacific BioLogic
Rhubarb rhizome • Salvia root • Sea Weed • Polygonum root • Polygonatum rhizome • Cassia seeds • Aucklandia root • Hawthorn fruit • Pseudoginseng root.

BRAND NAMES

© Copyright 2000, Natural Medicines Comprehensive Database (209) 472-2244. For updated data, go to www.NaturalDatabase.com. • 1297

Some Brand Name Natural Products - What they Contain
www.NaturalDatabase.com contains MANY more listings than appear here.

B R A N D   N A M E S

Arth Rx — Symmetry
Each packet contains: Glucosamine • Chondroitin Sulfate • Hydrolyzed gelatin • Boswellia • Curcumin • Bilberry • Grape Seed extract • Grape Skin extract • Tumeric extract.

Arth-9 — Rx Vitamins
Four capsules contain: Glucosamine Sulfate (Aminomonosaccharide) 1000 mg • Vitamin C (Ascorbic Acid) 250 mg • Bromelain 250 mg • Calcium (Citrate) 250 mg • Boswellin 250 mg • Curcumin 100 mg • Zinc (L-Monomethionine) 30 mg • Chondroitin Sulfate A (CSA) 25 mg • Copper (Glycinate) 2 mg.

Artho-Health Formula — Youngevity
Cosamin (Glucosamine Sulfate 200 mg, Chondroitin Sulfate 160 mg) • Vitamin C 15 mg • Manganese 500 mcg • Vilcabamba Mineral Essence: Potassium, Calcium, Magnesium, Zinc, Chromium, Selenium, Iron, Copper, Molybdenum, Vanadium, Iodine, Cobalt, Manganese.

Artho-Therapy — Phytopharmica
Each tablet contains: Active Ingredient: Capsaicin 0.025%. Other Ingredients: Purified water • Alcohol • Glycerin • Triethanolamine • Escin (Horse chestnut extract) • Glory lily • Methylparaben • Lavender essential oil. Cruelty-free-no animal testing. Contains no animal products.

Arthred-G — Richardson Labs
One rounded scoop contains: Arthred (enzymatically hydrolyzed collagen protein) 7 g • Glucosamine & Chondroitin complex [glucosamine HCL, glucosamine sulfate (potassium salt, sodium free), chondroitin sulfate].

Arth-Rid Us — The Herbalist
Devil's Claw root bark • Yucca root • Yerba Mansa root • Black Cohosh root • Wild Yam root.

Arthrimin GS Glucosamine Sulfate 500 mg — Jamieson
Each capsule contains: Glucosamine Sulfate (from Potassium Chloride Complex) 500 mg. Other Ingredients: Peppermint Leaf, and Betaine Hydrochloride.

Arthritis Guardian — Clinician's Choice
Three tablets contain: Shark Cartilage 1500 mg • Glucosamine Sulfate 450 mg • Linoleic Acid, Gamma Linolenic Acid (sunflower oil, borage oil) 150 mg • Boswellia 30 mg • Cayenne Fruit 30 mg • Glycosaminoglycan 30 mg • White Willow Bark 30 mg • Proprietary blend: Carrot Powder, Citrus Bioflavonoid Complex, Grape Powder 9 mg.

Arthro Herbal-Rx — Alternecare Health Products
Two capsules contain: Chondroitin Sulfate (Bovine Cartilage) 150 mg • Glucosamine Sulfate 350 mg • Cat's Claw 25 mg • Quercetin 50 mg • Bromelain 50 mg • Alfalfa 25 mg • Devil's Claw 10 mg • Yucca 20 mg • Pycnogenol 5 mg • Grape seed 5 mg • Suma 25 mg • Siberian Ginseng 25 mg • Lipoic Acid 25 mg.

Arthro-7 — Gero Vita
Each capsule contains: Chicken Collagen type II 400 mg • Methylsulfonylmethane (MSM) 50 mg • Cetyl Myristoleate (CMO) 50 mg • Bromelain (2400 GDU) 15 mg • Curcuma Longa Extract (root, 95% Curcumin) • Vitamin C (as Ascorbic Acid) 70 mg • Lipase (30 USP units) 50 mg.

Arthro-Glucosamine — Nutri-Quest
Each tablet supples: Glucosamine Sulfate 100 mg • N-Acetyl Glucosamine 50 mg • L-Glutathione 2 mg • N-Acetyl Cysteine 5 mg • L-Cysteine 50 mg • L-Glutamic Acid 50 mg • L-Glycine 50 mg • L-Taurine 25 mg • Vitamin C 50 mg • Vitamin E (Succinate) 25 IU • Pantothenic Acid 50 mg • Soluble Trachea (16% Chondroitin Sulfate-A) 25 mg • Silymarin 5 mg • Milk Thistle 100 mg • Green Lipped Mussel 25 mg (natural source of Mucopolysaccharides & Superoxide Dismutase).

Arthro-HCP — Met-Rx
Fourteen grams contain: Arthred (Hydrolyzed Collagen Protein) 10 g • Maltodextrin • Glucosamine Hydrochloride & Glucosamine Sulfate 1.5 g.

As-Comp — Enzymatic Therapy
Each capsule contains: Active Ingredient: Ephedrine (From Ma Huang extract (Ephedra sinensis) 200 mg) 12 mg • Other ingredients: Ginger root extract 6.5:1 (Zingiber officinale) 65 mg • Licorice root extract (Glycyrrhiza glabra) standardized to contain 5% Glycyrrhizic acid) 50 mg • Marshmallow root extract 4:1 (Althaea officinalis) (Mucilage

content 30-40%) 50 mg • Sundew Herb extract 4:1 (Drosera rotundifolia) 40 mg • Euphorbia Herb extract 4:1 (Euphorbia hirta) 40 mg • Senega root extract 4:1 (Polygala senega) 40 mg • Goldenseal root extract (Hydrastis canadensis) standardized to contain 5% total Alkaloids including Berberine, Hydrastine & Canadine 20 mg. Contains no sugar, salt, yeast, wheat, corn, soy, dairy products, coloring, flavoring, or preservatives.

Ascorbate-C — Atrium
Each teaspoon (5 gm) contains: Vitamin C (Calcium Ascorbate) 2000 mg • Rose Hips 1450 mg • Acerola 1000 mg • Lemon Bioflavonoids 500 mg • Rutin 25 mg • Hesperidin 25 mg • Calcium (from Calcium Ascorbate) 230 mg.

Aspen - Body Booster with Power — Aspen Group, Inc.
Each tablet contains: Raw Testicular concentrate (not an extract) of Bovine sources 300 mg • Multiple Glans Raw Gland concentrate (not an extract) containing Raw Liver Duodenum, Pancreas (porcine sources) & Raw Heart , Pituitary, Kidney, Spleen, Thymus & Adrenal concentrates of Bovine sources 225 mg • Cayenne 25 mg • Gotu-Kola 25 mg • Fo-Ti 25 mg • Damiana 32 mg • Guarana 50 mg.

Aspen - Candida — Aspen Group, Inc.
Each capsule contains: Pau D'Arco 4:1 extract 100 mg • Calcium Caprylate 100 mg • Goldenseal root extract 100 mg • Garlic extract (odorless) 50 mg • Licorice root extract 50 mg • Caprilic Acid 25 mg • Oregano 25 mg • Tea Tree oil 5 mg.

Aspen - Cardio- Health — Aspen Group, Inc.
Each caplet contains: Vitamin E (d-alpha tocopheryl acetate) 200 IU • Vitamin C 50 mg • Garlic extract (allium sativum) 300 mg • Hawthorn extract of leaf & flower (crategus laevigata) 50 mg • Co-Enzyme Q10 (ubiquinone) 5 mg.

Aspen - Daily Essentials — Aspen Group, Inc.
Three tablets contain: Vitamin E (d-alpha) 200 IU • Vitamin A 5000 IU • Beta Carotene 5000 IU • Vitamin D 400 IU • Vitamin C 400 mg • Folic Acid 400 mcg • Thiamine 1.5 mg • Riboflavin 1.7 mg • Niacin 20 mg • Vitamin B6 2 mg • Vitamin B12 6 mcg • Biotin 300 mcg • Pantothenic Acid 10 mg • Calcium (citrate) 600 mg • Phosphorus 450 mg • Iodine (kelp) 150 mcg • Magnesium (carbonate) 200 mg • Copper (gluconate) 2 mg • Zinc (gluconate) 15 mg • Vitamin K 100 mcg • Selenium (yeast) 75 mcg • Manganese (gluconate) 5 mg • Chromium (aspartate) 200 mcg • Molybdenum 150 mcg • Nickel 15 mcg • Tin 15 mcg • Vanadium 5 mg • Boron (citrate) 2 mg • Potassium (gluconate) 100 mg • Grape seed extract 10 mg • CoQ10 10 mg. Contains no sugar, starch, salt, wheat, corn, milk or soy derivatives.

Aspen - Flexile Plus — Aspen Group, Inc.
Three capsules contain: Glucosamine HCl 99% 1500 mg • Chondroitin Sulfate (purified chondritin sulfate 95%, mixed glycosominoglycans 5%) 1200 mg • Manganese Ascorbate 240 mg • Bromelain 100 mg • Boswellia Serrata extract 100 mg.

Aspen - Imun- Comp — Aspen Group, Inc.
Two tablets contain: Vitamin C: Ascorbic Acid 250 mg • Vitamin B1: Thiamin HCl 30 mg • Vitamin E: d-Alpha Tocopherol 200 IU • Beta Carotene 5000 IU • Copper: Gluconate 300 mcg • Selenium Chelate 25 mcg • Zinc: Gluconate 15 mg • Bone Marrow 65 mg • Lymph 65 mg • Papain 50 mg • Pituitary Whole 15 mg • Spleen 130 mg • Thymus 550 mg • Bromelain 50 mg • Echinacea extract 300 mg • L-Lysine HCl 250 mg • Trypsin 1:75 25 mg • Blue Flag 130 mg • Fennel 70 mg • Goldenseal herb 70 mg.

Aspen - Maximal Sterol Complex — Aspen Group, Inc.
Six tablets contain: Fucosterol 6963 mcg • Beta Sitosterol 5148 mcg • Campestrol 3.069 mcg • Stigmatero 1749 mcg • Other Naturally Occuring Sterols 9174 mcg • (26103 mcg of Sterols) • Liver 2600 mg • Orchic 1000 mg • Thymus 200 mg • Heart 200 mg • Lung 200 mg • Kidney 200 mg • Adrenal 150 mg • Prostate 120 mg • Pituitary 150 mg • Hypothalamus 60 mg • Pancreas 120 mg • Bee pollen 1000 mg • Korean Ginseng 100 mg • Royal Jelly 30 mg • Calcium 200 mg • Magnesium 100 mg • Potassium 99 mg • Octacosanol 1650 mcg • RNA 60 mg • DNA 30 mg • Linoleic Acid 1040 mg • Oleic Acid 698 mg • Palmitic Acid 263 mg • Linolenic Acid 109 mg • Stearic Acid 56 mg • Lignoceric Acid 14 mg • Arachidonic Acid 13 mg • Elcoanoic Acid 11 mg • Behenic C Acid 6 mg • Myristic Acid 5 mg • Capsicum 100 mg • Alfalfa 100 mg • Dandelion root 100 mg • Garlic 100 mg • Yellow Dock 100 mg • Gota Kola 100 mg • Licorice root 100 mg • Arginine 1200 mg • Lysine 600 mg • Ornithine 600 mg • Leucine 40 mg • Valine 38 mg • Lysine 34 mg • Isoleucine 30 mg • Phenylalanine

30 mg • Theronine 24 mg • Methionine 20 mg • Tryptophan 8 mg • Trace Minerals.

Aspen - Mega Max — Aspen Group, Inc.
Each tablet contains: Vitamin C 250 mg • Vitamin E 150 IU • Vitamin A 25,000 USP Units • Vitamin D 1000 USP Units • Vitamin B1 75 mg • Vitamin B2 75 mg • Vitamin B6 75 mg • Vitamin B12 75 mg • Niacinamide 75 mg • Choline 75 mg • Inositol 75 mg • Para Aminobenzoic Acid 75 mg • Pantothenic Acid 75 mg • Biotin 75 mg • Folic Acid 400 mcg • Rutin 25 mg • Citrus bioflavonoid complex 25 mg • Hesperiden complex 5 mg • Betaine HCl 25 mg • Glutamic Acid 25 mg • Iodine .15 mg • Calcium 50 mg • Potassium 10 mg • Iron 10 mg • Magnesium 7.2 mg • Manganese 6.1 mg • Zinc 15 mg • Selenium 10 mcg • Amino Acids: Arginine, Aspartic Acid, Alanine, Cystine, Glutamic Acid, Glycine, Histidine, Isoleucine, Lucine, Lysine, Methionine, Ornithine, Phenylalanine, Proline, Serine, Threonine, Tyrosine, Tryptophan & Valine in a natural base of Alfalfa • Parsley • Golden Seal root • Buckthorne root • Rosemary • Watercress • Mandrake root • Spinach • Lovage • Kelp • Kale • Ginseng & Rhubarb root.

Aspen - Mid-Life Plus — Aspen Group, Inc.
Each caplet contains: Vitamin E (as natural d-alpha tocopherol succinate) 30 IU • Vitamin C 60 mg • Thiamin (as thiamin mononitrate) 2 mg • Riboflavin 2 mg • Niacin (niacinamide) 20 mg • Vitamin B6 (as pyridoxine HCl) 10 mg • Vitamin B12 (as cyanocobalamin) 6 mcg • Folate (as folic acid) 400 mcg • Calcium (from calcium carbonate) 150 mg • Selenium (from L-Selenomethionine) 70 mcg • Boron (chelate) 1.5 mg • Purified Isoflavones (from soybean & pueraria root) 50 mg • Kava Kava root standardized extract (30% kavalactones) 100 mg • Black Cohosh root 40 mg.

Aspen - Muscle Builder — Aspen Group, Inc.
Four tablets contain: Gamma Oryzanol 50 mg • Inosine 200 mg • Testicular Glan 600 mg • L-Ornithine 700 mg • Beta-Sitosterol 200 mg • Adrenal 400 mg • Thymus 400 mg.

Aspen - Osteo — Aspen Group, Inc.
Each tablet contains: Calcium Orotate 376 mg • Magnesium Orotate 200 mg • Calcium Aspartate 24 mg • Vitamin D 400 mg.

Aspen - Primrose — Aspen Group, Inc.
Each softgel contains: Evening Primrose oil 500 mg • Vitamin E (d-alpha tocopherol) 10 IU • Gamma-Linoleic Acid 40 mg • Linoleic Acid 350 mg. Contains no sugar, starch, salt, wheat, corn, yeast or soy derivatives.

Aspen - Soy Special — Aspen Group, Inc.
Each tablet contains: Soy isoflavones 50 mg.

Aspen - Super Max 1600 Weight Gain — Aspen Group, Inc.
Each flavor (vanilla or chocolate) contains: Vitamin C 332 mg • Rose Hips 6.8 mg • Vitamin E 400 IU • Vitamin A 13332 USP Units • Vitamin D 532 USP Units • Vitamin B1 20 mg • Vitamin B2 16 mg • Vitamin B6 68 mg • Vitamin B12 8 mcg • Niacin 56 mg • Choline 40 mg • Inositol 26.8 mg • Para Aminobenzoic Acid 1600 mg • Pantothenic 132 mg • Biotin 400 mcg • Folic Acid 532 mcg • Rutin 1700 mcg • Glutamic Acid 880 mg • Iodine 200 mcg • Calcium 1280 mg • Phosphorus 1200 mg • Potassium 10 mg • Iron 36 mg • Copper 2800 mg • Magnesium 13.2 mg • Manganese 3200 mg • Zinc 20 mg • Amino Acids Arginine 7883 mg • Aspartic Acid 220 mg • Alanine 880 mg • Cystine 1100 mg • Glutamic Acid 880 mg • Glycine 1980 mg • Histidine 2332 mg • Isoleucine 7152 mg • Lucine 4840 mg • Lysine 5060 mg • Methionine 1100 mg • Phenylalanine 944 mg • Proline 328 mg • Serine 4840 mg • Threonine 3300 mg • Tyrosine 220 mg • Tryptophan 880 mg • Valine 4840 mg.

AspirActin — Nature's Plus
Three capsules contain: White Willow bark [(Salix alba) standardized 7-9% Salicin] 500 mg • Kava Kava [(Piper methysticum root) standardized 29-31% Kavalactones] 50 mg • Inositol Hexanicotinate (Flush-Free Niacin) 50 mg • Cayenne [(Capsicum frutescens fruit) standardized 100000 STU] 25 mg • Ginkgo Biloba leaf (standardized 24% Ginkgo Flavone-Glycosides, 6% Terpene Lactones) 10 mg.

AstaZanthin — Source Naturals
Marine Algae (Haematococcus pluvialis) 10 mg. Natural concentrate (AstaZanthin) yielding Astaxanthin complex 1 mg.

Astragalus Plus — The Herbalist
Astragalus root • Echinacea root • Lomatium root • Myrrh Gum • Poke root • Wild Indigo root • Yarrow flower • Cayenne pepper.

Astragalus-Shitake Virtue — Blessed Herbs
Astragalus root • Echinacea Angustifolia root • Licorice root • Shitake mycelium • Grain alcohol & Distilled Water.

Astragulus — Pharmanex
Each capsule Contains: Astragalus (Astragalus Membranaceus)(root extract)(10:1) 250 mg. Other Ingredients: Rice Flour, Gelatin, Magnesium Stearate, Silicon Dioxide.

A-Team: Adrenal Support — The Herbalist
Siberian Ginseng fresh-dried root (Eleuthero sent) • Oats fresh milky seed (Avena sativa) • Licorice fresh-dried root (Glycyrrhiza glabra) • Gotu Kola fresh herb (Hydrocotyle asiatica) • Cayenne fresh-dried pepper (Capsicum anuum).

Athero-Plus — Atrium
Two film coated tablets contain: Vitamin A Palmitate 3334 IU • Vitamin D3 (Fish oil) 67 IU • Vitamin B1 (Thiamine Mononitrate) 34 mg • Vitamin B2 (Riboflavin) 17 mg • Vitamin B6 (Pyridoxine HCL) 34 mg • Vitamin B12 (Cyanocobalamin) 34 mcg • Vitamin C (Ascorbic Acid, Sago Palm) 400 mg • Vitaimin E Succinate 134 IU • Beta Carotene 5000 IU • Biotin 100 mcg • Niacin-Niacinamide 67 mg • D-Calcium Pantothenate 167 mg • Folic Acid 267 mcg • Calcium Orotate 170 mg • Chromium Aspartate 67 mcg • Copper Gluconate 0.67 mg • Iodine (Kelp) 40 mcg • Iron (Ferrous Fumerate) 6.67 mg • Magnesium Orotate 170 mg • Magnesium Aspartate 6.67 mg • Molybdenum (Kelp) 34 mcg • Potassium Orotate 34 mg • Selenium Aspartate 67 mcg • Zinc Orotate 6.67 mg • Bromelain 50 mg • Choline Bitartrate 34 mg • L-Methionine 20 mg • PABA 17 mg • Rutin 17 mg.

Athle-Peak — The Herbalist
Jamaican Sarsaparilla root • Siberian Ginseng root • American Ginseng root • Licorice root • Wild Yam root • Cinnamon bark • Cayenne pepper.

Athletic Support — Amazon Support
Each capsule contains: Suma • Sarsaparilla • Maca • Catuaba • Chuchuhuasi • Guarana • Muira Puama • Yerba Mate • Tayuya • Iporuru.

Athletica — HerbaSway
Bitter Orange • Kudzu • Panax Ginseng • Siberian Ginseng • Astragalus • Schisandra • Ginger • Knotweed • Blackberry • Licorice • HerbaSwee (Cucurbitaceae fruit).

Atkins Allergy — Atkins
Six tablets contain: Pantethine (co-enzyme A precursor) 360 mg • Bioperine (Piperine) 5 mg • Citrus Bioflavonoids 1000 mg • Grape seed extract (Activin) 60 mg • Vitamin B12 (Cyanocobalamin) 1000 mcg • Vitamin B6 (Pyridoxine) 50 mg • Vitamin C (buffered) 2000 mg • Vitamin A (Acetate) 10000 IU • Quercitin (Flavonoid) 840 mg • Calcium (3-Phosphate, Ascorbate) 700 mg • Magnesium (Carbonate) 200 mg.

Atkins Basic #3 — Atkins
Each tablet contains: Magnesium Oxide 8 mg • Copper Sulfate 200 mcg • Vitamin E (d Alpha Tocopherol) 20 IU • Cyanocobalamin (Vitamin B12) 30 mcg • Biotin 75 mcg • Folic Acid 100 mcg • Pyridoxine (HCL) (Vitamin B6) 20 mg • Pyridoxal 5-Phosphate 2 mg • Calcium Pantothenate (Vitamin B5) 25 mg • Pantethine (80%) 25 mg • Niacinamide 5 mg • Niacin (Vitamin B3) 2 mg • Vitamin C (Calcium Ascorbate) 120 mg • Riboflavin (Vitamin B2) 4 mg • Thiamine (HCL) (Vitamin B1) 5 mg •Vitamin D2 15 IU • Beta Carotene 500 IU • Vitamin A 200 IU • L-Glutathione (reduced) 5 mg • N-Acetyl L-Cysteine 20 mg • Octacosanol 150 mcg • Selenium 40 mcg • Vanadyl Sulfate 15 mcg • Molybdenum (Sodium) 10 mcg • Chromium (Polynicotinate) 50 mcg • Zinc (Chelate) 10 mg • Manganese (Chelate) 4 mg • PABA 100 mg • Inositol 80 mg • Choline Bitartrate 100 mg.

Atkins Blood Pressure — Atkins
Six tablets contain: Taurine 1500 mg • Bioperine (Piperine) 5 mg • Hawthorn (1.5% Vitexin conc.) 300 mg • Calcium (from Ascorbate) 75 mg • Magnesium (Carbonate, Glycinate) 600 mg • Vitamin C (buffered) 600 mg • Pantethine (co-enzyme A precursor) 35 mg • L-Arginine base 100 mg • Inositol 600 mg • N-Acetyl-L-Cysteine 150 mg • Chromium (Picolinate) 200 mcg • Garlic 600 mg • Vitamin B6 (Pyridoxine) 150 mg • Potassium (Citrate) 99 mg.

Atkins Blood Sugar Tablets — Atkins
Six tablets contain: Chromium (Picolinate) 500 mcg • Bioperine (Piperine) 5 mg • Folic Acid (Folate) 800 mcg • Vitamin E natural

B R A N D N A M E S

**B
R
A
N
D

N
A
M
E
S**

150 IU • Manganese (Glycinate) 30 mg • Selenium (Selenomethionine) 120 mcg • Inositol 900 mg • Niacinamide 300 mg • Vitamin C buffered 1200 mg • Bis-Glycinato Oxovanadium Complex (BGOV) 15 mg • Biotin 4 mg • Taurine 600 mg • Alpha-Lipoic Acid 240 mg • Magnesium (Glycinate, Carbonate) 600 mg • Zinc (Monomethionine) 50 mg.

Atkins Cold & Flu — Atkins
Four tablets contain: natural Beta-Carotene 20000 IU • Bioperine (Piperine) 5 mg • Copper (Chelate) 4 mg • Vitamin B6 (Pyridoxine) 16 mg • Vitamin B3 (Niacinamide) 60 mg • Vitamin B2 (Riboflavin) 8 mg • Dimethylglycine (DMG) 80 mg • Folic Acid (Folate) 800 mcg • Garlic 640 mg • Magnesium (Aascorbate) 60 mg • Selenium (Selenate) 120 mcg • Citrus Bioflavonoids 320 mg • Calcium Pantothenate (Vitamin B5) 320 mg • Vitamin C buffered 2000 mg • Zinc (Monomethionine) 100 mg • Quercetin (Flavonoid) 320 mg • Vitamin A (Acetate) 13333 IU.

Atkins Dieters Advantage — Atkins
Four tablets contain: Citrin (55% Hydroxycitric Acid) 450 mg • Chromium (Polynicotinate) 200 mcg • Soy extract (containing active Saponins) 1500 mg • Methionine 250 mg • L-Carnitine Peptide Complex 500 mg • Vitamin B6 (Pyridoxine) 20 mg • Pantethine (Co-enzyme A precursor) 20 mg • Asparagus concentrate 50 mg • Parsley concentrate 50 mg • Kelp 20 mg • Spirulina 50 mg • Potassium (Citrate) 99 mg • Magnesium (Citrate/Carbonate) 60 mg • L-Glutamine 75 mg • DL-Phenylalanine 150 mg • L-Tyrosine 75 mg • Bioperine (Piperine) 5 mg.

Atkins Essential oils — Atkins
Each capsule contains: Flaxseed oil 400 mg • Vitamin E 5 IU • Fish oil (50% Omega-3 potency) 400 mg • Borage seed oil 400 mg.

Atkins Heart Care — Atkins
Eight tablets contain: Magnesium (Glycinate, Carbonate) 400 mg • Bioperine (Piperine) 5 mg • Cayenne 500 mg • Bromelain (Proteolytic Enzyme) 500 mg • Vitamin B6 (Pyridoxine) 10 mg • Folic Acid (Folate) 800 mcg • Selenium (Methionate) 150 mcg • Hawthorn (1.5% Vitexin conc.) 100 mg • Ginkgo Biloba (6% Terpene conc.) 60 mg • natural Beta-Carotene (Dunaliella salina) 12000 IU • Chromium (Picolinate) 200 mcg • Vitamin C buffered 1000 mg • Vitamin E natural 400 IU • Taurine 500 mg • Calcium (3-Phosphate) 500 mg.

Atkins Memory — Atkins
Eight tablets contain: Phosphatidylserine (PS) 160 mg • Bioperine (Piperine) 5 mg • Folic Acid (Folate) 800 mcg • Vitamin B12 (Cyanocobalamin) 1000 mcg • Vitamin B1 (Thiamine) 100 mg • N-Acetyl-L-Cysteine 1000 mg • Octacosanol 6 mg • Ginkgo Biloba (6% Terpene lactone conc.) 60 mg.

Atkins Menopause — Atkins
Four tablets contain: Black Cohosh (Cimicifuga rademosal) (2.5% Triterpenes) 25 mg • Vitamin E (d-Alpha-Tocopheryl) 200 IU • Bioperine (Piperine) 5 mg • Vitamin K 50 mg • Folic Acid 800 mcg • Tocotrienols mixed 3 mg • Boron (Boroglutamate) 3 mg • Alpha Lipoic Acid 10 mg • Pantethine (co-enzyme A precursor) 25 mg • Vitamin B6 (Pyridoxine) 50 mg • Calcium (Sulfate) 65 mg • Magnesium (Sulfate) 70 mg • Beta-Sitosterol 50 mg • Gamma Oryzanol 150 mg • Garlic (PurGar) 250 mg • Soy Phosphatidylcholine 400 mg • PABA (Para Amino Benzoic Acid) 500 mg • Soy Isoflavones concentrate (23.6% Genistein/Genistin; 3.8% Daidzin/Daldzein) 100 mg.

Atkins Shake Mix — Atkins
Chocolate shake mix contains: Protein 24 g • Carbohydrates 1g • Fat 9 g • Calories 180. Ingredients: Lipo-Pro Blend (special formulation containing: Calcium Caseinate, Milk Protein concentrate, Egg Whites, Glutamine Peptides, Hydrolyzed Whey Protein concentrate & Whey Protein Isolate) • Dutch Cocoa • High Oleic Sunflower oil • Polydextrose • Lecithin • Guar Gum • Vitamins & Minerals • Vanillin • Acesulfame Potassium • Beta-Carotene. Vanilla Shake Mix contains: Protein 23 g • Carbohydrates 1 g • Fat 8 g • Calories 170. Ingredients: Lipo-Pro Blend (special formulation containing: Calcium Caseinate, Milk Protein concentrate, Egg Whites, Glutamine Peptides, Hydrolyzed Whey Protein concentrate & Whey Protein Isolate) • High Oleic Sunflower oil • Lecithin • Guar Gum • Vitamins & Minerals • natural & artificial Flavors • Acesulfame Potassium • Beta-Carotene. Cappuccino Shake Mix contains: Protein 23 g • Carbohydrates 2 g • Fat 8 g • Calories 175 g. Ingredients: Lipo-Pro Blend (special formulation containing:Calcium Caseinate, Milk Protein concentrate, Egg Whites, Glutamine Peptides, Hydrolyzed Whey Protein concentrate & Whey Protein Isolate) • High Oleic Sunflower oil •

Lecithin • Enzyme Modified Soy Protein • Caramel Color • Guar Gum • Vitamins & Minerals • natural & artificial Flavors • Acesulfame Potassium • Beta-Carotene.

ATP Fuel — TwinLab
Three capsules contain: Creatine Monohydrate & Creatine Pyruvate 3000 mg • Potassium Phosphate 300 mg • ATP (Adenosine Triphosphate) 60 mg.

ATP Plus — Progressive Labs
Six tablets contain: Magnesium (as magnesium hydroxide) 300 mg • Malic Acid 1200 mg.

Atri A.S.F — Atrium
Each tablet contains: Raw Tissue concentrates (not extracts) of Bovine source of the following 200 mg: Thymus 80 mg • Partoid 80 mg • Adrenal 20 mg • Spleen 20 mg.

Atri CU- Chelate — Atrium
Each tablet contains: Spleen 28.5 mg • Brain 7.5 mg • Liver 5 mg • Heart 3.5 mg • Kidney 3.5 mg • Thymus 2 mg • Adrenal 2 mg • Pituitary 1 mg • Pancreas 1 mg • Duodenum 1 mg • Copper (Protein Chelated) 2 mg.

Atri E-Derm — Atrium
Each gram contains: Natural Vitamin E (d-Alpha Tocopheryl Acetate) 30 IU. In an absorbent base containing unsaturated fatty acids from Flax & Beet Lipids, Natural Vitamin A & Lecithin.

Atri Flexile — Atrium
Each capsule contains: Glucosamine Sulfate 500 mg • Uncaria tomentosa 200 mg • Curcumin 50 mg • Bromelain 25 mg. Contains no sugar, starch, salt, wheat, corn, yeast or soy derivatives.

Atri Free Amino — Atrium
Each 600 mg capsule contains: Free form Amino Acids: L-Alanine • L-Arginine • L-Aspartic Acid • L-Citruline • C-Cystine • L-Glutamic Acid • L-Glutamine • L-Glysine • L-Histidine HCL • L-Hydroxproline • L-Isoleucine • L-Leucine • L-Lysine • L-Methionine • L-Phenylalanine • L-Proline • L-Serine • L-Threonine • L-Tyrosine • L-Valine • L-Taurine.

Atri K-Chelate — Atrium
Each tablet contains: As chelated proteinates (Amino Acid Chelated Minerals): Potassium 100 mg • Raw Tissue concentrate from the following: (Spleen 28.5 mg, Brain 7.5 mg, Liver 5 mg, Heart 3.5 mg, Kidney 3.5 mg, Thymus 2 mg, Adrenal 2 mg, Pituitary 1 mg, Pancreas 1 mg & Duodenum 1 mg) 55 mg.

Atri Multi-Hypo — Atrium
Three tablets contain: Vitamin A (from Fish Liver oil) 10000 IU • Vitamin D3 400 IU • Vitamin B 10 mg • Vitamin B2 10 mg • Vitamin B6 10 mg • Vitamin B12 50 mcg • Niacinamide 100 mg • Pantothenic Acid 50 mg • Folic Acid 400 mcg • Vitamin C 120 mg • Vitamin E (d-Alpha Tocopherol Succinate) 15 mg • Biotin 30 mcg • Calcium 97 mg • Magnesium 72 mg • Manganese 15 mg • Potassium 53 mg • Zinc 15 mg • Iron (from Iron Sulfate) 18 mg • Iodine (from Kelp) 150 mcg • Choline Bitartrate 30 mg • Inositol 30 mg • PABA (Para Amino Benzoic Acid) 30 mg • Citrus Bioflavonoids 100 mg • Hesperidin 25 mg • Rutin 20 mg • Glutamic Acid 18 mg • L-Lysine (Monohydrochloride) 30 mg • L-Methionine 30 mg.

Atri- Stress-B+C — Atrium
Two tablets contain: Vitamin C (Ascorbic Acid) 500 mg • Vitamin B1 (Thiamine HCL) 100 mg • Vitamin B2 (Riboflavin) 100 mg • Vitamin B6 (Pyridoxine HCL) 100 mg • Vitamin B12 (Cyanocobalamin) 500 mcg • Niacinamide 100 mg • Pantothenic Acid 100 mg • Folic Acid 400 mcg • Biotin 100 mcg • Lemon Bioflavonoids 250 mg • Choline (Choline Bitartrate) 100 mg • Inositol 100 mg • PABA 50 mg.

Atri Zinc Plus — Atrium
Each tablet contains: Ascorbic Acid & Sodium Ascorbate 125 mg • Zinc Gluconate 25 mg • Rutin 25 mg.

Atri-770 — Atrium
Each capsule contains: Cold Pressed concentrated Wheat Germ oil 770 mg.

Atri-A + E Mulsion High concentrate — Atrium
Each drop contains: Emulsified Vitamin A Palmitate 15000 IU • Vitamin E (d-Alpha Tocopheryl Acetate) 10 IU.

Atri-A + E Mulsion Regular concentrate — Atrium
Each drop contains: Emulsified Vitamin A Palmitate 5000 IU • Vitamin E (d-Alpha Tocopheryl Acetate) 10 IU.

Some Brand Name Natural Products - What they Contain
www.NaturalDatabase.com contains MANY more listings than appear here.

Atri-Acidic — Atrium
Each tablet contains: Raw Stomach concentrate (Bovine) 50 mg • Raw Duodenum concentrate (Bovine) 50 mg • Betaine HCL 460 mg • Glutamic Acid HCL 200 mg • Pepsin 1:20000 25 mg • Potassium Chloride 25 mg.

Atri-Aloe-Lax — Atrium
Each capsule contains: Aloe 450 mg. Contains no sugar, starch, salt, wheat, corn, yeast or soy derivatives.

Atri-Aloe-V — Atrium
Each capsule contains: Aloe ferox (Aloe Vera resin) 430 mg • Aloe barbadensis (Aloe Vera leaf) 100 mg.

Atri-Amino — Atrium
Six tablets contain: Isoleucine 90 mg • Leucine 216 mg • Lysine 270 mg • Methionine 54 mg • Phenylalanine 132 mg • Threonine 132 mg • Valine 156 mg • Arginine 528 mg • Histidine 48 mg • Alanine 660 mg • Tyrosine 18 mg • Serine 252 mg • Aspartic Acid 402 mg • Cystine 18 mg • Glutamic Acid 684 mg • Glycine 1650 mg • Hydroxylysine 54 mg • Hydroxyproline 846 mg • Proline 984 mg. All of the Amino Acids in this preparation are of the natural (L) form.

Atri-Arthritis Spray — Atrium
Four fluid ounces contains: Oil of Wintergreen (Methyl Salicylate) 15% • Menthol 6% • IPA Alcohol. In a specially formulated, non-greasy base.

Atri-Bio-C — Atrium
Each tablet contains: Calcium Ascorbate 500 mg • Bioflavonoids 500 mg • Acerola 10 mg • Hesperidin 10 mg • Rutin 10 mg.

Atri-BLP — Atrium
Each capsule contains: Cayenne 200 mg • Parsley 90 mg • Ginger root 50 mg • Goldenseal root 40 mg • Garlic 35 mg • Siberian Ginseng 30 mg. Contains no sugar, starch, salt, wheat, corn, yeast or soy derivatives. Professional Formula.

Atri-Cal Chelate — Atrium
Three tablets contain: As Chelated Proteinates (AminoAcid Chelated Minerals) Calcium 450 mg • Raw Tissue concentrate from: (Spleen 74.1 mg, Brain 19.5 mg, Liver 13 mg, Heart 9.1 mg, Kidney 9.1 mg, Thymus 2 mg, Adrenal 2 mg, Pituitary 1 mg, Pancreas 2.6 mg, Duodenum 2.6 mg) 135 mg.

Atri-C-Flu — Atrium
Each capsule contains: Garlic 300 mg • Parsley 60 mg • Rose Hips 60 mg • Rosemary 25 mg • Watercress 20 mg. Professional Formula. Contains no sugar, starch, salt, wheat, corn, yeast or soy derivatives.

Atri-Daily Essentials — Atrium
Three tablets contain: Vitamin E (d-Alpha) 200 IU • Beta Carotene 5000 IU • Vitamin D 400 IU • Folic Acid 400 mcg • Thiamine 1.5 mg • Riboflavin 1.7 mg • Niacin 20 mg • Vitamin B6 2 mg • Vitamin B12 6 mcg • Biotin 300 mcg • Pantothenic Acid 10 mg • Calcium Citrate 600 mg • Phosphorous 450 mg • Iodine (Kelp) 150 mcg • Magnesium (Carbonate) 200 mg • Copper (Gluconate) 2mg • Zinc (Gluconate) 15 mg • Vitamin K 100 mcg • Selenium (yeast) 75 mcg • Manganese (Gluconate) 5 mg • Chromium (Aspartate) 200 mcg • Molybdenum 150 mcg • Nickel 15 mcg • Tin 15 mcg • Vanadium 5 mg • Boron (Citrate) 2 mg • Potassium (Gluconate) 100 mg • Grape seed extract 10 mg • CoQ10 10 mg. Contains no sugar, starch, salt, wheat, corn, milk or soy derivatives.

Atri-Detox — Atrium
Each capsule contains: Red Clover Blossoms 150 mg • Chaparral 80 mg • Licorice root 50 mg • Peach bark 50 mg • Oregon Grape root 40 mg • Stillingia 35 mg • Cascara Sagrada bark 30 mg • Sarsaparilla root 30 mg • Burdock root 15 mg • Buckthorn bark 10 mg. Professional Formula. Contains no sugar, starch, salt, wheat, corn, yeast or soy derivatives.

Atri-Disco — Atrium
Each tablet contains: First Phase (in Stomach) Manganese Sulfate 200 mg • Calcium Ascorbate 100 mg • Magnesium Aspartate 50 mg. Second Phase (in Duodenum) Alpha-Chymotrypsin 4 mg • Papain 100 mg • Bromelain 100 mg • Pancreatin 5x 50 mg.

Atri-DMG Plus — Atrium
Each tablet contains: NN Dimethyl Glycine 19.3 mg • Calcium Gluconate 30.7 mg • Glycine 25 mg • Lysine 25 mg.

Atri-EPA Plus — Atrium
Each capsule contains: Salmon oil [containing EPA (Eicosapentaenoic Acid)180 mg & DHA (Docosahexaenoic Acid) 120 mg] 1000 mg • Vitamin A (Fish oil) 100 IU • Vitamin E (Fish oil) 5 IU.

Atri-F — Atrium
Each capsule contains: Cold Processed Persic oil (yielding the following Lipid Acids referred to as Vitamin F factors: Oleic 192 mg, Linoleic 109 mg, Palmitic 18 mg, Stearic 4 mg, Linolenic 701 mcg, Heptodecanoic 400 mcg, Arachadic 330 mcg, Arachidonic 111 mcg) 370 mg • Potassium 113 mcg • Sodium 14 mcg • Magnesium 7 mcg • Phosphorus 4 mg • Calcium 4 mcg • trace amounts of: Manganese, Chromium, Zinc, Iron, Copper, Boron & Barium • Palmitoleic 5 mg.

Atri-Fem-Reg — Atrium
Each capsule contains: Goldenseal root 120 mg • Blessed Thistle 100 mg • Cramp bark 80 mg • Uva Ursi leaves 70 mg • False Unicorn 50 mg • Raspberry leaves 30 mg • Squaw Vine 20 mg • Ginger root 10 mg. Professional Formula. Contains no sugar, starch, salt, wheat, corn, yeast or soy derivatives.

Atri-Flav-1000 — Atrium
Three tablets contain: Vitamin C 1000 mg • Citrus Bioflavonoids 1000 mg • Rutin 100 mg. Other Ingredients: Rose Hips & Acerola, in a base containing Raw Spleen concentrate 4 mg.

Atri-FM-H — Atrium
Each capsule contains: Black Cohosh 200 mg • Sarsaparilla root 150 mg • Siberian Ginseng 40 mg • Licorice root 35 mg • False Unicorn 30 mg • Blessed Thistle 25 mg • Squaw Vine 20 mg. Professional Formula. Contains no sugar, starch, salt, wheat, corn, yeast or soy derivatives.

Atri-Gastro — Atrium
Each capsule contains: Colloidal Silica 200 mg • Irish Moss 50 mg • Beef Duodenum 20 mg • Pepsin 20 mg • Stomach Mucosa 10 mg • Di-Sodium Phosphate 10 mg. Glandulars are processed by freeze drying method. Contains no sugar, starch, salt, wheat, corn, yeast or soy derivatives.

Atri-GE-132 — Atrium
Each capsule contains: Germanium Sesquioxide 150 mg.

Atri-GE-132 Sub — Atrium
Each tablet contains: Germanium Sesquioxide 25 mg.

Atri-Gesic — Atrium
Three ounces contain: Lanolin • Menthol • Methyl Salicylate • Oil of Cassia • Stearic Acid • Spermwax • GMS • Tea • Methyl Gluceth E 10 • Camphor • Methyl Nicotinate • Propyl Parasept • Deionized Water.

Atri-Glucomannan — Atrium
Each capsule contains: Glucomannan Dietary Fiber (Konjac root source) 500 mg.

Atri-Greens Plus — Atrium
Each tablet contains: Vitamin A (Palmitate) 5000 IU • Vitamin C (Ascorbic Acid) 240 mg • Vitamin E (Acetate) 45 mg • Beta Carotene 150 mg • Selenium (Yeast) 50 mcg • Spirulina 25 mg • Chlorophyll 2 mg. In a base of cruciferous vegetables: Broccoli, Brussels Sprouts, Cabbage, Carrot, Cauliflower, Kale, Mustard Greens, Pumpkin, Spinach & Turnip Greens.

Atri-Herb-CLS — Atrium
Each capsule contains: Gentian root 50 mg • Valerian root 50 mg • Catnip 40 mg • Goldenseal root 40 mg • Barberry bark 30 mg • Cascara Sagrada 30 mg • Irish Moss 30 mg • Fenugreek seed 30 mg • Bugleweed 25 mg • Yellow Dock root 25 mg • St. John's Wort 25 mg • Brigham Tea 25 mg • Red Clover Blossoms 25 mg • Chickweed 25 mg. Professional Formula. Contains no sugar, starch, salt, wheat, corn, yeast or soy derivatives.

Atri-IBC — Atrium
Each capsule contains: Eyebright 100 mg • Goldenseal root • Barberry bark 100 mg • Red Raspberry leaves 100 mg • Cayenne 100 mg. Professional Formula. Contains no sugar, starch, salt, wheat, corn, yeast or soy derivatives.

Atri-INF — Atrium
Each capsule contains: Plantain 200 mg • Black Walnut leaves 100 mg • Goldenseal root 60 mg • Marshmallow root 50 mg • Bugleweed 40 mg. Professional Formula. Contains no sugar, starch, salt, wheat, corn, yeast or soy derivatives.

Atri-Kid-Uri — Atrium
Each capsule contains: Juniper berries 200 mg • Parsley 120 mg • Uva Ursi leaves 50 mg • Marshmallow root 45 mg • Ginger root 40 mg •

© Copyright 2000, Natural Medicines Comprehensive Database (209) 472-2244. For updated data, go to www.NaturalDatabase.com. • 1301

Some Brand Name Natural Products - What they Contain
www.NaturalDatabase.com contains MANY more listings than appear here.

B
R
A
N
D

N
A
M
E
S

Goldenseal root 20 mg. Professional Formula. Contains no sugar, starch, salt, wheat, corn, yeast or soy derivatives.

Atri-Lacto — Atrium
Each capsule contains: Lactobacillus Acidophilus & Bulgaras culture 400 mg. This nutrient culture media is Lactose, Whey & Milk solids. Contains a minimum two million total bacteria count.

Atri-Lax — Atrium
Each capsule contains: Psyllium husks 100 mg • Cascara Sagrada bark 100 mg • Prune concentrate 100 mg • Senna leaves 100 mg • Licorice root 45 mg • Chlorophyll 10 mg. Professional Formula. Contains no sugar, starch, salt, wheat, corn, yeast or soy derivatives.

Atri-LB-CLS — Atrium
Each capsule contains: Cascara Sagrada 150 mg • Bayberry root bark 75 mg • Cayenne 75 mg • Ginger root 50 mg • Goldenseal root 50 mg • Lobelia 30 mg • Red Raspberry leaves 30 mg • Turkey Rhubarb root 30 mg • Fennel seed 20 mg. Professional Formula. Contains no sugar, starch, salt, wheat, corn, yeast or soy derivatives.

Atri-Lipotropic — Atrium
Three capsules contain: Choline Bitartrate 1000 mg • Inositol 1000 mg • Methionine 300 mg.

Atri-Liv-GLB — Atrium
Each capsule contains: Barberry root bark 120 mg • Wild Yam 80 mg • Cramp bark 60 mg • Fennel seed 50 mg • Yellow Dock 40 mg • Ginger root 35 mg • Catnip 30 mg • Peppermint leaves 30 mg. Professional Formula. Contains no sugar, starch, salt, wheat, corn, yeast or soy derivatives.

Atri-Ly Poll — Atrium
Each tablet contains: Raw Bovine Tissue concentrate (not extracts) 20 mg: (Pituitary 5 mg • Adrenal 15 mg) • special blend of Bee Pollen 250 mg in a base of L-Lysine 400 mg (an Amino Acid known to be essential in human nutrition).

Atri-Lym-Inf — Atrium
Each capsule contains: Cayenne 150 mg • Echinacea 120 mg • Myrrh Gum 100 mg • Hawthorn berries 100 mg • Licorice root 30 mg. Professional Formula. Contains no sugar, starch, salt, wheat, corn, yeast or soy derivatives.

Atri-Mag Chelate Plus — Atrium
Each tablet contains: Amino Acid Chelated Minerals as: Magnesium 300 mg. Raw Tissue concentrates (Bovine source) from: Spleen 29 mg • Brain 8 mg • Liver 5 mg • Heart 4 mg • Kidney 4 mg • Thymus 2 mg • Adrenal 2 mg • Pituitary 1 mg • Duodenum 1 mg • Pancreas 1 mg.

Atri-Medicated Psoriasis Shampoo — Atrium
Eight fluid ounces contain: Active Ingredients: Coal Tar solution USP 5% • Colloidal Sulfur 2% • Salicylic Acid 2%. In a special base of Surface Active Cleansers, Wetting Agents & Lanolin.

Atri-Mega Plus — Atrium
Four tablets contain: Vitamin A Acetate 25000 IU • Vitamin D3 Cholecalciferol 1000 IU • Vitamin E Acetate 100 IU • Vitamin C (with Rose Hips) 500 mg • Folic Acid 0.1 mg • Thiamine (Vitamin B1) 50 mg • Riboflavin (Vitamin B2) 50 mg • Niacin 100 mg • Vitamin B6 50 mg • Vitamin B12 50 mcg • Biotin 50 mcg • Pantothenic Acid 50 mg • Choline Bitartrate 50 mg • Calcium (as Oyster Shell & Calcium Carbonate) 700 mg • Iodine (Kelp) 225 mcg • Iron (Ferrous Fumerate) 30 mg • Magnesium (as Oxide) 200 mg • Zinc (as Sulfate) 36 mg • Manganese (as Carbonate) 3mg • Potassium (Chloride & Kelp) 99 mg • Chromium (as Chelate) 20 mcg • Selenium (Yeast) 60 mcg • Betaine HCI 50 mg • Papain 200 mg • Para Aminobenzoic Acid 50 mg • Citrus Bioflavonoids 50 mg • Inositol 50 mg • Ribonucleic Acid (Yeast extract) 200 mg.

Atri-Mega-Lacto — Atrium
Each capsule contains: Lactobacillus Acidophilus with Bifidus Four Billion CFU (Colony Forming Units). Contains no preservatives artificial color. Contains no wheat, sugar, corn or soy.

Atri-Min 74 — Atrium
Each tablet contains: Sea Bed Montmorillonite (also known as Mineral 74100 mg Volcanic Montmorillonite) 900 mg.

Atri-Multi — Atrium
Each capsule contains: Vitamin A (from Fish Liver oil) 3333 IU • Vitamin D3 133 IU • Vitamin B1 4 mg • Vitamin B2 3 mg • Vitamin B6 3 mg • Vitamin B12 11 mcg • Niacinamide 34 mg • Pantothenic

Acid 17 mg • Folic Acid 134 mcg • Vitamin C 40 mg • Vitamin E (d-Alpha Tocopherol) 5 mg • Biotin 10 mcg • Calcium 32 mg • Magnesium 24 mg • Manganese 5 mg • Potassium 18 mg • Zinc 5 mg • Iron (from Sulfate) 6 mg • Iodine (from Kelp) 50 mcg • Choline Bitartrate 10 mg • PABA 9 mg • Citrus Bioflavonoids 100 mg • Hesperidin 9 mg • Rutin 7 mg • Glutamic Acid 6 mg • L-Lysine 10 mg • L-Methionine 10 mg • RNA (from Yeast) 15 mg. In a base of Watercress, Kelp, Alfalfa, Parsley.

Atri-Nerv — Atrium
Each capsule contains: Black Cohosh 100 mg • Cayenne 100 mg • Hops Flowers 80 mg • Scullcap 70 mg • Wood Betony 50 mg • Passiflora 40 mg • Valerian root 20 mg • Ladys Slipper 10 mg. Professional Formula. Contains no sugar, starch, salt, wheat, corn, yeast or soy derivatives.

Atri-Neuro — Atrium
Each tablet contains: Choline (Choline Bitartrate) 200 mg • L-Histidine 50 mg • L-Phenylalanine 50 mg • GABA (Amino Buteric Acid) 50 mg • L-Tyrosine 50 mg • Raw Brain concentrate 25 mg • Niacin 15 mg • Pyridoxine HCI 50 mg.

Atri-NTL-CA — Atrium
Each capsule contains: Horsetail grass 300 mg • Oat Straw 100 mg. Professional Formula. Contains no sugar, starch, salt, wheat, corn, yeast or soy derivatives.

Atri-Ortho-Phos — Atrium
Each drop contains: Ortho Phosphoric Acid 13 mg • Inositol 0.57 mg • Choline Bitartrate 0.27 mg. Thirty drops contain: Ortho Phosphoic Acid 390 mg • Inositol 17 mg • Choline Biartrate 8 mg.

Atri-Oxy — Atrium
Two tablets contain: Vitamin A (Beta Carotene) 25000 IU • Vitamin E (d-Alpha Tocopherol) 400 IU • Vitamin C 1000 mg • Bioflavonoid Complex 150 mg • Superoxide Dismutase 100 mg • Selenium 100 mcg • Zinc 25 mg • Copper 2 mg • Astragalus 50 mg • Rosemary 50 mg • Milk Thistle (Slymarin) 50 mg • Spirulina 100 mg • Chromium Picolinate 25 mcg • Grape seed extract 50 mg • Co-Enzyme Q-10 10 mg • L-Glutathione 10 mg • L-Cysteine 100 mg • Reishi Mushroom 50 mg • Curcumin 50 mg.

Atri-PMS — Atrium
Three tablets contain: Vitamin A Acetate 5000 IU • Vitamin B6 (Pyridoxine HCL) 100 mg • Adrenal concentrate 50 mg • Hypothalamus concentrate 10 mg • Ovary concentrate 50 mg • Pituitary concentrate 10 mg • Passion Flower 75 mg • Dong Quai 50 mg • Cramp bark 50 mg • Chionanthus 50 mg • Valerian 75 mg • Magnesium (Oxide) 200 mg • Iron (Peptonate) 20 mg • Red Raspberry 50 mg.

Atri-Pros — Atrium
Each capsule contains: Cayenne 160 mg • Uva Ursi leaves 70 mg • Parsley 60 mg • Goldenseal root 50 mg • Gravel root 50 mg • Juniper berries 30 mg • Marshmallow root 25 mg • Ginger root 20 mg • Siberian Ginseng 15 mg. Professional Formula. Contains no sugar, starch, salt, wheat, corn, yeast or soy derivatives.

Atri-Psoriasis Ointment — Atrium
Four ounces contains: Sulfur ppt 1.5% • Salicylic Acid 1.5%, Coal Tar Solution USP 2%. In a specially formulated base designed to retain the skin's moisure.

Atri-Res — Atrium
Each capsule contains: Marshmallow root 200 mg • Mullein 120 mg • Comfrey leaves 100 mg • Chickweed 50 mg. Professional Formula. Contains no sugar, starch, salt, wheat, corn, yeast or soy derivatives.

Atri-RNA/DNA — Atrium
Each tablet contains: Ribo-Nucleic Acid (RNA) 180 mg • Deoxy-Nucleic Acid (DNA) 40 mg.

Atri-SDT — Atrium
Each tablet contains: Trypsin 4 mg • Chymotrypsin 2 mg • Pancreatin 2 mg • Bromelain 3 mg • Papayotin 4 mg • Thymus concentrate (Bovine) 2 mg • Mannitol 13 mg. In a specially prepared natural spearmint flavored slow dissolving tablet base.

Atri-Selenium+E — Atrium
Each tablet contains: Vitamin C (Ascorbic Acid) 250 mg • Vitamin E (d-Alpha Tocopherol) 200 IU • Vitamin B1 (Thiamine HCL) 4 mg • Vitamin B2 (Riboflavin) 4 mg • Vitamin B6 (Pyridoxine HCL) 4 mg • Niacin 10 mg • Pantothenic Acid 50 mg • Selenium (Selenium Yeast) 50 mcg • Raw Heart concentrate 10 mg. In a base of Bone Meal.

Atri-S-G-V — Atrium
Each tablet contains: Selenium 50 mcg • Germanium 225 mcg • Vanadium 225 mcg, as Protein Chelates.

Atri-Statin — Atrium
Each tablet contains: Caprylic Acid 110 mg. Contains no sugar, starch, salt, wheat, corn, yeast or soy derivatives.

Atri-Thy-Kelp — Atrium
Each capsule contains: Mullein 140 mg • Parsley 90 mg • Watercress 80 mg • Kelp (Norwegian) 70 mg • Irish Moss 60 mg • Iceland Moss 40 mg. Professional Formula. Contains no sugar, starch, salt, wheat, corn, yeast or soy derivatives.

Atri-Trace — Atrium
Three tablets contain: Calcium (Egg & Oyster Shells) 250 mg • Magnesium (Gluconate) 50 mg • Manganese (Gluconate) 10 mg • Potassium (Gluconate) 50 mg • Zinc (Gluconate)15 mg • Vitamin D3 133 IU • Vitamin B6 50 mg • Glutamic Acid HCL 325 mg.

Atri-V&M+Complete — Atrium
Six tablets contains: Vitamin A (Fish oil) 10000 IU • Vitamin D (Fish oil) 400 IU • Vitamin C (Calcium Ascorbate, Acerola, Rose Hips) 400 mg • Vitamin E 60 IU • Vitamin B1 • Vitamin B2 10 mg • Vitamin B6 10 mg • Vitamin B12 25 mcg • Niacin 60 mg • Calcium (Bone Meal & Calcium Carbonate) 750 mg • Magnesium (Oxide) 375 mg • Phosphorus (Bone Meal) 700 mg • Iron (Amino Acid Chelate) 20 mg • Iodine (Kelp) 150 mcg • Potassium (Proteinate) 20 mg • Zinc (Amino Acid Chelate) 20 mg • Manganese (Amino Acid Chelate) 15 mg • Choline (Bitartrate) 50 mg • Inositol 500 mg • Lecithin 50 mg • Pantothenic Acid 50 mg • Folic Acid 400 mcg • PABA 30 mg • RNA-DNA 15 mg • Betaine HCL 25 mg • Biotin 100 mcg. In a base of Alfalfa, Kelp, Rose Hips, Acerola, Fish Liver oils, Bone Meal, Citrus Bioflavonoids, Papaya, Bromelain Enzymes & Essential Amino Acids.

Atri-Vana — Atrium
Each capsule contains: Vanadyl Sulfate 25 mg. Contains no wheat, sugar, starch, salt, corn, yeast, milk or soy.

Atri-Verm — Atrium
Each capsule contains: Pumpkin seed 100 mg • Culvers root 70 mg • Violet leaves 60 mg • Cascara Sagrada bark 50 mg • Slippery Elm bark 45 mg • Witch Hazel bark 40 mg • Mullein 30 mg • Echinacea 20 mg. Professional Formula. Contains no sugar, starch, salt, wheat, corn, yeast or soy derivatives.

Atri-Yeast — Atrium
Four tablets contain: Protein from a Special Yeast 1200 mg • Niacin 66 mg • Pantothenic Acid 13 mg • Vitamin B1 13 mg • Vitamin B2 13 mg • Vitamin B6 3 mg • Chromium 25 mcg • Selenium 7.5 mcg.

Atri-Zinc Chelate Plus — Atrium
Each tablet contains: Amino Acid Chelated Minerals as: Zinc 29 mg. Raw Tissue concentrates (Bovine source) from: Spleen 29 mg • Brain 8 mg • Liver 5 mg • Heart 4 mg • Kidney 4 mg • Thymus 2 mg • Andrenal 2 mg • Pituitary 1 mg • Duodenum 1 mg.

Attention! — Olympia Nutrition
Contains DHA 250 mg • Phosphatidylserine 20 mg • DMAE 100 mg • Choline 100 mg • TMG. No yeast, wheat, corn, milk, egg, soy glutens, preservatives, or artificial colors.

B/P Formula — Nature's Way
Two capsules contain: Proprietary Formula: Cayenne pepper fruit • Garlic bulb • Ginger • Goldenseal stem, leaf, flower • Parsley herb • Siberian Ginseng root. Other ingredients: Gelatin.

B100 Complex — Natrol
One tablet contains: Vitamin B1 (Thiamine) 100 mg • Vitamin B2 (Riboflavin) 100 mg • Vitamin B6 (Pyroxidoxine) 100 mg • Vitamin B12 (Cobalamin) 100 mcg • Niacinamide 100 mg • Folic Acid 400 mcg • Biotin 100 mcg • Pantothenic Acid 100 mg • Choline 100 mg • Inositol 100 mg • PABA 100 mg • ULTRAGREEN 150 mg. Other ingredients: Microcrystalline Cellulose, Calcium Carbonate, Croscarmellose Sodium, Stearic Acid, Silicon Dioxide, Magnesium Stearate.

B-12 Lingual — Progressive Labs
Each tablet contains: Vitamin B12 1000 mcg • Folate (folic acid) 400 mcg, in a base of Mannitol and Natural Cherry flavor.

B5 Facial Creme — Pharmacist Heldfond's eb5 Formulas for Younger Looking Skin
Water • Propylene Glycol • Tocopheryl Acetate • Stearic Acid • Mineral Oil • Cetyl Alcohol • Oat Flour • Retinyl Palmitate • Ergocalciferol • Propylparaben • Triethanolamine • Methylparaben • Potassium Sorbate • Allantoin • Imidazolidinyl • Urea • Panthenol • Cobomer-940 • Soluble Animal Collagen.

B-50 Caps With C — Now
Each capsule contains: Vitamin B1 (Thiamine) 50 mg • Vitamin B2 (Riboflavin) 50 mg • Vitamin B3 (Niacinamide) 50 mg • Vitamin B6 (Pyridoxine) 50 mg • Vitamin B12 100 mcg • Biotin 100 mcg • Folic Acid 400 mcg • Pantothenic Acid 100 mg • Vitamin C (Ascorbic Acid) 250 mg • PABA 50 mg • Choline (Bitartrate) 50 mg • Inositol 50 mg.

B-50 Complex — Now
Each capsule contains: Vitamin B1 (Thiamine HCL) 50 mg • Vitamin B2 (Riboflavin) 50 mg • Vitamin B3 (Niacinamide) 50 mg • Vitamin B5 (Pantothenic Acid) 50 mg • Vitamin B6 (Pyridoxine HCL) 50 mg • Vitamin B12 (Cyanocobalamin) 50 mcg • Biotin 50 mcg • Folic Acid 400 mcg • PABA 50 mg • Choline (Bitartrate) 50 mg • Inositol 50 mg.

B6 Min — Atrium
Each capsule contains: Vitamin B6 (Pyridoxine HCL) 200 mg • Magnesium Gluconate 120 mg • Potassium Gluconate 120 mg.

Barlean's Flax Oil — The Vitamin Shoppe
One teaspoon provides: Omega-3 7.7 g • Omega-6 2.3 g • Omega 9 2.2 g • VitaLox (a natural protectant blend of Ascorbic Acid and Rosemary extracts) 30 mg.

Barlean's Flax Oil High Lignin Formula — The Vitamin Shoppe
One tablespoon provides: Omega-3 6.1 g • Omega-6 1.8 g • Omega 9 1.7 g • Flaxseed Particles 2.6 g • VitaLox (a natural protectant blend of ascorbic acid and rosemary extracts) 30 mg.

Barlean's Vita-Flax — The Vitamin Shoppe
Certified Organic Flax Seed Powder containing: Protein (NX6.25) 34.7% • Fat 14.7% • Energy 435 Kcal/100 g. Vitamin E 0.01% • Dietary Fiber 34.2%. Total Fiber: Soluble Fiber 38%, Insoluble Fiber 62%.

B-Assure — The Vitamin Shoppe
Each capsule contains: 100 mg Champignon (Agaricus bisporus) stem and cap.

B-Complex — Nutri-Quest
Two tablets contain: Vitamin B1 100 mg • Vitamin B2 100 mg • Vitamin B6 50 mg • Niacinamide 100 mg • Pantothenic Acid 100 mg • Vitamin B12 100 mcg • Folic Acid 300 mcg • Biotin 100 mcg • Choline Bitartrate 100 mg • Inositol 100 mg • PABA 50 mg.

B-Complex 100 — The Vitamin Shoppe
Each capsule contains: Vitamin B1 100 mg • Vitamin B2 100 mg • Vitamin B6 100 mg • Vitamin B12 100 mcg • Niacinamide 100 mg • Folic Acid 400 mcg • Pantothenic Acid 100 mg • D-Biotin 100 mcg • Choline Bitartrate 100 mg • Inositol 100 mg • PABA 100 mg. No Yeast, Corn, Wheat, Soy, Salt, Sugar, Starch, Milk, Eggs, Preservatives, Artificial Colors or Flavors added.

B-Complex 50 mg — Nature's Life
Each tablet contains: Vitamin B1 (Thiamine HCl) 50 mg • Vitamin B2 (Riboflavin) 50 mg • Vitamin B6 (Pyridoxine HCl) 50 mg • Vitamin B12 (Cobalamin concentrate) 50 mcg • Niacinamide 50 mg • Pantothenic Acid (d-Calcium Pantothenate) 50 mg • Choline (Bitartrate) 50 mg • Inositol 50 mg • Biotin 50 mcg • Folic Acid 400 mcg • PABA (Para Aminobenzioc Acid) 50 mg • Lecithin 8 mg. In a natural base of Alfalfa, Parsley, Rice Bran & Watercress.

B-Complex with Folic Acid — Biodelivery
Two tablets contain: Choline Bitartrate 250 mg • D-Calcium Pantothenate 100 mg • Inositol 100 mg • Niacinamide 100 mg • PABA 50 mg • Riboflavin 50 mg • Thiamine HCL 50 mg • Pyridoxine HCL 45 mg • Pantethine 25 mg • Pyridoxal-5-Phosphate 5 mg • Biotin 200 mcg • Folic Acid 800 mcg • Cyanocobalamin 200 mcg • NT Factor tablet base 355 mg.

Be Sure — Wakunaga of America
Two caplets contain: Aspergillus Enzyme Complex 300 mg. Other Ingredients: Cellulose, Silica, Magnesium Stearate (vegetable source).

© Copyright 2000, Natural Medicines Comprehensive Database (209) 472-2244. For updated data, go to www.NaturalDatabase.com. • 1303

Some Brand Name Natural Products - What they Contain
www.NaturalDatabase.com contains MANY more listings than appear here.

Bee Complete — Futurebiotics
Two tablets contain: • Bee Pollen 1,000 mg • Royal Jelly 25 mg • Bee Propolis 500 mg.

Bee Pollen Chewable — Atrium
Each tablet contains: Bee Pollen 300 mg. Contains no sugar, starch, salt, wheat, corn, yeast or soy derivatives.

Bee Pollen Complex — Puritan's Pride
Each tablet contains: Bee Pollen 1000 mg • Bee Propolis 10 mg • Royal Jelly 10 mg.

Beef Liver 1500 mg — Nature's Life
Six tablets contain: Argentine Beef Liver (Defatted, Desicated & Pesticide Free) 9000 mg • Vitamin B12 (Cobalamin concentrate) 1000 mcg • Vitamin B2 457 mcg • Vitamin B6 224 mcg • Vitamin B12 1 mg • Niacin 2.2 mg • Choline 94 mg. Minerals: Calcium 2.7 mg • Copper 90 mcg • Iron 6.3 mg • Manganese 90 mcg • Potassium 94 mg • Sodium 28 mg • Zinc 1.3 mg. Amino Acids (naturally occurring): Alanine 747 mg • Arginine 297 mg • Aspartic Acid 99 mg • Cysteine 351 mg • Cystine 103 mg • Glutamic Acid 108 mg • Glysine 792 mg • Histidine (essential amino acid) 198 mg • Isoleucine (essential amino acid) 207 mg • Leucine (essential amino acid) 198 mg • Lysine (essential amino acid) 558 mg • Methionine (essential amino acid) 315 mg • Phenylalanine (essential amino acid) 369 mg • Proline 99 mg • Serine 441 mg • Threonine(essential amino acid) 306 mg • Tyrosine 396 mg • Tryptophan (essential amino acid) 36 mg • Valine (essential amino acid) 90 mg.

Benecol — McNeil Consumer Healthcare
Three softgels contain: Plant Stanol Esters 1.5 g. Other Ingredients: Gelatin, Glycerin, Sunflower Oil, Titanium Dioxide, Soybean Oil, Annatto Extract, Red 40, Yellow 8, Blue 1, Yellow 5.

Benefin — LaneLabs
Shark Cartilage 750 mg.

Benejoint — LaneLabs
Capsaicin • Shark Cartilage • Aloe Vera • Essential Oils.

Best Friends — Changes - TwinLab
One tablet contains: Vitamin A (as Alpha- and Beta-Carotene with mixed Carotenoids from D. Salina algae) 5000 IU • Vitamin C (as Ascorbic Acid with Sodium and Calcium Ascorbates) 100 mg • Vitamin D (as Cholecalciferol) 400 IU • Vitamin E (as mixed natural D-Alpha and DL-Alpha-Tocopherol Acetate) 80 IU • Thiamin (as Thiamin HCl) 1.5 mg • Riboflavin 1.7 mg • Niacin (as Niacinamide) 2 mg • Vitamin B6 (as Pyridoxine HCl) 2 mg • Folate (as Folic Acid) 400 mcg • Vitamin B12 (as Cyanocobalamin) 12 mcg • Biotin 75 mcg • Pantothenic Acid (as D-Calcium Pantothenate) 10 mg • Calcium (as Calcium Carbonate and Citrate) 125 mg • Iron (as Ferrous Fumarate) 5 mg • Iodine (as Potassium Iodide) 75 mcg • Magnesium (as Magnesium Oxide, Glycinate, and Citrate) 40 mg • Zinc (as Zinc Citrate and Glycinate) 5 mg • Selenium (as Selenomethionine) 25 mcg • Copper (as Coper Oxide, Citrate, Gluconate, and Glycinate) 2 mg • Manganese (as Manganese Sulfate, Citrate, Gluconate, and Glycinate) 1 mg • Chromium (as Chormium Dinicotinate Glycinate) 50 mcg • Molybdenum (as natural Molybdic Acid) 50 mcg • Fruit and vegatable phytonutrient concentrates 1500 mg: Dunaliela salina algae, Parsley, Tomato, Spinach, Kale, Yellow Squash, Turmeric, Orange, Cranberry, Lemon, Tangerine, Grapefruit, Red Grape, Strawberry, Cherry, Peach, Raspberry, Onion, Garlic, Leek, Broccoli, Cauliflower, Mustard Greens, Cabbage. Other ingredients: Fructose, Sorbitol, Natural and articial flavors, Microcrystalline Cellulose, Stearic Acid, Carrageenan, Glycine, Maltodextrin, Citric Acid, Magnesium Stearate, Silica, Frationated vegetable oil, Salt, and Carmine red.

Beta Fast GXR — Informulab
Concentrated, standardized, extended release extract formulation of Gymnema Sylvestre (GS).

Beta Glucans — Natrol
Two capsules contain: Oat Bran extract Seed (Avena sativa) 1500 mg, supplying Beta Glucan 185 mg. Other ingredients: Oat Bran powder, Magnesium Stearate, Gelatin.

BETA-C — Pharmagel
Beta Hydroxy Acid • Stabilized Vitamin C.

BetaGen — EAS
Each 6.6 gram serving contains: Ca HMB Monohydrate 1000 mg • Creatine Monohydrate 2000 mg • Potassium Phosphate 50 mg • L-Glutamine 400 mg • Taurine 200 mg. Ingredients: Dextrose, Phosphagen (HPCE pure Creatine Monohydrate) • Calcium b-Hydroxy b-Methylbutyrate Monohydrate • Citric Acid • L-Glutamine • Natural Flavors • Taurine • Potassium Phosphate • Aspartame • Beta-Carotene for color. Contains Phenylalanine.

Beta-Sea 10,000 IU — Holista
Each capsule contains: Beta Carotene (from Dunaliella salina algea) 10000 IU. Other Ingredients: Carotenoids.

Beta-Sea 25,000 IU — Holista
Each capsule contains: Beta Carotene (from Dunaliella salina algea) 25000 IU. Other Ingredients: Carotenoids.

Better BodyEnergy for Life — HealthWatchers System
Ma Huang • Chromium Picolinate • Brindel Berry • White Willow Bark • Ginger Root • Hawthorn Berry • Licorice Root • Gotu Kola • Passion Flower • Siberian Ginseng • Guarana • Rhemannia Root • Bladderwrack • Reishi Mushroom • Astragalus.

Better Living Multi Vitamins —
Health Center for Better Living
Each tablet contains: Vitamin A (Natural Fish Liver Oil) 10,000 IU • Beta Carotene (6 mg) 10,000 mg • Vitamin B1 (Thiamine HCl) 75 mg • Vitamin B2 (Riboflavin) 75 mg • Vitamin B3 (Niacinaide) 75 mg • Vitamin B5 (Pantothenic) 75 mg • Vitamin B6 (as pyridoxine HCl) 75 mg • Vitamin B12 (as cyanocobalamin) 100 mcg • Biotin 100 mcg • Folic Acid 400 mcg • Vitamin C (Ascorbic Acid) 250 mg • Vitamin D (Natural FLO) 400 IU • Vitamin E (100% Natural d-alpha) 150 IU • Calcium (Ostershell) 100 mg • Magnesium (Oxide, amino acid chelate) 60 mg • Zinc (Amino acid chelate) 1 mg • Iodine (Kelp) 150 mcg • Iron (Amino acid chelate • Chromium (Yeast Free GFT) 50 mcg • Boron (Amino acid chelate) 500 mcg • Molybdenum (Amino acid chelate) 50 mcg • Nucleic 50 mg.

Beyond Calcium — KAL - Nutraceutical
Five tablets contain: Vitamin D3 (as natural Cholecalciferol) 400 IU • Calcium (as Calcium Citrate) 1000 mg • Magnesium (as Magnesium Citrate) 400 mg • Boron (as Boron Amino Acid Chelate) 6 mg • Horsetail 20 mg • Guaranteed Potency Soy Isoflavones (from NovaSoy supplying 25 mg (40%) Isoflavones and 12.5 mg (20%) Genistin) 62.5 • Ipriflavone (as 7-Isopropoxy - Isoflavone from Ostivone) 200 mg • ActiSorb Base 10 mg: Bioperine extract (Black Pepper - Piper longum), Cayenne (Capsicum frutecens), Turmeric (Curcuma longa), Rosemary (Rosmarinus officinalis), Ginger (Zingiber officinale). Other ingredients: Cellulose, Stearic Acid, Silica, and Magnesium Stearate.

Beyond Echinacea — Flora
Echinacea • Balsam root • Peruvian Cat's Claw bark.

BF & SC — MMS Pro
Each capsule contains: Calendula flowers • White Oak bark • Marshmallow root • Mullein leaves • Black Walnut hulls • Gravel root • Slippery Elm bark • Wormwood • Scullcap.

Bifidus Balance +FOS — Jarrow Formulas
Each capsule contains: FOS (Fructo-Oligo-Saccharides) 210 mg • Bifidobacterium Breve R070 40% 800 million • Bifidobacterium Longum R023 40% 800 million • Bifidobacterium Bifidum R071 15% 300 million • Bifidobacterium Infantis R033 5% 100 million. Other Ingredients: Maltodextrin, Magnesium Stearate, Ascorbic Acid.

Bilberry — Progressive Labs
Each capsule contains: Bilberry leaf powder (Vaccinum myrtillus) 370 mg • Bilberry extract (Vaccinum myrtillus) 80 mg • Anthocyanids (from above) 25 mg.

Bilberry Formula — Quest
Each caplet contains: Bilberry (Vaccinium myrtillus) (provided by 50 mg P.E. 1:100 standardized to contain 25% anthocyanosides) 5000 mg • Citrus Bioflavonoids (providing Hesperidin 50 mg) 200 mg • Carrot powder (Daucus carota) 100 mg. Other Ingredients: Calcium Phosphate, Microcrystalline Cellulose, Vegetable Stearin, Croscarmellose Sodium, Magnesium Stearate (vegetable source).

Bilberry i sight — Nature's Life
Two capsules contain: Bilberry extract [(Viccinium myrtillus) standardized to 25% anthocyanosides] 360 mg • Vitamin C (Calcium Ascorbate) 300 mg • Vitamin B3 (Niacin) 40 mg • Vitamin B2 (Riboflavin) 3 mg • Vitamin E (d-Alpha Tocopheryl Succinate) 400 IU • Beta Carotene [(Dunaliella salina) equivalent to 15000 IU Vitamin A] 9 mg • Other naturally occurring carotenoids in D. salina: [Alpha Carotene 288 mcg, Cryptoxanthin 70 mcg, Zeaxanthin 58 mcg, Lutein 45 mcg].

1304 • © Copyright 2000, Natural Medicines Comprehensive Database (209) 472-2244. For updated data, go to www.NaturalDatabase.com.

Some Brand Name Natural Products - What they Contain
www.NaturalDatabase.com contains MANY more listings than appear here.

Bilberry-Go! — Wakunaga of America
Each caplet contains: Bilberry Standardized Extract (fruit) 120 mg. Other Ingredients: Cellulose, Starch, Magnesium Stearate (vegetable source), Silica.

Bile-Gest — Atrium
Each tablet contains: Ox Bile concentrate 195 mg • Collinsonia root 310 mg • Glycine 50 mg • Pepsin 30 mg • Raw Liver concentrate 30 mg.

Bio Berry Grape Seed Extract Plus — Flora
Grape Seed Extract 50 mg • Bilberry 10 mg. In a base of Cranberry powder.

Bio C-Complex 1000 — The Vitamin Shoppe
Each capsule contains: Pure Crystalline Vitamin C (fortified with Rose Hips) 1000 mg • Citrus Bioflavonoid Complex 100 mg. No Yeast, Wheat, Corn, Dairy, Soy, Salt, Sugar, Starch, Milk, Eggs, Gluten, Preservatives, Artificial Colors or Flavors added.

Bio C-Complex 500 — The Vitamin Shoppe
Vitamin C (fortified with Rose Hips Conc.) 500 mg • Citrus Bioflavonoid Complex 250 mg. No Yeast, Wheat, Corn, Dairy, Soy, Salt, Sugar, Starch, Milk, Eggs, Gluten, Preservatives, Artificial Colors or Flavors added.

Bio Ginkgo 27/7 — Pharmanex
Each tablet contains: Ginkgo (50:1) leaf extract (Ginkgo Biloba) 60 mg. Other Ingredients: Lactose Anhydrous, Microcrystaline Cellulose, Corn Starch, Sodium Starch Glycolate, Opadry Colors (which contain the Lakes of Yellow 5 and Blue 1), Colloidal Silicon Dioxide, Magnesium Stearate.

Bio St. John's — Pharmanex
Two capsules contain: St. John's Wort flowering tops and leaves (5:1) extract (Hypericum perforatum) 450 mg • Cordyceps Cs-4 Mushroom Mycleia (Cordyceps sinensis [Berk.] Sacc.) 750 mg. Other Ingredient: Gelatin.

Bio Trim — Dial Herbs
Ma Huang • Kola Nut • Ginger • White Willow • Ginkgo Biloba • Bladderwrack • Fo-Ti • Hawthorn berries • Saw Palmetto • Beet Powder • Chromium Proteinate • Zinc Picolinate • Boron Proteinate • Chromium Picolinate • Kola Nut extract.

BioChoice Immune Support — Legacy USA
Each packet contains: Vitamin A 5000 IU • Vitamin C 60 mg • Vitamin D3 400 IU • Vitamin E 30 IU • Niacin 20 mg • Folic Acid 0.4 mg • Pantothenic Acid 10 mg • Vitamin B6 2 mg • Vitamin B2 (Riboflavin) 1.7 mg • Vitamin B1 (Thiamin) 1.5 mg • Vitamin B12 6 mcg • Biotin 0.3 mg • Calcium 100 mg • Copper 0.6 mg • Iodine 45 mcg • Iron 5.4 mg • Magnesium 10 mg • Phosphorus 120 mg • Zinc 4.5 mg • Vitamin K1 80 mcg • Manganese 0.6 mg • Chromium 36 mcg. Other ingredients: DCV patented protein blend (egg powder, soy protein isolate, lactose free milk protein), fructose, sugar, cocoa (chocolate only), natural flavors, artificial flavors (strawberry only), oat fiber (chocolate only), maltodextrin (vanilla and strawberry only), soy lecithin, guar gum, salt, carrageenan, xantham gum. Available in Chocolate, Vanilla, and Strawberry flavors.

Bio-EFA Borage Oil 90 — Health From The Sun
Each capsule contains: Cis-Linoleic Acid (Omega-6) 190 mg • Gamma-Linolenic Acid (GLA) (Omega-6) 90 mg • Oleic Acids (Omega-9) 75 mg. Ingredients: 100% Pure Borage oil 500 mg. No sugar, starch, artificial preservatives, or colors.

Bioflora & Bioflora Powder — PhysioLogics
Each caplet contains: Fructooligosaccharides (FOS) 500 mg • Lactobacillus acidophilus 180 mg • Lactobacillus Bulgaricus 30 mg • Streptococcus Thermophilus 30 mg.

BioGinkgo 27/7 — Pharmanex
Ginkgo biloba leaf extract 50:1 concentration standardized to contain 27% ginkgo flavone glycosides and 7% terpene lactones 60 mg.

BioGreens — The Vitamin Shoppe
Three teaspoons contain: Organically grown wheatgrass, alfalfa 1923 mg • Soy Lecithin (99% oil-free, 97% phosphatides) 1862 mg • Royal Jelly, Bee Pollen, Honey Extract 1070 mg • Spirulina, Chlorella 700 mg • Vegetable Concentrate (carrot, spinach, bean sprout, celery, tomato, daikon) 700 mg • High Pectin Fruit Fibers (apple, banana, pineapple, papaya) 500 mg • Fructooligosacharides from Chicory root 400 mg • Dairy-Free Probiotic Cultures (Lactobacillus acidophilus, L. bifidus, L. plantarum, L. rhamnosus, S. thermopilus) 360 mg •

Wheat Germ Extract 350 mg • Vitamin E 120 IU • Acerola Berry Powder 120 mg • Licorice Root Extract 120 mg • Brown Rice 112 mg • Red Beet Extract 90 mg • Lipase 0.5 units • Amylase 0.5 skb units • Protease 10 hut • Aloe Vera 50 mg • Green Tea extract 30 mg • Reishi Mushroom 30 mg • Cat's Claw Extract 30 mg • Yucca Root Extract 30 mg • Ginger Root 30 mg • Ginkgo Biloba 20 mg • Bilberry Extract (25% anthocyanidins) 20 mg • Garcinia Extract 20 mg • Konjac Yam extract 20 mg • Maltodextrin 900 mg. Plus 60 mg of the following herbal extracts: Milk Thistle, Siberian Ginseng, Echinacea, American Ginseng.

Bio-Guard — Progressive Labs
Micellized antioxidant formula. Two mL contain: Vitamin A 10000 IU • Beta Carotene 2500 IU • Vitamin C 50 mg • Vitamin E 100 IU • Selenium (as selenomethionine) 50 mcg.

BioLax — Body Wise International, Inc.
Two caplets contain: Aloe Vera leaf extract 200:1 500 mg • Senna leaf 400 mg • Prune fruit 250 mg • Fig fruit 200 mg • Psyllium whole husks 100 mg • Celery seed 100 mg • Green Barley Grass 100 mg • Cruciferous Vegetables 100 mg • Lactobacillus Acidophilus 100 mg • Anise Seed

BioPectin — Flora
Modified citrus pectin.

Biopure E 400 — Dial Herbs
Natural Vitamin E (soy-free d-alpha tocopherol) • Medium Chain Triglycerides (coconut) • Oleic Acid (canola oil). Capsule Shell: (gelatin, vegetable glycerine, water).

Biovital Plus — Enzymatic Therapy
Vitamin A (Beta Carotene) non-toxic form of Vitamin A 40000 IU • Vitamin A Fish Liver oil 25000 IU • Vitamin E (D-Tocopherol Succinate) 800 IU • Vitamin D Fish Liver oil 600 IU • Vitamin C (Ascorbic Acid/Rose Hips) 3000 mg • Calcium (Carbonate, Citrate, Aspartate, Gluconate) 625 mg • Potassium Aspartate 375 mg • Magnesium Aspartate 375 mg • Pantothenic Acid (D-Calcium Pantothenate) 250 mg • Thiamine HCL (Vitamin B1) 250 mg • Niacin/ Niacinamide 250 mg • Manganese (Aspartate) 186 mg • Vitamin B6 (Pyridoxine HCL) 150 mg • Riboflavin (Vitamin B2/Liver) 100 mg • Zinc (Aspartate) 92 mg • Iron (Aspartate) 60 mg • Copper (Aspartate) 2 mg • Biotin 1 mg • Folic Acid 800 mcg • Chromium Aspartate 428 mcg • Iodine (Kelp) 225 mcg • Selenium (Aspartate) 120 mcg • Vitamin B12/Liver (Cyanocobalamin) 100 mcg • Other ingredients: Choline Bitartrate/Liver 750 mg • Bromelain (600 MCU) 400 mg • Pancreatic Enzymes (10X) 400 mg • PABA (Para Aminobenzoic Acid) 250 mg • Citrus Bioflavonoids 250 mg • Lipase 200 mg • L-Methionine 200 mg • Trace Mineral Complex Containing 72 trace minerals 200 mg • Alfalfa juice concentrate 200 mg • Liver concentrate (20X) 200 mg • Multi-Glandular concentrate 200 mg • Adrenal extract freeze-dried 200 mg • Thymus extract freeze-dried 200 mg • Saw Palmetto Berry extract 4:1 (Serenoa repens) 125 mg • Ma Huang extract (Ephedra sinensis) standardized to contain 6% Ephedrine 125 mg • Sarsaparilla root 4:1 (Smilax officinalis) 125 mg • Inositol 100 mg. Contains no sugar, salt, yeast, wheat, corn, dairy products, coloring, flavoring, or preservatives.

Bitters Virtue — Blessed Herbs
Aloe • Myrrh Gum • Senna • Camphor • Turkey Rhubarb root • Zedoary root • Manna • Carline Thistle • Angelica root • Licorice root • Fennel seed • Anise seed • Pomeranz peel • Gentian root • Galangal root & Peach brandy.

Black Cohosh Standardized Extract — Now
Two capsules contain: Black Cohosh root & rhizome 160 mg • (Cimicfuga racemosa) standardized to contain 2.5% total triterpene Glycosides, calculated as 27-Deoxyactein) 4 mg • Licorice root 250 mg • Dong Quai root (Angelica sinensis) 250 mg.

Black Cohosh-Blue Cohosh Virtue — Blessed Herbs
Black Cohosh root • Blue Cohosh root • Ginger root • Beth root • Grain alcohol & Distilled Water.

Black Currant 1000 — Health From The Sun
Each capsule contains: Alpha-Linolenic Acid (ALA) (Omega-3) 130 mg • Gamma-Linolenic Acid (Omega-6) 170 mg • Linoleic Acid (Omega-6) 430 mg • Oleic Acid (Omega-9) 90 mg • Stearidonic Acid (Omega -3) 25 mg. Ingredients: Black Currant seed oil, Gelatin, Glycerine, Water.

Black Currant 500 — Health From The Sun
Each capsule contains: Alpha-Linolenic Acid (ALA)(Omega-3) 65 mg

© Copyright 2000, Natural Medicines Comprehensive Database (209) 472-2244. For updated data, go to www.NaturalDatabase.com. • 1305

B R A N D   N A M E S

• Gamma-Linolenic Acid (GLA)(Omega-6) 85 mg • Linoleic Acid (Omega-6) 215 mg • Oleic Acid (Omega-9) 45 mg • Stearidonic Acid (Omega-3) 12 mg. Ingredients: Black Currant seed oil, Gelatin, Glycerine, Water.

Black Currant seed oil — Nutri-Quest
Each capsule contains: Black Currant seed oil 250 mg • Fatty Acid composition %: Gamma Linolenic 16.9% • Linoleic 45.2% • Oleic 12.7% • Alpha Linolenic 11.7% • Palmitic 7.4% • Stearidonic 2.9% • Stearic 1.6% • Eicosenoic Acid 1.1%. Other Ingredients: Myristic, Arachidic, Behenic, Lignoceric, Palmitoleic Acids with nautral Vitamin E 5 IU.

Black Ointment — 1st Herb Source
Chaparral herb • Lobelia herb • Comfrey herb • Red Clover herb • Plantain root • Golden Seal root • Myrrh gum • Marshmallow root • Mullein herb • Chickweed herb. In a base of Olive oil, Beeswax, Pine Tar, Vitamin E oil.

Blackstrap Molasses with Iron — Swanson
Each tablet contains: Blackstrap Molasses with 29 mg of Iron.

Bladderwrack-Dandelion Virtue — Blessed Herbs
Ma Huang • Guarana seed • Dandelion blend of flower, leaf & root • Bladderwrack • Grain alcohol & Distilled Water.

BLF # Breathe Easy Without Stimulants — Health Center for Better Living
Two tablets contain: Siberian Ginseng root extract (0.8% eleutherosides) 250 mg • American Ginseng root 250 mg • Ginger root standardized extract (5% gingerols) • Peppermint leaf 75 mg • Chickweed herb (aerial parts) 50 mg • Myrrh resin 50 mg • Mullein leaf 50 mg • Yerba Mate leaf (20% alkaloids) • MSM (methyisul-foraimethan, 36% organic sulfur) 1,000 mg.

BLF #1 Clear Complexion — Health Center for Better Living
Each capsule contains: Burdock Root 84 mg • Dandelion Root 84 mg • Red Clover tops 84 mg • Echinacea root 56 mg • Yellow Dock root 56 mg • Capsicum 28 mg • Alfalfa Leaf 28 mg • Valerian Root 28 mg.

BLF #12 Cholest-A Ingredients — Health Center for Better Living
Each capsule contains: Hawthorn Berry 113 mg • Fenugreek Seed 75 mg • Capsicum 75 mg • Plantain Herb 75 mg • Red Clover Blossom 75 mg • Black Cohosh Root 38 mg.

BLF #125 Woman's Balance — Health Center for Better Living
Each capsule contains: Dong Quai Root 102 mg • Damiana Leaf 61 mg • Kelp Atlantic 61 mg • Sarsaparilla Root 61 mg • Saw Palmetto Berry 41 mg • Chickweed Herb 41 mg • Capsicum 41 mg • Black Cohosh Root 41 mg.

BLF #13 Body Circulation — Health Center for Better Living
Each capsule contains Capsicum 84 mg • Bayberry Bark 34 mg • Hyssop Leaf 17 mg • Skullcap 17 mg • Witch Hazel Bark 17 mg.

BLF #16 Colon Helper — Health Center for Better Living
Each capsule contains: Slippery Elm Bark 145 mg • Aloe 145 mg • White Oak Bark 73 mg • Blue Vervain Herb 73 mg • Gentain Root 36 mg • Goldenseal Herb 15 mg.

BLF #17 Regularity Ingredients — Health Center for Better Living
Each capsule contains: Buckthorn Bark 113 mg • Cascara Sagrada Bark 113 mg • Chickweed Herb 75 mg • Elder Flower 75 mg • Oregon Grape Root 38 mg • Mandrake Root 38 mg.

BLF #2 Allergy First Aid — Health Center for Better Living
Each caplet contains: Allergy Herbal Blend (Hyssop whole plant, Mullein leaves, Thyme whole plant, Chrysanthemum flower, Magnolia flower, Angelica root, Vitex fruit, Atractylodes Rhizome, Bellflower root, Field Mint, Immature Tangerine peel, Ledebouriella root, Moutan bark, Perilla leaf and Schizonepeta stem) 200 mg • Boswellia Gum resin (40% boswellic acid) 100 mg • Yerba Mate leaf (20% alkaloids) 50 mg.• Meadowsweet 4:1 extract 50 mg • Eucalyptus leaf extract 25 mg • Fennel seed 25 mg.

BLF #21 Endless Energy — Health Center for Better Living
Each capsule contains: Ginseng Root 75 mg • Foti Root • Bee Pollen Granules 75 mg • Damiana Leaf 75 mg • Capsicum 50 mg • Kola Nut 50 mg • Echinacea Root 25 mg • Licorice Root 25 mg.

BLF #225 Man's Rejuvenator — Health Center for Better Living
Each capsule contains: Saw Palmetto Berry 75 mg • Cornsilk 75 mg • Gota Kola Herb 75 mg • Damiana Leaf 75 mg • Juniper Berry 38 mg • Kelp Atlantic 38 mg • Parsley Leaf 38 mg • Uva Ursi Leaf 38 mg.

BLF #23 Vision Booster — Health Center for Better Living
Vitamin A [as retinyl palmitate and 75% as beta-carotene with natural mixed carotenoids (alpha-carotene, beta-carotene, cryptoxanthin, zeaxanthin and lutein)] 10,000 IU • Vitamin C (as ascorbic acid) 250 mg • Vitamin E (as d-alpha-tocopheryl succinate and 50% as dl-alpha-tocopheryl acetate) 100 IU • Selenium (as selenomethionine) 100 mcg • Bilberry Herb blend [Bilberry leaf and Bilberry fruit standardized extract (25% anthocyanins)] 75 mg • Eyebright herb blend [Eyebright herb and eyebright herb 4:1 extract (whole plant)] 75 mg • Lutein (from marigold flower) 5 mg • L-Glutathione 5 mg • Taurine 5 mg • Quercetin dihydrate 75 mg • Lycium berry 5:1 extract 50 mg.

BLF #24 Fresh Start — Health Center for Better Living
Alfalfa • Hyssop • Chamomile • Cornsilk • Vitamins and minerals with antioxidant and diuretic qualities.

BLF #3 Love Formula — Health Center for Better Living
Two caplets contain: Tribulus terrestris extract (20% furanosterois) fruit and root 400 mg • Damiana 125 mg • Fo-ti root 125 mg • Gota Kola leaf extract (10% total asiaticosides) 50 mg • Saw Palmetto berry extract (85-95% sterols and fatty acid) 150 mg • Korean Ginseng root extract (10% ginsenosides) 200 mg.

BLF #30 Head-X — Health Center for Better Living
Each capsule contains: Fenugreek Seed 107 mg • Feverfew Herb 107 mg • Passion Flower Herb 43 mg • Rosemary leaf 43 mg • Peppermint Leaf 43 mg • Thyme leaf 21 mg • Marjoram leaf 21 mg • Blue Violet leaf 21 mg • Wood Betony Herb 21 mg • Lobelia Herb 21 mg.

BLF #31 Healthy Heart — Health Center for Better Living
Each capsule contains: Angelica Root 45 mg • Blue Cohosh Root 45 mg • Borage Herb 45 mg • Capsicum 45 mg • Blue Vervain Herb 45 mg • Peppermint Leaf 45 mg • Wood Betony Herb 45 mg • Sheep Sorrel Herb 23 mg • Garlic Bulb 23 mg • Barberry Bark 23 mg • Goldenseal Root 23 mg • Motherwort Herb 23 mg • Scullcap Herb 23 mg.

BLF #35 Sleep Like a Baby — Health Center for Better Living
Each capsule contains: Hops flower 113 mg • Passion flower 113 mg • Scullcap Herb 75 mg • Catnip Leaf 38 mg • Peppermint Leaf 38 mg • Rosemary Leaf 38 mg • Mullein Leaf 38 mg.

BLF #38 Kidney Flush — Health Center for Better Living
Each caplet contains: Vitamin B6 (as pyridoxine HCl) 5 mg • Magnesium (as magnesium oxide) • Potassium (as potassium citrate) • Uva Ursi Leaf standardized extract (20% arbutin) 100 mg • Chokeberry fruit standardized extract (35% quinic acid) 100 mg • Cranberry juice 10:1 concentrate 50 mg • Dandelion root standardized extract (20% taraxasterol) 50 mg • Aloe Vera 200x gel (25 mg) • Herbal Blend [Couchgrass (whole plant), Buchu leaf, Uva Uris leaf, Juniper berry, Hydrangea root, and Cornsilk stylus)] 200 mg.

BLF #41 Liver De-Tox — Health Center for Better Living
Each capsule contains: Fennel Seed 107 mg • Chicory Root 107 mg • Angelica Root 54 mg • Cleavers Herb 54 mg • Dandelion Root 27 mg • Gentian Root 27 mg • Hops Flower 27 mg • Elder Flower 27 mg • Wormwood Herb 11 mg • Lobelia Herb 11 mg.

BLF #42 Prime Lung — Health Center for Better Living
Each capsule contains: Mullein leaf 101 mg • Coltsfoot Herb 101 mg • Chickweed Herb 67 mg • Fenugreek Seed 34 mg • Pennyroyal Leaf 34 mg • Myrrh Gum 34 mg • Yarrow Flower 34 mg • Nettle Leaf 34 mg • Lobelia Herb 13 mg.

BLF #43 Bone & Nail Builder — Health Center for Better Living
Each Capsule contains: Bee Pollen Granules 87 mg • Horsetail 43 mg • Oatstraw 43 mg • Kelp Atlantic 43 mg • Ginseng root 43 mg • Foti root 43 mg • Chamomile flower 43 mg • Rose hips 43 mg • Red Clover blossom 43 mg • Lobelia Herb 17 mg.

BLF #44 Woman's Change — Health Center for Better Living
Two tablets contain: Black Cohosh root extract (2.5% triterpene glycosides) 160 mg • Dong Quai root extract 1% lingustilide) 200 mg

• Chaste Tree berry extract (5% vitexi cacpin) 100 mg • Licorice Root extract (13% glycyrrhizin) 100 mg • Soybean and Kudzu root extract (20% total isoflavones) 150 mg • Damiana leaf 100 mg • Wild Yam root extract (5% diosgenin) 150 mg • Red Clover flowers 100 mg.

BLF #47 Rest Ease Ingredients — Health Center for Better Living
Each capsule contains: Valerian Root 101 mg • Wintergreen Leaf 67 mg • Peppermint Leaf 67 mg • Spearmint Leaf 67 mg • Sassafras Root Bark 34 mg • Capsicum 34 mg • Burdock root 34 mg • Buckthorn bark 34 mg • Lobelia Herb 13 mg.

BLF #48 Anti-Stress — Health Center for Better Living
Each capsule contains: Hops flower 99 mg • Valerian root 99 mg • Scullcap Herb 66 mg • Catnip leaf 66 mg • Passion Flower Herb 66 mg • Red Clover Herb 33 mg • Black Cohosh Root 20 mg.

BLF #49 Stable Sugar — Health Center for Better Living
Each capsule contains: Juniper Berries 94 mg • Uva Ursi Leaf 94 mg • Garlic Bulb 94 mg • Dandelion Root 47 mg • Capsicum 47 mg • Mullein Leaf 47 mg • Licorice Root 28 mg.

BLF #52 Fatigue Fighter — Health Center for Better Living
Prime Ingredients: Capsicum • Ginseng.

BLF #53 Male Vigor — Health Center for Better Living
Two caplets contain: Yohimbe bark extract (2% yohimbe, 4% total alkaiods) 500 mg • Tribulus terrestris extract (20% furanosterols) fruit and root • Korean Ginseng root extract (10% ginsenosides) 200 mg • Yerba Mate leaf extract (20% total alkaloids) 125 mg • Saw Palmetto berry extract (85-95% sterols and fatty acid) 160 mg • Male support blend (Damiana leaf, Fo-ti root, Gota Kola leaf, and Pumpkin Seed concentrate) 250 mg.

BLF #54 Sinus & Hayfever Ingredients — Health Center for Better Living
Each capsule contains: Myrrh Gum 148 mg • Echinacea Root 74 mg • Bayberry Bark 74 mg • Plantain Herb 74 mg • Saw Palmetto Berry 22 mg • Licorice Root 22 mg • Goldenseal Herb.

BLF #55 Pro Skin Enhancer — Health Center for Better Living
Each capsule contains: Red Clover Blossom 115 mg • Spikenard root 115 mg • Dandelion root 58 mg • Chickweed Herb 29 mg • Plantain Herb 29 mg • Blue Vervain Herb 29 mg • Sarsaparilla root 29 mg • Buckthorn bark 29 mg • Goldenseal root 17 mg.

BLF #57 Vein Vanish — Health Center for Better Living
Each capsule contains: White Oak Bark 87 mg • Witch Hazel Bark 87 mg • Bayberry Bark 87 mg • Capsicum 87 mg • Kelp Atlantic 43 mg • Goldenseal Root 43 mg • Lobelia Herb 17 mg.

BLF #59 Weight Loss — Health Center for Better Living
Each capsule contains: Nettle Leaf 139 mg • Chickweed Herb 93 mg • Seawrack 93 mg • Kelp Atlantic 35 mg • Fennel Seed 23 mg • Hawthorn Berry 23 mg • Dandelion Root 12 mg • Echinacea Root 12 mg • Burdock Root 12 mg • Licorice Root 5 mg • Chia Seed 5 mg.

BLF #6 Healthy Joints — Health Center for Better Living
Burdock • Alfalfa • Kelp • Vitamin C • Vitamin E • Vitamin B6.

BLF #61 P.M.S. Stop — Health Center for Better Living
Each capsule contains: Black Cohosh Root 82 mg • Dong Quai Root 82 mg • Red Raspberry Leaf 82 mg • Chaste Tree Berry 57 mg • Ginger Root 49 mg • Dandelion Root 41 mg • Motherwort Herb 33 mg • Valerian Root 25 mg.

BLF #75 Prostate Support — Health Center for Better Living
Two tablets contain: Zinc (as zinc glycinate) 15 mg • Saw Palmetto berry extract (85-95% sterols and fatty acid) 320 mg • Pygeum bark 4:1 extract 100 mg • Pumpkin seed 10:1 concentrate 100 mg • Tomato lycopene concentrate (10,000 lycopene) 100 mg • Urinary tract support blend [Chokeberry extract (35% quinic acid), Cranberry juice 10:1 concentrate, Uva-Ursi leaf extract (20% arbutin)].

BLF #9: 120 Over 80 — Health Center for Better Living
Two tablets contain: Calcium (as calcium carbonate and calcium citratemalate-glycinate) 500 mg • Magnesium (as magnesium oxide and magnesium amino acid chelate) 200 mg • Potassium (as postassium citrate) • Ginger root extract (5% gingerols) 100 mg • Odor-controlled Garlic Extract (10,000 ppm allicin) 300 mg • Hawthorn berry extract (5% flavonoid glycosides) 250 mg • Capsicum pepper 50 mg • Panax Ginseng root extract (10% ginsenosides) 100 mg • Onion bulb 50 mg • Parsley leaf 50 mg.

Blood Pressure — Nutrivention
Three tablets contain: Vitamin B6 100 mg • Calcium 50 mg • Potassium 45 mg • Magnesium 30 mg • Manganese 15 mg • Vitamin D 50 IU • Hawthorne berries 500 mg • Apple Pectin 500 mg • Garlic powder concentrate 500 mg • Cayenne pepper 500 mg • Black Cohosh 300 mg • Valerian root (Star root) 200 mg • Hops 200 mg • L-Taurine 100 mg.

Blood Sugar Balance — ProHerbs
Two tablets contain: Biotin 600 mcg • Magnesium (as Oxide) 200 mg • Zinc (as Sulfate) 30 mg • Gymnema Sylvestre leaves (standardized to 24% Gymnemic Acid) 300 mg • Bitter Melon powder (Momordica charantia fruit) 200 mg • Ginkgo Biloba leaf (standardized to 24% flavonoids glycosides & 6% terpene lactones) 120 mg • Chromium Picolinate 400 mcg • Alpha Lipoic Acid 150 mg • Quercetin 50 mg • Vanadium (as Vanadyl Pentoxide) 40 mcg. Other ingredients: Dicalcium Phosphate, Microcrystalline Cellulose, Croscarmellose Sodium, Hydroxypropylmethylcellulose, Magnesium Stearate, Mineral Oil, Polyethylene Glycol, Stearic Acid, Titanium Dioxide, Sodium Lauryl Sulfate, FD&C Yellow #6 Lake, Red #40 Lake, Iron Oxide.

Blood Sugar Blues — The Herbalist
Devil's Club root bark • Blueberry leaf • Dandelion root • Oregon Grape root • Uva Ursi leaf • Juniper berry • Licorice root • Elecampane root.

Blood Sugar Formula — Nature's Way
Three capsules contain: Bilberry leaf 255 mg • Bitter Melon dried extract 150 mg • Caromix (Mixed Carotenoids) 30 mg • Chromium Polynicotinate 300 mcg • Fenugreek dried extract 210 mg • Gymnema sylvestre dried extract 66 mg • Prickly Pear leaf pad 420 mg. Other ingredients: Gelatin, Magnesium Stearate, Millet.

Blubberwack — The Herbalist
Bladderwrack • Gotu Kola herb • Kelp • Echinacea root • Kola Nut • Licorice root.

Blue Green Algae from Upper Klamath Lake — Futurebiotics
Blue-Green algae 500 mg.

Blue-Green Connection — HealthWatchers System
Spirulina• Chlorella• Klamath Lake Algae• Ginkgo Biloba• CoQ10. Wheatgrass • Alfalfa • Chlorophyll.

Body Guard — Jamieson
Chlorhexidine Gluconate • Glycerin • Nonoxynol-9 • Witch Hazel Herbal Extract.

Body Smoothing Lotion — Cellex-C
Ascorbic Acid • Vitamin E • Tomato extract • Evening Primrose oil • Tyrosine • Zinc • Glycine • Hyaluronic Acid • Aloe Vera extract • Chamomile extract • Allantoin • Bioflavonoids.

Bone & Joint Care — Natrol
Three capsules contain: Vitamin D (as cholecalciferol) 20 IU • Vitamin K (as Phytonadione) 10 mcg • Calcium (as calcium carbonate & calcium citrate) 250 mg • Magnesium (as Magnesium oxide) 125 mg • Zinc (as zinc citrate) 5 mg • Copper (as copper gluconate) 100 mcg • Glucosamine Sulfate 250 mg • MSM (Mehtyl Sulfonyl Methane) 250 mg • IpriFlavone 100 mg • Sea Cucumber 100 mg Mucopolysaccharides (26%) 26 mg • Horsetail grass 100 mg • Silica (8%) 8 mg • Bamboo 100 mg • Salicylic Acid 10 mg • Boron 2 mg. Other ingredients: Silicon Dioxide, Magnesium Stearate, Gelatin.

Bone & Joints — ProHerbs
Three tablets contain: Vitamin D (D3) 240 IU • Calcium (as Calcium Carbonate) 1005 mg • Isoflavones (as Soy standardized extract) 60 mg • Glucosamine Sulfate 510 mg • Chondroitin Sulfate 405 mg • Boron 4.5 mg. Other Ingredients: Croscarmellose Sodium, Hydroxypropylmethylcellulose, Magnesium Stearate, Mineral Oil, Polyethylene Glycol, Stearic Acid, Titanium Dioxide, Sodium Lauryl Sulfate, Iron Oxide.

Bone 350 Plus — Atrium
Each tablet contains: Raw Calf Bone concentrate 350 mg • Equisetum (Horsetail Rush) 150 mg.

Bone Builder — Schiff
Three tablets contain: Calcium (Carbonate, Chelate, Citrate-Malate) 1000 mg • Magnesium (Oxide, Chelate) 400 mg • Vitamin D3 (Cholecalciferol) 400 IU • Vitamin C (Ascorbic Acid) 150 mg • Vitamin K (Phytonadione) 25 mcg • Vitamin B6 (Pyridoxine,

BRAND NAMES

Coenzyme Pyridoxal-5-Phosphate) 10 mg • Vitamin B12 (Cyanocobalamin, Coenzyme Dibencozide) 25 mcg • Folic Acid (Folic Acid, Coenzyme Tetrahydrafolate) 200 mcg • Boron (Chelate) 1 mg • Zinc (Optizinc) 7.5 mg • Copper (Lysinate) 1 mg • Manganese (Glycinate) 10 mg • Molybdenum (Chelate) 50 mcg • Silica (Magnesium Trisillicate) 25mg • Strontium (Chloride) 100 mcg • Vanadium (Vanadyl Sulfate) 50 mcg • Sulphur (Vanadyl Sulfate) 30 mcg • Betaine HCl 50 mg • Glucose Polymers (Maltodextrin) 50 mcg • Citrus Bioflavonoids Complex 250 mg • Fennel (4:1 extract) 100 mg • Black Cohosh (4:1 extract) 100 mg • Blessed Thistle (4:1 extract) 100 mg. Natural base: Cellulose, Vegetable Sterates, Silica.

Bone Building Hair Teeth & Nails Formula — Youngevity
Calcium 250 mg • Magnesium 100 mg • Manganese 0.5 mg • Boron 240 mg • Vitamin D3 150 IU • Horsetail grass 25 mg • Rose Hips 25 mg • Vilcabamba Mineral Essence: Potassium, Calcium, Magnesium, Zinc, Chromium, Selenium, Iron, Copper, Molybdenum, Vanadium, Iodine, Cobalt, Manganese.

Bone Calcium — Now
Four tablets contain: Calcium (from 4000 mg Microcrystalline Hydroxyapatite) 1000 mg • Magnesium (from 835 mg Magnesium Oxide) 500 mg • Phosphorus (Hydroxyapatite) 500 mg • Zinc (Amino Acid Chelate) 15 mg • Copper (Amino Acid Chelate) 2 mg • Vitamin D (Cholecalciferol) 200 IU • Manganese (Amino Acid Chelate) 7 mg • Boron (Amino Acid Chelate) 3 mg.

Bone Formula — Pharmanex
Two capsules contain: Vitamin C (as Calcium Ascorbate Complex - Ester C) 60 mg • Vitamin D3 (as Cholecalciferol) 50 IU • Vitamin K1 (as Phytonadione) 20 mcg • Calcium (as Calcium Carbonate, Calcium Propionate) 250 mg • Magnesium (as Magnesium Asparate, Magnesium Oxide) 125 mg • Isoflavones (from Soy Extract) 12.5 mg • Silicon (as Sodium Metasilicate) 5 mg • Boron (as Boron Citrate) 1.5 mg. Other Ingredients: Magnesium Stearate, Sodium Carboxymethylcellulose.

Bone Health — Centrum Focused Formulas
Two tablets contain: Vitamin D 200 IU • Calcium Citrate 500 mg • Magnesium 40 mg • Zinc 7.5 mg • Copper 1 mg • Manganese 1.8 mg • Boron 250 mcg • Lycopene 1.5 mg • Saw Palmetto standardized Lipophilic fruit extract (Serenoa repens) 160 mg.

Bone Maximizer with MCHC — Metabolic Response Modifiers
Six capsules contain: Microcrystalline Hydroxyapatite (MCHC) 4000 mg • Calcium (from MCHC) 1000 mg • Protein (From MCHC) 1000 mg • Phosphorus (from MCHC) 500 mg • Magnesium Glycinate 500 mg • Zinc (Citrate) 18 mg • Boron (Citrate) 2 mg • Horsetail extract 25 mg • Vitamin D3 (Cholecalciferol) 480 IU • Vitamin K1 (Phylloquinone) 120 mcg • Vitamin C (Ascorbate) 72 mg • MSM (Kmethyl Sulfonyl Methane) 120 mg • Glucosamine 120 mg • Pregnenolone 10 mg.

Bone Protector with Ostivone — Natrol
Six capsules contain: Calcium (as calcium citrate) 1200 mg • 7-Isopropoxy-Isoflavone 600 mg. Other ingredients: Rice powder, Magnesium Stearate, Gelatin.

Bone Renew with Ostivone — Source Naturals
Four tablets contain: Calcium (as Calcium Citrate, Ethanolamine Phosphate and Malate) 800 mg • Ipriflavone (Ostivone) 600 mg.

Bone Support — TwinLab
Four tablets contain: Vitamin D (from Cholecalciferol) 800 IU • Calcium (from Calcium Citrate & Carbonate) 1500 mg • Magnesium (from Magnesium Aspartate & Oxide) 750 mg • Ostivone (Ipriflavone) (7-Isopropoxy Isoflavone) 600 mg • Novasoy Phytoestrogen extract (containing 40 mg of Soy Isoflavones) 100 mg • Boron (from Boron Citrate, Glycinate & Aspartate) 3 mg. Other Ingredients: Pharmaceutical Glaze, Cellulose, Stearic Acid Sodium Lauryl Sulfate, Magnesium Stearate, Colloidal Silicon Dioxide.

Borage oil 240 — Health From The Sun
Each capsule contains: Gamma-Linolenic Acid (GLA) (Omega-6) 240 mg • Linoleic Acid (Omega-6) 370 mg • Oleic Acid (Omega-9) 15 mg. Ingredients: Borage seed oil, Gelatin, Glycerine, Water.

Borage oil 300 — Health From The Sun
Each capsule contains: Gamma-Linolenic Acid (GLA) (Omega-6) 300 mg • Linoleic Acid (Omega-6) 480 mg • Oleic Acid (Omega-9) 190 mg. Ingredients: Borage seed oil, Gelatin, Glycerine, Water.

Borage-Licorice Virtue — Blessed Herbs
Borage • Astragalus root • Licorice root • Siberian Ginseng root • Wild American Ginseng root • Suma root • Reishi mycelium • Ginger root • Grain alcohol & Distilled water.

Boron Complex Plus — The Vitamin Shoppe
Four capsules contain: Boron 3 mg • Calcium 1000 mg • Magnesium 500 mg • Vitamin D3 400 IU • Zinc 15 mg • Manganese 5 mg • Copper 500 mcg • Betaine HCl 324 mg.

Botanaflor — Pharmanex
Each capsule contains: Jerusalem Artichole with Fructooligosaccharides 100 mg • Cellulose Powder 100 mg • Citrus Pectin 98 mg • Apple Pectin Fiber 66 mg • Konjac Root (Glucomannan) 59 mg • Date Fiber 52 mg • Prune Fiber 48 mg • Soybean Fiber 43 mg • Papaya Powder with Papain 30 mg • Pineapple Powder with Bromelain 30 mg • Bifidobacterium Bifidum 30 mg • Lactobacillus Acidophilus.

Botaname — Pharmanex
Two capsules contain: Garcinia Cambogia 500 mg • Peppermint powder 104 mg • Brewer's Yeast 100 mg • Cinnamon Ramulus powder 86 mg • Lemon Verabanae powder 86 mg • Chamomile flower powder 69 mg • Ginger root powder 69 mg • Chinese Licorice root extract 35 mg • Sweet Citrus Peel 35 mg • Chicory powder 16 mg.

Bovine Cartilage Plus — Atrium
Each capsule contains: Freeze Dried Bovine Cartilage 600 mg • Freeze Dried Soluble Trachea Substance 150 mg. Contains no sugar, starch, salt, wheat, corn or soy derivatives.

Bowel Support — Amazon Support
Each capsule contains: Cat's Claw • Macela • Jatoba • Jurubeba • Papaya • Carqueja.

Brain Actives — VitaStore
Six tablets contain: Gingko Biloba (24% Flavoneglycosides, 6% Terpene Lactones) 100 mg • Phosphatidylserine 300 mg • L-Methionine 300 mg • OPC Complex (Pine Bark & Grapeseed Extracts) 100 mg • Vitamin B1 (Thiamine) 1.5 mg • Vitamin B2 (Riboflavin) 1.5 mg • Vitamin B3 (Niacin) 20 mg • Vitamin B5 (Pantothenic Acid) 10 mg • Vitamin B6 (Pyridoxine) 2 mg • Vitamin B12 6 mcg • Lecithin 1000 mcg • Acetyl L-Carnitine 500 mg • L-Glutamine 250 mg • Manganese 35 mg.

Brain Alert — Nutrapathic
Two tabs contain: Vitamin B1 10 mg • Vitamin B6 20 mg • Vitamin B12 40 mcg • Niacin 10 mg • Niacinamide 10 mg • Biotin 30 mcg • Choline Bitartrate 20 mg • Inositol 10 mg • PABA 20 mg • Vitamin F 4 mg • Calcium 20 mg • Chloride 4 mg • Copper 4 mg • Magnesium 10 mg • Manganese 6 mg • Phosphorus 10 mg • Potassium 10 mg • Selenium 10 mcg • Silica 4 mg • Zinc 20 mg. Other Ingredients: Brain, Egg Lecithin, Rye Green, Red Clover, Peppermint leaves, L-Tyrosine, L-Arginine, Lecithin Granules, Barley Green, Bee Pollen, Gotu Kola, Ginkgo, Glutamic Acid, L-Phenylalanine, L-Glutamine, DNA, RNA, Hypothalamus, Pineal, Pituitary, Valerian, Ginseng, Spirulina, Wood Betony, Bupleurum Root, Chondroitin Sulfate, CoQ10.

Brain Booster — Optimum Nutrition
Ginkgo Biloba • Siberian Ginseng.

Brain Care — Quantum
Two tablets contain: Vitamin E (d-Alpha Tocopherol) 100 IU • Phosphatidylserine complex 100 mg • Phosphatidyl Choline 95 mg • Ginkgo leaf (Ginkgo Biloba) (24% Ginkgo Flavone Glycosides) 60 mg • Alpha-Linolenic Acid (Borage Oil) 50 mg • Coenzyme Q10 30 mg • DHA (Docosahexaenoic Acid) 10 mg • EPA (Eicosahexaenoic Acid) 10 mg. In a base of Stearic acid, Gura Gum, Magnesium Stearate.

Brain Essentials — Phytopharmica
Three tablets contain: Vitamin C (Ascorbic Acid) 300 mg • Magnesium Aspartate 100 mg • Potassium Aspartate 100 mg • Zinc Aspartate 30 mg • Manganese (Chelate) 15 mg • Folic Acid 800 mcg • Vitamin B12 (Cyanocobalamin) 500 mcg • Other ingredients: L-Glutamine 300 mg • L-Phenylalanine 300 mg • Brain extract freeze-dried 300 mg • Choline (Bitartrate) 200 mg • Gamma-Aminobutyric Acid (GABA) 100 mg • Alpha-Ketoglutaric Acid 100 mg • Glycine 100 mg • L-Tyrosine 100 mg • Pituitary extract freeze-dried 65 mg • L-Methionine 50 mg • RNA/DNA Complex 50 mg • L-Cysteine 50 mg • Pyridoxal Phosphate 15 mg. Contains no sugar, salt, yeast,

wheat, corn, soy, dairy products, coloring, flavoring or preservatives. All organs & glands derived from bovine sources.

Brain Fuel — Futurebiotics
Three tablets contain: Ginkgo Biloba (24% standardized extract) 45 mg • Korean Ginseng (7% ginsenoside extract) 15 mg • American Ginseng (7% ginsenoside extract) 10 mg • Gotu Kola extract (4:1 extract equivalent to) 150 mg • Ginkgo Biloba leaves 200 mg • Gotu Kola leaves 250 mg • Chinese Licorice extract (glycyrrhiza) 150 mg • Tyrosine 150 mg • Glutamine 275 mg • Phosphatidyl Choline (55% strength) 250 mg • Vitamin C 60 mg • Vitamin E (natural succinate) 5 IU • Vitamin B6 25 mg • Folic Acid 400 mcg • Vitamin B12 25 mcg • Vitamin B5 35 mg • Potassium 200 mg • Betaine HCl 50 mg • Bromelain 50 mg • Para Amino Benzoic Acid (PABA) 75 mg • L-Methionine 75 mg • Ribonucleic Acid (RNA) 50 mg.

Brain Link Complex — Pain & Stress Center
Five tablespoons contain: Vitamin A • Vitamin C • Calcium • Iron • Vitamin D • Vitamin E • Thiamin • Riboflavin • Niacin • Vitamin B6 • Folate • Vitamin B12 • Biotin • Pantothenic Acid • Iodine • Magnesium • Zinc • Selenium • Copper • Manganese • Chromium • Molybdenum. Amino Acid Profile: Alanine 290 mg • Arginine 149 mg • Aspartic Acid 473 mg • Cystine/Cysteine 167 mg • Glutamic Acid 837 mg • Glycine 2101 mg • Histidine 103 mg • Isoleucine 485 mg • Leucine 852 mg • Lysine 521 mg • Methionine 149 mg • Phenylalanine 335 mg • Proline 242 mg • Serine 202 mg • Threonine 252 mg • Tryptophan (from natural milk & egg protein) 111 mg • Tyrosine 898 mg • Valine 478 mg • Taurine 1500 mg • GABA 1500 mg • L-Glutamine 3000 mg • Inositol 50 mg • Choline 50 mg • PABA 2 mg.

Brain Nutrition — Enzymatic Therapy
Three tablets contain: Vitamin C (Ascorbic Acid) 300 mg • Magnesium Aspartate 100 mg • Potassium Aspartate 100 mg • Zinc Aspartate 30 mg • Manganese (Chelate) 15 mg • Folic Acid 800 mcg • Vitamin B12 (Cyanocobalamin) 500 mcg • Other ingredients: L-Glutamine 300 mg • L-Phenylalanine 300 mg • Brain extract freeze-dried 300 mg • Choline (Bitatrate) 200 mg • Gamma-Aminobutyric Acid (GABA) 100 mg • Alpha-Ketoglutaric Acid 100 mg • Glycine 100 mg • L-Tyrosine 100 mg • Pituitary extract freeze-dried 65 mg • L-Methionine 50 mg • RNA-NA Complex 50 mg • L-Cysteine 50 mg • Pyridoxal Phosphate 15 mg. Contains no sugar, salt, yeast, wheat, corn, soy, dairy products, coloring, flavoring or preservatives. All organs & glands derived from bovine sources.

Brain Pep — Pep Products, Inc.
One capsule contains: Gingko Biloba • Kola Nut • Gotu Kola • Siberian Ginseng • Schizandra • Ginger • L-Glutamine 130 mg.

Brain Plus — Progressive Labs
Each capsule contains: Raw Porcine Brain concentrate 100 mg • Choline (bitartrate) 100 mg • Inositol 100 mg. This product contains naturally occuring RNA/DNA qualitatively from the brain concentrate.

BrainStorm — Allergy Research Group
Two tablets contain: Vitamin B6 15 mg • Pyridoxal-Phosphate 5 mg • Dibencoside 50 mcg • Biotin 100 mcg • Folic Acid 100 mcg • Chromium (Nicotinate) 50 mcg • Zinc (Citrate) 10 mg • Selenium 50 mcg • Molybdenum 50 mcg • Boron (Citrate) 500 mcg • L-Glutamine 250 mg • Bacosides 100 mg • L-Tyrosine 200 mg • Choline (Bitartrate) 80 mg • Inositol 50 mg • DMAE 80 mg • Acetyl-L-Carnitine 50 mg • Phosphatidyl Serine 20 mg • Vitamin E 10 IU • Vitamin C 10 mg • Ginkgo Biloba 30 mg • Siberian Ginseng 40 mg • Korean Ginseng 40 mg • Gota Kola 100 mg • Phosphatidyl Choline 250 mg • Copper Sebacate 1 mg • Beta Carotene 2000 IU • Vitamin B1 10 mg • Thiamine Tetrahydro-Furfuryl Disulfide 5 mg • Vitamin B2 (Riboflavin) 10 mg • B2 Activated (Riboflavin 5 Phosphate) 5 mg • Vitamin B3 (Niacin) 5 mg • Vitamin B3 (Niacinamide) 30 mg • Calcium Pantothenate 40 mg.

Brainwash Shampoo — Evergreen Research
Active Ingredients: Ginkgo Biloba • Grape Seed Extract. Other Ingredients: Peppermint Oil, Calendula Oil, Arnica.

Brave Hart Deer Velvet Capsules — Hart Products
300 mg of pure Deer Velvet.

Breast Care System-3 — Natrol
Calcium 24 mg • Calcium D-Glucarate 200 mg. Breast Care Formula: Selenium 50 mcg • Green Tea Extract 50 mg • Garlic 50 mg • Grape Seed Extract 20 mg. Ultra Green Breast Care Ingredients: Rice Powder, Silica, Magnesium Stearate, Gelatin.

Breast Health — ProHerbs
Two tablets contain: Vitamin C (as Ascorbic Acid) 200 mg • Selenium (as Selenomethionine) 200 mcg • Broccoli extract (20:1 extract) 170 mg • Curcumin root extract (Curcuma longa standardized to 2% curcuminoids) 600 mg • Genistein (Soy extract) 20 mg • Citrus Bioflavonoid 100 mg • Flaxseed powder 400 mg. Other Ingredients: Dicalcium Phosphate, Microcrystalline Cellulose, Croscarmellose Sodium, Stearic Acid, Magnesium Stearate, Hydroxypropylmethylcellulose, Mineral Oil, Triacetin, Titanium Dioxide, FD&C Yellow #6 Lake.

Breast Health Formula — Great American Nutrition
Two capsules contain: Calcium (as calcium d-glucarate) 24 mg • Selenium (as selenomethionine, from SelenoMax) 100 mcg • Calcium D-Glucarate 200 mg • Green Tea leaf extract (Camellia sinensis, standardized to 48% polyphenols) 200 mg • Rosemary folia extract (Rosemarinus officialis, standardized to 6% rosemaric acid) 200 mg • Soy extract (standardized to 3% isoflavones) 400 mg • Citrus peel bioflavonoids (Citrus aurantium, standardized to 25% bioflavonoids) 100 mg • Boron Aspartate 3 mg. Other Ingredient: White Rice powder.

Breath Aid — D & E Pharmaceuticals
Each tablet contains: Ephedrine 12.5 mg • Guaifenesin 100 mg.

Breath Easy — Traditional Medicinals
Contains: Pseudoephedrine: 0.5 mg per cup as it naturally occurs in the whole Ma Huang herb (Ephedra sinisa) present in the blend. Other herbal ingredients: Peppermint leaf, Licorice root, Fennel seed, Eucalyptus leaf, Pleurisy root, Calendula flower, Ginger rhizome.

Breathe-Aid Formula — Nature's Way
Two capsules contain: Proprietary Formula: Chickweed leaf & stem • Ephedra HCL • Guaifenesin • Lobelia herb • Marshmallow root • Mullein leaf. Other ingredients: Gelatin, Magnesium Stearate, Millet.

Brewer's Yeast — Nature's Life
Twelve tablets contain: Vitamin B1 1 mg • Vitamin B2 1 mg • Vitamin B6 240 mg • Choline 23 mg • Folic Acid 120 mcg • Niacin 3 mg • Inositol 23 mg • Pantothenic Acid 600 mcg • Calcium 360 mcg • Chromium 9 mcg • Copper 300mcg • Iodine 18 mcg • Iron 2 mg • Magnesium 6 mg • Manganese 30 mcg • Phosphorus 8 mg • Potassium 10 mg • Selenium 12 mcg • Sodium 460 mcg • Zinc 600 mcg. Twelve tablets also supply 2.9 g of protein as follows: Alanine 216 mg • Arginine 155mg • Aspartic Acid 302 mg • Cysteine 72 mg • Glycine 148 mg • Glutamic Acid 402 mg • Histidine (essential amino acid) 78 mg • Isoleucine (essential amino acid) 140 mg • Leucine (essential amino acid) 222 mg • Lysine(essential amino acid) 234 mg • Methionine (essential amino acid) 43 mg • Phenylalanine (essential amino acid) 135 mg • Proline 140 mg • Serine 150 mg • Threonine (essential amino acid) 143 mg • Tryptophan (essential amino acid) 50 mg • Tyrosine 81 mg • Valine (essential amino acid) 179 mg • plus all the remaining nutrients found in yeast.

Brewer's Yeast — The Vitamin Shoppe
Typical analysis per six tablets: Vitamin B1 48 mg • Vitamin B2 16 mg • Niacin 1.6 mg • Folic Acid 13 mcg • Vitamin B6 160 mcg • Choline 15 mg • Pantothenic Acid 200 mcg • Biotin 20 mcg • Inositol 15 mg. No Corn, Wheat, Soy, Salt, Sugar, Starch, Milk, Eggs, Fish or Animal Derivatives, Preservatives, Artificial Colors of Flavors added.

Brighten-Up — Changes - TwinLab
Two caplets contain: St. John's Wort standardized extract aerial parts (0.3% hypericin) 300 mg • Panax Ginseng root standardized extract (4% ginsenosides) 200 mg • Ashwagandha root (Withania somnifera) 200 mg • Green Tea leaf standardized extract (20% methylxanthines) 150 mg • Kava Kava root standardized extract (30% kavalactones) 50 mg • Siberian Ginseng root standardized extract (0.8% eleutherosides) 50 mg • Schizandra berry standardized extract 50 mg - Schizandra berry standardized extract (9% schizandrins) 50 mg. Other ingredients: Dicalcium Phosphate, Vegetable Cellulose, Fractionated vegetable oil, Soy polysaccharides, Silica, and Vegetable resin glaze.

Bright-Eyes — Futurebiotics
Three tablets contain: Bilberry extract (standardized for 25% anthocyanidins) 10 mg • Eyebright (extract equivalent to) 500 mg • Chamomile (extract equivalent to) 250 mg • Rosemary (extract equivalent to) 200 mg • Beta Carotene 20,000 IU • Vitamin A 5000 IU • Quercetin 100 mg • Citrus bioflavonoids 100 mg • Vitamin C 1000 mg • Natural Vitamin E (d-alpha succinate) 200 IU • Vitamin B2 (riboflavin) 40 mg • Rutin 100 mg • Selenium (from selenomethionine) 100 mcg • Zinc (monomethionine) 15 mg •

B R A N D   N A M E S

© Copyright 2000, Natural Medicines Comprehensive Database (209) 472-2244. For updated data, go to www.NaturalDatabase.com.

Some Brand Name Natural Products - What they Contain
www.NaturalDatabase.com contains MANY more listings than appear here.

Vitamin B6 5 mg • Niacinamide 10 mg • Pantothenic Acid (B5) 40 mg • Chromium (GTF) 200 mcg • L-Cysteine 100 mg • L-Glutamine 75 mg. In a base of: (Alfalfa, Carrot, Parsley & Dandelion).

Bromelain Forte — Ortho Molecular Products
Each capsule contains: Bromelain 1200 GDU • Papain 110 MCU.

Bromelain Joint-Ease — Nature's Life
Four capsules contain: Bromelain [an enzyme from Pineapple fruit (Ananassa sativa) activity of 1500 mg = 3000 GDU (4500 MCU)] 1500 mg • Quercetin (Dimorphandra pod) 400 mg • Vitamin C (Ascorbic Acid) 750 mg • Zinc (Picolinate, Gluconate, Citrate) 15 mg • Copper (Gluconate, Citrate) 1 mg • Manganese (Citrate, Aspartate) 3 mg.

Bromelain Plus — Enzymatic Therapy
Each tablet contains: Vitamin C (Calcium Ascorbate) 225 mg • Pantothenic Acid (D-Calcium Pantothenate) 125 mg. Other ingredients: Bromelain (1800 MCU) pineapple enzyme 750 mg. Contains no sugar, salt, yeast, wheat, corn, soy, dairy products, coloring, flavoring or preservatives.

Bromezyme — Progressive Labs
Each capsule contains: Bromelain 50 mg • Papain 20 mg • Raw Spleen concentrate 20 mg • Raw Calf thymus 10 mg.

Bronchitis Remedy — Phytopharmica
Twenty drops contain: Antimonium tartaricum 4x • Ipecacuanha 4x • Pimpinella saxifraga 2x • Cetraria islandica 1x • Eucalyptus globulus 1x. In a base of 45% USP alcohol by volume.
Editor's Comments: This is a homeopathic product. It is so extremely diluted that its activity can not be explained by conventional scientific methods. Therefore this product can not be rated by the scientific criteria used in this Database. A patient receiving the extreme dilution of this product will not receive many, if any, molecules of the original active ingredient. Therefore, there are no harmful pharmacologic effects, and any beneficial effects are controversial and not due to a direct biochemical action of the ingredient on the body. Homeopathic products are allowed for sale in the U.S. due to legislation passed in the 19th century sponsored by a homeopathic physician who was also a Senator. The law still requires that the FDA allow the sale of products listed in this Homeopathic Pharmacopea of the United States.

Bronchoril — Phytopharmica
Active Ingredient: Glycerol Guaiacolate 200 mg. Other Ingredients: Fenugreek Seed Powder 4:1 (Trigonella foenum-graecum) 350 mg • Marshmallow Extract 4:1 (Althaea officinalis) (Mucilage content 30%-40%) 125 mg • PABA (Para-Aminobenzoic Acid) 50 mg • Mullein Leaf (Verbascum nigrum) 50 mg.

Buckley's Mixture Cough Suppresant — W.K. Buckley
Each teaspoonful (5 mL) contains: Dextromethorphan Hydrobromide 12.5 mg • Ammonium Carbonate • Camphor • Canada Balsam • Carrageenan • Glycerine • Menthol • Pine Needle Oil • Sodium Butylparaben • Sodium Propylparaben • Sodium Saccharin • Tincture of Capsicum • Water.

Buffered C Powder 2000 mg — The Vitamin Shoppe
One teaspoon contains: Vitamin C (calcium ascorbate) 2000 mg • Rose Hips 1450 mg • Acerola 1000 mg • Lemon Bioflavonoids 500 mg • Rutin 25 mg • Hesperidin 25 mg • Calcium (ascorbate) 230 mg. No Yeast, Wheat, Corn, Soy, Salt, Sugar, Starch, Gluten, Dairy, Milk, Eggs, Fish Or Animal Derivatives, Preservatives, Artificial Colors or Flavors added.

Buffered TLC — Jarrow Formulas
Two teaspoons contain: Vitamin C 3000 mg • Calcium 450 mg • Magnesium 250 mg • Potassium 99 mg • L-Taurine 1,000 mg • L-Lysine 250 mg • L-Proline 250 mg • Bromelain (2,000 mcu) 300 mg. Other Ingredients: Ribose, Mannitol, L-Glycine, Natural Lime and Mandarin flavors.

Burdock-Dandelion Formula — Quest
Each caplet contains: Burdock root powder (Arctium lappa) 90 mg • Dandelion root powder (Taraxacum officinale) 90 mg • Oregon Grape root powder (Mahonia aquifolium) 90 mg • Red Clover blossoms powder (Trifolium praetense) 90 mg • Echinacea angustifolia root powder (Echinacea angustifolia) 30 mg • Yellow Dock root powder (Rhumex) 30 mg • Cayenne powder (Capsicum) 20 mg • Kelp powder (Fucus vesiculosis) 20 mg • Licorice root powder (Glycirrhiza glabra) 5 mg. Other Ingredients: Calcium Phosphate, Microcrystalline Cellulose, Vegetable Stearin, Croscarmellose Sodium, Magnesium Stearate (vegetable source).

Burn It — ANS
Chromium Picolinate • Vitamin E • Selenium • Zinc.

C + Herbs — Jarrow Formulas
Each tablet contains: Silymarin (Silybum marianum) 30:1 Concentrate (standardized to 80% silybin) 75 mg • PicroLiv (3.5- 4% Kutkin from Picrorrhiza kurroa) 50 mg • Astragalus Root 6:1 Concentrate 150 mg • Schisandra 5:1 Concentrate 75 mg • Scutelluria root (Skullcap) 4:1 concentrate 150 mg • Vitamin C (Ascorbic Acid) 500 mg. Other Ingredients: Magnesium Stearate. Contains no soy, yeast, corn, sugar, starch, or artificial color, flavor, preservatives, or other common allergen.

C Aspa Scorb — Progressive Labs
Each teaspoon (5100 mg) supplies: Vitamin C 4000 mg • Magnesium (from magnesium ascorbate and magnesium aspartate) 250 mg • Zinc (from zinc ascorbate) 30 mg • Selenium (from selenium ascorbate) 50 mcg • Manganese (from manganese ascorbate) 4.2 mg • Potassium (from potassium ascorbate and potassium aspartate) 96 mg.

C&F Formula — Dial Herbs
Vinegar • Glycerine • Honey • the Tinctures of Garlic, Comfrey, Wormwood, Marshmallow , White Oak bark, Black Walnut, Mullein, Scullcap, Uva Ursi, Lobelia.

C-1000 — Atrium
Each tablet contains: Vitamin C 1000 mg • Naturally Associated Bioflavonoid Complex 100 mg.

C-1000 — Biodelivery
Each tablet contains: Vitamin C (Calcium Ascorbate-Niascorbate) 1000 mg • Bioflavonoids 100 mg • Pantethine 5 mg • NT Factor tablet base 50 mg.

C-1000-TR — Atrium
Each tablet contains: Vitamin C 1000 mg • Naturally Associated Bioflavonoid Complex 100 mg.

C-500 — Biodelivery
Each tablet contains: Vitamin C (Calcium Ascorbate-Niascorbate) 500 mg • Bioflavonoids 100 mg • Pantethine 5 mg • NT Factor tablet base 50 mg.

CAC Tabs — Dial Herbs
Cascara Sagrada • Buckthorn • Burdock • Chaparral • Dandelion • Licorice root • Barberry • Red Clover.

Cactus (Nopal) — Natural Dynamics
Each capsule contains: Nopal 650 mg.

Cactus Diet — Cactu-Life
Each capsule contains: Opuntia Streptacantha 500 mg.

Cal/Mag Balance — Nutri-Quest
Each tablet contains: Calcium Aspartate 175 mg • Calcium Citrate 175 mg • Magnesium Aspartate 175 mg • Magnesium Glycinate 175 mg • Vitamin C 25 IU • Vitamin D 20 mg of HCL.

Cal-Acid Complex — Atrium
Four tablets contain: Calcium (from Oyster Shell, Oyster Shell-Citrus Juice Complex, & Calcium Caseinate) 750 mg • Magnesium (from Magnesium Citrus Juice Complex & Oxide) 210 mg • Manganese (Manganese-Citrus Carbonate Juice Complex) 5 mg • Copper (as Gluconate) 0.1 mg • Vitamin D (Fish oil) 400 USP IU • Vitamin C with Rose Hips 40 mg • Vitamin E 10 IU • Betaine HCL & Glutamic Acid HCL sufficient to provide dilute HCL 10 min. Amino Acids, Peptids, & Polypeptids from Hydrolized Soy Protein with Lecithin & Alfalfa juice concentrate. Contains no sugar, starch, salt wheat or corn derivatives.

Cal-Acid Maxi — Atrium
Four tablets contain: Calcium (Calcium Citrate, Calcium Caseinate & Oyster Shell) 1500 mg • Magnesium (Magnesium Citrus Juice Complex & Oxide) 500 mg • Manganese (Manganese Citrus Carbonate Juice) 10 mg • Vitamin D (Fish oil) 500 IU • Vitamin C with Rose Hips 100 mg • Vitamin E (d-Alpha Tocopherol) 20 IU • Horsetail (Silica) 250 mg • Boron (Citrate) 3 mg. Betaine HCL & Glutamic Acid HCL sufficient to provide dilute HCL. Amino acids, peptids & polypeptids from hydrolyzed soy protein with Lecithin & Alfalfa juice concentrate. Contains no sugar, starch, salt, wheat, yeast or corn derivatives.

Calamacin — MMS Pro
Each capsule contains: Scullcap herb • Wood Betony • Black Cohosh root • Hops flowers • Valerian root • Cayenne.

B R A N D

N A M E S

Some Brand Name Natural Products - What they Contain
www.NaturalDatabase.com contains MANY more listings than appear here.

Cal-Chew Calcium 350 mg — Jamieson
Each tablet contains: Calcium (as Calcium Carbonate, Calcium Citrate, Calcium Malate, Calcium Succinate, Calcium Aspartate, Calcium Glutamate, Calcium Fumarate) 350 mg • Iron 0.4 mg.

Calcium — Natrol
Three tablets contain: Calcium 500 mg • Magnesium (Calcium & Magnesium are bound Krebs Cycle Carriers) 200 mg • Fruitbase 640 mg. Other ingredients: Mono- and Di-Glycerides, Croscarmellose Sodium, Silicon Dioxide, Stearic Acid, Magnesium Stearate.

Calcium Ascorbate — Atrium
Each tablet contains: Vitamin C (Ascorbic Acid) 1000 mg.

Calcium Ascorbate C-Complex 1000 mg — The Vitamin Shoppe
Each 1000 mg capsule contains: Vitamin C as calcium ascorbate 750 mg • Citrus Bioflavonoids 100 mg • Hesperidin 50 mg • Rutin 25 mg • Calcium 75 mg. No Yeast, Wheat, Corn, Dairy, Soy, Salt, Sugar, Starch, Milk, Eggs, Gluten, Preservatives, Artificial Colors or Flavors added.

Calcium Ascorbate Crystals — Nature's Life
Each teaspoon contains: Vitamin C (Calcium Ascorbate) 3240 mg • Calcium (Calcium Ascorbate) 360 mg.

Calcium Citrate Plus Vitamin D — Progressive Labs
Four tablets contain: Calcium (as calcium citrate) 3240 mg • Calcium (Calcium Ascorbate) 360 mg.

Calcium Citrate with Zinc & Magnesium — Now
Two tablets contain: Vitamin D (Fish oil) 100 IU • Calcium (Citrate) 600 mg • Magnesium (Oxide, Aspartate) 300 mg • Zinc (Amino Acid Chelate) 15 mg • Manganese (Amino Acid Chelate) 5 mg • Copper (Amino Acid Chelate) 1 mg.

Calcium Effervescent — Progressive Labs
Two tablets contain: Calcium (from calcium carbonate) 1000 mg • Vitamin D (as cholecaciferol) 400 IU. Ingredients: Citric Acid, Calcium Carbonate, Sorbitol, Sodium Bicarbonate, Sodium Carbonate, Magnesium Carbonate, Aspartame, Mineral oil, Natural Orange flavor, Cholecalciferol. Contains Phenylalanine.

Calcium Magnesium Phosphorus Superabsorbeze — Nature's Life
Each tablespoon contains: Calcium (Calcium Phosphate) 600 mg • Magnesium (Hydroxide, Carbonate) 300 mg • Vitamin D3 (Cholecalciferol) 200 IU. In a natural base of Purified Water, Citric Acid, Sorbital, natural Orange flavor & Cellulose.

Calcium Magnesium Superabsorbeze — Nature's Life
Each tablespoon contains: Calcium (Citrate, Lactate/ Gluconate) 600 mg • Phosphorus (Calcium Phosphate) 600 mg • Magnesium (Hydroxide, Carbonate) 300 mg • Vitamin D3 (Cholecalciferol) 200 IU. In a natural base of Purified Water, Citric Acid, Fructose, natural Orange flavor, Cellulose & Ascorbic Acid.

Calcium Magnesium Zinc — Nature's Life
Three tablets contain: Calcium (Carbonate, Citrate/Malate) 1000 mg • Magnesium (Oxide, Citrate) 600 mg • Zinc (Picolinate, Citrate) 15 mg • Copper (Gluconate, Citrate) 1 mg • Silicon (Dioxide) 20 mg • Boron (Citrate) 100 mcg • Glutamic Acid HCI 100 mg. In a natural base of Springtime Horsetail Herb (Equisetum arvense).

Calcium/Magnesium with Vitamin D — Jamieson
Each caplet contains: Vitamin D (as Cholecalciferol) 133 IU • Calcium (as Calcium Carbonate, Calcium Citrate, Calcium Succinate, Calcium Asparate, Calcium Glutamate, Calcium Furmarate) 333 mg • Magnesium (as Magnesium Oxide, Magnesium Citrate, Magnesium Malate, Magnesium Succiante, Magnesium Asparate, Magnesium Glutamate, Magnesium Fumarate) 167 mg.

Calcium-Magnesium — Biodelivery
Each tablet contains: Calcium (Citrate) 250 mg • Magnesium (Oxide) 250 mg • NT Factor tablet base 200 mg.

Calcium-Magnesium Complex — The Vitamin Shoppe
Four tablets provide: Calcium 1500 mg • Magnesium 420 mg • Vitamin D 1000 IU • Vitamin E 20 IU • Vitamin C 80 mg • Manganese 10 mg. Plus Betaine HCl and Glutamic Acid HCl. In a base containing: Hydrolyzed Soy Protein, Lecithin, and Alfalfa Powder.

Calcium-Magnesium for Children — The Vitamin Shoppe
Each tablet contains: Calcium 200 mg • Magnesium 100 mg.

Calcium-Magnesium-Zinc — The Vitamin Shoppe
Three tablets contain: Elemental Calcium 1500 mg • Elemental Magnesium 750 mg • Elemental Zinc 45 mg.

Calendula Oil — Blessed Herbs
Calendula flower • Organic Cold-Pressed Olive oil.

Calendula Salve — Dial Herbs
Calendula • Chamomile • Mullein. In a base of Bees Wax, Glycerine & Cold Pressed Olive oil.

Calm Aid Formula — Nature's Way
Two capsules contain: Blue Vervain stem, leaf, flower, fruit 150 mg • Chamomile flower 75 mg • Kava (dried extract 30% Kavalactones) 350 mg • L-5 Hydroxytryptophan (Griffonia bean extract) 5 mg • Niacin (Vitamin B3) 6.66 mg • Passion flower stem, leaf, flower, fruit 75 mg • Riboflavin (Vitamin B2) 568 mcg • Scullcap herb 60 mg • Thiamine (Vitamin B1) 500 mcg • Vitamin B12 (Cyanocobalamin) 2 mcg • Vitamin B6 (Pyridoxine HCL) 660 mcg • Wood Betony stem, leaf, flower 100 mg. Other ingredients: Gelatin, Magnesium Stearate, Millet.

Calm Thoughts — Source Naturals
Three tablets contain: Kava root extract (Piper methysticum) (Standardized to 30% kavalactones yielding 105 mg of kavalactones) 350 mg • Siberian Ginseng root 200 mg • Bacopa Monniera leaf extract (Standardized to 20% bacosides yielding 20 mg of bacosides) 100 mg • Lemon Balm herb 80 mg • St. John's Wort extract (Hypericum perforatum)(50 mg Standardized to 0.3% hypericin and 50 mg 4:1 extract) 100 mg • Valerian root 60 mg • Ashwagandha root 50 mg • Ginger root 50 mg • Licorice root extract (4:1) 50 mg • Ginkgo Biloba leaf extract (50:1) (Standardized to 24% Ginkgo flavone glycosides and 6% terpene lactones) 30 mg • Schizandra fruit 30 mg • Vitamin C (as Ascorbic Acid) 100 mg • Vitamin B1 (Thiamin) 25 mg • Vitamin B2 (Riboflavin) 25 mg • Niacinamide 25 mg • Vitamin B6 (Pyridoxine HCI) 25 mg • Vitamin B12 (Cyanocobalamin) 25 mcg • Vitamin B5 (Pantothenic Acid) 50 mg • Calcium (as Calcium Citrate) 100 mg • Magnesium 275 mg Magnesium Oxide and 25 mg Magnesium Taurinate) 300 mg • Zinc (as Zinc Citrate) 15 mg • Manganese (as Manganese Citrate) 3 mg • GABA (Gamma Amino Butyric Acid) 500 mg • Taurine (as Magnesium Taurinate) 300 mg • L-Tyrosine (200 mg as L-Tyrosine and 50 mg N-Acetyl L-Tyrosine) 250 mg.

CAL-MAG — The Vitamin Shoppe
Each tablet contains: Calcium 500 mg • Magnesium 250 mg.

Cal-Mag Chewable — Quest
Each tablet contains: Elemental Calcium (Citrate, Phosphate) 300 mg • Elemental Magnesium (Citrate, Oxide) 150 mg • Vitamin D3 100 IU. Other Ingredients: Sorbitol, Silicon Dioxide, Magnesium Stearate, Sucralose and Spearmint Flavor.

CAL-MAG w/Zinc and Vitamin D — Dial Herbs
Vitamin D • Calcium from Gluconate & Lactate • Magnesium • Zinc • Aqueous Extracts (from Hibiscus, Chamomille, Fennel, Spinach) • Fructose • Mango Juice • Orange Juice • Natural Flavor • Locust Seed Flour.

Cal-Min — Progressive Labs
Each tablet contains: Calcium (as calcium proteinate) 300 mg. In a base of mixed vegetable concentrate from: Cultured Peas, Lentils, Buckwheat, Millet, and Chlorophyll, carefully dried to preserve their natural trace nutrient and enzyme content.

Calorad — Essentially Yours Industries Corp.
Demineralized Water • Collagen Hydrolysat • Aloe Vera • Vegetal Glycerin • Potassium Sorbate • Citrus Extracts • Natural Peach Flavor.

Cal-Para — Atrium
Each tablet contains: Alkalinizing Calcium Calcium Lactate 325 mg • Calcium Aspartate (supplying Elemental Calcium 52) 80 mg • Magnesium Aspartate 75 mg • Magnesium Citrate (supplying Elemental Magnesium 21 mg) 70 mg.

Calsorb — PhysioLogics
Three caplets contain: Calcium (80% Citrate, 20% Carbonate) 500 mg • Magnesium (50% Citrate, 50% Glycinate) 250 mg.

Cal-Sym — Atrium
Each tablet contains: Acidifying Calcium Calcium Phosphate 100 mg

© Copyright 2000, Natural Medicines Comprehensive Database (209) 472-2244. For updated data, go to www.NaturalDatabase.com.

Some Brand Name Natural Products - What they Contain
www.NaturalDatabase.com contains MANY more listings than appear here.

• Calcium Ascorbate 50 mg • Calcium Aspartate (supplies Elemental Calcium 34 mg compounded to insure acidic pH) 35 mg • Ammonium Chloride 100 mg • Betaine HCL 12 mg • Glutamic Acid HCL 120 mg.

Caltrate 600 + Soy — Whitehall-Robbins Healthcare
Two tablets contain: Soy Isoflavones 50 mg • Calcium 1200 mg • Vitamin D 400 IU.

Canadian Ginseng — Jamieson
Each capsule contains: Canadian Ginseng whole root (Panax quinquefolium) containing a minimum of 5% Ginsenosides 250 mg.

Candid Care — Natrol
Two capsules contain: Zinc 9 mg • FOS 500 mg • Garlic 100 mg • Undecylenic Acid (as Zinc undecylenate acid) 50 mg • Citrus extract, dried powder from grapefruit Seed 25 mg. Other ingredients: Microcrystalline Cellulose, Silicon Dioxide, Magnesium Stearate, Gelatin.

Candida Formula — Enzymatic Therapy
Each capsule contains: Oregano oil extract (Origanum vulgare) 0.1 ml • Thyme oil extract (Thymus vulgaris) 0.05 ml • Peppermint oil extract (Mentha piperta) 0.05 ml • Goldenseal root (Hydrastis canadensis) standardized to contain 5% total Alkaloids including: Berberine, Hydrastine, & Canadine 50 mg. Developed in accordance with the recommendations & safety standards set forth by the German Kommission E. Contains no sugar, salt, yeast, wheat, corn, dairy products, flavoring or preservatives.

Candida Forte — Nature's Plus
Two softgels contain: Safflower oil 1000 mg, Vitamin C (Ascorbate) 500 mg • L-Cysteine free form amino acid 100 mg • Zinc (Ascorbate) 50 mg • Pau D'Arco 50 mg • Vitamin B6 (Pyridoxine HCL) 50 mg • Acidophilus (Lactobacillus) supplying 80 million viable cells 20 mg • Vitamin A Fish Liver oil 10000 IU • Beta Carotene supplying 15000 IU Vitamin A activity 9 mg • Garlic equivalent to 500 mg of fresh garlic 1 mg • Biotin 100 mcg • Free Form Amino Acid Complex containing 198.08 mg: L-Glutamine 40.8 mg, L-Lysine 25 mg, L-Leucine 20.2 mg, L-Proline 16.2 mg, L-Valine 14 mg, L-Serine 12.6 mg, L-Isoleucine 11 mg, L-Phenylalanine 9.32 mg, L-Threonine 8.64 mg, L-Arginine 7.3 mg, L-Alanine 6.28 mg, L-Aspartic Acid 7 mg, L-Methionine 6.08 mg, L-Histidine 5.74 mg, L-Glycine 3.52 mg, L-Tyrosine 3 mg, L-Cysteine 1.4 mg. In a natural herbal base of black walnut. Contains no yeast, wheat, corn, soy, milk, salt, sugar or starch.

Candimyacin — Phytopharmica
Each capsule contains: Oregano oil extract (Origanum vulgare) 0.1ml • Thyme oil extract (Thymus vulgaris) 0.05 ml • Peppermint oil extract (Mentha piperita) 0.05 ml • Goldenseal root extract (Hydrastis canadensis) 50 mg standardized to contain 5% total alkaloids including berberine, hydrastine & canadine. Contains no sugar, salt, yeast, wheat, corn, dairy products, flavoring or preservatives.

Candistatin — PhysioLogics
Two capsules contain: Calcium (as Calcium Caprylate) 65 mg • Magnesium (as 92% Magnesium Caprylate, 8% Magnesium Stearate) 79 mg • Caprylic Acid (as 63% Magnesium Caprylate, 37% Calcium Caprylate) 800 mg • Goldthread root (10% Alkaloids, 10 mg) 100 mg • Pau D'Arco bark & stem (3% Napthoquinones 1.8 mg) 60 mg.

Candistroy — Nature's Secret
Two tablets contain: Zinc tannates • Barberry root extract • Goldenseal root • Pau d'Arco bark • Oregon Grape root • Peppermint oil • Orange peel • Licorice root • Cinnamon bark • Clove buds • Thyme leaf • Allicin.

Canes Deer Velvet — Canes Deer Products
Each capsule contains: Whole stick dried Deer Velvet 250 mg. Contains no yeast, preservative, coloring or gluten.

Caprylate Complex — Progressive Labs
Three capsules contain: Caprylic Acid (as caprylate) 1290 mg • Calcium (as caprylate) 100 mg • Magnesium (as caprylate) 50 mg • Zinc (as caprylate) 5 mg.

CapsiCool Cayenne — Nature's Way
Two capsules contain: Proprietary Formula: Cayenne pepper fruit • Ginger • Glucomannan root. Other ingredients: Gelatin.

Carba-E-A-C — Atrium
Each rounded teaspoon contains approximately: Vitamin A Acetate 4000 IU • Vitamin C from Ascorbic Acid 100 mg • Vitamin E 33 IU. In a carrier of Carbamide (food grade).

Carbo Fuel (Complex Carbohydrate Peak Performance Energy Drink) — TwinLab
Each serving contains: Carbohydrates (from Glucose Polymers & Crystalline Pure Fructose) (no high fructose corn syrups are present) 80 grams. Other Ingredients: Vitamin B1 • Vitamin B2 • Vitamin B3 • Vitamin B6 • Pantothenic Acid • Biotin • Potassium • Magnesium • Yeast-Free GTF Chromium • Inosine • L-Carnitine • CoQ10 • Lipoic Acid • Pantetheine • Pyridoxine-Alpha-Ketoglutarate • Soluble Potassium (Phosphate & Succinates) • Citrates • Aspartates • Fumarates • Malates • Alpha-Ketoglutarates.

Carbo-Meta — Atrium
Each tablet contains: Pyridoxal-5-Phosphate 20 mg • Pyridoxine HCL 50 mg • Chromium Aspartate 500 mcg • Magnesium 50 mg • Manganese 5 mg • Zinc Aspartate 15 mg.

Cardio 150 — Atrium
Each tablet contains: Raw Heart concentrate (not an extract) of Bovine source 150 mg.

Cardio 20 — Futurebiotics
Six capsules supply: Beta-carotene 25,000 IU • Vitamin C (buffered ascorbate)1000 mg • Vitamin E (natural) 400 IU • Niacin (timed release, flush-free) 250 mg • Choline Bitartrate 150 mg • Inositol 75 mg • Calcium (ascorbate) 250 mg • Magnesium (oxide, chelate) 400 mg • Potassium (gluconate) 99 mg • Coenzyme Q10 15 mg • L-Carnitine 100 mg • Taurine 100 mg • Procyanidol 35 mg • Hawthorn berries (4:1 extract) 250 mg • Soy Isoflavone extract 100 mg • Cholestatin Beta-sitosterol complex 250 mg • Garlic (pure-gar 1500 deodorized concentrate) 400 mg • Cayenne 100 mg • Ginger 50 mg • Chlorella 250 mg. Procyanidol is a concentrated, solvent-free, whole grape extract containing high levels of flavonoid polyphenols.

Cardio Chelate — Nutri-Quest
Six tablets contain: Vitamin A (Palmitate) 3000 IU • Beta Carotene 7500 IU • Vitamin D3 100 IU • Vitamin C (Sago) 300 mg • Vitamin B1 30 mg • Vitamin B2 30 mg • Vitamin B6 75 mg • Vitamin B12 500 mcg • Biotin 200 mcg • Niacin 60 mg • D-Calcium Pantothenate (Pantothenic Acid) 150 mg • Folic Acid 300 mcg • Vitamin E (Succinate) 300 IU • Iodine (Kelp) 100 mcg • PABA 100 mg • Lecithin 120 mg • Choline Bitartrate 250 mg • Cysteine HCL 250 mg • L-Methionine 75 mg • L-Lysine 100 mg • Bromelain 30 mg • Lemon Bioflavonoid 900 mg • Rutin 30 mg • Inositol 75 mg • Garlic 120 mg • Cayenne 30 mg • Hawthorne berries 100 mg • Pancreatin 6X 25 mg • Thymus 30 mg • Spleen 30 mg • Heart 30 mg • Adrenal (Nutritrophic) 30 mg • Whole Pituitary 30 mg • Papain 30 mg • L-Glycine 75 mg • Calcium Gluconate 37 mg • Manganese Chelate 2.5 mg • Copper Gluconate 7.8 mcg • Molybdenum Chelate 12 mcg • Chromium Chelate 102 mcg • Selenium Chelate 30 mcg • Calcium Ascorbate 100 mg • Calcium Aspartate 100 mg • Potassium Aspartate 25 mg • Magnesium Ascorbate 75 mg • Magnesium Aspartate 75 mg • Ferrous Gluconate 15 mg • Zinc Aspartate 15 mg. In a base containing: Calcium Phosphate, Magnesium Phosphate, Calcium Flouride, Ferric Phosphate, Kali Phosphate, Silica, Chiorinum, Peppermint leaves, Black Cohosh, Scullcap, Licorice root, Watercress, Siberian Ginseng, Red Beet root, Parsley.

Cardio EDTA Chelate — Olympia Nutrition
EDTA 400 mg • MSM 100 mg • NAC 50 mg • Vitamin C 100 mg.

Cardio Flow — Progressive Labs
Six capsules contain: Vitamin A (retinyl palmitate) 10,000 IU • Vitamin C (ascorbic acid and zinc ascorbate) 640 mg • Elemental Potassium 210 mg (from Potassium Aspartate 684 mg, from Potassium Orotate 300 mg) • Elemental Magnesium 330 mg (from Magnesium Aspartate 1400 mg, from Magnesium Orotate 714 mg) • Elemental Zinc 25 mg (from Zinc Ascorbate 168 mg) • Elemental Selenium 70 mcg • Selenium Ascorbate 70 mcg • Sodium 28 mg • EDTA (Ethylenediamine tetra-acetic acid) 800 mg • Disodium EDTA 200 mg • L-Glutathione, reduced 20 mg • Bromelain (2000 GDU) 300 mg • Papain (525 TU/mg) 30 mg • Cilantro (coriander) 500 mg • Butcher's Broom 150 mg • Cardio Flow 600 mg: a proprietary blend of the following extracts: [Inula racemosa (root), Saussurea lappa (root), Terminalia arjuna (root), Desmodium gingatic (leaves), Commiphora mukul (resin), Bacopa monniera (leaves), Convolvulous pluricaulis (leaves)]. Other Ingredients: Rice flour, Magnesium Stearate.

Cardio Guardian — Clinician's Choice
Three tablets contain: Vitamin C (ascorbic acid) 180 mg • Vitamin E (dl-alpha tocopheryl acetate) 400 IU • Niacin (niacinamide) 300 mg • Niacin 100 mg • Vitamin B6 (pyridoxine hydrochloride) 23 mg •

 • © Copyright 2000, Natural Medicines Comprehensive Database (209) 472-2244. For updated data, go to www.NaturalDatabase.com.

Some Brand Name Natural Products - What they Contain

Folate (folic acid) 600 mcg • Vitamin B12 (cyanocobalmin) 150 mcg • Magnesium (glycinate) 15 mg • Zinc (gluconate) 15 mg • Selenium (aspartate) 120 mcg • RoseOx (patented, standardized process for an extract of Rosemary) 150 mg • Hawthorn 4:1 Extract 150 mg • Triphala Extract (Sstd. 40% tannin) 90 mg • White Willow Bark 60 mg • Motherwort 4:1 Extract 30 mg • L-Carnitine 30 mg • Seacol 30 mg • Linoleic Acid, Gamma Linolenic Acid (sunflower oil, borage oil) 30 mg • Proprietary blend: Grape Powder, Cayenne Fruit, Coenzyme Q10 45 mg.

Cardio Plus — Atrium
Three tablets contain: Vitamin E Acetate 300 IU • Vitamin C (with Rose Hips) 60 mg • Thiamine Mononitrate 15 mg • Vitamin B2 Riboflavin 2 mg • Niacin 100 mg • Vitamin B6 15 mg • Vitamin B12 2 mcg • Magnesium (as Citrus Juice Complex & Oxide) 100 mg • Zinc (as Gluconate) 5 mg • Potassium (as Citrus Juice Complex & Chloride) 99 mg • Chromium (amino acid complex) 10 mcg • Selenium(in yeast) 48 mcg • Choline Bitartrate 66 mg. In a base containing Lecithin 80 mg, Para Aminobenzoic Acid 30 mg, Inositol 4 mg, Cold Processed Heart Protein 90 mg.

Cardio ProtoChol — Fields of Nature
Each capsule contains: Vitamin E (as D-Alpha Tocopherly Acid Succinate) 10 IU • Niacin Powder 3 mg • Soybean Isoflavones extract (Novasoy) (Isoflavones 13 mg) 33 mg • Garlic bulb extract (Allicin 333 mcg) 33 mg • Guggulipids Extract (Guggulsterones 0.8 mg) 33 mg • Red Rice Yeast Extract (Lovastin 134 mcg) 33 mg • Lemon Bioflavonoids Complex 10 mg • Chitosan Powder 50 mg. Other Ingredients: Calcium Carbonate, Hydroxymethyl Propylcellulose, Magnesium Stearate, Silicon Dioxide.

Cardio Q10 — PhysioLogics
Each capsule contains: Vitamin E (as d-Alpha Tocopherol) 200 IU • Calcium (as Dicalcium Phosphate) 2 mg • Selenium (as Selenomethionine) 25 mcg • Coenzyme Q10 30 mg.

Cardio Results — Changes - TwinLab
Two caplets contain: Vitamin B6 (as Pyridoxine HCI) 15 mg • Folate (as Folic acid) 400 mcg • Vitamin B12 (as Cyanocobalamin) 250 mcg • Red Yeast rice (from fermentation of Monascus pupureus Went) 600 mg • Purified Soy phytosterols (45-55% Beta-Sitosterol) 50 mg. Other ingredients: Dicalcium phosphate, Vegetable cellulose, Fractionated vegetable oil, Soy polysaccharides, Silica, and Vita-Lok vegetable resin glaze.

Cardio Support Formula — The Vitamin Factory
Each tablet contains: Vitamin E (d-Alpha Tocopheryl-Succinate) 100 IU • Folic Acid 100 mcg • White Willow bark extract 4:1 100 mg • Hawthorne berry extract 50 mg • Coenzyme Q10 30 mg • Oat Beta Glucan powder (min 18%) 25 mg • Pycnogenol (Maritime Pine bark extract) 15 mg.

Cardiotrate — Progressive Labs
Each capsule contains: Raw Bovine heart concentrate 140 mg prepared by a special process which does not exceed physiological temperature (37° C). Guaranteed to be free of chemical pesticides and synthetic hormones.

Cardio-Vite — Atrium
Each tablet contains: Vitamin B1 2.2 mg • Vitamin B2 2.2 mg • Vitamin B6 50 mg • Pantothenic Acid 50 mg • Niacinamide 15 mg • Magnesium 50 mg • Potassium 50 mg.

Caribbean Tanning Secret — Futurebiotics
One tablet contains: Vitamin C 13 mg • Vitamin B 625 mg • Copper Gluconate 0.7 mg • Para Amino Benzoic Acid (PABA) 13 mg. In a base containing: (L-tyrosine, Aloe Vera, Carrot powder, & Yucca powder).

Carni Fuel — TwinLab
Each capsule contains: Carni Fuel L-Carnitine Magnesium Citrate 500 mg • L-Carnitine 200 mg • Magnesium 30 mg.

Carni Fuel (L-Carnitine Liquid Concentrate) — TwinLab
Each tablespoonful (15 ml) contains: L-Carnitine 1000 mg.

Carotenoid Complex — The Vitamin Shoppe
Each softgel contains: Phytofluene 0.033 mg • Lycopene (LYC-O-MATO) 5 mg • Lutein 5 mg • Beta-carotene (6251 IU Vitamin A) 3.75 mg • Alpha-carotene (1042 IU Vitamin A) 1.25 mg • Zeaxanthin 0.26 mg • Phytoene 0.098 mg. In a base of tomato and carrot concentrate.

Cartilade — BioTherapies, Inc.
Shark Cartilage.

Cartilage Care — PhysioLogics
Each capsule contains: Vitamin C (as Ascorbic Acid) 60 mg • Manganese (as Manganese Glycinate) 2 mg • Glucosamine Sulfate 200 mg • Chondroitin Sulfate 100 mg • Glucosamine Hydrochloride 100 mg • Sea Cucumber 100 mg.

Cartilage Companion — PhysioLogics
Each capsule contains: Glucosamine Sulfate 200 mg • Chondroitin Sulfate 67 mg • Methylsulfonylmethane (MSM) 333 mg.

Cartilage Formula — Pharmanex
Two capsules contain: Vitamin C (Ascorbic Acid) 100 mg • Vitamin E (d-Alpha Tocopheryl Succinate, Beta, Delta, Gamma Tocopherols) 50 IU • Zinc (Zinc Propionate) 7.5 mg • Boron (Boron Citrate) 3 mg • Glucosamine (Glucosamine Sulfate, Glucosamine Hydrochloride) 750 mg • Boswellia Serrata extract (Min. 95% Boswellic Acids) 150 mg • Tumeric extract (Min. 95% Curcumin) 100 mg • Quercetin 25 mg • Rutin 25 mg. Other Ingredients: Silicon Dioxide, Magnesium Stearate.

Cata-Comp — Enzymatic Therapy
Two capsules contain: Vitamin A (Beta Carotene) non-toxic form of Vitamin A 10000 IU • Vitamin E (D-Alpha Tocopherol Succinate) 75 IU • Vitamin C (Ascorbic Acid) 500 mg • Zinc (Picolinate) 10 mg • Manganese (Picolinate) 2 mg • Riboflavin (Vitamin B2) 2 mg • Selenium selenomethionine 75 mcg • Other ingredients: Hachimijiogan Herbal Complex 200 mg • Curcuma root extract (Curcuma longa) standardized to contain 97% Curcumin) 100 mg • L-Cysteine 50 mg • L-Glutamine 50 mg • L-Glycine 50 mg. Contains no sugar, salt, yeast, wheat, corn, dairy products, coloring, flavoring, or preservatives.

Catnip and Fennel — Dial Herbs
Catnip • Peppermint • Fennel • Lobelia.

Catnip and Peppermint — Dial Herbs
Catnip • Peppermint • Lobelia.

Cat's Claw Defense Complex — Source Naturals
Four tablets contain: Cat's Claw inner bark (Uncaria Tomentosa) 2000 mg • Whole-Leaf Aloe Vera powder (200:1 Concentrate) 200 mg • Proanthodyn (from Grape Seed extract) 60 mg • Quercetin 400 mg • Green Tea extract 40 mg • Turmeric Root Extract (Yielding 95% Curcumin) 400 mg • Silymarin (Milk Thistle seed extract) 50 mg • Reishi Mycelia biomass 200 mg • Shiitake Mycelia biomass 200 mg • Maitake Mycelia biomass 150 mg • Astragalus root 200 mg • St. John's Wort herb extract 100 mg • St. John's Wort herb powder 100 mg • Siberian Ginseng root 100 mg • Siberian Ginseng root extract 100 mg • Schizandra berries 200 mg • Pau d'Arco bark 100 mg • Pau d'Arco bark extract 100 mg • Isatis leaf 150 mg • Vitamin A (Beta Carotene) 10000 IU • Vitamin C (Ascorbic Acid, Magnesium and Zinc Ascorbates) 350 mg • Magnesium (Ascorbate) 10 mg • Zinc (Ascorbate) 12 mg • N-Acetyl Cysteine 600 mg.

Cayenne — Pharmanex
Each capsule contains: Cayenne (Capisicum Annum)(Pepper)(40000 Heat Units) 450 mg. Other Ingredients: Gelatin, Magnesium Stearate, Silicon Dioxide.

Cayenne Extra Hot — Nature's Way
Each capsule contains: Proprietary Formula: Cayenne pepper fruit • Ginger • Hawthorne berry. Other ingredients: Gelatin.

C-Complex/ Bioflavonoids/ Rutin — Nature's Life
Each tablet contains: Vitamin C 500 mg • Lemon Bioflavonoids Complex (natural whole unaltered TESTLAB concentrate containing Hesperidin, Eriocitrin, Flavonols, & Flavones derived from freshly dejuiced Lemons.) 500 mg • Acerola (Malpighia glabra) 50 mg • Hesperidin 50 mg • Rutin (Saphora japonica) 50 mg • Calcium (naturally buffering Calcium Carbonate) 12 mg. In a natural base of Bell Peppers & Rose Hips powder.

Celite-Complex 75 — Jamieson
Two capsules contain: Concentrated Citrus Bioflavonoids (Vitamin P) 100 mg • Ginkgo Biloba Extract Flavoglycoside-rich JGB24 250 mg • Bilberry Extract Anthocyanoside-rich JMF25 750 mg • Oil of Madagascar Cinnamon 20 mg • South Pacific Sea Kelp Extract 25 mg • Bromelain Enzyme (from Pineapple) 100 mg • Kola Nut Extract 250 mg. Other Ingredients: Soybean Oil, Vegetable Oil, Gelatin, Glycerin, Lecithin, Purified Water.

Celite-Complex 75-Firming Gel — Jamieson
Water • Glycerin • Butylene Glycol • Kola Nut (Cola acuminata) Extract • Coneflower (Echinacea purpurea) Extract • Propylene

© Copyright 2000, Natural Medicines Comprehensive Database (209) 472-2244. For updated data, go to www.NaturalDatabase.com.

BRAND NAMES

BRAND NAMES

Glycol • Butylene Glycol • Camellia oleifera Extract • Arnica montana Extract • Dimethylsilanol Hyaluronate • Jojoba Esters • Butcher's Broom (Rucus aculeatus) Extract • Kelp (Macrocystis pyrifera) Extract • Imidazolidinyl Urea • Triethanolamine • Carbomer • Methyl Paraben • Ethyl Paraben • Fragrance.

Cell Boost with IP-6 — TwinLab
Two capsules contain: Calcium 101 mg • Phosphorous 195 mg • Calcium Magnesium Phytate (Inositol Hexaphosphate) 1000 mg.

Cell Forte with IP-6 — Enzymatic Therapy
Each capsule contains: IP-6 (inositol hexaphosphate, from rice) 400 mg • Inositol (from rice) 110 mg. Contains no sugar, salt, yeast, wheat, gluten, corn, soy, dairy products, coloring, flavoring or preservatives.

Cella Free — Bodyonics
Six tablets contain: Herbal BioModulators (From Evening Primrose Oil (contains Gamma Linolenic Acid (GLA)), Borage (Seed Oil), Bladderwreck Extract, Dried Fucus Vesiculosus Extract, Fish Oil (containing the Omega-3 polyunsaturated fatty acids EPA (eicosapentaenoic acid) and DHA (docosahezaenoic acid)), Grape Seed Extract, Bioflavonoids, Soya Lecithin, Fatty Acids, Dried Sweet Red Clover Extract (Mellotus Officinals)(Tri Folium pratense)(Standardized to 1% biochanina), Dried Ginkgo Biloba Extract (Standardized to contain flavonglycosides) 1000 mg • Protein/Fiber BioModulators (From a mixture of Bioactive Oligopeptides prepared from food grade proteins by means of Enzymatic Hydrolysis of Bovine Globin Proteins, Casein and Wheat Protein. Plus Fibrabind (Chitosan) a naturally occuring fiber extracted from shellfish with vegetable pupl and citrus pectin (grapefruit)) 1750 mg • Therma/ Fluid Balance BioModulators (From UVA URSI Standardized to contain 120 mg of Hydroxyquinone and Yerba Mate Standardized to contain 300 mg Methyl Xanthines) 1000 mg. Other Ingredients: Calcium Carbonate, Stearic Acid, Croscarmellose, Magnesium Stearate.

Cellasene — Thompson Nutritional Products
Three softgels contain: Iodine 720 mcg • Cellasene Lipovascolen 702 mg • Cellasene support blend 1230 g. Other Ingredients: Bladderwrack extract, Grape seed extract, Sweet Clover extract, Ginko Biloba, Borage, Fish oil, Soya Lecithin.

Cell-FX — HerbTech
Each capsule contains: Shark Cartilage extract 200 mg.

Cell-FX (Bulk Powder) — HerbTech
Water-soluble concentrated Shark Cartilage 227 mg.

Cell-FX 500 mg — HerbTech
Each capsule contains: Shark Cartilage extract 500 mg.

CELL-Tech — Muscletech
Each serving contains: Creatine Monohydrate 10 g • Insulin-releasing Dextrose 75 g • Insulin-potentiating Lipoic Acid 200 mg • Chromium Picolinate 300 mcg • Potassium 150 mg • Phosphates 100 mg • Taurine • Magnesium.

Cellular Forte with IP-6 and Inositol — Phytopharmica
Each capsule contains: IP-6 as inositol hexaphosphate (rice) 400 mg • Inositol (rice) 110 mg. Contains no sugar, salt, wheat, gluten, corn, soy, dairy products, coloring, flvoring, or preservatives.

Cellu-Var Capsules — Enzymatic Therapy
Each capsule contains: Butchers Broom extract (Ruscus aculeatus) standardized to contain 10% Saponins calculated as Ruscogenin 100 mg • Gotu Kola extract (Centella asiatica) standardized to contain 70% of selected Triterpenic Acids: Asiaticoside, Asiatic Acid, & Madecassic Acid from Centella 30 mg • Escin extract (Aesculus hippocastanum) 10 mg. Contains no sugar, salt, yeast, wheat, corn, soy, dairy products, coloring, flavoring, or preservatives.

Cellu-Var Cream — Enzymatic Therapy
Deionized Water • Horse Chestnut (Escin) extract • Sea Ware extract • Cola vera extract • Rosemary extract in a base of Cholestanol (Dihydrocholesterol), a natural emulsifying agent. Contains no animal products.

Cerebra — DHM, Inc.
Each tablet contains: Huperzine A (Chinese club moss) 50 mcg • Vitamin E.

Cernilton Flower Pollen — Cernitin America
Two tablets contain: Cernitin Flower Pollen (Rye Grass Pollen) Extract Water-Soluble Pollen Extract (T60) 120 mg • Cernitin Flower

Pollen Extract Fat-Soluble Pollen Concentrate (GBX) 6 mg. Other Ingredients: Cellulose (Plant Fiber), Magnesium Stearate (vegetable source).

Cernilton T.S. Flower Pollen Triple Strength — Cernitin America
Two capsules contain: Cernitin Flower Pollen (Rye Grass Pollen) Extract Water-Soluble Pollen concentrate (T60) 360 mg • Cernitin Flower Pollen extract fat-soluble pollen concentrate (GBX) 18 mg. Other Ingredients: Cellulose (plant fiber), Magnesium Stearate (Vegetable Source).

CetylPure — Natrol
One capsule contains: Cetyl Myristoleate Proprietary Blend (CetylPure) 550 mg. Other Ingredients: Silica, Magnesium Stearate, Gelatin. Contains no yeast, wheat, milk, egg, soy, glutens, artificial colors or flavors, added sugar, starch, or preservatives.

Change-O-Life Formula — Nature's Way
Three capsules contain: Black Cohosh root • Blessed Thistle • False Unicorn root • Licorice root • Sarsaparilla root • Siberian Ginseng root • Squaw Vine vine, leaf, fruit. Other ingredients: Gelatin, Magnesium Stearate.

Changes Now — TwinLab
Two capsules contain: Vitamin C (Ascorbic acid) 50 mg • Lipase 300 LU • Calcium sulfate 100 mg • Multi-Source Fiber Complex 650 mg: Chitosan (Deacylated cellulose biopolymer), Glucomannan, Citrus Pectin, and Oat fiber. Other ingredients: Gelatin, Magnesium stearate, and Silica.

Changes Relief — Changes - TwinLab
Three caplets contain: Vitamin C (as Ascorbic Acid) 100 mg • Calcium (as Calcium Monohydrogen Phosphate) 300 mg • Phosphorus (as Calcium Monohydrogen Phosphate) 225 mg • Zinc (as Zinc Monomethionine) 13.75 mg • Copper (as Copper Gluconate) 500 mcg • Manganese (as Manganese Sulfate) 5 mg • Glucosamine Hydrochloride/Glucosamine Sulfate/N-Acetyl Glucosamine blend (with Chondroitin precursors) 750 mg • Turmeric rhizome standardized extract (12x) 300 mg • Boswellia serrata gum-resin 300 mg • Devil's Claw root standardized extract (5% harpagosides) 125 mg • Bromelain (80 GDU/g) 125 mg • White Willow bark 4:1 extract 150 mg • Ginger root standardized extract (5% gingerols) 125 mg • Alpine Snow Rose leaf (50% active polyphenolic proanthocyanidins) 213 mg. Other ingredients: Vegetable cellulose, Fractionated vegetable oil, Soy polysaccharides, Silica, and Vegetable resin glaze.

Changing Times — Nature's Plus
Two tablets contain: Wild Brazilian SUMA (Pfaffia paniculata [Martius] Kuntze) 300 mg • Calcium amino acid chelate/complex 200 mg • Magnesium amino acid chelate/complex 100 mg • Vitamin B6 (Pyridoxine HCL) 100 mg • Pantothenic Acid 100 mg • Phosphatidylcholine 100 mg • Siberian Ginseng (Eleutherococcus senticosus) 100 mg • Niacinamide 25 mg • Vitamin E nautral 200 IU • Vitamin B12 from Cobalamin 200 mcg • Selenium yeast free, amino acid complex 50 mcg. Yeast free. Sugar & starch free.

Chaparral and Red Clover — Dial Herbs
Chaparral • Red Clover • Echinacea • Buchu Leaves • Blood root.

Charco-Zyme — Atrium
Each capsule contains: Papaya leaf 65 mg • Papain 32.5 mg • Mycozyme 32.5 mg • Rennin NF 3.75 mg • Activated Charcoal 130 mg . In a base of Alfalfa & Peppermint. Contains no sugar, salt, wheat, corn, yeast or soy derivatives.

Chaste Tree-Siberian Ginseng Virtue — Blessed Herbs
Chaste Tree berry • Siberian Ginseng root • Hawthorn berry, leaf & flower • Lavender flower • Wild Yam root • Licorice root • Grain alcohol & Distilled Water.

Chem-Ex — Enzymatic Therapy
Two capsules contain: Pantothenic Acid (D-Calcium Pantothenate) 80 mg • Zinc (Chelate) 40 mg. Other ingredients: L-Cysteine 300 mg • L-Methionine 200 mg • Alpha-Ketoglutarate 60 mg • Taurine 50 mg • Glycine 40 mg. This exclusive formula also contains Licorice root extracts (Glycyrrhiza glabra). Contains no sugar, salt, yeast, wheat, corn, soy, dairy products, coloring, flavoring or preservatives.

Chew Chew Vites Multiple — Nature's Life
Two tablets contain: Vitamin A (Fish Liver oil) 5000 IU • Vitamin D3 (Cholecalciferol) 400 IU • Vitamin E (d-Alpha Tocopheryl with Beta, Gamma, & Delta Tocopherols) 30 IU • Vitamin B1 (Thiamine HCI) 5

Some Brand Name Natural Products - What they Contain
www.NaturalDatabase.com contains MANY more listings than appear here.

mg • Vitamin B2 (Riboflavin) 5 mg • Vitamin B6 Pyridoxine HCl 5 mg • Vitamin B12 (Cyanocobalamin) 10 mcg • Niacinamide 10 mg • Pantothenic Acid (d-Calcium Pantothenate) 10 mg • Folic Acid 0.1 mg • Choline (Bitartrate) 25 mcg • Inositol 25 mcg • PABA (Para Aminobenzoic Acid) 300 mcg • Biotin 75 mcg • Vitamin C (with Rose Hips) 150 mg • Calcium (Carbonate, Gluconate, Citrate) 28 mg • Chromium (Picolinate Nutrition 21) 50 mcg • Copper (Full ranged Amino Acid Chelate) 0.1 mg • Iodine (Kelp) 0.1 mg • Iron (Full ranged Amino Acid Chelate) 5 mg • Magnesium (Full ranged Amino Acid Chelate)15 mg • Manganese (Full ranged Amino Acid Chelate) 0.3 mg • Phosphorus (Proteinate) 4 mg • Potassium (Proteinate) 11.5 mg • Silicon (Dioxide) 5 mg • Zinc (Picolinate) 2 mcg • Essential Fatty Acids 5 mg • Hawaiian Spirulina 10 mg • Chlorophyll, Alfalfa 10 mg • Chlorella algae 10 mg. In a natural base of low Glycemic pure Crystalline Fructose, pasteurized Honey powder, natural Lemon flavor, Vegetarian Acidophilus powder, natural Pineapple flavor, Rose Hips powder, Lecithin, Lemon Bioflavonoids, Barley Grass, Sunflower Seed powder, Rice Bran, Wheat Germ, Alfalfa leaf, Watercress & Parsley.

Chewable Acerola C Complex 500 mg — The Vitamin Shoppe
Each wafer contains: Vitamin C (fortified with Acerola extract & Rose Hips Concentrate) 500 mg • Bioflavonoid complex 50 mg. Sweetened exclusively with fructose, a naturally occurring sweetener found in fruit, and all-natural Acerola cherry flavoring. No yeast, corn, wheat, salt, starch, soy, dairy, sucrose, fish or animal derivatives, preservatives, artificial colors or flavors added.

Chewable E — Country Life
Each wafer contains: Vitamin E (D-alpha tocopheryl succinate) 450 IU. No yeast, corn, wheat, soy, milk, salt, starch, or artificial colrs, sweeteners, flavors or preservatives.

Chewable Glucosamine Sulfate — Carlson
One tablet contains: Glucosamine Sulfate (providing Sulfur 4 g) 500 mg.

Chewable Orange Juice C 500 mg — The Vitamin Shoppe
Each chewable tablet contains: 500 mg Vitamin C, blend of natural Orange Juice concentrate, Orange Juice pulp, Orange peels, and natural fruit sugar. No Yeast, Wheat, Corn, Sucrose, Salt, Starch, Gluten, Milk, Eggs, Dairy, Fish or Animal Derivatives, Preservatives, Artificial Colors or Flavors added.

CHI Chinese Herbal Bar — Nature's Plus
Each 1.5 oz. bar contains: Ancient Chinese Herbs: Huang-Ch'i (Astragalus root) 312 mg • Dang Shen (Relative root) 228 mg • Ling Zhi (Reishi mushroom) 192 mg • Bai Zhu (Attractylodes root) 144 mg • Ji Xue Teng (Millettia stem) 144 mg • Tu Si Zi (Dodder seed) 144 mg • Shan Yao (Chinese Yam root) 144 mg • Nu Zhen zi (Privet fruit) 144 mg • Di Huang (Rehmannia root) 138 mg • Bei Sha Shen (Sand root) 136 mg • Wu Wei Zi (Schisandra fruit) 114 mg • Jiang (Ginger root) 114 mg • Suan Zao Ren (Jujube seed) 114 mg • Chieh Keng (Balloon Flower root) 114 mg • Gan Cao (Licorice root) 108 mg • Bai Shoa (Peony root) 72 mg • Ju Luo (Tangerine peel) 72 mg.

Chickweed Formula — Quest
Each caplet contains: Chickweed powder (Stellaria media) 120 mg • Fennel seed powder (Foeniculum vulgare) 80 mg • Burdock root powder (Actium lappa) 80 mg • Chia seeds powder (Salvia columbariae) 70 mg • Bladderwrack powder (Fucus Vesiculosis) 30 mg • Kelp powder (Fucus Vesiculosis) 30 mg. Other Ingredients: Calcium Phosphate, Microcrystalline Cellulose, Vegetable Stearin, Croscarmellose Sodium, Magnesium Stearate (vegetable source).

Child Lax — Dial Herbs
Senna • Fennel • Rhubarb.

Children Immu-C — Nutri-Quest
Each tablet contains: Vitamin C (Sago Palm) 125 mg • Biotin 20 mcg • Folic Acid 10 mcg • Vitamin A (Palmitate) 1500 IU • Rutin 7.5 mg • Lemon Bioflavonoids 10 mg • Hesperidin Complex 7.5 mg • Propolis 1 mg • Lymph 1 mg • Thymus 1 mg • Spleen 1 mg. In a base of Fructose & Maltodextrin, with pleasant tasting Tropical Fruit Flavoring.

Children's Echinacea+C+Zinc Raspberry Flavor — LiFizz Effervescent Vitamins
Each tablet contains: Vitamin C 400 mg • Zinc (Zinc Oxide, Zinc Sulfate) 10 mg • Echinacea extract (Echinacea purpurea) 67 mg. Other Ingredients: Citric Acid, Sodium Bicarbonate, Sorbitol, Mannitol, Red Beet Powder, Raspberry Flavor, Polyethylene Glycol 6000, Aspartame, Acesulfame Potassium, Wild Berry Powder, Magnesium Stearate, Silicon Dioxide.

Children's Multi-Vitamins — LiFizz Effervescent Vitamins
Each tablet contains: Vitamin A 2500 IU • Vitamin C 60 mg • Vitamin D 200 IU • Vitamin E 9 IU • Thiamin 1.05 • Riboflavin 1.19 mg • Niacinamide 14 mg • Vitamin B6 1.4 mg • Folic Acid 280 mcg • Vitamin B12 4.2 mcg • Biotin 210 mcg • Pantothenic Acid 7.9 mg • Calcium 200 mg. Available in Grape, Bubblegum, Orange, and Fruit Punch flavors.

Children's Chewable Vita-Bear — The Vitamin Shoppe
Each tablet contains: Vitamin C 200 mg • Citrus Bioflavonoid Complex 20 mg. No Yeast, Wheat, Corn, Sucrose, Salt, Starch, Soy, Gluten, Milk, Eggs, Dairy, Fish or Animal Derivatives, Preservatives, Artificial Colors or Flavors added.

Children's Chewable Vita-Bear — The Vitamin Shoppe
Each tablet contains: Calcium 200 mg • Magnesium 100 mg.

Chill Out — Pacific BioLogic
Gotu Kola • Peony root • Polygoni vine • Valerian root • Passion flower • Skullcap • Lemon Balm • Sweetflag rhizome • Polygala root • Citrus peel (unripened) • Salvia root • Schizandra fruit.

Chill Pill — Futurebiotics
Three tablets contain: Vitamin B1 (thiamin) 5 mg • Vitamin B2 (riboflavin) 5 mg • Niacinamide 200 mg • Calcium: (carbonate, phosphate, amino acid chelate) 150 mg • Vitamin B6 5 mg. In a balanced formula of Herbal extracts & powders including: Valerian root, Chamomile, Avena Sativa, Kava Kava, Hops, Skullcap, Spearmint, Nettles, Hawthorn, Fennel, Horsetail, Peppermint & Motherwort.

China Chlorella 200 Mg — Natrol
Fifteen tablets contain: Protein 2 mg • Vitamin A 1665 mg • Vitamin C 500 mg • Thiamine (B1) 45 mcg • Riboflavin (B2) 140 mcg • Niacin 714 mcg • Calcium 6.2 mg • Iron 5 mg • Vitamin E 0.03 IU • Vitamin B6 51 mcg • Folic Acid 0.8 mcg • Vitamin B12 4 mcg • Phosphorus 30 mg • Iodine 18 mcg • Potassium 27.3 mg • Magnesium 10 mg • Zinc 2.2 mg • Copper 3 mcg • Biotin 6 mcg • Pantothenic Acid 40 mcg • Chlorophyll 90.1 mg • RNA 89.1 mg • DNA 8.5 mg • Germanium 76 ppm.

Chinac Digestive Health Formula — Metabolife
Each caplet contains: Amomum longiligulare (Chinese Amomum) • Oryza sativa (Rice) • Artemisia annua (Sweet Wormwood) • Crataegus cuneata (Chinese Hawthorn) • Armeniaca amarum (Apricot) • Xanthium sibiricum (Xanthium) • Wolfiporia cocos (Poria) • Coix Lacryma-jobi (Job's Tears).

Chinac Immune Health Formula — Metabolife
Each caplet contains: Forsythia suspensa (Forsythia) • Isatis tinctoria (Isatis) • Astragalus membranaceus (Astragalus) • Lonicera dasystyla (Honeysuckle) • Belamcanda chinensis (Blackberry Lily) • Paeonia veitchii (Chinese Peony).

Chinac Joint Health Formula — Metabolife
Each caplet contains: Achryanthes bidentata (Achyranthes) • Wenyujin concisa (Wen Curcuma) • Erythrina variegata (Coral Tree) • Atractylodes macrocephala (Bai-Zhu Atractylodes) • Notopterygium incisum (Notopterygium) • Angelica pubescens (Pubescent Angelica).

Chinac Menstrual Health Formula — Metabolife
Each caplet contains: Lindera aggregata (Lindera) • Leonurus japonicus (Chinese Motherwort) • Angelica sinensis (Dong Quai) • Cyperus rotundus (Cyperus) • Corydalis yanhusuo (Corydalis).

Chinac Stress and Tension Formula — Metabolife
Each caplet contains: Corydalis yanhusuo (Corydalis) • Angelica dahurica (Fragrant Angelica) • Ligusticum sinense (Sichuan Lovage) • Saposhnikovia divaricata (Siler) • Arctium lappa (Burdock).

Chinese Herbal Formula — Futurebiotics
Four tablets contain: Extracts &/or Powders (Siberian Ginseng, Foti, Astragalus, Schizandra, LEM, Shiitake-Ganoderma Mushroom complex, Chinese Licorice, Codonopsis, Echinacea) equivalent to a minimum of 7000 mg • Beta Carotene 10,000 IU • Vitamin E (mixed tocopherols) 100 IU • Vitamin C 1000 mg • Selenium 100 mcg.

Chitosan — The Vitamin Shoppe
Each capsule contains: Chitosan, minimum 90% Deacetylated Chitin 250 mg • Aloe Vera 50 mg.

B R A N D   N A M E S

Chitosan Plus — Progressive Labs
Each capsule contains: Chitosan (marine fiber concentrate) 250 mg • Citric Acid 75 mg • Lipase (3000 units) 25 mg.

Chitosan-C with Biozan — Richardson Labs
Four caplets contain: BioZan: (Purified Chitosan, Betaine HCl, Oat bran, Aloe & Beta Glucan) 2500 mg • Chromium (picolinate) 200 mcg.

Chit-O-Slim Plus — Aspen Group, Inc.
Each capsule contains: Chitosan 500 mg • Chromium (picolinate) 50 mcg.

Chitosol — Sheldon Marketing
Four capsules contain: Chitosan 2000 mg • Vitamin C 400 mg.

Chlorophyll Liquid — Dial Herbs
Chlorophyllin Copper complex • Water • Oil of Mint • Glycerine, vegetable derived.

Chlorophyll Softgels — Dial Herbs
Chlorophyllin Copper complex • Water • Oil of Mint • Glycerine, vegetable derived.

Chloroplex — Progressive Labs
Each softgel contains: Chlorophyllin 50 mg.

Chloroplus — Atrium
Each capsule contains: Vitamin A 11000 IU • Vitamin D3 250 IU • Chlorophyll (oil soluble) 10 mg • Vitamin E (d-Alpha Tocopherol) 3 IU • Lecithin (Raw Unbleached) 210 mg • Pumpkin seed oil 45 mg • Sesame seed oil 22 mg • Halibut Liver oil • Skip Jack Liver oil.

Cholesta Balance — PhysioLogics
Each softgel contains: Pantethine (80% purity, 307 mg) 384 mg • Gamma Oryzanol (from Rice Bran) 100 mg.

Cholestaid — Omni Nutraceuticals
Two tablets contain: Esterin extract of Alfalfa 900 mg • Citric Acid 100 mg. Other ingredients: Microcrystalline, Croscarmellose Sodium, Stearic Acid, Silica.

Cholestain — Futurebiotics
One tablet contains: Beta Sitosterol 200 mg • Campesterol 100 mg • Stigmastero 180 mg.

Cholesta-Lo — Futurebiotics
Three tablets contain: Cholestatin 600 mg • Niacin (flush free) 200 mg • Chromium (polynicotinate) 100 mcg • Garlic (odorless) concentrate (2:1) 350 mg • Siberian Ginseng extract (10:1) 75 mg • Parsley 250 mg • Chickweed 200 mg • Hawthorn 150 mg • Ginger 200 mg • Cayenne 200 mg. (75 mg of 10:1 Siberian Ginseng extract is equal to 750 mg of raw Siberian Ginseng. 350 mg of 2:1 Garlic is equal to 875 mg of raw Garlic.)

CholesTame — Jarrow Formulas
Four tablets contain: Red Yeast Rice Extract (Monascus purpureus) (Xie Zhi Kang) 4% Statins 2400 mg • Coenzyme Q10 (Ubiquinone) 30 mg • Artichoke Leaf Extract (Cynara scolymus) 2% cynarine 400 mg • Guggul (Commiphora mukul) 4% guggulsterones 500 mg • Alpha Lipoic Acid 100 mg • Grape Seed Extract (Vitis vinifera) 95% polyphenols 50 mg • Pantethine 200 mg • Lutein 10 mg • Taurine 250 mg.

Cholesterol Metabolism — Nutrivention
Six tablets contain: Choline 500 mg • Inositol 500 mg • Niacinamide 200 mg • Unsaturated Fatty Acids (7% GAMA Linolenic Acid • 64% Linoleic Acid) 500 mg • Pantothenic Acid 200 mg • Magnesium 200 mg • Vitamin B6 100 mg • Vitamin D 600 IU • Lecithin 600 mg • Hawthorne berries 400 mg • Garlic powder concentrate 400 mg • Apple Pectin 360 mg • L-Methionine 340 mg • Capsicum 200 mg • Ginger root 200 mg • Butcher's Broom 100 mg • Betaine HCL 100 mg.

Cholesterol Support — Amazon Support
Each capsule contains: Artichoke • Mullaca • Annatto • Suma • Cat's Claw • Bitter Melon • Yerba Mate • Sarsaparilla.

Cholestin — Pharmanex
Each capsule contains: 600 mg of Cholestin, a proprietary strain of standardized Monascus purpureus Went yeast fermented on premium rice, which naturally contains HMG-CoA reductase inhibitors (0.4%) and unsaturated fatty acids. Other comprehensive testing show absence of heavy metals, residual solvents, and absence of microbial toxins.

Cholestoril — Enzymatic Therapy
Each tablet contains: Pantethine 300 mg. Contains no sugar, salt, yeast, wheat, corn, soy, dairy products, coloring, flavoring or preservatives.

Cholestra — HerbaSway
Soy • Hawthorn berry • Green Tea • He Sho Wu • Cassia tora • Blackberry • HerbaSwee (Cucurbitaceae fruit).

Cholestrex — Source Naturals
Nine tablets contain: Niacin 480 mg • Vitamin C (Calcium Ascorbate, Ascorbic Acid and Zinc Ascorbate) 900 mg • Vitamin E (D-Alpha Tocopheryl)(Natural) 100 IU • Calcium (Calcium Ascorbate) 100 mg • Zinc (Zinc Ascorbate) 6 mg • Copper (Copper Sevacate) 2 mg • Chromium (ChromeMate GTF Chromium Polynicotinate) 300 mcg • Oats (Bran and Fiber) 2500 mg • Grapefruit Pectin 1400 mg • Psyllium Seed Husk 1100 mg • Lecithin (with 24% Phosphatidyl Choline) 900 mg • Alfalfa Seed 600 mg • Beta Sitosterol 300 mg • L-Arginine 300 mg.

Chondroitin Plus — Atrium
Two capsules contain: Calcium Ascorbate 60 mg • Magnesium Ascorbate 60 mg • Vitamin C Content 100 mg • Thiamine HCL 25 mg • Pyridoxine HCL 10 mg • Niacinamide 60 mg • Manganese (Sulfate) 65 mg • Potassium (Citrate) 25 mg • Zinc (Citrate) 25 mg • Chondroitin Sulphates 125 mg • Mocopoly Saccharides 65 mg • Bioflavonoid Complex 50 mg • Betaine HCL 15 mg • Rutin 10 g • Black Cohosh 75 mg • Passiflora 75 mg • Valerian root 75 mg • Equestium 65 mg. Contains no sugar, starch, salt, wheat, corn, yeast or soy derivatives.

Chondroitin Sulfate — Jamieson
Each caplet contains: Chondroitin Sulfate (Equivalent to 400 mg Sodium Chondroitin Sulfate) 360 mg.

Chroma Slim for Men — Richardson Labs
Four capsules contain: Trace Mineral Blend: [Chromium (Picolinate) 400 mcg • Vanadium 120 mcg • Manganese (Picolinate) 2.5 mg]. Proprietary Lipotropic Blend: (Choline Bitartrate • L-Carnitine • Inositol • L-Methionine) 3000 mg. Essential Nutrient & Amino Acid Blend: (Ferulic Acid Esters • Taurine • L-Lysine HCl • L-Glutamic Acid • Base • Glycine USP • Cernitin flower pollen extract) 500 mg. Vitamin Blend: (Pantothenic Acid 10 mg • Vitamin B6 5 mg). Thermogenic Herbal Blend: (Panax Ginseng powdered extract • Cayenne • Mustard seed powder • Cinnamon powder • Ginger root powdered extract • Uva Ursi • Standardized White Willow bark powder) 424 mg. In a Base of: (Natural Peppermint • Saw Palmetto berries • Juniper berries & Spirulina).

Chroma Slim Plus — Richardson Labs
Four caplets contain: Trace Mineral Blend: [Chromium (Picolinate) 400 mcg • Vanadium 120 mcg • Manganese (Picolinate) 2.5 mg]. Proprietary Lipotropic & Lipid Transport Blend: (Choline Bitartrate • L-Carnitine • Inositol • L-Methionine) 3000 mg. Essential Nutrient & Amino Acid Blend: (Ferulic Acid Esters • Taurine • L-Lysine HCl • L-Glutamic Acid • Base • Glycine USP • Cernitin flower pollen extract) 500 mg. Vitamin Blend: [Potassium (Chloride) USP • Pantothenic Acid 10 mg • Vitamin B6 5 mg). In a Base of natural Peppermint & Bromelain.

Chrom-Adyl Surge — Biochem
Each capsule contains: Chromium 500 mcg • BMOV (Bis-Maltol OXO Vandium) 5 mg • Vanadyl Sulfate 5 mg.

ChromaSlim Biozan — Richardson Labs
Four caplets contain: BioZan: (Purified Chitosan, Betaine HCl, Oat bran, Aloe, Beta Glucan) 2500 mg • Chromium (Picolinate) 250 mcg.

Chromemate — Natrol
One capsule contains: Chromium (Polynicotinate) 200 mcg • L-Arginine 50 mg • L-Lysine 50 mg • Vitamin B6 (Pyridoxine) 10 mg. Other ingredients: Microcrystalline Cellulose, Magnesium Stearate, Gelatin.

Chromic Fuel (Chromium Picolinate) — TwinLab
Pure Crystalline Chromium Picolinate (supplying of Trivalent Chromium 200 mcg) 1.67 mg.

Chromium HCA — PhysioLogics
Each capsule contains: Calcium (as Calcium Salt of Hydroxy Citric Acid) 79 mg • Chromium (as Chromium Picolinate) 100 mcg • Garcinia cambogia [50% (-)- Hydroxy Citric Acid (HCA) 250 mg] 500 mg.

Chromium Nicotinate Complex — Progressive Labs
Each capsule contains: Niacin (as polynicotinate) 1300 mcg • Chromium (as polynicotinate) 200 mcg • Glutathione 250 mcg • Glycine 50 mcg • Cysteine 100 mcg • Aspartic Acid 100 mcg.

Chromium Picolinate — The Vitamin Shoppe
Each softgel contains: Chromium Picolinate, a compound of yeast-free Trivalent Chromium and Picolinic Acid 200 mcg.

Chromium Picolinate — Great American Nutrition
One tablet contains: Chromium (Picolinate) 200 mcg. Other Ingredients: Calcium Carbonate, Cellulose, Magnesium Stearate. Contains no added Sugar, Salt, Starch, Preservatives, Artificial Flavors, or Colors. Free of Corn, Soy, Wheat, Yeast, & Dairy Products. Suitable for vegetarians. Contains no animal products.

Chromium Picolinate — Richardson Labs
Each tablet contains: Chromium (Picolinate), derived from 3.2 mg of pure crystalline Chromium Picolinate. Contains no added sugar, salt, starch, preservatives, artificial flavors, or colors. Free of corn, soy, wheat, yeast, and dairy. Suitable for vegetarians. Contains no animal products.

Chromium Picolinate GTF — Atrium
Each capsule contains: Chromium (Chromium Picolinate) 200 mcg. Contains no sugar, starch, salt, wheat, corn, yeast, or soy derivatives.

Chromium Picolinate Plus — Progressive Labs
Each capsule contains: Chromium 200 mcg (from 1640 mg of chromium picolinate) • Gamma Oryzanol 15 mg • Boron (as boron aspartate) 2 mg.

Chromium Plus with Oxidative Factors — The Vitamin Shoppe
Each tablet contains: Zinc 30 mg • Chromium 100 mcg • Selenium 100 mcg.

Chrysin — ProLab
Each capsule contains: 5,7-Dihydroxyflanone (Chrysin) 250 mg.

Circulate Dietary Supplement Tablets — HealthWatchers System
Vitamin B6 • Vitamin B2 • Vitamin B12 • Vitamin B15 • Vitamin D • OrthoPhosphoric Acid or EDTA • Fenugreek Seed • Superoxide Dismutase • Rutin • Catalase • Beet Leaf • Phosphatidyl Choline • Alfalfa • Spanish Moss • Urea • Orchick Hyaluridase • Beta Carotene • Protomorphagens Pituitary • Heart Liver • Kidney • Brain.

Circulite Oil — The Herbalist
Oils of Sweet Almond, Eucalyptus, Camphor, St. John's Wort flower, Calendula flower, French Lavender, Peppermint, Sage & Extracts of Prickly Ash bark, Ginger root, Lobelia leaf.

Circuplex — Futurebiotics
Two tablets contain: Vitamin C 100 mg • Vitamin B1 (thiamin) 8 mg • Niacinamide 414 mg • Vitamin B2 (riboflavin) 8 mg • Niacin 20 mg • Vitamin B6 20 mg • Vitamin B12 10 mcg • Zinc (gluconate) 5 mg • Manganese (amino acid chelate) 5 mg. In a tablet base of: (Betaine HCl 20 mg, Citrus Bioflavonoids 50 mg, Alfalfa seed meal 200 mg, Oyster shell Calcium 50 mg, Cayenne 10 mg, Ginger 200 mg, Prickly Ash bark 200 mg & Peppermint) 100 mg.

Circutone — The Herbalist
Prickly Ash bark • Hawthorn berry, leaf & flower • Bayberry root bark • Ginger root • Yarrow flower • Cayenne pepper.

Citramannan — The Vitamin Shoppe
Each capsule contains: Citrimax (Hydroxy Citric Acid) 400 mg • Glucomannan (Konjac) root 400 mg.

Citratherm — MetPro
Citrus aurantium • Chromium Picolinate • Vitamin C • Niacin • St. John's Wort.

Citri-Caps — Progressive Labs
Each capsule contains: Malibar Tamarind (Garcinia cambogia, standardized to contain 50% (-) hydroxycitric acid) 333 mg • Atractylodes (Atractylodes lancea) 50 mg • Seville Orange flower (Citrus aurantii) 50 mg • Chromium (as chromium picolinate) 50 mcg • Chromium (as chromium arginate) 15 mcg.

Citri-Caps Plus — Progressive Labs
Each capsule contains: Malibar Tamarind (Garcinia cambogia, standardized to contain 50% (-) hydroxycitric acid) 333 mg • Ma Huang Extract (Ephedra sinica) 200 mg • Yerba Mate 75 mg •

Atractylodes (Atractylodes lancea) 50 mg • Seville Orange flower (Citrus Aurantii) 50 mg • Chromium (as chromium picolinate) 50 mcg • Chromium (as chromium arginate) 15 mcg.

CitriGenics — Roex
Six tablets contain: Citrimax Garcinia Cambogia 1500 mg • L-Carnitine 300 mg • Choline Bitartrate 100 mg • Inositol 100 mg • Betaine HCl 50 mg • Chromium 200 mcg • Green Tea extract 150 mg • Kola Nut extract 150 mg • Yerba Mate 100 mg • Ginger 100 mg • Spirulina 100 mg • Kelp with Trace Minerals 100 mg • Vitamin C 100 mg • Vitamin E 30 IU • Potassium 25 mg • Biotin 300 mcg • Niacinamide 50 mg • Vitamin A 5000 IU • Vitamin B6 20 mg • Vitamin B2 20 mg • Vitamin B12 6 mcg • Folic Acid 400 mcg • Iodine 150 mcg • Selenium 50 mcg.

CitriLean — Enzymatic Therapy
Each capsule contains: Garcinia cambogia extract (CitriMax) standardized to contain 50% (-) hydroxycitrate (125 mg/capsule) 250 mg • Ginger root extract 6.5:1 (Zingiber officinale) 50 mg • Fenugreek seed extract 4:1 (Trigonella foenum-graecum) 50 mg • Curcuma root extract (Curcuma longa) standardized to contain 4% curcumin 50 mg • Chromium Polynicotinate (ChromeMate) 25 mcg. Contains no sugar, salt, yeast, wheat, corn, soy, dairy products, coloring, flavoring, or preservatives.

Citrimate — Nature's Plus
Each tablet contains: Standardized Garcinia cambogia extract supplying 50% [-] Hydroxycitrate 500 mg • Chromium (Polynicotinate) 100 mcg. Contains no yeast, wheat, corn, soy, milk, salt, sugar or starch.

Citrimax — Nature's Plus
Each tablet contains: Standardized Garcinia cambogia extract supplying 50% [-] Hydroxycitrate 1000 mg. Contains no yeast, wheat, corn, soy, milk, salt, sugar or starch.

Citrimax — The Vitamin Shoppe
Standardized for 50% (-) Hydroxycitric Acid (HCA) • Chromium Picolinate 100 mcg.

Citrimax Fat Burners — Optimum Nutrition
Citrimax (H.C.A.).

CitrimaxPlus with ChromeMate — Natrol
One capsule contains: Chromium (Polynicotinate) 100 mcg • (-) Hydroxycitric Acid 250 mg • Uva Ursi 100 mg • Cascara Sagrada 75 mg. Other ingredients: Gelatin, Magnesium Stearate.

Citrin + Chromium — Olympia Nutrition
Hydroxycitrate (-) HCA + Chromium Picol.

CitriThin — Phytopharmica
Two capsules contain: Garcinia Cambogia extract (CitriMax) 500 mg standardized to contain 50% (-)hydroxycitrate (125 mg per capsule) • Ginger root extract 6.5:1 (Zingiber officinale) 100 mg • Fenugreek seed extract 4:1 (Trigonella foenum-graecum) 100 mg • Curcuma root extract (Curcuma longa) 100 mg standardized to contain 4% curcumin • Chromium Polynicotinate (ChromeMate) 50 mcg. Contains no sugar, salt, yeast, wheat, corn, soy, dairy products, coloring, flavoring, or preservatives.

Citrus Slender — Nature's Way
Each 14 g scoop contains: Arabinogalactan 2 g • Chromium Polynicotinate 100 mcg • Citrin 1.5 g • L-Carnitine l-Tartrate 800 mg. Other ingredients: Citric Acid, Fructose, Lemon Crystals, Lemon/Lime Crystals, Lime Crystals, Sodium Chloride, Sorbitol, Stevia, dried extract.

CLA — EAS
Each capsule contains: 1000 mg Vegetable oil with 60% conjugated Linoleic Acid (CLA) & 40% other Monounsaturated & Saturated Fatty Acid • 0.02% TBHQ (antioxidant) has been added to preserve freshness.

CLA 1000 — Human Development Technologies
Each softgel capsule contains: Tonalin 1000 mg yielding Conjugated Linoleic Acid 700 mg.

Classic Perfor-Max — Changes - TwinLab
One capsule contains: Proanthocyanidin Blend (85% Proanthocyanidins) Grape seed extract and Pine Bark 4:1 extract 50 mg • Turmeric rhizome extract 25 mg. Other ingredients: Maltodextrin, Calcium Sulfate, Gelatin, Cellulose, Magnesium Stearate, Silica, and Riboflavin color.

B R A N D   N A M E S

Some Brand Name Natural Products - What they Contain
www.NaturalDatabase.com contains MANY more listings than appear here.

B R A N D   N A M E S

Classic Thermo-Lift — Changes - TwinLab
Each capsule contains: Chromium (as Chromium picolinate) 200 mcg • MaHuang extract (aerial parts) (Standardized for 25 mg Ephedrine alkaloids) 310 mg • Proprietary herbal blend 260 mg: Guarana seed extract (39 mg Caffeine), White Willow bark, Siberian Ginseng root, Astragalus root, Bee Pollen, Bladderwrack kelp (Fucus vesiculosus), Ginger root, Gotu Kola leaf, Licorice root, Rehmannia root, and Reishi mushroom (fruiting body) • Other ingredients: Geltain, Maltodextrin, Magnesium stearate, Wheat Germ, Silica, and Turmeric extract.

CleanseSMART I — RenewLife
Artichoke leaf • Ashwaganda Root • Beet leaf (green rind) • Bupleurum root • Burdock root • Celandine • Chlorella • Corn silk • Dandelion root • Hawthorne berry • Larch gum • Milk Thistle seed • Mullein leaf • Red clover leaf and stem • Turmeric root.

CleanseSMART II — RenewLife
Magnesium Hydroxide • Cape aloe gel • Rhubarb • Slippery Elm bark • Marshmallow root • Fennel seed • Triphalia • Ginger root

Cleansing Herbs — Youngevity
Vitamin B2 • Cascara sagrada • Fennel • Peppermint • Yucca root • Pau d'Arco • Yellow Dock root • Vilcabamba Mineral Essence: Potassium, Calcium, Magnesium, Zinc, Chromium, Selenium, Iron, Copper, Molybdenum, Vanadium, Iodine, Cobalt, Manganese.

Cleansing Laxative — Zand
Each tablet contains: Active Ingredient: Cascara Sagrada bark 150 mg. Other Ingredients include : Chinese Rhubarb root, Frangula bark, Gentian root, Goldenseal root, Fennel seed, Kaolin clay, Anise seed, Oregon Grape root.

Clensa-Herb — Dial Herbs
Red Clover • Burdock • Echinacea • Chaparral • Mullein • Uva Ursi • Parsley • Marshmallow • Cascara Sagrada.

Clinical Nutrients for Senior Women — Phytopharmica
Six tablets contain: Vitamin A (Beta Carotene) 15000 IU • Vitamin A (Retinol) 2500 IU • Vitamin E 200 IU • Calcium (Citrate + Carbonate) 600 mcg • Vitamin C 300 mg • Magnesium (Aspartate) 300mg • Potassium (Aspartate) 99 mg • Vitamin B6 60 mg • Vitamin B1 60 mg • Vitamin B2 60 mg • Pantothenic Acid 50 mg • Niacin/Niacinamide 45 mg • Zinc (Picolinate) 15 mg • Manganese (Citrate) 15 mg • Copper (Gluconate) 1.5 mg • Folic Acid 800 mcg • Vitamin B12 800 mcg • Biotin 600 mcg • Iodine (Kelp) 300 mcg • Chromium (Polynicotinate) 200 mcg • Selenium 100 mcg • Vitamin K 60 mcg • Molybdenum 25 mcg • Flavonoids 100 mg • Alfalfa Juice concentrate 100 mg • Dong Quai extract 90 mg • Ginger root extract 60 mg • Fennel seed extract 30 mg • Green Tea extract 30 mg • Choline Bitartrate 30 mg • Inositol 30 mg • Betaine HCL 25 mg • PABA 30 mg • Glutamic Acid HCL 25 mg • Bromelain 15 mg • Papain 15 mg • Protease acid stable 5 mg • Lipase 5 mg • Boron 3 mg • Silica 1 mg • Vanadium (Sulfate) 50 mcg.

Clinical Nutrients Prenatal formula — Phytopharmica
Four tablets contain: Vitamin A (Beta Carotene) 15000 IU • Vitamin E (D-Alpha Tocopherol Succinate) 200 IU • Vitamin D 100 IU • Calcium (Citrate + Carbonate) 800 mg • Magnesium (Citrate) 400 mg • Vitamin C (Ascorbic Acid) 300 mg • Vitamin B6 (Pyridoxine HCL) 120 mg • Pantothenic Acid (D-Calcium Pantothenate) 100 mg • Potassium (Aspartate) 99 mg • Thiamine HCL (Vitamin B1) 60 mg • Riboflavin (Vitamin B2) 60 mg • Niacin/Niacinamide 45 mg • Iron (Ferrous Succinate) 30 mg • Zinc (Picolinate) 30 mg • Manganese (Citrate) 15 mg • Copper (Gluconate) 1.5 mg • Folic Acid 800 mcg • Vitamin B12 (Cyanocobalamin) 800 mcg • Biotin 600 mcg • Vitamin K (Phytonandione) 500 mcg • Iodine (Kelp) 300 mcg • Chromium (Polynicotinate) 200 mcg • Selenium (L-Selenomethionine) 100 mcg • Molybdenum (Sodium Molybdate) 25 mcg • Other ingredients: Ginger root extract 6.5:1 150 mg (Zingiber officinale) • Flavonoids (Mixed) 90 mg • Choline Bitartrate 90 mg • Inositol 90 mg • Dandelion root extract 4:1 (Taraxacum officinale) 60 mg • Red Raspberry leaves 60 mg • Boron (Sodium Tetraborate Decahydrate) 1 mg • Silica (Sodium Metasilicate) 1 mg • Vanadium (Sulfate) 50 mcg. Contains no sugar, salt, yeast, wheat, corn, dairy products, coloring, flavoring or preservatives.

CM Source — Now
Each 500 mg capsule contains : Cetyl Myristoleate 100 mg.

CMG — Natrol
Cetyl myristoleate 500 mg • MSM (Methyl sulfonyl methane) 500 mg • Glucosamine sulfate 500 mg • Sea Cucumber 25 mg.

C-M-K Citrate — Progressive Labs
Each capsule contains: Calcium (as calcium citrate) 100 mg • Magnesium (as magnesium citrate) 100 mg • Potassium (as potassium citrate) 25 mg.

Co Q10 — Pharmanex
Each softgel contains: Vitamin E (from Mixed Tocopherols) 30 IU • Coenzyme Q10 (Ubiquinone) 30 mg. Other Ingredients: Rice Bran Oil, Gelatin, Glycerin, Yellow Beeswax, Annatto Extract, Titanium Dioxide.

CoenZest — Holista
Each capsule contains: CoEnzyme Q10 (ubiquinone) 30 mg. Other Ingredients: Organic Flax Seed Oil.

Cognicine — Pacific BioLogic
DMAE • Bacopin • Ashwagandha extract • Black Pepper extract (bioperine).

Cold & Flu Support — Amazon Support
Each capsule contains: Picao Preto • Fedegosa • Amor Seco • Guaco • Bitter Melon • Clavillia • Mullaca • Samambaia • Quinine Bark • Gervao • Pau d'arco • Cat's Claw • Simarouba.

Cold Care P.M. — Traditional Medicinals
Contains: Menthol: 5 mg per cup as it naturally occurs in the Peppermint leaf (Mentha x piperia) present in the blend. Other herbal ingredients: Licorice root, Chamomile flower, Tilla Starflower, Yarrow flower, Passion flower herb, Eucalyptus leaf, Elder flower.

Cold-Eeze — Quigley Co.
Each lozenge contains: Zinc Gluconate 11.5 mg. Other ingredients: Glycine, corn syrup, sucrose, and natural flavors.

Cold-Eezer Plus — Quigley Co.
Each lozenge contains: Zinc Gluconate 14.5 mg. Other ingredients: Glycine, corn syrup, sucrose, and natural flavors.

Coldflua — HerbaSway
Bitter Orange • Kudzu • Ginger • Echinacea • Astragalus • Knotweed • Schisandra • Blackberry • Licorice • Skullcap • Cayenne pepper • HerbaSwee (Cucurbitaceae fruit).

Cold-FX - HerbTech — CV Technologies
Each capsule contains: Concentrated North American Ginseng (Panax quinquefolium) extract 200 mg.

Coleus Forskohlii extract — Enzymatic Therapy
One capsule contains: Coleus Forskohlii extract standardized to contain 18% Forskolin (9 mg per capsule) 50 mg. Contains no sugar, salt, yeast, wheat, corn, soy, dairy products, coloring, flavoring or preservatives.

Colloidal Magnesium Plus — Progressive Labs
Each capsule contains: Colloidal Calcium 25 mg • Colloidal Magnesium 50 mg • Colloidal Zinc 1.5 mg • Colloidal Copper 1 mg • Colloidal Manganese 0.1 mg • Colloidal Chromium 0.03 mg • Colloidal Molybdenum 0.012 mg.

Colloidal Minerals — Progressive Labs
One half ounce contains: Calcium 109 mg • Iron 0.24 mg • Phosphorus 109 mg • Iodine 180 mcg • Magnesium 56.9 mg • Zinc 16.3 mg • Selenium 0.09 mcg • Copper 1.24 mg • Manganese 2.8 mg • Chromium 0.4 mcg • Molybdenum 0.01 mcg • Chloride 0.1 mg • Sodium 0.74 mg • Potassium 171 mg • Sulfur 0.08 mg • Aluminum 2.15 mg • Silicon 0.4 mg • Lanthanum 0.1 mg • Thallium 0.02 mg • Cesium 0.4 mcg • Strontium 5.8 mcg • Vanadium 5.4 mcg • Boron 4.62 mcg • Nickel 4.45 mcg • Scandium 3.3 mcg • Ruthenium 3.13 mcg • Lithium 2.15 mcg • Titanium 1.57 mcg • Neodynium 0.15 mcg • Antimony 1.3 mcg • Cobalt 1.06 mcg • Flouride 0.94 mcg • Bismuth 0.33 mcg • Thallium 0.28 mcg • Zirconium 0.23 mcg • Beryllium 0.2 mcg • Cerium 0.2 mcg • Erbium 0.2 mcg • Bromine 0.16 mcg • Indium 0.13 mcg • Rubidium 0.13 mcg • Silver 0.1 mcg • Tin 0.1 mcg • Yttrium 0.1 mcg • Gallium 0.08 mcg • Tellurium 0.07 mcg • Praseodymium 0.05 mcg • Samarium 0.05 mcg • Barium 0.02 mcg • Cadmium 0.02 mcg • Dysprosium 0.02 mcg • Germanium 0.01 mcg • Gold < 0.01 mcg • Europium < 0.01 mcg • Niobium < 0.01 mcg • Palladium < 0.01 mcg • Ytterbium < 0.01 mcg • Hafnium < 0.01 mcg • Iridium < 0.01 mcg • Rhodium < 0.01 mcg • Terbium < 0.01 mcg • Holmium < 0.01 mcg • Lutetium < 0.01 mcg • Rhenium < 0.01 mcg • Tantalum < 0.01 mcg • Thorium < 0.01 mcg • Tungsten < 0.01 mcg • Plantium < 0.01 mcg • Carbon 7.8%. Other ingredients: Water, Glycerine, Natural Flavor, Grapefruit seed extract, Stevia.

Colloidal Silver — Changes - TwinLab
Four Droppersful (4 ml) contain: Colloidal Silver 20 mcg. Other ingredients: Demineralized water.

Colloidal Vitamins — Progressive Labs
One half ounce contains: Vitamin A (as beta carotene) 5000 IU • Vitamin C (ascorbic acid) 300 mg • Vitamin D 400 IU • Vitamin E 60 IU • Vitamin K 300 mcg • Thiamin (Vitamin B1) 3 mg • Riboflavin (Vitamin B2) 3.4 mg • Niacin (as niacinamide) 40 mg • Vitamin B6 4 mg • Folate (folic acid) 400 mcg • Vitamin B12 3 mcg • Biotin 300 mcg • Pantothenic Acid 20 mg • Choline Bitartrate 50 mg • Myonositol (inositol) 50 mg • Essential Fatty Acid complex 10 mg • Amino Acid complex 10 mg • Aloe powder 3 mg. Other Ingredients: Water, Glycerine, Natural Flavor, Grapefruit seed extract, Stevia.

Coloklysis — PhysioLogics
Each scoop contains: Psyllium seed & husk 10,000 mg • Oat fiber (Avena sativa) 1000 mg • Rice Bran 500 mg • Fructooligosaccharides (FOS) 250 mg • Alfalfa (Medicago sativa) 38 mg • Barley (Hordium vulgare) 38 mg • Apple Pectin (Malus sylvestris) 30 mg • Buckthorn bark (Rhamnus fangula) 38 mg • Papain (Carica papaya) 38 mg • Cascara sagrada (Rhamnus purshiana) 38 mg • Goldenseal (Hydrastis canadensis) 38 mg • Triphala 30 mg • natural Orange flavor 150 mg • Stevia extract 50 mg.

Coloklysis Daily — PhysioLogics
Each scoop contains: Psyllium 3400 mg • Oat fiber (Avena sativa) 2500 mg • Guar Gum 2500 mg • Acacia Gum 1200 mg • Apple Pectin 1000 mg • Rice Bran 500 mg • Fructooligosaccharides (FOS) 250 mg • L-Glutamine 100 mg • Aloe Vera 100 mg • Licorice 100 mg • Ginger 100 mg • Acesulfame Potassium 15 mg • Stevia 10 mg. Contains natural coloring and flavoring.

Colon Cleanse — Nature's Rx
Each capsule contains: Bentonita Clay • Micro-Crystalline Cellulose • Psyllium Seed • Senna Leaf • Citrus Pectin • Oat Bran • Nutra Flora FOS • Acidophilus Blend • Barley Grass • Golden Seal • Prune Concentrate • Slippery Elm Bark • Aloe Vera Leaf Extract • Bio-Perine • Cascara Sagrada.

Comfrey and Fenugreek — Dial Herbs
Comfrey • Fenugreek.

Comfrey/Aloe Capsules — Aloe Farms
Comfrey powder 100 mg • Aloe Vera powder 50 mg.

Commando 2000 — Nature's Plus
Two tablets contain: Commando Vitamin & Mineral Blend: Vitamin C corn free fortified with Rose Hips 1000 mg • Citrus Bioflavonoid Complex active flavonols, flavones, flavones & narigen - 44% 200 mg • Vitamin E natural 200 IU • Beta Carotene [carrot (Dunaliella salina) supplying 10000 IU Vitamin A activity] 60 mg • Zinc (Monomethionine) 20 mg • Selenium (Selenomethionine) 100 mcg. Commando Herbal Blend: Echinacea (Echinacea purpurea) 250 mg • Astragalus (Astragalus membranoceus) 150 mg • Garlic, odorless 70 mg • Ginkgo Biloba 50:1 standardized 24% ginkgo flavone-glycosides 5 mg. Commando Amino Acid Blend: NAC (N-Acetyl-Cysteine) 20 mg • L-Methionine free form amino acid 15 mg • L-Glutathione free form amino acid 10 mg. In a natural base of Pycnogenol (Pine bark extract), standardized 85-95% proanthocyanidins, antioxidant plant enzymes: catalase, glucose oxidase & peroxidase; & antioxidant vegetables : broccoli rich in sulforaphane, cabbage, cauliflower & tomato rich in lycopene. Contains no yeast, wheat, corn, soy, milk, salt, sugar or starch.

Complete Cleanse — PhysioLogics
Each caplet contains: Calcium (from Dicalcium Phosphate) 260 mg • Phosphorus (from Dicalcium Phosphate) 200 mg. Rapid Release Layer: Enzyme Activated Herbal Digestive extract blend containing: (Cellulose, Beet fiber root, Fenugreek seed, Licorice root, Fennel seed, Lipase (from Aspargillus cryzae), Date fruit, Fig fruit, Ginger root, Prune fruit) 500 mg • Herbal Detox extract blend 250 mg containing: (Tea Green leaf, Grapefruit seed, Burdock root, Chickweed aerial parts, Gentian root, Milk Thistle seed, Red Clover blossom, Dandelion root, Marshmallow root, Rosemary leaf, Yarrow flower, Yellow Dock root) 500 mg. Extended Release Layer: Enzyme-Activated Cleansing Fiber & Herb Blend containing: (Butternut bark, Beet fiber root, Licorice root, Flax seed, Peppermint oil) 250 mg • Probiotic Flora Replenishment Complex containing: (Lactic Culture of B.Coaugulins, Fructooligosaccharides & Inulides (from dahlia tuber & chicory root) 75 million cells • Intestinal Tract Immune Complex containing: (Black Walnut leaf, Methylsulonyimethane (MSM), Garlic bulb) 250 mg.

Complete Protein Diet — Optimum Nutrition
Each serving contains: Vanilla flavor Ingredients: Proprietary Protein Blend (Calcium Caseinate, Whey Protein Concentrate, Egg Albumen, Hydrolyzed Whey Peptides, Whey Protein Isolate, L-Glutamine) • Canola oil • Artificial Flavor • Complete Vitamin Mineral Blend (di-Potassium Phosphate, Magnesium Oxide, Potassium Chloride, Ascorbic Acid, dl-Alpha Tocopherol Acetate, Niacinamide, Vitamin A Palmitate, Zinc Oxide, Potassium Iodide, Vitamin K, D-Calcium Pantothenate, Copper Sulfate, Manganese Sulfate, Vitamin D3, Pyridoxine Hydrochloride, Thiamine Mononitrate, Riboflavin, Selenium Glycinate, Molybdenum Glycinate, Chromium Picolinate, Folic Acid, Biotin, Cyanocobalamin) • Lecithin • Cellulose Gum • Xanthan Gum • Aspartame • Acesulfame Potassium • Salt • FD&C Yellow #5 • FD&C Yellow #6.

Complexion Perfect — Aspen Group, Inc.
Four tablets contain: Vitamin A 5000 IU • Beta Carotene 5000 IU • Vitamin B1 (thiamine) 25 mg • Vitamin B2 (riboflavin) 25 mg • Vitamin B3 (niacin) 50 mg • Vitamin B5 (pantothenic acid) 25 mg • Vitamin B6 (pyridoxine HCl) 50 mg • Biotin 300 mcg • Vitamin C (calcium ascorbate) 500 mg • Vitamin E (succinate) 400 IU • Magnesium Oxide 200 mg • Zinc (gluconate) 12 mg • Burdock root 600 mg • L-Lysine HCl 500 mg • L-Proline 500 mg • Yellow Dock 500 mg • Silica (derived from horsetail extract) 400 mg • Grape seed extract (proanthodyn) 50 mg • Selenomethionine 200 mcg • Chromium Picolinate 50 mcg • GTF Chromium 25 mcg. Contains no sugar, starch, salt, wheat, corn, yeast or soy derivatives.

Composition 1 — Dial Herbs
Bayberry • White Pine bark • Clove • Cinnamon • Ginger • Cayenne.

Concentrated Broccoli — Jamieson
Each caplet contains: Concentrated Broccoli florets (Equivalent to 25000 mg fresh Broccoli) 450 mg • Concentrated Kale leaf and Radish root (Standardized to Active Isothiocyanates 450 mcg) 10 mg.

Connect-All — Nature's Plus
Two tablets contain: Glucosamine Sulfate (Aminomonosaccharide) 300 mg • Bromelain, proteolytic enzyme 600 GDU/gram, 200 mg • Calcium (Aminoate) 200 mg • Vitamin C corn free 60 mg • Aloe Vera leaf naturally rich in Mucopolysaccharide 50 mg • Chondroitin Sulfate A (CSA) 50 mg • Zinc (Monomethionine) 15 mg • Chinese Sea Cucumber (Microchele nobilis) 10 mg • Copper (Aminoate) 1 mg . In a highly active base of Alfalfa, Chlorella, Spirulina & low temperature dried Barley Grass juice, supplying naturally occuring chlorophyll & trace minerals. Contains no yeast, wheat, corn, soy, milk, salt, sugar or starch.

Continence with Flowtrol — Solaray - Nutraceutical
Two capsules contain: Butterbur root extract (Petasites hybridus) (Guaranteed to contain 15 mg sesquiterpenes) 100 mg • Flowtrol Proprietary Blend 870 mg: Cranberry berry extract (Vaccinium macrocarpon as CranActin Cranberry AF Extract) • Morinda root extract 5:1 • Psoralea fruit extract 5:1 • Raspberry fruit extract 5:1 (Rubus chingii) • Alpinia oxyphylla fruit and seed extract 5:1 • Lobelia (aerial). Other ingredients: Gelatin (capsule), Cellulose, Maltodextrin, Magnesium Stearate, Silica, and Magnesium Hydroxide.

Controlled-Release Melatonin — amni
Each tablet contains: Melatonin 2 mg.

COQ10 100 mg PLUS E — Progressive Labs
Each capsule contains: Co-Enzyme Q10 100 mg • Vitamin E (dl-alpha tocopheryl acetate) 100 IU.

CoQ10 Spray — Nature's Plus
Each spray contains: CoQ10 pharmaceutical grade Ubiquinone 30 mg. In a proprietary Liposomal Complex of Essential Metabolic Factors , Purified Water, Vegetable Glycerine, Purified Lecithin, Citrus seed extract (Citrus sinensis), Vitamin E & natural Mandarin Tangerine flavor.

Cordephrine XC — HealthDesigns
Each vegicap contains: Cordyceps Mycelia (Cordyceps sinensis) 450 mg. Other Ingredients: Pure plant cellulose (vegicaps). Does not contain ephedra or ephedrine.

Cordyceps (Caterpillar Fungus) — Olympia Nutrition
Caterpillar fungus 500 mg.

Cordyceps 500 — Pinnacle
Each tablet contains: 100% Purified Chinese Herbs 500 mg (Dong

© Copyright 2000, Natural Medicines Comprehensive Database (209) 472-2244. For updated data, go to www.NaturalDatabase.com. • 1319

BRAND NAMES

Some Brand Name Natural Products - What they Contain
www.NaturalDatabase.com contains MANY more listings than appear here.

Chong Zia Cao, Sha Shen, Wuwei Zi, Gan Jiang, Duhlulin). Free of yeast, corn, soy, wheat, lactose, citrus, milk, egg & fish products. No sugar, salt, starch, yeast, artificial coloring, flavoring, or preservatives.

Cordyceps 520 mg — Solaray
Each capsule contains: Cordyceps 520 mg. Other Ingredients: Gelatin, cellulose, & mangnesium stearate.

Cordyceps Power 800 mg — Planetary Formulations
Two capsules contain: Cordyceps Proprietary Blend 1600 mg. Other Ingredients: Dibasic calcium phosphate, colloidal silicon dioxide, magnesium stearate, modified cellulose gum, & stearic acid.

Cordyceps with Siberian Ginseng — Natrol
Each capsule contains: Cordyceps 300 mg • Siberian Ginseng 50 mg. Other Ingredients: Rice powder, silica, & gelatin. No yeast, wheat, corn, milk, egg, soy, glutens, artificial colors or flavors, added sugar, starch or preservatives.

CordyMax Cs-4 — Pharmanex
Two capsules contain: Cordyceps Cs-4 Mushroom Mycelia (Cordyceps sinensis [Berk.] Sacc.) 1050 mg. Other Ingredient: Gelatin.

Coreplex — Flora
Hawthorn blossoms & leaves • Passion Flower Herb • Hibiscus flowers • Hawthorn berry extract (1:4).

Coromega Orange Flavor —
European Reference Botanical Laboratories
Each packet contains: Vitamin C 45 mg • Vitamin E 7 IU • Folic Acid 100 mcg • Omega-3 fatty acids (EPA 350 mg • DHA 230 mg) 650 mg • Stevia Leaf extract 5 mg. Ingredients: Water, Egg Yolk, Natural Orange Flavor, Citric Acid, Sodium Benzoate, Vanillin, Beta Carotene, Potassium Sorbate, Menthol, Folic Acid.

Cortistat-PS — Champion Nutrition
Four capsules contain: Phosphatidylserine 100 mg • Phosphatidylcholine 105 mg • Phosphatidylethanolamine 70 mg • Phosphatidylinositol 30 mg • Arginine Aspartate 576 mg • Potassium Succinate 576 mg • Quercetin 100 mg • Feverfew 100 mg.

Coryza Forte — Progressive Labs
Each capsule contains: Vitamin A (as retinol & beta carotene) 4000 IU • Vitamin C (ascorbic acid) 300 mg • Vitamin B6 (pyridoxine HCl) 15 mg •Pantothenic Acid (as d-calcium pantothenate) 25 mg • Calcium (as calcium carbonate) 40 mg • Zinc (as zinc picolinate) 5 mg • Echinacea 50 mg • Citrus Bioflavonoid 5X complex (as undiluted hesperidin, naringin and rutin) 150 mg. Other ingredients: Pollen, Raw Bovine Trachea, Raw Bovine Thymus, Raw Bovine Adrenal, Raw Bovine Lymph, Raw Bovine Spleen, RNA, Rose Hips, Whey, Cellulose, Magnesium Stearate, Gelatin.

Coryza-Comp — Atrium
Each tablet contains: Vitamin A (Fish oil) 2000 IU • Vitamin C Ascorbic Acid 300 mg • Vitamin B6 Pyridoxine HCL 15 mg • Pantothenic Acid 25 mg • Calcium (Aspartate) 10 mg • Magnesium (Aspartate) 10 mg • Zinc (Aspartate) 2 mg • Citrus Bioflavonoids 150 mg • High-RNA Yeast 50 mg • Bee Pollen 10 mg • Raw Spleen concentrate (Bovine) 10 mg • Raw Thymus concentrate (Bovine) 10 mg • Raw Adrenal concentrate 5 mg • Raw Lymph concentrate (Bovine) 5 mg. In a base of Alfalfa & Rose Hips.

Cosamin — Nutramax Laboratories, Inc.
Each capsule contains: Glucosamine HCI (99%) 250 mg • Sodium Chondroitin Sulfate (95%) with Mixed Glycosaminoglycans (5%) 200 mg • Ascorbate (as manganese ascorbate) 33 mg • Manganese (as manganese ascorbate) 5 mg.

CosaminDS — Nutramax Laboratories, Inc.
Each capsule contains: Glucosamine HCI (99%) 500 mg • Sodium Chondroitin Sulfate (95%) with Mixed Glycosaminoglycans (5%) 400 mg • Ascorbate (as manganese ascorbate) 66 mg • Manganese (as manganese ascorbate) 10 mg.

Cosamine 500 mg — Kripps Pharmacy
Each capsule contains: Chondroitin Sulfate & Glucosamine powder (1:1 ratio) 500 mg.

Cotswold Deer Velvet — Cotswold
100% Deer Velvet.

Cough Syrup — Progressive Labs
Each 10 ml contains: Dextromethorphan Hydrobromide 10 mg •

Guaifenesin 100 mg • Potassium Citrate 85 mg • Citric Acid 35 mg. In a pleasant, mint-flavored, glycerin-sorbitol solution. Non-narcotic antitussive, expectorant, demulcent. Contains no sugar, alcohol, sodium, or antihistamine.

Cough-Eze Syrup — The Herbalist
Marshmallow root, Slippery Elm bark, Elecampane root, Wild Cherry bark, Mullein leaf, Horehound leaf, Licorice root, Cubeb berry, Orange peel, Cinnamon bark & Ginger root • Skunk Cabbage root & Lobelia leaf • Honey • Vegetable Glycerine • Peppermint Oil.

C-Plus-Citrus — Atrium
Each level teaspoon (3300 mg approx. wt.) contains: Vitamin C from: (Ascorbic Acid 900 mg & Sodium Ascorbate 625 mg) 1500 mg • Mannitol 1395 mg • Lemon Bioflavonoids 150 mg • Rose Hips 100 mg • Hesperidin Complex 50 mg • Rutin 30 mg. Contains natural Orange Juice flavor.

Cramp Bark-Catnip Virtue — Blessed Herbs
Cramp bark • Catnip flower & herb • Motherwort • Scullcap • Yarrow flower & herb • Grain alcohol & Distilled Water.

Cramp Free — Health Center for Better Living
Calcium • Magnesium • Potassium • other herbs.

Cran Support — Natrol
One capsule contains: Guaranteed Potency Cranberry extract supplying 90% solids 30-40% organic acids 400 mg • Uva Ursi leaves 115 mg • Vitamin C (Ascorbic Acid) 100 mg • FOS (Fruiti-Vin FructoOgligoSaccharides) 100 mg • Cat's Claw root 50 mg • Corn Silk 30 mg • Kava Kava root 8.5 mg. Other ingredients: Silica, Magnesium Stearate, Annatto, Gelatin.

Cran-Aid — Traditional Medicinals
Roselle Hibiscus flower • Cranberry Fruit concentrate • German Chamomile flower • Rose Hip • Uva Ursi leaf • Cleavers herb • Althea root • Peppermint leaf • Stevia leaf.

Cranberry — Aspen Group, Inc.
Each tablet contains: Cranberry extract (25:1 extract) 250 mg • Vitamin C 60 mg • Echinacea (4:1 extract) 30 mg • Buchu (4:1 extract) 15 mg • Juniper berry (4:1 extract) 15 mg • Uva Ursi (4:1 extract) 15 mg. Contains no sugar, starch, salt, wheat, corn, yeast or soy derivatives.

Cranberry — Pharmanex
Each capsule contains: Cranberry Fruit (15:1) concentrate (Vaccinium macrocarpon) 500 mg. Other Ingredients: Gelatin and Titanium Dioxide.

Cranberry + — PhysioLogics
Four tablets contain: Vitamin C (Ascorbic Acid) 300 mg • Cranberry extract (30% natural organic acids, 600 mg; 5% Anthocyanidins, 100 mg) 2000 mg • Goldenseal root (5% total Alkaloids, 10 mg) 200 mg.

Cranberry Juice Concentrate 1000 mg — Jamieson
Each capsule contains: Vitamin C (as Ascorbic Acid) 10 mg • Cranberry juice concentrate 1000 mg.

Cranberry Plus — Futurebiotics
Cranberry Extract (25:1 extract) 250 mg • Vitamin C 50 mg • Echinacea (4:1 extract equivalent to) 25 mg • Buchu (4:1 extract equivalent to) 12.5 mg • Juniper Berry (4:1 extract equivalent to) 12.5 mg • Uva Ursi (4:1 extract equivalent to) 12.5 mg.

Cran-C — Holista
Each capsule contains: Vitamin C 100 mg • Concentrated Cranberries (Vaccinum macrocarpon) of 25:1 extract (equivalent to 1132 mg of fresh cranberry juice) 45.3 mg.

Cran-Caps — Progressive Labs
Three softgels contain: Vitamin C 30 mg • Cranberry juice concentrate 3000 mg • Phosphatide complex 90 mg. Free of sugar and artificial sweeteners.

CranExtra — Enzymatic Therapy
Each capsule contains: Vitamin C (Ascorbic Acid) 1000 mg. Other ingredients: Cranberry extract (Vaccinium macrocarpon) standardized to contain 5% Anthocyanidins & 30% Organic Acids: Quinic, Malic, Citric & Hippuric Acid 100 mg • Uva Ursi (Arctostaphylos uva ursi) standardized to contain 20% Arbutin 100 mg. Contains no sugar, salt, yeast, wheat, corn, soy, dairy products, coloring, flavoring or preservatives.

1320 • © Copyright 2000, Natural Medicines Comprehensive Database (209) 472-2244. For updated data, go to www.NaturalDatabase.com.

Some Brand Name Natural Products - What they Contain
www.NaturalDatabase.com contains MANY more listings than appear here.

CranGuard — Phytopharmica
Each capsule contains: Vitamin C (ascorbic Acid) 100 mg • Other ingredients: Cranberry extract (Vaccinium macrocarpon) 100 mg standardized to contain 5% anthocyanidins & 30% organic acids (quinic, malic, citric & hippuric acid) • Uva Ursi (Arctostaphylos uva ursi) 100 mg standardized to contain 20% arbutin. Contains no sugar, salt, yeast, wheat, corn, soy, dairy products, coloring, flavoring, or preservatives.

Cravex — Natrol
Two tablets contain: Calcium 230 mg • Iodine (as Potassium Iodine) 150 mcg • Chromium (as Chromium Picolinate) 200 mcg • Gymnema Sylvestre powdered extract leaves 300 mg • Licorice root 250 mg Deglycyrrhizinated Licorice • powdered extract Glycerinic Acid (1%) 2.5 mg • L-Glutamine 250 mg • DL-Phenylalanine 250 mg • 5-Hydroxytryptophan (5-HTP) 10 mg. Other ingredients: Calcium Sulfate Dihydrate, Mono & Di-Glycerides, Microcrystalline Cellulose, Croscarmellose Sodium, Stearic Acid, Silicon Dioxide, Magnesium Stearate.

Creagen — ANS
Creatine Monohydrate.

Creagen Plus — ANS
Creatine Monohydrate • Dextrose • Taurine.

Creatine Blast — Pharmanex
Each scoop (42 g) contains: Phosphorus (as Dimagnesium Phosphate) 60 mg:Magnesium (as Dimagnesium Phosphate) 50 mg • Creatine Monohydrate 4 g • Taurine 1000 mg. Other Ingredients: Dextrose, Citric Acid, Natural Grape Flavor, Grape Skin Extract (color).

Creatine Chewable with FOS —
Natural Sport Supplements - Nutraceutical
Two wafers contain: Creatine Monohydrate 3 g • Proprietary FOS Fiber Blend (BeFlora) (265 mg Fructo-oligosaccharides) 530 mg. Other ingredients: Guar gum, Cellulose, Natural Tangerine flavor, Citric acid, Stearic acid, Maltose, Natural Orange flavor, Silica, and Magnesium Stearate.

Creatine Fuel — TwinLab
Each capsule contains: Creatine Monohydrate 700 mg. Each teaspoonful of powder contains: Creatine Monohydrate 5 g (5000 mg).

Creatine Fuel Loading Drink — TwinLab
HPLC Pure Creatine Monohydrate with added Dextrose (a high glycemic carbohydrate) • Chromium • Taurine • Magnesium • Alpha Lipoic Acid. Other Ingredients: L-Glutamine 2 g.

Creatine Fuel Plus — TwinLab
Creatine (Creatine Monohydrate) 7 g. It also contains muscle cell volumizers, insulin potentiators & anti-catabolic, lean body mass stimulators. Fat free.

Creatine Fuel Stack — TwinLab
Six capsules contain: Creatine Monohydrate 5000 mg • L-Glutamine 2000 mg • Taurine 200 mg.

Creatine Fuelchews — TwinLab
Each chew contains: Pure Creatine Monohydrate 1 g • Dextrose 3 g. No sucrose or fructose is present.

CreaVATE — ProLab
Each capsule contains: Creatine Pyruvate 750 mg.

Creavescent — GEN
Each serving contains: L-Glutamine 2 g • TCT TM (Total Creatine Transport) proprietary blend of: (Creatine Monohydrate) 5 g. Ingredients: Creatine Monohydrate • Fructose • L-Glutamine • Mono Poly-Saccharide • 2-Hydroxy-1, 2, 3-Propanetricarboxylic Acid • Sodium Hydrogen Carbonate • Orange Solids • Calcium Phosphate • Vitamin A • Vitamin D • Riboflavin.

CreaVol ATP — SportPharma
Each 41 g serving contains: 99% pure microfine Crystalline Creatine 5 g • Adenine Mucleotides including ATP • Vanadyl Sulfate • Taurine • Disodium & Potassium Phosphate • Dextrose (about 35 g per serving).

CTR Support — PhysioLogics
Each capsule contains: Turmeric (95% Curcumin) 250 mg • Boswellia (60% Boswellic Acids) 166.67 mg • Bromelain (2400 GDU)83.33 mg • Ginger (5% Gingerols) 33.33 mg • Yucca (14% Saponins) 16.67 mg • Devils Claw (3.5% Harpagosides) 16.67 mg • Quercetin (98% bioflavonoids) 16.67 mg.

Culturelle with Lactobacillus GG — Klaire Laboratories
Each capsule contains: Lactobacillus GG.

Curazyme — Enzymatic Therapy
Each capsule contains: Vitamin C (Ascorbic Acid) 50 mg • Pantothenic Acid (D-Calcium Pantothenate) 25 mg • Magnesium (Oxide) 25 mg • Curcuma root extract (Curcuma longa) standardized to contain 97% Curcumin 200 mg • Bromelain (2000 MCU) 200 mg • Butchers Broom extract (Ruscus aculeatus) standardized to contain 10% Saponins calculated as Ruscogenin 100 mg • Pancreatic Enzymes (10X) 50 mg • L-Cysteine 25 mg. Contains no sugar, salt, yeast, wheat, corn, soy, dairy products, coloring, flavoring, or preservatives.

CV-10 (Cardiovascular Nutritional Support) — Rx Vitamins
Six capsules contain: L-Taurine 500 mg • L-Carnitine 500 mg • Magnesium (Taurate) 400 mg • Hawthorne berry 100 mg • Potassium (Citrate) 99 mg • CoQ10 30 mg • Vitamin B3 (Niacin) 25 mg • Vitamin B6 (Pyridoxine) 25 mg • Folic Acid 400 mcg • Vitamin E 200 IU.

Cycla-Action — Nature's Plus
Each capsule contains: Blue Cohosh root 150 mg • Black Currant seed 125 mg • Mustard seed 75 mg • Red Raspberry leaves 75 mg • Cramp bark 75 mg • Squaw Vine 50 mg • False Unicorn 50 mg. Contains no yeast, wheat, corn, soy, milk, salt, sugar or starch.

Cycl-A-Vites — Nature's Plus
Two tablets contain: whole Black Currant seeds naturally supplying GLA 300 mg • Magnesium amino acid chelate/complex 250 mg • Vitamin B6 (Pyridoxine HCL) 200 mg • Bromelain natural pineapple 150 mg • Calcium amino acid chelate/complex 125 mg • Iron amino acid chelate/complex 18 mg . In a natural base of Red Raspberry leaves, Strawberry Leaves, Dong Quai, Uva Ursi, & Peppermint. Yeast free. Sugar & starch free.

Cyclo 3 Fort — Unknown
One capsule contains: Ruscus aculeatus root extract 150 mg • Trimethylhesperidin-chalcon 150 mg • ascorbic acid 100 mg.

CycloDiol-4 (Sports One Cycloplex Pro-Hormone) —
Sports One
Each lozenge contains: 4-Androstenediol Cycloplex (cyclodextrin complex) 25 mg.

CycloDiol-5 (Sports One Cycloplex Pro-Hormone) —
Sports One
Each lozenge contains: 5-Androstenediol Cycloplex (cyclodextrin complex) 25 mg.

CycloDiol-XS (Sports One Cycloplex Pro-Hormone) —
Sports One
Each lozenge contains: Nor-4-Androstenediol Cycloplex (cyclodextrin complex) 10 mg & 4-Androstenediol Cycloplex (cyclodextrin complex) 15 mg.

Cynara-SL Artichoke — Lichtwer Pharma
One capsule contains: Dried extract of Artichoke leaf. Other Ingredients: Gelatin, Magnesium Stearate, Silicon Dioxide, Talc, Titanium Dioxide, Sodium Lauryl Sulphate, FD&C Blue No. 1, FD&C Yellow No. 5.

Cytodyne — Cytodyne Technologies
Six capsules contain: Acetyl L-Carnitine1100 mg • Phosphatidylserine 175 mg • L-Alanine 200 mg • Alpha Ketoglutaric Acid 150 mg • L-Glutamine 2150 mg • Taurine 1050 mg • Ketoisocaporate 50 mg • Inositol 50 mg.

Cytolog — Allergy Research Group
Colostrum.

Cytomax — Champion Nutrition
Each 25 gram serving contains: Apple: Alpha-L-Polyactate • Energy 90 Kcal • Total Fat 0g • Sodium 100 mg • Potassium 120 mg • Total Carbohydrate 22 g • Sugars 10 g • Protein 0 g. Citrus: Energy 90 Kcal • Total Fat 0g • Sodium 100 mg • Potassium 120 mg • Total Carbohydrate 22 g • Sugars 10 g • Protein 0 g. Tangy-Orange: Energy 90 Kcal • Total Fat 0g • Sodium 100 mg • Potassium 120 mg • Total Carbohydrate 21 g • Sugars 11 g • Protein 0. Tropical: Energy 90 Kcal • Total Fat 0g • Sodium 100 mg • Potassium 100 mg • Total Carbohydrate 22 g • Sugars 11 g • Protein 0. Ingredients: Fructose • Alpha-L-Polyactate (our non-acidic patented L-Lactate formula combined with Sodium L-Lactate & Potassium L-Lactate) • Metacarb

© Copyright 2000, Natural Medicines Comprehensive Database (209) 472-2244. For updated data, go to www.NaturalDatabase.com. • 1321

**B
R
A
N
D

N
A
M
E
S**

(Champion Nutrition's original complex carbohydrate blend including Amylopectin Starches & Maltodextrins from Corn Hybrids) • Glucose • Citric Acid • Succinate ETF (Our Exclusive Succinate Compound containing: Potassium Succinate, L-Glutamic Acid, Inosine, Magnesium Succinate, Calcium Succinate) • Natural Flavoring • Malic Acid • L-Alanine • L-Glutamine • Ascorbic Acid • Natural Caramel Coloring • Potassium Citrate • Xanthan Gum • Sunett (Acesulfame-K) • Chromium Polynicotinate (Chromemate - GTF).

CytoPro — Cytodyne Technologies
Each rounded scoop contains: Cross Flow Micro/Ultra Filtered 100% pure Whey Protein Isolate (Beta Lactoglobulin 19100 MW/50% Alpha Lactoalbumin 14700 MW/20%, Glycomacropeptides 16200 MW/20%, Glutamine Peptides 6700 MW/5%, Immunoglobulin 95000 MW/3%, Bovine Serum Albumin 65000 MW/2%, Protease Peptone). CytoPro WPI (typical Amino Acid profile): L-Alanine 1071 mg • L-Arginine 538 mg • L-Aspartic Acid 2303 mg • L-Cystine 276 mg • L-Glutamic Acid 3870 mg • L-Glutamine 548 mg • L-Glycine 522 mg • L-Histidine 393 mg • L-Isoleucine 1433 mg • L-Leucine 2341 mg • L-Lysine 1999 mg • L-Methionine 409 mg • L-Phenylalanine 768 mg • L-Proline 1553 mg • L-Serine 1184 mg • L-Taurine 1000 mg • L-Threonine 1409 mg • L-Tryptophan 464 mg • L-Tyrosine 567 mg • L-Valine 1328 mg. Total amino profile in milligrams: 23976 mg.

CytoVol — EAS
Each 15 gram serving contains: L-Glutamine 2500 mg • Taurine 2000 mg • Manganese 50 mcg • Calcium AKG 1500 mg • Inositol 500 mg • Glycine 500 mg • RNA 250 mg • L-Alanine 2000 mg. Ingredients: Dextrose • L-Glutamine • Taurine • L-Alanine • Calcium Alpha-Ketoglutarate (AKG) • Citric Acid • Natural Flavors • Inositol • Glycine • Sodium Ribonucleic Acid (RNA) • Sodium Phosphate • Turmeric mixed with Maltodextrin for color • Aspartame • Manganese Glycinate. Contains Phenylalanine.

Daily 3 Complete — The Vitamin Shoppe
Each tablet contains: Vitamin D 400 IU • Vitamin A Activity 25000 IU • Vitamin C 500 mg • Vitamin E 400 IU • Vitamin B1 50 mg • Vitamin B2 50 mg • Vitamin B6 50 mg • Vitamin B12 500 mcg • Niacinamide 50 mg • PABA 50 mg • Pantothenic Acid 50 mg • Choline Bitartrate 50 mg • Inositol 50 mg • Biotin 50 mcg • Folic Acid 800 mcg • Vitamin K 30 mcg • Selenium 50 mcg • Green Tea extract 50 mg • CoQ10 100 mcg • L-Glutathione 10 mg • Pycnogenol 100 mcg • N-Acetyl Cysteine 15 mg • Molybdenum 50 mcg • Calcium 100 mg • Magnesium 50 mg • Potassium 50 mg • Zinc 15 mg • Iodine 150 mcg • Iron 10 mg • Manganese 5 mg • Chromium 100 mcg • Boron 3 mg • Apple pectin 50 mg • Papain 25 mg • Lipase 10 mg • Probiotics 10 mg • Betaine HCl 25 mg • Pepsin 25 mg • Protease 10 mg • Glutamic Acid 25 mg • Amylase 10 mcg • Chlorophyll 10 mg • Spirulina 45 mg • Bee Pollen 45 mg • Echinacea/Golden Seal 50 mg • Shiitake/Reishi mushrooms 45 mg • Barley grass 45 mg • Royal Jelly 15 mg • Alfalfa concentrate 45 mg • Siberian Ginseng 45 mg • Chlorella 45 mg • RNA/DNA 45 mg. A concentrated blend of: broccoli, tomato, garlic, onions, cauliflower, brussel sprouts, carrots, parsley, watercress. Pure dry, cold-pressed borage, flaxseed, safflower oils providing the essential fatty acids, Omega 3-6-9.

Daily Detox — M.D. Labs
Sarsaparilla • Milk Thistle • Red Clover • Dandelion • Yellow Dock • Burdock • Hibiscus • Echinacea • Fenugreek • Ginger • Cascara Sagrada. Other Ingredients: All Natural Fruit & Spice extracts.

Daily Enzyme Complex — Futurebiotics
Pancreas* 235 mg • Ox bile 35 mg • Duodenum 20 mg • Papaya enzyme 125 mg • Betaine 20 mg • Liver 20 mg • Vitamin B1 (thiamin) 3 mg • Bromelain 50 mg • Niacinamide 10 mg • Vitamin B2 (riboflavin) 3 mg • Peppermint 25 mg • Anise 25 mg • Chamomile 25 mg. *Whole dried pancreas, a source of Pancreatin, Trypsin, Amylase, Lipase, Lisotozyme, Diatase & Chymosin.

Daily Essentials — Aspen Group, Inc.
Three tablets contain: Vitamin E (d-alpha) 200 IU • Vitamin A 5000 IU • Beta Carotene 5000 IU • Vitamin D 400 IU • Vitamin C 400 mg • Folic Acid 400 mcg • Thiamine 1.5 mg • Riboflavin 1.7 mg • Niacin 20 mg • Vitamin B6 2 mg • Vitamin B12 6 mcg • Biotin 300 mcg • Pantothenic Acid 10 mg • Calcium (citrate) 600 mg • Phosphorus 450 mg • Iodine (kelp) 150 mcg • Magnesium (carbonate) 200 mg • Copper (gluconate) 2 mg • Zinc (gluconate) 15 mg • Vitamin K 100 mcg • Selenium (yeast) 75 mcg • Manganese (gluconate) 5 mg • Chromium (aspartate) 200 mcg • Molybdenum 150 mcg • Nickel 15 mcg • Tin 15 mcg • Vanadium 5 mcg • Boron (citrate) 2 mg • Potassium (gluconate) 100 mg • Grape seed extract 10 mg • CO Q10

10 mg. Contains no sugar, starch, salt, wheat, corn, milk or soy derivatives.

Daily Therapy 7-Vitamin Foaming Cleansing Gel — Orjene
Vitamin-packed antioxidant formula with Sea Minerals.

Daily Vits One-A-Day Multiple — Now
Each tablet contains: Vitamin A (100% as Beta Carotene) 5000 IU • Vitamin B1 (Thiamine HCL) 1.5 mg • Vitamin B2 (Riboflavin) 1.7 mg • Vitamin B3 (Niacinamide) 20 mg • Vitamin B5 (Pantothenic Acid) 10 mg • Vitamin B6 (Pyridoxine HCL) 3 mg • Vitamin B12 (Cyanocobalamin) 9 mcg • Biotin 300 mcg • Folic Acid 400 mcg • Vitamin C (Ascorbic Acid) 90 mg • Vitamin D (Calciferol) 400 IU • Vitamin E (natural d-Alpha Tocopherol) 30 IU • Calcium (Carbonate, Phosphate) 100 mg • Magnesium (Oxide) 80 mg • Zinc (Amino Acid Chelate) 15 mg • Iron (Ferrochel Bisglycinate) 9 mg • Copper (Amino Acid Chelate) 1 mg • Iodine (Kelp) 150 mcg • Potassium (Chloride) 50 mg • Manganese (Amino Acid Chelate) 2 mg • Selenium (Amino Acid Chelate) 70 mcg • Chromium (Chelavite Chelate) 120 mcg • Molybdenum (Amino Acid Chelate) 50 mcg • Choline (Bitartrate) 10 mg • Inositol 10 mg • PABA 10 mg • Boron (Amino Acid Chelate) 500 mcg • Vanadium (Amino Acid Chelate) 50 mcg • Panax ginseng (5% Ginsenosides) 100 mg.

Daily VM Caps — The Vitamin Shoppe
Each capsule contains: Vitamin A 10000 IU • Vitamin D 400 IU • Vitamin C 250 mg • Thiamin 8 mg • Riboflavin 8 mg • Niacin 25 mg • Vitamin B6 10 mg • Vitamin B12 25 mcg • Vitamin E 100 IU • Pantothenic Acid 25 mg • Biotin 300 mcg • Folate 400 mcg • Calcium 100 mg • Magnesium 50 mg • Iron 10 mg • Manganese 2 mg • Zinc 7 mg • Selenium 70 mcg • Chromium 50 mcg • Iodine 125 mcg • Citrus Bioflavonoids 25 mg • Para Aminobenzoic Acid 10 mg • Choline 10 mg • Inositol 10 mg • Potassium 10 mg • Betaine HCl 10 mg • Pepsin 10 mg • Papain 10 mg • Pancreatin 10 mg.

Damiana/Ginseng Formula — Nature's Way
Two capsules contain: Proprietary Formula: Damiana leaves • Fo-Ti root • Gotu Kola stem, leaf • Licorice root • Sarsaparilla root • Saw Palmetto berry • Siberian Ginseng root • Wild Yam root • Other ingredients: Gelatin.

Damiana-Sarsaparilla Formula — Quest
Each caplet contains: Damiana leaf powder (Tunera aphrodisiaca) 120 mg • Sarsaparilla root powder (Smilax officinalis) 90 mg • Saw Palmetto berry powder (Serenoa serrulata) 90 mg • Siberian Ginseng root powder (Eleutherococcus senticosus) 90 mg • Licorice root powder (Glycyrrhiza glabra) 60 mg • Kelp powder (Fucus versiculosis) 50 mg. Other Ingredients: Calcium Phosphate, Microcrystalline Cellulose, Vegetable Stearin, Croscarmellose Sodium, Magnesium Stearate (vegetable source).

Dandelion-Milk Thistle Virtue — Blessed Herbs
Dandelion blend of flower, leaf & root • Milk Thistle seed • Bladderwrack • Reishi mycelium • Scullcap • Licorice root • Prickly Ash bark • Grain alcohol & Distilled Water.

Deep Pore Cleanser — Jason
Vitamin C Complex • Alpha Lipoic Acid.

Deer Velvet — National Deer Horn, Ltd
Each capsule contains: Deer Velvet powder 250 mg.

Deer Velvet — Silberhorn
Each capsule contains: Deer Velvet 250 mg • Gelatine Capsule Shells.

Defender — Health Factor
Each tablet contains: Beta Carotene 5000 IU • Vitamin C (Ascorbic Acid) 60 mg • Vitamin E (d-Alpha Tocopheryl) 30 IU • Zinc (Amino Acid Chelate) 20 mg • Copper (Citrate) 2 mg • Selenium (Amino Acid Chelate) 100 mcg • Manganese (Citrate) 2 mg • Chromium (Nicotinate) 100 mcg • Boron (Citrate) 100 mcg • Vanadium (Citrate) 50 mcg • Molybdenum (Citrate) 50 mcg • Silicon (Citrate) 20 mcg • Grape seed (95% Polyphenols) 20 mg • Bilberry (25% Anthocyanidins) 5 mg.

Defender BVM — PhysioLogics
Two caplets contain: Vitamin A (as Beta Carotene) 5000 IU • Vitamin C (as Ascorbic Acid) 100 mg • Vitamin E (as d-Alpha Tocopherol Succinate) 240 IU • Selenium (as Selenomethionine) 400 mcg • Manganese (as Manganese Glycinate) 1.75 mg • Tea Green leaf (50% Polyphenols, 75 mg) 150 mg • N-Acetyl L-Cysteine 50 mg • Resveratrol (8% Resveratrol, 4 mg) 50 mg • Alpha Lipoic Acid 25 mg.

Some Brand Name Natural Products - What they Contain
www.NaturalDatabase.com contains MANY more listings than appear here.

Defy Your Age — Pharmagel
10% Alpha Hydroxy Acids • Stabilized Oxygen.

Dene-O-Lean — Pharmanex
Two capsules contain: Sunflower Oil 2000 mg • Conjugated Linoleic Acid 1200 mg • Capsaicin 100 mg.

Dentalgel — NutriBiotic
Contains 0.4% Grapefruit extract.

Derma Teen — Futurebiotics
MSM • Combination of vitamins • minerals, and horsetail.

Derma-Klear Akne Treatment Cream — Enzymatic Therapy
Contains: Sulfur 2.5%. Other ingredients: Purified Water, Zinc, Sage extract, Silymarin Phytosome, Hawthorne extract, Chamomile extract, 18-Beta-Glycyrrhetinic Acid, Essential Oil of Rosemary, Urea & Vitamin E (Tocopherol). Fragrance is natural & hypoallergenic. Contains no Benzoyl Peroxide.

DermaSlim TD — Alvin Last
Abies Canadensis • Ammonium Bromatum • Ammonium Carbonicum • Antimonium Crudem • Argentum Metallicum • Argentum Nitircum • Calcarea Carbonica • Capsicum Annuum • Cinchona Officinalis • Fucus Vesiculosus • Graphites • Kali Bichromicum • Kali Carbonicum • Kali Phosphoricum • Lycopodium Clavatum • Natrum Muriaticum • Phosphorus • Pulsatilla • Silicea • Spongia Tosta • Staphsagria • Sulphur • Thyroidunum • Veratrum Album.

Detox — Natrol
Two capsules contain: Zinc (as Zinc Chelate) 15 mg • Garlic (Pure-Gar) 250 mg • Dandelion powder root 200 mg • Yellow Dock powder root 200 mg • Sarsaparilla powder root 200 mg • Burdock powder root 150 mg • Cascara Sagrada powder 100 mg • Goldenseal powder root 75 mg • Licorice powder root 75 mg • Parsley powder leaf 50 mg • Milk Thistle extract Guaranteed Potency 80% Silymarin 28 mg • NAC (N-Acetyl Cysteine) 25 mg • Aloe Vera gel 200:1 extract 5 mg. Other ingredients: Silicon Dioxide, Magnesium Stearate, Gelatin.

Detox — The Herbalist
Oregon Grape root • Yellow Dock root • Dandelion root • Burdock root • Fennel seed.

Detox Formula — Gary Null
Each capsule contains: Apple Pectin 25 mg • Buckthorn bark 25 mg • Burdock root 25 mg • Cascara Sagrada bark 25 mg • Chrysanthemum 25 mg • Dandelion root 25 mg • Fennel seed 25 mg • Fiber 75 mg • Garlic 25 mg • Ginger root 25 mg • Goldenseal root 50 mg • Hibiscus 25 mg • Kelp 25 mg • Licorice root 25 mg • Marshmallow 25 mg • Orange peel 25 mg • Oregon Grape root 25 mg • Peppermint 25 mg • Prickly Ash bark 25 mg • Psyllium 50 mg • Red Clover 25 mg • Rose Hips 25 mg • Sarsaparilla root 25 mg • Stillingia 25 mg • Yellow Dock 25 mg.

Detox Support — Amazon Support
Each capsule contains: Graviola • Carquija • Erva Tostao • Fedegosa • Tayuya • Artichoke • Mutmaba • Espinheira Santa • Boldo • Chanca Piedra • Samambaia • Brazilian Peppertree • Sarsaparilla • Pau d'arco • Cat's Claw.

Detox Support — Now
Each capsule contains: Milk Thistle • Sodium Alginate • Chlorella • MSM as central ingredients.

Detoxinal — PhysioLogics
Two capsules contain: Vitamin C (Ascorbic Acid) 200 mg • Chlorella 200 mg • Garlic 100 mg • Milk Thistle (80% Silymarin, 80 mg) 100 mg • Burdock root 50 mg • Cascara sagrada 50 mg • Dandelion root 50 mg • Red Clover 50 mg • Algin 50 mg • Pectin 50 mg • Bromelain 50 mg.

Detoxygen — Nature's Plus
Two tablets contain: Botanical Blend: Hibiscus (Hibiscus sabdariffa) 250 mg • Red Clover (Trifolium pratense) 200 mg • Dandelion (Taraxacum officinale) 200 mg • Chinese Mushroom Complex 200 mg: Shiitake (Lentinus edodes) 150 mg • Reishi (Ganoderma lucidum) 50 mg • Echinacea (Echinacea purpurea) 100 mg • Cayenne (Capsicum frutescens) 75 mg • Yellow Dock (Rumex crispus) 50 mg • Milk Thistle (standardized 80% Silymarin) 50 mg • Celery Seed (Apium graveolens) 25 mg • Ginger root (Zingiber officinale) 25 mg • Juniper berries (Juniperus communis) 20 mg • Essential Cofactor blend: Creatine Monohydrate Energy Precursor 100 mg • Co-Enzyme Q10 (Ubiquinone) 10 mg • Vitamin B12 (Cobalamin concentrate) 250 mcg. Contains no yeast, wheat, corn, soy, milk, salt, sugar or starch.

Devil's Club-Bilberry Virtue — Blessed Herbs
Devil's Club Root bark • Bilberry leaf • Reishi mycelium • Siberian Ginseng root • Grain alcohol & Distilled Water.

Dexatrim — Chattem, Inc.
Each gelcap contains: Active Ingredient: Phenylpropanolamine HCl 75 mg. Inactive Ingredients: Carnauba wax, D&C Yellow No. 10 Aluminum Lake, FD&C Yellow No. 6. Aluminum Lake, Hydroxypropyl Methylcellulose, Iron Oxide, Magnesium Stearate, Microcrystalline Cellulose, Polyethylene Glycol, Polysorbate 80, Povidone, Silicon Dioxide, Stearic Acid, Titanium Dioxide.

Dexatrim Natural No Caffeine Formula — Chattem, Inc.
Each caplet contains: Chromium (as chromium dinicotinate glycinate) 250 mcg • Vanadium (as vanadium amino acid chelate) 100 mcg • Heartleaf Standardized Extract (Sida cordifolia, 12 mg naturally ocurring ephedrine) 120 mg • Thermonutrient Blend 100 mg: Steatite Atractylodes rhizome, Baikal Scullcap root, Balloon-Flower root, Licorice root, Terra Alba, Da Huang root, Mirabilite, Dong Quai root, Field Mint leaf, Forsythia fruit, Gardenia fruit, Ginger root, Lovage root, Schizonepeta stem, Siler root, White Peony root. Other Ingredients: Dicalcium Phosphate, Microchrystalline Cellulose, Croscarmellose Sodium, Stearic Acid, Hydroxypropyl Cellulose, & Polyethylene glycol.

Dexatrim No Caffeine — Chattem, Inc.
Each gelcap contains: Active Ingredient: Phenylpropanolamine HCl 75 mg. Inactive Ingredients: Carnauba wax, D&C Yellow No. 10 Aluminum Lake, Edetate Disodium, FD&C Blue No. 1., FD&C Red No. 40 Aluminum Lake, FD&C Yellow No. 6 Aluminum Lake, Gelatin, Glycerin, Hydroxypropyl Methylcellulose, Magnesium Stearate, Microcrystalline Cellulose, Pharmaceutical Glaze, Polyethylene Glycol, Polysorbate 80, Povidone, Propylene Glycol, Silicon Dioxide, Stearic Acid, Titanium Dioxide.

DGL — Enzymatic Therapy
Each chewable tablet contains: Licorice root extract 4:1 Deglycrrhizinated (Glycyrrhiza glabra) 380 mg • Glycine (Amino Acid) 50 mg • In a base of Fructose. Contains no sugar, salt, yeast, wheat, corn, soy, dairy products, coloring, flavoring or preservatives.

DGL Plus — Progressive Labs
Two capsules contain: Licorice root (Glycyrrhiza glabra): Deglycyrrhizinated Licorice extract 400 mg • NAG (N-Acetyl Glucosamine) 60 mg • Parotid Gland 10 mg • Gamma Oryzanol 50 mg • Glycine 50 mg.

DHA Neuromins — Source Naturals
Each softgel contains: Docohexaenoic acid 100 mg.

DHEA — Body Wise International, Inc.
Each capsule contains: DHEA (Dehydroepiandrosterone) 25 mg ¥ Calcium (from Dicalcium Phosphate) 6 mg.

DHEA -25- X-TRA — Progressive Labs
Each capsule contains: DHEA (dehydroepiandrosterone) 25 mg • Herbal Base: [Green Tea leaf extract (Camellia sinensis) - 35% polyphenols, Schizandra berry (Schizandra chinensis), Soybean extract (Glycine max) - 1% isoflavones (hypoallergenic), Ginkgo Biloba leaf extract (24% ginkgoflavonglycosides), Grape seed extract (Vitis vinifera) - 40% proanthocyanidins] 250 mg.

DHEA X-TRA — Progressive Labs
Each capsule contains: DHEA (dehydroepiandrosterone) 50 mg • Herbal Base: [Green Tea leaf extract (Camellia sinensis) - 35% polyphelols, Schizandra berry (Schizandra chinensis), Soybean extract (Glycine max) - 1% isoflavones (hypoallergenic), Ginkgo Biloba leaf extract (24% ginkgoflavonglycosides), Grape seed extract (Vitis vinifera) - 40% proanthocyanidins] 250 mg.

DHEAX — HealthWatchers System
Dioscorea Villosa • Alpha Ketoglutaric Acid • Phosphatidyl Serine • Pantothenic Acid • Gotu Kola Powder • Ginkgo Biloba Powder • Siberian Ginseng Pwder • L-Glutamine • L-Tyrosine • L-Glycine • L-Arginine-HCl • L-Ornithine • L-Lysine • Pantathine • Beta Sitosterol.

Diabest — PhysioLogics
Three tablets contain: Vitamin A (Palmitate) 2500 IU • Vitamin E (d-Alpha Tocopherol) 300 IU • Vitamin C (Ascorbic Acid) 300 mg • Magnesium (Glycinate) 300 mg • Niacin 150 mg • Zinc (Glycinate) 23 mg • Vitamin B6 (Pyridoxine HCl) 15 mg • Copper (Glycinate) 3 mg • Biotin 900 mcg • Chromium (Niacin/Glycine Chelate) 200 mcg • Selenium (as Selenomethionine) 50 mcg • Quercetin 150 mg • Ginkgo

B R A N D

N A M E S

B R A N D   N A M E S

leaf (24% Ginkgo flavonglycosides 75 mg, 6% terpene lactones 4.5 mg) 75 mg • Vanadyl Sulfate 750 mcg.

Diabest 2 — PhysioLogics
Each capsule contains: Chromium (33% Niacin/Glycine Chelate, 67% Picolinate) 300 mcg • Gymnema sylvestre (24% Gymnemic Acid 48 mg) 200 mg • Mormodica charantia 4:1 extract 100 mg • Bis (Glycinato) Oxovanadium (BGOV) 10 mg • Vanadyl Sulfate 10 mg.

Diabetic Support Formula — Nutrition Warehouse
Each tablet contains: Vitamin C (as Ascorbic Acid) 100 mg • Vitamin E (as dl-Alpha Tocopheryl Acetate) 30 IU • Biotin 350 mcg • Calcium (as Dicalcium Phosphate) 85 mg • Magnesium (as Magnesium Oxide) 250 mg • Zinc (as Zinc Oxide) 7.5 • Selenium (as Sodium Selenate) 70 mcg • Manganese (as Manganese Sulfate) 2 mg • Chromium (as Chromium Picolinate) 500 mcg • Lipoic Acid 30 mg • Vanadyl Sulfate 10 mg • Ginkgo Biloba 924% flavone glycosides) 20 mg • Coenzyme Q-10 5 mg • Taurine 50 mg • L-Carnitine 125 mg.

Diabetica Tea — HerbaSway
Panax Ginseng • Siberian Ginseng • Astragalus • Kudzu • Blackberry • Licorice • HerbaSwee (Cucurbitaceae fruit).

Dia-B-Tea — Amazon Support
One rounded teaspoon contains: Pata de Vaca • Pedra Hume Caa • Bitter Melon • Chanca Piedra • Stevia.

Di-Acid Dim — Atrium
Each tablet contains: First Phase (in Stomach): Glycine 32 mg • Pepsin 100 mg • Papain 50 mg. Second Phase (in Duodenum): Pancreatin 100 mg • Pancrelipase 50 mg • Amylase 30 mg • Bromelain 30 mg • Ox Bile extract 65 mg.

Di-Acid Stim - — Atrium
Each tablet contains: First Phase (in Stomach): Betaine HCL 100 mg • Glutamic Acid HCL 110 mg • Pepsin 100 mg • Papain 50 mg. Second Phase (in Duodenum): Pancreatin 100 mg • Pancrelipase 50 mg. Amylase 30 mg • Bromelain 40 mg • Ox Bile extract 60 mg.

Dia-Comp — Enzymatic Therapy
Two capsules contain: Vitamin E (Mixed Tocopherols) 50 IU • Magnesium (Chelate) 100 mg • Vitamin C (Ascorbic Acid) 100 mg • Vitamin B6 (Pyridoxine HCL) 10 mg • Manganese (Chelate) 10 mg • Zinc (Picolinate) 5 mg • Biotin 1000 mcg • Vitamin B12 (Cyanocobalamin) 250 mcg • Chromium (Picolinate) 50 mcg • Selenium (Aspartate) 40 mcg • Other ingredients: Blueberry extract 4:1 (Vaccinium myrtillus fructus) 300 mg • Gymnema sylvestre extract standardized to contain 24% Gymnemic Acid 150 mg • Bitter Melon extract (Momordica charanita) 100 mg • Fenugreek seed extract (4:1) (Trigonella foenum-Ggaecum) 100 mg.

Diet Fuel — TwinLab
Ma Huang 20 mg • Guarana 200 mg • HCA 500 mg • Chromium 200 mcg • L-Carnitine 100 mg • Green Tea.

Diet Fuel With Chitosan Formula — TwinLab
Two capsules contain: Chitosan (fiber) 1000 mg. Other Ingredients: Cellulose, Gelatin, Purified Water, Magnesium Stearate, MCT.

Diet Support — Now
Each capsule contains: Bitter Orange extract • L-Carnitine • Chromium.

Diet System 6 — Applied Nutrition
Six capsules contain: Super Citrimax : (Garcinia extract) 1500 mg. Energizing Herbs (Thermogenic Herbs): (Kola nut extract 550 mg • Guarana extract 100 mg • Ginger 100 mg). Three Lipotropics including: (Choline Bitartrate 100 mg • Inositol 100 mg • Betaine HCL 25 mg). Chromium: (Chromium Picolinate 150 mcg • ChromeMate 150 mcg). L-Carnitine: (L-Carnitine Complex) 300 mg. Vitamins & Minerals: 72 Trace Mineral Complex 100 mg: (Vitamin B3 20 mg, Vitamin B6 2 mg, Vitamin B12 6 mcg, Vitamin B2 1.7 mg, Vitamin E 15 IU, Folic Acid 400 mcg, Selenium 50 mcg , Vitamin C 60 mg, Potassium 25 mg, Iodine 150 mcg).

Diet Ultra III — The Vitamin Shoppe
Three tablets contain: Vitamin A (as acetate, beta-carotene) 10000 IU • Vitamin C (as ascorbic acid) 100 mg • Vitamin D (cholecalciferol) 400 IU • Vitamin E (as d-alpha tocopherol) 50 IU • Vitamin B1 (as thiamin hydrochloride) 25 mg • Vitamin B2 (as riboflavin) 25 mg • Vitamin B12 (as cobalamin) 25 mcg • Niacin (as nicotinic acid) 25 mg • Folic Acid 100 mcg • Biotin 100 mcg • Pantothenic Acid (as d-calcium pantothenate) 20 mg • Iron (as chelate) 10 mg • Calcium (as citrate) 100 mg • Iodine (from kelp) 150 mcg • Magnesium (as citrate)

50 mg • Zinc (as chelate) 15 mg • Selenium (as chelate) 25 mcg • Chromium (as chelate) 300 mcg • Gotu Kola (Centella asiatica) 50 mg • Siberian Ginseng (Eleutherococcus senticosus) root 50 mg • L-Carnitine 50 mg • Choline 150 mg • Inositol 150 mg • Omega-3 (fish) 15 mg.

Diet*Aid Caplets with Vitamin C — Rite Aid Corporation
Each Caplet Contains: Active Ingredient: Phenylpropanolamine Hydrochloride 75 mg. (appetite suppressant controlled release). Inactive Ingredients: Vitamin C (Ascorbic Acid) 180 mg, Calcium Sulfate, Croscarmellose Sodium, Ethylcellulose, FD&C Blue No. 1 Aluminum Lake, FD&C Red No. 40 Aluminum Lake, FD&C Yellow No. 6 Aluminum Lake, Hydroxypropyl Methylcellulose, Lactose, Magnesium Stearate, Polydextrose, Polyethylene Glycol, Propylene Glycol, Starch, Stearic Acid, Titanium Dioxide, Triacetin.

Diet-Metabo-7 — Source Naturals
Three tablets contain: Vitamin C (as Ascorbic Acid) 80 mg • Niacinamide 30 mg • Vitamin B6 (as Pyridoxine HCl) 30 mg • Pantothenic Acid (as Calcium-D-Pantothenate) 80 mg • Calcium 20 mg • Chromium (200 mcg Chromium 400 mcg Picolinate 200 mcg chromium polynicatinate) • Potassium (as Potassium Citrate) 20 mg • GABA (Gamma-Aminobutyric Acid) 500 mg • Phenylalanine (as L- & DL-Phenylalanine) 500 mg • Sida cordifolia extract (6% yielding 30 mg ephedrine alkaloids) 500 mg • Gymnema sylvestre extract (GS4) 400 mg • Green Tea leaf extract (20% yielding 60 mg of caffeine) 300 mg • Glutamine 200 mg • Guggul Yogaraj Gum Resin 200 mg • Kola Nut extract 20% yielding 30 mg of caffeine) 150 mg • Dandelion extract 4:1 (root & herb) 150 mg • Yerba Mate extract (8% yielding 10 mg of caffeine) 125 mg • Bupleurum root 100 mg • L-Tyrosine 100 mg • Horse Chestnut extract (Yielding 14 mg Aescin) 70 mg • Bladderwrack extract 30 mg • Ginkgo Biloba leaf extract (50:1) 30 mg • Ginger root 30 mg • N-Acetyl Cysteine 30 mg • Black Pepper fruit extract (Bioperine) 3 mg • Iodine (from Kelp) 100 mcg.

Digest RC — Cxresearch Inc.
Each tablet contains: Black Radish 75 mg • Charcoal 75 • Artichoke 47 mg • Calcium Phospate 45 mg • Cholic Acid 40 mg • Peppermint 15 mg.

Digest Support — Natrol
Two capsules contain: Proteolytic Enzymes: Protease I (20000 HUT) 200 mg • Protease II (16600 FCC) 8 mg • Amylolytic Enzymes: Amylase (10200 DU) 408 mg • Cellulase (410 CMC) 100 mg • Lactase (200 LAC) 20 mg • Lipolytic Enzymes: Lipase (300 LU) 100 mg • Maltase (90 DU) 90 mg • Sucrase (200 SU) 20 mg • Anti Gas Factor: Alpha Galactosidase (54 GAL) 54 mg. Other ingredients: TriCalcium Phosphate, Silica, Magnesium Stearate, Gelatin.

DigestEase — Pacific BioLogic
Ginger • Rhubarb • Elecampane • Gentian • Long Pepper • Tropical Almond • Emblic Myrobalan • Beleric Myrobalan • Glauber's Salt • Kaolin.

Di-Gest-Eze — Nutri-Quest
Each two-phase tablet contains: Phase One (Stomach): Betaine HCL 155 mg • L-Glutamic Acid HCL 100 mg • Pepsin 105 mg • Papain 50 mg. Phase Two (Duodenum): Pancreatin 100 mg • Pancrelipase 50 mg • Amylase 30 mg • Bromelain 30 mg • Ox Bile 65 mg • Parotid 2 mg.

Digestion Formula — Nature's Way
Two capsules contain: Angelica root 90 mg • Barberry bark 135 mg • Beet root 100 mg • Cayenne pepper fruit 25 mg • Dandelion root 315 mg • Fizyme Enzyme Formula 100 mg • Gentian root 135 mg. Other ingredients: Gelatin, Magnesium Stearate, Millet.

Digestion Support — Amazon Support
Each capsule contains: Boldo • Carqueja • Espinheira Santa • Sarsaparilla • Jurubeba • Gervao • Cat's Claw.

Digstive Enzyme Complex — Nutrilite
Each capsule contains: Lipase 31 mg • Lactase 40 mg • Amylase 20 mg • Alpha-Galactosidase 10 mg • Ginger Root Extract 150 mg • Nutrilite Parsley Concentrate with Phytofactors Plant Compounds.

Diol Stack — Substrate Solutions
Each tablet contains: Nor-4-Androstenediol 100 mg • 4-Androstenediol 100 mg.

Diurex Long Acting Water Capsules — Alva-Amco
Each capsule contains: Active Ingredients: Caffeine Anhydrous • Acetaminophen • Potassium Salicylate. Other Ingredients: Non-Pariell seeds, Magnesium Oxide, Titanium Dioxide, plus other coloring & coating ingredients.

Some Brand Name Natural Products - What they Contain
www.NaturalDatabase.com contains MANY more listings than appear here.

Diurex Water Caplets — Alva-Amco
Each caplet contains: Active Ingredient: Pamabrom 50 mg. Other Ingredients: Dicalcium Phosphate, FD&C Blue #1, Hydroxypropyl Methylcellulose, Magnesium Stearate, Polyethylene Glycol, Potassium Gluconate, Riboflavin, Stearic Acid, Titanium Dioxide. May also contain: Calcium Sulfate, Croscarmellose Sodium, Microcrystalline Cellulose, Mineral Oil, Polysorbate, Silicon Dioxide, Sodium Lauryl Sulfate.

Diurex Water Pills — Alva-Amco
Each pill contains: Active Ingredients: Potassium Salicylate • Caffeine Anhydrous • Salicylamide. Other Ingredients: Calcium Sulfate, Dicalcium Phosphate, Magnesium Trisilicate, Microcrystalline Cellulose, Starch, Magnesium Stearate, Stearic Acid, plus other fillers, coloring & coating ingredients.

Diutrate — Atrium
Each tablet contains: Buchu leaves 70 mg • Couch grass 70 mg • Hydrangea root 35 mg • Corn Silk 35 mg • Uva Ursi 10 mg • Hypothalamus 30 mg • Raw Kidney concentrate 60 mg • Vitamin B6 16 mg • Magnesium (Protein Chelated) 50 mg.

DMG-B15-Plus — Enzymatic Therapy
Each capsule contains: Potassium Aspartate 125 mg • Magnesium Aspartate 125 mg • Calcium Gluconate 31 mg • Other ingredients: Trimethylglycine (TMG) 100 mg • N,N-Dimethylglycine 100 mg • Glycine 25 mg. Contains no sugar, salt, yeast, wheat, corn, soy, dairy products, coloring, flavoring or preservatives.

D-MNS — Dial Herbs
Mistletoe • Blessed Thistle • Witch Hazel • Nettle • Shepherd's Purse • Red Raspberry • Cayenne.

DN-24 Hydracreme — Pharmagel
Vitamin Retinyl-A 25000 IU.

DNE Ephedrana 12.5 — D & E Pharmaceuticals
Each tablet contains: Ephedrine HCL 12.5 mg

Doctor's Choice Antioxidant — Enzymatic Therapy
Three capsules contain: Vitamin A (Beta Carotene) non-toxic form of Vitamin A 10000 IU • Vitamin E (D-Alpha Tocopherol) 200 IU • Vitamin C (Ascorbic Acid) 500 mg • Zinc (Picolinate) 15 mg • Manganese (Gluconate) 15 mg • Riboflavin (Vitamin B2) 6 mg • Selenium (L-Selenomethionine) 200 mcg • N-Acetylcysteine 100 mg • Cabbage extract (Brassica oleracea) 100 mg • Garlic extract, deodorized 100 mg • Ginger root extract 6.5:1 (Zingiber officinale) 100 mg • Green Tea extract (Camellia sinensis) 100 mg • Klamath Blue-Green Algae 100 mg • Curcuma root extract (Curcuma longa) standardized to contain 97% Curcumin 50 mg • Grape seed (PCO) extract (Procyanidolic oligomers (PCO) from grape seed extract) 10 mg. Other ingredients: Cellulose, Calcium Silicate, Silicon Dioxide, & Gelatin Capsule. Contains no sugar, salt, yeast, wheat, corn, dairy products, artificial coloring, artificial flavoring or preservatives.

Doctor's Choice Eye Formula — Enzymatic Therapy
Three tablets contain: Vitamin A (Fish Liver oil) 2500 IU • Vitamin A (Beta Carotene) non-toxic form of Vitamin A 2500 IU • Vitamin C (Ascorbic Acid) 600 mg • Vitamin E (D-Alpha Tocopheryl Acetate) 60 IU • Vitamin B2 (Riboflavin) 1.5 mg • Zinc (Picolinate) 9 mg • Selenium (L Selenomethionine) 50 mcg • Copper (Picolinate) 1 mg • Hachimijiogan Herbal Complex 400 mg • Bilberry (Vaccinium myrtillus fructus) Berry extract standardized to contain 25% Anthocyanosides (calculated as Anthocyanidins) 160 mg • Curcuma (Curcuma Longa) root extract standardized to contain 85-97% Curcumin) 50 mg • Grape (Vitis vinifera) seed (PCO) extract standardized to contain 95% Procyanidolic Oligomers (PCOs) 50 mg • Lutein (Marigold flower extract) 2 mg. Other ingredients: Cellulose, Calcium Carbonate, Cellulose Gum, Stearic Acid, Silicon Dioxide & Magnesium Stearate. Contains no sugar, salt, yeast, wheat, gluten, corn, dairy products, artificial coloring, artificial flavoring or preservatives.

Doctor's Choice Flax oil fortified with Borage & Pumpkin — Enzymatic Therapy
Flaxseed oil • Pumpkin seed oil • Borage seed oil • Rosemary Antioxidant S-327 • Average analysis per tablespoon: Omega-3 (LNA) 5250 mg • Omega-6 (LA) 2625 mg • Omega-9 (Oleic) 2600 mg • Gamma-Linolenic Acid (GLA) 325 mg. Contains no sugar, salt, yeast, wheat, corn, soy, dairy products, artificial coloring, artificial flavoring or preservatives.

Doctor's Choice for 45-Plus Women — Enzymatic Therapy
Six tablets contain: Vitamin A (Beta Carotene) 15000 IU • Vitamin A (Retinol) 2500 IU • Vitamin D 400 IU • Vitamin E (D-Alpha Tocopherol Succinate) 200 IU • Vitamin D 400 IU • Calcium (Citrate, Carbonate) 600 mg • Vitamin C (Ascorbic Acid) 300 mg • Magnesium (Aspartate) 300 mg • Potassium (Aspartate) 99 mg • Vitamin B6 (Pyridoxine HCL) 60 mg • Thiamine HCL (Vitamin B1) 60 mg • Riboflavin (Vitamin B2) 60 mg • Pantothenic Acid (D-Calcium Pantothenate) 50 mg • Niacin/Niacinamide 45 mg • Zinc (Picolinate) 15 mg • Manganese (Citrate) 15 mg • Copper (Gluconate) 1.5 mg • Folic Acid 800 mcg • Vitamin B12 (Cyanocobalamin) 800 mcg • Biotin 600 mcg • Vitamin K (Phytonadione) 60 mcg • Iodine (Kelp) 300 mcg • Chromium (Polynicotinate) 200 mcg • Selenium (L-Selenomet hionine) 100 mcg • Molybdenum (Sodium Molybdate) 25 mcg • Flavonoids mixed 100 mg • Alfalfa juice concentrate 100 mg • Dong Quai extract 4:1 (Angelica sinensis) 90 mg • Ginger root extract 6.5:1 (Zingiber officinale) 15 mg • Green Tea extract (Camellia sinensis) 30 mg • Choline Bitartrate 30 mg • Fennel seed extract 6:1 (Foeniculum vulgare) 30 mg • Inositol 30 mg • PABA (Para-Aminobenzoic Acid) 30 mg • Betaine HCL 25 mg • Glutamic Acid HCL 25 mg • Bromelain 15 mg • Papain 15 mg • Protease acid stable 5 mg • Lipase 5 mg • Boron (Sodium Tetraborate Decahydrate 3 mg • Silica (Sodium Metasilicate) 1 mg • Vanadium (Sulfate) 50 mcg. Other ingredients: Cellulose, Cellulose Gum, Stearic Acid, Silicon Dioxide & Magnesium Stearate. Contains no sugar, salt, yeast, wheat, corn, dairy products, artificial coloring, artificial flavoring, or preservatives.

Doctor's Choice for 50-Plus Men — Enzymatic Therapy
Four tablets contain: Vitamin A (Beta Carotene) 15000 IU • Vitamin A (Retinol) 2500 IU • Vitamin E (d-Alpha Tocopherol Succinate) 200 IU • Vitamin D (Ergocalciferol) 100 IU • Vitamin C (Ascorbic Acid) 300 mg • Magnesium (Aspartate) 250 mg • Calcium (Citrate • Carbonate) 250 mg • Niacin/Niacinamide 120 mg • Pantothenic Acid (D-Calcium Pantothenate) 100 mg • Potassium (Aspartate) 99 mg • Thiamine HCL (Vitamin B1) 60 mg • Riboflavin (Vitamin B2) 60 mg • Vitamin B6 (Pyridoxine HCL) 60 mg • Zinc (Picolinate) 30 mg • Manganese (Citrate) 15 mg • Copper (Gluconate) 1.5 mg • Folic Acid 800 mcg • Vitamin B12 (Cyanocobalamin) 800 mcg • Biotin 600 mcg • Iodine (Kelp) 300 mcg • Chromium (Polynicotinate) 200 mcg • Selenium (L-Selenomethionine) 100 mcg • Vitamin K (Phytonadione) 60 mcg • Molybdenum (Sodium Molybdate) 25 mcg • Mixed Flavonoids citrus 100 mg • Saw Palmetto Berry extract 4:1 (Serenoa repens) 80 mg • Ginger root extract 6.5:1 (Zingiber officinale) 60 mg • Alfalfa juice concentrate 60 mg • Choline Bitartrate 30 mg • Inositol 30 mg • PABA (Para-Aminobenzoic Acid) 30 mg • Green Tea extract (Camellia sinensis) 30 mg • Betaine HCL 25 mg • Glutamic Acid HCL 25 mg • Korean Ginseng root extract (Panax ginseng) standardized to contain 7% Saponins (calculated as Rg1) 15 mg • Bromelain 15 mg • Papain 15 mg • Protease acid stable 5 mg • Lipase 5 mg • Boron (Sodium Tetraborate Decahydrate) 2 mg • Vanadium (Sulfate) 50 mcg. Other ingredients: Cellulose, Stearic Acid, Cellulose Gum, Silicon Dioxide, & Magnesium Stearate. Contains no sugar, salt, yeast, wheat, corn, dairy products, artificial coloring, artificial flavoring or preservatives.

Doctor's Choice for Arthritics — Enzymatic Therapy
Two tablets contain: Niacin/Niacinamide 330 mg • Pantothenic Acid (D-Calcium Pantothenate) 100 mg • Magnesium (Oxide) 100 mg • Calcium Chloride 32 mg • Vitamin C (Ascorbic Acid) 30 mg • Zinc (Picolinate) 3 mg • Manganese (Chelate) 3 mg • Glucosamine Sulfate 500 mg • PABA (Para-Aminobenzoic Acid) 400 mg • Bio-Min TR8 a source of trace minerals 100 mg • Glutamic Acid HCL 40 mg • Ammonium Chloride 32 mg • Betaine HCL 20 mg • Chlorophyll 10 mg • Boron (Sodium Tetraborate Decahydrate) 3 mg. Other ingredients: Cellulose, Cellulose Gum, Stearic Acid, Silicon Dioxide, Magnesium Stearate, Alfalfa (Medicago sativa) leaves & stems juice concentrate, Black Cohosh (Cimicituga racemosa) root, Licorice (Glycyrrhiza glabra) root extract & Scullcap (Scutellaria baicalensis) whole plant. Contains no sugar, salt, yeast, wheat, corn, soy, dairy products, artificial coloring, artificial flavoring or preservatives.

Doctor's Choice for Bone Health — Enzymatic Therapy
Three tablets contain: Vitamin C (Ascorbic Acid) 100 mg • Vitamin D (Fish Liver oil) 300 IU • Vitamin K (Phytonadione) 300 mcg • Folic Acid 800 mcg • Vitamin B12 (Cyanocobalamin) 800 mcg • Calcium (Krebs Cycle Chelate) 600 mg • Magnesium (Krebs Cycle Chelate) 150 mg • Vitamin C (Ascorbic Acid) 100 mg • Zinc (Picolinate) 15 mg • Sodium 6 mg • Copper (Picolinate) 1 mg • Mixed Flavonoids (Citrus) 100 mg • Betaine HCL 30 mg • Soy Bean extract standardized to contain 25% Saponins & 13-17% Isoflavones calculated as

© Copyright 2000, Natural Medicines Comprehensive Database (209) 472-2244. For updated data, go to www.NaturalDatabase.com. • 1325

B R A N D   N A M E S

Genistein 20 mg • Boron (Sodium Tetrahydroborate) 3 mg • Silicon (Sodium Metasilicate) 1 mg • Strontium (Chloride) 500 mcg. Other ingredients: Cellulose, Cellulose Gum, Stearic Acid, Silicon Dioxide, & Magnesium Stearate.

Doctor's Choice for Diabetics — Enzymatic Therapy
Two tablets contain: Vitamin E (Mixed Tocopherols) 100 IU • Vitamin C (Ascorbic Acid) 300 mg • Magnesium (Krebs Cycle Chelate) 100 mg • Vitamin B6 (Pyridoxine HCL) 10 mg • Manganese (Krebs Cycle Chelate) 7.5 mg • Zinc (Picolinate) 7.5 mg • Copper (Picolinate) 0.5 mg • Biotin 1000 mcg • Folic Acid 400 mcg • Vitamin B12 (Cyanocobalamin) 400 mcg • Chromium (Picolinate) 200 mcg • Selenium (Aspartate) 50 mcg • Gymnema sylvestre leaves extract standardized to contain 25% Gymnemic Acid 200 mg • Bitter Melon extract (Momordica charantia) 200 mg • Fenugreek seed extract (4:1) (Trigonella foenum-graecum) 100 mg • Bilberry extract (Vaccinium myrtillus fructus) standardized to contain 25% Anthocyanosides calculated as Anthocyanidins 40 mg • Mixed Bioflavonoids (Citrus) 25 mg • Vanadyl Sulfate 5 mg. Other ingredients: Calcium Carbonate, Cellulose, Cellulose Gum, Silicon Dioxide, Dicalcium Phosphate, Magnesium Stearate & Calcium Silicate. Contains no sugar, salt, yeast, wheat, gluten, corn, dairy products, artificial coloring, artificial flavoring or preservatives.

Doctor's Choice for Female Teens — Enzymatic Therapy
Four tablets contain: Vitamin A (Beta Carotene) 15000 IU • Vitamin A (Retinol) 2500 IU • Vitamin E (D-Alpha Tocopherol Succinate) 200 IU • Vitamin D (Ergocalciferol) 100 IU • Calcium (Citrate, Carbonate) 500 mg • Vitamin C (Ascorbic Acid) 300 mg • Magnesium (Aspartate) 200 mg • Potassium (Aspartate) 99 mg • Vitamin B6 (Pyridoxine HCL) 90 mg • Niacin/Niacinamide 45 mg • Iron (Ferrous Succinate) 30 mg • Pantothenic Acid (D-Calcium Pantothenate) 30 mg • Thiamine HCL (Vitamin B1) 30 mg • Riboflavin (Vitamin B2) 30 mg • Zinc (Picolinate) 20 mg • Manganese (Citrate) 15 mg • Copper (Gluconate) 1.5 mg • Folic Acid 800 mcg • Vitamin B12 (Cyanocobalamin) 800 mcg • Biotin 300 mcg • Iodine (Kelp) 300 mcg • Chromium (Polynicotinate) 200 mcg • Selenium (L-Selenomethionine) 100 mcg • Vitamin K (Phytonadione) 60 mcg • Molybdenum (Sodium molybdate) 25 mcg • Mixed Flavonoids (Citrus) 100 mg • Alfalfa juice concentrate 60 mg • Choline Bitartrate 60 mg • Inositol 60 mg • Ginger root extract 6.5:1 (Zingiber officinale) 60 mg • Dandelion root extract 4:1 (Taraxacum officinale) 60 mg • Licorice root extract (Glycyrrhiza glabra) standardized to contain 5% Glycyrrhizic Acid 30 mg • Boron (Sodium Tetraborate Decahydrate) 2 mg • Silica (Sodium Metasilicate) 1 mg • Vanadium (Sulfate) 50 mcg. Other ingredients: Cellulose, Cellulose Gum, Stearic Acid, Magnesium Stearate & Silicon Dioxide. Contains no sugar, salt, yeast, wheat, corn, dairy products, coloring, flavoring, or preservatives.

Doctor's Choice for Healthy Cholesterol Levels — Enzymatic Therapy
Each capsule contains: Red Yeast Rice (Standardized to contain 1% Mevinolin) 475 mg • Artichoke (Cynara scolymus) leaf extract 50 mg • Ginger (Zingiber officinale) root extract 50 mg • Coenzyme Q10 (CoQ10) 8 mg. Other ingredients: Soybean oil, Vegetable oil, Beeswax, Lecithin, and Gelatin capsule.

Doctor's Choice for Heart Health — Enzymatic Therapy
Two tablets contain: Vitamin E (D-Alpha Tocopherol) 100 IU • Magnesium (Oxide) 150 mg • Niacin 100 mg • Vitamin C (Ascorbic Acid) 100 mg • Potassium (Chloride) 75 mg • Calcium Pangamate 20 mg • Vitamin B6 (Pyridoxine HCL) 10 mg • Sodium 6 mg • Folic Acid 200 mcg • Vitamin B12 (Cyanocobalamin) 200 mcg • Hawthorne berry extract (Crataegus oxyacantha) standardized to contain 1.8% Vitexin-2'-Rhamnoside 150 mg • Super Seven Complex Mixture of Herbs: Hydrangea, Black Cohosh (Cimicifuga racemosa), Buchu leaves, Couch Grass, Corn Silk, Dandelion leaf (Taraxacum officinale) & Ginger root (Zingiber officinale) 150 mg • Khella extract (Ammi visnaga) standardized to contain a minimum of 10% Pyrones calculated as Khellin 100 mg • L-Cysteine 100 mg • Carbamide 100 mg. Other ingredients: Cellulose, Cellulose Gum, Stearic Acid, Sodium Starch, Glycolate, Silicon Dioxide, Magnesium Stearate & Vanillin.

Doctor's Choice for Male Teens — Enzymatic Therapy
Four tablets contain: Vitamin A (Beta Carotene) 15000 IU • Vitamin A (Retinol) 2500 IU • Vitamin E (D-Alpha Tocopherol Succinate) 200 IU • Vitamin D (Ergocalciferol) 100 IU • Calcium (Citrate, Carbonate) 400 mg • Vitamin C (Ascorbic Acid) 300 mg • Magnesium (Aspartate) 200 mg • Potassium (Aspartate) 99 mg • Niacin/

Niacinamide 45 mg • Pantothenic Acid (D-CalciumPantothenate) 30 mg • Vitamin B6 (Pyridoxine HCL) 30 mg • Thiamine HCL (Vitamin B1) 30 mg • Riboflavin (Vitamin B2) 30 mg • Zinc (Picolinate) 30 mg • Manganese (Citrate) 15 mg • Copper (Gluconate) 1.5 mg • Folic Acid 800 mcg • Vitamin B12 (Cyanocobalamin) 800 mcg • Iodine (Kelp) 300 mcg • Chromium (Polynicotinate) 200 mcg • Selenium (L-Selenomethionine) 100 mcg • Vitamin K (Phytonadione) 60 mcg • Molybdenum (sodium Molybdate) 25 mcg • Biotin 300 mcg • Mixed Flavonoids (Citrus) 100 mg • Alfalfa juice concentrate 60 mg • Dandelion root extract 4:1 (Taraxacum officinale) 60 mg • Ginger root extract 6.5:1 (Zingiber officinale) 60 mg • Sarsaparilla root extract 4:1 (Simlax officinalis) 60 mg • Choline Bitartrate 30 mg • Inositol 30 mg • Boron (Sodium Tetraborate Decahydrate) 2 mg • Vanadium (Sulfate) 50 mcg.

Doctor's Choice for Men — Enzymatic Therapy
Three tablets contain: Vitamin A (Beta Carotene) non-toxic form of Vitamin A 15000 IU • Vitamin A (Retinol) 2500 IU • Vitamin E (D-Alpha Tocopherol Succinate) 200 IU • Vitamin D 100 IU • Magnesium (Aspartate, Chloride) 400 mg • Vitamin C (Ascorbic Acid) 300 mg • Calcium (Citrate, Carbonate) 200 mg • Potassium (Aspartate) 99 mg • Niacin 90 mg • Thiamine HCL (Vitamin B1) 60 mg • Riboflavin (Vitamin B2) 60 mg • Vitamin B6 (Pyridoxine HCL) 60 mg • Pantothenic Acid (D-Calcium Pantothenate) 60 mg • Zinc (Picolinate) 30 mg • Manganese (Citrate) 5 mg • Copper (Gluconate) 1 mg • Folic Acid 800 mcg • Vitamin B12 (Cyanocobalamin) 800 mcg • Biotin 600 mcg • Iodine (Kelp) 300 mcg • Chromium (Polynicotinate) 200 mcg • Selenium (Selenomethionine) 200 mcg • Vitamin K (Phytonadione) 60 mcg • Molybdenum (Sodium Molybdate) 25 mcg • Flavonoids mixed 50 mg • Alfalfa juice concentrate 50 mg • Choline Bitartrate 30 mg • Inositol 30 mg • Ginger root extract 6.5:1 (Zingiber officinale) 30 mg • Green Tea extract (Camellia sinensis) standardized to contain 70% Polyphenols 30 mg • Muira Puama extract 6:1 (Ptychopetalum olacoides) 30 mg • PABA (Para-Aminobenzoic Acid) 30 mg • Saw Palmetto Berry extract 4:1 (Serenoa repens) 30 mg • Korean Ginseng root extract (Panax ginseng) standardized to contain 7% Saponins (calculated as Ginsenoside Rg1) 15 mg • Carotenes from natural sources 5 mg • Boron (Sodium Tetraborate Decahydrate) 2 mg • Vanadium (Sulfate) 50 mcg. Other ingredients: Cellulose, Cellulose Gum, Stearic Acid, Silicon Dioxide & Magnesium Stearate. Contains no sugar, salt, yeast, wheat, corn, dairy products, artificial coloring, artificial flavoring, or preservatives.

Doctor's Choice for Women — Enzymatic Therapy
Four tablets contain: Vitamin A (Beta Carotene) non-toxic form of Vitamin A 15000 IU • Vitamin A (Retinol) 2500 IU • Vitamin E (D-Alpha Tocopherol Succinate) 200 IU • Vitamin D 100 IU • Calcium (Citrate, Carbonate) 400 mg • Vitamin C (Ascorbic Acid) 300 mg • Magnesium (Aspartate, Chloride) 300 mg • Potassium (Aspartate) 99 mg • Vitamin B6 (Pyridoxine HCL) 90 mg • Niacin/Niacinamide 90 mg • Thiamine HCL (Vitamin B1) 60 mg • Riboflavin (Vitamin B2) 60 mg • Pantothenic Acid (D-Calcium Pantothenate) 30 mg • Zinc (Picolinate) 20 mg • Iron (Ferrous Succinate) 18 mg • Manganese (Citrate) 5 mg • Vitamin B6 (Pyridoxal-5-Phosphate) 5 mg • Copper (Gluconate) 1 mg • Folic Acid 800 mcg • Vitamin B12 (Cyanocobalamin) 800 mcg • Biotin 600 mcg • Iodine (Kelp) 300 mcg • Chromium (Polynicotinate) 200 mcg • Selenium (Selenomethionine) 200 mcg • Vitamin K (Phytonadione) 60 mcg • Molybdenum (Sodium molybdate) 25 mcg • Flavonoids, mixed 50 mg • Alfalfa juice concentrate 50 mg • Choline Bitartrate 30 mg • Inositol 30 mg • Dong Quai extract 4:1 (Angelica sinensis) 30 mg • Ginger root extract (6.5:1) (Zingiber officinale) 30 mg • Licorice root extract (Glycyrrhiza glabra) standardized to contain 5% Glycyrrhizic Acid 30 mg • PABA (Para-Aminobenzoic Acid) 30 mg • Chaste Tree Berry extract 5:1 (Vitex agnus-castus) 15 mg • Fennel seed extract 6:1 (Foeniculum vulgare) 15 mg • Carotenes from natural sources 5 mg • Boron (Sodium Tetraborate Decahydrate) 3 mg • Silica (Sodium Metasilicate) 1 mg • Vanadium (Sulfate) 50 mcg. Other Ingredients: Cellulose, Cellulose Gum, Magnesium Stearate, Stearic Acid, & Silicon Dioxide. Contains no sugar, salt, yeast, wheat, corn, dairy products, artificial coloring, artificial flavoring or preservatives.

Doctor's Choice Prenatal Supplement — Enzymatic Therapy
Four tablets contain: Vitamin A (Beta Carotene) 15000 IU • Vitamin E (D-Alpha Tocopherol Succinate) 200 IU • Vitamin D (Ergocalciferol) 100 IU • Calcium (Citrate, Carbonate) 800 mg • Magnesium (Citrate) 400 mg • Vitamin C (Ascorbic Acid) 300 mg • Vitamin B6 (Pyridoxine HCL) 120 mg • Pantothenic Acid (D-Calcium Pantothenate) 100 mg • Potassium (Aspartate) 99 mg • Thiamine HCL (Vitamin B1) 60 mg • Riboflavin (Vitamin B2) 60 mg • Niacin/

Niacinamide 45 mg • Iron (Ferrous succinate) 30 mg • Zinc (Picolinate) 30 mg • Manganese (Citrate) 15 mg • Copper (Gluconate) 1.5 mg • Folic Acid 800 mg • Vitamin B12 (Cyanocobalamin) 800 mcg • Biotin 600 mcg • Vitamin K (Phytonadione) 500 mcg • Iodine (Kelp) 300 mcg • Chromium (Polynicotinate) 200 mcg • Selenium (L-Selenomethionine) 100 mcg • Molybdenum (Sodium Molybdate) 25 mcg • Ginger root extract 6.5:1 (Zingiber officinale) 150 mg • Mixed Flavonoids (Citrus) 90 mg • Choline Bitartrate 90 mg • Inositol 90 mg • Dandelion root extract 4:1 (Taraxacum officinale) 60 mg • Red Raspberry leaves 60 mg • Boron (Sodium Tetraborate Decahydrate) 1 mg • Silica (Sodium Metasilicate) 1 mg • Vanadium (Sulfate) 50 mcg. Other ingredients: Cellulose, Cellulose Gum, Stearic Acid, Silicon Dioxide & Magnesium Stearate.

Dolomite — The Vitamin Shoppe
Four tablets supply: Calcium 520 mg • Magnesium 312 mg.

Dong Quai — Fingerprint Botanicals
Each capsule contains: Dong Quai 500 mg.

Dong Quai — Nature's Way
Each capsule contains: Dong Quai 565 mg.

Dong Quai and Royal Jelly — General Nutrition Center
Each capsule contains: Dong Quai 300 mg • Agnus Castus berry 50 mg • Royal Jelly 50 mg • Wild Yam root 50 mg.

Dong Quai Extract — Montana Big Sky
Each capsule contains: Dong Quai 200 mg.

Dong Quai Extract in Vegetable Glycerin — Nature's Herbs
Each drop contains: Dong Quai 565 mg.

Dong Quai Root — Herbal Plus
Each capsule contains: Dong Quai 250 mg.

DopaBean 333 mg — Solaray - Nutraceutical
One capsule contains: Velvet Bean seed extract (Mucuna pruriens) 333 mg • Catecholamines 66 mg • L-dopa 50 mg. Other ingredients: Gelatin (capsule), Rice Flour, Maltodextrin, Magnesium Stearate, Silica, Alpha Galactosidase.

Down Size — Dial Herbs
Purified Water • Hydrolyzed Collagen • Glycerine • Natural Flavors • Aloe concentrate • Acesulfame Potassium • Citric Acid • Potassium Sorbate • Sodium Benzoate • Potassium Iodide.

Dream Sleep — The Herbalist
Hops blossom • Passionflower herb • Skullcap herb • Valerian root.

D-Snore — Quest
Sweet Almond Oil • Sesame Oil • Sunflower Oil • Olive Oil • Grape Seed Oil • Lecithin • Orange Seed Extract in a base of glycerin • Purified de-ionized Water • Natural Peppermint flavor.

Dymetadrine 25 — AST Sports Science
Each tablet contains: Ephedrine HCL 25 mg • Guaifenesin 200 mg.

Dymetadrine Xtrem — AST Sports Science
Two capsules contain: Ephedra extract 8% 600 mg • L-Phenylalanine 300 mg • L-Tyrosine 300 mg • Caffeine 200 mg • Willow Bark extract 100 mg.

E.T.-(Essiac Tonic) — The Herbalist
Burdock root • Sheep Sorrel leaf • Slippery Elm bark • Turkey Rhubarb root.

E-400 Sesame — Progressive Labs
Each softgel capsule contains: Vitamin E (d-alpha tocopherol) 400 IU • Sesame oil 200 mg. With Natural, Unesterified Mixed Tocopherols.

Ear Drops — NutriBiotic
Contains 0.1% grapefruit extract in a base of tea tree oil and vegetable glycerin.

Ear Oil — Blessed Herbs
Calendula flower • St. John's Wort flower • Mullein flower • Garlic & Organic Cold-Pressed Olive oil.

Easy Now — Traditional Medicinals
Contains: Peppermint leaf • Spearmint leaf • Passion flower herb • Valerian root • Licorice root • Catnip leaf • Chamomile flower • Rosemary leaf • Lavender flower • natural flavors.

Eater's Digest — Traditional Medicinals
Peppermint leaf • Ginger rhizome • Fennel seed • Rose Hip • Papaya leaf • Alfalfa Herb • Cinnamon bark.

EB5 Age Spot Formula —
Pharmacist Heldfond's eb5 Formulas for Younger Looking Skin
Hydroquinone 2% • Deionized Water • Mineral Oil • Cetearyl Alcohol • Cetearyl Phosphate • Glycerin • Petroleum • Steareth-2 • Stearyl Alcohol • Steareth-10 • Bilberry Extract • Sugar Cane Extract • Sugar Maple Extract • Orange Extract • Lemon Extract • Octyl Methoxcinnamate • Benzophenone-3 • Sodium Sulfite • Sodium Meta Bisulfite • Citric Acid • Propylene Glycol • Diazolidinyl Urea • Methylparaben • Propylparaben.

EB5 Body Formula —
Pharmacist Heldfond's eb5 Formulas for Younger Looking Skin
Purified Water • Methylsilanol Mannuronate • Mate Extract • Gotu Kola Extract • Thea Sinensis Extract • Butylene Glycol • Glyeryl Stearate • Stearic Acid • Cyclomehticome • Octyl Palmitate • Myristy Myristate • Dimethicone • Sunflower Oil • Isopropyl Lanolate • Soy Serol • Cetareth 20 • Tocopheryl Acetate • Choleth-24 • Ceteth 24 • Panthenol • Ivy Extract • Horsetail Extract • Kelp Extract • Algae Extract • Ginkgo Extract • Arnica Extract • Triethanolamine • Carbomer • Hydroxykpropyl • Methycellulose • Disodium EDTA • Methylparaben • Propylparaben • Imadazolidinyl Urea • Fragrance.

EB5 Body Lotion —
Pharmacist Heldfond's eb5 Formulas for Younger Looking Skin
Water • Tocopheryl Acetate • Stearic Acid • Propylene Glycol • Dicaprylate/Dicaprate • Mineral Oil • Butylene glycol • Glyeryl Stearate SE • Sorbitan Stearate • Polysorbate-60 • Squalane • Soy Sterol • Panthenol • Oat Flour • Lanolin Alcohol • Retinyl Palmitate • Ergocalciferol • Dimenthicone • Imidazolidinyl Urea • Disodium EDTA • Carbomer-940 • Polyamino Sugar • Condensate • Urea • Methylparaben • Propylparaben • Triethanolamine • Fragrance.

EB5 Cleansing Formula —
Pharmacist Heldfond's eb5 Formulas for Younger Looking Skin
Purified Water • Cycerin • Caprylic/Capric Triglyceride • Stearic Acid • Peg 8 • Glycol Distearate • Cetyl Alcohol • Triethanolamine • Tocopheryl Acetate • Lactic Acid • Polyquatemium-7 • Panthenol • Peg-10 • Soya Sterol • Oat Flour • Cetearyl Alcohol • Peg-40 Castor Oil • Sodium Cetearyl Sulfate • Cocamide DEA • Carbomer • Disodium • EDTA • BHA • Methylparaben • Propylparaben • Quantemium-15 • fragrance.

EB5 Footcare Formula —
Pharmacist Heldfond's eb5 Formulas for Younger Looking Skin
Deionized Water • Mineral Oil • Propylene Glycol • Stearic Acid • Microcystalline Wax • Cetyl Alcohol • PEG-100 Stearate • vitamin E Acetate • Oat Protein • Triethanolamine • Menthol • Eucalyptus Oil • Fragrance • DL Panthenol • Allantoin • Imidazolidiny Urea • Methylparaben • Propylparaben • Potassium Sorbate • Chamomile • Comfrey • Tea Tree Oil • White Lily Extract • Corn Flower Extract • Sandalwood Extract • Sunflower Extract • Basil Extract • Sage Extract • Jasmine Extract • Sugar Cane Extract • Maple Extract • Citrus Extract • Apple Extract • Vitamin A & D3 • Dipotassium • Glycyrrhzinate • Soluble Collagen • FD&C Blue #1 • FD&C Yellow #5.

EB5 Men's Facial Formula —
Pharmacist Heldfond's eb5 Formulas for Younger Looking Skin
Water • Propylene Glycol • Tocopheryl Acetate • Stearic Acid • Mineral Oil • Cetyl Alcohol • Oat Flour • Sodium PCA • Retinyl Palmiate • Ergocalciferol • Allantoin • Panthenol • Soluble Animal Collagen • Propylparaben • Triethanolamine • Methylparaben • Potassium Sorbate • Imidazolidinyl Urea • Carbomer-940 • Fragrance • FD&C Blue No. 1 and D&C Red No. 33.

EB5 Toning Formula —
Pharmacist Heldfond's eb5 Formulas for Younger Looking Skin
Purified Water • Hydrolyzed Wheat Protein • Arnica Extract • Barley Extract • Triethanolamine • Lactic Acid • Polysorbate 20 • Sodium PCA • Vitamin E Acetate • Allantoin • Panthenol • Witch Hazel Distillate • Sage Extract • Birch Leaf Extract • Comfrey Extract • Sambucus Extract • Blackberry Extract • Horsetail Extract • Tetrasodium EDTA • Methylparaben • Imidazolidinyl Uera • Quantemium-15 • Fragrance.

EB-C — MMS Pro
Each capsule contains: Eyebright • Golden Seal root • Bayberry root bark • Red Raspberry • Cayenne.

Echinacea — Nature's Way
Three capsules contain: Echinacea Purpurea stem, leaf, flower 1.20 g. Other ingredients: Gelatin.

BRAND NAMES

Some Brand Name Natural Products - What they Contain
www.NaturalDatabase.com contains MANY more listings than appear here.

B R A N D   N A M E S

Echinacea — Centrum Herbals
One capsule contains: Echinacea extract flower and root (Echinacea purpurea) 100 mg. Standardized to contain (based on extract weight): Total Phenols (marker) 3.0%, Cichoric Acid (natural active), Isobutyl Alkylamides (natural active), Activity Measure 15-lipoxygenase enzymatic assay. Other Ingredients: Dibasic Calcium Phosphate, Cellulose, Lactose Monohydrate, Hydroxypropy cellulose, Ethylcellulose, Castor Oil, Gelatin, Silicon Dioxide, Sodium Lauryl Sulfate, Proplene Glycol, Titanium Dioxide.

Echinacea — Gaia Herbs
Echinacea standardized for 1% isobutylamides and 4% phenolic compounds. Standardized Full Spectrum 90 mg of extract per capsule. Guaranteed Potency 45 mg of extract per capsule.

Echinacea — Pharmanex
Each capsule contains: Echinacea purpurea Root 6:1 Extract 225 mg. Other Ingredients: Rice Flour, Gelatin.

Echinacea & Goldenseal Combination — Atrium
Two fluid ounces contains: Echinacea • Goldenseal. In a synergistic base of Red Clover, Burdock, Parsley, Fennel, Ginger, Chamomille, Barberry & Cayenne. Contains 16-18% Grain Alcohol.

Echinacea 150 mg — Jamieson
Each capsule contains: Echinacea (Echinacea purpurea, powdered extract 1:3) 150 mg • Panax Ginseng (Standardized to 4% ginsenosides) 250 mg.

Echinacea 300 mg — Jamieson
Each capsule contains: Echinacea herb (Echinacea Purpurea, powdered 1:3) 300 mg • Allicin Rich Garlic bulb powder 300 mg • Ginger root (Zingiber Officinale, powdered Extract 1:6) 300 mg.

Echinacea and Golden Seal — Optimum Nutrition
Echinacea Angustifolia extract • Goldenseal powder.

Echinacea and Goldenseal — Dial Herbs
Echinacea • Goldenseal • Cayenne.

Echinacea Balance — HerbaSway
Echinacea • Green Tea • Ginger • Blackberry • HerbaSwee (Cucurbitaceae fruit).

Echinacea Extract — Progressive Labs
Each capsule contains: Echinacea 250 mg • Polysaccharides (from Echinacea) 37.5 mg • Phenolic compounds (from Echinacea) 10 mg.

Echinacea Extract — Jamieson
Each capsule contains: Echinacea herb 350 mg • (Echinacea purpurea 1:3 powdered extract). Other Ingredients: Dicalcium Phosphate, Micorcrystalline Cellulose, Magnesium Stearate, Silicon Dioxide.

Echinacea Extract — Ortho Molecular Products
Each capsule contains: Echinacea Angustifolia extract 200 mg • Echinacea Purpurea 200 mg.

Echinacea Goldenseal — Jamieson
Each capsule contains: Calcium (as Calcium Sulfate) 30 mg • Echinacea root extract 4:1 (Echinacea purpurea Moench.)(4% Phenolic Compounds) 185 mg • Goldenseal root extract 2:1 (Hydrastis canadensis L.)(5% Alkaloids and Hydrastine Compounds) 45 mg.

Echinacea Plus — The Herbalist
Echinacea fresh root (Echinacea angustifolia)• Echinacea fresh-dried seed (Echinacea pupurea).

Echinacea Plus — Traditional Medicinals
Echinacea purpurea herb • Lemongrass leaf • Spearmint leaf • Echinacea angustifolia herb • concentrated extract of E. Purpurea root.

Echinacea Root Complex — Nature's Way
Two capsules contain: Echinacea Angustifolia root • Echinacea Purpurea stem, leaf, flower • Proprietary Blend 900 mg. Other ingredients: Gelatin, Magnesium Stearate.

Echinacea Tincture — Jamieson
Each 2 ml (40 drops) contains: Echinacea angustifolia 1000 mg (1:2 pure tincture in 45% Ethanol) Derived from alcohol maceration of fresh plants (aerial parts).

Echinacea with Zinc — Aspen Group, Inc.
Each capsule contains: Echinacea Purpurea 380 mg • Zinc (citrate) 3 mg. Contains no sugar, starch, salt, wheat, yeast, corn or soy derivatives.

Echinacea/Astragalus/Reishi Formula — Nature's Way
Three capsules contain: Proprietary Formula: Astragalus root • Echinacea Purpurea stem, leaf, flower • Reishi (dried extract 10% Polysaccharides). Other ingredients: Gelatin.

Echinacea/Ester-C Formula — Nature's Way
Two capsules contain: Calcium 27 mg • Echinacea Purpurea stem, leaf, flower 722 mg • Ester-C (Patented form of Vitamin C) 207 mg. Other ingredients: Gelatin.

Echinacea/Ginseng Formula — Nature's Way
Two capsules contain: Proprietary Formula: Echinacea Angustifolia root • Echinacea Purpurea stem, leaf, flower • Siberian Ginseng root . Other ingredients: Gelatin, Magnesium Stearate, Millet.

Echinacea/Goldenseal — Gaia Herbs
Echinacea and Goldenseal standardized for 1% isobutylamides and 15% total alkaloids. Standardized Full Spectrum 100 mg of extract per capsule. Guaranteed Potency 50 mg of extract per capsule.

Echinacea/GSR Formula — Nature's Way
Three capsules contain: Proprietary Formula: Burdock root • Cayenne pepper fruit • Echinacea Angustifolia root • Echinacea Purpurea stem, leaf, flower • Gentain root • Goldenseal stem, leaf, flower • Wood Betony stem, leaf, flower. Other ingredients: Gelatin.

Echinacea-Go! — Wakunaga of America
Each capsule contains: Echinacea Standardized Extract (angustifolia & purpurea blend) leaf/root, standardized to 4% Phenolic Compounds. Other Ingredients: Cellulose, Colloidal Silica, Magnesium Stearate (vegetable source).

Echinacea-Goldenseal Formula — Quest
Each caplet contains: Echinacea angustifolia powder (provided by 100 mg P.E. 1:7 standardized to contain 4% echinacosides) 700 mg • Goldenseal root powder (Hydrastis canadensis) (provided by 50 mg P.E. 1:6 standardized to contain 5% hydrastine) 300 mg • Echinacea purpurea powder (Provided by 50 mg P.E. 1:5 standardized to contain 0.7% flavonoids) 250 mg • Astragalus root powder (Astragalus membranaceus) 100 mg. Other Ingredients: Calcium Phosphate, Microcrystalline Cellulose, Vegetable Stearin, Croscarmellose Sodium, Magnesium Stearate (vegetable source).

Echinacea-Reishi Virtue — Blessed Herbs
Astragalus root • Echinacea Angustifolia root • Pau d'Arco bark • Suma root • Siberian Ginseng root • Reishi mycelium • Licorice root • German Chamomile flower • Calendula flower • Grain alcohol & Distilled Water.

EchinaFresh — Enzymatic Therapy
Each capsule contains: Echinacea purpurea 50:1 concentration of powder from the fresh-pressed juice of stems, leaves, & flowers of organically grown Echinacea purpurea 50 mg.

Echinex — Chattem, Inc.
Each tablet contains: Standardized extract of Echinacea purpurea root & herb (4% total phenolic compounds) 250 mg • Standardized extract of Siberian Ginseng root (0.8% eleutherosides) 100 mg • Standardized extract of Ginger root (5% gingerols) 100 mg. Other ingredients: Cellulose, Croscarmellose Sodium, Stearic Acid, Magnesium Stearate, Silicon Dioxide, Hydroxypropyl Methylcellulose (aqueous film coating). Contains no sugar, starch, yeast, sodium, dairy or preservatives.

Eco-Green Multi — Now
Two tablets contain: Vitamin A (Beta Carotene) (15 mg) 25000 IU • Vitamin B1 (Thiamine HCL) 50 mg • Vitamin B2 (Riboflavin) 50 mg • Vitamin B3 (Niacinamide) 50 mg • Vitamin B5 (Pantothenic Acid) 50 mg • Vitamin B6 (Pyridoxine HCL) 50 mg • Vitamin B12 (Cyanocobalamin) 200 mcg • Biotin 100 mcg • Folic Acid 800 mcg • Vitamin C (Calcium Ascorbate) 500 mg • Vitamin D (Calciferol) 200 IU • Vitamin E (d-Alpha Succinate) 200 IU • Vitamin K (from green foods) 70 mcg • Calcium (Ascorbate, Citrate, Carbonate) 100 mg • Magnesium (50% Citrate, 50% Oxide) 100 mg • Zinc (Picolinate) 15 mg • Copper (Amino Acid Chelate) 500 mcg • Iodine (Kelp) 150 mcg • Potassium (Chloride) 25 mg • Manganese (Amino Acid Chelate) 5 mg • Selenium (L-Selenomethionine) 50 mcg • Chromium (Picolinate) 100 mcg • Molybdenum (Amino Acid Chelate) 50 mcg • Spirulina US grown 250 mg • Barley grass organically grown 250 mg • Chlorella (broken cell wall) 100 mg • Wheat grass organically grown 100 mg • Alfalfa juice concentrate 100 mg • Green Tea extract (40% Catechins) 50 mg • Choline (Bitartrate) 50 mg • Inositol 50 mg • PABA 30 mg • Trace Mineral concentrate 100 mg • Boron (Amino

Acid Chelate) 1 mg • Vanadium (Amino Acid Chelate) 50 mcg • Panax ginseng (5% Ginsenosides) 100 mg • Bioflavonoids (40%) 50 mg • Rutin 25 mg • Bromelain (2000 GDU from pineapple) 50 mg • Papain (140 MCU from papaya) 25 mg • Pepsin Enzymes (NF 1:10000) 25 mg • Lipase (3400 Usp Units) 25 mg • Amylase (20000 USP Units) 10 mg • Chlorophyll from green foods 8 mg • Amino Acids from green foods 350 mg. Vegetarian formula base ingredients contain: Di-Calcium Phosphate, Cellulose, Stearic Acid, Magnesium Stearate & Silica. Contains no yeast, soy, milk, corn, gluten or preservatives.

EFA Attention Formula — Health From The Sun
Each capsule contains: Vitamin E (as d-Alpha Tocopherol) 5 IU • Magnesium from Magnesium Oxide 55 mg • Zinc from Zinc Sulfate 0.5 mg • High DHA Fish oil (70 mg Omega-3 DHA) 175 mg • Arachidonic Acid (from Fish oil) 3 mg • Borage oil (16 mg Omega-6 GLA) 80 mg • Lecithin 50 mg • Ashwaganda root extract 25 mg • Bacopa Monnieri Whole Plant extract 25 mg. Other Ingredients: Gelatin, Glycerine, Beeswax (emulsifier), Water, Carob powder.

EFA Complex — PhysioLogics
Two soft gels contain: Vitamin E (as d-Alpha Tocopherol) 20 IU • Eicosapentaenoic Acid (from Marine Lipids)120 mg • Docosahexaenoic Acid (from Marine Lipids) 80 mg • Gamma-linolenic Acid (from Borage oil) 30 mg.

EFA Derma-Skin Formula — Health From The Sun
Each capsule contains: Vitamin A from Palmitate 3000 IU • Vitamin C from Ascorbic Acid 60 mg • Vitamin D as Cholecalciferol 100 IU • Vitamin E as d-Alpha Tocopherol 40 IU • Zinc from Zinc Sulfate 10 mg • Organic Flax seed oil (450 mg Omega-3 ALA) 800 mg • Borage seed oil (120 mg Omega-6 GLA) 600 mg • Burdock root extract 4:1 50 mg • Yellow Dock root extract 4:1 50 mg. Other Ingredients: Gelatin, Glycerine, Beeswax (emulsifier), Water, Carob powder, Lecithin.

EFA Heart Formula — Health From The Sun
Three capsules contain: Borage oil (180 mg GLA) 900 mg • Fish oil (18% EPA, 12% DHA) 1200 mg • Flax seed oil, organic 300 mg • Folic Acid 300 mcg • Garlic extract (0.8% Allicin) 300 mg • Gugulipid (10% Gugulsterone) 300 mg • Hawthorne extract (2% Vitexin) 105 mg • Tocopherols, mixed 3.9 mg • Tocotrienols 11 mg • Vitamin B6 from Pyridoxine Hydrochloride 1.2 mg. No sugar, starch, artificial preservatives, or colors.

EFA Joint Formula — Health From The Sun
Three capsules contain: Protein 1 g • Vitamin C as Ascorbic Acid 75 mg • Vitamin D3 as Cholecalciferol 100 IU • Vitamin E as d-Alpha Tocopherol 30 IU • Zinc from Zinc Sulfate 15 mg • Manganese from Manganese Gluconate 330 mcg • Borage seed oil 300 mg GLA 1500 mg • Glucosamine Sulfate 1200 mg • Organic Flax seed oil (250 mg ALA) 450 mg • Boswellic Acid from Boswellia Resin extract 100 mg. Ingredients: Gelatin, Glycerine, Beeswax (emulsifer), Water, Carob powder, Soy Lecithin.

Efalex — Efamol
Two capsules contain: Efamol Pure Evening Primrose Oil 280 mg • DHA 120 mg • GLA 24 mg • Arachidonic Acid 10.5 mg • Thyme Oil 2 mg • Vitamin E 15 IU. Other Ingredients: Tuna Oil, Gelatin, Glycerin.

Efalex Liquid — Efamol
Four teaspoons contain: Efamol Pure Evening Primrose Oil 1200 mg • DHA 480 mg • GLA 96 mg • Arachidonic Acid 42 mg • Thyme Oil 8 mg • Vitamin E 15 IU. Other Ingredients: Sunflower Oil, Tuna Oil, Flavoring (lemon oil, lime oil).

Efamol Fortify — Efamol
Two capsules contain: Efamol Pure Evening Primrose Oil 800 mg • EPA 14 mg • GLA 64 mg • Vitamin E 30 IU • Calcium 200 mg. Other Ingredients: Calcium Carbonate, Gelatin, Glycerin, Marine Fish Oil, Glyceryl Monostearate, Titanium Dioxide Color.

Efamol PMS Control — Efamol
Two capsules contain: Efamol Pure Evening Primrose Oil 500 mg • GLA 40 mg • Vitamin C 60 mg • Vitamin E 30 IU • Niacin 12 mg • Vitamin B6 40 mg • Biotin 80 mcg • Magnesium 40 mg • Zinc 4 mg. Other Ingredients: Gelatin, Sorbitol Syrup, Glyceryl Monostearate, Glycerin, Ascorbic Acid, Heavy Magnesium Oxide, Pyridoxine HCl, Lecithin, Nicotinamide, Zinc Sulphate Monohydrate, d-Biotin.

Efamol Pure Evening Primrose Oil — Efamol
Two capsules contain: Efamol Pure Evening Primrose Oil 1000 mg • Linoleic Acid 330 mg • Gamma Linolenic Acid 80 mg . Other Ingredients: Gelatin, Glycerin.

Efanatal — Efamol
Two capsules contain: Efamol Pure Evening Primrose Oil 500 mg • DHA (Docosahexaenoic Acid) 107 mg • Arachidonic Acid 9.4 mg • GLA 40 mg • Vitamin E 15 IU. Other Ingredients: Fish Oil, Gelatin, Glycerol, Carmine Color, Titanium Dioxide Color, Ammonium Phosphatide, Ascorbyl Palmitate.

Egg Fuel — TwinLab
Each serving contains: Calories 110 • Protein 25 g. Ingredient: Pure egg white protein. Fat free, sugar free, & lactose free.

Ela-Vites L-Phenylalanine Complex — Nature's Plus
Two tablets contain: L-Phenylalanine free form amino acid 600 mg • Vitamin C with Rose Hips 400 mg • L-Tyrosine free form amino acid 200 mg • Vitamin B6 (Pyridoxine HCL) 100 mg. In a natural herbal base containing Ginseng, Gotu Kola & Fo-Ti. Contains no yeast, wheat, corn, soy, milk, salt, sugar or starch.

Elderberry — Natrol
One lozenge contains: Vitamin C (as Calcium Ascorbate) 50 mg • Zinc (as Zinc Gluconate) 7.5 mg • Echinacea angustfolia entire plant 10 mg • Bee Propolis 10 mg • Slippery Elm Bark 10 mg • Elderberry 10 mg • Bee Pollen 10 mg. Other ingredients: Hydrogenated Starch, Hydrolysate, natural Elderberry flavor, Grape skin for color.

Elderberry - Extra Strength — Jamieson
Each capsule contains: Elderberry fruit (Sambucus Nigra L. 40 mg powdered extract 1:50) 2000 mg.

Elder-Zinc Lozenges — Now
Two lozenges contain: Vitamin C (Ascorbic Acid • Sodium Ascorbate) 300 mg • Zinc (as Zinc Gluconate) 24 mg • Elderberry (Sambucus nigra) 10:1 extract 200 mg • Echinacea purpurea root 50 mg • Bee Propolis 50 mg • Slippery Elm bark (Ulmus fulva) 50 mg.

Electrolyte Balance — The Vitamin Shoppe
Two tablets provide: Potassium 99 mg • Magnesium 500 mg • Calcium 250 mg • Boron 3 mg • Vitamin D 100 IU.

Elemax — Naturodoc
Each capsule contains: L-Glycine 200 mg • L-Tyrosine 150 mg • St. John's Wort (hypericum perforatum extract, .3% Hypericin) 150 mg • Niacin (Niacinol) 100 mg • 5-HTP (5-hydroxytryptophan) 25 mg • Siberian Ginseng (eleutherococcus senticosus, 1.2% eleutherosides) 25 mg • Ginkgo Biloba Extract (24% Ginkgo Extract) 25 mg • Colecus Forskohlii Extract (5-10% Forskolin) 25 mg • Coenzyme B6 (pyridoxal-5-phosphate) 5 mg • Folic Acid 500 mcg.

Elo-Plex — Progressive Labs
Each capsule contains: Vitamin C 100 mg • Vitamin B6 10 mg • Pantothenic Acid 50 mg • Zinc (as zinc proteinate) 3.3 mg • Copper (as copper proteinate) 0.3 mg • L-Tyrosine 150 mg • DL-Phenylalanine 80 mg • Adrenal 10 mg • Hypothalamus 15 mg.

E-mergen-C — Alacer
Each packet contains: Vitamin C 1000 mg • Vitamin B1 (Thiamine HCL) 0.38 mg • Vitamin B2 (Riboflavin) 0.43 mg • Special Niacin Complexes 5 mg • Vitamin B6 (Pyridoxine HCL) 10 mg • Folic Acid 12.5 mcg • Vitamin B12 (Cyanocobalamin) 25 mcg • Pantothenic Acid 2.5 mg • Calcium 50 mg • Magnesium 20 mg • Zinc 2 mg • Sodium 60 mg • Potassium 200 mg • Manganese 1.5 mg • Chromium (Ascorbate) 10 mg. Sweetened with Fructose. All nutrients in a base of Citric, Tartaric, Aspartic, & Malic (Apple) Acids. Naturally flavored with concentrates of Lemon & Lime.

Emerita — Transitions of Health
Aloe Vera gel • Distilled Water • D-Alpha Tocopherol • Mixed Tocopherols • Cetyl Alcohol • Almond oil • Octyl Palmitate • Panthenol • Peg 8 Stearate • Glycerine • Progesterone • Polysorbate 60 • Hyaluronic Acid, Oil of Lemon, Keratin, Carbomer 940 • Grapefruit seed extract.

Emulsified A Complex — Nature's Life
Each capsule contains: Vitamin A (Fish Liver oil) 7500 IU • Beta Carotene (Vitamin A equivalent to 7500 IU) 4.5 mg.

ENADA NADH — Menuco
Each micro tab provides: NADH 5.0 mg • Baking Soda (sodium bicarbonate) 3.0 mg • Vitamin C (sodium ascorbate) 0.3 mg. Other Ingredients: D-Mannitol, Microcrystalline Cellulose, Magnesium Stearate.

Some Brand Name Natural Products - What they Contain
www.NaturalDatabase.com contains MANY more listings than appear here.

B
R
A
N
D

N
A
M
E
S

Enada NADH — The Vitamin Shoppe
Each tablet contains: Vitamin C (as sodium ascorbate) 0.3 mg • NADH (reduced B-Nicotinamide Adenine Dinucleotide) 5 mg • Baking Soda (sodium bicarbonate) 3 mg. No yeast, corn, wheat, sugar, salt, starch, soy, milk.

EnadaNADH 2.5 Mg — Natrol
One micro tab contains: NADH (reduced 5-nicotinamide adenine dinucleotide) 2.5 mg • Baking Soda (Sodium Bicarbonate) 0.3 mg • Vitamin C (Sodium Ascorbate) 0.3 mg. Other ingredients: D-Mannitol, Microcrystalline Cellulose, Magnesium Stearate.

EnadaNADH 5 Mg — Natrol
One microtab contains: NADH (reduced 5-nicotinamide adenine dinucleotide) 5 mg • Baking Soda (Sodium Bicarbonate) 0.3 mg • Vitamin C (Sodium Ascorbate) 0.3 mg. Other ingredients: D-Mannitol, Microcrystalline Cellulose, Magnesium Stearate.

Endorphin+ — PhysioLogics
Each capsule contains: DL-Phenylalanine 450 mg • White Willow bark (7.5% Salicin, 1.9 mg) 25 mg • Feverfew flower, leaf (1.2% Parthenolide, 0.3 mg) 25 mg • Ginger root (5% Gingerols, 1.25 mg) 25 mg.

Endurox — PacificHealth Laboratories
Two Caplets Contains: Ciwujia root extract 800 mg • Calcium (sulfate) 130 mg. Other Ingredients: Microcrystalline Cellulose, Stearic Acid, Hydroxypropyl Cellulose, Magnesium Stearate, Titanium Dioxide, P.E.G., Caramel Color, Beet juice powder & Annatto extract.

Endurox Excel — Pacific Health Labs
Two caplets contain: Endurox (standardized root extract of the herb ciwujia) 1200 mg • Vitamin E 60 IU.

Endurox R4 — Pacific Health Labs
Two scoops contain: Vitamin C 470 mg • Vitamin E 400 IU • Calcium 100 mg • Iron 1.8 mg • Magnesium 250 mg • Chloride 270 mg • Sodium 230 mg • Potassium 140 mg • Ciwujia (Endurox) 600 mg • L-Glutamine 420 mg • L-Arginine 1420 mg. Other Ingredients: Complex Carbohydrates, Glucose, Whey Protein concentrate, Crystalline Fructose, L-Arginine, Vitamin E Acetate, Ciwujia, Ascorbic Acid, Sodium Chloride, Citric Acid, L-Glutamine, Magnesium Oxide, Artificial Flavor, Potassium Phosphate, FD&C Red #40.

Enerblast — Nature's Plus
Each tablet contains: Potassium Glycero-Phosphate 250 mg • Pyridoxal Alpha Ketoglutarate (PAK) 50 mg • Trimethylglycine (TMG) 25 mg • Inosine (HXR-Hypoxanthine Riboside) 25 mg • Creatine Phosphate 50 mcg. Contains no yeast, wheat, corn, soy, milk, salt, sugar or starch.

Energiza — HerbaSway
Bitter Orange • Panax Ginseng • Siberian Ginseng • Schisandra • Astragalus • Ginger • Kudzu • Blackberry • Licorice • HerbaSwee (Cucurbitaceae fruit).

Energizer Formula — Nature's Way
Two capsules contain: Proprietary Formula: Bee Pollen • Cayenne pepper fruit • Coenzyme Q10 (Ubiquinone) • Magnesium Stearate • Siberian Ginseng root • Spirulina • Thiamine (Vitamin B1) • Vitamin B12 (Cyanocobalamin). Other ingredients: Gelatin, Millet.

Energy — Nutrivention
Each tablet contains: Pantothenic Acid 100 mg • Vitamin B12 300 mcg • Folic Acid 200 mcg • Aspartic Acid 100 mg • Gotu Kola 100 mg • Licorice root 100 mg • Siberian Ginseng 100 mg.

Energy — Centrum Focused Formulas
One tablet contains: Thiamin (B1) 3 mg • Riboflavin (B2) 0.85 mg • Niacin (B3) 10 mg • Vitamin B6 1 mg • Vitamin B12 3 mcg • Biotin 15 mcg • Pantothenic Acid 5 mg • Taurine 100 mg • Panax Ginseng standardized root extract 62.5 mg.

Energy — ProHerbs
One tablet contains: Thiamin HCl (B1) 25 mg • Riboflavin (B2) 25 mg • Vitamin B6 (Pyridoxine HCl) 25 mg • Vitamin B12 (Cyanocobalamin) 50 mcg • Folic Acid 400 mcg • Korean Ginseng root (Panax Ginseng standardized to 10% ginsenosides) 100 mg • Kola Nut (3:1 extract) (Cola acuminata) 500 mg • Guarana root (Paullina cupana 3:1 extract) 200 mg • Royal Jelly 50 mg. Other Ingredients: Dicalcium Phosphate, Microcrystalline Cellulose, Croscarmellose Sodium, Hydroxypropylmethylcellulose, Magnesium

Stearate, Mineral Oil, Stearic Acid, Titanium Dioxide, Triacetin, FD&C Yellow #6 Lake.

Energy Elixir — Nature's Plus
Each serving contains: Royal Jelly lyophilized 3X-4.2% 10-HDA 250 mg • Guarana seed 125 mg • Spanish Bee Pollen 125 mg • Korean Ginseng 50 mg • Siberian Ginseng 50 mg • American Ginseng 12.5 mg. In a natural base of Purified Water, Wild Clover Honey, Citric Acid & Potassium Sorbate added to maintain freshness.

Energy Reserve — Clinician's Choice
Two tablets contain: Thiamin (mononitrate) 20 mg • Riboflavin 20 mg • Vitamin B12 (cyanocobalamin) 20 mcg • Siberian Ginseng Root 400 mg • Panax Ginseng Leaves 400 mg • Brazilian Guarana Seeds 200 mg • Green Tea Leaves 200 mg • Wild American Ginseng Root 100 mg • Red Chinese Ginseng Root 100 mg • Tienchi Ginseng Root 100 mg • Cayenne Fruit 20 mg • Proprietary blend 6 mg: Bee Pollen, Citrus Bioflavonoids, Soy Isoflavones.

Energy Support — Amazon Support
Each capsule contains: Jatoba • Guarana Extract • Yerba Mate Extract • Maca • Suma.

Ener-T — Atrium
Each tablet contains: Primary Yeast 705 mg. Specially grown & formulated because of its content of an accessory factor known as Termitin, Complex-T or Vitamin T. This yeast also typically contains 50% Protein, trace amounts of many B-Complex Vitamins & Inositol as well as trace amounts of many minerals.

EnerX — Quest
Niacin • Zinc • Yohimbe • Tribulus Terrestris • Panax Ginseng • Guarana • Ashwagandha • Arginine • Damiana • Muira Puama • Potent Herbal Blend.

Enviro-Gard — Aspen Group, Inc.
Four tablets contain: Vitamin A Palmitate 8000 IU • Beta Carotene 16,000 IU • Vitamin C 800 mg • Vitamin E 320 IU • Quercetin 160 mg • Zinc (gluconate) 12 mg • Copper Gluconate 0.1 mg • Yellow Dock 364 mg • Bupleurum 192 mg • Poria Cocos 192 mg • Gentian root 192 mg • Goldenseal 192 mg • Myrrh Gum 192 mg • Echinacea extract 192 mg • Milk Thistle extract (83% silymarin) 192 mg • N-Acetyl Cysteine 160 mg • Rosemary extract 160 mg • Hawthorn Berry extract 80 mg • Wild Yam root 80 mg • Wild Yam extract 77 mg • Marshmallow root 58 mg • Magnesium Ascorbate 24 mg • Grape seed extract 20 mg • Ginkgo Biloba 4 mg • Manganese Ascorbate 4 mg • Selenomethionine 80 mcg. Contains no sugar, starch, salt, wheat, yeast, corn or soy derivatives.

ENZOGENOL — Pharmacy Express Ltd.
Each tablet contains: Enzogenol (Pinus radiata bark extract) 50 mg • Citrus Bioflavonoids 100 mg • Betacarotene (ProVitA) 5 mg • Natural Vit E (80 IU) 66.7 mg • Ester C 250 mg • Selenium (from selenomethionine) 75 ug • Zinc (from OptiZinc) 7.5 mg • Pyridoxine Hydrochloride (Vitamin B6) 25 mg • Cysteine 50 mg • Methionine 50 mg • Folic Acid 100 ug. Contains no added yeast, gluten, artificial colors or preservatives.

Enzy-Derm — Atrium
Each gram contains: Pancreatin 12 mg • Papayotin 7 mg • Bromelain 6 mg • Trypsin 4 mg • Lipase 1.5 mg • Amylase 1.5 mg • Chymotrypsin 0.15 mg. In a base containing Vitamin A & Vitamin E.

Enzyme Aid Digestive Support — Nature's Life
Each tablet contains: Pancreatin (concentrate 4X NF) containing: (Protease activity 50000 USP IU; Amylase activity 50000 USP IU, Lipase activity 4000 USP IU) 500 mg • Glutamic Acid Hydrochloride 200 mg • Ox Bile extract 200 mg • Pepsin (NF 10000X) 200 mg • Lipase (activity 425 USP IU) 50 mg • Cellulase (activity 10 CMC-ASE IU) 10 mg.

Enzymes — Nutrivention
Each capsule contains: Pancreatin 100 mg • Papain 60 mg • Anise (Pimpinella anisum) 50 mg • Fennel (Foeniculum vulgare) 50 mg • Rutin 50 mg • Bromelain (natural Pineapple Enzyme) 45 mg • Trypsin 24 mg • Amylase 10 mg • Lipase 10 mg • L-Chymotrypsin 1 mg.

EPA-1000 — PhysioLogics
Each softgel contains: Vitamin E (d-Alpha Tocopherol) 10 IU • Marine Lipid concentrate (18% EPA, 12% DHA) 1000 mg.

EPAForte — Nature's Plus
Each softgel contains: Marine Lipid concentrate 900 mg supplying: Eicosapentaenoic Acid (EPA) 162 mg, Docosahexaenoic Acid (DHA)

108 mg, total Omega-3 Fatty Acids 270 mg • Magnesium Aspartate equivalent to 60 mg of elemental Magnesium 300 mg • Vitamin E natural 50 IU • Vitamin B6 (Pyridoxine HCL) 10 mg • Garlic equivalent to 500 mg of fresh garlic 1 mg • Selenium, Biotron yeast-free amino acid complex 25 mcg. Contains no yeast, wheat, corn, soy, milk, salt, sugar or starch.

EPH-833 — AST Sports Science
Each capsule contains: standardized 8% Ephedra extract 750 mg.

Ephedra Plus — Phytopharmica
Ephedrine 12 mg from 200 mg of Ma Huang extract (Ephedra sinensis) • Ginger root extract 6.5:1 (Zingiber officinale) 65 mg • Licorice root extract (Glycyrrhiza glabra) standardized to contain 5% glycyrrhizic acid 50 mg • Marshmallow root extract 4:1 (Althaea officinalis) (Mucilage content of 30-40%) 50 mg • Sundew Herb extract 4:1 (Drosera rotundifolia) 40 mg • Euphorbia Herb extract 4:1 (Euphorbia hirta) 40 mg • Senega root extract 4:1 (Polygala senega) 40 mg • Goldenseal root extract (Hydrastis canadensis) (standardized to contain 5% total alkaloids, including berberine, hydrastine & canadine) 20 mg.

Ephedra Super Cap — D & E Pharmaceuticals
Each capsule contains: 883 mg of pure Ephedra extract.

Ephedrine Formula 100 — D & E Pharmaceuticals
Each tablet contains: Ephedrine HCL 25 mg • Guaifenesin 100 mg.

Ephedrine Formula 200 — D & E Pharmaceuticals
Each tablet contains: Ephedrine HCL 25 mg • Guaifenesin 200 mg.

Ephedrine Formula 400 — D & E Pharmaceuticals
Each tablet contains: Ephedrine HCL 25 mg • Guaifenesin 400 mg.

Ephedrine HCL 25 mg — D & E Pharmaceuticals
Each tablet contains: Ephedrine HCL 25 mg.

Ephedrine Sulphate 25 mg — D & E Pharmaceuticals
Each tablet contains: Ephedrine Sulphate 25 mg.

Epresat Multivitamin — Flora
Each tablet contains: Vitamin A • Vitamin B1 • Vitamin B2 • Vitamin B6 • Vitamin C • Vitamin D • Vitamin E • Niacinamide.

Equal Ratio CAL-MAG — Quest
Each tablet contains: Calcium (HVP Chelate) 100 mg • Magnesium (HVP Chelate) 100 mg • Vitamin D3 200 IU. Other Ingredients: Croscarmellose Sodium, Magnesium Stearate (vegetable source), Microcrystalline Cellulose, Vegetable Stearin.

Erotikava — Pacific Sensuals
Each 1 oz. serving contains: Vanuatu Kava Kava • Honey • Ginger • Lycium • Epimedium • Polygala • Liquid Amber • Saigon Cinnamon bark • Licorice • Vegetable Glycerine • Cnidium seed.

Esberitox — Enzymatic Therapy
Each tablet contains: Baptisia tinctoria root extract (Wild Indigo root) 10 mg • Echinacea purpurea & pallida 1:1 root extract (Purple Coneflower root) 7.5 mg • Thuja occidentalis leaf extract (White Cedar leaf) 2 mg. Contains no salt, yeast, wheat, gluten, corn, soy, dairy products (except lactose), coloring, flavoring, or preservatives.

Escalation — Enzymatic Therapy
Each capsule contains: Cola Nut extract (Cola nitida) (contains Caffeine 35 mg) 250 mg • Green Tea extract (Camellia sinensis) (contains Caffeine 15 mg) 250 mg • Ma Huang extract (Ephedra sinensis) (contains Ephedrine 15 mg) 250 mg. Contains no sugar, salt, yeast, wheat, corn, soy, dairy products, coloring, flavoring, or preservatives.

Escalert — Enzymatic Therapy
Two capsules contain: Cola Nut extract (Cola nitida) (Contains 35 mg of Caffeine) 250 mg • Green Tea extract (Camellia sinensis) (contains 15 mg of Caffeine) 250 mg • Oat Straw extract 10:1 (Avena sativa) 50 mg • Schisandra extract standardized to contain 9% Schizandrin 50 mg • Siberian Ginseng extract (Eleutherococcus senticosus) standardized to contain greater than 1% Eleutherosides E 50 mg • Ginger root extract 6.5:1 (Zingiber officinale) 25 mg • Korean Ginseng root extract (Panax ginseng) standardized to contain 7% Saponins calculated as Ginsenoside Rg1 10 mg • Chromium (Polynicotinate) 100 mcg. Contains no sugar, salt, yeast, wheat, corn, soy, dairy products, coloring, flavoring or preservatives.

Especially for "Women" — The Vitamin Shoppe
Three capsules contain: Vitamin A Activity 10000 IU • Vitamin E 200 IU • Vitamin D 200 IU • Vitamin C 250 mg • Selenium 50 mcg • Vitamin B1 25 mg • Vitamin B2 25 mg • Niacinamide 25 mg • Vitamin B6 25 mg • Vitamin B12 250 mcg • Pantothenic Acid 25 mg • Citrus Bioflavonoids 100 mg • Biotin 100 mcg • Folic Acid 400 mcg • Choline Bitarate 25 mg • Inositol 25 mg • PABA 25 mg • Calcium 200 mg • Magnesium 100 mg • Potassium 25 mg • Phosphorus 50 mg • Manganese 15 mg • Zinc 15 mg • Iron 18 mg • Chromium 50 mcg • Iodine 225 mcg • Boron 3 mg • Silica 5 mg • Black Currant 100 mg • Dong Quai 50 mg • Royal Jelly 100 mg.

Especially for MEN — The Vitamin Shoppe
Two capsules contain: Vitamin A 5000 IU • Vitamin C 30 mg • Vitamin D 200 IU • Vitamin E 100 IU • Vitamin K 75 mcg • Niacin 30 mg • Vitamin B1 30 mg • Vitamin B2 30 mg • Vitamin B6 30 mg • Folic Acid 400 mcg • Vitamin B12 30 mcg • Biotin 250 mcg • Pantothenic Acid 30 mg • Calcium 200 mg • Iodine 150 mcg • Magnesium 100 mg • Zinc 25 mg • Selenium 100 mcg • Copper 2 mg • Manganese 5 mg • Chromium 50 mcg • Chloride 28 mg • Beta-carotene 3 mg • Potassium 30 mg • Silica 10 mcg • Choline 10 mg • Inositol 10 mg • PABA 10 mg • Citrus Bioflavonoids 25 mg • Korean Ginseng 70 mg • Damiana leaf 70 mg • Oat Straw 50 mg • Garlic 50 mg • Oyster extract 50 mg • Prostate Glandular 50 mg • Saw Palmetto 50 mg • L-Cysteine 50 mg • Nettles leaf 30 mg • Pumpkin seed 30 mg • L-Methionine 10 mg • Alpha Lipoic Acid 5 mg • Lycopene 1 mg.

Essential E — PhysioLogics
Each softgel contains: Vitamin E (d-Alpha Tocopheryl Acetate) 400 IU.

Essential Enzymes — Source Naturals
Each capsule contains: Vegetal analog of Pancreatin with acid-stable Protease (28652 FCC) 298 mg • Lipase (375 FCC) 125 mg • Alpha Amylase (630 FCC) 52 mg • Amyloglucosidase (2 FCC) 12.5 mg • Cellulase (100 FCC) 5 mg • Hemicellulase (650 FCC) 3 mg • Lactase (40 FCC) 5 mg.

Essential Fatty Acids — Nutri-Quest
Each capsule contains: Cod Liver 500 mg • Flaxseed oil 135 mg • Extra Virgin Olive oil 135 mg • Vitamin A 1190 IU • Vitamin D 124 IU. Also contains: Oleic, Linoleic, Palmitic, Arachidic & Linolenic, Eicosapentaenoic, & Docosahexaenoic.

Essential Meal — Gary Null
Fortified with branched chain amino acids.

Essential Minerals — Futurebiotics
Four tablets provide: Calcium: (carbonate, aspartate, citrate) 1000 mg • Magnesium: (oxide, aspartate, citrate) 800 mg • Vitamin D 200 IU • Boron (citrate) 3 mg • Iron (gluconate) 9 mg • Manganese (amino acid chelate) 5 mg • Copper (gluconate) 1.5 mg • Zinc (gluconate) 15 mg • Betaine HCl 250 mg • Potassium (chloride, proteinate) 75 mg.

Essential Nutrients — Progressive Labs
Six capsules contain: Vitamin A (retinyl palmitate) 10,000 IU • Vitamin A (beta carotene) 15,000 IU • Vitamin C (ascorbic acid) 1000 mg • Vitamin D (cholecalciferol) 80 IU • Vitamin E (d-alpha tocopheryl succinate) 400 IU • Thiamin (Vitamin B1) 50 mg • Riboflavin-5-Phosphate (Vitamin B2) 20 mg • Niacin 25 mg • Niacinamide 125 mg • Vitamin B6 (pyridoxine HCl with pyridoxal-5'-phosphate) 20 mg • Folate (folic acid) 800 mcg • Vitamin B12 (cyanocobalamin with adenosylocobalamin) 500 mcg • Biotin 800 mcg • Pantothenic Acid (d-calcium pantothenate) 500 mg • Calcium (aspartate & carbonate) 500 mg • Iodine (potassium iodide) 225 mcg • Magnesium (aspartate and oxide) 500 mg • Zinc (picolinate) 25 mg • Selenium (selenomethionine) 200 mcg • Copper (glycinate & oxide) 2 mg • Manganese (aspartate & sulfate) 20 mg • Chromium (as chromium picolinate) 200 mcg • Molybdenum (sodium molybdate) 100 mcg • Potassium (aspartate and chloride) 99 mg • Boron (chelate) 3 mg • Vanadium (vanadyl sulfate) 100 mcg • Choline Citrate 250 mg.

Essiac — Dial Herbs
Burdock • Sheep Sorrel • Rhubarb • Slippery Elm.

Essiac — Essiac Products Inc.
(Canadian) Turkish Rhubarb (Rheum palmatum) or Indian Rhubarb (Rheum officinale) • Sheep Sorrel (Rumex acetosella) • Slippery Elm bark (Ulmus fulva) • Burdock root (Arctium lappa).

Ester C — Derma E
Each tablet contains: Vitamin C • Vitamin E • Antioxidants and Skin Rejuvenators.

Ester C 1000 mg — The Vitamin Shoppe
Each tablet contains: Vitamin C (Calcium Ascorbate) 1000 mg •

BRAND NAMES

© Copyright 2000, Natural Medicines Comprehensive Database (209) 472-2244. For updated data, go to www.NaturalDatabase.com.

B R A N D   N A M E S

Calcium (as Ascorbate, Threonate) 125 mg. No yeast, corn, wheat, sugar, salt, starch, soy, citrus, milk, eggs, fish or animal derivatives, preservatives, artificial colors or flavors added.

Ester C 1000 mg with Bioflavonoids — The Vitamin Shoppe
Each tablet contains: Vitamin C (Calcium Ascorbate) (from 1250 mg Ester C) 1000 mg, plus Bioflavonoids Complex. No yeast, corn, wheat, sugar, salt, starch, soy, gluten, dairy, milk, eggs, fish or animal derivatives, preservatives, artificial colors or flavors added.

Ester C 500 mg — The Vitamin Shoppe
Each tablet contains: Vitamin C (Calcium Ascorbate) 500 mg • Calcium (as Ascorbate, Threonate) 60 mg. No yeast, corn, wheat, sugar, salt, starch, soy, citrus, milk, eggs, fish or animal derivatives, preservatives, artificial colors or flavors added.

Ester C 500 mg with Bioflavonoids — The Vitamin Shoppe
Each tablet contains: Vitamin C (Calcium Ascorbate) (from 625 mg Ester C) 500 mg, plus Bioflavonoids Complex. No yeast, corn, wheat, sugar, salt, starch, soy, gluten, dairy, milk, eggs, fish or animal derivatives, preservatives, artificial colors or flavors added.

Ester C Caps — Progressive Labs
Each capsule contains: Vitamin C (as calcium polyascorbate) 500 mg • Calcium (as calcium polyascorbate) 50 mg.

Ester C Plus Bioflavonoids and Pycnogenol 500 mg — The Vitamin Shoppe
Each capsule contains: Vitamin C (Calcium Ascorbate) (from 625 mg Ester C) 500 mg • Calcium (Calcium Ascorbate) 60 mg • Quercetin 25 mg • Pycnogenol 2.5 mg • Citrus Bioflavonoid Complex with Hesperidin and Rutin 200 mg. No yeast, corn, wheat, sugar, salt, starch, soy, dairy, preservatives, artificial colors or flavors added.

Ester C Powder 2000 mg with Bioflavonoids — The Vitamin Shoppe
Each teaspoon contains: Vitamin C (Calcium Ascorbate) 2000 mg, plus Bioflavonoids Complex. No yeast, corn, wheat, sugar, salt, starch, soy, gluten, dairy, milk, eggs, fish or animal derivatives, preservatives, artificial colors or flavors added.

Ester-C 1000 — Now
Each tablet contains: Vitamin C 1000 mg • Citrus Bioflavonoids (40%) 200 mg • Acerola powder 25 mg • Rose Hips powder 25 mg • Rutin 20 mg • Calcium 125 mg.

Ester-C 1000 Mg with Bioflavonoids — Natrol
Each tablet contains: Vitamin C (as calcium ascorbate) 1000 mg • Calcium (as calcium ascorbate) 100 mg • Lemon Bioflavonoid Complex consisting of extracts from lemon 200 mg. Other ingredients: Mono & Di-Glycerides, Stearic Acid, Croscarmellose Sodium, Silicon Dioxide, Magnesium Stearate.

Ester-C 250 Mg — Natrol
Each tablet contains: Vitamin C (as calcium ascorbate) 250 mg • Calcium (as calcium ascorbate) 25 mg. Other ingredients: Microcrystalline Cellulose, Stearic Acid, Mono & Di-Glycerides, Croscarmellose Sodium, Magnesium Stearate.

Ester-C 250 Mg Chewable — Natrol
Each wafer contains: Vitamin C (as calcium ascorbate) 250 mg • Calcium (as calcium ascorbate) 25 mg. Other ingredients: Fructose, Glycine, Mono & Di-Glycerides, Stearic Acid, natural Orange flavor, Citric Acid, Silicon Dioxide, Microcrystalline Cellulose, Gum Acacia, Magnesium Stearate.

Ester-C 250 Mg with Bioflavonoids — Natrol
Each tablet contains: Vitamin C (as calcium ascorbate) 250 mg • Calcium (as calcium ascorbate) 25 mg • Lemon Bioflavonoid Complex consisting of extracts from lemon 100 mg. Other ingredients: Microcrystalline Cellulose, Stearic Acid, Croscarmellose Sodium, Silicon Dioxide, Magnesium Stearate.

Ester-C 500 Mg capsule — Natrol
Each capsule contains: Vitamin C (as calcium ascorbate) 500 mg • Calcium (as calcium ascorbate) 50 mg. Other ingredients: Magnesium Stearate, Microcrystalline Cellulose, Gelatin.

Ester-C 500 Mg tablets — Natrol
Each tablet contains: Vitamin C (as calcium ascorbate) 500 mg • Calcium (as calcium ascorbate) 50 mg. Other ingredients: Microcrystalline Cellulose, Stearic Acid, Croscarmellose Sodium, Magnesium Stearate, Silicon Dioxide.

Ester-C 500 Mg with Bioflavonoids — Natrol
Each tablet contains: Vitamin C (as calcium ascorbate) 500 mg • Calcium (as calcium ascorbate) 50 mg • Lemon Bioflavonoid Complex consisting of extracts from lemon 200 mg. Other ingredients: Mono & Di-Glycerides, Stearic Acid, Croscarmellose Sodium, Silicon Dioxide, Magnesium Stearate.

Ester-C 500 Mg with Bioflavonoids Vegetarian capsules — Natrol
Each capsule contains: Vitamin C (as calcium ascorbate) 500 mg • Calcium (as calcium ascorbate) 50 mg • Citrus Bioflavonoid Complex consisting of extracts from: lemon, orange, grapefruit, lime, & tangerine 200 mg. Other ingredients: Magnesium Stearate, Silicon Dioxide, Vegetable Carbohydrate Gum, Glycerine.

Ester-C 500 Mg with Echinacea — Natrol
Each tablet contains: Vitamin C (as calcium ascorbate) 500 mg • Calcium (as calcium ascorbate) 50 mg • Echinacea extract (Phenolic compounds 4%) 50 mg • Echinacea (angustifolia) leaf powder 80 mg • Echinacea (Purpurea) leaf powder 80 mg • Echinacea (angustifolia) root powder 20 mg • Echinacea (Purpurea) root powder 20 mg. Other ingredients: Calcium Carbonate, Mono & Di-Glycerides, Croscarmellose Sodium, Stearic Acid, Silicon Dioxide, Magnesium Stearate.

Ester-C 500 Mg with Pycnogenol & Proanthocyanidis capsules — Natrol
Each capsule contains: Vitamin C (as calcium ascorbate) 500 mg • Calcium (as calcium ascorbate) 50 mg • Grape skin powder 50 mg • Rutin 50 mg • Hesperidin Complex 50 mg • Quercetin 25 mg • Pycnogenol (pine bark extract) 5 mg. Other ingredients: Silicon Dioxide, Magnesium Stearate, Gelatin.

Ester-C 500 Mg with Pycnogenol & Proanthocyanidis tablets — Natrol
Each tablet contains: Vitamin C (as calcium ascorbate) 500 mg • Calcium (as calcium ascorbate-carbonate) 70 mg • Grapeskin powder 50 mg • Rutin 50 mg • Hesperidin 50 mg • Quercitin 25 mg • Pycnogenol (pine bark extract) 5 mg. Other ingredients: Mono & Di-Glycerides, Calcium Carbonate, Croscarmellose Sodium, Silicon Dioxide, Stearic Acid & Magnesium Stearate.

Ester-C Antioxidant — Natrol
Two tablets contain: Vitamin A (as d-Salina beta carotene) 5000 IU • Vitamin C (as calcium ascorbate) 500 mg • Vitamin E (as d-alpha tocopheryl succinate with mixed tocopherols) 200 IU • Calcium (as ascorbate) 50 mg • Lemon Bioflavonoid Complex consisting of extracts from lemon 25 mg • a-Lipoic Acid 25 mg. Other ingredients: TriCalcium Phosphate, Microcrystalline Cellulose, Stearic Acid, Silicon Dioxide, Croscarmellose Sodium, Magnesium Stearate.

Ester-C Cold Season — Natrol
Two capsules contain: Vitamin C (as calcium ascorbate) 500 mg • Calcium (as calcium ascorbate) 50 mg • Zinc (chelate) 10 mg • Reishi/ Shiitake/ Maitake Blend, powdered extract (mushrooms) 150 mg • Echinacea 50:50 (purpurea & angustifolia), powdered extract supplying Phenolic compounds (4%) 75 mg • Citrus Bioflavonoid Complex extracts of: lemon, orange, grapefruit, lime & tangerine 50 mg • Black Elderberry extract, powdered 30 mg • Garlic, powdered extract bulb 30 mg • Licorice root extract supplying 25 % Glycerenic Acid 25 mg • Astragalus 25 mg • Cayenne supplying 40000 SCU 10 mg • Beta Glucans, oats 5 mg. Other ingredients: Silica, Magnesium Stearate, Rice powder, Gelatin.

Ester-C For Kids — Natrol
Each wafer contains: Vitamin C (as calcium ascrobate) 100 mg • Calcium (as calcium ascorbate) 10 mg • Citrus Bioflavonoids consisting of extracts from lemon 25 mg. Other ingredients: Fructose, Mono & Di-Glycerides, Glycine, Cellulose, natural Tropical fruit flavor, Stearic Acid, Silica, Magnesium Stearate, Guar Gum, Citric Acid.

Ester-C Nightime Formula — Natrol
Each tablet contains: Vitamin C (as calcium ascrobate) 500 mg • Calcium (as calcium ascorbate) 50 mg • Kava Kava root supplying 30% Kavalactones 100 mg • Valerian root supplying 0.8% Valerenic Acid 100 mg • Melatonin 1 mg. Other ingredients: TriCalcium Phosphate, Cellulose, Stearic Acid, Silica, Magnesium Stearate.

Ester-C Powder — Natrol
Each teaspoon contains: Vitamin C (as calcium ascorbate) 3200 mg • Calcium (as calcium ascorbate) 320 mg.

Some Brand Name Natural Products - What they Contain

www.NaturalDatabase.com contains MANY more listings than appear here.

Ester-C Powder with Bioflavonoids — Natrol
Each teaspoon contains: Vitamin C (as calcium ascorbate) 3000 mg • Calcium (as calcium ascorbate) 300 mg • Citrus Bioflavonoid Complex consisting of extracts from: lemon, orange, grapefruit, lime, & tangerine 300 mg.

Ester-C with Bioflavonoids — Natrol
Each capsule contains: Vitamin C (as calcium ascorbate) 500 mg • Calcium (as calcium ascorbate) 50 mg • Citrus Bioflavonoid Complex consisting of extracts from: lemon, orange, grapefruit, lime & tangerine 200 mg. Other ingredients: Magnesium Stearate, Gelatin.

Ester-C with Echinacea — Natrol
One capsule contains: Vitamin C (as calcium ascorbate) 500 mg • Calcium (as calcium ascorbate) 50 mg Echinacea extract (Phenolic compounds 4%) 50 mg • Echinacea (angustifolia) leaf powder 80 mg • Echinacea (Purpurea) leaf powder 80 mg • Echinacea (angustifolia) root powder 20 mg • Echinacea (Purpurea) root powder 20 mg. Other ingredients: Silicon Dioxide, Magnesium Stearate, Gelatin.

Ester-C Zinc Lozenges — Natrol
Each lozenge contains: Vitamin C (as calcium ascorbate) 150 mg • Calcium (as calcium ascorbate) 15 mg • Citrus Bioflavonoids consisting of extracts from lemon 25 mg • Zinc (Gluconate) 4.5 mg. Other ingredients: Fructose, Mono & Di-Glycerides, Glycine, Cellulose, natural fruit flavors, Stearic Acid, Silica, Magnesium Stearate, Guar Gum, Citric Acid.

EstroGentle — Pinnacle
Contains Black Cohosh • Soy germ • Red Clover leaf extract • Licorice root • Wild Yam • Chaste Tree Berry • Other botanicals.

Estroven — Amerifit
Each caplet contains: Vitamin E (as natural d-alpha tocopherol succinate) 30 IU • Thiamin (as thiamin mononitrate) 2 mg • Riboflavin 2 mg • Niacin (niacinamide) 20 mg • Vitamin B6 (as pyridoxine HCl) 10 mg • Vitamin B12 (as cyanocobalamin) 6 mcg • Folate (as folic acid) 400 mcg • Calcium (from calcium carbonate) 150 mg • Selenium (from l-selenomethionine) 70 mcg • Boron (chelate) 1.5 mg • Purified Isoflavones (from soybean & pueraria root) 50 mg • Kava Kava root standardized extract (30% kavalactones) 100 mg • Black Cohosh root 40 mg. Other Ingredients: Cellulose • Cellulose Gum • Fractionated Vegetable oil • Silica • Titanium Dioxide (natural mineral source) & Caramel Color.

Estroven Memory — Amerifit
Each tablet contains: Zinc 7.5 mg • Ginkgo Biloba leaf standardized extract 60 mg • Panax Ginseng root standardized extract 125 mg • Green Tea leaf standardized extract 250 mg • Isoflavones 10 mg • Grape skin standardized extract 75 mg.

E-TOCO 400 — Progressive Labs
Each softgel contains: Vitamin E (mixed tocopherols) 400 IU • Sesame seed oil 200 mg • Nutriene 100 mg • Mixed Tocotrienols from Nutriene 15 mg. Two softgels will supply 800 IU of Mixed Tocopherols and 30 mg of Tocotrienols.

Eucalyptus Salve — Dial Herbs
Eucalyptus • Camphor • Mint. In a base of Bees Wax , Glycerine & Cold Pressed Olive oil.

European Grape Seed Extract 50 mg — Jamieson
Each caplet contains: Calcium 30 mg • Grape Seed 60:1 Extract (Vitis vinifera)(Standardized to 95% Oligomeric Procyanidins) 50 mg.

Evening Primrose Deluxe — Health From The Sun
Each capsule contains: Gamma-Linolenic Acid (GLA) (Omega-6) 130 mg • Linoleic Acid (Omega-6) 950 mg • Oleic Acid (Omega-9) 80 mg. Ingredients: Evening Primrose seed oil, Gelatin, Glycerine, Water.

Evening Primrose Oil — Health From The Sun
Two capsules contains: Gamma-Linolenic Acid (GLA) (Omega-6) 100 mg • Linoleic Acid (Omega-6) 730 mg • Oleic Acid (Omega-9) 60 mg. Ingredients: Evening Primrose seed oil, Gelatin, Glycerine, Water.

Evening Primrose Oil — Jamieson
Each capsule contains: Vitamin E (as D-Alpha Tocopheryl Acetate) 13.6 IU • Gamma Linolenic Acid (GLA) 50 mg.

EverCLR — Herpes Relief, Ltd.
Each capsule contains: Burdock root • Ashwanganda root • Echinacea Angustifolia root • Echinacea Purpurea root • Hydrangea root.

Everyday Detox — Traditional Medicinals
Contains: Sweet Tea Vine herb (Gynostemma pentaphyllum) • Schisandra fruit dried aqueous extract • Licorice root • Ginger rhizome • Star Anise fruit • Lycium fruit dried aqueous extract • Schisandra fruit • Kukicha twig (Camellia sinensis).

Exandra Lean — The Kutting Edge
Two capsules contains: Citrus Aurantium 125 mg • Nor-Ephedrine 23 mg • L-Phenylalanin 300 mg • Citri Max 500 mg • Acetyl L-Carnitine 100 mg • L-Tyrosine 80 mg • Ginger Root 50 mg • Vitamin B5 40 mg.

Exec-U-Stress — Nature's Plus
Three tablets contain: Vitamin C with Rose Hips 600 mg • Niacinamide (Vitamin B3) 300 mg • Pantothenic Acid (Vitamin B5) 300 mg • L-Cysteine free form amino acid 200 mg • L-Glycine free form amino acid 200 mg • Vitamin B1 (Thiamine) 200 mg • Vitamin E natural 200 IU • Vitamin B6 (Pyridoxine HCL) 100 mg • Inositol 100 mg • PABA (Para-aminobenzoic acid) 75 mg • Zinc amino acid chelate/complex 50 mg • Vitamin B2 (Riboflavin) 50 mg • Choline (Bitartrate) 32 mg • Beta Carotene supplying 15000 IU Vitamin A activity 9 mg • Folic Acid 400 mcg • Vitamin B12 from Cobalamin 200 mcg • Selenium amino acid complex 100 mcg • Biotin 100 mcg. B-Complex vitamins in a fortified rice bran base. In a special base which provides for the gradual release of ingredients over a prolonged period of time for 40% better absorption & utilization. Sugar & starch free.

Expectorant — Dial Herbs
Garlic • Bayberry • Mullein • Blood root • Cayenne • Lobelia.

Ex-Stress Formula — Nature's Way
Two capsules contain: Proprietary Formula: Black Cohosh root • Cayenne pepper fruit • Hops flower • Scullcap herb • Valerian root • Wood Betony stem, leaf, flower. Other ingredients: Gelatin.

Ex-Tox — Progressive Labs
Three capsules contain: Vitamin C 600 mg • Bentonite 300 mg • L-Lysine 60 mg • DL-Methionine 600 mg • Sodium Alginate 450 mg • Chlorophyll 60 mg • Fruit pectin 150 mg • Garlic powder 30 mg.

Extreme Cordyceps —
Natural Sport Supplements - Nutraceutical
One capsule contains: Cordyceps CS-4 mycelial biomass (Cordyceps sinensis) (Minimum 36 mg Cordycepic acid) 525 mg • Cordyceps mycelial biomass (Cordyceps sinensis) (Minimum 10 mg Cordydepic acid, Minimum 1 mg Cordycepin) • Reishi mushroom (Ganoderma lucidum) 75 mg • Maitake mushroom (Grifola fondosa) 75 mg. Other ingredients: Gelatin, Magnesium Stearate, Silica, Brown Rice.

Extreme Power Plus — Dutch International Products
Green Tea • Kola Nut • 72 Trace Mineral Complex • Siberian Ginseng • Royal Jelly • White Willow bark • Ginger • Fo-Ti • Hawthorn berries • Saw Palmetto • Beet root powder • Chromium Picolinate • Guarana • Ma Huang • Zi Chi • Kelp • Citrimax • Calcium Carbonate • Magnesium Carbonate • Korean Ginseng • American Ginseng • Yerba Mate • Vitamin B12 • Bee Pollen.

Eye Beaute Pads — Pharmagel
Chamomile • Cucumber • Cornflower • Rosemary • Yarrow • Birch leaf • Sage • Nettle • Clover blossom.

Eye Contour Cream Plus — Cellex-C
Ascorbic Acid • Tyrosine • Zinc • Bioflavonoids • Vitamin E • Sodium Hyaluronate • Evening Primrose Oil • Glycine • Tomato oil • Aloe barbadensis gel • Chamomile extract • Allantoin.

Eye Contour Gel — Cellex-C
Ascorbic Acid • Tyrosine • Zinc • Bioflavonoids • Sodium Hyaluronate.

Eye Firming Gel — Pharmagel
Ginseng and plant extracts.

Eye Formula — Pharmanex
Each capsule contains: Beta-Carotene (Dunaliella Salina) 2500 IU • Vitamin C (Calcium Ascorbate, Ascorbic Acid) 150 mg • Vitamin E (d-Alpha Tocopheryl Succinate, Beta, Delta, Gamma Tocopherols) 75 IU • Zinc (Zinc Propionate) 2.5 mg • Selenium (L-Selenomethionine) 35 mcg • N-Acetyl-L-Cysteine 100 mg • Taurine 100 mg • Tumeric Extract (Min. 95% Curcumin) 50 mg • Ginkgo Biloba Extract (Min. 95% Flavonglycosides, Min. 6% Terpene Lactones) 30 mg • Alpha-Lipoic Acid 10 mg • Lutein (from Marigold flower exctract) 2.5 mg. Other Ingredients: Calcium Carbonate, Sodium Carboxymethylcellulose, Magnesium Stearate, Talc.

B R A N D   N A M E S

© Copyright 2000, Natural Medicines Comprehensive Database (209) 472-2244. For updated data, go to www.NaturalDatabase.com.

B R A N D   N A M E S

Eye Guard Plus — Nutrition Warehouse
Four capsules contain: Beta Carotene (pro-vitamin A) 40,000 IU • Natural Vitamin E (succinate) 400 IU • Vitamin C 1500 mg • Citrus Bioflavonoid Complex 250 mg • Quercetin (bioflavonoid) 100 mg • Bilberry extract (standardized 25%) 10 mg • Rutin 100 mg • Zinc (picolinate) 25 mg • Selenium (selenomethionine) 100 mcg • Taurine 200 mg • N-Acetyl Cysteine 200 mg • L-Glutathione 10 mg • Vitamin B2 (riboflavin) 50 mg • Chromium (GTF) 200 mcg • Lutein 20 mg.

Eye Support — Now
Three capsules contain: Vitamin A (natural Beta Carotene • D. salina) 15 mg/25 000 IU • Vitamin C (as Ascorbic Acid) 300 mg • Vitamin E (as d-Alpha-Tocopheryl Succinate) 200 IU • Riboflavin (Vitamin B2) 20 mg • Zinc (as L-OptiZinc) 25 mg • Selenium 100 mcg • Bilberry standardized extract (Vaccinum myrtillus) (25% Anthocyanidins) 100 mg • Lutein 10 mg • Green Tea extract (Camellia sinensis) (40% Catechins) 150 mg • N-Acetyl-Cysteine (NAC) 100 mg • Rutin 100 mg.

Eye Support — Olympia Nutrition
Bilberry • Lutein • Green Tea • Carotene • N-Acetyl Cysteine • Rutin.

Eye Treatment — Jason
Complete Vitamin C Complex • Vitamin E • Aloe Vera gel • Rose Hips.

Eyebright Formula — Nature's Way
Two capsules contain: Proprietary Formula: Bayberry bark • Cayenne pepper fruit • Eyebright stem, leaf, flower • Goldenseal root • Red Raspberry leaves. Other ingredients: Gelatin.

E-Z Vite Multiple — Nature's Life
Two tablets contain: Vitamin A (Fish Liver oil) 10000 IU • Vitamin D3 (Cholecalciferol) 400 IU • Vitamin B1 (Thiamine HCl) 10 mg • Vitamin B2 (Riboflavin) 10 mg • Vitamin B6 Pyridoxine HCl) 10 mg • Vitamin B12 (Cobalamin) 100 mcg • Niacin 30 mg • Pantothenic Acid (d-Calcium Pantothenate) 20 mg • Folic Acid 400 mcg • PABA (Para Aminobenzoic Acid) 30 mg • Biotin (d-Biotin) 3.5 mcg • Choline (Choline Bitartrate) 3 mg • Inositol 50 mg • Vitamin E (d-Alpha tocopherol, with Beta, Gamma & Delta Tocopherols) 10 IU • Vitamin C 100 mg • Lemon Bioflavonoids (TESTLAB) 30 mg • Rutin (Saphora japonica) 20 mg • Hesperidin Complex 5 mg • Calcium (Bone Meal) 40 mg • Copper (Gluconate) 100 mcg • Phosphorus (Bone Meal) 25 mg • Iodine (Icelandic Kelp) 100 mcg • Iron (Ferrous Fumarate) 10 mg • Magnesium (Oxide) 10 mg • Zinc (Gluconate) 2 mg • Potassium (Chloride) 10 mg • Manganese (Gluconate) 2 mg • Betaine HCl 25 mg • Liver (Defatted & Desiccated) 100 mg • RNA powder (Torula Yeast) 25 mg • Pancreatin (4 X N.F.) 25 mg. In a natural base of Raw Pancreas, Sodium Alginate, Torula B Yeast, Rose Hips & Acerola berries.

Fade Away Gel For Sun And Age Spots — Cellex-C
Glucosamine • Ascorbic Acid • Tyrosine • Zinc • Green Tea extract • Sodium Hyaluronate • Cucumber extract • Thyme extract.

Fade-Out Creme — Pharmagel
Vitamin C • Licorice Extract • PABA-free sunblock.

False Unicorn-Squaw Vine Virtue — Blessed Herbs
False Unicorn root • Squaw vine • Black Haw bark • Grain alcohol & Distilled Water.

Fat Binding Diet System 6 — Applied Nutrition
Two capsules contain: Vitamin C (ascorbic acid) 14 mg • Vitamin E (dl-alpha tocopheryl acetate) 4 IU • Riboflavin 0.5 mg • Niacin (niacinamide) 5 mg • Vitamin B6 (pyridoxine hydrochloride) 0.54 mg • Folic Acid 107 mcg • Vitamin B12 (cyanocobalamin) 2 mcg • Iodine (potassium iodide) 40 mcg • Selenium (sodium selenite) 14 mcg • Chromium (picolinate & 50% as polynicotinate) ChromeMate 80 mcg • Potassium (chloride) 6 mg • Garcinia Cambogia fruit (Super CitriMax, 60% Hydroxycitric acid extract) 460 mg • Chitosan (82% Deacetylated) 190 mg • Kola nut seed kernel extract (10% caffeine) 146 mg • Guarana seed extract (15% guaranine) 26 mg • Choline (bitartrate) 26 mg • Inositol 26 mg • Carnitine (L-Carnitine fumarate) 20 mg • Betaine (hydrochloride) 7 mg • Proprietary blend: (Ginger root, 72 Trace Minerals, Bioperine fruit (Piper nigrum extract, 95% Piperine) 60 mg. Other Ingredients: Gelatin, montnirollinite, silica & magnesium stearate.

Fat Burners — Amerifit
Two caplets contain: Vitamin B6 (as pyridoxine HCl) 10 mg • Iron (as ferrous fumarate) 4 mg • Chromium (chromium picolinate) 50 mcg • Choline complex: (Choline Citrate, Buchu leaves, Uva Ursi root &

fiber) 1000 mg • Inositol 250 mg • L-Carnitine (as carnitine tartrate, carnitine HCl) 50 mg • L-Lysine 100 mg • Methionine 200 mg • Lecithin (from glycine max) 100 mg • Betaine HCl 200 mg • Essential Fatty Acids: (Linoleic, Oleic) 100 mg. Other Ingredients: Dicalcium Phosphate, Microcrystalline Cellulose, Magnesium Stearate, Croscarmellose Sodium• Stearic Acid & Vegetable glaze.

Fat Busters — Nature's Plus
Two softgels contain: Plant Phytosterols 500 mg, supplying: Beta Sitosterol 200 mg • Campesterol 86 mg • Stigmasterol 80 mg • Safflower oil supplying 190 mg of free unsaturated fatty acids 240 mg • Lemon Grass oil 100 mg • Brindall berry extract 60 mg with naturally occuring [-] hydroxycitrate. Yeast free, sugar & starch free, no preservatives.

Fat Free Gainers Fuel 1000 — TwinLab
Each serving contains: Chromium (from Chromic Fuel Chromium Picolinate) 400 mcg. Other Ingredients: Branched Chain Amino Acids (L-Leucine, L-Isoleucine, L-Valine), Milk & Egg White Proteins, L-Carnitine & Kreb's Cycle Mineral Complexes (including Citrates, Aspartates, Succinates & Alpha-Ketoglutarates). Fat free with no added sugar.

Fat Free Gainers Fuel 2500 — TwinLab
Chromium (from patented Chromic Fuel Chromium Picolinate) 400 mcg • Kreb's Cycle Mineral Complexes (including Citrates, Aspartates, Succinates & Alpha-Ketoglutarates) • Milk & Egg White Proteins • Branched Chain Amino Acids (L-Leucine, L-Isoleucine & L-Valine), L-Carnitine. Fat free with no added sugar. Each serving supplies 2500 calories.

Fat Metabolizer 2000 — Youngevity
Cat's Claw • Siberian Ginseng • Bee Pollen • Kelp • Ephedra Sinica herb • White Willow bark • Licorice root • Hops flowers • Valerian root • Pantothenic Acid • Chromium Chelavite • Manganese Chelazome • Vilcabamba Mineral Essence: Potassium, Calcium, Magnesium, Zinc, Chromium, Selenium, Iron, Copper, Molybdenum, Vanadium, Iodine, Cobalt, Manganese.

Fat Metabolizer 2001+ — Youngevity
Cat's Claw • Ephedra Sinica herb • White Willow bark • Caffeine • Kelp • Pantothenic Acid • Chromium Chelavite • Manganese Chelazome • Vilcabamba Mineral Essence: Potassium, Calcium, Magnesium, Zinc, Chromium, Selenium, Iron, Copper, Molybdenum, Vanadium, Iodine, Cobalt, Manganese.

Fat Predator — Fat Predator Weight Loss Company, Inc.
Each capsule contains: Ephedra extract • Cola Nut extract • White Willow bark.

Fat Snatcher — Youngevity
Chitosan • Aloe Vera leaf • Citric Acid • Iso-Absorbic Acid (Vitamin C).

FATmelt - with Gymnema Sylvestre — Slimming and Nutrition Consultancy
Each capsule contains: L-Carnitine • Gymnema Sylvestre • Chromium Picolinate • Forskolii (4:1 extract) • Bioperine. In a Maltodextrin and Magnesium stearate base.

Fem Balance — The Vitamin Shoppe
Each capsule contains: Black Cohosh 20 mg.

FemActin — Nature's Plus
Three capsules contain: Dong Quai [(Angelica sinensis root) standardized 0.9% Ligustilide] 100 mg • Evening Primrose [(Oenothera biennis seed) standardized 4% Gamma-Linolenic Acid] 100 mg • Uva Ursi [(Arctostaphylos uva-ursi leaf) standardized 20-25% Arbutin] 75 mg • Suma [(Pfaffia paniculata root) standardized 5% Beta-Ecdysterone] 50 mg • Butcher's Broom [(Ruscus aculeatus L. rhizome) standardized 10% Saponin Glycosides] 50 mg • Nettle [(Urtica dioica leaf) standardized 1-2% Plant Silica] 50 mg • Goldenseal [(Hydrastis canadensis root & rhizome) standardized 10% Alkaloids, 5% Hydrastine]50 mg • Chasteberry [(Vitex agnus-castus fruit) standardized 0.5% Agnuside, 0.6% Aucubin] 50 mg • Vitamin B6 (Pyridoxine HCl) 25 mg • Iron (Amino Acid Chelate) 12 mg.

Female Advantage — Body Wise International, Inc.
Three capsules contain: Genestein (Soy Protein) 150 mg • Daidzein (Soy Protein) 80 mg • Black Cohosh root 50 mg • Bromelain substance 50 mg • Dong Quai 200 mg • Echinacea Purpurea root 20 mg • Oil of Evening Primrose 50 mg • Korean Ginseng 75 mg • Siberian Ginseng 75 mg • Goldenseal root 50 mg • Gotu Kola 50 mg •

Alpha-Ketoglutaric Acid 200 mg • Lady Slipper 25 mg • Licorice root 10 mg • Magnesium (Krebs Cycle Chelate) 15 mg • Passion Flower 50 mg • Suma root 50 mg • Valerian root 400 mg • Mexican Yam 100 mg • Zinc (Krebs Cycle Chelate) 10 mg • Flax Seed 100 mg • Kava Kava 250 mg.

Female Balance — Enzymatic Therapy
Three capsules contain: Vitamin A (Beta Carotene) (Non-toxic form of Vitamin A) 16665 IU • Vitamin E (D-Alpha Tocopherol Succinate) 200 IU • Vitamin C (Ascorbic Acid) 200 mg • Magnesium L-Aspartate 150 mg • Pantothenic Acid (D-Calcium Pantothenate) 100 mg • Thiamine HCL (Vitamin B1) 50 mg • Riboflavin (Vitamin B2) 50 mg • Calcium Citrate 50 mg • Iron (Ferrous Succinate) 18 mg • Zinc (Gluconate) 15 mg • Chromium (Polynicotinate) 250 mcg • Folic Acid 100 mcg • Vitamin B12 (Cyanocobalamin concentrate) 50 mcg • Selenium (L-Selenomethionine) 50 mcg • Other ingredients: Dong Quai extract (4:1) (Angelica sinensis) 75 mg • Licorice root extract (Glycyrrhiza glabra) standardized to contain 5% Glycyrrhizic acid) 60 mg • Milk Thistle extract (Silybum Marianum) standardized to contain 70% Silymarin calculated as Silybin) 50 mg • Black Cohosh extract (4:1) (Cimicifuga racemosa) 30 mg • Chaste Berry extract (5:1) (Vitex agnus-castus) 20 mg • Pyridoxal-5'-Phosphate 10 mg. Contains no sugar, salt, yeast, wheat, corn, dairy products, coloring, flavoring or preservatives.

Female Balance — Now
Three capsules contain: Vitamin B6 50 mg • Folic Acid 400 mcg • Borage oil powder (45 mg GLA) 325 mg • Wild Yam root extract (6% Diosgenin) 225 mg • Dong Quai root extract 5:1 150 mg • Vitex Agnus castus extract 10:1 150 mg.

Female Balance — Olympia Nutrition
Borage Oil powder • Wild Yam root • Dong Quai • Vitex Agnus • Vitamin B6.

Female Multi Vitamin — Health Center for Better Living
Each tablet contains: Vitamin A (as retinyl palmitate and 50% from beta-carotene) 3,000 IU • Vitamin C (as ascorbic acid) 100 mg • Vitamin D (as cholecalciferol) 200 IU • Vitamin E (as dl-alpha-tocopheryl acetate) 25 IU • Thiamin (as thiamin HCl) 7 mg • Riboflavin 7 mg • Niacin (as niacinamide) 25 mg • Vitamin B6 (as pyridoxine HCl) 25 mg • Folate (as folic acid) 200 mcg • Vitamin B12 (as cyanocobalamin) 50 mcg • Biotin 35 mcg • Pantothenic Acid (as D-calcium patothenate) 25 mg • Calcium (as dicalcium phosphate) 75 mg • Iron (as ferrous fumarate) 18 mg • Iodine (from Kelp) 25 mcg • Magnesium (as magnesium oxide) 75 mg • Zinc (as zinc citrate) 5 mg • Copper (as copper gluconate) 250 mcg • Manganese (as manganese gluconate) 1 mg • Chromium (as chromium dinicotinate glycinate) 50 mcg • Inositol 10 mg • Choline bitartrate 10 mg • Bioflavonoids complex: Citrus bioflavonoids, Hesperidin, Rutin, and Quercetin trace.

Female Remedy — Phytopharmica
Twenty drops contain: Aristolochia 6x • Mercurius corrosivus 6x • Aconitum napellus 4x • Bryonia 4x • Natrum muriaticum 4x • Sulphur 4x • Belladonna 3x • Cuprum aceticum 3x • Pulsatilla 3x • Lamium album 1x • In a base of 45% USP alcohol by volume.
Editor's Comments: This is a homeopathic product. It is so extremely diluted that its activity can not be explained by conventional scientific methods. Therefore this product can not be rated by the scientific criteria used in this Database. A patient receiving the extreme dilution of this product will not receive many, if any, molecules of the original active ingredient. Therefore, there are no harmful pharmacologic effects, and any beneficial effects are controversial and not due to a direct biochemical action of the ingredient on the body. Homeopathic products are allowed for sale in the U.S. due to legislation passed in the 19th century sponsored by a homeopathic physician who was also a Senator. The law still requires that the FDA allow the sale of products listed in this Homeopathic Pharmacopea of the United States.

Female Sage — Traditional Medicinals
Sage leaf • Chaste berry dry extract • Blue Vervain leaf • Oatstraw herb • Lemongrass leaf • Fennel seed • Rosemary leaf • Blessed Thistle leaf • Stevia leaf.

Female Toner — Traditional Medicinals
Spearmint leaf • Rose Hip • Red Rasberry leaf • Licorice root • Strawberry Leaf • Lemongrass leaf • Lemon Verbena leaf • Nettle leaf • Ginger rhizome • Chamomile flower • Angelica root • Blessed Thistle herb • Cramp bark.

Femdiol — Phytopharmica
Each capsule contains: Vitamin E (D-Alpha Tocopherol) 150 IU • Other ingredients: Barlean's Flaxseed oil 300 mg • Gamma-Oryzanol 100 mg • Pumpkin seed oil (Curcurbita pepo) 50 mg • Soy extract 20 mg standardized to contain 70% saponins & 10% isoflavones calculated as genistein. Contains no sugar, salt, yeast, wheat, corn, dairy products, flavoring or preservatives.

Fem-Gest — Progressive Labs
Ingredients: Stabilized Aloe Vera gel • Mexican Yam extract • Chamomile extract • Chaste Tree berry • Tocopheryl Acetate • Lavender extract • Jojoba oil • Safflower oil • Progesterone 950 mg • Carbomer 940 • Glyceryl Stearate (and) PEG-100 Stearate • C12-15 Alkyl Benzoate • Stearic Acid • Octyl Palmitate • Triethanolamine • Cetyl Alcohol • Methylparaben • Tetrasodium EDTA • Dimethicone • Propylparaben • Diazolidyl Urea.

FEM-H — MMS Pro
Each capsule contains: Black Cohosh root • Sarsaparilla root • Siberian Ginseng root • Licorice root • Blessed Thistle herb • Squaw Vine • False Unicorn root.

FeminEstra — Pacific BioLogic
Poria Plant Fungus (hoelen) • Polygonum root (thin) • Moutan Root bark • Chinese Yam • Cherry (cornelian asiatic) • Rehmannia root (fresh) • Rehmannia root (cooked in wine) • Curculigo rhizome • Alisma (water plantain rhizome) • Pearl - No Concentration.

Femme Advantage Creatine Serum — Muscle Marketing USA
Each serving comtains: Creatine Monohydrate • Vitamin B12 • Ginseng • Royal Jelly • Vitamin B5 • Soluable Bioflavonoids • Ginkgo extract • Wild Yam extract • Papain extract.

Fem-Mend Formula — Nature's Way
Two capsules contain: Proprietary Formula: Blessed Thistle • Cayenne pepper fruit • Cramp bark • False Unicorn root • Ginger • Goldenseal stem, leaf, flower • Red Raspberry leaves • Squaw Vine vine, leaf, fruit • Uva Ursi leaves. Other ingredients: Gelatin.

FemTone — Phytopharmica
Each two capsules contain: Vitamin C (Ascorbic Acid) 100 mg. Other ingredients: Dong Quai extract 4:1 (Angelica sinensis) 250 mg • Hesperidin Complex 200 mg standardized to contain 50% bioflavonoids • Licorice root extract (Glycyrrhiza glabra) 50 mg standardized to contain 5% glycyrrhizic acid • Chaste Tree berry extract 5:1 (Vitex agnus-castus) 50 mg • Black Cohosh extract 4:1 (Cimicifuga racemosa) 50 mg • False Unicorn root extract 4:1 (Helonias opulus) 50 mg • Fennel seed extract 6:1 (Foeniculum vulgare) 25 mg. Contains no sugar, salt, yeast, wheat, corn, soy, dairy products, coloring, flavoring or preservatives.

Femtrol — Enzymatic Therapy
Two capsules contain: Vitamin C (Ascorbic Acid) 100 mg. Other ingredients: Dong Quai extract 4:1 (Angelica sinensis) 250 mg • Hesperidin Complex standardized to contain 50% Bioflavonoids 200 mg • Licorice root extract (Glycyrrhiza glabra) standardized to contain 5% Glycyrrhizic Acid 50 mg • Chaste Tree Berry extract 5:1 (Vitex agnus-castus) 50 mg • Black Cohosh root extract 4:1 (Cimicifuga racemosa) 50 mg • False Unicorn root extract 4:1 (Helonias opulus) 50 mg • Fennel seed extract 6:1 (Foeniculum vulgare) 25 mg. Contains no sugar, salt, yeast, wheat, corn, soy, dairy products, coloring, flavoring or preservatives.

Fennel-Yam — Atrium
Each capsule contains: Fennel 250 mg • Wild Yam 250 mg. Contains no sugar, starch, salt, wheat, corn, yeast or soy derivatives.

Fen-Tastic — The Vitamin Shoppe
Two tablets contain: St. John's Wort root standardized for 3% hypericin 400 mg • Citrus Aurantium fruit 600 mg • 5-HTP 150 mg • Yerba Santa • Mate leaves standardized 20% methylzanthine 250 mg • White Willow bark 400 mg.

Fenu-Thyme Formula — Nature's Way
Two capsules contain: Proprietary Formula: Fenugreek seed • Thyme leaf. Other ingredients: Gelatin.

FerroComp — Phytopharmica
Each capsule contains: Vitamin C (Ascorbic Acid) 60 mg • Iron (Ferrous Succinate) 25 mg • Folic Acid 200 mcg • Vitamin B12 (Cyanocobalamin) 100 mcg • Other ingredients: Liquid Liver Fractions (predigested soluble concentrate) 250 mg • Chlorophyll

BRAND NAMES

**B
R
A
N
D

N
A
M
E
S**

(Fat-Soluble) 5 mg. Contains no sugar, salt, yeast, wheat, corn, dairy products, flavoring or preservatives. All organs & glands derived from bovine sources.

Fevera — HerbaSway
Cassia tora • Kudzu • Skullcap • Knotweed • Licorice • Blackberry • HerbaSwee (Cucurbitaceae fruit).

Feverfew — Now
Each capsule contains: Feverfew 0.9% 400 mg.

Feverfew — Pharmanex
Each capsule contains: Feverfew leaves and flowers (12:1) extract (Tanacetum parthenium) 125 mg. Other Ingredients: Rice Flour, Gelatin.

Feverfew (Nomigraine) Caplets — Life Brand
Dried Feverfew leaf (Tanacetum parthenium) 125 mg. This product is guaranteed to contain a minimum of 0.2% Parthenolide. Excipients: Dicalcium Phosphate, Microcrystalline Cellulose, Silicon Dioxide,Magnesium Stearate (plant source), Stearic Acid (plant source).

Fiber Clense — Nutri-Quest
Three tablets contain: Vitamin C 300 mg • Apple Pectin 150 mg • Garlic 150 mg • Rice Bran 600 mg • Sodium Alginate 300 mg • L-Cystine 200 mg • DL-Methionine 100 mg • L-Lysine 30 mg • Chlorophyll 10 mg • OatBran 600 mg • Red Beet root 100 mg.

Fiber Soy-Pro — The Vitamin Shoppe
SUPRO Soy Protein Isolate and BeneFiber Soluble Fiber. Orange citrus natural flavor. No yeast, corn, wheat, salt, starch, milk, gluten, eggs, fish or animal derivatives, preservatives, artificial colors or flavors added.

Fiberific — Nature's Plus
Each 1.4 oz. bar contains: Calories 120 • Calories from Fat 18 • Total Fat 2 g Saturated Fat 0 g • Cholesterol 0 mg • Total Carbohydrate 23 g • Complex Carbohydrate 14 g • Sugars 9 g • Dietary Fiber 8 g • Soluble Fiber 3.6 g • Insoluble Fiber 4.4 g • Protein 3 g • Sodium 43 mg • Potassium 196 mg. Ingredients include: Rolled Oats, Wheat Germ, Brown Rice, Apples, Prunes & Oat Bran. Naturally flavored with Friut Juice & Honey. No tropical oils.

Fibersol — TwinLab
Each rounded teaspoonful contains: Fiber Blend Concentrate (from Psyllium Seed Husks, Guar Gum, Apple Pectin) 4 g • Vitamin C 100 mg.

Fiber-Time — Atrium
Twelve ounces contain: Bran Fiber • Cascara Sagrada bark • Citrus Fiber • Karaya Gum • Apple Pectin • Prune powder • Psyllium Plantago Ovata Blond • Rhubarb root • Rice Fiber • Sweet Whey.

FibreNet — Pharmanex
Four capsules contain: Chitosan (from shellfish) PolmerPlex 1000 mg. Other Ingredients: Calcium Carbonate, Magnesium Stearate.

FibreNet Plus — Pharmanex
Each Scoop Contains: Vitamin A (85% Beta-Carotene) 6877 IU • Vitamin C 12 mg • Vitamin D 80 IU • Vitamin E 4 IU • Thiamin 0.30 mg • Riboflavin 0.34 mg • Niacin 4 mg • Vitamin B6 0.40 mg • Folate 80 mcg • Vitamin B12 1.2 mg • Biotin 60 mcg • Pantothenic Acid 2 mg • Calcium 187 mg • Iron 3.8 mg • Phosphorus 100 mg • Iodine 30 mcg • Magnesium 60 mg • Zinc 3 mg • Copper 0.40 mg • Sodium 60 mg • Potassium 190 mg • PolmerPlex 1000 mg • Crystalline Fructose, Oat Bran, Stabilized Rice Bran, Gum Arabic, Natural and Artificial Flavors, PolmerPlex, High Oleic Sunflower Oil, Corn Syrup Solids, Tricalcium Phosphate, Citric Acid, Beta-Carotene, Dipotassium Phosphate Cellulose Gum, Sugar Beet Fiber, Potassium Citrate, Sodium Caseinate, Magnesium Oxide, Soy Fiber, Salt, Pea Fiber, Xanthan Gum, Ground Psyllium Husks, Ascorbic Acid, dl-Alpha Tocopheryl Acetate, Dicalcium Phosphate, Soy Lecithin, Vitamin A Palmitate, Niacinamide, Zinc Oxide, Electric Iron, Copper Gluconate, d-Calcium Pantothenate, Cholecalciferol, Pyridoxine Hydrochloride, Riboflavin, Thiamine Mononitrate, Cyanocobalamin, Folic Acid, Biotin, Potassium Iodide.

Fibro Plus — Aspen Group, Inc.
Two capsules contain: Elemental Magnesium 200 mg • Malic Acid 300 mg • Glyciante 50 mg.

Fibromyalgin — Olympia Nutrition
Glucosamine, Collagen, Mag. Malate.

Fish Body Oil — Health Center for Better Living
Each softgel contains: EPA 180 mg • DHA 120 mg • Vitamin E 5 IU.

Flax Borage Combo — Health From The Sun
Three capsules contain: Alpha-Linolenic Acid (ALA)(Omega-3) 825 mg • Gamma-Linolenic Acid (Omega-6) 72 mg • Linoleic Acid (Omega-6) 320 mg • Oleic Acid (Omega-9) 260 mg. Ingredients: Certified Organic Flax seed oil, Borage seed oil, Gelatin, Glycerine, Water, Carob powder.

Flax Lignan Gold — Health From The Sun
One tablespoon contains: 100% Certified Organic Flax seed oil & Particulate with Rosemary extract • Mixed Tocopherols (Vitamin E) • Ascorbyl Palmitate (Vitamin C) • Citric Acid to protect freshness.

Flax Liquid Gold — Health From The Sun
One tablespoon contains: 100% Certified Organic Flax seed oil with Rosemary extract • Mixed Tocopherols (Vitamin E) • Ascorbyl Palmitate (Vitamin C) • Citric Acid to protect freshness.

Flax Seed Oil 1000 mg — Jamieson
Each capsule contains: Alpha Linolenic Acid (ALA) (from Flax seed oil) 500 mg.

Flax-O-Mega — Flora
Cold pressed Flax Seed oil 1000 mg.

Flexa-Herb — Dial Herbs
Kava Kava • Cramp bark • Cayenne • Ginger • Lobelia • Lady Slipper • Red Clover.

Flexaplex — Progressive Labs
Three capsules contain: Vitamin A 3000 IU • Vitamin B6 150 mg • Vitamin B12 300 mcg • Magnesium 300 mg • Copper 3 mg • Potassium 25 mg • Adrenal (Bovine) 30 mg • Valerian root 150 mg • Slippery Elm 30 mg • Gentian root 30 mg • Cape Aloes 30 mg • Skullcap 30 mg • Rue powder 30 mg.

Flor*Essence — Flora
Burdock root • Sheep Sorrel • Slippery Elm • Turkish Rhubarb • Watercress • Kelp • Blessed Thistle • Red Clover.

Flora Vision — Flora
Bilberry extract 250mg • Blueberry.

Floradix Iron and Herbs — Dial Herbs
Vitamin B1 • Vitamin B2 • Vitamin B6 • Folic Acid • Vitamin B12 • Vitamin C • Iron • Aqueous Extract from Carrot • Nettle Worth • Spinach • Quitch roots • Angelica roots • Fennel • Ocean Kelp • African Allow blossom • Orange peel • Juice concentrates: (Pear, Red Grape, Blackcurrant, Orange, Blackberry, Cherry, Beetroot) • Yeast (Saccharomyces cerevisiae) Extract • Honey • Rose Hip extract • Wheat Germ Extract • Natural Flavor.

Flush-Free HexaNiacin — Enzymatic Therapy
Each capsule contains: Niacin (Inositol hexaniacinate) contains 500 mg elemental Niacin 650 mg. Contains no sugar, salt, yeast, wheat, corn, soy, dairy products, coloring, flavoring, or preservatives.

Flush-free Niacin 500 mg — Nature's Life
Each tablet contains: Niacin (Inositol, Hexaniacinate) 500 mg.

Focus Child — Source Naturals
Two tablets contain: Magnesium (from Magnesium Aspartate and Oxide) 100 mg • Zinc (as Zinc Picolinate) 2 mg • L-Aspartate (from Magnesium Aspartate) 310 mg • DMAE (as DMAE Bitartrate) 100 mg • Standardized Soybean Lecithin (LECI-PS) 50 mg • Yielding 40% Phosphatidylserine 20 mg • Phosphatidylcholine 6 mg • Phosphatidylethanolamine 3.5 mg • Phosphatidylinositol 1 mg • DHA (Docosahexaenoic Acid (Neuromins)) 15 mg • Grape Seed extract 15 mg.

Folic Acid 400 mcg — Jamieson
Each tablet contains: Folate (as Folic Acid) 400 mcg.

Folic Acid Dophilus Plus B-12 — Dial Herbs
Two wafers contain: Folic Acid 800 mcg • Vitamin B12 400 mcg • Lactobacillus acidophilus • Lactobacillus plantarum • Lactobacillus bulgaricus • Lactobacillus casei 200 mcg.

For Men Only — Doctor's Best
Each tablet contains: L-Glycine 135 mg • L-Alanine 135 mg • L-Glutamic Acid 135 mg • Raw Prostate concentrate 100 mg • Saw Palmetto 100 mg • Golden Rod 50 mg • Pumpkin seed concentrate 10 mg • Vitamin E 10 IU • Zinc 5 mg • Flax Seed Oil 3 mg.

Some Brand Name Natural Products - What they Contain
www.NaturalDatabase.com contains MANY more listings than appear here.

Formula 600 Plus for Men — Nature's Life
Two capsules contain: Saw Palmetto berry (Serenoa repens B.) 600 mg • Active Aminos (l-Glutamic Acid • Glycine & L-Alanine) 170 mg • Zinc (Picolinate) 15 mg • Pumpkin seed (Curcurbita pepo) 50 mg • Pygeum africanum H. bark extract [(150:1) equivalent to 300 mg whole herb] 2 mg • Burdock root (Arctium lappa L.) 5 mg • Cayenne fruit (Capsicum annuum L. var. annuum) 5 mg • Goldenseal root (Hydrastis canadensis L.) 5 mg • Gravel root (Eupatorium purpureum L.) 5 mg • Juniper berry (Juniperus oxycedrus L.) 5 mg • Marshmallow root (Althaea officinalis L.) 5 mg • Parsley leaf (Petroselinum crispum(Mill) Nym.ex. A.W. Hill) 5 mg • White Pond Lily root (Nymphaea odorata) 5 mg • Vitamin B6 (Pyridoxine HCl) 5 mg • Copper (Gluconate) 1 mg • Nature's Life Active Aminos is an exclusive free-form blend of l-Glutamic Acid, l-Alanine & Glycine.

Formula 75 — Futurebiotics
Vitamin C (Rose hips) 250 mg • Vitamin A (palmitate 10,000 IU, beta carotene 7500 IU) 17,500 IU • Vitamin E (natural) 150 IU • Vitamin D (cholecalciferol) 400 IU • Riboflavin 75 mg • Thiamin 75 mg • Vitamin B6 (pyridoxine HCl) 75 mg • Niacinamide 75 mg • Vitamin B12 (cyanocobalamin) 75 mcg • Folic Acid 400 mcg • Pantothenic Acid 75 mg • Biotin 75 mcg • Iron (chelate) 1.3 mg • Calcium (chelate) 20 mg • Magnesium (chelate) 10 mg • Iodine (kelp) 150 mcg • Selenium (chelate) 25 mcg • Zinc (chelate) 10 mg • Manganese (chelate) 1 mg • Copper (chelate) 1 mg • Molybdenum (chelate) 25 mcg • Chromium (picolinate) 25 mcg • Boron (chelate complex) 0.5 mg • Potassium (chelate complex) 1.8 mg • Inositol 75 mg • Choline (bitartrate) 31 mg • Rutin 25 mg • Para Amino Benzoic Acid (PABA) 75 mg • Hesperidin complex 5 mg • Citrus bioflavonoid complex 25 mg • Betaine HCl 25 mg. In a Green Foods base of: (Alfalfa, Barley & Chlorella).

Forten-Zyme 550 — Atrium
Each tablet contains: Maxistrength Pancreatin 550 mg (which has been prepared by the lyophilization method to insure the preservation & concentration of natural occuring factors such as Amylase, Lipase & Protease enzyme activity. Proteolytic activity is ensured as specific Chymotrypsin & Trypsin content.). This formula is compounded in a buffered base of Amino Acids for maximum stability.

Four-In-One — Changes - TwinLab
One capsule contains: Vitamin C (as Calcium Ascorbate) 120 mg • Aloe 200:1 concentrate leaf gel 200 mg • Wild Yam root (Mexican Yam) 50 mg • Cat's Claw root bark (Uncaria tomentosa) 300 mg • DHEA (Dehydroepiandrosterone) 5 mg. Other ingredients: Gelatin, Magnesium Stearate, Calcium Stearate, and Silica.

Free Amino — Atrium
Full Spectrum - Composed of 22 Free Form Pure Amino Acids.

Free-B — Atrium
Each tablet contains: Vitamin B1 (Thiamine HCL) 100 mg • Vitamin B2 (Riboflavin) 50 mg • Vitamin B6 (Pyridoxine HCL) 50 mg • Vitamin B12 (Cyanocobalamin) 100 mcg • Niacinamide 150 mg • Pantothenic Acid 100 mg • Biotin 150 mcg • Calcium (Dicalcium Phosphate) 20 mg • Copper (Gluconate) 1 mg • Phosphorus (Dicalcium Phosphate) 20 mg • Zinc (Aspartate) 30 mg. In a base specially formulated to complement metabolic type concepts containing trace minerals in specific proportions. This product is completely yeast free & contains no sugar, starch, salt, corn, wheat or soy derivatives.

Fresh Nettle Leaf - Gaia Herbs — Gaia Herbs
Nettle leaf (2% caffeic acids and derivatives). Standardized Full Spectrum 100 mg of extract per capsule. Guaranteed Potency 50 mg of extract per capsule.

Friendly Flora — Nutri-Quest
Each capsule contains: Jerusalem Artichoke (rich source of Fructooligosaccarides) 200 mg • Cellulase 1200 CU • Lactobacillus Acidophilus 400 million • Acerola extract 25 mg • Rose Hips 25 mg • Bifidobacterium Bifidum 200 million • Bifidobacterium Longum 200 million • Protease 7500 HUT • Lipase 52 LU • Lactobacillus Casei 100 million • Lactobacillus Plantarum 100 million • Lactobacillus Rueteri 100 million • Lactobacillus Salicarius 100 million • Amylase 275 DU • EDS Mineral Mix (Kelp, Calcium Ascorbate, Magnesium Citrate, Zinc Gluconate, Manganese Gluconate). In a base of pure plant fiber.

From The Earth — The Vitamin Shoppe
Three tablets contain: Vitamin A 15000 IU • Vitamin D 400 IU • Vitamin E 200 IU • Vitamin C 1000 mg • Vitamin B1 25 mg • Vitamin

B2 25 mg • Vitamin B6 25 mg • Vitamin B12 500 mcg • Vitamin B3 25 mg • Inositol 25 mg • Choline 50 mg • PABA 25 mg • Pantothenic Acid 25 mg • Biotin 50 mcg • Folic Acid 400 mcg • Citrus Bioflavonoids Complex 125 mg • Rutin 25 mg • Quercetin 25 mg • Hesperidin 25 mg • Calcium 200 mg • Magnesium 100 mg • Potassium 99 mg • Zinc 15 mg • Manganese 5 mg • Molybdenum 50 mcg • Iodine 150 mcg • Copper 500 mcg • Selenium 50 mcg • Chromium 200 mcg • Boron 1 mg • Silica 5 mg • RNA 35 mg • DNA 10 mg • Carotenoids 4 mg • Chlorophyll 4 mg • Borage, Flax Seed, and Sunflower Oils 200 mg • L-Glutathione 5 mg • Spirulina 1000 mg • Wheat Grass 100 mg • Barley Grass 100 mg • Chlorella 100 mg • Bee Pollen 100 mg • Korean Ginseng root 50 mg • Garlic 10 mg • Bee Propolis extract 10 mg • Royal Jelly 5 mg • Bromelain 50 mg • Betaine HCl 50 mg • Papain 50 mg • Amylase 5 mg • Lipase 5 mg • Cellulase 5 mg • Lactobacillus Acidophilus, B. bifidum, L-bulgaricus (dairy free) 50 mg • Oat Bran 50 mg • Apple Pectin 50 mg • A unique blend of: Echinacea, Milk Thistle, Goldenseal, Ginger root, Ginkgo Biloba, Capsicum 50 mg.

From The Sea — Nutrition Warehouse
Three capsules contain: Glucosamine Sulfate (Aminomonosaccharide) 1000 mg • Sea Cucumber (Beche De-Mer) 1000 mg • Shark Cartilage 500 mg.

Fruit-Easy — Progressive Labs
Two tablets contain: A blend of the following 1400 mg: Apples • Cranberry powder • Orange juice powder • Pineapple juice powder • Siberian Ginseng • Gingko Biloba • Peaches • Dates • Bromelain • Papain • Lipase • Amylase • Protease • Cellulase • Powdered Cellulose • Apple pectin • Citris pectin • Prune powder • Glucomannan • Lactobacillus Acidophilus • Calcium Gluconate & Green Tea.

Fruitplex — HealthWatchers System
Apple • Lemon • Strawberry • Blueberry • Plum • Cantaloupe • Pear • Cherry • Grapefruit • Raspberry • Grape • Orange Peach • Watermelon • Pineapple • Papaya.

Fuel for Thought Neuro Nutrition — Nature's Plus
Two tablets contain: L-Glutamine free form amino acid 250 mg • Lecithin (Soya) 250 mg • RNA (Ribonucleic acid) 200 mg • L-Tyrosine free form amino acid 200 mg • L-Phenylalanine free form amino acid 100 mg • Phosphatidylcholine 100 mg • Raw Pituitary concentrate 25 mg • Vitamin B6 (Pyridoxine HCL) 10 mg. Sugar & starch free.

Full Spectrum Minerals — Now
Each tablet contains: Calcium (Carbonate, Amino Acid Chelate, Citrate) 1000 mg • Magnesium (Oxide, Amino Acid Chelate, Citrate) 500 mg • Zinc (Amino Acid Chelate) 22.5 mg • Iron (Amino Acid Chelate) 20 mg • Copper (Amino Acid Chelate) 1 mg • Potassium (Proteinate) 99 mg • Manganese (Amino Acid Chelate) 5 mg • Selenium (L-Selenium Methionine) 50 mcg • Chromium (yeast-free, Proteinate) 100 mcg • Molybdenum (Amino Acid Chelate) 59 mcg • Vanadium (Amino Acid Chelate) 50 mcg • Iodine (Kelp) 150 mcg • L-Glutamic Acid (HCL) 50mg • Vitamin D (Cholecalciferol) 200 IU • Boron 3 mg.

FX-Chrysin — GEN
Each capsule contains: Chrysin 250 mg • LPC (Lysophosphatidyl Choline) 200 mg.

G.I. Gel: Gastro-Intestinal Tonic — The Herbalist
Slippery Elm bark• Marshmallow root.

G.I. Support — Now
Three capsules contain: Vitamin A (as Retinol Palmitate) 5000 IU • Vitamin B3 (as Niacinamide) 40 mg • Vitamin B5 (as Calcium Pantothenate 50 mg • Biotin 1000 mcg • Folic Acid (Folate) 400 mcg • Zinc (as Zn Monomethionine) 15 mg • Selenium (as Selenomethionine) 140 mcg • L-Glutamine 500 mg • Apple Pectin 300 mg • N-Acetyl Glucosamine (NAG) 250 mg • Methylsulfonylmethane (MSM) 250 mg • Deglycyrrhizinated Licorice (DGL) 100 mg • Licorice extract 4:1 root 100 mg • Cat's Claw extract 15:1 bark 100 mg • Ginger powder root 100 mg • Aloe Vera concentrate 200:1 leaf (equivalent to 5000 mg fresh Aloe Vera) 25 mg • Pepsin Enzymes NF 1:10000) 50 mg • Pepsin (2000 USP papaya) 50 mg.

G/C 1000 — Progressive Labs
Each capsule contains: Vitamin C (from manganese ascorbate) 60 mg • Manganese (from manganese ascorbate) 15 mg • Glucosamine Hydrochloride 750 mg • Chondroitin Sulfate 250 mg.

© Copyright 2000, Natural Medicines Comprehensive Database (209) 472-2244. For updated data, go to www.NaturalDatabase.com.• 1337

Some Brand Name Natural Products - What they Contain
www.NaturalDatabase.com contains MANY more listings than appear here.

B
R
A
N
D

N
A
M
E
S

GABA Calm — Source Naturals
Gamma Amino Butyric Acid.

GABA-Val — Progressive Labs
Each capsule contains: Gamma Amino Butyric Acid (GABA) 50 mg • Valerian root extract (Valeriana officinalis) 300 mg • Thiamine HCl (Vitamin B1) 25 mg • Niacinamide 25 mg • Magnesium (amino acid chelate) 25 mg • Inositol 175 mg • Lupulin (hops pollen) 50 mg • Passion flower (Passiflora incarnata) 25 mg • Glutamic Acid 25 mg • Brain tissue 25 mg.

Gainers Fuel (Anabolic Weight Gain Formula) — TwinLab
Each serving contains: Calories 531. Each serving also contains Branched Chain Amino Acids (including Peptide Bonded & Free Amino Acids) 21 g, Essential Vitamins, Minerals, Trace Elements, Key Metabolic Optimizers & Lipotropic Factors.

Gainers Fuel 1000 (Super Anabolic Weight Gain Formula) — TwinLab
Each serving contains: Calories 1000 • Predigested Proteins & Amino Acids (Complex Carbohydrates, Anabolic Branched Chain Amino Acids) • Vitamins & Minerals • Pharmaceutical Grade Pancreatic digests of Whey Protein (Lactalbumin) & Egg White Protein (Albumin) • Chromium 400 mcg • Boron • L-Carnitine • Beta-Carotene • Kreb's Cycle Mineral Complexes (including Citrates, Aspartates, Succinates & Alpha-Ketoglutarates).

Gainers Fuel 2500 — TwinLab
Whey & Egg White Proteins • Branched Chain Amino Acids (L-Leucine, L-Isoleucine & L-Valine) • Essential Vitamins & Minerals • Chromium Picolinate & L-Carnitine (100% predigested). Low in fat without high levels of medium chain triglycerides that may cause gastrointestinal upset.

Gall & Liver Tablets — Life Brand
Agrimony herb 100.1 mg • Goose Grass 100.1 mg • Horehound herb 72.8 mg • Senna leaf 18.2 mg • Woodruff herb 81.25 mg • Wormwood herb 18.2 mg • Yarrow 81.9 mg. Excipients: Corn Starch, Sodium Bicarbonate, Silicon Dioxide, Magnesium Stearate, Methyl Paraben, Propyl Paraben.

Gallbladder Support — Amazon Support
Each capsule contains: Chanca Piedra • Boldo • Artichoke 4:1 Extract • Erva Tostao • Carqueja • Jurubeba.

Gallexier Herbal Bitters — Flora
Artichoke • Dandelion & other bitter herbs.

Garcinia Cambogia Plus — Atrium
Each capsule contains: Garcinia cambogia (standardized to contain 50% Hydroxycitric Acid) 340 mg • Atractylodes 80 mg • Citrus aurantii 80 mg • Chromium Picolinate 500 mcg • Chromium Arginate 160 mcg. Contains no sugar, starch, salt, wheat, corn or soy derivatives.

Garlic — Centrum Herbals
One capsule contains: Garlic bulb powder (Allium sativum) 300 mg • Allin (marker) allicin potential 45% 1300 mg. Standardized to contain: Gamma Glutamyl-S allyl-cysteine (natural active), Gamma Glutamyl-S-trans-1-propenyl-cysteine (natural active), Activity measure Angiotensin converting enzyme assay. Other Ingredients: Hydroxypropyl Cellulose, Hydroxpropyl Methylcellulose, Castor Oil, Gelatin, Silicon Dioxide, Sodium Lauryl Sulfate, Pharmaceutical Glaze, Riboflavin, FD&C Blue #1, Lecithin, Simethicone.

Garlic — Pharmanex
Each caplet contains: Garlic clove powder (Allium sativum) 650 mg. Other Ingredients: Excipients, Binders, Caplet Coating.

Garlic - Plus — Aspen Group, Inc.
Each tablet contains: High Potency Garlic (standardized to contain 2500 mcg of allicin) 300 mg • Enzyme Complex 60 mg • Rice Protein-Calcium complex 40 mg.

Garlic & Golden Seal — Nutrivention
Two fl oz contains: Garlic oil • Goldenseal root • Safflower oil • cold-pressed Olive oil • Tocopherol (natural Vitamin E).

Garlic (Allicin-Rich) — Life Brand
Garlic extract powder 500 mg (equivalent to 1500 mg of fresh Garlic cloves. Contains Allicin potential yield of 1.5 mg/g; Thiosulphonates 1.6 mg/g; Allicin 10 mg/g; Gamma Glutamylcysteines 20 mg/g. Excipients: Cellulose, Calcium Phosphate, Stearic Acid, Magnesium Stearate, aqueous base film coat.

Garlic HP — PhysioLogics
Each tablet contains: Garlic bulb (10000 mcg Allicin/gram) 400 mg.

Garlic/Parsley Formula — Nature's Way
Two capsules contain: Proprietary Formula: Garlic bulb • Parsley herb. Other ingredients: Gelatin.

Garlic-Go! — Wakunaga of America
Each caplet contains: Aged Garlic Extract Powder (bulb) 1000 mg. Other Ingredients: Cellulose, Silica, Magnesium Stearate (vegetable source).

Garlinase 4000 — Enzymatic Therapy
Each tablet contains: Garlic extract, equal to 4000 mg of fresh garlic, standardized to contain a minimum of 3.4% (11000 mcg) of Allicin per tablet by a unique patented process to assure maximum Allicin production in your body 320 mg. Contains no sugar, salt, yeast, wheat, corn, soy, dairy products, coloring, flavoring, or preservatives.

GarliPure Daily Formula — Natrol
One capsule contains: Garlic (Allium sativum) powdered extract bulb 600 mg containing: Gamma Glutamylcysteines 12000 mcg • Allicin 6000 mcg • Sulfur 4800 mcg • Thiosulfinates 1200 mcg • Allicin Yield 1200 mcg. Other ingredients: 100% Vegetarian capsule Shell made of Kosher Vegetable Cellulose & Water, Magnesium Stearate.

GarliPure Formula 500 — Natrol
Two tablets contain: Garlic (Allium sativum) powdered extract bulb 1000 mg containing: Gamma Glutamylcysteines 20000 mcg • Allicin 10000 mcg • Sulfur 8000 mcg • Thiosulfinates 1600 mcg • Allicin Yield 1500 mcg. Other ingredients: Dicalcium Phosphate, Microcrystalline Cellulose, Stearic Acid, Magnesium Stearate, aqueous base film coat.

GarliPure Maximum Allicin Formula — Natrol
One caplet contains: Garlic (Allium sativum) powdered extract bulb 600 mg containing: Gamma Glutamylcysteines 12000 mcg • Allicin 4800 mcg • Sulfur 3900 mcg • Thiosulfinates 3800 mcg • Allicin Yield 3600 mcg. Other ingredients: Microcrystalline Cellulose, Stearic Acid, Dicalcium Phosphate, Magnesium Stearate Silicon Dioxide, aqueous base film coat.

GarliPure Once Daily Potency — Natrol
One tablet contains: Garlic (Allium sativum) 600 mg Powdered extract bulb containing: Allicin 13800 mcg • Thiosulfinates 6060 mcg • Allicin Yield 6000 mcg • Gamma Glutamylcysteines 4800 mcg • Sulfur 3900 mcg. Other ingredients: Dicalcium Phosphate, Microcrystalline Cellulose, Croscarmellose Sodium, Silicon Dioxide, Stearic Acid, Magnesium Stearate.

GarliPure Organic Formula — Natrol
Two capsules contain: Garlic (Alium sativum), organically grown powdered extract bulb 1000 mg containing: Gamma Glutamylcysteines 15000 mcg • Allicin 10000 mcg • Sulfur 7000 mcg • Thiosulfinates 1600 mcg • Allicin Yield 1500 mcg. Other ingredients: 100% Vegetarian capsule Shell made of Kosher Vegetable Cellulose & Water, Silicon Dioxide, Magnesium Stearate.

GarliPure Selenium Plus Formulas — Natrol
One capsule contains: Selenium 67 mcg • Garlic (Allium sativum) powdered extract bulb 400 mg containing: Gamma Glutamylcysteines 8000 mcg • Allicin 4400 mcg • Sulfur 3200 mcg • Thiosulfinates 2040 mcg • Allicin Yield 2000 mcg. Other ingredients: Gelatin.

Garlique — SunSource
Each tablet contains: Garlic bulb powder (not less than 500 mcg of allicin yield) 400 mg. Other Ingredients: Dicalcium Phosphate, Microcrystalline Cellulose, Croscarmellose Sodium, Stearic Acid, Magnesium Stearate, Sodium Lauryl Sulfate, Colloidal Silicon Dioxide, Hydroxypropyl Methylcellulose Phthalate, Talc, Titanium Dioxide, Triacetin, Pharmaceutical glaze, (214-112). Contains no sugar, starch, yeast, caffeine, dairy or preservatives.

Garlite — Nature's Plus
Each Vegicap contains: Deodorized Garlic equivalent to a minimum of 2.5 times its weight in fresh garlic 500 mg. Contains no yeast, wheat, corn, soy, milk, salt, sugar or starch.

Gastritix Formula — Nature's Way
Two capsules contain: Chamomile flower 62.5 mg • Fennel seed 237.5 mg • Ginger 237.5 mg • Marshmallow root 50 mg • Slippery Elm bark 125 mg • Wild Yam root 237.5 mg. Other ingredients: Gelatin, Magnesium Stearate, Maltodextrin.

Some Brand Name Natural Products - What they Contain
www.NaturalDatabase.com contains MANY more listings than appear here.

Gastro-Relief — Phytopharmica
Active ingredient: Calcium Carbonate 250 mg Other ingredients: Deglycyrrhizinated Licorice (DGL) root extract (Glycyrrhiza glabra) 380 mg Glycine (Amino Acid) 50 mg No added sugar or fructose Contains no sugar, salt, yeast, wheat, corn, soy, dairy products, coloring, flavoring or preservatives.

GastroSoothe — Enzymatic Therapy
Each tablet contains: Active ingredient: Calcium Carbonate 250 mg. Other ingredients: Deglycyrrhizinated Licorice (DGL) root extract (Glycyrrhiza glabra) 380 mg Glycine (Amino Acid) 50 mg. No added sugar or fructose. Contains no sugar, salt, yeast, wheat, corn, soy, dairy products, coloring, flavoring or preservatives.

GastroSoothe Chocolate-Mint — Enzymatic Therapy
Each chewable tablet contains: Active ingredient: Calcium Carbonate 250 mg • Deglycyrrhizinated Licorice (DGL) root extract (Glycyrrhiza glabra) 380 mg • Glycine (Amino Acid) 50 mg. No added sugar or fructose. Flavored with Dutch Cocoa powder, Creme Flavor, & Peppermint.

GBLVR — Nutri-Quest
Proprietary blend 500 mg: Bayberry • Red Beet root • Yellow Dock • Dandelion root • Fennel seeds • Peppermint • Ginger root • Wild Yam • Blessed Thistle • Garlic 500 mg. In a base of 6X tissue salts: Calc Fluor.

GEN Andro*Gen — GEN
Each capsule contains: Androstenedione 100 mg.

GEN CM Relief — GEN
Each capsule contains: CMO (Cetyl-Myristoleate) 500 mg.

GEN Multi*GenX — GEN
Each six capsules contain: Antioxidants:Vitamin C (Ascorbic Acid) 1000 mg • Vitamin E (natural d-Alpha Tocopherol) 40 IU • Propanthocyanidins (Grape seed extract) 25 mg • Citrus bioflavinoids 100 mg • Lipoic Acid 50 mg. Vitamins: Vitamin A (Retinol Palmitate) 5000 IU • Vitamin A (Beta Carotene) 20000 IU • Vitamin D3 (Cholecalciferol) 400 IU • Vitamin B1 (Thiamine HCL) 50 mg • Vitamin B2 (Riboflavin) 50 mg • Vitamin B3 (Niacinamide) 50 mg • Vitamin B5 (Calcium d-Pantothenate) 50 mg • Vitamin B6 (Pyroxine HCL) 50 mg • Vitamin B12 (Cyanocobalamin) 40 mcg • Folic Acid 400 mcg • Biotin 300 mcg. Minerals: Calcium (from Citrate) 400 mg • Magnesium (from Citrate) 200 mg • Iron (from Fe glycinate) 9 mg • Potassium (from Chloride) 150 mg • Zinc (from Monomethionate-OptiZinc) 15 mg • Manganese (from Citrate) 10 mg • Iodine (from Kelp) 100 mcg • Copper (from Co Gluconate) 270 mcg • Chromium (from Cr Nicotinate/Glycinate) 200 mcg • Molybdenum (from Sodium Molybdate) 150 mcg • Selenium (from Amino Acid Chelate) 200 mcg. Lean Muscle Enhancement: RNA (Sodium Ribonucleic Acid) 150 mg • Inositol 40 mg • L-Carnitine 35 mg • Taurine (HCL) 75 mg • L-Glutamine 25 mg • MSM (Methyl Sulfonylmethane) 100 mg • Coenzyme Q10 (Ubiquinone) 30 mg.

GEN Pyruvate Burn — GEN
Each capsule contains: MED-PRO licensed Pyruvate, from a Pyruvic Acid Complex with Dihydroxyacetone 500 mg. Pyruvic Acid is stabalized with Calcium, Sodium, Potassium or Magnesium to form Pyruvate.

GEN Thermogen — GEN
Two capsules contain: Ma Huang extract standardized at 6%: 334 (334 x .06 = 20 mg) • Caffeine 200 mg • Naringin 40 mg • White Willow bark extract 75 mg • Potassium (Phosphate) 50 mg • Cayenne 35 mg.

Genistein — Source Naturals
Four tablets contain: Soybean powder 4000 mg • Genistein 11.6 mg • Daidzein 42.4 mg • Glycitein 32 mg • Total Isoflavones 86 mg.

Gest-Tonic — The Herbalist
Angelica root • Gentian root • Oregon Grape root • Bayberry root bark • Fennel seed • Prickly Ash bark • Ginger root.

GH Fuel — TwinLab
Six capsules contain: L-Ornithine Alpha-Ketoglutarate 3000 mg • Ma Huang extract (standardized for 6% Ephedrine) 334 mg • Kola extract (standardized for 12% Caffeine) 1000 mg • L-Carnitine 100 mg • Chromium (from Chromic Fuel patented Chromium Picolinate) 400 mcg.

GH Fuel Cocktail — TwinLab
Two tablespoonfuls contain: L-Arginine 6 g • L-Ornithine 1 g •

Taurine 250 mg • L-Carnitine 200 mg • Beta-Carotene 10000 IU • Vitamin D 100 IU • Vitamin C 1000 mg • Natural Vitamin E 400 IU • Vitamin B1 1.5 mg • Vitamin B2 1.9 mg • Vitamin B6 2 mg • Niacinamide 20 mg • Vitamin B12 12 mcg • Pantothenic Acid 500 mg • Folic Acid 400 mcg • Biotin 300 mcg • Choline 700 mg • Inositol 250 mg • Calcium (from KrebMins Calcium) 250 mg • Magnesium (from KrebMins Magnesium) 100 mg • Potassium (from KrebMins Potassium) 325 mg • Zinc (from Zinc Picolinate & KrebMins Zinc) 15 mg • Manganese (from KrebMins Manganese) 2 mg • Copper (from KrebMins Copper) 1 mg • Iodine (from Kelp) 10 mcg • Molybdenum (from KrebMins Molybdenum) 50 mcg • Chromium (from Chromium Picolinate) 100 mcg • Selenium (from KrebMins Selenium) 50 mcg • Boron (from Tri-Boron citrate, Aspartate & Glycinate) 1.5 mg. Natural orange flavor 100%.

GH Release — Nature's Plus
Two capsules contain: L-Ornithine free form amino acid 500 mg • L-Arginine free form amino acid 150 mg • Raw Pituitary concentrate 100 mg • Vitamin B6 (Pyridoxine HCL) 50 mg. Contains no yeast, wheat, corn, soy, milk, salt, sugar or starch.

GH3XL — HealthWatchers System
L-Glutamic Acid • L-Tyrosine • L-Taurine • Glucosamine HCL • Choline Bitartrate • Magnesium • Vitamin B6 • Vitamin Bee pollen • Kelp • Dulse • Irish Moss • Ginseng • Nettles • Alfalfa • Fo-Ti • Pau d'Arco • Fennel Seed • Schizandra • Barley Grass • Acacia Gum • Saussurea • Cat's Claw • Ginger • Licorice.

Ginger — Pharmanex
Each capsule contains: Ginger (Zingiber officinalis)(root extract)(20:1) 125 mg. Other Ingredients: Soybean Oil, Gelatin, Purified Water, Glycerin, Beeswax, Carob.

Ginger & Curcumin Joint-Ease — Nature's Life
Four capsules contain: Ginger root (Zingiber officinale) 1300 mg • Curcumin [from Turmeric root (Curcuma longa) providing 90-95% Curcuminoids] 1300 mg.

Ginger Aid — Traditional Medicinals
Ginger rhizome • Blackberry leaf • Stevia leaf • natural Lemon flavor.

Gingerall — Enzymatic Therapy
Each capsule contains: Ginger root extract (Zingiber officinale) standardized to contain 20% pungent compounds calculated as 6-Gingerol & 6-Shogaol 100 mg. Contains no sugar, salt, yeast, wheat, corn, dairy products, flavoring, or preservatives.

Gingko-Go! — Wakunaga of America
Each caplet contains: Ginkgo Biloba Standardized Extract 50:1 (leaf) standardized with 24% Ginkgo flavonglycosides & 6% Terpene lactones 120 mg. Other Ingredients: Cellulose, Vegetable Starch, Magnesium Stearate (vegetable source), Silica.

Ginkai — Lichtwer Pharma
Each tablet contains: LI 1370 Ginkgo Biloba leaf extract, standardized to 25% ginkgo flavonoids & 6% terpenoids 50 mg.

Ginkgo 5 — Pharmline
Active Ingredients: Ginkgo Biloba extract 24/6, standardized to not less than 24% total Ginkgo flavone glycosides & not less than 6% total terpene lactones.

Ginkgo Alert Formula — PhysioLogics
Each capsule contains: Niacin 5 mg • Vitamin B6 (Pyridoxine HCl) 5mg • Vitamin B12 (Cyanocobalamin) 250 mcg • DMAE 150 mg • L-Glutamine 150 mg • L-Pyroglutamic Acid 100 mg • L-Tyrosine 100 mg • Choline (Bitartrate) 50 mg • Ginkgo leaf (24% Ginkgo Flavonglycosides, 9.6 mg/ 6% Terpene Lactones, 2.4 mg) 40 mg • Panax ginseng (14% Ginsenosides, 3.5 mg) 25 mg.

Ginkgo Biloba — Centrum Herbals
One capsule contains: Ginkgo Biloba leaf extract 60 mg. Standardized to contain (based on extract weight): Ginkgo Flavone glycosides (marker) 24%, Terpene Lactones (marker) 6%, ginkgolide A (natural active), Ginkgolide B (natural active), Amentoflavone (natural active). Activity measure: GABA Central binding assay. Other Ingredients: Sucrose, Cellulose, Lactose, Monohydrate, Dibasic Calcium Phosphate, Hydroxypropy Cellulose, Ethylcellulose, Castor Oil, Flavor Extractives of St. John's Bread, Glucose, Caramel color, Silicon Dioxide, Sodium Lauryl Sulfate, Propylene Glycol, Tianium Dioxide.

BRAND NAMES

Some Brand Name Natural Products - What they Contain
www.NaturalDatabase.com contains MANY more listings than appear here.

BRAND NAMES

Ginkgo Biloba — Jamieson
Each tablet contains: Ginkgo extract (50:1)(Ginkgo biloba)(leaf)(24% flavoglycosides) 40 mg.

Ginkgo Biloba (50:1 extract) — Atrium
Each capsule contains: Ginkgo Biloba, 50:1 extract (24% Ginkgocides) 60 mg. Contains no sugar, starch, salt, wheat, corn, milk, yeast or soy.

Ginkgo Biloba Extract — The Vitamin Shoppe
Each capsule contains: Ginkgo Biloba leaf standardized to 24% ginkgoflavoglycosides and 6% ginkgolides-bilobalides.

Ginkgo Biloba Plus — Wakunaga of America
Each capsule contains: Aged Garlic Extract powder (bulb) 200 mg • Siberian Ginseng Extract 5:1 (root) 80 mg • Ginkgo Biloba Extract 50:1 (leaf) standardized to 24% ginkgoflavonglycosides & 6% terpene lactones 40 mg. Other Ingredients: Cellulose, Magnesium Stearate (vegetable source).

Ginkgo DHA Mind — The Vitamin Shoppe
Each capsule contains: Ginkgo Biloba leaf 24% ginkgoflavoglycosides 6% terpene 60 mg • DHA 50 mg.

Ginkgo Energizer — The Vitamin Shoppe
Each capsule contains: Ginkgo Biloba leaf standardized to 24% ginkgoflavoglycosides 6% ginkgolides-bilobalides 60 mg • CoQ10 30 mg.

Ginkgo Neuro-Mind — The Vitamin Shoppe
Each tablet contains: Vitamin B12 (as cyanocobalamin) 0.25 mcg • Vitamin B6 (as pyridoxine HCl) 10 mg • Ginkgo Biloba (Ginkgo biloba) leaf standardized to 24% ginkgoflavoglycosides 6% terpene lactones 50 mg • Phosphatidylserine (LECI-PS) 50 mg • DHA (Docosahexaenoic acid) (Neuromins) 50 mg. No yeast, corn, wheat, sugar, salt, starch, gluten, soy, milk, dairy, eggs, fish, citrus, preservatives, artificial colors or flavors added.

Ginkgo Phytosome — Phytopharmica
Each capsule contains: Ginkgo Phytosome 80 mg.

Ginkgo/Gotu Kola — Gaia Herbs
Ginkgo and Gotu Kola standardized for 12% flavonoid glycosides & 2.5% triterpenoids. Standardized Full Spectrum 100 mg of extract per capsule. Guaranteed Potency 50 mg of extract per capsule.

Ginkgo-Combo Ginkgo Biloba Complex in Vegetarian Capsules — Nature's Plus
Two Vegicaps contain: Ginkgo Biloba (8:1 extract Ginkgoaceae) 240 mg • Capsicum fruit 160 mg • Gotu Kola root 160 mg • Vitamin E natural 100 IU. Naturally rich in the flavonoids & bioflavonoids Quercetin, Kaempferol, Ginkgetin, Bilobetin, Isoginkgetin & Isorhamnetin. Contains no yeast, wheat, corn, soy, milk, salt, sugar or starch.

Ginkgold — Nature's Way
Each tablet contains: Egb 761 Ginkgo Biloba leaf extract; standardized to 24% Ginkgo flavone glycosides & 6% terpene lactones 60 mg.

Ginkgolidin — Phytopharmica
Each capsule contains: Ginkgo Biloba leaves extract (Ginkgo biloba folia) 40 mg standardized to contain 24% ginkgoflavonglycosides, 6% terpene lactones & 2% bilobalide.

Ginko Biloba — HealthWatchers System
Two capsules contain: Standard Ginkgo Biloba 120 mg • Ginko Biloba Powder equivalent to 6000 mg.

Ginkoba — Pharmaton
Each tablet contains: Standardized Ginkgo Biloba leaf extract (50:1) 40 mg. Other Ingredients: Hydroxypropyl Methylcellulose, Lactose, Talc, Polyethylene Glycol, Magnesium Stearate, Titanium Dioxide, Synthetic Iron Oxides. Contains no sugar, caffeine, or artificial stimulants.

Ginkoba M/E — Pharmaton
Each capsule contains: Panax Ginseng Extract (standardized G115) 100 mg • Ginkgo Biloba Extract (standarized GK501) 60 mg. Other Ingredients: Mannitol, Gelatin, Sicon dioxide, Magnesium Stearate.

Ginsana — Pharmaton
Each capsule contains: Standardized G115 Ginseng root extract (Panax Ginseng, C.A. Meyer) 100 mg. Other Ingredients: Sunflower oil, gelatin, glycerin, lecithin, beeswax, chlorophyll. Contains no sugar, caffeine, or artificial stimulants.

Ginsana Chewy Squares — Pharmaton
Each chewy square contains: Vitamin C • Standardized G115Ginseng root extract (Panax Ginseng, C.A. Meyer) 50 mg. Other Ingredients: Sucrose, Glucose, Palm kernel oil, Gelatin, Citric Acid, Ascorbic Acid, Lecithin, Natural Flavoring & Coloring.

GinsanaSport —
Boehringer Ingelheim Pharmaceuticals, Inc. Dist. by Pharmaton
Each capsule contains: Standardized G-115 Ginseng Extract (Panax Ginseng, C.A. Meyer) (root) 200 mg. Other Ingredients: Sunflower oil, gelatin, glycerin, beeswax, lecithin, tumeric, titanium dioxide, FD&C Green No. 3. Contains no sugar, caffeine, or atificial stimulants.

Ginseng — Centrum Herbals
One capsule contains: Ginseng root extract 100 mg. Standardized to contain (based on extract weight): Total Ginenosides (marker) 7.0%, Ginsenoside Rb1 (natural active), Ginsenoside Rg1 (natural active). Activity measure: Phospholipase A2 enzymatic assay. Other ingredients: Dibasic Calcium Phosphate, Cellulose, Lactose, Monohydrate, Hydroxyproply Cellulose, Ethylcellulose, Castor oil, Gelatin, Silicon Dioxide, Sodium Lauryl Sulfate, Propylene glycol, Titanium Dioxide.

Ginseng Complex — Puritan's Pride
Each capsule contains: American Panax Ginseng 200 mg • Korean Panax Ginseng 200 mg • Red Chinese Panax Ginseng 200 mg • Siberian Ginseng 200 mg • Royal Jelly 200 mg.

Ginseng Extract — The Vitamin Shoppe
Each softgel contains: 100 mg Panax Ginseng extract standardized for 8% ginsenosides.

Ginseng/Aloe Capsules — Aloe Farms
Siberian Ginseng powder 150 mg, Aloe Vera powder 100 mg.

Ginseng/Collagen Firming Creme — Derma E
Ginseng • Collagen (contains 22 amino acids).

Ginseng-Go! — Wakunaga of America
Each capsule contains: Korean Ginseng Extract Powder (root) 300 mg. Other Ingredients: Cellulose, Magnesium Stearate (vegetable source).

GinSting — Futurebiotics
Two tablets contain: Korean Ginseng 1000 mg • Bee Pollen 500 mg.

GinSwee Tea — HerbaSway
Ginger • Panax Ginseng • Blackberry • HerbaSwee (Cucurbitaceae fruit).

GKG — EAS
Each capsule contains: Alpha-Ketoglutaric Acid 250 mg • L-Glutamine 275 mg • Taurine 150 mg • Calcium 63 mg • Potassium 25 mg • Magnesium 25 mg • RNA 9.5 mg • Manganese 400 mcg.

GLA Forte — Nature's Plus
Two softgels contain: GLA (Gamma Linolenic Acid) from Borage & Black Currant Seed oils, 100 mg • Vitamin E (d-Alpha Tocopherol) 200 IU • Vitamin C corn free 100 mg • Vitamin B6 (Pyridoxine HCL) 50 mg • Niacinamide 25 mg • Zinc (Gluconate) 5 mg. In a base containing safflower oil, octacosanol, lecithin & rapeseed. Yeast free. Sugar & starch free.

GLA Mega-260 — Progressive Labs
Each softgel contains: Borage oil 1300 mg which supplies no less than Gamma Linolenic Acid (GLA) 260 mg and Vitamin E 1.5 IU: Fatty Acid Composition: Gamma Linolenic Acid 260 mg • Linoleic Acid 494 mg • Oleic Acid 221 mg.

Glan-Fem Plus — Atrium
Each tablet contains: Ovary 80 mg • Adrenal 20 mg • Thyroid (Thyroxin Free) 20 mg • Pituitary 10 mg • Vitamin B1 15 mg • Vitamin B2 17 mg • Vitamin B6 16 mg • Vitamin C 120 mg • Niacinamide 60 mg • Folic Acid 200 mcg • Vitamin E (d-Alpha Tocopherol) 60 IU • Manganese (Protein Chelated) 5 mg • Selenium 20 mcg.

Glan-Male Plus — Atrium
Each tablet contains: Orchic 80 mg • Adrenal 20 mg • Pituitary 10 mg • Vitamin B1 15 mg • Vitamin B2 17 mg • Vitamin B6 16 mg •

Vitamin C 120 mg • Niacinamide 60 mg • Folic Acid 200 mcg • Vitamin E (d-Alpha Tocopherol) 60 IU • Manganese (Protein Chelated) 5 mg • Selenium 20 mcg.

Gla-Plus — Atrium
Each capsule contains: Gamma Linolenic Acid (from Black Currant) 40 mg • Vitamin E (d-Alpha Tocopheryl Acetate) 10 IU.

Glenalan Deer Velvet — Glenalan
Each capsule contains: Pure NZ premium grade Red Deer Velvet Antler 500 mg.

Gluca-Herb — Dial Herbs
Cedar berries • Uva Ursi • Licorice • Mullein • Cayenne.

Glucogen Ace — ANS
Glucose • Vitamin A • Vitamin C • Vitamin E.

Glucomannan 500 Mg — Natrol
Two capsules contain: Hemicellulose 913 mg • Cellulose 61 mg • Pectin Substance 25 mg • Lignin 1 mg. From Amorphophallus Konjac root.

Glucomine — Body Wise International, Inc.
Three capsules contain: Glucosamine Sulfate 1500 mg • Chondroitin Sulfate 150 mg • Boswellia Gum Std. Extract (Boswellia serrata) 25 mg • White Willow Bark (Salix alba) 25 mg • Devils Claw-Inner Bark (Harpagophytum procumbens) 25 mg • Tea Tree Oil (Melaleuca alternifolia) 25 mg • Una de Gato (Uncaria tomentosa) 25 mg

Gluco-Pro 900 — Thompson Nutritional Products
Each tablet contains: Glucosamine HCl 500 mg • Chondroitin Sulfate 400 mg.

Glucosamine Chondroitin Sulfate — HealthWatchers System
Glucosamine Sulfate • Chondroitin Sulfate • Vitamin C.

Glucosamine Complex — Natrol
One capsule contains: Glucosamine Sulfate 100 mg • Glucosamine HCl 300 mg • Glucosamine N-Acetyl 100 mg. Other ingredients: Rice powder, Silicon Dioxide, Magnesium Stearate, Gelatin.

Glucosamine Formula — Symmetry
Each packet contains: Glucosamine • Chondroitin Sulfate • Hydrolyzed gelatin • Boswellia • Curcumin • Bilberry • Grape Seed extract • Grape Skin extract • Tumeric extract.

Glucosamine Fuel — TwinLab
Two tablets contain: Glucosamine Sulfate (Pure Pharmaceutical Grade) 1500mg • Chrondroitin Sulfate (Pure Pharmaceutical Grade) 1200mg • Glycerol Fuel (contains 99.7% Pure Pharmaceutical Grade Glycerol).

Glucosamine Plus Dietary Supplement — Dr. Art Ulene's Prescriptive Formulas
Two tablets contain: Niacin (B3) 100 mg • Curcumin 100 mg • Glucosamine Hydrochloride 730 mg • Frankincense Extract (boswellia serrata, roxb. excolabr, gum resin) 300 mg • Glucosamine Sulfate 50 mg • Quercetin 100 mg • Turmeric (Curcuma longa, rhizome powder) 100 mg.

Glucosamine Sulfate — Phytopharmica
Each capsule contains: Glucosamine Sulfate 500 mg Contains no sugar, yeast, wheat, corn, soy, dairy products, coloring, flavoring or preservatives. Each capsule contains 60 mg of sodium.

Glucosamine Sulfate Chondroitin Sulfate — Progressive Natural Products
One tablespoon contains: Glucosamine Sulfate 500 mg • Vitamin C 500 mg • Chondroitin Sulfate 150 mg • Shark Cartilage 50 mg • CMO 25 mg • Cherry extract 25 mg • Sea Cucumber 25 mg • Manganese Aspartate 5 mg • Zinc Citrate 5 mg • Boron Citrate 1 mg.

Glucosa-Plex — Progressive Labs
Each capsule contains: Vitamin C 50 mg • Vitamin E (succinate) 25 IU • Pantothenic Acid 50 mg • Glucosamine Sulfate 100 mg • N-Acetyl Glucosamine 50 mg • L-Glutathione 2 mg • N-Acetyl Cysteine 5 mg • L-Cysteine 50 mg • L-Glutamic Acid 50 mg • L-Glycine 50 mg • L-Taurine 25 mg • Soluble Trachea (16% pure chondroitin sulfate-A) 25 mg • Milk Thistle (Silybum marianum) 100 mg • Silymarin 5 mg • Green Lipped Mussel 25 mg (natural source of mucopolysaccharides and superoxide dismutase).

Glucos-Bal — Nutri-Quest
Each tablet contains: Vanadyl Sulfate 3 mg • Chromium (Picolinate)

200 mcg • Vitamin B1 10 mg • Vitamin B2 5 mg • Vitamin B6 5 mg • Vitamin B12 10 mcg • Folic Acid 200 mcg • Biotin 500 mcg • Pantothenic Acid (D-Calcium Pantothenate) 20 mg • Niacinamide 20 mg • Niacin 6 mg • Magnesium Aspartate 100 mg • Calcium Ascorbate 100 mg • Manganese Aspartate 4 mg • Zinc (Picolinate) 1 mg • Selenium (Chelate) 30 mcg.

Glucotize — MRI
Each tablet contains: a-Lipoic Acid (thioctic acid) 300 mg. Inactive Ingredients: Calcium Phosphate, Cellulose ethers & composites, Magnesium Stearate. Contains no yeast, corn, wheat, soy, sugar or sweeteners, artificial flavors, colors or preservatives.

Glutagen — ANS
Pure Glutamine.

Glutamine Capsules — Universal Nutrition
Each capsule contains: L-Glutamine 750 mg • Manganese Sulfate 400 mcg • Potassium Phosphate 30 mg.

Glutamine Flora — Nutri-Quest
Each tablet contains: Combined stabalized microencapsulated freeze-dried Lactobacillus Acidophilus, Bulgaricus & Bifidus 4.5 million IU • L-Glutamine 500 mg • Chlorophyll 20 mg • natural Vitamin E Succinate 5 IU.

Glutamine Fuel Capsules — TwinLab
Two capsules contain: L-Glutamine 1500 mg.

Glutamine Fuel Powder — TwinLab
Each teaspoonful contains: L-Glutamine 4500 mg (4.5 g).

Glutathione Plus — Atrium
Each capsule contains: L-Glutathione 50 mg • L-Glutamine 200 mg.

GLYCO-8 — Pharmagel
Glycolic Acid • Alpha Hydroxy Acids • Antioxidants.

Glyco-B — Atrium
Each tablet contains: Vitamin B1 35 mg • Vitamin B2 35 mg • Vitamin B6 35 mg • Vitamin B12 35 mcg • Vitamin C 180 mg • Pantothenic Acid 80 mg • Niacinamide 180 mg • Folic Acid 135 mcg • Choline Bitartrate 25 mg • Inositol 10 mg • Biotin 10 mcg • L-Lysine HCL 10 mg • Brewer's Yeast 50 mg • Pancrelipase 20 mg • Selenium 2 mcg • Adrenal 4 mg • Brain 4 mg • Liver 7 mg • Pancreas 2 mg.

Glycobar: Chocolate Chip — Pharmanex
Each bar contains: Honey • Peanut Butter (Peanuts, Salt) • Semi Sweet Chocolate Chips (Sugar, Chocolate Liquor, Coacoa Butter, Soy Lecithin, Vanilla) • Brown Sugar • Date Puree • Prune Puree • Rolled Oats • Sugar Beet Fiber • Brown Crisp Rice (Rice Flour, Rice Bran, Rosemary Extract) • Modified Guar Gum • Oat Bran • Peanuts • Barley Flakes • Rye Flakes • Soybean Oil • Soy Lecithin • Whey Powder.

Glycobar: Peanut Butter and Jelly — Pharmanex
Each bar contains: Honey • Peanut Butter (Peanuts, Salt) • Brown Sugar • Date Puree • Prune Puree • Rolled Oats • Strawberry and Blueberry Fruit Chips (Sugar, Strawberries, Blueberries, Glucose, Pectin, Citric Acid, Sodium Citrate, Natural Flavor) • Brown Crisp Rice (Rice Flour; Rice Bran, Rosemary Extract) • Modified Guar Gum • Oat Bran • Peanuts • Yogurt Chips (Sugar, Hydrogenated Palm Kernel Oil, Milk Solids, Color (Titanium Dioxide), Soy Lecithin, Vanilla) • Barley Flakes • Rye Flakes • Soybean Oil • Soy Lecithin • Whey Powder.

Glycoplex — Progressive Labs
Three capsules provide: Vitamin C 500 mg • Thiamin (Vitamin B1) 100 mg • Riboflavin (Vitamin B2) 100 mg • Niacinamide 500 mg • Vitamin B6 100 mg • Folate (folic acid) 300 mcg • Vitamin B12 50 mcg • Biotin 15 mcg • Pantothenic Acid (calcium pantothenate) 250 mcg • Chromium (chromium picolinate) 200 mcg • Inositol 50 mg • Pancrelipase 50 mg • Choline Bitartrate 50 mg • Pyloric substance 45 mg • Para Amino Benzoic Acid (PABA) 60 mg • L-Lysine Monohydrochloride 30 mg. Other ingredients: Raw Adrenal, Raw Pancreas, Raw Brain and Raw Liver concentrates.

GlyMordica — Amazing Herbs
Bitter Melon (Momordica Charantia).

Golden Flax Meal — Nature's Life
Two tablespoons (17 g) contain: Low fat Omegaflo Flax seed meal (certified organic by Farm Verified Organic). Naturally occuring fatty acids: Alpha Linolenic Acid (Omega-3) 1710 mg • LinoleicAcid

© Copyright 2000, Natural Medicines Comprehensive Database (209) 472-2244. For updated data, go to www.NaturalDatabase.com. • 1341

BRAND NAMES

(Omega-6) 480 mg • Oleic Acid (Omega-9) 50 mg • Lignin Fiber 1003 mg • Lignan 13.6 mg.

Golden Flax Oil — Nature's Life
One tablespoon contains: Lipid profile, based on a typical analysis of : Omega-3 as Alpha-Linolenic Acid EFA 8.6 g • Omega-6 as Alpha-Linoleic Acid EFA 2.7 g • Omega-9 as Oleic (Monounsaturated Fatty Acid) 2.4 g.

Golden Flax Oil 1000 mg — Nature's Life
Each capsule contains: 100% pure Flax oil (Certified Organically Grown) (Omegaflo Process fresh, unrefined, unfiltered, unbleached, virgin seed oil; Organically grown & processed according to California Organic Foods Act of 1990; Farm Verified Organic). Lipid profile based on a typical analysis: Omega-3 EFA as Alpha-Lenolenic Acid 570 mg • Omega-6 EFA as Leoleic Acid 180 mg • Omega-9 as Oleic Acid 160 mg • Vitamin A (from naturally occuring Beta Carotene) 286 IU • Vitamin E (from naturally occuring Tocopherols) 1 IU.

Golden Spleen 500 — Enzymatic Therapy
Each capsule contains: Spleen Polypeptides 375 mg: A mixture of highly purified bovine-derived spleen polypeptides naturally present in the spleen, including: Tuftsin, Splenopentin, Splenin, & Leukokinin • Goldenseal root extract 125 mg: (Hydrastis canadensis) standardized to contain 5% total Alkaloids including: Berberine, Hydrastine, & Canadine. Contains no sugar, salt, yeast, wheat, corn, dairy products, flavoring, or preservatives.

Goldenseal — Pharmanex
Each capsule contains: Goldenseal (Hydrastis canadensis) 4:1 root extract 250 mg. Other Ingredients: Rice Flour, Gelatin, Magnesium Stearate, Silicon Dioxide.

Goldenseal and Myrrh — Dial Herbs
Goldenseal • Myrrh.

Goldenseal Salve — Dial Herbs
Goldenseal • Myrrh • Shavegrass • Echinacea • Comfrey • Slippery Elm • Lobelia. In a base of Bees Wax , Glycerine & Cold Pressed Olive oil.

Goldenseal-Myrrh Virtue — Blessed Herbs
Goldenseal root • Myrrh Gum • Propolis • Grain alcohol & Distilled Water.

GO-lite/am (Appetite Manager) — Enviro-Tech Nutritionals
Griffonia simplicifolia (Containing 5-hydroxytryptophan) • St. John's Wort.

GO-lite/fm (Fat Metabolizer) — Enviro-Tech Nutritionals
Chitosan • Vitamin C • Iodine • Chromium • Thermal Herbal Blend (Sida Cordifolia and bitter orange peel) • Yerba mate leaf • Chitosan.

Good-Nite — Changes - TwinLab
One caplet contains: Melatonin 3 mg • Kava Kava root standardized extract (30% kavalactones) 250 mg • Herbal Extract Blend 275 mg: Valerian root standardized extract (0.8% valerenic acids), Catnip aerial parts, Chamomile flower, Hops stobile, Passion flower aerial parts, Skullcap root. Other ingredients: Dicalcium Phosphate, Vegetable cellulose, Fractionated vegetable oil, Silica, Soy polysaccharides, and Vegetalbe resin glaze.

GP Cordyceps — Solaray - Nutraceutical
Two capsules contain: Cordyceps (Cordyceps sinensis) 520 mg • Other ingredients: Gelatin (capsule), Cellulose, Magnesium.

Gram-Two Vitamin C — The Vitamin Shoppe
Two tablets contain: Vitamin C (as ascorbic acid and as mineral ascorbates of calcium, magnesium, zinc, and manganese) 2000 mg • Bioflavonoids (Hesperidin, Rose Hips, Acerola Cherry, Pectin, Orange, Grapefruit, Lemon, Rutin) 250 mg. No Yeast, Corn, Wheat, Sugar, Salt, Soy, Starch, Dairy, Milk, Eggs, gluten, Fish Or Animal Derivatives, Preservatives, Artificial Colors or Flavors added.

Grape Seed — Pharmanex
Each capsule contains: Grape (Vitis vinifera)(seed extract)(100:1) 75 mg. Other Ingredients: Rice Flour, Gelatin, Magnesium Stearate, Silicon Dioxide.

Grape Seed Antioxidant — Now
Each capsule contains: Grape seed extract (95%) 60 mg • Citrus Bioflavonoids (40%) 300 mg.

Grape Seed Extract Formula — Quest
Each caplet contains: Grape Seed powder (Vitis vinffera) (Provided by 25 mg P.E. 1:100 standardized to contain not less than 95% leucoanthocyanins) 2500 mg • Citrus Bioflavonoids 200 mg providing Hesperidin 50 mg • Rutin powder 25 mg. Other Ingredients: Calcium Phosphate, Microcrystalline Cellulose, Vegetable Stearin, Croscarmellose Sodium, Magnesium Stearate (vegetable source).

Grape seed extract Plus — Atrium
Each capsule contains: Grape seed extract (Leucocyanidins) 50 mg • Bioflavonoids 200 mg.

Grapefruit Concentrate With Fiber & Herbs — Natrol
Two capsules contain: Grapefruit concentrate 10:1 300 mg • Psyllium Husk fiber 100 mg • Rice Bran fiber 100 mg • Oat Bran fiber 100 mg • Licorice root 100 mg • Uva Ursi 100 mg • Apple Cider vinegar 50 mg • Deep Ocean Kelp 50 mg • Lecithin 50 mg • Spirulina 50 mg • Vitamin B6 (Pyridoxine HCL) 25 mg • L-Phenylalanine 25 mg • Cascara Sagrada 20 mg. This is a 10 time concentration of the equivalent of 3000 mg of Whole Grapefruit. Other ingredients: Silicon Dioxide, Magnesium Stearate, Gelatin, Microcrystalline Cellulose.

Grapefruit Extract — NutriBiotic
Grapefruit extract.

Green Multi — Nature's Life
Three tablets contain: Beta Carotene (equivalent to 25000 IU Vitamin A) 15 mg • Vitamin C 1000 mg • Vitamin E (d-Alpha Tocopheryl Succinate) 300 IU • Vitamin B1 (Thiamine Mononitrate) 25 mg • Vitamin B2 (Riboflavin, Riboflavin 5'-Phosphate) 25 mg • Vitamin B3 (Niacin) 25 mg • Pantothenic Acid (Calcium Pantothenate, Pantetheine-5' -Phosphate) 25 mg • Vitamin B6 (Pyridoxine HCl, Pyridoxal-5'-Phosphate) 25 mg • Folic Acid (Folacin) 400 mcg • Vitamin B12 100 mcg • Biotin (d-Biotin) 60 mcg • Choline (Bitartrate) 14 mg • Inositol (Niacinate) 20 mg • PABA (Para Aminobenzoic Acid) 25 mg • Boron (Citrate, Nature's Life Greens) 100 mg • Calcium (Carbonate, Citrate/Malate) 250 mg • Chromium (Picolinate, Polynicotinate) 100 mcg • Copper (Citrate, Gluconate) 1 mg • Iodine (Potassium Iodine, Nature's Life Greens) 75 mcg • Iron (Glycinate, Nature's Life Greens) 10 mg • Magnesium (Oxide, Nature's Life Greens) 125 mg • Manganese (Gluconate, Citrate) 6 mg • Molybdenum (Molybdate, Nature's Life Greens) 50mcg • Potassium (Gluconate, Iodide, Nature's Life Greens) 90 mg • Selenium (Selenite, Cysteine) 100 mcg • Vanadium (Vanadyl Sulfate) 25 mcg • Zinc (Picoliante, Monomethionine) 15 mg • Lemon Bioflavonoids Complex (50% active) 100 mg • Quercetin (Saphora japonica) 25 mg • Rutin (Sapora japonica) 25 mg • Hesperidin (Citrus fruit peel) 25 mg • Bromelain from Pineapple (2000 GDU/g) 25 mg • Papain from Papaya (2000 USP units/g) 25 mg • Betaine HCL, beets 25 mg • Amylase (30000 SKB IU/g) 6 mg • Lipase 10000 Usp IU/g) 6 mg • Cellulase (10000 USP IU/g) 6 mg • Nature's Life Greens powder 1000 mg.

Green Phytofoods — Now
Each nine gram serving contains: Lecithin fine powder 2000 mg • Spirulina (Hawaiian) 1000 mg • Alfalfa juice concentrate 700 mg • Wheat grass powder organic 500 mg • Barley grass powder organic 500 mg • Carrot powder 500 mg • Barley Malt powder 400 mg • Broccoli powder 350 mg • Brown Rice Bran 350 mg • Apple fiber 350 mg • Apple Pectin 300 mg • Oat Bran 300 mg • Chlorella powder 300 mg • Red Beet powder 300 mg • Panax ginseng root powder (min 5% Ginsenosides) 250 mg • Siberian Ginseng root powder (Eleutherococcus senticosus) 100 mg • Peppermint powder 150 mg • Green Tea extract (Camellia sinensis) (40% Catechins) 100 mg • Royal Jelly powder (min 5% 10-HDA) 100 mg • Fructo Oligo Saccharides (NutraFlora FOS) 100 mg • Trace Mineral concentrate 100 mg • Milk Thistle extract (80% Silymarin) 80 mg • Kelp powder 50 mg • Ginkgo Biloba extract (24% Ginkgo Flavonglycosides) 20 mg • Grape seed extract (95% Polyphenols) 20 mg • Bilberry extract (25% Anthocyanidins) 20 mg • Plant Based Enzymes 100 mg: Protease 12500 HUT, Lipase 200 LU, Lactase 200 LAC, Bromelain 5000 FCC, Amylase 2500 DU, Cellulase 500 CMC, Papain 6000 PU • Coenzyme Q10 10 mg • Alpha Lipoic Acid 10 mg • Stevia extract 10 mg.

Green Stuff — Gary Null
Contains a Green Mix (Green Kamut juice, Wheat Grass juice, Barley Green Juice, Alfalfa Leaf, Oat Grass Juice, Broccoli, Parsley, Kale), Flaxseed, Raw Brown Rice, Fruit Juice Mix (Pineapple, Lemon, Lime), Carrot juice, Earthrise Farms Spirulina, Yucca root, and Black Licorice root extract.

Some Brand Name Natural Products - What they Contain
www.NaturalDatabase.com contains MANY more listings than appear here.

Green Tea Extract — HealthWatchers System
Green Tea Extract • Green Tea Powder. Each capsule is the equivalent of 700 mg. of Green Tea Powder.

Gro Pro — Universal Nutrition
Ten capsules contain: Creatine Monohydrate 5000 mg • L-Glutamine 2000 mg • Acetyl L-Carnitine 500 mg • L-Leucine (BCAA) 250 mg • L-Isoleucine (BCAA) 250 mg • L-Valine (BCAA) 250 mg • N-Acetyl-Cysteine (NAC) 200 mg • Tribulus Terrestris L. 250 mg • DHEA 50 mg • Zinc 15 mg.

Growth Fuel — TwinLab
Nine capsules contain: B-Hydroxy B-Methylbutyrate Monohydrate (HMB) 3000 mg • L-Glutamine 2000 mg • Creatine Monohydrate 5000 mg • N-Acetyl-Cysteine (NAC) 200 mg • Acetyl-L-Carnitine 50 mg • Zinc (from Zinc Picolinate) 30 mg • DHEA (Dehydroepiandrosterone) 50 mg.

GSC (Glandular Stress Complex) — Progressive Labs
Each capsule contains: Vitamin B12 24 mcg • Raw Bovine Adrenal 15 mg • Raw Bovine Liver 15 mg • Raw Bovine Thymus 60 mg • Raw Bovine Spleen 15 mg • Raw Bovine Stomach 15 mg.

Guar Gum — Atrium
Each tablet contains: Pure Guar Gum 1000 mg.

Guarana Chai — Traditional Medicinals
Assam Black leaf Tea • Cardamom seed Ginger rhizome • Roasted Chicory root • Nutmeg seed • Organic Black Peppercorn • Guarana seed dry extract • Stevia leaf • Vanilla Bean dry extract • Clove stem • Rose petal • Cinnamon bark oil.

Guarana-Gotu Kola Virtue — Blessed Herbs
Ma Huang • Siberian Ginseng root • Guarana seed • Gotu Kola • Licorice root • Grain alcohol & Distilled Water.

Guggulbolic — Syn Trax
Each capsule contains: Guggulsterones 30 mg.

GugulPlex — Phytopharmica
Each tablet contains: Niacin 250 mg • Vitamin C 100 mg • Chromium 50 mcg • Guggul extract 250 mg • Ginger root extract 200 mg.

GugulPlus — Enzymatic Therapy
Each tablet contains: Niacin (Inositol hexaniacinate) 250 mg • Vitamin C (Potassium Ascorbate) 100 mg • Chromium (Chromium Polynicotinate) (ChromeMate brand of patented Niacin-bound GTF Chromium) 50 mcg • Other ingredients: Guggul extract (Commiphora Mukul) standardized to contain Guggulsterones 25 mg/gram) 250 mg • Ginger root extract 6.5:1 (Zingiber officinale) 200 mg. Contains no sugar, salt, yeast, wheat, corn, soy, dairy products, flavoring, or preservatives.

Gum Weed Salve — Dial Herbs
Gum Weed • Licorice • Myrrh • Goldenseal • Arnica • Strawberry • Lobelia • Cayenne. In a base of Bees Wax, Glycerine & Cold Pressed Olive oil.

Gum-Ease — The Herbalist
Echinacea root • Myrrh Gum • Blood root • Bayberry root bark • Essential oils of Peppermint, Cinnamon, Clove.

Gynecrine — Progressive Labs
Each capsule contains: Vitamin A 1000 IU • Vitamin C 100 mg • Vitamin E (dl-alpha tocopherol) 50 IU • Thiamin (Vitamin B1) 10 mg • Riboflavin (Vitamin B2) 10 mg • Vitamin B6 (pyridoxine) 18 mg • Iodine (as potassium iodide) 150 mcg • Magnesium (as magnesium oxide) 100 mg • Manganese (as manganese gluconate) 10 mg • Ovary concentrate (bovine) 20 mg • Mammary concentrate 10 mg • Pancreas concentrate 10 mg • Adrenal concentrate 10 mg • Pituitary concentrate 10 mg • Lecithin 10 mg • Flax seed oil 10 mg.

Gypsy Cold Care — Traditional Medicinals
Contains: Menthol: 5 mg per cup as it naturally occurs in the Peppermint leaf (Mentha x piperia) present in the blend. Other herbal ingredients: Rose Hip, Cinnamon bark, Yarrow flower, Ginger rhizome, Elder flower, Safflower petal, Clover stem, Hyssop herb, Licorice root dry extract.

Hair & Skin Formula — Nature's Way
Four capsules contain: Biotin (Biotin Triurate) 1.6 mg • Calcium 50 mg • Cayenne pepper fruit 160 mg • Fizyme Enzyme Formula 100 mg • Fo-Ti root 160 mg • Glucoamine HCL 400 mg • Horsetail grass 160 mg • Kelp (whole Thallus) 160 mg • MSM (Methyl Sulfonyl Methane) 600 mg • Nettle herb 160 mg • Oatstraw stem, leaf 160 mg • Rosemary herb 160 mg. Other ingredients: Gelatin, Magnesium Stearate, Millet.

Hair & Skin Nutrition — Enzymatic Therapy
Each capsule contains: Vitamin A (Fish Liver oil) 1666 IU • Vitamin D (Fish Liver oil) 333 IU • Vitamin E (D-Alpha Tocopherol) 33 IU • Vitamin C (Ascorbic Acid) 100 mg • Niacin/Niacinamide 33 mg • Zinc (Chelate) 15 mg • Vitamin B6 (Pyridoxine HCL) 10 mg • Pantothenic Acid (D-Calcium Pantothenate) 8.3 mg • Riboflavin (Vitamin B2) 1.7 mg • Biotin 333 mcg • Folic Acid 33 mcg • Other ingredients: Unsaturated Free Fatty Acids (Linoleic, Arachidonic & Linolenic from Unrefined Germ oil & Safflower seed oil) 300 mg • Lecithin (Soy) 200 mg • Choline Bitartrate 50 mg • Intrinsic Glandular Lipids 50 mg • Inositol 33 mg. In a base of L-Cysteine as a natural amino acid synergistic component. Contains no sugar, salt, yeast, corn, dairy products, flavoring or preservatives. All organs & glands derived from bovine sources.

Hair Formula — Pharmanex
Each capsule contains: Vitamin E (as D-Alpha Tocopheryl Acetate) 3 IU • Riboflavin (as Riboflavin-5-Phosphate) 0.75 mg • Vitamin B6 (as Pyridoxine Hydrochloride) 3 IU • Biotin (as Biotin) 200 mcg • Pantothenic Acid (as Calcium Pantothenate) 25 mg • DL-Methionine 200 mg • L-Cysteine 105 mg • Lactalbumin Hydrolysate 25 mg • Millet Extract 20 mg. Other Ingredients: Gelatin, Maltodextrin, Starch, Vanillin, Stearic Acid (Vegetable Derived), Silicon Dioxide.

Hair Genesis — Crawford Co.
Each softgel contains: BetaSitosterol 50 mg • Saw Palmetto Berry extract (85/95% liposterolic standardized) 200 mg • Lecithin 50 mg • Inositol 100 mg • Phosphatidyl Choline 25 mg • Niacin 15 mg • Biotin 100 mcg. Other Ingredients: Alcohol SDA-40, Propylene Glycol, Deionized Water, Polysorbate-80, Isoceteth-20, Hydrolyzed Mucopolysaccharides, Beta-Sitosterol, Biotin, and Citric Acid.

Hair Nutrients — Biotech
Three tablets contain: Shen Min (a proprietary blend of 12:1 standardized He Shou Wu (Fo Ti) root extract and He Shou Wu root powder) 1755 mg • BioPerine Black Pepper extract 3 mg.

Hair Support — Amazon Support
Each capsule contains: Nettles • Mutamba • Muira Puama • Sarsaparilla • Avenca • Gervao • Catuaba.

Hair, Skin & Nails — Health Factor
Each capsule contains: Choline Bitartrate 100 mg • DL Methionine 100 mg • Borage Seed 150 mg • Flax Seed 150 mg • Gelatin 150 mg • Lecithin 100 mg.

Hair, Skin & Nails for Men — Futurebiotics
Three tablets contain: • Beta Carotene 10,000 IU • Vitamin C 120 mg • Vitamin B2 (Riboflavin) 10 mg • Vitamin B1 (Thiamin) 10 mg • Calcium 600 mg • Iron (Amino Acid Chelate) 6 mg • Vitamin D (Fish Liver Oil) 200 IU • Vitamin E (Natural Mixed Tocopherols) 30 IU • Vitamin B6 (Pyridoxine) 10 mg • Folic Acid 400 mcg • Vitamin B12 16 mcg • Phosphorus 300 mg • Iodine (Kelp) 225 mcg • Magnesium (Oxide) 200 mg • Zinc (Gluconate) 25 mg • Biotin 400 mcg • Pantothenic Acid (Calcium Salt) 30 mg • Choline (Bitartrate) 150 mg • Inositol 60 mg • Para Amino Benzoic Acid • (PABA) 50 mg • Selenium (Amino Acid Chelate) 25 mcg • Manganese • (Amino Acid Chelate) 10 mg • Niacinamide 50 mg • In a special potentiating base containing: Gelatin, Cysteine, Methionine, Ribonucleic Acid (RNA), Bioflavonoids, Betaine HCl, Oat Straw, Horsetail Extract, Saw Palmetto Berry, Smilax Extract, Siberian Ginseng Extract, Standardized Panax Ginseng Extract & Rutin.

Hair, Skin & Nails for Women — Futurebiotics
Three tablets contain Vitamin A (Beta Carotene) 10,000 IU • Vitamin C 120 mg • Thiamin (B1) 10 mg • Riboflavin 10 mg • Niacinamide 50 mg • Calcium 600 mg • Iron (Amino Acid Chelate) 6 mg • Vitamin D (Fish Liver Oil) 200 IU • Vitamin E (Natural Mixed Tocopherols) 30 IU • Vitamin B6 (Pyridoxine) 10 mg • Folic Acid 400 mcg • Vitamin B12 16 mcg • Phosphorus 300 mg • Iodine (Kelp) 225 mcg • Magnesium (Oxide) 200 mg • Zinc (Gluconate) 15 mg • Biotin 400 mcg • Pantothenic Acid (Calcium Salt) 30 mg • Choline (Bitartrate) 150 mg • Inositol 60 mg • Para Amino Benzoic Acid (PABA) 50 mg • Selenium (Amino Acid Chelate) 25 mcg • Manganese (Amino Acid Chelate) 10 mg • Ribonucleic Acid (RNA) 60 mg • Bioflavonoids 50 mg Rutin 25 mg 50 mg • Rutin 25 mg • Betaine HCl 50 mg • In a base containing L-Cysteine, L-Methionine, Gelatin, Papain, Oat Straw, Echinacea, Horsetail, Asparagus.

BRAND NAMES

© Copyright 2000, Natural Medicines Comprehensive Database (209) 472-2244. For updated data, go to www.NaturalDatabase.com.

Some Brand Name Natural Products - What they Contain
www.NaturalDatabase.com contains MANY more listings than appear here.

B R A N D   N A M E S

Happy Camper — Natural Balance
Two capsules contain: Proprietary blend 840 mg: Passion Flower • Kava Kava • Siberian Ginseng • Gotu Kola • Schisandra • Wood Betony • Lavender.

Harmonex — Chattem, Inc.
Each caplet contains: Standardized St. John's Wort flower extract (0.3% hypericin) 450 mg • Standardized Siberian Ginseng root extract (0.8% eleutherosides) 90 mg. Other Ingredients: Microcrystalline Cellulose, Croscarmellose Sodium, Hydroxypropyl Methylcellulose, Sodium Carboxymethyl Cellulose, Magnesium Stearate, Dextrin, Dextrose, Mineral oil, Polyethylene Glycol, Caramel, Polysorbate 80, Propylene Glycol, Riboflavin, Silicon Dioxide, Sodium Citrate, Titanium Dioxide.

HAS Original Formula — Nature's Way
Two capsules contain: Proprietary Formula: Brigham Tea herb • Burdock root • Cayenne pepper fruit • Cleavers herb • Elecampane • Goldenseal root • Marshmallow root • Parsley herb • Rosemary herb. Other ingredients: Gelatin.

Hawaiian Noni Juice — Youngevity
Purified Water • Morinda citrifolia • Lecithin • Potassium Sorbate • Artificial Flavoring • Vilcabamba Mineral Essence: Potassium, Calcium, Magnesium, Zinc, Chromium, Selenium, Iron, Copper, Molybdenum, Vanadium, Iodine, Cobalt, Manganese.

Hawthorn — Pharmanex
Each capsule contains: Hawthorn flowers & leaves (5.5:1) extract (Crategus oxyacantha) 125 mg. Other Ingredients: Rice Flour, Gelatin.

Hay Relief — Rainbow Light
Each caplet contains: Nettle tops 260 mg • Golden seal rhizome and root powder 40 mg • Licorice root 40 mg • Lemon thyme herb 30 mg • Dong Quai root 20 mg • Eyebright herb 8 mg. Other ingredients: Cellulose or gum arabic, vegetable stearin, and silica.

H-Complex — Progressive Labs
Each capsule contains: Vitamin E 15 IU • Stone root (Collinsonia canadensis) 400 mg • Comfrey root (Symphytum officinale) 50 mg • Bayberry bark (Myrica cerifera) 50 mg • Goldenseal root (Hydrastis canadensis) 40 mg • Green Beet leaf powder 25 mg • Betony (Betonica officinalis) 10 mg.

HDT Andros-D 100 — Human Development Technologies
Each capsule contains: Androstenedione 100 mg • Zinc 15 mg • Bioperine 2.5 mg.

HDT GLX-37.5 — Human Development Technologies
Each capsule contains: Vanadyl Sulfate (yielding 7.5 mg elemental Vanadium) 37.5 mg • Taurine 600 mg • Magnesium 200 mg • Selenium 33 mcg • Ginger 20 mg • Cinnamon 20 mg • Chromium Picolinate 200 mcg.

Head Relief — Now
Two capsules contain: Feverfew leaf (Tanacetum parthenium) (min. 0.9% Parthenolide) 400 mg • Kava root extract (Piper methysticum) (30% Kavalactones) 100 mg • Ginger root extract (Zingiber officinale) 5% standardized 50 mg • Proprietary Blend of extracts 50 mg containing: Purple Willow Bark (Salix purpurea), Meadow Sweet (Filipendula ulmaria), Wintergreen (Gaultheria procumbens) to 25% standardized Salicin content.

Head Relief — Olympia Nutrition
Feverfew • Kava root • Ginger • Willow bark • Meadow Green • Wintergreen.

Headacha — HerbaSway
Ginkgo Biloba • Dong Quai • Ginger • Kudzu • Bupleurum • Coptis • Blackberry • HerbaSwee (Cucurbitaceae fruit).

Headache Remedy — Lehning Laboratories
Ruta graveolens 8X • Argentum nitricum 6X • Digitalis purpurea 6X • Cimicifuga racemosa 4X • Gelsemium sempervirens 4X • Sanguinaria canadensis 4X • Chelidonium majus 3X • Cyclamen europaeum 3X • Iris versicolor 3X • Melilotus 3X. In a base of 40% USP alcohol by volume.
Editor's Comments: This is a homeopathic product. It is so extremely diluted that its activity can not be explained by conventional scientific methods. Therefore this product can not be rated by the scientific criteria used in this Database. A patient receiving the extreme dilution of this product will not receive many, if any, molecules of the original active ingredient. Therefore, there are no harmful pharmacologic effects, and any beneficial effects are controversial and not due to a direct biochemical action of the ingredient on the body. Homeopathic products are allowed for sale in the U.S. due to legislation passed in the 19th century sponsored by a homeopathic physician who was also a Senator. The law still requires that the FDA allow the sale of products listed in this Homeopathic Pharmacopea of the United States.

Heal-All Salve — Blessed Herbs
Goldenseal root • Heal-All • Comfrey root • German Chamomile flower • Plantain leaf • Echinacea Angustifolia root • Yarrow flower • Gotu Kola • St. John's Wort flower • Calendula flower • Organic Cold-Pressed Olive oil & Essential oil of Lavender.

Healthy Hair, Skin, & Nails (60) — Rainbow Light
Each capsule contains: Beta-Carotene 5000 IU • Vitamin E natural 100 IU • Tomato Paste concentrate (Lycopene)300 mg • Vitamin C (Zinc & Copper Ascorbates) 180 mg • Rice Bran 150 mg • Inositol 150 mg • Horsetail herb 4:1 extract 150 mg • Nettles tops 4:1 extract 120 mg • Ginger rhizome 4:1 extract 120 mg • L-Cysteine 100 mg • Spirulina 100 mg • PABA (Para Aminobenzioc Acid) 75 mg • Red Pepper fruit 60 mg • Pantothenic Acid (Vitamn B5) 60 mg • Rosemary leaf 4:1 extract 50 mg • Maidenhair Fern 40 mg • Marine Mineral Complex 25 mg • Niacin (Vitamin B3) 20 mg • Zinc (Ascorbate)15 mg • Rosemary oil 3 mg • Pyridoxine (Vitamin B6) 2 mg • Biotin 1800 mcg • Copper (Ascorbate) 1500 mcg • Folic Acid 400 mcg • Cyanocobalamin (Vitamin B12) 6 mcg.

Healthy Heart with Folic Acid and B6 — Discount, Inc.
Each tablet contains: Vitamin B6 5 mg • Pyridoxal 5 Phosphate 0.5 mg • Folic Acid 600 mcg • Folinic Acid 1 mcg.

Healthy Soy Chocolate — Nature's Life
Each scoop (35 g) contains: Supro Soy Protein Isolate (with less than 2% Lecithin) • Rice Syrup Solids • Fructose • Cocoa powder (with less than 2% Lecithin) • Fructoligosaccharides • Magnesium Citrate • Calcium Carbonate • Glycine • Apple Pectin • Ascorbic Acid • d-Alpha Tocopherol Acetate • Zinc Citrate • Niacinamide • Copper Gluconate • d-Calcium Pantothenate • Manganese Gluconate • Vitamin A Palmitate • l-Selenomethionine • Cholecalciferol • Chromium Niacinate • Pyridoxine HCI • Thiamine Mononitrate • Riboflavin • Folic Acid • Biotin • Potassium Iodide • Sodium Selenite • Sodium Molybdate • Cyanocobalamin. Supro Soy Protein Isolate is 44% of the formula.

Healthy Soy Vanilla — Nature's Life
Each scoop (33 g) contains: Supro Soy Protein Isolate (with less than 2% lecithin) • Maltodextrin • Rice Syrup Solids • Fructose • Fructoligosaccharides • Magnesium Citrate • Calcium Carbonate • Glycine • Apple Pectin • natural Flavors • Ascorbic Acid • d-Alpha Tocopherol Acetate • Zinc Citrate • Niacinamide • Copper Gluconate • d-Calcium Pantothenate • Manganese Gluconate • Vitamin A Palmitate • l-Selenomethionine • Cholecalciferol • Chromium Niacinate • Pyridoxine HCI • Thiamine Mononitrate • Riboflavin • Folic Acid • Biotin • Potassium Iodide • Sodium Selenite • Sodium Molybdate • Cyanocobalamin. Supro Soy Protein Isolate is 44% of the formula.

Healthy Whey — Nature's Life
Three tablespoons or one rounded scoop (23 g) contain: Whey Protein concentrate • natural Flavor composed of Di, Tri, Oligo & Polypeptides (providing 58% B-lactoglobulin, 22% A-Lactalbumin, 10% Immunoglobulin, 10% Minor Proteins & Lactoferrin).

Healthy Woman Soy Menopause — Personal Products
Each tablet contains Soy Standardized extract 320 mg • Includes Isoflavones 55 mg.

Heart — Centrum Focused Formulas
One tablet contains: Vitamin E 200 IU • Vitamin B6 5 mg • Folate, Folic Acid, Folacin 200 mcg • Vitamin B12 200 mcg • Selenium 25 mcg • Manganese 1 mg • Garlic bulb powder (Allium sativum) 300 mg • Taurine 33 mg • Coenzyme Q10 4 mg.

Heart Actives — VitaStore
Six tablets contain: Coenzyme Q-10 5 mg • Chitosan 500 mg • Hawthorne 200 mg • Chromium 100 mcg • Green Tea Extract 200 mg • Fiber Complex (Oat Bran & Psyllium) 1000 mg • Lecithin 500 mg • Vitamin B3 (Niacin) 50 mg • Calcium 500 mg • L-Carnitine 250 mg • Ginger 200 mg • EFA Complex (Essential Fatty Acids) 500 mg • Selenium 150 mcg • Vitamin B1 (Thiamine) 1.5 mg.

Heart Formula — Nature's Way
Two capsules contain: Betaine Anhydrous 200 mg • Coenzyme Q10 (Ubiquinone) 15 mg • Folic Acid (Folate) 300 mc • Hawthorne dried

extract (1.8%-2.2% Vitexin) 350 mg • Niacin (Vitamin B3) 20 mg • Potassium (Aspartate, Chloride) 20 mg • Pyridoxine HCL 50 mg • Reishi dried extract (10% Polysaccharides) 25 mg • Siberian Ginseng root 250 mg • Vitamin B12 (Cyanocobalamin) 400 mcg • Vitamin E (d-Alpha Tocopheryl) 50 IU. Other ingredients: Gelatin, Magnesium Stearate, Millet.

Heart Science — Source Naturals
Six tablets contain: Vitamin A (Beta Carotene) 45000 IU • Vitamin B1 (Thiamin) 50 mg • Inositol Hexanicotinate 500 mg • Vitamin B6 (Pyridoxine HCI) 25 mg • Coenzymated B6 (Pyridoxal-5'-Phosphate)(Yielding 16.9 mg of Vitamin B6) 25 mg • Vitamin B12 (Cyanocobalamin) 500 mcg • Folic Acid 800 mcg • Vitamin C (Magnesium Ascorbate) 1500 mg • Vitamin E (D-Alpha Tocopheryl) (Natural) 400 IU • Chromium (ChromeMate Polynicotinate 150 mcg and Chromium Picolinate 150 mcg) 300 mcg • Copper (Sebacate) 750 mcg • Magnesium (Ascorbate, Taurinate and Oxide) 300 mg • Potassium (Citrate) 99 mg • Selenium (L-Selenomethionine) 200 mcg • Silica (from 400 mg of Horsetail Extract) 28 mg • Coenzyme Q10 (Ubiquinone) 60 mg • L-Carnitine L-Tartrate 500 mg • Hawthorn berry extract 400 mg • Proanthodyn (grape seed extract)(with a Proanthocyanidolic Value of 95) 100 mg • L-Proline 500 mg • L-Lysine (HCI) 500 mg • N-A-G (N-Acetyl Glucosamine) 500 mg • Bromelain (2000 GDU per g) 1200 mg • Taurine (Magnesium Taurinate) 500 mg • Inositol (Hexanicotinate) 50 mg.

Heart Support — Amazon Support
Each capsule contains: Abuta • Hawthorn • Bitter Melon • Chanca Piedra • Periwinkle • Mulungu • Artichoke.

Heart Support — Now
Three tablets contain: Vitamin B1 (Thiamine HCL) 50 mg • Vitamin B6 (Pyridoxine HCL) 50 mg • Vitamin B12 (Cyanocobalamin) 1000 mcg • Folic Acid 800 mcg • Magnesium (Oxide/Aspartate) 200 mg • Potassium (Chloride/Aspartate) 200 mg • Iodine (Kelp extract) 300 mcg • Selenium (Selenomethionine) 140 mcg • Coenzyme Q10, pure 30 mg • L-Carnitine 400 mg • Pure-Gar Garlic 1000 mg • Hawthorne berry extract (standardized to contain 1.25% Vitexin-4' Rhamnoside) 150 mg • Alpha Lipoic Acid 20 mg • Ginger root 250 mg • Cayenne pepper (40000 Heat units) 150 mg.

Heart Support — Nutri-Quest
Each tablet contains: Heart 100 mg • Spleen 40 mg • Co-Enzyme Q-10 2 mg • Vitamin C (Sago Palm) 100 mg • Vitamin E (Succinate) 100 IU • L-Carnitine HCL 20 mg.

Heart Support — Olympia Nutrition
CoQ10 • Alpha Lipoic Acid • Garlic • Hawthorn • Cayenne • Magnesium.

Heart's Ease — The Herbalist
Hawthorn berry, leaf & flower • Dandelion root, leaf & flower • Skullcap herb • Yarrow flower • Horsetail herb • Lemon Balm herb • Prickly Ash bark • Cayenne pepper.

Heavenly Skin & Hair Care — Gary Null
Whole leaf Aloe Vera concentrate, Jojoba oil, Licorice and Grape seed extracts, Tri-Silica complex, MSM, Antioxidant Botanical extracts, Liposomal Vitamins, Oat Bran glucan, Tissue Respiratory Factor, and more.

Heavyweight Gainer 900 — Champion Nutrition
Each serving contains: Metacarb-III (branching complex carbohydrates extracted from Corn Hybrids including Maltodextrins) • Peptol-III (pre-digested highly efficient protein blend consisting of Whey Protein Concentrate, Fat-Free, Cholesterol-Free, Red-Muscle Protein Complex, Debitterized Enzyme Digest of Lactalbumin, & Egg White Protein) • extra grade Whey • Fructose • low-fat Cocoa powder • MCT's • Metavite-III (Champion Nutrition's advanced Vitamin/Mineral formula consisting of di-Calcium Pantothenate, Potassium, Citrate, Magnesium Gluconate, Potassium Chloride, Choline Bitartrate, Inositol, Ascorbic Acid, D-Calcium Pantothenate, Niacin, Zinc Gluconate, d-Alpha Tocopherol Succinate, Molybdenum Aspartate, Selnium Aspartate, Manganese Gluconate, Chromemate-GTF (Chromium Polynicotinate), Copper Gluconate, Pyridoxal-5-Phosphate, Thiamine HCL, D-Biotin, Potassium Iodid, Ergocalciferol, Folic Acid, Cyanocobalamin) • Cellulose Gum • Xanthan • Natural & Artificial Flavors • Lecithin • Sunnette Brand of Acesulfame-K) • Carageenan • Aspartame. Contains Phenylalanine.

Hemaplex — Progressive Labs
Each capsule contains: Iron (from 200 mg iron peptonate) 32 mg • Vitamin C (ascorbic acid) 200 mg • Thiamin HCl (Vitamin B1) 2 mg •

Riboflavin (Vitamin B2) 2 mg • Niacin 13 mg • Niacinamide 15 mg • Vitamin B6 (pyridoxine HCl) 2 mg • Folate (folic acid) 400 mcg • Vitamin B12 (cyanocobalamin) 50 mcg • Base: (Raw Duodenum, Raw Liver, Raw Stomach, Red Bone Marrow, Beef Peptone, Citrus pectin, Betaine HCl, Bile Salts, Rose Hips, Alfalfa & Wheat germ) 50 mg.

Hem-Mend: Hemorrhoid Support — The Herbalist
Stone fresh dried root (Collinsonia canadensis)• Celandine fresh-flowering herb (Chaelidonium majus)• Witch Hazel fresh-dried leaf (Hamamelis virginiana)• Horsechestnut fresh nut (Aesculus hippocastanum).

Hemo-Plus — Atrium
Each tablet contains: Vitamin C 300 mg • Vitamin B1 10 mg • Vitamin B2 10 mg • Vitamin B6 10 mg • Vitamin B12 250 mcg • Folic Acid 800 mcg • Niacinamide 20 mg • Iron Peptonate 113 mg • Manganese (Proteinate Chelated) 5 mg • Liver 75 mg.

Hem-Tone — Enzymatic Therapy
Two capsules contain: Vitamin E (D-Alpha Tocopherol Succinate) 30 IU • Calcium Lactate 130 mg • Vitamin C (Ascorbic Acid) 100 mg • Phosphorus (Tricalcium Phosphate) 25 mg • Other ingredients: Colinsonia root (Stone root) 500 mg • Choline Bitartrate 150 mg • Butchers Broom extract (Ruscus aculeatus) standardized to contain 10% Saponins (calculated as Ruscogenin) 100 mg • Rutin (Buckwheat) 100 mg • Glycosaminoglycans 25 mg: A mixture of highly purified bovine-derived Glycosaminoglycans naturally present in the aorta including: Dermatan Sulfate, Heparan Sulfate, Hyaluronic Acid, Chondroitin Sulfate, & related Hexosaminoglycans. Contains no sugar, salt, yeast, wheat, corn, dairy products, coloring, flavoring, or preservatives. All organs & glands derived from bovine sources.

Hepato-C — Pacific BioLogic
Salvia root • Heydyotis • Scutellaria (barbat skullcap) • Peony root (red) • Codonopsis root (natural) • Lycium fruit • Dryopteris rhizome • Rhodiole Sachelanensi root • Polygonum root (thin) • Magnolia bark • Knotweed rhizome (bushy) • Astragalus root (Grade 1) • Capillaris shoots & leaves • Bitter Orange (ripened fruit) • Polyporus Sclerotium.

Hepato-Detox — Pacific BioLogic
Salvia root • Codonopsis root (natural) • Lycium fruit • Polygonatum rhizome • Astragalus root (Grade 1) • Reishi Mushroom • Privet fruit (ligustrum) • Ginseng root (red ji lin) • Cherry (cornelian asiatic).

Hepatox — Phytopharmica
Three tablets contain: Vitamin A (Fish Liver oil) 4500 IU • Niacin 40 mg • Vitamin C (Ascorbic Acid/Rose Hips) 25 mg • Biotin 200 mcg • Vitamin B12 (Cyanocobalamin) 3 mcg • Other ingredients: Choline Bitartrate 850 mg • Dehydrated Green Beet leaf juice powder 300 mg • L-Methionine 250 mg • Barberry bark of root 4:1 (Berberis vulgaris) 150 mg • Boldo extract (peumus boldo) 150 mg standardized to contain 1.52% essential oils • Greater Celandine extract (Chelidonium majus) 135 mg • Fringe Tree (Cheonanthus) 135 mg • Ox Bile extract 90 mg • Betaine HCL 75 mg • Inositol 50 mg • Liver (Desiccated) 40 mg • Unsaturated Free Fatty Acids 30 mg. Lipotrophic factors may provide support for normal fat metabolism. Chlorophyll is used in this product as a natural coloring agent. Contains no sugar, salt, yeast, wheat, corn, soy, dairy products, flavorings or preservatives. All organs & glands derived from bovine sources.

Herba Fuel — TwinLab
Three capsules contain: Ma Huang extract (standardized for 6% Ephedrine) 334 mg • Chinese Green Tea extract (standardized for 7% Caffeine & 20% Polyphenols) 1500 mg. In a natural base of Siberian Ginseng (Eleutherococcus senticosus).

Herbal Cold Relief — Jamieson
Each capsule contains: Ephedra stem extract (Ephedra since)(equivalent to 10.2 mg of ephedrine) 62.5 mg • Grindelia aerial parts 1:4 extract (Grindelia Camporum) 0.5 mg • Eucalyptus oil (Eucalypyus Globulus) 0.05 mg • Echinacea Root (Echinacea purpurea) 100 mg.

Herbal Decongestant Expectorant Capsules — Life Brand
Ma Huang (Ephedra) 50 mg as a standardized extract 1:10 (equivalent to 500 mg Ma Huang) with 4 mg of total Ephedrines • Wild Horehound leaf 150 mg • Thyme herb extract (1:4) 100 mg (equivalent to 400 mg of Thyme) •Coltsfoot leaf 50 mg • Mullein leaf 50 mg • Cayenne 1.125 mg • Marshmallow root 9 mg • Slippery Elm bark 9 mg. Excipients: Gelatin & water.

B R A N D   N A M E S

© Copyright 2000, Natural Medicines Comprehensive Database (209) 472-2244. For updated data, go to www.NaturalDatabase.com. • 1345

Some Brand Name Natural Products - What they Contain
www.NaturalDatabase.com contains MANY more listings than appear here.

BRAND NAMES

Herbal Diuretic — Progressive Labs
Each capsule contains: Active Ingredients: Proprietary blend 120 mg: Buchu leaves (Barsoma crenata) • Couch Grass root (Triticum repens). Other Herbs: Proprietary blend 330 mg: [Hydrangea root (Hydrangea arborescens), Corn Silk (Stigmata maidis), Juniper berry (Juniperus communis), Burdock root (Arctium lappa), Uva Ursi leaf (Arctostaphylos Uva-Ursi), Ginger root (Zingiber officinale) Parsley (Petroselium sativum), Marshlallow root (Althaea officinalis)].

Herbal Diuretic Formula — Quest
Each caplet contains: Uva Ursi leaf (Arctostaphylos uva-ursi) (Provided by 50 mg P.E. 1:4) 200 mg • Juniper berry extract (Junuperus communis) (Provided by 80 mg P.E. 1:4) 320 mg • Parsley root (Petroselinum crispum) (Provided by 40 mg P.E. 1:4) 160 mg. Other Ingredients: Buchu leaves, Cayenne, Corn Silk, Kelp, Parsley leaf, Pumpkin seed, Saw Palmetto berries, Calcium Phosphate, Vegetable Stearin, Croscarmellose Sodium, Magnesium Stearate (vegetable source).

Herbal Diuretic Tablets — Life Brand
Buchu leaf extract (1:4) 25 mg (equivalent to 100 mg Buchu leaf) • Uva Ursi leaf extract (1:3) 33.3 mg (equivalent to 100 mg Uva Ursi leaf) • Juniper berry extract (1:2) 50 mg (equivalent to 100 mg of Juniper berries) • Celery seed 75 mg • Parsley root 75 mg. Excipients: Micorcrystalline Cellulose, Tricalcium Phosphate, Corn Starch, Magnesium Stearate.

Herbal Douche — Dial Herbs
Mineral Water • Aloe Vera • White Oak bark • Slippery Elm • Uva Ursi • Cayenne.

Herbal Fem — Nutri-Quest
Golden Seal root, Dong Quai, Blessed Thistle, Red Raspberry leaves, Squaw Vine, Scullcap, Cayenne, Blue Cohosh, Licorice root, Wild Yam root, Passion Flower 408 mg. In a base of 6X tissue salts: Calc Fluor, Calc Phos, Calc Sulph, Kali Mur, Kali Phos, Kali Sulph, Mag Phos, Nat Mur, Nat Phos, Nat Sulph, Silica.

Herbal Gargle — Dial Herbs
Sage • Myrrh • Goldenseal • Bayberry • Cayenne • Ginger • pure Apple cider vinegar aged in wood.

Herbal GI — PhysioLogics
Each capsule contains: Glucosamine (HCl) 150 mg • Gamma Oryzanol 200 mg • Chamomile (1.2% Apigenin, 1.8 mg; 0.5% Essential oil, 0.75 mg) 150 mg • Aloe Vera 100 mg • Wild Yam (6% total Saponins, 4.5 mg) 75 mg.

Herbal Gold Cigarettes — Alternative Cigarettes Inc
Each cigarette contains: Marshmallow • Yerba Santa • Damiana • Passion Flower • Jasmine • Ginseng. Regular, menthol, vanilla, and cherry are available.
Editor's Comments: In April 2000, the Federal Trade Commission filed a complaint against manufacturers of natural or herbal cigarettes for making claims that these products were safer than conventional cigarettes. The labeling on these products is now required to state "Herbal cigarettes are dangerous to your health. They produce tar and carbon monoxide." If they use the term "No additives" they must also state "No additives in our tobacco does NOT mean a safer cigarette."

Herbal Grobust — HomeCure, Inc.
Sabal • Damiana • Dong Quai • Blessed Thistle • Kava Kava • Dandelion root • Oat Bran • Wild Yam • Mother's Wort.

Herbal Insomnia Tablets — Life Brand
Valerian root extract (1:4) 50 mg (equivalent to 200 mg Valerian root) • Passion Flower herb 80 mg • Chamomile flower extract (1:4) 15 mg (equivalent to 60 mg Chamomile flowers) • Mistletoe herb 50 mg • Hops flower 50 mg • Wild Lettuce leaf 40 mg. Excipients: Tricalcium Phospate, Corn Starch, Silicon dioxide, Magnesium Stearate.

Herbal Klenz — Progressive Labs
Each capsule contains: Vitamin A 3500 IU • Echinacea (Echinacea angustifolia) 200 mg • Golden Seal (Hydrastis canadensis) 125 mg • Irish Moss (Chondrus crispus) 40 mg • Ginger root (Zingiber officinale) 35 mg • Burdock root (Arctium lappa) 35 mg • Peony root (Paeonia officinalis) 35 mg • Peony root skin (Paeonia officinalis) 35 mg • Licorice root (Glycyrrhiza glabra) 25 mg • Red Clover flower (Trifolium pratense) 20 mg.

Herbal Laxative — Holista
Each capsule contains: Cascara Sagrada extract 200 mg • Senna leaves 250 mg.

Herbal Laxative (Stomach-Ease) Tablets — Life Brand
Senna leaves 240 mg • Cascara Sagrada bark 150 mg • Licorice root 30 mg • Juniper berries 8 mg • Rhubarb root 8 mg • Gentian root 8 mg • Buchu leaves 4 mg. Excipients: Corn Starch, Sodium Bicarbonate, Silicon Dioxide, Magnesium Stearate, oil of Peppermint.

Herbal Laxative Formula — Quest
Each caplet contains: Cascara Sagrada bark (Rhamnus purshiana) (Provided by 50 mg P.E. 7:1) 350 mg • Rhubarb root (Rheum officinale L.) (Provided by 30 mg P.E. 1:4) 120 mg. Other Ingredients: Cayenne, Ginger root, Licorice root, Marshmallow root, Calcium Phosphate, Croscarmellose Sodium, Microcrystalline Cellulose, Magnesium Stearate (vegetable source), Vegetable Stearin.

Herbal Migraine Formula — Quest
Each caplet contains: Feverfew powder (Tanacetum parthenium) (contains no less than 0.2% parthenolides) 125 mg. Other Ingredients: Calcium Phosphate, Croscarmellose Sodium, Microcrystalline Cellulose, Vegetable Stearin, Magnesium Stearate (vegetable source).

Herbal Nerve Tablets — Life Brand
Valerian root extract (1:4) 50 mg (equivalent to 200 mg Valerian root) • Skullcap herb 100 mg • Hops flowers 50 mg. Excipients: Tricalcium Phosphate, Corn Starch, Magnesium Stearate, Silicon Dioxide.

Herbal Nightcap — Trader Joe's
Passion flower 150 mg • Chamomile 4 mg • Hops 60 mg.

Herbal Pain and Fever Relief — Holista
Each capsule contains: White Willow bark powder 300 mg • Meadowsweet extract 250 mg.

Herbal Pain Relief Formula — Quest
Each caplet contains: White Willow bark (Salix alba) (Provided by 250 mg P.E. 1:12 standardized to contain 11% Salicin) 3000 mg. Other Ingredients: Blue Vervain, Kelp, Red Raspberry leaf, Skullcap and Wood Betony. Calcium Phosphate, Magnesium Stearate (vegetable source), Microcrystalline Cellulose, Vegetable Stearin.

Herbal Regulator — VitaStore
Two tablets contain: Potassium (as gluconate) 25 mg • Hydrangea root 100 mg • Graminis Rhizoma root 50 mg • Cornsilk 50 mg • Parsley whole herb 25 mg • Uva Ursi leaves 75 mg.

Herbal Relaxant Formula — Quest
Each caplet contains: Valerian root (Valeriana officinalis) (Provided by 100 mg P.E. 1:5 standardized to contain 0.8% Valerenic Acid) 500 mg • Chamomile flower (Chamomilla recutita L.) (Provided by 50 mg P.E. 1:4 standardized to contain 1% Apigenin) 200 mg. Other Ingredients: Ginger root, Hops, Marshmallow root, Skullcap, Calcium Phosphate, Croscarmellose Sodium, Magnesium Stearate (vegetable source), Microcrystalline Cellulose, Vegetable Stearin.

Herbal Seltzer — Dial Herbs
Sodium • White Willow bark • Fever Few • Ginger • Mint • Stevia • Potassium Bicarbonate • Sodium Bicarbonate • Citric Acid. Flavored & sweetened with natural orange flavorings, natural fruit flavors & dextrose.

Herbal Slim — Nature's Way
Four capsules contain: Proprietary formula: Black Walnut hulls • Burdock root • Chickweed leaf & stem • Echinacea Purpurea stem, leaf, flower • Fennel seed • Hawthorne berry • Kelp (whole Thallus) • Licorice root • Papaya leaves • Parsley herb • Safflower flower. Other ingredients: Gelatin.

Herbal Tranquility — Optimum Nutrition
Valerian Root • Passion-flower extract.

Herbal Up Formula — Nature's Way
Two capsules contain: Bee Pollen • Cayenne pepper fruit • Gotu Kola stem, leaf • Proprietary Blend (840 mg) • Siberian Ginseng root. Other ingredients: Gelatin.

Herbal UR-Kidney — Nutri-Quest
Proprietary blend 430 mg: Juniper Berries • Parsley • Uva Ursi, Marshmallow • Ginger • Golden Seal root • Corn Silk • Cleavers root. In a base of 6X tissue salts: Mag Phos, Nat Sulph, Calc Phos, Calc Sulph.

Herbal V: Women's Formula — VitaZip, Inc.
Avena Sativa 10:1 Extract • Kava Kava 30% • Muira Puama 4:1 Extract • St. John's Wort .3% • Ginkgo Biloba 24%/6%.

Some Brand Name Natural Products - What they Contain
www.NaturalDatabase.com contains MANY more listings than appear here.

Herbal Water Control — Jamieson
Two capsules contain: Calcium (as Calcium Sulfate) 54 mg • Uva Ursi leaf (Arctostaghylos uva-ursi (L) Spreng) 400 mg • Buchu leaf (Barosma Betulina Bartl. Et Wendl.) 200 mg.

Herbal Women's Formula — Quest
Each caplet contains: White Willow bark powder (Salix alba) (Provided by 85 mg P.E. 1:12 standardized to contain 11% Salicin) 1000 mg • Valerian root (Valeriana officinalis) (Provided by 40 mg P.E. 1:5 standardized to contain 0.8% Valerenic Acid) 200 mg • Chamomile flower (Chamomilla recutita L.) (Provided by 20 mg P.E. 1:4 standardized to contain 1% Apigenin) 80 mg • Uva Ursi leaf (Arctostaphylos uva-ursi) (Provided by 50 P.E. 1:4 standardized to contain 10% Arbutin) 200 mg • Juniper berry (Juniperus communis) (Provided by 80 mg P.E. 1:4) 320 mg • Parsley root (Petroselinum crispum) (Provided by 40 mg P.E. 1:4) 160 mg. Other Ingredients: Calcium Phosphate, Croscarmellose Sodium, Magnesium Stearate (vegetable source), Microcrystalline Cellulose, Silicon Dioxide.

Herbalax — Health Factor
Each capsule contains: Cascara Sagrada (Rhamnus purshiana) 260 mg • Peppermint (Menta piperita) 90 mg.

Herbal-Biotic — The Herbalist
Oregon Grape Root • Golden Seal root • Yerba Mansa root.

Herbal-F — Progressive Labs
Each capsule contains: Vitamin B6 (as pyridoxine HCl) 20 mg • Magnesium (as magnesium oxide/soy protein complex) 15 mg • Damiana leaf (Turnera aphrodisiaca) 60 mg • Passion flower (Passiflora incarnata) 40 mg • Black Cohosh root (Cimicifuga racemosa) 20 mg • Blue Cohosh root (Caulophyllum thalictroides) 20 mg • Ginger root (Zingiber officinale) 60 mg • Cramp bark (Viburnum opulus) 75 mg • Wild Yam root (Dioscorea villosa) 40 mg • False Unicorn root (Chamaelirium luteum) 40 mg • Squaw vine (Mitchella repens) 40 mg • Blackhaw bark (Viburnum punifolium) 40 mg • Prickly Ash bark (Zanthoxylum americanum) 40 mg • White Birch bark (Betula alba) 40 mg • Ovarian substance 10 mg.

Herbalife - Activated Fiber Tablets — Herbalife
Each tablet contains: Sodium Choleate • L-Carnitine.

Herbalife - Aminogen — Herbalife
Each tablet contains: Aminogen 250 mg.

Herbalife - Body Contouring Cream — Herbalife
Water • Cetyl Esters • Isopropyl Myristate • Stearyl Alcohol • Hydrogenated Coco-glycerides • Steareth-20 • Caffeine • Propylene Glycol • Lecithin • Aminophylline • Imidazolidinyl • Urea • Methylparaben • Carbomer • Propylparaben • Triethanolamine • Algae • Magnolia Bark Extract • Fragrance • Horsetail Extract • Rose Hips Extract • Mate.

Herbalife - Cell-U-Loss — Herbalife
Each tablet contains: Vitamin C 250 mg • Potassium 297 mg • Iron 9 mg • Exclusive Combination (Buchu, Couch Grass, Cornsilk, Hydrangea, Juniper Berry, & Uva Ursi) 1000 mg • Lecithin 50 mg • Kelp 100 mg • Cider Vinegar 100 mg.

Herbalife - Herbal Aloe Drink — Herbalife
Water • Aloe Vera Juice • Sodium Citrate • Citric Acid • Potassium Sorbate • Chamomile • Sodium Benzoate.

Herbalife - NRG-Nature's Raw Guarana Instant Tea — Herbalife
Maltodextrins • Roasted Guarana Seed Extract • Pekoe Tea Extract • Lemon Peel Extract • Citric Acid.

Herbalife - NRG-Nature's Raw Guarana Tablets — Herbalife
Each tablet contains: Guarana powder (contains 4% naturally occuring caffeine) 800 mg.

Herbalife - Thermo Bond — Herbalife
Each tablet contains: Sodium Choleate • Fiber Blend (natural fibers from apple, grains, citrus, & cellulose).

Herbalife - Thermojetics Beige — Herbalife
Each tablet contains: English Hawthorn Berry fruit 80 mg • Alfalfa leaves 70 mg • Parsley leaves 60 mg • Marshmallow root 55 mg • Uva Ursi leaves 50 mg • Corn cornsilk 50 mg • Magnolia Bark bark 30 mg • Fennel seed 25 mg • Astragalus root 20 mg • Pfaffia root 20 mg • Pau d'Arco bark 20 mg • European Goldenrod leaves 15 mg • Licorice root 15 mg. Other Ingredients: Microcrystalene cellulose, tapioca & corn starches, stearic acid, cross-linked sodium carboxymethylcellulose, sodium starch glyconate, silicon dioxide, magnesium stearate, food grade shellac, hydroxypropyl methylcellulose, titianium dioxide, & carmel.

Herbalife - Thermojetics Green Refresh — Herbalife
Each tablet contains: Balu • Yerba Mate Extract • Bladderwrack • Meadowsweet • Garcinia Cambogia • Valerian Root • Green Tea Extract • Fumitory Herb • Honeysuckle • FD&C Blue No. 1 Lake.

Herbalife - Thermojetics Herbal Concentrate — Herbalife
Each serving contains: Camellia sinensis (Green Tea & Orange Pekoe Tea) Extract • Maltodextrin • Fructose • Malva Sylvestris Extract • Cardamom Extract • Hibiscus Extract • Lemon Peel Extract.

Herbalife - Thermojetics Original Green — Herbalife
Each tablet contains: Calcium (as calcium carbonate) 58 mg • Iodine (from bladderwrack) 30 mg • Chinese Ephedra leaf 140 mg • Yerba Mate leaf 115 mg • Dried MaHuang Extract whole 70 mg • Bladderwrack whole 40 mg • Valerian root 40 mg • Fumaria Officinalis whole 30 mg • Dried Salix purpurea Extract bark 30 mg • Chondrus crispus whole 5 mg. Other Ingredients: Stearic acid, tapioca starch, microcrystalline cellulose, papain, cross-linked sodium carboxymethylcellulose, silicon dioxide, sodium starch glyconate, magnesium stearate, sodium laurel sulfate, food grade shellac, titianium dioxide, polyethylene glycol, riboflavin, & blue #1.

Herbalife - Thermojetics Yellow — Herbalife
Each tablet contains: Garcinia (Garcinia Cambogia Extract) 400 mg • GTF Chromium (Chomium Polynicotinate) 400 mg.

Herbalist's Choice — The Herbalist
Gotu Kola herb • Guarana seed • Kola Nut • American Ginseng root • Licorice root • Damiana leaf • Echinacea root • Osha root • Cinnamon bark • Ginger root • Cayenne pepper.

Herbal-M — Progressive Labs
Each capsule contains: Vitamin E 30 IU • Zinc (as zinc oxide) 15 mg • Damiana leaf (Turnera aphrodisiaca) 60 mg • Siberian/Korean Ginseng blend (Eleutherococcus senticosus & Panax ginseng) • Cayenne (Capsicum annuum) 50 mg • Dong Quai (Angelica sinensis) 25 mg • Yohimbe (Pausinystalia johimbe) 10 mg • Muira Puama (Pytchopetalum olacoides) 10 mg • Goldenrod (Solidago virguarea) 10 mg • Orchic Substance 10 mg.

HerbaSlim — HerbaSway
St. John's Wort • Bitter Orange • Green Tea • Cassia tora • Panax Ginseng • Kudzu • Knotweed • Lycium • Cayenne pepper • Blackberry • HerbaSwee (Cucurbitaceae fruit).

Herbs & Prunes Formula — Nature's Life
Each tablet contains: Senna leaf (Senna alexandrina) 400 mg • Rhubarb root (Rheum officinale) 10 mg • Chinese Asparagus root (Tian dong, Asparagus cochinchinensis) 5 mg • Beet leaf (Beta vulgaris rubra) 5 mg • Buckthorn bark (Rhamnus frangula) 5 mg • Cabbage leaf (Brassica oleracea capitata) 5 mg • Cascara Sagrada (Rhamnus purshiana) 5 mg • Celery leaf (Apium graveolens) 5 mg • Cranberry (Vaccinium macrocarpon) 5 mg • Culvers root (Leptandra virginica) 5 mg • Dried Prune (Prunus aractus) 5 mg • Parsley leaf (Petroselinum crispum) 5 mg • Spinach leaf (Spinacia oleracea) 5 mg.

Herpalieve — Phytopharmica
Active ingredient: Allantoin 1% Other ingredients: Melissa extract (Lemon balm) (70:1) & white soft paraffin with benzyl alcohol

Herpanacine — Diamond Formulas
Six capsules contain: L-Lysine 1500 mg • A-Beta-Carotene 25000 IU • L-Tyrosine 500 mg • E-D-Alpha 200 IU • Selenium 100 mcg • Dandelion leaf • Sarsaparilla • Astragulus • Ligustrum • Echinacea.

Herpilyn — Enzymatic Therapy
Each 0.18 oz tube contains: Active ingredient: Allantoin 1%. Other ingredients: Melissa extract (Lemon Balm) 70:1 • White Soft Paraffin with Benzyl Alcohol.

Hi Energy Multi for Men — Futurebiotics
Three tablets contain: Beta Carotene 25,000 IU • Vitamin C (Ascorbic Acid, Palmitate) 250 mg • Vitamin D 200 IU • Vitamin E 60 IU • Vitamin B1 (Thiamin) 25 mg • Vitamin B2 (Riboflavin) 25 mg • Niacinamide 50 mg • Pantothenic Acid 25 mg • Vitamin B6 25 mg • Vitamin B12 100 mcg • Biotin 300 mcg • Folic Acid 400 mcg • Phosphatidyl Choline 100 mg • Inositol 75 mg • Ribonucleic Acid (RNA) 75 mg • Para Amino Benzoic Acid (PABA) 75 mg • Zinc (Monomethionine) 30 mg • Calcium (Phosphate, Citrate, Amino Acid

BRAND NAMES

© Copyright 2000, Natural Medicines Comprehensive Database (209) 472-2244. For updated data, go to www.NaturalDatabase.com.

BRAND NAMES

Chelate) 200 mg • Magnesium (Citrate, Amino Acid Chelate) 200 mg • Iron (Gluconate) 6 mg • Potassium (Citrate) 99 mg • Chromium (Polynicotinate) 200 mcg • Copper (Gluconate) 2 mg • Iodine (Kelp) 200 mcg • Manganese (Proteinate) 5 mg • Molybdenum (Amino Acid Chelate) 25 mcg • Selenium (Selenomethionine) 200 mcg. In a base of herbal extracts, powders & nutritional concentrates equivalent to 2,000 mg: Active Ginsenosides (from Standardized Ginseng Extract), Saw Palmetto, Avena Sativa, Ginseng, Hawthorn, Garlic (Odorless Extract), Bee Pollen, Foti, Adrenal Concentrate, Octacosanol (Wheat Free), Alfalfa Juice Concentrate & Spirulina.

Hi-B-100 Complex - Tablet — Nature's Life
Each tablet contains: Vitamin B1 (Thiamine Hydrochloride) 100 mg • Vitamin B2 (Riboflavin) 100 mg • Vitamin B6 (Pyridoxine Hydrochloride) 100 mg • Vitamin B12 (Cobalamin concentrate) 100 mcg • Folic Acid 400 mcg • Biotin 100 mcg • Niacinamide 100 mg • Pantothenic Acid (d-Calcium Pantothenate) 100 mg • Choline (Bitartrate) 100 mg • PABA (Para Aminobenzoic Acid) 100 mg • Inositol 100 mg. In a natural base of Alfalfa, Parsley, Rice Bran & Watercress.

Hi-B-100 Complex - Capsule — Nature's Life
Each capsule contains: Vitamin B1 (Thiamine HCl) 100 mg • Vitamin B2 (Riboflavin) 100 mg • Vitamin B6 (Pyridoxine HCl) 100 mg • Vitamin B12 (Cobalamin concentrate) 100 mcg • Niacinamide 100 mg • Pantothenic Acid (d-Calcium Pantothenate) 100 mg • Choline (Bitartrate) 100 mg • Inositol 100 mg • Biotin 100 mcg • Folic Acid 400 mcg • PABA (Para-Aminobenzioc Acid) 100 mg. In a natural base of Rice Bran.

High Potency Cal-Mag Plus — Quest
Each tablet contains: Calcium (Citrate) 250 mg • Magnesium (Oxide) 250 mg • Vitamin C (Ascorbic Acid) 150 mg • Vitamin D3 100 IU • Zinc (Citrate) 10 mg. Other Ingredients: Croscarmellose Sodium, Magnesium Stearate (vegetable source), Microcrystalline Cellulose, Silicon Dioxide, Vegetable Stearin.

Higher Mind — Source Naturals
Four tablets contain: Phosphatidyl Serine (Leci-PS) 150 mg • Vitamin B1 (Thiamin) 100 mg • Vitamin B2 (Riboflavin) 25 mg • Vitamin B3 (Inositol Hexanicotinate 100 mg and Niacin 50 mg) 150 mg • Vitamin B5 (Pantothenic Acid) 50 mg • Vitamin B6 (PAK and Pyridoxine HCl) 100 mg • Vitamin B12 50 mcg • Folic Acid 800 mcg • Biotin 50 mcg • Vitamin C (Calcium and Zinc Ascorbates) 200 mg • Calcium (Ascorbate, Carbonate, Malate, Succinate) 100 mg • Magnesium (Malate, Succinate, Taurinate, Oxide) 200 mg • Zinc (Ascorbate) 10 mg • Manganese (Citrate) 5 mg • L-Pyroglutamic Acid 750 mg • L-Glutamine 500 mg • Acetyl L-Carnitine 300 mg • DMAE (Bitartrate) 100 mg • Taurine (Magnesium Taurinate) 200 mg • DLPA (DL-Phenylalanine) 200 mg • Phosphatidyl Choline 157.5 mg • Phosphatidyl Ethanolamine 105 mg • N-Acetyl L-Tyrosine 100 mg • GABA (Gamma Amino Butyric Acid) 100 mg • PAK (Pyridoxine Alpha-Ketoglutarate) 100 mg • Ginkgo Biloba extract 24% (50:1) 50 mg • Phosphatidyl Inositol 45 mg • Alpha-Lipoic Acid (Thioctic Acid) 20 mg • Coenzyme Q10 (Ubiquinone) 10 mg • Inositol 10 mg.

HighFive — Pharmanex
Each tablet contains: Boswellia Serrata Extract (stem) 125 mg • Fungal Protease (Aspergillus Oryzae) 100 mg • Bromelain (from pineapple extract) 50 mg • Quercetin 25 mg • Papain (from papaya extract) 10 mg. Other Ingredients: Dicalcium Phosphate, Microcrystalline Cellulose, Cellulose Powder, Silica, Magnesium Stearate.

High-Potency Serum — Cellex-C
Ascorbic Acid • Tyrosine • Zinc • Sodium Hyaluronate • Bioflavonoids.

Hi-Potent-C (powdered) — Nutri-Quest
Each level teaspoonful contains: Vitamin C 1500 mg • Mannitol 1355 mg • Rose Hips 250 mg • Lemon Bioflavinoids 130 mg • Hesperidin Complex 50 mg • Rutin 35 mg • Acerola concentrate 35 mg • natural Flavor.

HMB — EAS
Each 4 capsule serving contains: HMB 1000 mg • Potassium Phosphate 200 mg.

HMB — Pro Performance
Each tablet contains: HMB • Calcium Hydroxymethyl Butyrate Monohydrate (HMB) 250 mg • Monopotassium Phosphate 50 mg.

Holista Echinacea — Holista
Each capsule contains: Echinacea angustifolia/purpurea (root) (16:1 extract) 500 mg.

Holista Echinacea Tincture — Holista
Each mL contains: Echinacea angustifolia dried root 1:1 standardized extract in alcohol 45% 200 mg.

Holista Evening Primrose Oil 1000 mg — Holista
Each capsule contains: Evening Primrose Oil (not less than 100 mg of gamma-linolenic acid and 700 mg of lenoleic acid) standardized to 10% GLA 1000 mg.

Holista Evening Primrose Oil 500 mg — Holista
Each capsule contains: Evening Primrose Oil (not less than 50 mg of gamma-linolenic acid and 350 mg of lenoleic acid) standardized to 10% GLA 500 mg.

Holista Feverfew — Holista
Each capsule contains: Feverfew (Tanacetum parthenium) standardized to a minimum of 0.2% parthenolide 125 mg.

Holista Lactase enzyme — Holista
Each capsule contains: Food Chemical Codex Lactase 3000 units.

Holista Milk Thistle — Holista
Each capsule contains: Milk Thistle (Silybum marianum) standardized to silymarin 80% 150 mg.

Holista Milk Thistle Tincture — Holista
Each mL contains: Milk Thistle seed from 1:1 fluid extract in 65% alcohol 0.2 mg.

Holista Saw Palmetto — Holista
Each caplet contains: Saw Palmetto (Serenoa repens) extract from berries 10:1 160 mg.

Holista Saw Palmetto Tincture — Holista
Each mL contains: Saw Palmetto dried berries of Seronoa repens 1:1 in 45% alcohol 0.2 mg.

Holista Tea Tree Oil 20% Lotion — Holista
Tea Tree oil (Melaleuca alternifolia) 0.2 mL. Other Ingredients: Water, Alcohol.

Holista Valerian — Holista
Each capsule contains: Valerian Root Extract standardized to 0.8% Valerenic Acid 500 mg.

Holista Valerian Tincture — Holista
Each mL contains: Valerian Root from the rhizome and roots of Valeriana officianalis 1:1 in 60% alcohol 0.2 mg.

Holista Zinc Lozenges — Holista
Each lozenge contains: Zinc (citrate) 5 mg • Echinacea 50 mg • Vitamin C 50 mg.

Homocysteine De-Crease — Nutri-Quest
Each tablet contains: Trimethylglycine 300 mg • Pyridoxal 5 Phosphate 5 mg (enteric coated) • Vitamin B12 200 mcg • Dimethyl Gluyine 25 mg • Niacinamide 20 mg • Cysteine 15 mg • Molybdenum Chelate 30 mcg • Selenium Chelate 15 mcg • Vitamin B6 15 mg (enertic coated) • Folic Acid 275 mg • Vitamin E Succinate 10 IU • Red Beet root 25 mg • Choline Bitartrate 10 mg • Magnesium Chelate 100 mg • Zinc Chelate 10 mg.

Homocysteine Formula — Nature's Life
Each capsule contains: Vitamin B6 (Pyridoxine HCl) 10 mg • Folic Acid 800 mcg • Vitamin B12 400 mcg • Choline (Bitartrate) 50 mg • Betaine HCl 50 mg.

Homocysteine Regulators — Now
Each Vcap contains: Vitamin B6 (as Coenzyme Pyridoxyl-5-Phosphate) 20 mg • Vitamin B12 (as Cyanocobalamin) 250 mcg • Folic Acid 800 mcg • Trimethylglycine (Betaine) 400 mg.

HomocystexPlus with TMG & TroxeRutin — Natrol
One capsule contains: Riboflavin (Vitamin B2) 25 mg • Vitamin B6 (as pyridoxine HCl) 25 mg • Folic Acid 800 mcg • Vitamin B12 (as cobalamin) 500 mcg • Betaine TMG (as betaine trimethylglycine) 500 mg • TroxeRutin 100 mg • Choline (as choline bitartrate) 25 mg. Other ingredients: Silicon Dioxide, Magnesium Stearate, Gelatin.

Honey Apple Double Ginseng — Traditional Medicinals
Asian Ginseng root (Panax ginseng) • American Ginseng root (Panax quinquefolius) • Siberian Ginseng root (Eleutherococcus senticosus) •

Some Brand Name Natural Products - What they Contain
www.NaturalDatabase.com contains MANY more listings than appear here.

Chamomile flower • Licorice root • Orange peel • dried Apples • Prince Ginseng rootlets (Pseudostellada heterophylla) • Natural Honey & Apple flavors.

Honey C Chews Chewable C 100 mg — Nature's Life
Each wafer contains: Vitamin C (Buffered) 100 mg • Rose Hips powder (Rosa canina) 50 mg • Acerola berry powder (Malpighia glabra) 25 mg.

Honey C Chews Chewable C 300 mg — Nature's Life
Each wafer contains: Vitamin C (Buffered) 300 mg • Rose Hips powder (Rosa canina) 50 mg • Acerola berry powder (Malpighia glabra) 25 mg.

Hops, Valerian & Scullcap — Dial Herbs
Hops • Valerian • Scullcap.

Hormogen — Atrium
Each capsule contains: Lecithin 200 mg • Safflower oil 200 mg • Wheat Germ oil (Cold Pressed) 66.667 mg • Rice Bran oil 66.667 mg • Soybean oil 66.667 mg. Contains no sugar, starch, salt, wheat, corn, yeast, or soy derivatives.

Horse Chestnut Herbal Balm — Nature's Life
Deionized Water • Horse Chestnut seed extract [(Aesculus hippocastanum L.) standardized to 2% aescin] • Phospholipids from Safflower & Sunflower seed oil • Caprylic/Capric Triglyceride • Apricot Kernel oil • Soy Lecithin • Glycerine (Vegetable) • Tocopherol (natural Vitamin E) • Arnica extract • Panthenol • Saccharide Isomerate • Xanthan Gum • Carrageenan (Irish Moss) • Dimethicone • Lauroyl Lysine • Natural Fragrant Essential Oils Blend • Sodium Hydroxymethylglycinate.

Horsetail Extract Formula — Quest
Each caplet contains: Horsetail powder (Equisetum arvense) (provided by 125 mg 1:4 Aqueous Extract) 500 mg • Rosehips powder (Rose canina) 50 mg • Burdock root powder (Arctium lappa) 30 mg • Marshmallow root powder (Althaea officinalis) 30 mg • Parsley leaf powder (Plantago major) 30 mg • Slippery Elm bark powder (Ulmus fulva) 30 mg. Other Ingredients: Calcium Phosphate, Microcrystalline Cellulose, Croscarmellose Sodium, Magnesium Stearate (vegetable source), Vegetable Stearin.

Horsetail Plus Fo-Ti — The Herbalist
Horsetail fresh-dried herb (Equisetum arvense)• Fo-Ti fresh-dried root (Polygonum multiforum)• Nettles fresh-dried leaf (Urtica dioica)• Red Clover fresh-dried blossom (Trifolium pratense)• Burdock fresh-dried root (Arctium lappa).

Hot Flash — Source Naturals
Three tablets contain: Soy concentrate, yielding 65 mg Isoflavones 2100 mg • Black Cohosh 160 mg • Dong Quai extract 150 mg • Licorice root extract 150 mg • Vitex extract 100 mg.

Hot Flashex — Natrol
One tablet contains: Vitamin E (as d-alpha tocopherol) 50 IU • Calcium (as tri-calcium phosphate) 70 mg • Licorice 100 mg • Black Cohosh root 60 mg, Triterpenes (2.5%) 15 mg • Chamomile extract 50 mg • Kava Kava root 30 mg, Kavalactones (30%) 9 mg. Other ingredients: Mono & Di-Glycerides, Croscarmellose Sodium, Silicon Dioxide, Stearic Acid, Magnesium Stearate.

Hoxsey Formula — The Herbalist
Red Clover fresh-dried blossoms (Trifolium pratense)• Chapparal fresh-dried leaf (Larrea tridentata)• Licorice fresh-dried root (Glycyrrhiza glabra)• Oregon Grape fresh-dried root (Berberis nervosa)• Burdock fresh-dried root (Arcticum lappa)• Sarsaparilla fresh-dried root (Smilax ornata)• Echinacea fresh root (Echinacea angustifolia)• Prickly Ash fresh-dried bark (Zanthoxylum americanum).

Human Growth Hormone (HGH) — Youngevity
Each capsule contains: L-Lysine HCL • L-Arginine • L-Ornithine • L-Glutamine • L-Tyrosine • Vilcabamba Mineral Essence: Potassium, Calcium, Magnesium, Zinc, Chromium, Selenium, Iron, Copper, Molybdenum, Vanadium, Iodine, Cobalt, Manganese.

Huperzine A Ginkgo/Ginseng — Nutrapharm, Inc.
Each capsule contains: Huperzine A 50 mcg • Ginkgo biloba extract 60 mg • Panax ginseng extract 150 mg. Other Ingredients: Malto dextrin, magnesium stearate, microcrystalline cellulose, & silica. Free of sugar, yeast, milk, artificial colors, flavors & dyes.

Huperzine A w/Ginkgo — Nutrapharm, Inc.
Each capsule contains: Huperzine A 50 mcg • Ginkgo biloba extract 60 mg. Other Ingredients: Malto dextrin, magnesium stearate, microcrystalline cellulose, & silica. Free of sugar, yeast, corn, milk, artificial colors, flavors & dyes.

Huperzine A w/Ginseng — Nutrapharm, Inc.
Each capsule contains: Huperzine A 50 mcg • Panax ginseng extract (standardized to 8% ginsenosides) 150 mg. Other Ingredients: Malto dextrin, magnesium stearate, microcrystalline cellulose, & silica. Free of sugar, yeast, corn, milk products, artificial colors, flavors & dyes.

Huperzine A w/Vitamin E — Nutrapharm, Inc.
Each capsule contains: Huperzine A 50 mcg • Vitamin E (D-alpha tocopheryl acetate) 100 IU. Other Ingredients: Malto dextrin, magnesium stearate, & silica. Free of sugar, yeast, corn, milk, artificial colors, flavors & dyes.

HY 2 — Pacific BioLogic
St. John's Wort.

Hydra Cleanse — Pharmagel
Aloe Vera • A complex of marine-based extracts of Seaweed, Algae, and Spirulina • Oat extract • Beta Glucan • Panthenol.

Hydra Fuel (The Ultimate Fluid Replacement Sports Drink) — TwinLab
Glucose Polymers & Glucose (approximately 5%) • Fructose (about 2%). Replenishes important Electrolytes & Minerals (Sodium, Potassium, Magnesium, Chloride, Chromium & Phosphorus).

Hydroxycut — Muscletech
Four capsules contain: Hydroxagen (supplying 100 mg of Hydroxycitric Acid) 2000 mg • MaHuang extract 334 mg • Guarana extract 910 mg • Willow bark extract 100 mg • L-Carnitine 100 mg • Chromium Picolinate 300 mcg.

Hy-Gear — Met-Rx
Each 40 g serving contains: Creatine Monohydrate 5 g, Carbohydrate 34 g, Ingredients: Citrus Mist flavor: CeraSport (Rice Syrup Solids, Sodium Chloride, Potassium Chloride & Trisodium Citrate) • Fructose • Creatine Monohydrate • Glucose • Natural & Artificial Flavors • Citric Acid • Malic Acid • Beta Carotene & Beet juice powder for color. Strazzyberry Flavor: CeraSport (Rice Syrup Solids, Sodium Chloride, Potassium Chloride & Trisodium Citrate) • Fructose • Creatine Monohydrate • Glucose • Natural & Artificial Flavors • Beet juice powder for color.

HyperiCalm — Enzymatic Therapy
Each capsule contains: St. John's Wort (Hypericum perforatum) extract standardized to 0.3% hypericins (900 mcg) & 4% hyperforin (12 mg), verified by HPLC 300 mg. Contains no sugar, salt, yeast, wheat, corn, soy, dairy products, coloring, flavoring, or preservatives.

HyperiMed — Phytopharmica
Each capsule contains: St. John's Wort (Hypericum perforatum) extract standardized to 0.3% hypericins (900 mcg) & 4% hyperforin (12 mg), verified by HPLC 300 mg. Contains no sugar, salt, yeast, wheat, corn, soy, dairy products, coloring, flavoring, or preservatives.

Hypertension Support — Amazon Support
Each capsule contains: Abuta • Artichoke • Bitter Melon • Chanca Piedra • Graviola • Jurubeba • Mullaca • Suma • Periwinkle • Stevia • Pedra hume caa.

Hypo-Ade — Enzymatic Therapy
Two tablets contain: Vitamin A (Fish Liver oil) 5000 IU • Vitamin C (Ascorbic Acid) 200 mg • Niacin/Niacinamide 115 mg • Potassium Chloride 100 mg • Pantothenic Acid (D-Calcium Pantothenate) 100 mg • Thiamine HCL (Vitamin B1) 25 mg • Riboflavin (Vitamin B2) 25 mg • Vitamin B6 (Pyridoxine HCL) 25 mg • Zinc (Oxide) 10 mg • Manganese (Gluconate) 10 mg • Chromium (Polynicotinate) 267 mcg • Vitamin B12 (Cyanocobalamin) 25 mcg • Other ingredients: Inositol 200 mg • Pancreas extract 150 mg • Choline Bitartrate 100 mg • L-Methionine 100 mg • Green Beet leaf powder 100 mg • Adrenal extract 65 mg • Betaine HCL 50 mg • Wild Yam 50 mg • Pituitary extract 40 mg • Barberry, Bark of root extract (4:1) (Berberis vulgaris) 30 mg. This exclusive formulation also contains Dandelion (Taraxacum officinale), Goldenseal (Hydrastis canadensis), Raw Liver, Raw Lung, Raw Pancreas, Raw Heart, Raw Kidney, Raw Spleen, & Raw Brain. Contains no sugar, salt, yeast, wheat, corn, soy, dairy products, coloring, flavoring or preservatives.

BRAND NAMES

Some Brand Name Natural Products - What they Contain
www.NaturalDatabase.com contains MANY more listings than appear here.

B R A N D N A M E S

Hyporil — Phytopharmica
Two tablets contain: Vitamin A (Fish Liver oil) 5000 IU • Vitamin C (Ascorbic Acid) 200 mg • Niacin/Niacinamide 115 mg • Potassium Chloride 100 mg • Pantothenic Acid (D-Calcium Pantothenate) 100 mg • Thiamine HCL (Vitamin B1) 25 mg • Riboflavin (Vitamin B2) 25 mg • Vitamin B6 (Pyridoxine HCL) 25 mg • Zinc (Oxide) 10 mg • Manganese (Gluconate) 10 mg • Chromium (Polynicotinate) 267 mcg • Vitamin B12 (Cyanocobalamin) 25 mcg • Other ingredients: Inositol 200 mg • Pancreas extract 150 mg • Choline Bitartrate 100 mg • L-Methionine 100 mg • Green Beet leaf powder 100 mg • Adrenal extract 65 mg • Betaine HCL 50 mg • Wild Yam 50 mg • Pituitary extract 40 mg • Barberry bark of root extract 4:1 (Berberis vulgaris) 30 mg. This exclusive formulation also contains Dandelion (Taraxacum officinale), Goldenseal (Hydrastis canadensis), Raw Liver, Raw Lung, Raw Pancreas, Raw Heart, Raw Kidney, Raw Spleen & Raw Brain. Contains no sugar, salt, yeast, wheat, corn, soy, dairy products, coloring, flavoring, or preservatives.

Iberogast — Phytopharmica
Active Ingredients: Proprietary blend of the following herbal extracts 1 mL: Clown's mustard plant (Iberis amara) Chamomile flower (Matricariae flos) Angelica root (Angelicae radix) Caraway fruit (Carvi fructus) Milk thistle fruit (Cardui mariae fructus) Melissa leaf (Melissae folium) Celandine herbs (Chelidonii herba) Licorice root (Liquiritiae radix) Peppermint leaf (Menthae pipertae folium) Other Ingredients: Water & alcohol, 31%

IGF Fuel — TwinLab
Two capsules contain: DHEA (dehydroepiandrosterone) 50 mg • Zinc (from zinc picolinate) 50 mg • L-Glutamine 2000 mg.

Immortale for Men — Roex
Each tablet contains: Tribulus Terrestris 250 mg • Panax ginseng 50 mg • Damiana 50 mg • Avena sativa 100 mg • Sarsaparilla 50 mg.

Immortale for Women — Roex
Each tablet contains: Tribulus Terrestris 250 mg • Panax ginseng 50 mg • Damiana 50 mg • Avena sativa 100 mg • Dong Quai 50 mg.

IMMU-C — Nutri-Quest
Each tablet contains: Vitamin C (Sago Palm) 500 mg • Rutin 15 mg • Lemon Bioflavonoids 15 mg • Hesperidin Complex 15 mg • Tissue concentrates (not extracts) of Bovine Source from Lymph, Thymus, Spleen • 5X Propolis 2 mg.

Immuguard — Optimum Nutrition
Echinacea Angustifolia extract • Goldenseal root

Immumax-Rx — Alternecare Health Products
Each tablet contains: Bee Propolis 50 mg • Shiitake Mushroom 50 mg • Reishi Mushroom 50 mg • Garlic 25 mg • Suma 25 mg • Red Clover 25 mg • Pau d'Arco 25 mg • Milk Thistle 25 mg • Shark Cartilage 15 mg • Golden Seal 25 mg • Siberian Ginseng 25 mg • Echinacea 25 mg • Astralagus 25 mg • N-Acetyl Cysteine 15 mg • Zinc 15 mg • L-Glutathione 15 mg • CO Q10 5 mg.

ImmunACE — Nature's Plus
Two tablets contain: Vitamin C corn free 1000 mg • Vitamin E natural 400 IU • Beta Carotene pro-vitamin A, supplying Vitamin A 20000 IU • Zinc Amino Acid Chelate 300 mg, supplying Elemental Zinc 30 mg • L-Cysteine free form amino acid 200 mg • Iron Amino Acid Chelate 180 mg, supplying Elemental Iron 18 m • Selenium Amino Acid Complex 100 mg, supplying Elemental Selenium 200 mcg • Folic Acid 200 mcg. In a natural base of Pau D'Arco, Chlorophyll, Echinacea, Thyme, Juniper berry, Korean Ginseng, Irish Moss & Rosemary. Yeast free. Sugar & starch free.

ImmunActin Throat Syrup — Nature's Plus
Vegetable Glycerine • Exclusive Liposomal Herbal Complex [Elderberry extract (Sambucus canadensis fruit) (standardized 30% Falvonoids), Echinacea extract (Echinacea angustifolia root & rhizome) (standardized 4% Echinacosides), Slippery Elm (Ulmus rubra bark) (naturally rich in Phytosterols, Sesquitepenes & Mucilage), Goldenseal extract (Hydrastis canadensis root) (standardized 10% Alkaloids, 5% Hydrastine), White Willow extract (Salix alba bark) (standardized 7-9% Salicin), Astragalus extract (Astragalus membranaceus root) (standardized 0.4% 4'-Hydroxy-3'-Methoxyisoflavone 7-Sug), Schisandra extract (Schisandra chinensis fruit) (standardized 9% schisandrins), Zinc Gluconate] • Wild Clover • Honey • Methol • natural Cherry flavor.

ImmunActinB — Nature's Plus
Two capsules contain: Vitamin C corn free 300 mg • Vitamin E

natural 100 IU • Echinacea [(Echinacea angustifolia root & rhizome) standardized 4% Echinacosides] 50 mg • Astragalus [(Astragalus membranaceus root) standardized 0.4% 4'-Hydroxy-3'-Methoxyisoflavone 7-Sug] 50 mg • Chinese Green Tea [(Camellia sinensis leaf) decaffeinated, standardized 20% Polyphelols] 50 mg • Tumeric [(Curcuma longa rhizome) standardized 95% Curcumin] 50 mg • Garlic odor-modified [(Allium sativum clove) standardized 0.35% Allicin, 0.65% Allicin, 0.40% Thiosulfinates, 0.085% Allyl Mercaptan] 50 mg • Schisandra [(Schisandra chinensis fruit) standardized 9% Schisandrins] 25 mg • Pau D'Arco [(Tabebuia impetiginosa bark) standardized 3% Naphthoquinones] 25 mg • Goldenseal [(Hydrastis canadensis root & rhizome) standardized 10% Alkaloids, 5% Hydrastine] 25 mg • Shiitake Mushroom [(Lentinus edodes mycelia) standardized 3.2% KS-2 Polysaccharides (peptidomannan)] 15 mg • Zinc (Monomethionine) 15 mg • Beta Carotene (supplying 10000 IU of Vitamin A activity) 6 mg • Grape seed [(Vitis vinifera) standardized 95% Proanthocyanidins] 5 mg • Bioperine [(Piper nigrum fruit) standardized 95% 1-Piperoylpiperidine] 5 mg.

Immune Actives — VitaStore
Each tablet contains: Echinacea 500 mg • Goldenseal 250 mg • Beta Carotene (Vitamin A) 2500 IU • Zinc Gluconate 30 mg • Vitamin C 120 mg • Licorice 150 mg • Astralagus 145 mg • Grapeseed Extract 50 mg • Green Tea 200 mg • Garlic 300 mg • L-Lysine 500 mg.

Immune Defense — ProHerbs
Two tablets contain: Vitamin C (Ascorbic Acid) 500 mg • Vitamin E (DI-Alpha Tocopherol Acetate) 400 IU • Zinc (as Sulfate) 15 mg • Selenium (as Selenomethionine) 200 mcg • ActiVin Grape Seed extract (Vitis vinifera seeds standardized to 95% polyphenols) 100 mg • Echinacea root (Echinacea purpurea) 100 mg • Alpha Lipoic Acid (standardized to 4% phenolic compounds) 50 mg. Other Ingredients: Dicalcium Phosphate, Croscarmellose Sodium, Hydroxypropylmethylcellulose, Magnesium Stearate, Microcrystalline Cellulose, Mineral Oil, Polyethylene Glycol, Silicon Dioxide, Stearic Acid, Titanium Dioxide, Sodium Lauryl Sulfate, FD&C Yellow, #6 Lake, Yellow #10 Lake.

Immune Formula — Nature's Life
Three tablets contain: Antioxidant Vitamins: Beta Carotene [(Dunaliella salina) equivalent to 25000 IU Vitamin A] 15 mg • Other naturally occurring carotenoids in D. salina: Alpha Carotene (equivalent to 393 IU Vitamin A) 473 mcg • Cryptoxanthin (equivalent to 96 IU Vitamin A) 116 mcg • Zeaxanthin 95 mcg • Lutein 74 mcg • Vitamin C (Calcium Ascorbate) 1000 mg • Vitamin E (d-Alpha Tocopheryl Succinate) 200 IU. Other Nutrients: Vitamin A (Retinyl Palmitate) 8000 IU • Vitamin B6 (Pyridoxine HCl) 50 mg • Vitamin B12 (Cobalamin) 100 mcg • Folic Acid 400 mcg • Selenium (I-Selenomethionine) 100 mcg • Zinc (Citrate) 25 mg • Copper (Citrate) 2 mg • Medical Herbs: Echinacea purpurea root (Trout Lake Farm Certified Organically Grown) 500 mg •Korean Ginseng root extract [(Panax ginseng) standardized to 10% ginsenosides] 100 mg • Natural Base: Lemon Bioflavonoid Complex (50% active flavonols) 100 mg.

Immune Guardian — Clinician's Choice
Three tablets contain: Vitamin C (ascorbic acid, calcium ascorbate) 150 mg • Vitamin E (dl-alpha tocopheryl acetate) 90 IU • Zinc (amino acid chelate) 90 IU • Selenium (selenomethionine) 150 mcg • Echinacea Angustifolia 450 mg • Echinacea Purpurea Root 300 mg • Golden Seal Root 150 mg • Kudzu Root 150 mg • Odor Modified Garlic Bulb 150 mg • Bee Pollen 150 mg • RoseOx (patented, standardized process for an extract of Rosemary) 90 mg • Ascorbyl Palmitate 75 mg • Schizandra Fruit 75 mg • Proptietary blend 15 mg: Beta-Carotene, Reishi Mushroom, Shiitake Mushroom, Cinnamon Bark, Grape Powder.

Immune Support — Amazon Support
Each capsule contains: Cat's Claw • Suma • Avenca • Samambaia • Simauba • Chanca Piedra • Mullaca • Macela • Pau d'arco • Yerba Mate.

Immune System — Nutrivention
Each tablet contains: Vitamin A 5000 IU • Pantothenic Acid 25 mg • Vitamin B6 25 mg • Vitamin C 20 mg • Vitamin B1 18 mg • Vitamin B2 18 mg • Vitamin E 15 IU • Inositol 15 mg • Choline 8 mg • Magnesium 5 mg • Zinc 5 mg • Folic Acid 400 mcg • Selenium 50 mcg • Echinacea 100 mg • Astralagus 100 mg • L-Cysteine 100 mg • Suma 100 mg • Codonopis 75 mg • Rei-Shi Mushroom 75 mg • White Astractylodes 50 mg • Schizandra berries 50 mg • Privet berries 50

Some Brand Name Natural Products - What they Contain
www.NaturalDatabase.com contains MANY more listings than appear here.

mg • Watercress 50 mg • Shiitake Mushroom 50 mg • Juniper berries 50 mg.

Immune System Booster Formula — Cambridge Nutraceuticals
Each serving contains: Glutamine 10 g • Vitamin A (as mixed carotenoids) 6500 IU • Vitamin C 200 mg • Vitamin E 125 IU • Selenium 70 mcg • N-Acetyl-Cysteine 600 mg. Available in 650 g jar or single dose packets.

Immune-Action — Nature's Plus
Each capsule contains: Astragalus root 200 mg • Ligustrum berries 100 mg • Schisandra berries 100 mg • Shiitake Mushrooms 100 mg • Echinacea root 100 mg • Young Barley leaves 50 mg • Pau D'Arco bark 50 mg. Contains no yeast, wheat, corn, soy, milk, salt, sugar or starch.

Immunectar — Nature's Plus
Two tablespoons contain: Egg Yolk Lecithin 2000 mg & Phosphatidylcholine 250 mg, The above combination supplies: Neutral Lipids 60%, Phosphatidylcholine 20%, Phosphatidylethanolamine 3% • Colostrum Whey, naturally rich in immunoglobulins, nucleotides, gamma interferon, enzymes & vitamins 150 mg • SUMA (Pfaffia paniculata [Martius] Kuntze root) 150 mg • Chlorella 150 mg • Astragalus (Astragalus membranaceus root) 75 mg • Ligustrum (Ligustrum lucidum berries) 75 mg • Echinacea (Echinacea angustifolia root) 75 mg • Schisandra (Schisandra chinensis berries) 75 mg • Shiitake (Lentinus edodes mushrooms) 75 mg • Coenzyme Q10 15 mg.

Immun-Eeze — Allergy Limited
Each capsule and lozenge together contain: Vitamin C (as ascorbic acid) 250 mg • Thiamin (as thiamine mononitrate) 25 mg • Riboflavin 25 mg • Niacin (as niacinamide) 20 mg • Vitamin B6 (as pyridoxine HCL) 25 mg • Vitamin B12 (as cyanocobalamin) 3 mg • Manganese (as manganese citrate) 6 mg. Other ingredients: Maltodextrin, sucrose, gelatin, vegetable derived magnesium stearate, croscarmellose sodium, silicon dioxide.

Immunene — PhysioLogics
Each capsule contains: Cats Claw inner bark (Una de Gato) (2% Oxindole Alkaloids, 2 mg) 100 mg • Astragalus (70% Polysaccharides, 70 mg) 100 mg • Reishi (4% Triterpenes, 2 mg; 10% Polysaccharides, 5mg) 50 mg • Shiitake 50 mg • Shiitake extract (3.2% KS-2, 3.2mg) 10 mg • Maitake 10 mg.

Immunoboost — Shawnee Moon
Peony root • Gotu Kola • Chrysanthemum • Astragalus • Licorice • Kelp • Suma • Pau d'arco • Red Clover.

Immunocal — Immunotec
100% Milk Whey Protein.

ImmunoFin — LaneLabs
G-E Lipids 50 mg • Shark Liver Oil 250 mg.

IMMU-Power — Nutri-Quest
Each tablet contains: Tissue concentrate (not an extract) from Thymus 60 mg • Vitamin A (Palmitate) 300 IU • Vitamin B6 15 mg • Niacin 10 mg • Pantothenic Acid 55.5 mg • Vitamin B12 200 mcg • Folic Acid 150 mcg • Vitamin C (Sago Palm) 150 mg • Natural Vitamin E (Succinate) 70 IU • Suma 7 mg • ISB Complex 107 mg includes: Magnesium, Selenium, SOD Type G, Zinc, Echinacea purpurea, Goldenseal, L-Cysteine HCL, L-Ornithine, Ferric Phosphate, Garlic & L-Aspartic Acid & natural Flavor.

I-MNS — Dial Herbs
Black Cohosh • Blue Cohosh • Red Raspberry • Catnip • Wild Yam • Wild Carrot • Motherwort • Pennyroyal • St. John's Wort.

Imperial Green Tea — Jamieson
Each tea bag contains: Chinese Green Tea leaf (Camellia sinensis) • Ginger root (Singiber officinale) • Leechee fruit (Litchi chinensis).

InflamActin — Nature's Plus
Two capsules contain: Boswellin [(Boswellia serrata gum resin) (standardized 65% Boswellic Acids)] 250 mg • Bromelain (standardized 90 Gelatin Digesting Units) 150 mg • DLPA (dl-Phenylalanine) (Free Form Amino Acid) 100 mg • Turmeric [(Curcuma longa rhizome) standardized 95% Curcumin] 75 mg • Vitamin C corn free 60 mg • St. John's Wort [(Hypericum perforatum flower) (standardized 0.3-0.5% Hypericin)] 50 mg • Chamomile [(Matricaria recutita flower) standardized 1% Apigenin, 0.5% Essential oil] 50 mg • Feverfew [(Tanacetum parthenium leaf) standardized 0.7% Parthenolide] 50 mg • Goldenseal [(Hydrastis canadensis root & rhizome) standardized 10% Alkaloids, 5% Hydrastine] 25 mg • Ginger [(Zingiber officinale root) standardized 4% Volatile oils] 25 mg.

InflamActin Cream — Nature's Plus
Active ingredient: Methyl Salicylate 18%. Other Ingredients: Exclusive Liposomal Herbal Complex [Boswellin (Boswellia serrata gum resin extract) (standardized 65% Boswellic Acids), Tumeric rhizome extract (Curcuma longa) (standardized 95% Curcumin), Gorgonian extract (Pseudopterogoria elisbethae leaf) (standardized 4% Pseudopterosin), & natural Vitamin E] in a vanishing Liposomal Cream Base.

Inflamase — Progressive Labs
Each capsule contains: Enteric release phase: Pancreatin 100 mg • Lipase 10 mg • Amylase 10 mg • Trypsin 200 mg • Alpha Chymotrypsin 2 mg. Gastric release phase: Bromelain 100 mg • Catalase 25 mcg • Superoxide Dismutase 25 mcg. The two phase pH sensitive release of the ingredients in this product is due to its exclusive enteric matrix formulation.

Inholtra — Omni Nutraceuticals
Two Quicksorb gels contain: Vitamin C (as Ascorbyl Palmitate) 1 mg • Vitamin E (as D-Alpha Tocopherol) 7 IU • Manganese (as Manganese Aspartate) 0.60 mg • Omega-3 fatty acid (Eicosapentainoic Acid 400 mg and Docosahexaenoic Acid 300 mg) 465 mg • D-Glucosamine Sulfate 335 mg • N-Acetyl D-Glucosamine 335 mg • Omega-6 fatty acid (as Gamma-Linolenic Acid) 135 mg. Other Ingredients: Vegetable Oil, Fish Oil, Gelatin, Glycerin, Carob, Water.

Instant Soy'n Whey — Next Nutrition
One serving contains: Water-Extracted Soy Protein concentrate • Non-Denatured Whey Protein concentrate • Fructose • Natural Vanilla flavoring • Lecithin • Modified Food starch • Malic acid • Cellulose gum • Kudzu extract • Momordica extract • Stevia • Vitamin E.

Intensive Therapy Support — Amazon Support
Each capsule contains: Graviola • Cat's Claw (3% standardized extract) • Pau d'arco (4:1 extract) • Suma (5% standardized extract) • Bitter Melon (4:1 extract) • Espinheira Santa (leaf & bark) • Mullaca • Mutamba • Vassourinha.

IntestaLife — Holista
Each capsule contains: 4 billion active cells specially cultured strains of Lactobacillus Rhamnosus • Lactobacillus acidophilus • Bifido longum.

Intestamend — Health From The Sun
Three capsules contain: Protein 1 g • Calcium 24 mg • Glutamine 200 mg • Lysine 132 mg • Leucine 103 mg • Methionine 49 mg • Threonine 59 mg • Valine 69 mg • Trypophane 11 mg • Isoleucine 60 mg • Phenylalanine 48 mg. Ingredients: Deep-Ocean White Fish, Gelatin, Glycerine, Water, natural Rosemary flavor.

Intestinal Fortitude — Nutri-Quest
Each tablet contains: L-Glutamine 150 mg • Buffered Vitamin C (Sago) 25 mg • N-Acetyl Glucosamine 75 mg • Vitamin E Succinate 10 IU • Lipoic Acid 2 mg • Ginkgo Biloba extract 2 mg • Deglycerrized Licorice 50 mg • Slippery Elm 100 mg • Lactobacilus Acidophilus 1 million IU • Cats Claw 15 mg • Ginkgo Biloba herb 50 mg • Jerusalem Artichoke 25 mg • Zinc Chelate 5 mg • Lactobacillus Bifidus 1 million IU.

Intestinal Rescue — The Herbalist
Psyllium seed & husk • Guar gum • Ginger root • Medical Grade Pectin • Bentonite clay • Rhubarb root • Cinnamon bark.

INTLECS Huperzine A — Intlecs
Each tablet contains: Huperzine A (Chinese club moss, Huperzia serrata) 50 mcg.

Intrasound Cleanse Formula — TriStar Online
Each scoop contains: Maltodextrin • Calcium Citrate • Natural Flavors • Magnesium Citrate • Gum • Citric Acid • Beta Carotene Gum • Stevia • Rebaudiana Extract • Soy Lethicin • Beet Powder • Lactobacillus Acidophilus • Lactobacillus Bifidus • Frutooligosaccarides • Papaya Powder • Prune Powder • Ascorbic Acid • Barley Sprout Powder • Wheat Sprout Powder • Oat Sprout Powder • Fenugreek. Fiber blend: Oat Fiber, Cellulose Gel/Cellulose, Purified Cellulose, Partially Hydrolyzed Soy Fiber, Psyllium Husk, Rice Bran, Citrus Pectin.

© Copyright 2000, Natural Medicines Comprehensive Database (209) 472-2244. For updated data, go to www.NaturalDatabase.com. • 1351

Some Brand Name Natural Products - What they Contain
www.NaturalDatabase.com contains MANY more listings than appear here.

**B
R
A
N
D**

**N
A
M
E
S**

Intrasound Energy Drink — TriStar Online
Whole leaf aloe • Purified water • Natural Flavor • Fructose • Kaolin Clay • Trace Minerals • Citric Acid • Stevia • Xanthan Gum • Fiber • Ginseng Extract • Sage Extract • Dandelion Extract • Potassium Gluconate • Sodium Benzoate • Potassium Sorbate.

Intrasound Enzyme Formulas — TriStar Online
Each capsule contains: Amylase • Lipase • Protease • Cellulase • Intervase or Sucrase • Lactase • Malt Diastase • Calcium Citrate • Kaolin Clay • Beef Gelatin Capsule.

Intrasound Gel — TriStar Online
Generic Conductive Gel • Kaolin Clay

Intrasound Herbal Accelerator — TriStar Online
Each capsule contains: Lipase • Cellulase • Amylase • Protease • Chromium Picolinate • Chromium Polynicotinate • Garcinia Cambogia Extract • Sida Cordifolia Herb • Yerba Mate • Kola Nut • Bladderwrack Algae • Cayenne Pepper • Siberian Ginseng Root.

Intrasound Mouth Rinse — TriStar Online
Whole leaf aloe • Purified Water • Natural Flavor • Kaolin Clay • Chlorophyll • Stevia • Sodium Benzoate.

Intrasound Powder — TriStar Online
Kaolin Clay

Intrasound Tooth Gel — TriStar Online
Whole Leaf Aloe • Purified Water • Glycerin • Carrageenan (seaweed) • Hydrated Silica • Sodium Lauroyl Sarcosinate • Chlorophyll • Kaolin Clay • Natural Flavor • Stevia • Potassium Sorbate.

Intrinsic Plus — Progressive Labs
Each capsule contains: Vitamin B12 (cyanocobalamin) 500 mcg • Folate (folic acid) 800 mcg • Pancreatic enzyme concentrate 50 mg • Porcine Stomach 250 mg • Pyloric Substance 60 mg.

IP6 Capsule — Jarrow Formulas
Each capsule contains: Calcium-Magnesium Inositol Hexaphosphate 615 mg • IP6 50 mg • Calcium 85 mg • Magnesium 30 mg. Other Ingredients: Rice powder, Magnesium Stearate.

IP6 Powder — Jarrow Formulas
Each scoop contains: Calcium-Magnesium Inositol Hexaphosophate 1230 mg • IP6 (extracted from rice bran) 1000 mg • Calcium 170 mg • Magnesium 60 mg.

IpriBone — Preventive Nutrition GNC
Two tablets contain: Vitamin D (as Cholecalciferol) 400 IU • Calcium (as Calcimate Calcium Citrate Malate) 200 mg • 7-Isopropoxy Isoflavone (Ostivone) 600 mg.

Iron Complex — Nature's Life
Each capsule contains: Iron (Peptonate) 25 mg • Vitamin C 20 mg • Niacinamide 10 mg • Vitamin B1 (Thiamine HCl) 1 mg • Vitamin B2 (Riboflavin) 1 mg • Vitamin B6 (Pyridoxine HCl) 1 mg • Folic Acid 30 mcg • Vitamin B12 (Cobalamin concentrate) 15 mcg • Copper (Gluconate) 100 mcg • Manganese (Gluconate) 1 mg • Betaine HCl 15 mg. In a natural base of Rose Hips concentrate.

Iron Plex — PhysioLogics
Each capsule contains: Iron (from Ferrous Bisglycinate) 28 mg • Folic Acid 400 mcg • Dibencozide 250 mcg • Intrinsic Factor 20 mg.

Iron Plus — Nutri-Quest
Each tablet contains: Iron (Ferrous Fumarate) 50 mg • Vitamin C 100 mg • L-Glycine 100 mg • Niacinamide 15 mg • Betaine HCL 15 mg • Vitamin E (Succinate) 15 IU • D-Calcium Pantothenate (Pantothenic Acid) 13 mg • Vitamin B2 4 mg • Vitamin B1 3 mg • Vitamin B6 2 mg • Folic Acid 200 mcg • Vitamin B12 25 mcg • Choline Bitartrate 12.5 mg.

Iron Woman — Traditional Medicinals
Yellow Dock root • Burdock root • Dandelion root • Licorice root • Nettle leaf • Prune fruit • Astralagus root • Stevia leaf.

Iron-Folic Plus — Nutrilite
Each tablet contains: Folic Acid 33% DV • Ferrous Fumarate • Ferrous Gluconate • Nutrilite Spinach concentrate with phytofactors plant compounds.

Iron-Free MutliLogics — PhysioLogics
Each tablet contains: Vitamin A (Beta-Carotene) 12500 IU • Vitamin A (Palmitate) 2500 IU • Thiamine 75 mg • Riboflavin 75 mg • Niacin 75 mg • Pantothenic Acid 75 mg • Vitamin B6 (Pyridoxine HCl) 75 mg • Vitamin B12 (Cyanocobalamin) 75 mcg • Folic Acid 400 mcg • Biotin 300 mcg • Vitamin C (Ascorbic Acid) 250 mg • Vitamin D (Cholecalciferol) 400 IU • Vitamin E (d-Alpha Tocopherol) 150 IU • Calcium (Amino Acid Chelate) 20 mg • Magnesium (Amino Acid Chelate) 10 mg • Zinc (Amino Acid Chelate) 10 mg • Copper (Amino Acid Chelate) 1 mg • Manganese (Amino Acid Chelate) 1 mg • Chromium (Niacin/Glycine Chelate) 25 mcg • Iodine (Potassium Iodide) 150 mcg • Selenium (Amino Acid Chelate) 25 mcg • Molybdenum (Amino Acid Chelate) 25 mcg • Boron (Amino Acid Chelate) 500 mcg • Potassium (Amino Acid Complex) 1.8 mg • Bioflavonoids lemon 25 mg • Rutin 25 mg • Betaine (HCl) 25 mg • Choline (Bitartrate) 31 mg • Inositol 75 mg • PABA 75 mg • Hesperidin 5 mg.

IsoPure — Nature's Best
Each serving contains: Creamy Vanilla Ingredients: Ion Exchanged Whey Protein Isolate, Maltodextrin, Vitamin, Mineral & Amino Acid Blend, Natural & Artificial Flavor, Xanthan Gum, Aspartame, Acesulfame K. Dutch Chocolate Ingredients: Ion Exchange Whey Protein Isolate, Maltodextrin, Vitamin, Mineral & Amino Acid Blend, Cocoa, Xanthan Gum, Natural & Artificial Flavor, Aspartame, Acesulfame K. Orange Creamsicle Ingredients: Ion Exchange Whey Protein Isolate, Maltodextrin, Vitamin, Mineral & Amino Acid Blend, Natural & Artificial Flavor, Xanthan Gum, Aspartame, Acesulfame K, Artificial Color (Yellow #6). Strawberries & Cream Ingredients: Ion Exchange Whey Protein Isolate, Maltodextrin, Vitamin, Mineral & Amino Acid Blend, Natural & Artificial Flavor, Freeze-Dried Strawberry Crystals, Xanthan Gum, Aspartame, Acesulfame K, Artificial Color (Red #3). Chocolate Peanut Butter Swirl Ingredients: Ion Exchange Whey Protein Isolate, Maltodextrin, Vitamin, Mineral & Amino Acid Blend, Cocoa, Natural & Artificial Flavor, Xanthan Gum, Aspartame, Acesulfame K.

Isotonix OPC-3 — Isotonix
Grape Seed extract 25 mg • Red Wine extract 25 mg • Pine Bark extract 25 mg • Bilberry extract 25 mg • Bioflavonoids 25 mg. In a base of citric acid, fructose, dextrose, maltodextrin, apple pectin, silica, calcium sulfate, and potassium.

Jarro-Dophilus +Colostrum — Jarrow Formulas
Each capsule Contains: Lactobacillus Rhamnosus R049 20% 672 million • Lactobacillus Casei R215 20 % 672 million • Lactobacillus Plantarum R202 20% 672 million • Lactobacillus Acidophilus R052 10% 336 million • Bifidobacterium Longum R023 20% 672 million • Bifidobacterium Breve R070 10% 336 million • Colostrum 500 mg. Other Ingredients: Ascorbic Acid, Magnesium Stearate.

Jarro-Dophilus +FOS — Jarrow Formulas
Each capsule Contains: FOS (Fructo-Oligo-Saccharides) 210 mg • Lactobacillus Rhamnosus R049 20% 672 million • Lactobacillus Casei R215 20 % 672 million • Lactobacillus Plantarum R202 20% 672 million • Lactobacillus Acidophilus R052 10% 336 million • Bifidobacterium Longum R023 672 million • Bifidobacterium breve R070 10% 336 million • Vitamin C 1 mg. Other Ingredients: Maltodextrin, Magnesium Stearate.

Jarro-Dophilus +FOS Powder — Jarrow Formulas
Each capsule Contains: FOS (Fructo-Oligo-Saccharides) 4000 mg • Lactobacillus Rhamnosus R049 20% 2.4 billion • Lactobacillus Casei R215 20 % 2.4 billion • Lactobacillus Plantarum R202 20% 2.4 billion • Lactobacillus Acidophilus R052 10% 1.2 billion • Bifidobacterium Longum R023 2.4 billion • Bifidobacterium Breve R070 10% 1.2 billion • Vitamin C 1 mg. Other Ingredients: Maltodextrin, Magnesium Stearate.

Jarro-Dophilus +Lactoferrin — Jarrow Formulas
Each capsule Contains: Lactobacillus Rhamnosus R049 20% 672 million • Lactobacillis Casei R215 20 % 672 million • Lactobacillus Plantarum R202 20% 672 million • Lactobacillus Acidophilus R052 10% 336 million • Bifidobacterium Longum R023 20% 672 million • Bifidobacterium Breve R070 10% 336 million • Lactoferrin 200 mg. Other Ingredients: Ascorbic Acid, Magnesium Stearate.

Joint Actives — VitaStore
Six tablets contain: Glucosamine HCl 1500 mg • Shark Cartilage 500 mg • Salix Alba 200 mg • Boswellia 250 mg • Green-Lipped Mussel 250 mg • Quercetin 300 mg • Manganese 5 mg • L-Methionine 100 mg • Zinc Gluconate 25 mg • Turmeric 250 mg • Bromelain 200 mg • Vitamin C 300 mg • Vitamin E 90 IU.

Joint Cream — The Vitamin Shoppe
Glucosamine • Boswellin • Capsaicin.

Some Brand Name Natural Products - What they Contain
www.NaturalDatabase.com contains MANY more listings than appear here.

Joint Fuel — TwinLab
Six capsules contain: Glucosamine Sulfate 1500 mg • Chondroitin Sulfate A (CSA) 100 mg • Zinc (from Chelated Zinc Picolinate) 30 mg • Manganese (from Chelated Manganese Gluconate) 5 mg • Vitamin C 1000 mg • Natural Vitamin E (Succinate) 800 IU • Selenium (from Selenomethionine) 200 mcg • Turmeric extract (Curcuma longa) (standardized for 95% Curcumin) 1300 mg • Quercetin (Bioflavonoid) 100 mg • Bromelain 200 mg.

Joint Fuel Liquid Concentrate — TwinLab
Each tablespoonful contains: Glucosamine HCl 500 mg • Chondroitin Sulfate 400 mg • Betaine 166 mg • Hydrolyzed Collagen 33 mg • Chicken Type II Collagen 33 mg • Vitamin B6 3.3 mg • Folic Acid 400 mcg • Vitamin B12 166 mcg.

Joint Rescue — TwinLab
Three softgels contain: Vitamin E (from d-Alpha Tocopherols) 400 IU • Glucosamine HCl & Glucosamine Sulfate 750 mg • Chondroitin Sulfate 50 mg • Turmeric powder extract (standardized for 95% Curcumin) 650 mg • Boswellin (Boswellia serrata extract) (standardized for 65% Boswellic Acids) 13 mg • Ginger root extract 50 mg • EPA 750 mg • DHA 750 mg • Borage Oil 100 mg.

Joint Support — Futurebiotics
Four tablets contain: Devil's Claw 400 mg • Yucca 300 mg • Horsetail 200 mg • Ginger 200 mg • Alfalfa juice concentrate 200 mg • Chinese Cinnamon 250 mg • Magnesium: (oxide, chloride, ascorbate) 400 mg • Beta Carotene 250 mg • Vitamin C (ascorbic acid, Rose hips) 120 mg • Niacin 8 mg • Niacinamide 250 mg • Vitamin D (Fish oils) 200 IU • Vitamin E (natural) 25 IU • Vitamin B6 (pyridoxine HCl) 8 mg • Vitamin B12 (cyanocobalamin) 12 mcg • Zinc (sulfate) 15 mg • Copper (gluconate) 750 mcg • Biotin 80 mcg • Pantothenic Acid 35 mg • Selenium (methionate) 120 mcg • Glutamic Acid HCl 100 mg • Lecithin 100 mg • Betaine HCl 75 mg • Para Amino Benzoic Acid (PABA) 25 mg • Potassium (sulfate) 20 mg.

Joint Support — Now
Three capsules contain: Vitamin B3 (Niacinamide) 100mg • Vitamin B5 (Pantothenic Acid) 100 mg • Vitamin B6 (Pyridoxine HCl) 50 mg • Vitamin C (Ascorbic Acid) 100 mg • Magnesium (Oxide) 200 mg • Zinc (Picolinate) 15 mg • Manganese (Amino Acid Chelate) 7 mg • Copper (Amino Acid Chelate) 3 mg • Glucosamine HCL 1000 mg • Boswellin standardized herbal extract of Boswellia serrata 300 mg • Sea Cucumber 300 mg • Bromelain (2000 GDU activity from pineapple) 150 mg • PABA (Para-Aminobenzoic Acid) 10 mg • Devil's Claw (Harpagophytum procumbens) 100 mg.

Joint Support — Olympia Nutrition
Glucosamine • Boswellin • Sea Cucumber • Bromelain • Yucca • Alfalfa.

Joint Synergy — Olympia Nutrition
Glucosamine Sulfate • Sea Cucumber • MSM • Hydrolyzed Cartilage.

Joint/Arthritis Support — Amazon Support
Each capsule contains: Amor Seco • Cat's Claw Extract • Chuchuhasi • Tayuya • Iporuru • Pucao Preto • Mullaca • Sarsaparilla.

JointFlex — Eden Laboratories, Inc.
Active Ingredient: Camphor (3.1%). Inactive Ingredients: Acetylated lanolin, acrylates/C10-30, alkyl acrylate, crosspolymer, aloe vera, C12-15 alkyl benzoate, chondroitin sulfate, purified water, diazolidnyl urea, dimethicone, dimethiconol stearate, disodium EDTA, dl panthenol, glucosamine sulfate, glycerin, glycerol stearate, glycosaminoglycans, hydroxylated lanolin, hydroxypropylene methylcellulose, lodopropynyl, butylcarbomate, methyl gluceth-20, methyl glucose, sesquistearate, peppermint oil, polysorbate 20, potassium carbomer, tocopheryl acetate.

JointPower — Trimedica
Six capsules contain: Glucosamine Sulfate 1500 mg • Vitamin C 1000 mg • natural Vitamin E (Succinate) 800 IU • Manganese (Chelated Manganese Gluconate) 5 mg • Zinc (Chelated Zinc Picolinate) 15 mg • Copper (Chelated Copper Gluconate) 1.5 mg • Tumeric (Curcuma longa) extract (standardized for 95% Curcumin) 1300 mg • Boswellia serrata extract (standardized for 60-65 Boswellic Acids) 100 mg • Bromelain 100 mg • Selenium (from Selenomethionine) 200 mcg.

Joints Formula — Nature's Way
Three capsules contain: Alfalfa concentrate 125 mg • Boswellia dried extract 300 mg • Copper (Amino Acid Chelate) 1 mg • Glucosamine HCL 750 mg • Grape seed dried extract 48 mg • Manganese Amino Acid Chelate 5 mg • Nettle root 250 mg • Wild Yam root 75 mg • Zinc Amino Acid Chelate 7.5 mg. Other ingredients: Gelatin, Magnesium Stearate, Millet.

Jojoba & E Skin Oil — Derma E
90% Jojoba • 10% Vitamin E oil.

Just-Whey — SportPharma
Each serving contains: Calories 110 • Protein 23 g • Carbohydrates 2.5 g • Fat 1 g.

K & MG Aspartate — Atrium
Each tablet contains: Potassium Aspartate (which yields Potassium 78 mg & L-Aspartic Acid 209 mg) 261 mg • Magnesium Aspartate (which yields Magnesium 28 mg & L-Aspartic Acid 242 mg) 278 mg.

K & U — MMS Pro
Each capsule contains: Juniper berries • Parsley herb • Ginger root • Uva Ursi leaves • Marshmallow root • Cramp bark • Golden Seal root.

Kalm-Assure — Nature's Plus
Each tablet contains: Rapid Release Layer: Pantothenic Acid (Vitamin B5) 50 mg • GABA (Gamma Aminobutyric Acid) 25 mg • Magnesium (Citrate) 25 mg • Pyridoxal-5-Phosphate (P5P) 5 mg. Sustained Release Layer: Kava (Piper methysticum root) standardized 30% kavalactones 100 mg • Passion Flower (Passiflora incarnata) standardized 4% Isovitexin 75 mg • Hops fruit (Humulus lupulus) standardized 5.2% bitter acids 10 mg • Siberian Ginseng (Eleutherococcus senticosus) standardized 0.8% Eleutherosides 25 mg • Chamomile (Matricaria recutita flower) standardized 1% Apigenin 25 mg. Contains no yeast, wheat, corn, soy, milk, salt or starch.

Kan Jang, Kanjang — Swedish Herbal Institute
Andrographis paniculata • Echinacea angustifolia • Adathoda vasica • Acanthopanax s.

Kava 30% — Nature's Way
Each capsule contains: Kava Dried Extract (30% kavalactones) 350 mg • Passion Flower stem, leaf, fruit & flower 500 mg.

Kava Kava — Gaia Herbs
Kava Kava standardized for 5% kavalactones. Standardized Full Spectrum 136 mg of extract per capsule. Guaranteed Potency 68 mg of extract per capsule.

Kava Kava — Pharmanex
Each softgel contains: Kava Kava root (11:1) Extract (Piper methysticum) 175 mg. Other Ingredients: Soybean Oil, Gelatin, Glycerin, Maltodextrin, Beeswax, Lecithin, Carob.

Kava Kava 3000 mg — Jamieson
Each capsule contains: Kava Kava root 3000 mg (Piper methysticum, 250 mg powdered extract 1:12). Other Ingredients: Gelatin, Calcium Sulfate, Maltodextrin, Cellulose, Magnesium Stearate, Silica.

Kava Kava Plus — The Herbalist
Kava Kava root • Siberian Ginseng root • St. John's Wort flowering tops • Oat seed • Skullcap herb.

Kava Kava-Valerian Virtue — Blessed Herbs
Kava Kava root • Scullcap • Valerian root • St. John's Wort flower • Lobelia • Arnica flower & herb • Grain alcohol & Distilled Water.

Kavacin — Phytopharmica
Each capsule contains: Kava root extract (Piper methysticum) 200 mg standardized to contain 30% kavalactones (60 mg per capsule) • Oat Straw extract 10:1 (Avena sativa) 100 mg • Pyridoxine-Alpha-Ketoglutarate (PAK) 50 mg • Pantothenic Acid 50 mg • Nicotinamide 50 mg • Thiamine HCL (Vitamin B1) 25 mg. Contains no sugar, salt, yeast, wheat, corn, soy, dairy products, coloring, flavoring or preservatives.

Kavatime — Bodyonics
Each tablet contains: Kava Kava Root (Piper Methysticum) 350 mg • Kava Kava Powdered Extract 150 mg • Herbolics Support Complex (Derived from barley Malt Flour, Brewers Yeast (saccharomyces cerevisiae), Hops (humulus lupulus), and Ginger Root Extract (zingiber officinale) 50 mg. Other Ingredients: Calcium Phosphate, Magnesium Stearate, Gelatin.

KavaTone — Enzymatic Therapy
Each capsule contains: Kava Root Extract (Piper methysticum) (standardized to contain 30% Kavalactones 60 mg per capsule) 200 mg • Oat Straw Extract 10:1 (Avena sativa) 100 mg • Pyridoxine-Alpha-Ketoglutarate (PAK) 50 mg • Pantothenic Acid 50 mg,

© Copyright 2000, Natural Medicines Comprehensive Database (209) 472-2244. For updated data, go to www.NaturalDatabase.com. • 1353

B
R
A
N
D

N
A
M
E
S

Nicotinamide 50 mg • Thiamin HCL (Vitamin B1) 25 mg. Contains no sugar, salt, yeast, wheat, corn, soy, dairy products, coloring, flavoring, or preservatives.

Kavatrol - Capsule — Natrol
One capsule contains: Kava root extract (30% Kavalactones) 200 mg • In an exclusive base of complementary herbs: Passion flower, Chamomile flower, Hops flower, Schizandra fruit. Other ingredients: Magnesium Stearate, Silicon Dioxide, Gelatin.

Keto Pro — Met-Rx
Metamyosyn V.4 (unique blend of Milk Protein Isolates, Caseinate, Whey Protein Concentrate, Glutamine, Calcium-B-Hydroxy B-Methylbutyrate Monhydrate, Lactoferrin) • Medium Chain Triglycerides • Natural & Artifical Flavor • Cellulose Gum • Maltodextrin • Dipotassium Phosphate • Potassium Chloride • Potassium Citrate • Carrageenan • Salt • Sodium Citrate • Sucrolose.

KIC Fuel — TwinLab
Each capsule contains: KIC 500 mg.

Kid Vits — Now
Two tablets contain: Beta-Carotene 4000 IU • Vitamin A (as Palmitate) 1000 IU • Vitamin B1 (Thiamine HCL) 3 mg • Vitamin B2 (Riboflavin) 3.4 mg • Vitamin B3 (Niacinamide) 20 mg • Vitamin B5 (Pantothenic Acid) 15 mg • Vitamin B6 (Pyridoxine HCL) 4 mg • Vitamin B12 (Cyanocobalamin) 10 mcg • Biotin 100 mcg • Folic Acid 400 mcg • Vitamin C (Ascorbic Acid, Calcium Ascorbate) 120 mg • Vitamin D (Cholecalciferol) 200 IU • Vitamin E (d-Alpha Tocopheryl Succinate) 30 IU • Calcium (Carbonate, Ascorbate) 30 mg • Magnesium (Oxide, Amino Acid Chelate) 20 mg • Zinc (Amino Acid Chelate) 5 mg • Iron (Ferrochel Iron Bisglycinate) 5 mg • Copper (Amino Acid Chelate) 0.2 mg • Iodine (Kelp) 75 mcg • Manganese (Amino Acid Chelate) 1 mg • Selenium (Amino Acid Chelate) 10 mcg • Chromium (Chelavite) 60 mcg • Molybdenum (Amino Acid Chelate) 15 mcg • Acerola 25 mg • Bioflavonoids (40 % Hesperidin) 25 mg • Choline 10 mg • Inositol 10 mg • PABA 4 mg.

Kid-Alert — The Herbalist
Ginkgo fresh leaf (Ginkgo biloba) • Gotu Kola fresh herb (Hydrocotyle asiatica) • Lemon Balm fresh leaf (Melissa officinalis) • St. John's Wort fresh flower tops (Hypericum perf.) • Siberian Ginseng fresh-dried root (Eleuthero sent.) in a base of kosher glycerine and distilled water • grapefruit seed extract.

KidCalm St. John's Wort Complex — Enzymatic Therapy
Two capsules contain: Magnesium (Krebs Cycle Chelate) 50 mg • Vitamin B6 (Pyridoxal-5-Phosphate) 15 mg • Zinc (Krebs Cycle chelate) 15 mg. Other ingredients: St. John's Wort extract (Hypericum perforatum) standardized to contain 0.3% Hypericin, verified by HPLC 100 mg • Valerian root extract (Valerian officinalis) standardized to contain a minimum of 0.8% Valerenic acids 100 mg • GABA (Gamma-Aminobutyric Acid) 100 mg • L-Tyrosine 100 mg • Kava root extract (Piper methysticum) standardized to contain 30% Kavalactones 50 mg • Melissa extract (Melissa officinalis) standardized to contain a minimum of 5% Rosmarinic Acid 50 mg • Grape seed (PCO) extract standardized to contain 95% Procyanidolic Oligomers (PCOs) 20 mg. Contains no sugar, salt, yeast, wheat, gluten, corn, soy, dairy products, coloring, flavoring, or preservatives.

Kid-Ease — The Herbalist
Lemon Balm fresh leaf (Melissa officinalis) Valerian fresh root (Valeriana officinalis) • St. John's Wort fresh flower tops (Hypericum perf.). In a base of kosher glycerine and grapefruit seed extract.

Kidney Bladder Formula — Nature's Way
Two capsules contain: Proprietary formula: Cramp bark • Ginger • Goldenseal root • Juniper berries • Marshmallow root • Parsley herb • Uva Ursi leaves. Other ingredients: Gelatin.

Kidney Blend — The Herbalist
Dandelion root • Burdock seed • Uva Ursi leaf • Corn Silk • Echinacea root • St. John's Wort flower • Yarrow flower • Cayenne pepper.

Kidney Plus — The Herbalist
Uva Ursi leaf • Juniper berry • Buchu leaf • Echinacea root • Pipsessewa leaf • St. John's Wort flower • Yarrow flower • Cayenne pepper.

Kidney Support — Amazon Support
Each capsule contains: Chanca Piedra • Boldo • Cipo Cabeludo • Erva Tostao • Abuta • Jatoba.

Kidney Tea: Soothing Diuretic Tea — The Herbalist
Marshmallow root • Juniper berry • Plantain leaf • Dandelion root • Parsley root • Mullein leaf • Horsetail herb • Nettles leaf • Rosehips.

Kidneycare — PhysioLogics
Two capsules contain: Potassium 50 mg • Dandelion root 300 mg • Astragalus root (70% Polysaccharides, 175 mg) 250 mg • Corn silk 150 mg • Yarrow 150 mg.

Kidney-Liver Complex — Enzymatic Therapy
Two capsules contain: Kidney-Liver Complex (Predigested Soluble concentrate*) 500 mg • Artichoke extract (Cynara solymus) standardized to contain 15% Caffeylquinic Acids 100 mg • Multi-Glandular Complex: Raw Liver, Raw Lung, Raw Pancreas, Raw Heart, Raw Kidney, Raw Spleen & Raw Brain 100 mg. *Free-form concentrate predigested by enzymatic action, creating a highly absorbable form of glandular concentrate containing all the natural principles with a standardized content. Contains no sugar, salt, yeast, wheat, corn, soy, dairy products, coloring, flavoring, or preservatives.

Kids Be Well — The Herbalist
Astragalus fresh root (Astragalus membranaceous) • Echinacea fresh root (Echinacea angustifolia) • Lemon Balm fresh leaf (Melissa officinalis) • St. John's Wort fresh flower tops (Hypericum perf.) • Ginkgo fresh leaf (Ginkgo biloba) • in a base of kosher glycerine • and grapefruit seed extract.

Kid's Choice: Versatile Herbal for Children — The Herbalist
Echinacea root • Lemon Balm leaf • Goldenseal root.

Kinder Love Children's Multivitamin — Dial Herbs
Vitamin A • Vitamin C • Vitamin B from Yeast extract • Vitamin E • Thiamin • Niacin • Vitamin B6 • Calcium • Phosphorus • Magnesium • aqueous extract from: (Carrots, Anise, Licorice root, Milfoil herb, Horsetail herb, Chamomile flowers, Peppermint Leaves, Watercress, Wheat Germ, Coriander seeds, Nettles, Spinach, Orange peel) • Orange juice • Pear juice concentrate • Malt extract • Yeast extract • Maple Syrup • Honey • Rose Hip extract • Wheat Germ extract • Natural Flavor.

Kindervital — Flora
Multivitamin. Vitamin A • Vitamin B Complex • Vitamin C • Vitamin D • Vitamin E.

Kinder-Vites — Atrium
Two chewable tablets contain: Vitamins: Vitamin A (Palmitate) 2500 IU • Vitamin D3 200 IU • Vitamin E 10 IU • Vitamin K 10 mcg • Vitamin B1 3.2 mg • Vitamin B2 3 mg • Vitamin B6 3.2 mg • Vitamin B12 10 mcg • Vitamin C 100 mg • Niacinamide 13.5 mg • Folic Acid 200 mcg • Pantothenic Acid 5 mg • Biotin 60 mcg. Minerals: Calcium 12 mg • Magnesium 3.2 mg • Manganese 2.5 mg • Copper 100 mcg • Zinc 8 mg • Iron 12 mg • Iodine 100 mcg • Selenium 10 mcg • Chromium 10 mcg • Molybdenum 5 mcg • Vanadium 5 mcg. Associated Nutritional Factors: Citrus Bioflavonoids, Rutin, & Hesperidin 60 mg • Choline 10 mg • Inositol 2 mg • PABA 10 mg. Formulated in a base of pleasant tasting, natural source flavoring & excipients.

Kira St. John's Wort — Lichtwer Pharma
Each tablet contains: LI 160 St. John's Wort (Hypericum perforatum) standardized extract (with 92 mcg hypericin, 262 mcg pseudohypericin, & 18.37 mg hyperforin) 300 mg.

Knock Out — Schiff
Each caplet contains: Vitamin B6 (Pyroxidal-5-Phosphate) 0.5 mg • Magnesium (as Glycinate) 10 mg • Melatonin synthetic 3 mg • Kava Kava 2:1 extract 100 mg • Valerian extract (0.89% Valeric Acid) 100 mg • Gamma Aminobutyric Acid GABA 100 mg • Glycine 40 mg.

Korean Red Ginseng — Jamieson
Each caplet contains: Calcium 65 mg • Korean Red Ginseng Root (Panax Ginseng) 4% ginsenosides saponins 250 mg.

Kudja — HerbaSway
Kudzu • Ginkgo Biloba • Blackberry • Green Tea • HerbaSwee (Cucurbitaceae fruit).

Kwai Heart Fit — Lichtwer Pharma
One tablet contains: Garlic powder sucrose 300 mg • Vitamin C (Ascorbic Acid Sorbitol) 80 mg • Vitamin E (Tocopherol Acetate) 20 IU • Vitamin A (Acetate) 2640 IU. Other ingredients: Talc, Corn Starch, Hydroxypropylmethylcellulose, Polivinylpyrrolidone, Silicon Dioxide, Stearic Acid, Castor oil, Magnesium Stearate, Powdered

Cellulose, Glucose Syrup, Titanium Dioxide, Carnauba Wax/Bees Wax, Riboflavin, Beta-Carotene.

Kwai Odorfree Garlic — Lichtwer Pharma
Dried Garlic clove powder. Other Ingredients: Hydroxypropylmethylcellulose, Silicon Dioxide, Maltitol, Magnesium Stearate, Magnesium Silicate, Carnauba Wax, Powdered Cellulose, Castor Oil, Gum Arabic.

Kwik Size XXXL — Labrada Bodybuilding Nutrition
Each serving contains: Kwik Carb (Unique blend of Maltodextrin & Polydextrose) • Kwik Pro (Unique blend of cross flow ultrafiltered Whey Protein Concentrate, Calcium Caseinate, Specially Extracted & Spray-Dried Soy Protein Concentrate) • Cocoa powder (dutch processed) • Natural & Artificial flavors • Vitamin & Mineral Blend • Xanthan Gum • Dipotassium Phosphate • Aspartame • Peptigen (proprietary blend of Alpha Amylase, Malt Diatase, Protease, Lactase) • Medium Chain Triglycerides.

Kyo-Chlorella — Wakunaga of America
Six tablets contain: 100% pure broken cell wall Chlorella powder 3 g.

Kyo-Chrome Aged Garlic Extract Cholesterol Formula — Wakunaga of America
Two capsules contain: Aged Garlic extract powder 400 mg • Niacin 20 mg • Chromium (as Chromium Picolinate) 200 mcg. Other Ingredients: Microcrystalline Cellulose, Magnesium Stearate (vegetable source).

Kyo-Dophilus L. Acidophilus; B. Bifidum; B. Longum — Wakunaga of America
Each capsule contains: L. Acidophilus (Lactobacillus Acidophilus); B. Bifidum (Bifidobacterium Bifidum) and B. Longum (Bifidobacterium Longum) 1.5 billion cells. Other Ingredients: Vegetable Starch Complex.

Kyo-Green — Wakunaga of America
Each teaspoon contains: Kyo-Green Proprietary Blend 2.5 g • Barley Grass Powder • Cooked Brown Rice • Wheat Grass Powder • Bulgarian Chlorella • Pacific Kelp.

Kyolic — Wakunaga Consumer Products
Each caplet contains: Aged Garlic extract powder 600 mg • Microcrystalline Cellulose • Magnesium Stearate • Silicon Dioxide. Kyolic is free of dairy, sodium & yeast.

Kyolic Aged Garlic Extract Enriched with Vitamin B1 and B12 — Wakunaga of America
Each capsule contains: Vitamin B1 (Thiamine Hydrochloride) 8 mg • Vitamin B12(cyanocobalamin) 1 mcg. Other Ingredients: Aged Garlic Extract; Liver Extract, Water, Residual Alcohol from extraction.

Kyolic Aged Garlic Extract Garlic Plus — Wakunaga of America
Two capsules or tablets contain: Aged Garlic extract powder 540 mg • Brewer's Yeast 54 mg • Kelp 18 mg. Other Ingredients: Whey, Brewer's Yeast, Alginic Acid (seaweed), Kelp, Collodial Silica, Magnesium Stearate (vegetable source).

Kyolic Aged Garlic Extract Kyolic HI-PO — Wakunaga of America
Two capsules or tablets contain: Aged Garlic extract powder (bulb) 600 mg. Other Ingredients: Whey, Alginic Acid (seaweed), Silica, Cellulose, Magnesium Stearate (vegetable source).

Kyolic Aged Garlic Extract Plus Enzyme — Wakunaga of America
Two tablets contain: Aged Garlic powder 700 mg • KYOLIC Enzyme Complex (Amylase, Protease, Cellulose, and Lipase from Aspergillus oryzae and A. niger) 60 mg • Rice Protein-Calcium Complex 40 mg. Other Ingredients: Alginic Acid (seaweed), Collodal Silica, and Magnesium Stearate (vegetable source).

Kyolic Aged Garlic Extract Plus Lecithin — Wakunaga of America
Two capsules contain: Aged Garlic extract powder (bulb) 600 mg • Lecithin 380 mg. Other Ingredients: Silica, Magnesium Stearate (vegetable source).

Kyolic Aged Garlic Extract Vitamin A, C, E, Selenium — Wakunaga of America
Two capsules contain: Vitamin A (from 12 mg of Beta-Carotene) 20000 IU • Vitamin C (Calcium ascorbate) 240 mg • Vitamin E (d-alpha-Tocopheryl succinate) 120 IU • Selenium (L-Selenomethionine) 50 mcg • Aged Garlic Extract Powder (bulb) 400 mg • Green Tea Powder (leaf) 89 mg. Other Ingredients: Silica, Magnesium Stearate (vegetable source).

Kyolic Aged Garlic Extract Vitamin C, Astragalus — Wakunaga of America
Two capsules contain: Vitamin C (Ester C) 210 mg • Calcium (Citrate Polyascorbate) 46 mg • Aged Garlic extract powder (bulb) 440 mg • Astragalus extract powder (root) 200 mg. Other Ingredients: Calcium Citrate, Magnesium Stearate (vegetable source).

Kyolic Aged Garlic Extract Vitamin E, Cayenne, Hawthorn Berry — Wakunaga of America
Two capsules contain: Vitamin E (d-alpha-tocopheryl Succinate) 200 IU • Aged Garlic Extract Powder (bulb) 600 mg • Hawthorn Berry (fruit) 100 mg • Cayenne Pepper (fruit) 20 mg. Other Ingredients: Cellulose, Magnesium Stearate (vegetable source), Silica.

Kyolic Cardio Logic — Wakunaga of America
Each capsule contains: Vitamin E (as D-Alpha-Tocopheryl Acid Succinate) 50 IU • Vitamin B6 5 mg • Folate (as Folic acid) 200 mcg • Vitamin B12 100 mcg • Aged Garlic bulb extract powder 200 mg • L-Carnitine 30 mg • Coenzyme Q10 30 mg • Alpha-Lipoic Acid 30 mg. Other Ingredients: Cellulose, Collodial Silica, Magnesium Stearate (vegetable source).

Kyolic Echinacea Aged Garlic Extract — Wakunaga of America
Two capsules contain: Aged Garlic powder (bulb) 600 mg • Echinacea extract powder (root) 100 mg. Other Ingredients: Cellulose (pine), Magnesium Stearate (vegetable source).

Kyolic Estro Logic — Wakunaga of America
Each capsule contains: Black Cohosh root extract (standardized to 2.5% triterpene glycosides) 100 mg • Soybean Isoflavones (seed) (Standardized to 40% isoflavones) 50 mg • Wild Yam root extract (Standardized to 6% total saponins) 33.3 mg • Sage leaf extract 25 mg • Chaste Tree berry extract 12.5 mg • Vervain leaf extract 12.5 mg • Astragalus root extract 12.5 mg • Motherwort leaf extract 12.5 mg. Other Ingredients: Cellulose, Silica, Magnesium Stearate (vegetable source).

Kyolic Liquid Aged Garlic Extract — Wakunaga of America
1/4 teaspoon contains: Aged Garlic extract (bulb) 1 ml. Other Ingredients: Water and Residual Alcohol from Extraction.

Kyolic Neuro Logic — Wakunaga Consumer Products
Two capsules contain: Folate (as Folic acid) 200 mcg • Vitamin B12 100 mcg • Aged Garlic bulb powder 400 mg • Lecithin 200 mg • Ginkgo Biloba leaf extract 60 mg • Phosphatidylserine (30%) 50 mg • Acetyl-L-Carnitine 25 mg. Other Ingredients: Cellulose, Colloidal Silica, Magnesium Stearate (vegetable source).

Kyolic Prosta Logic — Wakunaga of America
Each capsule contains: Zinc (as Zinc Picolinate) 7.5 mg • Saw Palmetto berry extract 160 mg • Aged Garlic bulb extract powder 100 mg • Pumpkin seed oil extract 50 mg • Pygeum Africanum bark extract 50 mg • Lycopene (as tomato oleoresin 2.5 mg. Other Ingredients: Wheat Germ Oil, Beeswax, Soft Gelatin Capsule.

Kyolic Reserve Aged Garlic Extract — Wakunaga of America
Each capsule contains: Aged Garlic Extract powder (bulb) 600 mg. Other Ingredients: Vegetable Protein, Magnesium Stearate (vegetable source), Silica.

Kyolic-EPA Aged Garlic Extract — Wakunaga of America
Two capsules contain: EPA (Eicosapentaenoic Acid) 560 mg • DHA (Docosahexaenoic Acid) 240 mg • Aged Garlic powder 240 mg • Vitamin E mixed Tocopherol 10 mg. Other Ingredients: Glycerin, Soft gelatin capsule.

L & V Formula — Dial Herbs
Wild Lettuce • Valerian • Wood Betony.

L.B.T. Caps: Lower Bowel Tonic — The Herbalist
Cascara Sagrada fresh-dried bark (Rhamnus purshiana) • Barberry root bark (Berberis vulgaris) • Fennel fresh-dried seed (Foeniculum vulgare) • Bayberry fresh-dried root bark (Myrica cerifera) • Ginger fresh root (Zingiber officinale) • Turkey Rhubarb fresh-dried root (Rheum palmatum) • Lobelia fresh-dried herb (Lobelia inflata) • Cayenne fresh-dried pepper (Capsicum annum).

BRAND NAMES

Some Brand Name Natural Products - What they Contain
www.NaturalDatabase.com contains MANY more listings than appear here.

B
R
A
N
D

N
A
M
E
S

Lactobacillus Acidophilus Milk-Base — Nature's Life
Each capsule contains: Lactobacillus species (Combined L. Acidophilus, L. Bulgaricus & L. Caucasious) 250 mg.

Lactobacillus Acidophilus Milk-Free — Nature's Life
Each capsule contains: Lactobacillus Acidophilus 500 mg.

Lactoferrin with Colostrum — The Vitamin Shoppe
Each capsule contains: Lactoferrin (from whey) 100 mg • Colostrum (from bovine) providing 20% immunoglobulins 250 mg • Lysozyme (from whey) 5 mg. No yeast, corn, wheat, sugar, salt, starch, gluten, soy, eggs, fish or animal derivatives, citrus, preservatives, artificial colors or flavors added.

Lava — Universal Nutrition
Each 83 g serving contains: Creatine Monohydrate 5.5 g • Chromium 75 mcg • Glutamine 2.5 g • Taurine 1.2 g • Sodium 180 mg • Potassium 360 mg. Ingredients: Ultra & Micro-Filtrated Whey Protein Concentrate (Containing Whey Peptide-Rich Lactoglobulins, Lactalbumin, Immunoglobulins & Lactoferrin) • GlycoCarb Complex (Dextrose & Glucose Polymers) • Maltodextrin • 100% Pure Creatine Monohydrate • Glutamine • Taurine • Magnesium Oxide • Disodium Phosphate • Potassium Phosphate • Fruit Flavor • Lecithin • Ascorbic Acid • Vitamin E Succinate • Niacin • Citric Acid • Aspartame • Carmine (for color) •Chromium (GTF).

Laxaco — Jamieson
Each capsule contains: Calcium (as Calcium Sulfate) 25 mg • Senna leaf (Cassia senna L.) 240 mg • Cascara Sagrada bark (Rhamnus purshiana DC) 150 mg.

LaxActin — Nature's Plus
Each capsule contains: Cascara Sagrada (Rhamnus purshiana bark) (standardized 25-30% Hydroxyanthracene derivatives - HAD) 100 mg • Passion Flower [(Passiflora incarnata flower) standardized 3.5-4% Flavonoids] 100 mg • Senna [(Cassia senna leaf) standardized 5% Sennosides] 50 mg.

Laxaherb — Dial Herbs
Cascara Sagrada • Buckthorn • Ginger • Bayberry • Goldenseal • Raspberry • Fennel • Lobelia • Rhubarb.

L-Carnitine — New Hope Health Products
Each capsule contains: L-Carnitine 500 mg • Vitamin B5 15 mg • Vitamin B6 5 mg.

Lean "4" — The Vitamin Shoppe
Each six tablets contain: Lecithin 1200 mg • Vitamin B6 (pyridoxine HCl) 50 mg • Iodine (kelp) 210 mcg • Cider Vinegar Powder 240 mg • Grapefruit Powder 300 mg.

Lean Body — Labrada Bodybuilding Nutrition
Each 45 g serving contains: Vanilla: Calories 300 • Protein 45 g • Carbohydrates 28 g • Fat 1.5 g. Ingredients: Lean Pro unique blend of ProPlex (cross flow ultrafiltered Whey Protein Concentrate, Ion Exchange Whey Protein Isolate, Cross Flow Microfiltered Whey Protein Isolate, Hydrolyzed Whey Protein Isolate Peptides) • Milk Protein Isolate • Caseinate • L-Glutamine • Taurine • Magnesium Alpha Ketoglutarate • Maltodextrin • Vitamin & Mineral Blend • Polydextrose • Natural Flavors • Soy Lecithin • Xanthan Gum • Cellulose Fiber • Aspartame • L-Carnitine • Beta-Carotene for color. Chocolate Peanut Butter: Calories 300 • Protein 45 g • Carbohydrates 28 g • Fat 1.5 g. Ingredients: Lean Pro [Unique Blend of Proplete (Cross Flow Ultrafiltered Whey Protein concentrate, Ion Exchange Whey Protein Isolate, Cross Flow Microfiltered Whey Protein Isolate, Hydrolyzed Whey Protein Isolate Peptides), Caseinate, Milk Protein Isolate, L-Glutamine, Taurine, Magnesium Alpha Keto Glutarate] • Maltodextrin • Natural & Artificial Flavors including Hershey's Cocoa • Polydextrose • Cocoa (Dutch Processed) • Vitamin & Mineral Blend [Diacalcium Phosphate, Potassium Chloride, Magnesium Oxide, Vitamin C (Ascorbic Acid), Vitamin E (Alpha Tocopherol Acetate), Ferrous Fumarate, Beta Carotene, Vitamin B3 (Niacinamide), Zinc Oxide, Manganese Sulfate, Calcium Pantothenate, Vitamin A Palmitate, Zinc Picolinate, Copper Sulfate, Vitamin B6 (Pyridoxine Hydrochloride), Chromium Polynicotinate, Vitamin B2 (Riboflavin), Vitamin B1 (Thiamine Hydrochloride), Vitamin B12 (Cyanocobalamin), Vitamin D3 (Cholecalciferol), Folic Acid, Sodium Molybdate, Chromium Chloride, Biotin, Potassium Iodide, Sodium Selenite] • Xanthan Gum • Soy Lecithin • Aspartame • Salt • Cellulose Fiber. Wildberry: Calories 305 • Protein 45 g • Carbohydrates 28 g • Fat 1.5 g. Ingredients: Lean Pro [Unique Blend of Proplex+ (Cross Flow Ultrafiltered Whey Protein concentrate, Ion Exchange Whey Protein Isolate, Cross Flow Microfiltered Whey

Protein Isolate, Hydrolyzed Whey Protein Isolate Peptides), Milk Protein Isolate, Caseinate, L-Glutamine, Taurine, Magnesium Alpha Keto Glutarate], Maltodextrin, Vitamin & Mineral Blend (Diacalcium Phosphate, Magnesium Oxide, Ascorbic Acid, Vitamin E Acetate, Niacinamide, Electrolytic Iron, Riboflavin, Folic Acid, Biotin, Manganese Sulfate, Potassium Iodide, Chromium Picolinate, Cholecalciferol, Sodium Molybdate, Cyanocobalamin, Sodium Selenite) • Natural & Artificial flavors • Polydextrose • Medium Chain Triglycerides • Xanthan Gum • Cellulose Gum • Aspartame. Peanut Butter: Calories 300 • Protein 45 g • Carbohydrates 28 g, Fat 1.5 g.

Lean Gainer — Champion Nutrition
Each serving contains: Protein 50 g • Carbohydrates 12 g • Fat 4.5 g • Calories 280. Ingredients: Peptol-C (Whey Protein Concentrate, Creatine Monohydrate, Amino Acids, L-Leucine, L-Glutamine) • Metabarb-V (blend of Simple & Complex Carbohydrates containing Glucose Polymers & Whey) • Low Fat Cocoa powder • Natural & Artificial Flavors • Metavite IV (Vitamin-Mineral Complex) • FIBR3 (Cellulose, Oat Fiber, Psyllium husks) • Aspartame • Succinate ETF (Potassium Succinate, L-Glutamic Acid, Inosine, Magnesium Succinate, Calcium Succinate) • Bromelain • Papain • Defatted Peanut Flour • Sunette (Brand of Acesulfame-K) • Vanadyl Polynicotinate. Contains Phenylanine. No added sucrose or fructose.

Leci-Plus — Atrium
Each capsule contains: Raw Unbleached Lecithin 650 mg • Choline Bitartrate 50 mg • Inositol 50 mg • Biotin 60 mcg • Niacinamide 30 mg • Vitamin B6 2 mg • Magnesium Glycero Phosphate 100 mg • Magnesium 12 mg • Phosphorus 16 mg.

Lecithin — Health Center for Better Living
Rich source of choline, a B-complex nutrient, HCBL Lecithin. (Derived from soybeans).

Leci-Thin — Nature's Plus
Each wafer contains: Lecithin 1500 mg derived from natural Soybean, rich in Choline, Inositol & Phosphorus • Wheat Bran 500 mg • Vegetable Cellulose 200 mg • Protein, vegetable soy & peanut 150 mg. Made from the finest quality Lecithin, containing 95% Soy Phosphatides. In an all natural base of carob, coconut & vanilla bean. Each wafer contains approximately 16 calories. Yeast free; sweetened with VitaSweet.

Lecithin & Milk powder — Nature's Life
Two heaping tablespoons contain: Lipids: Linoleic Acid (Omega-6) 3681 mg • Linolenic Acid (Omega-3) 438 mg • Oleic Acid (Omega-9) 575 mg • Palmitic Acid 1269 mg • Stearic Acid 288 mg. Phospholipids: Phosphatidyl choline 2.8g • Phosphatidyl ethanolamine 2.5 g • Phosphatidyl inositol 1.8 g. Vitamins: Choline 378 mg • Inositol 275 mg. Minerals: Calcium 132 mg • Iron 1 mg • Magnesium 11 mg • Phosphorus 471 mg • Potassium 276 mg • Sodium 57 mg. Amino Acids: Alanine 103 mg • Arginine 137 mg • Aspartic Acid 213 mg • Cysteine 11 mg • Glutamic Acid 779 mg • Glycine 68 mg • Histidine (essential amino acid) 99 mg • Isoleucine (essential amino acid) 216 mg • Leucine (essential amino acid) 334 mg • Lysine (essential amino acid) 270 mg • Methionine (essential amino acid) 110 mg • Phenylalanine (essential amino acid) 190 mg • Proline 407 mg • Serine 209 mg • Threonine (essential amino acid) 148 mg • Tryptophan (essential amino acid) 49 mg • Tyrosine 209 mg • Valine (essential amino acid) 243 mg.

Lecithin-E — Nutrilite
Each Tablet Contains: Lecithin (from Soybean Oil) 290 mg • Vitamin E 30 IU.

Leg Vein & Circulation — ProHerbs
Two tablets contain: Vitamin C 240 mg • Green Tea leaves (Camellia sinensis standardized to 50% catechins) 100 mg • Horse Chestnut seed (Aesculus hippocastanum standardized to 18-20% total saponins) 300 mg • Butcher's Broom root (Ruscus aculeatus standardized to 10% saponins) 200 mg • Citrus Bioflavonoid complex 200 mg. Other Ingredients: Dicalcium Phosphate, Croscarmellose Sodium, Mineral Oil, Hydroxypropylmethylcellulose, Magnesium Stearate, Microcrystalline Cellulose, Polyethylene Glycol, Silicon Dioxide, Stearic Acid, Titanium Dioxide, FD&C Red #27 Lake and FD&C Blue #1 Lake.

Leg Veins Formula — Nature's Way
Two capsules contain: Butcher's Broom root 200 mg • Cayenne pepper fruit 50 mg • Dandelion leaf 250 mg • Grape seed dried extract 37.5 mg • Horse chestnut dried extract 200 mg • Prickly Ash bark 100 mg • Vitamin C (Ascorbic Acid) 30 mg. Other ingredients: Gelatin, Magnesium Stearate, Millet.

Some Brand Name Natural Products - What they Contain
www.NaturalDatabase.com contains MANY more listings than appear here.

Lemon-Lime Multi-Vitamin for Adults —
LiFizz Effervescent Vitamins
Each tablet contains: Magnesium 80 mg • Calcium 200 mg • Zinc 5 mg • Iron 6 mg • Vitamin A 5000 IU • Vitamin E 15 IU • Vitamin C 60 mg • Vitamin B2 (Riboflavin) 1.7 mg • Vitamin B6 (Pyridoxine) 2 mg • Vitamin B12 (Cyanocobalamin) 6 mcg • Vitamin B1 (Thiamin) 1.5 mg • Niacin (Vitamin PP or B3) 20 mg • Pantothenic Acid 10 mg • Free Folic Acid 400 mcg • Biotin 300 mcg • Vitamin D 400 IU.

L-Glutamine Plus — Atrium
Each tablet contains: L-Glutamine (an essential amino acid) 300 mg • L-Tryosine (an essential amino acid) 100 mg • Raw Bovine Adrenal concentrate 50 mg • Calcium Ascorbate (Vitamin C) 100 mg.

Lice Treatment & Prevention: Herbal Hair Oil —
The Herbalist
Pure essential oils of Rosemary• Lavender• Bay • Sage • Formulated with botanical extracts of Nettles leaf• Burdock root• Red Clover blossom• Chaparral leaf. In a base of cold-pressed oils of Sweet Almond and Jojoba.

Licorice Garlic — Atrium
Each capsule contains: Licorice root 250 mg • Garlic 260 mg. Contains no sugar, starch, salt, wheat, corn, yeast or soy derivatives.

Life Extension Mix — Olympia Nutrition
Multiple Vitamin • Mineral Enzyme • Antioxidant Flavonoid formula.

Life Spark — Source Naturals
Four tablets contain: Vitamin B1 (Thiamin) 30 mg • Vitamin B2 (Riboflavin) 30 mg • Niacin 25 mg and Niacinamide 125 mg 150 mg • Vitamin B5 (Pantothenic Acid) 100 mg • Vitamin B6 (Pyridoxine HCl) 25 mg • Vitamin B12 (Cyanocobalamin) 100 mcg • Vitamin E (D-Alpha Tocopheryl) (Natural) 150 IU • Magnesium (Oxide, Citrate) 250 mg • Potassium (Citrate) 99 mg • Glycine 500 mg • Tyrosine 250 mg • Coenzyme Q10 (Ubiquinone) 50 mg • Alpha-Lipoic Acid 25 mg • Herbal Blend 1170 mg: Siberian Ginseng, Panax Ginseng, Polygonum Multiflori (Fo Ti), Cyperus, Panax Ginseng extract, Tien Chi, and Siberian Ginseng extract.

Liga-Pane — Nutri-Quest
Each tablet contains: Shark Cartilage 50 mg • N-Acetyl Glucosamine 10 mg • Bromelain 10 mg • Valerian 50 mg • Feverfew 150 mg • Passion Flower 50 mg • Scullcap 25 mg • White Willow 100 mg • Magnesium Citrate 150 mg • Calcium Lactate 100 mg • Kava Kava 15 mg • Tumeric 10 mg • Vitamin B6 10 mg • Oregano 10 mg • Marjoram 10 mg • Thyme 10 mg • Basil powder 10 mg • Ginger 10 mg • Suma 10 mg • Manganese Chelate 15 mg • Molybdenum Chelate 50 mcg.

Line Assist Creme — Aspen Group, Inc.
Each gram contains: Tocopheryl Acetate 1% • Panthenol 1% • Ascorbyl Palmitate .3% • Water • Diisopropyl Adipate • Cetearyl Alcohol • Potassium Cetyl Phosphate • Retinyl Palmitate • Palmitate • Tocopherol • Dimethicone • Carbomer • Ammonium Hydroxide • Quaternium-15 • Disodium EDTA.

Liniment Virtue — Blessed Herbs
St. John's Wort flower • Comfrey root • Angelica root • Valerian root • Lobelia herb • Ginger root • Calendula flower • Arnica flower & herb • Cayenne pepper • Essential oils of Myrrh, Hyssop, Rosemary, Lavender & German Chamomile • Grain alcohol & Distilled Water.

Lipo Trim — Now
Three tablets contain: Choline 1000 mg • Inositol 1000 mg • L-Methionine 500 mg • Taurine 250 mg • L-Carnitine 100 mg • Pyridoxine (B6) 10 mg • Chromium Picolinate 200 mcg.

Lipo-Complex — Progressive Labs
Each capsule contains: Pancreatic enzyme concentrate 400 mg (equivalent in enzymatic activity to 4X USP) • Pepsin 1:3000 (from Pepsin 1:10,000) 100 mg • Green Beet leaf powder 100 mg • Raw Liver concentrate 10 mg • Ox bile 10 mg.

Lipoicare — PhysioLogics
Each capsule contains: Taurine 200 mg • Alpha-Lipoic Acid 25 mg • Calendula flower, Marigold (5% Lutein 3 mg; > 0.22% Zeaxanthin, 0.13 mg) 60 mg.

Lipotrope — Progressive Labs
Each capsule contains: Vitamin C 50 mg • Vitamin B6 5 mg • Folate (folic acid) 200 mcg • Vitamin B12 200 mcg • Pantothenic Acid 60 mg • Magnesium Aspartate 25 mg • Milk Thistle (Silybum marianum) 100 mg • Choline Bitartrate 150 mg • Inositol 75 mg • Betaine HCL 60 mg • DL-Methionine 50 mg • Black Radish (Raphanus nigra) 50 mg • Green Beet leaf powder 50 mg • Celandine (Chelidonium majus) 15 mg • Chionanthus (Chionanthus virginica) 15 mg • PABA 25 mg.

Lipotropic Complex — Nature's Life
Three tablets contain: L-Methionine (Free-Form Amino Acid) 1000 mg • Choline (from 2040 mg Choline Bitartrate) 1000 mg • Inositol 1000 mg • Betaine HCl (Sugar Beets) 250 mg • Milk Thistle (Silybum marianum) 50 mg • Vitamin B6 (Pyridoxine Hydrochloride) 10 mg • L-Taurine (Free-Form Amino Acid) 10 mg • L-Carnitine (Free-Form Amino Acid) 10 mg • Lecithin (Soy) (61% Phosphatides) 10 mg • Beet root powder (Beta vulgaris rubra) 5 mg • Dandelion root powder (Taraxacum officinale) 5 mg • Culvers root powder (Leptandra virginica) 5 mg • Apple Cider Vinegar 5 mg • Barberry root bark (Berberis vulgaris) 5 mg • Chromium (Nutrition 21 Picolinate) 25 mcg.

Lipotropic Fuel — TwinLab
Five capsules contain: Choline 500 mg • Inositol 250 mg • L-Methionine 100 mg • Vitamin B12 100 mcg • Betaine 100 mg • L-Carnitine 100 mg • Milk Thistle extract (standardized for 80% Silymarin) 500 mg • Natural Vitamin E (Succinate) 400 IU • Vitamin C 1000 mg • Vitamin B1 25 mg • N-Acetyl Cysteine (NAC) 250 mg • L-Glutathione 100 mg • Vitamin B2 25 mg • Selenium (from Selenomethionine) 150 mcg • Zinc (from Zinc Mono-Methionine) 15 mg.

Liquid Anti-Oxidant — Natrol
Two teaspoons (10 ml) contain: Anti-Oxidant Vitamins & Trace Minerals: Vitamin A (beta carotene) 10000 IU • Vitamin C (Calcium ascorbate) 500 mg • Vitamin E (acetate) 200 IU • Selenium (monomethionine) 90 mcg • Advanced Flavonoids: GP Complex+ 80 mg • Rutin, Quercetin, & Hesperidin 10 mg • Tropical fruit extracts from: Acerola, Cashew fruit, Passion fruit, Orange, Lime & Mango in a specially formulated base of: Purified Water, Brown Rice Syrup, Honey & Citric Acid.

Liquid Children's Multiple — Natrol
Two teaspoons contain: Essential Vitamins: Vitamin A (beta carotene) 2500 IU • Vitamin C (calcium ascorbate & ascorbic acid) 100 mg • Vitamin D3 (calciferol) 400 IU • Vitamin E (Acetate) 30 IU • Thiamine (Vitamin B1) 1 mg • Riboflavin(Vitamin B2) 1 mg • Niacin (Niacinamide) 12 mg • Vitamin B6 (pyridoxine HCl) 1.4 mg • Vitamin B12 (cyanocobalamin) 2.5 mcg • Pantothenic Acid (calcium d-pantothenate) 6 mg • Folic Acid 100 mcg • Biotin 20 mcg • Flavonoid: Hesperidin, Acerola, Cashew fruit, Passion fruit, Orange & Lime 10 mg • Tropical fruit extracts from: Lemon, Orange, Lime, Mango • Natural Vanilla Bean extract • Herbal extracts: Anise Seed, Licorice root, Millefolium plant, Horsetail Grass plant, Chamomile leaf & flowers, Peppermint leaf, Nettles plant, Spinach leaf & Sodium Benzoate (0.1% added to help protect flavor). In a base of Purified Water, Brown Rice Syrup, Glycerine & Citric Acid.

Liquid Children's Multi-Vitamin — Natrol
Two teaspoons (10 ml) contain: Essential Vitamins: Vitamin A (beta carotene) 2500 IU • Vitamin C (calcium ascorbate & ascorbic acid) 100 mg • Vitamin D3 (calciferol) 400 IU • Vitamin E (Acetate) 30 IU • Vitamin B1 (Thiamine) 1 mg • Vitamin B2 (Riboflavin) 1 mg • Niacin (Niacinamide) Vitamin B3 12 mg • Vitamin B6 (pyridoxine HCl) 1.4 mg • Vitamin B12 (cyanocobalamin) 2.5 mcg • Pantothenic Acid (calcium d-pantothenate) 6 mg • Folic Acid 100 mcg • Biotin 20 mcg • Flavonoid: Hesperidin 10 mg • Tropical fruit extracts from: Lemon, Orange, Lime, Mango • Other extracts from: natural Vanilla Bean extract • Herbal extracts: Anise Seed, Licorice root, Millefolium plant, Plantain root, Horsetail Grass plant, Chamomile leaf & flowers, Peppermint leaf, Nettles plant, Spinach leaf & Sodium Benzoate (0.1% added to help protect Flavor). In a base of: Purified Water, Brown Rice Syrup, Glycerine & Citric Acid.

Liquid Ester-C — Natrol
Two teaspoons (10 ml) contain: Vitamin C (from Ester-C calcium ascorbate) 250 mg • Calcium (from Ester-C calcium ascorbate) 25 mg • Pure Bioflavonoids containing: Rutin, Quercetin, & Hesperidin 10 mg • Tropical fruit extracts from: Acerola, Cashew fruit, Passion fruit, Orange, Lime & Mango. In a specially formulated base of: Purified Water, Brown Rice Syrup, Honey, natural Vanilla Bean extract, Citric Acid & Sodium Benzoate (0.1% added to help protect flavor). Ester-C is a unique ascorbate complex bound with calcium carbonate. It is naturally processed in purified water without the use of alcohol or acetone solvents.

BRAND NAMES

© Copyright 2000, Natural Medicines Comprehensive Database (209) 472-2244. For updated data, go to www.NaturalDatabase.com. • 1357

Some Brand Name Natural Products - What they Contain
www.NaturalDatabase.com contains MANY more listings than appear here.

B
R
A
N
D

N
A
M
E
S

Liquid Iron Ferrochel — Natrol
Four teaspoons (20 mL) contain: Iron & Vitamins: Iron (Ferrochel chelate) 14.5 mg • Vitamin C (Calcium Ascorbate) 100 mg • Vitamin B1 (Thiamine) 1 mg • Vitamin B6 (Pyridoxine HCl) 2 mg • Vitamin B12 (Cyanocobalamin) 3 mcg • Niacinamide 13 mg • Herbal extracts: Nettles, Kelp, Spinach, Yarrow, Angelica, Horsetail Grass, Siberian Ginseng, Yellow Dock, Burdock root, Pau D'Arco, Rose Hips & Alfalfa • Tropical fruit extracts from: Acerola, Pineapple, Cashew fruit, Passion fruit, Lime & Mango. In a specially formulated base of: Purified Water, Brown Rice Syrup, Honey & natural fruit flavors.

Liquid Kalm With Kava Kava root extract — Natrol
Two teaspoons (10 ml) contain: Guaranteed Potency Herbal extracts: Kava Kava root extract standardized to contain 30% Kavalactones 25 mg • Passion flower Herb extract standardized to Contain 3.5% Isovitexin 20 mg • Chamomile flower extract standardized to Contain 0.5% Apigenin 25 mg • Hops Cone extract standardized to Contain 0.35% Flavonoids 25 mg • Vitamin: Vitamin B6 2 mg • Herbal extract blend: Lemon Balm leaf, Oat Straw, Marjoram leaf, Cowslip herb, Rosemary leaf, Scullcap herb. Other ingredients: Honey & Brown Rice Syrup, natural Lemon & Ginger flavor, Cashew fruit & Passion fruit powder, Citric Acid, Sodium Benzoate (0.1% added to protect flavor).

Liquid Multi-Vitamin — Natrol
Two teaspoons (10 ml) contain: Vitamins & Minerals: Vitamin A (beta carotene) 10000 IU • Vitamin C (Calcium Ascorbate) 200 mg • Vitamin D (cholecalciferol) 400 IU • Vitamin E (Acetate) 100 IU • Vitamin B1 (Thiamine) 7.5 mg • Vitamin B2 (Riboflavin) 8.5 mg • Niacin (Niacinamide) Vitamin B3 20 mg • Vitamin B6 (Pyridoxine HCl) 17 mg • Vitamin B12 (cyanocobalamin) 50 mcg • Pantothenic Acid (calcium d-pantothenate) 50 mg • Inositol 25 mg • Folic Acid 400 mcg • Biotin 300 mcg. Advanced Flavonoids: GP Flavonoids Complex+ 50 mg • Rutin, Quercetin, & Hesperidin 10 mg • Herbal extracts: Nettles, Kelp, Parsley, Ginger, Oats, Alfalfa, Hops, Peppermint, Rose Hips, Spinach & Echinacea. natural Vanilla Bean flavor, natural Ginger flavor • Tropical fruit extracts from: Acerola, Pineapple, Cashew fruit, Passion fruit, Mango, Orange, Lime & Lemon. In a Specially Formulated Base of: Purified Water, Brown Rice Syrup, Honey, Glycerine, Citric Acid, Sodium Benzoate to help protect flavor, Milk Thistle & Citrus fruits.

Lithinase — Progressive Labs
Each capsule contains: Lithium Amino Acid Chelate 25 mg • Elemental Lithium 50 mcg • Pea powder 25 mg • Buckwheat 25 mg • Millet flour 25 mg • Lentil powder 25 mg (carefully dried to preserve their natural nutrient content).

Little One Children's Multiple — Metabolic Products
One tablet contains: Vitamin A (Palmitate) 2500 IU • Vitamin A (Natural Mixed Carotenoids) 2500 IU • Vitamin C (Hypoallergenic from Beet sugar and Ascorbyl Palmitate) 100 mg • Vitamin E (D-Alpha, Natural) 60 IU • Vitamin B1 (Thiamin Mononitrate) 5 mg • Vitamin B2 (Riboflavin) 5 mg • Vitamin B3 (Niacinamide) 25 mg • Vitamin B5 (D-Cal. Pantothenate) 25 mg • Vitamin B6 (Pyridoxine) 5 mg • Vitamin B12 (Cyanocobalamin) 10 mcg • Folic Acid 400 mcg • Biotin 300 mcg • Vitamin D (Cholecalciferol) 400 IU • Iron (Carbonyl) 9 mg • Iodine (K-Iodine) 100 mcg • Copper (Gluconate) 2 mg • Manganese (Gluconate) 1 mg • Zinc (Citrate) 15 mg • Molybdenum (Sodium Molybdate 25 mcg • Chromium (GTF-Polynicotinate) 100 mcg • Selenium (L-Selenomethionine, Sodium Selenite) 100 mcg .

Liv-A-Tox — Enzymatic Therapy
Three tablets contain: Vitamin A (Fish Liver oil) 4500 IU • Niacin 40 mg • Vitamin C (Ascorbic Acid/Rose Hips) 25 mg • Biotin 200 mcg • Vitamin B12 (Cyanocobalamin) 3 mcg • Other ingredients: Choline Bitartrate 850 mg • Dehydrated Green Beet leaf juice powder 300 mg • L-Methionine 250 mg • Barberry · bark of root 4:1 (Berberis vulgaris) 150 mg • Boldo extract (Peumus boldo) standardized to contain 1.52% essential oils 150 mg • Greater Celandine extract (Chelidonium majus) 135 mg • Fringetree (Cheonanthus) 135 mg • Ox Bile extract 90 mg • Betaine HCL 75 mg • Inositol 50 mg • Liver, desiccated 40 mg • Unsaturated Free Fatty Acids 30 mg. Chlorophyll is used in this product as a natural coloring agent. All organs & glands derived from bovine sources.

Liver — Nutrivention
Each tablet contains: Inositol 100 mg • Choline Bitartrate 100 mg • Vitamin E 50 IU • Vitamin B1 10 mg • Niacin 10 mg • Pantothenic Acid 10 mg • Vitamin A (Beta Carotene) 500 IU • Vitamin B12 100 mcg • Vitamin K 15 mcg • Lecithin 300 mg • Milk Thistle (Cardus

marianus) 200 mg • Dandelion root 200 mg • Burdock root 50 mg • L-Methionine 50 mg • L-Theronine 30 mg • Yellow Dock 25 mg • Butternut root bark 25 mg.

Liver Chelate — Atrium
Each tablet contains: Ferrous Fumarate as Chelated Proteinates 55 mg • Copper 1 mg • Folic Acid 40 mcg • Vitamin B12 20 mcg • Raw Liver concentrate (not an extract) of Bovine source 190 mg.

Liver Guard — Source Naturals
Two tablets contain: Vitamin B1 (Thiamin) 7.5 mg • Vitamin B2 (Riboflavin) 7.5 mg • Niacinamide and Niacin 50 mg • Vitamin B5 (Pantothenic Acid) 15 mg • Vitamin B6 (Pyridoxine HCl) 10 mg • Vitamin B12 (Cyanocobalamin) 25 mcg • Folic Acid 200 mcg • Vitamin C (Ascorbic Acid and Zinc Ascorbate) 527 mg • Fat-Soluble Vitamin C (from 238 mg of Ascorbyl Palmitate) 100 mg • Vitamin E (D-Alpha Tocopheryl) (Natural) 75 IU • Magnesium (Oxide, Malate) 60 mg • Potassium (Citrate) 49.5 mg • Selenium (as L-Selenomethionine) 50 mcg • Zinc (OptiZinc Zinc Monomethionine 10 mg and Zinc Ascorbate 5 mg) 15 mg • Silymarin (from Milk Thistle seed extract) 200 mg • N-Acetyl Cysteine 200 mg • Dandelion root extract 125 mg • Dandelion root 125 mg • Turmeric extract (95% Curcumin) 76 mg • Choline (Bitartrate) 50 mg • Inositol 50 mg • Alpha-Lipoic Acid (Thioctic acid) 25 mg • Coenzyme Q10 (Ubiquinone) 12.5 mg.

Liver Maintenance Formula — PhysioLogics
Each capsule contains: Milk Thistle (80% Silymarin, 80 mg) 100 mg • Dandelion (20% Taraxasterol, 20 mg; 3% Choline, 3 mg) 100 mg • Picrorhiza kurroa (4% Kutkin, 4 mg) 100 mg • Artichoke (5% Cynarin, 2.5 mg) 50 mg • Phylannthus amarus (4% Sesquiterpenes, 2 mg) 50 mg • Boldo (0.2% Boldine, 500 mcg) 25 mg • Black Radish 25 mg • Alpha Lipoic Acid 25 mg.

Liver Support — Amazon Support
Each capsule contains: Carqueja • Picao Preto • Erva Tostao • Tayuya • Tumeric • Artichoke • Mutamba • Boldo • Chanca Piedra • Sarsaparilla • Jurubeba • Gervao.

Liver-Enhancer — HerbaSway
Reishi • Poria • Cordyceps • Maitake Shiitake • Hericium • Schisandra • Lycium • Milk Thistle • Blackberry • HerbaSwee (Cucurbitaceae fruit).

Living Energy — Futurebiotics
Four tablets contain: Chlorella 500 mg • Bee Pollen 1000 mg • Ginseng 4:1 extract equivalent to 250 mg • Royal Jelly (freeze dried) 25 mg • Schizandra 4:1 extract equivalent to 250 mg • Astragalus 4:1 extract equivalent to 250 mg • Spirulina 500 mg • Alfalfa juice concentrate 1200 mg.

Livr D-Tox — Nutri-Quest
Each tablet contains: Glucuronic Acid 10 mg • Liver 5 mg • Vitamin A 1000 IU • Vitamin C 25 mg • Vitamin B1 5 mg • Vitamin E 10 IU • Black Currant seed oil 25 mg • Cellulase 50 mg • Amylase 50 mg • Lipase 50 mg • Protease 50 mg • Lipoic Acid 2 mg • Phosphatidyl Choline 5.75 mg • Choline Bitartrate 15 mg • DL-Methionine 5 mg • Calcium Chelate 50 mg • Magnesium 50 mg • Zinc Chelate 5 mg • Selenium Chelate 25 mcg • Manganese 1 mg • Milk Thistle 100 mg • Silymarin 5 mg • Garlic 50 mg • Beet root 25 mg • Beet leaf 25 mg.

Liv-R-Actin Milk Thistle Blend in Vegetarian Capsules — Nature's Plus
Two vegicaps contain: Herbal Blend containing: (Dandelion, Barberry, Goldenseal, Wild Oregon Grape & Celery seed) 600 mg • Milk Thistle extract, providing 70%, 98 mg of the active flavonoid Silymarin 140 mg. Contains no yeast, wheat, corn, soy, milk, salt, sugar or starch.

L-Lysine Plus — Atrium
Each tablet contains: L-Lysine HCL (an essential amino acid) 500 mg • Ascorbic Acid (Vitamin C) 100 mg.

Lobelia and Cayenne — Dial Herbs
Lobelia • Cayenne.

Lomatium-Goldenseal Virtue — Blessed Herbs
Lomatium root • Astragalus root • Osha root • Echinacea Angustifolia root • Goldenseal root • Siberian Ginseng root • Licorice root • Reishi mycelium • Shitake mycelium • Grain alcohol & Distilled Water.

Longest Living Acidophilus — Futurebiotics
Each capsule contains: Acidophilus fortified with Rhamnosus,

encapsulated in a base of Rice powder & Beet fiber. 1 billion Live Organisms per capsule.

Longe-Vit-E — Holista
Each capsule contains: Vitamin C (Ester-C) 250 mg • Beta Carotene 10000 IU • Vitamin E (d-alpha tocopherol) 200 IU • Selenium 50 mcg • Vitamin B6 25 mg • Magnesium 50 mg • Manganese 1.5 mg • Copper 1.0 mg.

Love-Berries — Nature's Plus
Each pill contains: Cranberry concentrate 45X 200 mg • Vitamin C corn free 60 mg. Sweetened with VitaSweet. Contains no yeast, wheat, corn, soy, milk, or salt.

LPC — OSMO Therapy
Each capsule contains: Lysophosphatidyl Choline 300 mg.

LPC Serum — The Vitamin Factory
One ounce contains: Pycnogenol • Liquid Vitamin C. Applied topically to the face. Using a highly stable derivative of Vitamin C called Magnesium Ascorbyl Phosphate (Mega-C), the Vitamin C and Pycnogenol are released into the skin by a liposomal delivery system which protects the ingredients.

Lung Support Formula — Gero Vita
Astragalus membranaceus • Cordyceps sinensis • Ophiopogon japonicus.

Lung-Mend — The Herbalist
Elecampane root • Grindelia herb • Pleurisy root • Butterbur root • Marshmallow root • Usnea lichen • Yerba Santa leaf • Lobelia leaf • Yerba Mansa root.

Lustre — Source Naturals
Six tablets contain: Vitamin A (Beta Carotene) 15000 IU • Vitamin A (Palmitate) 5000 IU • Vitamin B1 (Thiamin) 10 mg • Vitamin B2 (Riboflavin) 10 mg • Niacinamide 30 mg • Vitamin B5 (Calcium D-Pantothenate) 50 mg • Vitamin B6 (Pyridoxine HCI) 20 mg • Vitamin B12 (Cyanocobalamin) 30 mcg • Biotin 2000 mcg • Folic Acid 800 mcg • Vitamin C (Magnesium, Zinc and Manganese Ascorbates) 1000 mg • Vitamin E (D-Alpha Tocopheryl)(Natural) 200 IU • Copper (Sebacate) 1.5 mg • Magnesium (Ascorbate) 59 mg • Silica (Horsetail Silica Extract) 36 mg • Manganese (Ascorbate) 6 mg • Selenium (as L-Selenomethionine and Sodium Selenite) 200 mcg • L-Proline 600 mg • Inositol 500 mg • L-Cysteine (HCI) 400 mg • Choline (Bitartrate) 100 mg • L-Methionine 100 mg • N-Acetyl Cysteine 100 mg • PABA (Para Amino Benzoic Acid) 100 mg.

Lutein i care — Nature's Life
Each capsule contains: Lutein (FloraGLO) [from Marigold petals (Tagetes erecta)] 5 mg • Beta Carotene [(Dunaliella salina) equivalent to 5000 IU Vitamin A] 3 mg • Other naturally occurring carotenoids in D. salina: Zeaxanthin (T. erecta, D. salina) 370 mcg • Alpha Carotene 106 mcg • Cryptoxanthin 20 mcg • Zinc (Gluconate) 5 mg • Copper (Gluconate) 2.5 mg.

Lutein Plus — Nutrition Warehouse
Each capsule contains: Lutein (with 240- 600 mcg Zeaxanthin) 6 mg • In a 330 mg base of: Spinach, Blueberry Powder and Bilberry extract.

Lycopene — Nature's Life
Each capsule contains: Lycopene 6 mg • Carrot Carotenoids 2 mg providing: Beta Carotene (Vitamin A equivalent 2500 IU) 1500 mcg, Alpha Carotene (Vitamin A equivalent 417 IU) 500 mcg, Phytoene 39 mcg, Phytofluene 13 mcg.

Lycosoy — TwinLab
Two softgels contain: Vitamin D 400 IU • Vitamin E 200 IU • Selenium 200 mcg • Omega-3 Fish Oil conc. 460 mcg • Soy Bean extract 150 mg • Lycopene 5 mg • Green Tea leaf extract 2 mg.

Lymphatone — The Herbalist
Echinacea root • Red root • Cleavers herb • Yellow Dock root • Burdock root • Wild Indigo root • Poke root.

Lympho-Clear — Enzymatic Therapy
Each capsule contains: Red Clover extract 4:1 (Trifolium pratense) 200 mg • Burdock root extract 4:1 (Arctium lappa) 200 mg • Oregon Grape root extract 6:1 (Berberis aquifolium) 100 mg • Licorice root extract (Glycyrrhiza glabra) standardized to contain 5% Glycyrrhizic Acid 50 mg • Goldenseal root extract (Hydrastis canadensis) standardized to contain 5% total Alkaloids including: Berberine, Hydrastine & Canadine 50 mg. Contains no sugar, salt, yeast, wheat, corn, soy, dairy products, coloring, flavoring, or preservatives.

Lymph-Spleen Soluble Fractions — Phytopharmica
Each capsule contains: Lymph-Spleen Complex (predigested soluble concentrate) 250 mg • Multi-Glandular Complex 100 mg containing: Raw Liver, Raw Lung, Raw Pancreas, Raw Heart, Raw Kidney, Raw Spleen & Raw Brain. Contains no sugar, salt, yeast, wheat, corn, soy, dairy products, coloring, flavoring or preservatives. All organs & glands derived from bovine sources except raw pancreas (porcine).

Lysozyme Plus — Atrium
Each tablet contains: Pancreatin (maximum strength) 200 mg • Papain 100 mg • Bromelain 75 mg • Rutin 60 mg • Trypsin 35 mg • Thymus 35 mg • Amylase 15 mg • Lipase 15 mg • Lysozyme 10 mg • Cellulase 2 mg • Zinc Gluconate 4 mg • a-Chymotrypsin 1 mg.

M.C.H.C. Capsules — Progressive Labs
Each capsule contains: Calcium 250 mg, from 500 mg M.C.H.C. 125 mg, from 500 mg Calcium Citrate 125 mg • Iron (from M.C.H.C.) 0.3 mg • Vitamin K 20 mcg • Phosphorus (from M.C.H.C) 65 mg • Magnesium (from M.C.H.C.) 4 mg • Zinc (from M.C.H.C.) 0.075 mg • Copper (from M.C.H.C.) 0.01 mg • Manganese (from M.C.H.C.) 0.045 mg • Potassium (from M.C.H.C.) 0.035 mg • Protein (from M.C.H.C. as collagen glycosaminoglycans) 125 mg • Boron (as boron aspartate) 0.75 mg • Fluorapatite (from M.C.H.C.) 31 mcg • Silicon (from M.C.H.C.) 19 mcg • Strontium (from M.C.H.C.) 10 mcg.

M.C.H.C. Tablets — Progressive Labs
Each tablet contains: Calcium (elemental) 250 mg, from 500 mg M.C.H.C. 125 mg, from 500 mg. Calcium Citrate 125 mg • Iron (from M.C.H.C.) 0.3 mg • Vitamin K 20 mcg • Phosphorum (from M.C.H.C.) 65 mg • Magnesium (from M.C.H.C.) 4 mg • Zinc (fromM.C.H.C.) 0.075 mg • Copper (from M.C.H.C.) 0.01 mg • Manganese (from M.C.H.C.) 0.045 mg • Potassium (from M.C.H.C.) 0.035 mg • Protein (from M.C.H.C. as collagen glycosaminoglycans) 125 mg • Boron (as aspartate) 750 mcg • Fluorapatite (from M.C.H.C.) 31 mcg • Silicon (from M.C.H.C.) 19 mcg • Strontium (from M.C.H.C.) 10 mcg.

M.V. Teen — Futurebiotics
100% or more of the USRDA for 16 vitamins and minerals, 100 mcg of chromium and selenium.

Macro-Min — Atrium
Each tablet contains: Calcium Aspartate 600 mg • Magnesium Gluconate 300 mg • Potassium Aspartate 88.3 mg • Manganese Aspartate 50 mg • Vitamin D3 250 IU.

Macular Guardian — Clinician's Choice
Two tablets contain: Vitamin A (as retinyl acetate) 2000 IU • Vitamin C (as ascorbic acid) 120 mg • Vitamin E (as dl-alpha tocopheryl acetate) 200 IU • Riboflavin 6 mg • Selenium (as selenomethionine) 40 mcg • Manganese (as amino acid chelate) 10 mg • Eyebright Herb 200 mg • RoseOx (patented, standardized process for an extract of Rosemary) 100 mg • Ascorbyl Palmitate 20 mg • L-Lysine HCl 20 mg • Lutein 12 mg • L-Glutathione 10 mg • Lycopene 10 mg • Beta-Carotene 6 mg • Proprietary blend 8 mg: Cruciferex, Carrot Powder, Citrus Bioflavonoid Complex, Bilberry, Zeaxanthin.

Mag Link — Pain & Stress Center
Two tablets contain: Calcium (Calcium Carbonate) 225 mg • Magnesium (Magnesium Chloride Hexahydrate) 130 mg • Chloride 375 mg.

Magic Cigarettes — Alternative Cigarettes Inc
Each cigarette contains: Marshmallow • Yerba Santa • Damiana • Passion Flower • Jasmine • Ginseng. Regular and menthol are available.

Editor's Comments: In April 2000, the Federal Trade Commission filed a complaint against manufacturers of natural or herbal cigarettes for making claims that these products were safer than conventional cigarettes. The labeling on these products is now required to state "Herbal cigarettes are dangerous to your health. They produce tar and carbon monoxide." If they use the term "No additives" they must also state "No additives in our tobacco does NOT mean a safer cigarette."

MagnaCal — Holista
Each capsule contains: Calcium from citrate (equivalent to 625 mg) 125 mg • Magnesium from oxide (equivalent to 206 mg) 125 mg • Vitamin D3 100 IU.

Magnesium Complex — Klaire Laboratories
Each capsule contains: Magnesium Glycinate (Amino Acid Chelate) 100 mg.

© Copyright 2000, Natural Medicines Comprehensive Database (209) 472-2244. For updated data, go to www.NaturalDatabase.com. • 1359

Some Brand Name Natural Products - What they Contain
www.NaturalDatabase.com contains MANY more listings than appear here.

B R A N D   N A M E S

Magnesium Multi-Min — Nutri-Quest
Each tablet contains: As an Aspartic Acid Chelate (Amino Acid Chelate): Phosphorus 10 mg • Calcium 100 mg • Magnesium 500 mg • Iron 5 mg • Potassium 200 mg • Zinc 30 mg • Copper 250 mcg • Manganese 30 mg • Chromium 500 mcg • Molybdenum 10 mcg • Selenium 25 mcg • Vanadium 60 mcg • Silicon 0.33 mcg • Lithium 0.05 mcg.

Magnesium-Potassium Aspartate — The Vitamin Shoppe
Magnesium 100 mg • Potassium 100 mg.

Maharishi Amrit Kalash Ambrosia —
Maharishi Ayurveda Products
Meda Milkweed • Black Musale • Heart-Leaved Moonseed • East Indian Globe Thistle • Butterfly Pea • Licorice • Vanda Orchid • Elephant Creeper • Indian Wild Pepper.

Maharishi Amrit Kalash Nectar —
Maharishi Ayurveda Products
Whole Cane Sugar • Indian Gooseberry • Indian Gallnut • Ghee • Honey • Cardamom • Cinnamon • Dried Catkins • Indian Pennywort • Cyperus • Nutgrass • White Sandalwood • Aloeweed • Butterfly Pea • Shoe Flower • Licorice • Turmeric. Processed in the aqueous extract of: Castor Root • Country Mallow • Thatch Grass • Eragrostis cynosuroides • Sugar Cane • Indian Asparagus • Spreading Hogweed • Giant Potato • Winter Cherry • Indian Kudju • Trumpet Flower • Premna Integrifolia • Desmodium gangeticum • Uraria picta • Yellow-berried Night Shade • Small Caltrops • Phaseolus trilobus • Teramnus labialis • Bengal Quince • Cashmere bark.

Maharishi Amrit Kalash Sugar-Free Nectar —
Maharishi Ayurveda Products
Indian Gooseberry • Indian Gallnut • Cardamom • Cinnamon • Dried Catkins • Indian Pennywort • Cyperus • Nutgrass • White Sandalwood • Aloeweed • Butterfly Pea • Shoe Flower • Licorice • Turmeric. Processed in the aqueous extract of: Castor Root • Country Mallow • Thatch Grass • Eragrostis cynosuroides • Sugar Cane • Indian Asparagus • Spreading Hogweed • Giant Potato • Winter Cherry • Indian Kudju • Trumpet Flower • Premna Integrifolia • Desmodium gangeticum • Uraria picta • Yellow-berried Night Shade • Small Caltrops • Phaseolus trilobus • Teramnus labialis • Bengal Quince • Cashmere bark.

Male Advantage — Body Wise International, Inc.
Three capsules contain: Zinc (Krebs Cycle Chelate) 15 mg • Saw Palmetto Berry Fruit Extract 4:1 (Equivalent to 1000 mg Saw Palmetto) 250 mg • Kava Kava Root 250 mg • Alpha-Ketoglutaric Acid 200 mg • Flaxseed 100 mg • Pumpkin seed 75 mg • Korean Ginseng root 75 mg • Siberian Ginseng root 75 mg • Turmeric root extract (95% Curcumin) 50 mg • Damiana leaf 50 mg • L-Alanine 50 mg • L-Glutamic Acid 50 mg • Glycine 50 mg • Pygeum Africana Bark wet extract 150:1 50 mg • Gotu Kola whole plant 50 mg • Bromelain 50 mg.

Male Drive — Dial Herbs
Vitamin E • Yohimbe • Green Oats • Zinc • Siberian Ginseng • l-Histidine. In a base of Velvet Antler, Rehmanniae, Cormus Wolfberries, Astragalus seed, Epimedii, Vaccriae, Cyperi.

Male Fuel — TwinLab
Six capsules contain: Yohimbe bark extract (standardized for Yohimbine) 800 mg • L-Arginine HCL 2800 mg • Ginkgo Biloba extract (standardized for 24% flavonoid glycosides) 60 mg • Natural Vitamin E 400 IU • Zinc (from Zinc Picolinate) 30 mg • L-Tyrosine 100 mg • Vitamin B6 50 mg • Choline Bitartrate 200 mg • Vitamin B5 (Pantothenic Acid) 100 mg • Saw Palmetto (Serenoa repens) extract 120 mg • Phytosterol Complex (providing Beta-Sitosterol 60 mg) 120 mg.

Male Multi Vitamins — Health Center for Better Living
Each tablet contains: Vitamin A (as retinyl palmitate and 50% from beta-carotene) 5,000 IU • Vitamin C (as ascorbic acid) 150 mg • Vitamin D (as cholecalciferol) 100 IU • Vitamin E (as dl-alpha-tocopheryl acetate) 50 IU • Vitamin K (as phytonadione) 10 mcg • Thiamin (as thiamin HCl) 10 mg • Riboflavin 10 mg • Niacin (as niacinarnide) 30 mg • Vitamin B6 (as pyridoxine HCl) 5 mg • Folate (as folic acid) 100 mcg • Vitamin B12 (as cyanocobalamin) 10 mcg • Biotin 100 mcg • Pantothenic Acid (as D-calcium patothenate) 5 mg • Calcium (as calcium carbonate and dicalcium phosphate) 150 mg • Iodine (from Kelp) 50 mcg • Magnesium (as magnesium oxide) 25 mg • Zinc (as zinc citrate) 5 mg • Selenium (as selenomethionine) 100 mcg • Copper (as copper oxide) 1 mg • Manganese (as manganese

sulfate) 1 mg • Chromium (as chromium dinicotinate glycinate) 100 mcg • Molybdenum (as sodium molybdate) 20 mcg • Boron (as boron chelate) 300 mcg • Grape seed extract (40% proanthocyanidins) 10 mg • Citrus bioflavonoids complex 15 mg • Rutin 10 mg • Silica (from horsetail herb) 5 mg • Montmorillonite (source of 72 trace minerals) 25 mg • Octacosanol (from rice bran) 2 mg • Saw palmetto berry 50 mg.

Male Performax — PhysioLogics
Each capsule contains: Muira Puama root 500 mg • Oriental Ginseng root (Panax ginseng) (14% Ginsenosides, 3.5 mg) 25 mg • Ginkgo leaf (24% Ginkgo Flavonglycosides, 3.2 mg; 6% Terpene Lactones, 0.8 mg) 13 mg.

Male Power — Futurebiotics
Panax Ginseng (Active Standardized Ginsenosides) 5 mg • Siberian Ginseng (50:1 extract from) 750 mg • Avena Sativa (Wild Oats, extract from) 200 mg • Smilax (Sarsaparilla) 200 mg • Saw Palmetto (extract from) 200 mg • Mexican Yam (extract from) 200 mg • Polygonum Multiflorum (extract from) 250 mg • Astragalus (extract from) 250 mg • Schizandra (extract from) 250 mg • Alfalfa 500 mg • Licorice Root (extract from) 500 mg • Muira Puama 150 mg • Deer Antler 50 mg • Kelp 150 mg • Spirulina 100 mg • Black Cohosh 100 mg • Mullein 100 mg • Ginger 35 mg • Bee Pollen 500 mg • Royal Jelly 30 mg • Vitamin B12 500 mcg • Zinc (Citrate) 25 mg • Glandulars: Pancreas 100 mg • Orchic 90 mg • Thymus 90 mg • Adrenal 80 mg • Heart 75 mg • Lymph 35 mg • Prostate 35 mg • Spleen 20 mg • Pituitary 15 mg.

Male Response — Source Naturals
Three tablets contain: Vitamin E (as Natural D-Alpha Tocopheryl) 100 IU • Vitamin B6 (Pyridoxine HCl) 25 mg • Pantothenic Acid (Vitamin B5) 50 mg • Zinc (as OptiZinc Monomethionine) 15 mg • Selenium (as L-Selenomethionine and Selenium Chelate) 150 mcg • Copper (as Copper Sebacate) 1 mg • Tribulus leaf, stem and flower (Yielding 200 mg of Furostanol Saponins) 500 mg • Maca root extract (Lepidium Meyenii) 300 mg • Yohimbe bark standardized extract 4% (Yielding 9 mg of Yohimbine) 225 mg • Muira Puama stem extract 200 mg • Oat Straw leaf extract (Avena sativa) 200 mg • Siberian Ginseng root 200 mg • Damiana leaf and stem 200 mg • Saw Palmetto berry 200 mg • Mexican Sarsaparilla root 200 mg • Ashwagandha root 150 mg • Panax Ginseng root standardized extract 8% (Yielding 8 mg of Ginsenosides) 100 mg • Ginkgo Biloba leaf extract (50:1) (Yielding 14 mg of Ginkgo Flaconglycosides) 60 mg • Stinging Nettle root extract (16:1) 60 mg • Ginger root 60 mg.

Malic Acid Plus — Pain & Stress Center
Two capsules contain: Malic Acid 800 mg • Boswellia 300 mg • Magnesium 100 mg • Chromium Picolinate 50 mcg • Vitamin C 10 mg • Vitamin B6 5 mg.

Malic Acid+ — PhysioLogics
Each capsule contains: Magnesium (Oxide, Aspartate) 100 mg • Potassium (Aspartate) 10 mg • Malic Acid 250 mg • Coenzyme Q10 15 mg.

Maltsupex — Wallace Laboratories
Each level scoop contains: Malt Soup Extract derived from natural barley malt 8 g.

Mangaplex — Progressive Labs
Each tablet contains: Vitamin C (ascorbic acid) 80 mg • Vitamin D3 (cholecalciferol) 50 IU • Vitamin E (d-alpha tocopheryl succinate) 10 IU • Thiamin HCl (Vitamin B1) 5 mg • Vitamin B6 (pyridoxine HCl) 10 mg • Vitamin B12 (cyanocobalamin) 10 mcg • Calcium (calcium lactate 175 mg) 26 mg • Manganese (manganese sulfate 200 mg) 73 mg • Choline Bitartrate 30 mg • Bioflavonoids 20 mg • Horsetail 100 mg • Rose Hips 5 mg • Green Pea concentrate 200 mg • Raw Liver concentrate 10 mg.

Marine Beta Carotene — Jarrow Formulas
Each softgel contains: Beta Carotene (from Dunaliella salina) (Equivalent to 25000 IU of pro Vitamin A) activity 15 mg • Vitamin E 5 IU. Other Ingredients: Soybean Oil, Lecithin.

Marine Beta Carotene 25000 IU — Nature's Life
Each capsule contains: Beta Carotene (Dunaliella salina) (Vitamin A equivalent 25000 IU) (Other natural Carotenoids occuring in D. Salina) 15 mg • Alpha Carotene 500 mcg • Cryptoxanthin 130 mcg • Zeaxanthin 100 mcg • Lutein 86 mcg. Added as a naturally protective antioxidant: Vitamin E (d-Alpha Tocopherol) 1.5 IU.

B R A N D   N A M E S

Marine Carotene — The Vitamin Shoppe
Each softgel contains: 15 mg Natural Beta-carotene equivalent to 25000 IU Vitamin A activity along with other naturally occurring Carotenoids; Alpha-carotene, Lutein, Cryptoxanthin, and Zeaxanthin. No Yeast, Corn, Wheat, Fish, Dairy, Milk, Eggs, Salt, Sugar, Starch, Preservatives, Artificial Colors or Flavors added.

Martrim — VitaStore
Cayenne • Ginseng (Siberian) • Guarana (Paullinia Cupana) • Gymnema Sylvestre • Kelp • Phenylalanine • Pullulan • Sidacordifilia Extract • Zingiber • Vitamin A • Vitamin B1 • Vitamin B6 • Vitamin B12 • Vitamin C • Vitamin D • Vitamin E (d-alpha tocopherol) • Folic Acid • Iodine (Kelp) • Niacin • d-Biotin • Pantothenic Acid • Potassium Gluconate.

Masculex — Enzymatic Therapy
Two capsules contain: Vitamin E (D-Alpha Tocopherol) 100 IU. Other ingredients: Muira Puama Powdered extract 6:1 (Ptychopetalum olacoides) 250 mg • Liquid Liver Fractions (predigested soluble concentrate) 250 mg • Wheat Germ oil concentrate 100 mg • Beta-Sitosterol 100 mg • Mexican Damiana leaves extract (Tunera diffusa) 100 mg • Saw Palmetto Berry extract (Serenoa repens) standardized to contain 85%-95% fatty acids & biologically active sterols 40 mg • Cola Nut extract (Cola nitida) (contains 4.8 mg Caffeine) 40 mg • Panax ginseng extract standardized to contain 7% Saponins (calculated as Ginsenoside Rg1) 40 mg • Ginkgo Biloba leaves extract (Ginkgo biloba folia) standardized to contain 24% ginkgoflavonglycosides 20 mg. Contains no sugar, salt, yeast, corn, dairy products, flavoring or preservatives.

MascuPlex — Phytopharmica
Two capsules contain: Essential Vitamin: 100 IU Vitamin E (D-Alpha Tocopherol) • Other ingredients: Muira Puama powdered extract 6:1 (Ptychopetalum olacoides) 250 mg • Liquid Liver Fractions, predigested soluble concentrate 250 mg • Wheat Germ oil concentrate 100 mg • Beta-Sitosterol 100 mg • Mexican Damiana leaves extract (Turnera diffusa) 100 mg • Saw Palmetto berry extract (Serenoa repens) standardized to contain 85%-95% fatty acids & biologically active sterols 40 mg • Cola Nut extract (Cola nitida) contains 4.8 g caffeine 40 mg • Panax Ginseng extract 40 mg, standardized to contain 7% saponins calculated as ginsenoside Rg1 • Ginkgo Biloba leaves extract 20 mg (Ginkgo biloba folia) standardized to contain 24% ginkgoflavonglycosides. Contains no sugar, salt, yeast, corn, dairy, products, flavoring or preservatives.

Mass Action — Met-Rx
Each serving contains: Micronized Creatine 5 g • HMB 1.5 g • Trimethylglycine (TMG) 500 mg • Improved Nutrient Uptake. Ingredients: Glucose • Creatine Monohydrate • HMB • Trimethylglycine • Natural & Artificial Flavors • Beta Carotene & Beet juice powder for colors • Xanthan Gum • Aspartame.

Mass Fuel — TwinLab
High Biological-Quality Milk & Egg Proteins • Branched Chain Amino Acids (L-Leucine, L-Isoleucine & L-Valine) • L-Glutamine • Alpha-Ketoglutarates • Keto-Isocaproate (KIC) • L-Ornithine Alpha-Ketoglutarate • L-Carnitine • Creatine Monohydrate • High Potencies Of Vitamins & Minerals • Potassium 2000 mg • Chromium 300 mcg (from patented Chromic Fuel Chromium Picolinate). Mass Fuel is rich in complex carbohydrates. Contains no simple sugars & is fat free.

Masters — Pharmanex
Two capsules contain: Vitamin A (100% as Beta-Carotene)(Beta-Carotene, Dunaliella Salina) 3750 IU • Vitamin C (as Ascorbic Acid) 150 mg • Vitamin D3 (as Cholecalciferol) 200 IU • Vitamin E (as d-Alpha Tocopheryl Succinate) 150 IU • Riboflavin (as Riboflavin) 0.85 mg • Vitamin B6 (as Pyridoxine Hydrochloride) 1 mg • Folate (as Folic Acid) 200 mcg • Vitamin B12 (as Cyanocobalamin) 3 mcg • Calcium (Calcium Carbonate, Calcium Chelate, Calcium Citrate) 250 mg • Magnesium (Magnesium Oxide, Magnesium Chelate) 100 mg • Zinc (Zinc Chelate) 7.5 mg • Chromium (Chromium Chelate, Chromium Picolinate) 100 mcg • Korean Panax Ginseng with Ginsenosides 25 mcg • Siberian Ginseng extract with Eleutherosides 25 mcg • Ginkgo Biloba Powder with Ginkgoflavonglycosides 20 mg • Echinacea Purpurea Powder with Echinacosides 20 mg • Cranberry Concentrate with Quinnic Acid 12.5 mg • Bilberry Powder with Anthocyanosides 10 mg.

Max GLA — PhysioLogics
Each softgel contains: Linolenic Acid 375 mg • Gamma-Linolenic Acid (GLA) 229 mg • Oleic Acid 190 mg • Palmitic Acid 114 mg • Stearic Acid 41 mg • Palmitoleic Acid 3 mg.

Maxativa — Futurebiotics
Two tablets provide: Oat extract (4:1) 300 mg • Nettles extract (4:1) 150 mg • Glycine 100 mg • Vitamin C 100 mg • Smilax-Ginseng-Damiana Complex 400 mg • Bee Pollen (Lyophilized) 350 mg • Zinc (Oxide, Gluconate) 15 mg • Royal Jelly (Lyophilized) 45 mg • Niacinamide 15 mg.

MaxEPA 1000 mg — Nature's Life
Each capsule contains: MaxEPA 1000 mg providing the following naturally occuring essential nutrients: EPA (Eicosapentaneoic Acid) 180 mg • DHA (Docosahexaenoic Acid) 180 mg • Vitamin E (d-Alpha Tocopherol) 30 IU. In a natural base of certified organic Safflower oil.

Maxi-Complete — Atrium
Each tablet contains: Vitamin A Palmitate 10000 IU • Vitamin D2 Fish oil 400 IU • Vitamin B1 Thiamine HCL 10 mg • Vitamin B2 Riboflavin 10 mg • Vitamin B6 Pyridoxine HCL 10 mg • Vitamin B12 Cyanocobalamin 15 mcg • Vitamin C Ascorbic Acid 150 mg • Vitamin E Acetate 60 IU • Biotin 6 mcg • Niacin-Niacinamide 50 mg • Pantothenic Acid 25 mg • Folic Acid 400 mcg • Calcium Amino Acid Chelate 30 mg • Iodine 100 mcg • Iron Amino Acid Chelate 50 mg • Magnesium Amino Acid Chelate 20 mg • Manganese Amino Acid Chelate 6 mg • Phosphorus 20 mg • Zinc Amino Acid Chelate 5 mg • Choline Bitartrate 100 mg • Inositol 100 mg • PABA 30 mg • Rutin 25 mg. In a base of Alfalfa, Bone Meal, Bromelain, Kelp, Papaya, Rose Hips.

Maximum Strength Diet Aid Caplets Caffeine Free — Rite Aid Corporation
Each caplet contains: Active Ingredient: Phenylpropanolamine Hydrochloride 75 mg (appetite suppressant controlled release). Inactive Ingredients: Calcium Sulfate, D&C Yellow No. 10 Aluminum Lake, Ethylcellulose, FD&C Yellow No. 6 Aluminum Lake, Hydroxypropyl Cellulose, Hydroxypropyl Methylcellulose, Lactose, Magnesium Stearate, Polyethylene Glycol, Povidone, Propylene Glycol, Sorbitol, Stearic Acid, Titanium Dioxide.

Maxium Fat Burners — Optimum Nutrition
Citrimax(tm) 500 mg L-Carnitine • Choline • Inositol • Methionine.

MCH-Cal — Natrol
Two capsules contain: Vitamin D (as Cholecalciferol) 200 IU • Calcium (as calcium hydroxyapatite) 125 mg • Magnesium (as Magnesium oxide) 300 mg. Other ingredients: Magnesium Stearate, Silicon Dioxide, Gelatin.

MCT Fuel (Emulsified Medium-Chain Triglycerides) — TwinLab
Emulsified Medium Chain Triglycerides (MCTs) • Emulsified Vitamin E. Contains: 100% natural Orange flavor & small amounts of Lecithin & Apple Pectin. MCT Fuel's formula contains no chemical emulsifiers.

Medroid — Sports One
19-Nor-4-Androstenediol • 19-Norandrostenedione • Androstenedione • 4-Androstenediol • 5-Androstenediol • Tribulus Terrestris • Acetyl-L-Carnitine • Thermogenic Formula using a proprietary half-life enzymatic conversion excelerator. Capsule 1: (Tribulus Terrestris 250 mg, 5-Androstene-3B,17B-Diol 50 mg). Capsule 2: (Androstenedione 100 mg, Acetyl L-Carnitine 100 mg, 4-Androstene-3, 17-Diol 100 mg). Capsule 3 (Proprietary half-life excelerator): (Ma Huang herb 10:1 extract, Green Tea leaf 10:1 extract, White Willow bark, Secret Half Life Enzymatic Conversion Excelerator). Capsule 4: (5-Androstene-3B,17B-Diol 50 mg, 19-Nor-4-Androstene-3B, 17B-Diol 50 mg, 19-Norandrostenedione 100 mg).

Mega B-125 — The Vitamin Shoppe
Each sustained-release tablet contains: Vitamin B1 (Thiamin) 125 mg • Vitamin B2 (Riboflavin) 125 mg • Vitamin B6 (Pyridoxine Hcl) 125 mg • Vitamin B12 (Cobalamin Concentrate) 125 mcg • Niacinamide 125 mg • Folic Acid 400 mcg • Pantothenic Acid (d-Calcium Pantothenate) 125 mg • D-Biotin 125 mcg • Choline Bitartrate 125 mg • Inositol 125 mg • PABA 125 mg. In a base of Alfalfa, Watercress, Parsley, and Rice Concentrate. No Yeast, Corn, Wheat, Soy, Salt, Sugar, Starch, Milk, Eggs, Dairy, Fish or Animal Derivatives, Preservative, Artificial Colors of Flavors added.

Mega C-Complex 1000 — The Vitamin Shoppe
Each tablet contains: Vitamin C (fortified with Rose Hips) 1000 mg • Citrus Bioflavonoids 500 mg • Hesperidin Complex 50 mg • Rutin 50 mg • Acerola 10 mg. No Yeast, Wheat, Corn, Dairy, Milk, Eggs, Fish or Animal Derivatives, Soy, Salt, Sugar, Starch, Preservatives, Artificial Colors or Flavors added.

© Copyright 2000, Natural Medicines Comprehensive Database (209) 472-2244. For updated data, go to www.NaturalDatabase.com. • 1361

Some Brand Name Natural Products - What they Contain
www.NaturalDatabase.com contains MANY more listings than appear here.

B
R
A
N
D

N
A
M
E
S

Mega Chromic Fuel (Chromium Picolinate) 500 mcg —
TwinLab
Each capsule contains: Trivalent Chromium (from Pure Crystalline
Chromium Picolinate) 500 mcg.

Mega Creatine Fuel — TwinLab
Each capsule contains: University-Tested Pure Creatine Monohydrate
1200 mg.

Mega Manna 500 mg — Nature's Life
Each capsule contains: Glucomannan (Amorphophallus konjac)
500 mg.

Mega Mind — Source Naturals
Four tablets contain: Vitamin B1 (Thiamin) 500 mg • Vitamin B2
(Riboflavin) 50 mg • Vitamin B3 (150 mg Niacinamide and 50 mg
Niacin) 200 mg • Vitamin B5 (Pantothenic Acid) 50 mg • Vitamin B6
(Pyridoxine HCl) 50 mg • Vitamin B12 (Cyanocobalamin) 50 mcg •
Folic Acid 800 mcg • Biotin 500 mcg • Vitamin C (Calcium and Zinc
Ascorbates) 197 mg • Calcium (Ascorbate, Carbonate, Malate,
Succinate) 100 mg • Magnesium (Malate, Succinate, Taurinate,
Oxide) 200 mg • Zinc (Ascorbate) 10 mg • Manganese (Citrate) 5 mg
• L-Pyroglutamic Acid 1000 mg • L-Glutamine 500 mg • DMAE
(Bitartrate) 160 mg • Acetyl L-Carnitine 400 mg • N-Acetyl L-
Tyrosine 300 mg • Taurine (Magnesium Taurinate) 198 mg • Ginkgo
Biloba 24% with a Proanthocyanidolic value of 95 (50:1 Extract) 120
mg • Proanthodyn (from Grape Seed Extract) 100 mg • GABA
(Gamma Amino Butyric Acid) 100 mg • Coenzyme Q10 (Ubiquinone)
15 mg • Alpha-Lipoic Acid (Thioctic Acid) 15 mg.

Mega Minerals — Nature's Life
Four capsules contain: Boron (Citrate) 1 mg • Calcium (Carbonate,
Citrate/Malate) 1000 mg • Chromium (Picolinate {US Patent
#33988}, Polynicotinate) 200 mcg • Copper (Glyconate, Citrate) 1 mg
• Iodine (Kelp) 25 mcg • Iron (Fumerate, Peptonate) 15 mg •
Magnesium (Oxide, Citrate) 500 mg • Manganese (Citrate) 10 mg •
Molybdenum (Sodium Molybdate) 20 mcg • Potassium (Citrate) 99
mg • Selenium (l-Selenomethionine) 100 mcg • Silicon Dioxide 20
mg • Vanadium (Vanadyl Sulfate) 20 mcg • Zinc (Picolinate, Citrate)
15 mg • Vitamin D3 (Cholecalciferol) 200 IU • Betaine HCl 100 mg •
Glutamic Acid 100 mg.

Mega N-R-G Thirty — Progressive Labs
Four tablets contain: Vitamin A (50% as beta carotene) 15000 IU •
Vitamin C 600 mg • Vitamin D3 100 IU • Vitamin E 200 IU • Thiamin
(Vitamin B1) 25 mg • Riboflavin (Vitamin B2) 15 mg • Niacin (B3)
50 mg • Niacinamide (B3) 100 mg • Vitamin B6 25 mg • Folate (folic
acid) 400 mcg • Vitamin B12 100 mcg • Biotin 300 mcg • Pantothenic
Acid (as calcium pantothenate) 250 mg • Calcium (as aspartate) 120
mg • Iodine (from kelp) 150 mcg • Magnesium (as aspartate) 120 mg •
Zinc Gluconate 15 mg • Selenium (as aspartate) 200 mcg • Manganese
(as aspartate) 2 mg • Chromium (as aspartate) 200 mcg • Potassium
(as aspartate) 9.9 mg • Choline 100 mg • Inositol 100 mg •
Bioflavonoids 300 mg • PABA 100 mg • L-Methionine 75 mg •
L-Lysine 75 mg.

Mega Once-A-Day — Progressive Labs
Each tablet supplies: Vitamin A (as palmitate and beta carotene)
25000 IU • Vitamin C 250 mg • Vitamin D 500 IU • Vitamin E 150 IU
• Thiamin (Vitamin B1) 75 mg • Riboflavin (Vitamin B2) 75 mg •
Niacinamide 75 mg • Vitamin B6 (pyridoxine) 75 mg • Folate (folic
acid) 400 mcg • Vitamin B12 (cyanocobalamin) 75 mcg • Biotin 75
mcg • Pantothenic Acid 75 mg • Calcium (amino acid chelate) 50 mg •
Iron (amino acid chelate) 10 mg • Iodine (from kelp) 225 mcg •
Magnesium (amino acid chelate) 7 mg • Zinc (amino acid chelate) 15
mg • Selenium (amino acid chelate) 15 mcg • Copper (amino acid
chelate) 25 mcg • Manganese (amino acid chelate) 6 mg • Silicon
(amino acid chelate) 15 mg • Chromium (amino acid chelate) 10 mg •
Molybdenum (amino acid chelate) 5 mcg • Potassium 10 mg • Boron
(as boron gluconate) 750 mcg • Choline Bitartrate 75 mg • Inositol 75
mg • Para Amino Benzoic Acid (PABA) 75 mg • Betaine HCl 25 mg •
Glutamic Acid HCl 25 mg • Rutin 25 mg • Lemon bioflavonoid
complex 25 mg • Hesperidin complex 25 mg. Natural base of: Oat
fiber, Alfalfa, Lecithin, Parsley, Bee Pollen, Royal Jelly, and Albumin.

Mega Pak Multiple — Nature's Life
Each packet of nine capsules contains: Vitamin A (Fish Liver oil)
7500 IU • Beta Carotene (equivalent to 7500 IU Vitamin A) 4.5 mg •
Vitamin B1 (Thiamine HCl) 100 mg • Vitamin B2 (Riboflavin) 100
mg • Vitamin B6 (Pyridoxine HCl) 100 mg • Vitamin B12
(Cobalamin) 100 mcg • Folic Acid 400 mcg • Niacinamide 100 mg •
Pantothenic Acid (d-Calcium Pantothenate) 100 mg • Choline

(Bitartrate) 100 mg • Inositol 100 mg • Biotin (d-Biotin) 100 mcg •
PABA (Para Aminobenzoic Acid) 100 mg • Vitamin C 1000 mg •
Lemon Bioflavonoids Complex (TESTLAB) 25 mg • Rose Hips
(Rosa canina)15 mg • Acerola (Malpighia glabra) 5 mg • Hesperidin
Conplex (Citrus) 5 mg • Rutin (Saphora japonica) 5 mg • Vitamin E
(d-Alpha Tocopherol, Beta, Delta & Gamma Tocopherols) 400 IU •
Boron (Citrate) 1 mg • Calcium (Carbonate, Citrate/Malate) 1000 mg
• Chromium (Picolinate, Polynicotinate) 200 mcg • Copper
(Gluconate, Citrate) 1 mg • Iodine (Kelp) 25 mcg • Iron (Fumerate,
Peptonate) 15 mg • Magnesium (Oxide, Citrate) 500 mg • Manganese
(Citrate) 10 mg • Molybdenum (Sodium Molybdate) 20 mcg •
Potassium (Citrate) 99 mg • Selenium (l-Selenomethionine) 100 mcg •
Silicon Dioxide 20 mg • Vanadium (Vanadyl Sulfate) 20 mcg • Zinc
(Picolinate / Citrate) 15 mg • Vitamin D3 (Cholecalciferol) 200 IU •
Betaine HCl 100 mg • Glutamic Acid HCl 100 mg • Bromelain
(Proteolytic Enzyme from Pineapple, activity: 225 MCU) 250 mg •
Papain (Proteolytic Enzyme from Papaya, activity 17.5 MCU) 250
mg. In a natural base of Lecithin, Rice Bran & Soy oil.

Mega Potency Fat Burner — Optimum Nutrition
L-Carnitine • Citrimax Chromium Picolinate • Chromium
Polynicotinate.

Mega-16 Permathene Maximum Strength —
CCA Industries, Inc.
Each tablet contains: Active Ingredient: Phenylpropanolamine HCl 75
mg. Other Ingredients: Croscarmellose, D&C Yellow #10, Dicalcium
Phosphate, FD&C Blue #1, FD&C Yellow #6, Lactose, Magnesium
Stearate, Methylcellulose , Microcrystalline Cellulose, Stearic Acid,
Titanium Dioxide.

Mega-Cal Calcium 650 mg — Jamieson
Each caplet contains: Vitamin D (as Cholecalciferol) 200 IU •
Calcium (as Calcium Carbonate, Calcium Citrate, Calcium Fumarate,
Calcium Malate, Calcium Succinate, Calcium Glutamate) 650 mg.

MegaMind — Source Naturals
DMAE • Acetyl L-Carnitine • GABA • Pyroglutamic • Ginkgo •
Lipoic • CoQ10.

MegaMuscle — Life Extension
L-Arginine 5000 mg • L-Ornithine 2500 mg • Vitamin B6 •
Vitamin C.

Mega-Stress Complex — Nature's Plus
Each tablet contains: Vitamin C with Rose Hips 500 mg • Pantothenic
Acid 200 mg • Niacinamide 125 mg • Inositol 100 mg • Vitamin B6
(Pyridoxine HCL) 100 mg • Calcium amino acid chelate/complex 100
mg • Vitamin B1 (Thiamine) 60 mg • Vitamin B2 (Riboflavin) 60 mg
• Valerian root 50 mg • Magnesium amino acid chelate/complex 50
mg • Choline (Bitartrate) 32 mg • PABA (Para-aminobenzoic acid) 30
mg • Chamomile 25 mg • Zinc amino acid chelate/complex 25 mg •
Folic Acid 400 mcg • Vitamin B12 from Cobalamin 250 mcg • Biotin
75 mcg. B-Complex Vitamins in a fortified rice bran base. Yeast,
sugar, & starch free. In a special base which provides for the gradual
release of ingredients over a prolonged period of time for 40% better
absorption & utilization.

Mega-Vim 75 — Jamieson
Each caplet contains: Vitamin A (from Acetate) 8500 IU • Beta-
Carotene (Provitamin A) 1500 IU • Vitamin D 400 IU • Vitamin C
(Ascorbic Acid) 250 mg • Vitamin E (from Succinate) 150 IU •
Vitamin B1 (Thiamin Mononitrate) 75 mg • Vitamin B2 (Riboflavin)
75 mg • Vitamin B6 (Pyridoxine HCl) 75 mg • Vitamin B12
(Cyanocobalamin) 75 mcg • Niacinamide 75 mg • Vitamin B5
(Pantothenic Acid from Calcium D-Pantothenate) 75 mg • Biotin (D-
Biotin) 75 mcg • Folic Acid 0.4 mg • Chelated Calcium • Calicum
(Carbonate) 130 mg • Chelated Iron 4 mg • Chelated Copper 1 mg •
Iodine (from Kelp) 0.15 mg • Chelated Magnesium • Magnesium
(Oxide) 50 mg • Chelated Manganese 0.61 mg • Chelated Zinc 1.5 mg
• Chelated Potassium 2 mg • Chelated Chromium 10 mcg • Chelated
Selenium 10 mcg • Choline Bitartrate 75 mg • Inositol 75 mg.

Megavital Forte — Futurebiotics
One tablet contains: Vitamin C 60 mg • Vitamin B1 (thiamin HCl) 10
mg • Vitamin B2 (riboflavin) 10 mg • Niacinamide 25 mg • Vitamin E
15 IU • Vitamin B6 (pyridoxine Hcl) 10 mg • Folic Acid 400 mcg •
Vitamin B12 (cyanocobalamin) 50 mcg • Magnesium (oxide,
gluconate) 25 mg • Zinc (gluconate) 15 mg • Biotin 201 mcg •
Pantothenic Acid 20 mg • Choline Bitartrate 100 mg • Inositol 40 mg •
Iodine (potassium iodide) 180 mcg • Sodium Phosphate 500 mcg •
Phosphatidylcholine (55% strength) 50 mg • Papain 15 mg • Lecithin

© Copyright 2000, Natural Medicines Comprehensive Database (209) 472-2244. For updated data, go to www.NaturalDatabase.com.

Some Brand Name Natural Products - What they Contain

25 mg • Selenium (yeast) 100 mcg • Chromium (polynicotinate) 25 mcg • Betaine HCl 25 mg. In a biological base containing a special blend of: [Selenium Rich Yeast, Soy protein, Power Green complex (Barley grass, Chlorella, Alfalfa juice concentrate) & Para Amino Benzoic Acid (PABA)].

Mega-Vita-Min Multiple — Nature's Life
Each tablet contains: Beta Carotene (Vitamin A equivalent to 5000 IU) 3 mg • Vitamin B1 (Thiamine HCl) 10 mg • Vitamin B2 (Riboflavin) 10 mg • Vitamin B6 (Pyridoxine HCl) 10 mg • Vitamin B12 (Cobalamin concentrate) 100 mcg • Niacin 10 mg • Pantothenic Acid (D-Calcium Pantothenate) 20 mg • Folic Acid 400 mcg • Choline (Bitartrate) 90 mg • Inositol 90 mg • Biotin (D-Biotin) 50 mcg • PABA (Para Aminobenzoic Acid) 20 mg • Lemon Bioflavonoids Complex (Testlab) 15mg • Vitamin C 100 mg • Vitamin E (d-Alpha Tocopherol mixed with Tocopherols) 10 IU • Boron (Full-Ranged Amino Acid Chelated) 25 mg • Calcium (Full-Ranged Amino Acid Chelated) 50 mg • Chromium (Nutrition 21 Picolinate) 50 mcg • Copper (Full-Ranged Amino Acid Chelated) 200 mcg • Iodine (Icelandic Kelp) 225 mcg • Magnesium (Full-Ranged Amino Acid Chelated) 50 mg • Manganese (Full-Ranged Amino Acid Chelated) 2 mg • Molybdenum (Proteinate) 25 mcg • Phosphorus (Full-Ranged Amino Acid Chelated & Complexed) 19 mg • Potassium (Proteinate) 15 mg • Selenium (Nutrition 21 Selenomethionine) 25 mcg • Silicon (Dioxide) 25 mcg • Vanadium (Full-Ranged Amino Acid Chelated) 25 mcg • Zinc (Nutrition 21 Picolinate) 2 mg • Betaine HCl 30 mg • Nucleic Acids (RNA & DNA from Yeast) 30 mg • CoQ10 (Co-Enzyme Ubiquone) 500 mcg, Essential Fatty Acids (Soy, Spirulina) 25 mg • Super Green Pro 96 (Soy Protein Super Food) 330 Mg. In a natural base containing: Rose Hips concentrate, Acerola, Rutin, Hesperidin, Lecithin, Milk-Free Lactobacillus Acidophilus, Alfalfa leaf, Watercress, Parsley, 72 Trace Minerals, Rice Bran, Spirulina, Barley Green, Psyllium, Apple Pectin, Oat Bran, Bromelain, Papain, Chlorella & Chlorophyll.

Mega-Vites 75 — The Vitamin Shoppe
Each tablet contains: Vitamin D 400 IU • Vitamin A Activity 10000 IU • Vitamin C 250 mg • Vitamin E 150 IU • Vitamin B1 75 mg • Vitamin B2 75 mg • Vitamin B6 75 mg • Vitamin B12 75 mcg • Niacinamide 75 mg • PABA 75 mg • Pantothenic Acid 75 mg • Choline Bitartrate 75 mg • Inositol 75 mg • D-Biotin 75 mcg • Folic Acid 400 mcg • Rutin 25 mg • Citrus Bioflavonoid Complex 5 mg • Hesperidin 5 mg • Betaine Hydrochloride 25 mg • L-Glutamic Acid 25 mg • Iodine 150 mcg • Calcium 50 mg • Potassium 10 mg • Iron 10 mg • Magnesium 10 mg • Manganese 6.1 mg • Zinc 15 mg • Chromium 10 mcg • Selenium 10 mcg.

Mega-Zyme — Enzymatic Therapy
Two tablets contain: Pancreatic Enzymes 10X full strength, undiluted & uncut 325 mg: Units of Activity: Protease 96580, Amylase 98780, Lipase 24496 • Trypsin 75 mg • Papain 50 mg • Bromelain (1200 MCU) 50 mg • Amylase 10 mg • Lipase 10 mg • Lysozyme 10 mg • Chymotrypsin 2 mg. Potency levels found at time of manufacturing. In a base of other proteolytic enzymes in a special Bicarbonate Complex. Bicarbonates are key factors in triggering the release of Pancreatic Enzymes. Contains no sugar, salt, yeast, wheat, corn, soy, dairy products, coloring, flavoring or preservatives.

Melatonex — Chattem, Inc.
Each tablet contains: Vitamin B6 (as pyridoxine hydrochloride) 10 mg • Melatonin 3 mg. Other Ingredients: Dicalcium phosphate (binder and hardening agent), microcrystalline cellulose (binder and disintegrant), glyceryl monostearate (binder and disintegration retardant), magnesium stearate (lubricant).

Melatonin — BioDynamax
Each capsule contains: Melatonin 3 mg.

Melatonin — New Hope Health Products
Each capsule contains: Melatonin (5-Methoxy-tryptamine) 3 mg.

Melatonin — Optimum Nutrition
Each tablet contains: Melatonin 3 mg.

Melatonin 3 mg — TwinLab
Each tablet contains: Melatonin 3 mg.

Melatonin Controlled Release 2 mg — TwinLab
Each tablet contains: Melatonin 2 mg.

Melatonin PM Complex — Anabolic Laboratories
Each tablet contains: Melatonin 1 mg • Vitamin B6 (pyridoxine HCl) 5 mg • Vitamin B2 (riboflavin) 3 mg • Vitamin B3 (niacinamide) 10

mg • Vitamin B12 (ion-exchange resin) 12.5 mcg • Calcium (lactate) 40 mg • Magnesium (oxide) 30 mg • Chinese Herbal Complex 195 mg: Valerian Root extract, Zizyphus Spinosa seed, Salviae Miltiorrhiza root, Succinum (Amber), Biotae Orientalis seed, Coptis Chiensis rhizome, Chamomile flower, Hops Strobile, Passion Flower, Skullcap herb. Other Ingredients: Cellulose, Stearic Acid, Magnesium Stearate, Vanillin, Vegetable Oil, Silica.

Melatonin Spray — Nature's Plus
Each spray contains: Melatonin (N-Acetyl-5-Methoxytryptamine) 1.5 mg • GABA (Gamma Aminobutyric Acid) 2500 mcg • Pyridoxal-5-Phosphate (P5P) 2500 mcg. In a proprietary liposomal complex of Essential Metabolic Factors, Purified Water, Vegetable Glycerine, Purified Lecithin, Citrus seed extract (Citrus sinensis), Vitamin E & natural Peppermint flavor.

Melatonin Tablets, Accurate Release, 1 mg — Nature's Bounty
Each tablet contains: Melatonin (n-Acetyl-5 Methoxytryptamine) 1 mg. Inactive Ingredients: Dicalcium Phosphate, Microcrystalline, Cellulose, Vegetable Magnesium Stearate, Croscarmellose Sodium.

Melatonin Tablets, Accurate Release, 200 mcg — Nature's Bounty
Each tablet contains: Pure Melatonin 200 mcg.

Melatonin Time Release - 1 mg — Natrol
Each tablet contains: Calcium (as Dicalcium Phosphate) 40 mg • Melatonin 1 mg. Other Ingredients: Time Release Agent (Hydrogenated Vegetable Oil), stearic acid, silica, magnesium sterate.

Melatonin Time Release - 3 mg — Natrol
Each tablet contains: Calcium (as Calcium Carbonate) 63 mg • Melatonin 3 mg. Other Ingredients: Cellulose, silica, stearic acid, cellulose gum, magnesium stearate.

MemorActin — Nature's Plus
Two capsules contain: Phosphatidylcholine 250 mg • Inositol 125 mg • Ginkgo Biloba leaf (standardized 24% Ginkgo Flavone-Glycosides, 6% Terpene Lactones) 100 mg • Vitamin C corn free 100 mg • Pantothenic Acid (Calcium Pantothenate) 50 mg • Phosphatidylserine 25 mg • Bilberry [(Vaccinium myrtillus fruit) standardized 25% Anthocyanosides] 10 mg • Beta Carotene pro-Vitamin A (supplying 10000 IU of Vitamin A activity) 6 mg • Coenzyme Q10 (Ubiquinone) 2.5 mg.

Memorall — PharmAssure
One softgel contains: Vitamin E 50 IU • Huperzine A 50 mcg. Other Ingredients: Soybean Oil, Gelatin, Glycerin, Caramel Color, Titanium Dioxide as a natural mineral whitener.

Memory — ProHerbs
One tablet contains: Thiamin HCl (B1) 25 mg • Niacin (as Niacinamide) 10 mg • Vitamin B6 (Pyridoxine HCl) 25 mg • Vitamin B12 (Cyanocobalamin) 25 mcg • Ginkgo Biloba extract (Ginkgo biloba leaves standardized to 24% ginkgo flavonoid glycosides & 6% terpene lactones) 120 mg • Memorzine (Huperzia serrata moss extract) 25 mcg • Korean Ginseng (Panax Ginseng root standardized to 4% ginsenosides) 100 mg. Other Ingredients: Dicalcium Phosphate, Microcrystalline Cellulose, Croscarmellose Sodium, Hydroxypropylmethylcellulose, Magnesium Stearate, Mineral Oil, Polyethylene Glycol, Stearic Acid, Titanium Dioxide, Sodium Lauryl Sulfate, FD&C Yellow #10 Lake, FD&C Blue #1 Lake and FD&C Blue #2 Lake.

Memory 2000 — Natural Balance
Two tablets contain: Niacin 40 mg • Ginkgo leaf standardized extract 120 mg • Phosphatidylserine 100 mg • DMAE 100 mg • Acetyl-L-Carnitine 20 mg • Vinpocetine 5 mg.

Memory Formula — Youngevity
Ginkgo biloba leaf • Gotu Kola herb • Cayenne pepper • Siberian Ginseng • Magnesium • Lecithin • L-Glutamine • L-Tyrosine • Vitamin B6 • Vitamin B3 • Vilcabamba Mineral Essence: Potassium, Calcium, Magnesium, Zinc, Chromium, Selenium, Iron, Copper, Molybdenum, Vanadium, Iodine, Cobalt, Manganese.

Memory Power — The Vitamin Shoppe
Two tablets contain: Ginkgo Biloba extract standardized to contain 24% ginkgoflavonglycosides • L-Phenylalanine • L-Glutamine • RNA • Choline • Gotu Kola • Lecithin • Ginkgo Biloba leaf powder.

Memorya — HerbaSway
Ginkgo Biloba • Dong Quai • Kudzu • Rehmannia • Panax Ginseng •

© Copyright 2000, Natural Medicines Comprehensive Database (209) 472-2244. For updated data, go to www.NaturalDatabase.com.

**B
R
A
N
D

N
A
M
E
S**

Schisandra • Knotweed • Blackberry • HerbaSwee (Cucurbitaceae fruit).

Men Plus Ester C — Nutrivention
Two tablets contain: Vitamin C 300 mg • Vitamin E 200 IU • Choline Bitartrate 150 mg • Inositol 150 mg • Niacinamide 150 mg • Pantothenic Acid 150 mg • Essential Fatty Acids 100mg • Vitamin A 1500 IU • Vitamin B6 75 mg • Vitamin B2 75 mg • Vitamin B1 75 mg • Vitamin D 1000 IU • Biotin 500 mcg • Vitamin B12 500 mcg • Folic Acid 400 mcg • Iodine (Kelp) 150 mcg • Saw Palmetto berry 200 mg • Sarsaparilla 200 mg • Bioflavonoids 150 mg.

Men-Applause — The Herbalist
Dong Quai root • Black Cohosh root • Chaste Tree berry • Siberian Ginseng root • Oat seed • Wild Yam root.

Menopausal Formula — Nature's Herbs
Each capsule contains: Dong Quai 75 mg • Siberian Ginseng 100 mg.

Menopause — Nutrivention
Each tablet contains: Pantothenic Acid 50 mg • Vitamin B6 50 mg • Vitamin C 50 mg • Vitamin E 100 IU • PABA 50 mg • Calcium 50 mg • Iodine (Kelp) 150mcg • Borage GLA concentrate 150 mg • Mexican Wild Yam root 150 mg • Chaste Tree berry 150 mg • Dong Quai root 150 mg • Licorice root 100 mg • Unicorn root 100 mg • Black Cohosh root 50 mg • Passion flower 50 mg.

Menopause Formula — Natrol
Three capsules contain: Calcium (as calcium carbonate) 250 mg • Magnesium (as magnesium oxide) 125 mg • Soy Isoflavones 100 mg Genistein (10%) 10 mg • Kava Kava 100 mg Kavalactones (30%) 30 mg • Red Raspberry 100 mg • Wild Mexican Yam 50 mg • Licorice root 50 mg • Red Clover 50 mg • Horse Chestnut 50 mg • Dong Quai 50 mg • Black Cohosh root 40 mg • Damiana 30 mg • Vitex (agnus-castus) 25 mg • Gingko Biloba 24:6 25 mg • Gotu Kola 25 mg • Gamma Oryzanol 20 mg. Other Ingredients: Rice powder, Silicon Dioxide, Magnesium Stearate, Gelatin.

Menopause Formula — Nature's Life
Four capsules contain: Black Cohosh root extract (Cimicifuga racemosa) (standardized to provide 2.5% or 4 mg Triterpene Glycosides as 27-Deoxyactein) 160 mg • Vitamin C (Calcium Ascorbate) 1200 mg • Vitamin E (d-Alpha Tocopheryl Succinate) 200 IU • Hesperidin (plant source flavonols) 1200 mg • Women's Phyto-Estrogen Blend (Soy bean, Wild Yam, Rice Flour, Flax seed & Amaranth) 100 mg.

Menopause Formula — Pharmanex
Each capsule contains: Isoflavones (from Soy extract) 25 mg • Kava Lactones (from Kava Kava root extract) 25.5 mg • Black Cohosh root powder 50 mg. Other Ingredients: Calcium Carbonate, Maltodextrin, Magnesium Stearate, Silicon Dioxide.

Menopause Multiple — Source Naturals
Six tablets contain: SoyLife genistein-rich Soy concentrate (Yielding 62 mg of Isoflavones: Daidzein 34 mg, Glycitein 20 mg, Genistein 8 mg) • CimiPure Black Cohosh Standardized Extract 2.5% (Yielding 4 mg Triterpene Glycosides) (Containing 27-Deoxyactein) 160 mg • Vitex extract (Vitex Agnus-Castus) 150 mg • Dong Quai extract (Angelica sinensis) 100 mg • Licorice root extract (Glycyrrhiza glabra) 15 mg • Taurine (Magnesium Taurinate) 455 mg • N-Acetyl Cysteine 100 mg • Silymarin (Milk Thistle seed extract) 60 mg • Alpha-Lipoic Acid (Thioctic Acid) 30 mg • Ginkgo Biloba 24% (50:1 Extract) 20 mg • Coenzyme Q10 (Ubiquinone) 15 mg • Vitamin A (Beta Carotene) 13000 IU • Vitamin A (Palmitate) 7000 IU • Vitamin B1 (Thiamin) 50 mg • Vitamin B2 (Riboflavin) 50 mg • Niacinamide 50 mg • Vitamin B5 (Calcium D-Pantothenate) 70 mg • Vitamin B6 (Pyridoxine HCl) 50 mg • Vitamin B12 (Cyanocobalamin) 50 mcg • Biotin 200 mcg • Folic Acid 600 mcg • Vitamin C (Ascorbic Acid, Calcium and Magnesium Ascorbates) 1000 mg • Vitamin D3 (Cholecalciferol) 400 IU • Vitamin E (D-Alpha Tocopheryl)(Natural) 400 IU • Boron (Chelate) 3 mg • Calcium (Carbonate, Citrate and Ascorbate) 300 mg • Chromium (ChromeMate Polynicotinate 100 mcg and Chromium Picolinate 100 mcg) 200 mcg • Magnesium (Oxide, Taurinate, Malate, and Ascorbate) 400 mg • Manganese (Citrate) 2 mg • Selenium (L-Selenomethionine) 200 mcg • Zinc (OptiZinc Monomethionine) 12 mg.

Menopause Nutritional System 1 — Schiff
Four caplets contain: Vitamin A (as 50% Acetate & 50% Beta Carotene) 5000 IU • Vitamin C (as Ascorbic Acid) 500 mg • Vitamin D (as Cholecalciferol) 200 IU • Vitamin E (as d-Alpha Tocopheryl Succinate) 400 IU • Thiamin (as Thiamin Hydrochloride) 25 mg •

Riboflavin 25 mg • Niacin (Niacinamide) 25 mg • Vitamin B6 (as Pyridoxine Hydrochloride) 15 mg • Folate (as Folic Acid) • Vitamin B12 (as Cyanocobalamin) 25 mcg • Biotin 100 mcg • Pantothenic Acid (as d-Calcium Pantothenate) 25 mg • Calcium (as Citrate) 500 mg • Iron (as Ferrous Fumerate) 7.5 mg • Iodine (from Kelp) 75 mcg • Magnesium (as Oxide) 250 mg • Zinc (as Gluconate) 7.5 mg • Selenium (as L-Selenomethionine) 12.5 mg • Copper (as Gluconate) 1 mg • Manganese (as Gluconate 5 mg • Chromium (as Polynicotinate) 50 mcg. Potassium (as Gluconate) 50 mg • Choline (as Bitartrate) 25 mg • Inositol 25 mg • PABA (Para AminoBenzioc Acid) 25 mg • Boron (as Amino Acid Chelate) 1.5 mg • Bromelain 50 mg • Papain 32.5 mg • Bioflavonoids (from citrus) 400 mg • Rutin 100 mg. Other Ingredients: Cellulose, Maltodextrin, Stearic Acid, Sillica, Magnesium Sterate, Plyethylene Glycol.

Menopause Nutritional System 2 — Schiff
Four caplets contain: Fennel (Foeniculum vulgare)fruit 100 mg • Black Cohosh (Cimicifuga racemosa) root 100 mg • Anise (Pimpinella anisum) seed 100 mg • Blessed Thistle (Cnicus benedictus) whole herb 100 mg.

Menopause Remedy — Phytopharmica
Twenty drops contain: Lachesis mutus 10x • Glonoinum 8x • Kali carbonicum 6x • Bryonia 4x • Cactus grandiflorus 3x • In a base of 45% USP alcohol by volume.
Editor's Comments: This is a homeopathic product. It is so extremely diluted that its activity can not be explained by conventional scientific methods. Therefore this product can not be rated by the scientific criteria used in this Database. A patient receiving the extreme dilution of this product will not receive many, if any, molecules of the original active ingredient. Therefore, there are no harmful pharmacologic effects, and any beneficial effects are controversial and not due to a direct biochemical action of the ingredient on the body. Homeopathic products are allowed for sale in the U.S. due to legislation passed in the 19th century sponsored by a homeopathic physician who was also a Senator. The law still requires that the FDA allow the sale of products listed in this Homeopathic Pharmacopea of the United States.

Menopause Support — Amazon Support
Each capsule contains: Abuta • Chuchuhuasi • Muira Puama • Suma • Damiana • Maca • Wild Yam • Dong Quai • Mutamba • Licorice Root • Black Cohosh.

Menophase — Futurebiotics
Complex of 4:1 extracts & powders (equivalent to 1700 mg of raw herbs) 450 mg containing: Foti, Peony Root, Withania Somnifera, Dong Quai, Chinese Sage & Carlina Ancalis • Pantothenic Acid (Vitamin B5) 75 mg • Ribonucleic Acid (RNA) 40 mg • Pyridoxine (Vitamin B6) 15 mg • Zinc (from gluconate) 7.5 mg.

Menopryn — Rx Vitamins
Black Cohosh (standardized) 50 mg • Isoflavone complex.

Men's AM Multi — Clinician's Choice
Two tablets contain: Vitamin A (retinyl acetate & 26% as beta-carotene) 3900 IU • Vitamin C (ascorbic acid) 250 mg • Vitamin D (cholecalciferol) 400 IU • Vitamin E (dl-alpha tocopheryl acetate) 150 IU • Thiamin (mononitrate) 1 mg • Riboflavin 1 mg • Niacin (niacinamide) 10 mg • Vitamin B6 (pyridoxine hydrochloride) 1 mg • Folate (folic acid) 200 mcg • Vitamin B12 (cyanocobalamin) 4 mcg • Biotin 210 mcg • Pantothenic Acid (d-calcium pantothenate) 5 mg • Iodine (potassium iodide) 76 mcg • Calcium (amino acid chelate) 4 mg • Magnesium (oxide, amnio acid chelate) 9 mg • Potassium (chloride, amino acid chelate) 12 mg • Zinc (amino acid chelate, gluconate) 2 mg • Selenium (selenomethionine) 100 mcg • Copper (amino acid chelate) 1 mg • Manganese (amino acid chelate) 3 mg • Chromium (nicotinate, amino acid chelate, chelavite, picolinate) 40 mcg • Molybdenum (amino acid chelate) 4 mcg • RoseOx (patented, standardized process for an extract of Rosemary) 50 mg • Citrus Bioflavanoid Complex 10 mg •Saw Palmetto Berries 10 mg • Whole Oats 10 mg • Panax Ginseng Extract 4 mg • Proprietary blend 12 mg: Gingko Biloba Leaf, Echinacea Angustifolia, Panax Ginseng Root, Bee Pollen, Cruciferex, Grape Powder.

Men's Formula 800+ Prostate Support — Nature's Life
Two capsules contain: Saw Palmetto berry extract (Serenoa repens B. standardized to 85% Liposterolic Acids equivalent to 1600 mg whole herb) 160 mg • Stinging Nettle plant (Urtica dioica L.) 150 mg • Pygeum africanum H. bark extract (concentrated 130:1; equivalent to 6500 mg whole herb) 50 mg • Beta Sitosterol (Soy oil) 10 mg • Zinc (Gluconate, Citrate, Picolinate) 15 mg • Copper (Gluconate, Citrate) 1 mg •Flax seed oil (Linum usitatissimum L.) 235 mg • (Omegaflo

Some Brand Name Natural Products - What they Contain
www.NaturalDatabase.com contains MANY more listings than appear here.

Process Certified Organically Grown) Providing naturally occuring Omega 3 Essential Fatty Acid: Alpha Linolenic Acid 133 mg.

Men's Mood-Enhancer — HerbaSway
St. John's Wort • Ginkgo biloba • He Sho Wu • Horny Goat Weed • Schisandra • Knotweed • Astragalus • Lycium • Skullcap • Blackberry • Bupleurum • HerbaSwee (Cucurbitaceae fruit).

Men's PM Multi — Clinician's Choice
Two tablets contain: Vitamin A (retinyl acetate & 20% as beta-carotene) 1250 IU • Vitamin C (ascorbic acid) 450 mg • Vitamin D (cholecalciferol) 60 IU • Vitamin E (dl-alpha tocopheryl acetate) 150 IU • Thiamin (mononitrate) 0.5 mg • Riboflavin 0.7 mg • Niacin (niacinamide) 10 mg • Vitamin B6 (pyridoxine hydrochloride) 1 mg • Folate (folic acid) 200 mcg • Vitamin B12 (cyanocobalamin) 2 mcg • Biotin 90 mcg • Pantothenic Acid (d-calcium pantothenate) 5 mg • Calcium (carbonate, amino acid chelate) 84 mg • Iodine (potassium iodide) 74 mcg • Magnesium (oxide, amino acid chelate) 20 mg • Potassium (chloride, amino acid chelate) 16 mg • Zinc (oxide, amino acid chelate, gluconate) 32 mg • Selenium (selenomethionine) 100 mcg • Copper (amino acid chelate) 1 mg • Manganese (amino acid chelate) 1 mg • Chromium (nicotinate, picolinate, chelavite, amino acid chelate) 10 mcg • Molybdenum (amino acid chelate) 2 mcg • RoseOx (patented, standardized process for an extract of Rosemary) 50 mg • Citrus Bioflavanoid Complex 10 mg • Chamomile Flowers 10 mg • Passion Flower 10 mg • Valerian Root 10 mg • Mint Leaves 10 mg • Saw Palmetto Berries 10 mg • Whole Oats 10 mg • Hesperidin Complex 4 mg • Proprietary blend 8 mg: Reishi Mushroom, Shiitake Mushroom, Cruciferex, Grape Powder.

Men's Support — Rainbow Light
Each tablet provides: Sarsaparilla root 50 mg • Wild Oat green tops 100 mg • Damiana oxide 100 mg • Kava Kava rhizome 75 mg • Saw Palmetto fruit 50 mg • Pumpkin seed 25 mg • Ginseng 25 mg • Selenium 25 mg • Wood Betony 50 mg • Blue Vervain 50 mg • Ginger rhizome 100 mg • Vitamin A 1000 IU • Vitamin E 25 IU • Zinc 5 mg.

MenstraCalm — Jarrow Formulas
Four capsules contain: Vitamin C (calcium acsorbate) 100 mg • Vitamin D 100 IU • Vitamin E (natural d-alpha- tocopheryl succinate) 100 IU • Vitamin B6 (pyridoxine HCl) 25 mg • Folic Acid 200 mcg • Calcium (as calcium citrate) 132 mg • Magnesium (as magnesium oxide) 60 mg • Potassium (as potassium chloride) 99 mg • Dong Quai Root Extract 5:1 (Angelicae sinensis) 500 mg • Xiang Fu Tuber Extract 5:1 (Cyperus rotundus) 500 mg • Shu Di Huang 5:1 (Rehmannia glutinosa) 400 mg • Lindera 5:1 (Lindera strychnifolin) 200 mg • Chaste Tree Fruit Extract 5:1 (vitex agnus-castus) 300 mg • Dandelion Root (Taraxacum officinale) 200 mg.

Menstrual Support — Amazon Support
Each capsule contains: Abuta • Jatoba • Suma • Chuchuhuasi • Sarsaparilla • Picao Preto • Tayuya • Iporuru • Cramp Bark.

Menstru-Care — Natrol
Two tablets contain: Vitamin B12 (as cobalamin) 75 mcg • Folic Acid 100 mcg • Calcium (as calcium carbonate) 299 mg • Iron (as iron glycinate) 30 mg • Chasteberry 75 mg • CrampBark 4:1 (Viburnum opulus) 75 mg • Dong Quai 75 mg, Ferulic Acid (1%) 750 mcg • Uva Ursi 50 mg • Kava Kava 50 mg, Kavalactones (30%) 15 mg • Squaw Vine 50 mg • Black Cohosh 20 mg, Triterpenes (2.5%) 0.5 mg. Other ingredients: Mono & Di-Glycerides, Stearic Acid, Croscarmellose Sodium, Silicon Dioxide, Magnesium Stearate.

Menta-FX — HerbTech
St. John's Wort 200 mg • HT-1001 (extract of American Ginseng) 100 mg • Ginkgo Biloba 25 mg.

Mental Advantage — Phytopharmica
Each chewable tablet contains: Plumbum metallicum 8x • Ambra grisea 5x • Kali phosphoricum 5x • Ginkgo 1x • Magnesia muriatica 1x • Magnesia phosphorica 1x.
Editor's Comments: This is a homeopathic product. It is so extremely diluted that its activity can not be explained by conventional scientific methods. Therefore this product can not be rated by the scientific criteria used in this Database. A patient receiving the extreme dilution of this product will not receive many, if any, molecules of the original active ingredient. Therefore, there are no harmful pharmacologic effects, and any beneficial effects are controversial and not due to a direct biochemical action of the ingredient on the body. Homeopathic products are allowed for sale in the U.S. due to legislation passed in the 19th century sponsored by a homeopathic physician who was also a Senator. The law still requires that the FDA allow the sale of products listed in this Homeopathic Pharmacopea of the United States.

Mental Clarity — Centrum Focused Formulas
One tablet contains: Vitamin E 20 IU • Thiamin (B1) 0.55 mg • Riboflavin (B2) 0.85 mg • Niacin (B3) 10 mg • Vitamin B6 1 mg • Folate, Folic Acid, Folacin 200 mcg • Vitamin B12 3 mcg • Biotin 5 mcg • Pantothenic Acid 7.5 mg • Ginkgo Biloba standardized leaf extract 60 mg • Choline 8 mg.

Mental Edge — Source Naturals
Four tablets contain: Phosphatidyl Choline 350 mg • Choline (Bitartrate) 100 mg • DMAE (Bitartrate) 160 mg • Ginkgo Biloba leaf extract (50:1) 20 mg • Vitamin B1 (Thiamin) 50 mg • Vitamin B2 (Riboflavin) 20 mg • Vitamin B3 (80 mg Niacinamide and 40 mg Niacin) 120 mg • Vitamin B5 (Calcium D-Pantothenate) 120 mg • Vitamin B6 (Pyridoxine HCl) 25 mg • Vitamin B12 (Cyanocobalamin) 50 mcg • Folic Acid 400 mcg • Biotin 50 mcg • Inositol 30 mg • Vitamin C (Ascorbic Acid, Zinc and Magnesium Ascorbates) 150 mg • Calcium (Citrate) 60 mg • Magnesium (Oxide, Citrate) 120 mg • Potassium (Citrate) 99 mg • Zinc (Ascorbate) 10 mg • Manganese (Ascorbate) 5 mg • L-Pyroglutamic Acid 500 mg • L-Glutamine 500 mg • L-Tyrosine 275 mg • L-Phenylalanine 125 mg • Taurine 100 mg • Herbal Formula 595 mg: Siberian Ginseng 225 mg, Gotu Kola 150 mg, Schizandra 80 mg, Ginger root 80 mg, Cayenne 60 mg.

MESO-Tech — Muscletech
Each packet contains: MesoPro (Whey Protein concentrate, specially filtered & new Ion-Exchanged Whey Protein) • Maltodextrin • Glutamine Blend • natural & artificial Flavors • Cellulose Gums • Vitamin & Mineral Blend • Phenylalanine • Taurine • Guar Gum • Xanthan Gum • Acesulfame Potassium • Aspartame • Carrageenan • Essential Fatty Acid Blend (EFA's): (Borage oil, Lecithin, Flax seed oil). Phenylketonurics: Contains Phenylalanine.

Metabolic Thyrolean — ProLab
Each capsule contains: Phosphatidyl Choline 12.5 mg • Calcium Phosphate 125 mg • Dipotassium Phosphate 75 mg • Sodium Phosphate 37.5 mg • Disodium Phosphate 37.5 mg • Gum Guggul extract (Guggelsterone) 125 mg • Garcinia cambogia 125 mg • L-Tyrosine 125 mg.

Metabolife 356 — Metabolife
Each tablet contains: Guarana (contains caffeine 40 mg) • Ma Huang (contains ephedrine 12 mg) • Siberian Ginseng • Lecithin • Ginger root • Damiana • Sarsaparilla root • Goldenseal • Gotu Kola • Spirulina Algae • Bee Pollen • Nettle leaf • Royal Jelly • Bovine Complex. Other ingredients: Vitamin E 6 IU, Magnesium Chelate 75 mg, Zinc Chelate 5 mg, and Chromium Picolinate 75 mcg.

Metabolift — TwinLab
Two capsules contain: Ma Huang extract 334 mg • Guarana extract (standardized for 22% Caffeine) 910 mg • Chromium (from Chromic Fuel patented Chromium Picolinate) 200 mg. In a concentrated herbal base of White Willow bark extract & Cayenne.

Metab-O-Lite — Man-Richardson Labs
Each tablet contains: Vitamin E 6 IU • Magnesium (as magnesuim chelate) 75 mg • Zinc (as zinc chelate) 5 mg • Chromium (as chromium picolinate) 75 mcg • Proprietary Blend (Ephedra (Ma Huang) Concentrate (aerial part)(12 mg naturally occuring ephedrines), Bee Pollen, Siberian Ginseng (root), Ginger (root), Lecithin, Bovine Cartilage, Damiana (leaf), Sarsaparilla (root), Goldenseal (aerial part), Nettles (leaf), Gotu Kola (aerial part), Spirulina Algae, Royal Jelly). Other Ingredients: Cellulose, Croscarmellose Sodium, Hydroxypropyl Cellulose, Silica, Hydroxypropyl Methylcellulose, dl-Alpha-Tocopheryl Acetate, Magnesium Stearate, Maltodextrin, PEG.

Metabolol II — Champion Nutrition
Each serving contains: Chocolate: Calories 260 • Carbohydrates 40 g • Protein 18 g • Plain flavor: Calories 260 • Carbohydrates 39 g, Protein 21 g • Fat 2.5 g. Ingredients: Metacarb Plus (Champion Nutrition's new longer lasting blend of complex carbohydrates from corn hybrids) • Peptol PER4 + (our scientifically balanced, highest bio-availability protein formulation containing: Enzyme Modified Egg Albumin, Whey Protein Concentrate, Potassium Caseinate, Peptides from Enzyme Modified Lactalbumin, & Pharmaceutical Grade Amino Acids: L-Leucine, L-Isoleucine, L-Valine, L-Cystine, L-Phenylalanine, L-Methionine, L-Threonine, L-Lysine, L-Glutamic Acid) • Polylactate (Our revolutionary new liver energy source) • Medium Chain Triglycerides • Metavite (Our uniquely balanced, highest bioactive vitamin mineral formula containing: Calcium Carbonate, Pyridoxine Alpha-Ketoglutarate [PAK], Choline Bitartrate,

B R A N D

N A M E S

© Copyright 2000, Natural Medicines Comprehensive Database (209) 472-2244. For updated data, go to www.NaturalDatabase.com. • 1365

**B
R
A
N
D

N
A
M
E
S**

Inositol, Di-Calcium Phosphate, Calcium Lactate, Calcium Citrate, Magnesium Oxide, Magnesium Citrate, Zinc Picolinate, Ester-C, [Esterified Calcium Polyascorbate], Potassium Phosphate, D-Alpha Tocopherol Succinate Esterified Zinc Polyascorbate, Molybdenum Aspartate, Iron Succinate, Maganese Citrate, Niacin, Calcium Pantothenate, Copper Glycinate, Chromium-Polynicotinate) • Pyridoxal-5¢-Phosphate • Retinyl Palmitote, Riboflavin-5¢-Phosphate • Thiamine HCL • D-Biotin • Potassium Iodide • Ergocalciferol • Folic Acid • Cyanocobalamin • & Intrinsic Factor Complex • Succinate ETF Complex (Our exclusive Succinate Compound including: Potassium Succinate, Magnesium Succinate, Calcium Succinate, L-Glutamic Acid, Inosine, & Pyridoxine Alpha-Ketoglutarate [PAK] Inosine, Lecithin, Natural Flavors, L-Carnitine, Lipoic Acid, Selenium Aspartate).

Metaboloss — Metaboloss
Ginger • Magnesium • Vitamin E • Zinc • Ma Huang • Astragalus • Bee Pollen • Chromium Picolinate • Siberian Ginseng • Sarsaparilla • Goldenseal • Nettles • Gotu Kola • Lecithin • Damiana • Royal Jelly • Bladderwrack • Blue Green Algae • Licorice.

Metabotrim — Pharmanex
Each capsule contains: Vitamin C (Calcium Ascorbate) 75 mg • Niacin (Niacinamide) 10 mg • Vitamin B6 (Pyridoxine Hydrochloride, Pycodoxal-5-Phosphate) 3 mg • Vitamin B12 (Cyanocobalamin, Dibencozide) 6 mcg • Magnesium (Magnesium Asparate, Magnesium Citrate, Magnesium Chelate) 20 mg • Chromium (Chromium Chelate, Chromium Picolinate) 100 mcg • Potassium (Potassium Asparate, Potassium Citrate) 20 mg • Carnitine (L-Carnitine L-Tartrate) 100 mg. Other Ingredients: Cellulose, Magnesium Stearate, Vanillin, Silicon Dioxide.

MetaboTrim — VitaStore
Each tablet contains: Vitamin E 6 IU • Magnesium (as Magnesium Chelate) 75 mg • Zinc (as Zinc Chelate) 5 mg • Chromium (as Chromium Picolinate) 75 mcg. Blended Formula 728 mg: Guarana Concentrate (seed) (40 mg Naturally-occurring caffeine), Ma Huang Concentrate (herb: aerial part) (12 mg naturally-occurring ephedrine), Bee Pollen, Ginseng (root), Lecithin (vitamin), Bovine Complex, Damiana (leaf), Sarsaparilla (root), Goldenseal (aerial part), Nettles (leaf), Gotu Kola (aerial part), Spirulina Algae, Royal Jelly. Other Ingredients: Methocel, Silica, Croscarmellose Sodium, Magnesium Stearate.

Metalogic — PhysioLogics
Each capsule contains: Vitamin C (Ascorbic Acid) 250 mg • Zinc 15 mg • Copper (Glycinate) 500 mcg • N-Acetyl cysteine 200 mg • L-Methionine 30 mg • Alpha-Lipoic Acid 25 mg • L-Glutathione 5 mg • Selenium (Selenomethionine) 75 mcg.

Meta-Thin — New Hope Health Products
Two capsules contain: Garcinia cambogia (50%) HCA 750 mg • Ma Huang (8% ephedra) 225 mg • Green Tea (50% caffeine) 125 mg • Caffeine (anhydrous) 100 mg • White Willow bark (2% salicylates) 60 mg • Naringin 20 mg • L-Tyrosine 50 mg • Choline bitartrate 100 mg • Chromium (chelate 10%) 200 mcg • Vanadium (sulfate) 3 mg • Alpha-lipoic acid 50 mg • Vitamin B-5 (Pantothenic acid) 50 mg • Potassium (Phosphate) 74 mg • Iodine (as Potassium iodide) 750 mcg • Cayenne Pepper 10 mg.

MetaTox Oral — PhysioLogics
Each capsule contains: Vitamin C (Ascorbic Acid) 250 mg • N-Acetylcysteine 200 mg • L-Methionine (Zn/Se Monomethionine) 52.5 mg • Alpha-Lipoic Acid (USP) 5 mg • L-Glutathione (USP) 5 mg • Zinc (as Zinc Monomethionine) 15 mg • Copper (Glycinate) 0.5 mg • Selenium (Methionine) 75 mcg.

MET-Rx Meal Replacement For The Best Shape Of Your Life — Met-Rx
Each powdered packet contains: Extreme Chocolate: Glutamine 6 g • Calories 240 • Protein 38 g • Carbohydrates 19 g • Fat 2.5 g. Ingredients: METAMYOSYN (Unique blend of Milk Protein Isolates, Caseinate, Glutamine, Whey Protein Concentrate, Egg White) • Maltodextrin • Dutch Cocoa (alkali processed) • Vitamins & Minerals (Dicalcium Phosphate, Potassium Chloride, Dipotassium Phosphate, Potassium Citrate, Salt, Sodium Citrate, Magnesium Oxide, Choline Bitartrate, Ascorbic Acid, d- Alpha Tocopheryl Acetate, Ferrous Fumarate, Niacinamide, Vitamin A Palmitate, Zinc Oxide, Calcium Pantothenate, Vitamin K, Manganese Sulfate, Vitamin D3, Copper Sulfate, Pyridoxine Hydrochloride, Riboflavin, Thiamine Hydrochloride, Chromium Picolinate, Cobalamin Concentrate [Vitamin B12], Folic Acid, Biotin, Sodium Molybdate, Sodium

Selenite, Potassium Iodide) • Natural & Artificial Flavors • Partially Hydrogenated Coconut oil • Corn Syrup Solids • Cellulose Gum • Xanthan Gum • Aspartame • Carrageenan • Beta Carotene • Acesulfame Potassium • Lecithin • Mono & Diglycerides. Original: Calories 260 • Protein 37 g, • Carbohydrates 24 g • Fat 2 g. Ingredients: METAMYOSYN (Unique blend of Milk Protein Isolates, Caseinate, Glutamine, Whey Protein Concentrate, Egg White), Maltodextrin • Vitamins & Minerals (Dicalcium Phosphate, Potassium Chloride, Dipotassium Phosphate, Potassium Citrate, Salt, Sodium Citrate, Magnesium Oxide, Choline Bitartrate, Ascorbic Acid, d-Alpha Tocopheryl Acetate, Ferrous Fumarate, Niacinamide, Vitamin A Palmitate, Zinc Oxide, Calcium Pantothenate, Vitamin K, Manganese Sulfate, Vitamin D3, Copper Sulfate, Pyridoxine Hydrochloride, Riboflavin, Thiamine Hydrochloride, Chromium Picolinate, Cobalamin Concentrate [Vitamin B12], Folic Acid, Biotin, Sodium Molybdate, Sodium Selenite, Potassium Iodide) • Natural & Atrificial Flavors • Corn Syrup Solids • Cellulose Gum • Xanthan Gum • Aspartame • Carrageenan • Beta Carotene • Acesulfame Potassium • Lecithin • Mono & Diglycerides. White Chocolate Mocha: Calories 250 • Protein 37 g • Carbohydrates 22 g • Fat 2 g. Ingredients: METAMYOSYN (Unique blend of Milk Protein Isolates, Caseinate, Glutamine, Whey Protein Concentrate, Egg White), Maltodextrin • Vitamins & Minerals (Dicalcium Phosphate, Potassium Chloride, Dipotassium Phosphate, Potassium Citrate, Salt, Sodium Citrate, Magnesium Oxide, Choline Bitartrate, Ascorbic Acid, d-Alpha Tocopheryl Acetate, Ferrous Fumarate, Niacinamide, Vitamin A Palmitate, Zinc Oxide, Calcium Pantothenate, Vitamin K, Manganese Sulfate, Vitamin D3, Copper Sulfate, Pyridoxine Hydrochloride, Riboflavin, Thiamine Hydrochloride, Chromium Picolinate, Cobalamin Concentrate [Vitamin B12], Folic Acid, Biotin, Sodium Molybdate, Sodium Selenite, Potassium Iodide) • Natural & Artificial Flavors • Soluble Coffee • Dutch Cocoa (alkali processed) • Partially Hydrogenated Coconut oil • Corn Syrup Solids • Cellulose Gum • Xanthan Gum • Aspartame • Carrageenan • Beta Carotene • Acesulfame Potassium • Lecithin • Mono & Diglycerides.

MGN3 — LaneLabs
Two capsules contain: MGN-3 proprietary blend 500 mg: Rice Bran, Hyphomycetes Mycelia extract, Beet Root Fiber, Calcium Phosphate, Silica, Magnesium Stearate, Gelarin, Water, Glycerin.

Microhydrin — Royal BodyCare
Each capsule contains: Silica hydride powder 250 mg • Flanaga Microclusters (Silica, Potassium Carbonate, Magnesium Sulfate), Rice flour, Rice Bran oil.

Mid-Life — Aspen Group, Inc.
Each tablet contains: The compounds Triterpine Glycosides, standardized at 1 mg - derived from approximately 40 mg of Cimicufuga Racemosa root & rhizome. MID-LIFE contains natural plant extracts from Cimicufuga Racemosa.

Midlife Care — Health Factor
Each capsule contains: Oat Straw extract (10:1)(Avena sativa) 250 mg • Dong Quai extract (4:1)(Angelica sinensis) 100 mg • Black Cohosh extract (4:1)(Cimicifuga racemosa) 80 mg • Licorice extract (4:1)(Glycyrrhiza glabra) 70 mg • Chasteberry (Vitex agnus-castus) 50 mg • Pomegranate (Punica granatum) 39.5 mg.

Mid-Life Creme — Aspen Group, Inc.
Aloe Vera gel in Distilled Water with Catalyst Altered Normalizer • d-Alpha-Tocopherol & mixed Tocopherols • Cetyl Alcohol • Almond oil • Ociyl Palmitate • Panthenol • Peg 8 Stearate • Hydrogenated Vegetable oil • Glycerine • extract of Wild Yam • Micronized Progesterone • Polysorbate 60 • Propylene Glycol • Hyaluronic Acid • oil of Lemon • Keratin • Carbomer 940 • Grapefruit seed extract.

MigraActin — Nature's Plus
Two capsules contain: Feverfew [(Tanacetum parthenium leaf) standardized 1.2% Parthenolide] 700 mg • Pantothenic Acid 50 mg • Ginkgo Biloba leaf (standardized 24% Ginkgo Flavone-Glycosides, 6% Terpene Lactones) 10 mg • Bioperine [(Piper nigrum fruit) standardized 95% 1-Piperoylpiperidine] 5 mg • Trimethylglycine (TMG) 5 mg.

Migraban Feverfew — Jamieson
Each tablet contains: Dried Feverfew leaf (Tanacetum parthenium L.) (Equivalent to 250 mcg of Parthenolide with a complete active sesquiterpene lactone complex) 125 mg.

Migracare — Enzymatic Therapy
Each capsule contains: Feverfew extract (Tanacetum parthenium) standardized to contain 0.6% Parthenolide 100 mg.

Migra-Ease — Optimum Nutrition
Feverfew • White Willow.

Migra-Lieve — Natural Science Corp. of America
Two caplets contain: Feverfew Extract (Tanacetum parthenium, standardized to 0.7% Parthenolide) 100 mg • Magnesium (Citrate/Oxide 1:1) 300 mg • Riboflavin (Vitamin B2) 400 mg. Contains no yeast, milk, corn, wheat, gluten, soy sodium, salt, sugar, flavorings, preservatives, artificial colors.

Migraway — PhysioLogics
Each capsule contains: Riboflavin (Vitamin B2) 100 mg • Vitamin B6 (as Pyridoxine Hydrochloride) 20 mg • Ginger root (5% Gingerols, 7.5 mg) 150 mg • Feverfew leaf (1.2% Parthenolides, 0.6 mg) 50 mg • White Willow bark (7.5% Salicin, 3.75 mg) 50 mg • Ginkgo leaf (24% Ginkgoflavonglycosides, 9.6 mg; 6% Terpene Lactones, 2.4 mg) 40 mg.

Migrelief — Quantum
Each capsule contains: DHEA (Dehydroepiandrosterone) 25 mg • White Willow extract (4:1)(Salix alba) 125 mg • Meadowsweet extract (4:1) (Filipendula ulmaria) 125 mg • Feverfew (4:1) extract (Tanacetum parthenium) 75 mg. Standardized 4% Parthenolide I in a base of Vegetable Sterine & Magnesium Stearate.

Milagro For Men — Changes - TwinLab
Four caplets contain: Zinc (from Zinc Citrate) 30 mg • L-Arginine Hydrochloride 2800 mg • African Yohimbe bark standardized extract (2% yohimbine))Pausinystalia johimbe 800 mg • DHEA (Dehydroepiandrosterone) 50 mg • Global Male Herbal Blend 300 mg: Damiana leaf (Turnera aphrodisiaca), Muira Puama bark (Ptychopetalum olacoides), Jamaica Ginger root (Zingiber officinale), Mucuna pruriens seed, Withania somnifera root, Tinospora cordifolia leaf, Licorice root (Glycyrrhiza uralensis), Tribulus terrestris root, Nutmeg fruit (Myristica fragans), Korean Ginseng (Panax ginseng), Siberian Ginseng (Acanthopanax senticosus), Chinese Red Panax Ginseng (Panax ginseng), Manchurian Tienchi Ginseng (Panax notoginseng), Oat Straw (Avena sativa), Stinging Nettle (Urtica dioica). Other ingredients: Calcium Phosphate, Vegetable cellulose, Fractionated vegetable oil, Silica, and Vita-Lok vegetable resin glaze.

Milagro For Women — Changes - TwinLab
Four caplets contain: Vitamin E (as natural D-Alpha Tocopheral Succinate) 400 IU • Soy phytoestrogens concentrate (providing 80 mg isoflavones as daidzin and daidzein, genistin and genistein, glycitin and glycetein) 2670 mg • DHEA (Dehydroepiandrosterone) 50 mg • Global Female Herbal Blend 500 mg: Wild Yam (Discorea villosa), Red Clover blossom (Trifolium pratense), Damiana leaf (Turnera aphrodisiaca), Squaw Vine (Mitchella repens), Jamaica Ginger root (Zingiber officinale), Tribulus terrestris root, Licorice root (Glycyrrhiza uralensis), Fennel seed (Foeniculum vulgare), Magnolia bark (Magnolia officinalis), Korean Ginseng root (Panax ginseng), Siberian Ginseng root (Acanthopanax ginseng), Chinese Red Panax Ginseng root (Panax ginseng), Manchurian Tienchi Ginseng (Panax notoginseng), Black Cohosh root (Cimicifuaga racemosa), Oat Straw (Avena sativa), Stinging Nettle (Urtica dioica). Other ingredients: Dicalcium Phosphate, Vegatable cellulose, Fractionated vegetable oil, Silica, an Vita-Lok.

Mild Child — The Herbalist
Catnip leaf • Fennel seed • Chamomile flower • Lemon Balm leaf.

Milk Thistle — BioDynamax
Each tablet contains: Milk Thistle 175 mg.

Milk Thistle — Pharmanex
Each capsule contains: Milk Thistle (Silybum marianum)(seed extract)(30:1) 175 mg. Other Ingredients: Rice Flour, Gelatin, Magnesium Stearate, Silicon Dioxide.

Milk Thistle Formula — Quest
Each caplet contains: Milk Thistle seed powder (Silybum marianum) (provided by 60 mg of P.E. 1:8) 480 mg • Butternut bark of root powder (Juglans cineraria) 155 mg • Dandelion root powder (Taraxacum oficinale) 155 mg • Licorice root powder (Glycyrrhiza glabra) 40 mg • Wild Yam root powder (Dioscorea villosa) 10 mg. Other Ingredients: Calcium Phosphate, Microcrystalline Cellulose, Vegetable Stearin, Croscarmellose Sodium, Magnesium Stearate (vegetable source).

Milk Thistle Seed — Gaia Herbs
Milk Thistle seed (Standardized for 80% silymarins) Standardized Full Spectrum 150 mg of extract per capsule. Guaranteed Potency 75 mg of extract per capsule.

Milk-Based Soy-Free Lactobacillus Acidophilus — Nature's Life
Two tablespoons (1 fl.oz or 29.6 ml) contain: Purified Water, Non-fat Milk powder & viable Lactobacillus Acidophilus Culture.

Milk-Zyme — Atrium
Each capsule contains: Lactase 30 mg • Rennin 10 mg.

Mind & Memory — Health Factor
Each capsule contains: Ginkgo Biloba extract (4:1)(standardized extract to 24% Gingkoflavonglycosides) 160 mg • Gotu Kola extract (4:1)(Hydrocotyle asaitica) 150 mg • Rosemary (Rosmarinus officinalis) 150 mg.

Minerogen — ANS
Each capsule contains: Calcium 200 mg • Magnesium 75 mg • Copper 250 mcg • Chromium 25 mcg • Manganese 100 mcg • Molybdenum 50 mcg • Selenium 25 mcg • Potassium 100 mg • Vanadium 25 mcg • Boron 1 mg • Zinc 7.5 mg.

Mintacin — Enzymatic Therapy
Each capsule contains: Active ingredient: Simethicone 25 mg. Other ingredients: Peppermint oil extract (Mentha piperita) 0.2 mL. Contains no sugar, salt, yeast, wheat, corn, soy, dairy products, coloring, flavoring or preservatives. Chlorophyll is used as a natural coloring agent.

MI-T-Cell — Progressive Labs
Each capsule contains: Vitamin C (ascorbyl palmitate) 50 mg • Vitamin E Succinate 30 mg • Thiamin HCl (Vitamin B1) 5 mg • Riboflavin (Vitamin B2) 5 mg • Magnesium (as magnesium malate) 50 mg • L-Glutathione 50 mg • N-Acetyl-Carnitine 30 mg • N-Acetyl Cysteine 50 mg • CoEnzyme Q10 10 mg • Lipoic Acid 50 mg • L-Isoleucine 225 mcg • Red Grape skin (Vitis vinifera) 2% polyphenols 50 mg.

Mixed Vegetables — Nature's Plus
Three tablets contain: Broccoli floret (Brassica oleracea) naturally rich in sulorophane & indole-3-carbinol equivalent to 10000 mg fresh broccoli 1000 mg • Spinach leaf (Spinacia oleracea) naturally rich in monoterpenes equivalent to 1000 mg fresh Spinach 100 mg • Carrot root (Daucus carota) naturally rich in carotenoids, coumarins & Polyacetylenes equivalent to 1000 mg fresh Carrot 100 mg • Cabbage leaf (Brassica chinensis) naturally rich in Sterols, Phenolic Acids & Indoles equivalent to 1000 mg. fresh Cabbage 100 mg. Contains no yeast, wheat, corn, soy, milk, salt, sugar or starch.

Modrenal GF — PhysioLogics
Three caplets contain: Vitamin B1 (Thiamine HCI) 40 mg • Vitamin B2 (Riboflavin) 30 mg • Vitamin B5 (Calcium Pantothenate) 150 mg • Vitamin B6 (Pyridoxine HCI) 25 mg • Vitamin B12 (Cyanocobalamin) 30 mcg • Vitamin C (Ascorbic Acid) 200 mg • Vitamin E (D-Alpha Tocopherol) 100 IU • Vitamin B3 (Niacinamide) 50 mg • Iron (Ferrous Succinate) 10 mg • Magnesium (Citrate) 200 mg • Calcium (Citrate) 250 mg • Folic Acid 100 mcg • Biotin 20 mcg • Siberian Ginseng (Eleutherococcus senticosus; GPH: 0.3% eleutherosides b & e) 75 mg • Lemon Bioflavonoids 50 mg • Passion Flower 50 mg • Chamomile 50 mg • Skullcap 50 mg • Choline 40 mg • PABA 10 mg • Inositol 10 mg • Chromium GTF (Nicotinate) 250 mcg.

Moducare Sterinol — Dynapro
Each capsule contains: Plant Sterols 20 mg • Plant Sterolins 200 mcg. Other Ingredients: White Rice Flour, Magnesium Silicate, Gel Cap.

Moisturizing Cleansing Creme — Aspen Group, Inc.
Each gram contains: Tocopheryl Acetate 1% • Panthenol 1% • Water • Mineral Oil • Steareth-2 • PPG-15 • Stearyl Ether • Tocopheryl Acetate • Octyl Palmitate • Isoceteth-20 • Cetearyl Octanoate • Carbomer • Dimethicone • Ammonium Hydroxide • Propylene Glycol • Diazolidinyl Urea • Methylparaben • Propylparaben.

Molymin — Progressive Labs
Each capsule contains: Molybdenum (amino acid chelate) 50 mcg • Pea powder 150 mg • Lentil powder 75 mg • Buckwheat 75 mg • Millet flour 75 mg. Carefully dried to preserve their natural trace nutrient content.

Monolaurin (Coconut Extract) — Olympia Nutrition
Coconut extract 300 mg.

© Copyright 2000, Natural Medicines Comprehensive Database (209) 472-2244. For updated data, go to www.NaturalDatabase.com. • 1367

B R A N D   N A M E S

Monthly Comfort — Source Naturals
Six tablets contain: Vitamin A (Palmitate) 6000 IU • Vitamin C (Ascorbic Acid and Zinc Ascorbate) 600 mg • Vitamin E (D-Alpha Tocopheryl) (Natural) 150 IU • Vitamin B1 (Thiamin) 20 mg • Vitamin B2 (Riboflavin) 20 mg • Niacinamide 100 mg • Vitamin B5 (Calcium D-Pantothenate) 30 mg • Vitamin B6 (Pyridoxine HCl) 150 mg • Vitamin B12 (Cyanocobalamin) 30 mcg • Folic Acid 800 mcg • Calcium (Carbonate, Citrate) 200 mg • Chromium (ChromeMate GTF Yeast-Free Polynicotinate) 300 mcg • Magnesium (Oxide, Citrate) 450 mg • Zinc (Ascorbate) 20 mg • Taurine 500 mg • N-Acetyl Cysteine 300 mg • DLPA (DL-Phenylalanine) 250 mg • Choline (Bitartrate) 100 mg • Inositol 100 mg • Herbal Formula 1350 mg • Chasteberry 400 mgl Dong Quai root 200 mg • Black Cohosh root 175 mg • Blue Cohosh root 175 mg • Silymarin (Milk Thistle seed extract) 100 mg • Cyperus rhizome 100 mg • Dong Quai root extract 100 mg • Dandelion root extract 100 mg.

Mood Actives — VitaStore
Four tablets contain: St. John's Wort (0.3% Hypericin) 450 mg • Kava Kava 325 mg • Ginseng 200 mg • Valerian 200 mg • Licorice Root 150 mg • L-Methionine 100 mg • L-Phenylalanine 200 mg • L-Tyrosine 500 mg • L-Taurine 500 mg • Folic Acid 0.4 mg • Vitamin C 300 mg • Vitamin B6 (Pyridoxine) 4 mg • Vitamin B12 12 mcg • Zinc 50 mg.

Mood Aid Formula — Nature's Way
Each capsule contains: Korean Ginseng dried extract 33.3 mg • L-5 Hydroxytryptophan (Griffonia bean extract) 3.33 mg • Niacin (Vitamin B3) 3.33 mg • Riboflavin (Vitamin B2) 284 mcg • Scullcap herb 100 mg • St. John's Wort dried extract (0.3% Dianthrones measures as Hypercin) 300 mg • Thiamine (Vitamin B1) 350 mcg • Vitamin B12 (Cyanocobalamin) 1 mcg • Vitamin B6 (Pyridoxine HCL) 330 mcg. Other ingredients: Gelatin, Magnesium Stearate, Millet.

Mood Enhancer — Clinician's Choice
Three tablets contain: Valerian Root 300 mg • St. John's Wort Extract (std. 0.3% hypericin) 300 mg • Chamomile Flowers 300 mg • L-Tyrosine 30 mg • Proprietary blend 15 mg: Passion Flower, Sage Leaves, Isoflavones, Grape Powder, Acetyl-L-Carnitine.

Mood Support with St. John's Wort — Natrol
One capsule contains: Guaranteed Potency-St. John's Wort supplying 0.3% Hypericin 300 mg • Ginseng supplying 8% Ginsenosides 100 mg • L-Tyrosine 50 mg • Lemon Balm 25 mg • DMAE (Di Methyl Amino Ethanol Bitartrate) 25 mg • Vitamin E (d-Alpha Tocopheryl Acetate) 30 IU • Folic Acid 400 mcg • Vitamin B12 (Cyanocobalamin) 50 mcg • Selenium (l-Selenomethionine) 25 mcg. Other ingredients: Silica, Magnesium Stearate, Gelatin.

Mood Sync — Pain & Stress Center
Each capsule contains: St. John's Wort 175 mg • GABA 125 mg • Taurine 100 mg • Glutamine 75 mg • 5-HTP 25 mg • Vitamin B6 (Pyridoxine HCl) 5 mg.

Mor-Andro 200 — OSMO Therapy
Each capsule contains: 4-Androstene-3Beta,17Beta-Diol (androdiol) 100 mg • 4-Androstene 3, 17-Dione (androstenedione) 100 mg • Elemental Zinc Gluconate 5 mg • Niacin (nicotinic acid) 20 mg.

More than a Diet — American Health
Three duotabs contain: Chromium Factors: (Chromium Picolinate, Chromium Polynicotinate) 100 mg • Lipoactive Factors: L-Carnitine, Inositol, Choline L-Methionine, Lecithin, Phosphytidyl Choline (pc), Phosphytidyl Serine (ps), Taurine, Betaine HCI, Vanadium, Vanadyl Sulfate Amino Factors) 333mg • Herbal Thermal Factors 350 mg • Capsicum, Ginger, Licorice, Mustard seed, Green Tea, American Ginseng, Cinnamon, Korean Ginseng, Siberian Ginseng, Piper Longum, Gugulipid, Suma, Schizandra, Astragalus, Hawthorne, Kola Nut, Guarana 232 mg • Fiber Factors: Oat Bran Fiber, Citrus Pectin Fiber, Pulp Cellulose, Vegetable Cellulose, Beet Fiber 500 mg • Herbal Fluid Factors: Uva Ursi, Buchu Leaves, Couch Grass, Corn Silk, Hydrangea, Juniper berries 190 mg • Essential Fatty Acid Factors: Gotu Kola, Milk Thistle (Silymarin), Chickweed, Borage oil, Black Currant oil, Primrose oil, Flaxseed oil (CLA), Dandelion 80 mg • Appetite Factors : Citrimax (hca from Garnicia cambogia), Chitosan (Shellfish Fiber), OP's (Wheat Oligio Peptides), Gymenma, Sylvestre, Apple Cider Vinegar 450 mg • Green Super Food Factors: Spirulina, Chlorella, Barley Grass, Wheat Grass, Kelp 500 mg • Alfalfa Enzyme Factors: Bromelain, Bipase, Protease, Cellulase, Aspergillus niger, Aspergillus oryzae, FOS 215 mg • Pancreatin Fruit Extract Factors: Apple, Apricot, Banana, Cranberry, Orange, Lemon, Lime, Papaya,

Pineapple, Strawberry, Watermelon, Grapeseed (opc), Grapefruit 67.5 mg • Vegetable extract Factors: Cabbage, Celery, Broccoli, Brussels Sprouts, Yams, Carrots, Kale, Collard Greens, Spinach, Cauliflower 50 mg • Youth Factors: DHEA (does not contain more than 2 mg per tablet of DHEA), CoEnzyme Q10, Phaseolus vulgaris 109 mg.

Mother's Milk — Traditional Medicinals
Contains: Fennel seed • Anise seed • Coriander seed • Spearmint leaf • Lemongrass leaf • Lemon Verbena leaf • Althea root • Blessed Thistle leaf • Fenugreek seed.

Motion Mate Formula — Nature's Way
Two capsules contain: Ginger • Hyssop herb • Meadowsweet herb • Peppermint leaves • Red Raspberry leaves. Other ingredients: Gelatin, Magnesium Stearate, Millet.

Motion Sickness Remedy — Phytopharmica
Twenty drops contain: Cocculus indicus 8x • Plumbum aceticum 8x • Argentum nitricum 6x • Glonoinum 6x • Zincum valerianicum 6x • Belladonna 4x • Nux vomica 4x • Pulsatilla 4x • Vinca minor 3x • Artemesia vulgaris 1x. In a base of 45% USP alcohol by volume. Editor's Comments: This is a homeopathic product. It is so extremely diluted that its activity can not be explained by conventional scientific methods. Therefore this product can not be rated by the scientific criteria used in this Database. A patient receiving the extreme dilution of this product will not receive many, if any, molecules of the original active ingredient. Therefore, there are no harmful pharmacologic effects, and any beneficial effects are controversial and not due to a direct biochemical action of the ingredient on the body. Homeopathic products are allowed for sale in the U.S. due to legislation passed in the 19th century sponsored by a homeopathic physician who was also a Senator. The law still requires that the FDA allow the sale of products listed in this Homeopathic Pharmacopea of the United States.

Mouth-Mend — The Herbalist
Echinacea root • Golden Seal root • Myrrh Gum • Propolis • Spilanthes herb • Yerba Mansa root.

Movana — Pharmaton
Each tablet contains: St. John's Wort flower & leaves extract WS-5572 (Stabalized minimum hyperforin content 3%, Standardized Hypericin content 0.3%) 300 mg. Other Ingredients: Microcrystalline Cellulose • Corn Starch • Croscarmellose Sodium • Hydroxypropyl Methylcellulose, PEG-4000 • Magnesium Stearate • Silicon Dioxide • Ascorbic Acid • Synthetic Iron Oxide • Titanium Dioxide • Talc • Vanillin. Contains no artificial stimulants, caffeine, or sugar.

MPF — Progressive Labs
Six capsules contain: Vitamin A 25000 IU • Vitamin E 180 IU • Folic Acid 780 mcg • Zinc Picolinate 60 mg • L-Glutamine 1500 mg • N-Acetyl Glucosamine 1050 mg • Gamma Oryzanol 360 mg • Cat's Claw (Uncaria tomentosa) 450 mg.

MRP-44 — Human Development Technologies
Each serving contains: Calories 297 • Protein 44 g • Total Carbohydrate 26 g • Sugar 5 g • Total Fat 1.5 g • Saturated Fat 1 g • L-Glutamine 2 g • Taurine 1 g. Ingredients: MRP1000 (Micro Ultra Filtered Whey Protein concentrate • Egg Albumen • Micro Ultra Filtered Whey Protein Isolate, Ion Exchanged Whey Protein Isolate) • Maltodextrin • natural & artificial flavorings • L-Glutamine • Di-Calcium Phosphate • Taurine • Inulin • Cellulose Gum • Xanthan Gum • Magnesium Oxide • Lecithin • Fructose • Stevia • Acesulfame Potassium • Ascorbic Acid • Vitamin A Acetate • Vitamin E Acetate • Niacinamide • Iron Electrolytic • Zinc Oxide • D-Calcium Pantothenate • Ergocalciferol • Pyridoxine HCL • Copper Gluconate • Riboflavin • Thiamine Mononitrate • Folic Acid • Biotin • Potassium Ionide • Cyanocobalamin.

MSM — Trimedica
Each capsule contains: Methylsulfonylmethane 99.9% • Water 0.1%.

MSM 1000 — Aspen Group, Inc.
Each capsule contains: 100% pure MSM (Methyl Sulfonyl Methane) 1000 mg. Contains no sugar, starch, salt, wheat, corn, yeast or soy derivatives.

MSM Plus — Progressive Labs
Each capsule contains: Vitamin C (as magnesium ascorbate) 100 mg • Magnesium (as magnesium ascorbate) 7 mg • Methyl Sulfonyl Methane (MSM) 800 mg.

MSM Rejuvenator — Progressive Labs
Ingredients: Stabilized Aloe Vera gel • Methylsulfonyl Methane •

Glycerine • Caprylic/Capric Triglycerides • Jojoba oil • Polyquanterium-32 (colloidal polymers) • Evening Primrose oil • Cetyl Alcohol • Steryl Alcohol • Tetrahexyldecyl Ascorbate (lipid soluble Vitamin C) • Tocopheryl Acetate (Vitamin E) • Ginseng extract • Chamomile extract. Extracts of: Grape seed, Willow bark, Calendula, White Lily, Japanese Green Tea, Gum Mint, Cucumber, Soapbark, Balm of Gilead, Bee Propolis: Betaglucans. Essential oils of: Lemongrass, Rosemary, Sage, Cedarwood, Tetrasodium EDTA, Methylparaben, Propylparben, Diazolidiny Lurea.

Mucho Mate — Traditional Medicinals
Green & Roasted Yerba Mate leaf • Ginger rhizome • Lemon peel • Natural Lemon flavor • Stevia leaf.

Mucoplex — Progressive Labs
Each capsule contains: Comfrey root (Symphytum officinale) 225 mg • Pepsin (1:3000) 65 mg • Bromelain 50 mg • Raw Duodenum 10 mg.

Muco-Plex — Enzymatic Therapy
Two tablets contain: Niacin 30 mg • Vitamin B6 (Pyridoxine HCl) 10 mg • Iodine (Potassium Iodide) 75 mcg. Other Ingredients: Marshmallow extract 8:1 (Althea officinalis) mucilage content 30-40% 450 mg • Raw Duodenum Tissue 450 mg • Pancreatic Enzymes 3X 100 mg • L-Methionine 100 mg • Gastric Mucin powder 100 mg • Pepsin 1:10000 65 mg • Pituitary extract 15 mg. In a base of Crude Licorice extract (Glycyrrhiza glabra) & derivatives with an organically bound Allantoin-Methionine (Comfrey) Complex, Acidophilus, & Aloe Vera. Contains no sugar, salt, yeast, wheat, corn, soy, dairy products, coloring, flavoring or preservatives.

Mullein Lobelia — Atrium
Each capsule contains: Mullein leaves 375 mg • Lobelia 125 mg. Professional Formula. Contains no sugar, starch, salt, wheat, corn, yeast or soy derivatives.

Multi Caps — Progressive Labs
Three capsules contain: Vitamin A 10000 IU • Vitamin C 120 mg • Vitamin D3 400 IU • Vitamin E 15 IU • Thiamin (Vitamin B1) 10 mg • Riboflavin (Vitamin B2) 10 mg • Niacinamide 100 mg • Vitamin B6 10 mg • Folate (folic acid) 400 mcg • Vitamin B12 50 mg • Biotin 25 mcg • Pantothenic Acid 40 mg • Calcium 200 mg • Iron 15 mg • Magnesium 100 mg • Zinc 15 mg • Selenium 25 mcg • Manganese 20 mg • Iodine 150 mcg • Chromium 20 mcg • Potassium 99 mg • Choline 75 mg • Inositol 75 mg • PABA 30 mg • Citrus bioflavonoids 100 mg • Rutin 25 mg • Hesperidin 25 mg • Glutamic Acid 30 mg • L-Lysine 50 mg • DL-Methionine 50 mg • Pancreatin 60 mg • Bile Salts 5 mg • RNA (Brain) 50 mg • Unsaturated Fatty Acids 50 mg. Other ingredients: Rose Hips, Ginseng, Goldenseal, Fo Ti Teng, Gotu Kola, Sarsaparilla, Watercress, Kelp, Green Cabbage, Rice polishings, Raw Stomach substance (not an extract), Alfalfa, Parsley, Papaya.

Multi Chelate — Progressive Labs
Six capsules contain: Calcium 500 mg • Iron 15 mg • Magnesium 250 mg • Zinc 10 mg • Iodine 150 mcg • Selenium 25 mcg • Copper 1 mg • Manganese 10 mg • Chromium 50 mcg • Molybdenum 150 mcg • Potassium 99 mg • Vanadium 150 mcg • Silicone 2 mg • Raw Glandular concentrate 200 mg. The raw glandular materal in this product is prepared by a special process which does not exceed physiological temperature (37 Celcius). Guaranteed free of chemical pesticides and synthetic hormones.

Multi fiber Complex — Natrol
One capsule contains: Psyllium Seed husk 400 mg • Guar Gum 50 mg • Slippery Elm Bark 50 mg • Licorice root 50 mg • Apple Pectin 50 mg • Grapefruit Pectin 50 mg • Glucomannan 50 mg. Other ingredients: Magnesium Stearate, Silicon Dioxide, Gelatin.

Multi for Seniors — Health Center for Better Living
Each tablet contains: Vitamin A (as retinyl acetate and beta-carotene) 6,000 IU • Vitamin C (as ascorbic acid) 60 mg • Vitamin D (as cholecalciferol) 400 IU • Vitamin E (as dl-alpha-tocopheryl acetate) 45 IU • Vitamin K (as phytonadione) 10 mcg • Vitamin B1 (as thiamin mononitrate) 1.5 mg • Vitamin B2 (as riboflavin) 1.7 mg • Niacin (as niacinarnide) 20 mg • Vitamin B6 (as pyridoxine HCl) 3 mg • Folate (as folic acid) 200 mcg • Vitamin B12 (as cyanocobalamin) 25 mcg • Biotin 30 mcg • Pantothenic Acid (as D-calcium patothenate) 10 mg • Calcium (as calcium carbonate and dicalcium phosphate) 200 mg • Iron (as ferrous fumarate) 9 mg • Phosphorus (as dicalcium phosphate) 48 mcg • Iodine (as potassium iodide) 150 mcg • Magnesium (as magnesium oxide) 100 mg • Zinc (as zinc oxide) 15 mg • Selenium (as sodium selenate) 25 mcg • Copper (as cupric oxide) 2 mg • Manganese (as manganese sulfate (2.5 mg)) • Chromium

(as chromium amino acid chelate) 100 mcg • Molybdenum (as sodium molybdate) 25 mcg • Potassium (as postassium chloride) 80 mg • Nickel (as nickelous sulfate) 5 mcg • Silicon (as sodium metasilicate) 10 mcg • Vanadium (as sodium metavanadate) 10 mcg.

Multi Minerals — Nutrition Warehouse
Three tablets contain: Calcium (Carbonate, Citrate) 1000 mg • Magnesium (Oxide, Citrate) 500 mg • Zinc 22.5 mg • Iron 20 mg • Copper 1 mg • Potassium 99 mg • Manganese 5 mg • Selenium 50 mcg • Chromium (yeast-free) 100 mcg • Molybdenum 50 mcg • Vanadium 50 mcg • Iodine (Kelp) 150 mcg • L-Glutamic Acid (HCL) 50 mg • Vitamin D (Cholecalciferol) 200 IU • Boron Citrate 3 mg.

Multi Vitamin Energy Plus for Women — Futurebiotics
Two tablets contain: Beta Carotene 8500 IU • Vitamin C (Acerola, Ascorbic Acid) 225 mg • Thiamin 12.5 mg • Riboflavin 12.5 mg • Niacinamide 50 mg • Calcium (Phosphate, Carbonate) 625 mg • Iron (Amino Acid Chelate) 8 mg • Vitamin D 400 IU • Vitamin E (Natural Mixed Tocopherols) 30 IU • Vitamin B6 15 mg • Folic Acid 400 mcg • Vitamin B12 30 mcg • Biotin 300 mcg • Pantothenic Acid 25 mg • Para Amino Benzoic Acid (PABA) 85 mg • Choline 150 mg • Inositol 30 mg • Iodine (Kelp) 150 mcg • Magnesium (Oxide, Ascorbate) 150 mg • Zinc (Amino Acid Chelate) 15 mg • Ribonucleic Acid (RNA) 50 mg • Chromium (Polynicotinate) 60 mcg • Potassium (Amino Acid Chelate) 90 mg • Selenium (Selenomethionine) • In a base of Peony Root, Dong Quai, Aloe Vera, Methionine, Chamomile, Rosemary, American Ginseng, Chlorella, Bee Pollen, Sea Vegetable, Dandelion Root, Betaine HCl, Chinese Licorice & Raw Alfalfa Juice Concentrate.

Multi-Carotene — PhysioLogics
Each softgel contains: Carotenoids 306 mg • Beta Carotene (30000 IU) 18 mg • Alpha Carotene 10.8 mg • Gamma Carotene 0.9 mg • Lycopene 0.9 mg • Vitamin E (D-Alpha Tocopherol) 1 IU.

Multiglan Chelate — Atrium
Six tablets contain: Calcium 500 mg • Magnesium 250 mg • Potassium 99 mg • Manganese 10 mg • Iron 18 mg • Silicon 2 mg • Zinc 15 mg • Iodine (Kelp) 150 mcg • Chromium 200 mcg • Selenium 25 mcg • Molybdenum 150 mcg • Vanadium 150 mcg • As Chelated Proteinates, together in a base of of Raw Tissue concentrates (not extracts) from: [Spleen 144 mg, Brain 30 mg, Liver 20 mg, Heart 14 mg, Thymus 4 mg, Adrenal 4 mg, Pancreas 4 mg, Duodenum 4 mg, Pituitary 2 mg] 240 mg.

MultiLogics — PhysioLogics
Each tablet contains: Vitamin A (Beta-Carotene) 12500 IU • Vitamin A (Palmitate) 2500 IU • Thiamine 75 mg • Riboflavin 75 mg • Niacin 75 mg • Pantothenic Acid 75 mg • Vitamin B6 (Pyridoxine HCl) 75 mg • Vitamin B12 (Cyanocobalamin) 75 mcg • Folic Acid 400 mcg • Biotin 300 mcg • Vitamin C (Ascorbic Acid) 250 mg • Vitamin D (Cholecalciferol) 400 IU • Vitamin E (d-Alpha Tocopherol) 150 IU • Calcium (Amino Acid Chelate) 20 mg • Iron (Bisglycinate) 1.3 mg • Magnesium (Amino Acid Chelate) 10 mg • Zinc (Amino Acid Chelate) 10 mg • Copper (Amino Acid Chelate) 1 mg • Manganese (Amino Acid Chelate) 1 mg • Chromium (Niacin/Glycine Chelate) 25 mcg • Iodine (Potassium Iodide) 150 mcg • Selenium (Amino Acid Chelate) 25 mcg • Molybdenum (Amino Acid Chelate) 25 mcg • Boron (Amino Acid Chelate) 500 mcg • Potassium (Amino Acid Complex) 1.8 mg • Bioflavonoids lemon 25 mg • Rutin 25 mg • Betaine (HCI) 25 mg • Choline (Bitartrate) 31 mg • Inositol 75 mg • PABA 75 mg • Hesperidin 5 mg.

MultiLogics for Children — PhysioLogics
Two tablets contain: Vitamin A (as 67% Beta-Carotene, 33% Fish Liver oil) 7500 IU • Vitamin C (as Ascorbic Acid) 180 mg • Vitamin D3 (from Fish Liver oil) 200 IU • Vitamin E (as d-Alpha Tocopherol Succinate) 90 IU • Vitamin K (as Phytonadione) 30 mcg • Thiamine (as Thiamine Mononitrate) 3 mg • Riboflavin (Vitamin B2) 3.4 mg • Niacin (as Niacinamide) 20 mg • Vitamin B6 (as Pyridoxine HCI) 4 mg • Folic Acid 400 mcg • Vitamin B12 12 mcg • Biotin 300 mcg • Pantothenic Acid (as d-Calcium Panthothenate) 20 mg • Calcium (as Calcium Citrate-Aspartate Complex) 100 mg • Iron (as Iron Carbonyl) 4.5 mg • Iodine (as Potassium Iodide, Kelp) 75 mcg • Magnesium (as Magnesium Citrate-Aspartate Complex) 100 mg • Zinc (as Amino Acid Zinc Chelate) 5 mg • Selenium (as Amino Acid Selenium Complex) 50 mcg • Copper (as Copper Gluconate) 400 mcg • Manganese (as Amino Acid Manganese Chelate) 1 mg • Chromium (as Chromium Polynicotinate) 50 mcg • Molybdenum (as Amino Acid Molybdenum Chelate) 50 mcg • Black Currant seed 5 mg • Choline (Bitartrate) 5 mg • Boron (Aspartate-Citrate) 1 mg.

© Copyright 2000, Natural Medicines Comprehensive Database (209) 472-2244. For updated data, go to www.NaturalDatabase.com. • 1369

B R A N D   N A M E S

MultiLogics for Men — PhysioLogics
Three tablets contain: Vitamin E (d-Alpha Tocopherol Acetate) 250 IU • Calcium (Aquamins, Carbonate) 530 mg • Magnesium (Amino Acid Chelate/Oxide) 140 mg • Zinc (Amino Acid Chelate) 15 mg • Iron (Ferrous Bisglycinate) 5 mg • Copper (Amino Acid Chelate) 1 mg • Chromium (Amino Acid Chelate) 175 mcg • Selenium (Amino Acid Complex) 175 mcg • Tomato extract (1% Lycopene, 1.6 mg) 160 mg • Saw Palmetto berry (20-25% fatty acids & Lipid Sterols 15-18.75 mg) 75 mg • Bioflavonoids lemon 50 mg • Rutin 50 mg • Hesperidin 50 mg • Green Tea leaf (45% Polyphenols, 22.5 mg) 50 mg • Betaine HCl 50 mg • Ginkgo Biloba leaf (24% Ginkgo Flavonglycosides, 9.6 mg; 6% Terpene Lactones, 24 mg) 40 mg • Nettles (1-2% Silica, 300-600 mcg) 30 mg • Beta Sitosterol 30 mg • Black Cohosh root (Cimicifuga racemosa) 25 mg • Whole Grape/Wine Complex (45% Polyphenols, 11.25 mg) 25 mg • Bioperine (95% Piperine, 4.75 mg) 5 mg • Calendula flower Marigold (5% Lutein, 150 mg) 3 mg • Potassium (Amino Acid Chelate) 3.6 mg • Boron (Amino Acid Chelate) 500 mcg • Calendula flower Marigold (0.25% Zeaxanthin, 3.75 mcg) 150 mcg.

MultiLogics for Women — PhysioLogics
Three tablets contain: Vitamin E (d-Alpha Tocopherol Acetate) 250 IU • Calcium (Aquamins, Carbonate) 530 mg • Magnesium (Amino Acid Chelate/Oxide) 140 mg • Zinc (Amino Acid Chelate) 15 mg • Iron (Ferrous Bisglycinate) 5 mg • Copper (Amino Acid Chelate) 1 mg • Chromium (Amino Acid Chelate) 175 mcg • Selenium (Amino Acid Complex) 175 mcg • Tomato extract (1% Lycopene, 1.6 mg) 160 mg • Bioflavonoids lemon 50 mg • Rutin 50 mg • Hesperidin 50 mg • Green Tea leaf (45% Polyphenols, 22.5 mg) 50 mg • Betaine HCl 50 mg • Ginkgo Biloba leaf (24% Ginkgo Flavonglycosides. 9.6 mg; 6% Terpene Lactones, 24 mg) 40 mg • Black Cohosh root 25 mg • Whole Grape/Wine Complex (45% Polyphenols, 11.25 mg) 25 mg • Dong Quai (1% Ligustilides, 250 mcg) 25 mg • Chasteberry (0.5% Isoflavones, 125 mcg) 25 mg • Choline (Bitartate) 20 mg • Diadzein 13 mg • Bioperine (95% Piperine, 4.75 mg) 5 mg • Calendula flower Marigold (5% Lutein, 150 mg) 3 mg • Potassium (Amino Acid Chelate) 3.6 mg • Boron (Amino Acid Chelate) 500 mcg • Calendula flower Marigold (0.25% Zeaxanthin, 3.75 mcg) 150 mcg.

Multi-Mineral Citrate Complete — The Vitamin Shoppe
Eight capsules contain: Calcium 1000 mg • Magnesium 500 mg • Potassium 99 mg • Zinc 50 mg • Boron 3 mg • Copper 2 mg • Selenium 100 mcg • Chromium 200 mcg • Molybdenum 100 mcg • Iron 10 mg • Manganese 10 mg.

Multi-Minerals — The Vitamin Shoppe
Three tablets provide: Calcium 1000 mg • Zinc 22.5 • Copper 1 mg • Selenium 50 mcg • Chromium 100 mcg • Vanadium 50 mcg • Glutamic Acid 50 mg • Magnesium 500 mg • Iron 20 mg • Potassium 99 mg • Manganese 5 mg • Boron 3 mg • Molybdenum 50 mcg • Iodine 150 mcg • Vitamin D 200 IU.

Multi-Quest — Nutri-Quest
Three tablets contain: Vitamin A (Palmitate) 2000 IU • Vitamin D3 400 IU • Vitamin E (Succinate) 200 IU • Vitamin C (Sago Palm) 1000 mg • Lemon Bioflavonoids 100 mg • Rutin 25 mg • Hesperidin Complex 50 mg • Vitamin B6 25 mg • Vitamin B1 13 mg • Vitamin B2 10 mg • Niacin 45 mg • Vitamin B12 30 mcg • Pantothenic Acid (Calcium Pantothenate) 50 mg • Folic Acid 200 mcg • Choline Bitartrate 100 mg • Inositol 100 mg • Biotin 400 mcg • PABA 50 mg • L-Glycine 9.66 mg • Calcium Gluconate 15.36 mg • Vitamin F 5 mg • Chlorophyll 16 mg • Calcium Aspartate 500 mg • Magnesium Aspartate 250 mg • Phosphorus Chelate 200 mg • Potassium Proteinate 30 mg • Copper Chelate 1 mg • Zinc Aspartate 5 mg • Manganese Aspartate 15 mg • Molybdenum Chelate 50 mcg • Chromium Chelate 25 mcg • Selenium Chelate 30 mcg • Iodine (kelp) 50 mcg • Sodium Proteinate 30 mcg • Rubidium Chelate 15 mcg • Lithium Chelate 8 mcg • L-Phenylalanine 13 mg • L-Histidine 6 mg • L-Tyrosine 9 mg • L-Lysine 13 mg • L-Valine 15 mg • DL-Methionine 9 mg • L-Isoleucine 13 mg • L-Leucine 18 mg • L-Threonine 9 mg • L-Glutamic Acid 2 mg • Goldenseal root 45 mg • Siberian Ginseng 45 mg • Garlic 40 mg • Tillandsia 30 mg • Rice Bran 176 mg • Almond Meal 150 mg.

Multi-Scorb — Progressive Labs
Each tablet contains: Vitamin C (as mineral ascorbates) 1000 mg • Calcium (ascorbate) 50 mg • Magnesium (ascorbate) 30 mg • Zinc (ascorbate) 3 mg • Manganese (ascorbate) 3 mg • Potassium (ascorbate) 60 mg • Citrus BioFlavonoid 5X complex 125 mg (as undiluted hesperidin, naringin and rutin).

Munit-E — Holista
Each capsule contains: Beta Carotene 10000 IU • Vitamin A 5000 IU • Vitamin C 500 mg • Vitamin B6 25 mg • Zinc 20 mg • Echinacea (angustifolia/purpurea) 300 mg • Bioflavonoids 100 mg • Garlic 50 mg • Ginger 50 mg.

Muscle — Gary Null
Composed of plant sources. Fortified with Methionine, Leucine, Valine, Isoleucine, and Lysine.

Muscle Mass — Source Naturals
Two tablets contain: Vitamin C (Ascorbic Acid) 50 mg • Vitamin B5 (Calcium D-Pantothenate) 20 mg • Vitamin B6 (Pyridoxine HCl) 20 mg • Iodine (from kelp) 56 mcg. Other Ingredients: Arginine Pyroglutamate 718 mg, L-Lysine HCl 718 mg, L-Ornithine (Ornithine HCl) 200 mg, Branched Chain Amino Acids (BCAAs) 174 mg (L-Leucine 100 mg, L-Isoleucine 30 mg and L-Valine 44 mg), Lipotropic Factors 360 mg (Choline Bitartrate 200 mg. Inositol 100 mg, L-Methionine 30 mg and Betaine HCl 30 mg), Glycine 50 mg, Trans-Ferulic Acid 50 mg, L-Carnitine (L-Carnitine L-Tartrate) 10 mg, Special Herbal Blend 590 mg: Saw Palmetto, Sarsaparilla, Wild Yam Root, Astragalus, Kelp, Ginseng, Pueraria, Licorice Root.

Musclease — PhysioLogics
Two capsules contain: Magnesium (Aspartate) 100 mg • Calcium (Citrate) 50 mg • Valerian (0.8% Valernic Acids, 800 mcg) 100 mg • Kava Kava root (30% Kavalactones, 30 mg) 100 mg • Passion flower (3.5% Flavonoids, 3.5 mg) 100 mg.

MuscleTech — Muscletech
Six capsules contain: Acetyl-L-Carnitine 1000 mg • Glutamine 2000 mg • L-Leucine 1000 mg • L-Valine 250 mg • L-Isoleucine 250 mg • OKG 100 mg • Zinc 60 mg • Taurine 1000 mg.

Mustard Salve — Dial Herbs
Mustard • Wintergreen • Comfrey • Arnica • Camphor • Cayenne. In a base of Beeswax , Glycerine & Cold Pressed Olive oil.

Mutiglan Plus — Atrium
Each tablet contains: Spleen 256.5 mg • Brain 67.5 mg • Liver 45 mg • Heart 31.5 mg • Kidney 31.5 mg • Thymus 8 mg • Adrenal 8 mg • Pituitary 2 mg • Pancreas 9 mg • Duodenum 9 mg.

My Favorite Multiple Original - Capsules — Natrol
Six capsules contain: Vitamin A (as beta carotene & Vitamin A palmitate) 10000 IU • Vitamin C (as calcium ascorbate) 250 mg • Vitamin D (as cholecalciferol) 400 IU • Vitamin E (as d-alpha tocopheryl succinate) 400 IU • Thiamine (as thiamin HCl) (Vitamin B1) 50 mg • Riboflavin (Vitamin B2) 50 mg • Niacin (as niacin & niacinamide) 50 mg • Vitamin B6 (as pyridoxine HCl) 50 mg • Folic Acid 400 mcg • Vitamin B12 (as cyanocobalamin) 50 mcg • Biotin 300 mcg • Pantothenic Acid (as d-calcium pantothenate) 50 mg • Calcium (as calcium carbonate & calcium citrate) 1 g • Iron (as iron glycinate) 18 mg • Iodine (from kelp) 150 mcg • Magnesium (as magnesium citrate & magnesium oxide) 400 mg • Zinc 25 mg • Selenium 200 mcg • Copper 2 mg • Manganese (as manganese gluconate) 2 mg • Chromium 200 mcg • Molybdenum 50 mcg • Potassium (as potassium chloride) 99 mg • Betaine (as betaine TMG trimethylglycine) 300 mg • MultiEnzyme Blend: Amylase, Papain, Protease, Bromelain, Lipase 110 mg • GP Flavonoid Complex + 100 mg extracted from: Rose Hips fruit, Tumeric root, Acerola berries, Bilberry berries, Hawthorne berries, Grape skin, Milk Thistle seed, & Citrus fruit • PABA (as para amino benzoic acid) 50 mg • Choline (as choline bitartrate) 50 mg • Inositol 50 mg • Hesperidin 25 mg • Rutin 25 mg • Siberian Ginseng 4:1 extract root 1 mg • Boron 200 mcg. Other ingredients: Silicon Dioxide, Magnesium Stearate, Gelatin.

My Favorite Multiple Original - Tablets — Natrol
Four tablets contain: Vitamin A (as d-Salina beta carotene & Vitamin A palmitate) 10000 IU • Vitamin C (as calcium ascorbate) 250 mg • Vitamin D (as cholecalciferol) 400 IU • Vitamin E (as d-alpha tocopheryl succinate) 400 IU • Thiamine (asThiamine HCl) (Vitamin B1) 50 mg • Riboflavin (Vitamin B2) 50 mg • Niacin (as Niacin & Niacinamide) 50 mg • Vitamin B6 (as pyridoxine HCl) 50 mg • Folic Acid 400 mcg • Vitamin B12 (as cyanocobalamin) 50 mcg • Biotin 300 mcg • Pantothenic Acid (as d-calcium pantothenate) 50 mg • Calcium (as calcium carbonate & calcium citrate) 1 g • Iron (as iron glycinate) 18 mg • Iodine (from kelp) 150 mcg • Magnesium (as magnesium citrate & magnesium oxide) 400 mg • Zinc 25 mg • Selenium 200 mcg • Copper 2 mg • Manganese (as manganese gluconate) 2 mg • Chromium 200 mcg • Molybdenum 50 mcg • Potassium (as potassium chloride) 99 mg • Betaine (as betaine TMG

B R A N D **N A M E S**

trimethylglycine) 300 mg • Multi Enzyme Blend consisting of: amylase, papain, protease, bromelain, lipase 110 mg • GP Flavonoid Complex 100 mg extracted from: Rose Hips fruit, Tumeric root, Acerola berries, Bilberry berries, Hawthorne berries, Grape skin, Milk Thistle Seed, & citrus fruit • PABA (as para amino benzoic acid) 50 mg • Choline (as choline bitartrate) 50 mg • Inositol 50 mg • Hesperidin 25 mg • Rutin 25 mg • Siberian Ginseng 4:1 extract root 15 mg • Boron 200 mcg. Other ingredients: Microcrystalline Cellulose, Mono & Di-Glycerides, Silicon Dioxide, Magnesium Stearate, Stearic Acid, Croscarmellose Sodium.

My Favorite Multiple Take One — Natrol
One tablet contains: Vitamin A (as beta carotene) 10000 IU • Vitamin C (as calcium ascorbate)100 mg • Vitamin D (as cholecalciferol) 400 IU • Vitamin E (as d-alpha tocopheryl succinate) 100 IU • Thiamine (as thiamin HCl) (Vitamin B1) 15 mg • Riboflavin (Vitamin B2) 17 mg • Niacin 20 mg • Vitamin B6 (as pyridoxine HCl) 17 mg • Folic Acid 400 mcg • Vitamin B12 (as cyanocobalamin) 50 mcg • Biotin 300 mcg • Pantothenic Acid (as d-calcium pantothenate) 50 mg • Calcium 25 mg • Iron 18 mg • Iodine 150 mcg • Magnesium 10 mg • Zinc 15 mg • Selenium 200 mcg • Copper 2 mg • Manganese 5 mg • Chromium 200 mcg • Molybdenum 50 mcg • Potassium 5 mg • Silica 10 mg • Vanadium 10 mcg • Boron 3 mg • GP Flavonoid Complex + 100 mg, extracted from: Rose Hips fruit, Tumeric root, Acerola berries, Bilberry berries, Hawthorne berries, Grape skin, Milk Thistle Seed & Citrus fruit • UltraGreen Blend concentrate extract 100 mg from: Alfalfa juice leaf, barley grass, spirulina algae, parsley leaf, spinach leaf, peppermint leaf, & spearmint leaf • Lecithin 50 mg • Choline (as choline bitartrate) 50 mg • PABA (as para amino benzoic acid) 25 mg • Inositol 25 mg. Other ingredients: Mono & Di-Glycerides, Silicon Dioxide, Stearic Acid, Croscarmellose Sodium, Magnesium Stearate.

My Favorite Multiple Take One Without Iron - Tablets — Natrol
Each tablet contains: Vitamin A (as beta carotene) 10000 IU • Vitamin C (as calcium ascorbate) 100 mg • Vitamin D (as cholecalciferol) 400 IU • Vitamin E (as d-alpha tocopheryl succinate) 100 IU • Thiamine (as thiamin HCl) (Vitamin B1) 15 mg • Riboflavin (Vitamin B2) 17 mg • Niacin 20 mg • Vitamin B6 (as pyridoxine HCl) 17 mg • Folic Acid 400 mcg • Vitamin B12 (as cyanocobalamin) 50 mcg • Biotin 300 mcg • Pantothenic Acid (as d-calcium pantothenate) 50 mg • Calcium 25 mg • Iodine 150 mcg • Magnesium 10 mg • Zinc 15 mg • Selenium 200 mcg • Copper 2 mg • Manganese 5 mg • Chromium 200 mcg • Molybdenum 50 mcg • Potassium 5 mg • Silica 10 mg • Vanadium 10 mcg • Boron 3 mg • GP Flavonoids 100 mg, extracted from: Rose Hips fruit, Tumeric root, Acerola berries, Bilberry berries, Hawthorne berries, Grape skin, Milk Thistle seed, & Citrus fruit • UltraGreen Blend 100 mg concentrate extract from: Alfalfa juice leaf, Barley grass, Spirulina algae, Parsley leaf, Spinach leaf, Peppermint leaf, & Spearmint leaf • Lecithin 50 mg • Choline (as choline bitartrate) 50 mg • PABA (as para amino benzoic acid) 25 mg • Inositol 25 mg. Other ingredients: Mono & Di-Glycerides, Silicon Dioxide, Stearic Acid, Croscarmellose Sodium, Magnesium Stearate.

My Favorite Multiple Without Iron - Capsules — Natrol
Six capsules contain: Vitamin A (as beta carotene & Vitamin A palmitate) 10000 IU • Vitamin C (as calcium ascorbate) 250 mg • Vitamin D (as cholecalciferol) 400 IU • Vitamin E (as d-alpha tocopheryl succinate) 400 IU • Thiamine (as thiamin HCl) (Vitamin B1) 50 mg • Riboflavin (Vitamin B2) 50 mg • Niacin (as niacin & niacinamide) 50 mg • Vitamin B6 (as pyridoxine HCl) 50 mg • Folic Acid 400 mcg • Vitamin B12 (as cyanocobalamin) 50 mcg • Biotin 300 mcg • Pantothenic Acid (as d-calcium pantothenate) 50 mg • Calcium (as calcium carbonate & calcium citrate) 1 g • Iodine (from kelp) 150 mcg • Magnesium (as magnesium citrate & magnesium, oxide) 400 mg • Zinc 25 mg • Selenium 200 mcg • Copper 2 mg • Manganese (as manganese gluconate) 2 mg • Chromium 200 mcg • Molybdenum 50 mcg • Potassium(as potassium chloride) 99 mg • Betaine (as betaine TMG trimethylglycine) 300 mg • MultiEnzyme Blend 110 mg: amylase, papain, protease, bromelain & lipase • GP Flavonoid Complex + 100 mg extracted from: Rose Hips fruit, Tumeric root, Acerola berries, Bilberry berries, Hawthorne berries, Grape skin, Milk Thistle Seed & Citrus fruit • PABA (as para amino benzoic acid) 50 mg • Choline (as choline bitartrate) 50 mg • Inositol 50 mg • Hesperidin 25 mg • Rutin 25 mg • Siberian Ginseng 4:1 extract root 15 mg • Boron 200 mcg. Other ingredients: Silicon Dioxide, Magnesium Stearate, Gelatin.

My Favorite Multiple Without Iron - Tablets — Natrol
Four tablets contain: Vitamin A (as d-Salina beta carotene & Vitamin A palmitate) 10000 IU • Vitamin C (as calcium ascorbate) 250 mg • Vitamin D (as cholecalciferol) 400 IU • Vitamin E (as d-alpha tocopheryl succinate) 400 IU • Thiamine (as Thiamine HCl) (Vitamin B1) 50 mg • Riboflavin (Vitamin B2) 50 mg • Niacin (as Niacin & Niacinamide) 50 mg • Vitamin B6 (as pyridoxine HCl) 50 mg • Folic Acid 400 mcg • Vitamin B12 (as cyanocobalamin) 50 mcg • Biotin 300 mcg • Pantothenic Acid (as d-calcium pantothenate) 50 mg • Calcium (as calcium carbonate & calcium citrate) 1 g • Iodine (from kelp) 150 mcg • Magnesium (as magnesium citrate & magnesium oxide) 400 mg • Zinc 25 mg • Selenium 200 mcg • Copper 2 mg • Manganese (as manganese gluconate) 2 mg • Chromium 200 mcg • Molybdenum 50 mcg • Potassium (as potassium chloride) 99 mg • Betaine (as betaine TMG trimethylglycine) 300 mg • MultiEnzyme Blend 110 mg consisting of: Amylase, Papain, Protease, Bromelain & Lipase • GP Flavonoid Complex 100 mg extracted from: Rose Hips fruit, Tumeric root, Acerola berries, Bilberry berries, Hawthorne berries, Grape skin, Milk Thistle seed & Citrus fruit • PABA (as para amino benzoic acid) 50 mg • Choline (as choline bitartrate) 50 mg • Inositol 50 mg • Hesperidin 25 mg • Rutin 25 mg • Siberian Ginseng 4:1 extract root 15 mg • Boron 200 mcg. Other ingredients: Microcrystalline Cellulose, Mono & Di-Glycerides, Silicon Dioxide, Magnesium Stearate, Stearic Acid, Croscarmellose Sodium.

Mycelin3 — Allergy Research Group
Each capsule contains: Reishi (ganoderma lucidum) 300 mg • Shiitake (lentinus edodes) 300 mg • Cordyceps Sinensis 150 mg • Ascorbic Acid (vitamin C) 40 mg.

Myelin-MS — Olympia Nutrition
Spingomyelin- pharmaceutical grade.

MygraFew Standardized Feverfew Extract — Nature's Way
Each tablet contains: Dried Feverfew Extract (leaf, standardized Feverfew Extract delivering 600 mcg parthenolide, 5% parthenolide) 12 mg.

MygraFree — Phytopharmica
Each capsule contains: Feverfew extract (standardized to contain 0.6% Parthenolide) 100 mg.

MygrAid Formula — Nature's Way
Each capsule contains: Feverfew leaves 100 mg • Feverfew dried extract 33.3 mg • Lavender flower 50 mg • Linden leaf & flower 70 mg • Magnesium Amino Acid Chelate 33.3 mg. Other ingredients: Gelatin, Magnesium Stearate, Millet.

Myoplex Plus — EAS
Each 76 gram Vanilla Serving contains: Calories 280 • Protein 42 g • Carbohydrates 24 g • Fat 2 g Cholesterol 15 mg • Sodium 330 mg • Potassium 550 mg • Fiber < 1 g. Ingredients: Myopro (A unique blend of Whey Protein Isolate from specially filtered & ion-exchanged Whey Protein, Calcium Caseinate, Milk Protein Isolate, Taurine, L-Glutamine, Sodium Caseinate, Egg Albumin, & Calcium Alpha-Ketoglutarate [AKG]) • Maltodextrin • Corn Syrup Solids • Vitamin & Mineral Blend (Potassium Chloride, Disodium Phosphate, Calcium Phosphate, Magnesium Oxide, Potassium Citrate, Potassium Phosphate, Choline Bitartrate, Beta-Carotene, Ascorbic Acid, Dl-Alpha Tocopheryl Acetate, Ferrous Fumarate, Molybdenum Amino Acid Chelate, Boron Proteinate, Manganese Gluconate, Selenium Amino Acid Chelate, Niacinamide, Zinc Oxide, Calcium Pantothenate, Chromium Citrate, Copper Sulfate, Vitamin A Palmitate, Pyridoxine Hydrochloride, Riboflavin, Thiamine Hydrochloride, Vitamin D3, Folic Acid, Biotin, Potassium Iodide, & Cyanocobalamin) • Natural & Artificial Flavor • Partially Hydrogenated Canola oil • Aspartame • Citrimax (Garcinia cambogia), Salt • Medium-Chain Triglycerides • Xanthan Gum • Soy Lecithin • Cellulose Gum • Mono & Diglycerides • Borage oil. Contains Phenylalanine.

Myoplex Plus Deluxe — EAS
Each 83 gram Vanilla serving contains: Calories 300 • Protein 42 g • Carbohydrates 25 g • Fat 2 g • Cholesterol 5 mg • Sodium 450 mg • Potassium 550 mg • Fiber 1 g • Choline 100 mg • Molybdenum 50 mcg • Boron 1 mcg • Manganese 400 mcg • Selenium 33 mcg • Chromium 100 mcg • Vanadyl Sulfate 10 mg • Conjugated Linoleic Acid 1000 mg • Sodium RNA 9.5 mg. Ingredients: MyoPro (A proprietary protein blend containing Whey Protein Isolate from ion-exchanged Whey, Milk Protein Isolate, Calcium Caseinate, Sodium Caseinate, & Egg Albumin) • Maltodextrin GKG (A proprietary blend containing L-Glutamine, Calcium Alpha-Ketoglutarate [AKG], Taurine, Potassium Chloride, Potassium Phosphate, Magnesium Phosphate, Magnesium Oxide, Sodium RNA, & Manganese

© Copyright 2000, Natural Medicines Comprehensive Database (209) 472-2244. For updated data, go to www.NaturalDatabase.com.

Glycinate) • CLA (Calcium Conjugated Linoleic Acid from Sunflower oil) • Natural & Artificial Flavors • Partially Hydrogenated Canola oil • Xanthan Gum • V2G (A proprietary blend containing Taurine, Vanadyl Sulfate, & Sodium Selenate) • Vitamin & Mineral Blend (Choline Bitartrate, Beta-Carotene, Ascorbic Acid, Dl-Alpha Tocopheryl Acetate, Ferrous Fumarate, Molybdenum Amino Acid Chelate, Boron Proteinate, Niacinamide, Zinc Oxide, Calcium Pantothenate, Chromium Citrate, Copper Sulfate, Vitamin A Palmitate, Pyridoxine Hydrochloride, Riboflavin, Thiamine Hydrochloride, Vitamin D3, Folic Acid, Biotin, Potassium Iodide, & Cyanocobalamin) • Corn Syrup Solids • Salt • Soy Lecithin • Asparatame • Cellulose Gum • Carrageenan • Citrimax (Garcinia cambogia) • Medium-Chain Triglycerides • Mono & Diglycerides • Borage oil. Contains Phenylalanine.

Myoplex Plus Deluxe Bar — EAS
Each 90 gram Chocolate bar contains: Calories 340 • Protein 24 g • Carbohydrates 44 g • Fat 7 g • Cholesterol < 5 mg • Sodium 150 mg • Potassium 350 mg • Fiber 2 g • Sodium RNA 9.5 mg • Vanadyl Sulfate 7.5 mg. Ingredients: MyoPro (A proprietary protein blend containing Whey Protein Isolate from Ion-Exchanged Whey, Calcium Caseinate, & Milk Protein Isolate) • High-Fructose Corn Syrup • Sucrose • Low-Fat Cocoa (processed with Alkali), Partially Hydrogenated Vegetable oil (Cottonseed, Soybean) • Rice Flour • Natural & Artificial Flavors • Nonfat Milk • Milk • Cocoa • Unsweetened Chocolate • GKG (A proprietary blend containing L-Glutamine, Calcium Alpha-Ketoglutarate (AKG), Taurine, Potassium Chloride, Potassium Phosphate, Magnesium Oxide, Magnesium Phosphate, Sodium RNA, & Manganese Glycinate) • V2G (A proprietary blend containing Taurine, Vanadyl Sulfate, Sodium Selenate) • Vitamin & Mineral Blend (Dicalcium Phosphate, Sodium Ascorbate, Ferric Orthophosphate, Dl-Alpha Tocopherol Acetate, Niacinamide, Zinc Oxide, Copper Gluconate, Calcium Pantothenate, Chromium Citrate, Vitamin A Palmitate, Pyridoxine Hydrochloride, Riboflavin, Thiamine Mononitrate, Folic Acid, Chromium Chloride, Sodium Molybdate, Biotin, Potassium Iodide, Phylloquinone, Cholecalciferol, & Cyanocobalamin) • CLA (Calcium Conjugated Linoleic Acid from Sunflower oil) • Lecithin.

Myo-Tone — Enzymatic Therapy
Each tablet contains: Vitamin D (Fish Liver oil) 133 IU • Vitamin E succinate/Wheat Germ) 10 IU • Calcium (Bone Meal) 180 mg • Manganese (Chelate) 63 mg • Vitamin C (Ascorbic Acid/Rose Hips) 60 mg • Potassium Chloride 50 mg • Magnesium (Chelate) 30 mg • Vitamin B6 (Pyridoxine HCL) 6 mg • Thiamine HCL (Vitamin B1) 5 mg • Niacin 5 mg • Riboflavin (Vitamin B2) 5 mg • Vitamin B12 (Cyanocobalamin) 10 mcg • Other ingredients: Choline Bitartrate 50 mg • Muscle extract 50 mg • Inositol 50 mg • Betaine HCL 30 mg • Ammonium Chloride 30 mg, RNA Powder 3 mg. Contains no sugar, salt, yeast, corn, dairy products, coloring, flavoring or preservatives. All organs & glands derived from bovine sources.

Myrrh Salve — Dial Herbs
Myrrh • White Poplar • Balsam Fir • Black Walnut • Cayenne. In a base of Beeswax, Glycerine & Cold Pressed Olive oil.

Myrrh-Goldenseal Plus Formula — Nature's Way
Two capsules contain: Proprietary formula: Cayenne pepper fruit • Goldenseal root • Myrrh Gum (Oleo-Gum Resin from stems). Other ingredients: Gelatin.

Myrrh-Prickly Ash Bark Virtue — Blessed Herbs
Echinacea Angustifolia root • Goldenseal root • Myrrh Gum • Propolis • Prickly Ash bark • Grain alcohol & Distilled Water.

NAC Fuel — TwinLab
Each capsule contains: Highest Quality Pharmaceutical Grade NAC (N-Acetyl-Cysteine) 600 mg.

N-A-C Sustain — Jarrow Formulas
Each tablet contains: N-Acetyl-L-Cysteine 600 mg. Other Ingredients: Cellulose, Calcium Phosphate, Magnesium Stearate, Silicon Dioxide.

Nasal Spray — NutriBiotic
Contains 0.1% Grapefruit extract, combined with Sodium Ascorbate (buffered Vitamin C).

Natrol High Nutrition — Natrol
Each capsule contains: Vitamin C (as Ascorbic Acid) 60 mg • Niacin (as Niacinamide) (Vitamin B3) 2 mg • Vitamin B6 (as Pyridoxine HCl) 2 mg • Thiamine (Vitamin B1) 1.5 mg • In a specially formulated base containing: Winter Berry root 4:1, Country Malva

leaf 5:1, Siberian Ginseng root, Ginger root, Licorice root. Other ingredients: Silicon Dioxide, Magnesium Stearate, Gelatin.

Naturafed — Pacific BioLogic
Angelica root (dahurica) • Peppermint (field mint) • Bupleurum root (natural) • Ligusticum root (cnidium) • Ligusticum root (Chinese) • Astragalus root (Grade 1) • Scute root • Platycodon root • Honeysuckle flower • Schizonepta stem • Gentian root (Chinese) • Ephedra Herba (aerial) • Jasmine fruit (cape) • Magnolia flower • Houtuynia.

Natural Pain Relief Formula — Inholtra
Three gels contain: Glucosamine Sulfate 500 mg • N-Acetyl, D-Glucosamine 500 mg • Chondroitin Sulfates A & B 200 mg • EPA 400 mg • DHA 300 mg • GLA 300 mg • Vitamin E 10 IU • Ascorbyl Palmitate 5 mg • Manganese 1 mg.

Natural Quit — JBS Natural Products
Denicotizing Formula: Alfalfa leaf • Barberry bark • Buckthorn bark • Burdock root • Cascara Sagrada • Chaparral • Dandelion root • Goldenseal root • Hyssop • Kelp • Oregon Grape root • Pau D'Arco • Prickly Ash • Yellow Dock root • Yucca root. Anti-Addiction Formula: Anise seed • Barberry bark • Bee Pollen • Blue Cohosh root • Catnip herb • Cayenne 40M • Chamomile • Echinacea angustifolia herb • Eleutherococcus • Fennel seed • Gentian root • Gotu Kola • Hops flower • Lemongrass • Licorice root • Lobelia herb • Myrrh gum • Passionflower • Peppermint leaf • Safflower • Sarsaparilla • Skullcap herb • Slippery Elm bark • Valerian root • Wood Betony. Aromatherapy Formula: Camphor • Eucalyptus • Denatured Alcohol 40 • Peppermint • Rosemary • Ylang Ylang.

Natural Sterol Complex — Universal Nutrition
Two tablets contain: Mexican Wild Yam root 1000 mg • Smilax officinalis extract 1000 mg • Muira puama 1000 mg • Gotu Kola 515 mg • Boron 3 mg • Gamma Oryxanol 500 mg • Fucosterol 7959 mcg • Beta Sisterol 5663 mcg • Campesterol 3376 mcg • Stigmasterol 1924 mcg • other Sterols 1009 mcg • Bee Pollen 1000 mg • Guarana 500 mg • Korean Ginseng 100 mg • Cytochrome C 100 mg • Dimethylglycine 100 mg • Inosine 100 mg • Royal Jelly 30 mg • Kola Nut 25 mg • Calcium 200 mg • Magnesium 100 mg • Potassium 99 mg • Linoleic Acid 1040 mg • Oleic Acid 698 mg • Palmitic Acid 263 mg • Linoleic Acid 109 mg • Stearic Acid 56 mg • Lignoceric Acid 14 mg • Arachidonic Acid 13 mg • Behenic Acid 6 mg • Myristic Acid 5 mg • Octacosanol 1650 mcg • RNA 60 mg • DNA 30 mg • Capsicum 100 mg • Alfalfa 100 mg • Dandelion root 100 mg • Garlic 100 mg • Yellow Dock 100 mg • Licorice root 100 mg • Hops 100 mg • Milk Thistle 10 mg.

Natural Vitamin E — Biodelivery
Each tablet contains: Vitamin E 200 IU • Pantethine (Coenzyme A Precursor) 25 mg • Selenium 12.5 mg • NT Factor tablet base 47.5 mg.

Naturally Herbal Phen — Optimum Nutrition
St. John's Wort • Bitter Orange.

Naturally Phen — Optimum Nutrition
DL-Phenylalanine L-5-Hydroxytryptophan Tyrosine

Naturally Ripped — Optimum Nutrition
Ma Huang • Guarana • L-Carnitine • Chromium Picolinate.

Naturatussin 1 — Pacific BioLogic
Platycodon root (balloon flower) • Licorice root • Cynanchum root • Red Date (Chinese jujube) • Sophora root • Burdock fruit (great) • Fritillaria bulb (tendrilled) • Peppermint (field mint) • Ephedra Herba (aerial) • Apricot kernal (northern) • Aster root (purple).

Naturatussin 2 — Pacific BioLogic
Houttuynia Herba • Platycodon root (balloon flower) • Hogfennel root (peucedanum) • Aster root (purple) • Honeysuckle flower • Cynanchum root • Trichosanthes fruit peel • Peach kernal • Momordica Fruit (arhat) • Fritillaria bulb (tendrilled) • Burdock fruit (great).

Natura-UR — Pacific BioLogic
Angelica root (dahurica) • Citrus peel (tangerine) • Andrographis • Isatis leaves • Licorice root • Scute root • Platycodon root • Honey Suckle flower • Chrysanthemum flower • Forsynthia fruit • Burdock fruit • Notopterygium root & rhizome.

Nature Cleanse BotaniCleanse — Nature's Plus
Each tablet contains: Botanical Complex containing a proprietary blend of: [Butternut bark (Juglans cinera), Yellow Dock root (Rumex

B R A N D   N A M E S

crispus), Blessed Thistle flower (Cnicus benedictus), Red Clover leaf (Trifolium pratense), Clove bud (Eugenia caryophyllata), Milk Thistle seed (Silybum marianum), Uva Ursi leaf (Arctostaphylos uva-ursi), Cranberry fruit (Vaccinium macrocarpon), Ginger root (Zingiber officinale), Cascara Sagrada bark (Rhamnus purshiana)Hibiscus flower (Hibiscus abelmoschus), Juniper berry (Juniperus oxycedrus), Senna leaf (Cassia senna), Slippery Elm bark (Ulmus rubra), Fennel seed (Foeniculum vulgare), Cayenne fruit (Capsicum frutescens), Dandelion root (Taraxacum officinale), Parsley leaf (Petroselinum crispum), Alfalfa leaf (Medicago sativa), Fenugreek seed (Trigonella foenum-graecum), Aloe Vera & Apple Cider Vinegar • Green Food Complex 100 mg, a proprietary blend of Chlorophyll & trace mineral rich foods: Chlorella broken cell Blue-Green Micro-Algae, Spirulina Algae (Spirulina platensis), Irish Moss (Chondrus crispus), Barley grass juice (Hordeum vulgare), Pacific Kelp (Laminaria)] 500 mg • Vitamin C corn free 100 mg.

Nature Cleanse Fiber Diet — Nature's Plus
Nine capsules contain: Oat Bran (87% Fiber) 1912.5 mg • Psyllium husks (80% Fiber) 1912.5 mg • Apple pectin (84% Fiber) 180 mg • Vitamin C 157.5 mg • Butcher's Broom (15% Fiber) 135 mg • Bentonite U.S.P. grade 90 mg • Cellulose (100% Fiber) 90 mg • Lactobacillus acidophilus 90 million viable cells 22.5 mg. Contains no yeast, wheat, corn, soy, salt, sugar or starch.

Nature Cleanse PuriFiber Internal Cleansing & Revitalizing Powder — Nature's Plus
Each teaspoon (3.75g) contains: Fiber Complex 3500 mg containing a proprietary blend of fiber rich concentrates: Psyllium husks (Plantago ovata), Apple pectin (Malus sylvestris), Butcher's Broom rhizome (Ruscus aceleatus), Bentonite, modified citrus pectin, Cellulose, Rice fiber (Oryza sativa), Slippery Elm bark (Ulmus rubra), Oat bran (Avena sativa), Beet juice & fiber (Beta vulgaris), Prune fiber (Prunus) • Chitosan, vegetarian 50 mg • FOS (Fructooligosaccharides) Lactic flora growth accelerant 50 mg • Lipase fat-digesting enzyme 50 mg • Peptide FM bioactive oligopeptide 25 mg • Lactospor micro-encapsulated pure culture of B. Coagulans, provides 1 million viable cells 1.7 mg.

Nature's Fingerprint — Fingerprint Botanicals
Each capsule contains: Wild Yam root 150 mg • Evening Primrose 90 mg • Chaste Tree berry 50 mg.

Nature's Life Greens - Capsules — Nature's Life
Each 500 mg capsule contains: Green Peas (Pisum sativum) • Celery (Apium graveolens) Cabbage (Brassica oleracea capitata) • Cauliflower (Brassica oleracea botrutis) • Broccoli (Brassica oleracea italica) • Spinach (Spinacia oleracea) • Green Bell Peppers (Capsicum frutescens) • Green Onions (Allium cepa) • Hawaiian grown Spirulina plantesis • Parsley (Petroselinum crispum) • Green Chili Peppers (Capsicum annum) • Green Garlic sprouts (Allium sativum) • Jalepeno Peppers (Capsicum annum) • Green Tea leaves (Camellia sinensis) • Alfalfa (Medicago sativa) • Barley Grass (Hordeum vulgare) • Dunaliella salina • Chlorella • Pacific Alaria (Alaria marginata) • Kelp (Laminaria species) • Pacific Nori (Porphyra tenera) Dulse (Phodymenia palmata) • Kombu (Laminaria setchellii) • Sea Lettuce (Ulva lactuca) • Sea Palm (Pastelsi palmaeformis).

Nature's Life Greens - Powder — Nature's Life
Five grams of powder contain: Green Peas (Pisum sativum) • Celery (Apium graveolens) Cabbage (Brassica oleracea capitata) • Cauliflower (Brassica oleracea botrutis) • Broccoli (Brassica oleracea italica) • Spinach (Spinacia oleracea) • Green Bell Peppers (Capsicum frutescens) • Green Onions (Allium cepa) • Hawaiian grown Spirulina plantesis • Parsley (Petroselinum crispum) • Green Chili Peppers (Capsicum annum) • Green Garlic sprouts (Allium sativum) • Jalepeno Peppers (Capsicum annum) • Green Tea leaves (Camellia sinensis) • Alfalfa (Medicago sativa) • Barley Grass (Hordeum vulgare) • Dunaliella salina • Chlorella • Pacific Alaria (Alaria marginata) • Kelp (Laminaria species) • Pacific Nori (Porphyra tenera) Dulse (Phodymenia palmata) • Kombu (Laminaria setchellii) • Sea Lettuce (Ulva lactuca) • Sea Palm (Pastelsi palmaeformis).

Nature's Way Lycopene — Nature's Way
Each softgel capsule contains: Tomato seed oil standardized to (Lycopene) 5000 mcg • Canola oil • Beeswax • Lecithin • natural Vitamin E (d-Alpha Tocopheryl).

Nature's White Cross — D & E Pharmaceuticals
Each tablet contains: pure Ephedra extract 400 mg.

NeoProstate B-300 — BCN
Each caplet contains: Beta-sitosterol 300 mg • Zinc Citrate 15 mg. Ingredients: Mixed Sterols including Beta-sitosterol (at least 50%), Stig-masterol, Campesterol, Lupeol, Cycloartenon, Famesol, Phytol and Zinc.

Nerve Guard — Flora
St. John's Wort.

Nettle & Pygeum with Pumpkin — Enzymatic Therapy
Each capsule contains: Nettle root extract 16:1 (Urticae dioica radix) 300 mg • Pumpkin seed oil (Cucurbita pepo) 175 mg • Pygeum africanum extract standardized to contain 13% total sterols 25 mg.

Nettle-Reishi Virtue — Blessed Herbs
Nettle • Reishi mycelium • Chinese Ephedra • Yerba Santa leaf • Propolis • Ginkgo leaf • Licorice root • Grain alcohol & Distilled Water.

Neural Support Formula — The Vitamin Factory
Each tablet contains: Vitamin E (d-Alpha Tocopheryl-Succinate) 100 IU • Neuromins (13% DHA powder) 100 mg • Phosphatidylserine Complex 20% 50 mg • Ginkgo Biloba Leaf extract (24/6) 40 mg • Bacopin extract (Bacopa monniera, min. 20% Bacosides) 25 mg • Pycnogenol (Maritime Pine bark extract) 15 mg.

NeuRecover-DA (Depressant Abuse) — Natural Distributors International, Inc.
Six capsules contain: Vitamin A 2000 IU • Vitamin C 600 mg • Vitamin B1 14.5 mg • Vitamin B2 5 mg • Niacin (Niacinamide Ascorbate) 200 mg • Calcium (Chelate) 150 mg • Iron 9 mg • Vitamin E 30 IU • Vitamin B6 18 mg • Folic Acid 0.4 mg • Vitamin B12 0.03 mg • Magnesium 150 mg • Zinc 15 mg • Biotin 0.3 mg • Pantothenic Acid 90 mg • Chromium (Picolinate) 0.06 mg • DL-Phenylalanine 2760 mg • L-Glutamine 150 mg.

NeuRecover-SA (Stimulant Abuse) — Natural Distributors International, Inc.
Six capsules contain: Vitamin C (Ascorbate) 600 mg • Vitamin B1 10 mg • Vitamin B2 15 mg • Niacin (Niacinamide) 100 mg • Calcium (Chelate) 150 mg • Iron 9 mg • Vitamin B6 (Pyridoxal-5-Phosphate) 20 mg • Folic Acid 0.4 mg • Vitamin B12 0.03 mg • Magnesium (Oxide) 150 mg • Zinc (Chelate) 30 mg • Pantothenic Acid 90 mg • Chromium (Picolinate) 0.06 mg • DL-Phenylalanine 1500 mg • L-Tyrosine 900 mg • L-Glutamine 300 mg.

Neuro Care-Rx — Alternecare Health Products
Each capsule contains: Cayenne 125 mg • Ginger 125 mg • St. John's Wort 125 mg • Ginkgo Biloba 40 mg • Malic Acid 100 mg • Vitamin B3 100 mg • Vitamin C 60 mg • Manganese 10 mg • Copper 1 mg • Vitamin B6 50 mg.

Neuro Guardian — Clinician's Choice
Two tablets contain: Vitamin E (as dl-alpha tocopheryl acetate) 200 IU • Thiamin (as mononitrate) 10 mg • Riboflavin 10 mg • Niacin (as niacinamide) 50 mg • Pantothenic Acid (d-calcium pantothenate) 10 mg • Zinc (as amino acid chelate) 10 mg • Selenium (selenomethionine) 50 mcg • Chromium (as nicotinate, chelavite, picolinate) 100 mcg • Ginkgo Biloba Leaf Extract 4:1 150 mg • Lecithin 100 mg • Natural Beta Carotene 40 mg • Acetyl-L-Carnitine 30 mg • RoseOx (patented, standardized process for an extract of Rosemary) 30 mg • Lecithin (standardized to 30% phosphatidyl serine) 30 mg • Aminogen 20 mg • Cayenne Fruit Powder 200 mg • Choline (as choline bitartrate) 20 mg • L-Tyrosine 20 mg • Proprietary blend 8 mg: Astragalus, Carrot Powder, Pacific Kelp, Piper Longum Fruit Powder.

Neuro Optimizer — Jarrow Formulas
Four capsules contain: Cytidine 5'-diphoscholine (CDP Choline) 300 mg • Phosphatidyl Serine (PS) 100 mg • Acetyl L-Carnitine 500 mg • L-Glutamine 500 mg • Alpha Lipoic Acid 50 mg • Taurine 500 mg • Phosphatidylcholine 135 mg. Other Ingredients: Tricalcium Phosphate, Silicon Dioxide.

Neuro-Boost Spray — Nature's Plus
Each spray contains: Phosphatidylserine-rich purified Lecithin concentrate supplying Activated Phosphatides: [Phosphatidylserine (PS) 10 mg, Phosphatidylcholine (PC) 10 mg, Cephalin (Phosphatidylethanolamine) 6 mg, Phosphoinositides 3 mg] 50 mg • DMAE (2-Dimethylaminoethanol Bitartrate) 12.5 mg • N-Acetyl-Tyrosine pharmaceutical grade free form amino acid 5 mg • Pantothenic Acid 5 mg • Korean Ginseng root (Panax ginseng CA Meyer) standardized 15% ginsenosides 5 mg • Chinese Green Tea leaf

BRAND NAMES

© Copyright 2000, Natural Medicines Comprehensive Database (209) 472-2244. For updated data, go to www.NaturalDatabase.com. • 1373

Some Brand Name Natural Products - What they Contain
www.NaturalDatabase.com contains MANY more listings than appear here.

B R A N D   N A M E S

(Camellia sinensis) standardized 50% polyphenols 5 mg • Chinese Green Tea leaf standardized 24% ginkgo flavone glycosides, 6% terpene lactones 1000 mcg. In a proprietary Liposomal Complex of Essential Metabolic Factors , Purified Water, Vegetable Glycerine, Purified Lecithin, Citrus seed extract (Citrus sinensis), Vitamin E & natural Root Beer (Sarsaparilla) flavor.

NeuroGenic — Nature's Plus
Two tablets contain: Phosphatidyl Choline 250 mg • L-Glutamine free form amino acid 200 mg • Vitamin C corn free 150 mg • Pantothenic Acid 100 mg • L-Phenylalanine free form amino acid 100 mg • Ginkgo Biloba standardized 24% Ginkgo flavone-glycosides, 6% terpene lactones 60 mg • Ashwagandha (Withania somnifera) standardized 1.5% withanols 50 mg • Chinese Green Tea (Camellian sinensis) standardized 20% polyphenols 20 mg • Standardized Bilberry (Swedish Vaccinium myrtillus) standardized 25% Anthocyanosides 15 mg • PAK (Pyridoxal Alpha-Ketoglutarate) 10 mg • Co-Enzyme Q10 (Ubiquinone) 5mg. Contains no yeast, wheat, corn, soy, milk, salt, sugar or starch.

Neuro-Max — Metabolic Response Modifiers
Two capsules contain: Phospholipid Complex 500 mg • Ashwaganda extract 100 mg • Ginkgo Biloba extract 40 mg • Pregnenolone 50 mg.

Neuro-Max — New Hope Health Products
Two capsules contain: Phospholipid Complex (containing 100 mg Phosphatidylserine) 500 mg • Ashwagandha Extract 80 mg • Bacopa Monniera Extract 80 mg • Ginkgo Biloba Extract (28/11) 60 mg • Cytidine diphosphate choline 12 mg • Vinpocetine 5 mg • Niacin 10 mg.

Neuro-Max — Olympia Nutrition
Phosphatidylserine 50 mg • Ashwaghanda 50 mg • Ginkgo 20 mg • Pregnenolone 25 mg.

Neutra-Gas — Phytopharmica
Each enteric-coated capsule contains: Active Ingredient: Simethicone 25 mg. Other Ingredients: Peppermint oil extract (Mentha piperita) 0.2 ml. Chlorophyll is used as a natural coloring agent.

New Choice — The Herbalist
Gingko leaf • Gotu Kola herb • Guarana seed • American Ginseng root • Siberian Ginseng root • Jamaican Sarsaparilla root • Kola Nut • Licorice root • Cinnamon bark • Ginger root • Cayenne pepper.

New Life Colostrum — Symbiotics
100% Bovine Colostrum.

New Life Colostrum Capsules — Symbiotics
Two capsules contain: 100% Bovine Colostrum from New Zealand cows 960 mg • Vitamin A 336 IU • Vitamin C 2.8 mg • Iron 1.4 mg • Calcium 10 mg.

New Life Colostrum High-IG — Symbiotics
Two capsules contain: 100% Bovine Colostrum 960 mg • Vitamin A 504 IU • Vitamin C 4.2 mg • Iron 2.1 mg • Calcium 15 mg • Immunoglobulin 288 mg.

New Life Colostrum Powder — Symbiotics
One teaspoon contains: 100% Bovine Colostrum from New Zealand cows 1440 mg • Vitamin A 504 IU • Vitamin C 4.2 mg • Iron 2.1 mg • Calcium 15 mg • Immunoglobulin 246 mg.

New Man Tea — The Herbalist
Damiana leaf • Fo-ti root • Sassafras bark • Licorice root • Cinnamon bark • Saw Palmetto berry • Sarsaparilla bark • Parsley root • Marshmallow root • Orange peel.

New Woman Tonic — The Herbalist
Chaste Tree berry • Black Cohosh root • Black Haw bark • Motherwort herb • Cramp bark • Skullcap herb • Ginger root.

NewPhase — Chattem, Inc.
Each caplet contains: Multi-herbal blend 410 mg: Soy Protein Concentrate, Standardized Kudzu extract root, Standardized Red Clover Extract leaf • Standardized Chastetree Extract berry 75 mg • Standardized Black Cohosh Extract root 40 mg.

NFA-500 — Human Development Technologies
Each capsule contains: L-Tyrosine 500 mg • Acetylcholine 25 mg • DMAE 25 mg • St. John's Wort 60 mg. Additional Ingredients: DLPA, Ginkgo Biloba, Vitamin B12, Vitamin B6, Vitamin B1, Vitamin C, Copper Sulfate, Folic Acid, Phosphorus, Zinc, Bioperine.

N-FLAM Plus — Nutri-Quest
Each enteric coated tablet contains: Pancreatin 170 mg • Papain 100 mg • Bromelain 80 mg • Trypsin 40 mg (Chymotrypsin 8 mg) • Lipase 15 mg • Amylase 17 mg • Rutin 85 mg • Calf Thymus 45 mg • Zinc Gluconate 4 mg • Partoid concentrate 1 mg.

Niacin with Cholestatin — Futurebiotics
Each tablet contains: Niacin 400 mg • Cholestatin 400 mg.

Niacin+ — PhysioLogics
Each capsule contains: Niacin (Inositol Hexanicotinate) 400 mg • Vitamin C (Magnesium Ascorbate) 100 mg • Chromium (Niacinamide/Glycinate) 66 mcg.

Nico-End — Phytopharmica
Each tablet contains: Nux vomica 8x • Lobelia 6x • Staphysagria 6x • Tabacum 6x.
Editor's Comments: This is a homeopathic product. It is so extremely diluted that its activity can not be explained by conventional scientific methods. Therefore this product can not be rated by the scientific criteria used in this Database. A patient receiving the extreme dilution of this product will not receive many, if any, molecules of the original active ingredient. Therefore, there are no harmful pharmacologic effects, and any beneficial effects are controversial and not due to a direct biochemical action of the ingredient on the body. Homeopathic products are allowed for sale in the U.S. due to legislation passed in the 19th century sponsored by a homeopathic physician who was also a Senator. The law still requires that the FDA allow the sale of products listed in this Homeopathic Pharmacopea of the United States.

NightTime Complex with Melotonin — Pharmanex
Each capsule contains: Valerian root extract 75 mg • Passion Flower extract 37.5 mg • Kava Lactones (from Kava Kava root extract) 7.5 mg • Hops Strobile powder (fruit) 25 mg • Chamomile flower powder 25 mg • Melissa officinalis powder (leaf & flower) 25 mg • Mixed Tocopherols 0.5 mg • Melatonin 0.5 mg. Other Ingredients: Maltodextrin, Magnesium, Silicon Dioxide.

Nighty Night — Traditional Medicinals
Passionflower • Spearmint leaf • Chamomile herb • Lemon Verbena leaf • Licorice root • Lilia Star flower • Lemon peel • Lemongrass leaf • Catnip leaf • Hop Strobile.

Nitro Fuel (Ion Exchange Whey Protein Powder) — TwinLab
Each serving contains: Pure Protein 25 g.

Nitro Fuel (The Ultimate Anti-Catabolic Amino Acid Drink) — TwinLab
Protein (Amino Acids) & Carbohydrates • Whey Protein Concentrate [a source of Branched Chain Amino Acids (L-Leucine, L-Isoleucine, L-Valine)] • Chromium Picolinate • Alpha-Ketoglutarates. No preservatives or artificial flavors.

No. 1 GARLIC PLUS ESTER-C & FOS — Dial Herbs
Two capsules contain: Pure-Gar deodorized Garlic concentrate 300 mg • FOS Micro Flora Growth concentrate 300 mg • Vitamin C from Ester-C 200 mg.

No. 56 K KIDNEY — Systemic Formulas
Rose Hips • RNA/DNA Kidney Factors • Gelatin • Magnesium Sulfate • Vitamin C • Ch de Bugre • Fish Liver Oil (Source of Vitamins A and D) • Sete Sangrias • Calcium Carbonate • RNA/DNA Adrenal Factors • Hesperidin • Serine • RNA/DNA Thalamus Factors • Tyrosine • Spearmint Oil • Rose Petal Essence • Aloe Vera.

Nopal (Opuntia S.P.) — Concord
Each capsule contains: Nopal 500 mg.

Nopal Strepta (Prickly Pear Cactus) — Cactu-Life
Each capsule contains: 100% Opuntia Streptacantha 450 mg.

Nor Stack — Substrate Solutions
Each tablet contains: 19-Nor-4-Androstenediol 100 mg • 19-Nor-4-Androstenedione 100 mg.

NorCycloDiol-4 (Sports One Cycloplex Pro-Hormone) — Sports One
Each lozenge contains: Nor-4-Androstenediol Cycloplex (cyclodextrin complex) 10 mg.

NorCycloDione (Sports One Cycloplex Pro-Hormone) — Sports One
Each lozenge contains: 19-Nor-4-Androstenedione Cycloplex (cyclodextrin complex) 25 mg.

Some Brand Name Natural Products - What they Contain

www.NaturalDatabase.com contains MANY more listings than appear here.

Nordisk of Denmark Propolis — Health From The Sun
Each capsule contains: 50% Propolis • 50% Bee Pollen in a natural mineral base of Calcium Phosphate. No sugar added. No preservatives. No artificial coloring or flavoring.

N-R-G Protein Powder — Naturade
Each 1 oz serving contains: Isolated Soy Protein • Calcium Caseinate • Sweet Dairy whey • Carrageenan • Soy Lecithin • Enzymatically Predigested Lactalbumin • Egg albumin • Papian & Natural Vanilla flavor.

Nucleic Acid with RNA and DNA — Quest
Each tablet contains: RNA (Ribonucleic Acid) 200 mg • DNA (Deoxyribonucleic Acid) 60 mg • Brewer's Yeast 190 mg. Other Ingredients: Dibasic Calcium Phosphate, Microcrystalline Cellulose, Vegetable Stearin, Magnesium Stearate (vegetable source), Silicon Dioxide.

NutraFloraFOS — Natrol
One capsule contains: FOS (Fructooligosaccaharides) 500 mg. Other ingredients: Magnesium Stearate, Gelatin.

Nutramine — Calwood Nutritionals
L-Histidine 280 mg • L-Isoleucine 360 mg • L-Leucine 560 mg • L-Lysine 410 mg • L-Methionine 560 mg • L-Phenylalanine 560 mg • L-Threonine 250 mg • L-Tryptophan 130 mg • L-Valine 410 mg.

Nutramine T — Calwood Nutritionals
Two scoops contain: L-Histidine 220 mg • L-Isoleucine 290 mg • L-Leucine 440 mg • L-Lysine 310 mg • L-Methionine 440 mg • L-Phenylalanine 340 mg • L-Threonine 320 mg • L-Tryptophan 120 mg • L-Valine 360 mg • L-Tyrosine 660 mg.

NutraSleep — Source Naturals
Four tablets contain: Niacinamide 10 mg • Vitamin B6 (Pyridoxine HCl) 2 mg • Calcium (citrate and carbonate) 250 mg • Magnesium (citrate, oxide and taurinate) 450 mg • Taurine (Magnesium taurinate) 1000 mg • Inositol 700 mg • GABA (Gamma Amino Butyric Acid) 600 mg • Skullcap 250 mg • Passionflower 200 mg • Valerian root 200 mg • Chamomile extract 100 mg.

Nutri Fiber — Progressive Labs
One tablespoon contains: Calcium 10.2 mg • Iron 0.35% • Thiamin (Vitamin B1) 0.36 mg • Riboflavin (Vitamin B2) 0.18 mg • Niacin 1.89 mg • Vitamin B6 1.66 mg • Pantothenic Acid 044 mg • Phosphorus 11.5 mg • Magnesium 31.8 mg • Zinc 2.42 mg • Copper 0.26 mg • Manganese 0.13 mg • Sodium 0.6% • Potassium 34.2 mg • Linolenic Acid (omega 3) 1.36 g.

Nutri-1000 — The Vitamin Shoppe
Each tablet contains: Vitamin D 400 IU • Vitamin A 25000 IU • Vitamin C 100 mg • Vitamin E 100 IU • Vitamin B1 100 mg • Vitamin B2 100 mg • Vitamin B6 100 mg • Vitamin B12 100 mcg • Niacinamide 100 mg • PABA 100 mg • Pantothenic Acid 100 mg • Choline 100 mg • Inositol 100 mg • Biotin 100 mcg • Folic Acid 400 mcg • Rutin 25 mg • Citrus Bioflavonoid Complex 25 mg • Hesperidin Complex 5 mg • Betaine Hydrochloride 25 mg • Glutamic Acid 25 mg • Iodine 150 mcg • Calcium 50 mg • Potassium 15 mg • Iron 25 mg • Magnesium 20 mg Manganese 6.1 mg • Zinc 20 mg • Chromium 15 mcg • Selenium 10 mcg. In a whole-food base of rice concentrate, parsley, kelp, alfalfa, green cabbage, acerola, sarsaparilla, watercress, and golden seal.

Nutri-All Multiple Powder — Nature's Life
Each scoop (about 15 g) contains: Vitamin A (Beta Carotene) 20000 IU • Vitamin E (d-Alpha Tocopheryl Acetate) 390 IU • Vitamin B1 (Thiamine Mononitrate) 30 mg • Vitamin B2 (Riboflavin) 30 mg • Vitamin B3 (Niacinamide) 110 mg • Vitamin B6 (Pyridoxine HCl) 30 mg • Vitamin B12 (Cobalamin concentrate) 30 mcg • Folic Acid 400 mcg • Biotin 30 mcg • Pantothenic Acid (d-Calcium Pantothenate) 110 mg • Inositol 110 mg • Choline (Citrate) 110 mg • Vitamin C 510 mg • Lemon Bioflavonoids (TESTLAB 50% Flavonoids) 100 mg • Rutin 30 mg • Boron (Proteinate) 25 mcg • Calcium (Carbonate , Ascorbate, Citrate/Malate) 800 mg • Chromium (Polinicotinate, Aspartate) 60 mcg • Copper (Citrate) 1 mg • Iodine (Kelp) 22.5 mg • Iron (Fumerate) 8 mg • Magnesium (Oxide, Citrate) 400 mg • Manganese (Citrate) 4 mg • Molybdenum (Molybdate) 60 mcg • Potassium (Gluconate) 99 mg • Selenium (Selenomethionine) 60 mcg • Silicone (Dioxide) 10 mg • Zinc (Picolinate) 20 mg. In a natural base of Protein powder, Oat Fiber, Rice Syrup solids, Psyllium husks & natural Orange flavor. Contains 10 mg of naturally occurring Sodium.

Nutri-All Multiple Softgel — Nature's Life
Six softgel capsules contain: Beta Carotene (Vitamin A equivalent 10000 IU) 6 mg • Vitamin A (Fish Liver oil) 10000 IU • Vitamin D3 (Cholecalciferol) 400 IU • Vitamin B1 (Thiamine Mononitrate) 80 mg • Vitamin B2 (Riboflavin) 80 mg • Vitamin B3 (Niacinamide) 80 mg • Vitamin B6 (Pyridoxine HCl) 80 mg • Folic Acid 400 mcg • Vitamin B12 (Trituration of concentrate) 100 mcg • Biotin 50 mcg • Pantothenic Acid (d-Calcium Pantothenate) 80 mg • Choline Bitartrate 50 mg • Inositol 50 mg • Vitamin E (d-Alpha Tocopherol) 400 IU • Vitamin C (Ascorbic Acid & Rose Hips) 500 mg • Lemon Bioflavonoids (50% TESTLAB) 50 mg • Rutin Complex (Dimorphandra mollis) 25 mg • Hesperidin Complex (Citrus) 25 mg • Calcium (Carbonate) 1000 mg • Chromium (Picolinate, Nutrition 21) 200 mcg • Copper (Gluconate) 1 mg • Iodine (Potassium Iodide) 225 mcg • Magnesium (Oxide) 600 mg • Manganese (Citrate) 10 mg • Molybdenum (Molybdate) 20 mcg • Potassium (Citrate) 50 mg • Selenium (l-Selenomethionine) 50 mcg • Vanadium (Vanadyl Sulfate) 20 mcg • Zinc (Citrate) 15 mg • Betaine HCl 25 mg • CoEnzyme Q10 5 mg • Chlorophyll (oil-soluble) 100 mg. In a natural base of Safflower oil, Lecithin & Soy.

NutriBiotic Capsules Plus — NutriBiotic
100 mg of Grapefruit extract • Echinacea extract • Artemisa annua extract.

NutriBiotic Tablets — NutriBiotic
Grapefruit extract 100 mg.

NutriFi — Pharmanex
Each teaspoon contains: Oat Fiber • Maltodextrin • Dextrose (Glucose) • Cellulose • Citrus Pectin • Psyllium Fiber • Gum Arabic.

Nutrilite Antioxidant Complex with Pycnogenol — Nutrilite
Each capsule contains: Pycnogenol 60 mg • Grape Seed extract 30 mg • Green Tea extract (Decaffeinated) 300 mg • Alpha-Lipoic Acid 45 mg • Glutathione 60 mg • Turmeric extract 75 mg.

Nutrilite Bilberry with Lutein — Nutrilite
Each softgel contains: Bilberry extract • Lutein • Zeaxanathin • DHA.

Nutrilite Black Cohosh and Soy — Nutrilite
Each tablet contains: Black Cohosh extract 120 mg • Soy Protein 300 mg • Isoflavones 49.8 mg • Acerola Cherry Concentrate 30 mg • Calcium 60 mg.

Nutrilite Calcium Magnesium Plus — Nutrilite
Each tablet contains: Calcium 651 mg • Magnesium 324 mg • Zinc 10 mg • Copper 2 mg • Manganese 2.5 mg • Nutrilite Alfalfa Concentrate with Phytofactors Plant Compounds.

Nutrilite ChromPic Extra — Nutrilite
Each capsule contains: Chromium 300 mcg (providing Chromium picolinate 2400 mcg) • Vanadium 220 mcg • Gymnema sylvestre 100 mcg.

Nutrilite CoEnzyme Q10 Complex — Nutrilite
Each capsule contains: CoEnzyme Q10 30 mg • L-Carnitine 100 mg • Taurine 125 mg • Bioflavonoids 25 mg.

Nutrilite Digestive Enzyme Complex — Nutrilite
Each capsule contains: Lipase 31 mg • Lactase 40 mg • Amylase 20 mg • Alpha-galactosidase 10 mg • Ginger root extract 150 mg • Nutrilite Parsley Concentrate with Phytofactors Plant Compounds 50 mg.

Nutrilite Echinacea with Astragalus — Nutrilite
Each tablet contains: Echinacea extract 200.1 mg • Astragalus extract 50.1 mg • Chlorella powder 50.1 mg.

Nutrilite Garlic & Licorice — Nutrilite
Each tablet contains: Pure concentrated Garlic 1000 mg • Licorice extract 21 mg.

Nutrilite Ginkgo Biloba and DHA — Nutrilite
Each softgel contains: Standardized Ginkgo Biloba extract 160 mg • DHA 180 mg • Gotu Kola 68 mg.

Nutrilite Glucosamine HCL with Boswellia — Nutrilite
Four tablets contain: Glucosamine HCL 1500 mg • Boswellia 75.2 mg • Bromelain 160 mg • Nutrilite Acerola concentrate • Lemon Bioflavonoid concentrate with specific Phytofactors plant compounds.

Nutrilite LeadingEdge Heart Pack — Nutrilite
Each Packet Contains: CoEnzyme Q10 • Garlic • Licorice • Omega 3 Complex • Natural B Complex.

BRAND NAMES

© Copyright 2000, Natural Medicines Comprehensive Database (209) 472-2244. For updated data, go to www.NaturalDatabase.com. • 1375

Some Brand Name Natural Products - What they Contain
www.NaturalDatabase.com contains MANY more listings than appear here.

Nutrilite Milk Thistle and Dandelion — Nutrilite
Each tablet contains: Milk Thistle extract (Silybin Extract 228 mg) 468 mg • Dandelion root extract 375 mg • Turmeric extract 225 mg • Lemon Bioflavonoids • Acerola Cherry Concentrate.

Nutrilite Passionflower with Chamomile — Nutrilite
Each tablet contains: Passionflower 129.9 mg • Chamomile 81.3 mg • Hops 18.75 mg.

Nutrilite Saw Palmetto with Nettle Root — Nutrilite
Each softgel contains: Saw Palmetto 318 mg • Pumpkin Seed Oil 480 mg • Nettle Root 240 mg.

Nutrilite Siberian Ginseng with Ginkgo Biloba — Nutrilite
Each capsule contains: Siberian Ginseng extract 200 mg • Ginkgo Biloba extract 133.6 mg • Nutrilite Acerola Cherry and Citrus Bioflavonoid Concentrates.

Nutrilite St. John's Wort with Lemon Balm — Nutrilite
Each capsule contains: St. John's Wort (0.3% Hypericin) 900 mg • Lemon Balm 78 mg • Lemon Bioflavonoid Concentrate 72 mg • Vitamin C (from Acerola Cherry Concentrate) 10 mg.

Nutrilite Women's GLA Blend with Evening Primrose Oil — Nutrilite
Each softgel contains: Evening Primrose • Borage Oil • Black Currant Oil • Chasteberry • Dong Quai • Ginger Extract.

Nutrition Warehouse Boron Complex Plus — Nutrition Warehouse
Four capsules contain: Boron 3 mg • MCHA (microcrystalline hydroxyapatite) 2000 mg • Calcium (from MCHA) 520 mg • Phosphorous (from MCHA) 260 mg • Magnesium carbonate elemental 160 mg • Magnesium aspartate elemental 40 mg • Vitamin D3 260 IU • Vitamin K 120 mcg • Manganese 10 mg • Silica 100 mg. Other Ingredients: Magnesium, Potassium, Zinc, Selenium, Mangese, Iron, Collagen, Glycosaminoglycans, substituent Amino Acids.

Nutri-Vit — Progressive Labs
One tablespoon (15 ml) contains: Vitamin A 3750 IU • Vitamin C 60 mg • Vitamin D 600 IU • Vitamin E 15 IU • Thiamin (B1) 1.05 mg • Riboflavin (B2) 1.2 mg • Niacin 13.5 mg • Vitamin B6 1.05 mg • Folate (folic acid) 300 mcg • Vitamin B12 4.5 mcg • Biotin 225 mcg • Pantothenic Acid 7.5 mg • Iron 15 mg • Zinc 12 mg.

NxTrim — Nova Pharmaceutical, Inc.
Two tablets contain: Vitamin C (ascorbic acid) 200 mg • Niacin 10 mg • Vitamin B6 (as pyridoxine hydrochloride) 4 mg • Vitamin B12 (as cyanocobalamin) 166 mcg • Calcium (as dibasic calcium phosphate) 55 mg • Chromium (as chromium polynicotinate) 100 mcg • Phenylalanine (as L-phenylalanine hydrochloride) 300 mg • Glutamine (as L-glutamine hydrochloride) 50 mg • Tyrosine (as L-tyrosine hydrochloride)100 mg • St. John's Wort extract 50 mg • L-Carnitine 20 mg • Korean Ginseng powdered root 70 mg • Uva Ursi powdered leaves 50 mg. Other ingredients: Whey, Stearic Acid, Magnesium Stearate, Pharmaceutical Glaze.

O.U.T. (Ovarian Uterine Tonic) — The Herbalist
Chapparal leaf • Pipsissewa leaf • False Unicorn root • Prickly Ash bark • Cramp bark • Licorice root • Saw Palmetto berry • Red Clover blossom.

Oats-Scullcap Virtue — Blessed Herbs
Oats in milk stage • Scullcap • St. John's Wort flower • Lemon Balm • Lavender flower • Rosemary & Blackberry brandy.

OcuActin — Nature's Plus
Two capsules contain: Vitamin C corn free 100 mg • Citrus Bioflavonoid Complex 100 mg • Vitamin E natural 50 IU • Zinc (Monomethionine) 30 mg • Bilberry [(Vaccinium myrtillus fruit) standardized 25% Anthocyanosides] 25 mg • Goldenseal [(Hydrastis canadensis root & rhizome) standardized 10% Alkaloids, 5% Hydrastine] 25 mg • Echinacea [(Echinacea angustifolia root & rhizome) standardized 4% Echinacosides] 25 mg • Chinese Green Tea [(Camellia sinensis leaf) decaffeinated, standardized 50% Polyphenols] 25 mg • Grape Seed [(Vitis vinifera) standardized 95% Proanthocyanidins] 10 mg Glutathione (pharmaceutical grade Free Form Amino Acid) 10 mg • Beta Carotene (supplying 15000 IU of Vitamin A activity) 9 mg • Lutein (active Carotenoid from Marigold flower extract) 6 mg • Coenzyme Q10 (Ubiquinone) 5 mg • Copper (Glycinate) 2 mg • Zeaxanthin (active Carotenoid from Marigold flower extract) 263 mcg • Vitamin A (Retinol) 5000 IU • Selenium (Selenomethionine) 50 mcg.

Ocu-Care — Nature's Plus
Two tablets contain: Strengthening Nutrients: Bilberry standardized 25% Anthocyanosides 30 mg • Citrus Bioflavonoid Complex supplying: (Active Flavonones with Hesperidin & Eriocitrin 24%, Active Flavonols & Flavones, Pectin, Cellulose & Narigen 20%) 250 mg • Rutin (Saphora japonica) 100 mg. Protectant Nutrients: Pantothenic Acid 100 mg • L-Lysine free form amino acid 50 mg. Antioxidant Nutrients: Beta Carotene pro-Vitamin A, supplying 20000 IU Vitamin A activity • Vitamin A Fish Liver oil 5000 IU • Vitamin E natural 200 IU • NAC (N-Acetyl-Cysteine) 50 mg • Zinc (Monomethionine) 20 mg.

Ocular Defense — PhysioLogics
Two capsules contain: Vitamin A (Beta-Carotene) 10000 IU • Vitamin A (Palmitate) 2500 IU • Vitamin E (d-Alpha Tocopherol) 100 IU • Vitamin B2 (Riboflavin) 10 mg • Vitamin B6 (Pyridoxine HCl) 10 mg • Zinc (Glycinate) 15 mg • Copper (Glycinate) 2 mg • Chromium (Niacin/Glycine Chelate) 100 mcg • Selenium (Selenomethionine) 50 mcg • Taurine 200 mg • Bilberry fruit (36% Anthocyanosides, 36 mg) 100 mg • N-Acetylcysteine 100 mg • Quercetin (98% Bioflavonoids, 49 mg) 50 mg • Glutathione 25 mg.

Ocu-Plus — Aspen Group, Inc.
Two tablets contain: Beta-Carotene 25,000 IU • Vitamin E (d-alpha tocopherol) 400 IU • Vitamin C 1000 mg • Citrus bioflavonoid complex 250 mg • Quercetin 100 mg • Bilberry extract (25% anthocyanosides) 80 mg • Rutin 100 mg • Zinc (gluconate) 50 mg • Copper (gluconate) 2 mg • Selenium (selenomethionine) 50 mcg • N-Acetyl L-Cysteine (glutathione precursor) 200 mg • L-Glutathione 10 mg • Eyebright 50 mg • Alpha-Lipoic Acid 50 mg • Chromium Picolinate 200 mcg • Lutein (containing zeaxanthin) 6 mg • Ginkgo Biloba 25 mg.

Ocuvite — Bausch & Lomb
Each tablet contains: Vitamin A (100% as beta carotene) 5000 IU • Vitamin C (ascorbic acid) 60 mg • Vitamin E (dl-alpha tocopherol acetate) 30 IU • Zinc (from zinc oxide) 40 mg • Selenium (from sodium selenate) 40 mcg • Copper (from cupric oxide) 2 mg. Inactive Ingredients: Dibasic Calcium Phosphate, Microcrystalline Cellulose, Calcium Carbonate, Crospovidone, Hydroxypropyl Methylcellulose, Titanium Dioxide, Silica gel, Magnesium Stearate, Stearic Acid, FD&C Yellow No. 6, Triethyl Citrate, Polysorbate 80 & Sodium Lauryl Sulfate.

Ocuvite Extra — Bausch & Lomb
Each tablet contains: Vitamin A (100% as beta carotene) 6000 IU • Vitamin C (ascorbic acid) 200 mg • Vitamin E (dl-alpha tocopherol acetate) 50 IU • Riboflavin (Vitamin B2) 3 mg • Niacinamide (Vitamin B3) 40 mg • Zinc (from zinc oxide) 40 mg • Selenium (from sodium selenate) 40 mcg • Copper (from cupric oxide) 2 mg • Manganese 5 mg • L-Glutathione 5 mg. Inactive Ingredients: Dibasic Calcium Phosphate, Microcrystalline Cellulose, Calcium Carbonate, Crospovidone, Hydroxypropyl Methylcellulose, Titanium Dioxide, Silica Gel, Magnesium Stearate, Stearic Acid, FD&C Yellow No. 6, Triethyl Citrate, Polysorbate 80, & Sodium Lauryl Sulfate.

OKG Fuel Capsules OKG (L-Ornithine Alphaketoglutarate) — TwinLab
Each capsule contians: OKG 650 mg.

OKG Fuel Powder — TwinLab
Each teaspoonful contains: OKG 3.5 grams (3500 mg).

Olimmune — PhysioLogics
Three capsules contain: Licorice DGL (1% Glycyrrhizin, 7.6 mg) 760 mg • Astragalus (70% Polysaccharides, 140 mg) 200 mg • Ligusticum 200 mg • N-Acetyl-Cysteine (NAC) 135 mg • Olive leaf extract (17% Oleuropein, 17 mg) 100 mg.

Omega 3 Fatty Acids — Trader Joe's
EPA (eicosapentaenoic acid) 300 mg • DHA (docosahexaenoic acid) 200 mg • Calories 10. Contains no vitamin A, D, or cholesterol.

Omega 3-6-9 — The Vitamin Shoppe
Two softgels contain the Omega 3-6-9 essential fatty acids from 100% pure cold-pressed vegetable seed oils of: Borage 500 mg • Flaxseed 150 mg • Safflower 50 mg • Canola 200 mg • Olive 100 mg. Plus 150 mg of Omega-3 components (EPA-DHA) naturally present in Salmon Oil, providing the following: A/Gamma Linolenic Acid (Omega-3) 220 mg • Linoleic Acid (Omega-6) 290 mg • Oleic Acid (Omega-9) 306 mg.

1376 • © Copyright 2000, Natural Medicines Comprehensive Database (209) 472-2244. For updated data, go to www.NaturalDatabase.com.

Omega III Essential Fatty Acids — Nature's Life
Three capsules contain: Eicosapentaneoic Acid (EPA) (Fish Body oils) 540 mg • Docosahexaenoic Acid (DHA) (Fish Body oils) 360 mg • Garlic extract (1000:1)(Allium sativum) 150 mg • Vitamin C (Ascorbate Palmitate) 10 mg • Vitamin E (d-Alpha Tocopherol) 30 IU. In a natural base of certified organic Safflower oil.

Omega-3 — Natrol
Two softgels contain: Fish Oil concentrate 2 g • EPA (Eiicosapentaneoic Acid)(18%) 360 mg • DHA (Docosahexaenoic Acid) (12%) 240 mg • Total Omega-3; Fatty Acids (36%) 720 mg. Other Ingredients: Gelatin, Mixed Natural Tocopherols.

One Daily — The Vitamin Shoppe
Each tablet contains: Vitamin A 10000 IU • Vitamin D3 400 IU • Vitamin C 100 mg • Citrus Bioflavonoids 25 mg • Rutin 5 mg • Hesperidin Complex 5 mg • Vitamin E 150 IU • Vitamin B1 25 mg • Vitamin B2 25 mg • Vitamin B6 25 mg • Vitamin B12 100 mcg • Calcium Pangamate 25 mg • Pantothenic Acid 25 mg • Biotin 50 mcg • Folic Acid 400 mcg • Niacinamide 25 mg • Inositol 25 mg • Choline 25 mg • PABA 25 mg • Calcium 100 mg • Magnesium 50 mg • Potassium 25 mg • Manganese 5 mg • Zinc 15 mg • Iron 18 mg • Selenium 50 mcg • GTF Chromium 50 mcg • Iodine 150 mcg • Copper 2 mg • Molybdenum 100 mcg • Vitamin K 25 mcg • SOD 25 mcg • Octacosanol 100 mcg • L-Carnitine 5 mg • CoQ10 10 mcg • GLA 5 mg • Korean Ginseng 10 mg • Bee Pollen 10 mg • Royal Jelly 5 mg • Betaine HCl 10 mg • Pepsin 10 mg • Bromelain 10 mg • Papain 10 mg • Lecithin 25 mg • L-Glutathione 5 mg • L-Cysteine 5 mg • L-Methionine 5 mg • EPA & DHA 50 mg.

One Daily Multiple — Nature's Life
Each capsule contains: Beta Carotene (Vitamin A equivalent to 10000 IU) 6 mg • Vitamin D3 (Cholecalciferol) 200 IU • Vitamin E (d-Alpha Tocopheryl Succinate) 100 IU • Vitamin B1 (Thiamine Mononitrate) 25 mg • Vitamin B2 (Riboflavin & Riboflavin 5'-Phosphate) 25 mg • Vitamin B6 Pyridoxine HCI & Pyridoxine 5'-Phosphate) 25 mg • Niacinamide 50 mg • Vitamin B12 (Cyancobalamin) 100 mcg • Folic Acid 400 mcg • Pantothenic Acid (d-Calcium Pantothenate) 50 mg • Biotin (d-Biotin) 300 mcg • Choline (Bitartrate) 25 mg • Inositol 25 mg • PABA (Para Aminobenzoic Acid) 25 mg • Vitamin C 100 mg • Boron (Citrate) 50 mcg • Calcium (Carbonate, Citrate/ Malate) 50 mg • Chromium (Picolinate) 100 mcg • Copper (Gluconate, Citrate) 1 mg • Magnesium (Oxide , Citrate) 10 mg • Manganese (Gluconate) 5 mg • Molybdenum (Sodium Molybdate) 150 mcg • Potassium (Chloride) 5 mg • Selenium (Selenomethionine) 100 mcg • Silicon (Dioxide) 10 mg • Vanadium(Vandyl Sulfate) 25 mcg • Zinc (Picolinate) 15 mg.

One Daily without Iron — The Vitamin Shoppe
Each tablet contains: Vitamin A 10000 IU • Vitamin D3 400 IU • Vitamin C 100 mg • Citrus Bioflavonoids 25 mg • Rutin 5 mg • Hesperidin Complex 5 mg • Vitamin E 150 IU • Vitamin B1 25 mg • Vitamin B2 25 mg • Vitamin B6 25 mg • Vitamin B12 100 mcg • Calcium Pangamate 25 mg • Pantothenic Acid 25 mg • Biotin 50 mcg • Folic Acid 400 mcg • Niacinamide 25 mg • Inositol 25 mg • Choline 25 mg • PABA 25 mg • Calcium 100 mg • Magnesium 50 mg • Potassium 25 mg • Manganese 5 mg • Zinc 15 mg • Selenium 50 mcg • GTF Chromium 50 mcg • Iodine 150 mcg • Copper 2 mg • Molybdenum 100 mcg • Vitamin D 25 mcg • SOD 500 mcg • Octacosanol 100 mcg • L-Carnitine 5 mg • CoQ10 10 mcg • GLA 5 mg • Korean Ginseng 10 mg • Bee Pollen 10 mg • Royal Jelly 5 mg • Betaine HCl 10 mg • Pepsin 10 mg • Bromelain 10 mg • Papain 10 mg • Lecithin 25 mg • L-Glutathione 5 mg • L-Cysteine 5 mg • L-Methionine 5 mg • EPA & DHA 50 mg.

One Step — Progressive Labs
One level scoop (approx. 31 g.) contains: Calories 120 • Calories from fat 27 • Total Fat 3 g • Saturated Fat 0.625 g • Cholesterol 0 g • Sodium 28 mg • Potassium 419 mg • Total Carbohydrate 12 g • Dietary Fiber 6 g • Sugars 1 g • Protein 11 g • Vitamin A 5000 IU • Vitamin C 177 mg • Vitamin D 200 IU • Vitamin E 70 IU • Vitamin K 40 mcg • Thiamin (B1) 3 mg • Riboflavin (B2) 3 mg • Niacinamide (B3) 13 mg • Vitamin B6 30 mg • Folate (folic acid) 446 mcg • Vitamin B12 250 mcg • Biotin 150 mcg • Pantothenic Acid 23 mg • Calcium 326 mg • Iron 3 mg • Phosphorus 266 mg • Iodine 38 mcg • Magnesium 255 mg • Zinc (as ascorbate) 8 mg • Selenium 40 mcg • Copper (as amino acid chelate) 2 mg • Manganese (as ascorbate) 6 mg • Chromium (as nicotinate) 100 mcg • Molybdenum 13 mcg • Chloride 175 mg. Amino acids from Soy Protein & Rice Bran: Aspartic Acid 1583 mg, Threonine 551 mg, Serine 696 mg, Glutamic Acid 2491 mg, Proline 755 mg, Glycine 630 mg, Alanine 637 mg, Cysteine 378 mg, Valine 740 mg, Methionine 202 mg, Isoleucine 691 mg, Leucine 1109 mg, Tyrosine 499 mg, Phenylalanine 723 mg, Histidine 371 mg, Lysine 888 mg, Arginine 1028 mg, Tryptophan 173 mg. Ingredients: Arcon VF Hypoallergenic, Predigested Soy Protein concentrate, Rice bran, Lecithin, Colloidal Magnesium, Glucosamine HCl, Nopal (detoxifier and sugar regulator), Colloidal Calcium, MSM (methyl sulfonyl methane), Beta 1,3 Glucans, Inulin, Gamma Oryzanol, L-Glutamine, L-Ornithine, L-Taurine, Vitamin E Succinate, CitriMax, Globulin Protein, Ester C, Ascorbic Acid, Trimethylglycine, Citrus Bioflavonoid 5X complex, Aloe Isolate, Zinc Ascorbate, Pantothenic Acid, Pyridoxine HCl, Inositol, Creatine Pyruvate, Siberian Ginseng extract, Betatene(lycopene and mixed carotenoids), Alpha Lipoic Acid, Manganese Ascorbate, Borage Oil, NovaSoy (soy isoflavones), Gugulipid Extract, Leci-PS (phosphatidyl serine), Beta Carotene, Niacinamide, L-Glutathione, Querceitin, Copper Amino Acid Chelate, Seleno-L-Methionine, Atlantic Sea Kelp, Lutein, Pyridoxal-5'-Phosphate, Ginkgo Biloba leaf extract, Grape seed extract, Grape skin extract, Bioperine (black pepper extract), Mixed Tocotrienols, Coenzyme Q10, Pycnogenol, Boron, Natural Vanilla and other Natural Flavors, Stevia.

One-A-Day Bedtime & Rest — Bayer
Two tablets contain: Calcium 450 mg • Magnesium 80 mg • Lecithin 20 mg • Kava Kava Standardized extract (Piper methysticum) root 100 mg • Valerian Standardized extract (Valeriana officinalis) root 200 mg • Rosemary Standardized extract (Rosmannus officinalis) leaf 10 mg.

One-A-Day Bone Strength — Bayer
Each tablet contains: Vitamin D 100 IU • Calcium (precipitated) 500 mg • Soy Standardized extract (Glycine max or spp.) bean 28 mg.

One-A-Day Cholesterol Health — Bayer
Two tablets contain: Vitamin E 200 IU • Lecithin 100 mg • Garlic (Allium sativum) freeze dried/bulb 30 mg • Soy Standardized extract (Glycine max or spp.) bean 140 mg.

One-A-Day Cold Season — Bayer
Each tablet contains: Vitamin C 500 mg • Zinc 7.5 mg • Echinacea Standardized extract (Echinacea purpurea) whole plant/root 50 mg.

One-A-Day Energy Formula — Bayer
Each tablet contains: Thiamin (B1) 2.25 mg • Niacin 20 mg • Vitamin B6 3 mg • Folic Acid 200 mcg • Pantothenic Acid 10 mg • Chromium (as Picolinate) 100 mcg • Ginseng Standardized extract (Panex ginseng) root 200 mg.

One-A-Day Joint Health — Bayer
Each tablet contains: Vitamin C 30 mg • Vitamin E 30 IU • Manganese 1.5 mg • Lecithin 10 mg • Glucosamine Sulfate powder (includes Dipotassium CI 125 mg) 500 mg • Devil's Claw Standardized extract (Harpagophytum procumbens) root 134 mg.

One-A-Day Memory & Concentration — Bayer
Each tablet contains: Vitamin B6 1 mg • Vitamin B12 3 mcg • Choline 60 mg • Ginkgo Standardized extract (Ginkgo biloba) leaf 60 mg.

One-A-Day Menopause Health — Bayer
Each tablet contains: Vitamin E 15 IU • Calcium (precipitated) 250 mg • Lecithin 15 mg • Black Cohosh Standardized extract (Cimicifuga racemosa) root 10 mg • Soy Standardized extract (Glycine max or spp.) bean 42 mg.

One-A-Day Prostate Health — Bayer
Two softgels contain: Zinc 15 mg • Pumpkin Seed Oil Standardized extract 80 mg • Saw Palmetto Standardized extract (Serenoa repens) berry 320 mg.

One-A-Day Tension & Mood — Bayer
Each tablet contains: Vitamin C 60 mg • Thiamin (B1) 1.125 mg • Niacin 10 mg • Folic Acid 100 mcg • Pantothenic Acid 5 mg • Lecithin 15 mg • Kava Kava Standardized extract (Piper methysticum) rhizome/root 100 mg • St. John's Wort Standardized extract (Hypericum perforatum) leaves/flowers 225 mg.

Ophthaplus — Atrium
Each tablet contains: Raw Eye concentrate 120 mg • Raw Brain concentrate 20 mg • Eyebright 150 mg • Rutin 125 mg • Hesperidin Complex 20 mg.

Opti Fuel (The Ultimate Metabolic Optimizer) — TwinLab
Each serving contains: Pharmaceutical Grade Pep-Tide Bonded & Free Amino Acids [derived from the natural Pancreatic digests of Whey Protein (Lactalbumin) & Egg White Protein (Albumin)] 15 g • Branched Chain Amino Acids (L-Leucine, L-Isoleucine & L-Valine) •

B R A N D   N A M E S

Some Brand Name Natural Products - What they Contain

www.NaturalDatabase.com contains MANY more listings than appear here.

**B
R
A
N
D

N
A
M
E
S**

Carbohydrates & Medium Chain Triglycerides (MCTs) • High Potency Metabolic Activator Vitamins & Minerals • Electro-Lytes • Antioxidants • Stress B Complex • Lipotropic Factors • Methyl Donors • TMG-Trimethylglycine • Siberian Ginseng • Octacosanol • Gamma-Oryzanol & Synergistic Metabolic Optimizers (such as Inosine) • L-Carnitine • CoQ10 • Lipoic Acid • Pantetheine • Pyridoxine-Alpha-Ketoglutarate • Soluble Potassium Phosphate & Mineral Succinates • Aspartates • Citrates • Fumarates • Malates • Alpha-Ketoglutarates.

Opti Fuel 2 — TwinLab
Each serving contains: Carbohydrates (derived primarily from Glucose Polymers & Glucose with small amounts of 100% Pure Crystalline Fructose) 100 g • Predigested Whey Protein • Extra Branched Chain Amino Acids (L-Leucine, L-Isoleucine, L-Valine) • Vitamin C • Vitamin E • Beta-Carotene • Other Important Antioxidant Nutrients (such as Selenium, Coenzyme Q10 & Alpha Lipoic Acid, High Potency B Complex Vitamins, Calcium, Magnesium, Potassium, Zinc & Chromium Picolinate) • Carni Fuel, (L-Carnitine Magnesium Citrate). All predigested for easier digestion & assimilation.

Opti-Lean — Optimum Nutrition
Citrimax(tm) 500 mg • High Quality Protien 20 g • Carbohydrates 20 g.

OptimEyes — Body Wise International, Inc.
Three tablets contain: Beta Carotene (Dunaliella salina algae) 9 mg • Equivalent to Vitamin A 15000 IU • Vitamin C (as Ascorbic Acid) • Vitamin E (as D-Alpha Tocopheryl Succinate and Mixed Tocopherols-Alpha, Beta, Gamma and Delta) 100 IU • Zinc (Krebs Cycle Chelate) 20 mg • Selenium (as L-Selenomethionine) 250 mcg • Copper (Krebs Cycle Chelate) 2 mg • Taurine 500 mg • A-Acetyl-L-Cysteine 200 mg• Bilberry fruit extract 100:1 (25% Anthocyanidins) 80 mg • Gingko Biloba leaf extract 50:1 (24% Flavonglycosides) 60 mg • Alpha Lipoic Acid 25 mg • Lutein 6 mg.

Optimum Nutrition — Optimum Nutrition
Hawthorn Berry • Garlic Extract.

Optimum Omega — Pharmanex
Each capsule contains: Vitamin E (as d-Alpha Tocopheryl Acetate) 5 IU • Marine Lipid Concentrate 1000 mg (Omega 3 Fatty Acids: EPA 180 mg, DHA 120 mg, Other Omega 3 Fatty Acids 50 mg) • Deodorized Garlic Oil 1 mg. Other Ingredients: Gelatin, Glycerin, Purified Water.

Optimune — Biomune Systems
Patented Whey Protein concentrate.

Optimune — Rx Vitamins
Pharmaceutical Grade Arabinogalactan 250 mg • Phosphoric Nucleotides 4000 mcg.

OptiVision — PhysioLogics
Two capsules contain: Vitamin A (Beta-Carotene) 10000 IU • Vitamin A (Palmitate) 2500 IU • Taurine 200 mg • Bilberry (GPH: 36% anthocyanosides) 100 mg • Vitamin E (D-Alpha Tocopherol) 100 IU • N-Acetylcysteine 100 mg • Quercetin (GPH: 98% Bioflavonoids) 50 mg • Glutathione 25 mg • Vitamin B2 (Riboflavin) 10 mg • Vitamin B6 (Pyridoxine HCl) 10 mg • Zinc (Glycinate) 15 mg • Copper (Glycinate) 2 mg • Chromium (Niacin/Glycine Chelate) 100 mcg • Selenium (Selenomethionine) 50 mcg.

Opti-Vue — The Vitamin Shoppe
Two capsules contain: Vitamin A 10000 IU • Vitamin C 200 mg • Vitamin E 50 IU • Potassium 100 mg • Niacin 30 mg • Zinc 5 mg • Riboflavin 3 mg • Selenium 50 mcg • Lutein 6 mg • Zeaxanthin 240-600 mcg • Eyebright Extract 200 mg • Raw Eye Tissue 160 mg • Raw Muscle Tissue 100 mg • Inositol 100 mg • Alfalfa concentrate 50 mg • Citrus Bioflavonoids 50 mg • Quercitin 200 mg • Rutin 25 mg • Bilberry extract 40 mg • Glutathione 5 mg • N-Acetyl Cysteine 50 mg. In a special food base of rice carrot parsley, and spinach concentrates.

Optizinc — Natrol
Each capsule contains: Zinc (Monomethionine) 30 mg. Other ingredients: Microcrystalline Cellulose, Magnesium Stearate, Gelatin.

Opti-Zyme — Changes - TwinLab
One caplet contains: Calcium (from 500 mg Calcium Carbonate) 180 mg • Amylase 4250 DU • Protease 10255 HUT • Cellulase 630 CU • Lactase 350 Lac U • Lipase 65 LU • Invertase 0.6 IAU • Glucoamylase 15 AG • Multi-algae blend: Spirulina algae, Bladderwrack kelp, Klamath Lake algae, Canary Island algae, Chlorella algae, Maine coast kelp, and Sargassi seaweed • Supporting

herbal blend: Turmeric rhizome, Fennel seed, Ginger root, and Soy sprouts. Other ingredients: Vegetable cellulose, Fractionated vegetable oil, Soy polysaccherides, Silica, and Vegetable resin glaze.

Opti-Zyme Pro — Changes - TwinLab
One capsule contains: Amylase 3400 SKB • Lipase 2250 LU • Cellulase 5400 C-ase • Protease 10200 HUT • Amyloglucosidase 22 AG • Acid stable protease 340 APU • Invertase 102 Sumner U • Lactase 351 LAU • Lactobacillus acidophilus 100 million CFU • Bifidobacterium bifidum 50 million CFU • Dulse algae 50 mg • Trace mineral complex (Montmorillonite) 100 mg • Spirulina blue-green algae 50 mg • Bromelain 50 mg. Other ingredients: Gelatin, Calcium Sulfate, Magnesium Stearate, and Silica.

Organic Flax 1000 — Health From The Sun
Two capsules contain: Alpha-Linolenic Acid (ALA) (Omega-3) 1.1 g • Linoleic Acid (Omega-6) 280 mg • Oleic Acid (Omega-9) 290 mg. Ingredients: Certified Organic Flax seed oil, Gelatin, Glycerine, Water, Carob powder.

Orobronze — Biam
Canthaxanthine 0.30 g.

Oscillococcinum — Boiron
Each tube contains: Active Ingredients: Anas barbariae hepatis et cordis extractum HPUS 200 CK. Inactive Ingredients: Sucrose 0.85 g, Lactose 0.15 g.

Osha-Lomatium Virtue — Blessed Herbs
Osha root • Lomatium root • Pau d'Arco bark • Propolis • Shitake mycelium • Echinacea Angustifolia root • Goldenseal root • Licorice root • Grain alcohol & Distilled Water.

Osteo Formula — Quest
Each tablet contains: Calcium (HVP Chelate) 125 mg • Magnesium (HVP Chelate) 125 mg • Vitamin C 50 mg • Vitamin D3 50 IU • Silicon (HVP Chelate) 125 mcg • N-Acetyl Glucosamine (NAG) 125 mg • Betaine HCl 25 mg. Other Ingredients: Croscarmellose Sodium, Magnesium Stearate (vegetable source), Microcrystalline Cellulose, Vegetable Stearin.

Osteo Guard — Clinician's Choice
Four tablets contain: Vitamin C (ascorbic acid) 120 mg • Vitamin D (cholecalciferol) 400 IU • Calcium (carbonate, glycinate, gluconate, citrate, succinate, amino acid chelate, aspartate) 1000 mg • Magnesium (oxide, carbonate, citrate, amino acid chelate) 480 mg • Zinc (amino acid chelate) 10 mg • Manganese (amino acid chelate) 1 mg • L-Glutamic Acid 20 mg • Betaine Hydrochloride 20 mg • Proprietary blend 20 mg: Piper Longum Fruit, Pacific Kelp, Carrot Powder, Astragalus Membranaceus, Silica (horsetail herb), Boron (boron aspartate).

Osteo Protector — The Vitamin Shoppe
Each tablet contains: Vitamin D (as cholecalciferol) 100 IU • Calcium (as carbonate, hydroxyapatite) 500 mg • Magnesium (as oxide, citrate) 250 mg • Ipriflavone (7-Isopropoxy Isoflavone (Ostivone)) 200 mg. No yeast, corn, wheat, sugar, salt, starch, milk, gluten, soy, eggs, dairy, fish, citrus, preservatives, artificial colors or flavors added.

Osteo-Bi-Flex — Sundown Vitamins
Each tablet contains: Glucosamine HCl 500 mg • Chondroitin Sulfate 400 mg. Starch, salt & preservative free.

Osteologic — PhysioLogics
Four tablets contain: Vitamin D (as Cholecalciferol) 400 IU • Vitamin K (as Phytonadione) 80 mcg • Vitamin B6 (as Pyridoxine HCl) 2 mg • Folate (Folic Acid) 400 mcg • Pantothenic Acid (as D-Calcium Pantothenate) 10 mg • Calcium (as Calcium Carbonate) 1000 mg • Iodine (from Kelp) 471 mcg • Magnesium (as 58% Magnesium Oxide, 25% Magnesium Glycinate, 17% Magnesium Carbonate) 400 mg • Zinc (as Zinc Citrate) 15 mg • Selenium (from natural salts) 3 mcg • Copper (as Copper Aspartate) 2 mg • Manganese (as mixed Manganese salts) 378 mcg • Chromium (from natural salts) 38 mcg • Molybdenum (from natural salts) 115 mcg • Silicon (as Silicon Dioxide) 20 mg • Boron (as 98% Boron Aspartate, 2% natural salts) 3 mg.

Osteo-Plus — Nutri-Quest
Each tablet contains: Boron (special organic complex) 1 mg • Magnesium Chelate 400 mg • Calcium Chelate 100 mg • Calcium Aspartate 100 mg • Calcium Giuconate 50 mg • Calcium (Hydroxyapatite) 156 mg • Calcium (Veal Bone) 39 mg • Red Bone Marrow 10 mg • Calcium Citrate 50 mg • Vitamin C 25 mg • Vitamin D 50 IU • L-Glutamic Acid HCL 15 mg • Betaine HCL 10 mg •

Salmiac 10 mg • Parathyroid 2 mg. In a base containing Horsetail Rush (Shave grass), Source of Natural Silicon 15 mg, Calcium Fluoride (Cell Salt) Safflower herb 25 mg.

Osteoporosis Formula — Nature's Life
Each four capsules contain: Calcium (Citrate/Malate, Carbonate) 1000 mg • Magnesium (Oxide, Citrate) 500 mg • Vitamin C (Ascorbic Acid) 40 mg • Betaine HCl 40 mg • Zinc (Picolinate) 15 mg • Manganese (Gluconate) 5 mg • Boron (Citrate) 2 mg • Vitamin K1 mg • Copper (Gluconate) 1 mg • Silicon (Dioxide) 1 mg • Vitamin D3 (Cholecalciferol) 400 IU. In a natural base of Springtime Horsetail herb (Equisetum arvernse).

OsteoPrime — Enzymatic Therapy
Four tablets contain: Vitamin D 200 IU • Calcium (Aspartate, Citrate, Succinate, Fumarate, Carbonate, Lactate, Malate) 600 mg • Magnesium (Aspartate, Oxide) 250 mg • Vitamin C (Ascorbic Acid) 100 mg • Vitamin B6 (Pyridoxine) 25 mg • Niacinamide 20 mg 8 Zinc (Picolinate) 15 mg • Manganese (Aspartate) 15 mg • Thiamine HCL (Vitamin B1) 10 mg • Riboflavin (Vitamin B2) 10 mg • Pantothenic Acid (D-Calcium Pantothenate) 10 mg • Copper (Gluconate) 1.5 mg • Folic Acid 400 mcg • Vitamin K (Phytonadione) 150 mcg • Chromium (Aspartate) 100 mcg • Selenium sodium Selenite) 100 mcg • Molybdenum (Sodium Molybdate) 50 mcg • Vitamin B12 (Cyanocobalamin) 10 mcg. Other ingredients: Betaine HCL 20 mg • Silicon sodium Metasilicate) 1 mg • Boron (Chelated) 750 mcg • Strontium (Nonradioactice) 500 mcg. Contains no sugar, yeast, wheat, corn, soy, dairy products, coloring or preservatives.

OsteoPrime Forte — Phytopharmica
Four tablets contain: Vitamin D 200 IU • Calcium (aspartate, citrate, succinate, fumarate, carbonate, lactate, malate) 600 mg • Magnesium (aspartate, oxide) 250 mg • Vitamin C (ascorbic acid) 100 mg • Niacinamide 50 mg • Vitamin B6 (pyridoxine) 25 mg • Zinc (picolinate) 20 mg • Manganese (aspartate) 20 mg • Thiamine HCL (Vitamin B1) 20 mg • Riboflavin (Vitamin B2) 20 mg • Pantothenic Acid (D-Calcium pantothenate) 20mg • Copper (gluconate) 2 mg • Folic Acid 800 mcg • Vitamin K (phytonadione) 300 mcg • Chromium (aspartate) 200 mcg • Selenium (sodium selenite) 100 mcg • Molybdenum (sodium molybdate) 50 mcg • Vitamin B12 (cyanocobalamin) 20 mcg • Betaine HCL 20 mg • Boron (chelated) 2 mg • Silicon (sodium metasilicate) 1 mg • Strontium (nonradioactive) 500 mcg.

Osteosupport — Health Factor
Four tablets contain: Calcium (Citrate/Hydroxylapatite) 850 mg • Vitamin D3 (Cholecalciferol) 100 IU • Iodine (Kelp) 100 mcg • Magnesium (Citrate) 650 mg • Boron (Citrate) 2 mg • Silicon (Citrate) 500 mcg • Vanadium (Pentoxide) 75 mcg • Betaine HCl 65 mg • Glutamic Acid 65 mg.

Osteo-Support — The Vitamin Shoppe
Two tablets provide: Calcium 500 mg • Magnesium 250 mg • Vitamin D 100 IU.

OstiBone — NaturalMax - Nutraceutical
One capsule contains: Calcium (as Calcium Carbonate) 120 mg • Ostivone (as Isoproxy Isoflavone) 200 mg. Other ingredients: Gelatin, Cellulose, Magnesium Stearate.

Ostivone — Enzymatic Therapy
Each capsule contains: Ostivone(tm) (Ipriflavone) 200 mg. Contains no sugar, salt, yeast, wheat, gluten, corn, soy, dairy products, coloring, flavoring or preservatives.

Ostivone — Anabolic Laboratories
Each tablet contains: Ipriflavone (Ostivone 7-Isopropoxy Isoflavone) 200 mg.

Ostivone — Phytopharmica
Each capsule contains: Ostivone (Ipriflavone) 200 mg.

Ostivone — Source Naturals
One tablet contains: Ipriflavone (Ostivone) 300 mg.

Ostivone 100 mg — Natrol
Each capsule contains: 7-Isopropoxy-Isoflavone 100 mg. Other ingredients: Rice Powder, Magnesium Stearate, Gelatin.

Otrthoflex — Pacific BioLogic
Siberian Ginseng • Angelica root (Chinese) • Angelica root (pubescent) • Eucommia bark • Siler root • Cinnamon Twig • Astragalus root (Grade 1) • Homalomena rhizome • Notopterygium root & rhizome • Gentiana root • Pseudoginseng root (whole) • Teasal root • Ginger (Chinese Wild).

Ovary-Uterus Complex — Enzymatic Therapy
Each capsule contains: Ovary-Uterus Complex (Predigested Soluble concentrate*) 250 mg • Multi-Glandular Complex: Raw Liver, Raw Lung, Raw Pancreas, Raw Heart, Raw Kidney, Raw Spleen, & Raw Brain 100 mg. *Free-form concentrate predigested by enzymatic action, creating a highly absorbable form of glandular concentrate containing all the natural principles with a standardized content. Contains no sugar, salt, yeast, wheat, corn, soy, dairy products, coloring, flavoring or preservatives.

Overdrive — Pharmanex
Each capsule contains: Vitamin A (100% as Beta-Carotene from Dunaliella Salina, Beta-Carotene) 2500 IU • Vitamin C (as Ascorbic Acid) 300 mg • Vitamin E (d-Alpha Tocopheryl Succinate) 75 IU • Thiamin (as Thiamine Mononitrate) 0.75 mg • Riboflavin (as Riboflavin) 0.85 mg • Vitamin B6 (as Pyridoxine Hydrochloride) 1 mg • Folate (as Folic Acid) 100 mcg • Vitamin B12 (as Cyanocobalamin) 3 mcg • Pantothenic Acid (as d-Calcium Pantothenate) 5 mg • Magnesium (as Magnesium Asparate, Magnesium Oxide) 60 mg • Selenium (as L-Selenomethionine) 35 mcg • Chromium (as Chromium Chelate, Chrmium Picolinate) 100 mcg • Bromelain (from Pineapple extract) 50 mg • Papain (from Papaya extract) 50 mg • Citrus Bioflavonoid Complex 50 mg • Hydromins (from Sea Salt extract) 50 mg • N-Acetyl-L-Cysteine 20 mg • Quercetin 12.5 mg • Grape Seed Extract with Leucoanthocyanin 2.5 mg.

Oxy Shield — Futurebiotics
Three tablets contain: Vitamin E (natural d-alpha tocopherol) 400 IU • Beta Carotene 25,000 IU • Vitamin C 1000 mg • N-Acetyl Cysteine 125 mg • Cysteine 125 mg • Zinc (citrate, gluconate) 25 mg • Copper 1 mg • Selenium (selenomethionine) 150 mcg • Garlic (pure-gar) 400 mg • Green Tea 400 mg • Rosemary extract 50 mg • Licorice (extract from) 700 mg • Astragalus (extract from) 350 mg • Tricosanthes (extract from) 150 mg • Siberian Ginseng (extract from) 750 mg • Pau D'Arco 50 mg • Cayenne 30 mg • Methionine 50 mg • Red Clover flowers 100 mg • Barley grass powder 100 mg • Chamomile 100 mg • Ribonucleic Acid (RNA) 50 mg • Kelp 100 mg • Iodine (kelp) 150 mcg • Molybdenum 20 mcg.

Oxy-G2 — Body Wise International, Inc.
Two capsules contain: Beta Carotene (Vitamin A 6250 IU) 3.75 mg • Vitamin C 75 mg • Vitamin E (as d-alpha Tocopheryl Succinate) 30 IU • Pantothenic Acid (from Calcium Pantothenate) 50 mg • Selenium (as L-Selenomethionine) 100 mcg • Molybdenum (Krebs Cycle Chelate) 100 mcg • Organic Germanium 100 mg • Ginkgo Biloba Leaf 100 mg • Milk Thistle Seed Std. Extract (80% Silymarin) 50 mg • Echinacea Purpurea Root 50 mg • Cytochrome C Oxidase 50 mg • Krebs Cycle Chelated Replenished Factors 50 mg • L-Glutathione 50 mg • Ascorbyl Palmitate 50 mg • L-Cysteine 25 mg • L-Tyrosine 25 mg • Pau D'Arco (Taheebo Tea Bark) 25 mg • Chlorophyll 20 mg.

Oxy-Pro — Progressive Labs
Each capsule contains: Vitamin A (as beta carotene) 12500 IU • Vitamin C 150 mg • Vitamin E (d-alpha tocopheryl succinate) 100 IU • Riboflavin (B2) 12.5 mg • Niacinamide 12.5 mg • Vitamin B6 10 mg • Zinc (as zinc glycinate) 7.5 mg • Selenium (as selenomethionine) 100 mcg • Copper (as copper lysinate) 0.5 mg • Manganese (as manganese glycinate) 4 mg • Molybdenum (as sodium molybdate) 5 mcg • Quercitin 50 mg • N-Acetyl Cysteine 50 mg • Glutathione 2.5 mg.

Pacific Kelp — Quest
Each tablet contains: Pacific Kelp 650 mg. Other Ingredients: Calcium Carbonate, Silicon Dioxide, Magnesium Stearate (vegetable source).

Pain Relief Support — Amazon Support
Each capsule contains: Iporuru • Tayuya • Picao Preto.

Pain Stop — Flora
Willow bark.

Pain-Less — The Herbalist
White Willow bark • Feverfew herb • Jamaican Dogwood root bark • Black Cohosh root • Passionflower herb • Butterbur root • St. John's Wort flower.

Pain-Less Rub — The Herbalist
Oils of Sweet Almond, Aloe Vera, St. John's Wort flower, Calendula flower & Arnica flower • Essential oils of French Lavender,

© Copyright 2000, Natural Medicines Comprehensive Database (209) 472-2244. For updated data, go to www.NaturalDatabase.com. • 1379

B R A N D   N A M E S

Peppermint, Lemon Grass, Wintergreen, Nutmeg, Bergamot & Camphor • Extracts of Comfrey root, Echinacea root, White Willow bark & Cayenne pepper.

Palmitol — Flora
Saw Palmetto berries • Zinc 50 mg • Vitamin B6 120 mg.

Palmvitee — LaneLabs
Two capsules contain: Vitamin E 350 IU (as gamma tocotrienol, alpha tocotrienol, delta tocotrienol, & d-alpha tocopherol). Other Ingredients: Gelatin, water, & glycerin. Free of corn, yeast, wheat, & dairy products and contains no sugar, salt, starch, preservatives, artificial flavors or colors.

Panax Ginseng — Pharmanex
Each capsule contains: Ginseng Panax root (5:1) extract (Panax Ginseng C.A. Meyer) 100 mg. Other Ingredients: Rice Flour, Gelatin.

Pancreas Plus — Nutri-Quest
Each tablet contains: Pancretin 270 mg • Pancreas 130 mg [Tissue concentrate (not extract) of Bovine Source]. Natural occuring factors as well as concentrated forms of Protease, Lipase, & Amylase enzymes.

Pancreras Chelate Plus — Atrium
Each tablet contains: Zinc (Protein Chelated) 15 mg • Chromium (Protein Chelated) 200 mcg • Pancreas Substance (from total maxi strength Pancreatin 75 mg, Raw Pancreas concentrate 75 mg) 150 mg. To insure the naturally occuring factors as well as the concentrated forms of Lipase & Amylase Enzymes.

Pantethine Complex — The Vitamin Shoppe
Each tablet contains 300 mg of Pantethine Complex supplying: Pantethine (coenzyme A precursor) 150 mg • Pantothenic Acid (d-calcium pantothenate) 150 mg. No Yeast, Corn, Wheat, Salt, Sugar, Starch, Soy, Gluten, Milk, Eggs, Dairy, Fish or Animal Derivatives, Preservatives, Artificial Colors or Flavors added.

Para Thyrolate — Progressive Labs
Each capsule contains: Calcium 100 mg • Iodine 225 mcg • Phosphorus 40 mg • Parathyroid concentrate 500 mcg • Thyroid concentrate (thyroxin-free) 25 mg. Other Ingredients: Dicalcium Phosphate, Cellulose, Protein Conjugate, Pacific Sea Kelp, Calcium Carbonate, Papain, Guar Gum, Stearic Acid, Gelatin. The glandular material in this product is prepared by a special process which does not exceed physiological temperature (37° C). Guaranteed free of chemical pesticides and synthetic hormones.

Para-Cid — Atrium
Each tablet contains : Betaine HCL 250 mg • Pepsin 20 mg. In a slow release matrix.

Paraclear — PhysioLogics
Two capsules contain: Sweet Annie leaf, stem 400 mg • Garlic bulb (10000 mcg Allicin/g • 2 mg) 200 mg • Pau D'Arco bark, stem (3% Napthoquinone 6 mg) 200 mg • Goldthread root (10% Alkaloids, 15 mg) 150 mg • Black Walnut husk 100 mg • Ficin (from fig) 10 mg.

Para-Clens — Nutri-Quest
Each tablet contains: Artemisia Annua 50 mg • Garlic powder 50 mg • Black Walnut 50 mg • Pumpkin seed 50 mg • Oregano oil 1 mg • Tea Tree 2 mg • Grapefruit seed extract 50 mg • Bromelain 50 mg • Papain 50 mg.

Parathyroid — Atrium
Each tablet contains: Parathyroid (Bovine) 10 mg • Thyroid (Thyroxin free) 30 mg • Stomach (Bovine) 32 mg • Dulse 300 mg • Calcium 50 mg • Phosphorus 22 mg • Vitamin D3 100 IU • Vitamin B12 20 mcg • Folic Acid 440 mcg • Beet 50 mg • Carrot 50 mg. Calcium & Phosphorus from Bone Meal, Beet & Carrot powders, Iodine from Dulse powder.

Pau d'Arco-Black Walnut Virtue — Blessed Herbs
Pau d'Arco bark • Usnea lichen • Calendula flower • Echinacea Angustifolia root • Black Walnut hull • Goldenseal root • Myrrh Gum • Grain alcohol & Distilled Water.

PC-SPES — BotanicLab, Inc
Each capsule contains: Da Qing Ye (Isatis indigotica) • Licorice (Glycyrrhiza glabra, Glycyrrhiza uralensis) • San Qi (Panax Pseudoginseng) • Reishi Mushroom (Ganoderma lucidum) • Baikal Skullcap (Scutellaria baicalensis) • Chrysanthemum (Dendranthema morifolium) • Rabdosia Rebescens • Saw Palmetto (Serenoa repens). Editor's Comments: PC-SPES has been available commercially since 1996. "PC" stands for prostate cancer and "spes" is Latin for hope

(5548). Multiple very small clinical trials and a case report demonstrate that it can dramatically decrease serum prostate-specific antigen (PSA) levels (3576,5122,5548,5913), cause tumor cells to die (5913), and cause clinically significant reductions in serum testosterone (5548). In two reports, PSA levels fell significantly within 1 month of treatment (5122,5548). In another report, 100% of patients had a decline in PSA levels and 56% had undetectable levels at the end of the study period (3576,3577). Although PC-SPES does not contain estrogen, the licorice and Panax-pseudoginseng constituents have estrogenic activity. The saw palmetto constituent inhibits 5-alpha reductase, an enzyme involved in conversion of testosterone to the more biologically active dihydrotestosterone (5548). Reported side effects of PC-SPES include lowered libido, erectile dysfunction, hot flashes, breast tenderness/enlargement, reduction in overall body hair, pitting edema, significant drop in lipoprotein a, and venous thrombosis (5122,5548,5913). In one report, 92% of men had breast swelling or tenderness (3577). One expert reports that venous thrombosis occurs in just less than 4% of patients taking PC-SPES and that serious side effects are rare. Despite its relative safety, others recommend that PC-SPES should only be used under the care of a physician (5913). Some sources recommended starting with one capsule three times daily during the first week and 2 capsules three times daily during the second week. If this dose is tolerated, the dose can be increased to 3 capsules three times daily. Clinical trials have used 6-9 capsules daily. PC-SPES should be taken on an empty stomach and should not be administered concurrently with antacids or other medicines (3577). Depending on the dose required, cost is estimated to range from $162-$486/month (5233).

Pedi-Active Spray — Nature's Plus
Each spray contains: DMAE (2-Dimethylaminoethanol Bitartrate) 50 mg • LECI-PS Phosphatidylserine-rich purified Lecithin concentrate supplying Activated Phosphatides: [Phosphatidylserine 10 mg, Phosphatidylcholine 10 mg, Cephalin (Phosphatidylethanolamine) 6 mg, Phosphoinositides 3 mg] 50 mg. In a proprietary liposomal complex of Essential Metabolic Factors , Purified Water, Vegetable Glycerine, Purified Lecithin, Citrus seed extract (Citrus sinensis), Vitamin E & natural Wild Berry flavor.

Pedi-ADD — Aspen Group, Inc.
Each chewable tablet contains: Phosphatidylserine - Purified Lecithin concentrate supplying Activated Phosphatides 50 mg: Phosphatidylserine 10 mg • Phosphatidylcholine 10 mg • Cephalin (phosphatidylethanolamine) 6 mg • Phosphoinositides 5 mg • DMAE (2-dimethylaminoethanol bitartrate) 50 mg.

Pediatric Chewable — Clinician's Choice
One tablet contains: Vitamin A (as retinyl acetate & 50% as betacarotene) 2500 IU • Vitamin C (as ascorbic acid & sodium ascorbate) 60 mg • Vitamin D (as cholecalciferol) 200 IU • Vitamin E (as dl-alpha tocopheryl acetate) 15 IU • Thiamin (as mononitrate) 0.75 mg • Riboflavin 0.9 mg • Niacin (as niacinamide) 10 mg • Vitamin B6 (as pyridoxine hydrochloride) 1 mg • Folate (as folic acid) 200 mcg • Vitamin B12 (as cyanocobalamin) 3 mcg • Biotin 30 mcg • Pantothenic Acid (as d-calcium pantothenate) 5 mg • Calcium (as carbonate & gluconate) 85 mg • Iodine (as potassium Iodide) 75 mcg • Magnesium (as oxide) 15 mg • Zinc (as oxide) 7.5 mg • Copper (as cupric oxide) 1 mg • Manganese (as citrate) 0.5 mg • Chromium (as nicotinate) 10 mcg • Molybdenum (sodium molybdate) 5 mcg • Proprietary blend: Acerola powdered extract 4:1 • Carrot Powder, Spinach Powder 6 mg.

Pedia-Vit — Progressive Labs
Two teaspoons (10 ml) contain: Vitamin A 2500 IU • Vitamin C 40 mg • Vitamin D 400 IU • Vitamin E 10 IU • Thiamin (B1) 0.7 mg • Riboflavin (B2) 0.8 mg • Niacin (B3) 9 mg • Vitamin B6 0.7 mg • Folate (folic acid) 200 mcg • Vitamin B12 3 mcg • Biotin 150 mcg • Pantothenic Acid 5 mg • Iron 10 mg • Zinc 8 mg.

Pedi-Vites Multiple — Aspen Group, Inc.
Each tablet contains: Vitamin A Palmitate 180 IU • Vitamin D3 150 IU • Vitamin E 10 IU • Vitamin B1 2 mg • Vitamin B2 2 mg • Vitamin B6 2 mg • Vitamin B12 6 mcg • Vitamin C 60 mg • Niacinamide 5 mg • Folic Acid 100 mcg • Pantothenic Acid 3 mg • Biotin 30 mcg • Calcium (carbonate) 10 mg • Magnesium (gluconate) 2 mg • Manganese (gluconate) 1 mg • Selenium (selenium aspartate) 5 mcg • Chromium (chromium ACP) 5 mcg • Molybdenum (sodium molybdate) 2 mcg • Vanadium (vanadium sulfate) 2 mcg • Chlorophyll 1 mg • Boron (boron citrate) 50 mcg.

Peppermint Plus — Enzymatic Therapy
Each enteric-coated capsule contains: Peppermint oil extract (Mentha

Some Brand Name Natural Products - What they Contain
www.NaturalDatabase.com contains MANY more listings than appear here.

piperita) 0.2 ml • Rosemary oil extract (Rosemarinus officinalis) 0.02 ml • Thyme oil extract (Thymus vulgaris) 0.02 ml. Contains no sugar, salt, yeast, wheat, corn, dairy products, flavoring or preservatives.

Perfect Cal — Futurebiotics
Four tablets contain: Calcium (from Hydroxyappatite crystal) 400 mg • Calcium Complex (Citrate, Carbonate) 600 mg • Magnesium (Citrate, Oxide, Hydroxyappatite) 600 mg • Vitamin D 200 IU • Boron 1.5 mg • Horsetail (from extract) 750 mg.

PerfectRx — Nature's Best
Vanilla Perfect Rx Ingredients: Perfect Unique Protein Blend (Milk Protein Isolate, Calcium Caseinate, Whey Protein Concentrates, Egg Albumin), Maltodextrin, Potassium Chloride, Potassium Citrate, Sodium Chloride, Sodium Citrate, Dipotassium Phosphate, Natural & Artificial Flavors, Aspartame, Magnesium Oxide, Choline Bitartrate, Cellulose, Ascorbic Acid, d-Alpha Tocopheryl Acetate, Ferrous Fumarate, Niacin, Biotin, Xanthan Gum, Vitamin A Palmitate, Zinc, Oxide, D-Calcium Pantothenate, Vitamin K, Manganese Sulfate, Beta-Carotene, Copper Sulfate, Pyridoxine HCL, Riboflavin, Thiamine HCL, L-Glutamine, Chromium Picolinate, Cobalamin Concentrate (vitamin B12), Vitamin D-3, Folic Acid, Sodium Molybdate, Potassium Iodide, Sodium Selenite.

Perfor-Max — Changes - TwinLab
One caplet contains: Grape seed extract (vitis vinifera) 25 mg • Pine bark extract (Pinus pinaster) 25 mg • Turmeric rhisome extract 25 mg • Botanical Blend 50 mg: Green Tea leaf standardized extract (36% catechin & polyphenols), Hawthorn berry standardized extract (5% flavonoid glycosides), and Rosemary leaf extract. Other ingredients: Dicalcium Phosphate, Vegetable cellulose, Fractionated vegetable oil, Soy polysaccharides, Silica, and Vegetable resin glaze.

Peridin-C — Beutlich Pharmaceuticals
Each tablet contains: Ascorbic Acid (Vitamin C) 200 mg • Hesperidin Complex (Bioflavonoid) 150 mg • Hesperidin Methyl Chalcone (Bioflavonoid) 50 mg.

Perika St. John's Wort — Nature's Way
Each tablet contains: Perika (WS 5572) dried St. John's Wort extract 300 mg.

Permathene-16 Maximum Strength Caffeine Free — CCA Industries, Inc.
Each tablet contains: Active Ingredient: Phenylpropanolamine HCl 75 mg. Other Ingredients: Croscarmellose, D&C Yellow #10, Dicalcium Phosphate, FD&C Blue #1, FD&C Yellow #6, Lactose, Magnesium Stearate, Methylcellulose, Microcrystalline Cellulose, Stearic Acid, Titanium Dioxide.

Persic-GLA — Atrium
Each capsule contains: Borage oil 100 mg • Cold Processed Persic oil yielding to the following Lipid Acids: Referred to as Vitamin F Factors, (Oleic 192 mg, Linoleic 109 mg, Gamma Linolenic 30 mg, Palmitic 18 mg, Palmitoleic 5 mg, Stearic 4mg, Linolenic 701 mg, Heptodecanoic 409 mcg, Arachadic 330 mcg, Arachidonic 111 mcg) 370 mg • Potassium 113 mcg • Sodium 14 mcg • Magnesium 7 mcg • Phosphorus 4 mg • Calcium 4 mcg • trace amounts of Manganese, Chromium, Zinc, Iron, Copper, Baron, Barium. Contains no sugar, starch, salt, wheat, corn, yeast or soy derivatives.

PhenCal 106 — Great American Nutrition
Six tablets contain: Vitamin B6 (as pyridoxal-5-phosphate) 30 mg • Chromium (as picolinate) 200 mcg • DL-Phenylalanine 2700 mg • L-Tyrosine 300 mg • L-Glutamine 150 mg • L-5-Hydroxytryptophan 15 mg • L-Carnitine 60 mg.

Phen-Free — EAS
Four capsules contain: Caffeine 99 mg • Citrus aurantium 300 mg (standardized to 6% Synephrine) • Yohimbe 100 mg • Cordyceps 500 mg (standardized to 7% Cordyceptic Acid) • L-Tyrosine 500 mg • St. John's Wort 200 Mg (standardized to 0.3% Hypericin) • Cayenne Pepper powder 30 mg.

PhenSafe — Applied Nutrition
Three capsules contain: St. John's Wort (.3% hypericin) 300 mg • L-Glutamic Acid HCl 100 mg • B6 Pyridoxine HCl 20 mg • Niacinamide (B3) 10 mg • Zinc 8 mg • Folic Acid 200 mcg • ChromeMate 125 mcg • B12 100 mcg • Selenium 75 mcg. Each serving of the above nutrients is formulated with a special mixture containing these natural ingredients: [Advantra Z (citrus aurantium), Licorice root powder, Ginger root powder, Cayenne powder, Mustard

seed powder, Green Tea extract, Fennel seed powder, BioPerine] 640 mg.

Phos Fuel — TwinLab
Four capsules contain: Sodium Phosphate (Dibasic) 4000 mg • Potassium Bicarbonate 816 mg • L-Carnosine 50 mg • Lipoic Acid 100 mcg • Vitamin B1 1.5 mg • Vitamin B2 1.9 mg • Vitamin B3 (Niacinamide) 20 mg • Vitamin B6 2 mg • Pantothenic Acid 10 mg • Biotin 300 mcg.

Phosphagain 2 — EAS
Each 59 gram Vanilla serving contains: Calories 180 • Protein 25 g • Carbohydrates 13 g • Fat 1.5 g • Cholesterol 10 mg • Sodium 380 mg • Potassium 730 mg • Chromium 50 mcg • Selenium 30 mcg • Manganese 1 mg • Vitamin K 40 mcg • Molybdenum 60 mcg • Choline 80 mg. Ingredients: Nitrogenin 2 proprietary Protein/Nitrogen reinforcing matrix (Milk Protein Isolate, Calcium Caseinate, L-Glutamine, Taurine, Calcium Alpha-Ketoglutarate [AKG] & Egg Albumin) • Phosphagen (HPCE Pure Cratine Monohydrate) • Maltodextrin, Dextrose • Vitamin & Mineral Blend (Potassium Phosphate, Potassium Citrate, Salt, Magnesium Oxide, Choline Bitartrate, Disodium Phosphate, Beta-Carotene, Ascorbic Acid, Dl-Alpha Tocopheryl Acetate, Ferrous Fumarate, Niacin, Zinc Oxide, D-Calcium Pantothenate, Copper Sulfate, Vitamin A Palmitate, Manganese Sulfate, Chromium Citrate, Pyridoxine Hydrochloride, Riboflavin, Thiamine Hydrochloride, Sodium Molybdate, Vitamin D3, Folic Acid, Biotin, Potassium Iodide, Sodium Selenate, Vitamin K, & Cyanocobalamin) • Corn Syrup Solids • Partially Hydrogenated Canola oil • Xanthan Gum • Natural & Artificial Flavors • Sodium RNA • Soy Lecithin • Aspartame • Carrageenan. Contains Phenylalanine.

PhosphaGems — EAS
Each 42 gram serving contains: Calories 135 • Carbohydrates 35 g • Sodium 100 mg • Phosphagen (HPCE pure Creatine Monohydrate) 5.2 g. Ingredients: TriCarb Complex (Sucrose, High-Dextrose Corn Syrup & Dextrose) • Phosphagen (HPCE pure Creatine Monohydrate) • Modified Starch • Natural & Artificial Flavor • Disodium Phosphate • Malic Acid • colored with Cochineal extracts.

Phosphagen — EAS
Each 5 gram serving contains: Phosphagen 5 g.

Phosphagen HP — EAS
Each 43 gram Fruit Punch serving contains: Calories 140 • Carbohydrates 34 g • Sodium 95 mg • Potassium 80 mg • Phosphagen 5.25 g • Taurine 1000 mg. Ingredients: Dextrose • Phosphagen (HPCE pure Creatine Monohydrate), Taurine • Natural & Artificial Flavor • Citric Acid • Beet Powder for color • Magnesium Phosphate • Disodium Phosphate • Potassium Phosphate.

Phosphatide I-C-E — Progressive Labs
Each softgel contains: Phosphatidylcholine 420 mg • Phosphatidylethanolamine 210 mg • Phosphatidylinositol 120 mg • Total Phosphatides 750 mg. All phosphatides extracted from soybeans. This product contains the highest known concentration of naturally occuring phosphatides.

Phosphatidyl Choline Complex — Nature's Life
Each capsule contains: Phosphatidyl Choline Complex (Soy) 120 mg. Nutrient profile based on a typical analysis: Phosphatides: Phosphatidyl Choline (contains 65 mg Choline) 420 mg • Phosphatidyl Ethanolamine 108 mg • Phosphatidyl Inositol (contains 6 mg Inositol) 24 mg • Phosphatidic Acid 36 mg. Lipids: Linoleic Acid (Omega-6) 313 mg • Linolenic Acid (Omega-3) 24 mg • Oleic Acid (Omega-9) 73 mg • Palmitic Acid 78 mg • Stearic Acid 24 mg.

Phosphatidyl Serine — Progressive Labs
Each softgel contains: Phospholipids: Phosphatidylserene (soy phospholipid) 100 mg • Phosphatidylcholine (soy phospholipid) 45 mg • Phosphatidylethanolamine (soy phospholipid) 10 mg • Phosphatidylinositol (soy phospholipid) 10 mg. Fatty Acids: Linoleic Acid 113 mg • Linolenic Acid 11 mg • Oleic Acid 12 mg • Stearic Acid 1 mg • Palmitic Acid 24 mg • Capric Acid 49 mg • Caprylic Acid 130 mg. Minerals: Phosphorus 8 mg • Potassium 3 mg.

Phosphatidylserine — PhysioLogics
Two capsules contain: Phosphatidylserine Complex 500 mg. Phospholipids: Phosphatidylserine 100 mg • Phosphatidylcholine 100 mg • Phosphatidylethanolamine 60 mg • Phosphatidylinositol 30 mg. Fatty Acids: Linoleic Acid 135 mg • Linolenic Acid 30 mg • Oleic Acid 25 mg • Stearic Acid 15 mg • Palmitic Acid 45 mg. Minerals: Phosphorus 15 mg • Potassium 5 mg.

Some Brand Name Natural Products - What they Contain
www.NaturalDatabase.com contains MANY more listings than appear here.

BRAND NAMES

Phosphatidylserine Complex — The Vitamin Shoppe
Each softgel contains: 500 mg Phospholipids providing 100 mg of Phosphatidylserine and 400 mg other Phospholipids. No Yeast, Wheat, Salt, Sugar, Starch, Corn, Milk, Dairy, Eggs, Preservatives, Artificial Colors or Flavors added.

Phyto Estrogen Power — Nature's Herbs
Four capsules provide: Soy Germ Isoflavone conc. 1400 mg • Kudzu root extract 100 mg • Certified Potency Korean Ginseng extract 100 mg • Certified Potency Dong Quai extract 100 mg • Mexican Wild Yam extract 100 mg • Boron 3 mg • Natural Vitamin E 800 IU. In a base of Chasteberry powder and Arrowroot.

Phyto Flavonoids — Olympia Nutrition
Contains the extracts of Silymarin, Curcumin, Green Tea, Quercetin, Rosemary, Bilberry, Hawthorn, Ginger, Ginkgo Biloba, Bromelain, Cranberry.

Phyto Surge — Phytopharmica
One tablespoon contains: Arsenicum album 6x • Nux vomica 3x • Podophyllum peltatum 3x • Cinchona officinalis 2x • Rhamnus frangula 2x • Artemisia vulgaris 1x • Avena sativa 1x • Cinnamomum 1x • Gentiana lutea 1x • Sterculia acuminata 1x • In a base of 20% USP alcohol by volume.
Editor's Comments: This is a homeopathic product. It is so extremely diluted that its activity can not be explained by conventional scientific methods. Therefore this product can not be rated by the scientific criteria used in this Database. A patient receiving the extreme dilution of this product will not receive many, if any, molecules of the original active ingredient. Therefore, there are no harmful pharmacologic effects, and any beneficial effects are controversial and not due to a direct biochemical action of the ingredient on the body. Homeopathic products are allowed for sale in the U.S. due to legislation passed in the 19th century sponsored by a homeopathic physician who was also a Senator. The law still requires that the FDA allow the sale of products listed in this Homeopathic Pharmacopea of the United States.

Phyto-Biotic — Enzymatic Therapy
Each capsule contains: Barberry Bark of root extract 6:1 (Berberis vulgaris) 200 mg • Oregon Grape root extract 6:1 (Berberis aquifolium) 200 mg • Goldenseal root extract (Hydrastis canadensis) standardized to contain 5% total Alkaloids including Berberine, Hydrastine & Canadine 50 mg. Contains no sugar, salt, yeast, wheat, corn, soy, dairy products, coloring, flavoring, or preservatives.

Phytodolor — Phytopharmica
Active Ingredients: Common ash (Fraxinus excelsior) bark (4.5:1) 0.20 ml Aspen (Populus tremula) leaves & bark (4.5:1) 0.60 ml Goldenrod (Solidago virgaurea) aerial (4.8:1) 0.20 ml Other Ingredients: Water, Alcohol, 45.6%. This patented liquid formula is standardized to contain: Salicin-0.75 mg/ml, Salicylic alcohol-0.042 mg/ml, Isofraxidin-0.015 mg/ml & Rutin-0.06 mg/ml.

Phyto-Flavonoids — Futurebiotics
Two capsules contain: Procyanidol • Whole Grape extract* 50 mg • Green Tea powder concentrate 150 mg • Citrus bioflavonoids 500 mg • Rutin 75 mg • Quercetin 150 mg • Soy isoflavone extract 500 mg • Berry blend (Raspberry, Blackberry, Blueberry) 200 mg • Cruciferous Vegetable powder blend 200 mg. *Procyanidol is a concentrated solvent-free grape extract containing high levels of flavonoid polyphenols.

Phyto-Fruit — Olympia Nutrition
Guava • Papaya • Mango • Raspberry • Blueberry • Grapefruit • Grape • Ginseng.

PhytoFruit Concentrates — Now
Two V Caps contain: Grape seed extract (95% Polyphenols) 20 mg • Concentrated fruit extract powders: Acerola Cherry 50 mg, Cranberry 50 mg, Guava 50 mg, Papaya 50 mg, Raspberry 50 mg, Blueberry 50 mg, Grapefruit 50 mg, Mango 50 mg, Pineapple 50 mg, Strawberry 50 mg • Panax ginseng (5% Ginsenosides) 50 mg • Bromelain (2000 GDU from pineapple) 50 mg • Protease (100 SAP Units) 50 mg • Amylase (3000 DU Units) 50 mg • Lipase (100 LU Units) 50 mg • Cellulase (500 CMC Units) 50 mg.

Phytosterol Complex — Progressive Labs
Each capsule contains: Niacin (vitamin B3) 20 mg • Beta-Sitosterol 106 mg • Campesterol 52 mg • Stigmasterol 42 mg. This naturally derived vegetable product is produced without the use of harsh chemicals or solvents.

Phytotality — PhysioLogics
Each capsule contains: Broccoli extract (2% Glucosinolates, 2 mg) 100 mg • TeaGreen leaf (50 % Polyphenols, 50 mg) 100 mg • Tomato extract (1% Lycopene, 500 mcg) 50 mg • Calendula flower Marigold (5% Lutein, 150 mcg) 3 mg • Soy Isoflavones extract (5 % Isoflavones, 1.25 mg) 25 mg • Red Grape skin extract (30% Anthocyanidins, 7.5 mg) 25 mg • Garlic bulb (10000 mcg Allicin/g, 250 mcg) 25 mg • Turmeric (95% Curcumin, 1.9 mg) 2 mg • Ginger root (5% Gingerols, 100 mcg) 2 mg • Milk Thistle seed (80% Silymarin, 20 mg) 25 mg • Onion 2 mg • Carrot 2 mg • Beet root 2 mg • Celery 2 mg • Leek 2 mg • Garlic 2 mg • Cauliflower 2 mg • Asparagus 2 mg • Broccoli 2 mg • Cabbage 2 mg.

PhytoxyActin — Nature's Plus
Two capsules contain: Vitamin C corn free 250 mg • Broccoli [(Brassica oleracea floret) standardized 0.035% Lutein, 0.004% B-Cryptoxanthin, 0.0025% Lycopene, 0.0025% Alpha Carotene, 0.0025% Beta Carotene, 0.004% Sulforaphane] 100 mg • Carrot [(Daucus carota root) standardized 0.003% Lutein, 0.0010% Lycopene, 0.0063% Alpha Carotene, 0.0075% Beta Carotene] 100 mg • Vitamin E natural 100 IU • Spinach [(Spinacia oleracea leaf) standardized 0.0043% Lutein, 0.0024% Lycopene, 0.0043% Beta Carotene, 0.0038% B-Cryptoxanthin] 75 mg • Tomato [(Lycopersicon esculentum fruit) standardized 0.0075% Lutein, 0.0155% Lycopene, 0.0015% Beta Carotene] 75 mg • Echinacea[(Echinacea angustifolia root) standardized 4% Echinacosides] 75 mg • Astragalus [(Astragalus membranaceus root) standardized 0.4% 4'-Hydroxy-3'-Methoxyisoflavone 7-sug] 50 mg • Green Tea [(Camellia sinensis leaf) standardized 50% Polyphenols] 50 mg • Red Wine concentrate alcohol free [(Vitis vinifera fruit) standardized 20% Polyphenols] 50 mg • Turmeric [(Cuizome) standardized 95% Curcumin] 50 mg • Garlic odor-modified [(Allium sativum clove) standardized 0.35% Allicin, 0.65% Allicin, 0.40% Thiosulfinates, 0.085% Allyl Mercaptan] 50 mg • Shiitake Mushroom [(Lentinus edodes mycelia) standardized 3.2% KS-2 Polysaccharides] 25 mg • Grape seed extract [(Vitis vinifera) standardized 95% Proanthocyanidins] 25 mg • Beta Carotene pro-Vitamin A (naturally supplying 25000 IU of Vitamin A activity) 15 mg.

Pineal Concentrate — Progressive Labs
Each capsule contains: Veal bone concentrate 100 mg • Flaxseed oil 20 mg • Pineal concentrate 7 mg • Pituitary concentrate 3 mg. The glandular concentrate in this product is prepared by a special process which does not exceed physiological temperature (37° C). Guaranteed free of chemical pesticides and synthetic hormones.

Pineal Plus — Atrium
Each tablet contains: Raw Pineal Tissue concentrate (Bovine) 8 mg • Raw Whole Pituitary concentrate (Bovine) 20 mg • Raw Calf Bone concentrate (Bovine) 150 mg • Cold Pressed Flaxseed oil 10 mg.

Pinna-Cal — Changes - TwinLab
Six caplets contain: Vitamin D (as Cholecalciferol) 125 IU • Vitamin K (as Phytonadione) 80 mcg • Calcium (as purified Calcite, Hydroxyapatite, Calcium Citrate, and Calcium Lactate) 1000 mg • Magnesium (as Magnesium Citrate and Oxide) 400 mg • Boron (as Boron Citrate) 2 mg • Ipriflavone 600 mg • Other ingredients: Vegetable cellulose, Fractionated vegetable oil, Silica, Soy polysaccharides, and Vita-Lok vegetable resin glaze.

Pinnacle 5-HTP Tryptobol — Bodyonics
Two capsules contains: Griffonia Simplicifolia (providing 10% (100 mg) 5-HTP (5-Hydroxy-L-Tryptophan)) 1000 mg • Herbolics Support Complex (from Jatoba, Macca, Para Todo, Yerba Mate) 100 mg. Other Ingredients: Calcium Phosphate, Microcrystalline Cellulose, Magnesium Stearate, Gelatin.

Pinnacle Androstat 100 — Bodyonics
Each tablet contains Androstenedione 100 mg. Other Ingredients: Calcium Phosphate, Lecithin, Xanthan Gum, Stearic Acid, Magnesium Stearate.

Pinnacle Androstat Pro Six — Bodyonics
Each tablet contains balanced andro complex: 4-androstene-3, 17-diol (4-androstenediol) 125 mg • 4-androstenedione-3, 17-dione (4-androstenedione) 5 mg • 5-androstene-3, 17-dione (5-androstenedione) 5 mg • 5-androstene-3, 17-diol (5-androstenediol) 5 mg • 19-nor-5-androstene-3, 17-diol (19-nor 5-androstendiol) 5 mg. Other Ingredients: Calcium Phosphate, Lecithin, xanthan Gum, Stearic Acid, Magnesium Stearate, Inulinized in a bioactive complex of Phosepholrolytic Dahlin.

Some Brand Name Natural Products - What they Contain
www.NaturalDatabase.com contains MANY more listings than appear here.

Pinnacle Androstat100 Poppers Cool Mint Flavor — Bodyonics
Two tablets contain balanced andro complex: 4-androstene-3, 17-diol (4-androstenediol) 83.33 mg • 4-androstenedione-3, 17-dione (4-androstenedione) 3.33 mg • 5-androstene-3, 17-dione (5-androstenedione) 3.33 mg • 5-androstene-3, 17-diol (5-androstenediol) 3.33 mg • 19-nor-5-androstene-3, 17-diol (19-nor 5-androstenediol) 3.33 mg. Other Ingredients: Fructose, Sorbitol, Natural Flavor, Stearic Acid, Magnesium Stearate, Cellulose, Croscarmellose, Sucralose.

Pinnacle Androstat100 poppers Licorice Flavor — Bodyonics
Two tablets contain balanced andro complex: 4-androstene-3, 17-diol (4-androstenediol) 83.33 mg • 4-androstenedione-3, 17-dione (4-androstenedione) 3.33 mg • 5-androstene-3, 17-dione (5-androstenedione) 3.33 mg • 5-androstene-3, 17-diol (5-androstenediol) 3.33 mg • 19-nor-5-androstene-3, 17-diol (19-nor 5-androstendiol) 3.33 mg. Other Ingredients: Fructose, Sorbitol, Natural Flavor, Stearic Acid, Magnesium Stearate, Cellulose, Croscarmellose, Sucralose.

Pinnacle Androstat100 Poppers Wild Berry Flavor — Bodyonics
Two tablets contain balanced andro complex: 4-androstene-3, 17-diol (4-androstenediol) 83.33 mg • 4-androstenedione-3, 17-dione (4-androstenedione) 3.33 mg • 5-androstene-3, 17-dione (5-androstenedione) 3.33 mg • 5-androstene-3, 17-diol (5-androstenediol) 3.33 mg • 19-nor-5-androstene-3, 17-diol (19-nor 5-androstendiol) 3.33 mg. Other Ingredients: Fructose, Sorbitol, Natural Flavor, Stearic Acid, Magnesium Stearate, Cellulose, Croscarmellose, Sucralose.

Pinnacle Androstat6 — Bodyonics
Two tablet contains balanced andro complex: 4-androstene-3, 17-diol (4-androstenediol) 125 mg • 4-androstenedione-3, 17-dione (4-androstenedione) 5 mg • 5-androstene-3, 17-dione (5-androstenedione) 5 mg • 5-androstene-3, 17-diol (5-androstenediol) 5 mg • 19-nor-5-androstene-3, 17-diol (19-nor 5-androstendiol) 5 mg. Other Ingredients: Fructose, Sorbitol, Natural Licorice Flavor, Stearic Acid, Magnesium, Stearate and 100% Natural Beta Cyclodextrins.

Pinnacle Beta Activated Protein with HMB — Bodyonics
Twelve tablets contain: Calcium B-Hydroxy B-Methylbutyrate Monohydrate (HMB) 3 g • Beta Peptide (a proprietary blend of very distinct cosein, whey and aligopeptides) 12 g • Alanine 392 mg • Arginine 419 mg • Aspartic Acid 713 mg • Cystine 74 mg • Glutamic Acid 2806 mg • Glycine 232 mg • Isoleucine (BCAA) 635 mg • Leucine (BCAA) 1044 mg • Lysine 906 mg • Methionine 307 mg • Phenylalanine 556 mg • Proline 1178 mg • Serine 617 mg • Threonine 494 mg • Tryptophan 142 mg • Tyrosine 461 mg • Valine (BCAA) 732 mg. Other Ingredients: Calcium Phosphate, Stearic Acid, Magnesium Stearate, Croscarmellose, Silica.

Pinnacle BHP-5 — Bodyonics
Each tablet contains: Hydrolyzed BHP5 (Pregenolone) 15 mg. Other Ingredients: Calcium Phosphate, Stearic Acid, Magnesium Stearate, Croscarmellose.

Pinnacle Chrysinex 250 — Bodyonics
Each tablet contains: Chrysin Complex (Derived from a customized blend of 98% pure 5,7-Dihydroxyflavone and natural powered extract poplar bud (Populus candicans) 250 mg • Cruciferous Vegetable Concentrate (Standardized to contain 10% Indole 3-Carbinols) 25 mg. Other Ingredients: Calcium Phosphate, Stearic Acid, Magnesium Stearate, Lecithin, Xanthan Gum.

Pinnacle Cordyceps 500 — Bodyonics
Each tablet contains: Dong Chong Zia Cao (Cordyceps sinensis-winter bug, summer herb) • Sha Shen (Adenophora tetraphylla) • WuWei Zi (Schisandra chinensis) • Gan Jiang (Zingiber officinale) • Dahlulin (Dahlia inulin juice concentrate). Other ingredients: Dicalcium Phosphate, Croscarmellose, Magnesium Stearate, Stearic Acid.

Pinnacle Crea Glutide 2400 — Bodyonics
Each tablet contains: Crea-Glutide 2400 mg • Creatine Monohydrate 2 g • Glutamine Peptide 400 mg. Other Ingredients: Calcium Phosphate, Stearic Acid, Magnesium Stearate, Croscarmellose.

Pinnacle Crea-Glutide — Bodyonics
Two tablespoons contains: Dextrose • BioReacted Crea-Glutide Complex • Complex Carbohydrate • Dahlulin (Dry Dahlia Inulin Juice Complex) • Citric Acid • Natural Cranberry Flavor • Xanthan Gum • Stevia Extract • Beet Extract.

Pinnacle CreaRibose ATP Kichers — Bodyonics
Six tablets contain: Creatine Monohydrate 5 grams • D-Ribose 3 grams. Other Ingredients: Magnesium Stearate, Cellulose, Calcium Phosphate, Stearic Acid.

Pinnacle Fractionized CCK 100 — Bodyonics
Each tablet contains: Cholecystokinin (CCK) (Derived from a purified blend of edible bovine tissue fractions, providing 1000 picomotes of standardized Cholecystokinin (CCK) a bioactive substance) 100 mg. Other ingredients: Calcium Phosphate, Microcrystalline Cellulose, Stearic Acid, Magnesium Stearate, Croscarmellose Silica.

Pinnacle Gro Tropin — Bodyonics
Three capsules contains: Alpha GPC (Alpha-Glycerylphosarylcholine) 500 mg • AminoGlutein Peptide (standardized to provide 30% Glutamine Peptide) 500 mg • Colostrum (Colostral Isoform Extract) (standardized to provide 1300 nanograms of platelet derived growth factor) 500 mg • Tribulus Terrestris (standardized to provide 40% Furostanol Saponins) 500 mg • Phosphatidyl Serine 500 mcg • Chrysin (98% pure 5,7 Dehydroxyflavone) 750 mcg. Other Ingredients: Magnesium Strearate, Gelatin.

Pinnacle Horny Goat Weed — Bodyonics
Two capsules contain: Horny Goat Weed (Epimedium Grandiflorum) (Standardized 10% Icariin) 500 mg • Maca Pure (Lepidium Meyenii)(Standardized to contain 0.6% macamides and macaenes) 250 mg • Mucuna pruriens (Standardized 15% L-Dopa (L-Dihydroxyphenylalanine)) 33.3 mg • Polypodium vulgare (Standardized 8% 20-EDC (20-Hydroxyecdysone)) 25 mg. Other Ingredients: Calcium Phosphate, Magnesium Stearate, Gelatin.

Pinnacle P-ALC 500 — Bodyonics
Each tablet contains: Phosphorolytic Acetyl L-Carnitine (PALC) (Including Inulin and Succinates) 500 mg. Other Ingredients: Calcium Phosphate, Stearic Acid, Magnesium Stearate, Silica, Croscarmellose.

Pinnacle PS Complex 500 — Bodyonics
Each tablet contains: Cephalized PS (Phosphatidyl Serine Complex) (BioActivated Phospholipid fractions standardized to 55% cephalins phosphatidyl serine, choline, inositol and ethanolamine) 500 mg. Other Ingredients: Microcrystalline Cellulose, Calcium Phosphate, Stearic Acid, Magnesium Stearate, Croscarmellose, Silica.

Pinnacle PYRUVATE 1000 — Bodyonics
Each tablet contains: Sodium 60 mg • Potassium 40 mg • Calcium 100 mg • Stabilized Trimin Pyruvate Complex 1000 mg (From Calcium, Potassium, and Sodium salts of Pyruvic Acid, plus Dihydroxyacetone. Inulinized in a bioactive complex of Phosphorolytic Dahlia Inulin providing a long chain carbohydrate molecule). Other Ingredients: Calcium Phosphate, Stearic Acid, Magnesium Stearate, Silica, Croscarmellose.

Pinnacle PYRUVATE 500 — Bodyonics
Each tablet contains: Sodium 30 mg • Potassium 20 mg • Calcium 50 mg • Stabilized Trimin Pyruvate Complex 500 mg (From Calcium, Potassium, and Sodium salts of Pyruvic Acid, plus Dihydroxyacetone. Inulinized in a bioactive complex of Phosphorolytic Dahlia Inulin providing a long chain carbohydrate molecule). Other Ingredients: Calcium Phosphate, Stearic Acid, Magnesium Stearate, Silica, Croscarmellose.

Pinnacle Super Crea Glutide A-DS — Bodyonics
One scoop contains: Creaine Monohydrate 6 g • Glutamine Peptide 2 g • Taurine 2 g • Dahlulin (Dry Dahlia Inulin Juice Complex) 500 mg • Complex Carbohydrate • Natural Flavor • Xanthan Gum • Stevia Extract • Beta Carotene.

Pinnacle Thermophen — Bodyonics
Two tablets contain: St. John's Wort (0.3% hypericin) 150 mg • Citrus Aurantium (1.5- 3% synephrine) 200 mg • Kava Kava (40% Kavalactones) 100 mg • Yerba Mate (20% Methylxanthines) 200 mg. Other Ingredients: Calcium Phosphate, Microcrystalline Cellulose, Stearic Acid, Magnesium Stearate, Croscarmellose.

Pinnacle TRIBESTROL 250 — Bodyonics
Two captabs contain: Tribulus Terrestris (providing 40% (100 mg) Furostanol Saponins) 250 mg • Herbolics Support Complex (from Catuaga - Muira Puama - Chachuhuasu - Iporuru) 100 mg. Other Ingredients: Calcium Phosphate, Stearic Acid, Magnesium Stearate, Croscarmellose.

BRAND NAMES

B R A N D   N A M E S

Pinnacle Ultra Strength Volumax Chocolate Flavor — Bodyonics
Two scoops contain: Whey Protein Concentrate (Ion Exchange) • complex Carbohydrate (Maliodextrin) • Creatine Monohydrate • Dutch Cocoa Powder • Soy Fiber • Oat Fiber • Nat. & Art. Vanilla Flavor • Colostrum 20% • Glutamine Peptide • Dahluin (Dry Dahlia Inulin Juice Complex) • Whey Protein Hydrolysate • Tourine • Potassium Phosphate • Calcium Phosphate • Magnesium Oxide • Potassium Chloride • Xanthan Gum • Aspartame • Psyllium, Monosodium Phosphate • Ascorbic Acid • Beta Carotene • dl-Alpha Tocopheryl Acetate • ferrous Fumarate • Niacinamide • Zinc Oxide • Vitamin A • Palmitate • D-Calcium Pantothenate • Manganese Sulfate • RNA Powder • Soy Lecithin • Vitamin K-1 • Copper Sulfate • Pyridoxine Hydrochloride • Riboflavin • Thiamine Hydrochloride • Cyanocobalamin • Vitamin D-3 • Folic Acid • Chromium Chloride • Biotin • Selenomethionine • Chromium Picolinate • Sodium Molybdate • Potassium Iodide • Sodium Selenate.

Pinnacle Ultra Strength Volumax Vanilla Flavor — Bodyonics
Two scoops contain: Whey Protein Concentrate (Ion Exchange) • complex Carbohydrate (Maliodextrin) • Creatine Monohydrate • Soy Fiber • Oat Fiber • Nat. & Art. Vanilla Flavor • Colostrum 20% • Glutamine Peptide • Dahluin (Dry Dahlia Inulin Juice Complex) • Whey Protein Hydrolysate • Tourine • Potassium Phosphate • Calcium Phosphate • Magnesium Oxide • Potassium Chloride • Xanthan Gum • Aspartame • Psyllium, Monosodium Phosphate • Ascorbic Acid • Beta Carotene • dl-Alpha Tocopheryl Acetate • ferrous Fumarate • Niacinamide • Zinc Oxide • Vitamin A • Palmitate • D-Calcium Pantothenate • Manganese Sulfate • RNA Powder • Soy Lecithin • Vitamin K-1 • Copper Sulfate • Pyridoxine Hydrochloride • Riboflavin • Thiamine Hydrochloride • Cyanocobalamin • Vitamin D3 • Folic Acid • Chromium Chloride • Biotin • Selenomethionine • Chromium Picolinate • Sodium Molybdate • Potassium Iodide • Sodium Selenate.

Pinnacle Whey Ahead Chocolate Flavor — Bodyonics
One scoop contains: Whey Ahead Complex (a blend of Whey Protein Concentrates and Whey Protein Isolates, and Partially Pre-digested Ion Exchanged Whey Protein Hydrolysates) • Creatine Monohydrate • Glutamin Peptide • Dutch Cocoa Powder • Natural and Artifical Vanilla Flavor • Tourine • Dahlulin (Dry Dahlia Inulin Juice Complex) • Xanthan Gum • Beta Carotene • Aspartame.

Pinnacle Whey Ahead Vanilla Flavor — Bodyonics
One scoop contains: Whey Ahead Complex a blend of Whey Protein Concentrates and Whey Protein Isolates and partially Pre-digested Ion Exchanged Whey Protein Hydrolysates • Creatine Monohydrate • Glutamine Peptide • Natural and Artifical Vanilla Flavor • Tourine • Dahlulin (Dry Dahlia Inulin Juice Complex) • Xanthan Gum • Beta Carotene • Aspartame.

Pizazz — Nature's Plus
Each tablespoon contains: L-Phenylalanine free form amino acid 250 mg • Pantothenic Acid 75 mg • Inositol 50 mg • Niacinamide 40 mg • Vitamin B1 (Thiamine) 30 mg • Vitamin B2 (Riboflavin) 30 mg • Vitamin B6 (Pyridoxine HCL) 30 mg • Choline (Bitartrate) 21 mg • Vitamin B12 (from Cobalamin) 100 mcg • Biotin 30 mcg. In a natural high-energy base of Bee Pollen, Ginseng, Gotu Kola, & Fo-Ti. Sweetened with Honey & Blackstrap Molasses. Contains no yeast, wheat, corn, soy, milk or salt.

Plant Enzimase — Nutri-Quest
Each 360 mg capsule contains: Amylase 4500 DU • Protease 15000 HUT • Lipase 65 IU • Invertase 0.25 IAU • Malt Diastase 150 DPI • Lactase 200 LacU • Cellulase 60 CU. In a base of pure Beet root Fiber.

Plantain Salve — Dial Herbs
Plantain • Chickweed • Mint • Comfrey • Oat Straw. In a base of Bees Wax, Glycerine & Cold Pressed Olive oil.

PMS Formula — Nature's Way
Three capsules contain: Black Cohosh root 150 mg • Cramp bark 250 mg • Dandelion leaf 150 mg • L-5 Hydroxytryptophan (Griffonia bean extract) 5 mg • Lobelia herb 150 mg • Magnesium Amino Acid Chelate 50 mg • Niacin (Vitamin B3) 10 mg • Pyridoxine HCL 76 mg • Riboflavin (Vitamin B2) 852 mcg • Thiamine (Vitamin B1) 750 mcg • Vitamin B12 (Cyanocobalamin) 3 mcg. Other ingredients: Gelatin, Millet.

PMS Formula — The Vitamin Shoppe
Each capsule contains: Vitamin B12 25 mcg • Vitamin B6 10 mg • St. John's Wort 150 mg • Siberian Ginseng 100 mg • Korean Ginseng root 50 mg • Chamomile 100 mg.

PMS Forte — Futurebiotics
Two tablets contain: Thiamin HCl (B1) 12 mg • Riboflavin (B2) 12 mg • Pyridoxine HCl (B6) 65 mg • Niacinamide 50 mg • Vitamin C (Ascorbic Acid) 60 mg • Dong Quai (extract equal to) 300 mg • Choline Bitartrate 75 mg • Para Amino Benzoic Acid (PABA) 85 mg • Methionine 60 mg • Inositol 50 mg • Iron (Ferrous Fumarate) 8 mg • Potassium (Citrate, Gluconate) 60 mg • Magnesium (Oxide, Amino Acid Chelate) 350 mg • Vitamin B12 40 mg • Iodine (Potassium, Iodide) 150 mcg • Zinc (Gluconate) 15 mg • Pantothenic Acid 60 mg • Folic Acid 400 mcg • Calcium (Carbonate, Phosphate) 300 mg • Vitamin E 30 IU • Ribonucleic Acid (RNA) 40 mg • Biotin 300 mcg • In a base containing Vitex (Agnus Castus), Uva Ursi, Royal Jelly, Raw Alfalfa Juice Concentrate, Cramp Bark, Betaine HCl, Chamomile, Squawvine, American Ginseng Extract, Chinese Licorice, Melissa, Marjoram, Polygonum Multiflorum.

PMS Nutritional Sytems Part I — Schiff
Eight softgels contain: Beta Carotene (Vitamin A activity) 15000 IU • Vitamin D 100 IU • Vitamin E (d-Alpha Tocopheryl Acetate) 600 IU • Vitamin C (Ascorbic Acid) 1000 mg • Folic Acid 200 mcg • Thiamine Mononitrate (Vitamin B2) 50 mg • Riboflavin (Vitamin B2) 50 mg • Niacinamide 50 mg • Vitamin B6 (Pyridoxine HCI) 200 mg • Biotin 30 mcg • Pantothenic Acid (d-Calcium Pantothenate) 50 mg • Calcium (Calcium Chlelate) 150 mg • Magnesium (Magnesium Oxide) 300 mg • Iodine (Potassium Iodide) 150 mcg • Iron (Ferrous Chelate) 15 mg • Copper (Cupric Oxide) 0.5 • Zinc (Zinc Gluconate) 25 mg • Choline Bitartrate 500 mg • Manganese (Gluconate) 10 mg • Potassium (Potassuim Chloride) 100 mg • Selenium (Selenium Chelate) 100 mcg • Chromium (Chromium Chelate) 500 mg • Inositol 500 mg • Para Aminobenzioc Acid 50 mg.

PMS Nutritional Sytems Part II — Schiff
Each softgel contains: Sarsaparilla root 210 mg • Burdock root 210 mg • Ginger root 70 mg.

PMS Tea — Traditional Medicinals
One tea bag contains: Dandelion root (Tanaxacum officinale) 500 mg. Other herbal ingredients: Roasted Carob pod, Roasted Barley, Roasted Chicory root, Parsley leaf, Oat Straw herb, Nettle leaf, Chickweed herb, Uva Ursi leaf, Cramp bark, Cornsilk style & stigma.

PMSOS — Nature's Herbs
Four capsules contain: Vitamin B6 500 mg • natural Vitamin E (d-Alpha Tocopherol Succinate) 400 IU • Uva Ursi extract (concentrated standardized for 10% Arbutin equivalent to 1200 of dried herb) 400 mg • Valerian root extract (standardized for .72-.88% valernic acid = to 1600 mg of dried herb) 400mg • White Willow bark extract (standardized for 15% salicin - White Willow extract 5:1= to 1600 mg of dried herb) 200 mg • Chasteberry extract (Vitex agnus castus - standardized for 11k ppm Glycosides equivalent to 600 mg of dried herb) 100 mg • Ginger root 305 mg • Dong Quai root 200 mg.

PN-6 Formula — Nature's Way
Each capsule contains a proprietary blend 425 mg: Squaw Vine herb, Red Raspberry leaves, Blessed Thistle herb, Black Cohosh root, Pennyroyal herb, and False Unicorn.

Pneumotrate — Progressive Labs
Each capsule contains: Vitamin A 2500 IU • Beta Carotene 2500 IU • Vitamin C 90 mg • Bovine lung concentrate 200 mg.

PoisePlus — Atrium
Six tablets contain: Vitamin A 15000 IU • Vitamin E 140 IU • Vitamin C 1050 mg • Bioflavonoids 300 mg • Chlorophyll (oil) 60 mg • Along with the following Amino Acid chelated minerals: Calcium 500 mg • Magnesium 250 mg • Potassium 99 mg • Manganese 10 mg • Iron 15 mg • Zinc 10 mg • Copper 2 mg • Iodine 150 mcg • Chromium 200 mcg • Selenium 25 mcg • Molybdenum 150 mcg • Vanadium 150 mcg • Silicon 2 mcg. In a base of Raw Bovine Tissue concentrates (not extracts) from the following: (Spleen 150 mg, Brain 30 mg, Liver 25 mg, Heart 15 mg, Kidney 15 mg, Thymus 10 mg, Adrenal 10 mg, Pituitary 10 mg, Pancreas 10 mg, Duodenus 10 mg) 285 mg.

Polysorbate 80 — The Vitamin Shoppe
Contains 100% pharmaceutical-grade Polysorbate 80.

Positive Thoughts — Source Naturals
Three tablets contain: St. John's Wort (Hypericum Perforatum) 900

mg Yielding 0.3% Hypericin (2.7 mg) • Valerian root extract (Valeriana officinalis) 100 mg (Yielding 0.8% Valerenic Acids 800 mcg) • Kava Root Extract (Piper methysticum) 85 mg (Yielding 30% Kavalactones 25 mg) • Lemon Balm (Melissa officinalis) 100 mg • GABA (Gamma Amino Butyric Acid) 300 mg • Taurine (Magnesium Taurinate) 200 mg • Magnesium (oxide, taurinate) 200 mg • L-Tyrosine 200 mg • N-Acetyl L-Tyrosine 50 mg • L-Phenylalanine 100 mg • DMAE (Dimethylaminoethanol bitartrate) 60 mg • Vitamin C (Zinc ascorbate) 50 mg • Vitamin B1 (Thiamin) 25 mg • Vitamin B2 (Riboflavin) 25 mg • Niacinamide 50 mg • Vitamin B5 (Pantothenic Acid) 25 mg • Vitamin B6 (Pyridoxine HCl) 50 mg • Vitamin B12 (Cyanocobalamin) 25 mg • Biotin 300 mcg • Folic Acid 400 mcg • Manganese (citrate) 3 mg • Zinc (Zinc ascorbate) 10 mg.

Posture-D — S.C.P.I.
Two tablets contain: Calcium (as tribasic calcium phosphate) 1200 mg • Vitamin D (as cholecalciferol) 250 IU. Other Ingredients: Dextrose, Carboxymethylcellulose Sodium, Magnesium Stearate, Adipic Acid, Natural & Artificial Flavors, FD&C Red #40 Aluminum Lake, FD&C Blue #2 Aluminum Lake, FD&C Yellow #6 Aluminum Lake.

Potassium 50 mg — Jamieson
Each tablet contains: Potassium (as Potassium Gluconate) 50 mg.

Potassium Fuel — TwinLab
Two capsules contain: Potassium Alpha-Ketoglutarate (supplying Elemental Potassium 99 mg) 325 mg • Magnesium Alpha-Ketoglutarate (supplying Elemental Magnesium 100 mg) 700 mg.

Potassium Gluconate with Folic Acid — Quest
Each tablet contains: Potassium Gluconate 650 mg • Folic Acid 400 mcg. Other Ingredients: Croscarmellose Sodium, Calcium phosphate, Magnesium Stearate (vegetable source), Microcrystalline Cellulose, Vegetable Stearin.

Potassium Plus — Enzymatic Therapy
Each tablet contains: Potassium (Chloride/Citrate) 99 mg • Magnesium Citrate 10 mg • Magnesium Sulfate 5 mg • Pantothenic Acid (D-Calcium Pantothenate) 5 mg • Vitamin B6 (Pyroxidine HCL) 1 mg. Other ingredients: Colloidal Alkaline Ash Mineral concentrate: Alfalfa juice concentrate, Sea Plant extract, Bio-Min TR8 (Enzymatic Tract Mineral concentrate), Orange juice concentrate, Banana concentrate, & Sugar Cane juice concentrate (no sugar) 855 mg, Yucca 25 mg. Contains no sugar, salt, yeast, wheat, corn, soy, dairy products, coloring, flavoring or preservatives.

Power Fuel (Exercise & Recovery Drink) — TwinLab
Each serving contains: Carbohydrates (derived from Glucose Polymers & Glucose with small amounts of Fructose) 100 g • Anticatabolic Branched Chain Amino Acids (L-Leucine, L-Isoleucine, L-Valine) • L-Glutamine & Alpha-Ketoglutarates • Antioxidant Nutrients (Vitamin E, Vitamin C, & Beta-Carotene) • B Vitamins • Chromium (from patented Chromic Fuel Chromium Picolinate) • Coenzyme Q10 • L-Carnitine • Potassium • Magnesium • Phosphate & Creatine • Carni Fuel (a preferred form of L-Carnitine & Magnesium).

Power Herbs Migracin — Quantum
Two capsules contain: DHEA (Dehydroepiandrosterone) 25 mg • Feverfew extract 4:1 (equal to 200 mg of fresh Feverfew) 50 mg • White Willow bark extract: standardized for 15% Salicin 30 mg • extract 5:1 & powder of White Willow bark (equal to 1700 fresh Willow) 500 mg • DLPA (DL-Phenylalanine) 250 mg.

Power Nutrient — Changes - TwinLab
Two tablespoons (1 oz/30 ml) contain: Vitamin A (as 37% Beta-Carotene, 63% Retinyl palmitate) • Vitamin C (as Ascorbic acid) 60 mg • Vitamin D (as Cholecalciferol) 400 IU • Vitamin E (as DL-tocopherol) 30 IU • Thiamin (as Thiamine mononitrate) 1.5 mg • Riboflavin (as Riboflavin monophosphate) 1.7 mg • Niacin (as Niacinamide) 20 mg • Vitamin B6 (as Pyrodoxine HCL) 2 mg • Folate (as Folic acid) 400 mcg • Vitamin B12 (as Cyanocobalamin) 6 mcg • Biotin 300 mcg • Pantothenic acid (Vitamin B5) (as D-calcium pantothenate) 10 mg • Calcium (as Calcium lactate-gluconate) 40 mg • Iron 6 mg. Other ingredients: Purified water, Fructose, Citric acid, Colloidal mineral blend, Natural Cranberry flavor, Sodium benzoate, Potassium sorbate and Maltodextrin.

Power Nutrient Plus — Changes - TwinLab
One tablespoonful (15 ml) contains: Vitamin A (as 100% Beta-Carotene) 5000 IU • Vitamin C (Ascorbic acid) 60 mg • Vitamin D (as Cholecalciferol) 400 IU • Thiamin (as Thiamin HCl) 1.5 mg • Riboflavin (as Riboflavin-5-phosphate) 1.7 mg • Niacin (as

Niacinamide) 5 mg • Vitamin B6 (as Pyridoxine HCl) 2 mg • Folate (Folic acid) 400 mcg • Vitamin B12 (as Cyanocobalamin) 6 mcg • Biotin 300 mcg • Pantothenic acid (as D-calcium pantothenate) 10 mg • Calcium (as Calcium lactate-gluconate) 40 mg • Korean Ginseng root extract 50 mg. Other ingredients: Purified water, Fructose, Citric acid, Natural flavors, Aloe vera gel, Poly-colloidal organic minerals, Electrolyte complex (Potassium chloride, Magnesium citrate and Sodium citrate), Cellulose gum, Potassium sorbate, and Sodium benzoate.

Power Thin — Gold Star Nutrition
Ma Huang • Guarana • Magnesium • Chromium • Ginseng • Bladderwrack • Kola Nut • White Willow Bark • Fo-Ti • Ginger root • Gotu Kola • Licorice root • Hawthorne Berries • Saw Palmetto • Ginkgo Biloba • Boron • Spirulina • Potassium Citrate • Vitamin B12 • Folic Acid.

Power Vitamins for Men — Jamieson
Three caplets contain: Vitamin B1 (Thiamin Mononitrate) 20 mg • Vitamin B2 (Riboflavin) 20 mg • Vitamin B6 (Pyrodixine HCl) 20 mg • Niacinamide 150 mg • Vitamin B12 (Cyanocobalamin) 50 mcg • Panotothenic Acid (Calcium D-Panthenate) 30 mg • Folic Acid 0.2 mg • Vitamin A (Acetate) 7500 IU • Beta Carotene (Pro-Vitamin A) 1500 IU • Vitamin D 200 IU • Vitamin E (D-Alpha Tocopheryl Succinate) 30 IU • Vitamin C (Ascorbic Acid) 200 mg • Calcium (Carbonate) 250 mg • Magnesium (Oxide) 100 mg • Potassium 50 mg • Zinc 5 mg • Iodine (Kelp) 15 mg • Selenium 10 mcg • Chromium 10 mcg • Siberian Ginseng root (PE 1:8) 100 mg • Astragalus root (PE 1:4) 50 mg • Codonopsis root 50 mg • Damiana leaves (PE 1:6.5) 50 mg • Licorice root (PE 1:2) 50 mg • Fo-Ti root (PE 1:8) 50 mg • Grape Seed (PE 1:5) 50 mg • Citrus Bioflavoniods 50 mg • European Garlic 80 mg • Spirulina 80 mg • Chlorella 80 mg • Wheat Grass 80 mg • Borage 50 mg • Sunflower Oil 50 mg • Coenzyme Q10 (Ubiquinone) 10 mg • Seed Source Protein (Amaranth, Sunflower, Bean, Quinoa, Diu, Radish) 80 mg • Inositol 20 mg • Dl-Methionine 2.2 mg • Bromelain 48.5 mg • Papain 36.4 mg • Amylase 6.1 mg • Lipase 6.1 mg • Cellulase 3.0 mg.

PowerActin — Nature's Plus
Two capsules contain: Korean Ginseng [(Panax ginseng root) standardized 15% Ginsenosides] 250 mg • Siberian Ginseng [(Eleutherococcus senticosus root) standardized 0.8% Eleutherosides] 150 mg • Cayenne [(Capsicum frutescens fruit) standardized 100000 STU] 150 mg • Ashwagandha ([Withania somnifera root) standardized 1.5% Withanolids] 50 mg • Schisandra [(Schisandra chinensis fruit) standardized 9% Schisandrins] 50 mg • Coenzyme Q10 (Ubiquinone) 5 mg • Vitamin B12 (from Cobalamin) 500 mcg.

PoweRelief — Pain & Stress Center
Two capsules contain: DLPA (DL-Phenylalanine) 500 mg • GABA 200 mg • Boswellia 300 mg • Passion Flower 150 mg • Magnesium 10 mg • Vitamin B6 4 mg.

Pre. — Pacific BioLogic
Patrina • Peony root (white) • Bupleurum root (natural) • Ligusticum root • Jack-in-the-Pulpit rhizome • Angelica root (Chinese) • Hornet Nest • Vaccaria seeds • Argimony • Cyperus rhizome • Motherwort (Chinese) • Tumeric tuber • Bitter Orange ripened fruit.

Pregnancy Tea — Traditional Medicinals
Spearmint leaf • Red Rasberry leaf • Lemongrass leaf • Strawberry Leaf • Fennel seed • Nettle leaf • Rose Hip • Alfalfa herb • Lemon Verbena leaf.

Pregnancy-6 Formula — Nature's Way
Each capsule contains: Proprietary formula: Black Cohosh root • Blessed Thistle • False Unicorn root • Penny Royal flowering top • Red Raspberry leaves • Squaw Vine vine, leaf, fruit. Other ingredients: Gelatin.

Pregnenolone-15 — Phytopharmica
Each capsule contains: Pregnenolone 15 mg.

Prelieve PMS —
Boehringer Ingelheim Pharmaceuticals, Inc. Dist. by Pharmaton One mini-tablet contains: Standardized Vitex Agnus-Castus Extract (2:1) (fruit) 20 mg. Other Ingredients: Lactose, magnesium stearate, polyvidone, talc, PEG-100, polymethacrylic acid derivatives, FD&C blue #2, titanium dioxide, synthetic iron oxide.

Premenstra — HerbaSway
Dong Quai • Wild Yam • Knotweed • Ginger • Licorice • Blackberry • HerbaSwee (Cucurbitaceae fruit).

© Copyright 2000, Natural Medicines Comprehensive Database (209) 472-2244. For updated data, go to www.NaturalDatabase.com.

Some Brand Name Natural Products - What they Contain
www.NaturalDatabase.com contains MANY more listings than appear here.

B R A N D   N A M E S

Premium Echinacea — Holista
Each capsule contains: Echinacea angustifolia (root) from standardized 6.5:1 extract (4% echinacoside) 500 mg.

Pre-Natal — Aspen Group, Inc.
Each tablet contains: Vitamin A (from vitamin A acetate & beta carotene) 4000 IU • Vitamin D (cholecalciferol) 400 IU • Vitamin E (d2-alpha tocopherol acetate) 11 mg • Vitamin C (ascorbic acid) 100 mg • Folic acid 0.8 mg • Vitamin B1 (thiamine mononitrate) 1.84 mg • Vitamin B2 (riboflavin) 1.7 mg • Niacinamide 18 mg • Vitamin B6 (pyridoxine hydrochloride) 2.6 mg • Vitamin B12 (cyanocobalamin) 4 mcg • Calcium (calcium sulfate) 200 mg • Iron (ferrous fumerate) 20 mg • Zinc (zinc oxide) 25 mg.

Pre-Natal Caps — Now
Four capsules contain: Vitamin A (Beta Carotene) 10000 IU • Vitamin B1 (Thiamine HCL) 5 mg • Vitamin B2 (Riboflavin) 5 mg • Vitamin B3 (Niacinamide) 20 mg • Vitamin B5 (Pantothenic Acid) 20 mg • Vitamin B6 (Pyridoxine HCL) 5 mg • Vitamin B12 (Cyanocobalamin) 20 mcg • Biotin 300 mcg • Folic Acid 800 mcg • Vitamin C (Calcium Ascorbate) 120 mg • Vitamin D (Fish Liver oil) 400 IU • Vitamin E (d-Alpha Tocopheryl Succinate) 150 IU • Vitamin K 80 mcg • Calcium (Carbonate • Ascorbate) 1200 mg • Magnesium (Oxide) 500 mg • Zinc (Amino Acid Chelate) 15 mg • Iron (Bisglycinate) 36 mg • Copper (Amino Acid Chelate) 1 mg • Iodine (Kelp) 150 mcg • Manganese (Amino Acid Chelate) 3.5 mg • Selenium (L-Selenomethionine) 50 mcg • Chromium (Picolinate) 100 mcg • Molybdenum (Amino Acid Chelate) 80 mcg • Potassium (Chloride) 50 mg • Vanadium (Amino Acid Chelate) 25 mcg • Choline 10 mg • Inositol 10 mg • PABA 4 mg.

PreNatal Care — Natrol
Three tablets contain: Vitamin A (as Vitamin A palmitate & d-Salina beta carotene) 5000 IU • Vitamin C (calcium ascorbate) 100 mg • Vitamin D (as cholecalciferol) 200 IU • Vitamin E (as d-alpha tocopherol) 100 IU • Vitamin K 25 mcg • Thiamine (Vitamin B1) (as Thiamine HCI) 25 mg • Riboflavin (Vitamin B2) 25 mg • Niacinamide 25 mg • Vitamin B6 (pyridoxine HCI) 25 mg • Folic Acid 800 mcg• Vitamin B12 (as cobalamin) 50 mcg • Biotin 100 mcg • Pantothenic Acid (as calcium pantothenate) 50 mg • Calcium (as calcium carbonate) 250 mg • Iron 25 mg • Iodine (from kelp) 150 mcg • Magnesium (as magnesium oxide) 125 mg • Zinc (as zinc gluconate) 15 mg • Selenium (as l-Selenomethionine) 100 mcg • Copper (copper gluconate) 2 mg • Manganese (as manganese gluconate) 50 mcg • Potassium (as potassium proteinate) 99 mg • DHA (docosahexanoic acid) 100 mg • Choline (as choline bitartrate) 50 mg • Betaine (as betaine HCI) 50 mg • Ginger root extract 50 mg • Inositol 25 mg • PABA (para amino benzoic acid) 25 mg • Red Raspberry extract leaf 15 mg • Rosemary extract leaf 15 mg • Squaw Vine powdered aerial part 15 mg. Other ingredients: Mono & Di-Glycerides, Microcrystalline Cellulose, Stearic Acid, Silicon Dioxide, Magnesium Stearate.

Prenatal Daily — Health Factor
Three capsules contain: Beta Carotene (pro Vitamin A) 2500 IU • Vitamin A (Acetate) 4000 IU • Vitamin B1 (Thiamine HCI) 10 mg • Vitamin B2 (Riboflavin & R5'P) 10 mg • Vitamin B3 (Niacinamide) 20 mg • Calcium (Ascorbate & Carbonate) 250 mg • Iron (Feronyl) 40 mg • Vitamin D (Ergocalciferol) 400 IU • Vitamin E (d-Alpha Tocopheryl) 100 IU • Vitamin B6 (Pyridoxine HCI & P5'P) 30 mg • Folic Acid 800 mcg • Vitamin B12 (Cobalamin) 100 mcg • Iodine (Potassium Iodide) 150 mcg • Magnesium (Oxide) 125 mg • Zinc (Picolinate) 20 mg • Copper (Citrate) 2 mg • Biotin 300 mcg • Vitamin B5 (Pantothenic Acid) 25 mg • Vitamin B10 (PABA) 25 mg • Vitamin K (Phytonadione) 15 mcg • Choline (Bitartrate) 12.5 mg • Inositol 12.5 mg • Chromium (Nichrome-3) 200 mcg • Manganese (Citrate) 7 mg • Selenium (Amino Acid Chelate) 100 mcg • Lemon Bioflavonoids 25 mg • Rutin 5 mg • Hesperidin 5 mg • Lactobacillus Acidophilus (3 billion/gm) 20 mg.

Prenatal Multiple — Nature's Life
Six capsules contain: Beta Carotene (Vitamin A equivalent to 15000 IU) 9 mg • Vitamin D (Cholecalciferol) 200 IU • Vitamin B1 (Thiamine HCI) 50 mg • Vitamin B2 (Riboflavin) 50 mg • Vitamin B3 (Niacinamide) 50 mg • Vitamin B6 (Pyridoxine HCI) 75 mg • Vitamin B12 (Cyancobalamin concentrate) 50 mcg • Folic Acid 800 mcg • Pantothenic Acid (d-Calcium Pantothenate) 50 mg • Biotin (d-Biotin) 800 mcg • Inositol 50 mg • Choline (Bitartrate) 50 mg • PABA (Para Aminobenzoic Acid) 25 mg • Vitamin C 300 mg • Lemon Bioflavonoids Complex (Testlab 50%, Flavonoids, Flavones, Naringen & Eriocitrin) 50 mg • Rutin (Saphora japonica) 25 mg • Vitamin E (d-Alpha Tocopheryl Succinate) 200 IU • Vitamin K

(Phylloquinone) 5 mg • Boron (Citrate) 50 mcg • Calcium (Carbonate, Citrate/ Malate) 1000 mg • Chromium (Picolinate, Nutrition 21, US Patent #33988) 200 mcg • Copper (Gluconate, Citrate) 1.5 mg •Iodine (Potassium Iodide) 25 mcg • Iron (Fumarate, Peptonate) 18 mg • Magnesium (Oxide, Citrate) 500 mg • Manganese (Citrate) 10 mg • Molybdenum (Molybdate) 20 mcg • Potassium (Citrate, Iodide) 99 mg • Selenium (l- Selenomethionine) 100 mcg • Silicon (Dioxide) 20 mcg • Vanadium (Vanadyl Sulfate) 20 mcg • Zinc (Picolinate, Methionine) 15 mg • Red Raspberry leaf (Rubus idaeus) 100 mg • Betaine HCI 50 mg.

Prenatal Plus Optizinc — Nutrivention
Four tablets contain: Calcium (Chelate) 1200 mg • Magnesium (Chelate) 300 mg • Vitamin C 300 mg • Phosphorus (Chelate) 150 mg • Niacinamide 100 mg • Vitamin E 100 IU • Potassium 99 mg • Vitamin A 1500 IU • Pantothenic Acid 60 mg • Choline Bitartrate 60 mg • Inositol 50 mg • Vitamin B1 50 mg • Iron (Amino Acid Chelate) 45 mg • Vitamin B1 25 mg • Vitamin B2 25 mg • Zinc 25 mg • Manganese (Amino Acid Chelate) 10 mg • Vitamin D 400 IU • Copper 1 mg • Folic Acid 800 mcg • Biotin 300 mcg • Iodine (Kelp) 150 mcg • Chromium 100 mcg • Selenium 100 mcg • Vitamin B12 100 mcg • Vitamin K 100 mcg • Pumpkin seeds 200 mg • Yellow Dock 200 mg • Alfalfa 100 mg • Bioflavonoids 100 mg • Beet tops 100 mg • Horsetail grass 100 mg • Hesperidin 50 mg • PABA 30 mg • Rutin 25 mg.

Pre-Nate Oil — The Herbalist
Herbal oils of Sweet Almond, Safflower, Aloe Vera, Vitamin E, St. John's Wort flower, Calendula flower • Essential oils of French Lavender & Lemon.

Pressure-FX — HerbTech
Each capsule contains: Shark Cartilage 180 mg • Cordyceps extract 20 mg.

Pressur-Lo — Futurebiotics
Two tablets contain: Garlic (high potency, odorless, 2-1/2:1 concentrate equivalent to) 400 mg • Hawthorn berry (extract equivalent to) 375 mg • Horsetail 60 mg • Juniper berry 60 mg • Valerian 60 mg • Cayenne 50 mg • Beta Sitosterol complex 70 mg • Taurine160 mg • Calcium (carbonate, ascorbate) 160 mg • Magnesium (oxide, chloride, citrate) 120 mg • Selenium (methionate) 40 mcg • Chromium (polynicotinate) 60 mcg • Rutin 50 mg • Betaine HCl 50 mg • Niacinamide 60 mg • Zinc (gluconate) 6 mg • Ascorbic Acid 120 mg • Vitamin B1 (thiamin) 4 mg • Vitamin B2 (riboflavin) 4 mg • Vitamin B12 10 mcg • Vitamin D 50 IU • Vitamin B6 4 mg • Pantothenic Acid 40 mg • Beta Carotene 2000 IU.

Prevalin — VitaStore
Bee Pollen • Brindal Berry (Hydroxycitric Acid, HCA) • Chromium Picolinate • Ginger • Ginseng • Carnitine • White Willow Bark • Vitamin A • Vitamin B1 • Vitamin B6 • Vitamin B12 • Vitamin C • Vitamin D • Vitamin E (D-Alpha Tocopherol) • Folic Acid • Iodine (Kelp) • Niacin • d-Biotin • Pantothenic Acid • Potassium Gluconate.

Preventa Tea — HerbaSway
Soy • Green Tea • Ginger • Blackberry • HerbaSwee (Cucurbitaceae fruit).

Prevent-X — Cambridge Nutraceuticals
Each serving contains: L-Glutamine 10 g • N-Acetyl-Cysteine 4 g • Vitamin A (as mixed carotenoids) 4000 IU • Vitamin C 2000 mg • Vitamin E 700 IU • Folate 300 mcg • Magnesium 300 mg • Selenium 70 mcg • Zinc 10 mg • Copper 0.5 mg.

Prima-C — PhysioLogics
Each capsule contains: Vitamin C (as Calcium Ascorbate) 500 mg • Calcium (as Calcium Ascorbate) 57 mg • Bioflavonoids (from citrus) 7 mg • Hesperidin 10 mg • Rutin 10 mg.

Primaderm — Prime Pharmaceutical Corp. (Canadian)
Active Ingredient: Mahonia Aquifolium.

Primavar — Unknown
Each capsule contains: 19-Norandrostenedione 100 mg • 4-Androstenediol 100 mg.

Primavar II — Unknown
Each capsule contains: Bolandiol (Norandrostenediol) 100 mg • 4-Androstenediol 100 mg.

Prime Advantage Creatine Serum — Muscle Marketing USA
Each serving contains: Damiana • Yohimbe • Pygeum africanum • Glucosamine • Vitamin B12.

Some Brand Name Natural Products - What they Contain
www.NaturalDatabase.com contains MANY more listings than appear here.

Primrose Oil — Atrium
Each capsule contains: Oil of Evening Primrose 500 mg • Vitamin E (d-Alpha Tocopheryl Acetate) 10 IU • Gamma Linolenic Acid 40 mg • Lenoleic Acid 350 mg.

Pro Blend 55 — Human Development Technologies
Two scoops contain: Protein Blend (Micro Ultra Filtered Whey Protein concentrate, Egg Albumen, Calcium Caseinate, Micro Ultra Filtered Whey Protein Isolate, Ion Exchanged Whey Protein Isolate, Hydrolyzed Whey Protein Isolate) • natural & artificial Chocolate Flavorings • Acesulfame Potassium • Stevia.

Pro Fuel (Milk & Egg Protein Drink) — TwinLab
Each serving contains: Pure Milk & Egg Protein 40 g • Extra Branched Chain Amino Acids (L-Leucine, L-Isoleucine, L-Valine) • L-Glutamine • All Essential Vitamins & Minerals (including B Complex Vitamins plus Antioxidant VitaminC & Vitamin E, Calcium & Magnesium. Patented Chromic Fuel Chromium Picolinate (Potassium, Zinc & Chromium).

Pro Lite — Optimum Nutrition
L-Carnitine • Choline • Inositol.

Pro-50 — Enzymatic Therapy
Each capsule contains: Vitamin A (Fish Liver oil) 1500 IU • Zinc (Chelate) 20 mg • Vitamin B6 (Pyridoxine HCL) 10 mg • Other ingredients: EFA (unrefined Vegetable Lipids) 630 mg • Amino Acid Complex 150 mg • Prostate extract freeze-dried 150 mg • Saw Palmetto Berry extract 4:1 100 mg. Contains no sugar, salt, yeast, corn, dairy products, flavoring or preservatives. All organs & glands derived from bovine sources.

Pro-Antho Forte — Progressive Labs
Each capsule contains: Pycnogenol 10 mg • Grape seed extract (Vitis vinifera) (5:1 concentrate) 50 mg • Ginkgo leaf extract (Ginkgo biloba) (50:1 concentrate) 20 mg • Green Tea leaf extract (Camellia sinensis) (65% standardized extract) 75 mg • Quercetin 100 mg • Milk Thistle (Silibum marianum) (80% standardized extract) 10 mg. Pycnogenol is the registered trademark of Horphag Research Ltd. Pycnogenol is an extract of the bark of French Coastal Pine (Pinus maritime). Contains no animal products.

Probiata — Wakunaga of America
Each tablet contains: Lactobacillus acidophilus 1 billion live cells in a vegetable starch complex.

Probiotic A.Y. — Futurebiotics
Lactobacillus acidophilus 3 billion cells at formulation NutraFlora FOS (Fructooligosaccharides) 600 mg • Inulin FOS 200 mg • Garlic (Pure-Gar 1500TM deodorized concentrate) 75 mg • Pau D'Arco 25 mg • Licorice (4:1 extract) 25 mg • Caprylic Acid (MCT) 100 mg • Echinacea (4:1 extract) 25 mg.

Pro-Brom — Atrium
Each tablet contains: Bromelain 100 mg • Papayotin 30 mg.

Pro-Essence — Flora
Burdock root • Juniper Berry • Prickly Ash bark • Slippery Elm bark • Uva Ursi.

Pro-F Complex — Phytopharmica
Two tablets contain: Vitamin A (Fish Liver oil) 3000 IU • Vitamin D (Fish Liver oil) 100 IU • Calcium (Lactate) 82 mg • Zinc (Chelate) 20 mg • Magnesium (Citrate) 13 mg • Other ingredients: Pacific Sea Kelp 200 mg • Ovarian extract 90 mg • Whole Pituitary extract 60 mg • Adrenal extract 60 mg • Uterus extract 60 mg • RNA powder 60 mg. Contains no sugar, salt, yeast, wheat, corn, soy, dairy products, coloring, flavoring or preservatives. All organs & glands derived from bovine sources.

Pro-Gain — Nature's Life
Two scoops (28.35 g) contain: SUPRO brand soy protein isolate containing Lecithin • Whey • Fructose • Non-fat Dry Milk • natural Vanilla Flavor • Yeast • Egg Albumin • Eggshell powder • Kelp • natural Papain Enzyme concentrate • Cobalamin concentrate (B12). Pro-Gain also contains 34 mg of naturally occuring Isoflavones, including 21 mg Genistein & 10 mg Daidzen.

Progensa — Life-Flo
Each ounce contains: Natural Progesterone USP Grade 480 mg. Other Ingredients: Grape seed extract, aloe vera, vitamin E, & primrose.

ProgestaCare — Life-Flo
Aloe Vera gel • Caprylic/Capric Triglyceride • natural Progesterone

derived from the Mexican Wild Yam root • Evening Primrose oil (Oenothera biennis) • Vitamin E Acetate • Isostearic Acid • Glyceryl Stearate • Siberian Ginseng • Burdock root • Black Cohosh • MSM • Chamomile • Glycerin • Allantoin • Grape seed extract.

Pro-Gest-Ade — Enzymatic Therapy
Each tablet contains: Niacinamide 10 mg. Other ingredients: Betaine HCL 155 mg • Glutamic Acid HCL 155 mg • Bromelain (600 MCU) 100 mg • Papain 100 mg • Mylase (Lipase) 100 mg • Mycozyme (Fungal amylase) 25 mg • Ox Bile extract 16 mg • Pancreas extract 16 mg. Contains no sugar, salt, yeast, wheat, corn, soy, dairy products, coloring, flavoring or preservatives.

Progesterone Plus Creme — Nutri-Quest
Water • Stearic Acid • Cetyl Alcohol • Sesame oil • Progesterone USP (Homeopathic) • Triethanolame • Arnica oil • Evening Primrose oil • Zinc • Copper • Magnesium • Glyconucleopeptides • Peg 10 Soya Sterol • Hydroxyethylcellulose • Disodium EDTA • Cetyl Ricinoleate • Canola oil • Wild Yam • Dex-Panthenol (Vitamin B5) • Progesterone USP • Honey • Lecithin • NaPCA • Silicon • Iron • Peg 7 Glycerol Cocoate • Carrot oil • Carbomer • Phenyldimethicone • Sodium Hydroxymethylglycinate.

ProGram16: Chocolate — Pharmanex
One bar contains: Creatine 1 g • Taurine 250 mg • High Fructose Corn Syrup • Whey Protein Isolate • Soy Protein Isolate • Sugar • Milk Protein Isolate • Cocoa Butter • Unsweetened Chocolate • Lowfat Cocoa (Processed with Alkali) • Milk • Creatine Monohydrate • Glycerin • Maltodextrin • Dicalcium Phosphate • Natural and Artificial Flavors • Taurine • Magnesium Carbonate • Potassium Chloride • Potassium Citrate • Egg Whites • Ascorbic Acid • Lecithin • d-Alpha Tocopherol Acetate • Beta-Catrotene • Niacinamide • Calcium Pantothenate • Zinc Oxide • Chromium Chelate • Carbonyl Iron • Copper Gluconate • Manganese Sulfate • Pyridoxine Hydrochloride • Riboflavin • Thiamine Mononitrate • Folate (Folic Acid) • Biotin • Potassium Iodide • Sodium Molybdate • Sodium Selenitel Phytonadine • Cholecalciferol • Cyanocobalamin.

ProGram16: Coconut — Pharmanex
Each bar contains: High Fructose Corn Syrup • Whey Protein Isolate • Soy Protein Isolate • Sugar • Partially Defatted Peanut Flour • Milk Protein Isolate • Cocoa Butter • Unsweetened Chocolate • Milk • Creatine Monohydrate • Glycerin • Natural and Artificial Flavors • Maltodextrin • Dicalcium Phosphate • Potassium Chloride • Taurine • Magnesium Carbonate • Egg Whites • Ascorbic Acid • Lecithin • salt • d-Alpha Tocopherol Acetate • Beta-Catrotene • Niacinamide • Calcium Pantothenate • Zinc Oxide • Chromium Chelate • Carbonyl Iron • Copper Gluconate • Manganese Sulfate • Pyridoxine Hydrochloride • Riboflavin • Thiamine Mononitrate • Folate (Folic Acid) • Biotin • Potassium Iodide • Sodium Molybdate • Sodium Selenite • Phytonadine • Cholecalciferol • Cyanocobalamin.

ProGram16: Peanut Butter — Pharmanex
Each bar contains: High Fructose Corn Syrup • Whey Protein Isolate • Soy Protein Isolate • Sugar • Partially Defatted Peanut Flour • Milk Protein Isolate • Cocoa Butter • Unsweetened Chocolate • Milk • Creatine Monohydrate • Glycerin • Maltodextrin • Dicalcium Phosphate • Natural and Artificial Flavors • Taurine • Magnesium Carbonate • Potassium Chloride • Egg Whites • Ascorbic Acid • Lecithin • salt • d-Alpha Tocopherol Acetate • Beta-Catrotene • Niacinamide • Calcium Pantothenate • Zinc Oxide • Chromium Chelate • Carbonyl Iron • Copper Gluconate • Manganese Sulfate • Pyridoxine Hydrochloride • Riboflavin • Thiamine Mononitrate • Folate (Folic Acid) • Biotin • Potassium Iodide • Sodium Molybdate • Sodium Selenite • Phytonadine • Cholecalciferol • Cyanocobalamin.

Pro-Guard — Man-Nutra-Life Health and Fitness
Each tablet contains: Saw Palmetto Fruit 500 mg • Hydrangea Root and Rhiz. 100 mg • Golden Rod Herb 50 mg • Couch Grass Root 200 mg • Horsetail Herb 100 mg • Panax Ginseng Root 100 mg • Zinc Gluconate (Providing 15 mg zinc) 112.5 mg • Magnesium Amino Acid Chelate (Providing magnesium 15 mg) 75 mg • Calcium Ascorbate 250 mg • Pyridoxine Hydrocholoride (Vitamin B6) 15 mg • Glutamine 100 mg • Glycine 100 mg • Alanine 100 mg. No added sugar, yeast, artificial colours, gluten or animal products.

PRO-HGH Symbiotropin Growth Hormone Releasing Complex — Nutraceutics Co.
Two tablets contain: Anterior Pituitary Peptides • Aminotrope-7 (a sequenced glycoamino acid complex) 4200 mg • Novel Polyose complex (pharmaceutical mono, poly & oligo saccharides) 2230 mg. All in a base of: (L-Glutamine, L-Arginine, L-Pyroglutamate, GABA,

© Copyright 2000, Natural Medicines Comprehensive Database (209) 472-2244. For updated data, go to www.NaturalDatabase.com.

BRAND NAMES

**B
R
A
N
D

N
A
M
E
S**

L-Glycine, L-Lysine, L-Tyrosine & Vicia Faba Major. Naturally sweetened & flavored.

Prolab CarbPRO — ProLab
Granulated Medium Length Complex Carbohydrates (Maltodextrin) extracted from grains.

ProLab GlutaMASS — ProLab
Each capsule contains: L-Glutamine 275 mg • Alpha-Ketoglutaric Acid 250 mg • Taurine 150 mg • Calcium (AKG) 63 mg • Magnesium (oxide) 25 mg • Potassium (citrate) 25 mg • RNA 9.5 mg • Manganese 400 mcg.

ProLab Lean Rx — ProLab
Each 72 g packet contains: Protein Blend of Milk Protein Isolates • Caseinates • Whey Protein Concentrates & Egg Whites • Maltodextrin • Cocoa • Natural Flavors • Dicalcium Phosphate • Potassium Chloride • Dipotassium Phosphate • Potassium Citrate • Sodium Chloride • Sodium Citrate • Magnesium Oxide • Medium Chain Triglycerides • Choline Bitartrate • Vegetable Gum • Aspartame • Lecithin • Betaine • Beta Carotene • Manganese Sulfate • Canola oil • Glutamine • Inositol • Vitamin E Acetate • Vitamin B12 • Vitamin A Palmitate • Thiamine • Riboflavin • Vitamin D • Niacin • Pyridoxine HCL • Calcium Pantothenate • Potassium Iodide • Errous Gluconate • Copper Gluconate • Zinc Oxide • Biotin • Folic Acid • Selenium Chelate • Molybdenium Yeast • Vitamin K • Paba • Chromium Picolinate.

ProLab MSM — ProLab
Each capsule contains: MSM (Methyl-Sulfonyl-Methane) 1000 mg.

ProLab N-Large 2 — ProLab
Each serving (153 g) contains: Maltodextrin • Cross-Flow Micro-Filtered Cold Processed Ion Exchanged Whey • Fructose • Natural Flavoring.

ProLab Stoked — ProLab
Each rounded scoop contains: Caffeine 200 mg • Ephedra alkaloids 20 mg • Guarana 10 mg • Green Tea extract 10 mg • White Willow 75 mg. In a base of Yohimbe bark, Quercitin & Citrus aurantium.

Pro-Life Soy Protein — Nature's Life
Two scoops (28.35 g) contain: Supro brand soy protein isolate containing Lecithin • natural Vanilla Flavor • natural Papain Enzyme concentrate • Cobalamin concentrate.

Pro-Lite Soy Protein — Nature's Life
Two scoops (28.35 g) contain: Supro brand soy protein isolate containing Lecithin • natural Vanilla Flavor • natural Papain Enzyme concentrate • Cobalamin concentrate.

Promend — The Herbalist
Saw Palmetto berry • Goldenrod flower tops • Echinacea root • Horsetail herb • Plantain herb • Ginger root.

Promensil — Novogen
Each tablet contains: Isoflavone Phytoestrogens (as Red Clover leaf extract) 40 mg. Other Ingredients: Dicalcium phosphate, Microcrystalline cellulose, Hydroxypropyl methylcellulose, Magnesium stearate, Mixed tocopherols, Silica, Soy polysaccharide, Titanium dioxide, Polyethylene glycol, & Organic coloring containing: Red 40, Yellow 6, Yellow 5, Blue 1.

ProOmega — Nordic Naturals
EPA 173 mg • DHA 123 mg • Other Omega-3 49 mg.

Propalmex — Chattem, Inc.
Each softgel contains: Zinc (chelated from zinc gluconate) 75 mg • Standardized Saw Palmetto berry extract (85%-95% free fatty acids & phytosterols) 160 mg • Standardized Pumpkin seed oil extract (85%-95% free fatty acids) 40 mg.

Propax — Nutritional Therapeutics
Each multipack contains: Vitamin A (as acetate) 4375 IU • Vitamin A (as natural beta-carotene) 3750 IU • Vitamin C (as calcium ascorbate) 150 mg • Vitamin D3 (as cholecalciferol) 32 IU • Vitamin E (as d-alpha tocopherol) 145 IU • Vitamin K (as phytonadione) 2.5 mcg • Vitamin B1 6.25 mg • Vitamin B2 30 mg • Vitamin B3 (as niacinamide) 60 mg • Vitamin B6 (as pyridoxine/P-5-P) 40 mg • Folic Acid (as folate) 200 mcg • Vitamin B12 25 mcg • Biotin 25 mcg • Pantothenic Acid (as d-calcium) 25 mg • Calcium (as phosphate, ascorbate, citrate, sulfate, borogluconate) 360 mg • Iodine (as kelp) 18.75 mcg • Magnesium (as carbonate, oxide, glycinate, sulfate) 160 mg • Zinc (as methionate) 12.5 mg • Selenium (as selenomethionate)

75 mcg • Copper (as tyrosinate) 300 mcg • Manganese (as glycinate) 2.5 mg • Chromium (as nicotinate) 50 mcg • Molybdenum (as glycinate) 20 mcg • Potassium (as citrate) 12.8 mg • DHA (as Docosahexaenoic Acid) 120 mg • EPA (as Eicosopentaenoic Acid) 180 mg • Bioflavonoids (as citrus, rutin, rosehips, quercetin) 165 mg • Boron (as calcium borogluconate) 500 mcg • Co Enzyme Q 10 4 mg • Grape Seed Extract 5 mg • Inositol 24 mg • Pantethine (as coenzyme A precursor) 70 mg • Phosphoglycolipids 160 mg • Vanadium (as vanadyl sulfate) 12.5 mcg • Creatine - Monohydrate, Phosphate 122.5 mg • Alpha-Keto Glutarate 125 mg • Glutathione (as reduced) 5 mg • L-Tyrosine 60 mg • N-Acetyl-L-Cysteine 25 mg • Taurine 110 mg • Green Tea Extract 50 mg • Horsetail (as silica) 12.5 mg • Lactoferrin 4 mg • NT Factor (as tablet base) proprietary blend 1400 mg: defatted rice bran, arginine, beet root fiber, black strap molasses, glycine, magnesium sulfate, enriched polyunsaturated phosphatidyl choline (phospholipids), saponin (glycolipids), para-amino benzoate, leek, pantethine (bifidus growth factor), taurine, garlic, calcium borogluconate, omega-6 essential fatty acids, omega-3 essential fatty acids, artichoke, barley malt, potassium citrate, calcium sulfate, spirulina, bromelain, natural vitamin E, calcium ascorbate, alpha-lipoic acid, oligosaccharides, B-6, niacinamide, tocotrienols, riboflavin, inositol, niacin, calcium pantothenate, thiamin, B-12, bifidus, acidophilus, folic acid, chromium picolinate. Other Ingredients: Gelatin (soft gel capsules), microcrystalline cellulose, croscarmellose sodium, vegetable magnesium stearate, silica, water & glycerin.

Prophet 3H — Unknown.
Editor's Comments: The manufacturer refuses to disclose the ingredients of this product. Anecdotal evidence suggests that this product may have induced a seizure in one patient. Patients should be strongly encouraged to avoid using this product until more is known about its contents and safety.

Propo-Mune — Atrium
Each tablet contains: Propolis 5X 92 mg • Thymus 67 mg • Lymph 30 mg • Spleen 25 mg • Brain 25 mg • Folic Acid 400 mcg.

Prosta Glan — Progressive Labs
Each capsule contains: Magnesium (as magnesium gluconate) 10 mg • Zinc (as zinc gluconate) 3.3 mg • Raw Bovine prostate concentrate 80 mg • Saw Palmetto 4:1 extract Lipoic Sterolic (Serenoa repens) 100 mg • Pygeum (Prunus africanum) 25 mg • Glutamic Acid 135 mg • Alanine 135 mg • Glycine 135 mg • Uva Ursi leaf (Arctostaphylos uva-ursi) 10 mg • Unsaturated Fatty Acids 10 mg • Pumpkin seed concentrate (Curcurbita pepo) 10 mg • Pollen 5 mg. The glandular concentrate in this product is prepared by a special process which does not exceed physiological temperature (37° C). Guaranteed free of chemical pesticides and synthetic hormones.

Prosta Kit — Flora
Formula 1: Palmitol Saw Palmetto berries • Zinc 50mg • Vitamin B6 120 mg. Formula 2: Flax-O-Mega cold pressed flax seed oil 1000 mg. Formula 3: Pro-Essence Burdock root • Juniper Berry • Prickly Ash bark • Slippery Elm bark • Uva Ursi.

Prosta Support — Nutri-Quest
Each tablet contains: Vitamin C 10 mg • Vitamin B6 10 mg • Vitamin E (Succinate) 5 IU • Zinc Chelate 10 mg • L-Glycine 120 mg • L-Alanine 120 mg • L-Glutamic Acid 120 mg • Saw Palmetto 106 mg • Pygeum africanus extract 10 mg • Pygeum africanus herb 20 mg • Pumpkin seed 200 mg • Stinging Nettle leaves 75 mg • Echinacea 25 mg • Ginkgo Biloba 20 mg • Wild Yam 20 mg • Uva Ursi 10 mg.

Prostabs Plus — Futurebiotics
Three tablets contain: • Glutamic Acid 390 mg • Glycine 390 mg • Raw Prostate Concentrate 150 mg • Alanine 390 mg • Vitamin B6 7.5 mg • Vitamin C (Ascorbate) 15 mg • Zinc (Gluconate) 30 mg • Magnesium (Oxide) 105 mg • Saw Palmetto Berry Extract (4:1 extract equivalent to) 300 mg.

Prosta-Comp — Atrium
Each tablet contains: Saw Palmetto berry extract 100 mg • Pumpkin seed oil extract 50 mg • Pygeum africanum extract 25 mg • Uva Ursi 50 mg • Zinc Gluconate 25 mg • Hydrangea extract 150 mg • Panax ginseng extract 100 mg. Contains no sugar, starch, salt, wheat, corn, milk, yeast or soy derivatives.

Prost-Actin — Nature's Plus
Each tablet contains: Saw Palmetto berries 250 mg • Raw Prostate concentrate 140 mg • Zinc (Monomethionine) 50 mg • Vitamin A (Beta Carotene) 10000 IU • Vitamin E natural 200 IU. Contains no yeast, wheat, corn, soy, milk, salt, sugar or starch.

Some Brand Name Natural Products - What they Contain
www.NaturalDatabase.com contains MANY more listings than appear here.

Prostactive Plus Saw Palmetto — Nature's Way
Each softgel contains: Concentrated 12:1 Saw Palmetto Berry Extract 160 mg • Concentrated 10:1 Nettle Root Extract 120 mg.

ProstaMed — Enzymatic Therapy
Each capsule contains: Saw Palmetto Berry extract 160 mg standardized to contain 85%-95% fatty acids & sterols: 0.15% - 0.3% fatty alcohols, 0.2%-0.4% total sterols, 0.1%-0.3% beta-sitosterol. Contains no sugar, salt, yeast, wheat, corn, dairy products, flavoring or preservatives.

Prosta-Metto — The Vitamin Shoppe
Each softgel contains: Saw Palmetto extract 160 mg • Pumpkin seed oil 40 mg • Pygeum Africanum extract 10 mg • Bearberry extract 10 mg • Zinc 15 mg • Vitamin B6 5 mg.

ProstaPro — Phytopharmica
Each capsule contains: Saw Palmetto Berry extract 160 mg standardized to contain: Fatty Acids & Sterols 85%-95% • Fatty Alcohols 0.15%-0.3% • Total Sterols 0.2%-0.4% • Beta-Sitosterol 0.1%-0.3%. Contains no sugar, salt, yeast, wheat, corn, dairy products, flavorings or preservatives.

Prosta-Q — Farr Laboratories, LLC
Each capsule contains: Zinc (from zinc gluconate) 5 mg • Proprietary Blend (Quercetin, Cranberry (berry), Saw Palmetto (berry), Bromelain, Papain) 540 mg.

Prostata — Gero Vita
Urtica Dioica extract 16:1 150 mg • Serenoa Serrulata extract 106 mg • Apis Mellifica 83.33 mg • L-Alanine 66.67 mg • Glycine 66.67 mg • L-Glutamic Acid 66.67 mg • Pygeum Africanum extract 50 mg • Vitamin B6 15 mg • Panax Ginseng extract 8.33 mg • Zinc Arginate 7.5 mg • Hydrangea extract 5 mg • Copper 0.5 mg • Beta Carotene 8333 IU.

Prostate — Centrum Focused Formulas
One softgel contains: Vitamin A as Beta-carotene 5000 IU • Lycopene 1.5 mg • Saw Palmetto standardized Lipophilic fruit extract (Serenoa repens) 160 mg.

Prostate — ProHerbs
Two softgels contain: Vitamin E (Dl-Alpha Tocopheryl Acetate) 30 IU • Zinc (as Sulfate) 15 mg • Selenium (as Selenomethionine) 200 mcg • LycoPure (equivalent to 5 mg Lycopene) 71 mg • Saw Palmetto berries (Serenoa repens standardized to 85%-95% free fatty acids) 320 mg • Stinging Nettle root (Urtica dioca L. 2% minimum plant silica) 200 mg • Pumpkin Seed Oil (Cucurbita pepo seeds) 30 mg. Other Ingredients: Soybean Oil, Beeswax, Gelatin, Glycerin, Water, Chlorophylline, Sodium, Copper, Titanium Dioxide.

Prostate Formula — Nature's Way
Two capsules contain: Beta Glucan 2.2 mg • Calcium 26 mg • Dandelion leaf 230 mg • Lycopene 2.4 mg • Saw Palmetto dried extract 360 mg • Soy Isoflavone dried extract 25 mg • Zinc (Amino Acid Chelate) 7 mg. Other ingredients: Gelatin, Magnesium Stearate, Millet, Silica.

Prostate Formula — Youngevity
Saw Palmetto 400 mg • Pygeum bark 80 mg • Pumpkin seed 80 mg • Atractylodes herb • Licorice root 40 mg • Bupleurum root 40 mg • Vitamin E 100 IU • Vitamin C 60 mg • Vitamin B6 4 mg • Vilcabamba Mineral Essence: Potassium, Calcium, Magnesium, Zinc, Chromium, Selenium, Iron, Copper, Molybdenum, Vanadium, Iodine, Cobalt, Manganese.

Prostate Guardian — Clinician's Choice
Three tablets contain: Vitamin E (dl-alpha tocopheryl acetate) 150 IU • Zinc (glycinate) 15 mg • Niacin (niacinamide) 15 mg • Pygeum Bark Powder 30 mg • Saw Palmetto Berries 450 mg • Kudzu Root 450 mg • Pumpkin Seeds 360 mg • Panax Ginseng Root 150 mg • Siberian Ginseng Root 150 mg • Oat Straw Extract (10:1) 150 mg • Horny Goat Weed 90 mg • RoseOx (patented, standardized process for an extract of Rosemary) 75 mg • Cayenne Fruit • Proprietary blend 12 mg: Lycopene 1%, Citrus Bioflavanoid Complex, Horsetail Herb, Isoflavones.

Prostate Support — Amazon Support
Each capsule contains: Mutamba • Brazilian Peppertree • Jatoba • Nettles • Pau D'Arco • Chanca Piedra • Cipo Cabeludo • Sarsaparilla.

Prostate Support — Now
Each gelcap contains: Saw Palmetto • Pygeum • Stinging Nettle • Lycopene. Other ingredients: Pumpkin seed oil, Zinc & Vitamin B6.

Prostate Support Formula — PhysioLogics
Two capsules contain: Zinc (Glycinate) 15 mg • Copper (Glycinate) 2 mg • Vitamin B6 (Pyridoxine HCL) 100 mg • Beta Sitosterol 60 mg • Pygeum (2.5% Phytosterols 2.5 mg) 100 mg • Pumpkin seed powder 100 mg • Nettles (1-2% Plant Silica, 4-8 mg) 400 mg.

Prostate-Duo — Uronat Nutrition Company, Inc.
Each softgel contains: Saw Palmetto extract (minimun 85% free fatty acids & 5% sterols) 160 mg • Pygeum africanum extract (minimum 13% sterols) 50 mg. Other Ingredients: Gelatin, Glycerin, Pumpkin seed oil, Water, Carob. Free from sugar, salt, starch, artificial colors, preservatives, yeast, wheat, corn & milk.

Prostatonin — Pharmaton
Each capsule contains: Pygeum africanum 25 mg • Nettle Root 300 mg. Other Ingredients: Gelatin, triglycerides, glycerol, sorbitol, saya lecitin, synthetic iron oxides, & titanium dioxide.

Prostex — Metabolic Products
Two capsules contain: Proprietary Amino Acid blend: Glutamic Acid, Alanine, Aminoacetic Acid (glycine) 810 mg. Other ingredients: Gelatin, Polyethylene glycol 8000.

ProstGard — Holista
Each capsule contains: Zinc (from gluconate) 15 mg • Vitamin B6 (pyridoxine HCl) 5 mg • Saw Palmetto (Serenoa repens) extract of berries (10:1) 80 mg • Pumpkin Seed Oil 500 mg.

Prostoid — HealthWatchers System
Vitamin C • Vitamin A • Vitamin E • Vitamin B6; Serenoa Senulata • Pygeum Africanum Extract • Hydrangea Extract • Bee Pollen • Siberian Ginseng Extract • Glutamic Acid • L-Glycine • L-Alanine • Silica • Solidago Fragrans Extract • Zinc • Damiana • Dong Quai • Gotu Kola • Juniper • Copper.

Protazyme — Enzymatic Therapy
Each tablet contains: Potassium Chloride 32 mg • Niacinamide 10 mg • Vitamin B6 (Pyridoxine HCL) 500 mcg • Other Ingredients: Betaine HCL 325 mg • Glutamic Acid HCL 195 mg • Pepsin 1:10000 97 mg • Ammonium Chloride 32 mg • Papain 6X 30 mg • Ox Bile extract 15 mg • Pancreatic Enzymes 4X 10 mg. Contains no sugar, salt, yeast, wheat, corn, soy, dairy products, coloring, flavoring or preservatives.

Protector Caps — The Vitamin Shoppe
Three capsules contain: Vitamin A (Beta-carotene) 10000 IU • Vitamin E (d-alpha tocopheryl succinate) 200 IU • Ester C 500 mg • Pycnogenol 10 mg • Selenium (L-Selenomethionine) 50 mcg • CoQ10 10 mg • Green Tea extract (30% Polyphenols) 25 mg • Quercetin 25 mg.

Protector SPF 15 — Jason
Vitamin C Complex • Beta Hydroxy Acid.

Protein 95 Soy Protein — Nature's Life
Two 2 scoops (28.35 g) contain: SUPRO brand Soy Protein Isolate containing Lecithin • natural Vanilla Flavor • natural Papain Enzyme concentrate.

Protein Boost — Nutri-Quest
Two tablespoons contain: Alanine 646 mg • Arginine 1190 mg • Aspartic Acid 1853 mg • Cystine 187 mg • Glutamic Acid 3060 mg • Glycine 680 mg • Histidine 408 mg • Isoleucine 765 mg • Leucine 1275 mg • Lysine 986 mg • Methionine 221 mg • Phenylalanine 850 mg • Proline 901 mg • Serine 833 mg • Threonine 612 mg • Tyrosine 629 mg • Valine 782 mg. Ingredients: Isolated Soy Protein, Calcium & Sodium Caseinate, Tri Calcium Phosphate, Lecithin, Soybean oil, Magnesium Oxide, Papain, Ascorbic Acid, Ferrous Fumarate, Kelp, Niacin, Calcium Pantothenate, Vitamin A, Pyridoxine HCL, Thiamine HCL, Riboflavin, Vitamin D & natural Vanilla Flavor. All acids of (L) form.

ProtoChol Chewables — Fields of Nature
Each tablet contains: Phytosterol Concentrate 400 mg (as Beta-Sitosterol 172 mg, Campesterol 100 mg, Stigmasterol 44 mg). Other Ingredients: Dextrose, Magnesium Stearate, Adipic Acid, Aspartame, Natural and artificial flavors, Artificial colors (FD&C Red No. 40 Lake).

Protykin/ Reservatrol — Natrol
Two capsules contain: Polygonum cuspidatum extract root 50 mg • trans-Reservatrol 10 mg Total Reservatrols 12 mg • Emodin 5 mg. Other ingredients: Rice powder, Magnesium Stearate, Gelatin.

BRAND NAMES

Some Brand Name Natural Products - What they Contain
www.NaturalDatabase.com contains MANY more listings than appear here.

B
R
A
N
D

N
A
M
E
S

Provol — Upsher-Smith Laboratories
Pygeum africanum bark extract 50 mg.

ProXeed. — Sigma-Tau Pharmaceuticals, Inc.
Each packet contains: Active Ingredients: L-Carnitine Fumarate 1 g • Fructose • Acetyl L-Carnitine HCL .5 g • Citric Acid. Inactive Ingredients: Mannitol, polyethylene glycol, artificial flavorings, povidone, & silicone dioxide.

Proxylon — Syn Trax
Each capsule contains: 7-Isopropoxyisoflavone 250 mg.

PS Memory Care — Sundown Vitamins
Each softgel contains: Phosphatidylserine complex 500 mg Standardized to: Phosphatidylserine 100 mg • Phosphatidylcholine 45 mg • Phosphatidylethanolamine 10 mg • Phosphatidylinositol 5 mg. Other Ingredients: Soya Lecithin, Gelatin, Glycerine, Soybean Oil, Water.

Pseudo Ephedrine 30 mg — D & E Pharmaceuticals
Each tablet contains: Psuedo Ephedrine 30 mg.

Pseudo Ephedrine 60 mg — D & E Pharmaceuticals
Each tablet contains: Pseudo Ephedrine 60 mg.

Psoriasis Support — Amazon Support
Each capsule contains: Samambaia • Cat's Claw • Suma • Sarsaparilla • Bitter Melon • Chanca Piedra • Fedegosa • Gervao • Boldo.

Psyllium (Secrets of the Psyllium & Orange Flavored Psyllium Powder) — Trader Joe's
Psyllium husk fiber • Secrets of the Psyllium 85%: Fiber (per heaping tablespoon) 6 g • Orange flavored Psyllium powder 35%: Fiber (per heaping tablespoon) 3 g.

PTE Support — PhysioLogics
Two capsules contain: Bromelain (2400 GDU) 500 mg • Serratiopeptidase 10 mg.

Pure C Crystals — Nature's Life
Each 1/4 teaspoon contains: Vitamin C (Ascorbic Acid) 1250 mg.

Pure Citrimax — Natrol
One capsule contains: (-) Hydroxycitric Acid 250 mg. Other ingredients: Gelatin, Magnesium Stearate.

Pure Energy — Montana Big Sky
Each 800 mg caplet contains: Bee Pollen (Apis pollenus) • Dibaxic Calcium Phosphate • Gotu Kola (Centella asiatica) • Siberian Ginseng (Eleuterococcus senticosus) • Gotu Kola standardized extract • Royal Jelly • Siberian Ginseng standardized extract.

Pure Velvet — Velvet Health
100% premium quality pure Deer Velvet.

Pur-Gar — Now
Each tablet contains: Pur-Gar 600 mg.

Pycnogenol — Now
Each capsule contains: European Pine bark.

Pycnogenol — Olympia Nutrition
Proanthocyanidins from pine bark.

Pycnogenol 25 Mg — Natrol
One capsule contains: Pine Bark extract 25 mg. Other ingredients: Microcrystalline Cellulose, Magnesium Stearate, Gelatin.

Pycnogenol 50 Mg — Natrol
One capsule contains: Pine Bark extract 50 mg. Other ingredients: Microcrystalline Cellulose, Magnesium Stearate, Gelatin.

Pycnogenol Plus — Aspen Group, Inc.
Each capsule contains: Bioflavonoids 200 mg • Grape Seed extract 25 mg • Pycnogenol 25 mg.

Pycnogenol Plus — Atrium
Each capsule contains: Bioflavonoids 200 mg • Grape seed extract 25 mg • Pycnogenol 25 mg.

Pycnogenol with Vitamins C, E, & A — Derma E
Pycnogenol • Vitamin C • Vitamin E • Vitamin A.

Pycno-Plus Protection — HealthWatchers System
Grape Seed Extract • Pine Bark Pwder Plus • Beta Carotene • Vitamin C • Cat's Claw Powder • Bioflavonoids • Rutin • Acerola.

Pygeum — Nature's Way
Each capsule contains: Pygeum bark extract concentrate (standardized to 13% sterols 6.5 mg) 50 mg • B6 (Pyridoxine HCl)12.5 mg • Zinc (Citrate) 15 mg • Copper (Citrate) 1.5 mg • Selenium 50 mcg. In a base of Pumpkin seed oil.

Pyridoxal 5-Phosphate Plus — Klaire Laboratories
Each capsule contains: Pyridoxal 5-Phosphate 50 mg • Magnesium (as Magnesium Glycinate Chelate) 100 mg.

Pyruvate — Aspen Group, Inc.
Each capsule contains: Calcium Pyruvate 750 mg. Contains no sugar, starch, salt, wheat, yeast, corn, milk or soy derivatives.

Pyruvate 1000 — Pinnacle
Each tablet provides 1000 mg of Pyruvate 1000 from calcium and sodium salts of Pyruvic Acid, plus Dihydroxyacetone. Inulized in a bioactive complex of Phosphorolytic Dahlia Inulin providing a long chain carbohydrate molecule.

Pyruvate Fuel — TwinLab
Each capsule contains: Calcium Pyruvate Monohydrate 750 mg.

Pyruvate-C — Richardson Labs
Four caplets contain: Pyruvate: (Potassium Pyruvate, Calcium Pyruvate) 2 g • Chromium (picolinate) 400 mcg.

Python — Swedish Herbal Institute
One tablet contains: Damiana 100 mg • Gotu Kola 30 mg • Green Oat Straw seeds 100 mg • Muira Puama 100 mg • Saw Palmetto 100 mg • Ginkgo Biloba 30 mg • Siberian Ginseng 200 mg • Korean Ginseng root 200 mg • Guarana seeds 50 mg • Schisandra fruit/seed 100 mg • Stinging Nettle leaf 200 mg • Tribulus Terrestris 250 mg.

Q-Gel 15 mg — Tishcon
One softsule contains: Vitamin E 3 IU • Coenzyme Q-10 15 mg. Other ingredients: Gelatin, Glycerin, Purified water, Titanium dioxide, Annato seed extract, Proprietary Biosolv (Polysorbate 80, Lecithin, Sorbitan monoleate, Medium Chain Triglycerides).

Q-Gel Forte 30 mg — Tishcon
One softsule contains: Vitamin E 6 IU • Coenzyme Q-10 30 mg. Other ingredients: Gelatin, Glycerin, Purified water, Titanium dioxide, Annato seed extract, Proprietary Biosolv (Polysorbate 80, Lecithin, Sorbitan monoleate, Medium Chain Triglycerides).

Quanterra Emotional Balance — Warner-Lambert
Each tablet contains: LI 160 WS (hyperforin stabilized) St. John's Wort standardized extract 300 mg.

Quanterra Mental Sharpness, Ginkgo Biloba — Warner-Lambert
Each tablet contain: Egb 761 Ginkgo Biloba leaf extract; standardized to 24% Ginkgo flavone glycosides & 6% terpene lactones) 60 mg. Other Ingredients: Lactose, microcrystalline cellulose, maize starch, hydroxypropyl methylcellulose, croscarmellose sodium, polyethylene glycol, magnesium stearate, silicon dioxide, artificial color, talc, ferric oxide, & dimethicone.

Quanterra Prostate, Saw Palmetto — Warner-Lambert
Each softgel contains: Saw Palmetto Berry dried extract (Seronoa repens, berry, dried extract) 160 mg. Other Ingredients: Gelatin, Glycerol, & Ferric Oxide.

Quanterra Sinus Defense, Sinupret — Warner-Lambert
Each tablet contains: Gentian Root (Gentian lutea) 9 mg • Elder Flower (Sambucus nigra) 29 mg • European Vervain Aerial Parts (Verbena) 29 mg • Primrose Flower (Primula veris) 29 mg • Sorrel Aerial Parts (Rumex acesota) 29 mg. Other Ingredients: Sucrose, talc, lactose monohydrate, calcium carbonate, potato starch, maize starch, maize swell-starch flour, colloidal anhydrous silica, stearic palmitic acid, titanium dioxide, glucose syrup, gelatin, shellac, magnesium oxide, sorbitol, eudragit E 12.5, montan glycol wax, povidone, & castor oil.

Quanterra Sleep, Valerian — Warner-Lambert
Two tablets contain: Valerian (Valeriana officinalis, root, dried extract) 300 mg • Lemon balm (Melissa officinalis, leaf, dried extract) 150 mg. Other Ingredients: Sucrose, castor oil, talc, methylhydroxypropyl cellulose, microcrystalline cellulose, crospovidone, silicon dioxide, calcium carbonate, polyethylene glycol, titanium dioxide, eudragit L 30 D, glucose syrup, carmellose sodium, FD&C blue #2 aluminum lake, magnesium stearate, polyvidon, carnuba wax, & polysorbate 80.

B
R
A
N
D

N
A
M
E
S

Quanterra Stomach Comfort, Ginger — Warner-Lambert
Two capsules contain: Ginger (Zingiber Officinale, root) 500 mg.
Other Ingredients: Gelatin, colloidal anhydrous silica, & sodium laurel sulfate.

QueaseEase — Pacific BioLogic
Pinellia rhizome • Citrus peel • Fritillaria bulb • Poria Plant Fungus (hoelen) • Licorice root • Ginger rhizome • Chrysanthemum flower • Astragalus seed • Gastrodia rhizome • Bamboo shavings • Perilla leaf • Peppermint.

Quercetin-Bromelain — Doctor's Best
Each capsule contains: Quercetin 250 mg • Bromelain 125 mg.

Quercezyme-Plus — Enzymatic Therapy
Each capsule contain: Vitamin C (Ascorbic Acid) 100 mg • Magnesium (Carbonate) 25 mg • Other ingredients: Bromelain (1800 MCU) 125 mg • Quercetin 125 mg • Mixed Bioflavonoids Complex 50% concentrate 100 mg • L-Cysteine (HCL) 75 mg. Contains no sugar, salt, yeast, wheat, corn, soy, dairy products, coloring, flavoring or preservatives.

Quest Chromium GTF — Quest
Each capsule contains: Chromium (HVP Chelate) 200 mcg. Other Ingredients: Microcrystalline Cellulose, Magnesium Stearate (vegetable source).

Quest Ginkgo Biloba Extract — Quest
Each caplet contains: Ginkgo Biloba leaf extract (Ginkgo biloba) (provided by 60 mg P.E. 1:50 standardized to contain 24% Ginkgosides) 3000 mg • Citrus Bioflavonoids 200 mg providing Hesperidin 50 mg. Other Ingredients: Calcium Phosphate, Microcrystalline Cellulose, Croscarmellose Sodium, Vegetable Stearin, Magnesium Stearate (vegetable source).

Quest Green-Lipped Mussel — Quest
Each capsule contains: Freeze-Dried Green Lipped Mussel (Perna canaliculus) 625 mg.

Quest Kava Kava — Quest
Each capsule contains: Kava Kava (provided by 150 mg P.E. 1:12 standardized to 30% Kavalactones) 1800 mg. Other Ingredients: Microcrystalline Cellulose, Magnesium Stearate (vegetable source).

Quest Lycopene — Quest
Each capsule contains: Lyc-o-Mato brand Lycopene 5000 mcg. Other Ingredients: Rice Bran Oil, Sunflower Oil, Vegetable Stearin, Beeswax, Lecithin.

Quest MSM — Quest
Each caplet contains: Lignisul brand MSM 1000 mg. Other Ingredients: Croscarmellose Sodium, Silicon Dioxide, and Magnesium Stearate.

Quest SAM-e — Quest
Each capsule contains: S-adenosyl-methionine tosylate (providing 50 mg S-adenosyl-methionine) 100 mg. Other Ingredients: Croscarmellose Sodium, Microcrystalline Cellulose, Calcium Phosphate, Vegetable Stearin, Magnesium Stearate (vegetable source).

Quest Siberian Ginseng — Quest
Each capsule contains: Siberian Ginseng 500 mg.

Quick Trim — Cybergenics America Co.
Each caplet contains: Complex 1: Guarana seed extract • L-Tyrosine • L-Phenylalanine • Garcinia Cambogia (Citrimax) • Griffonia extract • Kola Nut powder • Chinese Ginseng • Cayenne pepper • Phenalgin • Astragalus root • Cinnamon bark • Green Tea • Pacific Kelp. Complex 2: Lecithin • Ginger • Cascara Sagrada • Buchu leaf extract • Uva Ursi leaf • Juniper berry extract • Choline Bitartrate • Inositol • L-Methionine • Chickweed herb • Red Clover powder • Dandelion root extract • Senna leaf extract • Cynarin complex. Complex 3: Chamomile flower • Valerian root extract • Hawthorne extract • Kava Kava root • Immature Orange peel • Lemon Verbena • Skullcap. Complex 4: Enzyme blend • Magnesium Oxide • Calcium Chelate • Selenium Yeast • Zinccitrata • Zinc Picolinate • Ascorbic Acid • Beta Carotene • Niacin • D Alpha Tocopheryl Acetate • Pyridoxine HCl • Riboflavin • Thiamin HCl • Potassium Iodide • Folic Acid • Cyanocobalamin • Chromium Picolinate • Phytonadione • Cholecalciferol.

Qu-up — Happy Families
Each capsule contains: Pure Deer Velvet extract (standardized at a ratio of 11:1 on IGF1 & IGF2) • Yerba Mate 200 mg • Damiana 200

mg • Guarana 100 mg • Natural Caffeine 50 mg • Vitamin B5 (Calcium D-Pantothenate) 20 mg • Vitamin B6 (Pyridoxine Hydrochloride) 20 mg • Vitamin B12 (Cobalamin) 20 mg. Contains no preservatives, sugars, milk, starch, wheat or yeast derivatives.

Raspberry — Natrol
Each single serving contains: Vitamin C (Ascorbic Acid) 250 mg • Acerola berry extract 20 mg • Echinacea (Purpurea extract 16:1) 12.5 mg • White Willow bark 100 mg • Slippery Elm bark 75 mg • Stevia powder 20 mg. Other ingredients: Lemon Juice powder, Fructose, natural Raspberry flavor, Honey powder, Citric Acid, Natural Elderberry flavor, Calcium Carbonate.

Raw Adrenal — Enzymatic Therapy
Two capsules contain: Vitamin C (Ascorbic Acid/Rose Hips) 250 mg • Pantothenic Acid (D-Calcium Pantothenate) 100 mg • Vitamin B6 (Pyridoxine HCL) 50 mg • Other ingredients: L-Tyrosine 250 mg • Betaine 250 mg • Pituitary extract freeze-dried 120 mg • Adrenal extract (Predigested Soluble concentrate*) 400 mg • Adrenal Cortex extract 33 mg. *Free-form concentrate predigested by enzymatic action, creating a highly absorbable form of glandular concentrate containing all the natural principles with a standardized content. All organs & glands derived from bovine sources.

Raw Adrenal II — Enzymatic Therapy
Each two tablets contain: Vitamin C (Ascorbic Acid/Rose Hips) 250 mg • Pantothenic Acid (D-Calcium Pantothenate) 250 mg • Vitamin B6 (Pyridoxine HCL) 50 mg • Other ingredients: L-Tyrosine 500 mg • Betaine 250 mg • Pituitary extract freeze-dried 120 mg • Adrenal extract (Predigested Soluble concentrate*) 100 mg • Ginger root extract 6.5:1 (Zingiber officinale) 100 mg • Adrenal Cortex extract 33 mg. *Free-form concentrate predigested by enzymatic action, creating a highly absorbable form of glandular concentrate containing all the natural principles with a standardized content. All organs & glands derived from bovine sources.

Recall Support — The Vitamin Shoppe
Two tablets contain: Ginkgo Biloba Extract 24% ginkgoflavoglycosides 25 mg • Phosphatidylserine 10 mg • L-Phenylalanine 250 mg • L-Glutamine 250 mg • Choline 250 mg • Gotu Kola 200 mg • RNA/DNA 100 mg • Magnesium (citrate, gluconate) 50 mg • Ginseng Extract (Panax Ginseng) 50 mg • B6 10 mg. In a base of Lecithin and Rice concentrate.

Red Clover Combination — Nature's Way
Each capsule contains: Barberry bark • Buckthorn bark • Burdock root • Cascara Sagrada bark • Echinacea Purpurea stem, leaf, flower • Licorice root • Peach bark • Prickly Ash bark • Red Clover blossoms • Rosemary herb • Sarsaparilla root • Sheep Sorrell. Other ingredients: Gelatin.

Red Dragon Cold & Flu Relief — Jamieson
Each capsule contains: Honeysuckle flower (Lonicera japonica Thunb. PE 1:2) 149.3 mg • Forsythia fruit (Forsythia suspensa Thunb. PE 1:2) 149.3 mg • White Mulberry Leaf (Morus Alba L.PE 1:2) 119.4 mg • Chrysanthemum flower (Chrysanthemum morifolium Ramat PE 1:2) 89.6 mg • Adenophora root (Adenophora Tetraphylla Thunb PE 1:2) 89.6 mg • Schizonepata stem (Schizonepata tenifolia Briq PE 1:2) 89.6 mg • Ningpo Figwort root (Scrophularia ninpoensis Hemsl PE 1:2) 74.6 mg • Great Burdock fruit (Arctium Lappa L PE 1:2) 74.6 mg • Hogfennel root (Peucedanum praeruptorum Dunn PE 1:2) 74.6 mg • Field Mint leaf (Mentha haplocalyx Briq PE 1:2) 44.8 mg • Licorice root (Glycyrrhiza uralensis Fischer PE 1:2) 44.8 mg. (PE = Powdered Extract).

Red Dragon Imperial Ginseng — Jamieson
Each caplet contains: Panax Ginseng (derived from Shiu Chu, Tien Chi and Red Kirin) • 500 mg Roots of: Prince Adenophorae, Salvia, Scrophulara, Codonopsis and Polygonum Ginsengs, Radix Astragail, Canodermae Lucidum, Fructus Lycii Berry.

Red Dragon Imperial Ginseng and Garlic — Jamieson
Each capsule contains: Panax Ginseng (derived from Shiu Chu, Tien Chi and Red Kirin) • Roots of: Prince Adenophorae, Salvia, Scrophulara, Codonopsis and Polygonum Ginseng, Radix Astragail, Canodermae Lucidum, Fructus Lycii Berry 250 mg • Tibetan Plateau Garlic 250 mg.

Red Dragon Imperial Ginseng and Royal Jelly — Jamieson
Each caplet contains: Panax Ginseng (derived from Shiu Chu, Tien Chi and Red Kirin) • Roots of: Prince Adenophorae, Salvia, Scrophulara, Codonopsis and Polygonum Ginsengs, Radix Astragail,

© Copyright 2000, Natural Medicines Comprehensive Database (209) 472-2244. For updated data, go to www.NaturalDatabase.com. • 1391

Some Brand Name Natural Products - What they Contain
www.NaturalDatabase.com contains MANY more listings than appear here.

B R A N D   N A M E S

Canodermae Lucidum, Fructus Lycii Berry 500 mg • Fresh Royal Jelly 250 mg.

Red Dragon Imperial Royal Jelly — Jamieson
Each capsule contains: Pure Royal Jelly concentrate equivalent to fresh Royal Jelly 500 mg.

Red Root-Cleavers Virtue — Blessed Herbs
Nettle • Horsetail Grass • Red Root • Cleavers • Sage leaf • Mullein leaf • Goldenseal root • Poke root • Ginger root • Grain alcohol & Distilled Water.

Red Stuff — Gary Null
Contains a fruit mix including Cranberries, Cherries, Pears, Watermelons, Pink Grapefruit, Lecithin, Apple Pectin, Papayas, and Peaches.

Reduced L-Glutathione 150 mg — Klaire Laboratories
Reduced L-Glutathione 150 mg.

Reduced L-Glutathione 75 mg — Klaire Laboratories
Reduced L-Glutathione 75 mg.

Regal Pro-Meal — Nature's Life
Two scoops (28.35 g) contain: Supro brand Soy Protein Isolate containing Lecithin • Whey • Fructose • Non-fat Dry Milk • natural Vanilla Flavor • Yeast • Egg Albumin • Eggshell powder • Kelp • natural Papain Enzyme concentrate & Cobalamin concentrate (B12). Regal Pro-Meal also contains 34 mg of naturally occuring Isoflavones including 21 mg Genistein & 10 mg Daidzein.

Rehab Forte — Progressive Labs
Two capsules contain: Vitamin C (ascorbic acid) 500 mg • Niacinamide 200 mg • Vitamin B6 (pyridoxine HCl) 50 mg • Calcium (amino acid chelate) 200 mg • Elemental Calcium 40 mg • Magnesium (amino acid chelate) 100 mg • Elemental Magnesium 20 mg • Zinc (amino acid chelate) 30 mg • Elemental Zinc 7.6 mg • Manganese (amino acid chelate) 50 mg • Elemental Manganese 5 mg • Copper (amino acid chelate) 2 mg • Elemental Copper 0.01 mg • Potassium Sulfate 200 mg • Elemental Potassium 90 mg • Chondroitin Sulfate 50 mg • Lemon bioflavonoids 500 mg • Rutin 50 mg.

Reishi Defense — Traditional Medicinals
Red Reishi Mushroom (Ganoderma lucidum) Mycclium & Fruit Body • Ginger rhizome • Astralagus root • Roasted Barley grain • Licorice root • Stevia leaf.

Rejoyn Veromax — American MedTech
Two capsules contain: L-Arginine 200 mg • Zizyphi fructus 200 mg • Siberian Ginseng 200 mg • Saw Palmetto 200 mg • Ginkgo Biloba 75 mg • L-Alanine 75 mg • Glutamic Acid 75 mg • L-Lysine 75 mg. Other Ingredients: Pvp, Di-Calcium Phosphate, Cellulose, Croscarmellose Sodium, Vegetable sterine, Magnesium stearate, Silicon dioxide and Pharmaceutical glaze.

Rejuveinate — PhysioLogics
Each capsule contains: Vitamin C (Ascorbic Acid) 60 mg • Horse Chestnut (15% Escin, 22.5 mg) 150 mg • Butcher's Broom (10% Ruscogenins, 10 mg) 100 mg • Gotu Kola (20% Terpenes, 12 mg) 60 mg • Hesperidin (35% Bioflavonoids, 14 mg) 40 mg • Bilberry fruit (36% Anthocyanosides, 7.2 mg) 20 mg.

Rejuvex — Chattem, Inc.
Each caplet contains: Vitamin E (as dl-alpha tocopherol acetate) 30 IU • Thiamin HCl (Vitamin B1) 2 mg • Riboflavin (Vitamin B2) 2 mg • Niacin (as Niacinamide) 10 mg • Vitamin B6 (as pyridoxine hydrochloride) 2 mg • Pantothenic Acid (as d-calcium pantothenate) 10 mg • Magnesium (as magnesium oxide) 500 mg • Selenium (as sodium selenate) 25 mcg • Manganese (as manganese sulfate) 2 mg • Standardized Dong Quai root extract 200 mg • Mammary gland powder 25 mg • Ovary gland powder 19 mg • Uterus gland powder 10 mg • Adrenal gland powder 10 mg • Pituitary gland powder 5 mg • Boron (chelated with citrate & aspartate) 3 mg. Other Ingredients: Microcrystalline Cellulose, Stearic Acid, Silicon Dioxide, Croscarmellose Sodium, Hydroxypropyl Methylcellulose, Magnesium Stearate, Polyethylene Glycol, Mineral oil, Shellac, & Talc.

Rejuvine — Metabolic Response Modifiers
Two teaspoons contain: DHEA 25 mg • Pregnenolone 25 mg.

Relax & Ease Tension — ProHerbs
Two tablets contain: Thiamine HCl (B1) 50 mg • Riboflavin (B2) 50 mg • Vitamin B6 (Pyridoxine HCl) 50 mg • Vitamin B12 (Cyanocobalamin) 100 mcg • Kava Kava root (Piper methysticum

standardized to 30% kavalactones) 300 mg • Passion Flower (Passiflora incarnata standardized to 4% flavonoids) 100 mg • Chamomile flower (Matricaria chamomilla standardized to greater than 1% apigenin) 100 mg. Other Ingredients: Dicalcium Phosphate, Microcrystalline Cellulose, Croscarmellose Sodium, Hydroxypropylmethylcellulose, Magnesium Stearate, Mineral Oil, Polyethylene Glycol, Stearic Acid, Titanium Dioxide, Sodium Lauryl Sulfate, Yellow #6 Lake, FD&C Blue #1 Lake, FD&C Red #40 Lake, FD&C Blue #2 Lake.

Relax & Sleep Formula 2 — Futurebiotics
Two tablets contain: Valerian root - A balanced blend of extract & powder equivalent to dried root 500 mg. • Chamomile - A balanced blend of extract & powder equivalent to dried blossoms 250 mg • Magnesium (oxide, amino acid chelate) 150 mg • Calcium (carbonate, phosphate, amino acid chelate) 150 mg. Specially formulated in a base of natural, time-tested herbs (in the form of extracts & powders) including: (Hawthorn berry, Fennel, Passion flower, Scullcap, Hops, Lemon Balm, Avena Sativa, Red Clover, Catnip, Spearmint leaves & Vanilla).

Relax Now — Health Factor
Each capsule contains: Kava Kava 100 mg • Valerian 100 mg • Scutellaria 100 mg • Passion flower (2:1 extract) 75 mg • Hops 25 mg • Chamomilla 6X • Lady Slipper 3X.

Relax-O-Comp — Phytopharmica
Each tablet contains: Vitamin D (Fish Liver oil) 50 IU • Calcium Citrate 162 mg • Niacin/Niacinamide 65 mg • Magnesium Gluconate 50 mg • Magnesium (Oxide) 50 mg • Vitamin B6 (Pyridoxine HCL) 10 mg • Zinc (Chelate) 10 mg • Other ingredients: Valerian extract Extra Strength (Valeriana officinalis) 75 mg • Chamomile extract (Matricaria chamomilla) 75 mg • Passion flower extract (Passiflora) 30 mg • Hops extract (Humulus lupulus) 30 mg • Unsaturated Free Fatty Acids 10 mg. In a base of Raw Crude Licorice extract, Anise seeds & Peppermint. Contains no sugar, salt, yeast, wheat, corn, soy, dairy products, flavoring or preservatives.

Relax-U — The Herbalist
Valerian root • Skullcap herb • Passionflower herb.

Relief Plus — Health Factor
Each capsule contains: Goldenseal extract (4:1)(Hydrastis canadensis) 125 mg • Chamomile (Matricaria chamomilla) 100 mg • Valerian (Valeriana officinalis) 85 mg • Feverfew (Tanacetum parthenium) 590 mg • Cayenne Pepper 50 mg.

Reliv Arthaffect — Reliv International
Each scoop (8.5 g) contains: Arthred (hydrolyzed collagen) • Glucosamine Sulfate • Ginkgo Biloba • Borage Oil Powder • Turmeric • Boswellia Serrata • Ashwagandha • Cat's Claw • Sarsaparilla Root • Licorice Root • Kelp • Burdock Root • Alfalfa • Barley Grass • Echinacea Root • Yucca Extract • Devil's Claw Extract • Bilberry Extract • Celery Seed • Capsicum • Aloe Vera • Bioperine (Piper nigrum extract) • Soy Lecithin.

Reliv Celleboost — Reliv International
Two capsules contain: (-)Hydroxycitric Acid 375 mg • Oatrim (Hydrolyzed Oat Flour) 360 mg • Chromium 50 mcg.

Reliv Cellebrate — Reliv International
Each scoop contains: (-) Hydroxycitric Acid 375 mg • L-Carnitine 75 mg • Chromium 50 mcg • Choline 50 mg • Inositol 50 mg • Gamma-Linolenic Acid (as Borage Oil Powder) 50 mg • Ginkgo Biloba Leaves 33 mg • Coenzyme Q10 15 mg. Other Ingredients: Maltodextrin, Soy Lecithin, & Quaker Oatrim (Hydrolyzed Oat Flour).

Reliv Classic — Reliv International
Each scoop (16 g) contains: Soy Protein Isolate • Soy Flour • Brewer's Yeast • Lecithin • Psyllium Fiber • Dicalcium Phosphate • Ascorbic Acid • Methionine • Potassium Chloride • Magnesium Phosphate • Natural Flavor • Licorice Root • Garlic Rhubarb Root • Rose Hips • Cayenne • Kelp • OptiZinc Brand of Zinc Momomethionine • Ferrous Fumarate • Calcium Pantothenate • Niacinamide • Vitamin E Acetate • Vitamin A Palmitate • Vitamin D • Copper • Gluconate • Papain • Bromelain • Thiamin HCL • Riboflavin • Beta Carotene • Pyridoxine HCL • Biotin • Folic Acid • Potassium Iodine • Vitamin B12 • Soldium Selenite • ChromeMate Brand of Niacin Bound Chromium Polynicotinate.

Reliv FibRestore — Reliv International
Each scoop (30 g) contains: Fructose • Fiber Blend (Oat Fiber, Corn

Bran, Apple Fiber, Soy Fiber, Pea Fiber, Citrus Fiber, Carrageenan Gum, Guar Gum, Xanthan Gum, Gum Arabic) • Maltodextrin • Natural Flavor • Herbal Blend (Oriental Ginseng, Garlic, Cayenne, Licorice Root, Kelp, Rhubarb Root, Hibiscus, Irish Moss, Siberian Ginseng, Aloe Vera Powder, Chicory Root, Dandelion Root, Chamomile Powder, Alfalfa Powder, Pearl Barley, Ginger Root, Celery Seed, Sarsaparilla, Passion Flower, Capsicum Fruit Powder, Fenugreek) • Lecithin • Ascorbic Acid • Citric Acid • Beta Carotene • Alpha Tocopheryl Acetate • Pepsin • Papain • Bromelain.

Reliv Innergize! — Reliv International
Each scoop (19 g) contains: Fructose • Maltodextrin • Citric Acid • Potassium Citrate • Natural Flavor • Tricalcium Phosphate • Sodium Chloride • Magnesium Oxide • Ascorbic Acid • Beta Carotene • OptiZinc Brand of Zinc Monomethionine • ChromeMate Brand of Niacin Bound Chromium Polynicotinate.

Reliv Now — Reliv International
Each scoop (15 g) contains: Whey • Soy Protein Isolate • Fructose • Dicalcium Phosphate • Magnesium Phosphate • Calcium Caseinate • Calcium Carbonate • Natural Flavor • Ascorbic Acid • Potassium Chloride • Lecithin • PABA (para-aminobenzoic acid) • Kelp • OptiZinc Brand of Zinc Monomethionine • Ferrous Fumarate • Calcium Pantothenate • Beta Carotene • Vitamin A Palmitate • Vitamin D3 • Thiamin HCL • Riboflavin • Niacinamide • Vitamin E Acetate • Pyridoxine HCL • Folic Acid • Vitamin B12 • Potassium Iodide • Copper Gluconate • Biotin • Sodium Selenite • ChromeMate Brand of Niacin Bound Chromium Polynicotinate • Sodium Molybdate • Vitamin K • Manganese Sulfate • Rutin • Garlic • Cayenne • Butternut Bark • Rhubarb Root • Blue Vervain • Licorice Root • Irish Moss.

Reliv ProVantage — Reliv International
Each scoop (26 g) contains: Soy Protein Isolate • Fructose • Medium Chain Triglycerides • Creatine Monohydrate • Tonalin (Conjugated Linoleic Acid-CLA) • Lecithin • L-Arginine • L-Glutamine • L-Leucine • L-Lysine • L-Carnitine • L-Alanine • Glycine • Ornithine Alpha Ketoglutarate • Coenzyme Q10 • Activin (Grapeseed extract) • Phosphatidylserine/Phosphatidylcholine Complex • Bioperine (Piper nigrum extract) • Natural & Artificial Flavors • Alpha-Lipoic Acid.

Reliv SoySentials — Reliv International
Each scoop (22 g) contains: Soy Protein Isolate • Fructose • Inulin • Dehydrated Cranberries • Calcium Carbonate • Dicalcium Phosphate • Lactobacillus Acidophilus • Lecithin • Natural & Artifical Flavors • Activin (Grape seed extract) • Protykin (Resveratrol) • Ipriflavone • Black Cohosh Root • Dong Quai Root • Wild Yam • Panax Ginseng • Green Tea Extract • Chasteberry • Horse Chestnut • Nettle Root • Hops • Licorice Root • Coenzyme Q10 • Folic Acid • Ascorbic Acid • Pyridoxine HCL • Alpha Tocopheryl Acetate • Beet Powder • Stevia Extract • Acesulfame Potassium • Alpha Lipoic Acid.

Reliv Ultrim-Plus — Reliv International
Each scoop (28 g) contains: Soy Protein Isolate • Whey • Fructose • Milk Protein • Nonfat Dry Milk • Xanthan Gum • Dicalcium Phosphate • Magnesium Phosphate • Calcium Carbonate • Natural & Artificial Flavor • Ascorbic Acid • Potassium Chloride • Lecithin • Aspartame • PABA (Para-aminobenzoic acid) • Kelp • OptiZinc Brand of Zinc Monomethionine • Ferrous Fumarate • Calcium Pantothenate • Vitamin A Palmitate • Vitamin D3 • Thiamin HCL • Riboflavin • Niacinamide • Vitamin E Acetate • Pyridoxine HCL • Folic Acid • Vitamin B12 • Potassium Iodide • Copper Gluconate • Biotin • Sodium Selenite • ChromeMate Brand of Niacin Bound Chromium Polynicotinate • Sodium Molybdate • Vitamin K • Manganese Sulfate • Rutin • Garlic • Cayenne • Butternut Bark • Rhubarb Root • Blue Vervain • Licorice Root • Irish Moss.

Remember-FX — HerbTech
North American Ginseng (Panax quinquefolium) 100 mg.

Remifemin — Enzymatic Therapy
Each tablet contains: Black Cohosh (Cimicifuga racemosa) & rhizome extract, standardized rhizome extract to contain Triterpene Glycosides calculated as 27-Deoxyacetin, approximately 20 mg.

Remifemin Plus — Enzymatic Therapy
Each tablet contains: Standardized Cimicifuga racemosa (Black Cohosh) root & rhizome extract standardized for Triterpene Glycosides content, calculated as 27-Deoxyactein 20 mg • St. John's Wort standardized to contain Hypericin 250 mcg. Contains no sugar, salt, yeast, wheat, gluten, corn, soy, dairy products (except lactose), coloring, flavoring, or preservatives.

Remotiv — Zeller
One tablet contains: Hypericum (St. John's Wort) extract of Ze 117 (standardized to a daily amount of 1 mg hypericin) 250 mg.

Renatrate — Progressive Labs
Each capsule contains: Vitamin A 5000 IU • Vitamin C 90 mg • Bovine kidney concentrate 300 mg. The glandular concentrate in this product is prepared by a special process which does not exceed physiological temperature (37º C). Guaranteed free of chemical pesticides and synthetic hormones.

Renew-U — The Herbalist
Milk Thistle seed • Echinacea root • Oregon Grape root • Dandelion herb • Burdock root • Yellow Dock root • Cleavers herb • Wild Indigo root • Ginger root • Fennel seed.

Repagene Emulsion — Atrium
Each teaspoon contains: Squalene 1 1/2 g in an Emulsified form. Contains no sugar or artificial flavor.

Resist — Pacific BioLogic
Astragalus root (Grade 1) • Ganoderma Fungus • Codonopsis root • Jujube fruit • Atractylodes (white) rhizome • Peony root (white) • Citrus peel (tangerine) • Cuscuta seeds • Dioscorea root • Schizandra fruit • Licorice root • Milletta root • Platycodon root • Ligustrum fruit • Glehnia root • Rehmannia root (prep.) • Ginger rhizome (fresh).

Resist 2 — Pacific BioLogic
Bitter Melon • St. John's Wort • Red Marine Algae • Echinacea Angustifolia • Tumeric rhizome • Licorice root (honey-baked) • Ligustrum root (Chinese) • Citrus peel (tangerine) • Viola (whole plant) • Prunella (selfheal spike) • Trichosanthis root • Knotweed rhizome (bushy) • Aucklandia root.

Respa-Herb — Dial Herbs
Ma Huang • Mullein • Goldenseal • Colts Foot • Comfrey • Marshmallow • Lobelia • Cayenne.

Resphora — PhysioLogics
Each capsule contains: Tylophora (GPH: 0.1% tylophorine alkaloids) 30 mg • Piper longum (GPH: 2% piperine) • Picrorhiza kurroa (GPH: 4% kutkin) 50 mg.

Respi-Oil — The Herbalist
Essential oils of Eucalyptus, Rosemary, Sage, Tea Tree & Nutmeg in a Sweet Almond oil base.

Respir-all — Now
Three tablets contain: Vitamin B5 (Pantothenic Acid) 100 mg • Vitamin B6 (Pyridoxine HCL) 20 mg • Vitamin C (as Magnesium Ascorbate) 500 mg • Magnesium (as Magnesium Ascorbate) 40 mg • Zinc (as L-OptiZinc Monomethionine) 10 mg • Quercetin 800 mg • Nettle root extract (Urtica dioica) (standardized 30 ppm Scopoletin) 500 mg • Bromelain (2000 GDU) 500 mg • Licorice root (Glycyrrhiza glabra) 4:1 extract 200 mg.

Respiratory Support — Amazon Support
Each capsule contains: Amor Seco • Embauba • Samambaia • Espinheira Santa • Fedegosa • Mullaca • Mutamba • Sarsaparilla • Jatoba • Vassourinha.

Respiratory Support Formula — PhysioLogics
Two capsules contain: Vitamin C (Ascorbic Acid) 130 mg • Ephedra root, stem (6% total Ephedrine Alkaloids, 12 mg) 200 mg • Lemon Bioflavonoids citrus 66 mg • Pleurisy root 45 mg • Mullein leaf 38 mg • Slippery Elm bark 38 mg • Licorice root 35 mg • Red Clover tops 35 mg • Ginkgo leaf (24% Ginkgo Flavonglycosides, 7.2 mg; 6 % Terpene Lactones, 1.8 mg) 30 mg.

Respi-Tea — The Herbalist
Wild Cherry bark • Slippery Elm bark • Coltsfoot leaf • Marshmallow root • Licorice root • Cinnamon bark • Yarrow blossom • Ginger root.

Respitonic — The Herbalist
Echinacea root • Golden Seal root • Osha root • Yerba Santa leaf • Horseradish root • Yarrow blossom • Cayenne pepper.

Restful — BioDynamax
Two capsules contain: Kava Kava root extract 300 mg • Chamomile 100 mg • Passion flower 100 mg • Calcium 100 mg • Magnesium 50 mg.

Restore-X — Cambridge Nutraceuticals
Each serving contains: L-Glutamine 10 g • N-Acetyl-Cysteine 600 mg • L-Arginine (from Zinc Arginate) 140 mg • Vitamin A (as mixed

© Copyright 2000, Natural Medicines Comprehensive Database (209) 472-2244. For updated data, go to www.NaturalDatabase.com. • 1393

**B
R
A
N
D

N
A
M
E
S**

carotenoids) 5000 IU • Vitamin C 500 mg • Vitamin E 200 IU • Thiamin 6 mg • Riboflavin 6.8 mg • Niacin 80 mg • Vitamin B6 8 mg • Pantothenic Acid 40 mg • Magnesium 200 mg • Zinc 20 mg • Selenium 100 mcg • Copper -0.75 mg • Folate 400 mcg • Vitamin B12 50 mcg.

Revenge — Champion Nutrition
Each 29 g serving contains: Vitamin C 60 mg • Vitamin E 60 IU • Thiamine 5 mg • Riboflavin 3 mg • Vitamin B6 5 mg • Pantothenic Acid 10 mg • Magnesium 12 mg • Chromium 240 mcg • Potassium 160 mg. Tropical Mango Blast Ingredients: Metacarb VII (proprietary carbohydrate blend which contains Amylopectin Food Starch Modified, Glucose Polymer [Maltodextrin]) • Fructose • Peptol-7 (proprietary Protein-Amino Acid Blend which contains: Whey Protein Concentrate, L-Leucine, Glycine, L-Glutamine, Taurine, L-Isoleucine & L-Valine) • Lactate Blend (Sodium Potassium Lactate, Creatine Lactate, Glycerol Stearate, Magnesium Lactate, Glycerol Lactate) • Glucose (Dextrose) • Natural & Artificial Flavoring • Cellulose • Malic Acid • Trutina Dulcem (Natural Kiwi extract) • Phosphatidylcholine • D-Ribose • Vitamin E Acetate • Talc • Ginseng Root extract • Proteoglycan Support (proprietary blend which includes Glucosamine Hcl & Glucosamine Ascorbate) • Creatine Alpha-Ketoglutarate • Citric Acid • Potassium Phosphate • Guarana seed extract (standardized to 50% Caffeine) • Potassium Citrate • Ascorbic Acid • Quercetin • Willow Bark extract (standardized to 50% Salycin) • Sunett (Acesulfame-K) • Sodium Citrate • Omega-3 Fatty Acids (Fish oil) • Xanthan Gum • Feverfew extract • Vitamin B Blend (Vitamin B1, Vitamin B2, Vitamin B3, Vitamin B5, Vitamin B6, Pantethine) • Curcumin • N-Acetylcysteine • Periwinkle standardized extract • Coenzyme Q10 • Lipoic Acid • Chromium Polynicotinate • Annatto & Carmine (natural colors).

ReVitalize — Rx Vitamins
Three PureCaps contain: Mixed Carotenoid complex (alpha, beta & gamma carotenes) 25000 IU • Vitamin C (ascorbic acid) 200 mg • Pantothenic Acid (calcium pantothenate) 100 mg • Calcium (amino acid chelate/complex) 50 mg • Magnesium (amino acid chelate/complex) 50 mg • Vitamin B1 (thiamine) 50 mg • Vitamin B2 (riboflavin) 50 mg • Vitamin B3 (niacin) 50 mg • Vitamin B6 (pyridoxine HCl) 50 mg • Citrus Flavonoid complex (active flavonols, flavonones, flavones & naringen-44%) 50 mg • Choline (bitartrate) 50 mg • Inositol 50 mg • Potassium (glycero-phosphate) 25 mg • Zinc (amino acid chelate/complex) 15 mg • Manganese (amino acid chelate/complex) 5 mg • Iron (amino acid chelate/complex) 4.5 mg • Copper (glycinate) 1 mg • Vanadium (as vanadyl sulfate) 1 mg • Vitamin D (calciferol) 400 IU • Vitamin E (d-alpha tocopherol) 200 IU • Folic Acid 400 mcg • Biotin 300 mcg • Iodine (kelp) 150 mcg • Vitamin B12 (cyanocobalamin) 100 mcg • Chromium (polynicotinate) 50 mcg • Selenium (amino acid complex) 50 mcg • Molybdenum (amino acid complex) 20 mcg • Korean Ginseng (Panax ginseng, standardized 5% ginsenosides) 50 mg • Chinese Green Tea extract (Camilla sinensis, standardized 40% polyphenols) 25 mg • Ginkgo Biloba (standardized 24% ginkgoflavoneglycosides, 6% terpene lactones) 10 mg • Bilberry (Vaccinium myrtillus, standardized 25% anthocyanosides) 5 mg • Wild Grape seed extract (Mahonia aquifolia, standardized 95-100% leucoanthocyanins) 5 mg • Oleoresin Tumeric (Curcuma longa, standardized 90-95% curcuminoids) 5 mg • Milk Thistle (Silybum marianum, standardized 80% Silymarin) 75 mg • Parsley Leaves (Petroselinum crispum, naturally rich in apiin & luteolin-7-apiolglucoside) 75 mg • Juniper Berries (juniperus communis, naturally rich in glucuronic acid) 50 mg • Celery seed 4x (Aplum graveolens, naturally rich in limonene) 50 mg • Cayenne (Capsicum frutescens, naturally rich in capsaicin) 50 mg • Glucosamine Sulfate (aminomonosaccharide) 30 mg • Borage Seed Oil (Borago officinalis, standardized 25% gamma linolenic acid) 25 mg.

Rezyme — Nature's Secret
Vegetarian Enzyme that contains a proprietary blend of Amylase, Glucoamylase, Cellulase, Lipase, Lactase, Alpha Galactosidase, Bromelain, Papain, Betaine HCl, Gentian, Licorice, and Ginger root. Enzyme Rebuilder, which contains Bitters, Lecithin, L-Glutamine, and Piper longum fruit.

Rhino Acidophilus — Dial Herbs
Lactobacillus acidophilus • Bifidobacterium bifidum • Bifidobacterium infantis • FOS, in a base of rice powder & natural flavors • Vitamin C from Ester-C. Flavored & sweetened with all-natural raspberry fruit juice crystals, dextrose & fructose.

Rhino Actalin Bars — Nutrition Now
Soy Protein Isolate, Calcium Sodium Caseinate, Whey Protein Concentrate, Glucose, High Fructose Glucose Syrup, Fractionated Vegetable Oils, Turbinado Sugar, Non-Fat Dry Milk, Yogurt Solids, Vanilla, Lecithin, Raisins, Apple Paste, Natural Flavors, Apple Fiber, Graham Flour, and Cinnamon.

Rhino Actalin Dietary Supplement — Nutrition Now
Each tablet contains: Magnesium 20 mg • Inosine 50 mg • Phosphatidylserine 50 mg • Amino Acid Blend 50 mg.

Rhino Chewy Vites — Dial Herbs
Vitamin A • Vitamin C • Vitamin D • Vitamin E • Vitamin B6 • VitaminB12 • Calcium • Thiamin • Riboflavin • Folic Acid • Biotin • Pantothenic Acid • Iodine • Magnesium • Zinc • Choline • Inositol • Fruitrim: (Fruit juice, Natural grain dextrins) • Evaporated Cane juice (natural milled sugar) • Gelatin • Lactate • Gluconate • Ascorbic Acid • d-Alpha Tocopheryl Acetate • Citrate Palmitate • Betartrate • Citric Acid • Lactic Acid • Natural Flavors • Natural Colors added (including Anatto, Tumeric, Carmine & Grape skin liquid) • Lightly polished with Fractionated Vegetable oil (Coconut origin) to prevent sticking • Beeswax.

Rhino Daily Pack — Nutrition Now
Each packet contains: Two Rhino Vites- 100% natural daily multi-vitamin • Two Rhino Calcium • One Rhino Ester-C (Vitamin C).

Rhino Echinacea — Dial Herbs
Two tablets contain: Echinacea 100 mg • Vitamin C 60 mg. Flavored & sweetened with all natural raspberry fruit juice crystals, dextrose & fructose.

Rhino Ester-C — Dial Herbs
Vitamin C from Ester-C • Calcium. Flavored & sweetened with all-natural cherry flavorings, natural fruit flavors, fructose, dextrose & bilberry.

Rhino Pops Box — Dial Herbs
Each lollipop contains: Isomalt • Maltitol • Citric Acid • Ascorbic Acid 50 mg • Natural Flavor • Color from Beet liquid • Echinacea • Goldenseal • Phosphorus 6x • Drosera 6x • Kali Carbonicum 6x • Belladonna 6x • Rumex Crispus 6x • Hydrastis 6x.
Editor's Comments: This is a homeopathic product. It is so extremely diluted that its activity can not be explained by conventional scientific methods. Therefore this product can not be rated by the scientific criteria used in this Database. A patient receiving the extreme dilution of this product will not receive many, if any, molecules of the original active ingredient. Therefore, there are no harmful pharmacologic effects, and any beneficial effects are controversial and not due to a direct biochemical action of the ingredient on the body. Homeopathic products are allowed for sale in the U.S. due to legislation passed in the 19th century sponsored by a homeopathic physician who was also a Senator. The law still requires that the FDA allow the sale of products listed in this Homeopathic Pharmacopea of the United States.

Rhino Support Pack — Nutrition Now
Each packet contains: Two Rhino Echinacea • Two Rhino Acidophilus • One Rhino Ester-C (Vitamin C).

Rice Bran Oil — Progressive Labs
Each tablespoon contains: Rice bran oil 14 g.

Ripped Fuel — TwinLab
Ma Huang 20 mg • Guarana 200 mg • Chromium 200 mcg • L-Carnitine 100 mg.

Ripped Fuel (Metabolic Enhancer) — TwinLab
Two capsules contain: Ma Huang extract (standardized for 6% Ephedrine) 334 mg • Guarana extract (standardized for 22% Caffeine) 910 mg • L-Carnitine 100 mg • Chromium (from Chromic Fuel patented Chromium Picolinate) 200 mcg.

Robert's Complex — Enzymatic Therapy
Each capsule contains: Niacinamide 5 m. Other ingredients: American Cranesbill (Geranium maculatum) 100 mg • Cabbage extract (Braccica oleracea) 100 mg • Marshmallow extract 4:1 (Althaea officinalis) mucilage content 30-40%)75 mg • Okra (Hibiscus esculentis) 75 mg • Slippery Elm (Ulma fulva) 75 mg • Duodenal Substance 75 mg • Echinacea root extract (Echinacea angustifolia) standardized to contain greater than 3.5% Echinacosides & 0.65% essential oils 25 mg • Goldenseal root extract (Hydrastis canadensis) standardized to contain 5% total Alkaloids including: Berberine, Hydrastine, & Canadine 25 mg • Pancreatic Enzymes 25 mg. Contains no sugar, salt, yeast, wheat, corn, soy, dairy products, coloring, flavoring or preservatives.

Some Brand Name Natural Products - What they Contain
www.NaturalDatabase.com contains MANY more listings than appear here.

RoseOx — Natrol
One capsule contains: Rosemary dried powdered extract leaf 250 mg. Other ingredients: Rice powder, Magnesium Stearate, Gelatin.

Royal Bee Power — Nature's Plus
Two tablets contain: Bee Pollen 500 mg • Propolis from extract 500 mg • Royal Jelly 50 mg. In a high energy natural base containing Gotu Kola, Ginseng & Fo-Ti. Contains no yeast, wheat, corn, soy, milk or salt.

Royal Jelly 2000 — Premier One - Nutraceutical
One capsule contains: Royal Jelly 3.5x (equivalent to 2000 mg) 572 mg.

Rubus-Ginger Tea — HerbaSway
Ginger • Green Tea • Blackberry • HerbaSwee (Cucurbitaceae fruit).

Rx Fuel Bio-Designed Food Formula — TwinLab
Two servings contain: Branched Chain Amino Acids (L-Leucine, L-Isoleucine, & L-Valine) • L-Glutamine1000 mg • L-Carnitine 100 mg • Chromium (from Chromic Fuel Chromium Picolinate) 200 mcg. No added sugar, fructose, corn syrup solids, artificial colors, artificial flavors, mono- & diglycerides, or salt. This unique formulation is rich in potassium, yet has only 200 mg of sodium per serving.

Rx-Bone Ostivone — Nutritional Dynamics
Two tablets contain: Vitamin D 100 IU • Calcium 1000 mg • Ostivone 200 mg. Other ingredients: Di-Calcium Phosphate, Microcrystalline Cellulose, Silica, Stearic Acid, Pharmaceutical glaze.

SAF for Kids — Natrol
Six capsules contain: Vitamin C (Ester-C brand) 60 mg • Calcium 100 mg • Vitamin B6 (pyridoxine HCI) 50 mg • Magnesium 50 mg • Additional ingredients: GABA 800 mg • Glycine 800 mg • Passion flower extract 6:1 500 mg • L-Taurine 500 mg • Other ingredients: Microcrystalline Cellulose, Magnesium Stearate, Gelatin. SAF Patent #1,540,075.

SAF The Stress Formula — Natrol
Four capsules contain: Vitamin C (Ester-C Brand) 100 mg • Thiamine (Vitamin B1) 3 mg • Riboflavin (Vitamin B2) 3.1 mg • Niacin (Niacinamide) 50 mg, • Vitamin B6 (Pyridoxine HCI) 4 mg • Magnesium 100 mg • GABA 650 mg • L-Tyrosine 650 mg • Siberian Ginseng 100 mg • Inositol 100 mg, Patent #4,973,467. Other ingredients: Calcium Carbonate, Magnesium Stearate, Microcrystalline Cellulose, Gelatin.

Salad-Tabs — Wakunaga Consumer Products
Two tablets contain: Vitamin A (as Palmitate and Beta-Carotene) 5000 IU • Vitamin C (as Asorbic Acid) 60 mg • Vitamin D (as Cholecalciferol) 400 IU • Vitamin E (as D-Alpha-Tocopherol Acid Succinate) 30 IU • Thiamine (Vitamin B1) 1.5 mg • Riboflavin (Vitamin B2) 1.7 mg • Niacin 20 mg • Vitamin B6 (as Pyridoxine Hydrochloride) 2 mg • Folate (as Folic Acid) 400 mcg • Vitamin B12 (as Cyanocobalamin) 6 mcg • Biotin 300 mcg • Pantothenic Acid (as Calcium Pantothenate) 10 mg • Iron (as Ferrous Fumarate) 18 mg • Iodine (as Potassium Iodide) 150 mcg • Zinc (as Zinc Oxide) 15 mg • Copper (as Copper Gluconate) 2 mg • Manganese (as Manganese sulfate) 2 mg • Young Barley and Wheat Grass powder 600 mg • Chlorella 180 mg. Other Ingredients: Cellulose, Silica, Magnesium Stearate (vegetable source).

Salmon Oil 1000 mg — Jamieson
Each capsule contains: EPA (Eicosapentaenoic Acid) 180 mg • DHA (Docosahexaenoic Acid) 120 mg.

Salusan Herbal Rest — Flora
St. John's Wort • Passion Flower • Valerian & other calming herbs.

Sambu — Flora
Elderberry.

Sambu Guard — Flora
Wildgrown elder fruit & flower • Echinacea • Acerola Cherry fruit powder) & Vitamin C.

Sambucol Black Elder — Jb Harris
Each lozenge contains: Vitamin C (as ascorbic acid) 100 mg • Elderberry dried extract (berries) 130 mg. Other Ingredients: Sorbitol, peppermint extract.

Sambucol Immune System — Jb Harris
Two teaspoons (10 mL) contain: Zinc 10 mg • Vitamin C 100 mg • Proprietary blend 4 g: Elderberry extract (berries), Propolis,

Echinacea angustifolia (root), Echinacea purpurea (stems, leaves, flowers). Other Ingredients: Glucose syrup, raspberry extract (berries), honey, citric acid, & natural flavors.

Sambucol Original — Jb Harris
Each lozenge contains: Black Elder Tree extract (sambucus nigra).

Sambucol-D (Sugar Free) — Jb Harris
Each tablespoon contains: Elderberry juice (Black Elder tree, sambucus nigra 1). Other Ingredients: Liquid sorbitol, water, citric acid, natural flavor, & raspberry.

SAMe — Pinnacle
Each tablet contains SAM-e 200 mg • Vitamin B12 50 mcg • Folic Acid 100 mcg.

SAM-e — Nature Made Nutritional Products
Two tablets contain: S-adenosylmethionine 1 400 mg • 4-butanedisulfonate • Cellulose • Sodium Starch Glycolate • Methacrylic Acid Copolymer • Talc • Polyethylene Glycol • Silica • Magnesium Stearate • Polysorbate 80 • Sodium Hydroxide • Iron Oxide • Simethicone.

Sandal Turmeric (soap) — Auromere Ayurvedic Soaps
Coconut oil • Palmyra oil • Rice Bran oil • Alkali • Water • Hydnocarpus (Cactus) oil • Castor oil • Neem oil • Indian Beech oil • Mohwa (Madhuca Indica) oil • Sesame oil • Sandalwood oil • Neem Bark • Dhub Grass (Cynodon Dactylon) • Indian Gooseberry (Amla) • Turmeric • Peepal (Bodhi Tree) • Licorice • Celastrus seed • Tulsi (Holy Basil) • Corallacarpus epigaeus • Nutgrass • Zedoary • Indian Madder Root • Costus • Mung Bean • Fenugreek.

Sandelios Beauty Caps — Health From The Sun
Each capsule contains: Wheat Germ oil 150 mg • Yeast 50 mg • Vitamin E (d-Alpha Tocopherol) 10 mg • Nicotinamide 10 mg • Vitamin B2 1 mg • Calcium D-Pantothenate 6.5 mg • Vitamin B1 1.2 mg • Vitamin B6 1 mg • Carotin 0.8mg • D-Biotin 20 mcg • Vitamin B12 2 mcg. No sugar, preservatives, artificial coloring or flavoring.

Sandelios Garlic Caps — Health From The Sun
Each capsule contains: Garlic oil with Allicin 270 mg. No sugar, preservatives, artificial coloring or flavoring.

Sanhelios Circu Caps with Butcher's Broom — Health From The Sun
Each capsule contains: natural Rusci aculeati (Butcher's Broom) extract 75 mg • Rosemary oil 2 mg. No sugar. No preservatives. No artificial coloring or flavoring.

Sanhelios Devil's Claw Caps — Health From The Sun
Each capsule contains: natural Devil's Claw extract 120 mg. No sugar, preservatives, artificial coloring or flavoring.

Sanhelios Garlic Forte — Health From The Sun
Each gelcap contains: Garlic oil, Maceration 2-3:1, 280 mg. No sugar, starch, salt, preservatives, coloring, or flavoring.

Sanhelios Kalm Caps — Health From The Sun
Each capsule contains: Valerian root extract 4:1 150 mg. No sugar, preservatives, artificial coloring or flavoring.

Sanhelios Onion Caps — Health From The Sun
Each capsule contains: natural etherial Onion oil from Allium Cepa Linne (1.5 mg). No sugar, preservatives, artificial coloring or flavoring.

Sanhelios Propolentum Capsules — Health From The Sun
Each capsule contains: Propolis 250 mg.

Sanhelios Propolentum Throat Lozenges — Health From The Sun
Each lozenge contains: Isomalt 1465 mg • Menthol Crystals 3 mg • Propolis powder 30 mg • Peppermint oil 2 mg.

Sanhelios Prosta Caps — Health From The Sun
Each capsule contains: Pumpkin seed oil with Cucurbitin 150 mg • Alpha-Tocopherolacetate equalling 40.8 IU • Vitamin E 30 mg. No sugar, preservatives, artificial coloring or flavoring.

Sanhelios Water Caps — Health From The Sun
Each capsule contains: natural Juniper berry oil 20 mg. No sugar, preservatives, artificial coloring or flavoring.

Satietrol — PacificHealth Laboratories
Each (18 g) packet contains: Casein from Whey Protein Isolate

BRAND NAMES

© Copyright 2000, Natural Medicines Comprehensive Database (209) 472-2244. For updated data, go to www.NaturalDatabase.com.

B R A N D   N A M E S

enriched with glycomacropeptides • Potato Fiber • Sunflower Oil • Corn Syrup Solids • Natural & Artificial Flavors • Konjac Flour • Maltodextrin • Guar Gum • Calcium Lactate • Sodium Caseinate • Soy Lecithin • Alfalfa Powder • Monoglycerides • Diglycerides • Dipotassium Phosphate • Sodium Silicoaluminate • Aspartame.

Saventaro — Phytopharmica
Each capsule contains: Saventaro (Uncaria tomentosa pentacylic chemotype) Standardized to contain a minimum of 1.3% pentacyclic oxindole alkaloids (POAs) and to be free of tetracyclic oxindole alkaloids (TOAs) 20 mg. Other Ingredients: Cellulose, Calcium Carbonate, Magnesium Stearate, Silicon Dioxide, Gelatin Capsule.

Saw Palmetto — Centrum Herbals
One softgel contains: Saw Palmetto berry extract (Serenoa repens) 160 mg. Total Fatty Acids (marker) 80%. Standardized to contain (based on extract weight): Linolenic Acid (natural active), Lauric Acid, Ethyl Ester (natural active), Linoleic Acid, Ethyl Ester (natural active), Activity measure: Adrenergic alpha 1B binding assay. Other ingredients: Corn oil, Yellow Wax, Gelatin, Propylene Glycol, Hydroxypropl methylcellulose, Titanium Dioxide, Carmine.

Saw Palmetto — Gaia Herbs
Saw Palmetto standardized for 90% fatty acids. Standardized Full Spectrum 150 mg of extract per capsule. Guaranteed Potency 75 mg of extract per capsule.

Saw Palmetto — Pharmanex
Each softgel contains: Saw Palmetto berries (10:1) extract (Serenoa repens) 160 mg. Other Ingredients: Olive Oil, Gelatin, Glycerin, Carob.

Saw Palmetto Complex — Enzymatic Therapy
Each capsule contains: Saw Palmetto Berry extract standardized to contain 85% to 95% fatty acids & sterols 80 mg • Pumpkin seed oil extract (Cucurbita pepo) 40 mg • Pygeum africanum extract standardized to contain 13% total sterols 10 mg • Bearberry extract (Uva Ursi) standardized to contain 10% Arbutin 5 mg. Contains no sugar, salt, yeast, wheat, corn, dairy products, flavoring or preservatives.

Saw Palmetto Extract — Jamieson
Each capsule contains: Pumpkin seed oil (Curcubita pepo) 100 mg • Saw Palmetto berry 4:1 extract (Serenoa repens) 50 mg • Pygeum bark 150:1 Extract (Pygeum africanum 50 mg • Cranberry fruit 25:1 extract (Viccinum macrocarpon) 10 mg.

Saw Palmetto Formula — Quest
Each caplet contains: Saw Palmetto berry powder (Serenoa serrulate/repens) 110 mg • Corn Silk powder (Zea mays) 110 mg • Pumpkin Seed powder 90 mg • Parsley leaf powder (Petroselinum crispu) 55 mg • Buchu leaf powder (Barosma betulina) 35 mg • Cayenne powder (Capsicum) 35 mg • Kelp powder (Fucus vesiculosis) 35 mg. Other Ingredients: Calcium Phosphate, Microcrystalline Cellulose, Vegetable Stearin, Croscarmellose Sodium, Magnesium Stearate (vegetable source).

Saw Palmetto Male Toner — Traditional Medicinals
Hibiscus flower • Saw Palmetto berry • Nettle root • Uva Ursi leaf • Ginger rhizome • Saw Palmetto berry dry extract • Althea root • Rose Hip • natural Lemon flavor • Stevia leaf.

Saw Palmetto Plus — Atrium
Each capsule contains: Saw Palmetto oil (50:1 extract) 160 mg • Olive oil 90 mg. Contains no wheat, sugar, starch, corn, salt, yeast, milk or soy.

Saw Palmetto-Suma Virtue — Blessed Herbs
Saw Palmetto berry • Siberian Ginseng root • Jamaican Sarsaparilla root • Suma root • Astragalus root • Damiana • Grain alcohol & Distilled Water.

Say Yes to Beans — Nature's Plus
Each Vegicap contains: Legumase (Saccharamyces cerevisae & Aspergillus enzyme complex) 125 mg • Licorice root (Glycyrrhiza glabra) standardized < 2% Glycyrrhizinic acid 75 mg • Ginger root (Zingiber officinale) standardized 5% gingerols 25 mg • Parsley seed (Petroselinum crispum) 20 mg. Contains no yeast, wheat, corn, soy, milk, salt, sugar or starch.

SB Normal Stool Formula — Shaman Botanicals
Each tablet contains: Croton lechleri extract (sap) (standardized to contain 250 mg of SP-303). Other Ingredients: Microcrystalline Cellulose, Coating (Methacrylic Acid Copolymer, Magnesium

Silicate, Triethyl Citrate), Glyceryl Monostearate, Sodium Starch Glycolate, Silicon Dioxide.

Schisandra — Pharmanex
Each capsule contains: Schisandra (Schisandra chinensis)(berry extract)(10:1) 200 mg. Other Ingredients: Rice Flour, Gelatin, Magnesium Stearate, Silicon Dioxide.

Sea & Earth — The Vitamin Shoppe
Sea-life protein • Vitamin C • Zinc • Silica • Green Tea extract • Red Wine extract • Red Cabbage extract • Grape Juice extract • Pine Bark extract • Citrus Bioflavonoids • Carotene.

Sea Cal Oyster Shell Calcium — Nature's Life
Two tablets contain: Calcium (Oyster Shell) 500 mg • Vitamin D3 (Cholecaciferol) 250 IU.

Sea Cucumber — Futurebiotics
Sea Cucumber 500 mg.

Sea Mussel — Futurebiotics
New Zealand Greenshell Mussel 500 mg.

Seaweed Virtue — Blessed Herbs
Kelp • Bladderwrack • Dulse & Other Seaweeds as Available. Grain alcohol & Distilled Water.

Secretagogue-One — MHP
Each packet contains: Anterior Pituitary Substance 25 mg • Glycoamino Acid-Glucose Complex 4200 mg • Novel polyose complex 2230 mg • Amino Acid Blend 500 mg • Broad Bean 10 mg.

Selenium 50 mcg — Jamieson
Each caplet contains: Selenium (Proteinate) 50 mcg • Beta-Carotene (Provitamin A) 5000 IU • Vitamin C (Ascorbic Acid) 60 mg • Vitamin E (Natural D-Alpha Tocopheryl Acetate) 10 IU.

Selenomax Selenium 200 Mcg — Nature's Life
Each tablet contains: Selenium (natural food yeast-based) (Nutrition 21 Selenomax) 200 mcg.

Senior-Vites Plus — The Vitamin Shoppe
Three tablets contain: Vitamin A Activity 20000 IU • Vitamin D 400 IU • Vitamin C 150 mg • Vitamin E 200 IU • Vitamin B1 35 mg • Vitamin B2 35 mg • Niacinamide 50 mg • Vitamin B6 35 mg • Vitamin B12 50 mcg • Pantothenic Acid 75 mg • Folic Acid 400 mcg • Biotin 300 mcg • PABA 35 mg • Inositol 100 mg • Choline 100 mg • Citrus Bioflavonoids 25 mg • Rutin 25 mg • Glutamine 100 mg • Taurine 100 mg • Glutamic Acid 50 mg • Pancreatin 25 mg • Ox Bile 10 mg • Calcium 100 mg • Magnesium 50 mg • Iron 18 mg • Zinc 15 mg • Manganese 6 mg • Potassium 45 mg • Iodine 225 mcg • Selenium 50 mcg • Chromium 25 mcg • Fo-Ti 50 mg • Gotu Kola 50 mg • Avena Sativa 25 mg • Siberian Ginseng 25 mg • Nettles extract 10 mg.

Sentinel Multi Vitamin — Health Center for Better Living
Each tablet contains: Vitamin A (as retinyl acetate and beta-carotene) 5000 IU • Vitamin C (as ascorbic acid) 60 mg • Vitamin D (as cholecalciferol) 400 IU • Vitamin E (as dl-alpha-tocopheryl acetate) 30 IU• Vitamin K (as phytonadione) 25 mcg • Thamin (as thiamin mononitrate) 1.5 mg • Riboflavin 1.7 mg • Niacin (as niacinamide) 20 mg • Vitamin B6 (as pyridoxine HCl) 2 mg • Folate (as folic acid) 400 mcg • Vitamin B12 (as cyancobalamin) 6 mcg • Biotin 30 mcg Pantothenic acid (as D-calcium pantothenate) 10 mg • Calcium (as dicalcium phosphate) 162 mg • Iron (as ferrous fumarate) 18 mg • Phosphorus (as dicalcium phosphate) 125 mg • Iodine (as potassium iodide) 150 mcg • Magnesium (as magnesium oxide) 100 mg• Zinc (as zinc oxide) 15 mg • Selenium (as sodium selenate) 25 mcg • Copper (as cupric oxide) 2 mg • Manganese (as manganese sulfate) 2.5 mcg • Chromium (as chromium chloride)• Molybdenum (as sodium moybdate) 25 mcg • Chloride (as potassium choride) 36.3 mg • Potassium (as potassium choride) 40 mg• Vanadium (as sodium metavandate) 10 mcg • Tin (as stannous chloride) 10 mcg • Silicon (as sodium metasilicate) 10 mcg • Nickel (as nickelous sulfate) 5 mcg.

SerenAid — Klaire Laboratories
Each capsule contains: Multi-Enzyme Complex (proprietary blend) 317 mg: L-Lysine, Peptidase FP, Papain (sulfite free), Protease, Acid-stable Protease, Lactase. Contains no gluten, casein, soy, corn, sugars, flavors, fragrances, preservatives, salicylates, artificial colors or other common allergenic substances.

Serenoa Repens — Progressive Labs
Each softgel contains: Saw Palmetto purified extract (95% free fatty acids) 160 mg • Olive oil 160 mg.

Serrapeptase (Serraflazyme) — Olympia Nutrition
Silk worm enzyme.

Serum For Sensitive Skin — Cellex-C
Ascorbic Acid • Tyrosine • Zinc • Sodium Hyaluronate • Pine Bark extract.

Shake and Bake — The Herbalist
Oils of Sweet Almond, Aloe Vera, Safflower, St. John's Wort flower, Calendula flower, & Vitamin E • Extracts of St. John's Wort flower, Calendula flower & Chamomile flower • Essential oils of Sandalwood, Lite Musk, French Vanilla.

Shark Oil — Futurebiotics
Shark liver oil 460 mg.

Sharp Thinking — Changes - TwinLab
Two caplets contain: Ginkgo Biloba leaf standardized extract (24% flavonglycosides, 6% terpene lactones) 120 mg • Huperine A (from Huperzia serrata extract whole plant) 50 mcg • Green Tea leaf standardized extract (30% polyphenols, 20% methylxanthines) 500 mg • Panax Ginseng root standardized extract (4% ginsenosides) 200 mg • Brahmi leaf standardized extract (10% asiaticosides)(Centella asiatica) 100 mg • Citrus aurantium fruit standardized extract (5-7% alkaloids) 50 mg. Other ingredients: Dicalcium Phosphate, Vegetable Cellulose, Fractionated vegetable oil, Soy polysaccharides, Silica, and Vegetable resin glaze.

Shen Min — Biotech
Three tablets contain: Shen Min (a proprietary blend of 12:1 standardized He Shou Wu (Fo Ti) root extract and He Shou Wu root powder providing a synergistic complex of chrysophanics and resveratrol) 1775 mg • Bioperine Black Pepper (Piper nigrum) 3.0 mg. Other ingredients: Dicalcium phoosphate, Microcrystalline Cellulose, Croscarmellose Sodium, Stearic Acid, Magnesium Stearate, Pharmaceutical glaze.

Ship-Assure — Nature's Plus
Two tablets contain: Ginger root [(Zingiber officinale) standardized 4% Volatile oils] 350 mg • Kava [(Piper methysticum) standardized 29-31% kavalactones] 50 mg • Chamomile flower [(Matricaria recutita) standardized 1% apigenin, 0.5% essential oil] 50 mg • Hops fruit [(Humulus lupulus) standardized 5.2% bitter acids, 4% flavonoids] 50 mg • Siberian Ginseng root [(Eleutherococcus senticosus) standardized 0.8% Eleutherosides] 50 mg • Passion Flower [(Passiflora incarnata) standardized 3.5-4% flavonoids, calculated as isovitexin] 50 mg • Wild Cherry (Prunus virginlana fruit) 50 mg. Contains no yeast, wheat, corn, soy, milk, salt, or starch.

SHN Skin-Hair-Nails — The Vitamin Shoppe
Three tablets contain: Vitamin A (beta carotene) 10,000 IU • Vitamin C 120 mg • Vitamin B1 10 mg • Vitamin B2 10 mg • Niacinamide 50 mg • Calcium 600 mg • Iron 6 mg • Vitamin D 200 IU • Vitamin E 30 IU • Vitamin B6 10 mg • Folic Acid 400 mcg • Vitamin B12 16 mcg • Phosphorus 300 mg • Iodine (kelp) 225 mcg • Magnesium 200 mg • Zinc 15 mg • Biotin 400 mcg • Pantothenic Acid 30 mg • Choline 150 mcg • Inositol 60 mg • PABA 50 mg • Selenium 25 mcg • Manganese 10 mg • RNA 60 mg • Bioflavonoids 50 mg • Rutin 25 mg • Betaine Hydrochloride 50 mg. In a base of L-Cysteine, Methionine, Gelatin, Papain, Oat Straw, Echinacea, Horse Tail, and Asparagus.

Siberian Ginseng — Gaia Herbs
Siberian Ginseng standardized for 0.8% eleutherosides B & E. Standardized Full Spectrum 200 mg of extract per capsule. Guaranteed Potency 100 mg of extract per capsule.

Siberian Ginseng — Pharmanex
Each capsule contains: Ginseng, Siberian (Eleutherococcus senticosus Max)(root extract)(10:1) 150 mg. Other Ingredients: Rice Flour, Gelatin, Magnesium Stearate, Silicon Dioxide.

Sil-150 — Phytopharmica
Each capsule contains: Milk Thistle extract (Silybum marianum) 150 mg standardized to contain 70% silymarin (105 mg per capsule) calculated as silybin. Contains no sugar, salt, yeast, wheat, corn, soy, dairy products, flavorings or preservatives. All organs & glands derived from bovine sources.

Silent Night Formula — Nature's Way
Four capsules contain: Proprietary Formula: Hops flower • Scullcap herb • Valerian root. Other ingredients: Gelatin.

Silica 10 mg — Jamieson
Each caplet contains: Standardized Silica 10 mg from pure spring Horsetail herb 3080 mg (Equisetum arvense L 770 mg powdered extract 1:4). With natural occurring flavonoids, saponins and minerals.

SiliCare — Holista
Each capsule contains Silicon (dioxide) derived from 410 mg 2.9% Spring Horsetail Equisetum arvense extract 5 mg.

Silybin Phytosome — Phytopharmica
Each capsule contains: Silybin Phytosome (milk thistle extract) 120 mg bound to phosphatidycholine under patent. Contains no sugar, salt, yeast, wheat, gluten, corn, dairy products, coloring, flavorings or preservatives.

Silymarin — Aspen Group, Inc.
Each capsule contains: Silymarin (Milk Thistle, standardized at 80%) 150 mg.

Simicort — Enzymatic Therapy
Active ingredient: Salicylic Acid 1.8%. Other ingredients: Purified Water, Organic Fatty Acid Complex (C11-C18), Glyceryl Stearate, Chamomile extract (0.5% Flavonoid Content), 18-Beta-Glycyrrhetinic Acid from Licorice root extract, Allantoin 2.0% from Comfrey root extract, Dimethicone, Vitamin E antioxidant, & Hypoallergenic Fragrance.

Sino-Lung Res-Q — Nutri-Quest
Each tablet contains: Lung 35 mg • Thymus 35 mg • Spleen 35 mg • Vitamin C 75 mg • Beta Carotene 12600 IU • Lemon Bioflavonoids 125 mg • Rutin 20 mg • Hesperidin Complex 75 mg • N-Acetyl Cysteine 35 mg • Propolis 20 mg • Cranberry 36 mg • Echinacea 30 mg • Goldenseal 35 mg • Elderberry 10 mg • Scullcap 35 mg.

SinuCheck — Enzymatic Therapy
Each capsule contains: Active ingredient: Pseudoephedrine HCl (from Ephedra sinensis) 30 mg • Other ingredients: Scullcap extract 4:1 (Scutellaria baicalensis) 100 mg • Chinese Thoroughwax extract (Bupleurum falcatum) 100 mg • Chinese Peony extract 4:1 (Paeonia Lactiflora) 100 mg • Dong Quai extract (4:1) (Angelica sinensis) 100 mg • Licorice root extract (Glycyrrhiza glabra) standardized to contain 5% Glycyrrhizic Acid 40 mg • Curcuma root extract (Curcuma longa) standardized to contain 4% Curcumin 20 mg • Ginger root extract 6.5:1 (Zingiber officinale) 20 mg. Contains no sugar, salt, yeast, wheat, corn, soy, dairy products, coloring, flavoring or preservatives.

SinuClear — Phytopharmica
Each capsule contains: Active ingredient: Pseudoephedrine HCL 30 mg (from Ephedra sinensis). Other ingredients: Scullcap extract 4:1 (Scutellaria baicalensis) 100 mg • Chinese Thoroughwax extract (Bupleurum falcatum) 100 mg • Chinese Peony extract 4:1 (Paeonia lactiflora) 100 mg • Dong Quai extract 4:1 (Angelica sinensis) 100 mg • Licorice root extract (Glycyrrhiza glabra) 40 mg standardized to contain 5% glycyrrhizic acid • Curcuma root extract (Curcuma longa) 20 mg standardized to contain 2.5% curcumin • Ginger root extract 6.5:1 (Zingiber officinale) 20 mg. Contains no sugar, salt, yeast, wheat, corn, soy, dairy products, coloring, flavoring or preservatives.

SinuComp — Phytopharmica
Each tablet contains: Cowslip flowers (Primula veris) 36 mg • Sour Dock (Rumex acetosa) 36 mg • Elder flowers (Sambucus nigra) 36 mg • Verbena (Verbena officinalis) 36 mg • Gentian root (Gentiana lutea) 12 mg. Product contains no sugar, salt, yeast, wheat, gluten, corn, soy, dairy products, coloring, flavoring, or preservatives.

SinuGuard — Enzymatic Therapy
Each tablet contains: Cowslip flower (Primula veris) 36 mg • Sour Dock (Rumex acetosa) 36 mg • Elder flower (Sambucus nigra) 36 mg • Verbena (Verbena officinalis) 36 mg • Gentian root (Gentiana lutea) 12 mg. Contains no sugar, salt, yeast, wheat, gluten, corn, soy, dairy products, coloring, flavoring or preservatives.

Sinus Ease — Nature's Life
Three capsules contain: Bromelain [an enzyme from Pineapple fruit (Ananassa sativa) activity of 1200 mg = 2,880 GDU (4320 MCU)] 1200 mg • Quercetin (a flavonoid from Pilocarpus gaborandi) 300 mg • Vitamin C (Buffered, as Calcium Ascorbic) 133 mg.

© Copyright 2000, Natural Medicines Comprehensive Database (209) 472-2244. For updated data, go to www.NaturalDatabase.com. • 1397

BRAND NAMES

**B
R
A
N
D

N
A
M
E
S**

Sinutone — The Herbalist
Eyebright herb • Golden Seal root • Bayberry root bark • Osha root • Yarrow flower • Horseradish root • Cayenne pepper.

Sitol — PharmaGen
Each capsule contains: Serenoa repens extract (standardized) 320 mg.

Sitol PA — PharmaGen
Each capsule contains: Serenoa repens extract (standardized) 320 mg • Pygeum africanum extract (standardized) 100 mg.

Skin Clear — The Herbalist
Echinacea root • Yellow Dock root • Oregon Grape root • Burdock root • Red Clover blossom • Jamaican Sarsaparilla root.

Skin Firming Cream Plus — Cellex-C
Ascorbic Acid • Tyrosine • Vitamin E • Zinc • Bioflavonoids • Sodium Hyaluronate • Evening Primrose oil • Glycine • Tomato extract • Aloe barbadensis gel • Chamomile extract • Allantoin.

Skin Tone Balancer — Jason
10% Complete Vitamin C Complex with Kojic Ester • Beta Hydroxy Acids • Barberry extract • Super Oxide Dismutase liposome.

Skin, Hair and Nails — Aspen Group, Inc.
Three tablets contain: Vitamin A 5000 IU • Vitamin C 60 mg • Vitamin B1 5 mg • Riboflavin 5 mg • Niacinamide 25 mg • Calcium 300 mg • Iron 3 mg • Vitamin D 100 IU • Vitamin E 15 IU • Vitamin B6 5 mg • Folic Acid 200 mcg • Vitamin B12 8 mcg • Phosphorus 150 mg • Iodine 112.5 mg • Magnesium 100 mg • Zinc 7.5 mg • Biotin 200 mcg • Pantothenic Acid 15 mg • Choline 75 mg • Inositol 30 mg • PABA 25 mg • Selenium 12.5 mcg • Manganese 5 mg • RNA 30 mg • Bioflavonoids 25 mg • Rutin 12.5 mg • Betaine HCI 25 mg • Horsetail Silica 50 mg. Contains no sugar, starch, salt, wheat, corn, yeast or soy derivatives.

Skin, Hair, Nails — Natrol
Two capsules contain: Vitamin A (as Vitamin A palmitate) 5000 mg • Vitamin C (ascorbic acid) 100 mg • Vitamin E (as d-alpha tocopherol succinate) 50 IU • Thiamine (Vitamin B1) (as Thiamine HCI) 10 mg • Riboflavin (Vitamin B2) 10 mg • Vitamin B6 (pyridoxine HCI) 20 mg • Vitamin B12 (as cobalamin) 50 mcg • Biotin 500 mcg • Zinc (as zinc oxide) 8 mg • Copper (as amino acid chelate) 2 mg • Manganese (as manganese carbonate) 2 mg • MSM (methyl sulfonyl methane) 250 mg • Trace Mineral Complex 100 mg • Cysteine (as L-cysteine hydrochloride) 75 mg • PABA (para amino benzoic acid) 50 mg • Burdock root 50 mg • Choline (as choline bitartrate) 25 mg • Inositol 25 mg • Silicon (as colloidal silicon) 20 mg • Glutathiione (as L-glutathione reduced) 2 mg. Other ingredients: Rice powder, Magnesium Stearate, Gelatin.

Sleep-Assure — Nature's Plus
Each tablet contains: Rapid Release Layer: Melatonin (N-Acetyl-5-Methoxytryptamine) 1.5 mg • GABA (Gamma Aminobutyric Acid) 10 mg • Pyridoxal-5-Phosphate (P5P) 10 mg. Sustained Release Layer: Melatonin (N-Acetyl-5-Methoxytryptamine) 1.5 mg • Herbal Blend containing equal proportions of: [Kava Kava root extract (Piper methysticum) standardized 29-31% kavalactones, Passion Flower extract (Passiflora incarnata) standardized 3.5-4% flavonoids calculated as isovitexin, Valerian root extract (Valeriana officinalis) standardized 1% Valerenic Acid, Chamomile flower (Matricaria recutita) standardized 1% Apigenin 0.5% essential oil] 25 mg. Contains no yeast, wheat, corn, soy, milk, salt, sugar or starch.

Slender Shaper — Pharmagel
E-L-A Complex.

Slender-Mist — Karemor
Vitamin B6 • Pantothenic Acid • Chromium • Hydroxy-Citric Acid • L-Carnitine. Available in Arctic Mint, Berry Supreme, Chocolate Fudge, and Tropical Delite flavors.

Slim Down GTF Chromium 200 mcg — Jamieson
Each tablet contains: Chromium (from brewer's yeast) 200 mcg.

Slim Smart — Health Center for Better Living
Chromium Pocolinate 200 mcg, other herbs.

Slim Trim(tm) — Life Extension
L- Arginine 500 mg L-Ornithine 250 mg.

Slimming Formula — Phytopharmica
One tablet contains: Thyroidinum 8x • Antimonium crudum 3x • Calcarea acetica 2x • Fucus vesiculosus 2x.
Editor's Comments: This is a homeopathic product. It is so extremely diluted that its activity can not be explained by conventional scientific methods. Therefore this product can not be rated by the scientific criteria used in this Database. A patient receiving the extreme dilution of this product will not receive many, if any, molecules of the original active ingredient. Therefore, there are no harmful pharmacologic effects, and any beneficial effects are controversial and not due to a direct biochemical action of the ingredient on the body. Homeopathic products are allowed for sale in the U.S. due to legislation passed in the 19th century sponsored by a homeopathic physician who was also a Senator. The law still requires that the FDA allow the sale of products listed in this Homeopathic Pharmacopea of the United States.

Slow Mag — Roberts
Two tablets contain: Calcium (from calcium carbonate) 212 mg • Magnesium 128 mg & Chloride 373 mg (from magnesium chloride hexahydrate) • Cellulose Acetate Phthalate • Pregelatinized Starch • Povidone • Diethylphthalate • Talc • Titanium Dioxide • Magnesium Stearate & FD&C Blue No. 2 Lake.

Slumber — Nutrivention
Two tablets contain: Calcium (Amino Acid Chelate) 500 mg • Magnesium (Amino Acid Chelate) 500 mg • Inositol 200 mg • Niacinamide 20 mg • Biotin 100 mcg • Passion flower 200 mg • Blue Vervain 200 mg • Hops 100mg • Valerian root (Star root) 100 mg • Wild Lettuce 100 mg.

SlumberActin — Nature's Plus
Three capsules contain: Chamomile [(Matricaria recutita root) standardized 1% Apigenin, 0.5% Essential oil] 200 mg • Valerian [(Valeriana officinalis root) standardized 1% Valernic Acids] 100 mg • Passion Flower [(Passiflora incarnata flower) standardized 3.5-4% Flavonoids] 75 mg • Hops [(Humulus lupulus fruit) standardized 5.2% Bitter Acids, 4% Flavonoids] 75 mg • Kava Kava [(Piper methysticum root) standardized 29-31% Kavalactones] 50 mg • English Hawthorne [(Crataegus laevigata berry) standardized 3.2% Vitexin] 50 mg • Magnesium (Amino Acid Chelate) 50 mg • Calcium (Amino Acid Chelate) 25 mg.

Smart Coffee w/ Ginkgo Biloba — Nature's Plus
Each 3 g serving contains: Instant herbal coffee blend: naturally decaffeinated Brazilian coffee (coffea), Ginkgo Biloba, standardized 24% ginkgo flavone-glycosides, 6% terpene lactones • Rosemary (Rosmarinus officinalis) • Fo-Ti (Polygonum multiflorum) • Wild Grape (Mahonia aquifolia) standardized 95-100% leucoanthocyanidins • Chinese Apricot (Prunus armeniaca). Contains no yeast, wheat, corn, soy, milk, salt, or starch.

Smart Pill — Only Natural, Inc.
Two tablets contain: Ginkgo Biloba leaf extract 10:1 250 mg • Gotu Kola 250 mg • Ginseng 100 mg • Capsicum 50 mg • L-Phenylalanine 200 mg • L-Glutamine 500 mg • L-Tyrosine 200 mg • GABA 300 mg • Vitamin B1 50 mg • Vitamin B3 50 mg • Vitamin B5 100 mg • Vitamin B6 50 mg • Vitamin B12 500 mcg • Folic Acid 200 mcg • Inositol 100 mg • Phosphatidylcholine 500 mg • RNA 100 mg • TMG 50 mg.

Smart Vitamins — Jamieson
Each capsule contains: Choline Bitartrate • Molasses cone • L-Glutamine • Brewers Yeast (a natural source of the B complex vitamin Family) • Acerola (a natural source of Vitamin C) • Taurine • Kola Nut • Korean Ginseng • Vegetable Magnesium Stearate • Wheat Germ Powder • Silica • Chromium Yeast • Turnera (Damiana aphrodesiaca) • Capsicum (Cayenne) • Gingko Biloba • Fo-Ti (Polygonum multiflorum).

Smoke-Less — The Herbalist
Lobelia leaf • Milk Thistle seed • Oat seed • Siberian Ginseng root • Licorice root.

Smooth Move — Traditional Medicinals
Sennosides A & B: 20 mg per cup as they naturally occur in Senna leaf (Casala angustifolia) present in the blend. Other herbal ingredients: Licorice root, Fennel seed, Orange peel, Cinnamon bark, Coriander seed, Ginger rhizome, natural Orange flavor.

Snooze — Pacific BioLogic
Valerian root • Dragon Bone (fossilized) • Oyster Shell (untreated) • Mimosa Tree flower • Chamomile • Gotu Kola • Hops • Polygala root • Jujube seed (sour) • Passion flower • Scullcap • Melatonin 1.5 mg per capsule.

Snorenz — MedGen, Inc.
Peppermint Oil • Sunflower Oil • Sesame Oil • Olive Oil • Almond Oil.

Some Brand Name Natural Products - What they Contain
www.NaturalDatabase.com contains MANY more listings than appear here.

SnoreStop — The Green Pharmacy
Each tablet contains: Nux vomica 4X • Nux vomica 6X • Belladonna 6X • Ephedra vulgaris 6X • Hydrastis canadensis 6X • Kali bichromicum 6X • Teucrium marum 6X • Histaminum hydrochloricum 12X.

Editor's Comments: This is a homeopathic product. It is so extremely diluted that its activity can not be explained by conventional scientific methods. Therefore this product can not be rated by the scientific criteria used in this Database. A patient receiving the extreme dilution of this product will not receive many, if any, molecules of the original active ingredient. Therefore, there are no harmful pharmacologic effects, and any beneficial effects are controversial and not due to a direct biochemical action of the ingredient on the body. Homeopathic products are allowed for sale in the U.S. due to legislation passed in the 19th century sponsored by a homeopathic physician who was also a Senator. The law still requires that the FDA allow the sale of products listed in this Homeopathic Pharmacopea of the United States.

Soft Gelatin Multiple — Nature's Life
Two capsules contain: Beta Carotene (Vitamin A equivalent 15000 IU) 9 mg • Vitamin A (Fish Liver oil) 10000 IU • Vitamin D3 (Cholecalciferol) 400 IU • Vitamin E (d-Alpha Tocopherol) 400 IU • Vitamin C 300 mg • Rose Hips 20 mg • Folic Acid 400 mcg • Vitamin B1 (Thiamine Mononitrate) 50 mg • Vitamin B2 (Riboflavin) 50 mg • Niacinamide 50 mg • Vitamin B6 (Pyridoxine HCl) 50 mg • Vitamin B12 (Cyanocobalamin) 100 mcg • Biotin (d-Biotin) 300 mcg • Pantothenic Acid(d-Calcium Pantothenate) 50 mg • Choline (Bitartrate) 25 mg • Inositol 25 mg • PABA (Para Aminobenzoic Acid) 25 mg • Boron (Calcium Boron Gluconate) 25 mcg • Calcium (Carbonate, Citrate, Aspartate) 200 mg • Chromium (Nutrition 21 Picolinate) 25 mcg • Copper (Gluconate) 2 mg • Iodine (Potassium Iodide) 150 mcg • Iron (Peptonate) 10 mg • Magnesium (Magnesium Oxide) 100 mg • Manganese (Amino Acid Chelate) 15 mg • Molybdenum (Free-Form Amino Acid Chelate) 25 mcg • Potassium (Phosphate & Iodide) 15 mg • Selenium (l-Selenomethionine, yeast-free) 15 mcg • Silicon Dioxide 20 mg • Vanadium (Vanadyl Sulfate) 25 mcg • Zinc (Citrate, Gluconate, Picolinate) 15 mg • Essential Fatty Acids (Safflower oil) 540 mg.

Soluble Enzyme Caps — Atrium
Each capsule contains: Papayotin 110 mg • Pancreatin (Bovine) 90 mg • Calf Thymus (Bovine) 50 mg • Bromelain 50 mg • Lipase 10 mg • Chymotrypsin 15 mg. Lemon flavor.

Solu-Min — Aspen Group, Inc.
Calcium • Phosphorus • Magnesium • Potassium • Sulfur • Iron • Iodine • Copper • Cobalt • Zinc • Chromium • Manganese • Molybdenum • Selenium • Aluminum • Antimony • Barium • Bismuth • Cadmium • Sodium • Cesium • Carbon • Lithium • Nickel • Platinum • Rubidium • Silver • Strontium • Silicon • Tungsten • Tin • Titanium • Tantalum • Thorium • Vanadium • Zirconium • Yttrium. Plus up to 30 other randomly occurring trace minerals in natural combinations.

Sore Throat Lozenge — Jamieson
Each lozenge contains: Slippery Elm bark 50 mg • White Horehound leaves 50 mg • Parsley root 20 mg • Thyme leaves 10 mg • Menthol 5 mg. Other Ingredients: Camphor 50 mcg, Acerola Cherry 40 mg, Sugar, Glucose, Honey, Anise Oil, and natural flavors.

Source of Life Oxygenic — Nature's Plus
Three tablets contain: Mixed Wild berry extract containing: (European Red Wine Grape, Bilberry, Blackberry, Black Raspberry, & Red Raspberry standardized 20% Polyphenols, 4% Anthocyanosides) 300 mg • Chinese Green Tea extract standardized 20% Polyphenols) 300 mg • Horseradish concentrate naturally rich in Peroxidase & Catalase 250 mg • Vitamin C fortified with Rose Hips, Mango, Guava & West Indian Cherry 100 mg • Beta Carotene (Dunaliella salina, Carrot) 2500 IU • Wild Grape seed extract standardized 95-100% Leucoanthocyanins 10 mg • Pycnogenol (Pine bark extract) standardized 85-95% Proanthocyanidins 5 mg. In a whole food base of Broccoli, Spinach, Cauliflower & Beet Greens. Contains no yeast, wheat, corn, soy, milk, salt, sugar or starch.

Source of Life Vibra-Gest — Nature's Plus
Each Vegicap contains: Brown Rice Fermentation: Amylase, 30000 units/gram 50 mg • Lactase, 1000 units/gram 50 mg • Lipase, 5000 units/gram 50 mg • Cellulase, 5000 units/gram 30 mg • Protease, 100000 units/gram 20 mg • Oxidase, 5000 units/gram 10 mg • Barley Malt: Diastase, 1000 units/gram 10 mg • Maltase, 1000 units/gram 10 mg • Sweet Potato: Phosphatase, 4000 units/gram 5 mg • Pineapple: Bromelain, 600 GDU/gram 35 mg • Papaya: Papain, 2 million units/gram 30 mg • Carrot Powder: Lactobacillus acidophilus 4 billion

viable cells/gram 100 mg • Natural Cultures: Bifidobacterium longum 1 billion viable cells/gram 50 mg • Lactobacillus bulgaricus 1 billion viable cells/gram 50 mg. Contains no yeast, wheat, corn, soy, milk, salt, sugar or starch.

Soy Defense — Changes - TwinLab
Two caplets contain: Vitamin E (as D-Alpha-Tocopheryl Succinate and Dl-Alpha-Tocopheryl Acetate) 200 IU • Mixed Soy phytosterols 50 mg • Tri-source isoflavone concentrate (defatted Soy Germ, Red Clover flower, and Kudzu root)(providing 40 mg total isoflavones) 1333 mg • Soy polysaccharides 150 mg. Other ingredients: Dicalcium Phosphate, Vegetable Cellulose, Fractionated vegetable oil, Silica, Calcium Sulfate, and Vegetable resin glaze.

Soy Essentials — Health From The Sun
Four tablets contain: Genistein (Aglycone) 2.88 mg • Diadzein (Aglycone) 2.20 mg • Beta Glucans 7.87 mg. Ingredients: Certified GMO-Free Fermented Soymeal (Soynatto), Microcrystalline Cellulose, Stearic Acid, HPC (cellulose), Croscarmellose Sodium, Magnesium Stearate, Silicon Dioxide, Pharmaceutical Glaze.

Soy Force Rx — Biotech
Two tablets contain: Soy Isoflavones 80 mg • Soy Protein Concentrate 500 mg • OPTiSOY Blend 300 mg.

Soy Isoflavone — Natrol
One capsule contains: Soy Isoflavone extract 100 mg containing: Isoflavones (10%) 10 mg • Daidzin & Daidzein (2%) 2 mg • Genistin & Genistein (9%) 9 mg • Glycitin & Glycitein (0.1%) 0.1 mg. Other ingredients: Rice powder, Magnesium Stearate, Gelatin.

Soy-Based Milk-Free Lactobacillus Acidophilus powder — Nature's Life
Each level tablespoon (6 g) contains: A freeze-dried blend of unrefined Apple Juice, Maltodextrin NF, SUPRO brand Soy Protein, pure Crystalline Fructose & our uniquely cultured probiotics Lactobacillus Acidophilus (95%), L. Bulgaricus (3%) & Bifidobacteria Bifidus (2%).

SoySwee Tea — HerbaSway
Soy • Ginger • Panax Ginseng • Siberian Ginseng • Blackberry • HerbaSwee (Cucurbitaceae fruit).

SP-500 — Phytopharmica
Each capsule contains: Spleen Polypeptides 375 mg, a mixture of highly purified bovine-derived spleen polypeptides naturally present in the spleen, including tuftsin, splenopentin, splenin & leukokinin • Goldenseal root extract (Hydrastis canadensis) 125 mg standardized to contain 5% total alkaloids including Berberine, Hydrastine & Canadine. Contains no sugar, salt, yeast, wheat, corn, dairy products, flavoring or preservatives. All organs & glands derived from bovine sources.

Speak Easy Throat Spray — The Herbalist
Yerba Mansa root • Echinacea root • Marshmallow root • Propolis • Myrrh Gum • Licorice root in a base of Vegetable Glycerine.

Special B-Complex 50 mg — Nature's Life
Each capsule contains: Vitamin C 50 mg • Vitamin B1 (Thiamine HCl) 50 mg • Vitamin B2 (Riboflavin) 50 mg • Niacinamide 50 mg • Vitamin B6 (Pyridoxine HCl) 50 mg • Folic Acid 800 mcg • Vitamin B12 (Cobalamin concentrate) 50 mcg • Biotin 50 mcg • Pantothenic Acid (d-Calcium Pantothenate) 50 mg • Choline (Choline Bitartrate) 50 mg • Inositol 50 mg • PABA (Para-Aminobenzioc Acid) 50 mg. In a natural base of Rice Bran, Alfalfa, Parsley, Watercress, Rose Hips & Acerola.

Special Two — Now
Two tablets contain: Vitamin A (Beta Carotene) (6 mg) 10000 IU • Vitamin B1 (Thiamine HCL) 50 mg • Vitamin B2 (Riboflavin) 50 mg • Vitamin B3 (Niacinamide) 50 mg • Vitamin B5 (Pantothenic Acid) 50 mg • Vitamin B6 (Pyridoxine HCL) 50 mg • Vitamin B12 (Cyanocobalamin) 100 mcg • Biotin 100 mcg • Folic Acid 400 mcg • Vitamin C (Calcium Ascorbate) 500 mg • Vitamin D (Calciferol) 200 IU • Vitamin E (d-Alpha Succinate) 200 IU • Vitamin K (from green foods) 70 mcg • Calcium (Ascorbate, Carbonate) 100 mg • Magnesium (Oxide , Amino Acid Chelate) 50 mg • Zinc (Amino Acid Chelate) 15 mg • Iron (Amino Acid Chelate) 10 mg • Copper (Amino Acid Chelate) 1 mg • Iodine (Kelp) 150 mcg • Potassium 50 mg • Manganese (Amino Acid Chelate) 5 mg • Selenium (Amino Acid Chelate) 50 mcg • Chromium (Yeast-free GTF) 100 mcg • Molybdenum (Amino Acid Chelate) 50 mcg • Boron (Amino Acid Chelate) 1 mg • Vanadium (Amino Acid Chelate) 50 mcg • Choline

BRAND NAMES

B R A N D   N A M E S

(Bitartrate) 50 mg • Inositol 50 mg • PABA 30 mg • Spirulina 250 mg • Chlorella (broken cell wall) 250 mg • Barley grass organic 250 mg • Alfalfa juice concentrate 100 mg • Octocosanol wheat-free 100 mg • Siberian Ginseng 50 mg • Bioflavonoids (40%) 50 mg • Rutin 25 mg • Psyllium husk fiber 50 mg • Echinacea 50 mg • Apple Pectin 25 mg • Betaine Hydrochloride 25 mg • Glutamic Acid 25 mg • Papain (Papaya) 25 mg • Lipase 10 mg • Amylase 10 mg • Chlorophyll 9 mg • 17 Amino Acids 380 mg (derived from Spirulina Chlorella , Barley grass & Alfalfa juice concentrate. Natural base includes Alfalfa, Rose Hips, Di-Calcium Phosphate, Cellulose, Stearic Acid & natural vegetable protein coating.

Spectro 3 — Solaray - Nutraceutical
Three tablets contain: Vitamin A (from Retinyl Palmitate, and 60% as natural Beta Carotene [Dunaliella salina algae]) 25000 IU • Vitamin C (as natural Ascorbic acid, Rose Hips, Acerola cherry) 1000 mg • Vitamin D (as Cholecalciferol D-3) 400 IU • Vitamin E (as natural d-Alpha Tocopheryl Succinate, d-Alpha Tocopheryl Acetate) 400 IU • Vitamin K 50 mcg • Thiamin (as Thiamine Mononitrate) (Vitamin B1) 25 mg • Riboflavin (Vitamin B2)25 mg • Niacin (as Niacinamide) 125 mg • Vitamin B6 (as Pyridoxine HCl) 50 mg • Folic Acid 400 mcg • Vitamin B12 (as Cyanocobalamin) 100 mcg • Biotin 300 mcg • Pantothenic Acid (as d-Calcium Pantothenate) 125 mg • Calcium (as Calcium Carbonate, Calcium Amino Acid Chelate) 500 mg • Iron (as Iron Fumarate, Iron Amino Acid Chelate) 18 mg • Phosphorous (as Potassium Phosphate) 23 mg • Iodine (from Kelp) 225 mcg • Magnesium (Magnesium Oxide, Magnesium Amino Acid Chelate) 250 mg • Zinc (as Zinc Citrate, Zinc Picolinate, Zinc Amino Acid Chelate) 15 mg • Selenium (as yeast free I-Selenomethionine) 100 mcg • Copper (as Copper Amino Acid Chelate) 0.5 mg • Potassium (as Potassium Phosphate, Potassium Chloride) 88 mg • Choline Bitartrate 50 mg • Inositol 50 mg • PABA (Para-Aminobenzoic Acid) 30 mg • Lecithin 50 mg • Bioflavonoid concentrate (from Citrus) 150 mg • Rutin concentrate 50 mg • Hesperidin concentrate 50 mg • Pectin 25 mg • Boron (as Tetra-Boron: Boron Citrate, Boron Glycinate, Boron Aspartate, Boron Lysinate) 1.5 mg • Spirulina (Spirulina platensis) 50 mg • Alfalfa juice (aerial) 125 mg • Carrot and Yam concentrate 100 mg • Barley Grass juice concentrate 75 mg • Rosemary leaf extract 25 mg • Aloe Vera gel concentrate 200x (equivalent to 400 mg) 2 mg • Parsley leaf 50 mg • Pancreatin 4x (equivalent to 120 mg) 30 mg • Diatase 20 mg • Papain (from Papaya) 50 mg • Ox Bile extract 20 mg • Glutamic Acid HCl 50 mg • Propolis 2x (equivalent to 50 mg) 25 mg • Royal Jelly 3.5x (equivalent to 14 mg) 4 mg • Bee Pollen. Other ingredients: Cellulose, Stearic Acid, Silica, Siberian Ginseng root, Calcium Phosphate, Whole Rice concentrate, Alfalfa herb, Montmorillonite Clay, Maltodextrin, Natural flavors and Natural food glazed coating.

Spirulina — Quest
Each capsule contains: Spirulina 500 mg.

SPL and PAN — Dial Herbs
Chamomile • Dandelion • Goldenseal • Parsley • Uva Ursi • Yellow Dock • Cayenne • Yarrow.

Sport Fuel — TwinLab
Six capsules contain: Beta-Carotene (pro-Vitamin A) 25000 IU • Vitamin D (from natural form Vitamin D3) 400 IU • Vitamin C 1000 mg • Natural Vitamin E (Succinate) 800 IU • CoQ10 (Coenzyme Q10) 30 mg • L-Glutathione 100 mg • N-Acetyl Cysteine (NAC) 200 mg • Alpha Lipoic Acid 100 mg • Vitamin B1 (Thiamine) 50 mg • Vitamin B2 (Riboflavin) 50 mg • Vitamin B6 (Pyridoxine) 50 mg • Vitamin B12 (Cobalamin) 100 mg • Folic Acid 400 mcg • Niacinamide 150 mg • Pantothenic Acid 250 mg • Biotin 300 mcg • PABA (Para-Aminobenzoic Acid) 25 mg • Choline Bitartrate 100 mg • Inositol 100 mg • L-Carnitine (from Carni Fuel L-Carnitine Magnesium Citrate) 100 mg • Magnesium (from L-Carnitine Magnesium Citrate, Aspartate, Alpha-Ketoglutarate & Oxide) 600 mg • Potassium (from Potassium Aspartate, Alpha-Ketoglutarate & Citrate) 100 mg • Zinc (from Zinc Picolinate) 30 mg • Manganese (from Manganese Gluconate) 5 mg • Copper (from Copper Gluconate) 2 mg • Iron (from Ferrous Fumarate) 10 mg • Iodine (from Potassium Iodide) 150 mcg • Selenium (from Selenomethionine & Selenate 50/50 mixture) 200 mcg • Chromium (from Chromic Fuel Chromium Picolinate) 400 mcg • Molybdenum (from natural Molybdic Acid) 150 mcg.

Sport Fuel With Iron — TwinLab
Six capsules contain: Beta-Carotene (pro-Vitamin A) 25000 IU • Vitamin D (from natural form Vitamin D3) 400 IU • Vitamin C 1000 mg • Natural Vitamin E (Succinate) 800 IU • CoQ10 (Coenzyme Q10) 30 mg • L-Glutathione 100 mg • N-Acetyl Cysteine (NAC) 200 mg •

Alpha ipoic Acid 100 mcg • Vitamin B1 (Thiamine) 50 mg • Vitamin B2 (Riboflavin) 50 mg • Vitamin B6 (Pyridoxine) 50 mg • Vitamin B12 (Cobalamin) 100 mcg • Folic Acid 400 mcg • Niacinamide 150 mg • Pantothenic Acid 250 mg • Biotin 300 mcg • PABA (Para-Aminobenzoic Acid) 25 mg • Choline Bitartrate 100 mg • Inositol 100 mg • L-Carnitine (from Carni Fuel L-Carnitine Magnesium Citrate) 100 mg • Calcium (from Calcium Citrate, Carbonate) 25 mg • Magnesium (from L-Carnitine Magnesium Citrate, Aspartate, Alpha-Ketoglutarate & Oxide) 600 mg • Potassium (from Potassium Aspartate, Alpha-Ketoglutarate & Citrate) 100 mg • Zinc (from Zinc Picolinate) 30 mg • Manganese (from Manganese Gluconate) 5 mg • Copper (from Copper Gluconate) 2 mg • Iron (from Ferrous Fumarate) 10 mg • Iodine (from Potassium Iodide) 150 mcg • Selenium (from Selenomethionine & Selenate‹50/50 mixture) 200 mcg • Chromium (from Chromic Fuel Chromium Picolinate) 400 mcg • Molybdenum (from natural Molybdic Acid) 150 mcg.

Sport Fuel Without Iron — TwinLab
Six capsules contain: Beta-Carotene (pro-Vitamin A) 25000 IU • Vitamin D (from natural form Vitamin D3) 400 IU • Vitamin C 1000 mg • Natural Vitamin E (Succinate) 800 IU • CoQ10 (Coenzyme Q10) 30 mg • L-Glutathione 100 mg • N-Acetyl Cysteine (NAC) 200 mg • Alpha Lipoic Acid 100 mg • Vitamin B1 (Thiamine) 50 mg • Vitamin B2 (Riboflavin) 50 mg • Vitamin B6 (Pyridoxine) 50 mg • Vitamin B12 (Cobalamin) 100 mcg • Folic Acid 400 mcg • Niacinamide 150 mg • Pantothenic Acid 250 mg • Biotin 300 mcg • PABA (Para-Aminobenzoic Acid) 25 mg • Choline Bitartrate 100 mg • Inositol 100 mg • L-Carnitine (from Carni Fuel L-Carnitine Magnesium Citrate) 100 mg • Calcium (from Calcium Citrate, Carbonate) 25 mg • Magnesium (from L-Carnitine Magnesium Citrate, Aspartate, Alpha-Ketoglutarate & Oxide) 600 mg • Potassium (from Potassium Aspartate, Alpha-Ketoglutarate & Citrate) 100 mg • Zinc (from Zinc Picolinate) 30 mg • Manganese (from Manganese Gluconate) 5 mg • Copper (from Copper Gluconate) 2 mg • Iodine (from Potassium Iodide) 150 mcg • Selenium (from Selenomethionine & Selenate‹50/50 mixture) 200 mcg • Chromium (from Chromic Fuel Chromium Picolinate) 400 mcg • Molybdenum (from natural Molybdic Acid) 150 mcg.

Sportalyte — Pharmanex
Twenty grams contain: Glucose • Fructose • Maltoextrin • Citric Acid • Natural Flavor • Sodium Chloride • Silicon Dioxide • Sodium Citrate • Magnesium Carbonate • Tricalcium Phosphate • Potassium Citrate • Magnesium Oxide • Ascorbic Acid • d- Alpha Tocopheryl Acetate • Potassium Chloride • Hydromins • Taurine • Fructooligosaccharides.

Sports One DIOL XS — Sports One
Each capsule contains: 4-Androstenediol 100 mg • Nor-4-Androstenediol 100 mg.

SS Cream — Cheil Jedang Corporation
70% ethanol extract of Bufonis venenum 10 mg • 100 mg extract of Angelicae gigantic radix, Cistanchis caulis, Torilidis semen, Ginseng radix alba, Zanthoxylli fructos • 100 mg extract of Asiasari radix, Caryophilli flos, Cinnamomi cortex.
Editor's Comments: In one controlled clinical trial in men suffering from premature ejaculation, SS Cream was applied to the glans penis 1-hour prior to intercourse and washed off immediately before intercourse. Men treated with the cream had significantly improved ejaculatory latency compared to placebo (2537).

St. John's Wort — Centrum Herbals
One capsule contains: St. John's Wort (Hypericum perforatum) flower and leaves 300 mg. Standardized to contain (based on extract weight): Total Hypericin compounds (marker) 0.3%, Hyperforin (marker), Quercetin (natural active), Amentoflavone (natural active), Gaba & Proline (natural actives). Activity measure: Muscarinic M1 binding assay. Other ingredients: Dibasic Calcium Phosphate, Maltodextrin, Cellulose, Lactose Monohydrate, Silicon Dioxide, Hydroxypropy cellulose, Ethycellulose, Castor Oil, Gelatin, Sodium Lauryl Sulfate, Propylene Glycol, Titanium Dioxide.

St. John's Complex — Body Wise International, Inc.
Each tablet contains: St. John's Wort Extract (0.3% Hypericin) 300 mg • Chamomile Flowers (Anthemis flores) 25 mg • Passion Flower (Passiflora incarnata) 25 mg.

St. John's Good Mood — Traditional Medicinals
Contains: St. John's Wort herb & dry extract • Lemon Balm leaf (Melissa) • Oatstraw herb • Damiana herb • Lavender flower • Berganot herb • Sage leaf • Spearmint leaf • Lemongrass leaf • Licorice root • Rose petals • Stevia leaf.

Some Brand Name Natural Products - What they Contain

St. John's Plus - Nutri-Quest — Nutri-Quest
Each tablet contains: St. John's Wort herb 400 mg • Pyridoxal-5-Phosphate 5 mg • Riboflavin-5-Phosphate 5 mg • Folic Acid 100 mcg • Vitamin B1 10 mg • Vitamin B12 250 mcg • Ginkgo Biloba extract 5 mg • Damiana herb 25 mg • Ginkgo Biloba herb 30 mg • Blue Vervain 25 mg • Kava Kava herb 10 mg • Hyssop herb 15 mg • Siberian Ginseng 10 mg • Niacinamide 50 mg • Calcium Citrate 100 mg • Magnesium Citrate 100 mg.

St. John's Plus - Rx Vitamins — Rx Vitamins
Each caplet provides: St. John's Wort flower (Hypericum perforatum, standardized 0.3-0.5 hypericin) 300 mg • Kava root (Piper methylsticum, standardized 29-31% kavalactones) 50 mg • Siberian ginseng root (Eleutherococcus senticosis, standardized 0.8% eleutherosides) 50 mg • Feverfew leaf (Tanacetum parthenium, standardized 0.7% parthenolide) 25 mg • L-Tyrosine (pharmaceutical grade, free form amino acid) 25 mg • Zinc (l-monomethionine) 10 mg • Vitamin B6 (pyridoxine HCl) 5 mg • Vitamin B12 (cyanocobalamin) 10 mcg.

St. John's Plus Kava Kava — Progressive Labs
Each capsule contains: Vitamin B6 (pyridoxine HCl) 25 mg • St. John's Wort 0.3% Hypericin 200 mg • Kava Kava 100 mg.

St. John's Wort — Gaia Herbs
St. John's Wort standardized for 0.5% hypericins. Standardized Full Spectrum 180 mg of extract per capsule. Guaranteed Potency 90 mg of extract per capsule.

St. John's Wort — Jamieson
Each tablet contains: Vitamin C 2.5 mg • St. John's Wort 4.4:1 extract (Hypericum perforatum L.)(Aerial parts of flower, stamen and leaf)(Containing 0.3% hypericin) 225 mg.

St. John's Wort — Metabolic Response Modifiers
Each capsule contains: Hypericum perforatum (0.3% Hypericin) 450 mg.

St. John's Wort — Nature's Way
Two capsules contain: St. John's Wort stem, leaf, flower 600 mg • St. John's Wort (dried extract 0.3% Dianthrones measures as Hypericin) 300 mg. Other ingredients: Gelatin, Magnesium Stearate, Millet.

St. John's Wort — Pharmanex
Each capsule contains: St. John's Wort (Hypericum perforatum) flower tops and leaves (5:1) 300 mg. Other Ingredients: Rice Flour, Gelatin, Magnesium Stearate, Silicon Dioxide.

St. John's Wort — Quest
Each caplet contains: St. John's Wort (Hypericum perfortum) (provided by 300 mg P.E. 1:5 standardized to contain 0.3% Hypercin) 1500 mg. Other Ingredients: Microcrystalline Cellulose, Calcium phosphate, Croscarmellose Sodium Dioxide, Vegetable Stearin, Magnesium Stearate.

St. John's Wort Blend — VitaStore
Each capsule contains: St. John's Wort (standardized for 0.3% Hypericin) • Kava Kava • Ginkgo Biloba.

St. John's Wort Forte — Phytopharmica
Each capsule contains: St. John's Wort extract 300mg • Valerian root extract 100 mg • Kava root extract 100 mg.

St. John's Wort Oil — Blessed Herbs
St. John's Wort flowering tops • organic cold-pressed Olive oil.

St. John's Wort Plus — Aspen Group, Inc.
Each capsule contains: St. John's Wort herb extract standardized to 0.3% Hypericin 300 mg • Kava Kava 100 mg • Vitamin B6 25 mg • Standardized extract St. John's Wort herb extract Hypericum Perforatum. No artificial colors, flavors or preservatives.

St. John's Wort Supreme — Gaia Herbs
St. John's Wort and Kava Kava standardized for 0.5% hypericins and 55% kavalactones. Standardized Full Spectrum 150 mg of extract per capsule. Guaranteed Potency 75 mg of extract per capsule.

St. John's Wort-Go! — Wakunaga of America
Each caplet contains: St. John's Wort Standardized Extract (herb with flower) standardized to 0.3% Hypericin 600 mg. Other Ingredients: Cellulose, Magnesium Stearate (vegetable source), Silica.

Stabilium — Smart Basics
Each capsule contains: Predigested Garum Armoricum 105 mg • Virgin Sunflower Oil 83 mg • Soya Lecithin Oil 12 mg.

Stamina — HerbaSway
Horny Goat Weed • Yohimbe • Dong Quai • Knotweed • Panax Ginseng • Licorice • Blackberry • HerbaSwee (Cucurbitaceae fruit).

Stamina 100 — Jamieson
Three caplets contain: Vitamin A (as Retinyl Acetate) 7500 IU • Vitamin C (as Ascorbic Acid) 125 mg • Vitamin D (as Cholecalciferol) 200 IU • Vitamin E (as Dl-Alpha Tocopheryl Acetate) 25 IU • Thiamin (as Thiamin Mononitrate) 12.5 mg • Riboflavin (Vitamin B2) 12.5 mg • Niacin (as Nicacinamide) 190 mg • Vitamin B6 (as Pyridoxine Hydrochloride) 12.5 mg • Folate (as Folic Acid) 200 mcg • Vitamin B12 (as Cyanocobalamin) 50 mcg • Pantothenic Acid (as Calcium D-Pantothenate) 30 mg • Caclium (as Calcium Carbonate) 600 mg • Iron (as Ferrous Fumarate) 10 mg • Iodine (as Potassium Iodide) 150 mcg • Magnesium (as Magnesium Oxide) 100 mg • Zinc (as Zinc Gluconate) 5 mg • Selenium (as Seleium Brown Rice Protein Chelate) 12.5 mcg • Manganese (as Manganese Gluconate) 3.5 mg • Chromium (as Chromium Brown Rice Protein Chelate) 10 mcg • Potassium (as Potassium Gluconate) 50 mg.

Stamina Beverage — Jamieson
Each bottle contains: Purified Water • Canadian Maple Syrup • Glucose • Natural Lemon and Orange Flavor (Tocopherols, Soybean Oil) • Canadian Ginseng Root (Panax Quinquegolium) • Citric Acid • Sodium Benzoate • Xanthan Gum • Caramel (natural color) • Potassium Sorbate.

Standardized Cider Vinegar with Apple Pectin — The Vitamin Shoppe
Each tablet has been standardized to provide 27 mg of acetic acid and 27 mg of apple pectin.

Standardized Feverfew Extract — Nature's Way
Each capsule contains: Feverfew leaves (standardized 0.7% Parthenolide) 370 mg.

Standardized Ginkgo Extract — Nature's Way
Each capsule contains: Ginkgo Biloba leaf extract; standardized to 24% Ginkgo flavone glycosides & 6% terpene lactones) 60 mg • Gotu Kola stem & leaf 400 mg. Other Ingredients: Gelatin & Millet.

Standardized Kava Extract — Nature's Way
Each softgel contains: Concentrated 10:1 Kava Extract (rhizome, standardized to 55% kavalactones) 128 mg.

Standardized Saw Palmetto Extract — Nature's Way
Each softgel contains: Saw Palmetto extract (berry, standardized to 85-95% Fatty Acids) 160 mg.

Stomach Plus — Atrium
Each tablet contains: Raw Stomach concentrate Bovine 323 mg • Folic Acid 100 mcg • Vitamin B12 50 mcg • Glycine 32 mg.

Stone Root-Corn Silk Virtue — Blessed Herbs
Stone root • Gravel root • Hydrangea root • Goldenrod • Corn Silk • Nettle • Grain alcohol & Distilled Water.

Strawberry-Apple Lactobacillus Acidophilus — Nature's Life
Two tablespoons (1 fl.oz or 29.6 ml) contain: Purified Water • Strawberry concentrate • Unfiltered Apple Juice • Pasteurized Honey • Soy Protein Isolate • Lactobacillus Acidophilus Culture.

ST-Res-Q — Nutri-Quest
Each tablet contains: Adrenal 25 mg • Thymus 70 mg • Spleen 20 mg • Stomach 10 mg • Parotid 80 mg (All bovine source). • Vitamin C 175 mg • Vitamin B2 15 mg • Vitamin B6 10 mg • Niacinamide 15 mg • Pantothenic Acid (D-Calcium Pantothenate) 105 mg • Grape seed extract 1 mg • Lemon Bioflavonoids 225 mg • L-Tyrosine 175 mg • Magnesium Oxide 75 mg • Zinc Chelate 5 mg • Chromium Chelate 50 mcg • Potassium Chelate 10 mg • Chlorella 50 mg.

Stress — Centrum Focused Formulas
One tablet contains: Vitamin C 150 mg • Vitamin E 22.5 IU • Thiamin (B1) 15 mg • Riboflavin (B2) 4.8 mg • Niacin (B3) 50 mg • Vitamin B6 5 mg • Folate, Folic Acid, Folacin 200 mcg • Vitamin B12 12.5 mcg • Biotin 15 mcg • Pantothenic Acid 12.5 mg • Zinc 7.5 mg • Copper 1 mg • Ginseng standardized root extract (Panax ginseng) 62.5 mg.

Stress Action — Nature's Plus
Two tablets contain: Vitamin C as Mineral Ascorbate 1000 mg • Desiccated Beef Liver 500 mg • Pantothenic Acid (Calcium Pantothenate) 125 mg • Vitamin B1 (Thiamine) 100 mg • Vitamin B2 (Riboflavin) 100 mg • Vitamin B6 (Pyridoxine HCL) 100 mg •

BRAND NAMES

BRAND NAMES

Niacinamide 100 mg • Vitamin E natural 100 IU • Choline (Bitartrate) 75 mg • Inositol 75 mg • PABA (Para-aminobenzoic acid) 50 mg • Bee Pollen 50 mg • Ginseng Korean 50 mg • Calcium ascorbate 50 mg • Zinc Ascorbate 25 mg • Magnesium Ascorbate 25 mg • L-Phenylalanine free form amino acid 20 mg • Iron (Gluconate) 20 mg • Potassium (Citrate) 15 mg • L-Cysteine free form amino acid 15 mg • L-Methionine free form amino acid 15 mg • Folic Acid 400 mcg • Vitamin B12 from Cobalamin 250 mcg • Biotin 100 mcg • Octacosanol 50 mcg • Chromium amino acid chelate 20 mcg • Selenium amino acid complex 10 mcg . In a natural rice bran base. In a special base which provides for the gradual release of ingredients over a prolonged period of time for 40% better absorption & utilization. Sugar & starch free.

Stress Away — Futurebiotics
Two tablets contain: Vitamin C (ascorbic acid/ascorbyl palmitate) 250 mg • Vitamin A (beta carotene) 5000 IU • Vitamin B1 (thiamin) 25 mg • Vitamin B2 (riboflavin) 25 mg • Niacinamide 200 mg • Calcium (phosphate, aspartate) 100 mg • Vitamin B6 5 mg • Folic Acid 400 mcg • Vitamin B12 50 mcg • Iodine (kelp) 75 mg • Magnesium (oxide, amino acid chelate) 100 mg • Zinc (oxide, picolinate) 15 mg • Biotin 300 mcg • Pantothenic Acid 50 mg • Choline Bitartrate 100 mg • Manganese (amino acid chelate) 3 mg • Chromium (amino acid chelate, polynicotinate) 40 mcg • Para Amino Benzoic Acid (PABA) 50 mg • Valerian 200 mg • Chamomile 100 mg • Skullcap 50 mg • Passion flower 50 mg • Methionine 50 mg • Ribonucleic Acid (RNA) 50 mg.

Stress B with C — Nature's Life
Two capsules contain: Vitamin B1 (Thiamine Mononitrate) 50 mg • Vitamin B2 (Riboflavin and Riboflavin 5'-Phosphate) 50 mg • Vitamin B6 (Pyridoxine HCl & Pyridoxal 5'-Phosphate) 50 mg • Vitamin B12 (Cobalamin concentrate) 250 mcg • Niacinamide 100 mg • Folic Acid 400 mcg • Pantothenic Acid (d-Calcium Pantothenate) 250 mg • Biotin (d-Biotin)100 mcg • PABA (Para Aminobenzoic Acid) 50 mg • Choline (Bitartrate) 100 mg • Vitamin C 1000 mg.

Stress Essentials — Phytopharmica
Each capsule contains: Vitamin C (Ascorbic Acid & Rose Hips) 100 mg • Calcium (Oyster Shell) 50 mg • Magnesium (Oxide) 30 mg • Potassium (Citrate) 25 mg • Pantothenic Acid (D-Calcium Pantothenate) 20 mg • Vitamin B6 (Pyridoxine HCL) 15 mg • Thiamine HCL (Vitamin B1) 12.5 mg • Riboflavin (Vitamin B2) 12.5 mg • Niacin 10 mg • Manganese (Chelate) 5 mg • Zinc (Chelate) 1.5 mg • Biotin 100 mcg • Folic Acid 75 mcg • Vitamin B12 (Cyanocobalamin) 25 mcg • Other ingredients: Inositol 50 mg • Siberian Ginseng extract 5:1 (Eleutherococcus senticosus) 50 mg • Valerian extract (Valeriana officinalis) 50 mg standardized to contain 0.2% to 0.8% valeric acids • L-Tyrosine 50 mg • Skullcap extract 4:1 (Scutellaria baicalensis) 50 mg • Passion flower extract (Passiflora) 50 mg • Hops extract (Humulus lupulus) 50 mg • PABA (Para-Aminobenzoic Acid) 5 mg. Contains no sugar, salt, yeast, wheat, corn, soy, dairy products, coloring, flavoring or preservatives.

Stress Plex — Nature's Plus
Two tablets contain: Vitamin C with Rose Hips 500 mg • Pantothenic Acid (Calcium pantothenate) 100 mg • Niacinamide 100 mg • Choline (Bitartrate) 100 mg • Inositol 100 mg • PABA (Para-aminobenzoic acid) 30 mg • Vitamin B1 (Thiamine) 10 mg • Vitamin B2 (Riboflavin) 10 mg • Vitamin B6 (Pyridoxine HCL) 10 mg • Folic Acid 100 mcg • Vitamin B12 (from Cobalamin) 25 mcg • Biotin 25 mcg. B-Complex vitamins in a fortified rice bran base. Contains no yeast, wheat, corn, soy, milk, salt, sugar or starch.

Stress Plus — Now
Each tablet contains: Vitamin B1 (Thiamine) 30 mg • Vitamin B2 (Riboflavin) 30 mg • Vitamin B3 (Niacinamide) 150 mg • Vitamin B6 (Pyridoxine) 30 mg • Vitamin B12 50 mcg • Pantothenic Acid 100 mg • Vitamin C (Ascorbic Acid) 500 mg • Biotin 300 mcg • Folic Acid 400 mcg • Magnesium (Oxide) 100 mg • PABA 40 mg • Choline (Bitartrate) 150 mg • Inositol 150 mg • Valerian root (50 mg of 4:1 extract) 200 mg.

Stress Tab B "600" — Nature's Life
Two tablets contain: Vitamin B1 (Thiamine HCl) 60 mg • Vitamin B2 (Riboflavin) 60 mg • Vitamin B6 (Pyridoxine HCl) 60 mg • Vitamin B12 (Cobalamin concentrate) 60 mcg • Vitamin C 600 mg • Niacin 30 mg • Niacinamide 30 mg • Folic Acid 600 mcg • Pantothenic Acid (d-Calcium Pantothenate) 600 mg • Biotin (d-Biotin) 600 mcg • Choline (Bitartrate) 60 mg • Inositol 60 mg • PABA (Para Aminobenzoic Acid) 60 mg.

Stressease — Jamieson
Each caplet contains: Thiamin (as Thiamin Mononitrate) 50 mg • Riboflavin (Vitamin B2) 50 mg • Niacin (as Niacinamide) 50 mg • Vitamin B6 (as Pyridoxine Hydrochloride) 50 mg • Folate (as Folic Acid) 400 mcg • Vitamin B12 (as Cyanocobalamin) 50 mg • Biotin 50 mg • Pantothenic Acid (as Calcium D-Pantothenate) 50 mg • Choline Bitartrate 50 mg • Inositol 50 mg.

Stress-End — Enzymatic Therapy
Each capsule contains: Vitamin C (Ascorbic Acid/Rose Hips) 100 mg • Calcium (Oyster Shell) 50 mg • Magnesium (Oxide) 30 mg • Potassium (Citrate) 25 mg • Pantothenic Acid (D-Calcium Pantothenate) 20 mg • Vitamin B6 (Pyridoxine HCL) 15 mg • Thiamine HCL (Vitamin B1) 12.5 mg • Riboflavin (Vitamin B2) 12.5 mg • Niacin 10 mg • Manganese (Chelate) 5 mg • Zinc (Chelate) 1.5 mg • Biotin 100 mcg • Folic Acid 75 mcg • Vitamin B12 (Cyanocobalamin) 25 mcg • Other ingredients: Inositol 50 mg • Siberian Ginseng extract 5:1 (Eleutherococcus senticosus) 50 mg • Valerian extract (Valeriana officinalis) standardized to contain 0.2% to 0.8% Valerenic Acids 50 mg • L-Tyrosine 50 mg • Skullcap extract 4:1 (Scutellaria baicalensis) 50 mg • Passion flower extract (Passiflora) 50 mg • Hops extract (Humulus lupulus) 50 mg • PABA (Para-Aminobenzoic Acid) 5 mg. Contains no sugar, salt, yeast, wheat, corn, soy, dairy products, coloring, flavoring, or preservatives.

Stresstabs — Unknown
Each tablet contains: Vitamin C 500 mg • Vitamin E 30 IU • Thiamin 10 mg • Riboflavin 10 mg • Nicanamide 100 mg • Vitamin B6 5 mg • Folic Acid 400 mcg • Vitamin B12 12 mcg • Biotin 45 mcg • Pantothenic Acid 20 mg. Ingredients: Ascorbic Acid • Calcium Carbonate • Cellulose • Riboflavin (Vitamin B2) • Thiamine Mononitrate (Vitamin B1) • Dicalcium Phosphate • Pyridoxine Hydrochloride (Vitamin B6) • Silicon Dioxide • Magnesium Stearate • Triethyl Citrate • Stearic Acid • Mineral oil • Folic Acid • Titanium Dioxide • FD&C Yellow #6 Aluminum Lake • Biotin • Cyanocobalamin (Vitamin B12).

Stresstabs + Zinc — Unknown
Each tablet contains: Vitamin C 500 mg • Vitamin E 30 IU • Thiamin 10 mg • Riboflavin 10 mg • Nicanamide 100 mg • Vitamin B6 5 mg • Folic Acid 400 mcg • Vitamin B12 12 mcg • Biotin 45 mcg • Pantothenic Acid 20 mg • Zinc 23.9 mg • Copper 3 mg. Ingredients: Ascorbic Acid • Calcium Carbonate • Cellulose • Niacinamide • dl-Alpha Tocopheryl Acetate (Vitamin E) • Starch • Zinc Oxide • d-Calcium Pantothenate • Hydroxypropyl Methylcellulose • Riboflavin (Vitamin B2) • Thiamine Mononitrate (Vitamin B1) • Dicalcium Phosphate • Pyridoxine Hydrochloride (Vitamin B6) • Silicon Dioxide • Triethyl Stearate • Stearic Acid • Magnesium Stearate • Cupric Oxide • Crospovidone • Providone • Mineral oil • Folic Acid • Titanium Dioxide • FD&C Yellow #6 Aluminum Lake • Biotin • Cyanocobalamin (Vitamin B12).

Substrate Solutions Di-Indolin — Substrate Solutions
Three tablets contain: Di-Indolin [proprietary blend of Diindolymethane, Vitamin E (as d-Alpha Tocopheryl Succinate), Phosphatidylcholine] 300 mg. Other Ingredients: Calcium Carbonate, Cellulose, Food Grade Starch, Magnesium Sterate, Tocophersolan, Silica.

Sun Pollen — Futurebiotics
Cracked Flower Pollen & Pollen Extract.

Super Anti-OX — Nutri-Quest
Each tablet contains: Grape seed extract 20 mg (92-95% Proanthocyanidins) • Ester-C (Zinc 2 mg) 14 mg • Vitamin C 100 mg • Vitamin E (Succinate) 50 IU • L-Glutathione 2 mg • N-Acetyl Cysteine 5 mg • Magnesium Aspartate 5 mg • Manganese Chelate 1 mg • Selenium Chelate 50 mcg • Chromium Chelate 50 mcg • Milk Thistle 150 mg • Silymarin 5 mg.

Super Antioxidant — Health Center for Better Living
Vitamin C 500 mg • Vitamin E 300 IU.

Super Antioxidant Capsules — The Vitamin Shoppe
Two capsules contain: Vitamin A (beta carotene and mixed carotenoids) 10,000 IU • Vit. E 200 IU • Vitamin C (Calcium ascorbate) 60 mg • Vitamin B1 25 mg • Vitamin B2 25 mg • Vitamin B3 25 mg • Vitamin B5 25 mg • Vitamin B6 25 mg • Vitamin B12 250 mcg • N-Acetyl Cysteine 50 mg • Glutathione 50 mg • Selenium 75 mcg • Zinc 15 mg • Green Tea Extract (30% Polyphenols) 25 mg •

Some Brand Name Natural Products - What they Contain
www.NaturalDatabase.com contains MANY more listings than appear here.

CoQ10 10 mg • Quercetin 25 mg • Alpha Lipoic Acid 10 mg • Garlic (odorless) 100 mg • Grape Seed Extract (minimum 85%-95% proanthocyanidins 10 mg • Manganese (Gluconate/Citrate) 15 mg.

Super Anti-Oxidant Complex — Nature's Plus
Two tablets contain: Vitamin C with Rose Hips 500 mg • Vitamin E natural 200 IU • Vitamin A (Beta Carotene) 10000 IU • Selenium amino acid complex 200 mcg • Chromium amino acid chelate 200 mcg. In a natural base of Carrots, Broccoli, Spinach & Beet Greens. In a special base which provides for the gradual release of ingredients over a prolonged period of time for 40% better absorption & utilization. Sugar & starch free.

Super Antioxidant tablets — Clinician's Choice
Two tablets contain: Vitamin C (as ascorbic acid) 120 mg • Vitamin E (as dl-alpha tocopheryl acetate) 200 IU • Zinc (as amino acid chelate) 4 mg • Selenium (selenomethionine) 100 mcg • RoseOx (patented, standardized process for an extract of Rosemary) 200 mg • Schizandra Fruit Powder 100 mg • Grape Powder 60 mg • Ascorbyl Palmitate 20 mg • Proprietary blend 10 mg: Astragalus, Beta Carotene, Carrot Powder, Coenzyme Q10, Cruciferex, Pycnogenol.

Super Antioxidants — Now
Two Vcaps contain: Green Tea extract (Camellia sinensis) (40% Catechins) 200 mg • Milk Thistle extract (Silybum marianum) (80% Silymarin) 100 mg • Curcumin extract (Curcuma longa) (min. 90% extract) 100 mg • Quercetin 100 mg • Bromelain from pineapple (2000 GDU) 100 mg • Cranberry powder extract 100 mg • Rosemary extract (Rosmarinus officinalis) 100 mg • Grape seed extract (95% Polyphenols) 30 mg • Ginkgo Biloba extract (24% Ginkgoflavoglycosides) 30 mg • Ginger root (Zingiber officinalis) 30 mg • Hawthorne berry extract (Crataegus oxyacantha) (1.8% Vitexin-4-Rhamnoside) 30 mg • Bilberry extract (Vaccimum myrtillus) (25% Anthocyanidins) 20 mg.

Super B Complex 100 — The Vitamin Shoppe
Each tablet contains: Vitamin B1 (Thiamin) 100 mg • Vitamin B2 (Riboflavin) 100 mg • Vitamin B6 (Pyridoxine HCl) 100 mg • Vitamin B12 (Cobalamin Concentrate) 100 mcg • Niacinamide 100 mg • Folic Acid 400 mcg • D-Biotin 100 mcg • Choline Bitartrate 100 mg • Inositol 100 mg • Pantothenic Acid (d-calcium pantothenate) 100 mg • PABA 100 mg. In a base of Alfalfa, Watercress, Parsley, Lecithin, and Rice Concentrate. No Yeast, Corn, Wheat, Soy, Salt, Sugar, Starch, Milk, Eggs, Fish or Animal Derivatives, Preservatives, Artificial Colors or Flavors added.

Super Cal-Mag — Nature's Life
Two tablets contain: Calcium (Chelated) (Carbonate, Aspartate, Aminoate, Citrate Complex) 1000 mg • Magnesium (Chelated) (Oxide, Aspartate, Aminoate, Citrate Complex) 500 mg.

Super C-Complex 500 — The Vitamin Shoppe
Each tablet contains: Vitamin C (with Rose Hips) 500 mg • Citrus Bioflavonoid Complex 100 mg • Hesperidin Complex 25 mg • Rutin 50 mg • Acerola 1 mg. No Yeast, Corn, Wheat, Dairy, Soy, Salt, Starch, Sugar, Gluten, Milk, Eggs, Fish or Animal Derivatives, Preservatives, Artificial Colors or Flavors added.

Super Complete Capsules — Ultimate Nutrition
Nine capsules contain: Vitamin A 10000 IU • Vitamin D 400 IU • Vitamin E 400 IU • Vitamin B1 100 mg • Vitamin B2 100 mg • Vitamin B6 100 mg • Vitamin B12 100 mcg • Niacinamide 100 mg • Pantothenic Acid 100 mg • Folic Acid 400 mcg • Biotin 300 mcg • Choline 100 mg • Inositol 100 mg • PABA 100 mg • Vitamin C 1500 mg • Bioflavonoids 250 mg • Rutin 50 mg • Rose Hips powder 20 mg • Hesperidin 20 mg • Acerola Cherry 10 mg • Glutamic Acid HCL 100 mg • Betaine HCl 100 mg • Calcium 1000 mg • Magnesium 500 mg • Iodine 150 mcg • Potassium 95 mg • Iron 30 mg • Zinc 22.5 mg • Manganese 10 mg • Copper 3 mg • Boron 3 mg • Chromium 200 mcg • Selenium 50 mcg.

Super Energy Up — The Vitamin Shoppe
Each capsule contains: Standardized Panax Ginseng extract, Fo-Ti root, Sukday, Licorice, Lycii Berries, and Damiana leaves in a base of Royal Jelly, Bee Pollen, Vitamin B12, and Octacosanol.

Super Enzymes — Now
Each tablet contains: Betaine HCL (from beet molasses) 200 mg • Bromelain (2000 GDU from pineapple) 50 mg • Papain (140 MCU uncoated from papaya) 50 mg • Pancreatin 4x (equivalent to 800 mg) 200 mg supplying: Amylase (20000 USP Units) 100 mg, Protease (20000 USP Units) (Trypsin & Chymotrypsin) 100 mg, Lipase (3400 USP Units) 25 mg • Pepsin Enzymes NF 1:10000 50 mg • Cellulase

10 mg • Ox Bile extract 100 mg • Papaya Enzymes 45 mg • Pineapple Enzymes 45 mg.

Super EPA DHA 500 mg — The Vitamin Shoppe
Each softgel contains: Vitamin E (as d-alpha tocopherol) 5 IU • EPA Eicosapentaenoic Acid (as marine fish oil) 300 mg • DHA Docosahexaenoic Acid (as marine fish oil) 200 mg.

Super Food — Youngevity
Phosphorus • Sulfur • Chloride • Sodium • Vitamin A • Vitamin B1 • Vitamin B2 • Vitamin B3 • Vitamin B5 • Vitamin B6 • Vitamin B12 • Vitamin C • Vitamin D • Vitamin E • Vitamin K • Folic Acid • Biotin • Soy Protein • Soybean Oil • Soy Lecithin • Lactobacillus Acidophilus • FOS • Papaya • Protease • Bromelain • Amylase • Lipase • Cellulase • Soy • Rice • Barley • Oats • Prunes • Citrus • Alfalfa • Capsicum fruit • Chlorella • Garcinia fruit • Licorice.

Super Gainers Fuel — TwinLab
Each serving contains: Calories 3000 • Milk & Egg Proteins 100 g • High Levels of Complex Carbohydrates • Branched Chain Amino Acids (L-Leucine, L-Isoleucine & L-Valine) • L-Glutamine • L-Carnitine • Alpha-Ketoglutarates • Creatine Monohydrate • High Potencies of Vitamins & Minerals (including Potassium 2000 mcg & Chromium 600 mcg) • Fat 29 g [from Medium Chain Triglycerides (MCTs)]. MCTs are lipids composed of Medium Chain Fatty Acids.

Super Ginseng — Dial Herbs
Siberian Ginseng • Korean Ginseng • Brazilian Ginseng • Chinese Ginseng • American Ginseng.

Super Growth Enhancer — Optimum Nutrition
L-Arginine • L-Ornithine • Vitamin B6 20 mg • Vitamin C 200 mg.

Super Herbal V — MD Healthline
Two capsules contain: Yohimbe Bark 250 mg • Damiana Extract 50 mg • Bilberry Powder 100 mg • Gingko Biloba Extract (24%) 60 mg • Siberian Ginseng Extract 100 mg • Schisandra Extract 200 mg • Avena Sativa Extract 10:1 250 mg • Saw Palmetto (30%) 100 mg.

Super Immuno-Comp — Enzymatic Therapy
Two capsules contain: Vitamin A (Beta Carotene) non-toxic form of Vitamin A 5000 IU • Vitamin C (Ascorbic Acid/Rose Hips) 100 mg • Vitamin B6 (Pyridoxine HCL) 5 mg • Zinc (Picolinate) 3 mg • Other ingredients: Astragalus extract (Astragalus membranaceus) 150 mg • Echinacea extract (Echinacea angustifolia) standardized to contain greater than 3.5% Echinacosides & 0.65% essential oils 150 mg • Goldenseal extract (Hydrastis canadensis) standardized to contain 5% total Alkaloids including: Berberine, Hydrastine & Canadine 150 mg • KS-2 (Peptidomannan Complex) Shiitake Mushroom, a purified extract of Lentinus Edodes 50 mg • Licorice root extract (Glycyrrhiza glabra) standardized to contain 5% Glycyrrhizic Acid 50 mg. Contains no sugar, salt, yeast, wheat, corn, soy, dairy products, coloring, flavoring, or preservatives.

Super Immuno-Tone — Phytopharmica
Two capsules contain: Vitamin A 5000 IU • Vitamin C 100 mg • Vitamin B6 5 mg • Zinc 3 mg • Astralagus extract 150 mg • Echinacea extract 150 mg • Goldenseal extract 150 mg • KS-2 (Shiitake Mushroom) 50 mg • Licorice root extract 50 mg.

Super Leci-Thins — Nature's Life
Three tablets contain: Lecithin (Soy) 1300 mg • Cider Vinegar 255 mg • Kelp 150 mg • Vitamin B6 (Pyridoxine HCI) 50 mg.

Super Male Plex — The Vitamin Shoppe
Two tablets contain: Yohimbe extract 10 mg • Raw Testicular 250 mg • Damiana 250 mg • Ginseng (Korean/Siberian) 500 mg • Octacosanol 250 mcg • Vitamin E 250 IU • Histidine 200 mg • Sarsaparilla 100 mg • Saw Palmetto 100 mg • Raw Prostate 100 mg • Bee Pollen 100 mg • Zinc 100 mg • Oyster extract 50 mg • Cayenne 50 mg • Gotu Kola 50 mg • Selenium 50 mcg • Niacin 15 mg • Royal Jelly 5 mg.

Super Malic — Optimox
Six tablets contain: Magnesium (Hydroxide) 300 mg • Malic Acid 1200 mg.

Super Mega Vite II Multiple — Nature's Life
Each tablet contains: Beta Carotene (Vitamin A equivalent to 10000 IU) 6 mg • Vitamin B1 (Thiamine HCI) 50 mg • Vitamin B2 (Riboflavin) 50 mg • Niacinamide 75 mg • Pantothenic Acid (Calcium Pantothenate) 75 mg • Vitamin B6 Pyridoxine HCI) 50 mg • Vitamin B12 (Cobalamin concentrate) 250 mcg • Folic Acid 400 mcg • Biotin (d-Biotin) 50 mcg • Choline (Bitartrate) 50 mg • Inositol 50mg • l-Methionine (free form) 25 mg • Vitamin E (d-Alpha Tocopherol plus

© Copyright 2000, Natural Medicines Comprehensive Database (209) 472-2244. For updated data, go to www.NaturalDatabase.com. • 1403

BRAND NAMES

**B
R
A
N
D

N
A
M
E
S**

mixed Tocopherols) 100 IU • Vitamin C 250 mg • Rutin 5 mg • Lemon Bioflavonoids Complex (TESTLAB 50%) 25 mg • Hesperidin Complex 5 mg • Calcium (Carbonate) 100 mg • Chromium (Chelate) 25 mcg • Copper (Chelate) 200 mcg • Iodine (Postassium Idodine) 100 mg • Iron (Chelate) 10 mg • Magnesium (Oxide) 40 mg • Manganese (Chelate) 7 mg • Phosporus (Potassium Phosphate) 45 mg • Potassium (Phosphate, Chloride, Iodide) 67 mg • Selenium (Nutrition 21) (l-Selenomethionine) 10 mcg • Silicon (Dioxide) 20 mg • Zinc (Chelate) 10 mg • Coenzyme Q-10 (Ubiquinone) 500 mcg • Betaine HCl 25 mg • Glutamic Acid HCl 25 mg. In a natural base of 72 Trace Minerals from an ancient sedimentary sea bed, Chamomile, Rice Bran & Rose Hips.

Super Mega Vite Multiple — Nature's Life
Each tablet contains: Vitamin A (Fish Liver oil) 25000 IU • Vitamin D3 (Cholecalciferol) 400 IU • Vitamin B1 (Thiamine HCl) 30 mg • Vitamin B2 (Riboflavin) 30 mg • Niacinamide 100 mg • Pantothenic Acid (d-Calcium Pantothenate) 100 mg • Vitamin B6 Pyridoxine HCl 30 mg • Vitamin B12 (Cyanocobalamin) 250 mcg • Folic Acid 400 mcg • PABA (Para Aminobenzoic Acid) 60 mg • Biotin (d-Biotin) 50 mcg • Choline (Choline Bitartrate) 100 mg • Inositol 100 mg • Vitamin E (d-Alpha Tocopheryl Succinate) 100 IU • Vitamin C 250 mg • Lemon Bioflavonoids Complex (50% Total Flavanones) 25 mg • Rutin 25 mg • Hesperidin Complex (50% Total Flavanones) 5 mg • Calcium (Bone Meal) 82.5 mg • Chromium (Chelate) 25 mcg • Copper (Gluconate) 200 mcg • Iodine (Potassium Iodide) 100 mcg • Iron (Ferrous Fumarate) 10 mg • Magnesium (Oxide) 40 mg • Manganese (Gluconate) 7 mg • Phosphorus (Bone Meal) 37.5 mg • Potassium (Iodide) 10 mg • Selenium (Nutrition 21 l-Selenomethionine) 10 mcg • Zinc (Gluconate) 10 mg • Super Oxide Dismutase 30 IU • Betaine HCl 25 mg • Glutamic Acid HCl 25 mg • Methionine 50 mg. In a natural base of Lecithin, Alfalfa, Watercress, Parsley, Duodenal Substance, Rose Hips powder, Chamomile, Molasses, Kale, Cabbage, Goldenseal, Sarsaparilla, 72 Trace Minerals, Pepsin & Kelp.

Super Nutrition Power — Mascot Enterprise
Velvet Deer Antler • Shark Cartilage • Salmon Oil • Royal Jelly • Albumin • Oyster extract • Orchic substance • Siberian Ginseng extract 5:1 • Cinnamon • Garlic • Noni • Muira Puama • Guarana extract 4:1 • Smilax • Avena Sativa 10:1 • Damiana leaf extract 4:1 • Vitamin E • Vitamin C • Vitamin B6 • Boron (Citrate) • Zinc (Sulfate) • Niacinamide.

Super Octacosanol — The Vitamin Shoppe
Each softgel contains: Octacosanol 3000 mcg • Wheat Germ Oil 235 mg • Lecithin 9 mg.

Super Odorless Garlic — Now
Each capsule contains: odorless Garlic extract 100:1 concentrate (equivalent to 5000 mg fresh Garlic) 50 mg • Hawthorne berry extract (standardized to contain 1.8% Vitexin-2-Rhamnoside) 100 mg • Hawthorne berry powder 250 mg • Cayenne pepper (40,000 Heat units) 100 mg.

Super Omega 3 — Nutri-Quest
Each capsule contains: Natural marine lipid concentrate 1 g • Omega-3 Fatty Acids 110 mg/1 g of Eicosapentaenoic Acid (EPA) • Omega-3 90 mg/1 g of Docosahexaenoic Acid (DHA).

Super Salve — The Herbalist
Oils of Sweet Almond, St. John's Wort flower, Plantain herb, Calendula flower, & Beeswax • Extracts of Poplar bud, Golden Seal root, Echinacea root, Plantain herb, Comfrey root, Marshmallow root, Yarrow flower.

Super Stress Formula — The Vitamin Shoppe
Two capsules contain: Vitamin C 1000 mg • Vitamin B1 (Thiamin) 50 mg • Vitamin B2 (Riboflavin) 50 mg • Vitamin B6 (Pyridoxine Hcl) 50 mg • Vitamin B12 (Cobalamin) 400 mcg • Niacinamide 100 mg • Folic Acid 400 mcg • Pantothenic Acid 250 mg • Biotin 100 mcg • Choline Bitartrate 100 mg • Inositol 100 mg • PABA 50 mg. No Yeast, Corn, Wheat, Soy, Salt, Sugar, Starch, Gluten, Milk, Eggs, Dairy, Preservatives, Artificial Colors or Flavors added.

Super Suppositories — The Herbalist
Tea Tree Oil • Herbal extracts of Usnea & Calendula in a base of Cocoa Butter & Purified Bees Wax.

Super Thistle X — Phytopharmica
Each capsule contains: Milk Thistle extract 100 mg bound to phosphatidylocholine under patent • Dandelion root extract 4:1 (Taraxacum officinale) 10 mg • Artichoke leaves extract (Cynara

scolymus) 10 mg standardized to contain 15% caffeylquinic acids • Licorice root extract (Glycyrrhiza glabra) 10 mg standardized to contain 5% glycyrrhizic acid. Contains no sugar, salt, yeast, wheat, corn, dairy products, coloring, flavorings or preservatives.

Super Vanadyl Fuel — TwinLab
Four capsules contain: Vanadyl Sulfate (supplying elemental Vanadium IV 4.87 mg) 25 mg • BMOV [Bis (maltolato) Oxovanadium] (supplying elemental Vanadium IV 320 mcg) 2 mg • Chromium (from Chromic Fuel Chromium Picolinate) 300 mcg • Chromium (from ChromeMate Chromium Nicotinate) 300 mcg • Natural Vitamin E 900 IU • Taurine 1000 mg • Selenium (from Sodium Selenate) 150 mcg • Zinc (from Zinc Picolinate) 30 mg • Manganese (from Manganese Gluconate) 5 mg • Magnesium (from Magnesium Oxide & Aspartate) 400 mg • Biotin 1000 mcg • Niacinamide 100 mg.

Super Vitamin E Creme — Aspen Group, Inc.
Each gram contains: Tocopheryl Acetate 25% • Panthenol 1% • Water • Glyceryl Stearate SE • Octyl Palmitate • Isoproyl Palmitate • Propylene Glycol • Cetearyl Alcohol • Cetyl Phosphate • Decyl Oleate • Aminomethyl Propanol • Carbomer • Allantoin • Diazolidinyl Urea • Methylparaben • Propylparaben.

Super Vita-Vim with Beta Carotene — Jamieson
Each caplet contains: Vitamin A (as Tetinyl Acetate and 15% [1500] IU as Beta-Carotene) 10000 IU • Vitamin C (as Ascorbic Acid) 200 mg • Vitamin D (as Cholecalciferol) 400 IU • Vitamin E (as Dl-Alpha Tocopheryl Acetate) 60 IU • Thiamin (as Thiamin Mononitrate) 30 mg • Riboflavin (Vitamin B2) 30 mg • Niacin (as Niacin and Nicacinamide) 60 mg • Vitamin B6 (as Pyridoxine Hydrochloride) 30 mg • Folate (as Folic Acid) 400 mcg • Vitamin B12 (as Cyanocobalamin) 60 mcg • Biotin 30 mcg • Pantothenic Acid (as Calcium D-Pantothenate) 30 mg • Calcium (as Calcium Carbonate) 140 mg • Iron (as reduced Iron) 4 mg • Iodine (from kelp) 100 mcg • Magnesium (as Magnesium Oxide) 100 mg • Zinc (as Zinc Gluconate) 10 mg • Selenium (from yeast) 10 mcg • Copper (as Copper Gluconate) 1 mg • Chromium (as Chromium Rice Protein Chelate) 50 mcg • Potassium (as Potassium Gluconate) 30 mg • Choline Bitartrate 30 mg • Inositol 30 mg • Dl- Methionine 2.2 mg.

Super Whey Fuel — TwinLab
Blend of Three key Whey Proteins: Micro-Filtered & Ion-Exchange Whey Protein Isolate, Modified Molecular Weight & Partially Pre-Digested Whey Protein, & Whey Protein Concentrate (enriched with Glutamine, Taurine, Arginine, Leucine, Isoleucine, Valine, Carnitine & Carnosine). Contains no added sugar, is low in lactose & contains Whey Protein 17 g per serving.

SuperCitriMax — Now
Each capsule contains: Calcium (from Citrimax) 90 mg • ChromeMate brand of Chromium (Chromium Polynicotinate) 100 mcg • Iodine (from Kelp) 150 mcg • CitriMax Garcinia cambogia extract 750 mg • Panax ginseng root powder 100 mg.

Super-Green Pro-96 Soy Protein — Nature's Life
Two scoops (28.35 g) contain: Full disclosure ingredients: SUPRO brand Soy Protein Isolate (including Lecithin) • Hawaiian Spirulina • natural Vanilla Flavor • Barley Grass • Psyllium seed husks • Apple Pectin • Oat Fiber • Chlorophyll • Lemon Bioflavonoids Complex • Bromelain • Papain • Kelp • Milk-free Lactobacillus acidophilus • Pyridoxine Hydrochloride (Vitamin B6).

Support Tonic For Men — Amazon Support
Each capsule contains: Muira Puama • Catuaba • Chuchuhuasi • Suma • Maca • Simarouba • Sarsaparilla • Jurubeba • Carqueja • Jatoba.

Support Tonic For Women — Amazon Support
Each capsule contains: Abuta • Catuaba • Suma • Maca • Simarouba • Sarsaparilla • Wild Yam • Chuchuhuasi • Espinheira Santa • Gervao • Jurubeba • Damiana.

Supra Renal 220 — Atrium
Each tablet contains: Raw Tissue concentrate from Bovine Sources (not extracts): (Adrenal 220 mg & Pituitary 15 mg) 235 mg • Vitamin C 175 mg • Bioflavonoid Complex 45 mg • Pantothenic Acid 70 mg • Methionine 60 mg • Choline 60 mg • Vitamin B1 25 mg • Vitamin B2 25 mg • Vitamin B6 25 mg • Niacinamide 50 mg • Magnesium 100 mg • Folic Acid 400 mcg • RNA 25 mg.

Supraene Creme — Atrium
Two ounces contains: Squalene 30 mg • Triethanolamine 5 mg • Ceresin Wax 5 mg • Glucam F-20 4 mg • Amerchol L-101 2.5 mg •

Some Brand Name Natural Products - What they Contain
www.NaturalDatabase.com contains MANY more listings than appear here.

Solulan 16 2.5 mg • Steral 2.5 mg • Cetyl Alcohol 2.5 mg • Carbopol 934 0.5 mg • Methyl Paraben 10 mg • Propyl Paraben 0.05 mg • Distilled Water 45.35 mg.

Suprema C Powder — Gary Null
One teaspoon contains Vitamin C 2500 mg • Selenium 65 mcg • Bioflavonoids 150 mg.

Suprema C Tablets — Gary Null
Each tablet contains: Vitamin C 500 mg • Selenium 6 mcg • Bioflavonoids 10 mg.

Swiss Herbal — The Vitamin Shoppe
Each tablet contains: Senna (Cassia senna) leaves standardized to 3% sennosides 100 mg • Strawberry (Fragaria vesca) leaves 50 mg • Peach (Prunus persica) leaves 50 mg • Anise (Pimpinella anisum) fruit and seeds 50 mg • Cranberry (Vaccinium macrocarpon) fruit 50 mg • Calendula (Calendula officinalis) flower and leaves 25 mg. No yeast, corn, wheat, sugar, salt, starch, milk, gluten, soy, eggs, dairy, fish or animal derivatives, citrus, preservatives, artificial colors or flavors added.

Swiss Kriss Tabs — Swiss Kriss
Each tablet contains: Active Ingredient: Finely powdered sun dried leaves of Senna. Also contains the following natural herbs: Finely powdered Strawberry Leaves • Peach Leaves • Anise seed • Caraway seed • Hibiscus & Calendula flowers for their flavoring & carminative principals.

Symbiotropin hGH — ASN
Each two tablets contain: Anterior Pituitary Peptides Aminotrope-7 (a sequenced glycoamino acid complex) 4200 mg • Novel Polyose Complex (pharmaceutical mono, poly & oligo saccharides) 2230 mg. In a base of L-Glutamine, L-Arginine, L-Pyroglutamate, GABA, L-Glycine, L-Lysine, L-Tyrosine & Vica faba major, all naturally sweetened & flavored.

Sympt-X Plus — Cambridge Nutraceuticals
Each serving contains: Glutamine 10 g • Vitamin A (as mixed carotenoids) 6500 IU • Vitamin C 330 mg • Vitamin E 100 IU • Selenium 50 mcg. Available in 650 g jar and Single Dose Packets.

Synadrene — Metaphysics - Pro-Soma Enterprises
One capsule contains: Citrus Aurantium 350 mg • Chromium Picolinate 400 mcg.

Synergistic Iron — Quest
Each capsule contains: Iron (HVP Chelate) 25 mg • Copper (HVP Chelate) 2 mg • Molybdenum (HVP Chelate) 50 mcg • Vitamin C (Ascorbic Acid) 100 mg • Niacin 10 mg • Vitamin B1 (Thiamine HCl) 5 mg • Vitamin B6 (Pyridoxine HCl) 5 mg • Vitamin B2 (Riboflavin) 2 mg • Pantothenic Acid (d-Calcium Pantothenate) 10 mg • Folic Acid 0.2 mg • Vitamin B12 (Cobalamin) 20 mcg • Biotin 50 mcg. Other Ingredients: Magnesium Stearate (vegetable source), Microcrystalline Cellulose.

Synergistic Magnesium — Quest
Each tablet contains: Magnesium (HVP Chelate) 150 mg • Calcium (HVP Chelate) 30 mg • Phosphorus (HVP Complex) 15 mg • Vitamin B6 (Pyridoxine HCl) 20 mg. Other Ingredients: Croscarmellose Sodium, Magnesium Stearate (vegetable source), Microcrystalline Cellulose, Vegetable Stearin.

Synergistic Manganese — Quest
Each capsule contains: Manganese (HVP Chelate) 50 mg • Vitamin B1 (Thiamine HCl) 20 mg • Vitamin C 100 mg. Other Ingredients: Magnesium Stearate (vegetable source), Microcrystalline Cellulose.

Synergistic Multiple Mineral — Quest
Each tablet contains: Calcium (HVP Chelate) 100 mg • Magnesium (HVP Chelate) 100 mg • Potassium (HVP Chelate) 33 mg • Iron (HVP Chelate) 5 mg • Manganese (HVP Chelate) 5 mg • Zinc (HVP Chelate) 5 mg • Copper (HVP Chelate) 1 mg • Iodine (Potassium Iodide) 50 mcg • Molybdenum (HVP Chelate) 50 mcg • Chromium (HVP Chelate) 10 mcg • Selenium (HVP Complex) 10 mcg. Other Ingredients: Croscarmellose Sodium, Magnesium Stearate (vegetable source), Mircocrystalline Cellulose, Vegetable Stearin.

Synergistic Selenium — Quest
Each capsule contains: Selenium (HVP Chelate) 200 mcg • Vitamin E (d-Alpha Tocopheryl Acetate) 25 IU • Vitamin C (Ascorbic Acid) 100 mg. Other Ingredients: Magnesium Stearate (vegetable source), Microcrystalline Cellulose.

Synergistic Zinc — Quest
Each tablet contains: Vitamin A (Palmitate) 5000 IU • Zinc (HVP Chelate) 20 mg • Copper (HVP Chelate) 1 mg. Other Ingredients: Calcium Phosphate, Croscarmellose Sodium, Magnesium Stearate (vegetable source), Microcrystalline Cellulose, Vegetable Stearin.

System D-Tox — Nutri-Quest
Six capsules contain: Vitamin A Palmitate 2000 IU • Vitamin C 750 mg • Vitamin B1 20 mg • Niacin 25 mg • Vitamin B12 50 mcg • Folic Acid 300 mcg • Calcium Aspartate 75 mg • Magnesium Glycinate 200 mg • Magnesium Aspartate 100 mg • Chromium Picolinate 50 mcg • Zinc Picolinate 20 mg • N-Acetyl Cysteine 30 mg • L-Glutamine 200 mg • Silymarin extract 5 mg • Quercetin 25 mg • L-Taurine 50 mg • L-Ornithine 20 mg • L-Glutamic Acid 20 mg • L-Carnitine 20 mg • Choline 50 mg • Propolis 20 mg • Yellow Dock 25 mg • Beta Carotene 7500 IU • Vitamin E Succinate Natural 200 IU • Vitamin B2 20 mg • Pyridoxal 5 Phosphate 20 mg • Pantothenic Acid 50 mg • Biotin 200 mcg • Calcium Gluconate 75 mg • Magnesium Citrate 100 mg • Selenomethionine 150 mcg • Manganese Aspartate 5 mg • Molybdenum Citrate 50 mcg • Reduced Glutathione 20 mg • Milk Thistle 50 mg • Beet root 50 mg • Glucaronic Acid 5 mg • L-Glycine 50 mg • L-Methionine 50 mg • L-Arginine 20 mg • L-Tyrosine 20 mg • Inositol 50 mg • Curcumin 5 mg • Chlorophyll 10 mg • Asparagus 15 mg • Dandelion root 25 mg • Siberian Ginseng 30 mg • Broccoli 15 mg • Mullein 25 mg • Co-Enzyme Q-10 1 mg.

Syste-Max — Changes - TwinLab
One heaping teaspoonful (6.8 g) contains: Vitamin A 668 IU • Vitamin C 100 mg • Vitamin E 60 IU • Psyllium seed husk 4000 mg • Soy Germ flour (providing 15 mg of isoflavones) 500 mg • Chitosan 100 mg • Phytosterol complex (providing 43 mg of beta-sitosterol) 100 mg • Oat flour 100 mg.

T-5W — Dial Herbs
Red Raspberry • Blue Cohosh • Bayberry • Squaw Vine • Blessed Thistle • Ginger • Motherwort • False Unicorn • Wild Yam • Lobelia • Cayenne.

T-ACN — Dial Herbs
Black Walnut • Burdock • Chaparral • Yellow Dock • Sassafras • Valerian.

Tadenan — European; Not available in the US.
Pygeum africanum extract standardized to contain 14% triterpenes and 0.5% n-docosanol usually in dosages of 100 - 200 mg.

T-AFT — Dial Herbs
Wild Lettuce • St. John's Wort • Valerian • Cayenne.

T-AIS — Dial Herbs
Rose Hips • Sage • Yarrow • Burdock • Echinacea • Goldenseal • Yellow Dock • Garlic • Nettle • Lemon Grass • White Oak bark • Black Cohosh • Fenugreek • Juniper berry • Oregon Grape • Plantain • Thyme.

T-AKE — Dial Herbs
Clove Oil • Oat Straw • Lobelia • Cayenne.

Take Control — Lipton
Water • Liquid Canola Oil • Vegetable Oil Sterol Esters • Liquid Sunflower Oil • Partially Hydrogenated Soybean Oil • Salt • Whey • Vegetable Mono- and Diglycerides • Potassium Sorbate • Lactic Acid • Calcium Disodium EDTA • Soy Lecithin • Artificial Flavor • Beta Carotene • Vitamin A (Palmitate).

T-ALER — Dial Herbs
Bayberry • Echinacea • Yarrow • Wild Cherry bark • Cayenne • Goldenseal.

T-ANEM — Dial Herbs
Comfrey root • Dandelion • Barberry • Parsley • Yellow Dock • Myrrh • Kelp.

Taraxatone — Cytodyne Technologies
Six capsules contain: Vitamin B6 24 mg • Magnesium 8.4 mg • Dandelion leaf powder 1500 mg • Uva Ursi leaf extract 900 mg • Guarana extract 600 mg • Taurine 115 mg.

T-ARTH — Dial Herbs
Yucca • Alfalfa • Buckthorn • Burdock • Parsley • Slippery Elm • Yarrow • Cayenne.

T-ASMA — Dial Herbs
Blood root • St. John's Wort • Mullein • Comfrey • Saw Palmetto • Wild Cherry bark • Goldenseal • Lobelia • Cayenne.

BRAND NAMES

© Copyright 2000, Natural Medicines Comprehensive Database (209) 472-2244. For updated data, go to www.NaturalDatabase.com. • 1405

Some Brand Name Natural Products - What they Contain
www.NaturalDatabase.com contains MANY more listings than appear here.

T-BB — Dial Herbs
Buckthorn • Yellow Dock • Garlic • Cayenne • Dandelion • Poke root.

T-BC — Dial Herbs
White Oak bark • Comfrey • Black Walnut • Marshmallow root •
Mullein • Gravel root • Wormwood • Lobelia • Scullcap • Glycerine.

T-BDW — Dial Herbs
Corn Silk • Plantain • St. John's Wort • Sanicle • Mullein •
Sarsaparilla • Cubeb berries • Watermelon seeds • Cayenne.

T-BF — Dial Herbs
Oat Straw • Shavegrass • Comfrey • Slippery Elm • Burdock •
Lobelia.

T-CAC — Dial Herbs
Buckthorn • Burdock • Chaparral • Dandelion • Cascara Sagrada •
Licorice • Red Clover • Barberry.

T-CIRC — Dial Herbs
Witch Hazel • Garlic • Ginger • Cayenne.

T-CS — Dial Herbs
Bayberry • Myrrh • Echinacea • Goldenseal • Cayenne.

T-DI — Dial Herbs
Hyssop • Garlic • Hydrangea • Catnip • Peppermint • Cayenne.

T-DIA — Dial Herbs
Yarrow • Juniper berries • Huckleberry • Cayenne • Goldenseal.

T-DREA — Dial Herbs
Witch Hazel • Slippery Elm • Ginger • Shepherd's Purse • Raspberry.

T-DRY — Dial Herbs
Sage • Yarrow.

T-DTX — Dial Herbs
Echinacea • Yellow Dock • Garlic • Lobelia • Cayenne.

Tea Tree Oil — Holista
Tea Tree oil (Melaleuca alternifolia) 100% pure.

T-EC — Dial Herbs
Eyebright • Bayberry • Passion flower • Goldenseal • Cayenne.

Teen Advantage Creatine Serum — Muscle Marketing USA
Each serving contains: Creatine Monohydrate • Glucosamine •
Vitamin B12 • L-Glutamine • Sodium Pyruvate • Royal Jelly •
Ginseng • Honey • Natural Glycerine • Natural Flavor • Distilled
Water.

Teen Link — Pain & Stress Center
Each capsule contains: 5-HTP 25 mg • St. John's Wort 165 mg •
GABA 120 mg • Glutamine 100 mg • Taurine 110 mg •
Vitamin B6 5 mg.

Tegreen 97 — Pharmanex
Each 250 mg capsule contains a 15:1 extract of Green Tea extract that
is standardized to contain a minimum of 97% pure polyphenols
including >160 mg of catechins of which >100 mg is EGC.

Ten Mushroom Combination — Smart Basics
Each capsule contains: Cordyceps • Reishi • Maitake • Shiitake •
Coriolus • Umbellatus Polyporus • Wood Ear • Tremella • Poria •
Hericium.

T-ENDO — Dial Herbs
Chaparral • Pipsessewa • Licorice • Prickly Ash • Cramp bark • False
Unicorn • Saw Palmetto • Red Clover.

T-ER — Dial Herbs
Eyebright • Bayberry • Passion flower • Goldenseal • Cayenne •
Mineral Water • Honey.

Testatropinol — ASN
Each tablet contains: Testatropinol is a 100% natural, non-herbal, non-
glandular, synergistic, homeopathic compound, consisting of:
Testosterone • Growth Hormone • Adrenalinum • Adrenocorticotropic
Hormone • Lutenizing Hormone • Follicle Stimulating Hormone •
Thyroid Stimulating Hormone • Progesterone • Estrone.
Editor's Comments: This is a homeopathic product. It is so extremely
diluted that its activity can not be explained by conventional scientific
methods. Therefore this product can not be rated by the scientific
criteria used in this Database. A patient receiving the extreme dilution
of this product will not receive many, if any, molecules of the original
active ingredient. Therefore, there are no harmful pharmacologic

effects, and any beneficial effects are controversial and not due to a
direct biochemical action of the ingredient on the body. Homeopathic
products are allowed for sale in the U.S. due to legislation passed in
the 19th century sponsored by a homeopathic physician who was also
a Senator. The law still requires that the FDA allow the sale of
products listed in this Homeopathic Pharmacopea of the United States.

Testosterone Fuel Booster — TwinLab
Two capsules contain: Natural Testosterone Boosters DHEA
(Dehydroepiandrosterone) (Pure Pharmaceutical Grade) 50 mg • Zinc
(from Zinc Picolinate) 50 mg • Natural LH Boosters Acetyl-L-
Carnitine 500 mg • Tribulus Terrestris extract 150 mg • Natural
Aromatase Inhibitor (anti-estrogen) • Novasoy Purified Soy extract
(providing 40% isoflavones)(providing isoflavones 80 mg including:
Genistein39 mg, Diadzein 34 mg & Glycitein 7 mg) 200 mg • Natural
DHT Inhibitors • Saw Palmetto (Serenoa repens) extract 120 mg •
Phytosterol Complex (providing 130 mg of Beta-Sitosterol) 250 mg.

T-FC1 — Dial Herbs
Red Raspberry • Black Cohosh • Lady Slipper • Blessed Thistle •
Damiana.

T-FC2 — Dial Herbs
Black Cohosh • Licorice root • Sarsaparilla • Ginseng • Goldenseal.

T-FC3 — Dial Herbs
Black Cohosh • Wood Betony • Blessed Thistle • Chamomile • Fennel
• Ginger • Cayenne.

T-FC4 — Dial Herbs
Wood Betony • Sarsaparilla • Valerian • Blessed Thistle • Dandelion •
Garlic • Chamomile.

T-FLO — Dial Herbs
Sanicle • Marshmallow • Fennel • Blessed Thistle • Ginger.

T-FVR — Dial Herbs
Peppermint • Garlic • Valerian • Yarrow • Echinacea • Goldenseal •
Cayenne • Lobelia.

T-GB — Dial Herbs
Dandelion • Oregon Grape • Rhubarb • Bayberry • Yellow Dock •
Lobelia.

T-GS — Dial Herbs
Catnip • Peppermint • Fennel • Cayenne • Lobelia.

T-H — Dial Herbs
White Willow bark • Valerian • Scullcap • Wood Betony.

T-HBP — Dial Herbs
Black Cohosh • Blue Cohosh • Wild Cherry bark.

T-HBRN — Dial Herbs
Sarsaparilla • Thyme • Valerian • Wood Betony • Peppermint • Catnip
• White Willow bark.

The Antioxidant Formula — Rx Vitamins
Three capsules contain: Vitamin C (Ascorbate) 500 mg • Beta
Carotene 25000 IU • Phytonutrient Blend (Broccoli, Spinach, Tomato)
150 mg • Citrus Bioflavonoid Complex 50 mg • Vitamin E 200 IU •
Selenium 50 mcg • Zinc 15 mg • NAC (N-Acetyl-Cysteine) 15 mg •
Bilberry 10 mg • L-Glutathione 10 mg • Wild Grape seed extract
10 mg.

The Antioxidant Phyters — The Vitamin Shoppe
Each tablet contains: Green and Red Wine 100 mg • Licorice 100 mg •
Pine bark and Grape seed 30 mg • Bilberry 50 mg • Ginkgo Biloba
50 mg • Marigold, Sunflowers 60 mg.

The AstaFactor — Aquasearch
Two softgels contain: Natural Astaxanthin (6 mg total carotenoids) 5
mg. Ingredients: Algal meal (Haematococcus pluvialis), Rice Bran
Oil, Natural Gelatin, Bee's Wax, Natural Vitamin E, Vegetal Glycerin.

The B-Total Solution with Extra B12 — Dial Herbs
Vitamin C • Vitamin B2 • Vitamin B3 • Vitamin B6 • Vitamin B12 •
Pantothenic Acid. In a base of Distilled Water, Glycerine, Sorbitol,
Sodium Bicarbonate, Citric Acid, Fruit flavors & Sodium Benzoate.

The Fat Metabolizer — The Vitamin Shoppe
Three tablets contain: Elemental Choline (from Chline Bitartrate)
1000 mg • Inositol 100 mg • L-Methionine 500 mg • Taurine 500 mg •
Vitamin B6 (Pyridoxine HCl) 30 mg • Betaine HCl 150 mg • Barberry
Extract (Berberis vulgaris) 100 mg.

1406 • © Copyright 2000, Natural Medicines Comprehensive Database (209) 472-2244. For updated data, go to www.NaturalDatabase.com.

BRAND NAMES

Some Brand Name Natural Products - What they Contain
www.NaturalDatabase.com contains MANY more listings than appear here.

The Fruit Phyters — The Vitamin Shoppe
Two tablets contain: Tomatoes, Red Grapefruit, Apricots, Watermelon 100 mg • Walnuts, Berries, Grapes, Apples, Tea • Orange, Lemons, Limes, Grapefruits, Tangerines, Cherries, Tomatoes, Strawberries 400 mg • Apricots, Cantaloupe, Citrus Fruits 150 mg • Citrus Fruits 100 mg • Papaya, Kiwi, Pineapples 50 mg • Mangoes, Citrus Fruits 100 mg.

The Green Phyters — The Vitamin Shoppe
Two tablets contain: Spirulina 200 mg • Chlorella 200 mg • Barley Juice 200 mg • Wheat Grass 200 mg • Alfalfa Leaf 200 mg • Chlorophyll 200 mg.

The Natural Choice Hepol — Allergon AB
Each tablet contains: Botanical Glutathione Yeast extract YH 85 mg • Aloe Vera extract 45 mg • Polbax extract 40 mg. Other Ingredients: Lacrose Alfa, Microcrystalline Cellulose, Magnesium Stearate, Colloidal Silicon Dioxide, Talc, Natural Resin.

The Natural Choice Probacillus Plus — Allergon AB
Each tablet contans: proprietary blend (Lacrobacillus Acidophilus • Bifidobacterium Bifidum) 4 Billion Cells. Other Ingredients: Insitol, Monoatril Glutamas, Ascorbate, Yeast extract, Polysaccharides, Skim Milk Powder, stearate, Dextrose.

The Natural Choice Profemme — Allergon AB
Each tablet contains: Flower Pollen extract WSI 72 mg • Flower Pollon extract LS1 4 mg. Other Ingredients: Microcrystalline Cellulose, Lactose, Magnesium stearate, Silicon Dioxide, Natural Resin, Polyethylene Glycol, Talc.

The Natural Choice Prostat — Allergon AB
Each tablet contains: Standardized extract of Graminae Pollen 70 mg • Fat soluble Gramanie extract EA 10 4 mg. Other Ingredients: Microcrystalline Cellulose, Lactose, Magnesium Stearate, Colloidal Silicon Dioxide, Natural Resin, Talc, Propylene Glycol.

The Ocular Formula — Rx Vitamins
Three capsules contain: Vitamin C (Ascorbate) 200 mg • Citrus Flavonoid Complex 100 mg • Vitamin E 100 IU • Zinc 30 mg • Glutathione 10 mg • Beta Carotene 9 mg • Vitamin A (Retinol) 5000 IU • Selenium 50 mcg • Lutein 6 mg • Zeaxanthin 260 mcg • Bilberry 100 mg • Grape seed 10 mg • Essential Cofactors: CoQ10 5 mg, Copper 3 mg.

The One-Minute Facial — Jason
Seven different Vitamin Cs • Alpha Lipoic Acid.

The Total EFA — Health From The Sun
Three capsules contain: Calories 35 • Calories from Fat 30 • Total Fat 3.5 g • Saturated Fat 0.5 g • Cholesterol 5 mg • Protein 1 g • Vitamin E 30 IU • Alpha-Linolenic Acid (ALA)(Omega-3) 699 mg • Docosahexaenoic Acid (DHA) (Omega-3) 138 mg • Eicosapentaenoic Acid (EPA)(Omega-3) 216 mg • Gamma-Linolenic Acid (GLA)(Omega-6) 288 mg • Lenoleic Acid (Omega-6) 620 mg • Oleic Acid (Omega-9) 520 mg. Ingredients: Certified Organic Flax seed oil, Borage seed oil, Fish oil, Gelatin, Glycerine, Water, Mixed Tocopherols.

The Total EFA — Health From The Sun
One tablespoon provides: High ALA (omega-3) 5872 mg • Evening Primrose oil • GLA (from Borage oil & Evening Primrose oil) 288 mg • Lignans 12 mg. Liquid version also contains special antioxidant complex: [Vitamin E (mixed tocopherols), Rosemary extract, Ascorbyl Palmitate (Vitamin C) & Citric Acid].

The Ultimate Anti-Oxidant Formula — Natrol
Two capsules contain: Vitamin A (Beta Carotene from d-Salina) 10000 IU • Vitamin E (d-alpha tocopheryl) 200 IU • Vitamin C (Ester-C Brand) 250 mg • Niacinamide 40 mg • Zinc (Krebs Cycle) 25 mg • Copper (Krebs Cycle) 2 mg • Selenium (Selenomethionine) 125 mcg • Flavonoids, Herbs, & other selected ingredients: Spirulina 300 mg GP Flavonoids Complex+ 200 mg, a 30% guaranteed potency extract of mixed flavonoids extracted from: Rose Hips, Tumeric, Acerola berry, Bilberry, Hawthorne berry, Grape skin, Milk Thistle, & Citrus fruits • Calendula 50 mg • Artichoke extract 10 mg. Other ingredients: Silicon Dioxide, Magnesium Stearate, Gelatin.

The Ultimate Calcium Formula — Roex
Six tablets contain: Calcium (Chelate, Citrate, Hydroxyapatite, Aspartate, Lactate) 1000 mg • Magnesium (Chelate, Oxide, Aspartate) 500 mg • Zinc (Gluconate , Citrate, Aspartate) 15 mg • Manganese 5 mg • Copper 2 mg • Vitamin D (Cholecalciferol) 400 IU • Boron 3 mg

• Trace Minerals 25 mg • Silica 150 mg • Selenium 50 mcg • Chromium 50 mcg • Molybdenum 10 mcg.

The Ultimate Weight Loss & Nutrition System — Nature's Secret
Three tablets provide: Vitamin B6 30 mg • Garcinia cambogia extract 600 mg • Pantothenic Acid 100 mg • Magnesium (aspartate) 25 mg • Chromium 300 mcg • Potassium (citrate) 128 mg • L-Carnitine 250 mg • Betaine HCl 100 mg • Lipotropic factors 800 mg • Choline, L-Methionine, Inositol, Lecithin, Triphala powder, Echinacea angustifolia, Cascara sagrada • Astragalus. Thermogenic support factors 757 mg: N-Acetyl Glucosamine, Uva Ursi leaf, Gotu Kola, Siberian Ginseng, L-Glutamine, Parsley leaf, Ginger root, Borage oil, Shave Grass herb, Piper longum, Licorice root. L-Phenylalanine, Corn Silk, Gugulipid, Pacific Kelp, L-Tyrosine, Atractylodes, Bladderwrack, Dulse, Chickweed herb, Dandelion root, Capsicum fruit, Lipase, Mustard seed, Protease, Cellulase.

The Vegi Phyters — The Vitamin Shoppe
Two tablets contain: Red, Yellow, and Dark vegetable, Carrots, Kale, Parsley, Spinach, Sweet Potatoes, Turnip Greens, Winter Squash, and Yams 300 mg • Cruciferous Vegetable 300 mg • Horseradish 100 mg • Chili Peppers 100 mg • Cabbage, Brussel Sprouts, Kale, Collard Greens, Broccoli, Mustard Greens 200 mg.

The Vitamin Shoppe Flax Seed Oil 1000 mg — The Vitamin Shoppe
Each softgel contains: 1000 mg of 100% pure, organically grown cold-pressed, unrefined virgin flax oil providing the following approximate essential fatty acids: Alpha-Linolenic Acid 550 mg • Linoleic Acid 150 mg • Oleic Acid 190 mg • natural Vitamin E 1 IU.

Thera Zinc Lozenges-Menthol — Natrol
One lozenge contains: Vitamin C (as Calcium Ascorbate) 50 mg • Zinc (as Zinc Gluconate) 7.5 mg • Echinacea angustifolia entire plant 10 mg • Bee Propolis 10 mg • Slippery Elm Bark 10 mg • Elderberry 10 mg • Bee Pollen 10 mg. Other ingredients: Hydrogenated Starch, Hydrolysate, natural Menthol Eucalyptus flavor.

Thera-C 3 Grams Lemon — Natrol
One single serving contains: Vitamin C (Ascorbic Acid) 250 mg • Acerola berry extract 20 mg • Echinacea (Purpurea extract 16:1) 12.5 mg • White Willow bark 100 mg • Slippery Elm bark 75 mg • Stevia powder 20 mg. Other ingredients: Lemon Juice powder, Citric Acid, Menthol from Peppermint, Honey powder, Fructose, Calcium Carbonate.

Theragran Heart Right — Bristol-Myers Squibb Co.
Two caplets contain: Vitamin A (8% as Beta-carotene, 2% as Alpha-carotene, Lutein, Lypcopene, Zeaxanthin, Cryptoxanthin) 5000 IU • Vitamin C 120 mg • Vitamin D 400 IU • Vitamin E 400 IU • Vitamin K 14 mcg • Thiamin (B1) 3 mg • Riboflavin (B2) 3.4 mg • Niacin (B3) 20 mg • Vitamin B6 16 mg • Folate, Folic Acid, Folacin 600 mcg • Vitamin B12 30 mcg • Biotin 30 mcg • Pantothenic acid 10 mg • Calcium 55 mg • Magnesium 150 mg • Zinc 15 mg • Selenium 70 mcg • Copper 1.5 mg • Manganese 2 mg • Chromium 50 mcg • Molybdenum 75 mcg • Proprietary Blend, 10 mg: Beta Carotene, Alpha Carotene, Lutein, Lycopene, Zeaxanthin, Cryptoxanthin.

Thermadrene — SportPharma
Each capsule contains: Ephedra Standardized extract 300 mg (equals 24 mg of Ephedrine) • USP Caffeine 80 mg • Guarana extract 150 mg (equals 15 mg of Caffeine) • Willow Bark extract 75 mg (natural Aspirin; equals less than 5 mg of Aspirin) • Cayenne 60 mg • Ginger root 40 mg.

Thermic Blast — Human Development Technologies
Four sprays contain: Caffeine 100 mg • Ephedra extract 8% aerial (Ephedrine 8 mg) 100 mg • Stevia extract 80% leaf (Steviosides 32 mg) 40 mg • White Willow bark 1% bark (Salicin 200 mcg) 20 mg • Green Tea extract 30% leaf (Polyphenols 6 mg) 20 mg • Guarana extract 10% seed (Caffeine 2 mg) 20 mg • Chromium Picolinate 400 mcg. Other Ingredients: Purified Water, Propylene Glycol, natural Cherry & Vanilla Flavors, Polysorbate 20, Benzyl Alcohol, Hydrochloric Acid Lecithin.

Thermicore — Met-Rx
Three capsules contain: Ma Huang extract 250 mg • Caffeine 200 mg • Bitter Orange extract 400 mg. Other Ingredients: Cellulose, Polyvinylpyrrolidone & Gelatin.

Thermo Cuts — Optimum Nutrition
Four capsules contain: Citrimax 2000 mg • MaHuang extract 334 mg

© Copyright 2000, Natural Medicines Comprehensive Database (209) 472-2244. For updated data, go to www.NaturalDatabase.com.

**B
R
A
N
D

N
A
M
E
S**

• Guarana extract 910 mg • Willow bark extract 100 mg • L-Carnitine 100 mg • Chromium Picolinate 300 mcg.

Thermo-Actives — Natrol
One capsule contains: Ginger extract roots (5% Gingerols) 150 mg • Sida cordifolia extract (0.8% Ephedrine) 100 mg • Mucuna pruriens 5:1 extract 100 mg • Cayenne Guaranteed Potency extract (90000 SHU) 50 mg • Mustard extract Seed (50% Saponins) 15 mg • Bioperine 4:1 extract 15 mg. Other ingredients: Rice powder, Silicon Dioxide, Magnesium Stearate, Gelatin.

ThermoDiet for Men — Futurebiotics
Two tablets contain: Spirulina 100 mg • MaHuang (Standardized Extract) 200 mg • Mustard Seed Powder 100 mg • Vitamin C 100 mg • Potassium (Citrate) 99 mg • Magnesium (Aspartate) 50 mg • Chromium (Picolinate) 200 mcg • Kelp 150 mg • Chinese Licorice 250 mg • Smilax.

ThermoDiet For Women — Futurebiotics
Two tablets contain: Spirulina 100 mg • MaHuang (Standardized Extract) 200 mg • Mustard Seed Powder 100 mg • Vitamin C 100 mg • Potassium (Citrate) 99 mg • Magnesium (Aspartate) 50 mg • Chromium (Picolinate) 200 mcg • Kelp 150 mg • Peony 250 mg • Foti 250 mg • Dong Quai 250 mg.

Thermogenics Original Formula — Silver Sage
Each capsule contains: Ephedrine alkaloids (from standardized Ma Huang plant extract 310 mg) 25 mg • Caffeine (16.8 mg from standardized Bissy Nut 140 mg) 50 mg • Acetylsalicylic Acid (Aspirin) 110 mg • Proprietary Blend of synergistic ingredients 249 mg: Siberian Ginseng root, Schizonepeta spica extract 5:1, Forsythia fruit extract 5:1, Green Tea leaf extract standardized for polyphenols/catechins content, Cayenne fruit, Ginger root • Vitamin C 50 mg • Pantothenic Acid 25 mg • Zinc amino acid chelate 7 mg • Selenium amino acid chelate 1 mcg • Manganese amino acid chelate 2.5 mg.

ThermoGenics Plus — Silver Sage
Each capsule contains: Ephedrine (in standardized whole Ma Huang extract) 14 mg • Caffeine (in standardized Bissy Nut) • Acetylsalicylic Acid • In a base of Vitamin C, Siberian Ginseng, Green Tea extract (standardized to 50% polyphenols/catechins), Schizonepeta spica extract (5:1), Forsythia fruit extract (5:1), White Willow bark, Cayenne, Pantothenic Acid, Ginger root, Zinc (Amino Acid Chelate), Manganese (Amino Acid Chelate), Selenium (Amino Acid Chelate).

Thermogenics Quick Start — Silver Sage
Each capsule contains: Ephedrine alkaloids (from standardized Ma Huang plant extract 250 mg) 20 mg • Caffeine (26 mg from standardized Bissy Nut 106 mg) 200 mg • Acetylsalicylic Acid (Aspirin) 324 mg • Proprietary Blend of synergistic ingredients 198 mg: Siberian Ginseng root, Schizonepeta spica extract 5:1, Forsythia fruit extract 5:1, Cayenne fruit, Ginger root • Vitamin C 40 mg • Pantothenic Acid 23 mg • Zinc amino acid chelate 14 mg • Selenium amino acid chelate 167 mcg • Manganese amino acid chelate 5 mg.

Thermo-Lift — Changes - TwinLab
One caplet contains: Chromium (Chromium dinicotinate glycinate, Chromium picolinate, and Niacin bound Chromium) 200 mcg • Vanadium (as bis(maltoalto)oxovanadium(iv)) 100 mcg • Mahuang stem standardized extract (Supplying 25 mg Ephedrine alkaloids) 310 mg • Thermogenic herbal blend 325 mg: Guarana seed standardized extract (20%) (Supplying 43 mg Caffeine), Citrus Peel standardized extract (5-7% alkaloids) (Citrus aurantium), White Willow bark, Siberian Ginseng root, Astragalus root, Bee Pollen, Bladderwrack kelp, Ginger root, Gotu Kola leaf, Licorice root, Rehmannia root, Reishi mushroom (Fruiting body). Other ingredients: Dicalcium phosphate, Vegetable cellulose, Fractionated Vegetable oil, Soy polysaccharides, Silica, and Vegetable resin glaze.

Thermo-Lift II — Changes - TwinLab
Each caplet contains: Niacin 10 mg • Chromium (as Chromium dinicotinate glycinate, Chromium polynicotinate and chromium picolinate) 100 mcg • Vanadium (as Vanadyl sulfate) 50 mcg • Panax Ginseng root standardized extract (8% ginsenosides) 100 mg • Guarana seed standardized extract (20% Caffeine) 225 mg • Yerba Mate leaf standardized extract 100 mg • L-Tyrosine 100 mg • Thermogenic herbal blend 75 mg: Standardized Citrus Peel extract (5% phenethylamines) (Citrus aurantium), Cayenne pepper, Cinnamon bark standardized extract, Ginger root, and White Willow bark• Supporting herbal blend 50 mg: Astragalus root, Bladderwrack kelp, Licorice root, Siberian Ginseng root, and Arctic root (Rhodiola rosea) standardized extract. Other ingredients: Dicalcium phosphate,

Vegetable cellulose, Fractionated Vegetable oil, Soy polysaccharides, Silica, and Vegetable resin glaze.

ThermoMax Warm Cream — Strategic Science & Technologies
Water • Choline chloride • L-arginine • Sodium Chloride • Mineral Oil • Glyceryl Stearate SE • Squalane • Cetyl Alcohol • Magnesium Chloride • Propylene Glycol Stearate SE • Wheat Germ Oil • Glyceryl Stearate • Isopropyl Myristate • Stearyl Stearate • Polysorbate-60 • Propylene Glycol • Oleic Acid • Tocopherol Acetate • Collagen • Sorbitan Stearate • Vitamin A • Vitamin D • Triethanolamine • O. Capsic • Methylparaben • Aloe Vera extract • Imidazolidinyl Urea • Propylparaben • BHA.

THERMOthin — Slimming and Nutrition Consultancy
Each capsule contains: Citrus aurantium • Citrin (HCA) • Guarana • Caffeine • White Willow bark • Chromium • Liquorice extract • Cayenne extract • Siberian Ginseng • Vitamin B6 • Iodine • Betaine HCL.

T-HFV — Dial Herbs
Bayberry • Cayenne • Mullein • Lobelia.

Think-02 — Traditional Medicinals
Contains: Peppermint leaf • Ginkgo leaf and Ginkgo dry leaf extract • Gotu Kola leaf • Sage leaf • Siberian Ginseng root • Lemon Balm leaf • Rosemary leaf • natural Lemon flavor • Stevia leaf.

Thinz Back-To-Nature — Alva-Amco
One tablet contains: Active Ingredient: Phenylpropanolamine HCl 75 mg. Other Ingredients: Apple powder • Brown Lake color blend • Dicalcium Phosphate • D&C Yellow #10 • FD&C Yellow #6 • Hydroxypropyl Methylcellulose • Magnesium Stearate • Mineral oil • Oat bran • Polyethylene Glycol • Titanium Dioxide • Wheat bran.

Thinz-Span — Alva-Amco
Each capsule contains: Phenylpropanolamine HCl 75 mg.

Thiodox — Allergy Research Group
Glutathione • N-Acetyl Cysteine • Lipoic Acid.

Thisilyn — Nature's Way
175 mg of Milk thistle extract standardized for a flavanoid content of 140 mg silymarin (80%), which includes silybinin, silychristin, and 85 mg of lactose.

ThistleComp — Phytopharmica
Each capsule contains: Artichoke leaves extract (Cynara scolymus) 250 mg standardized to contain 3% caffeylquinic acids • Curcuma root extract (Curcuma longa) 150 mg standardized to contain 2.5% curcumin • Boldo extract (Peumus boldo) 100 mg standardized to contain 1.52% essential oils • Milk Thistle extract (Silybum marianum) 70 mg standardized to contain 80% silymarin (56 mg) calculated as silybin. Contains no sugar, salt, yeast, wheat, corn, soy, dairy products, coloring, flavoring or preservatives.

ThistlePlex — Enzymatic Therapy
Each capsule contains: Artichoke leaves extract (Cynara scolymus) standardized to contain 3% Caffeylquinic Acids 250 mg • Curcuma root extract (Curcuma longa) standardized to contain 2.5% Curcumin) 150 mg • Boldo extract (Peumus boldo) standardized to contain 1.52% essential oils) 100 mg • Milk Thistle extract (Silybum marianum) standardized to contain 80% Silymarin (56 mg) calculated as Silybin 70 mg. Contains no sugar, salt, yeast, wheat, corn, soy, dairy products, coloring, flavoring, or preservatives.

ThistleRex — Phytopharmica
Each capsule contains: Milk Thistle extract 150 mg standardized to contain 80% silymarin (120 mg) calculated as silybin • Dandelion root extract 4:1 (Taraxacum officinale) 10 mg • Artichoke leaves extract (Cynara scolymus) 10 mg standardized to contain 3% caffeylquinic acids • Licorice root extract (Glycyrrhiza glabra) 10 mg standardized to contain 5% glycyrrhizic acid. Contains no sugar, salt, yeast, wheat, corn, soy, dairy products, coloring, flavoring or preservatives.

Thorene — Thorene Research Inc.
Each capsule contains: Tylophora asthmatica 30 mg • Boswellia serrata extract (60% Boswellin) 150 mg • Piper longa 100 mg • Hesperidin Methyl Chalcone 100 mg.

Three-In-One — Changes - TwinLab
One capsule contains: Vitamin C (as Calcium Ascorbate) 120 mg • Aloe Vera leaf gel 200:1 concentrate 200 mg • Mexican Yam root 4:1

(equivalent to 150 mg) 37.5 mg. Other ingredients: Gelatin, Maltodextrin, Calcium Sulfate, Magnesium Stearate, and Silica.

Throat Coat — Traditional Medicinals
Slippery Elm bark (Ulmus rubra). Other herbal ingredients: Licorice root, Wild Cherry bark, Fennel seed, Cinnamon bark, Orange peel, Althea root.

T-HRT — Dial Herbs
Hawthorne • Lecithin • Tansy • Fenugreek • Garlic • Cayenne.

T-HS — Dial Herbs
Ginseng • Damiana • Gotu Kola • Sarsaparilla • Sassafras • Saw Palmetto.

Thyme and Myrrh — Dial Herbs
Thyme • Myrrh.

Thymuril — Phytopharmica
Two tablets contain: Vitamin A (Beta Carotene) 25000 IU • Vitamin E 200 IU • Vitamin C (Ascorbate) 250 mg • Zinc (Chelate) 15 mg • Selenium (Chelate) 25 mcg • Enzymatic Polypeptide fractions 750 mg.

Thymus Cream — Atrium
Three fluid ounces contain: Extract of Thymus (Viobin) • Glycerin Hexadecenol • Sodium Laureth Sulfate • Stearic Acid • Methylparaben • Sodium Sulfate • Propylparaben • Natural Fragrance.

T-HYPO — Dial Herbs
Licorice • Juniper berry • Wild Yam • Dandelion • Ginger.

Thyro Complex — Progressive Labs
Each capsule contains: Raw Thyroid concentrate (thyroxin free) 60 mg • Raw Adrenal concentrate 30 mg • Raw Pituitary concentrate 10 mg • Raw Spleen concentrate 10 mg • Kelp 300 mg. This natural product is prepared by a special process which does not exceed physiological temperature (37° C). Guaranteed to be free of chemical pesticides and synthetic hormones.

Thyroid & L-Tyrosine Complex — Enzymatic Therapy
Each capsule contains: Magnesium (Oxide) 100 mg • Manganese (Chelate) 3 mg • Zinc (Chelate) 3 mg • Copper (Chelate) 150 mcg • Iodine (Kelp) 100 mcg • Molybdenum (Chelate) 50 mcg • Vitamin B12 (Cyanocobalamin) 50 mcg • Other ingredients: L-Tyrosine 124 mg • Multi-Glandular Complex: Raw Liver, Raw Lung, Raw Pancreas, Raw Heart, Raw Kidney, Raw Spleen, & Raw Brain 35 mg • Thyroid Substance (thyroxin-free) 4X. Contains no sugar, salt, yeast, wheat, corn, soy, dairy products, coloring, flavoring or preservatives.

Thyroid Complex — The Vitamin Shoppe
Each capsule contains: Thiamine (Vitamin B1) 10 mg • Riboflavin (Vitamin B2) 10 mg • Vitamin B6 (as pyridoxine HCl) 10 mg • Vitamin B12 (as cyanocobalamin) 25 mcg • Iodine (from kelp) 150 mcg • Magnesium (as magnesium oxide) 100 mg • Zinc (as zinc chelate) 3 mg • Selenium (as selenium chelate) 70 mcg • Copper (as copper chelate) 150 mcg • Manganese (as manganese chelate) 3 mg • Molybdenum (as molybdenum chelate) 150 mcg • L-Tyrosine 150 mg • Multi Gland Complex (from bovine liver, lung, pancreas, heart, kidney, spleen, brain) 35 mg. No yeast, corn, wheat, sugar, salt, starch, milk, gluten, eggs, fish, citrus, preservatives, artificial colors or flavors added.

Thyroid Support Formula — PhysioLogics
Each capsule contains: Riboflavin 20 mg • Niacin (as Niacinamide) 20 mg • Vitamin B6 (as Pyridoxine Hydrochloride) 1 mg • Iodine (from Kelp) 110 mcg • Zinc (as Zinc Gluconate) 5 mg • Copper (as Copper Glycinate) 300 mcg • Chromium (as Chromium Chelavite) 80 mcg • L-Tyrosine 300 mg • Coleus Forskohlii leaf (18% Forskolin, 9 mg) 50 mg.

Thyrosine Complex — Phytopharmica
Each capsule contains: Magnesium (Oxide) 100 mg • Manganese (Chelate) 3 mg • Zinc (Chelate) 3 mg • Copper (Chelate) 150 mcg • Iodine (Kelp) 100 mcg • Molybdenum (Chelate) 50 mcg • Vitamin B12 (Cyanocobalamin) 50 mcg • Other ingredients: L-Tyrosine 124 mg • Multi-Glandular Complex 35 mg containing: Raw Liver, Raw Lung, Raw Pancreas, Raw Heart, Raw Kidney, Raw Spleen, & Raw Brain • Thyroid Substance (Thyroxin-free) 4X. Contains no sugar, salt, yeast, wheat, corn, soy, dairy products, coloring, flavoring or preservatives. All organs & glands are derived from bovine sources except raw pancreas (porcine).

ThyroStart — Silver Sage
Two capsules contain: Kelp meal 500 mg • Vitamin C 20 mg • Magnesium 20 mg • L-Tryosine 20 mg • Vitamin B3 20 mg • Vitamin B2 10 mg • Zinc 10 mg • Vitamin B5 10 mg • Horsetail grass 5 mg • Gentian root 5 mg • Blue Flag 5 mg • Nettle leaf herb 5 mg • Radish extract 4:1 5 mg • Parathyroid substance 5 mg • Thymus substance 2.5 mg • Adrenal substance 2.5 mg • Pancreas substance 2.5 mg • Vitamin B6 2 mg • Vitamin B1 1.5 mg • Manganese 1 mg • Copper 0.02 mg • Vitamin A 2000 IU • Beta Carotene 2000 IU • Vitamin E 50 IU • Biotin 50 mcg • Folic Acid 50 mcg • Vitamin B12 10 mcg • Selenium 10 mcg • Molybdenum 10 mcg.

Tiger Vites — Body Wise International, Inc.
Beta Carotene (Dunaliella Salina Algae) (Equivalent to Vitamin A 5000 IU) 3 mg • Vitamin D3 (Cholecalciferol) 200 IU • Vitamin E (d-Alpha Tocopherol Acid Succinate and Mixed Tocopherols Beta, Gamma and Delta) 30 IU • Vitamin C 60 mg • Folic Acid 400 mcg • Vitamin B1 1.5 mg • Vitamin B2 1.7 mg • Vitamin B6 2 mg • Niacin (Niacinamide) 20 mg • Vitamin B12 6 mcg • Pantothenic Acid (d-Calcium Pantothenate) 5 mg • Biotin 150 mcg • Choline (Choline Bitartrate) 10 mcg • Inositol 10 mcg • Calcium (Krebs Cycle Chelate) 50 mg • Magnesium 40 mg • Copper 1 mg • Zinc 7.5 mg • Molybdenum 37.5 mcg • Iodine (Kelp) 75 mcg • Chromium 120 mcg • Selenium (L-Selenomethionine) 17.5 mcg • Manganese 0.5 mg • Potassium 0.5 mg • Iron 1.8 mg • PhytoNutrient Garden Blend* 25 mg • PhytoNutrient Orchard Blend* 25 mg • Pineapple 12.5 mg • Papaya 12.5 mg • Citrus Bioflavonoids 12.5 mg., *Blend of Broccoli, Bussels Sprout, Cabbage, Carrot, Cauliflower, Kale, Onion, Tomato, Acidophilus, Apple, Pectin, Bromelain, Cellulase, Cranberry, Date, Grape Seed extract, Grape Skin extract, Orange, Peach.

Tigra Pill — Universal Products, Performance Industries
Each tablet contains: Hydrolyzed protein rich in Arginine • D-Alpha-Tocopherol • Aromatic plant extract (Diamiana aphrodisiaca, Dioscorea villosa, Panax Ginseng, Smilax officinalis) • Choline sulfate • Vitamin B3 • Vitamin B1 • Zinc sulfate • Grape Seed extract • Essential oils of Peppermint • Savory • Clove • Magnesium stearate • Carboxymethylcellulosis • Magnesium silicate.

Time Fighters For Men — Changes - TwinLab
Four caplets contain: Vitamin A (as Beta-Carotene and mixed carotenoids from D. salina algae) 25000 IU • Vitamin C (as Ascorbic Acid) 500 mg • Vitamin D (as Cholecalciferol) 400 IU • Vitamin E (as Dl-Alpha-Tocopheryl and D-Alpha Tocopheryl Succinate) 200 IU • Vitamin B1 (as Thiamin HCl) 50 mg • Vitamin B2 (as Riboflavin) 50 mg • Niacin (as Niacinamide) 125 mg • Vitamin B6 (as Pyridoxine HCl) 50 mg • Folate (as Folic Acid) 800 mcg • Vitamin B12 (as Cyanocobalamin) 500 mcg • Biotin 300 mcg • Pantothenic acid (as D-Calcium Pantothenate) 50 mg • Calcium (as Calcium Carbonate and Citrate) 400 mg • Iodine (as Potassium Iodide) 150 mcg • Magnesium (as Magnesium Oxide and Aspartate) 500 mg • Zinc (as Zinc Citrate and Picolinate) 50 mg • Selenium (as Selenomethionine) 200 mcg • Copper (as Copper Gluconate) 2 mg • Manganese (as Manganese Gluconate) 2 mg • Chromium (as Chromium Dinicotinate Glycinate) 200 mcg • Molybdenum (as Sodium Molybdate) 150 mcg • Potassium (as Potassium Citrate and Chloride) 10 mg • Life Enhancement Men's Herbal Blend 360 mg: Soybean phytosterol complex (120 mg Beta-Sitosterol), Saw Palmetto berry 4:1 extract, Panax Ginseng extract (4% ginsenosides) • Marigold flower concentrate (2% Lutein) 50 mg • Tomato fruit concentrate (2% Lycopene) 50 mg • Choline Bitartrate 25 mg • Inositol 25 mg • PABA 10 mg • Whole Food Phytonutrient Concentrates 500 mg: Parsley, Dunaliela salina algae, Kale, Spinach, Cantoloupe, Carrot, Papaya, Red Peppers, Tomato, Yellow Squash, Turmeric, Cranberry, Tangerine, Grapefruit, Lemon, Orange, Pineapple, Leek, Onion, Garlic, Raspberry, Green Tea, Alfalfa, Soybean, Cherry, Peach, Pear, Red Grape, Strawberry, Asparagus, Broccoli, Bruessels Sprout, Cabbage, Cauliflower, Mustard Greens. Other Ingredients: Microcrystaline Cellulose, Croscarmellose Sodium, Stearic Acid, Silica, Caramel color, Magnesium Stearate, Vanillin, Pharmaceutical Glaze.

Time Fighters For Women With Iron — Changes - TwinLab
Four caplets contain: Vitamin A (as Beta-Carotene and mixed caotenoids from D. salina algae) 25000 IU • Vitamin C (as Ascorbic Acid) 500 mg • Vitamin D (as Cholecalciferol) 800 IU • Vitamin E (as Dl-Alpha-Tocopheryl Acetate and D-Alpha Tocopheryl Succinate) 200 IU • Thiamin (as Thiamin HCl) 25 mg • Riboflavin 25 mg • Niacin (as Niacinamide) 100 mg • Vitamin B6 (as Pyridoxine HCl) 25 mg • Folate (as Folic Acid) 800 mcg • Vitamin B12 (as Cyanocobalamin) 250 mcg • Biotin 300 mcg • Pantothenic Acid (as D-Calcium Pantothenate) 50 mg • Calcium (as Calcium Carbonate

© Copyright 2000, Natural Medicines Comprehensive Database (209) 472-2244. For updated data, go to www.NaturalDatabase.com. • 1409

BRAND NAMES

**B
R
A
N
D

N
A
M
E
S**

and Citrate) 500 mg • Iron (as Ferrous Fumarate) 18 mg • Iodine (as Potassium Iodide) 150 mcg • Magnesium (as Magnesium Oxide and Aspartate) 400 mg • Zinc (as Zinc Citrate and Picolinate) 30 mg • Selenium (as Selenomethionine) 200 mcg • Copper (as Copper Gluconate) 2 mg • Manganese (as Manganese Gluconate) 2 mg • Chromium (as Chromium Dinicotinate Glycinate) 200 mcg • Molybdenum (as Sodium Molybdate) 150 mcg • Potassium (as Potassium Citrate and Chloride) 10 mg • Boron (from Boron Citrate) 3 mg • Marigold flower concentrate (2% Lutein) 50 mg • Tomato fruit concentrate (2% Lycopene) 50 mg • Choline Bitartrate 25 mg • Inositol 25 mg • PABA 10 mg • Life Enhancement Women's Herbal Blend 200 mg : Panax Ginseng root extract, Black Cohosh root, Chaste Tree fruit • Whole Food Phytonutrient Concentrates 500 mg: Parsley, Dunaliela Salina Algae, Kale, Spinach, Cantaloupe, Carrot, Papaya, Tomato, Yellow Squash, Turmeric rhizome, Tangerine, Grapefruit, Lemon, Orange, Red Pepper, Alfalfa, Soybean, Cranberry, Green Tea, Raspberry, Cherry, Peach, Pear, Pineapple, Red Grape, Strawberry, Asparagus spear, Brussel sprouts, Garlic, Leek, Onion, Broccoli, Cauliflower, Mustard Greens, Cabbage. Other ingredients: Microcrystalline Cellulose, Croscarmellose Sodium, Stearic Acid, Silica, Magnesium Stearate, Vanillin, and Pharmaceutical Glaze.

Time Fighters For Women Without Iron — Changes - TwinLab
Four caplets contain: Vitamin A (as Beta-Carotene and mixed caotenoids from D. salina algae) 25000 IU • Vitamin C (as Ascorbic Acid) 500 mg • Vitamin D (as Cholecalciferol) 800 IU • Vitamin E (as Dl-Alpha-Tocopheryl Acetate and D-Alpha Tocopheryl Succinate) 200 IU • Thiamin (as Thiamin HCI) 25 mg • Riboflavin 25 mg • Niacin (as Niacinamide) 100 mg • Vitamin B6 (as Pyridoxine HCI) 25 mg • Folate (as Folic Acid) 800 mcg • Vitamin B12 (as Cyanocobalamin) 250 mcg • Biotin 300 mcg • Pantothenic Acid (as D-Calcium Pantothenate) 50 mg • Calcium (as Calcium Carbonate and Citrate) 500 mg • Iodine (as Potassium Iodide) 150 mcg • Magnesium (as Magnesium Oxide and Aspartate) 400 mg • Zinc (as Zinc Citrate and Picolinate) 30 mg • Selenium (as Selenomethionine) 200 mcg • Copper (as Copper Gluconate) 2 mg • Manganese (as Manganese Gluconate) 2 mg • Chromium (as Chromium Dinicotinate Glycinate) 200 mcg • Molybdenum (as Sodium Molybdate) 150 mcg • Potassium (as Potassium Citrate and Chloride) 10 mg • Boron (from Boron Citrate) 3 mg • Marigold flower concentrate (2% Lutein) 50 mg • Tomato fruit concentrate (2% Lycopene) 50 mg • Choline Bitartrate 25 mg • Inositol 25 mg • PABA 10 mg • Life Enhancement Women's Herbal Blend 200 mg : Panax Ginseng root extract, Black Cohosh root, Chaste Tree fruit • Whole Food Phytonutrient Concentrates 500 mg: Parsley, Dunaliela Salina Algae, Kale, Spinach, Cantaloupe, Carrot, Papaya, Tomato, Yellow Squash, Turmeric rhizome, Tangerine, Grapefruit, Lemon, Orange, Red Pepper, Alfalfa, Soybean, Cranberry, Green Tea, Raspberry, Cherry, Peach, Pear, Pineapple, Red Grape, Strawberry, Asparagus spear, Brussel sprouts, Garlic, Leek, Onion, Broccoli, Cauliflower, Mustard Greens, Cabbage. Other ingredients: Microcrystalline Cellulose, Croscarmellose Sodium, Stearic Acid, Silica, Magnesium Stearate, Vanillin, and Pharmaceutical Glaze.

T-ING — Dial Herbs
Valerian root • Chamomile • Lobelia • Arnica • Cayenne.

Titan Extra — Happy Families
Each capsule contains: 50 mg of standardized 33:1 Velvet extract (Equivalent to 165 mg of pure Deer Velvet).

T-JAUN — Dial Herbs
Barberry • Chamomile • Dandelion • Horehound • St. John's Wort • Tansy • Wood Betony • Yellow Dock.

T-KB — Dial Herbs
Peach bark • Marshmallow • Buchu Leaves • Corn Silk • Echinacea.

T-LB — Dial Herbs
Barberry • Cascara Sagrada • Licorice root • Senna Leaves • Red Raspberry • Lobelia • Cayenne.

T-LS — Dial Herbs
Prickly Ash • Sarsaparilla • Poke root • Stillingia • Red Clover • Burdock • Barberry • Peach bark • Licorice root • Chaparral • Echinacea • Cayenne.

T-MEM — Dial Herbs
Lady Slipper • Rosemary • Gotu Kola • Borage • Siberian Ginseng • Licorice • Lobelia.

TMG Plus — Progressive Labs
Each tablet contains: Trimethylglycine (anhydrous) 500 mg • Vitamin B6 (pyridoxine HCl) 37.5 mg • Vitamin B6 (pyridoxine-5'-phosphate) 7.5 mg • Folate (folic acid) 450 mcg • Vitamin B12 375 mcg • Selenium (from seleno-L-methionine) 7.5 mcg.

T-MISS — Dial Herbs
Wild Yam • Ginger • Red Raspberry • Catnip • False Unicorn • Squaw vine.

T-MSLE — Dial Herbs
Cleavers • Pleurisy root • Saffron • Valerian root • Yarrow • Bistort • Catnip • Cayenne • Lobelia.

T-MUSCL — Dial Herbs
Sarsaparilla • Saw Palmetto • Strawberry.

T-NAUS — Dial Herbs
Catnip • Peppermint • Cinnamon • Ginger • Alfalfa • Lobelia.

T-NRV — Dial Herbs
Black Cohosh • Blue Cohosh • Blue Vervain • Scullcap • Lobelia.

T-NSU — Dial Herbs
Cranesbill • Goldenseal • Marshmallow • Poke root • Echinacea.

Tocotrien-All — Natrol
One softgel contains: Tocotrienol Complex 50 mg containing alpha-tocopherols 30 IU • gamma-tocotrienols 45 mg • alpha-tocotrienols 4 mg • delta-tocotrienols 1 mg. Other ingredients: Gelatin, Nutriene (Rice oil).

Tocotrienols plus E-100 I.U. — The Vitamin Shoppe
Each softgel contains: Vitamin E (as d-alpha, d-gamma, d-beta, d-delta tocopherols) 100 IU • Tocotrienols (NuTriene) (as d-alpha, d-gamma, d-beta, d-delta tocopherols) 35 mg.

Tomentosin Plus — Atrium
Each capsule contains: Uncaris tomentosa 400 mg • Bromelain 100 mg • Salix alba 50 mg • Curcuma longa 40 mg.

Tonalin CLA 1000 Mg — Natrol
One softgel contains: Tonalin supplies 60-70% Conjugated Linoleic Acid from Sunflower oil 1000 mg. Other ingredients: Lecithin, Beeswax, Soybean oil, Gelatin.

Tonalin CLA 750 Mg — Natrol
One softgel contains: Tonalin supplies 60-70% Conjugated Linoleic Acid from Sunflower oil 750 mg • Chromium (Picolinate) 75 mcg • ThermoActives Capsicum (200 SCU) 100 mcg • Ginger root 100 mg. Other ingredients: Lecithin, Beeswax, Soybean oil, Gelatin.

Tonalin CLA for Men — Natrol
One capsule contains: Chromium (as Chromium Picolinate) 50 mcg • Sunflower oil 75 mg • CLA • Conjugated Linoleic Acid 150 mg • Alpha Lipoic Acid 8 mg • Vanadyl Sulfate 2 mg • Siberian Ginseng extract root 50 mg • Leucine (as L-Leucine Hydrochloride) 50 mg • Arginine (as L-Arginine Hydrochloride) 50 mg • Isoleucine (as L-Isoleucine Hydrochloride) 12 mg • Valine (as L-Valine Hydrochloride) 25 mg. Other ingredients: Silicon Dioxide, Magnesium Stearate, Gelatin.

Tone 'N' Trim — Optimum Nutrition
Citrimax(tm) • L-Carnitine • Chromium Picolinate

Tot Tonic — The Herbalist
Echinacea root • Golden Seal root • Lemon Balm herb • Yarrow flower • Yerba Santa leaf.

Total Immune — Allergy Research Group
Each serving scoop (20 g) provides: Co-Enzyme Q10 75 mg • Grape seed extract (95%) 250 mg • Alpha Carotene 5 mg • Beta Carotene (from mixed carotenoids) 7500 IU • Lycopene 1.5 mg • Vitamin E (mixed tocopherols) 200 IU • Vitamin C 1175 mg • Folic Acid 400 mcg • Vitamin A 2500 IU • Vitamin B1 23 mg • Vitamin B2 23 mg • Vitamin B3 (niacinamide) 150 mg • Vitamin B3 (niacin) 10 mg • Vitamin B5 150 mg • Vitamin B6 25 mg • Vitamin B12 200 mcg • Biotin 200 mcg • Inositol hexaphosphate 175 mg • Choline 63 mg • Germanium Sesquioxide 50 mg • N-Acetyl Cysteine 375 mg • Glutathione 175 mg • L-Carnitine 100 mg • Calcium (carbonate, glycinate) 50 mg • Magnesium (carbonate, glycinate) 75 mg • Vitamin D3 200 IU • Zinc (arginate) 15 mg • Copper (glycinate) 1 mg • Potassium (ascorbate) 50 mg • Chromium (picolinate) 100 mcg • Molybdenum 125 mcg • Manganese 1.25 mg • Selenium 100 mcg • EPA 500 mg • Iron (aspartate) 1.5 mg • Iodine 75 mcg • MSM 100 mg

• Borage oil 150 mg • Genestein (soy isolate) 5 mg • Tocotrienol 25 mg • Biofavonoid complex 50 mg • Trimethyl Glycine 250 mg • Sulforaphane (broccoli) 50 mg • Beta Glucan (1-3) 25 mg • Green Tea extract 50 mg • Mushroom extract 1500 mg • Bromelain 163 mg • Turmuric 100 mg • Panax Ginseng 50 mg • Astragalus 50 mg • Taurine 250 mg • Lactoferrin 50 mg • All in a base of: Wheat bran, Hydrolized Whey protein, Oat bran, Rice bran, Psyllium bran, Apple fiber, Lemon flavor, Stevia, Lemon oil & Lime oil.

Total Woman Formula — Youngevity
Damiana leaf (Turnera aphrodisiaca) • Dong Quai root (Angelica sinensis) • Saw Palmetto (Serenoa repens) • Fennel seed (Foeniculum vulgare) • Oat Bran (Avena sativa) • Vilcabamba Mineral Essence: Potassium, Calcium, Magnesium, Zinc, Chromium, Selenium, Iron, Copper, Molybdenum, Vanadium, Iodine, Cobalt, Manganese.

Toxoid OTC's Toxoid First Aid — HealthWatchers System
Zincboracyl crystals • Menthol • Denatured Ethyl Alcohol 60%.

Toxoid OTC's Toxoid Pain — HealthWatchers System
Zincboracyl crystals • Menthol • Camphor • Fang Fang Extract • Dong Quai Extract • Ling Man Zhin • Qin Jiu Extract.

Toxoid OTC's Toxoid Relief — HealthWatchers System
Trace Minerals • Zincboracyl crystals • Red Cabbage Extract • Aluminum Acetate.

Toxoid OTC's Toxoid Skin — HealthWatchers System
Salicylic Acid • Zincoracyl crystals • Purified Water.

T-PARA — Dial Herbs
Wormwood • Black Walnut • Senna • Wild Carrot.

T-PEP — Dial Herbs
Gotu Kola • Kelp • Alfalfa • Dandelion • Brigham Tea • Hydrangea • Saffron • Parsley.

T-PERSP — Dial Herbs
Pennyroyal • Cayenne • Catnip • Ginger • Chamomile • Mustard.

T-PNF — Dial Herbs
Wild Lettuce • Valerian • Scullcap • Blue Vervain • Arnica • Lobelia • Cayenne.

T-PR — Dial Herbs
Strawberry • Sassafras • Sarsaparilla • Echinacea • Garlic.

Trace-Min Plus — Progressive Labs
Three capsules contain: Vitamin B6 (pyridoxine HCl) 50 mg • Vitamin D (cholecalciferol) 50 IU • Calcium (as calcium carbonate and calcium citrate) 300 mg • Magnesium (as magnesium oxide and magnesium gluconate) 150 mg • Zinc (as zinc gluconate) 15 mg • Manganese (as manganese gluconate) 10 mg • Potassium (as potassium gluconate) 99 mg • Glutamic Acid HCl 325 mg.

Tranquility — Nature's Plus
Each tablet contains: Valerian root 200 mg • Magnesium amino acid chelate/complex 200 mg • Calcium Caseinate, amino acid chelate/ complex 100 mg • Chamomile 50 mg. In a base of milk protein concentrate (750 mg), containing 10 mg of naturally occuring L-Tryptophan. Yeast free. Sugar & starch free.

Transfer Factor Plus — 4 Life
Two capsules contain: Zinc Monomethionine 10 mg • Transfer Factor XF (concentrated transfer factor from bovine colostrum) 300mg • Proprietary blend: ThyRx (Thymus complex containing liposterolics, thymic T factor proteins and other proteinaceous compounds), Cordyvant polysaccharide complex (Inositol hexaphate IP6, Cordyceps sinensis (whole herb containing 7% cordyceptic acid), Beta glucan from Brewers Yeast, Saacharomyces cerevisiae (whole plant), Mannans from Aloe Vera leaf, Shiitake mushroom (Lentinus edodes whole plant 5:1 extract), Maitake mushroom (Grifola frondosa whole plant with concentrated D-fraction)) 580 mg.

T-RHU — Dial Herbs
Buchu Leaves • Oregon Grape • Cayenne • Black Cohosh • Buckthorn • Burdock • Hydrangea • Lobelia • Nettle • Scullcap • Wild Yam • White Willow bark • Yellow Dock • Arnica.

Tri-40 — Progressive Labs
Each capsule contains: Iodine (from kelp) 150 mcg • Thyroid concentrate (thyroxin free) 40 mg • Spleen concentrate 40 mg • Thymus concentrate 40 mg • Pacific Sea Kelp 100 mg. The glandular concentrate in this product is prepared by a special process which does not exceed physiological temperature (37º C). Guaranteed free of chemical pesticides and synthetic hormones.

TRIAX — Syn Trax
Each capsule contains: Tiratricol 1 mg. Other ingredients: Barley flour, gelatin, titanium dioxide, red #40, blue #1.

TRIBEST — New Hope Health Products
Each capsule contains: Tribulus terrestris (containing Furostanol and Protodioscin) 750 mg.

Tribestan — Sopharma
Each tablet contains: Tribestan from Tribulus Terrestris herb.

Tribestrone II — ASN
Each tablet contains: Tribulus Terrestris L. extract 450 mg • Ashwaganda extract 100 mg • Mucuna extract 100 mg • Bioperine standardized extract 1.5 mg.

Tribulus — The Vitamin Shoppe
Each caplet contains: Tribulus terrestris (fruit) standardized to 20% saponins 625 mg. No yeast, corn, wheat, sugar, salt, starch, milk, gluten, soy, eggs, dairy, fish, citrus, preservatives, artificial colors or flavors added.

Tribulus Fuel — TwinLab
Each capsule contains: Tribulus Terrestris extract (standardized for 20-29% steroidal saponins) 625 mg.

Tribulus Fuel Stack — TwinLab
Two capsules contain: Tribulus Terrestris extract 1250 mg • DHEA (dehydroepiandrosterone) 50 mg.

Trilean — VitaStore
Guarana (Paullinia Cupana) • Glutamine • Fennel • Choline • Spirulina • Hawthorne • Inositol • Bladderwrack • Vitamin A • Vitamin C • Vitamin D • Vitamin E • Vitamin B1 • Vitamin B2 • Vitamin B6 • Vitamin B12 • Folic Acid • Niacin • d-Biotin • Pantothenic Acid • Potassium • Calcium.

Trim Fit — Quest
Six caplets contain: Advantra-Z (Citrus aurantium) (Standardized to 4% Synephrine) 1050 mg • Green Tea extract (Camellia sinesis) (P.E. 1:6) 1050 mg • Tonalin (source of conjugated Linoleic Acid) 900 mg • Kelp (Fucus vesiculosus) 300 mg • St. John's Wort extract (Hypericum perforatum) (P.E. 1:5, Standardized to 0.3% Hypericin) 150 mg • Trim-zyme enzyme blend (Protease, Lipase, Amylase, Cellulase) 150 mg • Lipoic Acid 30 mg. Other Ingredients: Silicon Dioxide, Magnesium Stearate (vegetable source).

Trimax — Enzymatic Therapy
Each capsule contains: St. John's Wort extract (Hypericum perforatum) standardized to contain 0.15% Hypericins, verified by HPLC 500 mg • Valerian extract (Valeriana officinalis) standardized to contain a minimum of 0.8%, 15 mg • Passionflower extract (Passiflora) 15 mg. Contains no sugar, salt, yeast, wheat, corn, soy, dairy products, coloring, flavoring, or preservatives.

Trim-Plex — Nature's Plus
Three softgels contain: Lecithin (Soya) 600 mg • Kelp 300 mg • Apple Cider Vinegar 240 mg • Vitamin B6 (Pyridoxine HCL) 50 mg. In a natural blend of Vegetable (soy) oil & Chlorophyll. Sugar & starch free.

Trinovin — Novogen
Each tablet contains: Natural Isoflavones 40mg. Trinovin is made from red clover, which contains isoflavones (genistein, biochanin, daidzein, formononetin) with a high biochanin content. Other Ingredients: Dicalcium phosphate, Microcrystalline cellulose, Hydroxypropyl methylcellulose, Magnesium stearate, Mixed tocopherols, Silica, Soy polysaccharide, & Natural caramel color.

Trioxalon 500 — AST Sports Science
Each capsule contains: Tribulus Terrestris extract 500 mg.

Triple Stack — Crystal Springs
Each tablet contains: Tribulis 250 mg • DHEA 50 mg • Androstenendione 50 mg • Saw Palmetto 200mg • Pygeum 100 mg.

Triple Whey Fuel — TwinLab
Blend of three key Whey Proteins: Micro-Filtered & Ion-Exchange Whey Protein Isolate (with ~57% Beta-Lactoglobulin, ~24% Alpha-Lactalbumin, ~12% Immunoglobulins, ~7% Minor Peptones & Lactoferrin) • modified molecular weight & partially predigested (hydrolyzed) Whey Protein (providing di-, tri-, oligo- & poly-

Some Brand Name Natural Products - What they Contain
www.NaturalDatabase.com contains MANY more listings than appear here.

B
R
A
N
D

N
A
M
E
S

peptides) • Whey Protein Concentrate enriched with Glutamine. Contains no added sugar, is low in lactose & contains 20 g of whey protein per serving.

Tropical Noni — NutraMed
Morinda citrifolia.

Trym Tone 1200 — Futurebiotics
Four tablets contain: L-Arginine HCl 2100 mg • L-Glycine 1800 mg • L-Lysine HCl 300 mg • Vitamin C 30 mg • Pyridoxine HCl 15 mg • Chromium (polynicotinate) 75 mcg.

T-SEPT — Dial Herbs
Bayberry • Goldenseal • Myrrh • Mineral Water.

T-SHK — Dial Herbs
Lobelia • Cayenne • Mineral Water.

T-SKT — Dial Herbs
Myrrh • White Poplar bark • Balsam.

T-SLC — Dial Herbs
Comfrey • Mullein • Peppermint • Chickweed • Lobelia • Cayenne.

T-SS — Dial Herbs
Damiana • Licorice • Ginseng • Passion flower • Cayenne.

T-THD — Dial Herbs
Kelp • Parsley • Irish Moss • Cayenne • Licorice • Dulse • Bayberry • Bugleweed.

T-ULC — Dial Herbs
Goldenseal • Cayenne • Myrrh • Ginger • Comfrey • Poke root • Yellow Dock.

Tulsi-Neem (soap) — Auromere Ayurvedic Soaps
Coconut oil • Palmyra oil • Rice Bran oil • Alkali • Water • Neem oil • Hydnocarpus (cactus) oil • Castor Oil • Tulsi (Holy Basil) • Rose Petals • Zedoary • Turmeric • Fenugreek • Psoralea corlifolia (Babchi Seed) • Peepal (Bodhi Tree) • Alangium salviifolium • Costus • Indian Sarsaparilla • Shiva Neem (variety of Neem) • Hibiscus.

Tum-Ease — The Herbalist
Catnip leaf • Fennel seed • Angelica root • Gentian root • Oregon Grape root • Ginger root.

T-VV — Dial Herbs
Oat Straw • Buckthorn • Yarrow • Brigham Tea • Witch Hazel • St. John's Wort • Cayenne.

T-WRT — Dial Herbs
Garlic • Celandine • Mullein • Buckthorn.

Ty-Glute — Atrium
Each tablet contains: L-Glutamine 255 mg • L-Tyrosine 155 mg • Vitamin C 150 mg • Adrenal concentrate 45 mg.

T-YI — Dial Herbs
Echinacea • Goldenseal • Bayberry • Myrrh • Plantain • Slippery Elm • Wild Carrot.

Udo's Choice Beyond Greens — Flora
One tablespoon (8 g) contains: Udo's Choice perfected seed blend: (Certified Organic Flax seed & Defatted Flax, Certified Organic Sunflower seed & Defatted Sunflower seed, Certified Organic Sesame seed & Defatted Sesame seed, Rice germ & Bran powder, Oat germ & Bran powder) • Pines Barley Grass powder • Cracked Golden Flax seed • Pumpkin seed • Pines Alfalfa Grass powder • Rice bran • Dried Cane juice • Carrot • Soyforce Sprouted Soybeans • Tomato • Pines Oat Grass • Pines Rye Grass • Red Beet • Cinnamon • Peppermint • Ginger • Bilberry leaf • Spirulina • Bee pollen • Dulse • Chlorella • Broccoli • Parsley • Kelp • Hawthorne berry • Milk Thistle • Burdock root • Red Clover • Kale • Licorice root • Chrysanthemum • Yucca • Natural Almond flavor • Lemon Grass • Udo's Choice Digestive Enzyme blend: (Protease, Lipase, Amylase, Cellulase, Maltase, Glucoamylase, Invertase, Pectinase, with Phytase, Lactase) • Beet juice • American Ginseng • Ginkgo extract • Psyllium • Slippery Elm • Stevia leaf • Artichoke • Dandeloin root • Dandelion leaf • Rosemary • Thyme • Sage • Standardized Grape seed extract.

Udo's Choice Fast Food Blend — Flora
Certified Organic Flax • Sunflower & Sesame seeds • Pines Organic Cereal Grasses • Soyforce Powdered Sprouted Soybeans & much more.

Udo's Choice Oil Blend — Flora
Flax oil • Sunflower oil • Sesame oil • Medium Chain Triglycerides • Evening Primrose oil (12.6 mg GLA per tablespoon) • Rice germ & Bran oil • Soy Lecithin • d-Alpha Tocopheral (natural Vitamin E) • Oat germ & Bran oil. One table spoon LIQUID FORM contains: Calories 135 • Total Fat 14.5 g • Saturated Fat 1.5 g • Polyunsaturated Fat: (Omega-3 Fatty Acids 6.4 g, Omega-6 Fatty Acids 3.2 g) 10 g • Monounsaturated Fat (omega-9 fatty acids 3 g) 3 g • Medium Chain Triglycerides 231 mg. Two CAPSULES contain: Calories 20 • Total Fat 2 g • Saturated Fat .2 g • Polyunsaturated Fat : (Omega-3 Fatty Acids 920 mg, Omega-6 Fatty Acids 460 mg) 1.4 g • Monounsaturated Fat (omega-9 fatty acids 400 mg) .4g • Medium Chain Triglycerides 38 mg.

Udo's Choice Perfect Oil Blend — Flora
Flax oil • sesame seed oil • Sunflower oils & other unrefined oils • medium triglycerides • lecithin & d-alpha tocopherol.

Udo's Choice Super 5 — Flora
Each tablet contains: 1 billion plus viable organisms of Lactobacillus acidophilus DDS-1 • B. bifidum • L. bulgaricus • S. thermophilus & L. salivarius in a base of: (Maltodextrin, Fructose & Ascorbic Acid).

Ultimate Antioxidant II — Gary Null
Three capsules contain: Citrus Bioflavonoid Complex 300 mg • Rutin 25 mg • Bilberry extract 25 mg • Red Wine Concentrate 25 mg • Grape Skin extract 200 mg • China Green Tea 200 mg • Beta Carotene 10000 IU • L-Glutathione 5 mg • L-Cysteine 200 mg • Vitamin C 500 mg • Vitamin E 200 IU • Selenium 10 mcg • Zinc Picolinate 25 mg • CoQ10 10 mg • NAC 25 mg • Alpha Lipoic Acid 100 mg • Ascorbyl Palmitate 100 mg • SOD 25 mg • Vitamin B6 10 mg • Copper Lysinate 2 mg • Taurine 50 mg • Quercetin 50 mg • Pycnogenol 5 mg • Licorice 25 mg • Broccoli 25 mg • Lutein 25 mg • Cabbage 25 mg • Carrot powder 25 mg • Milk Thistle 25 mg.

Ultimate Athlete's Pain Formula — Biochem
Three softgel capsules contain: Boswellia serrata extract 500 mg • Omega-3 Fish oil concentrate 400 mg • Glucosamine HCL 250 mg • Glucosamine Sulfate 250 mg • Chondroitin Sulfate 200 mg • PolyNAG (N-Acetyl Glucosamine) 50 mg • Vitamin C (Ascorbyl Palmitate) 50 mg • Green-lipped Mussel extract 50 mg • CMO (Cetyl Myristoleate) 50 mg • Gamma-Lenolenic Acid (Borage seed oil) 50 mg • Vitamin E (d-Alpha Tocopheryl Acetate) 25 IU • Manganese (Sulfate) 5 mg • Boron (Borogluconate) 1.5 mg.

Ultimate Cleanse — Nature's Secret
Each tablet contains: Multi-Herb: Alfalfa Leaf • Fenugreek Seed • Ginger Root • Dandelion Root • Fennel Seed • Yarrow Flower • Hawthorne Berries • Horsetail Herb • Licorice Root • Marshmallow Root • Peppermint Leaf • Red Clover Tops • Red Raspberry Leaf • Safflower Oil • Scullcap Herb • Burdock Root • Chickweed Herb • Mullein Leaf • Papaya Leaf • Black Cohosh Root • Cayenne Fruit • Irish Moss • Pacific Kelp • Slippery Elm Bark • Yellow Dock Root • Plantain Herb • Echinacea Angustifolia Extract • Ginkgo Biloba Leaf Extract • Milk Thistle Extract. Multi-Fiber: Cascara Sagrada Bark • Fennel Seed • Psyllium Seed • Ginger Root • Acacia Gum • Alfalfa Leaf • Apple Pectin • Apple Powder • Barley Rice Fiber • Beet Root • Glucomannan • Gum Karaya • Peppermint Leaf • Lemon Peel • Oat Bran • Red Raspberry Leaf • Slippery Elm Bark • Shattered Cell Wall Chlorella • Lactobacillus Acidophilus (dairy free) • Guar Gum.

Ultimate Deer Antler Velvet — Ultimate Deer Products
Each capsule contains: Pure Deer Antler Velvet 250 mg.

Ultimate Fat Metabolizer — Biochem
Three tablets contain: Choline Bitartrate 500 mg • Inositol 500 mg • L-Carnitine 500 mg • L-Methionine 500 mg • Taurine 500 mg • Phosphatidyl Choline 200 mg • Betaine HCL 200 mg • Dandelion 100 mg • Milk Thistle 100 mg • Barberry 100 mg • Artichoke extract 50 mg • Vitamin B6 (Pyridoxine • Alpha-Ketoglutarate/Pyridoxal-5-Phosphate) 10 mg • Chromium 400 mcg.

Ultimate Fiber — Nature's Secret
Psyllium husks, Slippery Elm bark, Acidophilus powder, Fructooligosaccharides.

Ultimate Green — Nature's Secret
Each packet contain: Shattered Cell Wall Chlorella • Hawaiian Blue-Green Algae • Barley Grass • Wheat Grass • Alfalfa • Spinach.

Ultimate Libido Formula for Women — MD Healthline
Two capsules contain: Niacin 40 mg • Yohimbe Bark 500 mg • Dong Quai 150 mg • Sativari (Asparagus racemosus) 150 mg •

Ashwagandha 100 mg • L-Tyrosine 100 mg • L-Histidine 66 mg • Tree Peony 4:1 Extract 50 mg • Royal Jelly 50 mg • Wild Yam 10:1 Extract 40 mg • Quebracho Bark 20 mg • Ginger Root 5:1 Extract 20 mg • Sundew 20 mg • Guarana 20 mg • Damiana 20 mg • DHEA 10 mg.

Ultimate Multi Plus — Nature's Secret
Contains over 90 vitamins, minerals, amino acids, antioxidants, herbs, superfoods, digestive enzymes and Herbalgest.

Ultimate Oil — Nature's Secret
Blend of oils that offer a mixture of the essential fatty acids, Omega 3 and Omega 6.

Ultimate Sleep System — Rainbow Light
Two tablets contain: Valerian rhizome (standardized to 0.8% valernic acid) 160 mg • Kava Kava root(standardized to 30% kavalactones) 40 mg • Spirulina 100 mg • 4:1 Custom Herbal extracts: [Valerian rhizome, Hops strobiles, Kava Kava root, Passion flower herb, Valerian oil, Reishi fruiting body (providing 3200 mg herbal powder equivalent)] 800 mg. Nutritional Cofactors: N-Acetyl L-Carnitine (NAC) 10 mg • Niacin/Niacinamide (Vitamin B3)115 mg • Magnesium (Oxide, Pyroglutamate) 47.3 mg • Chromium (Polynicotinate) 30 mcg.

Ultimate Sports Multiple — Biochem
Four tablets contain: Vitamin A (Carotene Complex) 5000 IU • Vitamin D (Ergocalciferol) 200 IU • Vitamin E (d-Alpha Tocopheryl Succinate) 400 IU • Vitamin C (Ascorbic Acid) 1000 mg • Grape seed extract/Grape skin 100 mg • Vitamin B1 (Thiamine HCL/Thiamine Cocarboxylase) 100 mg • Vitamin B2 (Riboflavin/Riboflavin 5 Phosphate) 100 mg • Vitamin B3 (Niacin/Niacinamide) 200 mg • Vitamin B5 (d-Calcium Pantothenate/Pantethine) 200 mg • Vitamin B6 (Pyridoxine HCL/Pyridoxal 5 Phosphate) 100 mg • Folic Acid 400mcg • Vitamin B12 (Cyanocobalamine/ Didencozide) 200 mcg • d-Biotin 300 mcg • PABA 200 mcg • Selenium 100 mcg • Molybdenum 10 mcg • Choline Bitartrate 200 mg • Inositol 100 mg • Bromelain 100 mg • Betaine HCL 200 mg • L-Methionine 50 mg • Taurine 50 mg.

Ultimate Zinc-C Lozenges — Now
Each lozenge contains: Vitamin A (from Fish Liver oil) 1000 IU • Vitamin C (as Ascorbic Acid) 150 mg • Zinc (as Zinc Gluconate) 24 mg • Echinacea root powder 100 mg • Bee Propolis 100 mg • Slippery Elm bark powder (Ulmus fulva) 25 mg.

Ultra 30/20 Fish oil — Health From The Sun
Two capsules contain: Vitamin E 4 IU • Omega-3 Fatty Acids 1.2 g [EPA (600 mg) DHA (400 mg)]. Ingredients: All natural Fish Body oil concentrate, Gelatin, Glycerine, Mixed Tocopherols.

Ultra Bone Balance — Source Naturals
Four tablets contain: Vitamin C (as Calcium, Magnesium, Manganese Ascorbates) 52 mg • Vitamin D (as Cholecalciferol) 300 IU • Vitamin B6 (as Pyridoxine HCl) 20 mg • Folate (as Folic Acid) 200 mcg • Calcium (as Calcium Carbonate, Citrate, Ethanolamine Phosphate, Malate, Ascorbate) 1200 mg • Magnesium (as Magnesium Oxide, Citrate, Fumarate, Malate, Ascorbate) 600 mg • Zinc (as Zinc Chelate) 7.5 mg • Copper (as Copper Sebacate) 1 mg • Manganese (as Manganese Ascorbate) 6 mg • Ipriflavone (Ostivone) 600 mg • Genistein-Rich Soy concentrate (Yielding 50 mg total isoflavones) 125 mg • Silica (from Horsetail silica extract) 10 mg • Boron (as Boron Chelate) 3 mg.

Ultra Carotenoid Complex — The Vitamin Shoppe
Each softgel contains: Phytofluene 0.026 mg • Lycopene (LYC-O-MATO) 5 mg • Lutein 5 mg • Beta-carotene (25000 IU Vitamin A) 15 mg • Alpha-carotene (833 IU Vitamin A) 1 mg • Zeaxanthin 0.24 mg • Phytoene 0.055 mg.

Ultra Chondroitin 600 — Nature's Plus
Each protein coated tablet contains: Chondroitin Sulfate A - CSA (Glucuronic, N-Acetyl-D-Galactosamine 4-Sulfate) 600 mg • Bioperine bioavailability enhancing thermonutrient, (95% 1-piperoylpiperdine) 2.5 mg. Contains no yeast, wheat, corn, soy, milk, salt, sugar or starch.

Ultra Chroma Slim Plan with Biotrol — Richardson Labs
Three caplets contain: Manganese (as manganese picolinate) 1.25 mg • Chromium (as chromium picolinate) 200 mcg • Blood Sugar Support blend: [Manganese Picolinate, Chromium Picolinate, Vanadium (as vanadyl sulfate) 60 mcg] 10.4 mg • Lipotropic & Metabolic Support blend: (Choline Bitartrate, L-Carnitine Tartrate) 1.1 g • Appetite Control & Neurotransmitter Support blend: [Inulin, L-Phenylalanine, St. John's Wort extract leaves & flowers standardized to 0.3% hypercin, Capsicum fruit extract 10:1, Peppermint oil] 1.6 g • Energy Support blend: (Siberian Ginseng root, Calcium Pyruvate) 252 mg. Other Ingredients: Cellulose, Modified Cellulose Gum, Stearic Acid, Silica, Hydroxypropyl Methylcellulose, Magnesium Stearate, Peppermint leaves.

Ultra Chromium Picolinate — The Vitamin Shoppe
Each capsule contains: Chromium Picolinate, a compound of yeast-free trivalent chromium and picolinic acid 500 mcg.

Ultra Colloidal Silver — Olympia Nutrition
Deionized Water • Silver (10 ppm). Contains no animal proteins or artificial additives.

Ultra Cranberry 1000 — Nature's Plus
Each protein coated tablet contains: Cranberry concentrate 45X 1000 mg • Vitamin C corn free 100 mg. In a highly active herbal base of Juniper berries (Juniperus communis), Parsley (Petroselinum crispum), Uva Ursi (Arctostaphylos uva ursi) & Red Clover (Trifolium pratense). Contains no yeast, wheat, corn, soy, milk, salt, sugar or starch.

Ultra DHA 50 — Health From The Sun
Two capsules contain: Vitamin E 4 IU • Omega-3 Fatty Acids 700 mg [DHA (425 mg) EPA (200 mg)]. Ingredients: All natural Fish Body oil concentrate, Gelatin, Glycerine, Mixed Tocopherols.

Ultra Diet Pep — Natural Balance
Two tablets contain an herbal blend of Kola Nut, Ma Huang, Siberian Ginseng, Green Tea extract, Dandelion, Ginger, Passion Flower, Kelp, Gymnema Sylvestre, Pullulan and Fennel • Vitamin B6 15 mg • Vitamin B12 6 mcg • Pantothenic Acid 25 mg • Inositol 100 mg • DynaChrome Chromium 200 mcg • Bromelain 100 mg • Potassium 99 mg.

Ultra Fuel (The Ultimate Carbohydrate Energy & Recovery Drink) — TwinLab
Each 16 ounce serving contains: Carbohydrates 100 g • Carbohydrate & Energy Metabolizers (including Chromium) • Stress B Vitamins • Vitamin C. No added preservatives or sodium.

Ultra Garlite — Nature's Plus
Each tablet contains: Deodorized Garlic equivalent to a minimum of 2.5 times its weight in fresh garlic 1000 mg. In a special base which provides for the gradual release of ingredients over a prolonged period of time, for 40% better absorption & utilization. Contains no yeast, wheat, corn, soy, milk, salt, sugar or starch.

Ultra Hair — Nature's Plus
Two tablets contain: Vitamin C with Rose Hips 500 mg • Pantothenic Acid 500 mg • Inositol 500 mg • Choline (Bitartrate) 210 mg • L-Cysteine free form amino acid 100 mg • Vitamin B6 (Pyridoxine HCL) 100 mg • Vitamin B2 (Riboflavin) 100 mg • PABA (Para-aminobenzoic acid) 100 mg • Vitamin B1 (Thiamine) 30 mg • Niacinamide 30 mg • Zinc (Amino Acid Chelate) 5 mg • Vitamin A (Beta Carotene) 10000 IU • Biotin 2000 mcg • Folic Acid 400 mcg. In a natural base of unsaturated fatty acids from safflower oil, rice bran & spirulina ,naturally rich in RNA, DNA, amino acids & trace minerals. Yeast free. Sugar & starch free.

Ultra Inosine — Source Naturals
Two tablets contain: Vitamin C (Potassium and Sodium Ascorbates) 350 mg • Calcium (Carbonate) 100 mg • Vitamin B6 (Pyridoxine HCl) 10 mg • Magnesium (Oxide, Aspartate) 100 mg • Vitamin B5 (Pantothenic Acid) 50 mg • Potassium (Citrate, Ascorbate and Aspartate) 99 mg • Sodium (Ascorbate) 20 mg • Inosine (Pure Crystalline) 1000 mg • Aspartic Acid (Potassium and Magnesium Aspartates and L-Aspartic Acid) 200 mg • Branched Chain Amino Acids (BCAAs) 174 mg • (L-Leucine 100 mg, L-Isoleucine 30 mg, L-Valine 44 mg) • L-Carnitine L-Tartrate 20 mg • L-Lysine (HCl) 60 mg • Glycine 60 mg • Bee Pollen 200 mg • Octacosanol 4000 mcg • Spirulina 70 mg • Siberian Ginseng 100 mg • Tienchi Ginseng 100 mg.

Ultra Joint Response — Source Naturals
Three tablets contain: Vitamin A 5000 IU • Vitamin C 250 mg • Niacinamide 50 mg • Vitamin B6 12.5 mg • Zinc 15 mg • Selenium 100 mcg • Copper 1 mg • Manganese 10 mg • Molybdenum 130 mcg • MSM 1125 mg • Glucosamine Sulfate 900 mg • Boswellia serrata extract 321 mg • Quercetin 150 mg • Horse Chestnut extract 100 mg • Turmeric root extract 50 mg • Stinging Nettle leaf extract 50 mg •

Ashwagandha root extract 50 mg • N-Acetyl Cysteine 50 mg • Sea Cucumber 40 mg • Grape Seed extract 25 mg • Aloe Vera whole leaf concentrate 25 mg • Black Pepper fruit extract 1 mg.

Ultra Lipo-Plex — Nature's Plus
Two tablets contain: Choline Bitartrate equivalent to 1000 mg of choline 2381 mg • Inositol 1000 mg • L-Methionine free form amino acid 500 mg • Vitamin B6 (Pyridoxine HCL) 100 mg. In a natural herbal base containing Dandelion root, Fennel seed, Barberry bark, Parsley, Capsicum & Ginger. In a special base which provides for the gradual release of ingredients over a prolonged period of time, for 40% better absorption & utilization. Contains no yeast, wheat, corn, soy, milk, salt, sugar or starch.

Ultra Mega Vite Multiple — Nature's Life
Each tablet contains: Vitamin A (Fish Liver oil) 10000 IU • Vitamin D3 (Cholecalciferol) 400 IU • Vitamin E (d-Alpha Tocopherol) 200 IU • Vitamin B1 (Thiamine Mononitrate) 100 mg • Vitamin B2 100 mg • Vitamin B3 (Niacinamide) 100 mg • Vitamin B6 (Pyridoxine HCl • Pyridoxal 5'-Phosphate) 100 mg • Vitamin B12 (Cobalamin concentrate) 100 mg • Folic Acid 400 mcg • Biotin 300 mcg • Pantothenic Acid (d-Calcium Pantothenate) 100 mg • Inositol 10 mg • Choline (Bitartrate) 10 mg • PABA (Para Aminobenzoic Acid) 10 mg • Vitamin C 300 mg • Lemon Bioflavonoids (TESTLAB 50% Flavonoids) 50 mg • Rutin 25 mg • Hesperidin Complex (10% Flavonoids) 25 mg • Boron (Citrate) 25 mcg • Calcium (Carbonate, Citrate/Malate) 100 mg • Chromium (Amino-Nicotinate) 100 mcg • Copper (Gluconate, Citrate) 1 mg • Iodine (Potassium) 25 mcg • Iron (Fumerate, Peptonate) 10 mg • Magnesium (Oxide, Citrate) 60 mg • Manganese (Citrate, Gluconate) 5 mg • Molybdenum (Molybdate) 25 mcg • Potassium (Citrate) 15 mg • Selenium (Yeast) 50 mcg • Silicon (Dioxide) 10 mg • Vanadium (Sulfate) 25 mcg • Zinc (Citrate) 20 mg • Chlorophyll 5 mg • Betaine HCl 30 mg • Glutamic Acid HCl 30 mg • Nature's Life Greens 20 mg.

Ultra Nails — Nature's Plus
Two tablets contain: Calcium amino acid chelate/complex 500 mg • Gelatin 260 mg • Horsetail supplying natural silica 250 mg • Phosphorus amino acid complex 200 mg • L-Cysteine free form amino acid 100 mg • L-Methionine free form amino acid 100 mg • Vitamin B2 (Riboflavin) 50 mg • Sulphur from Sulphur containing amino acids 25 mg • Oat straw 25 mg • Magnesium amino acid chelate/complex 25 mg • Iron (Amino Acid Chelate) 5 mg • Vitamin A Fish Liver oil 10000 IU • Folic Acid 200 mcg • Vitamin B12 from Cobalamin 100 mcg • Vitamin D Fish Liver oil 400 IU. In a natural rice bran base, supplying a complete balance of B-Complex vitamins & trace minerals. Yeast free. Sugar & starch free.

Ultra Omega-3 Fish oil — Health From The Sun
Two capsules contain: Omega-3 Fatty Acids 600 mg [EPA (360) DHA (240 mg)]. Ingredients: All natural Fish Body oil, Gelatin, Glycerine, Water, Carob powder, Mixed Tocopherols (Vitamin E).

Ultra Power Nutrient — Changes - TwinLab
One packet (6g) contains: Vitamin A (as Retinyl palmitate with Lemongrass and Beta Carotene) 5000 IU • Vitamin C (as buffered mineral ascorbates) 60 mg • Vitamin D (as Cholecalciferol) 400 IU • Thiamin (Vitamin B1 as Thiamine hydrochloride) 1.5 mg • Riboflavin (Vitamin B2) 1.7 mg • Vitamin B6 (as Pyridoxine hydrochloride) 2 mg • Folate (as Folic acid) 400 mcg • Vitamin B12 (as Cyanocobalamin) 6 mcg • Biotin 300 mcg • Pantothenic acid (Vitamin B5) (as Calcium pantothenate) 10 mg • Calcium (as Calcium citrate ascorbate) 40 mg • Magnesium (as Magnesium citrate ascorbate) 20 mg • Sodium (as Sodium citrate ascorbate) 60 mg • Potassium (as Potassium citrate ascorbate) 200 mg • Sea minerals from Celtic marine algae 10 mg. Other ingredients: Crystalline fructose, Maltodextrin, Natural citrus flavors, Non-nutritive sweetener.

Ultra Prosta-Metto — The Vitamin Shoppe
Each softgel contains: Vitamin E 50 IU • Vitamin B6 5 mg • Zinc 15 mg • Saw Palmetto berries 160 mg • Pumpkin seed 40 mg • Pygeum Africanum bark 10 mg • Stinging Nettle leaf 50 mg • Lycopene 2.5 mg.

Ultra Skin — Nature's Plus
Two tablets contain: Unsaturated Fatty Acids from natural Safflower oil 500 mg • Vitamin C with Rose Hips 200 mg • Vitamin B2 (Riboflavin) 200 mg • Vitamin B6 (Pyridoxine HCL) 200 mg • Vitamin E natural 200 IU • Niacinamide 150 mg • PABA (Para-Aminobenzoic Acid) 150 mg • Pantothenic Acid 150 mg • Vitamin B1 (Thiamine) 100 mg • Zinc amino acid chelate/complex 50 mg • Vitamin A (Beta Carotene) 25000 IU • Biotin 400 mcg • Folic Acid

100 mcg • Vitamin B12 (from Cobalamin) 100 mcg • Vitamin D (Calciferol) 1000 IU. In a natural base of rice bran & spirulina (naturally rich in RNA, DNA, amino acids & trace minerals). In a special base which provides for the gradual release of ingredients over a prolonged period of time for 40% better absorption & utilization. Yeast free. Sugar & starch free.

Ultra Stress with Iron — Nature's Plus
Each tablet contains: Vitamin C with Rose Hips 500 mg • Pantothenic Acid 200 mg • Vitamin B1 (Thiamine) 125 mg • Vitamin B2 (Riboflavin) 125 mg • Vitamin B6 (Pyridoxine HCL) 125 mg • Niacinamide 125 mg • Inositol 75 mg • PABA (Para-aminobenzoic acid) 50 mg • Choline (Bitartrate) 32 mg • Iron amino acid chelate/complex 20 mg • Vitamin B12 from Cobalamin 500 mcg • Folic Acid 400 mcg • Biotin 125 mcg. B-Complex vitamins in a fortified rice bran base. In a special base which provides for the gradual release of ingredients over a prolonged period of time for 40% better absorption & utilization.

Ultra Sugar Control — Nature's Plus
Two tablets contain: CITRIMAX (Garcinia cambogia fruit) standardized 50% [-] hydroxycitrate 500 mg • Rehmannia Glutinosa root naturally rich in Beta-Sitosterol, Catalpol & Aucubin) 400 mg • L-Glutamine pharmaceutical grade free form amino acid 250 mg • L-Alanine pharmaceutical grade free form amino acid 250 mg • Gymnema Sylvestre leaf standardized 75% Gymnemic acids 200 mg • Chromium (Polynicotinate) 500 mcg. Contains no yeast, wheat, corn, soy, milk, salt, sugar or starch.

Ultra Virile-Actin — Nature's Plus
Two protein coated tablets contain: Vitamin E natural 200 IU • Korean Ginseng [(Panax ginseng root) standardized 15% Ginsenosides]100 mg • Siberian Ginseng [Eleutherococcus senticosus root) standardized 0.8% Eleutherosides] 100 mg • Bee Pollen, Spanish 75 mg • Saw Palmetto [(Serenoa repens berry) standardized 35%-45% free fatty acids] 60 mg • Brazilian Muirapuama (Phychopetalum olacoides root & rhizome) 50 mg • L-Histidine, pharmaceutical grade free form amino acid 50 mg • Zinc (Monomethionine) 50 mg • Cayenne [(Capsicum frutescens fruit) standardized 125000 STU/gram] 50 mg • L-Phenylalanine pharmaceutical grade free form amino acid 50 mg • St. John's Wort [(Hypericum perforatum flower) 0.3%-0.5% Hypericin] 50 mg • Royal Jelly 25 mg • L-Carnitine (L-Carnitine-L-Tartrate) 25 mg • Pacific Oyster extract [(Crassostreagis thunberg) naturally rich in trace elements & amino acids] 10 mg • Vitamin B6 (Pyridoxine HCL) 5 mg • Coenzyme Q10 (Ubiquinone) 2500 mcg. Contains no yeast, wheat, corn, soy, milk, salt, sugar or starch.

UltraAC — Great American Nutrition
Four capsules contain: Potassium (as potassium glycerophosphate) 112 mg • Chromium (as chromium picolinate) 200 mcg • Potassium Glycerophosphate 450 mg • DL-Phenylalanine 1000 mg • Zhi Shi fruit (Citrus aurantium, containing 10 mg synephrine from a 4% standardized extract) 250 mg • Kola Nut nut(Cola acuminata, containing 50 mg caffeine from a 10% standardized extract) 500 mg • Ginger root (Zingiber officinale) 100 mg. Other Ingredients: Rice powder, Magnesium Silicate & Magnesium Stearate.

UltraAP Activated Pyruvate — Great American Nutrition
Four capsules contain: Potassium (as potassium glycerophosphate) 125 mg • Potassium Glycerophosphate 500 mg • Caffeine (from caffeine citrate & Kola nut) 150 mg • Zhi Shi fruit (Citrus aurantium, synephrine from a 4% standardized extract 10 mg) 250 mg • Kola Nut nut (Cola acuminata) 500 mg • Siberian Ginseng root (Eleutherococcus senticosus) 200 mg • Quercetin 100 mg • Jing jie leaves(Schizonepeta divaricata, 5:1 extract) 10 mg • Fang feng leaves (Ledebouriella tenuifolia, 5:1 extract) 10 mg. Other Ingredients: Rice powder, Maltodextrin, Magnesium Silicate and Magnesium Stearate.

Ultra-Cal Night — Source Naturals
Four tablets contain: Calcium (Citrate, Carbonate, Malate, Fumarate, Ethanolamine Phosphate, and Ascorbate) 600 mg • Magnesium (Oxide, Citrate, Fumarate, Malate, and Ascorbate) 600 mg • SoyLife Genistein-Rich Soy Concentrate (Diadzein 13 mg, Glycitein 9 mg, Genistein 3 mg, total Isoflavones 25 mg) • Vitamin C (Magnesium and Calcium Ascorbates, Ascorbic Acid and Manganese Ascorbate) 285 mg • Vitamin B6 (Pyridoxine HCl) 20 mg • Vitamin D3 (Cholecalciferol) 200 IU • Folic Acid 200 mcg • L-Lysine (HCl) 60 mg • Silica (Horsetail Silica Extract) 10 mg • Zinc (Chelate) 7.5 mg • Manganese (Ascorbate) 6 mg • Boron (Amino Acid Chelate) 3 mg • Copper (Sebacate) 1 mg.

B
R
A
N
D

N
A
M
E
S

Ultra-Eyebright — Nutri-Quest
Each tablet contains: Eyebright 100 mg • Bilberry extract 6 mg • Ginkgo Biloba 6 mg • Siberian Ginseng 15 mg • Gymnema sylvestre 100 mg • Tumeric 25 mg • Quercetin 10 mg • Lemon Bioflavonoids 40 mg • Bromelain 30 mg • Pancreatin 30 mg • Papain 30 mg • Trypsin 40 mg (Chymotrypsin 8 mg) • Pancreolipase 15 mg • Amylase-Diastase 15 mg • Ox Bile 30 mg • Betaine HCL 10 mg • Rutin 50 mg • L-Glutathione 2.5 mg • L-Taurine 15 mg • N-Acetyl Cysteine 10 mg • Selenium Chelate 10 mcg • Zinc Chelate 15 mg • Chromium Aspartate 1 mg • Parotid 1 mg • Beta Carotene 1000 IU • Vitamin C 75 mg • Vitamin D 200 IU • Vitamin E (Succinate) 20 IU • Vitamin B2 20 mg • Vitamin B6 10 mg • Folic Acid 50 mcg.

Ultramet — Champion Nutrition
Each packet of Vanilla flavor contains: Peptol-EX protein 42 grams (Ion-Exchange Whey Protein Isolate, Calcium Caseinate, Milk Protein Isolate, Potassium Caseinate, Egg Albumen, Whey Protein Concentrate, Sodium Caseinate, L-Glutamine, Taurine, Calcium Alpha-Ketoglutarate & L-Arginine) • Carbohydrates 24 g (1.5 g Fiber) • Fat 2 g • Calories 280. Each packet of Chocolate flavor contains: Protein 41 g • Carbohydrates 23 g (3 g Fiber) • Fat 3 g • Calories 280 g. Vanilla Ingredients: Peptol-EX (New-Age Protein Amino Acid Blend consisting of high quality pure Ion-Exchange Whey Protein Isolate, Calcium Caseinate, Milk Protein Isolate, Potassium Caseinate, Egg Albumen, Whey Protein Concentrate, Sodium Caseinate, L-Glutamine, Taurine & Calcium Alpha-Ketoglutarate) • Maltodextrin • Corn Syrup Solids • Natural & Artificial Flavoring • Vitamin-Mineral Core • Partially Hydrogenated Canola oil • Soy Lecithin • Salt • Cellulose Gum • Aspartame • Xanthan Gum • Citrimax (Garcinia cambogia extract) • Medium-Chain Triglycerides • Carrageenan • Borage oil • Mono & Diglycerides. Phenylketonurics: contains Phenylalanine.

Ultra-Zyme — Nature's Plus
Two tablets contain: Pancreatin 4X quadruple strength 325 mg, supplying: Amylase 32500 USP Units, Protease (Trypsin & Chymotrypsin) 32500 USP Units, Lipase (Pancreatic lipase) 2600 USP Units • Glutamic Acid HCL 200 mg • Acidophilus (Lactobacillus, Bulgaricus, Bifidus) 150 mg • Ox Bile 120 mg • Bromelain, 1:10, pineapple, 100 mg • Pepsin NF 1:15000 65 mg • Malt Diastase 65 mg • Cellulase • Hemicellulase • 5 mg • Lactase 5 mg. In a natural herbal base of Peppermint, Fennel seed, Ginger & Rosemary. Contains no yeast, wheat, corn, soy, milk, salt, sugar or starch.

Una De Gato-Go! Cat's Claw Extract — Wakunaga of America
Each capsule contains: Cat's Claw standardized extract (Una De Gato)(bark) 250 mg. Other Ingredients: Cellulose, Collodial Silica, Magnesium Stearate (vegetable source).

UnDo — Lindsey Duncan's Home Nutrition
Blended Fiber Formula: Each tablet contains: Proprietary blend 495 mg: Fiber blend: (Apple pectin, Beet fiber, Barley fiber, Psyllium husk, Karaya Gum, Oat Bran) • Fennel seed • Buckthorn bark • Cascara Sagrada bark • Kava Kava root • Red Raspberry leaf • Ginger root • Capsicum Fruit. Blended Herb Formula: Each tablet contains: Proprietary blend 368 mg: Panax Ginseng root • Ginkgo Biloba leaf extract (50:1) • Garlic bulb • Milk Thistle extract (80% Silymarin) • Echinacea Angustifolia leaf extract (6:1) • Cat's Claw bark • Uva Ursi leaf • Alfalfa leaf • Hawthorn berries • Licorice root • Ginger root • Rosemary leaf • Oregon Grape root • Turmeric root • Dandelion leaf • Burdock root • Yellow Dock root • Mullein leaf • Fenugreek seed • Horsetail herb • Safflower flower • Butchers Broom root • Red root • Capsicum fruit • Schizandra fruit.

Upper Di-GST — Nutri-Quest
Each tablet contains: L-Glutamine 50 mg • Okra 25 mg • Stomach 125 mg • Folic Acid 250 mcg • Vitamin A 1500 IU • Parotid 10 mg • Aloe Vera 5 mg • N-Acetyl Glucosamine 50 mg • Bromelaine 25 mg • Duodenum 125 mg • Deglycerrized Licorice root 156 mg • Cabigen extract (Vitamin U) 20 mg • Slippery Elm 25 mg • Magnesium Chelate 75 mg.

Urban Air Defense — Source Naturals
Two tablets contain: Vitamin A (Beta Carotene 12500 IU and Palmitate 5000 IU) 17500 IU • Vitamin C (Magnesium Ascorbate, Vitamin C and Manganese Ascorbate) 500 mg • Fat-Soluble Vitamin C (from 186 mg of Ascorbyl Palmitate) 80 mg • Vitamin E D-Alpha Tocopheryl (Natural) 200 IU • Magnesium (Ascorbate) 30 mg • Zinc (OptiZinc Monomethionine) 15 mg • Manganese (Ascorbate) 5 mg • Copper (Sebacate) 750 mcg • Selenium (as L-Selenomethionine) 100 mcg • Quercetin 200 mg • N-Acetyl Cysteine 100 mg • Silymarin (Milk Thistle seed extract) 50 mg • Ginkgo Biloba extract 24% (50:1) 5 mg • Hawthorn berry 150 mg • Rosemary 150 mg • Schizandra 125 mg • Marshmallow root 85 mg • Astragalus 60 mg.

Urinary Formula — Nature's Way
Three capsules contain: Cleavers herb 180 mg • Corn Silk 150 mg • Cranberry concentrate fruit 600 mg • Dandelion leaf 180 mg • Goldenseal stem, leaf, flower 60 mg • Marshmallow root 180 mg. Other ingredients: Gelatin, Magnesium Stearate, Millet.

Urinary Support — Amazon Support
Each capsule contains: Chanca Piedra • Boldo • Cipo Cabeludo • Anamu • Jatoba • Brazilian Peppertree • Cha de Bugre.

Uriphron — Phytopharmica
Each tablet contains: Goldenrod extract 5.9:1 (Solidago virgaurea) 136 mg • Birch leaf extract 5.5:1 (Betula pendula) 109 mg • Orthosiphon leaf extract 6.2:1 (O. aristata) 97 mg. Contains no sugar, salt, yeast, wheat, gluten, corn, soy, dairy products, coloring, flavoring, or preservatives.

Uriplex — Enzymatic Therapy
Each tablet contains: Goldenrod extract 5.9:1 (Solidago virgaurea) 136 mg • Birch Leaf extract 5.5:1 (Betula pendula) 109 mg • Orthosiphon Leaf extract 6.2:1 (O. aristata) 97 mg. Contains no sugar, salt, yeast, wheat, gluten, corn, soy, dairy products, coloring, flavoring, or preservatives.

Usnea-Propolis Virtue — Blessed Herbs
Usnea lichen • Pau d'Arco bark • Echinacea Angustifolia root • Propolis • Goldenseal root • Myrrh Gum • Grain alcohol & Distilled Water.

Uva Ursi Formula — Quest
Each caplet contains: Uva Ursi leaf powder (Arctostaphylos uva-ursi) 85 mg • Dandelion root powder (Taraxacum officinale) 60 mg • Gentian root powder (Gentiana lutea) 55 mg • Huckleberry leaf powder (Vaccinium Myrtillus) 55 mg • Parsley leaf powder (Petroselinum crispum) 45 mg • Buchu leaf powder (Barosma betulina) 35 mg • Kelp powder (Fucus vesiculosis) 35 mg • Raspberry leaf powder (Rubus idaeus) 35 mg • Saw Palmetto berry powder (Serenoa serrulata/repens) 35 mg • Bladderwrack powder (Fuccus vesiculosis) 20 mg. Other Ingredients: Calcium Phosphate, Microcrystalline Cellulose, Vegetable Stearin, Croscarmellose Sodium, Magnesium Stearate (vegetable source).

U-Viva Vitamin E (Chewable) — Uviva
Each tablet contains: Vitamin E (d-alpha tocopheryl succinate) 400 IU. Other Ingredients: Sucrose, Wheat Starch, Talc Purified, Kaolin, CL 75470, Gelatin. No synthetic vitamin E, yeast, salt, preservatives, gluten, glucose, artifical colors & flavors.

V.H.G. — National Deer Horn, Ltd
Velvet 210 mg • Ginseng 210 mg • Angelica 210 mg • Licorice 75 mg • Carthamiseman 45 mg.

V2G — EAS
Each capsule contains: Vanadyl Sulfate 7.5 mg • Taurine 800 mg • Selenium (Sodium Selenate) 33 mcg.

Vag-Mend — The Herbalist
Golden Seal root • Thuja leaf • Usnea lichen • Bayberry root bark • Echinacea root • Red Raspberry leaf.

Valer-A-Somn — Phytopharmica
Each capsule contains: Valerian extract (Valeriana officinalis)(standardized to contain 0.2%-0.8% valerenic acids) 150 mg. Contains no sugar, salt, yeast, wheat, corn, soy, dairy products, coloring, flavoring or preservatives.

Valerian — Pharmanex
Each capsule contains: Valerian root extract (6:1) (Valerian officinalis) 350 mg. Other Ingredients: Gelatin, Rice Flour, Magnesium Stearate, Silicon Dioxide.

Valerian Plus — PhysioLogics
Each capsule contains: Valerian (0.8% Valerenic Acids, 1.52 mg) 190 mg • Chamomile 90 mg • Peppermint 90 mg • Propolis 45 mg • Passion flower 45 mg • American Ginseng 40 mg.

Valerian Root — Gaia Herbs
Valerian root standardized for 0.8% valerenic acid. Standardized Full Spectrum 100 mg of extract per capsule. Guaranteed Potency 50 mg of extract per capsule.

BRAND NAMES

© Copyright 2000, Natural Medicines Comprehensive Database (209) 472-2244. For updated data, go to www.NaturalDatabase.com. • 1415

Some Brand Name Natural Products - What they Contain
www.NaturalDatabase.com contains MANY more listings than appear here.

B R A N D   N A M E S

Valerian-Primrose Virtue — Blessed Herbs
Valerian root • Primrose flower & leaf • California Poppy flower & leaf • Hops strobile • Wild Lettuce • Passion flower • Scullcap • Grain alcohol & Distilled Water.

Val-Tran — Atrium
Each tablet contains: Valerian (standardized extract) 100 mg • Vitamin B6 5 mg • Magnesium Gluconate 50 mg • Magnesium Oxide 50 mg. In a base containing Chamomile, Anise & Peppermint.

Vanadyl Factors — Olympia Nutrition
Vanadyl Sulfate + 800 mg Taurine.

Vanadyl pH — SportPharma
Each capsule contains: Vanadyl Sulfate 7.5 mg.

Vanadyl Sulfate — Ultimate Nutrition
Each tablet contains: Vanadyl Sulfate 10 mg.

Vancol (Cholesterol Lowering Plan) — Omnicron International
Two chewable tablets contain: Beta Sitosterol 10 mg • Psyllium 200 mg • Chromium from Picolinate 50 mcg with natural Quinone Antioxidants. In a base of Calcium Carbonate & Magnesium Stearate.

VariCare — Enzymatic Therapy
Each tablet contains: Butcher's Broom extract (Ruscus aculeatus) standardized to contain 9 - 11% Saponins calculated as Ruscogenin 150 mg • Horse Chestnut extract (Aesculus hippocastanum) standardized to contain 20 - 22% Saponins calculated as Escin 125 mg • Gotu Kola Phytosome (Centella asiatica) standardized to contain 30 - 35% Centella Triterpenes 15 mg.

Varicosin — Phytopharmica
Each tablet contains: Butcher's Broom extract 150 mg • Horse Chestnut extract 125 mg • Gotu Kola Phytosome 15 mg.

Vascular Support Formula — The Vitamin Factory
Each tablet contains: Vitamin C (Ascorbic Acid) 500 mg • Pycnogenol (Maritime Pine bark extract) 100 mg.

VasoRect — Real Health Laboratories
Each capsule contains: L-Arginine 625 mg • Calcium 12.5 mg.

Vege Fuel — TwinLab
Pure Isolated Soy (All-Vegetable) Protein 100%. Contains no sugar, artificial sweeteners or flavors. It is fat free, cholesterol free & lactose free.

Vege Fuel (Aspartame Free) — TwinLab
Pure Isolated Soy (All-Vegetable) Protein 100%. Contains no sugar, artificial sweeteners or flavors. It is fat free, cholesterol free & lactose free.

Veg-Easy — Progressive Labs
Two tablets contain: Blend 1400 mg: Broccoli powder • Spirulina • Wheat Grass • Alfalfa powder • Spinach powder • Cabbage powder • Green Tea • Carrot • Barley grass • Parsley • Beet root powder • Kale • Oat fiber medium • Brussels Sprouts • Lipase • Amylase • Protease • Cellulase • Powdered Cellulose • Beet leaf powder • Barley fiber • Oat bran • Lactobacillus Acidophilus • Glucomannan & Calcium Gluconate.

Veg-Enzyme — Atrium
Each capsule contains: Protease Enzymes 150 mg • Amylase Enzymes 140 mg • Lipase Enzymes 25 mg • Cellulase Enzymes 10 mg.

VegeSil — Flora
Silica extract • Spring Horsetail.

Vegetarian Enzyme Complex — Futurebiotics
Protease 6500 HUT* • Amylase 2000 DU* • Cellulase 20 CU* • Lipase 14.5 LU* • Papaya enzyme (papain) 50 mg • Lactase 100 LacU* • Alfalfa powder 50 mg • Pineapple enzyme (bromelain) 50 mg • Betaine HCl3 mg*. Enzyme activity is determined & reported according to Standard Food Chemical Codex procedures accepted by the FDA.

Vegetarian Enzyme Complex 50 Plus — Futurebiotics
Protease 8000 HUT* • Amylase 4000 DU* • Cellulase 100 CU* • Lipase 40 LU* • Invertase 0.2 IAU* • Lactase 240 LacU* • Papain 10 mg • Maltase 15 AGU* • Gentian root 100 mg • Bromelain 10 mg • Fennel seed 50 mg. *Enzyme activity is determined & reported according to Standard Food Chemical Codex procedures accepted by the FDA.

Vegetarian Mega Minerals — Nature's Life
Two tablets contain: Boron (Citrate) 1 mg • Calcium (Carbonate, Citrate/Malate) 1000 mg • Chromium (Picolinate {US Patent #33,988}, Polynicotinate) 200 mcg • Copper (Glyconate, Citrate) 1 mg • Iodine (Kelp) 25 mcg • Iron (Fumerate, Peptonate) 15 mg • Magnesium (Oxide, Citrate) 500 mg • Manganese (Citrate) 10 mg • Molybdenum (Sodium Molybdate) 20 mcg • Potassium (Citrate) 99 mg • Selenium (l-Selenomethionine) 100 mcg • Silicon Dioxide 20 mg • Vanadium (Vanadyl Sulfate) 20 mcg • Zinc (Picolinate, Citrate) 15 mg • Betaine HCl 100 mg • Glutamic Acid HCl 100 mg.

Vegetarian Super Multi — Futurebiotics
Three tablets contain: Vitamin C 500 mg • Beta Carotene 15,000 IU • Vitamin B1 (thiamin) 20 mg • Vitamin B2 (riboflavin) 20 mg • Niacinamide 75 mg • Vitamin D 200 IU • Vitamin E (natural succinate) 100 IU • Vitamin B6 20 mg • Folic Acid 400 mcg • Vitamin B12 100 mcg • Biotin 300 mcg • Pantothenic Acid 50 mg • Inositol 50 mg. Minerals: Calcium: (carbonate, phosphate, ascorbate) 200 mg • Iron (gluconate) 8 mg • Phosphorus 100 mg • Iodine (kelp) 150 mcg • Magnesium: (oxide, ascorbate, amino acid chelate) 25 mcg • Zinc (gluconate, oxide) 25 mg • Copper (gluconate) 1 mg • Selenium (amino acid chelate) 200 mcg • Chromium (amino acid chelate) 200 mcg • Manganese (proteinate) 5 mg • Molybdenum (amino acid chelate) 25 mcg. Other ingredients: Choline 150 mg • Para Amino Benzoic Acid (PABA) 75 mg • Bioflavonoid complex 100 mg • Sodium Phosphate 1 mg • Methionine 75 mg • Betaine HCl 75 mg • Bromelain 75 mg • RNA/DNA (chlorella) 50 mg • Chlorella 400 mg. In a base of: (Sea Vegetable, Ginkgo Biloba, Milk Thistle, Golden Seal, Dandelion, Burdock root, Alfalfa & Horsetail) 500 mg.

Veggie Carotenoids — Now
Two VCaps contain: natural Beta-Carotene (D. salina) 12 mg/20000 IU • Alpha Carotene (D. salina) 400 mcg containing additional Carotenoids from D. salina algae: Xeaxanthin, Cryptoxanthin, Lycopene & Lutein • Lutein Floraglo Marigolds 3 mg • Lycopene natural source 3 mg • Broccoli concentrate (250 mcg Sulforaphane) 250 mg • Spinach concentrate (75 mcg Lutein) 100 mg • Tomato concentrate (140 mcg Lycopene) 100 mg • Kale powder 50 mg • Cabbage powder 50 mg • Brussels Sprouts powder 50 mg.

Veggie Carotenoids — Olympia Nutrition
Luteins • Broccoli • Spinach • Kale • Parsley • Cabbage • Asparagus.

Vegie-Tabs One — Dial Herbs
Parsley • Garlic • Black Walnut hulls • Red Beet • Kelp • Dulse • Wheat bran • Wheat germ • Oat straw • Honey • Spinach • Cabbage • Carrots • Squash • Onions • Broccoli • Yellow Dock • Chickweed • Echinacea • Ginger • Cloves • Alfalfa • Alfalfa seeds • Papaya seeds • Rice Bran Capsicum • Sweet Potato.

Vegie-Tabs Two — Dial Herbs
Parsley • Hawthorne • Black Walnut hulls • Red Beet • Kelp • Dulse • Millet • Oat Straw • Honey • Spinach • Cabbage • Carrots • Squash • Onions • Broccoli • Yellow Dock • Chickweed • Echinacea • Alfalfa • Alfalfa seeds • Papaya seeds • Rice Bran • Capsicum • Ginger • Cloves.

Vegiplex — HealthWatchers System
Brocolli • Kale • Sprouts • Spinach • Radish • Carrot • Beet • Tomato • Celery • Onion • Leek • Cauliflower • Brussel Sprouts. (all ingredients are whole and powdered.)

Vegzyme — Progressive Labs
Each 500 mg capsule contains: Protease 10000 NP Units • Lipase 3600 NL Units • Amylase 4000 NA Units • Cellulase 30 NC Units • Papaya leaf powder 25 mg. Other Ingredients: Plant fiber. All-vegetable source from cultures of Aspergillus Oryzae & Niger & Papaya. Naturally occurring Invertase, Maltase, Beta-Amylase, Hemicellulase, Phosphatase, Peroxidase, Catalase & Hydrolase are also present.

Vein Formula — Pharmanex
Each tablet contains: Vitamin C (as Calcium Ascorbate) 60 mg • Grape Seed Extract (as Masquelier's Original OPC's) 75 mg. Other Ingredients: Gelatin, Maltodextrin, Microcrystalline Cellulose, Magnesium stearate, Silicon dioxide.

Veinish — Quest
Sesame Oil • Emulsifying Wax • Stearic Acid • Marine Algae • Propylene Glycol • Cetyl Alcohol • Canola Oil • Calendula Oil • Marigold Extract • Chickweed Extract • Lecithin • Essence of Lemon.

Some Brand Name Natural Products - What they Contain
www.NaturalDatabase.com contains MANY more listings than appear here.

VelvaMax — Gold Mountain
Panax Ginseng • Reishi (Ganoderma lucidum) • Tienchi (Radix Pseudo-ginseng) • Astragalus (Astragalus membranaceus) • Licorice (Radix glycyrrhizae uralensis).

Venastat — Pharmaton
Each Supro Cap contains: Sustained Release Pellets of Standardized Horse Chestnut seed extract as Triterpene glycosides calculated as Escin (16%) 300 mg. Other Ingredients: Dextrin, Gelatin, Copolyvidone, Talc, Polymethacrylic Acid Derivatives, Titanium Dioxide, Dibutyl Phthalate, Synthetic Iron Oxide.

Venix — Pharmanex
Two capsules contain: Triacin, a proprietary blend of 1325 mg: Cs-4 Mushroom Mycelia (Cordyceps Sinensis [Berk.]Sacc.) • L-Arginine (as L-Arginine HCL) • Ginkgo Biloba Leaf Extract (50:1). Other Ingredients: Gelatin, Magnesium Stearate, Silicon Dioxide.

VHandC Tabs — Dial Herbs
Vinegar • Honey • Cayenne.

Viactiv Soft Calcium Chews — Mead Johnson Nutritionals
Each chew contains: Calcium (as calcium carbonate) 500 mg • Vitamin D 100 IU • Vitamin K 40 mcg • Potassium 15 mg • Phosphorus 8 mg • Lactose 0.5 mg • Caffeine 1.14 mg. Other Ingredients: Corn syrup, calcium carbonate, sugar, chocolate, nonfat milk, cocoa butter, salt, soy lecithin, glyceryl monostearate, artificial flavor, carrageenan, & sodium phosphate.

Vigorex Femme — New Hope Health Products
Each tablet contains: Sabal Serrulata (Saw Palmetto) • Avena Sativa (Common Oats).

Vigorex forte — Doc Johnson Enterprises
Active Ingredient: Avena sativa 1X. In a base of lactose. Editor's Comments: This is a homeopathic product. It is so extremely diluted that its activity can not be explained by conventional scientific methods. Therefore this product can not be rated by the scientific criteria used in this Database. A patient receiving the extreme dilution of this product will not receive many, if any, molecules of the original active ingredient. Therefore, there are no harmful pharmacologic effects, and any beneficial effects are controversial and not due to a direct biochemical action of the ingredient on the body. Homeopathic products are allowed for sale in the U.S. due to legislation passed in the 19th century sponsored by a homeopathic physician who was also a Senator. The law still requires that the FDA allow the sale of products listed in this Homeopathic Pharmacopea of the United States.

Vigorex Forte — New Hope Health Products
Each capsule contains: Avena Sativa Extract 300 mg.

Vincazine — Smart Basics
Each capsule contains: Vinpocetine 10 mg • (-) Huperzine A 50 mcg.

Vinpocetine — PhysioLogics
Each capsule contains: Vinpocetine 10 mg.

Vinpocetine — Amerifit
Each tablet contains: Vinpocetine 5 mg • Green Tea standardized extract 200 mg. Other Ingredients: Dicalcium posphate, croscamellose sodium, microcrystalline cellulose, magnesium stearate, silica stearic acid, & pharmaceutical glaze.

Vinpo-Zine — Smart Nutrition
Each capsule contains: Vinpocetine 10 mg • Huperzine A 50 mcg.

ViraMax — Solaray
Two capsules contain: Catuaba 500 mg • Yohimbe bark extract (supplying 10 mg of yohimbine) 500 mg • Muira Puama root 250 mg • Peruvian Maca root extract (4:1) 100 mg.

ViraPlex — Enzymatic Therapy
Each tablet contains: Vitamin A (Fish Liver oil) 10000 IU • Vitamin D (Fish Liver oil) 35 IU • Vitamin C (Ascorbic Acid/Rose Hips) 200 mg • Calcium (Lactate) 41 mg • Pantothenic Acid (D-Calcium Pantothenate) 25 mg • Zinc (Gluconate) 10.5 mg • Magnesium (Citrate) 6.7 mg • Vitamin B12 (Cyanocobalamin) 2.5 mcg • Other ingredients: RNA Powder 60 mg • Alfalfa juice powder 50 mg • Lemon Bioflavonoids 30 mg • Spleen extract 30 mg • Thymus extract 25 mg • Trace Mineral concentrate (Kelp) 25 mg • Unsaturated Free Fatty Acids 15 mg • Lung extract 10 mg. In a base of Chlorophyll, Lymph, & Fermentation extract. Contains no sugar, salt, yeast, wheat, gluten, corn, soy, dairy products, flavoring or preservatives.

Chlorophyll is used in this product as a natural coloring agent. All organs & glands derived from bovine sources.

Virility Support Formula — The Vitamin Factory
Each tablet contains: Niacin 10 mg • L-Arginine 250 mg • Marapuama root & bark extract 10:1 100 mg • Yohimbe bark extract (min 1% Yohimbe) 100 mg • Quebracho Branco bark extract (Aspidosperma • min. 6% Quebrachine) 25 mg • Catuaba bark extract 4:1 50 mg • Pycnogenol (Maritime Pine bark extract) 10 mg.

Virility-V — Aspen Group, Inc.
Two tablets contain: Yohimbe extract 2% 500 mg • Avena Sativa extract 10.1 150 mg • Androstenedion 90 mg • Saw Palmetto extract 4.1 100 mg • Guarana extract 22% 300 mg • Taurine 200 mg • Siberian Ginseng extract 35.1 30 mg • Tribulus Terrestris extract 40% 50 mg. Inactive ingredients: Dicalcium Phosphate, Microcrystaline Cellulose, Magnesium Stearte, Stearic Acid.

Virility-V Female — Aspen Group, Inc.
Three tablets contain: Vitamin D (as colecalcifero) 21 IU • Niacin (as xiacinamide) 20 mg • Vitamin B6 (as pyridoxine hydrochloride) 2.4 mg • Folic Acid (as folacin) 6.4 mg • Vitamin B12 (as cyanacolalamine) 6 mg. Other Ingredients: Avena Sativa (10:1) 150 mg, Kava Kava (30%) 10 mg, Mara Puama (4:1) 20 mg, St John's Wort (0.3%) 250 mg, Siberian Ginseng (35:1) 30 mg, Gingko Biloba (24%) 40 mg, Cordyceps 100 mg, Damiana 20 mg, L-Taurine 200 mg.

Virx — Nutri-Quest
Each tablet contains: Olive leaf 100 mg • L-Lysine 100 mg • Vitamin C 25 mg • Zinc Chelate 10 mg • Elderberry extract 100 mg • Selenium Chelate 50 mcg • Olive leaf extract 5 mg • Vitamin A 3333.33 IU • Echinacea 100 mg • Goldenseal 50 mg • Astragalus 100 mg • natural Beta Carotene 3333.33 IU.

Vision Essentials — Enzymatic Therapy
Each capsule contains: Vitamin A (Beta Carotene) non-toxic form of Vitamin A 5000 IU • Vitamin C (Ascorbic Acid) 100 mg • Riboflavin (Vitamin B2) 5 mg • Other ingredients: Bilberry extract (Vaccinium myrtillus Fructus) standardized to contain 25% Anthocyanosides (20 mg per capsule) calculated as Anthocyanidins 80 mg. Contains no sugar, salt, yeast, wheat, corn, soy, dairy products, coloring, flavoring, or preservatives.

Vision Formula — Nature's Way
Two capsules contain: Bilberry fruit (dried extract 25% Anthocyanins) 50 mg • Biotin (Biotin Triurate) 40 mcg • Cayenne pepper fruit 100 mg • Citrus Bioflavonoids 150 mg • Copper (Amino Acid Chelate) 1 mg • Lutein 6 mg • Niacin (Vitamin B3) 20 mg • Riboflavin (Vitamin B2) 8 mg • Siberian Ginseng root 50 mg • Taurine 150 mg • Tru-OPCs (dried Grape seed extract) 20 mg • Vitamin A (Retinol Palmitate) 2000 IU • Vitamin E (d-Alpha Tocopheryl) 80 IU • Zinc (Amino Acid Chelate) 16 mg. Other ingredients: Gelatin, Magnesium Stearate, Millet.

Vision Health — ProHerbs
Two tablets contain: Vitamin A (100% Beta Carotene) 2500 IU • Zinc (as Sulfate) 15 mg • Selenium (as Selenomethionine) 200 mcg • Copper (as Cupric Oxide) 2 mg • Bilberry extract (Vaccinium myrtillus fruit standardized to 25% anthocyanidins) 160 mg • Lutein 6 mg • Lycopene 5 mg. Other Ingredients: Dicalcium Phosphate, Microcrystalline Cellulose, Croscarmellose Sodium, Hydroxypropylmethylcellulose, Magnesium Stearate, Mineral Oil, Polyethylene Glycol, Stearic Acid, Titanium Dioxide, Sodium lauryl Sulfate, FD&C Red #40 Lake, FD&C Blue #1 Lake, FD&C Blue #2 Lake.

Visioplex — Progressive Labs
Each capsule contains: Vitamin A (acetate) 937 IU • Vitamin A (beta carotene) 3125 IU • Vitamin C 62.5 mg • Calcium (as calcium citrate) 12.5 mg • Vitamin E (dl-alpha tocopherol) 50 IU • Thiamin (vitamin B1) 2.5 mg • Riboflavin (vitamin B2) 3.1 mg • Niacin 1.25 mg • Niacinamide 6.25 mg • Vitamin B6 (pyridoxine HCl) 3.75 mg • Folate (folic acid) 100 mcg • Vitamin B12 6.25 mcg • Pantothenic Acid 12.5 mg • Magnesium (as magnesium citrate) 31.25 mg • Zinc (as zinc picolinate) 6.25 mg • Selenium (selenomethionine) 25 mcg • Copper (amino acid chelate) 0.375 mg • Raw Eye concentrate 8.75 mg • Eyebright (Euphrasia officinalis) 18.75 mg • Bilberry powder (Vaccinium myrtillis) 5 mg • Ginkgo extract (Ginkgo biloba) 7.5 mg • N-Acetyl-Cysteine (NAC) 31.25 • Quercetin 37.5 mg • Taurine 62.5 mg • L-Methionine 25 mg • Glutamic Acid 6.25 mg • Glycine 6.25 mg.

© Copyright 2000, Natural Medicines Comprehensive Database (209) 472-2244. For updated data, go to www.NaturalDatabase.com.

BRAND NAMES

Some Brand Name Natural Products - What they Contain
www.NaturalDatabase.com contains MANY more listings than appear here.

BRAND NAMES

Visual Eyes — Source Naturals
Four tablets contain: Vitamin A (Beta Carotene) 25000 IU • Vitamin A (Palmitate) 7500 IU (Total Vitamin A Activity) (32500 IU) • Vitamin B2 50 mg • Inositol Hexanicotinate 100 mg • Vitamin C (Magnesium Ascorbate) 1500 mg • Vitamin E (D-Alpha Tocopheryl Succinate) 400 IU • Chromium (ChromeMate(r) Polynicotinate 125 mcg 250 mcg and Chromium Picolinate 125 mcg) 250 mcg • Copper (Sebacate) 1 mg • Magnesium (Ascorbate, Taurinate) 164 mg • Selenium (L-Selenomethionine) 200 mcg • Zinc (Monomethionine) 30 mg • Bilberry extract (Yielding 37 mg of Anthocyanosides)100 mg • Lutein 10 mg • Alpha-Lipoic Acid 25 mg • Ginkgo Biloba 24% (50:1 Extract) 45 mg • Grape Seed extract (Proanthodyn with a Proanthocyanidolic Value of 95) 45 mg • Quercetin 320 mg • N-Acetyl Cysteine 400 mg • Taurine (Magnesium Taurinate) 500 mg • Inositol (Hexanicotinate) 10 mg.

Vita Fuel With Iron — TwinLab
Nine capsules contain: Beta-Carotene (pro-Vitamin A) 25000 IU • Vitamin D (from natural form Vitamin D3) 400 IU • Vitamin C 2000 mg • Natural Vitamin E (Succinate) 800 IU • CoQ10 (Coenzyme Q10) 30 mg • L-Glutathione 100 mg • N-Acetyl Cysteine (NAC) 200 mg • Alpha-Lipoic Acid 100 mg • Vitamin B1 (Thiamine) 50 mg • Vitamin B2 (Riboflavin) 50 mg • Vitamin B6 (Pyridoxine) 50 mg • Vitamin B12 (Cobalamin) 100 mcg • Niacinamide 75 mg • Pantothenic Acid 100 mg • Folic Acid 800 mcg • Biotin 600 mcg • PABA 10 mg • Choline Bitartrate 100 mg • Inositol 100 mg • L-Carnitine (from Carni Fuel L-Carnitine Magnesium Citrate) 100 mg • Creatine (Monohydrate) 1000 mg • Calcium (from Calcium Citrate & Carbonate) 500 mg • Magnesium (from L-Carnitine Magnesium Citrate, Aspartate, Alpha-Ketoglutarate & Oxide) 500 mg • Potassium (from Potassium Alpha-Ketoglutarate, Citrate & Aspartate) 500 mg • Zinc (from Zinc Picolinate) 50 mg • Manganese (from Manganese Gluconate) 10 mg • Iron (from Ferrous Fumarate) 10 mg • Copper (from Copper Gluconate) 2 mg • Iodine (from Potassium Iodide) 150 mcg • Selenium (from Selenomethionine & Selenate‹50/50 mixture) 200 mcg • Chromium (from Chromic Fuel patented Chromium Picolinate) 400 mcg • Molybdenum (from natural Molybdic Acid) 150 mcg.

Vita Fuel Without Iron — TwinLab
Nine capsules contain: Beta-Carotene (pro-Vitamin A) 25000 IU • Vitamin D (from natural form Vitamin D3) 400 IU • Vitamin C 2000 mg • Natural Vitamin E (Succinate) 800 IU • CoQ10 (Coenzyme Q10) 30 mg • L-Glutathione 100 mg • N-Acetyl Cysteine (NAC) 200 mg • Alpha-Lipoic Acid 100 mcg • Vitamin B1 (Thiamine) 50 mg • Vitamin B2 (Riboflavin) 50 mg • Vitamin B6 (Pyridoxine) 50 mg • Vitamin B12 (Cobalamin) 100 mcg • Niacinamide 75 mg • Pantothenic Acid 100 mg • Folic Acid 800 mcg • Biotin 600 mcg • PABA 10 mg • Choline Bitartrate 100 mg • Inositol 100 mg • L-Carnitine (from Carni Fuel L-Carnitine Magnesium Citrate) 100 mg • Creatine (Monohydrate) 1000 mg • Calcium (from Calcium Citrate & Carbonate) 500 mg • Magnesium (from L-Carnitine Magnesium Citrate, Aspartate, Alpha-Ketoglutarate & Oxide) 500 mg • Potassium (from Potassium Alpha-Ketoglutarate, Citrate & Aspartate) 500 mg • Zinc (from Zinc Picolinate) 50 mg • Manganese (from Manganese Gluconate) 10 mg • Copper (from Copper Gluconate) 2 mg • Iodine (from Potassium Iodide) 150 mcg • Selenium (from Selenomethionine & Selenate‹50/50 mixture) 200 mcg • Chromium (from Chromic Fuel patented Chromium Picolinate) 400 mcg • Molybdenum (from natural Molybdic Acid) 150 mcg.

Vita Male — Nutri-Quest
Each tablet contains: Yohimbe bark 250 mg • Damiana 40 mg • Gotu Kola 25 mg • Hawthorne berries 25 mg • Beet root.

Vita-Bear Children's Chewables — The Vitamin Shoppe
Each tablet contains: Vitamin C 200 mg • Citrus Bioflavonoid Complex 20 mg. Naturally flavored with freeze-dried fruit juices. No yeast, corn, wheat, sucrose, salt, starch, soy, gluten, milk, eggs, dairy, fish or animal derivatives, preservatives, artificial colors or flavors added.

VitaCardia — PhysioLogics
Three capsules contain: Vitamin B6 (as Pyridoxine HCl) 10 mg • Folic Acid 810 mcg • Vitamin B12 (as Cyanocobalamin) 510 mcg • Magnesium (as Magnesium Glycinate) 50 mg • Potassium (as Potassium Chloride) 100 mg • Hawthorne flower, leaf (1.8% Vitexin, 10.8 mg) 600 mg • Cordyceps (7% Cordyceptic Acid, 28 mg; 0.2% Adenosine, 800 mcg) 400 mg • Taurine 200 mg.

Vitacor Plus — Matthias Rath, Inc.
Each tablet contains: Ascorbic Acid 230 mg • Ascorbyl Palmitate 170 mg • Calcium Ascorbate 100 mg • Magnesium Ascorbate 100 mg • Vitamin E (d-Alpha-Tocopherol) 130 IU • Vitamin A (Beta-Carotene) 1665 IU • Vitamin B1 (Thiamine) 7 mg • Vitamin B2 (Riboflavin) 7 mg • Niacin 10 mg • Niacinamide 35 mg • Pantothenic Acid (d-Calcium Pantothenate) 40 mg • Vitamin B6 (Pyridoxal Phosphate) 10 mg • Vitamin B12 (Cyanocobalamin) 20 mcg • Vitamin D3 (Cholecalciferol) 130 IU • Folic Acid 90 mcg • Biotin 65 mcg • L-Proline 110 mg • L-Lysine 110 mg • L-Carnitine 35 mg • L-Arginine 40 mg • L-Cysteine 35 mg • Calcium (Glycinate, Ascorbate) 35 mg • Magnesium (Glycinate, Ascorbate) 40 mg • Potassium (Chelate) 20 mg • Zinc (Glycinate) 7 mg • Manganese (Chelate) 1.3 mg • Copper (Glycinate) 330 mcg • Selenium (L-Seleno Methionine) 20 mcg • Chromium (Glycinate) 10 mcg • Molybdenum (Glycinate) 4 mcg • Inositol 35 mg • Coenzyme Q10 7 mg • Phosphorous (Dicalcium Phosphate) 15 mg • Pycnogenol 7 mg • Citrus Bioflavonoids 100 mg • Vitamin E (Beta, Gamma & Delta Tocopherols) 22 mg • Carotenoids (Alpha-Carotene, Lutein, Zeaxanthin, & Cryptoxanthin) 50 mcg.

Vital K + Ginseng Capsules — Futurebiotics
Potassium • Calcium • Magnesium • 16 Herbal extracts Plus the Triple Ginseng Action of Korean, Siberian & American Ginsengs.

Vital K + Ginseng Extra — Futurebiotics
Siberian, Korean, & American Ginseng • 16 Invigorating Herbal extracts • Potassium • Calcium & Iron found in the Original Vital K.

Vital K Original with Magnesium — Futurebiotics
Potassium • Magnesium • Calcium • Iron & 17 Herbal extracts, including the major Chinese adaptogenic herbs: (Ginseng, Astragalus, Schizandra & Dong Quai).

Vitaliza — HerbaSway
Horny Goad Weed • Dong Quai • He Sho Wu • Panax Ginseng • Knotweed • Schisandra • Blackberry • HerbaSwee (Cucurbitaceae fruit).

Vitamin & Aloe Moisturizing Creme — Aspen Group, Inc.
Each gram contains: Tocopheryl Acetate 1% • Panthenol 1% • Water • Hydrogenated Polyisobutane • Octyl Methoxycinnamate • Mineral Oil • Ceteraryl Alcohol • Cetyl Phosphate • Dimethicone • Aloe Vera Gel • Aminomethyl Propanol • Fragrance • Carbomer • Propylene Glycol • Diazolidinyl Urea • Methylparaben • Propylparaben.

Vitamin 0 — R-Garden Internationale
Stabilized Oxygen in a solution of distilled water, Sodium Chloride, and trace minerals. Available in 4 oz, 2 oz, and 2 oz spray.

Vitamin A — Jamieson
Each capsule contains: Vitamin A (from Halibut liver oil) 10000 IU.

Vitamin A Retinyl Palmitate Wrinkle Treatment — Derma E
Vitamin A 10000 IU/100 gm, Vitamin E, Vitamin D, Allantoin.

Vitamin B 100 Complex — Jamieson
Each caplet contains: Thiamin (as Thiamine Mononitrate) 100 mg • Riboflavin (Vitamin B2) 100 mg • Niacin (as Niacinamide) 100 mg • Vitamin B6 (as Pyridoxine Hydrochloride) 100 mg • Folate (as Folic Acid) 400 mcg • Vitamin B12 (as Cyanocobalamin) 100 mcg • Biotin 100 mcg • Pantothenic Acid (as Calcium D-Pantothenate) 100 mg • Calcium 555 mg • Choline Bitartrate 100 mg • Inositol 100 mg.

Vitamin B12 — Jamieson
Each tablet contains: Vitamin B12 (as Cyanocobalamin) 1200 mcg • Calcium 80 mg.

Vitamin B12 100 mcg — Jamieson
Each tablet contains: Vitamin B12 (Cyanocobalamin) 100 mcg.

Vitamin B6 — Jamieson
Each tablet contains: Vitamin B6 (as Pyridoxine Hydrochloride) 100 mg.

Vitamin B-Complex — PhysioLogics
Each capsule contains: Thiamine (as Thiamine Mononitrate) 50 mg • Riboflavin 50 mg • Niacin 55 mg • Pantothenic Acid (as Calcium Pantothenate) 100 mg • Vitamin B6 (as Pyridoxine HCl) 50 mg • Vitamin B12 (as Cyanocobalamin) 50 mcg • Folic Acid 400 mcg • Biotin 300 mcg • Inositol 50 mg • Choline (Bitartrate) 50 mg • PABA 50 mg.

Vitamin C 1000 mg Timed Release — Jamieson
Each caplet contains: Vitamin C (as Ascorbic Acid) 1000. Other Ingredients: Rutin, Hesperidin, Lemon Bioflavonoids, Acerola, Rosehips.

Some Brand Name Natural Products - What they Contain
www.NaturalDatabase.com contains MANY more listings than appear here.

Vitamin C 200 mg — The Vitamin Shoppe
Each tablet contains: Vitamin C 200 mg • Citrus Bio-flavonoid Complex 20 mg.

Vitamin C 500 mg — Jamieson
Each tablet contains: Vitamin C (as Ascorbic Acid and Sodium Ascorbate) 500 mg • Sodium (as Sodium Ascorbate) 35 mg. Available in Chewable Orange, Grape Juice-Chewable, and Chewable Tropical Fruit flavors.

Vitamin C Skin Supplement Cream — Orjene
Antioxidants • Vitamin C • Ginkgo Biloba • Germanium • Chamomile.

Vitamin C Solution — Dial Herbs
Vitamin C • Vitamin B3 • Citrus bioflavonoids extract. In a base of Distilled Water, Fructose, Sorbitol, Vegetable Glycerine (kosher), Fruit flavors, Sodium Benzoate & Caramel color. Contains no fillers, binders, yeast, wheat, gluten, soy, dairy, artificial colors, or starch.

Vitamin C with Echinacea — Holista
Each tablet contains: Vitamin C 500 mg • Echinacea 100 mg.

Vitamin C, 500 mg (special) — Nature's Life
Vitamin C (Ascorbic Acid), 500 mg. In a natural base of Rose Hips Powder. Excipients: Cellulose, Magnesium stearate and Micro-Cellulose (tm) coating.

Vitamin C-1000 — PhysioLogics
Each tablet contains: Vitamin C (Ascorbic Acid) 1000 mg • Bioflavonoids lemon 30 mg.

Vitamin D 1000 IU — Jamieson
Each tablet contains: Vitamin D (as Cholecaliciferol) 1000 IU • Calcium (as Dicalcium Phosphate) 20 mg • Peanut oil.

Vitamin E - A&D Cream — Atrium
Three ounces contain: Vitamin E 1500 IU • Vitamin A 750 IU • Vitamin D 300 IU. In a Silicone Cream Base: Stearic Acid, Glycerol, Cetyl Alcohol, Beeswax, Apricot Kernel oil, Triethanolamine, Borax, Allantoin, Methyl Parasept.

Vitamin E 200 IU Supplement — Jamieson
Each tablet contains: Vitamin E (as Dl-Alpha Tocopheryl Acetate) 200 IU.

Vitamin E Essential Skin Cream — Orjene
Vitamin E 6000 IU • Vitamin A 20000 USP units • Vitamin D 5000 USP units.

Vitamin E Oil — Orjene
6000 IU of Vitamin E and Vitamin A and Vitamin D.

Vitamin Foundation Creme — Aspen Group, Inc.
Each gram contains: Tocopheryl Acetate • Panthenol • Water • Octyldodecyl Neopetanoate • Octyl Methoxycinnmate • Cetearyl Alcohol • Cetyl Phosphate • Dimethicone • Beeswax • Carbomer • Aminomethyl Propanol • Propylene Glycol • Diazolidinyl Urea • Methylparaben • Propylparaben.

Vitasana —
Boehringer Ingelheim Pharmaceuticals, Inc. Dist. by Pharmaton
Two gelcaps contain: Vitamin A (as beta carotene) 4000 IU • Vitamin C (as ascorbic acid) 120 mg • Vitamin D (as cholecalciferol) 400 IU • Vitamin E (as dl-aloha tocopheryl acetate) 30 IU • Vitamin B1 (as thiamine mononitrate) 2.4 mg • Vitamin B2 (riboflavin) 3.4 mg • Vitamin B3 (niacinamide) 30 mg • Vitamin B6 (as pyridoxine HCl) 4 mg • Folic Acid 400 mcg • Vitamin B12 (as cobalamin conc.) 2 mcg • Calcium (as calcium phosphate) 200 mg • Iron (as ferrous sulfate) 18 mg • Phosphorus (as calcium phosphate) 160 mg • Magnesium (as magnesium oxide) 20 mg • Zinc (as zinc sulfate) 2 mg • Copper (as copper sulfate) 2 mg • Manganese (as manganese sulfate) 2 mg • Standardized G115 Ginseng Extract (from Panax Ginseng, C.A. Meyer) (root) 80 mg.

Vita-Vim — Jamieson
Each caplet contains: Vitamin A (as Retinyl Acetate) 10000 IU • Vitamin C (as Ascorbic Acid) 150 mg • Vitamin D (as Cholecalciferol) 400 IU • Vitamin E (as Dl-Alpha Tocopheryl Acetate) 15 IU • Thiamin (as Thiamine Mononitrate) 4.5 mg • Riboflavin (Vitamin B2) 7.5 mg • Nicain (as Niacin and Nicacinamide) 65 mg • Vitamin B6 (as Pyridoxine Hydrochloride) 3 mg • Folate (as Folic Acid) 400 mcg • Vitamin B12 (as Cyanocobalamin) 14 mcg • Biotin 10 mcg • Pantothenic Acid (as Calcium D-Pantothenate) 15 mg •

Calcium (as Calcium Carbonate) 130 mg • Iron (as reduced Iron) 4 mg • Iodine (as from Kelp) 100 mcg • Magnesium (as Magnesium Oxide) 100 mg • Zinc (as Zinc Gluconate) 10 mg • Selenium (from yeast) 15 mcg • Copper (as Copper Gluconate) 1 mg • Choline Bitartrate 20 mg • Inositol 20 mg • Dl- Methionine 2.2 mg.

Vitex — Pharmanex
Each Capsule Contains: Vitex Fruit (20:1) Extract 175 mg. Other Ingredients: Rice Flour, Gelatin.

Vit-Min 100+ — Now
Each tablet contains: Vitamin A (6 mg Beta-Carotene) 10000 IU • Vitamin A (Acetate) 10000 IU • Vitamin B1 (Thiamine HCL) 100 mg • Vitamin B2 (Riboflavin) 100 mg • Vitamin B3 (Niacinamide) 100 mg • Vitamin B5 (Pantothenic Acid) 100 mg • Vitamin B6 (Pyridoxine HCL) 100 mg • Vitamin B12 (Cyanocobalamin) 100 mcg • Biotin 100 mcg • Folic Acid 400 mcg • Vitamin C (Calcium Ascorbate) 250 mg • Vitamin D (Calciferol) 400 IU • Vitamin E (d-Alpha Tocopheryl Succinate) 150 IU • Calcium (Ascorbate, Carbonate) 50 mg • Magnesium (Oxide • Amino Acid Chelate) 30 mg • Zinc (Amino Acid Chelate) 15 mg • Copper (Amino Acid Chelate) 500 mcg • Iodine (Kelp) 150 mcg • Iron (Amino Acid Chelate) 10 mg • Potassium 10 mg • Manganese (Amino Acid Chelate) 5 mg • Selenium (Amino Acid Chelate) 25 mcg • Chromium (Yeast-free GTF) 100 mcg • Molybdenum (Amino Acid Chelate) 50 mcg • Boron (Amino Acid Chelate) 500 mcg • Vanadium (Amino Acid Chelate) 50 mcg • Choline (Bitartrate) 100 mg • Inositol 100 mg • PABA 50 mg • Rutin 25 mg • Betaine (HCL) 25 mg • Glutamic Acid 25 mg • Spirulina 50 mg • Barley grass organic 50 mg • Citrus Bioflavonoids (40% Hesperidin) 25 mg • Psyllium husk fiber 25 mg. This timed release multiple is formulated in a base of 72 Trace Minerals, Dicalcium Phosphate, Cellulose, Stearic Acid, Silica & natural vegetable protein coating.

Vit-Min 75+ — Now
Each tablet contains: Vitamin A (natural Fish Liver oil) 10000 IU • Beta-Carotene (6 mg) 10000 IU • Vitamin B1 (Thiamine HCL) 75 mg • Vitamin B2 (Riboflavin) 75 mg • Vitamin B3 (Niacinamide) 75 mg • Vitamin B5 (Pantothenic Acid) 75 mg • Vitamin B6 (Pyridoxine HCL) 75 mg • Vitamin B12 (Cyanocobalamin) 100 mcg • Biotin 100 mcg • Folic Acid 400 mcg • Vitamin C (Ascorbic Acid) 250 mg • Vitamin D (natural Fish Liver oil) 400 IU • Vitamin E (100% d-Alpha) 150 IU • Calcium (Amino Acid Chelate, Oystershell) 100 mg • Magnesium (Oxide, Amino Acid Chelate) 60 mg • Zinc (Amino Acid Chelate) 15 mg • Copper (Amino Acid Chelate) 1 mg • Iodine (Kelp) 150 mcg • Iron (Amino Acid Chelate) 10 mg • Choline (Bitartrate) 100 mg • Inositol 75 mg • PABA 30 mg • Rutin 25 mg • Citrus Bioflavonoids (40%) 100 mg • Betaine (HCL) 25 mg • Glutamic Acid 25 mg • Potassium (Amino Acid Chelate) 10 mg • Manganese (Amino Acid Chelate) 5 mg • Selenium (Amino Acid Chelate) 25 mcg • Chromium (Yeast-free GTF) 50 mcg • Boron (Amino Acid Chelate) 500 mcg • Molybdenum (Amino Acid Chelate) 50 mcg • Nucleic Acid 50 mg. In a natural base containing Alfalfa, Parsley, Rice polishings, Lecithin & Rose Hips, Dicalcium Phosphate, Cellulose, Stearic Acid & Silica. Contains no sugar, salt, starch, yeast, wheat, corn, soy, milk or preservatives.

Vitor Velvet — St Leonards
Each capsule contains: 100% Deer Velvet.

Vitox — Pharmanex
Two capsules contain: Vitamin A (Vitamin A Palmitate) 3750 IU • Beta-Carotene (Beta-Carotene, Spirulina Pacifica) 6250 IU • Vitamin C (Calcium Ascorbate Comples-Ester-C, Acorbyl Palmitate) 250 mg • Vitamin D3 (cholecalciferol) 200 IU • Vitamin E (d-Alpha Tocopheryl Succinate, Beta, Gamma, Delta Tocopherols) 150 IU • Vitamin K (Phylloquinone) 35 mcg • Thiamin (Thiamine Mononitrate) 1.5 mg • Riboflavin (Riboflavin, Riboflavin-5-Phosphate) 1.7 mg • Niacin (Niacinamide Ascorbate) 20 mg • Vitamin B6 (Pyridoxine Hydrochloride, Pyridoxal-5-Phosphate) 2 mg • Folate (Folic Acid) 200 mcg • Vitamin B12 (Cyanocobalamin, Dibencozide) 6 mg • Biotin (Biotin) 150 mcg • Pantothenic Acid (d-Calcium Pantothenate) 25 mg • Calcium (Calcium Carbonate, Calcium Citrate, Calcium Chelate) 250 mg • Iron (Iron Chelate) 3 mg • Magnesium (Magnesium Oxide, Magnesium Citrate, Magnesium Chelate) 100 mg • Zinc (Zinc Chelate) 7.5 mg • Selenium (L-Selenomethionine) 50 mcg • Copper (Copper Chelate) 2.5 mg • Manganese (Manganese Chelate) 2.5 mg • Chromium (Chromium Chelate, Chromium Picolinate) 50 mcg • Boron (Boron) 0.5 mg • Reduced Glutathione 0.5 mg • Leucoanthocyanin (Grape Seed Extract) 0.5 mg.

BRAND NAMES

© Copyright 2000, Natural Medicines Comprehensive Database (209) 472-2244. For updated data, go to www.NaturalDatabase.com. • 1419

Some Brand Name Natural Products - What they Contain
www.NaturalDatabase.com contains MANY more listings than appear here.

B
R
A
N
D

N
A
M
E
S

Volumax — Pinnacle
Includes Colostrum 1000 mg, Super Crea-Glutide A-DS. Super Crea-Glutide tri-bonds pure Creatine Monohydrate with Glutamine Peptide and Taurine.

VP2 — AST Sports Science
Each serving contains: Calories 100 • Protein 24 g • Carbohydrates 1g • Fat 0.5 g. Ingredients: 100% Hydrolyzed Oligpeptide Isolated Whey Protein Fractions consisting of precision engineered Whey Protein Isolate Fractions (Beta-Lactoglobulin, Alpha-Lacalbumin, Immunoglobulin, Proteose-Peptone, Glycomacropeptides (GMP), Bovine Serum Albumin, Lactoferrin, Lactoperoxidase. Lysozyme, Relaxin, Lactollin, & Beta-Microglobulin), natural & artificial Flavors & Aspartame.

VPS Coriolus versicolor — JHS Natural Products
Each capsule contains: Coriolus extract 625 mg.

VS-10 Vanadyl Sulfate — Optimum Nutrition
Each tablet contains: Vanadyl Sulfate 10 mg.

VyoPro — AST Sports Science
Each serving contains: Fat-Free Whey Protein (L-Glutamine & B Vitamins) 18 g • Calories 82 • Protein 18 g • Carbohydrates 3 g • Fat per serving 1 g. Ingredients: 100% cool processed, (partially digested) amino-specific controlled Chymotrypsin/ Trypsin Hydrolyzed CCTH (Tryptic Hydrolysate) Oligopeptide Whey Protein from Micro Filtered & Stirred-Bed Reactor Ion-Exchange Whey Protein providing the highest percentage of Oligopeptides along with Di-, Tri-, & Poly-Peptides (multi-spectrum short & long amino acid chains) with specifically tailored & precision enginerred molecular weight profiles [isolate fractions 53% Beta-Lactalbumin (molecular weight - MW 18,400 - 36,800D), 24% Alpha-Lactalbumin (MW 14,200) 17% Immunoglobulin (MW 16,000-160,000D) 6% Minor Peptones {lactoferrin, lactoperoxidase, lysozyme, relaxin, lactollin, & Beta-microglobulin (MW 4,000 - 40,000D)}] • Dual Stage Glutamine Composite, consisting of low molecular weight Whey Glutamine Peptides (MW 500 - 10,000) & Microencapsulated Pure Crystalline L-Glutamine • Protein Absorption Enhancing Matrix (Cyanocobalamin, Pyridoxine HCL, Thiamin, Riboflavin, & Calcium Pantothenate) • natural Flavors • Aspartame.

Water Balance — Nutrivention
Three tablets contain: Vitamin B6 (Pyridoxine) 150 mg • Potassium (Amino Acid Complex) 149 mg • Corn Silk (Stigmata maidis) 900 mg • Buchu (Barosma betulina) 600 mg • Elder flowers (Sambuccua canadensis nigra) 300 mg • Hydrangea (Hydrangea arborescens) 300 mg • Uva Ursi (Arctostaphylos uva ursi) 300 mg • Parsley (Petroselinum sativum) 150 mg • Samphire (Crithmum maritimum) 150 mg • Watermelon seed (Citrullus vulgaris) 150 mg.

Water Pill — Natrol
Two tablets contain: Vitamin B6 (as Pyridoxine HCl) 150 mg • Potassium (as Potassium Gluconate) 99 mg • Buchu extract leaf 4:1 100 mg • Parsley extract leaf 4:1 100 mg • Uva Ursi extract leaf 4:1 100 mg • Juniper extract berry 4:1 20 mg. Other ingredients: Calcium Carbonate, Mono & Di-Glycerides, Stearic Acid, Croscarmellose Sodium, Silicon Dioxide, Magnesium Stearate.

Weight Loss Support — Amazon Support
Each capsule contains: Cha de Bugre • Carqueja • Guarana • Jurubeba • Mutamba • Picao Preto • Yerba Mate • Annatto.

Weightless Cinnamon-Spice — Traditional Medicinals
Cinnamon bark • Fennel seed • Roasted Chicory root • Uva Ursi leaf • Cleavers Herb • Flax seed • Licorice root • Red Clover Top • Clove stem • Star Anise seed • Hibiscus flower • Buchu leaf • natural flavors.

Weightless Cranberry — Traditional Medicinals
Contains: Hibiscus flower • Roasted Chicory root • Fennel seed • Red Clover top • Uva Ursi leaf • Parsley leaf • Cleavers herb • Cranberry • Other natural flavors.

Weightless Tea — Traditional Medicinals
Contains: Fennel seed • Hibiscus flower • Lemongrass leaf • Uva Ursi leaf • Lemon Verbena leaf • Flax seed • Spearmint leaf • Cleavers herb • Red Clover top • Parsley leaf • Buchu leaf • Natural flavors.

Welah Mide — Shawnee Moon
Buchu leaf • Red Clover • Saw Palmetto • Uva Ursi.

Wellness Formulas — Source Naturals
Three tablets contain: Vitamin A (Palmitate 4000 IU, Beta Carotene 1000 IU) 5000 IU • Vitamin C (Ascorbic Acid, and Zinc, Calcium, and Magnesium Ascorbates) 1075 mg • Calcium (Ascorbate) 7.5 mg • Copper (Sebacate) 300 mcg • Magnesium (Ascorbate) 3.8 mg • Selenium (Sodium Selenite) 25 mcg • Zinc (Ascorbate) 23 mg • Propolis 324 mg • Propolis extract 126 mg • Garlic clove 360 mg • Boneset leaf 328 mg • Polygonum Odoratum 200 mg • Echinacea Root 196 mg • Echinacea Extract 164 mg • Isatis (Root and Leaf) 159 mg • Horehound stems 150 mg • Bioflavonoids 120 mg • Astragalus root 90 mg • Angelica Archangelica root 87 mg • Mullein leaf 80 mg • Goldenseal root 75 mg • Siberian Ginseng root 66 mg • Hawthorn berry 55 mg • Oregon Grape root 55 mg • Siberian Ginseng extract 54 mg • Pau d'Arco extract 36 mg • Cayenne fruit 30 mg.

Wellness Source — HealthWatchers System
Vitamin A • Vitamin D • Vitamin E • Vitamin C • Vitamin B6 • Vitamin B2 • Vitamin B1 • Vitamin B12 • Vitamin U • Bioflavonoids • Choline Bitartrate • Niacin-Niacinamide • Pantothenic Acid • Inositol • Rutin • Papain • PABA • Lecithin • Quercetin • RNA • Hesperidin • DNA • CoQ10 • Folic Acid • Octacosanol • Biotin • Magnesium • Calcium • Zinc • Boron • Potassium • Manganese • Copper • Iodine (Kelp) • Selenium • Chromium.

Wellness Source Booster — HealthWatchers System
Beta Carotene • Vitamin E • Vitamin C • Calcium • Magnesium • Choline • Potassium • Silica • Niacinamide.

Wild Brazilian SUMA-750 — Nature's Plus
Each capsule contains: Wild Brazilian SUMA (Pfaffia paniculata [Martius] Kuntze) 750 mg. Naturally rich in the 6 Saponins, Pfaffosides A,B,C,D,E & F - average 6%; 100% pure. Contains no yeast, wheat, corn, soy, milk, salt, sugar or starch.

Wild Cherry Syrup — Dial Herbs
Wild Cherry bark • Cubeb berry • Mullein • Skunk Cabbage • Lobelia • Honey • Clove.

Wild Cherry Virtue — Blessed Herbs
Wild Cherry bark • Plantain leaf • Mullein leaf • Mullein flower • Licorice root • Black Cherry concentrate.

Wild Cherry-Slippery Elm Bark Formula — Quest
Each caplet contains: Wild Cherry bark powder (Prunus serotina) 60 mg • Slippery Elm bark powder (Ulmus fulva) 60 mg • Pleurisy Root powder (Asclepias tuberosa) 60 mg • Chickweed powder (Stellaria media) 40 mg • Horehound powder (Marrubium vulgare) 40 mg • Kelp powder (Fucus vesiculosus) 40 mg • Licorice root powder (Glycyrrhiza glabra) 40 mg • Mullein leaf powder (Verbascum thapsus) 40 mg • Cayenne powder (Capsicum minimum) 35 mg • Saw Palmetto berry powder (Serenoa serrulata) 15 mg. Other Ingredients: Calcium Phosphate, Microcrystalline Cellulose, Vegetable Stearin, Croscarmellose Sodium, Magnesium Stearate (vegetable source).

Wild Rose Nerve Formula — Dial Herbs
Valerian root • Mistletoe • Scullcap • Hops • Lady Slipper • Passion flower.

Wild Vites — Nature's Life
Each tablet contains: Vitamin A (Acetate) 5000 IU • Vitamin D3 (Cholecalciferol) 400 IU • Vitamin E (d-Alpha Tocopheryl acetate) 30 IU • Vitamin C (Ascorbic Acid) 60 mg • Vitamin B1 (Thiamine Monoitrate) 1.5 mg • Vitamin B2 (Riboflavin) 1.7 mg • Vitamin B3 (Niacinamide) 20 mg • Vitamin B5 (Pantothenic Acid) 10 mg • Vitamin B6 Pyridoxine HCl 2 mg • Vitamin B12 (Cobalamin) 6 mcg • Folic Acid 400 mcg • Biotin 300 mg. In a natural base of low-Glycemic pure Crystalline Fructose & Sorbitol.

Wild Yam — Alvin Last
Wild Yam extract • Aloe Vera gel • Soybean Oil • Stearic Acid • Cetyl Alcohol • Triethanolamine • Tocopheryl Acetate • Glycerin • Methylparaben • Propylparaben.

Wild Yam Cream — Youngevity
Wild Yam root extract (Dioscorea villosa) • Aloe Vera gel • Natural Emollients and Moisturizers • Avocado oil • Oat oil • Key Lime fragrance • Chamomile (Matricaria chamomilla) • Burdock root (Arctium lappa) • Black Cohosh (Cimicifuga racemosa) • Siberian Ginseng (Eleutherococcus senticosus) • D-Alpha Tocopherol Acetate • Methylparaben • Propylparaben.

Wild Yam/Dong Quai Formula — PhysioLogics
Each capsule contains: Wild Yam extract (6% Diosgenin, 12 mg) 200 mg • Dong Quai (1% Ligustilides, 2 mg) 200 mg • Soy bean (5% Isoflavones, 5 mg) 100 mg.

Some Brand Name Natural Products - What they Contain
www.NaturalDatabase.com contains MANY more listings than appear here.

Wild Yam-False Unicorn Virtue — Blessed Herbs
False Unicorn root • Black Haw bark • Wild Yam root • Lobelia • Grain alcohol & Distilled Water.

Winter Wellness — Now
Two tablets contain: Vitamin A 5000 IU • Vitamin C 500 mg • Potassium 20 mg • Zinc 15 mg • Bee Propolis 200 mg • Deodorized Garlic Extract 200 mg • Ginger root 200 mg • Oregon Grape root 150 mg • Peptizyme 125 mg • Echinacea angustifolia root extract 100 mg • Elderberry extract 100 mg • Olive leaf extract 100 mg • Quercetin 100 mg • Shitake mushroom extract 100 mg • Reishi mushroom 100 mg • American Ginseng root 100 mg • Licorice root extract 100 mg • Goldenseal root 75 mg • Cayenne pepper 50 mg.

Wobenzym N — Mucos
Each tablet contains: Pancreatin 100 mg • Chymotrypsin 1 mg • Bromelain 45 mg • Papain 60 mg • Rutoside 50 mg.

Woman's Choice — Phytopharmica
Three capsules contain: Vitamin A (Beta Carotene) (Non-toxic form of Vitamin A) 16665 IU • Vitamin E (D-Alpha Tocopherol Succinate) 200 IU • Vitamin C (Ascorbic Acid) 200 mg • Magnesium L-Aspartate 150 mg • Pantothenic Acid (D-Calcium Pantothenate) 100 mg • Thiamine HCL (Vitamin B1) 50 mg • Riboflavin (Vitamin B2) 50 mg • Calcium Citrate 50 mg • Iron (Ferrous Succinate) 18 mg • Zinc (Gluconate) 15 mg • Chromium (Polynicotinate) 250 mcg • Folic Acid 100 mcg • Vitamin B12 (Cyanocobalamin) 50 mcg • Selenium (L-Selenomethionine) 50 mcg • Other ingredients: Dong Quai extract 4:1 (Angelica sinensis) 75 mg • Licorice root extract (Glycyrrhiza glabra) 60 mg standardized to contain 5% glycyrrhizic acid • Milk Thistle extract 50 mg (Silybum marianum) standardized to contain 70% silymarin calculated as silybin • Black Cohosh extract 4:1 (Cimicifuga racemosa) 30 mg • Chaste Tree berry extract (Vitex agnus-castus) 20 mg standardized to contain 0.5% agnuside • Pyridoxal-5'-Phosphate 10 mg. Contains no sugar, salt, yeast, wheat, corn, dairy products, coloring, flavoring or preservatives.

Women's AM Multi — Clinician's Choice
Two tablets contain: Vitamin A (retinyl acetate & 26% as beta-carotene) 3900 IU • Vitamin C (ascorbic acid) 250 mg • Vitamin D (cholecalciferol) 400 IU • Vitamin E (dl-alpha tocopheryl acetate) 150 IU • Thiamin (mononitrate) 1 mg • Riboflavin 1 mg • Niacin (nianicamide) 10 mg • Vitamin B6 (pyridoxine hydrochloride) 2 mg • Folate (folic acid) 250 mg • Vitamin B12 (cyanocobalamin) 4 mcg • Biotin 200 mcg • Pantothenic Acid (d-calcium pantothenate) 5 mg • Calcium (carbonate, amino acid chelate, ascorbate, aspartate, citrate, gluconate) 220 mg • Iron (amino acid chelate) 12 mg • Iodine (potassium iodide) 76 mcg • Magnesium (oxide, amino acid chelate) 9 mg • Zinc (oxide, amino acid chelate, gluconate) 8 mg • Selenium (selenomethionine) 100 mcg • Copper (amino acid chelate) 1 mg • Manganese (amino acid chelate) 3 mg • Potassium (chloride, amino acid chelate) 12 mg • Chromium (nicotrate, picolinate, chelavite, amino acid chelate) 40 mcg • Molybdenum (amino acid chelate) 4 mcg • RoseOx (patented, standardized process for an extract of Rosemary) 60 mg • Citrus Bioflavanoid Complex 10 mg • Dong Quai 10 mg • Wild Yam 10 mg • Black Currant 10 mg • Red Raspberry Leaf 10 mg • Proprietary blend 12 mg: Panax Ginseng Extract, Schizandra Fruit, Echinacea Angustifolia, Grape Powder, Bee Pollen, Cruciferex.

Women's Daily Pack — YourLife/Leiner Health Products Inc.
Each packet contains: Vitamin A (acetate) 2500 IU • Vitamin A (Beta Carotene) 5000 IU • Vitamin C (ascorbic acid) 120 mg • Vitamin D (ergocalciferol) 200 IU • Vitamin E (dl-alpha tocopheryl acetate) 230 IU • Vitamin K (phytonadione) 10 mcg • Vitamin B1 (thiamine mononitrate) 2 mg • Vitamin B2 (riboflavin) 3 mg • Niacin (niacinamide) 20 mg • Vitamin B6 (pyridoxine HCl) 2 mg • Folate (folic acid) 400 mcg • Vitamin B12 (cyanocobalamin) 3 mcg • Biotin (d-biotin) 30 mcg • Pantothenic Acid (d-calcium pantothenate) 10 mg • Calcium: (Oyster Shell, Calcium Carbonate, Calcium Phosphate) 725 mg • Iron (ferrous fumarate) 4 mg • Phosphorus (calcium phosphate) 50 mg • Iodine (potassium iodide) 100 mcg • Magnesium (magnesium oxide) 100 mg • Zinc (zinc oxide) 20 mg • Selenium (selenium amino acid chelate) 30 mcg • Copper (copper oxide) 3 mg • Manganese (manganese sulfate) 4 mg • Chromium (chromium amino acid chelate) 20 mcg • Molybdenum (molybdenum amino acid chelate) 25 mcg • Chloride (potassium chloride) 36 mg • Evening Primrose oil (evening primrose seed) 500 mg. 7 day iron strip contains: Iron (ferrous sulfate) 18 mg. Contains no added yeast. Contains colors: (Titanium Dioxide, Yellow 6 Lake, Red 40 Lake, Blue 2 Lake).

Women's Guardian — Clinician's Choice
Two tablets contain: Vitamin B6 (pyridoxine HCl) 2 mg • Pantothenic Acid (calcium pantothenate) 50 mg • Beta-Sitosterol 300 mg • Dong Quai Herb 200 mg • Red Raspberry Leaf 160 mg • Kudzu Root 100 mg • Wild Yam 100 mg • Squaw Vine 50 mg • I-Isoleucine 40 mg • I-Leucine 40 mg • I-Valine 40 mg • Aminogen 20 mg • Black Cohosh Root 20 mg • Evening Primrose 20 mg • Lycopene (1%) 20 mg • Proprietary blend 12 mg: Lutein (5%), Chamomile Flowers, Passion Flower, Sage Leaves, Isoflavones, Grape Powder.

Women's Liberty — Traditional Medicinals
Licorice root • Orange peel • Wild Yam root • Ginger rhizome • Cinnamon bark • Dong Quai root • Clove stem • Fo Ti root • Angelica root.

Women's Mood-Enhancer — HerbaSway
St. John's Wort • Dong Quai • Rehmannia • Schisandra • Coptis • Ginkgo biloba • Cassia tora • Astragalus • Blackberry • HerbaSwee (Cucurbitaceae fruit).

Women's Nutritional System — Rainbow Light
Six tablets contain: Beta Carotene 10000 IU • Vitamin D 400 IU • Vitamin E natural 120 IU • Vitamin K 30 mcg • Thiamin (Vitamin B1) 36 mg • Riboflavin (Vitamin B2) 41 mg • Niacinamide 80 mg • Pantothenic Acid 80 mg • Pyridoxine (Vitamin B6) 48 mg • Folic Acid 800 mcg • Biotin (d-Biotin) 300 mcg • Cyanocobalamin (Vitamin B12) 144 mcg • Vitamin C 500 mg • Calcium (Amino Acid Chelate, Citrate) 200 mg • Magnesium (Amino Acid Chelate, Ascorbae, Oxide) 400 mg • Potassium (Aspartate, Choride) 99 mg • Manganese (Amino Acid Chelate) 2.5 mg • Iron (Amino Chelate) 22.5 mg • Zinc (Picolinate) 15 mg • Copper (Amino Acid Chelate) 1 mg • GTF Chromium (Polynicotinate) 30 mcg • Selenium (l-Selenomethionine) 40 mcg • Iodine (Kelp) 150 mcg • Molybdenum (Aspartate) 50 mcg • Choline (Bitartrate) 40 mg • Inositol 40 mg • PABA (Para Aminobenzioc Acid) 30 mg • Octacosanol (Spinach) 300 mcg • Black Currant (seed) 30 mg • Bioflavonoids 250 mg • Rutin 20 mg • L-Tyrosine 20 mg • Hesperidin Complex 15 mg • Protease 3600 HUT • Amylase 282 DU • Lipase 3 LU • Cellulase 3.2 CU. Superfood & Herbal Ingredients: Bee Pollen • Spirulina • Lemon juice powder • Wheatgrass • Dong Quai • Barley Grass • Echinacea agustifolia • Reishi (Ling Chi) • Rosemary oil • Blue Cohosh 4:1) 530 mg. Custom Herbal extracts: Vitex • Red Rasberry • Mulberry • Fo-Ti • Bladderwrack • Tumeric • Peony Cistanche • Cynomorium 270 mg.

Women's PM Multi — Clinician's Choice
Two tablets provide: Vitamin A (retinyl acetate & 20% as beta-carotene) 1250 IU • Vitamin C (ascorbic acid) 250 mg • Vitamin D (cholecalciferol) 60 IU • Vitamin E (dl-alpha tocopheryl acetate) 150 IU • Thiamin (mononitrate) 0.5 mg • Riboflavin 0.7 mg • Niacin (niacinamide) 10 mg • Folate (folic acid) 200 mcg • Vitamin B12 (cyanocobalamin) 2 mcg • Biotin 150 mcg • Pantothenic Acid (d-calcium pantothenate) 5 mg • Calcium (amino acid chelate, aspartate, citrate, gluconate) 16 mg • Iron (glycinate) 6 mg • Iodine (potassium iodide) 76 mcg • Magnesium (oxide, amino acid chelate) 20 mg • Potassium (chloride, amino acid chelate, gluconate) 16 mg • Zinc (oxide, amino acid chelate, gluconate) 12 mg • Selenium (selenomethionine) 100 mcg • Copper (amino acid chelate) 1 mg • Manganese (amino acid chelate) 1 mg • Chromium (nicotinate, picolinate, chelavite, amino acid chelate) 10 mcg • Molybdenum (amino acid chelate) 2 mcg • RoseOx (patented, standardized process for an extract of Rosemary) 50 mg • Citrus Bioflavonoid Complex 10 mg • Chamomile Flower 10 mg • Passion Flower 10 mg • Valerian Root 10 mg • Mint Leaves 10 mg • Dong Quai 10 mg • Wild Yam 10 mg • Black Currant 10 mg • Red Raspberry Leaf 10 mg • Hesperidin 4 mg • Proprietary blend: Isoflavones, Echinacea, Milk Thistle Fruit, Cruciferex, Grape Powder 10 mg.

Women's Stress System — Rainbow Light
Two tablets contain: Vitamin A (Beta Carotene) 250 IU • Vitamin E (d-Alpa Tocopheryl Acetate) 30 IU • Vitamin C (Ascorbic Acid) 120 mg • Magnesium (Citrate) 60 mg • Potassium (Chloride) 40 mg • Niacin-Niacinamide (Vitamin B3) 40 mg • Pantothenic Acid (Vitamin B5) 20 mg • Pyridoxine (Vitamin B6) 10 mg • Zinc (Glycinate) 8 mg • Riboflavin (Vitamin B2) 3 mg • Thiamin (Vitamin B1) 3 mcg • Copper (Glycinate) 750 mcg • Folic Acid 400 mcg • Biotin 300 mcg • Cyanocobalamin (Vitamin B12) 12 mcg • Soy extract 150 mg • Hawaiian Spirulina 70 mg • standardized to 1.5% Isoflavonoids Bioflavonoids citrus 50 mg • Wheat Grass 80 mg • 4:1 Custom Herbal extracts containing: [Siberian Ginseng (Eleuthero root), St. John's Wort herb, Kava root, Codonopis root, Vitex berry, Lavender oil] 302 mg. Other Nutritional Ingredients: L-Glutamine 50 mg, L-Taurine 20

B R A N D   N A M E S

B R A N D   N A M E S

mg, Alpha-Lipoic Acid 25 mg, L-Methionine 15 mg, L-Tyrosine 25 mg.

Women's Support Formula — PhysioLogics
Each capsule contains: Vitamin E (as d-Alpha Tocopheryl Acetate) 50 IU • Vitamin B6 (as Pyridoxine HCl) 25 mg • Folate (Folic Acid) 200 mcg • Magnesium (as Magnesium Oxide) 100 mg • Zinc (as Zinc Glycinate) 3.75 mg • Copper (as Copper Glycinate) 0.5 mg • Black Cohosh root 100 mg • Chastetree berry (5% Vitexicarpin, 5 mg) 100 mg • Dong Quai root (0.8% Ligustilides, 0.8 mg) 100 mg • Soy bean (5% Isoflavones, 2.5 mg) 50 mg • Kava Kava root (30% Kavalactones, 7.5 mg) 25 mg.

Xenadrine RFA-1 — Cytodyne Technologies
Two capsules contain: Citrus aurantium (standardized for 4% Synephrine) 125 mg • MaHuang (standardized for 6% Ephedrine) 335 mg • Guarana extract (standardized for 22% Caffeine) 910 mg • White Willow bark extract (standardized for 15% Salicin) 105 mg • Acetyl L-Carnitine 100 mg • L-Tyrosine 80 mg • Ginger root 50 mg • Vitamin B5 (Pathothenic Acid) 40 mg.

Xomatropin hGH Spray — ASN
Each two part formula contains: Part One: Secreatagoges • GH & IGF-1 Peptides. Part Two: Anti-Soatosatin called Revosatin (a power suppressor of an antagonistic hormone called somatosatin responsible for what is called the negative feedback loop for GH).

Xtra Advantage Creatine Serum — Muscle Marketing USA
Each 5 mL serving contains: Creatine Monohydrate • Glucosamine • L-Glutamine • L-Taurine • L-Carnitine • Magnesium • Zinc • Calcium • Vitamin B12 • Royal Jelly • Ginseng • Honey • Natural Glycerine • Natural Flavor • Distilled Water.

Xtra Fuel — TwinLab
Three capsules contain: Guarana extract (standardized for 22% Caffeine) 910 mg • Citrus aurantium extract (standardized for 4% Synephrine) 325 mg • L-Tyrosine 500 mg • Vitamin C 250 mg • Vitamin B6 10 mg • Ginkgo Biloba extract (standardized for 24% flavonoid glycoside) 60 mg • DMAE (2-Dimethylaminoethanol) 100 mg • Vitamin B5 (Pantothenic Acid) 100 mg.

Xtra-Mineral — The Herbalist
Yellow Dock root • Red Raspberry leaf • Nettles leaf • Dandelion root.

Yam Extract Plus 30 — Aspen Group, Inc.
Each capsule contains: Mexican Yam extract 500 mg • Adrenal substance (freeze dried) 200 mg.

Yam Extract Plus 30 — Atrium
Each capsule contains: Mexican Yam extract 500 mg • Adrenal Substance (freeze dried) 200 mg.

Yarrow-Pipsissewa Virtue — Blessed Herbs
Echinacea Angustifolia root • Yarrow flower • Pipsissewa • Oregon Grape root • Corn Silk • Kava Kava root • Hydrangea root • Grain alcohol & Distilled Water.

Yerba Manza-Eyebright Virtue — Blessed Herbs
Yerba Manza root • Yerba Santa leaf • Usnea lichen • Osha root • Eyebright • Propolis • Goldenseal root • Myrrh Gum • Licorice root • Grain alcohol & Distilled Water.

Yerba Santa-Echinacea Virtue — Blessed Herbs
Yerba Santa leaf • Osha root • Usnea lichen • Lomatium root • Pau d'Arco bark • Echinacea Angustifolia root • Goldenseal root • Myrrh Gum • Shitake mycelium • Propolis • Licorice root • Grain alcohol & Distilled Water.

Yin-Yang Athletic Tone — Flora
Chinese Red Ginseng • American Ginseng • Astragalus • Reishi Mushroom • Schisandra • Noto Ginseng • He Shou Wu • Codonopsis • Lycii berries • Licorice • Rehmania • Du Zhong • Prince Ginseng • Dodder Seed • Asparagus root.

Yin-Yang Beautiful Lady — Flora
Peony • Schisandra • Lycii berries • Licorice • He Shou Wu • Asparagus root • Noto Ginseng • Dang Gui • Codonopsis • Atractylodes • Poria.

Yin-Yang Crystal Clear Vision — Flora
Rehmania • Dodder Seed • Lycii berries • Chrysanthemum • He Shou Wu • Poria • Ligusticum • Acorus • Plantago Seeds.

Yin-Yang Golden Passage — Flora
Curculigo • Epimedii • Morinda root • Dang Gui • Phellodendron bark • Anemarrhena • Schisandra • Lycii berries • He Shou Wu • Licorice.

Yin-Yang Premenstrual Harmony — Flora
Bupleurum • Dang Gui • Peony • Poria • Atractylodes • Ginger • Licorice • Peppermint • Peony root bark • Cyperus berries • Ligusticum • Citrus Peel.

Yin-Yang Secret of Longevity — Flora
Chinese Red Ginseng • Astragalus • Noto Ginseng • Reishi Mushroom • Dang gui • Lycii berries • Asparagus root • Licorice • Poria • Prince Ginseng • Rehmania • Ligustrum Fruit • Schisandra • He Shou Wu.

Yin-Yang Tranquil Spirit — Flora
Zizyphus Jujube seed • Poria • Biota Seed • Anemarrhena • Licorice • Schisandra • Dang Gui.

YoHIMbe — HVL
Two capsules contain: Yohimbe 500 mg (Ultra Strength extract 4:1 equivalent to 2000 mg of Yohimbe) • Cellulose • Gelatin • Silica and Magnesium Stearate (vegetable source).

Yohimbe Fuel — TwinLab
Yohimbine (the active component in Yohimbe bark) 8 mg.

Young Again — Aspen Group, Inc.
Four tablets contain: Vitamin A Palmitate 500,000 IU/GR 8000 IU • Niacinamide 80 mg • Vitamin B6 20 mg • Vitamin C (magnesium ascorbate) 400 mg • Vitamin E (succinate) 100 IU • N-Acetyl Glucosamine 160 mg • L-Proline 360 mg • L-Lysine 320 mg • Glucosamine Sulfate 560 mg • Chondroitin Sulfate 160 mg • N-Acetyl Cysteine 120 mg • Quercetin Powder 80 mg • Grape seed extract (proanthodyn) 30 mg • Zinc (gluconate) 12 mg • Manganese Ascorbate 12 mg • Copper (gluconate) 0.5 mg • Selenomethionine 80 mcg. Contains no sugar, starch, salt, wheat, corn, yeast or soy derivatives.

Young Cha — National Deer Horn, Ltd
Dextrose • Lactose • Freeze dried Velvet • Herbal extract • Honey.

Youth-Assure — Nature's Plus
Two tablets contain: Rapid Release Layer: Melatonin (N-Acetyl-5-Methoxytryptamine) 3 mg. Sustained Release Layer: Pregnenolone pharmaceutical grade 50 mg • DHEA pharmaceutical grade Dehydroepiandrosterone 25 mg • LECI-PS, Phosphatidylserine-rich purified Lecithin concentrate supplying Activated Phosphatides: [Phosphatidylserine (PS) 5 mg, Phosphatidylcholine (PC) 5 mg, Cephalin (Phosphatidylethanolamine) 3 mg, Phosphoinositides 1.5 mg] 25 mg. Contains no yeast, wheat, corn, soy, milk, salt, or starch.

YST-RES-Q — Nutri-Quest
Two tablets contain: Lacto Bacillus 1 million IU • Caprylic Acid 50 mg • Grapefruit seed extract 100 mg • Garlic 25 mg • Berberis aquifolium 100 mg • Aloe Vera 25 mg • Undecenoic Acid 50 mg.

Yucca-AR Formula — Nature's Way
Two capsules contain: Proprietary Formula: Black Cohosh root • Black Walnut hulls • Brigham Tea herb • Burdock root • Cayenne pepper fruit • Hydrangea root • Rosemary herb • Sarsaparilla root • Valerian root • Wild Lettuce leaves • Wild Yam root • Yucca stalk. Other ingredients: Gelatin.

Zenibolin — Syn Trax
Each .25 mL contains: 19-Nor (5) Androstenediol • Isotonic Saline • Carboxymethylcellulose • Benzyl Alcohol.

Zicam Cold Remedy Nasal Spray — Gel Tech
Active Ingredients: Zincum Gluconium (Zinc) 2%. Inactive Ingredients: Benzalkonium chloride, glycerine, hydroxyethylcellulose, purified water, sodium chloride, & sodium hydroxide.

Zinaxin (HMP-33) — Eurovita A/S, Denmark
Each capsule contains: Zingiber Officinale Roscoe Extract (HMP-33 Extract) 255 mg. Recommended dosage is 2 capsules per day, in divided doses with liquid for the first month.

Zinaxin Rapid — Eurovita A/S, Denmark
Each capsule contains: Ginger Extract EV.EXT 77 (255 mg is equivalent to approximately 3000 mg of dried ginger rhizome and 1500 mg of dried galanga rhizome) • Sunflower Seed Oil • Gelatine • Glycerol • Beeswax Yellow • Lecithin • Titanium Dioxide • Copper Chlorophyllins. Recommended dosage is 2 capsules daily. Results should become noticeable within 2-4 weeks.

Zinc Chewable — Aspen Group, Inc.
Each tablet contains: Amino Acid Chelated Minerals as Zinc 29 mg • Raw Tissue concentrates (bovine source) from: Spleen 29 mg, Brain 8 mg, Liver 5 mg, Heart 4 mg, Kidney 4 mg, Thymus 2 mg, Adrenal 2 mg, Pituitary 1 mg, Duodenum 1 mg.

Zinc Citrate — Quest
Each tablet contains: Zinc (Citrate) 50 mg. Other Ingredients: Croscarmellose Sodium, Calcium Phosphate, Magnesium Stearate (vegetable source), Microcrystalline Cellulose, Silicon Dioxide, Vegetable Stearin.

Zinc Lozenge — Nutri-Quest
Each lozenge contains: Zinc Gluconate 75 mg.

Zinc Lozenges — Nature's Life
Each lozenge contains: Zinc (Gluconate) 10 mg • Vitamin C 100 mg • Beta Carotene (equivalent to 500 IU Vitamin A) 300 mcg • Purple Cone Flower root (Echinacea purpurea) 25 mg. In a natural base of low-Glycemic, pure Crystalline Fructose, pasteurized Honey powder, Hydrogenated Vegetable oil, natural Peppermint flavor, Eucalyptus leaf (Eucalyptus globulus) Licorice root (Glycyrrhiza glabra), Goldenseal root (Hydrastis canadensis), Slippery Elm bark (Ulmus ruba), & Fenugreek seed (Trigonella foenum-graecum).

Zinc Lozenges — Jamieson
Each lozenge contains: Vitamin C (as Ascorbic Acid) 50 mg • Zinc (as Zinc Gluconate) 5 mg. Other Ingredients: Eucalyptus, Anise Oil, Menthol, Camphor, Lemon.

Zinc Lozenges Plus — The Vitamin Shoppe
Each lozenge contains: Zinc 24 mg • Echinacea 100 mg • Vitamin C 150 mg • Propolis 100 mg • Vitamin A 1000 IU • Slippery Elm 25 mg. In a base of Golden Seal, Acerola, Fructose Cellulose, with Vanilla and Orange flavor.

Zinc Magnesium Aspartate — Substrate Solutions
Three capsules contain: Zinc (as L-OptiZinc & Aspartate) 30 mg • Magnesium (as Aspartate) 450 mg • Vitamin B6 (Pyridoxine Hydrochloride) 10.5 mg. Other Ingredients: Cellulose, Magnesium Stearate, Gelatin.

Zinc Plex — PhysioLogics
Each capsule contains: Zinc (as 50% Arginate, 25% Histidinate, 25% Glycinate) 30 mg • Copper (as 50% Glycinate, 50% Lysinate) 2 mg.

Zing! — Health Center for Better Living
Each capsule contains: Siberian Ginseng Root 106 mg.• Ginkgo Biloba Leaf 79 mg.• Gota Kola Herb 79 mg.• Kola Nut 79 mg.• Bee Pollen 53 mg.• Foti Root 26 mg.• Rehmannia Root 26 mg.• Spirulina 26 mg.

ZMA — SNAC (Balco Labs)
Each capsule contains: Zinc (Monomethionine/ Asparate) 10 mg • Magnesium (Aspartate) 150 mg • Vitamin B6 3.5 mg.

ZMA Rx-Strength — Advanced Therapeutics - Nature's Plus
Vitamin B6 (as Pyridoxine HCl) 0.5 mg • Magnesium (as Aspartate) 450 mg • Zinc (As Aspartate/Monomethionine) 30 mg • ZMA (Proprietary Anabolic Support Factor) 2424 mg.

ZonePerfect Fish Oil Capsules — ZonePerfect
Each capsule contains: Molecularly Distilled Fish oil • Natural Vitamin E 20 IU • EPA 160 mg • DHA 107 mg.

Zygest — PhysioLogics
Two capsules contain: Acid Protease (100 FCC/gm) 100 mg • Papain (6000 USP/mg) 100 mg • Protease (5000 FCC/gm) 80 mg • Amylase (5000 FCC/gm) 80 mg • Bromelain (2400 GDU/gm) 50 mg • Lipase (1000 LU/gm) 60 mg • Lactase (1000 FCC/gm) 20 mg • Cellulase (1000 FCC/gm) 10 mg • Hemicellulase (1000 FCC/gm) 10 mg.

Zymax — HealthWatchers System
Pancreatin • Papain • Rutin • Bromelain • Pancrelipase • Peppermint • Trypsin • Lipase • Amylase • Lysozyme • Cellulase • Chymotrypsin.

#100 ABC ACIDOPHILUS/BIFIDUM COMPLEX — Systemic Formulas
Each capsule contains: A minimum of one billion Lactobacillus acidophilus (NAS strain) and one billion Bifidobacterium bifidum (Malyoth strain) uniquely suspended in an anaerobic, sunflower oil matrix containing vitamin E as a natural antioxidant.

#101 ACP VITAMIN ACP — Systemic Formulas
Rose Hips • Orange Peel • Bone Meal • Vitamin C • RNA/DNA Liver Factors • Lemon Bioflavonoid • Vitamin E • RNA/DNA Thymus Factors • Pedra Hume Ca • Acacia Gum flower • Vitamin A.

#102 ACX VITAMIN DETOX — Systemic Formulas
Rose Hips • Vitamin C • RNA/DNA Liver Factors • Lemon Bioflavonoid • Pimiento • Vitamin E • Damiana • Pedra Hume Ca • RNA/DNA Thymus Factors • Vitamin A • Acacia Gum Flower • Hesperidin • RNA/DNA Spleen Factors • Peach Bark • Sun Dew.

#111 AZV Multi-Vitamin and Mineral Supplement — Systemic Formulas
RNA/DNA Liver Factors • Rose Hips • Kelp • Linseed Oil • Vitamin A • Vitamin D • Vitamin E • Vitamin C • Calcium • Niacin • Phosphorus • Iron • Vitamin B1 (Thiamine) • Vitamin B2 (Riboflavin) • Magnesium • Vitamin B6 (Pyridoxine HCl) • Pantothenic Acid • Potassium • Zinc • Manganese • Vitamin B12 (Cyanocobalamin) • plus Lemon Bioflavonoid, Autolyzed RNA/DNA Yeast.

#115 BSV VITAMIN B STRESS COMPLEX — Systemic Formulas
Abutua • Centaury • Red Bone Marrow • Nettle • Poke Root • Spearmint • RNA/DNA Liver and Parotid Factors • Guarana • Vitamin B2 • Fringe Tree • Choline Bitartrate • Inositol • Niacinamide • PABA • Vitamin B1 • Calcium Pantothenate • Vitamin B6 • Niacin • Vitamin B12 • Folic Acid • Biotin.

#12 B BRAIN — Systemic Formulas
RNA/DNA Brain Factors • Italian Pimiento • L-Alanine • Stevia • Tayuya • Vitamin B2 • Rutin • Niacin • Vitamin B6 • L-Glutamic Acid • Hydroxyproline • L-Proline • RNA/DNA Pituitary Factors • RNA/DNA Thalamus Factors.

#120 CAL CALCIUM PLUS — Systemic Formulas
Calcium (from Citrate, Lactate, Hydroxide, Bone Meal, Bone Ash, Carbonate, Oyster Shell, Lysinate, Methionate, and Aspartate) • Lecithin • Magnesium Oxide • Vitamin C • Vitamin E • Trace Minerals • Iron Chelate • Copper Carbonate • Vitamin D • Betaine HCl • Boron Chelate.

#126 CTV VITAMIN C THERAPEUTIC — Systemic Formulas
Ascorbic Acid • Sodium Ascorbate • Beta-carotene (source of Vit. A) • Sago Palm • Calcium Ascorbate • Calcium Carbonate • Bioflavonoids • Potassium Bitartrate • Hesperidin • Rose Hips • Thymol Iodide.

#130 EZV 200 IU VITAMIN E — Systemic Formulas
Lactose • Fructose • Vitamin E • Honey Bake.

#132 FLX VEGETABLE OMEGA-3 FLAX SEED OIL — Systemic Formulas
Superunsaturate (Alphalinolenic Acid, Omega-3) • Polyunsaturate (Linoleic Acid, Omega-6) • Monounsaturate (Oleic Acid) • Saturated Fatty Acid • Beta Carotene • Vit. E • Phytosterols • Lecithin and Traces of Fiber.

#134 LEV LECITHIN — Systemic Formulas
Lecithin • Inositol • Choline • Phospholipids.

#14 COLON — Systemic Formulas
Psyllium Husks • Cascara Sagrada • Licorice Root • Peach Bark • Stillingia • Dolomite • Calcium Carbonate • Citric Acid • Potassium Bicarbonate.

#140 Min Multi-Mineral Plus — Systemic Formulas
Great Salt Lake Water • Calcium Carbonate • Horse Tail • Magnesium Oxide • Calcium Lactate • Calcium Citrate • Irish Moss • Magnesium Chloride • Red Root • Zinc Chelate • Kelp • Manganese Chelate • Iron Chelate • Vitamin C • Iron Aspartate • Potassium Bitartrate • Copper Chelate • Manganese Picolinate • Zinc Picolinate • Molybdenum Chelate • Vanadium Chelate • Chromium Chelate • Selenium Chelate.

#150 PRO NUTRO PROTEIN — Systemic Formulas
Whey Protein • Pasteurized Saccharomyces Cerevisiae • Rice Protein • Green Lipped Mussel • RNA/DNA Trachea Factors • Dolomite • Dulse • Pimiento • Choline • Papain • Horse Tail (source of Silica) • Niacin • Pancreatin Enzyme • Vitamin C • Tyrosine • Valine • Aspartic Acid • Cystine • Methionine • Vitamin B6 • Vitamin E • RNA/DNA Thalamus Factors.

#155 PTM Potassium Stabilizer — Systemic Formulas
Potassium Bitartrate • Potassium Chloride • Magnesium Oxide • Boldo • Pfaffia • Kelp • Maracuja • Chamomile.

© Copyright 2000, Natural Medicines Comprehensive Database (209) 472-2244. For updated data, go to www.NaturalDatabase.com. • 1423

Some Brand Name Natural Products - What they Contain
www.NaturalDatabase.com contains MANY more listings than appear here.

B R A N D   N A M E S

#17 D DIGESTIVE — Systemic Formulas
Pancrelipase Enzyme • Golden Seal • RNA/DNA Oxbile Factors •
Aspartic Acid • Betaine HCl • L-Glutamic Acid • Echinacea • Lipase •
Amylase • Protease • Pepsin • Ammonium Chloride.

#18 Ds DIGESTIVE STABILIZER — Systemic Formulas
Kola Nut • Pancrelipase Enzyme • RNA/DNA Oxbile Factors •
Betaine HCl • Echinacea • Glutamic Acid • Spearmint • RNA/DNA
Liver Factors • Calcium • Papaya Leaves • Golden Seal • Aspartic
Acid • Ammonium Chloride • Pancreatin Enzyme • Gentian Root •
Guava Powder • Bromelain • Pepsin 1/3000.

#22 F+ Female Plus — Systemic Formulas
Sarsaparilla • Blue Cohosh • Dong Quai • Tayuya • False Unicorn •
Cana do Brejo • Carrapichinho • Pfaffia • Motherwort • Balm Mint •
Agoniada.

#31 GA ADRENAL — Systemic Formulas
RNA/DNA Adrenal Factors • Echinacea • Vitamin C • D-Calcium
Pantothenate • Inositol • Ma Huang • Sete Sangrias • RNA/DNA
Spleen Factors • Zinc Chelate • Selenium Aspartate.

#32 GB PITUITARY — Systemic Formulas
RNA/DNA Brain Factors • Whey Protein • RNA/DNA Pituitary
Factors • Peach Bark • Jaborandi • RNA/DNA Orchic Factors • L-
Methionine • Vitamin B6 • Superoxidedismutase.

#39 Gf THYROID — Systemic Formulas
Irish Moss • Thyroid-6x dilution • Pata de Vaca • Abutua Kelp •
Cucurbita Pepo • RNA/DNA Lung Factors • RNA/DNA Thymus
Factors.

#400 APHA pH CONTROL — Systemic Formulas
Rhubarb Root • Spearmint • Calcium Carbonate • Nettle • Seaweed •
Hyssop • Shave Grass • RNA/DNA Adrenal Factors • Potassium
Bitartrate.

#402 ARTA ARTHRO SUPPORT — Systemic Formulas
Chapu de Couro • Spearmint Leaves • Pomegranate • Vitamin B2 •
RNA/DNA Adrenal Factors • Potassium Bitartrate • Magnesium
Sulfate • Vitamin B6 • Niacin • Chaparral • Mistletoe • Yucca • Tayuya
• Burdock Seed • Lysine • Isoleucine • Methionine • Magnesium
Chelate • RNA/DNA Pituitary Factors • Zinc Chelate • Chromium
Chelate.

#403 ATAK SHIELD REJUVENATOR —
Systemic Formulas
Pau d'Arco • Yarrow • Stevia • Calcium Carbonate • Betaine HCl •
Tayuya • Gravel Root • Pimpinella Root • Yellow Dock • Echinacea •
Rose Hips.

#405 BLDB BLOOD BUILDER — Systemic Formulas
RNA/DNA Blood Factors • Burdock • RNA/DNA Liver Factors •
Wahoo • RNA/DNA Spleen Factors • L-Cystine • L-Leucine •
Chlorophyll.

#408 CLNZ TOXIN CHELATOR — Systemic Formulas
Dandelion Root • Pfaffia • Cinquefoil • Milk Thistle • Mountain
Mahogany • Yucca • Vitamin E • Wahoo • RNA/DNA Liver Factors •
L-Methionine.

#41 GT THYMUS — Systemic Formulas
Vitamin C • Sweet Basil • Golden Seal • RNA/DNA Thymus Factors •
Poke Root • Pau d'Arco • RNA/DNA Liver and Lung Factors •
Calcium Carbonate • Zinc Aspartate • RNA/DNA Spleen Factors •
Magnesium Chloride • Bitter Root • Beta Carotene • Thymol Iodide •
RNA/DNA Stomach Factors • Selenium Yeast • Chromium Chelate •
Vitamin B2 • Inositol • Niacinamide • PABA • Vitamin B1 • Calcium
Pantothenate • Vitamin B6 • Niacin • Vitamin B12 • Folic Acid •
Biotin.

#425 DIJS STOMACH ANTACID — Systemic Formulas
Oregon Grape • Golden Seal • Spearmint • Sodium Bicarbonate •
Potassium Bitartrate • Sodium Chloride • Spearmint Oil • Anise Oil •
Potassium Bicarbonate • Sodium Citrate • Malt Diastase •
Chlorophyll.

#428 DSIR DIGESTANT INTERNAL REGENERATOR —
Systemic Formulas
RNA/DNA Stomach and Duodenal Factors • Echinacea • Rose Hips •
Ma Huang • Stevia • Allantoin • RNA/DNA Thymus Factors •
Hesperidin • Vitamin C • L-Methionine • Senna Pod • L-Glutamic
Acid • Vitamin A • Pau d'Arco • Vitamin B6 • Spearmint Oil • Aloe
Vera • Sodium Copper Chlorophyll.

#435 GOLD SHIELD PLUS — Systemic Formulas
Golden Seal • Niacin • Vitamin B6 • Rose Hips • Vitamin C •
Fenugreek • Garlic • Vitamin B1 • Elder Berry • Spearmint Oil •
Lomatium Dissecutim.

#44 H HEART — Systemic Formulas
RNA/DNA Heart Factors • Lecithin • Chromium Chelate •
Phenylalanine • Sete Sangrias • Tayuya • RNA/DNA Thymus Factors
• Woodruff • RNA/DNA Spleen Factors • Tyrosine • Vitamin B2 •
Carnitine • Vitamin B1 • Niacin • Vitamin B6 • Calcium (from
Pantothenate) • Folic Acid • Biotin.

#45 Hcv HEART CARDIO VASCULAR —
Systemic Formulas
Sete Sangrias • RNA/DNA Heart Factors • Pimiento • Cassia Bark •
Stevia • Hawthorne Berries • Potassium Bitartrate.

#450 KDIR DIURETIC — Systemic Formulas
Manganese Chelate • Ch de Bugre • Juniper Berry • Peach Bark • Saw
Palmetto • Zinc Aminoate • Magnesium Sulfate • Peach Leaves • Uva
Ursi.

#46 Hn HEART NERVE — Systemic Formulas
RNA/DNA Brain and Spleen Factors • Hesperidin • RNA/DNA Lung
Factors • Calcium Pantothenate • Niacin • Tayuya • Vitamin B2 • L-
Threonine • RNA/DNA Aorta Factors • L-Methionine • Selenium
Chelate • RNA/DNA Heart Factors • Beta Carotene • Chromium
Chelate.

**#460 KYRO MUSCLE/LIGAMENT/TISSUE
STRENGTHENER** — Systemic Formulas
Orange Peel • Beta Carotene • Collagen • Bone Meal • Pfaffia •
Vitamin C • Manganese Chelate • Slippery Elm • RNA/DNA Liver
Factors • Vitamin B12 • Sete Sangrias • Vitamin E • Lemon
Bioflavonoid • Pimiento • RNA/DNA Heart Factors • Hesperidin •
Stevia • Cassia Bark • Potassium Bitartrate • Vitamin A • Hawthorne
Berry.

#481 OXAA CELL ORGANIZER — Systemic Formulas
Centaury Herb • Red Clover Blossom • Peach Bark • Stillingia •
Buckthorn Bark • Oregon Grape • Cascara Sagrada • Prickly Ash Bark
• Cinquefoil • Saw Palmetto • Burdock Root.

#482 OXCC CELL CLEANSER — Systemic Formulas
Choke Cherry • Irish Moss • Pimiento • Blessed Thistle • Peach Bark •
Oregon Grape • Fringe Tree • Red Clover • Burdock Root.

#483 OXOX CELL ACTIVATOR — Systemic Formulas
Fenugreek • Cyani Petals • Pulsatilla • Mandrake • Myrrh Gum •
Gentian Root • Primrose • Pfaffia • Bugleweed • Barberry • Prickly
Ash • Golden Seal • Blue Vervain • Catnip • Allantoin • Comfrey
Root.

#486 SENG RED GINSENG PLUS — Systemic Formulas
Red Ginseng • Pasteurized Saccharomyces Cerevisiae • Potassium
Phosphate (Source of Phosphorous and Potassium) • Yucca •
Chaparral.

#488 VIVI ANTI VIRO — Systemic Formulas
Pau D'Arco • Lomatium Dissecutim Oil • Vitamin E.

#491 VRM1 LARGE PATHOGENS — Systemic Formulas
Pau d'Arco • Rose Hips • Garlic • Valerian Root • Hops • Bromelain •
Zapilopatle Beans • Hojas de Jalapa • Dolomite • Worm Seed Oil.

#492 VRM2 SMALL PATHOGENS — Systemic Formulas
Black Walnut Husks • Wormseed Herb • Kamala • Quassia Chips •
Bromelain Enzyme • Bethyl Nut.

#493 VRM3 MICRO PATHOGENS — Systemic Formulas
Black Walnut Husks • Carrapichinho • Erva Tostao • Aniz Estrelado •
Bromelain Enzyme • Worm Seed Oil • Yerba Santa.

#494 VRM4 CELLULAR PATHOGENS —
Systemic Formulas
Kamala • Guarana • Carrapichinho • Maracuj • Wormseed Herb •
Papain • Alfazema.

#50 I EYES — Systemic Formulas
Rue Herb • Eye Bright • Vitamin A • Vitamin E • Chap,u de Couro •
Proline • Cystine • RNA/DNA Eye Factors • Vitamin B6 • Valine •
Niacin • RNA/DNA Brain Factors.

#58 Ks KIDNEY STABILIZER — Systemic Formulas
Rose Hips • Gelatin • RNA/DNA Kidney Factors • Magnesium

Sulfate • Juniper Berries • Vitamin C • Sete Sangrias • Spearmint Herb • Calcium Carbonate • Hesperidin Complex • Serine • Phenylalanine • RNA/DNA Adrenal and Thalamus Factors • Tyrosine • Vitamin A • Sodium • Copper • Chlorophyll.

#60 L LIVER — Systemic Formulas
RNA/DNA Liver Factors • Mountain Mahogany • Spearmint Leaves • Vitamin A • Vitamin D • Ragweed • Golden Seal • Quince Seed • Boldo • Vitamin C • Vitamin E.

#61 LB LIVER NORMALIZER — Systemic Formulas
Red Beet • Betaine HCl • Choline Bitartrate • Lipase 24.

#62 LS LIVER STIMULANT — Systemic Formulas
Rose Hips • Vitamin C • Chromium Chelate • Magnesium Chelate • Red Beet • Sete Sangrias • Ch de Bugre • Potassium Chelate • RNA/DNA Adrenal Factors • Choline Bitartrate • Iron Chelate • RNA/DNA Thymus Factors • Vitamin A • RNA/DNA Pituitary and Liver Factors.

#70 M+ MALE ENDOCRINE — Systemic Formulas
RNA/DNA Orchic Factors • Hops • Boldo (from Chile) • Cipó Caboclo • Abacateiro • Agoniada • Chinese Bamboo • Cipó Cravo • RNA/DNA Prostate Factors • African Yohimbe • Eucalyptus • Catuaba • Marapuama.

#72 Mpc Prostata Corrector — Systemic Formulas
Cucurbita Pepo Oil • Pau D'Arco • RNA/DNA Prostate Factors • Gingko Leaves • Pau D'Alho • RNA/DNA Orchic, Thymus, Pituitary & Hypothalamus Factors • Golden Seal • Echinacea Purpurea • Thyme.

#73 Mpr Prostata Ovatum — Systemic Formulas
Cucurbita Pepo Oil.

#75 N3 ANTI-TENSIVE — Systemic Formulas
Tayuya • Blue Vervain • Valerian Root Extract • Senna Leaves • L-Methionine • Passion Flower Extract • Calcium Chelate • Saw Palmetto • Sete Sangrias • Mandrake Root • Ephedra • Tyrosine.

#77 NC CALM — Systemic Formulas
Calcium Carbonate • Dulse • Passion Flowers • Marapuama • RNA/DNA Brain Factors • Tayuya • Boldo • Selenium Chelate • RNA/DNA Spleen and Lung Factors • Valerian • Niacin • Vitamin B12 • Vitamin B2 • Vitamin B1.

#78 P PANCREAS — Systemic Formulas
RNA/DNA Pancreas Factors • Catuaba • Cynita Cactus • Japecanga • Pata de Vaca • Pedra Hume Ca • Zinc Oxide.

#79 Ps PANCREAS STABILIZER — Systemic Formulas
RNA/DNA Pancreas Factors • Catuaba • Cynita Cactus • Japecanga • Pata de Vaca • Pedra Hume Ca • Zinc Oxide.

#80 R Lung — Systemic Formulas
Golden Seal • RNA/DNA Lung Factors • Pancreatin 4x • RNA/DNA Thymus Factors • L-Lysine • Aspartic Acid • Allantoin • Tayuya • Aloe Vera.
Editor's Comments: This is a homeopathic product. It is so extremely diluted that its activity can not be explained by conventional scientific methods. Therefore this product can not be rated by the scientific criteria used in this Database. A patient receiving the extreme dilution of this product will not receive many, if any, molecules of the original active ingredient. Therefore, there are no harmful pharmacologic effects, and any beneficial effects are controversial and not due to a direct biochemical action of the ingredient on the body. Homeopathic products are allowed for sale in the U.S. due to legislation passed in the 19th century sponsored by a homeopathic physician who was also a Senator. The law still requires that the FDA allow the sale of products listed in this Homeopathic Pharmacopea of the United States.

#82 S SPLEEN — Systemic Formulas
RNA/DNA Spleen Factors • Pedra Hume Ca • Nettle • Sweet Gum Tree • RNA/DNA Liver and Pancreas Factors • Lysine • L-Methionine • Leucine • Isoleucine.

#FPMS Female Premenses Syndrome — Systemic Formulas
Vitamin B6 • Cystine • Vitamin A • Magnesium Sulfate • Vitamin E • L-Thionine • Marapuama • Blue Malva • Pata de Vaca • RNA/DNA Pituitary Factors • L-Methionine • RNA/DNA Duodenal Factors • Choline • Motherwort • Angelica • Cyani Blossoms • Niacin • Inositol • Histidine • Superoxidedismutase • Dong Quai • Zinc Chelate • Vitamin B12 • Octacosanol.

@zit.gone — Pacific BioLogic
Kochia fruit • Licorice root • Phellodendron bark • Coptis rhizome •

Chrysanthemum flower • Forsythia fruit • Ophiopogonis tuber • Rehmannia root (fresh) • Trichosanthis root • Scrophularia root.

10 Mushroom Combination — Olympia Nutrition
Contains: Cordyceps, Reishi, Maitake, Shitake, Poria, Polyporus, Corialus, Tremella, Hericium, and Wood Ear mushrooms.

10% Plus Nighttime Cream — Jason
Alpha Hydroxy Acids.

100% Egg Protein — Healthy 'N Fit
100% pure extracted egg albumen (with a protein efficiency ratio of 3.9 or greater), enzymatic digest of egg albumia containing naturally occurring amino acids, vanilla flavoring, bromelain and papain.

100% Pure Red Deer Velvet — Glenfid
Pure Red Deer Velvet. No artificial preservatives of colourings.

12-1/2% Plus with SPF 12-1/2 Protective Moisturizer — Jason
Antioxidant Ester-C • Vitamin E.

19-Nor 250 — AST Sports Science
Each capsule contains: 19-Norandrostenedione 250 mg.

19-Nor-3-Andro — AST Sports Science
Each capsule contains: 19-Norandrostenedione 100 mg • Androstenediol 100 mg • Androstenedione 100 mg.

30 Day Beauty Secret — Futurebiotics
Formula I - Two tablets contain: • Royal Jelly (freeze dried) 50 mg • Horsetail (extract equivalent to) 300 mg • Dong Quai (extract equivalent to) 100 mg • Polygonum Multiflorum (extract equivalent to) 140 mg • Peony Root (extract equivalent to) 120 mg • Betaine HCl 75 mg • Selenium (Amino Acid Chelate) 50 mcg • Iodine (Kelp) 175 mcg • Iron (Amino Acid Chelate) 8 mg • Magnesium (Oxide, Amino Acid Chelate) 150 mg • Manganese (Amino Acid Chelate) 10 mg • Boron 3 mg • Zinc (Gluconate) 15 mg • Calcium (Carbonate, Phosphate, Casein) 300 mg • Phosphorus (Calcium Phosphate) 150 mg • Collagen 100 mg • Ribonucleic Acid (RNA) 50 mg • Sodium Phosphate 1 mg • Gelatin 200 mg • Papain 25 mg • Keratin 30 mg • Formula II - One caplet contains: Beta Carotene 10,000 IU • Vitamin C 150 mg • Vitamin B1 (Thiamin) 10 mg • Vitamin B2 (Riboflavin) 10 mg • Niacinamide 60 mg • Vitamin D (Fish Liver Oil) 200 IU • Vitamin E (Natural Mixed Tocopherols) 30 IU • Vitamin B6 (Pyridoxine) 10 mg • Vitamin B12 (Cyanocobalamin) 16 mcg • Folic Acid 400 mcg • Biotin 300 mcg • Pantothenic Acid 30 30 mg • Inositol 50 mg • Para Amino Benzoic Acid (PABA) 50 mg • Choline (Bitartrate) 150 mg.

30-Day Value Pack — Nature's Life
Mega-Vita-Min Vitamin C, 500 mg Each tablet contains: Beta Carotene (Vitamin A equivalent to 5000 IU) 3 mg • Vitamin B1 (Thiamine HCI) 10 mg • Vitamin B2 (Riboflavin) 10 mg • Vitamin B6 (Pyridoxine HCI) 10 mg • Vitamin B12 (Cobalamin concentrate) 100 mcg • Niacin 10 mg • Pantothenic Acid (d-Calcium Pantothenate) 20 mg • Folic Acid 400 mcg • Choline (Bitartrate) 90 mg • Biotin (d-Biotin) 50 mcg • PABA (Para Aminobenzoic Acid) 20 mg • LemonBioflavonoids Complex (TESTLAB) 15 mg • Vitamin C 100 mg • Vitamin E (d-Alpha Tocopheryl with mixed Tocopherols) 10 IU • Boron (Full-Range Amino Acid Chelated) 25 mcg • Calcium (Full-Range Amino Acid Chelated) 50 mg • Chromium (Nutrition 21 Picolinate) 50 mcg • Copper (Full-Range Amino Acid Chelated) 200 mcg • Iodine (Icelandic Kelp) 225 mcg • Magnesium (Full-Range Amino Acid Chelated) 50 mg • Manganese (Full-Range Amino Acid Chelated) 2 mg • Molybdenum (Proteinate) 25 mcg • Phosphorus (Full-Range Amino Acid Chelated & Complexed) 19 mcg • Potassium (Proteinate) 15 mg • Selenium (Nutrition 21 Selenomethionine) 25 mcg • Silicon (Dioxide) 25 mcg • Vanadium (Full-Range Amino Acid Chelated) 25 mcg • Zinc (Nutrition 21 Picolinate) 2 mg • Betaine HCI 30 mg • Nuclei Acids (RNA & DNA from Yeast) 30 mg • Co Q10 (Co-enzyme Ubiquinone) 500 mcg • Essential Fatty Acids (Soy, Spirulina) 25 mg • Super Green Pro 96 (Soy Protein Super Food) 330 mg. In a natural base containing: Rose Hips concentrate, Acerola, Rutin, Hesperidin, Lecithin, Milk-Free Lactobacillus Acidophilus, Alfalfa Leaf, Watercress, Parsley, 72 Trace Minerals, Rice Bran, Spirulina, Barley Green, Psyllium, Apple Pectin, Oat Bran, Bromelain, Papain, Chlorella & Chlorophyll.

3-Daily — The Vitamin Shoppe
Three capsules contain: Vitamin A Activity 25000 IU • Vitamin E 400 IU • Green Tea extract 50 mg • L-Glutathione 10 mg • Vitamin D 400 IU • Vitamin C 500 mg • CoQ10 100 mcg • Selenium 50 mcg •

© Copyright 2000, NATURAL MEDICINES COMPREHENSIVE DATABASE (209) 472-2244. For updated data, go to www.NaturalDatabase.com. • 1425

BRAND NAMES

BRAND NAMES

Pycnogenol 100 mcg • N-Acetyl Cysteine 15 mg • Molybdenum 50 mcg • Vitamin B1 50 mg • Vitamin B2 50 mg • Niacinamide 50 mg • Vitamin B6 50 mg • Vitamin B12 500 mcg • Folic Acid 800 mcg • Inositol 50 mg • Choline 50 mg • PABA 50 mg • Vitamin K 30 mcg • Biotin 50 mcg • Pantothenic Acid 50 mg • Calcium 100 mg • Magnesium 50 mg • Zinc 15 mg • Iron 10 mg • Iodine 150 mcg • Potassium 50 mg • Manganese 5 mg • Chromium 100 mcg • Boron 3 mg • Apple Pectin 50 mg • Betaine HCl 25 mg • Glutamic Acid 25 mg • Papain 25 mg • Pepsin 25 mg • Amylase 10 mcg • Lipase 10 mcg • Chlorophyll 10 mg • Spirulina 45 mg • Chlorella 45 mg • Barley Grass 45 mg • Alfalfa concentrate 45 mg • Bee Pollen 45 mg • Rutin 50 mg • Bioflavonoids 50 mg • Shark Cartilage 50 mg • Siberian Ginseng 45 mg • Royal Jelly 15 mg • Echinacea/Golden Seal 50 mg • Shiitake/Reishi Mushrooms 45 mg • RNA/DNA 45 mg. A concentrated blend of: broccoli, tomato, garlic, onions, cauliflower, brussel sprouts, carrots, parsley, watercress, and pure dry cold-pressed borage.

4-Diol 250 — AST Sports Science
Each capsule contains: 4-Androstenediol 250 mg.

50+ — Futurebiotics
Three capsules contain: Beta-carotene 10,000 IU • Vitamin C (buffered ascorbate) 300 mg • Vitamin E (natural) 100 IU • Vitamin D3 400 IU • Vitamin B1 25 mg • Vitamin B2 25 mg • Vitamin B3 (niacinamide) 25 mg • Vitamin B6 25 mg • Vitamin B12 100 mcg • Pantothenic Acid 25 mg • Biotin 300 mcg • Folic Acid 400 mcg • PABA 25 mg • Choline Bitartrate 50 mg • Inositol 25 mg • Calcium (ascorbate, carbonate, chelate) 200 mg • Magnesium (oxide, chelate) 3 mg • Potassium (chloride, iodide) 20 mg • Zinc (gluconate) 15 mg • Copper (gluconate) 2 mg • Manganese (amino acid chelate) 3 mg • Iodine (potassium iodide) 150 mcg • Selenium (amino acid chelate) 150 mcg • Chromium (amino acid chelate) 200 mcg • Molybdenum (amino acid chelate) 50 mcg • Siberian Ginseng 50 mg • Ginkgo Biloba 25 mg • Turmeric 25 mg • Garlic (Pure-Gar 1500 deodorized concentrate) 200 mg • Cayenne 25 mg • Gotu Kola 100 mg • Alfalfa 50 mg.

5-Diol 250 — AST Sports Science
Each capsule contains: 5-Androstenediol 250 mg.

7 Vitamin Treatment Cream — Orjene
Vitamin A • Vitamin B5, Vitamin C • Vitamin D • Vitamin E • Vitamin F • Vitamin H • Antioxidants. Fortified with Beta Carotene.

7-Keto — Enzymatic Therapy
Each capsule contains: 7-Keto DHEA 25 mg.

7-Keto DHEA — PhysioLogics
Each softgel contains: 3-Acetyl-7-Oxo Dehydroepiandrosterone 12.5 mg.

7-Keto Fuel — TwinLab
Each capsule contains: 7-Keto DHEA (3-Acetyl-7-Oxo-Dehydroepiandrosterone) 50 mg.

7-Keto Naturalean — Enzymatic Therapy
Each capsule contains: 7-Keto DHEA 100 mg • L-Tyrosine 100 mg • Asparagus Root Extract (Asparagus officinalis) standardized to contain 4.0-8.0% asparagosides 100 mg • Choline Bitartrate FCC 50 mg • Inositol 50 mg • Copper (Gluconate) 500 mcg • Manganese (Krebs Cycle Chelate) 500 mcg • Iodine (Potassium Iodine) 100 mcg. Other Ingredients: Magnesium stearate, Collodial Silicon dioxide, and Gelatin capsule.

8 Billion Acidophilus & Bifidus — Now
Each capsule contains: A guaranteed potency of: Lactobacillus Acidophilus 4 billion • Bifidobacterium Bifidum 3.2 billion •Bifidobacterium Longum 0.8 billion.

8% Plus Antioxidant Cuticle Cream — Jason
Vitamin A • Vitamin C • Vitamin E.

Potential Interactions Between
Drugs and Commonly Used Natural Medicines

This chart only contains those interactions that are likely to be clinically significant. It does not include all possible theoretical interactions nor does it include all incidents of case reports. For details on possible interactions between Drugs and Natural Medicines, see the listing for the specific natural medicine in the body of this database.

DRUGS	NATURAL MEDICINES
ANALGESICS/ANTI-INFLAMMATORIES	
Aspirin	Guar Gum • Licorice
Naloxone (*Narcan*)	Yohimbe
Narcotics	Gamma Hydroxybutyrate (GHB) • St. John's Wort
NSAIDs	Feverfew • Licorice
ANTI-INFECTIVES	
Antifungals	Brewer's Yeast
Itraconazole (*Sporanox*)	Grapefruit juice
Fluoroquinolones	Calcium • Iron • Magnesium • Zinc
Macrolide Antibiotics	Digitalis
Nonnucleoside Reverse Transcriptase Inhibitors (NNRTIs)	St. John's Wort
Penicillin	Guar Gum
Protease Inhibitors	St. John's Wort
Ritonavir (*Norvir*)	Gamma Hydroxybutyrate (GHB)
Saquinavir (*Fortovase, Invirase*)	Grapefruit juice • Gamma Hydroxybutyrate (GHB)
Quinine	Digitalis
Tetracyclines (*Achromycin, Sumycin*)	Calcium • Digitalis • Pectin
BLOOD MODIFIERS	
Anticoagulants/Antiplatelets	Acerola • American Ginseng • Bromelain • Chlorella • Danshen • Dong Quai • European Mistletoe • Fenugreek • Feverfew • Fish Oils • Gamma Linolenic Acid • Garlic • Ginger • Ginkgo leaf extract • Goldenseal • Guar Gum • Horse Chestnut seed • Panax Ginseng • Papain • Siberian Ginseng (Eleutherococcus) • Stinging Nettle above ground parts • Vitamin C • Vitamin E • Vitamin K
Heparin	Goldenseal
Warfarin	Acerola • Chlorella • Danshen • Devil's Claw • Dong Quai • Ginkgo leaf extract • Papain • Panax Ginseng • St. John's Wort • Vitamin C • Vitamin E • Vitamin K
CARDIOVASCULAR	
Antiarrhythmics	Aloe Latex
Antihypertensives	Devil's Claw • European Mistletoe • Fish Oils • Ginger • Goldenseal • Licorice • Stinging Nettle above ground parts • Yohimbe
Beta-Blockers	Coffee • Yohimbe

CHARTS

© Copyright 2000, Natural Medicines Comprehensive Database (209) 472-2244. For updated data, go to www.NaturalDatabase.com.

Potential Interactions Between
Drugs and Commonly Used Natural Medicines

This chart only contains those interactions that are likely to be clinically significant. It does not include all possible theoretical interactions nor does it include all incidents of case reports. For details on possible interactions between Drugs and Natural Medicines, see the listing for the specific natural medicine in the body of this database.

DRUGS	NATURAL MEDICINES
Calcium Channel Blockers (amlodipine, *Norvasc*; diltiazem, *Cardizem*; felodipine, *Plendil*; nicardipine, *Cardura*; nifedipine, *Procardia, Adalat*; nimodipine, *Nimotop*; nisoldipine, *Sular*)	Grapefruit juice • St. John's Wort
Cardiac Drugs	Devil's Claw • Digitalis • European Mistletoe • Ginger • Hawthorn
Carvedilol (*Coreg*)	Grapefruit juice
Cardiac Glycosides	Alder Buckthorn • Aloe Latex • Cascara • European Buckthorn
Digoxin (*Lanoxin*)	Digitalis • Ephedra • Guar Gum • Hawthorn • Licorice • Pectin • Psyllium • St. John's Wort
Cholesterol-Reducing Drugs	Gotu Kola
HMG-CoA Reductase Inhibitors ("statins")	Red Yeast (Monascus)
Lovastatin (*Mevacor*)	Grapefruit juice • Pectin
Simvastatin (*Zocor*)	Grapefruit juice
Clonidine (*Catapres*)	Yohimbe
Coronary Vasodilators	Hawthorn • L-Arginine
Diuretics	Aloe Latex
Potassium-Depleting Diuretics	Cascara • Gossypol • Licorice
Thiazide Diuretics	Ginkgo leaf extract
Guanabenz (*Wytensin*)	Yohimbe
Quinidine	Grapefruit juice
Reserpine	St. John's Wort

CENTRAL NERVOUS SYSTEM

DRUGS	NATURAL MEDICINES
5-HT1 Agonists ("Triptans")	St. John's Wort
Anesthetics	Evening Primrose Oil
Anticonvulsants	Sage
Carbamazepine (*Tegretol*)	Grapefruit juice • Psyllium
Antidepressants	European Mistletoe • SAMe • St. John's Wort
Clomipramine (*Anafranil*)	Grapefruit juice
Monoamine Oxidase Inhibitors (MAOIs)	American Ginseng • Black Tea • Brewer's Yeast • Caffeine • Cocoa • Coffee • Cola Nut • Ephedra • Fenugreek • Ginkgo leaf extract • Green Tea • Guarana • Panax Ginseng • Passion Flower • Phenylalanine • Wine • Yohimbe
Serotonin Agonists	5-HTP
Serotonin Antagonists	5-HTP
SSRIs	St. John's Wort • SAMe
Tricyclics	Yohimbe • St. John's Wort • SAMe

 © Copyright 2000, Natural Medicines Comprehensive Database (209) 472-2244. For updated data, go to www.NaturalDatabase.com.

Potential Interactions Between
Drugs and Commonly Used Natural Medicines

This chart only contains those interactions that are likely to be clinically significant. It does not include all possible theoretical interactions nor does it include all incidents of case reports. For details on possible interactions between Drugs and Natural Medicines, see the listing for the specific natural medicine in the body of this database.

DRUGS	NATURAL MEDICINES
Antipsychotics	American Ginseng • Coffee • Panax Ginseng • Siberian Ginseng (Eleutherococcus)
Carbidopa (*Lodosyn*)	5-HTP
Clozapine (*Clozaril*)	Black Tea • Caffeine • Cocoa • Coffee • Cola Nut • Green Tea • Guarana
CNS Depressants	German Chamomile • Hawthorn • Kava • Melatonin • Stinging Nettle above ground parts • Wine
Alcohol	Gamma Hydroxybutyrate (GHB) • Kava • Siberian Ginseng (Eleutherococcus) • Valerian
CNS Stimulants	American Ginseng • Panax Ginseng
Caffeine	Cocoa • Black Tea • Ephedra • Green Tea • Guarana • Panax Ginseng
Fenfluramine	St. John's Wort
Dopamine D2-Antagonists	Chasteberry
Levodopa (*Larodopa, Dopar*)	Kava
Lithium	Black Tea • Caffeine • Cocoa • Coffee • Green Tea • Guarana • Psyllium
Phenothiazines	Evening Primrose Oil • Yohimbe
Sedatives	Goldenseal • Gotu Kola • Kava • Passion Flower • Siberian Ginseng (Eleutherococcus) • Valerian
Barbiturates	Ginger • Goldenseal • Kava • Passion Flower • Siberian Ginseng (Eleutherococcus) • St. John's Wort • Valerian
Benzodiazepines	Kava • Melatonin • Valerian
Alprazolam (*Xanax*)	Kava
Midazolam (*Versed*), Triazolam (*Halcion*)	Grapefruit juice
Buspirone (*Buspar*)	Grapefruit juice

DIABETES

Insulin	Chromium • Coffee • Glucomannan
Oral Hypoglycemics	Alpha Lipoic Acid • American Ginseng • Coffee • Devil's Claw • Ephedra • Fenugreek • Garlic • Ginger • Gotu Kola • Glucomannan • Glucosamine Hydrochloride • Glucosamine Sulfate • Guar Gum • Horse Chestnut seed • Panax Ginseng • Psyllium • Siberian Ginseng (Eleutherococcus) • Stinging Nettle above ground parts
Metformin (*Glucophage*)	Guar Gum

© Copyright 2000, Natural Medicines Comprehensive Database (209) 472-2244. For updated data, go to www.NaturalDatabase.com. • 1429

Potential Interactions Between
Drugs and Commonly Used Natural Medicines

This chart only contains those interactions that are likely to be clinically significant. It does not include all possible theoretical interactions nor does it include all incidents of case reports. For details on possible interactions between Drugs and Natural Medicines, see the listing for the specific natural medicine in the body of this database.

DRUGS	NATURAL MEDICINES
GASTROINTESTINALS	
H2 Blockers	Iron • Peppermint Oil
Laxatives	Cascara
Stimulant Laxatives	Digitalis
Metoclopramide (*Reglan*)	Chasteberry
Proton Pump Inhibitors	Iron • Peppermint Oil
HORMONES	
Corticosteroids	Alder Buckthorn • Aloe Latex • Cascara • European Buckthorn • Fenugreek • Licorice
Hormone Therapy	American Ginseng • Chasteberry • Fenugreek • Licorice • Panax Ginseng • Saw Palmetto • Siberian Ginseng (Eleutherococcus)
Estrogenic Drugs	Androstenedione
Estrogens (17-beta-estradiol, ethinyl-estradiol)	Grapefruit juice • Soy
Oral Contraceptives	Chasteberry • Saw Palmetto • St. John's Wort
Oxytocin (*Pitocin*)	Ephedra
Thyroid Hormones	Bugleweed • Calcium • Horseradish • Red Yeast (Monascus)
IMMUNOSUPPRESSANTS	
Cyclosporine (*Neoral, Sandimmune*)	Grapefruit juice • St. John's Wort • Wine
Immunosuppressants	Andrographis • Astragalus • Echinacea • European Mistletoe
MISCELLANEOUS	
Bisphosphonates	Calcium • Coffee
Cytochrome P450-3A Inhibitors	Red Yeast (Monascus)
Photosensitizing Drugs	St. John's Wort
Penicillamine (*Cuprimine, Depen*)	Copper
Potassium-Depleting Drugs	Alder Buckthorn • Digitalis • European Buckthorn • Licorice
Protein-Bound Drugs	Horse Chestnut seed
Urine Acidifying Drugs	Uva Ursi
RESPIRATORY	
Beta-Adrenergic Agonists & Sympathomimetics	Black Tea • Caffeine • Cocoa • Cola Nut • Green Tea • Guarana • Yohimbe
Theophylline (*Theo-Dur*)	Black Tea • Caffeine • Cocoa • Cola Nut • Ephedra • Green Tea • Guarana • St. John's Wort

CHARTS

Potential Interactions Between
Commonly Used Natural Medicines and Drugs

This chart only contains those interactions that are likely to be clinically significant. It does not include all possible theoretical interactions nor does it include all incidents of case reports. For details on possible interactions between Natural Medicines and Drugs, see the listing for the specific natural medicine in the body of this database.

NATURAL MEDICINES	DRUGS
5-HTP	Carbidopa (*Lodosyn*) • Serotonin Agonists • Serotonin Antagonists
Acerola	Anticoagulants/Antiplatelets • Warfarin (*Coumadin*)
Alder Buckthorn	Cardiac Glycosides • Corticosteroids • Potassium-Depleting Drugs
Aloe Latex	Antiarrhythmics • Cardiac Glycosides • Corticosteroids • Diuretics
Alpha Lipoic Acid	Antidiabetes Drugs
American Ginseng	Anticoagulants/Antiplatelets • Antidiabetes Drugs • Antipsychotics • Hormone Therapy • Monoamine Oxidase Inhibitors (MAOIs) • Stimulants • Warfarin (*Coumadin*)
Andrographis	Immunosuppressants
Androstenedione	Estrogenic Drugs
Astragalus	Immunosuppressants
Black Tea	Beta-Adrenergic Agonists • Clozapine (*Clozaril*) • CNS Stimulants • Lithium • Monoamine Oxidase Inhibitors (MAOIs) • Theophylline (*Theo-Dur*)
Brewer's Yeast	Antifungals • Monoamine Oxidase Inhibitors (MAOIs)
Bromelain	Anticoagulants/Antiplatelets
Bugleweed	Thyroid Hormones
Caffeine	Beta-Adrenergic Agonists • Clozapine (*Clozaril*) • CNS Stimulants • Ephedrine • Lithium • Monoamine Oxidase Inhibitors (MAOIs) • Theophylline (*Theo-Dur*)
Calcium	Bisphosphonates • Fluoroquinolones • Levothyroxine • Tetracyclines
Cascara	Cardiac Glycosides • Corticosteroids • Laxatives • Potassium-Depleting Diuretics

C H A R T S

Potential Interactions Between
Commonly Used Natural Medicines and Drugs

This chart only contains those interactions that are likely to be clinically significant. It does not include all possible theoretical interactions nor does it include all incidents of case reports. For details on possible interactions between Drugs and Natural Medicines, see the listing for the specific natural medicine in the body of this database.

NATURAL MEDICINES	DRUGS
Chasteberry	Dopamine D2-Antagonists • Hormone Therapy • Metoclopramide (*Reglan*) • Oral Contraceptives
Chlorella	Anticoagulants/Antiplatelets • Warfarin (*Coumadin*)
Chromium	Insulin • Zinc
Cocoa	Beta-Adrenergic Agonists • Caffeine • Clozapine (*Clozaril*) • Lithium • Monoamine Oxidase Inhibitors (MAOIs) • Theophylline (*Theo-Dur*)
Coffee	Alendronate • Beta-Adrenergic Agonists • Caffeine • Clozapine (*Clozaril*) • CNS Stimulants • Ephedrine • Insulin • Lithium • Monoamine Oxidase Inhibitors (MAOIs) • Oral Hypoglycemics • Theophylline (*Theo-Dur*)
Cola Nut	Beta-Adrenergic Agonists • Caffeine • Clozapine (*Clozaril*) • CNS Stimulants • Ephedrine • Lithium • Monoamine Oxidase Inhibitors (MAOIs) • Theophylline (*Theo-Dur*)
Copper	Penicillamine (*Cuprimine, Depen*)
Danshen	Anticoagulants/Antiplatelets • Warfarin (*Coumadin*)
Devil's Claw	Antidiabetes Drugs • Antihypertensives • Antihypotensives (Vasopressors) • Cardiac Drugs • Warfarin (*Coumadin*)
Digitalis	Cardiac Drugs • Digoxin (*Lanoxin*) • Macrolide Antibiotics • Potassium-Depleting Drugs • Quinine • Stimulant Laxatives • Tetracyclines
Dong Quai	Anticoagulants/Antiplatelets • Warfarin (*Coumadin*)
Echinacea	Immunosuppressants
Eleutherococcus	See Siberian Ginseng

• © Copyright 2000, Natural Medicines Comprehensive Database (209) 472-2244. For updated data, go to www.NaturalDatabase.com.

CHARTS

Potential Interactions Between
Commonly Used Natural Medicines and Drugs

This chart only contains those interactions that are likely to be clinically significant. It does not include all possible theoretical interactions nor does it include all incidents of case reports. For details on possible interactions between Natural Medicines and Drugs, see the listing for the specific natural medicine in the body of this database.

NATURAL MEDICINES	DRUGS
Ephedra	Antidiabetes Drugs • Caffeine • Digoxin (*Lanoxin*) • Monoamine Oxidase Inhibitors (MAOIs) • Oxytocin (*Pitocin*) • Theophylline (*Theo-Dur*)
European Buckthorn	Cardiac Glycosides • Potassium-Depleting Drugs
European Mistletoe	Anticoagulants/Antiplatelets • Antidepressants • Antihypertensives • Antihypotensives (Vasopressors) • Cardiac Drugs • Immunosuppressants
Evening Primrose Oil	Anesthetics • Phenothiazines
Fenugreek	Anticoagulants/Antiplatelets • Antidiabetes Drugs • Corticosteroids • Hormone Therapy • Monoamine Oxidase Inhibitors (MAOIs)
Feverfew	Anticoagulants/Antiplatelets • NSAIDs
Fish Oils	Anticoagulants/Antiplatelets • Antihypertensives
Gamma Hydroxybutyrate (GHB)	Alcohol • Narcotic Analgesics • Ritonavir • Saquinavir
Gamma Linolenic Acid	Anticoagulants /Antiplatelets
Garlic	Anticoagulants/Antiplatelets • Antidiabetes Drugs
German Chamomile	Sedatives
Ginger	Anticoagulants/Antiplatelets • Antidiabetes Drugs • Antihypertensives • Antihypotensives (Vasopressors) • Barbiturates • Cardiac Drugs
Ginkgo leaf extract	Anticoagulants /Antiplatelets • Monoamine Oxidase Inhibitors (MAOIs) • Thiazide Diuretics • Warfarin (*Coumadin*)
Ginseng	See American Ginseng, Panax Ginseng and Siberian Ginseng
Glucomannan	Insulin • Oral Hypoglycemics

CHARTS

© Copyright 2000, Natural Medicines Comprehensive Database (209) 472-2244. For updated data, go to www.NaturalDatabase.com. • 1433

Potential Interactions Between
Commonly Used Natural Medicines and Drugs

This chart only contains those interactions that are likely to be clinically significant. It does not include all possible theoretical interactions nor does it include all incidents of case reports. For details on possible interactions between Drugs and Natural Medicines, see the listing for the specific natural medicine in the body of this database.

NATURAL MEDICINES	DRUGS
Glucosamine Hydrochloride	Antidiabetes Drugs
Glucosamine Sulfate	Antidiabetes Drugs
Goldenseal	Antihypertensives • Barbiturates • Heparin • Sedative Drugs
Gossypol	Potassium-Depleting Diuretics
Gotu Kola	Antidiabetes Drugs • Cholesterol-Reducing Drugs • Sedative Drugs
Grapefruit juice	Benzodiazepines (midazolam, *Versed*; triazolam, *Halcion*) • Buspirone (*BuSpar*) • Calcium Channel Blockers (amlodipine, *Norvasc*; diltiazem, *Cardizem*; felodipine, *Plendil*; nicardipine, *Cardura*; nifedipine, *Procardia, Adalat*; nimodipine, *Nimotop*; nisoldipine, *Sular*) • Carbamazepine (*Tegretol*) • Carvedilol (*Coreg*) • Clomipramine (*Anafranil*) • Cyclosporine (*Neoral, Sandimmune*) • Estrogens (17-beta-estradiol, ethinyl-estradiol) • HMG-CoA Reductase Inhibitors (lovastatin, *Mevacor*; simvastatin, *Zocor*) • Itraconazole (*Sporanox*) • Quinidine • Saquinavir (*Fortovase, Invirase*)
Green Tea	Beta-Adrenergic Agonists • Clozapine (*Clozaril*) • Ephedrine • Lithium • Monoamine Oxidase Inhibitors (MAOIs) • Theophylline (*Theo-Dur*)
Guar Gum	Anticoagulants/Antiplatelets • Antidiabetes Drugs • Aspirin • Digoxin (*Lanoxin*) • Metformin (*Glucophage*) • Penicillin
Guarana	Beta-Adrenergic Agonists • Clozapine (*Clozaril*) • CNS Stimulants • Lithium • Monoamine Oxidase Inhibitors (MAOIs) • Theophylline (*Theo-Dur*)
Hawthorn	Cardic Drugs • CNS Depressants • Coronary Vasodilators • Digoxin (*Lanoxin*)
Horse Chestnut seed	Anticoagulants/Antiplatelets • Antidiabetes Drugs • Protein-Bound Drugs
Horseradish	Thyroid Hormones

1434 • © Copyright 2000, Natural Medicines Comprehensive Database (209) 472-2244. For updated data, go to www.NaturalDatabase.com.

Potential Interactions Between
Commonly Used Natural Medicines and Drugs

This chart only contains those interactions that are likely to be clinically significant. It does not include all possible theoretical interactions nor does it include all incidents of case reports. For details on possible interactions between Natural Medicines and Drugs, see the listing for the specific natural medicine in the body of this database.

NATURAL MEDICINES	DRUGS
Iron	Fluoroquinolones • H2 Blockers • Proton Pump Inhibitors
Kava	Alcohol • Barbiturates • Benzodiazepines (alprazolam, *Xanax*) • CNS Depressants • Levodopa (*Larodopa, Dopar*) • Sedative Drugs
L-Arginine	Coronary Vasdodilators
Licorice	Antihypertensives • Aspirin • Corticosteroids • Digoxin (*Lanoxin*) • Hormone Therapy • NSAIDs • Potassium-Depleting Drugs
Magnesium	Fluoroquinolones
Melatonin	Benzodiazepines • CNS Depressants
Monascus	See Red Yeast
Panax Ginseng	Anticoagulants/Antiplatelets • Antidiabetes Drugs • Antipsychotics • Caffeine • Hormone Therapy • Monoamine Oxidase Inhibitors (MAOIs) • Stimulants • Warfarin (*Coumadin*)
Papain	Anticoagulants/Antiplatelets • Warfarin (*Coumadin*)
Passion Flower	Barbiturates • Monoamine Oxidase Inhibitors (MAOIs) • Sedative Drugs
Pectin	Beta-Carotene • Digoxin (*Lanoxin*) • Lovastatin (*Mevacor*) • Tetracyclines (*Achromycin, Sumycin*)
Peppermint Oil	H2 Blockers (*Zantac, Tagamet, Pepcid*) • Proton Pump Inhibitors (*Prilosec, Prevacid*)
Psyllium	Antidiabetes Drugs • Carbamazepine (*Tegretol*) • Digoxin (*Lanoxin*) • Insulin • Lithium • Warfarin (*Coumadin*)
Phenylalanine	Monoamine Oxidase Inhibitors (MAOIs)
Red Yeast	Cytochrome P450-3A Inhibitors • HMG-CoA Reductase Inhibitors ("statins") • Thyroid Hormones
Sage	Anticonvulsants

© Copyright 2000, Natural Medicines Comprehensive Database (209) 472-2244. For updated data, go to www.NaturalDatabase.com. • 1435

Potential Interactions Between
Commonly Used Natural Medicines and Drugs

This chart only contains those interactions that are likely to be clinically significant. It does not include all possible theoretical interactions nor does it include all incidents of case reports. For details on possible interactions between Drugs and Natural Medicines, see the listing for the specific natural medicine in the body of this database.

NATURAL MEDICINES	DRUGS
SAMe	Antidepressants • SSRIs • Tricyclics
Saw Palmetto	Hormone Therapy • Oral Contraceptives
Siberian Ginseng	Alcohol • Anticoagulants/Antiplatelets • Antidiabetes Drugs • Antipsychotics • Barbiturates • Hormone Therapy • Sedative Drugs
Soy	Estrogen
St. John's wort	5-HT1 Receptor Agonists ("Triptans") • Antidepressants • Barbiturates • Calcium Channel Blockers • Cyclosporine • Digoxin • Fenfluramine • Narcotics • Nonnucleoside Reverse Transcriptase Inhibitors (NNRTIs) • Oral Contraceptives • Photosensitizing Drugs • Protease Inhibitors • SSRIs • Theophylline • Tricyclics • Warfarin (*Coumadin*)
Stinging Nettle above ground parts	Anticoagulants/Antiplatelets • Antidiabetes Drugs • Antihypertensives • Antihypotensives (Vasopressors) • CNS Depressants
Uva Ursi	Urine Acidifying Drugs
Valerian	Alcohol • Barbiturates • Benzodiazepines • Sedative Drugs
Vitamin C	Anticoagulants/Antiplatelets • Warfarin (*Coumadin*)
Vitamin E	Anticoagulants/Antiplatelets • Warfarin (*Coumadin*)
Vitamin K	Anticoagulants/Antiplatelets • Warfarin (*Coumadin*)
Wine	CNS Depressants • Cyclosporine • Monoamine Oxidase Inhibitors (MAOIs)
Yohimbe	Antihypertensives • Beta-Blockers • Clonidine (*Catapres*) • Guanabenz (*Wytensin*) • Monoamine Oxidase Inhibitors (MAOIs) • Naloxone (*Narcan*) • Phenothiazines • Sympathomimetics • Tricyclic Antidepressants
Zinc	Fluoroquinolones

CHARTS

 © Copyright 2000, Natural Medicines Comprehensive Database (209) 472-2244. For updated data, go to www.NaturalDatabase.com.

THERAPEUTIC EFFICACY

This list shows which natural medicines are likely to be effective for certain medical conditions. The list is organized by disease state or by drug class. Under each heading natural medicines are listed according to their common names. This list was compiled by searching through this *Natural Medicines Comprehensive Database* to find each natural medicine that is identified as "LIKELY EFFECTIVE" or "EFFECTIVE" for a medical condition. For more information on any of the natural medicines identified in this list, review the listing for that medicine in the database.

ACETAMINOPHEN POISONING
N-Acetyl Cysteine

ACRYLONITRILE POISONING
N-Acetyl Cysteine

AMENORRHEA, SECONDARY
Progesterone

ANALGESIC, TOPICAL
Capsicum

ANESTHETIC, TOPICAL
Cocaine
Procaine

ANORECTAL DISORDERS
Witch hazel extract (Hamamelis water)

ANTIDEPRESSANTS
St. John's wort
S-Adenosylmethionine (SAMe)

ANTISEPTIC
Iodine (topically)

ANXIETY
Kava

ARIBOFLAVINOSIS
Riboflavin (Vitamin B2)

ARTHRITIS

Osteoarthritis
Capsicum
Chondroitin Sulfate
Glucosamine Sulfate
S-Adenosylmethionine (SAMe)

Rheumatoid Arthritis
Capsicum

BENIGN PROSTATIC HYPERPLASIA
Beta-Sitosterol
Pygeum
Saw Palmetto

BERIBERI
Thiamine (Vitamin B1)

BIOTIN DEFICIENCY
Biotin

BIRTH CONTROL (MALE)
Gossypol

BIRTH DEFECTS (NEURAL TUBE)
Folic Acid

BLOOD PRESSURE REDUCTION
Potassium

BRONCHOPULMONARY DISORDERS
N-Acetyl Cysteine

BURNS
Camphor (topically)

CALCIUM DEFICIENCY
Calcium
Dolomite

CATARACT SURGERY
Chondroitin

COLD SORES
Camphor (topically)

COLORECTAL CANCER (REDUCE RISK)
Calcium

**CONDYLOMATA ACUMINATA
(GENITAL AND ANAL WARTS)**
Podophyllum (topically)

CONGESTIVE HEART FAILURE
Coenzyme Q 10
Hawthorn (leaf, flower)
Hawthorn (leaf with flower extract)

CONSTIPATION
Alder Buckthorn
Apple
Black Psyllium
Blond Psyllium
Cascara
Castor Oil
European Buckthorn
Glycerol
Magnesium
Senna

CONTRACEPTION (MALE)
Gossypol

© Copyright 2000, Natural Medicines Comprehensive Database (209) 472-2244. For updated data, go to www.NaturalDatabase.com.

COPPER DEFICIENCY ANEMIA
Copper

CYSTATHIONINURIA
Pyridoxine (Vitamin B6)

CYSTIC FIBROSIS
N-Acetyl Cysteine

DEMENTIA
Ginkgo leaf extract

DEPRESSION
St. John's Wort
S-Adenosylmethionine (SAMe)

DERMATITIS
Lecithin

DIABETIC NEUROPATHY PAIN
Capsicum

DIARRHEA
Calcium
Pectin

DRY SKIN
Alpha Hydroxy Acids
Lecithin

ECLAMPSIA
Magnesium

EMETIC
Ipecac

ENCEPHALOPATHY (PORTOSYSTEMIC)
Branched-Chain Amino Acids

**ENCEPHALOPATHY
(SUBACUTE, NECROTIZING)**
Thiamine

ERYTHROPOETIC PROTOPORPHYRIA
Beta-carotene
Canthaxanthin

EXPECTORANT
Anise

FIBROIDS
Podophyllum (topically)

FLUORIDE (REDUCING EXCESS)
Calcium

FOLIC ACID DEFICIENCY
Folic Acid

GASTROINTESTINAL SPASM
Belladonna

GOITER
Iodine

HEART DISEASE RISK (REDUCING)
Oat bran

**HEMOLYTIC ANEMIA
(PREMATURE INFANTS)**
Vitamin E

HEMORRHOIDS
Camphor (topically)
Witch hazel

**HEPATIC DYSFUNCTION
(DUE TO PARENTERAL NUTRITION)**
Choline
Lecithin

HEREDITARY SIDEROBLASTIC ANEMIA
Pyridoxine (Vitamin B6)

HOMOCYSTINURIA
Betaine, anhydrous
Pyridoxine (Vitamin B6)

HORMONE THERAPY
Progesterone

HYPERCALCEMIA
Phosphate (sodium, potassium)

HYPERCALCIURIA
Potassium

HYPERCHOLESTEROLEMIA
Avocado
Blond Psyllium
Flaxseed
Guar Gum
Niacin
Oat Bran
Red Yeast
Sitostanol
Soy

High-Density Lipoprotein (HDL) Improvement
Avocado
Niacin

Low-Density Lipoprotein (LDL) Reduction
Avocado
Blond Psyllium
Guar Gum
Niacin
Oat bran
Sitostanol
Soy

**Very Low-Density Lipoprotein (VLDL)
Reduction**
Niacin

HYPERHOMOCYSTEINEMIA
Folic Acid

HYPEROXALURIA
Pyridoxine (Vitamin B6)

HYPERTENSION
Potassium

HYPERTHYROIDISM
Iodine

HYPERTRIGLYCERIDEMIA
Fish Oils
Niacin
Red Yeast

HYPOCALCEMIA
Calcium
Dolomite
Vitamin D (calcifediol, calcitriol,
dihydrotachysterol, ergocalciferol)

HYPOKALEMIA
Potassium

HYPOPHOSPHATEMIA
Phosphate salts
Vitamin D (calcitriol, dihydrotachysterol,
ergocalciferol) with phosphate

HYPOPROTHROMBINEMIA
Vitamin K (phytonadione, menadiol)

INFANT FORMULA REPLACEMENT
Whey Protein

INFERTILITY
Progesterone

INHALATION INJURY
N-Acetyl Cysteine

INSOMNIA
Melatonin

INTESTINAL FLORA RESTORATION
Lactobacillus acidophilus

IRON ABSORPTION (IMPROVING)
Vitamin C

IRON DEFICIENCY ANEMIA
Iron

ITCHING
Camphor (topically)

LACTOSE INTOLERANCE
Lactase

LAND-ADAMS SYNDROME
5-HTP

LAXATIVE
Alder Buckthorn
Blond Psyllium
Black Psyllium
Cascara
Castor Oil
European Buckthorn
Guar Gum
Magnesium
Olive Oil
Phosphate salts
Senna
Wheat Bran
Yellow Dock

L-CARNITINE DEFICIENCY
L-Carnitine

LIVER DISEASE
S-Adenosylmethionine (SAMe)

MAGNESIUM DEFICIENCY
Dolomite
Magnesium

MAPLE SUGAR URINE DISEASE
Thiamine (Vitamin B1)

MASTALGIA/MASTODYNIA
Evening Primrose Oil

MENOPAUSE SYMPTOMS
Black Cohosh

MENTAL ALERTNESS
Caffeine
Coffee
Guarana

METHEMOGLOBINEMIA, IDIOPATHIC
Acerola
Vitamin C

METHOTREXATE TOXICITY
Folic Acid

MUCOLYTIC ADJUNCT
N-Acetyl Cysteine

MUSCLE MASS (INCREASING)
Creatine

NERVOUSNESS
Kava

NEURAL TUBE DEFECTS
Folic Acid

CHARTS

NEURALGIAS
Capsicum

NEURITIS OF PREGNANCY
Thiamine (Vitamin B1)

NEURITIS, PERIPHERAL
Thiamine (Vitamin B1)

NIGHT BLINDNESS
Vitamin A

OPHTHALMOLOGY, ANESTHESIA
Cocaine

OPHTHALMOLOGY, SURGERY
Chymotrypsin

ORTHOPEDIC SURGERY
Coral

OSTEITIS FIBROSA
Vitamin D (calcitriol, dihydrotachysterol)

OSTEOARTHRITIS
Capsicum
Chondroitin Sulfate
Glucosamine Sulfate
S-Adenosylmethionine (SAMe)

OSTEODYSTROPHY (HEPATIC)
Vitamin D (calcifediol)

OSTEODYSTROPHY (RENAL)
Vitamin D (calcifediol, dihydrotachysterol)

OSTEOMALACIA
Vitamin D (cholecalciferol, ergocalciferol)

OSTEOPENIA
Vitamin D (calcifediol, calcitriol,
cholecalciferol)

OSTEOPOROSIS
Calcium
Ipriflavone
Vitamin D (calcifediol, cholecalciferol)

PANCREATIC INSUFFICIENCY
Pancreatin

PELLAGRA
Niacin
Niacinamide

PRETERM LABOR
Magnesium

POISONING
Activated Charcoal
Ipecac

PREMENSTRUAL SYNDROME
Calcium

PRIMARY HYPEROXALURIA
Pyridoxine (Vitamin B6)

PSORIASIS
Vitamin D (calcitriol, calcipotriene)

RADIOACTIVE IODIDES EMERGENCY
Iodine

RENAL FAILURE (PHOSPHATE BINDING)
Calcium

RENAL STONE (PREVENTION)
Phosphate salts

RESTLESSNESS
Kava

RHEUMATOID ARTHRITIS
Capsicum

RIBOFLAVIN DEFICIENCY
Riboflavin (Vitamin B2)

RICKETS
Vitamin D (calcitriol, cholecalciferol,
ergocalciferol)

SCURVY
Acerola
Vitamin C

SIDEROBLASTIC ANEMIA
Pyridoxine (Vitamin B6)

SLEEP DISTURBANCE
Melatonin

SORE THROAT
Slippery Elm

SPOROTRICHOSIS, CUTANEOUS
Iodine

SPORTS PERFORMANCE AID
Creatine

STRESS
Kava

STIMULANT
Caffeine
Coffee
Guarana

SUN-DAMAGED SKIN
Alpha Hydroxy Acids

C
H
A
R
T
S

THALLIUM-201 REDISTRIBUTION
Ribose

THIAMINE DEFICIENCY SYNDROMES
Thiamine (Vitamin B1)

THYROID HORMONE RESISTANCE (PITUITARY)
Tiratricol

THYROID STORM
Iodine

TYROSINEMIA
Acerola
Vitamin C

URINARY ALKALINIZATION
Potassium

VASOCONSTRICTOR, LOCAL
Cocaine

VENOUS INSUFFICIENCY SYMPTOMS
Horse Chestnut seed (standard extract)

VITAMIN A DEFICIENCY
Vitamin A

VITAMIN B6 DEFICIENCY
Pyridoxine (Vitamin B6)

VITAMIN C DEFICIENCY
Acerola
Vitamin C

VITAMIN E DEFICIENCY
Vitamin E

WARTS
Podophyllum (topically)

WATER PURIFICATION
Iodine

XANTHURENIC ACIDURIA
Pyridoxine (Vitamin B6)

XEROPHTHALMIA
Vitamin A

ZINC DEFICIENCY
Zinc

**C
H
A
R
T
S**

Drug Influences on Nutrient Levels and Depletion

Some medications can affect the levels of certain nutrients in the body. There is considerable interest in using nutritional supplements to counteract these possible drug-induced "nutrient depletions." The chart below shows the current scientific understanding of these relationships, and suggested actions.

DRUGS (includes some representative U.S. and Canadian Brand Names.)	NUTRIENT DEPLETED	POSSIBLE MECHANISM	COMMENTS & REFERENCES
ANTI-INFECTIVES			
Amphotericin B (*Abelcet, Amphotec, AmBisome, Fungizone Intravenous*)	Magnesium Potassium Sodium	The mechanism of nephrotoxicity involves direct cell membrane actions to increase permeability, as well as indirect effects secondary to activation of intrarenal mechanisms (tubuloglomerular feedback) and/or release of mediators (thromboxane A2). Consult individual product monographs for specific instructions on prevention of nephrotoxicity.	Sodium loading may be effective in reducing nephrotoxicity, but this may be a problem in patients with cardiac or hepatic disease. In some patients, hydration and sodium repletion prior to amphotericin B administration may reduce the risk of developing nephrotoxicity. Supplemental alkali medication may decrease renal tubular acidosis complications. Monitor renal function frequently during amphotericin B therapy. Consult individual product monographs for specific instructions. [4554-4555]
Antibiotics: Cephalosporins, Fluoroquinolones, Isoniazid, Macrolides, Penicillins, Sulfonamides, Tetracyclines, Trimethoprim/Sulfamethoxazole	Intestinal Micro Flora (B Vitamins, Vitamin K)	Destruction of normal intestinal microflora leads to decreased production of various B vitamins and vitamin K.	Various beneficial intestinal microflora are eliminated when antibiotics are taken. Some proponents of probiotics recommend taking them for 2-3 weeks during and after a course of antibiotics. Colonic bacteria are responsible for the production of various B vitamins and vitamin K. The nutritional importance of the quantity of vitamins produced by these organisms may not be clinically significant. Give supplements of these vitamins only if clinical judgment warrants it. [4434-4443]
Cycloserine (*Seromycin*)	Folic Acid	Folate antagonism. (Decreases the availability of substrates required for nucleic acid biosynthesis.)	Although the depletion of folic acid can be documented, it may or may not be clinically significant. Give supplements of this nutrient only if clinical judgment warrants it. [4453,4531]
Fluoroquinolones (Also See Antibiotics): Ciprofloxacin (*Cipro*), Enoxacin (*Penetrex*), Gatifloxacin (*Tequin*), Levofloxacin (*Levaquin*), Lomefloxacin (*Maxaquin*), Moxifloxacin (*Avelox*), Norfloxacin (*Noroxin*), Ofloxacin (*Floxin*), Sparfloxacin (*Zagam*), Trovafloxacin (*Trovan*)	Zinc	Decreases dietary zinc absorption.	The clinical significance is yet to be determined, and the need for supplementation has not been adequately studied. Give supplements of this vitamin only if clinical judgment warrants it. [506,828,2682]

© Copyright 2000, Natural Medicines Comprehensive Database (209) 472-2244. For updated data, go to www.NaturalDatabase.com. • 1443

CHARTS

Drug Influences on Nutrient Levels and Depletion

Some medications can affect the levels of certain nutrients in the body. There is considerable interest in using nutritional supplements to counteract these possible drug-induced "nutrient depletions." The chart below shows the current scientific understanding of these relationships, and suggested actions.

DRUGS (includes some representative U.S. and Canadian Brand Names.)	NUTRIENT DEPLETED	POSSIBLE MECHANISM	COMMENTS & REFERENCES
Isoniazid (*Laniazid*) (Also See Antibiotics)	Vitamin B6	Interferes with vitamin B6 metabolism.	Patients receiving > 10 mg/kg/day of INH should be supplemented with 50 - 100 mg of pyridoxine per day. [4480-4482]
Pentamidine (*NebuPent, Pentacarinat, Pentam 300*)	Folic Acid	Impairs folate absorption.	The need for supplementation has not been adequately studied. Give supplements of this vitamin only if clinical judgment warrants it. [4531]
Pyrimethamine (*Daraprim*)	Folic Acid	Folate antagonism. (Binds to dihydrofolate reductase)	At lower pyrimethamine doses, the need for supplementation has not been adequately studied. Give supplements of this vitamin only if clinical judgment warrants it. At larger pyrimethamine doses (those required to treat toxoplasmosis), if signs of folate deficiency develop, folinic acid (*Leucovorin*) should be administered in a dosage of 5 – 15 mg/day (orally, IV, or IM) until normal hematopoiesis is restored. [4425,4532]
Rifampin (*Rifadin, Rimactane, Rofact*)	Vitamin D	Inhibition of enzymes necessary for the formation of the most active metabolite of vitamin D (1,25-dihydroxyvitamin D).	There is no consensus that vitamin D supplementation is always required. Give supplements of this vitamin only if clinical judgment warrants it. [4513-4514]
Tetracyclines (Also See Antibiotics): Tetracycline (*Achromycin V, Panmycin, Robitet, Robicaps, Sumycin, Teline, Tetracap, Tetracyn, Tetralan*), Demeclocycline (*Declomycin*), Doxycycline (*Bio-Tab, Doryx, Doxy Caps, Doxychel, Doxychel Hyclate, Monodox, Periostat, Vibra-Tabs, Vibramycin*), Minocycline (*Dynacinn, Vectrin*), Oxytetracycline (*Terramycin, Uri-Tet*)	Calcium Iron Zinc	Tetracyclines may form complexes with calcium, iron and zinc in the GI tract and thus prevent absorption of adequate amounts of these elements. Doxycycline does not reduce zinc absorption.	Tetracycline doses should be staggered 2 hrs before or 2 hrs after calcium-containing foods or calcium, iron, or zinc supplements to avoid this interaction. Consider giving supplemental calcium doses of 0.8 - 1.5 g/day. Give supplements of these nutrients only if clinical judgment warrants it. [15,506,4412,4453,4531,4549-4550]
Trimethoprim (*Proloprim, Trimpex*)	Folic Acid	Folate antagonism. (Binds to dihydrofolate reductase.)	Mild folate deficiency may develop in patients on long-term or high-dose therapy. The need for supplementation has not been adequately studied. Give supplements of this vitamin only if clinical judgment warrants it. [4468]

1444 • © Copyright 2000, Natural Medicines Comprehensive Database (209) 472-2244. For updated data, go to www.NaturalDatabase.com.

Drug Influences on Nutrient Levels and Depletion

Some medications can affect the levels of certain nutrients in the body. There is considerable interest in using nutritional supplements to counteract these possible drug-induced "nutrient depletions." The chart below shows the current scientific understanding of these relationships, and suggested actions.

DRUGS (includes some representative U.S. and Canadian Brand Names.)	NUTRIENT DEPLETED	POSSIBLE MECHANISM	COMMENTS & REFERENCES
Trimethoprim/Sulfamethoxazole (Also See Antibiotics): (*Bactrim, Cotrim, Septra, Sulfatrim*)	Folic Acid	Folate antagonism. (Binds to dihydrofolate reductase.)	Mild folate deficiency may develop in patients on long-term or high-dose therapy (trimethoprim component). The need for supplementation has not been adequately studied. Give supplements of this vitamin only if clinical judgment warrants it. [4468]

ANTIGOUT/ANTIRHEUMATIC

DRUGS	NUTRIENT DEPLETED	POSSIBLE MECHANISM	COMMENTS & REFERENCES
Colchicine	Vitamin B12	Decreases intestinal absorption of vitamin B12.	There is evidence that patients on colchicine may have slightly lower levels of vitamin B12, but this does not represent a scientific consensus. Give supplements of this vitamin only if clinical judgment warrants it. [4543-4545]
Methotrexate (*Rheumatrex*)	Folic Acid	Folate antagonism. (Binds to dihydrofolate reductase.)	Recommend supplementation in patients receiving MTX for psoriasis, RA, and other indications requiring prolonged MTX therapy. Common but less serious toxicities of MTX include mucositis, mild alopecia, and GI disturbances, which may be caused by folate depletion. These toxicities are often treated or prevented with the use of folate supplementation. Folic acid at a dosage of 1 mg per day or 7 mg once a week is less expensive and less complicated than the use of folinic acid. Neither low-dose folate (1 mg per day) nor folinic acid ($\leq$ 5 mg per week) interferes with the beneficial effect of MTX. [4492-4494,4546]
Penicillamine (*Cuprimine, Depen*)	Copper Magnesium Vitamin B6 Zinc	Vitamin B6 - Formation of a complex between penicillamine and the reactive coenzyme PLP (pyridoxal-5'-phosphate). This leads to an inactivation of PLP. PLP is an enzyme necessary for the formation of vitamin B6. Copper, Magnesium, Zinc – Forms chelation complexes in the GI tract. Decreases absorption of these elements.	The need for supplementation has not been adequately studied. Give supplements of these nutrients only if clinical judgment warrants it. [4453,4531,4534-4535]

C H A R T S

Drug Influences on Nutrient Levels and Depletion

Some medications can affect the levels of certain nutrients in the body. There is considerable interest in using nutritional supplements to counteract these possible drug-induced "nutrient depletions." The chart below shows the current scientific understanding of these relationships, and suggested actions.

DRUGS (includes some representative U.S. and Canadian Brand Names.)	NUTRIENT DEPLETED	POSSIBLE MECHANISM	COMMENTS & REFERENCES
CARDIOVASCULAR			
ANTIHYPERTENSIVES			
Hydralazine (*Apresoline*)	Vitamin B6	Formation of a complex between hydralazine and the reactive coenzyme PLP (pyridoxal-5'-phosphate). This leads to an inactivation of PLP. PLP is an enzyme necessary for the formation of vitamin B6.	The need for supplementation has not been adequately studied. Give supplements of this mineral only if clinical judgement warrants it. [4453,4531,4533]
CARDIAC GLYCOSIDES			
Digoxin (*Lanoxicaps, Lanoxin*)	Magnesium	Limits reabsorption of magnesium in the renal tubule, leading to magnesium excretion.	The need for supplementation has not been adequately studied. Give supplements of this mineral only if clinical judgment warrants it. [4556]
CHOLESTEROL-REDUCING DRUGS			
HMG CoA Reductase Inhibitors ("Statins"): Atorvastatin (*Lipitor*), Cerivastatin (*Baycol*), Fluvastatin (*Lescol*), Pravastatin (*Pravacol*), Simvastatin (*Zocor*)	Coenzyme Q10	The enzyme HMG CoA reductase is also involved in the biosynthesis of coenzyme Q10. Inhibition of this enzyme leads to a decreased production of coenzyme Q10.	Clinical significance yet to be determined. Postulated potential decrease in cardiac function and possible contributor to liver dysfunction seen with HMG CoA reductase inhibitors. [4404-4410]
Cholestyramine (*LoCHOLEST, Prevalite, Questran*)	Beta-Carotene Folic Acid Vitamins A, D, E, K	All nutrients – Reduces gastrointestinal absorption, lowering of serum cholesterol and triglyceride levels.	It is likely that cholestyramine does bind with some of these nutrients but there has never been clinical proof that supplements are necessary. Supplementation may be valuable in some patients. [4454-4459,4551-4553]
Colestipol (*Colestid*)	Beta-Carotene Folic Acid Vitamins A, D, E, K	All nutrients – Reduces gastrointestinal absorption, lowering of serum cholesterol and triglyceride levels.	It is possible that supplementation with folic acid and vitamin D may be appropriate. In some cases it may be appropriate to supplement all nutrients depleted by colestipol. [4460-4461]

CHARTS

• © Copyright 2000, Natural Medicines Comprehensive Database (209) 472-2244. For updated data, go to www.NaturalDatabase.com.

Drug Influences on Nutrient Levels and Depletion

Some medications can affect the levels of certain nutrients in the body. There is considerable interest in using nutritional supplements to counteract these possible drug-induced "nutrient depletions." The chart below shows the current scientific understanding of these relationships, and suggested actions.

DRUGS (includes some representative U.S. and Canadian Brand Names.)	NUTRIENT DEPLETED	POSSIBLE MECHANISM	COMMENTS & REFERENCES
DIURETICS			
Loop Diuretics: Bumetanide (*Bumex, Burinex*), Ethacrynic acid (*Edecrin*), Furosemide (*Lasix*), Torsemide (*Demadex*)	Calcium Magnesium Potassium Sodium Thiamine Zinc	Increased urinary excretion.	Electrolyte disturbances more likely with higher doses or when used in combination with diuretics of another class. Hypokalemia and hypomagnesemia are most commonly clinically encountered. Supplementation may be appropriate in certain patients. Thiamine depletion might contribute to impaired heart function in some patients with congestive heart failure (CHF) treated with long-term furosemide. Supplementation with 200 mg thiamine (orally or intravenously) per day can replete thiamine, and in some cases, improve left ventricular function in these patients. Consider thiamine supplementation in patients using loop diuretics, especially long-term. [4412,4413-4425]
Thiazide and Thiazide Derivatives: Bendroflumethiazide (Naturetin), Benzthiazide (*Exna*), Chlorothiazide (*Diuril*), Chlorthalidone (*Hygroton, Thalitone*), Hydrochlorothiazide (*Esidrix, Hydrodiuril, Oretic*), Hydroflumethiazide (*Diucardin, Saluron*), Indapamide (*Lozide, Lozol*), Methyclothiazide (*Aquatensen, Enduron*), Metolazone (*Mykrox, Zaroxolyn*), Polythiazide (*Renese*), Quinethazone (*Hydromox*), Trichlormethiazide (*Diurese, Metahydrin, Naqua*)	Magnesium Potassium Sodium Zinc	Increased urinary excretion.	Electrolyte disturbances more likely with higher doses or when used in combination with diuretics of another class. Hypokalemia and hypomagnesemia are most commonly clinically encountered. Supplementation may be appropriate in certain patients. [4412,4416,4425,4444-4453]
Potassium Sparing: Triamterene (*Dyrenium*)	Folic Acid	Folate antagonism. (Binds to dihydrofolate reductase.)	The need for supplementation has not been adequately studied. Give supplements of this vitamin only if clinical judgment warrants it. [4425,4536-4537]

CHARTS

Drug Influences on Nutrient Levels and Depletion

Some medications can affect the levels of certain nutrients in the body. There is considerable interest in using nutritional supplements to counteract these possible drug-induced "nutrient depletions." The chart below shows the current scientific understanding of these relationships, and suggested actions.

DRUGS (includes some representative U.S. and Canadian Brand Names.)	NUTRIENT DEPLETED	POSSIBLE MECHANISM	COMMENTS & REFERENCES
CENTRAL NERVOUS SYSTEM			
ANTICONVULSANTS			
Carbamazepine (*Atretol, Epitol, Tegretol*)	Folic Acid Vitamin D (Ultimately may lead to decreases in serum calcium and potential bone loss.)	Folic Acid – Two mechanisms have been proposed: Induction of hepatic microsomal enzymes leading to increased folic acid metabolism and decreased intestinal absorption. Vitamin D – Increases the rate of vitamin D metabolism leading to decreased levels of various forms of vitamin D.	Studies of anticonvulsants in general demonstrate lower folic acid levels in treated patients. The necessity for supplementation to prevent peripheral neuropathies or red cell dyscrasias has not been adequately studied. The necessity for supplementation with vitamin D to potentially prevent osteomalacia has not been adequately studied: Give supplements of these vitamins only if clinical judgment warrants it. [4426-4433]
Phenytoin (*Dilantin*), Fosphenytoin (*Cerebyx*)	Folic Acid Vitamin D (Ultimately may lead to decreases in serum calcium and potential bone loss.)	Folic Acid - Several mechanisms have been proposed to explain the ability of phenytoin to deplete body folate. It appears to be more related to metabolic and distributional changes than decreases in dietary absorption. Vitamin D – Increases the rate of vitamin D metabolism leading to decreased levels of various forms of vitamin D. Phenytoin may also increase the renal excretion of polar vitamin D metabolites.	Based on patient specific circumstances, consider giving folic acid supplementation with the initial dose of phenytoin to prevent folate deficiency. Note that folic acid supplementation may alter phenytoin pharmacokinetics leading to lower serum concentrations and possible seizure breakthrough. Consider giving 400 – 800 IU/day of vitamin D to patients receiving long-term phenytoin therapy. Also recommend a diet rich in calcium.[4433,4471-4478]
Phenobarbital (*Luminal, Solfoton*)	Folic Acid Vitamin D (Ultimately may lead to decreases in serum calcium and potential bone loss.)	Folic Acid - Induces hepatic microsomal enzymes leading to an increase in folic acid metabolism. Vitamin D – Increases the rate of vitamin D metabolism leading to decreased levels of various forms of vitamin D.	The need for supplementation with folic acid has not been adequately studied. Give supplements of this vitamin only if clinical judgment warrants it. Consider giving 400 – 800 IU daily of vitamin D to patients receiving long-term phenobarbital therapy. Suggest a diet rich in calcium. Monitor vitamin D. Only give supplementation if deficiencies are noted. [4453,4530-4531]
Primidone (*Mysoline*)	Folic Acid	Folic Acid – Induces hepatic microsomal enzymes leading to an increase in folic acid metabolism.	The need for supplementation has not been adequately studied. Give supplements of this vitamin only if clinical judgment warrants it. [4453,4530-4531]
Valproic Acid (*Depakene, Depakote*)	L-Carnitine	Inhibits the biosynthesis of L-carnitine and possibly decreases the tissue uptake of L-carnitine.	Recommend oral L-carnitine supplementation in special subgroups of patients. See footnote at the end of the chart. [4523-4529]

CHARTS

 © Copyright 2000, Natural Medicines Comprehensive Database (209) 472-2244. For updated data, go to www.NaturalDatabase.com.

Drug Influences on Nutrient Levels and Depletion

Some medications can affect the levels of certain nutrients in the body. There is considerable interest in using nutritional supplements to counteract these possible drug-induced "nutrient depletions." The chart below shows the current scientific understanding of these relationships, and suggested actions.

DRUGS (includes some representative U.S. and Canadian Brand Names.)	NUTRIENT DEPLETED	POSSIBLE MECHANISM	COMMENTS & REFERENCES
PHENOTHIAZINES			
Phenothiazines: Chlorpromazine (*Thorazine*), Promazine (*Sparine*), Triflupromazine (*Vesprin*), Fluphenazine *(Moditen HCl, Permitil, Prolixin)*, Perphenazine (*Trilafon*), Prochlorperazine (*Compazine, Stemetil*), Trifluoperazine (*Stelazine*), Mesoridazine (*Serentil*), Thioridazine (*Mellaril*), Thiothixene (*Navane*)	Vitamin B2	Increases renal excretion and possibly inhibits synthesis.	Give 2 - 5 mg/day of riboflavin to patients on phenothiazines if clinical judgment warrants it. [4425]
DIABETES			
Glyburide (*Diabeta, Euglucon, Glynase, Micronase*), Acetohexamide (*Dymelor*), Tolazamide (*Tolinase*)	Coenzyme Q10	Inhibits NADH-oxidase, an enzyme necessary in the formation of coenzyme Q10.	Clinical significance is yet to be determined. Postulated potential decrease in cardiac function and possible impairment of insulin production and/or secretion. Give supplements of this nutrient only if clinical judgment warrants it. [4479]
Metformin (*Glucophage*)	Vitamin B12	Causes malabsorption of dietary vitamin B12.	The *Glucophage* package insert recommends obtaining hematological parameters annually and obtaining B12 at 2-3 year intervals in patients at increased risk for B12 deficiency. Give supplements of this vitamin only if clinical judgment warrants it. [4487-4491]
GASTROINTESTINALS			
ANTACIDS			
Aluminum Salts (*Amphojel, Alternajel, Gaviscon, Maalox, Riopan*)	Calcium Phosphorus	Binds calcium and phosphate in the gastrointestinal tract.	Prolonged administration of large doses may lead to hypocalcemia and/or hypophosphatemia. Avoid prolonged administration of large doses. [4400-4403]
Magnesium Salts (*Di-gel, Gelusil, Maalox, Mag-Ox, Milk of Magnesia, Mylanta, Riopan*)	Calcium Phosphorus	Binds calcium and phospate in the gastrointestinal tract.	Prolonged administration of large doses may lead to hypocalcemia and/or hypophosphatemia. Avoid prolonged administration of large doses. [4400-4403]
GI ANTI-INFLAMMATORIES			
p-Aminosalicylic Acid [aminosalicylic acid, PAS]	Folic Acid Vitamin B12	Inhibits absorption in the gastrointestinal tract.	The need for supplementation has not been adequately studied. Give supplements of these vitamins only if clinical judgment warrants it. [4557-4560]

© Copyright 2000, Natural Medicines Comprehensive Database (209) 472-2244. For updated data, go to www.NaturalDatabase.com.

CHARTS

Drug Influences on Nutrient Levels and Depletion

Some medications can affect the levels of certain nutrients in the body. There is considerable interest in using nutritional supplements to counteract these possible drug-induced "nutrient depletions." The chart below shows the current scientific understanding of these relationships, and suggested actions.

DRUGS (includes some representative U.S. and Canadian Brand Names.)	NUTRIENT DEPLETED	POSSIBLE MECHANISM	COMMENTS & REFERENCES
Sulfasalazine (*Azulfidine, Salazopyrin*)	Folic Acid	Inhibits folate absorption in the gastrointestinal tract.	Folate depletion is proposed to be involved in the various blood dyscrasias seen with sulfasalazine. Foods high in folic acid rather than folic acid supplements are recommended. Give supplements of this vitamin only if clinical judgment warrants it, and adequate amounts cannot be maintained by diet. [4515-4517]

HISTAMINE-2 BLOCKERS

H2 Blockers: Cimetidine (*Tagamet*), Famotidine (*Pepcid*), Nizatidine (*Axid*), Ranitidine (*Zantac*)	Iron Vitamin B12	Decreases iron and vitamin B12 absorption from the gastrointestinal tract.	The need for iron and vitamin B12 supplementation has not been adequately studied. B12 depletion may be particularly important in patients with inadequate diet, poor stores of the vitamin, and in patients receiving continuous therapy of more than two years. Give supplements of this vitamin if clinical judgment warrants it. [4538-4542]

LAXATIVES

Bisacodyl (*Bisacodyl Uniserts, Bisco-Lax, Correctol, Dulcagen, Dulcolax, Feen-a-mint, Fleet Laxative*)	Potassium	Increases gastrointestinal losses of potassium.	Reported in patients undergoing bowel-cleansing regimens. Use caution in patients who may be predisposed to hypokalemia (i.e. aggressive diuretic therapy). Give supplements of this mineral if clinical judgment warrants it. [4411-4412]
Mineral Oil	Beta-Carotene Calcium Vitamins A,D,E, K	Decreases gastrointestinal absorption.	May be avoided by limiting duration of use. [4495-4496]
Stimulant Laxatives: Cascara (*Various…*) Senna (*Senexon, Senolax, Senokot , Senna-Gen, Senokotxtra, Black-Draught, Gentlax, Dr. Caldwell Senna, Fletcher's Castoria, Dosalax*), Bisacodyl Tablets (*Bisacodyl Uniserts, Bisco-Lax, Correctol, Dulcagen, Dulcolax, Feen-a-mint, Fleet Laxative*)	Calcium Potassium Sodium Vitamin D	Calcium and Vitamin D - Decreases gastrointestinal absorption. Sodium and Potassium – Increases gastrointestinal losses.	Excessive use of stimulant laxatives may result in depletion of these essential elements and vitamin D. Limit to short-term use. [4411-4412,4425,4453]

PROKINETIC AGENTS

Metoclopramide (*Maxeran, Reglan*)	Vitamin B2	Decreases dietary vitamin B2 absorption from the gastrointestinal tract.	The need for supplementation has not been adequately studied. Give supplements of this vitamin only if clinical judgment warrants it. [4561]

C
H
A
R
T
S

Drug Influences on Nutrient Levels and Depletion

Some medications can affect the levels of certain nutrients in the body. There is considerable interest in using nutritional supplements to counteract these possible drug-induced "nutrient depletions." The chart below shows the current scientific understanding of these relationships, and suggested actions.

DRUGS (includes some representative U.S. and Canadian Brand Names.)	NUTRIENT DEPLETED	POSSIBLE MECHANISM	COMMENTS & REFERENCES
PROTON PUMP INHIBITORS			
Proton Pump Inhibitors: Lansoprazole (*Prevacid*), Omeprazole (*Losec, Prilosec*), Rabeprazole (*Aciphex*), Pantoprazole (*Pantoloc, Protonix*)	Beta-Carotene Iron Vitamin B12	Decreases beta carotene, iron and vitamin B12 absorption from the gastrointestinal tract.	The need for supplementation has not been adequately studied. Give supplementation of these vitamins only if clinical judgment warrants it. 31,4483-4486,4539-4541
HORMONES			
Corticosteroids [Glucocorticoids]: **Short-acting** Cortisone (*Cortone*), Hydrocortisone [Cortisol] (*Cortef, Hydrocortone*) **Intermediate-acting** Prednisone (*Deltasone, Meticorten, Orasone, Panasol-S*), Prednisolone (*Delta-Cortef, Prelone, Pediapred*), Triamcinolone (*Aristocort, Atolone, Kenacort*), Methylprednisolone (*Medrol*) **Long-acting** Dexamethasone (*Decadron, Dexameth, Dexone*), Betamethasone (*Celestone*)	Calcium (Indirectly – Vitamin D)	Calcium – Increases renal calcium excretion and decreases intestinal calcium absorption. Vitamin D - Depletion of calcium by steroids creates a greater need for vitamin D, which is necessary for appropriate GI absorption of calcium.	Steroid induced osteoporosis is a well-recognized consequence of long-term steroid administration. Supplement with calcium and vitamin D (calcitriol). Emerging data indicate that bisphosphonates may also be helpful. Depletion of calcium by steroids creates a greater need for vitamin D, which is necessary for appropriate GI absorption of calcium. It may be prudent to supplement these nutrients before, during, and after long-term and/or high-dose corticosteroids. 4462-4467
Estrogens: (*Cenestin, Estrace, Estratab, Ogen, Premarin, Premphase, Prempro*)	Magnesium Vitamin B6	Magnesium – Proposed shift of magnesium from plasma to other tissues. Vitamin B6 – Disturbance of tryptophan and vitamin B6 metabolism.	Although there has been much talk about giving vitamin B6 to people on estrogens, the need for supplementation has not been proven. Give supplements of these nutrients only if clinical judgment warrants it.4469-4470
Oral Contraceptives [Containing Estrogen]	Folic Acid Magnesium Vitamin B2 Vitamin B6 Vitamin B12	Folic Acid – Interferes with metabolism. Magnesium – Proposed shift of magnesium from plasma to other tissues. Vitamins B2, B6 – Interferes with metabolism. Vitamin B12 – Possibly due to increased metabolism and decreased B12 binding capacity.	Although there has been much talk about giving vitamin B6 to people on oral contraceptives, the need for supplementation has not been proven. Give supplements of these nutrients only if clinical judgment warrants it. 4497-4510,4547-4548

CHARTS

© Copyright 2000, Natural Medicines Comprehensive Database (209) 472-2244. For updated data, go to www.NaturalDatabase.com. • 1451

Drug Influences on Nutrient Levels and Depletion

Some medications can affect the levels of certain nutrients in the body. There is considerable interest in using nutritional supplements to counteract these possible drug-induced "nutrient depletions." The chart below shows the current scientific understanding of these relationships, and suggested actions.

DRUGS (includes some representative U.S. and Canadian Brand Names.)	NUTRIENT DEPLETED	POSSIBLE MECHANISM	COMMENTS & REFERENCES
MISCELLANEOUS			
Orlistat (*Xenical*)	Beta-Carotene Vitamin A Vitamin D Vitamin E Vitamin K	Beta-Carotene - Decreases the absorption of beta-carotene supplements from the gastrointestinal tract. Vitamin E - Decreases the absorption of vitamin E supplements by 60%. Vitamin A, vitamin D, and vitamin K - Possibly decreases the absorption from the gastrointestinal tract.	Separate administration of orlistat and beta-carotene, vitamin A, vitamin D, vitamin E, and vitamin K supplements by 2-hours to avoid this interaction. The effect of orlistat on the absorption of nutritionally derived vitamins is unknown. The need for supplementation has not been adequately studied. Give supplements of these vitamins only if clinical judgment warrants it. [1725-1727,1730, 6001]
Potassium Chloride (Extended Release) (*K-Dur, Micro K, Slow K*)	Vitamin B12	Malabsorption of dietary vitamin B12.	The need for supplementation has not been adequately studied. Give supplements of this vitamin only if clinical judgment warrants it. [4511-4512]
RESPIRATORY			
Theophylline (*Slobid, Theo-24, Theo-Dur, Theolair*)	Vitamin B6	Inhibits pyridoxal kinase leading to decreases in vitamin B6 levels.	There have been several studies looking at the possible depletion of vitamin B6 due to theophylline. There is no consensus yet. Give supplements of this vitamin only if clinical judgment warrants it. [4518-4522]

CHARTS (vertical sidebar)

Footnote: Oral L-carnitine supplementation is indicated for primary plasmalemmal carnitine transporter defect. In addition, oral L-carnitine supplementation is strongly suggested for the following groups: patients with certain secondary carnitine deficiency syndromes; symptomatic VPA-associated hyperammonemia; multiple risk factors for VPA-associated hepatotoxicity, or renal associated syndromes; infants and young children taking VPA; patients with epilepsy using the ketogenic diet who have hypocarnitinemia; patients on dialysis; and premature infants receiving TPN. An oral L-carnitine dosage of 100 mg/kg/day, up to a maximum of 2 g/day has been recommended.

GENERAL INDEX

(+)-chiroinositol .... see INOSITOL
1,2,3,4,5,6-Cyclohexanehexol .... see INOSITOL
1,2,5/3,4,6-inositol .... see INOSITOL
1,25-DHCC .... see VITAMIN D
1,25-dihydroxycholecalciferol .... see VITAMIN D
1,25-diOHC .... see VITAMIN D
1,25-hydroxycholecalciferol .... see VITAMIN D
1,25-hydroxyvitamin D3 .... see VITAMIN D
1,2-Butanolide .... see GAMMA BUTYROLACTONE
1,2-dithiolane-3-pentanoic acid ... see ALPHA-LIPOIC ACID
1,2-dithiolane-3-valeric acid .... see ALPHA-LIPOIC ACID
1,3,7-trimethylxanthine .... see CAFFEINE
1,4-BD .... see BUTANEDIOL
1,4-butanediol .... see BUTANEDIOL
1,4-butylene glycol .... see BUTANEDIOL
1,4-dihydroxybutane .... see BUTANEDIOL
1,4-tetramethylene glycol .... see BUTANEDIOL
13-Docosenoic acid .... see LORENZO'S OIL
17 beta-(1-ketoethyl)- delta 5-androsten-3 beta-ol
.... see PREGNENOLONE
19-nor-1, 25-dihydroxyvitamin D2 .... see VITAMIN D
1-Octacosanol .... see OCTACOSANOL
(1S)-1,2,4/3,5,6-inositol .... see INOSITOL
(1S)-inositol .... see INOSITOL
2(3H)-Furanone di-dihydro .... see BUTANEDIOL
2(3H)-Furanone Dihydro
.... see GAMMA BUTYROLACTONE
2,3 dihydro furanone ..... see GAMMA BUTYROLACTONE
2,3-Diphosphoglycerate .... see INOSINE
20-Dione .... see PROGESTERONE
22,23-dihydrostigmasterol .... see BETA-SITOSTEROL
24-alpha-ethylcholestanol .... see SITOSTANOL
24-beta-ethyl-delta-5-cholesten-3beta-ol
.... see BETA-SITOSTEROL
24-ethyl-cholesterol .... see BETA-SITOSTEROL
25-dihydroxycholecalciferol .... see VITAMIN D
25-dihydroxyvitamin D3 .... see VITAMIN D
25-HCC .... see VITAMIN D
25-hydroxycholecalciferol .... see VITAMIN D
25-OHCC .... see VITAMIN D
25-OHD3 .... see VITAMIN D
2-acetamido-2-deoxyglucose
.... See N-ACETYL GLUCOSAMINE
2-amino-2-deoxyglucose hydrochloride
.... see GLUCOSAMINE HYDROCHLORIDE
2-amino-2-deoxyglucose sulfate
.... see GLUCOSAMINE SULFATE
2-amino-3-methylbutanoic acid
.... see BRANCHED-CHAIN AMINO ACIDS
2-amino-3-methylvaleric acid
.... see BRANCHED-CHAIN AMINO ACIDS
2-amino-4-methylvaleric acid
.... see BRANCHED-CHAIN AMINO ACIDS
2-Amino-5-guanidinopentanoic acid .... see L-ARGININE
2-Dimethylaminoethanol .... see DEANOL
2-Methyl-1,4-Naphthoquinone .... see VITAMIN K
2-Methyl-3-Phytyl-1, 4-Naphthoquinone ..... see VITAMIN K
2-Oxoglutaric acid .... see ALPHA-KETOGLUTARATE
2-Oxopentanedoicic acid .. see ALPHA-KETOGLUTARATE
2-Oxopropanoate .... see PYRUVATE
2-oxopropanoic acid .... see PYRUVATE

2-Oxypropanoic Acid .... see PYRUVATE
3,3',4'5,7-Penthydroxyflavone .... see QUERCETIN
3,3',5-triiodothyroacetic acid .... see TIRATRICOL
3,3'-dihydroxy-4,4'-diketo-beta-carotene see MICROALGAE
3,4',5-stilbenetriol .... see RESVERATROL
3,4',5-trihydroxystilbene .... see RESVERATROL
3,5,4' -trihydroxystilbene .... see RESVERATROL
3-acetyl-7-oxo-dehydroepiandrosterone
.... see 7-KETO-DHEA
(3 beta)-3-hydroxypregn-5-en-20-one
.... see PREGNENOLONE
3-beta,5-alpha-stigmastan-3-ol .... see SITOSTANOL
3beta-acetoxy-androst-5-ene-7,17-dione
.... see 7-KETO-DHEA
3-beta-stigmast-5-en-3-ol .... see BETA-SITOSTEROL
3-carboxy-2-hydroxy-N,N,N trimethyl-1-propanaminium
.... see L-CARNITINE
(3-carboxy2-hydroxpropyl)trimethylammonium hydroxide
.... see L-CARNITINE
(3-carboxy-2-hydroxy-propyl)trimethylammonium
    hydroxide
.... see ACETYL-L-CARNITINE
3-dehydroretinol .... see VITAMIN A
3-hydroxy-4-N-trimethylaminobutyrate .. see L-CARNITINE
3-Hydroxybutyric Acid Lactone
.... see GAMMA BUTYROLACTONE
3-Pyridine Carboxamide
.... see NIACIN AND NIACINAMIDE
3R, 3'R-astaxanthin .... see MICROALGAE
3R,3'S-astaxanthin .... see MICROALGAE
3S, 3'S-astaxanthin .... see MICROALGAE
4,4-diketo-beta-carotene .... see CANTHAXANTHIN
4-AD .... see ANDROSTENEDIOL
4-Amino-2-Methyl-1-Naphthol .... see VITAMIN K
4-androstene-3,17-dione .... see ANDROSTENEDIONE
4-androstene-3beta,17beta-diol ..... see ANDROSTENEDIOL
4-Androstenediol .... see ANDROSTENEDIOL
4-butanolide .... see GAMMA BUTYROLACTONE
4-Butyrolactone .... see GAMMA BUTYROLACTONE
4-Hydroxy Butyrate
.... see GAMMA HYDROXYBUTYRATE
4-Hydroxybutanoic Acid Lactone
.... see GAMMA BUTYROLACTONE
4-hydroxybutyric acid
.... see GAMMA HYDROXYBUTYRATE
4-Pregnene-3 .... see PROGESTERONE
5-(1,2-dithiolan-3-yl) valeric acid
.... see ALPHA-LIPOIC ACID
5-AD .... see ANDROSTENEDIOL
5-androsten-3-beta-17-one-DHEA .... see 7-KETO-DHEA
5-androstene-3beta,17beta-diol ..... see ANDROSTENEDIOL
5-Androstenediol .... see ANDROSTENEDIOL
5-HTP .... see 5-HTP
5-hydroxytryptophan .... see 5-HTP
6,8-dithiooctanoic acid .... see ALPHA-LIPOIC ACID
6,8-thioctic acid .... see ALPHA-LIPOIC ACID
6,9-Dihydro-9-B-D-ribofuranosyl-1H-puin-6-one
.... see INOSINE
6-furfurylaminopurine .... see KINETIN
7-Isopropoxy Isoflavone .... see IPRIFLAVONE
7-Keto .... see 7-KETO-DHEA

© Copyright 2000, Natural Medicines Comprehensive Database (209) 472-2244. For updated data, go to www.NaturalDatabase.com. • 1453

7-keto dehydroepiandrosterone .... see 7-KETO-DHEA
7-ketodehydroepiandrostenedione .... see 7-KETO-DHEA
7-KETO-DHEA .... see 7-KETO-DHEA
7-ODA .... see 7-KETO-DHEA
7-oxo-dehydroepiandrosterone-3-acetate
.... see 7-KETO-DHEA
7-oxo-DHEA .... see 7-KETO-DHEA
7-oxo-DHEA-acetate .... see 7-KETO-DHEA
9-B-D-ribofuranosylhypoxanthine .... see INOSINE
A-Lan-Thus .... see TREE OF HEAVEN
A-Lipoic Acid .... see ALPHA-LIPOIC ACID
Aamalaki .... see INDIAN GOOSEBERRY
Aaron's Rod
.... see GOLDENROD, HOUSELEEK, MULLEIN
Abelmoschus moschatus .... see AMBRETTE
Abelmosk .... see AMBRETTE
Abies alba .... see FIR, FIR NEEDLE OIL
Abies balsamea .... see CANADA BALSAM
Abies excelsa .... see HEMLOCK SPRUCE
Abies pectinata .... see FIR
Abies sachalinensis .... see FIR NEEDLE OIL
Abies sibirica .... see FIR NEEDLE OIL
Abrojos .... see PUNCTURE VINE
Abrus pecatorius .... see PRECATORY BEAN
ABSCESS ROOT .... see ABSCESS ROOT
Absinth .... see WORMWOOD above ground parts
Absinthe .... see WORMWOOD above ground parts
Absinthii Herba .... see WORMWOOD above ground parts
Absinthites .... see WORMWOOD above ground parts
Absinthium .... see WORMWOOD above ground parts
ABUTA .... see ABUTA
Abyssinian Myrrh .... see MYRRH
Abyssinian Tea .... see KHAT
ACACIA .... see ACACIA
Acacia Catechu Heartwood Extract .... see CATECHU
Acacia farnesiana .... see CASSIE ABSOLUTE
Acacia senegal .... see ACACIA
Acanthopanax senticosus .... see GINSENG, SIBERIAN
Acedera Comœn .... see SORREL
Acer rubrum .... see RED MAPLE
ACEROLA .... see ACEROLA
Acetate Replacing Factor .... see ALPHA-LIPOIC ACID
Acetyl-Carnitine .... see ACETYL-L-CARNITINE
ACETYL-L-CARNITINE ...... see ACETYL-L-CARNITINE
Acetyl-Levocarnitine .... see ACETYL-L-CARNITINE
Acetylcarnitine .... see ACETYL-L-CARNITINE
Acetylcysteine .... see N-ACETYL CYSTEINE
Acetylformic Acid .... see PYRUVATE
Acetylglucosamine .... see N-ACETYL GLUCOSAMINE
Ache des Marais .... see CELERY
Achilee .... see YARROW
Achillea .... see YARROW
Achillea millefolium .... see YARROW
Achillea ptarmica .... see SNEEZEWORT
Achiote .... see ANNATTO
Achiotillo .... see ANNATTO
Achras sapota .... see CHICLE
Achras zapotilla .... see CHICLE
Achweed .... see GOUTWEED
Acidophilus .... see LACTOBACILLUS ACIDOPHILUS
Acidophilus Milk .... see YOGURT
ACKEE .... see ACKEE
Ackerkraut .... see AGRIMONY
ACONITE .... see ACONITE

Aconiti Tuber .... see ACONITE
Aconitum napellus .... see ACONITE
Acorus calamus .... see CALAMUS
Acrid Crowfoot .... see BUTTERCUP
Acrid Lettuce .... see WILD LETTUCE
Actaea alba .... see WHITE COHOSH
Actaea macrotys .... see BLACK COHOSH
Actaea pachypoda .... see WHITE COHOSH
Actaea racemosa .... see BLACK COHOSH
Actaea rubra .... see WHITE COHOSH
Actinidia chinensis .... see KIWI
Activated 7-dehydrocholesterol .... see VITAMIN D
ACTIVATED CHARCOAL
.... see ACTIVATED CHARCOAL
activated ergosterol .... see VITAMIN D
Acuilee .... see YARROW
Adam's Apple .... see LIME fruit, peel, LIME oil
Adam's Flannel .... see MULLEIN
ADAM'S NEEDLE .... see ADAM'S NEEDLE
Adam's Needle .... see YUCCA
Adder's Eyes .... see SCARLET PIMPERNEL
Adder's Root .... see ARUM
Adderwort .... see BISTORT
Ademetionine .... see SAMe
Adenosylcobalamin .... see DIBENCOZIDE
Adenosylmethionine .... see SAMe
Adermine Hydrochloride .... see PYRIDOXINE
Adiantifolia .... see GINKGO leaf extract
Adiantum capillus-veneris .... see MAIDENHAIR FERN
Adiantum pedatum .... see MAIDENHAIR FERN
Adiptam .... see BURNING BUSH leaf,
                                BURNING BUSH root
Adonis herba .... see PHEASANT'S EYE
Adonis vernalis .... see PHEASANT'S EYE
ADRUE .... see ADRUE
Adulsa .... see MALABAR NUT
Aegle marmelos .... see BAEL
Aegopodium podagraria .... see GOUTWEED
Aesculus hippocastanum
.... see HORSE CHESTNUT branch bark,
                 HORSE CHESTNUT flower,
                 HORSE CHESTNUT leaf,
                 HORSE CHESTNUT seed
Aetheroleum Pelargonii .... see ROSE GERANIUM
Aethusa cynapium .... see FOOL'S PARSLEY
Aframomum melegueta .... see GRAINS OF PARADISE
African Chillies .... see CAPSICUM
African Civet .... see CIVET
African Coffee Tree .... see CASTOR OIL, CASTOR seed
African Cucumber .... see BITTER MELON
African Ginger .... see GINGER
African Marigold .... see TAGETES
African Myrrh .... see MYRRH
African Pepper .... see CAPSICUM
African Plum Tree .... see PYGEUM
African Potato .... see AFRICAN WILD POTATO
AFRICAN WILD POTATO
.... see AFRICAN WILD POTATO
AGA .... see AGA
AGAR .... see AGAR
Agar-Agar .... see AGAR
Agarweed .... see AGAR
Agathosma betulina .... see BUCHU
Aged Garlic Extract .... see GARLIC

INDEX

Agnus Castus .... see CHASTEBERRY
Agracejo .... see EUROPEAN BARBERRY
Agriao .... see WATERCRESS
Agrimonia eupatoria .... see AGRIMONY
Agrimonia procera .... see AGRIMONY
Agrimoniae herba .... see AGRIMONY
AGRIMONY .... see AGRIMONY
Agromonia .... see AGRIMONY
AGROPYRON .... see AGROPYRON
Agropyron repens .... see AGROPYRON, COUCH GRASS
Agrostemma githago .... see CORN COCKLE
Ague Grass .... see ALETRIS
Ague Root .... see ALETRIS
Ague Tree .... see SASSAFRAS
Agueweed .... see BONESET
Ahuacate .... see AVOCADO
Ail .... see GARLIC
Ailanthus altissima .... see TREE OF HEAVEN
Ailanthus Glandulosa .... see TREE OF HEAVEN
Ailanto .... see TREE OF HEAVEN
Airelle .... see BILBERRY dried ripe fruit, BILBERRY leaf
Ajenjo .... see WORMWOOD above ground parts
Ajenuz .... see BLACK SEED
Ajo .... see GARLIC
Ajuga chamaepitys .... see GROUND PINE
Ajuga reptans .... see BUGLE
Akee .... see ACKEE
Aki .... see ACKEE
ALA .... see ALPHA-LIPOIC ACID
Alant .... see ELECAMPANE
ALC .... see ACETYL-L-CARNITINE
Alcachofa .... see ARTICHOKE
Alcacuz .... see LICORICE
Alcanna .... see HENNA
ALCAR .... see ACETYL-L-CARNITINE
Alcaucil .... see ARTICHOKE
Alcazuz .... see LICORICE
Alcea rosea .... see HOLLYHOCK
ALCHEMILLA .... see ALCHEMILLA
Alchemilla alpina .... see ALPINE LADY'S MANTLE
Alchemilla vulgaris .... see ALCHEMILLA
Alchemilla xanthochlora .... see ALCHEMILLA
Alchemillae alpinae herba
 .... see ALPINE LADY'S MANTLE
Alchornea castaneifolia .... see IPORURU
ALDER BUCKTHORN .... see ALDER BUCKTHORN
Alder Dogwood .... see ALDER BUCKTHORN
Alehoof .... see GROUND IVY
ALETRIS .... see ALETRIS
Aletris farinosa .... see ALETRIS
Aleurites cordata .... see TUNG SEED
Aleurites moluccana .... see TUNG SEED
Alexandrian-laurel .... see LAURELWOOD
Alexandrian Senna .... see SENNA
Alexandrinische Senna .... see SENNA
Alexandrinischer Lorbeer .... see LAURELWOOD
ALFALFA .... see ALFALFA
Algerian Geranium Oil .... see ROSE GERANIUM
ALGIN .... see ALGIN
Alginates .... see ALGIN
Alhucema .... see LAVENDER
Alisma plantago-aquatica .... see WATER PLANTAIN
Alkanet .... see ALKANNA
ALKANNA .... see ALKANNA

Alkanna Radix .... see ALKANNA
Alkanna tinctoria .... see ALKANNA
All-Heal .... see EUROPEAN MISTLETOE,
                            SELF-HEAL, VALERIAN
All Rac-Alpha-Tocopherol .... see VITAMIN E
All-Trans Lycopene .... see LYCOPENE
Alligator Pear .... see AVOCADO
Allii cepae bulbus .... see ONION
Allii Sativi Bulbus .... see GARLIC
Allium .... see GARLIC
Allium cepa .... see ONION
Allium sativum .... see GARLIC
Allium schoenoprasum .... see CHIVE
Allium ursinum .... see BEAR'S GARLIC
Allseed Nine-Joints .... see KNOTWEED HERB
ALLSPICE .... see ALLSPICE
Almond Oil .... see SWEET ALMOND
Alnus glutinosa .... see BLACK ALDER
Aloe .... see ALOE gel
Aloe africana .... see ALOE dried juice from leaf, latex,
                            ALOE gel
Aloe arborescens natalenis
 .... see ALOE dried juice from leaf,latex
Aloe barbadensis .... see ALOE dried juice from leaf, latex,
                            ALOE gel
Aloe Capensis .... see ALOE gel
ALOE dried juice from leaf, latex
 .... see ALOE dried juice from leaf, latex
Aloe ferox .... see ALOE dried juice from leaf, latex,
                            ALOE gel
ALOE gel .... see ALOE gel
Aloe Juice .... see ALOE dried juice from leaf, latex
Aloe Latex .... see ALOE dried juice from leaf, latex
Aloe Leaf Gel .... see ALOE gel
Aloe perfoliata .... see ALOE dried juice from leaf, latex
Aloe perryi .... see ALOE dried juice from leaf, latex
Aloe spicata .... see ALOE dried juice from leaf, latex,
                            ALOE gel
Aloe vera .... see ALOE dried juice from leaf, latex,
                            ALOE gel
Aloe Yucca .... see YUCCA
Aloerot .... see ALETRIS
Aloysia citriodora .... see LEMON VERBENA
Aloysia triphylla .... see LEMON VERBENA
Alpenkraut .... see HEMP AGRIMONY
Alpha-amino-4-imidazole propanoic acid ..... see HISTIDINE
Alpha-aminohydrocinnamic acid .... see PHENYLALANINE
Alpha-chymotrypsin .... see CHYMOTRYPSIN
ALPHA HYDROXY ACIDS
 .... see ALPHA HYDROXY ACIDS
ALPHA-KETOGLUTARATE
 .... see ALPHA-KETOGLUTARATE
Alpha-Ketoglutaric Acid
 .... see ALPHA-KETOGLUTARATE
Alpha-Ketopropionic Acid .... see PYRUVATE
Alpha KG .... see ALPHA-KETOGLUTARATE
ALPHA-LIPOIC ACID .... see ALPHA-LIPOIC ACID
Alpha-Lipoic Acid Extract .... see ALPHA-LIPOIC ACID
Alpha-tocopherol .... see VITAMIN E
Alpha tocotrienol .... see VITAMIN E
ALPINE CRANBERRY .... see ALPINE CRANBERRY
ALPINE LADY'S MANTLE
 .... see ALPINE LADY'S MANTLE
ALPINE RAGWORT .... see ALPINE RAGWORT

INDEX

Alpine Strawberry .... see STRAWBERRY
ALPINIA .... see ALPINIA
Alpinia officinarum .... see ALPINIA
Alquitran de Enebro .... see CADE OIL
Alraunwurzel .... see EUROPEAN MANDRAKE
Alstonia Bark .... see FEVER BARK
Alstonia constricta .... see FEVER BARK
Altamisa .... see FEVERFEW
Alteia .... see MARSHMALLOW
Althaea officinalis .... see MARSHMALLOW
Althaea rosea .... see HOLLYHOCK
Althaeae folium .... see MARSHMALLOW
Althaeae radi .... see MARSHMALLOW
Althea .... see MARSHMALLOW
Althea Rose .... see HOLLYHOCK
Aluminum Phosphate .... see PHOSPHATE SALTS
Amachazuru .... see JIAOGULAN
Amalaki .... see INDIAN GOOSEBERRY
Amanita muscaria .... see AGA
Amantilla .... see VALERIAN
AMARANTH .... see AMARANTH
Amaranthus hypochondriacus .... see AMARANTH
Amargo .... see QUASSIA
Amber .... see ST JOHN'S WORT
Amber Touch-and-Heal .... see ST JOHN'S WORT
Amblabaum .... see INDIAN GOOSEBERRY
Ambreine .... see LABDANUM
Ambretta .... see AMBRETTE
AMBRETTE .... see AMBRETTE
Ambroise .... see WOOD SAGE
AMERICAN ADDER'S TONGUE
.... see AMERICAN ADDER'S TONGUE
American Arborvitae .... see CEDAR leaf,
                                                    CEDAR LEAF OIL
American Aspidium .... see MALE FERN
AMERICAN BITTERSWEET
.... see AMERICAN BITTERSWEET
AMERICAN CHESTNUT ..... see AMERICAN CHESTNUT
American Cone Flower .... see ECHINACEA
American Cranberry .... see CRANBERRY
American Dill .... see DILL above ground parts, DILL seed
AMERICAN DOGWOOD .... see AMERICAN DOGWOOD
American Dwarf Palm Tree .... see SAW PALMETTO
AMERICAN ELDER .... see AMERICAN ELDER
American Elderberry .... see AMERICAN ELDER
American Ginseng .... see GINSENG, AMERICAN
American Greek Valerian .... see ABSCESS ROOT
AMERICAN HELLEBORE .... see AMERICAN
                                                    HELLEBORE
American Indigo .... see WILD INDIGO
American Ipecacuanha .... see INDIAN PHYSIC
AMERICAN IVY .... see AMERICAN IVY
American Liverleaf .... see LIVERWORT
American Mandrake .... see PODOPHYLLUM
AMERICAN MISTLETOE .. see AMERICAN MISTLETOE
American Mullein .... see MULLEIN
American Nightshade .... see POKEWEED berry,
                                                    POKEWEED root
AMERICAN PAWPAW .... see AMERICAN PAWPAW
American Pennyroyal .... see PENNYROYAL leaf,
                                                    PENNYROYAL oil
American Saffron .... see SAFFLOWER
AMERICAN SPIKENARD
.... see AMERICAN SPIKENARD

American Spinach .... see POKEWEED berry,
                                                    POKEWEED root
American Storax .... see STORAX
American Valerian .... see NERVE ROOT
American Veratrum .... see AMERICAN HELLEBORE
American White Hellebore .. see AMERICAN HELLEBORE
AMERICAN WHITE POND LILY
.... see AMERICAN WHITE POND LILY
American Woodbine .... see AMERICAN IVY
American Wormgrass .... see PINK ROOT
Amla .... see INDIAN GOOSEBERRY
Ammi .... see BISHOP'S WEED
Ammi daucoides .... see BISHOP'S WEED
Ammi majus .... see BISHOP'S WEED
Ammi visnagae .... see BISHOP'S WEED
Ammocallis rosea .... see MADAGASCAR PERIWINKLE
Amomum cardamomum .... see CARDAMOM
Amomum melegueta .... see GRAINS OF PARADISE
Amoraciae Rusticanae Radix .... see HORSERADISH
Amorphophallus konjac .... see GLUCOMANNAN
Amygdala Amara .... see BITTER ALMOND
Amygdala Dulcis .... see SWEET ALMOND
Anacardium occidentale .... see CASHEW
Anacyclus pyrethrum .... see PELLITORY
Anagallis arvensis .... see SCARLET PIMPERNEL
Anamirta cocculus .... see LEVANT BERRY
Anamirta paniculata .... see LEVANT BERRY
Ananas comosus .... see BROMELAIN
Ananas sativus .... see BROMELAIN
Anashca .... see MARIJUANA
Anchi Ginseng .... see GINSENG, AMERICAN
Anchusa .... see ALKANNA
Andira araroba .... see GOA POWDER
ANDIROBA .... see ANDIROBA
Andiroba-Saruba .... see ANDIROBA
ANDRACHNE .... see ANDRACHNE
Andrachne aspera .... see ANDRACHNE
Andrachne cordifolia .... see ANDRACHNE
Andrachne phyllanthoides .... see ANDRACHNE
Andro .... see ANDROSTENEDIONE
Androdiol .... see ANDROSTENEDIOL
ANDROGRAPHIS .... see ANDROGRAPHIS
Andrographis paniculata .... see ANDROGRAPHIS
Andrographolide .... see ANDROGRAPHIS
Andropogon citratus .... see LEMONGRASS
Andropogon nardus .... see CITRONELLA OIL
Androst-4-ene-3,17-dione .... see ANDROSTENEDIONE
Androstene .... see ANDROSTENEDIONE
ANDROSTENEDIOL .... see ANDROSTENEDIOL
ANDROSTENEDIONE .... see ANDROSTENEDIONE
Anemone a Lobes Aigus .... see LIVERWORT
Anemone acutiloba .... see LIVERWORT
Anemone americana .... see LIVERWORT
Anemone d'Amerique .... see LIVERWORT
Anemone hepatica .... see LIVERWORT
Anemone nemorosa .... see WOOD ANEMONE
Anemone nigricans .... see PULSATILLA
Anemone pratensis .... see PULSATILLA
Anemone pulsatilla .... see PULSATILLA
Anemopsis californica .... see YERBA MANSA
Anetheum graveolens .... see DILL above ground parts,
                                                    DILL seed
Anethi fructus .... see DILL seed
Anethi herba .... see DILL above ground parts

Anethum foeniculum ...... see FENNEL fruit, seed, FENNEL OIL

Aneurine Hydrochloride .... see THIAMINE

Angel Tulip .... see JIMSON WEED

Angelica archangelica ...... see ANGELICA herb, seed, ANGELICA root

Angelica atropurpurea .... see ANGELICA root

Angelica curtisi .... see ANGELICA root

ANGELICA herb, seed ...... see ANGELICA herb, seed

Angelica levisticum .... see LOVAGE

Angelica polymorpha sinensis .... see DONG QUAI

Angelica pubescens .... see ANGELICA root

ANGELICA root .... see ANGELICA root

Angelica rosaefolia .... see ANGELICA root

Angelica sinensis .... see DONG QUAI

Angelica sylvestris .... see ANGELICA root

Angelica Tree ...... see NORTHERN PRICKLY ASH

Angelicae Fructus .... see ANGELICA herb, seed

Angelicae Herba .... see ANGELICA herb, seed

Angelicin .... see BETA-SITOSTEROL

ANGEL'S TRUMPET .... see ANGEL'S TRUMPET

Angled Loofah .... see LUFFA

ANGOSTURA .... see ANGOSTURA

Angustura .... see ANGOSTURA

Anhydrous aluminum silicates
.... see COLLOIDAL MINERALS

Anhydrous Caffeine .... see CAFFEINE

Anhydrous Sodium Phosphate ...... see PHOSPHATE SALTS

Aniba rosaeodora .... see BOIS DE ROSE OIL

Animal Charcoal .... see ACTIVATED CHARCOAL

Anis des Vosges ...... see CARAWAY dried fruit, seed

ANISE .... see ANISE

Aniseed .... see ANISE

Aniseed Stars .... see STAR ANISE

Anisi Fructus .... see ANISE

Anisi stellati fructus .... see STAR ANISE

ANNATTO .... see ANNATTO

Annotta .... see ANNATTO

Annual Mugwort .... see SWEET ANNIE

Annual Wormwood .... see SWEET ANNIE

Antennaria dioica .... see CAT'S FOOT

Antennariase Dioicae Flos .... see CAT'S FOOT

Anthemis grandiflorum ...... see CHRYSANTHEMUM

Anthemis stipulacea ...... see CHRYSANTHEMUM

Anthoxanthum odoratum ...... see SWEET VERNAL GRASS

Anthriscus cerefolium .... see CHERVIL

Anthriscus longirostris .... see CHERVIL

Antialopecia Factor .... see INOSITOL

Antiberiberi Factor .... see THIAMINE

Antiberiberi Vitamin .... see THIAMINE

Anti-Blacktongue Factor .... see NIACIN AND NIACINAMIDE

Antineuritic Factor .... see THIAMINE

Antineuritic Vitamin .... see THIAMINE

Antipellagra Factor .... see NIACIN AND NIACINAMIDE

Antiscorbutic Vitamin .... see VITAMIN C

Antitumor Angiogenesis Factor
.... see BOVINE CARTILAGE

Antixerophthalmic Vitamin ...... see VITAMIN A

Anurine .... see THIAMINE

Aonla .... see INDIAN GOOSEBERRY

Aphanes arvensis .... see PARSLEY PIERT

Aphanizomenon flos-aquae ...... see BLUE-GREEN ALGAE

Apii Fructus .... see CELERY

Apis cerana .... see BEESWAX

Apis mellifera .... see BEESWAX, HONEY, HONEY BEE venom, ROYAL JELLY

Apis mellifera venom ...... see HONEY BEE venom

Apitoxin .... see HONEY BEE venom

Apium carvi ...... see CARAWAY dried fruit, seed, CARAWAY OIL

Apium graveolens .... see CELERY

Apium petroselinum ...... see PARSLEY leaf, root, PARSLEY seed

Apocynum cannabinum ...... see CANADIAN HEMP

APPLE .... see APPLE

APPLE CIDER VINEGAR ... see APPLE CIDER VINEGAR

APRICOT .... see APRICOT

Apricot Vine .... see PASSIONFLOWER

Aquilegia vulgaris .... see COLUMBINE

Ara-6 .... see LARCH ARABINOGALACTAN

Arabian Myrrh .... see MYRRH

Arachis .... see PEANUT OIL

Arachis hypogaea .... see PEANUT OIL

Aralia racemosa ...... see AMERICAN SPIKENARD

Arandano Americano .... see CRANBERRY

Arandano Trepador .... see CRANBERRY

Araoba .... see GOA POWDER

Aranuel .... see BLACK SEED

Arberry .... see UVA URSI

Arborvitae ...... see CEDAR leaf, CEDAR LEAF OIL

Arbutus uva-ursi .... see UVA URSI

Archangel ...... see WHITE DEAD NETTLE FLOWER

Archangelica officinalis ...... see ANGELICA root

Archangle .... see BUGLEWEED

Arcostaphylos .... see UVA URSI

Arctic Root .... see ROSEROOT

Arctium lappa .... see BURDOCK

Arctium minus .... see BURDOCK

Arctium tomentosum .... see BURDOCK

Arctostaphylos uva-ursi .... see UVA URSI

ARECA .... see ARECA

Areca catechu .... see ARECA

Areca Nut .... see ARECA

ARENARIA RUBRA ...... see ARENARIA RUBRA

Arg .... see L-ARGININE

Argasse .... see SEA BUCKTHORN

Argilla .... see KAOLIN

Arginine .... see L-ARGININE

Arginine Hydrocholoride ...... see L-ARGININE

Argousier .... see SEA BUCKTHORN

Argyreia nervosa ...... see HAWAIIAN BABY WOODROSE

Argyreia speciosa ...... see HAWAIIAN BABY WOODROSE

ARISTOLOCHIA .... see ARISTOLOCHIA

Aristolochia clematitis .... see ARISTOLOCHIA

Aristolochia serpentaria ...... see ARISTOLOCHIA

Arjuna .... see TERMINALIA

Armoise ...... see WORMWOOD above ground parts

Armoise Capillaire .... see YIN CHEN

Armoise Commune .... see MUGWORT

Armoracia lopathifolia .... see HORSERADISH

Armoracia rusticana .... see HORSERADISH

Armstrong .... see KNOTWEED HERB

ARNICA .... see ARNICA

Arnica cordifolia .... see ARNICA

Arnica Flos .... see ARNICA

Arnica Flower .... see ARNICA

I N D E X

Arnica fulgens .... see ARNICA
Arnica latifolia .... see ARNICA
Arnica montana .... see ARNICA
Arnica sororia .... see ARNICA
Arnikabluten .... see ARNICA
Arnotta .... see ANNATTO
ARRACH .... see ARRACH
ARROWROOT .... see ARROWROOT
Arrowwood .... see ALDER BUCKTHORN, WAHOO
Arruda Bravam .... see JABORANDI
Arruda Do Mato .... see JABORANDI
Arryan .... see CHEKEN
Arsesmart .... see SMARTWEED
Artemisia .... see MUGWORT
Artemisia absinthium
.... see WORMWOOD above ground parts,
WORMWOOD oil
Artemisia annua .... see SWEET ANNIE
Artemisia capillaris .... see YIN CHEN
Artemisia cina .... see WORMSEED
Artemisia dracunculus .... see TARRAGON
Artemisia scoparia .... see YIN CHEN
Artemisia vulgaris .... see MUGWORT
Artemisiae vulgaris herba .... see MUGWORT
Artemisiae vulgaris radix .... see MUGWORT
Artemisinin .... see SWEET ANNIE
Artesian Absinthium
.... see WORMWOOD above ground parts
Arthritica .... see COWSLIP
Artichaut Commun .... see ARTICHOKE
ARTICHOKE .... see ARTICHOKE
Artischocke .... see ARTICHOKE
ARUM .... see ARUM
Arum maculatum .... see ARUM
Arundinaria japonica .... see BAMBOO
Arusa .... see MALABAR NUT
Asa Foetida .... see ASAFOETIDA
Asafetida .... see ASAFOETIDA
ASAFOETIDA .... see ASAFOETIDA
ASARABACCA .... see ASARABACCA
Asaroun .... see ASARABACCA
Asarum .... see ASARABACCA
Asarum europaeum .... see ASARABACCA
Asclepias geminate .... see GYMNEMA
Asclepias incarnata .... see SWAMP MILKWEED
Asclepias tuberosa .... see PLEURISY ROOT
Ascophyllum nodosum ...... see ALGIN, BLADDERWRACK
Ascorbate .... see VITAMIN C
Ascorbic Acid .... see VITAMIN C
ASH .... see ASH
Ashangee .... see BUGLEWEED
Ashe Juniper
.... see CEDARWOOD bark, berry, leaf, seed, twig
Ashwaganda .... see WITHANIA
Ashwagandha .... see WITHANIA
Ashweed .... see GOUTWEED
Asian Ginseng .... see GINSENG, PANAX
Asiatic Ginseng .... see GINSENG, PANAX
Asimina triloba .... see AMERICAN PAWPAW
Aspalathus contaminata .... see RED BUSH TEA
Aspalathus linearis .... see RED BUSH TEA
Asparagi Rhizoma Root .... see ASPARAGUS
ASPARAGUS .... see ASPARAGUS
Asparagus officinalis .... see ASPARAGUS

Aspartate Chelated Minerals .... see ASPARTATES
Aspartate Mineral Chelates .... see ASPARTATES
ASPARTATES .... see ASPARTATES
ASPEN .... see ASPEN
Asperge .... see ASPARAGUS
Asperula odorata .... see SWEET WOODRUFF
Aspidosperma quebracho-blanco .... see QUEBRACHO
Ass Ear .... see COMFREY
Assant .... see ASAFOETIDA
Ass's Foot .... see COLTSFOOT
Astaxanthin .... see MICROALGAE
Aster helenium .... see ELECAMPANE
Aster officinalis .... see ELECAMPANE
Asthma Weed .... see LOBELIA
ASTRAGALUS .... see ASTRAGALUS
Astragalus gummifera .... see TRAGACANTH
Astragalus membranaceus .... see ASTRAGALUS
Astragalus mongholicus .... see ASTRAGALUS
Aswagandha .... see WITHANIA
Athemis nobilis .... see ROMAN CHAMOMILE
Athyrium filix-femina .... see LADY FERN
Atlantic Yam .... see WILD YAM
Atropa belladonna acuminata .... see BELLADONNA
Aubepine .... see HAWTHORN fruit,
HAWTHORN leaf, flower,
HAWTHORN leaf with flower extract
Auckland Costus .... see COSTUS OIL, COSTUS root
Aucklandia costus .... see COSTUS OIL, COSTUS root
Augentrostkraut .... see EYEBRIGHT
August Flower .... see GUMWEED
Aurantii Pericarpium .... see BITTER ORANGE peel
Australian Febrifuge .... see FEVER BARK
Australian Fever Bush .... see FEVER BARK
Australian Quinine .... see FEVER BARK
Australian Tea Tree Oil .... see TEA TREE OIL
AUTUMN CROCUS .... see AUTUMN CROCUS
Autumn Crocus .... see SAFFRON
Ava .... see KAVA
Avarada .... see WITHANIA
Aveleira .... see HAZELNUT
Avelinier .... see HAZELNUT
Avellano .... see HAZELNUT
Avena Fructus .... see OATS
Avena sativa .... see OAT above ground parts,
OAT BRAN, OATS, OAT STRAW
Avenae herba .... see OAT above ground parts
Avenae stramentum .... see OAT STRAW
AVENS .... see AVENS
AVOCADO .... see AVOCADO
Avocato .... see AVOCADO
Awa .... see KAVA
Axerophtholum .... see VITAMIN A
Axjun Argun .... see TERMINALIA
AY-27255 .... see VINPOCETINE
Ayak Chichira .... see MACA
Ayegreen .... see HOUSELEEK
Ayron .... see HOUSELEEK
Ayuk Willku .... see MACA
Azadirachta indica .... see NEEM
Azafron .... see SAFFRON
Azarum .... see ASARABACCA
Azeda-Brava .... see SORREL
Aztec Marigold .... see TAGETES
Azucacaa .... see STEVIA

INDEX

B .... see BORON, L-CARNITINE
B Complex Vitamin .... See FOLIC ACID,
NIACIN AND NIACINAMIDE,
PANTOTHENIC ACID, PYRIDOXINE,
RIBOFLAVIN, THIAMINE, VITAMIN B12
B-DPNH .... see NADH
B-hydroxy-N-trimethyl aminobutyric acid
.... see L-CARNITINE
B serratifolia .... see BUCHU
B-sitosterol 3-B-D-glucoside .... see BETA-SITOSTEROL
B-sitosterolin .... see BETA-SITOSTEROL
B(t) Factor .... see L-CARNITINE
BA JI TIAN .... see BA JI TIAN
Baby Hawaiian Woodrose
.... see HAWAIIAN BABY WOODROSE
Baby Wood-rose .... see HAWAIIAN BABY WOODROSE
Bac Ngu Vi Tu .... see SCHISANDRA
Baccae .... see EUROPEAN ELDER fruit
Bachelor's Button .... see FEVERFEW
Backache Root .... see MARSH BLAZING STAR
Bacopa monniera .... see BRAHMI
Bacopa monnieri .... see BRAHMI
Badiana .... see STAR ANISE
BAEL .... see BAEL
Bahama Cascarilla .... see CASCARILLA
Bahera .... see TERMINALIA
Bahia Powder .... see GOA POWDER
Bahira .... see TERMINALIA
Bai Dou Kou .... see CARDAMOM
Bai Guo Ye .... see GINKGO leaf, GINKGO leaf extract
Bai Qu Cai
.... see GREATER CELANDINE dried above ground parts
Baiguo .... see GINKGO seed
BAIKAL SKULLCAP .... see BAIKAL SKULLCAP
Baises De Sureau .... see EUROPEAN ELDER fruit
Bal .... see MYRRH
Bala .... see COUNTRY MALLOW
Bala Harade .... see TERMINALIA
Baldrian .... see VALERIAN
Baldrianwurzel .... see VALERIAN
Balera .... see TERMINALIA
Ballota .... see BLACK HOREHOUND
Ballota nigra .... see BLACK HOREHOUND
Balm .... see LEMON BALM
Balm of Gilead .... see CANADA BALSAM, POPLAR
Balm of Gilead Fir .... see HEMLOCK SPRUCE
Balmony .... see TURTLE HEAD
Balsam-Apple .... see BITTER MELON
Balsam Canada .... see CANADA BALSAM
Balsam Fir .... see CANADA BALSAM,
HEMLOCK SPRUCE
Balsam Fir Canada .... see CANADA BALSAM
Balsam Fir Oregon .... see OREGON FIR BALSAM
Balsam of Fir .... see CANADA BALSAM
Balsam of Peru .... see PERU BALSAM
Balsam of Tolu .... see TOLU BALSAM
Balsam Oregon .... see OREGON FIR BALSAM
Balsam Pear .... see BITTER MELON
Balsam Peru .... see PERU BALSAM
Balsam Poplar Buds .... see POPLAR
Balsam Styracis .... see STORAX
Balsam Tolu .... see TOLU BALSAM
Balsam-Weed .... see JEWELWEED
Balsambirne .... see BITTER MELON

Balsamo .... see BITTER MELON
Balsamodendron Myrrha .... see MYRRH
Balsamum Peruvianum .... see PERU BALSAM
Balsamum Styrax Liquidus .... see STORAX
Balsamum Tolutanum .... see TOLU BALSAM
Balucanat .... see TUNG SEED
BAMBOO .... see BAMBOO
Band Man's Plaything .... see YARROW
Baneberry .... see BLACK COHOSH, WHITE COHOSH
Banji .... see MARIJUANA
Bannal .... see SCOTCH BROOM flower,
SCOTCH BROOM herb
Bantu Tulip .... see AFRICAN WILD POTATO
Baptista tinctoria .... see WILD INDIGO
Baraka .... see BLACK SEED
Barbados Cherry .... see ACEROLA
Barbasco .... see WILD YAM
Barberry .... see OREGON GRAPE
Barber's Brush .... see TEAZLE
Bardana .... see BURDOCK
Bardanae Radix .... see BURDOCK
Bardane .... see BURDOCK
Bariar .... see COUNTRY MALLOW
BARLEY .... see BARLEY
Barosma betulina .... see BUCHU
Barosma crenulata .... see BUCHU
Barosmae Folium .... see BUCHU
Barrenwort .... see EPIMEDIUM
Barweed .... see CLIVERS
Basam .... see SCOTCH BROOM herb
BASIL .... see BASIL
Basil Thyme .... see CALAMINT
Basilici Herba .... see BASIL
Basket Willow .... see WILLOW BARK
Basking Shark Liver Oil .... see SHARK LIVER OIL
Bassora Tragacanth .... see KARAYA GUM
Basswood
.... see LINDEN CHARCOAL, LINDEN dried flower,
LINDEN dried leaf, LINDEN dried sapwood
Bastard Cinnamon .... see CASSIA
Bastard Ginseng .... see CODONOPSIS
Bastard Mahogany .... see ANDIROBA
Bastard Saffron .... see SAFFLOWER
Batavia Cassia .... see CINNAMON bark
Batavia Cinnamon .... see CINNAMON bark
Batchelor's Buttons ...... see BUTTERCUP, CORNFLOWER
Bauchweh .... see YARROW
Baurenlilien .... see WHITE LILY
Bay .... see SWEET BAY
Bay Laurel .... see SWEET BAY
Bay Tree .... see SWEET BAY
Bay Willow .... see WILLOW BARK
BAYBERRY .... see BAYBERRY
Bayberry .... see SWEET GALE
BCAAs .... see BRANCHED-CHAIN AMINO ACIDS
BD .... see BUTANEDIOL
Bdellium .... see MYRRH
BDO .... see BUTANEDIOL
Bead Tree .... see NEEM
Bead Vine .... see PRECATORY BEAN
Bean Herb .... see SUMMER SAVORY
BEAN POD .... see BEAN POD
Bean Trifoil .... see LABURNUM
Bear Grass .... see YUCCA

© Copyright 2000, Natural Medicines Comprehensive Database (209) 472-2244. For updated data, go to www.NaturalDatabase.com. • 1459

Bearberry .... see UVA URSI
Bearbind .... see GREATER BINDWEED
Beard Moss .... see USNEA
Bearded Darnel .... see TAUMELLOOLCH
Beargrape .... see UVA URSI
Bear's-Bind .... see GREATER BINDWEED
BEAR'S GARLIC .... see BEAR'S GARLIC
Bear's Grape .... see POKEWEED berry,
POKEWEED root, UVA URSI
Bear's Paw .... see MALE FERN
Bear's Weed .... see YERBA SANTA
Bearsgrape .... see UVA URSI
Beaumont Root .... see BLACK ROOT
Beaver Tree .... see MAGNOLIA bark
Beccabunga .... see BROOKLIME
Bedstraw .... see CLIVERS
Bedumil .... see VITAMIN B12
Bee Balm .... see OSWEGO TEA
Bee Glue .... see PROPOLIS
Bee Nettle .... see WHITE DEAD NETTLE FLOWER
Bee Plant ...... see BORAGE flower, dried above ground parts
BEE POLLEN .... see BEE POLLEN
Bee Propolis .... see PROPOLIS
Bee Sting Venom .... see HONEY BEE venom
Bee Venom .... see HONEY BEE venom
Beebread ..... see BORAGE flower, dried above ground parts,
RED CLOVER
Beeflower .... see WALLFLOWER
Beefsteak Plant .... see PERILLA
Beesnest Plant .... see WILD CARROT
BEESWAX .... see BEESWAX
BEET .... see BEET
Beg Kei .... see ASTRAGALUS
Beggar's Blanket .... see MULLEIN
Beggar's Buttons .... see BURDOCK
Beggarweed .... see DODDER, KNOTWEED HERB
Beggary .... see FUMITORY
Behada .... see TERMINALIA
Bei Chai Hu .... see BUPLEURUM
Bei Qi .... see ASTRAGALUS
Bei Wu Wei Zi .... see SCHISANDRA
Bejunco de Cerca .... see ABUTA
Bel .... see BAEL
Beleric Myrobalan .... see TERMINALIA
Belgium Valerian .... see VALERIAN
BELLADONNA .... see BELLADONNA
Belladonna .... see SCOPOLIA
Belladonna Scopola .... see SCOPOLIA
Bellflower .... see CODONOPSIS
Bellis perennis .... see WILD DAISY
Benedict's Herb .... see AVENS
Bengal Quince .... see BAEL
Bennet's Root .... see AVENS
Benzoe .... see BENZOIN
BENZOIN .... see BENZOIN
Berberidis cortex .... see EUROPEAN BARBERRY
Berberidis fructus .... see EUROPEAN BARBERRY
Berberidis radicis cortex .... see EUROPEAN BARBERRY
Berberidis radix .... see EUROPEAN BARBERRY
Berberis aquifolium .... see OREGON GRAPE
Berberis nervosa .... see OREGON GRAPE
Berberis repens .... see OREGON GRAPE
Berberis sonnei .... see OREGON GRAPE
Berberis vulgaris .... see EUROPEAN BARBERRY

Berberitze .... see EUROPEAN BARBERRY
Berberry .... see EUROPEAN BARBERRY
Berbis .... see EUROPEAN BARBERRY
Bergamot .... see BERGAMOT OIL, OSWEGO TEA
BERGAMOT OIL .... see BERGAMOT OIL
Bergamot Orange .... see BERGAMOT OIL
Bergamota .... see BERGAMOT OIL
Bergamotier .... see BERGAMOT OIL
Bergamoto .... see BERGAMOT OIL
Bergamotte .... see BERGAMOT OIL
Bergamotto Bigarade Orange ...... see BERGAMOT OIL
Bergwohlverleih .... see ARNICA
Berro .... see WATERCRESS
Berro Di Agua .... see WATERCRESS
Besenginaterkraut .... see SCOTCH BROOM flower
Besom .... see SCOTCH BROOM herb
Beta, beta-carotene-4,4-dione .... see CANTHAXANTHIN
BETA-CAROTENE .... see BETA-CAROTENE
Beta-D-fructofuranosidase
.... see FRUCTO-OLIGOSACCHARIDES
Beta-D-ribofuranose .... see RIBOSE
Beta, Epsilon-Carotene-3, 31-diol .... see LUTEIN
Beta-galactosidase .... see LACTASE
Beta-hydroxy-beta-methylbutyrate
.... see HYDROXYMETHYLBUTYRATE
Beta-hydroxy-gamma-trimethylammonium butyrate
.... see L-CARNITINE
(Beta-hydroxyethyl) trimethylethylammonium hydroxide
.... see CHOLINE
Beta-phenyl-alanine .... see PHENYLALANINE
Beta-sitostanol .... see SITOSTANOL
BETA-SITOSTEROL .... see BETA-SITOSTEROL
Beta-sitosterol glycoside .... see BETA-SITOSTEROL
Beta sitosterin .... see BETA-SITOSTEROL
Beta-tocopherol .... see VITAMIN E
Beta tocotrienol .... see VITAMIN E
Beta vulgaris .... see BEET
Betaine .... see BETAINE ANHYDROUS,
BETAINE HYDROCHLORIDE
BETAINE ANHYDROUS ..... see BETAINE ANHYDROUS
BETAINE HYDROCHLORIDE
.... see BETAINE HYDROCHLORIDE
Betel Nut .... see ARECA
Betel Quid .... see ARECA
BETH ROOT .... see BETH ROOT
Betonica officinalis .... see BETONY
BETONY .... see BETONY
Betula pendula .... see BIRCH
Betula pubescens .... see BIRCH
Betula verrucosa .... see BIRCH
Betulaceae family .... see HAZELNUT
Betulae folium .... see BIRCH
Bhang .... see MARIJUANA
Bianco spino .... see HAWTHORN fruit
Bibernellkraut .... see PIMPINELLA above ground parts
Bible Frankincense .... see FRANKINCENSE
Bidara .... see ANDROGRAPHIS
Bidens tripartitia .... see BURR MARIGOLD
Bifido .... see BIFIDOBACTERIUM BIFIDUM
BIFIDOBACTERIUM BIFIDUM
.... see BIFIDOBACTERIUM BIFIDUM
Big Marigold .... see TAGETES
Bignonia sempervirens .... see GELSEMIUM
BILBERRY dried ripe fruit ... see BILBERRY dried ripe fruit

BILBERRY leaf .... see BILBERRY leaf
Biletan .... see ALPHA-LIPOIC ACID
Biobran .... see MGN-3
Bioelectrical Minerals .... see COLLOIDAL MINERALS
Biota orientalis .... see ORIENTAL ARBORVITAE
BIOTIN .... see BIOTIN
Biowater .... see WILLARD WATER
Birangasifa .... see YARROW
BIRCH .... see BIRCH
Bird Bread .... see COMMON STONECROP
Bird Pepper .... see CAPSICUM
Birdlime Mistletoe .... see EUROPEAN MISTLETOE
Bird's Eye Maple .... see RED MAPLE
Bird's Foot .... see FENUGREEK
Bird's Nest Root .... see WILD CARROT
Bird's Tongue .... see ASH, KNOTWEED HERB
Birdweed .... see KNOTWEED HERB
Birthroot .... see BETH ROOT
Birthwort .... see ARISTOLOCHIA
Bis-carboxyethyl germanium sesquioxide
   .... see GERMANIUM
Bischofskrautfruchte .... see BISHOP'S WEED
Biscuits .... see TORMENTIL
Bishop Wort .... see BETONY
Bishop's Elder .... see GOUTWEED
BISHOP'S WEED .... see BISHOP'S WEED
Bishop's Weed Fruit .... see BISHOP'S WEED
Bishopsweed .... see BISHOP'S WEED, GOUTWEED
Bishopswort .... see BETONY, GOUTWEED
Bissy Nut .... see COLA NUT
BISTORT .... see BISTORT
BITTER ALMOND .... see BITTER ALMOND
Bitter Almond Oil .... see BITTER ALMOND
Bitter Apple .... see BITTER MELON, COLOCYNTH
Bitter Ash .... see WAHOO, QUASSIA
Bitter Bark .... see CASCARA
Bitter Buttons .... see TANSY
Bitter Cucumber .... see BITTER MELON, COLOCYNTH
Bitter Damson .... see SIMARUBA
Bitter Fennel .... see FENNEL fruit, seed
Bitter Gourd .... see BITTER MELON
Bitter Herb .... see CENTAURY, TURTLE HEAD
Bitter Lettuce .... see WILD LETTUCE
BITTER MELON .... see BITTER MELON
BITTER MILKWORT .... see BITTER MILKWORT
Bitter Nightshade .... see BITTERSWEET NIGHTSHADE
BITTER ORANGE flower, flower oil
   .... see BITTER ORANGE flower, flower oil
BITTER ORANGE peel .... see BITTER ORANGE peel
Bitter Redberry .... see AMERICAN DOGWOOD
Bitter Root .... see CANADIAN HEMP, GENTIAN
Bitter Winter .... see PIPSISSEWA
Bitter Wintergreen .... see PIPSISSEWA
Bittergurke .... see BITTER MELON
Bitterstick .... see CHIRATA
Bittersweet .... see BITTERSWEET NIGHTSHADE
BITTERSWEET NIGHTSHADE .... see BITTERSWEET
   NIGHTSHADE
Bitterwood .... see QUASSIA
Bitterwort .... see GENTIAN
Bixa orellana .... see ANNATTO
Bizzom .... see SCOTCH BROOM herb
BLACK ALDER .... see BLACK ALDER
Black Balsam .... see PERU BALSAM

Black-Berried Alder .... see EUROPEAN ELDER flower,
   EUROPEAN ELDER fruit
BLACK BRYONY .... see BLACK BRYONY
Black Caraway .... see BLACK SEED
Black Catechu .... see CATECHU
Black Cherry .... see WILD CHERRY
Black Choke .... see WILD CHERRY
BLACK COHOSH .... see BLACK COHOSH
Black Cumin .... see BLACK SEED
BLACK CURRANT berry ..... see BLACK CURRANT berry
BLACK CURRANT dried leaf
   .... see BLACK CURRANT dried leaf
BLACK CURRANT SEED OIL
   .... see BLACK CURRANT SEED OIL
Black Cutch .... see CATECHU
Black Date .... see JUJUBE
Black Dogwood .... see ALDER BUCKTHORN
Black Elder .... see EUROPEAN ELDER flower,
   EUROPEAN ELDER fruit
Black Elderberry .... see EUROPEAN ELDER fruit
Black-Eyed Susan .... see PRECATORY BEAN
Black Ginger .... see GINGER
Black Grape Raisins .... see GRAPE fruit, skin
BLACK HAW .... see BLACK HAW
BLACK HELLEBORE .... see BLACK HELLEBORE
BLACK HOREHOUND .... see BLACK HOREHOUND
BLACK MULBERRY .... see BLACK MULBERRY
BLACK MUSTARD oil .... see BLACK MUSTARD oil
BLACK MUSTARD seed .... see BLACK MUSTARD seed
BLACK NIGHTSHADE .... see BLACK NIGHTSHADE
Black Pepper
   .... see BLACK PEPPER AND WHITE PEPPER
BLACK PEPPER AND WHITE PEPPER
   .... see BLACK PEPPER AND WHITE PEPPER
BLACK PSYLLIUM .... see BLACK PSYLLIUM
BLACK ROOT .... see BLACK ROOT
Black Root .... see COMFREY
Black Sampson .... see ECHINACEA
BLACK SEED .... see BLACK SEED
Black Snakeroot .... see BLACK COHOSH
Black Stinking Horehound .... see BLACK HOREHOUND
Black Susans .... see ECHINACEA
Black Tang .... see BLADDERWRACK
BLACK TEA .... see BLACK TEA
BLACK WALNUT .... see BLACK WALNUT
Black Whortles .... see BILBERRY dried ripe fruit,
   BILBERRY leaf
BLACKBERRY leaf .... see BLACKBERRY leaf
BLACKBERRY root .... see BLACKBERRY root
Blackeye Root .... see BLACK BRYONY
BLACKTHORN berry .... see BLACKTHORN berry
BLACKTHORN flower .... see BLACKTHORN flower
Blackthorn Fruit .... see BLACKTHORN berry
Blackwort .... see COMFREY
Bladder Fucus .... see BLADDERWRACK
Bladderpod .... see LOBELIA
BLADDERWORT .... see BLADDERWORT
BLADDERWRACK .... see BLADDERWRACK
Blanc Poivre .. see BLACK PEPPER AND WHITE PEPPER
Blanket Herb .... see MULLEIN
Blanket Leaf .... see MULLEIN
Blasentang .... see BLADDERWRACK
Blatterdock .... see PETASITES leaf, PETASITES root

© Copyright 2000, Natural Medicines Comprehensive Database (209) 472-2244. For updated data, go to www.NaturalDatabase.com. • 1461

Blazing Star .... see ALETRIS, FALSE UNICORN, MARSH BLAZING STAR
Bleaberry .... see BILBERRY dried ripe fruit, BILBERRY leaf
Bleached Beeswax .... see BEESWAX
Bleeding Heart .... see NERVE ROOT, TURKEY CORN, WAHOO
BLESSED THISTLE .... see BLESSED THISTLE
Blighia sapida .... see ACKEE
Blind Nettle .... see WHITE DEAD NETTLE FLOWER
Blind Weed .... see SHEPHERD'S PURSE
Blisterweed .... see BUTTERCUP
Blond Plantago .... see BLOND PSYLLIUM
BLOND PSYLLIUM .... see BLOND PSYLLIUM
Blood Elder .... see DWARF ELDER
Blood Hilder .... see DWARF ELDER
Blood of the Dragon .... see SANGRE DE GRADO
BLOODROOT .... see BLOODROOT
Bloodroot ....see TORMENTIL
Bloodwood .... see LOGWOOD
Bloodwort .... see YARROW
Blooming Sally .... see PURPLE LOOSESTRIFE
Blowball .... see DANDELION above ground parts, DANDELION entire plant
Blue Balm .... see OSWEGO TEA
Blue Barberry .... see OREGON GRAPE
Blue Bells .... see ABSCESS ROOT
Blue Cap .... see CORNFLOWER
Blue Centaury .... see CORNFLOWER
BLUE COHOSH .... see BLUE COHOSH
Blue Curls .... see SELF-HEAL
BLUE FLAG .... see BLUE FLAG
Blue Flag .... see ORRIS
Blue Ginseng .... see BLUE COHOSH
BLUE-GREEN ALGAE .... see BLUE-GREEN ALGAE
Blue Gum .... see EUCALYPTUS dried leaf
Blue Mallow .... see MALLOW leaf
Blue Mallow Flower .... see MALLOW flower
Blue Monkshood Root .... see ACONITE
Blue Nightshade .... see BITTERSWEET NIGHTSHADE
Blue Pimpernel .... see SCULLCAP
Blue Sailors .... see CHICORY
Blue Vervain .... see VERBENA
Blueberry .... see BILBERRY dried ripe fruit, BILBERRY leaf
Bluebonnet .... see CORNFLOWER
Bluebottle .... see CORNFLOWER
Bluebow .... see CORNFLOWER
BNADH .... see NADH
Bobbins .... see ARUM
Bockshornsame .... see FENUGREEK
Bofareira .... see CASTOR OIL, CASTOR seed
BOG BILBERRY .... see BOG BILBERRY
Bog Myrtle .... see SWEET GALE
Bog Rhubarb .... see PETASITES leaf, PETASITES root
BOGBEAN .... see BOGBEAN
Bogshorns .... see PETASITES leaf, PETASITES root
Bohnenkraut .... see SUMMER SAVORY
BOIS DE ROSE OIL .... see BOIS DE ROSE OIL
Bois Douleur .... see MORINDA
Bol .... see MYRRH
Bola .... see MYRRH
Boldine .... see BOLDO
BOLDO .... see BOLDO

Boldo Folium .... see BOLDO
Boldoak Boldea .... see BOLDO
Boldus .... see BOLDO
Boletus Versicolor .... see CORIOLUS MUSHROOM
Bolivian Coca .... see COCA
Bolus Alba .... see KAOLIN
Bone Ash .... see PHOSPHATE SALTS
Bone Meal .... see CALCIUM
Bone Phosphate .... see PHOSPHATE SALTS
BONESET .... see BONESET
Bonnet Bellflower .... see CODONOPSIS
Bookoo .... see BUCHU
Boor Tree .... see EUROPEAN ELDER flower, EUROPEAN ELDER fruit
BORAGE flower, dried above ground parts .... see BORAGE flower, dried above ground parts
BORAGE SEED OIL .... see BORAGE SEED OIL
Borago .... see BORAGE flower, dried above ground parts
Borago officinalis .... see BORAGE flower, dried above ground parts, BORAGE SEED OIL
Borbonia pinfolia .... see RED BUSH TEA
Borneo-mahogany .... see LAURELWOOD
BORON .... see BORON
Boswellia carteri .... see FRANKINCENSE
Boswellia serrata .... see INDIAN FRANKINCENSE
Botfly Maggot .... see MAGGOTS
Bottle Brush .... see HORSETAIL
Bouncing Bess .... see RED-SPUR VALERIAN
Bouncing-Bet .... see RED SOAPWORT
Bountry .... see EUROPEAN ELDER flower, EUROPEAN ELDER fruit
Bourbon Geranium Oil .... see ROSE GERANIUM
Bourbon Vanilla .... see VANILLA
Bouillon Blanc .... see MULLEIN
BOVINE CARTILAGE .... see BOVINE CARTILAGE
BOVINE COLOSTRUM .... see BOVINE COLOSTRUM
Bovine Immunoglobulin .... see BOVINE COLOSTRUM
Bovine lactoferrin .... see LACTOFERRIN
Bovine Whey Protein Concentrate ...... see WHEY PROTEIN
Bovis and Soldier .... see RED-SPUR VALERIAN
Bovista .... see PUFF BALL
Bowman's Root .... see BLACK ROOT, INDIAN PHYSIC
Box Holly .... see BUTCHER'S BROOM
Box Tree .... see AMERICAN DOGWOOD
Boxberry .... see WINTERGREEN leaf, WINTERGREEN oil
BOXWOOD .... see BOXWOOD
Boxwood .... see AMERICAN DOGWOOD
BRAHMI .... see BRAHMI
Brake Root .... see LADY FERN
Bramble .... see BLACKBERRY leaf, BLACKBERRY root
Bran .... see WHEAT BRAN
BRANCHED-CHAIN AMINO ACIDS .... see BRANCHED-CHAIN AMINO ACIDS
Branching Phytolacca .... see POKEWEED berry, POKEWEED root
Brandlattich .... see COLTSFOOT
Brandy Mint .... see PEPPERMINT leaf
Brassica alba .... see WHITE MUSTARD
Brassica nigra .... see BLACK MUSTARD oil, BLACK MUSTARD seed
Brassica oleracea .... see CABBAGE
Brauneria Angustifolia .... see ECHINACEA
Brauneria Pallida .... see ECHINACEA

INDEX

Brazil Powder .... see GOA POWDER
Brazil Root.. see IPECAC
Brazilian Cocoa .... see GUARANA
Brazilian Ginseng .... see SUMA
Brazilian Ipecac .... see IPECAC
Brazilian Mahogany .... see ANDIROBA
Brazilian Rhatany .... see RHATANY
Brechnusssamen .... see NUX VOMICA
Breeam .... see SCOTCH BROOM herb
Breiapfelbaum .... see CHICLE
BREWER'S YEAST .... see BREWER'S YEAST
BREWER'S YEAST (HANSEN CBS 5926)
.... see BREWER'S YEAST (HANSEN CBS 5926)
Brideweed .... see YELLOW TOADFLAX
Bridewort .... see MEADOWSWEET
Brigham Tea .... see MORMON TEA
Brindal Berry .... see GARCINIA
Brindle Berry .... see GARCINIA
British Indian Lemongrass .... see LEMONGRASS
British Myrrh .... see SWEET CICELY
British Tobacco .... see COLTSFOOT
Brittle Willow .... see WILLOW BARK
Broad-Leafed Laurel .... see MOUNTAIN LAUREL
Broad-Leaved Dock .... see YELLOW DOCK
Broad-leaved Garlic .... see BEAR'S GARLIC
BROMELAIN .... see BROMELAIN
Bromelains .... see BROMELAIN
Bromelainum .... see BROMELAIN
Bromelin .... see BROMELAIN
Bromus hordeaceus .... see HAY FLOWER
Brook mint .... see JAPANESE MINT
BROOKLIME .... see BROOKLIME
Broom .... see SCOTCH BROOM herb
BROOM CORN .... see BROOM CORN
Broom Flower .... see DYER'S BROOM
Broom Tops .... see SCOTCH BROOM flower
Browme .... see SCOTCH BROOM herb
Brown Algae .... see LAMINARIA
Brown Psyllium .... see BLACK PSYLLIUM
Brownwort .... see SELF-HEAL
Bruchkraut .... see RUPTUREWORT
Bruisewort .... see COMFREY, WILD DAISY
Brum .... see SCOTCH BROOM herb
Brunfelsia hopeana .... see MANACA
Brunnenkresse .... see WATERCRESS
Brushes and Combs .... see TEAZLE
BRYONIA .... see BRYONIA
Bryonia alba .... see BRYONIA
Bryonia cretica .... see BRYONIA
Bryoniae Radix .... see BRYONIA
Bucco .... see BUCHU
BUCHU .... see BUCHU
Buck Qi .... see ASTRAGALUS
Buckbean .... see BOGBEAN
Buckels .... see COWSLIP
Buckeye .... see HORSE CHESTNUT branch bark,
                       HORSE CHESTNUT flower,
                       HORSE CHESTNUT leaf
BUCKHORN PLANTAIN .... see BUCKHORN PLANTAIN
Buckthorn berry .... see EUROPEAN BUCKTHORN
Buckthorn Bark .... see ALDER BUCKTHORN
Bucku .... see BUCHU
BUCKWHEAT .... see BUCKWHEAT
Buckwheat Pollen .... see BEE POLLEN

Buddhist Rosary Bead .... see PRECATORY BEAN
Budwood .... see AMERICAN DOGWOOD
Bugbane .... see AMERICAN HELLEBORE,
                                     BLACK COHOSH
BUGLE .... see BUGLE
Bugle .... see GROUND PINE
BUGLEWEED .... see BUGLEWEED
Bugloss .... see BORAGE SEED OIL
Bugula .... see BUGLE
Bugwort .... see BLACK COHOSH
BULBOUS BUTTERCUP ..... see BULBOUS BUTTERCUP
Bulgarian Yogurt .... see YOGURT
Bullock's Eye .... see HOUSELEEK
Bull's Eyes .... see MARSH MARIGOLD
Bullsfoot .... see COLTSFOOT
Bulnesia sarmienti .... see GUAIAC WOOD OIL
BUPLEURUM .... see BUPLEURUM
Bupleurum chinense .... see BUPLEURUM
Bupleurum exaltatum .... see BUPLEURUM
Bupleurum falcatum .... see BUPLEURUM
Bupleurum fruticosum .... see BUPLEURUM
Bupleurum longifolium .... see BUPLEURUM
Bupleurum multinerve .... see BUPLEURUM
Bupleurum octoradiatum .... see BUPLEURUM
Bupleurum rotundifolium .... see BUPLEURUM
Bupleurum scorzonerifolium ...... see BUPLEURUM
Burage .... see BORAGE SEED OIL
BURDOCK .... see BURDOCK
Burn Plant .... see ALOE dried juice from leaf, latex
Burnet Saxifrage .... see PIMPINELLA above ground parts,
                                     PIMPINELLA root
Burning Bush .... see WAHOO
BURNING BUSH leaf .... see BURNING BUSH leaf
BURNING BUSH root .... see BURNING BUSH root
BURR MARIGOLD .... see BURR MARIGOLD
Burr Seed .... see BURDOCK
Burrage .... see BORAGE flower, dried above ground parts,
                                     BORAGE SEED OIL
Burren Myrtle .... see BILBERRY dried ripe fruit,
                                     BILBERRY leaf
Burrwort .... see BUTTERCUP
Bursae Pastoris Herba .... see SHEPHERD'S PURSE
Bursting Heart .... see WAHOO
Bush Tree .... see BOXWOOD
Butane-1,4-diol .... see BUTANEDIOL
BUTANEDIOL (BD) .... see BUTANEDIOL (BD)
BUTCHER'S BROOM .... see BUTCHER'S BROOM
Butcher's-Broom .... see SCOTCH BROOM flower
Butter and Eggs .... see YELLOW TOADFLAX
Butter Bur .... see PETASITES leaf, PETASITES root
Butter Daisy .... see OX-EYE DAISY
Butter Rose .... see COWSLIP
BUTTERCUP .... see BUTTERCUP
Butter-Dock .... see PETASITES leaf, PETASITES root
Buttered Hayhocks .... see YELLOW TOADFLAX
Butterfly Dock ...... see PETASITES leaf, PETASITES root
Butterfly Weed .... see PLEURISY ROOT
Butternussbaum .... see BUTTERNUT
BUTTERNUT .... see BUTTERNUT
Button Snakeroot .... see MARSH BLAZING STAR
Buttonhole .... see HARTSTONGUE
Buttons .... see TANSY
Butua .... see ABUTA
Butylene glycol .... see BUTANEDIOL

INDEX

Butyrolactone .... see GAMMA BUTYROLACTONE
Butyrolactone Gamma ... see GAMMA BUTYROLACTONE
Buxus chinensis .... see JOJOBA
Buxus sempervirens .... see BOXWOOD
Ca .... see CALCIUM
Ca-A-Jhei .... see STEVIA
Ca-A-Yupi .... see STEVIA
Caa-He-E .... see STEVIA
CABBAGE .... see CABBAGE
Cabbage Palm .... see SAW PALMETTO
Cabernet Franc .... see GRAPE fruit, skin
Cabernet Sauvignon .... see GRAPE fruit, skin
Cacao .... see COCOA
Cachou .... see CATECHU
Cactus Flowers .... see PRICKLY PEAR CACTUS
Cactus grandiflorus .... see CEREUS
CADE OIL .... see CADE OIL
Caesalpinia bonducella .... see DIVI-DIVI
Cafe .... see COFFEE
Caffea .... see COFFEE
CAFFEINE .... see CAFFEINE
Caffeine and Sodium Benzoate .... see CAFFEINE
Caffeine Citrate .... see CAFFEINE
Caje Oil .... see NIAULI OIL
CAJEPUT OIL .... see CAJEPUT OIL
Cajeputi Aetheroleum .... see CAJEPUT OIL
Cajuput .... see CAJEPUT OIL
CALABAR BEAN .... see CALABAR BEAN
CALAMINT .... see CALAMINT
Calamintha ascendens .... see CALAMINT
Calamintha hortensis .... see SUMMER SAVORY
Calamintha montana .... see WINTER SAVORY
CALAMUS .... see CALAMUS
Calcifediol .... see VITAMIN D
calciferol .... see VITAMIN D
Calcii Pantothenas .... see PANTOTHENIC ACID
Calcipotriene .... see VITAMIN D
Calcipotriol .... see VITAMIN D
Calcitriol .... see VITAMIN D
Calcium .... see CALCIUM
Calcium Acetate .... see CALCIUM
Calcium Ascorbate .... see VITAMIN C
Calcium Aspartate .... see CALCIUM
Calcium Carbonate .... see CALCIUM
Calcium Carbonate Matrix .... see CORAL
Calcium Chelate .... see CALCIUM
Calcium Chloride .... see CALCIUM, PANGAMIC ACID
Calcium Citrate .... see CALCIUM
Calcium Citrate Malate .... see CALCIUM
CALCIUM D-GLUCARATE
.... see CALCIUM D-GLUCARATE
Calcium Glucarate .... see CALCIUM D-GLUCARATE
Calcium Gluconate .... see CALCIUM, PANGAMIC ACID
Calcium Lactate .... see CALCIUM
Calcium Lactogluconate .... see CALCIUM
Calcium Orotate .... see CALCIUM
Calcium Orthophosphate .... see PHOSPHATE SALTS
Calcium Pangamate .... see PANGAMIC ACID
Calcium Pantothenate .... see PANTOTHENIC ACID
Calcium Phosphate .... see CALCIUM,
                                                    PHOSPHATE SALTS
Calcium Phosphate Dibasic Anhydrous
.... see PHOSPHATE SALTS

Calcium Phosphate Dibasic Dihydrate
.... see PHOSPHATE SALTS
Calcium Phosphate Tribasic .... see PHOSPHATE SALTS
Calcium Pyruvate .... see PYRUVATE
CALENDULA .... see CALENDULA
Calendula officinalis .... see CALENDULA
Caley Pea .... see LATHYRUS
Calico Bush .... see MOUNTAIN LAUREL
California Buckthorn .... see CASCARA
California Poppies .... see CALIFORNIA POPPY
CALIFORNIA POPPY .... see CALIFORNIA POPPY
Calliphoridae .... see MAGGOTS
Calluna vulgaris .... see HEATHER
Calluna vulgaris flos .... see HEATHER
Callunae vulgaris herba .... see HEATHER
Calomba Root .... see COLOMBO
Calophyllum inophyllum .... see LAURELWOOD
CALOTROPIS .... see CALOTROPIS
Calotropis procera .... see CALOTROPIS
Caltha palustris .... see MARSH MARIGOLD
Caltrop .... see PUNCTURE VINE
Calumba .... see COLOMBO
Calumbo Root .... see COLOMBO
Calves' Snout .... see YELLOW TOADFLAX
Calystegia sepium .... see GREATER BINDWEED
Calzin .... see GRAPE fruit, skin
Camboge .... see GAMBOGE
Camellia sinensis .... see BLACK TEA, GREEN TEA
Camellia thea .... see BLACK TEA, GREEN TEA
Camellia theifera .... see BLACK TEA, GREEN TEA
Cammock .... see SPINY RESTHARROW
Camolea .... see MEZEREON
Camomilla .... see GERMAN CHAMOMILE
Camomille Allemande .... see GERMAN CHAMOMILE
CAMPHOR .... see CAMPHOR
Camphor of the Poor .... see GARLIC
Camphor Tree .... see CAMPHOR
Camphora .... see CAMPHOR
CANADA BALSAM .... see CANADA BALSAM
Canada Balsam .... see HEMLOCK SPRUCE
Canada Pitch .... see PINUS BARK
Canada Root .... see PLEURISY ROOT
Canada Tea .... see WINTERGREEN leaf,
                                                    WINTERGREEN oil
Canada Turpentine .... see CANADA BALSAM
Canadian Balsam .... see CANADA BALSAM
Canadian Beaver .... see CASTOREUM
CANADIAN FLEABANE .... see CANADIAN FLEABANE
Canadian Ginseng .... see GINSENG, AMERICAN
Canadian Hemlock .... see PINUS BARK
CANADIAN HEMP .... see CANADIAN HEMP
Canadian Trailing Arbutus ..... see CANADIAN FLEABANE
Canagnium odoratum macrophylla .... see CANANGA OIL
CANAIGRE .... see CANAIGRE
CANANGA OIL .... see CANANGA OIL
Canangium odoratum genuina ...... see YLANG YLANG OIL
Canarium commune .... see ELEMI
Canarium luzonicum .... see ELEMI
Cancer Jalap .... see POKEWEED berry, POKEWEED root
Candle-berry Tree .... see TUNG SEED
Candleberry .... see BAYBERRY, TUNG SEED
Candleflower .... see MULLEIN
Candlenut .... see TUNG SEED
Candlewick .... see MULLEIN

INDEX

CANELLA .... see CANELLA
Canella alba .... see CANELLA
Cangana odorata genuina .... see YLANG YLANG OIL
Cangana odorata macrophylla .... see CANANGA OIL
Cankerroot .... see GOLDTHREAD
Cankerwort .... see DANDELION above ground parts,
DANDELION entire plant,
TANSY RAGWORT
Cannabis .... see MARIJUANA
Cannabis sativa .... see MARIJUANA
CANTHAXANTHIN .... see CANTHAXANTHIN
Canton Cassia .... see CASSIA
Cao Mahuang.. see EPHEDRA
Capdockin .... see PETASITES leaf, PETASITES root
Cape Gooseberry .... see WINTER CHERRY
Cape Periwinkle.......... see MADAGASCAR PERIWINKLE
CAPERS .... see CAPERS
Capillary Wormwood...................................... see YIN CHEN
Capim-Cidrao .... see LEMONGRASS
Capim Doce .... see STEVIA
Capparis spinosa .... see CAPERS
Cappero... see CAPERS
Capsaicin .... see CAPSICUM
Capsella .... see SHEPHERD'S PURSE
Capsella bursa-pastoris .... see SHEPHERD'S PURSE
CAPSICUM.. see CAPSICUM
Capsicum annuum .... see CAPSICUM
Capsicum baccatum .... see CAPSICUM
Capsicum chinense .... see CAPSICUM
Capsicum Fruit .... see CAPSICUM
Capsicum frutescens .... see CAPSICUM
Capsicum pubscens .... see CAPSICUM
CARAMEL COLOR .... see CARAMEL COLOR
Caramuru .... see CATUABA
Carapa .... see ANDIROBA
Carapa guianensis .... see ANDIROBA
CARAWAY dried fruit, seed
.... see CARAWAY dried fruit, seed
CARAWAY OIL .... see CARAWAY OIL
Carbenia benedicta .... see BLESSED THISTLE
Carbon .... see ACTIVATED CHARCOAL
Carbonaceous Activated Water .... see WILLARD WATER
Carboxyethylgermanium Sesquioxide ..... see GERMANIUM
Card Thistle ....see TEAZLE
CARDAMOM ....see CARDAMOM
Cardo .... see ARTICHOKE
Cardo de Comer .... see ARTICHOKE
Cardo Santo .... see BLESSED THISTLE
Cardomomi Fructus ....see CARDAMOM
Cardon d'Espagne .... see ARTICHOKE
Cardoon .... see ARTICHOKE
Cardui mariae fructus .... see MILK THISTLE fruit, seed
Cardui mariae herba
............................see MILK THISTLE above ground parts
Carduus benedictus .... see BLESSED THISTLE
Carduus marainum
............................see MILK THISTLE above ground parts,
MILK THISTLE fruit, seed
Carex arenaria .... see GERMAN SARSAPARILLA
Carica papaya .... see PAPAIN, PAPAYA
Caricae Fructus .... see FIG
Caricae papayae folium .... see PAPAYA
Caricis rhizoma .... see GERMAN SARSAPARILLA
Carilla Gourd .... see BITTER MELON

CARLINA .... see CARLINA
Carlina acaulis .... see CARLINA
Carlinae Radix .... see CARLINA
Carline Thistle .... see MUGWORT
Carmantina .... see ANDROGRAPHIS
Carnitine .... see L-CARNITINE
Carnitine Acetyl Ester .... see ACETYL-L-CARNITINE
Carnitor .... see L-CARNITINE
CAROB .... see CAROB
Carolina Pink .... see PINK ROOT
Carolina Vanilla .... see DEERTONGUE
Caroline Jasmine .... see GELSEMIUM
Carony Bark .... see ANGOSTURA
Carophyll Red .... see CANTHAXANTHIN
Carosella .... see FENNEL fruit, seed
Carpenter's Herb .... see BUGLE, SELF-HEAL
Carpenter's Square ....see FIGWORT
Carpenter's Weed .... see SELF-HEAL, YARROW
Carphephorus odoratissimus .... see DEERTONGUE
CARRAGEENAN .... see CARRAGEENAN
Cartagena Ipecac .... see IPECAC
Carthamus tinctorius .... see SAFFLOWER
Carum carvi .... see CARAWAY dried fruit, seed,
CARAWAY OIL
Carum petroselinum .... see PARSLEY leaf, root,
PARSLEY seed
Carvi Fructus .... see CARAWAY dried fruit, seed
Caryophylli .... see CLOVE dried flowerbud, leaf, stem
Caryophyllum ....see CLOVE OIL
Caryophyllus .... see CLOVE dried flowerbud, leaf, stem,
CLOVE OIL
Caryophyllus aromaticus
.... see CLOVE dried flowerbud, leaf, stem,
CLOVE OIL
CASCARA .... see CASCARA
Cascara Sagrada .... see CASCARA
CASCARILLA .... see CASCARILLA
Caseweed .... see SHEPHERD'S PURSE
CASHEW .... see CASHEW
Cashou .... see CATECHU
Casis .... see BLACK CURRANT SEED OIL
Casse .... see SENNA
CASSIA .... see CASSIA
Cassia acutifolia .... see SENNA
Cassia angustifolia .... see SENNA
Cassia Aromaticum .... see CASSIA
Cassia Bark .... see CASSIA
Cassia Cinnamon .... see CASSIA
Cassia Lignea... see CASSIA
Cassia senna .... see SENNA
CASSIE ABSOLUTE .... see CASSIE ABSOLUTE
Cassis .... see BLACK CURRANT berry,
BLACK CURRANT SEED OIL
Castanea americana .... see AMERICAN CHESTNUT
Castanea dentata .... see AMERICAN CHESTNUT
Castanea sativa .... see EUROPEAN CHESTNUT
Castanea vesca .... see EUROPEAN CHESTNUT
Castanea vulgaris .... see EUROPEAN CHESTNUT
Castaneae Folium .... see EUROPEAN CHESTNUT
Castor... see CASTOR OIL
Castor Bean .... see CASTOR seed
Castor canadensis .... see CASTOREUM
Castor fiber .... see CASTOREUM
CASTOR OIL .... see CASTOR OIL

Castor Oil Plant .... see CASTOR OIL
CASTOR seed .... see CASTOR seed
CASTOREUM .... see CASTOREUM
Catalonina Jasmine .... see JASMINE
Catalyst Altered Water .... see WILLARD WATER
Catarrh Root .... see ALPINIA
Catchfly .... see CANADIAN HEMP
Catchweed .... see CLIVERS
CATECHU .... see CATECHU
Catechu nigrum .... see CATECHU
Caterpillar Fungus .... see CORDYCEPS
Catha edulis .... see KHAT
Catharanthus .... see MADAGASCAR PERIWINKLE
Catharanthus roseus ..... see MADAGASCAR PERIWINKLE
Catmint .... see CATNIP
CATNIP .... see CATNIP
Catrix .... see BOVINE CARTILAGE
Catrix-S .... see BOVINE CARTILAGE
CAT'S CLAW .... see CAT'S CLAW
Cat's Ear Flower .... see CAT'S FOOT
CAT'S FOOT .... see CAT'S FOOT
Cat's-Head .... see PUNCTURE VINE
Cat's-Paw .... see GROUND IVY
Cat's Tails .... see HAY FLOWER
Catsfoot .... see CAT'S FOOT, GROUND IVY
Catswort .... see CATNIP
CATUABA .... see CATUABA
Catuaba Casca .... see CATUABA
Caulophyllum .... see BLUE COHOSH
Caulophyllum thalictroides .... see BLUE COHOSH
Caulophyllum Tree .... see LAURELWOOD
Cavinton .... see VINPOCETINE
Cayenne .... see CAPSICUM
Cayenne Rosewood Oil .... see BOIS DE ROSE OIL
CDS .... see CHONDROITIN SULFATE
Ceanothus americanus .... see NEW JERSEY TEA
Cedar .... see CEDARWOOD bark, berry, leaf, seed, twig
CEDAR leaf .... see CEDAR leaf
CEDAR LEAF OIL .... see CEDAR LEAF OIL
CEDARWOOD bark, berry, leaf, seed, twig
.... see CEDARWOOD bark, berry, leaf, seed, twig
CEDARWOOD OIL .... see CEDARWOOD OIL
Cedoaria .... see ZEDOARY
Cedro .... see ANDIROBA
Celandine
.... see GREATER CELANDINE dried above ground parts
Celandine Herb
.... see GREATER CELANDINE dried above ground parts
Celandine Root
.... see GREATER CELANDINE rhizome, root
Celastrus scandens .... see AMERICAN BITTERSWEET
CELERY .... see CELERY
Celery Fruit .... see CELERY
Celery-Leafed Crowfoot ..... see POISONOUS BUTTERCUP
Celery Seed .... see CELERY
Cemphire .... see CAMPHOR
Centaurea cyanus .... see CORNFLOWER
Centaurium erythraea .... see CENTAURY
Centaurium minus .... see CENTAURY
Centaurium umbellatum .... see CENTAURY
CENTAURY .... see CENTAURY
Centella .... see GOTU KOLA
Centella asiatica .... see GOTU KOLA
Centella coriacea .... see GOTU KOLA

Centinode .... see KNOTWEED HERB
Centranthus ruber .... see RED-SPUR VALERIAN
Centraria .... see ICELAND MOSS
Centroporus squamosus .... see SHARK LIVER OIL
Cephaelis acuminata .... see IPECAC
Cephaelis ipecacuanha .... see IPECAC
Cephalin .... see PHOSPHATIDYLSERINE
Cerasomal-cis-9-cetylmyristoleate
.... see CETYL MYRISTOLEATE
Cerasus vulgaris .... see SOUR CHERRY
Ceratonia siliqua .... see CAROB
CEREUS .... see CEREUS
Cereus grandiflorus .... see CEREUS
Cerezo Acido .... see SOUR CHERRY
Cerisier Acide .... see SOUR CHERRY
Cervus elaphus .... see DEER VELVET
Cervus nippon .... see DEER VELVET
Cetoal .... see ZEDOARY
Cetorhinus maximus .... see SHARK LIVER OIL
Cetraria islandica .... see ICELAND MOSS
CETYL MYRISTOLEATE ... see CETYL MYRISTOLEATE
Cevitamic Acid .... see VITAMIN C
Ceylon Cinnamon .... see CINNAMON bark
Ceylon Citronella Grass .... see LEMONGRASS
Chaat .... see KHAT
Chamaelirium carolianum .... see FALSE UNICORN
Chamaelirium luteum .... see FALSE UNICORN
Chamaemelum nobile .... see ROMAN CHAMOMILE
Chamomile .... see GERMAN CHAMOMILE,
                                       ROMAN CHAMOMILE
Chamomilla recutita .... see GERMAN CHAMOMILE
Chamomillae ramane flos .... see ROMAN CHAMOMILE
Champaca Wood Oil .... see GUAIAC WOOD OIL
Champagne Of Life .... see KOMBUCHA TEA
CHANCA PIEDRA .... see CHANCA PIEDRA
Chanca-Piedra Blanca .... see CHANCA PIEDRA
Chandrika .... see INDIAN SNAKEROOT
Chanvrin .... see HEMP AGRIMONY
CHAPARRAL .... see CHAPARRAL
Charas .... see MARIJUANA
Charcoal .... see ACTIVATED CHARCOAL
Chardonnay .... see GRAPE fruit, skin
Charity .... see JACOB'S LADDER
Charnuska .... see BLACK SEED
Chaste Tree .... see CHASTEBERRY
CHASTEBERRY .... see CHASTEBERRY
CHAULMOOGRA .... see CHAULMOOGRA
Chaw .... see SMOKELESS TOBACCO
Cheat .... see TAUMELLOOLCH
Chebulic Myrobalan .... see TERMINALIA
Checkerberry ...... see SQUAWVINE, WINTERGREEN leaf,
                                      WINTERGREEN oil
Cheese Rennet .... see LADY'S BEDSTRAW
Cheese Renning .... see LADY'S BEDSTRAW
Cheeseflower .... see MALLOW flower
Cheiranthus cheiri .... see WALLFLOWER
Chekan .... see CHEKEN
CHEKEN .... see CHEKEN
Chelated Boron .... see CHELATED MINERALS
Chelated Calcium .... see CHELATED MINERALS
Chelated Chromium .... see CHELATED MINERALS
Chelated Cobalt .... see CHELATED MINERALS
Chelated Copper .... see CHELATED MINERALS
Chelated Iron .... see CHELATED MINERALS

INDEX

Chelated Magnesium .... see CHELATED MINERALS
Chelated Manganese .... see CHELATED MINERALS
CHELATED MINERALS ...... see CHELATED MINERALS
Chelated Molybdenum .... see CHELATED MINERALS
Chelated Potassium .... see CHELATED MINERALS
Chelated Selenium .... see CHELATED MINERALS
Chelated Trace Minerals .... see CHELATED MINERALS
Chelated Vanadium .... see CHELATED MINERALS
Chelated Zinc .... see CHELATED MINERALS
Chelidonii
.... see GREATER CELANDINE dried above ground parts
Chelidonii Herba
.... see GREATER CELANDINE dried above ground parts
Chelidonium majus
.... see GREATER CELANDINE dried above ground parts,
                        GREATER CELANDINE rhizome, root
Chelone .... see TURTLE HEAD
Chelone glabra .... see TURTLE HEAD
Chenopodium ambrosioides .... see CHENOPODIUM OIL
Chenopodium ambrosioides anthelminticum
.... see CHENOPODIUM OIL
CHENOPODIUM OIL .... see CHENOPODIUM OIL
Chenopodium vulvaria .... see ARRACH
CHEROKEE ROSEHIP .... see CHEROKEE ROSEHIP
CHERRY LAUREL WATER
.... see CHERRY LAUREL WATER
CHERVIL .... see CHERVIL
Chestnut .... see HORSE CHESTNUT seed
Chew .... see SMOKELESS TOBACCO
Chewing Tobacco .... see SMOKELESS TOBACCO
Chi Hu .... see BUPLEURUM
Chick-Pea .... see LATHYRUS
CHICKEN COLLAGEN .... see CHICKEN COLLAGEN
Chicken Toe .... see CORAL ROOT
Chickling Vetch .... see LATHYRUS
CHICKWEED .... see CHICKWEED
CHICLE .... see CHICLE
Chico Sapote .... see CHICLE
CHICORY .... see CHICORY
Chiendent Odorant .... see VETIVER
Ch'ih Shen .... see DANSHEN
Child Pick-a-Back .... see CHANCA PIEDRA
Chili Pepper .... see CAPSICUM
Chimaphila .... see PIPSISSEWA
Chimaphila corymbosa .... see PIPSISSEWA
Chimaphila umbellata .... see PIPSISSEWA
Chimney-Sweeps .... see BUCKHORN PLANTAIN
Chin Cups .... see CUPMOSS
China Bark .... see QUILLAIA
China Clay .... see KAOLIN
China Gooseberry .... see KIWI
China Root .... see ALPINIA, WILD YAM
China-Wood Oil .... see TUNG SEED
Chinarinde .... see CINCHONA
Chinchilla Enana .... see TAGETES
Chinese Almond .... see APRICOT
Chinese Angelica .... see DONG QUAI
Chinese Anise .... see STAR ANISE
Chinese Arborvitae .... see ORIENTAL ARBORVITAE
Chinese Cinnamon .... see CASSIA
CHINESE CLUB MOSS .... see CHINESE CLUB MOSS
Chinese Cornbind .... see FO-TI raw root
CHINESE CUCUMBER fruit
.... see CHINESE CUCUMBER fruit

CHINESE CUCUMBER root
.... see CHINESE CUCUMBER root
CHINESE CUCUMBER seed
.... see CHINESE CUCUMBER seed
Chinese Gelatin .... see AGAR
Chinese Ginger .... see ALPINIA
Chinese Ginseng .... see GINSENG, PANAX
Chinese Gooseberry .... see KIWI
Chinese Jujube .... see JUJUBE
Chinese Knotweed .... see FO-TI raw root
Chinese Licorice .... see LICORICE
Chinese Mint Oil .... see JAPANESE MINT
Chinese Parsley .... see CORIANDER
Chinese Privet .... see GLOSSY PRIVET
Chinese Rhubarb .... see RHUBARB
Chinese Rosehip .... see CHEROKEE ROSEHIP
Chinese Senega .... see SENEGA
Chinese Snake Gourd ...... see CHINESE CUCUMBER fruit,
                        CHINESE CUCUMBER root,
                        CHINESE CUCUMBER seed
Chinese Star Anise .... see STAR ANISE
Chinese Sumach .... see TREE OF HEAVEN
Chinese Tea .... see BLACK TEA, GREEN TEA
Chinese Thoroughwax .... see BUPLEURUM
Chinese Wormwood .... see SWEET ANNIE
Chinesischer Limonenbaum .... see SCHISANDRA
Ching-hao .... see SWEET ANNIE
Chinli-Chih .... see BITTER MELON
Chinwood .... see YEW
Chionanthus .... see FRINGETREE
Chionanthus virginicus .... see FRINGETREE
CHIRATA .... see CHIRATA
Chirayta .... see CHIRATA
Chiretta .... see ANDROGRAPHIS, CHIRATA
CHITOSAN .... see CHITOSAN
Chitosan Ascorbate .... see CHITOSAN
Chittem Bark .... see CASCARA
Chiu .... see YIN CHEN
CHIVE .... see CHIVE
CHLORELLA .... see CHLORELLA
Chlorella pyrenoidosa .... see CHLORELLA
Chlorella Vulgaris .... see CHLORELLA
CHLOROPHYLL .... see CHLOROPHYLL
Chlorophyll a .... see CHLOROPHYLL
Chlorophyll b .... see CHLOROPHYLL
Chlorophyll c .... see CHLOROPHYLL
Chlorophyll d .... see CHLOROPHYLL
CHLOROPHYLLIN .... see CHLOROPHYLLIN
Chocola .... see COCOA
Chocolate Root .... see WATER AVENS
Choke Cherry .... see WILD CHERRY
Cholecalciferol .... see VITAMIN D
CHOLINE .... see CHOLINE
Choline Bitartrate .... see CHOLINE
Choline Chloride .... see CHOLINE
Chondrodendron tomentosum .... see PAREIRA
Chondroitin 4- and 6-sulfate
.... see CHONDROITIN SULFATE
Chondroitin 4-sulfate .... see CHONDROITIN SULFATE
CHONDROITIN SULFATE
.... see CHONDROITIN SULFATE
Chondroitin Sulfate A .... see CHONDROITIN SULFATE
Chondroitin Sulfate C .... see CHONDROITIN SULFATE

© Copyright 2000, Natural Medicines Comprehensive Database (209) 472-2244. For updated data, go to www.NaturalDatabase.com. • 1467

I
N
D
E
X

Chondroitin Sulphate A Sodium
.... see CHONDROITIN SULFATE
Chondrus crispus .... see CARRAGEENAN
Chondrus Extract .... see CARRAGEENAN
Chongras .... see POKEWEED berry, POKEWEED root
Chop Nut .... see CALABAR BEAN
Chosen-Gomischi .... see SCHISANDRA
Chota-Chand .... see INDIAN SNAKEROOT
Christe Herbe .... see BLACK HELLEBORE
Christmas Flower .... see POINSETTIA
Christmas Rose Plant .... see BLACK HELLEBORE
Christ's Spear .... see ENGLISH ADDER'S TONGUE
Christ's Thorn .... see HOLLY
Chromic Chloride .... see CHROMIUM
CHROMIUM.................................... see CHROMIUM
Chromium Chloride .... see CHROMIUM
Chromium Nicotinate .... see CHROMIUM
Chromium Picolinate .... see CHROMIUM
Chrysanthemi vulgaris flos .... see TANSY
Chrysanthemi vulgaris herba .... see TANSY
CHRYSANTHEMUM .... see CHRYSANTHEMUM
Chrysanthemum cinerariifolium .... see PYRETHRUM
Chrysanthemum leucanthemum .... see OX-EYE DAISY
Chrysanthemum morifolium .... see CHRYSANTHEMUM
Chrysanthemum parthenium .... see FEVERFEW
Chrysanthemum sinense .... see CHRYSANTHEMUM
Chrysanthemum stipulaceum .... see CHRYSANTHEMUM
Chrysanthemum vulgare .... see TANSY
Chrysatobine .... see GOA POWDER
Chuan Xin Lian .... see ANDROGRAPHIS
Chuchuhuasha .... see CATUABA
Church Broom .... see TEAZLE
Church-Flower .... see MADAGASCAR PERIWINKLE
Churnstaff .... see YELLOW TOADFLAX
CHYMOTRYPSIN .... see CHYMOTRYPSIN
Chymotrypsin A .... see CHYMOTRYPSIN
Chymotrypsin B .... see CHYMOTRYPSIN
Chymotrypsinum .... see CHYMOTRYPSIN
CI Food Orange 8 .... see CANTHAXANTHIN
Cichorii Herba .... see CHICORY
Cichorii Radix .... see CHICORY
Cichorium intybus .... see CHICORY
Cicuta virosa .... see EUROPEAN WATER HEMLOCK
Cider Vinegar .... see APPLE CIDER VINEGAR
CIGUATERA .... see CIGUATERA
Ciguatera Poisoning .... see CIGUATERA
Cilantro .... see CORIANDER
Cimicifuga .... see BLACK COHOSH
Cimicifuga racemosa .... see BLACK COHOSH
Cinchol .... see BETA-SITOSTEROL
CINCHONA .... see CINCHONA
Cinchona calisaya .... see CINCHONA
Cinchona ledgeriana .... see CINCHONA
Cinchona pubescens .... see CINCHONA
Cinchona succirubra .... see CINCHONA
Cineraria maritima .... see DUSTY MILLER
Cinnamomi cassiae cortex .... see CASSIA
Cinnamomum aromaticum
.... see CASSIA, CINNAMON flower
Cinnamomum camphora .... see CAMPHOR
Cinnamomum cassia .... see CASSIA, CINNAMON flower
Cinnamomum verum .... see CINNAMON bark
Cinnamomum zeylanicum .... see CINNAMON bark
CINNAMON bark .... see CINNAMON bark

Cinnamon Flos................... see CINNAMON flower
CINNAMON flower .... see CINNAMON flower
Cinnamon Sedge .... see CALAMUS
Cinnamon Wood .... see SASSAFRAS
Cinquefoil .... see EUROPEAN FIVE-FINGER GRASS,
                                                        TORMENTIL
Cis-1,2,3,5-trans-4,6-Cyclohexanehexol .... see INOSITOL
Cis-9,trans-11 conjugated linoleic acid
.... see CONJUGATED LINOLEIC ACID
Cis-9-cetylmyristoleate .... see CETYL MYRISTOLEATE
Cis-9-Octadecenoic acid .... see LORENZO'S OIL
Cis-Resveratrol .... see RESVERATROL
Cissampelos pareira .... see ABUTA
Ciste .... see LABDANUM
Cistus incanus .... see LABDANUM
Cistus ladanifer .... see LABDANUM
Cistus ladaniferus .... see LABDANUM
Cistus polymorphus .... see LABDANUM
Cistus villosus .... see LABDANUM
Citrated Caffeine .... see CAFFEINE
Citri Sinensis .... see SWEET ORANGE
Citronella .... see LEMONGRASS, STONE ROOT
CITRONELLA OIL .... see CITRONELLA OIL
Citrullus colocynthis .... see COLOCYNTH
Citrus aurantifolia .... see LIME fruit, peel, LIME oil
Citrus aurantium
.... see BITTER ORANGE flower, flower oil,
                                                    BITTER ORANGE peel
Citrus aurantium amara
.... see BITTER ORANGE flower, flower oil,
                                                    BITTER ORANGE peel
Citrus aurantium bergamia .... see BERGAMOT OIL
Citrus aurantium dulcis .... see SWEET ORANGE
Citrus aurantium sinensis .... see SWEET ORANGE
Citrus bergamia .... see BERGAMOT OIL,
                                    BITTER ORANGE flower, flower oil,
                                                    BITTER ORANGE peel
Citrus bigaradia ... see BITTER ORANGE flower, flower oil,
                                                    BITTER ORANGE peel
Citrus decumana .... see GRAPEFRUIT OIL
Citrus maxima .... see GRAPEFRUIT OIL
Citrus medica var acida .... see LIME oil
Citrus paradisi .... see GRAPEFRUIT
Citrus racemosa .... see GRAPEFRUIT OIL
Citrus sinensis .... see SWEET ORANGE
Citrus vulgaris ..... see BITTER ORANGE flower, flower oil,
                                                    BITTER ORANGE peel
Citrus X paradisi .... see GRAPEFRUIT OIL
Civan Percemi .... see YARROW
Cives .... see CHIVE
CIVET .... see CIVET
Civettictis civetta .... see CIVET
Ciwujia .... see GINSENG, SIBERIAN
CLA .... see CONJUGATED LINOLEIC ACID
Cladonia pyxidata .... see CUPMOSS
Clarified Honey .... see HONEY
Clary .... see CLARY SAGE
CLARY SAGE .... see CLARY SAGE
Clary Wort .... see CLARY SAGE
Claviceps purpurea .... see ERGOT
Clay Suspension Products .... see COLLOIDAL MINERALS
Clear Eye .... see CLARY SAGE
Cleavers .... see CLIVERS
Cleaverwort .... see CLIVERS

INDEX

CLEMATIS .... see CLEMATIS
Clematis .... see WOODBINE
Clematis recta .... see CLEMATIS
Clematis virginiana .... see WOODBINE
Clematis vitalba .... see TRAVELER'S JOY
Climbing Knotweed .... see FO-TI raw root
CLIVERS .... see CLIVERS
Clot-Bur .... see MULLEIN
Clotbur .... see BURDOCK
Clous de Girolfe ..... see CLOVE dried flowerbud, leaf, stem,
CLOVE OIL
CLOVE dried flowerbud, leaf, stem
.... see CLOVE dried flowerbud, leaf, stem
Clove Garlic .... see GARLIC
CLOVE OIL .... see CLOVE OIL
Clove Pepper .... see ALLSPICE
Cloves .... see CLOVE dried flowerbud, leaf, stem
Clown's Lungwort .... see MULLEIN
CLUB MOSS .... see CLUB MOSS
CM .... see CETYL MYRISTOLEATE
CMO .... see CETYL MYRISTOLEATE
Cnici Benedicti Herba .... see BLESSED THISTLE
Cnicus .... see BLESSED THISTLE
Cnicus benedictus .... see BLESSED THISTLE
Co-Enzyme Q10 .... see COENZYME Q-10
CO Q10 .... see COENZYME Q-10
Coachweed .... see CLIVERS
Coakum .... see POKEWEED berry, POKEWEED root
Coakum-Chorngras .... see POKEWEED berry,
POKEWEED root
Coastal Douglas Fir .... see OREGON FIR BALSAM
Cobalamin Enzyme .... see DIBENCOZIDE
Cobalamins .... see VITAMIN B12
Cobamamide .... see DIBENCOZIDE
Cobamin .... see VITAMIN B12
Cobnut .... see HAZELNUT
COCA .... see COCA
Cocaine Plant .... see COCA
Cocash Weed .... see GOLDEN RAGWORT
Cocculus Indicus .... see LEVANT BERRY
Cocculus lacunosus .... see LEVANT BERRY
Cocculus suberosus .... see LEVANT BERRY
Cochin Ginger .... see GINGER
Cochin Lemongrass .... see LEMONGRASS
Cochlearia armoracia .... see HORSERADISH
Cochlearia officinalis .... see SCURVY GRASS
COCILLANA .... see COCILLANA
Cockle .... see CORN COCKLE
Cockle Buttons .... see BURDOCK
Cocklebur .... see AGRIMONY, BURDOCK
Cockspur Rye .... see ERGOT
Cockup Hat .... see QUEEN'S DELIGHT
Cocky Baby .... see ARUM
COCOA .... see COCOA
Cocoa Bean .... see COCOA
Cocoa Oleum .... see COCOA
Cocoa Seed .... see COCOA
Cocoa Semen .... see COCOA
Cocoa Testae .... see COCOA
Cocowort .... see SHEPHERD'S PURSE
Coculus Fructus .... see LEVANT BERRY
CODONOPSIS .... see CODONOPSIS
Codonopsis pilosula .... see CODONOPSIS
Codonopsis pilosula modesta .... see CODONOPSIS

Codonopsis tangsheng .... see CODONOPSIS
Codonopsis tubulosa .... see CODONOPSIS
Coenzyme 1 .... see NADH
Coenzyme B-12 .... see DIBENCOZIDE
COENZYME Q-10 .... see COENZYME Q-10
Coenzyme R .... see BIOTIN
Coffea arabica .... see COFFEE, COFFEE CHARCOAL
Coffea canephora .... see COFFEE, COFFEE CHARCOAL
Coffea liberica .... see COFFEE, COFFEE CHARCOAL
Coffea robusta .... see COFFEE
COFFEE .... see COFFEE
COFFEE CHARCOAL .... see COFFEE CHARCOAL
Cokan .... see POKEWEED berry, POKEWEED root
Cola acuminata .... see COLA NUT
Cola nitida .... see COLA NUT
COLA NUT .... see COLA NUT
Cola Seed .... see COLA NUT
Colchicum .... see AUTUMN CROCUS
Colchicum autumnale .... see AUTUMN CROCUS
Colchicum speciosum .... see AUTUMN CROCUS
Colchicum vernum .... see AUTUMN CROCUS
Cold-Pressed Grapefruit Oil .... see GRAPEFRUIT OIL
colecalciferol .... see VITAMIN D
Colewort .... see AVENS, CABBAGE
Colic Root .... see ALETRIS, ALPINIA, MARSH
BLAZING STAR, WILD YAM
Colle du Japon .... see AGAR
Collinsonia canadensis .... see STONE ROOT
COLLOIDAL MINERALS .... see COLLOIDAL
MINERALS
COLLOIDAL SILVER .... see COLLOIDAL SILVER
Colloidal Silver Protein .... see COLLOIDAL SILVER
Colloidal Trace Minerals ...... see COLLOIDAL MINERALS
COLOCYNTH .... see COLOCYNTH
Colocynth Pulp .... see COLOCYNTH
Colocynthidis Fructus .... see COLOCYNTH
COLOMBO .... see COLOMBO
Colostrum .... see BOVINE COLOSTRUM
Colour Index No 40850 .... see CANTHAXANTHIN
COLTSFOOT .... see COLTSFOOT
Coltstail .... see CANADIAN FLEABANE
COLUMBINE .... see COLUMBINE
Comb Flower .... see ECHINACEA
Combretum .... see OPIUM ANTIDOTE
Combretum micranthum .... see OPIUM ANTIDOTE
Combucha Tea .... see KOMBUCHA TEA
COMFREY .... see COMFREY
Cominho Negro .... see BLACK SEED
Commiphora .... see MYRRH
Commiphora abyssinica .... see MYRRH
Commiphora erythraea .... see MYRRH
Commiphora madagascariensis .... see MYRRH
Commiphora molmol .... see MYRRH
Commiphora mukul .... see GUGGUL
Commiphora myrrha .... see MYRRH
Common Alder .... see BLACK ALDER
Common Ash .... see ASH
Common Barberry .... see EUROPEAN BARBERRY
Common Basil .... see BASIL
Common Bean .... see BEAN POD
Common Bearberry .... see UVA URSI
Common Borage
.... see BORAGE flower, dried above ground parts

© Copyright 2000, Natural Medicines Comprehensive Database (209) 472-2244. For updated data, go to www.NaturalDatabase.com.

Common Bugloss

.... see BORAGE flower,
dried above ground parts
Common Centaury .... see CENTAURY
Common Cherry Laurel ...... see CHERRY LAUREL WATER
Common Chicory Root .... see CHICORY
Common Comfrey .... see COMFREY
Common Couch .... see HAY FLOWER
Common Dandelion .. see DANDELION above ground parts,
DANDELION entire plant
Common Dubbletjie .... see PUNCTURE VINE
Common Elder .... see EUROPEAN ELDER flower
Common Elderberry .... see AMERICAN ELDER
Common Fennel .... see FENNEL fruit, seed
Common Figwort .... see FIGWORT
Common Groundsel .... see GROUNDSEL
Common Guelder-Rose .... see CRAMP BARK
Common Hoarhound .... see WHITE HOREHOUND
Common Hops .... see HOPS
Common Jasmine .... see JASMINE
Common Juniper Berry .... see JUNIPER
Common Lavender .... see LAVENDER
Common Melilot .... see SWEET CLOVER
Common Nettle

.... see STINGING NETTLE above ground parts,
STINGING NETTLE root
Common Nightshade ...see BITTERSWEET NIGHTSHADE
Common Oak .... see OAK bark
Common Oleander .... see OLEANDER
Common Parsley .. see PARSLEY leaf, root, PARSLEY seed
Common Periwinkle .... see PERIWINKLE
Common Plantain .... see GREAT PLANTAIN
Common Polypod .... see LADY FERN
Common Ragwort .... see TANSY RAGWORT
Common Rue .... see RUE
Common Sage .... see SAGE
Common Sandspurry .... see ARENARIA RUBRA
Common Sassafras .... see SASSAFRAS
Common Shrubby Everlasting .... see IMMORTELLE,
SANDY EVERLASTING
Common Sorrel .... see WOOD SORREL
COMMON STONECROP ..... see COMMON STONECROP
Common Thyme ...... see THYME flower, leaf, THYME OIL
Common Valerian .... see VALERIAN
Common Vanilla .... see VANILLA
Common Verbena .... see VERBENA
Common Vervain .... see VERBENA
Common Wormwood

.... see WORMWOOD above ground parts
Common Yarrow...................................... see YARROW
Common Yew .... see YEW
Compass Plant .... see ROSEMARY
Compass Weed.................. see ROSINWEED, ROSEMARY
Compound Q .... see CHINESE CUCUMBER fruit,
CHINESE CUCUMBER root,
CHINESE CUCUMBER seed
Condroitin .... see CHONDROITIN SULFATE
CONDURANGO .... see CONDURANGO
Condurango Cortex .... see CONDURANGO
Coneflower .... see ECHINACEA
CONJUGATED LINOLEIC ACID ....see CONJUGATED
LINOLEIC ACID
Consolidae Radix .... see COMFREY
Consound .... see COMFREY

Constancy .... see LILY-OF-THE-VALLEY
Consumptive's Weed .... see YERBA SANTA
Continental Tea .... see LABRADOR TEA
CONTRAYERVA ....see CONTRAYERVA
Convall-Lily .... see LILY-OF-THE-VALLEY
Convallaria .... see LILY-OF-THE-VALLEY
Convallaria herba .... see LILY-OF-THE-VALLEY
Convallaria majalis .... see LILY-OF-THE-VALLEY
Convolvulus nervosus

.... see HAWAIIAN BABY WOODROSE
Convolvulus purga .... see JALAP
Convolvulus speciosus

.... see HAWAIIAN BABY WOODROSE
Cool Tankard

.... see BORAGE flower, dried above ground parts
COOLWORT .... see COOLWORT
Coon Root .... see BLOODROOT
Copaiba .... see COPAIBA BALSAM
COPAIBA BALSAM .... see COPAIBA BALSAM
Copaiba Oleoresin .... see COPAIBA BALSAM
Copaifera langsdorfii .... see COPAIBA BALSAM
Copaifera officinalis .... see COPAIBA BALSAM
Copaifera reticulata .... see COPAIBA BALSAM
Copaiva .... see COPAIBA BALSAM
Copal Tree .... see TREE OF HEAVEN
Copalm .... see STORAX
COPPER .... see COPPER
Copperose .... see CORN POPPY
Coptide .... see GOLDTHREAD
Coptis .... see GOLDTHREAD
Coptis groenlandica .... see GOLDTHREAD
Coptis trifolia .... see GOLDTHREAD
CoQ10 .... see COENZYME Q-10
Coqueret .... see WINTER CHERRY
CORAL .... see CORAL
CORAL ROOT .... see CORAL ROOT
Coralberry .... see WHITE COHOSH
Corallorhiza odontorihiza .... see CORAL ROOT
CORDYCEPS .... see CORDYCEPS
Cordyceps sinensis .... see CORDYCEPS
CORIANDER .... see CORIANDER
Coriandri Fructus .... see CORIANDER
Coriandrum sativum .... see CORIANDER
Coridothymus capitatus ...... see SPANISH ORIGANUM OIL
Coriolus .... see CORIOLUS MUSHROOM
CORIOLUS MUSHROOM .. see CORIOLUS MUSHROOM
Coriolus versicolor .... see CORIOLUS MUSHROOM
CORKWOOD TREE .... see CORKWOOD TREE
Corn Campion .... see CORN COCKLE
CORN COCKLE .... see CORN COCKLE
Corn Horsetail .... see HORSETAIL
CORN POPPY .... see CORN POPPY
Corn Rose .... see CORN COCKLE, CORN POPPY
CORN SILK .... see CORN SILK
Corn Sugar Gum .... see XANTHAN GUM
Cornel .... see AMERICAN DOGWOOD
Cornelian tree .... see AMERICAN DOGWOOD
CORNFLOWER .... see CORNFLOWER
Cornmint Oil .... see JAPANESE MINT
Cornsilk .... see CORN SILK
Cornu Cervi Parvum .... see DEER VELVET
Cornus florida .... see AMERICAN DOGWOOD
Corona De Cristo .... see PASSIONFLOWER
Corona Solis .... see SUNFLOWER OIL

INDEX

Corpus Luteum Hormone .... see PROGESTERONE
CORYDALIS .... see CORYDALIS
Corydalis... see TURKEY CORN
Corydalis cava .... see CORYDALIS
Corylaceae .... see HAZELNUT
Corylus avellana .... see HAZELNUT
Corylus heterophylla .... see HAZELNUT
Corynanthe johimbi .... see YOHIMBE
Corynanthe yohimbi .... see YOHIMBE
Cossoo .... see KOUSSO
COSTUS OIL .... see COSTUS OIL
COSTUS root .... see COSTUS root
COTTON .... see COTTON
Cotton Dawes .... see CUDWEED
Cotton Root .... see COTTON
Cotton Weed .... see CUDWEED
COUCH GRASS .... see COUCH GRASS
Couchgrass .... see AGROPYRON
Coudrier .... see HAZELNUT
Coughroot .... see BETH ROOT
Coughweed .... see GOLDEN RAGWORT
Coughwort .... see COLTSFOOT
Couhage .... see COWHAGE
Coumarouna Odorata .... see TONKA BEAN
COUNTRY MALLOW .... see COUNTRY MALLOW
Country Walnut .... see TUNG SEED
Covanamilpori .... see INDIAN SNAKEROOT
Cow Cabbage .... see AMERICAN WHITE POND LILY,
                                                       MASTERWORT
Cow Clover .... see RED CLOVER
Cow Grass .... see KNOTWEED HERB
Cow Milk Colostrum .... see BOVINE COLOSTRUM
Cow Parsnip .... see MASTERWORT
Cowbane .... see EUROPEAN WATER HEMLOCK
Cowberry .... see ALPINE CRANBERRY
COWHAGE .... see COWHAGE
Cowitch .... see COWHAGE
COWSLIP .... see COWSLIP
Cowslip .... see MARSH MARIGOLD
Cr .... see CHROMIUM
Crab's Eye .... see PRECATORY BEAN
Crabwood .... see ANDIROBA
Crack Willow .... see WILLOW BARK
CRAMP BARK .... see CRAMP BARK
Crampweed .... see POTENTILLA
CRANBERRY .... see CRANBERRY
Crataegi Flos .... see HAWTHORN leaf, flower
Crataegi Folium .... see HAWTHORN leaf, flower
Crataegi Folium Cum Flore
            .... see HAWTHORN leaf with flower extract
Crataegi Fructus .... see HAWTHORN fruit
Crataegus cuneata .... see HAWTHORN fruit
Crataegus laevigata .... see HAWTHORN fruit,
                                                  HAWTHORN leaf, flower,
                                  HAWTHORN leaf with flower extract
Crataegus monogyna .... see HAWTHORN fruit,
                                                  HAWTHORN leaf, flower,
                                  HAWTHORN leaf with flower extract
Crataegus oxyacantha .... see HAWTHORN fruit,
                                                  HAWTHORN leaf, flower,
                                  HAWTHORN leaf with flower extract
Crataegus pinnatifida .... see HAWTHORN fruit
Crawley .... see CORAL ROOT
Crawley Root .... see CORAL ROOT

Crawlgrass .... see KNOTWEED HERB
Creat .... see ANDROGRAPHIS
CREATINE .... see CREATINE
Creatine Monohydrate .... see CREATINE
Creeper .... see AMERICAN IVY
Creeping Barberry .... see OREGON GRAPE
Creeping Charlie .... see GROUND IVY
Creeping Jenny .... see MONEYWORT
Creeping Joan .... see MONEYWORT
Creeping Tom .... see COMMON STONECROP
Creosote Bush .... see CHAPARRAL
Crescione Di Fonte .... see WATERCRESS
Cresson au Poulet .... see WATERCRESS
Cresson De Fontaine .... see WATERCRESS
Cresson D'eau .... see WATERCRESS
Crest Marine .... see SAMPHIRE
Crewel .... see COWSLIP
Crithum maritimum .... see SAMPHIRE
Croci stigma .... see SAFFRON
Crocus .... see AUTUMN CROCUS
Crocus sativus .... see SAFFRON
Crosswort .... see BONESET
Croton eleuteria .... see CASCARILLA
Croton lechleri .... see SANGRE DE GRADO
CROTON SEEDS .... see CROTON SEEDS
Croton tiglium .... see CROTON SEEDS
Crow Corn .... see ALETRIS
Crowberry .... see POKEWEED berry, POKEWEED root
Crowfoot .... see BULBOUS BUTTERCUP,
                                                       WOOD ANEMONE
Crown-of-the-Field .... see CORN COCKLE
Crude Chrysarobin .... see GOA POWDER
Crystalline DMSO .... see MSM
Cs-4 .... see CORDYCEPS
CSA .... see CHONDROITIN SULFATE
CSC .... see CHONDROITIN SULFATE
Cu .... see COPPER
Cube Gambir .... see CATECHU
Cubeb Berries .... see CUBEBS
Cubeba .... see CUBEBS
Cubeba officinaliz......................... see CUBEBS
CUBEBS .... see CUBEBS
Cuckoo Bread .... see WOOD SORREL
Cuckoo Buds .... see BULBOUS BUTTERCUP
Cuckoo Flower .... see SALEP
Cuckoo Pint .... see ARUM
Cuckowes Meat .... see WOOD SORREL
Cucurbita pepo......................... see PUMPKIN
Cucurbitea peponis semen .... see PUMPKIN
Cuddy's Lungs......................... see MULLEIN
CUDWEED .... see CUDWEED
Cudweed .... see CAT'S FOOT
Cuivre .... see COPPER
Cukilanarpak......................... see DEVIL'S CLUB
Culveris Root .... see BLACK ROOT
Culver's Physic .... see BLACK ROOT
Culver's Root .... see BLACK ROOT
Culverwort .... see COLUMBINE
Cumaru .... see TONKA BEAN
CUMIN .... see CUMIN
Cumin des Pres .... see CARAWAY dried fruit, seed
Cuminum cyminum .... see CUMIN
Cuminum odorum .... see CUMIN
Cummin .... see CUMIN

© Copyright 2000, Natural Medicines Comprehensive Database (209) 472-2244. For updated data, go to www.NaturalDatabase.com. • 1471

Cundeamor .... see BITTER MELON
CUP PLANT .... see CUP PLANT
Cup-Puppy .... see CORN POPPY
CUPMOSS .... see CUPMOSS
Cupreol .... see BETA-SITOSTEROL
Cupressus sempervirens .... see CYPRESS
Curcuma .... see JAVANESE TURMERIC, TURMERIC
Curcuma aromatica .... see TURMERIC
Curcuma domestica .... see TURMERIC
Curcuma longa .... see TURMERIC
Curcuma xanthorrhiza .... see JAVANESE TURMERIC
Curcuma zedoaria .... see ZEDOARY
Curcumae longae rhizoma .... see TURMERIC
Curcumae xanthorrhizae rhizoma
.... see JAVANESE TURMERIC
Curcumin .... see TURMERIC
Curdwort .... see LADY'S BEDSTRAW
Cure All .... see LEMON BALM, WATER AVENS
Curled Dock .... see YELLOW DOCK
Curled Mint .... see SPEARMINT
Curly Dock .... see YELLOW DOCK
Cursed Crowfoot .... see POISONOUS BUTTERCUP
Cuscus .... see VETIVER
Cuscus Grass .... see VETIVER
Cuscuta epithymum .... see DODDER
Cusparia .... see ANGOSTURA
Cusparia Bark .... see ANGOSTURA
Custard Apple .... see AMERICAN PAWPAW
Cutch .... see AGROPYRON, CATECHU,
                                                      COUCH GRASS
Cutrus limon .... see LEMON
Cutweed .... see BLADDERWRACK
Cyamposis psoralioides .... see GUAR GUM
Cyamposis tetragonolobus .... see GUAR GUM
Cyani Flos .... see CORNFLOWER
Cyani Flower .... see CORNFLOWER
Cyanobacteria .... see BLUE-GREEN ALGAE
Cyanocobalamin .... see VITAMIN B12
Cyanocobalaminum .... see VITAMIN B12
CYCLAMEN .... see CYCLAMEN
Cyclamen europaeum .... see CYCLAMEN
Cyclohexitol .... see INOSITOL
Cycobemin .... see VITAMIN B12
Cydonia oblongata .... see QUINCE
Cymbopogon citratus .... see LEMONGRASS
Cymbopogon flexuosus .... see LEMONGRASS
Cymbopogon nardis .... see LEMONGRASS
Cymbopogon nardus .... see CITRONELLA OIL
Cymbopogon winterianus .... see CITRONELLA OIL
Cynanchum vincetoxicum .... see GERMAN IPECAC
Cynara cardunculus .... see ARTICHOKE
Cynara scolymus .... see ARTICHOKE
Cynoglossi herba .... see HOUND'S TONGUE
Cynoglossi radix .... see HOUND'S TONGUE
Cynoglossum officinale .... see HOUND'S TONGUE
Cynosbatos .... see ROSE HIP
Cyperus articulatus .... see ADRUE
CYPRESS .... see CYPRESS
Cypress Powder .... see ARUM
CYPRESS SPURGE .... see CYPRESS SPURGE
Cypripedium .... see NERVE ROOT
Cypripedium calceolus .... see NERVE ROOT
Cypripedium pubescens .... see NERVE ROOT
Cystadane .... see BETAINE ANHYDROUS

Cyste .... see LABDANUM
Cystisi scoparii flos .... see SCOTCH BROOM flower
Cystisus laburnum .... see LABURNUM
Cytisi scoparii herba .... see SCOTCH BROOM herb
Cytisus scoparius .... see SCOTCH BROOM flower,
                                                 SCOTCH BROOM herb
d-Alpha-Tocopherol .... see VITAMIN E
d-Alpha-Tocopheryl .... see VITAMIN E
d-Alpha-Tocopheryl Acetate .... see VITAMIN E
d-Alpha-Tocopheryl Succinate .... see VITAMIN E
d-Beta-Tocopherol .... see VITAMIN E
D-Biotin .... see BIOTIN
D-Calcium Pantothenate .... see PANTOTHENIC ACID
D-Carnitine .... see L-CARNITINE
D-chiro-inositol .... see INOSITOL
d-Delta-Tocopherol .... see VITAMIN E
d-Gamma-Tocopherol .... see VITAMIN E
D-Glucarate .... see CALCIUM D-GLUCARATE
D-glucaro-1,4-lactone .... see CALCIUM D-GLUCARATE
D-Panthenol .... see PANTOTHENIC ACID
D-pantothenic acid .... see PANTOTHENIC ACID
D-Pantothenyl Alcohol .... see PANTOTHENIC ACID
D-Phenylalanine .... see PHENYLALANINE
D-ribose .... see RIBOSE
d-Tocopherol .... see VITAMIN E
Da Huang .... see RHUBARB
DA QING YE .... see DA QING YE
Da Zao .... see JUJUBE
Daemonorops draco .... see DRAGON'S BLOOD
DAFFODIL .... see DAFFODIL
Dage of Jerusalem .... see LUNGWORT
Dagger Plant .... see YUCCA
Daggers .... see ORRIS
Daisy .... see TANSY
Dalmatian Sage .... see SAGE
Dalmation Insect Flowers .... see PYRETHRUM
Dalmation Pellitory .... see PYRETHRUM
Dambrose .... see INOSITOL
DAMIANA .... see DAMIANA
Damiana aphrodisiaca .... see DAMIANA
Damiana Herb .... see DAMIANA
Damiana Leaf .... see DAMIANA
Dan-Shen .... see DANSHEN
Dancing Mushroom .... see MAITAKE
DANDELION above ground parts
.... see DANDELION above ground parts
DANDELION entire plant ..... see DANDELION entire plant
Dandelion Herb .... see DANDELION above ground parts
Danewort .... see DWARF ELDER
Danggui .... see DONG QUAI
Dangshen .... see CODONOPSIS
DANSHEN .... see DANSHEN
Daphne .... see MEZEREON, SWEET BAY
Daphne mezereum .... see MEZEREON
Daphne Willow .... see WILLOW BARK
Dark Catechu .... see CATECHU
Darnel .... see TAUMELLOOLCH
Darri .... see BROOM CORN
DATE PALM .... see DATE PALM
Datura .... see JIMSON WEED
Datura sauveolens .... see ANGEL'S TRUMPET
Datura stramonium .... see JIMSON WEED
Daucus carota .... see WILD CARROT
Dead Man's Bells .... see DIGITALIS

Deadly Nightshade .... see BELLADONNA, BITTERSWEET NIGHTSHADE
Deaf Nettle .... see WHITE DEAD NETTLE FLOWER
DEANOL .... see DEANOL
Deanol aceglumate .... see DEANOL
Deanol acetamidobenzoate .... see DEANOL
Deanol benzilate .... see DEANOL
Deanol bisorcate .... see DEANOL
Deanol cyclohexylpropionate .... see DEANOL
Deanol hemisuccinate .... see DEANOL
Deanol pidolate .... see DEANOL
Deanol tartrate .... see DEANOL
Deep Sea Shark Liver Oil .... see SHARK LIVER OIL
Deer Antler .... see DEER VELVET
Deer Antler Velvet .... see DEER VELVET
Deer Balls ....see PUFF BALL
Deer Musk .... see MUSK
DEER VELVET .... see DEER VELVET
Deerberry .... see SQUAWVINE, WINTERGREEN leaf, WINTERGREEN oil
Deernut .... see JOJOBA
Deer's Tongue .... see DEERTONGUE
DEERTONGUE .... see DEERTONGUE
Dehydroepiandrosterone .... see DHEA
Dehydroretinol .... see VITAMIN A
Delicate Bess .... see RED-SPUR VALERIAN
Delphinii Flos .... see DELPHINIUM
DELPHINIUM .... see DELPHINIUM
Delphinium consolida .... see DELPHINIUM, LARKSPUR
Delphinium staphisagria .... see STAVESACRE
Delta 5-pregnen-3 beta-ol-20-one ..... see PREGNENOLONE
Delta tocotrienol .... see VITAMIN E
Delta-tocopherol .... see VITAMIN E
Demon Chaser .... see ST JOHN'S WORT
Dendranthema morifolium .... see CHRYSANTHEMUM
Deoxyribonucleic Acid .... see RNA AND DNA
Derriere Dos .... see CHANCA PIEDRA
Des Dos .... see CHANCA PIEDRA
Desert Herb .... see EPHEDRA
Desert Tea .... see MORMON TEA
Devil Tree .... see FEVER BARK
Devil's Apple .... see JIMSON WEED, PODOPHYLLUM
Devil's Bit .... see ALETRIS, FEVER BARK, PREMORSE
Devil's Bite .... see AMERICAN HELLEBORE
Devil's Bite Prairie-Pine .... see MARSH BLAZING STAR
Devil's Bones .... see WILD YAM
Devil's Bush .... see GINSENG, SIBERIAN
Devil's Cherries .... see BELLADONNA
DEVIL'S CLAW .... see DEVIL'S CLAW
Devil's Claw Root .... see DEVIL'S CLAW
DEVIL'S CLUB .... see DEVIL'S CLUB
Devil's-Darning-Needle .... see WOODBINE
Devil's Dung .... see ASAFOETIDA
Devil's Eye .... see HENBANE
Devil's Fuge .... see EUROPEAN MISTLETOE
Devil's Guts .... see DODDER
Devil's Head .... see YELLOW TOADFLAX
Devil's Herb .... see BELLADONNA
Devil's Nettle .... see YARROW
Devil's Plaything .... see YARROW
Devil's Ribbon .... see YELLOW TOADFLAX
Devil's Root .... see PEYOTE
Devil's Shrub .... see GINSENG, SIBERIAN
Devil's-Thorn .... see PUNCTURE VINE

Devil's Trumpet
.... see ANGEL'S TRUMPET, JIMSON WEED
Devil's Turnip .... see BRYONIA
Devil's Vine .... see GREATER BINDWEED
Devil's-Weed .... see PUNCTURE VINE
Dew Plant .... see SUNDEW
Dewberry ..... see BLACKBERRY leaf, BLACKBERRY root
Dexpanthenol .... see PANTOTHENIC ACID
Dexpanthenolum .... see PANTOTHENIC ACID
DHA (DOCOSAHEXAENOIC ACID)
.... see DHA (DOCOSAHEXAENOIC ACID)
Dhanburua .... see INDIAN SNAKEROOT
Dhar-Bu .... see SEA BUCKTHORN
DHEA .... see DHEA
DHT .... see VITAMIN D
Di-isopropylamine Dichloroacetate ... see PANGAMIC ACID
Dibasic Potassium Phosphate .... see PHOSPHATE SALTS
Dibasic Sodium Phosphate .... see PHOSPHATE SALTS
DIBENCOZIDE .... see DIBENCOZIDE
Dicalcium Phosphate .... see CALCIUM, PANGAMIC ACID, PHOSPHATE SALTS
Dicentra cucullaria .... see TURKEY CORN
Dichysterol .... see VITAMIN D
Dictamnus albus .... see BURNING BUSH leaf, BURNING BUSH root
Didin .... see MYRRH
Didthin .... see MYRRH
DIGITALIS .... see DIGITALIS
Digitalis lanata .... see DIGITALIS
Digitalis purpurea .... see DIGITALIS
Dihe .... see BLUE-GREEN ALGAE
Dihydro-2(3H)-Furanone
.... see GAMMA BUTYROLACTONE
Dihydro-beta-sitosterol .... see SITOSTANOL
Dihydrotachysterol .... see VITAMIN D
dihydrotachysterol 2 .... see VITAMIN D
Dihydroxysuccinic Acid ..... see ALPHA HYDROXY ACIDS
DILL above ground parts .... see DILL above ground parts
Dill Herb .... see DILL above ground parts
DILL seed .... see DILL seed
Dillweed .... see DILL above ground parts
Dilly .... see DILL above ground parts, DILL seed
Dimethyl Sulfone .... see MSM
(Dimethylamino)acetic Acid .... see DIMETHYLGLYCINE
Dimethylaminoethanol .... see DEANOL
Dimethylethanolamine .... see DEANOL
DIMETHYLGLYCINE .... see DIMETHYLGLYCINE
Dimethylglycine .... see PANGAMIC ACID
Dimethylsulfone .... see MSM
Dioscorea macrostachya .... see WILD YAM
Diosma .... see BUCHU
Dip .... see SMOKELESS TOBACCO
Dipotassium Hydrogen Orthophosphate .... see PHOSPHATE SALTS
Dipotassium Monophosphate .... see PHOSPHATE SALTS
Dipotassium Phosphate .... see PHOSPHATE SALTS
Dipsacus silvestris .... see TEAZLE
Dipteryx odorata .... see TONKA BEAN
Discorea composita .... see WILD YAM
Discorea floribunda .... see WILD YAM
Discorea mexicana .... see WILD YAM
Discorea villosa .... see WILD YAM
Dishcloth Sponge .... see LUFFA

INDEX

© Copyright 2000, Natural Medicines Comprehensive Database (209) 472-2244. For updated data, go to www.NaturalDatabase.com. • 1473

Disodium Hydrogen Orthophosphate Dodecahydrate
.... see PHOSPHATE SALTS
Disodium Hydrogen Phosphate ..... see PHOSPHATE SALTS
Disodium Phosphate .... see PHOSPHATE SALTS
Distilled Oil from Aniba rosaeodora wood
.... see BOIS DE ROSE OIL
Dita Bark .... see FEVER BARK
Dittany .... see BURNING BUSH leaf,
BURNING BUSH root
Divale .... see BELLADONNA
DIVI-DIVI .... see DIVI-DIVI
Dl-Alpha-Tocopherol .... see VITAMIN E
Dl-Alpha-Tocopheryl .... see VITAMIN E
Dl-Alpha-Tocopheryl Acetate .... see VITAMIN E
DL-Carnitine .... see L-CARNITINE
DL-Phenylalanine .... see PHENYLALANINE
Dl-Tocopherol .... see VITAMIN E
DMAE .... see DEANOL
DMG .... see DIMETHYLGLYCINE, PANGAMIC ACID
DMSO2 .... see MSM
Docosahexaenoic acid .... see DHA
Doctor Oje .... see FICIN
DODDER .... see DODDER
Dodder Of Thyme .... see DODDER
Dog-Bur .... see HOUND'S TONGUE
Dog Fish Liver Oil .... see SHARK LIVER OIL
Dog-Grass .... see AGROPYRON, COUCH GRASS
Dog Parsley ....see FOOL'S PARSLEY
Dog Poison ....see FOOL'S PARSLEY
Dog Standard .... see TANSY RAGWORT
Dog-Tree .... see AMERICAN DOGWOOD
Dogbane .... see CANADIAN HEMP
Doggies .... see YELLOW TOADFLAX
Doggrass .... see AGROPYRON, COUCH GRASS
Dog's Arrach .... see ARRACH
Dog's Tongue .... see HOUND'S TONGUE
Dog's Tooth Violet .... see AMERICAN ADDER'S TONGUE
Dogwood .... see ALDER BUCKTHORN,
AMERICAN DOGWOOD
Dogwood Bark .... see CASCARA
Dolichos lobatus ....see KUDZU
Dolloff .... see MEADOWSWEET
Doll's Eye .... see WHITE COHOSH
DOLOMITE .... see DOLOMITE
Dolomitic Limestone .... see DOLOMITE
Dong Chong Xia Cao .... see CORDYCEPS
Dong Chong Zia Cao .... see CORDYCEPS
Dong Qua .... see DONG QUAI
DONG QUAI .... see DONG QUAI
Dongqingzi .... see GLOSSY PRIVET
Donnerkraut .... see HEMP AGRIMONY
Doorweed .... see KNOTWEED HERB
Dorstenia contrayerva ....see CONTRAYERVA
Dostenkraut .... see HEMP AGRIMONY, OREGANO
Douglas Fir .... see OREGON FIR BALSAM
Douglas Spruce .... see OREGON FIR BALSAM
DOWN SYNDROME NUTRITIONAL SUPPLEMENTS
.... see DOWN SYNDROME
NUTRITIONAL SUPPLEMENTS
Downy Birch .... see BIRCH
Dr Sklenar's Kombucha Mushroom Infusion
.... see KOMBUCHA TEA
Drachenkraut .... see HEMP AGRIMONY
Draconis Resina .... see DRAGON'S BLOOD

Dracontium foetidum .... see SKUNK CABBAGE
Dracorubin .... see DRAGON'S BLOOD
Drago .... see SANGRE DE GRADO
Dragon Root .... see ARUM
Dragon-Bushes .... see YELLOW TOADFLAX
DRAGON'S BLOOD .... see DRAGON'S BLOOD
Dragon's Blood .... see HERB ROBERT,
SANGRE DE GRADO
Dragonwort .... see BISTORT
Drake .... see TAUMELLOOLCH
Drimia indica .... see SQUILL
Drimia maritima .... see SQUILL
Drimys winteri .... see WINTER'S BARK
Dromiceius nova-hollandiae .... see EMU OIL
Dropberry .... see SOLOMON'S SEAL
Dropsy Plant .... see LEMON BALM
Dropwort .... see MEADOWSWEET
Drosera .... see SUNDEW
Drosera intermedia .... see SUNDEW
Drosera longifolia .... see SUNDEW
Drosera Ramentacea .... see SUNDEW
Drosera rotundifolia .... see SUNDEW
Drudenfuss .... see EUROPEAN MISTLETOE
Drug Centaurium .... see CENTAURY
Drunken Sailor .... see RED-SPUR VALERIAN
Dry Ground Cranberry .... see ALPINE CRANBERRY
Dryopteris Filix-Mas .... see MALE FERN
Duboisia myoporoides .... see CORKWOOD TREE
Duck's Foot .... see PODOPHYLLUM
DUCKWEED .... see DUCKWEED
Dudgeon .... see BOXWOOD
Duffle .... see MULLEIN
Dukong Anak .... see CHANCA PIEDRA
Dulcarara ....see BITTERSWEET NIGHTSHADE
Dumb Nettle .... see WHITE DEAD NETTLE FLOWER
Dumpling Cactus .... see PEYOTE
Dun Daisy .... see OX-EYE DAISY
Dungkulcha .... see JIAOGULAN
Durfa Grass .... see AGROPYRON, COUCH GRASS
Durmast Oak .... see OAK bark
Durri .... see BROOM CORN
DUSTY MILLER .... see DUSTY MILLER
Dutch Agrimony .... see HEMP AGRIMONY
Dutch Eupatoire Commune .... see HEMP AGRIMONY
Dutch Myrtle .... see SWEET GALE
Dutch Rushes .... see HORSETAIL
Dutch Tonka .... see TONKA BEAN
Dutchman's Breeches .... see TURKEY CORN
Dwale .... see BELLADONNA
Dwarf Bay .... see MEZEREON
Dwarf Bilberry .... see BILBERRY dried ripe fruit,
BILBERRY leaf
Dwarf Carline .... see CARLINA
DWARF ELDER .... see DWARF ELDER
Dwarf Flax .... see MOUNTAIN FLAX
Dwarf Mallow .... see MALLOW leaf
Dwarf Marigold .... see TAGETES
Dwarf-Pine .... see PINE
DWARF PINE NEEDLE .... see DWARF PINE NEEDLE
Dwayberry .... see BELLADONNA
Dyeberry .... see BILBERRY dried ripe fruit,
BILBERRY leaf
DYER'S BROOM .... see DYER'S BROOM
Dyer's Bugloss .... see ALKANNA

I
N
D
E
X

Dyer's Greenwood .... see DYER'S BROOM
Dyer's Madder .... see MADDER
Dyer's Saffron .... see SAFFLOWER
Dyer's Weed .... see DYER'S BROOM
Dyer's Whin .... see DYER'S BROOM
Dysentery Bark .... see SIMARUBA
Dysentery Weed .... see CUDWEED
E Zhu .... see ZEDOARY
E161 .... see CANTHAXANTHIN
Eagle-Vine Bark .... see CONDURANGO
Early Fumitory .... see CORYDALIS
Earlyflowering .... see PERIWINKLE
Earth Gall .... see AMERICAN HELLEBORE
Earth-Nut .... see PEANUT OIL
Earth Smoke .... see FUMITORY
Earthbank .... see TORMENTIL
East India Catarrh Root .... see ALPINIA
East India Root .... see ALPINIA
East Indian Almond .... see CASHEW
East Indian Balmony .... see CHIRATA
East Indian Lemongrass .... see LEMONGRASS
East Indian Sandalwood
.... see WHITE SANDALWOOD wood
East Indian Sandalwood Oil
.... see WHITE SANDALWOOD oil
Easter Flower .... see POINSETTIA, PULSATILLA
Easter Giant .... see BISTORT
Easter Mangiant .... see BISTORT
Eastern Arborvitae ...... see CEDAR leaf, CEDAR LEAF OIL
Eastern Burning Bush .... see WAHOO
Eastern Fir .... see CANADA BALSAM
Eastern Hemlock .... see PINUS BARK
Eastern Red Cedar
.... see CEDARWOOD bark, berry, leaf, seed, twig
Eastern White Cedar ... see CEDAR leaf, CEDAR LEAF OIL
Eberesche .... see MOUNTAIN ASH
Ebereschenbeeren .... see MOUNTAIN ASH
Eberwurz .... see CARLINA
Eburnamenine-14-carboxylic acid, ethyl ester
.... see VINPOCETINE
ECHINACEA .... see ECHINACEA
Echinacea angustifolia .... see ECHINACEA
Echinacea pallida .... see ECHINACEA
Echinacea purpurea .... see ECHINACEA
Echiopanax horridum .... see DEVIL'S CLUB
Echte Kamille .... see GERMAN CHAMOMILE
Ecorce de Quina .... see CINCHONA
Ecuadorian Sarsaparilla .... see SARSAPARILLA
Edible Burdock .... see BURDOCK
Egg Lecithin .... see LECITHIN
Eggs and Bacon .... see YELLOW TOADFLAX
Eggs and Collops .... see YELLOW TOADFLAX
Egyptian Alcee .... see AMBRETTE
Egyptian Privet .... see HENNA
Ehrenpreiskraut .... see VERONICA
Eichenrinde .... see OAK bark
Eicosapentaenoic acid .... see EPA
Eight-Horned Anise .... see STAR ANISE
Eight Horns .... see STAR ANISE
Einbeere .... see HERB PARIS
Eira-Caa .... see STEVIA
Eisenkraut .... see VERBENA
Elder .... see EUROPEAN ELDER fruit
Elder Flower .... see AMERICAN ELDER

Elderberry .... see AMERICAN ELDER, EUROPEAN
ELDER flower, EUROPEAN ELDER fruit
Eldrin .... see RUTIN
ELECAMPANE .... see ELECAMPANE
Elemental Copper .... see COPPER
Elemental Iron .... see IRON
ELEMI .... see ELEMI
Elemi Oleoresin .... see ELEMI
Elemi Resin .... see ELEMI
Elephant-Climber ...... see HAWAIIAN BABY WOODROSE
Elephant Creeper .... see HAWAIIAN BABY WOODROSE
Elephant's Gall .... see ALOE dried juice from leaf, latex
Elettaria cardamomum .... see CARDAMOM
Eleuthera .... see GINSENG, SIBERIAN
Eleuthero .... see GINSENG, SIBERIAN
Eleuthero Ginseng .... see GINSENG, SIBERIAN
Eleutherococ .... see GINSENG, SIBERIAN
Eleutherococci radix .... see GINSENG, SIBERIAN
Eleutherococcus .... see GINSENG, SIBERIAN
Eleutherococcus senticosus .... see GINSENG, SIBERIAN
Elfdock .... see ELECAMPANE
Elfwort .... see ELECAMPANE
Ellanwood .... see EUROPEAN ELDER flower,
EUROPEAN ELDER fruit
Ellhorn .... see EUROPEAN ELDER flower,
EUROPEAN ELDER fruit
ELM BARK .... see ELM BARK
Eltroot .... see GOUTWEED
Elymus repens .... see AGROPYRON, COUCH GRASS,
HAY FLOWER
Elytrigia repens .... see AGROPYRON, COUCH GRASS
Emblic .... see INDIAN GOOSEBERRY
Emblic Myrobalan .... see INDIAN GOOSEBERRY
Emblica officinalis .... see INDIAN GOOSEBERRY
Emetic Herb .... see LOBELIA
Emperor .... see GRAPE fruit, skin
EMU OIL .... see EMU OIL
Enada .... see NADH
Enchanter's Plant .... see VERBENA
Enebro .... see JUNIPER
ENGLISH ADDER'S TONGUE
.... see ENGLISH ADDER'S TONGUE
English Chamomile .... see ROMAN CHAMOMILE
English Cowslip .... see COWSLIP
English Goatweed .... see GOUTWEED
English Green Valerian .... see JACOB'S LADDER
English Hawthorn .... see HAWTHORN fruit,
HAWTHORN leaf, flower,
HAWTHORN leaf with flower extract
ENGLISH HORSEMINT .... see ENGLISH HORSEMINT
ENGLISH IVY .... see ENGLISH IVY
English Lavender .... see LAVENDER
English Mandrake .... see BRYONIA
English Morello .... see SOUR CHERRY
English Oak .... see OAK bark
English Plantain .... see BUCKHORN PLANTAIN
English Sarsaparilla .... see TORMENTIL
English Tonka .... see TONKA BEAN
ENGLISH WALNUT hull ...... see ENGLISH WALNUT hull
ENGLISH WALNUT leaf .... see ENGLISH WALNUT leaf
English Watercress .... see HEDGE MUSTARD
English Yew .... see YEW
Englishman's Foot .... see BLOND PSYLLIUM
Enocianina .... see GRAPE fruit, skin

INDEX

EPA (EICOSAPENTAENOIC ACID)
.... see EPA (EICOSAPENTAENOIC ACID)
Epazote .... see CHENOPODIUM OIL
EPHEDRA .... see EPHEDRA
Ephedra distachya .... see EPHEDRA
Ephedra equisetina .... see EPHEDRA
Ephedra gerardiana .... see EPHEDRA
Ephedra intermedia .... see EPHEDRA
Ephedra nevadensis .... see MORMON TEA
Ephedra shennungiana .... see EPHEDRA
Ephedra sinensis .... see EPHEDRA
Ephedra sinica .... see EPHEDRA
Ephedrae herba .... see EPHEDRA
Epigaea repens .... see TRAILING ARBUTUS
Epilobium angustifolium .... see FIREWEED
EPIMEDIUM .... see EPIMEDIUM
Epimedium acuminatum .... see EPIMEDIUM
Epimedium brevicornum .... see EPIMEDIUM
Epimedium grandiflorum .... see EPIMEDIUM
Epimedium koreanum .... see EPIMEDIUM
Epimedium pubescens .... see EPIMEDIUM
Epimedium sagittatum .... see EPIMEDIUM
Epimedium wushanese .... see EPIMEDIUM
Epine Blanche .... see HAWTHORN fruit
Epine de Mai .... see HAWTHORN fruit
Epine-Vinette .... see EUROPEAN BARBERRY
EPO .... see EVENING PRIMROSE OIL
Equisetum arvense .... see HORSETAIL
Equisetum telmateia .... see HORSETAIL
Erba Da Cartentieri .... see YARROW
Erba Da Falegname .... see YARROW
Ergocalciferol .... see VITAMIN D
ergocalciferolum .... see VITAMIN D
ERGOT .... see ERGOT
Eriffe .... see CLIVERS
Erigeron canadensis .... see CANADIAN FLEABANE
Eringo ...... see ERYNGO above ground parts, ERYNGO root
Eriodictyon .... see YERBA SANTA
Eriodictyon californicum .... see YERBA SANTA
Eriodictyon glutinosum .... see YERBA SANTA
Erucic acid .... see LORENZO'S OIL
Erva Doce .... see STEVIA
Eryngii Herba .... see ERYNGO above ground parts
Eryngii Radix .... see ERYNGO root
Eryngium campestre .... see ERYNGO above ground parts,
ERYNGO root
Eryngium maritinum .... see ERYNGO root
Eryngium yuccifolium .... see ERYNGO root
ERYNGO above ground parts
.... see ERYNGO above ground parts
Eryngo-leaved Liverwort .... see ICELAND MOSS
ERYNGO root .... see ERYNGO root
Erysimum .... see HEDGE MUSTARD
Erysimum officinale .... see HEDGE MUSTARD
Erythraea centaurium .... see CENTAURY
Erythronium .... see AMERICAN ADDER'S TONGUE
Erythronium americanum
.... see AMERICAN ADDER'S TONGUE
Erythroxylon coca .... see COCA
Erythroxylum catuaba .... see CATUABA
Erythroxylum coca .... see COCA
Erythroxylum novogranatense .... see COCA
Eschscholzia californica .... see CALIFORNIA POPPY
Escine .... see HORSE CHESTNUT seed

Esere Nut .... see CALABAR BEAN
Espigon .... see PUNCTURE VINE
Espino Armarillo .... see SEA BUCKTHORN
Espino Cambron .... see EUROPEAN BARBERRY
Espino Falso .... see SEA BUCKTHORN
Espresso .... see COFFEE
Esrar .... see MARIJUANA
Estoraque Liquido .... see STORAX
Estragon .... see TARRAGON
Eternal Flower .... see IMMORTELLE,
SANDY EVERLASTING
Ethyl Apovincaminate .... see VINPOCETINE
Eucalypti Folium .... see EUCALYPTUS dried leaf
EUCALYPTUS dried leaf .... see EUCALYPTUS dried leaf
Eucalyptus fructicetorum .... see EUCALYPTUS OIL
Eucalyptus globulus .... see EUCALYPTUS dried leaf,
EUCALYPTUS OIL
EUCALYPTUS OIL .... see EUCALYPTUS OIL
Eucalyptus polybractea .... see EUCALYPTUS dried leaf
Eucalyptus smithii .... see EUCALYPTUS dried leaf,
EUCALYPTUS OIL
Eucalyptusblatter .... see EUCALYPTUS dried leaf
Eugenia aromatica
.... see CLOVE dried flowerbud, leaf, stem,
CLOVE OIL
Eugenia caryophyllata
.... see CLOVE dried flowerbud, leaf, stem,
CLOVE OIL
Eugenia caryophyllus
.... see CLOVE dried flowerbud, leaf, stem,
CLOVE OIL
Eugenia chequen .... see CHEKEN
Eugenia pimenta .... see ALLSPICE
Euonymus atropurpureus .... see WAHOO
Eupatorium .... see HEMP AGRIMONY
Eupatorium cannabinum .... see HEMP AGRIMONY
Eupatorium perfoliatum .... see BONESET
Eupatorium purpureum .... see GRAVEL ROOT
EUPHORBIA .... see EUPHORBIA
Euphorbia capitata .... see EUPHORBIA
Euphorbia cyparissias .... see CYPRESS SPURGE
Euphorbia hirta .... see EUPHORBIA
Euphorbia pilulifera .... see EUPHORBIA
Euphorbia poinsettia .... see POINSETTIA
Euphorbia pulcherrima .... see POINSETTIA
Euphraisiae herba .... see EYEBRIGHT
Euphrasia .... see EYEBRIGHT
Euphrasia officinalis .... see EYEBRIGHT
European Alder .... see EUROPEAN ELDER flower,
EUROPEAN ELDER fruit
European Angelica............................ see ANGELICA root
European Ash.................................... see ASH
European Aspidium .... see MALE FERN
EUROPEAN BARBERRY ... see EUROPEAN BARBERRY
European Beaver .... see CASTOREUM
European Bitter Polygala .... see BITTER MILKWORT
European Blackcurrant
.... see BLACK CURRANT SEED OIL
EUROPEAN BUCKTHORN
.... see EUROPEAN BUCKTHORN
EUROPEAN CHESTNUT .... see EUROPEAN CHESTNUT
European Cranberry................................. see CRANBERRY
European Cranberry-Bush .... see CRAMP BARK

INDEX

European Dill .... see DILL above ground parts, DILL seed

EUROPEAN ELDER flower
.... see EUROPEAN ELDER flower

EUROPEAN ELDER fruit .... see EUROPEAN ELDER fruit

European Elderberry .... see EUROPEAN ELDER fruit

European filbert .... see HAZELNUT

EUROPEAN FIVE-FINGER GRASS
.... see EUROPEAN FIVE-FINGER GRASS

European Goldenrod .... see GOLDENROD

European Hazel .... see HAZELNUT

European Hellebore .... see WHITE HELLEBORE

European Hops .... see HOPS

European Linden .... see LINDEN CHARCOAL, LINDEN dried flower, LINDEN dried leaf, LINDEN dried sapwood

EUROPEAN MANDRAKE
.... see EUROPEAN MANDRAKE

EUROPEAN MISTLETOE .. see EUROPEAN MISTLETOE

European Mountain-Ash .... see MOUNTAIN ASH

European Mullein .... see MULLEIN

European Oregano .... see OREGANO

European Pasqueflower .... see PULSATILLA

European Pennyroyal .... see PENNYROYAL leaf, PENNYROYAL oil

European Peony .... see PEONY flower, PEONY root

European Ragwort .... see TANSY RAGWORT

European Sanicle .... see SANICLE

European Senega .... see BITTER MILKWORT

European Squill .... see SQUILL

European Vervain .... see VERBENA

EUROPEAN WATER HEMLOCK
.... see EUROPEAN WATER HEMLOCK

European White Hellebore .... see WHITE HELLEBORE

European Wild Pansy .... see HEART'S EASE

Eurphrasia rostkoviana .... see EYEBRIGHT

EVENING PRIMROSE OIL .... see EVENING PRIMROSE OIL

Evening Trumpet Flower .... see GELSEMIUM

Evergreen .... see PERIWINKLE

Evergreen Snakeroot .... see BITTER MILKWORT

Everlasting .... see CUDWEED, SANDY EVERLASTING

Everlasting Friendship .... see CLIVERS

Everlasting Pea .... see LATHYRUS

Evernia prunastri .... see OAK MOSS

Eve's Cups .... see PITCHER PLANT

Ewe Daisy .... see TORMENTIL

Exogonium purga .... see JALAP

Expressed Almond Oil .... see SWEET ALMOND

Expressed Grapefruit Oil .... see GRAPEFRUIT OIL

Extrait De Pepins De Raisin .... see GRAPE seed

Eye Balm .... see GOLDENSEAL

Eye Root .... see GOLDENSEAL

EYEBRIGHT .... see EYEBRIGHT

Eyebright .... see CLARY SAGE

Eyrnigium planum .... see ERYNGO root

Fa Tha Lai Jone .... see ANDROGRAPHIS

Faba Calabarica ....see CALABAR BEAN

Faex Medicinalis .... see BREWER'S YEAST

Fagopyrum esculentum .... see BUCKWHEAT

Fairy Bells .... see WOOD SORREL

Fairy Cap .... see DIGITALIS

Fairy Caps .... see COWSLIP

Fairy Finger .... see DIGITALIS

Fairy Flax .... see MOUNTAIN FLAX

Fairy Herb .... see JIAOGULAN

Fairywand .... see FALSE UNICORN

Fake Saffron .... see SAFFLOWER

Fall Crocus .... see AUTUMN CROCUS

False Bittersweet .... see AMERICAN BITTERSWEET

False Box .... see AMERICAN DOGWOOD

False Cinnamon .... see CASSIA

False Coltsfoot .... see ASARABACCA

False Grapes .... see AMERICAN IVY

False Hellebore .... see AMERICAN HELLEBORE, PHEASANT'S EYE

False Indigo .... see WILD INDIGO

False Jacob's Ladder ....see ABSCESS ROOT

False Jasmin .... see GELSEMIUM

False Pareira .... see ABUTA

False Saffron .... see SAFFLOWER

FALSE UNICORN .... see FALSE UNICORN

False Valerian .... see GOLDEN RAGWORT

Farberrote .... see MADDER

Farfarae Folium leaf .... see COLTSFOOT

Farmer's Lily .... see WHITE LILY

Fatsia .... see DEVIL'S CLUB

Fe .... see IRON

Featerfoil .... see FEVERFEW

Featherfew .... see FEVERFEW

Feigen .... see FIG

Feldkamille .... see GERMAN CHAMOMILE

Fellen .... see BITTERSWEET NIGHTSHADE

Fellonwood .... see BITTERSWEET NIGHTSHADE

Felon Herb .... see MUGWORT

Felonwort .... see BITTERSWEET NIGHTSHADE

Feltwort .... see MULLEIN

Female Regulator .... see GOLDEN RAGWORT

Fen Ke .... see KUDZU

Fenge .... see KUDZU

Fennel Flower .... see BLACK SEED

FENNEL fruit, seed .... see FENNEL fruit, seed

FENNEL OIL .... see FENNEL OIL

FENUGREEK .... see FENUGREEK

Fer .... see IRON

Ferrous Carbonate Anhydrous .... see IRON

Ferrous Fumarate .... see IRON

Ferrous Gluconate .... see IRON

Ferrous Pyrophosphate .... see IRON

Ferrous Sulfate .... see IRON

Ferrula .... see SUMBUL

Ferula assa-foetida .... see ASAFOETIDA

Ferula foetida .... see ASAFOETIDA

Ferula gummosa .... see GALBANUM

Ferula rubricaulis .... see ASAFOETIDA

Ferula sumbul .... see SUMBUL

Festuca pratensis .... see HAY FLOWER

Fetid Nightshade .... see HENBANE

Feuille De Luzerne .... see ALFALFA

Feuilles d'Alchemille .... see ALCHEMILLA

Feuilles la Fievre .... see CHANCA PIEDRA

FEVER BARK .... see FEVER BARK

Fever Grass .... see LEMONGRASS

Fever Plant .... see EVENING PRIMROSE OIL

Fever Root .... see CORAL ROOT

Fever Twig .... see BITTERSWEET NIGHTSHADE

FEVERFEW .... see FEVERFEW

Fevertree .... see EUCALYPTUS dried leaf

© Copyright 2000, Natural Medicines Comprehensive Database (209) 472-2244. For updated data, go to www.NaturalDatabase.com. • 1477

INDEX

Feverwort .... see BONESET
Ficaria .... see LESSER CELANDINE
Fichtennadel_l .... see FIR NEEDLE OIL
FICIN .... see FICIN
Ficin anthelmintica .... see FICIN
Ficin glabrata .... see FICIN
Ficin laurfolia .... see FICIN
Ficus carica .... see FIG
Ficus insipida .... see FICIN
Fieberbaumblatter .... see EUCALYPTUS dried leaf
Fieberrinde .... see CINCHONA
Field Balm .... see CATNIP
Field Horsetail .... see HORSETAIL
Field Lady's Mantle .... see PARSLEY PIERT
Field Melilot .... see SWEET CLOVER
Field Mint Oil .... see JAPANESE MINT
Field Pansy .... see HEART'S EASE
Field Pumpkin .... see PUMPKIN
FIELD SCABIOUS .... see FIELD SCABIOUS
Field Seven .... see PANAX PSEUDOGINSENG
Field Sorrel .... see YELLOW DOCK
Fieldhove .... see COLTSFOOT
FIG .... see FIG
FIGWORT .... see FIGWORT
Figwort .... see LESSER CELANDINE
Filipendula .... see MEADOWSWEET
Filipendula ulmaria .... see MEADOWSWEET
Filuis Ante Patrem .... see COLTSFOOT
Finbar .... see SEA BUCKTHORN
Finnochio .... see FENNEL fruit, seed
FIR .... see FIR
FIR NEEDLE OIL .... see FIR NEEDLE OIL
Fir Tree .... see FIR, HEMLOCK SPRUCE
FIREWEED .... see FIREWEED
Fish Berries .... see LEVANT BERRY
Fish Killer .... see LEVANT BERRY
Fish Mint .... see SPEARMINT
Fish Oil Fatty Acid .... see DHA, EPA, FISH OILS
FISH OILS .... see FISH OILS
Fish Poison Bark .... see JAMAICAN DOGWOOD
Fish-Poison Tree .... see JAMAICAN DOGWOOD
Fish Wood .... see WAHOO
Fishfudle .... see JAMAICAN DOGWOOD
Fitch .... see BLACK SEED
Fitolaca .... see POKEWEED berry, POKEWEED root
Five-Finger Blossom .... see EUROPEAN
                                            FIVE-FINGER GRASS
Five-Finger Fern .... see MAIDENHAIR FERN
Five Fingers .... see EUROPEAN FIVE-FINGER GRASS
Five-Flavor-Fruit .... see SCHISANDRA
Five-Flavor-Seed .... see SCHISANDRA
Five Leaves .... see AMERICAN IVY
Fixed Almond Oil .... see SWEET ALMOND
FL-113 .... see IPRIFLAVONE
Flag .... see ORRIS
Flag Lily .... see ORRIS
Flaggon .... see ORRIS
Flake Manna .... see MANNA
Flame Seedless .... see GRAPE fruit, skin
Flannelflower .... see MULLEIN
Flapperdock .... see PETASITES leaf, PETASITES root
Flat-Podded Vetch .... see LATHYRUS
Flavin .... see RIBOFLAVIN
Flavine .... see RIBOFLAVIN

Flax .... see SENEGA
FLAXSEED .... see FLAXSEED
FLAXSEED OIL .... see FLAXSEED OIL
Flaxweed ..... see RUPTUREWORT, YELLOW TOADFLAX
Flea Wort .... see BLACK PSYLLIUM,
                                            CANADIAN FLEABANE
Fleaseed .... see BLACK PSYLLIUM
Fleischfarbige .... see PASSIONFLOWER
Flesh and Blood .... see TORMENTIL
Fleur de Camomile .... see GERMAN CHAMOMILE
Fleur De Camomille Romaine .. see ROMAN CHAMOMILE
Fleur De La Passion .... see PASSIONFLOWER
Fleur de Pied de Chat .... see SANDY EVERLASTING
Fleurs d'Arnica .... see ARNICA
Fliggers .... see ORRIS
Flor De Passion .... see PASSIONFLOWER
Florence Fennel .... see FENNEL fruit, seed
Florentine Iris .... see ORRIS
Flores Anthemidis .... see ROMAN CHAMOMILE
Flores Caryophylli .... see CLOVE OIL
Flores Caryophyllum
.... see CLOVE dried flowerbud, leaf, stem
Florist's Chrysanthemum .... see CHRYSANTHEMUM
Flos Magnoliae .... see MAGNOLIA flower bud
Flower Velure .... see COLTSFOOT
Flowering Ash .... see MANNA
Flowering Sally .... see PURPLE LOOSESTRIFE
Flowering Wintergreen .... see BITTER MILKWORT
Flowery Knotweed .... see FO-TI raw root
Fluelli .... see YELLOW TOADFLAX
Fluffweed .... see MULLEIN
Flux Root .... see PLEURISY ROOT
Fly Agaric .... see AGA
Fly-Catcher .... see PITCHER PLANT
Fly Larva .... see MAGGOTS
Fly-Trap .... see CANADIAN HEMP, PITCHER PLANT
FO-TI cured root .... see FO-TI cured root
FO-TI raw root .... see FO-TI raw root
Foal's Foot .... see COLTSFOOT
Foalswort .... see COLTSFOOT
Foam Flower .... see COOLWORT
Fodder Beet .... see BEET
Foeniculi antheroleum .... see FENNEL OIL
Foeniculum capillaceum .... see FENNEL fruit, seed,
                                            FENNEL OIL
Foeniculum officinale .... see FENNEL fruit, seed,
                                            FENNEL OIL
Foeniculum vulgare .... see FENNEL fruit, seed,
                                            FENNEL OIL
Foenugraeci Semen .... see FENUGREEK
Foenugreek .... see FENUGREEK
Folacin .... see FOLIC ACID
Folate .... see FOLIC ACID
Folia Vitis Viniferae .... see GRAPE leaf
FOLIC ACID .... see FOLIC ACID
Food of the Gods .... see ASAFOETIDA
Fool's-Cicely .... see FOOL'S PARSLEY
FOOL'S PARSLEY .... see FOOL'S PARSLEY
Forest Mushroom .... see SHIITAKE MUSHROOM
FORGET-ME-NOT .... see FORGET-ME-NOT
FOS .... see FRUCTO-OLIGOSACCHARIDES
Fossil Tree .... see GINKGO leaf, GINKGO leaf extract,
                                            GINKGO seed
FOTI, cured root .... see FO-TI cured root

FOTI raw root .... see FO-TI raw root
Foxberry .... see ALPINE CRANBERRY
Foxglove .... see DIGITALIS
Fox's Clote .... see BURDOCK
Foxtails .... see HAY FLOWER
Fragaria vesca .... see STRAWBERRY
Fragaria virginiana .... see STRAWBERRY
Fragaria viridis .... see STRAWBERRY
Fragariae folium .... see STRAWBERRY
Fragrant Agrimony .... see AGRIMONY
Fragrant Valerian .... see VALERIAN
Framboise .... see RASPBERRY
Frangula .... see ALDER BUCKTHORN
Frangula alnus .... see ALDER BUCKTHORN
Frangula Bark .... see ALDER BUCKTHORN
Frangula purshiana .... see CASCARA
Frangulae Cortex .... see ALDER BUCKTHORN
FRANKINCENSE .... see FRANKINCENSE
Frauenmantelkraut .... see ALCHEMILLA
Fraxinella .... see BURNING BUSH leaf,
                                                                  BURNING BUSH root
Fraxinus americana .... see ASH
Fraxinus excelsior .... see ASH
Fraxinus ornus .... see MANNA
French Honeysuckle .... see GOAT'S RUE
French Lavender .... see LAVENDER
French Lilac .... see GOAT'S RUE
French Marigold .... see TAGETES
French Psyllium .... see BLACK PSYLLIUM
French Thyme .... see THYME flower, leaf
French-Willow .... see FIREWEED
Fresh Water Leech .... see LEECH
Friar's Cowl .... see ARUM
Frijol de Soya .... see SOY
FRINGETREE .... see FRINGETREE
Frogsfoot .... see BULBOUS BUTTERCUP
Frogwort .... see BULBOUS BUTTERCUP
Frost Plant .... see FROSTWORT
Frostweed .... see FROSTWORT
FROSTWORT .... see FROSTWORT
FRUCTO-OLIGOSACCHARIDES
    .... see FRUCTO-OLIGOSACCHARIDES
Fructooligosaccharides Oligofructose
    .... see FRUCTO-OLIGOSACCHARIDES
Fructus Ammi Visnagae .... see BISHOP'S WEED
Fructus Cortex .... see ENGLISH WALNUT hull
Fructus Rosae Laevigatae .... see CHEROKEE ROSEHIP
Fruit de Celeri .... see CELERY
Fruits De Khella .... see BISHOP'S WEED
Fu Ling .... see PORIA MUSHROOM
Fucostanol .... see SITOSTANOL
Fucus .... see BLADDERWRACK
Fucus vesiculosis .... see BLADDERWRACK
Fuga Daemonum .... see ST JOHN'S WORT
Fum .... see ASAFOETIDA
Fumaria officinalis .... see FUMITORY
Fumiterry .... see FUMITORY
FUMITORY .... see FUMITORY
Fumus .... see FUMITORY
Funffing .... see AGRIMONY
Funffingerkraut .... see AGRIMONY
Fungus Japonicus .... see KOMBUCHA TEA
Furze .... see DYER'S BROOM
Fusanum .... see WAHOO

FuShen .... see PORIA MUSHROOM
Fusoria .... see WAHOO
Fytic Acid .... see IP-6
GABA (GAMMA-AMINOBUTYRIC ACID)
    .... see GABA (GAMMA-AMINOBUTYRIC ACID)
Gadrose .... see WAHOO
GAG .... see CHONDROITIN SULFATE
Gaga .... see MARIJUANA
Gaglee .... see ARUM
Gagroot .... see LOBELIA
Galactosaminoglucuronoglycan Sulfate
    .... see CHONDROITIN SULFATE
Galanga .... see ALPINIA
Galangal .... see ALPINIA
GALBANUM .... see GALBANUM
Galbanum Gum .... see GALBANUM
Galbanum Gum Resin .... see GALBANUM
Galbanum Oleogum Resin .... see GALBANUM
Galbanum Oleoresin .... see GALBANUM
Galbanum Resin .... see GALBANUM
Galega officinalis .... see GOAT'S RUE
Galegae officinalis herba .... see GOAT'S RUE
Galeopsidis Herba .... see HEMPNETTLE
Galeopsis ochroleuca .... see HEMPNETTLE
Galeopsis segetum .... see HEMPNETTLE
Galii odorati herba .... see SWEET WOODRUFF
Galipea officinalis .... see ANGOSTURA
Galium aparine .... see CLIVERS
Galium odorata .... see SWEET WOODRUFF
Galium verum .... see LADY'S BEDSTRAW
Gall Weed .... see GENTIAN
Gallium .... see CLIVERS
Gallwort .... see YELLOW TOADFLAX
Gambier .... see CATECHU
Gambierdiscus toxicus .... see CIGUATERA
Gambir .... see CATECHU
Gambir Catechu .... see CATECHU
Gambodia .... see GAMBOGE
GAMBOGE .... see GAMBOGE
Gamma Amino Butyric Acid .... see GABA
Gamma Butyrolactone ... see GAMMA BUTYROLACTONE
GAMMA BUTYROLACTONE (GBL)
    .... see GAMMA BUTYROLACTONE (GBL)
Gamma-Glutamylcysteinylglycine .... see GLUTATHIONE
Gamma Hydrate .... see GAMMA HYDROXYBUTYRATE
GAMMA HYDROXYBUTYRATE
    .... see GAMMA HYDROXYBUTYRATE
Gamma Hydroxybutyrate Sodium
    .... see GAMMA HYDROXYBUTYRATE
Gamma Hydroxybutyric Acid
    .... see GAMMA HYDROXYBUTYRATE
Gamma Hydroxybutyric Acid Lactone
    .... see GAMMA BUTYROLACTONE
Gamma-L-Glutamyl-L-cysteinylglycine
    .... see GLUTATHIONE
GAMMA LINOLENIC ACID
    .... see GAMMA LINOLENIC ACID
Gamma-OH .... see GAMMA HYDROXYBUTYRATE
GAMMA ORYZANOL .... see GAMMA ORYZANOL
gamma-tocopherol .... see VITAMIN E
gamma tocotrienol .... see VITAMIN E
Gamma-Trimethyl-Beta-Acetylbutyrobetaine
    .... see ACETYL-L-CARNITINE
Gamolenic Acid .... see GAMMA LINOLENIC ACID

INDEX

© Copyright 2000, Natural Medicines Comprehensive Database (209) 472-2244. For updated data, go to www.NaturalDatabase.com. • 1479

Gan Cao .... see LICORICE
Gan Zao .... see LICORICE
Ganga .... see MARIJUANA
Gange .... see KUDZU
Ganoderma lucidum .... see REISHI MUSHROOM
Garacilaria confervoides .... see AGAR
Garance .... see MADDER
GARCINIA .... see GARCINIA
Garcinia cambogia .... see GARCINIA
Garcinia hanburyi .... see GAMBOGE
Garden Angelica .... see ANGELICA root
Garden Artichoke.......................... see ARTICHOKE
Garden Asparagus .... see ASPARAGUS
Garden Balsam .... see JEWELWEED
Garden Basil .... see BASIL
Garden Beet .... see BEET
Garden Burnet .... see GREATER BURNET
Garden Chamomile .... see ROMAN CHAMOMILE
Garden Chervil .... see CHERVIL
GARDEN CRESS .... see GARDEN CRESS
Garden Fennel .... see FENNEL fruit, seed
Garden Heliotrope .... see VALERIAN
Garden Lavender .... see LAVENDER
Garden Marigold .... see CALENDULA
Garden Marjoram .... see MARJORAM
Garden Mint .... see SPEARMINT
Garden Nightshade .... see BLACK NIGHTSHADE
Garden Parsley ...... see PARSLEY leaf, root, PARSLEY seed
Garden Pepper .... see CAPSICUM
Garden Rhubarb .... see RHUBARB
Garden Rue .... see RUE
Garden Sage .... see SAGE
Garden Sorrel .... see SORREL
Garden Thyme .... see THYME flower, leaf
Garden Valerian .... see VALERIAN
GARDEN VIOLET .... see GARDEN VIOLET
Garden Violet .... see SWEET VIOLET
Gargaut .... see ALPINIA
Garget .... see POKEWEED berry, POKEWEED root
GARLIC .... see GARLIC
Garlic Clove .... see GARLIC
Garlic Sage .... see WOOD SAGE
Gartenmajoran .... see MARJORAM
Gas Black .... see ACTIVATED CHARCOAL
Gas Plant .... see BURNING BUSH leaf,
                            BURNING BUSH root
Gat .... see KHAT
Gatten .... see WAHOO
Gatter .... see WAHOO
Gattilier .... see CHASTEBERRY
Gaultheria Oil .... see WINTERGREEN oil
Gaultheria procumbens .... see WINTERGREEN leaf,
                            WINTERGREEN oil
Gay-Feather .... see MARSH BLAZING STAR
Ge .... see GERMANIUM
GE-132 .... see GERMANIUM
Gegen .... see KUDZU
Geissrautenkraut .... see GOAT'S RUE
Gelatin .... see AGAR
Gelidiella acerosa .... see AGAR
Gelidium amanasii .... see AGAR
Gelidium cartilagineum .... see AGAR
Gelidium crinale .... see AGAR
Gelidium divaricatum .... see AGAR

Gelidium pacificum .... see AGAR
Gelidium vagum .... see AGAR
Gelosa .... see AGAR
Gelosae .... see AGAR
Gelsemii Rhizoma .... see GELSEMIUM
Gelsemin .... see GELSEMIUM
GELSEMIUM .... see GELSEMIUM
Gelsemium nitidum .... see GELSEMIUM
Gelsemium sempervirens .... see GELSEMIUM
Gelsemiumwurzelstock Jessamine .... see GELSEMIUM
Gemeine Schafgarbe .... see YARROW
Gemeiner Beifuss .... see MUGWORT
Gemeiner Wasswedost .... see HEMP AGRIMONY
Gemnema melicida .... see GYMNEMA
Gemuseartischocke .... see ARTICHOKE
General Plantain .... see GREAT PLANTAIN
Genet............................ see SPANISH BROOM
Genet a Balais .... see SCOTCH BROOM flower
Genievre .... see JUNIPER
Genista juncea .... see SPANISH BROOM
Genista tinctoria .... see DYER'S BROOM
GENTIAN .... see GENTIAN
Gentiana .... see GENTIAN
Gentiana acaulis .... see GENTIAN
Gentiana lutea .... see GENTIAN
Gentianae radix .... see GENTIAN
Ge-Oxy 132 .... see GERMANIUM
Geranium robertianum .... see HERB ROBERT
GERMAN CHAMOMILE ..... see GERMAN CHAMOMILE
GERMAN IPECAC .... see GERMAN IPECAC
German Lactucarium .... see WILD LETTUCE
German Rue ....see RUE
GERMAN SARSAPARILLA
.... see GERMAN SARSAPARILLA
GERMANDER .... see GERMANDER
GERMANIUM .... see GERMANIUM
Germanium Lactate Citrate .... see GERMANIUM
Gero-Vita ....see PROCAINE
Gerovital ....see PROCAINE
Gerovital-H3 ....see PROCAINE
Geum .... see AVENS
Geum rivale .... see WATER AVENS
Geum urbanum .... see AVENS
Gewurznelken Nagelein
.... see CLOVE dried flowerbud, leaf, stem,
                            CLOVE OIL
GH-3 ....see PROCAINE
Giant Fennel .... see ASAFOETIDA
Gigartina mamillosa .... see CARRAGEENAN
Gill-Go-By-The-Hedge .... see GROUND IVY
Gill-Go-Over-The-Ground .... see GROUND IVY
Gillenia .... see INDIAN PHYSIC
Gillenia trifoliata .... see INDIAN PHYSIC
Gillyflower .... see WALLFLOWER
Ginepro .... see JUNIPER
Gingembre .... see GINGER
GINGER .... see GINGER
Gingko .... see GINKGO leaf,
                    GINKGO leaf extract, GINKGO seed
Ginjeira .... see SOUR CHERRY
Ginkgo Biloba .... see GINKGO leaf,
                    GINKGO leaf extract, GINKGO seed
Ginkgo Folium .... see GINKGO leaf,
                            GINKGO leaf extract

INDEX

GINKGO leaf .... see GINKGO leaf
GINKGO leaf extract .... see GINKGO leaf extract
GINKGO seed .... see GINKGO seed
Ginko Biloba .... see GINKGO leaf extract
Ginkyo .... see GINKGO leaf,
                          GINKGO leaf extract, GINKGO seed
Ginseng Asiatique .... see GINSENG, PANAX
Ginseng Radix .... see GINSENG, PANAX
Ginseng Root .... see GINSENG, PANAX
GINSENG, AMERICAN .... see GINSENG, AMERICAN
GINSENG, PANAX .... see GINSENG, PANAX
GINSENG, SIBERIAN .... see GINSENG, SIBERIAN
Ginsterkraut .... see SCOTCH BROOM flower
Giroflier .... see WALLFLOWER
GL701 .... see DHEA
GLA .... see GAMMA LINOLENIC ACID
Gladdon .... see CALAMUS
Gladyne .... see ORRIS
Glechoma hederacea .... see GROUND IVY
Glicerol .... see GLYCEROL
Globe Amaranth .... see BUTTERCUP
Globe Artichoke .... see ARTICHOKE
Globe Crowfoot .... see GLOBE FLOWER
GLOBE FLOWER .... see GLOBE FLOWER
Globe Ranunculus .... see GLOBE FLOWER
Globe Trollius .... see GLOBE FLOWER
Glockenbilsenkraut .... see SCOPOLIA
Glossy Buckthorn .... see ALDER BUCKTHORN
GLOSSY PRIVET .... see GLOSSY PRIVET
Glucerite .... see GLYCEROL
GLUCOMANNAN .... see GLUCOMANNAN
Gluconic Acid .... see PANGAMIC ACID
Gluconolactone .... see ALPHA HYDROXY ACIDS
Glucosamine .... see GLUCOSAMINE HYDROCHLORIDE,
                             GLUCOSAMINE SULFATE
GLUCOSAMINE HYDROCHLORIDE
.... see GLUCOSAMINE HYDROCHLORIDE
GLUCOSAMINE SULFATE
.... see GLUCOSAMINE SULFATE
GLUTAMINE .... see GLUTAMINE
GLUTATHIONE .... see GLUTATHIONE
Glycerin .... see GLYCEROL
GLYCEROL .... see GLYCEROL
Glycerol Trierucate Oil .... see LORENZO'S OIL
Glycerol Trioleate Oil .... see LORENZO'S OIL
Glycerol, 1,2,3-propanetriol .... see GLYCEROL
Glycerolum .... see GLYCEROL
Glyceryl Alcohol .... see GLYCEROL
Glycine .... see PANGAMIC ACID
Glycine max .... see SOY
Glycine soja .... see SOY, SOYBEAN OIL
Glycolic Acid .... see ALPHA HYDROXY ACIDS
Glycyrrhiza .... see LICORICE
Glycyrrhiza glabra .... see LICORICE
Glycyrrhiza glabra glandulifera .... see LICORICE
Glycyrrhiza glabra typica .... see LICORICE
Glycyrrhiza glabra violacea .... see LICORICE
Glycyrrhiza uralensis .... see LICORICE
Gnaphalium uliginosum .... see CUDWEED
GOA POWDER .... see GOA POWDER
Goathead .... see PUNCTURE VINE
Goatnut .... see JOJOBA
Goat's Arrach .... see ARRACH
Goat's Leaf .... see HONEYSUCKLE

Goat's Pod .... see CAPSICUM
GOAT'S RUE .... see GOAT'S RUE
Goat's Rue Herb .... see GOAT'S RUE
Goat's Thorn .... see TRAGACANTH
Goatweed .... see ST JOHN'S WORT
God's-Hair .... see HARTSTONGUE
Gokhru .... see PUNCTURE VINE
Gold-Bloom .... see CALENDULA
Gold Chain .... see COMMON STONECROP
Gold Cup .... see BULBOUS BUTTERCUP, BUTTERCUP
Gold Thread .... see GOLDTHREAD
Golden Chain .... see LABURNUM
Golden Daisy .... see OX-EYE DAISY
Golden Groundsel .... see GOLDEN RAGWORT
Golden Moss .... see COMMON STONECROP
GOLDEN RAGWORT .... see GOLDEN RAGWORT
Golden Rod .... see GOLDENROD, MULLEIN
Golden Root .... see GOLDENSEAL, ROSEROOT
Golden Senecio .... see GOLDEN RAGWORT
Golden Trumpet .... see CATUABA
GOLDENROD .... see GOLDENROD
GOLDENSEAL .... see GOLDENSEAL
Goldenseal .... see OX-EYE DAISY
Goldilocks ... see IMMORTELLE, SANDY EVERLASTING
Goldsiegel .... see GOLDENSEAL
GOLDTHREAD .... see GOLDTHREAD
Gomishi .... see SCHISANDRA
Gomme Arabique .... see ACACIA
Gomme de Senegal .... see ACACIA
Gommelaque .... see SHELLAC
Gonolobus condurango .... see CONDURANGO
Goose Tansy .... see POTENTILLA
Goosebill .... see CLIVERS
Goosefoot .... see ARRACH
Goosegrass .... see CLIVERS, POTENTILLA
Goosewort .... see POTENTILLA
Gorikapuli .... see GARCINIA
Gosling Weed .... see CLIVERS
Gossypium herbaceum .... see COTTON, GOSSYPOL
Gossypium hirsutum .... see COTTON, GOSSYPOL
GOSSYPOL .... see GOSSYPOL
Gota Kola .... see GOTU KOLA
GOTU KOLA .... see GOTU KOLA
Goudron de Cade .... see CADE OIL
Gout Herb .... see GOUTWEED
Goutberry ..... see BLACKBERRY leaf, BLACKBERRY root
GOUTWEED .... see GOUTWEED
Goutwort .... see GOUTWEED
Gracemere-Pear .... see PRICKLY PEAR CACTUS
Graine De Lin .... see FLAXSEED, FLAXSEED OIL
GRAINS OF PARADISE .... see GRAINS OF PARADISE
Grains of Paradise .... see CAPSICUM
Graminis Flos .... see HAY FLOWER
Graminis rhizoma .... see AGROPYRON
Granada .... see POMEGRANATE
Grape Bark .... see COCILLANA
GRAPE fruit, skin .... see GRAPE fruit, skin
Grape Juice .... see GRAPE fruit, skin
GRAPE leaf .... see GRAPE leaf
Grape Leaf Extract .... see GRAPE leaf
GRAPE seed .... see GRAPE seed
Grape Seed Extract .... see GRAPE seed
Grape Seed Oil .... see GRAPE seed
Grape Skin .... see GRAPE fruit, skin

INDEX

Grape Skin Extract .... see GRAPE fruit, skin
GRAPEFRUIT .... see GRAPEFRUIT, GRAPE fruit, skin
GRAPEFRUIT OIL .... see GRAPEFRUIT OIL
Grapple Plant .... see DEVIL'S CLAW
Grass .... see MARIJUANA, SWEET VERNAL GRASS
Grass Flower .... see HAY FLOWER
Grass Myrtle .... see CALAMUS
Grass Pollen Extract .... see RYE GRASS
Gratiola .... see HEDGE-HYSSOP
Gratiola officinalis .... see HEDGE-HYSSOP
Gravel Plant .... see TRAILING ARBUTUS
GRAVEL ROOT .... see GRAVEL ROOT
Gray Beard Tree .... see FRINGETREE
Greasewood .... see CHAPARRAL
Great Bur .... see BURDOCK
Great Burdocks .... see BURDOCK
Great Morel .... see BELLADONNA
Great Ox-Eye .... see OX-EYE DAISY
GREAT PLANTAIN .... see GREAT PLANTAIN
Great Raifort .... see HORSERADISH
Great Stinging Nettle
.... see STINGING NETTLE above ground parts,
STINGING NETTLE root
Great Willowherb .... see FIREWEED
GREATER BINDWEED .... see GREATER BINDWEED
GREATER BURNET .... see GREATER BURNET
Greater Burnet-Saxifrage .... see PIMPINELLA root
GREATER CELANDINE dried above ground parts
.... see GREATER CELANDINE dried above ground parts
GREATER CELANDINE rhizome, root
.... see GREATER CELANDINE rhizome, root
Greater Plantain .... see GREAT PLANTAIN
Grecian Laurel .... see SWEET BAY
Greek Hay .... see FENUGREEK
Greek Hay Seed .... see FENUGREEK
GREEK SAGE .... see GREEK SAGE
Green Arrow .... see YARROW
Green Bean .... see BEAN POD
Green Bell Pepper .... see CAPSICUM
Green Broom .... see DYER'S BROOM
Green Chili Pepper .... see CAPSICUM
Green Dragon .... see TRAGACANTH
Green Endive .... see WILD LETTUCE
Green Ginger .... see WORMWOOD above ground parts
Green Hellebore .... see AMERICAN HELLEBORE
Green Mint .... see SPEARMINT
Green Oil of Charity ..... see ENGLISH ADDER'S TONGUE
Green Onion .... see ONION
Green Ozier .... see AMERICAN DOGWOOD
Green Sauce .... see WOOD SORREL
GREEN TEA .... see GREEN TEA
Green Veratrum .... see AMERICAN HELLEBORE
Green Wolf's Foot .... see BUGLEWEED
Greenweed .... see DYER'S BROOM
Grenadier .... see POMEGRANATE
Griffe Du Chat .... see CAT'S CLAW
Griffe Du Diable .... see DEVIL'S CLAW
Grifola .... see MAITAKE
Grifola frondosa .... see MAITAKE
Grindelia .... see GUMWEED
Grindelia robusta .... see GUMWEED
Grindelia squarrosa .... see GUMWEED
Grindeliae herba .... see GUMWEED
Griottier .... see SOUR CHERRY

Grip Grass .... see CLIVERS
Grisset .... see SEA BUCKTHORN
Groats .... see OATS
Groseillier de Ceylan .... see INDIAN GOOSEBERRY
Grosse Kamille .... see ROMAN CHAMOMILE
Grosse Moosbeere .... see CRANBERRY
Ground Apple .... see ROMAN CHAMOMILE
Ground Berry .... see WINTERGREEN leaf,
WINTERGREEN oil
Ground Elder .... see GOUTWEED
Ground Furze .... see SPINY RESTHARROW
Ground Glutton .... see GROUNDSEL
Ground Holly .... see PIPSISSEWA
GROUND IVY .... see GROUND IVY
Ground Laurel .... see TRAILING ARBUTUS
Ground Lemon .... see PODOPHYLLUM
Ground Lily .... see BETH ROOT
GROUND PINE .... see GROUND PINE
Ground Raspberry .... see GOLDENSEAL
Ground Thistle .... see CARLINA
Groundbread .... see CYCLAMEN
Groundnuts .... see PEANUT OIL
GROUNDSEL .... see GROUNDSEL
Grub .... see MAGGOTS
Grundy Swallow .... see GOLDEN RAGWORT,
GROUNDSEL
GSH .... see GLUTATHIONE
Gua Lou .... see CHINESE CUCUMBER fruit
Gua Luo Ren .... see CHINESE CUCUMBER seed
Guaiac .... see GUAIAC WOOD resin, wood
Guaiac Heartwood .... see GUAIAC WOOD resin, wood
GUAIAC WOOD OIL .... see GUAIAC WOOD OIL
GUAIAC WOOD resin, wood
.... see GUAIAC WOOD resin, wood
Guaiacum .... see GUAIAC WOOD resin, wood
Guaiacum officinale .... see GUAIAC WOOD resin, wood
Guaiacum sanctum .... see GUAIAC WOOD resin, wood
Guajaci Lignum .... see GUAIAC WOOD resin, wood
Guapi .... see COCILLANA
Guar Flour .... see GUAR GUM
GUAR GUM .... see GUAR GUM
GUARANA .... see GUARANA
Guarana Bread .... see GUARANA
Guarana Gum .... see GUARANA
Guarana Seed Paste .... see GUARANA
Guarea rusbyi .... see COCILLANA
Guatemala Lemongrass .... see LEMONGRASS
GUAYULE .... see GUAYULE
Guelder Rose .... see CRAMP BARK
Guflatich .... see COLTSFOOT
Guggal .... see GUGGUL
Guggal Gum and Resin .... see MYRRH
GUGGUL .... see GUGGUL
Guggulu .... see GUGGUL
Guindo .... see SOUR CHERRY
Guinea Corn .... see BROOM CORN
Guinea Grains .... see GRAINS OF PARADISE
Guinea Rush .... see ADRUE
Guinea Sorrel .... see HIBISCUS
Gum Acacia .... see ACACIA
Gum Arabic .... see ACACIA
Gum Benjamin .... see BENZOIN
Gum Benzoin .... see BENZOIN
Gum Bush .... see YERBA SANTA

INDEX

Gum Camphor .... see CAMPHOR
Gum Dragon .... see TRAGACANTH
Gum Guggal .... see GUGGUL
Gum Guggulu .... see GUGGUL
Gum Ivy .... see ENGLISH IVY
Gum Myrrh .... see MYRRH
Gum Plant .... see COMFREY, YERBA SANTA
Gum Senegal .... see ACACIA
Gum Tragacanth .... see TRAGACANTH
Gum Tree .... see EUCALYPTUS dried leaf, STORAX
Gummae Mimosae .... see ACACIA
Gummi Tragacanthae .... see TRAGACANTH
Gummigutta .... see GAMBOGE
GUMWEED .... see GUMWEED
Gumweed Herb .... see GUMWEED
Gur-Mar .... see GYMNEMA
Gurmar .... see GYMNEMA
Gurmarbooti .... see GYMNEMA
Guru Nut .... see COLA NUT
Gutta Cambodia .... see GAMBOGE
Gutta Gamba .... see GAMBOGE
GYMNEMA .... see GYMNEMA
Gymnema sylvestre .... see GYMNEMA
Gynocardia Oil .... see CHAULMOOGRA
Gynostemma pedatum .... see JIAOGULAN
Gynostemma pentaphyllum .... see JIAOGULAN
Gypsophila paniculata .... see WHITE SOAPWORT
Gypsophilae radix .... see WHITE SOAPWORT
Gypsy Flower .... see HOUND'S TONGUE
Gypsyweed .... see BUGLEWEED, VERONICA
Gypsywort .... see BUGLEWEED
Haagdorn .... see HAWTHORN fruit
Haba Soya .... see SOY
Hackmatack .... see CEDAR leaf, CEDAR LEAF OIL
Haematoxylon campechianum .... see LOGWOOD
Haematoxylon lignum .... see LOGWOOD
Hagedorn .... see HAWTHORN fruit
Hagenia abyssinica .... see KOUSSO
Hag's Taper .... see MULLEIN
Hair of Venus .... see MAIDENHAIR FERN
Hairy Mint .... see WILD MINT
Hallelujah .... see WOOD SORREL
Hallfoot .... see COLTSFOOT
Hamamelis .... see WITCH HAZEL
Hamamelis virginiana .... see WITCH HAZEL
Hamburg Parsley .... see PARSLEY leaf, root
Handflower .... see WALLFLOWER
Hap Caps .... see DOWN SYNDROME
                    NUTRITIONAL SUPPLEMENTS
Happy Major .... see BURDOCK
Hara .... see TERMINALIA
Harada .... see TERMINALIA
Hardback .... see STONE ROOT
Hardhack .... see STONE ROOT
Hardhay .... see ST JOHN'S WORT
Hardock .... see BURDOCK
Harebur .... see BURDOCK
Hare's Beard .... see MULLEIN
Hare's Ear Root .... see BUPLEURUM
Haritaki .... see TERMINALIA
Harnblumen .... see SANDY EVERLASTING
HARONGA .... see HARONGA
Haronga madagascariensis .... see HARONGA
Harongabladder leaf .... see HARONGA

Harongarinde bark .... see HARONGA
Harpagophyti Radix .... see DEVIL'S CLAW
Harpagophytum .... see DEVIL'S CLAW
Harpagophytum procumbens .... see DEVIL'S CLAW
Harthorne .... see HAWTHORN fruit
Hart's Tree .... see SWEET CLOVER
Hart's Truffle .... see PUFF BALL
Hartshorn .... see EUROPEAN BUCKTHORN
HARTSTONGUE .... see HARTSTONGUE
Harunganae madagascariensis cortex bark .... see HARONGA
Harunganae madagascariensis folium leaf .... see HARONGA
Haselnuss .... see HAZELNUT
Haselstrauch .... see HAZELNUT
Hash .... see MARIJUANA
Hashish .... see MARIJUANA
Hauhechelwurzel .... see SPINY RESTHARROW
Haw .... see HAWTHORN fruit, HAWTHORN leaf, flower,
                    HAWTHORN leaf with flower extract
HAWAIIAN BABY WOODROSE
.... see HAWAIIAN BABY WOODROSE
HAWTHORN fruit .... see HAWTHORN fruit
HAWTHORN leaf, flower ...... see HAWTHORN leaf, flower
HAWTHORN leaf with flower extract
.... see HAWTHORN leaf with flower extract
Hawthorne .... see HAWTHORN fruit,
                    HAWTHORN leaf, flower,
                    HAWTHORN leaf with flower extract
HAY FLOWER .... see HAY FLOWER
Hay Flower .... see SWEET CLOVER
Hay Sack .... see HAY FLOWER
Haymaids .... see GROUND IVY
Hayriffe .... see CLIVERS
Hayruff .... see CLIVERS
Hazel .... see HAZELNUT, WITCH HAZEL
HAZELNUT .... see HAZELNUT
Hazelwort .... see ASARABACCA
HCA .... see GARCINIA
He-Shou-Wu .... see FO-TI raw root
He Zi .... see TERMINALIA
Headache .... see CORN POPPY
Headsman .... see BUCKHORN PLANTAIN
Headwark .... see CORN POPPY
Heal-all .... see FIGWORT, SELF-HEAL, STONE ROOT
Healing Herb .... see COMFREY
Heart of the Earth .... see SELF-HEAL
Heartleaf .... COUNTRY MALLOW
HEART'S EASE .... see HEART'S EASE
Heated Oyster Shell-Seaweed Calcium .... see CALCIUM
HEATHER .... see HEATHER
Heaven Tree .... see TREE OF HEAVEN
Heavy Kaolin .... see KAOLIN
Hedeoma pulegioides .... see PENNYROYAL leaf,
                    PENNYROYAL oil
Hedera helix .... see ENGLISH IVY
Hederae helicis folium .... see ENGLISH IVY
Hedge Bindweed .... see GREATER BINDWEED
Hedge-Burs .... see CLIVERS
Hedge Convolvulus .... see GREATER BINDWEED
Hedge Fumitory .... see FUMITORY
HEDGE-HYSSOP .... see HEDGE-HYSSOP
Hedge Lily .... see GREATER BINDWEED
HEDGE MUSTARD .... see HEDGE MUSTARD
Hedge Nettles .... see BETONY
Hedge Taper .... see MULLEIN

INDEX

Hedgeheriff .... see CLIVERS
Hedgehog .... see ECHINACEA
Hedgemaids .... see GROUND IVY
Hedgethorn .... see HAWTHORN fruit
Hediondilla .... see CHAPARRAL
Heeng .... see ASAFOETIDA
Heerabol .... see MYRRH
Hei Zao .... see JUJUBE
Helenium grandiflorum .... see ELECAMPANE
Helianthemum canadense .... see FROSTWORT
Helianthi Annui Oleum .... see SUNFLOWER OIL
Helianthus annuus .... see SUNFLOWER OIL
Helichrysum .... see SANDY EVERLASTING
Helichrysum arenarium .... see IMMORTELLE
Helichrysum augustifolium .... see SANDY EVERLASTING
Helichrysum italicum .... see SANDY EVERLASTING
Helichrysum oriental .... see SANDY EVERLASTING
Helichrysum stoechas .... see SANDY EVERLASTING
Helleborus niger .... see BLACK HELLEBORE
Hellweed .... see DODDER
Helmet Flower .... see SCULLCAP
Helonias .... see FALSE UNICORN
Helonias dioica .... see FALSE UNICORN
Helonias lutea .... see FALSE UNICORN
Hemicellulose Complex with Arabinoxylane .... see MGN-3
Hemlock Bark .... see PINUS BARK
Hemlock Gum .... see PINUS BARK
HEMLOCK SPRUCE .... see HEMLOCK SPRUCE
Hemlock Spruce .... see PINUS BARK
Hemlocktanne .... see PINUS BARK
Hemp .... see MARIJUANA
HEMP AGRIMONY .... see HEMP AGRIMONY
Hemp Tree .... see CHASTEBERRY
HEMPNETTLE .... see HEMPNETTLE
Hen Bell .... see HENBANE
Hen Of The Woods .... see MAITAKE
HENBANE .... see HENBANE
Hendibeh .... see CHICORY
HENNA .... see HENNA
Henna .... see ALKANNA
Hennae folium .... see HENNA
Henne .... see HENNA
Hens and Chickens .... see HOUSELEEK
Hepatica nobilis var acuta .... see LIVERWORT
Hepatica nobilis var obtusa .... see LIVERWORT
Hepatici noblis herba .... see LIVERWORT
Hepatique a Lobes Aigus .... see LIVERWORT
Hepatique d'Amerique .... see LIVERWORT
Heps .... see ROSE HIP
Heracleum lanatum .... see MASTERWORT
Heracleum sphondylium .... see MASTERWORT
Herb Bennet .... see AVENS
Herb Gerard .... see GOUTWEED
Herb Louisa .... see LEMON VERBENA
Herb Margaret .... see OX-EYE DAISY
Herb of Grace .... see RUE, VERBENA
Herb of the Cross .... see VERBENA
HERB PARIS .... see HERB PARIS
Herb Perter .... see COWSLIP
HERB ROBERT .... see HERB ROBERT
Herb Trinity .... see LIVERWORT
Herb Two-Pence .... see MONEYWORT
Herba .... see SWEET VIOLET
Herba de la Pastora .... see DAMIANA

Herba Dictamni Herba .... see BURNING BUSH leaf,
                                        BURNING BUSH root
Herba Epimedii .... see EPIMEDIUM
Herba eupatoriae .... see AGRIMONY
Herba fumariae .... see FUMITORY
Herba Malvae .... see MARSHMALLOW
Herbe Aux Charpentiers .... see YARROW
Herbe d'Absinthe ...... see WORMWOOD above ground parts
Herbe d'Aigremoine .... see AGRIMONY
Herbe de Hogweed .... see SCOTCH BROOM flower
Herbe de Sainte Cunegonde .... see HEMP AGRIMONY
Herbe de Saint-Guillaume .... see AGRIMONY
Herbed' Euphraise .... see EYEBRIGHT
Herbygrass .... see RUE
Hercules Woundwort .... see SELF-HEAL
Herniaria glabra .... see RUPTUREWORT
Herniaria hirsuta .... see RUPTUREWORT
Herniariae herba .... see RUPTUREWORT
Herniary .... see RUPTUREWORT
Herpestis monniera .... see BRAHMI
Hervea .... see MATE
Heshouwu .... see FO-TI raw root
Hexacosanol .... see OCTACOSANOL
Hexahydroxycyclohexane .... see INOSITOL
Hexanicotinoyl Inositol .... see INOSITOL NICOTINATE
Hexanicotinyl cis-1,2,3-5-trans-4,6-cyclohexane
                                 ...... see INOSITOL NICOTINATE
Hexenbesen .... see EUROPEAN MISTLETOE
HIBISCUS .... see HIBISCUS
Hibiscus abelmoschus .... see AMBRETTE
Hibiscus sabdariffa .... see HIBISCUS
Hierba Carmin .... see POKEWEED berry, POKEWEED root
Hierba de San Juan .... see MUGWORT
Hierba Santa .... see YERBA SANTA
High Balm .... see OSWEGO TEA
High Mallow .... see MALLOW flower, MALLOW leaf
High-bush Cranberry .... see CRAMP BARK
Highwaythorn .... see EUROPEAN BUCKTHORN
Higtaper .... see MULLEIN
Hilberry ...... see WINTERGREEN leaf, WINTERGREEN oil
Himalayan Mayapple .... see PODOPHYLLUM
Himalayan Rhubarb .... see RHUBARB
Hind Heal .... see TANSY, WOOD SAGE
Hind's Tongue .... see HARTSTONGUE
Hing Hua .... see SAFFLOWER
Hini .... see BLACK ROOT
Hip Fruit .... see ROSE HIP
Hip Sweet .... see ROSE HIP
Hipberry .... see ROSE HIP
Hippocastani Cortex ... see HORSE CHESTNUT branch bark
Hippocastani Flos .... see HORSE CHESTNUT flower
Hippocastani folium .... see HORSE CHESTNUT leaf
Hippocastani Semen .. see HORSE CHESTNUT branch bark,
                                    HORSE CHESTNUT seed
Hippophae rhamnoides .... see SEA BUCKTHORN
Hipposelinum levisticum .... see LOVAGE
Hirala .... see TERMINALIA
Hirshklee .... see HEMP AGRIMONY
Hirudo medicinalis .... see LEECH
HISTIDINE .... see HISTIDINE
Hive Dross .... see PROPOLIS
Hive Vine .... see SQUAWVINE
HMB .... see HYDROXYMETHYLBUTYRATE
Ho-Shou-Wu .... see FO-TI raw root

I
N
D
E
X

Hoarhound .... see BUGLEWEED, WHITE HOREHOUND
Hoary Plantain .... see BUCKHORN PLANTAIN
Hock-Heal.. see SELF-HEAL
Hockle Elderberry .... see LEVANT BERRY
Hoelen................................... see PORIA MUSHROOM
Hog Apple .... see MORINDA, PODOPHYLLUM
Hog Bean .... see HENBANE
Hog Gum .... see TRAGACANTH
Hogberry .... see UVA URSI
Hogweed .... see KNOTWEED HERB, MASTERWORT,
                                SCOTCH BROOM flower,
                                SCOTCH BROOM herb
Hoku-Gomishi .... see SCHISANDRA
Holligold .... see CALENDULA
HOLLY .... see HOLLY
Holly .... see PIPSISSEWA
Holly Barberry .... see OREGON GRAPE
Holly Bay .... see MAGNOLIA bark
Holly-Leaved Berberis .... see OREGON GRAPE
Holly Mahonia .... see OREGON GRAPE
HOLLYHOCK .... see HOLLYHOCK
Hollyhock Flower .... see HOLLYHOCK
Holm .... see HOLLY
Holme Chase .... see HOLLY
Holunderbeeren .... see EUROPEAN ELDER fruit
Holy Basil .... see BASIL
Holy Herb .... see YERBA SANTA
Holy Rope .... see HEMP AGRIMONY
Holy Thistle .... see BLESSED THISTLE,
                                MILK THISTLE above ground parts,
                                MILK THISTLE fruit, seed
Holy Tree .... see HOLLY, NEEM
Holy Weed .... see YERBA SANTA
Holywort .... see VERBENA
Honduras Sarsaparilla .... see SARSAPARILLA
HONEY .... see HONEY
HONEY BEE venom .... see HONEY BEE venom
Honey Plant .... see LEMON BALM
Honeybloom .... see CANADIAN HEMP
HONEYSUCKLE .... see HONEYSUCKLE
Hong Zao .... see JUJUBE
Honghua .... see SAFFLOWER
Honig .... see HONEY
Hoodwort .... see SCULLCAP
Hop Fruit .... see ROSE HIP
Hop Strobiles .... see HOPS
Hopfenzapfen .... see HOPS
HOPS .... see HOPS
Hordeum distychum .... see BARLEY
Hordeum vulgare .... see BARLEY
Horehound .... see WHITE HOREHOUND
Horns of Gold .... see DEER VELVET
Hornseed .... see ERGOT
Horny Goat Weed .... see EPIMEDIUM
Horse Balm .... see STONE ROOT
Horse Blobs .... see MARSH MARIGOLD
HORSE CHESTNUT branch bark
.... see HORSE CHESTNUT branch bark
HORSE CHESTNUT flower
.... see HORSE CHESTNUT flower
HORSE CHESTNUT leaf .... see HORSE CHESTNUT leaf
HORSE CHESTNUT seed ..... see HORSE CHESTNUT seed
Horse Daisy .... see OX-EYE DAISY
Horse-Elder .... see ELECAMPANE

Horse Gowan .... see OX-EYE DAISY
Horse Tongue .... see HARTSTONGUE
Horse Willow .... see HORSETAIL
Horsebane .... see WATER FENNEL
Horsefly Weed .... see WILD INDIGO
Horsefoot .... see COLTSFOOT
Horseheal .... see ELECAMPANE
Horsehoof .... see COLTSFOOT
HORSEMINT .... see HORSEMINT
HORSERADISH .... see HORSERADISH
HORSETAIL .... see HORSETAIL
Horsetail .... see LAMINARIA
Horsetail Grass .... see HORSETAIL
Horsetail Rush .... see HORSETAIL
Horseweed .... see STONE ROOT
Horsewood .... see CANADIAN FLEABANE
Hoshouwu .... see FO-TI raw root
Hot Pepper .... see CAPSICUM
Houblon .... see HOPS
HOUND'S TONGUE .... see HOUND'S TONGUE
Hound's Tongue .... see DEERTONGUE
Houndsbane .... see WHITE HOREHOUND
Houndsberry .... see BLACK NIGHTSHADE
HOUSELEEK .... see HOUSELEEK
Hsia Ts'Ao Tung Ch'Ung .... see CORDYCEPS
Hsiang-Dan .... see ALOE dried juice from leaf, latex
Hu Lu Ba .... see FENUGREEK
Hua Gu .... see SHIITAKE MUSHROOM
Huacatay .... see TAGETES
Huang Ken .... see DANSHEN
Huang qi .... see ASTRAGALUS
Huang Qin .... see BAIKAL SKULLCAP
Huang-T'eng Ken .... see THUNDER GOD VINE
Huangquin .... see BAIKAL SKULLCAP
Huanuco Coca .... see COCA
Huckleberry .... see BILBERRY dried ripe fruit,
                                                BILBERRY leaf
Huile De Bourrache .... see BORAGE SEED OIL
Huile D'Onagre .... see EVENING PRIMROSE OIL
Huisache .... see CASSIE ABSOLUTE
Hulm .... see HOLLY
Hulver Bush .... see HOLLY
Hulver Tree .... see HOLLY
Humic Shale .... see COLLOIDAL MINERALS
Hummingbird Tree .... see TURTLE HEAD
Humulus lupulus .... see HOPS
Hungarian Chamomile .... see GERMAN CHAMOMILE
Hungarian Pepper .... see CAPSICUM
Huntsman's Cup .... see PITCHER PLANT
Huo xiang .... see PATCHOULY OIL
HupA .... see HUPERZINE A
Huperazon .... see CHINESE CLUB MOSS
Huperzia serrata .... see CHINESE CLUB MOSS
Huperzine .... see HUPERZINE A
HUPERZINE A .... see HUPERZINE A
Hurtleberry .... see BILBERRY dried ripe fruit,
                                                BILBERRY leaf
Hurtsickle .... see CORNFLOWER
Husked Nut .... see EUROPEAN CHESTNUT
Hwanggi .... see ASTRAGALUS
Hwanggum .... see BAIKAL SKULLCAP
Hydnocarp .... see CHAULMOOGRA
Hydnocarpus .... see CHAULMOOGRA
HYDRANGEA .... see HYDRANGEA

INDEX

Hydrangea arborescens .... see HYDRANGEA
Hydrastis canadensis .... see GOLDENSEAL
Hydrated aluminum silicate .... see KAOLIN
Hydrazine .... see HYDRAZINE SULFATE
HYDRAZINE SULFATE .... see HYDRAZINE SULFATE
Hydrocotyle .... see GOTU KOLA
Hydrocotyle asiatica .... see GOTU KOLA
Hydroxocobalamin .... see VITAMIN B12
Hydroxocobalaminum .... see VITAMIN B12
Hydroxocobemine .... see VITAMIN B12
Hydroxyacetic Acid .... see ALPHA HYDROXY ACIDS
Hydroxyapatite .... see CALCIUM
Hydroxycitrate .... see GARCINIA
Hydroxycitric Acid .... see GARCINIA
HYDROXYMETHYLBUTYRATE (HMB)
.... see HYDROXYMETHYLBUTYRATE (HMB)
Hydroxypropionic Acid ...... see ALPHA HYDROXY ACIDS
Hydroxysuccinic acid .... see ALPHA HYDROXY ACIDS
Hyoscyami Folium .... see HENBANE
Hyoscyamus niger .... see HENBANE
Hypereikon .... see ST JOHN'S WORT
Hyperici Herba .... see ST JOHN'S WORT
Hypericum .... see ST JOHN'S WORT
Hypericum perforatum .... see ST JOHN'S WORT
Hyperimmune Bovine Colostrum
.... see BOVINE COLOSTRUM
Hypoxanthine Riboside .... see INOSINE
Hypoxanthosine .... see INOSINE
Hypoxis Plant .... see AFRICAN WILD POTATO
Hypoxis rooperi .... see AFRICAN WILD POTATO
HYSSOP .... see HYSSOP
Hyssopus officinalis .... see HYSSOP
Iandirova .... see ANDIROBA
IBOGA .... see IBOGA
Ice Vine .... see PAREIRA
Iceland Lichen .... see ICELAND MOSS
ICELAND MOSS .... see ICELAND MOSS
Ichthyomethia piscipula .... see JAMAICAN DOGWOOD
Ici Fructus .... see CAPSICUM
Idrossocobalamina .... see VITAMIN B12
Igelkopfwurzel .... see ECHINACEA
IGNATIUS BEAN .... see IGNATIUS BEAN
Ilex .... see MATE
Ilex aquifolium .... see HOLLY
Ilex opaca .... see HOLLY
Ilex paraguariensis .... see MATE
Ilex vomitoria .... see HOLLY
Illicium .... see STAR ANISE
Illicium verum .... see STAR ANISE
Imlee .... see TAMARIND
IMMORTELLE .... see IMMORTELLE
Impatiens balsamina .... see JEWELWEED
Impatiens biflora .... see JEWELWEED
Impatiens capensis .... see JEWELWEED
Impatiens pallida .... see JEWELWEED
In Chen .... see YIN CHEN
Inchinko .... see YIN CHEN
Inchin-Ko-To .... see YIN CHEN
India Root .... see ALPINIA
Indian Almond .... see TERMINALIA
Indian Apple .... see PODOPHYLLUM
Indian Arrowroot .... see WAHOO, ZEDOARY
Indian Arrowwood .... see WAHOO
Indian Bael .... see BAEL

Indian Balm .... see BETH ROOT
Indian Balsam .... see PERU BALSAM
Indian Bark .... see MAGNOLIA bark
Indian Bdellium-Tree .... see GUGGUL
Indian Bead .... see PRECATORY BEAN
Indian Berry .... see LEVANT BERRY
Indian Bolonong .... see CHIRATA
Indian Bread .... see PORIA MUSHROOM
Indian Chocolate .... see WATER AVENS
Indian Civet .... see CIVET
Indian Corn .... see CORN SILK
Indian Cress .... see NASTURTIUM, WATERCRESS
Indian Dye .... see GOLDENSEAL
Indian Echinacea .... see ANDROGRAPHIS
Indian Elm .... see SLIPPERY ELM
INDIAN FRANKINCENSE
.... see INDIAN FRANKINCENSE
Indian Gentian .... see CHIRATA
Indian Ginseng .... see WITHANIA
INDIAN GOOSEBERRY .... see INDIAN GOOSEBERRY
Indian Gum .... see CUP PLANT
Indian Head .... see ECHINACEA
Indian-Hemp .... see CANADIAN HEMP
Indian Hippo .... see INDIAN PHYSIC
Indian-laurel .... see LAURELWOOD
Indian Lilac .... see NEEM
INDIAN LONG PEPPER .... see INDIAN LONG PEPPER
Indian Mulberry .... see MORINDA
Indian Olibanum .... see INDIAN FRANKINCENSE
Indian Pennywort .... see GOTU KOLA
INDIAN PHYSIC .... see INDIAN PHYSIC
Indian Physic .... see CANADIAN HEMP
Indian Pink .... see PINK ROOT
Indian Plant .... see BLOODROOT, GOLDENSEAL
Indian Plantago .... see BLOND PSYLLIUM
Indian Podophyllum .... see PODOPHYLLUM
Indian Poke .... see AMERICAN HELLEBORE
Indian Red Paint .... see BLOODROOT
Indian Rhubarb .... see RHUBARB
Indian Root .... see AMERICAN SPIKENARD
Indian Saffron .... see SAFFRON, TURMERIC
Indian Sage .... see BONESET
Indian Senna .... see SENNA
Indian Shamrock .... see BETH ROOT
INDIAN SNAKEROOT .... see INDIAN SNAKEROOT
Indian Squill .... see SQUILL
Indian Tobacco .... see LOBELIA
Indian Tragacanth .... see KARAYA GUM
Indian Tumeric .... see GOLDENSEAL
Indian Valerian .... see VALERIAN
Indian Walnut........................... see TUNG SEED
Indian Water Navelwort .... see GOTU KOLA
Indigo Broom .... see WILD INDIGO
Inkberry .... see POKEWEED berry, POKEWEED root
Inorganic Germanium .... see GERMANIUM
Inose .... see INOSITOL
INOSINE .... see INOSINE
Inosite .... see INOSITOL
INOSITOL .... see INOSITOL
Inositol Hexaniacinate .... see INOSITOL NICOTINATE
Inositol Hexanicotinate .... see INOSITOL NICOTINATE
Inositol Hexaphosphate .... see IP-6
Inositol Monophosphate .... see INOSITOL
Inositol Niacinate .... see INOSITOL NICOTINATE

INOSITOL NICOTINATE ..... see INOSITOL NICOTINATE
Inositol Nicotinate .... see IP-6
Intoxicating Pepper .... see KAVA
Intrachol .... see CHOLINE
Intralipid .... see SOYBEAN OIL
Inula .... see ELECAMPANE
Inula helenium .... see ELECAMPANE
IODINE .... see IODINE
IP-6 .... see IP-6
Ipe .... see PAU D'ARCO
Ipe Roxo .... see PAU D'ARCO
IPECAC .... see IPECAC
Ipecacuanha .... see IPECAC
Ipes .... see PAU D'ARCO
Ipomoea .... see MEXICAN SCAMMONY ROOT
Ipomoea orizabensis ... see MEXICAN SCAMMONY ROOT
Ipomoea purga .... see JALAP
Iporoni .... see IPORURU
Iporuro .... see IPORURU
IPORURU .... see IPORURU
IPRIFLAVONE .... see IPRIFLAVONE
Ipurosa .... see IPORURU
Ipururo .... see IPORURU
Iris .... see BLUE FLAG, ORRIS
Iris caroliniana .... see BLUE FLAG
Iris florentina .... see ORRIS
Iris germanica .... see ORRIS
Iris pallida .... see ORRIS
Iris versicolor .... see BLUE FLAG
Iris virginica .... see BLUE FLAG
Iris x germanica var florentina .... see ORRIS
Irish Broom .... see SCOTCH BROOM herb
Irish Broom Tops .... see SCOTCH BROOM flower
Irish Moss Extract .... see CARRAGEENAN
Irish Potato .... see POTATO
IRON .... see IRON
irradiated ergosterol .... see VITAMIN D
Isatis indigota .... see DA QING YE
Isoflavone .... see RED CLOVER, SOY
Isoleucine .... see BRANCHED-CHAIN AMINO ACIDS
Ispaghula .... see BLOND PSYLLIUM
Ispagol .... see BLOND PSYLLIUM
Italian Fitch .... see GOAT'S RUE
Italian Jasmine .... see JASMINE
Italian Limetta .... see LIME fruit, peel, LIME oil
Itchweed .... see AMERICAN HELLEBORE
Ivy .... see AMERICAN IVY, ENGLISH IVY
Ivy-Leafed Cyclamen .... see CYCLAMEN
JABORANDI .... see JABORANDI
Jaborandi Pepper .... see INDIAN LONG PEPPER
Jack-Jump-About .... see GOUTWEED
Jack-of-the-Buttery .... see COMMON STONECROP
JACOB'S LADDER .... see JACOB'S LADDER
Jacob's Ladder .... see LILY-OF-THE-VALLEY
Jacob's Staff .... see MULLEIN
Jacob's Sword .... see ORRIS
Jaffa Orange .... see SWEET ORANGE
Jaguar Gum .... see GUAR GUM
Jalanimba .... see BRAHMI
JALAP .... see JALAP
Jalap .... see POKEWEED berry, POKEWEED root
Jalapa .... see JALAP
Jalape .... see JALAP
Jalnaveri .... see BRAHMI

Jamaica Dogwood .... see JAMAICAN DOGWOOD
Jamaica Ginger .... see GINGER
Jamaica Mignonette .... see HENNA
Jamaica Pepper .... see ALLSPICE
Jamaica Sorrel .... see HIBISCUS
JAMAICAN DOGWOOD ..... see JAMAICAN DOGWOOD
Jamaican Quassia .... see QUASSIA
Jamaican Sarsaparilla .... see SARSAPARILLA
JAMBOLAN bark .... see JAMBOLAN bark
JAMBOLAN seed .... see JAMBOLAN seed
Jambul .... see JAMBOLAN bark, JAMBOLAN seed
James' Tea .... see MARSH TEA
Jamestown Weed .... see JIMSON WEED
Jamguarandi .... see JABORANDI
Jamum .... see JAMBOLAN bark, JAMBOLAN seed
Japanese Arrowroot .... see KUDZU
Japanese Belladonna .... see SCOPOLIA
Japanese Epimedium .... see EPIMEDIUM
Japanese Ginseng .... see GINSENG, PANAX
Japanese Isinglas .... see AGAR
JAPANESE MINT .... see JAPANESE MINT
Japanese Silver Apricot ..... see GINKGO leaf, GINKGO leaf
                                                   extract, GINKGO seed
JASMINE .... see JASMINE
Jasminium grandiflorum .... see JASMINE
Jasminium officinale .... see JASMINE
Jateorhiza palmata .... see COLOMBO
Jaundice Berry .... see EUROPEAN BARBERRY
Jaundice Root .... see GOLDENSEAL
Java .... see COFFEE
Java Coca .... see COCA
Java Pepper .... see CUBEBS
Java Plum .... see JAMBOLAN bark, JAMBOLAN seed
JAVA TEA .... see JAVA TEA
JAVANESE TURMERIC .... see JAVANESE TURMERIC
Jequirity Bean .... see PRECATORY BEAN
Jequirity Seed .... see PRECATORY BEAN
Jersey Tea .... see NEW JERSEY TEA
Jesuit Tea .... see CHENOPODIUM OIL
Jesuit's Balsam .... see COPAIBA BALSAM
Jesuit's Bark .... see CINCHONA
Jesuit's Brazil Tea .... see MATE
Jesuit's Tea .... see MATE
Jewel Balsam Weed .... see JEWELWEED
Jewel Weed .... see JEWELWEED
JEWELWEED .... see JEWELWEED
Jew's Harp Plant .... see BETH ROOT
Jew's Myrtle .... see BUTCHER'S BROOM
JIAOGULAN .... see JIAOGULAN
JIMSON WEED .... see JIMSON WEED
Jintsam .... see GINSENG, PANAX
Jinyingzi .... see CHEROKEE ROSEHIP
Jinyinhua .... see HONEYSUCKLE
Joe Pye .... see GRAVEL ROOT
Joe-Pye Weed.. see GRAVEL ROOT
Johimbi .... see YOHIMBE
Johnny-Jump-Up .... see HEART'S EASE
Johns Wort .... see ST JOHN'S WORT
Joint Fir .... see EPHEDRA
Joint-Podded Charlock .... see WILD RADISH
JOJOBA .... see JOJOBA
Joshua Tree .... see YUCCA
Ju Hua .... see CHRYSANTHEMUM
Juarandi .... see JABORANDI

I
N
D
E
X

Juglandis Folium .... see ENGLISH WALNUT leaf
Juglandis Walnussfruchtschalen
.... see ENGLISH WALNUT hull
Juglans cinerea .... see BUTTERNUT
Juglans nigra .... see BLACK WALNUT
Juglans regia .... see ENGLISH WALNUT hull,
ENGLISH WALNUT leaf
JUJUBE .... see JUJUBE
Jujube Plum .... see JUJUBE
Jumbul .... see JAMBOLAN bark, JAMBOLAN seed
Jungle Weed .... see OPIUM ANTIDOTE
JUNIPER .... see JUNIPER
Juniper Tar .... see CADE OIL
Juniper Tar Oil .... see CADE OIL
Juniperi fructus .... see JUNIPER
Juniperus communis .... see JUNIPER
Juniperus oxycedrus .... see CADE OIL
Juniperus sabina .... see SAVIN TOPS
Juniperus virginiana
.... see CEDARWOOD bark, berry, leaf, seed, twig,
CEDARWOOD OIL
Juno's Tears .... see VERBENA
Jupiter's Bean .... see HENBANE
Jupiter's Beard .... see HOUSELEEK
Jupiter's Eye .... see HOUSELEEK
Jupiter's Nut .... see EUROPEAN CHESTNUT
Justicia Adhatoda .... see MALABAR NUT
Justicia paniculata .... see ANDROGRAPHIS
K .... see POTASSIUM
Kaa Jhee .... see STEVIA
Kadaya .... see KARAYA GUM
Kadeol .... see CADE OIL
Kadira .... see KARAYA GUM
Kaffree Tea .... see RED BUSH TEA
Kalmegh .... see ANDROGRAPHIS
Kalmia latifolia .... see MOUNTAIN LAUREL
KAMALA .... see KAMALA
Kamani Punna .... see LAURELWOOD
Kamcela .... see KAMALA
Kameela .... see KAMALA
Kamillen .... see GERMAN CHAMOMILE
Kansas Snakeroot .... see ECHINACEA
KAOLIN .... see KAOLIN
Karaya .... see KARAYA GUM
KARAYA GUM .... see KARAYA GUM
Kardone .... see ARTICHOKE
Karela .... see BITTER MELON
Kargasok Tea .... see KOMBUCHA TEA
Kariyat .... see ANDROGRAPHIS
Karkade .... see HIBISCUS
Kastanienblaetter .... see EUROPEAN CHESTNUT
Kat .... see KHAT
Katila .... see KARAYA GUM
Katsenpfotchenbluten .... see CAT'S FOOT
Katzenkrat .... see YARROW
Katzenpfotchenbluten .... see SANDY EVERLASTING
Kaugummibaum .... see CHICLE
KAVA .... see KAVA
Kava Kava .... see KAVA
Kava Pepper .... see KAVA
Kava Root .... see KAVA
Kava-kava .... see KAVA
Kawa .... see KAVA
Kawa Kawa .... see KAVA

Kawaratake .... see CORIOLUS MUSHROOM
Kawara-Yomogi .... see YIN CHEN
Keiri .... see WALLFLOWER
Kelp .... see BLADDERWRACK, LAMINARIA
Kelp-Ware .... see BLADDERWRACK
Kephalin .... see PHOSPHATIDYLSERINE
Kermesbeere .... see POKEWEED berry, POKEWEED root
Kew .... see KAVA
Kew Tree .... see GINKGO leaf, GINKGO leaf extract,
GINKGO seed
Key Flower .... see COWSLIP
Key Lime .... see LIME oil
Key of Heaven .... see COWSLIP
KH-3 .... see PROCAINE
Khareti .... see COUNTRY MALLOW
Khartoum Senna .... see SENNA
Khas-khas .... see VETIVER
KHAT .... see KHAT
Khella .... see BISHOP'S WEED
Khella Fruit .... see BISHOP'S WEED
Kher .... see ACACIA
Khus Khus .... see VETIVER
Khus-khus Grass .... see VETIVER
Kidney Bean .... see BEAN POD
Kidney Root .... see GRAVEL ROOT
Kidney Wort .... see LIVERWORT
Kif .... see MARIJUANA
Kinerase .... see KINETIN
Kinetase .... see KINETIN
KINETIN .... see KINETIN
King of Bitters .... see ANDROGRAPHIS
King Of Mushrooms .... see MAITAKE
Kingcups .... see MARSH MARIGOLD
Kings And Queens .... see ARUM
King's Clover .... see SWEET CLOVER
King's Crown .... see ROSEROOT
King's Cup .... see BULBOUS BUTTERCUP
King's Cure .... see PIPSISSEWA
King's Cureall .... see EVENING PRIMROSE OIL,
PIPSISSEWA
Kinnikinnik .... see UVA URSI
Kirta .... see ANDROGRAPHIS
Kita-Gomishi .... see SCHISANDRA
Kiwach .... see COWHAGE
KIWI .... see KIWI
Kiwi Fruit .... see KIWI
Klamath Blue/Green Algae .... see BLUE-GREEN ALGAE
Klamath Weed .... see ST JOHN'S WORT
Klapperschlangen .... see SENEGA
Kleine Kamille .... see GERMAN CHAMOMILE
Knackweide .... see WILLOW BARK
Knautia arvensis .... see FIELD SCABIOUS
Knee Holly .... see BUTCHER'S BROOM
Kneeholm .... see BUTCHER'S BROOM
Kniepp Hay Sack .... see HAY FLOWER
Knight's Spur .... see DELPHINIUM, LARKSPUR
Knitback .... see COMFREY
Knitbone .... see COMFREY
Knob Grass .... see STONE ROOT
Knob Root .... see STONE ROOT
Knobweed .... see STONE ROOT
Knotgrass .... see KNOTWEED HERB
Knotted Marjoram .... see MARJORAM
Knotted Wrack .... see BLADDERWRACK

INDEX

Knotty Brake .... see MALE FERN
KNOTWEED HERB .... see KNOTWEED HERB
Kojo-Kon .... see RESVERATROL
Kola Nut .... see COLA NUT
Koloquinthen .... see COLOCYNTH
Kombe .... see STROPHANTHUS
Kombe-Strophanthus Seeds .... see STROPHANTHUS
Kombucha Mushroom Tea .... see KOMBUCHA TEA
KOMBUCHA TEA .... see KOMBUCHA TEA
Konjac .... see GLUCOMANNAN
Konjac Mannan .... see GLUCOMANNAN
Kooso .... see KOUSSO
Korean Ginseng .... see GINSENG, PANAX
Korean Red .... see GINSENG, PANAX
Korean Red Ginseng .... see GINSENG, PANAX
Koriander .... see CORIANDER
Kosho .... see BLACK PEPPER AND WHITE PEPPER
Kosso .... see KOUSSO
KOUSSO .... see KOUSSO
Kraftwurz .... see ARNICA
Krameria .... see RHATANY
Krameria argentea .... see RHATANY
Krameria triandra .... see RHATANY
Kranbeere .... see CRANBERRY
Krestin .... see CORIOLUS MUSHROOM
Kreuzdornbeeren .... see EUROPEAN BUCKTHORN
K'u-Kua .... see BITTER MELON
Kua .... see ZEDOARY
Kuandong Hua .... see COLTSFOOT
Kudsu .... see KUDZU
KUDZU .... see KUDZU
Kudzu Vine .... see KUDZU
Kuguazi .... see BITTER MELON
Kukui .... see TUNG SEED
Kullo .... see KARAYA GUM
Kummel .... see CARAWAY dried fruit, seed
Kummich .... see CARAWAY dried fruit, seed
Kunigundendraut .... see HEMP AGRIMONY
Kuntze Saloop .... see SASSAFRAS
Kus es Salahin .... see KHAT
Kwaao Khruea .... see KUDZU
Kwassan .... see KOMBUCHA TEA
Kydney Root .... see GRAVEL ROOT
Kyunchinho .... see YIN CHEN
L-(+)-2-Aminoglutaramic acid .... see GLUTAMINE
L-2,5-diaminovaleric acid .... see ORNITHINE
L-2,6-diaminohexanoic acid .... see LYSINE
L-2-Amino-3- propionic acid .... see HISTIDINE,
                                            L-TRYPTOPHAN
L-2-amino-4-butyric acid .... see METHIONINE
L-3-hydroxy-4-(trimethylammonium)-butyrate
   .... see L-CARNITINE
L-5 hydroxytryptophan .... see 5-HTP
L-5-aminorvaline .... see ORNITHINE
L-acetylcarnitine .... see ACETYL-L-CARNITINE
L-ARGININE .... see L-ARGININE
L-Arginine Hydrochloride .... see L-ARGININE
L-CARNITINE .... see L-CARNITINE
L-carnitine Propionyl .... see PROPIONYL-L-CARNITINE
L-Glutamic Acid 5-Amide .... see GLUTAMINE
L-Glutamine .... see GLUTAMINE
L-Histidine .... see HISTIDINE
L-Isoleucine .... see BRANCHED-CHAIN AMINO ACIDS
L-Leucine .... see BRANCHED-CHAIN AMINO ACIDS

L-Lysine .... see LYSINE
L-Methionine .... see METHIONINE
L-Ornithine .... see ORNITHINE
L-ornithine alpha-ketoglutarate
   .... see ORNITHINE KETOGLUTARATE
L-Phenylalanine .... see PHENYLALANINE
L-trypt .... see L-TRYPTOPHAN
L-TRYPTOPHAN .... see L-TRYPTOPHAN
L-Valine .... see BRANCHED-CHAIN AMINO ACIDS
LABDANUM .... see LABDANUM
LABRADOR TEA .... see LABRADOR TEA
Labrador Tea .... see MARSH TEA
LABURNUM .... see LABURNUM
Lac .... see SHELLAC
Lacca .... see SHELLAC
Laccifer .... see SHELLAC
Laciniaria spicata .... see MARSH BLAZING STAR
LACTASE .... see LACTASE
Lactic acid .... see ALPHA HYDROXY ACIDS
LACTOBACILLUS ACIDOPHILUS
   .... see LACTOBACILLUS ACIDOPHILUS
Lactobacillus casei sp rhamnosus ..... see LACTOBACILLUS
                                                             GG
Lactobacillus Casei Strain GG .. see LACTOBACILLUS GG
LACTOBACILLUS GG .... see LACTOBACILLUS GG
Lactobacillus Rhamnosus GG ... see LACTOBACILLUS GG
LACTOFERRIN .... see LACTOFERRIN
Lactoflavin .... see RIBOFLAVIN
Lactuca virosa .... see WILD LETTUCE
Lactucarium .... see WILD LETTUCE
Ladder-To-Heaven .... see LILY-OF-THE-VALLEY
Ladies' Delight .... see HEART'S EASE
Ladies' Seal .... see BRYONIA
Lady Bleeding .... see AMARANTH
LADY FERN .... see LADY FERN
Lady Of The Meadow .... see MEADOWSWEET
LADY'S BEDSTRAW .... see LADY'S BEDSTRAW
Lady's Mantle .... see ALCHEMILLA
Lady's Nightcap .... see GREATER BINDWEED
Lady's Purse .... see SHEPHERD'S PURSE
Lady's Seals .... see SOLOMON'S SEAL
Lady's Slipper .... see NERVE ROOT
Lady's Thimble .... see DIGITALIS
Lady's Thistle .... see MILK THISTLE above ground parts,
                                 MILK THISTLE fruit, seed
Ladysmock .... see ARUM
Laetrile .... see APRICOT
Lai Margose .... see BITTER MELON
Lakritze .... see LICORICE
Lamb Mint .... see PEPPERMINT leaf, SPEARMINT
Lambkill .... see MOUNTAIN LAUREL
Lamb's Quarters .... see BETH ROOT
Lamb's Tongue .... see AMERICAN ADDER'S TONGUE
Lamii Albi Flos .... see WHITE DEAD NETTLE FLOWER
LAMINARIA .... see LAMINARIA
Laminaria digitata .... see ALGIN, LAMINARIA
Laminaria japonica .... see LAMINARIA
Lamium album .... see WHITE DEAD NETTLE FLOWER
Lamp Black .... see ACTIVATED CHARCOAL
Lan-Hiqui .... see SANGRE DE GRADO
Land Whin .... see SPINY RESTHARROW
Langer Pfeffer .... see INDIAN LONG PEPPER
Langwort .... see PETASITES leaf,
                         PETASITES root, WHITE HELLEBORE

INDEX

Laniqui .... see SANGRE DE GRADO
Lapacho .... see PAU D'ARCO
Lapacho Colorado .... see PAU D'ARCO
Lapacho Morado .... see PAU D'ARCO
Lappa .... see BURDOCK
Larch .... see LARCH ARABINOGALACTAN
LARCH ARABINOGALACTAN
.... see LARCH ARABINOGALACTAN
Larch Gum .... see LARCH ARABINOGALACTAN
LARCH TURPENTINE .... see LARCH TURPENTINE
Large Cranberry .... see CRANBERRY
Large Fennel .... see FENNEL fruit, seed
Large Indian Civet .... see CIVET
Large-Leaved Germander .... see WOOD SAGE
Larix .... see LARCH ARABINOGALACTAN
Larix dahurica .... see LARCH ARABINOGALACTAN
Larix decidua .... see LARCH TURPENTINE
Larix occidentalis .... see LARCH ARABINOGALACTAN
Lark Heel .... see DELPHINIUM, LARKSPUR
Lark's Claw .... see DELPHINIUM, LARKSPUR
Lark's Toe .... see DELPHINIUM, LARKSPUR
LARKSPUR .... see LARKSPUR
Larkspur .... see DELPHINIUM
Larkspur Lion's Mouth .... see YELLOW TOADFLAX
Larrea divaricata .... see CHAPARRAL
Larrea tridentata .... see CHAPARRAL
LATHYRUS .... see LATHYRUS
Lathyrus cicera .... see LATHYRUS
Lathyrus clymenu .... see LATHYRUS
Lathyrus hirsutus .... see LATHYRUS
Lathyrus incanus .... see LATHYRUS
Lathyrus odoratus .... see LATHYRUS
Lathyrus pusillus .... see LATHYRUS
Lathyrus sativus .... see LATHYRUS
Lathyrus sylvestris .... see LATHYRUS
Laurel .... see MOUNTAIN LAUREL, SWEET BAY
Laurel Camphor .... see CAMPHOR
Laurel Willow .... see WILLOW BARK
LAURELWOOD .... see LAURELWOOD
Laurocerasus Leaves .... see CHERRY LAUREL WATER
Laurocerasus officinalis ...... see CHERRY LAUREL WATER
Laurus nobilis .... see SWEET BAY
Laurus persea .... see AVOCADO
Lavandula angustifolia .... see LAVENDER
Lavandula dentata .... see LAVENDER
Lavandula latifolia .... see LAVENDER
Lavandula officinalis .... see LAVENDER
Lavandula pubescens .... see LAVENDER
Lavandula spica .... see LAVENDER
Lavandula stoechas .... see LAVENDER
Lavandula vera .... see LAVENDER
LAVENDER .... see LAVENDER
LAVENDER COTTON .... see LAVENDER COTTON
Lavose .... see LOVAGE
Lawsonia alba .... see HENNA
Lawsonia inermis .... see HENNA
Layor Carang .... see AGAR
Leberbluemchenkraut .... see LIVERWORT
Leberkraut .... see HEMP AGRIMONY
Leche de Higueron .... see FICIN
Leche de Oje .... see FICIN
LECITHIN .... see LECITHIN
Ledi palustris herba .... see MARSH TEA
Ledum groenlandicum .... see LABRADOR TEA

Ledum latifolium .... see LABRADOR TEA
Ledum palustre .... see LABRADOR TEA, MARSH TEA
LEECH .... see LEECH
Lei Gong Teng .... see THUNDER GOD VINE
Lei-Kung T'eng .... see THUNDER GOD VINE
Leimmistel .... see EUROPEAN MISTLETOE
Leinsamen .... see FLAXSEED
Lemna minor .... see DUCKWEED
LEMON .... see LEMON
LEMON BALM .... see LEMON BALM
Lemon Grass .... see LEMONGRASS
Lemon-Scented Verbena .... see LEMON VERBENA
LEMON VERBENA .... see LEMON VERBENA
Lemon Walnut .... see BUTTERNUT
LEMONGRASS .... see LEMONGRASS
Lent Lily .... see DAFFODIL
Lenticus edodes .... see LENTINAN,
                                         SHIITAKE MUSHROOM
LENTINAN .... see LENTINAN
Lentinan edodes .... see LENTINAN,
                                         SHIITAKE MUSHROOM
Lentinula edodes .... see LENTINAN,
                                         SHIITAKE MUSHROOM
Lentinus edodes .... see LENTINAN,
                                         SHIITAKE MUSHROOM
Lentisk .... see MASTIC
Leontodon taracum .... see DANDELION above ground parts
Leontodon taraxacum .... see DANDELION entire plant
Leontopodium .... see ALCHEMILLA
Leonuri cardiacae herba .... see MOTHERWORT
Leonurus .... see MOTHERWORT
Leonurus cardiaca .... see MOTHERWORT
Leopard's Bane .... see ARNICA
Leopard's Foot .... see MARSH MARIGOLD
Lepidium meyenii .... see MACA
Lepidium sativum .... see GARDEN CRESS
Leptandra virginica .... see BLACK ROOT
LESSER CELANDINE .... see LESSER CELANDINE
Lesser Centauru .... see CENTAURY
Lesser Dodder .... see DODDER
Lesser Hemlock .... see FOOL'S PARSLEY
Lesser Periwinkle .... see PERIWINKLE
Lettsomia nervosa ...... see HAWAIIAN BABY WOODROSE
Lettuce Opium .... see WILD LETTUCE
Leucanthemum parthenium .... see FEVERFEW
Leucine .... see BRANCHED-CHAIN AMINO ACIDS
Levacecarnine .... see ACETYL-L-CARNITINE
Levant .... see WORMSEED
LEVANT BERRY .... see LEVANT BERRY
Levant Nut .... see LEVANT BERRY
Levant Salep .... see SALEP
Levant Storax .... see STORAX
Levistici radix .... see LOVAGE
Levisticum officinale .... see LOVAGE
Levocarnitine .... see L-CARNITINE
Levoglutamide .... see GLUTAMINE
Levoglutamine .... see GLUTAMINE
Levo-Histidine .... see HISTIDINE
Levure De Biere .... see BREWER'S YEAST
Lian Fang .... see LOTUS flower
Lian Xu .... see LOTUS flower
Lian Zi .... see LOTUS seed
Liatris .... see DEERTONGUE
Liatris callilepis .... see MARSH BLAZING STAR

Liatris odoratis .... see DEERTONGUE
Liatris spicata .... see MARSH BLAZING STAR
Lichen Islandicus .... see ICELAND MOSS
Lichen Oak Moss .... see OAK MOSS
Lichwort .... see PELLITORY-OF-THE-WALL
LICORICE .... see LICORICE
Licorice Root .... see LICORICE
Life Everlasting .... see CAT'S FOOT
Life-giving Vine of Peru .... see CAT'S CLAW
Life of Man .... see AMERICAN SPIKENARD
Liferoot ... see ALPINE RAGWORT, GOLDEN RAGWORT
Light Kaolin .... see KAOLIN
Ligusticum levisticum .... see LOVAGE
Ligustro .... see GLOSSY PRIVET
Ligustrum .... see GLOSSY PRIVET
Ligustrum Fruit .... see GLOSSY PRIVET
Ligustrum lucidum .... see GLOSSY PRIVET
Lilium candidium .... see WHITE LILY
Lilium martagon .... see MARTAGON
Lily .... see LILY-OF-THE-VALLEY
Lily of the Desert .... see ALOE dried juice from leaf, latex
LILY-OF-THE-VALLEY .... see LILY-OF-THE-VALLEY
Lime Flower .... see LINDEN dried flower
LIME fruit, peel .... see LIME fruit, peel
LIME oil .... see LIME oil
Lime Tree .... see LINDEN CHARCOAL,
                                         LINDEN dried flower,
                                         LINDEN dried leaf,
                                         LINDEN dried sapwood
Limette .... see LIME fruit, peel, LIME oil
Limon .... see LEMON
Limonnik Kitajskij .... see SCHISANDRA
Linaria vulgaris .... see YELLOW TOADFLAX
LINDEN CHARCOAL .... see LINDEN CHARCOAL
LINDEN dried flower .... see LINDEN dried flower
LINDEN dried leaf .... see LINDEN dried leaf
LINDEN dried sapwood .... see LINDEN dried sapwood
Linden Tree .... see LINDEN dried flower
Linden Wood .... see LINDEN dried sapwood
Ling .... see HEATHER
Ling Chih .... see REISHI MUSHROOM
Ling Zhi .... see REISHI MUSHROOM
Lingen .... see ALPINE CRANBERRY
Lingenberry .... see ALPINE CRANBERRY
Lingon .... see ALPINE CRANBERRY
Lingonberry .... see ALPINE CRANBERRY
Lingum Vitae .... see GUAIAC WOOD resin, wood
Lini Semen .... see FLAXSEED
Linseed .... see FLAXSEED
Linseed Oil .... see FLAXSEED OIL
Lint Bells .... see FLAXSEED
Linum .... see FLAXSEED
Linum catharticum .... see MOUNTAIN FLAX
Linum usitatissimum ...... see FLAXSEED, FLAXSEED OIL
Lion's Ear .... see MOTHERWORT
Lion's Foot .... see ALCHEMILLA
Lion's Mouth .... see DIGITALIS
Lion's Tail .... see MOTHERWORT
Lion's Tooth .... see DANDELION above ground parts,
                                      DANDELION entire plant
LIPASE .... see LIPASE
Lipoic Acid .... see ALPHA-LIPOIC ACID
Lipoicin .... see ALPHA-LIPOIC ACID
Lipositol .... see INOSITOL

Lipotropic Factor .... see CHOLINE
Lippia citriodora .... see LEMON VERBENA
Liquid Amber .... see STORAX
Liquid Oxygen .... see VITAMIN O
Liquid Storax .... see STORAX
Liquidambar styraciflua .... see STORAX
Liquidamber orientalis .... see STORAX
Liquiritiae radix .... see LICORICE
Liquirizia .... see LICORICE
Liquorice .... see LICORICE
Little Dragon .... see TARRAGON
Little Pollom .... see BITTER MILKWORT
Live Culture Yogurt .... see YOGURT
Liveforever .... see HOUSELEEK
Liver Lily .... see ORRIS
Liverleaf .... see LIVERWORT
Liverweed .... see LIVERWORT
LIVERWORT .... see LIVERWORT
Liverwort .... see AGRIMONY
Liverwort-Leaf .... see LIVERWORT
Living Antiseptic .... see MAGGOTS
Lizard's Tail .... see YERBA MANSA
Lizzy-Run-Up-The-Hedge .... see GROUND IVY
Lobaria pulmonaria .... see LUNGMOSS
LOBELIA .... see LOBELIA
Lobelia inflata .... see LOBELIA
Lobster Flower Plant .... see POINSETTIA
Lobsterplant .... see POINSETTIA
Lochnera rosea .... see MADAGASCAR PERIWINKLE
Locoweed .... see JIMSON WEED
Locust Bean .... see CAROB
Locust Pods .... see CAROB
LOGWOOD .... see LOGWOOD
Lolium perenne .... see HAY FLOWER
Lolium temulentum .... see TAUMELLOOLCH
Long Birthwort .... see ARISTOLOCHIA
Long Pepper .... see INDIAN LONG PEPPER
Long Purples .... see PURPLE LOOSESTRIFE
Longwort .... see MULLEIN
Lonicera caprifolium .... see HONEYSUCKLE
Lonicera japonica .... see HONEYSUCKLE
Loofa .... see LUFFA
Loofah .... see LUFFA
LOOSESTRIFE .... see LOOSESTRIFE
Loosestrife .... see PURPLE LOOSESTRIFE
Lop Grass .... see HAY FLOWER
Lophophora williamsii .... see PEYOTE
Lorbeerweide .... see WILLOW BARK
Lords and Ladies .... see ARUM
LORENZO'S OIL .... see LORENZO'S OIL
LOTUS flower .... see LOTUS flower
LOTUS seed .... see LOTUS seed
Louisa .... see LEMON VERBENA
Louisiana Long Pepper .... see CAPSICUM
Louisiana Sport Pepper .... see CAPSICUM
Louseberry .... see LEVANT BERRY
Lousewort .... see STAVESACRE
LOVAGE .... see LOVAGE
Love Apple .... see TOMATO
Love Bean .... see PRECATORY BEAN
Love in a Mist .... see BLACK SEED
Love in Winter .... see PIPSISSEWA
Love Leaves .... see BURDOCK
Love-Lies-Bleeding .... see AMARANTH

© Copyright 2000, Natural Medicines Comprehensive Database (209) 472-2244. For updated data, go to www.NaturalDatabase.com. • 1491

Love Parsley .... see LOVAGE
Lovely Bleeding .... see AMARANTH
Love-Man .... see CLIVERS
Low Balm .... see OSWEGO TEA
Low Chamomile .... see ROMAN CHAMOMILE
Lowbush Cranberry .... see ALPINE CRANBERRY
LPC .... see PROPIONYL-L-CARNITINE
Lu-Hui .... see ALOE dried juice from leaf, latex
Lu Rong .... see DEER VELVET
Lucerne .... see ALFALFA
Lucilia sericata .... see MAGGOTS
Lucky Bean .... see PRECATORY BEAN
LUFFA .... see LUFFA
Luffa acutangula .... see LUFFA
Luffa aegyptiaca .... see LUFFA
Luffa cylindrica .... see LUFFA
Luffaschwamm .... see LUFFA
Lungenkraut .... see LUNGWORT
LUNGMOSS .... see LUNGMOSS
LUNGWORT .... see LUNGWORT
Lungwort .... see LUNGMOSS
Lupinus luteus .... see YELLOW LUPIN
Lupuli Strobulus .... see HOPS
Lurk-In-The-Ditch .... see PENNYROYAL leaf,
                                       PENNYROYAL oil
Lustwort .... see SUNDEW
Luteal Hormone .... see PROGESTERONE
LUTEIN .... see LUTEIN
Luteohormone .... see PROGESTERONE
Lutine .... see PROGESTERONE
LYCOPENE .... see LYCOPENE
Lycoperdon spp .... see PUFF BALL
Lycopersicon esculentum .... see TOMATO
Lycopi Herba .... see BUGLEWEED
Lycopodium clavatum .... see CLUB MOSS
Lycopus americanus .... see BUGLEWEED
Lycopus europaeus .... see BUGLEWEED
Lycopus virginicus .... see BUGLEWEED
Lyngbya wollei .... see BLUE-GREEN ALGAE
Lys .... see LYSINE
Lysimachia nummularia .... see MONEYWORT
Lysimachia vulgaris .... see LOOSESTRIFE
LYSINE .... see LYSINE
Lysine Hydrochloride .... see LYSINE
Lysine Monohydrochloride .... see LYSINE
Lythrum .... see PURPLE LOOSESTRIFE
Lythrum salicaria .... see PURPLE LOOSESTRIFE
M Mei Gee .... see SCHISANDRA
M viridis .... see SPEARMINT
Ma-Huang .... see EPHEDRA
MACA .... see MACA
Mace .... see NUTMEG AND MACE
Macis .... see NUTMEG AND MACE
Mackerel Mint .... see SPEARMINT
Macochihua .... see IPORURU
Macrocystis pyrifera .... see ALGIN
Mad-apple .... see JIMSON WEED
Mad-Dog Herb .... see SCULLCAP
Mad-Dog Weed .... see SCULLCAP, WATER PLANTAIN
Mad Weed .... see SCULLCAP
Madagascar Lemongrass .... see LEMONGRASS
MADAGASCAR PERIWINKLE .... see MADAGASCAR
                                       PERIWINKLE
Madagascar Vanilla .... see VANILLA

MADDER .... see MADDER
Madnep .... see MASTERWORT
Madonna Lily .... see WHITE LILY
Madre Selva .... see PASSIONFLOWER
Magdalena .... see MADAGASCAR PERIWINKLE
Maggi Plant .... see LOVAGE
MAGGOTS .... see MAGGOTS
MAGNESIUM .... see MAGNESIUM
Magnesium Aspartate .... see MAGNESIUM
Magnesium Carbonate .... see MAGNESIUM
Magnesium Chloride .... see MAGNESIUM
Magnesium Citrate .... see MAGNESIUM
Magnesium Gluconate .... see MAGNESIUM
Magnesium Hydroxide .... see MAGNESIUM
Magnesium Lactate .... see MAGNESIUM
Magnesium Orotate .... see MAGNESIUM
Magnesium Oxide .... see MAGNESIUM
Magnesium Pyruvate .... see PYRUVATE
Magnesium Sulfate .... see MAGNESIUM
Magnesium Trisilicate .... see MAGNESIUM
MAGNOLIA bark .... see MAGNOLIA bark
Magnolia biondii .... see MAGNOLIA flower bud
Magnolia denudata .... see MAGNOLIA flower bud
Magnolia emargenata .... see MAGNOLIA flower bud
Magnolia fargesii .... see MAGNOLIA flower bud
MAGNOLIA flower bud .... see MAGNOLIA flower bud
Magnolia glauca .... see MAGNOLIA bark
Magnolia heptaperta .... see MAGNOLIA flower bud
Magnolia salicifolia .... see MAGNOLIA flower bud
Magnolia sargentiana .... see MAGNOLIA flower bud
Magnolia sprengeri .... see MAGNOLIA flower bud
Magnolia Vine .... see SCHISANDRA
Magnolia wilsonii .... see MAGNOLIA flower bud
Mahonia aquifolium .... see OREGON GRAPE
Mahonia nervosa .... see OREGON GRAPE
Mahonia repens .... see OREGON GRAPE
Mahuang .... see EPHEDRA
Mahuanggen .... see EPHEDRA
Mai Ya .... see BARLEY
Maiden Fern .... see MAIDENHAIR FERN
MAIDENHAIR FERN .... see MAIDENHAIR FERN
Maidenhair Tree .... see GINKGO leaf,
                   GINKGO leaf extract, GINKGO seed
Maidis Stigma .... see CORN SILK
Maid's Hair .... see LADY'S BEDSTRAW
Maino .... see MACA
MAITAKE .... see MAITAKE
Maitake Mushroom .... see MAITAKE
Maize Pollen .... see BEE POLLEN
Maize Silk .... see CORN SILK
Majoran .... see MARJORAM
Majorana aetheroleum oil .... see MARJORAM
Majorana herb .... see MARJORAM
Majorana hortensis .... see MARJORAM
Maka .... see MACA
Makombu Thallus .... see LAMINARIA
MALABAR NUT .... see MALABAR NUT
Malabar Tamarind .... see GARCINIA
MALE FERN .... see MALE FERN
Malic Acid .... see ALPHA HYDROXY ACIDS
Mallaguetta Pepper .... see GRAINS OF PARADISE
Mallards .... see MARSHMALLOW
Mallotus philippinensis .... see KAMALA
MALLOW flower .... see MALLOW flower

MALLOW leaf .... see MALLOW leaf
Malpidnia glabra .... see ACEROLA
Malpidnia punicifolia .... see ACEROLA
Malus sylvestris ....see APPLE
Malva Flower .... see HOLLYHOCK
Malva neglecta .... see MALLOW leaf
Malva sylvestris .... see MALLOW flower, MALLOW leaf
Malvae arboreae flos .... see HOLLYHOCK
Malvae flos .... see MALLOW flower
Malvae folium .... see MALLOW leaf
Mamaerie .... see PAPAYA
MANACA .... see MANACA
Manchurian Fungus .... see KOMBUCHA TEA
Manchurian Mushroom Tea .... see KOMBUCHA TEA
Mandragora .... see EUROPEAN MANDRAKE
Mandragora officinarum ...... see EUROPEAN MANDRAKE
Mandragora vernalis .... see EUROPEAN MANDRAKE
Mandragore .... see EUROPEAN MANDRAKE
Mandrake .... see EUROPEAN MANDRAKE,
                                                            PODOPHYLLUM
MANGANESE .... see MANGANESE
Manganese Amino Acid Chelate .... see MANGANESE
Manganese Aminoate .... see MANGANESE
Manganese Ascorbate .... see MANGANESE
Manganese Aspartate Complex .... see MANGANESE
Manganese Chloride .... see MANGANESE
Manganese Chloridetetrahydrate .... see MANGANESE
Manganese Dioxide .... see MANGANESE
Manganese Gluconate .... see MANGANESE
Manganese Sulfate................................. see MANGANESE
Manganese Sulfate Monohydrate .... see MANGANESE
Manganese Sulfate Tetrahydrate .... see MANGANESE
Manganum .... see MANGANESE
Mangel ....see BEET
Mangold ....see BEET
Manila Elemi .... see ELEMI
Manilkara achras .... see CHICLE
Manilkara zapota .... see CHICLE
Manilkara zapotilla .... see CHICLE
MANNA .... see MANNA
Manna Ash .... see MANNA
Mannentake .... see REISHI MUSHROOM
Manzanilla .... see GERMAN CHAMOMILE,
                                                 ROMAN CHAMOMILE
Manzanita ....see UVA URSI
Mapato .... see RHATANY
Maranhao Jaborandi .... see JABORANDI
Maranta .... see ARROWROOT
Maranta arundinaceae .... see ARROWROOT
Marcory .... see QUEEN'S DELIGHT
Marginal Fern .... see MALE FERN
Margosa .... see NEEM
Marguerite .... see OX-EYE DAISY
Marian Thistle .... see MILK THISTLE above ground parts,
                                             MILK THISTLE fruit, seed
Marienmantel .... see ALCHEMILLA
Marigold .... see CALENDULA
Marigold of Peru.......................... see SUNFLOWER OIL
Mariguana .... see MARIJUANA
Marihuana .... see MARIJUANA
MARIJUANA.................................... see MARIJUANA
Marine Oils .... see FISH OILS
Marjolaine .... see MARJORAM
MARJORAM .... see MARJORAM

Markweed .... see POISON IVY
Marron Europeen .... see HORSE CHESTNUT branch bark,
                                         HORSE CHESTNUT flower,
                                         HORSE CHESTNUT leaf,
                                         HORSE CHESTNUT seed
Marrubii herba .... see WHITE HOREHOUND
Marrubium .... see WHITE HOREHOUND
Marrubium vulgare .... see WHITE HOREHOUND
Marsdenia condurango .... see CONDURANGO
MARSH BLAZING STAR .... see MARSH BLAZING
                                                            STAR
Marsh Citrus .... see MARSH TEA
MARSH MARIGOLD .... see MARSH MARIGOLD
Marsh Mint .... see WILD MINT
Marsh Penny .... see GOTU KOLA
Marsh Rosemary .... see LABRADOR TEA
MARSH TEA ....see MARSH TEA
Marsh Tea .... see LABRADOR TEA
Marsh Trefoil .... see BOGBEAN
MARSHMALLOW .... see MARSHMALLOW
MARTAGON .... see MARTAGON
Mary Thistle ....see MILK THISTLE above ground parts,
                                             MILK THISTLE fruit, seed
Marybud .... see CALENDULA
Maryland Pink .... see PINK ROOT
Master of the Wood .... see SWEET WOODRUFF
MASTERWORT .... see MASTERWORT
Masterwort .... see GOUTWEED
MASTIC .... see MASTIC
Mastranzo .... see WHITE HOREHOUND
Mate Folium .... see MATE
MATE .... see MATE
Matricaire .... see GERMAN CHAMOMILE
Matricaria chamomilla .... see GERMAN CHAMOMILE
Matricaria morifolia .... see CHRYSANTHEMUM
Matricaria recutita .... see GERMAN CHAMOMILE
Matricariae Flos .... see GERMAN CHAMOMILE
Matsbouza........................... see SCHISANDRA
Matsuhodo .... see PORIA MUSHROOM
Matteucccia struthiopteris .... see OSTRICH FERN
Matto Grosso Ipecac .... see IPECAC
Maudlin Daisy .... see OX-EYE DAISY
Maudlinwort .... see OX-EYE DAISY
Mauls .... see MALLOW flower
May .... see HAWTHORN fruit, HAWTHORN leaf, flower,
                             HAWTHORN leaf with flower extract
May Bells .... see LILY-OF-THE-VALLEY
May Lily .... see LILY-OF-THE-VALLEY
Mayapple .... see PODOPHYLLUM
Maybush ....see HAWTHORN fruit,
                                     HAWTHORN leaf,flower,
                            HAWTHORN leaf with flower extract
Mayflower .... see COWSLIP
Maypop .... see PASSIONFLOWER
Maypop Passion Flower .... see PASSIONFLOWER
Maythorn ....see HAWTHORN fruit
MCT .... see MEDIUM CHAIN TRIGLYCERIDES
Meadow Anenome .... see PULSATILLA
Meadow Cabbage .... see SKUNK CABBAGE
Meadow Clover .... see RED CLOVER
Meadow Fescue .... see HAY FLOWER
Meadow Lily .... see WHITE LILY
Meadow Queen .... see MEADOWSWEET
Meadow Routs .... see MARSH MARIGOLD

INDEX

Meadow Runagates .... see MONEYWORT
Meadow Saffran .... see AUTUMN CROCUS
Meadow Saffron .... see AUTUMN CROCUS
Meadow Sage .... see SAGE
Meadow-Wart .... see MEADOWSWEET
Meadow Windflower .... see PULSATILLA
Meadowbloom .... see BULBOUS BUTTERCUP,
                                                              BUTTERCUP
MEADOWSWEET .... see MEADOWSWEET
Mealy Kudzu ....see KUDZU
Mechoacan ....see JALAP
Medicago .... see ALFALFA
Medicago sativa .... see ALFALFA
Medicinal Charcoal .... see ACTIVATED CHARCOAL
Medicinal Leech .... see LEECH
Medicinal Rhubarb .... see RHUBARB
Medicinal Yeast .... see BREWER'S YEAST
Mediterranean Bay .... see SWEET BAY
Mediterranean Squill .... see SQUILL
MEDIUM CHAIN TRIGLYCERIDES (MCT)
.... see MEDIUM CHAIN TRIGLYCERIDES (MCT)
Meerdorn .... see SEA BUCKTHORN
Meereiche .... see BLADDERWRACK
Meerrettich ....see HORSERADISH
Mehlbeebaum .... see HAWTHORN fruit
Mehndi ....see HENNA
Meidorn .... see HAWTHORN fruit
Mejorana .... see MARJORAM
Mel ....see HONEY
MEL .... see MELATONIN
Melaleuca alternifolia .... see TEA TREE OIL
Melaleuca leucodendra .... see CAJEPUT OIL
Melaleuca leucodendron .... see CAJEPUT OIL
Melaleuca quinquenervia .... see CAJEPUT OIL
Melaleuca viridiflora .... see NIAULI OIL
Melampode .... see BLACK HELLEBORE
MELANOTAN-II ....see MELANOTAN-II
MELATONIN .... see MELATONIN
Melegueta Pepper .... see GRAINS OF PARADISE
Meletin .... see QUERCETIN
Melilot .... see SWEET CLOVER
Meliloti herba .... see SWEET CLOVER
Melilotus .... see SWEET CLOVER
Melilotus altissimus .... see SWEET CLOVER
Melilotus officinalis .... see SWEET CLOVER
Melissa .... see LEMON BALM
Melissa officinalis .... see LEMON BALM
Melissa pulegioides .... see PENNYROYAL leaf,
                                                              PENNYROYAL oil
Melissae folium .... see LEMON BALM
Melissenblatt .... see LEMON BALM
Melon Tree .... see PAPAYA
Melonenbaumblaetter .... see PAPAYA
Membranous Milk Vetch .... see ASTRAGALUS
Memeniran .... see CHANCA PIEDRA
Menadiol Acetate (K4) .... see VITAMIN K
Menadiol Sodium Diphosphate .... see VITAMIN K
Menadiol Sodium Phosphate .... see VITAMIN K
Menadiolum Solubile .... see VITAMIN K
Menadione (K3) .... see VITAMIN K
Menadione Sodium Bisulfite .... see VITAMIN K
Menaquinone (K2) .... see VITAMIN K
Menaquinone-6 .... see VITAMIN K
Menaquinone-7 .... see VITAMIN K

Menatetrenone .... see VITAMIN K
Mendee ....see HENNA
Mengkudu .... see MORINDA
Meniran .... see CHANCA PIEDRA
Menispermaceae .... see ABUTA
Menispermum cocculus .... see LEVANT BERRY
Menispermum Lacunosum .... see LEVANT BERRY
Menkoedoe .... see MORINDA
Mentha aquatica .... see WILD MINT
Mentha arvensis aetheroleum .... see JAPANESE MINT
Mentha arvensis var piperascens .... see JAPANESE MINT
Mentha canadensis .... see JAPANESE MINT
Mentha longifolia .... see ENGLISH HORSEMINT
Mentha piperita .... see PEPPERMINT leaf,
                                                              PEPPERMINT OIL
Mentha pulegium .... see PENNYROYAL leaf,
                                                              PENNYROYAL oil
Mentha spicata .... see SPEARMINT
Menthae piperitae aetheroleum .... see PEPPERMINT OIL
Menthae piperitae folium .... see PEPPERMINT leaf
Menthe Poivree .... see PEPPERMINT leaf,
                                                              PEPPERMINT OIL
MENTZELIA .... see MENTZELIA
Mentzelia cordifolia .... see MENTZELIA
Menyanthes .... see BOGBEAN
Menyanthes trifoliata .... see BOGBEAN
Merasingi .... see GYMNEMA
Mercurialis annua .... see MERCURY HERB
MERCURY HERB .... see MERCURY HERB
Merlot .... see GRAPE fruit, skin
Mescal Buttons .... see PEYOTE
Mescaline .... see PEYOTE
Meshashringi .... see GYMNEMA
Meso-inositol .... see INOSITOL
Meso-Inositol Hexanicotinate .... see INOSITOL
                                                              NICOTINATE
Metavanadate .... see VANADIUM
Methi .... see FENUGREEK
METHIONINE .... see METHIONINE
Methylcobalamin .... see VITAMIN B12
Methylphytyl Naphthoquinone .... see VITAMIN K
Methylsulfonylmethane .... see MSM
Mexican Chilies .... see CAPSICUM
Mexican Damiana .... see DAMIANA
Mexican Flameleaf .... see POINSETTIA
Mexican Marigold .... see TAGETES
Mexican Sarsaparilla .... see SARSAPARILLA
MEXICAN SCAMMONY ROOT
.... see MEXICAN SCAMMONY ROOT
Mexican Tea .... see CHENOPODIUM OIL
Mexican Valerian .... see VALERIAN
Mexican Vanilla .... see VANILLA
Mexican Yam .... see WILD YAM
Mexico Weed .... see CASTOR OIL, CASTOR seed
MEZEREON .... see MEZEREON
Mg .... see MAGNESIUM
MGN-3 .... see MGN-3
MICROALGAE .... see MICROALGAE
Microcystis aeruginosa .... see BLUE-GREEN ALGAE
Microcystis wesenbergii .... see BLUE-GREEN ALGAE
Middle Comfrey .... see BUGLE
Middle Confound .... see BUGLE
Midsummer Daisy .... see FEVERFEW
Miel Blanc .... see HONEY

Mignonette Tree .... see HENNA
Milefolio .... see YARROW
Milfoil .... see YARROW
Milk Ipecac .... see BETH ROOT, CANADIAN HEMP
MILK THISTLE above ground parts
.... see MILK THISTLE above ground parts
MILK THISTLE fruit, seed
.... see MILK THISTLE fruit, seed
Milk Vetch .... see ASTRAGALUS
Milk Willow-Herb .... see PURPLE LOOSESTRIFE
Milkweed .... see CANADIAN HEMP
Milkwort .... see SENEGA
Mill Mint .... see CALAMINT
Mill Mountain .... see MOUNTAIN FLAX
Millefeuille .... see YARROW
Millefolii flos .... see YARROW
Millefolii herba .... see YARROW
Millefolium .... see YARROW
Millegoglie .... see YARROW
Millepertuis .... see ST JOHN'S WORT
Mimosa farnesiana .... see CASSIE ABSOLUTE
Mineral Aspartates .... see ASPARTATES
Mineral-amino acid complex .. see CHELATED MINERALS
Minor Centaury .... see CENTAURY
Mint Oil .... see JAPANESE MINT
Minzol .... see JAPANESE MINT
Miracle Grass .... see JIAOGULAN
Miracle Plant .... see ALOE dried juice from leaf, latex
Mirobalano .... see INDIAN GOOSEBERRY
Mirobalanus embilica .... see INDIAN GOOSEBERRY
Mistlekraut .... see EUROPEAN MISTLETOE
Mistletein .... see EUROPEAN MISTLETOE
Mistletoe .... see AMERICAN MISTLETOE
Mitchella repens .... see SQUAWVINE
Mitoquinone .... see COENZYME Q-10
Mitrewort .... see COOLWORT
Mixed Tocopherols .... see VITAMIN E
Mizibcoc .... see DAMIANA
Mizu-Garashi .... see WATERCRESS
Mn .... see MANGANESE
Moccasin Flower .... see NERVE ROOT
Mocha .... see COFFEE
Mohave Yucca .... see YUCCA
Mokko .... see COSTUS OIL, COSTUS root
Mokkou .... see COSTUS root
Momordica charantia .... see BITTER MELON
Momordica murcata .... see BITTER MELON
Momordique .... see BITTER MELON
Monarda .... see OSWEGO TEA
Monarda didyma .... see OSWEGO TEA
Monarda Lutea .... see HORSEMINT
Monarda punctata .... see HORSEMINT
Monascus .... see RED YEAST
Monascus purpureus Went .... see RED YEAST
MONEYWORT .... see MONEYWORT
Mongolian Larch .... see LARCH ARABINOGALACTAN
Mongolian Larchwood
.... see LARCH ARABINOGALACTAN
Mongolian Milk .... see ASTRAGALUS
Moniera cuneifolia .... see BRAHMI
Monkey Flower .... see NERVE ROOT,
                                        YELLOW TOADFLAX
Monkey Nuts .... see PEANUT OIL
Monkey's Bench .... see MAITAKE

Monk's Pepper .... see CHASTEBERRY
Monkshood .... see ACONITE
Monkshood Tuber .... see ACONITE
Monobasic Potassium Phosphate .. see PHOSPHATE SALTS
Monohydroxysuccinic acid
.... see ALPHA HYDROXY ACIDS
Montmorency Cherry .... see SOUR CHERRY
Moon Daisy .... see OX-EYE DAISY
Moon Flower .... see OX-EYE DAISY
Moon Penny .... see OX-EYE DAISY
Moor Grass .... see POTENTILLA
Moose Elm .... see SLIPPERY ELM
Moosebeere .... see CRANBERRY
Mora De La India .... see MORINDA
Morello Cherry .... see SOUR CHERRY
MORINDA .... see MORINDA
Morinda .... see BA JI TIAN
Morinda citrifolia .... see MORINDA
Morinda officinalis .... see BA JI TIAN
Morinda Root .... see BA JI TIAN
Morindae radix .... see BA JI TIAN
MORMON TEA .... see MORMON TEA
Moroccan Geranium Oil .... see ROSE GERANIUM
Mortal .... see BITTERSWEET NIGHTSHADE
Mortification Root .... see MARSHMALLOW
Morus nigra .... see BLACK MULBERRY
Moschus moschiferus .... see MUSK
Mosquito Plant .... see PENNYROYAL leaf,
                                        PENNYROYAL oil
Moss Cranberry .... see ALPINE CRANBERRY
Mossberry .... see CRANBERRY
Moth Herb .... see MARSH TEA
Mother of Rye .... see ERGOT
Mother of Thyme .... see WILD THYME
Mother's-Heart .... see SHEPHERD'S PURSE
MOTHERWORT .... see MOTHERWORT
MOUNTAIN ASH .... see MOUNTAIN ASH
Mountain Balm .... see CALAMINT,
                                OSWEGO TEA, YERBA SANTA
Mountain Box .... see UVA URSI
Mountain Cranberry .... see UVA URSI
Mountain Damson .... see SIMARUBA
Mountain Everlasting .... see CAT'S FOOT
MOUNTAIN FLAX .... see MOUNTAIN FLAX
Mountain Grape .... see EUROPEAN BARBERRY,
                                        OREGON GRAPE
Mountain Hydrangea .... see HYDRANGEA
Mountain Ivy .... see MOUNTAIN LAUREL
MOUNTAIN LAUREL .... see MOUNTAIN LAUREL
Mountain Mint .... see CALAMINT,
                                OREGANO, OSWEGO TEA
Mountain Pink .... see TRAILING ARBUTUS
Mountain Polygala .... see SENEGA
Mountain Radish .... see HORSERADISH
Mountain Sorrel .... see WOOD SORREL
Mountain Strawberry .... see STRAWBERRY
Mountain-Sweet .... see NEW JERSEY TEA
Mountain Tea .... see WINTERGREEN leaf,
                                        WINTERGREEN oil
Mountain Tobacco .... see ARNICA
Mouse Antialopecia Factor .... see INOSITOL
MOUSE EAR .... see MOUSE EAR
Mouse Ear .... see CUDWEED
Mousetail .... see COMMON STONECROP

INDEX

Mousse D'Irlande .... see CARRAGEENAN
Mouth Root .... see GOLDTHREAD
Mouth-Smart.................................... see BROOKLIME
MSB Plus .... see DOWN SYNDROME
NUTRITIONAL SUPPLEMENTS
MSM (METHYLSULFONYLMETHANE)
.... see MSM (METHYLSULFONYLMETHANE)
MT-II ....see MELANOTAN-II
Mu Xiang .... see COSTUS OIL, COSTUS root
Mucara .... see KARAYA GUM
Mucuna pruriens .... see COWHAGE
Mudar Bark .... see CALOTROPIS
Muder Yercum .... see CALOTROPIS
Muguet .... see LILY-OF-THE-VALLEY
MUGWORT .... see MUGWORT
Mugwort .... see TARRAGON
MUIRA PUAMA .... see MUIRA PUAMA
MULLEIN .... see MULLEIN
Multiflora Preparata .... see FO-TI cured root
Mum .... see CHRYSANTHEMUM
Murillo Bark .... see QUILLAIA
Muscadier .... see NUTMEG AND MACE
Muscatel Sage .... see CLARY SAGE
Mushroom Of Immortality .... see REISHI MUSHROOM
Mushroom of Spiritual Potency ... see REISHI MUSHROOM
MUSK .... see MUSK
Musk Root .... see SUMBUL
Musk Seed .... see AMBRETTE
Muskat .... see GRAPE seed
Muskatbuam .... see NUTMEG AND MACE
Muskatnuss .... see NUTMEG AND MACE
Muskmallow .... see AMBRETTE
Mustard .... see BLACK MUSTARD seed
Mustard Oil .... see BLACK MUSTARD oil
Muster John Henry .... see TAGETES
Mutton Chops .... see CLIVERS
Muzei Mahuang .... see EPHEDRA
Myo-inositol .... see INOSITOL
Myo-inositol hexa-3-pyridine-carboxylate ..... see INOSITOL
NICOTINATE
Myosotis arvensis .... see FORGET-ME-NOT
Myrica .... see BAYBERRY
Myrica cerifera .... see BAYBERRY
Myrica gale .... see SWEET GALE
Myrica pensylvanica .... see BAYBERRY
Myristica .... see NUTMEG AND MACE
Myristica fragrans .... see NUTMEG AND MACE
Myristica officinalis .... see NUTMEG AND MACE
Myristicae Aril .... see NUTMEG AND MACE
Myristicae Semen .... see NUTMEG AND MACE
Myrobalan............................ see TERMINALIA
Myrobalan Emblic .... see INDIAN GOOSEBERRY
Myroxylan balsamum .... see TOLU BALSAM
Myroxylan toluiferum .... see TOLU BALSAM
Myroxylon balsamum .... see TOLU BALSAM
Myroxylon balsamum genuinum .... see TOLU BALSAM
Myroxylon balsamum pereirae .... see PERU BALSAM
Myroxylon pereirae .... see PERU BALSAM
MYRRH .... see MYRRH
Myrrhis odorata .... see SWEET CICELY
Myrti aetherolum .... see MYRTLE
Myrti folium .... see MYRTLE
Myrtilli Fructus .... see BILBERRY dried ripe fruit,
BILBERRY leaf

MYRTLE .... see MYRTLE
Myrtle .... see MADAGASCAR PERIWINKLE,
PERIWINKLE
Myrtle Flag .... see CALAMUS
Myrtle Flower .... see ORRIS
Myrtle Sedge .... see CALAMUS
Myrtus .... see CHEKEN
Myrtus communis .... see MYRTLE
Mysteria .... see AUTUMN CROCUS
Mystyldene .... see EUROPEAN MISTLETOE
N-(2furanylmethyl)-1H-purin-6-amine .... see KINETIN
N-3 Fatty Acid .... see DHA, EPA, FISH OILS
N3-polyunsaturated Fatty Acids .... see FISH OILS
N-6 Essential Fatty Acids ...... see OMEGA-6 FATTY ACIDS
N(6)furfuryladenine .... see KINETIN
N-(aminoiminomethyl)-N methyl glycine ..... see CREATINE
N-ACETYL CYSTEINE .... see N-ACETYL CYSTEINE
N-ACETYL GLUCOSAMINE
.......................see N-ACETYL GLUCOSAMINE
N-acetyl-5-methoxytryptamine .... see MELATONIN
N-Acetyl-B-Cysteine .... see N-ACETYL CYSTEINE
N-Acetylcysteine .... see N-ACETYL CYSTEINE
N-Acetyl-Cysteine .... see N-ACETYL CYSTEINE
N-Acetyl-D-Glucosamine
.......................see N-ACETYL GLUCOSAMINE
N-acetyl-L-cysteine .... see N-ACETYL CYSTEINE
N-amidinosarcosine .... see CREATINE
N-Carboxybutyl Chitosan .... see CHITOSAN
N-glycine .... see GLUTATHIONE
N-methylsarcosine ....see DIMETHYLGLYCINE
N-octacosanol .... see OCTACOSANOL
Nabin Chanvandi .... see ANDROGRAPHIS
NAC .... see N-ACETYL CYSTEINE
NAD .... see NADH
NADH .... see NADH
NAG ....see N-ACETYL GLUCOSAMINE
Naked Ladies .... see AUTUMN CROCUS
Nan Shanzha .... see HAWTHORN fruit,
HAWTHORN leaf, flower
Nanwuweizi .... see SCHISANDRA
Narcissus pseudonarcissus .... see DAFFODIL
Narrow Dock ....see YELLOW DOCK
Narrow-leaved Purple Cone Flower .... see ECHINACEA
Naseberry .... see CHICLE
Nasilord .... see WATERCRESS
Nasturtii herba .... see WATERCRESS
NASTURTIUM .... see NASTURTIUM
Nasturtium armoracia .... see HORSERADISH
Nasturtium officinale .... see WATERCRESS
Nature's Viagra .... see PUNCTURE VINE
Naughty Man's Cherries .... see BELLADONNA
Navel Orange ....see SWEET ORANGE
Navy Bean .... see BEAN POD
Neckweed .... see BROOKLIME
Nectar of the Gods .... see GARLIC
NEEM .... see NEEM
Nees .... see CASSIA
Neli .... see INDIAN GOOSEBERRY
Nelumbo nucifera .... see LOTUS flower, LOTUS seed
Nepeta cataria ....see CATNIP
Nepeta hederacea .... see GROUND IVY
Nerium oleander .... see OLEANDER
NERVE ROOT .... see NERVE ROOT
Netchweed .... see ARRACH

INDEX

Nettles .... see STINGING NETTLE above ground parts, STINGING NETTLE root
Neutral Calcium Phosphate .... see PHOSPHATE SALTS
NEW JERSEY TEA .... see NEW JERSEY TEA
NEW ZEALAND GREEN-LIPPED MUSSEL
.... see NEW ZEALAND GREEN-LIPPED MUSSEL
Ngu Mei Gee .... see SCHISANDRA
Nhau .... see MORINDA
Niacin .... see NIACIN AND NIACINAMIDE
NIACIN AND NIACINAMIDE (VITAMIN B3)
.... see NIACIN AND NIACINAMIDE (VITAMIN B3)
Niacinamide .... see NIACIN AND NIACINAMIDE
Niando .... see IPORURU
Niauli Aetheroleum .... see NIAULI OIL
NIAULI OIL .... see NIAULI OIL
Nicamid .... see NIACIN AND NIACINAMIDE
Nicaragua Ipecac .... see IPECAC
Nichol Seeds .... see DIVI-DIVI
Nicosedine .... see NIACIN AND NIACINAMIDE
Nicotiana tabacum .... see SMOKELESS TOBACCO
Nicotinamide .... see NIACIN AND NIACINAMIDE
Nicotinic Acid .... see NIACIN AND NIACINAMIDE
Nicotinic Acid Amide .... see NIACIN AND NIACINAMIDE
Nicotylamidum .... see NIACIN AND NIACINAMIDE
Nigella sativa .... see BLACK SEED
Nigelle de Crete .... see BLACK SEED
Night Blooming Cereus .... see CEREUS
Night Willow-Herb .... see EVENING PRIMROSE OIL
Nightshade .... see JIMSON WEED
Nikkar Nuts .... see DIVI-DIVI
Nim .... see NEEM
Nimba .... see NEEM
Nine Hooks .... see ALCHEMILLA
Ninety-Knot .... see KNOTWEED HERB
Ninjin .... see GINSENG, PANAX
Niruri .... see CHANCA PIEDRA
N,N-dimethylaminoacetic Acid ... see DIMETHYLGLYCINE
N,N-dimethylglycine .... see DIMETHYLGLYCINE
N,O-Sulfated Chitosan .... see CHITOSAN
No-Flush Niacin .... see INOSITOL NICOTINATE
Noah's Ark .... see NERVE ROOT
Noble Laurel .... see SWEET BAY
Noble Yarrow .... see YARROW
Nogal Americano .... see BLACK WALNUT
Nogal Ceniciento .... see BUTTERNUT
Nogueira-preta .... see BLACK WALNUT
Noisetier .... see HAZELNUT
Noix Muscade .... see NUTMEG AND MACE
Nokyong .... see DEER VELVET
Noni .... see MORINDA
Nono .... see MORINDA
Nonu .... see MORINDA
Noon Kie Oo Nah Yeah .... see SQUAWVINE
Nopol .... see PRICKLY PEAR CACTUS
North American Ginseng .... see GINSENG, AMERICAN
NORTHERN PRICKLY ASH
.... see NORTHERN PRICKLY ASH
Northern Schisandra .... see SCHISANDRA
Northern White Cedar .... see CEDAR leaf, CEDAR LEAF OIL
Norway Pine .... see HEMLOCK SPRUCE
Norway Spruce .... see FIR, HEMLOCK SPRUCE
Nosebleed .... see YARROW
Noyer Cerdre .... see BUTTERNUT

Noyer Noir .... see BLACK WALNUT
NSC-9704 .... see PROGESTERONE
N'spero .... see CHICLE
Nu Zhen .... see GLOSSY PRIVET
Nucleotides .... see RNA AND DNA
Nuez Moscada .... see NUTMEG AND MACE
Nutmeg .... see NUTMEG AND MACE
NUTMEG AND MACE .... see NUTMEG AND MACE
Nutmeg Flower .... see BLACK SEED
NuTriVene-D ..... see DOWN SYNDROME NUTRITIONAL SUPPLEMENTS
Nux Moschata .... see NUTMEG AND MACE
NUX VOMICA .... see NUX VOMICA
Nuzhenzi .... see GLOSSY PRIVET
Nymphaea odorata .... see AMERICAN WHITE POND LILY
NZGLM
.... see NEW ZEALAND GREEN-LIPPED MUSSEL
O-Sulfated N-Acetylchitosan .... see CHITOSAN
OAK bark .... see OAK bark
Oak Fern .... see LADY FERN
Oak Lungs .... see LUNGMOSS
OAK MOSS .... see OAK MOSS
OAT above ground parts .... see OAT above ground parts
OAT BRAN .... see OAT BRAN
Oat Fruit ....see OATS
Oat Grain .... see OATS
Oat Herb .... see OAT above ground parts
OAT STRAW .... see OAT STRAW
Oatmeal .... see OATS
OATS .... see OATS
Oblepikha .... see SEA BUCKTHORN
Ocimum basilicum .... see BASIL
OCTACOSANOL .... see OCTACOSANOL
Octacosyl alcohol .... see OCTACOSANOL
Oderwort .... see BISTORT
Oenanthe aquatica .... see WATER FENNEL
Oenothera biennis .... see EVENING PRIMROSE OIL
Ofbit .... see PREMORSE
Ogi .... see ASTRAGALUS
Ogon .... see BAIKAL SKULLCAP
Oil Nut .... see BUTTERNUT
Oil of Cade .... see CADE OIL
Oil of Clove ....see CLOVE OIL
Oil of Juniper Tar .... see CADE OIL
Oje .... see FICIN
Ojo De Pajaro .... see PRECATORY BEAN
OKG .... see ORNITHINE KETOGLUTARATE
Okra .... see AMBRETTE
Old Maid .... see MADAGASCAR PERIWINKLE
Old Man .... see ROSEMARY
Old Man's Beard .... see FRINGETREE, USNEA, WOODBINE
Old Man's Night Cap .... see GREATER BINDWEED
Old Man's Pepper .... see YARROW
Old Man's Root .... see AMERICAN SPIKENARD
Old Woman's Broom .... see DAMIANA
Olea europaea .... see OLIVE OIL
Oleae folium .... see OLIVE leaf
OLEANDER .... see OLEANDER
Oleanderblatter .... see OLEANDER
Oleandri folium .... see OLEANDER
Oleic acid .... see LORENZO'S OIL
Oleovitamin A .... see VITAMIN A
Oleum Bergamotte .... see BERGAMOT OIL

INDEX

Oleum Cadinum .... see CADE OIL
Oleum Chaulmoograe .... see CHAULMOOGRA
Oleum Geranii .... see ROSE GERANIUM
Oleum Juniperi Empyreumaticum .... see CADE OIL
Oleum Melaleucae .... see TEA TREE OIL
Olibanum .... see FRANKINCENSE
Oligomeric Proanthocyanidins .... see GRAPE seed
Oligomeric Procyanidins .... see GRAPE seed
Olivae oleum .... see OLIVE OIL
OLIVE leaf .... see OLIVE leaf
OLIVE OIL .... see OLIVE OIL
Olivier .... see OLIVE leaf
Omega 3 Fatty Acid .... see DHA, EPA, FISH OILS
OMEGA-6 FATTY ACIDS ... see OMEGA-6 FATTY ACIDS
Omega 6 Oils .... see OMEGA-6 FATTY ACIDS
Omega-6 polyunsaturated fatty acids .... see OMEGA-6
FATTY ACIDS
Omega Fatty Acid .... see DHA, EPA, FISH OILS
Omicha .... see SCHISANDRA
One-Berry .... see SQUAWVINE
Oneberry .... see HERB PARIS
Oneseed Hawthorn .... see HAWTHORN fruit,
HAWTHORN leaf, flower,
HAWTHORN leaf with flower extract
ONION .... see ONION
Ononidis radix .... see SPINY RESTHARROW
Ononis spinosa .... see SPINY RESTHARROW
Onopordum acanthium .... see SCOTCH THISTLE
Ontario Ginseng .... see GINSENG, AMERICAN
OPC .... see GRAPE seed
Ophioglossum vulgatum .... see ENGLISH ADDER'S
TONGUE
OPIUM ANTIDOTE .... see OPIUM ANTIDOTE
Oplopanax horridus .... see DEVIL'S CLUB
Opobalsam .... see TOLU BALSAM
Opopanax .... see MYRRH
Opossum Tree .... see STORAX
Opuntia .... see PRICKLY PEAR CACTUS
Opuntia streptacantha .... see PRICKLY PEAR CACTUS
Oraches .... see ARRACH
Oranda-Garashi .... see WATERCRESS
Orange Milkweed .... see PLEURISY ROOT
Orange Mullein .... see MULLEIN
Orange Root .... see GOLDENSEAL
Orange Swallow-Wort .... see PLEURISY ROOT
Orchanet .... see ALKANNA
Orchid .... see SALEP
Orchis morio .... see SALEP
Ordeal Bean .... see CALABAR BEAN
OREGANO .... see OREGANO
Oregon Balsam .... see OREGON FIR BALSAM
Oregon Barberry .... see OREGON GRAPE
OREGON FIR BALSAM .... see OREGON FIR BALSAM
OREGON GRAPE .... see OREGON GRAPE
Oregon Grape .... see EUROPEAN BARBERRY
Oregon Grape-Holly .... see OREGON GRAPE
Organic Germanium .... see GERMANIUM
Organy .... see OREGANO
Orgotein .... see SUPEROXIDE DISMUTASE
ORIENTAL ARBORVITAE .... see ORIENTAL
ARBORVITAE
Oriental Ginseng .... see GINSENG, PANAX
Origan De Marais .... see HEMP AGRIMONY
Origani vulgaris herba .... see OREGANO

Origano .... see OREGANO
Origanum .... see OREGANO
Origanum majorana .... see MARJORAM
Origanum Oil .... see SPANISH ORIGANUM OIL
Origanum vulgare .... see OREGANO
Orizaba Jalap .... see MEXICAN SCAMMONY ROOT
Ornicetil .... see ORNITHINE KETOGLUTARATE
ORNITHINE .... see ORNITHINE
Ornithine Alphaketoglutarate
.... see ORNITHINE KETOGLUTARATE
ORNITHINE KETOGLUTARATE
.... see ORNITHINE KETOGLUTARATE
Orozuz .... see LICORICE
ORRIS .... see ORRIS
Orthosiphon .... see JAVA TEA
Orthosiphon spicatus .... see JAVA TEA
Orthosiphon stamineus .... see JAVA TEA
Orthosiphonis folium .... see JAVA TEA
Orthovanadate .... see VANADIUM
Ortie .... see STINGING NETTLE above ground parts
Oryza sativa .... see RICE BRAN
Osier .... see AMERICAN DOGWOOD
Osier Rouge .... see WILLOW BARK
Osterick .... see BISTORT
OSTRICH FERN .... see OSTRICH FERN
OSWEGO TEA .... see OSWEGO TEA
Otaheite Walnut .... see TUNG SEED
Our Lady's Flannel .... see MULLEIN
Our Lady's Keys .... see COWSLIP
Our Lady's Mint .... see SPEARMINT
Our Lady's Tears .... see LILY-OF-THE-VALLEY
Our Lady's Thistle .... see MILK THISTLE fruit, seed
Our-Lord's-Candle .... see YUCCA
Ovolecithin .... see LECITHIN
Owler .... see BLACK ALDER
OX-EYE DAISY .... see OX-EYE DAISY
Oxadoddy .... see BLACK ROOT
Oxalis acetosella .... see WOOD SORREL
Oxerutin .... see RUTIN
Oxeye .... see PHEASANT'S EYE
Ox's Tongue
.... see BORAGE flower, dried above ground parts
Oxycoccus hagerupii .... see CRANBERRY
Oxycoccus macrocarpos .... see CRANBERRY
Oxycoccus microcarpus .... see CRANBERRY
Oxycoccus palustris .... see CRANBERRY
Oxycoccus quadripetalus .... see CRANBERRY
Oxykrinin .... see SECRETIN
Oyster Shell Calcium .... see CALCIUM
Pacific Valerian .... see VALERIAN
Pacific Yew .... see YEW
Padang-Cassia .... see CINNAMON bark
Paddock-Pipes .... see HORSETAIL
Paeonia mascula .... see PEONY flower, PEONY root
Paeonia officinalis .... see PEONY flower, PEONY root
Paeoniae flos .... see PEONY flower
Paeoniae Radix .... see PEONY root
Pagla-Ka-Dawa .... see INDIAN SNAKEROOT
PAGODA TREE .... see PAGODA TREE
Paigle .... see COWSLIP
Paigle Peggle .... see COWSLIP
Paintedleaf .... see POINSETTIA
Pale Catechu .... see CATECHU
Pale Gentian .... see GENTIAN

INDEX

Pale Mara .... see FEVER BARK
Pale Psyllium .... see BLOND PSYLLIUM
Pali-Mara .... see FEVER BARK
Palma Christi .... see CASTOR OIL, CASTOR seed
Palmier Nain .... see SAW PALMETTO
Palo de Santa Maria .... see LAURELWOOD
Palo Maria .... see LAURELWOOD
Palsy Root .... see MARSH MARIGOLD
Palsywort .... see COWSLIP
Panama Bark .... see QUILLAIA
Panama Ipecac .... see IPECAC
Panang Cinnamon .... see CINNAMON bark
Panax Ginseng .... see GINSENG, PANAX
Panax ginseng .... see GINSENG, PANAX
Panax horridum .... see DEVIL'S CLUB
Panax notoginseng .... see PANAX PSEUDOGINSENG
PANAX PSEUDOGINSENG .... see PANAX
PSEUDOGINSENG
Panax quinquefolius .... see GINSENG, AMERICAN
Panax schinseng .... see GINSENG, PANAX
Panax zingiberensis .... see PANAX PSEUDOGINSENG
PANCREATIN .... see PANCREATIN
Pancreatinum .... see PANCREATIN
Pancreatis pulvis .... see PANCREATIN
Pangamate .... see PANGAMIC ACID
PANGAMIC ACID .... see PANGAMIC ACID
Pansy .... see HEART'S EASE
PANTOTHENIC ACID .... see PANTOTHENIC ACID
Pantothenol .... see PANTOTHENIC ACID
Pantothenylol .... see PANTOTHENIC ACID
Papagallo .... see POINSETTIA
PAPAIN .... see PAPAIN
Papainum Crudum .... see PAPAIN
Papaver rhoeas .... see CORN POPPY
Papaw .... see PAPAYA
PAPAYA .... see PAPAYA
Paperbark Tree Oil .... see CAJEPUT OIL
Papoose Root .... see BLUE COHOSH
Pappelknospen .... see POPLAR
Paprika .... see CAPSICUM
Paracalcin .... see VITAMIN D
Paradisapfel .... see GRAPEFRUIT
Paradise Tree .... see TREE OF HEAVEN
Paraguay Tea .... see MATE
Paraguayan Sweet Herb .... see STEVIA
PAREIRA .... see PAREIRA
Pareira .... see ABUTA
Paricalcitol .... see VITAMIN D
Parietaria officinalis .... see PELLITORY-OF-THE-WALL
Paris quadrifolia .... see HERB PARIS
Pariswort .... see BETH ROOT
Parsley Breakstone .... see PARSLEY PIERT
Parsley Fern .... see TANSY
Parsley Fruit .... see PARSLEY seed
PARSLEY leaf, root .... see PARSLEY leaf, root
Parsley Piercestone .... see PARSLEY PIERT
PARSLEY PIERT .... see PARSLEY PIERT
PARSLEY seed .... see PARSLEY seed
PARSNIP above ground parts .... see PARSNIP above
ground parts
PARSNIP root .... see PARSNIP root
Parson and Clerk .... see ARUM
Parthenium argentatum .... see GUAYULE
Parthenocissus quinquefolia .... see AMERICAN IVY

Partridge Berry .... see ALPINE CRANBERRY,
SQUAWVINE, WINTERGREEN leaf,
WINTERGREEN oil
Pas d'Ane .... see COLTSFOOT
Pas Diane .... see COLTSFOOT
Pasania Fungus .... see SHIITAKE MUSHROOM
Pasqueflower .... see PULSATILLA
Passe Flower .... see PULSATILLA
Passiflora .... see PASSIONFLOWER
Passiflora incarnata .... see PASSIONFLOWER
Passiflorae herba .... see PASSIONFLOWER
Passiflore .... see PASSIONFLOWER
Passiflorina .... see PASSIONFLOWER
Passion Flower .... see PASSIONFLOWER
Passion Vine .... see PASSIONFLOWER
Passionaria .... see PASSIONFLOWER
Passionblume .... see PASSIONFLOWER
PASSIONFLOWER .... see PASSIONFLOWER
Passionflower Herb .... see PASSIONFLOWER
Passionsblumenkraut .... see PASSIONFLOWER
Password .... see COWSLIP
Pastinaca sativa .... see PARSNIP above ground parts,
PARSNIP root
Pastinacae herba .... see PARSNIP above ground parts
Pastinacae Radix .... see PARSNIP root
Patacon .... see ABUTA
Patalagandhi .... see INDIAN SNAKEROOT
Patchouli .... see PATCHOULY OIL
PATCHOULY OIL .... see PATCHOULY OIL
Patience Dock .... see BISTORT
Pattens and Clogs .... see YELLOW TOADFLAX
Pau-Azeitona .... see MORINDA
PAU D'ARCO .... see PAU D'ARCO
Pau de Arco .... see PAU D'ARCO
Pau De Reposta .... see CATUABA
Paullinia .... see GUARANA
Paullinia cupana .... see GUARANA
Paullinia sorbilis .... see GUARANA
Paul's Betony .... see BUGLEWEED
Pausinystalia johimbe .... see YOHIMBE
Pausinystalia yohimbe .... see YOHIMBE
Pauson .... see BLOODROOT
PCO .... see GRAPE seed
Pea Tree .... see LABURNUM
Peachwood .... see LOGWOOD
Peagle .... see COWSLIP
Peagles .... see COWSLIP
PEANUT OIL .... see PEANUT OIL
PEAR .... see PEAR
Pearl Barley .... see BARLEY
PECTIN .... see PECTIN
Pectinic Acid .... see PECTIN
Pedlar's Basket .... see YELLOW TOADFLAX
Pedunculate Oak .... see OAK bark
Pegu Catechu .... see CATECHU
Pegwood .... see WAHOO
Pelargonium graveolens .... see ROSE GERANIUM
Pelargonium Oil .... see ROSE GERANIUM
Pelican Flower .... see ARISTOLOCHIA
Pellagra Preventing Factor
.... see NIACIN AND NIACINAMIDE
PELLITORY .... see PELLITORY
PELLITORY-OF-THE-WALL
.... see PELLITORY-OF-THE-WALL

INDEX

Pellote .... see PEYOTE
PENNYROYAL leaf .... see PENNYROYAL leaf
PENNYROYAL oil .... see PENNYROYAL oil
Pennywort .... see YELLOW TOADFLAX
Pensee Sauvage .... see HEART'S EASE
Penta Tea .... see JIAOGULAN
PEONY flower .... see PEONY flower
PEONY root .... see PEONY root
Pepe .... see BLACK PEPPER AND WHITE PEPPER
Pepino Montero .... see BITTER MELON
Pepo .... see PUMPKIN
Pepper .... see BLACK PEPPER AND WHITE PEPPER
Pepper-And-Salt .... see SHEPHERD'S PURSE
Pepper Bark .... see WINTER'S BARK
Pepper Extract
.... see BLACK PEPPER AND WHITE PEPPER
Pepper Plant ... see BLACK PEPPER AND WHITE PEPPER
Pepper Wood .... see NORTHERN PRICKLY ASH
Peppercorn ..... see BLACK PEPPER AND WHITE PEPPER
PEPPERMINT leaf .... see PEPPERMINT leaf
PEPPERMINT OIL .... see PEPPERMINT OIL
Pepperrot .... see HORSERADISH
Pereira Brava .... see PAREIRA
Perennial Rye-Grass .... see HAY FLOWER
Pericarpium .... see SWEET ORANGE
PERILLA .... see PERILLA
Perilla frutescens .... see PERILLA
Periploca sylvestris .... see GYMNEMA
PERIWINKLE .... see PERIWINKLE
Periwinkle .... see MADAGASCAR PERIWINKLE
Perna canaliculus .... see NEW ZEALAND
                                      GREEN-LIPPED MUSSEL
Persea americana .... see AVOCADO
Persea gratissima .... see AVOCADO
Persely .... see PARSLEY leaf, root
Persian Lilac .... see NEEM
Persil .... see PARSLEY leaf, root, PARSLEY seed
Personata .... see BURDOCK
Peru-apple .... see JIMSON WEED
PERU BALSAM .... see PERU BALSAM
Peruvian Balsam .... see PERU BALSAM
Peruvian Bark .... see CINCHONA
Peruvian Coca .... see COCA
Peruvian Ginseng .... see MACA
Peruvian Rhatany .... see RHATANY
Petasites hybridus .... see PETASITES root
PETASITES leaf .... see PETASITES leaf
Petasites officinalis .... see PETASITES root
PETASITES root .... see PETASITES root
Petasites spp .... see PETASITES leaf
Petasitidis folium .... see PETASITES leaf
Petasitidis hybridus .... see PETASITES leaf
Petasitidis rhizoma .... see PETASITES root
Peter's Cress .... see SAMPHIRE
Petersylinge .... see PARSLEY leaf, root
Petite Sirah .... see GRAPE fruit, skin
Petroselini fructus .... see PARSLEY seed
Petroselini herba .... see PARSLEY leaf, root
Petroselinum crispum .... see PARSLEY leaf, root,
                                               PARSLEY seed
Petroselinum hortense .... see PARSLEY leaf, root,
                                               PARSLEY seed
Petroselinum sativum .... see PARSLEY leaf, root,
                                               PARSLEY seed

Petrosilini radix .... see PARSLEY leaf, root
Pettigree .... see BUTCHER'S BROOM
Petty Morel .... see BLACK NIGHTSHADE
Petty Mugget .... see LADY'S BEDSTRAW
Petty Mulleins .... see COWSLIP
Petty Whin .... see SPINY RESTHARROW
Pettymorell .... see AMERICAN SPIKENARD
Peumus boldus .... see BOLDO
Pewterwort .... see HORSETAIL
PEYOTE .... see PEYOTE
Pfaffia .... see SUMA
Pfaffia paniculata .... see SUMA
Pfeffer .... see BLACK PEPPER AND WHITE PEPPER
Pferdefut .... see COLTSFOOT
Phaseoli fructus .... see BEAN POD
Phaseolus vulgaris varieties .... see BEAN POD
PHEASANT'S EYE .... see PHEASANT'S EYE
PHENYLALANINE .... see PHENYLALANINE
Philanthropium .... see BURDOCK
Phoenix dactylifera .... see DATE PALM
Phoradendron flavescens ...... see AMERICAN MISTLETOE
Phoradendron leucarpum ...... see AMERICAN MISTLETOE
Phoradendron macrophyllum .... see AMERICAN
                                                 MISTLETOE
Phoradendron serontium .... see AMERICAN MISTLETOE
Phoradendron tomentosum ... see AMERICAN MISTLETOE
Phormia regina .... see MAGGOTS
Phosphate of Soda .... see PHOSPHATE SALTS
PHOSPHATE SALTS .... see PHOSPHATE SALTS
Phosphatidyl Choline .... see PHOSPHATIDYLCHOLINE
Phosphatidyl Serine .... see PHOSPHATIDYLSERINE
PHOSPHATIDYLCHOLINE
.... see PHOSPHATIDYLCHOLINE
PHOSPHATIDYLSERINE ... see PHOSPHATIDYLSERINE
Phragmites communis .... see REED HERB
Phyllanthus emblica .... see INDIAN GOOSEBERRY
Phyllanthus niruri .... see CHANCA PIEDRA
Phylloquinone (K1) .... see VITAMIN K
Physalis alkekengi .... see WINTER CHERRY
Physic Root .... see BLACK ROOT
Physostigma venenosum .... see CALABAR BEAN
Physotigma .... see CALABAR BEAN
Phytic Acid .... see IP-6
Phytoestrogen ... see ALFALFA, ANISE, BLACK COHOSH,
         DONG QUAI, FENNEL fruit, seed,
         FENNEL OIL, FLAXSEED,
         GINSENG, SIBERIAN,
         IPRIFLAVONE, LICORICE,
         RED CLOVER, RESVERATROL,
         SCARLET PIMPERNEL, SOY, WILD YAM
Phytolacca americana .... see POKEWEED berry,
                                               POKEWEED root
Phytolacca Berry .... see POKEWEED berry,
                                               POKEWEED root
Phytolacca decandra .... see POKEWEED berry,
                                               POKEWEED root
Phytomenadione .... see VITAMIN K
Phytonadione .... see VITAMIN K
Phytostanol .... see SITOSTANOL
Phytosterols .... see BETA-SITOSTEROL
Picea abies .... see FIR NEEDLE OIL,
                                         FIR, HEMLOCK SPRUCE
Picea aetheroleum .... see HEMLOCK SPRUCE

I
N
D
E
X

Picea excelsa .... see FIR NEEDLE OIL, FIR, HEMLOCK SPRUCE
Picea turiones recentes .... see HEMLOCK SPRUCE
Piceae aetheroleum .... see FIR NEEDLE OIL
Piceae turiones recentes .... see FIR
Pick-Pocket .... see SHEPHERD'S PURSE
Pickaway Anise .... see WAFER ASH
Picrasma .... see QUASSIA
Picrasma excelsa .... see QUASSIA
Pie Cherry .... see SOUR CHERRY
Pierce-Stone .... see SAMPHIRE
Pigeonberry .... see POKEWEED berry, POKEWEED root
Pigeon's Grass .... see VERBENA
Pigeonweed .... see VERBENA
Pignut .... see JOJOBA
Pigrush .... see KNOTWEED HERB
Pigweed .... see GOUTWEED, KNOTWEED HERB
Pigwood .... see WAHOO
Pilewort .... see AMARANTH, BULBOUS BUTTERCUP, LESSER CELANDINE
Piliolerial .... see PENNYROYAL leaf, PENNYROYAL oil
Pillbearing Spurge .... see EUPHORBIA
Pilocarpus microphyllus .... see JABORANDI
Pilosella officinarum .... see MOUSE EAR
Pilot Plant .... see CUP PLANT
Pilot Weed .... see ROSINWEED
Pimenta .... see ALLSPICE, BLACK PEPPER AND WHITE PEPPER
Pimenta dioica .... see ALLSPICE
Pimenta-Longa .... see INDIAN LONG PEPPER
Pimenta officinalis .... see ALLSPICE
Pimento .... see ALLSPICE, CAPSICUM
Pimienta .... see BLACK PEPPER AND WHITE PEPPER
Pimpernell .... see PIMPINELLA above ground parts, PIMPINELLA root
PIMPINELLA above ground parts
.... see PIMPINELLA above ground parts
Pimpinella anisum .... see ANISE
Pimpinella major ...... see PIMPINELLA above ground parts, PIMPINELLA root
PIMPINELLA root .... see PIMPINELLA root
Pimpinella saxifraga . see PIMPINELLA above ground parts, PIMPINELLA root
Pimpinellae herba ...... see PIMPINELLA above ground parts
Pimpinellae radix .... see PIMPINELLA root
Pin Heads .... see GERMAN CHAMOMILE
Pin-Ma Ts'ao .... see DANSHEN
Pinag .... see ARECA
PINE .... see PINE
Pine needle oil .... see BUTANEDIOL
Pine Oils .... see SCOTCH PINE NEEDLE
Pine Pollen .... see BEE POLLEN
Piney .... see PEONY flower, PEONY root
Pini Atheroleum .... see SCOTCH PINE NEEDLE
Pini Turiones .... see PINE
PINK ROOT .... see PINK ROOT
Pinlag .... see ARECA
Pinto Bean .... see BEAN POD
Pinus australis .... see TURPENTINE OIL
PINUS BARK .... see PINUS BARK
Pinus maritima .... see PYCNOGENOL
Pinus montana .... see DWARF PINE NEEDLE
Pinus mugo .... see DWARF PINE NEEDLE
Pinus mugo pumilio .... see DWARF PINE NEEDLE
Pinus palustris .... see TURPENTINE OIL
Pinus pinaster .... see PYCNOGENOL, TURPENTINE OIL
Pinus pumilio .... see DWARF PINE NEEDLE
Pinus sylvestris .... see PINE, SCOTCH PINE NEEDLE
Piper .... see BLACK PEPPER AND WHITE PEPPER
Piper cubeba .... see CUBEBS
Piper longum .... see INDIAN LONG PEPPER
Piper methysticum .... see KAVA
Piper nigrum
.... see BLACK PEPPER AND WHITE PEPPER
Pipperidge .... see EUROPEAN BARBERRY
Piprage .... see EUROPEAN BARBERRY
PIPSISSEWA .... see PIPSISSEWA
Piratancara .... see CATUABA
Piscidia communis .... see JAMAICAN DOGWOOD
Piscidia erythrina .... see JAMAICAN DOGWOOD
Piscidia piscipula .... see JAMAICAN DOGWOOD
Pissenlit .... see DANDELION above ground parts, DANDELION entire plant
Pistacia lentiscus .... see MASTIC
PITCHER PLANT .... see PITCHER PLANT
Pitirishi .... see CHANCA PIEDRA
Pituri .... see CORKWOOD TREE
Pix Cadi .... see CADE OIL
Pix Juniper .... see CADE OIL
Pix Liquida .... see PINE
Pix Oxycedri .... see CADE OIL
Plant-Derived Liquid Minerals .... see COLLOIDAL MINERALS
Plant Estrogen ....see SOY
Plant of Immortality ....see ALOE dried juice from leaf, latex
Plant Protease Concentrate .... see BROMELAIN, PAPAIN
Plant Stanol .... see SITOSTANOL
Plant sterols .... see BETA-SITOSTEROL
Plantaginis lanceolatae herba .... see BUCKHORN PLANTAIN
Plantaginis ovatae semen .... see BLOND PSYLLIUM
Plantaginis ovatae testa .... see BLOND PSYLLIUM
Plantago decumbens .... see BLOND PSYLLIUM
Plantago isphagula .... see BLOND PSYLLIUM
Plantago lanceolata .... see BUCKHORN PLANTAIN
Plantago major .... see GREAT PLANTAIN
Plantago ovata .... see BLOND PSYLLIUM
Plantago psyllium .... see BLACK PSYLLIUM
Plantain .... see BLACK PSYLLIUM, BUCKHORN PLANTAIN
Platycladus orientalis .... see ORIENTAL ARBORVITAE
PLC .... see PROPIONYL-L-CARNITINE
PLEURISY ROOT .... see PLEURISY ROOT
Plumrocks .... see COWSLIP
Pocan .... see POKEWEED berry, POKEWEED root
Pockwood .... see GUAIAC WOOD resin, wood
Podophylli pelati rhizoma/resina .... see PODOPHYLLUM
PODOPHYLLUM .... see PODOPHYLLUM
Podophyllum emodi .... see PODOPHYLLUM
Podophyllum hexandrum .... see PODOPHYLLUM
Podophyllum peltatum .... see PODOPHYLLUM
Poet's Jessamine .... see JASMINE
Pogostemon cablin .... see PATCHOULY OIL
Pogostemon heyneanus .... see PATCHOULY OIL
Pogostemon patchouly .... see PATCHOULY OIL
Pohl .... see MANACA
POINSETTIA .... see POINSETTIA
Poinsettia pulcherrima .... see POINSETTIA

INDEX

© Copyright 2000, Natural Medicines Comprehensive Database (209) 472-2244. For updated data, go to www.NaturalDatabase.com. • 1501

Poison Ash .... see FRINGETREE
Poison Black Cherries .... see BELLADONNA
Poison Flag .... see ORRIS
POISON IVY .... see POISON IVY
Poison Lettuce .... see WILD LETTUCE
Poison Nut .... see NUX VOMICA
Poison Tobacco .... see HENBANE
Poison Vine .... see POISON IVY
Poisonberry .... see BLACK NIGHTSHADE,
LEVANT BERRY

POISONOUS BUTTERCUP

.... see POISONOUS BUTTERCUP
Poivre .... see BLACK PEPPER AND WHITE PEPPER
Poivre Long .... see INDIAN LONG PEPPER
Poivre Noir .... see BLACK PEPPER AND
WHITE PEPPER
Poke .... see POKEWEED berry, POKEWEED root
Pokeberry .... see POKEWEED berry, POKEWEED root
POKEWEED berry .... see POKEWEED berry
POKEWEED root .... see POKEWEED root
Polar Plant .... see CUP PLANT,
ROSEMARY, ROSINWEED
Polecatweed .... see SKUNK CABBAGE
Polemonium coeruleum .... see JACOB'S LADDER
Polemonium reptans .... see ABSCESS ROOT
Poleo .... see JAPANESE MINT
POLICOSANOL .... see POLICOSANOL
Pollen D'Abeille .... see BEE POLLEN
Poly-NAG .... see N-ACETYL GLUCOSAMINE
Polygala amara .... see BITTER MILKWORT
Polygala glomerata .... see SENEGA
Polygala japonica .... see SENEGA
Polygala reinii .... see SENEGA
Polygala senega .... see SENEGA
Polygala senega latifolia .... see SENEGA
Polygala tenuifolia .... see SENEGA
Polygalae radix .... see SENEGA
Polygonatum multiflorum .... see SOLOMON'S SEAL
Polygoni Avicularis Herba .... see KNOTWEED HERB
Polygonum .... see FO-TI raw root
Polygonum aviculare .... see KNOTWEED HERB
Polygonum bistorta .... see BISTORT
Polygonum hydropiper .... see SMARTWEED
Polygonum multiflorum .... see FO-TI cured root,
FO-TI raw root
Polyporus .... see PORIA MUSHROOM
Polyporus Versicolor .... see CORIOLUS MUSHROOM
Polysaccharide Peptide .... see CORIOLUS MUSHROOM
Polysaccharide-K .... see CORIOLUS MUSHROOM
Polystictus Versicolor .... see CORIOLUS MUSHROOM
Polyunsaturated Fatty Acids .... see OMEGA-6 FATTY
ACIDS
POMEGRANATE .... see POMEGRANATE
Pomelo .... see GRAPEFRUIT
Poolroot .... see SANICLE
Poor Man's Parmacettie .... see SHEPHERD'S PURSE
Poor Man's Treacle .... see GARLIC
Poor Man's Weatherglass .... see SCARLET PIMPERNEL
Popinac Absolute .... see CASSIE ABSOLUTE
POPLAR .... see POPLAR
Popotillo .... see EPHEDRA, MORMON TEA
Poppy California .... see CALIFORNIA POPPY
Populi cortex .... see ASPEN
Populi folium .... see ASPEN

Populi Gemma .... see POPLAR
Populus balsamifera .... see POPLAR
Populus candicans .... see POPLAR
Populus tacamahacca .... see POPLAR
Populus tremula .... see ASPEN
Populus tremuloides .... see ASPEN
Porcelain Clay .... see KAOLIN
Poria .... see PORIA MUSHROOM
Poria cocos .... see PORIA MUSHROOM
PORIA MUSHROOM .... see PORIA MUSHROOM
Portland Arrowroot .... see ARUM
Pot .... see MARIJUANA
Pot Barley .... see BARLEY
Pot Marigold .... see CALENDULA
POTASSIUM .... see POTASSIUM
Potassium Acetate .... see POTASSIUM
Potassium Acid Phosphate .... see PHOSPHATE SALTS
Potassium Bicarbonate .... see POTASSIUM
Potassium Biphosphate .... see PHOSPHATE SALTS
Potassium Chloride .... see POTASSIUM
Potassium Citrate .... see POTASSIUM
Potassium Dihydrogen Orthophosphate
.... see PHOSPHATE SALTS
Potassium Gluconate .... see POTASSIUM
Potassium Iodide .... see IODINE
Potassium Phosphate .... see PHOSPHATE SALTS,
POTASSIUM
Potassium Pyruvate .... see PYRUVATE
POTATO .... see POTATO
Potency Wood .... see MUIRA PUAMA
POTENTILLA .... see POTENTILLA
Potentilla .... see TORMENTIL
Potentilla anserina .... see POTENTILLA
Potentilla erecta .... see TORMENTIL
Potentilla reptans .... see EUROPEAN FIVE-FINGER
GRASS
Poverty Weed .... see OX-EYE DAISY
Povidone Iodine .... see IODINE
Prairie Dock .... see CUP PLANT
Prairie Grub .... see WAFER ASH
Prasterone .... see DHEA
Prayer Beads .... see PRECATORY BEAN
Prayer Head .... see PRECATORY BEAN
PRECATORY BEAN .... see PRECATORY BEAN
Precipitated Calcium Phosphate .... see PHOSPHATE SALTS
Pregnancy Hormone .... see PROGESTERONE
Pregnanedione .... see PROGESTERONE
PREGNENOLONE .... see PREGNENOLONE
Prele .... see HORSETAIL
PREMORSE .... see PREMORSE
Premorse Scaboius .... see PREMORSE
Pretty Betsy .... see RED-SPUR VALERIAN
Prick Madam .... see COMMON STONECROP
Prickly Ash .... see NORTHERN PRICKLY ASH,
SOUTHERN PRICKLY ASH
PRICKLY PEAR CACTUS .... see PRICKLY PEAR
CACTUS
Prickly Yellow Wood .... see SOUTHERN PRICKLY ASH
Prickwood .... see WAHOO
Pride of China .... see NEEM
Prideweed .... see CANADIAN FLEABANE
Priest's Crown .... see DANDELION above ground parts,
DANDELION entire plant
Primrose .... see COWSLIP

I
N
D
E
X

Primula .... see COWSLIP
Primula elatier .... see COWSLIP
Primula officinalis .... see COWSLIP
Primula veris .... see COWSLIP
Prince's Feather .... see AMARANTH
Prince's Feathers .... see POTENTILLA
Prince's Pine .... see PIPSISSEWA
Proacemic Acid .... see PYRUVATE
Probiotic .... see BIFIDOBACTERIUM BIFIDUM,
BREWER'S YEAST,
LACTOBACILLUS ACIDOPHILUS,
LACTOBACILLUS GG,
SACCHAROMYCES BOULARDII,
YOGURT
PROCAINE .... see PROCAINE
Procaine Hydrochloride .... see PROCAINE
Processed Bovine Cartilage .... see BOVINE CARTILAGE
Procyanidolic Oligomers .... see GRAPE seed
Progestational Hormone .... see PROGESTERONE
PROGESTERONE .... see PROGESTERONE
Progesteronum .... see PROGESTERONE
PROPIONYL-L-CARNITINE
.... see PROPIONYL-L-CARNITINE
PROPOLIS .... see PROPOLIS
Propolis Balsam .... see PROPOLIS
Propolis Resin .... see PROPOLIS
Propolis Wax .... see PROPOLIS
Proteinase .... see TRYPSIN
Proteolytic Enzyme .... see TRYPSIN
Provitamin A .... see BETA-CAROTENE
Pruche de l'Est .... see PINUS BARK
Prunella .... see SELF-HEAL
Prunella vulgaris .... see SELF-HEAL
Pruni Spinosae Fructus .... see BLACKTHORN berry
Pruni Spinosae Llos .... see BLACKTHORN flower
Prunus africana .... see PYGEUM
Prunus amygdalus amara .... see BITTER ALMOND
Prunus amygdalus dulcis .... see SWEET ALMOND
Prunus armeniaca .... see APRICOT
Prunus Cerasus .... see SOUR CHERRY
Prunus dulcis amara .... see BITTER ALMOND
Prunus laurocerasus .... see CHERRY LAUREL WATER
Prunus serotina .... see WILD CHERRY
Prunus spinosa .... see BLACKTHORN berry,
BLACKTHORN flower
Prunus virginiana .... see WILD CHERRY
Prunus vulgaris .... see SOUR CHERRY
Pseudoginseng Root .... see PANAX PSEUDOGINSENG
Pseudotsuga douglasii .... see OREGON FIR BALSAM
Pseudotsuga menziesii .... see OREGON FIR BALSAM
Pseudotsuga mucronata .... see OREGON FIR BALSAM
Pseudotsuga taxifolia .... see OREGON FIR BALSAM
Psi .... see LYCOPENE
Psi-carotene .... see LYCOPENE
PSK .... see CORIOLUS MUSHROOM
Psoralea linearis .... see RED BUSH TEA
Psoriacin .... see BOVINE CARTILAGE
Psoriacin-T .... see BOVINE CARTILAGE
PSP .... see CORIOLUS MUSHROOM
Psychotria ipecacuanha .... see IPECAC
Psyllion .... see BLACK PSYLLIUM
Psyllios .... see BLACK PSYLLIUM
Psyllium .... see BLOND PSYLLIUM
Psyllium afra .... see BLACK PSYLLIUM

Psyllium arenaria .... see BLACK PSYLLIUM
Psyllium indica .... see BLACK PSYLLIUM
Psyllium Seed .... see BLACK PSYLLIUM
Ptarmigan Berry .... see UVA URSI
PtdSer .... see PHOSPHATIDYLSERINE
Ptelea trifoliata .... see WAFER ASH
Pterocarpus santalinus .... see RED SANDALWOOD
Pteroylglutamic acid .... see FOLIC ACID
Pteroylmonoglutamic acid .... see FOLIC ACID
pteroylpolyglutamate .... see FOLIC ACID
Ptychopetali lignum .... see MUIRA PUAMA
Ptychopetalum olacoides .... see MUIRA PUAMA
Ptychopetalum unicatum .... see MUIRA PUAMA
P'u-T'ao .... see BITTER MELON
Public House Plant .... see ASARABACCA
Pudding Grass .... see PENNYROYAL leaf,
PENNYROYAL oil
Pueraria lobata .... see KUDZU
Pueraria mirifica, Pueraria tuberosa .... see KUDZU
Pueraria montana var lobata .... see KUDZU
Pueraria montana var thomsonii .... see KUDZU
Pueraria pseudohirsuta .... see KUDZU
Pueraria Root .... see KUDZU
Pueraria thomsonii .... see KUDZU
Pueraria thunbergiana .... see KUDZU
Puerto Rican Cherry .... see ACEROLA
PUFA .... see FISH OILS
PUFAs .... see OMEGA-6 FATTY ACIDS
PUFF BALL .... see PUFF BALL
Pukeweed .... see LOBELIA
Pulegium .... see PENNYROYAL leaf, PENNYROYAL oil
Pulegium vulgare .... see PENNYROYAL leaf,
PENNYROYAL oil
Pulmonaria officinalis .... see LUNGWORT
Pulmonariae herba .... see LUNGWORT
PULSATILLA .... see PULSATILLA
Pulsatilla nigricans .... see PULSATILLA
Pulsatilla pratensis .... see PULSATILLA
Pulsatilla vulgaris .... see PULSATILLA
Pumacuchu .... see RHATANY
Pumilio Pine .... see PINE
PUMPKIN .... see PUMPKIN
PUNCTURE VINE .... see PUNCTURE VINE
Punica granatum .... see POMEGRANATE
Punk Tree .... see CAJEPUT OIL
Punnanga .... see LAURELWOOD
Pupurweide .... see WILLOW BARK
Purging Flax .... see MOUNTAIN FLAX
Purging Thorn .... see SEA BUCKTHORN
Purified Honey .... see HONEY
Purified Turpentine Oil .... see TURPENTINE OIL
Purines .... see RNA AND DNA
Purple Boneset .... see GRAVEL ROOT
Purple Clover .... see RED CLOVER
Purple Cockle .... see CORN COCKLE
Purple Cone Flower .... see ECHINACEA
Purple Foxglove .... see DIGITALIS
Purple Lapacho .... see PAU D'ARCO
Purple Leptandra .... see BLACK ROOT
PURPLE LOOSESTRIFE ...... see PURPLE LOOSESTRIFE
Purple Medick .... see ALFALFA
Purple Mulberry .... see BLACK MULBERRY
Purple Osier .... see WILLOW BARK
Purple Osier Willow .... see WILLOW BARK

INDEX

© Copyright 2000, Natural Medicines Comprehensive Database (209) 472-2244. For updated data, go to www.NaturalDatabase.com. • 1503

Purple Passion Flower .... see PASSIONFLOWER
Purple Pitcher Plant .... see PITCHER PLANT
Purple Side-Saddle Flower .... see PITCHER PLANT
Purple Turk's Cap Lily .... see MARTAGON
Purple Willow-Herb .... see PURPLE LOOSESTRIFE
Purshiana Bark .... see CASCARA
Putcha-Pat .... see PATCHOULY OIL
PYCNOGENOL .... see PYCNOGENOL
PYGEUM .... see PYGEUM
Pygeum africanum .... see PYGEUM
PYRETHRUM .... see PYRETHRUM
Pyrethrum parthenium .... see FEVERFEW
Pyridoxal .... see PYRIDOXINE
Pyridoxamine .... see PYRIDOXINE
PYRIDOXINE .... see PYRIDOXINE
Pyridoxine Hydrochloride .... see PYRIDOXINE
Pyrimidines .... see RNA AND DNA
Pyroleum Juniperi .... see CADE OIL
Pyroleum Oxycedri .... see CADE OIL
Pyrus communis .... see PEAR
PYRUVATE .... see PYRUVATE
Pyruvic acid .... see PYRUVATE
Qian Ceng Ta .... see CHINESE CLUB MOSS
Qinghao .... see SWEET ANNIE
Qinghaosu .... see SWEET ANNIE
Quackgrass .... see AGROPYRON, COUCH GRASS
Quaker .... see ARUM
Quaker Bonnet .... see SCULLCAP
Quaker Buttons .... see NUX VOMICA
QUASSIA .... see QUASSIA
Quassia amara .... see QUASSIA
Quassia Bark .... see QUASSIA
QUEBRACHO .... see QUEBRACHO
Quebracho Blanco .... see QUEBRACHO
Quebrachol .... see BETA-SITOSTEROL
Quebrapedra .... see CHANCA PIEDRA
Queen Anne's Lace .... see WILD CARROT
Queen Of The Meadow .... see GRAVEL ROOT,
                                                       MEADOWSWEET
QUEEN'S DELIGHT .... see QUEEN'S DELIGHT
Queen's Root .... see QUEEN'S DELIGHT
QUERCETIN .... see QUERCETIN
Quercetin-3-rhamnoglucoside .... see RUTIN
Quercetin-3-rutinoside .... see RUTIN
Quercus alba .... see OAK bark
Quercus cortex .... see OAK bark
Quercus Marina .... see BLADDERWRACK
Quercus petraea .... see OAK bark
Quercus robur .... see OAK bark
Quickbeam .... see MOUNTAIN ASH
Quick-In-The-Hand .... see JEWELWEED
QUILLAIA .... see QUILLAIA
Quillaja .... see QUILLAIA
Quillaja saponaria .... see QUILLAIA
Quimotripsina .... see CHYMOTRYPSIN
QUINCE .... see QUINCE
Quing Dai .... see DA QING YE
Quinina Criolla .... see CHANCA PIEDRA
Quinine .... see CINCHONA
Quinine Creole .... see CHANCA PIEDRA
Quitch Grass .... see AGROPYRON
Qut .... see KHAT
(R)-3-hydroxy-4-trimethylammonio-butyrate
.... see L-CARNITINE

Rabbits .... see YELLOW TOADFLAX
Raccoon Berry .... see PODOPHYLLUM
Race Ginger .... see GINGER
Racine de Carline Acaule .... see CARLINA
Racine De Guimauve .... see MARSHMALLOW
Racine d'echininacea .... see ECHINACEA
Radis .... see RADISH
RADISH .... see RADISH
Radix Anchusae .... see ALKANNA
Radix Cardopatiae .... see CARLINA
Radix Chamaeleontis Albae .... see CARLINA
Radix Codonopsis .... see CODONOPSIS
Radix Peurariae .... see KUDZU
Radix Pimpinelle Franconiae .... see MASTERWORT
Radix Polygoni Multiflori .... see FO-TI raw root
Radix Polygoni Shen Min .... see FO-TI cured root
Rag Paper .... see MULLEIN
Ragged Cup .... see CUP PLANT
Ragweed .... see TANSY RAGWORT
Ragwort .... see GOLDEN RAGWORT, TANSY
                                                       RAGWORT
Rainbow Weed .... see PURPLE LOOSESTRIFE
Raisin d'Amerique .... see POKEWEED berry,
                                                       POKEWEED root
Raisin D'Ours .... see UVA URSI
Raisins .... see GRAPE fruit, skin
Raiz Para Los Dientes .... see RHATANY
Ram-Goat Rose .... see MADAGASCAR PERIWINKLE
Rami Buah .... see CHANCA PIEDRA
Ramp .... see ARUM
Ramsons .... see BEAR'S GARLIC
Ramsted .... see YELLOW TOADFLAX
Ramsthorn .... see EUROPEAN BUCKTHORN
Ranunculus .... see LESSER CELANDINE
Ranunculus acris .... see BUTTERCUP
Ranunculus bulbosus .... see BULBOUS BUTTERCUP
Ranunculus ficaria .... see LESSER CELANDINE
Ranunculus sceleratus .... see POISONOUS BUTTERCUP
Raphani sativi radix .... see RADISH
Raphanus raphanistrum .... see WILD RADISH
Raphanus sativus .... see RADISH
RASPBERRY .... see RASPBERRY
Ratanhiae radix .... see RHATANY
Ratanhiawurzel .... see RHATANY
Rattle Pouches .... see SHEPHERD'S PURSE
Rattle Root .... see BLACK COHOSH
Rattlebush .... see WILD INDIGO
Rattlesnake Root .... see BETH ROOT,
                                       BLACK COHOSH, SENEGA
Rattlesnake Violet ..... see AMERICAN ADDER'S TONGUE
Rattleweed .... see BLACK COHOSH
Rauschpfeffer .... see KAVA
Raute .... see RUE
Rauvolfia serpentina .... see INDIAN SNAKEROOT
Rauwolfae radix .... see INDIAN SNAKEROOT
Rauwolfia .... see INDIAN SNAKEROOT
Rauwolfia Serpentina .... see INDIAN SNAKEROOT
Rauwolfiawurzel .... see INDIAN SNAKEROOT
Ray-Grass .... see TAUMELLOOLCH
Red American Ginseng .... see CANAIGRE
Red Bay .... see MAGNOLIA bark
Red Bearberry .... see UVA URSI
Red Beet .... see BEET
Red Bilberry .... see ALPINE CRANBERRY

RED BUSH TEA .... see RED BUSH TEA
Red Cedarwood
  .... see CEDARWOOD bark, berry, leaf, seed, twig
Red Cherry .... see SOUR CHERRY
Red Chickweed .... see SCARLET PIMPERNEL
Red Cinchona Bark .... see CINCHONA
RED CLOVER .... see RED CLOVER
Red Cockscomb .... see AMARANTH
Red Cole .... see HORSERADISH
Red Couchgrass .... see GERMAN SARSAPARILLA
Red Date .... see JUJUBE
Red Elm .... see SLIPPERY ELM
Red Fir .... see OREGON FIR BALSAM
Red Ginseng .... see GINSENG, PANAX
Red Globe .... see GRAPE fruit, skin
Red Gum .... see EUCALYPTUS dried leaf, STORAX
Red Indian Paint .... see BLOODROOT
Red-Ink Plant ...... see POKEWEED berry, POKEWEED root
Red Juniper .... see CEDARWOOD bark, berry,
  leaf, seed, twig
Red Lapacho .... see PAU D'ARCO
Red Legs .... see BISTORT
Red Malaga .... see GRAPE fruit, skin
RED MAPLE .... see RED MAPLE
Red Morocco .... see PHEASANT'S EYE
Red Pepper .... see CAPSICUM
Red Periwinkle .... see MADAGASCAR PERIWINKLE
Red Pimpernel .... see SCARLET PIMPERNEL
Red Plant .... see POKEWEED berry, POKEWEED root
Red Poppy .... see CORN POPPY
Red Puccoon .... see BLOODROOT
Red Raspberry .... see RASPBERRY
Red Rhatany .... see RHATANY
Red Rice Yeast .... see RED YEAST
Red Robin .... see KNOTWEED HERB
Red Root .... see BLOODROOT, NEW JERSEY TEA
Red Rooted Sage .... see DANSHEN
Red Rot .... see SUNDEW
Red Sage .... see DANSHEN, GERMAN
  SARSAPARILLA
RED SANDALWOOD .... see RED SANDALWOOD
Red Sanderswood .... see RED SANDALWOOD
Red Saunders .... see RED SANDALWOOD
RED SOAPWORT .... see RED SOAPWORT
RED-SPUR VALERIAN .... see RED-SPUR VALERIAN
Red Squill .... see SQUILL
Red Sunflower .... see ECHINACEA
Red Tea .... see HIBISCUS
Red Thyme Oil .... see THYME OIL
Red Vine Leaf AS 195 .... see GRAPE leaf
Red Vine Leaf Extract .... see GRAPE leaf
Red Weed .... see POKEWEED berry, POKEWEED root
Red Whortleberry .... see ALPINE CRANBERRY
RED YEAST .... see RED YEAST
Redberries .... see ALPINE CRANBERRY
Redberry .... see GINSENG, AMERICAN, UVA URSI
Reduced DPN .... see NADH
Reduced Nicotinamide Adenine Dinucleotide ...... see NADH
Reed .... see REED HERB
REED HERB .... see REED HERB
Reglisse .... see LICORICE
Regliz .... see LICORICE
Reifweide .... see WILLOW BARK
REISHI MUSHROOM .... see REISHI MUSHROOM

Ren Shen .... see GINSENG, AMERICAN,
  GINSENG, PANAX
Requia .... see ANDIROBA
Reseda .... see HENNA
Resin Tolu .... see TOLU BALSAM
Resina Tolutana .... see TOLU BALSAM
Restharrow .... see SPINY RESTHARROW
RESVERATROL .... see RESVERATROL
Retinol .... see VITAMIN A
Retinol Acetate .... see VITAMIN A
Retinol Palmitate .... see VITAMIN A
Retinyl Acetate .... see VITAMIN A
Retinyl Palmitate .... see VITAMIN A
RGH-4405 .... see VINPOCETINE
Rhamni cathartica fructus .. see EUROPEAN BUCKTHORN
Rhamni Purshianae Cortex .... see CASCARA
Rhamnol .... see BETA-SITOSTEROL
Rhamnus catharticus .... see EUROPEAN BUCKTHORN
Rhamnus frangula .... see ALDER BUCKTHORN
Rhamnus purshiana .... see CASCARA
Rhatanhia .... see RHATANY
Rhatania .... see RHATANY
RHATANY .... see RHATANY
Rhei radix .... see RHUBARB
Rheum australe .... see RHUBARB
Rheum emodi .... see RHUBARB
Rheum officinale .... see RHUBARB
Rheum palmatum .... see RHUBARB
Rheum rhabarbarum .... see RHUBARB
Rheum tanguticum .... see RHUBARB
Rheum x cultorum .... see RHUBARB
Rheumatism Root .... see WILD YAM
Rheumatism Weed .... see PIPSISSEWA
Rhizoma iridis .... see ORRIS
Rhizome Galangae .... see ALPINIA
Rhodiola rosea .... see ROSEROOT
Rhododendri Ferruginei Folium
  .... see RUSTY-LEAVED RHODODENDRON
Rhododendron ferrugineum
  .... see RUSTY-LEAVED RHODODENDRON
Rhoeados Flos .... see CORN POPPY
RHUBARB .... see RHUBARB
Rhus aromatica .... see SWEET SUMACH
Rhus Toxicodendron .... see POISON IVY
Ribes Nero .... see BLACK CURRANT SEED OIL
Ribes nigri folium .... see BLACK CURRANT dried leaf
Ribes nigrum .... see BLACK CURRANT berry,
  BLACK CURRANT dried leaf,
  BLACK CURRANT SEED OIL
Ribgrass .... see BUCKHORN PLANTAIN
RIBOFLAVIN .... see RIBOFLAVIN
Riboflavine .... see RIBOFLAVIN
Ribonucleic Acid .... see RNA AND DNA
RIBOSE .... see RIBOSE
Ribwort Plantain .... see BUCKHORN PLANTAIN
RICE BRAN .... see RICE BRAN
Rice Bran Oil .... see RICE BRAN
Rich Weed .... see STONE ROOT
Richleaf .... see STONE ROOT
Richmond .... see SOUR CHERRY
Ricinus communis .... see CASTOR OIL, CASTOR seed
Ricinus sanguines .... see CASTOR OIL, CASTOR seed
Ringworm Powder .... see GOA POWDER
Rio Ipecac .... see IPECAC

INDEX

Ripplegrass .... see BUCKHORN PLANTAIN
Rittterspornbluten .... see DELPHINIUM
RNA AND DNA .... see RNA AND DNA
Robbia .... see MADDER
Robin-Run-in-the-Grass .... see CLIVERS
Robin-Run-In-The-Hedge .... see GROUND IVY
Rock Brake .... see LADY FERN
Rock Cranberry .... see ALPINE CRANBERRY
Rock Fern .... see MAIDENHAIR FERN
Rock of Polypody .... see LADY FERN
Rock Parsley .... see PARSLEY leaf, root
Rock-Rose .... see FROSTWORT
Rock-Up-Hat .... see ECHINACEA
Rockberry .... see UVA URSI
Rockrose .... see LABDANUM
Rock's-Foot .... see HAY FLOWER
Rockweed .... see BLADDERWRACK
Rockwrack .... see BLADDERWRACK
Roga Mari .... see YARROW
Rokitnik .... see SEA BUCKTHORN
Rokujo .... see DEER VELVET
ROMAN CHAMOMILE .... see ROMAN CHAMOMILE
Roman-Coriander .... see BLACK SEED
Roman Laurel .... see SWEET BAY
Roman Motherwort .... see MOTHERWORT
Roman Plant .... see SWEET CICELY
Romarin Sauvage .... see MARSH TEA
Ronce d'Amerique .... see CRANBERRY
Rooibos Tea .... see RED BUSH TEA
Root of the Holy Ghost .... see ANGELICA root
Roripa armoracia .... see HORSERADISH
Rosa alba .... see ROSE HIP
Rosa camellia .... see CHEROKEE ROSEHIP
Rosa canina .... see ROSE HIP
Rosa cherokensis .... see CHEROKEE ROSEHIP
Rosa damascena .... see ROSE HIP
Rosa de castillo .... see ROSE HIP
Rosa gallica .... see ROSE HIP
Rosa laevigata .... see CHEROKEE ROSEHIP
Rosa nivea .... see CHEROKEE ROSEHIP
Rosa pomifera .... see ROSE HIP
Rosa rugosa .... see ROSE HIP
Rosa sinica .... see CHEROKEE ROSEHIP
Rosa ternata .... see CHEROKEE ROSEHIP
Rosa villosa .... see ROSE HIP
Rosae pseudofructus cum semen .... see ROSE HIP
Rosary Pea .... see PRECATORY BEAN
Rose-A-Rubie .... see PHEASANT'S EYE
Rose Apple .... see JAMBOLAN bark, JAMBOLAN seed
Rose-Colored Silkweed .... see SWAMP MILKWEED
ROSE GERANIUM .... see ROSE GERANIUM
ROSE HIP .... see ROSE HIP
Rose Hip with seed .... see ROSE HIP
Rose Laurel .... see MOUNTAIN LAUREL, OLEANDER
Rose Mallow .... see HOLLYHOCK
Rose Root .... see ROSEROOT
Rose Willow .... see AMERICAN DOGWOOD
Rosebay .... see FIREWEED, OLEANDER,
　　　　　　　　　　RUSTY-LEAVED RHODODENDRON
Rosehips .... see ROSE HIP
Roselle .... see HIBISCUS
ROSEMARY .... see ROSEMARY
Rosemary .... see DAMIANA

Rosenoble .... see FIGWORT
Rosenroot .... see ROSEROOT
ROSEROOT .... see ROSEROOT
Rosewood Oil .... see BOIS DE ROSE OIL
Rosin Rose .... see ST JOHN'S WORT
ROSINWEED .... ROSINWEED
Rosinweed .... see CUP PLANT, GUMWEED
Rosmarinus officinalis .... see ROSEMARY
Roter Wasserhanf .... see GRAVEL ROOT
Rottlera Tinctoria .... see KAMALA
Rou Gui .... see CASSIA
Round Buchu .... see BUCHU
Round-Leafed Sundew .... see SUNDEW
Round-Leaved Hepatica .... see LIVERWORT
Round-Lobe Hepatica .... see LIVERWORT
Rowan Tree .... see MOUNTAIN ASH
Roxanthin Red 10 .... see CANTHAXANTHIN
Royal Jasmine .... see JASMINE
ROYAL JELLY .... see ROYAL JELLY
RRR-Alpha-Tocopherol .... see VITAMIN E
Romische Kamille .... see ROMAN CHAMOMILE
Rubbed Thyme .... see THYME flower, leaf
Rubi Fruticosi Folium .... see BLACKBERRY leaf
Rubi Fruticosi Radix .... see BLACKBERRY root
Rubi idaei folium .... see RASPBERRY
Rubia tinctorum .... see MADDER
Rubiae tinctorum radix .... see MADDER
Rubus .... see RASPBERRY
Rubus fruticosus .... see BLACKBERRY leaf,
　　　　　　　　　　　　　　BLACKBERRY root
Rubus idaeus .... see RASPBERRY
Rubus strigosus .... see RASPBERRY
Rubywood .... see RED SANDALWOOD
Ruda .... see QUASSIA, RUE
RUE .... see RUE
Rue Officinale .... see RUE
Ruibarbo Caribe .... see MORINDA
Rum Cherry Bark .... see WILD CHERRY
Rumalon .... see BOVINE CARTILAGE
Rumex .... see YELLOW DOCK
Rumex acetosa .... see SORREL
Rumex aquaticus .... see WATER DOCK
Rumex crispus .... see YELLOW DOCK
Rumex hymenosepalus .... see CANAIGRE
Rumex obtusifolius .... see YELLOW DOCK
Rumput Roman .... see YIN CHEN
Run-By-The-Ground .... see PENNYROYAL leaf,
　　　　　　　　　　　　　　PENNYROYAL oil
Reunion Vanilla .... see VANILLA
Running Box .... see SQUAWVINE
Running Jenny .... see MONEYWORT
RUPTUREWORT .... see RUPTUREWORT
Rusci Aculeati Rhizoma .... see BUTCHER'S BROOM
Ruscus aculeatus .... see BUTCHER'S BROOM
Russian Formula .... see PANGAMIC ACID
Russian Krainer Tollkraut .... see SCOPOLIA
Russian Licorice .... see LICORICE
Russion Penicillin .... see PROPOLIS
Rust-Red Rhododendron
　　　　......... see RUSTY-LEAVED RHODODENDRON
Rust Treacle .... see GARLIC
RUSTY-LEAVED RHODODENDRON
　　　　......... see RUSTY-LEAVED RHODODENDRON

INDEX

Ruta graveolens .... see RUE
Rutae folium .... see RUE
Rutae herba .... see RUE
RUTIN .... see RUTIN
Rutine .... see RUTIN
Rutinum .... see RUTIN
Rutland Beauty .... see GREATER BINDWEED
Rutosid .... see RUTIN
Rutoside .... see RUTIN
Rutosidum .... see RUTIN
RYE GRASS .... see RYE GRASS
Rye Grass Pollen .... see RYE GRASS
Rye Grass Pollen Extract .... see RYE GRASS
Rye Pollen Extract .... see RYE GRASS
S-Adenosyl Methionine .... see SAMe
S-Adenosyl-L-Methionine .... see SAMe
Sabal Fructus .... see SAW PALMETTO
Sabal serrulata .... see SAW PALMETTO
Sabina .... see SAVIN TOPS
Sabline Rouge .... see ARENARIA RUBRA
Sabojira .... see CHICLE
SACCHAROMYCES BOULARDII
.... see SACCHAROMYCES BOULARDII
Saccharomyces cerevisiae .... see BREWER'S YEAST
Saccharomyces cerevisiae Hansen CBS 5926
.... see BREWER'S YEAST (HANSEN CBS 5926)
Sacha Foster .... see CHANCA PIEDRA
Sacred Bark .... see CASCARA
Sacred Herb .... see YERBA SANTA
Sacred Mushroom .... see PEYOTE
Sadilata .... see ANDROGRAPHIS
SAFFLOWER .... see SAFFLOWER
SAFFRON .... see SAFFRON
Saffron Crocus .... see SAFFRON
Saffron Marigold .... see TAGETES
Safran .... see SAFFRON
Sagackhomi .... see UVA URSI
SAGE .... see SAGE
Sage of Bethlehem .... see SPEARMINT
Sagrada Bark .... see CASCARA
Sahlep .... see SALEP
Saigon Cassia .... see CINNAMON bark
Saigon Cinnamon .... see CINNAMON bark
Sailor's Tobacco .... see MUGWORT
Saint John's Wort .... see ST JOHN'S WORT
Sakau .... see KAVA
Salad Chervil .... see CHERVIL
Salad Oil .... see OLIVE OIL
Salai Guggal .... see INDIAN FRANKINCENSE
SALEP .... see SALEP
Salicare .... see PURPLE LOOSESTRIFE
Salicis cortex .... see WILLOW BARK
Salisburia .... see GINKGO leaf extract
Salisburia Adiantifolia .... see GINKGO leaf
Salix alba .... see WILLOW BARK
Salix daphnoides .... see WILLOW BARK
Salix fragilis .... see WILLOW BARK
Salix pentandra .... see WILLOW BARK
Salix purpurea .... see WILLOW BARK
Sallow Thorn .... see SEA BUCKTHORN
Saloop .... see SALEP
Salsaparilha .... see SARSAPARILLA
Salsepareille .... see SARSAPARILLA
Salsify .... see COMFREY

Salt-rheum Weed .... see TURTLE HEAD
Salvia .... see ALOE gel
Salvia lavandulaefolia .... see SAGE
Salvia miltiorrhiza .... see DANSHEN
Salvia officinalis .... see SAGE
Salvia Root .... see DANSHEN
Salvia sclarea .... see CLARY SAGE
Salvia triloba .... see GREEK SAGE
Salvia yunnanensis .... see DANSHEN
SAM-e .... see SAMe
Sambilata .... see ANDROGRAPHIS
Sambrani Chettu .... see BRAHMI
Sambuci Sambucus .... see EUROPEAN ELDER fruit
Sambucus ....see AMERICAN ELDER,
                               EUROPEAN ELDER flower
Sambucus canadensis ....see AMERICAN ELDER
Sambucus ebulus .... see DWARF ELDER
Sambucus nigra .... see EUROPEAN ELDER flower,
                               EUROPEAN ELDER fruit
Samch'il .... see PANAX PSEUDOGINSENG
SAMe .... see SAMe
Samento .... see CAT'S CLAW
Sammy .... see SAMe
SAMPHIRE .... see SAMPHIRE
Sampier .... see SAMPHIRE
San Qi .... see PANAX PSEUDOGINSENG
San Qui .... see PANAX PSEUDOGINSENG
Sand Plantain .... see BLOND PSYLLIUM
Sand Sedge .... see GERMAN SARSAPARILLA
Sandalwood .... see WHITE SANDALWOOD wood
Sandalwood Padauk .... see RED SANDALWOOD
Sandberry ....see UVA URSI
Sanddorn .... see SEA BUCKTHORN
Sanderswood .... see WHITE SANDALWOOD oil
Sandriedgraswurzelstock ... see GERMAN SARSAPARILLA
Sandwort ....see ARENARIA RUBRA
SANDY EVERLASTING ...... see SANDY EVERLASTING
Sang .... see GINSENG, AMERICAN, GINSENG, PANAX
Sangre de Drago .... see SANGRE DE GRADO
Sangre de Dragon .... see SANGRE DE GRADO
SANGRE DE GRADO .... see SANGRE DE GRADO
Sangrel .... see ARISTOLOCHIA
Sangue de Agua .... see SANGRE DE GRADO
Sangue de Drago .... see SANGRE DE GRADO
Sanguinaria .... see BLOODROOT
Sanguinaria canadensis .... see BLOODROOT
Sanguinary .... see SHEPHERD'S PURSE, YARROW
Sanguis Draconis .... see DRAGON'S BLOOD
Sanguisorba .... see GREATER BURNET
Sanguisorba officinalis .... see GREATER BURNET
SANICLE .... see SANICLE
Sanicula europaea .... see SANICLE
Saniculae herba .... see SANICLE
Sanshichi .... see PANAX PSEUDOGINSENG
Santa Maria .... see FEVERFEW
Santal Oil .... see WHITE SANDALWOOD oil
Santali Lignum Albi ..... see WHITE SANDALWOOD wood
Santali lignum rubrum .... see RED SANDALWOOD
Santalum album .... see WHITE SANDALWOOD oil,
                               WHITE SANDALWOOD wood
Santolina .... see LAVENDER COTTON
Santolina chamaecyparissias ...... see LAVENDER COTTON
Santonica .... see WORMSEED
Sapodilla .... see CHICLE

© Copyright 2000, Natural Medicines Comprehensive Database (209) 472-2244. For updated data, go to www.NaturalDatabase.com. • 1507

INDEX

Sapodillbaum .... see CHICLE
Saponaria officinalis .... see RED SOAPWORT
Saponariae rubrae radix .... see RED SOAPWORT
Sapota achras .... see CHICLE
Sapote .... see CHICLE
Sapotier .... see CHICLE
Sapotillier .... see CHICLE
Sappan .... see RED SANDALWOOD
Sarapin .... see PITCHER PLANT
Sardian Nut .... see EUROPEAN CHESTNUT
Sarothamnus scoparius .... see SCOTCH BROOM flower,
                                              SCOTCH BROOM herb
Sarothamnus vulgaris .... see SCOTCH BROOM flower,
                                              SCOTCH BROOM herb
Sarpagandha .... see INDIAN SNAKEROOT
Sarracenia purpurea .... see PITCHER PLANT
Sarsa .... see SARSAPARILLA
SARSAPARILLA .... see SARSAPARILLA
Sarsaparillae radix .... see SARSAPARILLA
Sarsaparillewurzel .... see SARSAPARILLA
Sasha Foster .... see CHANCA PIEDRA
SASSAFRAS .... see SASSAFRAS
Sassafras ablidum .... see SASSAFRAS
Sassafras officinale .... see SASSAFRAS
Sassafras varifolium .... see SASSAFRAS
Sassafrax .... see SASSAFRAS
Satan's Apple .... see EUROPEAN MANDRAKE
Satureja capitata .... see SPANISH ORIGANUM OIL
Satureja hortensis .... see SUMMER SAVORY
Satureja montana .... see WINTER SAVORY
Satureja obovata .... see WINTER SAVORY
Satyrion .... see SALEP
Sauerdorn .... see EUROPEAN BARBERRY
Sauerkirsche .... see SOUR CHERRY
Sauerkirschenbaum .... see SOUR CHERRY
Sauge .... see SAGE
Saussurea lappa .... see COSTUS OIL, COSTUS root
Sauvignon Blanc .... see GRAPE fruit, skin
SAVIN TOPS .... see SAVIN TOPS
Savine .... see SAVIN TOPS
Savory .... see SUMMER SAVORY, WINTER SAVORY
SAW PALMETTO .... see SAW PALMETTO
Saw Palmetto Berry .... see SAW PALMETTO
Sawi .... see MARIJUANA
Saxifrage .... see PIMPINELLA above ground parts,
                                              PIMPINELLA root
Saxifrax .... see SASSAFRAS
Saynt Johannes Wort .... see ST JOHN'S WORT
Scabiosa succisa .... see PREMORSE
Scabish .... see EVENING PRIMROSE OIL
Scabwort .... see ELECAMPANE
Scaldweed .... see DODDER
Scaley Dragon's Claw .... see CORAL ROOT
Scarlet Berry .... see BITTERSWEET NIGHTSHADE
Scarlet Monarda .... see OSWEGO TEA
SCARLET PIMPERNEL .... see SCARLET PIMPERNEL
Scarlet Sage .... see SAGE
Sceau D'Or .... see GOLDENSEAL
Sceitbezien .... see SEA BUCKTHORN
Scented Fern .... see TANSY
SCHISANDRA .... see SCHISANDRA
Schisandra Berry .... see SCHISANDRA
Schisandra chinensis .... see SCHISANDRA
Schisandra splenanthera .... see SCHISANDRA

Schizandra .... see SCHISANDRA
Schollkraut .... see GREATER CELANDINE
                                      dried above ground parts
Schwarze Walnuss .... see BLACK WALNUT
Schwarzkummel .... see BLACK SEED
Schweintang .... see BLADDERWRACK
Scilla indica .... see SQUILL
Scilla maritima .... see SQUILL
Sclerutin .... see RUTIN
Scoke .... see POKEWEED berry, POKEWEED root
Scolopendrium vulgare .... see HARTSTONGUE
Scoparium .... see SCOTCH BROOM herb
Scoparius .... see SCOTCH BROOM flower,
                                      SCOTCH BROOM herb
Scopola .... see SCOPOLIA
SCOPOLIA .... see SCOPOLIA
Scopolia carniolica .... see SCOPOLIA
Scopoliae Rhizoma .... see SCOPOLIA
Scotch Barley .... see BARLEY
SCOTCH BROOM flower ..... see SCOTCH BROOM flower
SCOTCH BROOM herb .... see SCOTCH BROOM herb
Scotch Fir .... see PINE
Scotch Heather .... see HEATHER
Scotch Mercury .... see DIGITALIS
Scotch Pine .... see PINE
SCOTCH PINE NEEDLE ...... see SCOTCH PINE NEEDLE
Scotch Quelch .... see AGROPYRON, COUCH GRASS
SCOTCH THISTLE .... see SCOTCH THISTLE
Scouring Rush .... see HORSETAIL
Scratchweed .... see CLIVERS
Scrophula Plant .... see FIGWORT
Scrophularia .... see FIGWORT
Scrophularia mailandica .... see FIGWORT
Scrophularia nodosa .... see FIGWORT
Scrubby Grass .... see SCURVY GRASS
Scubby Trefoil .... see WAFER ASH
SCULLCAP .... see SCULLCAP
SCURVY GRASS .... see SCURVY GRASS
Scurvy Grass .... see WATERCRESS
Scurvy Root .... see ECHINACEA
Scutellaria baicalensis .... see BAIKAL SKULLCAP
Scutellaria lateriflora .... see SCULLCAP
Se .... see SELENIUM
Sea Ash .... see SOUTHERN PRICKLY ASH
SEA BUCKTHORN .... see SEA BUCKTHORN
Sea Coral .... see CORAL
Sea Fennel .... see SAMPHIRE
Sea Girdles .... see LAMINARIA
Sea Grape .... see EPHEDRA
Sea Holly .... see ERYNGO above ground parts,
                                      ERYNGO root
Sea Holme .... see ERYNGO above ground parts,
                                      ERYNGO root
Sea Hulver .... see ERYNGO above ground parts,
                                      ERYNGO root
Sea Onion .... see SQUILL
Sea Parsley .... see LOVAGE
Sea Sedge .... see GERMAN SARSAPARILLA
Sea Squill Bulb .... see SQUILL
Sea Wormwood .... see WORMSEED
Seabuckthorn .... see SEA BUCKTHORN
Seagirdle Thallus .... see LAMINARIA
Sealroot .... see SOLOMON'S SEAL
Sealwort .... see SOLOMON'S SEAL

Seawrack .... see BLADDERWRACK
Secale cereale .... see RYE GRASS
Secale cornutum .... see ERGOT
SECRETIN .... see SECRETIN
Sedum acre .... see COMMON STONECROP
Sedum rhodiola .... see ROSEROOT
Sedum rosea .... see ROSEROOT
See Bright .... see CLARY SAGE
Seed-Free Bean Pods .... see BEAN POD
Seed on the Leaf .... see CHANCA PIEDRA
Seedorn .... see SEA BUCKTHORN
Segg .... see ORRIS
Sehydrin .... see HYDRAZINE SULFATE
Selada-Air .... see WATERCRESS
Selagine .... see HUPERZINE A
Selenicereus grandiflorus .... see CEREUS
SELENIUM .... see SELENIUM
SELF-HEAL .... see SELF-HEAL
Self-Heal .... see SANICLE
Selleriefruchte .... see CELERY
Selleriesamen .... see CELERY
Semen Anisi .... see ANISE
Semen Cumini Pratensis ...... see CARAWAY dried fruit, seed
Semences de Carvi .... see CARAWAY dried fruit, seed
Seminole Bead .... see PRECATORY BEAN
Sempervivum tectorum .... see HOUSELEEK
Sena Alejandrina .... see SENNA
Senaga Snakeroot .... see SENEGA
Seneca .... see SENEGA
Seneca Snakeroot .... see SENEGA
Senecio aureus .... see GOLDEN RAGWORT
Senecio cineraria .... see DUSTY MILLER
Senecio Herb .... see ALPINE RAGWORT
Senecio jacoboea .... see TANSY RAGWORT
Senecio nemorensis .... see ALPINE RAGWORT
Senecio vulgaris .... see GROUNDSEL
SENEGA .... see SENEGA
Senega Snakeroot .... see SENEGA
Seneka .... see SENEGA
Seng .... see GINSENG, PANAX
Sengreen .... see HOUSELEEK
SENNA .... see SENNA
Senna Alexandrina .... see SENNA
Sennae folium .... see SENNA
Sennae fructus .... see SENNA
Sennae fructus acutifoliae .... see SENNA
Sennae fructus angustifolia .... see SENNA
Septfoil .... see TORMENTIL
Serenoa repens .... see SAW PALMETTO
Serenoa serrulata .... see SAW PALMETTO
Serpent's Tongue ..... see AMERICAN ADDER'S TONGUE,
                          ENGLISH ADDER'S TONGUE
Serpentaria .... see ARISTOLOCHIA, MONEYWORT
Serpyllum .... see WILD THYME
Serratula spicata .... see MARSH BLAZING STAR
Seso Vegetal .... see ACKEE
Sessile Oak .... see OAK bark
Seven Barks .... see HYDRANGEA
Shaddock Oil .... see GRAPEFRUIT OIL
Shamrock .... see WOOD SORREL
Shanzha .... see HAWTHORN fruit,
                          HAWTHORN leaf, flower
SHARK CARTILAGE .... see SHARK CARTILAGE
Shark Liver .... see SHARK LIVER OIL

SHARK LIVER OIL .... see SHARK LIVER OIL
Shark Oil .... see SHARK LIVER OIL
Sharp-Lobe Hepatica .... see LIVERWORT
Shatter Stone .... see CHANCA PIEDRA
Shave Grass .... see HORSETAIL
Sheep Laurel .... see MOUNTAIN LAUREL
Sheep-Lice .... see HOUND'S TONGUE
Sheep Sorrel .... see YELLOW DOCK
Sheggs .... see ORRIS
Shelf Fungi .... see MAITAKE
SHELLAC .... see SHELLAC
Shellflower .... see TURTLE HEAD
Shen Min .... see FO-TI raw root
Shepherd's Barometer .... see SCARLET PIMPERNEL
Shepherd's Club .... see MULLEIN
Shepherd's Heart .... see SHEPHERD'S PURSE
Shepherd's Knapperty .... see TORMENTIL
Shepherd's Knot .... see TORMENTIL
Shepherd's Needle .... see SWEET CICELY
SHEPHERD'S PURSE .... see SHEPHERD'S PURSE
Shepherd's Scrip .... see SHEPHERD'S PURSE
Shepherd's Sprout .... see SHEPHERD'S PURSE
Shepherd's Staff .... see MULLEIN
Shepherd's Thyme .... see WILD THYME
Shi Liu Gen Pi .... see POMEGRANATE
Shi Liu Pi .... see POMEGRANATE
Shield Fern .... see MALE FERN
Shigoka .... see GINSENG, SIBERIAN
Shih Yin Ch'en .... see YIN CHEN
SHIITAKE MUSHROOM ..... see SHIITAKE MUSHROOM
Shitake .... see SHIITAKE MUSHROOM
Sho-saiko-to .... see BUPLEURUM
Shore Cranberry .... see ALPINE CRANBERRY
Short Buchu .... see BUCHU
Shoti .... see ZEDOARY
Shou Wu .... see FO-TI raw root
Shovelweed .... see SHEPHERD'S PURSE
Shoyu .... see SOY
Shrubby Hare's-ear .... see BUPLEURUM
Shu-Wei Ts'ao .... see DANSHEN
Siberian Beaver .... see CASTOREUM
Siberian Ginseng .... see GINSENG, SIBERIAN
Sicilian Thyme .... see SPANISH ORIGANUM OIL
Sickle-leaf Hare's-ear .... see BUPLEURUM
Sicklewort .... see BUGLE, SELF-HEAL
Siclewort .... see SELF-HEAL
Sida cordifolia .... see COUNTRY MALLOW
Side-Saddle Plant .... see PITCHER PLANT
Sigualuo .... see LUFFA
Silberdistelwurz .... see CARLINA
Silberweide .... see WILLOW BARK
Silerkraut .... see ALCHEMILLA
Silky Cornel .... see AMERICAN DOGWOOD
Silky Loofah .... see LUFFA
Silphium laciniatum .... see ROSINWEED
Silphium perfoliatum .... see CUP PLANT
Silver Birch .... see BIRCH
Silver in suspending agent .... see COLLOIDAL SILVER
Silver Leaf .... see QUEEN'S DELIGHT
SILVER LINDEN .... see SILVER LINDEN
Silver-Morning-Glory .... see HAWAIIAN BABY
                                              WOODROSE
Silver Protein .... see COLLOIDAL SILVER
Silverweed .... see JEWELWEED, POTENTILLA

© Copyright 2000, Natural Medicines Comprehensive Database (209) 472-2244. For updated data, go to www.NaturalDatabase.com. • 1509

INDEX

Silybum .... see MILK THISTLE fruit, seed
Silybum marianum
.... see MILK THISTLE above ground parts,
MILK THISTLE fruit, seed
Silymarin .... see MILK THISTLE above ground parts,
MILK THISTLE fruit, seed
SIMARUBA .... see SIMARUBA
Simaruba amara .... see SIMARUBA
Simmondsia chinensis .... see JOJOBA
Simpler's Joy .... see VERBENA
Simson .... see GROUNDSEL
Sinapis alba .... see WHITE MUSTARD
Sinapis albae semen .... see WHITE MUSTARD
Sine Semine .... see BEAN POD
Singer's Plant .... see HEDGE MUSTARD
Singletary Pea .... see LATHYRUS
Sinsemilla .... see MARIJUANA
Sisymbrium officinale .... see HEDGE MUSTARD
SITOSTANOL .... see SITOSTANOL
Sitosterin .... see BETA-SITOSTEROL
Sitosterol .... see BETA-SITOSTEROL
Sitosterolins .... see BETA-SITOSTEROL
Sitosterols .... see BETA-SITOSTEROL
Sium sisarum .... see SKIRRET
SJW .... see ST JOHN'S WORT
Skewerwood .... see WAHOO
SKIRRET .... see SKIRRET
Skoke .... see POKEWEED berry, POKEWEED root
Skullcap .... see BAIKAL SKULLCAP, SCULLCAP
SKUNK CABBAGE .... see SKUNK CABBAGE
Skunkweed .... see SKUNK CABBAGE
Slave Wood .... see SIMARUBA
Slipper Root .... see NERVE ROOT
Slipper Weed .... see JEWELWEED
SLIPPERY ELM .... see SLIPPERY ELM
Slippery Root .... see COMFREY
Sloe .... see BLACKTHORN berry
Sloe Berry .... see BLACKTHORN berry
Sloe Flower .... see BLACKTHORN flower
Slough-Heal .... see SELF-HEAL
Small Cranberry .... see CRANBERRY
Small Hemlock .... see FOOL'S PARSLEY
Small Nettle
.... see STINGING NETTLE above ground parts,
STINGING NETTLE root
Small Periwinkle .... see PERIWINKLE
Small Radish .... see RADISH
Small Spikenard .... see AMERICAN SPIKENARD
Smallage .... see CELERY, LOVAGE
Smallpox Plant .... see PITCHER PLANT
Smallwort .... see LESSER CELANDINE
SMARTWEED .... see SMARTWEED
Smell Fox .... see WOOD ANEMONE
Smellage .... see LOVAGE
Smilax aristolochiaefolii .... see SARSAPARILLA
Smilax aristolochiifolia .... see SARSAPARILLA
Smilax febrifuga .... see SARSAPARILLA
Smilax medica .... see SARSAPARILLA
Smilax officinalis .... see SARSAPARILLA
Smilax regelii .... see SARSAPARILLA
SMOKELESS TOBACCO .... see SMOKELESS TOBACCO
Smooth Hydrangea .... see HYDRANGEA
Smooth Lawsonia .... see HENNA
Smooth-Leaved Elm .... see ELM BARK

Smooth Loofah .... see LUFFA
Smut Rye .... see ERGOT
Sene d'Egypte .... see SENNA
Snake Butter .... see SHIITAKE MUSHROOM
Snake Leaf .... see AMERICAN ADDER'S TONGUE
Snake Lily .... see ORRIS
Snake Root .... see BITTER MILKWORT, SENEGA
Snakeberry .... see BITTERSWEET NIGHTSHADE,
WHITE COHOSH
Snakebite .... see BETH ROOT, BLOODROOT
Snakehead .... see TURTLE HEAD
Snakeroot .... see ASARABACCA, ECHINACEA
Snakeweed .... see ARISTOLOCHIA,
BISTORT, EUPHORBIA
Snap Bean .... see BEAN POD
Snapdragon .... see YELLOW TOADFLAX
Snapping Tobacco Wood .... see WITCH HAZEL
SNEEZEWORT .... see SNEEZEWORT
Snow Rose .... see RUSTY-LEAVED RHODODENDRON
Snowball Bush .... see CRAMP BARK
Snowdrop Tree .... see FRINGETREE
Snowflower .... see FRINGETREE
Snuff .... see SMOKELESS TOBACCO
Soap Tree .... see QUILLAIA
Soap Tree Bark .... see QUILLAIA
Soapbark .... see QUILLAIA
Soapweed .... see YUCCA
Soapwort .... see RED SOAPWORT, WHITE SOAPWORT
SOD .... see SUPEROXIDE DISMUTASE
Sodium 4-hydroxybutyrate ....
see GAMMA HYDROXYBUTYRATE
Sodium Alginate .... see ALGIN
Sodium Ascorbate .... see VITAMIN C
Sodium gamma-hydroxybutyrate .... see GAMMA
HYDROXYBUTYRATE
Sodium Gluconate .... see PANGAMIC ACID
Sodium Orthophosphate .... see PHOSPHATE SALTS
Sodium Oxybate ...... see GAMMA HYDROXYBUTYRATE
Sodium Oxybutyrate
.... see GAMMA HYDROXYBUTYRATE
Sodium Phosphate .... see PHOSPHATE SALTS
Sodium Pyruvate .... see PYRUVATE
Soja .... see SOY
Sojabohne .... see SOY
Solanum dulcamara ..... see BITTERSWEET NIGHTSHADE
Solanum nigrum .... see BLACK NIGHTSHADE
Solanum tuberosum .... see POTATO
Soldiers .... see PURPLE LOOSESTRIFE
Soldier's Herb .... see BUCKHORN PLANTAIN
Soldier's Wound Wort .... see YARROW
Solidago virgaurea .... see GOLDENROD
SOLOMON'S SEAL .... see SOLOMON'S SEAL
Solsequia .... see MARSH MARIGOLD
Soma .... see AGA
Somalien Myrrh .... see MYRRH
Sonnenhutwurzel .... see ECHINACEA
Sophora japonica .... see PAGODA TREE
Sophorin .... see RUTIN
Sophretin .... see QUERCETIN
Sorb Apple .... see MOUNTAIN ASH
Sorbi acupariae fructus .... see MOUNTAIN ASH
Sorbus aucuparia .... see MOUNTAIN ASH
Sorghum .... see BROOM CORN
Sorghum vulgare .... see BROOM CORN

I
N
D
E
X

Sorosi .... see BITTER MELON
SORREL .... see SORREL
Sorrel .... see YELLOW DOCK
Sorrel Dock .... see SORREL
SOUR CHERRY .... see SOUR CHERRY
Sour Dock .... see SORREL, YELLOW DOCK
Sour Trefoil .... see WOOD SORREL
Souring Rush .... see HORSETAIL
South African Star Grass ...... see AFRICAN WILD POTATO
Southern Bayberry .... see BAYBERRY
Southern Black Haw .... see BLACK HAW
Southern Ginseng .... see JIAOGULAN
SOUTHERN PRICKLY ASH .... see SOUTHERN
                                                              PRICKLY ASH
Southern Schisandra .... see SCHISANDRA
Southern Wax Myrtle .... see BAYBERRY
Southernwood Root .... see CARLINA
Sow Berry .... see EUROPEAN BARBERRY
Sowbread .... see CYCLAMEN
SOY .... see SOY
Soy Fiber .... see SOY
Soy Milk .... see SOY
Soya .... see SOY
Soybean .... see SOY
Soybean Curd .... see SOY
Soybean Lecithin .... see LECITHIN
SOYBEAN OIL .... see SOYBEAN OIL
Soyca .... see SOYBEAN OIL
Soy-Protein .... see SOY
SP 303 .... see SANGRE DE GRADO
Spadic .... see COCA
Spanish Bayonet .... see YUCCA
SPANISH BROOM .... see SPANISH BROOM
Spanish Chestnut .... see EUROPEAN CHESTNUT,
                                    HORSE CHESTNUT branch bark,
                                        HORSE CHESTNUT flower,
                                              HORSE CHESTNUT leaf
Spanish Jasmine .... see JASMINE
Spanish Lavender .... see LAVENDER
Spanish Licorice .... see LICORICE
SPANISH ORIGANUM OIL
            .... see SPANISH ORIGANUM OIL
Spanish Psyllium .... see BLACK PSYLLIUM
Spanish Saffron .... see SAFFRON
Spanish Sage .... see SAGE
Spanish Thyme .... see SPANISH ORIGANUM OIL,
                          THYME flower, leaf, THYME OIL
Spanish Vetchling .... see LATHYRUS
Spargelkraut .... see ASPARAGUS
Spargelwurzelstock .... see ASPARAGUS
Sparrow Grass .... see ASPARAGUS
Sparrow Tongue .... see KNOTWEED HERB
Spartium junceum .... see SPANISH BROOM
Spartium scoparium .... see SCOTCH BROOM flower,
                                    SCOTCH BROOM herb
Spathyema Foetida .... see SKUNK CABBAGE
SPEARMINT .... see SPEARMINT
Speckled Jewels .... see JEWELWEED
Speedwell .... see BROOKLIME, VERONICA
Spergularia rubra .... see ARENARIA RUBRA
Spiceberry .... see WINTERGREEN leaf,
                                    WINTERGREEN oil
Spigelia marilandica .... see PINK ROOT
Spignet .... see AMERICAN SPIKENARD

Spike Lavender .... see LAVENDER
Spiked Loosestrife .... see PURPLE LOOSESTRIFE
SPINACH .... see SPINACH
Spinacia oleracea .... see SPINACH
Spinaciae folium .... see SPINACH
Spinatblatter .... see SPINACH
Spindle Tree .... see WAHOO
Spiny Dogfish Shark .... see SQUALAMINE
SPINY RESTHARROW .... see SPINY RESTHARROW
Spiraea ulmaria .... see MEADOWSWEET
Spiraeae flos .... see MEADOWSWEET
Spire Mint .... see SPEARMINT
Spireae herba .... see MEADOWSWEET
Spirit Plant .... see REISHI MUSHROOM
Spirits Of Turpentine .... see TURPENTINE OIL
Spirulina .... see BLUE-GREEN ALGAE
Spirulina maxima .... see BLUE-GREEN ALGAE
Spirulina platensis .... see BLUE-GREEN ALGAE
Spitzwegerichkraut .... see BUCKHORN PLANTAIN
Spogel .... see BLOND PSYLLIUM
Sponge Cucumber .... see LUFFA
Sponsa Solis .... see MARSH MARIGOLD
Spoon Laurel .... see MOUNTAIN LAUREL
Spoonwood .... see KAMALA
Spoonwort .... see SCURVY GRASS
Spotted Elder .... see WITCH HAZEL
Spotted Monarda .... see HORSEMINT
Spotted Thistle .... see BLESSED THISTLE
Spotted Touch-Me-Not .... see JEWELWEED
Spotted Wintergreen .... see PIPSISSEWA
Spring Grass .... see SWEET VERNAL GRASS
Spruce .... see FIR, HEMLOCK SPRUCE
Spruce Fir .... see FIR, HEMLOCK SPRUCE
Spumonto .... see KOMBUCHA TEA
Spurge Flax .... see MEZEREON
Spurge Laurel .... see MEZEREON
Spurge Olive .... see MEZEREON
Spurred Rye .... see ERGOT
Sqaulus acanthias .... see SHARK LIVER OIL
SQUALAMINE .... see SQUALAMINE
Squalus acanthias .... see SHARK CARTILAGE,
                                          SQUALAMINE
Squaw Balm .... see PENNYROYAL leaf,
                                    PENNYROYAL oil
Squaw Berry .... see SQUAWVINE
Squaw Root .... see BLUE COHOSH
Squaw Tea .... see MORMON TEA
Squaw Vine .... see SQUAWVINE
Squaw Weed .... see ALPINE RAGWORT,
                                    GOLDEN RAGWORT
Squawmint ..... see PENNYROYAL leaf, PENNYROYAL oil
Squawroot .... see BLACK COHOSH
SQUAWVINE .... see SQUAWVINE
Squawweed .... see ALPINE RAGWORT,
                                    GOLDEN RAGWORT
SQUILL .... see SQUILL
Squirrel Corn .... see CORYDALIS, TURKEY CORN
St Anthony's Turnip .... see BULBOUS BUTTERCUP
St Barbara's Hedge Mustard .... see HEDGE MUSTARD
St Bartholemew's Tea .... see MATE
St Benedict Thistle .... see BLESSED THISTLE
St James' Weed .... see SHEPHERD'S PURSE
St James Wort .... see TANSY RAGWORT
St James's Tea .... see LABRADOR TEA

INDEX

St John's Bread .... see CAROB
St John's Herb .... see HEMP AGRIMONY
St John's Plant .... see MUGWORT
ST JOHN'S WORT .... see ST JOHN'S WORT
St Josephwort .... see BASIL
St Mary Thistle ...... see MILK THISTLE above ground parts,
                            MILK THISTLE fruit, seed
St Mary's Seal .... see SOLOMON'S SEAL
ST-200 .... see ACETYL-L-CARNITINE
Stabilized Liquid Oxygen .... see VITAMIN O
Stabilized Oxygen .... see VITAMIN O
Stabilized Rice Bran .... see RICE BRAN
Stachys officinalis .... see BETONY
Staff Vine .... see BITTERSWEET NIGHTSHADE
Stag Bush .... see BLACK HAW
Staggerweed .... see DELPHINIUM,
                            LARKSPUR, TURKEY CORN
Staggerwort .... see TANSY RAGWORT
Stags Horn .... see CLUB MOSS
Stammerwort .... see TANSY RAGWORT
STAR ANISE .... see STAR ANISE
Star-Bu .... see SEA BUCKTHORN
Star Chickweed .... see CHICKWEED
Starbloom .... see PINK ROOT
Starchwort .... see ARUM
Starflower .... see BORAGE SEED OIL
Stargrass .... see ALETRIS
Starweed .... see CHICKWEED
Starwort .... see ALETRIS, FALSE UNICORN
Staunchweed .... see YARROW
Stave Oak .... see OAK bark
Stave Wood .... see SIMARUBA
STAVESACRE .... see STAVESACRE
Stay Plough .... see SPINY RESTHARROW
Stellaria .... see ALCHEMILLA
Stellaria media .... see CHICKWEED
Stemless Carlina Root .... see CARLINA
Stemless Gentian .... see GENTIAN
Sterculia acuminata .... see COLA NUT
Sterculia Gum .... see KARAYA GUM
Sterculia tragacanth .... see KARAYA GUM
Sterculia urens .... see KARAYA GUM
Sterculia villosa .... see KARAYA GUM
Sterinol .... see BETA-SITOSTEROL
Sterolins .... see BETA-SITOSTEROL
Sterretjie .... see AFRICAN WILD POTATO
STEVIA .... see STEVIA
Stevia eupatorium .... see STEVIA
Stevia rebaudiana .... see STEVIA
Stick-a-Back .... see CLIVERS
Stickwort .... see AGRIMONY, WOOD SORREL
Stigma Maydis .... see CORN SILK
Stigmastanol .... see SITOSTANOL
Stillingia .... see QUEEN'S DELIGHT
Stillingia sylvatica .... see QUEEN'S DELIGHT
Stillingia treculeana .... see QUEEN'S DELIGHT
STINGING NETTLE above ground parts
        .... see STINGING NETTLE above ground parts
STINGING NETTLE root ...... see STINGING NETTLE root
Stingless Nettle .... see WHITE DEAD NETTLE FLOWER
Stinking Arrach .... see ARRACH
Stinking Balm see PENNYROYAL leaf, PENNYROYAL oil
Stinking Benjamin .... see BETH ROOT
Stinking Goosefoot .... see ARRACH

Stinking Motherwort .... see ARRACH
Stinking Nanny .... see TANSY RAGWORT
Stinking Nightshade .... see HENBANE
Stinking Prairie Bush .... see WAFER ASH
Stinking Roger .... see TAGETES
Stinking Rose .... see GARLIC
Stinking Tommy .... see SPINY RESTHARROW
Stinking Willie .... see TANSY
Stinkweed .... see JIMSON WEED
Stinkwort .... see JIMSON WEED
Stone Oak .... see OAK bark
STONE ROOT .... see STONE ROOT
Stonebreaker .... see CHANCA PIEDRA
STORAX .... see STORAX
Storkbill .... see HERB ROBERT
Stractan .... see LARCH ARABINOGALACTAN
Strained Honey .... see HONEY
Stramonium .... see JIMSON WEED
Strangle Tare .... see DODDER
Straw .... see OAT STRAW
STRAWBERRY .... see STRAWBERRY
Strawberry Bush .... see WAHOO
Strawberry Tomato .... see WINTER CHERRY
Strawberry Tree .... see WAHOO
String Bean .... see BEAN POD
String Of Sovereigns .... see MONEYWORT
Stringy Bark Tree .... see EUCALYPTUS dried leaf
Strong-Scented Lettuce .... see WILD LETTUCE
Strophanthi Grati Semen .... see STROPHANTHUS
Strophanthi Kombe Semen .... see STROPHANTHUS
STROPHANTHUS .... see STROPHANTHUS
Strophanthus gratus .... see STROPHANTHUS
Strophanthus kombe .... see STROPHANTHUS
Strophanthus Seeds .... see STROPHANTHUS
Strychni Semen .... see NUX VOMICA
Strychnos ignatii .... see IGNATIUS BEAN
Strychnos nux-vomica .... see NUX VOMICA
Strychnos Seed .... see NUX VOMICA
Stubwort .... see WOOD SORREL
Styrax .... see STORAX
Styrax benzoin .... see BENZOIN
Styrax paralleloneurus .... see BENZOIN
Subholz .... see LICORICE
Succory .... see CHICORY
Sudanese Tea .... see HIBISCUS
Sugar Maple .... see RED MAPLE
Sugar Pods .... see CAROB
Sugarbeet .... see BEET
Sulfated N-Carboxymethylchitosan .... see CHITOSAN
Sulfated O-Carboxymethylchitosan .... see CHITOSAN
Sulfonyl Sulfur .... see MSM
Sultanas .... see GRAPE fruit, skin
SUMA .... see SUMA
Sumaruba .... see SIMARUBA
Sumatra Benzoin .... see BENZOIN
SUMBUL .... see SUMBUL
SUMMER SAVORY .... see SUMMER SAVORY
Sumpfporst .... see MARSH TEA
Sun Drop .... see EVENING PRIMROSE OIL
Sun Rose .... see FROSTWORT
SUNDEW .... see SUNDEW
SUNFLOWER OIL .... see SUNFLOWER OIL
Sunkfield............. see EUROPEAN FIVE-FINGER GRASS

INDEX

SUPEROXIDE DISMUTASE .... see SUPEROXIDE DISMUTASE
Surelle .... see WOOD SORREL
Surgical Maggot .... see MAGGOTS
Surinam Quassia .... see QUASSIA
Surinam Wood .... see QUASSIA
Swallow-Wort .... see PLEURISY ROOT
Swamp Cabbage .... see SKUNK CABBAGE
Swamp Cedar .... see CEDAR leaf, CEDAR LEAF OIL
Swamp Dogwood .... see AMERICAN DOGWOOD, WAFER ASH
Swamp Laurel .... see MAGNOLIA bark
Swamp Maple .... see RED MAPLE
SWAMP MILKWEED .... see SWAMP MILKWEED
Swamp Root .... see YERBA MANSA
Swamp Sassafras .... see MAGNOLIA bark
Swamp Silkweed .... see SWAMP MILKWEED
Swamp Tea .... see MARSH TEA
Sweating Plant .... see BONESET
Sweatroot .... see ABSCESS ROOT
Sweet Acacia .... see CASSIE ABSOLUTE
SWEET ALMOND .... see SWEET ALMOND
Sweet Almond Oil .... see SWEET ALMOND
SWEET ANNIE .... see SWEET ANNIE
Sweet Balm .... see LEMON BALM
Sweet Bark .... see CASCARILLA
Sweet Basil .... see BASIL
SWEET BAY .... see SWEET BAY
Sweet Bay .... see MAGNOLIA bark
Sweet Bracken .... see SWEET CICELY
Sweet Broom .... see BUTCHER'S BROOM
Sweet Bugle .... see BUGLEWEED
Sweet Cane .... see CALAMUS
Sweet Chamomile .... see ROMAN CHAMOMILE
Sweet Chervil .... see SWEET CICELY
Sweet Chestnut .... see EUROPEAN CHESTNUT
SWEET CICELY .... see SWEET CICELY
Sweet Cinnamon .... see CALAMUS
SWEET CLOVER .... see SWEET CLOVER
Sweet Cumin .... see ANISE
Sweet-Cus .... see SWEET CICELY
Sweet Dock .... see BISTORT
Sweet Elder .... see AMERICAN ELDER, EUROPEAN ELDER flower
Sweet Elm .... see SLIPPERY ELM
Sweet False Chamomile .... see GERMAN CHAMOMILE
Sweet Fennel .... see FENNEL fruit, seed
Sweet-Fern .... see SWEET CICELY
Sweet Flag .... see BLUE FLAG, CALAMUS
SWEET GALE .... see SWEET GALE
Sweet Grass .... see CALAMUS
Sweet Gum .... see STORAX
Sweet-Humlock .... see SWEET CICELY
Sweet Leaf of Paraguay .... see STEVIA
Sweet Lucerne .... see SWEET CLOVER
Sweet Mandulin .... see HEMP AGRIMONY
Sweet Marjoram .... see MARJORAM
Sweet Mary .... see LEMON BALM
Sweet Melilot .... see SWEET CLOVER
Sweet Myrtle .... see CALAMUS
Sweet Oil .... see OLIVE OIL
SWEET ORANGE .... see SWEET ORANGE
Sweet Pea .... see LATHYRUS
Sweet Pepper .... see CAPSICUM
Sweet Root .... see CALAMUS, LICORICE
Sweet Rush .... see CALAMUS
Sweet Scented Cactus .... see CEREUS
Sweet Sedge .... see CALAMUS
Sweet Slumber .... see BLOODROOT
Sweet-Smelling Trefoil .... see HEMP AGRIMONY
SWEET SUMACH .... see SWEET SUMACH
Sweet Vernal .... see PHEASANT'S EYE
SWEET VERNAL GRASS .. see SWEET VERNAL GRASS
Sweet Vernal Grass .... see HAY FLOWER
SWEET VIOLET .... see SWEET VIOLET
Sweet Violet Herb .... see SWEET VIOLET
Sweet Violet Root .... see SWEET VIOLET
Sweet Weed .... see MARSHMALLOW
Sweet Wood Bark .... see CASCARILLA
SWEET WOODRUFF .... see SWEET WOODRUFF
Sweet Wormwood .... see SWEET ANNIE
Sweethearts .... see CLIVERS
Sweetleaf .... see STEVIA
Sweets .... see SWEET CICELY
Swertia chirata .... see CHIRATA
Swine Snout .... see DANDELION above ground parts, DANDELION entire plant
Swinebread .... see CYCLAMEN
Swine's Grass .... see KNOTWEED HERB
Swiss Mountain Pine .... see PINE
Swynel Grass .... see KNOTWEED HERB
Sycocarpus rusbyi .... see COCILLANA
Symphytum officinale .... see COMFREY
Symphytum Radix .... see COMFREY
Symplocarpus foetidus .... see SKUNK CABBAGE
Synkfoyle .... see EUROPEAN FIVE-FINGER GRASS
Syrian Tragacanth .... see TRAGACANTH
Syxygii cumini cortex .... see JAMBOLAN bark
Syxygii cumini semen .... see JAMBOLAN seed
Syzugium cumini .... see JAMBOLAN bark
Syzugium jambolana .... see JAMBOLAN bark
Syzygium aromaticum .... see CLOVE dried flowerbud, leaf, stem, CLOVE OIL
Syzygium cumini .... see JAMBOLAN seed
Syzygium cumini jambolana .... see JAMBOLAN seed
Tabasco Pepper .... see CAPSICUM
Tabebuia avellanedae .... see PAU D'ARCO
Tabebuia heptaphylla .... see PAU D'ARCO
Tabebuia impetiginosa .... see PAU D'ARCO
Tabernanthe iboga .... see IBOGA
Table Grapes .... see GRAPE fruit, skin
Tag Alder .... see BLACK ALDER
TAGETES .... see TAGETES
Tagetes erecta .... see TAGETES
Tagetes glandulifera .... see TAGETES
Tagetes minuta .... see TAGETES
Tagetes patula .... see TAGETES
Taheebo .... see PAU D'ARCO
Taheebo Tea .... see PAU D'ARCO
Tahiti Vanilla .... see VANILLA
Tahitian Noni Juice .... see MORINDA
Tahitian Vanilla .... see VANILLA
Tailed Chubebs .... see CUBEBS
Tailed Pepper .... see CUBEBS
Take Control .... see SOYBEAN OIL
Takila .... see ANDROGRAPHIS
Talepetrako .... see GOTU KOLA

© Copyright 2000, Natural Medicines Comprehensive Database (209) 472-2244. For updated data, go to www.NaturalDatabase.com. • 1513

INDEX

Tall Melilot .... see SWEET CLOVER
Tall Nasturtium .... see WATERCRESS
Tall Speedwell .... see BLACK ROOT
Tall Veronica .... see BLACK ROOT
Tallow Shrub .... see BAYBERRY
Tamalaka .... see CHANCA PIEDRA
TAMARIND .... see TAMARIND
Tamarindo .... see TAMARIND
Tamarindus indica .... see TAMARIND
Tamus .... see BRYONIA
Tamus communis .... see BLACK BRYONY
Tan Kue Bai Zhi .... see DONG QUAI
Tan-Shen .... see DANSHEN
Tan Xiang .... see WHITE SANDALWOOD wood
Tanaceti parthenii .... see FEVERFEW
Tanacetum parthenium .... see FEVERFEW
Tanacetum vulgare .... see TANSY
Tang .... see BLADDERWRACK
Tang Kuei .... see DONG QUAI
Tangantangan Oil Plant ... see CASTOR OIL, CASTOR seed
Tanner's Bark .... see OAK bark
Tanner's Oak .... see OAK bark
TANNIC ACID .... see TANNIC ACID
TANSY .... see TANSY
Tansy Flower .... see TANSY
Tansy Herb .... see TANSY
TANSY RAGWORT .... see TANSY RAGWORT
Taraxaci herba .... see DANDELION above ground parts
Taraxacum .... see DANDELION above ground parts,
                                      DANDELION entire plant
Taraxacum officinale
      .... see DANDELION above ground parts,
                                      DANDELION entire plant
Taraxacum vulgare
      .... see DANDELION above ground parts,
                                      DANDELION entire plant
Tare .... see TAUMELLOOLCH
Target-Leaved Hibiscus .... see AMBRETTE
TARRAGON .... see TARRAGON
Tart Cherry .... see SOUR CHERRY
Tartaric Acid .... see ALPHA HYDROXY ACIDS
Tarweed .... see GUMWEED, YERBA SANTA
Tasmanian Blue Gum .... see EUCALYPTUS dried leaf
Taso-Ho-Hua .... see THUNDER GOD VINE
Taspine .... see SANGRE DE GRADO
Tatuaba .... see CATUABA
TAUMELLOOLCH .... see TAUMELLOOLCH
Tausendaugbram .... see YARROW
Taxus bacatta .... see YEW
Taxus brevifolia .... see YEW
TC-80 .... see IPRIFLAVONE
Tchaad .... see KHAT
T'Chai from the Sea .... see KOMBUCHA TEA
TCV-3b .... see VINPOCETINE
Tea .... see BLACK TEA, GREEN TEA
TEA TREE OIL .... see TEA TREE OIL
Teaberry .... see WINTERGREEN leaf,
                                      WINTERGREEN oil
Teamster's Tea .... see EPHEDRA, MORMON TEA
Teasel .... see BONESET, TEAZLE
TEAZLE .... see TEAZLE
Tecuitlatl .... see BLUE-GREEN ALGAE
Teinturiere .... see POKEWEED berry, POKEWEED root
Temu Kuning .... see ZEDOARY

Temu Lawak .... see JAVANESE TURMERIC
Temu Lawas .... see JAVANESE TURMERIC
Temu Putih .... see ZEDOARY
Terebinthina Laricina .... see LARCH TURPENTINE
Terebinthina Veneta .... see LARCH TURPENTINE
Terebinthinae aetheroleum .... see TURPENTINE OIL
TERMINALIA .... see TERMINALIA
Terminalia arjuna .... see TERMINALIA
Terminalia belerica .... see TERMINALIA
Terminalia bellirica .... see TERMINALIA
Terminalia chebula .... see TERMINALIA
Terra Japonica .... see CATECHU
Tertiary Calcium Phosphate .... see PHOSPHATE SALTS
Tetrahydro-2-Furanone .... see GAMMA
                                      BUTYROLACTONE
Tetramethylene glycol .... see BUTANEDIOL
Tetramethylene-1,4-diol .... see BUTANEDIOL
Tetterberry .... see BRYONIA
Tetterwort .... see BLOODROOT,
      GREATER CELANDINE dried above ground parts
Teucrium chamaedrys .... see GERMANDER
Teucrium scordium .... see WATER GERMANDER
Teucrium scorodonia .... see WOOD SAGE
Tewon Lawa .... see JAVANESE TURMERIC
Texas Cedarwood .... see CEDARWOOD bark,
                                  berry, leaf, seed, twig
Thalictroc .... see HEDGE MUSTARD
The Roman Plant .... see SWEET CICELY
Thea bohea.......................... see BLACK TEA, GREEN TEA
Thea sinensis .... see BLACK TEA, GREEN TEA
Thea viridis .... see BLACK TEA, GREEN TEA
Theobroma .... see COCOA
Theobroma cacao .... see COCOA
Thevetia peruviana .... see OLEANDER
Thiamin .... see THIAMINE
Thiamin Chloride .... see THIAMINE
Thiamin Hydrochloride .... see THIAMINE
THIAMINE .... see THIAMINE
Thiamine Chloride .... see THIAMINE
Thiamine Hydrochloride .... see THIAMINE
Thiaminium Chloride Hydrochloride .... see THIAMINE
Thick-Leaved Pennywort .... see GOTU KOLA
Thimbleberry .... see BLACKBERRY leaf,
                                      BLACKBERRY root
Thioctacid .... see ALPHA-LIPOIC ACID
Thioctan .... see ALPHA-LIPOIC ACID
Thioctic Acid .... see ALPHA-LIPOIC ACID
Thomas Balsam .... see TOLU BALSAM
Thompson Seedless .... see GRAPE fruit, skin
Thormantle .... see TORMENTIL
Thorn-apple .... see JIMSON WEED
Thorny Burr .... see BURDOCK
Thoroughwax .... see BUPLEURUM
Thoroughwort .... see BONESET, HEMP AGRIMONY
Thor's Beard .... see HOUSELEEK
Thousand-Leaf.................................. see YARROW
Three-Leafed Ivy .... see POISON IVY
Three-Leafed Nightshade .... see BETH ROOT
Three-Leaved Grass .... see WOOD SORREL
Three-Leaved Hop Tree .... see WAFER ASH
Three Seven .... see PANAX PSEUDOGINSENG
Threewingnut....................... see THUNDER GOD VINE
Throat Root .... see WATER AVENS
Throatwort .... see DIGITALIS, FIGWORT

INDEX

Throw-Wort .... see MOTHERWORT
Thuga .... see CEDAR leaf
Thuja .... see CEDAR leaf, CEDAR LEAF OIL
Thuja occidentalis .... see CEDAR leaf, CEDAR LEAF OIL
Thuja Oil .... see CEDAR LEAF OIL
Thuja orientalis .... see ORIENTAL ARBORVITAE
THUNDER GOD VINE .... see THUNDER GOD VINE
Thunder Plant .... see HOUSELEEK
Thyme Aetheroleum .... see THYME OIL
THYME flower, leaf .... see THYME flower, leaf
THYME OIL .... see THYME OIL
Thyme-Leave Gratiola .... see BRAHMI
Thymi herba .... see THYME flower, leaf
Thymus capitatus .... see SPANISH ORIGANUM OIL
Thymus serpyllum .... see WILD THYME
Thymus vulgaris ...... see THYME flower, leaf, THYME OIL
Thymus zygis .... see THYME flower, leaf, THYME OIL
Tian Hua Fen .... see CHINESE CUCUMBER root
Tian Qi .... see PANAX PSEUDOGINSENG
Tiarella cordifolia .... see COOLWORT
Tickleweed Veratro Verdesee
.... AMERICAN HELLEBORE
Tickweed .... see PENNYROYAL leaf, PENNYROYAL oil
Tienchi Ginseng .... see GINSENG, AMERICAN
Tiglium .... see CROTON SEEDS
Tiglium Seeds .... see CROTON SEEDS
Tilia argentea .... see SILVER LINDEN
Tilia cordata .... see LINDEN CHARCOAL,
                                                  LINDEN dried flower,
                                                  LINDEN dried leaf,
                                                  LINDEN dried sapwood
Tilia platyphyllos .... see LINDEN CHARCOAL,
                                                  LINDEN dried flower,
                                                  LINDEN dried leaf,
                                                  LINDEN dried sapwood
Tilia tormentosa .... see SILVER LINDEN
Tiliae carbo .... see LINDEN CHARCOAL
Tiliae flos .... see LINDEN dried flower
Tiliae folium .... see LINDEN dried leaf
Tiliae lignum .... see LINDEN dried sapwood
Tiliae tormentosae flos .... see SILVER LINDEN
Tilki Uzumu .... see HERB PARIS
Timothy .... see HAY FLOWER
Tindved .... see SEA BUCKTHORN
Tinnevelly Senna .... see SENNA
Tipton Weed .... see ST JOHN'S WORT
TIRATRICOL .... see TIRATRICOL
To-Nezumimochi .... see GLOSSY PRIVET
Toadpipe .... see HORSETAIL, YELLOW TOADFLAX
Tobacco .... see SMOKELESS TOBACCO
Tocopherol .... see VITAMIN E
Tocopheryl Acetate .... see VITAMIN E
Tocopheryl Acid Succinate .... see VITAMIN E
Tocopheryl Succinate .... see VITAMIN E
Tocotrienol .... see VITAMIN E
Tofu .... see SOY
Tohai .... see KHAT
Tohat .... see KHAT
Toliufera balsamum .... see TOLU BALSAM
Tolu .... see TOLU BALSAM
TOLU BALSAM .... see TOLU BALSAM
Toluiferum Balsamum .... see TOLU BALSAM
Tom Rong .... see GAMBOGE
TOMATO .... see TOMATO

Tonga .... see KAVA
Tonka .... see TONKA BEAN
TONKA BEAN .... see TONKA BEAN
Tonka Seed .... see TONKA BEAN
Tonquin Bean .... see TONKA BEAN
Tonquin Musk .... see MUSK
Toothache Bark .... see NORTHERN PRICKLY ASH
Toothache Tree .... see SOUTHERN PRICKLY ASH
Torch Weed .... see MULLEIN
Torches .... see MULLEIN
TORMENTIL .... see TORMENTIL
Tormentilla .... see TORMENTIL
Tormentillae rhizoma .... see TORMENTIL
Toronja .... see GRAPEFRUIT
Torquin Bean .... see TONKA BEAN
Touch-Me-Not ... see GINSENG, SIBERIAN, JEWELWEED
Toute Epice .... see BLACK SEED
Toxicodendron radicans .... see POISON IVY
Toywort .... see SHEPHERD'S PURSE
Trackleberry .... see BILBERRY dried ripe fruit,
                                                  BILBERRY leaf
TRAGACANTH .... see TRAGACANTH
Tragacanth Gum .... see TRAGACANTH
TRAILING ARBUTUS .... see TRAILING ARBUTUS
Trailing Mahonia .... see OREGON GRAPE
Trailing Swamp Cranberry .... see CRANBERRY
Trailing Tansy .... see POTENTILLA
Trametes versicolor .... see CORIOLUS MUSHROOM
Trans-10,cis-12 conjugated linoleic acid . see CONJUGATED
                                                  LINOLEIC ACID
Trans-Resveratrol .... see RESVERATROL
TRAVELER'S JOY .... see TRAVELER'S JOY
Traveler's-Joy .... see WOODBINE
Travmulsion .... see SOYBEAN OIL
Tree Moss .... see OAK MOSS, USNEA
TREE OF HEAVEN .... see TREE OF HEAVEN
Tree of Life .... see CEDAR leaf, CEDAR LEAF OIL
Tree's Dandruff .... see USNEA
Trefoil .... see LIVERWORT, RED CLOVER
Triac .... see TIRATRICOL
Triacylglycerol lipase .... see LIPASE
Tribule terrestre .... see PUNCTURE VINE
Tribulus .... see PUNCTURE VINE
Tribulus terrestris .... see PUNCTURE VINE
Tricalcium Phosphate .... see CALCIUM,
                                                  PHOSPHATE SALTS
Tricholomopsis edodes .... see LENTINAN,
                                                  SHIITAKE MUSHROOM
Trichosanthes .... see CHINESE CUCUMBER fruit,
                                                  CHINESE CUCUMBER root,
                                                  CHINESE CUCUMBER seed
Trichosanthes kirilowii .... see CHINESE CUCUMBER fruit,
                                                  CHINESE CUCUMBER root,
                                                  CHINESE CUCUMBER seed
Trifolium .... see RED CLOVER
Trifolium pratense .... see RED CLOVER
Trigonella .... see FENUGREEK
Trigonella foenum-graecum .... see FENUGREEK
triiodothyroacetic acid .... see TIRATRICOL
Trilisa odoratissima .... see DEERTONGUE
Trillium erectum .... see BETH ROOT
Trimethylethanolamine .... see CHOLINE
Trimethylglycine .... see BETAINE ANHYDROUS

INDEX

Trimethylglycine hydrochloride
.... see BETAINE HYDROCHLORIDE
Tripsin .... see TRYPSIN
Tripterygium wilfordii .... see THUNDER GOD VINE
Triticum .... see AGROPYRON
Triticum aestrivum .... see WHEAT BRAN
Triticum repens .... see AGROPYRON, COUCH GRASS
Trollius europaeus .... see GLOBE FLOWER
Trompillo .... see COCILLANA
Troene De Chine .... see GLOSSY PRIVET
Tropaeolum majus .... see NASTURTIUM
True Angostura .... see ANGOSTURA
True Bay .... see SWEET BAY
True Chamomile .... see GERMAN CHAMOMILE
True Ivy .... see ENGLISH IVY
True Lavender .... see LAVENDER
True Saffron .... see SAFFRON
True Sage .... see SAGE
True Senna .... see SENNA
Trueno .... see GLOSSY PRIVET
Trumpet Bush .... see PAU D'ARCO
Trumpet Weed .... see GRAVEL ROOT
Truxillo Coca .... see COCA
TRYPSIN .... see TRYPSIN
Tryptophan .... see L-TRYPTOPHAN
Tschambucco .... see KOMBUCHA TEA
Tschut .... see KHAT
Tsuga canadensis .... see PINUS BARK
Tsuru-kokemomo .... see CRANBERRY
Tuber Root .... see PLEURISY ROOT
Tuckahoe .... see PORIA MUSHROOM
Tumeric .... see TURMERIC
Tun-Hoof .... see GROUND IVY
Tuna Cardona .... see PRICKLY PEAR CACTUS
Tung .... see TUNG SEED
TUNG SEED .... see TUNG SEED
Turangi-Ghanda .... see WITHANIA
Turi Hutan .... see CHANCA PIEDRA
Turkey Claw .... see CORAL ROOT
Turkey Corn .... see CORYDALIS
TURKEY CORN .... see TURKEY CORN
Turkey Grass .... see VERBENA
Turkey Rhubarb .... see RHUBARB
Turkey Tail .... see CORIOLUS MUSHROOM
Turk's Cap .... see MARTAGON
TURMERIC .... see TURMERIC
Turmeric .... see ZEDOARY
Turmeric Root .... see GOLDENSEAL, TURMERIC
Turnera aphrodisiaca .... see DAMIANA
Turnera diffusa .... see DAMIANA
Turnera microphylla .... see DAMIANA
Turnerae diffusae folium .... see DAMIANA
Turnerae diffusae herba .... see DAMIANA
Turnhoof .... see GROUND IVY
Turnip Radish .... see RADISH
TURPENTINE OIL .... see TURPENTINE OIL
Turpentine Weed .... see CUP PLANT
TURTLE HEAD .... see TURTLE HEAD
Turtlebloom .... see TURTLE HEAD
Tussilage .... see COLTSFOOT
Tussilago farfara .... see COLTSFOOT
Twinberry .... see SQUAWVINE
Twitchgrass .... see AGROPYRON
Two-Eyed Berry .... see SQUAWVINE

Twopenny Grass .... see MONEYWORT
Tyosen-Azami .... see ARTICHOKE
Tzu Tan-Ken .... see DANSHEN
Una De Gato .... see CAT'S CLAW
Ubidecarenone .... see COENZYME Q-10
Ubiquinone .... see COENZYME Q-10
Ulmaria .... see MEADOWSWEET
Ulmus fulva .... see SLIPPERY ELM
Ulmus minor .... see ELM BARK
Ulmus rubra .... see SLIPPERY ELM
Umbellate Wintergreen .... see PIPSISSEWA
Umbrella Leaves .... see PETASITES leaf
Uncaria Gambier Leaf/Twig Extract .... see CATECHU
Uncaria guianensis .... see CAT'S CLAW
Uncaria tomentosa .... see CAT'S CLAW
Undi .... see LAURELWOOD
Unicorn Root .... see ALETRIS
Upas .... see COCILLANA
Upright Virgin's Bower .... see CLEMATIS
Upstart .... see AUTUMN CROCUS
Uragoga granatensis .... see IPECAC
Uragoga ipecacuanha .... see IPECAC
Urginea indica .... see SQUILL
Urginea maritima .... see SQUILL
Urginea scilla .... see SQUILL
Urtica .... see STINGING NETTLE above ground parts,
                    STINGING NETTLE root
Urtica dioica .. see STINGING NETTLE above ground parts,
                    STINGING NETTLE root
Urtica urens .... see STINGING NETTLE above groundparts,
                    STINGING NETTLE root
Urticae herba et folium
.... see STINGING NETTLE above ground parts
Urticae Radix .... see STINGING NETTLE root
USNEA .... see USNEA
Usnea barbata .... see USNEA
Usnea florida .... see USNEA
Usnea hirta .... see USNEA
Usnea Lichen .... see USNEA
Usnea plicata .... see USNEA
Ussuri .... see GINSENG, SIBERIAN
Ussurian Thorny Pepperbrush ..... see GINSENG, SIBERIAN
Utricularia vulgaris .... see BLADDERWORT
Uva De Raposa .... see HERB PARIS
UVA URSI .... see UVA URSI
Uvae ursi folium .... see UVA URSI
UZARA .... see UZARA
Uzarae radix .... see UZARA
V .... see VANADIUM
V fragrans .... see VANILLA
V tahitensis .... see VANILLA
va Capitata .... see CABBAGE
Vaccinium hagerupii .... see CRANBERRY
Vaccinium macrocarpon .... see CRANBERRY
Vaccinium microcarpum .... see CRANBERRY
Vaccinium myrtillus .... see BILBERRY dried ripe fruit,
                                BILBERRY leaf
Vaccinium oxycoccos .... see CRANBERRY
Vaccinium palustre .... see CRANBERRY
Vaccinium uliginosum .... see BOG BILBERRY
Vaccinium vitis-idaea .... see ALPINE CRANBERRY
Valencia Orange .... see SWEET ORANGE
VALERIAN .... see VALERIAN
Valeriana .... see VALERIAN

Valeriana edulis .... see VALERIAN
Valeriana jatamansii .... see VALERIAN
Valeriana officinalis .... see VALERIAN
Valeriana rhizome .... see VALERIAN
Valeriana sitchensis .... see VALERIAN
Valeriana wallichii .... see VALERIAN
Valerianae radix .... see VALERIAN
Valeriane .... see VALERIAN
Valine .... see BRANCHED-CHAIN AMINO ACIDS
Vanadate .... see VANADIUM
VANADIUM .... see VANADIUM
Vanadium Pentoxide .... see VANADIUM
Vanadyl .... see VANADIUM
Vanadyl Sulfate .... see VANADIUM
VANILLA .... see VANILLA
Vanilla Leaf .... see DEERTONGUE
Vanilla planifolia .... see VANILLA
Vanilla Plant .... see DEERTONGUE
Vanilla tahitensis .... see VANILLA
Vanilla Trilisa .... see DEERTONGUE
Vapor .... see FUMITORY
Varech .... see BLADDERWRACK
Varnish Tree .... see TREE OF HEAVEN, TUNG SEED
Vegetable Antimony .... see BONESET
Vegetable Caterpillar .... see CORDYCEPS
Vegetable Gelatin .... see AGAR
Vegetable Mercury .... see MANACA, PODOPHYLLUM
Vegetable Pepsin .... see PAPAIN
Vegetable Sponge .... see LUFFA
Vegetable Sulfur .... see CLUB MOSS
Vegetable Tallow .... see BAYBERRY
Vegilecithin .... see LECITHIN
Vellorita .... see AUTUMN CROCUS
Velvet Antler .... see DEER VELVET
Velvet Dock .... see ELECAMPANE
Velvet Flower .... see AMARANTH
Velvet Leaf .... see ABUTA, PAREIRA
Velvet of Young Deer Horn .... see DEER VELVET
Velvet Plant .... see MULLEIN
Venastat .... see HORSE CHESTNUT seed
Venetian Turpentine .... see LARCH TURPENTINE
Venostasin Retard .... see HORSE CHESTNUT seed
Venostat .... see HORSE CHESTNUT seed
Venus' Basin .... see TEAZLE
Venus Hair .... see MAIDENHAIR FERN
Venus Shoe .... see NERVE ROOT
Veratrum album .... see WHITE HELLEBORE
Veratrum luteum .... see FALSE UNICORN
Veratrum viride .... see AMERICAN HELLEBORE
Verbasci flos .... see MULLEIN
Verbascum densiflorum .... see MULLEIN
Verbascum phlomides .... see MULLEIN
Verbascum thapsiforme .... see MULLEIN
Verbascum thapsus .... see MULLEIN
VERBENA .... see VERBENA
Verbena citriodora .... see LEMON VERBENA
Verbena officinalis .... see VERBENA
Verbena triphylla .... see LEMON VERBENA
Verbenae herba .... see VERBENA
Vernis de Japon .... see TREE OF HEAVEN
VERONICA .... see VERONICA
Veronica beccabunga .... see BROOKLIME
Veronica Herb .... see VERONICA
Veronica officinalis .... see VERONICA

Veronica Virginica Root .... see BLACK ROOT
Veronicae herba .... see VERONICA
Veronicastrum Virginicum .... see BLACK ROOT
Verrucaria .... see MARSH MARIGOLD
Vervain .... see VERBENA
VETIVER .... see VETIVER
Vetivergras .... see VETIVER
Vetiveria zizanoides .... see VETIVER
Viable Antiseptic .... see MAGGOTS
Viburnum .... see BLACK HAW
Viburnum opulus .... see CRAMP BARK
Viburnum prunifolium .... see BLACK HAW
Viburnum prunifolium ferrugineum .... see BLACK HAW
Viburnum rufidulum .... see BLACK HAW
Vinca minor .... see PERIWINKLE
Vinca rosea .... see MADAGASCAR PERIWINKLE
Vincae minoris herba .... see PERIWINKLE
Vine Bower .... see WOODBINE
Vine of Mount Ida .... see ALPINE CRANBERRY
Vinettier .... see EUROPEAN BARBERRY
VINPOCETINE .... see VINPOCETINE
Viola odorata ...... see GARDEN VIOLET, SWEET VIOLET
Viola tricolor .... see HEART'S EASE
Violae Odoratae Rhizoma .... see SWEET VIOLET
Violae Tricoloris Herba .... see HEART'S EASE
Violet .... see SWEET VIOLET
Violet Bloom .... see BITTERSWEET NIGHTSHADE
Violet Willow .... see WILLOW BARK
Viosterol .... see VITAMIN D
Virginia Cedarwood
.... see CEDARWOOD bark, berry, leaf, seed, twig
Virginia Creeper .... see AMERICAN IVY
Virginia Serpentary .... see ARISTOLOCHIA
Virginia Snakeroot .... see ARISTOLOCHIA
Virginia Water Horehound .... see BUGLEWEED
Virginian Poke .... see POKEWEED berry, POKEWEED root
Virginian Prune .... see WILD CHERRY
Virginian Strawberry .... see STRAWBERRY
Virgin's Bower .... see WOODBINE
Visci .... see EUROPEAN MISTLETOE
Visci albi folia .... see EUROPEAN MISTLETOE
Visci albi fructus .... see EUROPEAN MISTLETOE
Visci albi herba .... see EUROPEAN MISTLETOE
Visci albi stipites .... see EUROPEAN MISTLETOE
Viscum album .... see EUROPEAN MISTLETOE
Visnaga Fruit .... see BISHOP'S WEED
Visnagafruchte .... see BISHOP'S WEED
Vitacarn .... see L-CARNITINE
Vitadurin .... see VITAMIN B12
VITAMIN A .... see VITAMIN A
Vitamin A1 .... see VITAMIN A
Vitamin A2 .... see VITAMIN A
Vitamin B Complex .... See FOLIC ACID,
                        NIACIN AND NIACINAMIDE,
                        PANTOTHENIC ACID,
                        PYRIDOXINE, RIBOFLAVIN,
                        THIAMINE, VITAMIN B12
Vitamin B(t) .... see L-CARNITINE
Vitamin B(t) Acetate .... see ACETYL-L-CARNITINE
Vitamin B1 .... see THIAMINE
VITAMIN B12 .... see VITAMIN B12
Vitamin B15 .... see PANGAMIC ACID
Vitamin B17 .... see APRICOT
Vitamin B2 .... see RIBOFLAVIN

INDEX

Vitamin B3 .... see IP-6, NIACIN AND NIACINAMIDE
Vitamin B6 .... see PYRIDOXINE
Vitamin B8 .... see INOSITOL
Vitamin B9 .... see FOLIC ACID
VITAMIN C (ASCORBIC ACID)
.... see VITAMIN C (ASCORBIC ACID)
VITAMIN D .... see VITAMIN D
Vitamin D2 .... see VITAMIN D
Vitamin D3 .... see VITAMIN D
VITAMIN E .... see VITAMIN E
Vitamin G .... see RIBOFLAVIN
Vitamin H .... see BIOTIN
VITAMIN K .... see VITAMIN K
Vitamin K1 .... see VITAMIN K
Vitamin K2 .... see VITAMIN K
Vitamin K3 .... see VITAMIN K
Vitamin K4 .... see VITAMIN K
Vitamin K5 .... see VITAMIN K
VITAMIN O .... see VITAMIN O
Vitamin PP .... see NIACIN AND NIACINAMIDE
Vitaminum A .... see VITAMIN A
Vitellin .... see LECITHIN
Vitex agnus-castus .... see CHASTEBERRY
Vitis coignetiae .... see GRAPE seed
Vitis pentaphylla .... see JIAOGULAN
Vitis vinifera .... see GRAPE fruit, skin, GRAPE leaf,
                                                    GRAPE seed, WINE
Viverra civetta .... see CIVET
Viverra zibetha .... see CIVET
Vizra Ufar .... see ANDROGRAPHIS
Vogelknoeterichkraut .... see KNOTWEED HERB
Vogelmistel .... see EUROPEAN MISTLETOE
Volatile Almond Oil .... see BITTER ALMOND
Vomit Wort .... see LOBELIA
W-3 Fatty Acid .... see DHA, EPA, FISH OILS
W Factor .... see BIOTIN
Wacholderbeeren .... see JUNIPER
Wacholderteer .... see CADE OIL
WAFER ASH .... see WAFER ASH
WAHOO .... see WAHOO
Wake Robin .... see ARUM, BETH ROOT
Waldmeister .... see SWEET WOODRUFF
Walewort .... see DWARF ELDER
Wall Germander .... see GERMANDER
Wall Ginger .... see COMMON STONECROP
WALLFLOWER .... see WALLFLOWER
Wallflower .... see CANADIAN HEMP
Wallpepper .... see COMMON STONECROP
Wallstock-Gillofer .... see WALLFLOWER
Wallwort .... see COMFREY
Walnussblatter .... see ENGLISH WALNUT leaf
Walnut Hull .... see ENGLISH WALNUT hull
Walnut Leaf .... see ENGLISH WALNUT leaf
Walpole Tea .... see NEW JERSEY TEA
Wandering Jenny .... see MONEYWORT
Wandering Tailor .... see MONEYWORT
Wang Sun .... see HERB PARIS
Warnera .... see GOLDENSEAL
Wartwort .... see CUDWEED
Wasserkresse .... see WATERCRESS
Wasshanf .... see HEMP AGRIMONY
Wateorhiza palmata .... see COLOMBO
Water Agrimony .... see BURR MARIGOLD
WATER AVENS .... see WATER AVENS

Water Blobs .... see MARSH MARIGOLD
Water Bugle .... see BUGLEWEED
Water Cabbage .... see AMERICAN WHITE POND LILY
Water Chisch .... see WATER AVENS
Water-cup .... see PITCHER PLANT
WATER DOCK .... see WATER DOCK
Water Dragon .... see MARSH MARIGOLD
Water Dropwort .... see WATER FENNEL
WATER FENNEL .... see WATER FENNEL
Water Flag .... see ORRIS
Water Flower .... see WATER AVENS
WATER GERMANDER .... see WATER GERMANDER
Water Gourd .... see LUFFA
Water Hoarhound .... see BUGLEWEED
Water-Holly .... see OREGON GRAPE
Water Horehound .... see BUGLEWEED
Water Lemon .... see PASSIONFLOWER
Water Lily .... see AMERICAN WHITE POND LILY
Water Maudlin .... see HEMP AGRIMONY
Water Mint .... see WILD MINT
Water Nymph .... see AMERICAN WHITE POND LILY
Water Pepper .... see SMARTWEED
Water Pimpernel .... see BROOKLIME
Water Pink .... see TRAILING ARBUTUS
WATER PLANTAIN .... see WATER PLANTAIN
Water Purslane .... see BROOKLIME
Water Shamrock .... see BOGBEAN
WATERCRESS .... see WATERCRESS
Waterhemp .... see HEMP AGRIMONY
Waterkres .... see WATERCRESS
Wax Bean .... see BEAN POD
Wax Cluster .... see WINTERGREEN leaf,
                                                    WINTERGREEN oil
Wax Dolls .... see FUMITORY
Wax Myrtle .... see BAYBERRY
Waxberry .... see BAYBERRY
Waxwork .... see AMERICAN BITTERSWEET
Waythorn .... see EUROPEAN BUCKTHORN
Weather Plant .... see PRECATORY BEAN
Weaver's Broom .... see SPANISH BROOM
Weed .... see MARIJUANA
Weeping Ash .... see ASH
Weibe Senfsamen .... see WHITE MUSTARD
Weidenrinde .... see WILLOW BARK
Weissdorn .... see HAWTHORN fruit
Wermut .... see WORMWOOD above ground parts
Wermutkraut .... see WORMWOOD above ground parts
West Indian Bay .... see ALLSPICE
West Indian Cherry .... see ACEROLA
West Indian Dogwood .... see JAMAICAN DOGWOOD
West Indian Lemongrass .... see LEMONGRASS
Western Larch .... see LARCH ARABINOGALACTAN
Western Shisandra .... see SCHISANDRA
Western Yew .... see YEW
Westwood-Pear .... see PRICKLY PEAR CACTUS
Weyl Ash .... see GOUTWEED
WHEAT BRAN .... see WHEAT BRAN
WHEATGRASS .... see WHEATGRASS
WHEY PROTEIN .... see WHEY PROTEIN
Whig Plant .... see ROMAN CHAMOMILE
White Archangel ..... see WHITE DEAD NETTLE FLOWER
White Ash .... see ASH, GOUTWEED
White Baneberry .... see WHITE COHOSH
White Bay .... see MAGNOLIA bark

White Beeswax .... see BEESWAX
White Birch .... see BIRCH
White Bole .... see KAOLIN
White Bryony ....see BRYONIA
White Cedar .... see CEDAR leaf, CEDAR LEAF OIL
White Cinnamon .... see CANELLA
WHITE COHOSH .... see WHITE COHOSH
White Daisy .... see OX-EYE DAISY
WHITE DEAD NETTLE FLOWER .... see WHITE DEAD
NETTLE FLOWER
White Dragon Flower .... see ORRIS
White Fringe .... see FRINGETREE
White Gum .... see STORAX
WHITE HELLEBORE .... see WHITE HELLEBORE
WHITE HOREHOUND .... see WHITE HOREHOUND
White Laurel .... see MAGNOLIA bark
WHITE LILY .... see WHITE LILY
White Mulberry .... see BLACK MULBERRY
WHITE MUSTARD .... see WHITE MUSTARD
White Pepper .... see BLACK PEPPER AND
WHITE PEPPER
White Potato ....see POTATO
White Quebracho .... see QUEBRACHO
White Root .... see PLEURISY ROOT
White Rot .... see GOTU KOLA
WHITE SANDALWOOD oil
.... see WHITE SANDALWOOD oil
WHITE SANDALWOOD wood
.... see WHITE SANDALWOOD wood
White Saunders .... see WHITE SANDALWOOD wood
White Saunders Oil .... see WHITE SANDALWOOD oil
WHITE SOAPWORT .... see WHITE SOAPWORT
White Sorrel .... see WOOD SORREL
White Spruce Oil .... see FIR NEEDLE OIL
White Squill .... see SQUILL
White Thyme Oil .... see THYME OIL
White Walnut .... see BUTTERNUT
White Wax .... see BEESWAX
White Waxtree .... see GLOSSY PRIVET
White Weed .... see OX-EYE DAISY
White Willow.................................. see WILLOW BARK
White Wood .... see CANELLA
Whitehorn .... see HAWTHORN fruit,
HAWTHORN leaf, flower,
HAWTHORN leaf with flower extract
Whitetube Stargrass .... see ALETRIS
Whitlockite .... see PHOSPHATE SALTS
Whorlywort................................... see BLACK ROOT
Whortleberry....................... see BILBERRY dried ripe fruit,
BILBERRY leaf
Wiesen-Feldkummel .... see CARAWAY dried fruit, seed
Wiesensauerampfer .... see SORREL
Wigandia californicum .... see YERBA SANTA
Wild Agrimony .... see POTENTILLA
Wild Angelica .... see ANGELICA root
Wild Balsam .... see JEWELWEED
Wild Bergamot .... see HORSEMINT
Wild Black Cherry .... see WILD CHERRY
Wild Boar Fruit .... see ROSE HIP
WILD CARROT .... see WILD CARROT
Wild Celandine .... see JEWELWEED
Wild Chamomile .... see GERMAN CHAMOMILE
WILD CHERRY .... see WILD CHERRY
Wild Chicory .... see CHICORY

Wild Cinnamon .... see CANELLA
Wild Clover .... see RED CLOVER
Wild Coleus .... see PERILLA
Wild Cotton .... see CANADIAN HEMP
Wild Crane's-Bill .... see HERB ROBERT
Wild Cucumber .... see BITTER MELON
Wild Curcuma .... see GOLDENSEAL
WILD DAISY .... see WILD DAISY
Wild Endive .... see DANDELION above ground parts,
DANDELION entire plant
Wild Fennel .... see FENNEL fruit, seed
Wild Garlic .... see BEAR'S GARLIC
Wild Gentian .... see GENTIAN
Wild Germander .... see GERMANDER
Wild Ginger .... see ASARABACCA
Wild Hops .... see BRYONIA
Wild Hydrangea .... see HYDRANGEA
Wild Ice Leaf .... see MULLEIN
WILD INDIGO .... see WILD INDIGO
Wild Iris .... see ORRIS
Wild Laburnum .... see SWEET CLOVER
Wild Lady's Slipper .... see JEWELWEED
Wild Lemon .... see PODOPHYLLUM
WILD LETTUCE .... see WILD LETTUCE
Wild Liquorice .... see SPINY RESTHARROW
Wild Mandrake .... see PODOPHYLLUM
Wild Marjoram .... see OREGANO
Wild Mexican Yam .... see WILD YAM
WILD MINT .... see WILD MINT
Wild Nard .... see ASARABACCA
Wild Nep .... see BRYONIA
Wild Oat Herb .... see OAT above ground parts
Wild Pansy .... see HEART'S EASE
Wild Passion Flower .... see PASSIONFLOWER
Wild Pea .... see LATHYRUS
Wild Pepper .... see GINSENG, SIBERIAN, MEZEREON
Wild Pine .... see MORINDA
Wild Plum Flower .... see BLACKTHORN flower
WILD RADISH .... see WILD RADISH
Wild Red American Ginseng .... see CANAIGRE
Wild Red Desert Ginseng .... see CANAIGRE
Wild Rosemary .... see LABRADOR TEA, MARSH TEA
Wild Snowball .... see NEW JERSEY TEA
Wild Strawberry .... see STRAWBERRY
Wild Sunflower.......................... see ELECAMPANE
WILD THYME.............................. see WILD THYME
Wild Tobacco .... see LOBELIA
Wild Vanilla .... see DEERTONGUE
Wild Vine .... see BRYONIA
Wild Woodbine .... see AMERICAN IVY
Wild Woodvine .... see AMERICAN IVY
Wild Wormwood .... see MUGWORT
WILD YAM .... see WILD YAM
WILLARD WATER .... see WILLARD WATER
WILLOW BARK .... see WILLOW BARK
Willow Herb .... see FIREWEED
Willow Sage .... see PURPLE LOOSESTRIFE
Willowherb .... see FIREWEED
Wind Flower .... see PULSATILLA, WOOD ANEMONE
Wind Root.......................... see PLEURISY ROOT
WINE .... see WINE
Wine Grapes .... see GRAPE fruit, skin
Wineberry .... see BILBERRY dried ripe fruit,
BILBERRY leaf

INDEX

© Copyright 2000, Natural Medicines Comprehensive Database (209) 472-2244. For updated data, go to www.NaturalDatabase.com. • 1519

Wingseed .... see WAFER ASH
Winter Bloom .... see WITCH HAZEL
WINTER CHERRY .... see WINTER CHERRY
Winter Cherry .... see WITHANIA
Winter Clover .... see SQUAWVINE
Winter Marjoram .... see OREGANO
Winter Pink .... see TRAILING ARBUTUS
WINTER SAVORY .... see WINTER SAVORY
Wintera .... see WINTER'S BARK
Wintera Aromatica .... see WINTER'S BARK
Wintergreen .... see PERIWINKLE
WINTERGREEN leaf .... see WINTERGREEN leaf
WINTERGREEN oil .... see WINTERGREEN oil
Winterlien .... see FLAXSEED
WINTER'S BARK .... see WINTER'S BARK
Winter's Cinnamon .... see WINTER'S BARK
Wintersweet .... see OREGANO
Wisconsin Ginseng .... see GINSENG, AMERICAN
Witch Grass .... see AGROPYRON
WITCH HAZEL .... see WITCH HAZEL
Witch Meal .... see CLUB MOSS
Witchazel .... see WITCH HAZEL
Witchen .... see MOUNTAIN ASH
Witches' Pouches .... see SHEPHERD'S PURSE
Witch's Bells .... see DIGITALIS
WITHANIA .... see WITHANIA
Withania coagulans .... see WITHANIA
Withania somnifera .... see WITHANIA
Wogon .... see BAIKAL SKULLCAP
Wolfiporia cocos .... see PORIA MUSHROOM
Wolf's Bane .... see ARNICA
Wolfs Claw .... see CLUB MOSS
Wolfsbane .... see ACONITE
Wolfstrapp .... see BUGLEWEED
Wolly Foxglove .... see DIGITALIS
Woman's Long Hair .... see USNEA
Wonder Bulb .... see AUTUMN CROCUS
Wonder Tree .... see CASTOR OIL, CASTOR seed
WOOD ANEMONE .... see WOOD ANEMONE
Wood Betony .... see BETONY
Wood Gum .... see LARCH ARABINOGALACTAN
Wood-Rose .... see HAWAIIAN BABY WOODROSE
WOOD SAGE .... see WOOD SAGE
Wood Sanicle .... see SANICLE
WOOD SORREL .... see WOOD SORREL
Wood Sour .... see WOOD SORREL
Wood Spider .... see DEVIL'S CLAW
Wood Strawberry .... see STRAWBERRY
Wood Sugar .... see LARCH ARABINOGALACTAN
Wood Vine .... see BRYONIA
Wood Waxen .... see DYER'S BROOM
Woodbind .... see ENGLISH IVY
WOODBINE .... see WOODBINE
Woodbine .... see GELSEMIUM
Woodbine .... see HONEYSUCKLE
Woodruff .... see SWEET WOODRUFF
Woody .... see BITTERSWEET NIGHTSHADE
Woody Climber .... see AMERICAN IVY
Woody Nightshade ...... see BITTERSWEET NIGHTSHADE
Woolen .... see MULLEIN
Woolly Morning Glory .... see HAWAIIAN BABY
WOODROSE
Woolly Parsnip .... see MASTERWORT

Woolly Thistle .... see SCOTCH THISTLE
Woolmat .... see HOUND'S TONGUE
Wordward .... see SWEET WOODRUFF
Wormgrass .... see PINK ROOT
WORMSEED .... see WORMSEED
WORMWOOD above ground parts
.... see WORMWOOD above ground parts
WORMWOOD oil .... see WORMWOOD oil
Wound Wort .... see GOLDENROD, SELF-HEAL,
YARROW
Wu-jia .... see GINSENG, SIBERIAN
Wu Jia Pi .... see GINSENG, SIBERIAN
Wu Wei Zi .... see SCHISANDRA
Wundkraut .... see ARNICA
Wurmkraut .... see WORMWOOD above ground parts
Wurzelstock .... see KAVA
Wymote .... see MARSHMALLOW
XANTHAN GUM .... see XANTHAN GUM
Xanthomonas campestris .... see XANTHAN GUM
Xanthophyll .... see LUTEIN
Xanthoxylum .... see NORTHERN PRICKLY ASH,
SOUTHERN PRICKLY ASH
Xian Ling Pi .... see EPIMEDIUM
Xiwuweizi .... see SCHISANDRA
Xue Jie .... see DRAGON'S BLOOD
XueZhiKang .... see RED YEAST
Xysmalobium undulatum .... see UZARA
Yagona .... see KAVA
YARROW .... see YARROW
Yaw Root .... see QUEEN'S DELIGHT
Yege .... see KUDZU
Yellow Astringent .... see EPHEDRA
Yellow Bark .... see CASCARA
Yellow Beeswax .... see BEESWAX
Yellow Beet .... see BEET
Yellow Broom .... see WILD INDIGO
Yellow Bugle .... see GROUND PINE
Yellow Chaste Weed .... see IMMORTELLE, SANDY
EVERLASTING
Yellow Cleavers .... see LADY'S BEDSTRAW
YELLOW DOCK .... see YELLOW DOCK
Yellow Flag .... see ORRIS
Yellow Galium .... see LADY'S BEDSTRAW
Yellow Gentian .... see GENTIAN
Yellow Ginseng .... see BLUE COHOSH
Yellow Horse .... see EPHEDRA
Yellow Indian Paint .... see GOLDENSEAL
Yellow Indigo .... see WILD INDIGO
Yellow Iris .... see ORRIS
Yellow Jasmine .... see GELSEMIUM
Yellow Jessamine Root .... see GELSEMIUM
YELLOW LUPIN .... see YELLOW LUPIN
Yellow Melilot .... see SWEET CLOVER
Yellow Oleander .... see OLEANDER
Yellow Paint .... see GOLDENSEAL
Yellow Pheasant's Eye .... see PHEASANT'S EYE
Yellow Puccoon .... see GOLDENSEAL
Yellow Rod .... see YELLOW TOADFLAX
Yellow Sandalwood ...... see WHITE SANDALWOOD wood
Yellow Sandalwood Oil ..... see WHITE SANDALWOOD oil
Yellow Saunders .... see WHITE SANDALWOOD wood
Yellow Saunders Oil .... see WHITE SANDALWOOD oil
Yellow Snakeleaf ...... see AMERICAN ADDER'S TONGUE
Yellow Snowdrop ..... see AMERICAN ADDER'S TONGUE

INDEX

Yellow Starwort .... see ELECAMPANE
Yellow Sweet Clover .... see SWEET CLOVER
YELLOW TOADFLAX .... see YELLOW TOADFLAX
Yellow Vine .... see THUNDER GOD VINE
Yellow Wax .... see BEESWAX
Yellow Willowherb .... see LOOSESTRIFE
Yellow Wood .... see NORTHERN PRICKLY ASH
Yellowroot .... see GOLDENSEAL, GOLDTHREAD
Yellows .... see BUTTERCUP, NERVE ROOT
Yellowweed .... see BUTTERCUP
Yemen Myrrh .... see MYRRH
Yerba buena .... see SPEARMINT
Yerba Dulce .... see STEVIA
YERBA MANSA .... see YERBA MANSA
Yerba Mate .... see MATE
YERBA SANTA .... see YERBA SANTA
YEW .... see YEW
YIN CHEN .... see YIN CHEN
Yin Chen Hao .... see YIN CHEN
Yin Yang Huo .... see EPIMEDIUM
Yinhsing .... see GINKGO leaf,
                          GINKGO leaf extract, GINKGO seed
YLANG YLANG OIL .... see YLANG YLANG OIL
Yoghurt .... see YOGURT
YOGURT .... see YOGURT
YOHIMBE .... see YOHIMBE
Yohimbehe .... see YOHIMBE
Yohimbehe cortex .... see YOHIMBE
Youthwort .... see MASTERWORT, SUNDEW
YUCCA .... see YUCCA
Yucca aloifolia .... see YUCCA
Yucca arborescens .... see YUCCA
Yucca brevifolia .... see YUCCA
Yucca filamentosa .... see ADAM'S NEEDLE, YUCCA
Yucca glauca .... see YUCCA
Yucca mohavensis .... see YUCCA
Yucca schidigera .... see YUCCA
Yucca whipplei .... see YUCCA
Yuma .... see WILD YAM
Yun-Zhi .... see CORIOLUS MUSHROOM
(Z,Z,Z)-Octadeca-6,9,12-trienoic acid .... see GAMMA
                                          LINOLENIC ACID
Zacate Violeta .... see VETIVER
Zaffer .... see SAFFLOWER
Zafran .... see SAFFLOWER
Zanthoxylum .... see NORTHERN PRICKLY ASH,
                          SOUTHERN PRICKLY ASH
Zanthoxylum americanum ....
                          see NORTHERN PRICKLY ASH
Zanthoxylum clava-herculis ....
                          see SOUTHERN PRICKLY ASH
Zanzibar Pepper .... see CAPSICUM
Zao .... see JUJUBE
Zapote .... see CHICLE
Zapotillo .... see CHICLE
Zea .... see CORN SILK
Zea mays .... see CORN SILK
Zeaxanthin .... see LUTEIN
Zedoaire .... see ZEDOARY
Zedoaria .... see ZEDOARY
Zedoarie rhizoma .... see ZEDOARY
ZEDOARY .... see ZEDOARY
Zhihe-Sho-Wu .... see FO-TI cured root
ZhiTai .... see RED YEAST

Zhong Mahuang .... see EPHEDRA
Zi Shou Wu .... see FO-TI cured root
Zibeth .... see CIVET
Zimblòten .... see CINNAMON flower
Zimbro .... see JUNIPER
ZINC .... see ZINC
Zinc Acetate .... see ZINC
Zinc Aspartate .... see ZINC
Zinc Gluconate .... see ZINC
Zinc Methionine .... see ZINC
Zinc Monomethionine .... see ZINC
Zinc Oxide .... see ZINC
Zinc Sulfate .... see ZINC
Zingiber officinale .... see GINGER
Zishouwu .... see FO-TI cured root
Zitwer .... see ZEDOARY
Zitwerwirtzelstock .... see ZEDOARY
Zn .... see ZINC
Zoom .... see GUARANA
Zyzyphus jujube .... see JUJUBE

INDEX

" Tell the Editors . . . "

This *Database* is constantly evolving. Our research and editorial team analyzes new studies every day and makes updates to the Web version of this *Database* every day. We view our work as similar to a clearing house of information on natural medicines. If you spot a statement that needs to be changed, or updated, you can use this form, or a copy of it, to communicate directly with the editors. Feel free to mail, e-mail, or fax. We appreciate your help!

1. What part of the database are you commenting about?

Page number _____ Section _____ .

_____

2. What wording should be added?

Please be specific about exact wording that you propose adding. Use additional pages if needed.

_____

_____

_____

_____

3. What wording should be deleted?

Please tell us which words you think should be removed. _____ .

_____

_____

4. What reference citations support this change?

Please give us specific reference citations. We base entries into this *Database* on reliable studies published in peer-reviewed professional literature. Please give us enough information so that we can find the reference.

_____

_____

Name _____

Address _____

_____

Phone # _____

E-mail _____

Please send this information to:

NATURAL MEDICINES
COMPREHENSIVE DATABASE

3120 W. March Lane
P.O. Box 8190, Stockton CA 95208
TEL: 209-472-2244
FAX: 209-472-2249
E-mail: Mail@NaturalDatabase.com

© Copyright 2000, Natural Medicines Comprehensive Database (209) 472-2244. For updated data, go to www.NaturalDatabase.com. • 1523

Get additional copies of

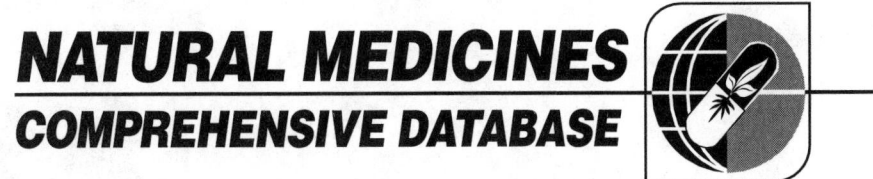

NATURAL MEDICINES
COMPREHENSIVE DATABASE

❏ I want to START a new subscription to *Natural Medicines Comprehensive Database*.
- ❏ Printed version at $92
- ❏ Web version at $92 per year
- ❏ BOTH versions $132 (This is the best deal.)

❏ I want to EXTEND my subscription to *Natural Medicines Comprehensive Database*.
- ❏ Send me a new printed version at $92
- ❏ Extend my web subscription at $92 per year
- ❏ Give me BOTH a new printed version and one more year of the web version for $132

❏ I want to get Continuing Education credits. Send me the next two CE Booklets. 4 credits each. Total of $19.

Indicate your profession so we can send you the Booklet that is accredited for you:

❏ Physician ❏ Pharmacist ❏ Nurse Practitioner ❏ Physician Assistant ❏ Dietitian

In California add 7.75% sales tax. For printed versions shipped outside the U.S. add $18.

If you prefer, you can sign up online at www.NaturalDatabase.com.

❏ Payment enclosed (make check payable to Natural Database)
❏ Please charge my VISA, Mastercard, or American Express

Card number _____ Exp date _____

Signature _____

❏ Bill my business or institution on this purchase order number _____

Ship to:

Name _____

Address _____

City _____ State _____ Zip Code _____

Phone _____ E-mail _____

Send this order form to:

Natural Medicines Comprehensive Database
Pharmacist's Letter / Prescriber's Letter
3120 W. March Lane
P.O. Box 8190
Stockton, CA 95208

Telephone: 209-472-2244 • Fax: 209-472-2249
E-mail: mail@NaturalDatabase.com • Website: www.NaturalDatabase.com

© Copyright 2000, Natural Medicines Comprehensive Database (209) 472-2244. For updated data, go to www.NaturalDatabase.com. • 1525

Get additional copies of

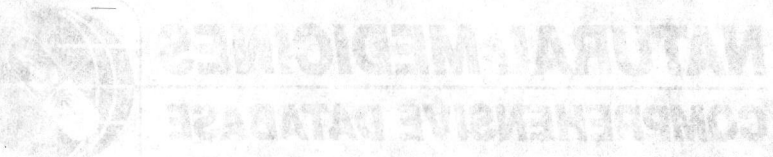

NATURAL MEDICINES
COMPREHENSIVE DATABASE

☐ I want to START a new subscription to Natural Medicines Comprehensive Database.
   ☐ Printed version for $92.
   ☐ Web version for $92 per year.
   ☐ BOTH versions for $172. This is the best deal!

☐ I want to EXTEND my subscription to Natural Medicines Comprehensive Database.
   ☐ Send me a new printed version at $92.
   ☐ Extend my web subscription for $92 per year.
   ☐ Give me BOTH a new printed version at the best price and the
      web version for $172.

☐ I am an accredited provider offering Continuing Education credits. Send me the next two CE modules at a reduced rate. Total of $96.

☐ If there is anything else we can do to serve you better. Please let us know...

☐ California add 7.75 sales tax. Not prepaid. For printed version shipped outside the U.S. add $18 S&H.

☐ We make it easy for you. Order/sign up online at www.NaturalDatabase.com.

☐ My payment enclosed. (my check payable to Natural Database)
☐ Please charge my VISA, MasterCard or American Express.

Natural Medicines Comprehensive Database
Pharmacist's Letter/Prescriber's Letter
3120 W. March Lane
P.O. Box 8190
Stockton, CA 95208
Telephone: 209-472-2244   Fax: 209 472-2249
E-mail: mail@NaturalDatabase.com   Website: www.NaturalDatabase.com

Get Continuing Education Credits

Accredited for physicians, pharmacists, nurse practitioners, and physician assistants.*

You can earn Continuing Education credits as a part of your subscription to this *Natural Medicines Comprehensive Database*. The editors compile Continuing Education Booklets based on this *Database*. When you sign up for the CE you get your first Booklet right away, then a new Booklet every six months. Each Booklet gives you up to 4 hours of credit. This CE is accredited for physicians, pharmacists, nurse practitioners, and physician assistants.*

The CE series is entitled *"Natural Medicines in Clinical Management."*
Each Booklet delves into the use of natural medicines in the clinical management of several specific disease states and compares the use of the natural medicines to conventional drugs. Clinical pearls and cautions appear frequently. Many useful charts are included too.

The fifth Booklet in this ongoing series is *"Natural Medicines in the Clinical Management of Depression, Headache, Arthritis, Menopausal Symptoms, and Atherosclerosis"* Fall 1999.

The sixth Booklet is *"Natural Medicines in the Clinical Management of Alzheimer's Disease, Diabetes, and Men's Health"* Spring 2000.

The price per Booklet is only $9.50 each for health professionals who have purchased either a current version of the Book or current access to the Web version of this *Database*. This price includes everything, including grading and certificate.

❑ Send me the current CE Booklet and a new Booklet in six months. $9.50 per Booklet. $19 per year.

❑ Send me the six prior Booklets in the series. $9.50 per Booklet. $57 total.

Indicate your profession so we can send you the Booklet that is accredited for you:
❑ Physician ❑ Pharmacist ❑ Nurse Practitioner ❑ Physician Assistant ❑ Dietitian

Your subscription to the *Database* is under what name? _____

❑ Payment enclosed (make check payable to Natural Database)
❑ Bill my business or institution on this purchase order number _____
❑ Please charge my VISA, Mastercard, or American Express

Card number _____ Exp date _____

Ship to:

Name _____

Address _____

City _____ State _____ Zip Code _____

Phone _____ E-mail _____

Send this order form to:

Natural Medicines Comprehensive Database
Pharmacist's Letter / Prescriber's Letter
3120 W. March Lane
P.O. Box 8190
Stockton, CA 95208
Telephone: 209-472-2244 • Fax: 209-472-2249
E-mail: mail@NaturalDatabase.com • Website: www.NaturalDatabase.com

*Physicians: Prescriber's Letter is accredited by the Accreditation Council for Continuing Medical Education (ACCME) to provide continuing medical education for physicians.

Prescriber's Letter designates each Booklet for up to 4 hours in category 1 credit towards the AMA Physician's Recognition Award. Each physician should claim only those hours of credit that he/she actually spent in the educational activity.

Pharmacists: Pharmacist's Letter is approved by the American Council on Pharmaceutical Education as a provider of continuing pharmaceutical education.

Nurse Practitioners: The individual Booklets in the series have been granted 4.0 contact hours of continuing education by the American Academy of Nurse Practitioners.

Physician Assistants: The American Academy of Physician Assistants accepts AMA category 1 CME credit for the Physician's Recognition Award from organizations accredited by the ACCME. *Prescriber's Letter* is accredited by ACCME.

Dietitians: Accreditation applied for. Please contact our office.

© Copyright 2000, Natural Medicines Comprehensive Database (209) 472-2244. For updated data, go to www.NaturalDatabase.com. • 1527

You can sign up for access to www.NaturalDatabase.com

This printed version of *Natural Medicines Comprehensive Database* was current the day the data were extracted from www.NaturalDatabase.com, but each day the site is updated with new data.

If you have not yet purchased your access to the site, now is a good time to do so. You can sign up by phone, mail, fax, or by going to the site.

Everything in this printed version - plus more - is in the Website. More brand name products are listed. (There's just not space to list them all here.) The site also does terrific searches for you. You can have it search for interactions...uses...names...and search by many other criteria. You can even have the site help you find products or names for which you don't know the correct spelling. You get the latest additions and updates. For each ingredient, you can click to see which brand name products contain it. For each monograph you can click to see all the references used to compile the data for that monograph. In addition, you can click on thousands of these references and read the original abstract originally printed in the scientific journal. You can also post questions and comments and interact with the editors and with health professionals who post their comments.

Since you have already purchased this printed version you get the Web access for ONE-THIRD OFF. Access lasts one year and is for either one user or one computer.

ONE-THIRD OFF!
Only $59 for one year of access
Price valid on orders placed prior to June 30, 2001.

❏ **YES,** please send me an access code so I can use www.NaturalDatabase.com

    ❏ Payment enclosed (make check payable to Natural Database)

    ❏ Please charge my VISA, Mastercard, or American Express

        Card number _____ Exp date _____

        Signature _____

    ❏ Bill my business or institution on this purchase order number _____

    Ship to:

        Name _____

        Address _____

        City _____ State _____ Zip Code _____

        Phone _____ E-mail _____

If you have already had access and are using this special price to extend your access for another year, please write your passcode and member number here:

Access # _____

Member # _____

Send this order form to:

Natural Medicines Comprehensive Database
Pharmacist's Letter / Prescriber's Letter
3120 W. March Lane
P.O. Box 8190
Stockton, CA 95208
Telephone: 209-472-2244 • Fax: 209-472-2249
E-mail: mail@NaturalDatabase.com • Website: www.NaturalDatabase.com

© Copyright 2000, Natural Medicines Comprehensive Database (209) 472-2244. For updated data, go to www.NaturalDatabase.com. • 1529

You can sign up for access to www.NaturalDatabase.com

This printed version of *Natural Medicines Comprehensive Database* was current the day the data were extracted from www.NaturalDatabase.com, but each day the site is updated with new data.

If you have not yet purchased your access to the site, now is a good time to do so. You can sign up by phone, mail, fax, or by going to the site.

Everything in this printed version - plus more - is in the Website. More brand name products are listed. (There's just not space to list them all here.) The site also does terrific searches for you. You can have it search for interactions...uses...names...and search by many other criteria. You can even have the site help you find products or names for which you don't know the correct spelling. You get the latest additions and updates. For each ingredient, you can click to see which brand name products contain it. For each monograph you can click to see all the references used to compile the data for that monograph. In addition, you can click on thousands of these references and read the original abstract originally printed in the scientific journal. You can also post questions and comments and interact with the editors and with health professionals who post their comments.

Since you have already purchased this printed version you get the Web access for ONE-THIRD OFF. Access lasts one year and is for either one user or one computer.

ONE-THIRD OFF!

Only $59 for one year of access

Price valid on orders placed prior to June 30, 2001.

❐ **YES,** please send me an access code so I can use www.NaturalDatabase.com

    ❐ Payment enclosed (make check payable to Natural Database)

    ❐ Please charge my VISA, Mastercard, or American Express

        Card number _____ Exp date _____

        Signature _____

    ❐ Bill my business or institution on this purchase order number _____

    Ship to:

        Name _____

        Address _____

        City _____ State _____ Zip Code _____

        Phone _____ E-mail _____

    If you have already had access and are using this special price to extend your access for another year, please write your passcode and member number here:

    Access # _____

    Member # _____

Send this order form to:

Natural Medicines Comprehensive Database
Pharmacist's Letter / Prescriber's Letter
3120 W. March Lane
P.O. Box 8190
Stockton, CA 95208
Telephone: 209-472-2244 • Fax: 209-472-2249
E-mail: mail@NaturalDatabase.com • Website: www.NaturalDatabase.com

1530 • © Copyright 2000, Natural Medicines Comprehensive Database (209) 472-2244. For updated data, go to www.NaturalDatabase.com.